EMERGENCY MEDICINE PROCEDURES

Eric F. Reichman, PhD, MD, FAAEM, FACEP

Attending Physician
Assistant Residency Director
Director of Surgical Techniques and Skills Laboratory
Department of Emergency Medicine
Cook County Hospital
Assistant Professor of Emergency Medicine
Director of Surgical Techniques and Skills Laboratory
Rush Medical College
Chicago, Illinois

Robert R. Simon, MD, FAAEM

Chairman
Department of Emergency Medicine
Cook County Hospital and Provident Hospital
Chairman
Department of Emergency Medicine
Rush-Presbyterian-St. Luke's Medical Center
Professor of Emergency Medicine
Rush Medical College
Chairman of the Board
International Medical Corps
Chicago, Illinois

With over 1500 illustrations by Susan Gilbert, CMI
Additional illustrations by Laurel Lhowe

McGraw-Hill
Medical Publishing Division

New York Chicago San Francisco Lisbon London Madrid Mexico City
Milan New Delhi San Juan Seoul Singapore Sydney Toronto

EMERGENCY MEDICAL PROCEDURES

1 2 3 4 5 6 7 8 9 0 KGP/KGP 0 9 8 7 6 5 4 3

ISBN 0-07-136032-8

This book was set in Times New Roman
by Clarinda, Clarinda, IA, and GTS Global Companies, York Campus, PA
The editors were Andrea Seils, Susan Noujaim, and Karen Davis.
The production supervisor was Richard Ruzycka.
The interior designer was Joan O'Connor.
The cover designer was Aimée Nordin.
The illustrations were done by Susan Gilbert, with the assistance of Faith Cogswell.
Additional illustrations were done by Laurel Lhowe.
The indexers are Jerry Ralya and Marilyn Rowland.
Quebecor World Kingsport was printer and binder.

This book is printed on acid-free paper.

Library of Congress Cataloging-in-Publication Data

Reichman, Eric.
    Emergency medicine procedures / Eric Reichman,
  Robert Simon ; with illustrations by Susan Gilbert and
  Laurel C. Lhowe.
        p. ; cm.
    Includes bibliographical references and index.
    ISBN 0-07-136032-8
      1. Emergency medicine—Handbooks, manuals, etc.
  I. Simon, Robert R. (Robert Rutha)   II. Title
      [DNLM: 1. Emergency Medicine—methods—
    Handbooks. WB 39 R352e 2003]
  RC86.8 .R45 2003
  616.02′5—dc21   2002075365

CONTENTS

CONTRIBUTORS

Ikem Ajaelo, MD
Attending Physician
Valley Emergency Physicians
Oakland, California
(Chapter 116)

Steven E. Aks, DO, FACMT
Fellowship Director
Medical Toxicology
Toxicon Consortium
Attending Physician
Department of Emergency Medicine
Cook County Hospital
Associate Professor of Emergency Medicine
Rush Medical College
Chicago, Illinois
(Chapter 50)

Joseph P. Allegretti, MD
Attending Physician
Department of Otolaryngology and Bronchoesophagology
Rush-Presbyterian–St. Luke's Medical Center
Assistant Professor
Department of Otolaryngology and Bronchoesophagology
Rush Medical College
Chicago, Illinois
(Chapter 146)

Gary An, MD
Attending Physician
Department of Trauma Surgery
Cook County Hospital
Chicago, Illinois
(Chapter 169)

Michael J. Armstrong, MD
Attending Physician, Emergency Department
St. Michael's Hospital
Attending Physician
Emergency Department
St. Francis Hospital
Milwaukee, Wisconsin
(Chapter 105)

Bashar M. Attar, MD
Chairman
Division of Gastroenterology
Cook County Hospital
Associate Professor of Medicine
Rush Medical College
Chicago, Illinois
(Chapters 51, 52)

Jamil D. Bayram, MD
Attending Physician
Department of Emergency Medicine
Rush-Presbyterian-St. Luke's Medical Center
Assistant Professor of Emergency Medicine
Rush Medical College
Chicago, Illinois
(Chapter 58)

Robert Bilkovski, MD, FAAEM
Attending Physician
Department of Emergency Medicine
Advocate Christ Medical Center
Assistant Clinical Professor of Emergency Medicine
University of Illinois
Oak Lawn, Illlinois
(Chapters 42, 108)

David J. Bird, MA, DO
Attending Physician
Department of Anesthesiology
Cook County Hospital
Assistant Professor of Anesthesiology
Rush Medical College
Chicago, Illinois
(Chapters 2, 10)

Katherine Blossfield
Tachyarrhythmia Field Engineer
Medtronic Incorporated
Downers Grove, Illlinois
(Chapter 24)

Faran Bokhari, MD
Attending Physician
Department of Trauma Surgery
Cook County Hospital
Assistant Professor of Surgery
Rush Medical College
Chicago, Illinois
(Chapters 31–35)

Brenna Born, MD
Attending Physician
Department of Emergency Medicine
Holy Cross Hospital
Chicago, Illinois
(Chapter 130)

Michael Bourn, DO
Attending Physician
Department of Emergency Medicine
Grant/Riverside Methodist Medical Center
Westerville, Ohio
(Chapter 48)

Steven H. Bowman, MD, FACEP
Attending Physician
Program Director
Department of Emergency Medicine
Cook County Hospital
Assistant Professor of Emergency Medicine
Rush Medical College
Chicago, Illinois
(Chapters 84–86)

Dudley Brown, Jr., MD
Resident
Department of Obstetrics and Gynecology
Cook County Hospital
Chicago, Illinois
(Chapter 110)

Jennifer A. Cabel, MD
Attending Physician
Northwestern University Medical School
Division of Emergency Medicine
Chicago, Illinois
(Chapter 13)

David D. Caldarelli, MD
Chairman
Department of Otolaryngology and Bronchoesophagology
Rush-Presbyterian–St. Luke's Medical Center
Professor
Department of Otolaryngology and Bronchoesophagology
Rush Medical College
Chicago, Illinois
(Chapter 148)

Angelique S. Kelly Campen, MD, FACEP
Emergency Physician
Southern California Permanente Medical Group
Adjunct Assistant Professor of Medicine
Division of Emergency Medicine
UCLA Medical Center
Los Angeles, California
(Chapter 68)

Kenneth D. Candido, MD
Associate Professor of Anesthesiology
Department of Anesthesiology
Northwestern University Medical School
Chicago, Illinois
(Chapters 1, 17, 107)

John R. Canning, MD
Attending Urologist
Provident Hospital of Cook County
Professor of Urology
Department of Urology
Loyola University Medical Center
Maywood, Illinois
(Chapter 126)

Hazel Cebrun, MD
Attending Physician
West Houston Medical Center
Houston, Texas
(Chapter 78)

Austen Chai, MD
Attending Physician
Department of Emergency Medicine
Cook County Hospital
Assistant Professor of Emergency Medicine
Rush Medical College
Chicago, Illinois
(Chapters 104, 156, 157)

Steven Charous, MD
Director
Center for Voice Disorders
Rush-Presbyterian–St. Luke's Medical Center
Assistant Professor
Department of Otolaryngology and Bronchoesophagology
Rush Medical College
Glenview, Illinois
(Chapter 149)

George Chiampas, DO
Attending Physician
Department of Emergency Medicine
Rush-Presbyterian-St. Luke's Medical Center
Clinical Instructor of Emergency Medicine
Rush Medical College
Chicago, Illinois
(Chapter 147)

Wendy A. Cole, MD
Department of Emergency Medicine
Alameda County Medical Center/Highland Hospital
Oakland, California
(Chapter 120)

Jim Comes, MD
Assistant Clinical Professor of Medicine
Department of Emergency Medicine
UCSF–Fresno Medical Education Program
University Medical Center
Fresno, California
(Chapter 74)

Karen S. Cosby, MD
Attending Physician
Department of Emergency Medicine
Cook County Hospital
Assistant Professor of Emergency Medicine
Rush Medical College
Chicago, Illinois
(Chapters 8, 15, 53, 95)

Eileen Frances Couture, DO
Director of Emergency Services
Cermak Health Service
Attending Physician
Department of Emergency Medicine
Cook County Hospital
Assistant Professor of Emergency Medicine
Rush Medical College
Chicago, Illinois
(Chapter 170)

Holly H. Cromwell, MD
Attending Physician
Department of Emergency Medicine
Sturdy Memorial Hospital
West Warwick, Rhode Island
(Chapter 9)

M. Chris Decker, MD
Assistant Professor of Emergency Medicine
Department of Emergency Medicine
Medical College of Wisconsin
Milwaukee, Wisconsin
(Chapter 29)

Mark Doucette, MD
Attending Physician
Department of Emergency Medicine
Holy Cross Hospital
Denver, Colorado
(Chapter 129)

Rami Doukky, MD
Attending Physician
Division of Cardiology
Cook County Hospital
Assistant Professor of Medicine
Rush Medical College
Chicago, Illinois
(Chapter 20)

Martin Ehrlich, MD
Attending Emergency Physician
Ventura County Medical Center
Ventura, California
(Chapter 167)

Maher Fattouh, MD
Resident Physician
Department of Anesthesiology and Pain Management
Cook County Hospital
Chicago, Illinois
(Chapter 4)

Robert Feldman, MD
Attending Physician
Assistant Director
Adult Emergency Services
Department of Emergency Medicine
Cook County Hospital
Assistant Professor of Emergency Medicine
Rush Medical College
Chicago, Illinois
(Chapters 36–40)

Angela Flippin, MD
Resident Physician
Department of Obstetrics and Gynecology
Cook County Hospital
Chicago, Illinois
(Chapter 115)

Ardena L. Flippin, MD, MT, ASCP, FAAEM, MBA
Attending Physician
Associate Director of Academic Affairs
Department of Emergency Medicine
Cook County Hospital
Assistant Professor of Emergency Medicine
Rush Medical College
Chicago, Illinois
(Chapters 77, 78)

Brian Fong, MD
Department of Emergency Medicine
St. Mary's Hospital and Medical Center
Long Beach, California
(Chapter 96)

Arani Forghani, DO
Resident Physician
Department of Obstetrics and Gynecology
Cook County Hospital
Chicago, Illinois
(Chapter 111)

Cory Franklin, MD
Attending Physician
Division of Critical Care
Medical Intensive Care Unit
Cook County Hospital
Assistant Professor of Medicine
Rush Medical College
Chicago, Illinois
(Chapter 41)

Michael Friedman, MD, FACS
Chairman
Section of Head and Neck Surgery
Department of Otolaryngology and Bronchoesophagology
Rush-Presbyterian–St. Luke's Medical Center
Chairman
Department of Otolaryngology and Bronchoesophagology
Rush Medical College
Chicago, Illinois
(Chapter 147)

Bassen Ghaly, MD
Resident
Department of Anesthesiology and Pain Management
Cook County Hospital
Chicago, Illinois
(Chapter 3)

Yogesh Ghandi, MD
Attending Physician
Department of Neurosurgery
Cook County Hospital
Assistant Professor of Neurosurgery
University of Illinois at Chicago
Chicago, Illinois
(Chapters 97, 98, 101, 102)

Rick Gimbel, MD
Attending Physician
Division of Emergency Medicine
Northwestern University Medical School
Chicago, Illinois
(Chapter 12)

Jeffrey Gordon, MD, FACEP
Attending Physician
Department of Emergency Medicine
Resurrection Medical Center
Chicago, Illinois
(Chapter 82)

Thomas P. Graham, MD, FACEP
Assistant Professor of Medicine/Emergency Medicine
UCLA School of Medicine
Los Angeles, California
(Chapter 88)

Lauren S. Grossman, MD, MS
Attending Physician
Resident Research Director
Department of Emergency Medicine
Cook County Hospital
Assistant Professor of Emergency Medicine
Rush Medical College
Chicago, Illinois
(Chapters 99, 100)

David D. Gummin, MD, FACEP, ABMT
Attending Physician
Infinity Healthcare, Inc.
Clinical Associate Professor of Emergency Medicine
Medical College of Wisconsin
Associate Medical Director
Wisconsin Poison Center, Milwaukee
Elm Grove, Wisconsin
(Chapters 49, 50)

Samuel J. Gutman, MD, CCFP (EM)
Department of Family Practice
University of British Columbia
St. Paul's Hospital
Vancouver, British Columbia, Canada
(Chapters 81, 89)

David A. Harter, MD
Attending Physician
Department of Emergency Medicine
Cook County Hospital
Assistant Professor of Emergency Medicine
Rush Medical College
Chicago, Illinois
(Chapter 80)

Ronald F. Hayden, MD, FACEP
Medical Director
Department of Emergency Medicine
Berkshire Medical Center
Pittsfield, Massachusetts
(Chapter 109)

Susan K. Hendricks, MD
Maternal-Fetal Medicine
Department of Obstetrics and Gynecology
Rockford Memorial Hospital
Rockford, Illinois
(Chapters 110–115)

Heather Herbolsheimer, MS, DO
Resident Physician
Department of Obstetrics and Gynecology
Cook County Hospital
Chicago, Illinois
(Chapter 112)

H. Gene Hern, Jr., MD, MS
Assistant Clinical Professor of Medicine
University of California, San Francisco
Attending Physician
Emergency Department
Highland Hospital
Alameda County Medical Center
Oakland, California
(Chapter 16)

Mark E. Hoffmann, MD
Attending Staff Physician
Department of Emergency Medicine
St. Cloud Hospital
St. Cloud, Minnesota
(Chapters 6, 44)

Teresita M. Hogan, MD, FACEP
Associate Professor of Emergency Medicine
University of Illinois
Program Director
Emergency Medicine Residency Program
Resurrection Medical Center
Chicago, Illinois
(Chapters 62, 71)

R. Harold Holbrook, Jr., MD
Associate Professor
Director, Prenatal Diagnosis
Department of Obstetrics and Gynecology
Stanford University School of Medicine
Palo Alto, California
(Chapter 114)

Amy M. Hutson, MD
Attending Physician
Department of Emergency Medicine
Kauai Medical Clinic
Lihue, Kauai, Hawaii
(Chapters 63, 64, 76)

Shawn Janes, MD
Attending Physician
Department of Emergency Medicine
Royal Columbian Hospital
Westminister, British Columbia, Canada
(Chapter 66)

Mark E. Johnson, MD, PhD
Attending Physician
Department of Emergency Medicine
Community Hospital
Munster, Indiana
(Chapter 75)

Michael P. Jones, MD
Attending Physician
Racine Emergency Physicians, SC
Department of Emergency Medicine
All Saints-St. Mary's Medical Center
Racine, Wisconsin
(Chapter 125)

Paul J. Jones, MD
Assistant Professor
Director of Resident Education
Department of Otolaryngology and Bronchoesophagology
Rush-Presbyterian–St. Luke's Medical Center
Rush Medical College
Chicago, Illinois
(Chapter 143)

Kimberly T. Joseph, MD, FACS, CNSP
Attending Physician
Associate Director
Trauma Intensive Care Unit
Department of Trauma Surgery
Cook County Hospital
Chicago, Illinois
(Chapter 28)

Iksoo Kang, MD, FAAP, FACEP
Attending Physician
Department of Emergency Medicine
Western Medical Center, Santa Ana
Santa Ana, California
(Chapter 45)

Zach Kassutto, MD
Chief, Department of Emergency Medicine
St. Christopher's Hospital for Children
Associate Professor of Emergency Medicine and Pediatrics
Medical College of Pennsylvania
Philadelphia, Pennsylvania
(Chapter 73)

Stephen M. Kelanic, MD
Attending Physician
Department of Otolaryngology and Bronchoesophagology
Rush-Presbyterian–St. Luke's Medical Center
Instructor
Department of Otolaryngology and Bronchoesophagology
Rush Medical College
Chicago, Illinois
(Chapter 148)

Russell F. Kelly, MD
Attending Physician, Program Director
Division of Cardiology
Cook County Hospital
Assistant Professor of Cardiology
Rush Medical College
Attending Physician, Section of Cardiology
Rush-Presbyterian–St. Luke's Medical Center
Chicago, Illinois
(Chapter 41)

Kevin P. Kern, DO
Attending Physician
Department of Emergency Medicine
Cook County Hospital
Assistant Professor of Emergency Medicine
Rush Medical College
Chicago, Illinois
(Chapter 154)

Mark P. Kling, MD, FAAEM, CSCS
Attending Physician
Department of Emergency Medicine
Cook County Hospital
Assistant Professor of Emergency Medicine
Rush Medical College
Chicago, Illinois
(Chapters 69, 72)

Lacy Knight, MD
Attending Physician
Department of Emergency Medicine
Community Hospital
Munster, Indiana
(Chapter 131)

Lukas Kolm, MD, MPH
Attending Physician
Department of Emergency Medicine
Wentworth-Douglass Hospital
Dover, New Hampshire
(Chapters 79, 171)

Anita Kulkarni, MD
Attending Physician
Department of Emergency Medicine
Northwest Memorial Hospital
Houston, Texas
(Chapter 122)

Roy Landsberg, MD
Attending Physician
Department of Otolaryngology and Bronchoesophagology
Rush-Presbyterian–St. Luke's Medical Center
Instructor
Department of Otolaryngology and Bronchoesophagology
Rush Medical College
Chicago, Illinois
(Chapter 147)

Charles M. Lash, MD
Attending Physician
Division of Urology
Cook County Hospital
Clinical Instructor of Urology
Rush Medical College
Chicago, Illinois
(Chapters 124, 127)

John K. Lee, MD
Attending Physician
Kansas City Cardiology Associates
Research Medical Office Tower
Kansas City, Missouri
(Chapter 24)

Moses S. Lee, MD, FACEP
Attending Physician
Director of Emergency Medical Services
Department of Emergency Medicine
Cook County Hospital
Assistant Professor of Emergency Medicine
Rush Medical College
Chicago, Illinois
(Chapter 172)

Robert R. Leschke, MD
Assistant Professor
Associate Program Director
Department of Emergency Medicine
Medical College of Wisconsin
Froedtert Hospital
Milwaukee, Wisconsin
(Chapters 47, 48)

David L. Levine, MD, FACEP
Associate Director Adult Emergency Services
Department of Emergency Medicine
Cook County Hospital
Assistant Professor of Emergency Medicine
Rush Medical College
Chicago, Illinois
(Chapters 118, 119)

John E. Lewis, Jr., MD, MS
Attending Physician
Department of Emergency Medicine
Cook County Hospital
Clinical Instructor of Emergency Medicine
Rush Medical College
Chicago, Illinois
(Chapter 113)

Krystaleah Lindsay, HBSc, MD, FACEP
Attending Physician
Associate Education Director
Department of Emergency Medicine
St. Paul's Hospital
Clinical Instructor
Emergency Medicine
Department of Family Practice
University of British Columbia
Vancouver, British Columbia, Canada
(Chapter 117)

O. John Ma, MD
Research Director
Vice Chair for Academic Advancement
Department of Emergency Medicine
Truman Medical Center
Associate Professor of Emergency Medicine
University of Missouri–Kansas City School of Medicine
Kansas City, Missouri
(Chapters 6, 44)

Ritu Malik, MD
Attending Physician
Department of Emergency Medicine
UCLA Medical Center
Instructor of Medicine/Emergency Medicine
Los Angeles, California
(Chapter 70)

Khursheed A. Mallick, MD
Senior Attending Physician
Division of Urology
Cook County Hospital
Assistant Professor of Urology
Rush Medical College
Chicago, Illinois
(Chapter 128)

James R. Markey, MD
Chairman, Division of Adult Anesthesia
Department of Anesthesiology
Cook County Hospital
Assistant Professor of Anesthesiology
Rush Medical College
Chicago, Illinois
(Chapters 2, 10)

Steve L. Meeks, MD, FACEP
Assistant Professor of Emergency Medicine
Rush Medical College
Chairman and Medical Director
Department of Emergency Medicine
Westlake Hospital
Melrose Park, Illinois
(Chapter 17)

Jehangir Meer, MD
Department of Emergency Medicine
London Health Sciences Center
University of Western Ontario Hospital
London, Ontario, Canada
(Chapter 121)

Shayle Miller, MD
Attending Physician
Director, Adult Emergency Services
Cook County Hospital
Assistant Professor of Emergency Medicine
Rush Medical College
Chicago, Illinois
(Chapter 80)

Stephen E. Miller, MD
Attending Physician
Department of Emergency Medicine
Alameda County Medical Center/Highland Hospital
Clinical Instructor in Emergency Medicine
University of California San Francisco
Oakland, California
(Chapter 166)

Mark Morocco, MD
Clinical Instructor of Emergency Medicine
David Geffen School of Medicine at UCLA
UCLA Emergency Medicine Center
Los Angeles, California
(Chapter 5)

Kimberly Nagy, MD, FACS
Director of Research and Education
Department of Trauma Surgery
Cook County Hospital
Associate Professor of General Surgery
Rush Medical College
Chicago, Illinois
(Chapters 14, 55)

Isam F. Nasr, MD
Attending Physician
Associate Director Adult Emergency Services
Department of Emergency Medicine
Cook County Hospital
Assistant Professor of Emergency Medicine
Rush Medical College
Chicago, Illinois
(Chapters 3, 4, 11)

Ned F. Nasr, MD
Attending Physician
Department of Anesthesiology
Cook County Hospital
Assistant Professor of Anesthesiology
Rush Medical College
Chicago, Illinois
(Chapters 1, 3, 4, 11)

Jacqueline A. Nemer, MD, FACEP
Attending Physician
Division of Emergency Medicine
University of California, San Francisco
Assistant Clinical Professor of Medicine
University of California, San Francisco
San Francisco, California
(Chapter 167)

Ann Nguyen, MD
Attending Physician
Department of Emergency Medicine
Bellevue Hospital Center
New York, New York
(Chapter 127)

Flavia Nobay, MD
Assistant Clinical Professor of Medicine
Division of Emergency Medicine
University of California, San Francisco
San Francisco, California
(Chapter 43)

Justin Onzuka, MD, Honours BSc
Chief Resident
Department of Emergency Medicine
McMaster University Medical Centre
Hamilton, Ontario, Canada
(Chapters 163–165)

Charles Orsay, MD
Associate Chairman
Department of Surgery
Chairman
Division of Colon and Rectal Surgery
Cook County Hospital
Chicago, Illinois
(Chapters 57, 59–61)

Lisa R. Palivos, MS, MD
Attending Physician
Department of Emergency Medicine
Cook County Hospital
Assistant Professor of Emergency Medicine
Rush Medical College
Chicago, Illinois
(Chapters 90, 91)

Sharad Pandit, MD
Attending Physician
Transport Director
Assistant Program Director
Emergency Medicine
Department of Emergency Medicine
St. Christopher's Hospital for Children
Assistant Professor of Emergency Medicine and Pediatrics
Medical College of Pennsylvania
Philadelphia, Pennsylvania
(Chapter 73)

Kenneth Pearlman, MD
Attending Physician
EMS Medical Director
Northwestern Memorial Hospital Division of
    Emergency Medicine
Assistant Professor of Emergency Medicine
Northwestern University Medical School
Chicago, Illinois
(Chapter 9)

Eric L. Pedicini, DO, MHPE
Attending Anesthesiologist
Department of Anesthesiology and Pain Management
Cook County Hospital
Assistant Professor of Anesthesiology
Rush Medical College
Chicago, Illinois
(Chapters 1, 4, 107)

Don W. Penney, MD, MSC, FACEP
Professor of Emergency Medicine
Medical College of Georgia
Neurological Surgeon
Gwinnett Medical Center
Lawrenceville, Georgia
(Chapters 97, 98, 101, 102)

Roland Petri, MD, MPH
Attending Physician
Division of Emergency Medicine
Northwestern University Medical School
Chicago, Illinois
(Chapter 12)

Susan B. Promes, MD, FACEP
Residency Program Director
Department of Emergency Medicine
Associate Clinical Professor of Surgery
Department of Surgery
Duke University Medical Center
Durham, North Carolina
(Chapter 54)

Margaret J. Provenza, MD
Member, Associates in Head and Neck Surgery, S.C.
Clinical Instructor of Otolaryngology
Department of Otolaryngology and Bronchoesophagology
Rush Medical College
Chicago, Illinois
(Chapter 145)

Yanina Purim-Shem-Tov, MD
Attending Physician
Department of Emergency Medicine
Rush-Presbyterian–St. Luke's Medical Center
Clinical Instructor of Emergency Medicine
Rush Medical College
Chicago, Illinois
(Chapter 124)

Ratnakar S. Rajanahally, MD, FACC
Attending Physician
Pacemaker Clinic Director
Division of Cardiology
Cook County Hospital
Assistant Professor of Cardiology
Rush Medical College
Chicago, Illinois
(Chapters 20, 21, 23)

Paul S. Ray, DO
Chairman
Department of Urology
Cook County Hospital
Professor of Urology
Rush Medical College
Chicago, Illinois
(Chapters 121, 124)

Eric F. Reichman, PhD, MD, FAAEM, FACEP
Attending Physician
Assistant Residency Director
Director of Surgical Techniques and Skills Laboratory
Department of Emergency Medicine
Cook County Hospital
Assistant Professor of Emergency Medicine
Director of Surgical Techniques and Skills Laboratory
Rush Medical College
Chicago, Illinois
(Chapters 5, 7,11, 22, 45, 58, 65–67, 69, 75, 78, 79, 83, 104, 106, 144, 154, 157, 171)

Rebecca R. Roberts, MD
Attending Physician
Co-Director Research Division
Department of Emergency Medicine
Cook County Hospital
Assistant Professor of Emergency Medicine
Rush Medical College
Chicago, Illinois
(Chapters 138, 141, 142)

Roxanne Roberts, MD, FACS
Associate Director of Trauma Surgery
Director, Trauma Intensive Care Unit
Chair, Division of Clinical Services
Department of Trauma Surgery
Cook County Hospital
Chicago, Illinois
(Chapters 27, 30)

Robert Rodriguez, MD, FACEP
Assistant Clinical Professor of Emergency Medicine
Department of Emergency Medicine
Alameda County Medical Center
Oakland, California
(Chapter 46)

Mark Rolain, MD
General Ophthalmologist
St. Joseph Mercy Hospital
Pontiac, Michigan
(Chapter 135)

John S. Rose, MD
Associate Residency Director
Assistant Professor of Medicine
Division of Emergency Medicine
University of California, Davis
Sacramento, California
(Chapter 168)

Daniel J. Ross, MD, DDS
Attending Physician and Clinical Faculty
Department of Emergency Medicine
Resurrection Medical Center
Clinical Assistant Professor of Emergency Medicine
University of Illinois
Chicago, Illinois
(Chapters 155, 158–160)

David Rovinsky, MD
Orthopedic Surgeon
Kauai Medical Clinic
Lihue, Kauai, Hawaii
(Chapters 63, 64, 76)

Dino P. Rumoro, DO, FACEP
Clinical Chairman
Department of Emergency Medicine
Rush-Presbyterian–St. Luke's Medical Center
Assistant Professor of Emergency Medicine
Rush Medical College
Chicago, Illinois
(Chapters 133, 136, 137)

Joseph A. Salomone III, MD, FAAEM
Residency Program Director
Department of Emergency Medicine
Truman Medical Center
Associate Professor
University of Missouri–Kansas City School of Medicine
Kansas City, Missouri
(Chapter 18)

Steven Salzman, MD
Attending Physician
Department of Trauma Surgery
Christ Hospital
Chicago, Illinois
(Chapter 33)

Payman Sattar, MD, MS
Attending Physician
Director of Echocardiography
Director, Cardiology Clinics
Department of Adult Cardiology
Cook County Hospital
Assistant Professor of Emergency Medicine
Rush Medical College
Chicago, Illinois
(Chapters 19, 26)

Eric Savitsky, MD
Assistant Professor of Medicine/Emergency Medicine
UCLA Emergency Medicine Residency Program
Los Angeles, California
(Chapter 139)

Shari Schabowski, MD
Attending Physician
Department of Emergency Medicine
Cook County Hospital
Assistant Professor of Emergency Medicine
Rush Medical College
Chicago, Illinois
(Chapter 132)

Jeff Schaider, MD
Attending Physician, Associate Chairman
Department of Emergency Medicine
Cook County Hospital
Associate Professor of Emergency Medicine
Rush Medical College
Chicago, Illinois
(Chapter 162)

Jeffrey S. Schlab, MD
Attending Physician
Department of Emergency Medicine
Seton Medical Center
Attending Physician
Department of Emergency Medicine
Seton Northwest Hospital
Austin, Texas
(Chapter 140)

Peter T. Schubel, MD
Attending Physician
Department of Emergency Medicine
Grand Strand Regional Medical Center
Myrtle Beach, South Carolina
(Chapter 7)

Julio C. Silva, MD, FACEP
Associate Clinical Chairman
Department of Emergency Medicine
Rush-Presbyterian–St. Luke's Medical Center
Assistant Professor of Emergency Medicine
Rush Medical College
Chicago, Illinois
(Chapters 151–153)

Sanford Scot Sineff, MD
Attending Physician
Barnes–Jewish Hospital
Assistant Professor of Emergency Medicine
Washington University School of Medicine
St. Louis, Missouri
(Chapter 67)

Andreas Skoubis, DO
Attending Physician
Department of Emergency Medicine
Rush-Presbyterian–St. Luke's Medical Center
Clinical Instructor of Emergency Medicine
Rush Medical College
Chicago, Illinois
(Chapter 129)

Erik Sloan, MD
Attending Physician
Department of Emergency Medicine
St. Anthony Medical Center
Chicago, Illinois
(Chapter 112)

Robert F. Smith, MD, MPH
Chair, Division of Prehospital Care and Prevention
Department of Trauma Surgery
Cook County Hospital
Chicago, Illinois
(Chapter 25)

Eric R. Snoey, MD
Associate Clinical Professor
University of California, San Francisco
Residency Director
Department of Emergency Medicine
Alameda County Medical Center/Highland Hospital
Oakland, California
(Chapters 120, 166)

Steven J. Socransky, MDCM, FRCP
Attending Physician
Department of Emergency Medicine
Sudbury Regional Hospital
Sudbury, Ontario, Canada
(Chapter 134)

Julia H. Sone, MD
Chairman, Section of Surgical Endoscopy
Division of Colon and Rectal Surgery
Cook County Hospital
Clinical Instructor of Surgery
University of Illinois
Chicago, Illinois
(Chapter 56)

Sam Stokes III, MD
Attending Physician
The Urology Institute and Continence Center
Thomasville, Georgia
(Chapters 121–123)

Geraldine L. Stratton, MD
Attending Physician
Department of Emergency Medicine
Torrance Memorial Medical Center
Torrance, California
(Chapter 70)

Susan Stroud, MD
Clinical Instructor, Department of Emergency Services
San Francisco General Hospital
San Francisco, California
(Chapter 46)

Brian C. Sullivan, MD
Attending Physician
Department of Emergency Medicine
Resurrection Medical Center
Chicago, Illinois
(Chapter 87)

Mark Tanaka, MD
Emergency Medicine Resident
Department of Emergency Medicine
Cook County Hospital
Chicago, Illinois
(Chapter 114)

James T. Thomas, MD
Fellow, Division of Cardiology
Cook County Hospital
Chicago, Illinois
(Chapters 21, 23)

Alfred E. Tober, MD
Department of Emergency Medicine
University of Manitoba Health Science Center
St. Boniface Hospital
Winnipeg, Alberta, Canada
(Chapter 83)

Dedra R. Tolson, MD
Acting Instructor, Attending Physician
Emergency Medical Services
University of Washington Medical Center
Seattle, Washington
(Chapters 62, 106)

Neil Troost, MD
Attending Physician
Department of Emergency Medicine
St. Mary's Hospital
Evansville, Indiana
(Chapter 128)

Atilla B. Üner, MD
Visiting Assistant Clinical Professor
UCLA Emergency Medicine Center
Associate Medical Director
UCLA Center for Prehospital Care
Associate Medical Director
Department of Emergency Medicine
Coalinga Regional Medical Center
Los Angeles, California
(Chapters 103, 173)

Suneel Upadhye, BSc, MD, FRCP
Staff Emergency Physician
McMaster University
Hamilton, Ontario, Canada
(Chapters 159–161)

Jeffrey M. VanBendegom, MD
Attending Physician
St. Mary's Hospital
Racine, Wisconsin
(Chapter 96)

Michelle M. Verplanck, DO
Clinical Assistant Professor of Ophthalmology
College of Osteopathic Medicine
Michigan State University
Byrd Eye Clinic
Lincoln Park, Michigan
(Chapter 135)

Patricia Vidal, MD
Attending Physician
Division of Urology
Cook County Hospital
Assistant Professor of Urology
Rush Medical College
Chicago, Illinois
(Chapters 125, 129–131)

Richard Waddell, MD, LT, USN
Staff Physician
Emergency Medicine Department
U.S. Naval Hospital Roosevelt Roads
Puerto Rico
(Chapter 65)

Anthony Waechter, MD
Attending Physician
Department of Emergency Medicine
Kaiser-Walnut Creek Hospital
Walnut Creek, California
(Chapter 110)

David L. Walner, MD
Attending Physician
Department of Otolaryngology and Bronchoesophagology
Rush-Presbyterian–St. Luke's Medical Center
Assistant Professor
Department of Otolaryngology and Bronchoesophagology
Rush Medical College
Chicago, Illinois
(Chapter 150)

Paula L. Ward, MD
Assistant Professor
Division of Emergency Medicine
University of Texas Southwestern Medical Center
Dallas, Texas
(Chapters 92–94)

Daryl D. Wilson, MD
Attending Physician
Department of Emergency Medicine
Provident Hospital of Cook County
Chicago, Illinois
(Chapter 22)

Alon P. Winnie, MD
Chairman
Department of Anesthesiology and Pain Management
Cook County Hospital
Professor of Anesthesiology
Rush Medical College
Chicago, Illinois
(Chapter 107)

Daniel Wu, MD
Assistant Professor
Department of Emergency Medicine
Emory University School of Medicine
Attending Physician
Department of Emergency Medicine
Grady Memorial Hospital
Attending Physician
Department of Emergency Medicine
Crawford W. Long Hospital
Atlanta, Georgia
(Chapter 123)

FOREWORD

We first met Bob Simon in the late 1970's when we were all new Emergency Medicine faculty at UCLA and the University of Chicago. Things were very different in Emergency Medicine back then, but Bob already had a clear vision of what the specialty could and must become. He believed that if we were ever to fulfill our promise, we had to teach ourselves, and however many generations of students, to be true experts in the field we were hoping to develop.

This meant that we had to be as good at everything we did as any of the so-called consultants with whom we would interact on a daily basis. If we were going to intubate patients, we would need to be able to intubate, in an emergency, at least as well as any anesthesiologist. If we were going to diagnose patients with pulmonary embolism, we would by god have to know at least as much about the differential diagnosis of shortness of breath, or chest pain, as any pulmonologist or critical care specialist. And so on and so forth.

Bob devoted himself to that process—of learning to be an expert himself, and more importantly teaching his students with legendary zeal and dedication—right from the very beginning. He published, almost single-handedly, textbooks in emergency orthopedics as well as emergency medical procedures—books which not only reflected his personal fascination with these topics, but which also demanded of his readers that they too be committed to expertise and excellence.

The settings in which the discipline of Emergency Medicine is practiced vary widely, from suburban urgent care centers to urban trauma centers, from basic hospitals in rural areas to tertiary university medical centers in our largest cities. While the approach to evaluating and medically treating patients remains largely the same regardless of location, the types of procedures per-

formed at a patient's bedside vary greatly by practice setting. For almost all of us, there will come a time when we are faced with the need to do a procedure about which we were not trained, or which we have not performed in quite some time. Hence, there will always be a need for excellent procedure texts. This particular book covers the large majority of procedures that are likely to be performed in any ED practice setting. The well-organized table of contents divides the book into many relatively short chapters, which makes it user friendly for a busy clinician. The chapters themselves are well written and contain many clear, useful diagrams—a critically important component of any procedure book. The chapter format is consistent and includes discussions of anatomy and pathophysiology, procedure indications and contraindications, necessary equipment, patient preparation, procedural techniques, alternative treatments, aftercare instructions, and complications. Important concepts are highlighted and controversial issues are discussed and well referenced.

We are especially delighted to have been asked to write the Foreword for this new text. Rather than producing a solo effort, Bob has worked with an extremely knowledgeable lead editor and many contributing authors. Multi-authored texts of necessity sacrifice some element of personal wisdom, but gain so much more from the evidence-based input from a wide array of talented authors. Thus this book reflects the evolution of our specialty from a place where a few giants like Bob Simon pushed and kicked and prodded the specialty into being, to a place where legions of talented, dedicated, and knowledgeable young academicians demonstrate why Emergency Medicine has now attained a place of honor and respect in the larger world of Medicine (not to mention the larger society in general), and why the very best medical sudents compete to join us.

This book will take its place alongside other excellent texts in Emergency Medicine, but what makes it more special in our minds is both the unique person from whose vision, 25 years ago, it first sprung, and the way in which it represents the growth and maturation of a specialty. It's hard to improve on the work of a Bob Simon, but we are sure there is no one prouder than Bob of the fact that this text is indeed an improvement on even his solo efforts.

Jerome R. Hoffman, MD
Professor of Medicine/Emergency Medicine
UCLA School of Medicine

Robert S. Hockberger, MD
Chairman
Department of Emergency Medicine
Harbor-UCLA Medical Center
Professor of Medicine/Emergency Medicine
UCLA School of Medicine

PREFACE

The scope of Emergency Medicine is extremely broad; it covers the care of the neonate through the geriatric, surgical, and medical patients, and encompasses all organ systems. Emergency Medicine is rapidly evolving to reflect our increasing experience, knowledge, and research. Procedural skills must supplement our cognitive skills. Achieving proficiency in procedural skills is essential for the daily practice of Emergency Medicine. In this textbook, we have produced a clear, complete, and easy-to-understand guide to procedures. It will provide all practitioners, from the medical student to the seasoned Emergentologist, with a single procedural reference on which to base their clinical practices and technical skills.

The primary purpose of this text is to provide a detailed, step-by-step approach to procedures performed in the Emergency Department—and it is expressly about procedures. While well referenced, it is not meant to be a comprehensive reference but an easy-to-use and clinically useful text that should be at hand in every Emergency Department. The content and information are complete. The book is organized and written for ease of access and use. The detail is sufficient to allow the reader to gain a thorough understanding of each procedure. When available, alternative techniques or hints are presented. Each chapter provides the reader with clear and specific guidelines for performing every procedure. Although some may use this text as a library reference, its real place is in the Emergency Department where the procedures are performed. Despite its size, we hope that this book will find its way to the bedside to be used by medical students, residents, and practicing clinicians.

This book will satisfy the needs of physicians with a variety of backgrounds and training. While it is primarily written for Emergentologists, many other practitioners will find this a valuable reference. This book is written for those who care for people with acute illnesses or injuries. Medical students and residents will find this an authoritative work on procedural skills. Medical students, residents, and practitioners with limited experience will find all the information in each chapter to learn a complete procedure. Family Physicians, Internists, and Pediatricians will find this text useful to review procedures infrequently performed in the clinic, office, or urgent care center. Intensivists and Surgeons involved in the care of acutely ill patients will also find this book a wonderful resource. Experienced clinicians can get a quick refresher on the procedure while enhancing their knowledge and skills. Physicians actively involved in the education of medical students and residents will find this text an easy-to-understand and well-illustrated source of didactic material.

The text has 15 sections containing 173 chapters. The contents are organized into sections, each representing an organ system, an area of the body, or a surgical specialty. Each chapter is devoted to a single procedure. This should allow quick access to complete information. Most of the chapters follow a similar format, thus allowing information to be retrieved as quickly and as efficiently as possible. There are often several acceptable methods to perform a procedure. While alternative techniques are described in many chapters, we have not exhaustively included all alternative techniques. Key information, cautions, and important facts are highlighted throughout the text in **bold** type.

Each chapter, with a few exceptions, follows a standard format. The relevant anatomy and pathophysiology are discussed, followed by the indications and contraindications for the procedure. A list of the necessary equipment is provided. Preparation of the patient—including consent, anesthesia, and analgesia—is addressed. The procedure is then described step by step.

Cautions are placed where problems commonly occur. Alternative techniques and helpful hints for each procedure are presented. Aftercare and follow-up are discussed. Any potential complications are described, including the methods to reduce and care for the complications. Finally, a summary contains a review of any critical or important information.

This book covers a wide variety of procedures. We have made an effort to think of most procedures that may be performed in a rural or urban Emergency Department and have incorporated them into this text. This includes procedures performed routinely or rarely. It also includes procedures that are often performed in the acute care, clinic, and office setting. Some of the procedures in this book may be performed frequently in the daily practice of Emergency Medicine, such as laceration repair or endotracheal intubation. Other procedures, such as cricothyroidotomy, are seldom to rarely performed but critical to the practice of Emergency Medicine. While many of the procedures are well known to the Emergentologist, some are uncommon and may not be so widely known. This gives the reader an opportunity to acquire new information that may be converted, with proper practice and training, into a useful skill. A few of the procedures are performed only by Surgeons. They are included to promote understanding by those who may later see the patients in the Emergency Department and have to provide emergent care for a complication.

We have drawn on a wide variety of authors. The majority of authors are residency-trained, board-certified, practicing Emergentologists. We have the honor of having many contributors from outside the field of Emergency Medicine who are experts in their own specialties. Many of them are from Cook County Hospital, including the trauma surgeons. The authors do have biases because of differences in education, experience, and training. We have tried to base all recommendations on sound clinical and scientific data. However, we have not excluded personal experience or preferences when appropriate. In these cases, the authors also present alternative techniques.

Hopefully, this book will grow and change with time. Suggestions from you, the reader, would be most appreciated. Let us know what additional procedures should be included or excluded in future editions.

Eric F. Reichman, PhD, MD
Robert R. Simon, MD

ACKNOWLEDGMENTS

This has been an educational, sometimes fun, and time-consuming process. I must thank my wife, Kristi, for all her patience during this endeavor that took thousands of hours and 4 years. Thanks too to Joey, who was FAB and always kept me entertained, day and night. To Jake, who spent endless hours sleeping at my feet, keeping me company, and waiting to be taken for a walk. Even Gizmo helped, although he constantly interrupted my work by rolling on top of the desk and throwing papers about the room.

I would like to acknowledge the support of friends, colleagues, current residents, and former residents in the Department of Emergency Medicine at Cook County Hospital. They provided friendship, encouragement, and the drive to finish this work. A special thanks goes to Bob Simon and Jeff Schaider. Their friendship, patience, mentoring, advice, and always being available were invaluable throughout this process. The editorial assistance, hard work, and devotion of Mishelle Taylor is well respected and treasured.

I must also thank those who helped me get to this point in my career. Their friendship, mentoring, and efforts have not gone unappreciated. Graduate school training in Gross Anatomy and Neuroanatomy at the Uniformed Services University of the Health Sciences (USUHS) has formed a framework for everything that I do. This was due to the efforts of Malcolm Carpenter, Rosemary Borke, and Dave Beebe. Emergency Medicine Residency at the Medical College of Wisconsin was a fantastic experience. I always looked forward to an ED shift, taking care of "room 9" patients, and the helicopter flight experiences. I couldn't have done this without the support, advice, and friendship of Tom Aufderheide, Dan Debehnke, and Mike Keefer.

Finally, I want to thank the authors. Many of you are good friends whom I cherish. They gave of themselves and their time—even after I would call or e-mail them week after week asking, "Where's my chapter?"

Eric F. Reichman

I would like to acknowledge Mishelle Taylor, my administrator. Her work on this project was truly immense.

Robert R. Simon

EMERGENCY MEDICINE PROCEDURES

Section One

RESPIRATORY PROCEDURES

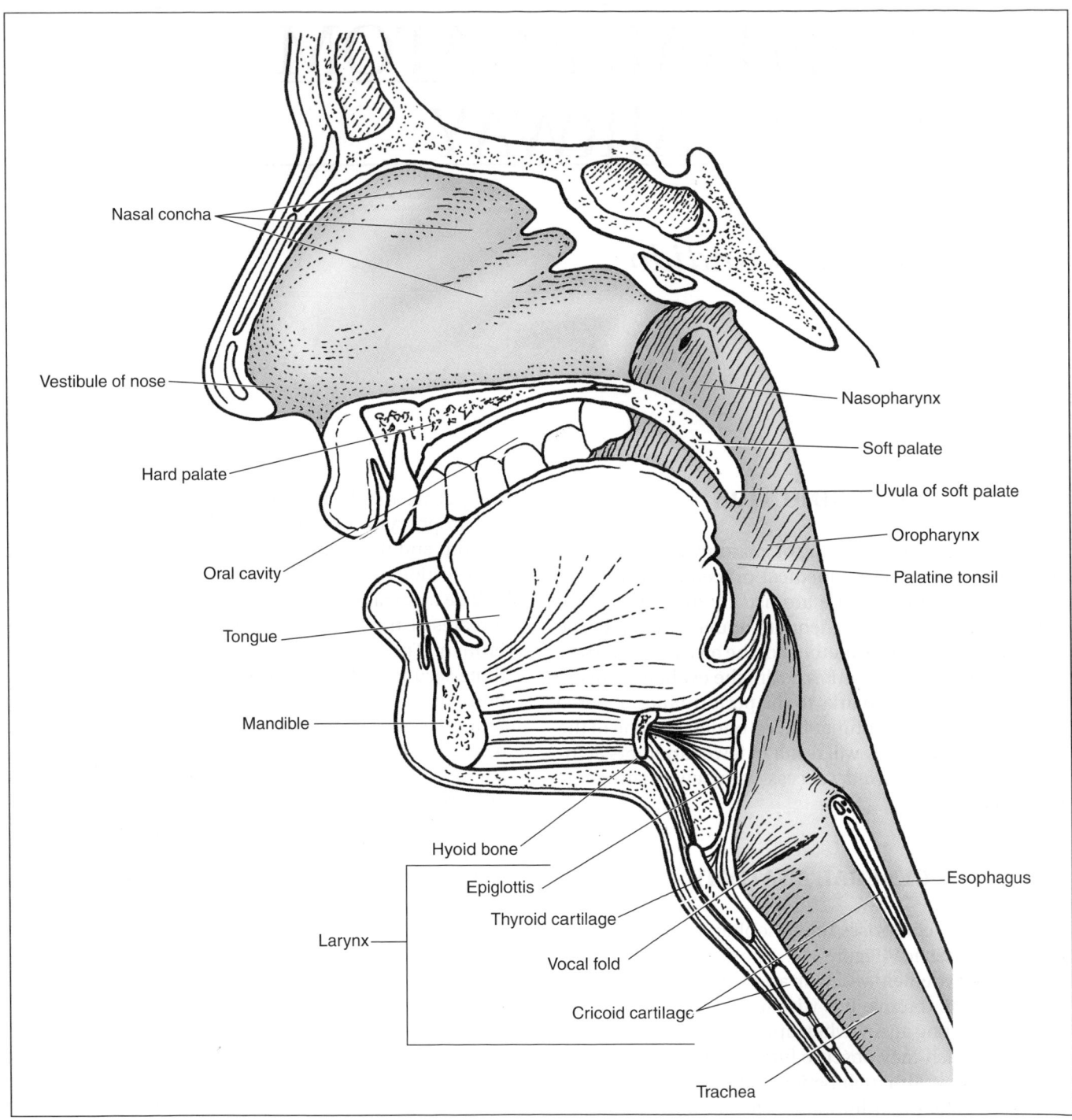

FIGURE 1-1 Anatomy of the airway. The drawing is a midsagittal section through the head and neck.

rent laryngeal nerve supplies sensation below the vocal cords. The recurrent laryngeal nerve provides the motor input to all of the intrinsic muscles of the larynx except to the cricothyroid muscle, which is supplied by the external branch of the superior laryngeal nerve. Bilateral injury to the recurrent laryngeal nerve will result in total airway closure due to unopposed stimulation of the vocal cord adductor, the cricothyroid muscle.[1]

There are three paired and three unpaired cartilages of the larynx.[2] The paired cartilages are the smaller arytenoid, corniculate, and cuneiform cartilages (Figure 1-2). The unpaired cartilages are the larger thyroid, cricoid, and epiglottic cartilages. Although not part of the larynx, the hyoid bone has many attachments to the larynx. The cricoid cartilage is signet ring–shaped, as opposed to the C-shaped cartilages of the trachea (Figure 1-2). Because

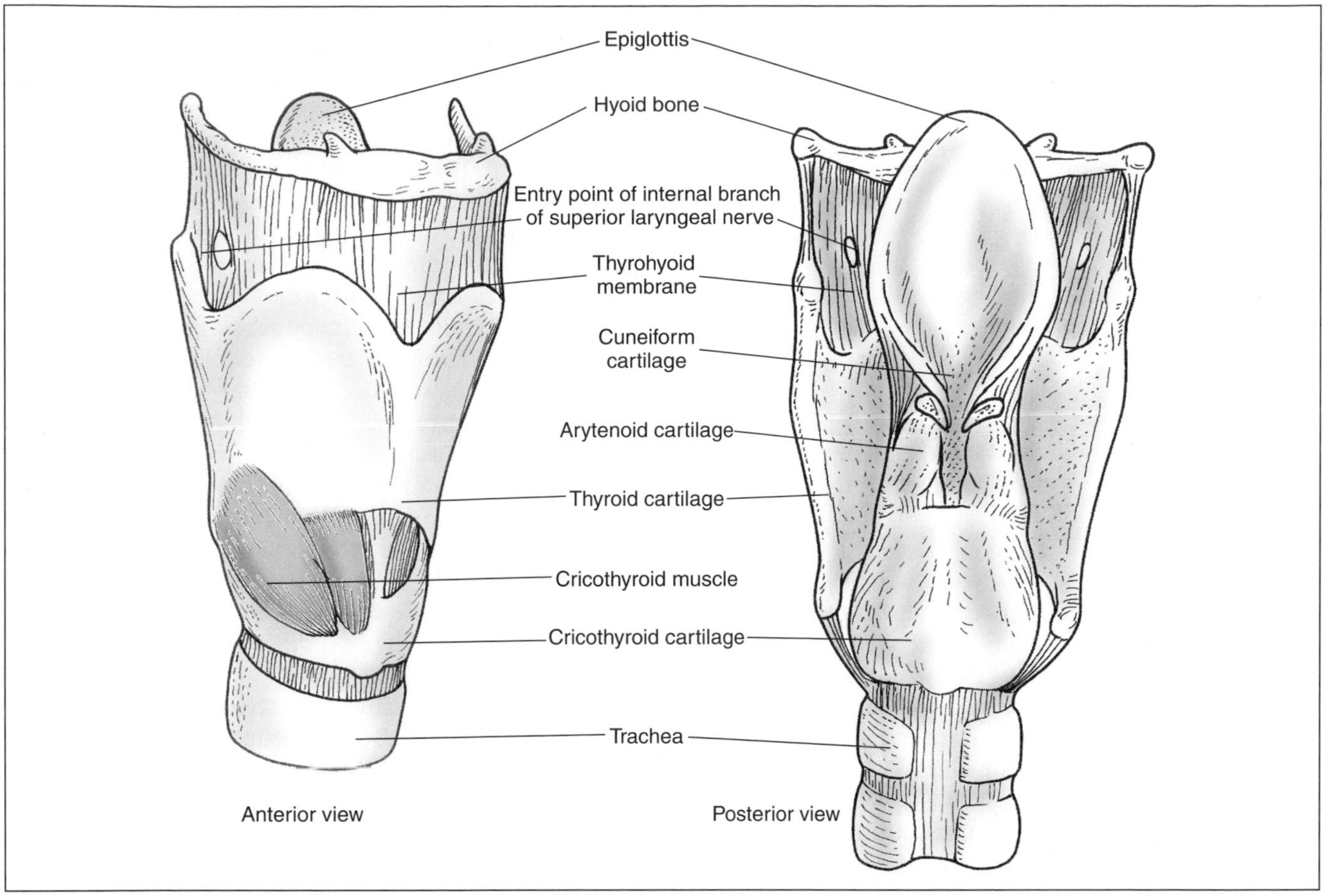

Epiglottis

Hyoid bone

Entry point of internal branch
of superior laryngeal nerve

Thyrohyoid
membrane

Cuneiform
cartilage

Arytenoid cartilage

Thyroid cartilage

Cricothyroid muscle

Cricothyroid cartilage

Trachea

Anterior view

Posterior view

FIGURE 1-2 Right anterolateral and posterior views of the skeleton of the larynx. The thyroid cartilage shields the smaller cartilages of the larynx.

it forms a complete circle, depression of the cricoid cartilage will put pressure on structures located posteriorly (e.g., the esophagus) without occluding the airway. **The application of posteriorly directed pressure on the cricoid cartilage during intubation is known as the Sellick maneuver (Figure 1-3). The Sellick maneuver will not prevent regurgitation from active vomiting.** It has been shown to be effective in the prevention of passive regurgitation and subsequent aspiration.[3] The cricoid cartilage is also an important landmark for locating the cricothyroid membrane, which lies inferior to the thyroid cartilage and superior to the cricoid cartilage (Figure 1-2). The cricothyroid membrane is usually located at the level of the sixth cervical vertebra. The cricothyroid membrane is the location where emergency cricothyroidotomies and recurrent laryngeal nerve blocks are performed.

The three paired cartilages are located on the posterior aspect of the larynx (Figure 1-2). This position renders them vulnerable to injury during intubation.[2] By staying anterior and by not inserting a laryngoscope blade too deeply during intubation attempts, it is less likely that these cartilages will become dislocated or oth-

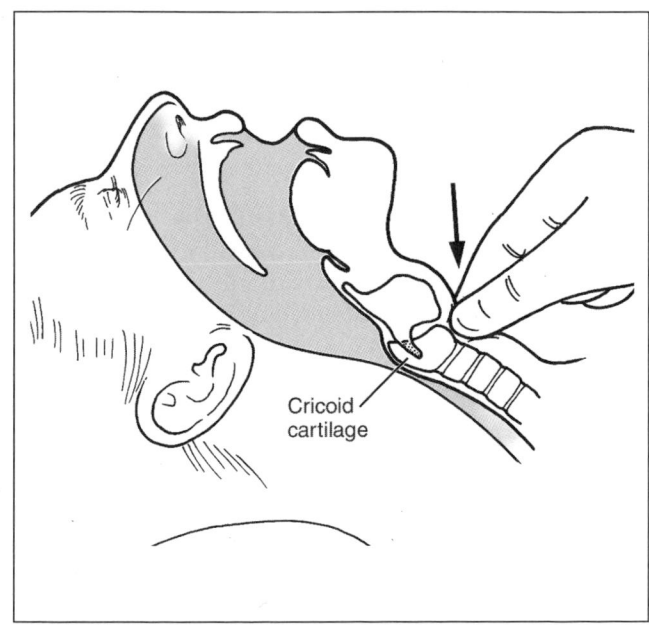

Cricoid
cartilage

FIGURE 1-3 The Sellick maneuver. Cricoid pressure is applied to the cricoid cartilage to occlude the esophagus and prevent regurgitation and subsequent aspiration of gastric contents.

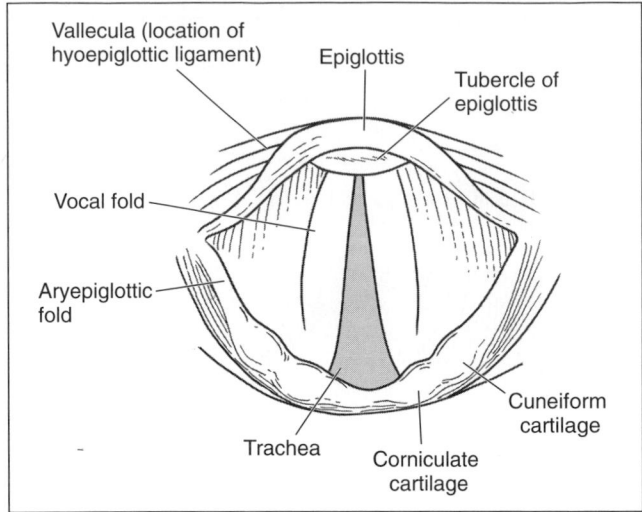

FIGURE 1-4 Laryngoscopic view of the larynx.

erwise injured. This is particularly true if a straight laryngoscope blade is being used.

One of the attachments of the hyoid bone to the larynx is the hyoepiglottic ligament located at the base of the vallecula (Figure 1-4). This ligament is important because it is where the tip of the curved Macintosh laryngoscope blade is placed to move the epiglottis anteriorly and out of the path of vision during intubation. Another attachment of the hyoid bone to the larynx is the thyrohyoid membrane (Figure 1-2). As its name implies, it runs from the inferior border of the hyoid bone to the superior aspect of the thyroid cartilage. Just inferior to the lateral border of the hyoid bone, the internal branch of the superior laryngeal nerve passes through the thyrohyoid membrane (Figure 1-2). At this point, the internal branch of the superior laryngeal nerve is superficial enough to be easily anesthetized with an injection of local anesthetic solution.

AIRWAY EVALUATION

The evaluation of the airway should always start with a thorough history. It should include whether the patient has ever required intubation and if there was any difficulty. Additional history should focus on the patient's dentition and any surgery on or near the airway. There are many congenital syndromes (Table 1-1) and acquired conditions (Table 1-2) that can complicate airway management. These should be kept in mind when performing the airway history and physical examination.

External evaluation of the airway is a critical step to a successful intubation. Several brief evaluations are helpful in predicting a difficult intubation. External inspection should include mouth opening, atlantooccipital extension, and thyromental distance. Internally, inspect the teeth, palate, tongue, and other soft tissue for abnormal anatomy or masses. External inspection should identify obvious problems (cervical collars, face and/or neck trauma, severe micrognathia, massive obesity, etc.).

The next three steps in evaluating the airway may help to identify patients with potentially difficult airways. In adults, the distance between the thyroid cartilage ("Adam's apple") and the inside of the anterior aspect of the mandible is known as the thyromental distance. It should be at least 5 cm or about three large finger breadths.[1] **Distances less than 5 cm may indicate that visualization of the larynx during intubation may be difficult or impossible due to a lack of space in which to displace the tongue.** The next evaluation requires the patient to open his or her mouth maximally. Ideally, the patient will be in a seated or semisitting position. The distance between the maxillary and mandibular incisors in an average adult is 3 to 4 cm or about two large finger breadths.[5] Limited mouth opening may impair visualization of the airway as well as expose the teeth to damage during intubation. Adults should be able to flex their cervical spine 35 degrees and extend the cervical spine (atlantooccipital joint) 80 degrees from a neutral position.[6] This range of neck movement allows for the alignment of the oral, pharyngeal, and laryngeal axes (Figure 1-5). This alignment of the axes provides the greatest chance for a successful intubation.

The internal examination should evaluate the patient's dentition, palate, and tongue. Note any protuberant incisors, loose teeth, broken teeth, dental work, and

TABLE 1-1. SELECTED CONGENITAL SYNDROMES ASSOCIATED WITH DIFFICULT ENDOTRACHEAL INTUBATION

Syndrome	Description
Down	Cervical spine spondylolisthesis; large tongue, small mouth make laryngoscopy difficult; small subglottic diameter possible; frequent laryngospasm
Goldenhar (oculoauriculovertebral anomalies)	Mandibular hypoplasia and cervical spine abnormality make laryngoscopy difficult
Klippel-Feil	Neck rigidity because of cervical vertebral fusion
Pierre Robin	Small mouth, large tongue, mandibular anomaly; awake intubation essential in neonate
Treacher Collins (mandibulofacial dysostosis)	Laryngoscopy difficult
Turner	High likelihood of difficult intubation

SOURCE: Modified from Barash et al.[1]

TABLE 1-2. ACQUIRED CONDITIONS AFFECTING THE AIRWAY AND ASSOCIATED WITH DIFFICULT ENDOTRACHEAL INTUBATION

Condition	Principal pathologic clinical features of the airway
Acromegaly	Macroglossia; prognathism
Acute burns	Edema of airway (worsens with time, secure airway early!)
Angioedema	Obstructive swelling renders ventilation and intubation difficult
Arthritis	
Rheumatoid arthritis	Temporomandibular joint ankylosis, cricoarytenoid arthritis, deviation of larynx, restricted mobility of cervical spine
Ankylosing spondylitis	Ankylosis of cervical spine; less commonly ankylosis of temporomandibular joints; lack of mobility of cervical spine
Benign tumors	Stenosis or distortion of airway
Cystic, hygroma, lipoma, adenoma	
Diabetes mellitus	May have reduced mobility of atlantooccipital joint
Foreign body	Airway obstruction
Hypothyroidism	Large tongue, abnormal soft tissue (myxedema) make ventilation and intubation difficult
Infectious	
Supraglottitis	Laryngeal edema
Croup	Laryngeal edema
Abscess (intraoral, retropharyngeal)	Distortion and stenosis of airway and trismus
Ludwig's angina	Distortion and stenosis of airway and trismus
Malignant tumors	Stenosis or distortion of airway; fixation of larynx or adjacent tissues secondary to infiltration or fibrosis from irradiation
Carcinoma of tongue, larynx, or thyroid	
Morbid obesity	Short, thick neck and large tongue are likely to be present
Pregnancy	Edema of airway
Sarcoidosis	Airway obstruction (lymphoid tissue)
Scleroderma	Tight skin and temporomandibular joint involvement make mouth opening difficult
Temporomandibular joint syndrome	Severe impairment of mouth opening
Thyromegaly	Goiter may produce extrinsic airway compression or deviation
Trauma	Cerebrospinal rhinorrhea, edema of airway; hemorrhage; unstable fracture(s) of maxillae and mandible; intralaryngeal damage; dislocation of cervical vertebrae
Head, face, or cervical spine injury	

SOURCE: Modified from Miller.[4]

dental devices. Determine if the palate is normal, high and arched, or cleft. Determine if the tongue is elevated, larger, or wider than normal in comparison to the oral cavity. Any abnormality can make the procedure of orotracheal intubation more difficult. A common classification used by Anesthesiologists to grade the difficulty of laryngoscopy and intubation involves the identification of the size of the tongue in relation to the faucial pillars, the soft palate, and the uvula.[7] It is important to perform this evaluation by first instructing patients to open their mouths and protrude their tongues maximally in the sitting position. The patient should not say "ahhh," as this distorts the anatomy and may falsely improve the airway classification. The Mallampati classification, named after its author, has three grades.[7] Class 1 is when the faucial pillars, soft palate, and uvula can be fully visualized (Figure 1-6). In class 2, the faucial pillars and soft palate can be visualized but the uvula is partially masked by the base of the tongue. Class 3 is when only the soft palate can be visualized (Figure 1-7). The predictive value of this classification is that during direct laryngoscopy, the entire glottis can be exposed in 100 percent of class 1, 65 percent of class 2, and 0.1 percent of class 3 airways.[7]

ANATOMIC DIFFERENCES BETWEEN THE ADULT AND THE INFANT

There are numerous differences between the airway of an adult and that of a child. The head-to-body ratio is larger in the child. This causes the neck to be flexed when the child is supine. Placing a rolled towel under the child's shoulders will correct the flexion. A child has a small mouth with a relatively large tongue as compared to an adult. This can make orotracheal intubation difficult. The presence of adenoidal tissue in the child makes nasotracheal intubation difficult and orotracheal intubation the preferred method.

The anatomic differences between the larynx of an adult and that of a young child are summarized in Table 1-3 and Figure 1-8.[1] **The most important difference is that the narrowest portion of the infant airway is below the level of the vocal cords at the cricoid cartilage. In an adult, the narrowest point is the vocal cords.** An endotracheal tube may therefore pass through the vocal cords of a young child but might not advance past the cricoid cartilage due to normal anatomy. Forcing an endotracheal tube past the vocal cords in a young child

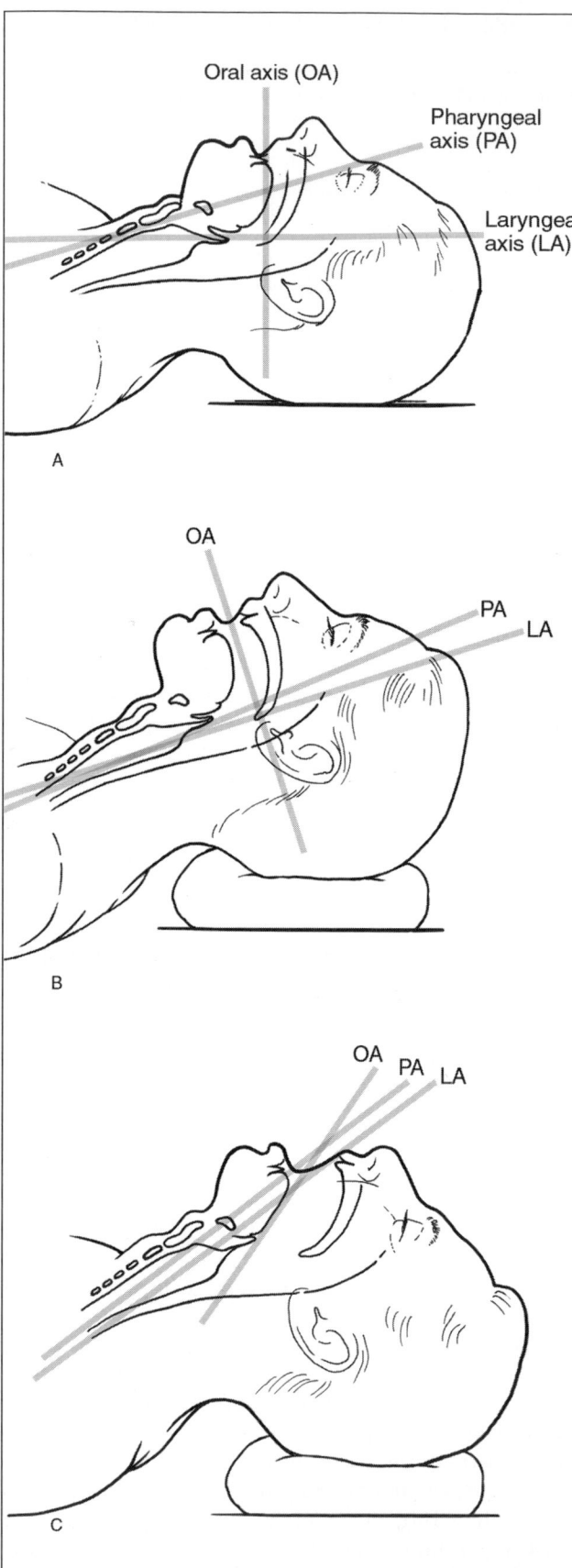

Oral axis (OA)

Pharyngeal axis (PA)

Laryngeal axis (LA)

A

OA

PA LA

B

OA PA LA

C

◄ **FIGURE 1-5** Schematic diagram demonstrating head positioning for endotracheal intubation. *A.* The normal alignment of the oral, pharyngeal, and laryngeal axes. *B.* Elevation of the head about 10 cm with pads below the occiput, while the shoulders remain on the table, aligns the laryngeal and pharyngeal axes. *C.* Subsequent head extension, at the atlantooccipital joint, serves to create the shortest distance and most nearly straight line from the incisor teeth to glottic opening.

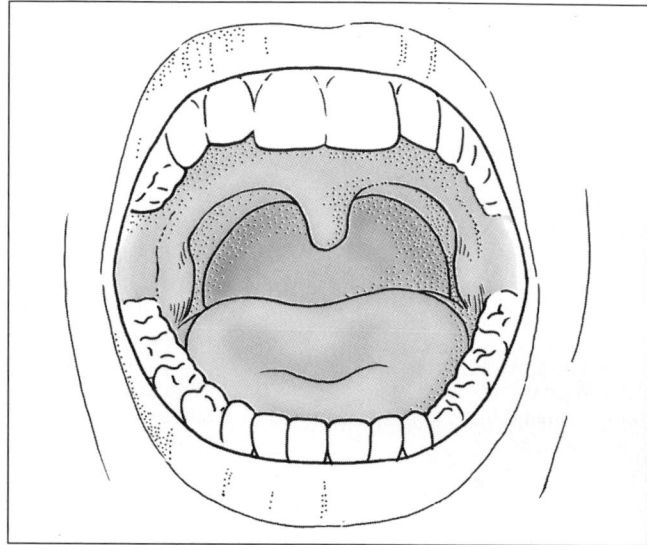

FIGURE 1-6 Illustration of a patient in whom faucial pillars, soft palate, and uvula are fully visible (Mallampati class 1).

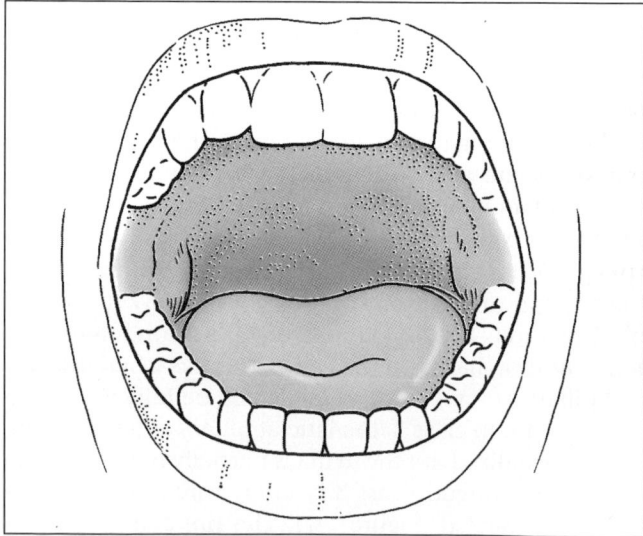

FIGURE 1-7 Illustration of a patient in whom none of the three pharyngeal structures are visible (Mallampati class 3).

TABLE 1-3. ANATOMIC DIFFERENCES BETWEEN THE CHILD'S AND ADULT'S LARYNX

	Child's larynx	Adult's larynx
Size	Smaller	Larger
Shape	Lumen is funnel-shaped with the narrowest part below the vocal cords and within the cricoid ring	Narrowest part of lumen is at the vocal cords
Location	Higher, closer to the tongue base; vertical extent is opposite C3, C4, C5 vertebrae; more anterior	Vertical extent is lower, opposite C4, C5, C6 vertebrae
Epiglottis	Longer, narrower, and "U" shaped; the angle between glottis and epiglottis is more acute; increased chance of airway obstruction (see Figure 1-8)	Shorter and wider
Vocal cords	Angled in relation to the axis of trachea; shorter; more cartilaginous; more distensible; more likely to be injured	Perpendicular to the axis of trachea
Rigidity	The laryngeal cartilages are softer and more pliable	More rigid
Response to trauma	Mucous membrane is more loosely attached and swells more readily when traumatized or infected	Less vulnerable to trauma and infection

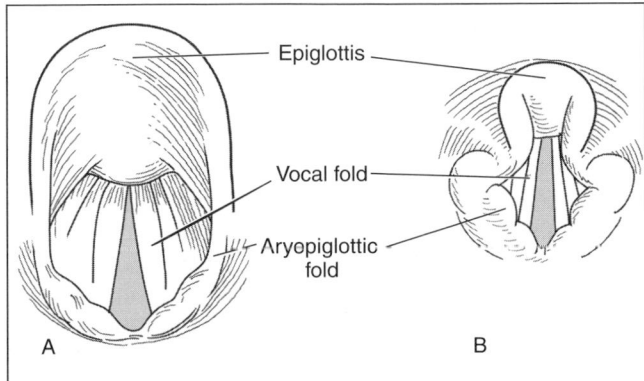

FIGURE 1-8 Differences between the adult's larynx (*A*) and the child's larynx (*B*).

may result in trauma to the airway and subsequent tracheal stenosis. The child's laryngeal inlet is narrow and more susceptible to obstruction. The U-shaped epiglottis and a more acute angle between the epiglottis and glottis cause the aryepiglottic folds to be more in the midline (Figure 1-8*B*).[1]

Differences also exist in the trachea. Children have a relatively shorter trachea. This makes both right main bronchial intubation and accidental extubation much easier. The narrower diameter of the trachea with smaller spaces between the cartilaginous rings makes a tracheostomy more difficult to perform. To avoid injury and subsequent subglottic stenosis, uncuffed endotracheal tubes should be used in children less than 8 years of age.

REFERENCES

1. Barash PG, Cullen BF, Stoelting RK: *Clinical Anesthesia.* Philadelphia: Lippincott-Raven, 1997:573–577.
2. Moore KL, Dalley AF: *Clinically Oriented Anatomy.* Baltimore: Lippincott Williams & Wilkins, 1999:1038–1053.
3. Sellick BA: Cricoid pressure to control regurgitation of stomach contents during induction of anaesthesia. *Lancet* 1961; 2:404–406.
4. Miller RD: *Anesthesia.* Philadelphia: Churchill Livingstone, 2000:1417–1419.
5. Block C, Brechner VL: Unusual problems in airway management. II. The influence of the temporomandibular joint, the mandible, and associated structures on endotracheal intubation. *Anesth Analg* 1971; 50(1):114–123.
6. Nichol HC, Zuck D: Difficult laryngoscopy— the "anterior" larynx and the atlanto-occipital gap. *Br J Anaesth* 1983; 55:141–143.
7. Mallampati SR, Gugino LD, Desai SP, Freiberger D: A clinical sign to predict difficult tracheal intubation: a prospective study. *Can Anaesth Soc J* 1985; 32(4):429–434.

Chapter 2
BASIC AIRWAY MANAGEMENT

David J. Bird
James R. Markey

INTRODUCTION

Airway management is one of the most basic and important aspects of Emergency Medicine. The concepts and techniques described in this chapter can be applied to a variety of environments. Understanding the following concepts and having an opportunity to practice them will allow one to provide the most fundamental of all medical care, support of a patient's airway.

Airway management is crucial. Without oxygen the brain begins to die within minutes.[1] The primary purpose of airway management is to facilitate the transport of oxygen to the lungs. The secondary purpose is to protect the airway from contamination with blood, fluids, or food. Airway management can be as simple as lifting a snoring patient's chin or as involved as awake fiberoptic-guided endotracheal intubation.

Time is always critical when a patient needs airway support. A healthy individual having maximally breathed 100% oxygen will begin to desaturate and have brain injury after 5 minutes of apnea. However, a sick patient breathing room air will desaturate almost immediately upon becoming apneic.[1]

The fundamental importance of airway management is reflected by the fact that two-thirds of Basic Life Support taught by the American Heart Association is concerned with this vital function.[2] **The mission of airway management is "to ensure a patent airway, provide supplemental oxygen, and institute positive-pressure ventilation when spontaneous breathing is inadequate or absent."**[3] These three key aspects of airway management warrant repeating. Ensure a patient airway. Provide supplemental oxygen. Provide positive-pressure ventilation.

Inadequate ventilation may occur for a variety of reasons. Spontaneously breathing patients may develop an airway obstruction due to food, blood, secretions, or tissue obstruction from the loss of the normal pharyngeal tone. Unconscious patients should have their airway secured as well as receiving mechanical ventilation. Despite spontaneous respiration, the unconscious patient is at risk for aspiration of gastric contents. The conscious patient with airway obstruction will be in obvious distress and is more likely to have obstruction due to a foreign body, tissue swelling from an infection, laryngeal edema, cancer, or laryngospasm.

ANATOMY AND PATHOPHYSIOLOGY

The "airway" includes the nasal, oral, pharyngeal, and laryngeal anatomy and physiology. This highly complex system is responsible for conveying warmed and filtered air to the trachea and lungs while simultaneously allowing for passage of liquids and solids to the esophagus. Phonation is actually a secondary physiologic function of the larynx.[4] This highly sophisticated system allows us to drink liquid, eat food, breathe, and talk simultaneously. However, if a small drop of liquid or a particle of food enters the airway, a profound system of reflexes is activated to protect its integrity.[5]

The nasal cavity and the nasopharynx is the area from the tip of the nose to the palate. It is highly innervated by the ophthalmic and maxillary branches of the trigeminal nerve. The mucosa of the nasal cavity and the nasopharynx is highly vascular. It is this high degree of vascularity that allows cool air from the environment to be warmed prior to entering the lungs. It also dictates that care be taken when nasal airways are placed. It takes very little trauma to the nasal mucosa to cause significant epistaxis. Polyps or mucus can obstruct the nasopharynx, as can congestion due to an upper respiratory infection. The nasopharynx is oriented in an anteroposterior plane. In a supine patient, nasal airways or nasogastric tubes should always be passed perpendicular to the horizontal axis and not in a cephalad direction.

The primary structure contained within the oropharynx is the base of the tongue. The anterior two-thirds of the tongue is innervated by the lingual nerve, a branch of the facial nerve. The posterior one-third of the tongue, the tonsils, and the palate are innervated by the glossopharyngeal nerve.[6] Salivary glands located in the oropharynx can produce a significant volume of saliva, creating potential problems for mask ventilation or intubation. Loose teeth can be inadvertently dislodged, becoming potentially hazardous foreign bodies in the airway.

Edentulous patients present a unique set of problems for mask ventilation.[7] The lack of a maxillary alveolar ridge allows the face mask to collapse into the airway. Redundant tissue, due to lack of teeth, tends to collapse into the airway as well as making mask ventilation without an oral or nasal airway extremely difficult. An appropriately sized and placed oral airway is the best way to overcome the problem of upper airway obstruction in the unconscious and edentulous adult patient.

The larynx acts as the sphincter of the pulmonary system and is made up of nine cartilages to support this function.[6] There are three paired and three unpaired cartilages. The unpaired cartilages are the epiglottis, the thyroid cartilage, and the cricoid cartilage. The paired cartilages are the arytenoids, the corniculates, and the cuneiforms. **The cricoid cartilage is the only complete ring in the entire airway.** This presents a unique opportunity for the practitioner to help prevent gastric aspiration. **The cricoid cartilage can be firmly pressed posteriorly to pinch the esophagus against the cervical spine and prevent the passive regurgitation of gastric contents. This is known as the Sellick maneuver.[8]**

The sensory and motor innervation of the larynx is derived from the vagus nerve.[6] The superior laryngeal nerve is a branch of the vagus nerve and gives rise to the internal branch, which provides the sensory innervation of the upper larynx. The superior laryngeal nerve also gives rise to the external branch, which provides the motor innervation to the cricothyroid muscle (a vocal cord adductor). The recurrent laryngeal nerve provides the sensory innervation to the larynx below the vocal cords and motor innervation to all other laryngeal muscles.[6] The cricothyroid membrane stretches from the thyroid cartilage to the cricoid cartilage and is a key landmark for airway management.

The trachea is approximately 15 cm long in an adult. It is composed of 17 or 18 C-shaped cartilaginous rings.[6] The rings are essential to prevent the trachea from collapsing during the negative intrathoracic pressures generated on inspiration.

INDICATIONS

The decision to institute airway support must often be made very quickly and frequently without the aid of laboratory results or pulmonary function studies. **The decision to institute emergent airway support is usually based on clinical judgment and signs and symptoms of inadequate oxygenation and ventilation.** The signs of impending respiratory failure are tachypnea, dyspnea, cyanosis, agitation, and the use of accessory muscles.[9] In the case of partial airway obstruction, the patient will demonstrate extreme anxiety, audible wheezing or stridor, as well as aggressive attempts to clear the obstruction. If the obstruction is complete, there may be no audible breath sounds at all.

If time permits, a more formal evaluation of the indicators that warrant respiratory assistance should be performed (Table 2-1). The ultimate signs indicating the necessity for airway assistance are hypoxia and hypercarbia. The most common etiologies resulting in the need for airway support are cardiopulmonary arrest, drug overdose, toxic reactions, and obstruction (food, vomit, or foreign body). Impending ventilatory failure due to congestive heart failure, severe asthma, or pneumonia are also common indications for intubation.

CONTRAINDICATIONS

There are no absolute contraindications for basic airway management. The contraindications for the various methods of endotracheal intubation are discussed in subsequent chapters.

EQUIPMENT

Bag-valve-mask device
Oxygen source
Clear face masks, various sizes and shapes
Oropharyngeal airways
    Large, 100 mm (size 5)
    Medium, 90 mm (size 4)
    Small, 80 mm (size 3)
Nasopharyngeal airways
    Large, 8.0 to 9.0 mm inner diameter
    Medium, 7.0 to 8.0 mm inner diameter
    Small, 6.0 to 7.0 mm inner diameter
Head strap
Yankauer suction catheter
Suction source
Pulse oximetry
Tongue blade
Water-soluble lubricant or anesthetic jelly

TABLE 2-1. INDICATORS THAT WARRANT RESPIRATORY ASSISTANCE

$SaO_2 < 90\%$
$PaO_2 < 60$ mmHg on 40% O_2
Respiratory rate > 35
$PaCO_2 > 55$ mmHg
Vital capacity < 15 mL/kg
A-a gradient > 350 mmHg on 100% O_2

SOURCE: From Shapiro et al.[10]

TECHNIQUES

PATIENT POSITIONING

The first goal of airway management, regardless of a patient's ability to breathe spontaneously, is the establishment of a patent airway. This may be all that is required in a patient who has an upper airway foreign body or a patient who has suffered a loss of consciousness with loss of pharyngeal tone. **The importance of proper positioning cannot be overemphasized.** The success of airway management is predicated on this very basic but often overlooked issue. Placing the patient in the "sniffing" position, or lateral decubitus position, may correct many upper airway obstructions due to soft tissue impingement.[11] **The "sniffing" position is achieved by flexing the cervical spine approximately 15 degrees and extending the atlantooccipital joint maximally** (Figure 2-1). This is the position one subconsciously adopts in order to sniff and smell. **This position can also be achieved with the chin-lift and/or jaw-thrust maneuvers.**

If the patient is obese or has large breasts, they often cannot be effectively managed supine on a bed. The normal sniffing position in an obese person is often not sufficient to relieve an airway obstruction (Figure 2-2A).

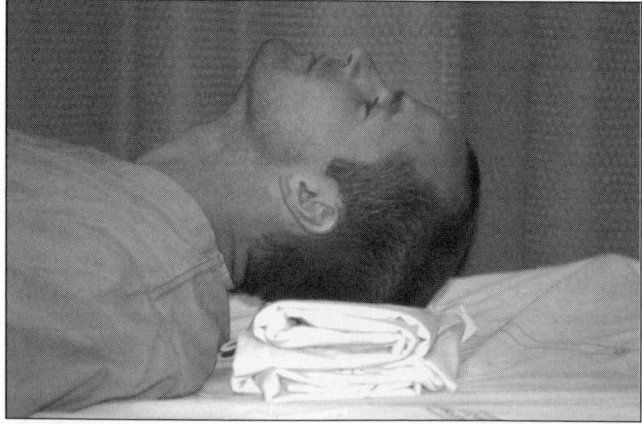

FIGURE 2-1 The "sniffing" position for successful airway management.

Place a ramp or shoulder roll under the patient's upper back to achieve the sniffing position (Figure 2-2B).

JAW-THRUST MANEUVER

The jaw thrust is one of the most basic maneuvers and an initial method of establishing a patent airway.[12] The jaw-thrust maneuver is a two-handed technique used with the face mask and a second person to provide positive-pressure ventilation. The operator is positioned at the head of the patient and places their fingers on the angles of the mandible bilaterally, then displaces the mandible anteriorly (Figure 2-3).

CHIN-LIFT MANEUVER

The chin lift is also one of the most basic maneuvers and an initial method of establishing a patent airway.[12] The chin lift is performed by placing the fingers under the mandible (Figure 2-4). **Do not place the fingers on the soft tissues of the submandibular space, as this will elevate the tongue and cause further obstruction.** Lift the chin in an anterior and cephalic direction. The head may also be tilted slightly posterior to aid in opening the airway.

NASOPHARYNGEAL AIRWAYS

The majority of airway obstruction occurs in the pharynx.[13] In addition to proper positioning, one can use various aids to overcome this site of obstruction and facilitate effective ventilation. The most commonly used devices are oropharyngeal (oral) and nasopharyngeal (nasal) airways. Regardless which device is chosen, it is important to place a large enough airway to bridge the area of soft tissue impingement on the pharynx. Nasopharyngeal airways are soft rubber or plastic tubes that are inserted through the nostril and into the oropharynx, just above the epiglottis. Nasopharyngeal airways are available in numerous sizes (Figure 2-5). The larger the inner diameter, the longer the tube. Once positioned, the nasopharyngeal airway is more comfortable for the patient than an oropharyngeal airway but nasopharyngeal airways carry the significant risk that their placement may result in epistaxis.[3,10] A size 30 or 32 French airway is appropriate for most adults. It can be safely placed in the conscious, semiconscious, or unconscious patient. It can also be used when an oropharyngeal airway cannot be placed (oral trauma, braces, seizures, trismus, etc.). **It is imperative to also perform the jaw thrust and/or chin lift to prevent the tongue from obstructing the airway.**

Insertion of a nasopharyngeal airway is a rapid procedure. Choose the proper size oropharyngeal airway. Place the flared end of the airway near the tip of the patient's nose. The distal end of the nasopharyngeal airway should be at the external auditory canal. Liberally apply water-soluble lubricant or anesthetic jelly to the na-

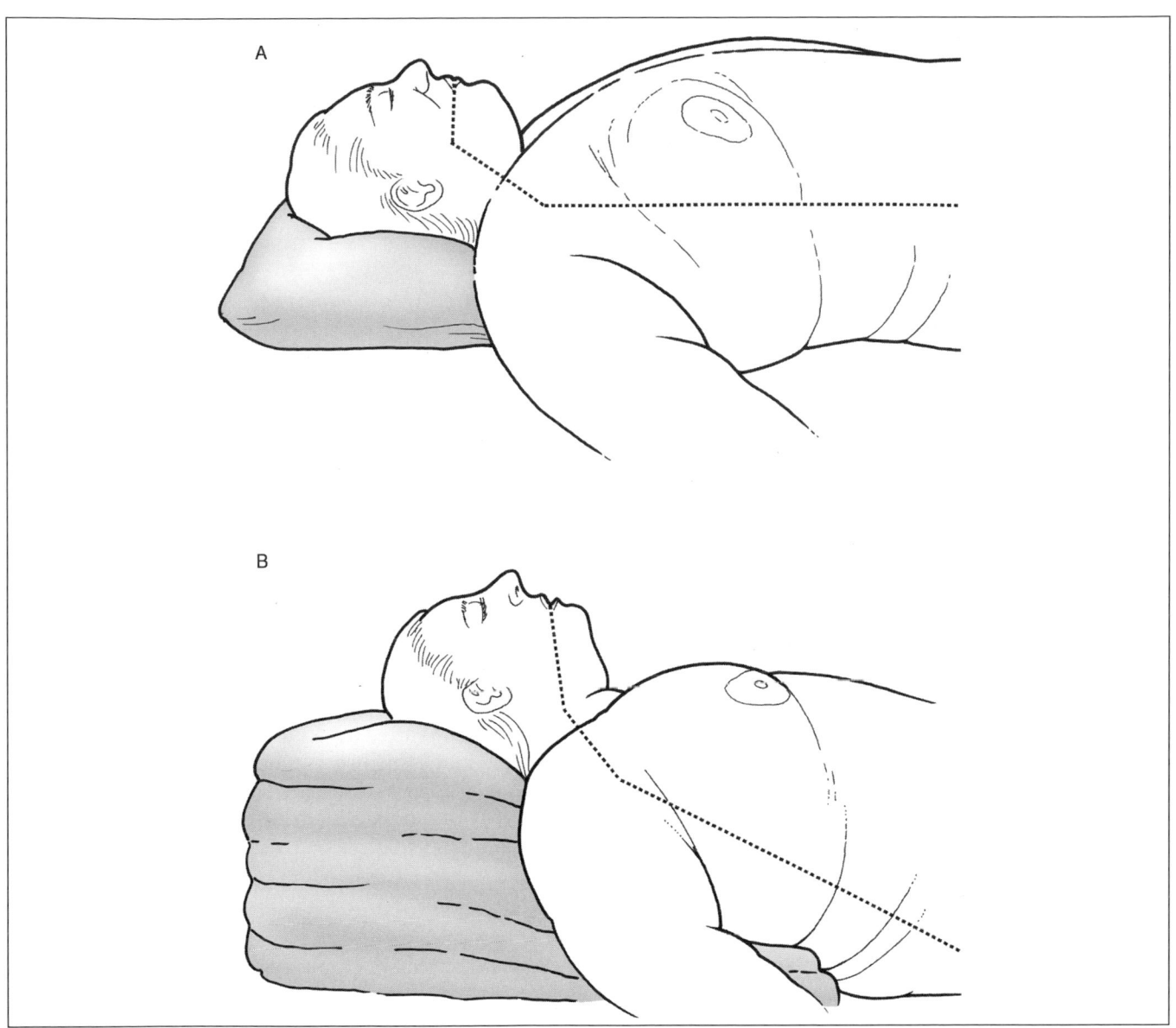

FIGURE 2-2 Airway management in the obese patient. *A.* The normal "sniffing" position is inadequate to open the airway. The dotted line represents the axis of the airway. *B.* A ramp placed under the head and shoulders will achieve the "sniffing" position.

sopharyngeal airway. If not contraindicated, apply a vasoconstrictor to the patient's nasal mucosa. Gently insert the nasopharyngeal airway with the beveled tip against the nasal septum (Figure 2-6). This will prevent the tip from getting caught on the inferior or middle turbinate and causing epistaxis. Insert it completely until the flared end is against the nostril. Rotate the nasopharyngeal airway 90 degrees so it is concave upward. If resistance is encountered during insertion, slight rotation will often facilitate the passage of the airway. Supplementary oxygen or positive-pressure ventilation with a bag-valve-mask device can be started after insertion of the airway.

Insertion of a nasopharyngeal airway is associated with complications. If the device is too long, it may cause laryngospasm and vomiting. It may also be placed with its tip in the esophagus, resulting in gastric distention and subsequent aspiration. Nasal mucosal injury upon insertion can cause epistaxis and aspiration of blood.

OROPHARYNGEAL AIRWAYS

The oropharyngeal airway is a semicircular plastic device that holds the tongue up and away from the posterior pharyngeal wall (Figure 2-7). These airways cause less trauma and are more easily placed than nasopha-

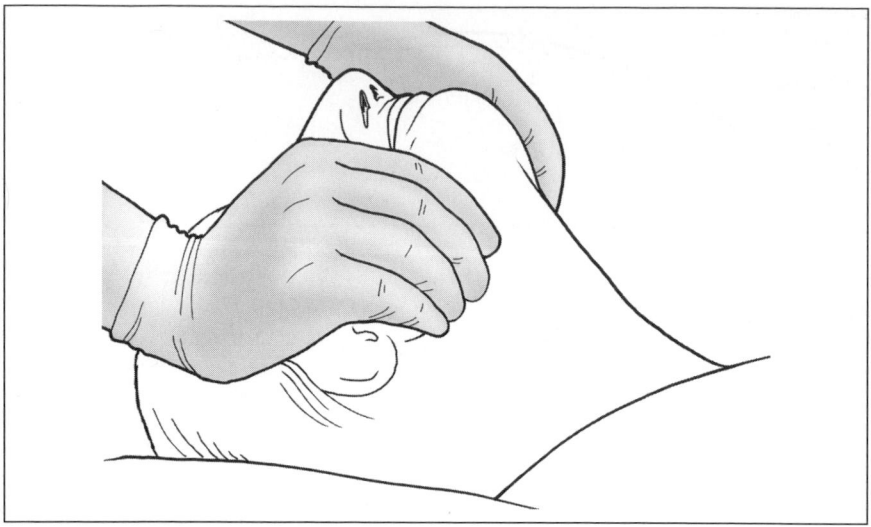

FIGURE 2-3 The jaw-thrust maneuver.

ryngeal airways. **Oropharyngeal airways must be used only in unconscious patients. They may result in laryngospasm and vomiting if placed in a conscious or semiconscious patient.**[14] An 8.0, 9.0, or 10.0 cm oral airway is appropriate for most adults.

Insertion of the oropharyngeal airway is a quick and simple procedure. Choose the proper size oropharyngeal airway. The correct size is estimated by placing the airway next to the patient's mouth. The distal tip should lie just above the angle of the mandible. Clear the mouth and oropharynx of any blood, secretions, or vomit with the Yankauer suction catheter. Open the patient's jaw with the left hand. Separate the teeth with a "scissors-like" action of the thumb on the lower teeth and the index or middle finger on the upper teeth. Insert the oropharyngeal airway curved side down (Figure 2-8A). The tip will slide along the palate. After insertion, rotate it 180 degrees, so that the curve of the oropharyngeal airway follows the curvature of the tongue. An alternative method is to use a tongue blade to depress the tongue and then insert the oropharyngeal airway as above. If the tongue blade is used, the oropharyngeal

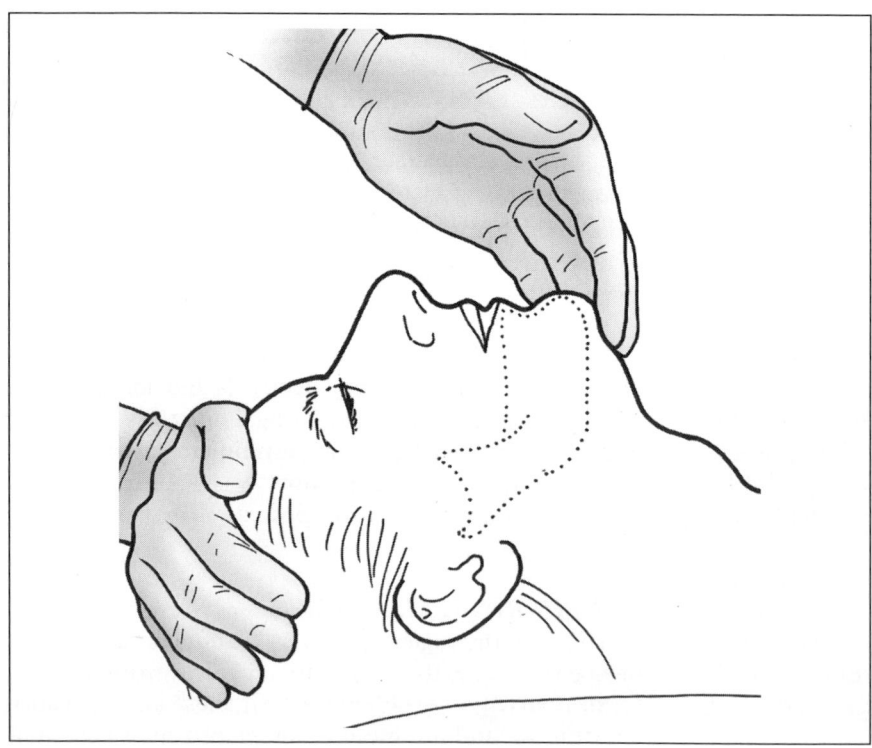

FIGURE 2-4 The chin-lift maneuver.

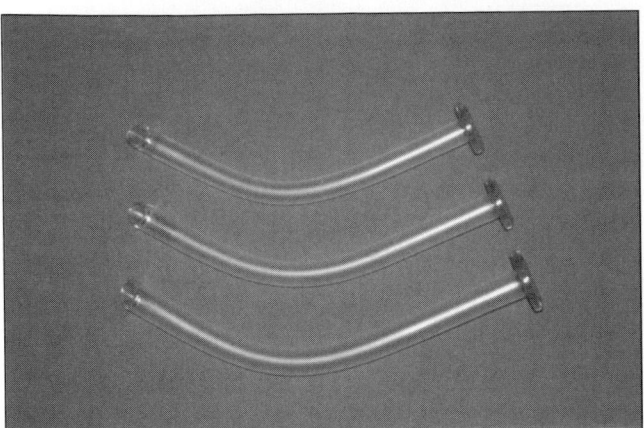

FIGURE 2-5 Nasopharyngeal airways.

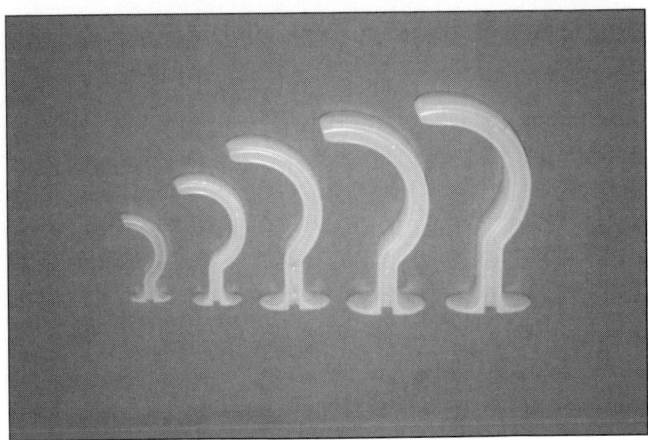

FIGURE 2-7 Oropharyngeal airways.

airway may also be inserted with the curve side upward (Figure 2-8*B*). Supplementary oxygen or positive-pressure ventilation with a bag-valve-mask device can be started after the insertion of the airway.

Insertion of an oropharyngeal airway is not a benign procedure. If the airway is not inserted properly, it can push the tongue posteriorly and further obstruct the oropharynx. If the lips or tongue are caught between the teeth and the oropharyngeal airway, significant lacerations can occur. If the oropharyngeal airway is too long, it can force the epiglottis closed against the vocal cords and produce a complete airway obstruction. Too small an airway will force the tongue against the pharynx and produce an obstruction.

Oropharyngeal airways have many uses. The primary indication is to maintain a patent airway. It will prevent the patient from biting, occluding, and lacerating an endotracheal tube. It facilitates oropharyngeal suctioning by removing the tongue from the airway. It will also protect the tongue from bites during seizure activity.

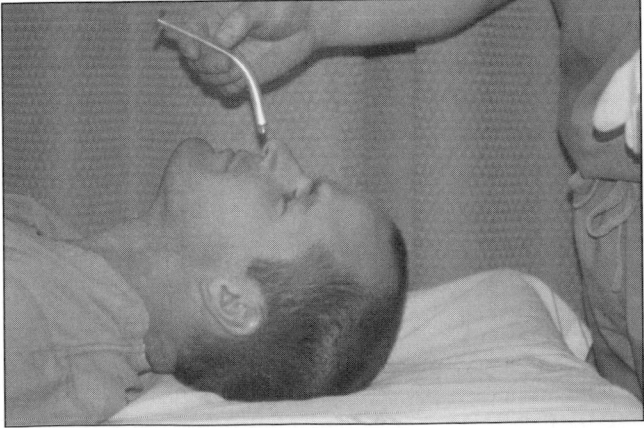

FIGURE 2-6 Insertion of the nasopharyngeal airway.

MASK VENTILATION

The likelihood of success in airway management is almost always predictable, given enough time to fully assess a patient's history and anatomy.[15] The ease of mask ventilation and intubation is directly related to anatomy. Anesthesiologists rely on a series of classification criteria to help predict the success of airway management. The most widely used is the Mallompatti classification.[16] This evaluation—coupled with an examination of the patient's body habitus, thickness of the patient's neck, temporomandibular joint function, ability to fully open the mouth, dental structures, cervical range of motion, and thyromental distance—can predict the ease or difficulty of airway management.[15–21]

The distinction must be made between ease of mask ventilation and ease of oral endotracheal intubation. The two are often correlated but can, at times, be completely unrelated. For example, a patient with a normal body habitus who is in a cervical halo may be very easy to ventilate by mask but impossible to intubate orally via direct laryngoscopy. Conversely, the patient who is obese, suffers from sleep apnea, but has a Mallompatti class 1 airway may be very easy to intubate but virtually impossible to ventilate by mask.

After achieving the proper positioning, the presence of spontaneous respirations must be evaluated. If the patient is not breathing and there is no evidence of a foreign body, positive-pressure ventilation must be initiated. In the awake patient with complete airway obstruction due to a foreign body, the Heimlich maneuver is the method of choice.[2] If the patient has become unconscious and the foreign body is clearly visible, remove it. However, caution must be used to prevent forcing the object further into the airway. Instrument removal of airway foreign bodies with a McGill forceps is possible if the foreign body is visible and within reach of the forceps.

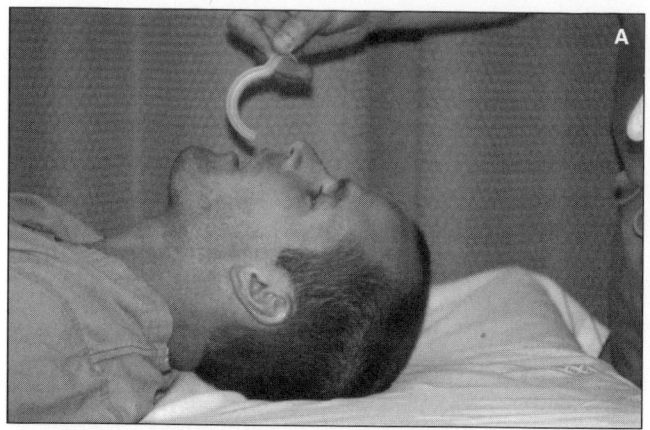

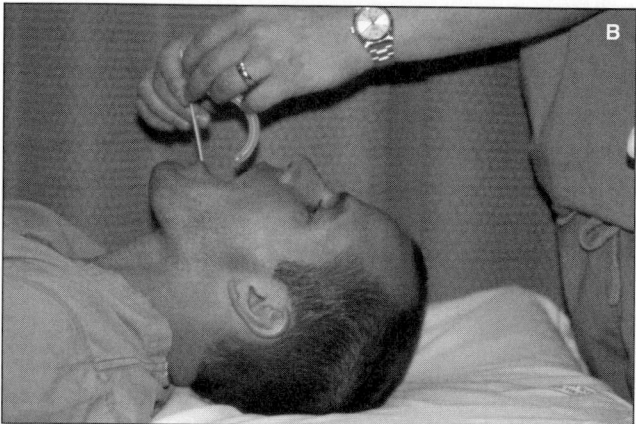

FIGURE 2-8 Insertion of the oropharyngeal airway. *A.* It is inserted with the curve toward the tongue. After insertion, it is rotated 180 degrees. *B.* It is inserted with the curve toward the palate. A tongue blade is used to depress the tongue and facilitate insertion.

Once the airway is patent, the options for positive-pressure ventilation include mouth-to-mouth, mouth-to-mask, and bag-valve devices (mask ventilation). **The key to effective mask ventilation is ensuring a continually patent airway. This is initially achieved by placing the patient in the sniffing position, coupled with a combination of chin lift and jaw thrust. Neglect of this key maneuver leads to excessive use of positive-pressure ventilation in an attempt to compensate for an obstructed upper airway.** It will force gas into the stomach, increasing intraabdominal pressure and resulting in the need for ever-increasing positive pressure on the airway. Eventually, rising intraabdominal pressure will make ventilation difficult or impossible and significantly increases the risk of gastric aspiration. When called upon to mask ventilate a patient, **always keep in mind the importance of proper positioning and the use of an appropriately sized oral or nasal airway as an adjunct.**

Face masks should be made of clear plastic and/or silicone, have a soft seal, and have an anatomic shape that conforms to the contours of the patient's face. Typical adult sizes are 3, 4, and 5. **The mask must be large enough to completely cover the nose and mouth but not so large as to allow a leak.** There are two ways to properly hold a face mask. The one-handed technique is performed with the left hand (Figure 2-9). Place the little, ring, and middle fingers under the left side of the patient's mandible. Place the index finger and thumb on the bottom and top portions of the mask. **This technique allows the operator to simultaneously lift the mandible and extend the atlantooccipital joint while applying enough downward pressure to create an airtight seal.** An elastic head strap is a very helpful device to aid in sealing the mask tightly. The right hand is used to ventilate the patient through the bag-valve device.

A two-handed technique may be necessary in patients with facial hair and those who are obese, elderly, or edentulous. Two people are required to perform this technique, in which both of the operator's hands are applied to the face mask to aid in the creation of a tight seal and align the airway properly (Figure 2-10). Place the index, middle, ring, and small fingers of the left hand on the body of the left half of the mandible. Position the right hand similarly on the right half of the mandible. Place the face mask on the patient's face. Apply both thumbs to the mask and apply pressure to create a seal. Anteriorly elevate the mandible to perform the jaw-thrust maneuver. This makes it necessary to have an assistant apply positive pressure through the bag-valve device.

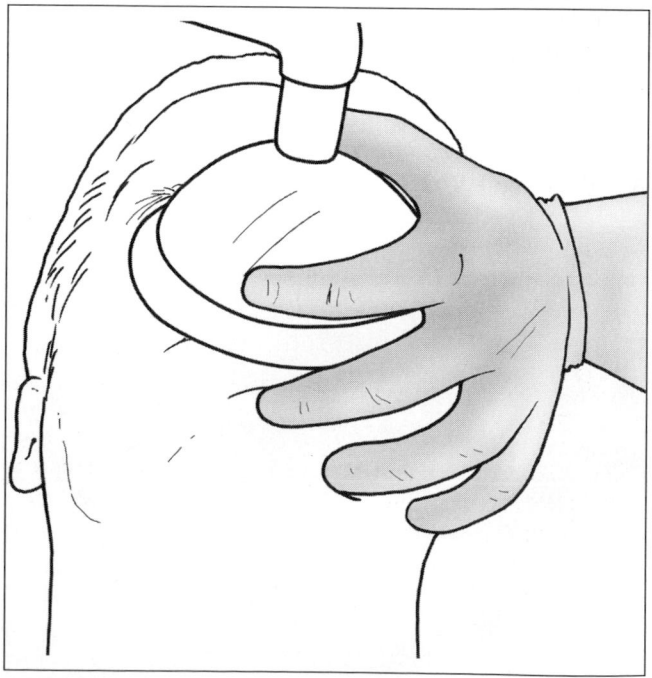

FIGURE 2-9 The one-handed, one-person mask ventilation technique.

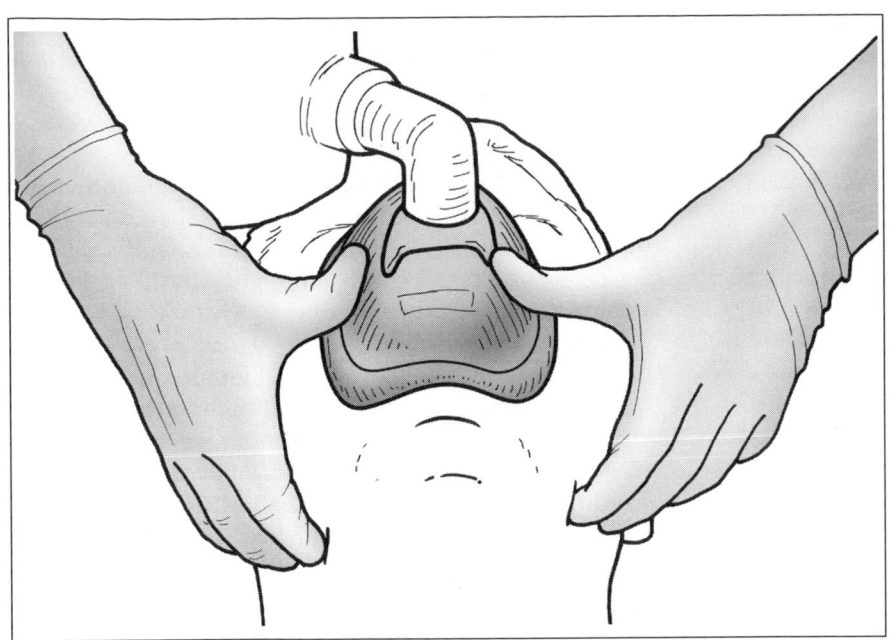

FIGURE 2-10 The two-handed, two-person mask ventilation technique.

A bag-valve device is used to provide positive-pressure ventilation. It consists of a self-inflating bag connected to oxygen on one end and a one-way (non-rebreathing) valve on the other. The valve is connected to the mask, or other airway device, to allow one-way flow of oxygen. This device can also force air into the esophagus and stomach and place the patient at risk for aspiration.

Stand above the patient's head. Place the patient in the sniffing position. Apply a face mask. Attach the bag-valve device to the mask and begin positive-pressure ventilation. If ventilation is difficult, apply the jaw-thrust and/or chin-lift maneuvers. If ventilation is still difficult, insert an oropharyngeal or nasopharyngeal airway. If ventilation is still difficult, the patient requires an invasive airway device immediately.

The American Society of Anesthesiologists has published an algorithm to facilitate decision making in the face of airway management problems. A detailed discussion of the various intubation options is contained in following chapters.

COMPLICATIONS

The most serious complication of basic airway management is aspiration of gastric contents. The aspiration of acidic gastric contents can result in an acute chemical pneumonitis. This phenomenon is known as the Mendelson syndrome and has an associated 50 percent mortality.[22] It is a significant risk when airway management is needed emergently or routinely in the pregnant, trauma, diabetic, or obese patient.

Less serious complications include soft tissue trauma to the lips, tongue, oral cavity, and eyelids. Tooth fractures or avulsions are uncommon but possible. A dermatitis or allergic reaction to the plastic material is rarely seen. Facial nerve dysfunction due to pressure effects of the mask are transient. Corneal abrasions, conjunctival chemosis, and increased intraocular pressure are common with masks that are too large.

SUMMARY

Basic airway management is a fundamental skill that must be mastered by all caregivers. With an oxygen source, a means to deliver positive-pressure ventilation, attention to detail in positioning, and the use of airway adjuncts, it is usually possible to prevent hypoxia and hypercarbia in the apneic patient. The ultimate measure of the efficacy of ventilation and oxygenation is a normal $PaCO_2$ and PaO_2. The various methods of securing the airway are discussed elsewhere in this text.

REFERENCES

1. Farmery AD, Roe PG: A model to describe the rate of oxyhaemoglobin desaturation during apnoea. *Br J Anaesth* 1996; 76(2):284–291.
2. American Heart Association: Standards and Guidelines for Cardiopulmonary Resuscitation and Emergent Cardiac Care. *JAMA* 1986; (255):2184–2202.

3. Cummins ROA: Adjuncts for airway control, ventilation, and oxygenation, in *American Heart Association Textbook of Advanced Cardiac Life Support.* Dallas, TX: American Heart Association, 1994:2.1–2.17.

4. Negus VE: *The Comparative Anatomy and Physiology of the Larynx.* New York: Grune & Stratton, 1949:192–200.

5. Petcu LG, Sabaki CT: Laryngeal anatomy and physiology. *Clin Chest Med* 1991; 12(3):415–423.

6. Pansky B: *Review of Gross Anatomy,* 5th ed. New York: Macmillan, 1984:64–67.

7. Dorsch JA, Dorsch SE: *Understanding Anesthesia Equipment,* 3rd ed. Baltimore: Williams & Wilkins, 1994:363–398.

8. Sellick BA: Cricoid pressure to control regurgitation of stomach contents during induction of anesthesia. *Lancet* 1961; 2:404–406.

9. Honig EG, Ingram HR: Chronic bronchitis, emphysema, and airways obstruction, in Braunwald E, Fauci AS, Kasper DL, Hauser SL, et al (eds): *Harrison's Principles of Internal Medicine,* 15th ed. New York: McGraw–Hill, 2001:1491–1498.

10. Shapiro BA, Harrison RA, Cane RD, et al: *Clinical Application of Blood Gases,* 4th ed. Chicago: Year Book, 1989:77–98.

11. Gillespie NA: *Endotracheal Anesthesia,* 2nd ed. Madison, WI: University of Wisconsin Press, 1950.

12. Stone DJ, Gal JT: Airway management, in Miller RD (ed): *Anesthesia,* vol 2. New York: Churchill Livingstone, 1990:1265–1292.

13. Nandi PR, Charlesworth CH, Taylor SJ, et al: Effects of general anesthesia on the pharynx. *Br J Anaesth* 1991; 66:157–162.

14. Stauffer JL: Medical management of the airway. *Clin Chest Med* 1991; 12(3):449–482.

15. Frerk CM: Predicting difficult intubation. *Anaesthesia* 1991; 46:1005–1008.

16. Mallompatti SR, Gatt SP, Gugino LD, et al: A clinical sign to predict difficult tracheal intubation: a prospective study. *Can Anaesth Soc J* 1985; 32:429–434.

17. Cass NM, James NR, Lines V: Difficult direct laryngoscopy complicating intubation for anesthesia. *Br Med J* 1956; 1:488–489.

18. White A, Kander PL: Anatomical factors in difficult direct laryngoscopy. *Br J Anaesth* 1975; 47: 469–474.

19. Nichol HC, Zuck D: Difficult laryngoscopy: the "anterior" larynx and the atlanto-occipital gap. *Br J Anaesth* 1983; 55:141–143.

20. Bannister FB, MacBeth RG: Direct laryngoscopy and intubation. *Lancet* 1944; 2:651–654.

21. Samsoon GLT, Young JRB: Difficult tracheal intubation: a retrospective study. *Anesthesia* 1987; 42:487–490.

22. Mendelson CL: Aspiration of stomach contents into the lungs during obstetric anesthesia. *Am J Obstet Gynecol* 1946; 52:191–205.

Chapter 3
PHARMACOLOGIC ADJUNCTS TO INTUBATION

Ned F. Nasr
Isam F. Nasr
Bassen Ghaly

INTRODUCTION

Oral endotracheal intubation without pharmacologic assistance should be reserved for the unresponsive and apneic patient. Unconscious patients capable of resisting laryngoscopy or those with spontaneous respiratory effort should be intubated with the assistance of pharmacologic adjuncts. A rapid sequence induction optimizes intubation conditions while minimizing the risk of aspiration for the patient. It can be performed with a high rate of success and minimal complications.[1] Rapid sequence intubation requires the use of several pharmacologic adjuncts (Tables 3-1 and 3-2). This includes a potent anesthetic agent to induce unconsciousness and a neuromuscular blocking agent to produce paralysis.

INDUCTION AGENTS

The ideal induction agent has an extremely rapid onset of action, produces predictable deep anesthesia, has a short duration of action, and has no adverse effects.[2] Unfortunately such an agent does not yet exist. However, there are at least six drugs that can safely be used for induction of anesthesia and intubation. These include thiopental, methohexital, etomidate, ketamine, and propofol. Midazolam and fentanyl may also be used alone or in conjunction with the above agents.[2] The decision as to which induction agent is the most suitable is largely dependent on the physician's experience and his or her understanding of each drug's properties. In this section, each of these drugs is briefly detailed as to its pharmacokinetics, mechanism of action, pharmacodynamics, administration, and adverse effects.

BARBITURATES

For more than 50 years, barbiturates have been a mainstay in the induction of anesthesia. They rapidly produce sedation and hypnosis in a dose-dependent fashion. They are also less expensive than many of the newer induction agents.[3] Because of their high potency, rapid onset, and short duration of action, the most commonly used barbiturates are thiopental (Pentothal™) and methohexital (Brevital™).

PHARMACOKINETICS

When injected intravenously, these ultra-short-acting barbiturates can produce effects in one arm-brain circulation time, or less than 30 seconds.[4] They are readily bound to plasma proteins. The onset of central nervous system (CNS) depression is primarily due to the rapid distribution of thiopental or methohexital to well-perfused, low-volume tissue. This so-called central compartment consists mainly of the brain and liver. Approximately 15 percent of these lipid-soluble drugs remain unbound and free to diffuse across the blood-brain barrier at high initial concentrations. Brain levels peak in about 1 minute. The duration of a single dose of thiopental is approximately 5 to 10 minutes, while an equipotent dose of methohexital lasts approximately 4 to 6 minutes.[5] The short duration of action is due to the redistribution of the drugs from the small-volume central compartment to the large-volume peripheral compartment, which is predominantly made up of lean muscle. Both thiopental and methohexital are metabolized in the liver and excreted by the kidneys. Methohexital has a substantially higher hepatic extraction ratio, which may account for its shorter duration of action. Clearance of the drugs has little to do with the cessation of CNS effects in single or multiple small doses. If barbiturates are given in mul-

TABLE 3-1. RECOMMENDED ANESTHETIC DOSES FOR RAPID SEQUENCE INDUCTION

Medication	Adult dose (mg/kg)	Pediatric dose (mg/kg)	Onset (sec)	Duration (min)
Thiopental	3–6	5–6	< 30	5–10
Methohexital	1–3	1–2	< 30	5–10
Etomidate	0.2–0.3	0.2–0.3	15–45	3–12
Ketamine	1–2	1–3	45–60	10–20
Propofol	1.5–2.5	2.5–3.5	15–45	5–10
Midazolam	0.2–0.4	0.5–1.0	30–90	10–30
Fentanyl	0.005–0.015	0.005–0.015	15–45	30–60

tiple high doses or in an infusion, the concentration in the peripheral tissue approaches the plasma concentration and the rate of redistribution is greatly diminished.[6] This prolongs their anesthetic effects.[6]

MECHANISM OF ACTION

Barbiturates, along with other common intravenous (IV) anesthetic agents, are postulated to act on the γ-aminobutyric acid receptor complex (GABA). Specifically, these drugs work on the GABA$_A$ receptor.[7] GABA is the principal inhibitory neurotransmitter in the CNS. The GABA receptor complex forms a transmembrane chloride channel when activated. The influx of chloride ion causes hyperpolarization and functional inhibition of the postsynaptic neurons. Barbiturates can act on the GABA receptor in two ways. At lower doses, they may potentiate the action of endogenously produced GABA by decreasing the rate of its dissociation from the receptor complex. At higher doses, barbiturates may directly activate the chloride ion channels and inhibit neuronal activity.[3] It is important to note that barbiturates do not inhibit sensory impulses and therefore have no analgesic effect. In fact, they may produce hyperalgesia (increased response to painful stimuli) when given in subhypnotic doses.[3]

PHARMACODYNAMICS

Barbiturates produce dose-dependent depression of cerebral oxygen metabolism (CMRO$_2$), cerebral blood flow (CBF), and electroencephalogram (EEG) activity. A flat EEG tracing correlates to a maximal barbiturate suppression of CMRO$_2$ to 55 percent of normal.[3] The diminished CMRO$_2$ and CBF lead to a decrease in intracranial pressure (ICP). Since barbiturates lower mean arterial pressure less than they lower ICP, cerebral perfusion pressure (CPP) is usually enhanced. Barbiturates are commonly used in neuroanesthesia and in treatment of acute brain injury.

The cardiovascular effects of barbiturates include decreased cardiac output, decreased systemic arterial pressure, and a direct negative inotropic effect on the myocardium. Barbiturates decrease cardiac output primarily by depressing the vasomotor center, causing peripheral vasodilatation and decreasing venous return to the heart. Both thiopental and methohexital have a positive chronotropic effect on the heart. Methohexital produces a greater increase in heart rate, which may explain why an equipotent dose of methohexital produces significantly less hypotension than does thiopental.[3] Though the increase in heart rate mitigates the drop in blood pressure, myocardial oxygen demand is increased while coronary vascular resistance is decreased. If the aortic pressure remains stable, coronary blood flow will increase to meet the increased demand. Therefore barbiturates must be used cautiously in any patient whose condition is sensitive to tachycardia or a decrease in preload (hypovolemia, congestive heart failure, ischemic heart disease, or pericardial tamponade). Methohexital has less cardiovascular depressant effects and a shorter duration of action; it may be more useful than thiopental in the Emergency Department setting.

Barbiturates cause dose-dependent central respiratory depression characterized by diminished tidal volume and minute ventilation. The rate and depth of respiration may be suppressed to the point of apnea. The physiologic response to hypercarbia and hypoxemia may also be blunted, even after the hypnotic effects have dissipated. All of these effects may be greatly exaggerated with the concomitant use of opioids and in patients with chronic obstructive pulmonary disease.[8]

TABLE 3-2. RECOMMENDED NEUROMUSCULAR BLOCKING AGENTS FOR INTUBATION AND RAPID SEQUENCE INDUCTION

Medication	Adult dose (mg/kg)	Pediatric dose (mg/kg)	Onset (min)	Duration (min)
Succinylcholine	0.6–1.0	1–2	1	2–3
Succinylcholine for RSI	1.5	2	1	3–5
Pancuronium	0.1	0.07–0.10	2–5	40–60
Atracurium	0.5	0.5	3	20–35
Vecuronium	0.1	0.05–0.10	3	30–40
Vecuronium for RSI	0.3–0.5	0.3–0.5	1	60–120
Rocuronium	0.6	1.0	4–6	15–85
Rocuronium for RSI	0.9–1.2	1.0–1.2	1.0–1.5	30–110

ADMINISTRATION

Thiopental and methohexital are available as sodium salts and should be dissolved in 0.9% saline. The recommended dose of thiopental is 3 to 5 mg/kg (5 to 6 mg/kg in children and 6 to 8 mg/kg in infants) IV given over 1 minute. The recommended dose of methohexital is 1 to 3 mg/kg IV over 30 seconds. The induction dose should be reduced in patients premedicated with fentanyl or midazolam. Doses may have to be adjusted in patients with known hepatic or renal disease because decreased plasma albumin levels leave a greater fraction of barbiturate available to cross the blood-brain barrier. A 30 to 40 percent reduction should be made in the geriatric population since their diminished muscle mass slows the rate of redistribution and lengthens the duration of CNS effects.[3]

ADVERSE EFFECTS

The most significant complications of barbiturate therapy stem from their cardiopulmonary depressant effects. As stated above, these agents should be used with caution in patients who are hypovolemic, have significant cardiovascular disease, or have reactive airway disease. Thiopental can raise plasma histamine levels, which may be associated with a transient skin rash and bronchospasm. Its use should be avoided in patients with a history of hypersensitivity to barbiturates. Severe anaphylactic reactions are extremely uncommon.[3] Laryngeal reflexes appear to be more active with thiopental than with propofol. Thiopental should be avoided in people with asthma.[3] Laryngospasm following induction with thiopental is more likely the result of airway manipulation in a "lightly" anesthetized patient.[3] Methohexital has known epileptogenic effects and is frequently associated with myoclonic tremors and other CNS excitatory side effects, such as hiccups.[3] Barbiturates stimulate the production of porphyrins and thus are contraindicated in patients with acute intermittent porphyria, variegate porphyria, and hereditary coproporphyria.[3] Pain at the site of intravenous injection is more common with the administration of methohexital than thiopental. Due to their high alkalinity (pH 10), extravascular or intraarterial injection of these drugs may cause severe pain, tissue necrosis, and thrombosis. Intraarterial injection should be treated promptly with heparinization, papaverine, and lidocaine injections.[3]

ETOMIDATE

Etomidate (Amidate™) is an ultra-short-acting hypnotic unrelated to any other intravenous anesthetic agent. Like barbiturates, it is highly potent and produces a rapid onset of anesthesia. It lacks the barbiturates' cardiodepressant side effects. Given its favorable profile, etomidate has become a popular induction agent. In many Emergency Departments, it is now the induction agent of choice for rapid sequence intubation.[9]

PHARMACOKINETICS

Etomidate is a carboxylated imidazole agent that undergoes a molecular rearrangement at physiologic pH, which grants it greater lipid-solubility. Approximately 75 percent of the drug is plasma protein–bound. The free fraction accumulates readily in the CNS. Unconsciousness is produced within one arm-brain circulation. Peak brain concentration is achieved within 1 minute. Redistribution of the drug is quite rapid. A single bolus dose produces hypnosis in 10 seconds and lasts approximately 3 to 5 minutes. Since it has a high extraction ratio and undergoes rapid hydrolysis by liver, clearance of etomidate is dependent on hepatic blood flow, with inactive metabolites excreted in the urine.[10]

MECHANISM OF ACTION

By modulating GABA receptors to produce hyperpolarization and functional inhibition of the postsynaptic neurons, etomidate (like barbiturates, propofol, and benzodiazepines) produces dose-dependent CNS depression. GABA antagonists may attenuate its effects. Etomidate has no analgesic properties.[11]

PHARMACODYNAMICS

Etomidate produces dose-dependent depression of $CMRO_2$, CBF, and EEG activity analogous to that of the barbiturates. Since it does not affect mean arterial pressure, etomidate decreases ICP with minimal effect on CPP. It is useful in patients with elevated ICP, especially those who are hemodynamically unstable.[12] Etomidate causes minimal cardiovascular depression. Even in the presence of significant cardiac disease, the patient's heart rate, blood pressure, and cardiac output are adequately maintained. The respiratory depressant effects of etomidate appear to be substantially less than those for thiopental or propofol. It may be safer than barbiturates in patients with diminished pulmonary function. Etomidate is considered to be the induction agent of choice in patients with severe cardiopulmonary disease and high-risk patients in whom maintenance of blood pressure is crucial.[13] Etomidate does not blunt the sympathetic response to laryngoscopy and intubation. It should be combined with an opioid for analgesia in patients who would be at risk from a transient elevation of blood pressure or heart rate.[14] **Etomidate is the only available intravenous anesthetic that does not induce the release of histamine and thus is safe for patients with reactive airways.[15]**

ADMINISTRATION

Etomidate is formulated in a 0.2% solution with 35% propylene glycol. The standard induction dose is

0.3 mg/kg IV. There is virtually no accumulation of the drug. Emergence time is dose-dependent but remains short, even after repeated boluses of etomidate.[16] Dose adjustments for elderly patients or those with hepatic or renal disease may be required.

ADVERSE EFFECTS

The most common side effects of etomidate are nausea, vomiting, myoclonus during the induction phase, and injection-site pain. Myoclonic activity has been reported in about one-third of cases and is attributed to interruption of inhibitory synapses in the thalamocortical tract rather than CNS excitation.[2] Pretreatment with an opioid analgesic or a benzodiazepine has been reported to diminish the frequency of myoclonic movements.[11] Vein irritation and pain at the intravenous site can be attributed to the propylene glycol. Use of a large vein with simultaneous analgesic and saline infusion reduces the incidence of injection pain.[17] A single induction dose of etomidate suppresses adrenocortical hormone synthesis for 5 to 8 hours. The significance of this is unknown. In critically ill patients on an etomidate infusion, increased mortality has been attributed to suppression of cortisol synthesis.[18]

KETAMINE

Ketamine (Ketalar™, Ketaject™) is a phencyclidine derivative that is unique among induction agents. It produces a dissociative anesthetic state characterized by profound analgesia and amnesia. Patients may appear awake with their eyes open. They may make spontaneous nonpurposeful movements. Patients' protective reflexes are usually maintained. This agent has been widely used since 1970.[19] Ketamine is fast-acting and has a brief duration of action.

PHARMACOKINETICS

Ketamine has a pKa of 7.5. Approximately 12 percent is plasma protein–bound. Therefore roughly half of the unbound fraction is available to accumulate rapidly in the CNS. A single induction dose produces anesthesia within 30 seconds and brain concentration peaks at 1 minute. Like barbiturates and etomidate, ketamine follows the three-compartment model, with rapid redistribution to the peripheral tissues.[19] Its CNS effects last approximately 10 to 15 minutes. Recovery of full orientation and function may take an additional 60 minutes. Ketamine is readily metabolized by hepatic microsomal enzymes to norketamine. Norketamine is one-fourth as potent as its precursor. The active metabolite may explain the prolonged recovery time. Norketamine is hydroxylated and excreted by the kidneys. Ketamine has a high extraction ratio, and its clearance is dependent on hepatic blood flow.[2]

MECHANISM OF ACTION

At the molecular level, ketamine acts by binding to the N-methyl-D-aspartate (NMDA) receptors on postsynaptic neurons. This receptor is a gated ion channel that allows depolarization and initiation of an action potential when activated by glutamate or NMDA. Ketamine blocks the flux of ions through this channel and inhibits the stimulatory effects of these neurotransmitters. Ketamine depresses neuronal activity in the cerebral cortex and the thalamus. It stimulates the limbic system. Analgesia is produced by interrupting the association pathways responsible for the interpretation of painful stimuli that run from the thalamocortical and limbic systems.[20]

PHARMACODYNAMICS

Although ketamine produces dose-dependent CNS depression, it increases $CMRO_2$ and CBF, leading to an increase in ICP. Ketamine has a potent sympathomimetic effect. Its use often produces an increase in heart rate and arterial blood pressure. It has a direct negative inotropic effect on the myocardium, which is evident in the critically ill patient with depleted catecholamines. Ketamine produces minimal to no respiratory depression and has a potent bronchodilatory effect. It increases both bronchial and oral secretions. In contrast to other anesthetic agents, ketamine is likely to preserve protective airway reflexes. Skeletal muscle tone is also increased, resulting in the occurrence of random movements.[19]

ADMINISTRATION

Ketamine is available in 1% and 5% aqueous solutions for intravenous administration and a 10% aqueous solution for intramuscular (IM) injection. The induction dose of ketamine is 1 to 2 mg/kg IV over 1 minute or 5 to 10 mg/kg IM.[2]

In the Emergency Department, ketamine is indicated for the intubation of asthmatic patients due to its bronchodilatory properties. Ketamine may also be therapeutic for these patients, because the increase in bronchial secretions may decrease the incidence of mucous plugging.[21] Due to its cardiostimulatory effects, ketamine may also be useful in the hemodynamically unstable patient. **Ketamine should not be used in those with suspected head trauma or intracranial pathology because it may increase ICP. It should not be used in patients with ischemic heart disease because it can increase blood pressure, heart rate, and myocardial oxygen demand.**

ADVERSE EFFECTS

The most significant side effect of ketamine is the postanesthetic emergence reactions. Up to 30 percent of patients treated with ketamine have reported unpleasant sensations, agitation, hallucinations, restlessness, or nightmares.[2] Those patients most affected were elderly, females, and those receiving more than 2 mg/kg. Children seem less adversely affected than adults. These reactions can be attenuated or eliminated by the coadministration of a benzodiazepine or propofol. Other side effects include hypersalivation, random movements, nystagmus, and increased intraocular pressure. Ketamine may activate epileptogenic foci in patients with seizure disorder.[19]

PROPOFOL

Introduced in 1989, propofol (Diprivan™) is a sedative-hypnotic agent used for conscious sedation or the induction and maintenance of anesthesia. Although unrelated to any of the other induction agents, it has a profile similar to that of thiopental. Despite its cardiopulmonary depressant effects, the use of propofol has greatly expanded. It is well suited for ambulatory surgery performed on relatively healthy outpatients. Recovery after propofol anesthesia is rapid and is accompanied by less residual sedation, fatigue, and confusion than any other induction agent. Propofol is associated with a low incidence of postanesthetic emesis.[22] Its role as an adjunct to emergency airway management in the Emergency Department is still unfolding.

PHARMACOKINETICS

Propofol is an alkyl-phenol compound that is insoluble in water. It is 98% plasma protein–bound. Since it is highly lipophilic, any unbound drug rapidly accumulates in the brain and liver. A single bolus produces hypnosis in as little as 15 to 45 seconds. Its duration of action, like that of thiopental, is 5 to 10 minutes and reflects a rapid redistribution to lean muscle mass. Propofol is cleared from the central compartment by hepatic metabolism. Its metabolites are water-soluble and excreted in the urine.[2]

MECHANISM OF ACTION

Propofol produces CNS depression by modulating the $GABA_A$ receptor by the same mechanism as barbiturates.[2]

PHARMACODYNAMICS

Propofol produces a dose-dependent CNS depression without analgesia. It does have a strong amnestic effect. It decreases $CMRO_2$, CBF, and ICP. Since its cardiodepressant effects are greater than those of thiopental, CPP may be affected at high doses. Propofol is a myocardial depressant and potent vasodilator that lowers blood pressure and cardiac output. These effects attenuate the hemodynamic pressor response to laryngoscopy and intubation. Propofol blunts the baroreflex, so that heart rate does not increase in proportion to a drop in blood pressure. Decreased respiratory rate and

tidal volume are seen with propofol. Ventilatory response to hypercarbia is diminished; however, propofol may produce bronchodilation in patients with chronic obstructive pulmonary disease (COPD).[23] Propofol appears to have a strong anticonvulsant effect and may be used to terminate status epilepticus.[24]

ADMINISTRATION

Propofol is prepared as a 1% oil-in-water emulsion that contains egg lecithin, soybean oil, glycerol, and EDTA. The adult dose for induction is 2.0 to 2.5 mg/kg IV. For sedation, an infusion rate of 25 to 75 μg/kg/min is titrated to effect. Dosages should be reduced to 1.0 to 1.5 mg/kg IV in the elderly, in high-risk patients, and in anyone premedicated with an opioid or a benzodiazepine.[23] Propofol supports bacterial growth, and any unused portion should be discarded.

ADVERSE EFFECTS

Propofol produces pain on injection in up to 75 percent of patients. This may be reduced or prevented by pretreatment with an opioid or the addition of 0.01% lidocaine to the emulsion. Propofol may cause mild CNS excitation in the form of myoclonus, tremors, or hiccups.[2]

BENZODIAZEPINES

Benzodiazepines are a large class of drugs with anxiolytic, sedative, hypnotic, and amnestic properties. Of these, diazepam (Valium™), lorazepam (Ativan™), and midazolam (Versed™) are most used to facilitate intubation. They have a relatively short time of onset when given intravenously. Compared to midazolam, diazepam and lorazepam have longer times of onset and less predictable dose-effect relationships. They are all insoluble in water and are formulated in propylene glycol, which can produce a high rate of venous irritation.[25]

Midazolam is the newest of the three drugs. It has become the standard choice for preinduction anxiolysis, sedation, and amnesia. Midazolam is well suited and widely used as an induction agent.[26] It may be administered alone or in combination with an opioid. There is considerable hypnotic synergy when midazolam is used in combination with an opioid. The opioids provide excellent analgesia, which is a property lacking in midazolam.[2] When midazolam is used as the sole induction agent, recovery of consciousness takes longer than with thiopental, methohexital, etomidate, or propofol as a single agent. Midazolam is often used as a coinduction agent with ketamine or propofol, as it facilitates the onset of anesthesia without prolonging emergence times.[2] When combined with ketamine, midazolam attenuates ketamine's cardiostimulatory side effects as well as the incidence, severity, and recall of emergence reactions.[27]

PHARMACOKINETICS

Midazolam is formulated at a pH of 3.5, as it is water-soluble in an acidic environment. At physiologic pH, it undergoes a molecular rearrangement that makes it highly lipophilic. It is 94 percent protein-bound in the plasma. Unbound midazolam rapidly accumulates in the CNS, where it produces dose-dependent sedation or unconsciousness in 30 to 90 seconds. The drug redistributes less rapidly than many of the other hypnotics. This is reflected in the 10 to 30 minute duration of its CNS effects.[28] Midazolam is oxidized by the liver and excreted in the urine. Changes in hepatic blood flow can influence the clearance of midazolam.[29] Age has little effect on the elimination half-life.[29] Fentanyl has been shown to competitively inhibit the hepatic metabolism of midazolam in vitro and to decrease its clearance.[30]

MECHANISM OF ACTION

Benzodiazepines bind to a specific site on the alpha subunit of the $GABA_A$ receptor and enhance inhibitory neurotransmission. Midazolam has the greatest affinity for the receptor.[2] It has been proposed that the percentage of benzodiazepine receptor occupancy accounts for its effects. A 20 percent occupancy provides anxiolysis. A 30 to 50 percent occupancy causes sedation. Greater than 60 percent occupancy produces unconsciousness. It is unknown how the benzodiazepines produce amnesia.[2]

PHARMACODYNAMICS

Like thiopental and propofol, midazolam decreases $CMRO_2$ and CBF. Midazolam has a ceiling effect with respect to cerebral metabolism. The cerebrovascular response to carbon dioxide is unaffected by midazolam. It is also a potent anticonvulsant. Midazolam is a mild cardiodepressant and can decrease systemic vascular resistance and cardiac output.[28] The cardiac index and coronary blood flow are usually not affected by midazolam.[31] The drop in blood pressure is often masked by the sympathetic response to laryngoscopy. However, it may be pronounced in hypovolemic patients or in those who were given large doses.

Midazolam's respiratory effects also have a ceiling. It produces a mild and dose-dependent respiratory depression. In relatively healthy patients, the respiratory depression is insignificant. The respiratory depression is enhanced in patients with pulmonary disease. Hypoxemia is seen more frequently in patients who receive midazolam in combination with an opioid, such as fentanyl, than with either drug alone.[32]

ADMINISTRATION

An induction dose of midazolam is 0.2 to 0.4 mg/kg IV. When used as a coinduction agent (with ketamine, propofol, or fentanyl), the dose of midazolam is reduced to 0.1 to 0.2 mg/kg. For sedation, the dose is 0.04 to 0.1 mg/kg IV. It can also be administered intramuscularly at a dose of 0.07 to 0.1 mg/kg when rapid onset is not required.[2] Doses may have to be lowered in older patients because sensitivity to the hypnotic effects of midazolam increases with age, independent of pharmacokinetic factors.[33]

ADVERSE EFFECTS

Midazolam has relatively few adverse effects. It is a mild cardiorespiratory depressant. When it is combined with an opioid, a synergistic respiratory depressant effect may result in hypoxemia, apnea, and death. Those patients receiving this combination should be monitored with pulse oximetry while being given oxygen supplementation.[32] Unlike diazepam, midazolam produces little venous irritation and pain upon injection. It may precipitate a psychotic episode in patients taking valproate. It does cross the placenta and is associated with birth defects, especially involving the lip and palate, when administered in the first trimester.[28]

OPIOIDS

Opioids produce dose-dependent analgesia, sedation, and respiratory depression by mimicking the effects of endogeneous opiopeptins.[34] Morphine is the standard to which all opioids are compared. However, fentanyl (Sublimaze™) is the opioid of choice for use in the Emergency Department due to its rapid onset and short duration of action.[35] It has been in use since 1968 and its effects are well documented. Unlike morphine, fentanyl is rarely associated with a significant release of histamine.[36] Fentanyl has a remarkable hemodynamic stability profile.[36] If given in a large dose, fentanyl will produce anesthesia adequate for intubation. It is more often used as a sedative-analgesic or as a pretreatment adjuvant with one of the previously mentioned induction agents. Fentanyl is a synthetic opioid that is 50 to 100 times more potent than morphine. Structurally related to the phenylpiperidines, it is highly lipophilic and produces excellent short-term analgesia and sedation.[37]

Alfentanil (Alfenta™) is a structural derivative of fentanyl. It has a more rapid onset of action than fentanyl and half the duration of effect. Alfentanil is between one-sixth and one-ninth as potent as fentanyl. Its uses are analogous to those of fentanyl. It has been in use in the United States since 1982.[38] Recent data have shown alfentanil to be safe and effective for use in emergent rapid sequence intubation.[39] In cardiac patients, it was associated with a greater degree of cardiovascular depression than fentanyl.[40] Alfentanil is associated with a greater incidence of nausea and vomiting than fentanyl.[41] There are no data to suggest that alfentanil is more efficacious than fentanyl for use in the Emergency Department.

PHARMACOKINETICS

Upon intravenous injection, plasma fentanyl is 85 percent protein-bound. Its lipophilic nature allows it to enter highly perfused tissues rapidly, including the brain, heart, and lungs. After a single bolus dose of fentanyl, effects may be seen in as little 10 seconds, and they peak in 3 to 5 minutes. Morphine's effects peak in 20 to 30 minutes. Fentanyl has a high affinity for adipose tissue and redistribution accounts for the cessation of effects, which can take up to 30 to 60 minutes. An equipotent dose of morphine has a duration of 3 to 4 hours. Redistribution of fentanyl from peripheral tissues to the central compartment after large or repeat doses may prolong its effects. Clearance of morphine and fentanyl is by hepatic metabolism. These drugs have a high extraction ratio, and changes in hepatic blood flow can influence the clearance of fentanyl.[38]

MECHANISM OF ACTION

Fentanyl binds to the μ opioid receptor found throughout the CNS. Activation of the opioid receptor causes hyperpolarization and inhibition of neurotransmitter release.[34] It has been suggested that fentanyl may also be a low-affinity NMDA receptor antagonist.[42]

PHARMACODYNAMICS

Fentanyl decreases CBF and cerebral oxygen consumption. In patients with head trauma, a relatively small dose (3 μg/kg) produced an elevation of ICP.[43] Fentanyl has little effect on cardiac contractility and can produce a mild reduction in heart rate. Systemic vascular resistance and blood pressure may be slightly reduced, but they are usually unaffected in patients without cardiac pathology.[44] Respiratory depression induced by fentanyl is dose-dependent. The respiratory rate first decreases, followed by the tidal volume and subsequent apnea. The patient's response to hypercarbia is blunted when sedated with fentanyl.[45]

ADMINISTRATION

Fentanyl can be used in several ways to facilitate emergency intubation. Given purely for analgesia, as little as 3 to 5 μg/kg IV over 2 minutes may allow for an awake intubation. For adults, incremental doses of fentanyl from 25 to 50 μg can be titrated to produce the desired effect.[37] Fentanyl has a more stable hemodynamic profile during rapid sequence induction than either thiopental or midazolam.[35] In hemodynamically unstable patients and those with poor cardiac reserve, 5 to 15 μg/kg of fentanyl may be used as the sole induction agent.[35]

The most prudent role for fentanyl is as an adjunct to an induction agent. Three minutes prior to intubation, premedication with 2 to 4 μg/kg of fentanyl IV over 2 minutes provides excellent analgesia and attenuates the transient hypertension and tachycardia associated with laryngoscopy and intubation.[46] Although lidocaine and beta-blockers have also been shown to blunt the pressor response, opioids are more effective and reliable and do not produce rebound hypotension and bradycardia.[47,48]

ADVERSE EFFECTS

Other than the respiratory depression that is common to all opioids, fentanyl has relatively few adverse side effects. It may produce nausea and vomiting. Compared to other opioids such as morphine, nausea and vomiting are uncommon side effects.[37] Fentanyl is not associated with a significant release of histamine, which is reflected in its hemodynamic stability. Muscular rigidity, frequently involving the chest wall and diaphragm, may occur. This happens more often at higher doses, typically greater than 15 μg/kg, and may be prevented or relieved by neuromuscular blockade or by opioid antagonism with naloxone.[49] Myoclonic movements may occur, but these do not reflect seizure activity on the EEG. As with all opioids, biliary colic and urinary retention are associated with fentanyl administration.[37]

NEUROMUSCULAR BLOCKING AGENTS

Neuromuscular blockade is an integral part of the rapid sequence induction and intubation protocol. The combination of a paralytic agent and a sedative or analgesic is superior to the use of any single agent. The use of a neuromuscular blocking (NMB) agent to facilitate intubation provides for control of the airway and better visualization of the vocal cords than does sedation without paralysis.[50] It is also well documented that, in the Emergency Department setting, rapid sequence induction with an NMB agent allows for faster intubations with fewer complications than sedation alone.[1] The use of a sedative without NMB should be reserved for the awake oral intubation of a patient with a difficult airway.

NMBs are classified as either depolarizing or nondepolarizing, depending on their action on the nicotinic acetylcholine receptor of the motor end plate. The optimal NMB agent has a rapid onset of action, a predictably short duration of action, and no side effects. As with induction agents, the optimal NMB agent has yet to be found. Until a better agent is developed, succinylcholine (Anectine™) remains the standard NMB agent for Emergency Department intubations.[51]

SUCCINYLCHOLINE

Succinylcholine is the only depolarizing NMB agent in clinical use. Introduced in 1952, it is a chemical combination of two acetylcholine molecules. **It is the most widely used NMB in the Emergency Department because its onset of action is faster and its duration of action is shorter than those of any other NMB agent. This is particularly important in patients who cannot be intubated after neuromuscular blockade and where the resumption of spontaneous respirations is vital.**

MECHANISM OF ACTION

The structure of succinylcholine allows it to bind noncompetitively to acetylcholine receptors, causing depolarization of the postjunctional neuromuscular membrane. This initial depolarization is seen as a brief period of fasciculation following the administration of the drug. Unlike acetylcholine, which is hydrolyzed within milliseconds, succinylcholine remains intact for several minutes. It produces paralysis by occupying the acetylcholine receptors, and making the motor end plates refractory, so that muscle contraction cannot occur. Muscle relaxation proceeds from the distal muscles to the proximal muscles, and thus the diaphragm is one of the last muscles to become paralyzed.[52]

PHARMACOLOGY

After a paralytic dose of succinylcholine, adequate intubating conditions are almost always achieved within 1 minute. Since succinylcholine is rapidly hydrolyzed by plasma pseudocholinesterase to succinylmonocholine, only a small fraction of the administered dose reaches the neuromuscular junction. Succinylmonocholine, which also has some neuromuscular blocking properties, is further hydrolyzed to succinic acid and choline. These end products are rapidly taken up by cells and reused in various biochemical molecules. The rapid degradation of succinylcholine provides a concentration gradient that causes the diffusion of succinylcholine off of the Ach receptors and allows repolarization of the myocyte membrane. The duration of apnea following a single dose of succinylcholine is 3 to 5 minutes and reflects the activity of plasma pseudocholinesterase.[53] Repeated doses or infusion of succinylcholine may produce tachyphylaxis, prolonged paralysis, and repolarization of the neuromuscular membrane known as a phase II block.[53] **If paralysis of greater than 3 to 5 minutes is desired, a nondepolarizing agent can be administered after the patient is intubated.**

ADMINISTRATION

The recommended dose of succinylcholine to produce optimal intubating conditions is 1.0 to 1.5 mg/kg IV as a bolus. This dose should be increased to 1.5 to 2.0 mg/kg in children. Succinylcholine can also be administered intramuscularly, which may become important for use in an emergency when control of the airway is necessary and the patient has no IV access. The intramuscular dose is twice the intravenous dose.[54]

ADVERSE EFFECTS

Although relatively uncommon, a number of potential adverse effects are associated with the administration of succinylcholine. These include muscular fasciculations and myalgia, autonomic stimulation, histamine release, prolonged apnea, elevated intracranial and intraocular pressure, hyperkalemia, and malignant hyperthermia.[53] **The use of succinylcholine is recommended for rapid sequence induction and intubation as the risk of a compromised airway far outweighs the potential harm from these side effects.**

The fine, chaotic muscle contractions that are often observed at the onset of paralysis are associated with several side effects, most commonly myalgia but also increased IOP, increased ICP, and increased intragastric pressure. Muscle pain 24 to 48 hours after the administration of succinylcholine is most prominent in young, muscular men, while it is unlikely in children, the elderly, and those with undeveloped or diminished muscle mass. Muscle fasciculations may be prevented by the administration of a defasiculating dose (10 percent of the paralytic dose) of a nondepolarizing NMB agent given 3 to 5 minutes prior to the succinylcholine.[55]

In most patients, muscle fasciculations are a benign phenomenon and precurarization is unnecessary. In patients with eye injuries or suspected intracranial pathology, it is prudent to use a nondepolarizing NMB agent.[56] Rocuronium is a nondepolarizing agent that has been shown to significantly decrease IOP during rapid sequence induction.[57] Its use may be indicated in patients with penetrating eye injuries.[57]

In fact, the transient increase in intraocular and intracranial pressure during laryngoscopy and intubation may be even greater without the use of succinylcholine. Increased ICP may also occur with the use of succinylcholine. While the magnitude and clinical significance of this increase remains unclear, defasciculation with a nondepolarizing NMB agent has been shown to prevent this rise in ICP.[58]

Increased intragastric pressure may increase the risk of aspiration. Precurarization decreases this rise in pressure. Succinylcholine increases the tone of the lower esophageal sphincter and may mitigate the risk of aspiration.[59] Regurgitation of stomach contents is more likely the result of distention from overzealous mask ventilation.

Succinylcholine binds to acetylcholine receptors throughout the body, including those of the autonomic ganglia. Succinylcholine may also have direct muscarinic effects on the heart. It is difficult to characterize a specific cardiovascular effect typical of succinylcholine. It may produce tachycardia, bradycardia, or dysrhythmias.[53] Children are particularly susceptible to bradycardia following succinylcholine administration. It is recommended that all children be given 0.01 mg/kg IV of atropine prior to administration of succinylcholine.[54]

Prolonged apnea following succinylcholine is a sign of decreased plasma pseudocholinesterase levels. This may occur in patients with hepatic disease, anemia, renal failure, or cancer; those on cytotoxic drugs; patients with connective tissue disorders; pregnant patients; patients with cocaine intoxication; and those with genetically deficient enzyme activity. In most cases this is of little significance because apnea rarely exceeds 20 minutes.[60]

Succinylcholine may produce an increase in serum potassium level, which is typically less than 0.5 meq/L. It should be used with caution in patients with significant hyperkalemia. Its use is not contraindicated in patients with renal failure. It has been associated with cases of massive hyperkalemia (> 5 meq/L) and cardiac arrest in patients who have had massive muscle trauma, severe burns, and major nerve or spinal cord injury at least 1 week prior to receiving succinylcholine.[53] In such patients, succinylcholine should not be used starting 24 hours after the insult.

Malignant hyperthermia is an extremely rare adverse reaction to inhaled anesthetics and/or succinylcholine. It has an autosomal dominant inheritance pattern and affects 1 in 15,000 children as well as 1 in 50,000 adults. Malignant hyperthermia is characterized by a rapid elevation in temperature and aggressive rhabdomyolysis shortly after administration of the offending agent. Treatment involves aggressive cooling measures, volume replacement, correction of acid-base and electrolyte disturbances, and administration of dantrolene.[53] Masseter muscle rigidity is a benign side effect in most cases that has been reported in children receiving succinylcholine. In several reported cases of fatal malignant hyperthermia, masseter muscle rigidity was the first sign of an abnormal reaction.[61] **Despite the lengthy list of potential adverse effects, the benefits of intubation with a rapidly acting, short-lasting paralytic agent such as succinylcholine provides the safest conditions for intubation in the Emergency Department.**

NONDEPOLARIZING AGENTS

Nondepolarizing NMB agents act by competitive inhibition of the Ach receptors at the motor end plate. They weakly bind to the receptor and block the binding site for acetylcholine without producing any effect on the postsynaptic neuromuscular membrane. Following the kinetics of competitive inhibition, this blockade is dependent on the relative concentrations of acetylcholine and NMB available in the synaptic cleft. As the ratio returns in favor of acetylcholine, normal neuromuscular transmission is restored. Thus, return of muscle function can be hastened by the use of a cholinesterase inhibitor such as neostigmine or edrophonium, but only after some muscular contraction can be observed. Nondepolarizing agents have not only the potential for reversal but also far fewer side effects than succinylcholine. Their longer time to onset and much longer duration of action make them less useful for rapid sequence induction.[53]

Nondepolarizing NMB agents can be grouped by chemical structure. The steroid-based agents include pancuronium, vecuronium, rocuronium, and rapacuronium. The oldest nondepolarizing agent, d-tubocurarine, is a benzylisoquinoline, as are atracurium, cisatracurium, and mivacurium.[53] Pancuronium, atracurium, vecuronium, and rocuronium have been extensively studied for use in rapid sequence intubation.[62]

Pancuronium, in use since 1972, is classified as a long-acting agent. It produces paralysis in 2 to 5 minutes and lasts 40 to 60 minutes. It is associated with an increased heart rate, blood pressure, and cardiac output through a postganglionic vagolytic effect. It is not associated with the release of histamine. Pancuronium's low cost and familiarity have made it popular. Its slow onset of action limits its usefulness in facilitating emergent endotracheal intubation. More rapid-acting, albeit more expensive, agents such as vecuronium and rocuronium are now widely available.

Vecuronium can produce good intubating conditions within 1 minute at 2.5 times the normal dose. Unfortunately, this produces paralysis for 1 to 2 hours. The normal intubating dose of vecuronium (0.1 mg/kg) takes 3 minutes to produce adequate paralysis for intubation, and the patient will remain apneic for 30 to 35 minutes.

Rocuronium is considered the best nondepolarizing agent for use in the Emergency Department because it produces intubating conditions in roughly 60 to 90 seconds and is comparable to succinylcholine. However, the intubating dose of 0.9 to 1.2 mg/kg maintains paralysis for 20 to 25 minutes. This still far exceeds the 3 to 5 minutes provided by succinylcholine.[63] **If prolonged paralysis is required in an agitated patient, a nondepolarizing agent should be used after intubation with succinylcholine.**

Despite the relatively few side effects of nondepolarizing NMBs, rapid sequence intubation with succinylcholine is the safest course of action. The short duration of paralysis provides a measure of security in case the patient cannot be intubated quickly. Rapacuronium is a new nondepolarizing NMB agent. It has been developed as a replacement for succinylcholine in the rapid sequence protocol. It has onset times and duration of action similar to those of succinylcholine. Rapacuronium remains to be proven to have any significant benefit over succinylcholine in the Emergency Department. At present, succinylcholine is firmly in place as the muscle relaxant of choice for rapid sequence emergency intubations.[64]

MISCELLANEOUS AGENTS

LIDOCAINE

Lidocaine is a local anesthetic agent that, in low doses, has an antiarrhythmic effect on the heart. It also blocks the rise in ICP associated with laryngoscopy.[65–68] It attenuates the hypotensive and tachycardic response to laryngoscopy. It does not affect myocardial contractility in therapeutic doses. It is usually administered to patients with head injuries to blunt the ICP response to laryngoscopy.[67,68] The dose is 1 to 2 mg/kg IV.

ATROPINE

Atropine is an acetylcholine receptor antagonist that is rapid-acting. It prevents bradycardia during rapid sequence induction and intubation. It is frequently administered in children, as they can develop a significant bradycardia and possible asystole during laryngoscopy. It has a secondary effect of reducing secretions produced in the respiratory tract and the salivary glands. The dose is 0.01 mg/kg IV with a minimum dose of 0.10 mg IV and a maximum dose of 0.40 mg IV.

REFERENCES

1. Dufour DG, Larose DL, Clement SC: Rapid sequence intubation in the emergency department. *J Emerg Med* 1995; 13(5):705–710.
2. Reves JG, Glass P, Lubarsky DA: Nonbarbiturate intravenous anesthetics, in Miller RD (ed): *Anesthesia,* 5th ed. Philadelphia: Churchill Livingstone, 2000:228–272.
3. Fragen RJ, Avaram MJ: Barbiturates, in Miller RD (ed): *Anesthesia,* 5th ed. Philadelphia: Churchill Livingstone, 2000:209–227.
4. Olson RW: Barbiturates. *Int Anesthesiol Clin* 1988; 26:245.
5. Price HL, Kovnat PJ, Safer JN, et al: The uptake of thiopental by body tissues and its relation to the duration of narcosis. *Clin Pharmacol Ther* 1960; 1(1):16–22.
6. Bischoff KB, Dedrick RL: Thiopental pharmacokinetics. *J Pharm Sci* 1968; 57(8):1346–1351.
7. Franks NP, Lieb WR: Molecular and cellular mechanisms of general anesthesia. *Nature* 1994; 367:607–613.
8. Blouin RT, Conard PF, Gross JB: Time course of ventilatory depression following induction doses of propofol and thiopental. *Anesthesiology* 1991; 75(6):940–944.
9. Laurin EG, Sakles JC, Prosser B, et al: Safety of etomidate for rapid-sequence intubation (abstr). SAEM 1996 Annual Meeting, Davis, California.
10. Van Hamme MJ, Ghoneim MM, Amber JJ: Pharmacokinetics of etomidate, a new intravenous anesthetic. *Anesthesiology* 1978; 49(4):274–277.
11. Giese JL, Stanley TH: Etomidate: a new intravenous anesthetic induction agent. *Pharmacotherapy* 1983; 3(5):251–258.
12. Modica PA, Tempelhoff R: Intracranial pressure during induction of anesthesia and tracheal intubation with etomidate-induced EEG burst suppression. *Can J Anaesth* 1992; 39(3):236–241.
13. Gooding JM, Weng J, Smith RA, et al: Cardiovascular and pulmonary responses following etomidate induction of anesthesia in patients with demonstrated cardiac disease. *Anesth Analg* 1979; 58(1):40–41.
14. Harris CE, Murray AM, Anderson JM, et al: Effects of thiopentone, etomidate, and propofol on hemodynamic response to tracheal intubation. *Anaesthesia* 1988; 43(suppl):32–36.
15. Nimmo WS, Miller M: Pharmacology of etomidate. *Contemp Anesth Pract* 1983; 7:83–95.
16. Bird TM, Edbrooke DL, Newby DM, et al: Intravenous sedation for the intubated and spontaneously breathing patient in the intensive care unit. *Acta Anesth Scand* 1984; 28:640–643.
17. Holdcroft A, Morgan M, Whitman JG, et al: Effect of dose and premedication on induction complications with etomidate. *Br J Anesth* 1976; 49:199–204.
18. Wagner RL, White PF: Etomidate inhibits adrenocortical function in surgical patients. *Anesthesiology* 1984; 61(6):647–651.
19. White PF, Way WL, Trevor AJ: Ketamine—its pharmacology and therapeutic uses. *Anesthesiology* 1982; 56(2):119–136.
20. Wong DHW, Jenkins LCP: An experimental study of the mechanism of action of ketamine on the central nervous system. *Can Anaesth Soc J* 1974; 21(1):57–67.
21. Lundy PA, Gowdey DW, Calhoun EH: Tracheal smooth muscle relaxant effect of ketamine. *Br J Anaesth* 1974; 46:333–336.
22. Borgeat A, Wilder-Smith OHG, Suter PM: The nonhypnotic therapeutic applications of propofol. *Anesthesiology* 1994; 80(3):642–656.
23. Sebel PS, Lowdon JD: Propofol: a new intravenous anesthetic. *Anesthesiology* 1989; 71(2):260–277.
24. Ebrahim ZY, Schubert A, Van Ness P, et al: The effects of propofol on the electroencephalogram of patients with epilepsy. *Anesth Analg* 1994; 78:275–279.

25. Whitwam JG, Al-khudhairi, McCloy RF: Comparison of midazolam and diazepam in doses of comparable potency during gastroscopy. *Anaesthesiology* 1983; 55:773–777.

26. Dickinson ET, Cohen JE, Mechem CC: The effectiveness of midazolam as a single pharmacologic agent to facilitate endotracheal intubation by paramedics. *Prehosp Emerg Care* 1999; 3:191–193.

27. White PF: Comparative evaluation of intravenous agents for rapid sequence induction—thiopental, ketamine, and midazolam. *Anesthesiology* 1982; 57(4):279–284.

28. Reves JG, Fragen RJ, Vinik HR, et al: Midazolam—pharmacology and uses. *Anesthesiology* 1985; 62(3):310–324.

29. Kanto J, Analtonen L, Himberg JJ, et al: Midazolam as an intravenous induction agent in the elderly: a clinical and pharmacokinetic study. *Anesth Analg* 1986; 65:15–20.

30. Oda Y, Mizutani K, Hase I, et al: Fentanyl inhibits metabolism of midazolam: competitive inhibition in vitro. *Br J Anaesth* 1999; 82(6):900–903.

31. Marty J, Nitenberg J, Blanchet S, et al: Effects of midazolam on the coronary circulation in patients with coronary artery disease. *Anesthesiology* 1986; 64(2):206–210.

32. Bailey PL, Pace NL, Ashburn MA, et al: Frequent hypoxemia and apnea after sedation with midazolam and fentanyl. *Anesthesiology* 1990; 73(5):826–830.

33. Jacobs JR, Reve JG, Marty J, et al: Aging increases pharmacodynamic sensitivity to the hypnotic effects of midazolam. *Anesth Analg* 1995; 80:143–148.

34. Pasternak GW: Pharmacological mechanisms of opioid analgesics. *Clin Neuropharmacol* 1993; 16(1):1–18.

35. Silivotti ML, Ducharme J: Randomized double-blind study on sedatives and hemodynamics during rapid-sequence intubation in the emergency department: the SHRED study. *Ann Emerg Med* 1998; 31:313–324.

36. Flacke JW, Flacke WE, Bloor BC, et al: Histamine release by four narcotics: a double blind study in humans. *Anesth Analg* 1987; 66:723–730.

37. Bailey PL, Egan TD, Stanley TH: Intravenous opioid anesthetics, in Miller RD (ed): *Anesthesia,* 5th ed. Philadelphia: Churchill Livingstone, 2000:273–355.

38. Mather LE: Clinical pharmacokinetics of fentanyl and its newer derivatives. *Clin Pharmacokinet* 1983; 8:422–446.

39. Groener R, Moyes DG: Rapid tracheal intubation with propofol, alfentanil and a standard dose of vecuronium. *Br J Anaesth* 1997; 79:384–385.

40. Spiss CK, Coraim F, Haider W, et al: Haemodynamic effects of fentanyl or alfentanil as adjutants to etomidate for induction of anaesthesia in cardiac patients. *Acta Anaesthesiol Scand* 1984; 28:554–556.

41. Kay B, Stephenson DK: Alfentanil (R39209): initial clinical experience with a new narcotic analgesic. *Anaesthesia* 1980; 35:1197–1201.

42. Yamakura T, Sakimura, Shimoji K: Direct inhibition of the *N*-methyl-D-aspartate receptor channel by high concentrations of opioids. *Anesthesiology* 1999; 91(4):1053–1063.

43. Sperry RJ, Bailey, Reichman MV, et al: Fentanyl and sufentanil increase intracranial pressure in head trauma patients. *Anesthesiology* 1992; 77(3):416–420.

44. Bailey PL, Wilbrink J, Zwanikken P, et al: Anesthetic induction with fentanyl. *Anesth Analg* 1985; 64:48–53.

45. Cartwright P, Prys-Roberts C, Gill K, et al: Ventilatory depression related to plasma fentanyl concentrations during and after anesthesia in humans. *Anesth Analg* 1983: 62:966–974.

46. Martin DE, Rosenberg H, Aukberg SJ, et al: Low-dose fentanyl blunts the circulatory response to tracheal intubation. *Anesth Analg* 1982; 61(8):680–684.

47. Pathak D, Slater RM, Ping SS, et al: Effects of alfentanil and lidocaine on the hemodynamic responses to laryngoscopy and tracheal intubation. *J Clin Anesth* 1990; 2:81–85.

48. Helfman SM, Gold MI, DeLisser EA, et al: Which drug prevents tachycardia and hypertension associated with tracheal intubation: lidocaine, fentanyl, or esmolol? *Anesth Analg* 1991; 72:482–486.

49. Streisand JB, Bailey PL, LeMaire L, et al: Fentanyl-induced rigidity and unconsciousness in human volunteers. *Anesthesiology* 1993; 78(4):629–634.

50. Li J, Murphy-Lavoie H, Bugas C, et al: Complications of emergency intubation with and without paralysis. *Am J Emerg Med* 1999; 17(2):141–144.

51. Walls RM: Airway management. *Emerg Med Clin North Am* 1993; 11(1):53–57.

52. Katz RL, Ryan JF: The neuromuscular effects of suxamethonium in man. *Br J Anaesth* 1969; 41:381–390.

53. Savarese JJ, Caldwell JE, Lien CA, et al: Pharmacology of muscle relaxants and their antagonists, in Miller RD (ed): *Anesthesia,* 5th ed. Philadelphia: Churchill Livingstone, 2000:412–477.

54. Yamamoto LG: Rapid sequence anesthesia induction and advanced airway management in pediatric patients. *Emerg Med Clin North Am* 1991; 9(3):611–623.

55. Martin R, Carrier J, Pirlet M, et al: Rocuronium is the best non-depolarizing relaxant to prevent succinylcholine fasciculations and myalgia. *Can J Anaesth* 1998; 45(6):521–525.

56. Konchigeri HN, Lee YE, Venugopal K: Effect of pancuronium on intraocular pressure changes induced by succinylcholine. *Can Anaesth Soc J* 1979; 26(6):479–481.

57. Vinik HR: Intraocular pressure changes during rapid sequence induction and intubation: a comparison of rocuronium, atracurium, and succinylcholine. *J Clin Anesth* 1999; 11:95–100.

58. Stirt JA, Grosslight KR, Bedford RF, et al: "Defasciculation" with metocurine prevents succinylcholine-induced increases in intracranial pressure. *Anesthesiology* 1987; 67(1):50–53.

59. Smith G, Dalling R, Williams TIR: Gastro-oesophageal pressure gradient changes produced by induction of anesthesia and suxamethonium. *Br J Anaesth* 1978; 50:1137–1142.

60. Whittaker M: Plasma cholinesterase variants and the anaesthetist. *Anaesthesia* 1980; 35:174–197.

61. Ramerirez JA, Cheetham ED, Laurence AS, et al: Suxamethonium, masseter spasm, and later malignant hyperthermia. *Anaesthesia* 1998; 53:1109–1116.

62. Magorian T, Flannery KB, Miller RD: Comparison of rocuronium, succinylcholine, and vecuronium for rapid-sequence induction of anesthesia in adult patients. *Anesthesiology* 1993; 79(5):913-918.

63. Sakles JC, Laurin EG, Rantapaa AA, et al: Rocuronium for rapid sequence intubation in emergency department patients. *J Emerg Med* 1999; 17(4):611–616.

64. Fleming NW, Chung F, Glass PS, et al: Comparison of intubation conditions provided by rapacuronium (ORG 9487) or succinylcholine in humans during anesthesia with fentanyl and propofol. *Anesthesiology* 1999; 91(5):1311–1317.

65. White PF, Schlobohm RM, Pitts LH, et al: A randomized study of drugs for preventing increases in intracranial pressure during endotracheal suctioning. *Anesthesiology* 1982; 57:242–244.

66. Yano M, Nishiyama H, Yokota H, et al: Effect of lidocaine on ICP response to endotracheal suctioning. *Anesthesiology* 1986; 64:651–653.

67. Hamill JF, Bedford RF, Weaver DC, et al: Lidocaine before endotracheal intubation: intravenous or laryngotracheal? *Anesthesia* 1981; 55:578–581.

68. Splinter WM: Intravenous lidocaine does not attenuate the hemodynamic response of children to laryngoscopy and tracheal intubation. *Can J Anaesth* 1990; 37:440–443.

Chapter 4
RAPID SEQUENCE INDUCTION

Ned F. Nasr
Isam F. Nasr
Maher Fattouh
Eric L. Pedicini

INTRODUCTION

Rapid sequence induction (RSI) of anesthesia, sometimes referred to as "crash" induction, has become a safe and effective method of establishing emergent airway control in patients with suspected life-threatening emergencies. It ensures optimal patient compliance in a well-controlled environment. RSI involves the near simultaneous administration of a potent sedative-hypnotic agent and a neuromuscular blocking agent.[1] Various pretreatment drug regimens have been advocated to prevent potentially deleterious side effects, such as aspiration of gastric contents, cardiovascular excitation or depression, and intracranial pressure elevation.

The first endotracheal tubes were developed for the resuscitation of the newborn and victims of drowning in the nineteenth century but were not used in anesthesia until 1878.[13] Muscle relaxants were not prepared until some 60 years later. Succinylcholine was prepared by the Nobel Laureate Daniel Bovet in 1949, after which it gained the widespread usage it still enjoys today. The RSI technique did not come into modern day practice until the end of World War II.

Patients can be hypoxic, confused, uncooperative, unstable, and unknowing of their medications or medical conditions and can require airway control within minutes of arrival at the Emergency Department. **RSI is the preferred method for securing the airway in the Emergency Department, as these patients are at risk for aspiration.** These risks include vomiting from gastrointestinal obstruction, opioids, or hypotension; regurgitation from diabetic gastroparesis, gastroesophageal reflux, increased gastric pressure, or decreased lower esophageal sphincter tone; impaired laryngeal protective reflexes; and difficult airway management.[7] Conditions such as recent meal ingestion, pain, obesity, and pregnancy place patients at higher risk as well.

INDICATIONS

The primary indication for RSI is to quickly protect and secure the airway. The rationale behind RSI is to create an environment in which the trachea can be intubated as quickly and with as little difficulty as possible. The clinical conditions occurring at the time of attempted intubation are therefore of great importance. During RSI of anesthesia, the drugs used to produce hypnosis and muscle relaxation interact together to produce the intubating conditions. A complete list of the indications for RSI appears in Table 4-1.

CONTRAINDICATIONS

There are few contraindications to RSI. It should not be performed by an inexperienced intubator. If the operator has doubts about his or her ability to intubate the patient, an awake intubation should be considered. The unavailability of equipment, contraindications to muscle relaxants, and critically ill patients in whom the airway can be secured by other methods (fiberoptic intubation, topical anesthesia, or minimal sedation with a benzodiazepine and/or narcotic) are also contraindications to RSI. Table 4-2 lists the many common contraindications to the use of succinylcholine.

TABLE 4-1. INDICATIONS FOR RAPID SEQUENCE INTUBATION (RSI) IN THE EMERGENCY DEPARTMENT

Head trauma with the need for airway control
Head trauma with the need for ventilation
Head trauma with a decreased Glasgow Coma Scale score
Uncooperative or combative patient with compromised airway
Uncontrolled seizure activity requiring airway control
Depressed level of consciousness and questionable ability to maintain a patent airway
Airway protection and risk for pulmonary aspiration (e.g., full stomach, pregnancy, and obesity)
Potentially difficult intubation after airway evaluation
Definitive maintenance of airway patency
Respiratory failure
Emergency surgery and requirement for general anesthesia
Application of advanced cardiac life support and administration of drugs

SOURCE: Adapted from references 2 and 7.

TABLE 4-2. CONTRAINDICATIONS TO THE USE OF SUCCINYLCHOLINE

Cardiac arrhythmia
Children and adolescents unless no other option exists
Exaggerated hyperkalemia in susceptible patients
    More than 24 hours after major burns and trauma
    Crush injuries
    Denervation
    Prolonged immobilization
    Paraplegia
    Hemiplegia
    Disuse atrophy
    Severe abdominal infection
    Muscular atrophy
History of malignant hyperthermia
Increased intracranial pressure (relative)
Increased intragastric pressure (relative)
Increased intraocular pressure (relative)
Masseter muscle spasm or rigidity
Plasma cholinesterase deficiency (relative)

SOURCE: Adapted from references 1, 2, and 8.

EQUIPMENT

Supplemental oxygen with appropriate tubing and connectors
Laryngoscope handle with extra batteries
Laryngoscope blades, various sizes and types
Endotracheal tubes, various sizes
Wire stylet, malleable type
Nonrebreather oxygen masks, various sizes
Oropharyngeal airways, various sizes
Nasopharyngeal airways, various sizes
Suction source with appropriate tubing
Suction catheters for endotracheal tubes
Yankauer suction catheter
Bag-valve-mask devices, various sizes
Face masks, various sizes
Stethoscope
Water-soluble lubricant or anesthetic jelly
Tape
Benzoin adhesive
Syringes, 10 and 20 mL
Medications drawn up and labeled
Pulse oximeter
Cardiac monitor
Automatic sphygmomanometer
End-tidal carbon dioxide (CO_2) monitor/device
Crash cart
Resuscitation medications
Personnel (respiratory technician, medication nurse, recorder, in-line stabilization assistant)

The equipment required for RSI is the same as that for any intubation.[10,13] Complete details regarding the selection of properly sized equipment can be found in Chapter 5. In addition, backup equipment should be readily available if the patient cannot be intubated. This can be a laryngeal mask airway, cricothyroidotomy tray, retrograde guidewire kit, or percutaneous jet ventilation system to name a few.

PATIENT PREPARATION

RSI can be performed with little or no preparation. If possible, a few steps can be performed while the patient is being evaluated. Administer supplemental oxygen to the patient with a nonrebreather mask and apply continuous pulse oximetry and cardiac monitoring. Obtain intravenous access. If time permits, pharmacologic agents can be used to increase gastric pH and motility (nonparticular antacid, H_2-receptor blockers, and metoclopramide). An antisialagogue (atropine or glycopyrrolate) may also be administered for excessive oral secretions.

Evaluate the airway (Chapter 1). **If, after evaluation of the airway, there is sufficient doubt as to the possibility of intubating the patient successfully, a neuromuscular relaxant should not be administered.** Consideration should be given to securing the airway in another fashion (e.g., awake intubation).

TECHNIQUE

The three main characteristics of RSI are preoxygenation, application of cricoid pressure, and the avoidance of positive-pressure ventilation (if possible) prior to securing the airway with a cuffed endotracheal tube. In addition, RSI requires the presence of ancillary equipment and experienced assistance. The details of timing, drug choice, and dosage are not rigidly defined. A RSI protocol is described below from start to finish.

Preoxygenate the patient with 100% O_2 by nonrebreather mask, or ventilate with a bag-valve-mask device using cricoid pressure, to build an oxygen reserve and prevent hypoxemia during induction. Traditionally, preoxygenation for 5 minutes is the routine practice. If this is not practical, attempt to preoxygenate the patient for 3 minutes.[6] However, four maximal inspirations are equally effective in the cooperative patient.[6]

While an assistant is preoxygenating the patient, evaluate the airway to anticipate any difficulties during the intubation (Chapter 1). Assemble all required equipment. Connect the bag-valve device to a mask and an oxygen supply. Lubricate and place the malleable stylet into the endotracheal tube. Attach a syringe to the inflation port of the endotracheal tube cuff. Inflate the cuff to look for any air leaks. Deflate the cuff and leave the syringe attached to the inflation port. Attach the laryngoscope blade to the handle and make sure that the light is functional. Simultaneously, the nurses should apply continuous pulse oximetry and cardiac monitoring to the patient, draw up and label the required medications, establish intravenous access, set up the suction, record all events, and continuously observe the cardiac monitor and pulse oximeter.

If there is no suspicion of a cervical spine injury, position the patient in the optimum "sniffing" position. If there is suspicion of a cervical spine injury, an assistant should provide manual in-line axial stabilization of the head and neck during the intubation sequence and remove the anterior aspect of the cervical spine collar to allow for maximal mouth opening and access to the neck.

Premedicate the patient (Table 4-3). Atropine (0.01 mg/kg, minimum 0.1 mg) should be given to children to prevent bradycardia. Fentanyl (2 to 3 μg/kg) or one of its derivatives can be given to blunt the intracranial pressure response, transient hypertension, and tachycardia associated with intubation. Lidocaine (1.0 to 1.5 mg/kg) can also be given for the same purposes. Phenylephrine (50 μg) can be given to attenuate the hypotensive response to the procedure. Administer a defasciculating dose of a nondepolarizing neuromuscular blocking agent. This is one-tenth of the intubating dose (Table 4-4). Administer an appropriate induction agent as indicated by the clinical setting and patient's hemodynamic status (Tables 4-5 and 4-6). Flush the intravenous line with 10 mL of crystalloid solution after each drug to ensure delivery.

Administer a neuromuscular blocking agent.[1,2,5] Numerous agents are available (Table 4-4). The most commonly used medications are succinylcholine (1.0 to 1.5 mg/kg) or rocuronium (1.0 to 1.2 mg/kg). **Succinylcholine is the preferred agent. Its effects are short-lasting (4 to 6 minutes). This is especially useful if the patient cannot be intubated, as he or she will need to be ventilated with a bag-valve-mask device until the succinylcholine wears off.** Rocuronium allows the same intubating conditions as succinylcholine except that it lasts for 30 to 60 minutes. This is problematic if the patient cannot be intubated.

An assistant should apply cricoid pressure as soon as the patient loses consciousness and maintain it until successful oral endotracheal intubation has been confirmed. Avoid mask ventilation if possible. If hypoxemia or hypercarbia ensues, begin mask ventilation to a

TABLE 4-3. PHARMACOLOGIC ADJUNCTS TO INTUBATION IN THE PREMEDICATION PHASE

Agent	Standard dose	Trauma dose	Blood pressure	Cerebral perfusion pressure
Fentanyl*	2.0–8.0 μg/kg	1.0–3.0 μg/kg	Stable	Stable
Sufentanil[†]	0.25–1.0 μg/kg	0.1–0.2 μg/kg	Stable	Stable
Alfentanil[‡]	5.0–25.0 μg/kg	5 μg/kg	Stable	Stable
Remifentanil[¶]	0.25–1.0 μg/kg/min	0.05–0.5 μg/kg/min	Stable	Stable
Lidocaine[§]	1.0–1.5 mg/kg	1.0–1.5 mg/kg	Stable	Stable or increased

*Minimal hemodynamic or cerebrovascular effects. Useful agents for blunting the noxious stimuli of direct laryngoscopy or intubation. The half-time of equilibration between the effect and plasma is relatively slow (5 to 6 minutes). May cause central vagal stimulation with resultant bradycardia and occasionally hypotension in patients with high sympathetic tone.

[†]Similar to fentanyl, but more potent and faster offset.

[‡]Similar to fentanyl, but faster onset and duration of action. Half-time of equilibration between the effect site and the plasma is 1.5 minutes, making this opioid a very appropriate drug to provide a transient peak effect after a single bolus dose. May prevent the increase in intraocular pressure caused by succinylcholine.[8]

[¶]Similar to alfentanil in terms of fast onset. Extremely rapid clearance (3 to 4 L/minute) due to esterase metabolism, resulting in a rapid and predictable recovery.

[§]Useful adjuvant agent for blunting airway reflexes. Also blunts blood pressure, intracranial pressure, and intraocular pressure responses to intubation, involuntary muscle movements after etomidate, and injection site pain from propofol and etomidate. Topical lidocaine is also effective in blunting reflexes.

SOURCE: Adapted from Chapter 3.

3. Groener R, Moyes DG: Rapid tracheal intubation with propofol and alfantanil and a standard dose of vecuronium. *Br J Anesth* 1997; 79:384–385.

4. Sackles JC, Laurin EG, Rantapaa AA, et al: Rocuronium for rapid sequence intubation of emergency department patients. *J Emerg Med* 1999; 17(4): 611–616.

5. Silverman SM, Culling RD, Middaugh RE: Rapid-sequence orotracheal intubation: a comparison of three techniques. *Anesthesiology* 1990; 73(2):244–248.

6. Gambee MA, Hertzka RE, Fisher DM: Preoxygenation techniques: comparison of three minutes and four breaths. *Anesth Analg* 1987; 66:468–470.

7. Smith, CE: Rapid sequence intubation in trauma. The 10th Annual Trauma Anesthesia and Critical Care Society Symposium, May 1997 (poster).

8. Zimmerman AA, Funk KJ, Tidwell JL: Propofol and alfentanil prevent the increase in intraocular pressure caused by succinylcholine and endotracheal intubation during rapid sequence induction of anesthesia. *Anesth Analg* 1996; 83:814–817.

9. Kirkegaard-Nielsen H, Caldwell JE, Berry PD: Rapid sequence intubation with rocuronium. *Anesthesiology* 1999; 91:131–136.

10. Thwaites AJ, Rice CP, Smith I: Rapid sequence induction: a questionnaire survey of its routine conduct and continued management during a failed intubation. *Anaesthesia* 1999; 54:376–381.

11. Muir JD, Randalls PB, Smith GB, et al: Disposable carbon dioxide detector. *Anesthesia* 1991; 46:323.

12. Rosenberg M, Block CS: A simple, disposable end-tidal carbon dioxide detector. *Anesth Prog* 1991; 38:24–26.

13. Dorsch, JA, Dorsch SE: *Understanding Anesthesia Equipment,* 4th ed. Baltimore: Williams & Wilkins, 1999:711–713.

Chapter 5
OROTRACHEAL INTUBATION

Mark Morocco
Eric F. Reichman

INTRODUCTION

Airway control is the first and most critical action of the Emergency Physician. The "A" in the ABCs demands that no other action may take place until the airway is secure. Endotracheal intubation inserts an artificial airway connecting the respiratory system to the outside world and gives definitive control of the airway. Once the tube is in place, all methods of support can be applied. If the airway is not secure, nothing can help the patient. Endotracheal intubation can be accomplished by a variety of methods. The method of choice will be dictated by physician preference and experience, the patient's condition, and the type of equipment available. The most common method of endotracheal intubation is orotracheal intubation. There are no good alternatives to intubation when oxygenation and ventilation are threatened. All actions should be focused on two objectives: to get the tube in quickly and in the right place. The proper preparation, practice, and personnel can assure that the "nightmare airway" is an extremely rare event.[1]

ANATOMY AND PATHOPHYSIOLOGY

For the purposes of intubation, our discussion of the anatomy starts at the lips and travels inward to end at the right mainstem bronchus. As you approach the patient, visualize the normal structures expected and match them with what is seen. Distortion occurs from edema or trauma. Structures may be hidden by vomit or blood. Since all structures are viewed upside-down, from the position over the head of the patient, the potential for disorientation multiplies.

Begin at the face and move inward (Figures 5-1 and 5-2). The philtrum of the upper lip will be located at the 6 o'clock (bottom) position. Symmetrical swelling, carbon deposits, blistering, or signs of trauma to the lips can indicate that the inner anatomy of the airway may be altered and the intubation more difficult. Moving inward, open the patient's mouth and check the teeth for fractures, size, and the presence of removable dental devices. Large upper incisors and/or limited jaw opening will make endotracheal intubation more difficult. The tongue hangs down from the floor of the lower jaw (mandible) and ends with the tip against the upper (maxillary) incisors (Figure 5-2). Visualize the tongue as a hanging oval of tissue with two "tips" (Figure 5-2). The first is the anterior tip of the tongue proper. The second is the epiglottis. The anatomic "floor" of this view is formed by the hard and soft palates, which end at the palatopharyngeal arch (Figure 5-2). The uvula is located inferiorly and in the midline. The palatoglossal arch and palatopharyngeal arch form twin vertical pillars that lie posterior to the molars of the upper teeth (Figure 5-2). All of these structures are potential sources of obstruction and must be evaluated for swelling, deformity, or trauma. The "back wall" is the posterior wall of the pharynx (Figure 5-2).

At the posterior wall of the pharynx, the airway bends 90 degrees to run parallel to the bed. Visualized from the perspective of the top of the patient's head, the root of the tongue and the lingual tonsils are located at the 12 o'clock position (Figures 5-3 and 5-4). The tongue continues into a blind pocket known as the vallecula. Following the vallecula posteriorly, it is continuous with the epiglottis. The epiglottis hangs with its tip pointing downward. Directly behind and protected by the epiglottis is the entry to the remainder of the airway (Figure 5-4). The esophagus lies at the 6 o'clock position. From the viewpoint of the intubator, the hypopharynx appears like the numeral 8. The top half is the airway and the bottom half the esophagus.

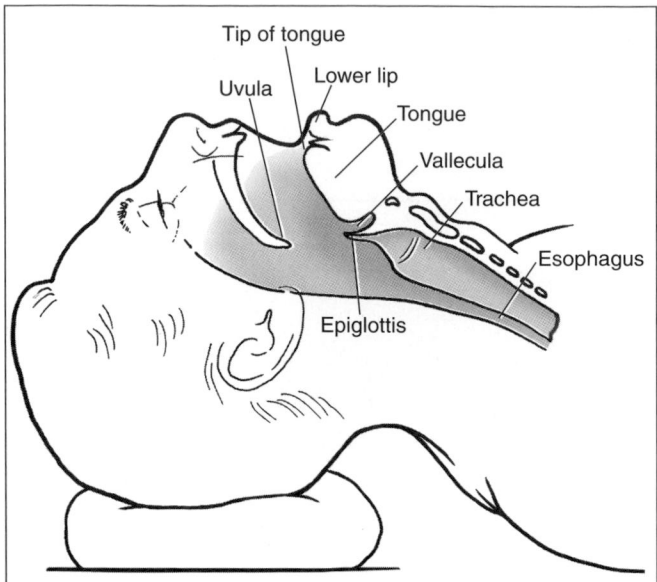

FIGURE 5-1 Schematic representation of the airway.

Under the epiglottis is the larynx (Figure 5-5). The vocal cords are located in the midline and form an "A" shape, with its apex toward the epiglottis. **Identifying the vocal cords is important, since the visualization of the endotracheal tube passing between the cords is proof of a successful endotracheal intubation.** The arytenoid cartilages are paired structures. One lies at the posterior aspect of each vocal cord. The aryepiglottic folds are paired structures that span from the lateral edge of the epiglottis to the arytenoid cartilages. They contain muscles that move the arytenoid cartilages and subsequently open and close the vocal cords. The trachea bifurcates at the carina into the right and left mainstem bronchi. In some patients the tracheal rings are easily visible through the vocal cords.

INDICATIONS

Any threat to oxygenation and/or ventilation is a relative indication for endotracheal intubation. If the threat is simple and easily removed, remove it. **If there is uncertainty that the patient's airway patency, respiratory drive, or oxygenation cannot be maintained without intervention, endotracheal intubation is required.** Time is of the essence. The decision to intubate early can make the difference between a controlled, successful procedure and a chaotic, "crashing" nightmare. Endotracheal intubation can be performed to administer resuscitation medications, ensure a patent airway, deliver oxygen, isolate the airway, reduce the risk of aspiration of gastric or oral contents, suction the trachea, ventilate the patient, and apply positive-pressure ventilation. Other indications include altered mental status,

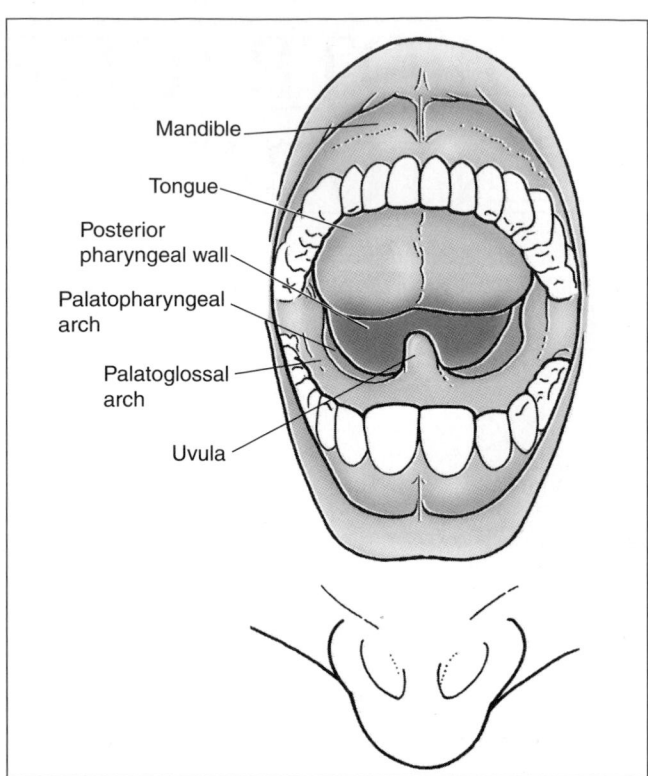

FIGURE 5-2 The oral structures as viewed from above the supine patient's head.

head injury requiring hyperventilation, hypoxemia, hypoventilation, apnea, lack of a gag reflex, and unconsciousness.

CONTRAINDICATIONS

Orotracheal intubation is relatively contraindicated in patients who do not need it, who are likely to be injured by the procedure, or whose injuries make success unlikely. Spontaneous breathing with adequate ventilation and normal mental status may allow less invasive techniques such as continuous positive airway pressure (CPAP) in patients whose medical conditions are likely to respond quickly to interventions, such as cardiogenic pulmonary edema or pneumonitis.[2] Trauma patients, with likely cervical spine injury or anterior neck wounds, as well as severely immobile arthritis patients may be injured by the manipulation required during oral endotracheal intubation.[3] Severe orofacial injuries, bleeding, deep airway obstruction, or gross deformity of the head and neck may make successful intubation impossible. A quickly changing obstruction, such as edema or an expanding hematoma, may require a surgical airway if oral endotracheal intubation is delayed. **Choose a surgical airway if the manipulation or time required for oral endotracheal intubation puts the patient at risk for spinal injury or hypoxia.[4]** Orotracheal intubation

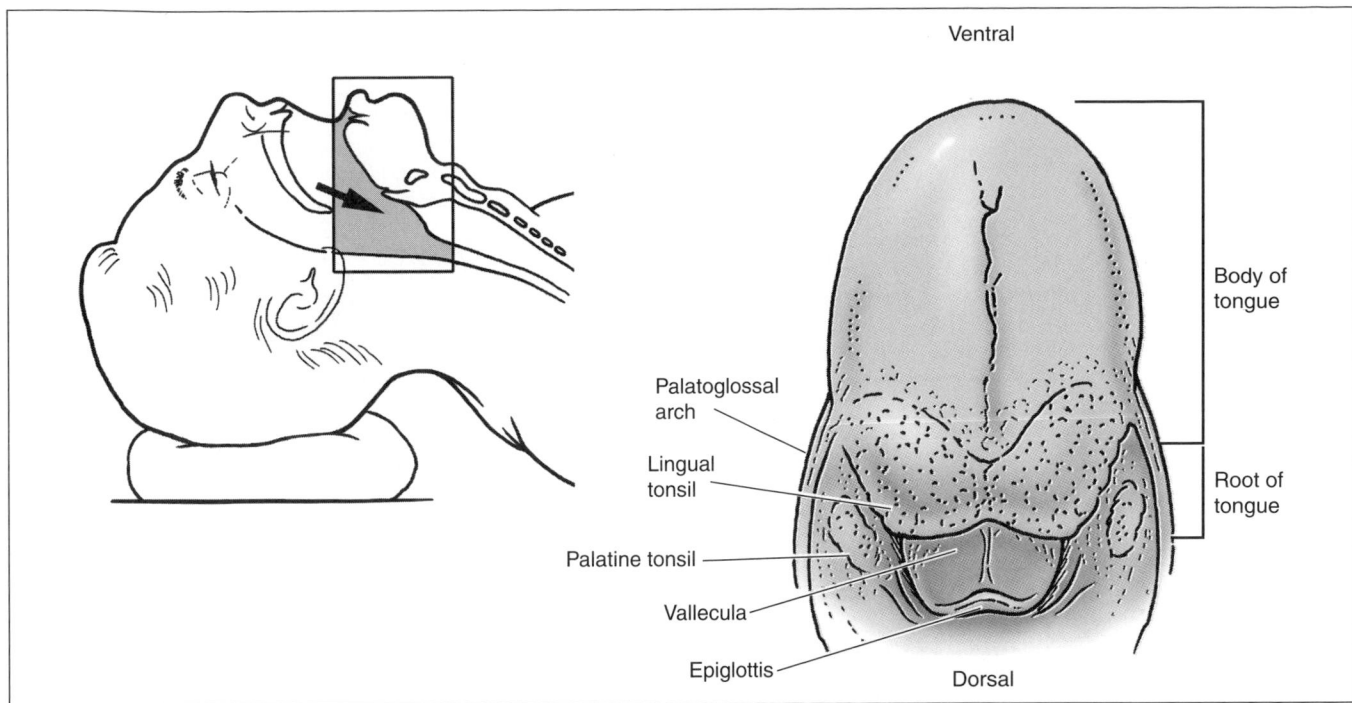

FIGURE 5-3 The tongue and adjacent structures as viewed from above the supine patient's head.

should not be performed by individuals unfamiliar with the equipment and technique.

EQUIPMENT

Endotracheal tubes, various sizes
10 mL syringe
Water-soluble lubricant or anesthetic jelly
Wire stylet, malleable type
Laryngoscope handle
Fresh batteries for the laryngoscope
Laryngoscope blades, various sizes and shapes
Supplemental oxygen with appropriate tubing and connectors
Nonrebreather oxygen masks, various sizes
Wall suction with appropriate tubing
Yankauer suction catheter
Bag-valve device, sizes: infant, child, adult small, adult medium, adult large
Oral airways, sizes: infant, child, adult 3 to 5
Nasal airways, various sizes
Benzoin adhesive
Tape
Pulse oximeter
Cardiac monitor
Automatic sphygmomanometer
End-tidal carbon dioxide (CO_2) monitor/device
Cricothyrotomy backup tray
Crash cart
Resuscitation medicines

Personnel (respiratory technician, medication nurse, in-line stabilization assistant, recorder)
Medications (premedications, induction, anesthetics, paralytics), see Table 5-1

Many institutions make an "intubating/airway kit" (Figure 5-6). It contains a combination of laryngoscope handles, laryngoscope blades, oropharyngeal airways, nasopharyngeal airways, tongue blades, a malleable stylet, various sizes of endotracheal tubes, syringes, tape, and commercially available devices to secure the endotracheal tube.

ENDOTRACHEAL TUBES

The choice of endotracheal tube size will vary based on the patient's age, anatomic anomalies, body habitus, and airway anatomy (Table 5-1). The endotracheal tube is sized based on the internal diameter (ID) measured in millimeters. The size is printed onto the surface of the endotracheal tube for reference. The sizes begin with 2.5 mm and increase in 0.5 mm increments. Some generalities hold true in most patients. Adult males usually require a size 7.5 to 9.0 cuffed endotracheal tube. Adult females usually require a size 7.0 to 8.0 cuffed endotracheal tube. Endotracheal tube selection in children can be made by one of several methods. A Broselow tape will identify the proper size tube. Visually select a tube with an inside diameter that matches the size of the width of the nail of the patient's little finger. If time allows, the following formula may be used to confirm the tube size:

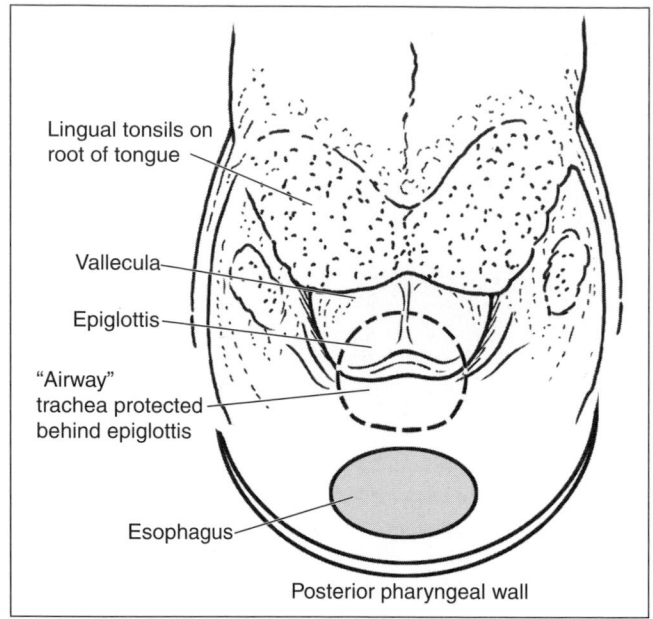

FIGURE 5-4 Structures of the hypopharynx as viewed from above the supine patient's head.

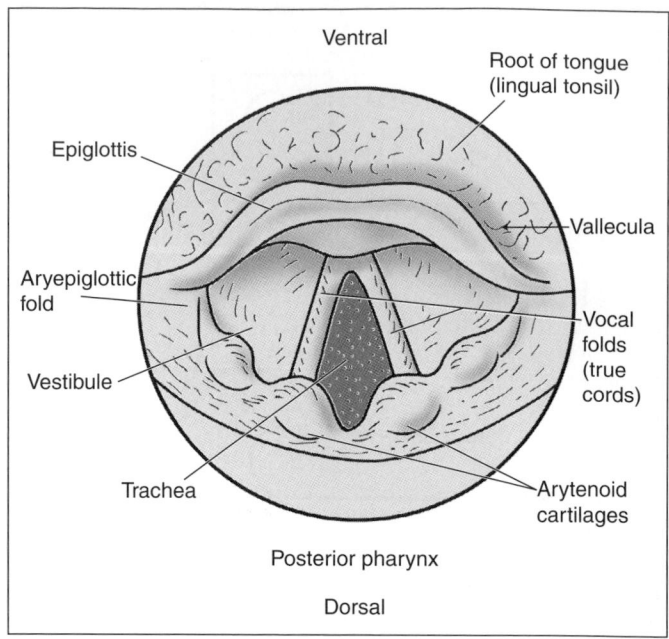

FIGURE 5-5 The structures of the glottis as viewed from above the supine patient's head.

tube size = (4 + child's age in years)/4. An uncuffed endotracheal tube should be used in children under 8 years of age to prevent the complications of subglottic and tracheal stenosis. After determining the proper size endotracheal tube, also select and prepare a tube that is one size smaller in case the airway is smaller than expected.

The endotracheal tube is a clear polyvinyl chloride disposable tube that is open on both ends (Figure 5-7). The proximal end contains a standard size (15 mm) connector that will attach to the bag-valve device, a ventilator, and other sources of positive-pressure ventilation. The distal end is beveled. It has a perforation, located approximately 0.5 to 0.75 cm from the tip and opposite the bevel, known as the Murphy eye. Printed on the tube are the size, a radiopaque line to aid in radiographic visualization, and 1 cm incremental marks beginning at the tip. An inflatable cuff is positioned proximal to the Murphy eye. An inflation port, to inflate the cuff, hangs from the proximal third of the endotracheal tube. A syringe, filled with air, attaches to the inflation port to inflate and deflate the cuff.

The endotracheal tube's cuff is a high-volume, low-pressure balloon. It is designed to accommodate a high volume of air before the intracuff pressure rises. This is

TABLE 5-1. ORAL ENDOTRACHEAL TUBE SIZES AND POSITION BASED ON PATIENT'S AGE

Patient's age	Size* (French)	Internal diameter (mm)	External diameter†(mm)	Distance inserted from lips (cm)
Premature	10	2.5	3.3	10
Full-term/newborn	12	3.0	4.0–4.2	11
1–6 months	14	3.5	4.7–4.8	11
6–12 months	16	4.0	5.3–5.6	12
1–2 years	18	4.5	6.0–6.3	13
3–4 years	20	5.0	6.7–7.0	14
5–6 years	22	5.5	7.3–7.6	15–16
7–8 years	24	6.0	8.0–8.2	16–17
9–10 years	26	6.5	8.7–9.3	17–18
11–13 years	28–30	7.0	9.3–10.0	18–20
Female ≥ 14 years	28–30	7.0	9.3–10.0	20–22
Male ≥ 14 years	32–34	8.0	10.7–11.3	22–24

*Calculated as follows: External diameter (mm) × π.

†Varies by manufacturer.

SOURCE: Modified from Stone and Gal.[6]

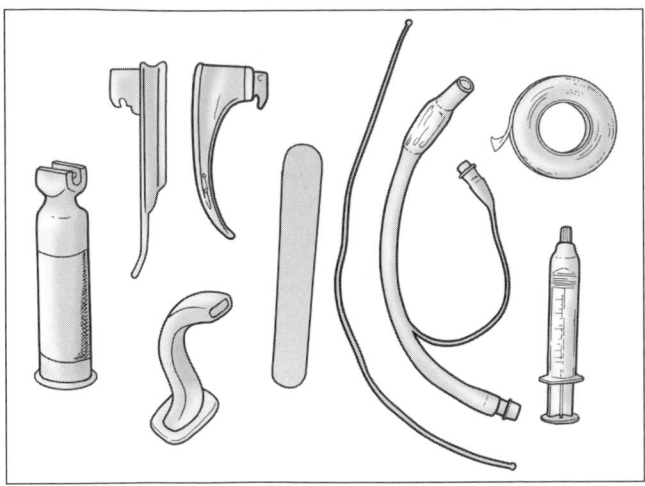

FIGURE 5-6 An airway/intubation kit. It contains the items most commonly needed for orotracheal intubation. *From left to right:* laryngoscope handle, laryngoscope blades, oropharyngeal airways, tongue blade, malleable stylet, endotracheal tubes, tape, and syringe.

an extremely important feature. If the intracuff pressure rises, it is transmitted to the delicate tracheal mucosa where it can cause pressure necrosis and ischemia.

All endotracheal tubes should be examined for defects before use. Attach a 10 mL syringe filled with air to the inflation port. Inject the air to inflate the cuff. The cuff should inflate symmetrically and have no air leak. Deflate the cuff completely. Leave the syringe attached to the inflation port in order to inflate the cuff later on, after the endotracheal tube has been inserted into a patient's airway. If a tube is defective, discard it and open a new endotracheal tube.

LARYNGOSCOPES

The laryngoscope is a handheld device that is used to elevate the tongue and epiglottis to expose the glottis (Figure 5-8). **It is a device that is held in the left hand re-**

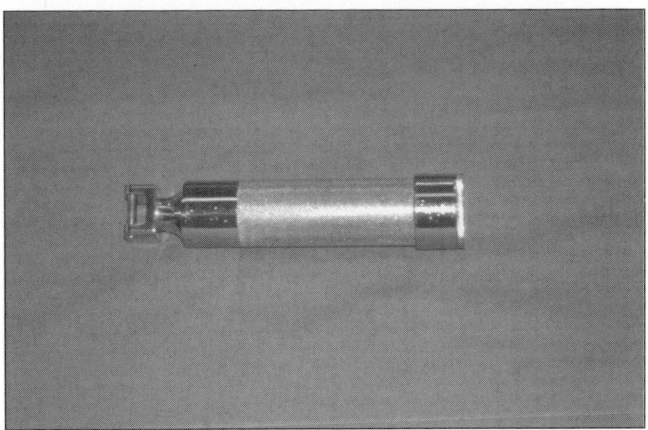

FIGURE 5-8 The laryngoscope handle.

gardless of which hand of the user is dominant. It consists of a handle and a blade. The handle contains the battery for the light source. The distal end of the handle has a fitting where the handle connects to the blade. A transverse bar indicates where the indentation on the proximal blade attaches to the handle.

The laryngoscope blade has a removable bulb attached to its distal third. A fiberoptic bundle within the blade transfers power from the handle to the bulb. The choice of the type and size of laryngoscope blade will vary with physician experience and preference. **The best blade is one that the intubator feels comfortable and confident using.** The curved Macintosh blade is most commonly used (Figure 5-9). It is the easier blade to use for those with little experience with orotracheal intubation. Many feel that it requires less forearm strength to use as compared to the straight blade. The straight Miller blade is often reserved for those experienced with the blade and with orotracheal intubation (Figure 5-10).

The tip of the curved Macintosh blade fits into the vallecula and indirectly lifts the epiglottis to expose the

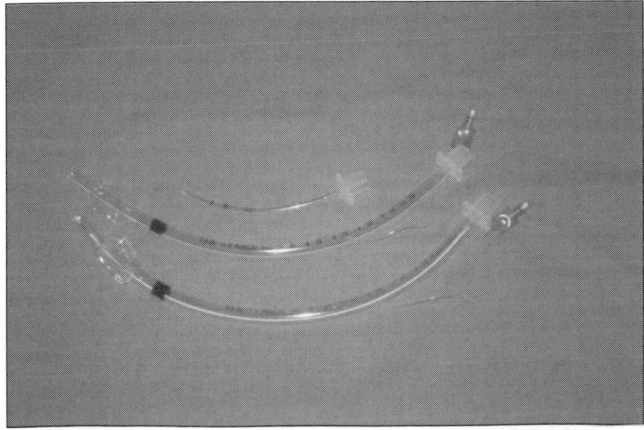

FIGURE 5-7 The endotracheal tube.

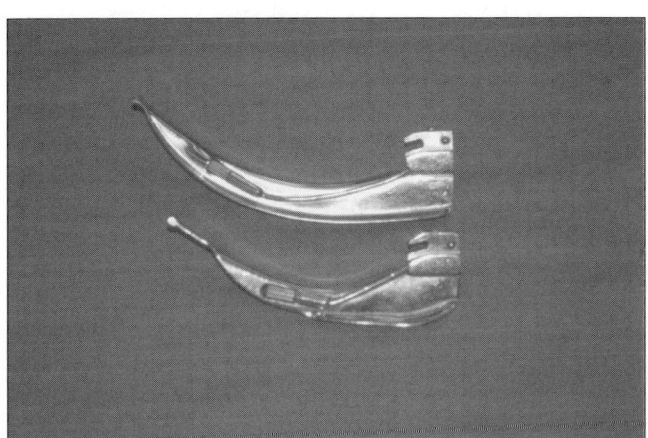

FIGURE 5-9 The Macintosh laryngoscope blade.

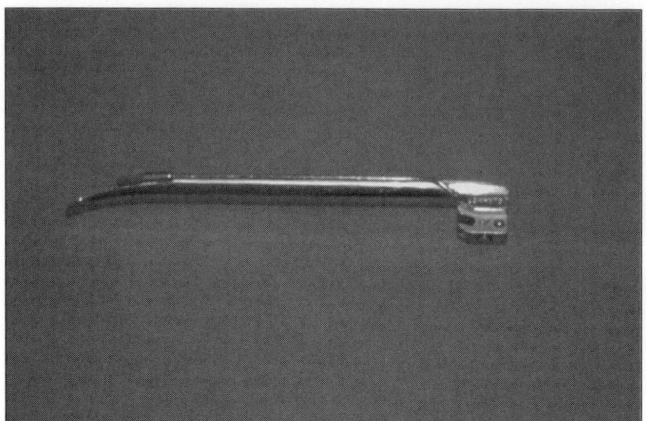

FIGURE 5-10 The Miller laryngoscope blade.

vocal cords (Figure 5-11). A size 2 blade is used for 3- to 6-year-olds. A size 3 blade is used for children starting at about age 6, for women, and for small to average-size males. A size 4 blade is usually reserved for large males.

The tip of the straight Miller blade goes directly under the epiglottis to expose the vocal cords (Figure 5-12). A size 0 to 1.0 blade is used for neonates, infants, and toddlers up to 2 years of age. A size 2 blade is used for children 3 to 6 years of age. A size 3 blade is used for women and average-size males. A size 4 blade is rarely used, and then mainly for large males.

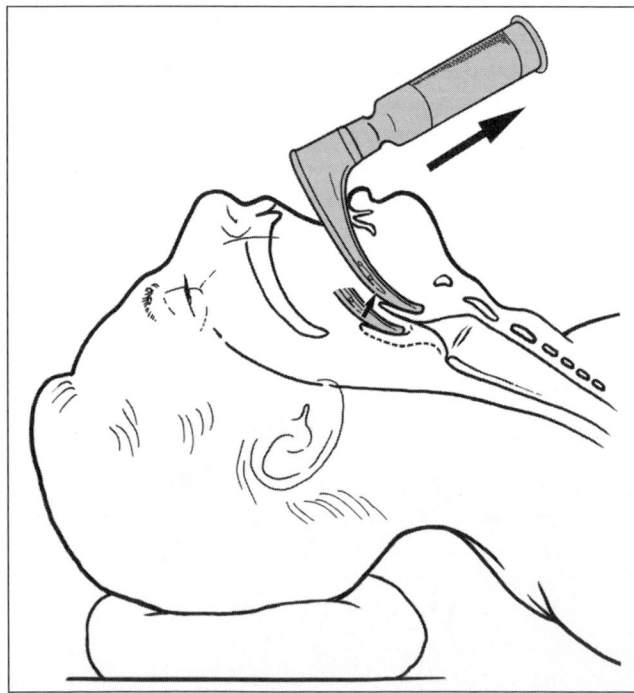

FIGURE 5-11 Use of the Macintosh blade. It is inserted into the vallecula to elevate the mandible, tongue, and epiglottis as a unit.

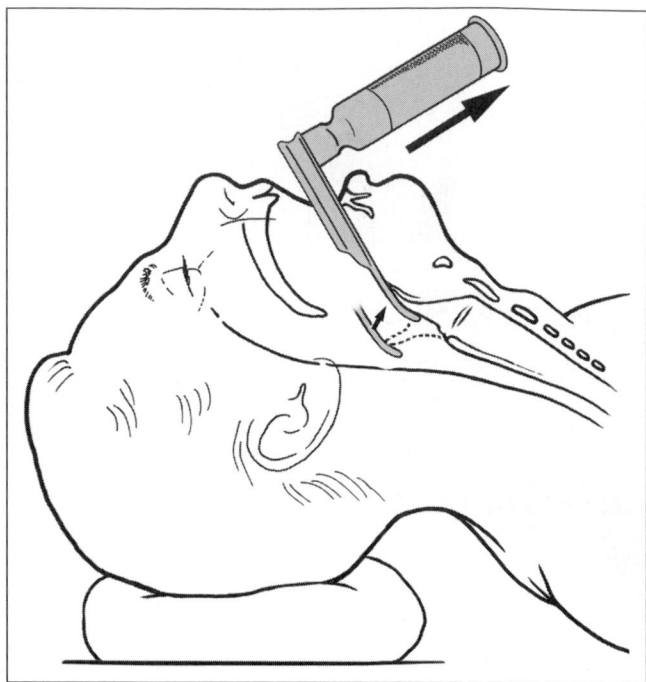

FIGURE 5-12 Use of the Miller blade. It is inserted below the epiglottis to elevate the mandible, tongue, and epiglottis as a unit.

STYLETS

The stylet is a semirigid piece of metal that is bendable (Figure 5-13). It is often plastic-coated. It inserts into the lumen of the endotracheal tube. It should be lubricated with water-soluble lubricant or anesthetic jelly prior to insertion into the endotracheal tube. **The tip of the stylet should be 1 cm proximal to the tip of the endotracheal tube to prevent injury to the patient's airway.** The endotracheal tube, with a stylet, can be bent to maintain a specific shape. This is used to facilitate passage of the endotracheal tube through the vocal cords. It is commonly bent into a "hockey-stick" or "J" shape for most intubations. A greater curvature is often used for intubations when the larynx is "anterior," in difficult intubations, and in "blind" intubations.

PREPARATION

PHYSICIAN

Once the decision to intubate has been made, the physician must use training and experience to begin leading the team toward a successful intubation. Although the process must move quickly, the physician must, by example, ensure a calm and orderly environment. Making the decision to intubate earlier allows the team to follow a shorter and easier time line. The physician must visualize this time line and identify actions and potential problems before they occur. A backup

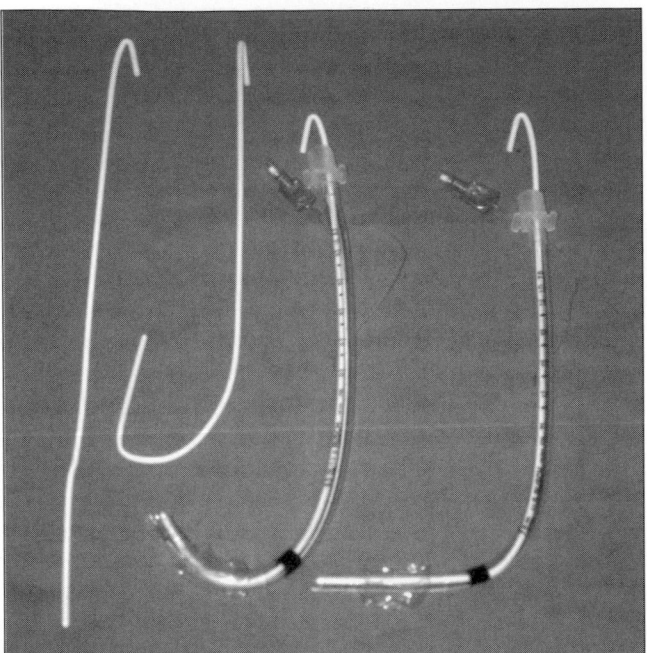

FIGURE 5-13 The intubating stylet. It may be bent into any required shape. When inserted into an endotracheal tube, it will form the endotracheal tube into the desire shape. The most common shapes are the "J" and the "hockey stick."

plan should also be available in case orotracheal intubation is impossible. Any Emergency Department patient about to be intubated is a high priority, so do not be afraid to use resources liberally. Obtain assistants to help as soon as the decision to intubate is made.

PERSONNEL

Shortly before the procedure begins, assemble the entire team near the bed and go over "the game plan" calmly and quickly. All personnel should be gloved, gowned, and masked. Eye protection should be worn by all personnel to protect against splash injury from blood and secretions. **Explicitly identify assistants and assign their roles early.** Give instructions clearly and calmly before the procedure begins. It is helpful to write down medications with doses in the order that they will be given and to review them quickly with the medication nurse. Emphasize that it will be the nurse's job to draw up, label, and administer the medications, followed by a saline flush. Reinforce that during the procedure this will be a particular nurse's only job. The respiratory assistant has three important tasks: helping to ventilate the patient, applying cricoid pressure, and handing the endotracheal tube to the intubator so that visual contact with the vocal cords is not lost. If cervical spine immobilization is needed, a third assistant should be explicitly instructed as to how and when the team leader would like the patient's neck secured.

EQUIPMENT

Check that the room is ready and all equipment is within arm's reach. Turn on the suction and the oxygen. Confirm that both systems work. Attach the suction tip and check to see whether there is a small finger hole in the barrel that must be covered for the suction to work. If so, close it with a piece of tape so that the suction is "always on." This is not a concern if a Yankauer suction catheter is being used. Ensure that the suction tubing is long enough to reach the center of the bed. Place the suction catheter under the mattress to the right of the patient's head and within easy reach. Place the spare suction tip nearby. Set the oxygen flow regulator to 15 L/min. Apply a nonbreather mask to the oxygen and the patient. Place the bag-valve device near the head of the bed and within easy reach. Confirm that the noninvasive blood pressure cuff, cardiac monitor, and pulse oximeter are working and attached to the patient. Confirm that the end-tidal CO_2 monitor is nearby and working. If such a monitor is unavailable, a disposable in-line monitoring device should be available. Ensure that the patient has at least one working intravenous line.

Assemble the intubation equipment. Place the laryngoscope blade on the handle. Open the blade and confirm that the light works. Close the blade into the ready position, flat against the handle, to keep the bulb cool and not drain the batteries. Take the endotracheal tube and the backup smaller one and prepare them. Insert the 10 mL syringe into the inflation port for the endotracheal tube cuff. Inject enough air to inflate the balloon. If there is no leak, deflate the balloon until it is completely flat against the endotracheal tube. **Leave the syringe attached.** Liberally lubricate the stylet. Insert the stylet into the endotracheal tube until its tip is 1 cm proximal to the distal tip of the endotracheal tube. Place a bend in the stylet as it enters the proximal end of the endotracheal tube to keep the stylet from advancing. Bend the stylet/endotracheal tube assembly into a curve roughly approximating a "hockey stick" or "J" (Figure 5-13). Lubricate the tip of the endotracheal tube and the collapsed cuff. Place the assembly back into the endotracheal tube package. Place the endotracheal tubes, laryngoscope, backup laryngoscope handle and blades, oral airways, and tape on a tray within easy reach of the bed. Check the room lighting. Raise the bed to minimize excessive bending and better visualize the patient's airway.

PATIENT PREPARATION

If the patient is competent and awake, explain the procedure, clarify advance directives, and obtain consent. If time permits, a history is especially helpful. The mnemonic AMPLE can help to provide quick information: allergies, medications, past medical history, last meal, and events leading to the current problem.

Confirm again that the appropriate monitoring sources are working and attached to the patient. Confirm adequate intravenous access. Place the patient, with a normal neck, in the "sniffing" position, with the head extended at the atlantooccipital joint while the neck is relatively flexed. A folded towel under the occiput helps to gently raise and tilt the head back into the proper position (Figure 5-14). **Correct positioning is probably the most important preparation of the patient.** Dentures should be left in place temporarily, as they help to stabilize the mouth and prevent occlusion during preoxygenation and bag-valve-mask ventilation.

If the patient is breathing spontaneously, begin preoxygenation for 5 minutes before the procedure (if time permits). Use a well-fitting nonrebreather mask with the oxygen flow regulator set at 15 L/min. This displaces nitrogen from the lungs and gives the patient a physiologic reservoir of oxygen for approximately 5 minutes while apneic. **Remember: 5 minutes of preoxygenation provides 5 minutes of protection.**[5] If bag-valve-mask ventilation is required, have an assistant apply posteriorly directed cricoid pressure to minimize gastric distention and decrease the chance of vomiting and aspiration. Have assistants ready to turn the patient onto his or her left side to minimize the risk of aspiration if vomiting occurs. Monitor the pulse oximeter to assure good oxygenation and ventilation. It should rise to the high 90s and remain there. If not, check the O_2 circuit from the wall to the patient and confirm that spontaneous breathing is still occurring.

TECHNIQUE

The evaluation and preparation for orotracheal intubation are complex and essential. If done well, the intubation will hopefully be quick and anticlimactic. Position the respiratory assistant to the right side near the patient's head. The intubator should stand at the head of the bed. Adjust the bed to place the mattress level with the intubator's umbilicus. Pull the bed away from the wall at least 2 feet and clear a "maneuvering space" of tubes, lines, and equipment to prevent distractions. If in-line cervical immobilization is needed, the assistant should stand at the intubator's left hip, ready to remove the collar and hold the neck in position.

Grasp the laryngoscope with the left hand. **It is a left-handed instrument regardless of the handedness of the intubator.** Pull it open and lock the blade onto the handle. Confirm that the light is functioning. The tip of the laryngoscope blade should be pointed toward the patient's chin. Pass the prepared endotracheal tube and suction catheter to the respiratory assistant, who will place them into the right hand when asked. This allows the intubator to keep visual contact with the patient's airway during the procedure.

Induction of anesthesia is the final preparation for orotracheal intubation. The choice of drug sequence is based on the physician's experience and the patient's condition (Table 5-2). A typical sequence begins with a defasciculating dose of a nondepolarizing neuromuscular blocking drug. After 2 to 3 minutes, induce anesthesia with a sedative followed immediately by a paralytic agent (i.e., succinylcholine). Apply cricoid pressure. Once the patient's muscles are relaxed, perform the intubation as described below. Refer to Chapters 3 and 4 regarding the complete details of rapid sequence induction and the pharmacology of the induction agents. **Some patients, especially the old and sick, may stop breathing earlier than anticipated. Be prepared to intubate before the expected time of drug onset.**

Observe the patient's chest. Watch it rise. When it stops, note the time. Place your right thumb on the patient's jaw. Gently pull down the lower lip and open the mouth. Reinspect the oral cavity. Remove any dentures or foreign bodies. Compare what you see with what you expect to see. Fix any problems as you go further into the airway. If blood or vomit is seen, ask for the suction catheter. **Apply the suction catheter without removing your gaze from the patient's airway.** When done suctioning, hold the suction catheter up for the assistant to take.

Firmly grasp the laryngoscope in the left hand (Figure 5-14A). Insert the tip of the laryngoscope blade into the right side of the patient's mouth. Smoothly advance the blade inward while keeping pressure against the tongue. Use the blade to trap and push the tongue to the left as the blade is simultaneously moved to the midline, "clearing a path" for your gaze. Keep the left wrist firm. **Use the forearm, wrist, and hand as a single unit and avoid bending or flexing the wrist. It is essential to move the patient's tongue up and to the left.** The tongue will protect the mandibular teeth from being injured by the laryngoscope blade. It allows the laryngoscope blade to be moved away from the maxillary teeth. It also opens a path to visualize the patient's airway.

When the blade has been inserted all the way, lift the patient's airway up and forward exactly along the long axis of the laryngoscope handle, which should be aimed toward a point directly above the patient's chin (Figures 5-11, 5-12, and 5-14B). **Do not "cock" or "crank back" on the laryngoscope handle with your wrist, or the back of the laryngoscope blade may break the incisors.** The epiglottis should be seen at the base of the tongue.

INTUBATING WITH THE (CURVED) MACINTOSH BLADE

Advance the tip of the laryngoscope blade into the vallecula—the space between the base of the tongue

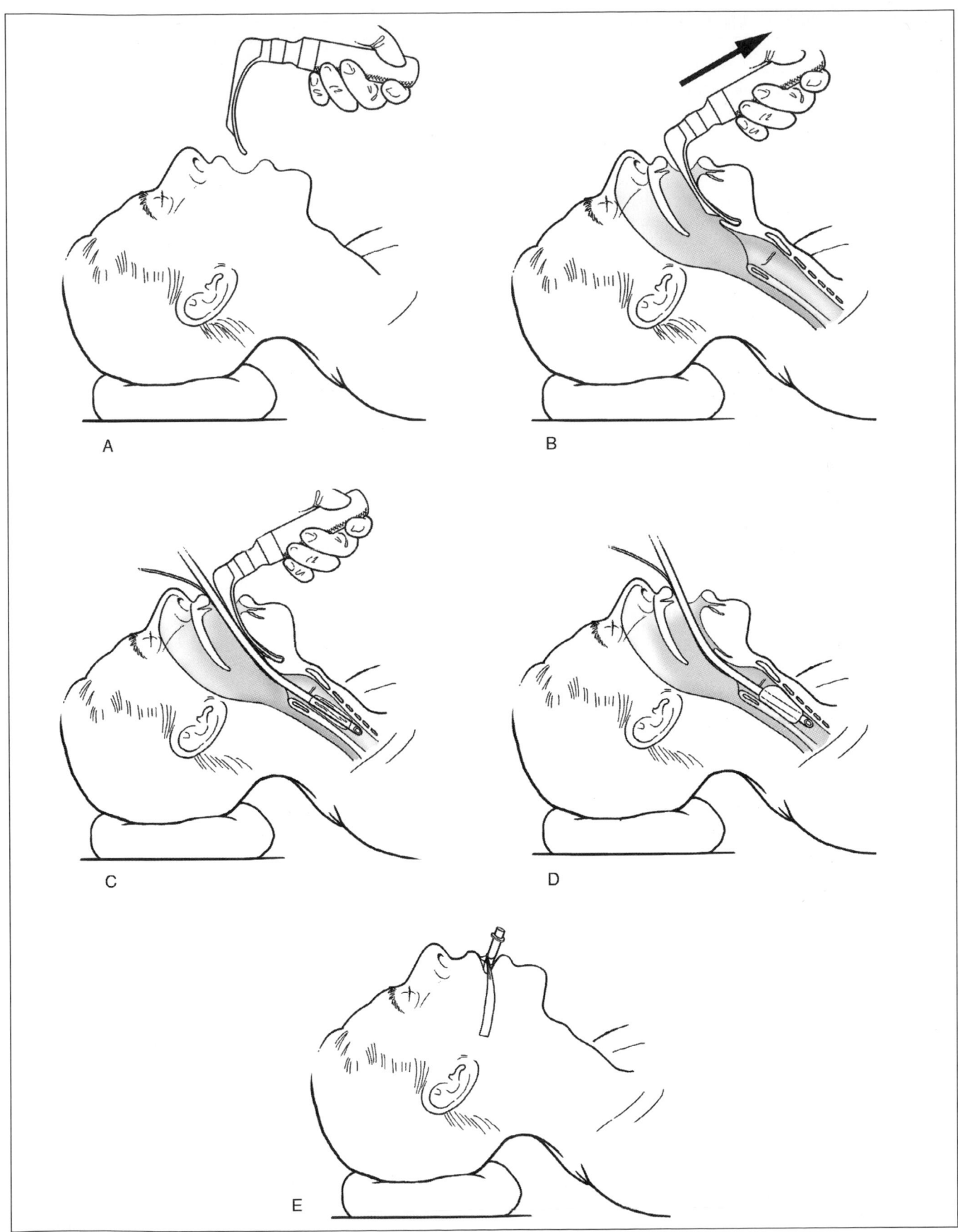

FIGURE 5-14 Orotracheal intubation. *A.* Proper positioning of the laryngoscope blade above the patient's mouth. *B.* The blade is inserted into the vallecula. The handle is lifted anteriorly and inferiorly to elevate the mandible, tongue, and epiglottis (*arrow*). The glottis will be visible. *C.* The endotracheal tube is inserted into the trachea until the cuff is below the vocal cords. *D.* The laryngoscope has been removed and the cuff inflated. *E.* The endotracheal tube is secured.

TABLE 5-2. RAPID SEQUENCE INDUCTION MEDICATIONS FOR SPECIFIC PATIENT PROFILES

Patient type	Premedication*	Induction and paralysis†
"Normal adult"	Vecuronium (0.01 mg/kg)	Etomidate (0.3 mg/kg) or propofol (1– 2.5 mg/kg) or thiopental (3 mg/kg) and succinylcholine (2 mg/kg)
"Normal child"	Vecuronium (0.01 mg/kg) and atropine (0.02 mg/kg, min dose 0.1 mg)	Thiopental (5 mg/kg) and succinylcholine (2 mg/kg)
Asthma, adult	Lidocaine (1.5 mg/kg) and atropine (0.5 mg)	Ketamine (1–2 mg/kg) and succinylcholine (2 mg/kg)
Asthma, child	Lidocaine (1.5 mg/kg) and atropine (0.02 mg, min 0.1 mg)	Ketamine (1–2 mg/kg) and succinylcholine (2 mg/kg)
Head injury, adult	Vecuronium (0.01 mg/kg) and lidocaine (1.5 mg/kg) and fentanyl (3–5 μg/kg)	Etomidate (0.3 mg/kg) and succinylcholine (2 mg/kg)
Head injury, child	Vecuronium (0.01 mg/kg) and atropine (0.02 mg/kg, min 0.1 mg) and lidocaine (1.5 mg/kg) and fentanyl (3–5 μg/kg)	Thiopental (5 mg/kg) and succinylcholine (2 mg/kg)
Head injury, adult, hypotensive	Vecuronium (0.01 mg/kg) and fentanyl (3 μg/kg) and lidocaine (1.5 mg/kg)	Etomidate (0.2 mg/kg) and succinylcholine (1.5 mg/kg)
Head injury, child, hypotensive	Vecuronium (0.01 mg/kg) and atropine (0.02 mg/kg, min 0.1 mg) and lidocaine (1.5 mg/kg) and fentanyl (2–3 μg/kg)	Midazolam (0.15 mg/kg) or etomidate (0.3 mg/kg) and succinylcholine (2 mg/kg)
Hyperkalemia or renal failure, adult	None	Etomidate (0.3 mg/kg) or propofol (1.0–2.5 mg/kg) or thiopental (3 mg/kg) and rocuronium (0.6 mg/kg) or vecuronium (0.01 mg/kg)
Hyperkalemia or renal failure, child	None	Thiopental (5 mg/kg) and rocuronium (0.6 mg/kg) or vecuronium (0.01 mg/kg)
Status epilepticus, adult	None	Thiopental (3 mg/kg) and succinylcholine (2 mg/kg)
Status epilepticus, child	None	Thiopental (5 mg/kg) and succinylcholine (2 mg/kg)
Pregnancy	Atropine (0.5 mg)	Ketamine (1–2 mg/kg) and rocuronium (0.6 mg/kg) or vecuronium (0.01 mg/kg)

*Given 3 min before intubating (T−3).

†Given simultaneously at the beginning of intubation (T=0) and wait for 45 to 60 seconds for onset of paralysis.

and the body of the epiglottis (Figures 5-11 and 5-14*B*). Lift the laryngoscope handle to raise the tongue, jaw, and epiglottis as a unit (Figure 5-11). Observe carefully as the epiglottis pivots upward and uncovers the glottis (Figure 5-5). The amount of upward/forward force needed to lift the airway structures can be surprisingly large. The vocal cords should be visualized. The application of cricoid pressure by pressing the cricoid cartilage back, upward, rightward, and posteriorly (in this sequence) can help bring the vocal cords into view when the intubator cannot apply more lifting force due to lack of strength or reluctance to lift the airway, as in suspected neck injury. **This is known as the BURP maneuver.**

INTUBATING WITH THE (STRAIGHT) MILLER BLADE

Insert the laryngoscope blade completely. If the epiglottis is seen, insert the tip directly under and slightly beyond it. Lift the epiglottis and airway as above by raising your hand along the long axis of the laryngoscope handle toward a point above the patient's chin (Figure 5-12). **If neither the epiglottis nor the vocal cords are seen, the tip of the laryngoscope blade is in the esophagus.** Locate the airway by lifting as above while slowly withdrawing the laryngoscope blade. As the

tip slides back, it will "catch" the epiglottis and the airway should "fall down" into view. The BURP maneuver may now be applied if necessary. Some physicians use a variation of this to localize the epiglottis by inserting the blade deeply and lifting, then withdrawing while feeling for the "give" as the epiglottis tip falls off of the retreating blade, and then readvancing a small distance to "scoop up" the epiglottis, exposing the airway.

When the vocal cords are visualized, ask the assistant to pass the endotracheal tube into your right hand. This allows you to keep a "visual lock" on the vocal cords. Insert the endotracheal tube into the right side of the patient's mouth. Advance the endotracheal tube so that the tip reaches the vocal cords without letting the body of the tube block the view. Continue to advance the endotracheal tube through the vocal cords until the cuff passes through them and into the trachea (Figure 5-14*C*). Advance the tube an additional 2 to 3 cm. **The tip and cuff of the endotracheal tube must be visualized passing through the vocal cords to assure placement in the trachea.**

The fit of the endotracheal tube through the vocal cords always seems to be tight, even in larger patients. A well-lubricated tip with the cuff completely collapsed is essential. Rolling the tube gently between the thumb and index finger at the moment of insertion can also help pilot the tip between the vocal cords. If the endotracheal tube is too large or the vocal cord opening narrow, ask the assistant to pass the smaller tube, which has already been prepared.

Once the endotracheal tube has been inserted, the intubator's right hand must hold the tube in place continuously until it is properly taped and secured. The assistant should inflate the endotracheal tube cuff with the attached 10 mL syringe of air (Figure 5-14*D*) and then remove the syringe and stylet. **The intubator must hold the endotracheal tube firmly to make sure that it does not become dislodged.** The assistant should attach the end-tidal CO_2 monitor and the bag-valve device to the endotracheal tube. If symmetrical lung sounds are heard on auscultation and if pulse oximetry and CO_2 monitoring appear appropriate, secure the endotracheal tube in position in the right corner of the patient's mouth (Figure 5-14*E*).

ASSESSMENT

In the Emergency Department, simple common-sense methods will quickly and accurately assess endotracheal tube placement. **The assessment must be made quickly!** An endotracheal tube in the wrong place, the esophagus, is as quickly dangerous as a properly placed one is lifesaving. Was the endotracheal tube visualized passing through the "A frame" of the vocal cords? **This is the most important assessment.** If it was directly visualized being placed and continuously held in place, it is properly positioned. Is the pulse oximeter reading in the high 90s and steady or rising? Is the CO_2 monitoring appropriate? Be familiar with the monitor in your institution. Electronic monitors will show a respiratory waveform and a numerical value. In-line monitors connected between the endotracheal tube and the respiratory circuit will change color with inspiration and expiration to indicate the flow of CO_2 passed the device.

Evaluate the patient. Symmetrical upper chest rise without increasing abdominal size suggests proper placement. Persistent "fogging" or condensation inside the endotracheal tube with each breath for at least six ventilations will also confirm proper placement. Auscultate lateral to the nipples for strong and symmetrical breath sounds during positive-pressure breaths. Avoid auscultating in the midline, where "normal" breath sounds can be heard from a misplaced endotracheal tube in the esophagus. Auscultate at the lateral apices and bases of the lungs. Auscultate over the epigastrium. Correct placement will give strong, symmetrical sounds except in the epigastrum. If epigastric sounds are strongest or "gurgling" or vocalization is heard, assume

incorrect endotracheal tube placement. Breath sounds that are asymmetrical and stronger on the right indicate a right mainstem intubation. Deflate the cuff and gently withdraw the endotracheal tube in 1 cm increments while auscultating. Continue to withdraw the endotracheal tube until equal breath sounds are heard. Secure the tube and reinflate the cuff.

Obtain a chest radiograph after clinically confirming the placement of the endotracheal tube. The tip of the radioopaque stripe of the endotracheal tube should be over the third or fourth thoracic vertebra and 3 to 4 cm above the carina of the trachea. Always inspect the radiograph for any signs of a pneumomediastinum, pneumothorax, or hemothorax.

Clinical assessment of the endotracheal tube's position should take less than 15 seconds. If you are unsure of the endotracheal tube's position, leave the first tube in place while applying cricoid pressure. If the patient's pulse oximetry is in the mid- to high 90s, the endotracheal tube can be removed and intubation reattempted. If the pulse oximetry is low, remove the endotracheal tube and ventilate the patient with a bag-valve-mask device for 30 to 60 seconds to allow the pulse oximetry to rise into the high 90s before making a second attempt at intubation. **Do not ventilate the patient by bag-valve-mask without the application of cricoid pressure. The stomach will inflate with air and increase the risk of aspiration.** Some physicians prefer to leave the misplaced endotracheal tube in place. Leaving the first tube might seem to complicate subsequent attempts but can serve to vent gastric vomit out of the oropharynx as well as to locate the esophageal entrance during the next attempt at direct visualization of the airway.

As long as ventilation is possible with the bag-valve-mask device and pulse oximetry can be maintained above 92% ($Po_2 = 60$ mmHg), two or three attempts can be made at orotracheal intubation. If 30 seconds elapse or pulse oximetry falls to 92%, stop the intubation attempt and ventilate the patient for 30 to 60 seconds, as above. In training programs, the third attempt should be made by the most skilled person available. Three failed attempts define a "failed airway" and call for rescue intubation by an alternative method. **Any patient in whom bag-valve-mask ventilation becomes impossible must be given a surgical airway.**

COMPLICATIONS

Hypoxia is the most destructive complication. It often results from prolonged intubation attempts, with or without proper preoxygenation, and unrecognized misplaced endotracheal tubes. Without adequate oxygenation, irreversible brain injury begins to occur within 2 to 3 minutes. Hypoxia can also cause cardiac arrhythmias.

An unrecognized esophageal intubation will result in significant morbidity and mortality. After intubation, the proper endotracheal tube placement should be confirmed by auscultation, chest rise, fogging in the endotracheal tube, end-tidal CO_2 monitoring, and chest radiography. **Any manipulation or movement of the endotracheal tube or the patient's upper body (head, neck, and torso) should be followed by an assessment of the endotracheal tube's position. It can easily become dislodged and migrate into the hypopharynx and esophagus.** Other methods to confirm endotracheal tube placement include inserting a fiberoptic bronchoscope through the tube and visualizing the tracheal rings and carina (Chapter 10) or inserting a lighted stylet and following the illumination into the trachea (Chapter 8).

Bradycardia can be produced by pharyngeal manipulation. It may be especially pronounced in children because of their higher vagal tone. Pretreatment with atropine (0.02 mg/kg with a minimum dose of 0.15 mg) in children under 6 years of age can avoid this. It will also serve to decrease airway secretions.

Increased intracranial pressure can occur as a result of the direct laryngoscopy. The exact cause of this transient rise is unknown. Lidocaine has been postulated as being of benefit in blunting this but is so far unproven. A dose of 1.5 to 2.0 mg/kg IV may be used as a premedication if time allows and the patient's condition warrants its use.

Direct mechanical complications from the laryngoscope include lacerations of the lips, trauma to the pharyngeal wall, broken teeth, or dentures that may be aspirated and require later removal. Vomiting can cause subsequent chemical and bacterial pneumonitis. Pneumothorax is a rarely seen complication of laryngoscopy. It is more often associated with positive-pressure ventilation. It may also cause apnea, bronchospasm, and/or laryngospasm due to prolonged stimulation of the pharynx.

Laryngospasm may result from insertion of the laryngoscope blade or attempts to advance the endotracheal tube through the vocal cords. This occurs more often in patients who are awake, semiconscious, not paralyzed, and not anesthetized. It may be prevented by the application of nebulized lidocaine, topical anesthetic spray, transtracheal injection of lidocaine, or laryngeal nerve blocks. If laryngospasm occurs during intubation, remove the laryngoscope and begin positive-pressure ventilation. **Positive-pressure ventilation will often overcome the laryngospasm. If not, consider paralyzing the patient immediately with succinylcholine or performing a surgical airway.**

A "leak" of air out the patient's mouth or nose during ventilation signifies a mechanical problem with the endotracheal tube. If the cuff is damaged, the endotracheal tube must be removed and replaced. Check the position of the endotracheal tube by direct laryngoscopy. If the cuff is located between or above the vocal cords, it will not secure the airway properly. Deflate the cuff, advance it through the vocal cords, and reinflate the cuff. If the cuff slowly deflates, there may be a leak in the inflation port. Reinflate the cuff and apply a hemostat to the tubing attached to the inflation port or attach a closed stopcock to the inflation port.

The risk of aspiration increases in patients with difficult airways or full stomachs. This includes obese and pregnant patients. The use of an awake endotracheal intubation or rapid sequence induction will minimize the risk of aspiration. **A properly placed endotracheal tube with the cuff inflated will decrease, but not totally eliminate, the risk of aspiration.**

SUMMARY

Orotracheal intubation is both common and lifesaving. It is the primary and preferred method of airway management. Every Emergency Physician must master this skill. With proper preparation, definitive control of the airway can be obtained. This assures that patients can be oxygenated and ventilated when they cannot do this on their own. Good team leadership skills are nearly as important as physical dexterity and assure an orderly and quick procedure. Rapid patient assessment is important to prevent complications. If orotracheal intubation is unsuccessful, another form of intubation or a surgical airway should be performed.

REFERENCES

1. Sakles JC, Laurin EG: Airway management in the emergency department: a one-year study of 610 tracheal intubations. *Ann Emerg Med* 1998; 31:325–332.
2. Falk JL, O'Brien JF, Shesser R: Heart failure, in Rosen P, Barkin R, Danzl DF, et al (eds): *Emergency Medicine: Concepts and Clinical Practice,* 4th ed. St. Louis: Mosby–Year Book, 1998:1645–1646.
3. Thierbach AR: Airway management in trauma patients. *Anesth Clin North Am* 1999; 17(1):70–71.
4. Walls RM: Management of the difficult airway in the trauma patient. *Emerg Med Clin North Am* 1998; 16(1):47–55.
5. Gerardi MJ, Sacchetti AD, Cantor RM, et al: Rapid sequence intubation of the pediatric patient. *Ann Emerg Med* 1996; 28:58–59.
6. Stone DJ, Gal TJ: Airway management, in Miller RD (ed): *Anesthesia,* vol 2. New York: Churchill Livingstone, 1990:1265–1292.

Chapter 6
DIGITAL (TACTILE) OROTRACHEAL INTUBATION

O. John Ma
Mark E. Hoffmann

INTRODUCTION

For patients who require orotracheal intubation, digital (tactile) intubation is an alternative airway technique. This procedure involves using the index and middle fingers as a guide to blindly place the endotracheal tube into the larynx. Digital tracheal intubation has been demonstrated to be a safe, simple, and rapid method.[1] It should be considered as a secondary method of intubation when other methods prove difficult or impossible.[1] It is particularly suited for prehospital and aeromedical use, where equipment and alternate intubation techniques are limited or unavailable. One study demonstrated an 88 percent success rate among paramedics who intubated with this technique.[2]

ANATOMY AND PATHOPHYSIOLOGY

For this procedure, the only two significant anatomic structures that the intubator will encounter are the tongue and the epiglottis. The epiglottis is the cartilaginous structure that is located at the root of the tongue and serves as a valve over the superior aperture of the larynx during the act of swallowing.[3]

INDICATIONS

Digital orotracheal intubation is an ideal alternative technique for intubating the comatose or chemically paralyzed patient when other more conventional methods for intubation have failed. In particular, this procedure is useful when oral secretions or blood inhibit the direct visualization of the upper airway.[1] Since this technique involves minimal movement of the head and neck, it may be a suitable method for intubating patients with known or suspected cervical spine injuries. Digital intubation may be a useful procedure for paramedics and aeromedical personnel in the out-of-hospital setting, when trapped patients require intubation but are not in a position for more conventional methods.[2] It is an alternative technique for out-of-hospital intubation where other techniques and equipment are unavailable or limited. This procedure also has been performed successfully in intubating neonates.[4]

CONTRAINDICATIONS

There are no absolute contraindications to digital intubation. The main danger of this procedure is to the health care worker performing the intubation, who is at risk for having his or her fingers bitten by the patient. **This technique should not be performed on any patient who is awake or semiconscious. It should be performed only on patients who are paralyzed or unconscious.** A relative contraindication would be performing this procedure on a patient with multiple fractured teeth that may abrade or cut the intubator's fingers.

EQUIPMENT

Endotracheal tubes, various sizes
Wire stylet, malleable (optional)
10 mL syringe
Water-soluble lubricant or anesthetic jelly
Bag-valve device
Oxygen source and tubing
Gauze, 4×4 squares

PATIENT PREPARATION

Endotracheal intubation in the Emergency Department is commonly performed on an emergent or urgent basis. If there is time, the risks, benefits, and complications of the procedure should be explained to the patient and/or the patient's representative.

The use of gloves, a bite block, and gauze over the teeth as guards are recommended when performing this procedure. The patient should be lying supine. If the patient has sustained a concerning mechanism of injury, the cervical spine should be immobilized. An assistant can help hold the patient's head to maintain in-line immobilization. The patient should be placed on continuous cardiac monitoring, pulse oximetry, and supplemental oxygen.

TECHNIQUE

Prepare the endotracheal tube. Attach a 10-mL syringe to the cuff's inflation port. Inflate the cuff and inspect it for any air leaks. Deflate the cuff and leave the syringe attached to the inflation port. The use of a stylet is optional. It may be used if the patient's larynx is anterior, the intubator has short fingers, or it is the physician's preference. Lubricate and insert the stylet until it is 1 cm proximal to the distal end of the endotracheal tube. Bend the malleable stylet just as it enters the endotracheal tube. This will prevent it from migrating distally and injuring the patient. Gently bend the distal end of the endotracheal tube into a "J." Liberally lubricate the distal end of the endotracheal tube. Induce anesthesia (Chapters 3 and 4) if the patient is conscious.

The intubator should stand at the patient's right side and be facing the patient. Insert the right index and middle fingers into the right angle of the patient's mouth (Figure 6-1). Slide the fingers along the surface of the tongue until the epiglottis is palpated. The metacarpophalangeal joints of the index and middle fingers will usually be at the level of the patient's incisors. The tip of the epiglottis is approximately 8 to 10 cm from the incisors. Elevate the epiglottis with the index finger (Figure 6-2).

Insert the endotracheal tube into the patient's mouth and between the two fingers (Figure 6-2). Alternatively, the endotracheal tube can be advanced between the two fingers and the tongue. Advance the tip of the endotracheal tube into the trachea (Figure 6-2). Have an assistant withdraw the stylet if one was used. Advance the endotracheal tube 3 to 4 cm with the left hand.[1,5] While securely holding the endotracheal tube with the left hand, gently withdraw the right hand. Inflate the cuff. Begin ventilating the patient.

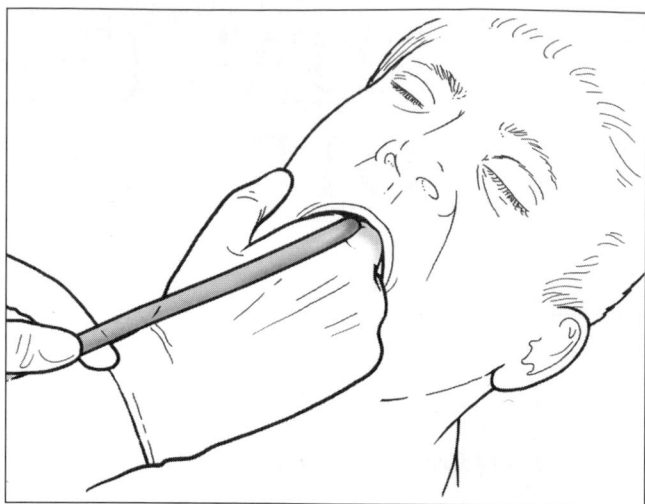

FIGURE 6-1 The index and middle fingers are placed in the right side of the patient's mouth and advanced until the epiglottis is palpated.

ASSESSMENT

The placement of an endotracheal tube should be followed by an assessment to ensure its proper positioning. This includes visual inspection of chest rise and lack of abdominal movement with ventilation, fogging in the endotracheal tube for at least six breaths, auscultation, and end-tidal CO_2 monitoring. This should be followed by a chest radiograph.

AFTERCARE

The steps of ensuring proper placement of the endotracheal tube and securing the tube are the same as for any patient who has undergone orotracheal intubation (Chapter 5).

COMPLICATIONS

No significant complications to the patient have been identified with digital intubation. One study involving a small number of cadavers found that digital intubation predisposes to left mainstem intubation. The investigators concluded that decreased right-sided breath sounds after tactile intubation may represent an easily corrected left mainstem intubation rather than other pathology.[6] An awake or semiconscious patient may gag, with subsequent vomiting and aspiration and injury to the intubator's fingers. The possibility of esophageal intubation is significant, especially if the intubator has small fingers or the airway is anterior.

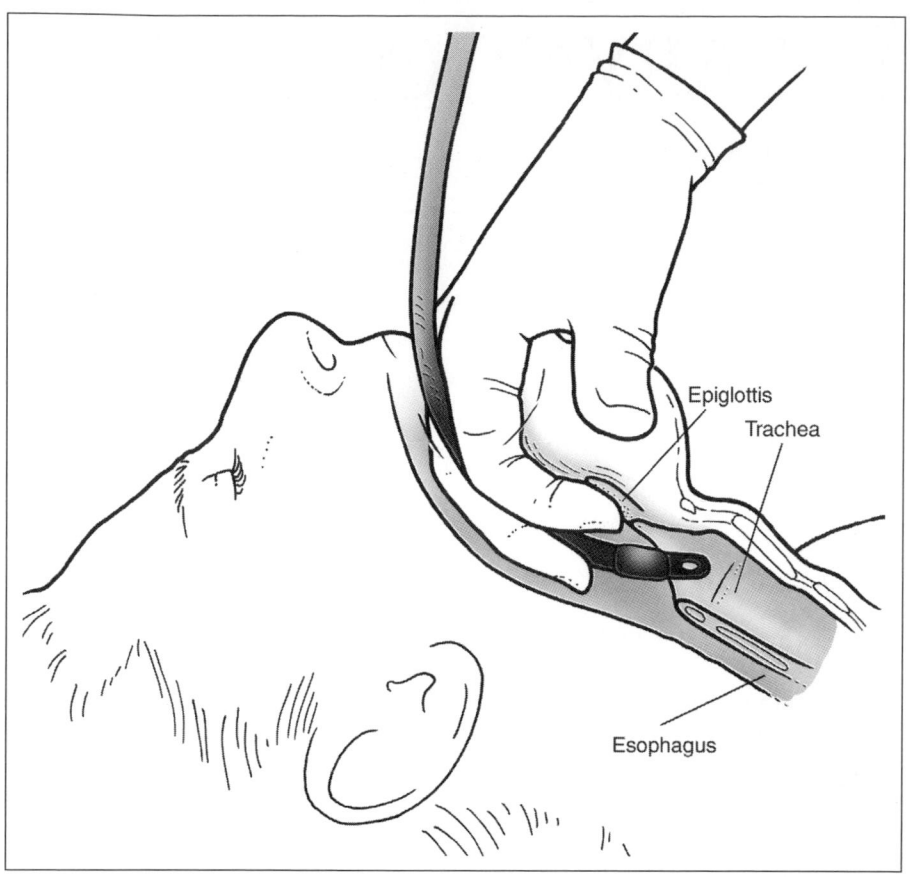

Epiglottis

Trachea

Esophagus

FIGURE 6-2 Advancing the endotracheal tube. The epiglottis is elevated with the index finger. The endotracheal tube is advanced between the fingers and into the larynx.

SUMMARY

Digital (tactile) intubation remains a viable alternative technique for management of the airway; every practitioner of Emergency Medicine should become familiar with it. It is a rapid and safe method to intubate a patient. It is an ideal method for intubating a comatose or paralyzed patient if the upper airway cannot be visualized because of secretions or blood. Digital intubation should also be considered when intubating the patient with a known or suspected cervical spine fracture, since this technique requires minimal head and neck movement. It is also a viable method for out-of-hospital intubation.

REFERENCES

1. Stewart RD: Tactile orotracheal intubation. *Ann Emerg Med* 1984; 13:175–178.
2. Hardwick WC, Bluhm D: Digital intubation. *J Emerg Med* 1984; 1:317–320.
3. Snell RS, Smith MS: *Clinical Anatomy for Emergency Medicine.* St. Louis: Mosby, 1993.
4. Hancock PJ, Peterson G: Finger intubation of the trachea in newborns. *Pediatrics* 1992; 89:325–326.
5. Cook RT: Digital endotracheal intubation. *Am J Emerg Med* 1992; 10:396.
6. White SJ: Left mainstem intubation with digital intubation technique: an unrecognized risk. *Am J Emerg Med* 1994; 12:466–468.

Chapter 7
BULLARD LARYNGOSCOPE INTUBATION

Peter T. Schubel
Eric F. Reichman

INTRODUCTION

The Bullard laryngoscope (CIRCON ACMI, Stamford, CT) was designed by Dr. Roger Bullard; former Director of Obstetrical Anesthesia at the Medical College of Georgia. It can be an important device in the management of the difficult airway. It is a rigid laryngoscope that combines a curved blade with fiberoptic visualization into a simple and easy-to-use handheld unit (Figure 7-1).

ANATOMY AND PATHOPHYSIOLOGY

The contoured handle is the central structure of the Bullard laryngoscope (Figure 7-2). The proximal handle contains an 11 French (3.7 mm) working port, a site to attach the light source, and a visualization port. A traditional laryngoscope handle attaches to the Bullard's handle and is used as the light source. Alternatively, a fiberoptic light source may be used by attaching an adapter to this site. Incorporated into the handle is an 11 French port, which allows oxygen insufflation, suctioning, administration of pharmaceuticals, or the passage of a guidewire to promote tracheal intubation.[1,2] An optical port on the Bullard's handle allows a 55 ± 5 degree field of view from the tip of the blade.[1,2] Attached to the distal handle is a curved metal blade for intubating. The curved blade is designed to conform to the shape of the oropharnyx. It is similar in shape to a Macintosh blade. A fiberoptic bundle runs through the handle and along the contour of the blade to allow visualization of the vocal cords and tracheal intubation without a direct line of sight.

The intubating mechanism involves a dedicated stylet that attaches to the handle (Figure 7-3). The Bullard laryngoscope comes with an accessory stylet, which attaches to the fiberoptic bundle between the eyepiece and the handle. The stylet aligns beneath the flange of the blade. There is a small central opening in the dedicated stylet (4.5 mm in the adult model, 3.6 mm in the pediatric long model) large enough to allow the passage of a guidewire.

The Bullard laryngoscope comes in three sizes (Figure 7-4). The largest model has a blade 2.5 cm wide, which extends 2.7 cm beyond the fiberoptic bundle and is used for adults and children over 10 years of age. The pediatric model is used for neonates, infants, and small children. It has a blade that is 1.3 cm wide and extends 0.6 cm beyond the fiberoptic bundle. The pediatric long model is used in larger children up to 10 years of age. The blade is 1.6 cm wide and extends 1.4 cm beyond the fiberoptic bundle.[1,2]

This unique design gives the Bullard laryngoscope several advantages to promote successful intubation (Figures 7-1 and 7-2). The device is handheld, readily portable, self-contained, and it allows direct visualization of the airway. It is operated as quickly as a traditional laryngoscope with a Macintosh blade. The simple design, related to that of traditional laryngoscopes, makes the Bullard laryngoscope easy to use. Physicians skilled in oral intubation had a high rate of successful intubation during the first attempt and gained proficiency after three to five attempts.[1,2] **The ability to visualize the vocal cords without aligning the oral, pharyngeal, and laryngeal axes allows successful intubation with a minimum of cervical spine movement.** This makes the Bullard laryngoscope a valuable tool in the intubation of patients with actual or potential cervical spine injuries.[1–6] The ease of insertion, despite limited mouth opening, lends itself to airway management in patients with congenital malformations (Pierre

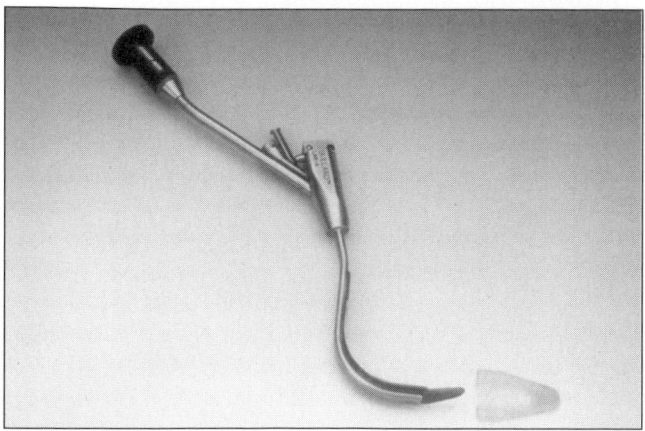

FIGURE 7-1 The Bullard laryngoscope.

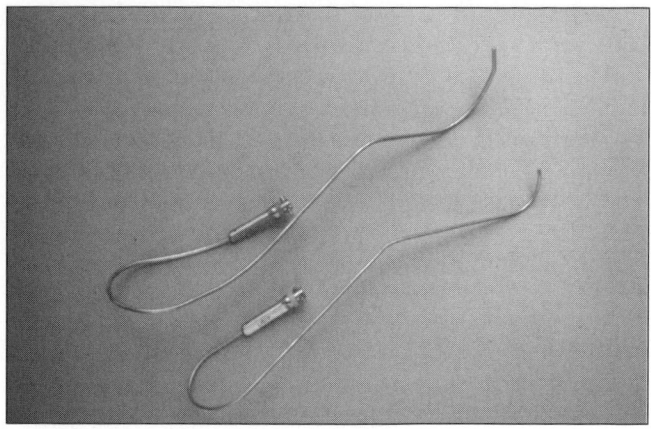

FIGURE 7-3 The intubating stylet.

Robin, micrognathia, etc.), cervical spine immobilization, oromaxillofacial trauma, and trismus of any etiology.[2,6] The large working port provides the ability to insufflate oxygen and suction during intubation. The Bullard laryngoscope has a potential salvage role in failed intubations prior to the creation of a surgical airway.[1,2,4]

INDICATIONS

The Bullard laryngoscope may be used for routine intubation or in the management of difficult airways, including anatomic abnormalities and traumatic injuries. It is useful for the intubation of patients with actual or potential cervical spine injuries, patients with difficulty opening their mouths wide enough to provide direct visualization, anatomically challenging airways (American Society of Anesthesiologists classes 3 and 4), oromaxillofacial trauma, and in rescue situations when other methods of intubation have failed.[1–7]

CONTRAINDICATIONS

The ability to intubate easily with traditional laryngoscopes would be a relative contraindication. As with any airway adjunct, the Bullard laryngoscope should be used by individuals trained in airway management and comfortable with its proper use. **Any proximal obstruc-**

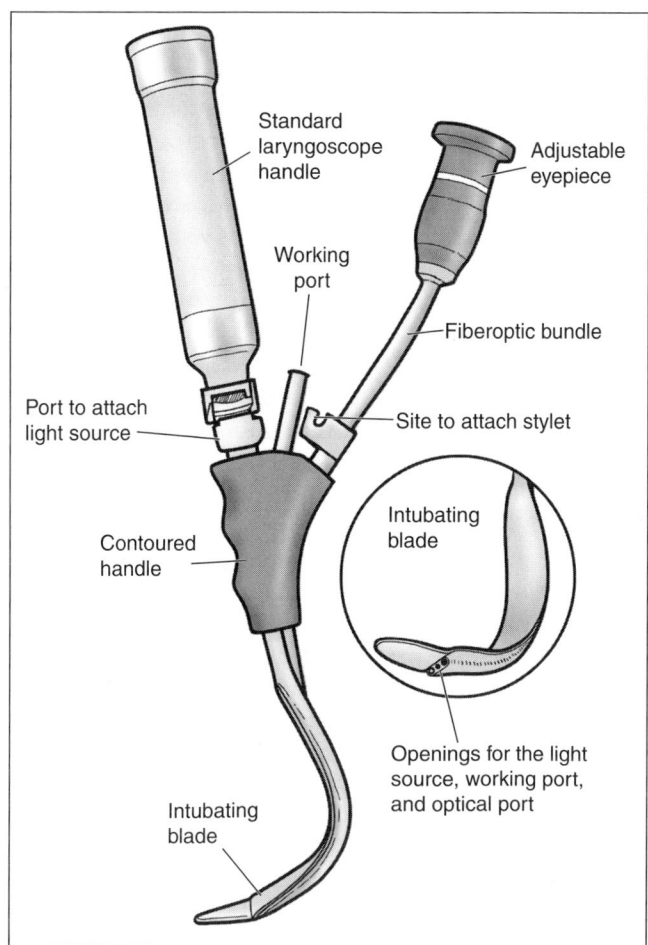

FIGURE 7-2 Anatomy of the Bullard laryngoscope.

Standard laryngoscope handle

Adjustable eyepiece

Working port

Fiberoptic bundle

Port to attach light source

Site to attach stylet

Contoured handle

Intubating blade

Openings for the light source, working port, and optical port

Intubating blade

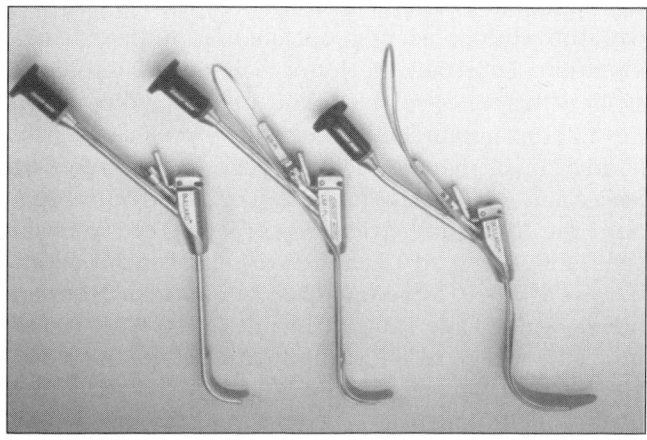

FIGURE 7-4 Three versions of the Bullard laryngoscope. *From left to right:* the pediatric model, the pediatric long model, and the standard model.

tion that would prevent passage of an endotracheal tube would preclude using the Bullard laryngoscope.

The optical port may become obstructed by particulate matter, thick secretions, or vomitus and make visualization difficult. In these cases, a standard laryngoscope and a Yankaur catheter attached to wall suction may be more appropriate.

EQUIPMENT

Bullard laryngoscope (size appropriate for the patient)
Accessory stylet
Blade extender (optional)
Standard laryngoscope handle (or optional fiberoptic light source and adapter)
Video camera (optional)
Endotracheal tube
10 mL syringe
Bag-valve-mask device
Oxygen source
Suction source

PATIENT PREPARATION

The patient preparation and pharmacologic adjuncts are similar to those used for rapid sequence intubation. Refer to Chapters 3 and 4 for complete details.

TECHNIQUE

Assemble the Bullard laryngoscope when the possible need for airway intervention is recognized (Figure 7-1). The working port can be fitted with a three-way stopcock to provide intermittent suction and oxygen insufflation. Attach a traditional laryngoscope handle as the light source. If available, a fiberoptic light source, with the required adapter, may be used to provide illumination. Lubricate the lower half of the intubating stylet with a water-soluble lubricant. Attach the stylet to the fiberoptic bundle, between the eyepiece and the handle, on the right side of the laryngoscope (Figure 7-1). Select and load the appropriate size endotracheal tube onto the intubating stylet (Figure 7-5). The tip of the stylet should extend 0.5 cm past the distal end of the endotracheal tube. Place the tip of the stylet beneath the flange of the blade. If a video camera is used, it should now be attached to the eyepiece and secured. It is recommended, but not required, that a disposable plastic blade extender be placed on the tip of the metal blade for adult intubations.

The intubator should stand above the head of the bed. Open the patient's mouth. A minimum opening of

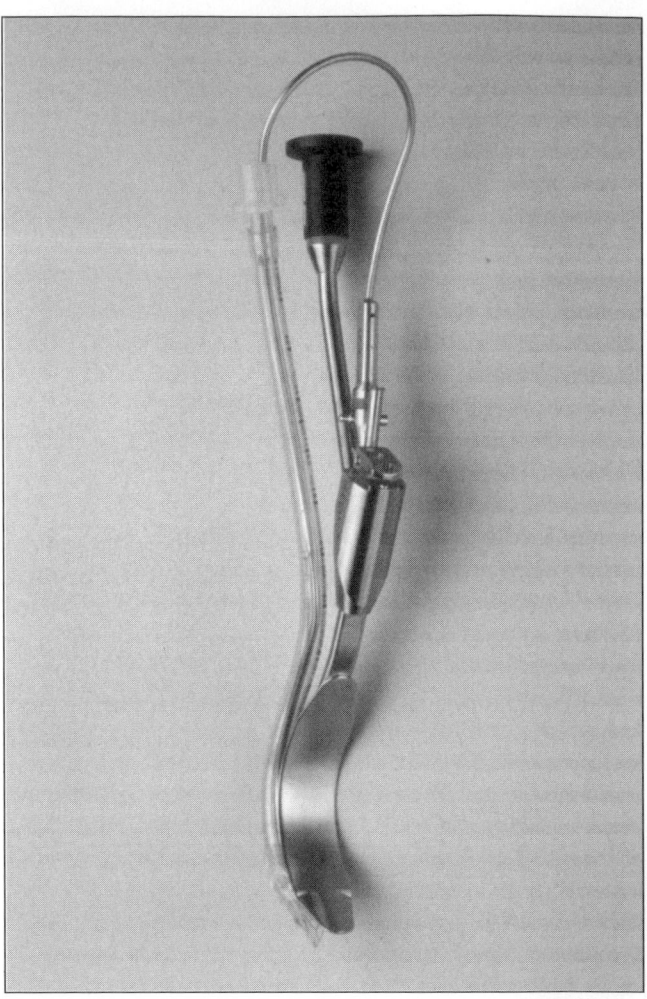

FIGURE 7-5 The Bullard laryngoscope with an endotracheal tube loaded on the stylet.

0.6 cm between the mandibular incisors and the maxillary incisors is required. **The blade is introduced similar to that of an oral airway rather than a traditional Macintosh blade.** Hold the handle of the Bullard laryngoscope parallel to the patient and toward the patient's feet (Figure 7-6A). Center the tip of the laryngoscope blade over the patient's mouth and tongue. Insert the blade directly into the center of the patient's mouth. **The Bullard blade, unlike that of a traditional laryngoscope with a Macintosh blade, should not be placed lateral to the tongue.** Lift the laryngoscope handle upward (Figure 7-6B). Slightly elevate the Bullard laryngoscope to lift up the tongue (Figure 7-6C). The blade will follow the contour of the tongue and pharynx with minimal effort.

The blade of the laryngoscope should be underneath the epiglottis and elevating it (Figures 7-6C and D). Visualize the airway through the fiberoptic port. The view can be focused by turning the eyepiece. If the blade is not beneath the epiglottis, it can be repositioned by moving it toward the posterior pharynx in an attempt to

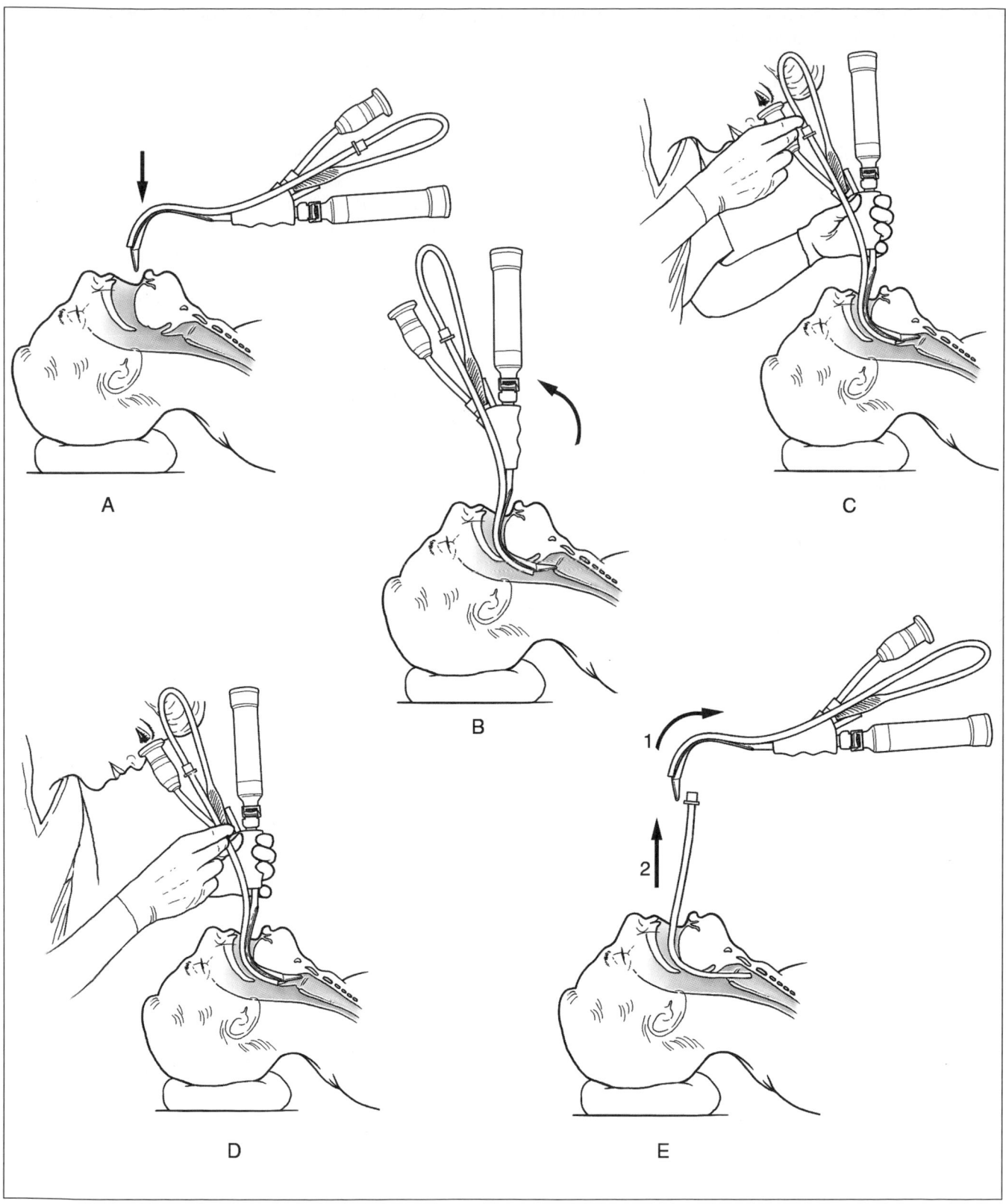

FIGURE 7-6 Intubating with the Bullard laryngoscope. *A.* Inserting the laryngoscope. *B.* Rotation of the handle 90 degrees properly positions the laryngoscope. *C.* Slight elevation of the laryngoscope moves the tongue and epiglottis out of the visual axis. *D.* Advancement of the endotracheal tube under direct visualization. *E.* Removal of the laryngoscope. It is first rotated 90 degrees toward the patient's feet (*curved arrow*), then lifted out of the mouth (*straight arrow*).

catch the epiglottis. If blood, debris, or secretions limit the view, apply suction through the working port. When the vocal cords are visualized, advance the endotracheal tube under direct visualization (Figure 7-6*D*). Secure the endotracheal tube at the patient's teeth with your non-dominant hand.

Remove the Bullard laryngoscope with your dominant hand by reversing the technique of insertion (Figure 7-6*E*). Tilt the handle of the laryngoscope toward the patient's feet until it is parallel to the patient's body. Lift the laryngoscope blade straight up and out of the oral cavity. Inflate the endotracheal tube cuff. Attach a bag-valve-mask device to the endotracheal tube and begin ventilating the patient.

ALTERNATIVE TECHNIQUES

The most common difficulty in passing the endotracheal tube is that the right arytenoid cartilage can block its passage. This can be overcome by directing the laryngoscope slightly toward the patient's left side. Alternatively, rotate the endotracheal tube until the bevel is facing the viewing channel. An endotracheal tube with a Murphy eye can be used instead of a standard endotracheal tube. Load it on the intubating stylet with the tip of the stylet exiting through the Murphy eye.

The Bullard laryngoscope allows for other options. The stylet has a central opening (4.5 mm in the adult, 3.6 mm in the pediatric long), which can be used to pass an intubating guidewire through the vocal cords.[2] An intubating guidewire may also be passed through the working port and through the vocal cords. In either case, after inserting the guidewire, remove the Bullard laryngoscope and pass the endotracheal tube over the guidewire and into the trachea.

It is also possible to pass an endotracheal tube with a standard stylet. Bend the endotracheal tube, with the stylet, into a shape similar to that of the Bullard laryngoscope blade. Insert the Bullard laryngoscope without the endotracheal tube attached. Visualize the vocal cords through the Bullard laryngoscope. Insert the endotracheal tube, free-handed, while the cords are visualized through the scope.

AFTERCARE

After intubation has been achieved, the endotracheal tube should be secured, its proper position confirmed, and ventilation of the patient begun.

The Bullard laryngoscope must be cleaned. Wipe off any blood, debris, food, or vomitus. Dispose of the plastic blade extender. Rinse the laryngoscope under running water. The older version of the Bullard laryngoscope requires soaking in a sterilizing agent. The newer versions of the Bullard laryngoscope can be sterilized by numerous methods. Refer to the manufacturer's instructions for complete details.

COMPLICATIONS

The majority of complications mirror those of endotracheal intubation. These include failure to intubate, esophageal intubation, right mainstem bronchus intubation, and all of the hemodynamic consequences of intubation. Refer to Chapter 5 for a complete description of these complications.

Potential problems may arise that are specific to the Bullard laryngoscope. The vocal cords may not be visualized. First, confirm that the laryngoscope is in midline. If the blade is above the epiglottis and the view obscured, reposition it by moving the blade into the posterior pharynx and attempt to capture the epiglottis. To avoid this difficulty, use a disposable plastic blade extender. If the view is obscured by blood, fluid, or vomitus, suction through the working port. Once positioned, the stylet with the loaded endotracheal tube should be visualized through the scope. If not, it may have slipped underneath the blade. Reposition the stylet and endotracheal tube without removing the laryngoscope.[2] The stylet, if extended too far beyond the endotracheal tube, may cause abrasions, bleeding, and lacerations to the walls of the oral cavity, oropharynx, and laryngopharynx. These can be prevented with proper assembly of the Bullard laryngoscope.

SUMMARY

The Bullard laryngoscope is a rigid structure composed of a handle, blade, and fiberoptic bundle. It allows for direct visualization of the vocal cords and endotracheal tube placement despite no direct line of sight. It may be used for routine and difficult intubations. This includes patients with congenital malformations, cervical spine immobilization, actual or potential cervical spine injuries, oromaxillofacial trauma, and trismus. It allows endotracheal tube placement with little manipulation of the cervical spine and minimal mouth opening. Its similarity in structure and use to traditional laryngoscopes make it easier to master and faster to use than flexible fiberoptic intubating bronchoscopes. It allows for several methods of intubation. The primary limitation of the Bullard laryngoscope may be one of initial cost. Prices range from $4000 to $8000, depending on the size and accessories. The Bullard laryngoscope is a valuable tool in the management of both routine and difficult airways.

REFERENCES

1. Borland L, Casselbrant C: The Bullard laryngoscope. A new indirect oral laryngoscope (pediatric version). *Anesth Analg* 1990; 70:105–108.
2. Gutstein HB: The difficult pediatric airway. Use of the Bullard laryngoscope and lightwand in pediatric patients. *Anesth Clin North Am* 1998; 16(4):795–813.
3. Hastings RH, Vigil AC, Hanna R, et al: Cervical spine movement during laryngoscopy with the Bullard, Macintosh, and Miller laryngoscopes. *Anesthesiology* 1995; 82(4):859–869.
4. Cohn AI, Zornow MH: Awake endotracheal intubation in patients with cervical spine disease: a comparison of the Bullard laryngoscope and the fiberoptic bronchoscope. *Anesth Analg* 1995; 81:1283–1286.
5. Watts AD, Gelb AW, Bach OB, Pelz DM: Comparison of the Bullard and Macintosh laryngoscopes for endotracheal intubation of patients with a potential cervical spine injury. *Anesthesiology* 1997; 87(6): 1335–1342.
6. Ghouri AF, Bernstein CA: Use of the Bullard laryngoscope blade in patients with maxillofacial injuries. *Anesthesiology* 1996; 84:490.

Chapter 8
LIGHTED STYLET
INTUBATION

Karen S. Cosby

INTRODUCTION

Direct laryngoscopy for orotracheal intubation requires direct visualization of the vocal cords and glottis. It is a time-honored method that is effective for securing most airways. Occasionally, difficulties may be encountered where the airway cannot be properly visualized. Airways may be difficult because of anatomic variations, disease processes, trauma, or particular clinical settings (Table 8-1). These airway challenges require alternative approaches. The lighted stylet is an innovative alternative that provides a safe, rapid, relatively easy, and indirect approach for airways that cannot be easily visualized by direct laryngoscopy.

The concept of using a light-guided introducer for orotracheal intubations first appeared in print in the late 1950s. Several authors described rather ingenious devices to tunnel a lightbulb attached to an introducer through the endotracheal tube and power it with a pocket battery, penlight, or laryngoscope handle.[1–4] These primitive devices were simple and effective. Although intriguing, further development of this technology was stagnant until the late 1970s, when several authors described use of the Flexium surgical light as a lighted stylet or "lightwand."[5,6] After a few problems with bulb dislodgment, the makers of the Flexium light revised the design and marketed the first lighted stylet, known as the Tube-Stat (Concept, Inc.).[7,8] A similar design is still available as the Tube-Stat lighted intubating stylet (Medtronic Xomed, Jacksonville, FL). In the mid-1990s, Laerdal introduced the more sophisticated Trachlight. It was an improvement over previous lighted stylets with a more intense light source, a more flexible lightwand, and a separate retractable stylet that adjusts to a variety of endotracheal tube lengths.[9]

There are two models of lighted stylets available today. The Tube-Stat (Medtronic Xomed, Jacksonville, FL) is the simplest. It incorporates a stylet, power source, and lightbulb all in a single piece. The unit is inserted into the endotracheal tube in place of the stylet. A switch on the handle activates the light. The second available model is the Trachlight (Laerdal Medical Corporation, Wappingers Falls, NY). It comprises a battery-powered handle, the lightwand, and a separate stylet that inserts into the lightwand (Figure 8-1). It is a simple device to operate (Figure 8-2). It is likely that further developments will continue to make these and similar models attractive options in airway management.

ANATOMY AND PATHOPHYSIOLOGY

The Trachlight is a simple and easy-to-use device (Figure 8-1). It has an L-shaped handle that is easy to hold, with a "pencil-grip" near the base. The front of the "L" has a channel that holds the stylet. The bottom of the handle has a connecting bracket and clamp that attach to the connector on the proximal portion of the endotracheal tube. The disposable wand attaches to the handle and contains a stylet.

The trachea lies anterior to most structures of the neck and is covered anteriorly only by skin, subcutaneous tissue, and pretracheal fascia. A light source positioned within the trachea will transilluminate a bright and discrete glow that can easily be seen on the surface of the neck (Figure 8-3*A*). In contrast, the esophagus lies posteriorly and is surrounded by numerous soft tissue structures. A light source directed within the pharynx and esophagus will be diffused by the surrounding tissue and appear dull (Figure 8-3*D*). At the bedside, the ex-

TABLE 8-1. INDICATIONS FOR INTUBATING WITH A LIGHTED STYLET

Anatomic abnormalities	**Limited jaw mobility**
Congenital head and neck anomalies	Temporomandibular immobility
Pierre Robin syndrome	Trismus
Treacher Collins syndrome	
Midface hypoplasia	**Trauma**
	Dental trauma
Excessive secretions	Maxillofacial trauma
Blood	
Vomitus	**Miscellaneous**
	Unable to intubate by other methods
Limited cervical spine movement	
Known or suspected cervical spine injury	
Cervical arthritis	
Burn strictures of the neck	

aminer can easily discriminate between the dull, diffuse transillumination of an esophageal light source and the more discrete, intense signal transmitted from within the trachea. A submental, superior to the hyoid bone, glowing light indicates that the tip is positioned in the vallecula (Figure 8-3*B*). A lateral glowing light indicates placement in the pyriform sinus (Figure 8-3*C*).

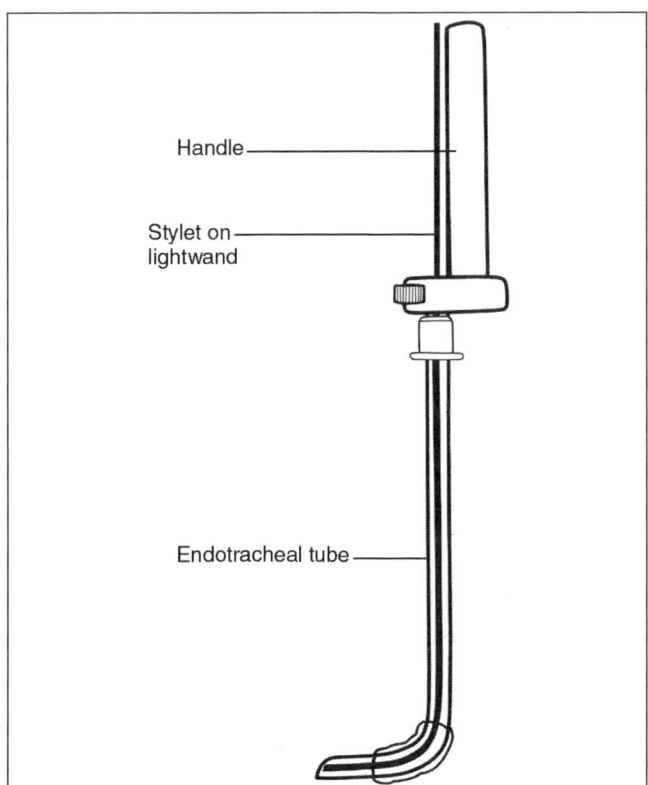

Handle

Stylet on lightwand

Endotracheal tube

FIGURE 8-1 The Trachlight lighted stylet.

INDICATIONS

Light-guided intubation is primarily used in difficult airways when direct laryngoscopy is likely to fail. It is a blind and indirect technique that is particularly useful when anatomic variations prevent easy visualization of the vocal cords, the cervical spine is immobilized or its movement restricted, there is limited mobility of the jaw, there is significant maxillofacial trauma in the presence of extensive dental work or loose teeth, or when excess secretions impair direct visualization (Table 8-1).[10–16] Lighted stylets are generally considered an adjunct to other, more traditional airway approaches.

Lighted stylets have been used and described in a variety of clinical settings. They have been used for routine intubations as well as in emergent intubations. The technique can be used on awake patients who are breathing on their own or in apneic patients. Originally described in adults, the technique and equipment have been modified for children and infants.[12–14] Although primarily described as an orotracheal technique, the use of the lighted stylet has also been modified for nasotracheal intubation.[17,18] Lighted stylets have been used in the Operating Room, the Emergency Department, and in the prehospital setting. The technique is relatively simple and easy to learn, while the equipment is inexpensive and portable. These characteristics make this technique adaptable to most clinical situations.

When direct methods of intubation fail because of the inability to visualize the glottis, there are a number of options. These include nasotracheal intubation, blind digital (tactile) intubation, esophageal obturators, retrograde guidewires, fiberoptic bronchoscopy, laryngeal mask airways, lighted stylets, and surgical approaches. There have been no significant studies directly comparing these methods. However, there are a number of specific advantages to use of the lighted stylets. In experienced hands, intubations with lighted stylets are faster and have fewer complications than those done by the nasotracheal route or by bronchoscopy.[11,15,19,20] Lighted stylets are simpler, less expensive, and more portable than fiberoptic bronchoscopes.[15,20] Lighted stylet intubations are faster, and certainly less invasive, than surgical approaches. The choice of techniques will ultimately depend upon the skill and experience of the intubator. A sound argument can be made for keeping lighted stylets available for those skilled in their use, particularly for the occasional difficult airway.

CONTRAINDICATIONS

Intubation with lighted stylets is relatively safe and simple. **Patients with laryngeal trauma should have**

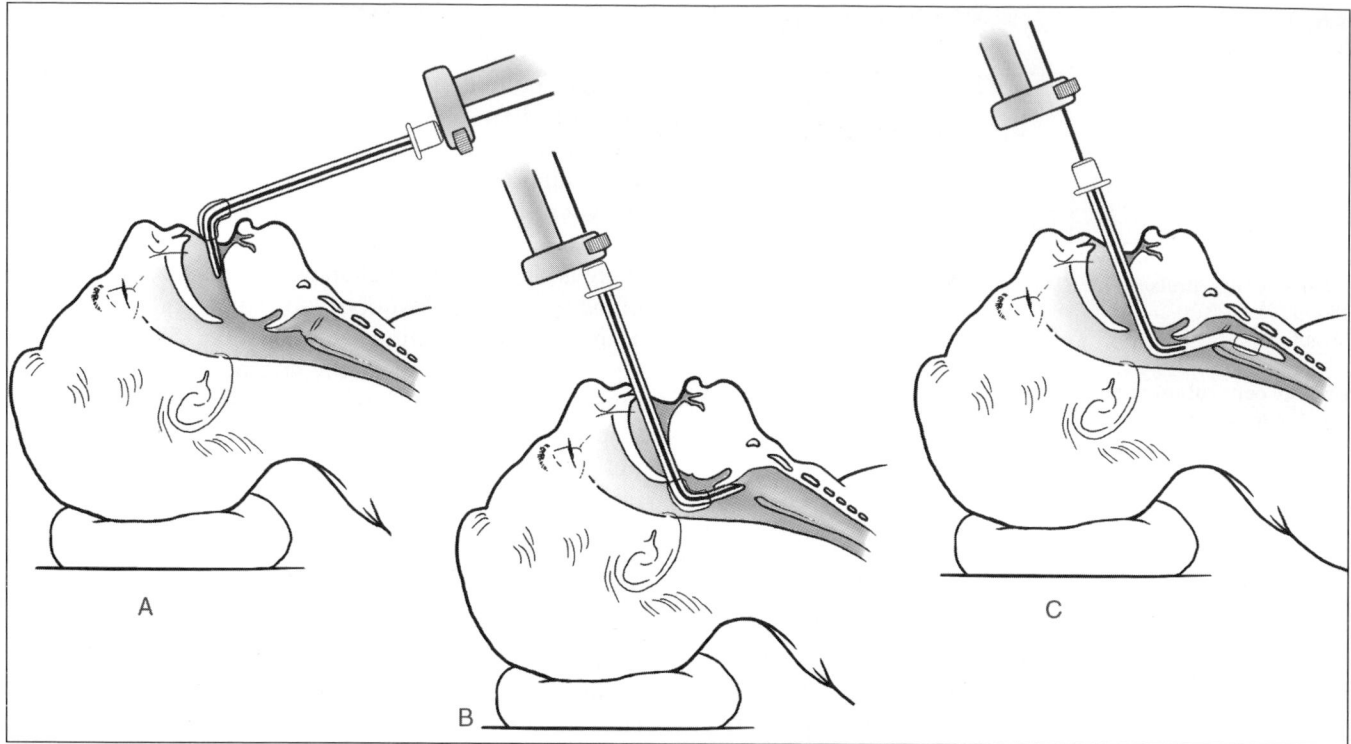

FIGURE 8-2 Insertion of the lighted stylet. *A.* Insert the hockey stick–shaped endotracheal tube and stylet over the tongue. *B.* Move the tube in a vertical arc toward the patient's head. As the lighted stylet approaches the trachea, the bright light transilluminates the anterior neck. *C.* The endotracheal tube is advanced.

direct laryngeal visualization for intubation rather than a blind technique that may cause additional trauma. There are few contraindications to this technique. As a blind technique, it should not be used if there is any active infection or known tumor of the posterior pharynx or upper airway. The presence of epiglottitis, a retropharyngeal abscess, tracheal stenosis, a laryngeal polyp or tumor, or an airway foreign body precludes the use of this technology. It may be less successful in bright sunlight, particularly in the obese patient.[10,11,15,21] If the lighted stylet meets resistance, it should be withdrawn, redirected, and advanced only if it passes with ease. **Should unexpected difficulty occur during passage of the lighted stylet, the technique should be abandoned and an alternative method used to intubate the patient.** As with any clinical procedure, lighted stylets should be used only by clinicians who have sufficient experience and training with the equipment and the technique.

EQUIPMENT

Lighted stylet
Endotracheal tubes, various sizes
10 mL syringe
Water-soluble lubricant or anesthetic jelly
Bag-valve device

PATIENT PREPARATION

Once the decision is made to intubate, the patient should be prepared as for any other intubation. The patient should have intravenous access secured and routine hemodynamic monitoring, including an automatic blood pressure monitor, cardiac monitor, and continuous pulse oximetry. Suction should be immediately available. The choice of anesthetic will be determined by the clinical setting. General anesthesia with paralytics will most commonly be used to optimize control of the situation. However, this technique can be used with topical anesthesia alone in cooperative patients.

As with all intubations, the patient should be preoxygenated prior to airway manipulation. Unlike the case with other techniques, the position of the neck can be neutral. The "sniffing" position is not required for this technique. If the patient is in a cervical collar, the anterior half must be opened or removed to be able to visualize the glowing light. An assistant can maintain in-line stabilization of the cervical spine when the collar is opened.

TECHNIQUE

The exact technique will depend upon the type of lighted stylet or lightwand used. Since this technology varies by manufacturer, anyone employing these airway adjuncts should be familiar with the equipment and manufacturer's instructions prior to adopting them for use clinically. This text describes the general guidelines for the lighted stylets available at the time of this writing. The reader is urged to take advantage of the teaching videos supplied by some manufacturers.[22]

Assemble the lighted stylet and check the light source. Liberally apply lubricant to the stylet. Select an appropriate-size endotracheal tube. Attach a 10 mL syringe to the cuff's inflation port and check the integrity of the cuff. Load the endotracheal tube over the lighted stylet (Figure 8-1).

Measure the mandibular-hyoid distance in the patient. Place the index finger in the submental space below the chin and determine the number of finger breadths between the mandible and the hyoid bone.[23,24] Typical measurements are one to three finger breadths. Bend the tip of the endotracheal tube and stylet sharply at a site that approximates the mandibular-hyoid distance between the bend and the junction of the lighted tip of the stylet. This is usually 3 to 6 cm from the distal end of the endotracheal tube and just above the cuff. Be sure the bend is 90 to 120 degrees. This allows the maximal light intensity to be directed anteriorly.

Stand above or to the side of the patient's head. The lighted stylet, unlike the traditional laryngoscope, can be held in either hand. Lower the bed to facilitate insertion of the lighted stylet. Grasp the patient's jaw with your nondominant hand. Place your thumb on the mandibular molars and your fingers under the body of the mandible. Lift upward and inferiorly to open the jaw, elevate the tongue, and elevate the epiglottis. Grasp the lighted stylet with your dominant hand and turn it on. It is best held with a "pencil-grip" over the proximal endotracheal tube.

Introduce the endotracheal tube from the side of the patient's mouth and bring it to the midline. As the hockey stick–shaped tip is placed over the tongue, the handle will project toward the patient's feet (Figure 8-2A). Advance the tip by moving the handle in a vertical arc towards the patient's head (Figure 8-2B). This will bring the endotracheal tube toward the vocal cords. A bright light will be seen in the midline of the neck just below the hyoid bone (Figure 8-3A). **If the light is in the submental space, the tip of the endotracheal tube is in the vallecula (Figure 8-3B). If the light is lateral, the tip of the endotracheal tube is lodged in the pyriform sinus (Figure 8-3C). A dull, faint light in the midline signifies that the tip of the endotracheal tube is in the esophagus (Figure 8-3D).** If the glowing light is malpositioned, simply withdraw the endotracheal tube, reposition it in the midline, and advance it again.

Once a bright and discrete light is detected in the midline at the level of the thyroid cartilage (Adam's apple), it is safe to advance the endotracheal tube. If you are using the Trachlight, the manufacturer suggests withdrawing the stylet 10 cm before advancing the endotracheal tube. This makes the distal tip of the endotracheal tube more flexible and helps it make the acute turn before advancing down the trachea.

Advance the endotracheal tube while observing the transilluminating light march down the neck to the suprasternal notch (Figure 8-3A). The light will disappear as the tube passes behind the suprasternal notch. If the glowing light is in the midline and the endotracheal tube is resistant to advancement, the epiglottis is obstructing its advancement. Slightly rock the unit in the sagittal plane (from the patient's head to the feet) to slip the tip of the endotracheal tube under the epiglottis. If resistance is still encountered, remove the lighted stylet. Ventilate the patient with a bag-valve-mask device. Load a smaller endotracheal tube onto the lighted stylet and try again. At the point the light is lost, the tip of the endotracheal tube is appropriately positioned midway between the vocal cords and carina.[25] Remove the stylet, inflate the endotracheal tube cuff, secure the endotracheal tube at the lips, and begin ventilating the patient.

Special caution should be used in very thin or very obese patients. In the thin patient, a bright light may be visible even when the stylet is in the esophagus. When the patient is thin, gently rock the light off midline to compare the diffuse dull light to that seen when the light is truly midline. In the obese patient, the extra soft tissue may dull the light. Dim the room lights to facilitate adequate visualization.

The glowing light must maintain a continual brightness to demonstrate tracheal intubation. If the glowing light is briefly lost or dulls and then returns, the endotracheal tube has been misplaced in the esophagus. The brief loss or dulling of the glowing light corresponds to its passage behind the larynx. The return of the bright glowing light corresponds to the endotracheal tube advancing past the larynx and into the esophagus. This is commonly seen in infants, small children, and very thin adults. Gently withdraw the lighted stylet while applying anteriorly directed traction to the tip of the stylet. Stop withdrawing the lighted stylet when the glowing light suddenly intensifies after it exits the esophagus. Readvance the lighted stylet, as previously described, while applying anterior traction on the unit to help it enter the larynx.

ASSESSMENT

The position of the endotracheal tube should be confirmed by end-tidal CO_2 monitoring, fogging in the endotracheal tube for at least six ventilations, auscultation, and chest x-ray. The patient should be assessed and reassessed at every step to assure adequate oxygenation and ventilation.

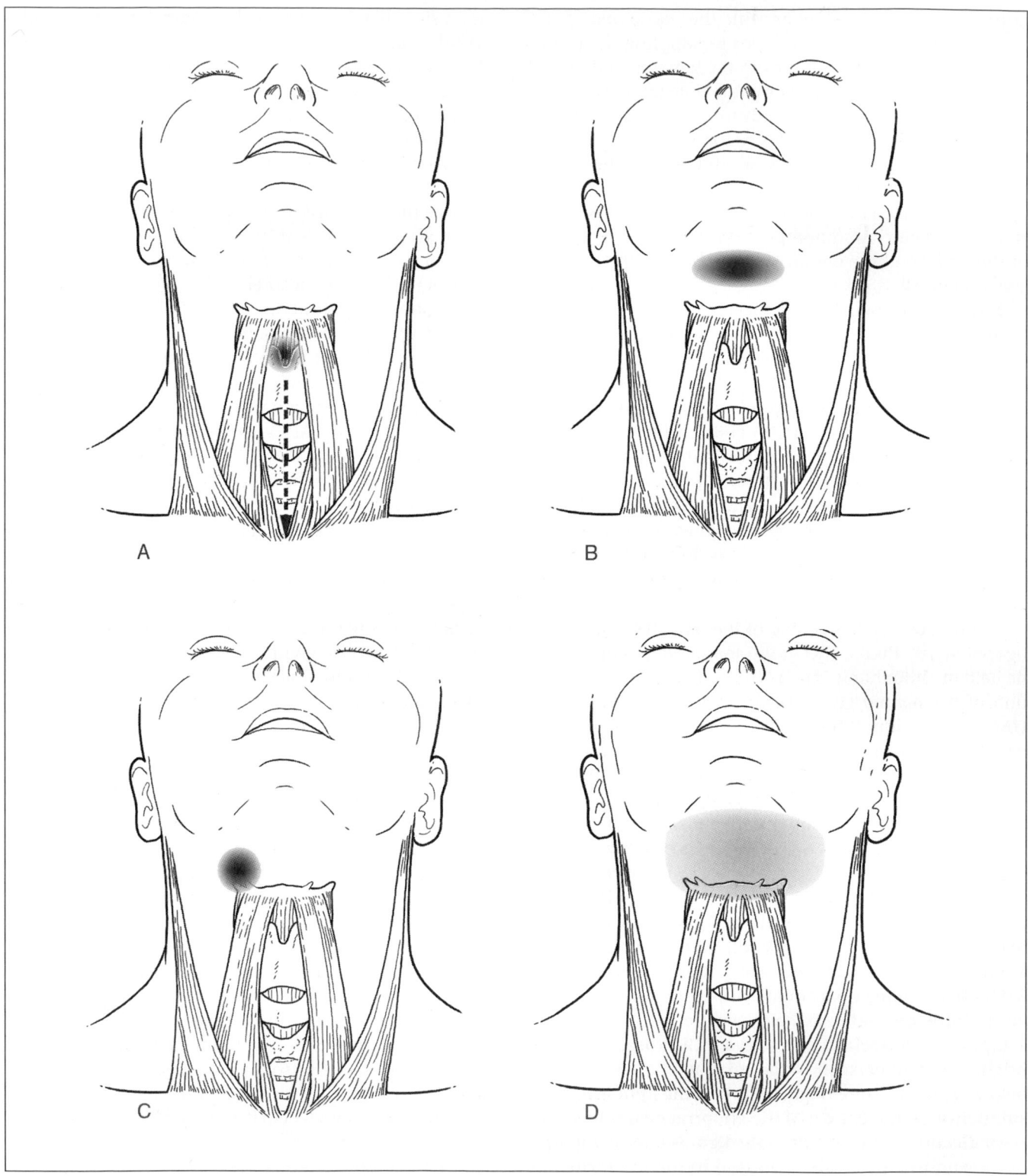

FIGURE 8-3 Appearance of the transilluminated light of the lighted stylet based on the position of the tip. *A.* Proper placement in the larynx with a bright distinct light in the midline at the level of the thyroid cartilage (Adam's apple). With advancement of the endotracheal tube, the light marches down the anterior neck and disappears behind the sternal notch (*arrow*). *B.* Incorrect placement in the vallecula causes a submental glow, superior to the hyoid. *C.* Incorrect placement in the pyriform sinus causes a glow off the midline. *D.* Incorrect esophageal placement causes a diffuse, dull, or absent light.

AFTERCARE

The ongoing care of the patient should proceed as with any other intubation technique. Routine care of the endotracheal tube is no different. The manufacturer's guidelines should be followed for maintenance of the equipment.

COMPLICATIONS

Lighted intubating stylets are relatively free of complications. In over 30 years of development and use, the literature cites only a handful of complications. This includes two reports of accidental bulb dislodgment, two arytenoid dislocations, one case of stylet fracture, a lacerated frenulum, and varied reports of mild soft tissue trauma, sore throat, and hoarseness that are not statistically different from those after intubations done by direct laryngoscopy.[7–9,21,26–30] The newer models have been revised to minimize these problems and have been remarkably free of adverse events. In experienced hands, complications with this technique are unusual. Weiss reported no complications in 253 patients intubated with a lighted stylet.[11]

Success rates with lighted stylet intubation are comparable to those with other techniques. Success rates on first attempts are reported as low as 70 percent with the Tube-Stat and as high as 92 percent with the Trachlight.[9,16,20,31] When multiple attempts are allowed, success rates approach 100 percent.[20,23] In the prehospital setting, under adverse and emergent conditions, success rates of 88 percent have been reported.[21] More importantly, rates of successful intubation remain high for difficult airways. Hung reported the successful intubation in 95 of 96 known difficult airways.[10] This included patients with prior difficult or failed intubations by direct laryngoscopy, patients with unstable cervical spines or ankylosing temporomandibular joints, and the morbidly obese. Holzman reported successful intubation in 30 of 31 children with anatomic airway abnormalities.[12]

Intubation times with lighted stylets are comparable to those with other techniques and range from 15.7 to 45 seconds.[9–11,20,21,23,26] Recent evidence suggests that intubation with a lighted stylet may cause fewer hemodynamic alterations when compared to direct laryngoscopy.[32,33]

The skill level of the intubator is an important factor in success rates, time to intubation, and possibly complications.[12] The best success rates are reported by those who have devoted a great deal of time to the technique and use it regularly. There is a definite learning curve, and time to intubation improves with experience.[14,21,26] Skills may improve with practice in a cadaver lab.[23,26]

Manikins designed as intubation teaching models can be modified for use with lighted stylets.[31] Proper training, use of teaching videos, didactics, formal practice with training manikins and in cadaver labs, and supervised clinical experience are all important means of developing and maintaining a skill level and decreasing complication rates.

SUMMARY

Lighted stylets are a valuable adjunct in airway management, particularly in difficult airways. The American Society of Anesthesiologists includes use of lighted stylets in its recommendations for the management of difficult airways.[34] The American Heart Association encourages instruction in alternative airway approaches, including lighted stylets, for difficult airways.[35] The use of lighted stylets has proven to be rapid, safe, and effective in emergent and difficult settings.

The success of lighted stylet techniques is determined by the experience of the clinician. Since this technique is likely to be of greatest benefit in the occasional unexpected airway emergency, maintaining sufficient skills to use it in the emergent setting is a challenge. In order to be of use in the acute situation, clinicians will need to devote time and effort to developing and maintaining the skills they will need to cope with an airway emergency when it presents.

REFERENCES

1. Macintosh SR, Richards H: Illuminated introducer for endotracheal tubes. *Anaesthesia* 1957; 12(2):223–225.
2. Richards H, Hooper ERS: Flexometallic tube and bougie. *Anaesthesia* 1957; 12:111–113.
3. Yamamura H, Yamamoto T, Kamiyama M: Device for blind nasal intubation. *Anesthesiology* 1959; 20(2):221.
4. Berman RA: Lighted stylet. *Anesthesiology* 1959; 20(3):382–383.
5. Ducrow M: Throwing light on blind intubation. *Anaesthesia* 1978; 33:827–829.
6. Raymond RL: "Light wand" intubation. *Anaesthesia* 1979; 34:677–678.
7. Stewart RD, Ellis DG: Lighted stylet and endotracheal intubation: I. *Anesthesiology* 1987; 66:851.
8. Williams RT, Stewart RD: Transillumination of the trachea with a lighted stylet. *Anesth Analg* 1986; 65:542–543.
9. Hung OR, Pytka S, Morris I, et al: Clinical trial of a new lightwand device (Trachlight) to intubate the trachea. *Anesthesiology* 1995; 83(3):509–514.

10. Hung OR, Pytka S, Murphy MF, et al: Clinical trial of a new lightwand device for intubation in patients with difficult airways. *Anesthesiology* 1993; 79(3A):A498.

11. Weis FR, Hatton MN: Intubation by use of the light wand: experience in 253 patients. *J Oral Maxillofac Surg* 1989; 47:577–580.

12. Holzman RS, Nargozian CD, Florence FB: Light-wand intubation in children with abnormal upper airways. *Anesthesiology* 1988; 69(5):784–787.

13. Krucylak CP, Schreiner MS: Orotracheal intubation of an infant with hemifacial microsomia using a modified lighted stylet. *Anesthesiology* 1992; 77:826–827.

14. Berns SD, Patel RI, Chamberlain JM: Oral intubation using a lighted stylet vs direct laryngoscopy in older children with cervical immobilization. *Acad Emerg Med* 1996; 3(1):34–39.

15. Hung OR, Murphy M: Lightwands, lighted-stylets, and blind techniques of intubation. *Anesthesiol Clin North Am* 1995; 14(2);477–489.

16. Graham DH, Dell WA, Robinson AD, et al: Intubation with lighted stylet (letter). *Can J Anaesth* 1991; 38(2):261–262.

17. Verdile VP, Chiang J, Bedger R, et al: Nasotracheal intubation using a flexible lighted stylet. *Ann Emerg Med* 1990; 19(5):506–510.

18. Stewart RD, LaRosee A, Stoy WA, et al: Use of a lighted stylet to confirm correct endotracheal tube placement. *Chest* 1987; 92(5):900–903.

19. Fox DJ, Castro T, Rastrelli AJ: Comparison of intubation techniques in the awake patient: the Flexi-lum surgical light (lightwand) versus blind nasal approach. *Anesthesiology* 1987; 66:69–71.

20. Saha AK, Higgins M, Walker G, et al: Comparison of awake endotracheal intubation in patients with cervical spine disease: the lighted intubating stylet versus the fiberoptic bronchoscope. *Anesth Analg* 1998; 87:477–479.

21. Vollmer TP, Stewart RD, Paris PM, et al: Use of a lighted stylet for guided orotracheal intubation in the prehospital setting. *Ann Emerg Med* 1985; 14(4):324–328.

22. *Trachlight Stylet and Tracheal Lightwand Teaching Video.* Wappingers Falls, NY: Laerdal Medical Corporation, 1995.

23. Ellis DG, Stewart RD, Kaplan RM, et al: Success rates of blind orotracheal intubation using a transillumination technique with a lighted stylet. *Ann Emerg Med* 1986; 15(2):138–142.

24. Clinton JE, Ruiz E: Emergency airway management procedures, in Roberts JR, Hedges JR (eds): *Clinical Procedures in Emergency Medicine.* Philadelphia: Saunders, 1985:1–29.

25. Stewart RD, LaRosee A, Kaplan RM, et al: Correct positioning of an endotracheal tube using a flexible lighted stylet. *Crit Care Med* 1990; 18(1):97–99.

26. Ellis DG, Jakymec A, Kaplan RM, et al: Guided orotracheal intubation in the operating room using a lighted stylet: a comparison with direct laryngoscopic technique. *Anesthesiology* 1986; 64:823–826.

27. Stone DJ, Stirt JA, Kaplan MJ, et al: A complication of lightwand-guided nasotracheal intubation. *Anesthesiology* 1984; 61:780–781.

28. Szigeti CL, Baeuerle JJ, Mongan PD: Arytenoid dislocation with lighted stylet intubation: case report and retrospective review. *Anesth Analg* 1994; 78:185–186.

29. Debo RF, Colonna D, Dewerd G, et al: Cricoarytenoid subluxation: complication of blind intubation with a lighted stylet. *Ear Nose Throat J* 1989; 68:517–520.

30. Cohen AI, Joshi S: Lighted stylet intubation: greasing your way to success. *Anesth Analg* 1994; 78:1205–1206.

31. Eyck RPT, Vayer JS: Airway management: a new look at old models. *J Emerg Med* 1987; 5:563–566.

32. Hung OR, Pytka S, Murphy MD, et al: Comparative hemodynamic changes following laryngoscopic or lightwand intubation. *Anesthesiology* 1993; 79(3A):A497.

33. Hung OR, Pytka S, Murphy MF, et al: An improved intubation technique for novice intubators: clinical trial of a new lightwand. *Acad Emerg Med* 1994; 1(3):319.

34. Practice guidelines for management of the difficult airway. A report by the American Society of Anesthesiologists Task Force on Management of the Difficult Airway. *Anesthesiology* 1993; 7(3):597–602.

35. Reed AP: Current concepts in airway management for cardiopulmonary resuscitation. *Mayo Clin Proc* 1995; 70:1172–1184.

Chapter 9
ESOPHAGEAL-TRACHEAL COMBITUBE INTUBATION

Kenneth Pearlman
Holly H. Cromwell

INTRODUCTION

The Esophageal-Tracheal Combitube (ETC; Kendall Sheridan, Mansfield, MA) is a double-lumen airway device that can be blindly inserted into the unconscious and unresponsive patient. An ETC functions to adequately ventilate and oxygenate a patient while simultaneously protecting the airway from aspiration.[1,2] It is most often used in the prehospital setting by emergency medical technicians not trained in standard orotracheal intubation and by paramedic-level rescuers as an alternative when standard orotracheal intubation fails.[3–5]

ANATOMY AND PATHOPHYSIOLOGY

The ETC is a double-tubed, double-lumen, double-cuffed device (Figure 9-1). The ETC starts as two distinct tubes that fuse into one but remain functionally separated by a partition. The shorter-lumen tube is continuous with the distal open port, also known as the tracheoesophageal lumen. The longer-lumen tube is continuous with the eight perforations known as the proximal ports. The distal tracheoesophageal cuff is similar to that of an endotracheal tube. It is a high-volume, low-pressure balloon. A large proximal pharyngeal cuff is designed to be positioned between the base of the tongue and the palate. Upon inflation, it separates the oral and nasal cavities from the remainder of the airway. The longer tube, proximal cuff inflation port, and the proximal (pharyngeal) cuff are color-coded blue. The shorter tube, distal tracheoesophageal cuff, and its inflation port are clear in color.

The ETC is inserted blindly into a patient's airway. If the distal tip enters the trachea, the patient is ventilated through the shorter tube and the distal cuff prevents aspiration of gastric contents into the trachea. If the distal tip enters the esophagus, the patient is ventilated through the longer tube, whose proximal ports lie in the hypopharynx, while the distal cuff will occlude the esophagus.

The ETC is available in two sizes. The 37F SA model is meant for small adults. The manufacturer recommends its use in patients with a height of 122 to 168 cm (4 to 5.5 ft). The 41F model is meant for larger adults with a height of 152 cm (5 ft) and greater. Patients in the intermediate range of 152 to 168 cm (5 to 5.5 ft) can use either model. A recent study demonstrated that the 37F SA model can be used in patients up to 183 cm (6 ft, 1 in) in height.

Several advantages of the ETC contribute to its usefulness in the acute situation. The ETC is effective as either a primary or backup airway management device. A patient can be ventilated with the tip in the esophageal or tracheal position. Minimal training is necessary to use the ETC. There is no need for a laryngoscope during the placement of the ETC. These attributes, and the fact that the tube is easily inserted with neutral head and neck positioning, make it suitable for rescuers of all skill levels. The dual lumens and balloons also offer certain advantages. When placed in the esophageal position, the distal lumen design allows for gastric suctioning. The balloons firmly secure the tube, making dislodgment unlikely. The oral balloon can functionally tamponade oropharyngeal bleeding and serve to minimize the risk of aspirating oral debris.[6]

INDICATIONS

The primary indication for an ETC is as a backup device for airway management in and out of the hospital.

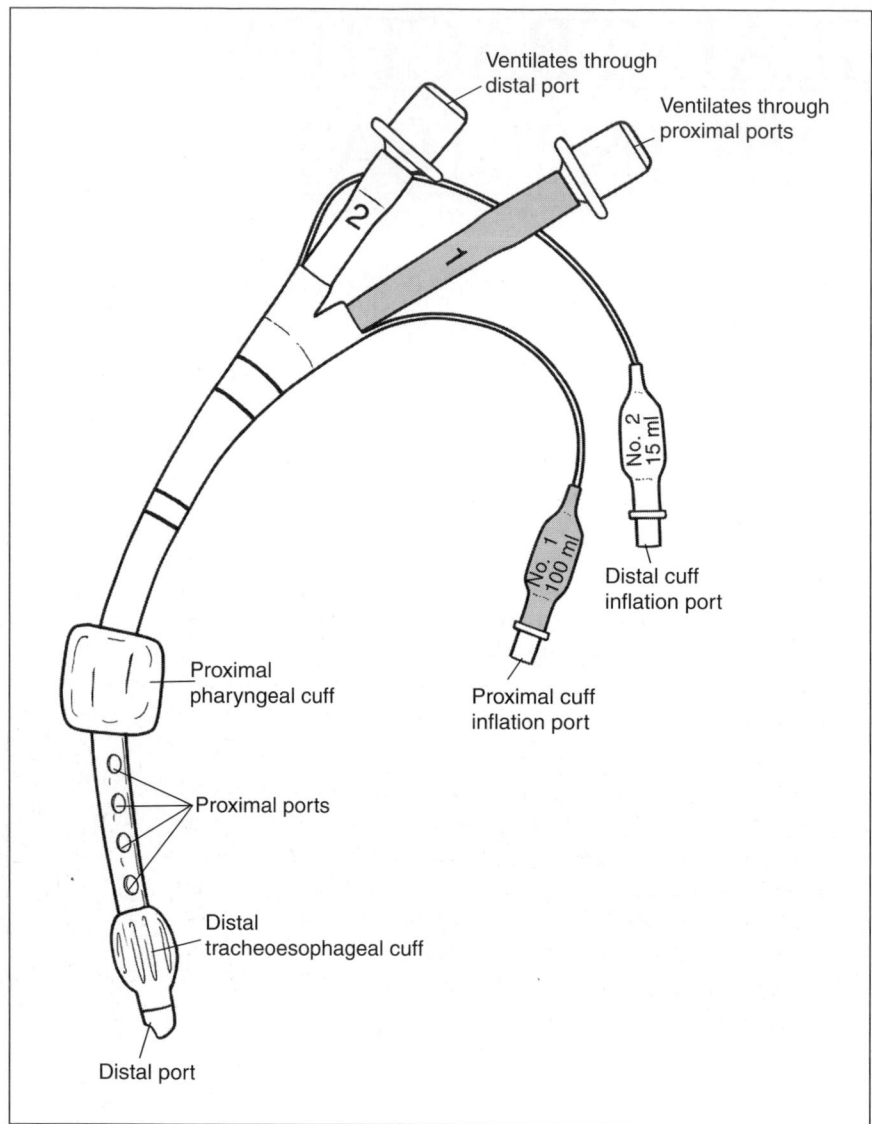

Ventilates through distal port

Ventilates through proximal ports

No. 2 15 ml

No. 1 100 ml

Distal cuff inflation port

Proximal pharyngeal cuff

Proximal cuff inflation port

Proximal ports

Distal tracheoesophageal cuff

Distal port

FIGURE 9-1 Anatomy of the Esophageal-Tracheal Combitube.

It can be used for difficult or failed orotracheal intubations. It should be placed on crash carts for use by individuals not skilled with orotracheal intubation. In situations with limited access to the patient's head (e.g., extrication situations), the ETC can be used where standard orotracheal intubation cannot be performed. Since it can be inserted with the patient's head and neck in a neutral position, the ETC should be considered in situations of potential cervical spine injury. The ETC is an appropriate device for management of the airway when visualization is limited due to bleeding or secretions. All Emergency Medicine Physicians should become familiar with the ETC if it is used by emergency medical technicians in their region as well as considering it as an alternative airway device for difficult airways.[6,7]

CONTRAINDICATIONS

Certain contraindications exist and should be addressed. **The ETC should not be used on patients with an intact gag reflex.** If intubation is anticipated, there should be enough time to premedicate the patient and induce anesthesia before inserting the ETC. The size limits of the standard ETC prevent its use in patients under 5 feet tall. The smaller SA model can be used in shorter adults and adolescent patients from 4 to 5.5 feet in height. **Neither model can be used in people less than 4 feet in height.** It should not be used if the patient has a latex allergy or has ingested a caustic substance.

The ETC is contraindicated if the patient has known esophageal disease or airway obstruction. Patients with known esophageal disease (those who have strictures or cancer or who are victims of caustic ingestions) are at an increased risk of complications such as perforation and failed performance of device. Patients with known upper airway obstruction (secondary to congenital disorders, cancer, or other anatomic abnormalities) are also at increased risk for complication and performance failure.

EQUIPMENT

The ETC comes prepackaged in kit form with the dual lumen airway, two syringes for balloon inflation, a vomit deflector, and a flexible suction catheter (Figure 9-2). The vomit deflector is not routinely used, as it may be associated with significant complications. The suction catheter is 12 French in size and designed to be inserted through the smaller tube and to exit the tracheo-esophageal port. As in any emergent situation, an oxygen source should be available, as well as equipment and supplies for advanced life support (e.g., those obtainable in a standard crash cart). Additionally, it is optimal to have equipment available for placement of a surgical airway if necessary.

PATIENT PREPARATION

Preoxygenate the patient with a bag-valve-mask device using 100% oxygen. Intravenous access should be established. The patient can be supine or in any position that may be required. The neutral position is not required. Prepare the equipment while an assistant is ventilating the patient. Remove the ETC and equipment from the package. Attach the syringes to their respective ports and inflate the cuffs (Figure 9-3). If a leak of air is present or if the cuff does not inflate properly, discard the ETC and open another packaged ETC. Deflate the

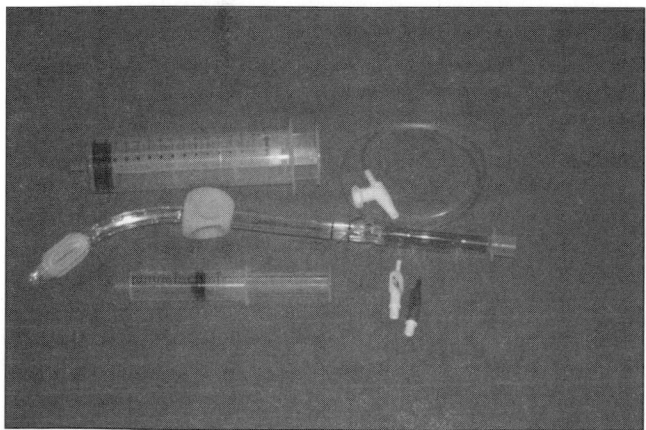

FIGURE 9-2 The Esophageal-Tracheal Combitube kit from Kendall-Sheridan, Mansfield, MA.

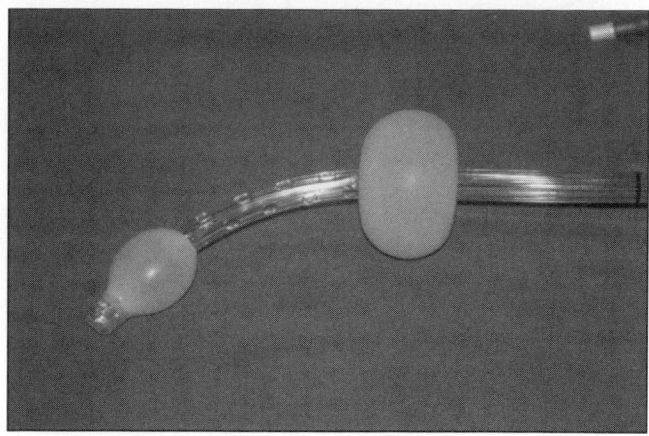

FIGURE 9-3 The Esophageal-Tracheal Combitube with the cuffs inflated.

cuffs and leave the syringes attached to the ports. Lubricate the tip of the ETC liberally.

TECHNIQUE

Insert the thumb of your nondominant hand into the patient's mouth and over the tongue (Figure 9-4*A*). Place your fingers under the chin. Depress the tongue and open the jaw simultaneously. Remove any dental devices and foreign bodies. Grasp the ETC with your dominant hand. The curve of the ETC should be in the same direction as the natural curve of the pharynx. Insert the ETC into the midline of the patient's mouth. Advance the ETC in a downward curved motion until the patient's teeth or alveolar ridge lies between the two printed bands (Figure 9-4*B*). **Do not insert the ETC forcefully as significant injury can occur**. If it does not advance easily, redirect it and then reinsert the device. Inflate the pharyngeal cuff with 100 mL of air (85 mL in the SA model). The ECT will withdraw slightly from the patient's mouth as the pharyngeal cuff is inflated. Inflate the distal cuff with 15 mL of air.

Because most intubations are esophageal, begin ventilation through the longer blue tube labeled #1 (Figure 9-4*C*). Auscultation of breath sounds, symmetric rise of the chest, fogging in the tube for more than six breaths, and lack of gastric insufflation confirm placement within the esophagus and ventilation through the proximal ports (Figure 9-4*C*). If no breath sounds are auscultated and gastric insufflation occurs, the trachea is intubated (Figure 9-4*D*). Begin ventilation through the shorter clear tube and verify by auscultation the presence of breath sounds.

If breath sounds cannot be auscultated when ventilating through either tube, the ETC may be too far into the pharynx. Deflate the pharyngeal cuff and withdraw

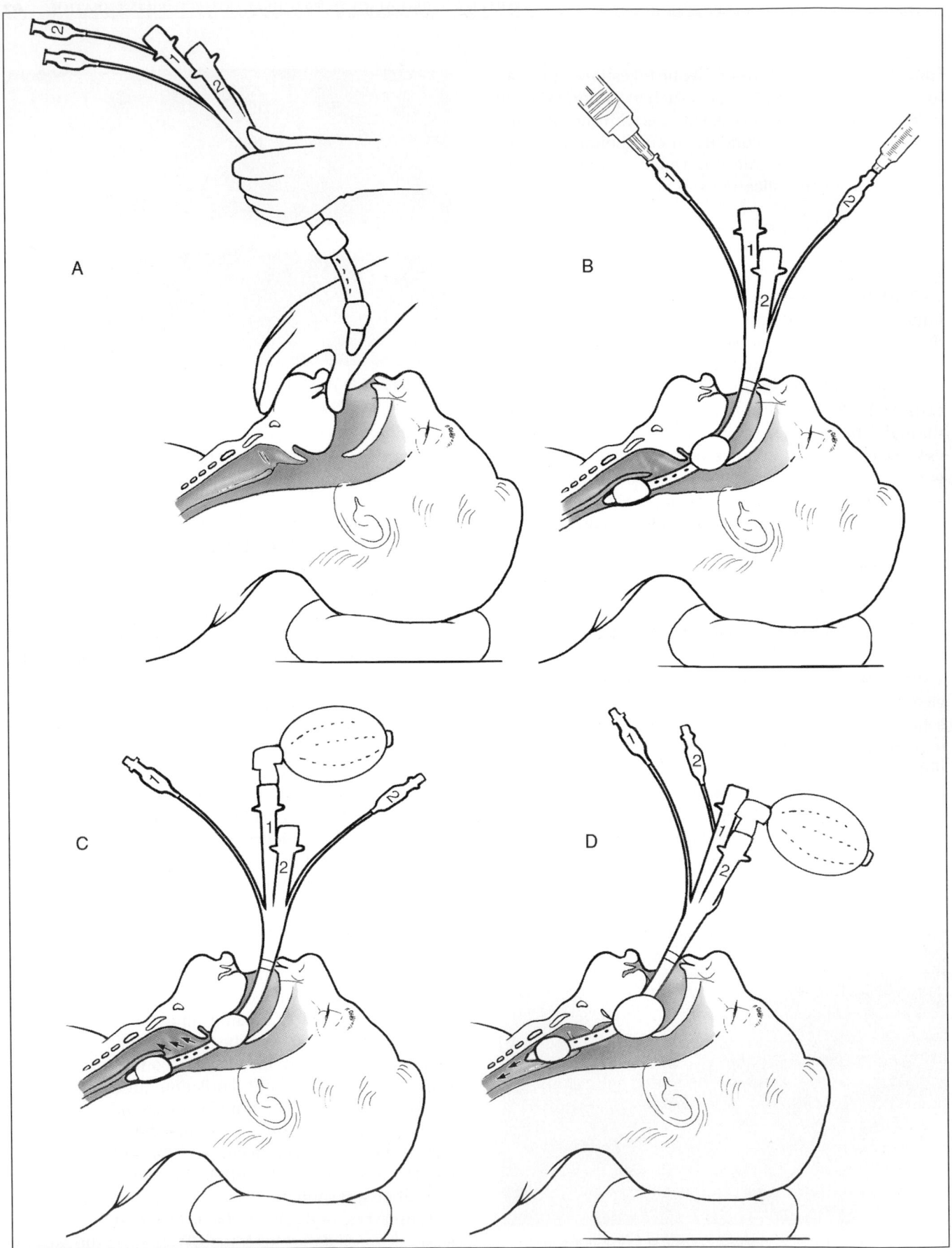

FIGURE 9-4 Insertion of the Esophageal-Tracheal Combitube. *A.* Positioning of the patient and the physician. *B.* The tube is inserted until the patient's teeth are between the black lines and the cuffs are inflated. *C.* The tube is inserted into the esophagus. The patient is ventilated through the longer tube (1) and air is directed from the proximal ports (*arrows*). *D.* The tube is inserted into the trachea. The patient is ventilated through the shorter tube (2) and air is directed through the distal port (*arrows*).

the ETC 2 to 3 cm. Reinflate the pharyngeal cuff. Ventilate through the longer tube and confirm tube placement as noted above.

AFTERCARE

Secure the ETC. This is accomplished using the standard method of taping or a commercially available endotracheal tube holder. Although there are reports of short-term (4 to 6 hours) ventilator use with the Combitube, most practitioners will choose to replace the ETC with a standard endotracheal tube for long-term ventilation.[8] Several methods for replacing the ETC are available.

The first is to remove the ETC entirely and intubate the patient orotracheally. Deflate the pharyngeal cuff. Suction the patient's mouth and oropharynx. Tilt the ETC to the left side of the patient's mouth. Deflate the distal cuff. Remove the ETC. Intubate the patient orotracheally by the standard method.[9]

Alternative methods of intubation are also possible. Deflate the pharyngeal cuff. Suction the mouth and oropharynx. Tilt the ETC to the left side of the patient's mouth. Insert the laryngoscope and visualize the tip of the ETC. If it is in the esophagus, intubate the patient, deflate the distal cuff, and remove the ETC. This method will prevent aspiration, especially if endotracheal intubation is unsuccessful. If the tube is in the trachea, an assistant should deflate the distal cuff and remove the ETC. After the ETC clears the patient's vocal cords, immediately insert the endotracheal tube.

COMPLICATIONS

Despite the potential utility of the ETC in acute situations, several disadvantages must be kept in mind. These include its high cost, bulky packaging, and the fact that the detachable "vomit deflector" can be a biohazard if improperly managed. It is best not to use the vomit deflector, as it is associated with aspiration. Several risks are also inherent to the insertion and mechanics of the ETC. It should be recognized that the presence of a rigid cervical collar can cause great difficulties in the proper placement of this device.[10] The ETC is most frequently inserted into the esophagus. Therefore there is a risk of esophageal injury.[11] **There is no way to suction the trachea with the open distal port in the esophagus. It is important to note that resuscitation drugs that can be routinely given through an endotracheal tube cannot be given through the ETC positioned with the tip in the esophagus.** Drugs will accumulate in the blind end of the tube and not reach the circulatory system. Significant soft tissue injury can occur due to the tip of the de-

vice or if the balloons contain too much air.[10,12] If forced, the tip can perforate the esophagus, piriform sinus, or vallecula.

SUMMARY

The Esophageal-Tracheal Combitube can adequately ventilate a patient whether it is placed in the esophageal or tracheal position. It is relatively simple to use and requires minimal training. It offers an additional technique for emergency care providers to secure the airway in both the prehospital and hospital environment. It should be included in every armamentarium dedicated to the difficult airway.

REFERENCES

1. Doerges V, Sauer C, Ocker H: Airway management during cardiopulmonary resuscitation: comparative study of bag-valve-mask, laryngeal mask airway and Combitube in a bench model. *Resuscitation* 1999; 41(1):63–69.
2. Rumball CJ, MacDonald D: The PTL, Combitube, laryngeal mask, and oral airway: a randomized prehospital comparative study of ventilatory device effectiveness and cost-effectiveness in 470 cases of cardiorespiratory arrest. *Prehosp Emerg Care* 1997; 1(1):1–10.
3. Levitan RM, Kush S, Hollander JE: Devices for difficult airway management in academic emergency departments: results of a national survey. *Ann Emerg Med* 1999; 33(6):694–698.
4. Calkins MD, Robinson TD: Combat trauma airway management: endotracheal intubation versus laryngeal mask airway versus Combitube use by Navy SEAL and reconnaissance combat corpsmen. *J Trauma* 1999; 46(5):927–932.
5. Yardy N, Hancox D, Strang T: A comparison of two airway aids for emergency use by unskilled personnel. The Combitube and laryngeal mask. *Anaesthesia* 1999; 54(2):181–183.
6. Klauser R, Roggla G, Pidlich J: Massive upper airway bleeding after thrombolytic therapy: successful airway management with the Combitube. *Ann Emerg Med* 1992; 21(4):431–433.
7. Blostein PA, Koestner AJ, Hoak S: Failed rapid sequence intubation in trauma patients: esophageal tracheal Combitube is a useful adjunct. *J Trauma* 1998; 44(3):534–537.
8. Frass M, Frenzer R, Mayer G: Mechanical ventilation with the Esophageal Tracheal Combitube (ETC) in the intensive care unit. *Arch Emerg Med* 1987; 4(4):219–225.

9. Urtubia RM, Aguila CM, Cumsille MA: Combitube: a study for proper use. *Anesth Analg* 2000; 90(4):958–962.

10. Mercer MH, Gabbott DA: Insertion of the Combitube airway with the cervical spine immobilized in a rigid cervical collar. *Anaesthesia* 1998; 53(10):971–974.

11. Oczenski W, Krenn H, Dahaba AA, et al: Complications following the use of the Combitube, tracheal tube and laryngeal mask airway. *Anaesthesia* 1999; 54(12):1161–1165.

12. Wafai Y, Salem MR, Baraka A, et al: Effectiveness of the self-inflating bulb for verification of proper placement of the Esophageal Tracheal Combitube. *Anesth Analg* 1995; 80:122–126.

Chapter 10
FIBEROPTIC ENDOSCOPIC INTUBATION

James R. Markey
David J. Bird

INTRODUCTION

The flexible fiberoptic bronchoscope has become a popular and useful instrument for placing endotracheal tubes in awake and nonparalyzed patients. **It is unique in that its flexible cord allows it to conform to the patient's anatomy, making intubation possible in a variety of clinical situations when intubation by direct laryngoscopy is likely to be difficult or impossible.** When performed properly, awake fiberoptic tracheal intubation is more accepted by patients and is associated with fewer hemodynamic changes than awake laryngoscopy.[1] It may be used to intubate a patient orally or nasally. It provides excellent visualization of the airway.

Proficiency in the skills required for fiberoptic intubation requires both instruction and practice.[2] In most instances, it is a lack of expertise with the fiberoptic bronchoscope as well as inadequate patient preparation that results in technical problems and prevents the successful completion of fiberoptic intubation. Successful intubation is also prevented when blood and/or secretions obstruct the fiberoptic port.

ANATOMY AND PATHOPHYSIOLOGY

A more detailed description of airway anatomy is provided in Chapters 1 and 2, on airway anatomy and basic airway management. Interested readers are referred to other sources for a more detailed description of the fiberoptic bronchoscope's anatomy.[3]

The basic anatomy of the fiberoptic bronchoscope is shown in Figure 10-1. The major components are the handle, the insertion cord, and a light source. The handle contains the eyepiece for image viewing and a dial to bring the image into focus. A lever controls an angulation wire, which allows for movement of the bronchoscope's insertion cord tip in one plane.

The bronchoscope's insertion cord is composed of thousands of glass fibers, each approximately 10 μm in diameter, which transmit an image to a more proximal viewing lens. These fiber bundles are fragile and break easily, resulting in deterioration of the visual image; thus they should be handled with care. There is a side port that can be used for the insufflation of oxygen, instillation of local anesthetic or saline solution, limited suction (due to the small size of the port), passage of a guidewire, and end-tidal CO_2 monitoring.[4,5] Any fiberoptic bronchoscope used for intubation should have a length of at least 55 to 60 cm. Although fiberoptic nasopharyngoscopes have been successfully used for endotracheal intubation, they are typically unsuitable because of their short length.[6,7]

INDICATIONS

Fiberoptic intubation of the airway is indicated in situations where it becomes necessary to secure a patient's airway, and an awake intubation technique is preferable to one that renders the patient unconscious. This would include patients who are at increased risk for aspiration of their gastric contents (e.g., uncertain about food intake, less than 8 hours fasting, alcohol intoxication, parturient, bowel obstruction). A fiberoptic intubation is indicated when it is anticipated that direct laryngoscopy might be difficult to perform. This would include morbidly obese patients, those having limited mandibular opening, an unstable or immobile cervical spine, macroglossia, micrognathia, patients who appear to have pathologic airway anatomy (tracheal deviation, stenosis, tumors, trauma), and those who appear to be at increased risk for dental damage.[4]

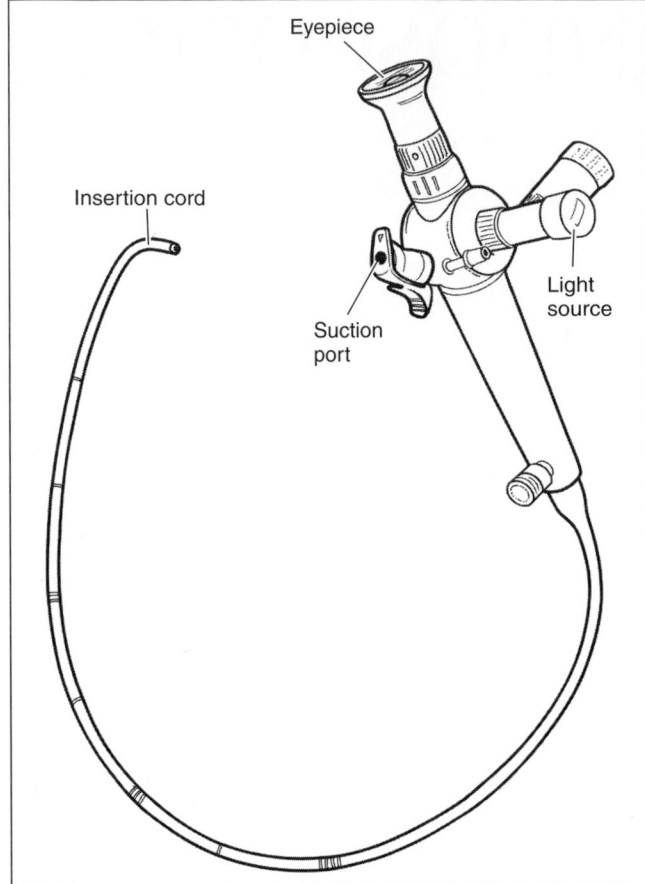

FIGURE 10-1 Anatomy of the fiberoptic intubating bronchoscope.

CONTRAINDICATIONS

Fiberoptic intubation is not recommended for those patients who are actively vomiting or have significant oropharyngeal bleeding. These fluids will cover the fiberoptic port and prevent visualization through the bronchoscope. Patients who are hypoxic or require assisted ventilation by mask are poor candidates for fiberoptic intubation, since the technique can require several minutes to perform. An exception might be when a patient can be ventilated by laryngeal mask airway through which fiberoptic endotracheal intubation may be performed.[8,9] Contraindications specific to nasal fiberoptic intubation would include coagulopathy, significant midface trauma, severe intranasal pathology, fracture of the cribriform plate, and leakage of cerebrospinal fluid.[4]

Relative contraindications to fiberoptic intubation of the airway are situations when instrumentation of the airway may further compromise airway patency, such as stridor resulting from airway edema, infection, or epiglottitis. **Some authors advocate fiberoptic intubation as an option to consider in these circumstances, but only by individuals extremely proficient at fiberop-**tic intubation and only with an Otolaryngologist standing by to perform an emergency tracheostomy if the need arises.[7,10] Otherwise, it might be prudent to first proceed with establishing an airway by utilizing a different method, including a surgical airway. Occasionally, an emergency tracheostomy cannot be successfully performed in these patients before complete airway obstruction occurs. Therefore, one should always be prepared to provide oxygen emergently by another route (e.g., transtracheal jet ventilation) to prevent brain damage due to hypoxia.

EQUIPMENT

Nasal Anesthesia

Cotton-tipped applicators
4% lidocaine
0.25% phenylephrine
4% cocaine

Oropharyngeal Anesthesia

2% viscous lidocaine or benzocaine spray
Cotton 4×4 swabs soaked in 4% lidocaine
Emesis basin
Yankauer suction
Tongue blade

Laryngeal Anesthesia

Alcohol swabs
10 mL syringes
21 gauge needle, 1½ inches
4% lidocaine, for transtracheal injection or nebulizer administration
1% lidocaine anesthetic solution
Nebulizer device with tubing

Fiberoptic Bronchoscopy and Intubation

An assistant
Fiberoptic bronchoscope with working channel
Light source
Endotracheal tubes, various sizes
Suction source and catheters
Cuffed tracheal tubes of various sizes
Oxygen source
Oxygen tubing
Bag-valve device
Face masks
Water-soluble lubricant or anesthetic jelly
Gauze 4×4 squares
Antisialagogue (glycopyrrolate 0.3 to 0.4 mg IV or IM, atropine 0.5 mg IV)

Miscellaneous Supplies

Alternative invasive intubation kit/device
Cricothyroidotomy tray/kit
Medications (paralytics, sedatives, etc.)
Crash cart
Cardiac monitor
Pulse oximetry

PATIENT PREPARATION

Fiberoptic intubation is best performed on awake and spontaneously breathing patients. Rendering the patient unconscious might relax and distort the airway anatomy, placing the patient at risk for more serious complications including apnea, airway obstruction, and aspiration of gastric contents.[11] **Proper patient preparation is essential to the successful completion of a fiberoptic intubation.** Proper patient preparation includes counseling the patient, clearing the airway of secretions and blood, judicious sedation, and anesthetizing the mouth, pharynx, larynx, and trachea.[4]

Counseling is an important and often underestimated part of patient preparation. The bronchoscopist can gain the patient's confidence and cooperation, which are invaluable aids for the performance of a successful fiberoptic intubation. Thoroughly explain the necessity for the procedure and the technique.

Before proceeding with fiberoptic bronchoscopy, monitors for electrocardiogram, blood pressure, and pulse oximetry should be placed along with an intravenous line for the administration of drugs. Supplemental oxygen should be administered and can be delivered either by nasal cannula, "blow-by," or through the side port of the fiberoptic bronchoscope. Delivering oxygen through the side port offers the additional advantage of blowing airway secretions away from the fiberoptic bronchoscope's tip. Unfortunately it has the potential disadvantage of causing gastric distention.[12]

Instrumentation of the airway may cause the patient to produce copious secretions, making an otherwise straightforward fiberoptic bronchoscopy extremely difficult. Bronchoscopy via a dry airway devoid of secretions can be accomplished in most instances by administering 0.3 to 0.4 mg of glycopyrrolate. This is a potent antisialagogue and should be administered intravenously 20 minutes before or intramuscularly 30 minutes before fiberoptic bronchoscopy.

Sedation can be extremely beneficial in gaining patient cooperation during the performance of fiberoptic bronchoscopy.[13] Sedative drugs, if used at all, should be judiciously titrated to the desired effect with continual assessment of the patient's level of consciousness, while at the same time avoiding respiratory depression. Midazolam given in small doses (0.015 to 0.075 mg/kg) has the advantage of producing minimal respiratory depression and may be preferable to opioids. Sedation should be avoided if, at the time of fiberoptic bronchoscopy, the patient has a tenuous airway, labored respirations, a distended abdomen, or is vomiting.

The patient may be in a sitting, semirecumbent, or supine position during fiberoptic bronchoscopy. In morbidly obese patients, the sitting position will, by virtue of gravity, displace redundant pharyngeal tissue anteriorly and open the pharyngeal space.[14] However, use of the sitting position also requires the bronchoscopist to stand at the patient's side, thus inverting the image seen through the fiberoptic bronchoscope. Alternatively, the bronchoscopist can stand on a platform in order to be of sufficient height to correctly perform the procedure. When performing the procedure with the patient in the supine position, the patient's head should lie flat against the table surface with the neck extended (if it is safe to do so). This head position brings the tracheal axis more in line with the nasal and oral passageways and elevates the epiglottis from the posterior pharyngeal wall. The "sniffing position," while optimal for direct laryngoscopy, increases obstruction of the glottis by the epiglottis during fiberoptic bronchoscopy and makes the passage of the fiberoptic bronchoscope more difficult.[14] Maneuvers performed by an assistant, such as the jaw thrust or pulling the tongue forward with a cotton swab, can help to move the pharyngeal tissue anteriorly and allow increased maneuverability of the fiberoptic bronchoscope's tip.[4]

AIRWAY ANESTHESIA

In order to establish a quiet larynx devoid of reflexes, it is extremely helpful, prior to attempting fiberoptic bronchoscopy, to provide regional anesthesia of the airway. This will also gain the patient's acceptance and cooperation during the procedure. It is especially effective in improving the success rate of individuals who are less experienced at performing fiberoptic intubation. Whether to abolish the laryngeal reflexes of a patient considered to have a "full stomach" remains an unresolved controversy. In considering this option, one must weigh the risk of abolishing the laryngeal reflexes and rendering the patient potentially vulnerable to gastric aspiration versus leaving the laryngeal reflexes intact and thus also maintaining the associated discomfort for the patient. When deliberating whether or not to proceed with a regional block of the larynx in a patient considered to be at risk for gastric aspiration, bear in mind that aspiration of gastric contents can and occasionally does occur in patients with intact laryngeal reflexes. Also, instrumentation of the airway in patients with an intact gag reflex is very likely to induce vomiting.

If the nasal passageways are the anticipated route for intubation, they should be prepared by shrinking and anesthetizing the nasal mucosa. Cocaine (4%) applied topically (maximum dose 200 mg) has the advantage of providing profound vasoconstriction and anesthesia to the nasal passageways. The same effect can be provided by applying 0.25 to 1.0% phenylephrine topically to the nasal mucosa, followed by 4% lidocaine via cotton-tipped applicators. These applicators should be gently placed, one at a time, through the middle meatus and back to the inferior turbinate. A nasal passage that accommodates four to five single cotton-tipped applicators will usually allow passage of a 7.0 mm endotracheal tube.[4]

Once the antisialagogues have taken effect, the tongue and pharynx can be anesthetized. Place a tongue blade on the patient's tongue and apply topical anesthetic spray. While the manufacture of 10% lidocaine spray has recently ceased, benzocaine spray remains available and will usually provide effective anesthesia for the posterior pharynx within 30 seconds. There are numerous reports of methemoglobinemia from the overzealous use of benzocaine.[15] It should be limited to several short sprays.

Alternatively, the patient can swish viscous 2% lidocaine in their mouth for several minutes to provide effective anesthesia. There are several methods of block-ing the glossopharyngeal nerve, the simplest of which, if the patient is not at risk for aspiration, is to apply lidocaine-soaked cotton swabs to the palatoglossal arch for 5 minutes.

Bilateral blockade of the superior laryngeal nerve will provide effective anesthesia of the supraglottic structures (Figure 10-2). These nerves can be blocked by contacting the superior cornua of the hyoid bone with the tip of a 21 gauge needle. Contact with the bone can be made easier by extending the patient's head and gently palpating the hyoid bone with the thumb and forefinger of one hand. By applying gentle pressure to one side, the opposite cornua comes into closer contact with the skin and is subsequently easier to contact with the needle. Walk the needle tip off the bone inferiorly and advance it 3 to 4 mm through the thyrohyoid membrane. **Aspiration should be performed before injecting the anesthetic solution to confirm that the needle has not entered the external carotid artery.** Inject 2 mL of 1% lidocaine.

Occasionally, the hyoid bone cannot be palpated due to obesity, infections, or masses. In those instances, a superior laryngeal nerve block should not be attempted. As an alternative, nebulized 4% lidocaine administered for at least 20 minutes prior to fiberoptic bronchoscopy

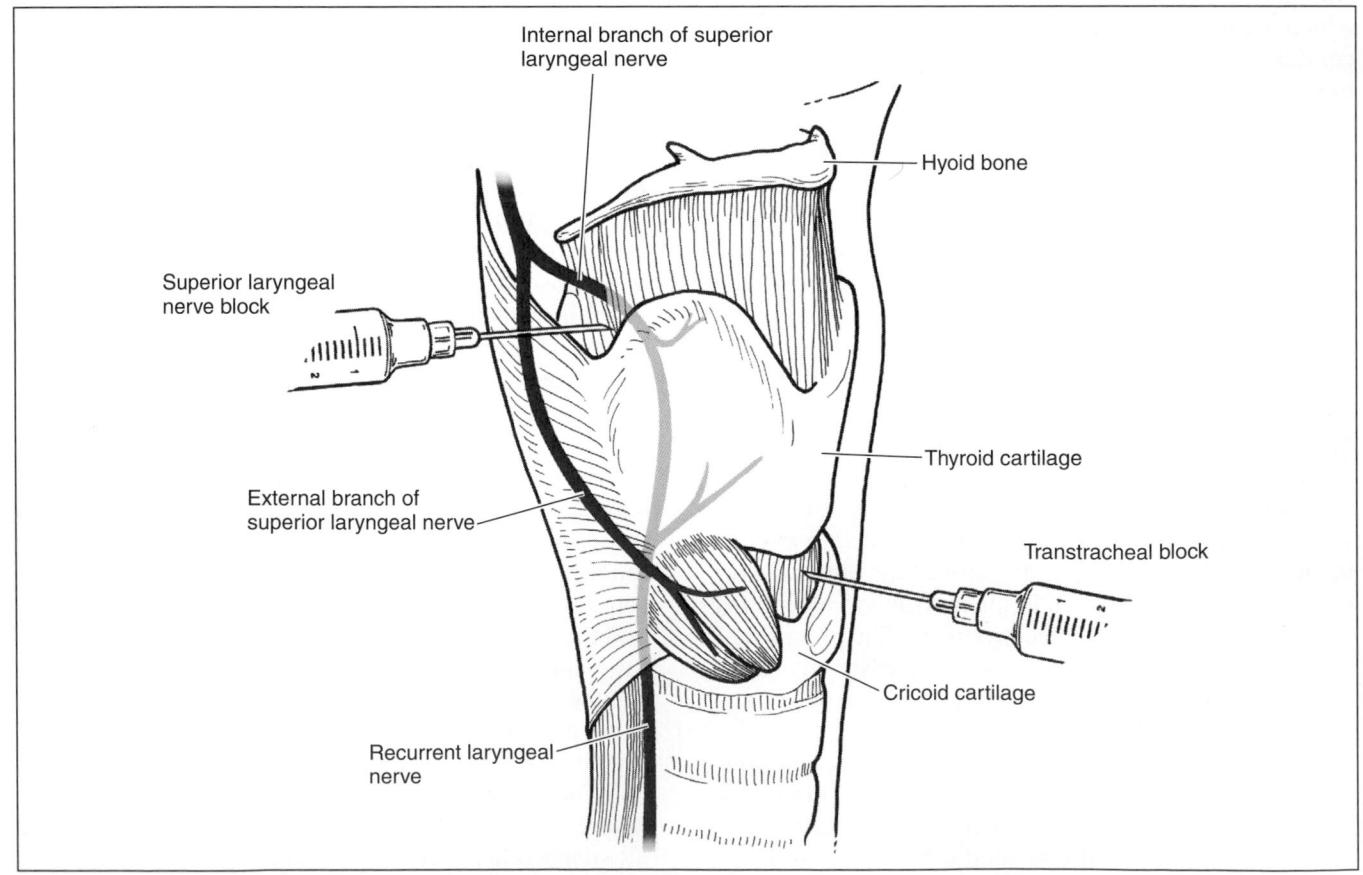

FIGURE 10-2 Anatomy of the larynx. The syringes demonstrate the superior laryngeal nerve block and the transtracheal block.

will usually provide adequate anesthesia of the supraglottic structures. A second alternative is the "spray as you go" technique. Once the epiglottis is visualized through the fiberoptic bronchoscope, instill 3 to 4 mL of 4% lidocaine through the working channel of the scope and onto the epiglottis and the surface of the vocal cords.[4] This will induce coughing and temporarily obliterate the view of the laryngeal structures. Allow 2 to 3 minutes for the anesthetic solution to exert its effect before proceeding with fiberoptic bronchoscopy.

The right and left recurrent laryngeal nerves provide sensory innervation to the trachea and the laryngeal structures below the vocal cords. They can be effectively blocked by performing a transtracheal injection of 4 mL of 4% lidocaine (Figure 10-2). Clean the surface of the skin over the cricothyroid membrane. Advance a 20 gauge intravenous catheter-over-the-needle on a 5 mL syringe containing 2 to 3 mL of sterile saline, perpendicularly through the cricothyroid membrane. Advance the unit until it is in the trachea (1 to 2 cm). The lumen of the trachea is identified by the loss of resistance. Aspiration of air, as evidenced by the presence of bubbles in the syringe, also signifies that the trachea has been entered. **Care should be taken to not pass entirely through the trachea, as this could result in a pneumomediastinum.**[16] Once the trachea has been entered, advance the catheter over the needle and into the trachea. Withdraw the needle and syringe. Attach a syringe containing 3 to 4 mL of 4% lidocaine to the catheter. Briskly inject the lidocaine through the catheter and into the tracheal lumen. This will cause the patient to cough and disperse the local anesthetic solution throughout the trachea.

After completion of the blocks, a suction catheter should be passed into the oropharyngeal cavity. This will clear the airway of secretions and blood that can impair the visual image. It will also determine the adequacy of topical anesthesia for preventing coughing and gagging.

TECHNIQUES

Prepare the fiberoptic bronchoscope. Attach the light source. Check the focus of the image by holding the tip of the insertion cord 1 to 2 cm over a printed page. Adjust the eyepiece until the letters on the image are clear. Note how the image appears as you move toward and away from the page. Briefly use the angulation lever to move the tip of the insertion cord and learn its movements. **The most difficult aspect of mastering fiberoptic bronchoscopy is learning to simultaneously angulate the tip, rotate the scope, and advance the insertion cord.**[7] It requires repetition and practice to develop these skills before attempting to intubate a patient.

Before insertion of the fiberoptic bronchoscope into the endotracheal tube, let the fiberoptic strands hang toward the floor. Identify the plane in which the angulation lever moves the tip. When fiberoptic bronchoscopes are stored coiled in a case, over time the insertion cord may develop a curve. Slightly rotate the fiberscope to the right or left until the angulation of the tip is in the midline plane. Look through the eyepiece and note the position of the directional arrow (▼) on the anterior edge of the image that correlates with midline.

To prevent fogging, apply antifog solution to the insertion cord tip or place the tip in warm water before inserting the fiberoptic bronchoscope into the patient's airway. Warming the endotracheal tube with warm water just prior to placing it on the insertion cord will soften the tube and may make the later advancement of the endotracheal tube through the nares easier.

Apply a thin film of silicone spray or water-soluble lubricant over the insertion cord to facilitate passage of the endotracheal tube over the flexible cord. Insert the flexible insertion cord completely through the endotracheal tube, taking care not to get any of the lubricant on the lens tip. The insertion tip should exit the distal tip of the endotracheal tube. Do not place the tip of the insertion cord through the Murphy eye of the endotracheal tube. Lubricate the endotracheal tube liberally.

Hold the fiberoptic bronchoscope in your dominant hand with the angulation lever operated by the thumb and the suction port (if used) covered by the index finger (Figure 10-3). The other end of the scope should be held between the index finger and thumb of the nondominant hand. Place the nondominant hand at the patient's nose or mouth. There should be no slack in the fiberoptic bronchoscope between the two hands. The removal of slack from the insertion cord makes more precise rotary movements of the tip possible.

NASAL INTUBATION

Nasal fiberoptic intubation has advantages over the oral route. For those less experienced at fiberoptic bronchoscopy, nasal fiberoptic bronchoscopy is usually easier to perform because less angulation of the tip is required.[10] Once inserted, nasal endotracheal tubes are better tolerated by patients and are associated with a lower incidence of accidental extubation. Disadvantages include a higher incidence of bacteremia, middle ear infection, epistaxis, and alar necrosis.[4] **Nasal intubation, unlike oral intubation, may produce bacteremia; therefore appropriate endocarditis prophylaxis should be provided for those at risk.**

Through inspection, determine which is the most patent nostril. Remove the insertion cord from the endotracheal tube. Advance the endotracheal tube through the nares until the tip is just past the soft palate. This is usually at a depth of 10 to 12 cm. Pass the insertion cord through the endotracheal tube. This approach has the advantage of bringing the tip of the fiberscope directly

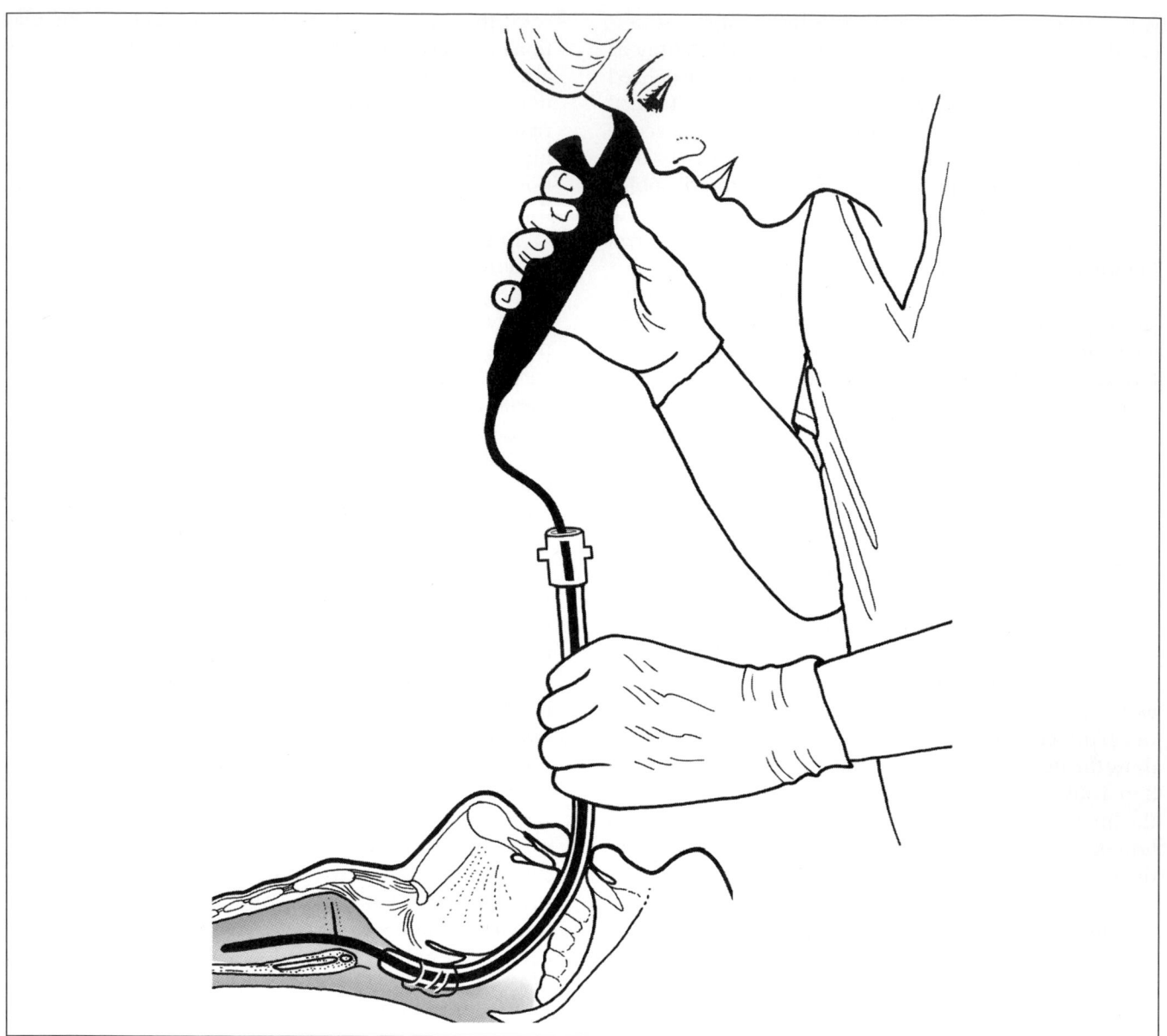

FIGURE 10-3 After the tip of the fiberoptic bronchoscope is placed in the trachea, the endotracheal tube is advanced.

midline and toward the epiglottis. The disadvantage here is that of causing some patient discomfort very early on in the procedure and possibly decreasing patient cooperation before the insertion cord has entered the trachea. There is the potential for epistaxis, making visualization of laryngeal structures difficult if not impossible. Despite the application of topical anesthesia to the nasal passages, they are difficult to anesthetize completely. For the awake patient, passage of the tracheal tube is often the most uncomfortable part of the fiberoptic intubation procedure.

A second preferred approach is to temporarily affix the endotracheal tube to the fiberoptic bronchoscope handle with tape. Insert and navigate the insertion cord's tip along the posterior floor of the nares. Continue to advance the insertion cord until the endotracheal tube enters the oropharynx. This will serve to minimize patient discomfort and the risk of epistaxis early in the procedure. Occasionally, loss of view and maneuverability of the fiberscope's tip occurs in the velopharyngeal area as the tip of the fiberscope encounters the pharyngeal mucosa. Pulling the tongue forward with gauze, using the jaw-thrust maneuver, or simply advancing the insertion cord a few centimeters further will usually bring pharyngeal structures back into view.

The distance from the nares to the epiglottis is usually about 15 cm, and at this point the epiglottis will come into view.[7] **If the 15 cm mark has been passed, it**

is very likely that the fiberoptic bronchoscope has entered the esophagus. If that is the case, withdraw it to 12 cm and redirect the tip upward with a slight downward movement of the angulation lever. This will usually bring the glottic opening into view. Occasionally, the epiglottis will obscure the glottic opening. Position the tip of the fiberoptic bronchoscope just above the tip of the epiglottis, then advance it a few millimeters posterior to the epiglottis while angulating the tip of the fiberoptic bronchoscope slightly anterior by pressing down on the angulation lever. This will bring the glottic opening into view. Simultaneously rotate, angulate, and advance the fiberoptic bronchoscope tip toward and past the vocal cords.

Once the fiberoptic bronchoscope tip has passed the vocal cords, bring the tip into neutral position with a light downward motion of the angulation lever. Occasionally, some operators have difficulty passing the fiberscope through the vocal cords. There are several common causes for this. The tip of the scope may remain angulated and abutting the wall of the trachea. The vocal cords may not be properly anesthetized and may therefore have closed reflexively.[17] Finally, the fiberoptic bronchoscope's tip may be abutting the arytenoid cartilages or the pyriform sinus. If inadequate anesthesia is the cause, inject 2 mL of 4% lidocaine through the working channel of the fiberscope and wait several minutes for it to take effect. Additionally, having the patient inspire deeply will bring the vocal cords into greater opposition.

Once past the vocal cords, advance the insertion cord tip further to bring the bifurcation of the trachea at the carina into view. The trachea can easily be identified anteriorly by the cartilaginous rings and posteriorly by the smooth mucosa of the posterior wall. Advance the endotracheal tube over the fiberoptic bronchoscope and into the trachea (Figure 10-3).

Occasionally, when the trachea is not anesthetized, the patient's subsequent coughing and the associated muscular contractions of the trachealis muscle will collapse the trachea almost completely. This makes it difficult to discern if the insertion cord tip is actually in the trachea or whether to advance the insertion cord or endotracheal tube into the trachea. Wait until the trachealis muscle relaxes and then continue with the procedure.

To prevent endobronchial intubation in adults, which can occur with flexion of the head, confirm that the tip of the endotracheal tube is 3 cm above the carina.[18] This is accomplished by advancing the tip of the fiberoptic bronchoscope to the carina with the thumb and forefinger of the nondominant hand. Mark the point on the insertion cord where it exits the endotracheal tube. Look through the eyepiece while withdrawing the fiberoptic bronchoscope until the tip of the tracheal tube is visualized. Note the distance on the insertion cord between the marked point and the tracheal tube connector. This

difference in length correlates with the distance between the tracheal tube tip and the carina.

Occasionally, difficulty is encountered while attempting to pass the endotracheal tube through the nares and nasal cavity. This might be caused by a deviated nasal septum, enlarged turbinates, a nasal spur (which can also tear the endotracheal tube cuff), or nasal polyps. Selection of an endotracheal tube that is too large, inadequate lubrication, or failure to presoften the endotracheal tube can be the cause. Reattempt insertion with a well-lubricated, presoftened endotracheal tube that is 0.5 to 1.0 mm smaller.

Inability to pass the endotracheal tube past the vocal cords is usually related to the endotracheal tube becoming caught on the epiglottis, aryepiglottic folds, or corniculate cartilages.[17,19] This occurs with greater frequency when the diameter of the fiberoptic bronchoscope is significantly smaller than that of the endotracheal tube or with oral fiberoptic intubation, due to the greater curve that the endotracheal tube must assume for it to enter the trachea.[7] When this occurs, withdraw the endotracheal tube slightly, rotate it 15 degrees, and reattempt to pass it over the insertion cord and into the trachea.[10] If this maneuver fails, rotate the endotracheal tube so that its bevel faces either posteriorly or to the left and laterally. Reattempt to advance the tube. If these maneuvers are unsuccessful, consider substituting either a smaller endotracheal tube or a spiral-bound endotracheal tube. The latter usually passes on the first attempt, most likely because of its flexibility and the more obtuse angle of its bevel.[20]

ORAL INTUBATION

Begin by noting any loose or broken teeth. After ensuring an adequate sensory block by absence of a gag reflex, one of several oral intubating airways available on the market (Ovassapian, Patil, Wilkes) can be inserted into the patient's mouth. These devices are placed in the patient's mouth like any other oral airway. They allow for the midline passage of the endotracheal tube and fiberoptic bronchoscope. These devices also serve to protect the delicate glass fibers within the insertion cord from the patient's teeth.

Technical problems exist in attempting oral fiberoptic intubation. As stated earlier, oral fiberoptic intubation requires that the insertion cord tip traverse a more acute angle to reach the vocal cords than it would by the nasal route. If one can safely do so, maximally extending the patient's head at the atlantooccipital joint will bring the oropharyngeal and laryngeal axes more closely in line. This maneuver will reduce the angle that the fiberoptic bronchoscope tip must traverse.

In performing oral intubation, the endotracheal tube becomes hung up on the vocal cords more frequently than with the nasal route. A technique believed to significantly improve the first-time pass rate with oral fiberoptic bronchoscopic intubation is to pass a lubricated 5.0 mm inner diameter (ID) endotracheal tube through a 7.0 mm ID endotracheal tube that has been cut to 24 cm. This should leave 2 cm of the 5.0 mm ID endotracheal tube protruding from distal end. It is believed that the close approximation of the diameters of the 5.0 mm ID endotracheal tube and the fiberoptic bronchoscope allows easier passage of the scope. After the 5.0 mm ID/7.0 mm ID endotracheal tube complex is in place, withdraw the 5.0 mm ID endotracheal tube, leaving the 7.0 mm ID endotracheal tube in the trachea.[21]

ALTERNATIVE TECHNIQUES

Alternative techniques that have been shown to be as effective as fiberoptic intubation for intubating patients with unstable cervical spines include the Bullard laryngoscope[22] and the lighted stylet.[23] Blind nasotracheal intubation has been shown to be as successful as nasal fiberoptic intubation in anesthetized patients with unstable cervical spines, but the comparison has yet to be made for awake patients.[24]

A combined technique using oral fiberoptic intubation through a laryngeal mask airway (LMA) can be extremely helpful in instances where there is severe oropharyngeal bleeding or when a patient is unconscious and direct laryngoscopy is not possible.[8,10] After confirming successful placement of the LMA (Chapter 17), place a self-sealing bronchoscopy elbow over the proximal end of a 6.0 mm ID endotracheal tube. Advance the endotracheal tube tip through the LMA until the LMA grille is encountered (resistance will be felt). Inflate just enough air into the endotracheal tube cuff to provide a seal for positive-pressure ventilation via the endotracheal tube. Advance the insertion cord through the endotracheal tube and into the trachea under direct visualization. Deflate the endotracheal tube cuff. Advance the endotracheal tube over the fiberoptic bronchoscope and into the trachea until the endotracheal tube adapter meets the adapter of the LMA. Inflate the endotracheal tube cuff and confirm ventilation through the endotracheal tube.

Because standard endotracheal tubes are not long enough to allow removal of the LMA, longer endotracheal tubes have been developed. If you do not have access to a specially made endotracheal tube, use a nasal Rae tube, which is 6 cm longer than a standard endotracheal tube. If a longer endotracheal tube is not available, another endotracheal tube can be temporarily lengthened by removing the adapter of the 6.0 mm ID endotracheal tube and placing the tip of a 5.0 mm ID endotracheal tube into the lumen of the 6.0 mm ID endotracheal tube. This maneuver lengthens the endotracheal tube

enough that the LMA cuff can be deflated and withdrawn, leaving the 6.0 mm ID endotracheal tube correctly placed in the trachea. Additionally, ventilation can be maintained the entire time simply by using a bagvalve device connected to the 5.0 mm ID endotracheal tube adapter. After removing the LMA, remove the 5.0 mm ID endotracheal tube from the 6.0 mm ID endotracheal tube, replace the adapter, and resume ventilation.[25] After removing the LMA and establishing ventilation, always confirm by fiberoptic bronchoscopy that the endotracheal tube is correctly positioned.

ASSESSMENT

Always verify that the endotracheal tube lies in the trachea. This can be reliably accomplished by both fiberoptic means and by the presence of expired end-tidal CO_2. After properly securing the tracheal tube, confirm that it is properly positioned above the carina by either fiberoptic bronchoscopy or a chest radiograph.

COMPLICATIONS

While the fiberscope is passed through the glottis and into the trachea under direct vision, the tracheal tube is passed blindly over the bronchoscope's tip. It is thus possible to cause injury to the arytenoids, resulting in permanent hoarseness, particularly if the tracheal tube's bevel faces anteriorly.[26]

The tracheal tube may also be blocked in the nasal cavity or larynx, resulting in epistaxis, nasal turbinate fracture, and tearing of the tracheal tube's cuff.[1,4] Sinusitis and otitis media are also known complications from nasal intubation.[4]

SUMMARY

Awake intubation under direct visualization in spontaneously breathing patients by either the oral or nasal route is possible with the fiberoptic bronchoscope. Intubation by means of the fiberoptic bronchoscope is an option to consider when direct laryngoscopy is risky, difficult, or impossible. In some instances, awake fiberoptic intubation may be preferable to other emergency intubation techniques that render the patient unconscious and apneic.

Fiberoptic intubation is associated with a high success rate when performed by appropriately trained individuals. Training and practice are required to develop and master the necessary skills. Appropriate patient selection, preparation, and operator patience are essential for a safe and successful fiberoptic intubation.

The benefits of performing regional anesthesia of the oropharynx, larynx, and trachea prior to fiberoptic intubation are a quiet visual field and improved patient acceptance.

Fiberoptic intubation may be performed in conjunction with an LMA. It should be emphasized that while in most instances fiberoptic intubation is an extremely safe and effective means of securing the airway, one must be prepared to implement an alternate plan for securing the airway and for providing oxygen to the lungs in the case of failure or sudden deterioration of the patient's condition.

REFERENCES

1. Imai M, Matsumura C, Hanaoka Y, et al: Comparison of cardiovascular responses to airway management: fiberoptic intubation using a new adapter, laryngeal mask insertion, or conventional laryngoscopic intubation. *J Clin Anesth* 1995; 7: 14–18.
2. Ovassapian A, Yelich SJ, Dykes MHM, Golman ME: Learning fiberoptic intubation: use of simulators v. traditional teaching. *Br J Anesth* 1988; 61:217–220.
3. Ovassapian A: *Fiberoptic Endoscopy and the Difficult Airway.* Philadelphia: Lippincott-Raven, 1996.
4. Ovassapian A, Randel GI: The role of the fiberscope in the critically ill patient. *Crit Care Clin* 1995; 11(1):29–51.
5. Wolf LH, Gravenstein D: Capnography during fiberoptic bronchoscopy to verify tracheal intubation. *Anesth Analg* 1997; 85:701–703.
6. Guzman JL: Use of a short flexible fiberoptic endoscope for difficult intubations. *Anesthesiology* 1997; 87:1563–1564.
7. Mason RA: Learning fiberoptic intubation: fundamental problems. *Anaesthesia* 1992; 47:729–731.
8. Benumof JL: Laryngeal mask airway and the ASA difficult airway algorithm. *Anesthesiology* 1996; 84:686–699.
9. Preis CA, Hartmann T, Zimpfer M: Laryngeal mask airway facilitates awake fiberoptic intubation in a patient with severe oropharyngeal bleeding. *Anesth Analg* 1998; 87:728–729.
10. Dellinger RP: Fiberoptic bronchoscopy in adult airway management. *Crit Care Med* 1990; 18:882–887.
11. Nandi PR, Charlesworth CH, Taylor SJ, et al: Effect of general anesthesia on the pharynx. *Br J Anesth* 1991; 66:157–162.
12. Hershey MD, Hannenberg AA: Gastric distension and rupture from oxygen insufflation during fiberoptic intubation. *Anesthesiology* 1996; 85:1479–1480.
13. Reed AP: Preparation of the patient for awake flexible fiberoptic bronchoscopy. *Chest* 1992; 101:244–253.
14. Roberts J: Anatomy and patient positioning for fiberoptic laryngoscopy. *Anesthesiol Clin North Am* 1991; 9:53–67.
15. Ellis FD, Seiler JG, Palmore MM: Methemoglobinemia: a complication after fiberoptic orotracheal intubation with benzocaine spray. *J Bone Joint Surg* 1995; 77:937–939.
16. Bowes WA, Johnson JO: Pneumomediastinum after planned retrograde fiberoptic intubation. *Anesth Analg* 1994; 78:795–797.
17. Ovassapian A, Yelich SJ, Dykes MH, et al: Fiberoptic nasotracheal intubation—incidences and causes of failure. *Anesth Analg* 1983; 62:692–695.
18. Sugiyama K, Yokoyama K, Satoh K, et al: Does the Murphy eye reduce the reliability of chest auscultation in detecting endobronchial intubation? *Anesth Analg* 1999; 88:1380–1383.
19. Katnelson T, Frost EAM, Farcon E, et al: When the endotracheal tube will not pass over the flexible fiberoptic bronchoscope. *Anesthesiology* 1992; 76:151–152.
20. Brull SJ, Wiklund R, Ferris C, et al: Facilitation of fiberoptic orotracheal intubation with a flexible tracheal tube. *Anesth Analg* 1994; 78:746–748.
21. Marsh NJ: Easier fiberoptic intubations. *Anesthesiology* 1992; 76:860–861.
22. Cohn AI, Zornow MH: Awake endotracheal intubation in patients with cervical spine disease: a comparison of the Bullard laryngoscope and the fiberoptic bronchoscope. *Anesth Analg* 1995; 81:1283–1286.
23. Saha AK, Higgins M, Walker G, et al: Comparison of awake endotracheal intubation in patients with cervical spine disease: the lighted intubation stylet versus the fiberoptic bronchoscope. *Anesth Analg* 1998; 87:477–479.
24. Van Elstraete AC, Mamie JC, Mehdaoui H: Nasotracheal intubation with immobilized cervical spine: a comparison of tracheal tube cuff inflation and fiberoptic bronchoscopy. *Anesth Analg* 1998; 87:400–402.
25. Reynolds PI, O'Kelly SW: Fiberoptic intubation and the laryngeal mask airway. *Anesthesiology* 1993; 79:1144.
26. Nakayama M, Kataoka N, Usui Y, et al: Techniques of nasotracheal intubation with the fiberoptic bronchoscope. *J Emerg Med* 1992; 10:729–734.

Chapter 11
NASOTRACHEAL INTUBATION

Isam F. Nasr
Ned F. Nasr

INTRODUCTION

Nasotracheal intubation is a relatively simple procedure that is performed rapidly without the aid or risks of neuromuscular blockade.[1] This method of intubation is sometimes favored in difficult airway cases, especially when oral access is limited or impossible. Such conditions include trismus, oral injuries, and obstructive oral processes such as angioedema. Nasotracheal intubation is also the method of intubation preferred by some authors for acute epiglottitis.[2]

Nasotracheal intubation is well tolerated by most patients and produces less reflex salivation than orotracheal intubation, thus leading to fewer attempts at self-extubation. The nasotracheal tube is more easily stabilized and is generally easier to care for than an orotracheal tube. This method prevents biting of the tube by the patient and manipulation by the patient's tongue.[2,3]

INDICATIONS

Nasotracheal intubation is indicated in any patient with spontaneous respirations, especially those whose period of intubation is anticipated to be brief.[1–3] It is indicated in patients who are unable to lie supine due to respiratory distress from severe asthma, chronic obstructive pulmonary disease (COPD), or congestive heart failure. It is also indicated in patients who are unable to open their mouths due to facial trauma, mandibular trauma, or trismus. Nasotracheal intubation can be performed in patients with limited airway patency due to obstruction from neoplasm or tongue swelling. Nasotracheal intubation is an appropriate method of intubation in patients who require neck immobilization for suspected cervical spine injuries as well as patients who are unable to move their necks due to cervical kyphosis, severe arthritis, or post-radiation fibrosis. Because they are often intubated for a short time, patients with severe alcohol intoxication or drug overdose whose level of consciousness is decreased are good candidates for nasotracheal intubation.[1–3] Nasotracheal intubation may be performed in patients who have contraindications to paralytic agents.

CONTRAINDICATIONS

Nasotracheal intubation is contraindicated in patients with apnea, severe facial or maxillofacial fractures, basilar skull fractures, head injury with an elevated intracranial pressure, nasal or nasopharyngeal obstruction, patients receiving thrombolytics or parenteral anticoagulants, and in the presence of a coagulopathy.[1–3] It is also contraindicated in patients with neck injuries, as the procedure may increase morbidity and mortality.

Nasotracheal intubation should not be performed in neonates, infants, or young children. The more anterior and cephalic position of the airway in these age groups makes blind passage of an endotracheal tube almost impossible. A patient must provide a degree of cooperation during the procedure. A crying, kicking, and struggling child who must be restrained is not a candidate for nasotracheal intubation.

EQUIPMENT

Nasal mucosa vasoconstrictor (4% cocaine, oxymetazoline, phenylephrine)

Nasal mucosa anesthetic (viscous lidocaine, cocaine, benzocaine spray, xylocaine spray)

Nasopharyngeal airways, multiple sizes

Laryngoscope handle

Laryngoscope blades, various sizes and types

Endotracheal tubes, various sizes

Endotrol tubes, various sizes (Mallinckrodt Medical, St. Louis, MO)

Magill forceps

Suction apparatus

Topical anesthetic (4% cocaine or 2% lidocaine with epinephrine)

Gauze strips

Water-soluble lubricant or anesthetic jelly

Bag-valve device

Face mask

Oxygen source and tubing

PATIENT PREPARATION

Explain the risks, benefits, and potential complications of the procedure to the patient and/or their representative if time permits. All procedural steps should be clearly outlined, with the understanding that an orotracheal intubation may be necessary should the physician fail to secure the airway nasotracheally. Since this is a lifesaving procedure, a signed consent may not be necessary, but a procedure note should be included in the medical record.

Prepare the patient with preoxygenation, hemodynamic monitoring, pulse oximetry, and intravenous access. Place the patient supine and in the "sniffing" position if there is no suspicion of a cervical spine injury. If the patient needs to remain sitting due to respiratory distress, also place them in the sniffing position. Examine the patient's nostrils. Choose the larger and more patent nostril for the intubation.

Prepare the mucous membranes. Apply a topical vasoconstrictor to shrink the nasal mucosa. Apply a topical anesthetic to the nasal mucosa. Cocaine is preferred if not contraindicated, because it is a single agent that acts as both a vasoconstrictor and an anesthetic. Dilate the nasal passage. Liberally lubricate a series of increasingly larger-size nasopharyngeal airways. Insert and then remove the smallest nasopharyngeal airway. Continue to insert and remove each successively larger nasopharyngeal airway until the nasal passage is dilated. This procedure can take 2 to 3 minutes. If time is an issue, insert a gloved and lubricated pinky finger into the nostril to dilate it. Apply topical anesthetic spray to the palate and oropharynx.

Choose an endotracheal tube. The proper size tube should be at least 0.5 to 1.0 mm smaller than the size chosen for orotracheal intubation of the same patient. Apply a 10 mL syringe to the inflation port and inflate the cuff. Check the integrity of the cuff. Deflate the cuff and leave the syringe attached. Lubricate the endotracheal tube liberally.

TECHNIQUES

BLIND PLACEMENT OF AN ENDOTRACHEAL TUBE

The technique of blind nasotracheal intubation was first described by Magill in 1930. The technique essentially remains the same with some modifications to increase the success rate and limit complications. This technique is technically more difficult than the placement under direct vision described below. **Its major advantages are that the patient's mouth does not have to be opened and minimal to no cervical spine movement is required.** This procedure may be performed while the patient is sitting or supine. Prepare the patient as mentioned previously.

Insert the endotracheal tube into the nostril with the bevel facing the septum (Figures 11-1 and 11-2A). If the patient's right nostril is being used, insert the endotracheal tube concave side down (Figure 11-1A). If the patient's left nostril is being used, insert the endotracheal tube concave side up (Figure 11-1B). Advance the endotracheal tube with gentle pressure along the nasal floor to pass it through the nasal cavity (Figure 11-2B). If any resistance is felt, slightly withdraw the endotracheal tube. Readvance the tube with a slight twisting motion to bypass the obstruction. If resistance is still met, withdraw the endotracheal tube, prepare the other nostril, and insert the tube into the other nostril.

When the endotracheal tube is inserted approximately 5 to 7 cm, the tip will be past the choana and in the nasopharynx (Figure 11-2B). Continue advancing the tube as resistance is met while the tube makes a 90 degree change of direction into the oropharynx. A slight twisting motion may be required to advance the endotracheal tube. A loss of resistance signifies that the endotracheal tube has made the curve. Stop advancing the tube and rotate it so that the tube's natural curve is concave upward and in the same curvature of the airway. If the tube will not curve from the nasopharynx into the oropharynx, several options are available. These include trying the other nostril, using an endotracheal tube 0.5 mm smaller and reattempting intubation through the original nostril, or using an Endotrol tube (described in the next section).

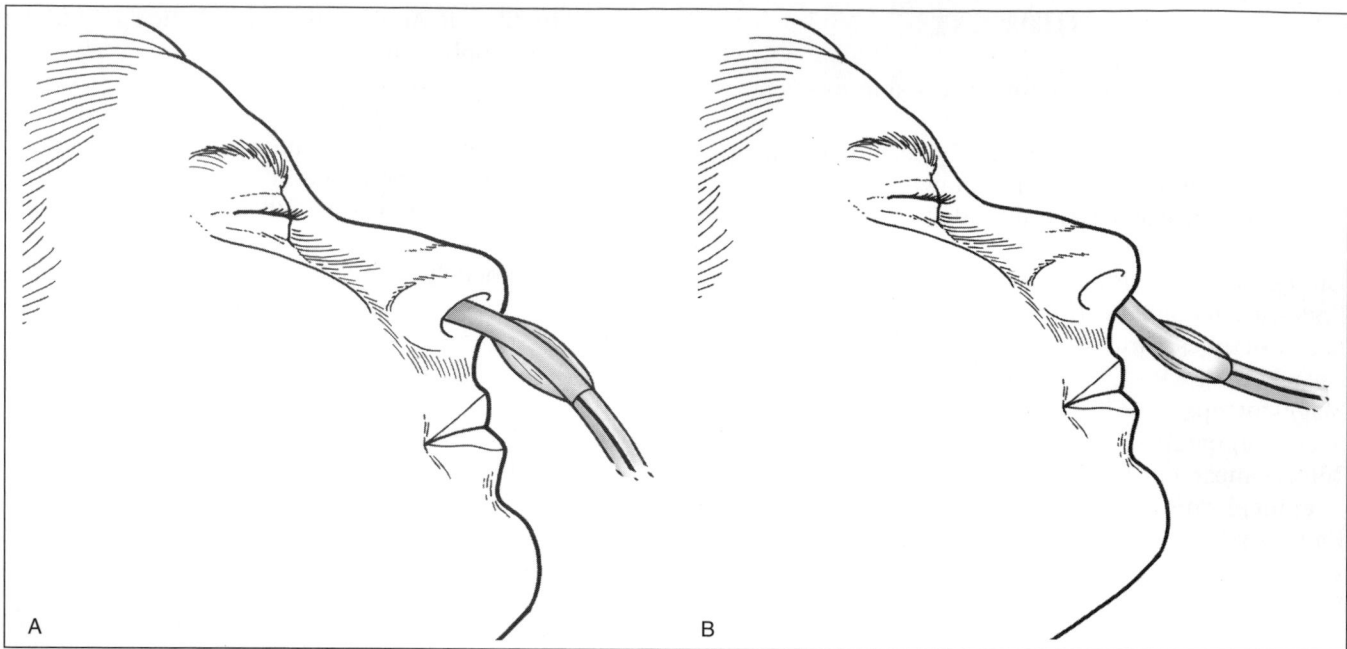

FIGURE 11-1 Insertion of the nasotracheal tube. The bevel of the endotracheal tube should face the septum. *A.* Placement in the right nostril with the concave side of the tube downward. *B.* Placement in the left nostril with the concave side upward. When the tip of the tube enters the nasopharynx, rotate it 180 degrees.

Advance the endotracheal tube through the oropharynx and into the laryngopharynx (Figure 11-2*C*). Listen for breath sounds through the proximal end of the endotracheal tube while advancing it. The breath sounds and air movement will be maximal when the tip of the tube is just above the glottis. As soon as an exhalation is heard, the patient will take a breath and advance the endotracheal tube. The vocal cords are opened their widest during inspiration, and this will facilitate passage of the endotracheal tube.

The patient will often cough or gag as the endotracheal tube traverses the vocal cords. At this point, breath sounds should be audible from the proximal end of the endotracheal tube and it should fog with each breath. If the patient is able to groan or speak, the esophagus has been intubated. Withdraw the tube and reinsert it during inspiration. The application of posteriorly applied pressure on the trachea (Sellick's maneuver) will occlude the esophagus and may allow easier endotracheal intubation. The use of an Endotrol tube can also aid in endotracheal intubation.

If resistance to the advancement of the endotracheal tube is felt, it may be caught in the hypopharynx. Common sites for the tip of the endotracheal tube to get caught are the arytenoid cartilage, piriform sinus, vallecula, and the vocal cords. Withdraw the endotracheal tube 3 to 4 cm, slightly rotate the tube, and readvance it.

Inflate the endotracheal tube cuff. Confirmation of tube placement should be done by auscultating both lungs while ventilating the patient with a bag-valve device through the nasotracheal tube. Adjust the position of the tube until both lungs are being ventilated equally and secure the tube (Figure 11-2*D*). Continue to ventilate the patient.

BLIND PLACEMENT OF THE ENDOTROL TUBE

The indications, contraindications, and patient preparation are the same as described above. The Endotrol tube is an endotracheal tube whose tip can be controlled. It looks like a cuffed endotracheal tube but has a plastic ligature along the inner side that is connected to a ring at the proximal tube. Pulling of the ring exerts tension on the plastic ligature, leading to an increase in the curvature of the tip of the endotracheal tube (Figure 11-3). This will project the tip anteriorly and inferiorly (Figure 11-3). The procedure for inserting the Endotrol tube is the same as that for inserting an endotracheal tube. Changing the curvature of the tip will aid in passage of the tube from the nasopharynx to the oropharynx and from the hypopharynx into the trachea. If the ring is sitting firmly against the nares after intubation, the tip of the tube may be exerting continuous pressure on the anterior tracheal mucosa. Cut the ligature and remove the ring.

PLACEMENT UNDER DIRECT VISION

The technique begins with nasotracheal intubation, followed by direct laryngoscopy. The placement of a na-

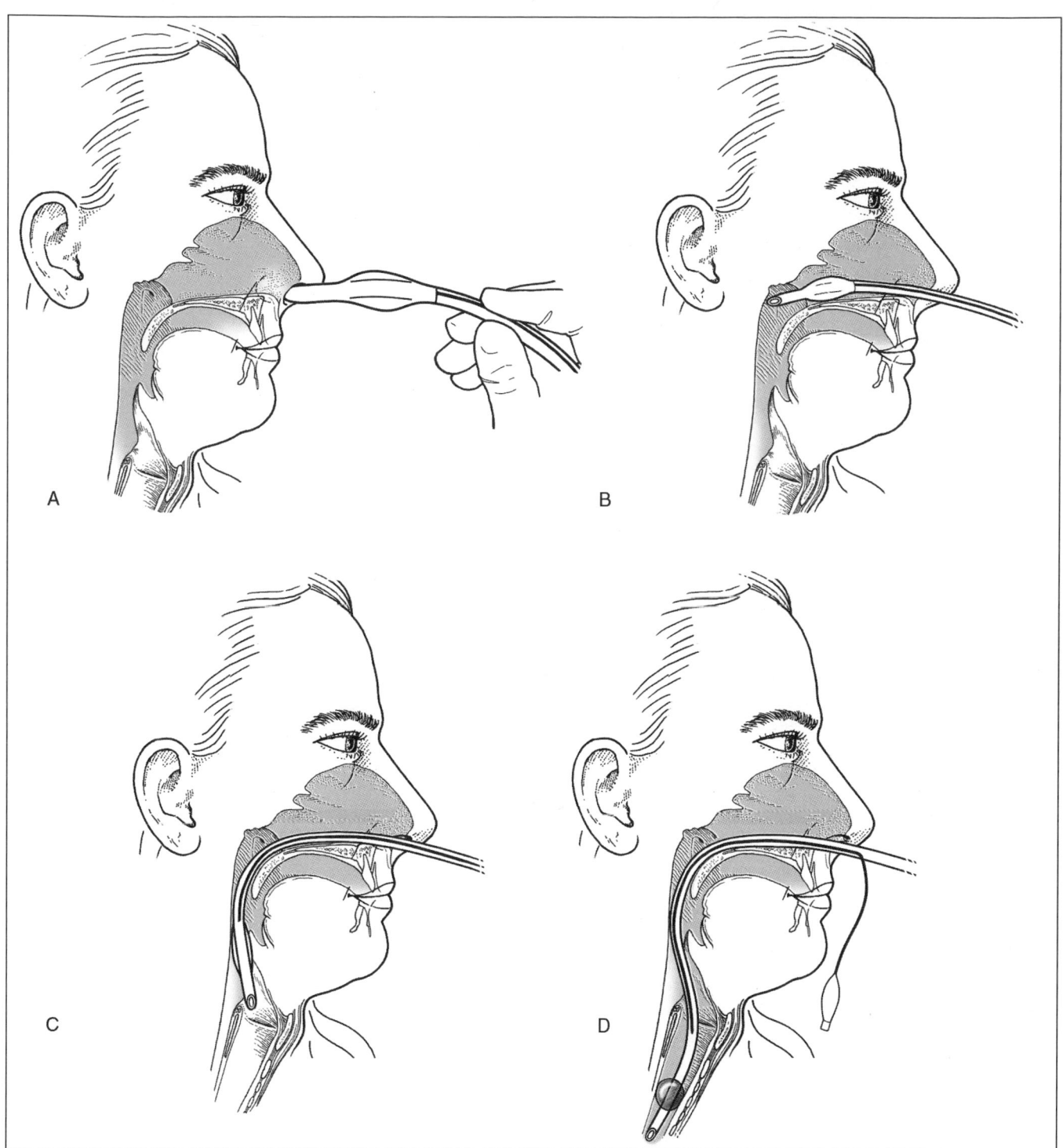

FIGURE 11-2 Blind nasotracheal placement. *A.* The nasotracheal tube is placed within the nasal cavity. *B.* The tube is advanced along the floor of the nasal cavity and into the nasopharynx. *C.* The tube is advanced into the laryngopharynx. *D.* At the start of inspiration, the tube is advanced through the vocal cords and into the trachea.

sotracheal tube using direct visualization must be performed with the patient supine. The indications and precautions are similar to those for orotracheal intubation. This method should be considered in the event of an oral injury that renders an orotracheal tube a nuisance. It may be useful if blind nasotracheal intubation is unsuccessful.

This procedure is initially performed as previously described. Once the tube is inserted into the hypopharynx, direct laryngoscopy is performed. Using the left

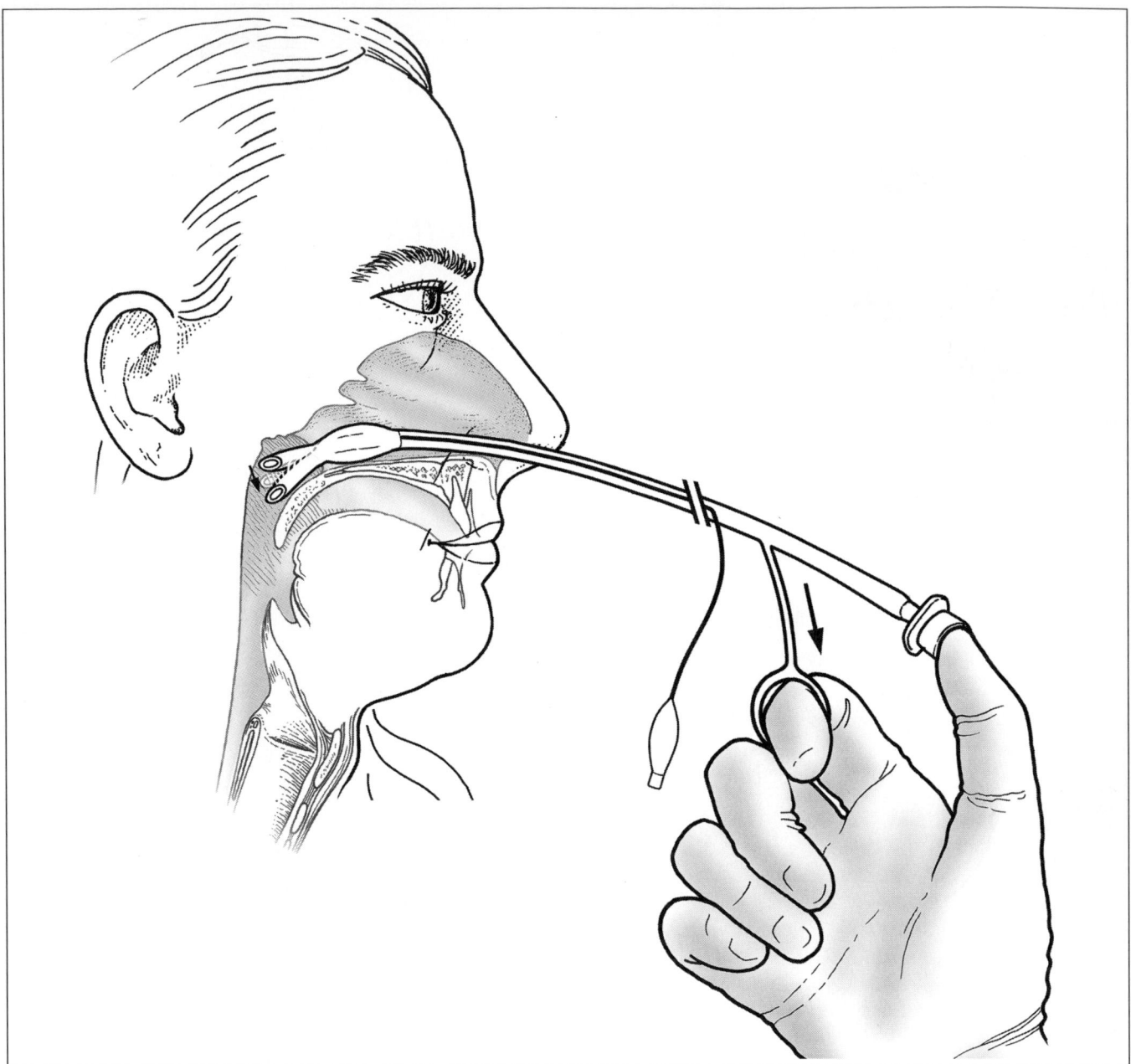

FIGURE 11-3 Blind nasotracheal placement of an Endotrol tube. Tension exerted on the ring of the tube causes the curvature of the tube to increase (*arrow*).

hand, grasp the laryngoscope and insert the blade. Visualize the patient's epiglottis and vocal cords as well as the endotracheal tube. Using a Magill forceps with the right hand, grasp the endotracheal tube just above the cuff (Figure 11-4). **Never grasp the cuff, as it is delicate and can easily be damaged by the Magill forceps.** Have an assistant grasp the proximal end of the endotracheal tube and gently advance it while the physician simultaneously guides the tip through the vocal cords (Figure 11-4). Remove the Magill forceps and the laryngoscope. Inflate the cuff, secure the tube, and ventilate the patient.

ASSESSMENT

The position of the endotracheal tube should be confirmed by end-tidal CO_2 monitoring, fogging in the endotracheal tube for at least six ventilations, auscultation, and chest x-ray.

AFTERCARE

The ongoing care of the patient should proceed as with any other intubation technique.

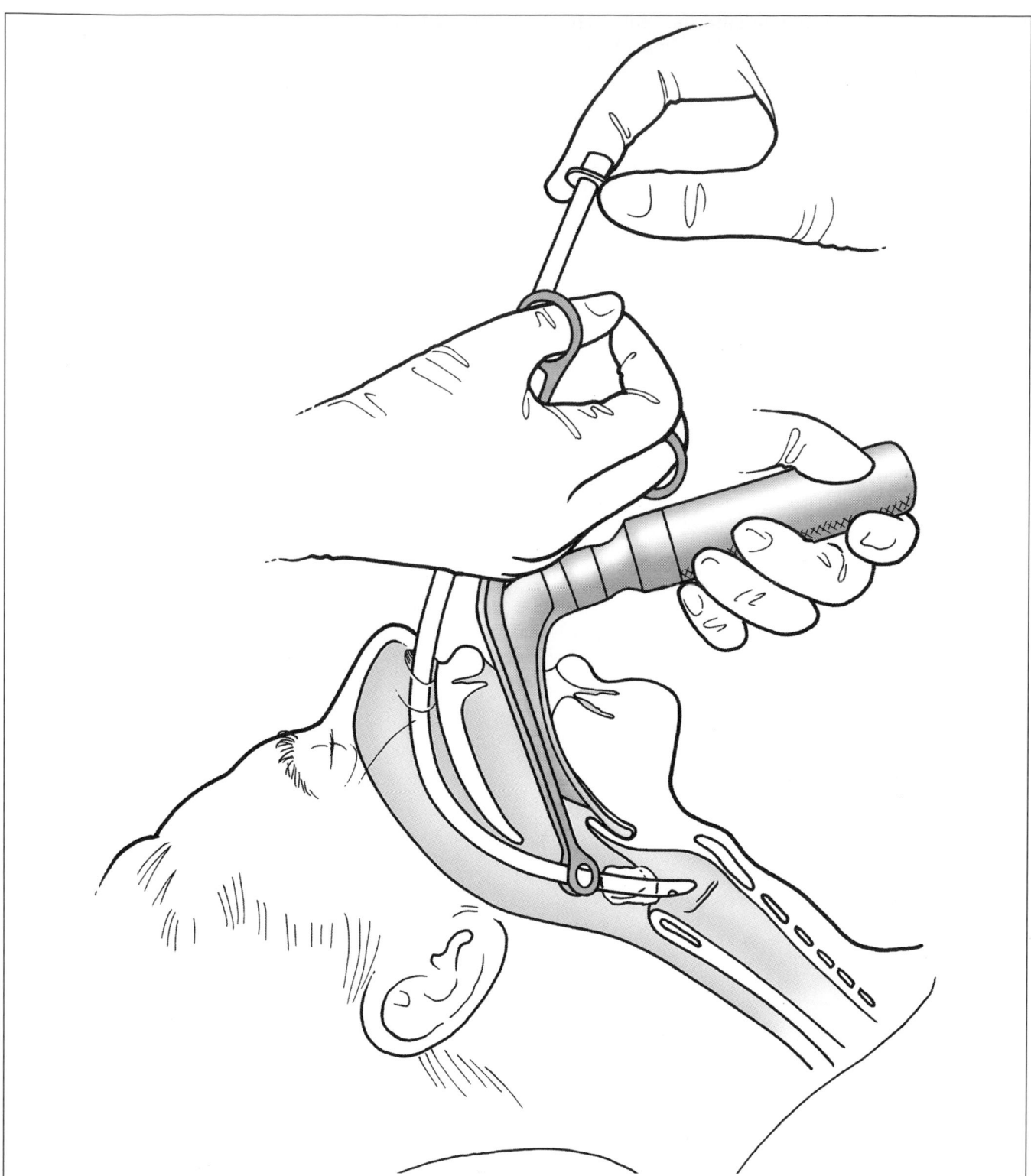

FIGURE 11-4 Nasotracheal intubation under direct visualization.

COMPLICATIONS

The immediate complications of nasotracheal intubation include epistaxis, laryngeal and tracheal trauma, mucosal avulsion, retropharyngeal laceration, turbinate avulsion, intracranial placement, bacteremia, esophageal intubation, and prolonged attempts to place the tube.[4,5] Many of these can be prevented by choosing the appropriate size endotracheal tube, ensuring adequate nasal mucosal vasoconstriction, and applying a liberal amount of lubricant to the endotracheal tube. Long-term complications include maxillary sinusitis, retropharyngeal abscess, mediastinitis, nasal mucosal necrosis, and cellulitis.[4,5]

SUMMARY

Nasotracheal intubation is an alternative to orotracheal intubation to secure an airway in the spontaneously breathing patient. It allows awake intubations while the patient maintains protective airway reflexes, and it avoids the risks of paralytic agents. It is a fairly simple procedure that should be considered in patients in whom an oral airway is considered difficult and in those with an anticipated short intubation period.

REFERENCES

1. Roppolo LP, Vilke GM, Chan TC, et al: Nasotracheal intubation in the emergency department, revisited. *J Emerg Med* 1999; 17(5):791–799.
2. McGill JW, Clinton JE: Tracheal intubation, in Roberts JR, Hedger JR (eds): *Clinical Procedures in Emergency Medicine*, 3rd ed. Philadelphia: Saunders, 1998:3–34.
3. Anderson DM: Airway management, in Howell J, Alfieri M, Jagoda A, et al (eds): *Emergency Medicine*. Philadelphia: Saunders, 1998:50–51.
4. Holdgaard HO, Pedersen J, Schurizek BA, et al: Complications and late sequelae following nasotracheal intubation. *Acta Anaesthiol Scand* 1993; 37:475–480.
5. Seaman M, Ballinger P, Sturgill TD, et al: Mediastinitis following nasal intubation in the emergency department. *Am J Emerg Med* 1991; 9:37–39.

Chapter 12
RETROGRADE GUIDEWIRE INTUBATION

Rick Gimbel
Roland Petri

INTRODUCTION

Failure to establish a definitive airway is a significant cause of death and disability among emergency patients. While oral endotracheal intubation via direct laryngoscopy remains the "gold standard" of airway management, difficult situations arise in which oral endotracheal intubation is impossible, is contraindicated, or fails. Retrograde guidewire intubation is an alternative airway management technique that should be familiar to those involved with emergency airway management.[1]

Retrograde intubation was first described in 1960 by Butler and Carillo.[2] In 1963, Waters described insertion of an epidural catheter through a cricothyroid puncture as an alternative means of establishing an airway.[3] Powell and Odzil reported a series of 15 patients in whom retrograde intubation was employed without complications using a plastic catheter rather than an epidural catheter as a guide into the trachea.[4] The current technique of retrograde intubation varies little from these original descriptions.

Retrograde intubation represents one of several alternative maneuvers for securing the difficult airway. While mouth tumors, cervical arthritis, and jaw ankylosis represent rare cases of difficult-to-control airways, maxillofacial trauma continues to represent the most common indication for alternative airway management. Retrograde intubation has proven to be an effective method used by Emergency Physicians and prehospital personnel to establish an airway.

Completion times for retrograde intubation vary based upon physician experience. Among health care professionals who had no prior experience with the technique but who had just completed a mannequin-aided training course, the mean length of time to intubation was 71 +/− 4 seconds.[1] In a second study involving resident physicians after a brief instruction course, 36 of 40 residents (90 percent) completed retrograde intubation within 150 seconds, with a mean intubation time of 56 +/− 6 seconds.[10]

INDICATIONS

The American Society of Anesthesiologists defines a difficult airway "as the clinical situation in which a conventionally trained anesthesiologist experiences difficulty with mask ventilation, difficulty with tracheal intubation or both."[5] **Retrograde intubation should be considered in any patient in whom endotracheal intubation may be difficult, is contraindicated, or has failed.** It is indicated when airway control is required and less invasive methods have failed. Maxillofacial trauma and cervical spine fractures represent the most common etiologies of a difficult airway.[6] In one report of 19 patients with either maxillofacial trauma or fractures of the cervical spine, 6 had prior, failed orotracheal intubation attempts. In all of these patients, retrograde intubation was successful on the first attempt.[6] Jaw ankylosis, cervical arthritis, mouth tumors, and muscular dystrophy represent less common but equally challenging airway situations.[4,7]

Another clinically important situation arises when a patient presents with impending ventilatory failure. While retrograde intubation is generally a longer procedure than orotracheal intubation, oxygenation and ventilation can be maintained with a bag-valve-mask device during the procedure. It is useful when bleeding obstructs visualization of the glottis.

A less common indication includes retrograde intubation of a difficult airway in a patient being ventilated with a laryngeal mask airway. This indication exists because withdrawal of the laryngeal mask airway over a blindly placed catheter can result in dislodgement of the catheter, necessitating replacement of the laryngeal mask airway.[8]

CONTRAINDICATIONS

The major contraindication to retrograde intubation is the ability to control the airway with less invasive techniques. Other contraindications include an anterior neck mass, infections, or cancerous process overlying the cricothyroid membrane. Trismus, or the inability to open the mouth, is a contraindication to this technique. Apneic patients who cannot be ventilated with a bag-valve-mask device should receive a cricothyroidotomy and not a retrograde guidewire intubation. Those unfamiliar with the equipment and/or technique should not attempt this procedure. While one case report presents the successful use of a mannequin to teach retrograde intubation to emergency caregivers, familiarity with the procedure is required for optimum patient management.[1]

EQUIPMENT

68 to 80 cm spring guidewire with a J tip
16 to 18 gauge catheter-over-the-needle (angiocatheter)
Endotracheal tubes, various sizes
Sterile saline
10 mL syringes
18 gauge needles
Hemostats, 2
Magill forceps
Sterile drape
20 mL syringe
Povidone iodine solution
Face mask
Bag-valve device
Oxygen source and tubing
Suction source and tubing
Yankauer suction catheter
1% lidocaine
4% viscous lidocaine (optional)
Spray anesthetic (lidocaine or benzocaine)
Tape (or a commercially available endotracheal tube holder)

Retrograde intubation can be performed using a standard commercial retrograde intubation kit (Cook C-Retro-11.0-70-38E-110 Retrograde Intubation Set, Cook Incorporated, Bloomington, IN). It consists of an 18 gauge needle set, 68 to 80 cm spring guidewire, and an

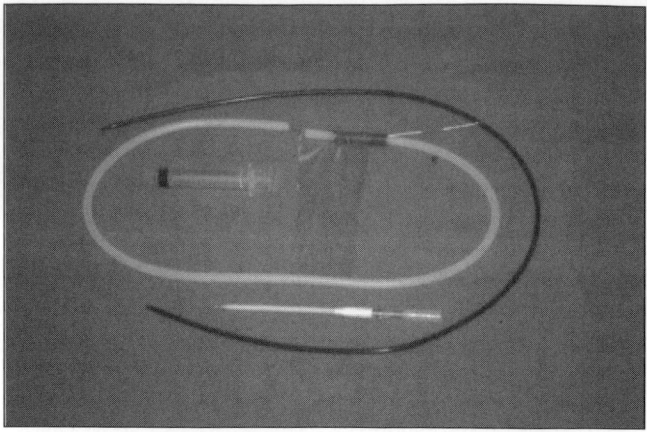

FIGURE 12-1 The retrograde guidewire intubation kit.

11 French introducer catheter (Figure 12-1). The remainder of the material must be supplied as listed above.

PATIENT PREPARATION

If time permits, and the patient is aware of pain, anesthetize the airway. Nebulized viscous lidocaine will anesthetize the airway in 15 to 20 minutes. Alternatively, inject 2 mL of 1% lidocaine percutaneously through the cricothyroid membrane and into the trachea.[6] This may cause the patient to cough and gag, with the subsequent possibility of aspiration. Lidocaine or benzocaine may be sprayed into the pharynx. An alternative anesthetic method includes a superior laryngeal nerve block.[9] Refer to Chapter 10 for details regarding this nerve block.

Clean the patient's neck of any dirt and debris. Identify, by palpation, the hyoid bone, thyroid cartilage, cricoid cartilage, and cricothyroid membrane. Apply povidone iodine to the patient's neck, followed by sterile drapes.

TECHNIQUE

The procedure is relatively simple in theory but difficult to perform "in the heat of battle."[1,10–13] Prepare the equipment. Place the 16 to 18 gauge catheter-over-the-needle onto a 10 mL syringe containing 3 to 5 mL of sterile saline. Select an appropriate size endotracheal tube for the patient. Check the integrity of the cuff. Lubricate the inside and outside of the distal tip of the endotracheal tube liberally. Open the retrograde guidewire kit and/or assemble all equipment. The equipment should be preassembled, prepackaged, sterilized, and stored in an easily accessible site.

Stabilize the patient's larynx with the thumb and middle finger of the nondominant hand. Identify the cricothyroid membrane with the index finger of the nondominant hand. Leave the index finger on the cricothyroid membrane. Insert the 16 to 18 gauge catheter-over-the-needle guided along the index finger, at a 20 to 30 degree angle upward and through the cricothyroid membrane (Figure 12-2A). Some physicians prefer to use the needle without the catheter. **Care should be taken to puncture the cricothyroid membrane just above the cricoid cartilage to avoid injury to the cricothyroid arteries.** The loss of resistance signifies that the needle is in the larynx. Aspirate air through the saline-filled syringe to confirm correct needle placement (Figure 12-2A). Advance the catheter until the hub is against the skin. Remove the needle and syringe, leaving the catheter pointed upward and through the cricothyroid membrane. If this has not already been done and the patient is awake, inject 2 mL of 1% lidocaine through the catheter.

Advance the guidewire through the catheter and into the oropharynx (Figures 12-2B and 12-3). The guidewire may exit the mouth or nose. If it is not visualized, insert the laryngoscope and look for the guidewire. It is often in the oropharynx or hypopharynx. Retrieve it with a Magill forceps. The preferred site of exit is the mouth, but the nose is acceptable. Continue to advance the guidewire through the mouth (or nose) until only 4 to 5 cm of the wire is protruding from the patient's neck. **Carefully remove the catheter while firmly holding the guidewire in place.** Place a hemostat on the guidewire where it enters the skin of the neck (Figure 12-2C). This will ensure that the tip does not pull through the skin and into the trachea.

If the kit is being used, select the introducer catheter contained in it. Pass the introducer catheter over the guidewire that is exiting the mouth (or nose). Advance the catheter until resistance is met. This signifies that the tip of the introducer catheter is at the inside of the cricothyroid membrane (Figure 12-2C). Advance the well-lubricated endotracheal tube over the introducer and guidewire (Figure 12-2D). Continue to advance the endotracheal tube until resistance is met. The tip of the endotracheal tube should be at the inside of the cricothyroid membrane (Figure 12-2D). While securely holding the endotracheal tube at the patient's mouth, remove the hemostat from the guidewire. Pull on the proximal end of the guidewire until the distal tip is through the skin and just into the trachea (5 to 6 cm). **Simultaneously withdraw the guidewire and introducer catheter while advancing the endotracheal tube into the trachea** (Figure 12-2E). Inflate the endotracheal tube cuff and confirm proper placement (auscultation, detection of end-tidal CO_2, fogging in the endotracheal tube, etc.).

A second method can also be used to insert the endotracheal tube. This follows the same technique described above to the point of the guidewire exiting the mouth (or nose), being secured with a hemostat at the neck, and passing the introducer catheter over the guidewire. Remove the hemostat from the guidewire. **While securely holding the introducer catheter at the patient's mouth (or nose), remove the guidewire through the mouth (or nose).** Advance the introducer catheter an additional 2 to 3 cm into the trachea. Lubricate the endotracheal tube liberally. Place the endotracheal tube over the introducer catheter. While holding the introducer catheter securely, advance the endotracheal tube into the patient's trachea. Remove the introducer catheter. Inflate the endotracheal tube cuff and confirm proper placement (auscultation, detection of end-tidal CO_2, fogging in the endotracheal tube, etc.).

ALTERNATIVE TECHNIQUES

This technique may be performed without a formal retrograde intubation kit as the introducer catheter is not required.[7,12,13] This follows the same technique described above to the point of the guidewire exiting the mouth (or nose) and being secured with a hemostat at the neck (Figure 12-2C). Lubricate the endotracheal tube liberally. Insert the guidewire through the Murphy eye and into the endotracheal tube. This allows the distal tip of the endotracheal tube to project approximately 1 cm distal to the site at which the guidewire enters the larynx. As an alternative, some physicians prefer to load the guidewire through the tip of the endotracheal tube (Figure 12-4). **Always hold the proximal end of the guidewire to maintain control during the procedure.** Advance the endotracheal tube over the guidewire until resistance is felt. The tip of the endotracheal tube should be at the inside of the cricothyroid membrane. **Hold the proximal end of the guidewire firmly.** Release the hemostat over the neck. Pull the guidewire through the skin and just into the trachea (5 to 6 cm). Advance the endotracheal tube until it is at 20 to 21 cm at the teeth for an adult female or 22 to 23 cm at the teeth for an adult male. Hold the endotracheal tube securely at the patient's lips. Withdraw the guidewire through the patient's mouth. Inflate the endotracheal tube cuff and confirm proper placement (auscultation, detection of end-tidal CO_2, fogging in the endotracheal tube, etc.).

When the endotracheal tube is advanced over the guidewire until resistance is met, the tip should be situated against the inside of the cricothyroid membrane. It is imperative to determine if the tip of the tube is in the trachea or caught on the epiglottis, arytenoid cartilage, pyriform recess, vallecula, or vocal cords. If concern exists as to the position of the tip, withdraw the endotracheal tube 2 cm, rotate it 90 degrees, and readvance it into the trachea. As an alternative, a laryngoscope or fiberoptic broncho/nasopharyngoscope can be inserted

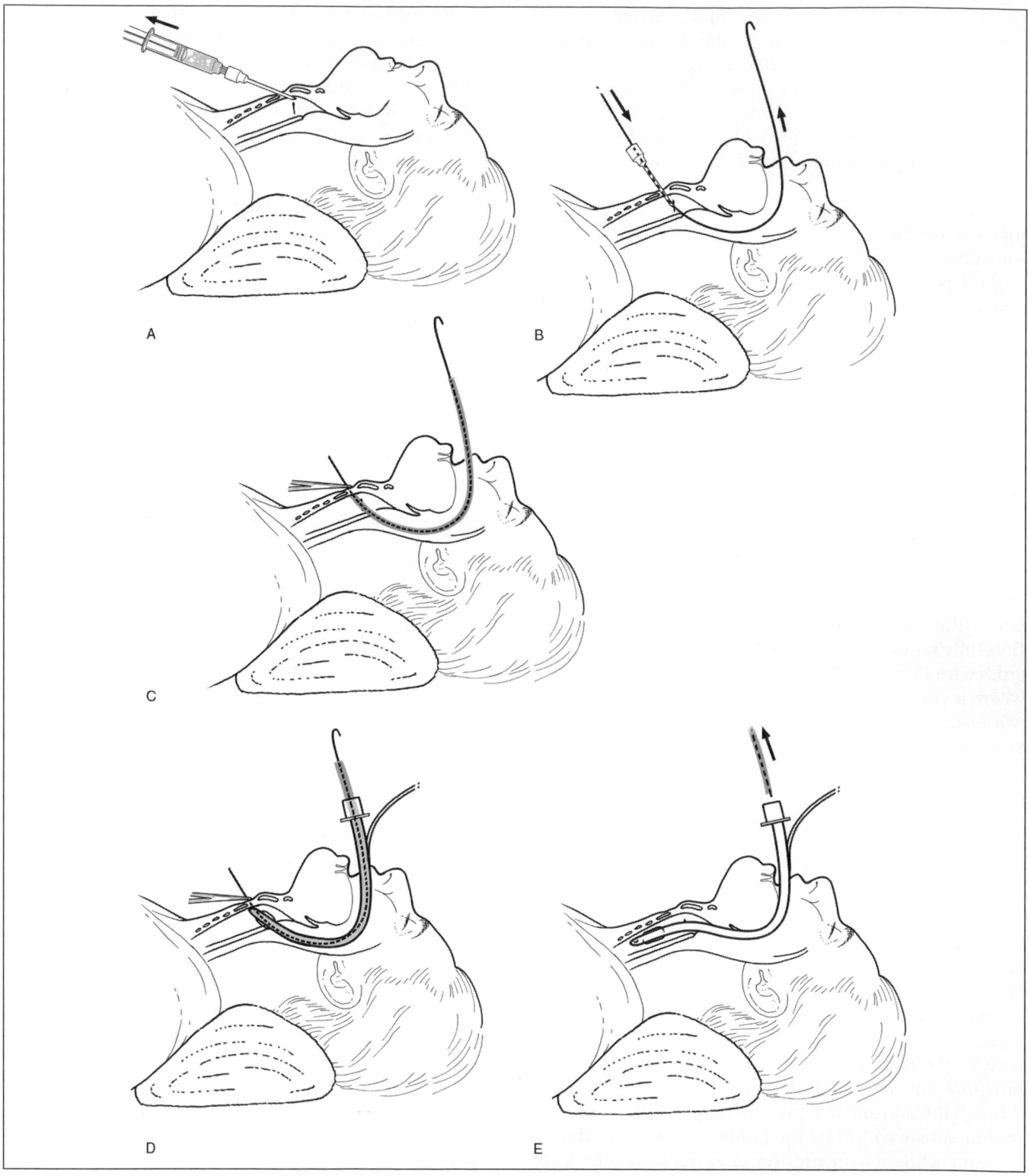

FIGURE 12-2 Retrograde guidewire intubation. *A.* A syringe containing saline is attached to the catheter-over-the-needle. The catheter-over-the-needle is inserted cephalad through the cricothyroid membrane and at a 20 to 30 degree angle to the skin. The air bubbles in the syringe indicate air aspirated from the trachea. *B.* The needle and syringe have been removed and the catheter remains. The guidewire is fed through the catheter and out the patient's mouth. *C.* The distal guidewire is clamped with a hemostat as it exits the skin of the neck. The introducer catheter is fed over the guidewire and advanced to the cricothyroid membrane. *D.* An endotracheal tube is advanced over the guidewire and introducer catheter until its tip is at the cricothyroid membrane. *E.* The hemostat is removed. The endotracheal tube is advanced as the guidewire and introducer catheter are removed.

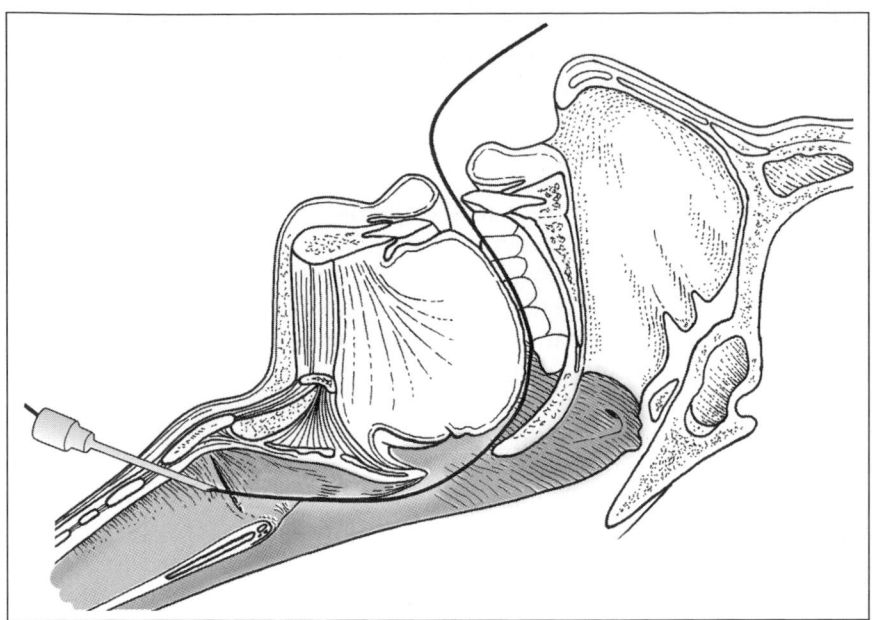

FIGURE 12-3 The guidewire is inserted through the needle (or catheter depending on physician preference) until it exits the mouth.

to help visualize the placement of the endotracheal tube.

Another variation involves the use of the guidewire sheath as an introducer catheter.[12,13] Shorten the sheath by 3 to 5 cm using sterile scissors. The remainder of the technique is the same as described above. The only drawback to this technique is that the curvature of the sheath must be straightened before use to allow easy threading over the guidewire.

In another description, a central venous catheter is used rather than a guidewire.[6] It allows the physician to inject air through the catheter retrogradely to help locate the catheter in the mouth of severely injured patients with significant intraoral blood or secretions. This technique requires a relatively long central venous catheter. It does allow retrograde intubation without the use of a formal retrograde intubation kit.

Finally, another version uses a lighted stylet attached to the endotracheal tube.[14] The lighted stylet acts as a guide to indicate the tube's location. When the tip of the endotracheal tube enters the glottic opening, a bright, circumscribed glow is readily seen in the anterior neck,

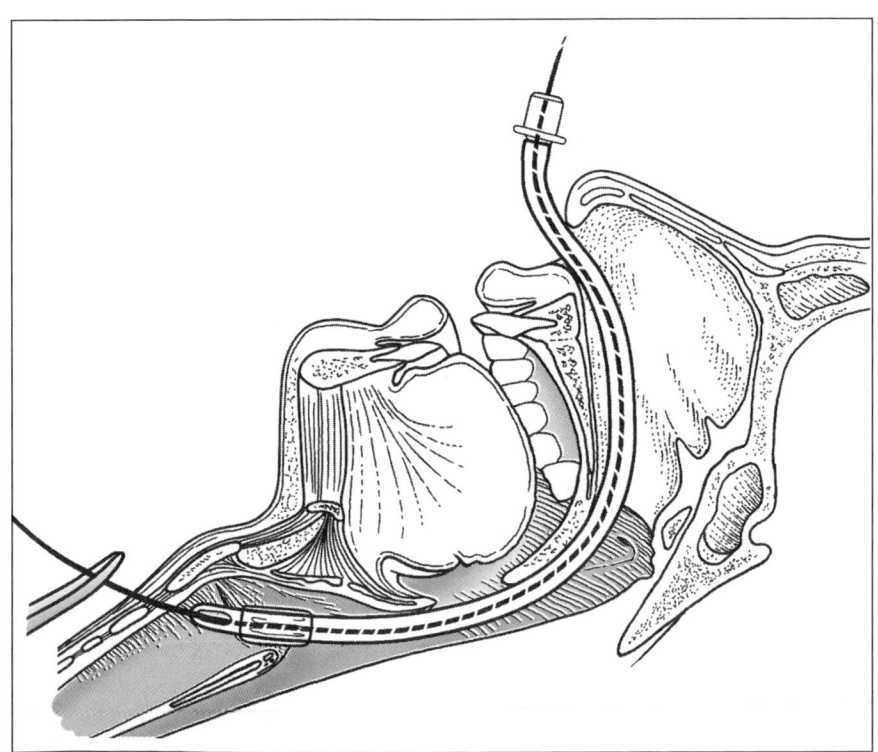

FIGURE 12-4 The endotracheal tube is advanced over the guidewire until the tip is against the cricothyroid membrane.

below the thyroid prominence. This glow acts as an indicator of correct endotracheal tube placement.

When continuous oxygenation is required throughout the procedure, two possibilities exist.[12] A T-adapter (1260, Deseret, Sandy, UT) can be connected to the needle hub with its side arm for oxygen insufflation. Alternatively, a swivel adapter with a fiberoptic bronchoscopic cap (1/25/09, Portex, Wilmington, MA) can be interposed between the endotracheal tube and the anesthesia breathing circuit.

ASSESSMENT

Auscultation of both lungs will confirm proper placement of the endotracheal tube and minimize the risk of intubation into the right mainstem bronchus. End-tidal CO_2 has also become part of the postintubation routine. After the procedure is completed, a chest radiograph will confirm the placement of the endotracheal tube tip in relation to the clavicles and carina.

AFTERCARE

The patient should receive standard wound care and dressing of the skin at the neck entrance site. Wound checks and infection monitoring should continue as with any other surgical procedure. The risk of skin, tracheal, or pharyngeal infection is minimal if sterile technique was followed. If infection develops, wound evaluation and treatment with appropriate antibiotics is warranted.

COMPLICATIONS

Complications of retrograde guidewire intubation include those of standard endotracheal intubation. Complications can occur when the needle traverses the cricothyroid membrane.[10] Hypoxia due to prolonged intubation time or incorrect endotracheal tube placement remains an important complication. Drug reactions or side effects secondary to administered medications must always be considered.

Retrograde intubation is associated with additional complications due to use of the guidewire. One case report discusses a patient with a past history of retrograde intubation for coronary bypass surgery who experienced a foreign-body sensation and bloody sputum 2 years after the procedure.[15] Upon radiographic examination, the patient was found to have a 10 cm segment of guidewire fixed in the soft tissue of the puncture site and extending cephalad 2 cm past the true vocal cords.

In one cadaveric study, numerous complications were noted during 40 cricothyroid punctures. Two punctures (5 percent) occurred below the cricothyroid membrane. One was between the cricoid cartilage and first tracheal ring. The other was between the first and second tracheal rings. Four cases (10 percent) showed minor injuries to the thyroid or cricoid cartilage. Three cases (7.5 percent) showed injuries to the posterior wall of the larynx, epiglottis, or soft palate. No posterior tracheal perforations were found in this study. The clinical importance of these injuries is unclear given the nature of this postmortem study.

Three technical complications from retrograde guidewire intubation have been identified.[10,12] Difficulties inserting the guidewire can be prevented by first aspirating air into a saline-filled syringe to confirm the intratracheal needle tip position. Endotracheal intubation over a flexible guidewire necessitates keeping the guidewire taut to minimize the risk of kinking. Unfortunately, this moves the guidewire anteriorly toward the narrowest portion of the glottis and may prevent passage of the endotracheal tube, as the tip can become caught on the epiglottis or the vocal cords. This problem is obviated by the use of the introducer catheter in the retrograde guidewire intubation kit. It lies in the posterior pharynx and glottis and allows for easier passage of the endotracheal tube into the trachea. The tip of the endotracheal tube may flip out of the larynx when the introducer is being removed, because the distance between the vocal cords and the point where the introducer enters and anchors the larynx averages only 1.0 to 1.3 cm in adults.

While complications may occur in association with retrograde intubation, the rate of complications is relatively low. In one study, 20 resident physicians performed retrograde intubation twice each on 40 cadavers.[10] In two cases (5 percent), the wire was fed caudad into the trachea due to improper angling of the needle. The remaining intubations were performed without complications.

SUMMARY

Retrograde tracheal intubation requires little operator experience or equipment. Multiple reports suggest that this technique is safe, relatively easy to learn, and routinely successful. All physicians involved in the airway management of critically ill and injured patients should be aware of this technique as a potential method to overcome the challenge of a difficult airway. Within the armamentarium of management techniques for the difficult airway, retrograde guidewire intubation should be given due consideration in any situation in which orotracheal intubation is impossible or contraindicated.

REFERENCES

1. Van Stralen D, Rogers M, Perkin R, et al: Retrograde intubation training using a mannequin. *Am J Emerg Med* 1995; 13:50–52.
2. Butler FS, Cirillo AA: Retrograde tracheal intubation. *Anesth Analg* 1960; 39:333–338.
3. Waters DJ: Guided blind endotracheal intubation. *Anesthesia* 1963; 18:158–162.
4. Powell WF, Ozdil T: A translaryngeal guide for tracheal intubation. *Anesth Analg* 1967; 46:231–233.
5. American Society of Anesthesiologists: Practice guidelines for management of the difficult airway. *Anesthesiology* 1993; 78:597–602.
6. Barriot P, Riou B: Retrograde technique for tracheal intubation in trauma patients. *Crit Care Med* 1988; 16:712–713.
7. Van Stralen D, Perkin RM: Retrograde intubation difficulty in an 18-year-old muscular dystrophy patient. *Am J Emerg Med* 1995; 13:100–101.
8. Harvey S, Fishman R, Edwards S: Retrograde intubation through a laryngeal mask airway. *Anesthesiology* 1996; 85:1503–1504.
9. Gotta AW, Sullivan CA: Anaesthesia of the upper airway using topical anaesthetic and superior laryngeal nerve block. *Br J Anaesth* 1981; 53:1055–1058.
10. Stern Y, Spitzer T: Retrograde intubation of the trachea. *J Laryngol Otol* 1991; 105:746–747.
11. Borland LM, Swan DM, Lett S: Difficult pediatric endotracheal intubation: a new approach to the retrograde technique. *Anesthesiology* 1981; 55:577–578.
12. King HK, Wank LF, Khan AK, et al: Translaryngeal guided intubation for difficult intubation. *Crit Care Med* 1987; 15:869–871.
13. Lau HP, Yip KM, Liu CC: Rapid airway access by modified retrograde intubation. *J Formosan Med Assoc* 1996; 95(4):347–349.
14. Hung OR, Al-Qatari M: Light-guided retrograde intubation. *Can J Anaesth* 1997; 44(8):877–882.
15. Contrucci RB, Gottlieb JS: A complication of retrograde intubation. *ENT J* 1990; 69:776–778.

Chapter 13
PERCUTANEOUS TRANSTRACHEAL JET VENTILATION

Jennifer A. Cabel

INTRODUCTION

Percutaneous transtracheal jet ventilation (PTTJV) provides emergency ventilatory support in patients who cannot be adequately ventilated with a bag-valve-mask device (with oral or nasal airways) or endotracheally intubated.[1,2] This includes patients with upper airway foreign bodies or neoplasms, maxillofacial trauma, laryngeal edema, or infection.[2,3] It is also used electively with general anesthesia for surgery involving the larynx and subglottic areas.[4] PTTJV involves placement of a percutaneous catheter into the trachea and ventilation via a cyclic delivery of tidal volume to the lungs.[5]

ANATOMY AND PATHOPHYSIOLOGY

Early studies of transtracheal ventilation done by Jacoby used transtracheal catheters connected to 4 to 5 L/min of oxygen.[6] Oxygenation with this apparatus was adequate, but patients quickly developed hypercarbia due to lack of ventilation.[5] This "apneic oxygenation" also occurs in ventilation through a catheter attached to a bag-valve device.[7] The low pressure and flow of oxygen generated by the bag-valve device results in increases in $PaCO_2$ of 4 mmHg/min and the rapid development of respiratory acidosis.[1,8]

Numerous studies have since demonstrated that intermittent jets of pressurized 100% oxygen at 50 pounds per square inch (psi) allows for both oxygenation and adequate ventilation.[8,9] Inspiration occurs with insufflation of pressurized oxygen through the transtracheal catheter. Exhalation occurs passively secondary to the elastic recoil of the lungs and chest wall.[10] This passive exhalation is sufficient to maintain adequate gas exchange.

The anterior neck provides direct access to the airway via the trachea as it extends from the larynx into the lungs (Figure 13-1). At the top of the laryngeal skeleton is the thyroid cartilage, which lies at the level of the fourth and fifth cervical vertebrae. The laryngeal prominence of the thyroid cartilage (more prominent in men) is easily palpated with the thumb and index finger. The cricoid cartilage lies just inferior to the thyroid cartilage at the level of the sixth cervical vertebra. It serves as the junction of the larynx and trachea. Multiple cartilaginous rings support the trachea. Between the cricoid and thyroid cartilages lies the cricothyroid membrane. The cricothyroid membrane is a palpable membranous depression just inferior to the laryngeal prominence and is the access site for PTTJV.[11] The cricothyroid artery is a branch of the superior thyroid artery. It travels transversely across the cricothyroid membrane just below the thyroid cartilage. Placement of the catheter through the lower half of the cricothyroid membrane will prevent injury to this small artery.

Once the catheter is placed and appropriately connected to an oxygen source, oxygen is delivered via bulk flow through the cannula into the trachea and lungs. Entrainment of room air translaryngeally via the Venturi principle is negligible, even with minimal upper airway obstruction.[1] Therefore, near 100% O_2 is delivered with each insufflation.

Inhalation occurs through the catheter via a pressurized flow of oxygen. Exhalation occurs passively through the elastic recoil of the lungs and chest wall. The minute ventilation delivered during PTTJV is proportional to the volume of air injected, the driving air pressure, and the degree of upper airway obstruction.[2,12] Animal studies demonstrate that PTTJV delivers more tidal volume than positive-pressure mask ventilation with the same tracheal and transpulmonary pressures despite delivery of oxygen from a pressurized source.[2]

INDICATIONS

Transtracheal jet ventilation is indicated as a backup emergent airway in any patient who cannot be endotracheally intubated or ventilated with a bag-valve-mask device despite the use of a jaw-thrust maneuver, oropharyngeal airway, or nasopharyngeal airway.[1,2,5] It serves as a simple, relatively safe, and effective alternative to cricothyroidotomy.[1,6] This is especially true in pediatric patients below 5 years of age, in whom a cricothyroidotomy is contraindicated. PTTJV is the procedure of choice in the pediatric age group for establishing an emergent airway when endotracheal intubation fails.[7] PTTJV can serve as a quick alternative to a difficult intubation. It is especially valuable in cases of maxillofacial trauma, suspected cervical spine injury, or when nasal intubation is contraindicated or unsuccessful.[5,6,13] PTTJV is also used routinely by Anesthesiologists in the operating room. Electively, transtracheal catheters are placed in patients undergoing surgery of the upper airway, including the larynx and subglottic structures.[7]

PTTJV is also indicated in cases of upper airway obstruction due to foreign bodies, laryngeal edema, neoplasm, or infection.[2,3] In cases of upper airway foreign bodies, PTTJV not only serves as an emergent airway but can also assist in dislodging the foreign body.[6,7] Animal studies have demonstrated that the expulsion of foreign bodies from the hypopharynx and upper trachea is possible with high-frequency jet ventilation, in effect similar to the Heimlich maneuver.[13] Yealy demonstrated that approximately 30 percent of the air flow from transtracheal jet ventilation is directed cephalad and can therefore assist in the expulsion of airway foreign bodies.[14]

PTTJV has a large number of advantages when compared to an emergent cricothyroidotomy.[1–21] It is easier and faster to perform. The technique is simpler to learn. The need for a large number of instruments, surgical preparation and technique, and an assistant is eliminated. The complications of bleeding, glottic stenosis, subglottic stenosis, and tracheal erosion are significantly lessened. If the patient survives, PTTJV causes less cosmetic disfigurement. Finally, PTTJV can direct secretions and foreign bodies out of the proximal trachea.

CONTRAINDICATIONS

Percutaneous transtracheal jet ventilation is contraindicated in patients who can be orally or nasally intubated. Anterior neck trauma may be a contraindication to PTTJV. Damage to the larynx or cricoid cartilage is a contraindication to PTTJV. If laryngeal trauma is suspected, catheter placement may result in laryngeal disruption.[5,12] It should not be performed in patients with partial or complete transection of the trachea. Lower tracheal or proximal bronchial tree disruption can result in an increased risk of pneumothorax and pneumomediastinum with high-pressure ventilation.[5,7,12]

Complete airway obstruction is also an absolute contraindication to PTTJV.[5,8,12] Exhalation requires passive recoil of the lungs and chest wall, and a patent airway for outflow of gas. A patient with a complete upper airway obstruction is at an increased risk for barotrauma (pneumothorax and pneumomediastinum). Numerous studies have been performed to evaluate PTTJV with varying degrees of upper airway obstruction. Ward et al. found that progressively increasing airway obstruction up to 80 percent did not cause barotrauma.[20] **With upper airway obstruction, less air is allowed to escape and more volume is forced into the lungs.** Therefore, tidal volume increases with increasing airway obstruction. Once a patient develops complete upper airway obstruction, auto-PEEP (end-expiratory alveolar pressure above the set level of positive end-expiratory pressure) will develop as air is trapped within the thoracic cavity with no outlet and insufflation of air under pressure continues. This will ultimately result in barotrauma and decreased mean arterial pressure.[19]

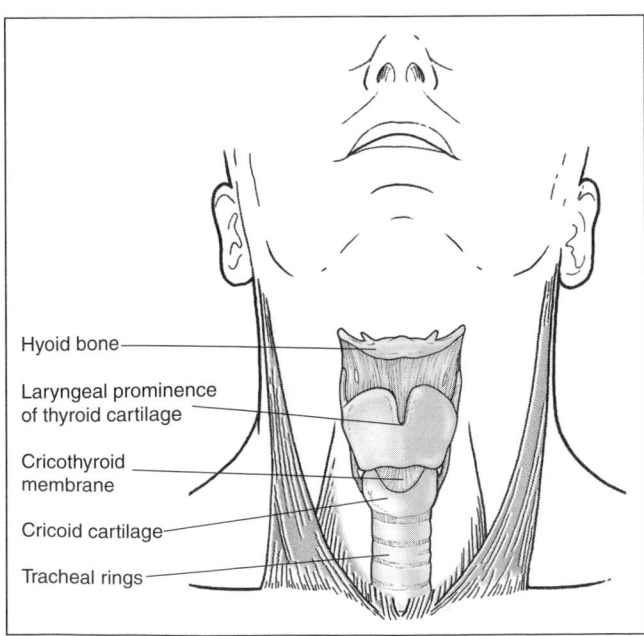

Hyoid bone

Laryngeal prominence of thyroid cartilage

Cricothyroid membrane

Cricoid cartilage

Tracheal rings

FIGURE 13-1 Airway structures of the neck.

EQUIPMENT

Povidone iodine solution
Oxygen source
Pressurized oxygen source, wall source or tank at 50 psi
Noncompressible high-pressure oxygen tubing
Valve device (manual push valve, Y connector, T piece)
12 to 16 gauge 2 to 3 inch catheter-over-the-needle
    (angiocatheter)
10 mL syringe
Sterile saline
Sterile drapes
Local anesthetic solution (1% lidocaine)
3–0 nylon suture
Needle driver
Bag-valve device
3 mL syringe
Adult endotracheal tube connector

A percutaneous transtracheal jet ventilation system can be purchased from a commercial company. It may also be assembled with individual parts.[1] Examples of two PTTJV systems are shown in Figure 13-2. The oxygen source may be a wall supply or tank. It should have a pressure regulator that can provide 100% O_2 at 50 psi through noncompressible and high-pressure tubing. Along the tubing there must be a valve (Y connector or manual push valve) to allow intermittent flow of oxygen.[5] The flow into the trachea is regulated by manual control of this valve. Ventilations should be delivered at a rate of 12 to 20 breaths per minute. Oxygen flow rates will vary with catheter size. Flow rates for 20, 16, and 14 gauge catheters at 50 psi are 400, 500, and 1600 mL/sec respectively.[9] The inspiratory time is brief compared to the expiratory time by a ratio of 1:2 to 1:9 seconds.[2,10,15]

If a high-pressure system is unavailable, the patient may still be ventilated through a transtracheally placed

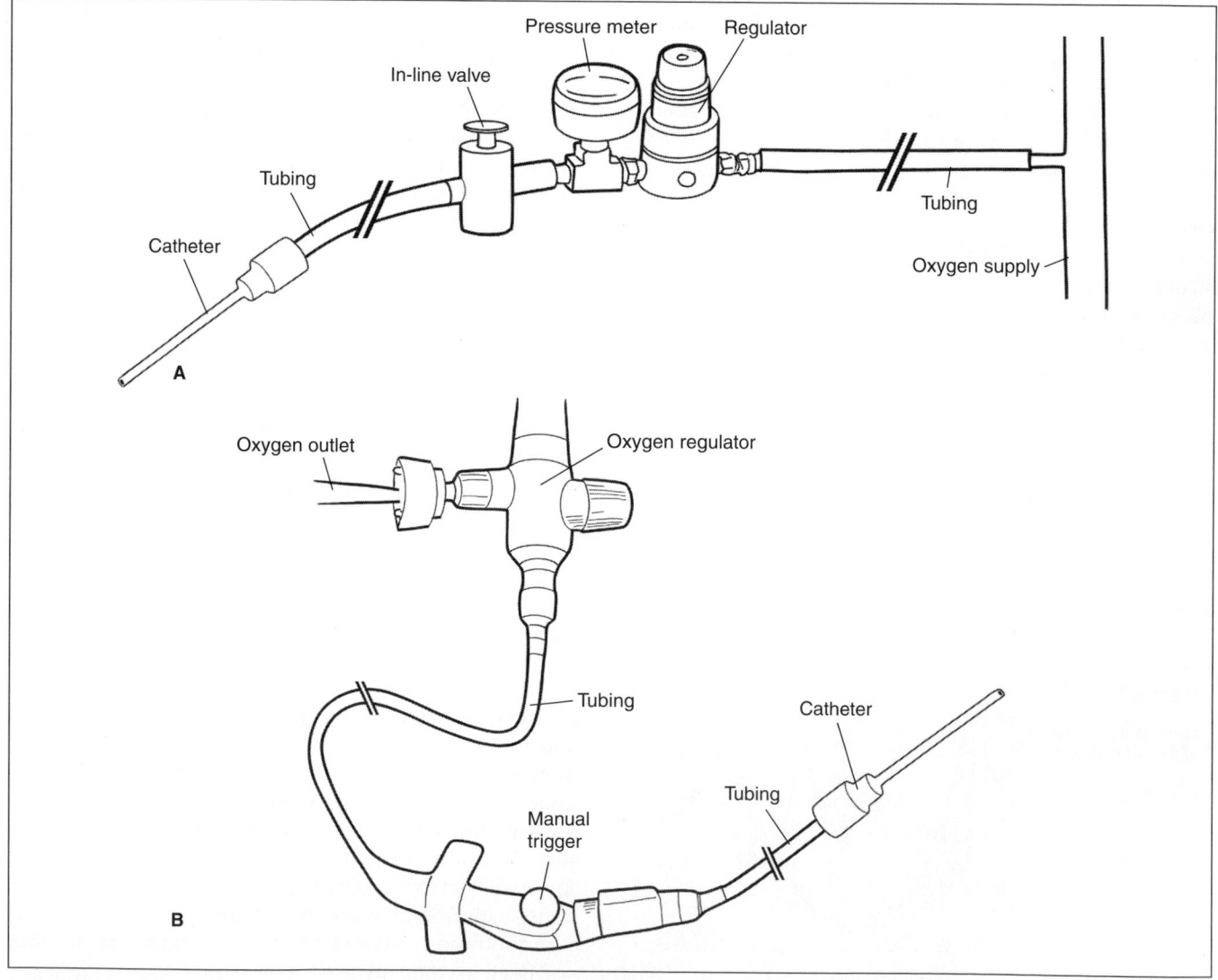

FIGURE 13-2 Examples of high-pressure jet ventilation systems. *A.* Modified from Greenfield.[21] *B.* Modified from Patel.[10]

catheter. Attach a 3 mL syringe without the plunger to the catheter. Insert a standard endotracheal tube connector, from a size 5 to 9 endotracheal tube, into the barrel of the syringe. Connect the bag-valve device to the connector and begin ventilation.

PATIENT PREPARATION

The establishment of transtracheal jet ventilation requires not only proper insertion of the transtracheal catheter but also proper setup of the ventilatory equipment. The required equipment should be prepackaged and placed where it is readily accessible. Ensure that the fittings are secure and the tubing is not damaged. Place the patient supine and in the "sniffing" position if no contraindications exist. The patient is most likely already in the proper position, as this technique is most often performed on apneic patients in whom other intubation techniques have failed. Place a rolled towel behind the middle of the neck to hyperextend the neck and allow for better access. Identify by palpation the hyoid bone, thyroid cartilage, cricoid cartilage, and cricothyroid membrane. Clean the anterior neck of any dirt and debris. Apply povidone iodine solution to the anterior neck.

TECHNIQUE

Stand at the side of the bed and adjacent to the patient's head and neck. **Reidentify the anatomic landmarks. This is crucial to perform this procedure.** Using the nondominant hand, place the thumb on one side of the thyroid cartilage and the middle finger on the other side. Use these fingers to stabilize the larynx. Use the index finger to identify the anatomic landmarks.[5,10] Start at the laryngeal prominence (Adam's apple) and work inferiorly. The soft membranous defect inferior to the laryngeal prominence is the cricothyroid membrane. Below this is the cartilaginous ring of the cricoid cartilage.

Attach a 12 to 16 gauge catheter-over-the-needle (angiocatheter) to a 10 mL syringe containing 5 mL of sterile saline. Insert the catheter-over-the-needle through the skin, subcutaneous tissue, and inferior aspect of the cricothyroid membrane. **The inferior aspect of the cricothyroid membrane is the preferred site as it avoids injury to the cricothyroid arteries.**[7] Direct the catheter-over-the-needle inferiorly and at a 30 to 45 degree angle (Figure 13-3A). Maintain constant negative pressure within the syringe as it is advanced (Figure 13-3B). Continue to advance the catheter-over-the-needle while maintaining negative pressure until air bubbles are visible in the syringe and a loss of resis-

tance is felt.[5,10] These both signify that the catheter-over-the-needle is within the trachea.

Once placement within the trachea is confirmed, securely hold the needle and advance the catheter until the hub is against the skin (Figure 13-3C). Remove the needle and syringe (Figure 13-3C). Reattach the syringe without the needle to the catheter. Aspirate once again to reconfirm placement of the catheter within the trachea. The 2 to 3 cm catheter should be long enough to pass into the tracheal lumen without sitting against the posterior wall. If the catheter tip directly touches or faces the posterior tracheal wall, there is the risk of forcing air submucosally.[12] Firmly grasp and hold the catheter hub at the skin of the neck. Remove the syringe. Attach the oxygen tubing to the catheter (Figure 13-3D). Begin ventilation and continue until a more permanent and secure airway is established.[5]

ASSESSMENT

Transtracheal jet ventilation requires continuous cardiac and pulse oximetry monitoring. Arterial blood gas samples should be obtained periodically to look for hypoxia and hypercarbia. Careful attention must be paid to maintaining a patent upper airway to allow for expiration. Oropharyngeal and/or nasopharyngeal airways, or a jaw-thrust maneuver, are often adequate.

AFTERCARE

The catheter and tubing must be secured to prevent accidental dislodgement.[10] There are three ways to secure the equipment. The first and preferred method is to suture it in place. Place a skin wheal of local anesthetic solution (1% lidocaine) next to the catheter hub. Using 3–0 nylon suture, place a stitch through the skin wheal and tie it securely. Do not cut the suture. Wrap the long end of the suture around the catheter hub two or three times and tie it securely to the tail of the suture. Wrap the long end of the suture around the oxygen tubing, just above the attachment to the catheter hub, two or three times and tie it securely to the tail of the suture. Alternatively, wrap a piece of umbilical or plain tape around the patient's neck, the catheter hub, and the oxygen tubing. A second alternative is to attach a commercially available endotracheal tube holder around the patient's neck and connect it to the oxygen tubing. The catheter will still have to be secured with suture or by being taped to the oxygen tubing and skin.

The catheter, oxygen tubing, and patient must be continually assessed during PTTJV. Check the catheter tubing at regular intervals for signs of dislodgement or kinking. Examine the patient for crepitus in the neck and

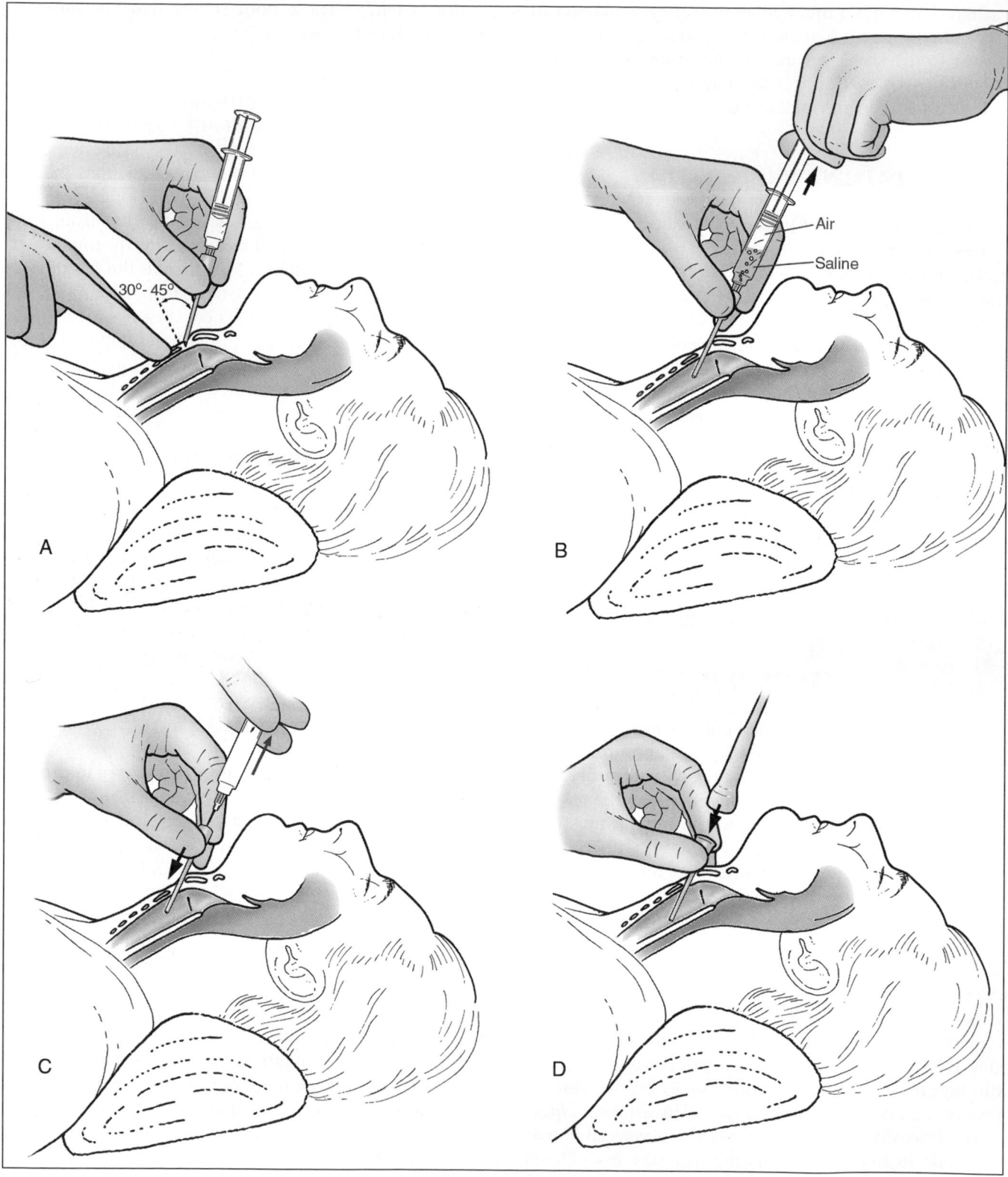

FIGURE 13-3 Insertion of the transtracheal catheter. *A.* The catheter-over-the-needle is inserted 30 to 45 degrees to the perpendicular (*dotted line*) and aimed inferiorly. *B.* Application of negative pressure to a saline-containing syringe during catheter insertion (*arrow*). Air bubbles in the saline confirm intratracheal placement of the catheter. *C.* The catheter is advanced until the hub is against the skin. The needle and syringe are then removed. *D.* High-pressure oxygen tubing is attached to the catheter and ventilation is begun.

torso. If crepitus is present, the catheter tip is most likely directly against or directed toward the mucosa of the posterior tracheal wall. Oxygen is being forced into the submucosal tissues and tracking subcutaneously. Remove the catheter and reinsert a new one. Obtain a chest radiograph to assess the patient for a pneumomediastinum, pneumopericardium, or pneumothorax that may require decompression. Pulse oximetry and cardiac monitoring should also be continuously monitored.

COMPLICATIONS

Percutaneous transtracheal jet ventilation is a relatively safe and effective means of establishing an emergent airway in a patient who cannot be intubated. Complications are fewer than with a cricothyroidotomy, but they do occur and must be anticipated.

Subcutaneous emphysema occurs most commonly when the transtracheal catheter is misplaced, becomes dislodged into the soft tissues of the neck during ventilation, or is placed against the mucosa of the posterior tracheal wall.[1,5,6] It may also occur if catheter placement is unsuccessful on the first attempt, creating a port for leakage of pressurized air into the subcutaneous tissue of the neck.[5] Frequent examination of the catheter site for evidence of subcutaneous emphysema may provide the earliest clue to catheter malfunction.

Barotrauma may present as a pneumothorax, pneumomediastinum, or pneumopericardium. It may be a result of upper airway obstruction. The exhalation of air is passive and depends on a patent upper airway. **It is therefore important to monitor chest rise and fall as evidence of continued air exchange.**[1] An oropharyngeal airway, nasopharyngeal airway, or jaw-thrust maneuver will often provide adequate upper airway patency.[5] **Assume, until proven otherwise, that any sudden change in the patient's heart rate or blood pressure during PTTJV is secondary to a tension pneumothorax.** There has been a case report of laryngospasm with PTTJV use during an elective surgical procedure.[16] It resulted in sudden desaturation and hypotension that were easily resolved with the administration of a paralytic agent.

Catheter obstruction is another potential complication. Most commonly, the catheter will kink as it traverses the soft tissues of the neck.[1,5] This may occur if the catheter is dislodged or as a result of high-pressure ventilation. The use of a commercially available kink-resistant catheter greatly reduces this risk.

The catheter may be inappropriately placed. Misplacement of the catheter into the submucosa of the larynx can lead to a laryngeal pneumatocele. If this is suspected or identified, remove the catheter and reinsert a new one. The pneumatocele can be aspirated with a

needle and syringe after placement of a new catheter.[5] Misplacement of the catheter posteriorly through the back of the trachea and perforation of the esophagus is a theoretical concern that has never been reported.[1,5,6]

Pulmonary aspiration is another potential complication in PTTJV. The epiglottis provides no airway protection, and the small transtracheal catheter does not prevent aspiration of secretions or gastric contents into the lungs. Animal studies have demonstrated that pulmonary aspiration in fact did not occur despite variable frequencies of ventilation, variable oxygen flow pressure, and cardiac compressions during cardiopulmonary resuscitation (CPR).[17,18] Studies have shown that the pressurized flow of air through the catheter provides an adequate forceful gas outflow from the lungs.[17,18] This may prevent pulmonary aspiration. Secretions and foreign bodies have been shown to stay above the jetting catheter while PTTJV is in progress. **If PTTJV is to be discontinued, great care must be taken to assure complete suctioning and cleansing of the upper airway above the catheter.**[18]

Less serious complications include local hematoma formation at the catheter insertion site, hemoptysis, and cough.[1,5,6] The use of nonhumidified oxygen in the catheter has been reported to cause irritation and erosion to the tracheal mucosa.[1]

SUMMARY

Percutaneous transtracheal jet ventilation is an effective and easy method for establishing an emergent airway in patients who cannot be ventilated with a bag-valve-mask device or intubated. The indications for PTTJV are the same as those for a cricothyroidotomy. Placement of a catheter through the cricothyroid membrane and attached to a high-pressure oxygen source will provide adequate oxygenation and ventilation until a more definitive airway can be established. This is a rapidly performed airway management technique that should be considered as a backup rescue technique.

REFERENCES

1. Benumof JL, Scheller MS: The importance of transtracheal jet ventilation in the management of the difficult airway. *Anesthesiology* 1989; 71(5):769–778.
2. Carl ML, Rhee KJ, Schelegle ES, et al: Pulmonary mechanics of dogs during transtracheal jet ventilation. *Ann Emerg Med* 1994; 24(6):1126–1135.
3. Jacobson S: Upper airway obstruction. *Emerg Med Clin* 1989; 7(2):205–217.

4. Depierraz B, Ravussin P, Brossard E, et al: Percutaneous transtracheal jet ventilation for paediatric endoscopic laser treatment of laryngeal and subglottic lesions. *Can J Anaesth* 1994; 41(12):1200–1207.

5. Jorden RC: Percutaneous transtracheal ventilation. *Emerg Med Clin* 1988; 6(4):745–752.

6. Frame SB, Timberlake GA, Kerstein MD, et al: Transtracheal needle catheter ventilation in complete airway obstruction: an animal model. *Ann Emerg Med* 1989; 18(2):127–133.

7. Mace SE: Cricothyrotomy and translaryngeal jet ventilation, in Roberts JR, Hedges JR (eds): *Clinical Procedures in Emergency Medicine*. Philadelphia: Saunders, 1998:66–74.

8. Neff CC, Pfister RC, Sonnenberg EV: Percutaneous transtracheal ventilation: experimental and practical aspects. *J Trauma* 1983; 23(2):84–90.

9. Yealy DM, Stewart RD, Kaplan RM: Myths and pitfalls in emergency translaryngeal ventilation: correcting misimpressions. *Ann Emerg Med* 1988; 17(7):690–692.

10. Patel R: Percutaneous transtracheal jet ventilation: a safe, quick, and temporary way to provide oxygenation and ventilation when conventional methods are unsuccessful. *Chest* 1999; 116(6):1689–1694.

11. Moore KL: *Clinically Oriented Anatomy*. Baltimore: Williams & Wilkins, 1992:816–817.

12. Tinker JH, Rogers MC, Covino BJ: *Principles and Practice of Anesthesiology*. St. Louis: Mosby–Year Book, 1993:226–231.

13. Klain M, Keszler H, Brader E: High frequency jet ventilation in CPR. *Crit Care Med* 1981; 9(5):421–422.

14. Yealy DM, Plewa MC, Reed JJ, et al: Manual translaryngeal jet ventilation and the risk of aspiration in a canine model. *Ann Emerg Med* 1990; 19:1238–1241.

15. Stothert JC, Stout MJ, Lewis LM, et al: High pressure percutaneous transtracheal ventilation: the use of large gauge intravenous–type catheters in the totally obstructed airway. *Am J Emerg Med* 1990; 8(3):184–189.

16. Schumacher P, Stotz G, Schneider M, et al: Laryngospasm during transtracheal high frequency jet ventilation. *Anaesthesia* 1992; 47:855–856.

17. Jawan B, Cheung HK, Chong ZK, et al: Aspiration and transtracheal jet ventilation with different pressures and depths of chest compression. *Crit Care Med* 1999; 27(1):142–145.

18. Jawan B, Lee JH: Aspiration in transtracheal jet ventilation. *Acta Anaesthesiol Scand* 1996; 40:684–686.

19. Carl ML, Rhee KJ, Schelegle ES, et al: Effects of graded upper-airway obstruction on pulmonary mechanics during transtracheal jet ventilation in dogs. *Ann Emerg Med* 1994; 24(6):1137–1143.

20. Ward KR, Menegazzi JJ, Yealy D, et al: Translaryngeal jet ventilation and end–tidal Pco_2 monitoring during varying degrees of upper airway obstruction. *Ann Emerg Med* 1991; 20(11):1193–1197.

21. Greenfield RH: Percutaneous transtracheal ventilation, in Henretig FM, King C, et al (eds): *Textbook of Pediatric Emergency Procedures*. Baltimore: Williams & Wilkins, 1997:239–250.

Chapter 14
CRICOTHYROIDOTOMY

Kimberly Nagy

INTRODUCTION

Establishment of an airway is of prime importance to survival. The most predictive factor of survival from cardiac arrest is establishment of an airway.[1] Unfortunately, the Emergentologist is occasionally confronted with an airway that is extremely difficult or even impossible to obtain by endotracheal intubation. Between 1 and 4 percent of all emergent airways require a cricothyroidotomy.[2–5] Up to 7 percent of trauma patients who present in cardiopulmonary arrest will require a cricothyroidotomy.[3]

The technique of cricothyroidotomy has been in use since the early 1900s. In 1921, Chevalier Jackson condemned its use because of fears of subglottic stenosis.[6,7] Jackson's technique involved incising the cricoid cartilage, which led to the subglottic stenosis. The technique was popularized again in 1966 by Brantigan and Grow, but it was considered primarily an elective procedure.[6,7] **Cricothyroidotomy has since evolved into the surgical airway of choice for emergent situations in which other intubation methods have failed or are contraindicated.**[2,8] The physician using rapid sequence induction to intubate patients should be knowledgeable and skilled in performing a cricothyroidotomy.[3] The success rate of a cricothyroidotomy is between 96 and 100 percent.[4,9]

A cricothyroidotomy has numerous advantages over a tracheostomy.[6,10,11] A cricothyroidotomy is easier, faster, and safer to perform. It can be performed in less than 2 minutes. It can be performed by those with little or no surgical training. It does not require the support of an operating room and a large amount of equipment. The anatomic landmarks are superficial, easily seen, and easily palpated. The procedure does not require a deep dissection, as the structures are located subcutaneously.

The cricothyroid membrane is not covered by any structures that would interfere with the procedure. Because the cricothyroid membrane is in the upper part of the neck, there is less chance of injuring the esophagus. A cricothyroidotomy can be performed with the patient's neck in a neutral position. This is especially important in those with potential cervical spine injuries. The procedure has fewer associated complications than a tracheostomy. Although not a concern when securing an airway, the skin incision will heal with a smaller and less noticeable scar.

ANATOMY AND PATHOPHYSIOLOGY

The cricothyroid membrane is located between the thyroid cartilage superiorly and the cricoid cartilage inferiorly (Figure 14-1). **The cricothyroid membrane must be identified by palpation of the surrounding cartilaginous structures.** Using the nondominant hand, place the thumb on one side of the thyroid cartilage and the middle finger on the other side (Figure 14-2). Palpate the laryngeal prominence (Adam's apple) with the index finger. Moving inferiorly, the index finger will fall into a hollow, which is the location of the cricothyroid membrane. The next structure palpated is the firm cartilaginous ring of the cricoid cartilage, followed by the tracheal rings. In a thin patient, it is important to locate the hyoid bone superiorly to be sure that you are not making your incision superior to the vocal cords.

The cricothyroid membrane itself is a thin membrane measuring 2 to 3 cm in width and only 9 to 10 mm in height.[8,11] It is located approximately 1 cm below the true vocal cords.[11] There is relatively little subcutaneous tissue overlying the cricothyroid membrane. There are few to no vascular structures overlying the cricothyroid

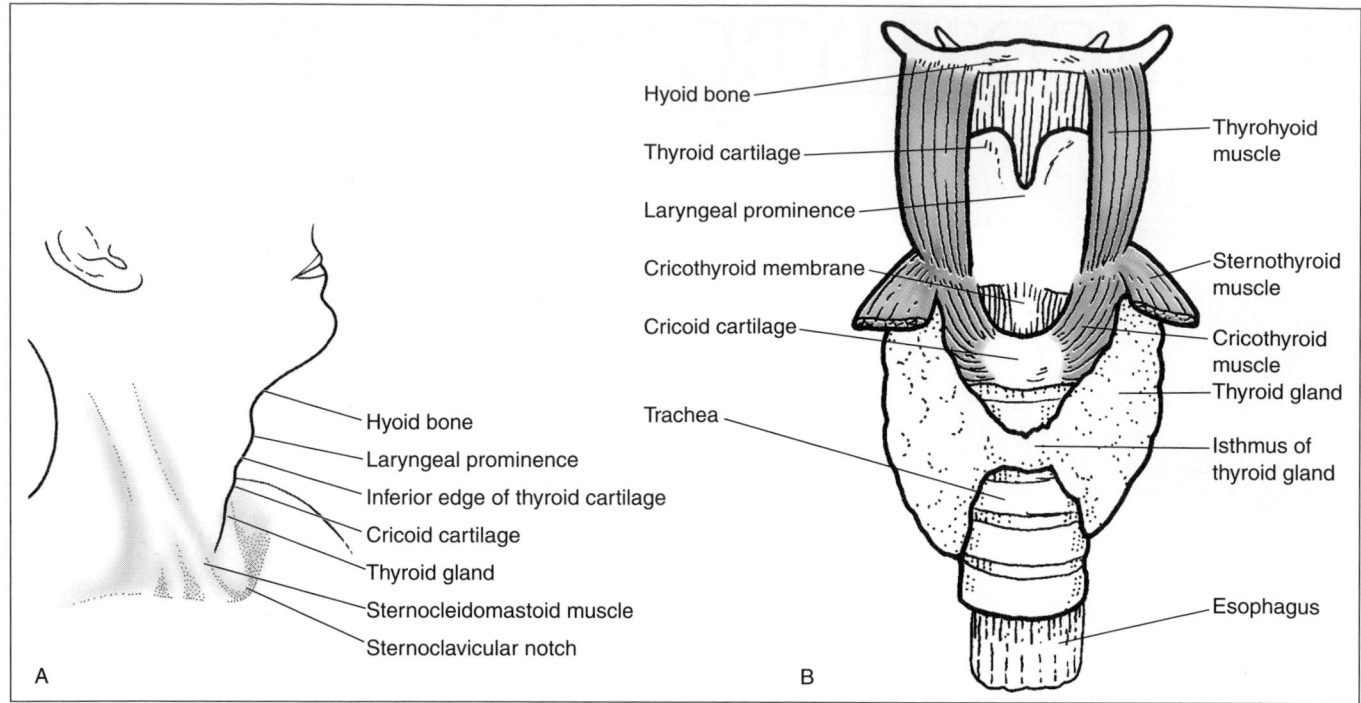

FIGURE 14-1 Anatomy of the airway in the neck region. *A.* Topographic anatomy. *B.* The framework of the airway.

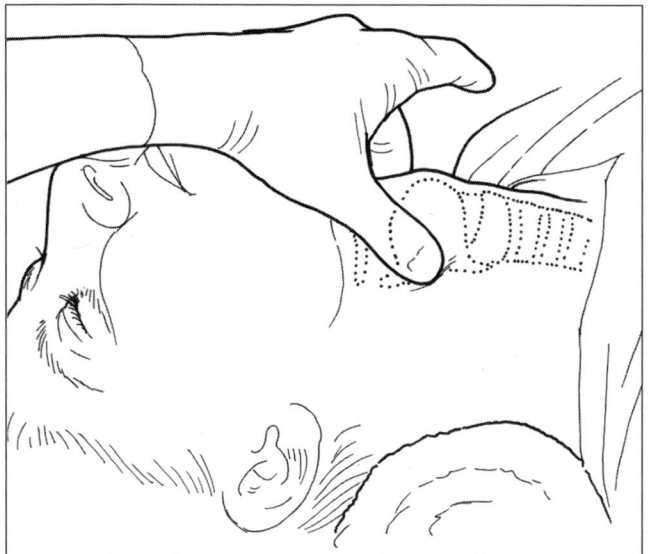

FIGURE 14-2 Proper hand positioning to identify the airway structures of the neck.

membrane. The anterior cricothyroid arteries travel from lateral to medial over the superior border of the cricothyroid membrane. The anterior jugular veins may lie immediately superior and lateral to the cricothyroid membrane. Farther lateral and posterior are the great vessels of the neck. Posterior to the larynx and trachea is the esophagus. It is therefore important not to make the incision too deep, thus risking an esophageal intubation or injury.

INDICATIONS

The most frequent indication for an emergent or urgent surgical airway is the inability to intubate endotracheally with less invasive techniques. These less invasive techniques may have failed or been contraindicated.[10] **Attempts at orotracheal or nasotracheal intubation should be made prior to attempts at creating a surgical airway.**[4,8] A common reason for the failure of orotracheal intubation is not using rapid sequence induction and the patient's clenched teeth precluding intubation.[9] Other common reasons for failure to establish endotracheal intubation include severe neck or facial injury resulting in distortion of the normal anatomy, edema, masseter spasm, laryngospasm, cervical spine injury, deformities of the mouth and/or pharynx, upper airway hemorrhage, large amounts of vomitus in the oropharynx, and upper airway obstruction.[8,9,11] **Although endotracheal intubation should be attempted first, it is prudent to have the surgical airway supplies nearby if you suspect that the patient will have a difficult airway.**

Needle cricothyroidotomy is the emergent "surgical" airway of choice in a patient younger than 8 to 10 years of age.[11,12] In young children, the cricothyroid membrane as well as its surrounding structures are much smaller and more difficult to access. It is easier to injure one of the cervical vessels or the esophagus when a standard cricothyroidotomy is performed in a child. In addition, subglottic stenosis is a common late complication following cricothyroidotomy in children.[12] A needle cricothyroidotomy is a safer alternative and allows for adequate oxygenation and ventilation until a formal tracheostomy or other method of endotracheal intubation can be performed. Unfortunately, the small caliber of the catheter does not often provide adequate oxygenation and ventilation in an adult.

CONTRAINDICATIONS

There are a few absolute contraindications to performing a cricothyroidotomy. The most important is if the patient can be endotracheally intubated by less invasive methods. Partial or complete transection of the airway is a contraindication to a cricothyroidotomy. In these cases, a tracheostomy is the preferred method to secure the airway. Finally, this procedure should not be performed in cases of significant injury or fracture of the cricoid cartilage, larynx, and/or thyroid cartilage.

There are some situations where the performance of a cricothyroidotomy may be less desirable. The presence of laryngeal pathology (tumor, fracture) may preclude the performance of a cricothyroidotomy and necessitate a high tracheostomy.[11,13] If a patient has been previously intubated endotracheally for a prolonged period, there is a higher incidence of long-term complications following cricothyroidotomy.[13] While this does not prevent the performance of a cricothyroidotomy, one should consider an early revision to a tracheostomy to minimize these complications. Other relative contraindications to performing a cricothyroidotomy are the presence of a coagulopathy, massive neck swelling, or a hematoma in the neck, all of which increase the risk of bleeding and distortion of the anatomy. Finally, unfamiliarity with the technique may lead to increased complications.[11]

EQUIPMENT

General Supplies

Sterile gloves, gowns, and drapes
Face mask and eye protection
Local anesthetic solution (1% lidocaine)
5 mL syringes
21 and 25 gauge needles
Bag-valve-mask device
Oxygen source and tubing

Surgical Cricothyroidotomy

Povidone iodine solution
#11 scalpel blade on a scalpel handle

Trousseau tracheal dilator or curved 6 inch hemostat
Tracheal hook
Hemostats, 4 small
Needle driver
Suture scissors
Tracheostomy tubes, sizes #4 and #6
Endotracheal tubes, various sizes
Tracheostomy tape (twill tape)
3–0 sutures for hemostasis (Dexon, Vicryl, or chromic)
3–0 nylon sutures for skin closure
1 inch tape (or a commercially available endotracheal tube holder)
Gauze, 4×4 squares
Iodoform gauze ribbon
Percutaneous cricothyroidotomy kit

Needle Cricothyroidotomy

Povidone iodine solution
14 gauge catheter-over-the-needle (angiocatheter), 2 inch
5 mL syringe
Endotracheal tubes, various sizes
High-flow oxygen tubing with a small hole cut in the side
Tape

The equipment should be prepackaged in a sterile tray that is readily accessible. Some institutions maintain separate cricothyroidotomy and tracheostomy trays. Others have one tray that has all the equipment necessary to perform both procedures. If a cricothyroidotomy tray is not immediately available, a thoracotomy tray usually contains all the required equipment to perform this procedure.

PATIENT PREPARATION

Since a cricothyroidotomy is most commonly an emergent procedure, there is little if any time to explain this to the patient and obtain their consent. If there is sufficient probability that an awake and stable patient will require a surgical airway, informed consent may be obtained.

Place the patient supine with their head in a neutral position. Place a rolled towel under the patient's upper shoulders and neck if no contraindications exist (Figure 14-3). This position offers excellent exposure, prevents the airway structures from moving, and lengthens the cricothyroid membrane. While it is not impossible to perform a cricothyroidotomy with a cervical collar on the patient, it is very difficult. If the patient is at risk for a cervical spine injury, it is preferable to remove the collar while an assistant maintains in-line stabilization of the neck in a neutral position. An additional assistant

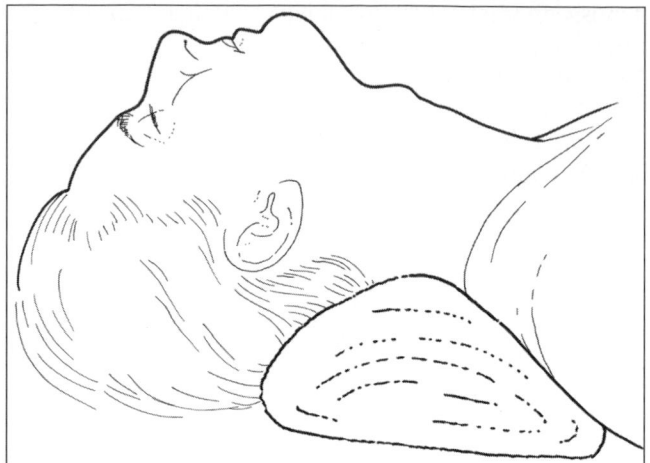

FIGURE 14-3 The patient is positioned with a rolled towel under the upper shoulders. This position offers excellent exposure, stabilizes the airway structures, and lengthens the cricothyroid membrane.

should maintain the airway and provide ventilatory support with a bag-valve-mask device.

In the ideal situation, the skin of the anterior neck should be prepped with povidone iodine and sterile drapes placed to isolate a surgical field. The physician performing the procedure should be clad in a mask, sterile gown, and gloves. The circumstances in which the procedure is usually performed often require that the airway be obtained rapidly. In these cases, a quick spray of povidone iodine and sterile gloves will suffice.

TECHNIQUES

During the performance of this procedure, one or two assistants should be maintaining the airway and providing ventilation and oxygenation with a bag-valve-mask device. The right-handed physician should be standing at the patient's right side.[11] The position is reversed for the left-handed physician.

Stabilize the large thyroid cartilage in place with the thumb and middle finger of the nondominant hand[8,14] (Figure 14-2). **The immobilization of the larynx cannot be overemphasized. If the larynx is not secure and thus the landmarks are lost, the procedure will fail. Identify the anatomic landmarks necessary to perform this procedure. This is critical to the performance of a cricothyroidotomy.** Place the index finger over the laryngeal prominence (Adam's apple). Move the index finger inferiorly to identify the cricothyroid membrane, cricoid cartilage, and tracheal rings. Move the index finger superiorly until it falls back into the cricothyroid membrane. Leave the index finger over the cricothyroid membrane. Using the index finger of the dominant

hand, confirm that the nondominant index finger is situated over the cricothyroid membrane. If the patient is awake and stable, the area of the incision should be infiltrated with local anesthetic solution.

TRADITIONAL TECHNIQUE

Make a 2 to 3 cm transverse incision, centered in the midline, through the skin and subcutaneous tissue (Figures 14-4 and 14-5A). Continue the incision through the cricothyroid membrane. As one gains skill with this procedure, all layers may be incised simultaneously with one incision. The beginner should proceed with some caution because there is a small risk of incising through the posterior wall of the airway.[8,11] **The incision should be no longer than 2 or 3 cm, as this represents the width of the membrane.**[7,14] Longer incisions risk injury to the anterior jugular veins that lie just lateral to the thyroid cartilage.[11]

Longitudinal incisions in the midline are not recommended. They take longer to perform and require repositioning after the skin incision. The primary indication for a longitudinal skin incision is in the patient with a suspected laryngeal injury and distortion of the anatomic landmarks.[11] In these cases, the longitudinal incision permits the extension of the incision inferiorly in order to perform a high tracheostomy.

Once the cricothyroid membrane has been incised and the airway entered, bubbling should be noted through the wound. This is true if the patient is ventilating spontaneously or with the assistance of a bag-valve-mask device. **Do not remove the scalpel.** Insert the tracheal hook along the scalpel and grasp the inferior border of the thyroid cartilage (Figure 14-5B). Elevate the tracheal hook to retract the thyroid cartilage anteriorly and superiorly.[4,5] The scalpel may now be removed. Insert a Trousseau tracheal dilator or a large (6 inch) hemostat through the cricothyroid membrane while maintaining control of the thyroid cartilage (Figure 14-5C). Spread the jaws of the dilator to further enlarge the opening in the cricothyroid membrane.[4,5,7,8] Remove the dilator while continuing to maintain control of the airway with the tracheal hook.

Select a tracheostomy tube that is of an appropriate size for the patient. Have an assistant lubricate the obturator and outer cannula, then insert the obturator into the outer cannula. While maintaining control of the airway with the tracheal hook, insert the tracheostomy tube perpendicularly (90 degrees) to the skin (Figure 14-5D). Continue to advance the tracheostomy tube with a semicircular motion and inferiorly until the flange is against the skin. The tracheostomy tube should pass with minimal difficulty. Remove the tracheal hook. Remove the obturator, insert the inner cannula, connect the bag-valve device, and ventilate the patient.[4] Inflate

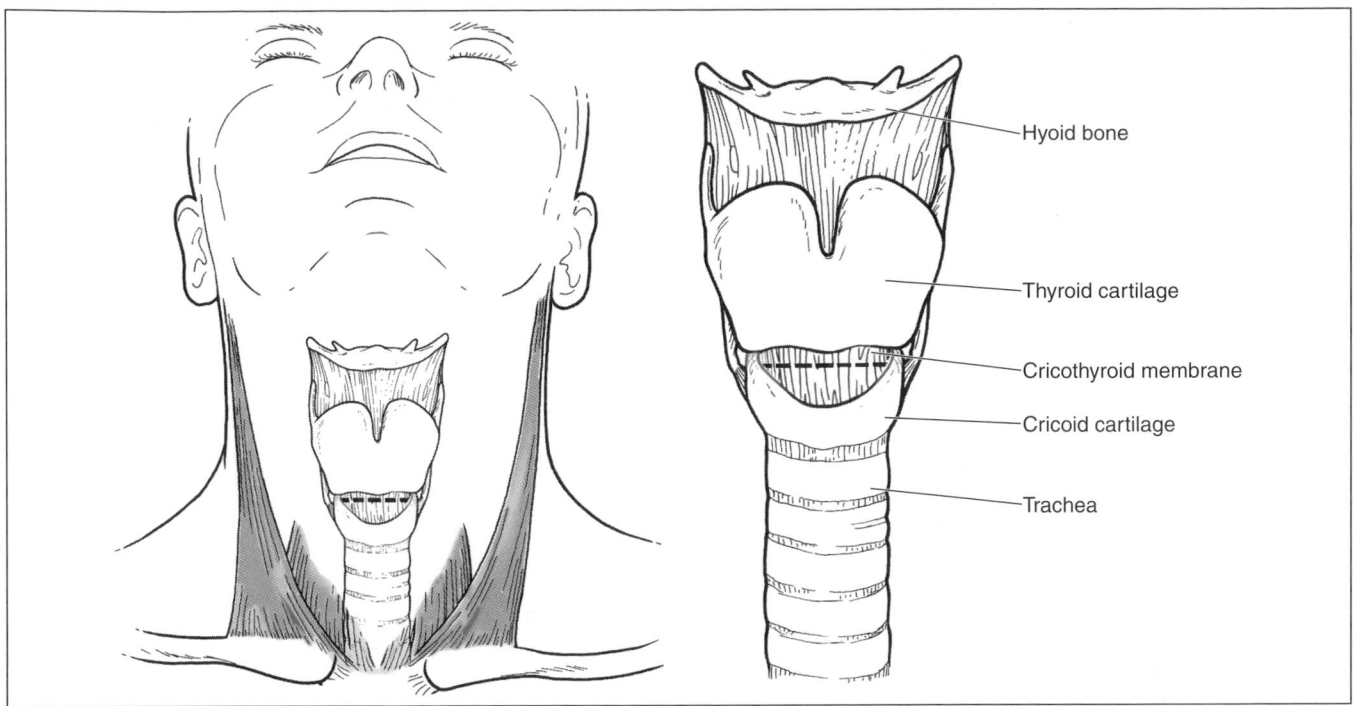

FIGURE 14-4 The cricothyroidotomy site. The dotted line represents the incision site over the cricothyroid membrane.

Hyoid bone

Thyroid cartilage

Cricothyroid membrane

Cricoid cartilage

Trachea

the cuff of the tracheostomy tube. Confirm the intratracheal position of the tube by auscultating bilateral breath sounds and noting the absence of breath sounds over the stomach.

If a tracheostomy tube is not available, an endotracheal tube can be used. The endotracheal tube is much longer than is needed. Remove the 15 mm connector from the proximal end of the endotracheal tube. Cut the endotracheal tube with scissors just above where the tubing to inflate the cuff enters the tube. Place the 15 mm connector on the shortened endotracheal tube. The procedure to insert an endotracheal tube is the same as that for a tracheostomy tube.

ALTERNATIVE SURGICAL TECHNIQUE

An alternative surgical approach to a cricothyroidotomy was first developed by Oppenheimer.[17] It is simpler, more rapid, and easier to perform than the traditional technique described above (Figures 14-6 and 14-7). The technique has been modified from the original description.[18]

Clean, prepare, and drape the neck as mentioned previously. Position the nondominant hand with the thumb on one side of the thyroid cartilage and the middle finger on the other side (Figures 14-6A and 14-7A). Identify the anatomic landmarks as described previously. Leave the nondominant index finger over the cricothyroid membrane. If the patient is awake, infiltrate local anes-

thetic solution subcutaneously over the cricothyroid membrane.

Guide a #11 surgical blade along the nondominant index finger and into the cricothyroid membrane using a stab incision (Figures 14-6A and B, Figure 14-7B). **Do not insert the scalpel blade more than 1.5 to 2.0 cm to prevent it from injuring the esophagus.** It is recommended to hold the scalpel just above the blade with the thumb and index finger to prevent it from plunging too deep.[18] Air or bubbles from the incision signify that the tip of the scalpel blade is inside the trachea. **Do not remove the scalpel blade.** Move it laterally 0.75 cm to extend the incision (Figures 14-6C and 14-7C). Rotate the scalpel blade 180 degrees and extend the incision 0.75 cm in the opposite direction (Figures 14-6D and 14-7D). **Do not remove the scalpel blade.** Removing the scalpel from the incision will make you lose your landmarks and the location of the incision through the cricothyroid membrane.

With the scalpel blade in place, insert a tracheal hook into the midline of the incision (Figures 14-6E and 14-7E). Grasp the inferior border of the thyroid cartilage with the tracheal hook. Lift the tracheal hook upward and superiorly to elevate and control the airway (Figures 14-6F and 14-7F). **Remove the scalpel from the incision only after the airway is controlled with the tracheal hook.**

The incision site must be expanded to accommodate the passage of an endotracheal tube or a tracheostomy

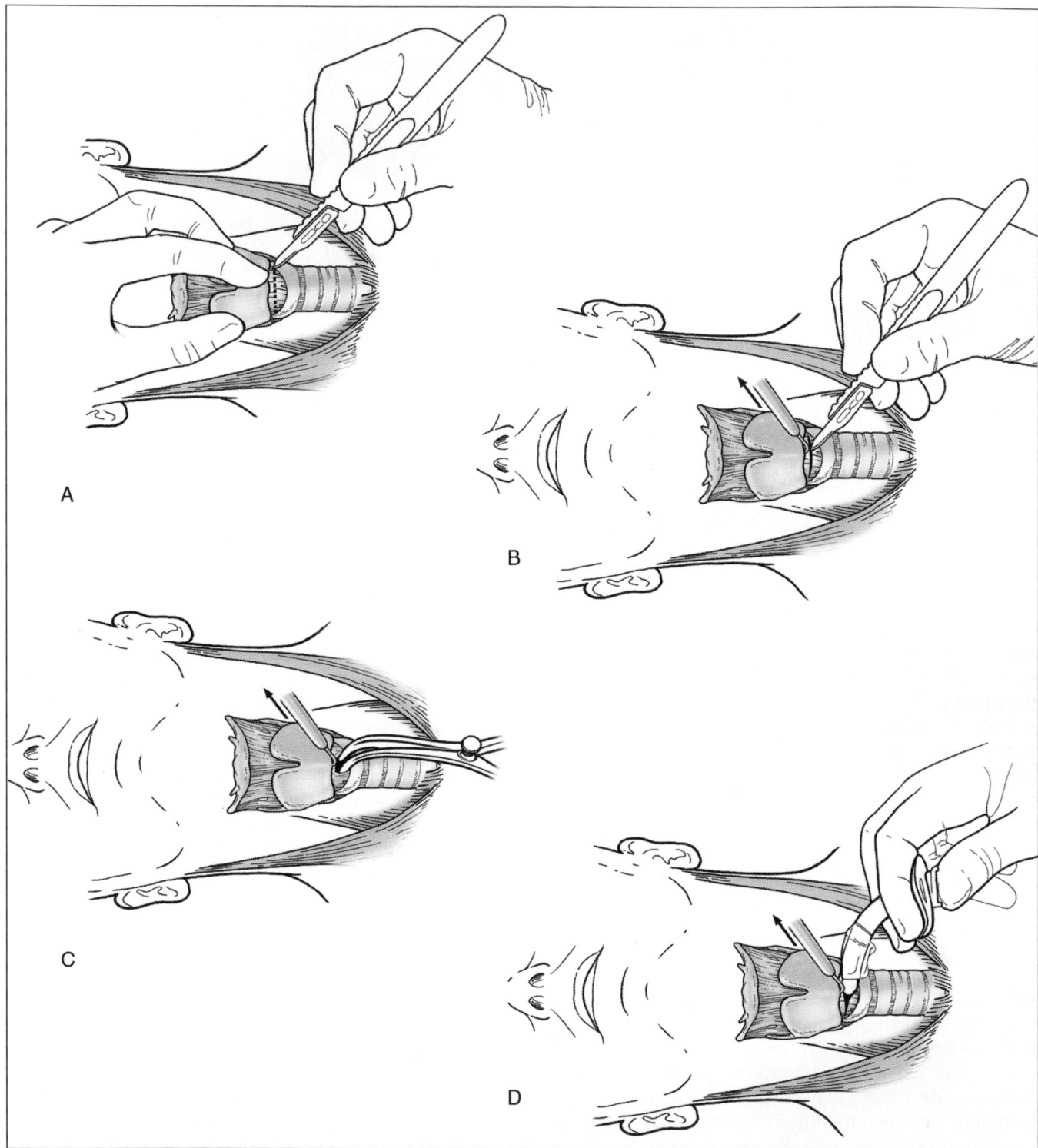

FIGURE 14-5 A surgical cricothyroidotomy. *A.* The nondominant hand stabilizes the cricothyroid membrane. A transverse incision is made through the skin, subcutaneous tissue, and cricothyroid membrane. *B.* A tracheal hook is inserted over the scalpel blade to grasp the inferior border of the thyroid cartilage. The hook is lifted anteriorly and superiorly to control the airway (*arrow*). *C.* A Trousseau dilator is inserted into the incision and opened to dilate the incision site. *D.* A tracheostomy tube is inserted through the cricothyroid membrane.

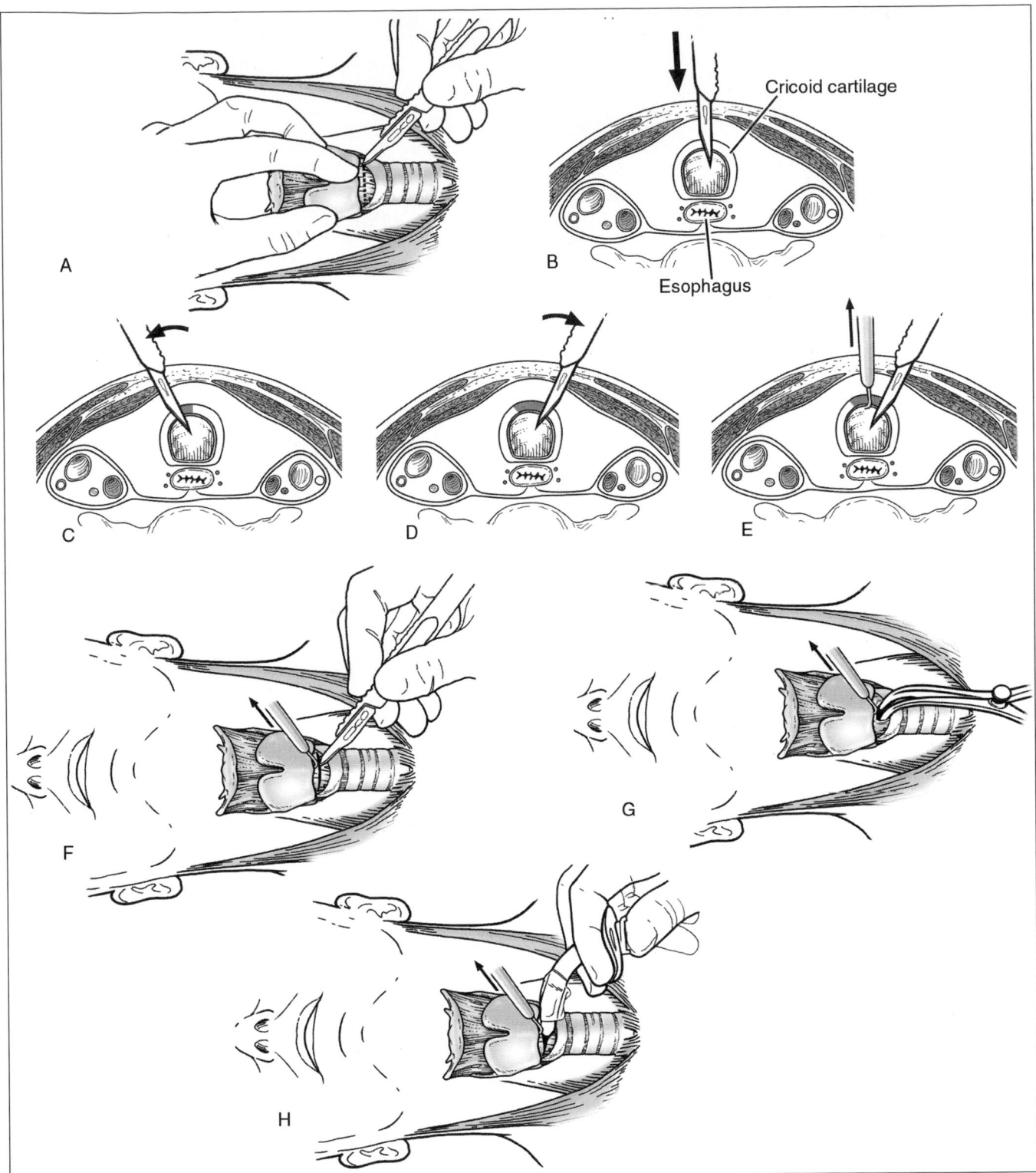

FIGURE 14-6 An alternative method to perform a surgical cricothyroidotomy. *A.* The thyroid cartilage is secured while a stab incision is made in the cricothyroid membrane. *B.* The scalpel blade penetrates the midline and enters the airway. *C.* The incision is extended laterally from the midline. *D.* The scalpel is rotated 180 degrees and extends the incision to the other side. *E.* A tracheal hook is inserted in the midline and grasps the inferior border of the thyroid cartilage. *F.* The thyroid cartilage is lifted anteriorly and superiorly to control the airway (*arrow*). After the airway is controlled, the scalpel is removed. *G.* A Trousseau dilator is inserted into the incision. The jaws are opened to dilate the incision. *H.* A tracheostomy tube is inserted into the trachea using a semicircular motion.

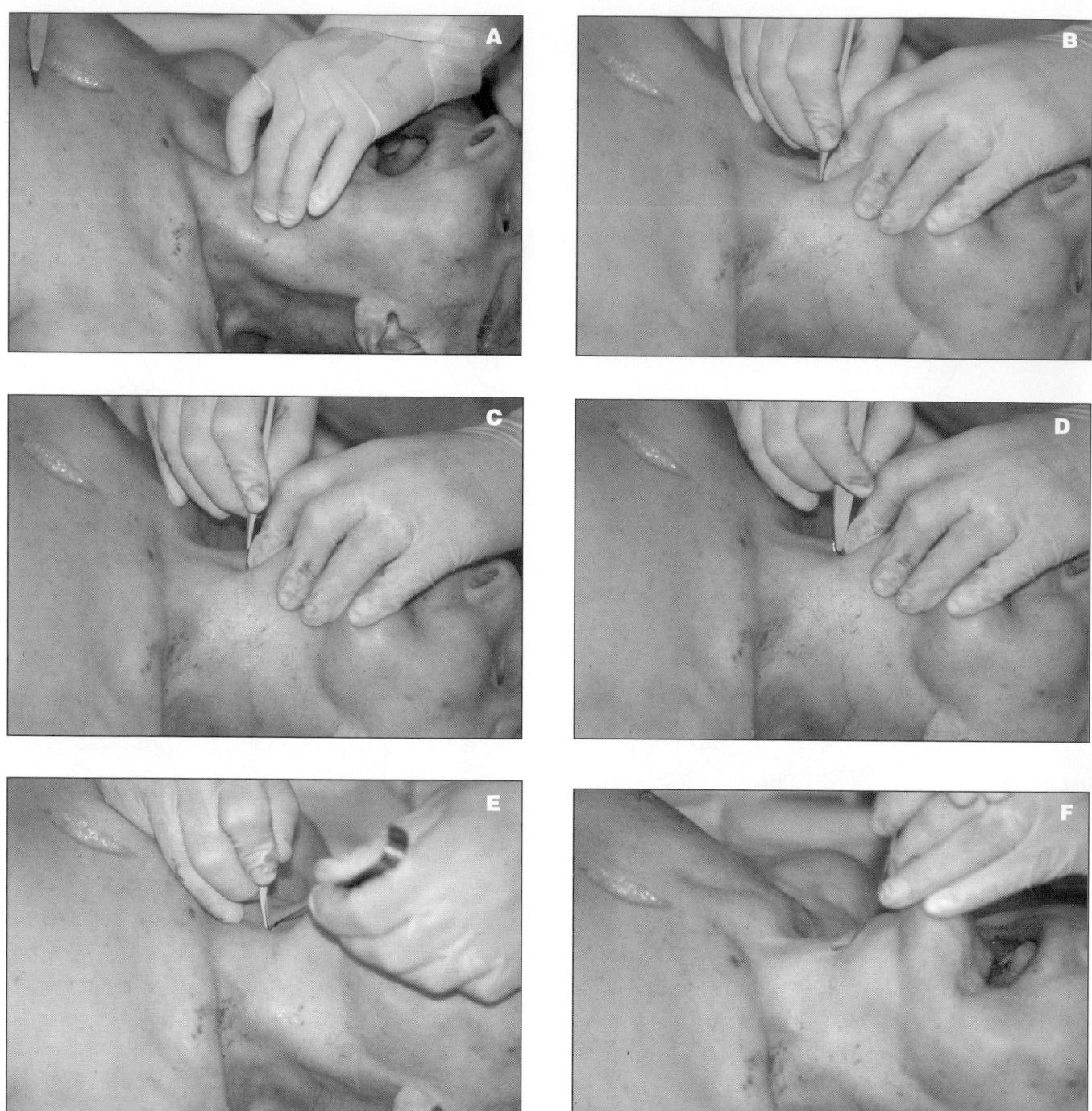

FIGURE 14-7 The alternative method performed on a cadaver. *A.* The larynx is stabilized and the physician's index finger overlies the cricothyroid membrane. *B.* A stab incision is made into the cricothyroid membrane using the finger as a guide. *C.* The incision is extended toward the physician. *D.* The scalpel is rotated 180 degrees and the incision is extended away from the physician. *E.* A tracheal hook is inserted over the scalpel blade to grasp the inferior border of the thyroid cartilage. *F.* The tracheal hook is lifted upward and superiorly to control the airway. The scalpel has then been removed.

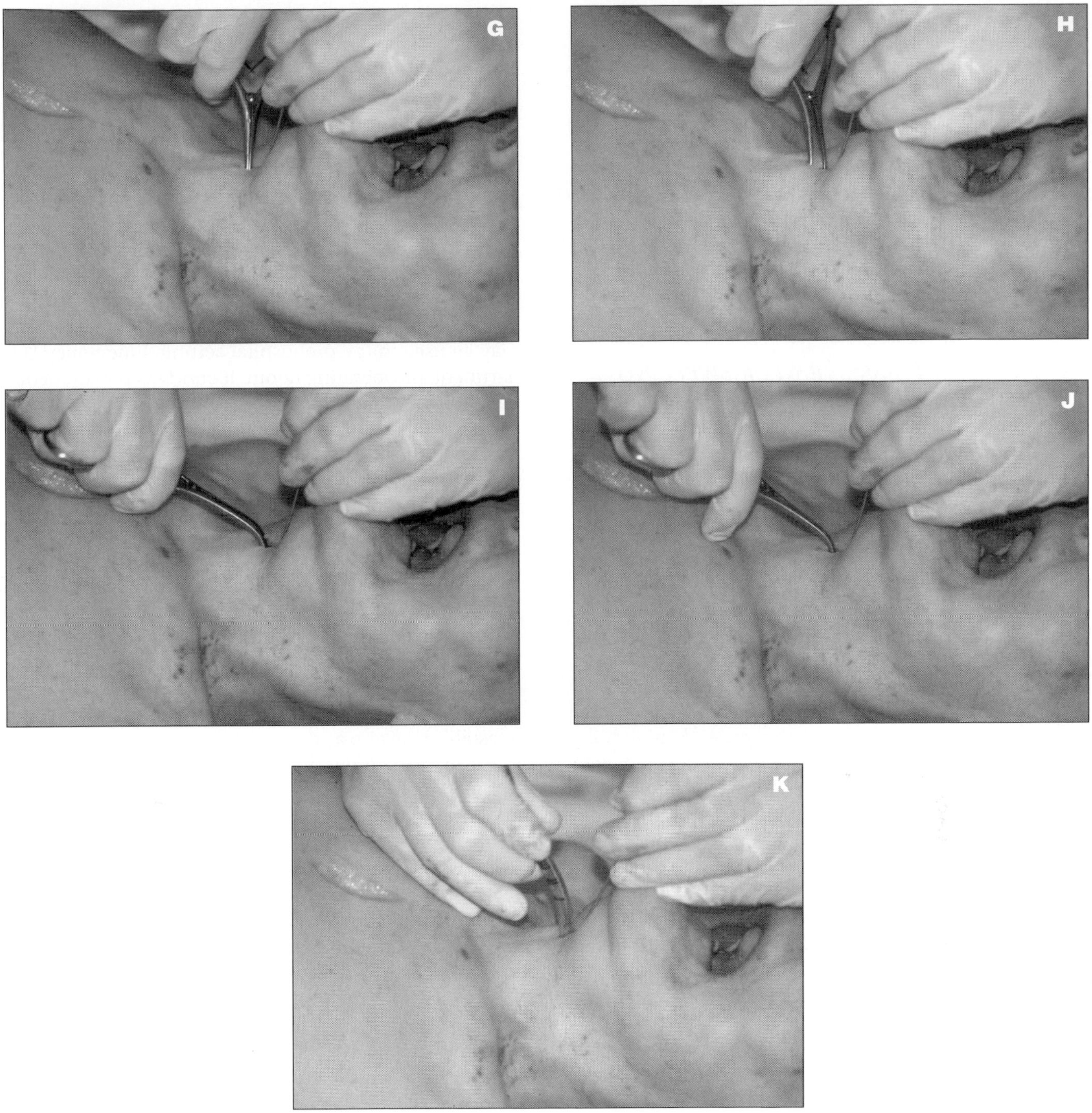

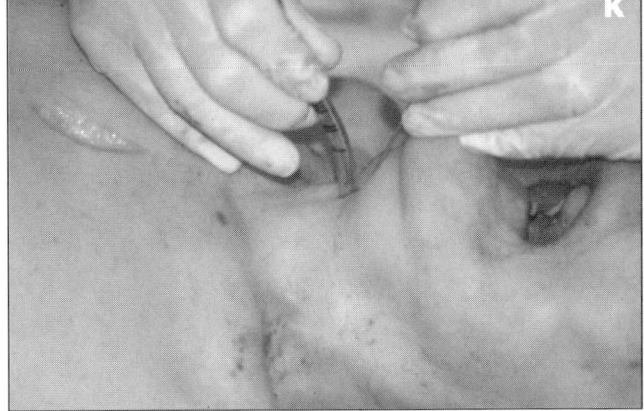

G. The Trousseau dilator is inserted into the cricothyroid membrane. *H.* The jaws of the dilator are opened to widen the incision. *I.* The dilator is rotated 90 degrees. *J.* The jaws of the dilator are opened to open the incision in a second plane. *K.* An endotracheal tube is inserted through the incision and into the trachea.

tube. While controlling the airway with the tracheal hook, insert the jaws of a Trousseau dilator (or 6 inch hemostat) through the cricothyroid membrane in the midsagittal plane (Figures 14-6G and 14-7G). Open the jaws of the instrument to dilate the opening (Figure 14-7H). Rotate the dilator 90 degrees within the incision (Figure 14-7I). Open the jaws of the dilator to dilate the incision in the transverse plane (Figure 14-7J). Insert an endotracheal tube or a tracheostomy tube through the incision and into the trachea (Figures 14-6H and 14-7K). Hold the tube securely against the skin and remove the tracheal hook. The remainder of the procedure is as described previously.

PATIENTS WITH MASSIVE NECK SWELLING

Patients may present with massive neck swelling secondary to hemorrhage, hematoma, edema, or subcutaneous emphysema after trauma.[19] These patients often have no palpable anatomic landmarks in the neck, making it difficult to create a surgical airway. The traditional surgical methods used to perform a cricothyroidotomy are not usable due to hemorrhage and difficulty in identifying the anatomic landmarks. However, a technique has been developed to perform a cricothyroidotomy in these patients.[20–22]

To use this technique, the location of the hyoid bone must be determined (Figure 14-8A). A piece of suture, string, or tracheal tie is required. Place one end of the suture at the angle of the patient's mandible. Stretch the suture along the mandible and note where it contacts the tip of the chin (Figure 14-8A, line 1). Cut the suture at the point where it contacts the tip of the chin. Fold the suture in half. Place one end of the folded suture on the tip of the chin. Pull the other end of the folded suture tight to make a 90 degree angle to line 1 (Figure 14-8A, line 2). An imaginary line should be drawn from the free end of the folded suture to the angle of the patient's mandible (Figure 14-8A, line 3). This third line is the line used to identify the hyoid bone.

Insert a #11 scalpel blade through the midline of the neck in an upward and posterior direction along line 3 (Figure 14-8B). Advance the scalpel blade until it meets resistance as it contacts the hyoid bone. Alternatively, a spinal needle can be inserted along line 3 until it contacts the hyoid bone (Figure 14-8C). Then insert the #11 scalpel along the track of the spinal needle until the hyoid bone is also contacted. **Do not remove the scalpel.** Insert a tracheal hook along the scalpel blade until the hyoid bone is contacted. Move the tip of the tracheal hook under the hyoid bone. Lift the tracheal hook anteriorly and superiorly to elevate and control the airway (Figure 14-8D). **Do not release the hold of the tracheal hook on the hyoid bone.** Remove the scalpel from the incision.

Make an incision inferiorly and in the midline starting at the site the tracheal hook exits the skin. **The incision should extend directly inferiorly without regard to the anatomy of the neck. Do not release the tension on the tracheal hook.** Identify the cricothyroid membrane. Make a transverse incision through the cricothyroid membrane. Dilate the opening and insert a tracheostomy tube into the trachea as described previously.

SELDINGER TECHNIQUE

A percutaneous cricothyroidotomy kit is available from several manufacturers (one source is Cook Critical Care, Bloomington, IN). It is a self-contained kit that may be used in the prehospital setting, Emergency Department, or Operating Room. It contains percutaneous needles, a catheter-over-the-needle, a syringe, a #15 scalpel blade, adult and pediatric airway catheters, dilators that fit inside the airway catheters, a 30 cm flexible guidewire, and a tracheal tie (Figure 14-9). The dilator was developed to fit inside the airway catheter (Figure 14-10). The dilator and airway catheter are inserted as a unit during the procedure.

The percutaneous cricothyroidotomy kit can be used to establish an airway using a modification of the Seldinger technique.[23–25] This technique can be used to establish an airway in about the time it takes to create a surgical cricothyroidotomy.[23,24] For those with little surgical experience, it may be a simpler method with which to establish an airway than traditional surgical methods.

Clean, prep, drape, and anesthetize the patient's neck as mentioned previously. Lubricate the dilator liberally and insert it through the airway catheter (Figure 14-10). Lubricate the airway catheter and dilator after it has been assembled into a unit. Stabilize the trachea with the nondominant hand and identify the landmarks as previously described. Leave the nondominant index finger over the center of the cricothyroid membrane.

Make a stab incision in the skin over the center of the cricothyroid membrane with the #15 scalpel blade (Figure 14-11A). Insert the catheter-over-the-needle attached to a 5 mL syringe containing saline through the skin incision and aimed inferiorly (Figure 14-11B). The catheter-over-the-needle should be inserted at a 30 to 45 degree angle to the skin (Figure 14-11B). Advance the catheter-over-the-needle while applying negative pressure to the syringe. Stop advancing the catheter-over-the-needle when the airway has been entered. This will be signified by a loss of resistance and air bubbles in the syringe (Figure 14-11B).

While holding the syringe securely, advance the catheter until the hub is at the skin of the neck. Hold the catheter hub securely against the skin of the neck and remove the needle and syringe. Insert and advance the guidewire through the catheter and into the trachea (Figure 14-11C). Grasp the guidewire securely and re-

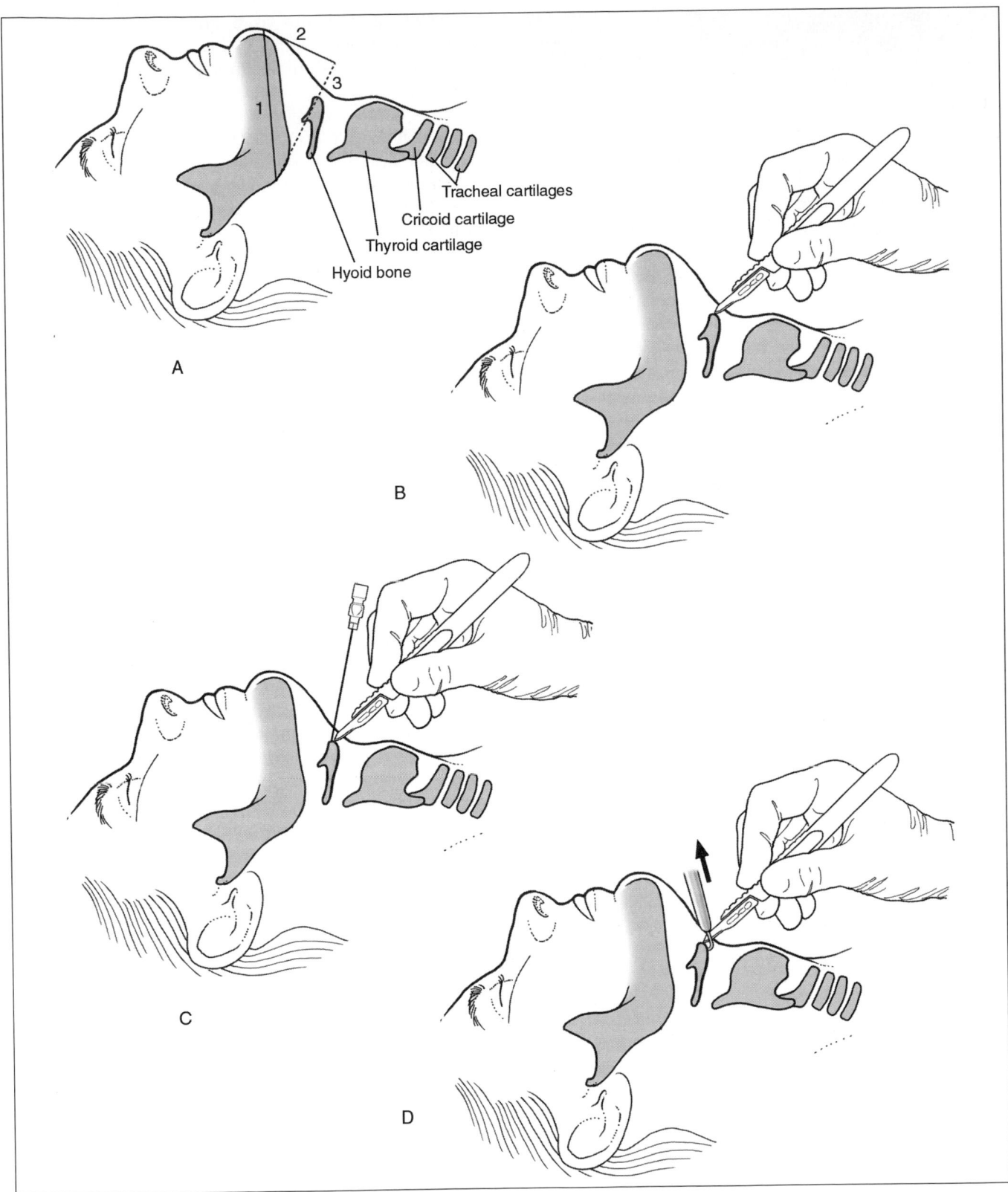

FIGURE 14-8 Cricothyroidotomy in a patient with neck swelling. *A.* Locate the hyoid bone. Line 1 is from the angle of the mandible to the tip of the chin. Line 2 is half the length of line 1 and perpendicular to it. Line 3 is from the tip of line 2 to the angle of the patient's mandible. *B.* A #11 scalpel blade is inserted in the midline and aimed along line 3 until it contacts the hyoid bone. *C.* An alternative method. A spinal needle is used to locate the hyoid bone. A #11 scalpel blade is inserted along the tract of the spinal needle until the hyoid bone is contacted. *D.* A tracheal hook is inserted along the scalpel blade and used to grasp the hyoid bone. The tracheal hook is lifted anteriorly and superiorly to elevate and control the airway.

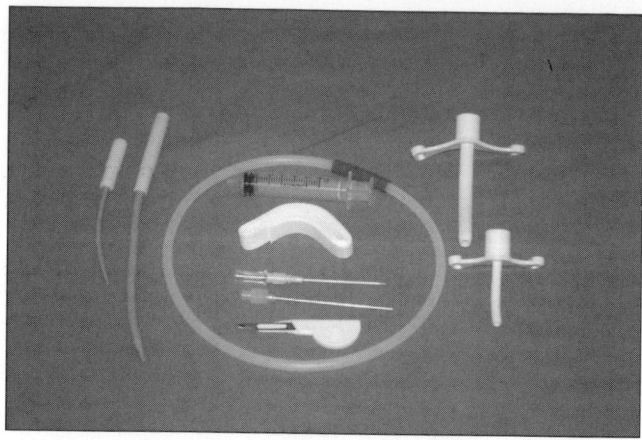

FIGURE 14-9 The percutaneous cricothyroidotomy kit (Cook Critical Care, Bloomington, IN).

move the catheter over the guidewire (Figure 14-11*D*). **Do not release your grasp on the guidewire in order to prevent it from completely entering the patient's airway.**

Insert the dilator/airway catheter unit over the guidewire and into the trachea (Figure 14-11*E*). The tip of the dilator is rigid. **Insert it gently to prevent injury to or perforation of the posterior tracheal wall.** Continue to advance the unit until the flange is against the skin of the neck. Hold the airway catheter securely. Remove the

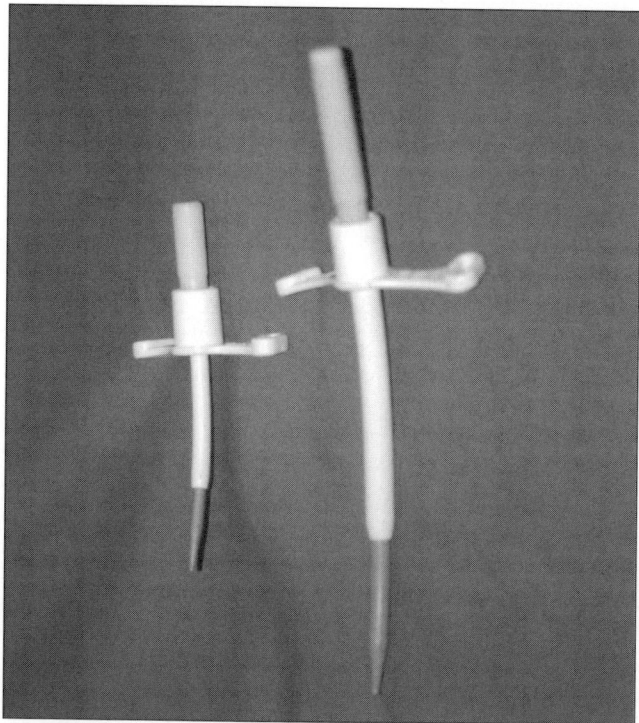

FIGURE 14-10 The dilator is placed inside the airway catheter to form a unit. The pediatric unit (*left*) and the adult unit (*right*) are both contained within each percutaneous cricothyroidotomy kit.

guidewire and dilator as a unit, leaving the airway catheter in place (Figure 14-11*F*). Begin ventilation of the patient and secure the airway catheter as previously described.

NEEDLE CRICOTHYROIDOTOMY

A needle cricothyroidotomy, rather than a surgical cricothyroidotomy, should be performed in children less than 8 years of age. The latter is technically more difficult. The child has a laryngeal prominence that is difficult to palpate, since it is not well developed. The cricothyroid membrane is small and often will not allow the passage of an airway tube. The larynx is anatomically positioned relatively higher than in an adult and is more difficult to access.

Stand at the side of the bed and adjacent to the patient's head and neck.[11] **Reidentify the anatomic landmarks. This is crucial to performing this procedure.** Using the nondominant hand, place the thumb on one side of the thyroid cartilage and the middle finger on the other side. Use these fingers to stabilize the larynx.[8,14] Use the index finger to identify the anatomic landmarks.[4,5,11] Start at the laryngeal prominence (Adam's apple) and work inferiorly. The soft membranous defect inferior to the laryngeal prominence is the cricothyroid membrane. Below this is the cartilaginous ring of the cricoid cartilage.

Attach a 12 to 16 gauge catheter-over-the-needle (angiocatheter) to a 10 mL syringe containing 5 mL of sterile saline. Insert the catheter-over-the-needle through the skin, subcutaneous tissue, and inferior aspect of the cricothyroid membrane. The inferior aspect of the cricothyroid membrane is the preferred site, as use of it avoids injury to the cricothyroid arteries. Direct the catheter-over-the-needle inferiorly and at a 30 to 45 degree angle (Figure 14-12*A*). Maintain constant negative pressure within the syringe as it is advanced (Figure 14-12*B*). Continue to advance the catheter-over-the-needle while maintaining negative pressure until air bubbles are visible in the syringe and a loss of resistance is felt. These both signify that the catheter-over-the-needle is within the trachea.

Once placement within the trachea is confirmed, securely hold the needle and advance the catheter until the hub is against the skin (Figure 14-12*C*). Remove the needle and syringe (Figure 14-12*C*). Reattach the syringe without the needle to the catheter. Aspirate once again to reconfirm placement of the catheter within the trachea. The 2 to 3 cm catheter should be long enough to pass into the trachea without sitting against the posterior wall. If the catheter tip directly touches or faces the posterior tracheal wall, there is the risk of forcing air submucosally. Grasp and hold the catheter hub firmly at the skin of the neck. Remove the syringe. Attach the oxygen tubing to the catheter (Figure 14-12*D*). Begin

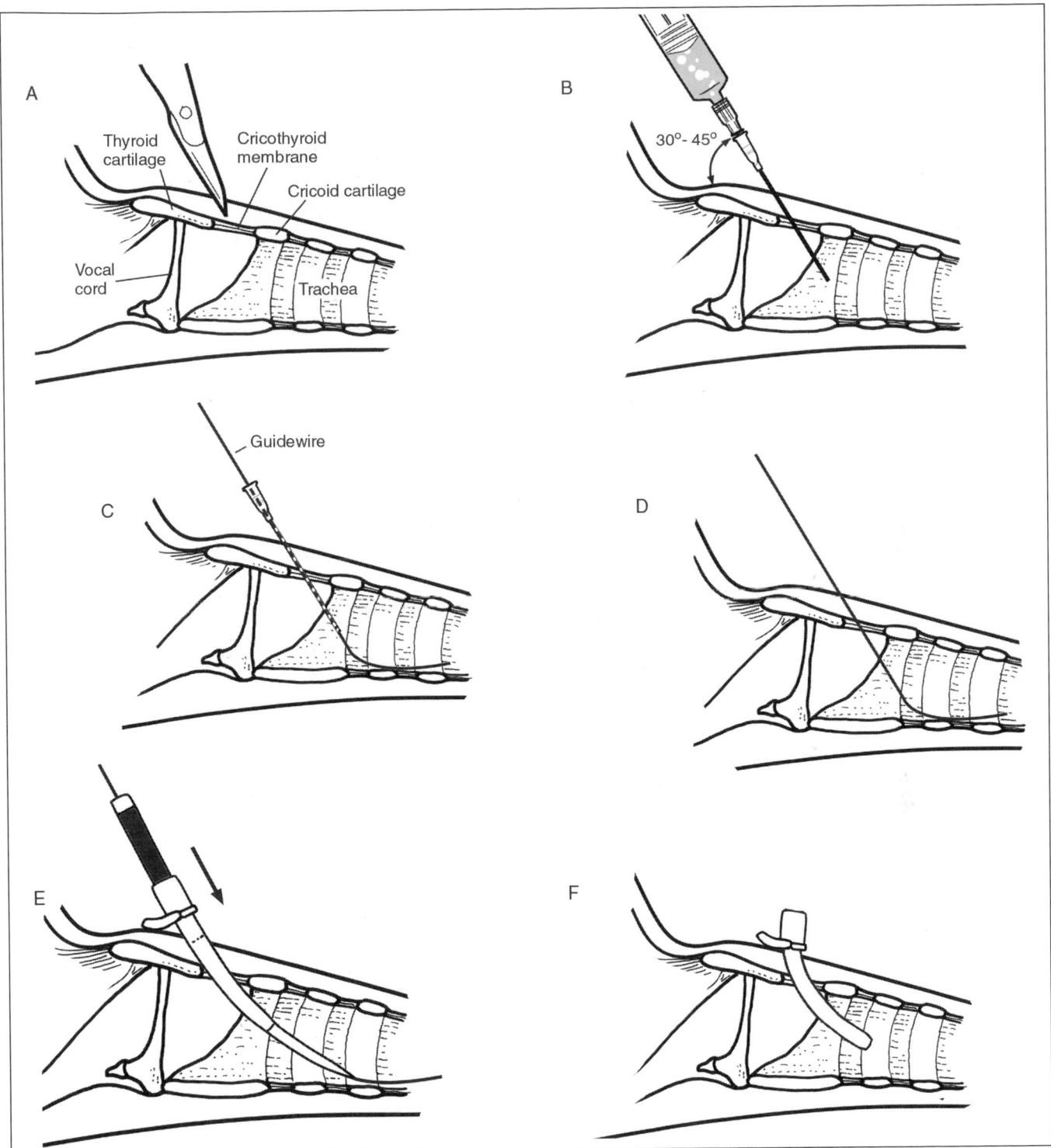

FIGURE 14-11 The percutaneous cricothyroidotomy. *A.* A stab incision is made in the midline over the cricothyroid membrane. *B.* A catheter-over-the-needle is inserted at a 30 to 45 degree angle to the skin and advanced in a caudal direction. Negative pressure is applied to a saline-containing syringe during catheter insertion (*arrow*). Air bubbles in the saline confirm intratracheal placement of the catheter. *C.* The catheter has been advanced until the hub is against the skin. The needle and syringe have been removed. A guidewire is inserted through the catheter. *D.* The catheter has been removed, leaving the guidewire in place. *E.* The dilator/airway catheter unit is advanced over the guidewire. *F.* The guidewire and dilator have been removed, leaving the airway catheter in place.

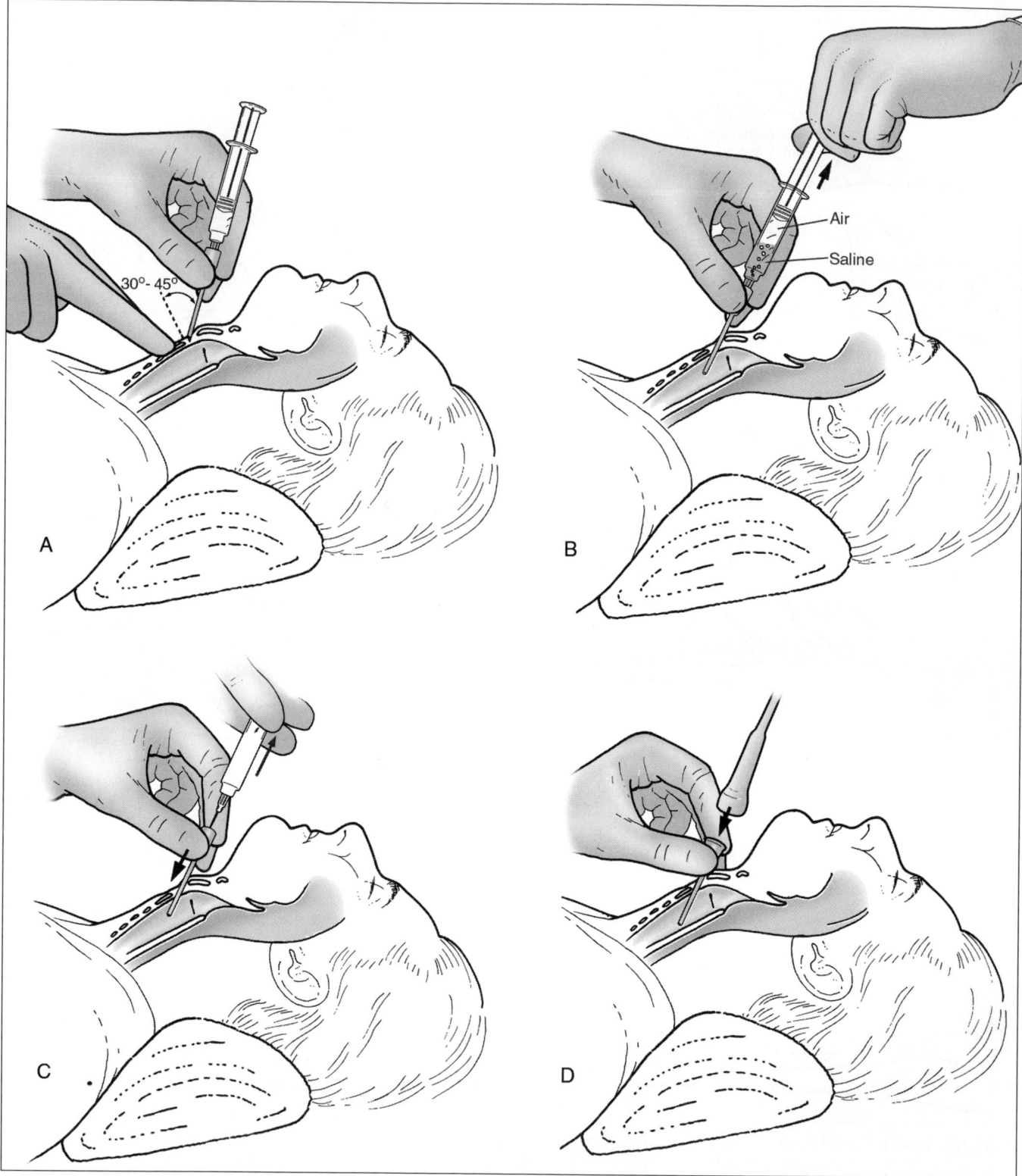

FIGURE 14-12 Insertion of the transtracheal catheter. *A.* The catheter-over-the-needle is inserted 30 to 45 degrees to the perpendicular (*dotted line*) and aimed inferiorly. *B.* Application of negative pressure to a saline-containing syringe during catheter-over-the-needle insertion (*arrow*). Air bubbles in the saline confirm intratracheal placement of the catheter. *C.* The catheter is advanced until the hub is against the skin. The needle and syringe are then removed. *D.* High-pressure oxygen tubing is attached to the catheter and ventilation is begun.

ventilation and continue until a more permanent and secure airway is established.

At this point, the patient may be oxygenated and ventilated by two methods. The first involves inserting the adapter piece from a #3.0 endotracheal tube to the catheter hub and then connecting it directly to the bag-valve device or a ventilator. This method allows for the confirmation of breath sounds and provides better ventilation of the patient.

The second method of oxygenation involves direct connection of the high-flow oxygen tubing to the hub of the catheter. This method requires cyclic ventilation for 1 to 2 seconds followed by exhalation for 4 to 5 seconds.[12] This method provides adequate oxygenation but less adequate ventilation and is more labor-intensive. The complete details of this technique can be found in Chapter 13, on percutaneous transtracheal jet ventilation.

Once breath sounds are confirmed, the catheter can be secured to the skin. This may be done with nylon sutures or strips of adhesive dressing tape. The patient should undergo a formal tracheostomy as soon as possible because of the risk of dislodging the catheter and the suboptimal ventilation associated with this technique.

ASSESSMENT

Immediately after securing the tracheostomy tube, the physician should confirm proper positioning by auscultation of bilateral breath sounds, chest rise, and end-tidal CO_2 monitoring. Obtain a chest radiograph to confirm the position of the tube and rule out the presence of a pneumothorax.[12]

AFTERCARE

The tracheostomy tube should be held in place firmly while the patient is ventilated with a bag-valve device or a ventilator.[11] **Do not release the hold on the tracheostomy tube until it is secured.** Obtain hemostasis of the wound edges by grasping any bleeding vessels with a hemostat and place an absorbable 3–0 suture over the vessel. If the skin incision is significantly larger than the tracheostomy tube, pack the wound with iodoform gauze. Secure the tracheostomy tube by placing twill tape (tracheostomy tape) through one end of the flange, around the patient's neck, and through the other end of the flange.[11,12] Suture the four corners of the tracheostomy flange to the patient's skin using 3–0 nylon suture.

If an endotracheal tube was inserted, it should also be secured. Wrap tape around the endotracheal tube as it exits the tracheostomy site. Wrap the tape around the patient's neck and back onto the endotracheal tube. Alternatively, a commercially available endotracheal tube holder can be used to secure the tube.

The cricothyroidotomy tube can be removed easily when the indication for airway control no longer exists. This usually occurs after the patient is orotracheally intubated, nasotracheally intubated, or has a tracheostomy performed. After removal of the tube, place an occlusive dressing, such as petroleum gauze, over the incision until it heals. If the patient is predicted to require ventilatory management for more than 7 days, it is advised that the cricothyroidotomy be converted to a formal tracheostomy to minimize the risk of long-term complications.

COMPLICATIONS

Complications following a cricothyroidotomy can be classified as early or late based on when they occur. Early complications will be recognized either immediately after insertion of the tracheostomy tube or within a few hours. Late complications may not be apparent for weeks to months following the procedure.

The most serious early complication is malposition of the tracheostomy tube within the soft tissues of the neck. If the tube is not within the trachea, the patient cannot be ventilated or oxygenated. This, fortunately, is easily recognized on auscultating the chest. It can be remedied by removing the tracheostomy tube and replacing it in its proper location. The tube may also be misplaced above or below the cricothyroid membrane. Placement above the cricothyroid membrane often results from inadequate palpation of landmarks and is associated with an incision into the larynx. The airway should be converted to a tracheostomy once this malposition is recognized.[6] Placement below the cricoid cartilage has been estimated to occur in 10 percent of cricothyroidotomies.[2] There is no specific treatment required for this other than the recognition that the patient actually has a high tracheostomy.

Laryngeal injury may occur if the tracheostomy tube that is inserted is larger than the cricothyroid membrane. The cricothyroid membrane is only 9 to 10 mm in height in the average adult.[8,11] Placement of a tracheostomy tube with a larger outer diameter may cause a fracture of the thyroid cartilage. It is important that the tracheostomy tube to be placed be no larger than a #6.0 or a #7.0.[8,11] Placement of a larger tube is also associated with an increased incidence of subglottic granulation and stenosis.[2,4]

Incisional bleeding occurs in 4 to 8 percent of patients following a cricothyroidotomy.[2,4,6,8,15] This may result from transection of the anterior jugular veins if the incision extends too far laterally. Bleeding is usually easily treated by point ligation of the bleeding vessels and packing around the tracheostomy tube with iodoform gauze. A small amount of bleeding or oozing from the cricothyroid arteries can be tamponaded by packing iodoform gauze around the tracheostomy tube.

Because the cricothyroidotomy is usually performed in less than sterile circumstances, there is a risk of wound infection.[15] This is usually the result of skin flora. It can be treated with wet-to-dry saline dressing changes. Occasionally, the infection will not resolve until the cricothyroidotomy tube has been removed, either by decannulation or conversion to a formal tracheostomy. Antibiotics are usually not required.

Late complications take two general forms: progressive airway obstruction and chronic voice changes. Patients with progressive airway obstruction present with slowly increasing stridor and dyspnea weeks to months after the procedure. This usually results from subglottic stenosis and granulation tissue formation at the site of the stoma.[2,6,13] It is unclear whether this complication results from the cricothyroidotomy or the tracheostomy tube. The majority of these patients have had prolonged endotracheal intubations before the cricothyroidotomy or prolonged tracheostomy placement after the cricothyroidotomy.[2,13,14,16] In one series,[16] patients with a cricothyroidotomy for a prolonged period (average 72 days) had a 52 percent incidence of chronic obstruction compared to no obstruction in patients with cricothyroidotomy for a shorter period (average 27 days). Jacobson recommends that the tracheostomy tube be removed by the fourth day to minimize these long-term complications.[9]

A final late complication is that of voice changes. This has been described in 2.5 to 25 percent of patients with a cricothyroidotomy.[6,13–15] Again, many of these patients had other methods of airway management either before or after the cricothyroidotomy. Voice changes tend to be somewhat nonspecific. Patients will complain of hoarseness, decreased volume, and fatigue. These changes may be due to small amounts of granulation tissue at the stoma site and generally resolve over time.[4]

SUMMARY

Cricothyroidotomy is a potentially lifesaving technique. It is an important procedure for the Emergency Physician to be skilled in, as it may represent the only access to the patient's airway. It can be used to provide oxygenation and ventilation to a patient when other less invasive airway control methods have failed or are contraindicated. It is a relatively safe, simple, and reliable procedure that can be performed within a few minutes. Knowledge of the anatomy of the anterior neck is essen-

tial in order to minimize early complications. A self-contained percutaneous cricothyroidotomy kit is available for use in the prehospital setting, Emergency Department, or Operating Room.

REFERENCES

1. Copass MK, Oreskovich MR, Bladergroen MR, et al: Prehospital cardiopulmonary resuscitation of the critically injured patient. *Am J Surg* 1984; 148: 20–26.
2. Erlandson MJ, Clinton JE, Ruiz E, et al: Cricothyrotomy in the emergency department revisited. *J Emerg Med* 1989; 7:115–118.
3. Ligier B, Buchman TG, Breslow MJ, et al: The role of anesthetic induction agents and neuromuscular blockade in the endotracheal intubation of trauma victims. *Surg Gynecol Obstet* 1991; 173:477–481.
4. Salvino CK, Dries D, Gamelli R, et al: Emergency cricothyroidotomy in trauma victims. *J Trauma* 1993; 34:503–505.
5. Hawkins ML, Shapiro MB, Cué JI, et al: Emergency cricothyrotomy: a reassessment. *Am Surg* 1995; 61:52–55.
6. Boyd AD, Romita MC, Conlan AA, et al: A clinical evaluation of cricothyroidotomy. *Surg Gynecol Obstet* 1979; 149:365–368.
7. Gleeson MJ, Pearson RC, Armistead S, et al: Voice changes following cricothyroidotomy. *J Laryngol Otol* 1984; 98:1015–1019.
8. McGill J, Clinton JE, Ruiz E: Cricothyrotomy in the emergency department. *Ann Emerg Med* 1982; 11:361–364.
9. Jacobson LE, Gomez GA, Sobieray RJ, et al: Surgical cricothyroidotomy in trauma patients: analysis of its use by paramedics in the field. *J Trauma* 1996; 41:15–20.
10. Mulder DS, Marelli D: The 1991 Fraser Gurd lecture: evolution of airway control in the management of injured patients. *J Trauma* 1992; 33:856–862.
11. Walls RM: Cricothyroidotomy. *Emerg Med Clin North Am* 1988; 6:725–736.
12. *Advanced Trauma Life Support,* 6th ed. Chicago: American College of Surgeons, 1997.
13. Cole RR, Aguilar EA: Cricothyroidotomy versus tracheotomy: an otolaryngologist's perspective. *Laryngoscope* 1988; 98:131–135.
14. DeLaurier GA, Hawkins ML, Treat RC, et al: Acute airway management: role of cricothyroidotomy. *Am Surg* 1990; 56:12–15.
15. Holst M, Hertegård S, Persson A: Vocal dysfunction following cricothyroidotomy: a prospective study. *Laryngoscope* 1990; 100:749–755.

16. Kuriloff DB, Setzen M, Portnoy W, et al: Laryngotracheal injury following cricothyroidotomy. *Laryngoscope* 1989; 99:125–130.

17. Oppenheimer RP: Airway . . . instantly. *JAMA* 1974; 230(1):76.

18. Simon RR, Brenner BE: *Emergency Procedures and Techniques,* 3rd ed. Baltimore: Williams & Wilkins, 1994:71–88.

19. Alonso WA, Pratt LL, Zollinger WK, et al: Complications of laryngotracheal disruption. *Laryngoscope* 1974; 84:1276–1290.

20. Simon RR, Brenner BE: Emergency cricothyroidotomy in the patient with massive neck swelling: Part 1. Anatomical aspects. *Crit Care Med* 1983; 11(2):114–118.

21. Simon RR, Brenner BE, Rosen MA: Emergency cricothyroidotomy in the patient with massive neck swelling: Part 2. Clinical aspects. *Crit Care Med* 1983; 11(2):119–123.

22. Simon RR: Emergency tracheotomy in patients with massive neck swelling. *Emerg Med Clin North Am* 1989; 7(1):95–101.

23. Eisenburger P, Laczika K, List M, et al: Comparison of conventional surgical versus Seldinger technique emergency cricothyroidotomy performed by inexperienced clinicians. *Anesthesiology* 2000; 92(3):687–690.

24. Ala-Kokko TI, Kyllönen M, Nuutinen L: Management of upper airway obstruction using a Seldinger minitracheotomy kit. *Acta Anaesth Scand* 1996; 40:385–388.

25. Walls RM: Cricothyroidotomy. *Emerg Med Clin North Am* 1988; 6(4):725–736.

Chapter 15
TRACHEOSTOMY

Karen S. Cosby

INTRODUCTION

Control of the airway is the first priority in the resuscitation of a critically ill patient. Tracheostomy has long been relied upon in desperate moments to secure an airway. Modern Emergency Physicians have many options for airway management. They are skilled in a variety of invasive, noninvasive, and surgical procedures to optimize the management of a patient's airway. The role of tracheostomy for emergent airway access has diminished as newer, safer, and equally effective techniques have evolved. Familiarity with the methods for tracheostomy is still valuable. Knowledge of proper techniques, possible indications, limitations, and likely complications will guide one's judgment in critical moments, when it most counts. Understanding the procedure for a tracheostomy will allow Emergency Physicians to properly care for a problem or complication when a patient with a tracheostomy tube presents to the Emergency Department.

ANATOMY AND PATHOPHYSIOLOGY

A surgical approach to the airway relies upon a sound knowledge of the anatomy of the neck and a safe approach to the trachea. **A careful review of this anatomy illustrates how critical it is to remain in the midline in order to avoid morbidity and mortality.** External landmarks are useful in identifying the significant structures of the airway[1,2] (Figure 15-1). The laryngeal prominence is a useful guide to the thyroid cartilage. The cricoid cartilage can be identified as a ring just inferior to the thyroid cartilage. In the absence of edema or a hematoma, a finger marched down the midline from the cricoid cartilage can palpate and identify the cartilaginous rings of the trachea. In an emergent situation, these external landmarks may be all a physician has to guide the establishment of a surgical airway.

The neck is a complex three-dimensional structure with numerous vital structures coursing through a small space (Figures 15-2 through 15-6). The cervical portion of the airway is anterior, superficial, and midline. It is covered by skin, subcutaneous tissue, and numerous muscles (Figure 15-2). The basic cartilaginous framework of the airway begins superiorly at the hyoid bone and continues inferiorly with the larynx and trachea (Figure 15-3). The external skeleton of the larynx comprises the hyoid bone, thyroid cartilage, and cricoid cartilage.[3] The hyoid bone is a U-shaped structure attached to the mandible, tongue, and base of the skull by muscles. It is the most stable portion of the airway. Even in the presence of pathology, the hyoid bone is remarkably constant in position and can be considered a stable landmark.[4–6]

The larynx is easy to identify externally. The prominent thyroid cartilage forms the laryngeal prominence (Adam's apple) at its inferior pole (Figure 15-3). It is a freely mobile structure that is anchored by muscles and moves with deglutition. Airway manipulation done on an awake patient will need to fix the larynx to avoid involuntary movement of the larynx from reflex swallowing. The thyroid cartilage is attached to the cricoid cartilage via the cricothyroid membrane (Figure 15-3). This is the site for a cricothyroidotomy. The cricoid is signet ring–shaped and is the only complete cartilaginous ring in the airway. Procedures should avoid damage to the cricoid cartilage, fearing a loss of stability in the airway. The cricotracheal ligament attaches the cricoid cartilage to the trachea.

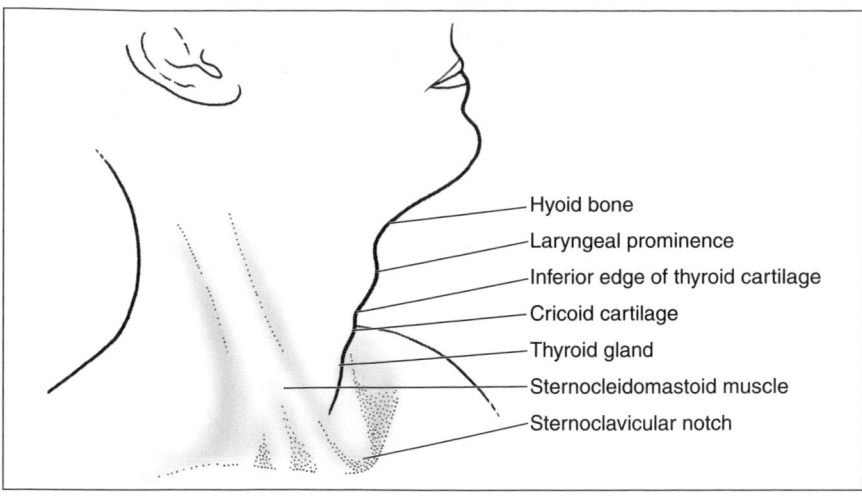

FIGURE 15-1 Lateral view of the topographic anatomy of the neck.

The trachea is a cartilaginous and membranous tube that is approximately 10 to 11 cm long and 2 to 2.5 cm wide in the average adult. It extends from the neck into the thorax, where it ends at the carina by dividing into the right and left mainstem bronchi (Figure 15-4). It is made up of 16 to 20 incomplete U-shaped cartilaginous rings. It is remarkably elastic. Full extension of the neck adds significant length to the supraclavicular trachea. This feature should be taken advantage of during a tracheostomy.[7]

The trachea is bordered anteriorly by skin, subcutaneous tissue, platysma muscle, pretracheal fascia, and the thyroid gland (Figure 15-5). The pretracheal fascia is the anterior portion of the deep cervical fascia. It descends from the thyroid and cricoid cartilages and splits to enclose the thyroid gland, trachea, and esophagus. The pretracheal fascia continues downward into the thorax and mediastinum. Anterior to the trachea, it is very thin and inconsequential. Laterally, it is extremely thick and blends with the carotid sheath.

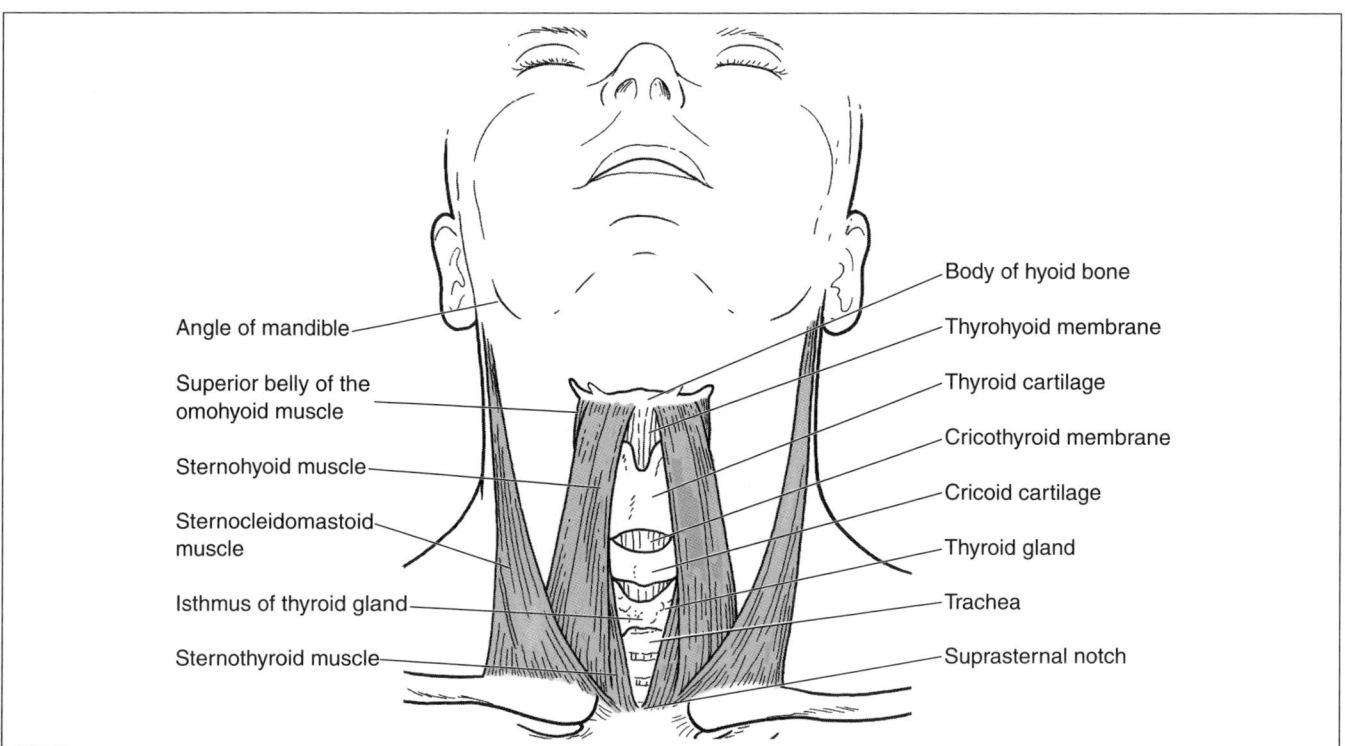

FIGURE 15-2 The superficial muscles and airway structures in the neck.

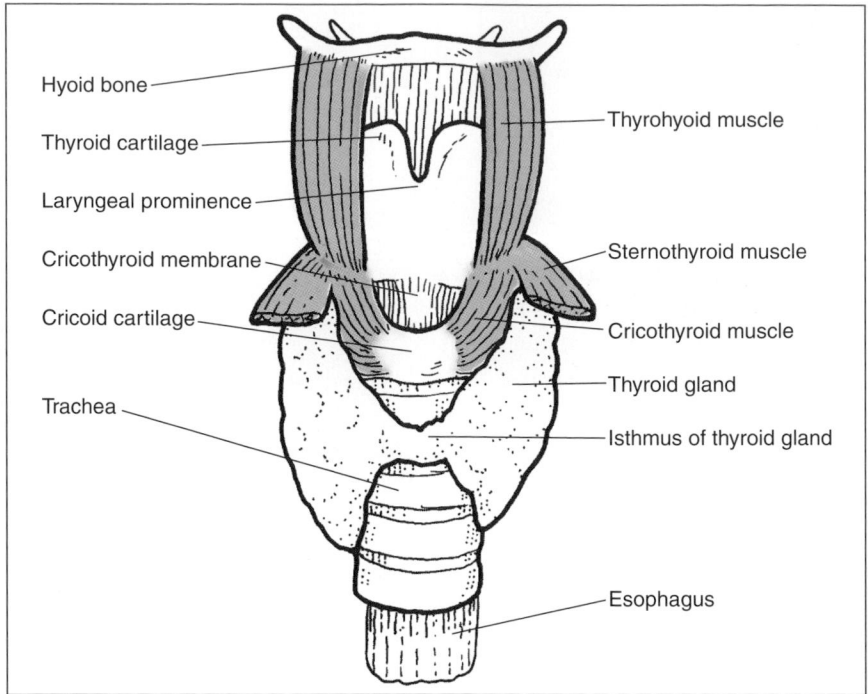

Hyoid bone

Thyroid cartilage

Laryngeal prominence

Cricothyroid membrane

Cricoid cartilage

Trachea

Thyrohyoid muscle

Sternothyroid muscle

Cricothyroid muscle

Thyroid gland

Isthmus of thyroid gland

Esophagus

FIGURE 15-3 The framework of the airway in the neck.

The thyroid gland lies anterior to the second through fourth tracheal rings and is inevitably encountered during a tracheostomy. It is a richly vascular structure (Figure 15-6) that receives its blood supply from the superior thyroid artery (a branch of the external carotid artery) and the inferior thyroid artery (a branch of the thyrocervical trunk). These vessels anastomose into a rich plexus on the anterior surface of the thyroid gland. These major arteries do not usually cross the midline. Unfortunately, the midline is not always free of blood vessels. An unpaired thyroid ima artery will occasionally be found in the midline to supply the isthmus of the thyroid gland. The anterior thyroid veins often form a vascular arch across the midline and just inferior to the thyroid gland. A hastily performed tracheostomy or one carried out under difficult conditions may encounter significant hemorrhage from transected vessels.

A number of vital structures surround the trachea and are at risk for injury during a tracheostomy. Their positions relative to one another are best appreciated in a cross-sectional view of the neck (Figure 15-5). The deep strap muscles, the sternohyoid and sternothyroid, run adjacent to the trachea and may have to be reflected away for adequate visualization (Figure 15-2). The right and left lobes of the thyroid gland encase the upper trachea (Figure 15-6). The recurrent laryngeal nerves lie posterolateral to the trachea. The trachea forms the medial border of the anterior triangle of the neck. The common carotid artery, internal jugular vein, and vagus nerve are adjacent to the thyroid gland. The esophagus lies immediately posterior to the trachea. Any of these structures may be damaged during a tracheostomy.

INDICATIONS

The tracheostomy is an ancient and time-honored technique for securing and maintaining an artificial airway. The American Academy of Otolaryngology–Head and Neck Surgery has proposed specific clinical indicators for the use of a tracheostomy[8] (Table 15-1). A number of indications for tracheostomy are widely accepted[8–15] (Table 15-2). Formal tracheostomy is generally considered an elective procedure done under nonemergent conditions after the airway has been secured by other techniques.[16–20] Its use as an emergency procedure is controversial. Used by battlefield surgeons during wartime, its reputation as a procedure of last resort is not without reason. When performed under emergency circumstances, it is fraught with danger.

A tracheostomy is frequently considered in the treatment of upper airway obstructions including epiglottitis, deep space neck infections, angioedema, airway foreign bodies, multiple lacerations to the floor of the mouth, and complex facial fractures. Although these conditions can create serious and immediate airway compromise, the airway can be managed in most cases with orotracheal intubation. **An emergency tracheostomy is not the treatment of choice but rather the choice of last resort.**

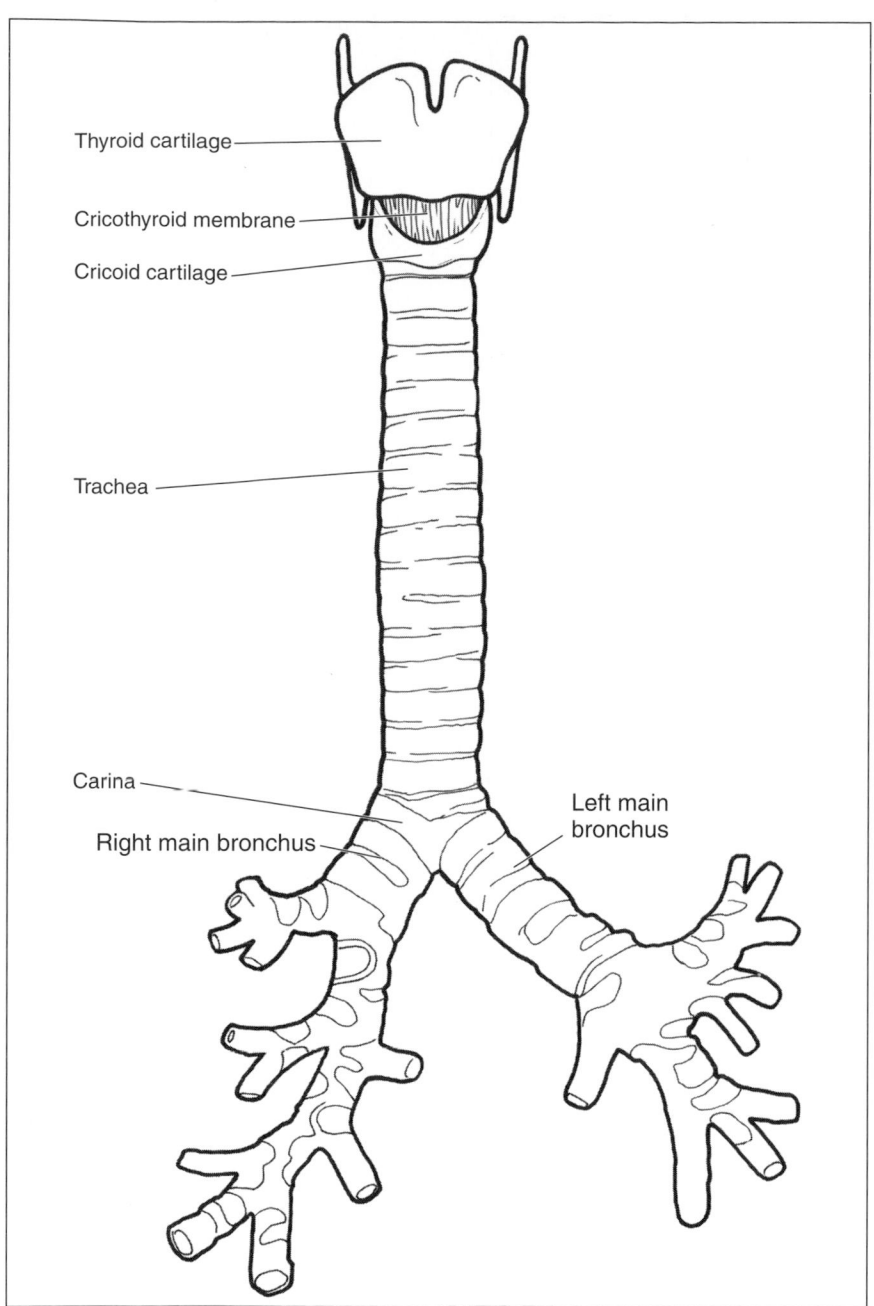

Thyroid cartilage

Cricothyroid membrane

Cricoid cartilage

Trachea

Carina

Right main bronchus

Left main bronchus

FIGURE 15-4 The cartilaginous framework of the airway in the neck.

There are only three clinical settings in which emergency tracheostomy should be considered: laryngotracheal injury with airway disruption[15,25,26]; the need for a surgical airway in an infant or small child[27,28]; and the need for an airway when all other methods have failed (the notorious "slash-trach"). With the exception of these limited applications, an emergency tracheostomy is discouraged.[15,29,30]

LARYNGOTRACHEAL TRAUMA

Most head and neck trauma patients can be managed with nonsurgical airway techniques. There are a number of options available, including orotracheal intubation, nasotracheal intubation, intubation guided by a lighted stylet or "lightwand," retrograde guidewire intubation, and fiberoptic-assisted intubation. If a surgical airway is necessary, cricothyroidotomy is usually the procedure of choice.

Laryngotracheal disruption is an unusual injury. This is the one injury in which a tracheostomy is the undisputed method for establishing and securing the airway. This rare injury has been described in high-speed accidents when the anterior neck strikes a fixed cable or rope. It has also been reported in unrestrained passen-

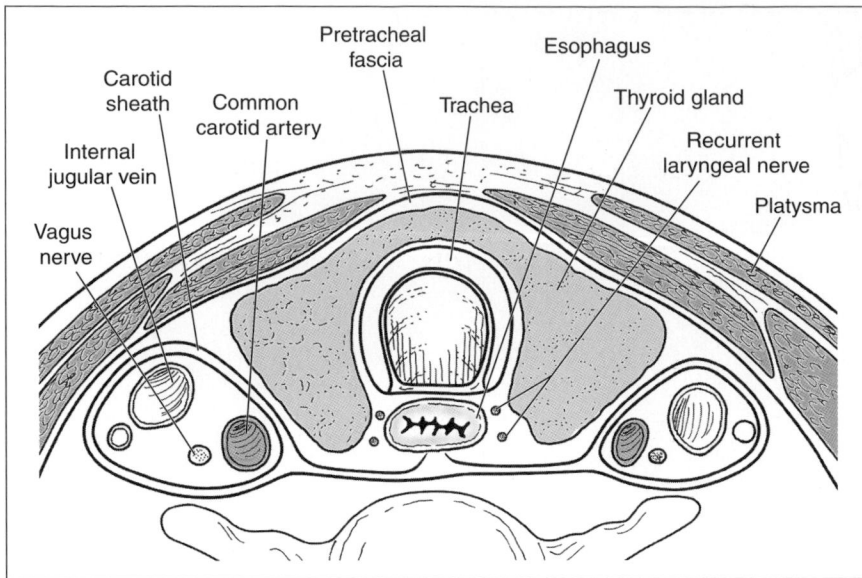

FIGURE 15-5 Cross-sectional anatomy of the neck at the level of the isthmus of the thyroid gland.

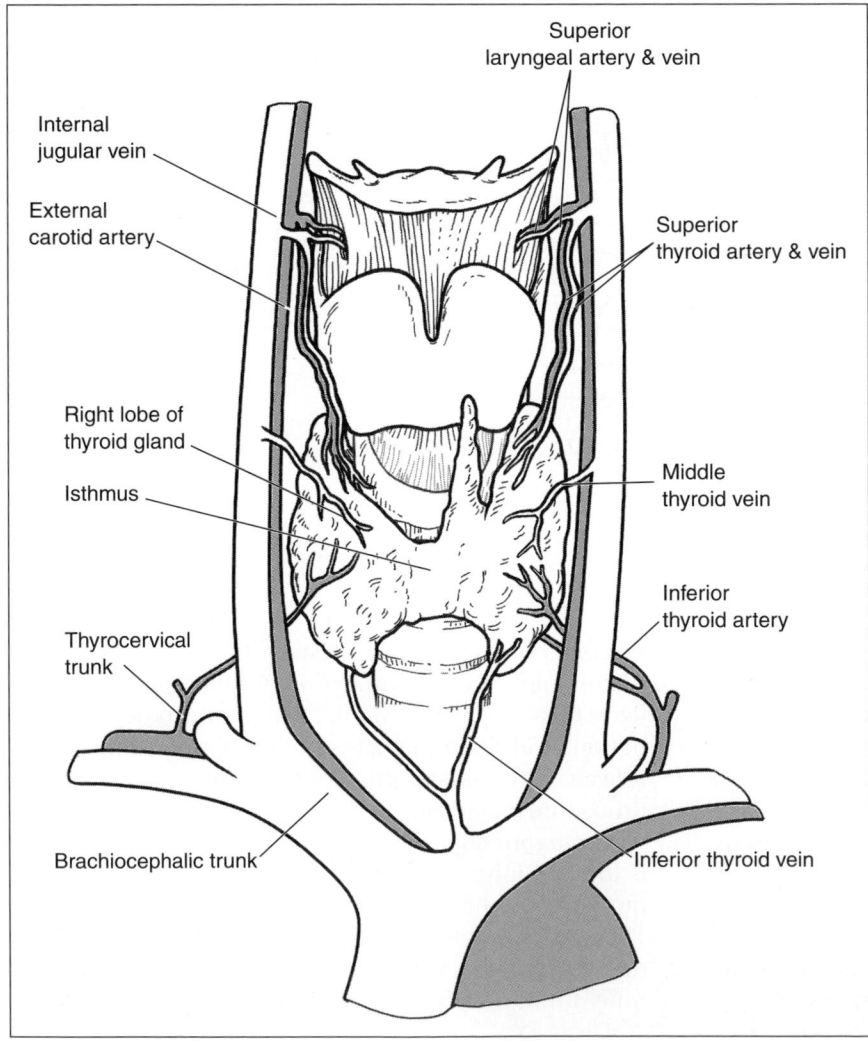

FIGURE 15-6 Vascular structures supplying and surrounding the thyroid gland.

TABLE 15-1. CLINICAL INDICATORS FOR PERFORMING A TRACHEOSTOMY, AS PROPOSED BY THE AMERICAN ACADEMY OF OTOLARYNGOLOGY–HEAD AND NECK SURGERY

Upper airway obstruction, including
 Obstructive sleep apnea
 Bilateral vocal cord paralysis
Need for prolonged mechanical ventilation
Inability of patient to manage his or her secretions
Facilitation of ventilation support
Adjunct to manage head and neck surgery
Adjunct to manage head and neck trauma
Difficulty with intubation and need for airway

SOURCE: Adapted from Weissler.[8]

gers who strike the dashboard with the neck extended ("padded-dash syndrome"). Most patients with laryngo-tracheal disruption die at the scene of the injury. Those who survive present with varying degrees of respiratory distress, visible bruising over the anterior neck, hoarseness or aphonia, subcutaneous emphysema over the neck and chest wall, and blood-streaked sputum. A defect may be palpable in the neck. Soft tissue radiographs of the neck may show an interrupted air column. When this injury is suspected, immediate efforts should focus on getting the patient to the operating room. Visual inspection of the airway by laryngoscopy should be performed once the surgical team is present and prepared to explore the neck.

A tracheostomy may need to be performed immediately if the patient is in extremis. If the airway is disrupted, a "low tracheostomy" between the fourth and fifth tracheal rings should be performed. The severed airway will tend to retract into the thorax, and a low tracheostomy will offer the best chance of securing the dismembered segment. Misguided attempts to visualize the airway, intubate orally, or perform a cricothyroidot-

TABLE 15-2. COMMONLY CITED INDICATIONS FOR PERFORMING A TRACHEOSTOMY

Airway obstruction[9,10,11,13]
 Tumor, trauma, hemorrhage
 Edema, foreign body, infection
 Congenital airway anomalies
Trauma to face and neck with airway compromise[9,10,12]
Inability to open mouth
 Maxillomandibular fixation, trismus[14]
 Angioedema[11,13]
 Need for prolonged ventilatory support[10]
 Impaired clearance of secretions
 Need for aggressive pulmonary toilet[11]
 Laryngeal injury[5,7,11]
 Unstable cervical spine[12]
 Laryngospasm[13]
 Surgical airway in an infant[5]
 Inability to intubate by other measures[12]

omy may further damage the already precarious airway. This is fortunately a rare injury with only a few case reports in the literature.[25,26] A tracheostomy performed in this setting is more treacherous than usual. Although a tracheostomy may be the only way to secure the airway, this airway intervention has a better chance of success when performed in the operating room.

SURGICAL AIRWAY IN THE PEDIATRIC PATIENT

Surgical approaches to the airway are more difficult and complicated in pediatric patients, especially newborns and infants. The infant's cricothyroid membrane, unlike that of the adult, is extremely narrow and cannot easily be used for access to the airway. The pediatric trachea is more floppy and mobile, and the working area is substantially smaller than in an adolescent or an adult. Attempts at creating emergency invasive airways in children are typically acts of desperation. A calm, reasoned approach to the pediatric airway and common respiratory problems is essential. Efforts should first be made to suction the airway clear of secretions, followed by ventilation with a bag-valve-mask device. **Direct visualization by laryngoscopy and orotracheal intubation should be attempted before resorting to a surgical airway.** If an unstable patient cannot be ventilated, a needle cricothyroidotomy can serve as a temporizing measure until a surgical team can be assembled and better control achieved.

Attempts at emergency tracheostomy may be heroic, but they are associated with a greater risk of failure. Every other available alternative should be considered first. The best approach to an airway crisis is anticipation of potential airway compromise and early intervention before tracheostomy becomes the only remaining option.

THE "CRASH TRACHEOSTOMY"

The need for emergent surgical airways has been reduced by the improved training and skills of Emergency Physicians, the use of a wider variety of pharmacologic aids for sedation and paralysis, and the development of innovative approaches and technology for airway management. Even in the face of dire circumstances, clinicians should first attempt the techniques with which they are most experienced. Common noninvasive techniques may be surprisingly effective, even in difficult settings.

CONTRAINDICATIONS

Simply stated, emergency tracheostomy is contraindicated when other methods can be used to secure the airway. There are a few instances when an immediate surgical airway is necessary. **Cricothyroidotomy is the**

procedure of choice when an invasive approach to the airway is needed. Compared to tracheostomy, cricothyroidotomy is faster and more direct; it relies predominantly on external landmarks, requires only a single operator, can be done with ambient lighting, and requires a limited amount of equipment.[8,21] In contrast, tracheostomy is a procedure requiring multiple steps. It involves direct visualization to dissect through vascular structures and requires better light than is commonly present at the bedside. It is easier and therefore faster to execute if one has an assistant, proper suctioning equipment, and electrocautery. Without these advantages, the technique is difficult and likely to be complicated. A "timely trach" can be performed within 5 to 10 minutes.[8] The average times to establish an airway by open tracheostomy in elective procedures range from 13.5 to 105 minutes.[21–24] Although this time frame may be adequate for urgent situations, it is too slow for the true emergency in a patient who lacks an airway.

EQUIPMENT

A tracheostomy requires an extensive amount of equipment. Appropriate supplies should be sterilized and assembled in a prepackaged tray. A list of required equipment is given in Table 15-3. If such a tray is not available, supplies that are immediately on hand have to suffice. A thoracotomy or major procedure tray will contain most of the required equipment.

PATIENT PREPARATION

Patient preparation will depend largely on the circumstances dictating the procedure. If the patient is uncooperative, hypoxic, or thrashing about, rapid control will have to be established with a sedative. The ideal agent is one that sedates with minimal hemodynamic consequences, preserves spontaneous respirations, and leaves an intact gag reflex (e.g., ketamine). If the patient is awake and cooperative, calm reassurance may allow the procedure to be performed under local anesthesia. If the patient is unconscious, a local anesthetic is sufficient.

Place a rolled towel under the patient's shoulders and neck if no contraindications exist (Figure 15-7). This detail cannot be emphasized enough. Full neck extension brings the airway anterior and increases the length of the supraclavicular trachea by as much as 2.6 cm.[7] It enlarges the surgical field for improved access. Neck extension tends to fix the airway in position and pull it taut. When the neck is in a neutral or flexed position, the trachea lies more posteriorly and is more "floppy." In this situation, it is easier for the operator to stray off midline. When the neck is flexed, the surgical field may be reduced to a dark hole with poor visibility.

Prior to beginning the incision, the operator should check the equipment. A tracheostomy tube that is appropriate for the patient's size should be selected. An average male will accommodate a size 7 or 8 Shiley tracheal tube. An average-size female will accommodate a

TABLE 15-3. THE SUPPLIES REQUIRED TO PERFORM A TRACHEOSTOMY

Patient preparation	Setup
Cardiac monitor	Povidone iodine solution
Pulse oximeter	Surgical drapes to enclose the field
Intravenous line with saline	Sterile gown, gloves, and mask
Oxygen	
Ambu bag for ventilating patient	

Procedure	
Local anesthesia	Two pairs of scissors, one straight and one curved
10 mL syringe	Two tissue forceps without teeth
1% lidocaine	Two Allis forceps, to grasp the trachea
18 gauge needle	Two small rakes, for exposure
25 gauge needle	Mastoid retractor
#10 scalpel blade and handle	Trousseau dilator
#11 scalpel blade and handle	Two tracheal hooks
Two skin forceps	10 mL syringe
Eight small curved hemostats	Umbilical tape
Sterile 4×4 gauze squares, two dozen	Needle holder
Two Kocher forceps (if needed, to clamp the thyroid)	
Frazier suction catheter with suction tubing	
Suture ligatures (3–0 chromic, 3–0 silk, 3–0 nylon)	
Tracheostomy tube, appropriate size for patient	
Water-soluble lubricant or anesthetic jelly	
Suction source and tubing	

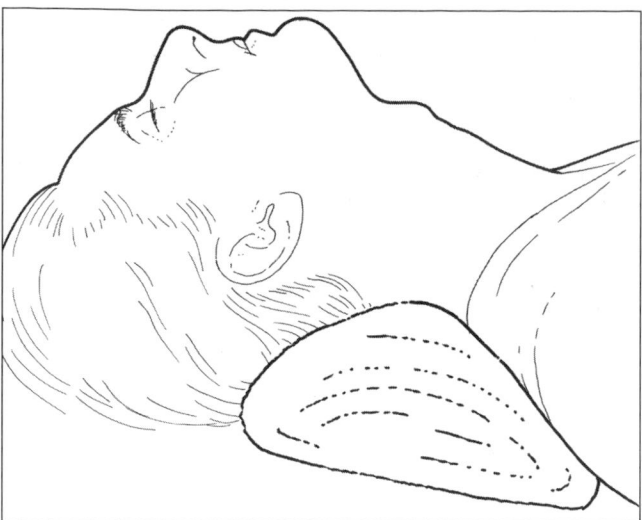

FIGURE 15-7 Optimal patient positioning for a tracheostomy with the neck extended.

size 6 or 7 Shiley tracheal tube. The cuff of the tracheal tube should be tested prior to use. As an alternative, an endotracheal tube can be used.

Identify the anatomic landmarks required to perform this procedure. Using the nondominant hand, place the thumb on one side and the middle finger on the other side of the patient's trachea (Figure 15-8). Identify the laryngeal prominence (Adam's apple) with the index finger. Slide the index finger caudally to identify the cricothyroid membrane, cricoid cartilage, and tracheal rings.

Clean the neck of any dirt and debris. Apply povidone iodine to the anterior neck. Even during the resuscita-

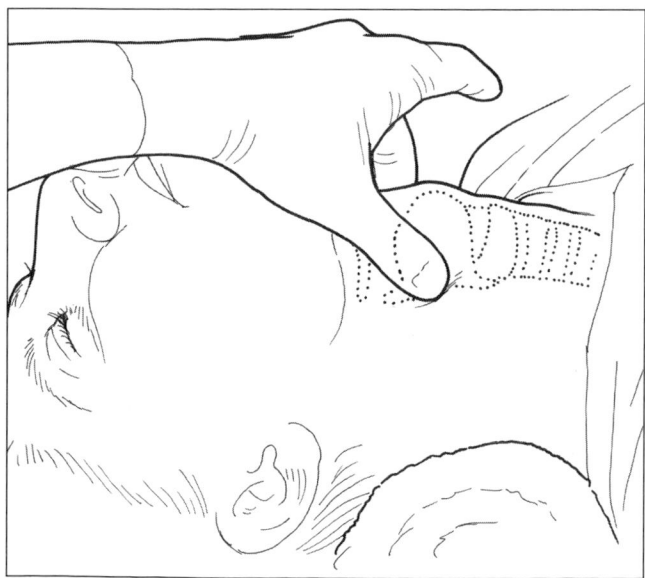

FIGURE 15-8 Hand positioning to palpate the anatomic landmarks.

tion of an unstable patient, there should be adequate time to prep the neck with an aseptic solution. Prepare yourself by applying a mask, eye protection, sterile gown, and sterile gloves. Apply a sterile drape to isolate a surgical field. Infiltrate local anesthetic solution (1% lidocaine) along the planned incision line. Insert a needle through the cricothyroid membrane and inject 2 mL of local anesthetic solution into the trachea to blunt the cough reflex. Insertion of a needle into the airway to administer local anesthetic provides a valuable sense of depth of the airway.

Once the patient is positioned, prepped, and anesthetized, establishment of the airway should be just 2 to 3 minutes away. **The last step in preparation should be the mental decision that no other technique will suffice and the commitment to proceed with confidence.**

TECHNIQUE

In the most critical situation, the simplest technique is likely to be the most successful.[31] The right-handed operator should stand to the patient's right and fix the airway with their left hand (Figure 15-8). Left-handed operators should adjust their technique based on their preference for handedness. Apply the thumb and third digit of the nondominant hand on the thyroid cartilage while the index finger palpates the cricoid and tracheal rings (Figure 15-8). An awake or lightly anesthetized patient may swallow or gulp during the procedure, thereby moving the landmarks. Fixing the left hand firmly on the upper airway will minimize this distraction.

Make a 3 or 4 cm vertical midline incision through the skin and subcutaneous tissues beginning just below the cricoid cartilage and extending inferiorly to the supraclavicular notch (Figure 15-9). A larger skin incision causes no harm as long as it remains superficial, to avoid damaging the cricoid cartilage. **The incision should be exactly in the midline.**

Once the skin and subcutaneous tissue have been incised, attention should be directed toward clearing the pretracheal space and defining the tracheal rings. Divide the superficial and deep strap muscles in the midline and retract them away from the trachea (Figure 15-10). Bluntly dissect free and reflect away any blood vessels in front of the trachea. If they impede progress, they can be clamped with hemostats and divided. The thyroid gland lies above the trachea. Bluntly dissect between it and the trachea with a hemostat to mobilize the thyroid gland (Figure 15-11). Retract the thyroid gland upward (Figure 15-12). If this becomes difficult, it may be faster to divide the isthmus between two hemostats (Figure 15-13). The divided edges can be oversewn after the tracheostomy tube is in place. Once the thyroid has been divided, how-

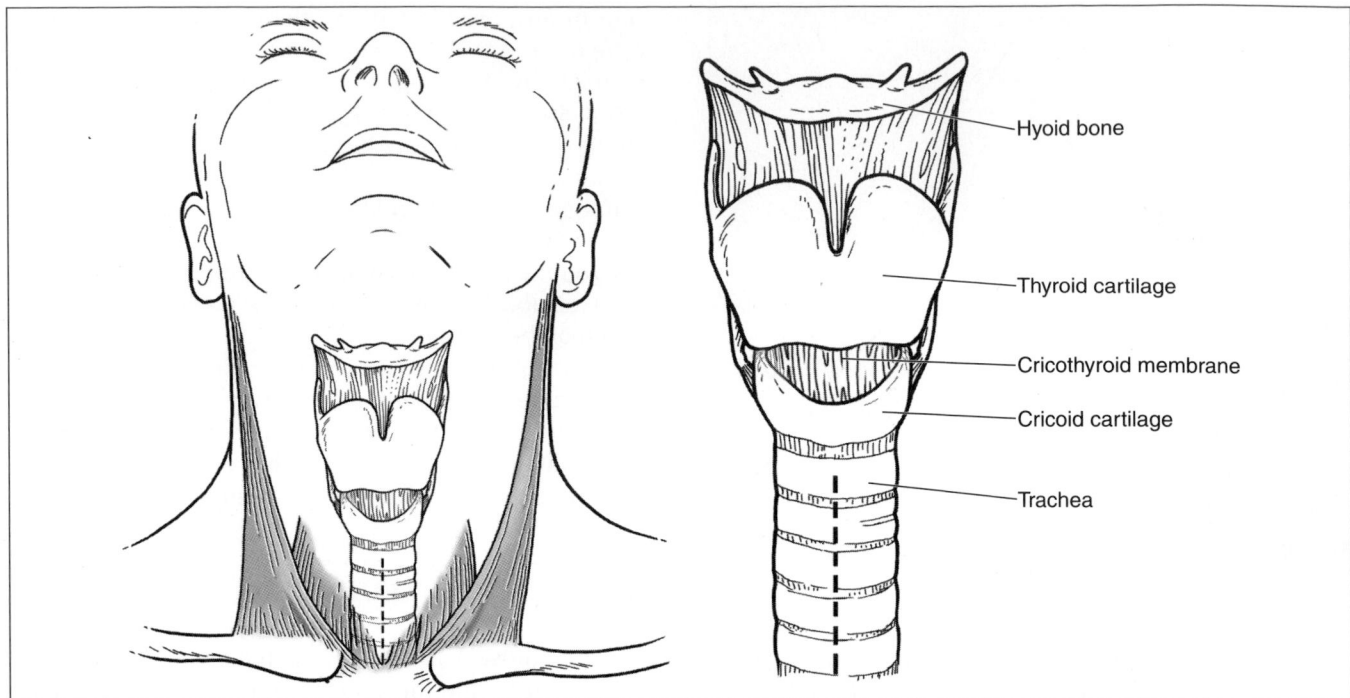

FIGURE 15-9 The skin incision is made in the midline, beginning below the cricoid cartilage and extending down toward the supraclavicular notch. An incision made with these landmarks will lie over the second through fourth tracheal rings.

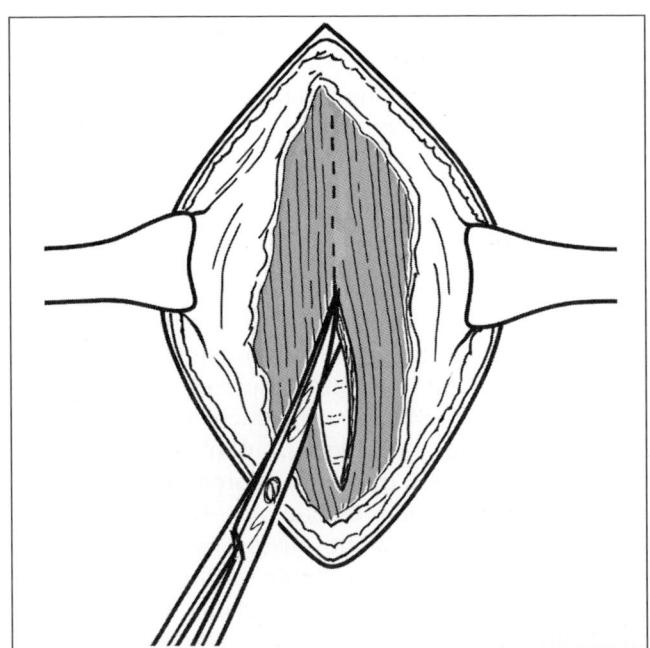

FIGURE 15-10 The skin and subcutaneous tissues have been retracted. The strap muscles are divided in the midline to expose the pretracheal space.

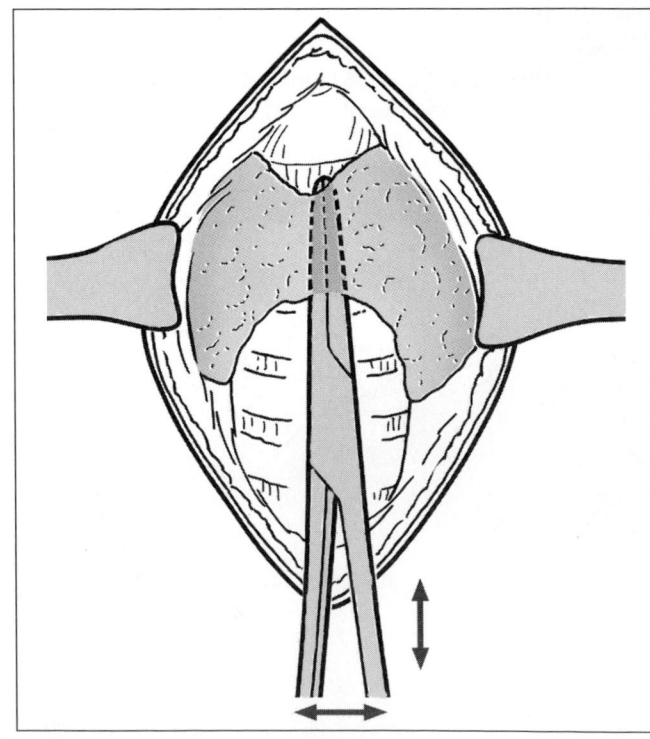

FIGURE 15-11 The thyroid gland is bluntly dissected from the trachea. Arrows represent movement of the hemostat.

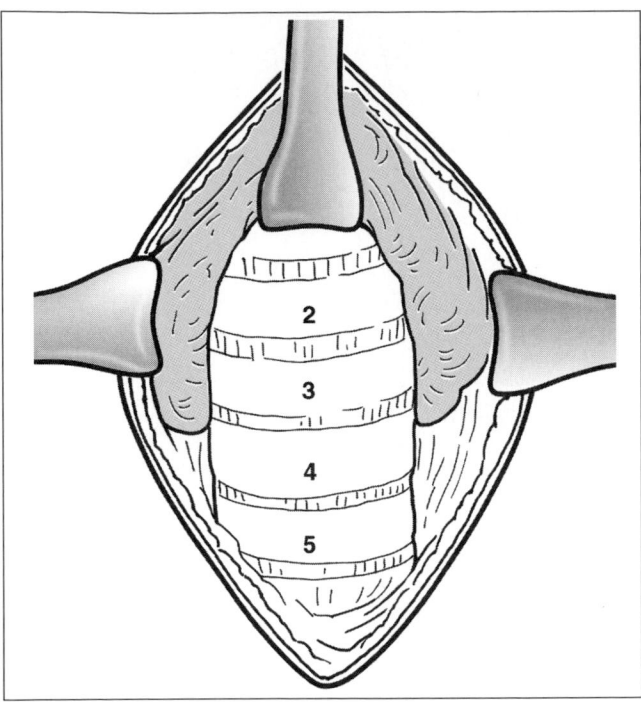

FIGURE 15-12 The thyroid gland is retracted upward and out of the surgical field.

ever, the operating field will be cluttered with hemostats and may be partially obscured. Do not apply traction to the instruments, as this can avulse tissue, leading to bleeding and further obstruction of the surgical field. An alternative option to consider in the emergent setting is to use the nondominant index finger to dissect the pretracheal space bluntly and reflect the thyroid isthmus. This minimalist blunt approach lacks finesse but is effective and timely.[10]

When ready to make the tracheal incision, it may be helpful to have an assistant place a tracheal hook under the first tracheal ring and apply traction superiorly and anteriorly (Figure 15-14). Have the assistant hold the tracheal hook in position. This will elevate and immobilize the trachea. The assistant should direct their hands superior to the wound to keep the field unobstructed. If the neck is properly extended, this may be unnecessary.

Make an incision in the trachea. The preferred tracheotomy is a midline vertical incision extending from the second through the fourth tracheal rings (Figure 15-15A). There are other options, but they are discouraged in the emergent setting because they stray from the midline (Figures 15-15B to D). Insert a Trousseau dilator or hemostat into the incision. Use the dilator to open and widen the incision. Alternatively, the sides of the tracheal incision can be grasped and held open with Allis forceps (Figure 15-16A).

Lubricate the appropriate size tracheostomy tube liberally. Place the tracheostomy tube, with its obturator,

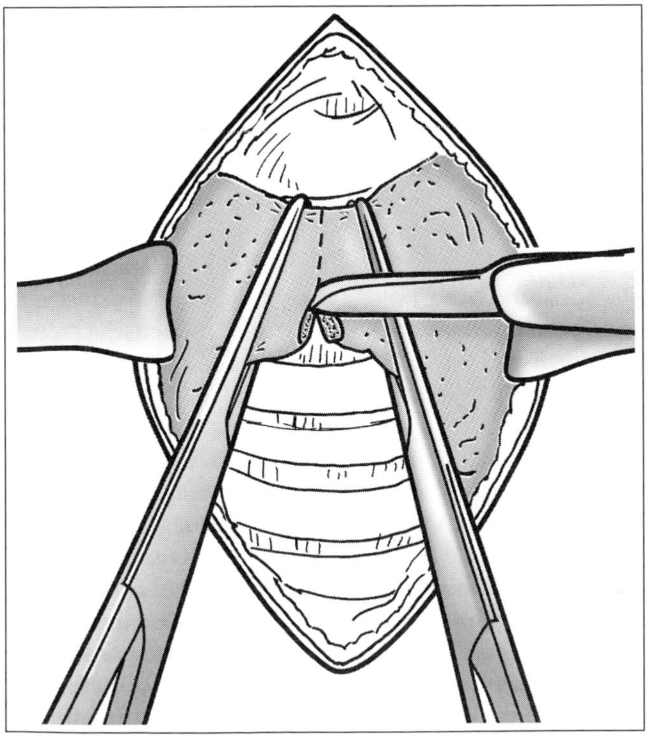

FIGURE 15-13 An alternative method of clearing the thyroid gland from the surgical field. The isthmus is clamped and transected.

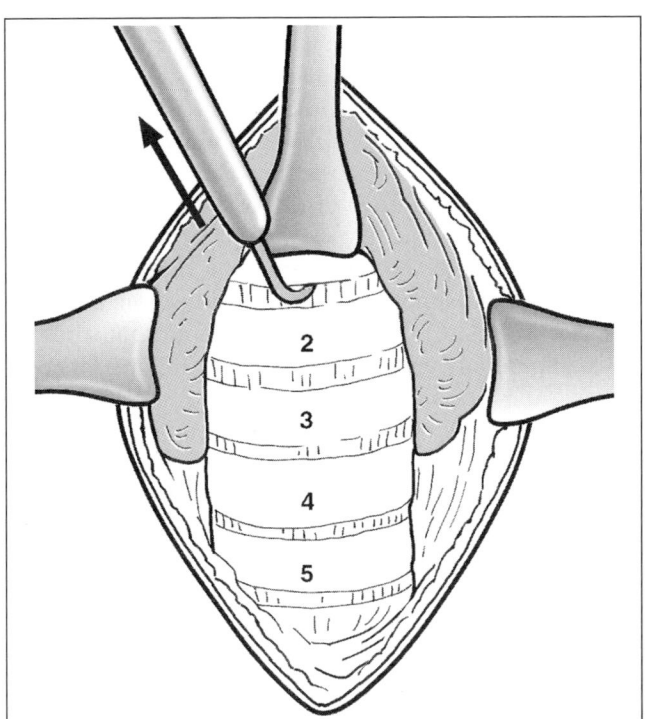

FIGURE 15-14 A tracheal hook is placed below the first tracheal ring to elevate and immobilize the trachea.

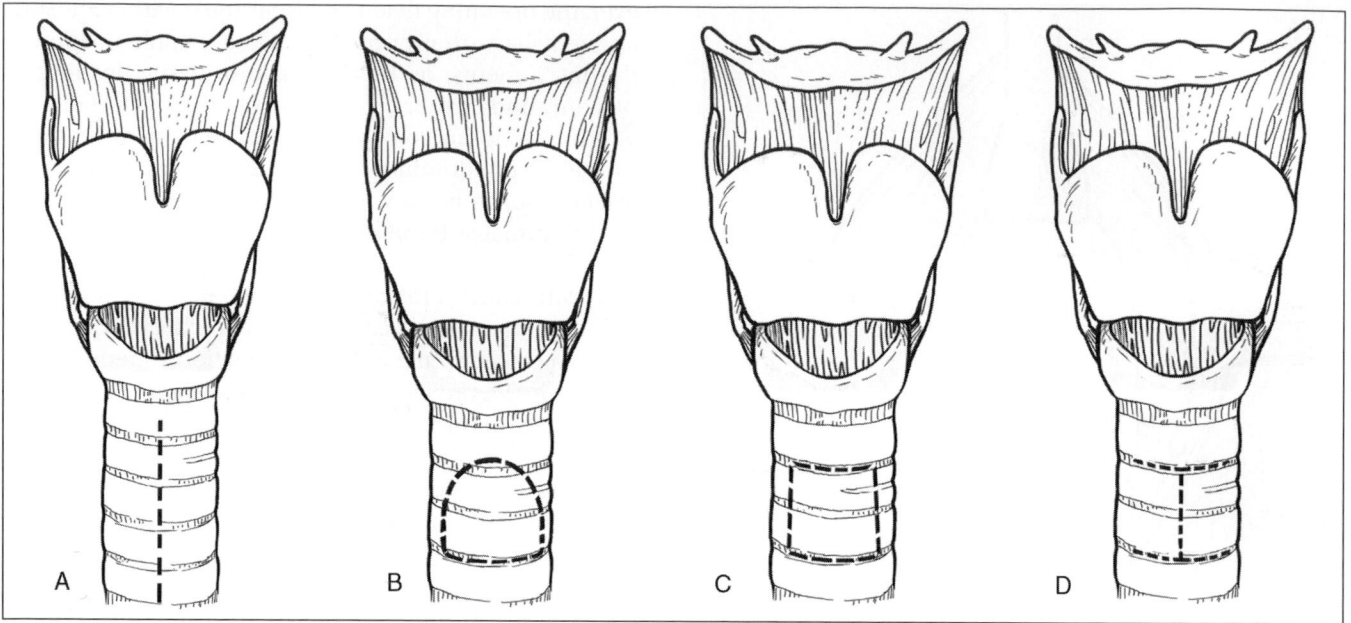

FIGURE 15-15 Types of tracheal incisions. *A.* A midline vertical incision through the second, third, and fourth tracheal rings. This is the preferred technique in an emergent procedure. *B.* A U-shaped inferiorly based window. *C.* A window has been created by excising the second and third tracheal rings. *D.* A T flap.

through the tracheotomy while the incision is held open (Figure 15-16*A*). Advance the tracheostomy tube and inflate the cuff (Figure 15-16*B*). Hold the tracheostomy tube in place securely. Remove the obturator and insert the inner cannula. Attach a bag-valve device and begin ventilating the patient.

ALTERNATIVE TECHNIQUES

Since 1969, a number of authors have described a third invasive option for airway control, the percutaneous dilatational tracheostomy. The first commercial kits for percutaneous tracheostomies became available in 1985. Although techniques vary somewhat, they all rely on an initial puncture of the airway followed by progressive dilatation of a tract. Once a sufficiently large tract is formed, an airway tube is placed. There is now enough evidence to argue that percutaneous tracheostomies are competitive with, and perhaps preferable to, formal open tracheostomies done under elective conditions.[22,23,32-44] Several large series of percutaneous tracheostomies are now complete, but significant results are available only for elective tracheostomies done in patients who have already been intubated.[33,35,36,41] Even enthusiastic supporters of percutaneous techniques agree that the need for emergent airway control is a contraindication to the percutaneous route. Cricothyroidotomy remains the procedure of choice for emergency

surgical access to the airway. In those few circumstances in which cricothyroidotomy cannot be performed (e.g., laryngotracheal disruption, loss of external landmarks), percutaneous tracheostomies are even less likely to succeed. Percutaneous dilatational tracheostomy should not be used as emergent procedures.

ASSESSMENT

Once the airway is established, tracheostomy tube positioning should be confirmed by auscultation, ease of ventilation, and pulse oximetry. Obtain a chest and neck radiograph to also confirm the tracheostomy tube position.

AFTERCARE

Once the airway has been established, inspect the wound to ensure hemostasis. Any clamped vessels or thyroid tissue should be tied. If the thyroid isthmus has been ligated, oversew it with a running 3–0 chromic suture. The skin edges do not need to be closed unless the skin incision was overly zealous. If the skin is reapproximated, close it loosely to avoid the development of subcutaneous emphysema. Secure the tracheostomy tube with umbilical tape wrapped around the neck. Suture the flange of the tracheostomy tube to the skin using 3–0

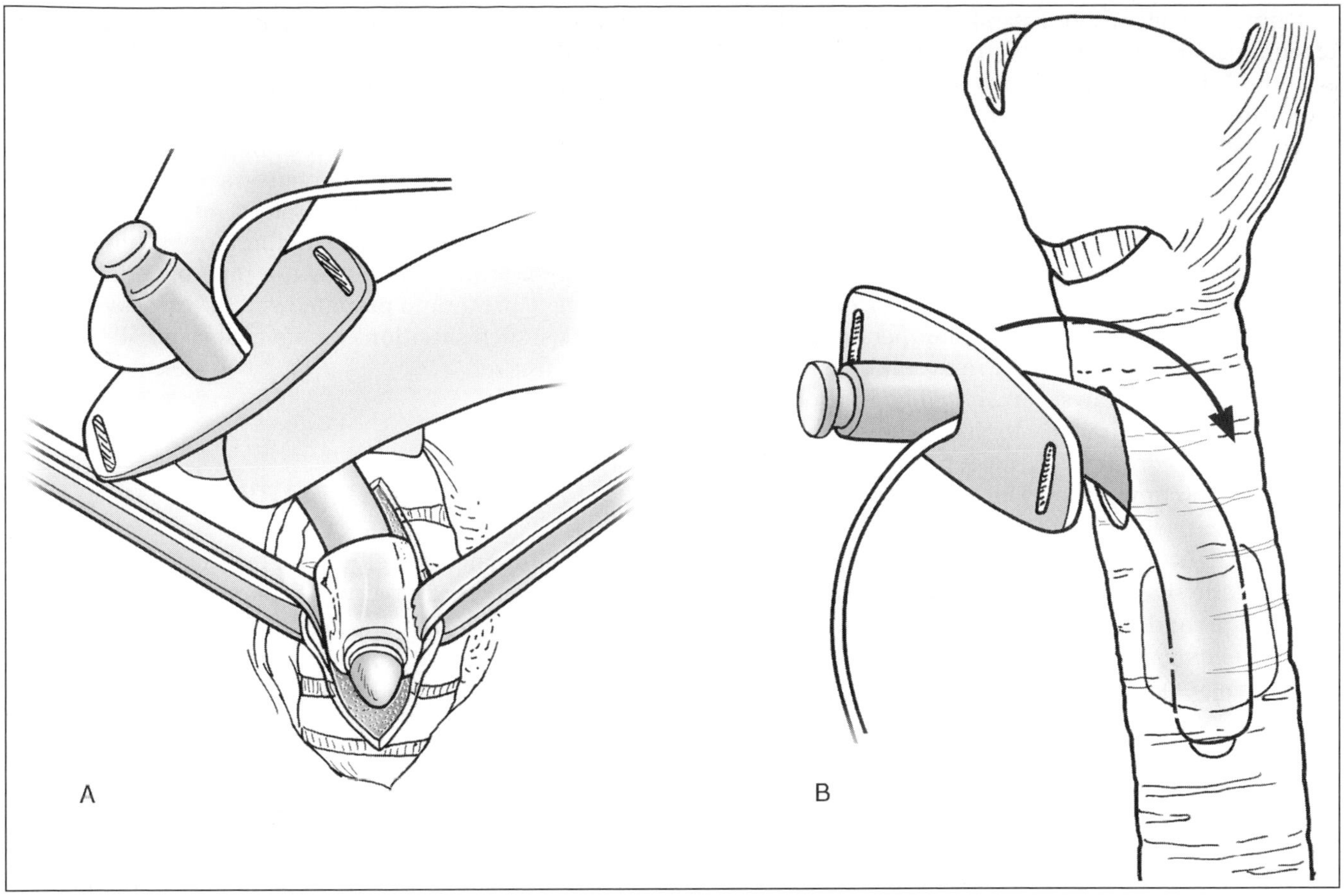

FIGURE 15-16 Insertion of the tracheal tube. *A.* The incision is held open with a Trousseau dilator, hemostat, or Allis forceps (shown here) as the tracheostomy tube is inserted. *B.* The tracheostomy tube is advanced and the cuff inflated.

silk as an additional safeguard (Figure 15-17). If the wound is oozing, place a loose gauze pad between the skin and the tracheostomy.

Special care should be taken to protect the artificial airway. Suction the lumen frequently and as necessary to prevent obstruction from blood or secretions. Admin-

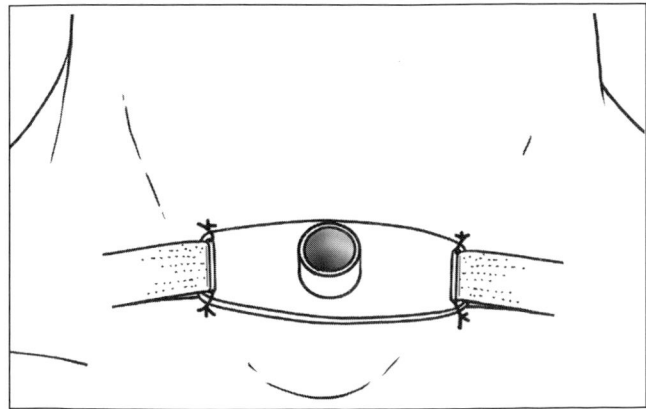

FIGURE 15-17 The tracheostomy tube is secured in place with umbilical tape ("tracheal tie"), then sutured.

ister humidified oxygen through the tube to prevent dried and inspissated secretions from occluding it.

COMPLICATIONS

Tracheostomy is a relatively basic and common surgical procedure. Despite this, it has an unusually high complication rate. Authors report widely different morbidity rates, perhaps determined in part by the clinical settings if not their own biases. Reported morbidity ranges from 6 to 58 percent, with procedures done emergently having the highest rates.[17,18,20,21] However discomforting these numbers may be, the risk is certainly acceptable in the face of an unstable airway in a dying patient.

Under emergent circumstances, a variety of things can and do go wrong. It is best if one has thought about these possibilities and considered alternative strategies prior to experiencing them. The most common problem with a hastily performed tracheostomy is hemorrhage. Most bleeding can be controlled by direct pressure. An assistant may be invaluable in providing sufficient control until the airway is established. The search for a bleeding source during a tracheostomy will cost valuable time. The best way to avoid this difficulty is strict hemostasis during the procedure and being careful to avoid the transection of any blood vessels. The next most likely problem is inadvertent injury to adjacent structures. This can be avoided by remaining strictly in the midline, positioning the patient properly, and using a tracheal hook. If proper technique has not been used, insertion of the tracheostomy tube can create a false passage. This should not occur if the operator has visualized the trachea and remained in the midline.

The Emergency Physician should be cautious not to adopt methods for tracheostomies learned from elective procedures performed in the operating room under controlled circumstances. **The emergent tracheostomy must be carried out with the simplest, fastest, and most straightforward technique possible.** Tracheostomies done under elective conditions may use rescue stay sutures and more elaborate tracheal incisions. The added benefits of these features do not offset the additional time required to perform them.

Other complications from a tracheostomy can be divided into immediate operative complications, postoperative complications, and delayed complications. A summary of reported complications is given in Table 15-4. **Immediate operative complications are for the most part due to damage to surrounding structures or passage of the tube in a false tract. These complications can be avoided by staying in the midline.** No single detail is as important in ensuring success and avoiding problems. Postoperative complications can be minimized by maintaining strict attention to and proper care of the site and tube. **The best way to avoid these complications is to avert the need for a tracheostomy in the first place.** Expertise in alternative airway techniques, including cricothyroidotomy, is ultimately the only way to avoid the very high-risk emergent tracheostomy.

Any physician who cares for patients under emergency circumstances should think through the clinical scenarios in which an emergent tracheostomy may be necessary. Expertise in surgical airway techniques should first be obtained in a laboratory setting. Unless one is poised to respond with a plan of action for the emergent airway and prepared with the necessary surgical skills, such situations create chaos and all too often end in disaster.

SUMMARY

A well-trained Emergency Physician must be prepared for any kind of airway emergency and should be skilled in a variety of approaches. Optimal airway management begins with optimal medical management of the patient, including the early identification of possible airway compromise and aggressive preventive treatment. Many airway problems can be averted with anticipatory action. In the armamentarium of airway procedures, tracheostomy will be (and should be) a rare solution. The physician who is knowledgeable about and comfortable with alternative airway techniques, including surgical access, will be prepared to act decisively yet appropriately upon encountering a challenging airway crisis. While a cricothyroidotomy is the surgical airway procedure of choice, a tracheostomy should be considered for laryngeal injuries with airway disruption, a surgical airway in an infant or child, or when all other methods have failed.

TABLE 15-4. COMPLICATIONS OF TRACHEOSTOMIES

Immediate	Delayed	Postoperative
Hemorrhage	Hemorrhage	Disrupted tract
False passage	Tracheal stenosis	Displaced tube
Damage to surrounding structures	Subglottic stenosis	Obstructed tube, mucus plugging
Recurrent laryngeal nerve	Tracheoinnominate artery fistula	Delayed hemorrhage
Esophagus	Tracheoesophageal fistula	Subcutaneous emphysema
Posterior tracheal perforation	Fused vocal cords	Mediastinal emphysema
Common carotid artery	Delayed wound problems	Infection: wound, tracheitis, mediastinitis, pneumonia
Internal jugular vein	Excess granulation tissue	Aspiration
Anterior jugular vein	Persistent stoma	
Pleura, pneumothorax		
Cricoid		
Air embolism		
Apnea		
Cardiac dysrhythmias		
Cardiac arrest		

SOURCE: Adapted from references 8, 10, 13, 16–18, 24, 29, 30, and 45.

REFERENCES

1. Moore KL: *Clinically Oriented Anatomy.* Baltimore: Williams & Wilkins, 1980:1103.
2. McMinn RMH, Hutchings RT: *Color Atlas of Human Anatomy.* Chicago: Year Book, 1977:33–43.
3. Morris IR: Functional anatomy of the upper airway. *Emerg Med Clin North Am* 1988; 6(4):639–669.
4. Simon RR, Brenner BE: Emergency cricothyroidotomy in the patient with massive neck swelling: Part 1. Anatomical aspects. *Crit Care Med* 1983; 11(2):114–118.
5. Simon RR, Brenner BE, Rosen MA: Emergency cricothyroidotomy in the patient with massive neck swelling: Part 2. Clinical aspects. *Crit Care Med* 1983; 11(2):119–123.
6. Simon RR: Emergency tracheotomy in patients with massive neck swelling. *Emerg Med Clin North Am* 1989; 7(1):95–101.
7. Mathisen DJ: Surgery of the trachea. *Curr Probl Surg* 1998; 35(6):455–542.
8. Weissler MC: Tracheotomy and intubation, in Bailey BJ (ed): *Head and Neck Surgery-Otolaryngology.* Philadelphia: Lippincott, 1993:711–724.
9. Wenig BL, Applebaum EL: Indications for and techniques of tracheotomy. *Clin Chest Med* 1991: 12(3):545–553.
10. Lewis RJ: Tracheostomies: indications, timing, and complications. *Clin Chest Med* 1992; 13(1):137–149.
11. Tayal VS: Tracheostomies. *Emerg Med Clin North Am* 1994; 12(3):707–727.
12. Walls RM: Airway management. *Emerg Med Clin North Am* 1993; 11(1):53–60.
13. Hemenway WG: The management of severe obstruction of the upper air passages. *Surg Clin North Am* 1961; 41(1):201–212.
14. Taicher S, Givol N, Peleg M, et al: Changing indications for tracheostomy in maxillofacial trauma. *J Oral Maxillofac Surg* 1996; 54:292–295.
15. Piotrowski JJ, Moore EE: Emergency department tracheostomy. *Emerg Med Clin North Am* 1988; 6(4):737–744.
16. Arjmand EM, Spector JG: Airway control and laryngotracheal stenosis, in Ballenger JJ, Snow JB (eds): *Otorhinolaryngology—Head and Neck Surgery,* 15th ed. Baltimore: Williams & Wilkins, 1996:466–497.
17. Timmis HH: Tracheostomy: an overview of implications, management and morbidity. *Adv Surg* 1973; 7:199–233.
18. Chew JY, Cantrell RW: Tracheostomy: complications and their management. *Arch Otolaryngol Head Neck Surg* 1972; 96:538–545.
19. Vender JS, Shapiro BA: Essentials of artificial airway management in critical care. *Acute Care* 1987; 13:97–124.
20. Linscott MS, Horton WC: Management of upper airway obstruction. *Otolaryngol Clin North Am* 1979; 12(2):351–373.
21. Bernard AC, Kenady DE: Conventional surgical tracheostomy as the preferred method of airway management. *J Oral Maxillofac Surg* 1999; 57:310–315.
22. Griffen MM, Kearney PA: Percutaneous dilatational tracheostomy as the preferred method of airway management. *J Oral Maxillofac Surg* 1999; 57:316–320.
23. Leinhardt OJ, Mughal M, Bowles B, et al: Appraisal of percutaneous tracheostomy. *Br J Surg* 1992; 79:255–258.
24. Selecky PA: Tracheostomy: a review of present day indications, complications, and care. *Heart Lung* 1974; 3(2):272–283.
25. Alonso WA, Pratt LL, Zollinger WK, et al: Complications of laryngotracheal disruption. *Laryngoscope* 1974; 84(8):1276–1290.
26. Butler RM, Moser FH: The padded dash syndrome: blunt trauma to the larynx and trachea. *Laryngoscope* 1968; 78(7):1172–1182.
27. McLaughlin J, Iverson KV: Emergency pediatric tracheostomy: a usable technique and model for instruction. *Ann Emerg Med* 1986; 15(4):463–465.
28. Lynn HB, van Heerden JA: Tracheostomy in infants. *Surg Clin North Am* 1973; 53(4):945–952.
29. Hamilton PH, Kang JJ: Emergency airway management. *Mt Sinai J Med* 1997; 64(4&5):292–301.
30. Simon RR, Brenner BE: *Emergency Procedures and Techniques,* 3rd ed. Baltimore: Williams & Wilkins, 1994:32–89.
31. Weymuller EA: Acute airway management, in Cummings CC, Fredrickson JM, Harker LA, et al (eds): *Otolaryngology—Head and Neck Surgery,* 2nd ed. St Louis: Mosby, 1993:2382–2395.
32. Sheldon GF, Fakhry SM, Messick WJ: Respiratory failure and ventilatory support, in Nyhus LM, Baker RJ, Fischer JE (eds): *Mastery of Surgery,* 3rd ed. Boston: Little, Brown, 1997:99–115.
33. Moe KS, Schmid S, Stoeckli S, et al: Percutaneous tracheostomy: a comprehensive evaluation. *Ann Otol Rhinol Laryngol* 1999; 108:384–391.
34. Bobo ML, McKenna SJ: The current status of percutaneous dilational tracheostomy: an alternative to open tracheostomy. *J Oral Maxillofac Surg* 1998; 56:681–685.
35. Powell DM, Price PD, Forrest LA: Review of percutaneous tracheostomy. *Laryngoscope* 1998; 108:170–177.
36. Berrouschot J, Oeken J, Steiniger L, et al: Perioperative complications of percutaneous dilational tracheostomy. *Laryngoscope* 1997; 107:1538–1544.

37. Hill BB, Zweng TN, Maley RH, et al: Percutaneous dilational tracheostomy: report of 356 cases. *J Trauma* 1996; 40(8):238–244.

38. Graham JS, Mulloy RH, Sutherland FR, et al: Percutaneous versus open tracheostomy: a retrospective cohort outcome study. *J Trauma* 1996; 42(2):245–250.

39. Toursarkissian B, Zweng TN, Kearney PA, et al: Percutaneous dilational tracheostomy: report of 141 cases. *Ann Thorac Surg* 1994; 57:862–867.

40. Ciaglia P, Graniero KD: Percutaneous dilational tracheostomy: results and long-term follow-up. *Chest* 1992; 101(2):464–467.

41. Anderson HL, Bartlett RH: Elective tracheotomy for mechanical ventilation by the percutaneous technique. *Clin Chest Med* 1991; 12(3):555–560.

42. Ciaglia P, Firsching R, Syniec C: Elective percutaneous dilational tracheostomy: a new simple bedside procedure; preliminary report. *Chest* 1985; 87(6):715–719.

43. Toye FJ, Weinstein JD: Clinical experience with percutaneous tracheostomy and cricothyroidotomy in 100 patients. *J Trauma* 1986; 26(11):1034–1040.

44. Schachner A, Ovil Y, Sidi J, et al: Percutaneous tracheostomy—a new method. *Crit Care Med* 1989; 17(10):1052–1056.

45. Kirchner JA: Tracheotomy and its problems. *Surg Clin North Am* 1980; 60(5):1093–1104.

Chapter 16
TRACHEOSTOMY CARE

H. Gene Hern, Jr.

INTRODUCTION

All Emergency Physicians should be familiar with tracheostomy care and the management of tracheostomy complications. Rapid assessment and understanding of tracheostomies and their potential complications can be lifesaving in the critically ill and tracheostomy-dependent patient.

Although tracheostomies have been performed since ancient times, they were perfected only during the past century. A Greek physician named Asclepiades of Bismuth has been credited with performing the first successful tracheostomy in 100 B.C.[1] Two of the four physicians summoned to President George Washington's deathbed were said to have argued for tracheostomy as his only means of survival. In the 1800s, Trousseau reported successful tracheostomies in more than 2000 cases of upper airway obstruction secondary to diphtheria.[2] Chevalier Jackson, in the twentieth century, perfected the tracheostomy technique and reduced the operative mortality from 25 percent to below 1 percent.[3] This is roughly what it remains today.

The important aspects of tracheostomy care include the assessment of respiratory distress in the tracheostomy patient, proper suctioning techniques, and assessment and evaluation of possible complications arising from the tracheostomy itself or its placement. For the purposes of this chapter, tracheostomy care is divided into routine care and emergent care.

ANATOMY AND PATHOPHYSIOLOGY

The trachea is a fibromuscular tube with approximately 18 to 20 cartilaginous arches extending from the cricoid cartilage to the division into right and left main-

stem bronchi (Figure 15-4). The surface of the tracheal mucosa is covered with respiratory epithelium. This epithelium is responsible for the formation of secretions, mucociliary "elevator" movement of secretions and debris, and humidification. Of note, the remaining part of the upper respiratory tract (which is bypassed by the tracheostomy) plays a major role in the warming and humidification of inspired air.

The terms tracheostomy and tracheotomy are widely interchanged in current parlance. Tracheotomy refers to the actual incision through the skin and the trachea, which is then kept open by a tracheotomy tube. Tracheostomy refers to the procedure whereby the tracheal opening is actually sutured to the skin incision. This creates a more permanent orifice. The term tracheostomy is used in the remaining sections of this chapter.

A tracheostomy is created by an incision at the level of the second and third tracheal rings. After the subcutaneous tissue is divided, an incision is made into the trachea. A hook is inserted into the incision and used to stabilize the trachea while a tube is placed in its lumen. The trachea is secured to the overlying skin and the tube is secured in place. Further details can be found in Chapter 15.

EQUIPMENT

Tracheostomy tubes vary in their composition, angles, and types and the presence or absence of a cuff. The basic tube consists of an outer cannula and an inner cannula (Figure 16-1). The size of the tracheostomy tube is usually defined by its inner diameter. The outer cannula is the more permanent fixture in the tracheostomy. The inner cannula is a low-profile tube that inserts into the outer cannula. It can easily be removed and re-

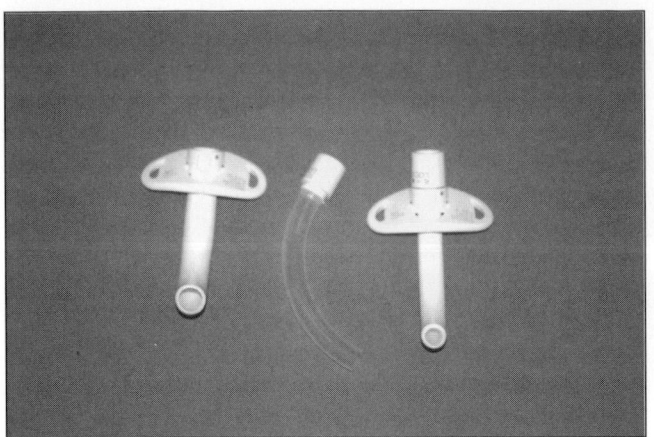

FIGURE 16-1 The tracheostomy tube consists of an outer cannula (*left*) and an inner cannula (*middle*). The inner cannula inserts and locks into the outer cannula (*right*).

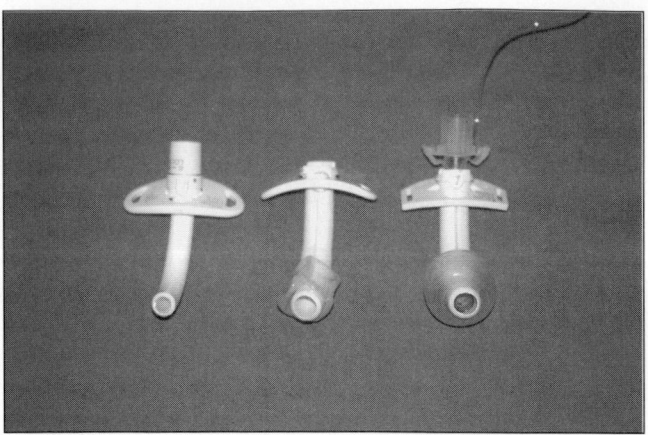

FIGURE 16-3 Tracheostomy tubes may be uncuffed (*left*) or cuffed (*middle*). The inflated cuff is a high-volume, low-pressure system (*right*).

placed. The inner and outer cannulas contain a locking mechanism by which the inner cannula is secured into the outer cannula. The proximal end of the inner cannula contains a standard 15 mm connector that allows direct connections to a ventilator or bag-valve device.

Pediatric tracheostomy tubes, it must be noted, have a much smaller inner diameter and do not accommodate inner cannulas (Figure 16-2). Since pediatric tracheostomy tubes are not made with an inner cannula, they require more frequent suctioning and changing.

Tracheostomy tubes are manufactured with and without cuffs (Figure 16-3). Older high-pressure, low-volume cuffs produced tracheal mucosal injury within hours. They have been replaced by high-volume, low-pressure cuffs that can be used for extended periods with minimal mucosal injury.

Obturators are solid devices that aid in the smooth insertion of the tracheostomy tube (Figure 16-4). When placed inside the outer cannula, an obturator will totally occlude the cannula and extend a few millimeters be-

yond the distal end. The smooth tip of the obturator allows the inner cannula to be inserted with minimal effort and prevents the edges of the cannula from getting caught and damaging tissue. Once the outer cannula has been inserted, the obturator is removed and replaced with a low-profile inner cannula.

ROUTINE CARE

The routine care of the patient with a tracheostomy includes humidification of air as well as cleaning and suctioning of the tracheostomy. Inspired air that bypasses the upper respiratory tract in patients with tracheostomies is not as warm or humidified as air inspired through the nose or mouth. When cold, dry air is inspired into the trachea, the mucociliary "elevator" becomes impaired, resulting in thicker secretions. It is important, especially in the postoperative period, to warm

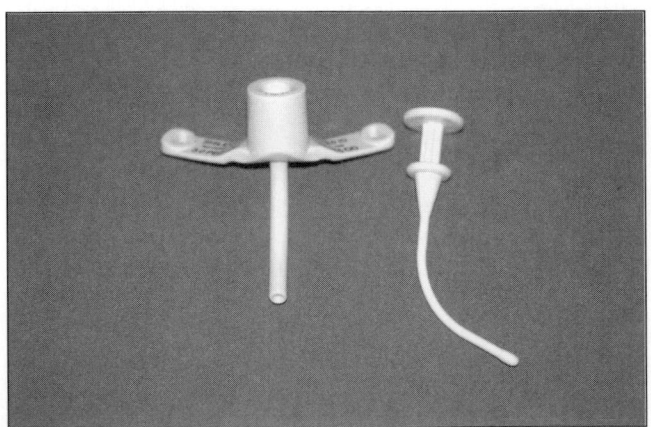

FIGURE 16-2 The pediatric tracheostomy tube.

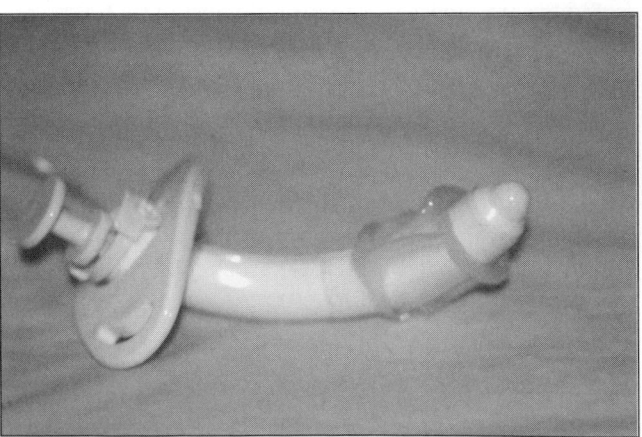

FIGURE 16-4 The obturator is a solid device (*left*) that inserts into and projects from the distal end of the outer cannula (*right*).

and humidify the inspired air for the patient with a tracheostomy.[4]

Care of the tracheostomy must include ensuring adequate cleanliness of the tube. Cleanse the skin site with diluted hydrogen peroxide, at a 50% concentration, applied to cotton-tipped swabs or other similar absorbent devices.[5] The skin surrounding the tracheostomy should be kept dry between cleanings with tracheal bandages or gauze sponges. It is important to note the underlying skin condition. Erythematous or macerated skin can become eroded or infected. Proper skin-care techniques should be used to ensure skin viability. Tracheal bandages or tape used to secure the tracheostomy in place should not be so tight as to compromise skin perfusion. A good rule of thumb is to have two finger breadths of laxity between the skin and the securing ties.[5]

SUCTIONING

Suctioning of the tracheostomy should be conducted when there are thick and tenacious secretions at the tracheostomy lumen or when the patient is having difficulty clearing secretions. Suctioning through the tracheostomy will eliminate debris and infectious agents, improve oxygenation, and prevent atelectasis. Other indications for suctioning include diminished or coarse breath sounds, unexplained decreases in oxygen saturation levels, or increased airway pressures.[6] Suctioning should not be done as part of "routine care" when there are few secretions or if the patient is adequately able to generate enough force to clear the secretions.[7] While the suctioning of tracheostomies is often essential to proper pulmonary toilet, it can also be hazardous. Known complications to tracheal suctioning include hypoxia, hypotension, atelectasis, infections, tracheal mucosal damage, vagus stimulation, arrhythmias, and even cardiac arrest.[6,8]

Suctioning can also be very frightening to the patient and must be done with some expediency and professionalism. These patients' anxiety levels are quite high, as their ability to breathe may be compromised by secretions, they may be hypoxic, and they have a decreased ability to communicate freely at baseline.[4]

EQUIPMENT
Protective clothing (disposable gowns, gloves, face shields, goggles, shoe covers)
Bag-valve device
Flexible multieyed suction catheter, less than half the diameter of the inner cannula
Saline bullets
Continuous wall suction
Pressure regulator to maintain suction pressure

PATIENT PREPARATION
Place the patient in an upright or semirecumbent position. If possible, hyperextend the patient's neck. Preoxygenate the patient with 100% oxygen prior to suctioning. **Hypoxia is a common complication of suctioning and can be virtually eliminated with proper preoxygenation.** In addition, proper preoxygenation often prevents cardiac arrhythmias from occurring during suctioning.[8] Pretreatment with atropine in neonates and children has been suggested to minimize bradycardic episodes.[9]

It has been debated which technique of preoxygenation is best. Options include hand ventilation with a bag-valve device for five to eight breaths, hyperventilation with 100% O_2 via a nonrebreathing mask, or hyperventilation with 100% O_2 via a ventilator. The advantage of hand ventilation is that there is faster delivery of oxygen to the lungs rather than waiting for the higher percentage of oxygen to bleed down the ventilator tubing into the lungs. However, maintaining tidal volumes and positive end-expiratory pressure may be more important in particular settings. The bag-valve device may result in decreased cardiac output and hypotension secondary to increased intrathoracic pressures.[6] The method of preoxygenation is left up to the physician.

Assemble and prepare the equipment. Set the pressure regulator to 60 to 80 mmHg for infants, 80 to 100 mmHg for children, and 100 to 120 mmHg for adolescents and adults. Higher pressures may cause injury to the tracheal mucosa. The suction catheter chosen should be approximately one-half the diameter of the tracheostomy tube. The catheter has an open valve that must be covered to apply suction through the tip of the catheter. If available, apply cardiac monitoring and pulse oximetry to the patient prior to suctioning.

TECHNIQUE
The procedure should be performed with aseptic technique. The physician should wash his or her hands and apply sterile gloves. The use of a face mask, eye protection, and a gown is highly recommended. The insertion of the suction catheter often induces the patient's cough reflex. Proper protective clothing will prevent the physician from being exposed to respiratory secretions.

Gently insert the suction catheter into the trachea (Figure 16-5). Advance it approximately 8 to 10 cm until the tip is at the level of the carina. **Suction pressure should never be applied during insertion of the suction catheter.** Withdraw the catheter approximately 2 to 3 cm and apply suction by placing a finger over the catheter's open valve.[10] Continue to apply suction as the catheter is simultaneously rotated and withdrawn. This technique will limit the amount of mucosal damage from the suction catheter. If the catheter is not being withdrawn when suction is applied, the mucosal surface will invaginate into the holes in the catheter tip. The re-

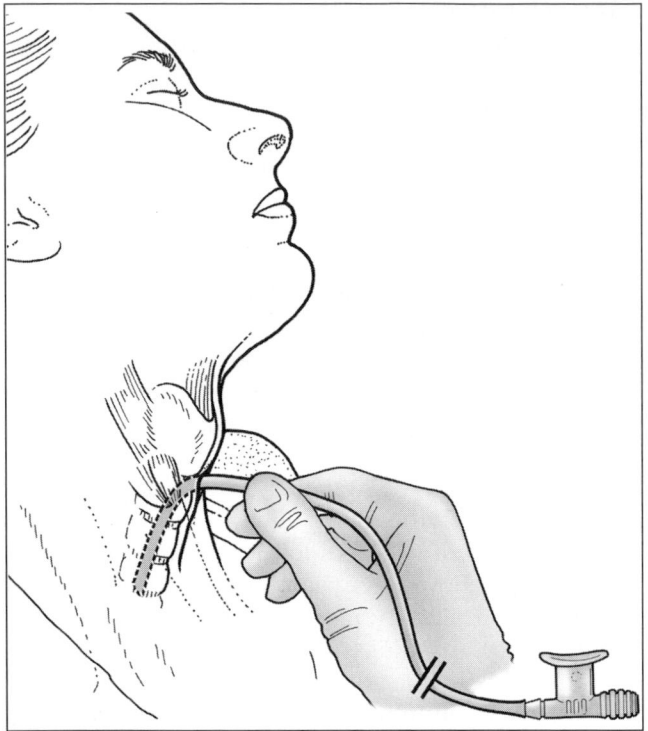

FIGURE 16-5 Insertion of a suction catheter. The vent is uncovered during insertion to prevent tracheal mucosal injury.

sulting trauma may cause bleeding or erosion of the tracheal mucosal surface.[7]

Suction the airway for no more than 10 to 15 seconds.[7] This will ensure that the patient experiences a minimal amount of hypoxia. If the suctioning must be repeated, preoxygenation with 100% oxygen must precede each suctioning episode.

The standard use of saline to loosen secretions is somewhat controversial. Some authors have suggested that saline is used to break up thick and tenacious sputum and mucus.[9] There is little support for this assertion. It has been shown that saline instillation increases the cough reflex and stimulates a cough response, which may increase mucus clearance. Others have noted that little saline is actually recovered with suctioning and that saline itself may cause a gradual decrease in oxygen saturation.[6] The instillation of saline into the tracheostomy cannot be recommended at this time.

EMERGENT CARE

When a patient with a tracheostomy presents to the Emergency Department complaining of shortness of breath or respiratory distress, he or she must receive immediate attention. Obstruction and hypoxia are frequent causes of morbidity in this patient population.

What follows is a discussion of the algorithm for airway obstruction and respiratory distress in the patient with a tracheostomy.[9]

EQUIPMENT
Protective clothing (disposable gowns, gloves, face shields, goggles, shoe covers)
Bag-valve device
Red rubber catheter
Flexible multieyed suction catheter, less than half the diameter of the inner cannula
Saline bullets
Continuous wall suction
Pressure regulator to maintain suction pressure
Continuous electrocardiographic (ECG) monitor
Pulse oximetry
Tracheostomy tubes of various sizes, at least the current size of the tube and one smaller
Water-soluble lubricant
Tracheal airway kit (hook, dilator, forceps)
Endotracheal tubes
Laryngoscope and blades
Access to advanced airway equipment, including a fiberoptic scope

PATIENT PREPARATION
The evaluation of any patient with a tracheostomy who is in respiratory distress begins with placing the patient in a room capable of advanced airway management. Place the patient on 100% oxygen and obtain intravenous access, cardiac monitoring, and continuous pulse oximetry. Equipment should be readily available and accessible. This includes endotracheal and tracheostomy tubes of various sizes as well as a laryngoscope and laryngoscope blades.

The practitioner must evaluate the type of tracheostomy tube present. Recognition of the type of tube will aid in the evaluation of possible complications and the management of the respiratory distress. For instance, if the tube has no inner cannula (pediatric tubes), the entire tracheostomy tube may have to be removed for further cleaning after suctioning is performed. If the tracheostomy tube has no cuff, the patient's respiratory distress may be due to aspiration of secretions or gastric contents.

TECHNIQUE
Inspect the tracheostomy tube for obvious signs of obstruction. The degree of obstruction will increase exponentially as the cross-sectional diameter of the tracheostomy tube decreases. As dried secretions, blood, or aspirated material gathers in the inner cannula, the amount of force required to create airflow through the tube increases dramatically. In addition, secretions may

act as a ball-valve mechanism, allowing air to move inward but not outward.

An obvious obstruction or foreign body, if visible at the tracheostomy tube opening, must be removed. The practitioner must then suction the patient through the inner cannula using the technique described above. Keep in mind the importance of preoxygenation. If this does not adequately relieve the patient's respiratory distress, remove the inner cannula. Inspect it for dried secretions and clean it later if necessary. The patient may again be suctioned, this time through the outer cannula. If no diminution of symptoms is noted, the outer cannula may need to be removed.

Before removing the outer cannula, it is important to have all the necessary equipment to replace it at the bedside. If the outer cannula has a cuff, deflate it. Remove the outer cannula with a smooth circular motion. Inspect it for a foreign body and dried secretions. The outer cannula may be cleaned then replaced or may be replaced with an entirely new tracheostomy tube. The practitioner may elect to use a fiberoptic scope or red rubber catheter to aid in tube placement. Each of these devices allows the tracheostomy tube to be placed over it and guided into the tracheal lumen.

If the tracheostomy is relatively new, less than 4 weeks old, it should be removed over a red rubber catheter (Figure 16-6). This will ensure that the tracheostomy tube is inserted into the trachea and not a false passage. Lubricate the red rubber catheter. Insert the catheter through the outer cannula and into the trachea (Figure 16-6A). Advance the catheter 8 or 9 centimeters. While holding the catheter securely, remove the outer cannula over the catheter (Figure 16-6B). Lubricate a new outer cannula. Insert the outer cannula over the catheter and advance it into the trachea (Figure 16-6C). Remove the catheter and insert the inner cannula into the outer cannula.

A suction catheter can be used as an alternative to a red rubber catheter. Attach the suction catheter to an oxygen source. Lubricate the end of the suction tubing. Advance an outer cannula over the distal end of the suction tubing. Insert the suction catheter into the tracheostomy to a depth of 8 or 9 centimeters. Place a finger over the open valve to provide oxygen to the patient through the catheter. This will prevent the patient from becoming hypoxemic during the procedure. Advance the outer cannula over the catheter and into the trachea. Remove the suction catheter and insert the inner cannula into the outer cannula.

If no assist device is used, the tracheostomy tube can be replaced manually (Figure 16-7). Lubricate the obturator and insert it into the outer cannula. Inflate the cuff and check its integrity. Deflate the cuff. Lubricate the outer cannula liberally. Place the tip of the obturator perpendicular to the neck and insert it with a semicircu-

lar motion (Figure 16-7A). Continue advancing the outer cannula with a semicircular motion as it curves into the trachea (Figure 16-7B). Remove the obturator and insert the inner cannula into the outer cannula. Begin ventilation of the patient if necessary.

If the new tracheostomy tube will not advance into the trachea, repeat the procedure with a tracheostomy tube one size smaller. **Do not force the tube, as this can create a false passage in the subcutaneous tissues of the neck.** If it still will not advance, attempt to insert an uncuffed tube. Alternatively, insert the tracheostomy tube over a catheter (Figure 16-8). Lubricate a red rubber catheter (or oxygen catheter) and insert it 8 or 9 cm through the tracheostomy (Figure 16-8A). Insert a lubricated outer cannula over the catheter and into the trachea (Figure 16-8B). Remove the catheter and insert the inner cannula. As a last resort, a tracheostomy hook and Trousseau dilator can be used to lift and open the tracheostomy site to allow the insertion of a tracheostomy tube.

ASSESSMENT

The adequacy of airway maneuvers in the patient with a tracheostomy resides in the patient's response to the interventions. If the patient's pulse oximetry and heart rate return to baseline and the patient appears more comfortable, secure the tracheostomy tube. Take care to ensure adequate skin care beneath the tracheostomy tube site.

If a patient remains in respiratory distress despite all appropriate actions, then further causes of respiratory distress must be evaluated. Obtain a chest radiograph. Consult a Pulmonologist for fiberoptic bronchoscopy to evaluate the patient for mucus plugging or foreign-body aspiration. Do not forget to consider other causes of respiratory distress in the patient with a tracheostomy. This includes but is not limited to pneumothorax, pneumonia, pulmonary embolus, cardiac failure, and myocardial infarction.

AFTERCARE

The patient should be observed for a few hours to ensure the stability of the airway. During this time, further suctioning can be performed as required. Educate the patient and family about preventive measures regarding tracheostomy care.

Once the patient's respiratory distress has been addressed, the patient should be evaluated for further conditions that may preclude him or her from being discharged. Were there just some dried secretions in the inner cannula? Does the patient have a new source of secretions (bacterial pneumonia) that could not be managed at home? Are the caregivers at home knowledgeable about the tracheostomy and trained to deal with

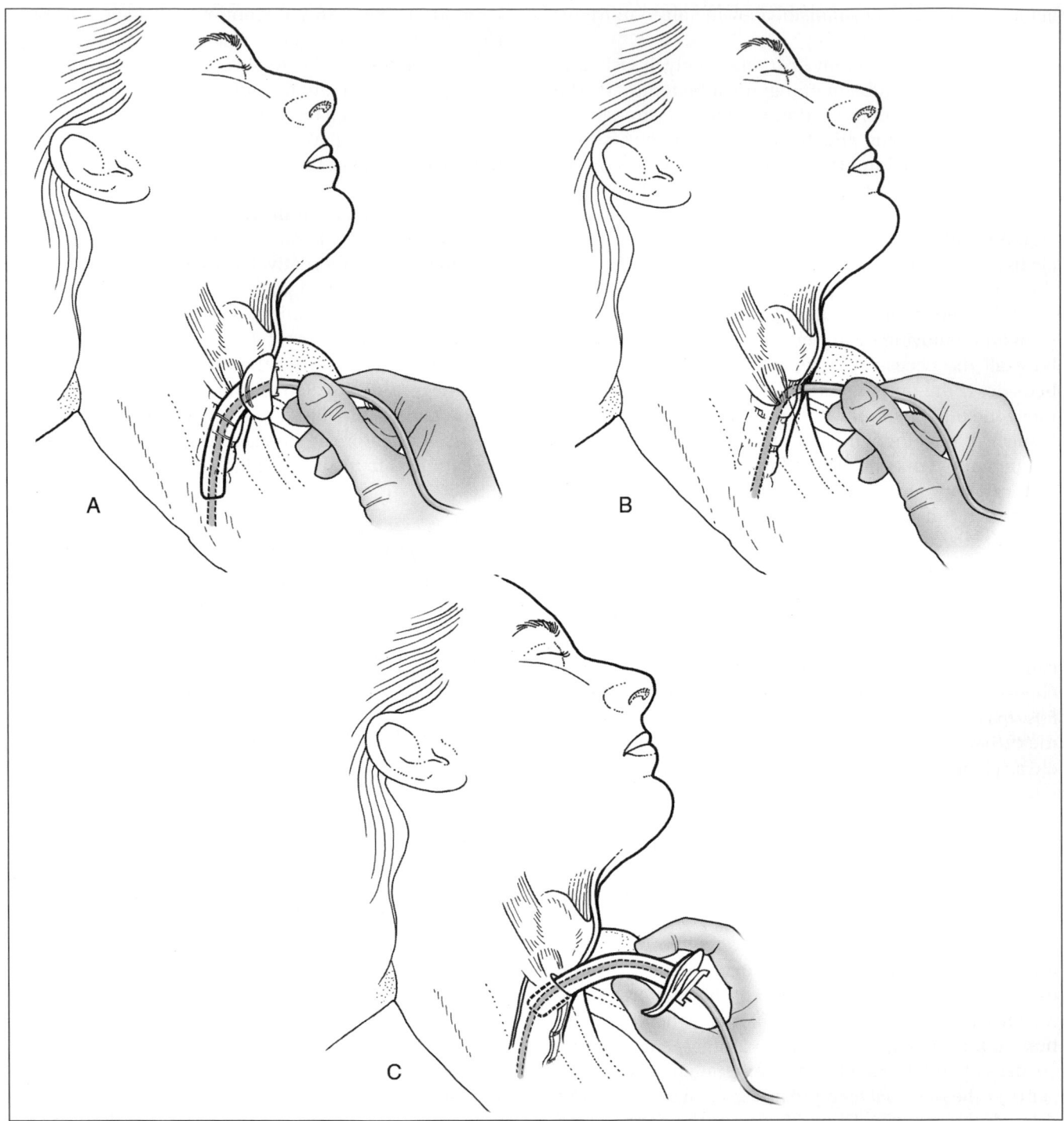

FIGURE 16-6 Removal of the outer cannula over a catheter. *A.* The catheter is inserted through the outer cannula to a depth of 8 to 9 centimeters. *B.* The outer cannula has been removed over the catheter. *C.* The new outer cannula is inserted over the catheter and into the trachea.

complications? If there is any question about the patient's ability to deal with further episodes of respiratory compromise, the patient should be admitted for further evaluation by an Otolaryngologist. The patient may require skilled home care or a skilled nursing facility in order to care for the tracheostomy fully.

COMPLICATIONS OF THE TRACHEOSTOMY

In addition to respiratory compromise from plugging of the tracheostomy with secretions, other complications may cause the patient to present to the Emergency

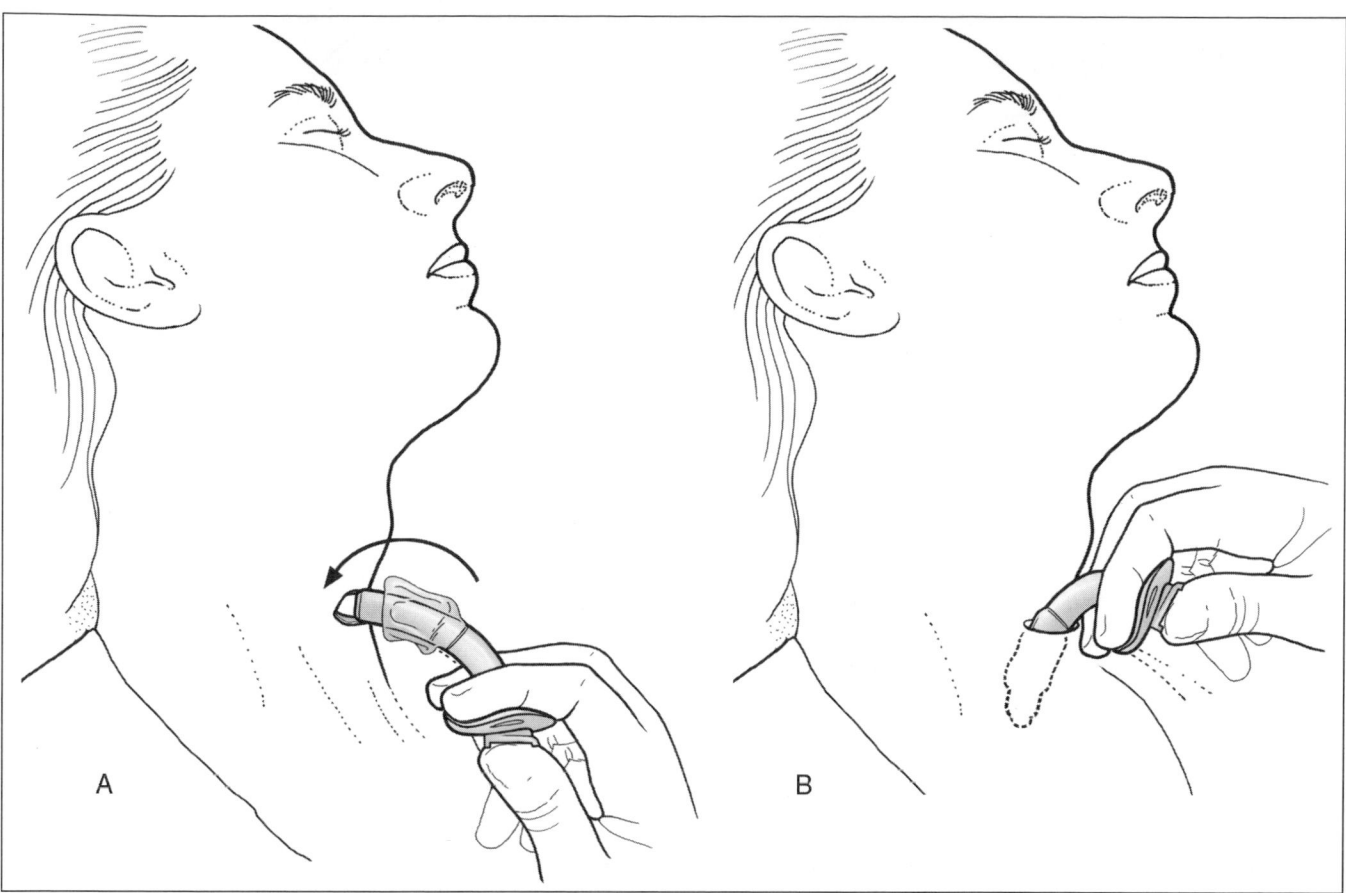

FIGURE 16-7 Manual insertion of a tracheostomy tube. *A.* It is positioned 90 degrees to the tracheostomy site and advanced with a semicircular motion (*arrow*). *B.* The system continues to be advanced, following the curve of the tube, until the flange is against the skin.

Department. One retrospective review over a 7-year period showed that 33 percent of patients presented with dislodged tracheal tubes, 30 percent presented with infection (one-quarter of these had cellulitis around the tracheostomy, the rest had bronchitis or pneumonia), 18 percent had plugged tracheal tubes, 11 percent had bleeding, 5 percent had tracheal or stomal stenosis, and 3 percent had a pneumothorax.[2]

Bleeding is a significant concern in the patient with a tracheostomy. While bleeding at the site of a recent tracheostomy may be a frequent complication, it may also be extremely serious. Bleeding can arise from granulation tissue, venous sources, or arterial sources including the great vessels. Tracheoinnominate fistulas are quite rare, occurring in less than 2 percent of cases, but they carry a mortality rate of 25 to 50 percent.[9] They may present as the classic "exsanguinating bleed" but often present with a less impressive sentinel bleed. Any bleeding of more than a few milliliters of blood should raise concern for a possible fistula of the innominate artery. Prompt critical resuscitation measures and emergent consultation with a Vascular Surgeon and Otolaryngologic Surgeon is required. Techniques for controlling bleeding from the innominate artery include local digital pressure, hyperinflation of the tracheostomy tube cuff, and traction on the tracheostomy tube. **When bleeding occurs, the tracheostomy tube should not be removed until the airway is secured by another means.**

Pneumothoraces and subcutaneous air occur in a small number of patients.[9] Pediatric patients are at a higher risk, as the dome of the pleura in a child is closer to the site of the operation. As patients "fight" a ventilator or attempt to inspire against an obstructed airway, they generate tremendous negative inspiratory pressures. This can result in the dissection of air between the tissue planes and into the thoracic cavity, causing a pneumothorax. The possibility of a tension pneumothorax must always be considered in patients with tracheostomies and respiratory distress or hypotension.

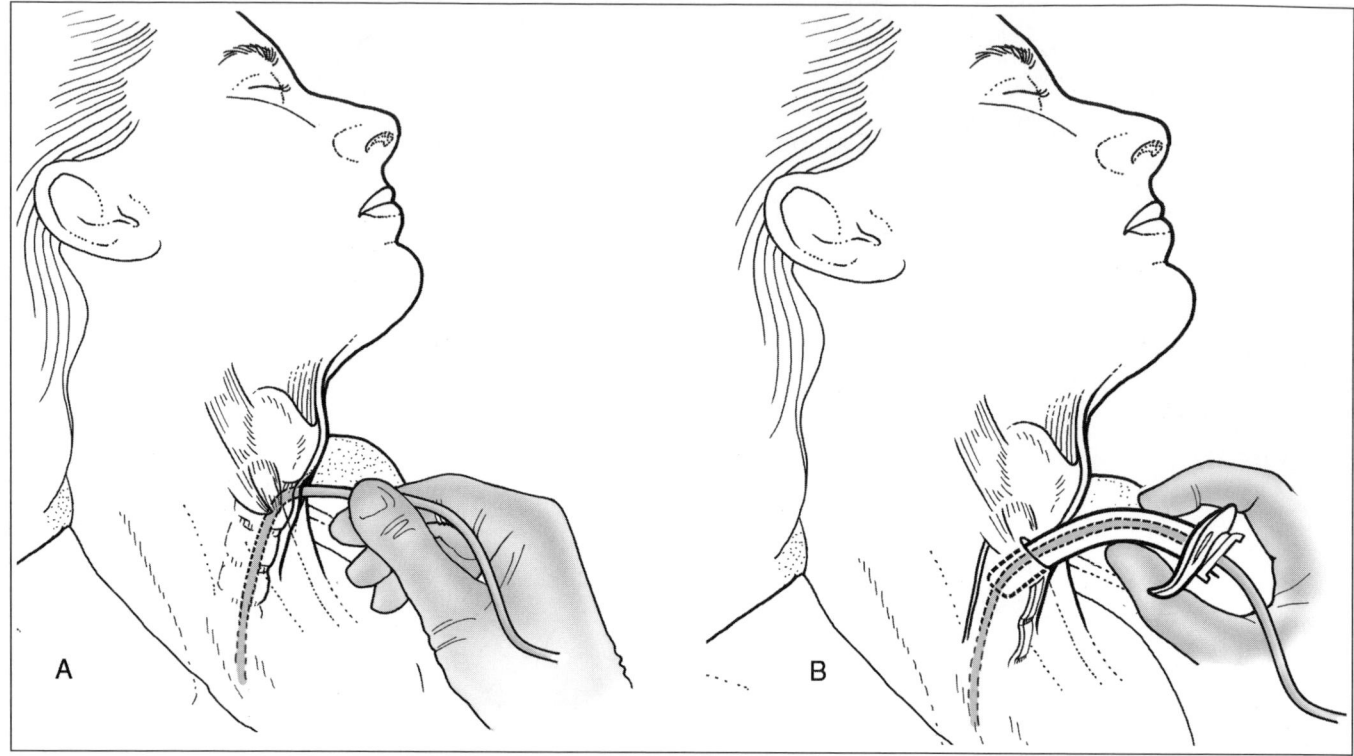

FIGURE 16-8 Insertion of the tracheostomy tube over a catheter. *A.* Insert the catheter through the tracheostomy to a depth of 8 to 9 centimeters. *B.* Advance the outer cannula over the catheter.

SUMMARY

Clinicians should be familiar with tracheostomy equipment and its management. Patients presenting to an Emergency Department may require immediate and critical intervention to resuscitate them. Familiarity with various techniques to evaluate the patient with a tracheostomy should include tracheal suctioning, removal of inner and outer cannulas, replacement of a tracheostomy tube, and evaluation for other emergent conditions relating to tracheostomies. This would include bleeding, infection, and pneumothorax at the very minimum. In addition, the clinician should be mindful of other conditions of the esophagus, trachea, or soft tissues that might complicate the care of the patient with a tracheostomy. The ultimate goal is to provide the patient with adequate oxygenation and ventilation.

REFERENCES

1. Chew JY, Cantrell RW: Tracheostomy. Complications and their management. *Arch Otolaryngol* 1972; 96(6):538–545.
2. Hackeling T, Triana R, Ma OJ, et al: Emergency care of patients with tracheostomies: a 7-year review. *Am J Emerg Med* 1998; 16(7):681–685.
3. Jackson C: Tracheotomy. *Laryngoscope* 1909; 19:285–290.
4. Quigley RL: Tracheostomy—an overview. Management and complications. *Br J Clin Pract* 1988; 42(10):430–434.
5. Fowler S, Knapp-Spooner C, Donohue D: The ABC's of tracheostomy care. *J Pract Nurs* 1995; 45(1):44–48.
6. Clarke L: A critical event in tracheostomy care. *Br J Nurs* 1995; 4(12):676–681.
7. Buglass E: Tracheostomy care: tracheal suctioning and humidification. *Br J Nurs* 1999; 8(8):500–504.
8. Shim C, Fine N, Fernandez R, Williams MH Jr: Cardiac arrhythmias resulting from tracheal suctioning. *Ann Intern Med* 71(6):1149–1153.
9. Tayal VS: Tracheostomies. *Emerg Med Clin North Am* 1994; 12(3):707–727.
10. Mapp CS: Trach care: are you aware of all the dangers? *Nursing* 1988; 18(7):34–43.
11. Young CS: A review of the adverse effects of airway suction. *Physiotherapy* 1984; 70(3):104–108.
12. Weissler MC: Tracheotomy and intubation, in Bailey BJ (ed): *Head and Neck Surgery—Otolaryngology.* Philadelphia: Lippincott, 1993:711–717.

Chapter 17
LARYNGEAL MASK AIRWAYS

Steve L. Meeks
Kenneth D. Candido

INTRODUCTION

The laryngeal mask airway (LMA) is a novel device that fills the gap in airway management between that of endotracheal intubation and the use of a face mask. It was introduced in the United Kingdom in 1983 by British anesthesiologist A. I. J. Brain. His goal was to develop an airway apparatus that could rapidly overcome an obstructed airway, is simple to use, and is atraumatic to insert. In 1991, the LMA was approved for use in the United States by the U.S. Food and Drug Administration.

The LMA was designed primarily as a means of providing ventilatory support while avoiding the fundamental disadvantage of the need to visualize and penetrate the vocal cords with an endotracheal tube.[1] The LMA is introduced into the hypopharynx without visual control. It forms a low-pressure seal around the laryngeal inlet and permits positive-pressure ventilation. In fact, with the introduction of the new LMA Proseal, pressures of up to 30 cmH$_2$O may be administered safely (A. I. Brain, M.D., personal communication). Once inserted, the LMA may be used as a conduit for fiberoptically guided endotracheal intubation or to place an endotracheal tube blindly.[2] Since it was initially described, the LMA has come to be viewed as a viable method of airway management, with over 800 articles and case reports describing the advantages and disadvantages of the device.[3]

Many disadvantages of the standard LMA became apparent with widespread use of the device. More than 10 years after its introduction, Brain et al began to work on a new airway system with better intubation characteristics than the standard LMA. The intubating laryngeal mask airway (ILMA) was developed through the aid of analysis of magnetic resonance images of the human pharynx and laboratory testing of endotracheal tubes.[4] The new and more "anatomically correct" ILMA effects more precise placement. The design of the ILMA also avoids head and neck manipulation and insertion of the intubator's fingers in the patient's mouth, both of which occur during the placement of the standard LMA.[4,5]

There are currently five models of the LMA. The LMA-Classic is the original and most commonly used version. It is the model referred to in this chapter as the LMA. The LMA-Flexible is a wire-reinforced version of the LMA that is more flexible than the original version and resists kinking. It is used by Anesthesiologists for patients undergoing head and neck procedures. It is not used in the Emergency Department. The LMA-Fastrach is a modified version of the LMA that allows endotracheal intubation through the unit. It is also referred to as the intubating laryngeal mask airway (ILMA). It allows ventilation during intubation attempts. Its advantages include the following: no manipulation of the head and neck is required, it can accommodate up to a size 8 endotracheal tube, it facilitates one-handed insertion, it can be inserted from the patient's side or from above the head, and it can be used in conjunction with fiberoptic intubation. The LMA-Proseal is the latest version. It features a cuff deflator, modified cuff design, dual tubes, and a bite block.

Given that either the standard LMA or the ILMA may be available in the Emergency Department, the techniques for inserting both of these devices are discussed in this chapter. The anatomic differences between the two devices produce subtle differences in their insertion methods. The indications, contraindications, assessment, and complications associated with the LMA and ILMA are largely identical.

ANATOMY AND PATHOPHYSIOLOGY

The anatomy of the airway is briefly reviewed below (Figure 17-1). The oral cavity is bounded by the hard and soft palate above and the anterior portion of the tongue and the reflection of its mucosa onto the floor of the mouth below. Posteriorly, the mouth opens into the oropharynx through the oropharyngeal isthmus. The pharynx is a U-shaped tube extending from the base of the skull to the level of the cricoid cartilage, at which point it becomes continuous with the esophagus.[6] The larynx extends from its oblique opening bordered by the aryepiglottic folds, the tip of the epiglottis, and the posterior commisure to the base of the cricoid cartilage.[6] The esophagus lies posterior to the airway. When inflated and properly positioned, the tip of the device will lie in the esophagus at the level of the upper esophageal sphincter and directly posterior to the cricoid cartilage (Figure 17-2).

INDICATIONS

The indications for the use of the LMA and the ILMA parallel the general indications for active airway management. These include the correction of hypoxemia or hypercarbia, the provision of controlled hyperventilation, the provision of a secure airway in the presence of obstruction, and the provision of airway access for pulmonary hygiene and bronchoscopy. For those patients presenting to an Emergency Department who require airway management, the LMA and the ILMA may aid in supporting airways that are difficult to manage as well as being an invaluable aid to blind and fiberoptic intubation. Since the success rate in inexperienced hands approaches 90 percent, the device is superbly suited for use by medical personnel who have had only a minimum of training in airway management.[7]

Airway control also facilitates emergent radiographic investigations [e.g., computed tomography (CT) or mag-

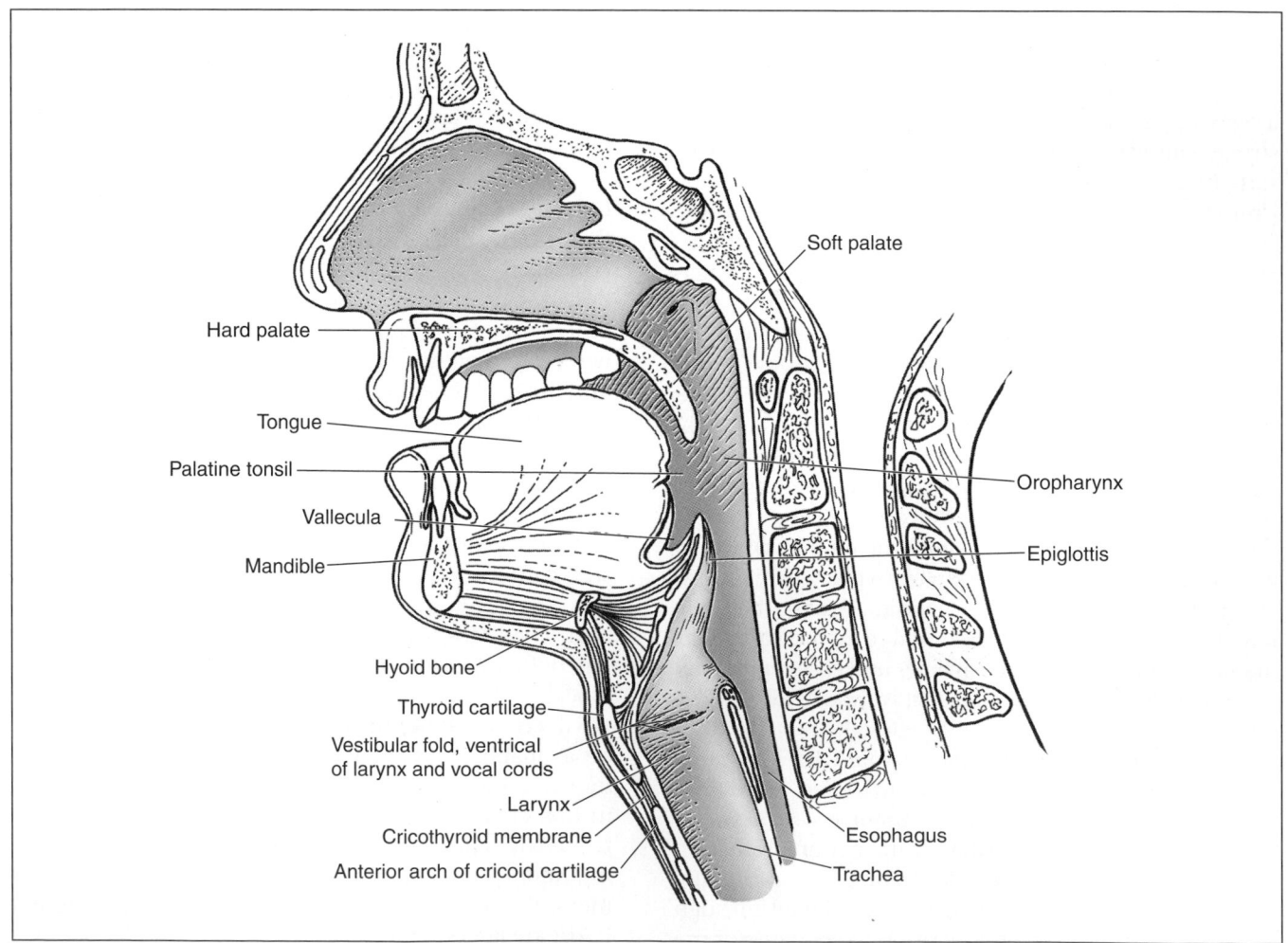

FIGURE 17-1 Midsagittal section of the head and neck demonstrating the airway.

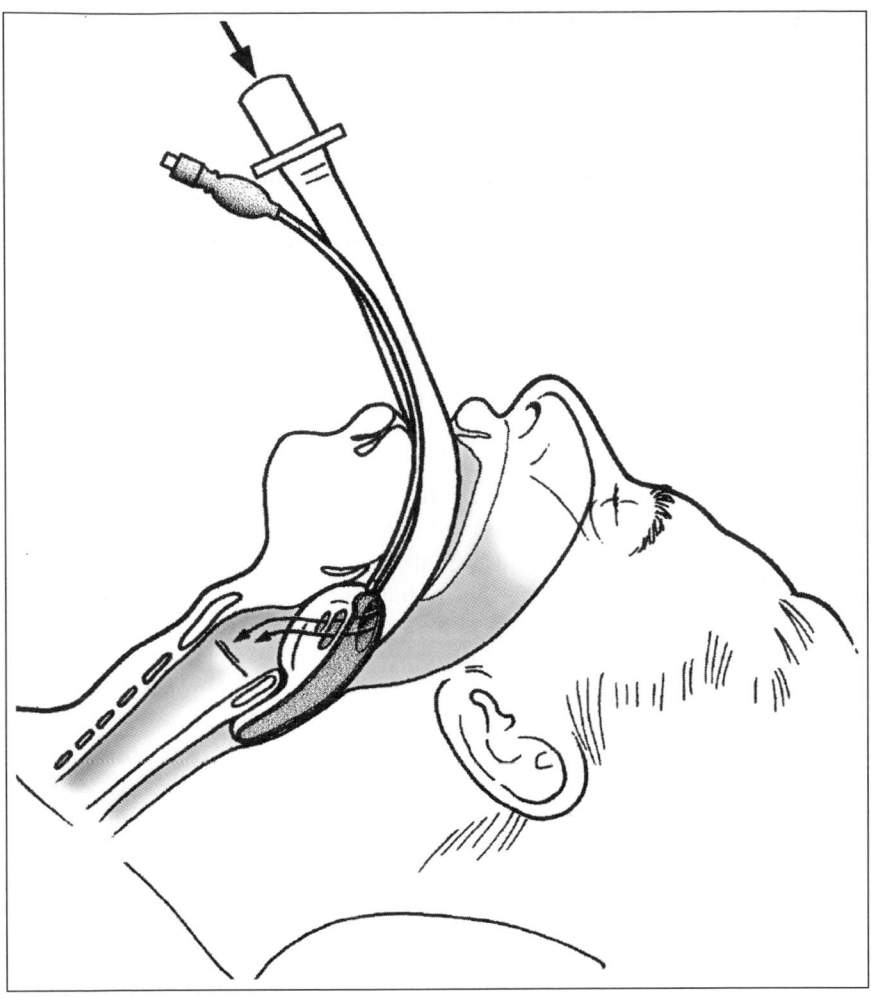

FIGURE 17-2 Sagittal view of the airway demonstrating correct placement of the laryngeal mask airway.

netic resonance imaging (MRI) scans] without motion artifact.[6] The standard LMA contains no ferromagnetic components and is a suitable alternative to an endotracheal tube in many situations. It is ideal for use in patients emergently requiring diagnostic MRI scans. Use of the LMA does not require a metal laryngoscope, which is contraindicated if a patient requires airway management in the MRI suite.

Either the LMA or the ILMA may be used in the event of failed endotracheal intubation. They have a role in securing the airway preemptively in patients with an "anteriorly" situated larynx, a situation whereby direct laryngoscopy and endotracheal intubation are historically difficult. In emergent situations, the LMA is a safe alternative to the esophageal obturator airway, which it has largely supplanted in clinical use. The LMA has also proved to be useful in burn patients requiring repeated dressing changes, especially of the face. Finally, the LMA may well be the airway technique of choice for professional singers who require short-term airway management, since there is less likelihood of causing vocal cord or laryngeal nerve injury with this approach.[7]

However, in all its uses, there is a conspicuous absence of airway protection from aspiration. The newest prototype, the LMA Proseal, is being marketed as having addressed these limitations and includes an improved laryngeal seal (for permitting positive-pressure ventilation at pressures up to 30 cmH_2O) and a drain tube in tandem with the airway tube. The drain tube facilitates blind insertion of a gastric tube for decompressing the stomach. An introducer aids insertion of Proseal while obviating the need to introduce the operator's fingers into the mouth.

CONTRAINDICATIONS

There are no absolute contraindications to the use of the LMA or the ILMA. However, there are several relative contraindications. These devices should not be used in individuals who are at an increased risk of regurgitation or aspiration unless other techniques for securing the airway have failed. This is supported by uncontrolled studies using fiberoptic bronchoscopy, which have shown that the esophagus is visible within the LMA mask in 6 to 9 percent of patients.[7] Patients at high risk for aspiration include those with previous upper gastrointestinal surgery, known or symptomatic hiatal hernia, gastroesophageal reflux disease, women more than 10 weeks pregnant, patients with intestinal ileus or peptic ulcer disease, obese patients, or those individuals who are not fasted.[5,8,9]

These devices should not be used in individuals with severe respiratory diseases.[2,8,9] Specifically, individuals with airway obstruction at or below the larynx and those with low pulmonary compliance or high airway resistance (morbid obesity, bronchospasm, pulmonary edema, pulmonary fibrosis, or thoracic trauma) are not appropriate candidates for the LMA or ILMA.

Patients must be able to assume the "sniffing" position, analogous to that of individuals positioned for direct laryngoscopy prior to endotracheal intubation. If they cannot extend their head and flex their neck (passively or actively), they should not be considered as candidates for the LMA. The ILMA is more appropriate in these patients. If patients cannot open their mouth at least 1.5 cm due to anatomic limitations (ankylosing spondylitis, severe rheumatoid arthritis, cervical spine instability, etc.), they should not receive these devices.[7] This is one situation where blind nasotracheal intubation or fiberoptically guided nasotracheal tube placement has an advantage over the LMAs.

In emergent situations where cricoid pressure is needed to prevent active or passive regurgitation of stomach contents prior to airway placement, the LMA is not an appropriate airway choice. It will not prevent subsequent aspiration of stomach contents as efficiently as will a cuffed endotracheal tube. The act of placing an LMA after the application of cricoid pressure (Sellick maneuver) has been shown to have a significantly high failure rate.[7] The newly developed LMA Proseal, which features dual tubes (airway and drain) as well as a modified cuff designed to provide separation of the respiratory and alimentary tracts, may prove invaluable in negating this "Achilles' heel" of the standard LMA.

Finally, the LMA is relatively contraindicated in cases of pharyngeal pathology. This includes but is not limited to abscesses, hematomas, and tissue disruptions. These processes make the use of the LMA difficult. Additionally, the device may rupture abscesses and hematomas, causing the patient to aspirate.

EQUIPMENT

LMA, various sizes
ILMA, various sizes
Endotracheal tubes
Water-soluble lubricant or anesthetic jelly
Syringes, 10 and 20 mL
Oxygen source, tubing, and regulator
Face mask
Pulse oximeter
Cardiac monitor
Noninvasive blood pressure monitor
Advanced Cardiac Life Support (ACLS) medications
Access to advanced airway equipment

THE LMA

The standard LMA preceded the ILMA by more than a decade. The prototype of the LMA was constructed by forming a shallow mask with an inflatable rubber cuff joined to a tube communicating with the lumen of the mask at an angle.[1,2] The modern LMA is made of flexible silicone, is completely latex-free, and has a more tapered appearance (Figure 17-3). It has a variably sized, internally ridged tube fused at a 30 degree angle to a spoon-shaped mask with a flexible rim.

The LMA is a disposable unit that can be used multiple times. It must be sterilized between uses, following specific recommendations provided by the manufacturer. It is designed to conform to the contours of the hypopharynx, with its lumen facing the glottic opening (Figure 17-2). It consists of an airway tube, inflation line, and mask (Figure 17-3). Overall, it looks like a giant spoon.

The airway tube has a large bore and is clear, like an endotracheal tube.[2] The proximal end contains a standard 15 mm airway adapter that can connect to a bag-valve device or a ventilator. A black line along the posterior border is used as a marker for proper positioning. The distal end of the airway tube connects to the mask.

The mask is elliptical in shape (Figure 17-4). The outer rim of the mask contains an inflatable cuff. When inflated and properly positioned, the tip of the LMA will lie in the esophagus at the level of the upper esophageal sphincter and directly posterior to the cricoid cartilage

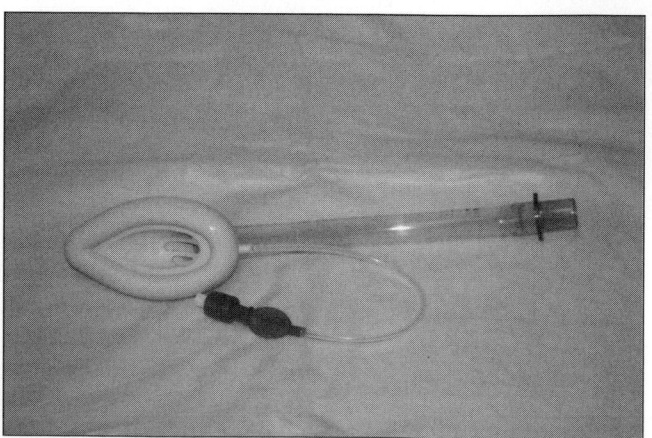

FIGURE 17-3 The laryngeal mask airway.

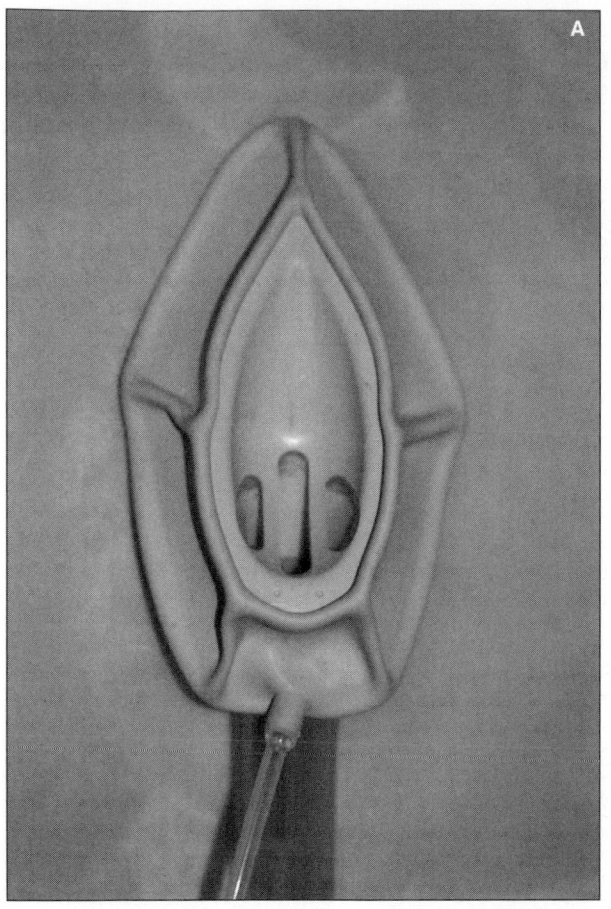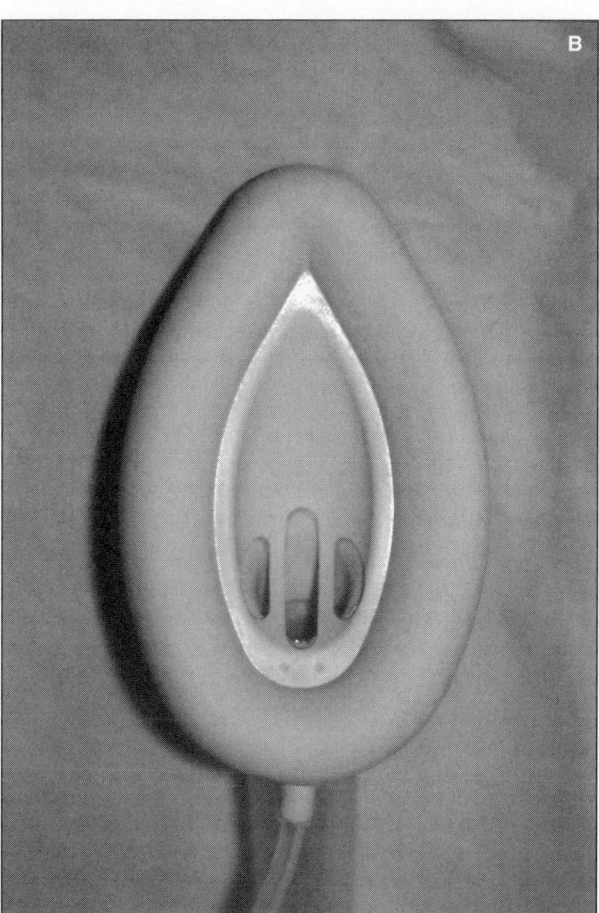

FIGURE 17-4 The distal end or mask of the laryngeal mask airway. *A.* The cuff in the deflated state. *B.* The cuff in the inflated state.

(Figure 17-2). The lateral edges of the mask rest in the pyriform fossae. The upper edge rests against the base of the tongue. The LMA provides a seal against the upper esophageal sphincter, aryepiglottic folds, and distal epiglottis so as to direct air into the trachea and avoid insufflation of the stomach[2,3] (Figure 17-2).

The distal end of the airway tube opens into the mask. This opening is covered by two vertical aperture bars (Figure 17-4) that prevent the epiglottis from obstructing the lumen of the airway tube. The aperture bars should be cut off prior to inserting the LMA if an endotracheal tube is to be inserted through the LMA.

The inflation line is used to inflate and deflate the cuff (Figure 17-4). The distal end of the inflation line attaches to the upper border of the cuff. The proximal end contains an inflation port and balloon, similar to an endotracheal tube. An air-filled syringe attaches to the inflation port to inflate the cuff.

The correct size of the LMA is based upon the weight of the patient (Table 17-1).[2] The distal end assumes a different shape when the cuff is inflated and deflated (Figure 17-4). When deflated, the distal end is pentagon-shaped (Figure 17-4A). When inflated, it is oval-shaped (Figure 17-4B).

THE ILMA

The form of the ILMA (Figure 17-5) was derived from head and neck sagittal MRI studies in 50 normal subjects whose heads were held in a neutral position. The convex radius of the curve of the silicone-covered steel tube represents a value close to the best-fit curve derived from the MRI studies.[4] The new prototype consists of an anatomically curved steel tube connected to the standard LMA cuff sizes 3, 4, and 5.[5,8]

The ILMA has several significant modifications that make it different from the LMA (Figure 17-5). The airway tube is stainless steel covered with silicone rubber. The proximal end has a handle fused to the airway tube to facilitate insertion, manipulation, and removal of the ILMA. It is curved to follow the curve of the hypopharynx and position the mask aperture over the glottic aperture. It has a larger inner diameter (13 mm versus 9 mm) than the LMA.[8] This allows the ILMA to accommodate a cuffed endotracheal tube with an inner diameter up to

TABLE 17-1. LARYNGEAL MASK AIRWAY (LMA) SIZE SELECTION

Patient's weight (kg)	LMA size	Maximum cuff inflation volume (mL)	Largest endotracheal tube size*	Fiberoptic bronchoscope size (mm)
< 5	1.0	4	3.5	2.7
5–10	1.5	7	4.0	3.0
10–20	2.0	10	4.5	3.5
20–30	2.5	14	5.0	4.0
30–50	3.0	20	6.0 (cuffed)	5.0
50–70	4.0	30	6.0 (cuffed)	5.0
70–100	5.0	40	7.0 (cuffed)	5.0
> 100	6.0	50	7.0 (cuffed)	5.0

*The inner diameter in millimeters.

9.0 mm[5,10] (Figure 17-6). It is significantly shorter (14.5 versus 20 cm) than the LMA.[8]

The mask of the ILMA is similar to that of the LMA with two major modifications. In the ILMA, there is a ramp inside the distal away tube as it meets the mask that continues into the mask aperture. It is designed to direct the endotracheal tube into the center of the aperture and into the patient's airway. It has a large, single, stiff epiglottic elevating bar (EEB) vertically oriented over the mask aperture (Figures 17-5B and 17-6). The EEB is designed to lift the epiglottis away from the path of the advancing endotracheal tube.

The ILMA was designed to be used with a wire-reinforced cuffed silicone endotracheal tube, with an 8.0 mm inner diameter[5] (Figure 17-7). It has a transverse block line along its posterior surface, which serves as a marker to let the intubator know when the tip of the endotracheal tube is positioned at the epiglottic elevating

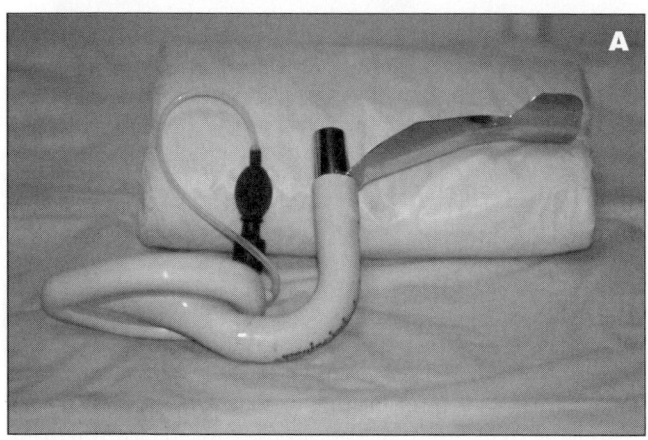

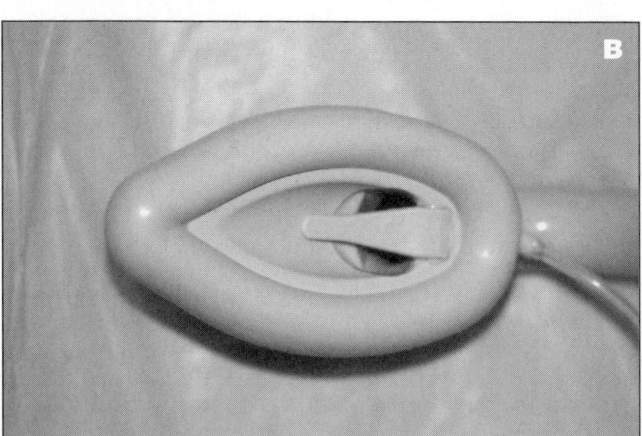

FIGURE 17-5 The intubating laryngeal mask airway. *A.* Overall view of the device. *B.* The mask.

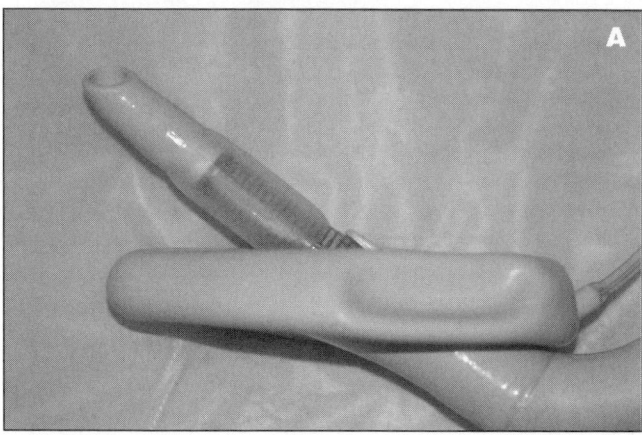

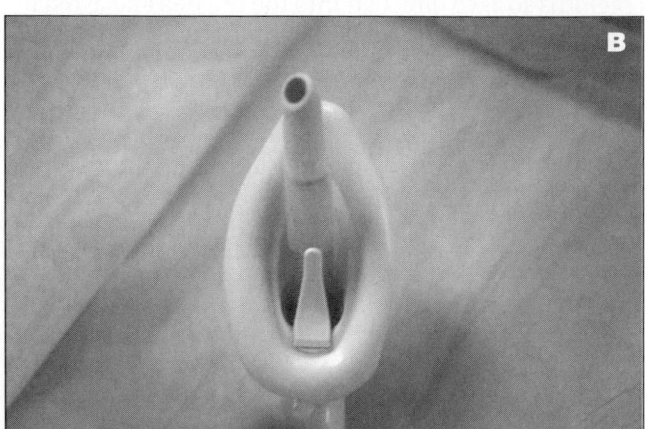

FIGURE 17-6 An endotracheal tube is inserted through the intubating laryngeal mask airway. The tip of the endotracheal tube is guided by the V-shaped epiglottic elevator bar. *A.* Lateral view. *B.* View of the mask.

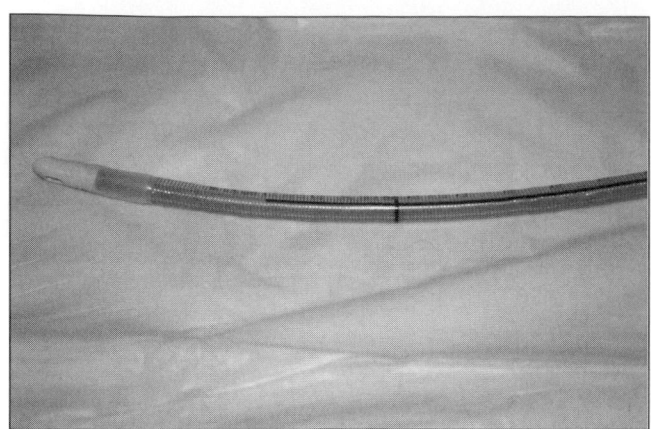

FIGURE 17-7 Prototype of the silicone endotracheal tube used with the intubating laryngeal mask airway.

bar. This occurs when the endotracheal tube is inserted through the ILMA and the transverse bar is located at the proximal end of the airway tube. While it is ideal to use the wire-reinforced silicone endotracheal tube, a standard endotracheal tube may also be used with the ILMA.

PATIENT PREPARATION

The patient should be appropriately monitored with electrocardiography (ECG), end-tidal CO_2 monitoring, and pulse oximetry. The patient preparation is exactly the same as that for orotracheal intubation. See Chapter 5 for the full details. As for any situation where airway manipulation is to occur and the patient's protective airway reflexes are blunted or ablated, a fully functioning suction apparatus with a variety of catheters must be immediately available. Insertion of the LMA requires an anesthetic depth similar to that which allows placement and acceptance of an oropharyngeal airway.[7] Successful placement of the standard LMA is much more likely if the patient is premedicated. In the case of the ILMA, the successful placement of the endotracheal tube is highly dependent on adequate sedation and/or muscle relaxation. The optimal induction agent should produce jaw relaxation and attenuation of airway reflexes, permitting insertion of the LMA or the ILMA within 30 to 60 seconds of loss of consciousness. A variety of induction agents may be used. Refer to Chapters 3 and 4 for complete details.

There is some controversy as to what physical examination findings represent the endpoint for judging when to insert the LMA or ILMA. The consensus is that the first attempt at insertion should occur following the loss of the eyelash reflex (seventh cranial nerve) and when the jaw is relaxed.[9,11] This typically occurs 30 to 60 seconds after administration of the ultra-short-acting induction agents. Some practitioners also rely on the onset of ap-

nea and/or loss of response to verbal stimuli as signs of adequate depth of anesthesia.[11]

TECHNIQUES

LARYNGEAL MASK AIRWAY

Prior to insertion, carefully inspect the cuff for leaks with the cuff slightly overinflated. Completely deflate the cuff. The newest LMA, the LMA-Proseal, features a cuff deflator, which is a compact, portable instrument for assuring complete removal of air without causing the silicone to wrinkle.

The technique for inserting the LMA is rather simple (Figure 17-8). Lubricate the posterior surface of the LMA with a water-soluble lubricant. Care must be taken to avoid lubricating the anterior surface of the device, as the gel might obstruct the distal aperture or trickle into the larynx, provoking laryngospasm.[7] Position the patient's head as for endotracheal intubation in the sniffing position. Place the nondominant hand behind the patient's head to stabilize the occiput and slightly flex the neck (Figure 17-8*A*). Allow the patient's jaw to fall open. An assistant may be required to help open it. A topical local anesthetic or spray, such as benzocaine (Hurricaine Spray, Beutlich Pharmaceuticals, Waukegan, IL), may permit insertion in the awake patient.

Insert the LMA into the oral cavity with the aperture facing but not touching the tongue (Figure 17-8*A*). It is essential that the leading edge of the cuff be smooth, wrinkle-free, and shaped like a wedge. This facilitates passage of the cuff around the posterior pharyngeal curvature and into the hypopharynx while avoiding the epiglottis. Place the index and middle fingers of the dominant hand against the junction between the LMA tube and the cuff (Figure 17-8*B*). Advance the LMA in one smooth movement following the curvature of the pharynx until it enters the hypopharynx (Figure 17-8*B*). The fingers should lie almost horizontally when the LMA is properly positioned.[12,13] Grasp and stabilize the airway tube with the nondominant hand, then remove the index and middle fingers of the intubating hand (Figure 17-8*C*). **Slightly advance the LMA further downward until resistance is felt. At this point, it is important not to push further.** If difficulty is encountered, a rotational movement of the tube, slight inflation of the cuff, a jaw-thrust maneuver, or, in rare cases, the use of a laryngoscope may be helpful.[7]

Inflate the cuff with the recommended volume of air (Figure 17-8*D*). **Do not overinflate the cuff. Inflation usually causes a characteristic outward movement of the airway tube of up to 1.5 cm as the cuff centers itself around the laryngeal inlet.** A slight forward movement of both the thyroid and cricoid cartilages will be noted. **The longitudinal black line on the shaft of the tube**

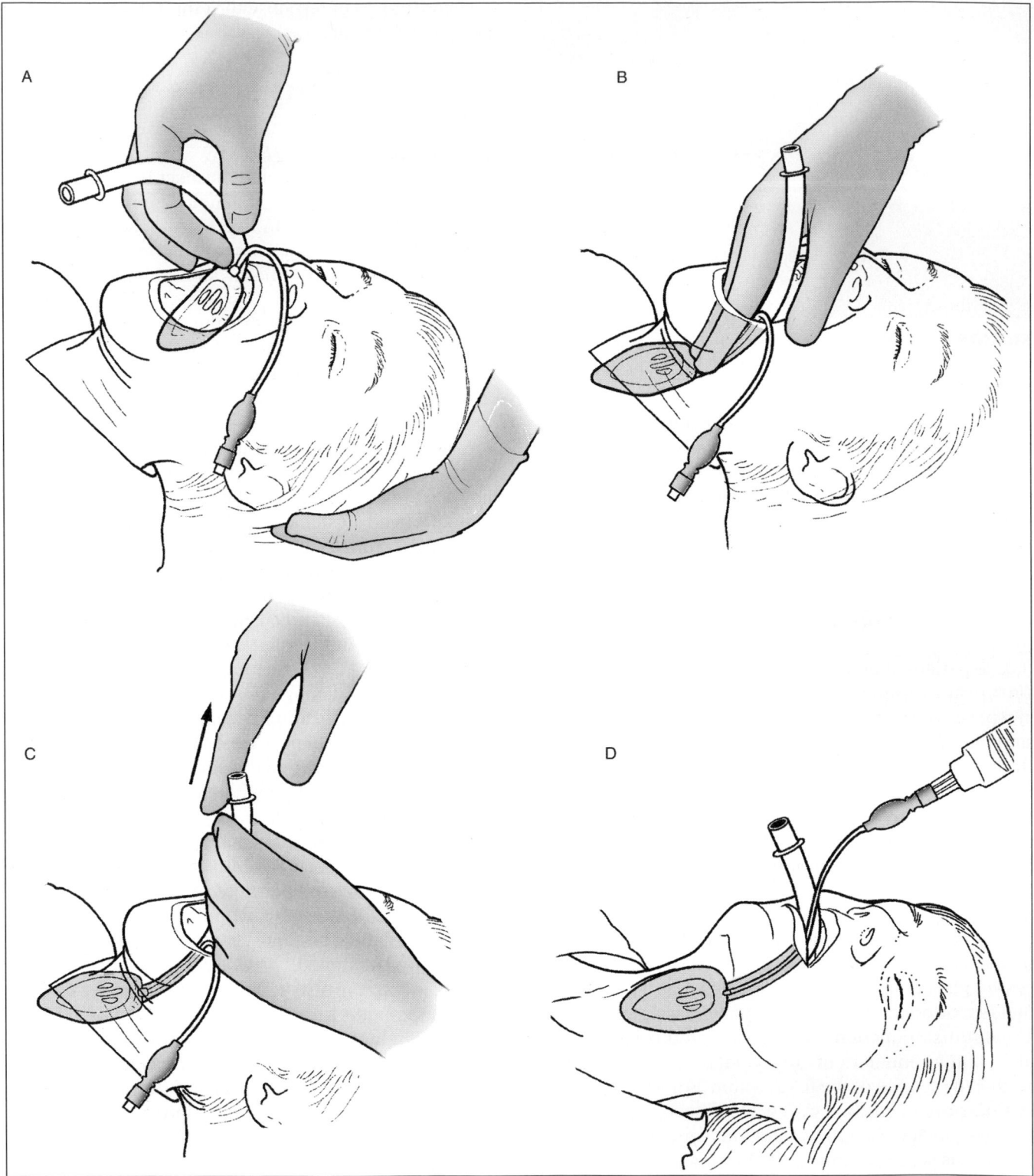

FIGURE 17-8 Insertion of the laryngeal mask airway. *A.* The patient's head is properly positioned and the LMA is inserted into the patient's mouth. *B.* The LMA is advanced with two fingers. *C.* The LMA is stabilized while the insertion hand is removed. *D.* The cuff is inflated.

should lie in the midline against the upper lip. Any deviation may indicate misplacement of the cuff and partial airway obstruction.[7] When correctly positioned, the tip of the LMA cuff lies at the base of the hypopharynx against the upper esophageal sphincter, the sides lie in the pyriform fossae, and the upper border of the mask lies at the base of the tongue, pushing it forward.[7] Even when grossly malpositioned, the mask may still create a useful airway. This is one characteristic that clearly distinguishes the LMA from both the endotracheal tube and the oropharyngeal airway. Secure the LMA with tape, like an endotracheal tube. A commercially available endotracheal tube holder may also be used to secure the LMA.

INTUBATING LARYNGEAL MASK AIRWAY

The technique for inserting the ILMA is not very different from that for the standard LMA (Figure 17-9). It involves a one-handed rotational movement in the sagittal plane with the patient's head supported to achieve a neutral position.[5] The ILMA may be inserted from above the patient's head (like the LMA) or standing to the side of the patient's head. It may be inserted with the right or left hand.

Prior to insertion, slightly overinflate the cuff and check it for leaks. Completely deflate the cuff. Lubricate the posterior surface of the airway tube and the mask liberally. Grasp the ILMA by its handle. Place the patient in the sniffing position if no contraindications exist. Open the patient's mouth with the nondominant hand. Position the ILMA over the patient with the tip of the mask in the patient's mouth (Figure 17-9A). Slowly insert the mask while the posterior aspect of the mask maintains constant contact with the hard palate. When the entire mask is inside the patient's mouth and against the hard palate, rotate the ILMA inward along the natural curve of the hard palate and pharynx (Figure 17-9B). The airway tube should maintain constant contact with the upper central incisors as the unit is advanced. Stop advancing the unit when resistance is felt. This signifies that the tip of the mask is in the upper esophagus (Figure 17-9B).

Inflate the cuff with the recommended volume of air (Figure 17-9C). **Inflation usually causes a characteristic outward movement of the airway tube, up to 1.5 cm, as the cuff centers itself around the laryngeal inlet.** A slight forward movement of the thyroid and cricoid cartilages will be noted. The airway tube should lie in the midline against the upper central incisors. Any deviation may indicate misplacement of the cuff and partial airway obstruction. When correctly positioned, the tip of the ILMA cuff lies at the base of the hypopharynx against the upper esophageal sphincter, the sides lie in the pyriform fossae, and the upper border lies at the base of the tongue, pushing it forward.

Confirm proper placement of the ILMA. Have an assistant attach a bag-valve device to the proximal end of the airway tube and ventilate the patient. Observe the upper chest rise, auscultate bilateral breath sounds, and observe end-tidal CO_2 monitoring to confirm proper placement. An anterior movement, or bulging, of the cricoid and thyroid cartilages during or after cuff inflation also indicates correct positioning of the ILMA.[1]

Insert an endotracheal tube. Lubricate the wire-reinforced silicone endotracheal tube (or standard endotracheal tube) liberally. Insert the silicone tube into the ILMA until the transverse black line on its posterior surface is at the proximal end of the airway tube (Figure 17-9D). At this point, the tip of the silicone tube will be just inside the distal end of the airway tube. If necessary, an assistant can connect a bag-valve device to the silicone tube and ventilate the patient. Make sure that the longitudinal black line on the posterior surface of the silicone tube is facing upward.

Slowly and gently advance the silicone tube 1.5 cm beyond the transverse black line. If no resistance is felt, the tip of the silicone tube is just past the vocal cords. Continue to advance the silicone tube an additional 4 cm (Figure 17-9E). The patient can be ventilated by an assistant during this procedure if necessary. Inflate the cuff of the silicone tube and ventilate the patient through the silicone tube (Figure 17-9F). Confirm proper tube placement by the auscultation of breath sounds, observation of chest rise, and end-tidal CO_2 monitoring.

The ILMA should now be withdrawn. Deflate the cuff of the ILMA. Have an assistant remove the bag-valve device and the 15 mm adapter on the proximal end of the silicone tube. Withdraw the ILMA by gently reversing the ILMA over the silicone tube (Figure 17-9G). **Simultaneously apply slight pressure to the proximal end of the silicone tube so it does not become dislodged (Figure 17-9G).** When the mask begins to exit the patient's mouth, stop withdrawing the ILMA. **Grasp the silicone tube firmly at the patient's mouth and hold it securely.** Withdraw the ILMA over the silicone tube in a smooth curved motion (Figure 17-9H). Reattach the standard respiratory connector, ventilate the patient, and reconfirm proper placement of the silicone endotracheal tube.

Some physicians like to use a "pusher" to prevent accidental extubation while the ILMA is being withdrawn. Cut a 25 cm length from a second silicone endotracheal tube. Insert this into the ILMA as it is being removed. Apply slight pressure so it pushes against the first endotracheal tube and prevents it from moving proximally. When the ILMA exits the patient's mouth, remove the ILMA and pusher as a unit. Secure and assess the proper positioning of the endotracheal tube, as mentioned previously.

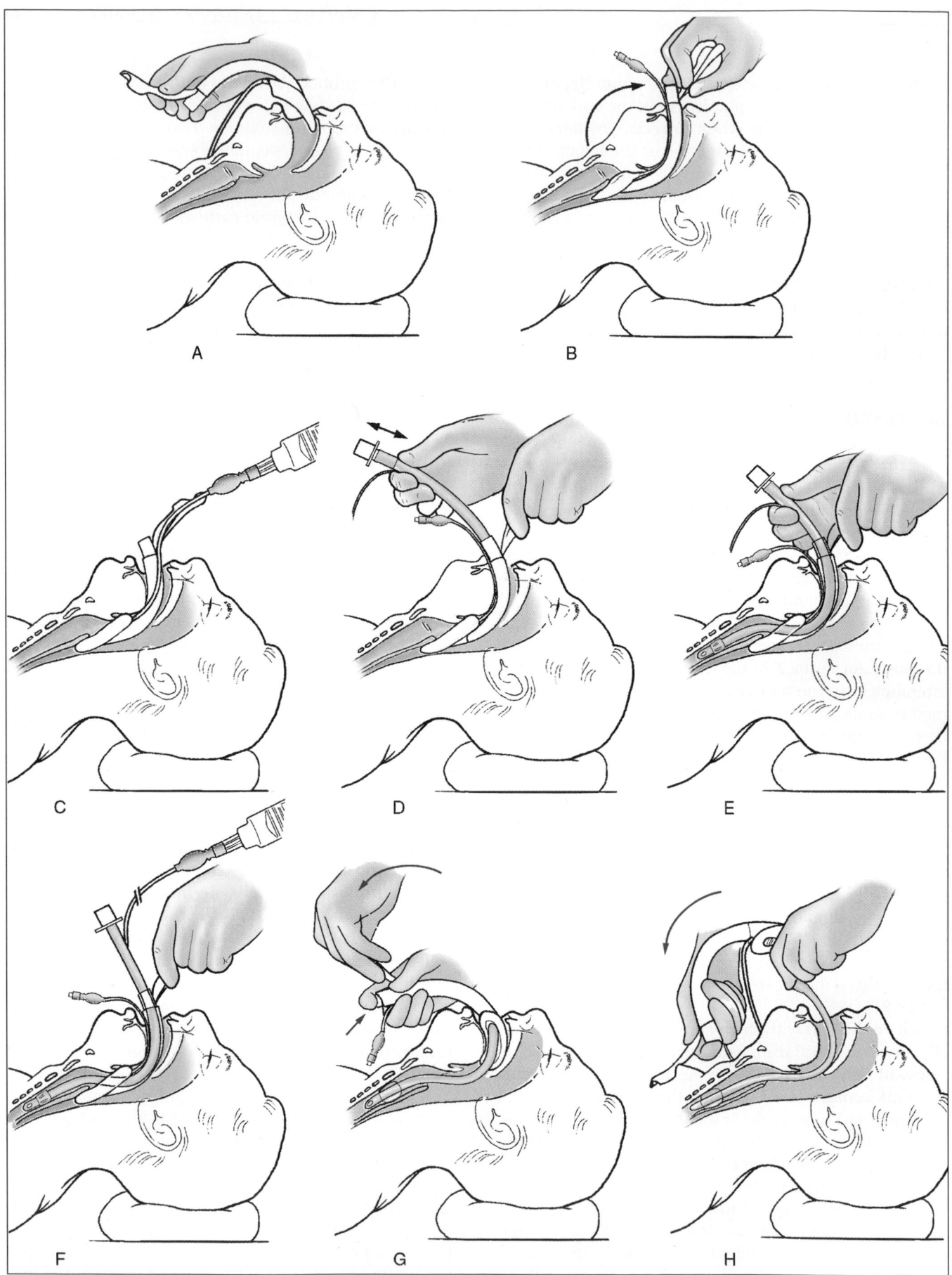

FIGURE 17-9 Insertion of the intubating laryngeal mask airway. *A.* The ILMA is inserted. *B.* The ILMA is advanced until resistance is encountered. *C.* The cuff is inflated. *D.* The ILMA is stabilized and the endotracheal tube is inserted. *E.* The endotracheal tube is advanced into the trachea. *F.* The endotracheal tube cuff is inflated. *G.* The ILMA is carefully removed. *H.* When the ILMA has exited the patient's mouth, grasp and stabilize the endotracheal tube. Completely remove the ILMA.

ALTERNATIVE TECHNIQUES

It is generally held that difficulty in insertion of the standard LMA occurs most frequently at the point where the tip of the mask passes just behind the tongue as it changes direction towards the hypopharynx.[14] Most of the suggested alternative methods of inserting the LMA involve the negotiation of direction change from the pharynx to the hypopharynx. Some authors suggest that a partially inflated mask is easier to place in the correct position.[14] Others employ a jaw-thrust maneuver. After adequate jaw relaxation has been established, the mask is positioned firmly and flatly against the hard palate, as recommended. Perform the jaw-thrust maneuver with the nondominant hand while firmly thrusting the mask into place with the dominant hand, in one motion.[15] The jaw thrust creates a space in the hypopharynx for the mask. In rare cases, the use of a laryngoscope may help facilitate LMA placement, though this reduces the inherent simplicity of the technique of LMA insertion.

Given that there is less experience with the ILMA, few alternative methods of insertion exist. However, one must remember that the metal handle on the tip of the ILMA tube may be used to modify the position of the cuff within the hypopharynx.[8] Pulling back on the metal handle toward the intubator rotates the tube caudally in the sagittal plane. Pushing on the metal handle away from the intubator rotates the tube cephalad in the sagittal plane.

ASSESSMENT

Successful placement of the LMA or the ILMA is most accurately demonstrated by the auscultation of bilateral breath sounds, chest wall movement, and end-tidal CO_2 monitoring.[5,8] One may also gain a sense of accuracy of placement during insertion. During observation of the front of the neck while inserting the LMA or the ILMA, one may see a bulging of the tissues overlying the larynx. Visualization of this bulge, in addition to increased resistance to forward motion of the mask, indicates that the device is in the correct position.[1] A chest radiograph should be obtained if an endotracheal tube has been placed through the LMA or the ILMA.

COMPLICATIONS

There are numerous documented complications associated with the use of the LMA and ILMA. One of the most obvious of these and potentially the most devastating is the failure to place the device successfully or to obtain a satisfactory laryngeal seal. Fortunately, even in in-experienced hands, the incidence of failure to achieve satisfactory ventilation is quite low. One large study, a retrospective review of 11,910 surgical cases where the standard LMA was used, noted an overall success rate of 99.81 percent.[16] Success rates have been classified as success on one single attempt and overall success. The overall success rate allows up to three attempts to be considered for successful placement. One investigator claimed a 95.5 percent single-attempt success rate in a retrospective analysis of 1500 cases.[9] Most studies imply correct LMA placement in 88 to 90 percent of first attempts.[7] ILMA failure rates, due to the relative newness of the technique, have not been clearly delineated. They would be expected to be somewhat higher than with the standard LMA due to the increased technical skill required for its placement. Besides failure, there are other complications, which may be divided into minor complications and major complications.

MINOR COMPLICATIONS

Minor complications are those that may result in significant patient morbidity but are usually not associated with mortality or extremely deleterious outcomes. Stomach inflation can occur during positive-pressure ventilation at pressures greater than 20 cmH_2O for the standard LMA. Cuff herniation secondary to overinflation may result in failure of the cuff to seal effectively. Partial airway obstruction may occur in up to 10 percent of adults and 25 to 50 percent of pediatric patients when standard LMA cuffs are examined by fiberoptic bronchoscopy.[7] Trapping of the epiglottis in the distal aperture of the LMA may result in edema of the epiglottis. Air leaks around the cuff can occur during positive-pressure ventilation at pressures greater than 20 cmH_2O for the standard LMA. Forceful attempts to pass the LMA around the posterior pharyngeal curvature can result in uvular bruising.[7] Lingual nerve injury, tongue numbness, parotid gland swelling, and hypoglossal nerve palsy are sometimes noted. Unilateral vocal cord paralysis can occur secondary to traumatic insertion. Bilateral vocal cord paralysis has not been reported. Dental trauma may occur during the insertion of the LMA or during maintenance of the airway.

MAJOR COMPLICATIONS

Major complications are those from which significant patient morbidity may be expected, including patient mortality. Fortunately, as regards the LMA, major complications are exceedingly rare. In a report of 11,910 surgical cases where the standard LMA was used, there were a total of 18 critical events related to the LMA, for an overall incidence of 0.15 percent.[16] These events included regurgitation of stomach contents (0.03 percent), vomiting of stomach contents (0.017 percent), pulmonary aspiration (0.009 percent), laryngospasm (0.07

percent), bronchospasm (0.025 percent), cardiac dysrhythmias (0.09 percent), and cardiac arrest (0.06 percent). While there appears to be a higher incidence of critical events when the device is used for controlled ventilation and positive-pressure ventilation, the incidence has not proved to be statistically significant.

In general, the complication rate (defined as events not attributable to the patient's underlying condition or to surgical or other interventions) should be equivalent to that seen during placement of either a Guedel or Berman type oropharyngeal airway. Referring to standard anesthesiology textbooks, one realizes that the complication rate in each of the aforementioned categories when using the LMA is statistically significantly lower than that occurring during direct laryngoscopy and endotracheal intubation, potentially due to the intense autonomic nervous system stimulation occurring with the latter procedure.

SUMMARY

A major advancement in airway management was made with the introduction of the LMA. It is superior to a face mask in that it prevents supraglottic obstruction and reduces the likelihood of gastric insufflation.[2] However, it does not provide protection from aspiration. The newest model, the LMA-Proseal, recently developed and soon to be put into clinical practice, may ameliorate some of the fears associated with use of standard LMAs in patients at moderate risk for regurgitation and pulmonary aspiration.

The standard LMA clearly has earned a valuable place in the armamentarium of clinicians who provide airway management. The technique is easy to learn, easy to teach, and requires no specialized equipment. The LMA causes minimal autonomic nervous system activation and less of a response from the cardiovascular system than with direct laryngoscopy. The LMA is not associated with a risk of esophageal or endobronchial intubation. Both, however, are possible complications following use of the ILMA. The LMA has minimal effects on the intraocular pressure response to airway manipulation. The LMA may be of use in cases of suspected cervical spine injury.

The use of an LMA in place of a face mask avoids many risks, such as injury to the eyes, supraorbital and facial nerves, nose, and lips. There is less of a risk of operator hand fatigue than with the bag-valve-mask device. The LMA provides a safer and more secure airway in children and adults than does a face mask, with fewer episodes of hypoxemia as detected by pulse oximetry.[7]

The introduction of the ILMA more than a decade after the standard LMA further defined and expanded the role of this apparatus in airway management. It allows for precise endotracheal tube placement, therefore ensuring airway protection. It is anatomically designed to ensure more accurate placement of the cuff. Given the ease of placement of the new ILMA without the need for the rescuer to be positioned behind the head, there may be a significant place for the ILMA in future airway management algorithms.[4]

The newest LMA device, the LMA-Proseal, may help solve the greatest limitation to LMA use, that of assuring an air- and watertight seal around the laryngeal inlet while isolating it from the esophagus and minimizing the risk of pulmonary aspiration. Its efficacy in doing so will certainly be the subject of many future papers and debates.

REFERENCES

1. Brain AIJ: The laryngeal mask—a new concept in airway management. *Br J Anaesth* 1983; 55:801–805.
2. Roman AM: Noninvasive airway management, in Tintinalli J, Kelen GD, Stapczynski JS (eds): *Emergency Medicine: A Comprehensive Study Guide*, 5th ed. New York: McGraw-Hill, 2000:83.
3. Weiler N, Eberle B, Heinrichs W: The laryngeal mask airway: routine, risk, or rescue? *Intens Care Med* 1999; 25:761–762.
4. Brain AIJ, Verghese C, Addy EV, et al: The intubating laryngeal mask. I: Development of a new device for intubation of the trachea. *Br J Anaesth* 1997; 79:699–703.
5. Brain AIJ, Verghese C, Addy EV, et al: The intubating laryngeal mask. II: A preliminary clinical report of a new means of intubating the trachea. *Br J Anaesth* 1997; 79:704–709.
6. Walls RM: Airway management, in Rosen P, Barkin R (eds): *Emergency Medicine: Concepts and Clinical Practice*, 4th ed. St. Louis: Mosby–Year Book, 1998:14–15.
7. Pennant JH, White PF: The laryngeal mask airway. Its uses in anesthesiology. Review article. *Anesthesiology* 1993; 79:144–163.
8. Kapila A, Addy EV, Verghese C: The intubating laryngeal mask airway: an initial assessment of performance. *Br J Anaesth* 1997; 79:710–713.
9. Brimacombe J: Analysis of 1500 laryngeal mask uses by one anaesthetist in adults undergoing routine anaesthesia. *Anaesthesia* 1996; 51:76–80.
10. Patel A, Bailey PM, Wakeling HG: The intubating laryngeal mask and distorted airway anatomy. *Br J Anaesth* 1999; 82(5):809–811.
11. Nanson J: Avoiding movement at a laryngeal mask airway insertion. *Br J Anaesth* 1999; 83(1):194–195.

12. *Insertion of the Re-enforced LMA. Step by Step.* 2000. http://www.saga.nl/lma/steps.html.

13. *The Laryngeal Mask.* 2000. http://gasbone.herston. uq.edu.au/teach/su602/docs/cl3laryg.html.

14. Dingley J, Asai MD: Insertion methods of the laryngeal mask airway. *Anaesthesia* 1996; 51:596–599.

15. Cass L: Inserting the laryngeal mask. *Anaesth Intens Care* 1991; 19(4):615.

16. Verghese C, Brimacombe JR: Survey of laryngeal mask airway usage in 11,910 patients: safety and efficacy for conventional and nonconventional usage. *Anesth Analg* 1996; 82:129–133.

Chapter 18
TRANSTRACHEAL ASPIRATION

Joseph A. Salomone III

INTRODUCTION

Transtracheal aspiration is a technique for the collection of bronchial secretions for laboratory evaluation and culture. This technique is useful when standard sputum collection has not provided adequate material or determination of the infective agent(s). Specimens collected by this technique are free of contamination from nasal, oral, and pharyngeal secretions. Pecora first described this technique in 1959.[1] Several modifications to the original technique have been made.[2–5] This technique may be more properly named transcricothyroid membrane aspiration.

ANATOMY AND PATHOPHYSIOLOGY

The most superficial portion of the cervical airway begins at the inferior thyroid cartilage and extends inferiorly to the thyroid isthmus (Figure 18-1). The inferior border of the thyroid cartilage is attached to the cricoid cartilage by the cricothyroid ligament. This is formed by a thicker central conus elasticus and laterally by thinner ligaments that are covered by the cricothyroid muscles (Figure 18-1B). The internal surface is covered by the mucous membrane of the larynx. Collectively, this is often referred to as the cricothyroid membrane or cricovocal membrane. The paired cricothyroid arteries cross from lateral to medial to form an arch that anteriorly crosses the upper one-third of the cricothyroid membrane. The pyramidal lobe of the thyroid occasionally extends superiorly to this level.

INDICATIONS

Transtracheal aspiration is indicated for the collection of tracheobronchial secretions for laboratory evaluation. Often, previous attempts to collect standard coughed and expectorated sputum samples have failed to yield adequate samples or reveal the etiology of a pulmonary infection. Patients who do not appear to be responding to the appropriate antibiotic regimen that was indicated by evaluation and culture of sputum samples may benefit from this technique to better determine the pathogen(s). This is particularly true in cases of atypical or mixed flora, as in suspected aspiration pneumonias, where this technique may yield superior culture results when compared to sputum samples.[6]

CONTRAINDICATIONS

Patients who are unable to cooperate with or tolerate the required positioning should not be selected for this technique.[7] Agitated patients requiring sedation that may affect respiratory effort should be avoided. Traumatically injured patients should have the cervical spine cleared for possible injury prior to performing the procedure. Patients with known or suspected blood dyscrasias (abnormal platelet counts, elevated prothrombin or partial thromboplastin times) should not be subjected to this technique due to the increased risk of tracheal hemorrhage. The operator must be able to easily identify the patient's anatomic landmarks, including the thyroid and cricoid cartilages and the intervening membrane space. Patients with abnormal or dis-

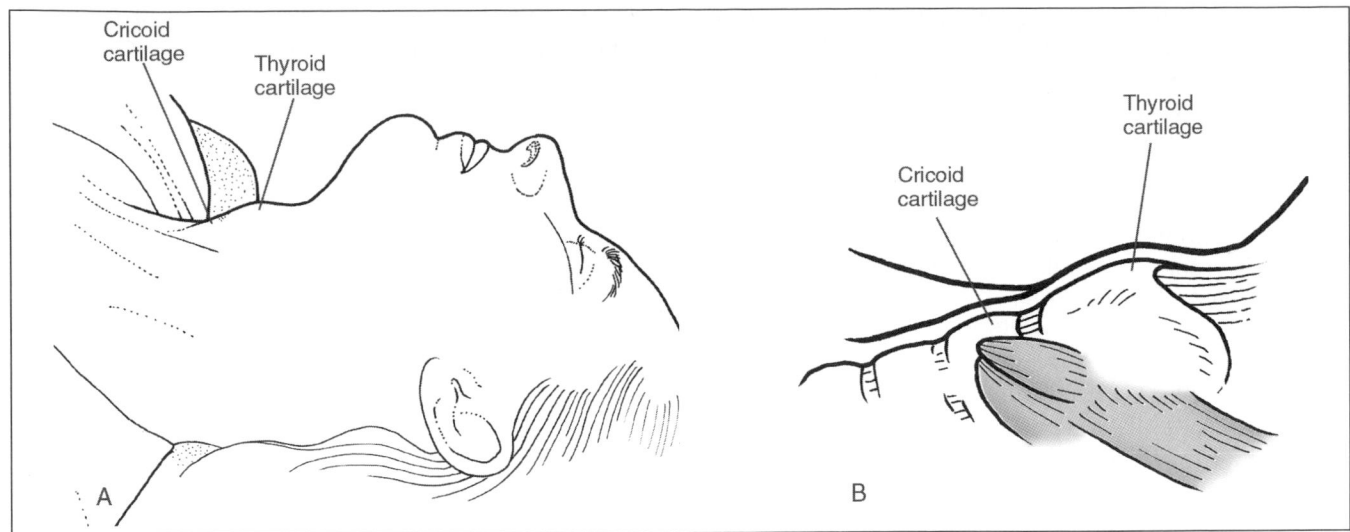

FIGURE 18-1 Anatomy of the airway structures of the neck. *A.* Topographic anatomy. *B.* The cartilaginous structures.

torted anatomy should be excluded. Patients who are endotracheally intubated or have a tracheostomy do not require this procedure.

EQUIPMENT

Sterile gown, gloves, and mask
Pillow or padding for shoulders
Povidone iodine solution or alternative cleansing
  solution
Sterile gauze squares
Normal saline solution, sterile and preservative-free
Local anesthetic solution, 3 mL (1% lidocaine HCl)
3 mL syringes
30 mL syringe
25 to 27 gauge needles, ½ inch
18 to 22 gauge catheter-through-the-needle
18 to 22 gauge catheter-over-the-needle, 3 inch long
18 to 19 gauge needles, 1½ inch
Pulse oximeter
Cardiac monitor
Sterile specimen container
Bandage, 1 inch wide
Resuscitation equipment including emergent airway
  management supplies

PATIENT PREPARATION

Explain the procedure, its risks, and its benefits to the patient and/or their representative. Obtain an informed consent. Place the patient on cardiac monitoring and continuous pulse oximetry. Administer supplemental oxygen and establish intravenous access.

Sedation is not generally required. A small dose of midazolam (1 to 5 mg IV) may be used, if appropriate, for light sedation. Deep sedation should be avoided, as it may compromise respiratory effort and increase the risk of aspiration of gastric contents.

Place the patient supine in bed. Place a pillow or appropriate padding under the patient's shoulders and upper back to allow for comfortable hyperextension of the neck. Identify by palpation the thyroid cartilage, laryngeal prominence (Adam's apple), cricoid cartilage, and cricothyroid membrane. These are the anatomic landmarks that will be used to identify the proper site for performing the procedure.

TECHNIQUE

The operator should wear a mask, appropriate eye protection, sterile gown, and sterile gloves. Using sterile technique, prepare the equipment. Draw 3 to 5 mL of sterile and preservative-free normal saline solution into a 30 mL syringe with a sterile needle. Attach an appropriately sized needle from a catheter-through-the-needle set (18 to 20 gauge for an adult, 20 to 22 gauge for a child) to a 3 mL syringe. Draw up 1 to 3 mL of local anesthetic solution into a 3 mL syringe armed with a 25 to 27 gauge needle. Position the patient as noted above. Clean the anterior neck of any dirt and debris. Apply povidone iodine solution and allow it to dry. Palpate the anterior neck and reidentify the thyroid cartilage, laryngeal prominence, cricoid cartilage, and cricothyroid membrane. Leave the nondominant index finger over the cricothyroid membrane for reference.

Apply a small intradermal wheal of local anesthetic solution at the anterior midpoint of the cricothyroid membrane (Figure 18-2). Inject 0.5 to 1.0 mL of local anesthetic solution into the subcutaneous tissue over the cricothyroid membrane, taking care not to distort the anatomy. Reidentify the cricothyroid membrane by palpation. Insert the needle on the syringe, directed caudally and at a 45 degree angle to the skin (Figure 18-3). Continue to advance the needle while applying negative pressure to the syringe (Figure 18-3A). Stop advancing the needle when air is aspirated. This signifies that the needle is inside the trachea. Hold the needle securely and remove the syringe. Insert the catheter through the needle (Figure 18-3B). While holding the catheter securely, withdraw the needle until the tip has exited the skin of the neck (Figure 18-3C). **Place the needle guard over the needle.** This will prevent shearing off of the catheter. Apply the 30 mL syringe containing saline to the catheter (Figure 18-3C).

Ask the patient to cough if they are not already doing so. Aspirate with the 30 mL syringe as the patient coughs. If no specimen is obtained, instill the sterile saline. Once again, ask the patient to cough if not stimulated by the saline. Aspirate until a specimen is acquired. An alternative to using a large syringe for aspiration is the use of low wall suction and a Lukens tube or similar trap device to collect the specimen. Remove the catheter, needle, and syringe as one unit. Hold direct pressure on the puncture site for 3 to 5 minutes. Apply a bandage or sterile dressing to the puncture site. Place the specimen in a sterile container and have it transported to the laboratory.

ALTERNATIVE TECHNIQUES

Many physicians are reluctant to use the catheter-through-the-needle system as there is the possibility of shearing off the catheter within the trachea. **This can be prevented by applying the needle guard over the needle immediately after it is withdrawn from the skin.**

An alternative is to use a catheter-over-the-needle (angiocatheter) system. Cleanse, prepare, and anesthetize the patient as above. Apply the catheter-over-the-needle onto a 3 or 5 mL syringe. Insert the catheter-over-the-needle while applying negative pressure to the syringe. When the trachea has been entered, advance the catheter until the hub is against the skin. Remove the needle and syringe. Attach the 30 mL syringe containing saline to the catheter. The remainder of the procedure is described above.

AFTERCARE

The patient should be observed for bleeding at the puncture site, the development of subcutaneous emphysema, any changes in sputum production, or hemoptysis. The patient should remain on continuous pulse oximetry to monitor possible deterioration in respiratory status. Obtain a chest radiograph immediately after the procedure and in 24 hours to look for subcutaneous air and/or a pneumothorax. Any procedure that might stimulate coughing should be avoided for at least 24 hours.

COMPLICATIONS

The complications range from minimal hemoptysis and localized subcutaneous emphysema to massive pulmonary hemorrhage and death.[8-13] Minimal hemoptysis was seen in 15 percent of pediatric patients in one study and commonly in several adult studies. Localized subcutaneous emphysema in the anterior neck occurred in 5 to 18 percent of patients. There are rare reports of fatal

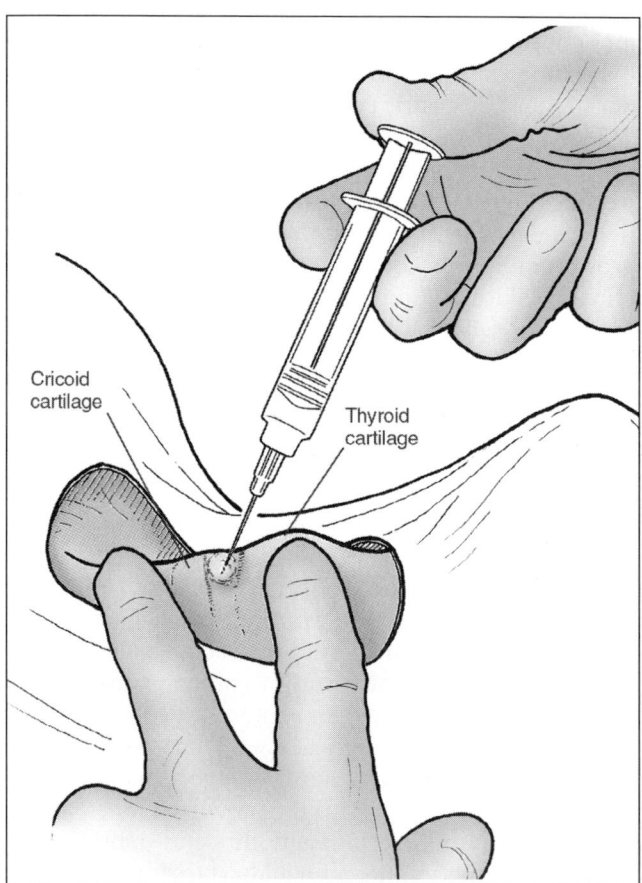

Cricoid cartilage

Thyroid cartilage

FIGURE 18-2 An intradermal wheal of local anesthetic solution is placed over the middle of the cricothyroid membrane.

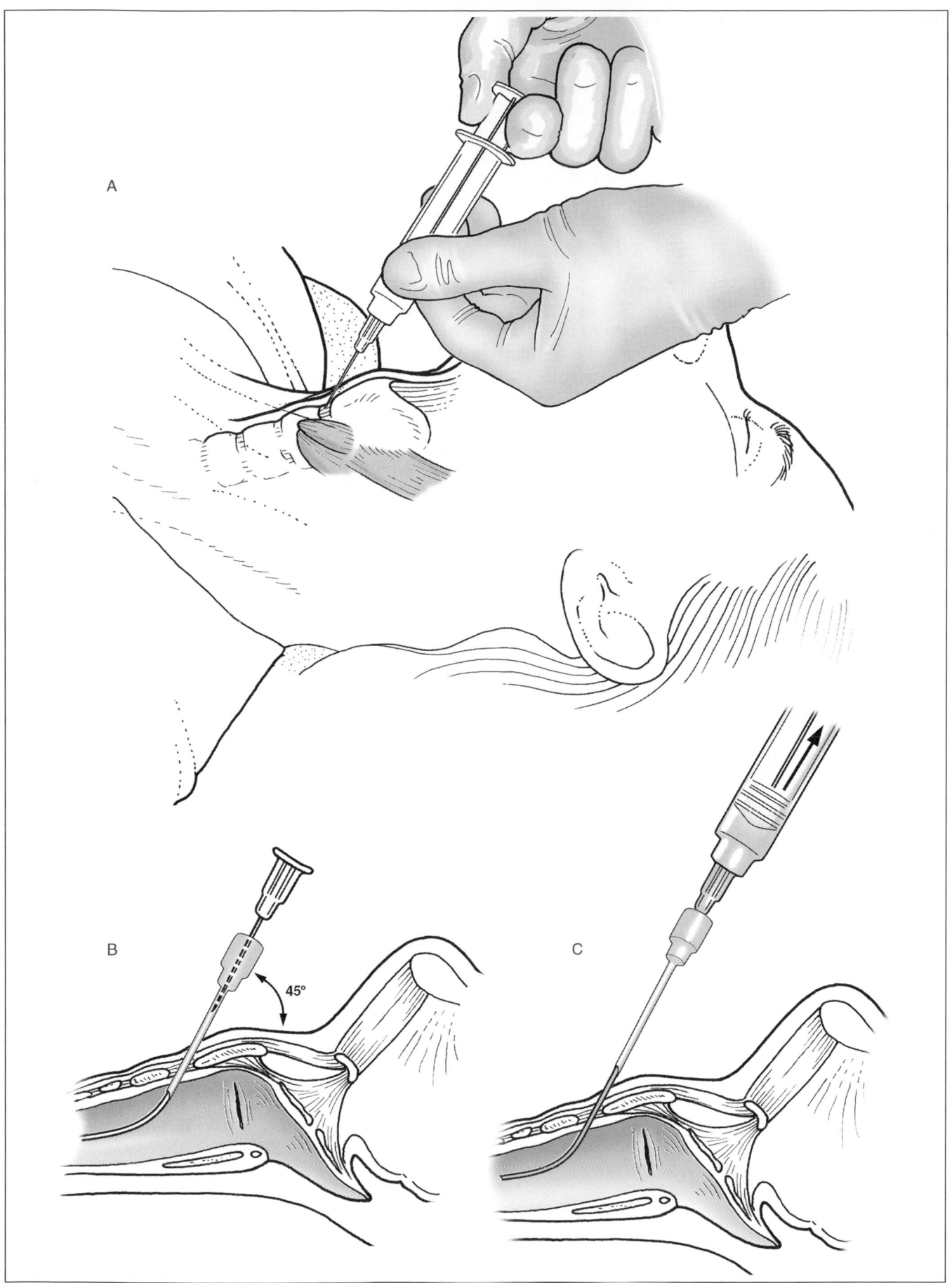

FIGURE 18-3 The transtracheal aspiration technique with a catheter-through-the-needle system. *A.* The needle is inserted through the cricothyroid membrane while negative pressure is applied to the syringe. *B.* The syringe has been removed and the catheter advanced through the needle. *C.* The needle has been withdrawn until its tip exits the skin. A syringe containing saline is attached to the hub of the catheter.

endotracheal hemorrhage, profound coughing with development of massive subcutaneous and mediastinal emphysema, vomiting and aspiration of gastric contents, cardiac dysrhythmias, and sudden cardiac death. There is at least one case of fatal gastrointestinal hemorrhage from ruptured esophageal varices and Mallory-Weiss tears following "unrestrainable" coughing.

SUMMARY

Transtracheal aspiration is a useful technique for obtaining uncontaminated specimens for analysis and culture. The procedure is best used in those patients who have complicated courses or are failing to respond to appropriate treatment or when there is a high index of suspicion for aspiration pneumonia and more atypical infectious agents.

REFERENCES

1. Pecora DV: A comparison of securing uncontaminated tracheal secretions for bacterial examination. *J Thorac Surg* 1959; 37:653–654.
2. Kalinski RW, Parker RH, Brandt D, et al: Diagnostic usefulness and safety of transcutaneous aspiration. *N Engl J Med* 1967; 276(11):604–608.
3. Hahn HH, Beaty HN: Transtracheal aspiration in the evaluation of patients with pneumonia. *Ann Intern Med* 1970; 72:183–187.
4. Brooks I: Percutaneous transtracheal aspiration in the diagnosis and treatment of aspiration pneumonia in children. *J Pediatr* 1980; 96(6):1000–1004.
5. Lieberman D, Lieberman D, Alroy G, et al: Transtracheal aspiration: reduction in complication rate by using a modified technique. *Isr J Med Sci* 1984; 20:641–642.
6. Reis K, Levison M, Kaye D: Transtracheal aspiration in pulmonary infection. *Arch Intern Med* 1974; 133:453–458.
7. Pratter MR, Irwin RS: Transtracheal aspiration: guidelines for safety. *Chest* 1979; 76(11):518–520.
8. Spencer CD, Beaty HN: Complications of transtracheal aspiration. *N Engl J Med* 1972; 286(6):304–305.
9. McCartney RD, McMurty RJ: Complications of transtracheal aspiration. *N Engl J Med* 1973; 287:1094.
10. Schillaci RF, Iacavoni VE, Conte RS: Transtracheal aspiration complicated by fatal endotracheal hemorrhage. *N Engl J Med* 1976; 295(9):488–490.
11. Bartlett JG: Diagnostic accuracy of transtracheal aspiration bacteriologic studies. *Am Rev Respir Dis* 1977; 115:777–782.
12. Holt GR, Davis WE, Ailor EI, et al: Massive airway hemorrhage after transtracheal aspiration. *South Med J* 1978; 71(3):325–327.
13. Schmerber J, Deltenre M: A new fatal complication of transtracheal aspiration. *Scand J Respir Dis* 1978; 59:232–235.

Section Two

CARDIOTHORACIC PROCEDURES

Chapter 19
CARDIOVERSION AND DEFIBRILLATION

Payman Sattar

INTRODUCTION

The application of electricity to the heart induces depolarization of the myocardial cells in uniform fashion. This may interrupt reentry circuits that are inducing an arrhythmia. Once depolarization of the myocardium has been achieved, the sinus node may then resume its normal pacing function.

The techniques of cardioversion and defibrillation are relatively straightforward and practically identical. The main differences are the indications and use of synchronization with cardioversion. **The purpose of cardioversion is to deliver a precisely timed electrical current to the heart to convert an organized rhythm to a more hemodynamically stable rhythm. The purpose of defibrillation is to deliver a randomly timed high-energy electrical current to the heart that is fibrillating to restore a normal sinus rhythm.** These techniques are currently performed by emergency medical technicians, nurses, paramedics, physicians, and a variety of other health care workers on a daily basis. This chapter discusses the techniques of manual cardioversion and defibrillation. A discussion of Advanced Cardiac Life Support, cardiac rhythms, chemical cardioversion, and pediatric advanced life support is beyond the scope of this work. The technique of automatic external defibrillation is not discussed.

INDICATIONS

CARDIOVERSION

In general, electrical cardioversion is performed either electively or emergently. In the Emergency Department, the role of electrical cardioversion is usually limited to urgent or emergent situations or when medical therapy has failed.[1,2] This includes reentry tachycardias (supraventricular tachycardia, atrial fibrillation, atrial flutter, and Wolf-Parkinson-White syndrome) associated with acute myocardial infarctions, altered levels of consciousness, chest pain, congestive heart failure, dizziness, dyspnea, hypotension, presyncope, pulmonary edema, shock, or syncope.

In the Emergency Department, electrical cardioversion is often preferred to chemical cardioversion for many reasons. Electrical cardioversion is simple and quick to perform. It is effective—in most cases almost immediately. It may be more successful than chemical cardioversion. The complications are usually minimal. Potential allergic reactions and toxic effects are nonexistent with electrical cardioversion.

DEFIBRILLATION

Defibrillation is indicated when ventricular fibrillation or ventricular tachycardia has not spontaneously converted to an organized rhythm. Ventricular fibrillation and ventricular tachycardia are rarely spontaneously reversible and are not compatible with life. Cardioversion may be performed immediately if the patient is found pulseless, unconscious and apneic, or during the Advanced Cardiac Life Support (ACLS) protocol. "Fine" ventricular fibrillation can be present and may be confused with asystole. It may be secondary to low gain amplitude or improper lead positioning. If "quick-look" paddles are being used, they may be rotated 90 degrees. If a monitor is being used, select a different lead and/or increase the gain to determine if the cardiac rhythm is fine ventricular fibrillation or asystole. Ventricular fibrillation or ventricular tachycardia secondary to myocardial ischemia or infarct, electrolyte abnormalities, long-QT syndromes, hypothermia, or drug toxicity (digoxin, tricyclic antidepressants, antiarrhythmics, antihistamine and macrolide antibiotic combinations) may convert to a more stable rhythm with defibrillation.

CONTRAINDICATIONS

CARDIOVERSION

Cardioversion is contraindicated for several cardiac rhythms or conditions. **Elective cardioversion of atrial fibrillation should not be attempted unless it is known with certainty that the rhythm initiated within the last 48 hours.** Cardioversion of chronic atrial fibrillation, or atrial fibrillation having lasted longer than 48 hours, may dislodge atrial thrombi, resulting in embolization and end organ injury. There is some controversy in the literature regarding the cardioversion of atrial flutter greater than 48 hours old without anticoagulation.[3,4] **Cardioversion in patients with digoxin toxicity should be avoided.** Cardioversion in digoxin toxicity is usually ineffective and has been associated with postshock ventricular tachycardia and ventricular fibrillation.[5] Cardioversion is also contraindicated when the patient is without a pulse or has an underlying cardiac rhythm of asystole, ventricular fibrillation, or ventricular tachycardia.

Alterations in the chemical or metabolic milieu of the myocardium may cause subsidiary pacemakers to become more dominant and overtake the sinus mode. This is referred to as enhanced automaticity and can be due to drugs (e.g., digoxin), hypoxia, or electrolyte abnormalities (e.g., hypokalemia or hypomagnesemia). Uniform depolarization with electricity does not terminate this abnormality, as uniform depolarization already exists. The rhythms that may occur are sinus tachycardia, ectopic atrial tachycardia, multifocal atrial tachycardia, and the digoxin toxic rhythms. Treatment of the underlying etiology is the treatment of choice.

DEFIBRILLATION

There are few contraindications to defibrillation. The main contraindication is in a patient who has made it clear that he or she does not wish to be resuscitated. Defibrillation should not be used for arrhythmias other than ventricular tachycardia or ventricular fibrillation.

EQUIPMENT

Defibrillator/cardioversion unit
Conductive jelly or pads
Suction source, tubing, and catheter
Airway management supplies
Advanced Cardiac Life Support (ACLS) medications
Intravenous sedative agents
Cardiac monitor
Noninvasive blood pressure monitor
Pulse oximeter
Oxygen source and tubing
Nasal cannula or face mask to deliver oxygen

The typical defibrillator/cardioversion unit performs both cardioversion and defibrillation (Figure 19-1). A list of available features is given in Table 19-1. Newer models feature lower power outputs to accommodate their use in children, pediatric and adult paddles, biphasic waveforms, and cardiac pacing capabilities. Each operator should be familiar with the specific unit at their facility. The general features of the unit are discussed below.

The unit is self-contained. It plugs into a standard electrical outlet. The unit also contains rechargeable batteries, which allow it to be portable. An oscilloscope provides real-time monitoring of the patient's cardiac rhythm. A continuous electrocardiographic (ECG) rhythm strip providing documentation on paper is standard with each unit, producing a hard copy to attach to the patient's medical record. Numerous dials or electronic touchpads with digital displays allow the operator to set the working mode, energy level, pacemaker settings, and oscilloscope input (ECG leads or "quick-look" paddles). The depolarizer within the machine provides direct electric current for cardioversion and defibrillation.

The synchronizer permits the discharge of electric current based on the patient's ECG waveform. It searches for the R and S waves of the ECG tracing to determine the proper time to discharge the current. It avoids delivering the current during the repolarization phase of the myocardial action potential, when the heart may convert to ventricular fibrillation or ventricular tachycardia. When the operator pushes the button to discharge the unit, a brief delay is noted while the syn-

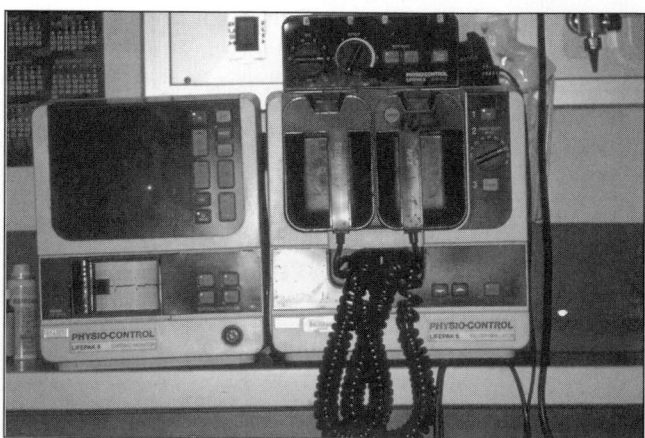

FIGURE 19-1 The defibrillator/cardioversion unit.

TABLE 19-1. CHARACTERISTICS OF A TYPICAL DEFIBRILLATOR/CARDIOVERSION UNIT

Adult and pediatric paddles
Cardioversion capability
Continuous ECG rhythm-strip documentation on paper
Defibrillator capability
Depolarizer
On/off switch
Oscilloscope to monitor cardiac rhythms
Pacing capabilities
Portability
"Quick-look" paddles
Safety mechanism to prevent accidental electrical discharge
Synchronizer
Standard ECG leads (three) to attach to the shoulders and lower extremity
Wide range of energy selection

chronizer searches for an appropriate time to discharge the current.

The paddles must be firmly applied to the patient's torso. They allow a "quick look" and transmit the patient's cardiac rhythm to the oscilloscope, letting the operator make medical decisions before the ECG leads are attached to the patient. Each paddle has a button on which a thumb is to be placed. This serves as a safety mechanism. Both buttons must be depressed simultaneously to discharge the current. This prevents accidental and premature discharge of current, which may injure the patient, the operator, or bystanders. Some units use self-adhesive disposable patches as an alternative to paddles. These are not often used because of their significant cost.

Paddles come in various shapes and sizes. Adult paddles are round, oval, or rectangular in shape. They measure 8 to 10 cm in greatest diameter. They can be used on children weighing more than 10 kg or over 1 year of age, adolescents, and adults. Pediatric paddles also come in a variety of shapes and measure 4 to 6 cm in greatest diameter. The pediatric paddles are to be used in children weighing less than 10 kg or less than 1 year of age. Some units contain both adult and pediatric paddles. In these units, the adult electrode slides off the paddle handle to reveal the pediatric-size electrode.

In choosing the proper paddle for a small child, the cutoff of 10 kg and 1 year of age is relative. Choose the largest paddle that will achieve complete and full contact with the child's chest wall. Larger paddles will allow a greater amount of myocardium to be depolarized while decreasing the current density applied, so as to minimize myocardial injury. The paddles must be at least 2 to 3 cm apart to prevent electrical bridging and burn injury to the child. Using paddles that are too large will deliver the electric current over too great an area and decrease its effectiveness. The opposite is true in adults (using paddles that are too small will deliver the

electric current over a small area, which makes it too intense and increases the damage to the myocardium).

The paddles may be positioned in several different patterns.[6,7] The most commonly used positions are anterolateral (Figure 19-2) followed by anteroposterior (Figure 19-3). Anterolateral paddles are positioned with the anterior paddle at the right upper sternal border over the second and third intercostal spaces. The lateral paddle is placed in the left midaxillary line centered over the fourth and fifth intercostal spaces. Anteroposterior placement is often used with disposable patches rather than paddles (Figure 19-3). The anterior patch is centered over the sternum and the posterior patch is placed between the scapulae. If pediatric paddles are required but not available, adult paddles can be substituted.[6] Roll the child onto their right side and place the paddles in the anteroposterior position. Other paddle positions include the laterolateral (axilla-to-axilla) position and the parasternal-infraclavicular (oblique, left anterior chest to right posterior infrascapular) position.[7]

Electrically conductive contact medium should always be applied between the electrode and the patient's chest wall. The most commonly used material is in the form of a gel or paste. Conductive pads are commercially available but significantly more expensive than gel or paste. The contact material helps to maximize current flow, minimize resistance, reduce transthoracic impedance, and prevent thermal or electrical burns to the chest wall. The contact medium should be applied to the paddles generously. It should not connect the paddles, because then it would divert the electric current along the chest wall, away from the heart, and cause burns to

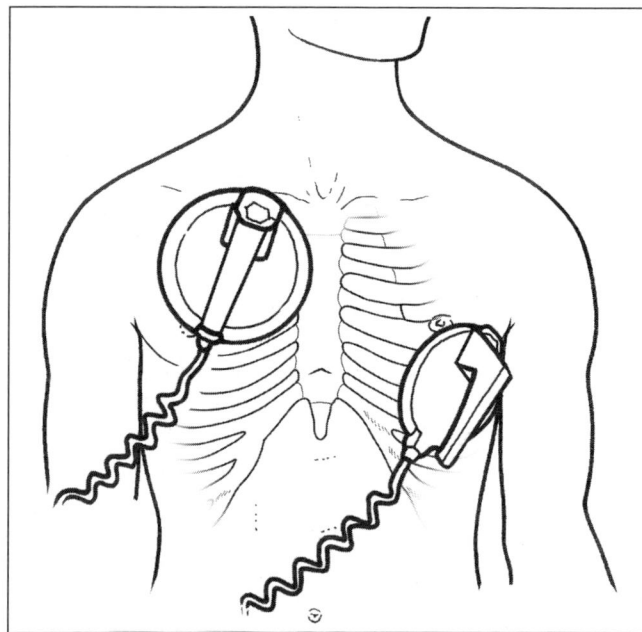

FIGURE 19-2 Anterolateral pad and paddle positioning.

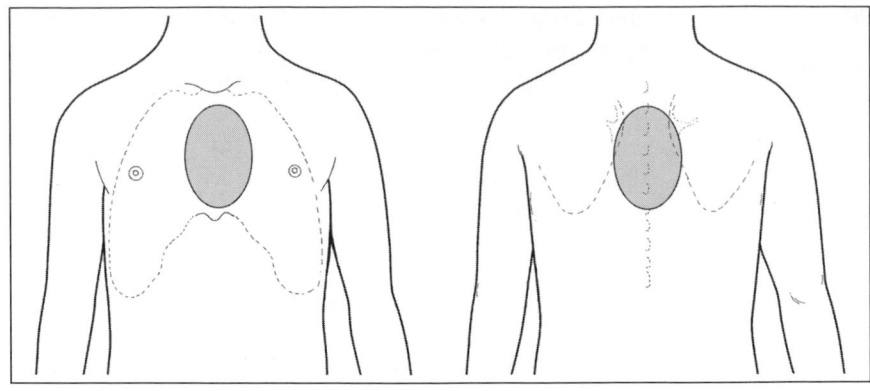

FIGURE 19-3 Anteroposterior pad and paddle positioning.

the chest wall. The self-adhesive disposable patches are prelubricated with contact medium and need no additional contact medium. If contact medium is not available, saline-soaked gauze squares can be used in an emergency. The saline must be squeezed out of the gauze squares to prevent the accumulation of liquid on the chest wall, which could bridge the two paddles.

PATIENT PREPARATION

Place the patient supine on a bed. Attach the cardiac monitor, noninvasive blood pressure monitor, pulse oximetry, and oxygen to the patient. Obtain intravenous access. Suction and resuscitation equipment should be readily available in case it is needed. Cardioversion is scary and extremely uncomfortable for patients. Briefly explain the procedure to the patient, including the risks, benefits, and complications. Premedicate the patient prior to cardioversion if no contraindications exist, the patient is hemodynamically stable, and he or she can tolerate a delay to cardioversion. The choice of the appropriate sedative agent is physician-dependent. Commonly used agents include etomidate, ketamine, midazolam, methohexital, propofol, and thiopental. Diazepam and lorazepam are not often used because of the long delay to onset of action.

TECHNIQUE

Stand at the patient's left side. Turn on the defibrillator/cardioversion unit. Set the display to the "quick-look" paddles. Instruct the nurses to apply the ECG leads to the patient. Grasp the left paddle (sternum) with the left hand and the right paddle (apex) with the right hand. This is the anterolateral paddle position. Apply the paddles and observe the patient's cardiac rhythm. Set the mode as asynchronous (defibrillation) or synchronous (cardioversion) based on the patient's cardiac rhythm. Set the energy level (Table 19-2). Apply conduc-

tive pads to the patient's torso in the anterolateral position. Alternatively, apply conductive jelly to the paddles liberally and rub them together to coat the electrode surface completely. Apply the paddles firmly to the torso in the anterolateral position. **The paddles should be separated from each other by at least 2 to 3 cm to prevent arcing of the current and injury to the patient.**

Prepare to deliver the electric current to the patient. Charge the paddles. This must be done on the unit or the paddles before the initial and each subsequent discharge. It takes approximately 2 to 5 seconds to charge the paddles following activation of the charge button. **Ensure that nurses and other assistants are not touching the patient or the stretcher.** The assistant ventilating through a bag-valve device attached to an endotracheal tube does not need to drop the bag, as plastic is nonconductive. **The person who will deliver the charge to the patient should ensure that their body is not in direct contact with the patient or the stretcher.**

TABLE 19-2. RECOMMENDED INITIAL AND SUBSEQUENT ENERGY LEVELS FOR CARDIOVERSION OR DEFIBRILLATION

Cardiac rhythm	Initial energy setting	Subsequent energy settings*
Atrial fibrillation, adults	100 J	200, 300, 360 J
Atrial flutter, adults	50 J	100, 200, 300, 360 J
Supraventricular tachycardia, adults	50 J	100, 200, 300, 360 J
Ventricular tachycardia, adults	200 J	300, 360 J
Ventricular fibrillation, adults	200 J	300, 360 J
Supraventricular tachycardia, children	0.5 J/kg	1.0 J/kg
Ventricular tachycardia, children	2.0 J/kg	4.0 J/kg
Ventricular fibrillation, children	2.0 J/kg	4.0 J/kg

*To be performed sequentially in this order.

Reevaluate the patient's cardiac rhythm. If still required, deliver the charge by simultaneously pressing the discharge buttons on each paddle. Observe the monitor and reevaluate the patient's cardiac rhythm. The unit can be recharged to deliver another electric charge to the patient if indicated.

The technique using self-adhesive disposable patches is similar with a few exceptions. Apply the patches in the anterolateral or anteroposterior position. No supplemental contact medium is required. Charge the patches by pressing the charge button on the defibrillator/cardioversion unit. Press the discharge button on the defibrillator/cardioversion unit to deliver the charge to the patient.

COMPLICATIONS

Complications of cardioversion can range from none to death. Thermal and electrical burns are potential injuries. Skin burns may result, the severity of which increases depending on the energy level utilized and the number of shocks delivered. Care must be taken to avoid contact between the ECG monitor leads and the paddles, or of the paddles with each other, as sparks or fire may result. Burns can be minimized by utilizing electrically conductive contact media and firmly applying the paddles to the patient. Remove any fluid materials on the chest wall (conductive jelly, saline, sweat, urine, water), as they can form a bridge between the paddles and result in arcing and thermal burns to the thorax. Also remove any nitroglycerin patches or ointments from the patient's torso. Ensure that there are no open oxygen sources that could ignite when the unit is discharged. If performed properly, repeated shocks will produce only a mild erythema to the chest wall.

Occasionally hypertension, other arrhythmias, or heart block may develop. If a shock is delivered on the T wave, ventricular fibrillation may result.[9-11] This usually occurs immediately and can be corrected with another nonsynchronized countershock. Ensure that the unit is in synchronous mode, not asynchronous mode, when cardioverting an organized cardiac rhythm. Always observe the monitor before delivering a countershock to ensure that it is required. If the T wave is large, change the monitor lead so that the T wave is smaller than the R wave and the unit will not cardiovert during a vulnerable period. Ventricular fibrillation that occurs within 30 to 60 seconds after the delivery of a synchronous shock is often due to digoxin toxicity and is difficult or impossible to correct. Transient ST-segment elevation may occur.[12] Creatine kinase enzyme elevations may occur, most being skeletal in origin.[10] The higher the energy level used and the more countershocks given, the greater the muscle damage that may result. Usually no

significant permanent myocardial damage occurs. Systemic emboli may occur from clots in the left atrium becoming dislodged if the underlying rhythm prior to the cardioversion or defibrillation is atrial fibrillation. **Do not apply the paddles directly over an implanted defibrillator or pacemaker.** The electric discharge can permanently damage these devices. Adjust the position of the paddles so they are not directly over these devices.

Avoid injury to yourself or others by ensuring that no one is in contact with the bed or the patient when the shock is administered. Such injuries can range from mild shocks and burns to cardiac dysrhythmias. An improperly functioning unit can cause injury despite being used properly. Periodic maintenance and calibration of the unit is necessary.

SUMMARY

Cardioversion and defibrillation are the processes of applying electric current to a patient's chest to terminate a dysrhythmia. Cardioversion is a safe and effective method of converting reentry arrhythmias. If the patient is stable, a trial of medical therapy is warranted. If the patient is "unstable," cardioversion should be initiated as soon as possible. Consider administering parenteral sedation, as cardioversion is anxiety-provoking and painful for the patient. Cardioversion should be performed in the synchronized mode. Always be prepared for ventricular fibrillation or ventricular tachycardia as a result of cardioversion of an organized rhythm. ACLS medications and airway support must be readily available. Defibrillation is essentially cardioversion of ventricular fibrillation. It is performed like cardioversion except that synchronization and sedation are not required.

REFERENCES

1. Sanchez-Diaz CJ, Gonzalez-Carmona VM, Ruesga Zamora E, et al: Electrical cardioversion in the emergency service: experience in 1000 cases. *Arch Inst Cardiol Mex* 1987; 57(5):387–394.
2. Mancini GBJ, Goldberger AL: Cardioversion of atrial fibrillation: consideration of embolization, anticoagulation, prophylactic pacemaker, and long term success. *Am Heart J* 1982; 104(3):617–621.
3. Lanzarotti CJ, Olshansky B: Thromboembolism in chronic atrial flutter: is the risk underestimated? *J Am Coll Cardiol* 1997; 30(5):1506–1511.
4. Arnold AZ, Mick MJ, Mazurek RP, et al: Role of prophylactic anticoagulation for direct current cardioversion in patients with atrial fibrillation or atrial flutter. *J Am Coll Cardiol* 1997; 19(4): 851–855.

5. Kleiger R, Lown B: Cardioversion and digitalis. II. clinical studies. *Circulation* 1966; 33:878–887.
6. Foltin G: Basic life support, in Dieckmann RA, Fiser DH, Selbst SM (eds): *Illustrated Textbook of Pediatric Emergency and Critical Care Procedures*. St. Louis: Mosby, 1997:288–291.
7. Moulton C, Dreyer C, Dodds D, et al: Placement of electrodes for defibrillation—a review of the evidence. *Eur J Emerg Med* 2000; 7(2):135–143.
8. Dalzell GW, Anderson J, Adgey AAJ: Factors determining success and energy requirements for cardioversion of atrial fibrillation. *Q J Med* 1990; 76(281):903–913.
9. Aberg H, Cullhed I: Direct current countershock complications. *Acta Med Scand* 1968; 183:415–421.
10. Ross EM: Cardioversion causing ventricular fibrillation. *Arch Intern Med* 1964; 114: 811–813.
11. Ebrahimi R, Rubin SA: Electrical cardioversion resulting in death from synchronization failure. *Am J Cardiol* 1994; 74:100–102.
12. Cantor A, Stein B, Keynan A: "Intermittent" and transient ST-segment elevation following direct current cardioversion. *Int J Cardiol* 1988; 20:403–405.

Chapter 20
TRANSCUTANEOUS CARDIAC PACING

Rami Doukky
Ratnakar S. Rajanahally

INTRODUCTION

Transcutaneous cardiac pacing was introduced in 1952 by Zoll as a means of treating asystole and significant bradyarrhythmias.[1] The high current densities at the skin surface that were required to pace the cardiac tissue in these early devices caused painful stimulation of the cutaneous nerves and underlying skeletal muscles.[1] It was also difficult to determine when the heart was capturing due to significant muscular artifact. With the development of transvenous cardiac pacing leads in the 1950s, interest in external cardiac pacing waned. Although transvenous cardiac pacing has traditionally served as the mainstay of urgent temporary pacing, it requires significant time and operator skill to implement. This makes transvenous cardiac pacing less than ideal. As a result, in the 1980s, noninvasive pacing reemerged as a therapy for bradycardia and asystole.[2,3] Technologic advances, including large adhesive electrodes and electrocardiographic (ECG) filtering, have largely overcome the early problems of extreme discomfort and interpretation of capture on the ECG.

Noninvasive transcutaneous cardiac pacing offers several advantages over invasive cardiac pacing techniques. It is comparatively easy to perform and requires minimal training. Thus, physicians, nurses, and paramedics can institute temporary cardiac pacing. Because it can be performed quickly, noninvasive cardiac pacing can be initiated almost immediately, eliminating the setup and the insertion time of invasive techniques. Noninvasive cardiac pacing carries none of the risks and complications associated with the invasive techniques. It is also more cost-effective than invasive pacing.

ANATOMY AND PATHOPHYSIOLOGY

The heart is the only muscle of the body that generates its own electrical impulses. Its automaticity and subsequent rhythmic contractions propel blood to the tissues of the body. The initial cardiac impulse starts in the right atrium of the heart at the sinoatrial (SA) node. The sympathetic and parasympathetic nervous systems control the rate of impulse generation at the SA node. Once the electric stimulus is generated, it is conducted along the internal conduction pathways of the heart to the muscular atrial and ventricular walls. A delicate balance between electrolyte flux to create action potentials, myocardial integrity to allow impulses to become contractions, and an intact conduction system must be maintained. Conduction system problems are often the result of inadequate blood flow to the heart due to ventricular infarction and coronary artery occlusion. The blood supply to the conduction system of the heart originates from the right coronary artery. Occlusion of the right coronary artery can result in arrhythmias and conduction delays.

INDICATIONS

Transcutaneous cardiac pacing is a temporary method of cardiac pacing that is widely used in various clinical settings.[4-9] It serves as a bridge to temporary transvenous cardiac pacing or to permanent pacemaker placement in patients with severe, symptomatic, or hemodynamically unstable bradyarrhythmias that do not respond to pharmacologic therapy. In bradysystolic cardiac arrest, pacing is not routinely recommended but should be used as early as possible after the onset of arrest.[10–15] In patients with bradyarrhythmias that are expected to be transient, digoxin toxicity, or atrioventricular (AV) block in the setting of inferior wall myocardial infarction, transcutaneous cardiac pacing is quick, simple, and not associated with the morbidity or mortality of transvenous cardiac pacing.

It is indicated in patients with AV conduction blocks and sinus node dysfunction. It should be performed in symptomatic patients (syncope, presyncope, dizziness, fatigue, etc.) with complete or third-degree AV block, asystolic pauses exceeding 3 seconds, or an escape pacemaker rate less than 40 beats per minute. Patients with type I or type II second-degree AV block who are symptomatic should be transcutaneously paced. Symptomatic bifascicular block is also an indication for temporary transcutaneous cardiac pacing. Patients with sinus node dysfunction are candidates for pacing. Sinus node dysfunction includes sinus pause with symptoms of cerebral hypoperfusion (syncope, presyncope, dizziness), chronic sinus node dysfunction with or without symptoms but with escape rates of less than 40 beats per minute, or symptomatic sinus bradycardia.

Transcutaneous cardiac pacing leads can be applied and the system set up as prophylaxis, or standby, when bradyarrhythmias are expected.[10] If the patient develops bradyarrhythmias, the pacer can be immediately activated without the delays associated with obtaining the equipment and setting up the system. This includes patients with acute anterior or inferior wall myocardial infarctions and digoxin overdose.[16] Transcutaneous pacing can also be prophylactically applied before surgery, as anesthesia can increase preexisting cardiac conduction blocks. It can also be applied before cardiac diagnostic studies.

Transcutaneous cardiac pacing can be used to overdrive-pace the myocardium to suppress ventricular or supraventricular tachyarrhythmias.[17–19] This is very rarely indicated, as the rates required to overdrive-pace the heart are difficult to obtain on a transcutaneous pacing system. Patients do not usually tolerate transcutaneous overdrive pacing due to the accompanying chest wall contractions and discomfort. The transvenous or transthoracic routes should be used for overdrive pacing of the myocardium.

CONTRAINDICATIONS

There are no absolute contraindications to transcutaneous cardiac pacing. Severe hypothermia is a relative contraindication for transcutaneous cardiac pacing in patients with bradycardia. In these patients, bradycardia may be physiologic due to a decreased metabolic rate.[20] The ventricles are more prone to fibrillation and more resistant to defibrillation as body temperature de-

creases.[21] Pacing is relatively contraindicated in patients with bradysystolic cardiac arrest for more than 20 minutes due to poor resuscitation rates in these patients.[10–15]

EQUIPMENT

Pulse generator and monitor unit
Pacing cable
Pacemaker patches
ECG electrode patches
ECG monitor and cable
Soap and water for skin preparation (for nonemergent treatment or prophylaxis)
Intravenous analgesics and sedatives

In hospitals, this equipment is usually available on a preprepared "crash cart."[22] The transcutaneous pacing unit is an integral component of a standard defibrillator/cardioversion unit (Figure 20-1). The pacemaker patches are either round or rectangular in shape. The electrodes are packaged in pairs, with one being positive and the other negative. The negative electrode may be labeled "front," "apex," or "anterior." It should be placed over the apex of the heart. The positive electrode may be labeled "back" or "posterior." It should be placed between the patient's scapulae.

PATIENT PREPARATION

If the clinical situation permits, explain the purpose of transcutaneous cardiac pacing to the patient and/or their representative.[22] Discuss the equipment, the procedure, potential sensations the patient may experience, and the interventions to relieve discomfort. A signed

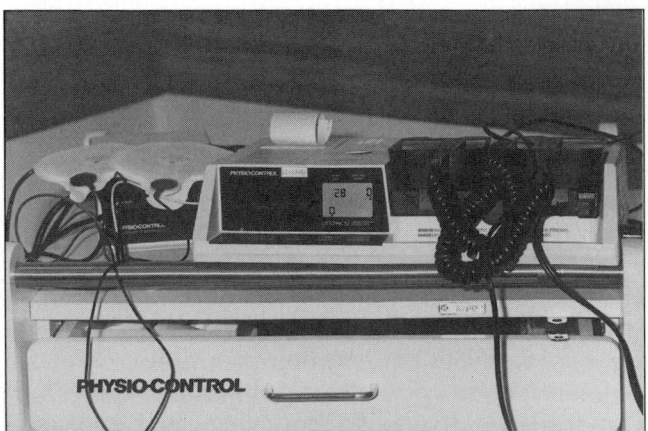

FIGURE 20-1 The transcutaneous cardiac pacing generator and surface patch electrodes. This is an integral component of the defibrillator/cardioversion unit.

consent is not required to perform this procedure. Simply document in the medical record that "the risks and benefits have been explained to the patient, who agrees with the procedure."

Prepare the skin for placement of the electrode patches. Clean any dirt and debris from the skin. If necessary, use soap and water to clean the skin. Avoid flammable cleaning liquids, such as alcohol-containing solutions. If the patient is extremely hirsute, shaving may be necessary, so that the electrode patches will adhere to the skin.

TECHNIQUE

Two pacing electrodes must be applied to the thorax (Figure 20-2). Place the negative (anterior) electrode on the anterior chest wall, centered over the apex of the heart (Figure 20-2A) or over the lead V_3 position (Figure 20-2B). Place the positive (posterior) electrode directly behind the anterior electrode and to the left of the thoracic spine, between the spine and the left scapula[4,5] (Figure 20-2C). As an alternative, the positive electrode may be placed on the right upper chest and the negative electrode over the apex of the heart (Figure 20-3).

In patients with excessive body hair, shaving may be required to ensure good skin-electrode contact.[4] In conscious patients, trimming rather than shaving excessive hair is recommended to avoid tiny nicks in the skin that can increase pain and skin irritation.

Connect the electrodes to the pacing generator. Turn on the pacing unit. Set the pacing rate to 80 beats per minute. In the setting of a bradysystolic arrest or with unconscious patients, it is recommended to turn the stimulating current to maximal output (200 mA) to ensure ventricular capture. Once capture is achieved, the current may be gradually decreased until loss of capture, which defines the pacing current threshold. In conscious bradycardic patients or when used prophylactically, pacing is begun in the demand mode at rates slightly faster than the native rhythm and at minimal current output. Gradually increase the current by 5 to 10 mA at a time until cardiac capture is documented, which defines the pacing threshold, or until intolerable discomfort develops (Figure 20-4). The final current output should be set at the pacing threshold or 5 to 10 mA above it. When transcutaneous pacing is used as standby technique, the physician should first document that capture is possible by initiating a brief period of pacing at a rate slightly faster than the patient's intrinsic rate and then return the device to the standby mode.[4]

ASSESSMENT OF SUCCESSFUL PACING

Assess electrical capture by monitoring the ECG on the oscilloscope of the pacemaker unit or the cardiac monitor. Successful capture is usually characterized by a widening QRS complex and, especially, a broad T wave. It is easy to mistake the wide, slurred afterpotential following an external pacing spike for electrical capture. **The only sure sign of electrical capture is the presence of a consistent ST segment and T wave after each pacer spike.** The hemodynamic response to transcutaneous pacing must also be assessed, either by palpable pulse rate, noninvasive blood pressure monitoring, or arterial catheter blood pressure monitoring. The pulse should be taken at the right carotid or right femoral artery to avoid confusion between the jerking muscle contractions caused by the pacer and a pulse. The pulse count taken manually should match the paced heart rate read by the generator monitor. A significantly lower pulse rate

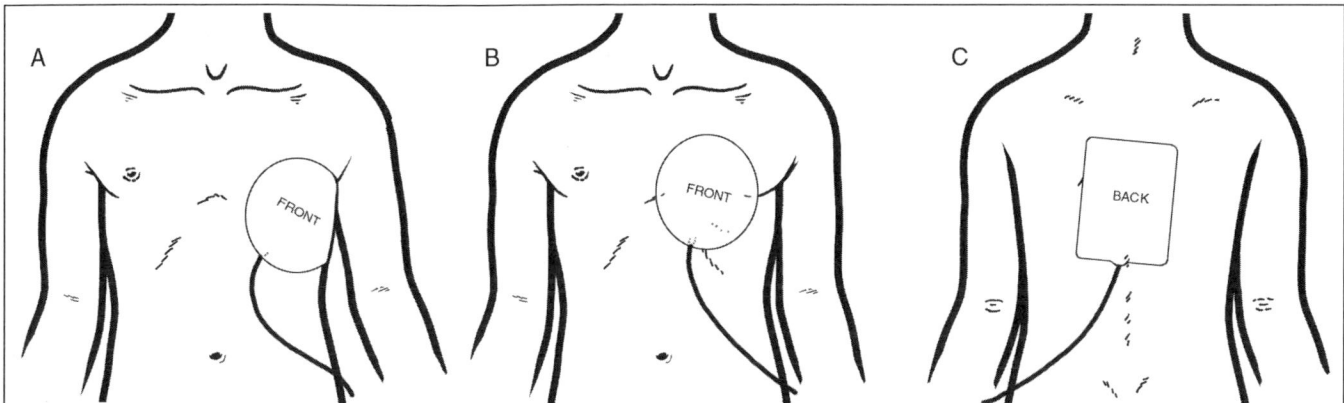

FIGURE 20-2 Placement of the transcutaneous pacing electrodes. *A.* Anterior (negative) electrode position centered over the cardiac apex. *B.* Anterior (negative) electrode position centered over the V_3 lead position. *C.* Posterior (positive) electrode position.

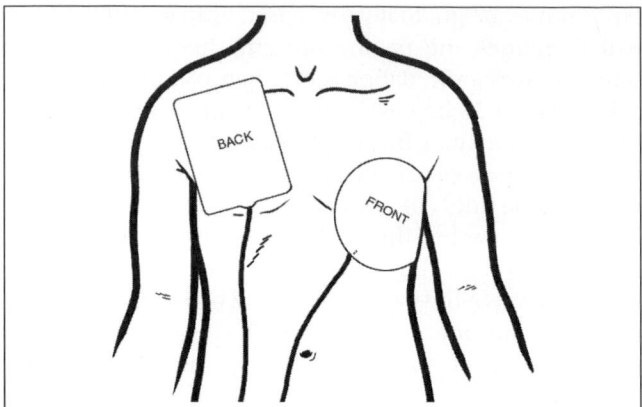

FIGURE 20-3 Alternative transcutaneous pacing electrode positions The negative electrode is positioned over the cardiac apex. The positive electrode is positioned on the right anterior chest wall.

than that observed on the monitor may indicate failure to capture. It is recommended to confirm capture on a standard 12-lead ECG.

Transcutaneous pacing thresholds tend to be lowest in healthy individuals or in patients with minimal hemodynamic compromise. In these settings, the threshold is usually in the range of 40 to 80 mA.[10,24] Most patients are paced using a current in the range of 20 to 140

mA.[10] No clear correlation has been established between the pacing threshold and patient age, weight, body size, chest diameter, or etiology of heart disease.[10,25,26] However, thresholds are usually elevated following thoracic surgery, in patients with emphysema or pericardial effusion, and after positive-pressure ventilation.[10]

Success rates in achieving ventricular capture vary widely depending on the setting where transcutaneous cardiac pacing is being used. Success rates appear to be highest when transcutaneous cardiac pacing is used prophylactically or early (within 5 minutes of bradycardic arrest). In these settings, success rates may exceed 90 percent.[10] Zoll reported a 78 percent success rate in diverse clinical situations.[10] The time to the initiation of transcutaneous cardiac pacing largely determines the success rate. With prolonged pacing, there can be changes in pacing threshold leading to capture failure. Failure to capture may be encountered due to a variety of reasons. Table 20-1 illustrates the most common causes of failure to capture, with suggested solutions to these problems.

AFTERCARE

Patients should be evaluated periodically to ensure that they are comfortable during transcutaneous cardiac

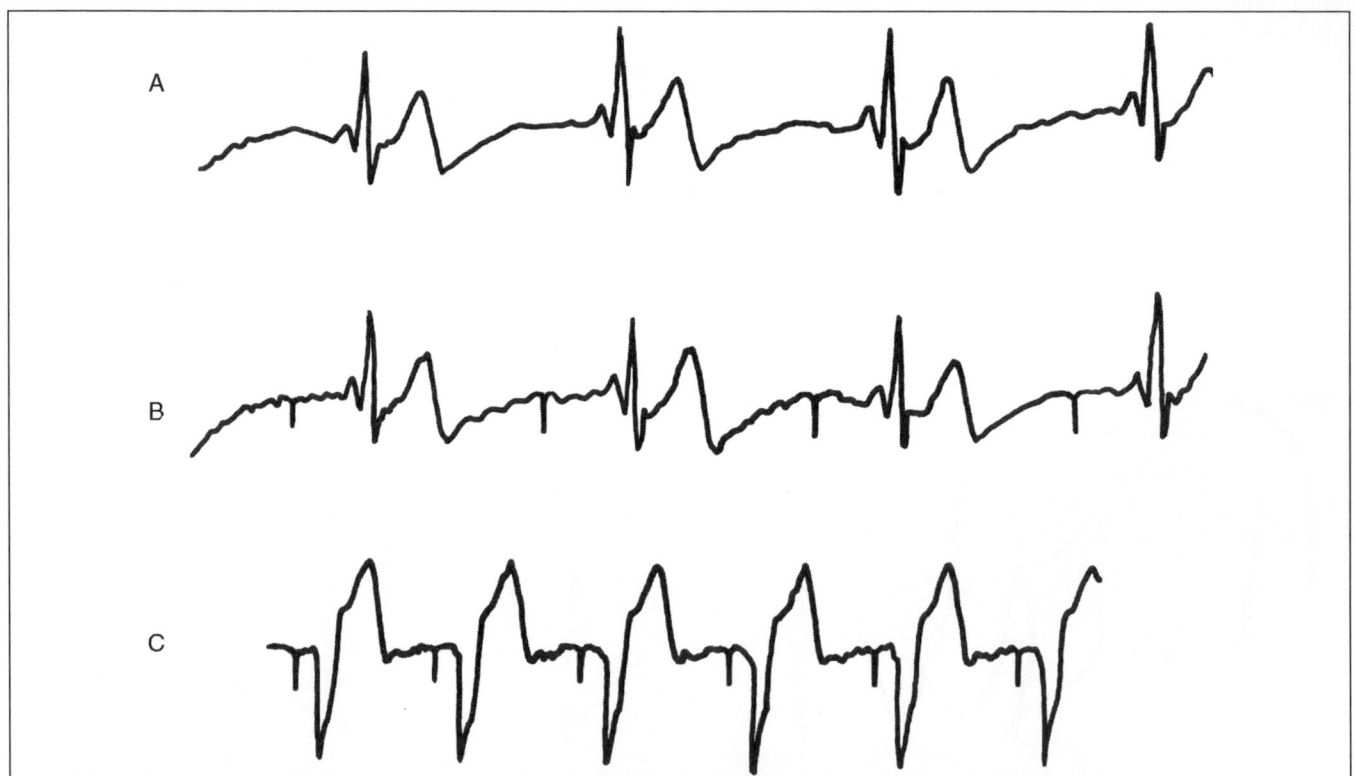

FIGURE 20-4 Assessing electrocardiographic capture with transcutaneous pacing. *A.* Native patient bradycardic rhythm. *B.* No capture as pacing is below the threshold level. *C.* Capture and pacing is above the threshold level.

TABLE 20-1. COMMON CAUSES OF FAILURE TO CAPTURE AND SUGGESTED SOLUTIONS

Etiology	Solution
Suboptimal electrode placement	Reposition electrodes, avoiding the spine, scapula, and sternum
Negative electrode placed posteriorly	Place negative electrode anteriorly over the cardiac apex or the V_3 lead position
Poor skin-electrode contact	Clean skin of sweat and debris; dry skin thoroughly; trim hair
Faulty electrical contact	Check electrical connections
Generator battery depletion	Change battery; plug generator into an electric outlet
Increased intrathoracic air	Reduce positive-pressure ventilation; relieve pneumothorax
Pericardial effusion	Pericardiocentesis; pericardial window
Myocardial ischemia/metabolic derangement	CPR; ventilation; correct acidosis; correct hypoxia; correct electrolyte abnormalities
High threshold	Use stimuli of longer pulse width

SOURCE: Modified from Ellenbogen.[4]

pacing. If not contraindicated, consider using parenteral analgesics and/or sedatives. Capturing should be evaluated periodically, as pacing thresholds may increase with prolonged pacing. The skin of the thorax under the pacemaker patches should be evaluated periodically. If erythema or signs of thermal burns are present, reposition the electrodes. This is especially important in patients who are unconscious or have an altered mental status, as they cannot complain of pain.

COMPLICATIONS

Patients who are conscious or who regain consciousness during transcutaneous pacing will experience discomfort because of pectoral muscle contractions. On higher levels of current output, the patient may experience strong, painful "knocks" on the chest. Table 20-2 lists some common causes for painful transcutaneous pacing, with suggested solutions.

Coughing may occur due to diaphragmatic pacing. Analgesia with narcotics and sedation with benzodiazepines may be necessary to make this discomfort more tolerable until transvenous cardiac pacing can be instituted. This discomfort has been minimized with

TABLE 20-2. CAUSES OF PAINFUL TRANSCUTANEOUS PACING AND SUGGESTED SOLUTIONS

Etiology	Solution
Conductive foreign body beneath electrode	Remove foreign body
Electrode over skin abrasions (shaved)	Reposition electrodes; avoid shaving beneath electrodes
Apprehensive patient or low pain tolerance	Administer parenteral narcotics and/or benzodiazepines
Sweat or salt deposits, saline, conductive jelly, blood, or vomitus on skin	Cleanse and dry skin
High threshold to pacing	Use longer pulse-width stimuli

SOURCE: Modified from Ellenbogen.[4]

newer designs for pacemakers and electrodes. Up to two-thirds of patients describe their experience with transcutaneous pacing as tolerable.

Third-degree burns have been reported in pediatric patients where improper or prolonged transcutaneous cardiac pacing was used. Frequent skin inspection with electrode repositioning can minimize this complication.

SUMMARY

Transcutaneous cardiac pacing is a temporary method of cardiac pacing in patients with severe symptomatic bradyarrhythmias due to high-grade AV blocks, sinus node dysfunction, bradysystolic cardiac arrest, or rarely for overdrive pacing to suppress ventricular and supraventricular tachyarrhythmias. It is comparatively easy to perform and requires minimal training. Transcutaneous cardiac pacing is contraindicated in bradycardic patients due to severe hypothermia. Once capture is achieved, the current output should be set at a level slightly higher (5 to 10 mA) than the pacing threshold. Successful transcutaneous cardiac pacing can be established in 80 to 90 percent of patients. Discomfort and pain due to muscle contraction are the most common side effects of transcutaneous cardiac pacing. Most patients will require sedation to tolerate transcutaneous cardiac pacing for a significant length of time.

REFERENCES

1. Zoll PM, Linethal AJ, Norman LR: Treatment of unexpected cardiac arrest by external electric stimulation of the heart. *N Engl J Med* 1956; 254:541–546.
2. Syverud SA, Hedges JR, Dalsey WC, et al: Hemodynamics of transcutaneous cardiac pacing. *Am J Emerg Med* 1986; 4:17–20.
3. Dalsey WC, Syverud SA, Trott A: Transcutaneous cardiac pacing. *J Emerg Med* 1984; 1:201–205.
4. Ellenbogen KA: *Cardiac Pacing*, 2nd ed. Cambridge, MA: Blackwell, 1996:168–173.

5. Cummins RO: *Advanced Cardiac Life Support.* Dallas American Heart Association, 1997, chap 5, 1–8.

6. Gregoratos G, Cheitlin MD, Conill A, et al: ACC/AHA Guidelines for implantation of cardiac pacemakers and antiarrhythmic devices. *J Am Coll Cardiol* 1998; 31(5):1175–1209.

7. Hedges JR, Feero S, Shltz B, et al: Prehospital transcutaneous cardiac pacing for symptomatic bradycardia. *PACE Pacing Clin Electrophysiol* 1991; 14:1473–1478.

8. Syverud SA: Cardiac pacing. *Emerg Med Clin North Am* 1988; 6:197–215.

9. Syverud SA, Dasley WC, Hedges JR: Transcutaneous and transvenous cardiac pacing for early bradysystolic cardiac arrest. *Ann Emerg Med* 1986; 15:121–124.

10. Zoll PM, Zoll RH, Falk RH, et al: External noninvasive temporary cardiac pacing: clinical trials. *Circulation* 1985; 71:937–944.

11. Eitel DR, Guzzardi LJ, Stein SE, et al: Noninvasive transcutaneous cardiac pacing in prehospital cardiac arrest. *Ann Emerg Med* 1987; 16:531–534.

12. Barthell E, Troiano P, Olson D, et al: Prehospital external cardiac pacing: a prospective, controlled clinical trial. *Ann Emerg Med* 1988; 17:1221–1226.

13. Hedges JR, Syverud SA, Dasely WC, et al: Prehospital trial of emergency transcutaneous cardiac pacing. *Circulation* 1987; 76:1337–1343.

14. Cummins RO, Graves JR, Halstrom A, et al: Out-of-hospital transcutaneous pacing by emergency medical technicians in patients with asystolic cardiac arrest. *N Engl J Med* 1993; 328:1377–1382.

15. Paris PM, Stewart RD, Kaplan RM, et al: Transcutaneous pacing for bradysystolic cardiac arrests in prehospital care. *Ann Emerg Med* 1985; 14:320–323.

16. Ryan TJ, Anderson JL, Antman EM, et al: ACC/AHA guidelines for management of patients with acute myocardial infarction. *J Am Coll Cardiol* 1996; 28(5):1328–1428.

17. Estes NA III, Deering TF, Manolis AS, et al: External cardiac programmed stimulation for noninvasive termination of sustained supraventricular and ventricular tachycardia. *Am J Cardiol* 1989; 63:177–183.

18. Rosenthal ME, Samato NJ, Marchlinski FE, et al: Noninvasive cardiac pacing for termination of sustained, uniform ventricular tachycardia. *Am J Cardiol* 1986; 58:561–562.

19. Altamura G, Bianconi, Boccaamo R, et al: Treatment of ventricular and supraventricular tachyarrhythmias by transcutaneous cardiac pacing. *PACE Pacing Clin Electrophysiol* 1989; 12:331–338.

20. Best R, Syverud SA, Nowak RM: Trauma and hypothermia. *Am J Emerg Med* 1985; 3:48–55.

21. Zoll PM, Zoll RH, Belgard AH: External noninvasive electric stimulation of the heart. *Crit Care Med* 1981; 9:393–394.

22. *Cook County Hospital Policy: Application of Temporary External Chest Pacing.* Chicago: Cook County Hospital, 1997:1–5.

23. Syverud SA, Hedges JA: Emergency transcutaneous cardiac pacing, in Roberts JR, Hedges JR (eds): *Clinical Procedures in Emergency Medicine.* Philadelphia: Saunders, 1998:225–231.

24. Falk RH, Ngai STA, Kumanki DJ, et al: Cardiac activation during external cardiac pacing. *PACE Pacing Clin Electrophysiol* 1987; 10:503–506.

25. Klein LS, Miles WM, Heger JJ, et al: Transcutaneous pacing: patient tolerance, strength-interval relations and feasibility for programmed electrical stimulation. *Am J Cardiol* 1988; 62:1126–1129.

26. Kelly JS, Royster RL, Argent KC, et al: Efficacy of noninvasive transcutaneous cardiac pacing in patients undergoing cardiac surgery. *Anesthesia* 1989; 70:747–751.

Chapter 21
TRANSTHORACIC CARDIAC PACING

James T. Thomas
Ratnakar S. Rajanahally

INTRODUCTION

The survival rates for all types of cardiac arrest with standard Advanced Cardiac Life Support (ACLS) regimens ranges from 8.5 to 28.5 percent.[1-3] Survival rates for patients with asystolic or pulseless idioventricular rhythm are quite low, with mortality rates close to 100 percent.[4-6] Obviously, any technique or therapy that improves these statistics would be highly desirable and expected to be associated with poor results.

Transthoracic cardiac pacing is the technique of pacing the heart with an electrode introduced percutaneously into the ventricular cavity using a needle trocar introducer. Bipolar pacing wires are commonly used today. The transthoracic cardiac pacing technique is faster and simpler to implement than transvenous cardiac pacing. It requires no venous access, blood flow, fluoroscopy, or electrocardiograph for guidance.

Although the history of electrical stimulation of the heart dates back to the mid-eighteenth century, Zoll accomplished the first successful clinical application of external cardiac pacing in 1952, utilizing externally applied closed chest pacing for a Stoke-Adams attack.[7] Transthoracic cardiac pacing was introduced in 1957 and became popular in the 1960s. With the development of sophisticated transvenous pacemaker electrodes, the technique of transthoracic cardiac pacing fell out of vogue. Recent improvements in the design of the transcutaneous cardiac pacing unit will allow this noninvasive device to be well tolerated by patients. The capture rates for transcutaneous pacing is over 80 percent and hence preferred as the initial mode of cardiac pacing. There is limited literature on transthoracic cardiac pacing; it comprises mostly anecdotal data and retrospective analysis rather than prospective randomized trials. The benefits and complications of transthoracic pacing are not well defined.

ANATOMY AND PATHOPHYSIOLOGY

The heart is the only muscle of the body that generates its own electrical impulses. Its automaticity and subsequent rhythmic contractions propel blood to the tissues of the body. The initial cardiac impulse starts in the right atrium of the heart at the sinoatrial (SA) node. The sympathetic and parasympathetic nervous system controls the rate of impulse generation at the SA node. Once the electrical stimulus is generated, it is conducted along the internal conduction pathways of the heart to the muscular atrial and ventricular walls. A delicate balance between electrolyte flux to create action potentials, myocardial integrity to allow impulses to become contractions, and an intact conduction system must be maintained. Conduction system problems are often the result of inadequate blood flow to the heart due to ventricular infarction and coronary artery occlusion. The blood supply to the conduction system of the heart originates from the right coronary artery. Occlusion of the right coronary artery can result in arrhythmias and conduction delays.

INDICATIONS

The indications for transthoracic cardiac pacing are not well described. General guidelines suggest that when the time and clinical situation permits, cardiac pacing should be done using the transvenous route, employing fluoroscopy or a flow-directed pacemaker catheter.[9] **When time is a factor, transthoracic cardiac pacing may be performed if a transcutaneous pacemaker is not available or its use has been unsuccessful.**

Transthoracic cardiac pacing can be used in asystole, although no clear-cut indication or guidelines exist.

There are no prospective studies addressing the success rates and it is therefore impossible to comment on changes in survival rate, percentage of capture, or frequency of complications if the procedure was used routinely. Preston et al estimated a 40 percent success rate in achieving pacing by the transthoracic route.[10] Asystole and slow idioventricular rhythm as causes of cardiac arrest are associated with mortality rates close to 100 percent[12] and are indications for emergency cardiac pacing.[17–19] We would expect that transthoracic cardiac pacing would be most effective following cardiac arrest from primary cardiac disease.[9] Transthoracic cardiac pacing may not be effective in cardiac arrest secondary to hypovolemia (trauma), severe electrolyte or acid-base abnormalities, sepsis, or drug intoxication. Transthoracic cardiac pacing may be lifesaving when bradycardia or asystole secondary to prolonged ischemia during hypovolemic shock persists despite correction of the underlying pathology.

The use of transthoracic cardiac pacing in unstable patients is more controversial. Transthoracic cardiac pacing may be considered in patients with unstable sinus bradycardia, junctional bradycardia, atrial fibrillation with high-degree atrioventricular (AV) block, and AV dissociation with inadequate ventricular response, producing pulmonary edema, seizures, ventricular fibrillation, or ventricular tachycardia.[9] Transthoracic cardiac pacing is a simple procedure and can be accomplished rapidly. It should be considered if a transcutaneous pacemaker is not available or has been unsuccessful in pacing unstable patients.

CONTRAINDICATIONS

Transthoracic cardiac pacing should not be performed in stable, awake patients. It is also contraindicated if the patient has abnormalities that could be quickly and easily corrected by medication. In stable and awake patients, transcutaneous or transvenous cardiac pacing is the preferred mode of pacing.

Transthoracic cardiac pacing may be ineffective in electromechanical dissociation and ventricular fibrillation. In ventricular fibrillation, the heart becomes insensitive to pacemaker activity, and in electromechanical dissociation, any mode of pacing is ineffective.[11,13–15] Bellet et al[16] demonstrated that a pacemaker was ineffective in patients with prolonged cardiac arrest. Patients with cardiac arrest for more than 5 to 10 minutes could not be resuscitated with the use of cardiac pacing; but patients who had pacemakers placed within 2 to 4 minutes after cardiac standstill were successfully resuscitated. Hence, as shown in many studies, transthoracic cardiac pacing may be ineffective if used as a last alternative, as any technique of pacing would be.

EQUIPMENT

Transthoracic cardiac pacing wires/kit
Pacemaker generator
10 mL syringe
Povidone iodine solution
Water-soluble lubricant
Sterile gauze squares
Sterile drapes
Sterile gloves
Mask
Cap

The widely used instrumentation for transthoracic cardiac pacing is a sterile, one-time-use, prepackaged kit. One example is the Elecath 11-KTM1 kit (Figure 21-1). The apparatus consists of a 37 cm bipolar J-shaped pacing wire, a 6 inch 18 gauge blunt-end steel canula with a pointed inner trocar, and a plastic electrical connector that accepts the pacing wire and can be attached to a battery-powered external pacemaker generator. The canula and trocar function as a catheter-over-the-needle.

PATIENT PREPARATION

Explain to the patient the risks and benefits of the procedure if they are awake and alert. A signed consent is not required and time is often lacking to obtain a signature. Document in the medical record that the patient was informed of the risks and benefits of the procedure. Place the patient supine. Clean the chest and subxiphoid area of any dirt and debris. Apply povidone iodine to the chest and subxiphoid area. Allow it to dry if time permits. Apply sterile drapes to delineate a sterile field.

Cardiopulmonary resuscitation (CPR) can be continued during most of the procedure but should be stopped while the intracardiac needle is being inserted to avoid possible damage to the lung or myocardium. Full ventilation of the lungs is recommended during subxiphoid cannula placement to depress the diaphragm and thus minimize the risk of injury to the liver and stomach. Insert a nasogastric tube to decompress the stomach prior to performing the procedure.

The physician should prepare themself and the equipment. If time permits, put on a cap, mask, sterile gloves, and sterile gown. Open the transthoracic cardiac pacing kit onto a sterile field. Lubricate the trocar liberally and insert it securely into the steel cannula.

TECHNIQUE

Quickly identify the anatomic landmarks necessary to perform this procedure and determine the approach

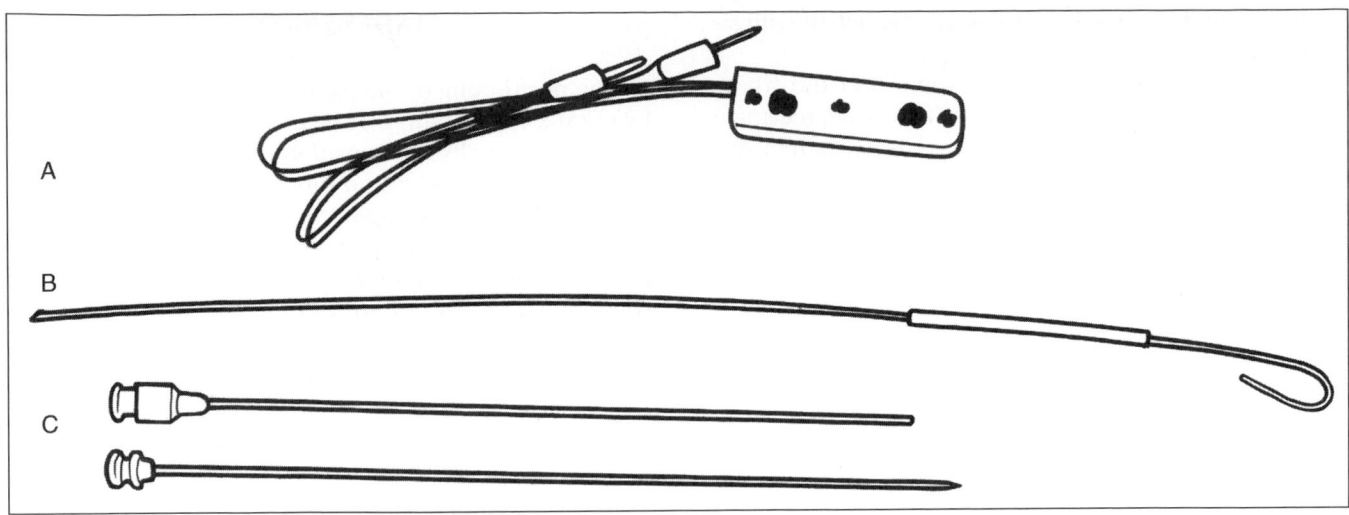

FIGURE 21-1 Equipment required for transthoracic cardiac pacing. *A.* Electrical connector. *B.* Bipolar pacing wire with a sleeve. *C.* Blunt steel cannula with pointed trocar.

to be used. The cannula-over-the-trocar can be inserted through the left fifth intercostal space either parasternally, 4 cm lateral to the midsternal line, or 6 cm lateral to the midsternal line (Figure 21-2*A*). The tip of the cannula-over-the-trocar should be aimed toward the second costal cartilage. Alternatively, the cannula-over-the-trocar can

be inserted through the left xiphocostal junction and aimed toward either the right shoulder, left shoulder, or sternal notch (Figure 21-2*B*). The simplest landmarks to identify and the quickest approach is to insert the cannula-over-the-trocar at the left xiphocostal junction and aimed toward the sternal notch. The preferred

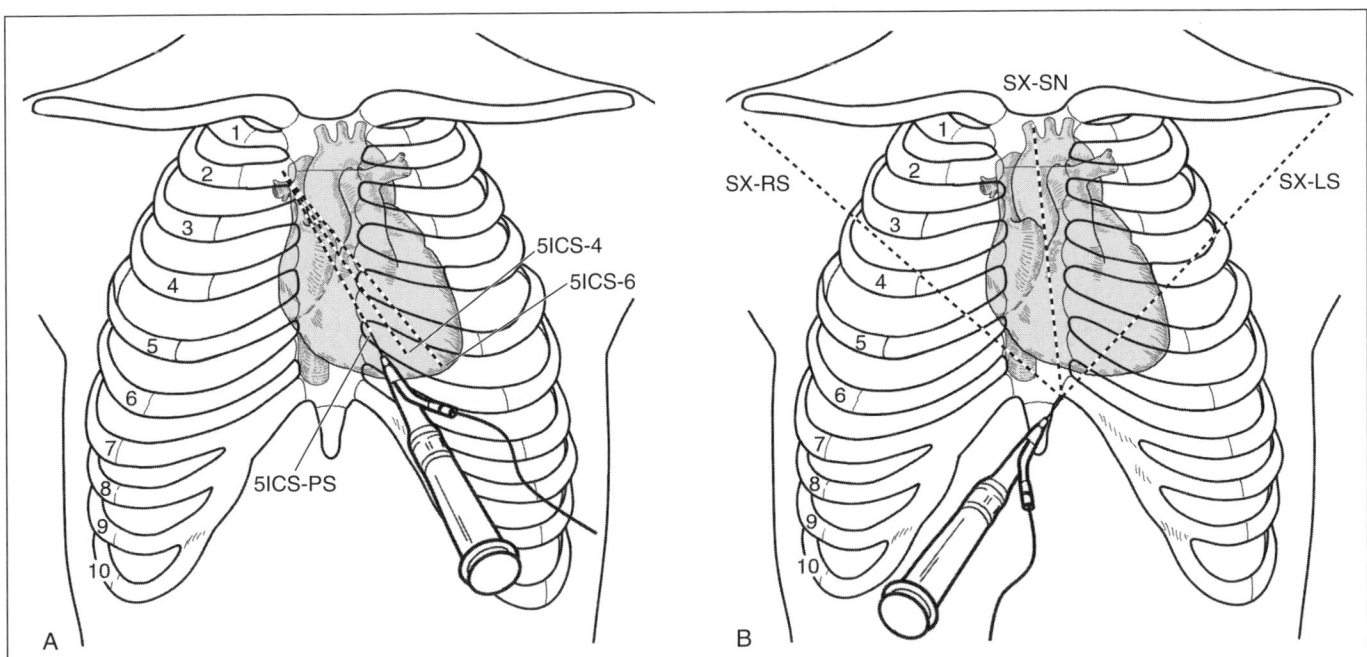

FIGURE 21-2 Placement of a percutaneous transthoracic cardiac pacemaker. *A.* Parasternal approaches. 5ICS-PS = fifth intercostal space immediately to the left of the sternum, 5ICS-4 = fifth intercostal space, 4 cm from the midsternal line, 5ICS-6 = fifth intercostal space, 6 cm from the midsternal line. *B.* Subxiphoid approaches. SX-RS = subxiphoid–right shoulder, SX-SN = subxiphoid–sternal notch, SX-LS = subxiphoid–left shoulder.

landmarks and approach are those with which the physician is most comfortable.

Briefly stop CPR. Insert the cannula-over-the-trocar from the left xiphocostal region at a 30 to 40 degree angle to the skin and directed toward the sternal notch. Advance the cannula-over-the-trocar approximately three-fourths of its length. Hold and stabilize the cannula and withdraw the trocar. Attach a 10 mL syringe to the cannula. Apply negative pressure to the syringe. If the cannula is within the ventricle, the aspiration of blood into the syringe confirms proper positioning. If blood is not aspirated, withdraw the cannula and restart the procedure.

Insert the transcutaneous pacing wire. Advance the plastic sheath over the pacing wire until it straightens out and covers the J-shaped end of the pacing wire. Insert the plastic sheath into the cannula hub. Advance the pacing wire through the cannula and into the ventricle. Stop advancing the pacing wire when 4 to 5 cm remains outside the cannula. **No resistance should be felt while the pacing wire is being advanced.** If resistance is felt, the cannula is not within the ventricle. Remove the cannula and pacing wire as a unit and restart the procedure. When it is inside the ventricle, the pacing wire will reform its J shape. Hold the pacing wire securely. Withdraw the cannula over the pacing wire. **Do not release the hold on the proximal end of the pacing wire outside the patient's thorax, so as to prevent it from slipping inside the thorax.**

Insert the proximal end of the pacing wire into the plastic connector. Secure it with the screws in the body of the connector. Connect the positive and negative terminals of the plastic connector to the pacemaker generator. Turn on the pacemaker generator. Set the pacing rate at 70 to 90 beats per minute in an asynchronous mode. Set the current output to the maximum milliampere rate on the pacemaker generator. After myocardial capture of the electrical stimulus is demonstrated (each pacer spike followed by a QRS complex), lower the current output until 1:1 pacing is lost. Gradually increase the current output to attain stimulation threshold when 1:1 capture is regained. The optimal current output is two to three times the stimulation threshold. Change the mode of the pacemaker to a demand pacemaker with a backup rate of 60 to 70 beats per minute. A complete description of the functioning of the pacemaker generator is presented in Chapter 22.

Pacer spikes should be seen on the electrocardiogram (ECG). If not, check the contact between the pacer wire and electrical connector. Check the batteries in the pacemaker energy source. Pacer spikes not followed by myocardial capture usually indicate inadequate positioning of the pacing electrode. Gently manipulate the transthoracic pacemaker wire to change its position.

ASSESSMENT

The positioning of the pacing wire should be verified by chest x-ray. Obtain a 12-lead ECG to document capture and to verify the positioning of the pacing wire based on the QRS configuration in the ECG. A left bundle-branch-block configuration will be demonstrated on the ECG if the pacing wire is in the right ventricle. If the pacing wire is in the right atrium or left ventricle, it will still pace the myocardium but the ECG will have a different QRS configuration. If the patient is in AV block, an atrially positioned pacing wire will be ineffective.

AFTERCARE

If the patient survives, secure the pacing wire to the skin with 3–0 nylon suture. A transvenous or permanent pacemaker should be inserted as soon as possible. Consult a Cardiologist immediately and admit the patient to an intensive care unit.

COMPLICATIONS

Analysis of the complications of transthoracic cardiac pacing is greatly limited by the paucity of short-term survivors and the absence of radiographic or pathologic evaluation of nonsurvivors. Potential complications include laceration of the right atrium, ventricles, coronary arteries, great vessels, vena cava, stomach, liver, and lung. Hemopericardium is a ubiquitous finding in some autopsy studies, and cardiac tamponade has been reported.[20] Pneumothorax has been reported and is a particular concern in persons receiving positive-pressure ventilation.[21]

SUMMARY

The technique of transthoracic cardiac pacing has been clinically feasible for more than 30 years. Yet, the procedure remains controversial and is limited by the paucity of prospective randomized clinical trials and guidelines. There is no clear understanding of the effect of transthoracic cardiac pacing on the outcome of cardiac arrest and the complications associated with the procedure. Most of the available information comes from animal studies, retrospective analysis, and anecdotal data.

The technique of transthoracic cardiac pacing is simple and can be performed in less than a minute. Transthoracic cardiac pacing may be useful in the setting of cardiac arrest with asystole or a pulseless idioventricular rhythm. It may be performed if a transcutaneous cardiac pacing system is not available or not effective. In unstable patients with drug-resistant bradycardia producing cardiovascular collapse or lethal escape rhythms whose clinical condition does not warrant a delay to insert a transvenous pacing catheter, transthoracic cardiac pacing can be initiated promptly.

REFERENCES

1. Roberts JR, Greenberg MI, Crisanti JW, et al: Successful use of emergency transthoracic pacing in bradyasystolic cardiac arrest. *Ann Emerg Med* 1984; 13:277–283.
2. Hollingsworth JH: The results of cardiopulmonary resuscitation: a 3 year university hospital experience. *Ann Intern Med* 1969; 71:459–466.
3. Lemire JG, Johnson AL: Is cardiac resuscitation worth while—a decade of experience. *N Engl J Med* 1972; 286:970–972.
4. Iseri LT, Humphrey SB, Siner EJ: Pre-hospital bradyasystolic cardiac arrest. *Ann Intern Med* 1978; 88:741–745.
5. White JD: Transthoracic pacing in cardiac asystole. *Am J Emerg Med* 1983; 1:264–266.
6. Myerberg RJ, Conde CA, Sung RJ, et al: Clinical, electrophysiologic and hemodynamic profile of patient resuscitated from pre-hospital cardiac arrest. *Am J Med* 1980; 68:568–576.
7. Zoll PM: Resuscitation of the heart in ventricular stand still by external electric stimulation. *N Engl J Med* 1952; 247:768–771.
8. Thevenet A, Hodges PC, Lillehei CW: The use of myocardial electrode inserted percutaneously for control of complete A-V block by an artificial pacemaker. *Dis Chest* 1958; 34:621–631.
9. Roberts JR, Greenberg MI: Emergency transthoracic pacemaker. *Ann Emerg Med* 1981; 10:600–612.
10. Preston TA: The use of pacemaker for the treatment of acute arrhythmias. *Heart Lung* 1977; 6(2):249–255.
11. Raizes G, Wagner G, Hackel D: Instantaneous non-arrhythmic cardiac death in acute myocardial infarction. *Am J Cardiol* 1977; 39:1–6.
12. Brown CG, Gurley HT, Hutchins GM, et al: Injuries associated with percutaneous placement of transthoracic pacemaker. *Ann Emerg Med* 1985; 14:223–228.
13. Gottlieb R, Chung EK: Techniques of temporary pacing, in Chung EK (ed): *Artificial Cardiac Pacing—A Practical Approach.* Baltimore: Williams & Wilkins, 1978:150–160.
14. Daicel GR, Miscia VF: Shock, pacemakers and surgical therapy, in Eliot RS (ed): *Acute Cardiac Emergency.* Mount Kisco, NY: Futura, 1972:253.
15. Dreifus LS, Chaudry KR, Otawa S: Temporary and emergency cardiac pacing, in Naclerio E (ed): *Cardiac Pacing.* Philadelphia: Lea & Febiger, 1979:133–143.
16. Bellet S, Muller OF, DeLeon AC, et al: The use of an internal pacemaker in the treatment of cardiac arrest and slow heart rates. *Arch Intern Med* 1960; 105:361–371.
17. Johnson RA, Haber E, Austen WG: *The Practice of Cardiology.* Boston: Little, Brown, 1981:28.
18. Meltzer LE, Cohen HE: The incidence of arrhythmias associated with acute myocardial infarction, in Meltzer LE, Dunning AJ (eds): *Textbook of Coronary Care.* Philadelphia: Charles Press, 1972.
19. White JD, Brown CG: Immediate transthoracic pacing for cardiac asystole in an emergency department setting. *Am J Emerg Med* 1985; 3:125–128.
20. Tintinalli JE, White BC: Transthoracic pacing during CPR. *Ann Emerg Med* 1981; 10:113–116.
21. Le K, Goldschlager N: Temporary cardiac pacing in the intensive care unit. *J Intens Care Unit* 1996; 11(2):57–78.

Chapter 22
TRANSVENOUS CARDIAC PACING

Daryl D. Wilson
Eric F. Reichman

INTRODUCTION

Emergency cardiac pacing can be accomplished by several methods. These include epicardial, esophageal, transcutaneous, transthoracic, and transvenous pacing. pacing can be a temporizing and lifesaving technique that should be familiar to physicians working in an Emergency Department. It will allow the patient to maintain a cardiac rhythm while providing oxygen and nutrients to the vital organs.

The earliest use of electricity to stimulate the heart can be found in an essay written in the late 1700s.[1] It discusses the use of electric current and artificial ventilation to revive victims of drowning. Transvenous pacing was first attempted on dogs in 1905 by Floresco. The technology and technique have since been developed to allow successful transvenous pacing in humans. It involves the placement of a pacing wire through the central venous circulation and into direct contact with the myocardium of the right ventricle.

ANATOMY AND PATHOPHYSIOLOGY

The heart is the only muscle of the body that generates its own electric impulses. Its automaticity and subsequent rhythmic contractions propel blood to the tissues of the body. The initial cardiac impulse starts in the right atrium of the heart at the sinoatrial (SA) node. The sympathetic and parasympathetic nervous systems control the rate of impulse generation at the SA node. Once the electric stimulus is generated, it is conducted along the internal conduction pathways of the heart to the muscular atrial and ventricular walls. A delicate balance between electrolyte flux to create action potentials, myocardial integrity to allow impulses to become contrac-

tions, and an intact conduction system must be maintained. Conduction system problems are often the result of inadequate blood flow to the heart due to ventricular infarction and coronary artery occlusion. The blood supply to the conduction system of the heart originates from the right coronary artery. Occlusion of the right coronary artery can result in arrhythmias and conduction delays.

A transvenous pacing catheter may be introduced through the femoral, internal jugular, or subclavian vein. **In the Emergency Department, the right internal jugular vein or left subclavian vein are the primary sites (Figure 22-1). These routes allow a more direct and easy access for the pacing catheter to enter the right ventricle.** The right internal jugular vein is preferred, as it allows a relatively straight line of access through the superior vena cava and right atrium into the right ventricle.[2] The other routes are technically more difficult to use and often require fluoroscopy for proper placement of the pacing catheter.

In children, the femoral vein is often used to insert a transvenous cardiac pacing catheter (Figure 22-2). The child's relatively large head and short neck makes access to the internal jugular vein difficult. The subclavian vein in a child is situated more posterior to the clavicle than in an adult. This makes it more difficult to access the subclavian vein while increasing the chance of causing a pneumothorax. Insertion of the pacing catheter via the femoral vein often requires fluoroscopy.

INDICATIONS

The indications for transvenous pacing are the same as for other methods of cardiac pacing. Patients with symptomatic bradycardia unresponsive to drug therapy,

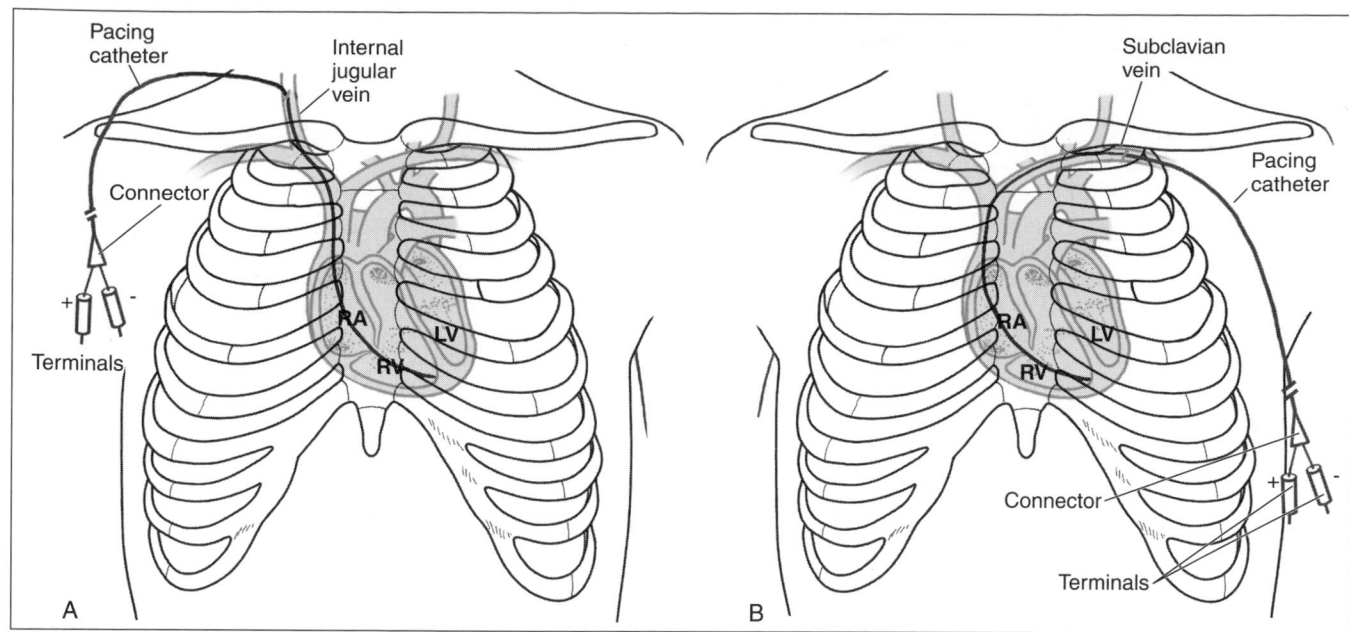

FIGURE 22-1 Common sites for introducing a transvenous pacing catheter. *A.* The right internal jugular vein. *B.* The left subclavian vein.

conduction delays that may degenerate into complete heart block, atrioventricular dissociation, and ventricular arrhythmias that require overdrive pacing can benefit from transvenous pacing.[1–3] Transvenous pacing may be used in patients who do not tolerate or whose heart does not capture with transcutaneous pacing. If a permanent pacemaker is not functioning, a transvenous pacing catheter may be temporarily inserted to pace the myocardium. A more complete discussion on the indications for cardiac pacing is presented in Chapter 20, on transcutaneous cardiac pacing.

CONTRAINDICATIONS

Patients who are hypothermic should not have a transvenous pacing catheter inserted into the heart. These patients have increased irritability of the myocardium and are prone to life-threatening ventricular fibrillation if the pacing wire contacts the heart muscle.[1,2] Digoxin toxicity and other drug ingestions that may increase the irritability of the myocardium are relative contraindications to the placement of a transvenous pacing catheter. Patients who are asystolic for extended periods of time have a low likelihood of successful resuscitation.[2] These patients are not candidates for transvenous pacer placement.

EQUIPMENT

Flexible transvenous cardiac pacing catheter (Figure 22-3)
Pacemaker generator (Figure 22-4)
Spare battery for pacemaker
Sterile drapes, gloves, and gown
Povidone iodine solution
Cordis or Swan introducer catheter kit, one size larger than the pacing catheter
Cardiac monitor
Local anesthetic solution
3–0 nylon suture
Gauze squares
Skin tape
Alligator clips and connecting wire
Towels for shoulder rolls
Defibrillator
Airway management equipment
Resuscitative drugs

The pacemaker generator is a simple device (Figure 22-4). An example is the Medtronic 5375 demand pulse generator (Figures 22-4*A* and *B*). Newer models of pacemaker generators (Figures 22-4*C* and *D*) have digital displays and other more sophisticated pacing options but function essentially the same as older models. **The**

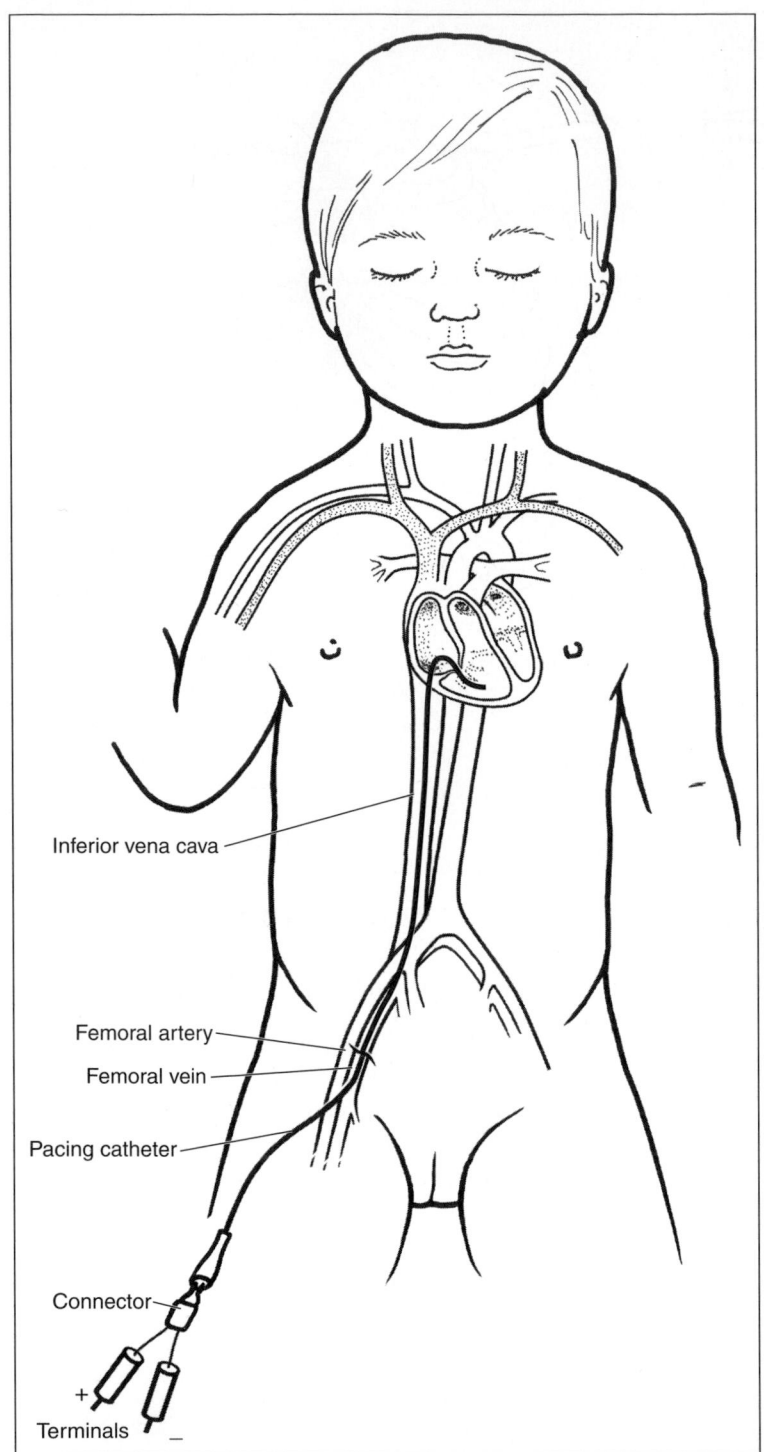

Inferior vena cava

Femoral artery
Femoral vein

Pacing catheter

Connector

+
Terminals _

FIGURE 22-2 The femoral vein is used in children to access the central venous circulation and introduce a transvenous pacing catheter.

Emergency Physician must be familiar with the pacemaker generator and its use prior to needing it in an emergent situation. The on/off switch is used to turn the unit on. In the "on" position, a spring-loaded safety prevents the unit from accidentally being turned off. The rate-control dial allows the physician to adjust the number of pacing stimuli per minute. The upper rate limit is often inadequate if overdrive pacing is required. The pace indicator light is illuminated whenever a pacing stimulus is generated. The sense indicator light is illuminated whenever a cardiac impulse is sensed. The battery test button is used to determine if the battery has sufficient voltage to operate the pacemaker generator. Depress the battery test button to check the battery voltage. If both the pacing and sensing indicator lights illuminate simultaneously, the battery has sufficient

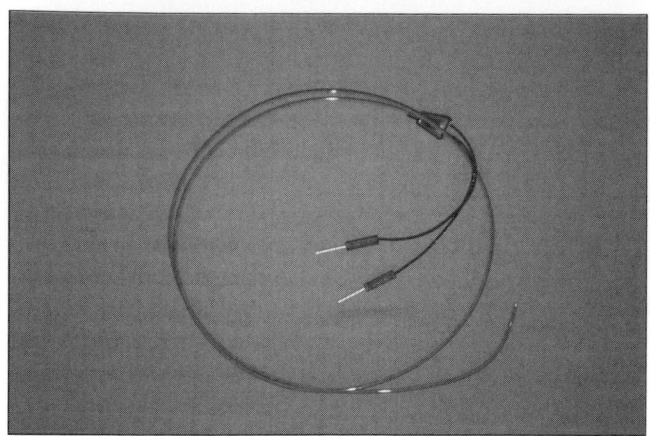

FIGURE 22-3 The flexible transvenous pacing catheter.

voltage. The output control dial is used to adjust the amplitude of the stimulus current. The sensitivity control dial is used to suppress the pulse generator. The bottom of the pacemaker has an access panel under which the battery is located. The top of the pacemaker has positive and negative terminals where the electrodes of the pacemaker catheter insert.

The pacemaker wires are enclosed in a catheter and come in a variety of lengths and sizes. They are typically 1 m in length with markings at intervals of 10 centimeters. They come in both flexible and rigid styles. The rigid catheters are not often used due to the possibility of myocardial perforation. The flexible catheters have a balloon at the tip, which allows the catheter to flow with the blood into the chambers of the heart.

The pacemaker catheter should be inserted under electrocardiographic (ECG) guidance. An insulated wire with an alligator clip at each end is required. One end is attached to the pacemaker wire and the other to the ECG lead. This allows the physician to observe the ECG waveforms as they change while the catheter is - advanced.[2–4] This technique is known as ECG positioning. It requires the patient to have intrinsic cardiac activity.

PATIENT PREPARATION

As with all procedures, the risks, benefits, and possible complications must be explained to the patient. If the patient is unable to consent, an appropriate representative may accept for the patient. The patient may also give verbal consent if they are unable to sign but fully understands the risks and benefits of the procedure. The physician should wear sterile surgical gloves and a gown, cap, and mask to decrease the risk of contamination and subsequent infection.

Place the patient supine and, if possible, in the Trendelenburg position. Place the patient on continuous pulse oximetry, cardiac monitoring, and supplemental oxygen. Establish peripheral intravenous access. Clean and prep the skin in a sterile fashion with povidone iodine at the site chosen to access the central venous system. If the internal jugular vein or the subclavian vein is being used as the site of vascular access, place rolled towels under the patient's shoulders. Turn the patient's head to the opposite side of venous access.

TECHNIQUE

Access the central venous circulation by placing a Swan or Cordis introducer. Refer to Chapter 38 for the complete details on inserting these catheters.

Prepare the pacing catheter (Figure 22-5). Attach the precordial lead V_1 to the pacemaker catheter negative terminal. This is accomplished using an insulated wire with an alligator clip at each end. Attach one alligator clip to the negative pacemaker wire. Attach the other alligator clip to the V_1 lead of the ECG monitor. Inflate the balloon with 1.5 mL of air in a container of sterile saline to assess the integrity of the balloon. The presence of bubbles in the saline indicates a balloon leak. Turn on the ECG monitor and set it to lead V_1. Touch the tip of the pacing catheter and observe the monitor to confirm that the monitor is recording. A large pressure wave should be seen that soon returns to baseline.

Insert the pacemaker catheter through the rubber diaphragm of the central venous introducer sheath. Advance the catheter 10 centimeters. This ensures that the balloon is past the introducer catheter and within the vascular system. Inflate the balloon with 1.5 mL of sterile saline. **Slowly advance the catheter while observing the ECG monitor (Figure 22-6).** In the subclavian or internal jugular vein, the P wave and the QRS complex are both small in amplitude and inverted (Figure 22-6A). In the superior vena cava, the P wave increases in amplitude but is still inverted while the QRS complex is unchanged (Figure 22-6B). When the pacing catheter reaches the right atrium, a large P wave with a negative polarity and a small QRS complex will be observed (Figure 22-6C). Continue to advance the catheter. As the lower atrium is entered, the P waves become upright and the QRS complex increases in amplitude (Figure 22-6D). Continue to advance the catheter into the right ventricle. The QRS complex should appear normal on the V_1 lead. When the catheter is floating freely in the right ventricle, the P waves are upright with a large-amplitude QRS complex (Figure 22-6E). Deflate the balloon and advance the catheter until ST-segment elevation is observed (Figure 22-6F). This indicates that the catheter is abutting the right ventricular wall.

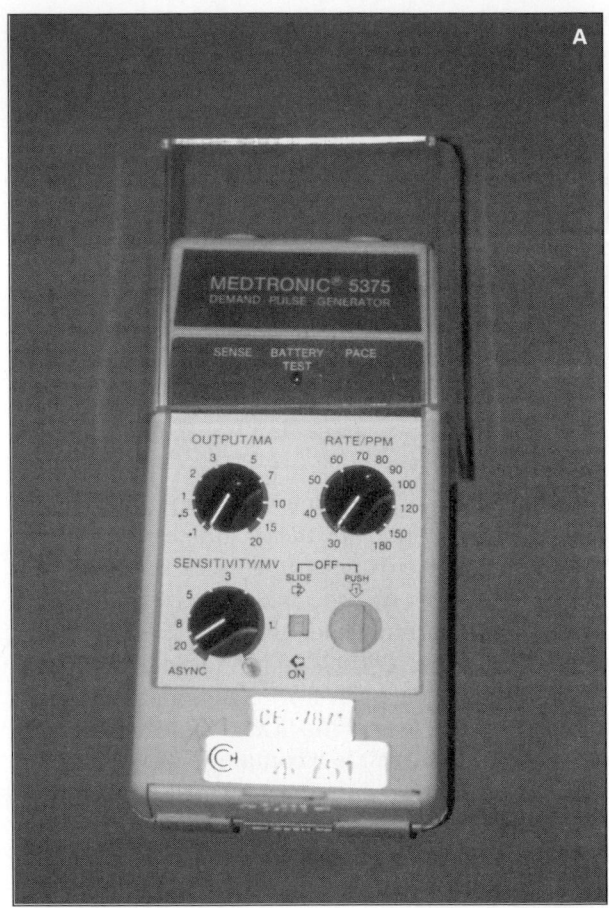

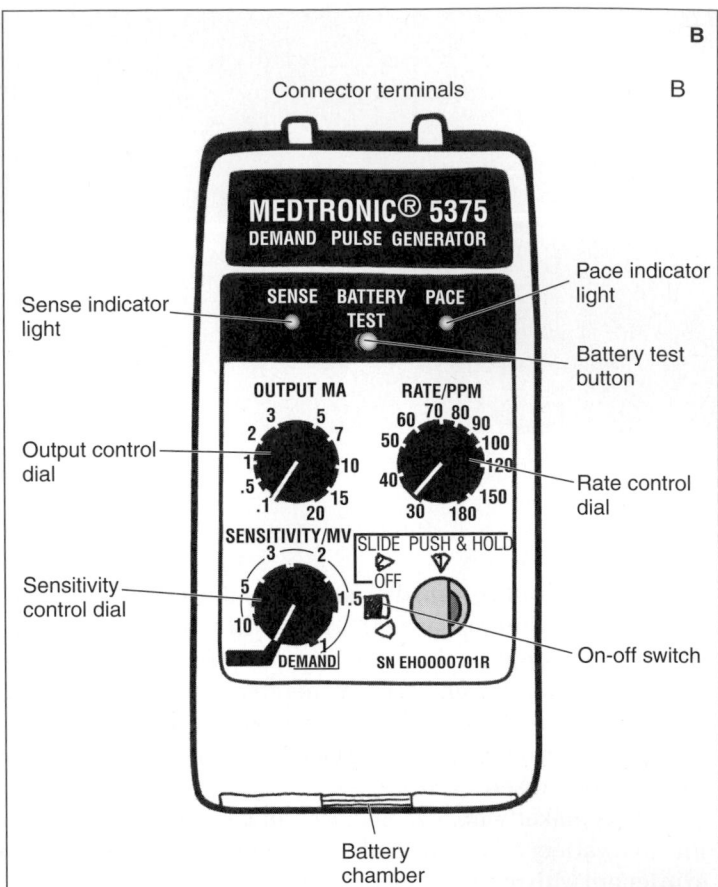

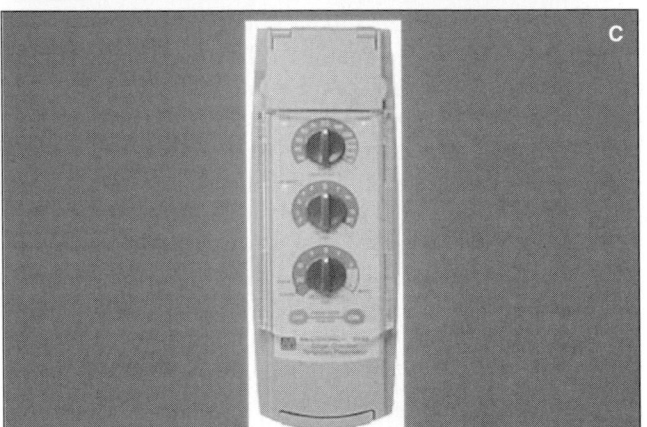

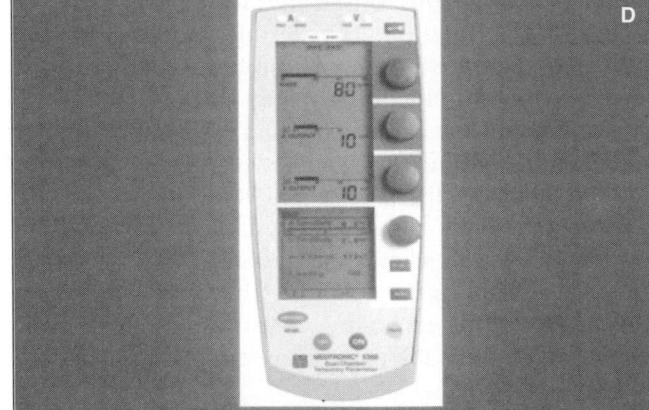

FIGURE 22-4 Examples of pacemaker generators.

Occasionally, the catheter may not enter the right ventricle or advance past the right ventricle. If the catheter exits the right atrium and enters the inferior vena cava, the amplitude of the P wave and QRS complex will decrease (Figure 22-6*G*). Withdraw the catheter several centimeters until the atrial waveforms are seen, then readvance the catheter. If the catheter exits the right ventricle and enters the pulmonary artery, the P wave will become negative and the QRS amplitude will decrease (Figure 22-6*H*). Withdraw the catheter several centimeters until the right ventricle waveforms are seen, then readvance the catheter.

Connect the pacemaker generator to the catheter (Figure 22-7). Disconnect the negative terminal of the pacemaker catheter from the ECG lead. Connect the pacemaker catheter terminals on the proximal end of the catheter to the negative and positive terminals of the pacemaker generator. Set the pacemaker generator on demand mode with a rate of 70 beats per minute. Start with 5 mA of energy on the output dial. Turn on the pace-

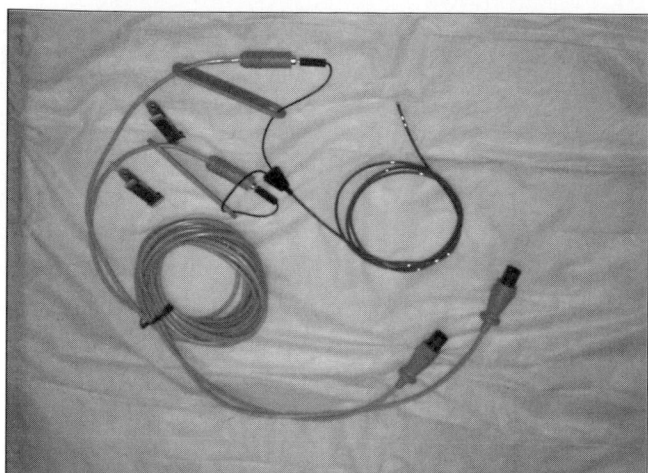

FIGURE 22-5 The negative pacemaker terminal is connected to an insulated wire. The insulated wire will be connected to the ECG lead V_1.

maker. Increase the energy until capture is seen on the monitor. This is signaled by pacing spikes and a wide QRS complex in lead V_1. **Once capture is attained, decrease the pacemaker generator output to just below where pacing stops. This is known as the threshold point. Resume pacing at 2 mA above the threshold point.**[2]

ALTERNATIVE TECHNIQUE

Blind transvenous catheter placement is an alternative to the above method. The pacing catheter is inserted without ECG guidance. This technique is often used when alligator clips are not available to connect the pacing catheter terminals to the ECG monitor. A flexible catheter should be used. **Never place a rigid catheter blindly due to the risk of myocardial perforation.**

Prepare the catheter. Test the balloon as mentioned previously. Make sure the pacemaker generator is off. Connect the pacemaker catheter terminals to the pacemaker generator. Insert the pacemaker catheter through the rubber diaphragm of the central venous introducer sheath. Advance the catheter 10 centimeters. Inflate the balloon with 1.5 mL of sterile saline.

Turn on the pacemaker. **Set the pacemaker on demand mode with a rate twice the patient's native heart rate.** This usually ranges from 80 to 120 beats per minute. Set the output dial to 1.5 to 2.0 mA.

Advance the catheter while observing the sensing indicator light. When the catheter enters the right ventricle, the sensing indicator will illuminate with every other native heartbeat. Stop advancing the catheter. Deflate the balloon. Increase the output dial to 5 mA. Slowly advance the catheter until ventricular capture occurs. **Do not advance the catheter more than 10 cm past the**

point where the sensing indicator began to illuminate. If ventricular capture is not successful within 10 cm, withdraw the catheter and rotate it 90 degrees. Readvance the catheter up to 10 centimeters. Continue to repeat the process until ventricular capture is successful. Once this occurs, slowly decrease the ventricular rate to 70 beats per minute.

AFTERCARE

Secure the pacing catheter by suturing it to the chest wall. Infiltrate subcutaneously with 2 mL of local anesthetic solution 1 cm from where the catheter exits the central venous sheath. Using 3–0 nylon, secure the catheter to the skin. Apply antibacterial ointment to the site where the pacing catheter exits the central venous sheath. Apply an adhesive dressing, such as Tegaderm, over the sheath and catheter. Obtain an ECG. It will show the characteristic left bundle branch block pattern. Obtain a postprocedural chest radiograph to assess the catheter position and rule out any pneumothorax. Admit the patient to an intensive care unit. Consult a Cardiologist for possible permanent pacemaker placement.

COMPLICATIONS

Perforation of the ventricular septum, the myocardium of the atria, or the free wall of the ventricle may take place during catheter placement. This is more commonly seen with the rigid catheters. If the pattern on the ECG changes from a left to a right bundle branch block, septal perforation should be suspected.[2,5] If there is an increase in the pacing threshold, septal perforation should also be suspected. Ventricular perforation can present as a failure to capture or as cardiac tamponade. When perforation is present, a friction rub may be audible on cardiac auscultation. Perforation of the inferior wall could stimulate and pace the diaphragm.[2,5] The treatment for these complications is to withdraw and reposition the pacing catheter. The patient must then be evaluated and observed for the possibility of cardiac tamponade.

Cardiac arrhythmias may occur during insertion of the pacing catheter. Ventricular arrhythmias can occur during the procedure and even after the procedure is completed. Immediately withdraw the catheter a few centimeters and observe the rhythm. If that resolves, readvance the catheter. A defibrillator and cardiac resuscitation drugs must be available to facilitate immediate treatment of any rhythm disturbance.[2,5]

In transvenous pacing, as with any procedure, infection can be a delayed complication. The most common organisms are skin flora. The types of infection can

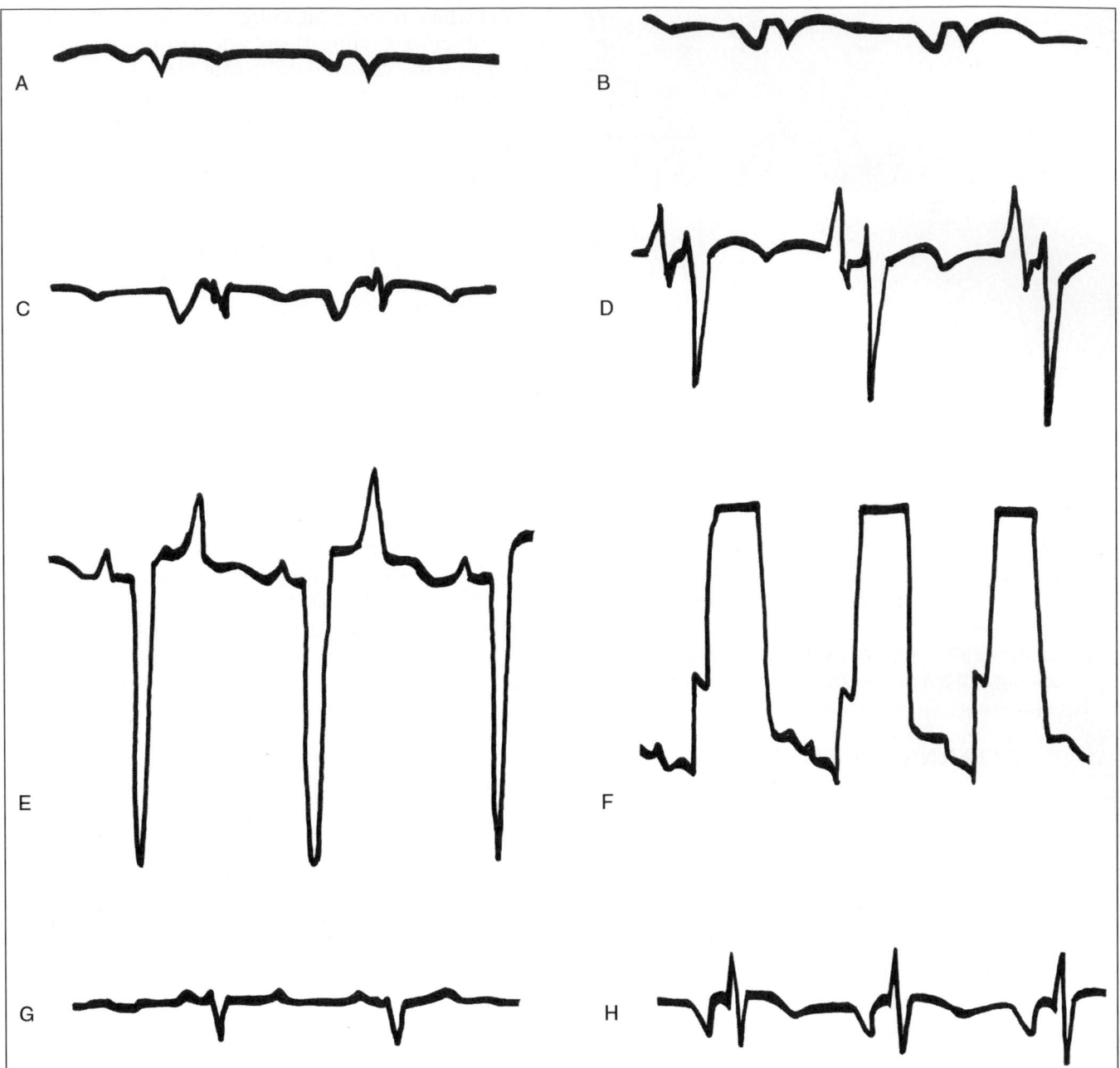

FIGURE 22-6 Typical ECG tracings seen with the transvenous pacing catheter within the different anatomic sites. *A.* The subclavian or internal jugular vein. *B.* The superior vena cava. *C.* The high right atrium. *D.* The low right atrium. *E.* Free-floating in the right ventricle. *F.* Abutting the right ventricular wall. *G.* The inferior vena cava. *H.* The pulmonary artery.

range from cellulitis at the puncture site to myocarditis and florid septicemia.[2,3,5] Antibiotic therapy should be started and the catheter removed and cultured. If the pacing catheter is absolutely required, a new puncture site should be selected and a new pacing catheter inserted.

The balloon can be a source of complications.[6,7] Air embolism has been reported. This can be prevented by assessing the balloon for leaks prior to inserting the catheter. Do not overinflate the balloon. An air em-

bolism or a piece of ruptured balloon may obstruct part of the pulmonary circulation. Do not inflate the balloon after it is inserted more than 10 to 15 cm into the ventricle. If the balloon is inflated when the catheter tip is in a branch of the pulmonary artery, the vessel may rupture.

The pacing circuit (catheter, wires, pacemaker) can also be a source of complications. The catheter may become dislodged or fractured. The pacemaker may fail due to battery drainage, generator failure, or electrical interference.

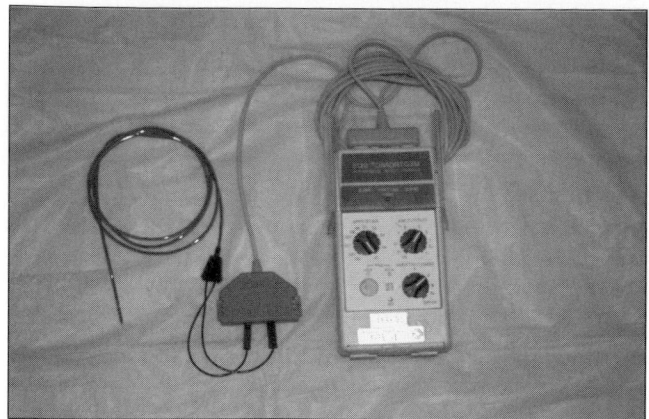

FIGURE 22-7 The transvenous pacing catheter connected to the pacemaker generator.

Complications related to obtaining central venous access are discussed in Chapter 38. They include air embolism, infection, sepsis, cellulitis, pneumothorax, improper placement, arterial puncture, venous thrombosis, venous thrombophlebitis, and guidewire complications.

SUMMARY

Placement of a transvenous cardiac pacing catheter can be a lifesaving procedure. It is a safe method to electrically stimulate the heart. It is indicated when an unstable rhythm of the heart is refractory to medications and transcutaneous pacing. This procedure should be mastered by all physicians caring for critically ill and/or injured patients.

Proper placement of the pacing catheter is cardinal to its functioning. Recognition of the ECG changes that occur in the different anatomic areas helps to guide its placement. One must also be aware of the potential complications and the treatment that should be administered if a complication occurs.

REFERENCES

1. Vukmir RB: Emergency cardiac pacing. *Am J Emerg Med* 1993; 11(2):166–176.
2. Simon RR, Brenner BE: *Emergency Procedures and Techniques,* 3rd ed. Baltimore: Williams & Wilkins, 1994:426–430.
3. Chen H, Sola JE, Lillemoe KD, et al: *Manual of Common Bedside Surgical Procedures.* Baltimore: Williams & Wilkins, 1996:86–88.
4. Goldberger J, Kruse J, Ehlert FA, et al: Temporary transvenous pacemaker placement: what criteria constitute an adequate pacing site? *Am Heart J* 1993; 126(2):488–493.
5. Murphy JJ: Current practice and complications of temporary transvenous cardiac pacing. *Br Med J* 1996; 312(7039):1134.
6. Campo I, Garfield GJ, Escher DJW, et al: Complications of pacing by pervenous subclavian semifloating electrodes including extraluminal insertions. *Am J Cardiol* 1970; 26:627–634.
7. Foote GA, Schabel SI, Hodges M: Pulmonary complications of the flow-directed, balloon-tipped catheter. *N Engl J Med* 1974; 290:927–931.

Chapter 23
PACEMAKER ASSESSMENT

James T. Thomas
Ratnakar S. Rajanahally

INTRODUCTION

Pacemakers are common among Emergency Department patients. Patients may present due to symptoms referable to pacemaker malfunction or symptoms unrelated to the pacemaker, and its presence may modify the investigation and therapeutic approach. It is important for the Emergency Physician to understand the workings of a pacemaker, the problems that may be encountered, the etiologies of the problems, and the assessment of a patient with a pacemaker.

There are numerous indications for the implantation of a cardiac pacemaker.[1-7] However, a detailed discussion regarding the indications for permanent pacemaker insertion is beyond the scope of this chapter.[6,7] The most common indication for permanent pacemaker placement is symptomatic bradycardia. Mortality rates can be decreased in these patients with pacing. A permanent pacemaker is inserted prophylactically when intrinsic cardiac rhythms can degenerate to higher-degree blocks or in patients who may develop symptoms in the near future even though the initial presentation was asymptomatic. An example would be the Mobitz type 2 second-degree atrioventricular (AV) block. In addressing the treatment modalities for cardiac rhythm disturbances, the decision to implant a pacemaker can be difficult and must be reached by careful review of each patient on an individual basis.

The pacemaker unit is implanted by a Cardiologist in the cardiac catheterization laboratory. The pacemaker unit consists of the pacemaker generator, the pacemaker wires or leads, and the terminal electrodes. The square or rectangular pacemaker generator is implanted subcutaneously in the left or right upper chest; it is responsible for the functioning of the unit and contains the battery that powers it. A reed switch in the pacemaker generator can be used to inactivate its sensing mechanism and cause it to perform in an asynchronous mode. The pacemaker wires are embedded in plastic catheters and attached to the pacemaker generator. The wires are inserted through the subclavian vein or, less commonly, through the cephalic vein and into the right side of the heart. The terminal electrodes are at the distal end of the pacing wires and are designated as unipolar or bipolar. The terminal electrodes are placed in the right ventricle or the right atrium and right ventricle under fluoroscopic guidance. After insertion, the unit is programmed and tested.

The North American Society for Pacing and Electrophysiology and the British Pacing and Electrophysiology Group have accepted a five-letter pacemaker code, which is also followed by the pacemaker industry (Table 23-1). The code is generic in nature. The character position is labeled in Roman numerals I through V. The first letter designates the chamber(s) in which pacing occurs. The second letter designates which cardiac chamber(s) the pacemaker uses to sense intrinsic electrical cardiac activity. The third letter designates how the pacemaker responds to sensed intrinsic electrical activity. A sensed event may inhibit (I), trigger (T), both inhibit and trigger (D), or cause no response (O) from the pacemaker generator. To have a designation other than O, the pacemaker must be a dual-chamber system. The fourth letter reflects the programmability and rate modulation of the unit. The fifth letter designates the antitachyarrhythmia function(s) of the pacemaker. The fourth and fifth letters are rarely used, as these functions are not often required. The code does not describe the characteristics, specific functions, or unique functions that are specific to each pacemaker unit or the manufacturer of the unit. The most common mode for a pacemaker is VVI. The reader is referred to other

TABLE 23-1. THE GENERIC AND STANDARD PACEMAKER CODES

Position	I	II	III	IV	V
Interpretation	Chamber(s) paced	Chamber(s) sensed	Response to sensing	Programmability rate modulation	Anti-tachyarrhythmia function(s)
Variable	0	0	0	0	0
	A	A	T	P^1	P^2
	V	V	I	M	S
	D (A+V)	D (A+V)	D (T+I)	C	D (P+S)
				R	

KEY: A = atria, C = communicating, D = dual, I = inhibited, M = multiprogrammable, 0 = none, P^1 = simple programmable, P^2 = pacing, R = rate modulation, S = shock, T = triggered, V = ventricle.

references for a more complete discussion of pacemaker modes.[6,7]

EVALUATION OF PACEMAKER FUNCTION

Pacemaker patients who present to the Emergency Department with a complaint that may be associated with their pacemaker require a thorough evaluation. Place the patient on the pulse oximeter and cardiac monitor and apply a noninvasive blood pressure cuff. Provide supplemental oxygen via a nasal cannula or face mask. A history and physical examination should be performed while simultaneously obtaining a 12-lead electrocardiogram (ECG). Obtain posteroanterior and lateral chest radiographs if the patient is stable. If not, a portable anteroposterior chest radiograph will suffice. Perform a magnet examination of the pacemaker. **A Cardiologist should always be consulted regarding a patient with an actual or potential pacemaker problem.**

HISTORY AND PHYSICAL EXAMINATION

The initial evaluation begins with a complete history. Palpitations, dizziness, presyncope, syncope, or any symptom that may resemble those prior to pacemaker implantation may reflect a potential pacemaker malfunction. In patients who have had their pacemaker placed recently, the complaints related to potential pacemaker infection should also be explored. Determine if the patient is taking medications that can raise the myocardial threshold to pacing. Traumatic injury to the torso can cause the leads to displace or fracture. Direct trauma over the pacemaker generator can render it inoperable. Ask the patient if they have a "pacemaker card." This is a business card–size piece of paper that is given to the patient after pacemaker implantation to identify the pacemaker type, manufacturer of the unit, programmed rate, the five-letter code programmed in the pacemaker, and the manufacturer's phone number. The patient should be questioned regarding any known

changes in the pacemaker settings since receiving the pacemaker card.

Perform a thorough examination of the patient. Observe the vital signs for bradycardia, fever, hypertension, hypotension, or tachycardia. Evaluate the veins of the head and neck for venous engorgement suggesting a central venous thrombosis or a superior vena cava syndrome. Edema of the ipsilateral upper extremity indicates thrombosis and possible occlusion of the subclavian vein. Identify the location of the pacemaker pocket and implantation scar on the skin. Note if the pacemaker generator has moved from its original position. This can cause a partial or complete disconnection of the pacemaker wires from the generator. Inspect the pacemaker pocket for signs of infection, including a discharge, edema, skin erosion, erythema, redness, tenderness, and/or warmth.

ELECTROCARDIOGRAM

A 12-lead ECG should be obtained. This recording will disclose whether the patient is presently being paced and in what manner (e.g., ventricular or atrioventricular pacing). If not, the underlying rhythm and PR interval of an intrinsic cardiac beat can be readily established (Figure 23-1). Bipolar spikes tend to be smaller, and examination of various leads of the ECG tracing may clarify the presence or absence of capture. A paced beat occurs when ventricular depolarization is secondary to pacer stimulation (Figure 23-1). The pacer spike is seen immediately preceding the QRS complex. A fusion or pseudofusion beat can occur due to pacemaker firing on an intrinsically occurring P wave or QRS complex. A fusion beat is a QRS complex that has been formed by depolarization of the myocardium and was initiated by both the pacemaker spike and the patient's intrinsic electrical activity (Figure 23-1). The QRS configuration of the fusion beat is different from the paced QRS morphology and the intrinsic cardiac QRS morphology. It is a hybrid of the paced and intrinsic QRS complex morphology. A pseudofusion beat is a QRS complex that is formed by

Intrinsic beat
Paced beat
Fusion beat
Pseudofusion beat

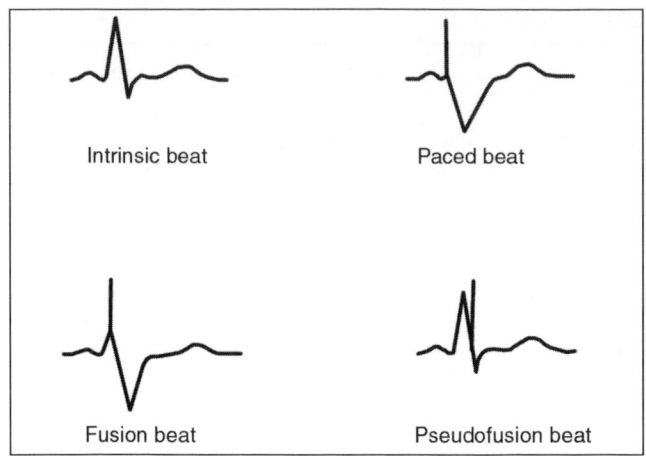

FIGURE 23-1 Schematic of typical electrocardiographic beats.

the depolarization of the myocardium initiated by the patient's intrinsic electrical activity, and a pacemaker spike is present distorting the terminal QRS complex. The morphology is similar to that of the intrinsic QRS complex (Figure 23-1). It is often due to the pacemaker firing during the refractory period of an intrinsic P wave or during the beginning of the QRS complex before intracardiac voltage increases to activate the sensing circuit and inhibit the pacemaker. Pseudofusion beats can be normal occurrences in pacemaker patients.

A properly functioning pacemaker will sense intrinsic cardiac electrical activity. If the intrinsic cardiac activity is below the programmed rate, a pacemaker spike will be seen followed by a QRS complex in a single-chamber or ventricular pacemaker (Figure 23-2). If the patient has a dual-chamber pacemaker, a pacemaker spike will be followed by a P wave; then a second pacemaker spike will be seen followed by a QRS complex (Figures 23-3 and

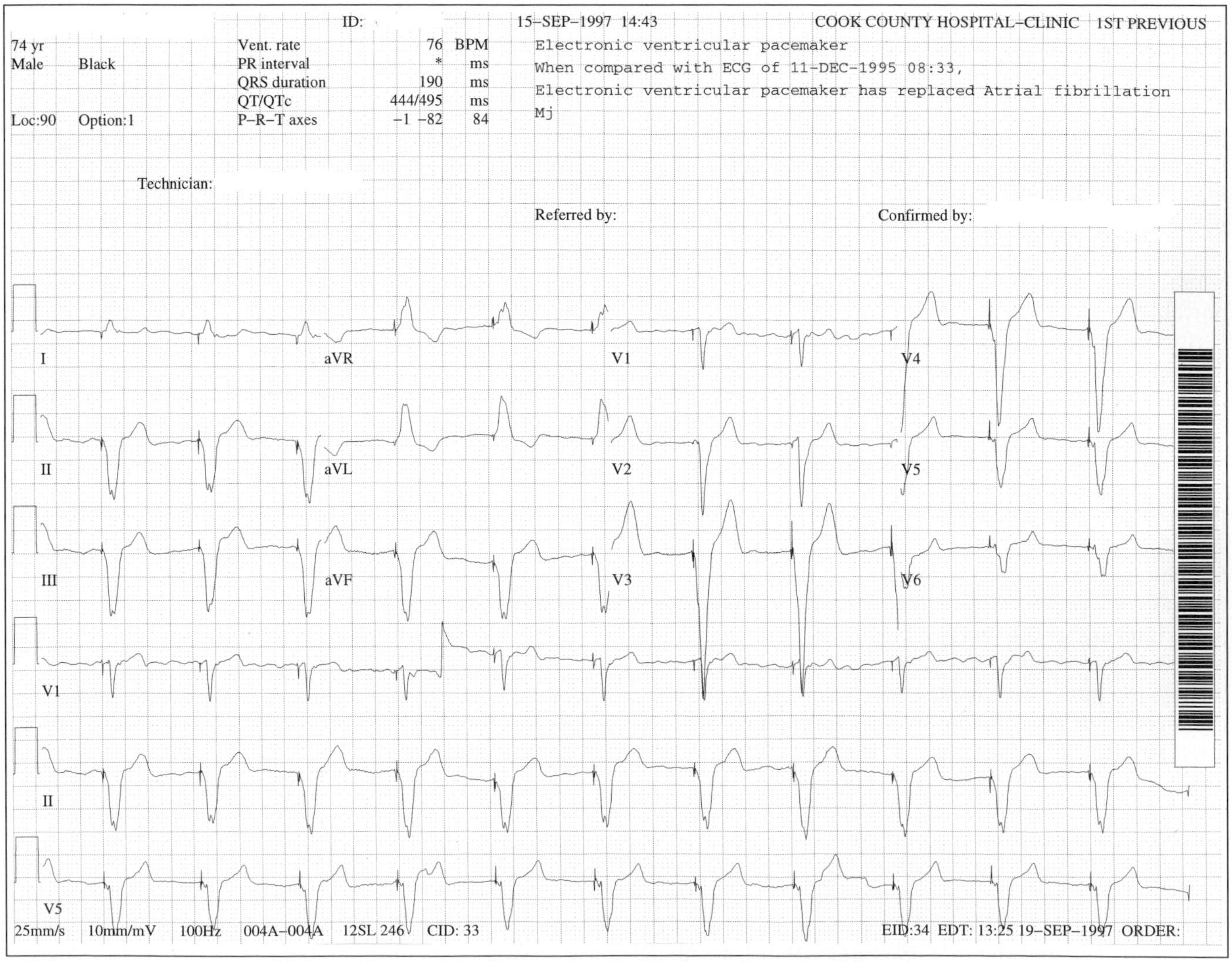

ID:
15-SEP-1997 14:43
COOK COUNTY HOSPITAL-CLINIC
1ST PREVIOUS
74 yr
Male Black
Loc:90 Option:1
Vent. rate 76 BPM
PR interval * ms
QRS duration 190 ms
QT/QTc 444/495 ms
P-R-T axes -1 -82 84
Electronic ventricular pacemaker
When compared with ECG of 11-DEC-1995 08:33,
Electronic ventricular pacemaker has replaced Atrial fibrillation
Mj
Technician:
Referred by:
Confirmed by:
I
aVR
V1
V4
II
aVL
V2
V5
III
aVF
V3
V6
V1
II
V5
25mm/s 10mm/mV 100Hz 004A-004A 12SL 246 CID: 33
EID:34 EDT: 13:25 19-SEP-1997 ORDER:

FIGURE 23-2 A 12-lead electrocardiogram of a single-chamber or ventricular pacemaker.

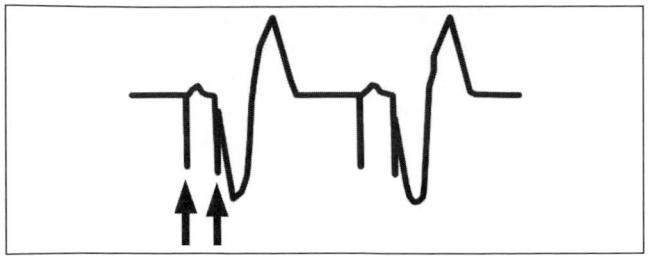

FIGURE 23-3 Schematic of an electrocardiographic monitor strip of a dual-chamber pacemaker. Atrial (*first arrow*) and ventricular (*second arrow*) pacing spikes are clearly visible.

23-4). If the intrinsic cardiac electric activity is above the programmed rate, no pacemaker spike should be seen on the ECG. Since the pacemaker wire is usually implanted in the right ventricle, a typical paced QRS complex will have a left bundle branch pattern (Figures 23-1, 23-2, 23-3, and 23-4). Occasionally, the pacing wire will

be implanted in the left ventricle and the QRS complex will have a right bundle branch pattern.

Examine the current ECG and determine the electrical axis of the pacemaker spike, the electrical axis of the QRS complex, and the morphology of the QRS complex. These must be compared to the same features on previously obtained ECGs. A change in the axis of the pacemaker spike may be seen in cases of lead migration. A change in the ECG morphology from a left bundle branch pattern to a right bundle branch pattern suggests that the lead has perforated the interventricular septum and is now within the left ventricle.

MAGNET EXAMINATION

A magnet may be used to assess battery depletion, failure of a component of the system, or the possibility of oversensing. It can also be used in an attempt to terminate pacemaker-mediated tachycardia (discussed

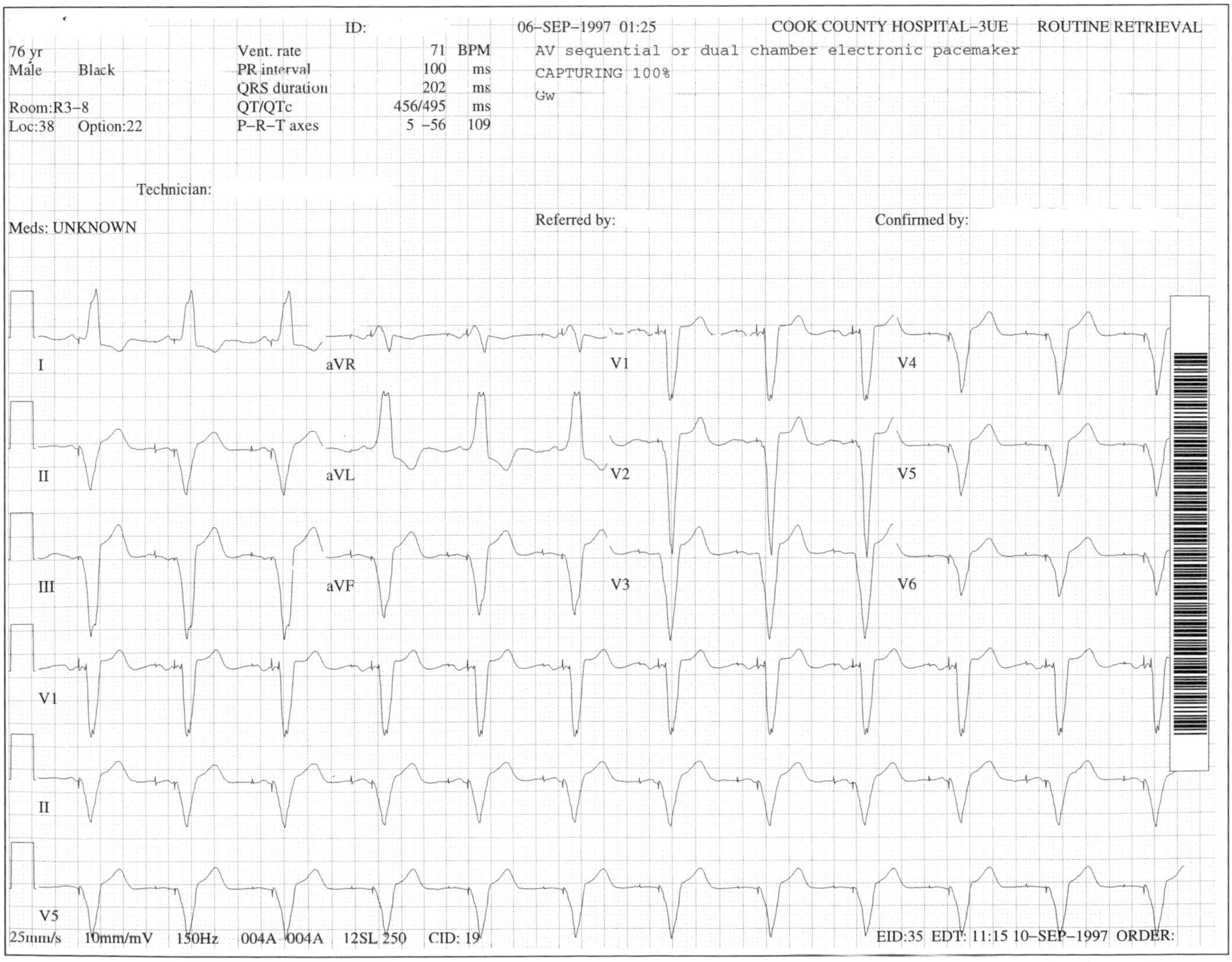

76 yr		ID:			06–SEP–1997 01:25	COOK COUNTY HOSPITAL–3UE	ROUTINE RETRIEVAL
76 yr		Vent. rate	71	BPM	AV sequential or dual chamber electronic pacemaker		
Male	Black	PR interval	100	ms	CAPTURING 100%		
		QRS duration	202	ms	Gw		
Room:R3–8		QT/QTc	456/495	ms			
Loc:38	Option:22	P–R–T axes	5 –56 109				

Technician:

Meds: UNKNOWN   Referred by: Confirmed by:

I   aVR   V1   V4

II   aVL   V2   V5

III   aVF   V3   V6

V1

II

V5

25mm/s   10mm/mV   150Hz   004A 004A   12SL 250   CID: 19   EID:35 EDT: 11:15 10–SEP–1997 ORDER:

FIGURE 23-4 A 12-lead electrocardiogram of a dual-chamber or atrioventricular sequential pacemaker.

further on in this chapter). A doughnut-shaped magnet is required for this procedure. A standard or generic magnet may be used. Occasionally, but rarely, a brand-specific magnet may be required to evaluate a pacemaker. A transcutaneous pacemaker generator, cables, and skin electrodes must be available in case of an emergency.

To obtain the magnet rate, place a standard magnet over the pacemaker generator while obtaining a 12-lead ECG and rhythm strip. **The magnetic field causes the reed switch to close and temporarily convert the pacemaker into the asynchronous (VOO or DOO) mode (Figure 23-5). This essentially turns off the sensing mode and the pacemaker fires at the programmed rate.** The magnet rate may be slower or faster than the program rate and depends on the model of the pacemaker. Pacemaker spikes occurring during the refractory period of an intrinsic QRS complex will not be captured (Figure 23-5*B*). Theoretically, a pacing spike occurring on the T wave could induce ventricular arrhythmias, but this is rarely a practical problem.

The application of the magnet over the pacemaker generator can have a variety of results. If it is working properly, the pacemaker will fire at the programmed rate. This indicates that the failure to pace the myocardium in a patient with bradycardia is due to oversensing. The unit may be sensing a large T wave as a QRS complex. Alternatively, it may be sensing a normal T wave as a QRS complex if the QRS complexes are small in amplitude. If a patient's bradycardia is corrected, tape the magnet in place over the pacemaker generator. If the generator is pacing intermittently, the magnet may not be directly over the pacemaker generator. Reposition the magnet and observe the results. If no pacemaker spikes are seen on the ECG, a component of the system (generator, battery, leads) has failed. If the pacemaker spikes occur at less than the programmed rate, the battery may be depleted or the set rate has been changed.

CHEST RADIOGRAPHY

Obtain overpenetrated posteroanterior and lateral chest radiographs. This is helpful in locating the pacemaker generator and lead positions. Look for a loose connection where the lead connects to the pacemaker generator. Manipulation of the pulse generator within the pocket may relieve or reproduce the patient's problem. A pneumothorax and/or hemothorax may be detected in patients whose pacemakers have been recently implanted.

The pacemaker lead may have become dislodged from its implantation site. This is extremely uncommon with current systems, as they have safety mechanisms to prevent lead dislodgement. Ensure that the distal end of the pacing wire is within the cardiac silhouette and against the myocardium. It may be free-floating within the ventricle or may have perforated the ventricular wall. Previous chest radiographs should be obtained and compared to the current radiographs to help determine if the leads have been displaced.

Lead fractures can occur anywhere along the length of the pacing wire. They most often occur at stress points adjacent to the pacemaker or just under the clavicle as the pacing wire enters the subclavian vein. The lead also has a J-shaped retention wire to help maintain its shape. The tip of the retention wire may occasionally protrude from the plastic-coated lead. This protruding wire has the potential to puncture the right atrium or superior vena cava and cause a hemorrhagic pericardial effusion that may result in cardiac tamponade.

ELECTROCARDIOGRAPHIC ABNORMALITIES

LACK OF CAPTURE OR INTERMITTENT CAPTURE (FAILURE TO CAPTURE)

Failure to capture is noted by the lack of a QRS complex after an appropriately timed and placed pacemaker spike on the ECG (Figure 23-6). Lack of capture

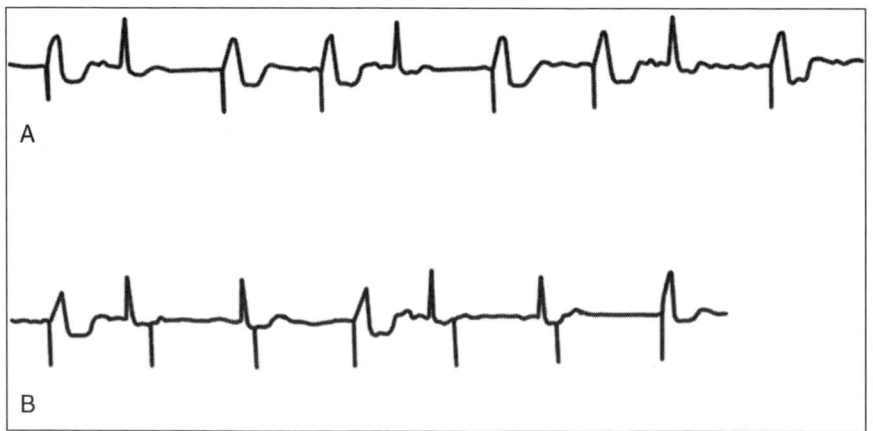

FIGURE 23-5 Schematic of a pacemaker's electrocardiographic monitor strip. *A.* Pacemaker activity without a magnet applied. *B.* Pacemaker activity with a magnet applied.

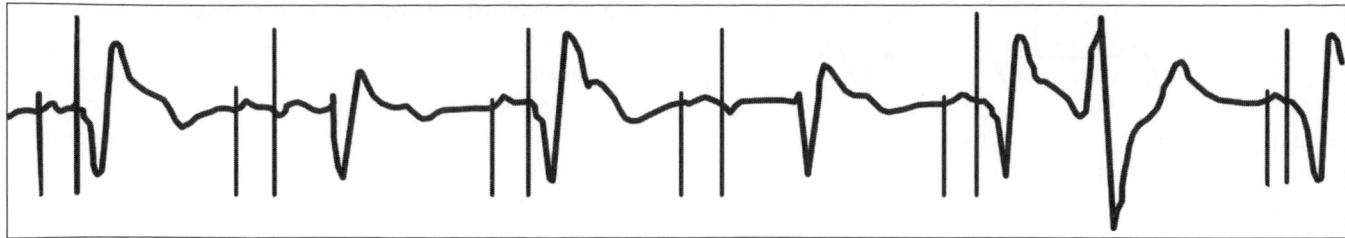

FIGURE 23-6 Schematic of an electrocardiographic monitor strip of an AV sequential pacemaker demonstrating lack of capture or intermittent capture.

or intermittent capture may be due to poor electrode position, a dislodged electrode, perforation of the myocardium by the electrode, or accidental placement of the electrode into the coronary sinus. A poor threshold may be present from the time of implantation. A chronic rise in threshold can be related to fibrosis around the tip of the lead, causing lack of capture or intermittent capture. Severe metabolic abnormalities and drugs can increase the pacing threshold. A myocardial infarction involving the myocardium at the tip of the pacer leads will cause a rise in the pacing threshold. Lead fracture and poor connections between the electrode and generator can present as lack of capture or intermittent capture. The pacemaker generator battery may fail and present with too low a voltage to capture the heart but enough voltage to generate a pacemaker spike. Insulation breaks in the pacemaker lead allow parallel electrical circuits to occur in the system and may cause various pacemaker abnormalities.

TOTAL LACK OF PACEMAKER STIMULUS (FAILURE TO PACE)

Failure to pace is noted by a lack of the pacemaker spike on the ECG and the failure to deliver a stimulus to the myocardium when there is a pause in the intrinsic cardiac electrical activity. The ECG tracing obtained showing no pacemaker spikes points to a total lack of pacemaker stimulus. Total or nearly total battery failure, complete inhibition of a demand pacemaker by skeletal muscle contraction or electrical magnetic interference, oversensing, insulation failure, lead fracture, or an improper connection between the electrode and the pulse generator can all cause total lack of pacemaker stimulus. The incorrect diagnosis of lack of pacemaker stimulus can be made if the patient's pacemaker spike is very small. The observation of multiple leads of the ECG tracing usually prevents misdiagnosis. If the patient's intrinsic heart rate is faster than the minimum set rate for the pacemaker, it is normal not to see any pacer spikes or paced beats.

RATE CHANGE

Rate change is defined as a stable change in the pacemaker's rate of firing compared to the pacemaker's

rate at the time of implantation. Minor chronic changes in the pacemaker rate of one or two beats per minute can occur in some patients. The most common cause for a marked drop in the paced rate is battery depletion. This is a sign that the elective battery replacement time is nearing. Inappropriate sensing of the preceding T wave as a QRS complex can also result in a paced rate several beats per minute slower than the programmed rate.

INTERMITTENT OR ERRATIC PROLONGATION OF THE PACING SPIKE INTERVAL

A prolongation of the pacing spike interval can be due to inappropriate sensing of the T wave, pacemaker afterpotential, or skeletal muscle activity (Figure 23-7). Intermittent fracture of leads, poor electrode–generator connection, breaks in the insulation of the leads, external electromagnetic interference, or radiofrequency interference can also cause this malfunction.

LACK OF APPROPRIATE SENSING (FAILURE TO SENSE)

Failure to sense is recognized by noting pacemaker spikes on the ECG despite the patient's intrinsic cardiac rate being higher than the pacemaker's programmed rate (Figure 23-8). The demand pacemaker may not sense the preceding QRS complex appropriately and fire. This may be due to poor electrode position, lead dislodgement, reed switch malfunction, magnet use, breaks in insulation of the lead, battery failure, and inappropriate programming of the sensitivity of the pulse generator. Low-amplitude QRS complexes or broad QRS complexes with a low slew rate, as in a bundle branch block, may be responsible for pacemaker sensing problems.

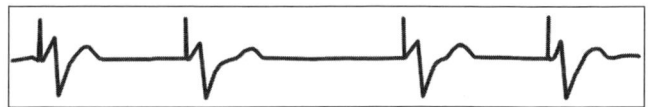

FIGURE 23-7 Schematic of an electrocardiographic monitor strip demonstrating intermittent or erratic prolongation of the pacing spike interval.

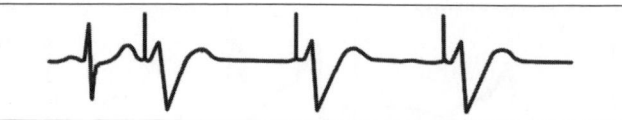

FIGURE 23-8 Schematic of an electrocardiographic monitor strip demonstrating lack of appropriate sensing or failure to sense.

PACEMAKER-MEDIATED TACHYCARDIA

Pacemaker-mediated tachycardia is a paced rhythm in which the pacemaker is firing at a very high rate (Figure 23-9). The paced rhythm can occur only when the pacemaker is programmed to an atrial synchronized pacing mode (e.g., DDD). The rhythm is synchronized to the retrograde P waves. The retrograde P wave is sensed after ventricular pacing and causes the pacemaker to fire at or near the upper rate limit programmed into the pacemaker. This rhythm must be terminated by automatic extension of the atrial refractory period, magnet application, reprogramming the pacemaker, isometric pectoral exercises, a precordial thump, transcutaneous pacing, or cutting of the leads as they exit the pacemaker. A Cardiologist should be consulted and at bedside prior to performing these maneuvers.

PACEMAKER INTERROGATION

Pacemaker interrogation by personnel trained in cardiology and/or electrophysiology should be carried out if any abnormality is seen in the initial evaluation in the Emergency Department. The pacemaker should be interrogated to obtain generator life, lead information (atrial and/or ventricular), pulse amplitude, current, and impedance. The above measured data and program parameters can be used in further defining the malfunction.

COMPLICATIONS OF CARDIAC PACING UNRELATED TO ELECTROCARDIOGRAPHIC ABNORMALITIES

IMPLANTATION-RELATED COMPLICATIONS

Complications may occur from the implantation procedure. Discomfort and ecchymosis at the incision site or the pacemaker pocket are common in the first few days. Nonsteroidal anti-inflammatory drugs, excluding aspirin, are adequate and appropriate to alleviate the discomfort. Assure the patient that the discomfort and ecchymosis will resolve spontaneously. The patient should not be taking aspirin in the immediate postimplantation period unless authorized and/or prescribed by the Cardiologist.

The most common insertion site for the pacemaker wires is through the subclavian vein using a blind insertion technique. Complications include air embolism, arteriovenous fistula formation, brachial plexus injury, hemothorax, pneumothorax, subclavian artery puncture, subcutaneous emphysema, and thoracic duct injury. Refer to Chapter 38 for complete details on complications related to the placement of a central venous line.

A hematoma may form at the site of the subcutaneous pacemaker generator. This can be due to anticoagulation therapy, aspirin therapy, or an injury to a subcutaneous artery or vein. A hematoma can be managed with the application of dry, warm compresses to the area and oral analgesics. The hematoma may be evacuated by the Cardiologist if it continues to expand and threatens to compromise the incision site. Otherwise, a hematoma is self-limited and resolves spontaneously.

The ventricular wall may be perforated during the implantation of the pacemaker lead or postimplantation. The patient may be asymptomatic, complain of chest pain and/or dyspnea, or have signs and symptoms of cardiac tamponade. Other signs suggestive of ventricular perforation include diaphragmatic contraction or hiccups, friction rub, intercostal muscle contraction, pericardial effusions, pericarditis, or a right bundle branch pattern on the ECG. The evaluation may include chest radiography, echocardiography, and/or pacemaker interrogation and evaluation.

PACEMAKER SYNDROME

The pacemaker syndrome is defined as adverse hemodynamic effects that cause the patient to become symptomatic or limit their ability to be fully functional even though the pacemaker system is functioning normally. Patients may complain of anxiety, apprehension, dizziness, fatigue, pulsations in the neck, or shortness of breath. Ventricular pacing can cause lack of atrioventricular synchrony, leading to decreased left ventricular filling and subsequent decreased cardiac output. Syncope and presyncope are thought to be associated with a vagal reflex initiated by elevated right and/or left atrial pressures caused by dissociation of the atrial and ventricular contractions. The high wedge pressure can result in shortness of breath. Patients with

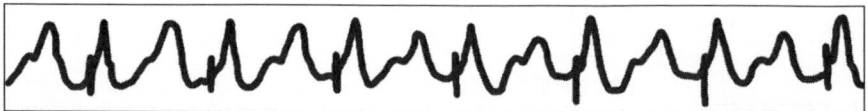

FIGURE 23-9 Schematic of an electrocardiographic monitor strip demonstrating pacemaker-mediated tachycardia.

the pacemaker syndrome most commonly have documented one-to-one ventricular-to-atrial conduction during ventricular pacing. Patients with retrograde AV conduction are more symptomatic. However, a pacemaker syndrome can occur in the absence of retrograde atrioventricular conduction.

INFECTION

Infection often occurs shortly after implantation and is usually localized to the pacemaker pocket area. However, endocarditis has also been reported in association with pacemakers. Infection may present as localized erythema and tenderness, localized inflammation, purulent discharge from the skin incision, skin erosion, sepsis, and/or bacteremia. The pacemaker generator and leads usually have to be removed to eradicate an infection. In some instances, the infection has been treated successfully with parenteral antibiotics and the unit did not require removal.

The pacemaker electrode becomes endothelialized in a few weeks postimplantation. Patients do not require prophylactic antibiotics when they undergo a procedure that is likely to produce transient bacteremia. Prophylactic antibiotics are given only in the first few weeks after permanent pacemaker implantation.

STIMULATION OF THE DIAPHRAGM AND PECTORAL MUSCLE

Stimulation of the diaphragm may be caused by perforation of the right ventricular wall by the pacing wire and can occur with very few complications. Diaphragmatic stimulation can also occur without perforation of the right ventricular wall. Decreasing the pulse width and/or voltage output can minimize the stimulation until the defective component can be replaced.

Pectoral muscle stimulation is less common with the currently available bipolar pacemakers. An insulation break or defect in the pacing wire before it enters the subclavian vein will allow the current to flow in the area of the pacemaker generator and cause skeletal muscle stimulation. This can also be seen with current leakage from the connector of the pacing wires or sealing plugs. In rare instances, erosion of the protective coating of the pacemaker generator can cause this phenomenon. Decreasing the pulse width and/or voltage output can minimize the stimulation until the defective component can be replaced.

THROMBOSIS

Thrombosis of the vein (subclavian or cephalic) containing the pacemaker lead occurs commonly but rarely causes clinical symptoms. Patients with symptomatic thrombosis and occlusion of the subclavian vein may present with ipsilateral edema and pain in the upper extremity. Occlusion of the superior vena cava can result in a superior vena cava syndrome. Thrombus formation in the right atrium and/or right ventricle can result in pulmonary embolic and hemodynamic compromise. Fortunately, these events are extremely rare.

ALLERGIC REACTIONS

Allergic reactions to the metal components of the pacemaker have been noted in the past. Current pacemaker generators and leads are coated with a substance to prevent the body from being exposed to the metal. Allergic reactions to the pacemaker covering are very rare but have been reported.

SUMMARY

Routine follow-up of patients with pacemakers in the pacemaker clinic helps to identify pacemaker malfunction earlier and before problems occur. Patients presenting to the Emergency Department with symptoms referable to pacemaker malfunction should have a history and physical examination, chest radiograph, routine ECG, and ECG recording with a magnet over the pacemaker. This helps to identify patients with pacemaker malfunction who require detailed pacemaker interrogation. A Cardiologist should be consulted on every patient who presents with an actual or potential pacemaker problem.

REFERENCES

1. Moses HW, Moulton KP, Miller BD, et al: *A Practical Guide to Cardiac Pacing,* 4th ed. Boston: Little, Brown, 2000.
2. Griffin JC, Schuenemeyer TD, Hess KR, et al: Pacemaker follow-up: its role in the detection and correction of pacemaker system malfunction. *PACE Pacing Clin Electrophysiol* 1986; 9:387–391.
3. Hayes DL, Vlietstra RE: Pacemaker malfunction. *Ann Intern Med* 1993; 119(8):828–835.
4. Phibbs B, Marriott HJL: Complication of permanent transvenous pacing. *N Engl J Med* 1985; 312(22):1428–1432.
5. Schuller H, Brandt J: The pacemaker syndrome: old and new causes. *Clin Cardiol* 1991; 14:336–340.
6. Hayes DL, Zipes DP: Cardiac pacemakers and cardioverter-defibrillators, in Braunwald E, Zipes DP, Libby P (eds): *Heart Disease: A Textbook of Cardiovascular Medicine.* Philadelphia: Saunders, 2001:775–802.
7. Gregoratos G, Cheitlin MD, Conill A, et al: ACC/AHA guidelines for implantation of cardiac pacemakers and antiarrhythmia devices: a report of the American College of Cardiology/American Heart Association Task Force on Practice Guidelines (Committee on Pacemaker Implantation). *J Am Coll Cardiol* 1998; 31(5):1175–1209.

Chapter 24

AUTOMATIC IMPLANTABLE CARDIOVERTER-DEFIBRILLATOR ASSESSMENT

John K. Lee
Katherine Blossfield

INTRODUCTION

The treatment of individuals at high risk for sudden death has changed dramatically with the introduction of implantable cardioverter-defibrillator (ICD) technology. The superiority of the ICD device over antiarrhythmic therapy has been confirmed in randomized trials.[1-3] Expanding clinical indications for the implantation of these devices arose with the publication of the MADIT (Multi-center Autonomic Defibrillator Implantation Trial) trial, the results of which have been validated by the MUSTT (Multicenter UnSustained Tachycardia Trial) trial. These studies demonstrated a survival benefit of ICDs in patients with nonsustained ventricular tachycardia.[4,5] The number of ICD implants continues to increase. In 1999 alone, based on industry statistics, close to 50,000 ICDs were implanted in the United States.[6]

The Emergency Department will often be the contact point for these patients. This requires Emergency Physicians to be familiar with the problems that can be encountered by a patient with an ICD. This chapter deals with technical aspects of an ICD, basic interrogation of the device, and the general approach to a patient who presents to the Emergency Department with an implantable defibrillator.

TECHNICAL CONSIDERATIONS

ICD technology has progressed exponentially since its introduction by Mirowski and colleagues in the early 1980s.[7] Early devices were true "shock boxes," capable of detecting a tachycardia and delivering a shock without the ability to pace.[8] The ICD system is comprised of a pulse generator, a battery, and a lead system. The lead system is required for sensing, pacing, and the delivery of therapy. Earlier systems required that the pulse generators be placed abdominally due to their large size (Figure 24-1). Defibrillation was delivered via two epicardial patches positioned anteriorly and posteriorly. Occasionally, a transvenous spring electrode in the superior vena cava was utilized with an epicardial patch. Sensing was achieved through separate epicardial screw-in electrodes. Initial lead placement required either a sternotomy, lateral thoracotomy, or a subxiphoid approach, making early implants quite cumbersome.[9]

ICD implantation has evolved quite rapidly due to advancements in lead technology, generator technology, and the development of biphasic defibrillation waveforms which lowered the energy requirements necessary for successful defibrillation.[10] The creation of a (bipolar) lead combining pacing and sensing capabilities with a high-voltage electrode coil allowed for nonthoracotomy system implants, which reduced surgical morbidity and mortality.[11] The leads were now positioned transvenously via the subclavian vein and fixed to the inside of the right ventricle. However, the leads still had to be tunneled subcutaneously to the abdomen, as the generators remained fairly large. Technology has advanced the development of more compact generators. The smallest commercially available devices today are under 40 cm^3 and weigh well under 100 grams. Smaller generators allow for subcutaneous pectoral implantation and simplification of the implantation process[12] (Figure 24-2).

The ICD generator houses the batteries, high-voltage capacitors, and microprocessors necessary to process sensed intrinsic cardiac electrical activity. In essence, the generator is a minicomputer within a hermetically

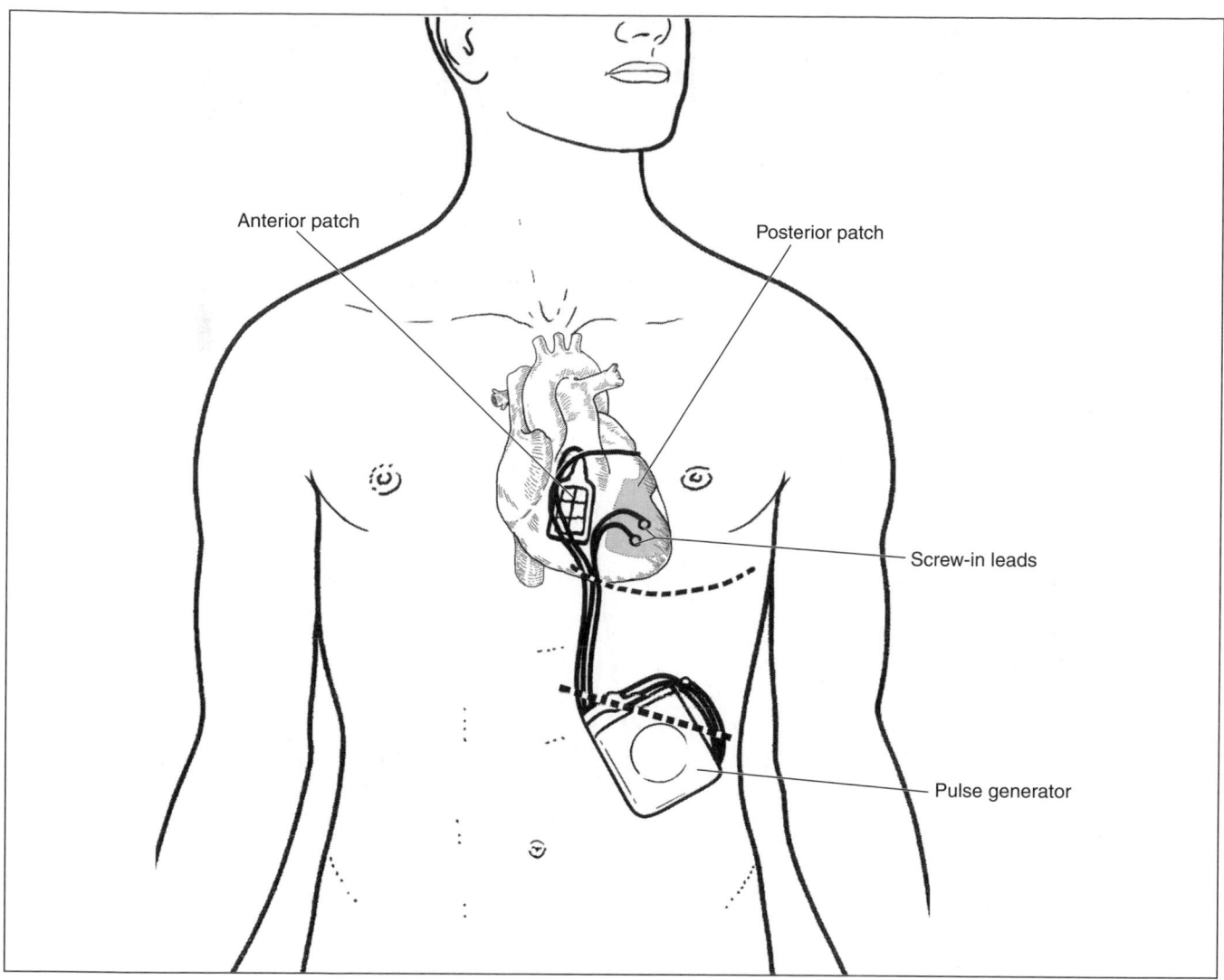

FIGURE 24-1 Abdominal placement of the ICD generator. Initial implants required a thoracotomy to position the epicardial patches needed for defibrillation as well as the screw-in sensing leads. The leads were tunneled abdominally to the ICD generator.

sealed titanium can (a.k.a. case) capable of generating shocks. Typical ICDs contain lithium silver vanadium oxide cells that store between 2 and 7 volts.[12] The high voltages necessary for defibrillation are generated with the aid of high-voltage capacitors that are able to generate 700 to 800 volts of defibrillation energy in under 20 seconds.

Current devices allow extensive programmability for tiered antitachycardia pacing, tiered high-voltage therapies, bradycardia pacing, supraventricular tachycardia discrimination algorithms, and detailed diagnostics of tachycardic and bradycardic episodes.[13,14] They also allow physicians to conduct completely noninvasive programmed stimulation. The most recent iterations provide dedicated dual-chamber and antitachycardia pacing as well as options for atrial defibrillation.[15]

ROUTINE ICD FOLLOW-UP

A systematic follow-up procedure to assess the integrity of the ICD system is recommended (Table 24-1). The device should be interrogated with the appropriate system analyzer. The system components should be assessed to assure battery voltage, lead and electrode integrity, and capacitor charge times. These data are used to reveal when the device's batteries have reached their end of life (EOL), indicating the need for standard replacement. System integrity test results can reveal malfunctions that may compromise the device's ability to treat an arrhythmia effectively.[16,17] Once the system's integrity has been verified, each recorded arrhythmic episode should be analyzed to determine the appropriateness and effectiveness of therapies. This is achieved by exam-

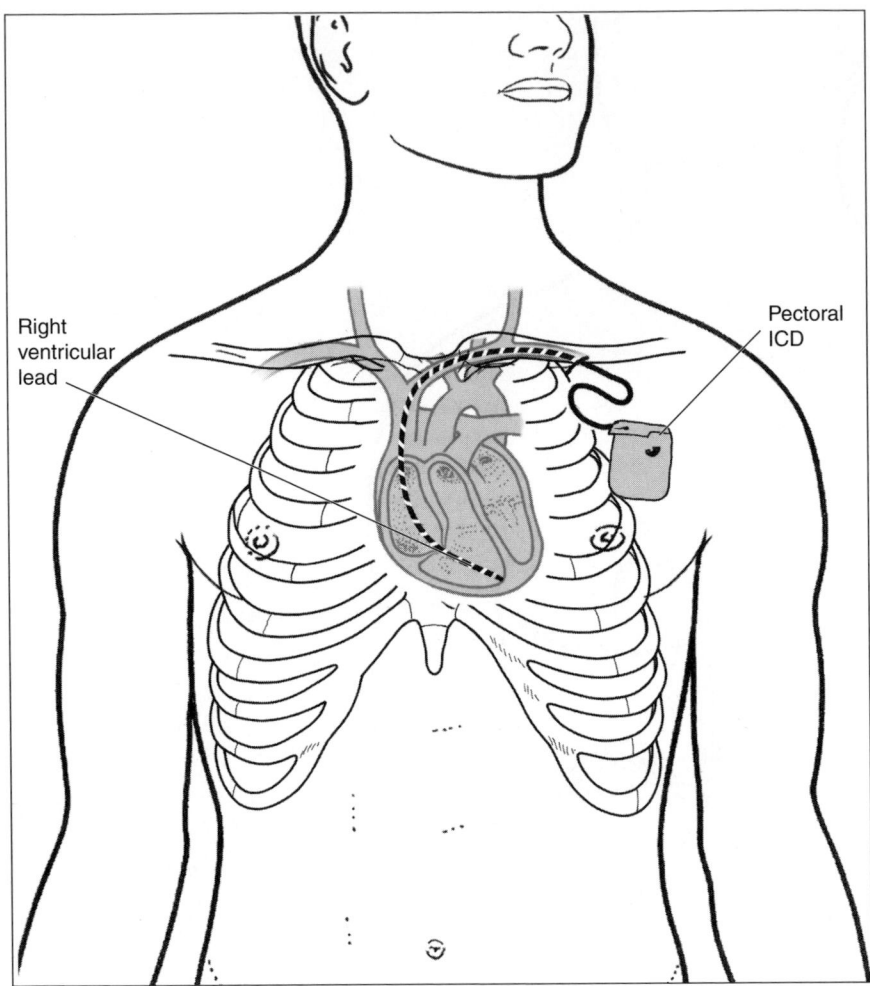

Right ventricular lead

Pectoral ICD

FIGURE 24-2 The current nonthoracotomy system. The development of smaller generators and biphasic waveforms for defibrillation allowed for transvenous positioning of the ICD leads and a pectorally located generator.

TABLE 24-1. THE ICD FOLLOW-UP CHECKLIST

1. Detailed history and physical examination. Question patient about shocks, palpitations, light-headedness, syncope, chest pains, or symptoms of congestive heart failure. Note any changes in medications (antiarrhythmic therapy). Examine incision site for any indication of infection.
2. Interrogate device with appropriate system analyzer.
3. Check lead parameter including pacing thresholds and lead impedances. Sensing is established by examining intracardiac R waves.
4. Determine capacitor reformation times.
5. Check battery voltage.
6. Measure impedance of the high-voltage coil. In older ICDs, this may require the administration of a subthreshold shock.
7. Analyze arrhythmia counters. Examine corresponding intracardiac electrograms to determine appropriateness of therapy.
8. Make the necessary program changes. These include adjusting the tachycardia zones, changing the detection cutoff rates, turning on special features to aid tachycardia discrimination (stability, sudden-onset criteria, electrogram width), and adjusting the sensitivities.
9. Confirm changes and reinterrogate device.

ining the stored diagnostic information contained within the ICD, which may include intracardiac electrograms, arrhythmic interval values, classification markers for each interval, episode plots, textual episode descriptions, energy, charge time and impedance values for shocks, and device classifications of therapy success. This diagnostic information can be extremely valuable to determine whether programming changes should be made.

BATTERY AND CAPACITORS

Battery voltages and capacitor charge times must be noted. Generator replacement is usually recommended when voltages fall below the elective replacement indicator (ERI), which is approximately 2.6 volts. When battery voltage falls below 2.2 volts, the battery has reached EOL. This signifies a more urgent need for battery replacement. The need to replace a generator is also dependent on capacitor charge times. Two consecutive charge times greater than 16 seconds is considered prolonged and may warrant urgent replacement regardless of the battery voltage. The capacitors should be reformed periodically to replenish their charge. This function can be programmed automatically at preset time intervals. Automatic capacitor reformation is usually set to 6 months. More frequent reformation is performed as the device reaches the end of its battery voltage.

LEAD INTEGRITY

Various parameters are checked to ensure lead integrity, including pacing thresholds, lead impedance, and the size of intracardiac R waves. At the time of implantation, a pacing threshold of ≤ 1.0 volt at a pulse width of 0.5 milliseconds is desired. An acute rise in threshold may be seen initially; it generally falls with time. Chronic thresholds range between 0.5 and 2.0 volts. Epicardial leads generally exhibit higher thresholds. Any change in thresholds must be compared with prior trends to assess its significance. Pacing thresholds may also change with the administration of antiarrhythmic drug therapy.

Lead impedances will vary based on the type of lead. Normal impedances range from 300 to 1200 ohms. A sudden change in impedance may signal a problem with lead integrity. A high impedance reading suggests the possibility of lead or patch fracture. A low impedance indicates a problem with the insulation. The impedance of the high-voltage coil must also be evaluated. In older-generation devices, this requires the administration of a small shock and may be difficult to perform in the Emergency Department setting. Epicardial and active can systems demonstrate lower impedance values compared to endocardial systems due to their larger surface area. Normal values generally range between 20 and 80 ohms. High impedance values, as with the pace/sense leads, usually indicate a fracture in the defibrillation system. Any stark changes in impedance levels may suggest a patch problem. This includes crinkling, seroma formation, or migration. Any impedance change in an endocardial system may indicate lead dislodgement.

R-wave amplitude is a direct measure of intracardiac electrogram activity and determines the device's ability to sense. At implantation, an R wave of ≥ 5 millivolts is desired to ensure adequate detection of ventricular fibrillation. The most common explanations for a decrease in R-wave amplitude after an implant is lead dislodgment or local factors such as edema or fibrosis. This change may be associated with an increase in lead impedance and pacing thresholds.

ANALYZING APPROPRIATENESS OF THERAPY

Current ICDs have simultaneous marker channels with real-time intracardiac electrograms (Figure 24-3). It is important to document intracardiac activity during sinus rhythm. These electrograms can be used as a basis of comparison with tachycardia events. The signals should be examined for evidence of noise, which may be an indicator of sensing problems, a connector issue, or a faulty adaptor. In the event of noise detection, electro-

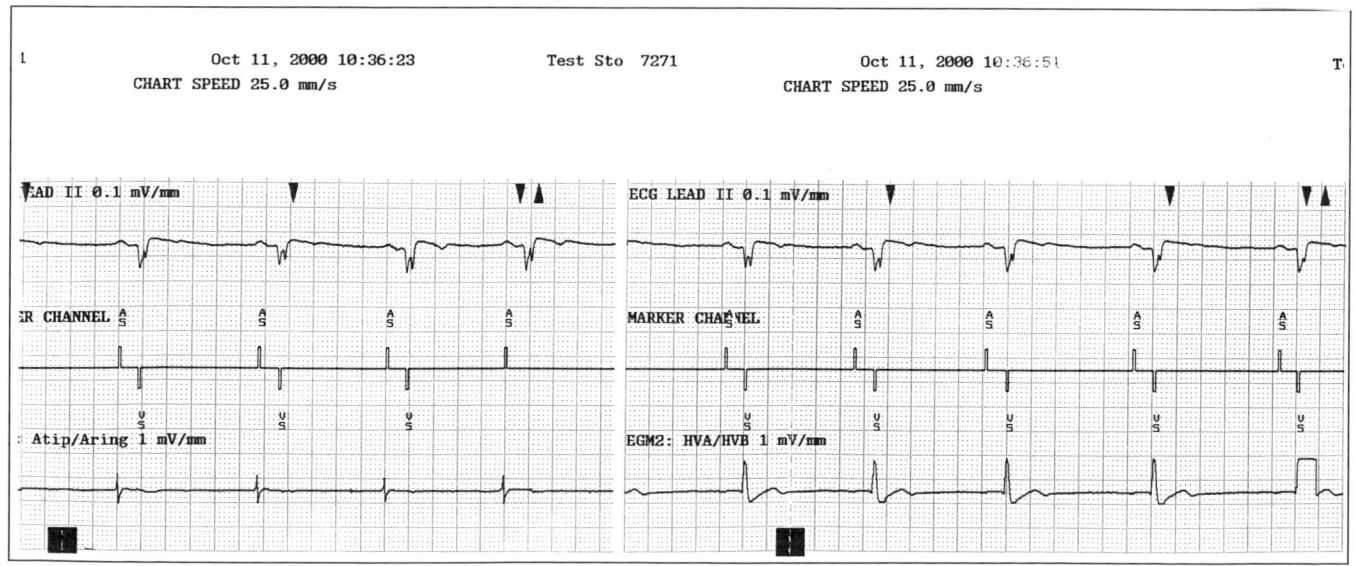

FIGURE 24-3 The intracardiac electrogram as recorded by the ICD. Printouts were obtained from a Medtronic Gem II DR dual-chamber ICD. The first line shows an ECG rhythm strip (lead II). The marker channel directly under the rhythm strip indicates behavior (sensing/pacing) in each chamber. The third line represents the intracardiac electrogram from the atrium (*left*) and ventricle (*right*). Measured in millivolts per millimeter, larger signals imply better sensing.

grams must be examined during various maneuvers including deep breathing, arm maneuvers, and bending. Intracardiac electrograms should be examined for T-wave oversensing or detection of pacemaker spikes as ventricular signals. In dual-chamber devices, oversensing by the atrial lead should be ruled out. Wide variations in electrogram size may suggest that the lead is not stable or well fixed.

THE ICD IN THE EMERGENCY DEPARTMENT

A patient with an implantable defibrillator may present to the Emergency Department for various reasons. Individuals with recently implanted devices may be quite anxious and may seek medical attention even after single discharges. Patients may also present after multiple ICD discharges or in full cardiac arrest, requiring cardiopulmonary resuscitation. The warmth, local redness, and pain associated with a potential infection of the ICD pocket may prompt the individual to seek medical attention. Questions regarding interactions between ICDs and electromagnetic interference (EMI) will arise more frequently. These clinical situations are discussed in greater detail below.

Patients with ICDs must be placed on continuous telemetry. A detailed history and physical examination should be performed. The patient should be questioned regarding the number of shocks received, symptomatic palpitations, presyncope, symptoms of congestive heart failure, or symptoms consistent with angina. The pocket site must be examined for evidence of local infection, including warmth, tenderness, and discharge. Upper extremity or neck swelling ipsilateral to the inserted endocardial lead suggests the possibility of a subclavian vein or superior vena cava thrombosis.[18] Bilateral head edema and neck vein swelling suggests the possibility of a superior vena cava thrombosis or a superior vena cava syndrome. It is important to document any changes in medications or whether antiarrhythmic therapy has recently commenced. Routine blood work should be obtained, including a complete blood count, serum electrolytes, magnesium level, renal function indices, and quantitative levels of measurable medications.

The ICD model should be identified. Patients are generally given identification cards that list the manufacturer, lead system, generator model, and a 24 hour emergency contact number. Often this information is not available. However, in an emergency situation, an overpenetrated chest radiograph showing the generator will demonstrate the radiopaque identifier of the manufacturer.

The chest radiograph is not only important for device identification but can also give useful information about lead integrity. In a recent implant, a chest radiograph is routinely performed to assure lead positioning, slack in the lead, and to rule out a pneumothorax. In patients with epicardial patches, it is an excellent tool for demonstrating patch crinkling, fracture, or migration. With endocardial systems, the lead can again be assessed for fractures or discontinuities. Fractures can occur anywhere along the lead. They are most commonly seen near the junction of the first rib and the clavicle—a condition referred to as "subclavian crush."

If the patient presents with a ventricular arrhythmia and is hemodynamically stable, attempts should be made to obtain a 12-lead electrocardiogram (ECG) before any interventions are made to terminate the arrhythmia. Often this may be difficult due to concomitant discharges from the device, an anxious staff, and an anxious patient. Antiarrhythmic medications such as amiodarone, procainamide, and beta-blockers may have to be considered in the event of recurrent ventricular tachycardia. Despite the absence of clinical trials examining the efficacy of lidocaine, it is generally considered the treatment of choice in the setting of an acute myocardial infarction or acute ischemia if the patient is experiencing a ventricular arrhythmia.

EMERGENCY DEACTIVATION (MAGNET BEHAVIOR)

The ability of an ICD to identify and treat tachyarrhythmias can be temporarily disabled with the use of a magnet. This situation may arise in the setting of multiple ICD discharges where the shocks are not tolerated or prior to a surgical procedure where electrocautery is necessary. **The application of a magnet overlying the ICD pulse generator forms a magnetic field that trips a reed switch in the ICD generator circuit. This results in a suspension of tachycardia detection and therapy delivery.** Magnets can be obtained from industry manufacturers and are usually doughnut-shaped. Generally, a single magnet will suffice. In obese patients or in pockets with significant edema, two or more magnets may be required to achieve deactivation.[19] **A cardioverter-defibrillator unit must be readily available if an ICD is deactivated.**

The magnet response of an ICD varies subtly from manufacturer to manufacturer. In Medtronic devices, the application of a magnet temporarily disables tachycardia detection and therapy with no effect on bradycardia pacing. Removal of the magnet will resume arrhythmia detection. When activated, newer Medtronic devices (Gem II DR, patient alert function) will elicit a continuous beep lasting for 15 seconds if a magnet is placed directly over the ICD. A magnet applied over Guidant (CPI) defibrillators also inhibits tachycardia therapy with no effect on bradycardic pacing. These devices will generate beeping tones, which change to a continuous tone. The constant tone indicates that the device is off and will not deliver tachycardia therapy. The device can be turned back on by reapplying the magnet over the ICD for 30 seconds. Tones will now change from continuous to beeping synchronous with R waves, signifying that the device is on again. Newer-generation Guidant ICDs (Prism II) have a built-in electrocautery feature that can be activated by use of the Guidant programmer. This will suspend tachyarrhythmia therapies and pace in the DOO mode. Regular functioning of the ICD is restored by turning this feature off.

MULTIPLE ICD DISCHARGES

Emergency Department patients presenting with multiple ICD discharges require immediate attention. From a psychological perspective, multiple discharges are usually not well tolerated and can be emotionally devastating to the patient.[18] Myocardial injury and transient reduction in left ventricular function can occur as a result of multiple shocks. This has been associated with a poorer long-term prognosis. Multiple discharges can lead to premature depletion of battery life.

ESTABLISHING THE ETIOLOGY

It is important to establish the etiology of the shocks in order to administer proper and prompt management (Table 24-2). **It is of the utmost importance to determine whether the shocks are appropriate for ventricular tachycardia or fibrillation.** Recurrent ventricular tachyarrhythmia is a common cause of repeated ICD firing. Ineffective termination of a tachyarrhythmia in this situation can be the result of an increase in defibrillation thresholds secondary to concomitant antiarrhythmic

TABLE 24-2. CAUSES OF FREQUENT ICD DISCHARGES

Sustained ventricular tachyarrhythmias
    Frequently recurring episodes, each one terminated by a shock
    One shock needed to terminate each episode of sustained ventricular tachyarrhythmia
Nonsustained ventricular tachyarrhythmias
Supraventricular rhythms satisfying detection criteria
    Atrial fibrillation
    Sinus tachycardia
    Paroxysmal supraventricular tachycardia
Oversensing of signals
    Sensing lead failure
    Double and triple counting of pacing artifacts
    P-wave oversensing
    T-wave oversensing
    Electromagnetic interference
Random component failure

SOURCE: Reproduced from Pinski et al.,[19] with permission.

drug therapy and lead migration or lead dislodgement. Inefficient termination can occur if inappropriately low amounts of energy are programmed for the initially administered shock. Shocks may also be the result of inappropriate detection of supraventricular tachycardias (SVTs), the most frequent of which include sinus tachycardia and atrial fibrillation.[20] The administration of a low-energy shock may convert a benign SVT into an unstable ventricular arrhythmia resulting in ICD proarrhythmia. The introduction of an atrial lead in dual-chamber devices has aided in the discrimination process between SVTs and ventricular tachyarrhythmias. Inappropriate ICD firing can occur because of the erroneous detection of noise or interference that can be the result of insulation breakdown or a loose set screw (Figure 24-4). Oversensing of T waves, pacing artifacts, R waves, and electromagnetic interference may also lead to inappropriate detection and discharge. Finally, random component failure should be considered if all other causes have been ruled out.

APPROACH TO THE PATIENT WITH MULTIPLE DISCHARGES

These patients must be under constant ECG monitoring. In devices with limited stored diagnostic capabilities, this may be the only means of establishing shock-rhythm correlation. Sedation is reasonable in extremely anxious patients. Once the patient is stabilized, the device should be interrogated and stored electrograms obtained for analysis.[21] An electrophysiology consultation should be obtained for assistance in interrogating the ICD and troubleshooting. The patient's history may offer subtle clues. For instance, it is often useful to inquire about the pattern of ICD discharge. Consecutive shocks occurring within a few seconds suggest an inappropriate SVT, oversensing, or device failure. On the other hand, isolated shocks occurring every few minutes may be indicative of recurrent ventricular tachycardia. Increasing shortness of breath, orthopnea, or paroxysmal nocturnal dyspnea suggests worsening heart failure, which can precipitate ventricular arrhythmias.

Careful examination of the 12-lead ECG is crucial. ST-segment elevations imply an acute myocardial infarction and will require a primary intervention or thrombolysis. An ECG obtained during an actual shock may establish whether the culprit arrhythmia is a supraventricular or ventricular tachycardia.

If the discharges are inappropriate, the ICD should be emergently deactivated, as previously described. Paroxysmal SVTs should be terminated with appropriate measures such as intravenous adenosine or verapamil. In the situation where discharges are secondary to rapid atrial fibrillation, attempts must be made to control the patient's ventricular response with atrioventricular (AV) nodal blocking agents such as diltiazem, ver-

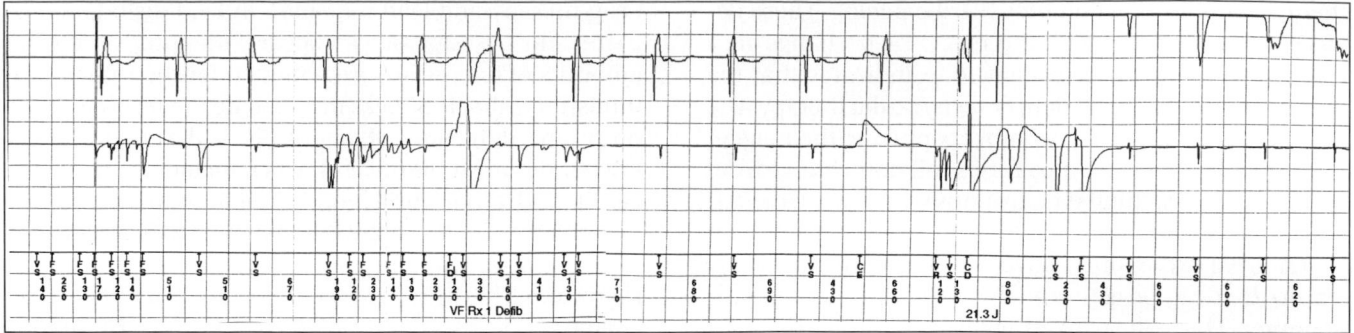

FIGURE 24-4 Inappropriate ICD discharge. Intracardiac electrogram of a patient with a Ventak Mini III presenting with repetitive ICD discharges. Examination of the intracardiac electrograms (line 2) demonstrates noise sensed as ventricular fibrillation (FS) resulting in an inappropriate shock (CD). Noise was traced to an insulation break in the ICD lead. Lead replacement corrected the problem.

apamil, beta-blockers, and digoxin. Chemical cardioversion or electrical conversion may be attempted in the event of hemodynamic instability. Shocks secondary to prolonged episodes of nonsustained ventricular tachycardia can be prevented by adjusting initial detection parameters coupled with the addition of antiarrhythmic drug therapy.

Patients in electrical storm require immediate attention. This condition involves recurrent, hemodynamically unstable ventricular tachycardia or fibrillation occurring two or more times in a 24 hour period.[22] An Electrophysiologist should be promptly consulted and the patient stabilized prior to transfer to the intensive care unit (ICU). Defibrillator pads should be applied in anticipation of the development of unstable cardiac arrhythmias. Potential reversible causes, such as electrolyte abnormalities, need to be identified and promptly corrected. If torsades de pointes is established, the treatment of choice is magnesium and/or temporary cardiac pacing. Thrombolysis or urgent catheterization/intervention may be needed in the setting of an acute infarction. If analysis of stored electrograms demonstrates ineffective discharges, the ICD should be deactivated. Attempts to terminate the arrhythmia in the hemodynamically stable patient via antitachycardia pacing (ATP) is a useful option.

Intravenous antiarrhythmic drugs are a necessary adjunct in these situations. The administration of amiodarone in combination with beta-blocker therapy has been shown to be successful in the management of electrical storm.[23] Often a combination of antiarrhythmic drugs will be required. Bretylium should be reserved until other antiarrhythmic agents have failed.

ICDs AND CARDIAC RESUSCITATION

In the situation where an ICD recipient requires resuscitation, Advanced Cardiac Life Support (ACLS) guidelines should be followed and the device considered inactive.[24,25] If the clinical situation permits and an ICD programmer is readily available, the device should be deactivated. This will prevent the reinduction of ventricular fibrillation or tachycardia due to concomitant ICD discharges that may occur during cardiopulmonary resuscitation (CPR). **There is often some hesitation to initiate resuscitative measures in patients with an ICD for fear of getting shocked. This fear is understandable but unwarranted.** Although a mild electric shock might be perceived, these discharges do not pose a risk to persons administering CPR, nor do they damage external monitoring devices.

External defibrillation is permissible, although the paddles should be positioned away from the device. Individuals with epicardial patches may require higher energies for defibrillation. Current can be shunted from the myocardium through the patches. Moreover, the insulated portion of the patch serves as a shield from the administered shock. In patients with epicardial patches, an anteroposterior paddle configuration has been suggested for changing the defibrillation vector.[26]

The defibrillator may be reset after external defibrillation is delivered, especially if the paddles are located in close proximity to the generator. It is important that devices be reinterrogated after the successful completion of a resuscitation to ensure that programmed parameters have not been altered, including the pacing thresholds.

INFECTION OF AN IMPLANTABLE DEFIBRILLATOR

An infected ICD system represents a serious medical situation that should be dealt with urgently. The incidence of infection ranges from 2 to 11 percent in systems that were implanted via thoracotomy or sternotomy. The infection rates for nonthoracotomy implants approach those of pacemakers and range from 0.8 to 1.5 percent.[27–29] Infections generally present clinically within 6 months of the implant, but more typically within the first 3 months. Infection should be suspected when local and systemic signs and symptoms of inflammation are apparent. Systemic symptoms are seen in up to 50 percent of patients, especially in those with infections caused by *Staphylococcus aureus*.[30] The pocket and/or incision site is often visibly erythematous, warm, and tender. A fever may be present. Blood work often reveals a leukocytosis. Frank suppuration or device erosion may be seen. Pericarditis may be evident if epicardial patches are infected. Blood cultures may aid in documenting the culprit organism. Infections occurring late are generally indolent and rarely present with fever or leukocytosis; moreover, blood cultures are generally negative.

The most common microorganisms include *S. aureus* and coagulase-negative staphylococci. Other common organisms include *Escherichia coli, Pseudomonas, Serratia, Corynebacterium, Proprionibacterium acnes, Candida* spp., streptococci, and atypical mycobacteria. Infection is generally the result of skin contamination during surgery. It can also occur due to hematogenous seeding from distant intravenous sites or indwelling catheters or from concomitant respiratory or urinary tract infections.

APPROACH TO AN INFECTED ICD

The goals of therapy include identifying the culprit organisms, establishing the extent of the infection, and containment of the infection. In the Emergency Department, routine laboratory tests should be obtained that include a complete blood count and differential. Blood for cultures should also be drawn, but it must be kept in mind that they are often negative. Wound cultures may be helpful in differentiating an infection from a pocket hematoma, sterile subcutaneous fluid accumulation, or an inflammatory reaction to pacemaker components. Attempts to aspirate the pocket should be performed in consultation with an Electrophysiologist and/or Surgeon. Often, a sterile pocket or hematoma can become infected after aspiration.

There is no single diagnostic modality that can determine the extent of the infection. Defibrillator infections should never be assumed to be localized, as organisms can migrate from the leads into the heart. In patients with epicardial patches, a chest radiograph may reveal patch deformities or wrinkling, suggesting distal migration of the infection. A computed tomography (CT) scan can also detect localized fluid accumulation and patch wrinkling. Echocardiography has been utilized to confirm the presence of vegetations on the leads or coil. Gallium and indium scans may be helpful in localizing infection.

Although a few reports suggest that infection of a defibrillator system may be controlled, the treatment of choice continues to be explanting the entire system, followed by the administration of parenteral antibiotic agents. Some localized infections restricted to the ICD generator have been managed with the removal of the generator, debridement, and systemic antibiotic therapy. Vancomycin is frequently used as an empiric agent when cultures are still pending given its good coverage against coagulase-negative staphylococci and methicillin-resistant *Staphylococcus aureus* (MRSA).

ELECTROMAGNETIC INTERFERENCE AND ICDs

The ability of ICDs (and pacemakers) to function is dependent on their ability to sense intrinsic cardiac electrical activity. Hermetic shielding, filtering, interference rejection circuits, and bipolar sensing have safeguarded ICDs (and pacemakers) against the effects of common electromagnetic sources. However, exposure to electromagnetic interference (EMI) may still result in oversensing, asynchronous pacing, ventricular inhibition, and spurious ICD discharges. EMI may also lead to loss of output, increased pacing thresholds, and decreased R-wave amplitude. Common sources of EMI include cellular phones, electronic article surveillance (antitheft) devices, and metal detectors. Occupational sources of EMI include high-voltage power lines, electrical transformers, arc welding, and electric motors. Interference can also be encountered through medical equipment and procedures such as magnetic resonance imaging, electric cautery, spinal cord stimulators, transcutaneous electric nerve stimulator units, radiofrequency catheter ablation, therapeutic diathermy, and lithotripsy.[32]

Patients with ICDs and pacemakers should be instructed to avoid environments with large magnetic fields. The use of cellular phones is permissible. The U.S. Food and Drug Administration (FDA) recommends that direct contact of the phone with the device should be avoided. Use of the contralateral ear while using the phone is suggested. Although inappropriate shocks have been documented through electronic article surveillance systems, recent studies have deemed it safe for patients to walk through these systems as long as they avoid lingering around these devices.

SUMMARY

Expanding clinical indications and the increasing number of annual implants will require Emergency Department Physicians to become familiar with problems typically encountered by the patient with an implantable defibrillator. Complications associated with ICDs are not uncommon. Troubleshooting and programming should ideally be performed in conjunction with a trained Electrophysiologist. Patients presenting with cardiopulmonary arrest may require the device to be deactivated and external defibrillation performed. Do not apply external defibrillation paddles directly over the ICD.

REFERENCES

1. The Antiarrhythmic versus Implantable Defibrillators (AVID) Investigators: A comparison of antiarrhythmic-drug therapy with implantable defibrillators in patients resuscitated from near-fatal ventricular arrhythmias. *N Engl J Med* 1988; 319:661–666.

2. Connolly SJ, Gent M, Roberts RS, et al: Canadian implantable defibrillator study (CIDS): a randomized trial of the implantable cardioverter defibrillator against amiodarone. *Circulation* 2000; 101(11):1297–1302.

3. Kuck KH, Cappato R, Siebels J, et al: Randomized comparisons of antiarrhythmic drug therapy with implantable defibrillators in patients resuscitated from cardiac arrest: the Cardiac Arrest Study Hamburg (CASH). *Circulation* 2000; 102:748–754.

4. Moss AJ, Hall WJ, Cannom DS, et al: Improved survival with an implanted defibrillator in patients with coronary disease at high risk for ventricular arrhythmia. *N Engl J Med* 1996; 335:1933–1940.

5. Buxton AE, Lee KL, Fisher JD, et al: A randomized study of the prevention of sudden death in patients with coronary artery disease. *N Engl J Med* 1999; 341:1882–1890.

6. Medical Data International: *U.S. Markets for Arrhythmia Management Devices.* Englewood, CO: IHS Health, 1999:4–22.

7. Mirowski M, Reid PR, Winkle RA, et al: Mortality in patients with implanted automatic defibrillators. *Ann Intern Med* 1983; 98:585–588.

8. Mirowski M: The automatic implantable cardioverter-defibrillator: an overview. *J Am Coll Cardiol* 1985; 6:461–466.

9. Mahomed Y: Surgical techniques for implantation of the implantable cardioverter defibrillator, in Zipes DP, Jalife J (eds): *Cardiac Electrophysiology: From Cell to Bedside,* 2nd ed. Philadelphia: Saunders, 1995:1412–1425.

10. Raviele A, Gasparini G (for the Italian Endotak Investigator Group): Italian multicenter clinical experience with endocardial defibrillation: acute and long-term results in 307 patients. *PACE Pacing Clin Electrophysiol* 1995; 18(2):599–608.

11. Shahian DM, Williamsom WA, Svensson LG, et al: Transvenous versus transthoracic cardioverter-defibrillator implantation: a comparative analysis of morbidity, mortality and survival. *J Thorac Cardiovasc Surg* 1995; 109:1066–1074.

12. Nierbauer MJ, Wilkoff BL: Implantable cardioverter-defibrillators: technical aspects, in Zipes DP, Jalife J (eds): *Cardiac Electrophysiology: From Cell to Bedside,* 3rd ed. Philadelphia: Saunders, 2000:949–957.

13. Leitch JW, Gillis AM, Wyse DG, et al: Reduction in defibrillator shocks with an implantable device combining antitachycardia pacing and shock therapy. *J Am Coll Cardiol* 1991; 18:145–151.

14. Bardy GH, Troutman C, Polle JE, et al: Clinical experience with a tiered-therapy multiprogrammable antiarrhythmia device. *Circulation* 1992; 85:1689–1698.

15. Swerdlow CD, Schsls W, Dijknam B, et al: Detection of atrial fibrillation and flutter by a dual-chamber implantable-cardioverter defibrillator. *Circulation* 2000; 101(8):878–885.

16. Wilbur SL, Marchlinski FE: Implantable cardioverter-defibrillator follow-up. *Cardiol Rev* 1999; 7:176–190.

17. Nisam S, Fogoros RN: Troubleshooting of patients with implantable cardioverter-defibrillators, in Singer I (ed): *Interventional Electrophysiology.* Baltimore: Williams & Wilkins, 1997:793–823.

18. Kowey PR: The calamity of cardioversion of conscious patients. *Am J Cardiol* 1988; 61:1106–1107.

19. Pinski SL, Trohman RG: Implantable cardioverter-defibrillators: implications for the nonelectrophysiologist. *Ann Intern Med* 1996; 122:770–777.

20. Grimm W, Flores BF, Marchlinski FE: Electrocardiographically documented unnecessary, spontaneous shocks in 241 patients with implantable cardioverter-defibrillators. *PACE Pacing Clin Electrophysiol* 1992; 15:1667–1673.

21. Hook BG, Marchlinski FE: The value of ventricular electrogram recording in the diagnosis of arrhythmias precipitating electrical device therapy. *J Am Coll Cardiol* 1991; 17:985–990.

22. Dorian P, Cass D: An overview of the management of electric storm. *Can J Cardiol* 1997; 13:13A–17A.

23. Credner SC, Klingenheben T, Mauss O, et al: Electrical storm in patients with tranvenous implantable cardioverter defibrillators. *J Am Coll Cardiol* 1998; 32:1909–1915.

24. Chapman PD, Veseth-Rogers JL, Duquette SE: The implantable defibrillator and the emergency physician. *Ann Emerg Med* 1989; 18:579–585.

25. White RD, Feldman RA: The automatic internal cardioverter defibrillator (AICD): description and guidelines for interaction during cardiac arrest. *Ann Emerg Med* 1989; 18:586–588.

26. Pinski SL, Arnold AZ, Mick M, et al: Safety of external cardioversion/defibrillation in patients with internal defibrillation patches and no device. *PACE Pacing Clin Electrophysiol* 1991; 14:7–12.

27. Smith PN, Vidaillet HJ, Hayes JJ: Infections with non-thoracotomy implantable cardioverter-defibrillators: can these be prevented? *PACE Pacing Clin Electrophysiol* 1998; 21:42–55.

28. Gold MR, Peters RW, Johnson JW: Complications associated with pectoral implantation of cardioverter defibrillators. *PACE Pacing Clin Electrophysiol* 1997; 20:208–211.

29. Karchmer AW: Infections of prosthetic valves and intravascular devices, in Mandell GL, Bennett JE, Dolin R (eds): *Principles and Practice of Infectious Diseases,* 5th ed. New York: Churchill Livingstone, 2000:903–917.

30. O'Nunain S, Perez I, Roelke M, et al: The treatment of patients with infected implantable cardioverter-defibrillator systems. *J Thorac Cardiovasc Surg* 1997; 113:121–129.

31. Lai KK, Fontecchio SA: Infections associated with implantable cardioverter-defibrillators placed transvenously and via thoracotomies: epidemiology, infection control, and management. *Clin Infect Dis* 1998; 27:265–269.

32. Pinski SL, Trohman RG: Interference with cardiac pacing. *Cardiol Clin* 2000; 18(1):219–239.

Chapter 25
PERICARDIOCENTESIS

Robert F. Smith

INTRODUCTION

Pericardiocentesis is the removal of fluid from the pericardial space surrounding the heart. The fluid is usually aspirated with a needle and syringe. Occasionally, a catheter is placed within the pericardium or a surgical approach is used. This may be performed for diagnosis, to obtain pericardial fluid; to relieve a pericardial effusion and improve cardiac output; or as a lifesaving measure to relieve a cardiac tamponade. **The technique is relatively simple to perform yet has a significant rate of complications.**

Since humanity's earliest times, penetrating cardiac injuries have held a dramatic place in both romantic and medical literature.[1-8] In 1649, Riolanus first described pericardial tamponade.[3] He noted that "an abundance of moisture is collected therein [the pericardium], which causes suffocation, and overwhelms the heart." In 1827, Thomas Jowett described the first use of pericardiocentesis as an intervention for pericarditis.[4] In 1829, Baron Larrey, Napoleon's Surgeon, is reported to have performed the first successful pericardiocentesis.[5] By 1939, Bigger had suggested that some patients with cardiac tamponade could be managed with pericardial tubes alone, with prompt operation for recurrence.[7]

ANATOMY AND PATHOPHYSIOLOGY

The pericardium is an inverted cone-shaped sack surrounding the heart and lying on top of the diaphragm (Figure 25-1). The inner portion, or visceral pericardium, is a single layer of mesothelial cells covering the epicardium. The outer layer is composed of a dense outer fibrous tissue with an inner layer of mesothelial cells known as the parietal pericardium. The fibrous peri-

cardium is attached to the central tendinous portion of the diaphragm inferiorly. Superiorly, the outer fibrous layer blends with the sheath covering the great vessels. Anteriorly, it attaches to the posterior surface of the sternum. Posteriorly, it is attached to the thoracic vertebral column, esophagus, bronchi, and aorta.

The heart is contained within the pericardial sac. Numerous portions of the heart are exposed behind the anterior chest wall (Figure 25-2). This includes the right ventricle, left ventricle, right atrium, left atrium, aorta, pulmonary artery, and inferior vena cava. These structures are vulnerable to injury behind the anterior chest wall[9,10] (Table 25-1). The surface area that each of these structures contributes to the anterior cardiac silhouette is also listed in this table. These numbers reflect, roughly, the anatomic incidence of injury with cardiac trauma.[11] Traumatic injury to any of these structures can result in a pericardial effusion and cardiac tamponade.

The pericardial cavity is a potential space between the visceral and parietal layers of the pericardium. Normally 20 to 50 mL of fluid is contained within this space. The fluid acts as a lubricant to the motion of the heart. Accumulation of fluid in the pericardial space requiring drainage can have a variety of etiologies. From a review of several retrospective series, the estimated causes and relative frequencies of pericardial effusions are listed in Table 25-2.[12-18]

Cardiac tamponade is a life-threatening condition that must be diagnosed and treated emergently. The diagnosis of cardiac tamponade is primarily clinical. It may easily be overlooked unless a high index of suspicion is maintained in both medical and trauma patients. Sauer and Murdock describe a "danger zone" for penetrating torso trauma[19] (Figure 25-3). The superior border is bounded by a line through the sternal notch. The lateral borders are bound by a line through the

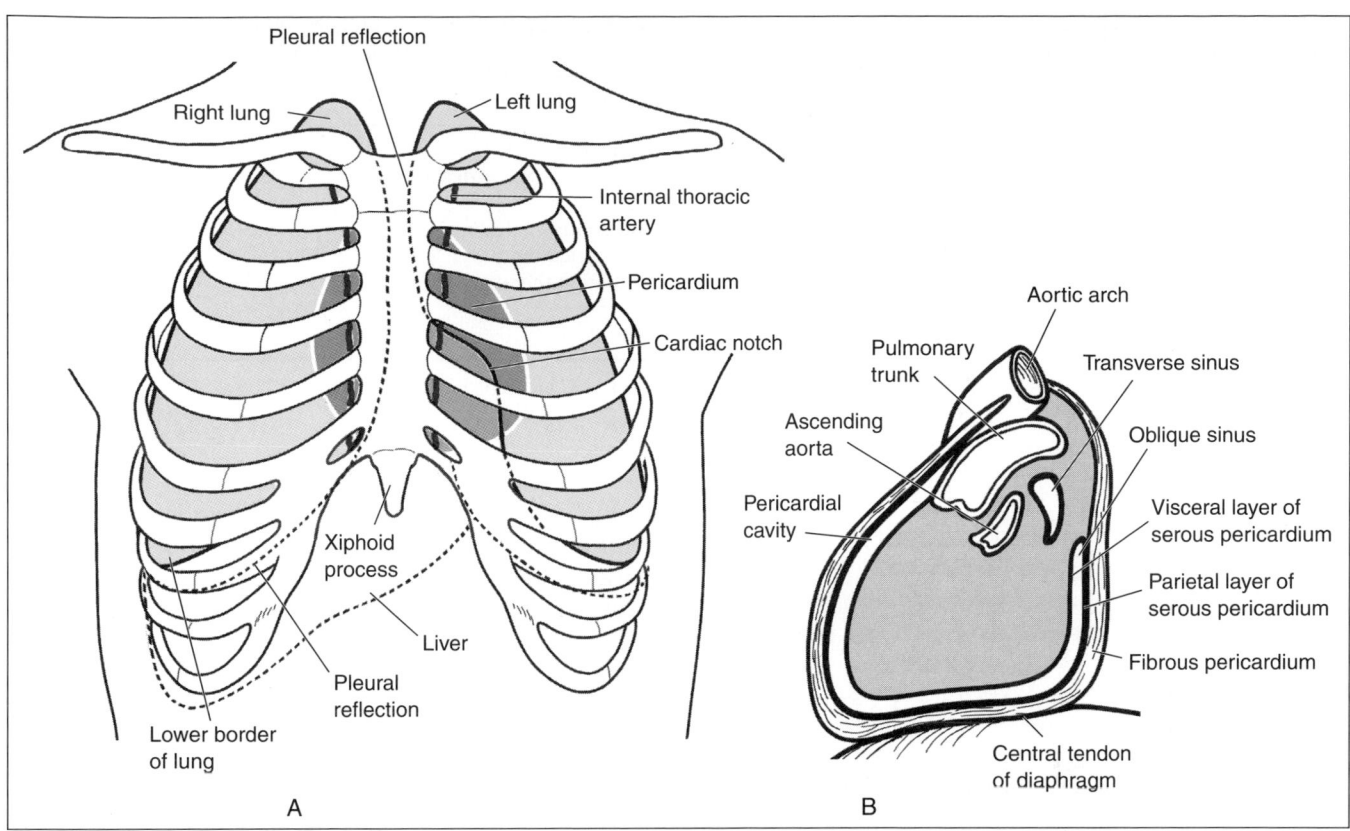

FIGURE 25-1 The pericardium. *A.* Relationship of the pericardium to the major thoracic structures. *B.* Midsagittal section through the heart and pericardium.

midclavicle. The inferior border is identified by a line through the epigastric area. Any penetrating injury in the danger zone or through it has the potential to cause a cardiac injury and pericardial tamponade.

The clinical effects of cardiac tamponade occur due to accumulation of fluid under pressure in the pericardial space. This space can become quite large over time. In some chronic disease states, pericardial effusions of 1 to 2 L can occur without signs of cardiac tamponade.[14,20] The ability of the pericardial sac to stretch acutely is limited. Estimates of the volume of fluid required to acutely accumulate and produce a cardiac tamponade range from 60 to 200 milliliters.

Cardiac tamponade should always be considered as a cause of shock in the medical patient. This includes patients who are taking oral or parenteral anticoagulants, have known cancer, have known pericardial disease, are suspected of having an aortic dissection, or have had a recent myocardial infarction. Cardiac tamponade can also be due to iatrogenic causes, including central venous line placement, transthoracic cardiac pacing, transvenous cardiac pacing, and cardiopulmonary resuscitation.

The pressure-volume relationship between the size of the pericardial effusion and the pressure imposed on the cardiac chambers is exponential. The initial accumulation of fluid produces little or no clinical effect. The initial physiologic strategies of compensation include an increase in the systemic venous pressure, catecholamine release, and tachycardia. At some point the ability of the pericardial space to distend and accommodate more fluid is overwhelmed. From this point on, even small amounts of fluid generate significant and increasing pressure on the heart chambers. As the pericardial pressure rises, venous filling of the right heart is drastically impaired. The interventricular septum bulges into the left ventricle. Left ventricular filling becomes compromised from the lack of flow from the right ventricle and the bulging inward of the interventricular septum. Eventually, cardiac perfusion decreases and the heart suffers injury.

A progressive decline in cardiac output occurs as pericardial fluid accumulates and intrapericardial pressure increases.[21] Initially, the right atrial pressure is greater than the intrapericardial pressure as the body compensates by increasing venous return. This is followed by the equilibration of the right atrial and intrapericardial pressures. Eventually, as the heart chambers cannot achieve a pressure lower than the surrounding pericardial fluid pressure, equilibration of

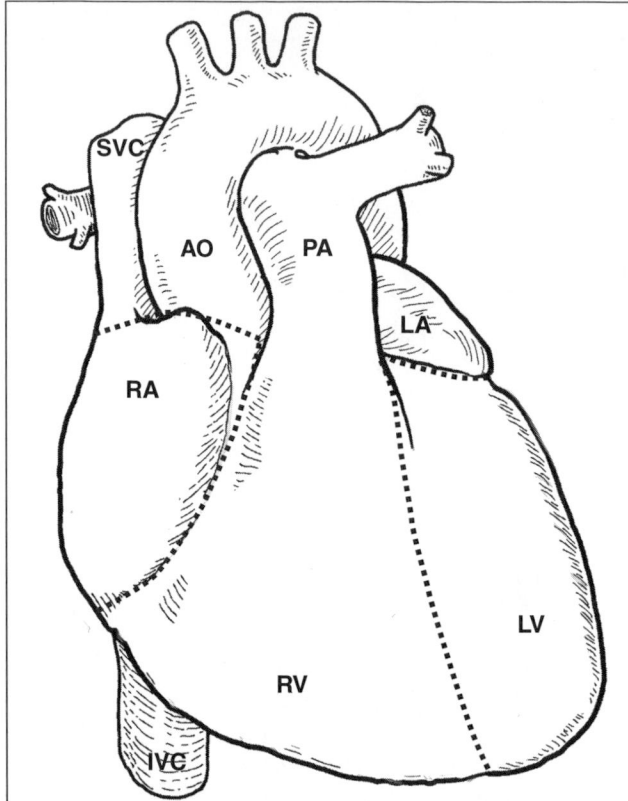

FIGURE 25-2 View of the heart and great vessels, which can become injured behind the anterior chest wall. (AO = aorta, IVC = inferior vena cava, LA = left atrium, LV = left ventricle, PA = pulmonary artery, RA = right atrium, RV = right ventricle, SVC = superior vena cava.)

diastolic pressure in each heart chamber occurs and produces the greatest drop in cardiac output. As the intrapericardial pressure continues to increase, the cardiac chambers collapse, resulting in intractable hypotension and death. The disproportionate effects of the later small amounts of fluid explain why withdrawal of even a small amount of fluid from the pericardial cavity can produce dramatic temporary improvements in the clinical status of the patient. It also explains why "moni-

TABLE 25-1. STRUCTURES VULNERABLE TO INJURY BEHIND THE ANTERIOR CHEST WALL*

Anatomic structure	%
Right ventricle	55
Left ventricle	20
Right atrium	10
Left atrium	1
Aorta and pulmonary artery	10
Inferior vena cava	4

*The percentages represent the surface area of each structure and the estimates of incidence of injury with cardiac trauma.[9–11]

TABLE 25-2. THE ETIOLOGIES AND RELATIVE FREQUENCIES OF PERICARDIAL EFFUSIONS

Etiology	Relative frequency (%)
Cancer	15–40
Connective tissue diseases	2–11
Idiopathic	13–14
Infectious (including HIV)	2–14
Postpericardiotomy	2–16
Radiation therapy	4–7
Trauma	7–9
Uremia	5–10

SOURCE: Adapted from references 12–18.

toring" patients for the evolution of cardiac tamponade with central venous pressure lines is dangerous, as the patient will proceed from stable and compensated to profoundly unstable quite suddenly.

Several clinical findings are associated with cardiac tamponade. These findings may be absent if the patient is hypovolemic due to hemorrhage. **Beck's triad of muffled heart sounds, hypotension, and jugular venous distention is associated with cardiac tamponade.** Almost all patients with cardiac tamponade will have at least one of these signs. **Unfortunately, very few patients with cardiac tamponade will have all three signs.** Restlessness, fatigue, tachycardia, and tachypnea are often present. These can progress to shock, coma, and eventually death.

Changes in the jugulovenous waveforms may be seen in cardiac tamponade. Instead of the normal systolic X

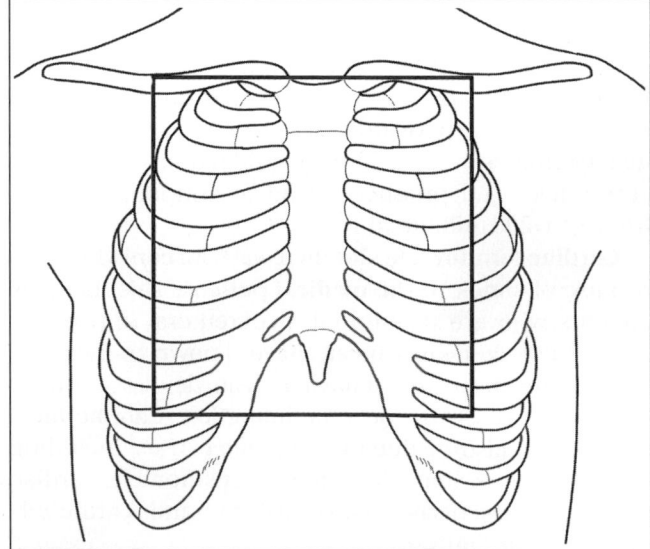

FIGURE 25-3 The "danger zone" for penetrating chest trauma.[19]

descent and diastolic Y descent, only the systolic X descent occurs in cardiac tamponade. This is a result of the increased diastolic pressure being exerted by the accumulating pericardial fluid. The only time the right heart can fill is during systole, when the internal volume of the heart is reduced.

Kussmaul's two signs, paradoxical increase of the jugulovenous pressure during inspiration and pulsus paradoxus, may be seen in patients with cardiac tamponade. Pulsus paradoxus is a drop in systolic blood pressure of ≥ 10 mmHg during inspiration. To measure this, inflate the blood pressure cuff to greater than the systolic pressure. Slowly release the cuff pressure until beats are heard only during expiration. Keep deflating the cuff pressure until beats are heard continuously in both inspiration and expiration. The difference between these two physiologic points is the amount of pulsus paradoxus. This normal physiologic finding is exaggerated by the accumulation of pericardial fluid, forcing the right heart and interventricular septum into the left ventricle.

Electrocardiographic and radiographic signs of cardiac tamponade are often not present. Changes on the electrocardiogram (ECG) may be present in patients with cardiac tamponade. Electrical alternans is a change in the morphology or amplitude of the QRS complexes on the ECG as the heart swings to and fro within the pericardial fluid (Figure 25-4). It may be associated with pericardial tamponade but is not pathognomonic. Pulseless electrical activity in the absence of hypovolemia or a tension pneumothorax is highly suggestive of cardiac tamponade. Authors differ as to the clinical significance of these findings. The finding of an enlarged cardiac silhouette on a chest radiograph may be useful in chronic pericardial effusions but is usually absent or nonspecific in the acute setting.

Traumatic cardiac tamponade can be caused by a variety of agents and etiologies. This includes bullets, knives, ice picks, displaced fractured ribs, central venous line placement, pacemaker insertion, pericardiocentesis, intracardiac injection, surgery, migrating pins or needles, nails ejected from machinery, and venous bullet embolization. **Cardiac tamponade is the most common presentation of penetrating cardiac injuries overall. It occurs in 80 to 90 percent of stab wounds and 20 percent of gunshot wounds.[11]**

Cardiac ultrasound is rapidly becoming the diagnostic procedure of choice to identify cardiac tamponade. A prospective study at Cook County Hospital showed that ultrasound performed by emergency personnel was 96 percent accurate and 90 percent sensitive.[22] Cardiac ultrasonography performed on trauma patients can be 98 to 100 percent accurate in diagnosing pericardial fluid and cardiac tamponade.[23–25] The series of 261 patients had no false negatives. Other studies have demonstrated false-negative rates in the range of 5 to 40 percent.[19,26,27] Other ultrasonographic findings in pericardial tamponade include a swinging heart, collapse of the right and left ventricular chambers, and marked inspiratory changes in ventricular dimensions.[10] Some authors advocate using transesophageal echocardiography, even in unstable patients, because of its superior imaging when compared to transthoracic echocardiography.[28] Other methods of imaging the pericardium include computed tomography (CT), helical CT, and MRI. These modalities should be used only for stable patients in whom the diagnosis of a pericardial effusion and not cardiac tamponade is being considered.

INDICATIONS

Significant controversy exists over the role of pericardiocentesis.[9] The only indication for emergent pericardiocentesis would be in a patient in whom the life-threatening physiologic changes of cardiac tamponade were present and the diagnosis was consistent with known prior disease or mechanism of injury. Pericardiocentesis is also performed in the cardiac catheterization laboratory or the intensive care unit to obtain pericardial fluid for diagnostic testing. It may also be performed in a resuscitation patient with pulseless electrical activity (PEA) when other etiologies for PEA have been ruled out.

CONTRAINDICATIONS

There are no absolute contraindications to performing a pericardiocentesis in the unstable patient with signs of cardiac tamponade. Uncorrected bleeding disorders in a stable medical patient would be an absolute contraindication to performing the procedure. Small, loculated, or posteriorly located effusions in a stable patient are also considered contraindications.

While the dramatic beneficial effects of withdrawing even a small amount of pericardial fluid are well documented, many authors feel that there is little or no role for pericardiocentesis in the trauma patient. These authors argue that once the diagnosis of a pericardial effusion is made, the patient should receive a prompt sternotomy.[11] If the patient is too unstable for transport to the operating room, an emergent thoracotomy should be performed. In the trauma patient, aggressive fluid replacement with crystalloid and blood as well as needle thoracostomy to rule out a tension pneumothorax should be done before pericardiocentesis is contemplated.[29]

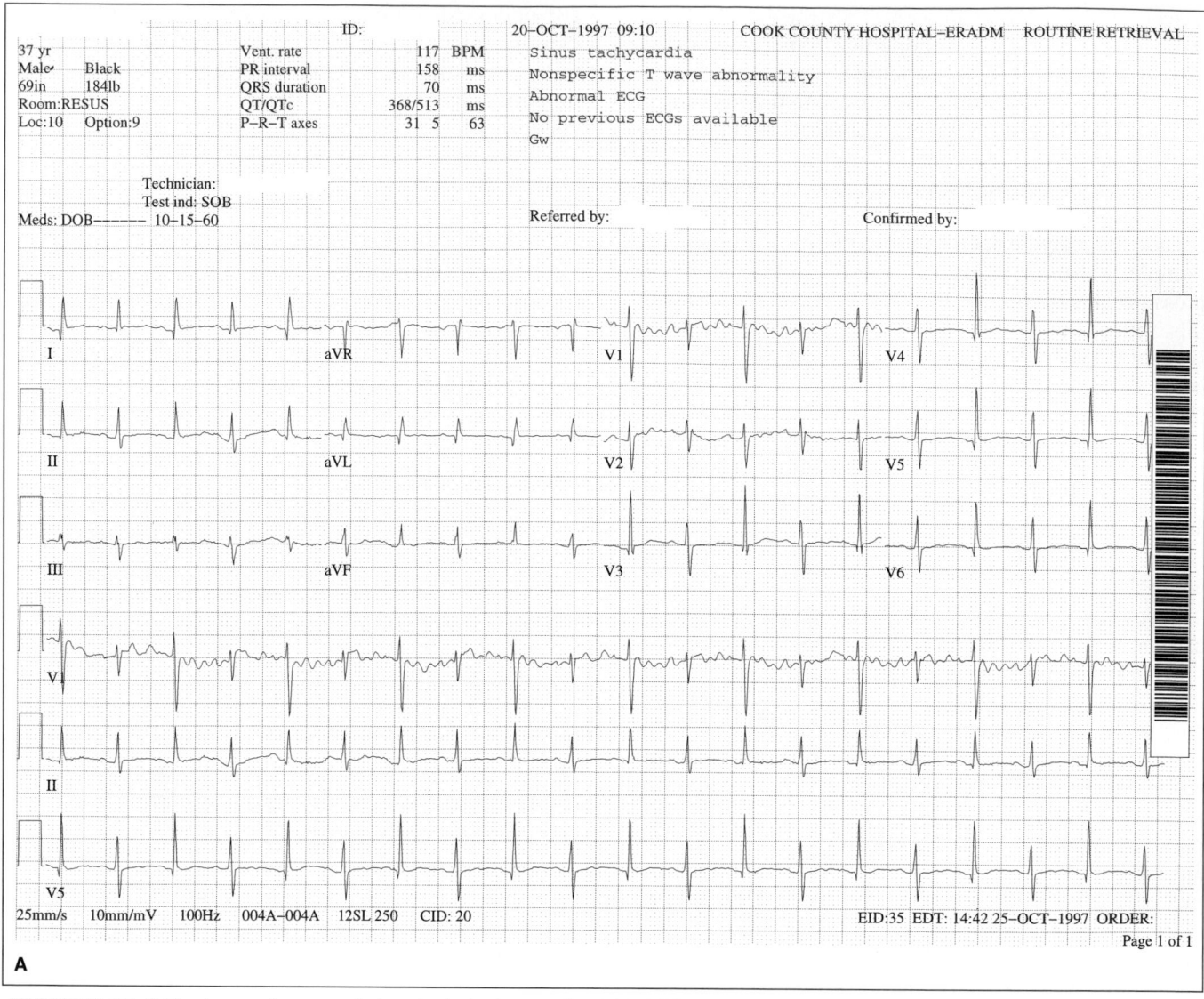

FIGURE 25-4 Electrocardiogram of electrical alternans. *A.* Initial ECG in the Emergency Department. Bedside echocardiography revealed a large pericardial effusion with right ventricular diastolic collapse.

EQUIPMENT

Pericardiocentesis

Povidone iodine solution
Local anesthetic solution (1% lidocaine)
25 gauge needle, 5/8 inch long
18 gauge needle, 1½ inches long
Syringes (10, 20, and 60 mL)
Sterile drapes
Towel clips
18 gauge spinal needle, 7.5 to 12.5 cm long
#11 scalpel blade
4×4 gauze squares
Alligator clips connected by a wire
Collection basin
ECG monitor
J-tipped guidewire, 0.035 mm in diameter

Size 6 to 10 French flexible multihole catheter, 5 to
  6 inches long, with or without a pigtail
Three-way stopcock
Plastic tubing
Ultrasound machine
Sterile cover for the ultrasound probe (can be sterile glove)
Variable-angle needle guide attachment if available
Nasogastric tube

Subxiphoid Pericardial Window

Electrocautery set
Forceps
Small retractor
Small rib spreaders
Sutures, 2–0 Vicryl and 3–0 nylon
Sterile suction device
Yankauer suction catheter
Suction tubing

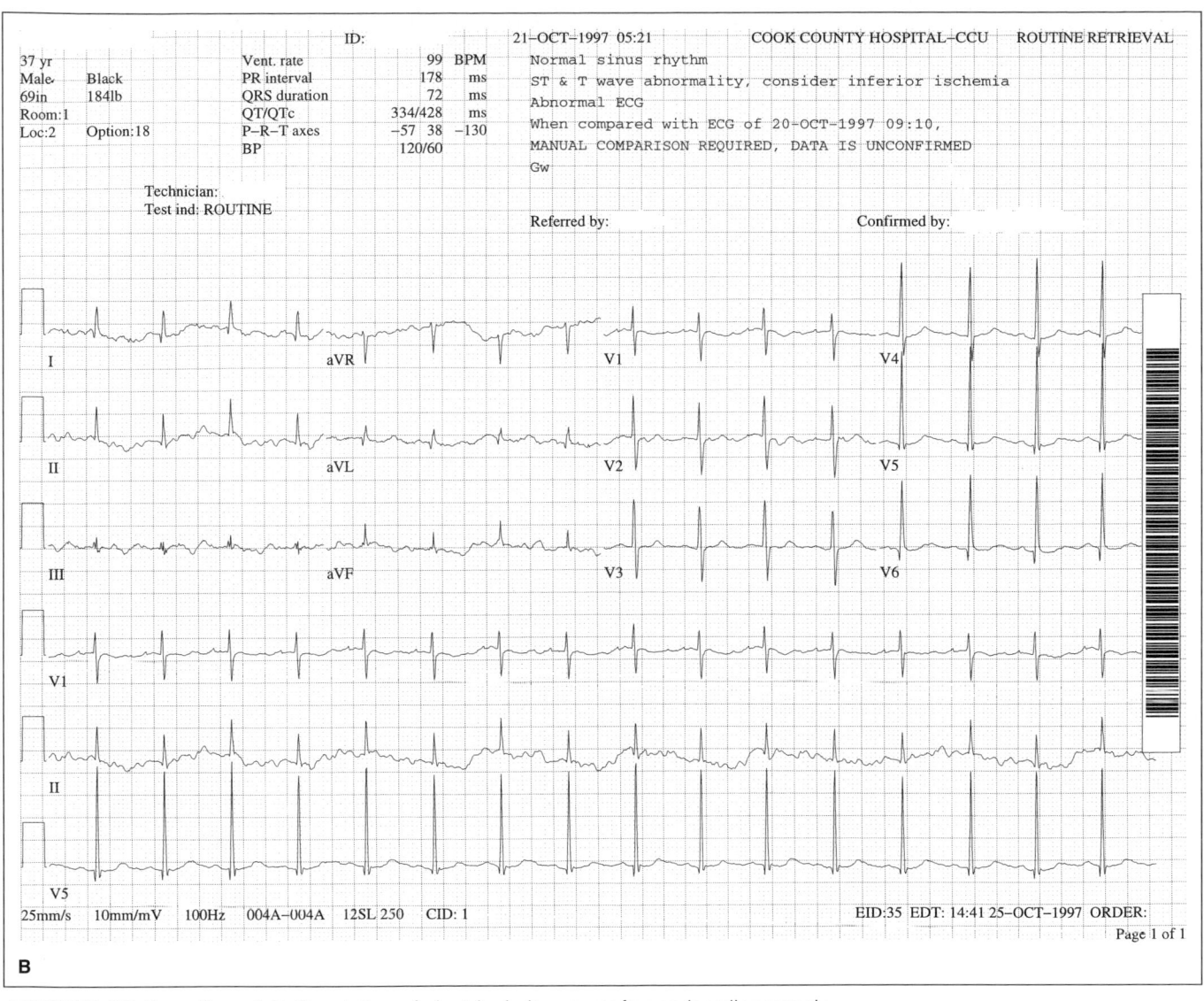

ID: 21-OCT-1997 05:21   COOK COUNTY HOSPITAL-CCU   ROUTINE RETRIEVAL

37 yr   Vent. rate   99 BPM   Normal sinus rhythm
Male   Black   PR interval   178 ms   ST & T wave abnormality, consider inferior ischemia
69in   184lb   QRS duration   72 ms   Abnormal ECG
Room:1   QT/QTc   334/428 ms   When compared with ECG of 20-OCT-1997 09:10,
Loc:2   Option:18   P-R-T axes   -57 38 -130   MANUAL COMPARISON REQUIRED, DATA IS UNCONFIRMED
                      BP   120/60   Gw

                Technician:
                Test ind: ROUTINE
                                                       Referred by: Confirmed by:

I   aVR   V1   V4

II   aVL   V2   V5

III   aVF   V3   V6

V1

II

V5
25mm/s   10mm/mV   100Hz   004A-004A   12SL 250   CID: 1   EID:35 EDT: 14:41 25-OCT-1997 ORDER:
                                                                                                   Page 1 of 1

B

FIGURE 25-4 *continued. B.* Resolution of electrical alternans after pericardiocentesis.

Most Emergency Departments do not have single guidewires and 6 to 10 French flexible catheters readily available to use for a pericardiocentesis. A commercially produced pericardiocentesis kit is available from numerous manufacturers and contains all the required equipment. In an emergency situation, a 6 to 10 French single-lumen central venous line access kit may be substituted.

PATIENT PREPARATION

Explain the procedure to the patient and/or their representative. A signed consent is not necessary as this is an emergent procedure. If possible, place the patient semirecumbent at a 30 to 45 degree angle (Figure 25-5). This position brings the heart closer to the anterior chest wall. The supine position is an acceptable alternative. Assess the patient for any mediastinal shift by physical examination and chest radiography (if time permits).

Apply the cardiac monitor, pulse oximeter, and supplemental oxygen to the patient. While the placement of an arterial line is ideal, such a line may not be available. Place the noninvasive blood pressure monitor on the patient's arm. **Insert a nasogastric tube to decompress the stomach.** This will decrease the possibility of gastric perforation during the procedure.

Identify the anatomic landmarks necessary to perform this procedure. The needle can be inserted at numerous sites (Figure 25-6). These include the following: below the xiphoid process, at the right sternocostal margin, at the left sternocostal margin (subxiphoid approach), in the left or right fifth intercostal space parasternally (parasternal approach), or in the left fifth intercostal space at the midclavicular line (apical approach). The most commonly used site is at the left sternocostal margin or the subxiphoid approach. This is the approach described throughout the "Techniques" section of this chapter.

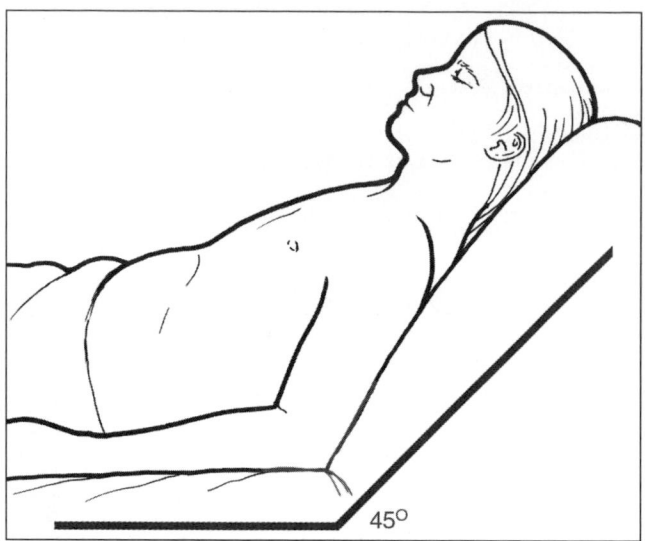

FIGURE 25-5 Ideal patient positioning for performing a pericardiocentesis.

Surgically prepare the xiphoid and subxiphoid areas. Clean any dirt, debris, and fluid from the area. Apply povidone iodine solution to the xiphoid and subxiphoid areas and allow it to dry. Apply sterile drapes to delineate a sterile surgical field. Reidentify the anatomic landmarks. If the patient is awake, anesthetize the needle tract with local anesthetic solution. Place a subcutaneous wheal of local anesthetic solution at the site chosen to insert the needle. Inject local anesthetic solution through the skin wheal and into the subcutaneous and muscular tissues of the wall of the torso.

Prepare the equipment. Set up a sterile field on a bedside table. Open all required equipment and place it on the sterile field. Put on sterile gloves and a mask. If time permits, dress in a sterile gown. Attach the spinal needle onto a 20 mL syringe containing 5 mL of sterile saline.

TECHNIQUES

BLIND INSERTION TECHNIQUE

Puncture the skin with a #11 scalpel blade between the xiphoid process and the left costal margin. Grasp the syringe with the dominant hand. Insert the spinal needle through the skin incision and at a 45 degree angle to the midsagittal plane (Figure 25-7*A*) and at a 45 degree angle to the abdominal wall (Figure 25-7*B*). Aim the tip of the spinal needle toward the patient's left shoulder. Alternatively, the spinal needle can be aimed toward the patient's left midclavicle, right midclavicle, or sternal notch to theoretically lessen the chance of iatrogenic damage to the coronary arteries.

Advance the spinal needle 4 to 5 cm while applying negative pressure to the syringe and observing the cardiac monitor. While advancing the needle, inject 0.25 to 0.50 mL of saline occasionally to ensure that the needle remains patent. Continue advancing the spinal needle while applying negative pressure until there is a return of blood, cardiac pulsations are felt, or an abrupt change in the ECG waveform occurs. **If the ECG waveform shows an injury pattern, withdraw the needle in 1 to 2 mm increments until the ECG pattern normalizes.** This indicates that the needle is touching or has penetrated the myocardium. Stop advancing the needle. Aspirate with the syringe. If a large volume of blood is quickly and easily withdrawn, it often means that the tip of the spinal needle is within the ventricle. Techniques to

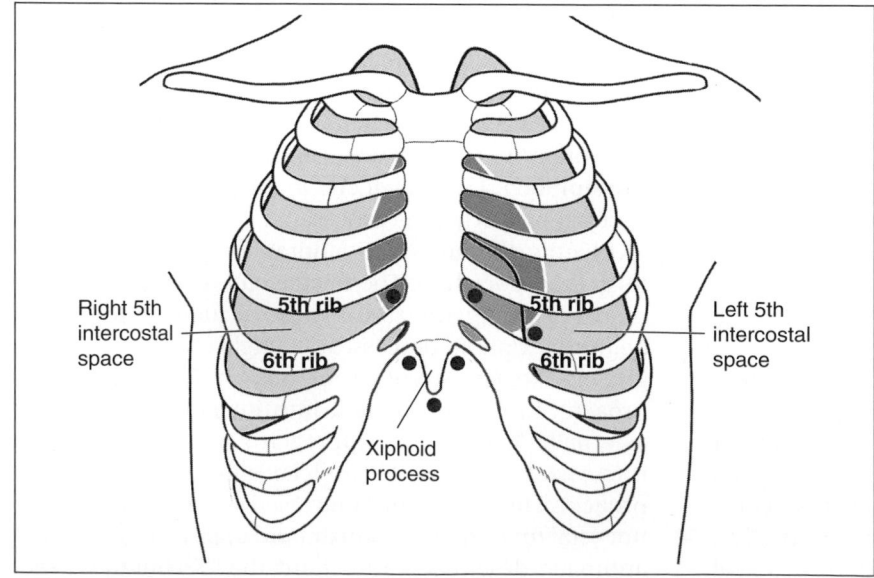

FIGURE 25-6 Potential sites to perform a pericardiocentesis.

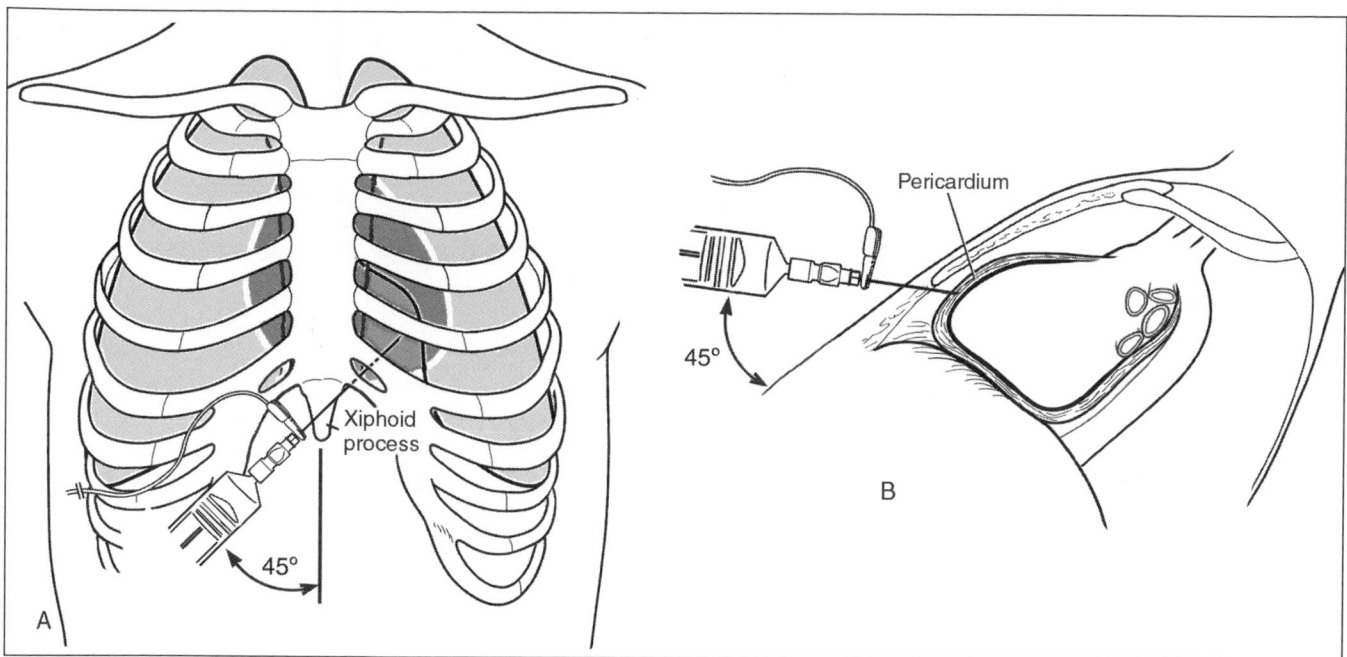

FIGURE 25-7 The subxiphoid approach. The needle is inserted at a 45 degree angle to the midsagittal plane (*A*) and at a 45 degree angle to the abdominal wall (*B*).

confirm intraventricular needle-tip placement have been described and include the following: observing that the aspirate does not form a clot, comparing the patient's hemoglobin to that of the aspirate, injecting fluorescein and looking for a fluorescent flush under the skin of the eyelids, or injecting 3 mL of dehydrocholic acid (Decholin) and asking whether the patient experiences a bitter taste. These are time-consuming and less reliable than ultrasound, if available.

When the pericardial space is entered and fluid is aspirated, there should be a marked improvement in the patient's clinical status. Withdraw as much fluid as possible. When the syringe is filled with fluid, stop withdrawing the plunger. Stabilize the spinal needle against the patient's torso and remove the syringe. Replace the syringe with a new one and continue the procedure. Alternatively, attach a three-way stopcock between the spinal needle and the syringe. Attach intravenous extension tubing to the stopcock. An assistant can open and close the stopcock while the physician aspirates fluid and ejects it through the intravenous extension tubing and into a basin. As the pericardial space is drained, the epicardium will approach the needle tip. If an injury pattern appears on the cardiac monitor, withdraw the needle slightly and continue to aspirate fluid. Remove the needle when fluid can no longer be aspirated.

ECG-MONITORED TECHNIQUE

The purpose of ECG monitoring is to prevent accidental ventricular puncture with the spinal needle. Attach one alligator clip to the base of the spinal needle and the other to the V_1 lead of the ECG machine (Figure 25-8). The V_1 lead will serve as an active electrode based at the tip of the spinal needle. As the spinal needle is advanced, an injury pattern noted by ST-segment elevation will be seen if the myocardium is contacted or penetrated by the spinal needle. The presence of a premature ventricular contraction or a ventricular arrhythmia can also signify contact with the myocardium.

Prepare the patient as previously described. Prepare the equipment (Figure 25-8). Turn on the ECG machine. Insert and advance the spinal needle, as described previously, while observing the ECG monitor. If an injury pattern or premature ventricular complexes are seen on the ECG monitor, withdraw the needle in 1 to 2 mm increments until the injury pattern disappears. Aspirate the pericardial fluid as described in the preceding section.

SELDINGER TECHNIQUE

An indwelling catheter may be placed in the pericardial cavity to drain the pericardial fluid (Figure 25-9). This may be done in cases of medical or traumatic pericardial effusions, since the pericardial fluid often reaccumulates. An indwelling catheter allows intermittent drainage of pericardial fluid without the potential complications associated with repeated needle sticks from a pericardiocentesis. This procedure can "buy time" if an operating room and/or Surgeon is not immediately available to perform a pericardial window.

The technique is similar to that of placing an indwelling central venous line. Clean and prepare the pa-

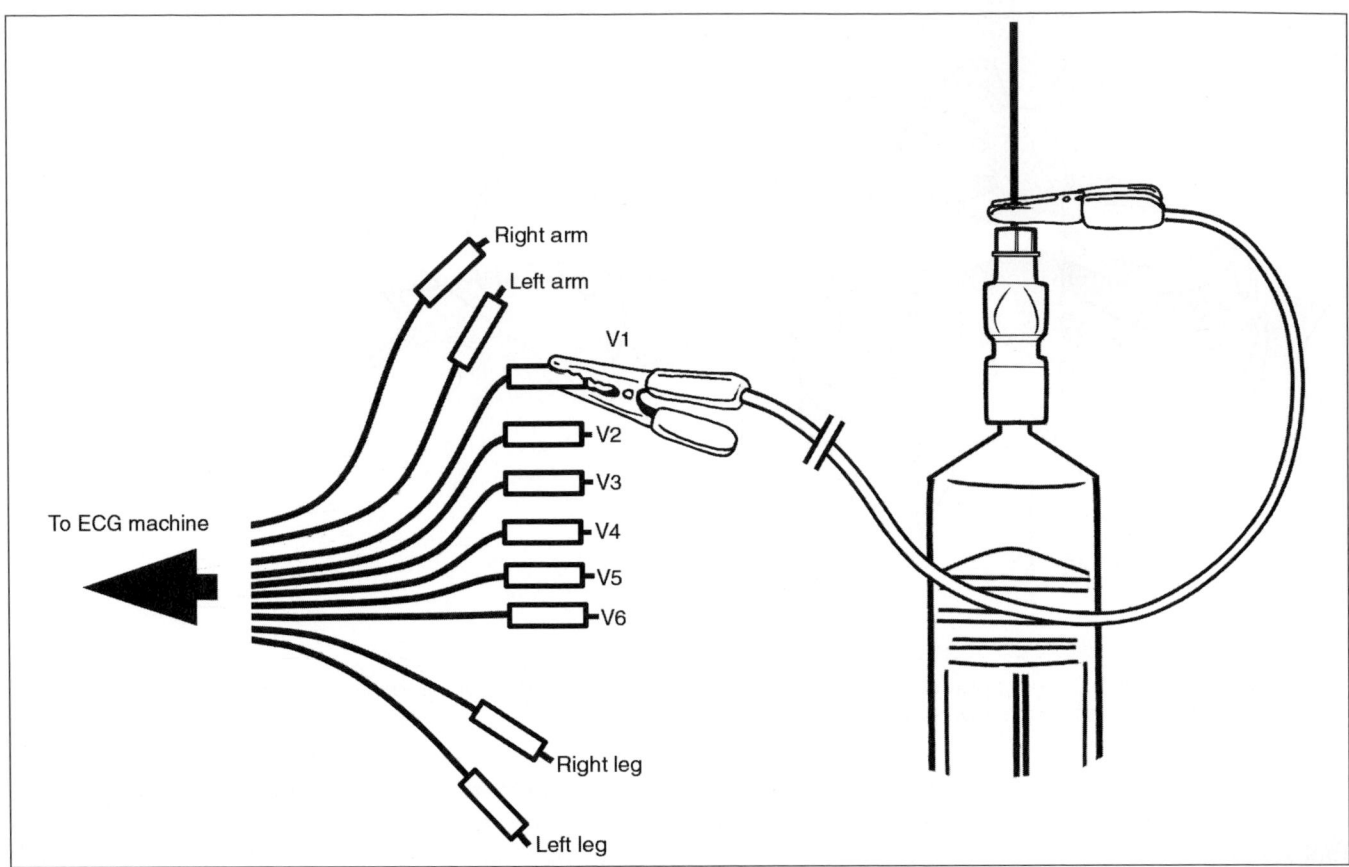

FIGURE 25-8 Equipment preparation for the ECG-monitored technique.

tient. Insert the spinal needle, blindly or with ECG monitoring, as described in the previous sections (Figure 25-7). Aspirate to confirm that the tip of the spinal needle is within the pericardial cavity (Figure 25-9A). **It is imperative that the tip of the spinal needle be within the pericardial cavity and not within the cardiac chamber. If intracardiac placement of the needle is suspected, the position of the needle must be verified by one of the methods described in the section on blind insertion technique or by fluoroscopy or ultrasonography.**

Grasp and stabilize the spinal needle with the nondominant hand. Gently remove the syringe from the spinal needle with the dominant hand. Insert the guidewire through the needle and into the pericardial cavity (Figure 25-9B). Advance the guidewire until approximately one-third of its length is within the patient. Stabilize the guidewire with the nondominant hand. Remove the needle over the guidewire while leaving the guidewire within the pericardial cavity (Figure 25-9C).

Stabilize the guidewire with the nondominant hand. Advance the dilator over the guidewire and into the pericardial cavity (Figure 25-9D). **If the guidewire is within the heart, dilating a tract through the myocardium can result in cardiac tamponade and/or exsanguination. It**

is therefore imperative to know that the guidewire is within the pericardial cavity and not within the heart. Remove the dilator while leaving the guidewire within the pericardial cavity. Advance the soft multihole catheter over the guidewire and into the pericardial cavity (Figure 25-9E). Remove the guidewire while leaving the catheter within the pericardial cavity (Figure 25-9F). Secure the catheter at the skin with the nondominant hand. Attach a syringe to the catheter and aspirate pericardial fluid. This should cause a rapid improvement in the patient's clinical status. Detach the syringe and attach a three-way stopcock to the catheter.[20] Secure the catheter to the skin with nylon sutures.

ULTRASOUND-GUIDED TECHNIQUE

Many authors feel that ultrasound-guided pericardiocentesis is now the standard of care.[14,20,30,31] The exact techniques will vary. The echocardiogram is used to localize the area of the largest effusion. The point of needle insertion will be where the pericardial fluid is maximal. The location and direction of the ultrasound waves should be fixed in the mind of the person performing the pericardiocentesis, and the needle is advanced simi-

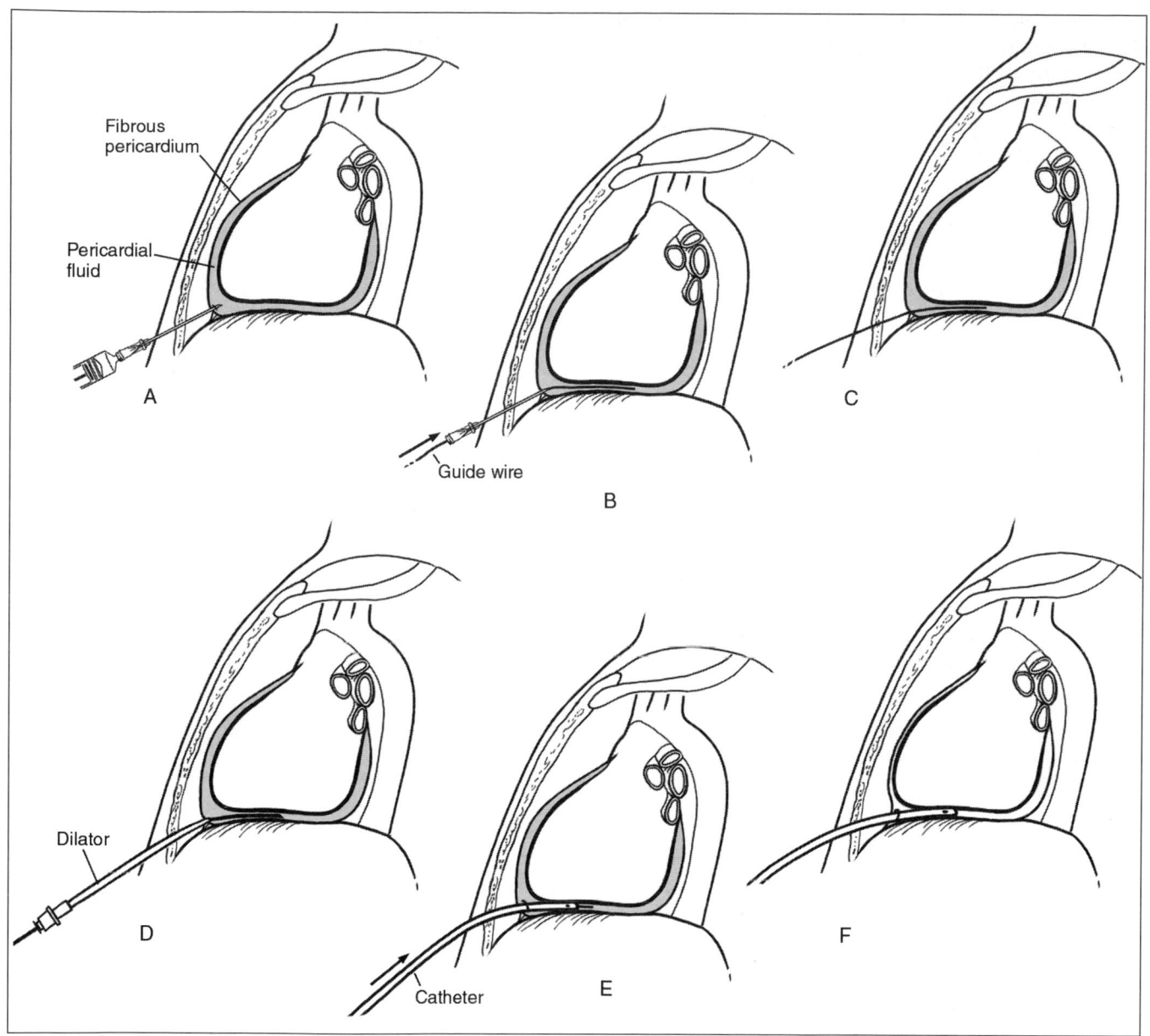

FIGURE 25-9 The Seldinger technique. *A.* The spinal needle is inserted into the pericardial space. *B.* The guidewire is inserted through the needle. *C.* The needle has been removed and the guidewire remains within the pericardial cavity. *D.* The dilator is advanced over the guidewire to dilate the needle tract. *E.* The catheter is advanced over the guidewire. *F.* The guidewire has been removed and the catheter remains within the pericardial cavity.

larly.[32] Alternatively, the transducer may be used to actively guide the placement of the needle.[33] The transducer is used to locate the area of largest effusion and the needle is inserted suitably close by and advanced toward the maximal effusion. Proper needle placement can be further confirmed by injecting saline that has been shaken to produce bubbles.[32] The bubbles will show well on the ultrasound. Some transducers now come with central lumens designed to accept a pericardiocentesis needle, while others have attachable variable-angle needle guides.[30,34]

SUBXIPHOID PERICARDIAL WINDOW

A pericardial window will minimize false-negative results seen with a pericardiocentesis, iatrogenic bleeding, and cardiac tamponade from myocardial injury by the pericardiocentesis needle. Prepare the patient as previously described. Inject local anesthetic solution subcutaneously from the xiphoid process across the confluence of the lower ribs and 6 cm down the midline. Inject local anesthetic solution into the muscular layers in the midline over the xiphoid process and 8 cm inferiorly.

Make a midline longitudinal incision from the xiphisternal junction to about 8 cm below the tip of the xiphoid process (Figure 25-10A). Incise down to the linea alba. Bluntly dissect the space behind the lower sternum to separate the anterior diaphragm from the sternum. Lift the lower sternum with a retractor (Figure 25-10B). Use an electrocautery unit for hemostasis. Bluntly divide the fatty tissue and retrosternal attachments of the diaphragm to reveal the diaphragm beneath the angle of the xiphoid and the left costal margin. It will often appear blue in color due to underlying blood.

Grasp the pericardium with a forceps. Incise the pericardium with a scissors or with shallow strokes of a scalpel (Figure 25-10B). Fluid should rush out rapidly. Remove a piece of the pericardium to make sure that it remains open. Gently explore the pericardial space digitally and with the suction device to remove any clot and fluid. Allow the skin to stay open to permit free drainage of the pericardial space. Alternatively, place a 28 French chest tube in the pericardial space and secure it with a purse-string suture through the pericardium (Figure 25-10C). The chest tube may exit the skin incision or a separate incision in the skin. Attach the chest tube to a suction source. Close the linea alba with interrupted 2–0 Vicryl sutures. Close the subcutaneous tissue and skin with 3–0 nylon sutures.

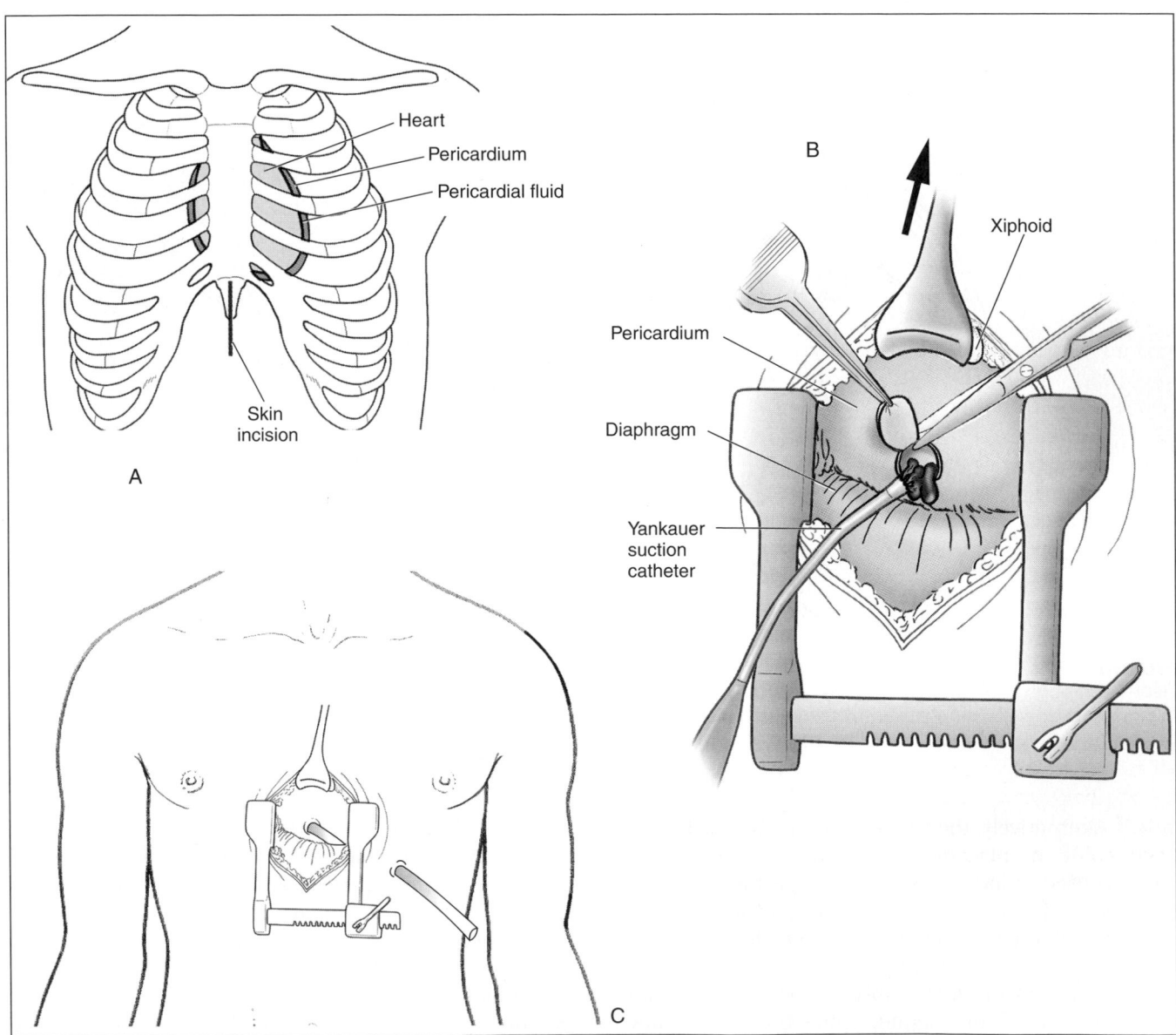

FIGURE 25-10 The pericardial window. *A.* The site of the skin incision. *B.* The xiphoid and sternum are lifted upward to expose the pericardium. An incision is made and a piece of the pericardium is removed. *C.* A chest tube is inserted into the pericardial space to allow continuous drainage of fluid.

ASSESSMENT

It must be emphasized that the lack of blood return does not rule out the diagnosis of cardiac tamponade. False-negative aspirations from a pericardiocentesis are well documented and are described at rates as high as 80 percent.[29] The occurrence of false-negative aspirations is often due to clotted blood in the pericardial space that cannot be aspirated or from failure to enter the pericardial space.

As mentioned, a dramatic improvement in the patient's clinical status should be observed after successful drainage of the pericardial space. The patient's blood pressure and cardiac output should increase while intracardiac pressure and intrapericardial pressure decrease. Obtain a chest radiograph after the procedure to rule out a hemothorax and/or pneumothorax.

AFTERCARE

Secure the catheter with sutures to the skin and check for stability. If not already done, consult a Surgeon for definitive care of trauma patients. Prepare these patients for rapid transport to the operating room. Monitor patients for reaccumulation of pericardial fluid and for hemodynamic instability. If fluid reaccumulates, the procedure should be repeated or the stopcock opened and the pericardial space reaspirated. Flush with sterile saline after each aspiration to maintain the patency of the catheter. Consult a Thoracic Surgeon if purulent fluid is aspirated in medical patients. All patients must be admitted to an intensive care unit for further monitoring, evaluation, and treatment.

COMPLICATIONS

Complication rates vary from 4 to 40 percent.[14,35] The complication rates of echocardiographically guided aspirations have been reported to be less than 5 percent.[14] Death may result from recurrence or occurrence of tamponade, bleeding, or dysrhythmias. Few if any deaths have been reported with echocardiographically guided aspirations. Reaccumulation of pericardial fluid may occur in up to 70 percent of blind aspirations.[14] Continuous drainage with a pericardial catheter can reduce this to 25 percent.[14] Bleeding, hemothorax, and/or cardiac tamponade can occur due to injury of the myocardium, coronary arteries, pericardial vasculature, or internal mammary vessels by the spinal needle. **To minimize injury, do not rock the spinal needle or change its direction once it is inserted into the patient.** A pneumothorax or pneumopericardium can form from penetration of the lung by the spinal needle. Dysrhyth-mias, ventricular fibrillation, ventricular tachycardia, or asystole can occur if the needle penetrates the myocardium. Hepatic damage leading to leakage of bile or blood can be seen if the needle penetrates the liver. If the patient is awake and alert, a vasovagal reaction can occur. False-negative aspirations (dry tap) occur if the blood in the pericardial cavity is clotted or if the needle is not within the pericardial cavity. False-positive aspirations may be seen if the needle is within the heart chamber or a vascular structure.

SUMMARY

Pericardiocentesis is an infrequently performed procedure. It can be lifesaving when a patient has a pericardial tamponade. The procedure is relatively simple yet has a significant rate of complications, morbidity, and mortality. The use of echocardiography to assist in making the diagnosis and in guiding the placement of the pericardiocentesis needle dramatically reduces false diagnoses and complications. The exact role of pericardiocentesis in trauma remains controversial, but it may be lifesaving in the unstable patient before they are able to receive definitive surgical therapy.

REFERENCES

1. Celsus AC: *De Medicina,* vol II (Spencer WG, trans). Cambridge, MA: Harvard University Press; London: Heinemann, 1938.
2. De Vigo G: *The Most Excelent Worckes of Chirurgery* (Traheron B, trans). London: E Whytchurch, 1550.
3. Riolanus J: *A Sure Guide: Or the Best and Nearest Way to Physick and Chyrurgery* (Culpepper N, trans). London: P Cole, 1657.
4. Jarcho S: Thomas Jowett on pericardiocentesis (1827). *Am J Cardiol* 1973; 31:273–276.
5. Larrey DJ: *Clin Chir* 1829; 15:108.
6. Hill LL: A report of a case of successful suturing of the heart, and a table of thirty-seven other cases of suturing by different operators with various terminations, and the conclusions drawn. *Med Rec* 1902; 62:846–848.
7. Bigger IA: Heart wounds: a report of seventeen patients operated upon in the Medical College of Virginia hospitals and a discussion of the treatment and prognosis. *J Thorac Cardiovasc Surg* 1939; 8:239–253.
8. Blalock A, Ravitch MM: A consideration of the nonoperative treatment of cardiac tamponade resulting from wound of the heart. *Surgery* 1943; 14:157–162.
9. Symbas PN: *Cardiothoracic Trauma.* Philadelphia: Saunders, 1989:16–55.

10. Chong HH, Plotnick GD: Pericardial effusion and tamponade: evaluation, imaging modalities, and management. *Comp Ther* 1995; 21(7):378–385.

11. Thourani VH, Feliciano DV, Rozycki G, et al: Penetrating cardiac trauma at an urban trauma center: a 22 year perspective. *Am Surg* 1999; 65(9):811–818.

12. Lee KS, Marwick T: Hemopericardium and cardiac tamponade associated with warfarin therapy. *Cleve Clin J Med* 1993; 60(4):336–338.

13. Kwan T, Karve MM, Emerole O: Cardiac tamponade in patients infected with HIV. *Chest* 1993; 104(4):1059–1062.

14. Ball JB, Morrison WL: Cardiac tamponade. *Postgrad Med J* 1997; 73(857):141–145.

15. Krikorian JG, Nancock EW: Pericardiocentesis. *Am J Med* 1978; 65:808–814.

16. Wong B, Murphy J, Chang CJ, et al: The risk of pericardiocentesis. *Am J Cardiol* 1979; 44:1110–1114.

17. Guberman BA, Fowler NO, Engel PJ, et al: Cardiac tamponade in medical patients. *Circulation* 1981; 64:633–640.

18. Callahan JA, Sweward JB, Nishimura RA, et al: Two-dimensional echocardiography guided pericardiocentesis: experience in 117 consecutive cases. *Am J Cardiol* 1985; 55:476–479.

19. Sauer PE, Murdock CE: Immediate surgery for cardiac and great vessel wounds. *Arch Surg* 1967; 95(7):7–11.

20. John RM, Treasure T: How to aspirate the pericardium. *Br J Hosp Med* 1990; 43(3):221–223.

21. Reddy PS, Curtiss EI, Uretsky BF: Spectrum of hemodynamic changes in cardiac tamponade. *Am J Cardiol* 1990; 66:1487–1491.

22. Jimenez E, Martin M, Krukencamp I, et al: Subxiphoid pericardotomy versus echocardiography: a prospective evaluation of the diagnosis of occult penetrating cardiac injury. *Surgery* 1990; 108:676–680.

23. Rozycki GS, Feleciano DV, Schmidt JA, et al: The role of surgeon performed ultrasound in patients with possible cardiac wounds. *Ann Surg* 1996; 223:737–746.

24. Rozycki GS, Feliciano DV, Ochsner MG, et al: The role of ultrasound in patients with possible penetrating cardiac wounds: a prospective multicenter study. *J Trauma* 1999; 46(4):543–552.

25. Rozycki GS, Ballard RB, Feliciano DV, et al: Surgeon-performed ultrasound for the assessment of truncal injuries: lessons learned from 1540 patients. *Ann Surg* 1998; 228(4):557–567.

26. American College of Surgeons: *Advanced Trauma Life Support for Doctors,* 6th ed. Chicago: American College of Surgeons, 1997.

27. Titus AA, Schinco MA, Scannell G, et al: Demystifying traumatic pericardial tamponade: the effect of expeditious ultrasound, 1999. http://www.aast.org/99abstracts/99abs096.html.

28. Shon DW, Shin GJ, Oh JK, et al: Role of transesophageal echocardiography in hemodynamically unstable patients. *Mayo Clin Proc* 1995; 70:925–931.

29. Wilson RF: Thoracic trauma, in Tintinalli JE, Krome RL, Ruiz E (eds): *Emergency Medicine: A Comprehensive Study Guide,* 4th ed. New York: McGraw-Hill, 1996:1156–1182.

30. Jouriles NJ: Pericardial and myocardial disease, in Rosen P, Barkin R, Danzl DF, et al (eds): *Emergency Medicine: Concepts and Clinical Practice,* 4th ed. St Louis: Mosby, 1998:1716–1744.

31. Kirkland LL, Taylor RW: Pericardiocentesis. *Crit Care Clin* 1992; 8(4):699–712.

32. Tsang SM, Freeman WK, Sinak LJ, et al: Echocardiographically guided pericardiocentesis: evolution and state-of-the-art technique. *Mayo Clin Proc* 1998; 73:647–652.

33. Clarke DP, Cosgrove DO: Real-time ultrasound scanning in the planning and guidance of pericardiocentesis. *Clin Radiol* 1987; 38:119–122.

34. Hanaki Y, Kamiya H, Todoroki H, et al: New two-dimensional, echocardiographically directed pericardiocentesis in cardiac tamponade. *Crit Care Med* 1990; 18(7):750–753.

35. Simon RR, Brenner BE: *Emergency Procedures and Techniques,* 2nd ed. Baltimore: Williams & Wilkins, 1982.

Chapter 26
INTRACARDIAC
INJECTION

Payman Sattar

INTRODUCTION

The practice of intracardiac injection seems to have originated in the 1800s. It was quite common throughout the 1960s, as it was thought to be the most expeditious route of drug delivery during a cardiac arrest.[1,2] By the mid-1970s, the practice of intracardiac injection declined. Safer and simpler routes of medication administration (intravenous, endotracheal, intraosseous) became available. Experimental data suggested that there was no advantage to intracardiac injection over intravenous administration of medications. Cardiopulmonary resuscitation (CPR) must be interrupted to perform an intracardiac injection. In difficult patients or in inexperienced hands, the time required for this procedure may be too prolonged. Finally, many serious complications may occur as a result of an intracardiac injection.[2]

ANATOMY AND PATHOPHYSIOLOGY

The technique of intracardiac injection is similar to that of a pericardiocentesis (Chapter 25). Both techniques use the same anatomic landmarks, the same anatomic approach, and the transthoracic insertion of a needle through the pericardium. In performing a pericardiocentesis, the tip of the needle is inserted into the pericardial space. Intracardiac injection requires the tip of the needle to be inserted through the myocardium and into a cardiac chamber.

The technique of intracardiac injection is easy to teach, is rapid and simple to perform, and requires no special equipment. It begins with identification of the anatomic landmarks required to perform the procedure.

For the subxiphoid approach, palpate the xiphoid process of the sternum and the left costosternal angle. For the left parasternal approach, palpate the left fourth or fifth intercostal spaces immediately adjacent to the sternum.

INDICATIONS

The primary indication for an intracardiac injection is when vascular access is not readily available or unobtainable in an arrested patient with asystole, pulseless electrical activity, pulseless ventricular tachycardia, or ventricular fibrillation. If the endotracheal route of medication administration has failed to achieve resuscitation, the intracardiac injection of resuscitative medications may be warranted and can be attempted as a last effort to resuscitate the patient.

CONTRAINDICATIONS

As candidates for this route of medicinal delivery have undergone cardiac arrest, there are no absolute or relative contraindications to performing this procedure. A few clinical conditions may make the procedure more difficult to perform. Chronic obstructive pulmonary disease can shift the heart from its normal position and increase the risk of a pneumothorax (with or without tension). Therapeutic or overanticoagulation may result in a hemopericardium and cardiac tamponade. Dextrocardia will require some alterations in needle positioning.

EQUIPMENT

Povidone iodine solution or swabs
18 gauge spinal needle or 18 gauge 3½ inch needle (for adults)
22 gauge spinal needle (for children)
Syringes, 5 and 10 mL
Nasogastric tube
Epinephrine, 1:1000 and 1:10,000

Epinephrine is the only resuscitative medication that should be administered by intracardiac injection. Administer 1 mg of epinephrine as the initial and subsequent doses in an adult patient. Administer 0.01 mg/kg (or 0.1 mL/kg) of the 1:10,000 concentration of epinephrine as the initial dose in children. Administer 0.1 to 0.2 mg/kg (or 0.1 to 0.2 mL/kg) of the 1:1000 concentration of epinephrine for subsequent doses in children.

PATIENT PREPARATION

This procedure is often performed on a patient who is clinically "dead" and as a last effort at resuscitation. A consent form is not required to perform this procedure. The patient will be supine with CPR in progress. If time permits, insert a nasogastric tube to decompress the stomach. Apply povidone iodine solution to the area around the lower sternum, xiphoid process of the sternum, upper epigastric, and left costosternal angles. Identify, by palpation, the anatomic landmarks required to perform the procedure. Draw up the required dose of epinephrine into a syringe or use prefilled syringes. Attach a spinal needle to the syringe containing the epinephrine.

TECHNIQUES

The two routes for intracardiac injection are the subxiphoid and the left parasternal approaches. Both are utilized in a similar fashion. The left parasternal approach offers a more direct and shorter route. However, it is associated with a higher rate of complications. Both approaches require cessation of CPR in order to perform the procedure. **The procedure of intracardiac injection should be performed as rapidly as possible to avoid prolonged cessation of CPR, but not at the expense of safety to the physician or the assistants.** It should take less than 10 seconds to perform an intracardiac injection.

SUBXIPHOID APPROACH

Stop performing CPR. Stop ventilating the patient and allow the lungs to deflate passively. Identify the spot

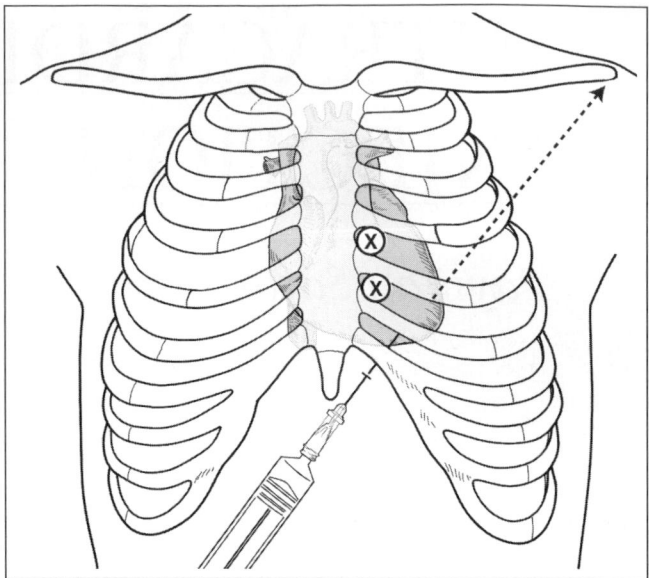

FIGURE 26-1 Intracardiac injection. The needle is inserted 1 cm to the left of the xiphoid process and aimed toward the left shoulder. The needle may also be inserted parasternally in the left fourth or fifth intercostal space (as denoted by the ⊗).

1 cm to the left of the patient's xiphoid process in the costosternal angle (Figure 26-1). Insert the needle with the bevel up at a 30 to 45 degree angle to the skin of the abdominal wall and aimed toward the left shoulder. Apply negative pressure to the syringe as it is advanced. Stop advancing the needle when blood flows freely into the syringe. This signifies that the tip of the needle is within the cardiac chamber. Quickly inject the epinephrine, then withdraw the needle. Resume CPR and ventilation of the patient.

If the attempt at intracardiac injection is unsuccessful, the needle should be withdrawn and flushed and intracardiac injection reattempted. **CPR and ventilation must be resumed after each attempt at intracardiac injection, whether successful or not.** Variations on the direction of the needle can be made for subsequent attempts. The needle may be directed toward the suprasternal notch, left midclavicle, or right midclavicle.

As an alternative, the spinal needle can be inserted through the skin and into the subcutaneous tissue with its obturator in place. Remove the obturator when the tip of the spinal needle is in the subcutaneous tissue. Attach the syringe containing epinephrine to the spinal needle. Gently depress the plunger of the syringe to expel the air within the needle into the subcutaneous tissues. Advance the needle while applying negative pressure. Stop advancing the needle when blood flows freely into the syringe. Quickly inject the epinephrine, then withdraw the needle. Resume CPR and ventilation of the patient.

LEFT PARASTERNAL APPROACH

This approach utilizes the fourth or fifth intercostal space, approximately 1 cm (or 1 finger breadth) lateral to the left sternal border (Figure 26-1). Stop performing CPR. Stop ventilating the patient and allow the lungs to deflate passively. Insert the needle perpendicular to the chest wall. Stabilize the needle with one hand and the syringe with the other. **Advance the needle with both hands and without excessive force.**[3] It is very easy to plunge into the heart if too much force is applied to the needle. Apply negative pressure to the syringe as it is advanced. Stop advancing the needle when blood flows freely into the syringe. Quickly inject the epinephrine, then withdraw the needle. Resume CPR and ventilation of the patient.

INFANTS AND CHILDREN

The technique of intracardiac injection for infants and children is essentially the same as that described above for the adult patient.[4] While the subxiphoid approach has been "adopted as the standard," the left parasternal approach can also be effectively utilized. A 22 gauge spinal needle should be used in infants and children. **Use caution when inserting and advancing the spinal needle since the pediatric skin and subcutaneous tissue are thin and easily penetrated.** The dose of epinephrine administered is weight-based and varies from the initial dose to subsequent doses (see "Equipment," above, for discussion).

COMPLICATIONS

Overall, according to pooled data, complications are rare.[2,5,6] Pneumothorax is the most common complication, especially with the parasternal approach. Other reported complications include coronary artery laceration, myocardial laceration, hemopericardium, cardiac tamponade, pulmonary artery laceration, and perforation of the stomach or liver. Intramyocardial injection has been reported and is associated with intractable ventricular fibrillation. **Identification of the appropriate anatomic landmarks for needle insertion and direction can minimize complications. Careful adherence to** **proper technique can also minimize complications.** The use of a small-gauge spinal needle and the subxiphoid approach may result in fewer complications versus a large-gauge needle and the left parasternal approach.[7]

SUMMARY

Although intracardiac injection is an effective route of medication delivery to a patient in cardiac arrest, its popularity has declined due to safer, simpler, and more effective methods of vascular access. When intravenous access is not readily accessible or when the endotracheal administration has not provided the desired effect, intracardiac injection should be considered as an alternative technique. It is important not to permit prolonged cessation of CPR during the procedure.

REFERENCES

1. Davison R, Barresi V, Parker M, et al: Intracardiac injections during cardiopulmonary resuscitation. *JAMA* 1980; 244:1110–1111.
2. Spivey WH, Lathers CM, Malone DR, et al: Comparison of intraosseous, central, and peripheral routes of sodium bicarbonate administration during CPR in pigs. *Ann Emerg Med* 1985; 14(12):1135–1140.
3. Tarantino Q: *Pulp Fiction.* Los Angeles: Buena Vista Studios, 1994.
4. Ledwith CAW: Intracardiac injections, in Dieckmann RA, Fiser DH, Selbst SM (eds): *Illustrated Textbook of Pediatric Emergency and Critical Care Procedures.* St Louis: Mosby, 1997:272–273.
5. Bjork VO, Cullhed I, Hallen A, et al: Sequelae of left ventricular puncture with angiography. *Circulation* 1961; 24:204–212.
6. Sabin HI, Khunti K, Coghill SB, et al: Accuracy of intracardiac injections determined by a post mortem study. *Lancet* 1983; 2:1054–1055.
7. Simon RR, Brenner BE: *Emergency Procedures and Techniques,* 3rd ed. Baltimore: Williams & Wilkins, 1994:143–144.

Chapter 27
NEEDLE THORACOSTOMY

Roxanne Roberts

INTRODUCTION

A tension pneumothorax is a unilateral progressive collection of air in the pleural space. If not treated, it results in increasing intrapleural pressures, shifting of intrathoracic structures, hypoxemia, and death. It occurs from a one-way air leak into the pleural cavity from the airway conduits, the lung, or the thoracic wall. The air leak causes air to enter the pleural cavity and become trapped, without a method of egress. Rapid decompression of the tension pneumothorax with a catheter-over-the-needle is known as a needle thoracostomy and is lifesaving.

A tension pneumothorax is an immediate life-threatening condition that requires prompt recognition and treatment to prevent the patient's imminent demise. The diagnosis must be suspected based upon the patient's prior medical history, the mechanism of injury, physical examination findings, and a patient in extremis. **Importantly, treatment must not be delayed to obtain further diagnostic testing (e.g., chest radiograph).** These patients most often present with acute and dramatic cardiopulmonary compromise, which may be manifest by a combination of the following signs and symptoms: respiratory distress, chest pain, air hunger, hypotension, tachycardia, diaphoresis, unilateral absence of or decrease in breath sounds, hyperresonance to percussion, increased central venous pressure, hypoxemia, cyanosis, deviation of the cardiac point of maximal impulse, and tracheal deviation.

ANATOMY AND PATHOPHYSIOLOGY

The most common cause of a tension pneumothorax is mechanical ventilation with positive pressure in a patient with a visceral pleural injury.[1] A tension pneumothorax is present in 50 percent of ventilator-associated pneumothoraces.[2] When this occurs in intensive care unit (ICU) patients, they often have minimal functional reserve. To further cloud the issue, they are frequently on other supports (inotropic agents, complex ventilator settings, etc.), making their physical examination difficult and confusing. They may also have a number of other coexisting factors that are making them unstable. This group of patients has a particularly disastrous course if a tension pneumothorax develops. Rapid diagnosis and treatment are imperative.[3]

The placement of a central venous catheter has been associated with the development of a pneumothorax. The incidence of this is approximately 3 to 6 percent with use of the subclavian approach. Tension pneumothorax may be delayed in approximately 0.4 percent of attempts to gain central venous access. In one case report, a patient developed a tension pneumothorax while under general anesthesia 10 days after the placement of a subclavian central venous line.[4]

A tension pneumothorax may also occur in the setting of blunt or penetrating trauma of the lung. It may occur uncommonly following a tracheobronchial or esophageal injury. It may complicate a simple pneumothorax if the parenchymal lung leak does not seal spontaneously. In this case, the site of the lung injury acts as a one-way valve, allowing air entry into the pleural space and not allowing it to escape. Occasionally, chest wall defects may result in a tension pneumothorax if the wound is completely covered by an occlusive dressing or if the wound itself acts as a ball-valve mechanism. More rarely, it may occur following markedly displaced fractures of the thoracic spine. In the past, based on studies using the canine model, the pathophysiology of this disease was considered to be associated primarily with a mechanical pressure–related phenomenon.[5] Air accumulated in the involved pleural space and caused an increasing intrapleural pressure. This pressure caused compression of the ipsilateral lung, displacement of the diaphragm caudally, movement of the mediastinum and heart toward the uninjured side, kinking of the great vessels, and compression of the contralateral lung. This anatomic shift of structures would result in impaired filling of the heart and a disastrous fall in cardiac output.[6] Unfortunately, the canine model is not as similar to the human as was once thought. The mediastinum in the dog is more mobile. It is fenestrated, so that air communicates from one hemithorax to the other. Therefore elevations of intrapleural pressure in dogs would affect central structures and cause cardiovascular compromise more readily than in humans.

Recently, this pressure-related mechanism has come into question as the primary event. Experiments have been performed in goats, monkeys, sheep, and swine; all of which have a mediastinum that is more similar to that of the human than the dog.[7–10] These studies support the hypothesis that central hypoxemia is the primary factor in the lethality of a tension pneumothorax and occurs prior to the development of significant hypotension. In this hypothesis, the mechanical pressure–related phenomenon is a late event.

These mechanisms become more confusing and mixed in the ventilator-dependent patient. There is a lack of studies documenting hemodynamic changes in the human subject with a tension pneumothorax.[11–14] In one case report, three ventilated ICU patients demonstrated decreased cardiac output as the first sign of a tension pneumothorax.[12] The authors proposed that the absence of spontaneous breathing did not allow increased variations in negative intrathoracic pressure to act as a compensatory mechanism to prevent hemodynamic compromise. In another similar case, decreased cardiac output and mixed venous oxygen saturation were the dominant signs of a tension pneumothorax.[13] Hemoglobin desaturation via pulse oximetry was shown to be the earliest sign in a ventilator-dependent patient with a tension pneumothorax.[14]

Electrocardiographic (ECG) changes may be seen in association with a tension pneumothorax. In a left-sided tension pneumothorax, the more commonly described ECG changes are a rightward shift of the mean frontal QRS axis, precordial T-wave inversions, reduced R-wave voltage, and decreased and/or alternating QRS amplitude.[15–17] Other unique changes include PR-segment elevation in the inferior leads and reciprocal PR-segment depression in the aV_R lead.[18] A case report cited transient bradycardia, hypotension, and precordial ST-segment elevation; all of which reversed after treatment of a right-sided tension pneumothorax.[19] Numerous mechanisms have been proposed as the causes of these ECG changes. They include simple displacement of the heart, rotation of the heart around its anteroposterior or longitudinal axis, transient hypoxia, changes in coronary artery blood flow, changes in pleural pressure, pulmonary resistance, pericardial tension, acute ventricular dilatation, alterations in ventricular repolarization, pressure-induced atrial injury, and insulation of the chest wall from the associated air.[15–20] The vast majority of ECG changes have been noted with left-sided rather than right-sided tension pneumothoraces. **The degree of pneumothorax and the severity of symptoms do not seem to correlate with the magnitude of the ECG abnormalities. In summary, ECG changes are not uncommon in tension pneumothorax and should not distract from the true diagnosis.**

INDICATIONS

A tension pneumothorax must be considered in the differential diagnosis of any patient in extremis. If it is a possible etiology for the patient's cardiopulmonary collapse, needle decompression should be performed without delay. In every circumstance, and especially in the emergent setting, one may not be able to be 100 percent certain of the diagnosis. However, needle decompression is a relatively low-risk procedure with great lifesaving potential.

One setting that may be particularly confusing is in the dying patient with left precordial penetrating trauma. The immediate differential would be tension pneumothorax versus pericardial tamponade versus massive hemothorax. Physical examination findings are usually helpful but may also be confusing, mixed, or difficult to elicit in a noisy resuscitation. **Needle decompression should be the first maneuver in this situation.** It may be lifesaving and will aid in the diagnosis. It is less invasive, quicker, and easier to perform than a pericardiocentesis. A tension pneumothorax is more common than pericardial tamponade in this setting. As for a massive hemothorax, a chest tube setup requires some time but should be requested at the time needle decompression is proceeding.

CONTRAINDICATIONS

There are no absolute contraindications to performing a needle thoracostomy to decompress a tension pneumothorax. It is imperative to identify the anatomic landmarks properly and perform this procedure carefully if the patient has a known or suspected coagulopathy.

EQUIPMENT

Povidone iodine solution
12 to 16 gauge catheter-over-the-needle
5 or 10 mL syringe

PATIENT PREPARATION

Briefly describe the procedure to the patient if they are competent, able to understand, and cooperative. Place the patient supine. Some physicians place the patient supine with the head of the bed elevated to 30 degrees. This will allow the air to rise to the anterior upper chest. Unfortunately, this is not the most functional position. It is from the supine position that the patient can most easily be accessed and controlled by the greatest number of practitioners. This position is optimal to allow for other lifesaving maneuvers (airway management, cardiopulmonary resuscitation, etc.). Simultaneous with the performance of this procedure, other interventions should be requested: 100% face-mask oxygen (if the patient is not already intubated), pulse oximetry, cardiac monitoring, chest tube setup, intravenous access, and stat chest radiography.

TECHNIQUE

The safest, easiest, and most reliable site for a needle thoracostomy to decompress a tension pneumothorax is the second intercostal space in the midclavicular line[1,2,6,21] (Figure 27-1). Apply a 12, 14, or 16 gauge catheter-over-the-needle onto a 5 or 10 mL syringe without the plunger. Identify the second intercostal space in the midclavicular line. Apply povidone iodine solution to the needle insertion site if time permits. Place the nondominant index finger over the needle insertion site. Grasp the syringe with the dominant hand. Insert the catheter-over-the-needle perpendicular to the skin and just above the superior border of the third rib (Figure 27-2*A*). This will avoid injury to the neurovascular bundle underlying the inferior border of the second rib. Advance the catheter-over-the-needle until a rush of air, with or without blood, is heard escaping from the syringe. Stop advancing the catheter-over-the-needle. Advance the catheter until the hub is against the skin while simultaneously withdrawing the needle (Figure 27-2*B*).

ALTERNATIVE TECHNIQUES

Other sites have been described for performing a needle thoracostomy. These include the fourth or fifth inter-

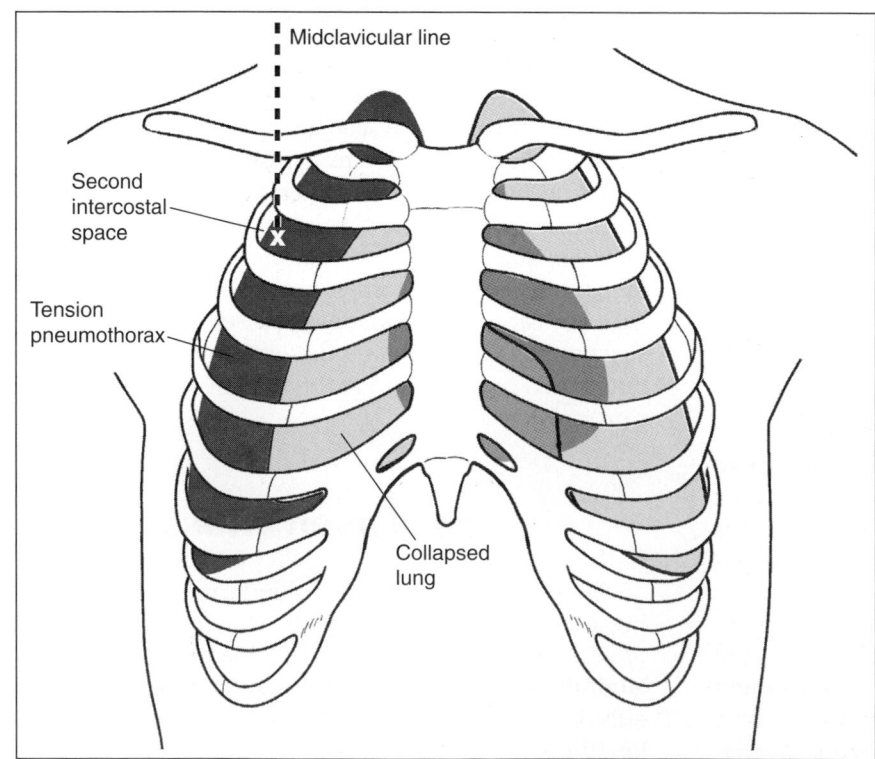

FIGURE 27-1 A right-sided tension pneumothorax. The preferred site for a needle thoracostomy is the second intercostal space in the midclavicular line.

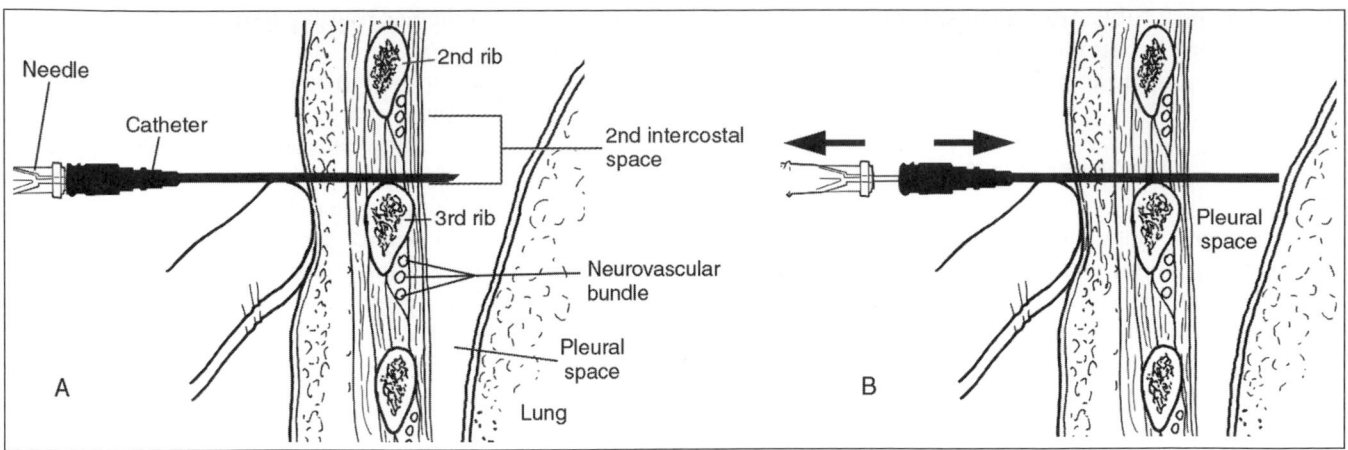

FIGURE 27-2 Decompression of a tension pneumothorax with a catheter-over-the-needle. *A.* The catheter-over-the-needle is inserted through the second intercostal space and into the pleural cavity. *B.* The catheter is advanced while the needle is removed.

costal space in the midaxillary line or the second intercostal space in the anterior axillary line.[22–25] There are several problems with these alternative approaches. In the fourth or fifth intercostal space, the ribs are close together, with narrower interspaces making needle placement more difficult. There is more rib motion with breathing and arm movement can make catheter dislodgment more likely. In the supine patient, air will rise ventrally rather than laterally. Practically speaking, during the resuscitation of the unstable patient, the most important position for the Emergency Physician is at the patient's head. Insertion of a catheter in the second intercostal space in the anterior axillary line is easier from this position than inserting a laterally placed catheter. The fourth or fifth intercostal space in the midaxillary line is the ideal space for a chest tube. Placement of the catheter in these alternative sites would mean having to penetrate more tissue, especially in the obese patient, making reaching the pleural space more difficult and dislodgment of the catheter more likely. The major drawback to using the fourth or fifth intercostal space is the risk of inserting the catheter-over-the-needle below the diaphragm and into the liver (on the right) or the spleen (on the left).

If the patient is in extremis, a definitive chest tube should not be the primary therapy for a tension pneumothorax. The setup and performance of a tube thoracostomy takes much longer than rapid decompression with a catheter-over-the-needle.

ASSESSMENT

Once the catheter has been placed into the pleural space, a gush of air should rush out of the syringe. **The procedure will have converted a tension pneumotho-**

rax into a simple pneumothorax requiring a tube thoracostomy. The patient should improve hemodynamically and symptomatically. Saturations on pulse oximetry should rise after the decompression. If this does not occur, too short of a catheter-over-the-needle may have been used, in which case the procedure should be repeated with a longer one. If that is not available, rapidly perform a tube thoracostomy. The other possibility is that the pleural space was entered appropriately but the diagnosis was incorrect. In this event, another cause of the patient's shock state should be sought and consideration should be given to "prophylactic" chest tube placement. This may prevent later sequelae from the iatrogenic catheter stab wound to the chest and simplify the further workup and monitoring of this unstable patient.

AFTERCARE

After insertion of the catheter and improvement in the patient's clinical status, the immediate life threat has been treated. Secure the catheter against the skin with a suture or an assistant holding it in place. **The patient should continue to be observed and monitored closely for recurrence of the tension pneumothorax and procedural complications.** The patient should be hooked up to a pulse oximeter and cardiac monitor if this has not already been done. Intravenous access should be established. Obtain baseline laboratory studies, an arterial blood gas, and a chest radiograph. The patient should have a thorough history and physical examination to search for the etiology of the tension pneumothorax. **A definitive chest should be placed using sterile technique to prevent recurrence of the tension pneumothorax and to treat the simple pneumothorax.** Refer to Chapter 28 for complete details regarding the placement of a chest tube. After a chest tube is inserted, remove the needle thoracostomy catheter and place a bandage over the puncture site.

COMPLICATIONS

An incorrect diagnosis of a tension pneumothorax in an unstable patient is always a possibility, even in the best of hands. If this is the case, the cause of the patient's shock state must still be aggressively sought and treated. A prophylactic chest tube should be considered for a presumed parenchymal lung injury from the needle thoracostomy. This is especially true if the patient is going to be transported out of the resuscitation area, will be given a general anesthetic, or is to be placed on positive-pressure ventilation.

Depending on the patient's body habitus and the catheter length, the pleural space may not have been reached to be decompressed. In one study from the United Kingdom, the chest wall thickness was estimated to be 1.3 to 5.2 cm by ultrasound in the second intercostal space.[26] A 3.0 cm cannula would fail to penetrate into the pleural cavity in 57 percent of the patients in this study. A 4.5 cm cannula would fail to penetrate into the pleural cavity in 4 percent of the patients. In this case, the procedure should be repeated with a longer catheter-over-the-needle. If one is not immediately available, a tube thoracostomy should be performed immediately.

Even in the case of initial effective decompression of a tension pneumothorax, the catheter may become dislodged, clotted, kinked, or its tip may retract from the pleural space into the surrounding soft tissues. **If the tension pneumothorax recurs, immediately repeat the procedure.** Once needle decompression is reaccomplished, immediately perform a tube thoracostomy. If possible, a tube thoracostomy can be initiated by one physician while other members of the resuscitation team continue with other interventions. This would hopefully prevent recurrence of the tension pneumothorax secondary to a delay in chest tube placement because other interventions (e.g., CPR, intubation, venous access, etc.) must also be performed.

There may be complications secondary to the catheter placement. A local hematoma or underlying lung laceration may occur. Infectious agents may be introduced into the pleural cavity. If the catheter-over-the-needle is introduced too close to the sternum, the underlying mediastinal vessels or internal mammary artery may be penetrated or lacerated. If the catheter-over-the-needle is introduced under the inferior border of the second rib instead of over the superior border of the third rib, the intercostal vessels or nerve may be lacerated. Proper technique in placing the catheter-over-

the-needle should be observed to minimize preventable complications.

The standard approach to relieving a tension pneumothorax is the placement of a large-bore needle in the ipsilateral second intercostal space. This works well in the standard patient where there are no adhesions or scarring in the pleural space. However, this may not be the proper needle location in the patient with prior pulmonary disease, pleural disease, or pleural adhesions. The classic hospital patient in this category is the patient with adult respiratory distress syndrome on positive end-expiratory pressure (PEEP) with high airway pressures who develops loculated tension pneumothoraces. The needle placed in the standard manner often fails to reach the affected pleural area. Stat chest radiographs are often required to help guide placement of the needles and/or chest tubes in these more complex patients.[6] Bedside ultrasonography is also useful to help guide the procedure.

SUMMARY

Tension pneumothorax is a clinical diagnosis that is often made in an agonal patient with respiratory distress, absent (or decreased) breath sounds over a hemithorax, and severe cardiopulmonary compromise. Needle thoracostomy to decompress the tension pneumothorax should be performed immediately in the second intercostal space in the midclavicular line. This is a lifesaving procedure that is quick, simple to perform, easy to learn, and requires no special equipment. Needle thoracostomy should be followed as soon as feasible by a definitive tube thoracostomy.

REFERENCES

1. American College of Surgeons: *Advanced Trauma Life Support Instructor Manual*, 6th ed. Chicago: American College of Surgeons, 1997:150.
2. Taylor RW, Civetta JM, Kirby RR: *Techniques and Procedures in Critical Care*. Philadelphia: Lippincott, 1990:306.
3. Steier M, Ching N, Roberts EB, et al: Pneumothorax complicating continuous ventilator support. *J Cardiovasc Surg* 1974; 67(1):17–23.
4. Plewa MC, Ledrick D, Sferra JJ: Delayed tension pneumothorax complicating central venous catheterization and positive pressure ventilation. *Am J Emerg Med* 1995; 13(5):532–535.
5. Bennett RA, Orton EC, Tucker A, et al: Cardiopulmonary changes in conscious dogs with induced progressive pneumothorax. *Am J Vet Res* 1989; 50(2):280–284.

6. Symbas PN: *Cardiothoracic Trauma*. Philadelphia: Saunders, 1989:314–317.

7. Rutherford RB, Hurt Jr JJ, Brickman RD, et al: The pathophysiology of progressive tension pneumothorax. *J Trauma* 1968; 8:212–227.

8. Gustman P, Yerger L, Wanner A: Immediate cardiovascular effects of tension pneumothorax. *Am Rev Respir Dis* 1983; 127(2):171–174.

9. Carvalho P, Hildebrandt J, Charan NB: Changes in bronchial and pulmonary arterial blood flow with progressive tension pneumothorax. *J Appl Phys* 1996; 81(4):1664–1669.

10. Barton ED, Rhee P, Hutton KC, et al: The pathophysiology of tension pneumothorax in ventilated swine. *J Emerg Med* 1997; 15(2):147–153.

11. Connolly JP: Hemodynamic measurements during a tension pneumothorax. *Crit Care Med* 1993; 21(2):294–296.

12. Beards SC, Lipman J: Decreased cardiac index as an indicator of tension pneumothorax in the ventilated patient. *Anaesthesia* 1994; 49(2):137–141.

13. Woodcock TE, Murray S, Ledingtham IM: Mixed venous oxygen saturation changes during tension pneumothorax and its treatment. *Anaesthesia* 1984; 39(10):1004–1006.

14. Laishley RS, Aps C: Tension pneumothorax and pulse oximetry. *Br J Anaesth* 1991; 66(2):250–252.

15. Walston A, Brewer D, Kitchens C, et al: The electrocardiographic manifestations of spontaneous left pneumothorax. *Ann Intern Med* 1974; 80:375–379.

16. Botz G, Brock-Utne JG: Are electrocardiogram changes the first sign of impending peri-operative pneumothorax? *Anaesthesia* 1992; 47(12):1057–1059.

17. Kuritzky P, Goldfarb AL: Unusual electrocardiographic changes in spontaneous pneumothorax. *Chest* 1976; 70(4):535–537.

18. Strizik B, Forman R: New ECG changes associated with a tension pneumothorax. *Chest* 1999; 115(6):1742–1744.

19. Slay RD, Slay LE, Luehrs JG: Transient ST-elevation associated with tension pneumothorax. *J Am Coll Emerg Phys* 1979; 8(1):16–18.

20. Feldman T, January CT: ECG changes in pneumothorax: a unique finding and proposed mechanism. *Chest* 1984; 86(1):143–145.

21. Green G: *Chest Injuries*, 2nd ed. Bristol, England: Wright, 1984:48–52.

22. McEwin JI: Pleural disease, in Rosen P, Barkin R, Danzl DF, et al (eds): *Emergency Medicine: Concepts and Clinical Practice*, 4th ed. St. Louis: Mosby, 1998:1511–1528.

23. Society of Critical Care Medicine: *Fundamentals of Critical Care Support: Provider Manual*, 2nd ed. Anaheim, CA: Society of Critical Care Medicine, 1998:253–255.

24. Carrero R, Wayne M: Chest trauma. *Emerg Med Clin North Am* 1989; 7(2):389–418.

25. Barton ED, Epperson M, Hoyt DB, et al: Prehospital needle aspiration and tube thoracostomy in trauma victims: a six-year experience with aeromedical crews. *J Emerg Med* 1995; 13(2):155–163.

26. Britten S, Palmer SH, Snow TM: Needle thoracentesis in tension pneumothorax: insufficient cannula length and potential failure. *Injury* 1996; 27(5):321–322.

Chapter 28
TUBE THORACOSTOMY

Kimberly T. Joseph

INTRODUCTION

A tube thoracostomy is the placement of a tube through the thoracic wall and into the pleural cavity. It is commonly referred to as a chest tube. It is placed in order to evacuate air, blood, or other fluid that collects within the pleural space. The etiology of the air or fluid collections can be due to iatrogenic complications, infection, lung disease, malignancy, or trauma.

Thoracic trauma continues to account for nearly one-quarter of all trauma-related mortality.[1,2] Although some injuries require surgical intervention, the majority may be treated nonoperatively. Injuries to the chest wall, lung, trachea, bronchi, or esophagus may lead to the presence of abnormal air and/or fluid in the pleural space. The use of a tube thoracostomy (chest tube) in these situations may be both diagnostic and therapeutic. Historically, closed-tube drainage of the pleura has been used for various indications for more than a century.[3] This chapter deals primarily with the use of tube thoracostomy following trauma.

ANATOMY AND PATHOPHYSIOLOGY

On inspiration, the diaphragm and accessory muscles of respiration contract and generate negative pressure within the pleural space. Penetration of the visceral or parietal pleura due to injury disrupts this pressure gradient and allows air to enter the "potential space" between the parietal and visceral pleurae, resulting in a pneumothorax.[1,2] **A simple pneumothorax is the accumulation of air that is not under pressure within the pleural space.** It may cause the ipsilateral lung to collapse. As air continues to accumulate and if there are no adhesions, the increased pressure in the thoracic cavity may push the mediastinum toward the noninjured side. This can cause angulation of the atriocaval junction, impairment of atrial filling, and a subsequent decrease in cardiac output manifest by hypotension. **The presence of a pneumothorax under pressure accompanied by respiratory and/or circulatory compromise is termed a tension pneumothorax and is an immediate life threat.**

There are two important points to remember about a tension pneumothorax. First, it is a clinical diagnosis based on the patient's presenting signs and symptoms. Do not wait for a chest film to establish the diagnosis. Second, the initial treatment of this entity is needle decompression followed by tube thoracostomy. A large-bore needle is inserted in the second intercostal space in the midclavicular line at the superior border of the rib. If the patient has a tension pneumothorax, a gush of air will ensue and the patient's symptoms will improve. Thus, the tension pneumothorax is converted to a simple pneumothorax and a chest tube may be inserted for more definitive management. Refer to Chapter 27 for complete details regarding the needle thoracostomy procedure.

An open pneumothorax is caused by a traumatic chest wall injury that results in a defect that is greater than or equal to two-thirds the diameter of the patient's trachea. Air passes via the path of least resistance (the defect) and leads to equilibration of the intra- and extrathoracic pressures, thus compromising both oxygenation and ventilation. Like a tension pneumothorax, this is an immediate life threat. Initial treatment may consist of a nearly occlusive "three-sided" dressing creating a one-way valve for egress of air from the pleural cavity. Alternatively, the patient may be placed on positive-pressure ventilation. The chest tube can then be inserted at a site remote from the actual defect. Refer to Chapter 30 for complete details regarding the management of open chest wounds.

Injury to the chest may also result in laceration of vascular structures, including the lung parenchymal vessels, intercostal vessels, internal mammary arteries, great vessels, or heart. Although the body can absorb small amounts of free blood from the pleural space, the presence of free blood over a prolonged period of time leads to increased risk of infection and fibrosis.[3,4] The body cannot effectively clear large quantities of blood or clot from the pleural cavity. Blood in the pleural space, otherwise known as a hemothorax, can in most cases be treated with chest tube insertion. However, when a major systemic or pulmonary vessel has been injured, resulting in massive hemothorax (greater than 1500 mL of blood in the pleural space), tube thoracostomy is usually followed by urgent surgical intervention.

Penetrating wounds or blunt rupture of the thoracic esophagus may result in a pneumomediastinum, pneumothorax, hydrothorax, or some combination thereof. Esophageal injury should be suspected in any patient with a knife or ice pick wound in a suspicious location, a transmediastinal bullet trajectory, or a severe and sudden compression of the chest or abdomen.[2] If a pneumothorax or hydrothorax is a presenting finding, tube thoracostomy is used as part of the treatment. However, these patients require urgent surgical attention. Tube thoracostomy may also be used in the treatment of traumatic chylothorax resulting from injury to the thoracic duct.

One special circumstance deserves mention. Certain patients who have sustained significant blunt trauma to the torso may have a diaphragmatic rupture. Chest radiographs may reveal an air density in the hemithorax that could be mistaken for a pneumothorax. However, this may actually represent the presence of the stomach or colon in the thoracic cavity. When a chest tube is inserted in such a case, extra care must be taken in entering the pleura so as not to injure a hollow viscus inadvertently.

INDICATIONS

The indications for a tube thoracostomy following blunt or penetrating trauma to the chest include the presence of a simple pneumothorax, hemothorax, hemopneumothorax, hydrothorax, or chylothorax. A chest tube is placed prophylactically in patients with penetrating injuries to the chest who do not have evidence of a pneumothorax on initial chest radiographs but are ex-

pected to undergo general anesthesia. The medical indications for a tube thoracostomy include a pneumothorax, empyema, recurrent pleural effusion, pleurodesis, or a malignant pleural effusion. A tube thoracostomy should also be performed after the needle decompression of a tension pneumothorax into a simple pneumothorax.

With the advent of computed tomography (CT), traumatic pneumothoraces that are not evident on chest radiographs may be detected. The question then arises as to whether or not these pneumothoraces should be treated. One study looked at 40 patients who sustained chest trauma and were discovered by CT scan to have pneumothoraces.[5] The study concluded that patients undergoing positive-pressure ventilation should have placement of a chest tube. However, the study could not confirm that patients with small pneumothoraces who were not going to be ventilated could safely be observed. In the Trauma Unit at Cook County Hospital, tube thoracostomy is not used for patients with evidence of pneumothorax visible only on CT scan unless they require assisted ventilation or general anesthesia.

CONTRAINDICATIONS

The only absolute contraindication to performing a tube thoracostomy is in the patient who requires an open thoracotomy. Although there are no firm contraindications to performing a tube thoracostomy in a trauma patient, there are some areas of controversy. It has been suggested that a patient with a small (< 20 percent) pneumothorax without an associated hemothorax following trauma may be managed with close observation rather than a chest tube, especially in the case of blunt injuries. If observation is selected for such a patient, chest radiographs should be repeated within 3 to 6 hours to rule out an enlarging pneumothorax or the delayed manifestation of a hemothorax.[2,6]

There are several relative contraindications to performing a tube thoracostomy in the medical patient. These include the presence of a coagulopathy, large pulmonary blebs or bullae, pulmonary adhesions, loculated pleural effusions, tuberculosis, or previous tube thoracostomies. These patients may require CT or ultrasound guidance to place the chest tube. A coagulopathy should be corrected before the chest tube is inserted if such placement is not required emergently.

There has been some suggestion in the literature that there may be a role for the prehospital placement of chest tubes by physicians.[7] While this has not gained widespread acceptance, aeromedical crews frequently perform tube thoracostomies in the field.

EQUIPMENT

Povidone iodine solution
10 to 20 mL syringe
Local anesthetic solution (10 to 20 mL of 1% lidocaine
    with epinephrine)
25 or 27 gauge needle
#10 surgical scalpel blade on a handle
Kelly clamps, large and medium
Chest tubes, sizes 12 to 42 French
Sterile water
Chest tube drainage apparatus with a water seal
Christmas tree connector
Suction source and tubing
Needle driver
Mayo scissors, large curved
Size 0 or 1–0 suture, silk or nylon
Petrolatum-impregnated gauze
4×4 gauze squares
Adhesive tape, 3 to 4 inches wide
Sterile drapes
Sterile gloves
Tincture of benzoin spray or swabs
0.25% bupivacaine

Most hospitals and Emergency Departments have prepared "chest tube trays" that contain all the equipment required to place a chest tube except the chest tubes, local anesthetic solution, and a collection system. These last three items will vary based on the etiology of the air and/or fluid in the pleural cavity, the age and size of the patient, and physician preference.

Chest tubes are available in numerous sizes and from multiple manufacturers. The lower the number, the smaller the size of the chest tube. A spontaneous pneumothorax may be drained with an 18 to 26 French tube in adults and a 14 to 16 French tube in children. Traumatic pneumothoraces are usually drained with a 32 to 36 French tube in adults and a 16 to 20 French tube in children. Traumatic hemothoraces, traumatic hemopneumothoraces, and empyemas require larger-size tubes. A 36 to 40 French tube in adults and a 20 to 24 French tube in children will provide adequate drainage without becoming occluded by blood clots or purulent material.

Chest tubes used in the Emergency Department are hollow, clear, straight plastic tubes (Figure 28-1). The distal end of the chest tube has numerous fenestrations or holes that allow the passage of air and/or fluid into and through the tube. A radiopaque stripe allows for radiographic localization of the chest tube after it is inserted into the patient. The proximal end of the chest tube is beveled to allow it to fit better on a plastic connector.

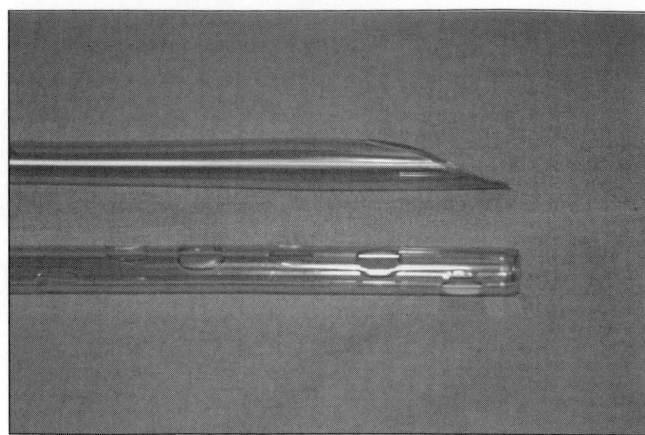

FIGURE 28-1 The chest tube. The proximal end is beveled while the distal end is fenestrated.

DRAINAGE SYSTEMS

It is important to know how to use the drainage system available at your institution to prevent any complications arising from the use of these devices. The classic glass bottle system with rubber corks is rarely, if ever, used today in the Emergency Department. Commer-

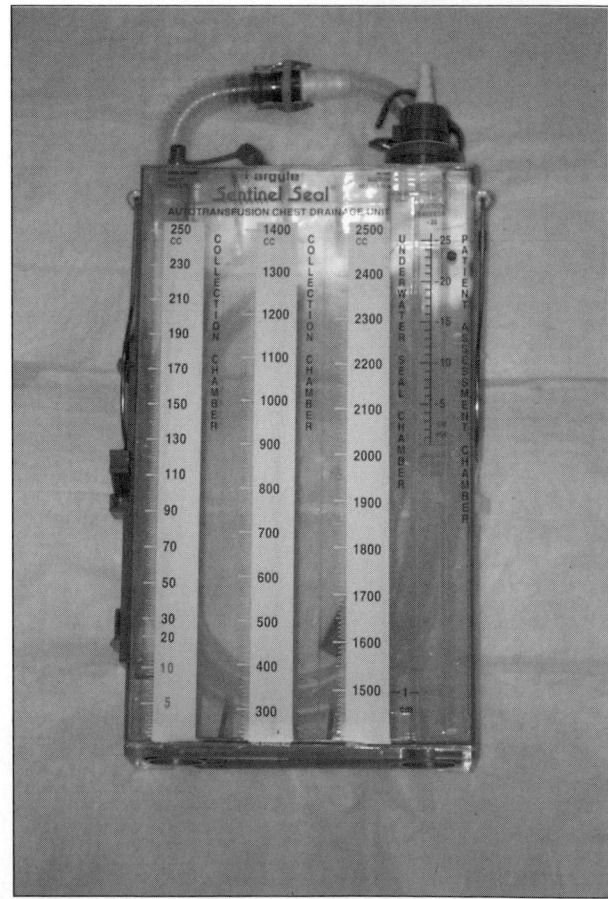

FIGURE 28-2 A commercially available chest tube drainage system.

cially available drainage systems are currently available in most hospitals (Figure 28-2). They are made of lightweight plastic and intended for single-patient use. They are preassembled, are disposable, and may be used for autotransfusions. They have clear plastic covers to allow easy visualization of the fluid within the unit.

The system is a single unit that consists of three or four chambers, depending on the manufacturer. The first chamber connects to the chest tube with flexible rubber tubing. It collects blood clots and/or other fluid expressed through the chest tube. The second chamber is the water seal. It allows one-way flow of air away from the patient and maintains a negative intrathoracic pressure gradient compared to the atmosphere. The third chamber is the suction regulator, which attaches to the wall suction. It draws in atmospheric air when needed to limit the negative pressure of the vacuum. One manufacturer has included a fourth chamber to assess the patient's intrapleural pressure (Sentinal Seal, Sherwood Medical, Ireland).

PATIENT PREPARATION

As with all invasive procedures, an informed consent for a tube thoracostomy should be obtained from the patient or their representative and documented in the medical record whenever possible. This should include a discussion of the risks of organ injury, infection, and other complications to be described further on in this chapter. It should be understood that following trauma, tube thoracostomy is often performed under urgent or emergent conditions. Lifesaving care should always proceed on the patient's behalf with the appropriate documentation in the medical record after the patient is resuscitated.

Place the patient supine or semierect with the arm on the involved side raised away from the chest (Figure 28-3). A soft restraint may be placed around the wrist to prevent the arm from moving during the procedure. Apply povidone iodine solution to the chest wall and allow it to dry. Apply sterile drapes to demarcate a sterile field. Sterile technique should be observed and followed by all involved personnel, who should be fully gowned, masked, and gloved.

Identify the fifth intercostal space (ICS) in the mid-to anterior axillary line. This is the preferred site for chest tube insertion. The reasons for this are twofold. The diaphragm rises during respiration to the level of the nipple. Chest tube insertion below the fifth ICS unnecessarily risks puncture of the diaphragm or abdominal organs. The area of the midaxillary line is the least muscular area of the chest wall and is thus an easier area from which to gain access to the pleural cavity.[1–3]

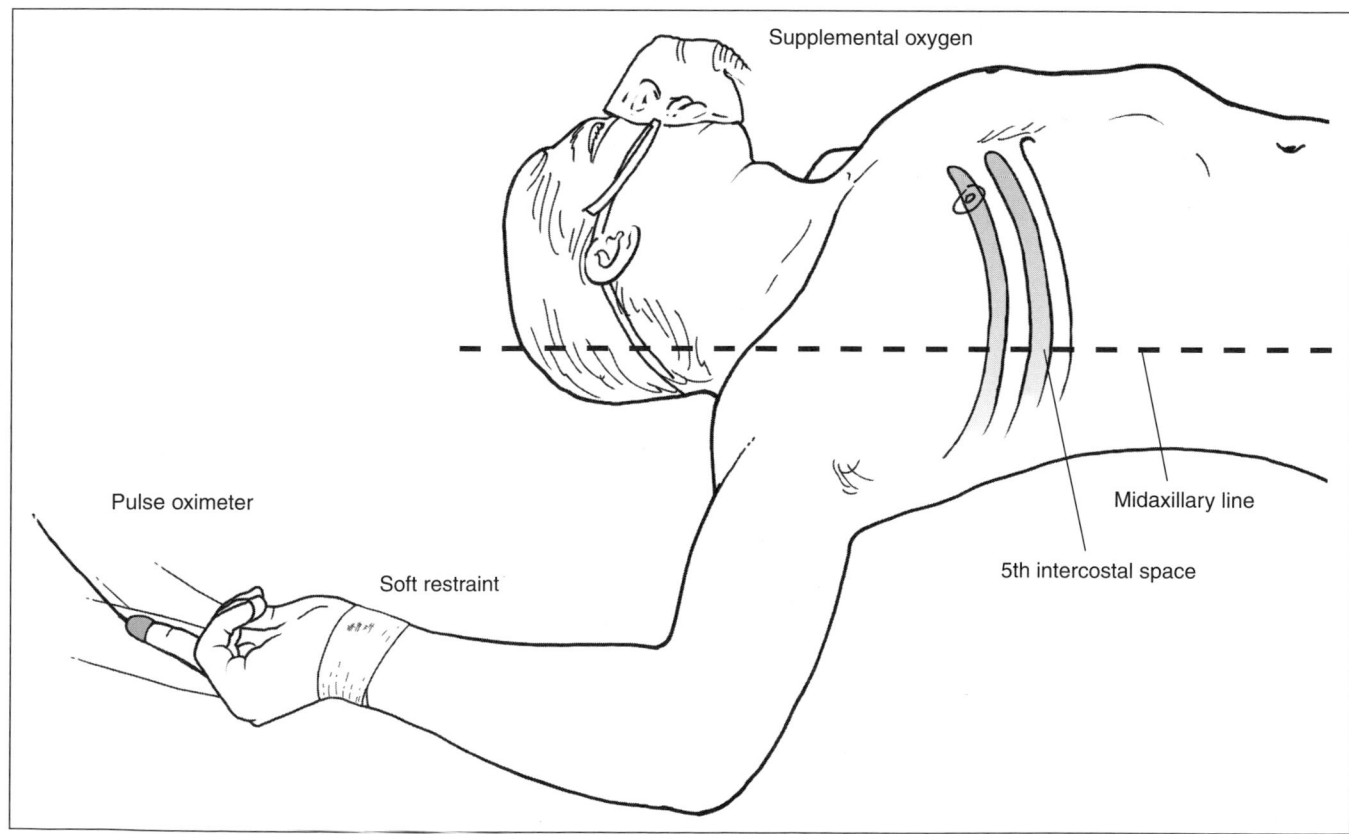

FIGURE 28-3 Patient positioning for a tube thoracostomy. Note the application of supplemental oxygen, pulse oximetry, and a soft restraint.

If not contraindicated, the administration of parenteral analgesics, sedatives, and/or conscious sedation will be greatly appreciated by the patient, as the procedure is quite painful. Appropriate protocols for patient monitoring should be employed. At minimum, the patient should have supplemental oxygen applied, continuous pulse oximetry, and frequent checks of vital signs. Continuous cardiac monitoring should also be employed and monitored.

If the patient is awake and aware of their surroundings, infiltrate local anesthetic solution into the chest wall and pleural cavity. This should be performed regardless of whether the patient receives parenteral analgesics, sedatives, and/or conscious sedation. Approximately 10 to 20 mL of 1% lidocaine with epinephrine is required to provide adequate analgesia. Raise a subcutaneous wheal of local anesthetic solution one interspace below the one to be used to insert the chest tube (i.e., sixth ICS). Infiltrate local anesthetic solution subcutaneously and upward to a point above the fifth ICS. Redirect the needle to anesthetize the intercostal muscles and parietal pleura of the fifth ICS. Advance the needle into the pleural cavity and inject 2 to 3 mL of local anesthetic solution to adequately anesthetize the pleura (Figure 28-4).

TECHNIQUE

The technique described here is an "open" technique, as opposed to that employing the use of a trocar. Trocar-aided insertion of chest tubes is associated with a higher incidence of complications and does not result in any significant saving of time.[1–3] For these reasons, a trocar should not be used.

Make a 3 to 5 cm incision with the #10 scalpel blade over the rib one ICS below the desired ICS (Figures 28-5 and 28-6A). Bluntly dissect a tract or tunnel with the 6 inch Kelly clamp in the subcutaneous tissue in a cephalic direction to the rib above. Orient the clamp with the tips curved toward the skin. Advance the closed tips of the clamp in 1 cm increments and open the jaws to dissect the tract (Figure 28-6B). The tract should terminate at the upper border of the above rib. **This will avoid injury to the neurovascular bundle lying under the inferior border of the rib.** Rotate the clamp 180 degrees such that the tip is aimed just above the superior border of the rib and toward the pleural cavity. Briskly push the closed tips of the clamp through the intercostal muscles and parietal pleura and into the pleural cavity (Figure 28-6C). **This maneuver requires a significant amount of force to enter the pleural cavity.** A twisting motion as the clamp is advanced may facilitate penetration into the pleural cavity. If the clamp is advanced slowly, the intercostal muscles will stretch and entering the pleural cavity will be difficult.

A loss of resistance associated with a rush of air or fluid should occur as the pleural cavity is entered with the closed tips of the clamp (Figure 28-6C). If under pressure, the fluid contained within the pleural cavity may exit the tract forcibly. **It is important not to plunge too deeply with the clamp as the pleural cavity is entered.** The tips of the clamp can injure the diaphragm, great vessels, heart, or lung. The forward motion of the clamp can be partially opposed by bracing the nondominant hand on the underside of the clamp and applying counterpressure away from the patient as the clamp enters the pleural cavity.

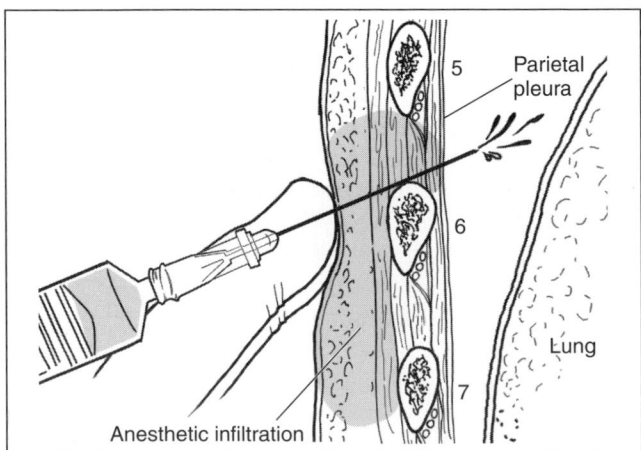

FIGURE 28-4 Infiltration of local anesthetic solution into the chest wall and pleural cavity.

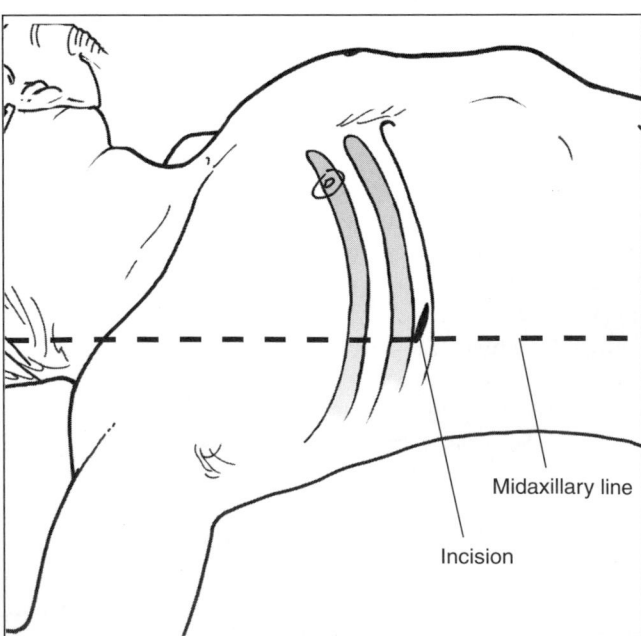

FIGURE 28-5 The initial skin incision is made over the rib one interspace below the desired chest tube insertion site.

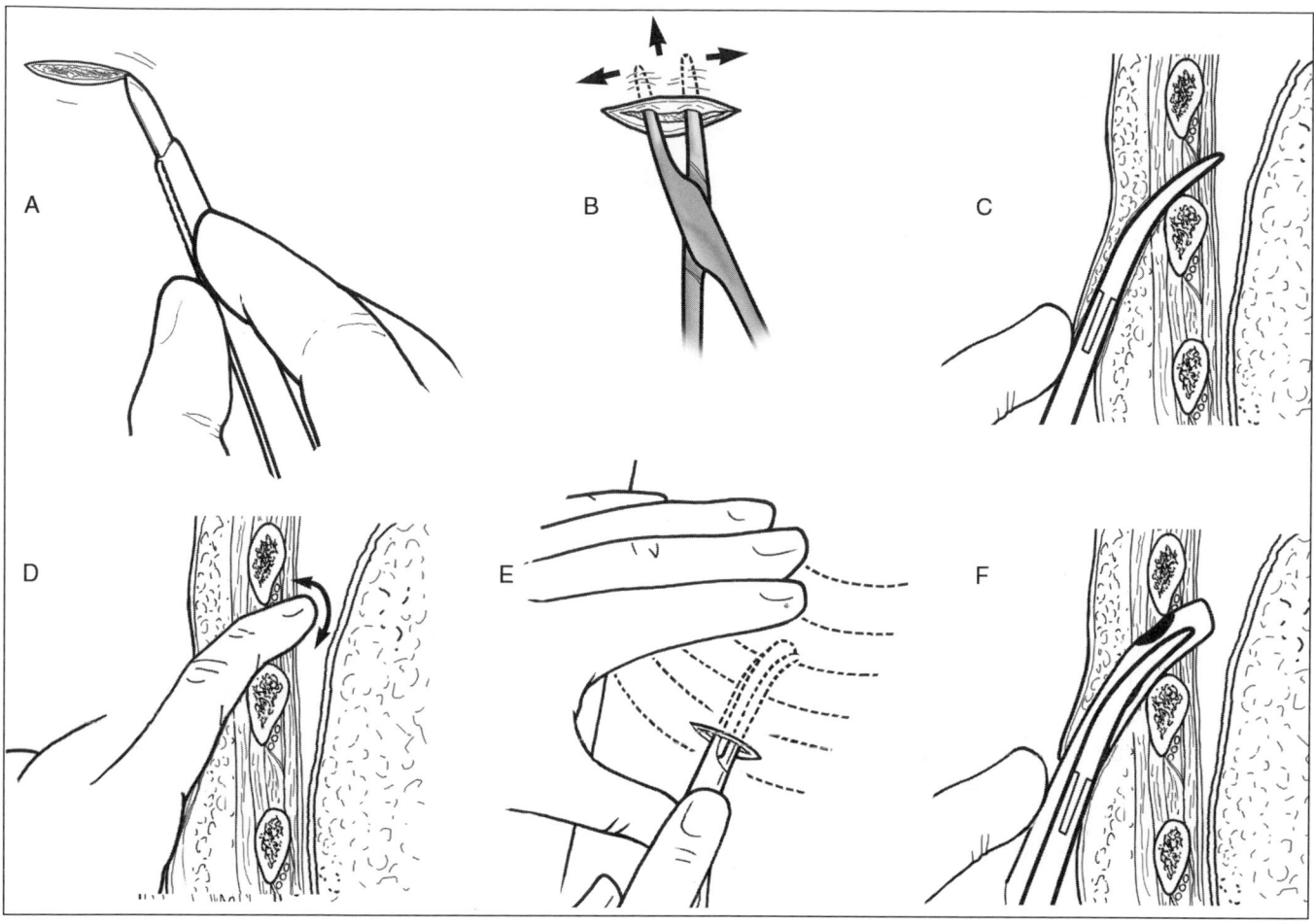

FIGURE 28-6 The tube thoracostomy. *A.* The skin incision is made. *B.* A tract is bluntly dissected in the subcutaneous tissues. *C.* The Kelly clamp is forced into the pleural cavity. *D.* A finger is inserted through the tract to feel for adhesions. *E.* The chest tube is held in the Kelly clamp and inserted through the tract. *F* The chest tube is guided into the pleural cavity.

Spread the jaws of the clamp to enlarge the tract through the subcutaneous tissue, intercostal muscles, and parietal pleura. Insert a finger through the tract and into the pleural cavity (Figure 28-6D). Rotate the finger to ascertain the presence or absence of adhesions. Gently break any loose adhesions between the lung and thoracic cage with the finger. Dense adhesions require the chest tube to be inserted at another site.

Prepare to insert the chest tube. Estimate the distance from the skin incision to the apex of the lung by laying the chest tube over the patient. Apply a clamp onto the chest tube at the estimated site at which it should exit the skin incision. This location should be 4 to 5 cm proximal to the fenestrations in the chest tube. Cut off the beveled end of the chest tube just above the bevel.

Grasp and clamp the tips of the large Kelly clamp onto the distal end of the chest tube. Insert the tips of the clamp and chest tube through the tract and into the pleural cavity (Figures 28-6E and F). Use the clamp to direct the tip of the chest tube posteriorly and superiorly. Alternatively, the dominant index finger can be placed

through the tract to direct the chest tube. The use of the finger in the tract is the preferred method to guide the chest tube. The finger will be able to confirm the proper intrapleural placement of the chest tube. Release the Kelly clamp and advance the chest tube until all the fenestrations are within the pleural cavity and the preplaced clamp on the chest tube is at the skin incision. Hold the chest tube securely in place. Remove the Kelly clamp from the incision. Release the clamp on the chest tube.

Secure the chest tube with 0 or 1–0 silk or monofilament nylon suture (Figure 28-7). The many techniques that have been described for securing chest tubes are idiosyncratic and probably equivalent. Suffice it to say that the tube should be sewn in such a way that the incision is closed fairly tightly around the tube to assure a better seal and that routine movements of the patient should not dislodge it.

Place the first stitch as a simple interrupted stitch at one end of the skin incision (Figure 28-7A). Leave both ends of the suture long after tying the knot in the first stitch. Wrap the needle end of the suture firmly around

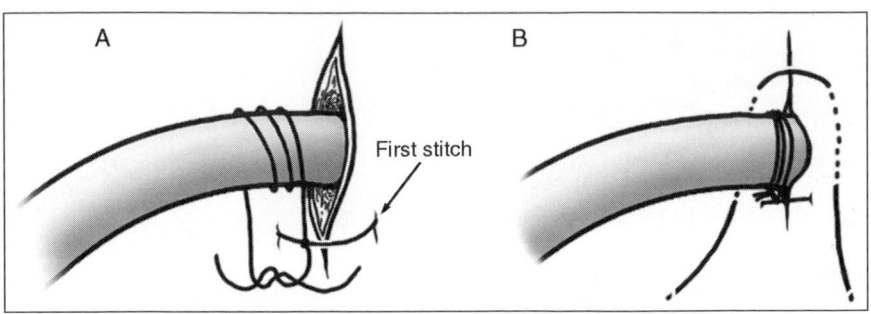

FIGURE 28-7 Securing the chest tube to the thoracic wall. *A.* The stay suture. *B.* The purse-string suture.

the chest tube three or four times. Tie a knot in the suture to secure the chest tube to the skin (Figure 28-7*A*). Place the second stitch as a purse-string suture encompassing the chest tube (Figure 28-7*B*). Leave both ends of the suture long. Wrap both ends of the suture around the chest tube and tie a bow, not a knot. This stitch will be used later to close the skin incision after the chest tube is removed. Place simple interrupted or horizontal mattress sutures to close the remainder of the skin incision.

Apply an occlusive dressing over the incision site (Figure 28-8). Apply petrolatum gauze over the incision site and around the chest tube as it exits the incision. Place gauge squares over the incision site. Apply tincture of benzoin to the chest wall surrounding the gauze squares. Tape the gauze and chest tube to the torso. The ends of the tape should be adherent to the tincture of benzoin. **Do not place tape over the patient's nipple. If the tape must cover the nipple, protect it with a piece of gauze.**

Immediately connect the chest tube to a drainage system (Figure 28-9), which is a self-contained multi-chamber device.[3] The first chamber is a collecting chamber that connects directly to the chest tube. The second chamber contains a small amount of saline or water and acts as a one-way valve. This assures flow only in the direction away from the patient. The third chamber controls suction, with a capability of at least 20 cm of water suction, and attaches to the wall suction system. Commercially available systems encompass all three chambers in one container.

ASSESSMENT

Obtain an anteroposterior portable chest radiograph. Observe the position of the chest tube. Remove the chest tube and insert a new one if it is bent, kinked, or in the fissure of the lung. If its tip is against the mediastinum, unsecure the tube, withdraw it a few centimeters, resecure the tube, and obtain a repeat radiograph. If the chest tube is located in the subcutaneous tissue, remove it and insert a new one. Observe the fenestrations on the

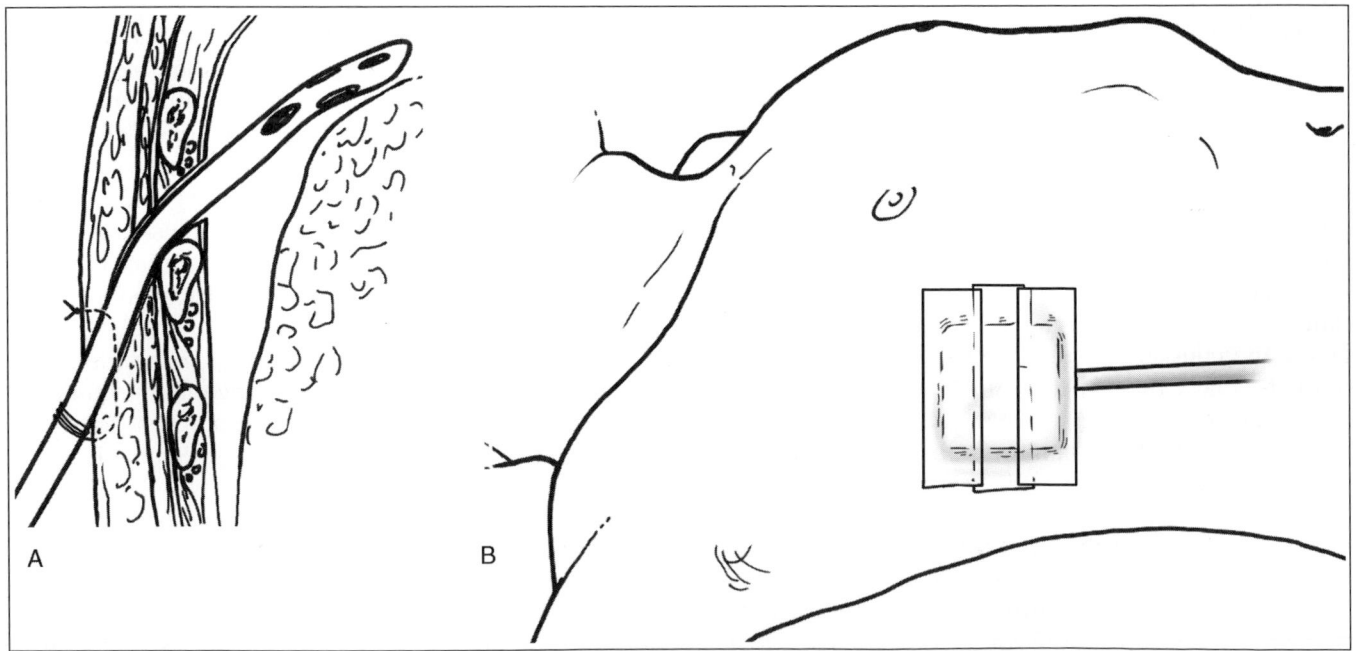

FIGURE 28-8 Securing the chest tube. *A.* The chest tube has been secured with suture to the chest wall. *B.* An occlusive dressing has been placed over the incision and taped to the chest wall.

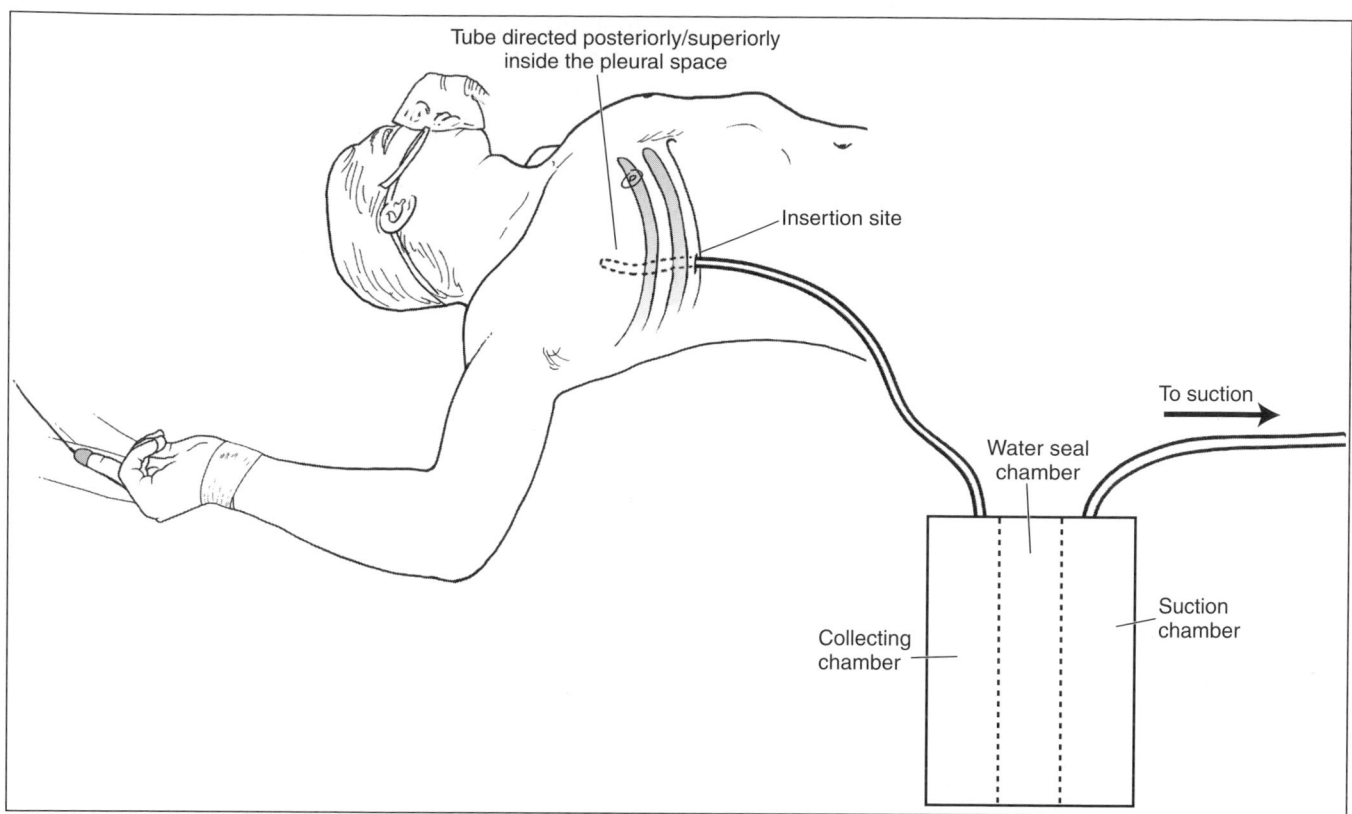

FIGURE 28-9 The chest tube is connected to a drainage system.

distal end of the chest tube in the radiograph. They all must be within the thoracic cavity. If not, remove the chest tube and insert a new one. **Never advance a chest tube further into the thoracic cavity after obtaining a chest radiograph, as this may track infectious material into the pleural cavity.**

Persistent bubbling in the system or failure of the lung to reexpand indicates a leak in the system. Check the system to ensure that all connections are secure. Place tape over the connections to eliminate leaks and prevent the components from becoming dislodged. Check the tubing for any holes or fissures. Examine the chest tube and the radiograph to confirm that all fenestrations are within the thoracic cavity. If not, replace the chest tube. An injury to the trachea, mainstem bronchus, a large bronchiole, or the esophagus can cause a persistent air leak. Insert a second chest tube to keep up with the leak and prepare the patient for bronchoscopy and/or esophagoscopy to diagnose the etiology of the persistent air leak.

AFTERCARE

Patients with chest tubes require close monitoring. Serial chest radiographs should be obtained to monitor resolution of the inciting process. The presence of air

leaks from the chest tube indicates that the injury has not completely healed and the seal between the parietal and visceral pleurae has not yet been restored. Suction should be maintained until there is no evidence of an air leak. The acceptable minimal daily output from a chest tube as a criterion for removal varies according to the institution, the practitioner, and the reason for insertion. It is also unclear whether a trial period of water seal following suction is strictly necessary. There is literature to suggest that both suction and water seal protocols for removing chest tubes are effective and have similar incidences of recurrent pneumothoraces.[8] However, there is also literature supporting an abbreviated trial of water seal following suction, as it may allow time for occult pneumothoraces to manifest themselves and thus alleviate the need for reinsertion of a chest tube.[9] The chest tube insertion site should be monitored for signs of infection.

The chest tube and collection tubing should be checked periodically for blockage. If blocked, the tubing may be milked or stripped to alleviate the blockage and avoid the need to replace the chest tube. Milking refers to forcing air, fluid, or clots back into the chest. Stripping refers to creating negative pressure within the tubing to move fluid or clots distally and into the collecting chamber. To milk the tube, clamp or pinch the tubing shut distally while using the other hand to compress the tubing and move proximally to force the contents back into the thoracic cavity. To strip the tube, clamp or pinch the tubing shut proximally while using the other hand to compress the tubing and move distally followed by the sudden release of the proximal tubing.

CHEST TUBE REMOVAL

In planning to remove a chest tube, one must be prepared to replace it. All the necessary equipment and supplies should be readily available in case the patient urgently requires a new chest tube.

Place the patient supine or semirecumbent. The use of parenteral sedation and soft restraints is rarely necessary when removing a chest tube. Carefully remove the tape securing the chest tube to the chest wall. Be cautious when removing the tape if it covers the patient's nipple, so as to prevent any injury. Remove the gauze squares and petrolatum gauze covering the incision site. Untie the bow securing the free ends of the purse-string suture that was previously placed. Cut the suture that is holding the chest tube to the chest wall. Remove this suture. Place the first half of a surgeon's knot in the free ends of the purse-string suture. Pass the ends of the suture to an assistant. **Instruct the patient to exhale fully and hold their breath. This will prevent ambient air from being drawn through the chest wall and into the pleural cavity.** Quickly and smoothly remove the chest tube while the assistant cinches down the knot of the suture to seal the skin incision. Tie additional knots to secure the purse-string suture. Place petrolatum jelly or topical antibiotic ointment over the incision. Cover the site with gauze squares and tape it securely.

The patient should be observed for 4 to 6 hours for any signs of cardiovascular or respiratory compromise. If the patient remains asymptomatic, obtain expiratory posteroanterior and lateral chest radiographs. Evaluate the radiograph for the recurrence of the pneumothorax, hemothorax, pyothorax, and/or hydrothorax. The dressing may be removed in 24 to 48 hours. Remove the chest wall sutures in 8 to 10 days.

COMPLICATIONS

Tube thoracostomy is often described as a simple procedure. But if it is not performed with care and attention, it can result in serious complications, including injuries to thoracic and abdominal organs.[1,2] An unusual occurrence of sudden death following chest tube insertion has been reported.[10] It was attributed to hemorrhage near the vagus nerve, causing irritation and stimulation of the vague nerve and refractory bradycardia. Injury to the heart and great vessels can occur if the chest tube is placed anteriorly. Lung injury can occur if the clamp plunges inward on entering the pleural cavity. **It is imperative that the Kelly clamp be controlled as it enters the pleural cavity.** If the lung is adherent to the chest wall, it may be penetrated by the Kelly clamp or the chest tube. **A trocar should never be used to insert a chest tube, as it can cause significant injury to the lung.**

Other complications associated with chest tube placement and removal include recurrent, residual, and loculated pneumothoraces. These may require the placement of additional chest tubes. A retained hemothorax may require decortication and may develop into an empyema.[4,11,12]

Posttraumatic empyema remains a serious complication of thoracic trauma with incidences ranging from 2 to 25 percent.[1,2,4,12] The etiology of the infection is not always clear. A break in sterile technique on chest tube insertion, nosocomial pneumonia, superinfected pulmonary contusion, and undrained hemothoraces have all been implicated. In recent years there has been considerable discussion in the literature regarding the use of antibiotics in patients requiring tube thoracostomy for trauma in the hope of reducing the incidence of empyema.[13–15] Although there is much evidence in support of the concept, opinion remains divided. One thing remains clear: empyemas that can be attributed to the chest tube insertion process are completely preventable complications that can be avoided by strict adherence to aseptic technique.

Bleeding can occur from several sites. Incision site bleeding is often due to superficial venules and arterioles. The application of pressure and the suturing of the incision closed will alleviate this bleeding. If the dissection or penetration into the pleural cavity occurs along the inferior surface of a rib, an intercostal artery or vein can be lacerated. Securing the chest tube against the inferior surface of the rib may tamponade the bleeding. If the bleeding continues, attempt to tamponade it with a Foley catheter. Insert the catheter into the pleural cavity, inflate the cuff, and withdraw the catheter to lodge the cuff against the posterior surface of the rib. A final option is to extend the incision to expose and ligate the bleeding vessel. Lung injury and bleeding from penetration into the pleural cavity is often self-limited and minor. A trocar should never be used, as risk of injury to intrathoracic structures is significantly increased. An anteriorly placed chest tube should be at least 3 cm from the lateral border of the sternum to prevent injury to the internal mammary artery.

The chest tube can become occluded and stop functioning. A large tube should always be inserted if its purpose it to drain blood, clots, or purulent material. Attempt to milk and/or strip the tubing, as described previously. Obtain a chest radiograph to determine if the chest tube is kinked. If the occlusion cannot be dislodged or the tube is kinked, the chest tube should be removed and a new one inserted.

Subcutaneous emphysema results from air from an inadequately decompressed pneumothorax that tracks into the subcutaneous tissues. Ensure that the chest tube, drainage system, and suction source are functioning properly. Replace any component that is not functioning.

Reexpansion pulmonary edema occurs from the rapid expansion of a lung that has been collapsed for over 48 to 72 hours or from the removal of a large pleural effusion. Patients will begin to experience increasing shortness of breath and hypoxemia within a few hours of the procedure. Repeat chest radiographs will show an expanded lung with pulmonary edema. The exact etiology of this complication is unknown. This complication may be prevented by the slow expansion of a lung and the removal of pleural fluid in increments. Treatment includes supportive care, supplemental oxygenation, and positive-pressure ventilation (BiPAP, CPAP, intubation). Diuretics have no role in relieving the edema.

The sources of pain for a patient with a tube thoracostomy are numerous. These include the skin incision, intercostal muscle transection, the chest tube, and the underlying injury. Pain can often be managed with parenteral analgesics and sedation. Intrapleural bupivacaine has been found to be effective in reducing pain.[16–18] Administer 20 to 40 mL of 0.25% bupivacaine through the chest tube and into the pleural cavity. Clamp the chest tube or the tubing for up to 10 minutes to allow the bupivacaine to thoroughly coat the pleural cavity. **Carefully monitor and observe the patient to ensure that they do not develop a tension pneumothorax while the chest tube is clamped.** Unclamp the chest tube and allow the excess anesthetic to drain into the collection system. This can provide several hours of pain relief to a patient who may have limits on or contraindications to parenteral analgesics.

SUMMARY

Tube thoracostomy is useful in the treatment of thoracic injuries resulting in pneumothoraces, hemothoraces, hydrothoraces, and chylothoraces. Attention must be paid to observe sterile technique, choose the proper insertion site, carefully enter the pleura, and verify entry via digital exam. Appropriate drainage systems should be employed to assure maintenance of a closed, watertight system. The patient should be monitored regularly while the chest tube is in place. Practitioners performing this procedure should be cognizant of the serious complications that may be associated with tube thoracostomies, some of which are directly related to technique.

Adherence to the principles described above will assist in avoiding many of these complications and provide optimal care for victims of thoracic trauma.

REFERENCES

1. Richardson JD, Spain DA: Injury to the lung and pleura, in Mattox KL, Feliciano DV, Moore EE (eds): *Trauma*, 4th ed. New York: McGraw-Hill, 2000:523–544.
2. Symbas PN: *Cardiothoracic Trauma.* Philadelphia: Saunders, 1989.
3. Symbas PN: Chest drainage tubes. *Surg Clin North Am* 1989; 69(1):41–46.
4. Mandal AK, Thadepalli H, Mandal AK, et al: Post-traumatic empyema thoracis: a 24-year experience at a major trauma center. *J Trauma* 1997; 43(5):764–771.
5. Enderson BL, Abdalla R, Frame SB, et al: Tube thoracostomy for occult pneumothorax: a prospective randomized study of its use. *J Trauma* 1993; 35(5):726–729.
6. Kiev J, Kerstein MD: Role of three hour roentgenogram of the chest in penetrating and nonpenetrating injuries of the chest. *Surg Gynecol Obstet* 1992; 175:249–253.
7. Schmidt U, Stalp M, Gerich T, et al: Chest tube decompression of blunt chest injuries by physicians in the field: effectiveness and complications. *J Trauma* 1998; 44(1):98–101.
8. Davis JW, Mackersie RC, Hoyt DB, et al: Randomized study of algorithms for discontinuing tube thoracostomy drainage. *J Am Coll Surg* 1994; 179:553–557.
9. Martino K, Merrit S, Boyakye K, et al: Prospective randomized trial of thoracostomy removal algorithms. *J Trauma* 1999; 46(3):369–371.
10. Ward EW, Hughes TS: Sudden death following chest tube insertion: an unusual case of vagus nerve irritation. *J Trauma* 1994; 36(2):258–259.
11. Helling TS, Gyles NR, Eisenstein CL, et al: Complications following blunt and penetrating injuries in 216 victims of chest trauma requiring tube thoracostomy. *J Trauma* 1989; 29(10):1367–1370.
12. Eddy AC, Luna GK, Copass M: Empyema thoracis in patients undergoing emergent closed tube thoracostomy for thoracic trauma. *Am J Surg* 1989; 157:494–497.
13. Nichols RL, Smith JW, Musik AC, et al: Preventive antibiotic usage in traumatic thoracic injuries requiring tube thoracostomy. *Chest* 1994; 106(5):1493–1498.

14. Brunner RG, Vinsant GO, Alexander RH, et al: The role of antibiotic therapy in the prevention of empyema in patients with an isolated chest injury (ISS 9-10): a prospective study. *J Trauma* 1990; 30(9):1148–1153.

15. Evans JT, Green JD, Carlin PE, et al: Meta-analysis of antibiotics in tube thoracostomy. *Am Surg* 1995; 61(3):215–219.

16. Seltzer JL, Larijani GE, Goldberg ME, et al: Intrapleural bupivacaine—a kinetic and dynamic evaluation. *Anesthesiology* 1987; 67(5):798–800.

17. Knottenbelt JD, James MF, Bloomfield M: Intrapleural bupivacaine analgesia in chest trauma: a randomized double-blind controlled trial. *Injury* 1991; 22(2):114–116.

18. Engdahl O, Boe J, Sandstedt S: Intrapleural bupivacaine analgesia during chest drainage treatment for pneumothorax. A randomized double-blind study. *Acta Anesth Scand* 1993: 37(2):149–153.

Chapter 29
THORACENTESIS

M. Chris Decker

INTRODUCTION

Thoracentesis is a term derived from the Greek meaning "to pierce the chest." It is used today to refer to the removal of air or fluid from the thoracic cavity. Accumulation of pleural fluid is not a specific diagnosis but rather a reflection of an underlying process. In almost all newly discovered pleural effusions, thoracentesis should be performed to aid in the diagnosis and management of the underlying etiology.

Hippocrates first described thoracentesis in the management of empyema.[1] Thoracentesis was used widely in World War II and the Korean conflict in lieu of a thoracotomy for chest drainage. By the time of the Vietnam War, this practice was replaced by thoracostomy tubes. Today, thoracentesis is used in the diagnosis and therapy of pleural effusions, emergent and temporizing treatment of a tension pneumothorax, and the management of small, nontraumatic pneumothoraces.[1–4]

A pleural effusion can be identified clinically and radiologically. Clinically, the patient may develop pain related to irritation of the parietal pleura, compromised pulmonary mechanics, or interference with gas exchange.[3] The pain may be located in the chest, abdomen, or ipsilateral shoulder. Another common symptom is a cough; its mechanism is unclear. Dyspnea occurs secondary to the space-occupying effect of the fluid and alterations in gas exchange. In extreme cases, pleural effusions can reduce cardiac output. On physical examination, tactile fremitus is absent or attenuated and there is dullness to percussion. Auscultation reveals decreased breath sounds on the involved hemithorax.

Radiographically, on a posteroanterior (PA) chest radiograph, an effusion can be diagnosed when there is homogeneous opacification in the hemithorax, absent air bronchograms, and clouded vesicular vascular markings. In a cadaveric study, the minimum fluid volume needed to blunt the costophrenic angle was 175 mL.[5] More than 500 mL had to be injected into some cadavers to blunt the costophrenic angle.[5] A lateral decubitus film is often necessary and will determine whether the fluid is loculated or free-flowing. It will also be helpful if one of these signs is present on the PA chest radiograph: a clear costophrenic angle, an elevated hemidiaphragm, a blurred contour of the diaphragmatic dome, or the gastric bubble seen more than 2 cm from the lung border in patients with left-sided pleural effusions.[2] If the fluid collection is 10 mm thick on the lateral decubitus film, thoracentesis can most likely be performed using clinical skills to locate the fluid.[6] If it is less than 10 mm thick, ultrasound may be needed for localization.[3]

A pneumothorax may be simple or under pressure (also known as tension). A simple pneumothorax may present clinically with chest pain, dyspnea, hypoxia, and tachycardia. Physical examination may reveal, on auscultation, decreased breath sounds on the affected side. Performance of a thoracentesis to relieve a tension pneumothorax is based on the mechanism of lung injury, the patient's symptoms, and physical examination findings. Mechanisms of injury to the lung include mechanical ventilation, chest trauma, instrumentation of the chest, and spontaneous lung rupture. Classically, the patient has a clinical presentation of hypotension, tachycardia, and absent breath sounds on the affected side. Other symptoms may include a deviated trachea, acute change in mental status, air hunger, chest pain, cyanosis, diaphoresis, hypoxia, and cardiorespiratory arrest.[1,4] Sometimes a patient with a tension pneumothorax may have a normal physical examination due to subtle auscultation findings often missed in a noisy

Emergency Department. Tactile fremitus may be absent and percussion is typically hyperresonant over the hemithorax with the tension pneumothorax.

There are two major indications for performing a thoracentesis.[1–3,7] The first is for the evacuation of air. This includes a simple pneumothorax and the emergent diagnosis and temporizing treatment of a tension pneumothorax. The second is for the evacuation of fluid. This may be done to help diagnose the etiology of pleural effusion or for the treatment of a symptomatic pleural effusion.

PLEURAL EFFUSIONS

ANATOMY AND PATHOPHYSIOLOGY

The pleura is a serous membrane that covers the lungs, mediastinum, diaphragm, and thoracic cavity. The pleural space is a potential space between the lung and the thoracic cavity. A thin layer of fluid exists between the visceral pleura covering the organs and the parietal pleura covering the chest wall. This fluid acts as a lubricant.[3] Pleural fluid originates from three sources: parietal capillaries, visceral capillaries, and the interstitium. Hydrostatic and oncotic forces govern the flow of fluid in the pleural space. These forces are summarized in Figure 29-1. In a healthy person, the protein free fluid enters the pleural space from the parietal pleura and is absorbed by the visceral pleura. Small amounts of protein leak into the pleural space. Approximately 10 percent of the pleural fluid and large proteins are removed by the lymphatics at a rate of up to 20 mL/h for each

hemithorax.[2] Ventilation and muscular activity facilitate the action of the lymphatics.[3]

Alterations in pleural fluid homeostasis will lead to pleural effusions. Hydrostatic changes result in protein free effusions (transudates). Changes in oncotic pressure (abnormality in the lung or pleura) lead to effusions. The differential diagnosis of transudates and exudates is listed in Table 29-1.

INDICATIONS

A thoracentesis may be performed to remove pleural fluid for analysis to diagnose the etiology of the fluid (e.g., malignancy, infection). It may also be performed to relieve the patient's symptom of dyspnea.

CONTRAINDICATIONS

The only absolute contraindications are an uncooperative patient or a patient who refuses to give informed consent for the procedure.[7] Uncooperative patients or patients with altered levels of consciousness may require sedation for the procedure.

There are numerous relative contraindications to performing a thoracentesis. Patients receiving anticoagulants or with a bleeding diathesis, whether known or suspected, have a significant risk of bleeding.[2,7] Consider reversing the anticoagulant or the bleeding disorder prior to performing the thoracentesis. A small volume of pleural fluid may make the procedure difficult to perform and increase the risk of complications.[7] Patients on mechanical ventilators are at an increased risk of developing a pneumothorax and a tension pneumothorax.[1] One study has shown that a thoracentesis

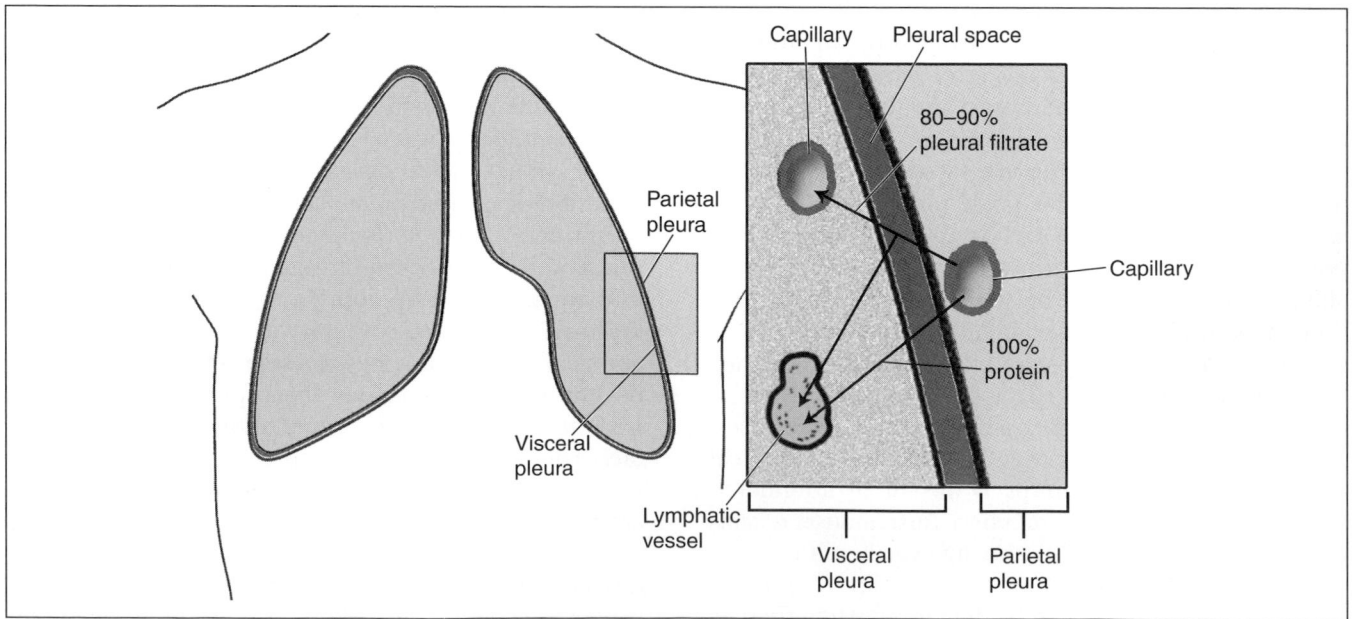

FIGURE 29-1 Schematic of pleural fluid homeostasis in a normal lung.

TABLE 29-1. DIFFERENTIAL DIAGNOSIS OF FLUID EXUDATES AND FLUID TRANSUDATES IN THE PLEURAL SPACE

Exudates	Transudates
Asbestos exposure	Atelectasis
Collagen vascular disease	Cirrhosis of the liver with ascites
Drug-induced	Congestive heart failure
Empyema	Nephrotic syndrome
Esophageal rupture	Peritoneal dialysis
Idiopathic	
Malignancy	
Pancreatitis	
Parapneumonic	
Pulmonary embolism	
Thoracic duct exposure	
Tuberculosis	
Viral	

can be done as safely in a ventilator-dependent patient as in patients not being mechanically ventilated.[8] Pleural adhesions may limit the amount of fluid obtained or require multiple thoracenteses to drain the fluid.[1] Areas of cellulitis or other infection on the chest wall should be avoided unless no alternate site can be identified for the procedure.[1,3] Unsupervised physicians with little or no experience should not be performing this procedure, as the risk of complications is increased.[6] Patients with chronic obstructive pulmonary disease are at increased risk for complications.

EQUIPMENT

Diagnostic Thoracentesis for Pleural Effusions

Local anesthetic solution, 1 to 2% lidocaine
Heparin, 1000 U/mL
Atropine, 1 mg
Alcohol pads
Antiseptic solution
Gauze pads, 4×4
Sterile drapes
Sterile towels
Sterile gloves
Band-Aids
25 or 27 gauge needle
21 and 22 gauge needles, 1.5 inches long
10 mL syringes
50 mL syringe
18 or 20 gauge needle

Therapeutic Thoracentesis for Pleural Effusions

The supplies listed above
16 to 18 gauge catheter-over-the-needle
14 to 18 gauge catheter-through-the-needle

Three-way stopcock
Connector tubing (connects to three-way stopcock and sterile container)
Sterile container for pleural fluid
50 mL syringe
Intravenous extension tubing

Commercial kits have been developed and are available to provide the equipment needed to perform a thoracentesis. The kits are disposable, are intended for single-patient use, and contain the required equipment. They save time in that the equipment does not have to be found and set up. Disadvantages include potential increased cost and limited equipment in the kit.[9] The most common kits include the Pharmaseal, distributed by Baxter (Jacksonville, TX); the Arrow Clark Thoracentesis Kit, distributed by Arrow (Reading, PA); and the Argyle Turkel Safety Thoracentesis Kit, distributed by Boston Scientific (Miami, FL).[3]

PATIENT PREPARATION

Explain the procedure, risks, and benefits to the patient or their representative and obtain a signed consent form.[1] The position of the patient can vary depending on their clinical condition. Patients who are ambulatory and cooperative should sit up at the edge of a bed with their feet on the floor or a stool (Figure 29-2). Place the patient's head and arms on an elevated bedside tray. The patient's back should be as vertical as possible so that the lowest part of the hemithorax is posterior. This will ensure that the free-flowing fluid remains posteriorly.[1–3,7]

In debilitated patients, one of three other positions is recommended. Place the patient in the lateral decubitus position, lying on the side of the pleural effusion. The patient's back should be along the edge of the bed. The procedure would then be performed in the midscapular line or the posterior axillary line. Place a ventilator-dependent patient into the lateral decubitus position, lying on the side with the pleural effusion.[8] Second, place the patient supine and elevate the head of the bed maximally. The patient would then be sitting with the assistance of the bed and the procedure would be performed in midaxillary or posterior axillary line.[3] Finally, the patient can be placed supine. The procedure would then be performed at the posterior or midaxillary line. With the patient supine, ultrasonography may be required to locate the pleural fluid. Sedation or paralysis may be needed for optimal positioning.

After positioning the patient, clean any dirt or debris from the skin. Identify the anatomic landmarks required to perform the procedure. After viewing the chest radiograph and estimating the amount of pleural fluid, percuss from superior to inferior starting at the midscapular or posterior axillary line. **The site chosen for**

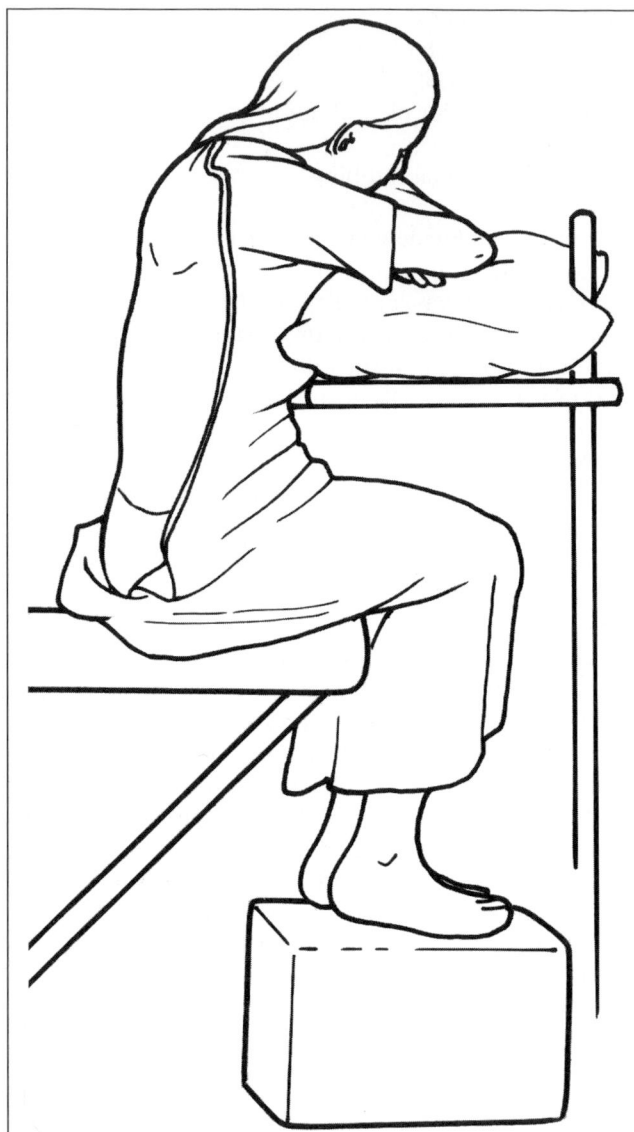

FIGURE 29-2 Recommended positioning of an ambulatory patient for a diagnostic or therapeutic thoracentesis for the evacuation of fluid.[2]

aspiration should be a single interspace below the top of the dullness to percussion. If the fluid thickness is less that 10 mm on decubitus radiographs, ultrasound may be used to locate the fluid.[5,7] Although not required, some physicians place the patient on the cardiac monitor, noninvasive blood pressure cuff, pulse oximetry, and supplemental oxygen. Apply povidone iodine solution to the skin surface and allow it to dry. Apply sterile drapes around the site of the procedure. Atropine should be at the bedside. It can be administered (1.0 mg subcutaneously or intramuscularly or 0.5 mg intravenously) to patients who develop symptomatic bradycardia during the procedure.

Place a skin wheal of local anesthetic solution over the thoracentesis site using a 25 or 27 gauge needle on a 10 mL syringe containing the local anesthetic solution. Remove the 25 or 27 gauge needle from the syringe. Apply a 21 or 22 gauge, 1.5 to 3.0 inch needle to the syringe containing the local anesthetic solution. Anesthetize the subcutaneous tissues and the periosteum of the rib (Figure 29-3). Walk the needle up the rib while simultaneously injecting local anesthetic solution. Gently aspirate prior to injecting each time the needle is advanced to ensure that the needle is not within a blood vessel. When the superior border of the rib is located, slowly and carefully advance the needle over the rib while applying negative pressure on the syringe. When the pleural space has been entered, fluid will flow into the syringe. Inject and aspirate small volumes (1 to 2 mL) while the needle is within the pleural cavity. This will distribute the local anesthetic solution into the pleural fluid and ensure anesthesia of the pleura. Withdraw the needle from the pleural cavity and out the skin.

DIAGNOSTIC THORACENTESIS TECHNIQUE FOR PLEURAL EFFUSIONS

Attach an 18 gauge needle to a 50 mL syringe containing 1 mL of heparin. The heparin will ensure accurate pH and cell counts as it prevents the fluid from clotting. Introduce the needle through the anesthetized track and into the pleural cavity (Figure 29-4B). Aspirate up to

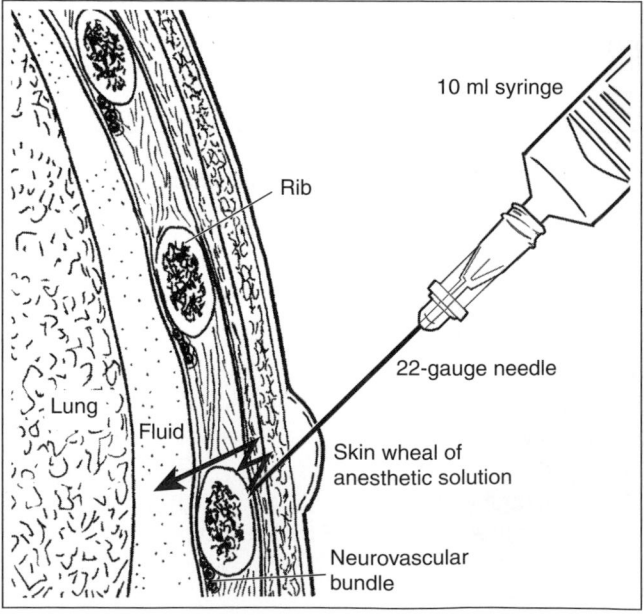

FIGURE 29-3 Administration of local anesthesia. A skin wheal is made. The needle is inserted through the skin wheal while local anesthetic solution is injected to anesthetize the subcutaneous tissues and the periosteum of the rib. The needle is "walked" above the upper border of the rib so as to avoid the neurovascular bundle inferior to the rib. The pleura and pleural space is then infiltrated with local anesthetic solution.

50 mL of fluid. Withdraw the needle and place the fluid into the appropriate sterile containers.

If pleural fluid cannot be aspirated, also known as a dry tap, four possibilities must be considered. The needle may be too short, positioned too high to reach the fluid (Figure 29-4A), positioned too low to reach the fluid (Figure 29-4C), or there may not actually be an effusion. Repeat the physical examination and review the chest radiograph to reconfirm the presence of a pleural effusion. Penetration of the lung with the needle is rarely catastrophic but can result in a pneumothorax.[3]

For debilitated patients, the principles are the same with the exception of the site for the procedure. If the patient is supine, use the midaxillary line or the posterior axillary line. Be cautious of the diaphragm, as it can be as high as the fifth interspace on expiration at the anterior axillary line. If the patient is in the lateral decubitus position, use the midscapular line or the posterior axillary line for the procedure.

THERAPEUTIC THORACENTESIS TECHNIQUES FOR PLEURAL EFFUSIONS

The same sterile preparation, location of fluid, positioning, and anesthesia considerations apply for therapeutic thoracentesis as with the diagnostic procedures. However, there is one difference between a diagnostic and a therapeutic thoracentesis—that is, the quantity of fluid removed. Up to 1.5 L is removed in a therapeutic

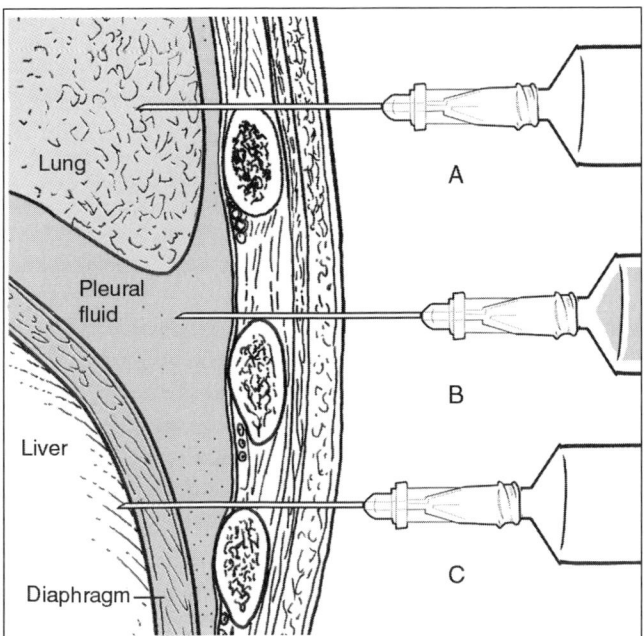

FIGURE 29-4 Needle positioning for a diagnostic thoracentesis. A. The pleural space is entered above the effusion (too high). B. The pleural space is entered properly over the rib and into the fluid. C. The needle is too low and enters the abdominal cavity below the diaphragm.

thoracentesis. A diagnostic thoracentesis requires approximately 10 to 20 mL of pleural fluid.

Catheter-over-the-Needle Technique

Two types of catheters can be used to perform this procedure. They are the catheter-over-the-needle and the catheter-through-the-needle (Figures 29-5 and 29-6). The catheter-over-the-needle technique is most commonly used (Figure 29-5). Make a small "nick" in the skin with a #11 surgical blade at the needle insertion site. Attach a 14 to 18 gauge catheter-over-the-needle to a 10 mL syringe as a handle. Insert the catheter-over-the-needle into the nick and advance it, reproducing the original anesthetized tract (Figure 29-5A). Apply negative pressure to the syringe as the catheter-over-the-needle is advanced. When fluid is encountered, angle the catheter-over-the-needle caudally. Advance the catheter until the hub is against the skin. Withdraw the needle while the catheter remains in the pleural cavity (Figure 29-5B). **When the needle is removed, quickly cover the catheter with a gloved finger. This will prevent ambient air from entering the pleural cavity.** Attach intravenous catheter extension tubing to the hub of the catheter. Place a three-way stopcock attached to a 50 mL syringe onto the extension tubing. Hold the catheter hub against the skin securely. Aspirate fluid into the syringe and then advance the fluid into the sterile container by adjusting the three-way stopcock.

An alternative option is to set up a siphon through the three-way stopcock. Prime the tubing with pleural fluid. Place the end of the tubing into a sterile container that is located below the site of the catheter. This allows the fluid to flow freely into the sterile container. Fluid can be removed in 50 mL aliquots up to 1.5 L. As a general rule, this is the limit, due to the risk of postevacuation pulmonary edema and excessive protein loss.[1]

Catheter-through-the-Needle Technique

The second option is to utilize the catheter-through-the-needle system (Figure 29-6), known as the Bardig Intracath system. It is not as popular as the catheter-over-the-needle systems. Place the needle on a tuberculin syringe. Insert the needle and advance it through the anesthetized tissues (Figure 29-6A). A small "nick" in the skin with a #11 surgical blade will facilitate needle entry. Apply negative pressure to the syringe as the needle is advanced along the anesthetized tract and into the pleural cavity. When fluid is aspirated, stop advancing the needle. **Remove the syringe and cover the needle hub with a gloved finger. This will prevent ambient air from entering the pleural cavity.** Angle the needle slightly caudally and advance the catheter through the needle (Figure 29-6B). Withdraw the needle, leaving the catheter

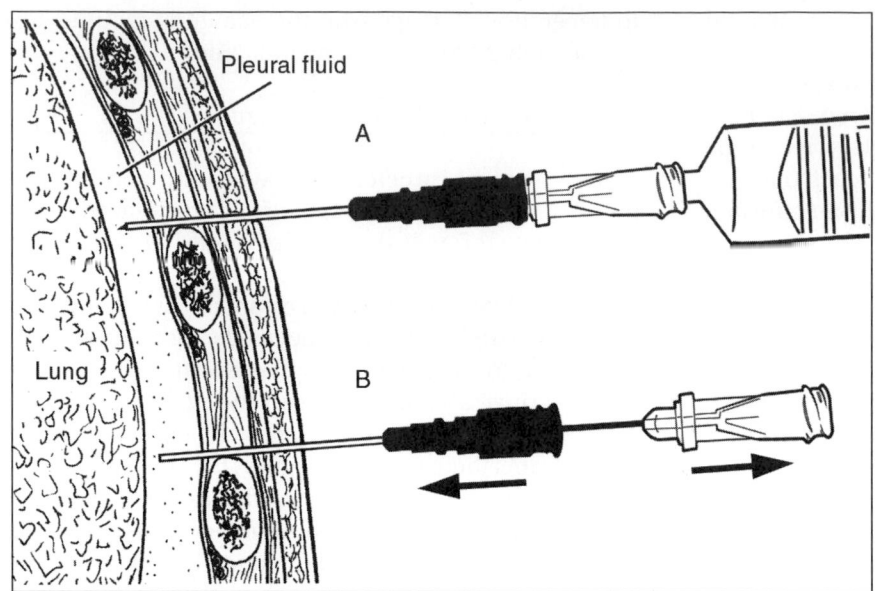

FIGURE 29-5 The catheter-over-the-needle technique. *A.* The needle and catheter are inserted over the rib and aimed slightly caudally into the pleural cavity. *B.* The needle is removed and the catheter remains within the pleural cavity.

within the pleural cavity (Figure 29-6*C*). **Once the needle is removed, do not readvance the needle, as the catheter may shear off and fall into the pleural cavity.** Place the needle guard on the needle. Secure the catheter by taping it to the skin. Withdraw fluid as previously described. Fluid can be removed in 50 mL aliquots up to 1.5 L. As a general rule, this is the limit, due to the risk of postevacuation pulmonary edema and excessive protein loss.[1]

ASSESSMENT

Fluid analysis criteria have been established to separate transudates and exudates.[10] If the fluid fits one of the criteria in Table 29-2, it is an exudate. These parameters have been confirmed to have 98 percent sensitivity and 83 percent specificity in detecting exudates.[11] Color and odor can be helpful. If the fluid has a putrid odor, consider an infection. White or yellow fluid suggests an empyema or chylothorax. The fluid's white blood cell

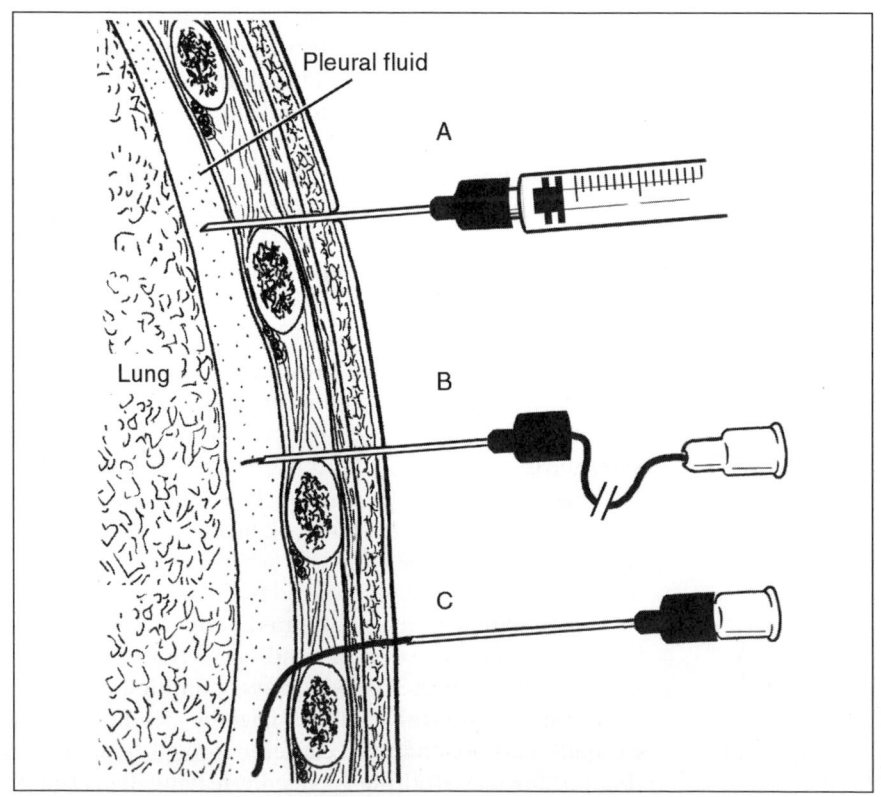

FIGURE 29-6 The catheter-through-the-needle technique. *A.* The needle is inserted over the rib and aimed slightly caudally into the pleural space. *B.* The catheter is inserted through the needle and into the pleural cavity. *C.* The needle is removed and the catheter remains within the pleural cavity.

TABLE 29-2. LABORATORY FEATURES OF A PLEURAL FLUID EXUDATE

Fluid/serum lactate dehydrogenase (LDH) > 0.6

Fluid/serum protein > 0.5

Pleural fluid LDH > 200 IU/mL

TABLE 29-3. POTENTIAL COMPLICATIONS ASSOCIATED WITH A THORACENTESIS

Cough	Intrapleural infection
Hemothorax	Pneumothorax
Hypovolemia	Reexpansion pulmonary
Hypoxemia	edema
Inadequate yield	Tension pneumothorax
Laceration of the liver or spleen	Vasovagal reactions
Pain at the procedure site	

count is of limited benefit. If it is > 10,000, the fluid likely represents a parapneumonic effusion. If the fluid is grossly bloody, consider a hemothorax. If the pleural fluid's hematocrit is > 50 percent of the serum hematocrit, a hemothorax is likely and chest tube placement should be considered. Other helpful tests include a fluid pH. If the pH is below 7.25 to 7.30, consider it the result of a parapneumonic process, rheumatologic process, esophageal rupture, or malignancy. Cytology is important to search for an underlying malignancy. Up to 50 percent of patients with a pulmonic malignancy will have neoplastic cells in the pleural fluid.[3] Bacteriologic information such as Gram's stain, acid-fast, and fungal preparations are also important; although the yield can be below 30 percent.[7] Fluid should always be sent for aerobic and anaerobic cultures to rule out an infectious etiology for the pleural effusion.

AFTERCARE

When done aspirating fluid, remove the catheter and apply a bandage to the puncture site. A follow-up chest radiograph should be obtained upon completion of the procedure to assess for a pneumothorax. An expiratory film is the best film to look for a pneumothorax, especially if it is small. A chest radiograph should be repeated in 4 to 6 hours to look for a delayed pneumothorax. If no pneumothorax is present and if appropriate for his or her clinical condition, the patient may be discharged with good instructions and close follow-up.

The procedure site should be evaluated two to three times a day for signs of infection. These patients should be educated about the signs, symptoms, and significance of an infection. They should return to their primary physician or the Emergency Department immediately if they develop fever, chills, shortness of breath, redness or pus at the puncture site, or if any concerns arise.

COMPLICATIONS

The potential complications of a thoracentesis are listed in Table 29-3.[1,3,7,11,12] Complication rates range from 20 to 50 percent. The major complications are a 5 to 19 percent incidence of pneumothorax and a 1 to 7 percent incidence of pneumothorax requiring a chest tube.[13] One author recommends ultrasound-guided thoracentesis for all patients as the safest approach, al-

though this is disputed by others.[13,14] The use of the proper technique and operator experience are important in reducing the rate of complications.[15–17] Quereshi compiled methods to reduce the incidence of pneumothorax.[7] They are direct supervision of inexperienced operators, removal of small amounts of fluid, use of small-gauge needles, use of ultrasound for small effusions, and use of a needle-catheter system for a therapeutic procedure.

PNEUMOTHORAX

ANATOMY AND PATHOPHYSIOLOGY

A thoracentesis can be performed to relieve a simple pneumothorax or a tension pneumothorax. Primary spontaneous pneumothoraces occur in otherwise healthy people without antecedent trauma. Secondary spontaneous pneumothoraces occur as a complication of underlying lung disease, most commonly chronic obstructive pulmonary disease.[1,3] A traumatic pneumothorax occurs as a result of penetrating or blunt trauma to the thoracic cavity. An iatrogenic pneumothorax is a subcategory of the traumatic pneumothorax, with the three most common etiologies being pleural biopsy, subclavian vein catheterization, and thoracentesis.

The pressure in the pleural space is negative in reference to the atmosphere. This is due to the tendency of the lung to collapse and the chest wall to expand. The alveolar pressure is greater than the pleural space pressure due to the elastic recoil of the lung. As a result, if a communication occurs between the alveolar and pleural space, the air will preferentially move into the pleural space until the pressure equalizes. The physiologic consequence is a decrease in vital capacity and PaO_2. This may be well tolerated in otherwise healthy people but not in patients with underlying cardiac and/or pulmonary disease. If a one-way valve develops such that air can only enter the pleural space from the alveolus but not return, the intrapleural pressure will eventually exceed atmospheric pressure, with a progressive increase in air occupying the pleural space. Clinical deterioration may occur due to a decreasing PaO_2 and cardiac output.[18–20] Other data point to hypoxia and hypercarbia as the cause of clinical deterioration.[9]

INDICATIONS

All tension pneumothoraces require needle drainage followed by tube thoracostomy. Patients usually present with respiratory distress, tachycardia, unilateral absence of breath sounds, hypotension, and neck vein engorgement. Although difficult to assess, these patients have tracheal deviation that is often limited to the thoracic cavity.

Not all simple pneumothoraces require drainage, as they may resolve spontaneously. Conservative management has shown a spontaneous resorption rate of 1.25 percent per day.[17] A pneumothorax should be drained if the patient complains of dyspnea, dyspnea on exertion, pain, or if the pneumothorax is estimated to be 15 percent or greater.

CONTRAINDICATIONS

There are no absolute or relative contraindications to relieving a tension pneumothorax, as it is a life-threatening emergency.

Contraindications to thoracentesis to relieve a simple pneumothorax are few. These include infection at the site of the procedure, in which case an alternate site should be selected.[3] A traumatic pneumothorax or a pneumothorax associated with a hemothorax or pyothorax requires tube thoracostomy. Any pneumothorax that is expanding or expanding despite thoracentesis also requires a tube thoracostomy. Any patient on anticoagulation or with a suspected bleeding diathesis, whether known or suspected, may require reversal of the condition before the procedure.[1]

EQUIPMENT

Pneumothorax—Tension

Alcohol swab or povidone iodine solution
12 to 16 gauge catheter-over-the-needle, 2 inches long

Pneumothorax—Stable

Povidone iodine solution
Sterile gauze sponge
Sterile towels
Sterile basin
Syringes for anesthesia infiltration, 5 and 10 mL
25 gauge needle for anesthesia infiltration of the skin
21 or 23 gauge needle for infiltration of subcutaneous
     tissue, periosteum, and pleura
16 or 18 gauge catheter-over-the-needle
14 to 18 gauge catheter-through-the-needle
Three-way stopcock
50 mL syringe
Intravenous extension tubing

Commercial kits have been developed and are available to provide the equipment needed to perform a thoracentesis. These kits are disposable, intended for single-patient use, and contain all the required equipment. They save time in that the equipment does not have to be found and set up. Disadvantages include potentially increased cost and limited equipment in the kit.[9] The most common kits include the Pharmaseal, distributed by Baxter (Jacksonville, TX); the Arrow Clark Thoracentesis Kit, distributed by Arrow (Reading, PA); and the Argyle Turkel Safety Thoracentesis Kit, distributed by Boston Scientific (Miami, FL).[3]

PATIENT PREPARATION

Explain the procedure, its risks, and benefits to the patient or their representative and have a consent form signed.[1] Place the patient supine on the bed. Alternatively, the patient may be supine with the head of the bed elevated to 30 degrees (Figure 29-7). Clean any dirt or debris from the skin. Identify the anatomic landmarks required to perform the procedure. Although not required, it is recommended to place the patient on the car-

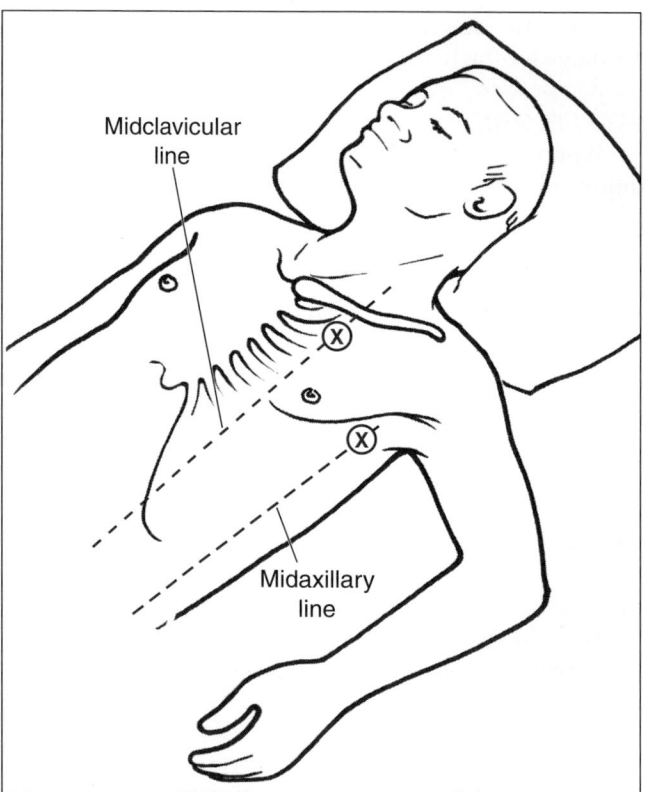

FIGURE 29-7 Relief of a tension pneumothorax. The patient should be in the supine position, with the head of the bed elevated 30 degrees if not contraindicated. The second intercostal space in the midclavicular line is the recommended site. For pleural effusions or a debilitated patient, the midaxillary line or posterior axillary line may be used at the level of the fourth or fifth intercostal space.

diac monitor, noninvasive blood pressure cuff, pulse oximetry, and supplemental oxygen. Apply povidone iodine solution to the skin surface and allow it to dry. Apply sterile drapes around the site of the procedure. Atropine should be at the bedside. It may be administered (1.0 mg subcutaneously or intramuscularly or 0.5 mg intravenously) to patients who develop symptomatic bradycardia during the procedure. The most common approach is the second intercostal space in the midclavicular line (Figure 29-7). An alternate site is the fourth or fifth intercostal space in the midaxillary line.

TENSION PNEUMOTHORAX TECHNIQUE

If the patient has a tension pneumothorax, thoracentesis is both a diagnostic and therapeutic procedure. A tension pneumothorax is a true life threat. Identify by palpation the second intercostal space in the midclavicular line. **Insert the catheter-over-the-needle over the superior border of the third rib to avoid the neurovascular bundle, which is located on the inferior border of the second rib.** Advance the catheter-over-the-needle into the pleural space. If time permits, a 5 to 10 mL syringe without the plunger can be attached to the catheter-over-the-needle. The syringe barrel can be used as a handle to advance the catheter-over-the-needle.

When the pleural cavity is entered, a release of pressure and a small "pop" may be felt. Stop advancing the needle and advance the catheter until the hub is against the skin. Remove the needle. If the patient has a tension pneumothorax, a continuous rush of air will be heard or felt. **Needle thoracentesis for a tension pneumothorax is a temporizing measure, therefore a tube thoracostomy should be performed immediately after this lifesaving procedure.** Refer to Chapter 28 for complete details regarding this procedure.

SIMPLE PNEUMOTHORAX TECHNIQUES

A primary spontaneous pneumothorax occupying over 15 percent of the hemithorax is the indication for simple aspiration via a thoracentesis.[3] The same sterile preparation, location of fluid, positioning, and anesthesia considerations apply to the evacuation of a simple pneumothorax as to a diagnostic thoracentesis.

Catheter-over-the-Needle Technique

Two types of catheters can be used to perform this procedure. They are the catheter-over-the-needle and the catheter-through-the-needle (Figures 29-5 and 29-6). The catheter-over-the-needle technique is most commonly used (Figure 29-5). Make a small "nick" in the skin with a #11 surgical blade at the needle insertion site. Attach a 14 to 18 gauge catheter-over-the-needle to a 10 mL syringe as a handle. Insert the catheter-over-

the-needle into the nick and advance it, reproducing the original anesthetized tract (Figure 29-5A). Apply negative pressure to the syringe as the catheter-over-the-needle is advanced. When air is encountered, angle the catheter-over-the-needle superiorly. Advance the catheter until the hub is against the skin. Withdraw the needle while the catheter remains within the pleural cavity (Figure 29-5B). **When the needle is removed, quickly cover the catheter with a gloved finger. This will prevent ambient air from entering the pleural cavity.** Attach intravenous catheter extension tubing to the hub of the catheter. Place a three-way stopcock attached to a 50 mL syringe onto the extension tubing. Hold the catheter hub against the skin securely. Aspirate air into the syringe and then advance the air into the room by adjusting the three-way stopcock. Air is then withdrawn manually. This process should be continued until resistance is felt. **If no resistance is felt after 4 L of aspiration, it is presumed that expansion has not occurred and a continual leak of air exists from the lung into the pleural cavity; therefore a tube thoracostomy should be performed.** After no more air is aspirated, close the stopcock and secure it to the chest wall. The success rate for the aspiration of a pneumothorax is 64 percent.[21,22]

Catheter-through-the-Needle Technique

The second option utilizes the catheter-through-the-needle system (Figure 29-6), which is known as the Bardig Intracath system. It is not as popular as the catheter-over-the-needle systems. Place the needle on a tuberculin syringe. Insert the needle and advance it through the anesthetized tissues (Figure 29-6A). A small "nick" in the skin with a #11 surgical blade will facilitate the needle entry. Apply negative pressure to the syringe as the needle is advanced along the anesthetized tract and into the pleural cavity. When air is aspirated, stop advancing the needle. Remove the syringe and cover the needle hub with a gloved finger. This will prevent ambient air from entering the pleural cavity. Angle the needle slightly superiorly and advance the catheter through the needle (Figure 29-6B). Withdraw the needle, leaving the catheter within the pleural cavity (Figure 29-6C). **Once the needle is removed, do not readvance the needle, as the catheter may shear off and fall into the pleural cavity.** Place the needle guard on the needle. Secure the catheter by taping it to the skin. Withdraw air as previously described.

Seldinger Technique

Drainage can also be accomplished using a pigtail or straight catheter and the Seldinger technique (Figure 29-8). Attach a 16 gauge, 2 inch catheter-over-the-needle to a 5 or 10 mL syringe. Insert the catheter, as described above, aimed superiorly. Remove the needle and syringe. **Quickly cover the catheter hub with a gloved finger.** Insert the guidewire through the catheter (Figure 29-8*A*). **Hold the guidewire securely to prevent it from falling completely into the pleural cavity.** Remove the catheter over the guidewire, leaving the guidewire in place (Figure 29-8*B*). Extend the skin incision with a #11 scalpel blade by 3 to 5 mm to allow the catheter to enter into the pleural space without "crumpling" (Figure 29-8*C*). Advance the dilator over the guidewire and into the pleural cavity to dilate the tract (Figures 29-8*C* and *D*). A gentle twisting motion of the dilator as it is

advanced will aid in its insertion into the pleural cavity (Figure 29-8*D*). Hold the guidewire securely. Remove the dilator while leaving the guidewire in place. Insert the catheter over the guidewire and into the pleural cavity (Figure 29-8*E*). Remove the guidewire and attach a three-way stopcock to the catheter. Aspirate the air as described previously.

Drainage Systems

Drainage systems for a pneumothorax vary in style but function with the same "one-way valve" principle. The simplest method is a flutter valve. It is best illus-

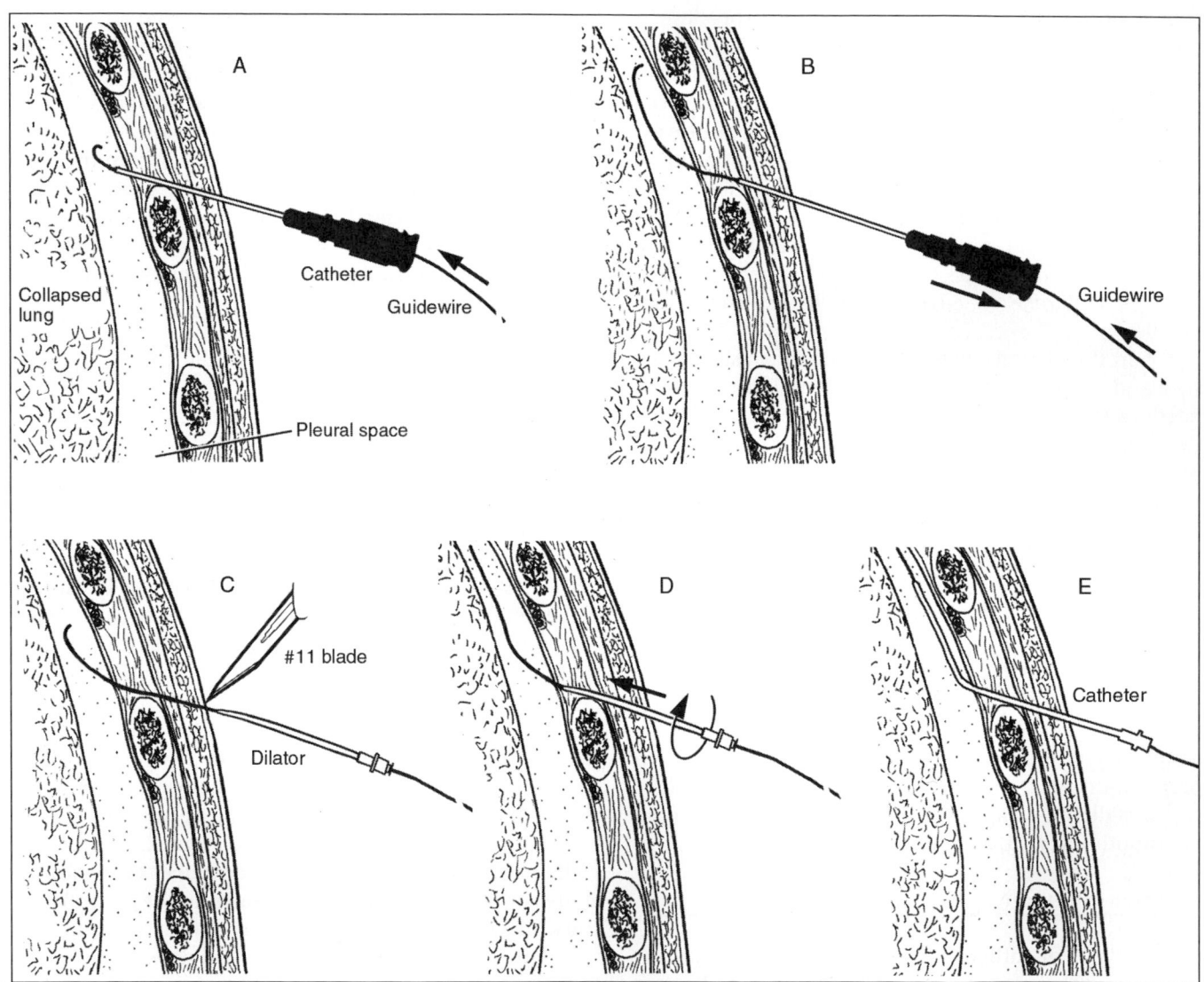

FIGURE 29-8 The Seldinger technique for inserting a catheter to aspirate a pneumothorax. A catheter-over-the-needle is placed into the pleural cavity and aimed superiorly. The needle is removed while the catheter remains in the pleural cavity. *A.* A guidewire is inserted through the catheter. *B.* The catheter is removed while the guidewire remains in the pleural cavity. *C.* The skin incision is enlarged with a #11 scalpel blade. A dilator is placed over the guidewire. *D.* The dilator is advanced over the guidewire and into the pleural cavity. A gentle twisting motion will help guide the dilator through the tract. *E.* The dilator has been removed while the guidewire remains inside the pleural cavity. The catheter is advanced over the guidewire and into the pleural cavity. The guidewire is then removed while the catheter remains inside the pleural cavity.

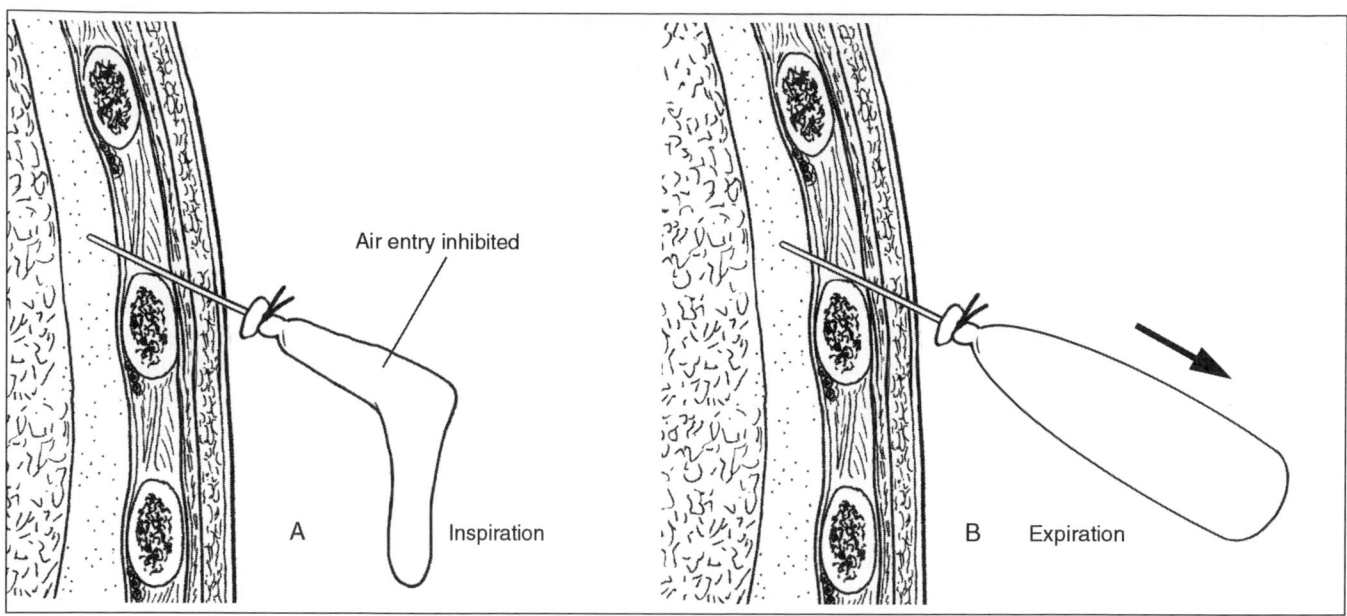

FIGURE 29-9 Use of a finger from a sterile glove as a one-way valve. Place the proximal end of the finger on the drainage system and cut the distal tip. It will act as a one-way valve.

trated by the following noncommercial method. Cut a premoistened finger from a sterile glove. Tie the proximal end to the thoracentesis catheter with a silk suture and cut the distal end open to the air[1] (Figure 29-9). This creates a flutter valve and allows air to escape with coughing or expiration and prevents air from reentering the pleural space on inspiration.

A commercial kit often contains a Heimlich flutter valve[1] (Figure 29-10). **The arrow on the clear protective tube covering the Heimlich valve must point away from the patient.** Suction is usually not needed. Stable patients can be sent home with this setup. This includes patients with a primary spontaneous pneumothorax and a small apical pneumothorax with initial reexpansion and good apposition of the lung with the lateral chest wall. Up to 30 percent of patients with a secondary pneumothorax can be treated on an ambulatory basis. Additional requirements include good residual lung function, normal oxygen saturation, and an air leak adequately treated by thoracentesis.[12] **A contraindication to using the flutter valve is a hemothorax.** A closed underwater seal system is recommended in these cases. Refer to Chapter 28 for details regarding the use of a closed underwater seal system and the other indications for its use.

ASSESSMENT

Relief of a tension pneumothorax will equalize the pressure between the atmosphere and the pleural space. The patient will now have a simple pneumothorax. The vitals signs should begin to normalize, the pulse oximetry improves, and the respiratory distress improves. If the patient had a tension pneumothorax, he or she will need a tube thoracostomy followed by a chest radiograph. The patient may begin to cough when the lung reexpands. Breath sounds should be present bilaterally upon reexpansion.

If the patient does not improve clinically after needle decompression for a tension pneumothorax, there are two possibilities. First, the pleural space may not have been entered with the needle. This occurs when the patient is obese or very muscular. The procedure may then be repeated with a longer needle. Second, the patient may not have had a tension pneumothorax. Reevaluate the patient by physical examination and review the chest radiograph to determine if a tension pneumothorax is present.

After relief of a simple pneumothorax, a chest radiograph is indicated. It will allow the physician to determine the success or lack thereof of the procedure. If at

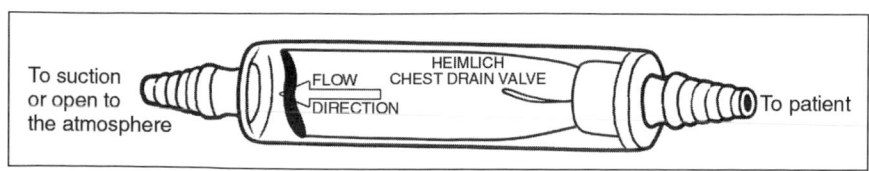

FIGURE 29-10 The Heimlich valve.

any point the pneumothorax is not improving with a thoracentesis or if the patient's symptoms worsen, a tube thoracostomy should be performed.

AFTERCARE

Obtain a follow-up chest radiograph upon completion of the procedure to assess for a pneumothorax. An expiratory film should be obtained, especially if the pneumothorax was small. A chest radiograph should be repeated 4 to 6 hours after the procedure to look for a delayed pneumothorax. If no pneumothorax is present and if appropriate for his or her clinical condition, the patient may be discharged with good instructions and close follow-up.

The procedure site should be evaluated two to three times a day for signs of infection. These patients should be educated about the signs, symptoms, and significance of an infection. They should return to their primary physician or Emergency Department immediately if they develop fever, chills, shortness of breath, redness or pus at the puncture site, or if any concerns arise.

A patient may be a candidate for outpatient management with a Heimlich valve under the following conditions: a stable primary spontaneous pneumothorax, close apposition of the lung to the lateral chest wall with initial thoracentesis and aspiration and drainage procedures, physician satisfaction with the position of the catheter, and an air leak that is manageable with one thoracentesis. Contraindications for outpatient management include traumatic pneumothoraces, secondary pneumothoraces, a patient with poor residual function, a large air leak requiring tube thoracostomy, a hemothorax, unacceptable residual collapse defined as poor apposition of the lateral lung to the lateral chest wall, or if the patient is not reliable.[23]

Instructions to the patient should include the following: clean the thoracentesis site with mild soap daily; apply a split dressing around the catheter and tape it to the skin; make sure that the tubing is taped firmly to the valve to prevent accidental dislodgment; the arrow on the valve should point away from the patient; the sound of air exiting the valve is expected; and showers are permitted but not a bath or swimming. If these patients experience shortness of breath, chest pain, or difficulty breathing, they should call 911 and immediately return to the Emergency Department. They should be provided with instructions on dealing with signs of infection.

The patient should follow-up daily for radiographic evaluation. Upon complete inflation of the lung, the thoracentesis catheter can be removed. The patient should be observed for 4 to 6 hours and a repeat chest radiograph obtained. The patient can be discharged if the lung is completely expanded. If not, a thoracostomy tube should be reinserted and the patient admitted.

COMPLICATIONS

Complications associated with this procedure can be numerous. Clinically, a pneumothorax can become worse. Causes include lacerating the lung with the needle, inadequate coverage of the hub of the needle or catheter with a gloved finger after entering the pleural space, and an air leak in the drainage system. A tension pneumothorax can occur from a lung laceration along with inadvertent plugging of the drainage system (e.g., fluid in tube, kinking). A hemothorax is possible if the lung, intercostal artery, or mammary artery is lacerated with the needle. Less common complications include cardiac or great vessel perforation due to poor positioning of the needle upon insertion. Infection occurs about 2 percent of the time if sterile technique is observed. Catheter shearing is possible with the catheter-through-the-needle system if the needle guard is not placed on the needle or the catheter is withdrawn through the needle. Reexpansion hypotension has been reported following rapid evacuation of persistent unilateral pneumothoraces of at least 1 week's duration. The mechanism is unclear, but it is associated with reexpansion pulmonary edema that precipitates intravascular volume depletion. Myocardial depletion may also be a contributing factor.[1] Many of these complications can be prevented by the use of proper and careful technique.

SUMMARY

A thoracentesis can help differentiate between transudates and exudates. Together with the clinical presentation, the information can be useful in diagnosing the patient's condition. It can be lifesaving if the patient has a tension pneumothorax. It offers an alternative to tube thoracostomy for patients with stable spontaneous primary pneumothoraces. Outpatient management can be considered in some cases with the addition of a Heimlich valve. Regardless of what method is used, physicians in training should be supervised until competency with this procedure is demonstrated.

REFERENCES

1. Ross DS: Thoracentesis, in Roberts JR, Hedges JR (eds): *Clinical Procedures in Emergency Medicine*, 3rd ed. Philadelphia: Saunders, 1998:130–147.
2. Quigley RL: Thoracentesis and chest tube drainage. *Crit Care Clin* 1995; 11(1):111–126.
3. Light RW: *Pleural Diseases*, 3rd ed. Baltimore: William & Wilkins, 1995:7–17, 242–278, 311–327.

4. American College of Surgeons Committee on Trauma: *Advanced Trauma Life Support for Doctors,* 6th ed. Chicago: American College of Surgeons, 1997:127–156.

5. Ruskin JA, Gurney JW, Thorsen MK, et al: Detection of pleural effusions on supine chest radiograph. *Am J Roentgenol* 1987; 148(4):681–683.

6. Health and Public Policy Committee, American College of Physicians: Diagnostic thoracentesis and pleural biopsy in pleural effusions. Position paper. *Ann Intern Med* 1987; 103:799–802.

7. Qureshi N, Momin ZA, Brandstetter RD: Thoracentesis in clinical practice. *Heart Lung* 1994; 23(5):376–383.

8. Godwin JE, Sahn SA: Thoracentesis: a safe procedure in mechanically ventilated patients. *Ann Intern Med* 1990; 115:800–802.

9. Rutherford RB, Hurt HH Jr, Brickman RB, et al: The pathophysiology of progressive, tension pneumothorax. *J Trauma* 1968; 8(2):212–227.

10. Light RW, Macgregor I, Luchinger PC, et al: Pleural effusions. The diagnostic separation of transudates and exudates. *Ann Intern Med* 1972; 77(4):507–513.

11. Burgess LJ, Marith FJ, Taljeard FJ: Comparative analysis of the biochemical parameters used to distinguish between pleural transudates and exudates. *Chest* 1995; 107(6):1604–1609.

12. Ponn RB, Silverman HJ, Federico JA: Outpatient chest tube management. *Ann Thorac Surg* 1997; 64:1437–1440.

13. Swineburne AJ, Bixby K, Fedullo AJ, et al: Pneumothorax after thoracentesis. *Arch Intern Med* 1991; 151:2095

14. Grogan DR, Irwin RC, Channick R, et al: Complications associated with thoracentesis: a prospective randomized study comparing three different methods. *Arch Intern Med* 1990; 150:873–877.

15. Seneff MW, Corwin W, Gold LH, et al: Complications associated with thoracentesis. *Chest* 1986; 90(1):97–100.

16. Bartter T, Mayo PD, Pratter MR, et al: Lower risk and higher yield for thoracentesis when performed by experienced operators. *Chest* 1993; 103(6):1873–1876.

17. Stradling P, Poole G: Conservative management of spontaneous pneumothorax. *Thorax* 1966; 21:145–149.

18. Light RW: Tension pnuemothorax. *Intens Care Med* 1994; 20:468–469.

19. Connally JP: Hemodynamic measurements during a tension pneumothorax. *Crit Care Med* 1993; 21(2):294–296.

20. Brann BS, Mayfield SR, Goldstein M, et al: Cardiovascular effects of hypoxia/hypercarbia, and tension pneumothorax in newborn piglets. *Crit Care Med* 1994; 22(9):1453–1460.

21. Talbot-Stern J, Richardson H, Tomlanovich MC, et al: Catheter aspiration for simple pneumothorax. *J Emerg Med* 1986; 4:437–442.

22. Valles P, Sullivan M, Richardson H, et al: Sequential treatment for simple pneumothorax. *Ann Emerg Med* 1988; 17(9):936–942.

Chapter 30

OPEN CHEST WOUND MANAGEMENT

Roxanne Roberts

INTRODUCTION

Open chest wounds come in a variety of shapes and sizes. Their one commonality is an open communication between the pleural space and the external environment. The wounds have often been sealed by the soft tissues of the chest wall in the vast majority of patients with penetrating injuries to the chest. The primary concern with these patients is the diagnosis and treatment of underlying thoracic, cervical, or abdominal injuries. **Rarely, small perforations may produce a valve-like entry into the pleural space, enabling air to be sucked in during inspiration but blocking air egress during expiration. Thus air will continue to accumulate, leading to a tension pneumothorax requiring needle decompression followed by the tube thoracostomy.** Larger, more destructive wounds of the chest may also occur. These are most common in combat injuries. In civilian practice they are often secondary to shotgun injuries. The larger wounds are also caused by high-velocity weapons, explosions, propeller injuries, or fencepost impalements, to name a few. Clothing, wadding, shell fragments, and pieces of the chest wall may all be driven into the thoracic cavity. Such injuries are associated with physical loss of a portion of the chest wall itself, making adequate ventilation impossible.[1] These wounds are called open chest wounds, open pneumothoraces, sucking chest wounds, and communicating pneumothoraces.

Wounds of the chest are described in the earliest of medical documents, the Edwin Smith papyrus. This document dates from the time of Imhotep (3000 B.C.). It contains descriptions of 58 cases, 3 of which involved chest injuries per se. One was actually an open chest wound, case number 40. The patient sustained a penetrating injury to the anterior thorax through the manubrium.

Treatment consisted of binding the wound with fresh meat on the first day and, later, with grease, honey, and lint.

During Greco-Roman times, open chest wounds were universally fatal. In 362 B.C., Epaminondas was wounded by a spear to the chest at the battle of Mantinea. Once he discovered that the Thebans had been victorious, he pulled the spear out, knowing that he would die.

Galen cared for chest wounds in gladiators. Treatment consisted of a poultice and leaving the wound open. This treatment did not change until the time of Theodoric, who advised the closing of chest wounds. In 1267, he was quoted as saying, "The stitches should be placed in accordance with the size of the wound so that the natural heat cannot escape in any way nor the air outside be able to enter." His advice was not accepted by all. The master military surgeon Paré left the wounds open for 2 to 3 days to allow drainage of blood, after which he would close them.

During the Battle of Crecy in 1346, firearms and firearm injuries were first introduced. In 1382, small guns were used against the Venetians. Injuries from these weapons were documented in the chronicles of these battles.

Techniques of managing chest wounds have improved with each subsequent war. The most important treatable aspect of these chest wounds was the associated open pneumothorax. The question of whether to manage such injuries open or closed remained controversial. In Rome in 1514, John de Vigo was the first surgeon to present his views on gunshot wounds of the chest. He thought them to be universally fatal and, in most part, untreatable. William Hewson, in 1767, observed that a patient with a large open chest wound was not able to breathe but could do so easily once the injury was closed.

It took another 40 years for Baron Larrey, Napoleon's surgeon, to confirm Hewson's observation in a wounded soldier. He gave one of the best descriptions of an open pneumothorax, shock, and air hunger in his memoirs of the Napoleonic wars:

"A soldier was brought to the hospital at the Fortress of Ibrahym Bey, immediately after a wound penetrated the thorax between the fifth and sixth true ribs. It was 8 cm in extent. A large quantity of frothy and vermillion blood escaped from it with a hissing noise at each inspiration. His extremities were cold, pulse scarcely perceptible, countenance discolored, and respiration short and laborious: In short he was every moment threatened with a fatal suffocation. After having examined the wound, the divided edges of the part, I immediately approximated the two lips of the wound and retained them by means of adhesive plaster, and a suitable bandage around the body. In adopting this plan I intended only to hide from the sight of the patient and his comrades, the distressing spectacle of the hemorrhage, which would soon prove fatal; and I therefore thought that the effusional blood into the cavity of the thorax, could not increase the danger. But the wound was scarcely closed, when he breathed more freely, and felt easier. The heat of the body soon returned, and the pulse rose. In a few hours he became quite calm, and to my great surprise, grew better. He was cured in a very few days, and without difficulty."

Another famous accounting of an open chest wound was by William Beaumont in 1825. He attended Alexis St. Martin in 1822, who was shot in the lower chest. Beaumont arrived within one-half hour of the injury and noted that the wound had been caused by a short-range blast, within a yard of St. Martin's chest: "fracturing and carrying away the anterior half of the sixth rib, fracturing the fifth, lacerating the lower portion of the left lobe of the lungs, the diaphragm and perforating the stomach. The whole mass of materials forced from the musket, together with fragments of clothing and pieces of fractured ribs, were driven into the muscles and cavity of the chest."

Upon Beaumont's arrival, he found lung and stomach herniating from the wound. "After cleaning the wound from the discharges and other extraneous matter, and replacing the stomach, and the lung as far as practicable, I applied the carbonated fermenting poultice and kept the surrounding parts constantly wet with a lotion of muriate of ammonia and vinegar." After an hour, Beaumont returned expecting to find his patient dead. To his pleasure and surprise, the patient was, in fact, improved. He had saved his life by closing his chest wound.

By the final years of World War I the controversy of "to close or not to close" was resolved in favor of immediate wound closure. However, when closing these wounds it was important to understand the physiology of negative intrathoracic pressure. The German internist Buelau introduced closed underwater seal drainage of an empyema in 1875. In 1889, T. Holmes, a consulting surgeon at St. George's Hospital in London, introduced intercostal drainage for large chest wounds. However, he did not advocate an underwater seal. It was not until World War II that closed tube drainage was added to the treatment of an open pneumothorax as a routine measure. Positive-pressure ventilation was introduced in the early 1900s. The most recent advancement in the treatment of these injuries came from the Scandinavians, who invented respirators in the early 1950s. Mortality from chest wounds steadily decreased in each war. It was 79 percent in the Crimean War, 62.5 percent in the Civil War, 55.7 percent in the Franco-Prussian War, 24.6 percent in World War I, 12 percent in World War II, and in recent civilian experience is now 4 to 7 percent.[2]

ANATOMY AND PATHOPHYSIOLOGY

The pathophysiology of an open pneumothorax has not much been improved upon since the days of Hewson and Larrey. The pathophysiologic changes of a sucking chest wound depend on the size of the wound and the intactness of the pleural space and lung. A defect in the chest wall is usually of no major clinical significance if the pleural space is obliterated.[3] However, most commonly, the pleural space is free and the air and/or blood moves in and out through the chest wall defect, making a "sucking" sound. In larger injuries, this air movement causes the ipsilateral lung to move inward and collapse on inspiration (Figure 30-1A). The lung may expand slightly or remain completely collapsed upon expiration, depending on the size of the chest wall defect (Figure 30-1B). There may also be mediastinal motion toward the noninjured lung during inspiration and toward the injured lung during expiration. This to-and-fro motion compromises the function of the healthy lung as well as the injured lung because it prevents its full expansion during inspiration. During expiration, some of the air from the noninjured lung may shift to the injured lung, and the reverse may happen during inspiration (an element of the "pendelluft" phenomenon). This entire mechanism results in a large functional dead space in the noninjured lung and loss of ventilation of the injured lung, causing severe ventilatory derangement, asphyxia, hypoxemia, and hypercarbia.[2–4]

The patient with an open pneumothorax may manifest a spectrum of presentations, ranging from asymptomatic and stable to severely dyspneic and agonal. The presentation depends on the size of the chest wall defect, the extensiveness of the injuries to the lung and other structures, the preinjury pulmonary status, and whether the pleural space is free or has adhesions. The

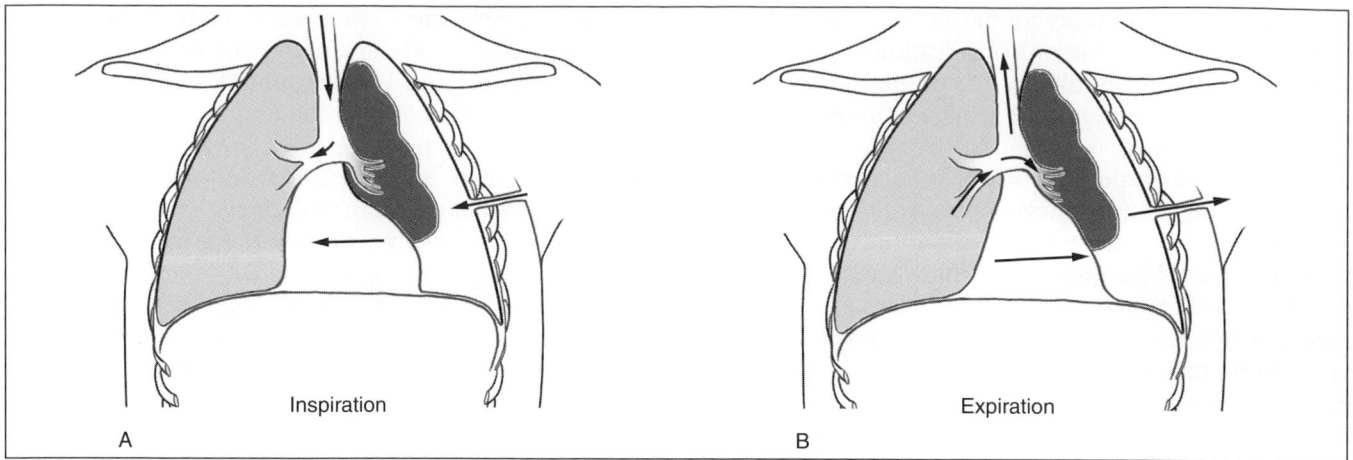

FIGURE 30-1 The effects of an open chest wound. *A.* Air moves into the pleural cavity and the lung collapses with inspiration. *B.* Air exits the pleural cavity and the lung expands slightly with expiration. The arrows represent the direction of airflow.

patient may present with progressive respiratory insufficiency leading to a rapid demise if not treated. **The critical diameter of the chest wall wound has been described as two-thirds (or greater) the diameter of the trachea.[5] It is thought that at this size, air moves preferentially through the chest wall rather than through the glottis.**

INDICATIONS

Diagnosis of these injuries can be made easily based upon the obvious presence of the chest wall defect and the noise produced as the air moves in and out through the wound. In the symptomatic patient, all open chest wounds should be treated immediately.[3,6] Treatment techniques should be selected based on the patient's clinical condition and stability (Figure 30-2).

Most experts agree that only the symptomatic patients should be treated in the field. An occlusive dressing should be placed over the wound but taped on only three sides. **The three-sided dressing allows air within the pleural cavity to be expelled into the atmosphere while preventing atmospheric air from entering the pleural cavity. If the wound is taped on all four sides, an open pneumothorax may quickly be converted into a tension pneumothorax.[4,5,7–10]**

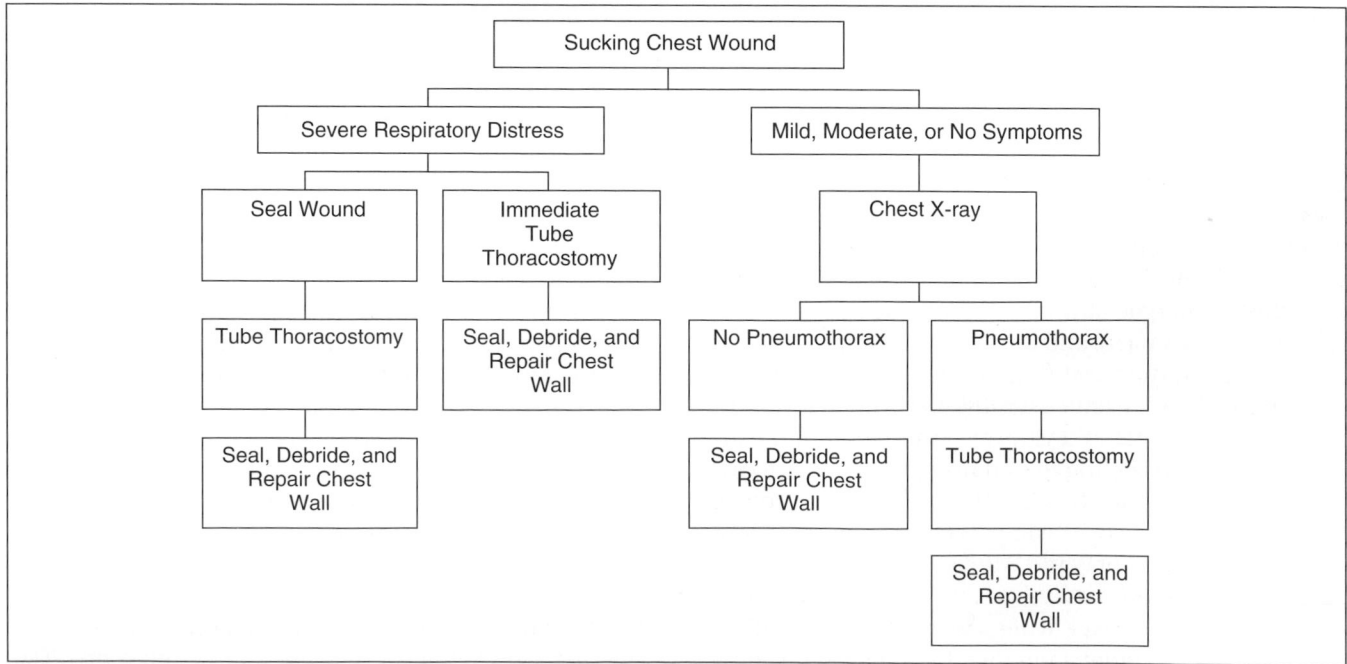

FIGURE 30-2 Algorithm for the diagnosis and treatment of an open pneumothorax. Modified from Symbas.[3]

In the hospital setting, the very symptomatic patient should be treated as in the field. However, a completely occlusive dressing may be placed over the wound if a chest tube is subsequently to be placed. There should be continuous and close monitoring of the patient for the development of a tension pneumothorax if the wound is completely sealed prior to the tube thoracostomy. If a tension pneumothorax occurs, removal of the occlusive dressing on one side should relieve it.

Obtain a rapid, portable anteroposterior chest radiograph if the patient is asymptomatic, mildly symptomatic, or moderately symptomatic. If a pneumothorax is present, a tube thoracostomy should be performed and the wound sealed. If the patient becomes severely symptomatic, the practitioner should default to the other limb of the algorithm.

CONTRAINDICATIONS

There are no contraindications to the placement of a three-sided occlusive dressing, as this is a treatment for a life-threatening emergency. It must be properly placed to prevent the accidental conversion to a totally occlusive dressing and the progression of an open pneumothorax to a tension pneumothorax.

EQUIPMENT

Povidone iodine solution
Petrolatum gauze
Gauze, 4×4 squares
Reinforcing sterile dressings
Tincture of benzoin
Adhesive tape
Sterile gloves

PATIENT PREPARATION

The amount and timing of patient preparation will be dictated by the location of the patient and his or her physiologic status. An informed consent is not required, as this is a noninvasive and lifesaving procedure. Such procedures should occur emergently with minimal patient preparation. If time permits, place the patient on the cardiac monitor and pulse oximeter and provide supplemental oxygen by face mask.

If the patient has severe respiratory insufficiency, orotracheal intubation should be performed before or simultaneously with the application of the three-sided occlusive dressing. Positive-pressure ventilation through the endotracheal tube will expand the collapsed lung and force the intrapleural air out the wound and into the atmosphere.

Prepare the chest wall if the patient is asymptomatic, mildly symptomatic, or moderately symptomatic. Clean the wound and surrounding chest wall of any dirt and debris. Apply povidone iodine solution to the skin surrounding the wound and allow it to dry. Do not place the povidone iodine into the wound, as this has been shown to inhibit wound healing. Apply the three-sided occlusive bandage as described below. **If the patient is moderately to severely symptomatic, no preparation is required, as this wastes valuable time. Immediately apply the three-sided occlusive bandage.**

TECHNIQUE

The safest initial therapy for symptomatic sucking chest wounds is careful application of a petrolatum gauze–based dressing taped on three sides (Figure 30-3). Apply three or four layers of petrolatum gauze over the wound. The dressing should extend 6 to 8 cm beyond the margins of the wound so that it will not be sucked into the pleural cavity in the spontaneously breathing patient. Cover the petrolatum gauze with dry 4×4 gauze squares. Apply tincture of benzoin around three sides of the dressing. Apply tape to secure the three sides of the dressing to the chest wall.

ALTERNATIVE TECHNIQUES

An alternative to the three-sided dressing is one that is totally occlusive. **This should be done only in the setting where rapid placement of a chest tube will be undertaken.** This occurs most commonly in the hospital. It may be considered in the field when tube thoracostomy is included in the prehospital standing medical orders.[23]

ASSESSMENT

Once the three-sided dressing has been placed, the patient should continue to be monitored for associated complications and investigated for underlying injuries. **Paramount among the complications is conversion of a simple pneumothorax to a tension pneumothorax.** These patients have typically sustained an injury comprising great kinetic energy, whether from a blunt or penetrating event. Associated injuries will be very common. A head-to-toe secondary survey is imperative.

AFTERCARE

The aftercare of these patients consists of a tube thoracostomy followed by aggressive wound care, pain management, pulmonary toilet, continued monitoring, and investigation for other underlying injuries. **Once the**

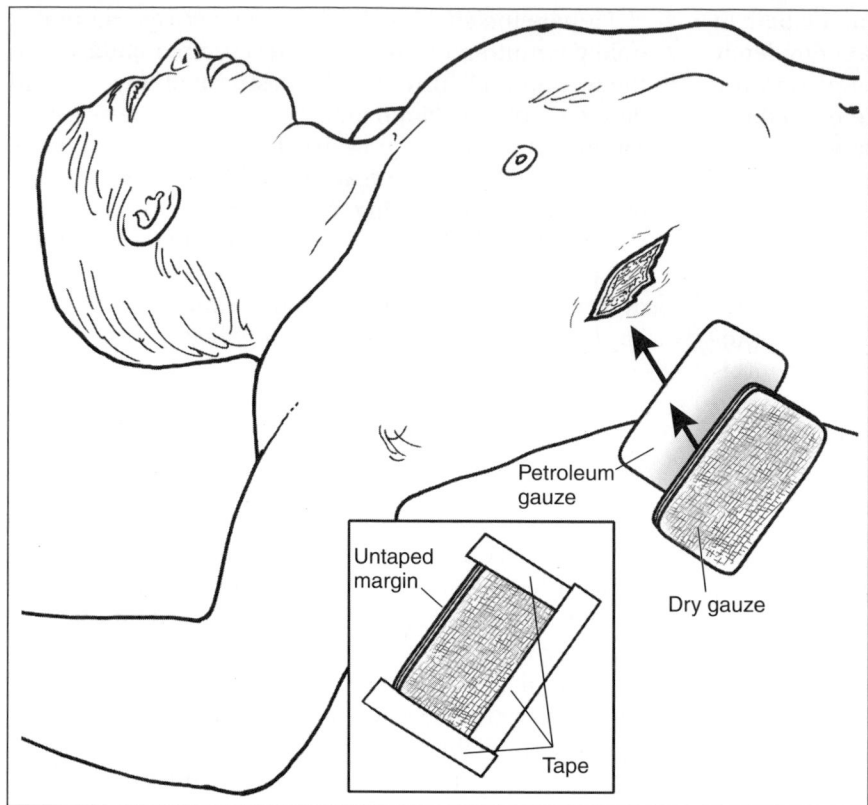

FIGURE 30-3 The three-sided occlusive dressing.

wound is closed, the underlying pneumothorax or hemopneumothorax should be treated with placement of a chest tube. This should be placed through a separate stab wound, away from the injury site.

Pain will be a major problem for these patients. Trauma to the parietal pleura, bony structures, and intercostal nerves is very painful. It is imperative that these patients be able to make adequate ventilatory efforts, cough, deep breathe, perform incentive spirometry, and have aggressive pulmonary toilet. These are all necessary to prevent atelectasis, retained secretions, and pneumonia.[11] Various pain-relieving techniques may be utilized. Infiltration of long-acting local anesthetic solution may give initial relief, especially during wound debridement. Parenteral analgesics are the initial treatment modality. Advanced techniques to consider include regional blocks, intercostal blocks, or delivery via intrapleural or epidural catheters.

Once the patient is stabilized in the hospital setting, more definitive wound care should be considered. Small, clean wounds may be managed simply with changes of occlusive dressings. Local irrigation and debridement may be added if there is a limited amount of contamination. Large, grossly contaminated, and/or complex wounds are best managed in the operating room. Optimally, these wounds should be debrided and closed primarily. However, some wounds may be contaminated or complex, such that closure is not possible initially. In such cases, the wound should be debrided

and left open. Large, occlusive dressings are placed along with chest tubes for removal of air, fluid, and blood. Multiple operative debridements may be required. When the wound is clean and the patient is optimized, secondary closure may be performed.[11]

Closure of large wounds may require a combination of complex techniques. These may include various skin, subcutaneous tissue, and muscle flaps.[12] Free rib grafts, pectoral muscle flaps, latissimus dorsi muscle flaps, abdominal muscle flaps, omentum flaps, skin grafts, or a myocutaneous flap can be utilized.[12–19] If using these is not possible, closure may be accomplished with a prosthetic material such as Prolene or Marlex, either temporarily or definitively.[20–22] In wounds of the lower chest, detachment of the diaphragm with reattachment at a higher level may be utilized. This converts an open chest wound to an intraabdominal wound and alleviates the ventilatory problems.

COMPLICATIONS

Complications may occur acutely or may be delayed. **Occlusion of the chest wall defect and decompensation of the patient from a simple pneumothorax being converted to a tension pneumothorax is the primary early complication. The patient must be closely monitored until a chest tube can be inserted.** A tension pneumothorax can result if the wound is completely occluded by a blood clot, a dressing that has been sucked into the wound, soft tissue, or a bandage that is adherent on all four sides. **Immediately remove the bandage to relieve a tension pneumothorax.** Some physicians and authors remove only one side of the occlusive bandage to relieve the pneumothorax. The choice to remove part or all of the bandage is physician-dependent. If the patient is still symptomatic, ensure that the wound is not occluded by a blood clot or soft tissue.

Other complications would ensue from the failure to seek, diagnose, and treat other underlying, potentially life-threatening injuries. The patient may develop respiratory insufficiency secondary to multiple causes, some of which may be preventable with optimal care. These causes include inadequate pulmonary toilet, inadequate pain management, pulmonary contusion, pneumonia, and/or adult respiratory distress syndrome. Wound complications may include infection, fasciitis, osteomyelitis, empyema, hemothorax, and loculated hemothoraces or pneumothoraces. These wounds require frequent evaluation and aggressive care to prevent these sequelae.

SUMMARY

Open chest wounds are easily diagnosed by the evident chest wall defect and the auscultation of air moving into and out of the pleural cavity. This is a true life-threatening emergency. Treatment is dictated by the patient's clinical presentation. Lifesaving therapy should be undertaken with the simple application of a three-sided petrolatum gauze dressing. The three-sided dressing allows air within the pleural cavity to be expelled into the atmosphere while preventing atmospheric air from entering the pleural cavity. This converts the open pneumothorax to a closed pneumothorax and eliminates the major physiologic derangement. Once the patient is stabilized, more definitive care should be carried out with chest tube placement and appropriate wound care.

REFERENCES

1. Keen G: *Chest Injuries,* 2nd ed. Bristol, England: Wright, 1984:124–132.
2. Blaisdell FW, Trunkey DD (eds): *Trauma Management:* vol III. *Cervicothoracic Trauma.* New York: Thieme, 1986:129–151.
3. Symbas PN: *Cardiothoracic Trauma.* Philadelphia: Saunders, 1989:364–366.
4. Vukich DJ, Markovchick V: Thoracic trauma, in Rosen P, Barkin R, Danzl DF, et al (eds): *Emergency Medicine: Concepts and Clinical Practice,* 4th ed. St. Louis: Mosby, 1998:514–527.
5. American College of Surgeons: *Advanced Trauma Life Support Instructor Manual,* 6th ed. Chicago: American College of Surgeons, 1997:151.
6. Shardey G: Management of traumatic pneumothorax. *Aust Fam Physician* 1984; 13(4):296–299.
7. Feliciano DV, Mattox KL (eds): *Trauma,* 3rd ed. Stamford, CT: Appleton & Lange, 1996:397–398.
8. Mattox KL, Allen MK: Emergency department treatment of chest injuries. *Emerg Med Clin North Am* 1984; 2(4):783–797.
9. Mattox KL: Prehospital care of the patient with an injured chest. *Surg Clin North Am* 1989; 69(1):21–29.
10. Carrero R, Wayne M: Chest trauma. *Emerg Med Clin North Am* 1989; 7(2):389–418.
11. Pate JW: Chest wall injuries. *Surg Clin North Am* 1989; 69(1):59–70.
12. Coleman JJ III: Complex thoracic wounds: muscle and musculocutaneous anatomy in closure. *South Med J* 1985; 78(2):125–129.
13. Arnold PG, Pairolero PC: Chondrosarcoma on the manubrium: resection and reconstruction with the pectoralis major muscle. *Mayo Clin Proc* 1978; 53(1):54–57.
14. Brown RG, Fleming WH, Jurkiewicz MJ: An island flap of the pectoralis major muscle. *Br J Plast Surg* 1977; 30(2):161–165.
15. Arnold PG, Pairolero PC: Use of pectoralis major muscle flaps to repair defects of anterior chest wall. *Plast Reconstr Surg* 1979: 63(2):205–213.
16. Chaikhouni A, Dyas CL Jr, Robinson JH, et al: Latissimus dorsi free myocutaneous flap. *J Trauma* 1981; 21(5):398–402.
17. Parkash S, Palepu J: Rectus abdominus myocutaneous flap—clinical experience with ipsilateral and contralateral flaps. *Br J Surg* 1983; 70(2):68–70.
18. Jurkiewicz MJ, Arnold PG: The omentum: an account of its use in the reconstruction of the chest wall. *Ann Surg* 1977; 185(5):548–554.
19. Boyd AD, Shaw WW, McCarthy JG, et al: Immediate reconstruction of full-thickness chest wall defects. *Ann Thorac Surg* 1981; 32(4):337–346.
20. Eschapasse H, Gaillard J, Henry F, et al: Repair of large chest wall defects: experience with 23 patients. *Ann Thorac Surg* 1981; 32(4):329–336.
21. Hubbard SG, Todd EP, Carter W, et al: Repair of chest wall defects with prosthetic material. *Ann Thorac Surg* 1979; 27(5):440–444.
22. Romero LH, Nagamia HF, Lefemine AA, et al: Massive impalement wound of the chest: a case report. *J Thorac Cardiovasc Surg* 1978; 75(6):832–835.
23. Barton ED, Epperson M, Hoyt DB, et al: Prehospital needle aspiration and tube thoracostomy in trauma victims: a six-year experience with aeromedical crews. *J Emerg Med* 1994; 13(2):155–163.

Chapter 31
EMERGENCY DEPARTMENT THORACOTOMY

Faran Bokhari

INTRODUCTION

With an increase in urban violence, there has been an increase in the number of critically injured patients seen in inner-city Emergency Departments. This increase in violence has been combined with better triage and transport systems, resulting in the arrival of sicker patients at the Emergency Department. Previously, these patients might not have survived long enough to make it to the Emergency Department.[1]

The majority of individuals with penetrating chest injuries arrive in the Emergency Department in stable condition and are managed without major operative procedures.[2] A subset of individuals, however, arrive in extremis and may require a thoracotomy. The purpose of the thoracotomy may be to control hemorrhage within the chest, to relieve a pericardial tamponade that cannot be decompressed by a needle thoracotomy, to redistribute cardiac output to the brain and the heart, or to provide more effective cardiac massage.[3]

ANATOMY AND PATHOPHYSIOLOGY

The structures within the chest include the heart, esophagus, lungs, bronchi, pulmonary hilar vessels, and numerous other vascular structures. The heart is located in the anterior mediastinum. The aorta and esophagus are located in the posterior mediastinum. The internal mammary arteries course along the posterior aspect of the anterior chest wall just lateral to the sternum. The intercostal vessels run along the inferior aspect of the ribs. The subclavian vessels are at the very superior aspect of the thorax. They course directly under the clavicles and can be very difficult to visualize via an anterolateral thoracotomy. The azygos vein can be found coursing along the posterior right hemithorax and emptying into the superior vena cava.

The heart is covered by the tough pericardial sac. **The phrenic nerves run superiorly to inferiorly on the pericardiac sac bilaterally.** They can be visualized as white or yellow strands on either side of the pericardium. Once the pericardial sac is opened, the left anterior descending coronary artery can be visualized on the anterior surface of the heart. It overlies the interventricular septum. Injuries to the left of this artery denote left ventricular damage, while injuries to the right denote right ventricular damage. The majority of the anterior surface of the heart is occupied by the right ventricle.

The posterior mediastinum contains the aorta. It is located posterior to the esophagus and runs lateral to the vertebral bodies. The thoracic aorta gives off the intercostal vessels. If torn during the mobilization of the aorta, the intercostals vessels can cause troublesome bleeding.

Beall et al originally introduced the Emergency Department thoracotomy for penetrating chest wounds.[4] This procedure was subsequently used for patients with penetrating abdominal wounds and victims of blunt trauma. **In recent years, several studies have shown an abysmal survival rate associated with Emergency Department thoracotomy in victims of blunt trauma.** When vital signs are present in the field, the survival rates for such individuals range from 0.6 to 6.0 percent.[5,6] Patients who undergo an Emergency Department thoracotomy for penetrating abdominal injuries have survival rates of approximately 5 percent.[12] In these cases, the thoracotomy is performed for resuscitation purposes.

Patients with penetrating chest trauma who present without signs of life in the field have a poor prognosis. Survival for these patients ranges from 0 to 9 percent.[7,8] If the patient sustains penetrating chest trauma and has signs of life in the field, survival averages 14 percent, with a range of 0 to 36 percent.[1] The reason for the wide range probably lies in the small numbers of patients in the studies and the varying definitions of "signs of life."

The best survival for penetrating chest injury and Emergency Department thoracotomy is in patients with stab wounds resulting in cardiac tamponade. The survival for this entity ranges from 21 to 71 percent.[6,9,10] It should be noted that 90 percent of patients who receive an Emergency Department thoracotomy for penetrating chest injuries survive and have good neurologic outcomes.[9] This must be contrasted with a 50 percent incidence of good neurologic outcome in survivors of blunt trauma who receive a thoracotomy.[11]

INDICATIONS

Signs of life, if present at the scene or at any time during the transport or resuscitation, should prompt an Emergency Department thoracotomy in patients with penetrating chest trauma. These signs include a palpable pulse, a blood pressure, pupil reactivity, any purposeful movement, an organized cardiac rhythm, or any respiratory effort. **Thus the patient must have signs of life on presentation or have lost them en route to the hospital if a thoracotomy is to be considered.** A thoracotomy should be performed to control hemorrhage within the thoracic cavity, to decompress a pericardial tamponade unrelieved by a needle thoracostomy, to cross-clamp the aorta and redistribute the cardiac output to the brain and heart, and to provide open cardiac massage. Patients who are in shock or rapidly deteriorating clinically after penetrating chest trauma and are not responding to aggressive fluid resuscitation are also candidates for a thoracotomy.

CONTRAINDICATIONS

There are a few well-supported contraindications to performing an Emergency Department thoracotomy. **A thoracotomy should not be performed in patients with penetrating chest trauma who have no vital signs in the field.** In the absence of field vitals, the survival rates are at the lower end of the range. The few that survive have severe neurologic impairment. **Victims of blunt trauma with or without field vitals should not undergo Emergency Department thoracotomy.**

EQUIPMENT

Povidone iodine solution
Sterile towels
Sandbags or towels

#3 scalpel handle
#10 scalpel blade
U.S. Army retractors, 1 set
Curved Mayo scissors, 8¾ and 6¾ inches
Curved Metzenbaum scissors, 5½ inches
Toothed forceps
Finochietto rib retractor, 12 inch spread
Suction source
Suction tubing
Yankauer suction catheter
2–0 silk suture on a large curved needle
Hemostats
Needle driver, 10 inches
Gauze 4×4 squares
Sternal saw, hand-operated
Liebsche knife (sternal osteotome) and hammer

All hospitals and Emergency Departments have pre-prepared, prepackaged sterile thoracotomy trays. Review the equipment available on the trays at your institution to become familiar with their contents before the tray is required emergently.

PATIENT PREPARATION

The patient should be supine, intubated, and ventilated. Abduct the left upper extremity 180 degrees (Figure 31-1). The extremity should be held in position by an assistant or with the use of a soft restraint. Place sandbags or towels under the patient's left scapula. This will elevate the torso off the bed to allow for more complete access. Apply povidone iodine solution to the patient's left chest. Apply sterile drapes over the chest to demarcate a surgical field.

An Emergency Department thoracotomy is primarily performed on patients who are unresponsive. As such, there is no immediate need for analgesics, sedatives, or local anesthetic solution. If the patient is resuscitated, they will experience significant postprocedural pain. **Parenteral analgesics and sedatives should be available and administered in that event.**

Set up the required equipment. Open the prepackaged, sterile thoracotomy tray on a bedside table. The tray should contain all the equipment required for the procedure. The physician and assistants performing the thoracotomy should be wearing sterile gloves, sterile gowns, goggles, and masks.

TECHNIQUES

LEFT-SIDED THORACOTOMY

Apply the scalpel blade to the handle. Identify the site to be used to make the initial skin incision. This is the

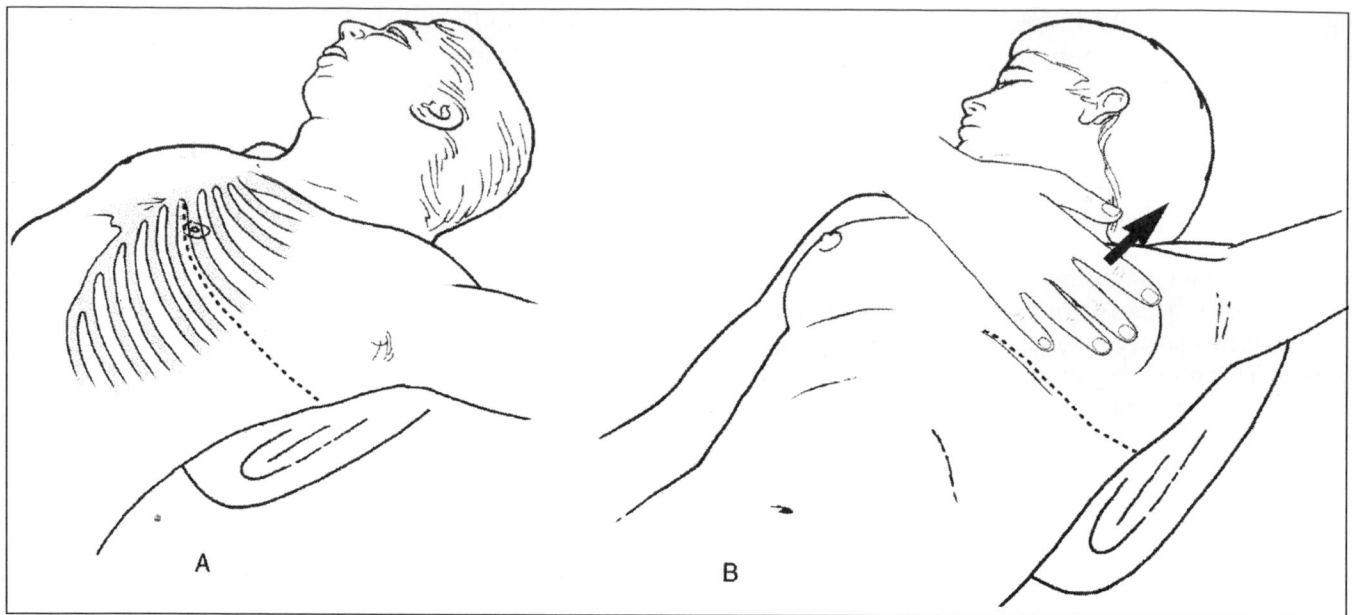

FIGURE 31-1 Patient positioning. Place a sandbag or towel under the left shoulder and abduct the left arm 180 degrees. Identify the fifth intercostal space in the male (*A*) or the inframammary line in the female (*B*).

left fourth or fifth intercostal space, corresponding to the intercostal space below the nipple in a male and below the inframammary fold in a female (Figure 31-1). **Using one stroke of the scalpel, make an incision extending from the sternum to the posterior axillary line (Figure 31-2*A*).** Carry the incision through the skin, subcutaneous tissues, and superficial chest musculature down to and through most of the intercostal muscles (Figure 31-2*A*). An Army retractor may be used to open and separate the edges of the incision. This step is based on physician preference and is not required.

Discontinue mechanical ventilation. This will allow the lung to deflate and minimize injury on entering the thoracic cavity. Puncture through the intercostal muscles in the anterior axillary line with the curved Mayo scissors. Carefully extend the puncture 2 to 3 cm using the curved Mayo scissors. Insert the nondominant index and middle fingers through the incision and separate the lung from the chest wall. Advance the fingers and Mayo scissors simultaneously superiorly then inferiorly to cut the intercostal muscles along the entire inner space (Figure 31-2*B*). Resume mechanical ventilation.

Insert the Finochietto retractor with the arm and crank positioned near the bed (Figure 31-2*C*). Turn the crank to open the arms of the rib spreader. Clear any blood from the left hemithorax and inspect for any brisk bleeding. If extensive bleeding is observed, it must be controlled. Use digital pressure initially to control intercostal artery bleeding. Apply a hemostat to the bleeding vessel. Subsequently place 2–0 silk stitches to tie off the bleeding vessels. For subclavian vessels, digital control must be followed by rapid transport to the operating room, since these vessels are difficult to control through an anterolateral thoracotomy.

OPENING THE PERICARDIUM

Move the left lung superiorly and laterally to expose the pericardial sac. **A pericardiotomy should be performed if blood is seen within the pericardial sac, if the heart cannot be visualized through the pericardium, or if there is no other obvious injury within the chest and a potential cardiac injury may exist. Many physicians will routinely open the pericardium when they are performing a thoracotomy, as a pericardial tamponade is difficult to detect visually.**

Open the pericardial sac anterior to the phrenic nerve. Grasp and elevate the pericardium with a toothed forceps anterior to the phrenic nerve, which appears as a white or yellow strand along the lateral aspect of the pericardium (Figure 31-2*D*). Make an incision in the pericardium near the apex of the heart. Note the color of the fluid that is expressed from the pericardial sac. It should normally be straw-colored without any hint of red. Insert the jaws of the Mayo scissors into the pericardial sac. **Extend the incision with the Mayo scissors parallel to the phrenic nerve,** from the apex of the heart to the root of the aorta. Deliver the heart from the pericardium and inspect it for any injury. Internal cardiac massage may be performed for asystole, bradycardia, and/or hypotension. The technique is described in Chapter 32.

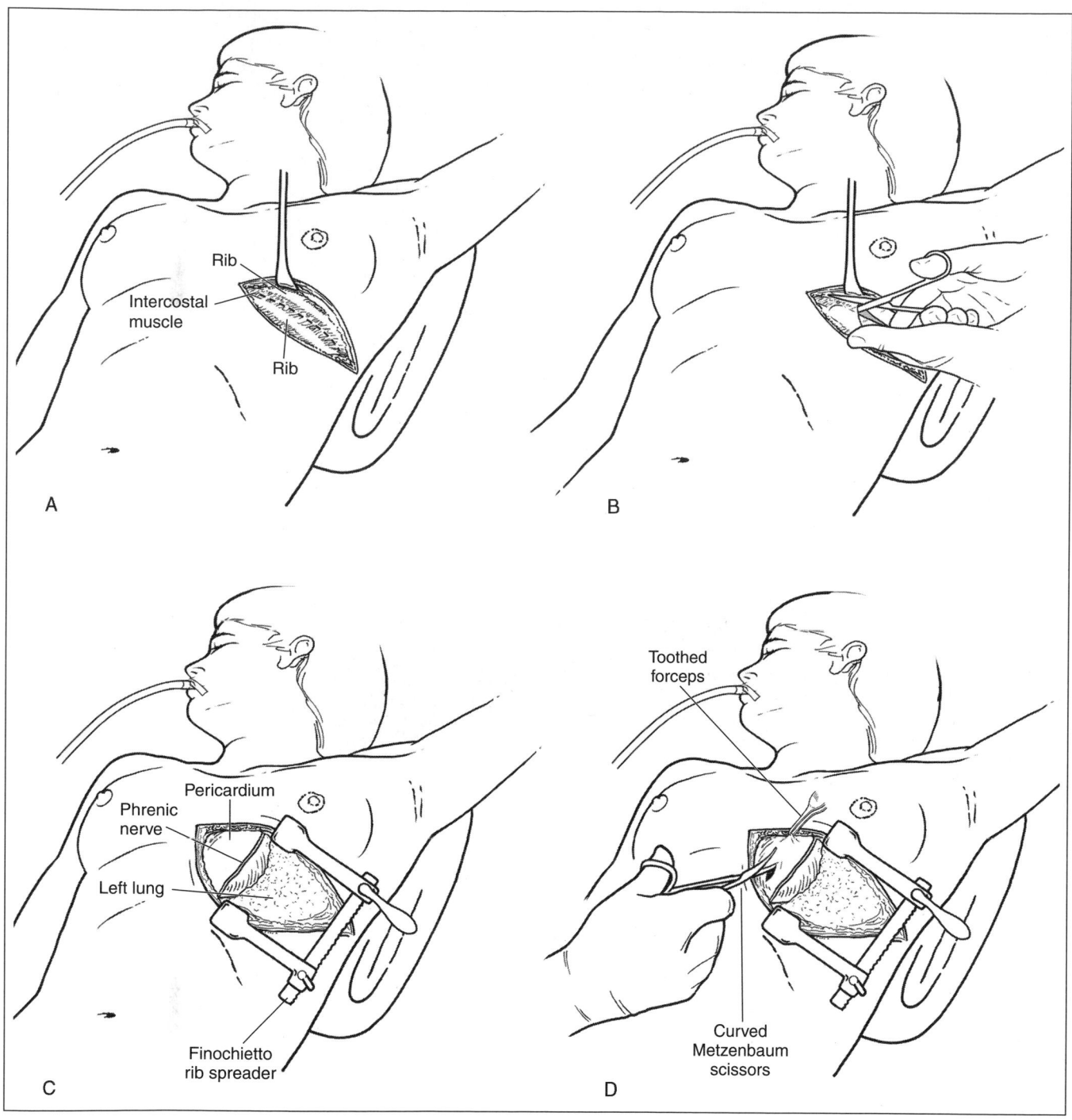

FIGURE 31-2 Emergency Department thoracotomy. *A.* The initial incision is made through the skin, subcutaneous tissue, and superficial muscles. *B.* The intercostal muscles are incised with a Mayo scissors. *C.* The Finochietto rib spreader is inserted and opened. *D.* The pericardium is grasped and opened.

RIGHT-SIDED THORACOTOMY

If there is a high index of suspicion of injury in the right hemithorax with minimal or no injury found in the left hemithorax, the thoracotomy must be extended to the right side. If possible, extend the incision through the sternum using a curved Mayo scissors and continue it to the right posterior axillary line (Figure 31-3). Remove the Finochietto rib spreaders from the left side and apply them to the patient's right fifth intercostal space. Examine the right hemithorax for injury. When the sternum is cut, the internal mammary arteries on both sides will be lacerated. Apply hemostats to the transected vessels to obtain hemostasis. They may later be tied off if the patient is resuscitated.

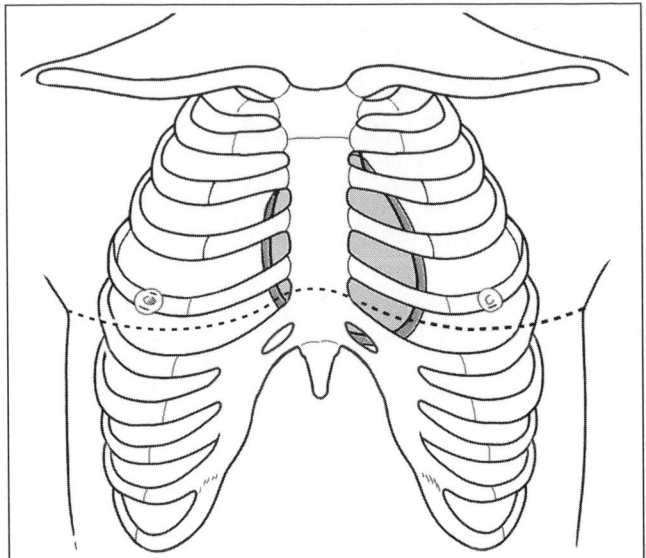

FIGURE 31-3 The left-sided incision is continued across the sternum and the right fifth intercostal space to perform a right-sided thoracotomy.

Occasionally, the large curved Mayo scissors cannot transect the calcified sternum. Perform a right-sided thoracotomy similar to that on the left. If further access is required, cut the sternum with a hand-held sternal saw or Liebsche knife (Figure 31-4). Pass one end of the sternal saw from the left fifth intercostal space, behind the sternum, and out of the right fifth intercostal space (Figure 31-4A). Place an index finger through the loop on each end of the sternal saw. Move the hands toward and away from the patient in a to-and-fro motion until the

sternum is transected. Alternatively, a Liebsche knife can be used to transect the sternum (Figure 31-4B). Place the hooked portion of the knife under the sternum with the sharp blade against the lateral border of the sternum. Lift up the handle of the Liebsche knife to lock it against the posterior surface of the sternum. This will prevent the tip of the knife from cutting the heart. Hit the flat knob on the back of the knife with a hammer to drive the knife through the sternum.

ASSESSMENT

Any bleeding should be controlled with the application of pressure, hemostats, and/or sutures. Any injuries to the heart (Chapter 33) or the hilum and great vessels (Chapter 34) should be managed. Cross-clamping of the proximal aorta will prevent further exsanguination from more distal injuries (Chapter 35). Open cardiac massage can be performed while the resuscitative efforts continue (Chapter 32).

AFTERCARE

If a patient is resuscitated in the Emergency Department, they should be transported to the operating room for definitive care as soon as the Anesthesiologist and Surgeon are available. Continue the administration of fluids, packed red blood cells, and inotropic agents as necessary until the patient is hemodynamically stable.

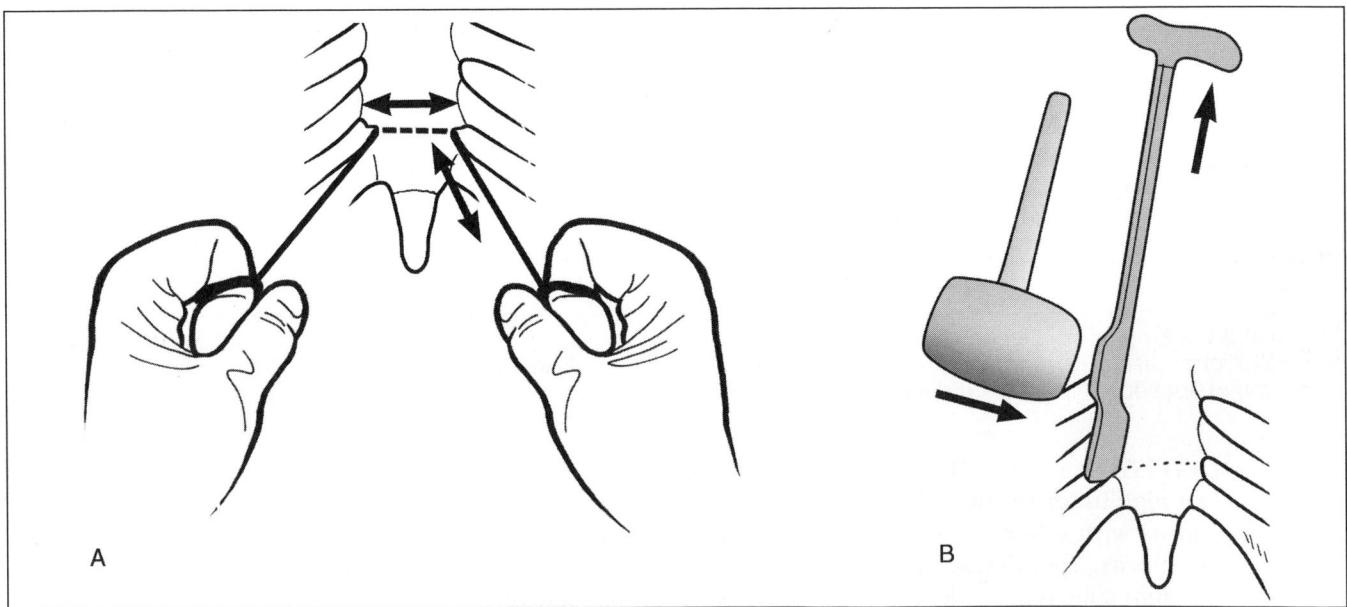

FIGURE 31-4 The sternum is cut with a sternal saw (A) or a Liebsche knife (B). The arrows represent movement of the instruments.

Administer parenteral analgesics and/or sedation if not contraindicated.

COMPLICATIONS

The Emergency Department thoracotomy has many potential and serious complications. Fortunately, this procedure is often being performed as a last effort at resuscitation of a "dead patient." The complications are, therefore, not significant when the alternative to this procedure is death.

The thoracotomy is never performed under sterile conditions. Time is often of the essence in performing this procedure. Povidone iodine solution and sterile drapes are rarely applied before an emergent thoracotomy. If applied, the povidone iodine does not have time to dry before the skin incision is made. Parenteral antibiotics should be administered if the patient is resuscitated.

The complications of the thoracotomy include vascular and organ injury. Lacerations of the internal mammary or intercostal arteries can be ligated with silk suture. There is also the possibility of inadvertent laceration of the lung or the myocardium during the initial incision. By temporarily halting mechanical ventilation while performing the thoracotomy, injury to the underlying lung can often be prevented. These injuries will need repair at the appropriate time.

A pericardiotomy can result in significant complications. The left phrenic nerve may be transected. The myocardium or a coronary artery can be lacerated. The heart may be fixed by adhesions to the pericardium from pericardial disease or pericarditis. Attempting to remove the heart from the pericardium can result in avulsion of the atrial or ventricular myocardium. Performance of the pericardiotomy adds another delay in initiating cardiac compressions.

Care should be taken to prevent injury to any of the health care providers. Universal precautions should be followed by all personnel. The use of gloves, goggles, masks, and gowns will protect against exposure to the patient's blood. All needles, scalpels, and scissors should be returned to the bedside tray immediately after use and not left on the patient or the bed. Use extreme caution when placing your hands inside the patient's hemithorax. Fractured ribs from the trauma or the Finochietto rib spreader can easily penetrate gloves and skin.

SUMMARY

An Emergency Department thoracotomy is a lifesaving procedure when used on patients in extremis secondary to penetrating chest or abdominal trauma. To be considered for this procedure, the patient must have signs of life when brought to the Emergency Department, must have lost them en route, or have lost them on the scene. This procedure should not be used in patients who are moribund due to blunt trauma. The Emergency Physician must have the appropriate surgical backup before performing a thoracotomy, since this procedure does not provide definitive therapy.

REFERENCES

1. Millham FH, Grindlinger GA: Survival determinants in patients undergoing emergency room thoracotomy for penetrating chest injury. *J Trauma* 1993; 34:332–336.
2. Thompson DA, Rowlands BJ, Walker WE, et al: Urgent thoracotomy for pulmonary or tracheobronchial injury. *J Trauma* 1988; 28(3):276–280.
3. Ledgerwood AM, Kazmers M, Lucas CE: The role of thoracic aortic occlusion for massive hemoperitoneum. *J Trauma* 1976; 16(8):610–615.
4. Beall AC, Diethrich EB, Crawford HW, et al: Surgical management of penetrating cardiac injuries. *Am J Surg* 1966; 112:686–692.
5. Velmahos GC, Degiannis E, Souter I, et al: Outcome of a strict policy on emergency department thoracotomies. *Arch Surg* 1995; 130:774–777.
6. Kavolius J, Golocovsky M, Champion HR: Predictors of outcome in patients who have sustained trauma and who undergo emergency thoracotomy. *Arch Surg* 1993; 128:1158–1162.
7. Mazzorana V, Smith RS, Morabito DJ, et al: Limited utility of emergency department thoracotomy. *Am Surg* 1994; 60:516–521.
8. Baker CC, Thomas AN, Trunkey DD: The role of emergency room thoracotomy in trauma. *J Trauma* 1980; 20:848–855.
9. Lorenz HP, Steinmetz B, Liebeman J, et al: Emergency thoracotomy: survival correlates with physiologic status. *J Trauma* 1992; 32:780–787.
10. Schwab CW, Adcock OT, Max MH: Emergency department thoracotomy (EDT): a 26 month experience using an "agonal" protocol. *Am Surg* 1986; 52:20–29.
11. Branney SW, Moore EE, Feldhaus KM, et al: Critical analysis of two decades of experience with post injury emergency department thoracotomy in a regional trauma center. *J Trauma* 1998; 45(1): 87–95.
12. Feliciano DV, Burch JM, Spjut-Patrinely V, et al: Abdominal gunshot wounds: an urban trauma center's experience with 300 consecutive patients. *Ann Surg* 1988; 208(3):362–370.

Chapter 32
OPEN CARDIAC MASSAGE

Faran Bokhari

INTRODUCTION

The purpose of cardiopulmonary resuscitation (CPR) during cardiac arrest or hypovolemic shock is to provide adequate cardiac output. This can be done using either closed or open chest cardiac massage. Open cardiac massage may on rare occasions be performed in the Emergency Department. It is performed on patients who have had an emergent thoracotomy after penetrating chest trauma and have inadequate cardiac activity. It may also be performed, in rare instances, after a thoracotomy to decompress a pericardial tamponade in a medical patient.

ANATOMY AND PATHOPHYSIOLOGY

The efficacy of cardiac massage can be established by measuring the cardiac output, coronary perfusion pressure, and cerebral perfusion pressure. Guercio et al showed a higher cardiac index with open than with closed cardiac massage.[1] A minimal coronary perfusion pressure of 15 mmHg must be maintained for return of spontaneous circulation. While not all patients with this pressure will have a return of spontaneous circulation, a pressure of less than 15 mmHg predicts a uniformly fatal outcome.[2] While closed chest CPR generated only 1 to 9 mmHg of pressure, Boczar et al. found that their patients all had a coronary perfusion pressure of almost 20 mmHg throughout open chest massage.[3] Open chest CPR produces improved cerebral perfusion and better neurologic recovery.[4]

INDICATIONS

Open cardiac massage is indicated if absent or inadequate cardiac activity is noted after a thoracotomy.

CONTRAINDICATIONS

The only absolute contraindication to performing open cardiac massage is the presence of a palpable pulse. Open cardiac massage is ineffective if the patient has a pericardial tamponade. Perform a pericardiotomy and remove any clots from the pericardial sac. The heart may then begin to beat spontaneously. If not, repair any lacerations to the myocardium prior to performing cardiac compressions.

EQUIPMENT

No equipment is required to perform open cardiac massage other than that needed to perform the thoracotomy and pericardiotomy (Chapter 31).

PATIENT PREPARATION

The preparation and positioning of the patient is exactly the same as that for a thoracotomy (Figure 32-1). A thoracotomy must first be performed (Figure 32-1). Refer to Chapter 31 for complete details on thoracotomy. A pericardiotomy should be performed only if absolutely

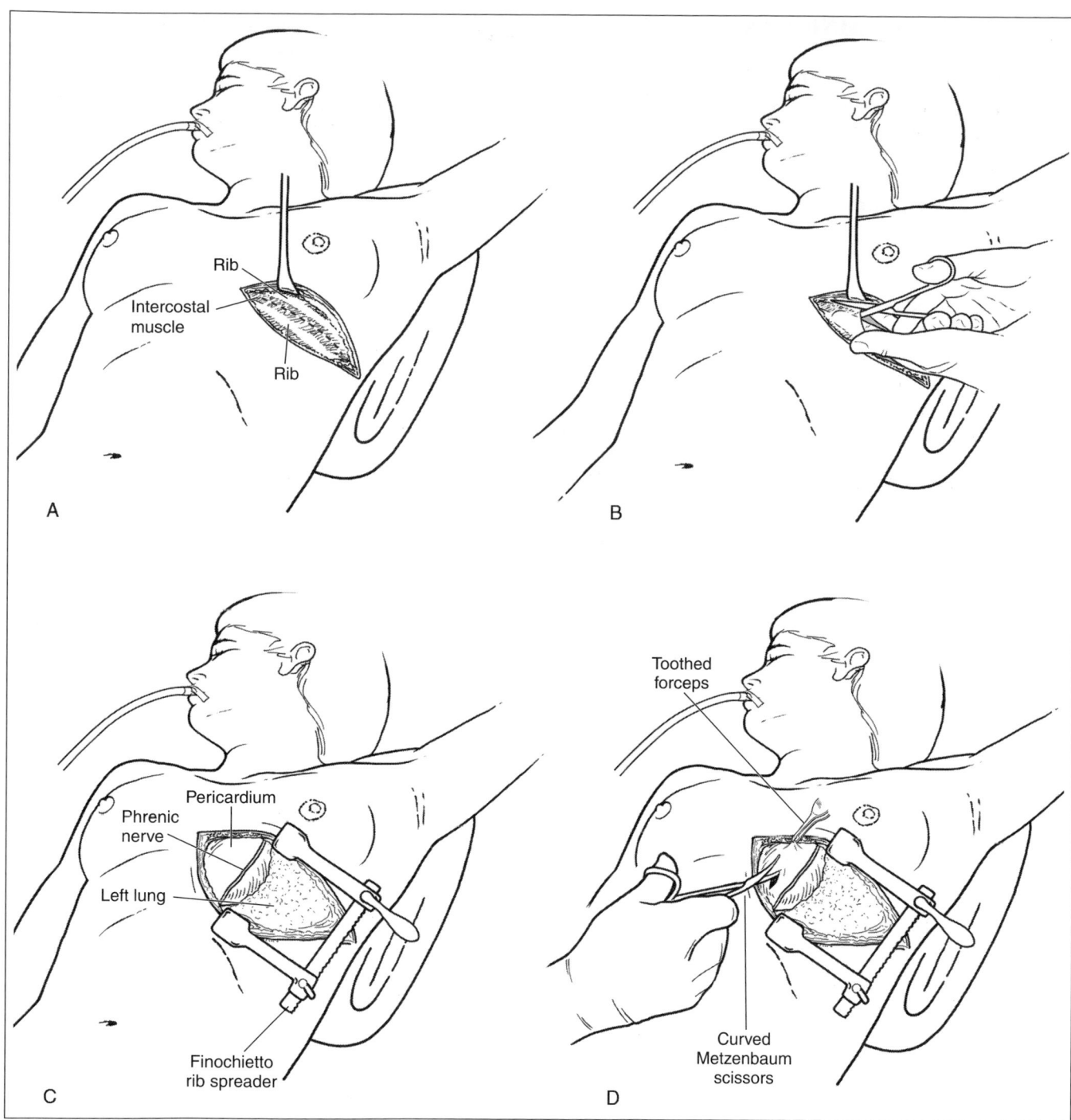

FIGURE 32-1 The anterolateral thoracotomy.

necessary—that is, if blood is seen within the pericardial sac or cardiac tamponade is suspected. Remove any blood and clots from the pericardial sac, deliver the heart from the pericardial sac, and repair any myocardial lacerations.

An intact pericardium is preferable if open cardiac massage is to be performed. It prevents the fingertips from inadvertently rupturing the atria or ventricles should the heart be grasped incorrectly. The pressure from open cardiac massage is distributed over a larger area if the pericardium remains intact. The heart will move within the pericardial sac, prevent the fingers from compressing one spot for a prolonged time, and may decrease the chance of myocardial rupture.

TECHNIQUES

Several important principles must be kept in mind prior to performing open cardiac massage. The heart must be angled not more than 20 to 30 degrees into the left hemithorax (Figure 32-2A). Angulation of more than 30 degrees may crimp the pulmonary veins and vena cava closed and thus minimize cardiac output. The compressive forces should be applied perpendicular to the interventricular septum. Your hands should be placed directly behind and in front of the heart. The left anterior descending artery can be used as a landmark, as it runs above the interventricular septum. Do not place the fingers over the coronary arteries so that their flow is occluded. The fingertips should never be used to compress the heart, as they may rupture the myocardium. Use only the palm, volar surfaces of the fingers, and pads of the fingers to perform cardiac compressions. The fingers should always be held tightly together to form a flat surface. This allows the force of compression to be spread out and not concentrated over one finger. Each compression of the heart must be followed by complete relaxation of the heart.

It is during this relaxation phase (diastole) that the cardiac chambers fill with blood and the coronary arteries perfuse the myocardium.

Three techniques have been described to perform open cardiac massage (Figures 32-2 and 32-3). These include the one-handed massage with sternal compression, one-handed compression, and two-handed compression. Two-handed compression has been shown to be consistently superior to the other two techniques in generating cardiac output.[5]

ONE-HANDED MASSAGE WITH STERNAL COMPRESSIONS

Tightly adduct the fingers of the dominant hand to make a flat surface. Insert the hand into the thoracotomy incision and against the posterior surface of the heart (Figures 32-2A and B). Angle the heart 20 to 30 degrees into the left hemithorax. Compress the heart against the sternum, beginning with the heel of the hand, then the palm, then fingers in sequence. This method is difficult to perform in children because of the plasticity of the sternum.[6]

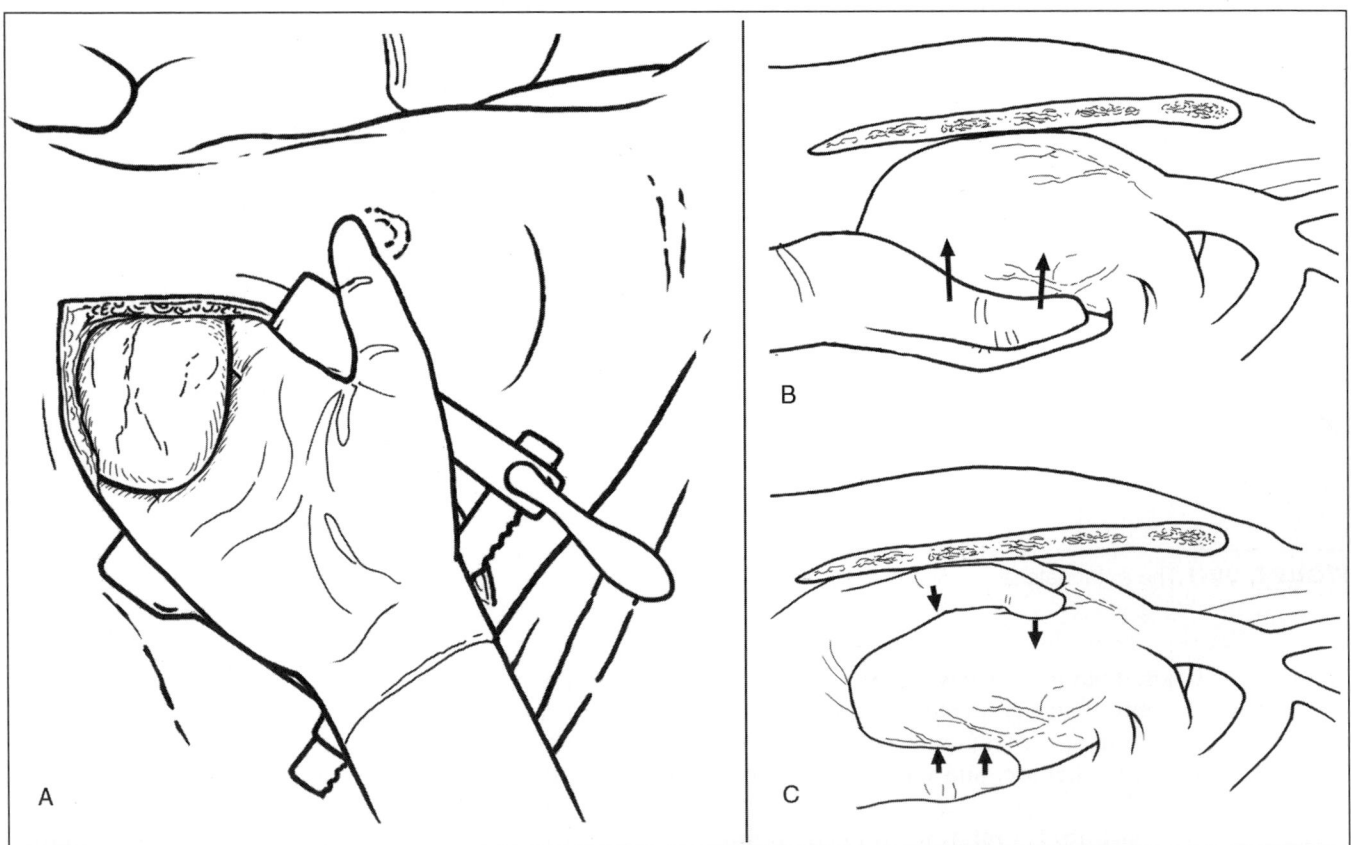

FIGURE 32-2 One-handed open cardiac massage. *A*. The dominant hand angles the heart 20 to 30 degrees into the left hemithorax. *B*. One-handed cardiac massage with sternal compression. *C*. The one-handed compression technique.

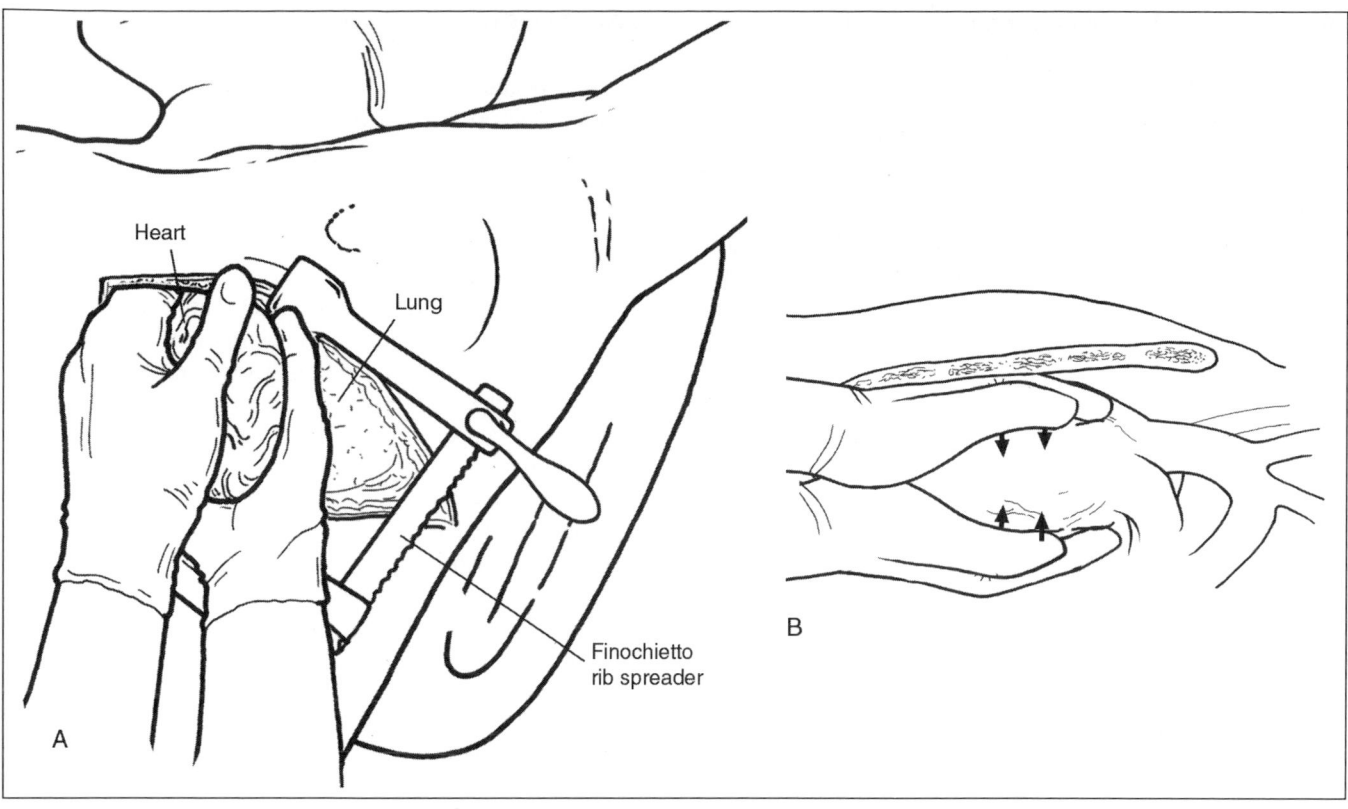

FIGURE 32-3 Two-handed open cardiac massage. *A.* The hands are positioned on the anterior and posterior surfaces of the heart. *B.* Compressions begin at the cardiac apex with the palms and progress toward the base of the heart with the fingers.

ONE-HANDED COMPRESSIONS

Tightly adduct the fingers of the dominant hand to make a flat surface. Insert the hand into the thoracotomy incision and against the anterior surface of the heart (Figure 32-2*C*). Place the thumb against the posterior surface of the heart. The apex of the heart will lie in the palm of the hand. Angle the heart 20 to 30 degrees into the left hemithorax. Appose the thumb and fingers to compress the heart. This is not the preferred method, as the thumb can place significant pressure on the left ventricle and possibly cause it to rupture.

TWO-HANDED COMPRESSIONS

Tightly adduct the fingers and cup the left hand. Insert the left hand into the thoracotomy incision and against the anterior surface of the heart (Figure 32-3*A*). Tightly adduct the fingers of the right hand to make a flat surface. Insert the right hand into the thoracotomy incision and against the posterior surface of the heart (Figure 32-3*A*). Angle the heart 20 to 30 degrees into the left hemithorax. Appose the hands to compress the heart (Figure 32-3*B*). Compressions should ideally begin with the heel of the hands and progress toward the fingers.

ASSESSMENT

Compressions should begin at a rate appropriate for the patient's age as specified by the American Heart Association (Pediatric Advanced Life Support and Advanced Cardiac Life Support). Assess the effectiveness of the cardiac compressions by noting a palpable carotid pulse. A radial or femoral arterial line can be placed to monitor the effectiveness of the compressions. This line allows for repeated blood and blood gas sampling. The arterial line will also allow the physician to ensure that the heart is completely relaxed between compressions.

AFTERCARE

If a spontaneous cardiac rhythm and a peripheral pulse return, the patient must be taken to the operating room emergently for definitive treatment.

COMPLICATIONS

The major complication of open cardiac massage is myocardial rupture or perforation. This can occur from compression of the heart against a jagged and fractured rib or sternum. Incorrect technique with too vigorous a massage can result in perforation of the ischemic myocardium by the fingertips. Other complications include decreased cardiac output with compressions if the heart is angled more than 30 degrees into the left hemithorax and kinks shut the vena cava or pulmonary veins. If the patient survives, parenteral antibiotics should be administered to prevent infection and sepsis. The complications associated with the thoracotomy and the pericardiotomy are discussed in Chapter 31.

SUMMARY

Open cardiac massage is a more efficient way of maintaining circulation than closed chest massage. Cardiac compressions can be performed with one or two hands, depending on physician preference. The two-handed technique is preferred, as it generates greater cardiac output than the one-handed techniques. Once a cardiac rhythm and blood pressure are restored, definitive treatment for injuries must be provided expeditiously in the operating room.

REFERENCES

1. Del Guercio LRM, Feins NR, Cohn JD, et al: Comparison of blood flow during external and internal cardiac massage in man. *Circulation* 1965; 319(suppl 1):171–179.
2. Sanders AB, Ogle M, Ewy GA: Coronary perfusion pressure during cardiopulmonary resuscitation. *Am J Emerg Med* 1985; 3:11–14.
3. Boczar ME, Howard MA, Rivers EP, et al: A technique revisited: hemodynamic comparison of closed and open chest cardiac massage during human CPR. *Crit Care Med* 1995; 23(3):498–503.
4. Alifimoff JK, Safar P, Bircher, N, et al: Cerebral recovery after prolonged closed chest, MAST augmented, and open chest CPR. *Anesthesiology* 1980; 53(suppl):S147.
5. Barnet WM: Comparison of open-chest cardiac massage techniques in dogs. *Ann Emerg Med* 1986; 15(4):408–411.
6. King BR, Wagner DK: Emergency thoracotomy, in Henretig FM, King C, Joffe MD, et al (eds): *Textbook of Pediatric Emergency Procedures*. Baltimore: Williams & Wilkins, 1997:415–427.

Chapter 33
CARDIAC WOUND REPAIR

Steven Salzman
Faran Bokhari

INTRODUCTION

Wounds of the heart are highly lethal. Traumatic cardiac penetration carries a 70 to 80 percent fatality rate.[1] Major factors determining survivability include whether or not cardiac standstill has occurred as well as the amount of tissue destruction sustained from the injury.[2]

Penetrating wounds can be caused by knives, bullets, ice picks, and (infrequently) rib or sternal fragments. **Regardless of the offending agent, repair must be done as expeditiously as possible.** The right ventricle is the most frequently injured chamber. However, injury to the heart may occur at more than one site. This is especially true with bullet wounds.

The goal of treatment in the Emergency Department is temporary hemostasis. Many different techniques of cardiorrhaphy have been described. We will limit our discussion to five possible approaches to dealing with these injuries (i.e., digital or Foley catheter occlusion, vascular clamps, staples, and sutures).

ANATOMY AND PATHOPHYSIOLOGY

The heart is contained within the pericardial sac. Numerous portions of the heart are exposed behind the anterior chest wall (Figure 25-2). This includes the right ventricle, left ventricle, right atrium, left atrium, aorta, pulmonary artery, and inferior vena cava. These structures are vulnerable to injury behind the anterior chest wall.[3,4] The surface areas that each of these structures contributes to the anterior cardiac silhouette are as follows: 55 percent right ventricle, 20 percent left ventricle, 10 percent right atrium, 10 percent aorta and pulmonary artery, 4 percent inferior vena cava, and 1 percent left atrium.[5] These numbers also reflect, roughly, the ana-

tomic incidence of injury with cardiac trauma.[5] Traumatic injury to any of these structures can result in a pericardial effusion and cardiac tamponade.

INDICATIONS

Any penetrating injury to the heart requires immediate and temporary repair to prevent the patient from exsanguinating. A bluish hue behind the pericardium or a tense pericardial sac after penetrating trauma suggests an underlying cardiac injury. A pericardiotomy should be performed, any blood and clot removed from the pericardial sac, and the heart explored for the site of injury.

CONTRAINDICATIONS

The only absolute contraindication to performing a cardiorrhaphy is if the patient has obvious signs of death. It should not be performed if the patient has not had any vital signs for over 15 minutes, as anoxic brain injury is irreversible. It is also contraindicated in patients with penetrating chest trauma who do not meet the criteria for performing an anterolateral thoracotomy (Chapter 31).

EQUIPMENT

Silk suture, 4–0 and 5–0 (or Prolene)
2-0 silk, on a semicircular atraumatic needle
10 inch needle driver
Foley catheter, sizes 14 to 20 French
Satinsky vascular clamp
Allis clamps

Defibrillator with internal cardiac paddles
Mayo scissors
Metzenbaum scissors, curved
Teflon pledgets
Sterile saline
20 mL syringe
Standard skin stapler, 6 mm wide staples
Laparotomy pads
Gauze, 4×4 squares
Hemostats

PATIENT PREPARATION

No preparation is required other than that of performing a thoracotomy and a pericardiotomy (Chapter 31). The patient should be intubated and ventilated with 100% oxygen. The patient should be monitored by telemetry, a noninvasive blood pressure cuff, and pulse oximetry.

TECHNIQUES

Bleeding from a cardiac wound should ideally be stopped by placing a finger over the wound and immediately transporting the patient to the Operating Room for definitive repair. Unfortunately, the Anesthesiologist, Surgeon, and/or Operating Room may not be immediately available. If the Emergency Physician performs a thoracotomy, they should be versed in methods of temporary cardiac wound repair. Several techniques are available to control hemorrhage from a cardiac wound.

CONTROL OF THE HEART

It is extremely difficult to maintain a finger over a cardiac wound or to stitch a cardiac wound if the heart is beating. An apical traction suture known as Beck's suture can be placed to control the heart (Figure 33-1). The apex of the heart is the ideal site because it is often away from most lacerations, is a thick portion of the heart, and is away from any major coronary arteries. Place a 2–0 silk suture through the apex of the heart and remove the needle from the suture. The ends of the suture can be grasped to elevate and control the heart while it is beating.

SAUERBRUCH MANEUVER

Large cardiac wounds and wounds with significant bleeding are difficult to repair, as the blood obscures the surgical field. Experienced Surgeons may temporarily clamp the inferior and superior vena cava to maintain a bloodless field. **Clamping the vena cava should not be performed by an Emergency Physician, as it is time-consuming and can injure other structures.** A quicker

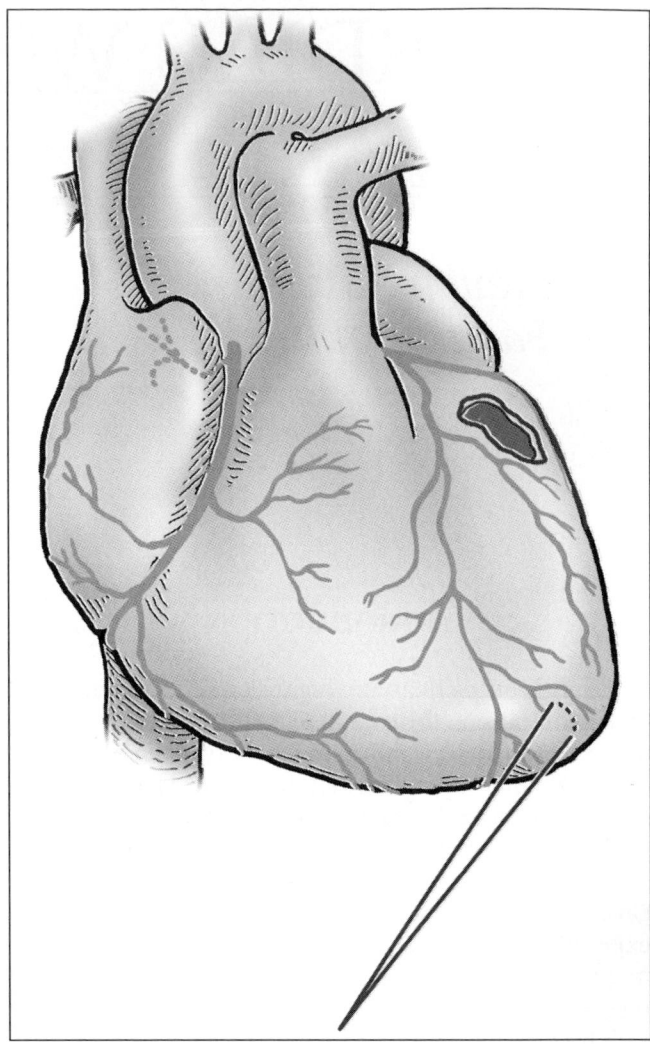

FIGURE 33-1 The apical traction suture known as Beck's suture may be placed to control the heart.

and safer alternative is the Sauerbruch maneuver, or grip, to partially occlude venous inflow through the inferior and superior vena cava (Figure 33-2). This technique will stabilize the heart for wound repair and allow the bleeding site to be identified and repaired.

Insert the nondominant hand in the pericardial cavity and toward the vena cava. Place the middle finger behind the vena cava and the index finger in front of the vena cava (Figure 33-2). The thumb should be on the anterior surface of the heart. The ring and little fingers should be on the posterior surface of the heart. Use the thumb and the ring and little fingers to cradle the heart while apposing the middle and index fingers to partially occlude the vena cava. This technique can be used to control hemorrhage from the heart, great vessels, or hilum. **While effective at controlling hemorrhage, this technique will significantly reduce cardiac output and result in cardiac arrest. The grip should be released**

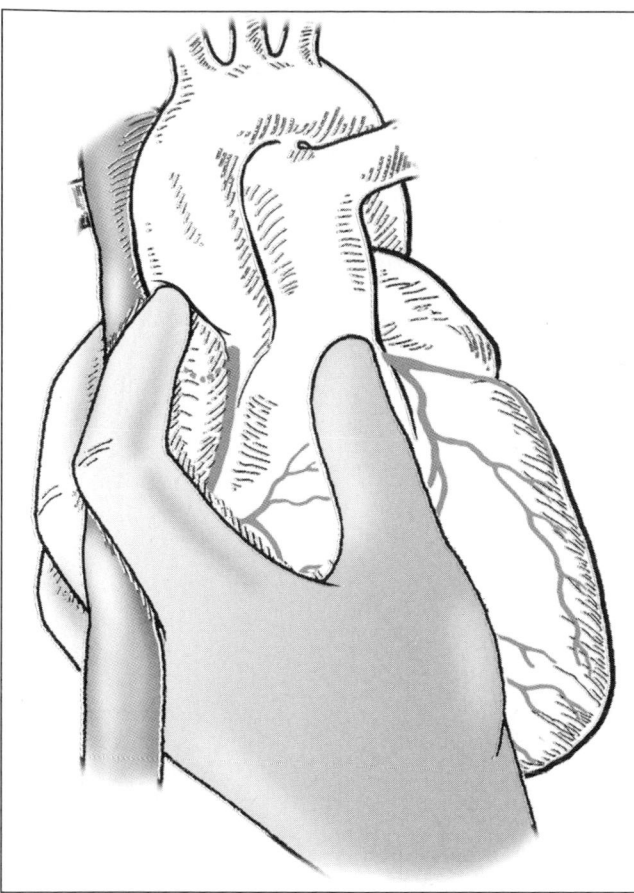

FIGURE 33-2 The Sauerbruch maneuver to partially occlude venous inflow from the superior and inferior vena cava.

every 30 to 60 seconds to ensure coronary artery perfusion.

DIGITAL OCCLUSION

Digital occlusion of small cardiac wounds can provide excellent hemostasis while awaiting definitive repair. Once a finger is placed on or over the defect, it must remain there until the appropriate materials to perform cardiorrhaphy are available. **Do not place a finger into the defect as this may increase the size of the wound.** Unfortunately, the fingertip often slips off the wound if the heart is beating. The fingertip interferes with visualization and repair of the wound. It also places the health care worker at risk for a needle-stick injury while attempting to repair the wound.

FOLEY CATHETER TECHNIQUE

A Foley catheter may be used to provide temporary hemostasis. As with digital occlusion, this is only a temporizing measure. Inflate the cuff of the Foley catheter with sterile saline to check its integrity and look for leaks. **Deflate the cuff. Place a hemostat on the Foley catheter just proximal to the cuff. This will prevent air**

from being drawn through the catheter and causing an air embolism.

Identify the location of the cardiac wound (Figure 33-3A). Insert the catheter through the cardiac wound until the balloon is within the cardiac chamber (Figure 33-3B). Open the hemostat, inflate the cuff with 20 to 30 mL of sterile saline, and reclamp the Foley catheter (Figure 33-3C). **This step should be done quickly to prevent air from being drawn through the catheter.**

Apply gentle traction to the catheter (Figure 33-3D). Apply just enough traction to mostly occlude the wound and slow the bleeding. A small amount of bleeding is adequate and acceptable to visualize the wound and perform a temporary repair. Do not try to provide complete hemostasis. This will result in excessive traction on the catheter, causing the cuff to pull through the wound, enlarge the wound, and further lacerate the myocardium.

Repair the cardiac wound. Place a purse-string suture around the wound (Figure 33-3E). **Use caution when placing the suture so that the needle does not pierce and rupture the cuff of the Foley catheter.** The catheter may be advanced into the cardiac chamber temporarily while the suture is being placed. This will prevent the needle from piercing the cuff. **Do not advance the cuff too far into the heart and for too long a time period. The cuff may occlude blood flow through the valves and result in cardiac arrest.** After the purse-string suture is placed, deflate the cuff and quickly remove the Foley catheter (Figure 33-3F). Tie the ends of the suture to close the cardiac wound (Figure 33-3G). Place additional knots to secure the suture.

The Foley catheter technique is simple and effective. It avoids the problems associated with digital occlusion. The catheter may be placed in posterior cardiac wounds that are difficult to visualize and where it is hard to maintain digital occlusion. The Foley catheter does not interfere with visualization of the wound, wound repair, or the simultaneous performance of cardiac massage. Intravenous catheter tubing may be inserted into the lumen of the Foley catheter to infuse crystalloid solutions or red blood cells directly into the heart and central circulation. This technique is especially valuable in repairing wounds at the junction of the right atrium and vena cava.

CLAMP TECHNIQUE

Atrial wounds can bleed profusely and are difficult to control. The thin walls do not allow digital occlusion to be effective. The atrial wound can be grasped and compressed between the thumb and index finger. An atraumatic Satinsky vascular clamp can be placed around the wound to provide hemostasis (Figure 33-4). The wound may then be repaired with 4–0 or 5–0 interrupted silk sutures.

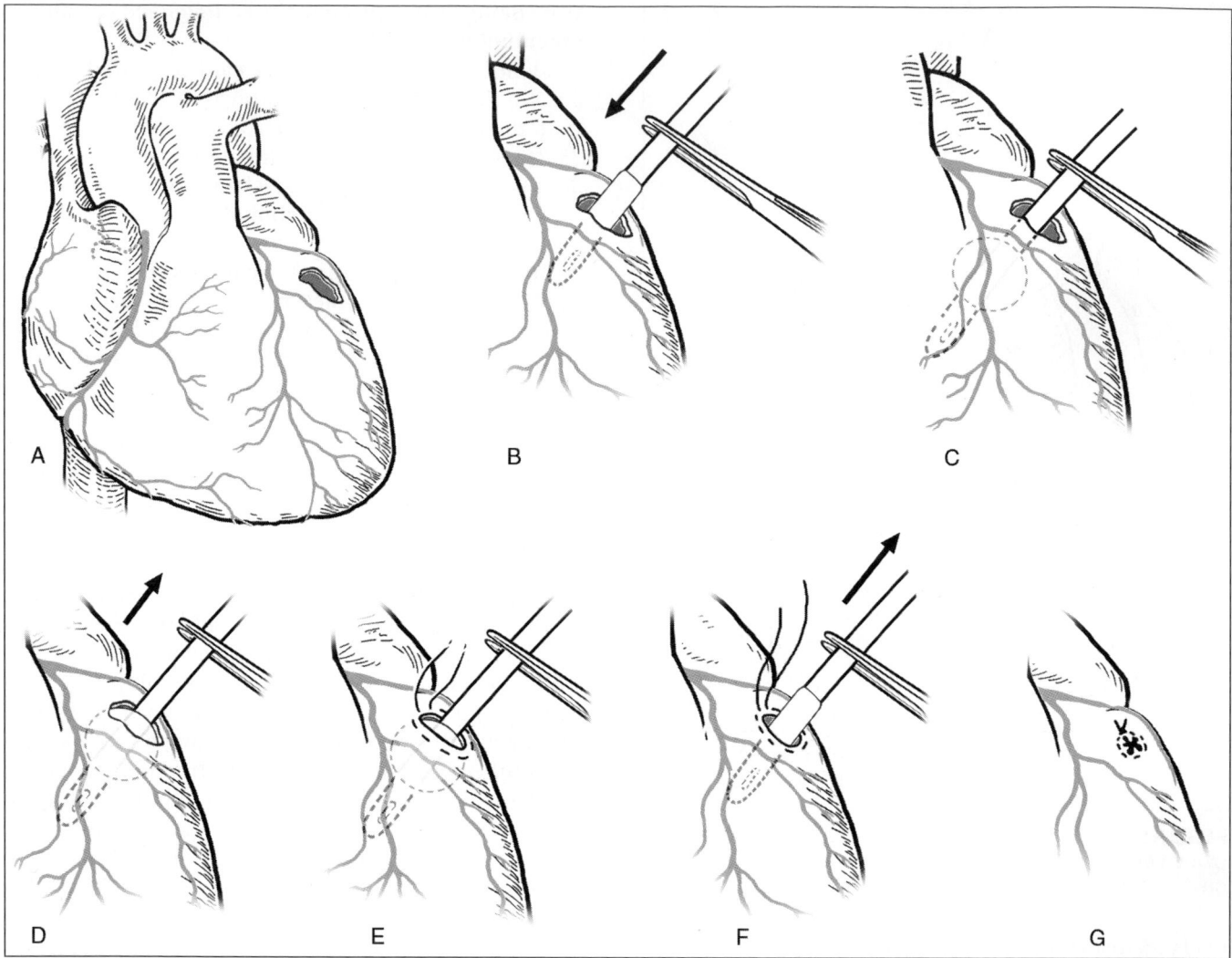

FIGURE 33-3 The Foley catheter technique to occlude and repair a cardiac wound. *A.* The cardiac wound is identified. *B.* The Foley catheter is inserted through the wound. *C.* The cuff is inflated. *D.* Gentle traction is applied to occlude the wound with the cuff. *E.* A purse-string suture is placed around the wound. *F.* The cuff is deflated and the Foley catheter is removed. *G.* The purse-string suture is tightened and tied to occlude the wound.

Allis clamps may be substituted if a Satinsky clamp is not available. Place a clamp on each of the opposing edges of the atrial wound. Apply upward traction, then cross the Allis clamps to approximate the wound edges. The wound may now be sutured closed. The Allis clamps do not provide as bloodless a field as does the Satinsky clamp.

STAPLE TECHNIQUE

Skin staples provide a quick and easy method to repair cardiac wounds. Careful approximation and stapling of the wound will rapidly close the defect and aid in controlling massive blood loss. Staples may be used to close small, large, or multiple lacerations. It avoids the potential complications of a needle stick to the physician.

Cardiac wounds are closed similarly to skin lacerations (Figure 33-5). Obtain a standard skin stapler with 6 mm wide staples. These are readily available in most Emergency Departments for wound closure. Use the nondominant hand to appose the wound edges. Grasp the stapler with the dominant hand. Place staples at 5 mm intervals until the wound is closed.

SUTURE TECHNIQUES

Suturing of cardiac wounds is more time consuming than the other methods previously described. It requires technical proficiency and understanding of the heart's

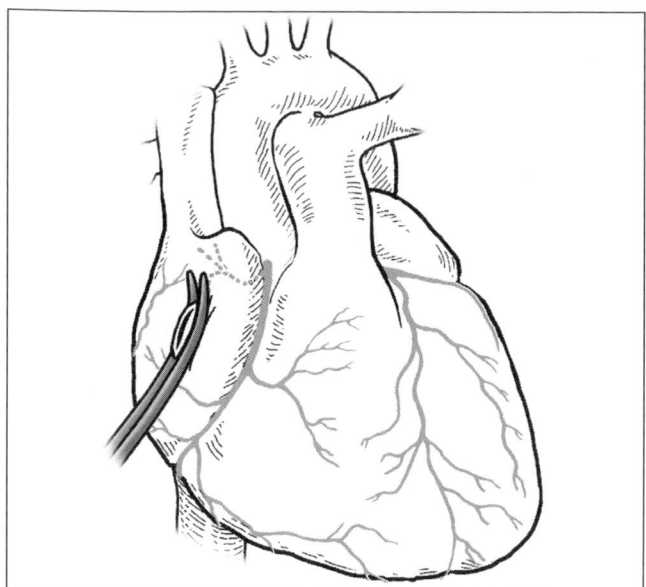

FIGURE 33-4 A Satinsky vascular clamp provides hemostasis for atrial wounds.

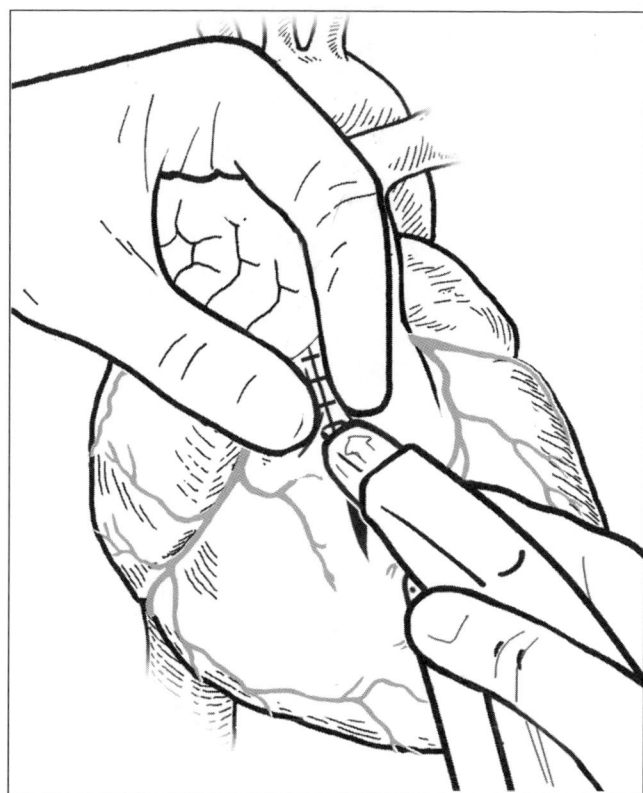

FIGURE 33-5 The cardiac stapling technique provides temporary hemostasis.

surface anatomy. Place horizontal mattress sutures using 2–0 or 3–0 silk or Prolene suture material (Figure 33-6). **The sutures should not be tied tightly. It is easy to inadvertently tear through the myocardium.** Teflon pledgets should be used to reinforce the repair and prevent cutting through the heart tissue (Figures 33-6*A* and *B*). This is especially important when the wound edges are irregular or tattered. Care should be taken to avoid injury to the coronary vessels, which may lie in close proximity to a cardiac wound. Ensure that the sutures are placed adjacent to and underneath the coronary vessels (Figure 33-6*C*).

Large cardiac wounds are difficult to repair. They bleed profusely. The digital occlusion and Foley catheter techniques are ineffective on large wounds. The wound edges are difficult to grasp and appose so that they can be repaired with a skin stapler. Place an incomplete horizontal mattress stitch on each side of the wound (Figure 33-7). Grasp the free ends of the sutures and cross them across the wound to appose the wound edges. Instruct an assistant to hold the suture ends while the cardiac wound is repaired with 2–0 or 3–0 silk, Prolene, or staples. The incomplete mattress sutures may then be removed or tied to each other.

FIBRILLATION

The myocardium can be deliberately placed in fibrillation to halt myocardial contractions and repair large ventricular wounds. **This should be performed only if other techniques of cardiac wound repair are unsuccessful.** Place the internal cardiac paddles on the anterior and posterior surfaces of the heart. Apply 20 J through the paddles to fibrillate the heart. Repair the cardiac wound. **Perform intermittent cardiac massage while repairing the fibrillating myocardium. Do not allow the heart to fibrillate for more than 3 minutes.** Defibrillate the heart with the internal paddles using 20 J of energy. Repeat the defibrillation with 20 J of energy until the heart begins beating. **Do not use more than 20 J to defibrillate the heart with the internal cardiac paddles as myocardial necrosis can occur.**

AFTERCARE

If the patient is resuscitated, immediately transport them to the operating room for definitive repair of the cardiac wound and any other injuries.

COMPLICATIONS

The complications associated with digital pressure include further destruction of tissue. If pulled too tightly, Foley catheters can become dislodged and restart troublesome bleeding. They can also enlarge a cardiac

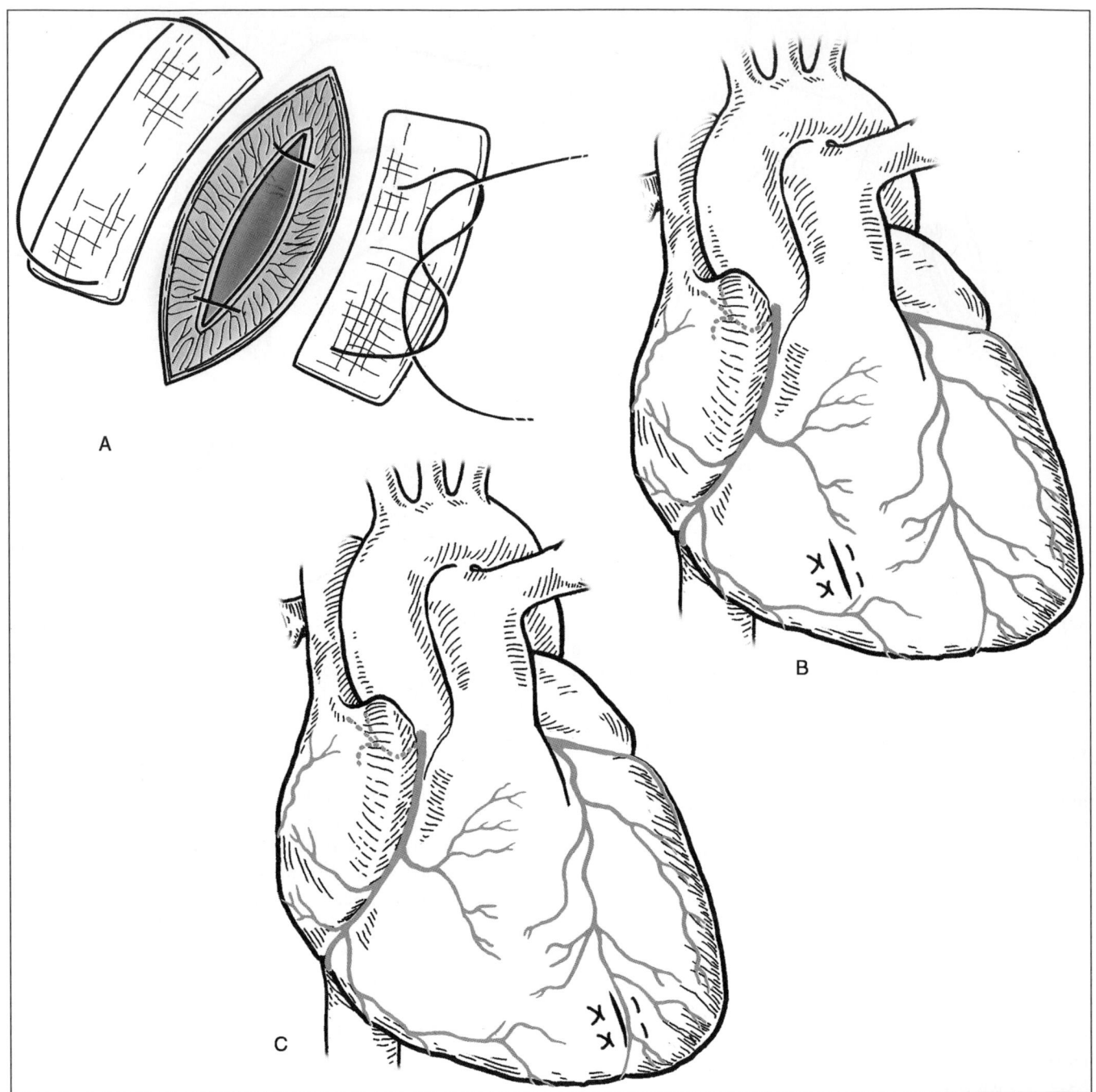

FIGURE 33-6 Horizontal mattress sutures used to close cardiac wounds. *A.* Teflon pledgets are placed on either side of the wound to prevent the suture from pulling through the myocardium. *B.* Wounds are closed with multiple horizontal mattress sutures. *C.* When suturing near a coronary artery, ensure that the sutures pass completely below the artery.

wound if the cuff pulls through the wound. A drop in cardiac output can result if the cuff obstructs the cardiac valves, impinges on the chordae tendineae, or occupies space within the cardiac chamber. Suturing is probably associated with the greatest rate of complications. Tearing of the myocardium is a frequently encountered problem. The suture should be tied just tight enough to

stop the bleeding. Care should be exercised to avoid ligation of the major coronary vessels and their branches. Dysrhythmias can result from occlusion of venous inflow (Sauerbruch maneuver) or injury to the coronary vasculature. If the patient is resuscitated, administer broad-spectrum antibiotics to prevent any potential infectious complication.

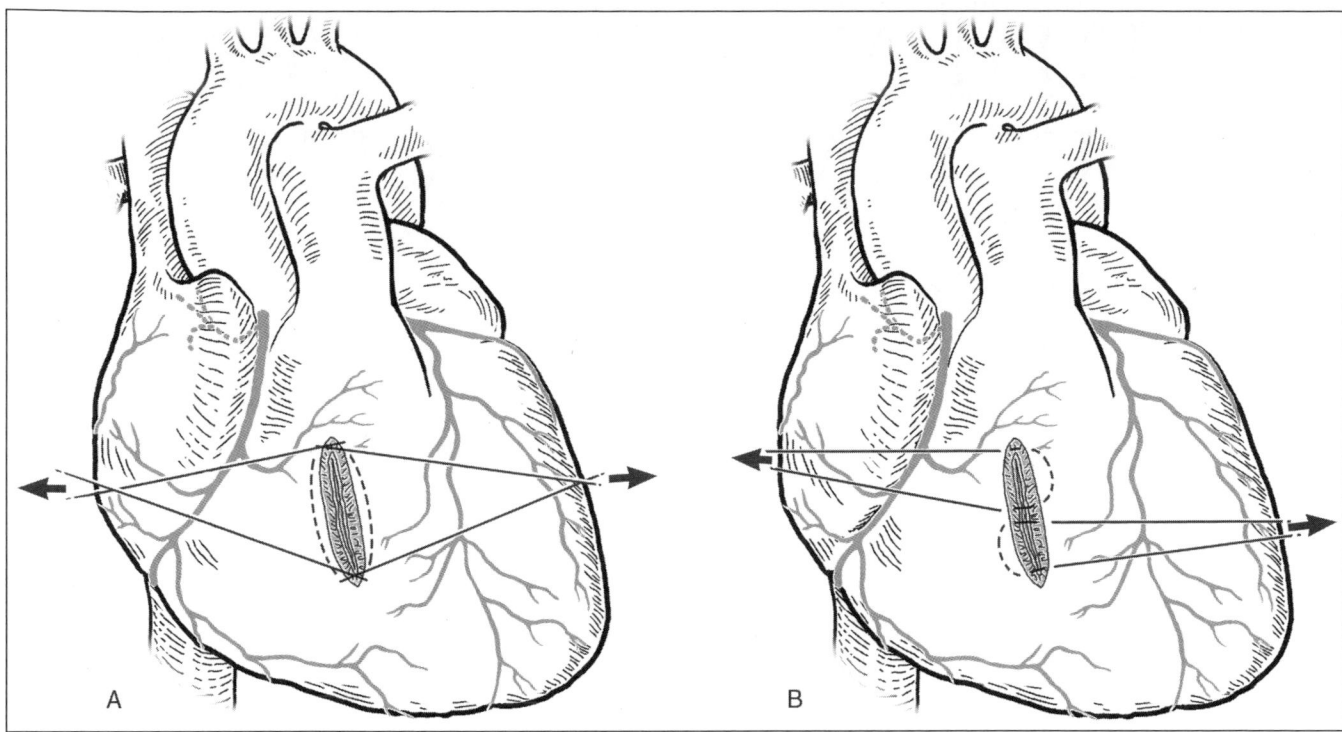

FIGURE 33-7 Incomplete horizontal mattress stitches may be placed on each side of a large wound. Tension applied to the sutures will appose the wound edges (*arrows*).

SUMMARY

Injuries to the heart can be devastating. The role of Emergency Department management is to temporarily control bleeding and rapidly transport the patient to the operating room for definitive repair. If there is a delay in transporting the patient to the operating room, the Emergency Physician must be versed in the techniques used to repair cardiac wounds.

REFERENCES

1. Buckman RF Jr, Buckman PD, Badellino MM: Heart, in Invatury RR, Cayten CG, Cayton CG (eds): *The Textbook of Penetrating Trauma.* Baltimore: Williams & Wilkins, 1996:499–511.
2. Ivatury RR: Injury to the heart, in Mattox KL, Feliciano DV, Moore EE (eds): *Trauma,* 4th ed. New York: McGraw-Hill, 2000:409–423.
3. Symbas PN: *Cardiothoracic Trauma.* Philadelphia: Saunders, 1989:16–55.
4. Chong HH, Plotnick GD: Pericardial effusion and tamponade: evaluation, imaging modalities, and management. *Comp Ther* 1995; 21(7):378–385.
5. Thourani VH, Feliciana DV, Rozycki G, et al: Penetrating cardiac trauma at an urban trauma center: a 22 year perspective. *Am Surg* 1999; 65(9):811–818.

Chapter 34

HILUM AND GREAT VESSEL WOUND MANAGEMENT

Faran Bokhari

INTRODUCTION

Injuries to the thoracic great vessels can be a significant cause of morbidity and mortality. Large vessels in the hilum of the lung include the pulmonary artery and vein. The great vessels also include the vena cava, aorta, innominate artery, subclavian artery, and subclavian vein. The mortality from injuries to the subclavian artery is approximately 5 percent if patients who are moribund on admission to the Emergency Department are excluded.[1] However, the mortality from injury to the vena cava and the pulmonary vessels is over 60 percent.[2] While over 85 percent of patients with penetrating injuries to the thorax are stable, the remainder present in varying levels of hypovolemic shock. They may have bled externally or into the chest. Each hemithorax can hold up to one-half of an individual's blood volume. In these cases, an Emergency Department thoracotomy may be performed for hypovolemic shock.

ANATOMY AND PATHOPHYSIOLOGY

Injury to the thoracic great vessels may be due to blunt trauma, diagnostic procedures, iatrogenic causes, or penetrating trauma. Crush injuries, deceleration injuries, motor vehicle versus pedestrian collisions, and penetrating thoracic injuries may all signify an injury to a thoracic great vessel. The vessels that are most commonly injured include the aorta, innominate artery, pulmonary vein, and venae cavae.

The portable anteroposterior chest radiograph is the initial radiographic screening. It may reveal loss of the aortic knob contour, left-sided pleural effusions, mediastinal widening, nasogastric tube deviation, or tracheal deviation, all of which suggest injury to a great vessel. Other findings suggestive of such an injury include depression of the left mainstem bronchus, left apical capping, narrowing of the carinal angle, sternal fractures, opacification of the aortopulmonary window, and widening of the paraspinous stripe.

Numerous physical examination findings are suggestive of a thoracic great vessel injury. Asymmetric pulses or unequal blood pressures between the extremities are quick and simple to evaluate. Hypotension may be due to internal or external hemorrhage. Steering wheel contusions, sternal fractures, thoracic spine fractures, and a left-sided flail chest signify potential intrathoracic injury. A thoracic outlet hematoma or a hoarse voice can occur from injury to the aorta or one of its major branches. Paraplegia may be due to hypotension or an aortic disruption.

INDICATIONS

Attempts should be made to control any laceration or rupture of the thoracic great vessels.

CONTRAINDICATIONS

There are no absolute contraindications to temporarily controlling any hemorrhage from a thoracic great vessel after performing a thoracotomy (Chapter 31). The thoracotomy should not be performed if the patient has obvious signs of death, no vital signs in the field, or no vital signs for over 15 minutes. A pericardial tamponade or cardiac injury may require management prior to managing a great vessel injury.

EQUIPMENT

3–0 Prolene suture
Foley catheters, sizes 14 to 20 French
10 inch needle driver
Satinsky vascular clamps
Sterile saline
20 mL syringe
Laparotomy pads
Gauze, 4×4 squares
Umbilical clamp
Hemostats

PATIENT PREPARATION

There is no preparation required other than performing an anterolateral thoracotomy (Chapter 31). The patient should be intubated, ventilated, and monitored with telemetry, pulse oximetry, and a noninvasive blood pressure cuff.

TECHNIQUES

DIGITAL OCCLUSION

Digital pressure may be used to control small lacerations of the thoracic vena cava. It will provide adequate hemostasis while repairing the wound. **Place a fingertip over the defect.** Do not place a finger in the defect. Place horizontal mattress sutures using 3–0 Prolene to close the defect. Unfortunately, the fingertip interferes with visualization of the wound and places the physician at risk for a needle-stick injury. The fingertip will have to be intermittently removed to place the sutures.

Digital pressure and rapid transport to the operating room is the most practical method of dealing with injuries to the subclavian vessels. These vessels are extremely difficult to control through a traditional anterolateral thoracotomy incision. If digital pressure is ineffective, pack the apex of the thoracic cavity with laparotomy pads or gauze squares and apply compression from below.

FOLEY CATHETER TECHNIQUE

By inserting a Foley catheter into the vessel, inflating the cuff, and placing it under gentle traction, one may occlude a wound to a great vessel (Figure 34-1). As with digital occlusion, this is only a temporizing measure. Inflate the cuff of the Foley catheter with sterile saline to check its integrity and look for leaks. Deflate the cuff. **Place a hemostat on the Foley catheter proximal to the cuff. This will prevent air from being drawn through the catheter and causing an air embolism.**

Identify the location of the vascular injury. Insert the catheter through the wound until the cuff is within the vessel (Figure 34-1A). Open the hemostat, inflate the cuff with 10 to 20 mL of sterile saline, and reclamp the Foley catheter. **This step should be completed quickly to prevent air from being drawn through the catheter. Do not overinflate the cuff so that it occludes flow through the vessel. Apply gentle traction to the catheter (Figure 34-1B). Apply just enough traction to mostly occlude the wound and slow the bleeding. Do not try to provide complete hemostasis.** This will result in excessive traction on the catheter, causing the cuff to pull through the

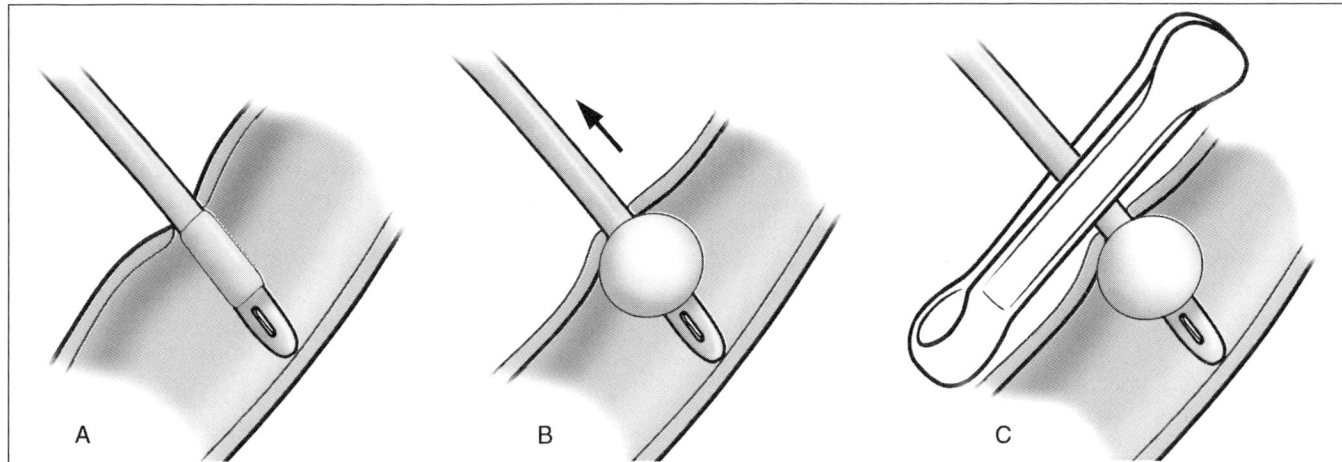

FIGURE 34-1 The Foley catheter technique to occlude an injury to a great vessel. *A.* The catheter is inserted through the wound and into the vessel. *B.* The cuff is inflated and gentle traction (*arrow*) is applied to occlude the wound with the cuff. *C.* An umbilical clamp is placed to prevent the catheter from migrating inward.

wound, enlarge the wound, and further injure the vessel. Place an umbilical clamp or hemostat on the catheter just outside the vessel to prevent it from migrating into the vessel (Figure 34-1C).

The Foley catheter technique is simple and effective. It avoids the problems associated with digital occlusion. It does not interfere with visualization of the wound or the simultaneous performance of cardiac massage. Intravenous catheter tubing may be inserted into the lumen of the Foley catheter to infuse crystalloid solutions or red blood cells directly into the heart and central circulation.

CROSS-CLAMPING TECHNIQUE

Injuries to the thoracic great vessels can bleed profusely and are difficult to control. Digital occlusion is often ineffective. An atraumatic Satinsky vascular clamp can be placed to partially occlude the great vessel and isolate the injury (Figure 34-2). This will provide temporary hemostasis until definitive repair in the operating room can take place.

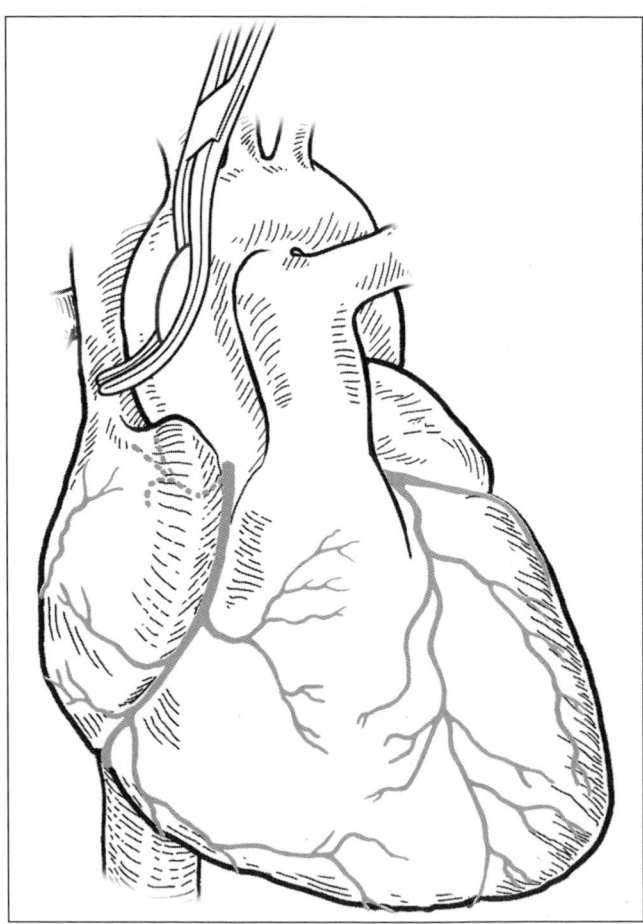

FIGURE 34-2 A Satinsky vascular clamp may be used to partially occlude the great vessel and isolate the injury.

Large wounds and complete transections are difficult to manage. Injuries to the pulmonary vasculature in the region of the hilum are most expeditiously controlled by placing a Satinsky vascular clamp across the respective hilum. Grasp the hilum between the thumb and the forefinger. Place the clamp carefully around the entire hilum. Take care not to injure the pulmonary parenchyma or the vessels any further. Vascular injuries may be controlled by placing a cross-clamp proximal to the injury and occluding the backbleeding with additional clamps (Figure 34-3). These patients should be immediately transported to the operating room to be placed on bypass and repair the injuries. It is generally not recommended for the Emergency Physician to suture great vessel injuries in an attempt to repair them.

AFTERCARE

If the patient is resuscitated, they should immediately be transported to the operating room for definitive repair of the injury to the great vessels and any other injuries.

COMPLICATIONS

The complications associated with digital pressure include extending the injury if the procedure is not performed carefully. Inaccurate digital control can lead to unnecessary loss of blood during transport of the patient to the operating room. Foley catheters, if pulled too tightly, can become dislodged and restart troublesome bleeding. They can also enlarge a wound if the cuff pulls through the wound. The cuff may obstruct flow through the vessel and compromise cardiac output. An overly rough mobilization and clamping can increase the size of the injury and cause massive bleeding. Cross-clamping of the aorta and/or pulmonary artery will obstruct peripheral blood flow. The vessel must be repaired or the patient placed on bypass to prevent anoxia and permanent neurologic dysfunction.

SUMMARY

Injuries to the thoracic great vessels carry a high mortality as bleeding occurs unimpeded into the pleural space. The survival of the patient depends on their presenting condition as well as the speed and accuracy with which the intrathoracic hemorrhage is controlled.

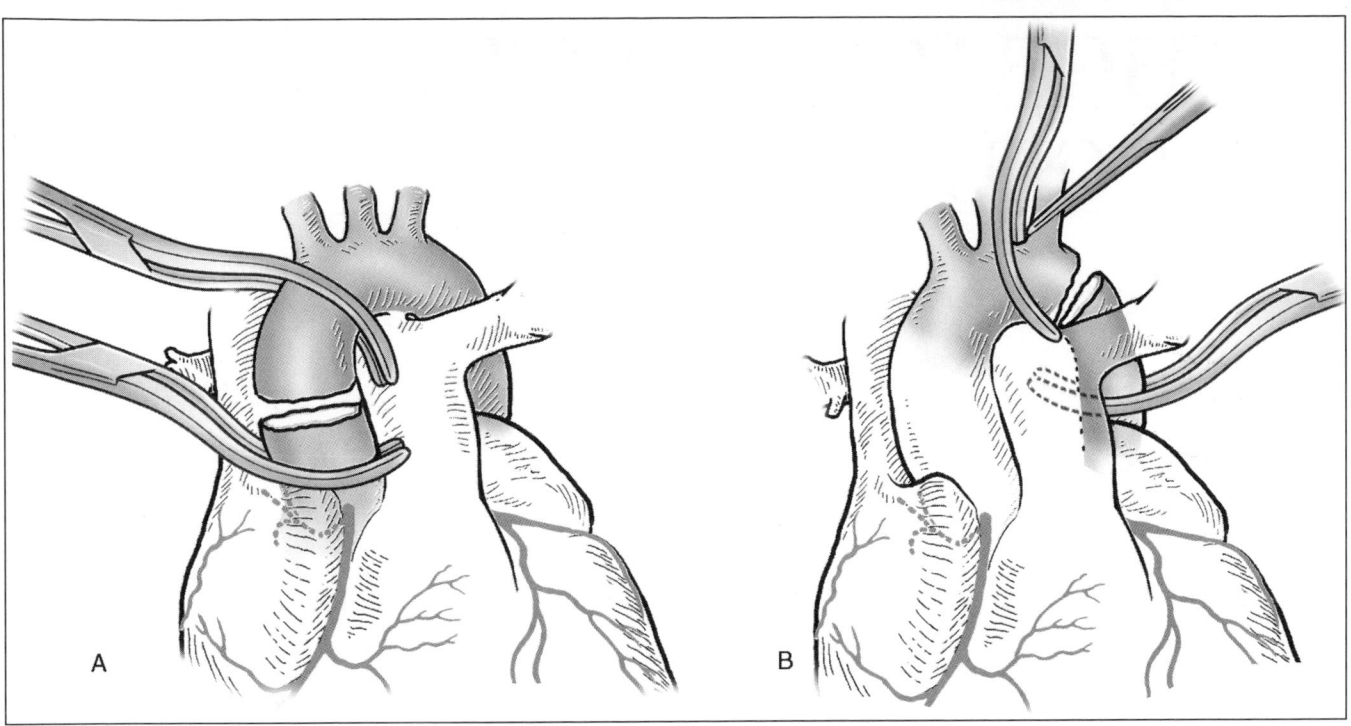

FIGURE 34-3 Cross-clamping of vascular injuries. *A.* Cross-clamp the great vessels to provide temporary hemostasis. *B.* Distal vessels must also be cross-clamped to prevent backbleeding.

REFERENCES

1. Mattox KL, Wall MJ, LeMaire SA: Injuries to the thoracic great vessels, in Mattox KL, Feliciano DV, Moore F.F. (eds): *Trauma,* 4th ed. New York: McGraw-Hill, 2000:559–582.

2. Mattox KL, Feliciano DV, Burch J, et al: Five thousand seven hundred sixty cardiovascular injuries in 4459 patients: epidemiologic evolution 1958–1987. *Ann Surg* 1989; 209(6):698–707.

Chapter 35
THORACIC AORTIC OCCLUSION

Faran Bokhari

INTRODUCTION

Temporary thoracic aortic occlusion should be performed during an Emergency Department thoracotomy for hypovolemic shock. It preserves cerebral and coronary artery perfusion pressure.[1] The blood flow to the viscera below the cross clamp, however, falls to less than 10 percent of baseline flow.[2] This can be advantageous since it stops distal hemorrhage, but it can later result in the undesired metabolic consequences of acidosis, hyperkalemia, and multiple organ system failure.[3,4]

ANATOMY AND PATHOPHYSIOLOGY

The aorta begins at the left ventricle and gives rise to the arteries of the body, directly or indirectly (Figure 35-1). It leaves the ventricle and is directed upward as the ascending aorta. It arches to the left and backwards at the level of the sternal angle to become the aortic arch. The arch gives rise to the brachiocephalic trunk, left common carotid artery, and left subclavian artery. The aortic arch is directed inferiorly after giving rise to the left subclavian artery and is known as the descending aorta. The descending aorta is subdivided into the thoracic portion above the diaphragm and the abdominal portion below the diaphragm. It descends through the posterior mediastinum, lying first against the left side of the fifth thoracic vertebral body. As it descends, it gradually approaches the midline of the 12th thoracic vertebral body, at which point it passes through the diaphragm.

The esophagus is a thin, muscular tube measuring approximately 2.0 to 2.5 cm in diameter. It descends along the vertebral bodies. It travels forward, away from the vertebral bodies, and to the right at the level of the ninth thoracic vertebral body. It traverses the diaphragm at the level of the 10th thoracic vertebral body. It lies posterior and medial to the descending thoracic aorta throughout most of its course. It migrates as it travels distally, so that its lower part lies in front of the aorta just above the diaphragm (Figure 35-1).

INDICATIONS

The primary reason to occlude the descending thoracic aorta is to temporarily direct blood flow from below the diaphragm to preserve flow to the brain and heart. The descending thoracic aorta may be occluded in patients with penetrating thoracic or abdominal trauma in which hypovolemic shock and clinical deterioration are not responsive to aggressive fluid resuscitation and blood transfusion. These patients should have the appropriate indications to perform an anterolateral thoracotomy (Chapter 31). The thoracic aorta may also be occluded immediately prior to laparotomy if the patient has a tense abdomen filled with blood. The abdominal incision will decompress the abdomen and result in hypotension, decreased coronary and cerebral perfusion pressure, exsanguination, and death. Uncontrollable hemorrhage below the diaphragm can be controlled by temporarily occluding the descending thoracic aorta.

CONTRAINDICATIONS

There are no absolute contraindications to temporarily occluding the descending thoracic aorta after performing an anterolateral thoracotomy. The thoracotomy should not be performed if the patient has obvious signs of death, no vital signs in the field, or no vital signs for over 15 minutes.

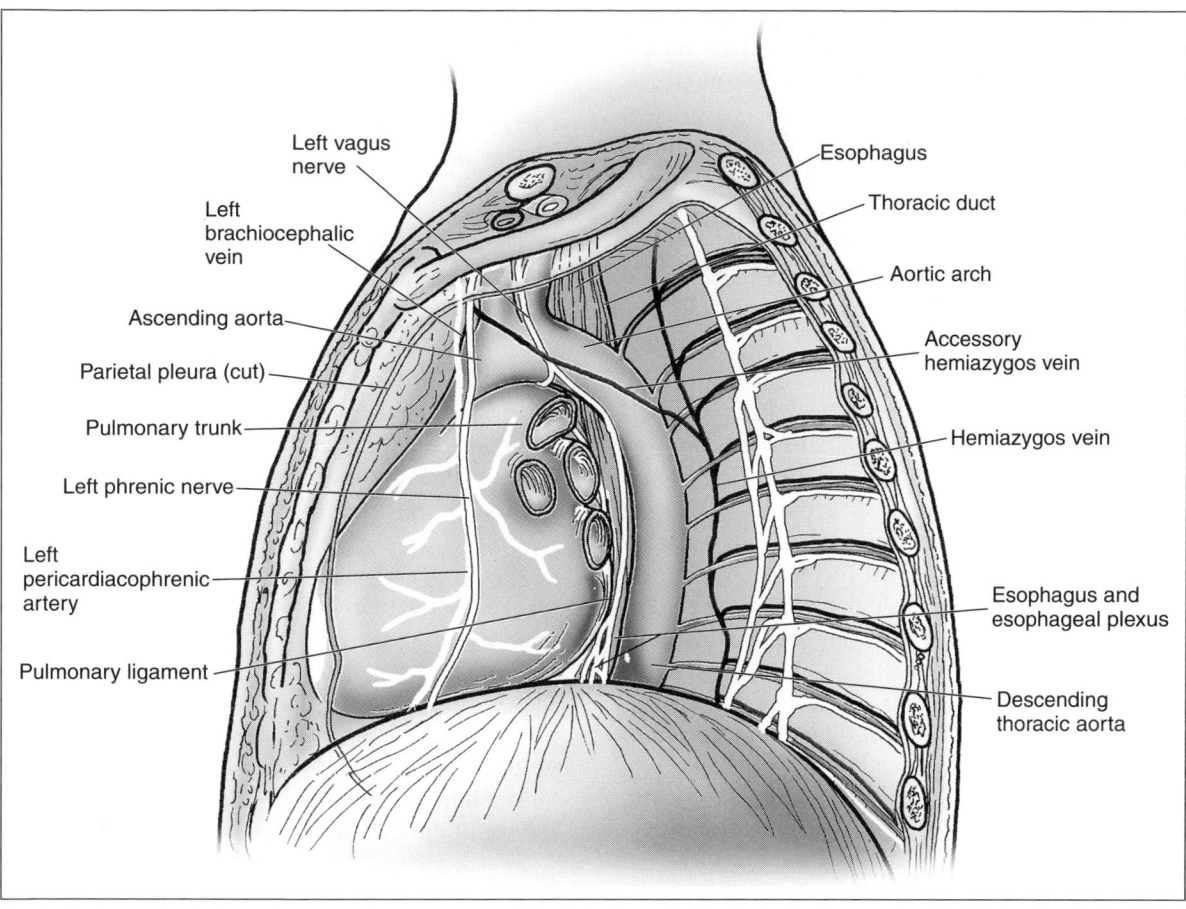

FIGURE 35-1 Anatomy of the aorta and surrounding structures of the mediastinum and left hemithorax. The mediastinal pleura has been removed to visualize the underlying structures.

EQUIPMENT

Satinsky vascular clamp
Metzenbaum scissors
DeBakey or large Kelly clamp
Nasogastric tube
Aortic compressor, Conn or homemade
Gauze, 4×4 squares

PATIENT PREPARATION

There is no preparation required other than performing an anterolateral thoracotomy (Chapter 31). The patient should be intubated, ventilated, and monitored with telemetry, pulse oximetry, and a noninvasive blood pressure cuff. Insert a nasogastric tube.

TECHNIQUE

Identify the aorta by palpation. It is often easier to identify and isolate the aorta just above the diaphragm. In this location, the aorta is slightly separated from the adjacent esophagus. Elevate the left lung with the nondominant hand superiorly and medially. Instruct an assistant to maintain the lung out of the way. Place the dominant hand through the thoracotomy incision and into the posteroinferior recess of the thoracic cavity. Advance the hand along the diaphragm and toward the midline. The fingers will first encounter the vertebral bodies. The next palpable structure is the aorta. It lies anterior to the vertebral bodies. The aorta may be difficult to palpate if it is collapsed in the patient with hypovolemic shock. In the elderly, the aorta may be significantly calcified, which helps to identify it despite hypovolemia. The aorta is covered by the mediastinal pleura. Place the thumb and index finger of the nondominant hand over the aorta just above the diaphragm.

Isolate the aorta. Bluntly dissect open the mediastinal pleura overlying the aorta with a DeBakey clamp or a large curved Kelly clamp. **Never use a scalpel to open the mediastinal pleura, as it may lacerate the aorta.** Some physicians may prefer to use a Metzenbaum scissors to dissect and open the mediastinal pleura. Identify the aorta by palpation. Bluntly separate the aorta from the esophagus with the dominant hand. It may be extremely difficult to separate the aorta from the esophagus in the patient with hypotension, hypovolemia, and/or shock. Place a nasogastric tube if this has not been done previously. The nasogastric tube will be palpable within the esophagus and can be used to identify the esophagus. Hook the dominant index finger around the aorta. **Use the finger to separate the aorta from the vertebral bodies. The dissection should not be extensive. It should free approximately 3 to 4 cm of the descending thoracic aorta.**

DIRECT COMPRESSION

Direct compression of the aorta is fast and simple, it does not interfere with the operative field, and it causes less damage than the application of a clamp. Digital compression is often ineffective. Aortic compression devices have a unique shape to occlude the aorta atraumatically by compressing it against the vertebral bodies. It may be applied before or after the aorta is isolated. Homemade compression devices may use rubber tubing to occlude the aorta[5] (Figure 35-2A). The Conn compressor is commercially available and uses a metal plate to occlude the aorta (Figure 35-2B). Place the distal end of the compression device against the distal descending thoracic aorta (Figure 35-2C). Apply downward pressure to occlude the aorta. The degree of occlusion can be controlled by increasing or decreasing the pressure applied to the aorta.

CROSS-CLAMPING

The descending thoracic aorta is most commonly occluded with an atraumatic or Satinsky vascular clamp. Aortic compression devices are rarely available in Emergency Departments or on thoracotomy trays. The aorta must first be separated and isolated from the esophagus, as described above. Place an index finger behind the descending thoracic aorta to elevate it away from the underlying esophagus (Figure 35-3A). Place the Satinsky vascular clamp over the aorta. One jaw should be posterior to the aorta and adjacent to the index finger while the other jaw is anterior to the aorta. Clamp the aorta and remove the index finger (Figure 35-3B).

It is imperative not to clamp the esophagus. Do not clamp the aorta before it is dissected from the esophagus. Esophageal injury can lead to perforation, ischemia, and sepsis if the patient is resuscitated. Ideally, the clamp should be placed under direct visualization of the aorta. Unfortunately, this is not always practical. The index finger under the aorta can confirm the proper isolation of the aorta and the proper position of the jaws of the clamp before the aorta is occluded.

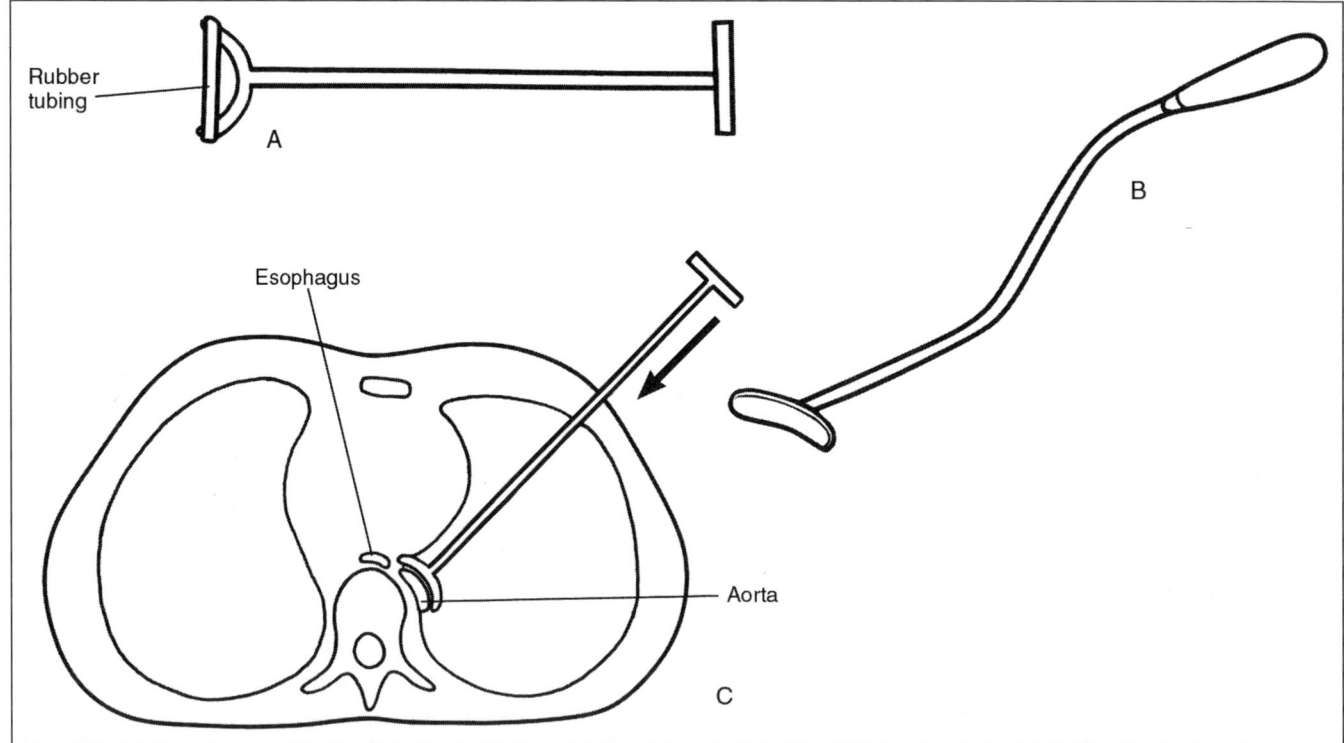

FIGURE 35-2 Aortic compression. *A.* The homemade aortic compression device.[5] *B.* The commercially available Conn compressor. *C.* The aorta is compressed between the distal end of the compression device and the thoracic vertebral body.

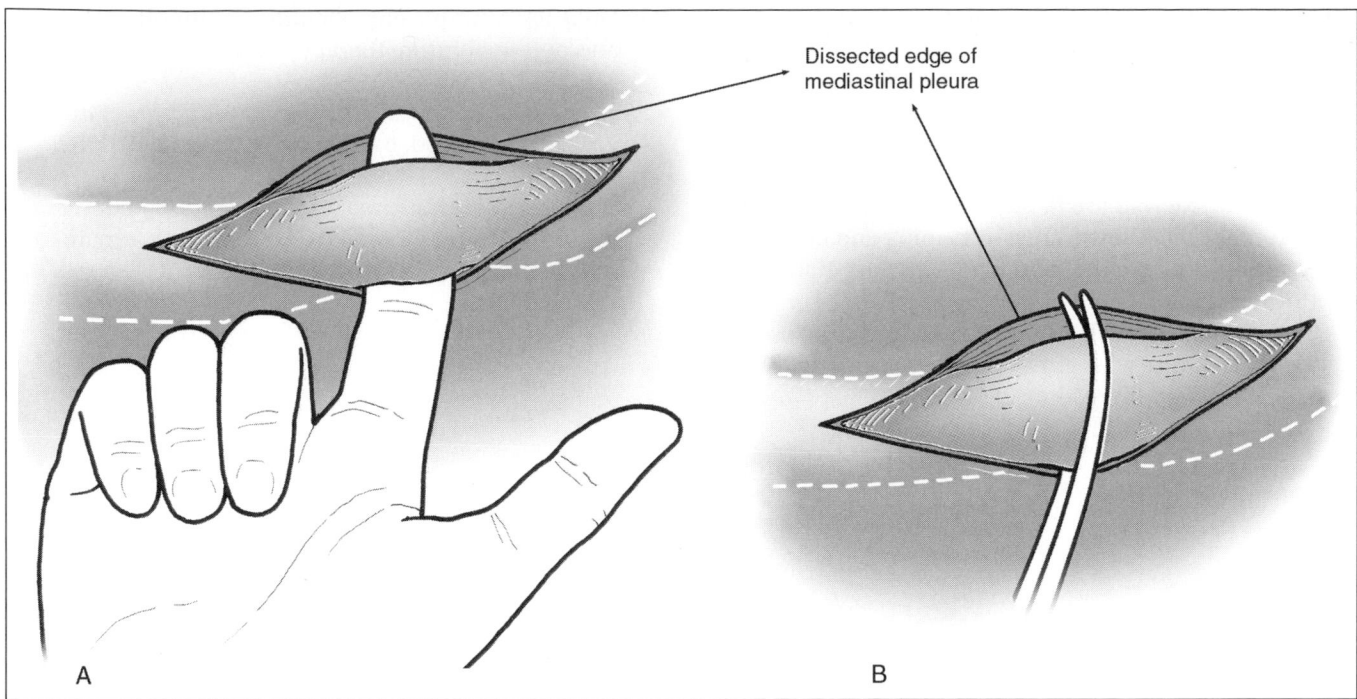

FIGURE 35-3 Aortic cross-clamping. *A.* The mediastinal pleura has been bluntly opened and the aorta isolated from the esophagus. *B.* The Satinsky clamp is placed across the aorta to occlude distal blood flow.

AFTERCARE

If—after the thoracotomy, open cardiac massage, and aortic cross-clamping—there is return of a cardiac rhythm and a carotid pulse, the patient must be taken immediately to the operating room for definitive treatment. The patient's blood pressure in the upper extremity should be monitored every 30 to 60 seconds after the aorta is occluded. An elevated blood pressure can result in a hemorrhagic stroke or left ventricular failure. Elevated blood pressure will require intermittent release of the aortic occlusion and/or pharmacologic management. Parenteral broad-spectrum antibiotics should be administered to prevent infection.

COMPLICATIONS

Intercostal arteries arising from the thoracic aorta can be damaged during mobilization of the aorta. This will result in troublesome bleeding that requires operative control. The aorta, vena cava, or the esophagus can be damaged by the clamp. Aortic cross-clamping can precipitate hypertension, stroke, and left-sided heart failure. If the patient is successfully resuscitated, this should be dealt with by periodically releasing the clamp. Lack of blood flow through the artery of Adamkiewicz will cause ischemia of the distal spinal cord. There is a 5 percent incidence of paraplegia when the blood supply to the distal aorta and spinal cord is disrupted. This incidence increases dramatically when the spinal cord is ischemic for more than 30 minutes.[6]

Aortic cross-clamping causes visceral ischemia. The gut loses its barrier function and becomes a cytokine-generating organ, which leads to a systemic inflammatory response and multiple organ failure. Renal and liver failure can result from a lack of blood flow.

The organs distal to the aortic clamp become severely ischemic and receive only 10 percent of the basal cardiac output. The anaerobic metabolism in these organs generates lactic acid. When the aortic clamp is released, acid and potassium are released into the central circulation and can cause a cardiac arrest. Thus bicarbonate must be given at this time and the cardiac rhythm monitored carefully.

SUMMARY

Aortic cross-clamping is a useful adjunct to open cardiac massage in hypovolemic shock. It can help salvage patients by increasing coronary and cerebral perfusion. It may be performed as a lifesaving and temporizing measure until the patient can be taken to the operating room for definitive management.

REFERENCES

1. Michel JB, Bardou A, Tedgui A, et al: Effect of descending thoracic aorta clamping and unclamping on phasic coronary blood flow. *J Surg Res* 1984; 36:17–24.
2. Oyama M, McNamara JJ, Suehiro GT, et al: The effects of thoracic aortic cross-clamping and declamping on visceral organ blood flow. *Ann Surg* 1983; 197:459–463.
3. Grotz MRW, Deitch EA, Ding J, et al: Intestinal cytokine response after gut ischemia—role of gut barrier failure. *Ann Surg* 1999; 229(4):478–486.
4. Deitz EA: Multiple organ failure—pathophysiology and potential future therapy. *Ann Surg* 1992; 216(2):117–134.
5. Simon RR, Brenner BE: *Emergency Procedures and Techniques,* 4th ed. Baltimore: Williams & Wilkins, 1994:144–145.
6. Safi HJ, Miller CC: Spinal cord protection in descending thoracic and thoracoabdominal aortic repair. *Ann Thorac Surg* 1999; 67:1937–1939.

Section Three
VASCULAR PROCEDURES

Chapter 36
GENERAL PRINCIPLES OF INTRAVENOUS ACCESS

Robert Feldman

INTRODUCTION

The practice of Emergency Medicine frequently requires access to a patient's venous circulation. Venous access allows sampling of blood as well as administration of medications, nutritional support, and blood products. Devices such as cardiac pacing wires and pulmonary artery catheters can be introduced into the patient's central venous circulatory system.

Percutaneous, as opposed to surgical, venous access is usually rapid, safe, and well tolerated. An understanding of the various techniques available, patient anatomy, and indications for the procedure allows the practitioner to choose the appropriate site and method of venous access.

ANATOMY AND PATHOPHYSIOLOGY

Veins, like arteries, have a three-layered wall composed of an internal endothelium surrounded by a layer of muscle then a layer of connective tissue[1] (Figure 36-1). The muscular layer of a vein is much weaker than that of an artery. While veins can dilate and constrict somewhat on their own, they do so mostly in response to the pressure within them. Veins with high pressures become engorged and are easier to access. The use of venous tourniquets, dependent positioning, "pumping" via muscle contraction, and the local application of heat or nitroglycerin ointment all contribute to venous engorgement.[2] These maneuvers can be used to aid in the performance of a venipuncture or peripheral venous access.

The connective tissue surrounding veins can be a help or a hindrance during attempts at peripheral venous access. Deficient connective tissue permits the vein to "roll" from side to side and evade the needle. Tough connective tissue can impede the entry of a flexible catheter through the soft tissues and into the vein.

This tissue also serves to stabilize the vein and prevent its collapse.

Venous valves are an important aspect of peripheral venous anatomy[1] (Figure 36-2). They encourage unidirectional flow of blood back towards the heart. Venous valves prevent blood from pooling in the dependent portions of the extremities due to gravitational forces. Valves can impede the passage of a catheter through and into a vein. Forcing a catheter past venous valves may damage them and contribute to later venous insufficiency. Valves are more numerous at the points where tributaries join larger veins and in the lower extremities. Valves are almost totally absent within the large central veins, the veins of the head, and the veins of the neck.

Veins can be subdivided into central veins and peripheral veins. The important central veins with regard to venous access are the internal jugular, subclavian, and femoral veins. Central veins are usually larger than peripheral veins and have fewer tributaries.

Superficial peripheral veins are generally visible beneath the surface of the skin of the extremities and neck. They are often tortuous and continually merge and divide. Peripheral veins are easiest to access at the apex of the "Y" formed when two tributaries merge into a larger vein or where the vein is straight and free of branches (and hence valves) for 2 cm or so proximal to the site of puncture (Figure 36-3). These sites tend to be anchored and "roll" less than other sites. The superficial veins of the upper extremity are preferred to those of the lower extremity for peripheral venous access. Indwelling catheters in the upper extremity interfere less with patient mobility and the risk of phlebitis is lower.[1]

The depth of the vein beneath the epidermis will affect the ease with which it may be accessed. Very superficial veins are often small, fragile, and easily passed "through and through" with a needle, resulting in a hematoma. The deeper veins are often not visible and

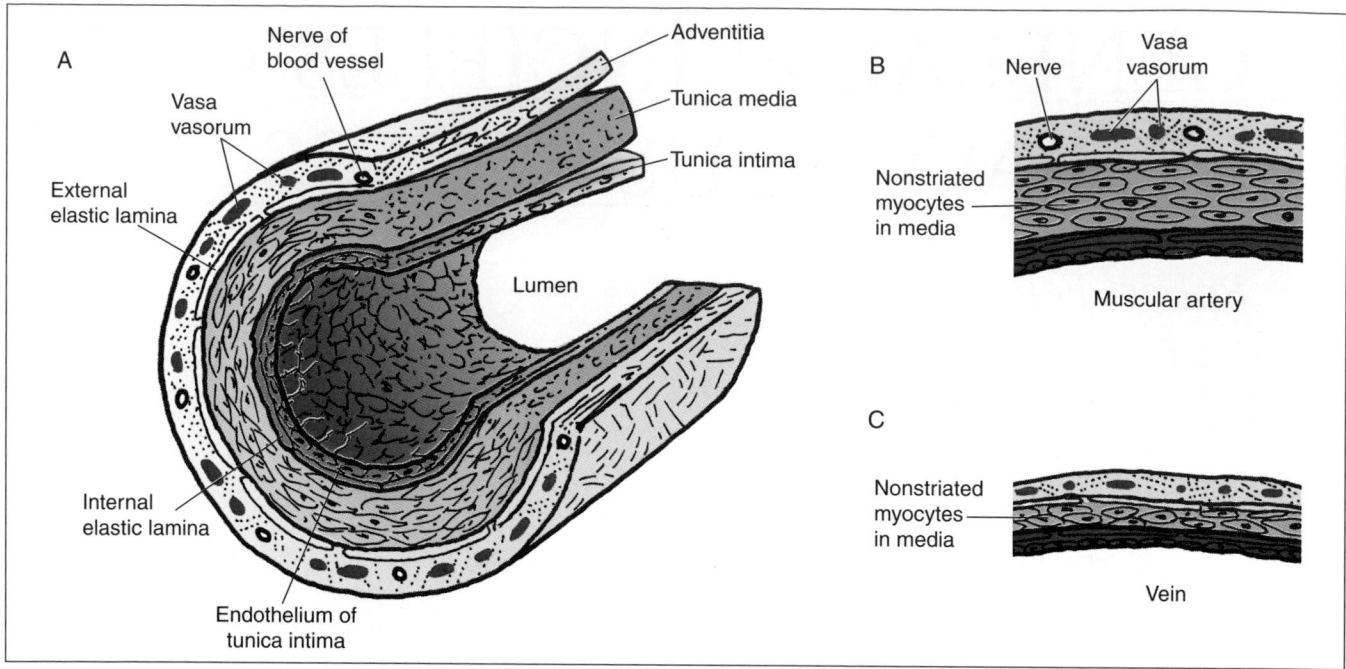

FIGURE 36-1 Comparative anatomy of an artery and a vein. Note the vein's thinner wall with fewer myocytes and elastic fibers. This is indicative of the lower pressure within veins compared to arteries.

must be located by surface landmarks and palpation. The angle of insertion of the needle must be varied depending on the depth of the vein being punctured (Figure 36-4). A shallow angle (30 to 45 degrees) should be used for small and superficial veins (Figure 36-4A). A more obtuse angle (60 degrees) should be used to access deeper veins (Figure 36-4B). This steeper angle allows the vein to be penetrated within a reasonable horizontal distance from the skin puncture site. Very small and superficial veins should be entered at a very acute (15 to 30 degrees) angle (Figure 36-4C).

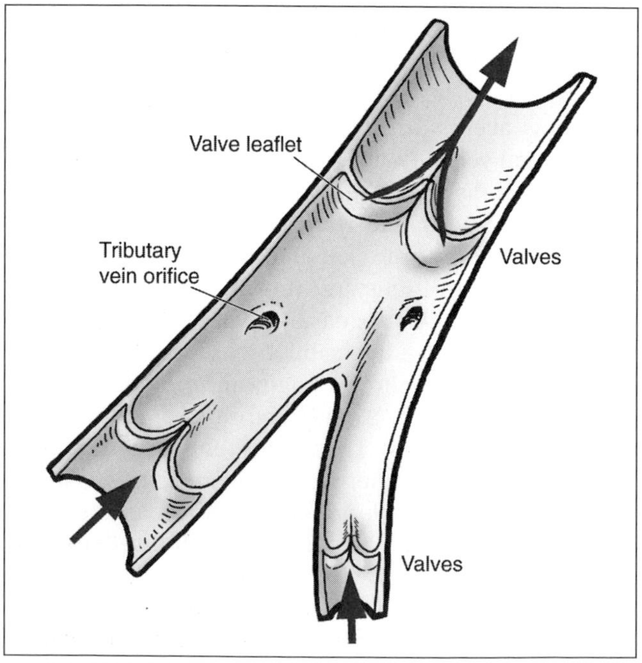

INDICATIONS

Venous puncture (venipuncture) with a needle is indicated only for the sampling of venous blood. Medications may be administered as a one-time dose via this technique. The risk of medication extravasation with this technique is high, and it has therefore fallen out of favor.

Venous cannulation is indicated for repeated sampling of venous blood. It is also performed for the administration of intravenous medications, fluid solutions, blood products, and nutritional support. The specific indications for peripheral venous access, central venous access, and the various techniques of venous cannulation are discussed below and in Chapters 37 and 38.

CONTRAINDICATIONS

Veins should not be accessed through infected skin. A vein proximal to a running venous infusion should not be used for venous blood sampling. The blood sample will be tainted or diluted by the infused solution. The

FIGURE 36-2 Venous valves. Cross-section of converging veins demonstrating the valve leaflets that only permit forward flow, proximally, toward the right heart. The arrows represent the directional flow of blood.

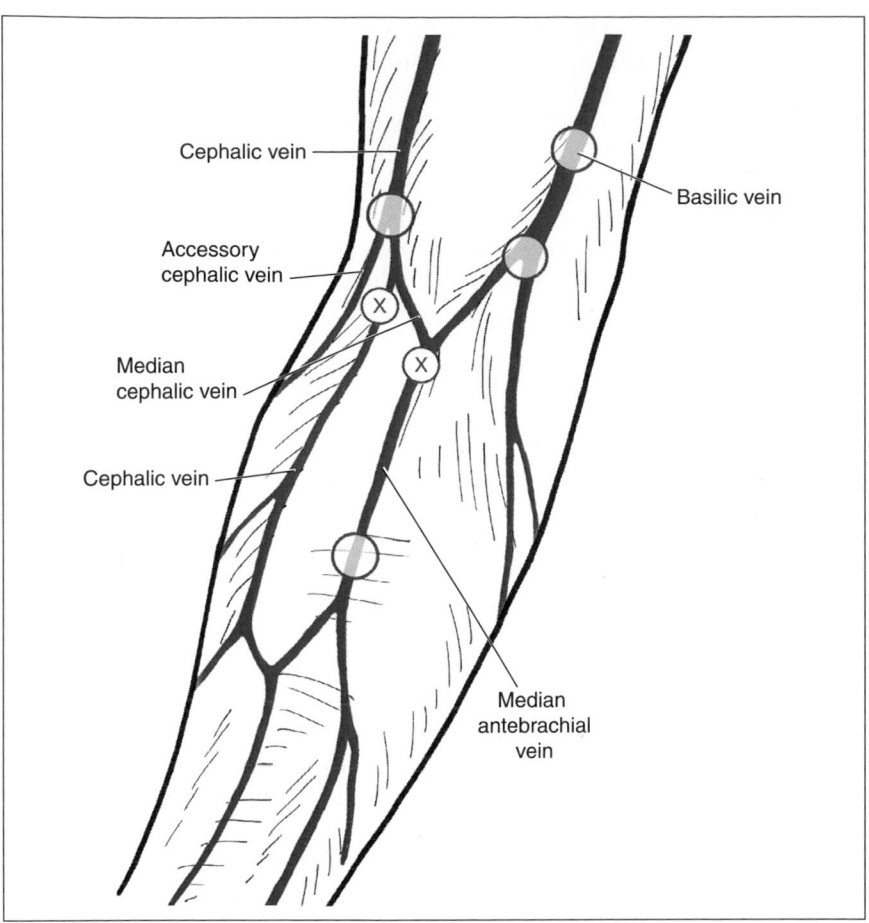

FIGURE 36-3 Preferred venous access sites. Preferred sites (red "O") are at the apex of converging veins or in the middle of a long straight vein. Sites just distal to branching or convergence of veins (red "X") are best avoided due to the presence of valves and the difficulty in threading a cannula.

hole in the vein may allow blood, infused solutions, and medications to extravasate into the surrounding tissues.

Venipuncture and venous cannulation of veins in an extremity with an arteriovenous fistula should be avoided. Veins in the upper extremity that may be needed for arteriovenous fistula construction for hemodialysis in the near future should not be punctured unless absolutely necessary. Scarring of the vein may complicate later surgical procedures.

CATHETER MATERIALS

Indwelling catheters are made of flexible polymers that are less likely to break or erode through the vessel wall than more rigid materials such as steel or glass. Polymer resins, Teflon, and polyurethane are commonly used materials. Latex-containing products should be avoided due to the risk of allergic reactions. Polyurethane catheters may be weakened by alcohol-based solutions.[1] Thus, such solutions should not be infused through polyurethane catheters.

All catheters are potentially thrombogenic. They should be left in place only as long as needed. Catheters impregnated with antiseptics, such as chlorhexidine and silver sulfadiazine, are commercially available and may decrease the incidence of catheter-related sepsis.[4] Chlorhexidine has been associated with immediate hypersensitivity reactions, most commonly in persons of Japanese descent.[5] Silver sulfadiazine has not been proven safe to use in sulfa-sensitive patients. Catheters are also available that, when immersed in an antibiotic solution prior to insertion, allow an antibiotic to bind to their surface. These catheters may reduce the risk of infection with organisms susceptible to the chosen antibiotic, which is usually vancomycin.

FLUID-FLOW CONSIDERATIONS

Both the diameter and the length of the infusion device will affect the flow rate through the catheter. Viscous fluids (e.g., blood products and albumin) will infuse more slowly than less viscous fluids (e.g., saline). These relationships can be seen in the solution of Poiseuille's equation for ideal fluid flow through a cylindrical tube:

$$\text{Flow rate} \propto (\pi \times \text{catheter radius}^4 \times \text{pressure gradient along the tube})$$
$$\div (8 \times \text{tube length} \times \text{dynamic fluid viscosity})$$

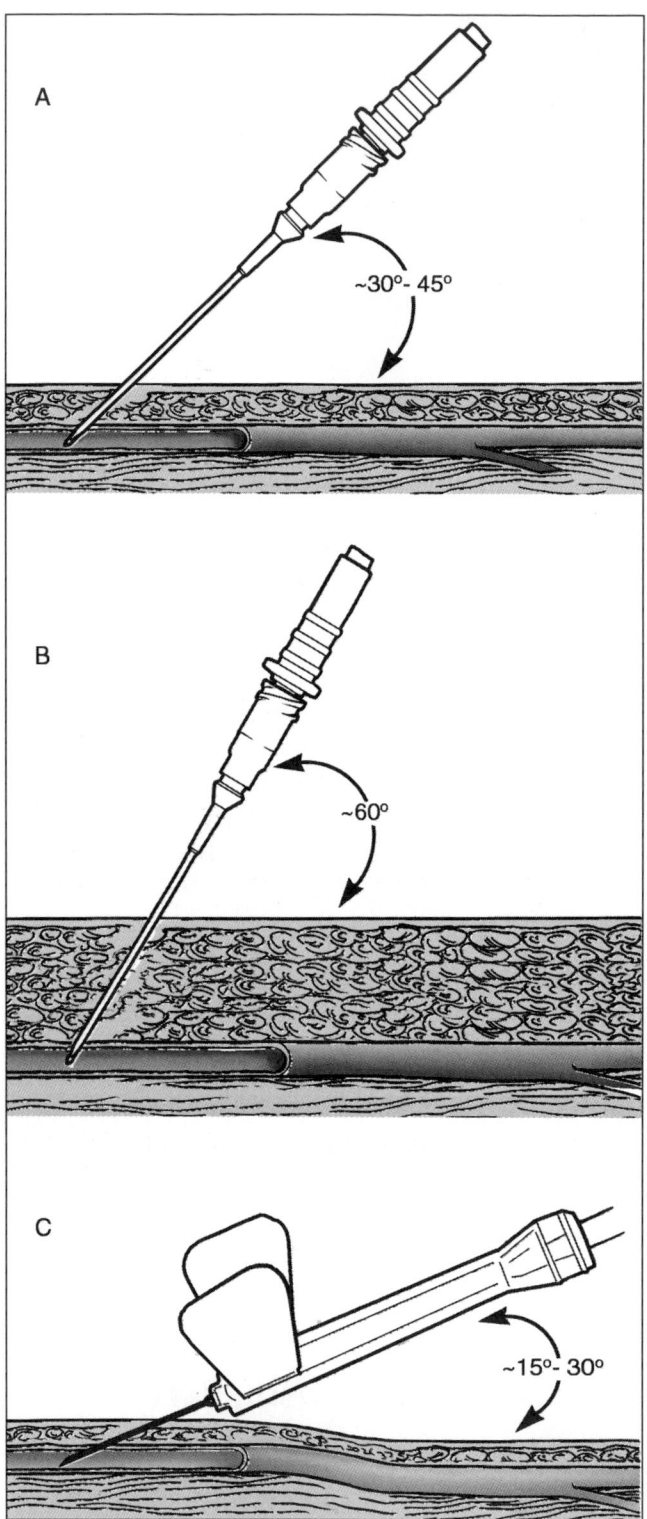

FIGURE 36-4 The angle between the needle and the skin must be varied based upon the depth and diameter of the target vein. *A.* A shallow angle must be used for small and superficial veins. *B.* A steeper angle must be used for deeper veins. *C.* A butterfly-type needle permits the shallowest angle of entry for very small and superficial veins.

The pressure gradient and resistance to flow is inversely proportional to the length of the tubing. Changes in catheter diameter will have the most effect on flow rates. The flow rate increases to the fourth power as the catheter's internal radius increases. Flow rates can be maximized by using the largest internal diameter (smallest-gauge) catheter that will fit inside the chosen vein. Large-bore venous catheters are preferred for the highest-volume rapid fluid resuscitations, particularly of viscous blood products. Flow rates decrease as catheter length increases. Use of the shortest possible catheter to access the chosen vein will permit the highest fluid infusion rates. External pressure applied to the bag of infusion solution will linearly increase the flow rate.

VENIPUNCTURE

Five types of devices are used for vascular access (Figure 36-5). There are numerous variations of these devices. The butterfly needle and hollow needle are used for venipuncture. Blood may be withdrawn using a butterfly-type needle (Figure 36-6) or a standard hypodermic needle. The butterfly needle, attached to a short length of plastic tubing, allows for greater control while accessing small and superficial veins. It is often too short to reach deeper veins. Versions with an integral sheath to minimize accidental needle sticks are available (Figure 36-7A).

Venous blood sampling can be accomplished by one of several methods. Blood may be allowed to drip from the open end of the butterfly extension tubing into small-volume collection tubes in small pediatric patients. Some form of suction is used to withdraw the blood more rapidly in older children and adults. A syringe or vacuum tube may be used (Figure 36-8). Vacuum tubes reduce the risk of needle-stick injuries. The amount of suction provided is fixed and may result in hemolysis of the specimen and cause small veins to collapse. Syringe aspiration allows greater control over the amount of suction applied. Large syringes can be difficult to manipulate while maintaining the tip of the needle in the vein. Use a 5 to 10 mL syringe, as larger syringes result in hemolysis of the specimen and collapse of the vein. Use caution, as the needle used to transfer the specimen from the syringe to the laboratory tubes can cause a needle-stick injury.

VENOUS CANNULATION

There are four main techniques of vein cannulation.[6-8] The first is the needle-only, using a butterfly-type needle. This is seldom used today. The catheter-over-the-needle technique is the one most commonly

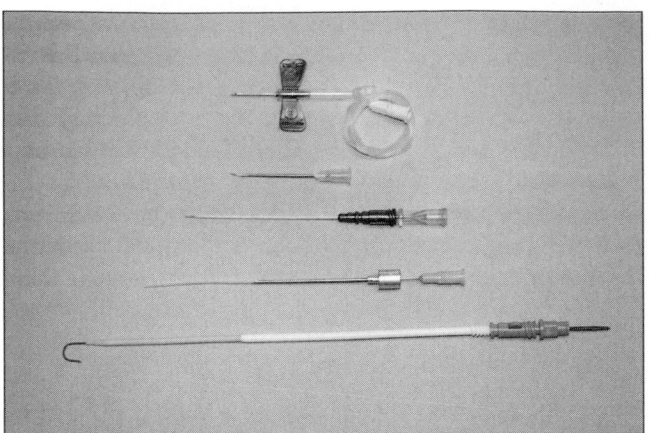

FIGURE 36-5 Venous access devices. *From top to bottom:* butterfly needle with extension tubing, hollow needle, catheter-over-the-needle, catheter-through-the-needle, and the wire-guided catheter.

used for peripheral venous cannulation. The catheter-through-the-needle technique is occasionally used but not very popular. The Seldinger wire-guided technique is most commonly used for central venous access. The major advantages and disadvantages of each technique are summarized in Table 36-1.

Identify the vein to be cannulated and the site of the skin puncture. Clean the area of any dirt and debris. Cleanse the skin with isopropyl alcohol or povidone iodine. Apply a tourniquet to the extremity, proximal to the venous cannulation site, to engorge the vein. Additional engorgement of the vein can be accomplished by placing the extremity in a dependent position, "pumping" via muscle contractions of the extremity, and applying heat or nitroglycerin ointment over the vein. **Do not attempt cannulation if the vein cannot be seen or palpated in the engorged state.** A small subcutaneous wheal of local anesthetic solution may be placed at the skin puncture site to provide some comfort to the patient. The next step is to cannulate the vein by one of the methods described below.

NEEDLE-ONLY TECHNIQUE

This technique is used occasionally for short-term venous access in young children and elderly patients with fragile veins. This system is prone to malposition and infiltration. The tip of the needle can easily lacerate the vein if the needle is not secure and allowed to move.

Grasp and fold the wings of the butterfly needle with the dominant index finger and thumb (Figure 36-6B). Briskly insert the needle through the skin and into the vein. A flash of blood will be seen in the tubing when the tip of the needle enters the vein. Carefully advance the needle an additional 3 to 5 mm into the vein. Attach a 5 mL syringe to the extension tubing and aspirate blood. The flow of blood into the syringe confirms proper

intravascular placement of the needle. Remove the tourniquet from the extremity. Securely tape the wings of the butterfly needle to the patient's skin. Remove the 5 mL syringe, attach intravenous tubing to the catheter, and begin the intravenous infusion.

CATHETER-OVER-THE-NEEDLE TECHNIQUE

The catheter-over-the-needle systems are the ones most commonly used for venous access. The infusion catheter fits closely over a hypodermic needle. The needle and the catheter are advanced as a unit into the vein. These devices are inexpensive (about $1 to $4 each), come in a variety of diameters (12- to 24-gauge) and lengths, and are widely available. Versions designed to minimize accidental needle-stick injuries are available and their use is encouraged[10] (Figure 36-7B).

Insert the catheter-over-the-needle through the skin and into the vein (Figure 36-9A). A flash of blood in the hub of the needle confirms that the tip of the needle is within the vein. Advance an additional 2 to 3 mm to ensure that the catheter is within the vein. Hold the hub of the needle securely. Advance the catheter over the needle until its hub is against the skin (Figure 36-9B). Apply pressure, with the nondominant index finger, over the catheter to prevent blood from exiting the catheter. Remove the tourniquet from the extremity. Withdraw the needle (Figure 36-9C). Attach intravenous tubing to the hub of the catheter and begin the infusion (Figure 36-9D). Secure the catheter to the skin with tape.

Placement of these catheters is usually quick and simple. Several considerations should always be kept in mind when using the catheter-over-the-needle technique. Intravascular placement of the system is indicated by a flash of blood in the hub of the needle. If the patient's venous pressure is very low or if the needle is long and narrow, both sides of the vessel may be traversed (through and through) before the practitioner realizes that the needle was within the vein (Figure 36-10A). If the tip of the needle is withdrawn from the vein, the catheter will not advance. If the catheter is advanced when the tip of the needle but not the catheter is within the vein, the catheter will not advance. The catheter will push the vein off the needle (Figure 36-10B). Place a finger just distal to the puncture site. Depress the skin and pull it distally to prevent the vein from "rolling" as the catheter-over-the-needle is inserted into the vein (Figures 36-10C and D).

CATHETER-THROUGH-THE-NEEDLE TECHNIQUE

As opposed to the over-the-needle approach, this technique eliminates the need for a needle that is as long as the catheter and eliminates the possibility of pushing the vein off the end of the needle when the catheter is advanced.[11] This system is used most

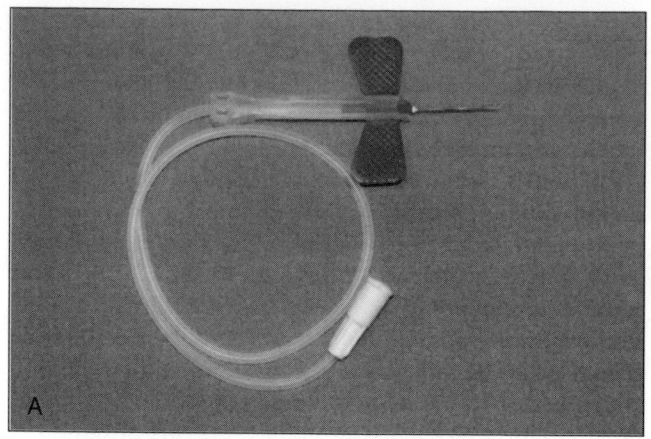

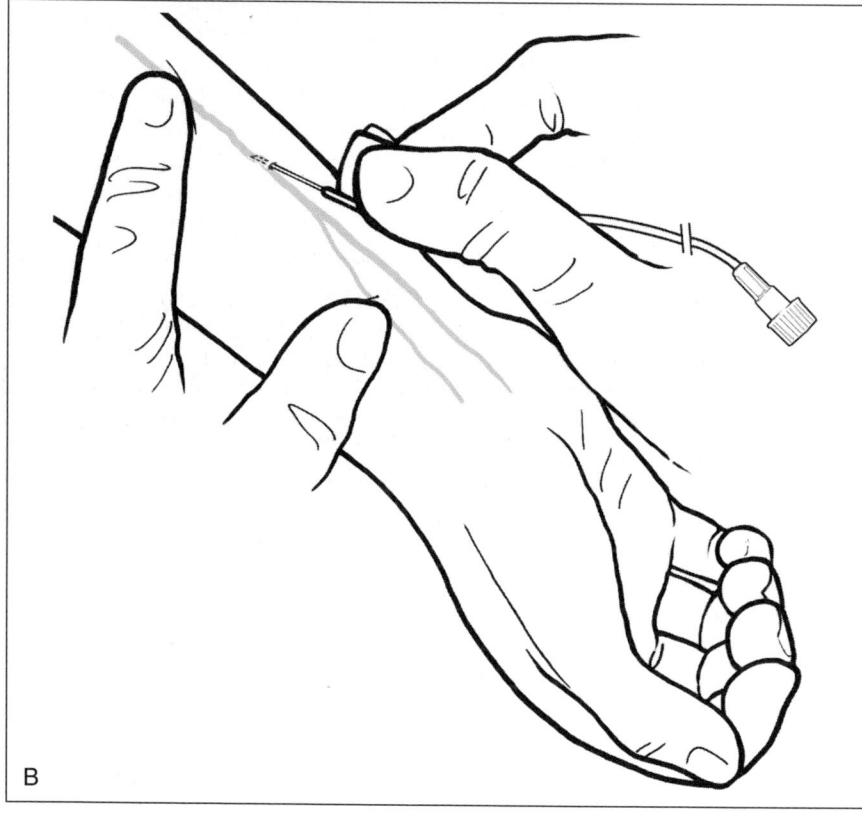

FIGURE 36-6 The butterfly–type needle. *A.* Butterfly needle with attached extension tubing. *B.* The wings of the catheter are folded together and used to direct the needle into the superficial vein. The needle may be secured within the vein and used as an infusion cannula or removed after blood samples are collected.

commonly for central, rather than peripheral, venous access. Catheters up to 61 cm (24 inches) long are available and allow central venous access from the antecubital vein or the femoral vein. Select a catheter size that is appropriate for the patient and the site of entry. Packaged with each catheter is a needle and a needle guard. The needle will have an inner diameter that is slightly larger than the outer diameter of the catheter. The needle guard has a beveled channel in which the needle can reside. The needle guard hinges closed over the needle to hold it securely and prevent the needle from shearing the catheter. Holes in the corners of the needle guard allow it to be sewn to the patient's skin.

Place the needle on a tuberculin syringe. Insert the needle through the skin and into the vein while applying negative pressure to the syringe (Figure 36-11*A*). A flash of blood in the syringe confirms that the tip of the needle is within the vein. Advance the needle an additional 2 mm to ensure that the tip of the needle is completely within the vein. Grasp and hold the needle securely with the nondominant hand. Remove the syringe with the dominant hand. Immediately place the nondominant thumb over the needle hub to prevent air from entering the vein. Remove the tourniquet from the extremity.

Insert the catheter through the hub of the needle (Figure 36-11*B*). Advance the catheter through the needle

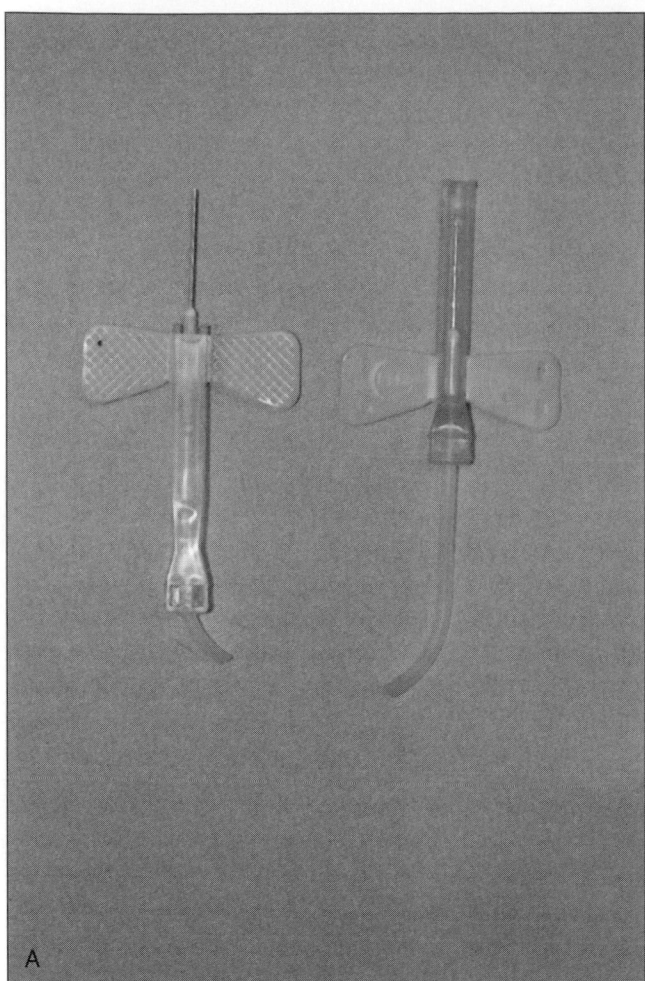

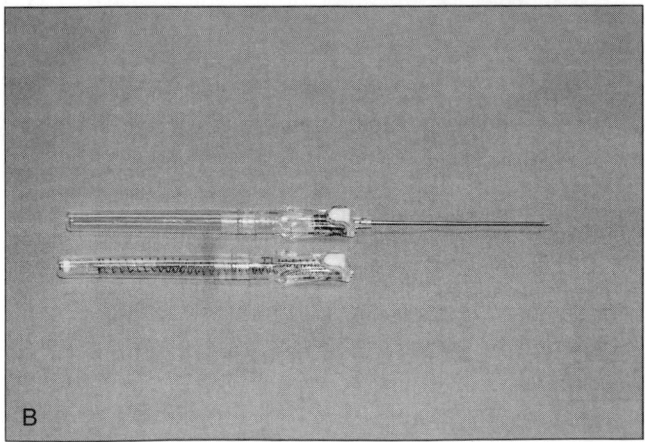

FIGURE 36-7 Needle-stick prevention devices.
A. Butterfly needle with an integral needle sheath. The left figure demonstrates the sheath retracted and the needle exposed. The right figure demonstrates the needle safety sheathed. *B.* The spring-loaded catheter-over-the-needle system. The top figure demonstrates the catheter-over-the-needle. The bottom figure demonstrates the needle inside the safety handle.

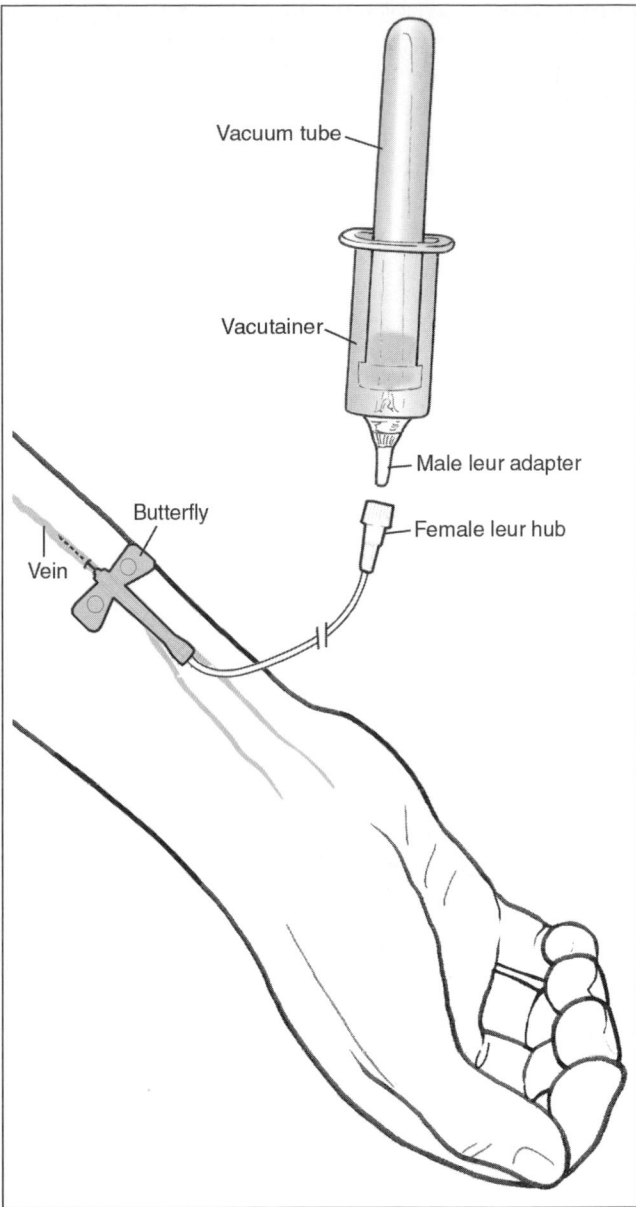

FIGURE 36-8 The Vacutainer. Once the needle is inserted into the vein, a Vacutainer adapter is connected to the female Luer hub. Specimens can be collected into different types of vacuum tubes without the risk of an accidental needle stick. However, the suction applied by the vacuum tube, unlike a syringe, cannot be controlled and may cause hemolysis and/or a small vein to collapse.

until the desired length of catheter is within the vein. **If the catheter will not advance, remove the catheter and needle as a unit. Never withdraw the catheter through the needle. The sharp bevel of the needle may cut the catheter as it is being withdrawn and result in a catheter embolism in the central venous circulation.**

Withdraw the needle over the catheter (Figure 36-11*C*). **Do not allow the catheter to be withdrawn through the needle.** Continue to withdraw the needle

TABLE 36-1. FEATURES OF VENOUS CATHETERIZATION TECHNIQUES

	Butterfly needle	Catheter-over-the-needle	Catheter-through-the-needle	Seldinger
Diameter of vein punctured compared to catheter diameter	Same	Slightly smaller	Larger	Smaller
Catheter length compared to needle	Same	Slightly shorter	Longer, up to 61 cm (24 inches)	Unlimited
Speed of insertion	Rapid	Rapid	Slower	Slowest
Risk of extravasation	Highest	Low, higher with shorter catheters	Low	Very low
Security of catheter with patient movement	Lowest	Fair to good	Good	Excellent when sutured
Best choice for	Peripheral venous sampling	Peripheral venous infusion	Central venous access	Central venous access
Can change catheter without new venous puncture?	No	Can use small wire and Seldinger technique	No	Yes

until the tip is completely outside the skin. Apply the needle guard over the needle (Figure 36-11D). Attach intravenous tubing to the hub of the catheter and begin infusing fluids through the catheter. Secure the catheter and needle guard to the skin with tape and/or sutures.

The main disadvantage of this technique is the possibility of the needle tip shearing off the catheter, causing a catheter embolism in the venous circulation. **This can be prevented by not withdrawing the catheter through the needle and applying the needle guard immediately after the needle is withdrawn from the skin.** The contaminated needle must be handled to some extent, creating a potential risk for needle-stick injuries. The needle used for the venipuncture must be larger in diameter

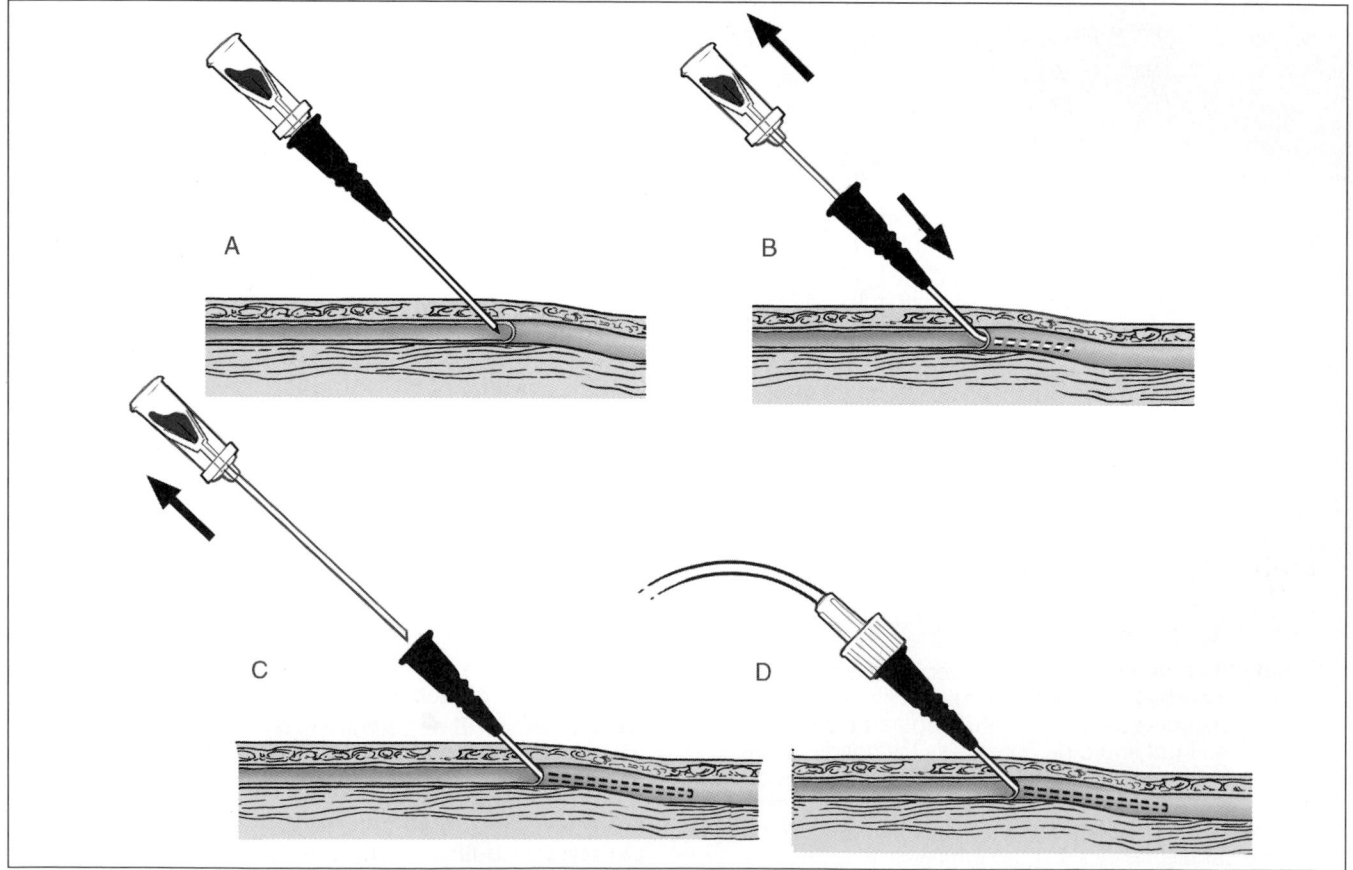

FIGURE 36-9 The catheter-over-the-needle technique. *A.* The vein is punctured and blood returns in the needle hub. *B.* The catheter is advanced over the needle and into the vein. *C.* The needle is removed. *D.* Intravenous extension tubing is attached to the catheter.

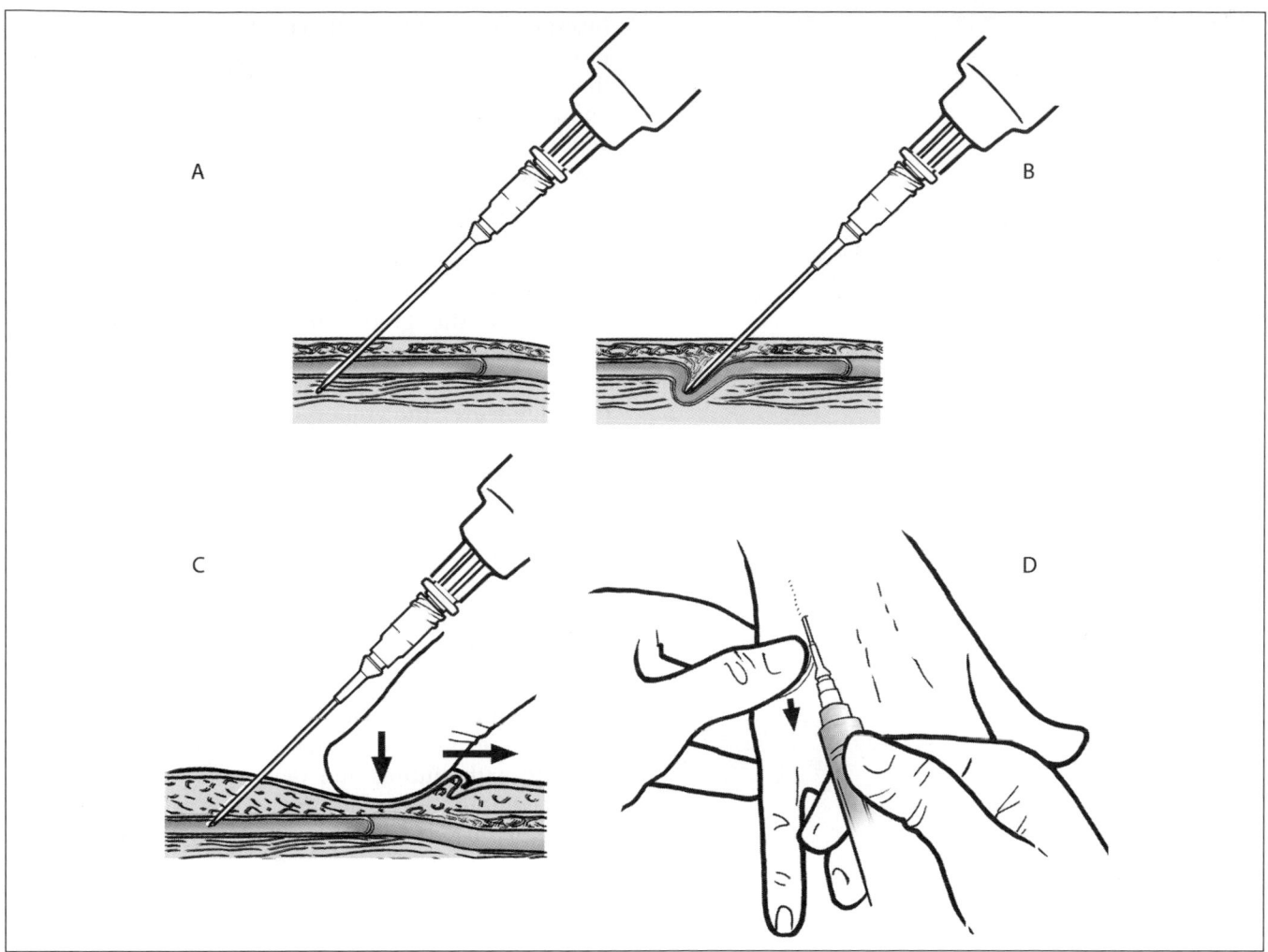

FIGURE 36-10 Pitfalls of the catheter-over-the-needle technique. *A.* Through-and-through puncture of the vein. *B.* The catheter can push the vein off the needle and prevent cannulation. *C.* Push a finger into the skin distal to the puncture site and pull back (*arrow*) to keep the vein straight and prevent it from moving. *D.* The nondominant thumb is used to pull the skin and stabilize the vein.

than the catheter. This limits the practical diameter of the catheter. The needle punctures a hole in the vessel larger than the catheter and increases the risk of hematoma formation.

SELDINGER TECHNIQUE

First described by Seldinger in 1953, this technique allows for the placement of a catheter over a wire rather than directly over a needle.[12,13] The wire used must be longer than the catheter. The needle used to insert the wire can be short and of a smaller gauge than the catheter. If desired, the catheter type may be changed later without the need for a new venous puncture. Materials needed for catheter insertion are commercially available in a prefabricated kit (Arrow International, 800-523-8446; Cook Inc., 800-457-4500).

The Seldinger technique is most commonly used for central venous catheter insertion. It can be used for pe-

ripheral venous access if a short, thin guidewire is available. All-in-one kits are available from Arrow (product RA-04020). They are intended for peripheral arterial line placement but can also be used to place catheters in the brachial veins and the external jugular veins.

The Seldinger technique for venous catheter insertion is described briefly here. Refer to Chapter 38 (central venous access techniques) for a more complete discussion. Choose the puncture site. Prepare the patient for the procedure. Cleanse the area of the puncture site of any dirt and debris. The vein may first be located with a small "finder" needle if there is doubt about its exact location. Insert a 25 or 27 gauge needle attached to a 5 mL syringe through the skin. Advance the needle while applying negative pressure to the syringe. A flash of blood signifies that the tip of the needle is within the vein. Note the depth and location of the vein based on the depth and direction of the "finder" needle.

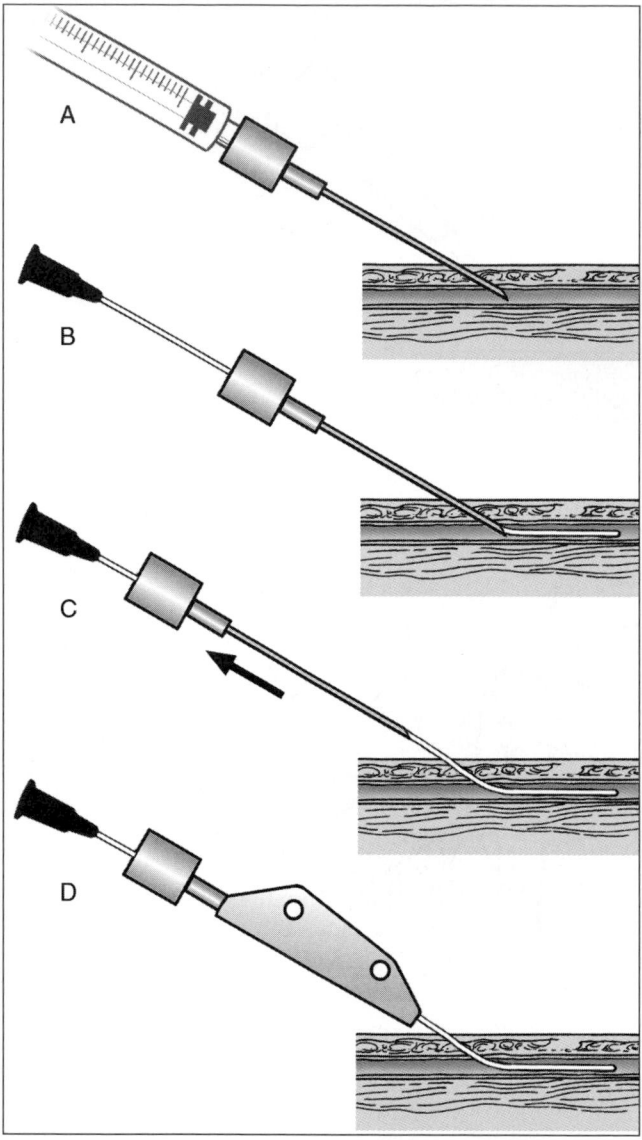

FIGURE 36-11 The catheter-through-the-needle technique.[9,11] *A.* The vein is punctured with the needle. *B.* The syringe has been removed. The catheter is inserted through the needle and into the vein. *C.* The needle is withdrawn over the catheter and completely outside the skin. *D.* The needle guard is attached to secure the needle and prevent it from shearing the catheter.

Insert the thin-walled introducer needle while applying negative pressure to the syringe. The introducer needle has a tapered hub on the proximal end to guide the wire into the needle lumen. Avoid using a standard hypodermic needle, as it does not allow for the passage of the guidewire. A flash of blood in the needle hub signifies that the tip of the needle is within the vein (Figure 36-12*A*). Advance the needle an additional 1 to 2 mm into the vein. Hold the needle securely in place and remove the syringe.

Occlude the needle hub with a sterile gloved finger. This will prevent air from entering the venous system.

Insert the guidewire through the hub of the needle (Figure 36-12*B*). Advance it to the desired depth, ensuring that it is at least several centimeters beyond the beveled end of the needle. **To prevent loss of the wire into the venous circulation, never let go of the guidewire with both hands at the same time.** Hold the guidewire securely in place. Remove the needle over the guidewire (Figure 36-12*C*). Make a small nick in the skin adjacent to the guidewire with a #11 scalpel blade (Figure 36-12*D*). **Direct the sharp edge of the scalpel blade away from the guidewire to prevent nicking the guidewire.**

Place the plastic dilator over the guidewire. Advance the dilator over the guidewire to enlarge the subcutaneous passage for the catheter. Continue to advance the dilator until the hub is against the skin. Withdraw the dilator over the guidewire while leaving the guidewire in place. Advance the catheter over the guidewire and to the desired depth (Figure 36-12*E*). A twisting motion of the catheter may aid in its advancement through the skin and into the vein. Remove the guidewire through the catheter (Figure 36-12*F*).

Aspirate blood from the catheter with a syringe to confirm intravenous placement. Flush the catheter with sterile saline or begin an infusion. Secure the catheter to the skin with sutures and tape. While this technique seems complicated at first glance, it is easy to learn and can be performed in a few minutes by an experienced physician.

COMPLICATIONS

Complications specific to each technique and site are discussed more fully in the following chapters. Venous catheters should be assessed immediately after their placement and also be reassessed frequently. The assessment must include the skin puncture site, catheter function, the extremity distal to the catheter, and the patient's overall condition. Some of the common problems are noted in Table 36-2. Other specific complications of peripheral and central venous access are discussed in the following chapters.

SUMMARY

Venous access is an essential skill for all providers of care to the acutely ill and injured. As with most procedures, success rates increase and complication rates decrease with experience. Successful venipuncture or cannulation is not the end of the provider's obligation to the patient. Frequent reassessment of the venous access site, the equipment, and the patient is essential to prevent serious complications.

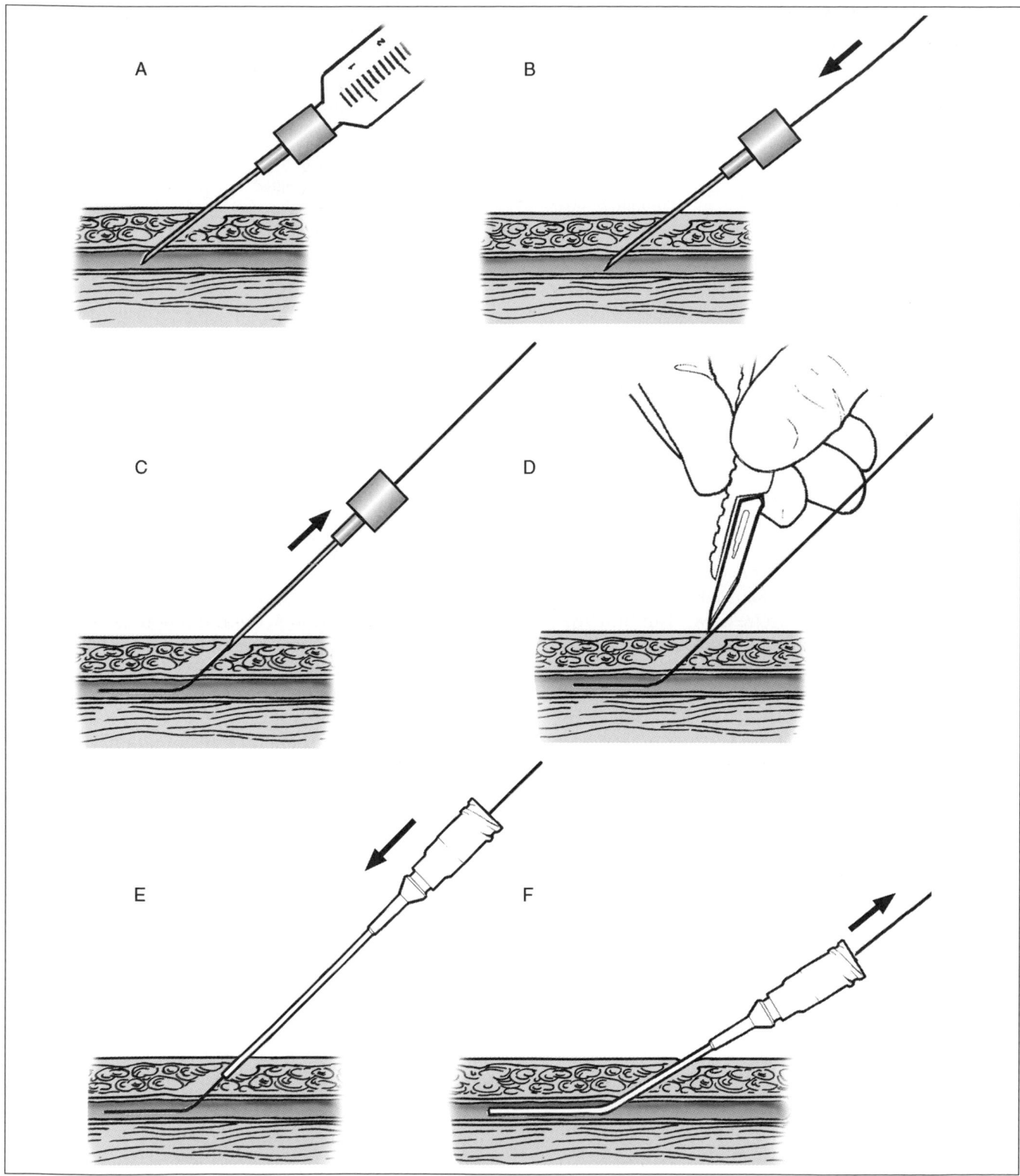

FIGURE 36-12 The Seldinger technique. *A.* The vein is punctured by the needle and blood is aspirated. *B.* The syringe has been removed. The guidewire is inserted through the needle and into the vein. *C.* The needle is withdrawn over the guidewire. *D.* The skin puncture site is enlarged to permit catheter passage. *E.* The catheter is advanced over the guidewire and into the vein. *F.* The guidewire is withdrawn through the catheter.

TABLE 36-2. COMPLICATIONS OF VENOUS CATHETERIZATION

	Observation	Complications	Errors in technique	Response
Skin puncture site	Immediate swelling	Hematoma	Laceration or through-and-through puncture	Remove catheter, apply pressure
Skin puncture site	Delayed swelling	Extravasation or hematoma	Catheter dislodged or damaged, vein lacerated	Remove catheter, apply pressure
Skin puncture site	Erythema or discharge	Infection	Catheter in place too long, catheter or skin contaminated	Remove catheter, give parenteral antibiotics
Catheter	Cannot infuse	Thrombosis or kinking	Catheter not flushed enough, catheter not secured properly	Flush catheter, check position, remove catheter
Catheter	Blood runs up IV tubing	Arterial placement	Arterial puncture not recognized	Remove catheter, apply pressure
Catheter	Cannot aspirate from proximal lumens of multi-lumen line	Extravascular placement or migration of proximal lumens	Not enough catheter inserted; patient movement; catheter not properly secured	Change catheter over a wire if distal port is intravascular
Systemic	Fever	Line sepsis	Catheter left in place too long or contaminated	Remove catheter once infection is verified
Systemic	Hemodynamic or respiratory compromise	Pneumothorax, pericardial tamponade	Pleura punctured during insertion; catheter tip malpositioned	Chest radiograph, auscultate chest; pericardial or pleural drainage

REFERENCES

1. Williams PL, Warwick R: *Gray's Anatomy,* 36th ed. Philadelphia: Saunders, 1980:629–765.
2. Vaksmann G, Rey C, Breveire G-M, et al: Nitroglycerine ointment as aid to venous cannulation in children. *J Pediatr* 1987; 111(1):89–91.
3. Bledsoe BE: *Atlas of Paramedic Skills.* Engelwood Cliffs, NJ: Prentice-Hall, 1987:124–142.
4. *Arrow Single-Lumen Central Venous Catheterization,* product manual. Reading, PA: Arrow International, 1995.
5. Maki DG, Stolz SM, Wheeler S, et al: Prevention of central venous catheter–related bloodstream infection by use of an antiseptic-impregnated catheter: a randomized, controlled trial. *Ann Intern Med* 1997; 127:257–266.
6. Oda T, Hamasaki J, Kanda N, et al: Anaphylactic shock induced by an antiseptic-coated central venous catheter. *Anesthesiology* 1997; 87:1242–1244.
7. Hambrick EL, Georges GC: Peripheral intravenous access, in Roberts JR, Hedges JR (eds): *Clinical Procedures in Emergency Medicine,* 3rd ed. Philadelphia: Saunders, 1998:322–333.

8. Bhende MS: Venipuncture and peripheral venous access, in Henretig FM, King C: *Textbook of Pediatric Emergency Procedures.* Baltimore: Williams & Wilkins, 1997:797–810.
9. Lavelle J, Costarino A: Central venous access and central venous pressure monitoring, in Henretig FM, King C (eds): *Textbook of Pediatric Emergency Procedures.* Baltimore: Williams & Wilkins, 1997:251–278.
10. Orenstein R: The benefits and limitations of needle protectors and needleless intravenous systems. *J Intraven Nurs* 1999; 22(3):122–128.
11. *Intracath: Directions for Use.* Sandy, UT: Deseret Medical, 1987.
12. Seldinger SI: Catheter replacement of the needle in percutaneous arteriography: a new technique. *Acta Radiol* 1953; 39:368–376.
13. Dailey RH: Use of wire-guided (Seldinger-type) catheters in the emergency department. *Ann Emerg Med* 1983; 12(8):489–492.

Chapter 37
VENIPUNCTURE AND PERIPHERAL INTRAVENOUS ACCESS

Robert Feldman

INTRODUCTION

Puncture of a peripheral vein is the most common invasive procedure performed in the Emergency Department. While some newer point-of-care testing techniques require only capillary blood, the vast majority of laboratory studies require venous blood. Cannulation of a peripheral vein is performed on a daily basis and is the cornerstone of circulatory resuscitation; it is an essential skill for all emergency personnel, from phlebotomists to nurses to physicians. A variety of approaches for obtaining peripheral venous access are described in this chapter.

ANATOMY AND PATHOPHYSIOLOGY

Veins and arteries are composed of a three-layered wall of internal endothelium surrounded by a layer of muscle then a layer of connective tissue[1] (Figure 37-1). The muscular layer of a vein is much thinner and weaker than that of an artery. While veins can dilate and constrict somewhat on their own, they do so mostly in response to the pressure within them. Veins with high internal pressures become engorged and are easier to access. The use of venous tourniquets, dependent positioning, "pumping" via muscle contraction, and the local application of heat or nitroglycerin ointment all contribute to venous engorgement.[2] These maneuvers can be used to aid in the performance of a venipuncture or cannulation of a peripheral vein.

The connective tissue surrounding veins can be a help or a hindrance during attempts at gaining peripheral venous access. Deficient connective tissue permits the vein to "roll" from side to side and evade the needle.

Tough connective tissue can impede the entry of a flexible catheter through the soft tissues and into the vein. This tissue also serves to stabilize the vein and prevent its collapse.

Venous valves are an important aspect of peripheral venous anatomy[1] (Figure 37-2). Venous valves encourage unidirectional flow of blood back to the heart. Because of gravitational forces, they prevent blood from pooling in the dependent portions of the extremities. Valves can impede the passage of a catheter through and into a vein. Forcing a catheter past venous valves may damage them and contribute to later venous insufficiency. Valves are more numerous at the points where tributaries join larger veins and in the lower extremities. Valves are almost totally absent within the large central veins, the veins of the head, and the veins of the neck.

Veins can be subdivided into central veins and peripheral veins. The important central veins with regard to venous access are the internal jugular, subclavian, and femoral veins. Central veins are usually larger than peripheral veins and have fewer tributaries.

Superficial peripheral veins are generally visible beneath the surface of the skin of the extremities and neck. They are often tortuous and continually merge and divide. Peripheral veins are easiest to access at the apex of the "Y" formed when two tributaries merge into a larger vein or where the vein is straight and free of branches (and hence valves) for 2 cm or so proximal to the site of puncture (Figure 37-3). These sites tend to be anchored and hence "roll" less than other sites. The superficial veins of the upper extremity are preferred to those of the lower extremity for peripheral venous access. Indwelling catheters in the upper extremity interfere less with patient mobility, and they pose a lower risk of phlebitis.[2] The superficial veins of the extremities are shown in

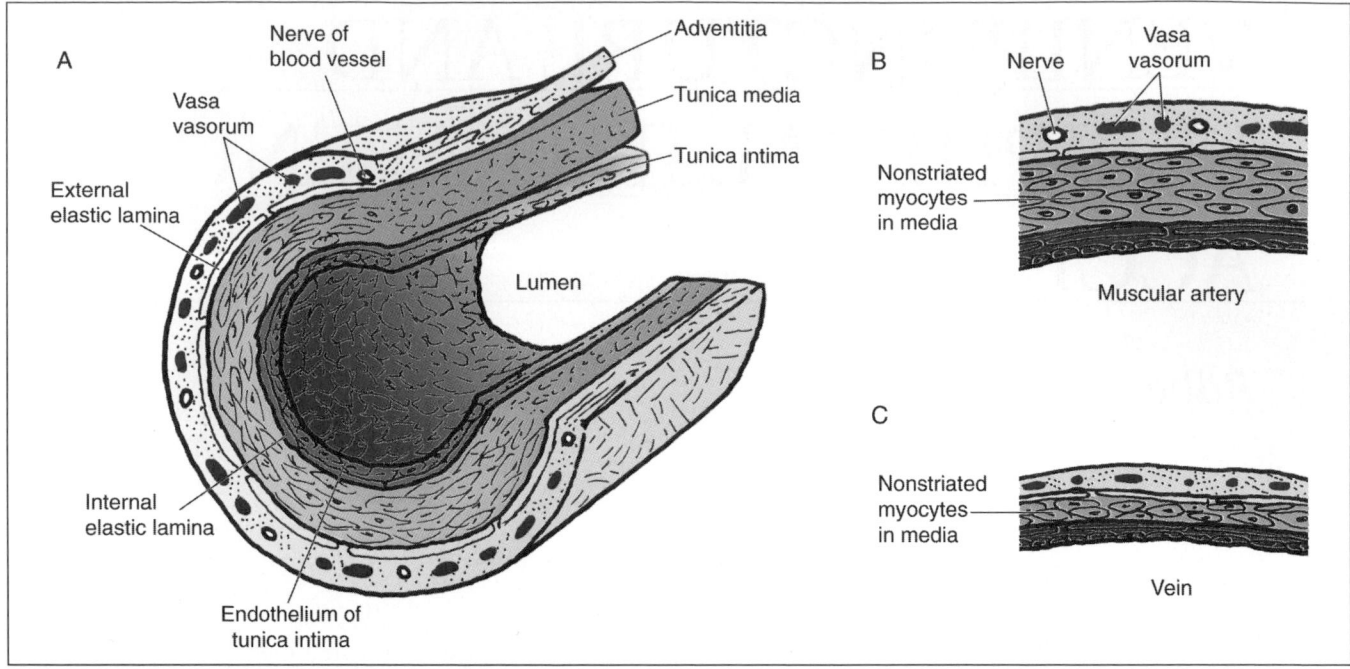

FIGURE 37-1 Comparative anatomy of an artery and a vein. Note the vein's thinner wall with fewer myocytes and elastic fibers. This is indicative of the lower pressure within veins compared to arteries.

Figures 37-4 and 37-5. The veins most commonly used for venous sampling are the basilic and cephalic veins as well as their branches and tributaries (Figure 37-4). The veins of the dorsal foot and the distal saphenous veins

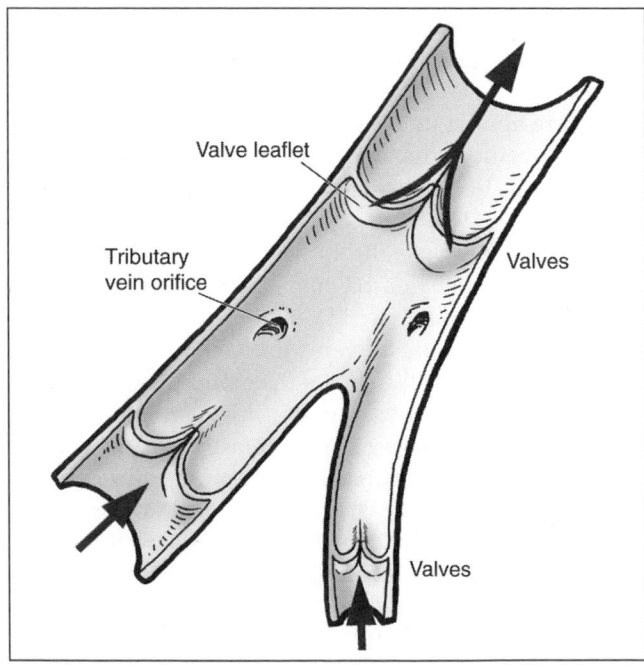

FIGURE 37-2 Venous valves. Cross section of converging veins demonstrating the valve leaflets that permit only forward flow, proximally, toward the right heart. The arrows represent the directional flow of blood.

are the most commonly used veins in the lower extremity (Figure 37-5).

The depth of the vein beneath the epidermis will affect the ease with which it may be accessed. Very superficial veins are often small, fragile, and easily passed "through and through" with a needle, resulting in a hematoma. The deeper veins are often not visible and must be located by surface landmarks and palpation. The angle of insertion of the needle must be varied depending on the depth of the vein being punctured (Figure 37-6). A shallow angle (30 to 45 degrees) should be used for small and superficial veins (Figure 37-6*A*). A more obtuse angle (60 degrees) should be used to access deeper veins (Figure 37-6*B*). This angle allows the vein to be penetrated within a reasonable horizontal distance from the skin puncture site. Very small and very superficial veins should be entered at a very acute (15 to 30 degree) angle (Figure 37-6*C*).

The upper extremity is preferred to the lower for vein cannulation, and distal placement should be attempted before moving more proximally.[3] Avoid veins overlying a joint if possible. Adherence to these simple principles will allow the patient maximum mobility and increase the chance of successfully cannulating a vein in the chosen extremity. Any solutions or medications infused distally can extravasate and injure the surrounding tissues once a proximal vein has been punctured unsuccessfully. It is easiest to insert a venous cannula where two tributaries merge and form a "Y." Choose a straight portion of vein without branches to minimize the chance of hitting valves within the vein; this also makes it easier to thread the catheter (Figure 37-3).

The deep brachial veins are variably located alongside the brachial artery, running lateral and/or medial to the artery[4,5] (Figure 37-7). The brachial veins are relatively small, not visible to the practitioner, have a close relationship to the brachial artery, and are thus not normally punctured. **It is important to prevent injury to the brachial artery when cannulating or puncturing the brachial veins.** The brachial artery is the sole arterial supply of the forearm, hand, and median nerve. The deep brachial veins may be used when superficial veins have been destroyed by scarring due to intravenous drug abuse, chemotherapy, or prior infusions. The location and cannulation of the brachial veins can be aided through the use of ultrasound.[6]

The neck is an important potential site for peripheral venous access through the external jugular vein (Figure 37-8). This vein begins at the level of the mandible and runs obliquely across the sternocleidomastoid muscle. It dives beneath the fascia in the subclavian triangle of the neck to join with the subclavian vein.[5] Some patients have double external jugular veins on one or both sides. The external jugular vein has two sets of valves (Figure 37-8). One is located where the external jugular vein joins the subclavian vein and the other is located about 4 cm above the clavicle. These valves are not fully competent but may prevent the passage of a guidewire or catheter.[5,7]

INDICATIONS

Peripheral venous access is indicated for venous blood sampling. It is also performed for the administration of intravenous medications, fluid solutions, and blood products. Peripheral venous lines may be used for

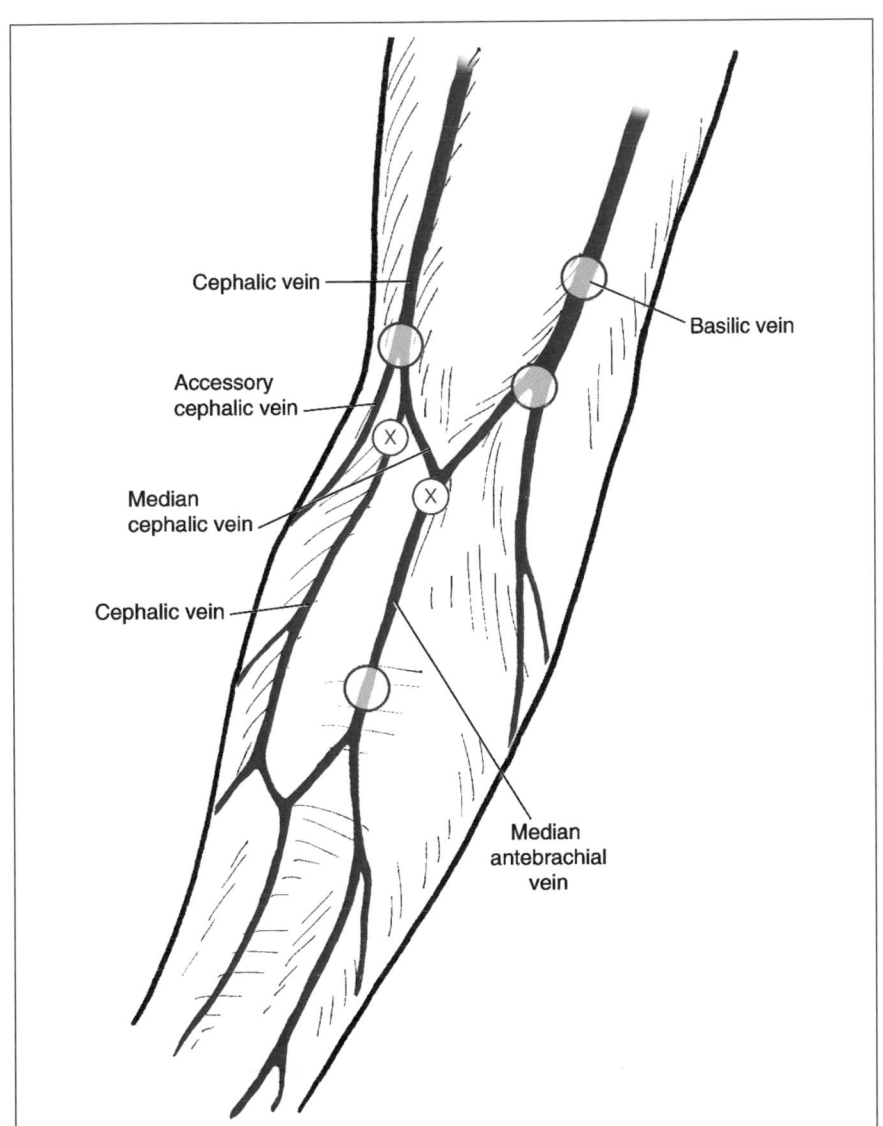

Cephalic vein

Accessory cephalic vein

Median cephalic vein

Cephalic vein

Basilic vein

Median antebrachial vein

FIGURE 37-3 Preferred vein entry points. Preferred sites (red "O") are at the apex of converging veins or in the middle of a long straight vein. Sites just distal to branching or convergence of veins (red "X") are best avoided due to the presence of valves and the difficulty in threading a cannula.

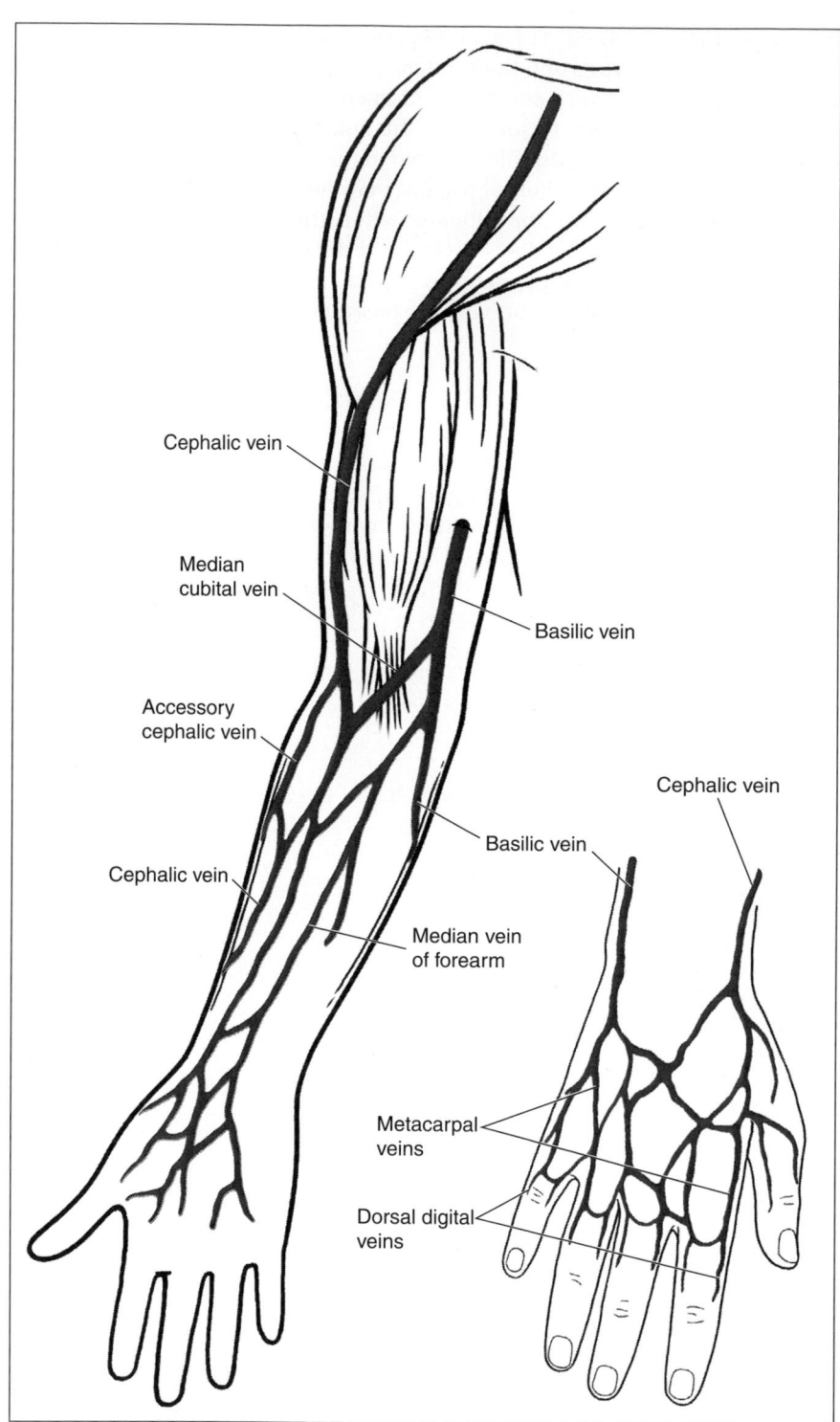

FIGURE 37-4 Superficial veins of the upper extremity. *A.* Volar surface of the upper extremity. *B.* Dorsal surface of the hand and wrist.

short-term partial nutritional support; full nutritional support requires central venous access.

CONTRAINDICATIONS

Sclerosing solutions, vasopressors, concentrated solutions of electrolytes or glucose, and chemotherapeutic agents are more safely infused into a central vein. Peripheral venous access in an injured extremity should be avoided, if possible, so as not to interfere with care of the injury and venous drainage of the limb. Avoid using the veins of an upper extremity for peripheral venous access if they may be used for the construction of an arteriovenous fistula for future dialysis. If possible, venipuncture should not be performed through infected or burned skin.

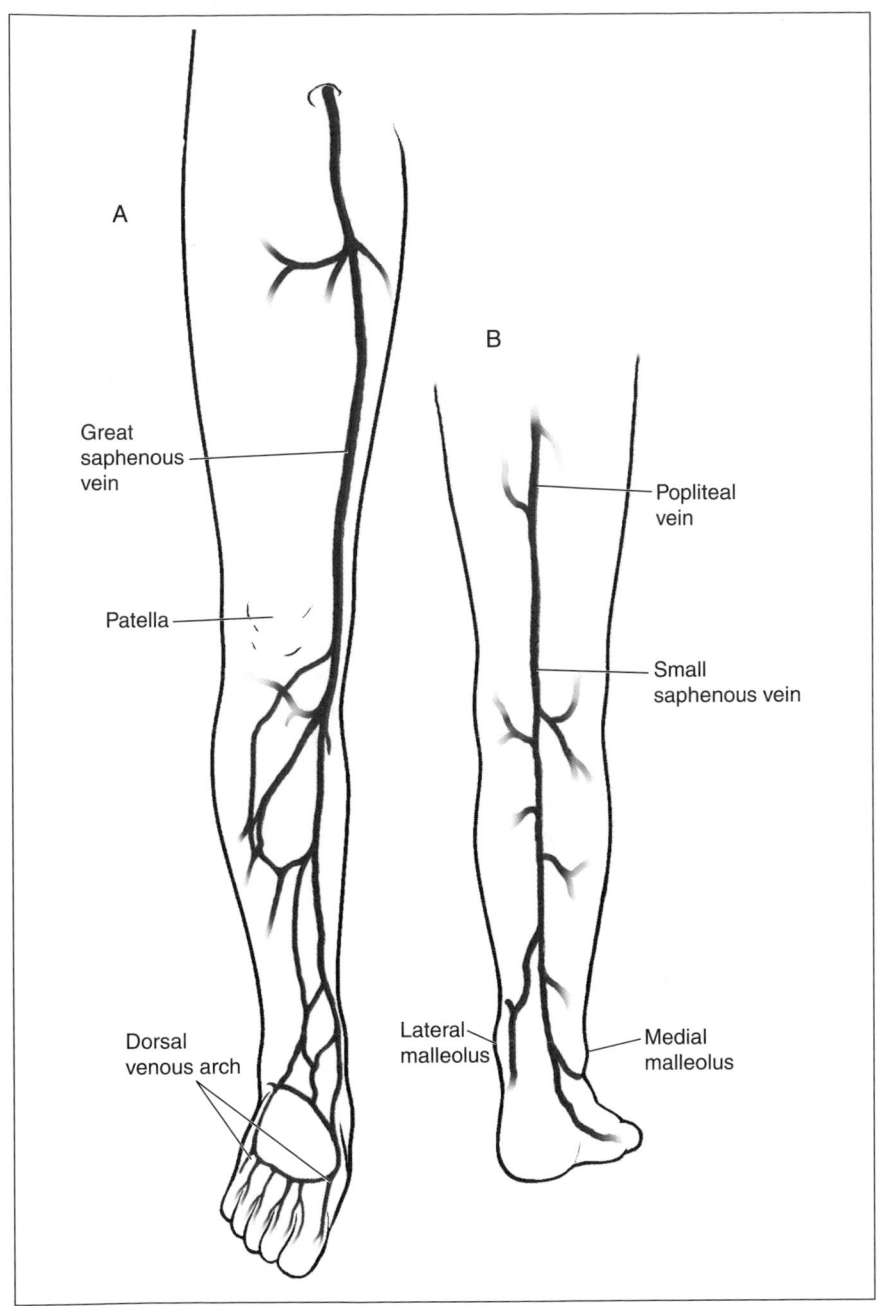

FIGURE 37-5 Superficial veins of the lower extremity. *A.* Anterior surface. *B.* Posterior surface.

EQUIPMENT

Antiseptic solution (antibacterial soap, 70% isopropanol, povidone iodine)
Local anesthetic solution
25 gauge needle
1 mL syringe
Gloves
Immobilization supplies if necessary
1 inch tape, waterproof or plastic
Transparent dressing
Gauze, 4×4 squares
Tourniquet
Desired venous access device (catheter and needle system)
Heparin lock or infusion set
Intravenous fluids
Vacuum blood collection tubes
Heparin
Medicine cup
Scissors
Gauze roll or stockinette

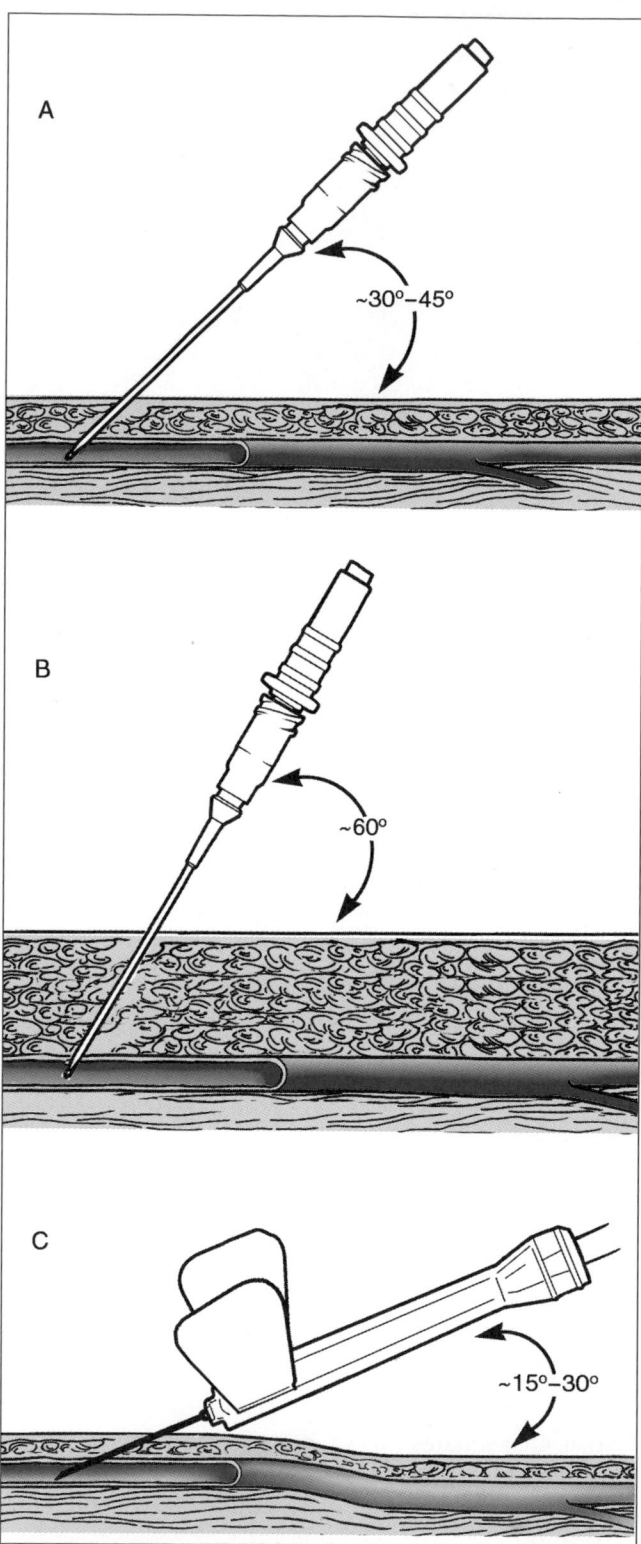

FIGURE 37-6 The angle between the needle and the skin must be varied based upon the depth and diameter of the target vein. *A.* A shallow angle must be used for small and superficial veins. *B.* A steeper angle must be used for deeper veins. *C.* A butterfly-type needle permits the shallowest angle of entry for very small and superficial veins.

PATIENT PREPARATION

Explain the procedure to the patient and/or their representative. Obtain verbal consent for the venipuncture unless it is an emergency. Select a site for the venipuncture. A site in the upper extremity is preferred. While a satisfactory vein is usually evident upon inspection, the placement of a venous tourniquet will aid the process greatly. It is easiest to place the tourniquet a few inches proximal to the elbow when first trying to locate a vein in the upper extremity. This restricts venous return from the entire extremity distal to the tourniquet and allows rapid inspection of the entire limb. Release the tourniquet once the site is chosen.

If difficulty is encountered in finding a vein, the use of dependent positioning, "pumping" via muscle contraction, and the local application of heat or nitroglycerin ointment will all contribute to venous engorgement.[2] These maneuvers can be used to aid in the performance of a venipuncture or peripheral venous access.

Clean the puncture site of any dirt and debris. Apply 70% isopropanol or povidone iodine to the area and allow it to dry.[8] Iodine-containing antiseptics are usually cleaned off with alcohol after they dry to lessen the chance of a local skin reaction. A small amount of local anesthetic may be infiltrated subcutaneously, with a 25 gauge needle, over the puncture site. Take care not to puncture the target vein accidentally. Reapply the tourniquet.

TECHNIQUES

PERIPHERAL VENIPUNCTURE

Stabilize the vein with the nondominant hand (Figure 37-9). Insert the needle attached to a syringe or vacuum tube adapter, with the bevel upward, into the vein at a 45 to 60 degree angle (Figure 37-6A). Lower angles, at times nearly parallel to the skin, may be needed to enter very narrow or superficial veins. This is easiest to achieve with a butterfly-type needle (Figure 37-6C). Apply negative pressure to the syringe. A flashback of blood in the hub of the needle indicates that the tip of the needle is within the vein. Pulsatile blood that pushes back the syringe plunger indicates an arterial puncture. Unless venous blood is specifically needed for a test, collect the necessary samples before removing the needle. No additional harm will be done by withdrawing a blood sample from an artery that has already been punctured.

If no blood is obtained, slowly advance the needle until it is deeper than the judged depth of the vein. Apply negative pressure to the syringe and slowly withdraw the needle. The vein will often have been punctured through-and-through (Figure 37-10B) and the specimen will be obtained as the needle is withdrawn (Figure 37-10C). If no blood is obtained by the time the needle is

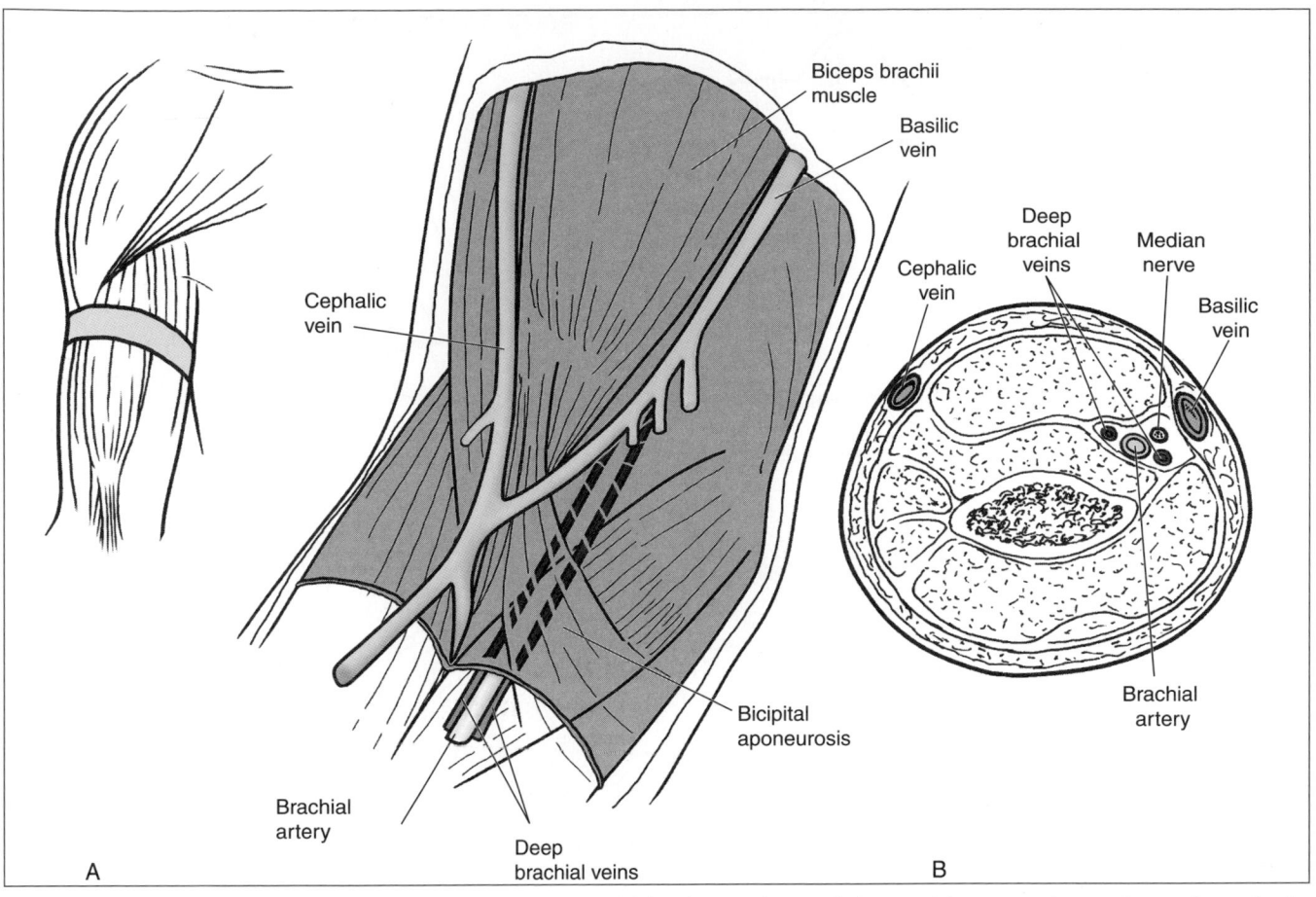

FIGURE 37-7 The deep brachial veins. *A.* The deep brachial veins are located deep to biceps tendon and muscle and adjacent to the brachial artery. *B.* Cross section of the arm 2 cm above the elbow. Note the two deep brachial veins, one on each side of the brachial artery.

withdrawn to just beneath the skin, redirect the needle and make another attempt at puncturing the vein. Before redirecting the needle, it must be withdrawn to just beneath the skin. **Never sweep the point of the needle around without withdrawing it, as the sharp bevel of the needle can lacerate nearby structures.** If swelling develops, indicating hematoma formation, remove the tourniquet and apply direct pressure for 5 to 10 minutes. Search for another venous access site.

Release the tourniquet. Apply direct pressure to the puncture site with sterile gauze or cotton once the specimen is obtained. Remove the needle from the patient's skin and continue direct pressure for 5 minutes. Peripheral arterial punctures should have direct pressure applied for at least 10 minutes.

PERIPHERAL INTRAVENOUS CANNULATION

Cannulation of a vein begins with a successful venipuncture with the desired device, as described above. This section focuses on the use of the catheter-over-the-needle technique of peripheral venous access, as it is the most commonly used method.

Insert the catheter-over-the-needle through the skin and into the vein (Figure 37-11*A*). A flash of blood in the hub of the needle confirms that the tip of the needle is within the vein. Advance the catheter-over-the-needle an additional 2 to 3 mm to ensure that the catheter is within the vein. An alternative is to drop the hub of the needle nearly parallel to the skin before advancing the catheter-over-the-needle (Figure 37-12*A*). This will prevent the needle from puncturing the far wall of the vein (Figure 37-12*B*) and the catheter from pushing the vein away from the needle (Figure 37-12*C*). Hold the hub of the needle securely. Advance the catheter over the needle until its hub is against the skin (Figure 37-11*B*). Withdraw the needle (Figure 37-11*C*). Apply pressure, with the nondominant index finger, over the catheter to prevent blood from exiting the catheter.

While applying digital pressure over the catheter, apply a device or intravenous tubing to the hub of the catheter. A syringe or vacuum device may be attached to the catheter to draw blood samples (Figure 37-13*B*). Intravenous tubing can be attached to the catheter to begin a fluid infusion (Figure 37-13*C*). A saline or

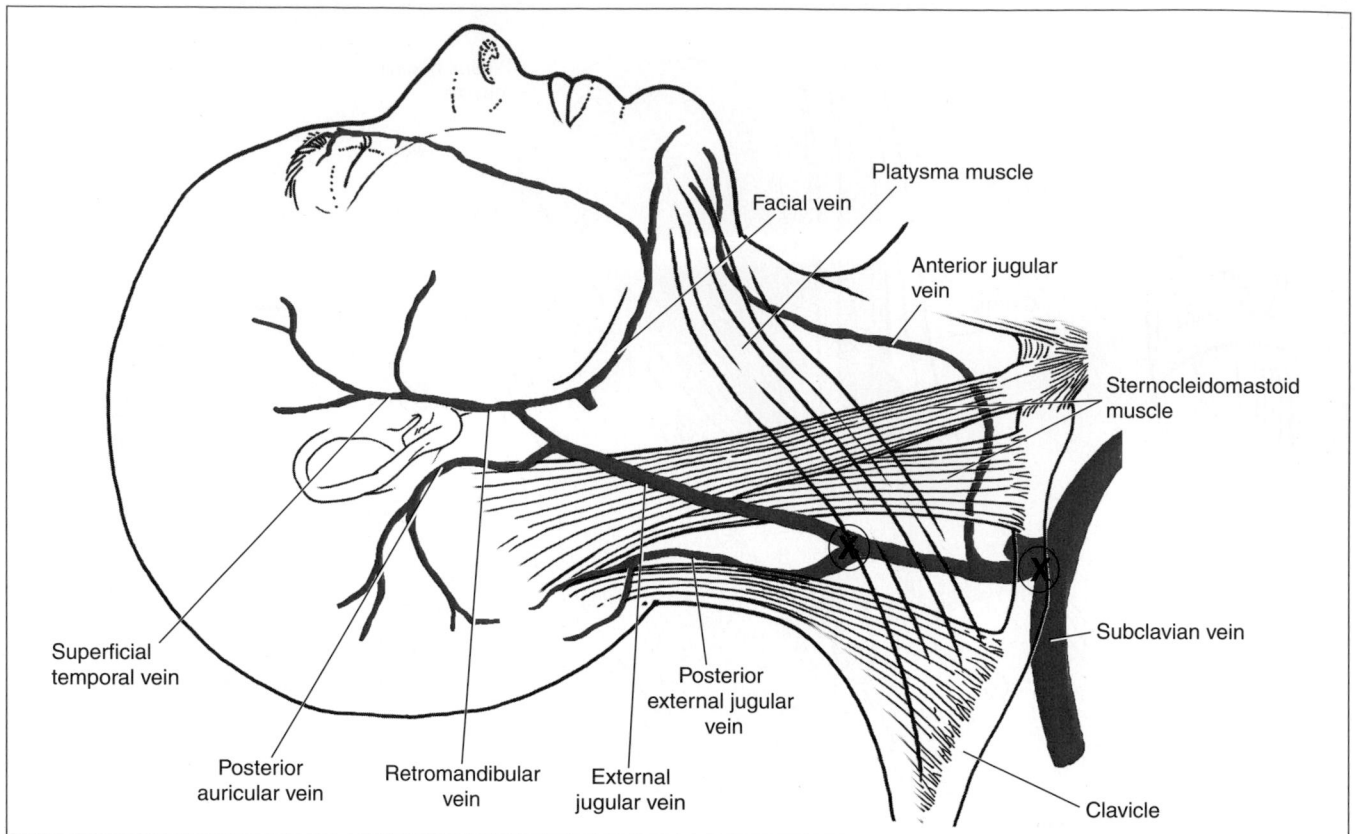

FIGURE 37-8 The external jugular veins. The anterior external jugular vein is usually larger than the posterior and runs deep to the platysma muscle. Note its relationship to the internal jugular vein. Valves (noted by the "X") are normally present in the external jugular vein where it enters the subclavian vein and about 4 cm superior to the clavicle.

heparin lock may be attached to the catheter to be used later for intravenous access (Figure 37-13D).

Secure the intravenous catheter to the skin (Figure 37-14). There are numerous methods to tape the catheter to the skin; only two are described here. Place a 2 inch piece of adhesive tape sticky side up under the catheter hub (Figure 37-14A). Fold the ends of the adhesive tape over the catheter and onto the skin to form a "chevron" (Figure 37-14B). Alternatively, fold the adhesive tape to form a "U" (Figure 37-14C). Apply a 2 inch piece of adhesive tape over the catheter hub (Figure 37-14D). Place a transparent dressing over the catheter hub and distal intravenous tubing (Figure 37-14E). Some prefer to use the transparent dressing without the adhesive tape. The catheter may be sutured to the skin when vascular access is essential and when the catheter may be pulled out by a young child or combative patient. It is very rare that a peripheral intravenous catheter must be sewn into place.

ALTERNATIVE TECHNIQUES

ARTERIAL LINE KIT

The modified Seldinger technique, used with a radial artery catheterization kit (Arrow International, 800-523-

8446, product RA-04020), is very useful for the catheterization of deep brachial and external jugular veins. The kit is commonly available in Emergency Departments and Intensive Care Units. It consists of a one-piece unit that incorporates a catheter-over-the-needle, a guidewire in a feed tube, and a lever to advance the guidewire (Figure 37-15). The black mark on the feed tube is a reference mark. The tip of the guidewire is positioned at the tip of the needle when the advancement lever is at the reference mark.

The integral guidewire and soft 2 inch 20 gauge catheter found in the Arrow kit can ease the process of catheterization considerably. The depth of the deep brachial vein combined with overlying skin (which is often scarred from previous venipunctures) makes catheterization with the usual 1¼ inch catheter difficult. The external jugular vein is quite mobile and the overlying tissues are fairly tough. This can make it quite difficult to thread an over-the-needle catheter into the vein without pushing the vein off the end of the needle.

Select a vein to cannulate. Clean and prep the skin overlying the puncture site. Place a tourniquet on the extremity. Open the package and remove the unit. Advance the guidewire through the needle and then retract it. Do not use the catheterization unit if the guidewire does not

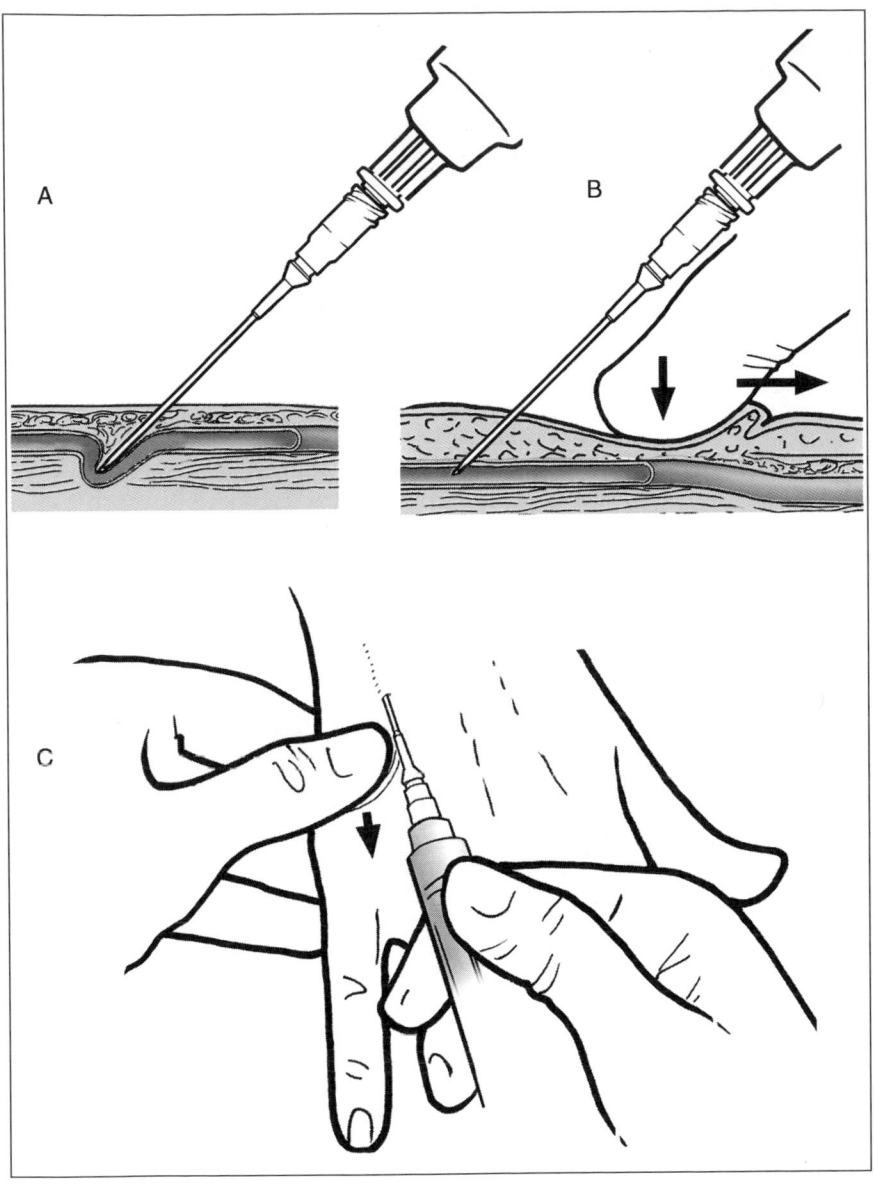

FIGURE 37-9 Stabilization of the vein during venipuncture. *A.* Without stabilization, the vein may kink or roll away from the tip of the hypodermic needle. *B.* Gentle stabilizing pressure with the operator's fingertip allows entry into the vein, as shown in *C.*

advance and retract smoothly. Ensure that the guidewire advancement lever is retracted as far as possible so that the guidewire is not within the needle. **The flashback of blood will not be seen if the guidewire is not fully retracted and out of the needle.**

Stabilize the vein with the nondominant hand. Insert the catheter-over-the-needle through the skin and into the vein (Figure 37-16*A*). A flash of blood in the hub of the needle indicates that the tip of the needle is within the vein. Hold the needle hub securely. Advance the guidewire, using the advancement lever, into the vein (Figure 37-16*B*). Continue to advance the guidewire as far as possible into the vein. The advancement lever must be distal to the reference mark to ensure that the guidewire is past the tip of the needle. **Stop advancing the guidewire if resistance is encountered. Do not force the guidewire against resistance. Do not retract the guidewire if resistance to advancement is encountered. Doing so may damage the vein or shear off a piece of the guidewire. Withdraw the entire unit and repeat the procedure with a new unit.**

The guidewire should be advanced as far as possible into the vein. Advance the catheter-over-the-needle an additional 1 to 2 mm into the vein. This will ensure that the catheter tip is within the vein. Hold the hub of the needle securely. Advance the catheter over the needle and guidewire until its hub is against the skin (Figure 37-16*C*). A twisting motion may help to advance the catheter against resistance. Release the tourniquet. Hold the catheter hub firmly against the skin. Remove the needle and guidewire through the catheter as a unit. Attach a syringe, vacuum blood collection system, intravenous line, or saline (heparin) lock onto the catheter hub. Secure the catheter with adhesive tape.

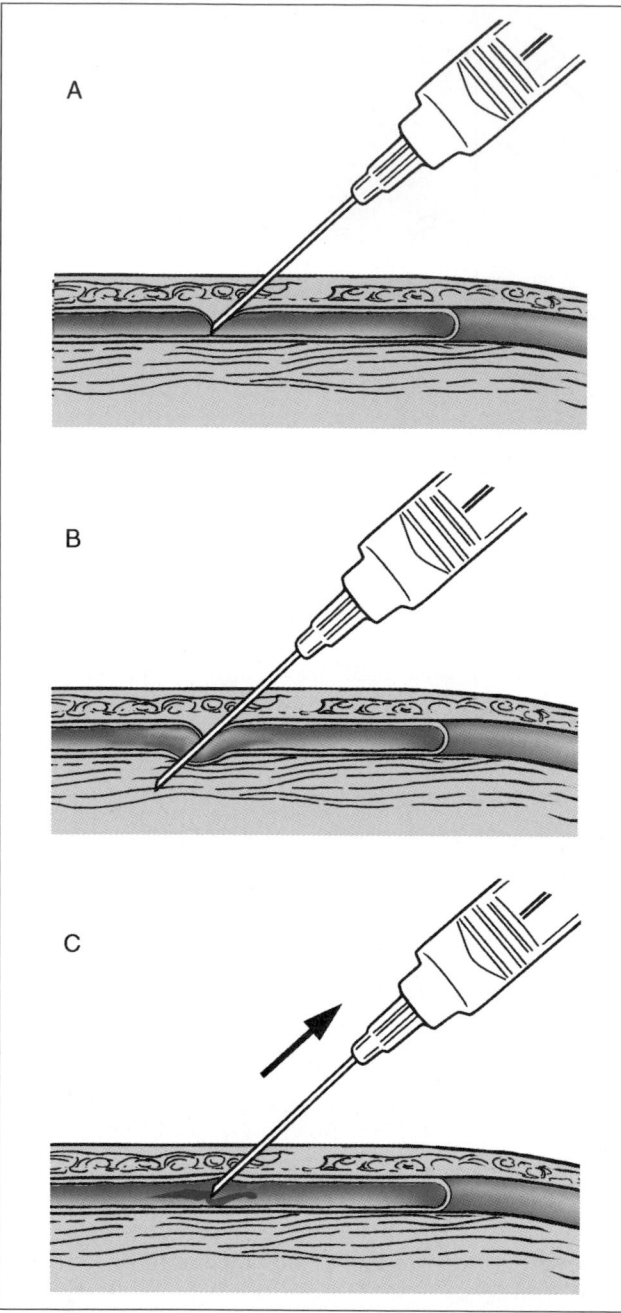

FIGURE 37-10 Through-and-through puncture of the vein. *A.* The tip of the hypodermic needle can collapse the vein, preventing a flashback of blood in the syringe. *B.* The vein may then be punctured through-and-through without the operator's knowledge. *C.* Slow withdrawal of the needle permits the vein to open, and blood returns into the syringe.

EXTERNAL JUGULAR VEIN CANNULATION

Place the patient in the Trendelenburg position to distend the external jugular vein. Turn the patient's head to the opposite side. Clean and prep the skin of the neck. Place the nondominant thumb or index finger above the midportion of the clavicle to obstruct outflow and dis-

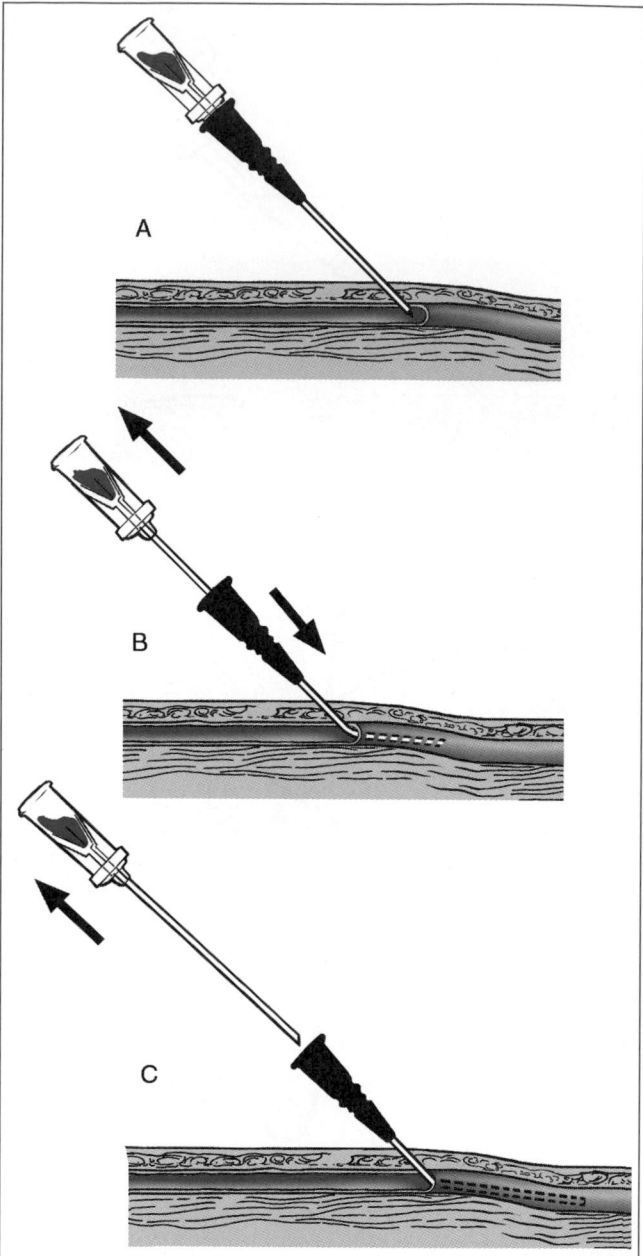

FIGURE 37-11 The catheter-over-the-needle technique. *A.* The vein is punctured and blood returns in the needle hub. *B.* The catheter is advanced over the needle and into the vein. *C.* The needle is removed.

tend the external jugular vein. Align the catheter-over-the-needle parallel to the vein with the bevel of the needle upward and the tip of the needle pointing toward the clavicle. Enter the vein midway between the angle of the mandible and the midclavicle. Insert the catheter-over-the-needle during inspiration, when the valves of the external jugular vein are open. Be sure to cover the open hub of the needle and/or catheter with a finger at all times to prevent an air embolism. The remainder of the technique is similar to that described previously.

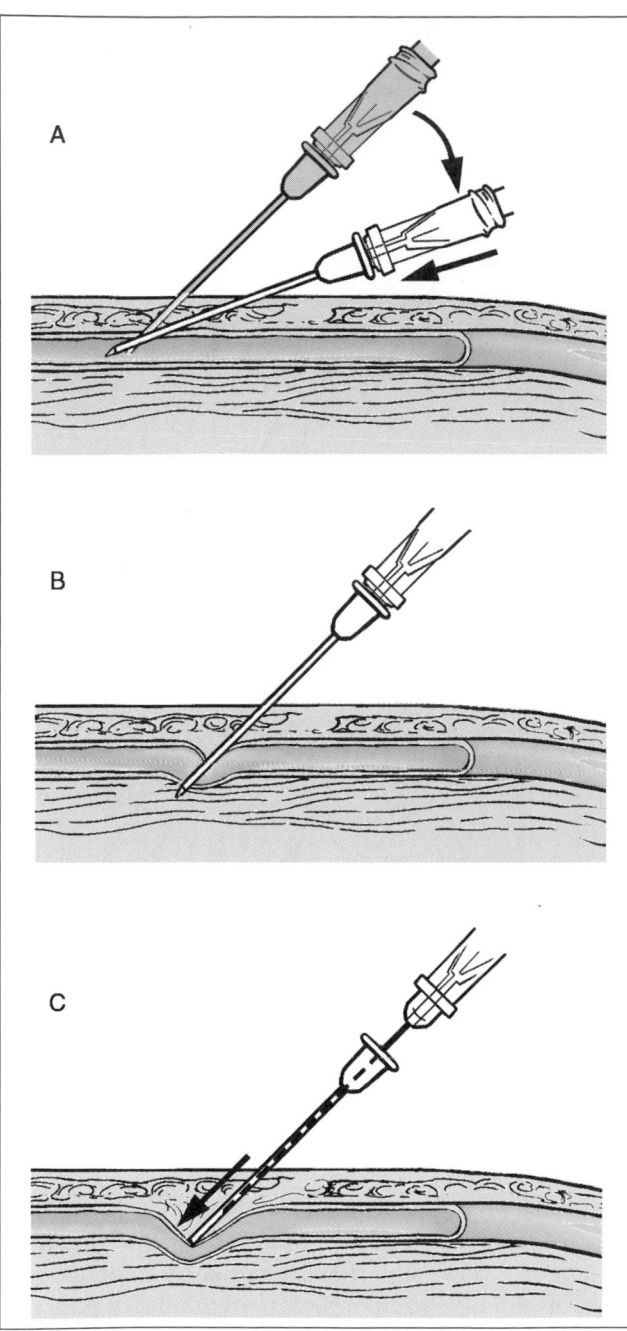

FIGURE 37-12 Advancing the catheter-over-the-needle. *A.* Drop the catheter hub toward the skin, then advance the catheter-over-the-needle 2 to 3 mm into the vein. *B.* If it is advanced at the original angle to the skin, the far wall of the vein may be punctured. *C.* If the catheter is advanced over the needle as soon as the vein is entered, the catheter may push the vein off the end of the needle, resulting in unsuccessful venous cannulation.

DEEP BRACHIAL VEIN CANNULATION

Extend the patient's arm. By palpation, identify the brachial artery pulse in the antecubital fossa. Clean and prep the skin of the antecubital fossa. Place a tourniquet on the upper arm. Reidentify the brachial artery pulse.

Place a catheter-over-the-needle onto a 5 mL syringe and insert it just medial or lateral to the brachial artery pulse and at a 30 to 45 degree angle to the skin with the tip of the needle pointing cephalad. Advance the catheter-over-the-needle while applying negative pressure to the syringe. A flash of blood in the syringe indicates that the vein has been entered. The remainder of the technique is similar to that described previously.

PEDIATRIC CONSIDERATIONS

Venipuncture and peripheral venous access can be quite a challenge in the infant and small child. Proper restraint of the extremity by a board or an assistant will greatly aid the process. Aside from the techniques discussed above, there are a few techniques that can facilitate pediatric vascular access.[9,10] The scalp veins can be used for venous access in newborns. They are most easily cannulated with a small (23 or 25 gauge) butterfly needle or catheter. A rubber band can be placed about the baby's head as a tourniquet (Figure 37-17). Other veins commonly used include those of the antecubital fossa, dorsal hand, dorsal foot, external jugular vein, and saphenous vein at the knee or groin. For small and superficial veins, it can be helpful to place a small bend at the hub of the catheter-over-the-needle assembly (Figure 37-18). This allows for the use of a less acute angle and easier entry into the vein without puncturing the far wall.

The best guide to the gauge (diameter) of catheter to use is to compare the catheter to the vein. The catheter should be at least slightly smaller than the vein. In practice, the smallest readily available catheters are 24 gauge. A 22 gauge catheter will allow a much higher flow rate if it can be inserted successfully.

Keeping a peripheral intravenous line from being pulled out by an active toddler is quite a challenge. Each institution has its own "recipe" for securing pediatric IVs. The catheter is taped to the skin in the usual manner. Several strips of tape can be placed to secure the tubing to the skin and act as "strain reliefs" to prevent traction applied to the tubing from being transmitted to the catheter. Half of a medicine cup can be used as a shield for the catheter itself (Figure 37-19*A*). The clear medicine cup acts as a window, so that the catheterization site can easily be inspected without removing all the dressings. The whole assembly can then be covered with a gauze roll or stockinette (Figure 37-19*B*). A cup with one-quarter or one-third cut away may be used to protect a scalp vein access site (Figure 37-19*C*).

ASSESSMENT

Refer to Table 36-2, in the preceding chapter, for some general principles of intravenous line assessment. The

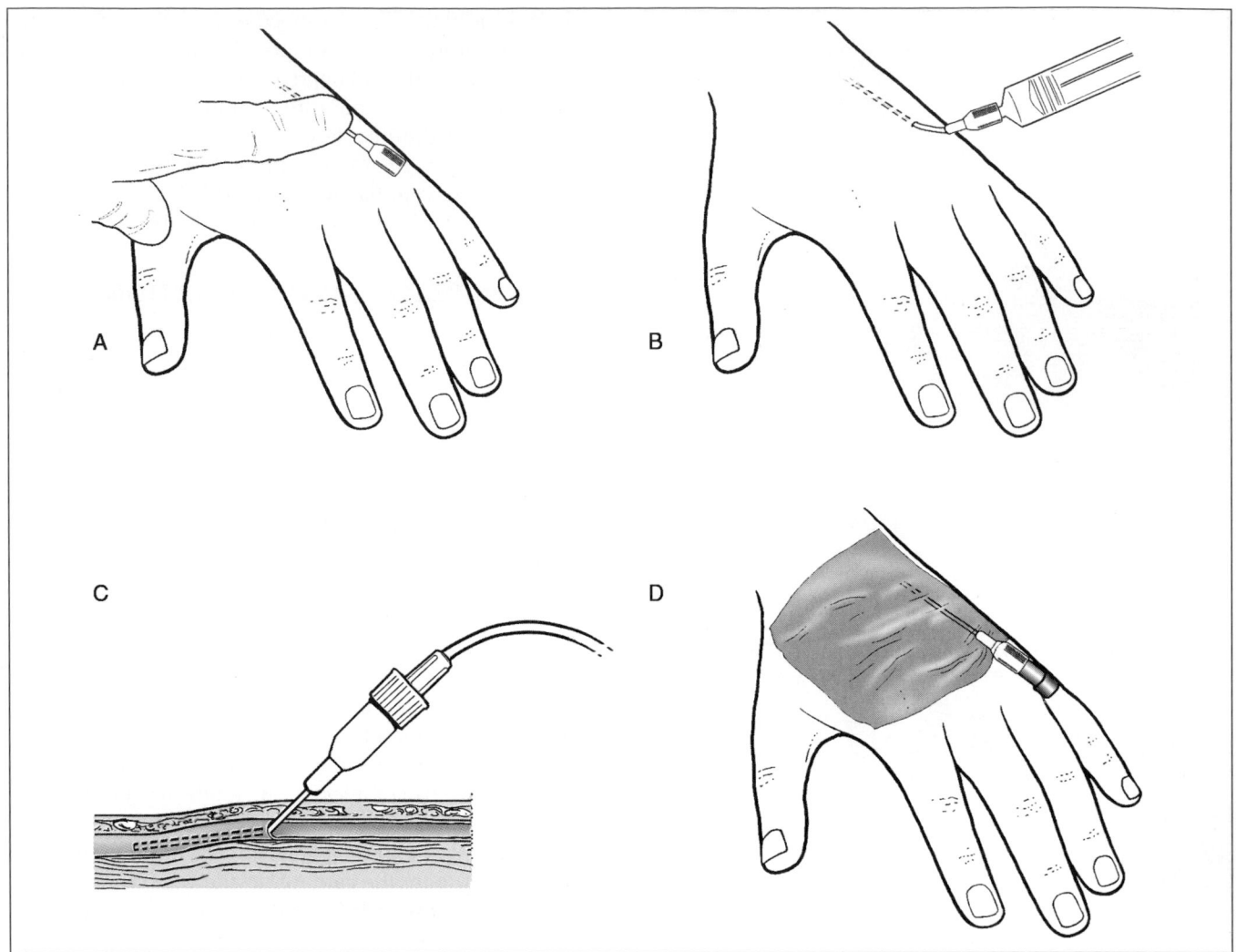

FIGURE 37-13 Peripheral intravenous cannulation. *A.* Apply gentle pressure over the catheter with a gloved finger to prevent hemorrhage from the catheter hub. *B.* Blood samples may be withdrawn from the cannula via syringe or vacuum tubes. *C.* Intravenous infusion tubing is attached to the catheter. *D.* A saline (heparin) lock is attached to the catheter.

line should flush easily. Any infusions should flow by gravity alone. Progressive swelling at the catheterization site indicates the formation of a hematoma or extravasation of infused fluids. Peripheral infusions of vasopressors and caustic solutions require the skin puncture site to be assessed frequently and carefully, since extravasation may lead to extensive local soft tissue necrosis. Pain at the intravenous access site must be taken seriously and should prompt a search for the cause. Pinched skin, extravasation, or thrombosis must be looked for and ruled out.

AFTERCARE

Most authorities recommend changing peripheral infusion sites at least every three days, although this is probably overly cautious.[11,12] It may be impractical if the patient has poor superficial veins. Any cannula with signs of venous thrombosis, skin erythema, or puncture site discharge must be removed at once. Heparin or saline locks that have not been accessed should be flushed regularly, usually every 8 hours. Saline works as well as heparin solutions for most applications.[13] About 1 mL of flush is adequate for peripheral venous catheters.

Dressings should be inspected and changed if they have become moist or contaminated. Routine dressing changes are probably unnecessary.[13] The transparent dressings are widely used despite some studies suggesting that transparent occlusive dressings are associated with higher rates of infection than plain gauze dressings.[14] Transparent dressings have the advantages of allowing easy inspection of the catheter site and holding the catheter securely in place. Individual institutions

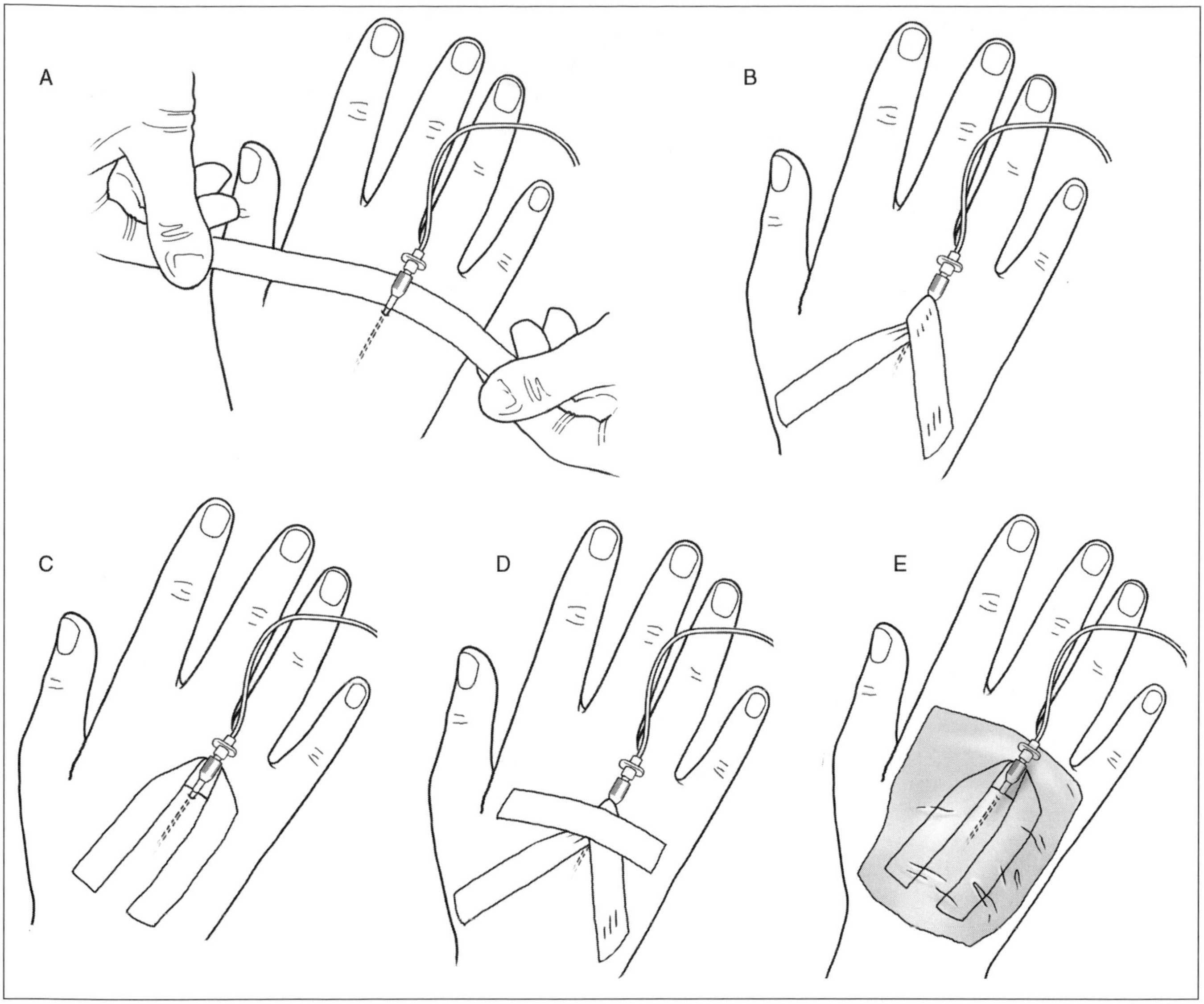

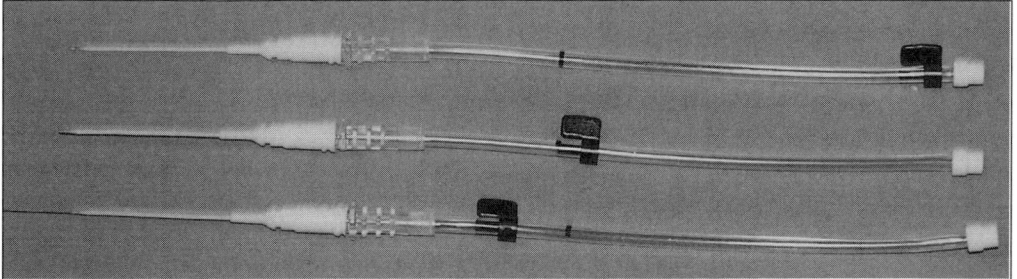

FIGURE 37-14 Securing the intravenous catheter. *A.* Place a narrow strip of adhesive tape sticky side up under the catheter hub. *B.* Fold the tape over the catheter to form a "chevron." *C.* Alternatively, the tape with the sticky side up can be folded to form a "U." *D.* A second piece of tape is applied to better secure the catheter to the skin. *E.* A transparent dressing is applied over the catheter.

FIGURE 37-15 The Arrow radial artery catheterization set. Note the different positions of the guidewire. The guidewire is within the feed tube (*top*). The tip of the guidewire is at the tip of the needle when the advancement lever is at the reference mark (*middle*). The guidewire is advanced through the catheter-over-the-needle (*bottom*).

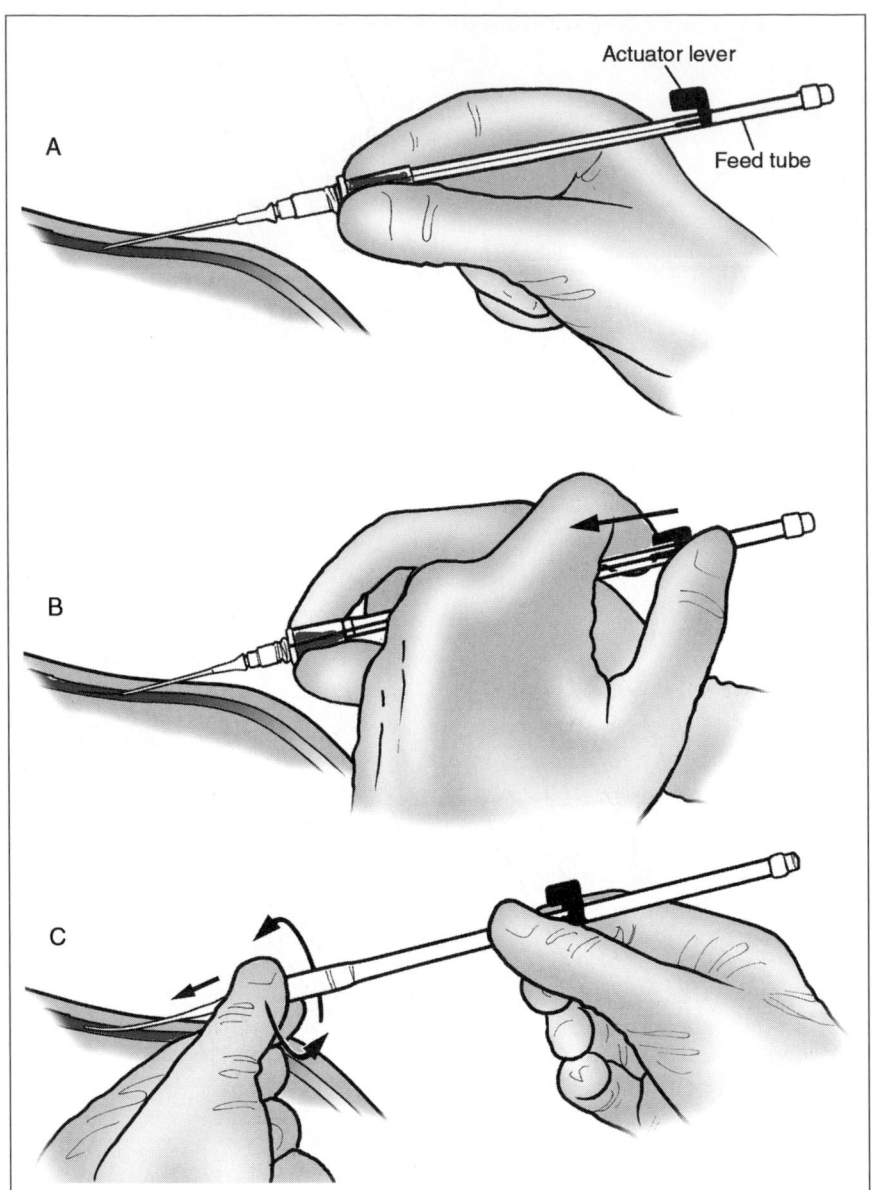

Actuator lever

Feed tube

A

B

C

FIGURE 37-16 The Arrow radial artery catheterization set. *A.* The vein is punctured and blood returns into the hub of the needle. *B.* The guidewire is advanced into the vein. *C.* The catheter is advanced over the needle and guidewire with a back-and-forth rotating motion. The needle and guidewire are then removed as a unit.

often have their own nursing guidelines and infection control statistics to support their choice of dressing.

REMOVAL OF INTRAVENOUS CATHETERS

Turn off any intravenous infusions and clamp the tubing. Place the infusion site in a dependent position below the right atrium to prevent a venous air embolism. Remove any tape and dressings from the infusion site. Apply direct pressure to the skin puncture site with a gauze pad. Briskly remove the catheter or needle. Hold firm direct pressure for 5 to 10 minutes, then apply a bandage. The patient should be instructed to check for signs of thrombophlebitis and cellulitis for the next several days.

COMPLICATIONS

PERIPHERAL VENIPUNCTURE

The main complications of venipuncture are pain and hematoma formation. Pain during venipuncture can be minimized by using small-gauge needles and minimizing the number of attempts at venipuncture. Hematomas and bleeding can be prevented by removing the tourniquet before removing the needle and applying direct pressure after removal of the catheter. Hematomas are self-limited and easily treated with mild analgesics and cool packs. Other complications include nerve injury, usually reversible paresthesias. Arterial puncture is common with deep brachial lines and may rarely be catastrophic if it causes thrombosis of the

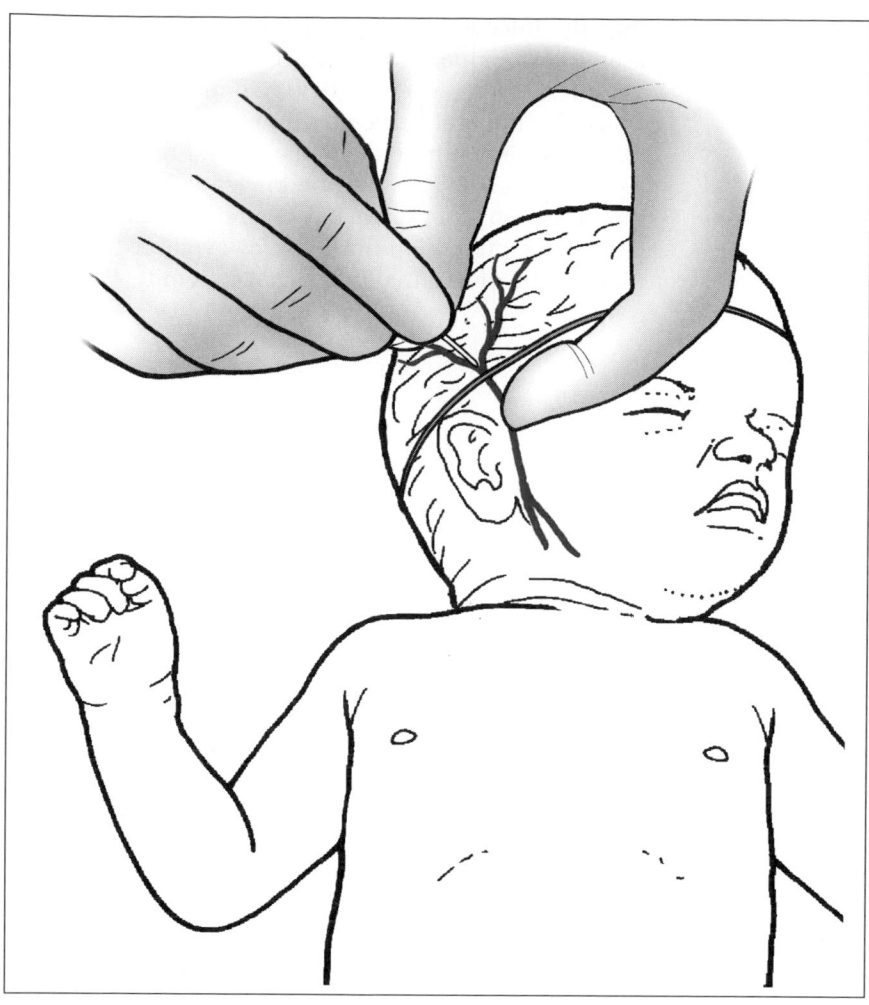

FIGURE 37-17 Scalp vein cannulation in the neonate. A rubber band makes a convenient tourniquet.

brachial artery, the sole arterial supply of the forearm and hand.[14] Infection from simple venous sampling is uncommon.

PERIPHERAL INTRAVENOUS CANNULATION

In addition to the complications described for venipuncture, indwelling venous catheters pose additional risks. Some of these are summarized in Table 36-2 of the preceding chapter. Steel needle cannulas can move easily, causing lacerations of the vein and neighboring structures. The risk of infection is greater the longer a catheter is left in place. Intravenous catheters increase the risk of superficial venous thrombosis and thrombophlebitis. This may be prevented by limiting catheter manipulation during tubing changes and by using extension tubing at the catheter hub. It is possible to injure a number of structures in the neck during external jugular vein cannulation. This includes the carotid artery, internal jugular vein, and trachea. It is also possible to cause a pneumothorax. None of these complications should occur as long as deep penetration with the needle is avoided. Extravasation of vasopressors or caustic solutions can cause local skin necrosis. Extravasation of

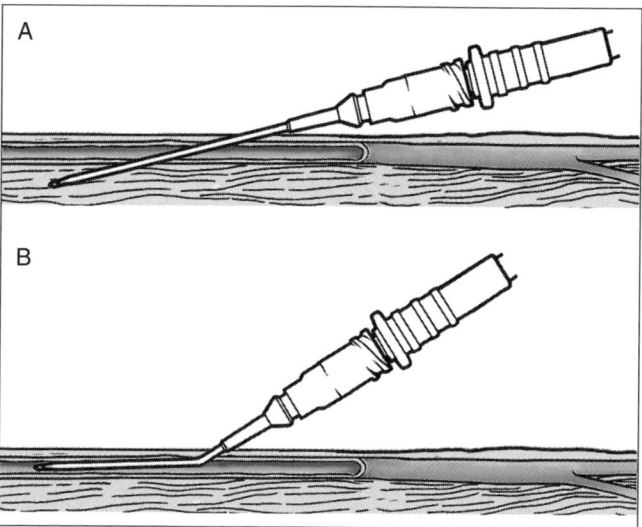

FIGURE 37-18 Cannulation of a small superficial vein with a catheter-over-the-needle. *A.* The "shoulder" of the catheter hub prevents the needle from being placed nearly parallel to the skin. *B.* A slight bend at the base of the needle permits the needle to run nearly parallel to the skin surface, enabling the subcutaneous vein to be cannulated. Always make sure that the catheter can be advanced over the needle before puncturing the patient's skin.

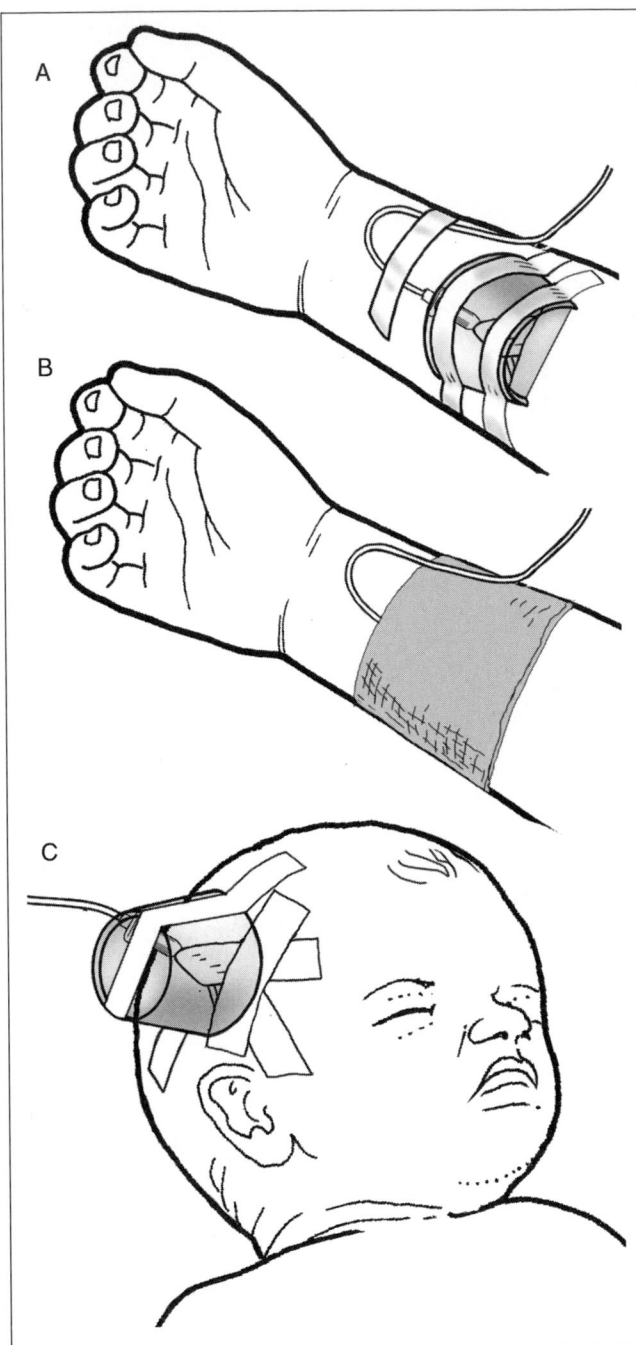

FIGURE 37-19 Securing pediatric intravenous lines. *A.* Use a clear plastic medicine cup, cut in half lengthwise, to protect the skin puncture site. *B.* A stockinette or gauze roll can be used to further protect the site from manipulation. *C.* Protecting a scalp vein cannula with tape and a clear plastic medicine cup.

large volumes into a muscle compartment can lead to a compartment syndrome, although this is rare with superficial peripheral venous lines. Extravasation and tissue injury may be prevented by using a small-gauge catheter in a large vein, diluting medications before administration, and observing intravenous access sites fre-

quently. Infections can often be prevented by using aseptic technique and sterile dressings, and changing peripheral catheters every 48 to 72 hours. The complications of peripheral nerve palsies, pressure necrosis, and compromised peripheral circulation are rare but do occasionally occur. They can be prevented with frequent neurovascular checks to any restrained extremity, by padding all pressure points, and by avoiding the placement of circumferential tape on an extremity.

SUMMARY

The gaining of peripheral venous access is an essential skill for nearly all medical practitioners, from paramedics to physicians. The only way to become proficient at these techniques is to master them during training and to practice them regularly. Equally important is frequent reassessment of venous cannulas so that complications can be detected and treated early, before they become major problems for the patient and the practitioner.

REFERENCES

1. Bledsoe BE: *Atlas of Paramedic Skills.* Englewood Cliffs, NJ: Prentice-Hall, 1987:124–142.
2. Roseman JM: Deep, percutaneous antecubital venipuncture: an alternative to surgical cutdown. *Am J Surg* 1983; 146(2):285.
3. Keyes LE, Frazee BW, Snoey ER, et al: Ultrasound-guided brachial and basilic vein cannulation in emergency department patients with difficult intravenous access. *Ann Emerg Med* 1999; 34(6):711–714.
4. Williams PL, Warwick R: *Gray's Anatomy*, 36th ed. Philadelphia: Saunders, 1980:629–765.
5. Elliott TS, Faroqui MH, Armstrong RF, et al: Guidelines for good practice in central venous catheterization. *J Hosp Infect* 1994; 28:163–176.
6. Blitt CD, Wright WA, Petty WC, et al: Central venous catheterization via the external jugular vein—a technique employing the J-wire. *JAMA* 1974; 229(7):817–818.
7. Cunningham FJ Jr, Engle WA, Rescorla FJ: Pediatric vascular access and blood sampling techniques, in Roberts JR, Hedges JR (eds): *Clinical Procedures in Emergency Medicine*, 3rd ed. Philadelphia: Saunders, 1998:281–290.
8. Bhende MS: Venipuncture and peripheral venous access, in Henretig FM, King C (eds): *Textbook of Pediatric Emergency Procedures*. Baltimore: Williams & Wilkins, 1997:797–810.
9. Bregenzer T, Conen D, Sakmann P, et al: Is routine replacement of peripheral intravenous catheters necessary? *Arch Intern Med* 1998; 158:151–156.

10. Homer LD, Holmes KR: Risks associated with 72- and 96-hour peripheral intravenous catheter dwell times. *J Intraven Nurs* 1998; 21(5):301–305.

11. Maki DG, Ringer M: Evaluation of dressing regimens for prevention of infection with peripheral intravenous catheters. *JAMA* 1987; 258(17):2396–2403.

12. Hoffmann KK, Weber DJ, Samsa GP, et al: Transparent polyurethane film as an intravenous catheter dressing—a meta-analysis of the infection risks. *JAMA* 1992; 267(15):2072–2076.

13. Epperson EL: Efficacy of 0.9% sodium chloride injection with and without heparin for maintaining indwelling intermittent injection sites. *Clin Pharmacol* 1984; 3:626–629.

14. Kramer DA, Staten-McCormick M, Freeman SB: Percutaneous brachial vein catheterization: an alternate site for IV access. *Ann Emerg Med* 1983; 12(4):247.

Chapter 38
CENTRAL VENOUS ACCESS

Robert Feldman

INTRODUCTION

Percutaneous cannulation of the central veins is an essential technique for both long-term and emergent medical care. Access to the major veins of the torso allows rapid high-volume fluid resuscitation, administration of concentrated ionic and nutritional solutions, and hemodynamic measurements.

ANATOMY AND PATHOPHYSIOLOGY

The tip of the central venous catheter must lie in the superior or inferior vena cava and never in the right atrium. The thin wall of the right atrium may easily be perforated by the catheter tip, resulting in hemorrhage and cardiac tamponade. The central venous anatomy is shown in Figure 38-1. The superior vena cava is accessed through the internal jugular veins, the subclavian veins, and less commonly via the external jugular veins. The inferior vena cava is accessed through the femoral veins. These access routes are discussed in greater detail in the corresponding sections below. The advantages and disadvantages of each route for central venous access are summarized in Table 38-1.

INTERNAL JUGULAR VEIN

The internal jugular vein is not directly visible from the surface of the skin. A thorough knowledge of its anatomic relationships is essential for successful cannulation. The internal jugular vein exits the skull through the jugular foramen, just anteromedial to the mastoid process.[1] It joins the subclavian vein deep and just lateral to the head of the clavicle[1] (Figure 38-2). The surface projection of the internal jugular vein runs from the earlobe to the medial clavicle, between the sternal and clavicular heads of the sternocleidomastoid muscle. The internal jugular vein increases in diameter as it descends. It is joined by tributary veins in the upper neck, making it easier to cannulate below the level of the cricoid cartilage.

The internal jugular vein is collapsible (Figure 38-3). It has a very small diameter in low-flow states, as during cardiopulmonary resuscitation (CPR) and when the patient is upright. The vein is easily compressible and will collapse with gentle external pressure from a palpating finger or a large-diameter needle indenting the skin (Figure 38-3B). Fortunately, the vein is also very distensible. Placing the patient in the Trendelenburg position or having the patient perform the Valsalva maneuver will distend the vein and help to locate the vessel (Figure 38-3C).

The common carotid artery travels alongside the internal jugular vein and is an important anatomic landmark for locating the internal jugular vein. The carotid artery runs deep and slightly anterior to the internal jugular vein. The left internal jugular vein usually overlaps the carotid artery in the lower neck (Figure 38-3A). The right internal jugular vein and the right carotid artery are usually separated slightly.

The right internal jugular vein is generally preferred to the left internal jugular vein as the site of central venous cannulation. The right internal jugular vein provides a nearly direct route to the superior vena cava. The dome of the right lung is somewhat lower than that of the left lung and thus decreases the chance of a pneumothorax. The thoracic duct is relatively large and lies high in the left chest. These favor the right internal jugular approach to central venous cannulation to minimize complications.[1,2]

There are three main approaches to the internal jugular vein as defined by their relationship to the sternocleidomastoid muscle. These are the anterior, central, and

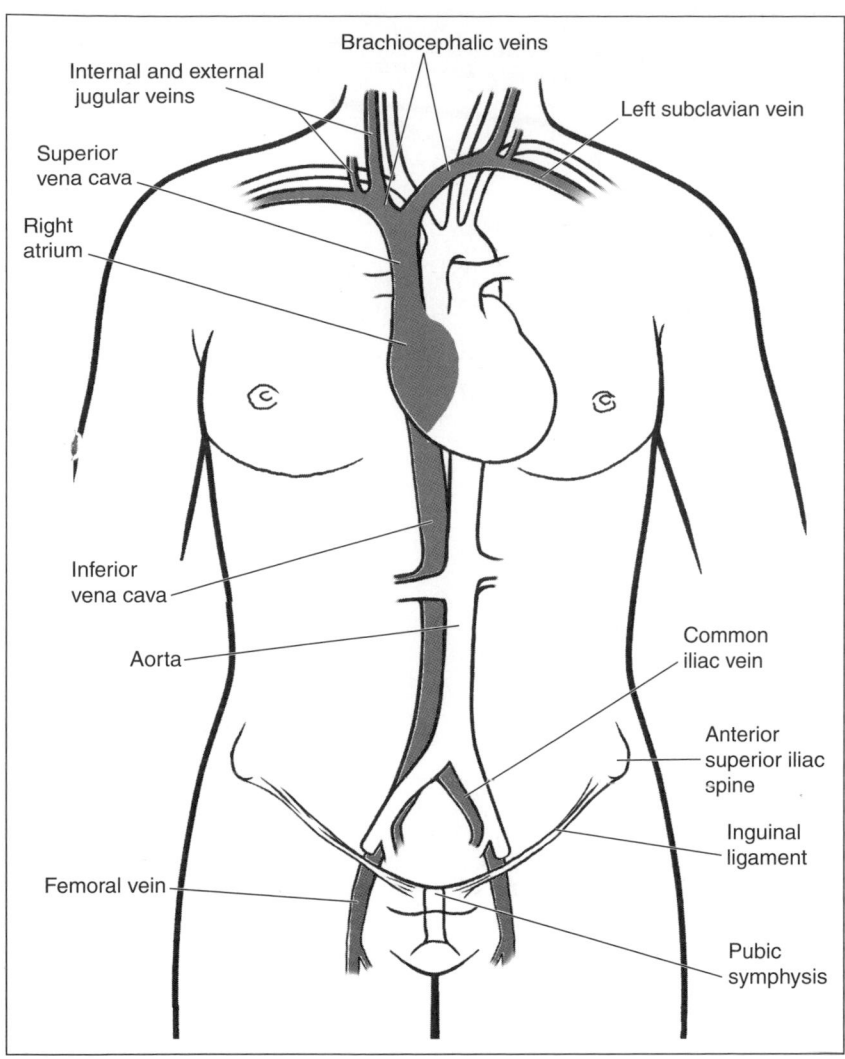

FIGURE 38-1 The anatomy of the central venous system.

posterior approaches (Figures 38-4, 38-5, and 38-6). The central approach is most commonly used. These three approaches are summarized in Table 38-2.

SUBCLAVIAN VEIN

The subclavian vein begins as the continuation of the axillary vein at the lateral edge of the first rib[1,3-5] (Figure 38-7). The subclavian vein courses anterior to the anterior scalene muscle, which separates it from the subclavian artery. The subclavian vein descends to join the in-

ternal jugular vein and form the brachiocephalic trunk, which empties into the superior vena cava.

The subclavian veins are 1 to 2 cm in diameter in an adult. Fibrous connective tissue joins the subclavian vein to the clavicle and first rib, preventing collapse of the vessel even in the event of a cardiac arrest. Anatomically associated structures include the thoracic duct, which joins the left subclavian vein at its junction with the left internal jugular vein. The right subclavian vein is preferred to the left for central venous access for this

TABLE 38-1. CHARACTERISTICS OF THE VARIOUS ROUTES OF CENTRAL VENOUS CANNULATION

	Internal jugular vein	External jugular vein	Subclavian vein	Femoral vein
Risk of infection	Low	Low	Low	High
Patient mobility	Fair	Poor	Good	Bedridden
Trendelenburg required?	Yes	Yes	Yes	No, best for CHF or dyspnea
Need to stop CPR?	Probably	Probably	Yes	No, may continue CPR
Suitable for long-term use?	Yes, but not if ambulatory	No	Yes—best choice	No, remove within 2–3 days
Risk of venous thrombosis	Low	Low	Low	High

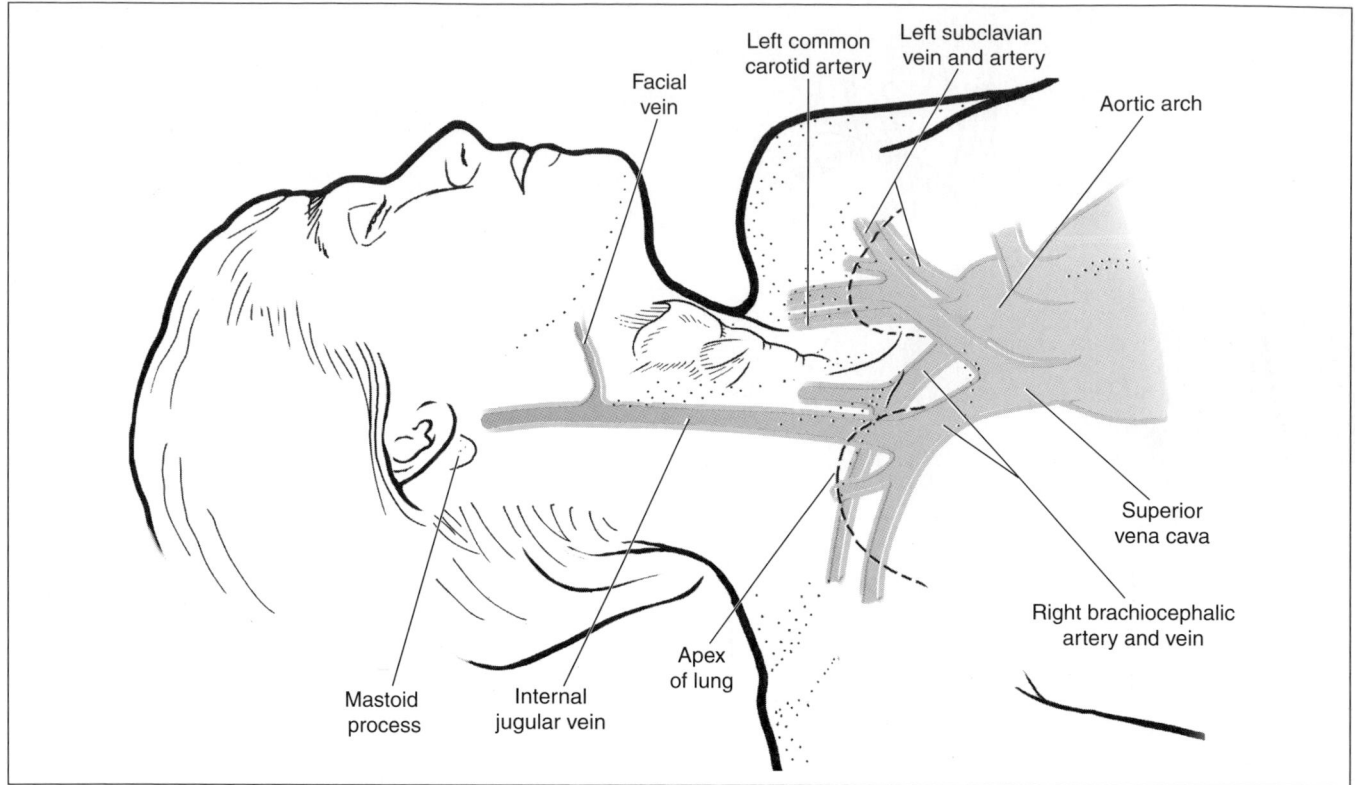

FIGURE 38-2 Anatomy and surface relationships of the internal jugular vein.

reason. The domes of the pleura lie posterior and inferior to the subclavian veins and medial to the anterior scalene muscles. The subclavian arteries lie immediately posterior to the veins.

Subcutaneous fatty tissue, chest morphology, the close proximity of the pleura, and the close proximity of the subclavian artery make the subclavian vein the least favored site for central venous access in children. This is especially true in infants. An experienced practitioner should perform the procedure if this route must be used in a neonate, infant, or small child.

FEMORAL VEIN

The puncture site for femoral vein cannulation lies medial to the femoral artery and inferior to the inguinal ligament[1,2,6] (Figure 38-8). The femoral vein lies within the femoral sheath and just medial to the femoral artery in the groin. This relationship can be remembered by the mnemonic "toward the NAVEL." This describes, from lateral to medial, the contents of the femoral sheath (femoral Nerve, femoral Artery, femoral Vein, Empty space, and Lymphatics). The femoral artery lies at the midpoint of a line connecting the symphysis pubis and the anterior superior iliac spine.[1,6] The femoral vein lies approximately 1 cm medial to the femoral artery pulse in an adult.[3,7] It lies approximately 5 mm medial to the femoral artery in infants and young children.[3,7] The femoral venous pulse may be felt instead of the arterial

pulse. During CPR chest compressions, attempt puncture directly over the pulsations if an initial attempt at femoral vein cannulation medial to the pulse fails.

The puncture site to enter the femoral vein must be at least 1 to 2 cm inferior to the inguinal ligament, depending on the patient's size. The femoral vein becomes the external iliac vein superior to the inguinal ligament (Figure 38-8). **Blood can flow freely into the retroperitoneal space, forming a potentially large and externally invisible hematoma if the posterior wall of the femoral vein is punctured by a through-and-through needle track above the inguinal ligament. It is imperative to puncture the femoral vein inferior to the inguinal ligament!**

INDICATIONS

The internal jugular route is acceptable for central venous access in most cases. It allows ready access to the superior vena cava for long-term central venous access, caustic infusions, and monitoring of central venous pressure. Pulmonary artery catheters and transvenous pacing wires can be introduced through the right internal jugular vein. The internal jugular vein is accessible without terminating CPR efforts, although chest compressions and the lack of carotid pulsations make accessing it difficult. The risk of a pneumothorax is probably

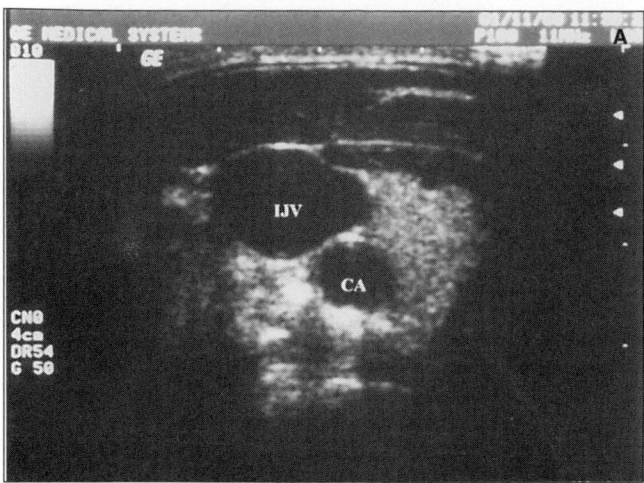

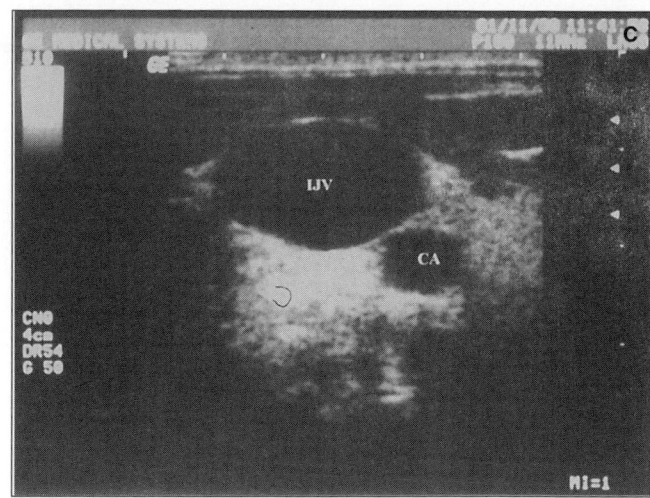

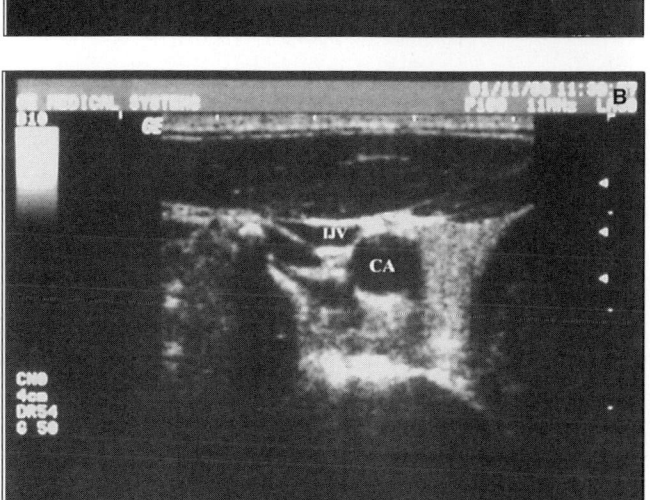

FIGURE 38-3 Ultrasonic cross sections of the left internal jugular vein (IJV) and carotid artery (CA). *A.* The patient is supine. *B.* With gentle external pressure applied, the low-pressure internal jugular vein collapses easily while the carotid is still patent. *C.* The Valsalva maneuver or placement of the patient in the Trendelenburg position dilates the internal jugular vein.

less with the internal jugular vein cannulation as opposed to the subclavian vein route, although patient mobility is less and discomfort is greater. In a coagulopathic patient, the internal jugular vein puncture site is compressible, but hematoma formation may lead to compromise of the airway.

The subclavian vein is the preferred route for longer-term central venous access. This site allows for ambulation (unlike a femoral line) and neck movement without discomfort (unlike a jugular line). The catheter is concealable under clothing, making outpatient use more acceptable.

The femoral vein is often the preferred route for emergency central venous cannulation in many patients. The indications are the same as for any central venous access with a few exceptions. The femoral vein is not a suitable route for ambulatory patients beyond the initial resuscitation and stabilization period, as patients with femoral central venous lines must be confined to bed. Femoral venous access is easily obtained in patients with respiratory distress and pulmonary edema, since they do not need to be placed in the Trendelenburg

position. Femoral venous access is relatively easy during CPR and often does not require the cessation of chest compressions. The femoral vein is easily compressible. This makes it preferable to the subclavian vein in coagulopathic patients or those undergoing thrombolysis, although peripheral access would be preferred in these cases.[8] There is no risk of injury to the airway, pleura, or carotid arteries in very young or combative patients. Femoral central venous lines are generally preferred for initial central venous access in the very young or combative patient if deep sedation or neuromuscular paralysis is contraindicated or otherwise unnecessary.[3]

CONTRAINDICATIONS

The usual contraindications to any invasive procedure apply to central venous access. Cellulitis or overlying infection at the puncture site is a contraindication to central venous access. An alternative should be sought if the patient is combative, agitated, or uncooperative. These patients require sedation and/or paralysis prior to

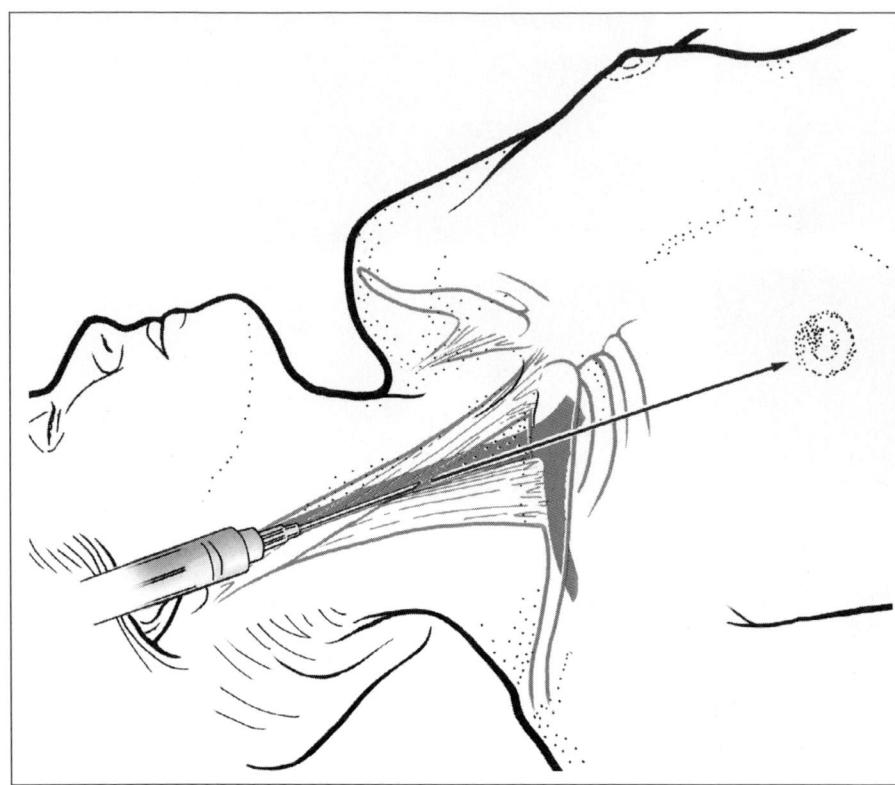

FIGURE 38-4 Central approach to the right internal jugular vein.

insertion of the central venous line. Distorted anatomic landmarks due to fractures, deformities, obesity, previous catheterization at the site, surgery, or trauma are relative contraindications. There is a small but real risk of serious morbidity and even death due to the procedure. **Do not place a central venous line unless a peripheral line is inadequate or unobtainable and unless person-** **nel capable of managing complications are immediately available.**

INTERNAL JUGULAR VEIN CANNULATION

Anatomic distortion of the neck, such as from subcutaneous emphysema or a hematoma, may make placement of an internal jugular line difficult and hazardous.

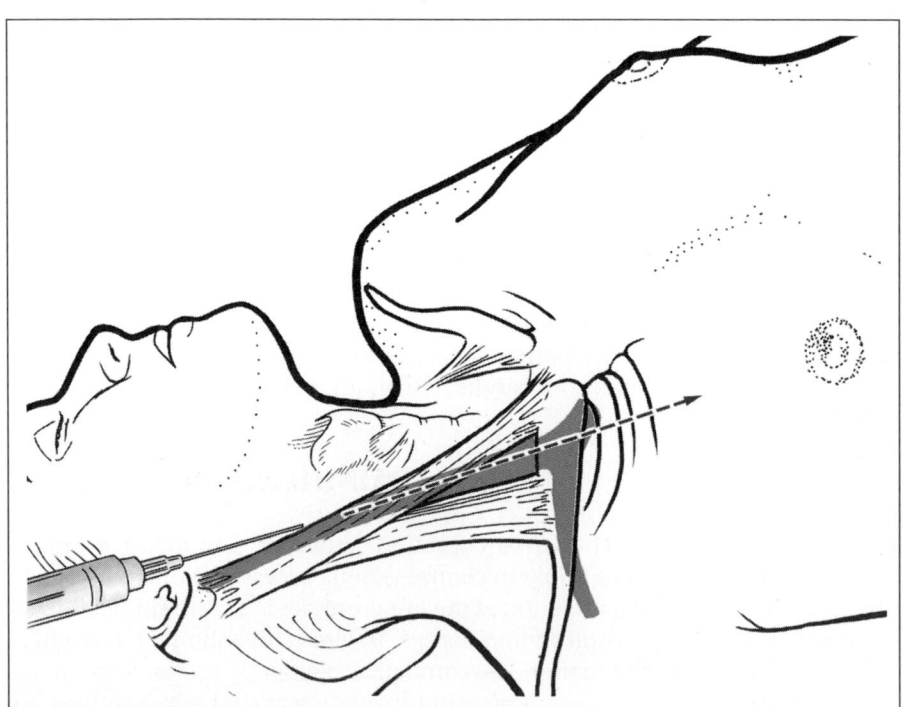

FIGURE 38-5 Anterior approach to the right internal jugular vein.

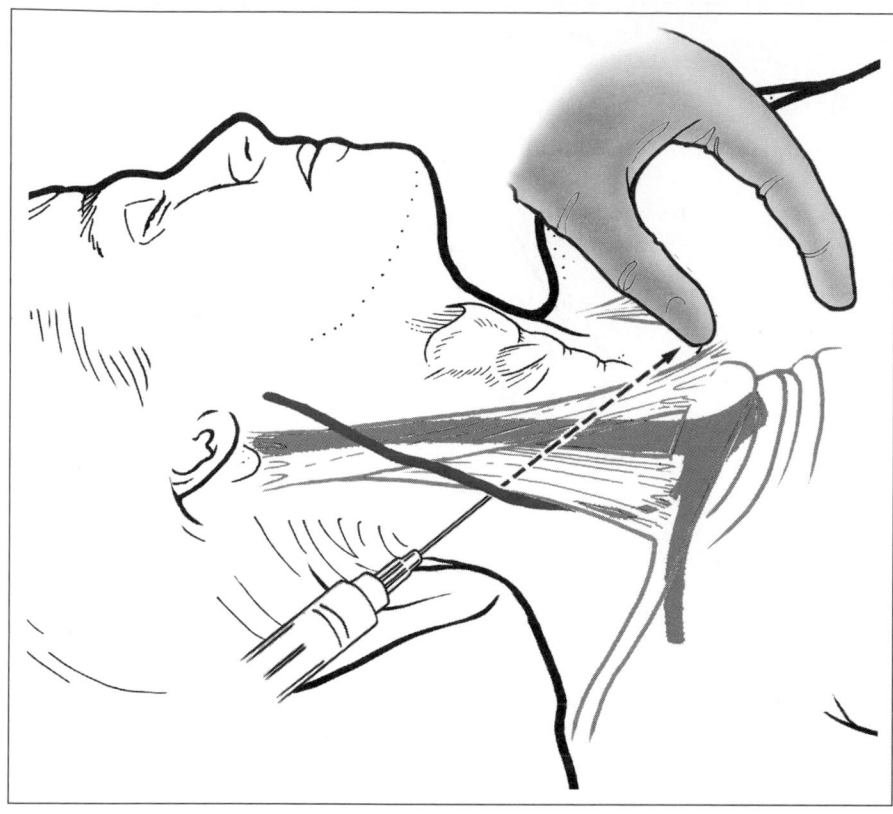

FIGURE 38-6 Posterior approach to the right internal jugular vein.

Known severe carotid artery stenosis or atherosclerosis on the desired side of cannulation is a relative contraindication to internal jugular vein cannulation. Accidental carotid artery puncture during line placement may result in plaque rupture and subsequent stroke. The vein may be collapsed and difficult to access in the hypovolemic patient. Other contraindications to cannulating the internal jugular vein include cervical spine fractures (actual or suspected) or penetrating neck injuries.

The subclavian or femoral route may be preferable in some circumstances. The subclavian route is probably a better choice for long-term lines in ambulatory patients, as for hemodialysis. The limited neck mobility due to an internal jugular line is very uncomfortable. Ongoing or impending thrombolytic administration is a contraindication to internal jugular puncture. A femoral central

venous line is preferable in this case. Successful internal jugular cannulation requires the patient to be placed supine and preferably in 15 to 30 degrees of Trendelenburg tilt. This may be impossible in a patient with severe pulmonary compromise. The femoral route is preferred in this case. Internal jugular vein cannulation is difficult in children under 1 year of age due to poor landmarks and a very short neck.[3] Internal jugular cannulation is contraindicated in any child who cannot be adequately immobilized or paralyzed after insertion of the central venous line. Internal jugular cannulation will be more difficult if the patient's neck cannot be turned.

A left bundle branch block is a relative contraindication to central venous cannulation. The guidewire can induce complete heart block when it enters the right ventricle.[9] Extreme caution should be used if an internal

TABLE 38-2. APPROACHES TO THE INTERNAL JUGULAR VEIN

	Central	Anterior	Posterior
Insertion landmark	Superior apex of the triangle formed by the two heads of the sternocleidomastoid muscle and the clavicle	Medial edge of the sternocleidomastoid muscle at level of thyroid cartilage	Lateral edge of sternocleidomastoid muscle, 1/3 of the way from the clavicle to the mastoid process
Angle with skin	30° (child), 45–60° (adult)	30° (child), 45° (adult)	30–45°, dive under the border of the sternocleidomastoid muscle
Aim toward	Ipsilateral nipple	Ipsilateral nipple	Sternal notch
Internal jugular vein depth in an adult	Within 3 cm	Within 3 cm	Within 5 cm

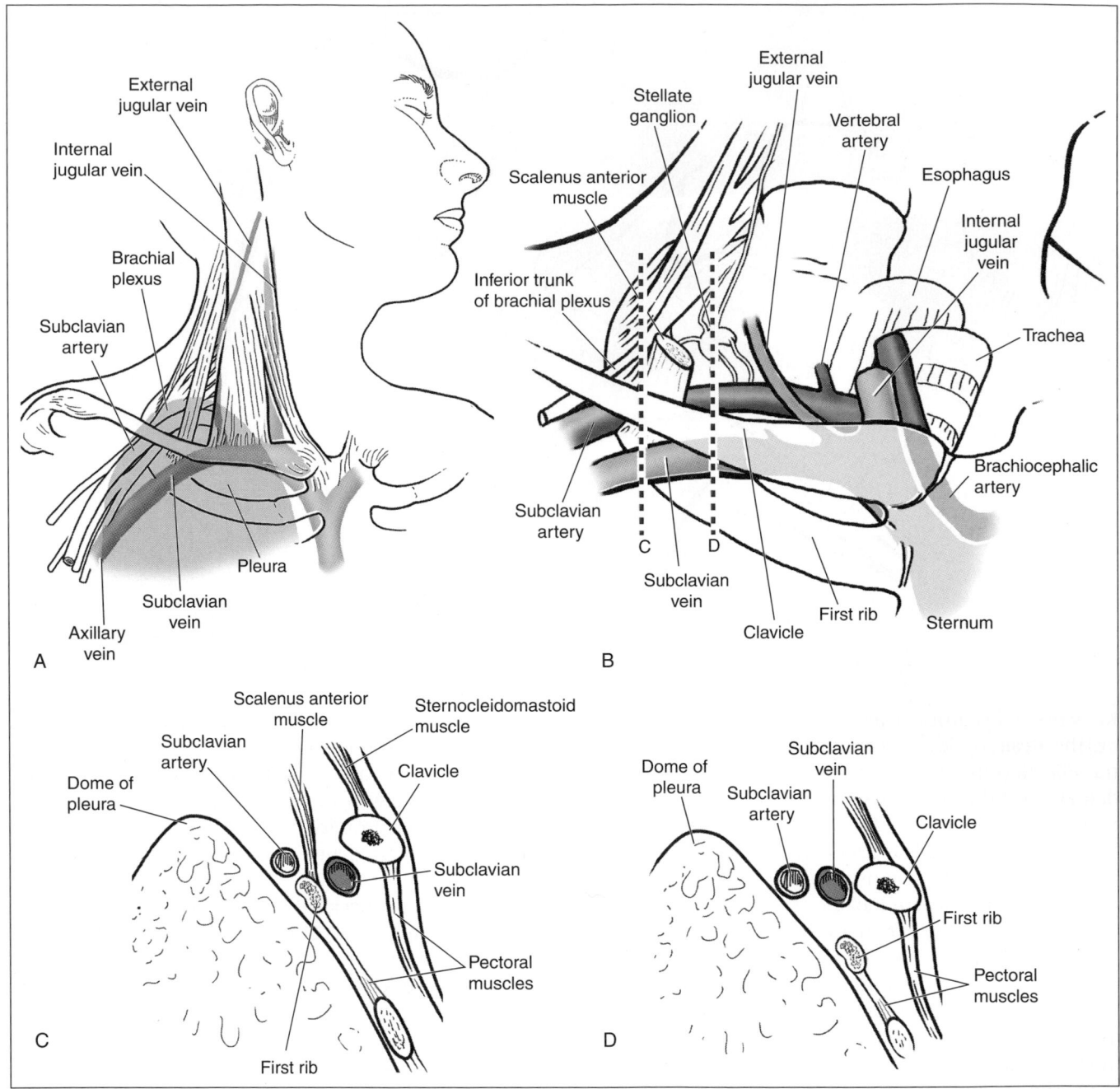

FIGURE 38-7 The anatomy of the subclavian vein. *A.* The right subclavian vein. *B.* Magnified view of the right subclavian vein demonstrating adjacent structures that may be injured during attempted cannulation. *C.* Sagittal section through the midclavicle. Note that the first rib protects the subclavian artery during an infraclavicular approach to the subclavian vein. *D.* Sagittal section through the medial third of the clavicle. Note the proximity of the subclavian artery and pleural dome to the subclavian vein.

jugular or subclavian central line is necessary. Avoid inserting the guidewire into the heart. Transcutaneous and transvenous cardiac pacing equipment should be readily available.

SUBCLAVIAN VEIN CANNULATION

The subclavian vein is incompressible and should be accessed with care in any patient who is coagulopathic.

Current or imminent systemic thrombolysis is an absolute contraindication to placing a subclavian vein catheter.[8] Subclavian vein cannulation should be performed on the contralateral side if the patient is relying on a single lung. Chest wall deformities, distorted anatomy, and suspected vascular injury to the chest or ipsilateral upper extremity are also contraindications. This route should also be avoided if the patient has had

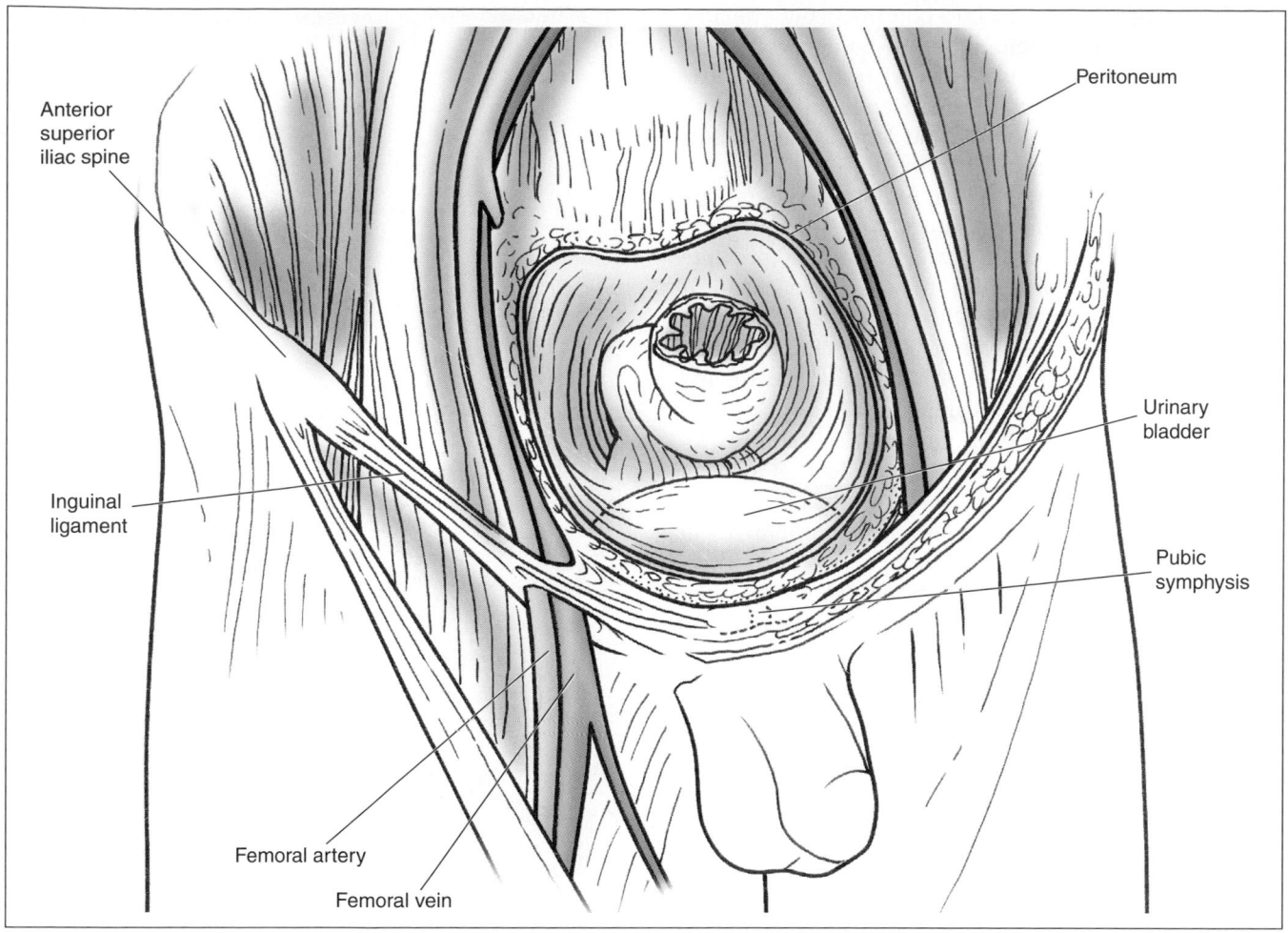

FIGURE 38-8 Anatomy of the femoral vein.

prior surgery or trauma to the clavicle, the first two ribs, or the subclavian vessels.

FEMORAL VEIN CANNULATION

Contraindications to femoral line placement include infection, venous thrombosis, or significant trauma to the ipsilateral lower extremity or groin area. Abdominal trauma may result in an interruption of the inferior vena cava, allowing any infused fluid or blood to flow into the abdomen rather than into the central circulation. During CPR, blood return below the diaphragm is reduced and a femoral catheter must end near the level of the diaphragm for medications to be most effective.[6]

Catheterization via the internal jugular vein or subclavian vein is usually easier if the purpose of central venous access is pulmonary artery catheterization or transvenous cardiac pacing. These procedures often require fluoroscopy when they are performed through the femoral vein. Central venous pressures measured through a femoral vein catheter may be inaccurate unless the patient is perfectly supine.

EQUIPMENT

Povidone iodine solution
Sterile drapes or towels
Local anesthetic solution
25 gauge needle
5 mL syringes
"Finder" needle, usually 22 gauge for an adult
5 mL syringe with a nonlocking hub
Thin-walled introducer needle or catheter-over-the-needle
Guidewire
Gauze 4×4 squares
Sterile gloves
Central venous line
Dilator
#11 scalpel blade
Nylon or silk suture, 3–0 or 4–0
Sterile saline
Needle driver
Tape and catheter site dressing material
Catheter clamp, if supplied with the kit

A variety of standard kits are commercially available (Figure 38-9). They contain all required equipment except local anesthetic solution and sterile gloves. The appropriate catheter should be chosen based on the patient's needs. The optimal catheter lengths for patients of different ages are summarized in Table 38-3.

Catheters with between one and four lumens are available. Multiple-lumen catheters are available in a variety of sizes and allow simultaneous venous pressure measurement, administration of numerous medications, and venous sampling without disconnecting the infusion apparatus. Disadvantages of multiple-lumen catheters over single-lumen catheters include smaller lumen sizes for a given catheter's outside diameter, greater cost, and the need to maintain unused lumens. There is probably no increased risk of infection in using triple-lumen versus single-lumen catheters.[10–12] Some comparisons between these devices are summarized in Table 38-4.

Percutaneous sheaths are intended primarily for the introduction of intravascular devices, such as pulmonary artery catheters and transvenous pacing wires. They are most often used in the Emergency Department as a large-bore line for the rapid resuscitation of hypotensive and hypovolemic patients. Sheaths are available in many sizes and configurations. Many models have an adjustable hemostasis valve that may be removed and a side port that allows infusion while the main lumen is being used for monitoring.

The equipment required for subclavian vein cannulation is the same as that for internal jugular vein cannulation. Subclavian vein catheters must be slightly longer or inserted farther than internal jugular vein catheters. Left-sided catheters must be a few centimeters longer or inserted farther than right-sided catheters. The longer needle should be used for subclavian vein cannulation if the kit used has two different lengths of introducer needles.

PATIENT PREPARATION

The procedure, its risks, and its benefits should be explained to the patient and/or their representative. Obtain an informed consent for the procedure unless it is being performed emergently. Place the patient in the Trendelenburg position if catheterization of the internal jugular vein is being attempted. Position the patient in at least 15 degrees of Trendelenburg to prevent an air embolism. Rotate the patient's head toward the side opposite that to be cannulated.

The subclavian vein is fixed to the surrounding tissues and will neither collapse nor distend; therefore the Valsalva maneuver or extreme Trendelenburg position is not necessary. Head rotation is neither necessary nor helpful. On the side to be cannulated, place the patient's arm

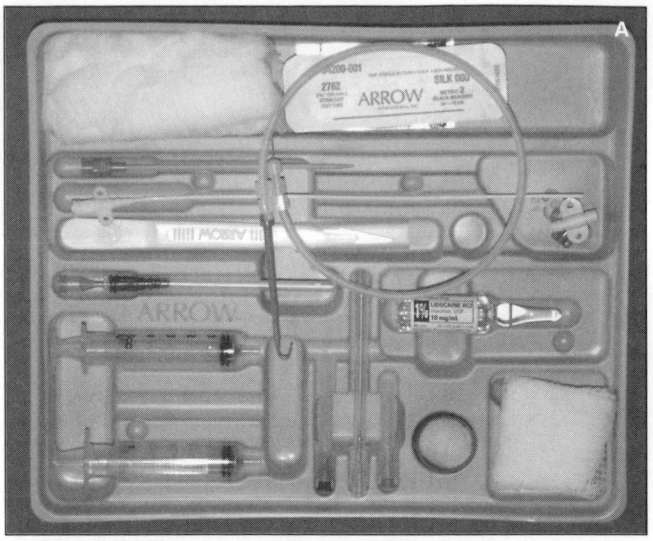

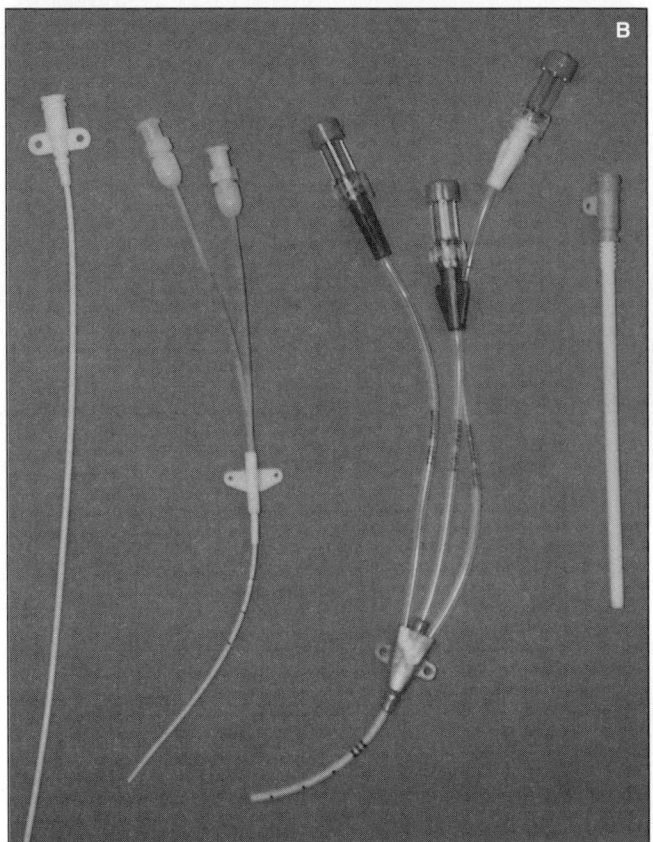

FIGURE 38-9 Equipment needed for central venous catheterization. *A.* A commercially available central venous line kit. *B.* Examples of different catheter types available. From left to right: single-lumen, double-lumen, triple-lumen, and introducer sheath (Cordis).

adducted to the torso or in slight abduction if the deltoid muscle is very large. Avoid placing rolled towels between the shoulder blades, as this can decrease the distance between the clavicle and first rib, compress the subclavian vein, and make the procedure more difficult.[13]

TABLE 38-3. CATHETER SIZES AND TYPES

Catheter size (French)	Number of lumens	Patient size	Venous access site	Minimum catheter length (cm)*
2	1	Infant	Femoral, internal jugular, external jugular, or subclavian	5
3	1	< 5 kg	Femoral, internal jugular, external jugular, or subclavian	5
4	1, 2	5–10 kg	Femoral	5
		10–15 kg	Femoral, internal jugular, external jugular, or subclavian	8–12
5	1, 2, 3	> 15 kg	Femoral, internal jugular, external jugular, or subclavian	12–15
7	1 (sheath), 2, 3	> 40 kg	Femoral, internal jugular, external jugular, or subclavian	15–25
8 and larger	1 (sheath), 2, 3, 4	Adult	Femoral, internal jugular, or subclavian	15–25

* The longer end of the catheter length range is for use in the subclavian veins, with the longest catheters needed for the left subclavian vein.
SOURCE: Adapted from references 3, 7, and 37.

Place the patient supine or in slight reverse Trendelenburg if femoral vein catheterization is being attempted. The Trendelenburg position is contraindicated due to the risk of venous air embolism. Slight external rotation and abduction of the extremity may be helpful. It is easier for a right-handed operator to perform the procedure on the patient's right side.

Identify the anatomic landmarks for the procedure after positioning the patient. Clean any dirt and debris from the area of the puncture site. Apply povidone iodine solution and allow it to dry.[14] **It is recommended to prepare the entire neck and clavicular area if the internal jugular or subclavian routes are attempted so that, if access to one site is unsuccessful, another site may by accessed without reprepping and draping. Due to the risk of inducing a pneumothorax, attempts at contralateral internal jugular or subclavian vein cannulation after an unsuccessful attempt must be delayed until a chest radiograph is checked to prevent bilateral pneumothoraces.**

Infiltrate the subcutaneous tissues at the needle puncture site with a generous volume of local anesthetic solution, including any areas that will be used for suturing the catheter in place. This allows the local anesthetic to diffuse throughout the area and take effect before the main procedure begins. Any distortion of anatomic landmarks caused by anesthetic infiltration decreases as the anesthetic is absorbed into the subcutaneous tissues.

Apply electrocardiographic monitoring, pulse oximetry, and noninvasive blood pressure monitoring to the patient and administer supplemental oxygen. Electrocardiographic monitoring during insertion of a central line is recommended due to the risk of ventricular dysrhythmias should the guidewire or catheter enter the right ventricle. It is preferable to have a designated person—physician or nurse—whose only job is to watch the monitoring equipment. The patient's face and chest will be draped for the internal jugular or subclavian vein cannulation procedure. The operator will be focused on the procedure and unaware of any sudden patient deterioration, ventilator disconnect, or other irregularities. Resuscitation equipment should be immediately available. A postinsertion chest radiograph to verify line placement and the lack of a pneumothorax must be immediately available.

TABLE 38-4. COMPARISONS BETWEEN CENTRAL VENOUS CATHETER TYPES

	Single-lumen	Multiple-lumen	Sheath (Cordis)
Minimum outer diameter	Smallest	Intermediate	Largest
Infusion rate	Moderate	Lowest (resuscitation catheters with larger lumen available)	Fastest (for central lumen; side port is slower)
Simultaneous infusions, or infusion while monitoring	No	Yes	Yes, if central lumen and side port both used
Length	Varies, fairly long	Long	Short
Allows device insertion (pulmonary artery lines and transvenous pacemakers)	No	No	Yes

Prepare for the procedure. Apply sterile gloves, a sterile gown, and a face mask if the situation is not a life-threatening emergency. Some physicians prefer to double-glove. If one glove becomes contaminated, it can be discarded and the procedure continued without interruption. Open the desired venous access kit. Perform a quick inventory and identify all necessary equipment before beginning the procedure. Set up a sterile field next to the patient and within easy reach. Place the equipment that must be immediately at hand on the sterile field. This includes a sterile drape, syringe, large-bore hollow needle, guidewire, and gauze squares. Any other equipment, including the catheter itself, may be temporarily set aside on a bedside stand.

INTERNAL JUGULAR VEIN CATHETERIZATION TECHNIQUES

CENTRAL APPROACH TO THE INTERNAL JUGULAR VEIN

While an internal jugular vein cannula can be inserted using the over-the-needle and through-the-needle techniques, the Seldinger technique is often preferred.[15,16] See Chapter 36 and Table 38-5 for a more complete discussion. The Seldinger technique uses a flexible guidewire, inserted through a special thin-walled hollow needle, to guide a catheter of any desired length through the skin and into the central circulation. This technique is described below and summarized in Table 38-6.[2]

Clean, prep, and drape the area as described previously. Place the patient in the Trendelenburg position with the head down 15 to 30 degrees. Rotate the patient's head away from the side that will be cannulated. Excessive rotation will distort the anatomic landmarks and may bring the internal jugular vein closer to the carotid artery.

Several cardinal rules for the insertion of the catheter should be observed. Always occlude the open hub of a needle or catheter in a central vein to prevent an air embolism. Never let go of the guidewire, so as to prevent its embolization into the central venous circulation. Never apply excessive force to the guidewire on insertion or removal. Doing so may injure the vessel, break the guidewire, and/or embolize the guidewire.

Attach the thin-walled introducer needle to a 5 mL syringe containing 1 mL of sterile saline or local anesthetic solution. The specially designed introducer needle included with the catheter should be used, as it has a relatively thin wall and a larger internal diameter relative to its external diameter. It has a shorter bevel than a conventional hypodermic needle. It also has a tapered hub to guide the guidewire into the needle proper.

If there is doubt about the exact location of the vein, it may first be located with a small "finder" needle. Insert a 25 or 27 gauge needle attached to a 5 mL syringe through the skin puncture site previously chosen. Advance the needle at a 30 to 60 degree angle to the skin while applying negative pressure to the syringe. A flash of blood signifies that the tip of the needle is within the vein. Note the depth and location of the vein. Remove the finder needle. Alternatively, the finder needle may be left in place for reference.

Insert the introducer needle at a 30 to 60 degree angle at the apex of the triangle formed by the sternal and clavicular heads of the sternocleidomastoid muscle and the clavicle (Figure 38-4). This point is just lateral to the carotid artery pulse.[2,3] Direct the introducer needle toward the ipsilateral nipple. Shallower angles make it necessary to traverse a greater amount of subcutaneous tissues and structures before entering the vessel. Steeper angles make insertion of the catheter over the guidewire difficult, as the guidewire tends to kink. Shallower angles are generally necessary in children whose vessels are smaller. Inject a small amount of the fluid in the syringe to remove any skin plug that may block blood return once the vein has been penetrated.

Apply negative pressure to the syringe by withdrawing the plunger. Advance the introducer needle into the vein (Figure 38-10A). If the vein is not located within 3 to 5 cm of the skin—this distance will vary depending on the patient's size and the target vessel's location—stop advancing the introducer needle. Withdraw the needle slowly while continuing to aspirate. Often, the vessel will have been completely traversed and no blood will return due to collapse of the vein by the pressure of the skin

TABLE 38-5. COMPARISON OF CATHETERIZATION METHODS

	Seldinger	Catheter-over-the-needle	Catheter-through-the-needle
Insertion needle	Small	Large	Largest
Speed	Slowest	Fastest	Fast
Number of steps	4+	1	2
Risk of catheter shear	None	Low	Highest
Catheters and lumens available	Single- or multiple-lumen, sheath/introducer	Single-lumen only	Single-lumen only
Rate of infusion	Highest (with sheath)	Moderate	Low to moderate

TABLE 38-6. SUMMARY OF THE SELDINGER METHOD OF CENTRAL VENOUS CANNULATION*

Step	Action	Tips and caveats
1	Prep and drape the skin puncture site.	For internal jugular vein, prepping down to the clavicle and up to the jaw will enable an attempt at the ipsilateral subclavian vein (or vice versa).
2	Anesthetize the puncture site if not already done.	Anesthetize the suture sites also.
3	Uncap the distal lumen.	Additional lumens may be flushed at this point or after insertion, as desired.
4	Locate the vein using the finder needle and aspirating syringe.	Internal jugular vein should be reached within 3 cm. Stop advancing after 4–5 cm if the vein is not located.
5	Remove the finder needle, noting the direction and depth of the internal jugular vein. Or withdraw the needle slightly so it is outside the internal jugular vein and leave it in place as a guide.	A few drops or a line of blood may be left on the skin as the finder is withdrawn to show the proper direction.
6	Insert introducer needle on a syringe along the "finder's" path until venous blood is aspirated. Alternatively, an introducer catheter and needle assembly can be used to cannulate the internal jugular vein; the needle is then withdrawn.	Syringe must have a nonlocking hub. A little saline in the syringe allows any occluding skin plug to be ejected. The vein is often located on withdrawal of the needle, since the friction of the large needle in the tissues can compress the internal jugular vein.
7	Disconnect the syringe from the needle, immediately occluding the open needle hub to prevent air embolism.	Do not move the needle at all! Keep the hand holding the needle in contact with the patient's skin to prevent movement.
8	Insert the guidewire through the introducer needle and into the vein.	Do not move the needle! Do not force the guidewire—it should pass easily!
9	Advance the guidewire into the vein to the desired depth or until ventricular ectopy is seen on the ECG monitor.	The guidewire must be securely in the vein, not just in the subcutaneous tissue.
10	Withdraw the introducer needle a few millimeters and use the scalpel to enlarge the puncture site slightly.	Keeping the needle in place eliminates any possibility of cutting the guidewire.
11	Remove the introducer needle.	Never let go of the guidewire!
12	Thread the dilator over the guidewire until it can be grasped outside the hub, then insert and withdraw the dilator.	Always keep a firm grip on the guidewire!
13	Thread the catheter tip over the guidewire and withdraw the guidewire from the skin until it can be grasped at the infusion hub.	Never let go of the guidewire.
14	Insert the catheter to the desired depth; most catheters are marked in centimeters, with larger markings every 5 and 10 cm. Introducer sheaths should be inserted completely.	The tip of the catheter should be in the superior vena cava, at the level of the manubriosternal angle.
15	Holding the catheter in place, remove the guidewire. Occlude the open hub with a gloved finger to prevent air embolism.	Do not apply excessive force to the guidewire. If it is trapped, withdraw the catheter a few centimeters and try again. Do not break the wire!
16	Attach a syringe to the catheter hub and aspirate blood, taking samples as desired; then flush the lumen with saline and begin the desired venous infusion.	Other lumens may be aspirated, flushed, and clamped.
17	Verify intravenous placement before suturing the catheter in place.	If the patient's blood travels up the intravenous tubing, the catheter is in the carotid artery!
18	Remove the patient from the Trendelenburg position.	
19	Suture the catheter to the skin with sutures and tape.	Take care not to puncture the catheter or to occlude it with a tight suture.
20	Apply a dressing to the catheter site.	
21	Verify catheter tip position by chest x-ray.	Catheter tip must be in the superior vena cava, not in the right atrium. Tip should be above the azygos vein and the carina, with the tip parallel to the vessel wall.

* The central approach to the internal jugular vein is used as an example, although the same technique is used for other approaches and central veins.

being forced inward as the introducer needle passes through it. Under normal physiologic conditions, veins have very low pressures within them and are easily collapsed by external pressure. If no blood is aspirated while withdrawing the needle, withdraw the introducer needle to the subcutaneous plane and redirect it slightly medially. Avoid putting continuous pressure on the

carotid artery pulse, as even gentle pressure may collapse the internal jugular vein (Figure 38-3B).

Stabilize and hold the introducer needle perfectly still with the nondominant hand once blood returns in the syringe. The carotid artery has been entered if the blood is bright red and/or forces the plunger of the syringe back. Remove the syringe. Blood should flow slowly and

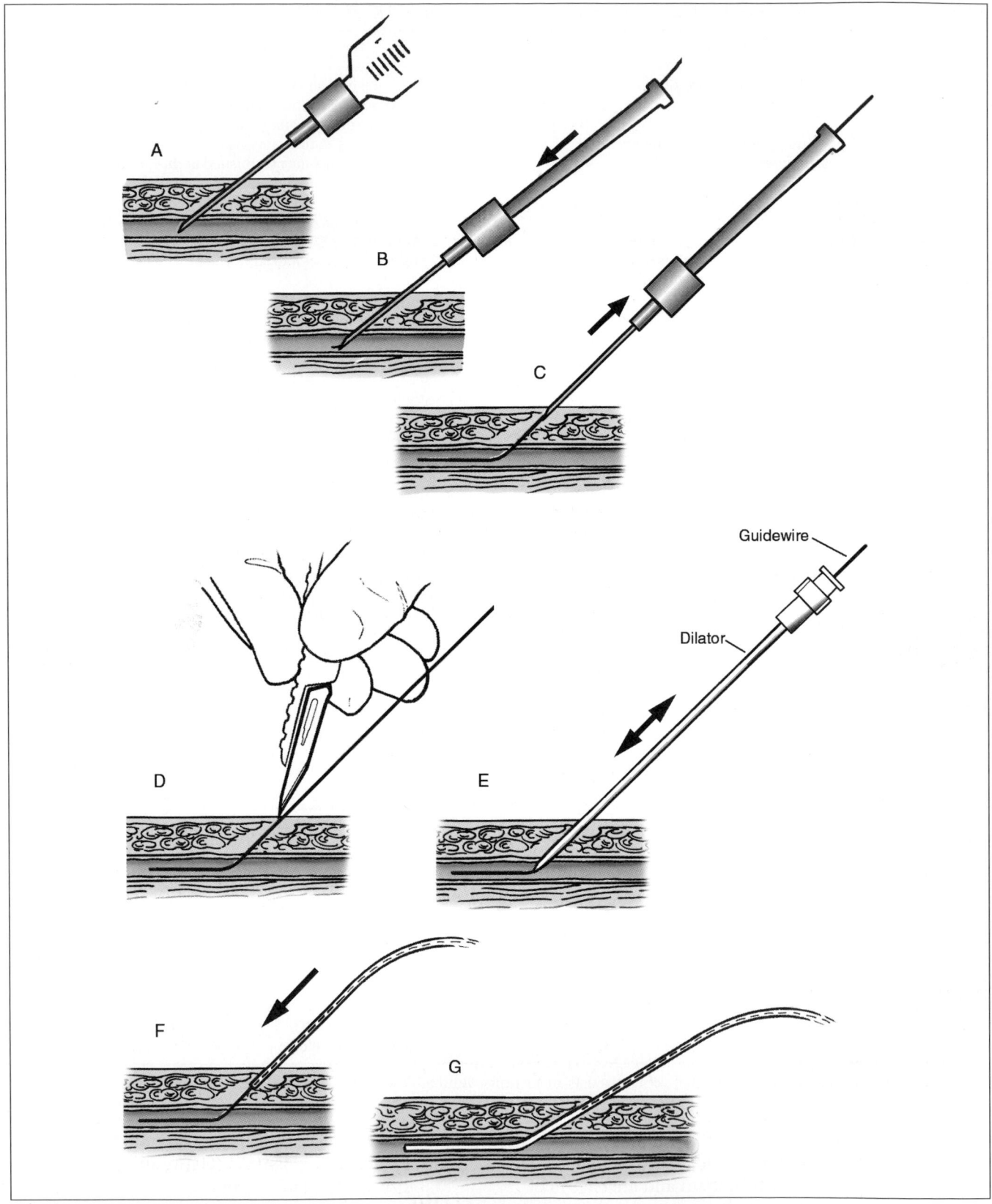

FIGURE 38-10 The Seldinger technique. *A.* The vein is punctured by the introducer needle and blood is aspirated. *B.* The syringe has been removed. The guidewire is inserted through the introducer needle and into the vein. *C.* The introducer needle and guidewire sleeve are withdrawn over the guidewire. *D.* The skin puncture site is enlarged. *E.* The dilator is advanced over the guidewire until the hub is against the skin; then it is removed. *F.* The catheter is advanced over the guidewire and into the vein. *G.* The guidewire is withdrawn through the catheter.

freely from the hub of the needle. The introducer needle is in the carotid or subclavian artery if blood squirts out the introducer needle hub. If blood dribbles out or does not flow from the hub and the patient has spontaneous circulation, reattach the syringe and reposition the introducer needle until free flow is obtained. Occlude the open hub of the introducer needle with the thumb of the nondominant hand while keeping the small finger of the hand in contact with the patient's skin. The operator's proprioceptive reflexes will prevent movement of the introducer needle by maintaining contact with the patient's skin. Even a millimeter of movement may result in failure to stay within the lumen of the vein.

Prepare the guidewire (Figure 38-11). Grasp the guidewire and its sleeve with the dominant hand. The tip of the guidewire has a "J" shape when the sleeve is retracted (Figure 38-11A). Slide the sleeve forward to straighten out the "J" of the guidewire (Figure 38-11B). Insert the wire sleeve into the hub of the introducer needle (Figure 38-11C). Advance the guidewire through the sleeve and into the introducer needle. **Never let go of the guidewire! One end of the wire must always be held to prevent loss of the wire and embolization into the central circulation.**

Do not simply reverse the guidewire if the sleeve used to straighten the curved end of the guidewire is lost. The straight end of the guidewire can puncture the wall of the vein. Grasp the guidewire between the fourth and fifth fingers and the palm of the dominant hand

(Figure 38-12A). Apply gentle traction on the curved guidewire tip with the thumb and the second and third fingers in order to straighten the guidewire (Figure 38-12B). The guidewire can then be inserted into the introducer needle hub without the use of the sleeve.

Advance the guidewire through the introducer needle and into the vein (Figure 38-10B). The guidewire should advance easily into the vein. **Never force the guidewire.** Guidewire resistance may indicate that the introducer needle is not within the vein, is against the wall of a vessel, or is caught as the vessel bends. Slightly withdraw the guidewire, rotate it slightly, and readvance it. **The use of force will kink the guidewire and may cause it to damage the vein and adjoining tissues.** Advance the guidewire 5 to 10 cm into the vessel or until ectopic beats are seen on the cardiac monitor. Withdraw the introducer needle and guidewire sheath while securely holding

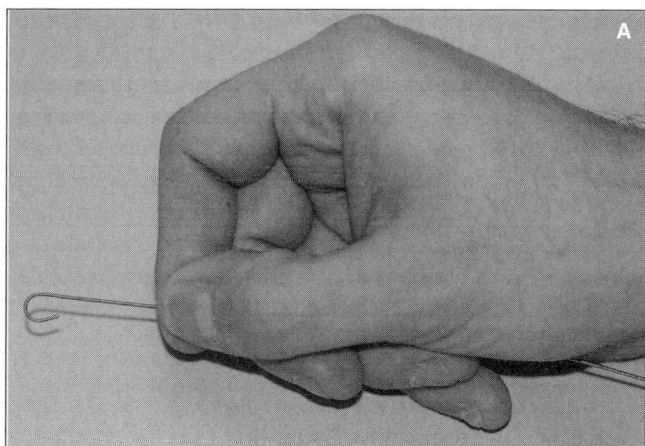

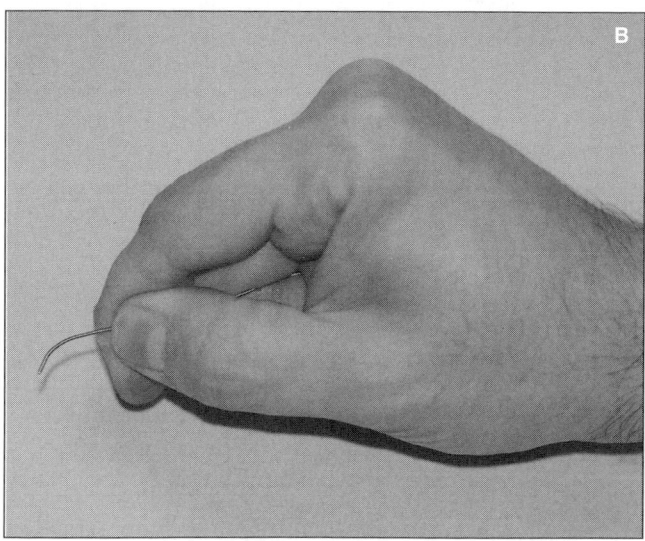

FIGURE 38-12 Straightening the "J" tip. *A.* Grasp the guidewire between the ring and small fingers and the palm. *B.* Apply traction using the thumb and index fingers, stretching the outer coil of the wire over the solid core to straighten the "J" tip.

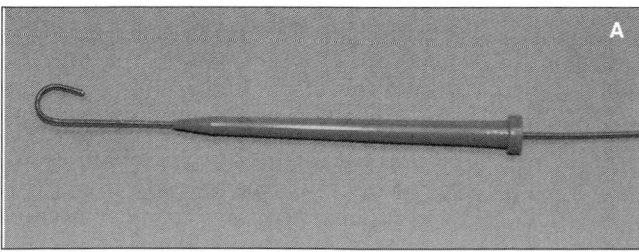

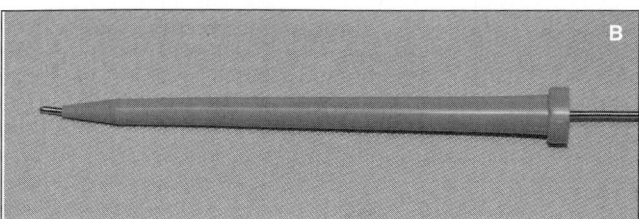

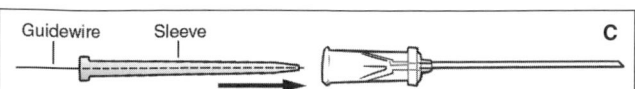

FIGURE 38-11 Guidewire preparation. *A.* The plastic sleeve is retracted, showing the "J" tip. *B.* The plastic sleeve is advanced to cover the guidewire tip, allowing the wire to be threaded into the introducer needle. *C.* The sleeve is inserted into the hub of the introducer needle.

the guidewire (Figure 38-10*C*). Grasp the guidewire with the nondominant hand as soon as the guidewire is visible between the tip of the introducer needle and the skin. Finish removing the needle over the guidewire.

Make a small incision in the skin adjacent to the guidewire using a #11 scalpel blade (Figure 38-10*D*). Place the dilator over the straight end of the guidewire (Figure 38-10*E*). Advance the dilator over the guidewire, through the skin, and into the vein. Continue to advance the dilator until its hub is against the skin. **Do not release hold of the guidewire at any time.** Remove the dilator over the guidewire.

Place the catheter tip over the guidewire. Advance the catheter over the guidewire and into the vein to the desired depth (Figure 38-10*F*). **Do not release hold of the guidewire.** Gently rolling or twisting the catheter between the thumb and forefinger may aid in its advancement. Hold the catheter securely in place and remove the guidewire (Figure 38-10*G*). Occlude the open catheter lumen with a sterile-gloved finger to prevent air embolization and excessive blood loss.

Attach a syringe to the catheter hub and aspirate blood to confirm that the catheter is within the vein.

Withdraw any necessary blood samples from the catheter. Attach infusion tubing or a heparin lock to the port and flush the catheter to prevent a blood clot from obstructing the lumen. If a multilumen catheter is inserted, flush any other lumens after first withdrawing any air (Figure 38-13). Securely attach the catheter to the skin with nylon or silk sutures. Cover the skin puncture site with a sterile dressing.

ANTERIOR APPROACH TO THE INTERNAL JUGULAR VEIN

The skin puncture site is at the anterior border of the sternal head of the sternocleidomastoid muscle, just lateral to the carotid artery[2,4,6] (Figure 38-5). Enter the skin at a 45 to 60 degree angle. Direct the introducer needle toward the ipsilateral nipple. The internal jugular vein in an adult should be encountered within 3 to 5 cm. If the vein is not encountered by 5 cm, withdraw the tip of the introducer needle to the subcutaneous space and redirect it slightly medially. The remainder of the procedure is as described for the central approach above and in Table 38-6.

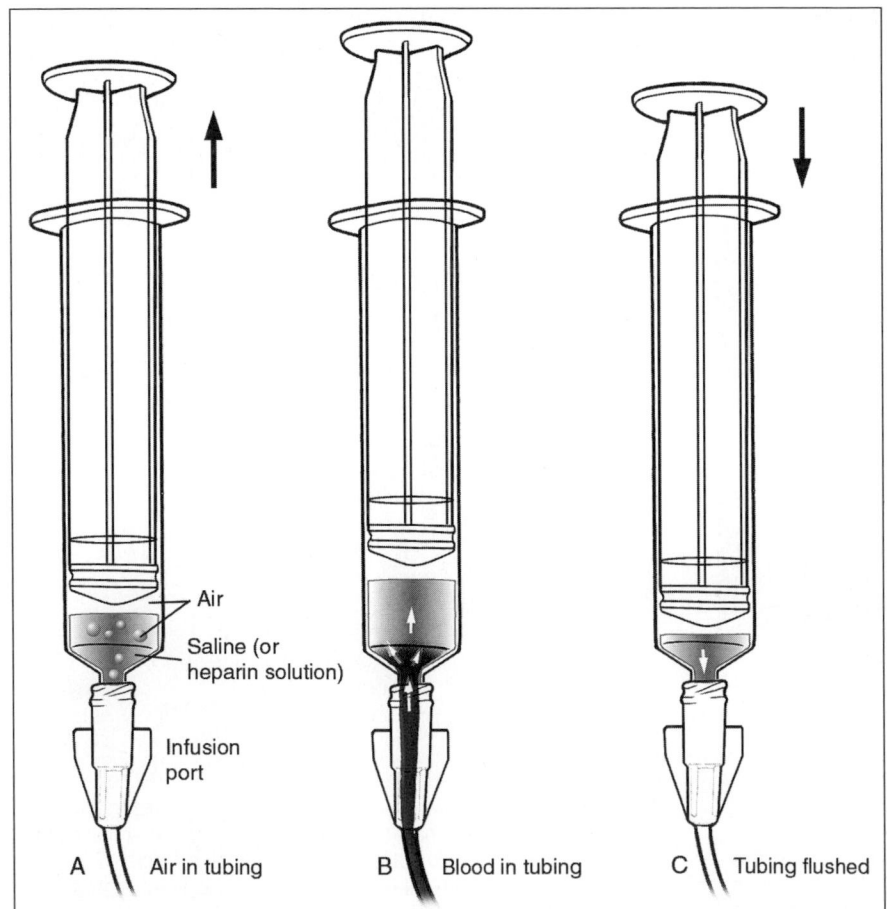

FIGURE 38-13 Aspiration and flushing of catheters. *A.* Any air in the lumen of the tubing is aspirated into the syringe of flush solution. The syringe must be held upright, as shown. *B.* Stop aspirating once all the air is removed from the catheter and blood begins to enter the syringe. *C.* Flush solution is injected until the lumen is filled and contains no blood. This usually requires 2 to 4 mL of flush solution.

POSTERIOR APPROACH TO THE INTERNAL JUGULAR VEIN

Enter the skin at the posterior edge of the sternocleidomastoid muscle, one-third of the way from the clavicle to the mastoid process[2,4,6] (Figure 38-6). Alternatively, the point where the external jugular vein crosses the lateral border of the sternocleidomastoid muscle can be used. Direct the introducer needle under the muscle at a 30 to 45 degree angle to the skin and toward the sternal notch. Place the index finger of the nondominant hand in the sternal notch to provide a landmark with the patient draped. In an adult, the internal jugular vein should be encountered within 5 centimeters. This approach is not recommended in children.[3] The remainder of the procedure is as described for the central approach above and in Table 38-6.

SUBCLAVIAN VEIN CATHETERIZATION TECHNIQUES

The technique is identical to that described above for internal jugular vein cannulation except for the puncture site. Two techniques, infraclavicular and supraclavicular, are described below and summarized in Table 38-7.

INFRACLAVICULAR APPROACH TO THE SUBCLAVIAN VEIN

The infraclavicular approach to the subclavian vein is most often used. It is commonly thought to be easier to perform and less likely to result in a pneumothorax than the supraclavicular approach, although data for this belief are lacking.[17] Some physicians prefer not to use a finder needle for infraclavicular subclavian vein cannulation as there is no danger of penetrating the carotid artery. This also makes as few needle passes near the pleura as possible in order to decrease the risk of a pneumothorax. Estimate the distance from the skin puncture site to the superior vena cava (i.e., the manubriosternal junction).

Several different skin entry sites are described in the literature. Some feel that the preferred entry site is 1 cm caudal to the junction of the medial and middle thirds of the clavicle. The subclavian vein lies just posterior to the clavicle at this site. The first rib lies between the pleural dome and the subclavian vein. Direct the introducer needle just superior and posterior to the suprasternal notch while staying as close to the frontal (coronal) plane as possible. The needle and syringe should be parallel to the bed (Figure 38-14). Placing the nondominant index finger in the sternal notch will help to guide placement (Figure 38-14).

Some practitioners prefer to enter the skin inferior to the clavicle at the deltopectoral groove, or the point just lateral to the midclavicular line along the inferior surface of the clavicle. This is the point where the skin may be maximally depressed. Direct the introducer needle parallel to the bed and toward the sternal notch. This entry site may make it easier to keep the introducer needle in the coronal plane. The distance before entering the subclavian vein is longer than in the preceding approach and the protection offered by the first rib is lost.

One of the editors (R.R.S.) prefers to use a different landmark. Palpate the bony tubercle, or protrusion, on the inferior surface of the clavicle and approximately one-third to one-half the length of the clavicle from the sternoclavicular joint. The advantage of this site is that it is a definitive landmark and avoids approximating distances, as described for the other sites above. Insert the introducer needle parallel to the bed and aimed just posterior to the sternal notch.

The bevel of the introducer needle should be oriented caudally, as should the "J" in the guidewire. This position will allow the guidewire to enter the innominate vein and superior vena cava rather than being directed upward into the internal jugular vein or across to the contralateral subclavian vein (Figure 38-15). Once venous blood is aspirated, the Seldinger technique for catheter insertion is otherwise the same as previously described for internal jugular vein cannulation. Aspiration of bright red blood under pressure indicates subclavian artery puncture, which will be incompressible. Remove

TABLE 38-7. COMPARISON OF SUBCLAVIAN VEIN CANNULATION ROUTES

	Infraclavicular approach	Supraclavicular approach
Entry site	Just inferior to the clavicle at the midclavicular line	1 cm lateral to the clavicular head of the sternocleidomastoid muscle, 1 cm posterior to the clavicle
Needle orientation	Keep as close to the coronal plane as possible	Tip aimed 10 degrees anterior to the coronal plane
Needle bevel and "J" wire directed (FIG)	Medially and caudally	Medially
Aim toward	Just posterior to the sternal notch	Contralateral nipple, needle bisects angle formed by the clavicle and the clavicular head of the sternocleidomastoid muscle
Distance from skin to subclavian vein	3–4 cm	2–3 cm

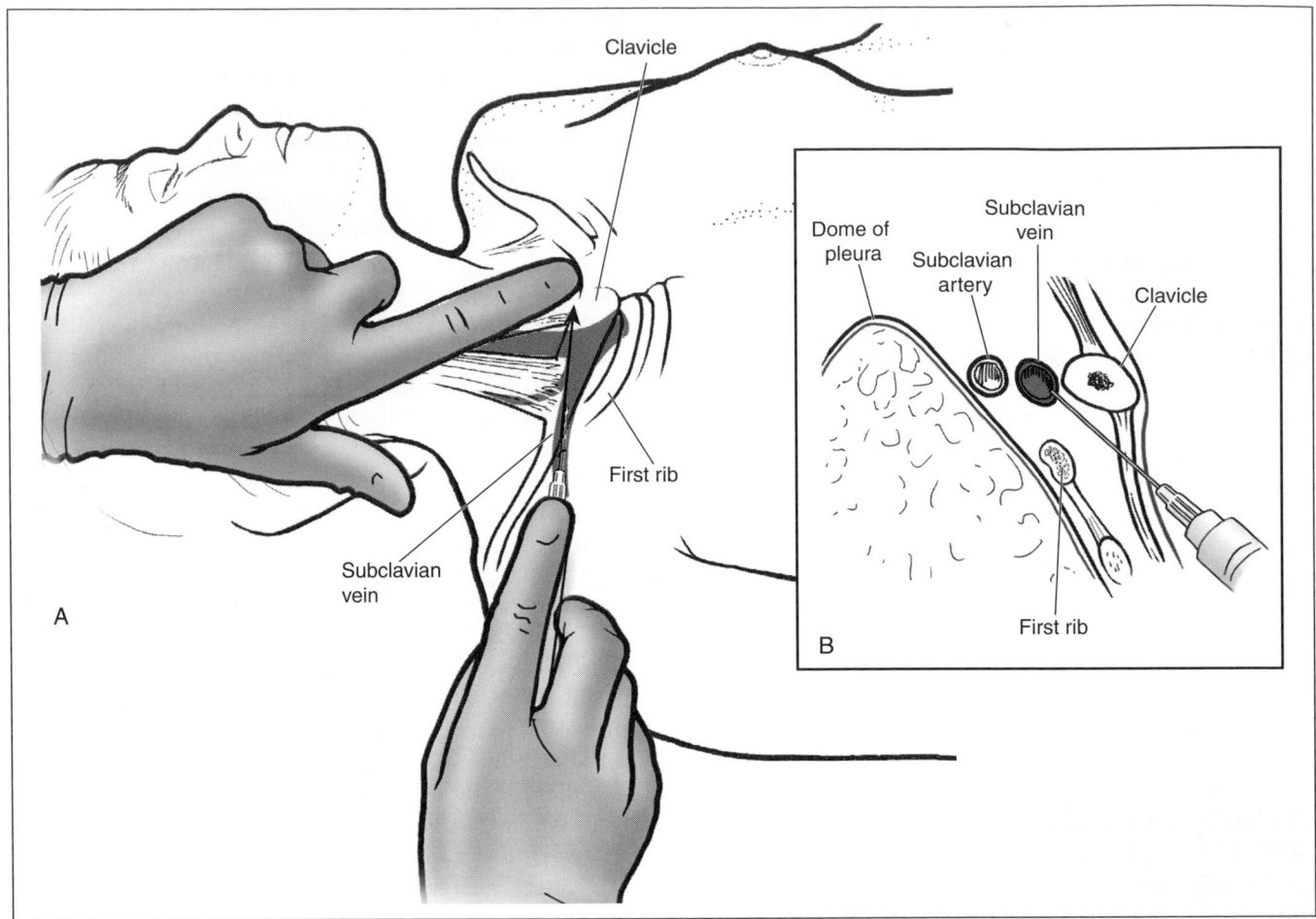

FIGURE 38-14 Infraclavicular approach to subclavian vein cannulation. *A.* Frontal (oblique) view of the procedure. *B.* Sagittal section through the medial third of the clavicle. Note the proximity of the pleura and subclavian artery.

the introducer needle and observe the patient for signs of significant hemorrhage over the next several hours. Aspiration of air indicates penetration of the pleura. Observation with serial chest radiographs for at least the next 6 to 24 hours is essential to evaluate the size of the resulting pneumothorax.

SUPRACLAVICULAR APPROACH TO THE SUBCLAVIAN VEIN

While most practitioners are more comfortable with the infraclavicular approach to the subclavian vein, the supraclavicular approach offers some advantages. The subclavian vein is closer to the skin. The route from a right-sided skin puncture site to the superior vena cava is more direct. It allows easier access to the superior vena cava while avoiding the hazards of a left-sided puncture (i.e., the thoracic duct). The skin entry site is more accessible during CPR and requires less interruption of external chest compressions.[18] With experience, the complication rate for the supraclavicular approach is probably lower than that for the infraclavicular approach.[17,19]

Estimate the distance from the skin puncture site to the superior vena cava to guide the catheter insertion depth. The skin is entered at a point 1 cm lateral to the lateral border of the clavicular head of the sternocleidomastoid muscle and 1 cm superior to the clavicle[20] (Figure 38-16). The introducer needle should bisect the angle formed by the clavicle and the lateral border of the sternocleidomastoid muscle (Figure 38-16*A*). Direct the introducer needle toward the contralateral nipple or a point just superior and posterior to the sternal notch. Orient the introducer needle bevel medially (Figure 38-15). The subclavian vein should be entered within 2 to 3 cm in an adult. The length of catheter inserted will be a few centimeters less than that for the infraclavicular approach.

Alternative skin entry sites and approaches have been described. Enter the skin 1 cm medially and 1 cm superiorly to the midpoint of the clavicle with the introducer needle directed toward the ipsilateral sternoclavicular joint.[21] The skin can be entered just posterior to the clavicle, at the junction of the medial and middle third of the

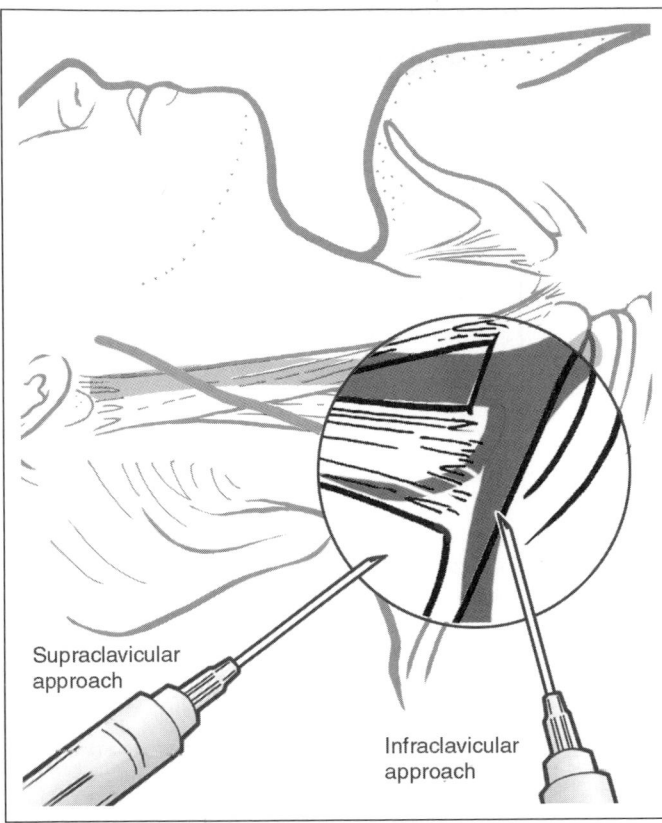

FIGURE 38-15 Introducer needle bevel orientation for subclavian vein cannulation. Varying the orientation of the introducer needle bevel for infraclavicular and supraclavicular techniques helps guide the "J" shaped guidewire into the superior vena cava.

clavicle, with the introducer needle directed toward the ipsilateral sternoclavicular joint and parallel to the coronal plane.[22] This last approach is probably the simplest, although the study cited was performed on cadavers rather than live patients.

FEMORAL VEIN CATHETERIZATION TECHNIQUE

The use of an ECG monitor is still recommended even though the short guidewire may not reach the heart. Particular care must be taken if the patient has a preexisting left bundle branch block, as complete heart block may result if the guidewire or catheter enters the right ventricle.[9] Premeasuring from the insertion site to the xiphoid process will give the maximum depth of catheter insertion.

The introducer needle should enter the skin 2 to 4 cm inferior to the midpoint of the inguinal ligament and 1 cm medial to the femoral artery pulse (Figure 38-17). In an infant or young child, the introducer needle should

enter the skin 1 to 2 cm inferior to the inguinal ligament and 0.5 cm medial to the femoral artery pulse. The cannulation technique is as described previously for the internal jugular vein.

Two site-specific considerations deserve mention.[2,3,6] The use of a finder needle is unnecessary, since there are no vital structures in the area other than the femoral artery that is compressible if it is punctured. The introducer needle is directed at a 45 to 60 degree angle to the skin and parallel to the long axis of the thigh. Shallower angles may be necessary in very small and thin patients. **Use caution to avoid puncturing the posterior wall of the vein above the inguinal ligament, since this can result in a retroperitoneal hemorrhage.**

ALTERNATIVE TECHNIQUES

USE OF THE SELDINGER-HUB INTRODUCER CATHETER

Some central venous access kits, including some manufactured by Arrow (Arrow International, 800-523-8446), include a catheter-over-the-needle with a tapered hub that can be used in place of the thin-walled introducer needle. This technique has the advantage of allowing the introducer catheter to remain in place while venous placement is verified. It provides less likelihood of the vein being lost as the aspiration syringe is removed and the guidewire advanced. A guidewire advanced through the introducer catheter cannot become sheared off, as when it is inserted through the needle.

The vein is entered with the catheter-over-the-needle assembly attached to an aspirating syringe, as described previously. Once the flashback of blood is obtained, advance the catheter-over-the-needle 2 mm further into the vein. This will ensure that the tip of the introducer catheter is within the vein. Hold the hub of the needle securely. Advance the catheter into the vein until its hub is against the skin. Withdraw the needle. If necessary, the introducer catheter may be attached to a pressure transducer and the venous waveform verified to confirm venous rather than arterial placement. Blood gas measurements may also be performed. Advance the guidewire through the introducer catheter and into the vein. The remainder of the procedure is as previously described.

MULTIPLE-LUMEN CATHETERS

Prior to skin puncture, remove the cap from the distal port's injection hub. It is usually marked "distal." It is colored brown in the Arrow kits. The other lumens may be flushed with saline or heparin solution and recapped or left capped and flushed later (Figure 38-13). Heparin concentrations no higher than 100 U/mL should be used to avoid temporarily anticoagulating the patient.[23]

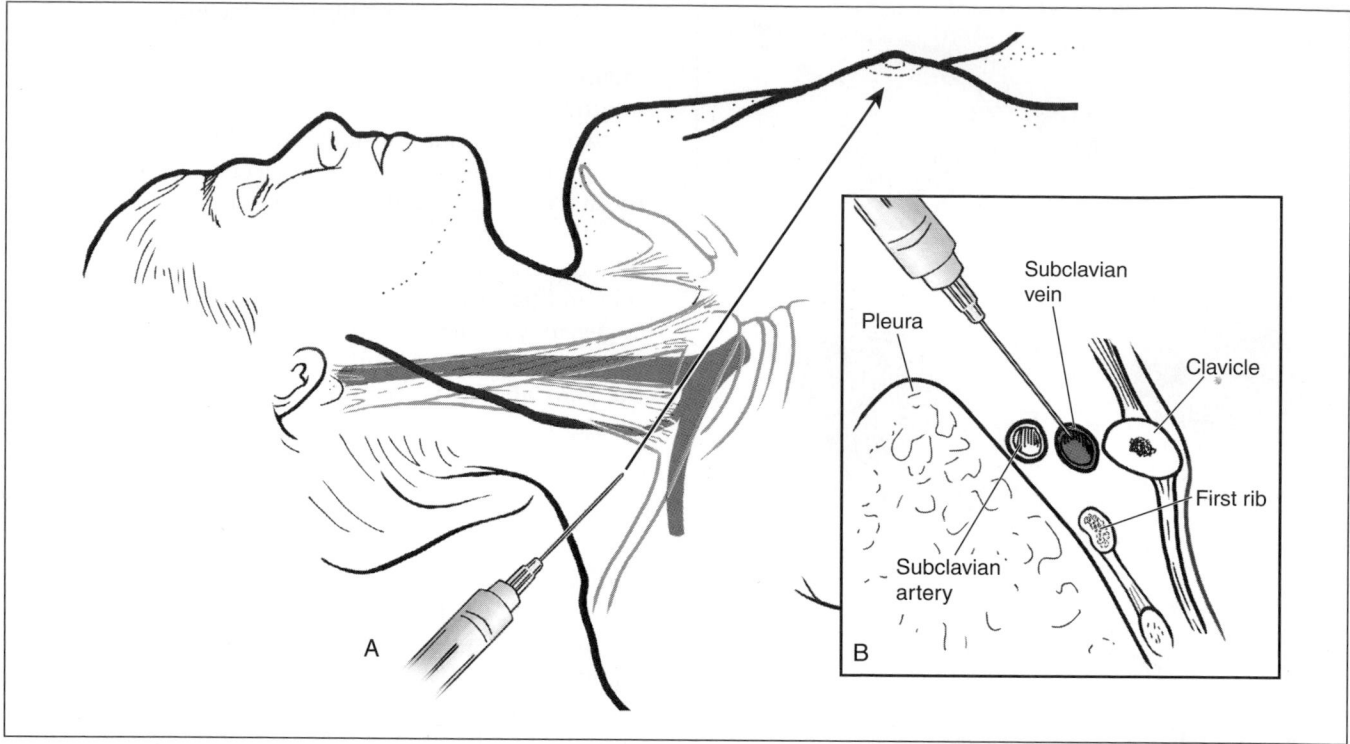

FIGURE 38-16 Supraclavicular approach to subclavian vein cannulation. *A.* From the insertion point 1 cm superior to the clavicle and 1 cm lateral to the border of the sternocleidomastoid muscle, direct the introducer needle tip at a 45 degree angle to the transverse and sagittal planes and slightly anterior toward the contralateral nipple. *B.* Sagittal section through the medial third of the clavicle. Note that the introducer needle track must be directed anteriorly to avoid the subclavian artery and the dome of the pleura.

The introducer needle and guidewire are inserted as described previously. Place the multiple-lumen catheter tip over the guidewire. Advance the catheter until the guidewire emerges from the distal port hub (Figure 38-18). Insert the catheter to the desired depth. Remove the guidewire. Flush the distal lumen and connect it to the desired infusion. If not done previously, aspirate and flush the other lumens with the desired solution (Figure 38-13).

PERCUTANEOUS INTRODUCER SHEATH (CORDIS)

The insertion technique differs slightly from those described above (Figure 38-19). Insert the plastic dilator into the lumen of the sheath. The entire assembly must be advanced over the guidewire as a unit rather than utilizing separate dilation and insertion steps (Figure 38-19C). A correspondingly larger skin nick must be made with the scalpel, since the sheath is usually of larger diameter than a catheter. Advance the dilator-sheath unit over the guidewire and into the vein (Figure 38-19D). A twisting motion may aid in its advancement. Continue to advance the unit until the hub of the sheath is against the skin (Figure 38-19E). Remove the guidewire and dilator as a unit (Figure 38-19E). The remainder of the procedure is as described previously.

PEDIATRIC CONSIDERATIONS

The anterior or central approach to the internal jugular vein is preferred for children.[3] Appropriate catheter sizes and lengths are shown in Table 38-3. The child must be sedated and immobilized prior to attempts at cannulation of the internal jugular or subclavian vein. The femoral vein is the vein of choice if central venous access is needed in a combative child who cannot be completely restrained. The patient need not be in Trendelenburg position, the consequences of a misdirected needle are less severe, and the procedure is less threatening as the face is not draped.[7] A shallower angle of skin entry than in an adult is necessary to access the femoral vein. Enter the skin 1 to 2 cm inferior to the inguinal ligament and 0.5 mm medial to the femoral artery.

ASSESSMENT

Examine the patient. Examine the lung fields carefully to exclude a significant pneumothorax. Vital signs should be rechecked. Obtain a portable anteroposterior chest radiograph to verify line tip placement in the superior vena cava and rule out a procedure-related pneumothorax. Check the catheter site for hematoma formation or

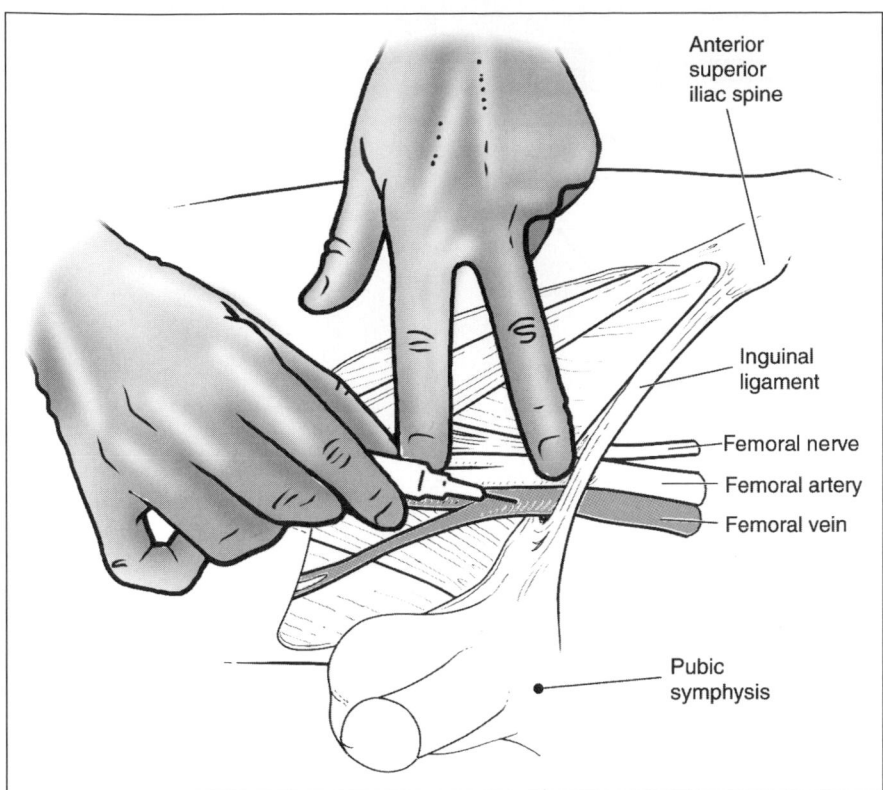

FIGURE 38-17 Femoral vein cannulation. The skin puncture site is 1 cm medial to the femoral artery pulse and 2 to 4 cm inferior to the inguinal ligament. Direct the introducer needle posteriorly at a 45 to 60 degree angle while aspirating.

hemorrhage along the dilated catheter track. Control any hemorrhage with direct pressure.

Check the function of the catheter by aspiration and infusion through all ports, as discussed above. A proximal lumen may be extravascular if it fails to aspirate blood easily. A catheter may be exchanged over a guidewire as long as the distal tip of the catheter is definitely intravascular. Do not attempt to advance the catheter once the guidewire has been removed.

Check the position of the catheter tip on the chest radiograph. The catheter must not be in the heart due to the risk that erosion through the thin right atrial wall will result in a pericardial hemorrhage and tamponade.[24,25] Landmarks for an internal jugular or sub-

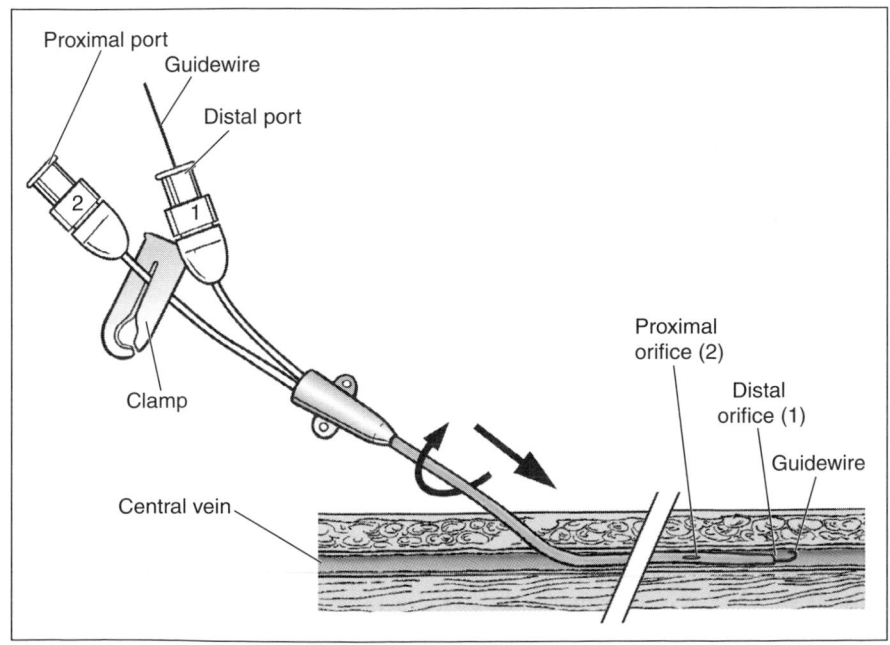

FIGURE 38-18 Inserting a multiple-lumen catheter. The guidewire exits through the uncapped distal port. The proximal port(s) must be clamped or capped to prevent air embolism.

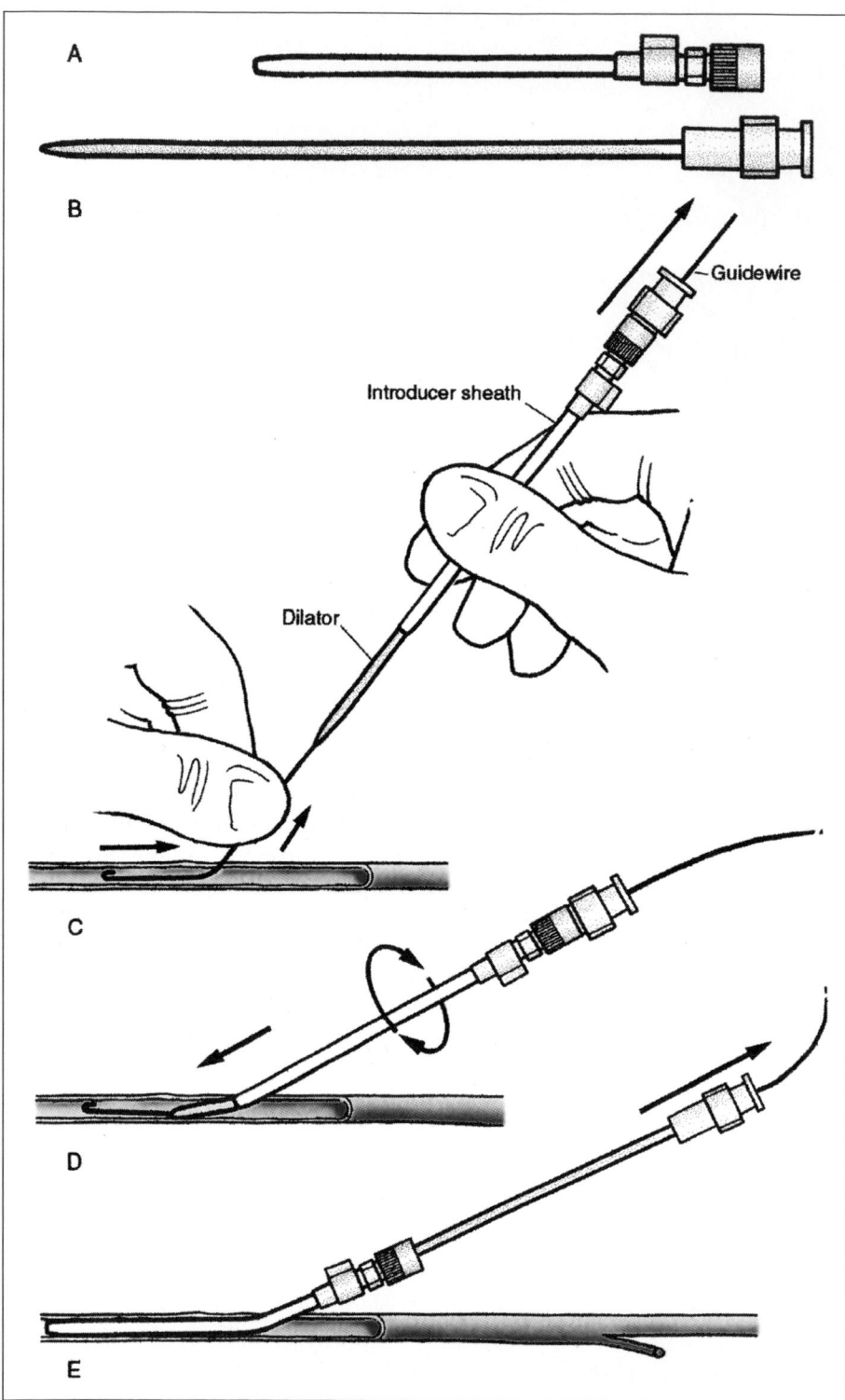

FIGURE 38-19 Inserting an introducer sheath. *A.* The sheath. *B.* The dilator. *C.* The dilator is inserted into the sheath and the unit is threaded over the guidewire. *D.* Advance the unit over the guidewire and into the vein using a twisting motion (*arrow*). *E.* The dilator and guidewire are removed as a unit, leaving the sheath in place.

clavian vein catheter tip include the following: above the level of the carina, above the azygos vein, and at/above the manubriosternal junction. The tip of the catheter should be parallel to the vein to prevent erosion through the wall of the vein. If the catheter crosses over to the opposite subclavian vein and the patient cannot tolerate an attempt at repositioning, it may be

used for intravenous infusion. Lines placed from the subclavian vein into the jugular system must be replaced. Catheters in or below the right atrium must be pulled back immediately to prevent perforation of the myocardium.

Most femoral vein catheters can be fully inserted. Premeasurement is recommended to make sure that the catheter tip will not reach the right atrium. If there is any doubt about the catheter position, postinsertion abdominal and chest radiographs should be obtained. The tip of the catheter must be at or below the xiphoid process of the sternum. Reassess the distal neurovascular status of the lower extremity after line placement.

AFTERCARE

The catheter must be sutured in place to prevent malpositioning of the line. Tie a surgeon's knot at the skin, then secure the suture to the hole(s) provided in the catheter wings. A catheter clamp is often provided in the kit for longer catheters. It too should be sutured in place. The clamp holds the catheter in place by friction. It is not a guarantee that the catheter will not move. Catheter depth should be checked daily by inspection and by frequent chest radiographs. Movement of the patient's head and neck may move the tip of the internal jugular vein catheter by as much as 4 cm.[26]

Introducer sheaths have large lumens and present a significant risk of causing an air embolism. Cap the main lumen if it is not being used for an infusion. Any built-in diaphragm is not a reliable means of preventing an air embolism.[27] Do not use the dilator as an occluder or infusion port, as the stiff plastic can easily erode through the wall of the vein. An occlusive dressing can be used if no occluder is available.

The skin puncture site should be checked regularly for signs of infection. Cellulitis or purulent drainage requires a new central venous line at another site. Remember to restrain any patient who is uncooperative so as to prevent inadvertent removal of the central line.

While the short-term infection rate of femoral lines compares favorably with that in other central lines, some precautions are necessary to prevent soilage of the site.[28,29] Consider the judicious use of bladder catheterization in patients who are incontinent of urine and of rectal tubes in patients with loose stools. Patients with percutaneous femoral vein catheters must be confined to bed to prevent catheter dislodgment and hemorrhage around the catheter. Frequent assessment for venous thombosis in the lower extremity is essential. It is recommended that femoral lines be discontinued when an alternative venous access site is available or within 3 days, whichever is sooner.[30]

REMOVAL OF THE CENTRAL VENOUS CATHETER

When removing a central venous catheter from the internal jugular or subclavian vein, place the patient in the Trendelenburg position. To remove a femoral vein catheter, place the patient supine. Remove the dressing overlying the skin puncture site. Cut the suture securing the catheter to the skin. Ask the patient to exhale and hold his or her breath. Briskly remove the catheter and cover the puncture site with a gauze dressing. The track from the skin surface to the vein can be a source of a fatal venous air embolism.[31] If the catheter had a large diameter or remained in place for more than 2 to 3 days, apply an occlusive dressing to the site for the first 1 to 2 days after the catheter has been removed. The skin puncture site should be observed for signs of infection twice a day for 48 hours.

COMPLICATIONS

INTERNAL JUGULAR VEIN CATHETERIZATION

Internal jugular venous access has a myriad of potential complications.[24,32–35] Infection can be either at the local site or in a systemic line due to bacteremia and sepsis. A pneumothorax can occur during line placement. A hemothorax may be life-threatening, especially if a venopleural fistula is created. A chylothorax occurs if the thoracic duct is lacerated. Occasionally, carotid artery puncture can result. It may be complicated by a stroke if the blood supply to the brain is interrupted or if a plaque embolizes. Airway compromise can occur due to the formation of a hematoma and compression of the airway. An air embolism can occur if the catheter lumens are left open to the air during insertion or if connections loosen and separate at a later time. Right ventricular irritation from the catheter tip can cause cardiac dysrhythmias. Puncture of the right atrial wall can lead to pericardial tamponade and death. The guidewire can become entrapped, necessitating surgical or interventional radiology removal. Embolization of the guidewire or catheter parts occurs with improper use of the equipment. Anaphylactic reactions to antibiotic-impregnated catheters have been reported. The cardiac monitors should be observed during the procedure to prevent the death of a critically ill patient from being unnoticed while the catheter is being inserted. Thrombosis of the catheter or vein may lead to pulmonary embolism.

Many of these complications can be prevented if the procedure outlined above is followed carefully. Complications during catheterization occur in proportion to the operator's inexperience.[33] If the patient is unlikely to survive a mistake, the most experienced person available should perform the procedure!

SUBCLAVIAN VEIN CATHETERIZATION

Complications of subclavian vein cannulation are similar to those of internal jugular vein cannulation, as described above. While there is no risk of carotid artery injury if the procedure is performed correctly, the subclavian artery can be lacerated if the needle is advanced too deeply. Malposition of the catheter tip, usually due to overinsertion of the catheter, is common. Lacerations of the thoracic duct can be avoided by performing the procedure on the right side, avoiding overpenetration with the introducer needle, and avoiding directing the needle too superiorly toward the junction of the subclavian vein and internal jugular vein. Other complications, such as injury to the brachial plexus and phrenic nerve, are uncommon. They can be prevented by avoiding overinsertion of the needle during the procedure and avoiding needle paths superior and posterior to the subclavian vein.

A pneumothorax is a very real risk with subclavian vein catheterization. The procedure should not be performed unless personnel are immediately available who can deal with this complication.[36] The risk of a pneumothorax is probably higher in obese patients, who may have distorted anatomic landmarks and in whom a more acute angle is required to enter the subclavian vein. Patients with emphysema may have higher pleural domes and less pulmonary reserve in the event of a pneumothorax.

FEMORAL VEIN CATHETERIZATION

Deep venous thrombosis of the femoral and more distal veins is a recognized complication of femoral venous lines.[30] Inadvertent cannulation of the femoral artery may occur. This is particularly true during an episode of severe hypotension or cardiac arrest. If such an episode goes unrecognized, infusion of vasopressors into the artery may result in ischemic injury to the distal limb.

SUMMARY

Central venous access is often necessary in critically ill patients and in those with poor peripheral veins. Mastery of these techniques is essential for anyone who will be caring for acutely ill and unstable patients. While all approaches to the central circulation have acceptably low complication rates (1 to 5 percent) when performed by experienced providers, they all carry real risks to the patient.[17,24] Be certain that there is no safer peripheral access alternative before placing a central venous line.

The internal jugular vein is a good choice for central venous access in nonambulatory patients. The right internal jugular vein provides easy access to the superior vena cava for monitoring and for infusion of solutions too concentrated or irritating for peripheral veins. This route poses a slightly lower risk of complications than the subclavian route.[33,35]

The subclavian vein provides easy access to the central circulation. Subclavian vein catheters are more easily tolerated by awake and ambulatory patients than are internal jugular or femoral catheters. Subclavian vein cannulation does present very real risks to the patient that must be balanced against the need for the procedure and other alternatives. Subclavian vein access is the least preferred route in young children due to their small size, the proximity of the pleura, and the proximity of the subclavian artery.[3]

Femoral vein cannulation is an essential emergency skill. It allows the easiest central venous access in most patients with the lowest risk of catastrophic immediate complications compared to jugular and subclavian access procedures.

REFERENCES

1. Williams PL, Warwick R: *Gray's Anatomy,* 36th ed. Philadelphia: Saunders, 1980:629–765.
2. Barker WJ: Central venous catheterization: internal jugular approach and alternatives, in Roberts JR, Hedges JR (eds): *Clinical Procedures in Emergency Medicine,* 2nd ed. Philadelphia: Saunders, 1991:340–351.
3. Lavelle J, Costarino A: Central venous access and central venous pressure monitoring, in Henretig FM, King C (eds): *Textbook of Pediatric Emergency Procedures.* Baltimore: Williams & Wilkins, 1997:251–278.
4. Sutariya BB, Berk WA: Vascular access, in Tintinalli JE, Kelen GD, Stapczynski JS (eds): *Emergency Medicine: A Comprehensive Study Guide,* 5th ed. New York: McGraw-Hill, 2000:102–111.
5. Dronen SC: Central venous catheterization: subclavian vein approach, in Roberts JR, Hedges JR (eds): *Clinical Procedures in Emergency Medicine,* 2nd ed. Philadelphia: Saunders, 1991:325–340.
6. Cummins RO: *Advanced Cardiac Life Support.* Dallas: American Heart Association,1994, chap 6:1–13.
7. Yeh TS: Deep venous lines, in Yeh TS, Hanson JH (eds): *My Way—A Resident Handbook for the Pediatric ICU,* 2nd ed. Oakland, CA: Children's Hospital Oakland, 1992:19–22.
8. Lee HS, Quinn T, Boyle RM: Safety of thrombolytic treatment in patients with central venous cannulation. *Br Heart J* 1995; 73:359–362.
9. Eissa NT, Kvetan V: Guide wire as a cause of complete heart block in patients with preexisting left bundle branch block. *Anesthesiology* 1990; 73:772–774.
10. Gil RT, Kruse JA, Thill-Baharozian MC, et al: Triple- vs. single-lumen central venous catheters. *Arch Intern Med* 1989; 149:1139–1143.
11. Farkas J-C, Liu N, Bleriot J-P, et al: Single- versus triple-lumen central catheter-related sepsis: a prospective randomized study in a critically ill population. *Am J Med* 1992; 93:277–282.

12. Miller JJ, Venus B, Mathru M: Comparison of the sterility of long-term central venous catheterization using single lumen, triple lumen, and pulmonary artery catheters. *Crit Care Med* 1984; 12(8):634–637.

13. Jesseph JM, Conces DJ, Augustyn GT: Patient positioning for subclavian vein catheterization. *Arch Churg* 1987; 122:1207–1209.

14. Elliott TS, Faroqui MH, Armstrong RF, et al: Guidelines for good practice in central venous catheterization. *J Hosp Infect* 1994; 28:163–176.

15. Seldinger SI: Catheter replacement of the needle in percutaneous arteriography: a new technique. *Acta Radiol* 1953; 39:368–376.

16. Dailey RH: Use of wire-guided (Seldinger-type) catheters in the emergency department. *Ann Emerg Med* 1983; 12(8):489–492.

17. Sterner S, Plummer DW, Clinton J, et al: A comparison of the supraclavicular approach and the infraclavicular approach for subclavian vein catheterization. *Ann Emerg Med* 1986; 15(4):421–423.

18. Dronen S, Thompson B, Nowak R, et al: Subclavian vein catheterization during cardiopulmonary resuscitation. *JAMA* 1982; 247(3):3227–3230.

19. Nevarre DR, Domingo OH: Supraclavicular approach to subclavian catheterization: review of the literature and results of 178 attempts by the same operator. *J Trauma* 1997; 42(2):305–309.

20. Yoffa D: Supraclavicular subclavian venepuncture and catheterization. *Lancet* 1965; 2:614–617.

21. Conroy JM, Rajagopalan PR, Baker JD, et al: A modification of the supraclavicular approach to the central circulation. *South Med J* 1990; 83(10):1178–1181.

22. MacDonnell JE, Perez H, Pitts SR: Supraclavicular subclavian vein catheterization: modified landmarks for needle insertion. *Ann Emerg Med* 1992; 21(4):421–424.

23. Fry B: Intermittent heparin flushing protocols. *J Intraven Nurs* 1992; 15(3):160–163.

24. Carr M, Jagannath A: Hemopericardium resulting from attempted internal jugular vein catheterization: a case report and review of complications of central venous cannulation. *Cardiovasc Intervent Radiol* 1986; 9:214–218.

25. Collier PE, Ryan JJ, Daimond DL: Cardiac tamponade from central venous catheters: case report and review of the English literature. *Angiology* 1984; 35:595–600.

26. Curelaru I, Linder L-E, Gustavsson B: Displacement of catheters inserted through internal jugular veins with neck flexion and extension. *Intens Care Med* 1980; 6:179–183.

27. Bristow A, Batjer H, Chow V, et al: Air embolism via a pulmonary artery catheter introducer. *Anesthesiology* 1985; 63:340–341.

28. Stenzel JP, Green TP, Fuhrman BP: Percutaneous femoral venous catheterizations: a prospective study of complications. *J Pediatr* 1989; 114(3):411–415.

29. Williams JF, Seneff MG, Friedman BC: Use of femoral venous catheters in critically ill adults: prospective study. *Crit Care Med* 1991; 19(4):550–553.

30. Meredith JW, Young JS, O'Neil EA, et al: Femoral catheters and deep venous thrombosis: a prospective evaluation with venous duplex sonography. *J Trauma* 1993; 35(2):187–191.

31. Phifer TJ, McIntyre B, Conrad SA: The residual central venous catheter track—an occult source of lethal air embolism: case report. *J Trauma* 1991; 31(11):1558–1560.

32. Richet H, Hubert B, Nitemberg G, et al: Prospective multicenter study of vascular–catheter-related complications and risk factors for positive central-catheter cultures in intensive care unit patients. *J Clin Microbiol* 1990; 28:2520–2525.

33. Sznajder JI, Zveibil FR, Bitterman H, et al: Central vein catheterization: failure and complication rates by three percutaneous approaches. *Arch Intern Med* 1986; 146:259–261.

34. Arnold IR, Brack MJ, Verma PK, et al: Infected right atrial thrombi: a complication of central venous cannulation. *Int J Cardiol* 1994; 43:101–104.

35. Eisenhauer ED, Derveloy RJ, Hastings PR: Prospective evaluation of central venous pressure (CVP) catheters in a large city-county hospital. *Ann Surg* 1982; 196:560–564.

36. Walker MM, Sanders RC: Pneumothorax following supraclavicular subclavian venepuncture. *Anaesthesia* 1969; 24(3):453–460.

37. *Cook Double Lumen Central Venous Catheter Instructions.* Cook Critical Care, PO Box 489, Bloomington, IN 47402, USA, 800-457-4500. Cook Inc., 1995.

Chapter 39

TROUBLESHOOTING INDWELLING CENTRAL VENOUS LINES

Robert Feldman

INTRODUCTION

Implanted venous access devices are essential for the long-term care of many chronically ill patients. These patients may have poor peripheral venous access due to the many venipunctures they have previously suffered. When a patient's long-term venous access device cannot be easily aspirated or flushed, the Emergency Physician must act quickly and intelligently to diagnose and correct the malfunction without further damaging the device.

ANATOMY AND PATHOPHYSIOLOGY

Indwelling central venous catheters allow access to the central venous circulation from a peripheral site. This access to the central circulation is via the end of a partially implanted catheter that protrudes from the body or through the skin into a subcutaneous reservoir of a fully implanted catheter.[1,2] The proximal tip of the central venous line may reside in either the superior vena cava or in the right atrium.

Indwelling central venous access devices may malfunction for a variety of reasons. The catheter tip may be lodged against the wall of the blood vessel. The catheter may become obstructed by an intraluminal or external clot. The catheter tubing may be obstructed mechanically or by precipitated medications. Phenytoin and diazepam cannot be given through silicone indwelling lines as they can crystallize and permanently obstruct the catheter lumen.[3] Calcium and phosphate can form an insoluble precipitate within the catheter lumen. Infused lipids can form waxy casts within the catheter lumen.

INDICATIONS

Any catheter that cannot be easily flushed or aspirated must be investigated further. If peripheral venous access is readily available, and the patient is not acutely ill due to catheter sepsis or central venous thrombosis, catheter troubleshooting can be deferred to the Primary Care Provider. The Emergency Physician will have to correct the problem, if possible, if emergent or urgent access to the device is needed.

CONTRAINDICATIONS

Any device that is obviously displaced from the central circulation is not salvageable and should not be used. Dislodging a clot or septic thrombus from a catheter tip can lead to a fatal pulmonary embolism. Catheter manipulation should be avoided if signs of sepsis or central venous thrombosis are present.[4] Unfortunately, such a diagnosis is often possible only in retrospect. The use of indwelling dialysis lines for other purposes is discouraged. Manipulation of a dialysis line should only be undertaken in a true emergency or if the line is malfunctioning and is needed for hemodialysis.

EQUIPMENT

Povidone iodine solution
Sterile alcohol prep pads
Thrombolytic agent
Syringes, 5 mL and 10 mL
18 gauge needles
Noncoring (Huber) needle
70% ethanol solution
0.1 N hydrochloric acid (HCl) solution
Sterile saline
Heparinized saline flush solution (100 U/mL)
Sterile gauze squares
Sterile gloves

The use of a specific thrombolytic agent is institution- and physician-specific. Streptokinase, recombinant tissue plasminogen activator (t-PA), and urokinase have all been successfully used to dissolve a clot within a central venous catheter.[3,5–9] Urokinase and recombinant tissue plasminogen activator are most commonly used. Streptokinase is more likely to lead to a hypersensitivity reaction, especially if the patient has prior exposure to it, and is therefore not recommended. Urokinase is the thrombolytic agent used by most institutions because it is much less expensive than t-PA. Urokinase may be purchased in concentrations of 5000 U/mL and 250,000 U/5 mL (50,000 U/mL). The concentration of 5000 U/mL is used for dissolving a clot within a catheter. Our institution prefers to use t-PA for this process. Our pharmacy dilutes a 50 mg vial of t-PA with 50 mL of sterile water to produce 25 syringes containing 2 mg of t-PA in 2 mL (1 mg/mL). The syringes of t-PA are then frozen until needed. The Groshong catheters have a slit valve at their proximal end that alleviates the need for heparin. Refer to Chapter 38 for a complete discussion of the use of heparinized saline in central venous lines.

Repair kits are available for damaged partially implanted catheters. The kits avoid the need to remove the device and implant a new catheter. If the external tubing of the device is damaged, apply a smooth catheter clamp proximal to the damaged area and arrange to have the device repaired. The use of these kits is beyond the scope of this chapter.

PATIENT PREPARATION

Discuss the procedure with the patient and/or their representative. Most patients with indwelling central venous access devices are very familiar with their use and idiosyncrasies. The patient will often be able to tell the practitioner if the line has had problems in the past and the method used to correct the problem. Some patients will be able to suggest postural changes (e.g., raising an arm or lying in the Trendelenburg posi-

tion) that will help the catheter function better. Obtain a posteroanterior and lateral chest radiograph to confirm that the tip of the catheter is in a proper location. **Any manipulation, injection, or aspiration of a central venous line must be done using strict sterile techniques.** Clean any dirt and debris from the distal port of a partially implanted device or the skin overlying the reservoir of a fully implanted device. Apply povidone iodine and allow it to dry. Wipe off the iodine with a sterile alcohol prep pad. **This process must be performed every time a needle is inserted into a central venous access device.**

TECHNIQUES

An algorithmic approach to the occluded indwelling central venous catheter is summarized in Figure 39-1.[5] **The key principle is that forced irrigation of the catheter, especially with a 1 mL syringe, is never performed as the catheter may rupture.**

A catheter that flushes easily but cannot be aspirated may have a fibrin sheath around the catheter tip forming a one-way valve. The tip may also be lodged against the wall of the superior vena cava or the right atrium. Repositioning the patient may alleviate the problem. The catheter may be cautiously used for an infusion if there are no signs of infection (new heart murmur, fever, erythema or discharge at the catheter or subcutaneous reservoir site) and the catheter tip is in good position. Refer the patient to their Primary Care Provider or a consultant for follow-up of the malfunction.

The problem is more serious if the catheter does not easily flush. Attempt to obtain peripheral intravenous access while attempting to correct the problem with the central venous catheter. If there are no signs of infection, and the catheter is not ruptured or malpositioned, the Emergency Physician must decide if a prolonged effort at resolving the occlusion is necessary. If so, proceed as described below and in Figure 39-1.

PARTIALLY IMPLANTED CATHETERS

A clot or small amount of precipitate within the partially implanted catheter may be able to be aspirated if the catheter bore is large enough to permit passage. Remove the Luer-lock cap from the catheter. Connect a 10 mL syringe with 2 to 3 mL of sterile saline directly to the occluded port's Luer adapter. Any clot large enough to occlude the catheter will not pass through a needle. Apply negative pressure to the syringe. The catheter is probably occluded by a clot or a precipitate if the obstruction cannot be aspirated. Remove the syringe and attach a new Luer-lock cap.

If a precipitate is seen in the catheter aspirate, determine if it is waxy or solid. Waxy precipitates are due to the lipid component of parenteral nutrition fluids.

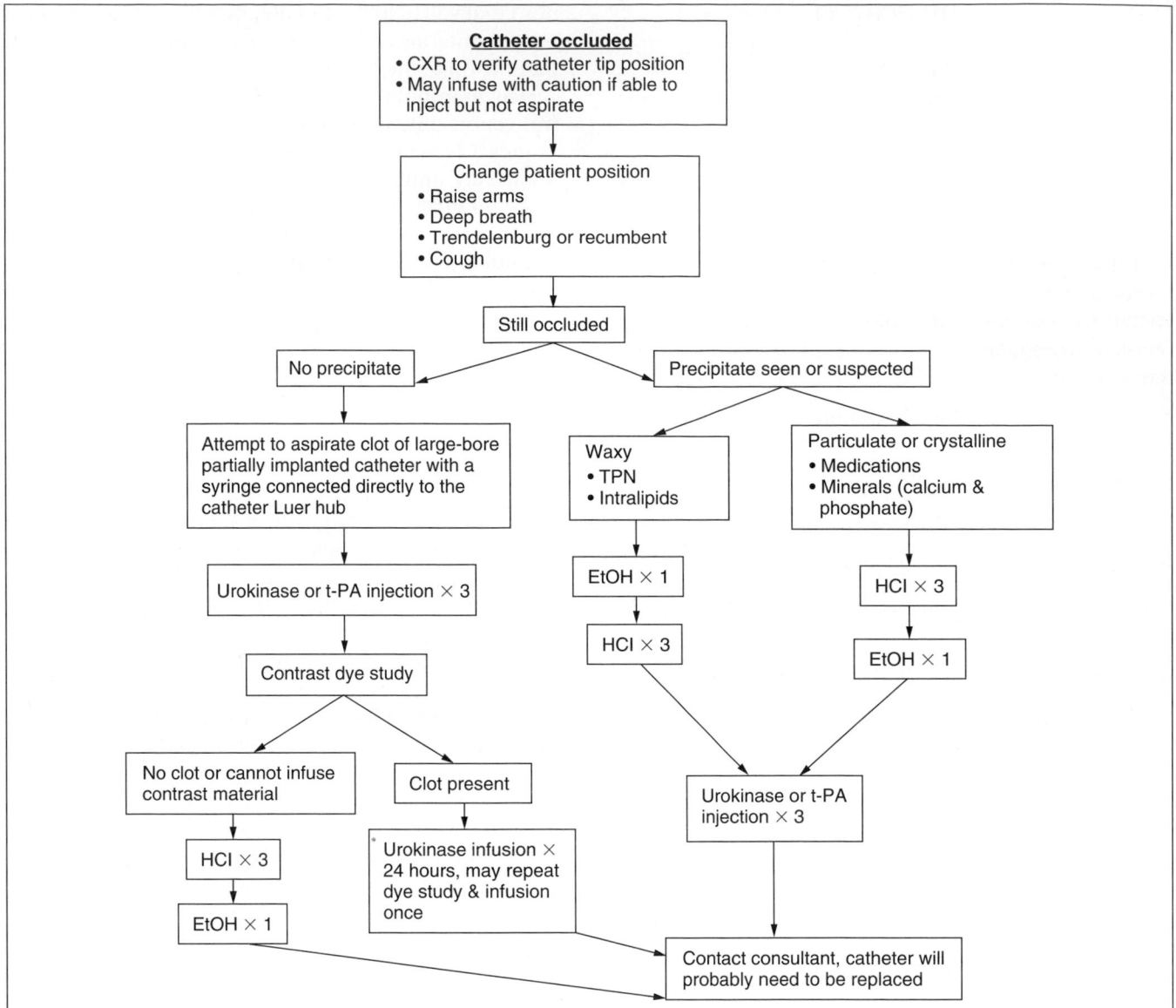

FIGURE 39-1 An algorithmic approach to the occluded central venous catheter. Continue to work down the protocol until the occlusion is resolved. (CXR = chest radiograph, EtOH = 70% ethanol in water, HCl = 0.1 normal hydrochloric acid solution, TPN = total parenteral nutrition.)

Waxy precipitates may be dissolved with a solution of 70% ethanol in water. Inject 1 to 2 mL of this alcohol-water solution and allow it to dwell in the catheter for 1 hour. Aspirate the catheter to determine patency. If still occluded, inject 1 to 2 mL of 0.1 N hydrochloric acid solution. Allow the solution to dwell in the catheter for 20 minutes. Aspirate the catheter to determine patency. Attempt to infuse 0.1 N hydrochloric acid solution two more times. The next step is to infuse a thrombolytic agent, as described below, or to replace the catheter.

Solid precipitates are due to precipitation of medications or minerals. Dilute 0.1 hydrochloric acid solution may be used to dissolve precipitated calcium and phosphate crystals. Infuse 1 to 2 mL of 0.1 N HCL and allow it to dwell in the catheter 20 minutes. Aspirate the catheter

to determine patency. The process may be repeated up to 3 times. If still occluded, inject 1 to 2 mL of 70% ethanol in water and allow it to dwell in the catheter for 1 hour. Aspirate the catheter to determine patency. The next step is to inject a thrombolytic agent, as described below, or to replace the catheter.

If no precipitate is present, or if efforts to clear the precipitate fail, a clot may be present within the catheter lumen. Clots probably form to some extent in the majority of implanted central venous catheters. The clots may obstruct the catheter lumen.[10] Thrombosis of the central veins, superior vena cava, or right atrium may also occur. Suspect a major vein thrombosis if there is swelling, pain, or edema of anatomic structures that are drained by the cannulated vein(s).

Small clots may be dissolved by a bolus or infusion of a thrombolytic agent. Inject 1 mL of urokinase (5000 U/mL) or 2 mL of t-PA (1 mg/mL) into the catheter. Allow the solution to dwell in the catheter for 30 minutes. Aspirate the catheter to determine patency. This process may be repeated up to 3 times. If still occluded, inject 2 mL of intravenous contrast dye under fluoroscopy or inject the dye and obtain a radiograph. If no clot is present or if the contrast material will not infuse, attempt to clear the catheter with hydrochloric acid solution (up to 3 times) and 70% ethanol in water. If a clot is present within the catheter, a urokinase infusion may be begun over a 24-hour period. Administer the urokinase at a dose of 200 U/Kg-hr mixed to run at a rate of at least 20 mL/hr.[8,9] The infusion should occur through an intravenous line equipped with a 0.22 micron or 0.45 micron filter. Thrombolytic infusions should be undertaken in consultation with the patient's Primary Care Provider as the patient will require hospital admission. If these methods do not successfully clear the catheter, or if a thrombolytic infusion is contraindicated, remove the catheter and replace it with another one if the patient requires immediate vascular access.

FULLY IMPLANTED CATHETERS

The procedure is the same for a fully implanted central venous access device with one exception. The subcutaneous reservoir will not be able to be initially cleared by aspiration. Any clot or precipitates large enough to occlude a catheter will not pass through a noncoring (Huber) needle. **Always use a noncoring (Huber) needle when aspirating or injecting through a fully implanted catheter.**

AFTERCARE

Indwelling central venous lines must be flushed with saline, followed by the appropriate heparin solution if necessary, after clearing the obstruction. Refer to Chapter 38 for the complete details. Patients given thrombolytics must be assessed for bleeding at the catheter site and elsewhere prior to discharge, if they do not require hospital admission. Patients receiving thrombolytic infusions must be admitted for the infusion and for monitoring of complications. Patients and their care providers must be made aware of any catheter malfunctions and the attempts made at restoring catheter patency.

COMPLICATIONS

The complications associated with attempts to deocclude a catheter include catheter rupture, disconnection of the catheter from any implanted reservoir, hemorrhage, and contamination of the catheter with subsequent infection. Assessment for these complications is discussed in Chapter 38.

SUMMARY

In the course of their treatment, a number of patients with indwelling central venous access devices will present to the Emergency Department with malfunctioning catheters. Familiarity with the strategies for diagnosis and correction of the catheter dysfunction will enable the Emergency Physician to restore the function of some, but not all, indwelling lines. Early consultation with the patient's Primary Care Provider, Vascular Surgeon, or interventional Radiologist is essential if the procedures outlined do not promptly restore the catheter's function.

REFERENCES

1. Howell JM: Accessing indwelling lines, in Roberts JR, Hedges JR (eds): *Clinical Procedures in Emergency Medicine*, 3rd ed. Philadelphia: Saunders, 1998:385–393.
2. Fuchs SM: Accessing indwelling central lines, in Henretig FM, King C (eds): *Textbook of Pediatric Emergency Procedures*. Baltimore: Williams & Wilkins, 1997:811–820.
3. Taylor JP, Talor JE: Vascular access devices: uses and aftercare. *J Emerg Nurs* 1987; 13(3):160–167.
4. Rockoff MA, Gang DL, Vacanti JP: Fatal pulmonary embolism following removal of a central venous catheter. *J Pediatr Surg* 1984; 19(3):307–309.
5. Dyer BJ, Weiman MG, Ludwig S: Central venous catheters in the emergency department: access, utilization, and problem solving. *Pediatr Emerg Care* 1995; 11(2):112–117.
6. Rodenhuis S, van't Hek LGFM, Vlasveld LT, et al: Central venous catheter associated thrombosis of major veins: thrombolytic treatment with recombinant tissue plasminogen activator. *Thorax* 1993; 48:558–559.
7. Suarez CR, Ow EP, Lambert GH, et al: Urokinase therapy for a central venous catheter thrombus. *Am J Hematol* 1989; 31:269–272.
8. Bagnall HA, Gomperts E, Atkinson JB, et al: Continuous infusion of low dose urokinase in the treatment of central venous catheter thrombosis in infants and children. *Pediatrics* 1989; 83:963–966.
9. Haire WD, Liebermann RP, Lund GB, et al: Obstructed central venous catheters: restoring function with a 12-hour infusion of low-dose urokinase. *Cancer* 1990; 66:2279–2285.
10. Anderson AJ, Krasnow SH, Boyer MW, et al: Hickman catheter clots: a common occurrence despite daily heparin flushing. *Cancer Treat Rep* 1987; 71(6):651–653.

Chapter 40

ACCESSING INDWELLING CENTRAL VENOUS LINES

Robert Feldman

INTRODUCTION

Venous access for medication administration, nutritional support, and blood sampling is essential for the management of many chronic diseases. A variety of indwelling central venous access devices have been developed to avoid repeated venipunctures and permit direct access to the central circulation. These devices may be partially or completely implanted under the patient's skin. The Emergency Physician must be able to access these devices to administer medications and withdraw blood samples without damaging the device or causing it to clot off. The necessary procedures for successfully accessing indwelling central venous lines are described in this chapter.

ANATOMY AND PATHOPHYSIOLOGY

Indwelling central venous lines allow access to the central venous circulation from a peripheral site.[1,2] This is accomplished through either the end of a partially implanted catheter or through the skin into a subcutaneous reservoir of a fully implanted catheter (Figure 40-1). The proximal tip of the central venous line may lie in the superior vena cava or in the right atrium. Catheters designed for right atrial placement are made of softer and more pliable material than are catheters used for short-term transcutaneous central venous access. These catheters are unlikely to erode through the thin right atrial wall.

The internal jugular, subclavian, and femoral veins can all be utilized as a route for a central venous line to access the superior vena cava or right atrium. The subclavian veins are most commonly used to maximize patient comfort and mobility. When the line is initially inserted, the vein is punctured transcutaneously, the catheter is inserted into the vein, and its distal end is

tunneled under the skin. If the line is partially implanted, the distal end of the catheter is brought external to the skin through a small puncture (Figure 40-1A). If the line is fully implanted, its distal end is connected to a subcutaneous reservoir that is placed in a pocket dissected under the skin of the chest wall (Figure 40-1B).

PARTIALLY IMPLANTED CATHETERS

Partially implanted central venous catheters (Figures 40-1A and 40-2) are those whose distal end emerges from the skin via a subcutaneous tunnel.[3] This tunnel helps prevent the spread of skin flora along the outside of the catheter and toward the central circulation. Most partially implanted catheters use a subcutaneous Dacron cuff to further insulate the proximal catheter from skin flora and help anchor the catheter in place.[4]

A variety of models are in use, including the Broviac,[5] Hickman,[6] and Groshong[7] catheters. All are available in single- or multiple-lumen versions. Broviac and Hickman catheters must be flushed with heparin solution daily. The Groshong catheter is unique in that it has a slit valve at its proximal end that prevents blood from reentering the catheter once it has been flushed (Figure 40-3). Groshong catheters need only a weekly saline flush to prevent clot formation.

FULLY IMPLANTED CATHETERS

Fully implanted central venous catheters are those that are entirely embedded and do not exit the skin (Figures 40-4 and 40-5). The catheter's distal end is attached to a subcutaneously implanted reservoir.[4] Various catheters, including Hickman and Groshong catheters, can be attached to a subcutaneous reservoir. Most fully implanted central venous access systems are known by the brand names Port-A-Cath and Infusaport. These catheters must be flushed with heparin solution monthly when not in use.[7] The reservoir's infusion port is covered with a self-sealing silicone rubber membrane

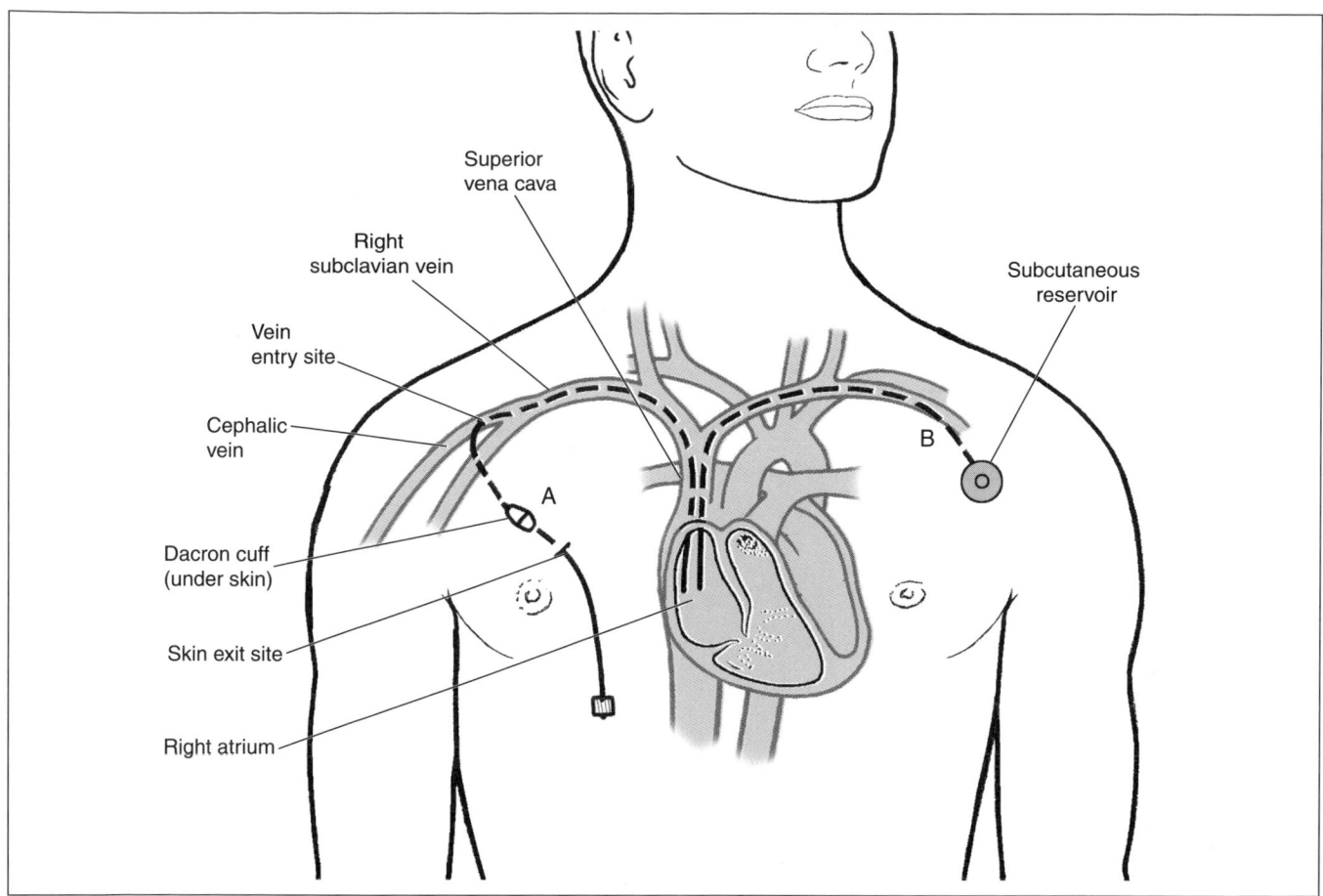

Superior
vena cava

Right
subclavian vein

Vein
entry site

Cephalic
vein

A

Subcutaneous
reservoir

B

Dacron cuff
(under skin)

Skin exit site

Right atrium

FIGURE 40-1 Indwelling central venous lines. *A.* The partially implanted central venous line. The distal end of the line emerges from the chest wall. Contamination of the implanted portion is prevented by a subcutaneous tunnel and a Dacron cuff around the catheter. *B.* The fully implanted central venous line. The catheter is connected to a reservoir that is contained in a subcutaneous pocket.

(Figures 40-4 and 40-5). Specially designed noncoring or Huber needles must be used when accessing the subcutaneous reservoir to avoid permanently damaging the self-sealing membrane.

INDICATIONS

PATIENTS REQUIRING INDWELLING CENTRAL VENOUS LINES

Patients of all ages and with a variety of diagnoses may present with an indwelling central venous line. Some examples of such presentations are chronic painful conditions requiring parenteral analgesia (e.g., sickle cell disease), chronic infections requiring long-term parenteral antibiotics (e.g., endocarditis, osteomyelitis), the need for prolonged hyperalimentation, and cancer patients required chemotherapy and blood sampling. Any patient who will require several weeks of repeated intravenous blood sampling and/or drug administration is a candidate for an indwelling central venous line.

ACCESS OF INDWELLING CENTRAL VENOUS LINES

Fully or partially implanted central venous access devices may be accessed routinely when phlebotomy is required, medications must be administered, or intravenous fluids must be administered.

CONTRAINDICATIONS

Fully implanted devices should not be accessed through infected skin. Catheters known or suspected to be infected should be used cautiously, as they may be a source of septic emboli, although it is sometimes possible to treat catheter sepsis without removing the device.[8,9] Phenytoin and diazepam cannot be given via silicone indwelling central venous lines as they can crystallize and permanently obstruct the catheter lumen.[10]

Devices used for hemodialysis should be accessed only in a true emergency and if no other method of venous access can be readily obtained. This guideline is intended to prevent loss of the patient's dialysis ac-

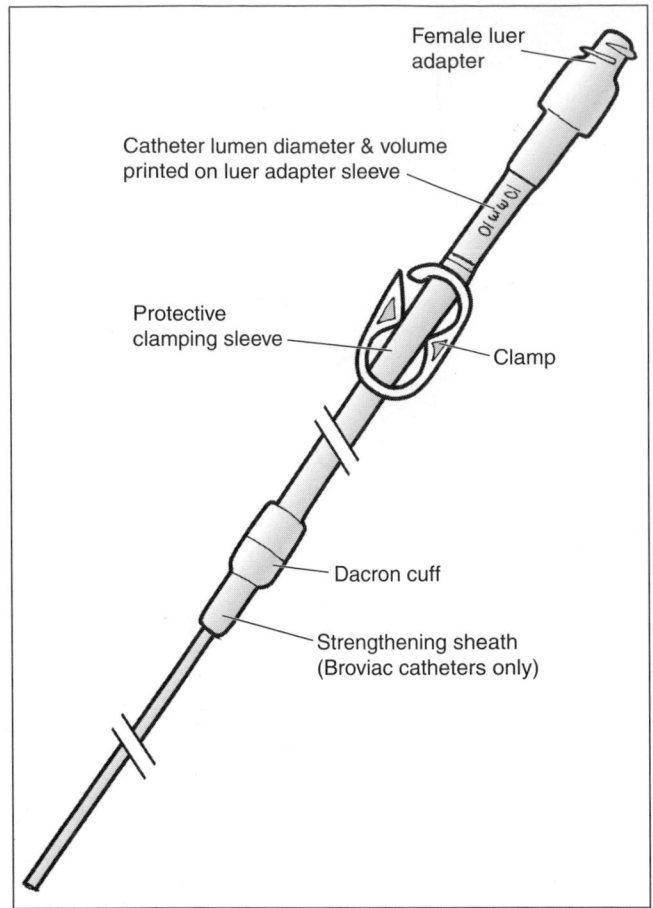

FIGURE 40-2 The partially implanted central venous catheter. A single-lumen (Hickman or Broviac) line is shown schematically. The Dacron cuff lies in the subcutaneous tissue just proximal to the skin entry site. The catheter tip lies in either the proximal superior vena cava or the right atrium.

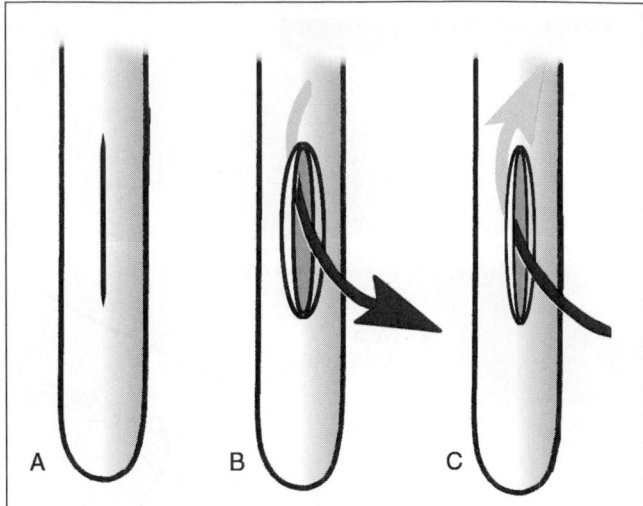

FIGURE 40-3 The Groshong central venous catheter tip. Detail of the Groshong three-position slit valve that prevents venous blood from passively entering the catheter when it is not in use. *A.* The closed or resting position of the slit valve. *B.* The valve opens outward from positive pressure when the catheter is flushed or infused. *C.* The valve opens inward from negative pressure when the catheter is aspirated.

cess due to device damage, clotting, or an infection. An inability to dialyze the patient will lead to significant morbidity and mortality. There are a finite number of veins available for dialysis access.

EQUIPMENT

Povidone iodine solution
Sterile gauze, 4×4 squares
Syringes, 5 and 10 mL
20 gauge needles
Sterile saline, 0.9%
Heparinized saline flush (100 and 1000 U/mL)
Adhesive tape
Luer-lock caps
Blood collection tubes
Infusion set
Any intravenous fluids or medications to be injected
Huber needle, noncoring right angle or straight angle

Topical anesthetic (EMLA cream, ethynyl chloride
   spray, or ice)
Injectable anesthetic without epinephrine, 1% lidocaine
Sterile alcohol prep pads
Sterile gloves
Sterile drapes

PATIENT PREPARATION

Discuss the necessary procedure with the patient and/or their representative. Obtain informed consent for accessing the device. Patients with indwelling central venous lines are usually very familiar with their care and use. They can often advise the practitioner on the correct procedure, appropriate flush solution, and any anatomic manipulations necessary to optimize flow through the line (e.g., raising the arms, turning the head, etc.). **Sterile technique is required at all times when accessing indwelling central venous catheters.**

TECHNIQUES

PARTIALLY IMPLANTED CATHETERS

Accessing a partially implanted central venous catheter is simple and similar to accessing a heparin-locked peripheral intravenous catheter.[7,10] Remove any adhesive tape and gauze wrapped around the distal end of the lumen to be accessed. Fasten the catheter clamp on the desired lumen (Figure 40-2). Clean the catheter cap

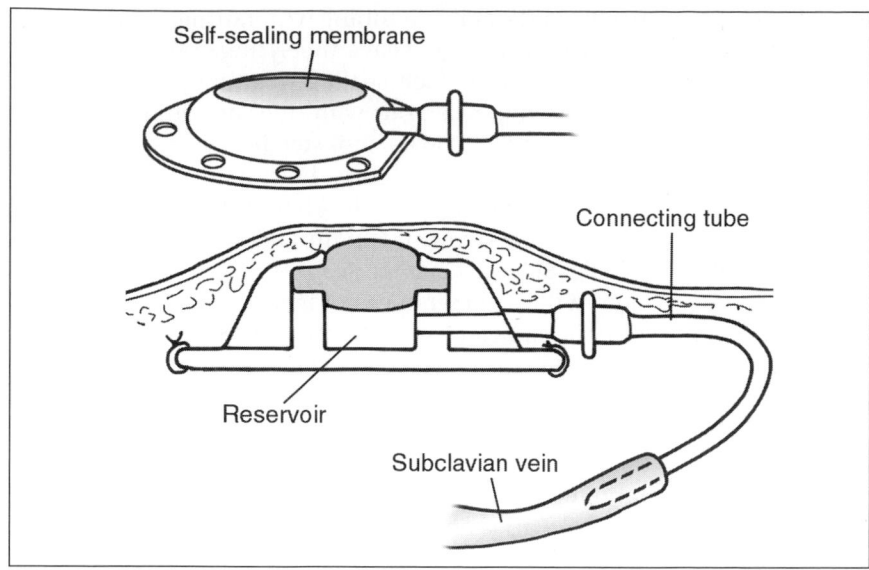

FIGURE 40-4 The fully implanted central venous catheter. The reservoir lies in the subcutaneous tissue and is anchored with sutures to keep the diaphragm facing the skin surface.

and Luer adapter with povidone iodine solution and allow it to dry. The technique for accessing the catheter will vary depending on whether blood sampling with or without a subsequent infusion is required.

BLOOD SAMPLING FROM PARTIALLY IMPLANTED CATHETERS

Blood samples may be withdrawn through the catheter cap using a 20 gauge hypodermic needle attached to a 5 or 10 mL syringe if blood is to be sampled without beginning an infusion. Insert the needle through the Luer cap. Open the catheter clamp. Withdraw 5 mL of blood from the catheter. Discard the blood sample, needle, and syringe. This blood sample is diluted by the catheter

contents (i.e., saline or heparinized saline) and does not truly represent the circulating blood. This step is essential when accessing dialysis catheters as they contain a dose of concentrated heparin (1000 U/mL). If unable to aspirate blood, gently flush the catheter with 2 to 3 mL of sterile saline. **Avoid using a syringe smaller than 5 mL to inject as pressure high enough to damage the catheter can be generated.** Refer to Chapter 39 for troubleshooting instructions if the catheter does not flush easily.

Withdraw the required blood samples using a new needle and syringe. Transfer the blood samples into collection tubes for the laboratory. The catheter must now be flushed to prevent it from clotting off. Flush the catheter with the appropriate solution in a 5 or 10 mL

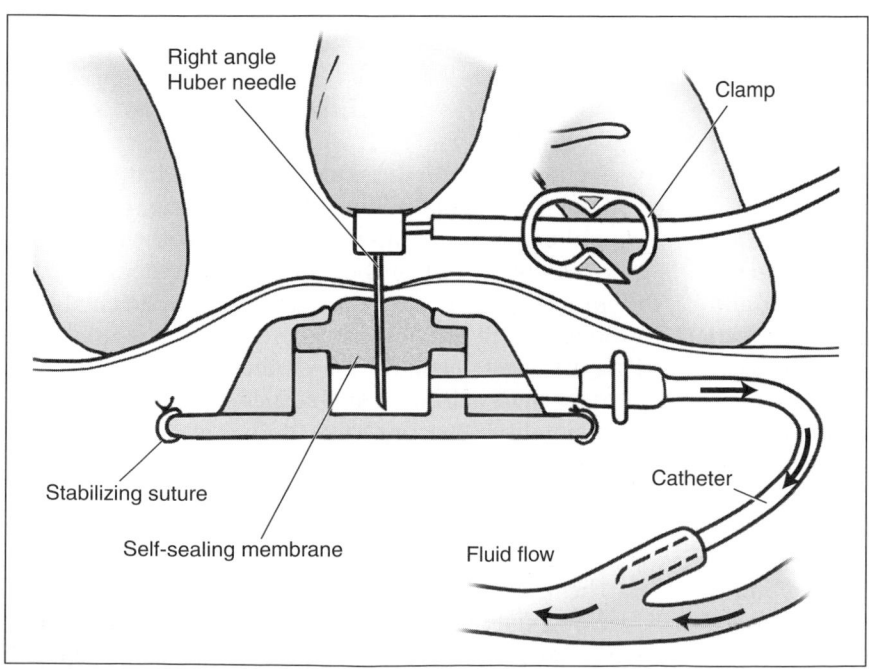

FIGURE 40-5 Accessing the fully implanted central venous catheter system. The reservoir is stabilized between the fingers of the operator's nondominant hand as a noncoring (Huber) needle is used to penetrate the skin and reservoir.

syringe armed with a 20 gauge needle. Inject 3 to 5 mL of heparinized saline (100 U/mL) into Broviac and Hickman catheters. Inject 5 mL of normal saline into a Groshong catheter. Inject dialysis catheters with the volume printed on the catheter, usually ≤ 2 mL, of heparinized saline (1000 U/mL).

Secure the free end of the catheter. Tape the catheter to the patient's chest wall to prevent accidental traction on the catheter. Evaluate the skin puncture site. Reapply a dressing over the skin puncture site if necessary.

BLOOD SAMPLING AND INFUSION THROUGH PARTIALLY IMPLANTED CATHETERS

The Luer cap can be removed entirely and the catheter lumen accessed directly with a Leur-hub syringe if an infusion is to be subsequently started. **Ensure that the catheter clamp is securely closed.** Remove the cap from the catheter. Attach a 5 or 10 mL syringe to the hub of the catheter. Open the catheter clamp. Withdraw 5 mL of blood into the syringe. Close the catheter clamp. Remove and discard the syringe with the original blood sample. Apply a new syringe, open the catheter clamp, and withdraw the blood sample. Close the catheter clamp. Remove the syringe. Continue this sequence of events until all required blood samples are obtained. **It is imperative to make sure that the catheter is clamped when the cap or syringe is removed to prevent an air embolism.** Secure attached primed intravenous tubing to the hub of the catheter and begin the infusion.

Clamp the catheter lumen when terminating the infusion or if no infusion is to be started. Remove the intravenous tubing or the syringe from the catheter. Attach a syringe containing the appropriate flush solution, open the catheter clamp, and flush the catheter. Close the catheter clamp. Remove the syringe. Apply a new sterile cap onto the hub of the catheter. **Never use "needle-less" caps, as they are a potential source of air emboli.** Open the catheter clamp to prevent catheter damage from long-term clamping. Secure the catheter to the patient's chest wall.

FULLY IMPLANTED CATHETERS

A noncoring Huber-type needle must be used to access subcutaneous injection ports (Figures 40-5 and 40-6). A small-gauge standard hypodermic needle can be used in a dire emergency if a noncoring needle is not available. The diaphragm covering the injection reservoir can be damaged by a standard hypodermic needle, leading to subcutaneous hemorrhage and necessitating surgical replacement of the implanted device.

Clean the skin overlying the injection port with povidone iodine solution and allow it to dry. The application of a topical or injectable anesthetic over the reservoir is optional but greatly appreciated by the patient. Remove the iodine solution with an alcohol pad. Flush the Huber needle and extension tubing with normal saline using a 5 or 10 mL syringe. Leave the syringe attached. Locate the center of the self-sealing membrane (diaphragm). Stabilize the reservoir with the nondominant hand (Figure 40-5). Slowly and steadily insert the needle through the skin and into the reservoir (Figure 40-5). Stop advancing the needle when it touches the far wall of the device. Gently flush 2 to 3 mL of saline through the needle. Refer to Chapter 39 for troubleshooting instructions if the catheter does not flush easily.

If the catheter can be flushed easily, secure the Huber needle in place by stabilizing it with gauze squares and tape. Withdraw 5 to 10 mL of blood. Close the clamp on the tubing (Figure 40-5). Remove and discard the syringe. Attach a new syringe, open the clamp, and withdraw the required blood samples. Clamp the tubing and remove the syringe. If an infusion is to be started, attach the primed intravenous tubing set and begin the infusion. If no infusion is desired or when discontinuing an infusion, clamp the tubing and disconnect the infusion set. Attach a 5 or 10 mL syringe containing heparinized saline (100 to 200 U/mL). Open the clamp and flush the device with 3 to 5 mL of heparinized saline. Use only saline if a Groshong catheter is attached to the reservoir. Remove the Huber needle from the skin. Control any skin bleeding with direct pressure. Apply a sterile dressing.

ASSESSMENT

Assessment of line function after accessing a central venous access device will not occur until the next access attempt. This procedure is described above. Troubleshooting nonfunctioning indwelling central venous lines is discussed in Chapter 39.

AFTERCARE

Secure the line to the skin with tape so that the tubing will not get caught on the patient's clothing. The patient should be given a written record of how the access device was used and flushed in the Emergency Department to convey to their primary care physician should problems with the line become evident at a later time. Patients must regularly assess their indwelling access sites for signs of infection. This includes erythema, pain, purulent discharge, or serous discharge.

COMPLICATIONS

The most important elements after accessing indwelling lines are to not allow the central venous line to clot off and not to contaminate the line. Strict adherence

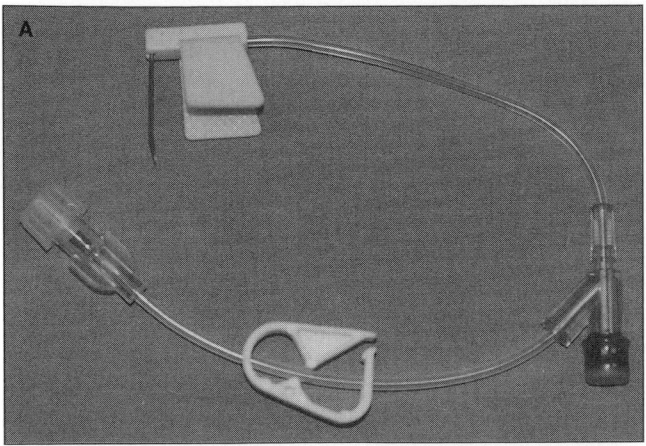

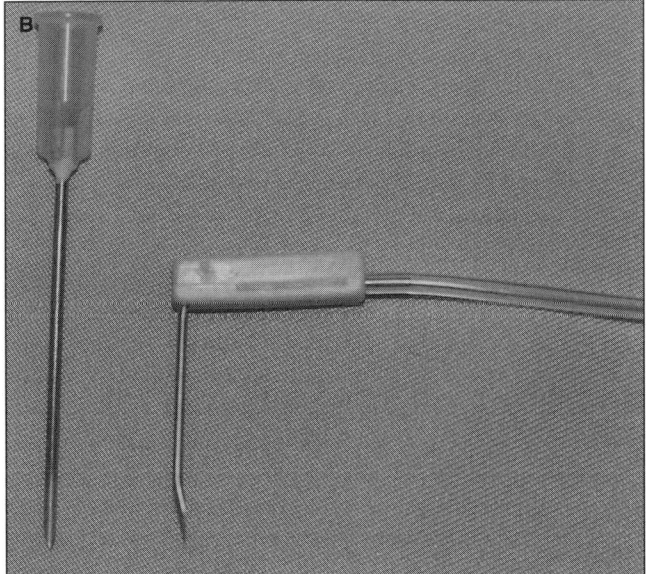

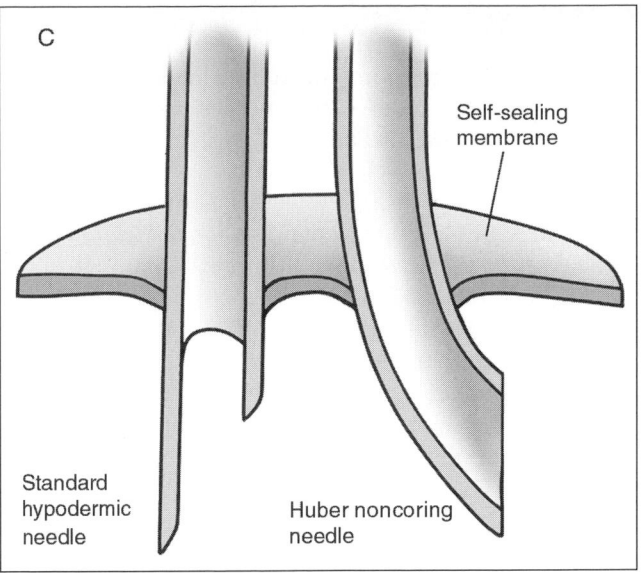

FIGURE 40-6 The Huber needle. *A.* Photo of a complete right-angle Huber needle set, including the extension tubing and clamp. *B.* Photo showing the right-angle Huber needle compared with a standard hypodermic needle. *C.* Drawing showing the key difference between a standard hypodermic needle and the Huber needle. The hypodermic needle tip can cut a cylindrical core of subcutaneous tissue and the diaphragm sealing the subcutaneous reservoir. The Huber needle pushes the subcutaneous tissue and the diaphragm material aside without removing any of it.

to the procedures described above will minimize the chances of these problems occurring. Complications associated with the catheter include right atrial thromboses, right atrial erosion with pericardial tamponade (rare with implanted lines), and pulmonary embolism.[7,9,11,12] Fully implanted catheters may become disconnected from the subcutaneous reservoir or may leak into the subcutaneous tissue due to diaphragm failure. Any hematoma formation near the reservoir must be assessed promptly to prevent major hemorrhage. Infection and line sepsis can be prevented using strict sterile technique.

An air embolism should be suspected if the patient becomes confused, hypotensive, and/or tachycardic while accessing the central venous access device. This complication is 100 percent preventable by ensuring that the catheter tubing is clamped closed whenever the end of the tubing is without a cap. Immediately place the patient in the Trendelenburg position and on his or her left side (left lateral decubitus position). This will

hopefully cause any air emboli to collect in the apex of the right ventricle and not enter the pulmonary artery.

Repair kits are available for damaged partially implanted catheters. These can serve to avoid the need to remove the device and implant a new catheter. If the external tubing of the partially implanted catheter is damaged, apply a smooth catheter clamp proximal to the damaged area and arrange to have the device repaired. Instructions for the use of these kits are beyond the scope of this chapter.

SUMMARY

The Emergency Physician will encounter many patients with indwelling central venous lines. Careful adherence to sterile technique and proper technique will allow access for phlebotomy, medication administration, and fluid administration while preserving the indwelling line for future use.

REFERENCES

1. Howell JM: Accessing indwelling lines, in Roberts JR, Hedges JR (eds): *Clinical Procedures in Emergency Medicine,* 3rd ed. Philadelphia: Saunders, 1998:385–394.
2. Fuchs SM: Accessing indwelling central lines, in Henretig FM, King C (eds): *Textbook of Pediatric Emergency Procedures.* Baltimore: Williams & Wilkins, 1997:811–820.
3. Schanzer H, Kaplan S, Bosch J, et al: Double-lumen, silicone rubber, indwelling venous catheters. *Arch Surg* 1986; 121:229–232.
4. Bothe A, Piccione W, Ambrosino JJ, et al: Implantable central venous access system. *Am J Surg* 1984; 147:565–569.
5. Broviac JW, Cole JJ, Scribner BH: A silicone rubber catheter for prolonged parenteral alimentation. *Surg Gynecol Obstet* 1973; 136:602–606.
6. Hickman RO, Buckner CD, Clift RA, et al: A modified right atrial catheter for access to the venous system in marrow transplant recipients. *Surg Gynecol Obstet* 1979; 148:871–875.
7. Dyer BJ, Weiman MG, Ludwig S: Central venous catheters in the emergency department: access, utilization, and problem solving. *Pediatr Emerg Care* 1995; 11(2):112–117.
8. Tenney JH, Moody MR, Newman KA, et al: Adherent microorganisms on lumenal surfaces of long-term intravenous catheters. *Arch Intern Med* 1986; 146:1949–1954.
9. Rockoff MA, Gang DL, Vacanti JP: Fatal pulmonary embolism following removal of a central venous catheter. *J Pediatr Surg* 1984; 19(3):307–309.
10. Taylor JP, Talor JE: Vascular access devices: uses and aftercare. *J Emerg Nurs* 1987; 13(3):160–167.
11. Marcoux C, Fisher S, Wong D: Central venous access devices in children. *Pediatr Nurs* 1990; 16(2):123–133.
12. Greene FL, Moore W, Strickland G, et al: Comparison of a totally implantable access device for chemotherapy (Port-A-Cath) and long-term percutaneous catheterization (Broviac). *South Med J* 1988; 81(5):580–583.

Chapter 41
PULMONARY ARTERY (SWAN-GANZ) CATHETERIZATION

Russell F. Kelly
Cory Franklin

INTRODUCTION

The routine clinical catheterization of the pulmonary artery was made possible by the pioneering work of H.J.C. Swan and William Ganz. Together they developed the soft, balloon-tipped, flow-directed pulmonary artery catheter (PAC) that bears their names.[1] Prior to the work of Swan and Ganz, pulmonary artery catheterization was performed using a stiff catheter that required fluoroscopic guidance and was associated with a high complication rate. The Swan-Ganz PAC allows reliable and continuous measurement of hemodynamic parameters to be performed safely, even in critically ill patients.[2–4] While complications are uncommon, they can occur. The optimal application of the PAC, both its insertion and interpretation of the data, requires appropriate training and skill.[5–7]

This chapter concentrates on the technique of PAC insertion. Obtaining central venous access is a necessary prerequisite for this technique and is discussed in Chapter 38. A detailed discussion of the interpretation of the abundant variety of data that the PAC may provide is beyond the scope of this chapter.[8] The interpretation of data is discussed primarily as it concerns PAC insertion and associated complications.

ANATOMY AND PATHOPHYSIOLOGY

The PAC is advanced into the right atrium from a venous access site in the neck, chest, upper extremity, or lower extremity. The balloon near the tip of the catheter is inflated during its insertion. The balloon follows the flow of blood through the right heart—from the right atrium through the tricuspid valve into the right ventricle, then up the right ventricular outflow tract through the pulmonic valve into the pulmonary artery, and from there into a branch of the pulmonary artery (Figure 41-1).

When the PAC is correctly positioned, inflating the balloon near its tip will occlude the forward blood flow to that arterial segment (Figure 41-2). The lumen opening at the tip of the PAC will therefore measure the downstream pressure in that vessel, rather than pulmonary artery pressure. Because the pulmonary circulation has no valves, the pressure that the PAC tip measures beyond the inflated balloon is equal to the pressure in the pulmonary capillaries. This pressure is, in turn, equal to the pressures in the pulmonary veins and the left atrium. During diastole, when the mitral valve is open, this pressure is equal to the left ventricular diastolic pressure. The left ventricular end-diastolic pressure is a very important parameter because it is the best clinical indicator of preload. Thus, measurement of the pulmonary capillary wedge pressure (or pulmonary artery occlusion pressure, as it is sometimes called) provides an excellent assessment of left ventricular filling without the need to catheterize the left side of the heart.

The PAC may also be used to measure cardiac output using the thermodilution method. The tip of the PAC has a temperature-sensitive probe. When a given volume of cold saline is injected into the right atrial port of the PAC, it cools the temperature of the blood flowing past the catheter tip. If the cardiac output is high, the cold saline is mixed with and carried along by a larger flow of blood so that the temperature change detected at the PAC tip is smaller and dissipates faster. If cardiac output is low, the cold saline mixes with a smaller volume of blood and the temperature change is more apparent and slower to dissipate.

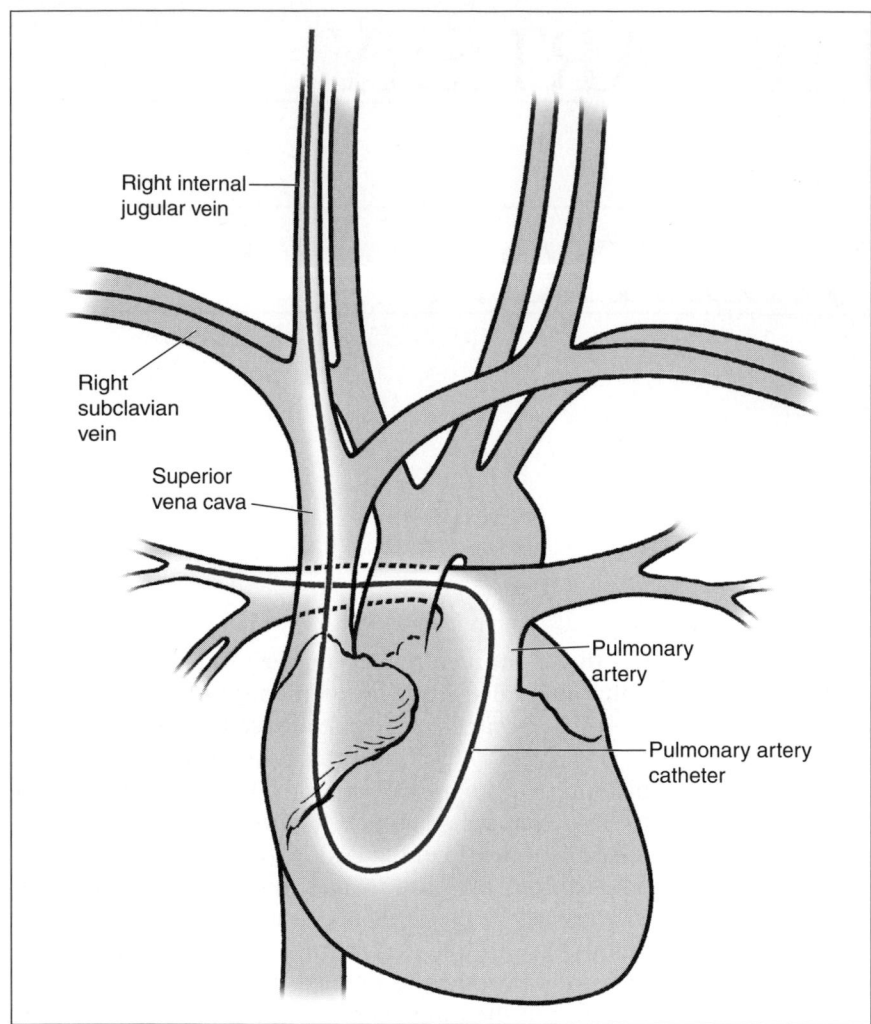

FIGURE 41-1 Cardiac anatomy as it pertains to pulmonary artery catheter insertion. The PAC enters the right atrium from the superior vena cava, crosses the tricuspid valve into the right ventricle, and then crosses the pulmonic valve into the pulmonary artery. The catheter tip lies in a branch of the right pulmonary artery.

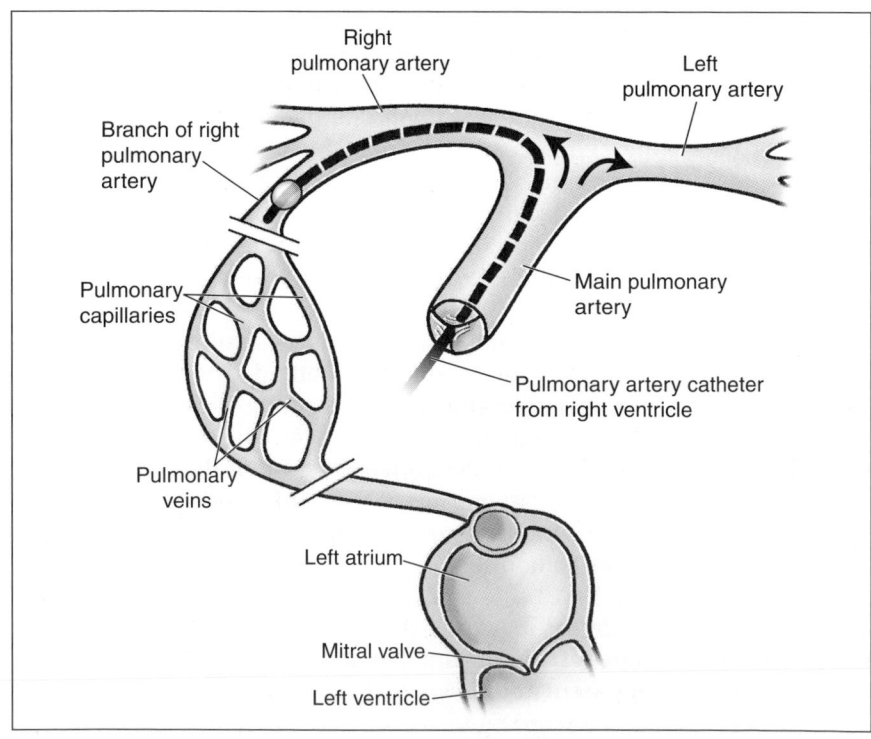

FIGURE 41-2 Diagram of the principle underlying pulmonary capillary wedge pressure. Balloon inflation blocks transmission of the forward pulmonary artery pressure to the tip of the catheter. The catheter tip therefore measures the downstream pressure of the pulmonary circulation. Because the pulmonary circulation has no valves, the pressure measured at the catheter tip is equal to the pressure in the left ventricle when the mitral valve is open (diastole).

INDICATIONS

The major advantage of the PAC is that it provides accurate measurements of hemodynamic parameters such as pulmonary capillary wedge pressure and cardiac output. This is particularly useful in critically ill patients, as the clinical estimation of these parameters is frequently incorrect.[9–13] The PAC may be used for diagnostic or therapeutic purposes. Diagnostically, the PAC is usually used in situations where clinical judgment alone cannot reliably determine the physiologic basis for hemodynamic instability, pulmonary edema, or reduced urine output. Therapeutically, the PAC may help to direct therapy in patients in whom noninvasive clinical parameters are insufficient guides of treatment efficacy. The most common clinical indications for the PAC in medical and surgical patients are listed in Table 41-1.

It should be noted that despite the prevalence of PAC use, few prospective studies have documented improved clinical outcomes with the PAC except in perioperative surgical patients. Retrospective studies have suggested that the use of the PAC may be associated with worse outcomes.[14–17] These studies are open to question because of their retrospective nature and tendency toward selection bias (i.e., sicker patients are more likely to receive a PAC).[18] This issue is the subject of ongoing studies and analysis. As with any intervention, the physician must carefully assess the potential benefits and risks in making the decision to place a PAC.

CONTRAINDICATIONS

There are no circumstances in which PAC insertion is absolutely contraindicated. Insertion of a PAC may be relatively contraindicated in cases where the risks of obtaining vascular access (e.g., severe bleeding diathesis) or of passing the catheter (e.g., a mobile thrombus in the right heart or right-sided endocarditis) outweigh the potential benefits of obtaining the data the PAC provides.

A PAC is not indicated in situations where it will provide no diagnostic information that cannot be acquired by less invasive means. For example, while a PAC may be helpful in diagnosing or treating patients with mitral regurgitation or ventricular septal defects following myocardial infarction, echocardiography may be sufficiently diagnostic and may obviate the need for a PAC. The same can be true in cases of cardiac tamponade. The PAC may also be superfluous in situations where it will provide little or no therapeutic guidance. The insertion of a PAC is not necessary if a therapeutic trial of fluid administration restores urine output and blood pressure in a hypovolemic patient who has normal cardiac function. A PAC should not be inserted if the appropriate equipment is unavailable or if personnel experienced with the insertion and interpretation of the PAC data are not present.[19,20]

TABLE 41-1. COMMON CLINICAL INDICATIONS FOR PULMONARY ARTERY CATHETER PLACEMENT IN MEDICAL AND SURGICAL PATIENTS

Cardiac
A. Complicated myocardial infarction
   i. Management of refractory hypotension or left ventricular failure
   ii. In presence of hemodynamic deterioration due to a mechanical complication, to differentiate mitral regurgitation from acute ventricular septal defect
B. Other cardiac conditions
   i. Diagnose/manage cardiac tamponade
   ii. Distinguish cardiogenic from noncardiogenic pulmonary edema
   iii. Management of severe cardiomyopathy
   iv. Diagnose/manage severe pulmonary hypertension

Medical/Surgical
In the setting of sepsis, trauma, burns, multiple organ failure, pulmonary embolus, or drug overdose.

If any of the following is found to be unresponsive to conventional medical management:
A. Hypotension
B. Low urine output
C. Hypoperfusion (evidenced by cool skin, mental obtundation, lactic acidosis)
D. Severe hypoxemia requiring high levels of PEEP (> 10 cm)

Preoperative
A. High-risk cardiac surgery (e.g., CABG in elderly patients, multiple valve replacement, ventricular aneurysm resection)
B. Complicated vascular surgery (dissecting aneurysm, resection of thoracic or abdominal aneurysm)
C. Other surgical patients with multiple risk factors
   i. Myocardial infarction within 6 months
   ii. Poor left ventricular function
   iii. Elevated Goldman or ASA score

EQUIPMENT

Povidone iodine solution
Saline or dextrose solution with or without heparin (1 to 2 U/mL)
Pressure bag with manometer
Pressure tubing
Pressure transducer for distal port (CVP port optional)
Stopcocks and occlusive caps for each port of PAC
Fluid infusion tubing for sheath sideport and for PAC ports
PAC
Balloon inflation syringe
Catheter sleeve
Sterile dressing for site
Electrocardiogram (ECG) and pressure monitor

The materials required to place a percutaneous introducer sheath are available in commercially prepared prepackaged kits. Refer to Chapter 38 for the details regarding the placement of the introducer sheath. Note that many PACs require an 8.5 French introducer sheath. In addition, it is desirable to use an introducer sheath that allows the sterile protective sleeve over the PAC to be affixed securely to the sheath.

The PAC consists of a balloon lumen that ends in a balloon just proximal to the catheter tip, a distal lumen that opens at the end of the PAC, a lumen that opens approximately 30 cm proximal to the tip, and a thermister (Figure 41-3). Many PACs have one or more additional lumens opening proximal to the tip. Some of these lumens are designed to accommodate a cardiac pacing wire. A 3 mL syringe with a safety stop at 1.5 mL is supplied with each PAC. This syringe is used to inject air into the balloon. Distances from the tip of the PAC are indicated by linear markings on the shaft. By the standard designation, each thin line represents 5 cm increments and each thick line 10 cm increments.

PATIENT PREPARATION

Routine laboratory studies are advisable prior to PAC insertion in nonemergent circumstances. Hematologic abnormalities (severe anemia, thrombocytopenia, coagulation system deficiencies) can increase the risk or adverse consequences of bleeding. Electrolyte derangements (hyperkalemia, hypokalemia, hypomagnesemia) that may predispose to arrhythmias should be identified and corrected when possible.

Explain to the patient and/or their representative the risks, benefits, and complications of the procedure. Obtain informed consent for the procedure if possible. The use of mild sedation may be advantageous in some patients. Place the patient supine if possible. Continuous ECG monitoring is essential. Pulse oximetry should be routinely monitored. Arterial pressure monitoring is often desirable in patients receiving a PAC. Apply supplemental oxygen. Equipment and personnel necessary for assisting with the PAC insertion procedure and for managing potential complications should be immediately available. This should include equipment for emergency airway management and emergency cardiac pacing.

The choice of which central venous access site to use for PAC insertion must be individualized. The preferred sites are the right internal jugular vein or the left subclavian vein. The PAC tends to float into the desired position more easily from these sites. The left internal jugular vein and the right subclavian vein are acceptable alternatives. The femoral vein may also be used. The femoral approach may be quite difficult without fluoroscopic guidance of the catheter. The external jugular veins, basilic veins, and axillary veins are additional alternatives that carry the same difficulty.

It is essential that strict sterile technique be maintained throughout the insertion procedure. A large sterile field is necessary, as is close attention to the long PAC, which can easily become contaminated. It is also very important to take all necessary precautions with syringe needles, scalpel blades, and suture needles to prevent injury to the physician.

Insert a percutaneous introducer sheath into the central venous system. Refer to Chapter 38 for details regarding the insertion of the sheath. If the patient already has a single-lumen or multi-lumen central venous catheter inserted, it may be exchanged for an introducer sheath. Remove any bandages and dressings on the catheter and skin access site. Thoroughly prep the catheter, skin access site, and surrounding skin with povidone iodine solution and allow it to dry. Drape a sterile field. Discon-

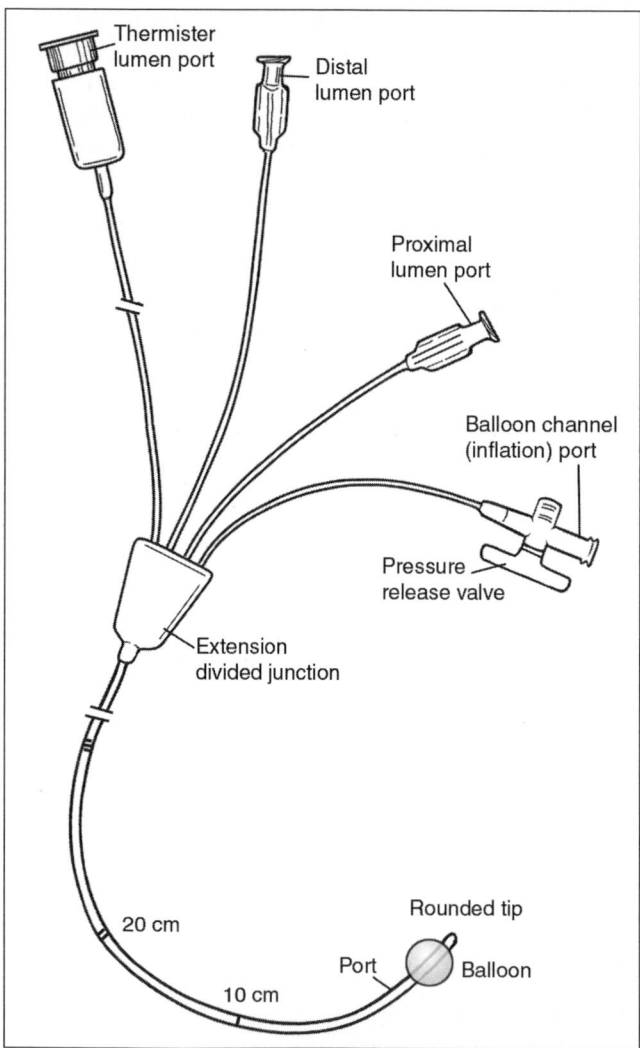

FIGURE 41-3 The pulmonary artery catheter.

tinue any infusions through the catheter. Open an introducer sheath kit. Cut any sutures securing the catheter to the skin. Insert a guidewire through the hub of the distal port and into the central venous circulation. Withdraw the catheter over the guidewire. Insert and secure the percutaneous sheath over the guidewire as described in Chapter 38.

TECHNIQUE

Set up a sterile table and open the PAC kit. Remove the protective sleeve. It allows later repositioning of the PAC while maintaining sterility. Place the sleeve over the catheter and slide it far back (> 60 cm) from the catheter tip. Attach the balloon inflation syringe to the PAC. Inflate the balloon once to confirm the integrity of the balloon. It is a good idea to inflate the balloon in a full bowl of sterile saline and observe for air bubbles to ensure that there are no leaks or gross eccentricities. Allow the balloon to deflate passively. **Deflation by aspirating air from the balloon should be avoided as it places undue stress on the balloon.** Flush the PAC ports with sterile saline and attach a stopcock to each port. Attach the pressure tubing to the distal port. The entire apparatus, including the PAC and the pressure monitoring system, should be flushed with sterile saline to ensure that no air remains in any part of the system. Have an assistant set up, calibrate, and level the transducer.

Hand the proximal end of the PAC to an assistant to attach to the ECG monitor. Finally, shake the tip of the PAC while observing the pressure waveform on the monitor to confirm that the monitoring system is operative.

Insert the PAC through the diaphragm on the introducer sheath, taking care to orient the natural curve of the catheter toward the right ventricular outflow tract. Continue to advance the PAC. Inflate air into the balloon and lock the pressure release valve when the PAC is passed far enough, typically 10 to 15 cm, to exit the sheath. **The PAC should never be advanced with the balloon deflated, as this may provoke ectopy or injure the heart or other vascular structures. Conversely, the PAC should always be withdrawn with the balloon deflated.**

Pay close attention to the distance markings on the catheter and to the pressure waveform on the monitor when advancing the PAC. Typical pressure waveforms are illustrated in Figure 41-4. The average distances from the different catheter insertion sites into each chamber of the heart are listed in Table 41-2. Advance the PAC into the right atrium (Figure 41-4A). Continue to advance the PAC into the right ventricle, which will be apparent by an abrupt change in the pressure waveform (Figure 41-4B). Continue to advance the PAC into the pulmonary artery outflow tract, again confirmed by a change in the pressure waveform (Figure 41-4C). Passing the PAC through the right ventricle may produce some ventricular ectopy, which is generally uncomplicated.

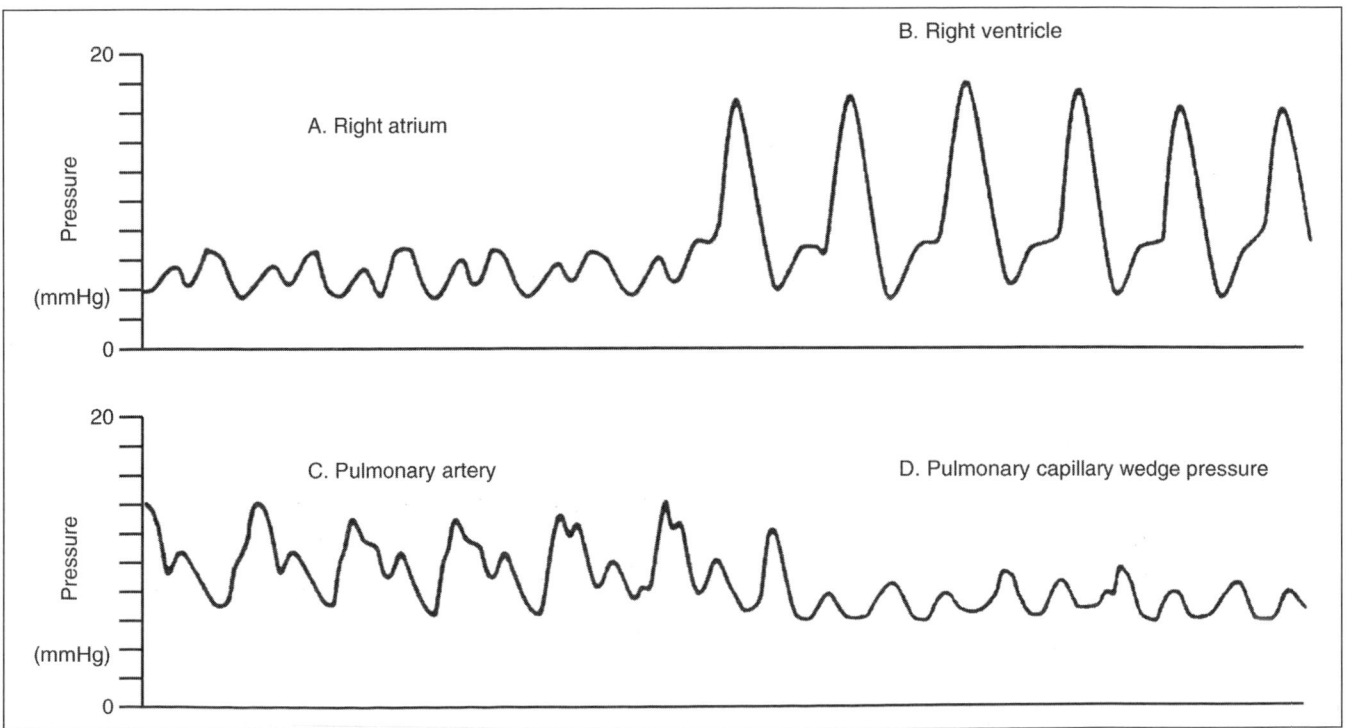

FIGURE 41-4 Typical pressure waveforms recorded by the pulmonary artery catheter during insertion.

TABLE 41-2. AVERAGE DISTANCES IN CENTIMETERS FROM THE CATHETER INSERTION SITE TO THE CATHETER TIP POSITION*

	Right atrium distance	Right ventricle distance	Pulmonary artery distance	Wedge distance
Subclavian vein	10	20	30–40	40–45
Right internal jugular vein	15	25	35–45	45–50
Left internal jugular vein	20	30	40–50	50–55
Right antecubital vein	45	60	70–80	80–85
Left antecubital vein	50	65	75–85	85–90

* These distances are considered the common estimates for uncomplicated PAC placement in patients with normal-sized hearts. The distances will vary in patients and may be greater, especially in the patient with a dilated right ventricle. Any time there is a gross discrepancy between these distances and the actual observed placement distance, the physician should consider catheter misplacement, catheter looping, or catheter knotting. An immediate portable anteroposterior chest radiograph should be obtained to evaluate the situation.

Advance the PAC a few centimeters further to produce a wedge tracing (Figure 41-4D). Deflate the balloon. This will result in the reappearance of the pulmonary artery waveform. If the wedge tracing persists, withdraw the PAC with the balloon deflated until the pulmonary artery waveform reappears. Whenever it is unclear where the tip of the PAC is located, deflate the balloon and withdraw the PAC to a spot where the waveform is recognizable. Take notice of the distance marking. Inflate the balloon and advance the PAC until the desired tracing is obtained.

Difficulties in passing the PAC into the pulmonary artery may occur in patients with pulmonary hypertension, significant tricuspid regurgitation, or markedly dilated right heart chambers. In such cases, having the patient inspire slowly and deeply will increase venous return to the right heart and may allow the PAC to be advanced successfully. Tilting the patient's head upward and repositioning the patient on their left side may also be helpful. Fluoroscopic guidance may be necessary if repeated attempts are unsuccessful.

Pull up the protective sleeve over the catheter and secure it to the introducer sheath. It is important not to advance the PAC itself during this manipulation. Begin any infusions through the PAC. Secure the PAC and dress the access site in standard fashion. After the PAC is secured, it is mandatory to document correct positioning by obtaining an anteroposterior chest radiograph. Assessment and aftercare of the skin puncture site is described in Chapter 38.

DATA INTERPRETATION

As mentioned in the introduction to this chapter, a detailed discussion of PAC data interpretation cannot be undertaken here. However, anyone who places or uses PACs in the management of critically ill patients should be familiar with the standard information provided by the PAC. The data generated by the PAC can be divided into two categories. The first set of information comprises data that are directly measured and include the right-sided heart pressures, thermodilution cardiac output, and blood gas obtained from a mixed venous sample from the distal pulmonary artery port. These data, including normal values, are listed in Table 41-3. The second set of data comprises the variables that are mathematically derived from the measured data (Tables 41-4 and 41-5). These provide information crucial to understanding cardiac and pulmonary physiology and pathology. Today, this information is routinely available on an instantaneous basis as part of computer software packages that accompany the monitoring equipment. PAC users should become familiar with both sets of information and their application in different clinical situations. The reader is advised to consult a current textbook of cardiology or critical care medicine for a more detailed description of the hemodynamic data provided by the PAC.

TABLE 41-3. VARIABLES OBTAINED FROM THE PULMONARY ARTERY CATHETER THROUGH DIRECT MEASUREMENT

Variable	Normal values	Main utility	Comments
Cardiac output (CO)	4–6 L/min	Diagnosis of shock (high output versus low output); titration of vasoactive medications	Measurement is prone to error; should be indexed to patient's size
Pulmonary capillary wedge pressure (PCWP)	5–15 mmHg	Volume status, diuresis, fluid challenges	Often overinterpreted; must be used with other values
Right atrial pressure (RAP)	0–10 mmHg	Status of right ventricle	Less useful than PCWP
Pulmonary artery pressure (PAP)	15–25 mmHg systolic; 8–15 mmHg diastolic	Status of right ventricle and pulmonary circuit	Pulmonary artery diastolic can be substituted for PCWP in most patients
Mixed venous oxygen saturation ($S\bar{v}O_2$)	70–80%	Evaluation of oxygen delivery; pulmonary shunt fraction	Best obtained by blood gas from distal pulmonary artery

TABLE 41-4. DERIVED VARIABLES OBTAINED FROM THE PULMONARY ARTERY CATHETER

Variable	Normal values	Main utility	Comments
Systemic vascular resistance (SVR)	800–1600 dynes/sec/cm^{-5}	Shock states, vasodilator versus vasopressor therapy (afterload)	Unclear whether value should be indexed to patient's size
Pulmonary vascular resistance (PVR)	20–200 dynes/sec/cm^{-5}	Pulmonary hypertension; acute and chronic lung disease	Unclear whether value should be indexed to patient's size
Left ventricular stroke work index (LVSWI)	56 ± 6 gm-m/m^2	Left ventricular performance	Clinical utility uncertain
Right ventricular stroke work index (RVSWI)	8.8 ± 0.9 gm-m/m^2	Right ventricular performance	Clinical utility uncertain
Oxygen delivery ($\dot{D}O_2$)	900–1100 mL/min	Shock states, anemia, low cardiac output	Often amenable to therapy, but controversial
Oxygen consumption ($\dot{V}O_2$)	200–250 mL/min	Sepsis, burns, trauma, ventilator patients	Affected by many variables; use is controversial
Pulmonary shunt fraction (Q_s/Q_t)	3–5%	Acute and chronic lung disease	Underused in the evaluation of pulmonary disease

COMPLICATIONS

In addition to the complications associated with obtaining venous access and with prolonged use of indwelling catheters (Chapter 38), complications may occur during or after the insertion of the PAC. The complications directly related to the PAC may be divided into those that are associated with catheter insertion and those associated with long-term maintenance (Table 41-6). Both sets of complications can be further divided into those problems where there has been systematic study and the incidence of complications has been published and those that have been observed and published as case reports but the actual incidence of which is unknown.

Problems with tracing quality may occur due to problems involving the catheter itself or other parts of the system. Catheter problems include positioning too distal or not distal enough, balloon rupture, or clot formation at the tip. Problems elsewhere in the system include air in the lines, loose connections, failure of the transducer, failure of the wires, or failure of the monitor. The system should be zeroed and calibrated again to confirm the accuracy of the pressure values if abnormally high or low values are obtained. Sometimes it is just not possible to obtain a good wedge tracing despite repeated attempts. In such cases, the pulmonary diastolic pressure may be used as a surrogate for the wedge.

A right bundle branch block may occur due to impact of the PAC with the right side of the septum during insertion. This is usually transient. Even if it persists for hours, it is well tolerated in most patients. However, superimposition of a right bundle branch block in the presence of a preexisting left bundle branch block leaves the patient with complete heart block. This complication can result in severe bradycardia and hemodynamic embarrassment. **It is important to be prepared to institute temporary pacing when placing a PAC in patients with a left bundle branch block.**

Arrhythmias during insertion, most commonly premature ventricular beats, are usually due to irritation of the right ventricle. This is especially true of the outflow tract. Premature ventricular contractions are usually well tolerated unless sustained ventricular tachycardia or ventricular fibrillation occurs. Slight withdrawal and redirection of the PAC is usually adequate. Arrhythmias after insertion may be due to catheter loops in the right heart, which will be apparent on the chest radiograph and can be corrected by careful withdrawal of the PAC until the loop is removed. Arrhythmias may also occur if the PAC tip slips back into the right ventricle. In this case, the pressure tracing will show a typical right ventricular waveform. Readvancement of the PAC into the pulmonary artery should eliminate the arrhythmias.

Other potentially serious but rare complications during placement include injuries to the great vessels,

TABLE 41-5. FORMULAS FOR THE DERIVATION OF VARIABLES

SVR = (mean arterial pressure − mean arterial pressure) × 80 cardiac output

PVR = (mean pulmonary artery pressure − pulmonary capillary wedge pressure) × 80 cardiac output

LVSWI = SV × (mean arterial pressure − pulmonary capillary wedge pressure) × 0.0136 body surface area

RVSWI = SV × (mean arterial pressure − right atrial pressure) × 0.0136 body surface area

(DO_2) = [(cardiac output × hemoglobin) × (13.4) × (% O_2 saturation)] + (PO_2 × 0.0031)

(VO_2) = (cardiac output × hemoglobin) × (13.4) × ($SaO_2 - SvO_2$)

$(Q_s/Q_t) = \dfrac{\text{(pulmonary capillary } O_2 \text{ content} - CaO_2)}{\text{(pulmonary capillary } O_2 \text{ content} - CvO_2)}$

KEY: CaO_2, arterial oxygen content; CvO_2, mixed venous oxygen content; PO_2, partial pressure of oxygen; SaO_2, arterial oxygen saturation; SV, stroke volume. Other terms are defined in Tables 41-3 and 41-4.

TABLE 41-6. RECOGNIZED COMPLICATIONS OF PULMONARY ARTERY CATHETERIZATION

Related to catheter insertion (published incidence)
Complete heart block (0–2.6%)
Ventricular arrhythmias requiring treatment (0–3%)
Hematoma (0–3%)
Air embolism (0.1%)
Pneumothorax (0.1–1.5%)
Inability to place catheter with multiple attempts (1.7%)
Injury to great vessels (0.1–13%)
Ventricular arrhythmias (20–50%)

**Related to catheter insertion (reported, but incidence
   unpublished)**
Hemothorax
Hemomediastinum
Lymphatic duct perforation
Injury to trachea
Injury to phrenic or vagus nerve
Guidewire embolism
Catheter knotting (requiring surgical removal)
Cardiac perforation

Related to long-term maintenance (published incidence)
Pulmonary artery rupture (0–0.5%)
Pulmonary infarction (0–0.5%)
Catheter infection (1–5%)

**Related to long-term maintenance (reported, but incidence
   unpublished)**
Catheter shearing with embolization
Misreading or misunderstanding of data
   provided by catheter

trachea, lymphatic duct, vagus nerve, or phrenic nerve as well as a pneumothorax, hemothorax, hemomediastinum, and cardiac perforation. On occasion, the PAC has become knotted during placement, necessitating surgical removal.

The most serious complications related to long-term maintenance of the PAC are pulmonary artery rupture, pulmonary artery infarction, and catheter infection. Pulmonary artery rupture is usually the result of the catheter becoming overwedged and/or the balloon over-inflated. Pulmonary infarction has been seen primarily in patients with mitral regurgitation or pulmonary hypertension and may be avoided if the duration of balloon inflation is kept to a minimum. Catheter infection occurs in 1 to 5 percent of PAC placements and can be minimized by strict sterile maintenance of the PAC as well as continually reevaluating the need for the PAC and keeping the placement time as short as possible. The majority of PACs should be used for 72 hours or less.

SUMMARY

Since its introduction three decades ago, the PAC has proved an invaluable aid in the management of critically ill patients. Despite having its detractors, the PAC has not only proven useful in the diagnosis and treatment of intensive care problems but has also taught a generation of physicians and nurses about the pathophysiology of cardiopulmonary diseases. Those who criticize the PAC for failing to change the outcome of certain diseases must remember that it is only as good an intervention as those who use it. Furthermore, by itself, the PAC merely provides information—not judgment and certainly not wisdom. These are left to the practitioner. Those who manage patients with the PAC must learn to integrate the data they obtain with the clinical findings and other laboratory information they collect. It is axiomatic that PAC data should never be interpreted in the absence of clinical context. In this respect, how the current generation of physicians learns to manage patients with the PAC will presage, in many ways, how the next generation of physicians will learn to manage patients with technologies still undiscovered, when much of the information provided by the PAC will be available through noninvasive techniques such as advanced ultrasound equipment and sophisticated body scanners.

REFERENCES

1. Swan HJC, Ganz W, Forrester JS, et al: Catheterization of the heart in man with use of a flow-directed balloon-tipped catheter. *N Engl J Med* 1970; 283:447–451.
2. Ganz W, Donoso R, Marcus HS, et al: A new technique for measuring cardiac output by thermodilution in man. *Am J Cardiol* 1971; 27:392–396.
3. Forrester JS, Diamond G, McHugh TJ, Swan HJC: Filling pressures in the right and left sides of the heart in acute myocardial infarction. *N Engl J Med* 1971; 285:190–192.
4. Forrester JS, Diamond G, Chatterjee K, Swan HJC: Medical therapy of acute myocardial infarction by application of hemodynamic subsets. *N Engl J Med* 1976; 295:1356–1362, 1404–1412.
5. Mathay MA, Chatterjee K: Bedside catheterization of the pulmonary artery: risk compared with benefit. *Ann Intern Med* 1988; 109:826–834.
6. Shah KB, Rao TL, Laughlin S, El-Etr AA: A review of pulmonary artery catheterization in 6,245 patients. *Anesthesiology* 1984; 61:271–275.
7. Boyd KD, Thomas SJ, Gold J, et al: A prospective study of complications of pulmonary artery catheterization in 500 consecutive patients. *Chest* 1983; 83:245–249.
8. Sharkey SW: Beyond the wedge: clinical physiology and the Swan-Ganz catheter. *Am J Med* 1987; 83:111–121.

9. Forrester JS, Diamond GA, Swan HJC: Correlative classification of clinical and hemodynamic function after acute myocardial infarction. *Am J Cardiol* 1977; 39:137–145.

10. Bayliss J, Norell M, Ryan A, et al: Bedside haemodynamic monitoring: experience in a general hospital. *Br Med J* 1983; 287:187–190.

11. Connors AFJ, McCaffree DR, Gray BA: Evaluation of right-heart catheterization in patients without acute myocardial infarction. *N Engl J Med* 1983; 308:263–267.

12. Eisenberg PR, Jaffe AS, Schuster DP: Clinical evaluation compared to pulmonary artery catheterization in the hemodynamic assessment of critically ill patients. *Crit Care Med* 1984; 12:549–553.

13. Fein AM, Goldberg SK, Wahlenstein MD, et al: Is pulmonary artery catheterization necessary for the diagnosis of pulmonary edema? *Am Rev Respir Dis* 1984; 129:1006–1009.

14. Gore JM, Goldberg RJ, Spodick DH, et al: A community-wide assessment of the use of pulmonary artery catheters in patients with acute myocardial infarction. *Chest* 1987; 92:721–727.

15. Zion MM, Balkin J, Rosemann D, et al: Use of pulmonary artery catheters in patients with acute myocardial infarction. *Chest* 1990; 98:1331–1335.

16. Connors AF, Speroff T, Dawson NV, et al: The effectiveness of right heart catheterization in the initial care of critically ill patients. *JAMA* 1996; 276:889–897.

17. Mimoz O, Rauss A, Rekik N, et al: Pulmonary artery catheterization in critically ill patients: a prospective analysis of outcome changes associated with catheter-prompted changes in therapy. *Crit Care Med* 1994; 22:573–579.

18. American College of Cardiology Consensus Document: Present use of right heart catheterization in patients with cardiac disease. *J Am Coll Cardiol* 1998; 32:840–864.

19. Iberti TJ, Fischer EP, Leibowitz AB, et al: A multicenter study of physicians' knowledge of the pulmonary artery catheter. *JAMA* 1990; 264:2928–2932.

20. Komadina KH, Shenk DA, LaVeau P, et al: Interobserver variability in the interpretation of pulmonary artery catheter pressure tracings. *Chest* 1991; 100:1647–1654.

Chapter 42

NONINVASIVE CARDIAC OUTPUT MONITORING

Robert Bilkovski

INTRODUCTION

It has been widely accepted that determination of cardiac output (CO) is a useful and often lifesaving adjunct in the resuscitation of critically ill patients. Monitoring of these patients typically occurs within the intensive care unit (ICU), operating room, cardiac catheterization lab, or Emergency Department. Cardiac output determination has conventionally been obtained by thermodilution or dye dilution measurements that are invasive and associated with potential risk to the patient. Complication rates up to 7.2 percent using the invasive pulmonary artery (PA) catheter have been reported.[1-3] There is wide variability in CO measurements using a PA catheter as well. Stetz and Miller identified error rates between 4 and 10 percent with triplicate CO measurements, while single CO measurements had a wider variability, ranging between 7 and 17 percent.[4] Other disadvantages to use of the PA catheter include risk of sepsis, intermittent cardiac output determinations, expense, and restricted use to "monitored" facilities within a hospital (i.e., ICU or operating room).

Noninvasive devices that measure cardiac output have been slowly gaining acceptance in the medical community and have shown very good agreement with the "gold standard" thermodilution technique. Transesophageal Doppler (TED) and thoracic electrical bioimpedance (TEB) are two modalities that can measure CO noninvasively and continuously. Furthermore, they can measure other hemodynamic variables such as preload, contractility, and systemic vascular resistance in real time. This provides the physician with the ability to follow trends as well as the response to interventions such as the institution of vasopressors or following the administration of a fluid bolus. The measurements obtained require little training, are highly reproducible, and pose little risk to the patient. Another advantage lies in their ability to identify hemodynamic compromise before it becomes clinically apparent and when therapy may be most beneficial. Most Emergency Departments utilize noninvasive devices to measure blood pressure, heart rate, oxygen saturation, and, on rare occasions, central venous pressure. These noninvasive devices may allow the Emergency Physician to monitor the hemodynamic status of a patient more closely and to institute therapy earlier.

TRANSESOPHAGEAL DOPPLER

INTRODUCTION

In 1842, Christian Doppler identified that the velocity of a moving object is proportional to the shift in reflected frequency of an optic wave of known frequency. This principle has been adapted to sound waves and is now the basis for Doppler devices that measure the velocity of blood flow and related hemodynamic variables continuously. The first use of Doppler to measure the velocity of red blood cells in humans or animals occurred in 1969.[5,6] Cardiac output determination was first conducted via the suprasternal approach, but this was cumbersome, and it was difficult to obtain data continuously.[7,8] The device currently in use involves Doppler measurements through a transesophageal approach, directly measuring the blood velocity in the descending aorta. The esophageal Doppler monitor (EDM; CardioQ, Deltex Medical Inc.) is one such device that will display continuous hemodynamic data (cardiac output, peak velocity, and corrected flow time) in addition to the characteristic flow-velocity waveform (Figure 42-1).

ANATOMY AND PATHOPHYSIOLOGY

Cardiac output is a product of heart rate (HR) and stroke volume (SV), where CO = HR × SV. Stroke volume can be determined by multiplying the spatial average blood velocity within the aorta during systole (V),

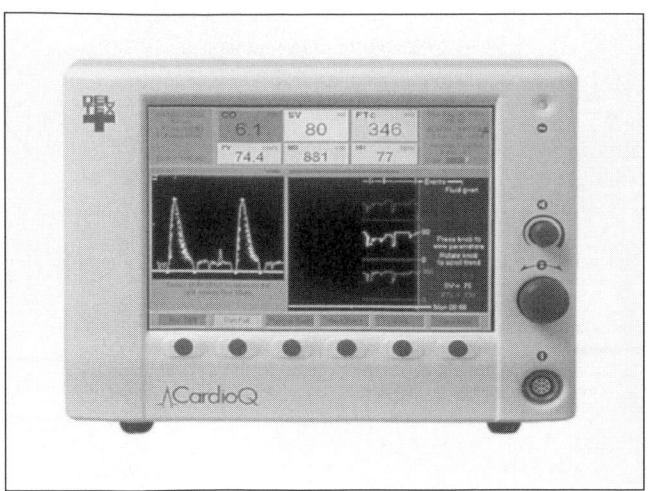

FIGURE 42-1 The CardioQ esophageal Doppler recorder. (Photo courtesy of Deltex Medical Incorporated.)

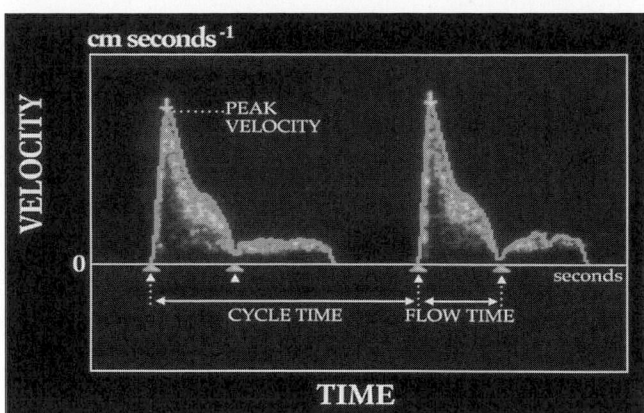

FIGURE 42-2 The flow-velocity waveform from an esophageal Doppler probe. The graphs demonstrate peak velocity and flow time.

ejection time (ET), and the cross-sectional area of the aorta (CSA), where SV = V × ET × CSA. The descending aorta CSA is related to the height, age, and weight of the patient; thus cardiac output determination produces only an estimate and not a precise measurement.

Once the device is inserted and the flow-velocity waveform is obtained, the EDM will display the peak velocity (PV) and flow time (FT). The peak velocity is the apex of the waveform, and the flow time is the length of the waveform base (Figure 42-2). The flow time is dependent upon heart rate. Given that most hemodynamic interventions will affect heart rate, the FT must be corrected. Like the corrected QT interval on an electrocardiogram (ECG), the FT is corrected using a modification of Bazett's equation, yielding the corrected flow time (FTc).

The normal range for peak velocity is age-dependent: 90 to 120 cm/sec for a 20-year-old, 70 to 100 cm/sec for a 50-year-old, and 50 to 80 cm/sec for a 70-year-old. Values lying above or below this range correspond to a hyperdynamic or hypodynamic state, respectively. The peak velocity is therefore an indicator of cardiac contractility. Tall waveforms indicate increased contractility, while short waveforms represent depressed contractility.

The corrected flow time represents left ventricular filling (preload) and systemic vascular resistance. A normal FTc is approximately 330 to 360 milliseconds. Values below this indicate hypovolemia and/or systemic vasoconstriction. Values above the normal range typify states of vasodilatation. To summarize, changes in the peak velocity correlate with changes in inotropy and to a lesser extent SVR, while changes in FTc represent changes in preload. Applying Starling principles, improving FTc (preload) will also result in greater peak velocity. Singer studied normal volunteers and monitored their hemodynamic response to increasing infu-

sions of dobutamine and esmolol (inotropic changes); phentolamine, metaraminol, and methoxamine (afterload); and plasma removal (preload) and was able to corroborate the above effects.[9] The waveform changes associated with alterations in preload are shown in Figure 42-3. The waveform changes associated with alterations in inotropy are shown in Figure 42-4. The waveform changes associated with alterations in afterload are shown in Figure 42-5. An overview of flow-velocity waveform changes from normal that are expected with various hemodynamic variations are shown in Figure 42-6.

INDICATIONS

The present-day use of the esophageal Doppler has been predominantly within the ICU and operating room. The Emergency Department is beginning to utilize this technology in trauma resuscitation and septic shock. The indications can be broadened to include patients with occult hemodynamic compromise. For instance, patients who are manifesting a systemic inflammatory response syndrome (SIRS) may benefit from early recognition and treatment of deviations in contractility or preload that have not resulted in hypotension. The patient with congestive heart failure may also benefit from an esophageal Doppler. The titration of medications to clinical symptoms as well as hemodynamic parameters may convert an admission into a discharge. The most apparent application for TED technology is with trauma resuscitations where aggressive fluid administration can be monitored beat-to-beat in attempts to normalize hemodynamic parameters.

In general, the esophageal Doppler may be used under the following conditions: to allow recognition of circulatory compromise at the earliest possible time, to gain a better understanding of pathophysiologic conditions, and to provide real-time monitoring of interventions applied to patients with hemodynamic compromise or those at high risk for deterioration.

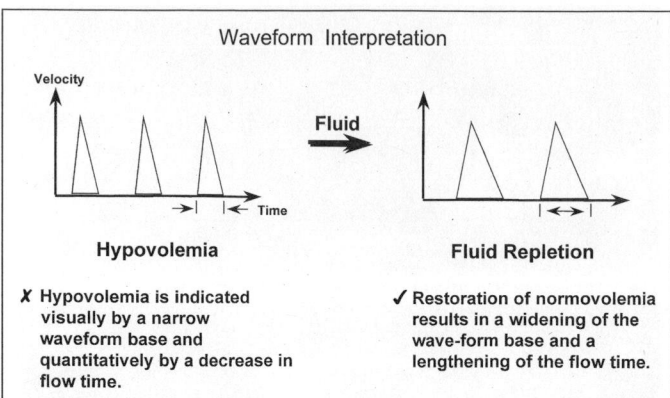

FIGURE 42-3 The flow-velocity waveform changes following a fluid bolus (alteration in preload).

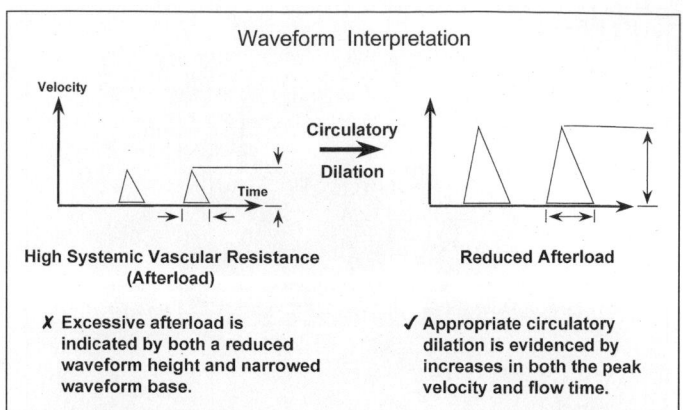

FIGURE 42-5 The flow-velocity waveform changes following the use of a systemic vasodilating agent (alteration in afterload).

CONTRAINDICATIONS

The primary limitation to the use of the esophageal Doppler is that it requires placement within the esophagus. The probe is similar in size to a nasogastric tube but is more rigid and less tolerable by the awake individual. The TED should not be used in patients with oropharyngeal or midface injuries. Extreme caution should be exercised for patients with portal hypertension complicated by esophageal varices. Moreover, the TED is relatively contraindicated in patients with esophageal strictures, recent esophagogastric operations, or caustic ingestions.

EQUIPMENT

The only equipment required is the TED machine with a probe and a willing patient. The probe has a beveled end from which the Doppler signal is emitted. This beveled surface must be facing the posterior surface of the esophagus during insertion in order to capture the blood flow of the descending aorta. The use of a nasal decongestant (cocaine, oxymetazoline, phenylephrine), if not contraindicated, is highly recommended.

TECHNIQUE

The TED can be inserted via the orogastric or nasogastric approach (refer to Chapter 47 for complete details). The nasogastric approach is preferred in the awake patient. Apply a nasal decongestant. Apply lubricant to the probe. Gently insert the probe through either naris until it reaches the nasopharynx. Gradually advance the probe, while maintaining its correct position, until a distinct and clear flow-velocity curve is obtained on the TED machine output display. The image quality may be improved by slight rotation of the probe, either in a clockwise or counterclockwise direction. Secure the probe to the patient once a proper waveform has been obtained. The orogastric application is similar to above with the exception of applying an aerosolized anesthetic to the posterior oropharynx.

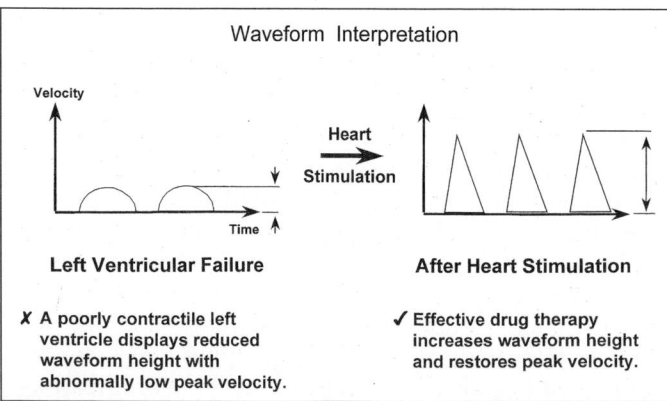

FIGURE 42-4 The flow-velocity waveform changes associated with the institution of an inotropic agent.

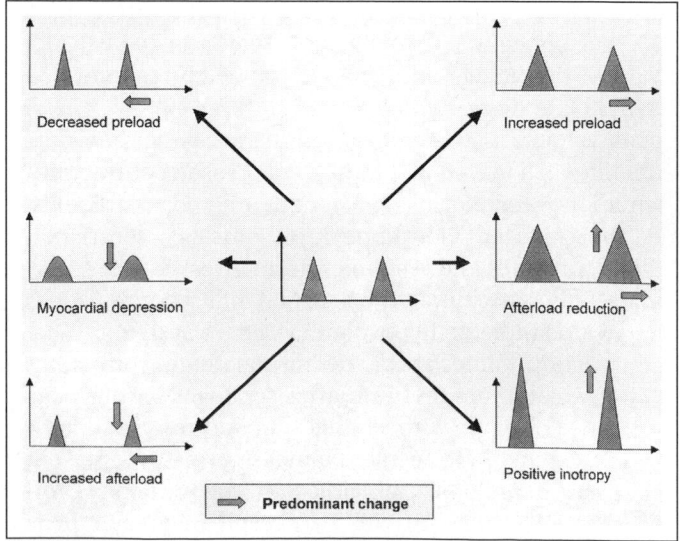

FIGURE 42-6 Waveform changes from baseline following hemodynamic modifications.

AFTERCARE

Radiographic confirmation of TED probe placement is not necessary as the waveform output corresponds to proper positioning. Unlike the PA catheter, the esophageal Doppler may remain in position for many days without fear of inducing harm or injury to the patient. Once it has been decided to discontinue monitoring with the TED, simply remove the probe in a manner similar to removing a nasogastric tube. The probe is not reusable and must be discarded.

COMPLICATIONS

The complications associated with use of the TED is minimal. Minor bleeding from the nares may occur. Packing is effective if direct pressure fails to control epistaxis. Sinusitis may develop with prolonged use. Prevention with nasal decongestants may minimize this complication. Chapter 47 provides a more detailed discussion of the complications associated with the use of a nasogastric tube.

SUMMARY

The esophageal Doppler monitor has been shown in numerous studies to correlate well with the cardiac output determination obtained by thermodilution.[10–14] The corrected flow time provides a measure of preload. The peak velocity represents inotropy and, to a lesser extent, systemic vascular resistance. The device is relatively inexpensive compared to a pulmonary artery catheter and has a better safety profile. TED can provide continuous cardiac output readings that have less interrater variability than transthoracic Doppler and thus allow for more effective trending of resuscitative interventions. The drawbacks include its low compliance in the awake patient and its inaccurate readings in patients with valvular abnormalities (i.e., aortic stenosis or mitral regurgitation). More importantly, cardiac output determinations are estimates, and the trends are more helpful as opposed to absolute values. The esophageal Doppler is not intended to replace the PA catheter. It may, however, prove to be an important adjunct in the resuscitation of critically ill patients and the identification of occult hemodynamic compromise in high-risk patients.

THORACIC ELECTRICAL BIOIMPEDANCE

INTRODUCTION

Thoracic electrical bioimpedance (Z) was first developed by NASA to monitor hemodynamic changes in astronauts during the 1960s. The first clinical use of bioimpedance to determine cardiac output was by Nyober.[15] Kubicek utilized the first derivative of impedance (dZ/dt) to better estimate cardiac output calculations in astronauts and labeled it the Kubicek equation.[16,17] Application to a heterogeneous population with varying illnesses and body habitus generated poor correlation of stroke volume calculated by bioimpedance to other established methods for stroke volume measurement.[18] A new set of equations that circumvented the false assumptions of the Kubicek equation was proposed by Sramek and further modified by Bernstein.[19–22] The Sramek-Bernstein equation has been incorporated in the software of current bioimpedance monitoring devices such as the NCCOM3-R7 (Bomed Corp., Irving, CA). The Kubicek equation is the foundation for the CIC-1000 (Sorba Medical Systems Inc., Brookfield, WI).

The application of bioimpedance cardiography is minimally invasive, affordable, and has very good reproducibility.[23] Cardiac output determination by thermodilution provides only a "snapshot" of a patient's hemodynamic status. Bioimpedance allows for continuous, real-time data acquisition that enables a physician to follow a response to therapy. Such a device can be utilized not only in the ICU or the operating room but also in the Emergency Department. This may allow the Emergency Physician to recognize hemodynamic compromise earlier and thus to expedite initiation of therapy when it is likely to be most effective.

ANATOMY AND PATHOPHYSIOLOGY

With electrical bioimpedance, the patient interfaces with the transducer through a series of disposable surface electrodes that allow for measurements of current flowing parallel to the spine. The electric current transmitted is of low frequency (50 to 100 kHz), high-amplitude (0.2 to 5.0 mA) alternating current, it cannot be sensed by the patient, and is totally safe. The voltage is sensed by the pairs of electrodes at the beginning and end of the thorax. These electrodes can also sense the ECG, which is necessary in order to determine hemodynamic variables such as cardiac output and stroke volume.

The electrical resistance (Z = impedance) to this electric current is directly proportional to the content of fluid within the thoracic cavity. The lungs and thoracic wall are of low conductance for electric current. The majority of the impedance is derived from the plasma within the heart and great vessels. The average baseline impedance (Z_o) of the thorax changes due to respiration and the accumulation of interstitial fluid. Since air is a poor conductor of electricity compared to plasma, Z_o will rise with inspiration due to increased resistance within the chest. On the other hand, increased interstitial volume (i.e., pulmonary edema) will cause Z_o to fall. The bioimpedance device will monitor Z_o and has an inverse relationship with thoracic intravascular fluid volumes (thoracic fluid volume index, or TVFI), where

$TVFI = 1/Z_o$. This index provides a way to assess central fluid status of a patient noninvasively and continuously and will aid the physician in making appropriate treatment decisions.

The change in electrical bioimpedance (ΔZ) primarily reflects velocity and volumetric changes of aortic blood flow during each cardiac cycle. The first derivative of impedance (dZ/dt) is reflective of aortic blood flow. The maximum rate of change [(dZ/dt)$_{max}$] is proportional to the peak velocity of aortic blood flow. The timing of dZ/dt in correlation with the ECG allows for measurement of systolic time intervals such as the ventricular ejection time and the preejection period.

The stroke volume determined by Nyober utilized ΔZ but was found to have excessive respiratory variability. Kubicek utilized dZ/dt in the stroke volume equation, which was calculated as $SV = Rho \times L^2/Z_o^2 \times (dZ/dt)_{max} \times LVET$, where Rho = the specific resistance of blood, L = thorax length, and LVET = left ventricular ejection time. Sramek proposed that $Rho \times L^2/Z_o^2$ be replaced by $VEPT/Z_o$, where VEPT = volume of thoracic electrically participating tissue and is equal to $L^3/4.25$. This is based on the premise that the thorax is a truncated cone as opposed to a cylinder and the resistance of blood is negligible in the total resistance. Bernstein further elaborated on the equation by correcting the VEPT calculation due to differences in body habitus and using a nomogram that incorporates the patient's sex, height, and weight.[21]

The bioimpedance device can be used to determine other hemodynamic variables, such as systolic and diastolic time intervals. The description of the cardiac cycle was pioneered by Lababidi et al and is shown in Figure 42-7.[24] The A wave is at or shortly after the beginning of the fourth heart sound and just before the ECG Q wave. The B wave occurs at the first heart sound at the apex, coincident with aortic valve opening. The X wave signals aortic valve closure. The O wave occurs at mitral valve opening. The preejection period (PEP) represents isovolumic contraction (A→B). The left ventricular ejection time (LVET) begins at the end of the PEP and ends at the closure of the aortic valve (B→X). The PEP and LVET comprise the systolic interval. The isovolumic relaxation time (IVRT) begins when the aortic valve closes and ends on the beginning of mitral flow (X→O). The filling time (FT) is the interval between mitral valve flow and the beginning of the next cardiac cycle (O→A). The diastolic time interval comprises both the IVRT and the FT.

Contractility was first determined utilizing bioimpedance 30 years ago utilizing the ratio of PEP/LVET to reflect cardiac ejection fraction.[25] Currently there are several formulas used to calculate contractility, including the Heather index, Minnesota index, and acceleration contractility index (ACI). The Heather index [HI = (dZ/dt)$_{max}$/QZ1, QZ1 = time from beginning of the Q wave to peak dZ/dt] has been shown to be the most accurate for determining contractility, and all three calculations are based on dZ/dt$_{max}$.[26,27] The ability of physicians to categorize patients with congestive heart failure into those with systolic or diastolic dysfunction has been problematic. With the use of bioimpedance, however, Summers et al identified patients with a HI < 5 to have predominantly systolic dysfunction, while an IVRT > 0.125 correlated with diastolic dysfunction.[28] The use of TEB may facilitate the management of this difficult subset of patients.

INDICATIONS

The indications for the use of thoracic electrical bioimpedance are similar to those for transesophageal Doppler monitoring—namely, the management of patients with hemodynamic compromise (i.e., shock) and the recognition of occult hemodynamic compromise. TEB can also be utilized to recognize diastolic dysfunction, determine hypovolemia during tilt testing, monitor exercise tolerance, or gauge the adequacy of hemodialysis. Due to the noninvasive nature of TEB, it may become a useful adjunct in the resuscitation of critically ill patients prior to the insertion of a pulmonary artery catheter.

CONTRAINDICATIONS

There are no contraindications to the use of a bioimpedance device. There are, however, situations that will result in inaccurate measurements. Anything that creates noise within the system (i.e., shivering, excessive movement, and extreme obesity) will affect stroke volume determination as well as measurement of other hemodynamic variables. Current systems incorporate waveform averaging in order to minimize the effect of system noise. Poor skin electrode contact has been problematic, notably with excessive diaphoresis. The CIC-1000 (Sorba Medical Systems Inc., Brookfield, WI) has devised electrodes that minimize noise and optimize impedance waveform analysis (Figure 42-8).

Other limitations include valvular abnormalities and extremes in heart rate or rhythm. Aortic regurgitation can lead to falsely elevated stroke-volume estimates. Bradycardia (< 60 beats per minute) or tachycardia (> 140 beats per minute) can lead to inaccurate results. Patients with paced rhythms can alter calculation of the preejection period due to an altered QRS morphology. Algorithms have been created to overcome many of these flaws. It is nonetheless important to identify circumstances when TEB measurements may be less reliable. Electrode placement can also significantly alter hemodynamic measurements. A 1 cm difference in thoracic length has been shown to result in a 10 percent error in stroke volume.[29]

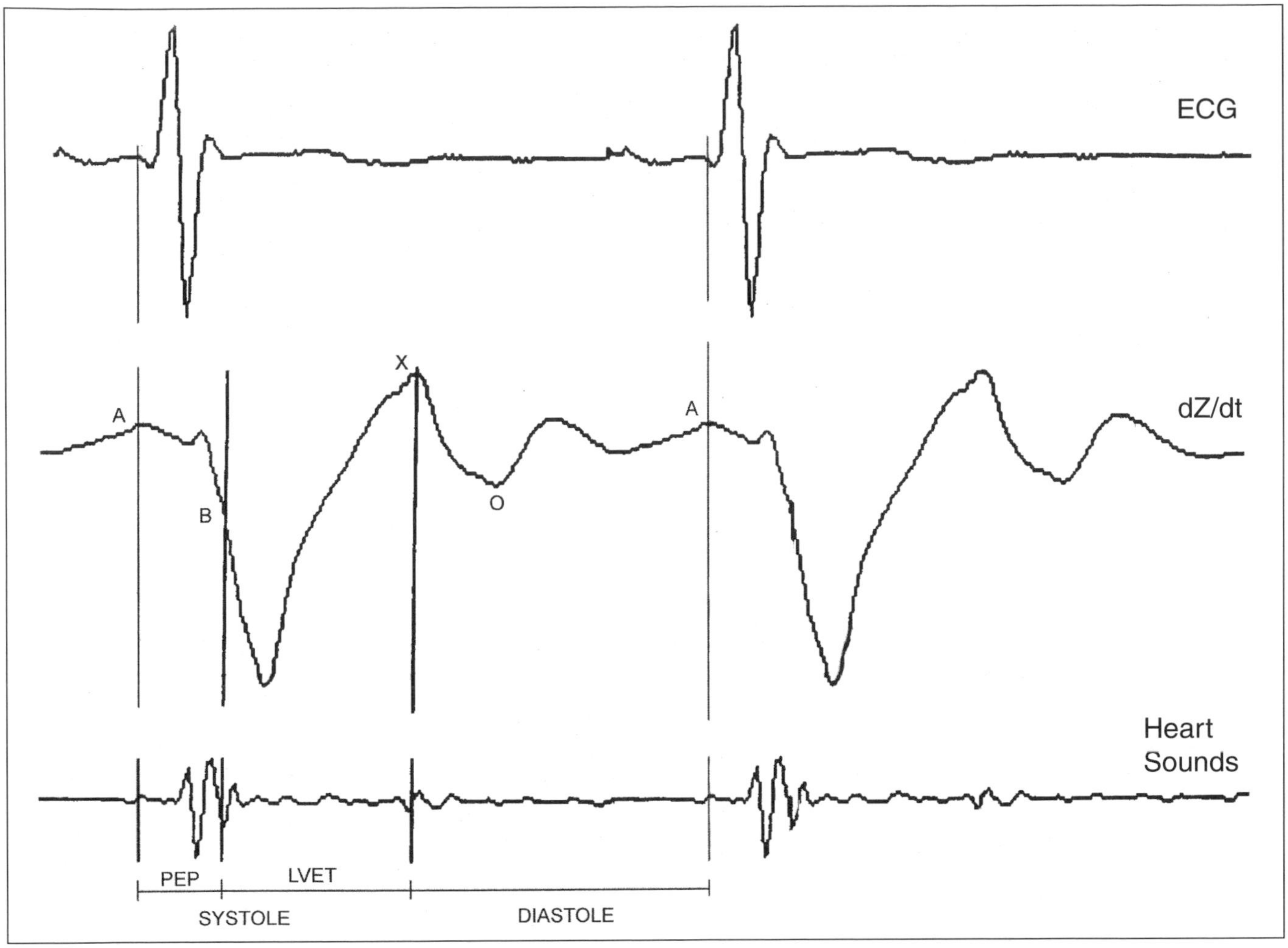

ECG

dZ/dt

Heart Sounds

PEP   LVET

SYSTOLE   DIASTOLE

FIGURE 42-7 The description of the cardiac cycle.[24] Refer to the text for a full description of the cardiac cycle.

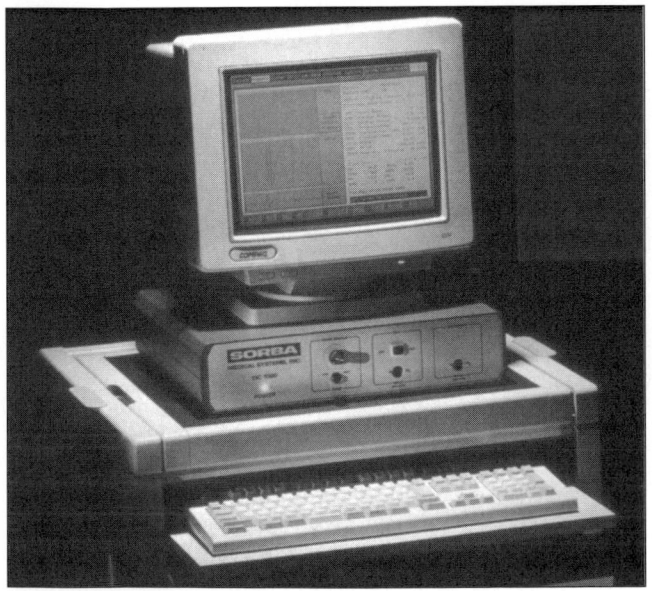

FIGURE 42-8 The CIC-1000 bioimpedance device. (Photo courtesy of Sorba Medical Systems.)

EQUIPMENT

Regardless on the TEB device used, the amount of equipment necessary is limited. The TEB device and electrodes are the mainstays of the equipment. Other materials needed include electrode preparation gel and a tape measure. The recommended electrode setup for the CIC-1000 from Sorba Medical Systems is shown in Figure 42-9. A sample screen display of measured hemodynamic values is shown in Figure 42-10.

SUMMARY

Given the growing safety concerns regarding the pulmonary artery catheter, thoracic electrical bioimpedance has been found to be safe, inexpensive, and simple to use. There is good correlation between TEB and thermodilution-derived cardiac output measurements.[30] Compared to cardiac output obtained via a PA catheter, the TEB values tend to underestimate slightly, as these are indirect measurements. The ability to provide continuous and beat-to-beat output of hemodynamic data

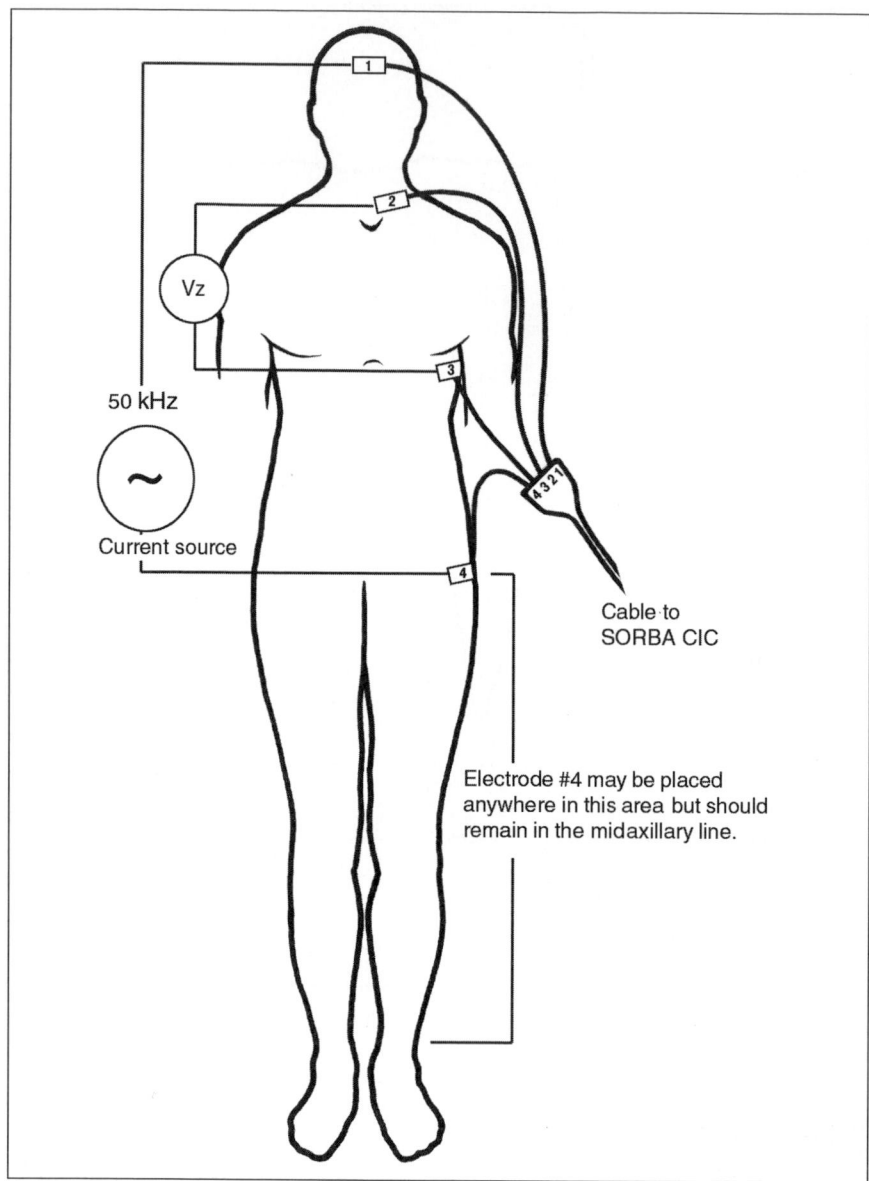

FIGURE 42-9 Recommended electrode placement for the Sorba CIC-1000 bio-impedance device. (Courtesy of Sorba Medical Systems.)

is a distinct advantage despite this limitation. The ability to follow trends in real time gives the physician an opportunity to monitor disease progression as well as response to therapeutic interventions. Bioimpedance may be used to identify abnormal hemodynamics in patients with normal blood pressure and heart rate. While pulse oximetry has become recognized as the "fifth" vital sign, TEB may provide the physician a potential "sixth" vital sign to be used in the care of emergent patients. The Emergency Physician has up to the present relied upon vital signs, mentation, and urine output as clues to hemodynamic embarrassment. He or she can now greatly benefit from the use of TEB. The ability to use TEB as a diagnostic tool may prove to be of great benefit in differentiating between systolic and diastolic dysfunction or identifying hypovolemia during tilt testing.

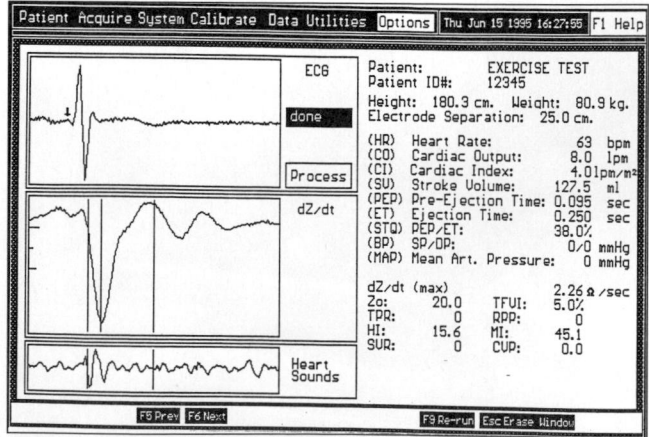

FIGURE 42-10 Sample output of hemodynamic data from a bioimpedance device.

CHAPTER SUMMARY

The pulmonary artery catheter remains the mainstay for the determination of hemodynamic variables such as cardiac output, stroke volume, and pulmonary artery wedge pressure. The mounting evidence of increased morbidity and mortality with its use has forced many physicians to refocus. There is a growing body of evidence suggesting that noninvasive devices such as transesophageal Doppler or thoracic electrical bioimpedance can function as adjuncts to more invasive hemodynamic monitoring devices. While noninvasive devices provide estimates of cardiac output, their ability to provide continuous data may prove invaluable. The ability to monitor the response to therapy and/or disease progression as well as to recognize occult hemodynamic derangement will be of great value to the Emergency Physician. Until recently, the Emergency Physician has had to rely on parameters such as blood pressure, pulse, or mentation as markers of abnormal circulation; these are known to be unreliable and typically change significantly only late in the disease process. Earlier institution of resuscitative therapy may translate into decreased ICU utilization, decreased morbidity, and decreased mortality.

REFERENCES

1. Elliot CG, Zimmerman GA, Clemmer TP: Complications of pulmonary artery catheterization in the care of critically-ill patients. A prospective study. *Chest* 1979; 76(6):647–652.
2. Foote GA, Schabel SI, Hodges M: Pulmonary complications of the flow-directed balloon-tipped catheter. *N Engl J Med* 1974; 290(17):927–931.
3. Robin ED: Death by pulmonary artery flow-directed catheter—time for a moratorium? *Chest* 1987; 92(4):727–731.
4. Stetz CW, Miller RG, Kelly GE, et al: Reliability of the thermodilution method in the determination of cardiac output in clinical practice. *Am Rev Respir Dis* 1982; 126:1001–1004.
5. Satomura S: A study of the flow patterns in superficial arteries by ultrasonics. *J Acoust Soc Jpn* 1969; 15:151–158.
6. Franklin DW, Schlegel WA, Rushmer R: Blood flow measured by Doppler ultrasound frequency shift of back-scattered ultrasound. *Science* 1969; 134:564–565.
7. Kumar A, Minagoe S, Thangathurai D, et al: Noninvasive measurement of cardiac output during surgery using a new continuous-wave Doppler esophageal probe. *Am J Cardiol* 1989; 64(12):793–798.
8. Huntsman LL, Stewart DK, Barnes SR, et al: Noninvasive Doppler determination of cardiac output in man. Clinical validation. *Circulation* 1983; 67(3):593–602.
9. Singer M, Allen MJ, Webb AR, et al: Effects of alterations in left ventricular filling, contractility and systemic vascular resistance on the ascending aortic blood velocity waveform of normal subjects. *Crit Care Med* 1991; 19(9):1138–1145.
10. Madan AK, Uybarreta VV, Alaibadi-Wahle S, et al: Esophageal Doppler ultrasound monitor versus pulmonary artery catheter in the hemodynamic management of critically ill surgical patients. *J Trauma* 1999; 46(4):607–612.
11. Leone D, Servillo G, De Robertis E, et al: Monitoring cardiac output: esophageal Doppler vs thermodilution. *Minerva Anesthesiol* 1998: 64(7–8):351–356.
12. Freund PR: Transesophageal Doppler scanning versus thermodilution during general anesthesia. An initial comparison of cardiac output techniques. *Am J Surg* 1987: 153(5):490–494.
13. Singer M, Clarke J, Bennett ED: Continuous hemodynamic monitoring by esophageal Doppler. *Crit Care Med* 1989; 17(5):447–452.
14. Wong DH, Watson T, Gordon I, et al: Comparison of changes in transit time ultrasound, esophageal Doppler, and thermodilution cardiac output after changes in preload, afterload, and contractility in pigs. *Anesth Analg* 1991; 72(5):584–588.
15. Nyober J: *Electrical Impedance Plethysmography.* Springfield, IL: Charles C Thomas, 1959:243.
16. Kubicek WG, Karnegis JN, Patterson RP, et al: Development and evaluation of an impedance cardiac output system. *Aerospace Med* 1966; 37(12):1208–1212.
17. Kubicek WG, From AH, Patterson RP, et al: Impedance cardiography as a noninvasive means to monitor cardiac function. *J Assoc Adv Med Instr* 1970; 4(2):79–84.
18. Keim HJ, Wallace JM, Thurston H, et al: Impedance cardiography for determination of stroke index. *J Appl Physiol* 1976; 41(5 Pt 1):797–799.
19. Sramek BB, Rose DM, Miyamoto A: Stroke volume equation with a linear base impedance model and its accuracy, as compared to thermodilution and magnetic flow meter techniques in humans and animals. Proceedings of the Sixth International Conference on Electrical Bioimpedance 1983. Zadar, Yugoslavia.
20. Sramek BB: Noninvasive technique for measuring cardiac output by means of electrical impedance. Proceedings of the Fifth International Conference on Electrical Bioimpedance 1981. Tokyo, Japan.

21. Bernstein DP: A new stroke volume equation for thoracic electrical bioimpedance: theory and rationale. *Crit Care Med* 1986; 14(10):904–909.

22. Bernstein DP: Continuous noninvasive real-time monitoring of stroke volume and cardiac output by thoracic electrical bioimpedance. *Crit Care Med* 1986; 14(10):898–901.

23. Salandin V, Zussa C, Risica G, et al: Comparison of cardiac output estimation by thoracic electrical bioimpedance, thermodilution, and Fick methods. *Crit Care Med* 1988; 16(11):1157–1158.

24. Lababidi Z, Ehmke DA, Durnin RE, et al: The first derivative thoracic impedance cardiogram. *Circulation* 1970; 41(4):651–658.

25. Garrard CL Jr, Weissler AM, Dodge HT: The relationship of alterations in systolic time intervals to ejection fraction in patients with cardiac disease. *Circulation* 1970; 42(3):455–462.

26. Hill DW, Merrifield AJ: Left ventricular ejection and the Heather index measured by non-invasive methods during postural changes in man. *Acta Anaesthesiol Scand* 1976; 20(4):313–320.

27. Mancini R, Kottke FJ, Patterson R, et al: Cardiac output and contractility indices: establishing a standard in response to low-to-moderate level exercise in healthy men. *Arch Phys Med Rehabil* 1979; 60(12):567–573.

28. Summers RL, Kolb JC, Woodward LH, et al: Differentiating systolic from diastolic heart failure using impedance cardiography. *Acad Emerg Med* 1999; 6(7):693–699.

29. Appel PL, Kram HB, Mackabee J, et al: Comparison of measurements of cardiac output by bioimpedance and thermodilution in severely ill surgical patients. *Crit Care Med* 1986; 14(11):933–935.

30. Fuller HD: The validity of cardiac output measurement by thoracic impedance: a meta-analysis. *Clin Invest Med* 1992; 15(2):103–112.

Chapter 43
PERIPHERAL VENOUS CUTDOWN

Flavia Nobay

INTRODUCTION

Venous access in the critically ill patient is of the utmost importance. The literature regarding peripheral venous cutdowns extends back to 1940 when Keeley introduced the venous cutdown as an alternative to venipuncture in patients with shock.[1] Interestingly, there has been a noticeable lack of recent investigations regarding this procedure, most likely because Dr Keeley's indications for peripheral venous cutdowns have not changed. The steps outlined in 1940 for exposing the peripheral vein and its cannulation are remarkably unchanged. The peripheral cutdown indications and technique have withstood the test of time.

Peripheral venous access can be extremely difficult due to vascular collapse from shock, previous injury to the vessel, obesity, or scars. Direct visualization of the vein to be cannulated will frequently be quicker and more fruitful than indirect visualization with central venous lines. Although this procedure has become less utilized with the increasing popularity of central venous access, familiarity with this procedure allows for large-bore access and the rapid infusions required in the critically ill trauma patient or medical code with difficult access. It is not uncommon to be managing a critically ill patient who cannot be cannulated peripherally or centrally and the venous cutdown becomes the procedure of choice for resuscitation. All Emergency Physicians should be familiar with the peripheral venous cutdown in order to effectively manage resuscitations in the trauma or medical setting. This technique can only be successfully performed if one understands the anatomy and details of venous cannulation. Practicing the cutdown technique before its critical need will help one to perform optimally in the emergent setting.

ANATOMY AND PATHOPHYSIOLOGY

There are three critical areas for venous cutdowns (Figure 43-1). All Emergency Physicians should be knowledgeable of the anatomy of the saphenous vein at the ankle, the saphenous vein at the groin, and the basilic vein at the elbow. **The potential injury to the patient can be significant if one approaches this procedure without regard to the clinical anatomy.**

GREATER SAPHENOUS VEIN

The greater saphenous vein is the longest vein in the body. It is the ideal vein for a peripheral venous cutdown due to its anatomical regularity and superficiality (Figure 43-2). The saphenous vein begins at the medial dorsal venous arch of the foot. It passes upward and 1.5 to 2.5 cm directly anterior to the medial malleolus (Figure 43-2A). At the level of the medial malleolus, the saphenous vein lies just above the periosteum of the tibia.[2] It continues to ascend in the leg, along with the saphenous nerve, in the superficial fascia over the medial aspect of the leg. The vein passes posteromedially to the knee. Above the knee, it curves forward onto the anteromedial thigh. It passes over the falciform margin of the deep investing fascia to join the femoral vein approximately 4 cm below and 3 cm lateral to the pubic tubercle (Figure 43-2B).

The superficial and consistent position of the saphenous vein, in both adults and children, makes this the ideal location for a peripheral venous cutdown. It allows the Emergency Physician to perform the procedure while not interfering with concurrent resuscitative efforts at the neck, thorax, and abdomen.

The greater saphenous vein is easily identified at the ankle. It will be found, approximately, 2.5 cm anterior

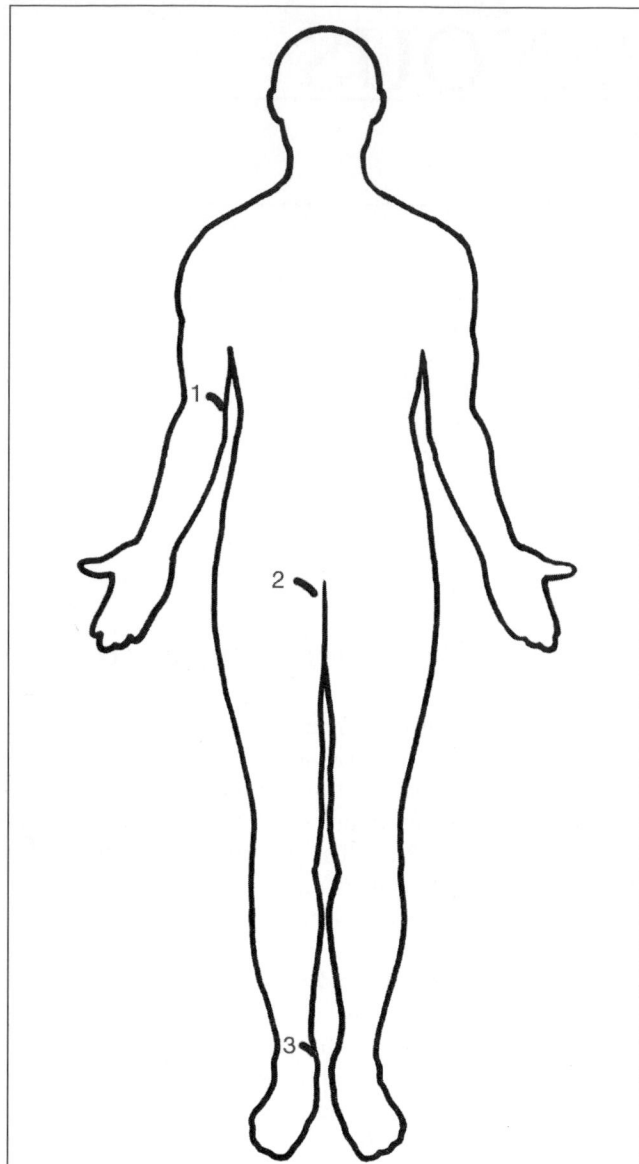

FIGURE 43-1 Common sites for peripheral venous cutdowns include the inner arm above the elbow (1), the inner thigh (2), and the inner ankle (3).

ment. This is approximately 2 cm below the approach for the placement of a femoral central venous line, level with where the scrotal or labial fold meets the thigh. The greater saphenous vein is also at its largest diameter in this same location. At the level of the scrotal or labial fold meeting the thigh, the greater saphenous vein is easily isolated from the surrounding subcutaneous tissue. If the deep investing fascia of the thigh muscles is visible, the dissection is too deep to find the greater saphenous vein.

BASILIC VEIN

The basilic vein is the site of choice for a peripheral venous cutdown in the upper extremity (Figure 43-3). It can be traced starting from the dorsal venous arch of the hand. It ascends on the posteromedial forearm to become anteromedial on the forearm. It continues to ascend to the midportion of the arm where it pierces the deep fascia. The basilic vein runs in the groove between the biceps and triceps muscles in the distal one-third of the arm. The vein can always be found in the groove between the biceps and triceps muscles. A peripheral venous cutdown should be performed in this location. The basilic vein is more consistently found 2 cm cephalad and 1 to 2 cm lateral to the medial epicondyle of the humerus on the volar (anterior) surface of the arm. The brachial artery and median nerve lie deep to the basilic vein in this location and are unlikely to be injured if the dissection remains superficial.

Simon et al recommend the approach to the basilic vein through the groove between the biceps and triceps muscles in the distal one-third of the arm.[5,8] They feel that locating the vein above and lateral to the medial epicondyle of the humerus will result in difficult cannulation secondary to the surrounding dense venous plexus. There is a significant risk of injury to the medial antebrachial cutaneous nerve and the deep brachial artery if one tries to find the basilic vein in the middle third or proximal third of the arm. Injury to the median antebrachial cutaneous nerve will result in sensory loss to the ulnar aspect of the forearm.

BRACHIAL VEIN

Brachial vein cutdowns should not be performed in the Emergency Department. The brachial vein is small in diameter. It is located relatively deep and would require significant time-consuming steps to locate it. The anatomical structures surrounding the brachial vein include major arteries and nerves that can easily become injured while isolating the vein. Patients in hypovolemic shock will often not have a brachial artery pulse. This can lead to confusion as to which vessel is the artery and which is the vein.[2] Inadvertent cannulation of the

and 2.5 cm superior to the medial malleolus. It may be palpable if the patient is not hypovolemic or obese. The saphenous nerve, a branch of the femoral nerve, travels with the greater saphenous vein. It supplies sensory innervation to the skin of the medial leg and foot as far as the first metatarsal. This nerve is often transected when isolating the greater saphenous vein at the ankle. Fortunately, this nerve is of minimal clinical significance.

The saphenous vein in the thigh travels on the anteromedial surface and enters the fossa ovalis to join the femoral vein (Figure 43-2B). The femoral vein is at its largest diameter 3 to 4 cm distal to the inguinal liga-

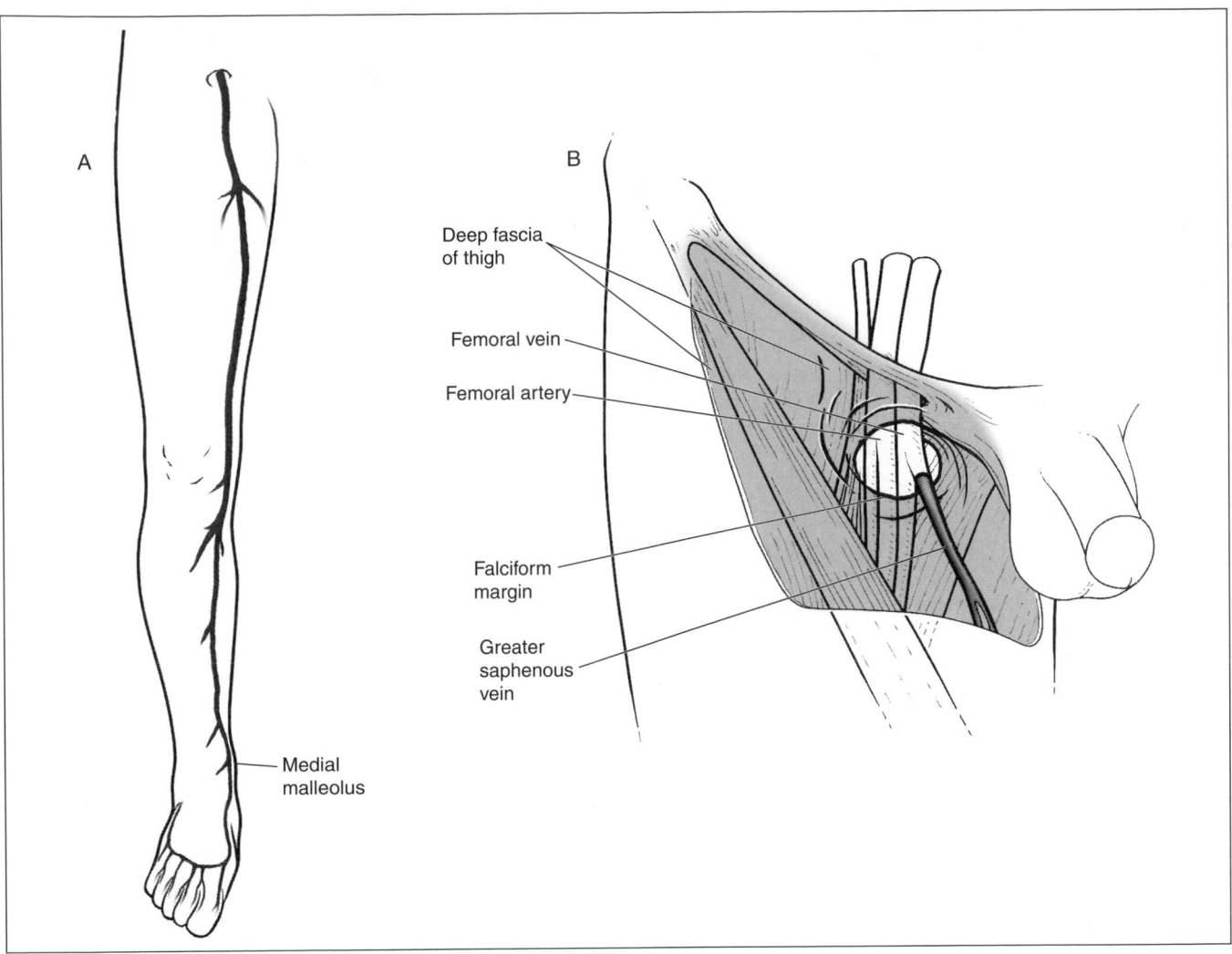

FIGURE 43-2 Anatomy of the greater saphenous vein. *A.* The subcutaneous course of the vein in the lower extremity. *B.* Detail of the greater saphenous vein at the groin.

brachial artery can result in a brachial artery thrombosis and upper extremity ischemia.

INDICATIONS

The primary indication for a peripheral venous cutdown is the need for venous access in a patient with no peripheral access and in whom central access is not obtainable or contraindicated. This is the ideal procedure for the intravenous drug user with no peripheral veins and scarred central access sites, the burn patient with peripheral venous collapse and scarring, the patient in cardiorespiratory arrest, or the hypovolemic trauma patient that requires definitive and life-saving volume resuscitation.[3] Hypovolemic shock is well treated with peripheral venous cutdowns because a unit of blood can be infused in less than three minutes with intravenous extension tubing inserted directly into the vein.[4]

This is also an excellent technique for emergent pediatric vascular access. Direct visualization of the vein will aid in cannulation of a vessel that may be collapsed secondary to hemorrhage, hypovolemia, and/or shock. This technique should only be used after other access attempts (interosseous access, central venous access, peripheral venous access—including scalp veins) have failed.[4]

CONTRAINDICATIONS

The only contraindication to a peripheral venous cutdown is if a vascular injury or long bone fracture is present proximally in the extremity. Relative contraindications include infection overlying the cutdown site, bleeding disorders, or severely distorted anatomy in the area of the cutdown or the limb.

EQUIPMENT

Local anesthetic solution
10 mL syringe
22 gauge needle
#10 scalpel blade
#11 scalpel blade
#3 scalpel handle
Curved Kelley hemostat
Small mosquito hemostat
Vein pick
Fine tooth forceps
Iris scissors
Sharp tissue-cutting scissors
Povidone iodine solution
Sterile drapes
Towel clips
Sterile polyethylene intravenous tubing
Sterile intravenous extension tubing
Central line kit (for Seldinger method)
Catheter-over-the-needle, 16 or 18 gauge
Sterile 4×4 sponges
5 mL syringe
18 gauge needles
Self-retaining skin retractors
Small rake, two
Needle driver
Silk suture, 3–0 and 4–0
Injectable sterile saline
Intravenous tubing and solution
Dressing
Antibiotic ointment

PATIENT PREPARATION

The patient is usually in extremis and positioned supine if a peripheral venous cutdown is to be performed. They may also be in the Trendelenburg position. While this position is not optimal for performing a peripheral venous cutdown, it may be the best position for the patient. The limb selected for the peripheral venous cutdown should be secured to the bed with a restraint, tape, or by an assistant. **Although this is an emergent procedure, time should be taken to perform it in as sterile a manner as possible.** Identify the landmarks for the procedure. Clean the skin of any dirt and debris. If the patient is awake and aware of the surroundings, the area of the cutdown should be anesthetized. Infiltrate local anesthetic solution into the subcutaneous tissue where the incision will be made. Prepare the skin with povidone iodine solution and allow it to dry. Apply sterile drapes to isolate a surgical field.

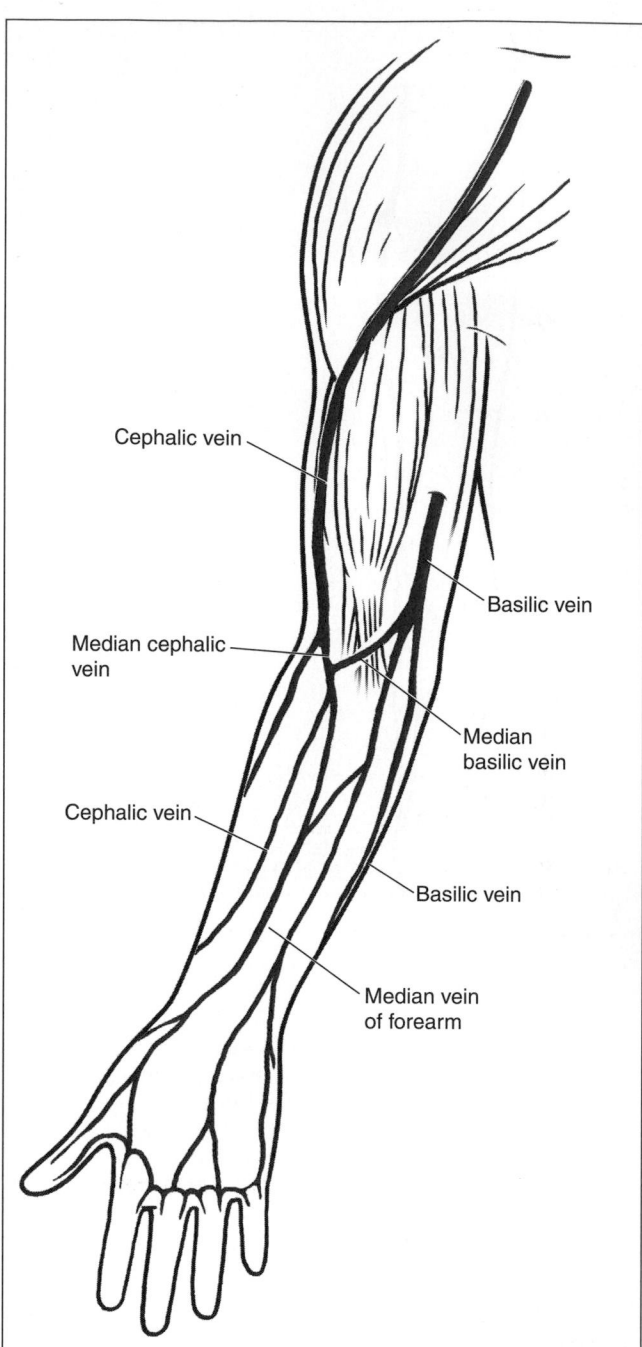

FIGURE 43-3 The superficial veins of the upper extremity.

TECHNIQUES TO ISOLATE THE VEINS

The technique of cannulation is the same regardless of the vein chosen. The methods to isolate the saphenous vein and the basilic vein will be discussed in this section. A discussion of three different techniques to cannulate the isolated vein will be presented in the following section.

GREATER SAPHENOUS VEIN ISOLATION AT THE ANKLE

The saphenous vein is easily found and isolated at the ankle (Figure 43-4). Extend and externally rotate the lower extremity. Identify the medial malleolus of the tibia. Find the spot 2.5 cm anterior and 2.5 cm superior to the medial malleolus. The greater saphenous vein will be found at this site. Alternatively, place the index and middle fingers at the level of the malleolus (Figure 43-4*A*). The vein will be found two finger breadths above and two finger breadths in front of the medial malleolus. The vein may be palpable if the patient is not hypovolemic or obese.

Stretch the skin taught over the distal tibia with the nondominant hand (Figure 43-4*B*). Note the position of the hands in the illustration. **The nondominant hand is placed with the fingertips pointing toward the physician.** This will prevent inadvertent injury while making the skin incision. Transversely incise the skin overlying the great saphenous vein using a #10 scalpel blade, from the anterior tibial border to the posterior tibial border (Figure 43-4*B*). **This incision should be superficial to only expose the subcutaneous tissue.** An incision into the subcutaneous tissue may transect the vein causing significant bleeding, difficulty visualizing the surgical field, and difficulty finding the ends of the vein that can retract proximally and distally. Apply tension to the skin on either side of the incision to expose the underlying structures. This can be accomplished with the nondominant hand, a self-retaining retractor, or skin rakes held by an assistant.

Isolate the greater saphenous vein.[5] Grasp and hold a curved hemostat (Kelly clamp) with the tip facing downward. Insert the hemostat along the posterior border of the tibia and scrape the tip along the tibia. Advance the hemostat along the tibia while scraping the periosteum until the tip reaches the anterior border of the tibia (Figure 43-4*C*). If done properly, all of the tissue between the skin and the tibia will be above the hemostat. Rotate the hemostat 180 degrees (Figure 43-4*C*). The tip of the hemostat will be facing upward (Figure 43-4*D*). Widely open the arms of the hemostat (Figure 43-4*D*). This will open the jaws of the hemostat and separate the saphenous vein from the saphenous nerve and fibrous strands of connective tissue. The saphenous vein should be visible between the jaws of the hemostat. If there is difficulty identifying the vein, squeeze the foot to backfill the vein with blood. Insert a straight hemostat (Kelly clamp) between the jaws of the curved hemostat and below the greater saphenous vein (Figure 43-4*E*). Remove the curved hemostat to leave the straight hemostat elevating the greater saphenous vein (Figure 43-4*F*). This straight hemostat will be useful as a "cutting board" to later transect the vein by allowing more manual control of the vein.

An alternative technique to isolate the vein is used by some physicians. **This technique is not recommended by the editors but is briefly described for the sake of completeness.** Make the transverse skin incision. Place the jaws of a curved hemostat parallel to the greater saphenous vein. Open the arms of the hemostat to allow the jaws to dissect through the subcutaneous tissue. Continue placing the hemostat and opening the jaws until the vein is isolated. This technique is harder to perform because the vein is less likely to be identified given the white background of the periosteum.[1,4,7] Additionally, this technique takes significantly longer to find and isolate the vein.

GREATER SAPHENOUS VEIN ISOLATION AT THE GROIN

The groin vasculature offers the potential for massive infusion of blood or fluids in a matter of minutes. These vessels are closer to the central circulation and large enough to easily accommodate intravenous tubing, cut off at a 45 degree angle, as a catheter. The greater saphenous vein is superficial at the groin and lies in a meshwork of subcutaneous tissue. It is superficial to the femoral artery and vein. The saphenous vein travels on the anteromedial surface of the thigh and enters the fossa ovalis to join the femoral vein (Figure 43-2*B*). The greater saphenous vein is at its largest diameter 3 to 4 cm distal to the inguinal ligament. This is approximately 2 cm below the site for placement of a femoral central venous line and level with where the scrotal or labial fold meets the thigh.

Identify the location where the scrotal or labial fold meets the thigh (Figure 43-5). Identify the lateral edge of the mons pubis. Identify the point where a vertical line from the lateral edge of the mons pubis meets a horizontal line from the scrotal/labial fold. Make a transverse, medial to lateral, incision with a #10 scalpel blade on the patient's thigh starting where the scrotal or labial fold meets the thigh. Extend the incision laterally until it meets the vertical line from the lateral edge of the mons pubis.

Dissect the subcutaneous tissue to locate the greater saphenous vein. Place the jaws of a curved hemostat parallel to the greater saphenous vein. Open the arms of the hemostat to allow the jaws to dissect through the subcutaneous tissue. Continue placing the hemostat and opening the jaws until the vein is isolated. **The dissection is too deep if the deep investing fascia or the muscle bellies of the thigh muscles are encountered.** Stop, reidentify the landmarks, and adjust the skin incision as necessary.

Alternatively, the subcutaneous tissues can be bluntly dissected using 4×4 gauze squares. Grasp 2 or 3 gauze squares in each hand. Put the fingertips of both hands, covered with gauze, in the center of the incision. Move

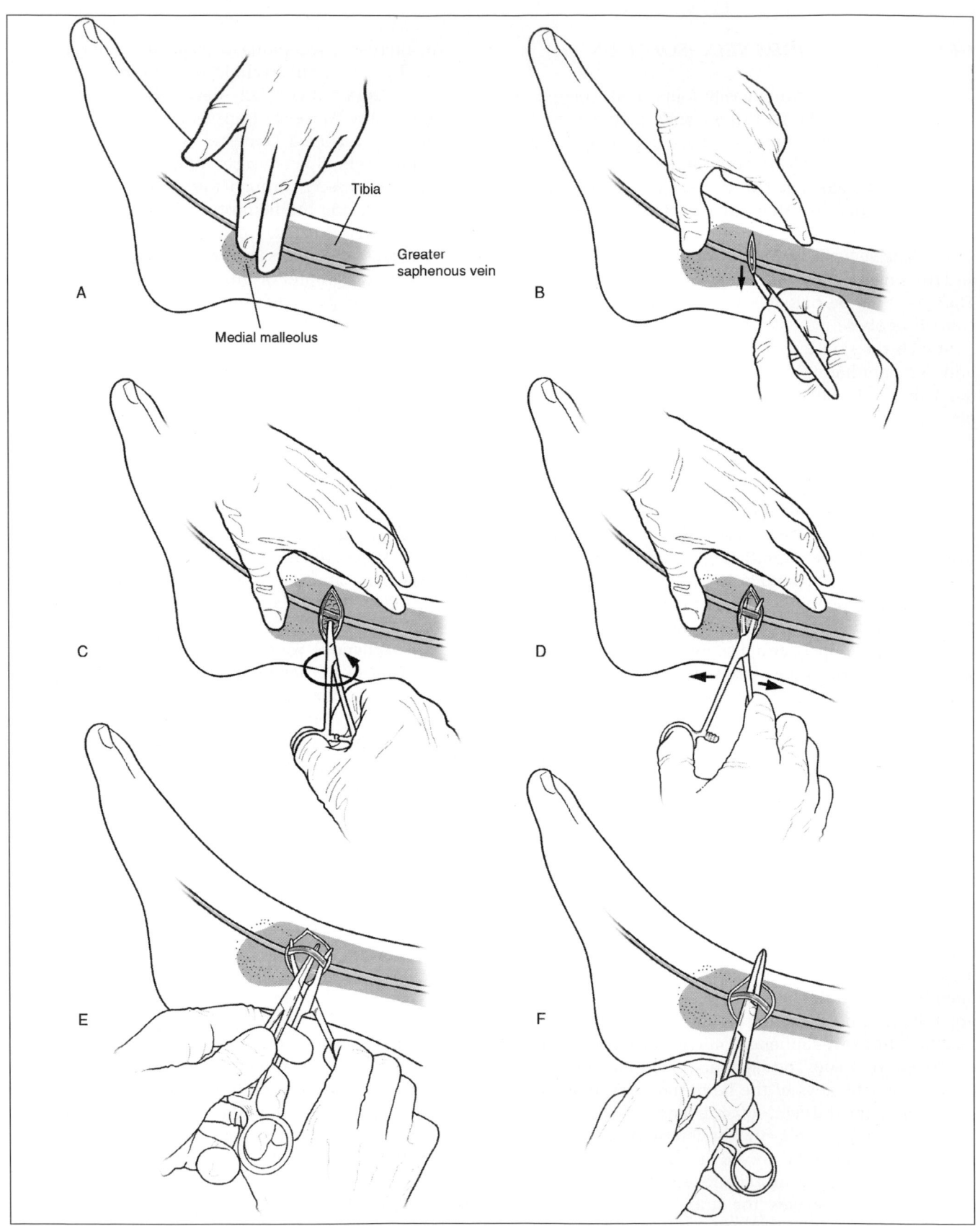

FIGURE 43-4 Isolation of the greater saphenous vein at the ankle. *A.* Identifying the vein. *B.* A transverse skin incision is made from the anterior to the posterior border of the medial tibia. *C.* A curved hemostat is scraped along the tibia then rotated 180 degrees (*curved arrow*). *D.* The hemostat is spread to separate the tissues. *E.* A straight hemostat is inserted between the jaws of the curved hemostat to elevate the vein. *F.* The curved hemostat has been removed.

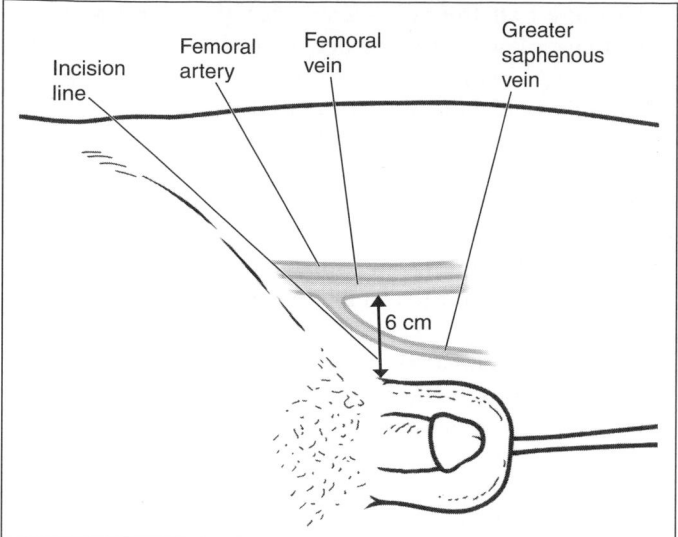

FIGURE 43-5 Isolation of the greater saphenous vein at the groin. The skin incision should begin where the scrotal or labial fold meets the thigh. Extend the incision laterally until it meets a vertical line from the lateral edge of the mons pubis.

the hands in opposite directions, cephalad and caudad, while scraping the subcutaneous tissue with the gauze. Reapply the hands in the incision and repeat the motion until the greater saphenous vein is exposed. This technique applies pressure parallel to the greater saphenous vein and will not injure the vein.

BASILIC VEIN ISOLATION AT THE ELBOW

The basilic vein may be used for a peripheral venous cutdown. This is often performed when the greater saphenous vein cannot be accessed due to lower extremity amputation, deformity, injury, or trauma. This site is not ideal as it may interfere with resuscitative efforts while the basilic vein is being exposed. The basilic vein is consistently found 2 cm cephalad and 1 to 2 cm lateral to the medial epicondyle of the humerus on the volar (anterior) surface of the arm. It may also be found in the groove between the biceps and triceps muscles. There is controversy in the literature as to where the incision for the basilic vein cutdown should be performed. The simple answer is that if one fails in isolating the vein in one location, make an incision in the second location and isolate the vein.

Position the patient to allow exposure of the basilic vein. Abduct the patient's arm 90 degrees with the elbow flexed 90 degrees and the palm facing upward (Figure 43-6). This positioning is required to access the basilic vein by either location.

Identify the point 2 cm cephalad and 2 cm lateral from the medial epicondyle of the humerus. This is the location of the basilic vein. Make a 4 to 6 cm transverse incision with a #10 scalpel blade centered around the reference point. The incision should only cut through the epidermis. Bluntly dissect the subcutaneous tissue with a curved hemostat or 4×4 gauze squares, as described previously, to locate the basilic vein. **The dissection is**

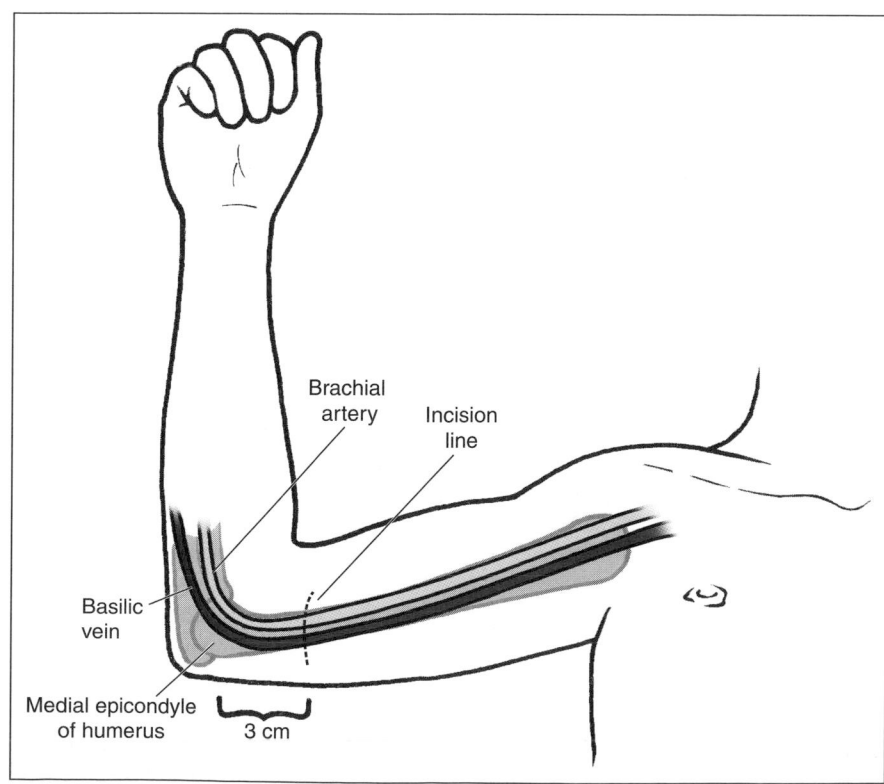

FIGURE 43-6 Isolation of the basilic vein.

too deep if the brachial artery, median nerve, or muscle fibers are encountered. Stop, reidentify the landmarks, and adjust the skin incision as necessary.

Alternatively, the basilic vein can be isolated in the middle of the distal third of the arm. Palpate the groove between the biceps and triceps muscles. This is the location of the basilic vein. Make a 4 to 6 cm horizontal incision centered about the groove. Bluntly dissect with a curved hemostat until the vein is located. The basilic vein is superficial to the muscle fascia and the brachial artery.

TECHNIQUES FOR CANNULATION OF THE VEIN

There are a number of techniques to cannulate a vein after it has been isolated. Either of the following techniques can be used to cannulate the greater saphenous vein or basilic vein. It is important to realize that this may be a lifesaving procedure in an emergent setting, and the rapid and definitive cannulation of the vessel is the primary goal and not the technique chosen.

SURGICAL TECHNIQUE USING INTRAVENOUS TUBING

Isolate the chosen vein as described previously. Place a straight hemostat (Kelly clamp) under the midportion of the vein (Figure 43-7A). Slightly elevate the hemostat. Pass a silk suture under the vein at its proximal end and a second silk suture at its distal end (Figure 43-7B). Grasp the silk sutures with a hemostat to maintain the position of the tie and to allow for manipulation of the vein. Tie the distal suture to occlude inflow of blood from distal veins (Figure 43-7C). Do not cut either of these two sutures. The proximal suture will be left untied at this time to allow for control and manipulation of the vein.

Have an assistant prepare the catheter. Attach sterile intravenous polyethylene tubing to a bag of sterile saline. Cut the angiocatheter attachment hub off the end of the tubing at a 45 degree angle. Some authors suggest using a feeding tube instead of intravenous tubing.[4] This is not recommended. Intravenous tubing is ubiquitously available. With a feeding tube, the rounded tip may be more difficult to advance into the vein. The only advantage to using a feeding tube is that the rounded tip has less chance of puncturing the posterior wall of the vein.

Incise the vein. With the nondominant hand, grasp the hemostat holding the proximal suture. Raise the hemostat to flatten the vein and prevent back bleeding. Make an incision through half of the vein with the tip of a #11 scalpel blade (Figure 43-7D). **Do not cut the entire vein as this will cause significant bleeding and loss of the proximal end. If the incision is too large, greater** than one-half the vein's diameter, the vessel may be torn completely and retract from the surgical field.[4] The straight hemostat below the vein will act as a cutting board and prevent injury to underlying structures from the scalpel blade. As an alternative, the jaws of the straight hemostat can be opened and the vein cut with an iris scissors (Figure 43-7E).

Insert the intravenous tubing into the vein. Gently relax the tension on the proximal suture to allow the vein to open. Advance the intravenous tubing 2 to 3 cm into the vein (Figure 43-7F). Often times, there is considerable difficulty advancing the catheter. **Do not force the catheter through the vein as it is very delicate.** Troubleshoot by removing the catheter and make sure that the lumen of the vein has been cannulated. This is sometimes difficult to accomplish. If so, have an assistant control the proximal suture. Using a mosquito hemostat, grasp the cut edge of the vein and lift upward to expose the vein's lumen and insert the intravenous tubing (Figure 43-7G). For small veins, a mosquito hemostat may be too large to grasp the cut edge of the vein. Insert a vein pick or an 18 gauge needle with the tip bent into a 90 degree angle into the lumen of the vein (Figure 43-7H). Lift upward to expose the vein's lumen and insert the intravenous tubing.

After inserting the intravenous tubing, palpate the posterior aspect of the vein for penetration of the catheter. **The catheter must be removed if it penetrates through the posterior wall of the vein.** Release the proximal suture and allow the intravenous fluid to flow into the vein if the tubing has not penetrated the posterior wall of the vein. Tie the proximal suture to secure the intravenous tubing within the vein if the fluid flow is unobstructed and the fluid is not extravasating into the surrounding tissues (Figure 43-7I). **Do not tie the suture too tight to occlude the tubing.** If the tubing is within the lumen of the vein and the fluid is not flowing, the tubing may be against a venous valve. Gently advance the catheter 2 to 3 mm or withdraw it 2 to 3 mm and observe the fluid for flow. It is not necessary to close the skin incision at this time. Place saline moistened gauze over the incision site. Wrap a sterile dressing (Kerlix) around the extremity and the skin incision site.

If the patient survives the episode for which a venous cutdown was performed, the skin incision must be closed. If the intravenous tubing was inserted as above, the skin incision will be sutured closed and the tubing will exit the incision. This is not optimal, according to some physicians, as it may allow access of bacteria through the wound and into the underlying vein. An alternative method is available (Figure 43-8). After exposing the vein, grasp and elevate the distal skin edge with a hemostat. Make a stab incision with a #11 scalpel blade approximately 1 cm distal to the previously made skin incision (Figure 43-8A). Use caution not to cut the underlying

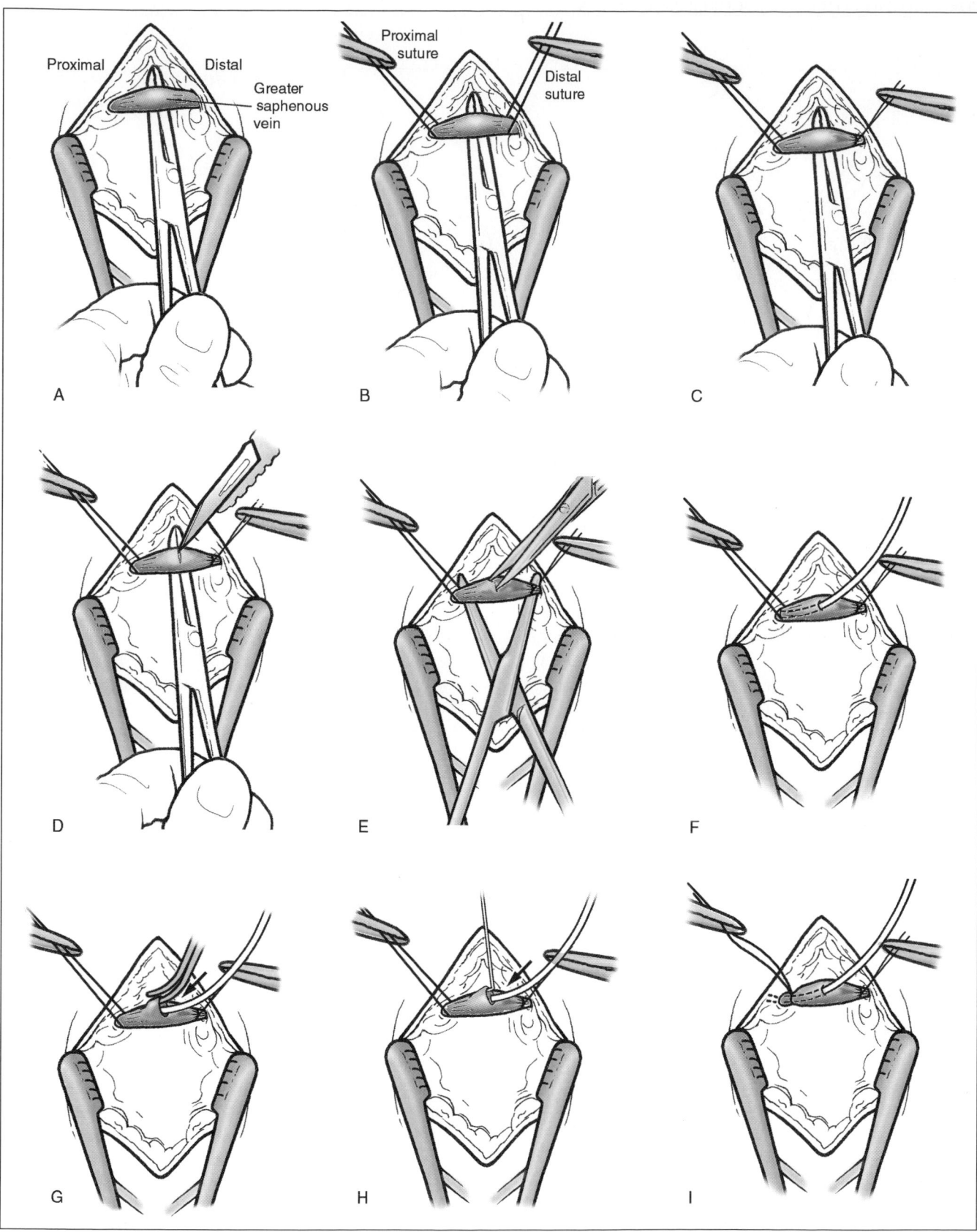

FIGURE 43-7 Venous cannulation using intravenous tubing. *A.* The vein has been isolated. *B.* A silk suture has been placed proximally and distally around the vein. *C.* The distal suture is tied. *D.* An incision is made through half of the vein with a #11 scalpel blade. *E.* Alternatively, the hemostat is opened and an iris scissors is used to cut half of the vein. *F.* The catheter is inserted into the vein and advanced. *G.* A mosquito hemostat can be used to grasp the vein and hold it open while the tubing is inserted. *H.* For small veins, a vein pick or 18 gauge needle with the tip bent can be used to hold open the vein. *I.* The proximal suture is tied to secure the tubing.

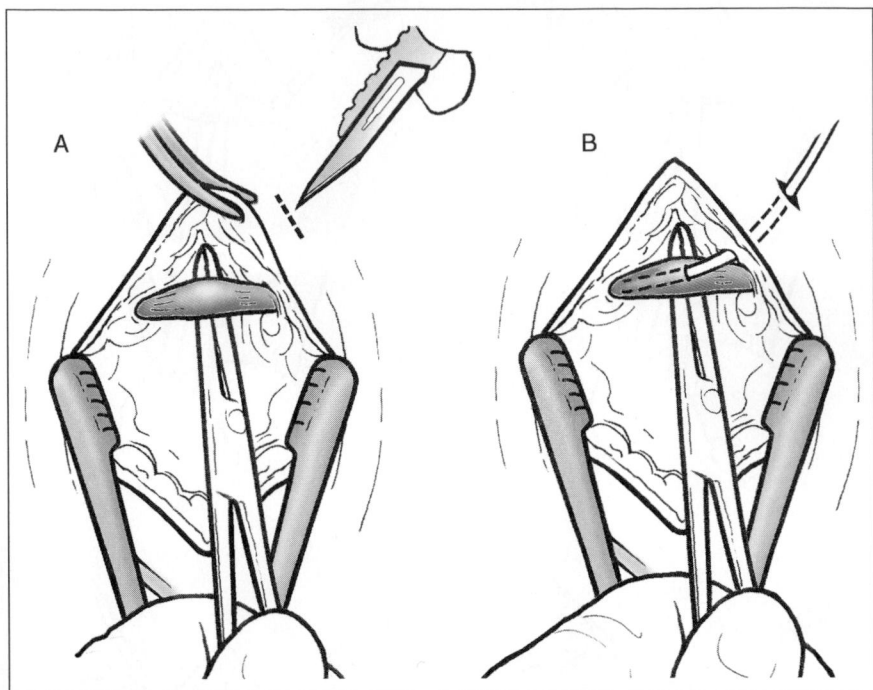

FIGURE 43-8 Alternative technique of venous cannulation with intravenous tubing. *A.* The distal skin edge is elevated. A #11 scalpel blade is used to make a stab incision in the skin and subcutaneous tissues. *B.* The tubing is fed through the stab incision and into the vein.

vein. Insert the intravenous tubing through the stab incision and pull it through the skin incision. Incise the vein and insert the tubing as described previously. This allows the tubing to be tunneled through the subcutaneous tissue before cannulating the vein (Figure 43-8*B*).

SELDINGER TECHNIQUE

Another technique of venous cannulation uses the Seldinger method.[6,7] All of the required equipment can be found in a prepackaged central venous line access kit. This includes the guidewire, introducer sheath, dilator, and the venous catheter. A large caliber line, such as an 8 or 9 French introducer sheath, is recommended. This technique may save 1 to 2 minutes on cannulation time by eliminating the ligature and tie off steps.

Isolate the chosen vein as described previously. Place a straight hemostat (Kelly clamp) under the midportion of the vein and open the jaws (Figure 43-9*A*). This technique will insert the catheter as if cannulating a central vein. Refer to Chapter 38 for complete details. Insert the catheter-over-the-needle into the vein (Figure 43-9*A*). Stop advancing the unit when a flash of blood is seen in the needle hub. Advance the catheter into the vein while removing the straight clamp. Remove the needle. Insert the guidewire through the catheter. Remove the catheter while the guidewire remains in the vein. Place the dilator through the introducer sheath. Insert the tip of the guidewire into the dilator. Feed the guidewire through the dilator until it comes out the proximal end (Figure 43-9*B*). Advance the dilator and introducer sheath into

the vein with a twisting motion while holding the tip of the guidewire (Figure 43-9*C*). Continue to advance the unit until the hub of the introducer sheath is just above the vein. Remove the guidewire and dilator as a unit (Figure 43-9*D*). Attach intravenous tubing to the introducer sheath and begin instilling fluids. It is not necessary to close the skin incision at this time. Place saline-moistened gauze over the incision site. Wrap a sterile dressing (Kerlix) around the extremity and the skin incision site.

MODIFIED SELDINGER TECHNIQUE

An alternative and quicker method can be used to insert the introducer sheath into the vein (Figure 43-10). Isolate the chosen vein as described previously. Place a straight hemostat (Kelly clamp) under the midportion of the vein and open the jaws (Figure 43-10*A*). Assemble the unit by placing the dilator through the sheath and insert the guidewire through the dilator (Figure 43-10*B*). The guidewire should protrude 3 to 4 mm beyond the tip of the dilator. Make an incision in the lateral half of the vein (Figure 43-10*C*). While holding the proximal guidewire and catheter hub, insert the distal guidewire into the vein. Continue to insert the entire unit with a twisting motion into the vein (Figure 43-10*D*). Continue to advance the unit until the hub of the introducer sheath is just above the vein. Remove the guidewire and dilator as a unit (Figure 43-10*E*). Attach intravenous tubing to the introducer sheath and begin instilling fluids.

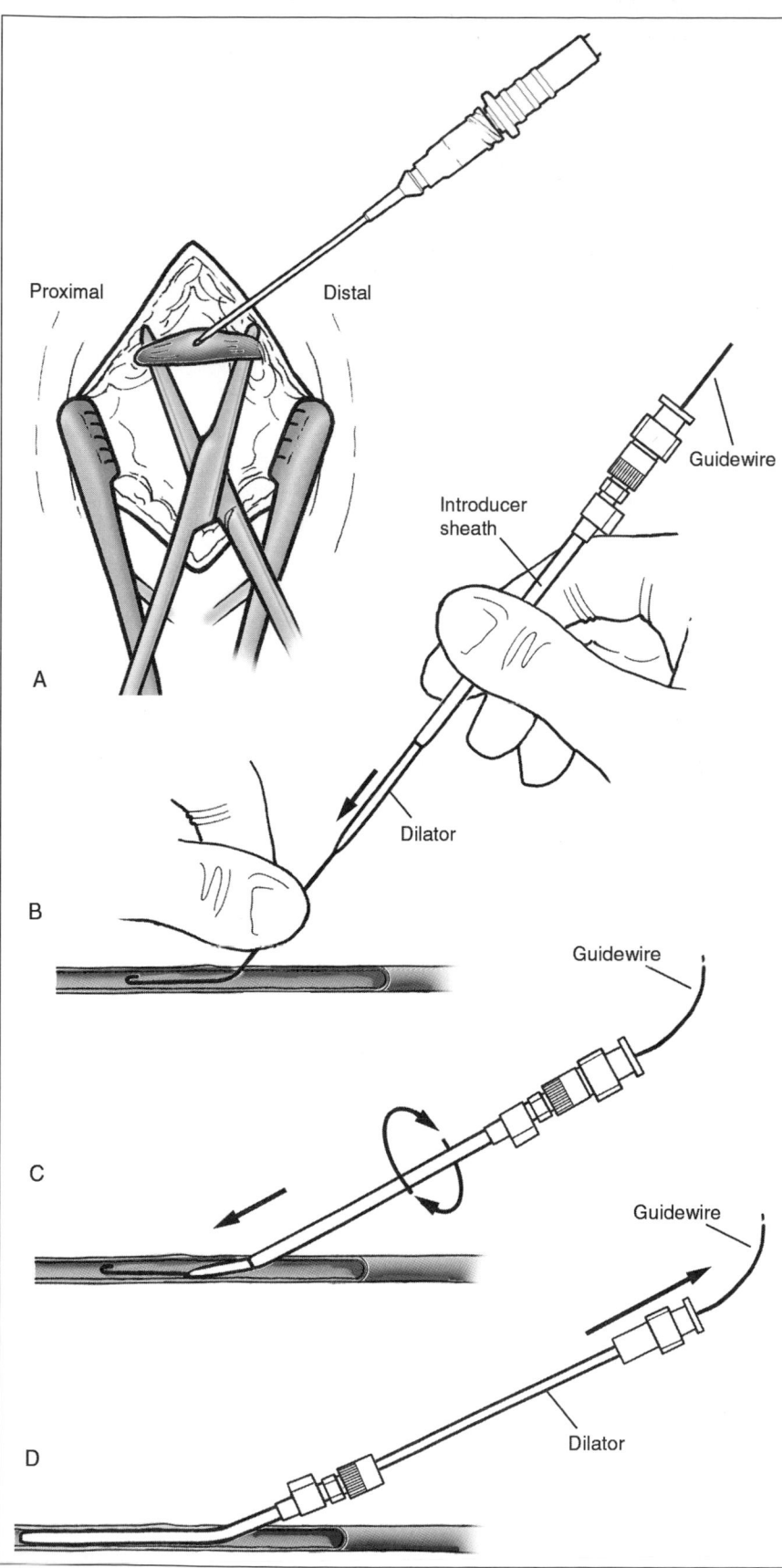

Proximal

Distal

Guidewire

Introducer
sheath

Dilator

A

B

Guidewire

C

Guidewire

D

Dilator

FIGURE 43-9 The Seldinger technique
of venous cannulation. *A.* The vein has
been isolated. The catheter-over-the-
needle is inserted into the vein. *B.* A
guidewire has been placed into the vein.
The dilator and sheath are fed over the
guidewire. *C.* The dilator and sheath are
advanced into the vein with a twisting
motion. *D.* The guidewire and dilator are
removed as a unit.

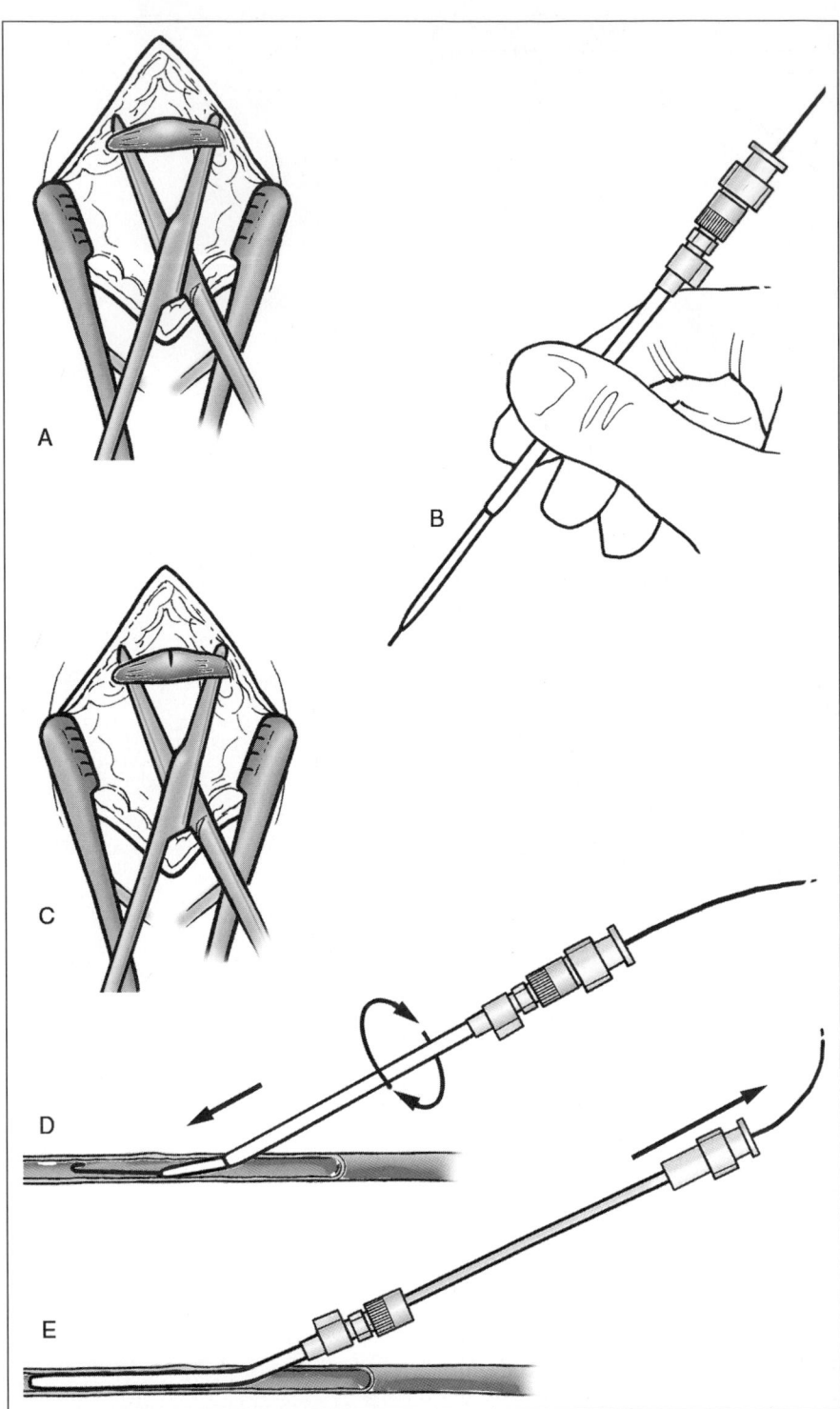

FIGURE 43-10 A modified Seldinger technique of venous cannulation. *A.* The vein has been isolated. *B.* The dilator, guidewire, and sheath are assembled as a unit. *C.* An incision has been made in the vein. *D.* The unit is inserted into the vein, guidewire first. A twisting motion will aid in its insertion. *E.* The guidewire and dilator are removed as a unit.

INTRAVENOUS CATHETER TECHNIQUE

This final technique involves the insertion of a standard, 16 to 18 gauge, intravenous catheter-over-the-needle into the vein (Figure 43-11). This method is very quick, provides a more secure cannulation, and potentially decreases the chance of infection.

Isolate the chosen vein as described previously. Place a straight hemostat (Kelly clamp) under the midportion of the vein and open the jaws (Figure 43-11*A*). This technique will insert the catheter as if cannulating a peripheral vein. Refer to Chapters 36 and 37 for complete details. Insert the catheter-over-the-needle into the vein

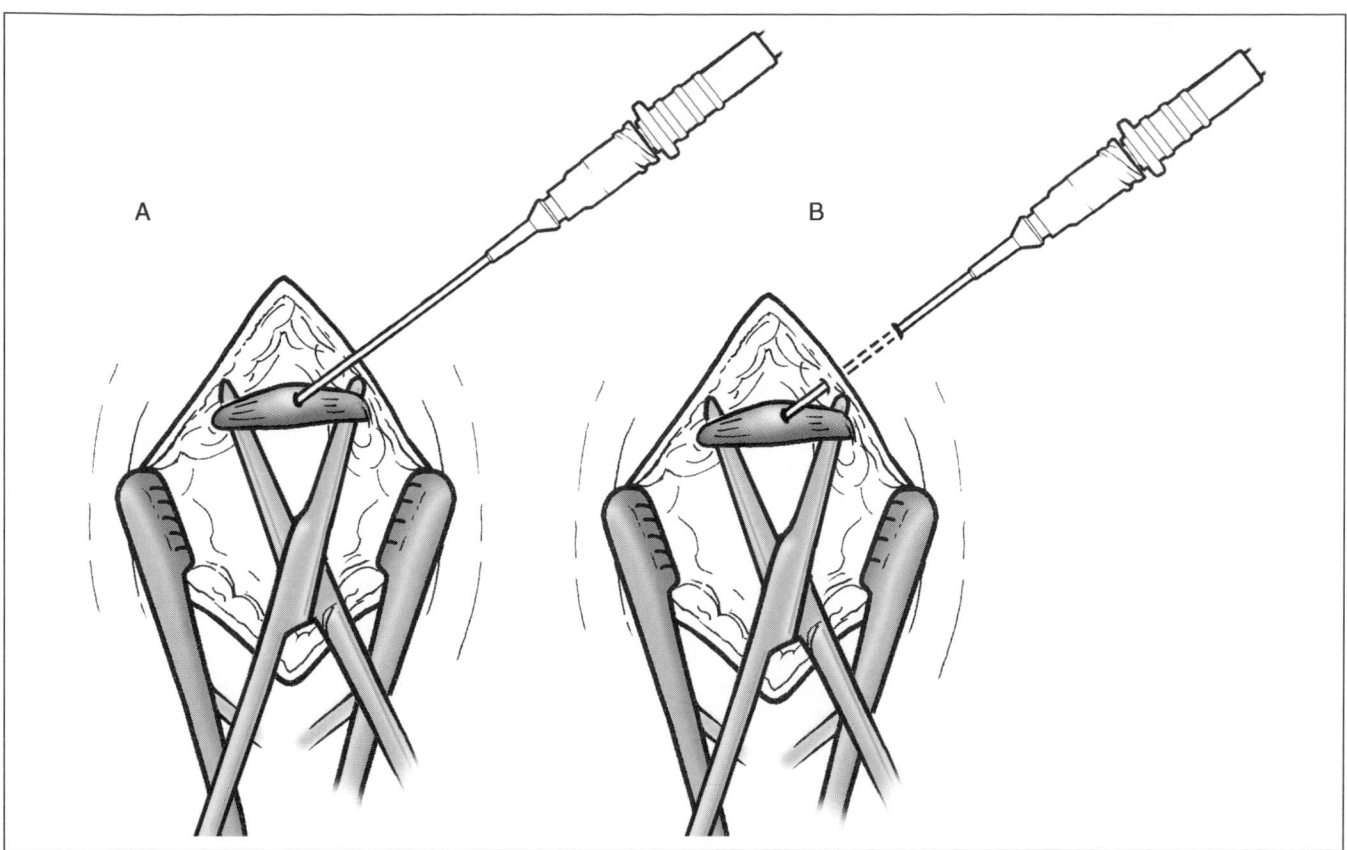

FIGURE 43-11 Intravenous catheter technique of venous cannulation. *A.* A catheter-over-the-needle is inserted into the vein. *B.* A catheter-over-the-needle is inserted through the skin and into the vein.

under direct visualization (Figure 43-11*A*). Stop advancing the unit when a flash of blood is seen in the needle hub. Advance the catheter into the vein while removing the straight clamp. Advance the catheter until the hub is just above the vein. Remove the needle. Attach intravenous tubing to the catheter hub and begin instilling fluids. Tie the proximal suture to secure the catheter within the vein. It is not necessary to close the skin incision at this time. Place saline-moistened gauze over the incision site. Wrap a sterile dressing (Kerlix) around the extremity and the skin incision site.

Alternatively, insert the catheter-over-the-needle through the skin, 1 cm distal to the distal skin edge, until the tip is visualized in the incision (Figure 43-11*B*). Insert the catheter-over-the-needle into the vein under direct visualization. Stop advancing the unit when a flash of blood is seen in the needle hub. Advance the catheter into the vein while removing the straight clamp. Advance the catheter until the hub is against the skin. Remove the needle. Attach intravenous tubing to the catheter hub and begin instilling fluids. The advantage of this method is that the catheter goes through the skin, which will stabilize the catheter and prevent it from becoming dislodged.

AFTERCARE

Suture the wound closed with simple interrupted 4–0 nylon sutures (Figure 43-12). Place a suture through the skin, wrap it around the catheter and tie it to secure the catheter to the skin. Apply antibacterial ointment to the incision, the sutures, and the site where the catheter exits the skin. Secure the intravenous tubing (Figure 43-13). The catheter can be looped around the toe, for a cutdown at the ankle, and secured with gauze wrap or an elastic wrap (Figure 43-13*A*). The catheter can be secured by taping it to the skin (Figure 43-13*B*). The limb can be immobilized on a board, after the catheter is secured at the ankle or elbow, for added security from inadvertent dislodgement of the catheter (Figure 43-13*C*).

COMPLICATIONS

The complications of a peripheral venous cutdown include arterial injury, nerve injury, phlebitis, thromboembolism, wound dehiscence, and wound infection. The incidence of complications ranges from 2 to 15 percent.[9,10] The difficulty in reporting complications is that

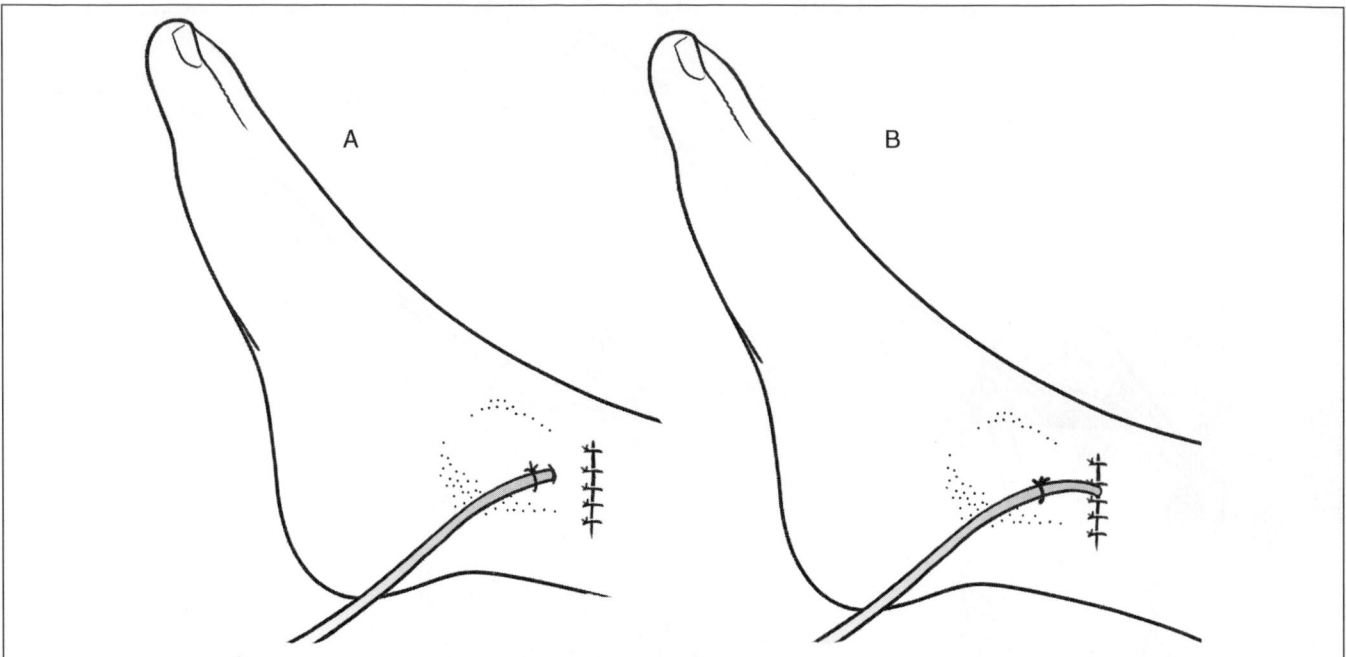

FIGURE 43-12 The skin incision is closed with interrupted 4–0 nylon sutures. The catheter exits a separate skin incision (*A*) or the original skin incision (*B*) and is secured with a suture.

there is a high mortality rate in patients undergoing this procedure due to the primary problem (e.g., hypovolemia, sepsis, shock, trauma, etc.).

PHLEBITIS

It is generally agreed that phlebitis occurs more commonly in the lower extremity than the upper extremity. However, there is little data to support this. Phlebitis usually results from prolonged catheterization. It may be seen within hours of catheter placement and as long as 18 days after the removal of the catheter.[10] In 1960, Bogen looked at 234 ankle cutdowns and found a 4 percent phlebitis rate.[11] He felt this was secondary to infection. The strength of the correlation was attributed to a previous nonrelated study that found *Staphylococcus aureus* on almost all catheter tips in patients with phlebitis as opposed to catheter tips in patients without phlebitis. Interestingly, these cases of phlebitis all resolved without the use of antibiotics. Moran et al cultured 89 cutdown sites and observed that the pathogenic species causing infection were *S. aureus*, *Enterococcus*, and *Proteus*.[10] These organisms were cultured more frequently in patients that had cutdowns that were left in place for longer periods of time. Moran et al did not find a correlation between infection and phlebitis and postulated that phlebitis occurred because of irritation of the vein wall by the catheter.[10] Regardless of the rates and species, it is clear from all of these studies that **early removal of the intravenous catheter within 12 hours of placement will significantly decrease the incidence of phlebitis.**

INFECTION

Moran et al did not find that prophylactic antibiotics reduced infection rates.[10] They found that daily topical antibiotic ointment, in particular Neosporin™, reduced positive local wound cultures from a rate of 78 to 18 percent. In 1968, Collins et al studied polyethylene catheters and found a 2 percent bacteremia rate and a 1 percent death rate from *Pseudomonas* species in debilitated patients.[12] Rhee et al in 1988 found only one case of cellulitis in their study of 78 patients.[9] Regardless of the rates and species, it is clear from all of these studies that **early removal of the intravenous catheter within 12 hours of placement will significantly decrease the incidence of infection and subsequent complications.** Obviously, sterile technique is also encouraged with this procedure in order to minimize complications related to infection.

ASSOCIATED INJURIES

Injury to adjacent arteries, nerves, and veins can be avoided by a detailed understanding of the local anatomy and careful procedural technique. Aggressive and forceful dissection without an understanding of the anatomy or the procedure will increase the incidence of complications. Injury to adjacent cutaneous nerves is unavoidable and inconsequential. Venous spasm, which

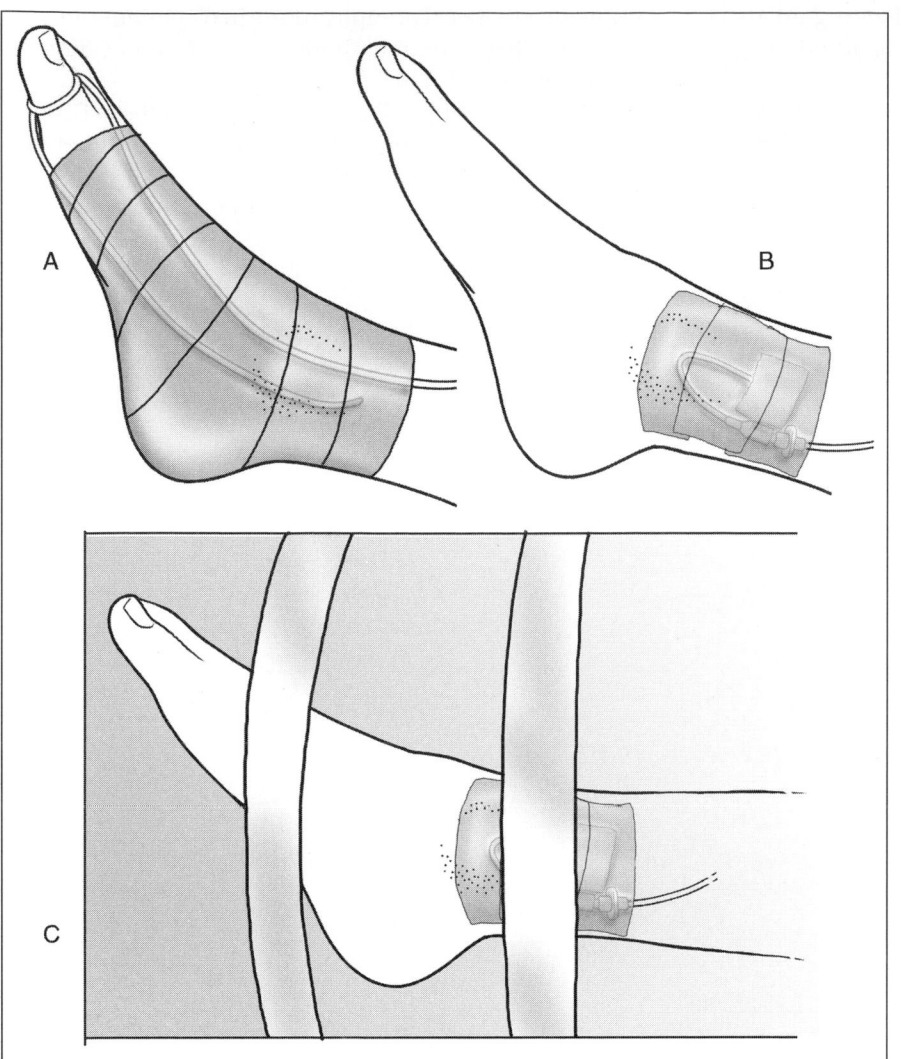

FIGURE 43-13 Securing the intravenous catheter. *A.* The catheter is looped around the great toe, for an ankle cutdown, and secured with gauze or elastic wrap. *B.* The catheter is secured with tape. *C.* The ankle or elbow can be secured to a board for additional security.

causes nonuniform acceptance of the intravenous extension tubing, may also occur.[13]

SUMMARY

The peripheral venous cutdown is an excellent technique for rapid fluid or blood product infusion in the emergent setting. This is usually performed when other methods of venous access are unavailable or have failed. It is a relatively simple procedure. If learned properly, it can be lifesaving in the critically ill and/or injured patient. It is imperative to understand the relevant local anatomy and identify the clinical landmarks before this procedure is performed. Strict adherence to sterile technique and the early removal of the catheter will decrease the rate of infection and complications.

REFERENCES

1. Keeley JL: Intravenous injections and infusions. *Am J Surg* 1940; 50:485–490.
2. Knopp R: Venous cutdowns in the emergency department. *JACEP* 1978; 7(12):439–443.
3. Snell RS: *Clincial Anatomy for Medical Students,* 4th ed. Boston: Little, Brown, 1992.
4. Dronen SC, Lanter P: Venous cutdown, in Roberts JR, Hedges JR (eds): *Clinical Procedures in Emergency Medicine,* 3rd ed. Philadelphia: Saunders, 1998:341–351.
5. Simon RR, Hoffman JR, Smith M: Modified new approaches for rapid intravenous access. *Ann Emerg Med* 1987; 16(1):44–48.
6. Klofas E: A quicker saphenous vein cutdown and a better way to teach it. *J Trauma* 1997; 43(6):985–987.

7. Shockley LW, Butzier DJ: A modified wire-guided technique for venous cutdown access. *Ann Emerg Med* 1990; 19(4):393–395.

8. Simon RR, Brenner BE: *Emergency Procedures and Techniques,* 3rd ed. Baltimore: Williams & Wilkins, 1994:405–412.

9. Rhee KJ, Derlet RW, Beal SL: Rapid venous access using saphenous vein cutdown at the ankle. *Am J Emerg Med* 1988; 7(3):263–266.

10. Moran JM, Atwood RP, Rowe MI: A clinical and bacteriological study of infections associated with venous cutdowns. *N Engl J Med* 1965; 272(11):545–560.

11. Bogen JE: Local complications in 67 patients with indwelling venous catheters. *Surg Gynecol Obstet* 1960; 110:112–114.

12. Collins RN, Braun PA, Zinner SH, et al: Risk of complications with polyethylene intravenous catheters. *N Engl J Med* 1968; 279(7):340–343.

13. Nowak RM: Venous cutdowns in the emergency room. *JACEP* 1979; 8(6):245.

Chapter 44
INTRAOSSEOUS INFUSION

Mark E. Hoffman
O. John Ma

INTRODUCTION

Obtaining peripheral vascular access in the critically ill pediatric patient may be difficult and time-consuming. It may be difficult because of the small size of the peripheral veins, the increased subcutaneous tissue, and vascular collapse that may accompany severe dehydration or cardiac arrest. Administration of endotracheal medications may not provide rapid and reliable drug absorption during a cardiorespiratory arrest.[1,2]

An alternative route for blood, drug, and fluid administration is via an intraosseous line. This previously abandoned technique was reintroduced in the mid-1980s in response to the need for more immediate vascular access during cardiopulmonary resuscitation.[3,4] Studies have demonstrated that peripheral venous access during pediatric cardiac arrest constituted the fastest way of obtaining vascular access (mean time of 3.0 minutes). However, it was only successful in 17 percent of patients. This was in stark contrast to the 83 percent success rate for intraosseous lines, 81 percent for peripheral venous cutdowns, and 77 percent for central venous lines.[5,6] The time required to place an intraosseous line was 4.7 minutes compared to 8.4 minutes for a central venous line and 12.7 minutes for a peripheral venous cutdown. The insertion of an intraosseous line was recently studied in the prehospital arena, where it was shown to be safe and effective.[7,8] Intraosseous infusion is quick, safe, and effective in compromised neonates.[9] There has also been interest in its role in the resuscitation of adult patients when vascular access is unobtainable.[10]

ANATOMY AND PATHOPHYSIOLOGY

Long bones are composed of a dense outer cortex and inner soft, spongy (cancellous) bone (Figure 44-1). The nutrient artery supplies the bone with a rich vascular network. It pierces the cortex and divides into ascending and descending branches that further divide into arteri-

oles and then capillaries. Venous drainage from the capillaries into the medullary venous sinusoids, located at the proximal and distal portions of the long bone, flows into the central venous channel located in the shaft of the long bone.[11]

The intraosseous needle is inserted through the cortex and into the bone marrow (medullary) cavity of a long bone. Numerous anatomic sites can be used to access the medullary cavity. The most traditional site, which is favored in pediatric patients, is the flat anteromedial surface of the proximal tibia (Figure 44-2). The distal tibia just above the medial malleolus is the preferred site in adult patients (Figure 44-3). In the adult, it is easier to penetrate the cortex of the medial malleolus than the thicker cortex of the proximal tibia. A third site for intraosseous access is the flat anterior surface of the distal femur (Figure 44-4).

Crystalloid infusion studies through an intraosseous line in animals have demonstrated an infusion rate of approximately 10 to 20 mL/min with gravity and up to 40 mL/min under pressure.[12,13] Fluids and medications administered through an intraosseous line are immediately absorbed into the systemic circulation. Sodium bicarbonate infusion, even during a cardiac arrest, was shown to have superior buffering capacity when administered via an intraosseous line than by a peripheral intravenous line.[14] Medications and fluids that may be administered by the intraosseous route are listed in Table 44-1.[15,16] The medication concentrations, dosages, and infusion rates through an intraosseous line are the same as those through a peripheral intravenous line. Succinylcholine has been effectively infused by the intraosseous route for muscle paralysis prior to endotracheal intubation.[17]

INDICATIONS

The placement of an intraosseous line is indicated when vascular access is rapidly required for the resuscitation of a patient and standard vascular access is unob-

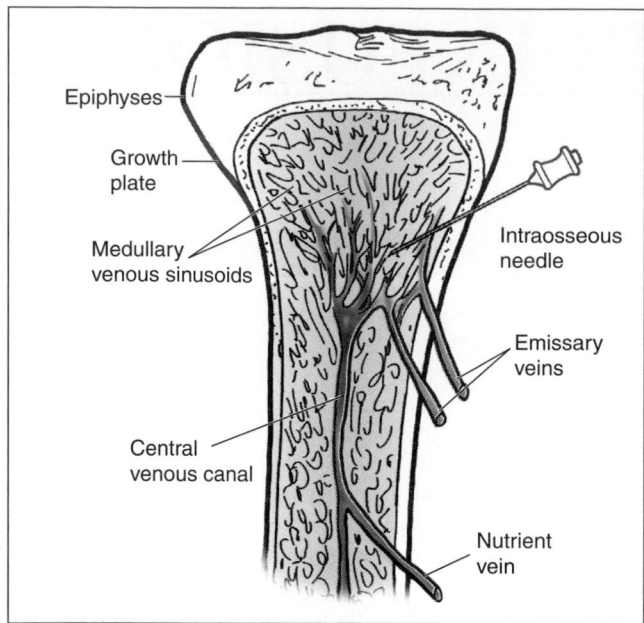

FIGURE 44-1 Venous anatomy of a long bone.

tainable or delayed. Traditionally, this procedure has been utilized in the pediatric population during a cardiac arrest. It may be used in the adult population as well. Situations that may require the placement of an intraosseous line are cardiac arrest, shock, trauma, severe dehydration, extensive burns, status epilepticus, or any condition that requires urgent administration of fluids, medications, or blood products.[18] In addition to resuscitation, the intraosseous needle can provide the resuscitators with blood for typing, crossmatching, and

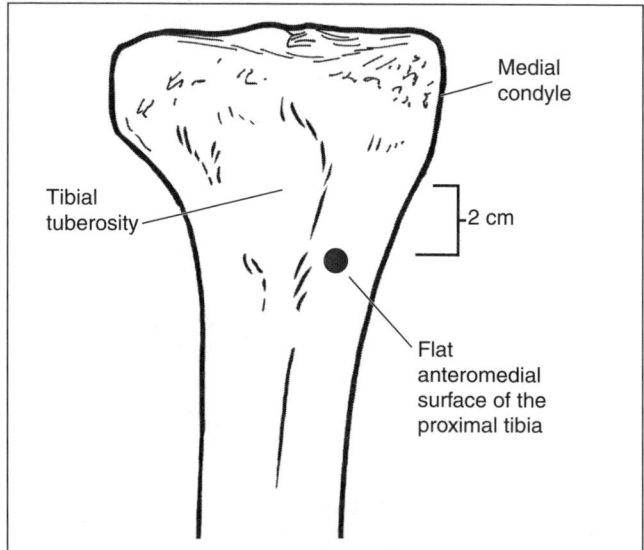

FIGURE 44-2 The proximal tibia is the traditional site used in pediatrics for intraosseous access. The red circle represents the site of insertion of the intraosseous needle.

laboratory analysis. Electrolytes, creatinine, blood urea nitrogen (BUN), glucose, calcium, and arterial blood gas values from blood samples obtained through an intraosseous needle are similar to those from samples taken via traditional routes.[19,20]

CONTRAINDICATIONS

Placement of an intraosseous line is contraindicated in diseased or osteoporotic bone. The placement of an intraosseous line through areas of cellulitis, abscesses, or burns should be avoided.[21] Fractures in the ipsilateral bone increase the risk of extravasation-induced compartment syndrome and nonunion of the fractures.[22] Failed placement of an intraosseous line in the same bone is a relative contraindication.

EQUIPMENT

Sandbag or towel
Povidone iodine solution
Local anesthetic solution, 1% lidocaine
Intraosseous needle
Aspiration syringe, 5 to 10 mL
Primed intravenous tubing with normal saline
Tape
Plastic protective cup
Leg board for immobilization

Intraosseous needles are available in a number of sizes and styles (Figure 44-5). These include the Cook intraosseous needle (Cook Critical Care, Bloomington, IN), the Illinois sternal/iliac aspiration needle (Sherwood Medical, St. Louis, MO), the Jamshidi disposable sternal/iliac aspiration needle (Baxter Healthcare, Valencia, CA), and the MedSurg Industries Illinois sternal/iliac aspiration needle (MedSurg Industries, Rockville, MD). The unit consists of a detachable handle, an intraosseous needle, an obturator, and a sleeve to prevent the needle from penetrating too deeply. The intraosseous needle ranges in size from 12 to 20 gauge. Those needles available today are variations of the basic unit, including adjustable-length shafts to decrease the risk of penetrating too deeply, a variety of tips on the obturator (lancet, pencil point, trocar), threaded versus nonthreaded shafts, needle side ports to increase flow rates, numerous lengths, and numerous handle types. **Only specifically designed intraosseous needles should be used for this procedure.** Spinal needles often bend and do not penetrate the cortex of the bone. Their long length causes increased resistance to fluid flow. Standard hypodermic needles also often bend and do not penetrate the cortex of the bone. Both these types of

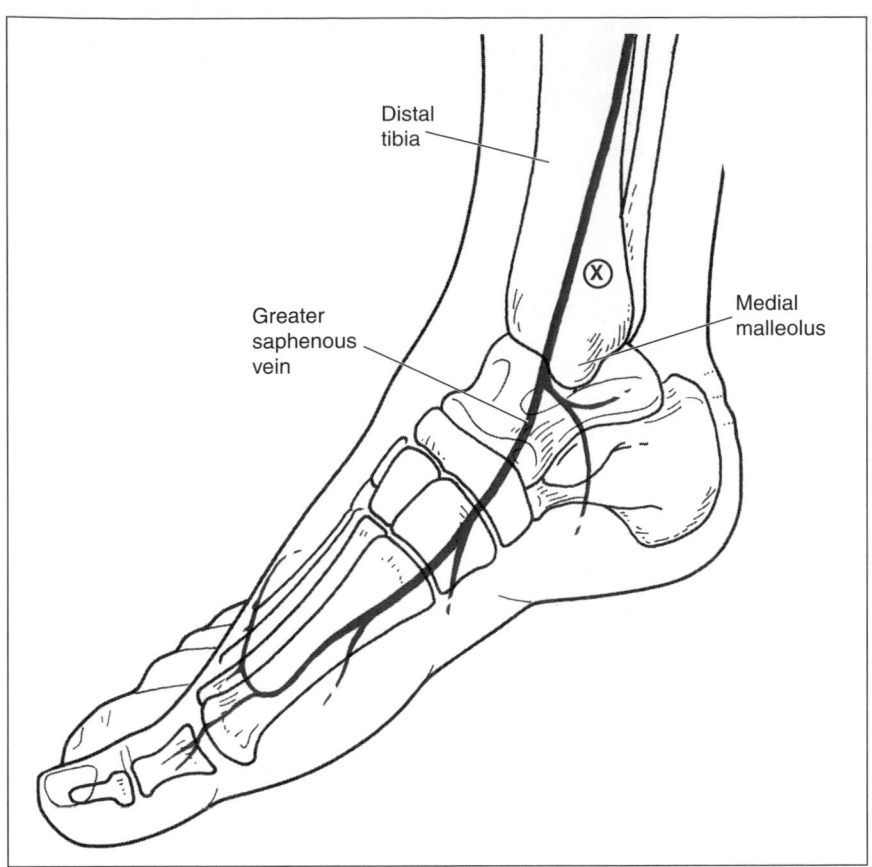

FIGURE 44-3 The distal tibia is the preferred site for intraosseous access in adult patients. The ⊗ represents the site of insertion of the intraosseous needle.

needles may break while being inserted and injure the health care provider.

A new system has recently been developed to perform intraosseous infusion through the sternum (Pyng Medical, Richmond, BC, Canada). It is a multiple-component kit to be used for sternal intraosseous access in the adult patient. A special introducer limits the depth to which the needle can be inserted. This prevents injury to the underlying great vessels, heart, lung, and mediastinum. This system cannot be recommended until further information and trials of its effectiveness and safety are available.

PATIENT PREPARATION

Explain the procedure, its risks, and benefits to the patient and/or their representative if time permits. This procedure is often performed in emergencies; therefore informed consent can be waived. Place the patient supine with the lower extremity supported behind the knee with a towel or sandbag. Identify by palpation the landmarks required to perform the procedure.

Currently, the primary site of choice for intraosseous line placement is the proximal tibia. Alternate sites include the distal tibia and distal femur. Palpate the bony landmarks with the nondominant hand. The bony landmarks for the approach via the proximal tibia are the tibial tuberosity and the flat anteromedial surface of the proximal tibia. The site of intraosseous needle placement is approximately 2 cm below the tuberosity on the flat anteromedial surface of the proximal tibia (Figure 44-2). The bony landmark for the approach via the distal tibia is the junction of the medial malleolus and the flat anteromedial surface of the distal tibia just posterior to the greater saphenous vein[18] (Figure 44-3). This is the preferred site in the adult patient. The bony landmarks for the approach via the distal femur are the medial and lateral condyles of the femur and the patella. The intraosseous needle should be positioned approximately 2 cm above these structures (Figure 44-4). This site is utilized less often due to the abundance of muscle and soft tissue structures.

Prepare the patient. Clean any dirt and debris from the skin. Apply povidone iodine solution to the skin and allow it to dry if time permits. This procedure is extremely painful. If time permits, the use of a local anesthetic solution in the conscious or semiconscious patient will be greatly appreciated. Infiltrate local anesthetic solution into the skin, subcutaneous tissues, and periosteum overlying the bone puncture site.

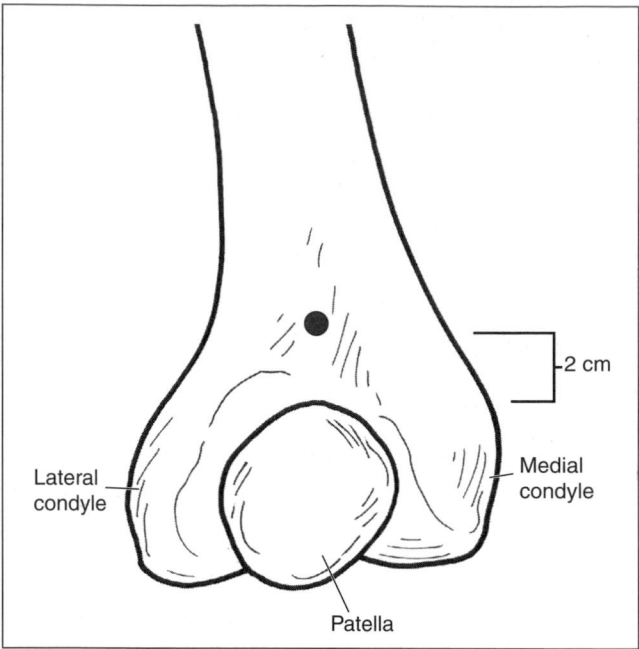

FIGURE 44-4 The distal femur is an alternative site for intraosseous access. The red circle represents the site of insertion of the intraosseous needle.

TECHNIQUE

Examine the intraosseous needle to ensure that it is functioning properly. Reidentify the landmarks with the nondominant hand. Stabilize the extremity with the nondominant hand (Figure 44-6A). Grasp the intraosseous needle firmly with the dominant hand. The

TABLE 44-1. MEDICATIONS AND FLUIDS THAT MAY BE ADMINISTERED THROUGH AN INTRAOSSEOUS LINE[13–18]

Medications

Adenosine	Diazoxide	Lorazepam
Antibiotics	Digoxin	Mannitol
Antitoxins	Dobutamine	Morphine
Anesthetics	Dopamine	Naloxone
Atracurium besylate	Ephedrine	Pancuronium
Atropine	Epinephrine	Phenobarbital
Calcium gluconate	Heparin	Phenytoin
Calcium chloride	Insulin	Propranolol
Contrast media	Isoproterenol	Sodium bicarbonate
Dexamethasone	Levarterenol	Succinylcholine
Diazepam	Lidocaine	Thiopental
		Vecuronium

Fluids

Dextrose solutions
Sodium chloride solutions
Lactated Ringer's solution
Packed red blood cells
Plasma
Blood products

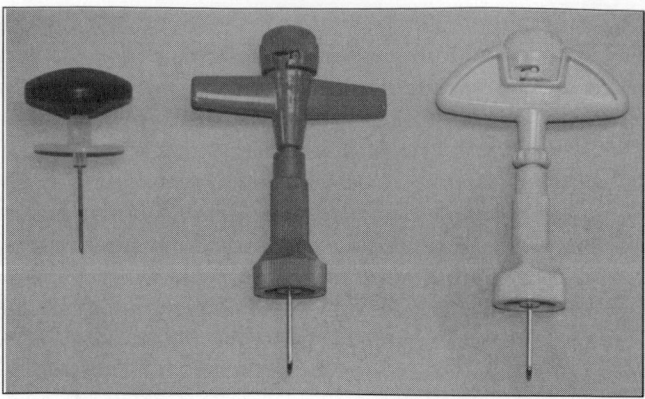

FIGURE 44-5 Intraosseous infusion needles. *From left to right*: the Cook intraosseous infusion needle and two models of the Illinois sternal/iliac aspiration needle.

handle of the intraosseous needle should be firmly planted in the palm of the dominant hand. Insert the needle perpendicularly or slightly angulated (at a 10 to 15 degree angle) to the long axis of the bone (Figure 44-6). **The intraosseous needle should always be directed away from the growth plate to avoid injuring it.** Direct the needle caudad in the proximal tibial approach and cephalad in the distal tibial and distal femoral approaches.

Advance the needle through the skin and subcutaneous tissue until the bone is contacted. Advance the intraosseous needle through the bone. A twisting or rotary motion should be used to cut through the cortex of the bone (Figure 44-6A). A significant reduction in the resistance to forward motion will be encountered when the cortex is penetrated and the needle enters the medullary canal. This distance is rarely greater than 1 cm in most patients. An index finger may be placed 1 cm from the bevel of the intraosseous needle prior to advancement. This will help prevent overpenetration into and through the cortex on the opposite side of the bone.[23] Alternatively, adjust the sleeve so that only 1 cm of the intraosseous needle is exposed. Stop advancing the intraosseous needle when it enters the medullary canal.

Remove the stylet when the medullary canal is entered (Figure 44-6B). Attach a 5 to 10 mL syringe to the hub of the intraosseous needle (Figure 44-6C). Aspirate blood from the medullary canal to confirm proper placement of the needle. Any samples obtained may be sent to the laboratory for subsequent analysis. The aspiration of more than 2 to 3 mL of blood may not be possible in cardiac arrest situations. Attach intravenous tubing to the hub of the intraosseous needle and begin the infusion of fluids. Medications can be administered through the injection port of the intravenous tubing. Place a sterile dressing around the skin puncture site and apply pressure for 5 minutes.[24]

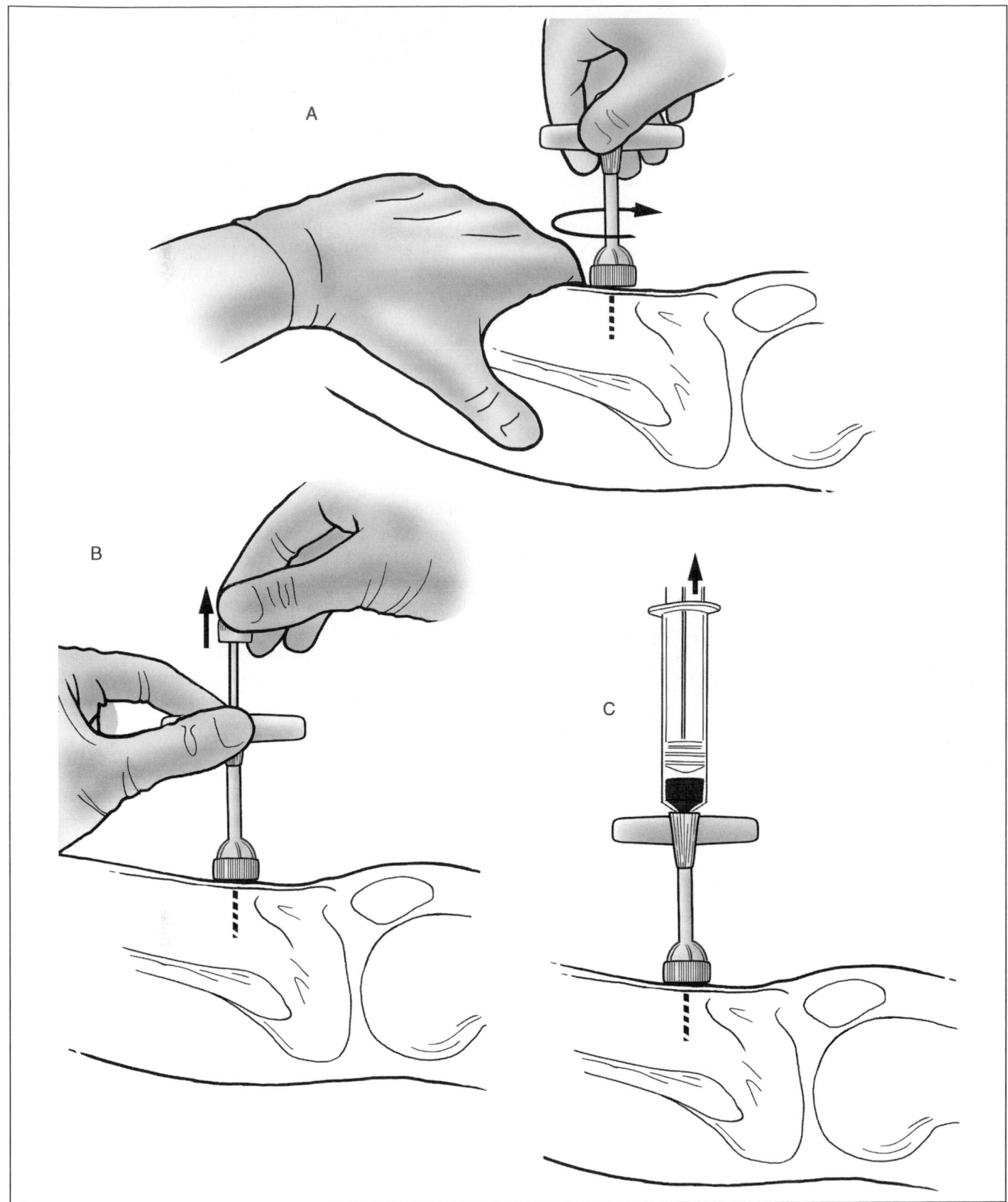

FIGURE 44-6 Placement of an intraosseous line. *A.* The nondominant hand is used to support the extremity. The intra-osseous needle is inserted with a twisting motion to cut through the cortex of the bone. *B.* The handle and obturator are removed. *C.* A syringe is attached to the hub of the intraosseous needle and bone marrow is aspirated.

ASSESSMENT

Assess whether the intraosseous needle is correctly positioned within the medullary cavity. First aspirate blood from the marrow cavity. This may not be possible because of poor circulation in patients with a cardiac arrest. A second sign of correct placement is to assess whether the intraosseous needle will stand erect without support. Finally, flush the intraosseous line. The ability of the fluid to flow without inducing soft tissue swelling can also be used to confirm proper placement. A C-arm fluoroscopic imaging device may be used at the bedside to confirm accurate placement of the intraosseous needle.[25]

AFTERCARE

Secure the intraosseous needle by taping it in place. It may be easier to apply 4×4 gauze squares on two sides of the intraosseous needle to support it and then tape the needle and gauze in place. Tape the intravenous tubing securely at several points. This will prevent traction on the tubing from pulling the intraosseous needle out of the bone. Tape a plastic cup over the intraosseous needle to avoid inadvertent disruption during patient resuscitation or positioning. Immobilize the extremity with a "leg board" on the posterior aspect of the extremity. The intraosseous line should be removed once the resuscitation is complete and another form of secure vascular access has been obtained.

COMPLICATIONS

The most common complication of intraosseous infusions are subcutaneous and subperiosteal extravasation of fluid due to technical difficulty.[4] Under ideal circumstances, the type of intraosseous needle used should not affect extravasation rates.[26] Extravasation is usually due to under- or overpenetration of the cortex. There have been cases of tibial fracture due to overpenetration of the cortex.[27,28] A compartment syndrome may occur when there is extravasation or when intraosseous lines are placed in fractured bones.[22] Necrosis and sloughing of the skin at the insertion site of the intraosseous needle are due to extravasation of fluid or medication.[29]

Localized infections may occur after intraosseous needle placement. Cellulitis or the formation of subcutaneous abscesses occur in 0.7 percent of patients.[21] Osteomyelitis has been reported in 0.6 percent of patients with intraosseous needles and in 10 percent of those receiving hypertonic solutions by the intraosseous route.[3,30]

Injury to the growth plate is a commonly mentioned complication; however, the literature does not support this.[31,32] Fat embolism has also been mentioned as a possible complication. The use of an intraosseous line for the infusion of emergency drugs and fluids does not increase the magnitude of fat embolization during cardiopulmonary resuscitation.[33,34] In recent animal studies, the rate of the intraosseous infusion and the osmolarity of the infused fluid did not adversely affect the bone marrow or bone development.[35]

The flow rate of fluid through an intraosseous line is slower than that through a peripheral intravenous line. This may be due to a small marrow cavity, a fibrous marrow cavity, and/or the replacement of red marrow with yellow marrow. Fluid flow rates can be increased by applying a pressure bag onto the intravenous fluid bag or using a level-one infuser. The placement of a second intraosseous line may be required to further increase the amount of fluid that can be infused.

SUMMARY

The placement of an intraosseous line is a viable option in the resuscitation of a patient when traditional vascular access techniques have failed. The procedure is technically straightforward and has been demonstrated to be successful in the hands of trained health care workers, including prehospital personnel. Complications have been related mostly to technical mistakes and can be avoided if care is taken to correctly identify landmarks, avoid the growth plate, regulate the depth of intraosseous needle placement, and ensure the early removal of the intraosseous line.

REFERENCES

1. Ralston SH, Tacker WA, Showen L, et al: Endotracheal versus intravenous epinephrine during EMD with dogs. *Ann Emerg Med* 1985; 14(11):1044–1048.
2. Orlowski JP, Gallagher JM, Porembka DT: Endotracheal epinephrine is unreliable. *Resuscitation* 1990; 19:103–113.
3. Rossetti VA, Thompson BM, Miller J, et al: Intraosseous infusion: an alternative route of pediatric intravascular access. *Ann Emerg Med* 1985; 14(9):885–888.
4. Bohn D: Intraosseous vascular access: from the archives of to the ABC. *Crit Care Med* 1999; 27(6):1053–1054.
5. Brunette DD, Fisher R: Intravascular access in pediatric cardiac arrest. *Am J Emerg Med* 1988; 6(6):577–579.

6. Orlowski JP: Emergency alternatives to intravenous access: intraosseous, intratracheal, sublingual, and other-site drug administration. *Pediatr Clin North Am* 1994; 41(6):1183–1199.

7. Fuchs S, LaCovey D, Paris P: A prehospital model of intraosseous infusion. *Ann Emerg Med* 1991; 20(4):371–374.

8. Anderson TE, Arthur K, Kleinman M, et al: Intraosseous infusion: success of a standardized regional training program for prehospital ACLS providers. *Ann Emerg Med* 1994; 23(1):52–55.

9. Ellemunter H, Simma B, Trawoger R, et al: Intraosseous lines in preterm and full term neonates. *Arch Dis Child Fetal Neonatal Ed* 1999; 80(1):F74–F75.

10. Waisman M, Waisman D: Bone marrow infusion in adults. *J Trauma* 1997; 42(2):288–293.

11. Williams PL, Warwick R: *Gray's Anatomy,* 35th ed. Philadelphia: Saunders, 1973.

12. Hodge D, Delgado-Paredes C, Gleisher G: Intraosseous infusion flow rates in hypovolemic "pediatric" dogs. *Ann Emerg Med* 1987; 16(3):305–307.

13. Schoffstall JM, Spivey WH, Davidheiser S, et al: Intraosseous crystalloid and blood infusion in a swine model. *J Trauma* 1989; 29(3):384–387.

14. Spivey WH, Lathers CM, Malone DR, et al: Comparison of intraosseous, central, and peripheral routes of sodium bicarbonate administration during CPR in pigs. *Ann Emerg Med* 1985; 14(12):1135–1140.

15. Getschman SJ, Dietrich AM, Franklin WH, et al: Intraosseous adenosine: as effective as peripheral or central venous administration? *Arch Pediatr Adolesc Med* 1994; 148:616–619.

16. Sawyer RW, Bodai BI, Blaisdell FW, et al: The current status of intraosseous infusion. *J Am Coll Surg* 1994; 179:353–360.

17. Tobias JD, Nichols DG: Intraosseous succinylcholine for orotracheal intubation. *Pediatr Emerg Care* 1990; 6(2):108–109.

18. Iserson KV: Intraosseous infusion in adults. *J Emerg Med* 1989; 7:587–591.

19. Orlowski JP, Porembka DT, Gallagher JM, et al: The bone marrow as a source of laboratory studies. *Ann Emerg Med* 1989; 18(12):1348–1351.

20. Johnson L, Kissoon N, Fiallos M, et al: Use of intraosseous blood to assess blood chemistries and hemoglobin during cardiopulmonary resuscitation with drug infusions. *Crit Care Med* 1999; 27(6): 1147–1152.

21. Fiser DH: Intraosseous infusion. *N Engl J Med* 1990; 322(22):1579–1581.

22. Simmons CM, Johnson NE, Perkin RM, et al: Intraosseous extravasation complication reports. *Ann Emerg Med* 1994; 23(2):363–366.

23. Spivey WH: Intraosseous infusions. *J Pediatr* 1987; 111(5):639–643.

24. Mofenson HC, Tascone A, Caraccio TR: Guidelines for intraosseous infusions. *J Emerg Med* 1988; 6:143–146.

25. Garcia CT, Cohen DM: Intraosseous needle: use of the miniature C-arm imaging device to confirm placement. *Pediatr Emerg Care* 1996; 12(2):94–97.

26. LaSpada J, Kissoon N, Melker R, et al: Extravasation rates and complications of intraosseous needles during gravity and pressure infusion. *Crit Care Med* 1995; 23(12):2023–2028.

27. La Fleche FR, Slepin MJ, Vargas J, et al: Iatrogenic bilateral tibial fractures after intraosseous infusion attempts in a 3-month-old infant. *Ann Emerg Med* 1989; 18(10):1099–1101.

28. Katz DS, Wojtowyez AR: Tibial fracture: a complication of intraosseous infusion. *Am J Emerg Med* 1994; 12(2):258–259.

29. Rimar S, Westry JA, Rodriquez RL: Compartment syndrome in an infant following an emergency intraosseous infusion. *Clin Pediatr* 1988; 27(5):259–260.

30. Barron BJ, Tran HD, Lamki LM: Scintographic findings of osteomyelitis after intraosseous infusion in a child. *Clin Nucl Med* 1994; 19(4):307–308.

31. Dedrick DK, Mase C, Ranger W, et al: The effects of intraosseous infusion on the growth plate in a nestling rabbit model. *Ann Emerg Med* 1992; 21(5):494–497.

32. Brickman KR, Rega P, Koltz M, et al: Analysis of growth plate abnormalities following intraosseous infusion through the proximal tibial epiphysis in pigs. *Ann Emerg Med* 1998; 17(2):121–123.

33. Fiallos M, Kissoon N, Abdelmoneim T, et al: Fat embolism with the use of intraosseous infusion during cardiopulmonary resuscitation. *Am J Med Sci* 1997; 314(2):73–79.

34. Plewa MC, King RW, Fenn-Buderer ND, et al: Hematologic safety of intraosseous blood transfusion in a swine model of pediatric hemorrhagic hypovolemia. *Acad Emerg Med* 1995; 2(9):799–809.

35. Brickman KR, Rega P, Schoolfield L, et al: Investigation of bone developmental and histopathologic changes from intraosseous infusion. *Ann Emerg Med* 1996; 28(4):430–435.

Chapter 45
UMBILICAL VESSEL CATHETERIZATION

Iksoo Kang
Eric F. Reichman

INTRODUCTION

Umbilical vessel catheterization can be used as a reliable method of obtaining rapid vascular access in the neonate. Umbilical vessel catheters may be used for fluid resuscitation, blood transfusion, medication administration, frequent blood sampling, and cardiovascular monitoring.[1–4] Either the umbilical artery or vein may be used for vascular access. The artery can usually be accessed within the first 24 hours of life. It is occasionally possible to use the umbilical artery up to 7 days after birth.[1] The umbilical vein can be accessed for up to 2 weeks of age.[1,5]

Umbilical artery catheterization is more desirable than umbilical vein catheterization because it allows frequent arterial blood gas sampling and continuous blood pressure monitoring, in addition to fluid, blood, and medication administration. Unfortunately, umbilical artery catheterization is more difficult and time consuming to perform, especially in unskilled hands. Therefore, umbilical vein catheterization is the preferred procedure for the infant in shock and in need of rapid resuscitation. Arterial access can be obtained later in a more controlled environment, such as in the neonatal intensive care unit. **Umbilical vessel catheterization can lead to serious complications and should be reserved for the patient in whom peripheral venous access attempts have been unsuccessful.**[4,6]

ANATOMY AND PATHOPHYSIOLOGY

The fetal circulatory system is quite different from that of the neonate or infant (Figure 45-1). Oxygenated blood from the placenta travels via the umbilical vein, through the ductus venosus in the liver, to the inferior vena cava, and into the right atrium. Oxygenated blood from the inferior vena cava preferentially enters the left atrium through the foramen ovale. It then enters the left ventricle, then the aorta. This oxygen-rich blood supplies the brain prior to mixing with the oxygen-poor blood coming through the ductus arteriosus. Deoxygenated blood from the superior vena cava enters the right ventricle and is pumped to the pulmonary artery. It then passes through the ductus arteriosus to meet the oxygenated blood in the aorta.

Pulmonary vascular resistance decreases dramatically as the infant takes its first breaths. The systemic vascular resistance increases when the umbilical cord is clamped. The foramen ovale closes with the combination of decreased pulmonary artery pressure and increased systemic resistance. The ductus arteriosus closes within 24 to 48 hours due to the release of prostaglandins and increased oxygen tension. The ductus venosus closes when the umbilical cord is clamped.

The umbilical vein and arteries can easily be differentiated by examination of a cross section of the umbilical cord (Figure 45-2). The umbilical vein is a single vessel with thin walls and a large lumen. It is usually flattened in one direction. There are two thick-walled umbilical arteries that are significantly smaller in diameter than the umbilical vein. Occasionally, only a single umbilical artery is present.

INDICATIONS

Umbilical artery catheterization is indicated when frequent arterial blood gas determinations and blood pressure monitoring are required in the first few days of life.[3] Umbilical artery catheters can be used for delivering blood, fluids, total parenteral nutrition, and medica-

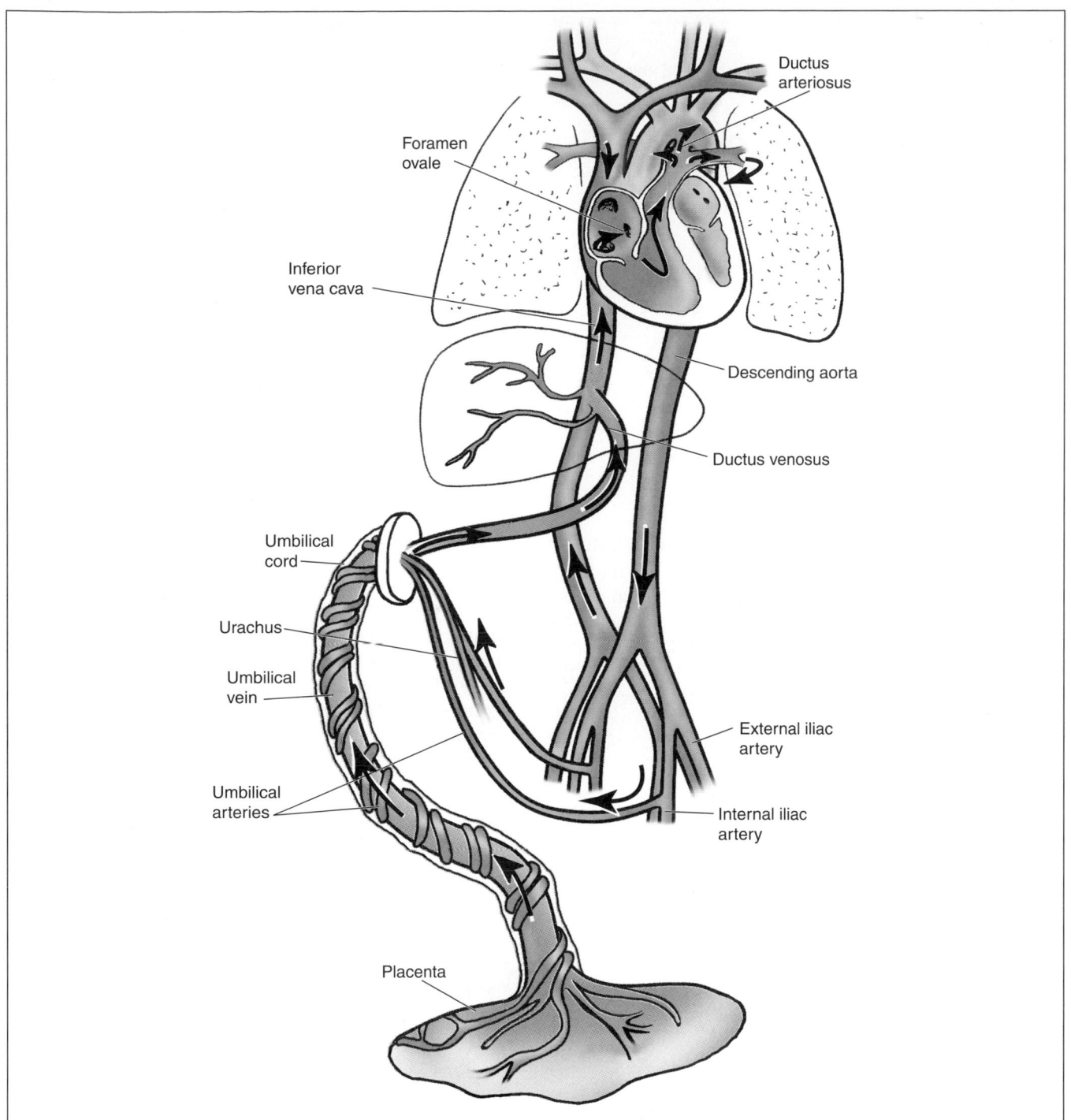

FIGURE 45-1 The fetal circulation.

tions, and for exchange transfusions.[1,2] Neonates under 24 hours of age can usually be catheterized without much difficulty. Skilled clinicians can sometimes perform this up to 7 days after delivery.[1]

Umbilical vein catheterization is easier to perform than umbilical artery catheterization. It is the preferred procedure for the neonate in shock needing rapid administration of intravenous fluids, blood, or medications.[1] The vein can be used to monitor central venous pressure. This procedure is possible in neonates up to 2 weeks of age.[1]

CONTRAINDICATIONS

Umbilical vessel catheterization in the Emergency Department should be performed only on severely ill neonates in whom peripheral vascular access attempts

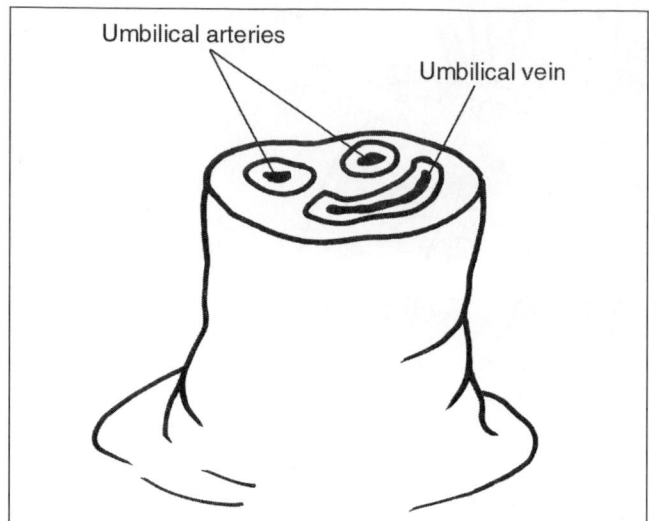

FIGURE 45-2 Anatomy of the umbilical cord.

have failed. Never insert an umbilical catheter if there are any signs of infection on or around the remnant of the umbilical cord. Umbilical vessel catheterization is contraindicated if a neonate is older than the previously stated ages. An alternate route of vascular access is required if the possibility of an abdominal abnormality exists, as manifested by a distended abdomen or visible defects.[1]

EQUIPMENT

Umbilical catheters, 5.0 French for full-term and 3.5
   French for preterm neonates
Umbilical tape
Povidone iodine solution
Sterile gauze
Sterile drapes
Sterile gown, sterile gloves, cap, and mask
Adhesive tape
Radiant warmer with light
Cardiac monitor
Pulse oximeter
3–0 or 4–0 silk suture with a needle
Needle driver
Smooth-curved iris forceps
Iris scissors
2 small, smooth-curved hemostats
Straight Crile forceps
#10 scalpel blade and handle
3-way stopcock
10 mL syringe filled with normal saline
Heparinized sterile saline solution, 1 unit of heparin/
   1 mL of saline

PATIENT PREPARATION

Attempts at peripheral venous access should have failed in a sick neonate prior to attempting umbilical vessel catheterization. All equipment should be readily available on a pre-prepared sterile tray. Place the tray with the instruments on a Mayo stand next to the neonate's bed. Place the neonate under a radiant warmer with a light source. Place the neonate on a cardiac monitor, continuous pulse oximeter, and supplemental oxygenation. Place the neonate supine with the lower extremities in the frog-leg position (Figure 45-3). The physician performing the procedure should wear a cap, mask, sterile gloves, and sterile gown. Scrub the umbilical cord and abdomen with povidone iodine solution and allow it to dry. Place sterile drapes around the umbilical area, ensuring the neonate's head is exposed for observation.

TECHNIQUES

After the patient has been positioned and prepped, the procedure can begin. **Sterile technique must be maintained throughout this procedure.** Loosely tie a piece of umbilical tape around the base of the umbilical cord (Figure 45-4). Place a 3–0 or 4–0 silk purse-string suture through the base of the umbilical cord and just above the umbilical tape (Figure 45-4). **Avoid piercing the umbilical vessels and the skin of the abdominal wall.** Leave the suture untied and the ends uncut. This will be used later to secure the umbilical vessel catheter. Gently grasp the distal umbilical cord, using the straight forceps, approximately 0.5 to 2.0 cm from its base. Cut the cord transversely across the top edge of the forceps with a #10 scalpel blade (Figure 45-4). **Do not cut the cord too close to the base in case it needs to be recut for a repeat attempt.** Grasp the cord with forceps or fingers and identify the two arteries and larger single vein. The umbilical artery or vein may now be catheterized as described in the following sections.

UMBILICAL ARTERY CATHETERIZATION

Determine the desired position of the catheter tip (Figure 45-5). There are two possible positions for the umbilical artery catheter tip. The low position, catheter tip at L3 to L5, corresponds to the level just above the aortic bifurcation.[1,7] The high position, catheter tip at T6 to T9, corresponds to the level above the diaphragm, between the ductus arteriosus and origins of the mesenteric arteries.[1,7] Controversy exists over which position is the preferred site for the catheter tip. Some authors believe the high position is prone to fewer complications.[3,4]

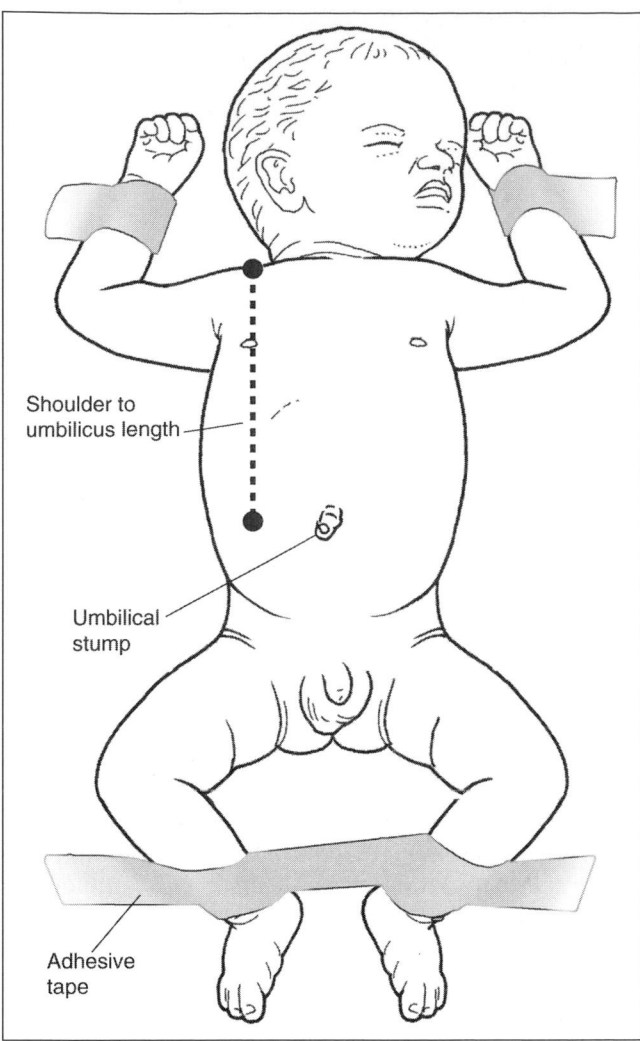

FIGURE 45-3 Positioning of the neonate. The dotted line represents the shoulder-umbilical length.

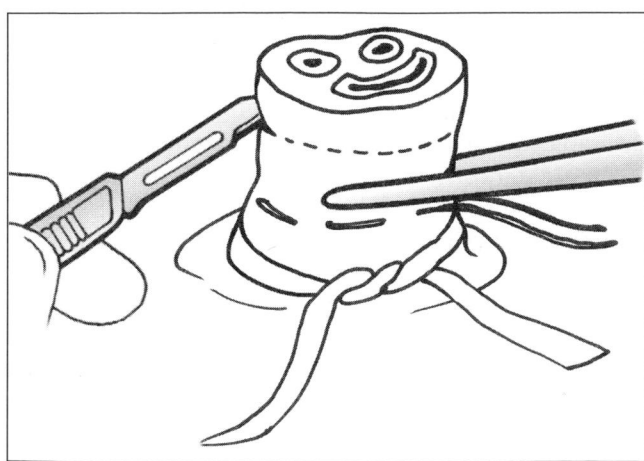

FIGURE 45-4 Preparing the umbilical cord stump. Umbilical tape has been placed at the base and tied loosely. A purse-string suture has been placed through the stump and just above the umbilical tape. The distal end of the umbilical cord is removed along the dotted line.

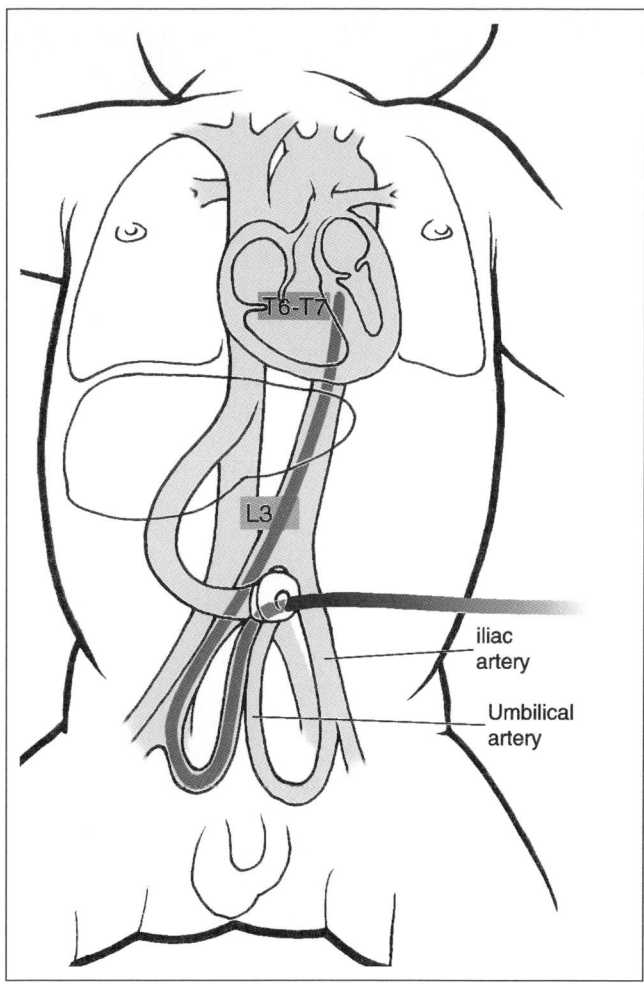

FIGURE 45-5 Positioning of the tip of the umbilical artery catheter. The low position, between L3 and L5, is just above the aortic bifurcation. The high position, between T6 and T9, is above the diaphragm, between the ductus arteriosus and the mesenteric arteries. The shaded boxes represent the vertebral bodies in the midline.

Measure the shoulder to umbilicus length by measuring the distance between the tip of the shoulder to the level perpendicular to the umbilicus (Figure 45-3). Using the shoulder-umbilical length and the desired position of the catheter tip, determine the umbilical catheter length to be inserted into the artery (Figure 45-6). Add the length of the umbilical stump to the umbilical artery catheter length found on the y-axis of the graph to determine the corrected length of catheter to be inserted.

Flush the catheter with the heparinized saline solution, if there are no contraindications to heparin. Attach the 3-way stopcock, in the closed position, to the hub of the catheter. Identify the arteries and choose one for catheterization. Grasp the distal portion of the umbilical cord with the two smooth-curved hemostats to stabilize the end of the umbilical cord (Figure 45-7). Instruct an assistant to hold the hemostats. **Do not apply traction**

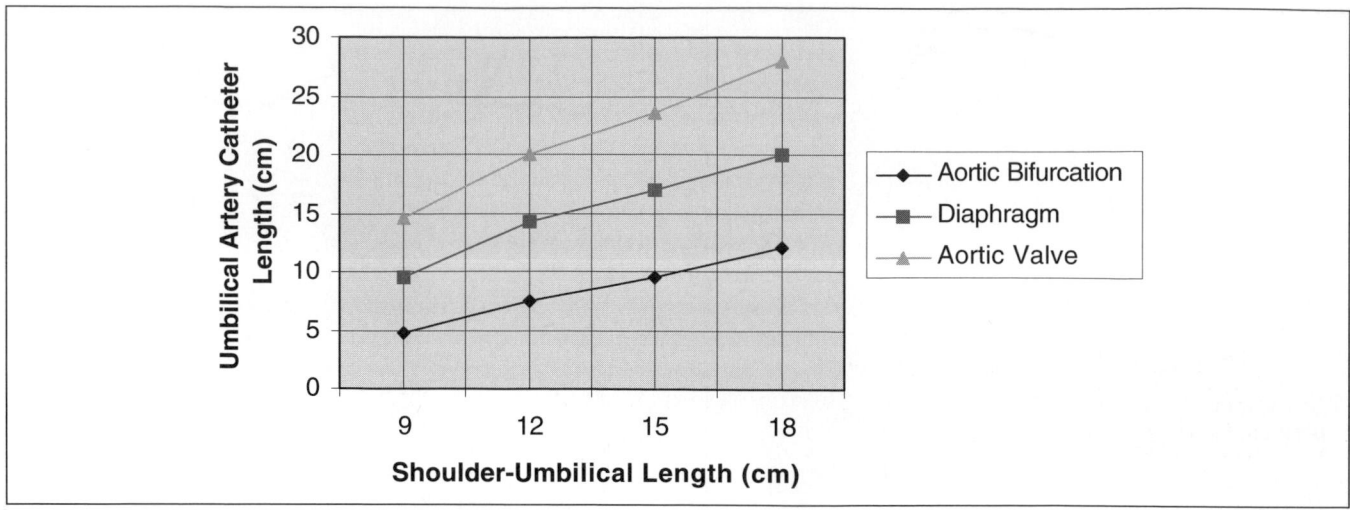

FIGURE 45-6 Graph to determine the correct length of catheter to insert into the umbilical artery. Using the shoulder-umbilical length and the desired position of the catheter tip, determine the length of catheter on the y-axis to be inserted into the artery. Add the length of the umbilical stump to the umbilical artery catheter length found on the y-axis of the graph to determine the corrected length of catheter to be inserted. Adapted and modified from Roberts.[7]

to the hemostats to prevent injury to the umbilical cord. Insert the tips of the smooth-curved iris forceps into the lumen of the artery and gently allow the jaws of the forceps to open (Figure 45-7). This will dilate the arterial wall. Repeatedly insert and open the tips of the curved iris forceps within the arterial lumen to a depth of 0.5 to 1.0 centimeter.[1]

Grasp the catheter approximately 1.0 cm from the tip. Gently insert the tip of the catheter into the artery

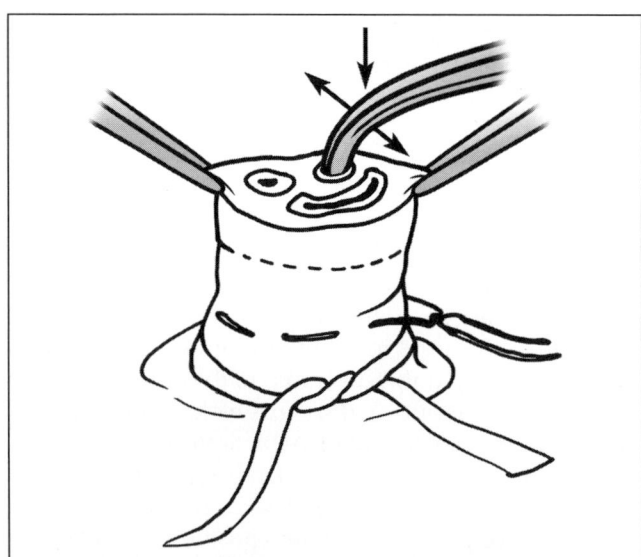

FIGURE 45-7 Preparation for catheter insertion. The upper edges of the umbilical cord stump are stabilized with two smooth-jaw curved hemostats. A smooth-jaw curved iris forceps is placed into one umbilical artery and allowed to open and dilate the artery.

(Figure 45-8). Apply gentle pressure for about 30 seconds. The muscles of the artery may spasm and prevent the catheter from advancing. If the spasm persists, remove the catheter. Place 0.1 mL of a 2% lidocaine solution into the catheter tip.[1] Reinsert the catheter and flush the lidocaine into the artery at the level of the spasm. If the catheter still will not advance, a twisting motion may allow it to advance. Catheterize the other umbilical artery if this fails. Advance the catheter to the predetermined length. Tighten the umbilical tape to temporarily secure the catheter. Obtain radiographic confirmation of placement prior to using the catheter.

UMBILICAL VEIN CATHETERIZATION

Catheterizing the umbilical vein is much easier than the umbilical artery. The lumen is larger and easier to negotiate. This quality makes the umbilical vein more desirable for vascular access in emergency situations.[6,8]

First determine the desired position of the catheter tip. Ideally, it should be located at the junction of the inferior vena cava and the right atrium (Figure 45-9). Measure the shoulder-umbilical length (Figure 45-3). Using the shoulder-umbilical length and the desired position of the catheter tip, determine the umbilical catheter length to be inserted into the vein (Figure 45-10). Add the length of the umbilical stump to the umbilical vein catheter length found on the y-axis of the graph to determine the corrected length of catheter to be inserted.

Umbilical vein catheterization is similar to that of the artery with three exceptions. Any visible clots must be removed from the lumen of the vein prior to inserting the catheter. **The vein requires no dilating. In an emer-**

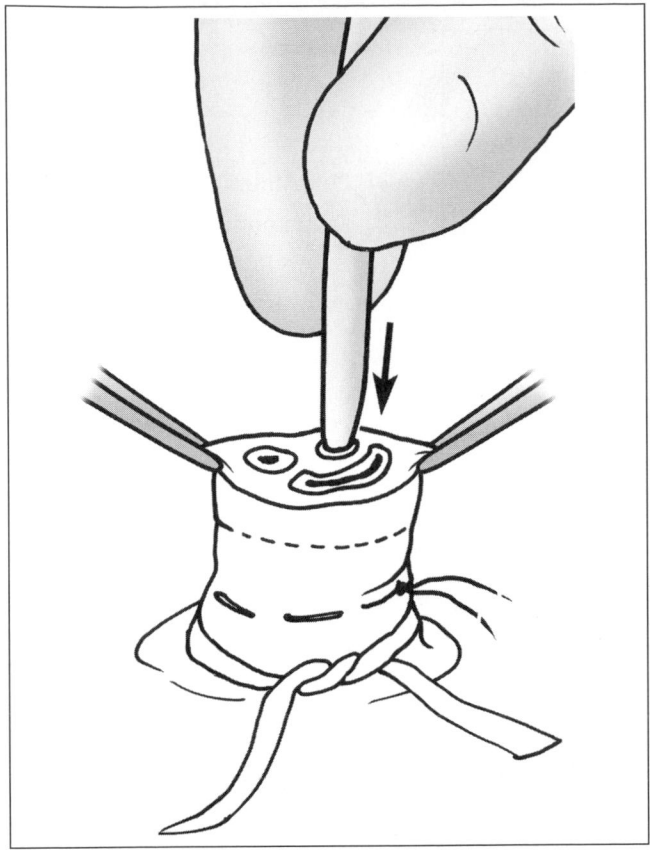

FIGURE 45-8 The catheter is inserted into the umbilical artery and advanced to the desired depth.

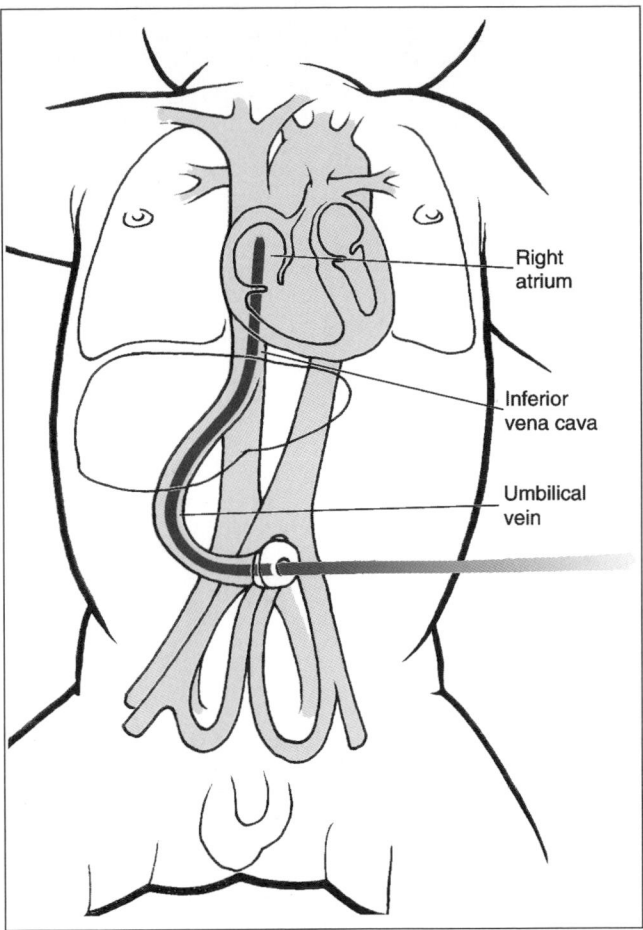

FIGURE 45-9 Positioning of the tip of the umbilical vein catheter. The tip should be above the diaphragm, at the junction of the inferior vena cava and the right atrium.

gency, when awaiting radiographic confirmation is not feasible, the umbilical vein catheter should only be inserted 4 to 5 cm until there is free flow of blood to avoid potential placement of the tip into the portal system.[1,4,5,6] The catheter can be replaced with a more permanent line once the patient has been stabilized.[8] The nonemergent umbilical venous catheter should be placed with the tip above the diaphragm, at the junction of the inferior vena cava and right atrium as determined previously. Tighten the umbilical tape to temporarily secure the catheter. Obtain radiographic confirmation of placement prior to using the catheter.

ASSESSMENT

Confirm the proper placement of the catheter tip. The umbilical tape has been tightened to temporarily secure the catheter within the umbilical cord. **Do not infuse anything through the line until proper placement is confirmed radiographically.** This can be accomplished with plain radiographs or, if available, fluoroscopy. If the catheter is in too far, withdraw it and reevaluate the new catheter tip position radiographically. **If the catheter is not in far enough, do not ad-**

vance the catheter. Withdraw the catheter and restart the procedure with a new catheter.

AFTERCARE

Secure the catheter more permanently after confirming that the catheter tip is in the desired location (Figure 45-11). Tighten and tie a knot in the previously placed purse-string suture. Wrap the loose ends of the suture around the catheter as it enters the umbilical vessel, then secure it with several square knots. **Loosen and remove the umbilical tape to avoid umbilical cord necrosis.**[3] Secure the catheter to the abdominal wall with adhesive tape.

COMPLICATIONS

Prevention of complications requires strict adherence to sterile technique, flushing of the catheter prior to insertion, gentle catheter manipulation during in-

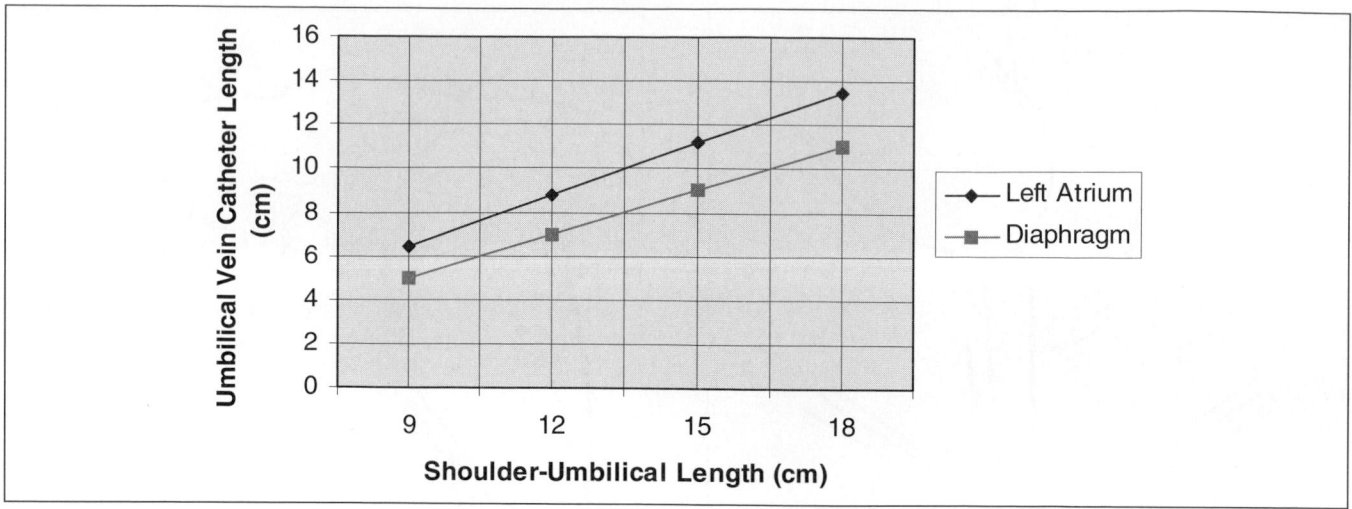

FIGURE 45-10 Graph to determine the correct length of catheter to insert into the umbilical vein. Using the shoulder-umbilical length and the desired position of the catheter tip, determine the length of catheter on the y-axis to be inserted into the vein. Add the length of the umbilical stump to the umbilical vein catheter length found on the y-axis of the graph to determine the corrected length of catheter to be inserted. Adapted and modified from Roberts.[7]

sertion, and accurate positioning of the catheter. It is essential that no air be allowed to enter the catheter. An air bubble can enter the central circulation, pass through the foramen ovale, and lodge in an end artery. The air bubble can cause a stroke if it ends up in a central nervous system artery or a myocardial infarction if it ends up in a coronary artery.

Even if all precautions are observed, complications are still unavoidable.[4] Complication rates as high as 20 percent for venous catheters and 10 percent for arterial catheters have been reported.[9] A venous catheter placed in the portal system may lead to hepatic necrosis, hemorrhage, and thrombus formation, which may lead to a pulmonary embolus or portal hypertension.[2–5] Phlebitis or sepsis can ensue if strict aseptic technique is not followed.[9] Umbilical artery catheterization may be complicated by vasospasm or thrombosis, causing ischemia of the lower extremities or intraabdominal organs.[1,4,5,9,10] Embolization of clots can cause loss of digits, organ infarcts, or skin ulceration.[1,9] Vessel and bowel perforation from forceful manipulation of the catheter, an air embolus from an unflushed catheter prior to insertion, false track formation, cardiac arrhythmias, damage to cardiac valves, and myocardial perforation have all been reported.[2,5,6,9,11] Necrotizing enterocolitis, biliary venous fistula, pericardial effusion,

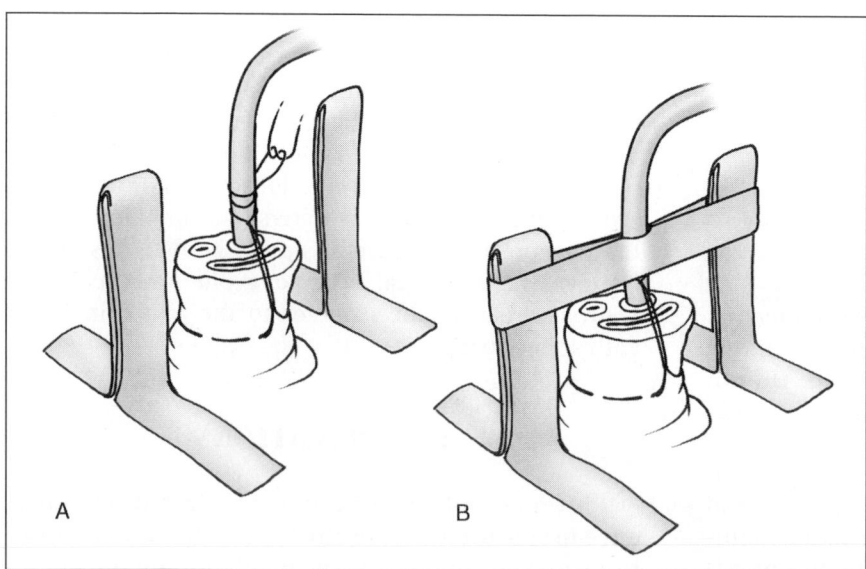

A   B

FIGURE 45-11 Securing the umbilical vessel catheter. *A.* The purse-string suture is tied about the umbilical cord and the umbilical tape is removed. The ends of the suture are wrapped around the catheter, as it enters the umbilical vessel, and secured with square knots. *B.* Tape is applied to secure the catheter to the abdominal wall.

hypoglycemia from high positioning of an umbilical artery catheter, and bladder rupture have also been reported.[11-16] Occasionally, a persistent urachus in the umbilical cord stump may be mistaken for an umbilical vein. Catheterization of the urachus will result in the flow of urine, not blood, and is easily identified and corrected.

SUMMARY

Umbilical vessel catheterization is a readily available method of obtaining vascular access in the sick newborn. These vessels can be used for fluid resuscitation, blood transfusion, medication administration, frequent blood sampling, and cardiovascular monitoring. Because serious complications may result from using this route, it should be reserved for infants in whom peripheral vascular access is unsuccessful.

REFERENCES

1. Lipton JD, Schafermeyer RW: Umbilical vessel catheterization, in Henretig FM, King C (eds): *Textbook of Pediatric Emergency Procedures.* Baltimore: Williams & Wilkins, 1997:515–523.
2. Wilkinson A, Calvert S: Procedures in neonatal intensive care, in Robertson, NRC (ed): *Textbook of Neonatology,* 2nd ed. Edinburgh: Churchill Livingstone, 1992:1175–1176.
3. Feick HJ, Donn SM: Vascular access and blood sampling, in Donn SM, Faix RG (eds): *Neonatal Emergencies.* New York: Futura, 1991:38–44.
4. McAneney C: Umbilical vessel catheterization, in Dieckmann RA, Fiser DH, Selbst SM (eds): *Illustrated Textbook of Pediatric Emergency and Critical Care Procedures.* St. Louis: Mosby, 1997:503–505.
5. Christopher NC, Cantor RM: Venous and arterial access, in Barkin RM (ed): *Pediatric Emergency Medicine: Concepts and Clinical Practice,* 2nd ed. St. Louis: Mosby, 1997:153–154.
6. Ruddy RM: Illustrated techniques of pediatric emergency procedures, in Fleisher GR, Ludwig S (eds): *Textbook of Pediatric Emergency Medicine,* 3rd ed. Baltimore: Williams & Wilkins, 1993:1581–1585.
7. Roberts WB: Procedures, in Siberry GK, Iannone R (eds): *The Harriet Lane Handbook,* 15th ed. St. Louis: Mosby, 2000:51–55.
8. Burke-Strickland M: Technique for placing umbilical catheters. *Minn Med* 1972; 55(11):1021–1024.
9. Weber AL, DeLuca S, Shannon DC: Normal and abnormal position of the umbilical artery and venous catheter on the roentgenogram and review of complications. *Am J Roentgenol* 1974; 120(2): 361–367.
10. Kumar RK, Coulthard MG: Renal infarction due to umbilical artery catheters. *Indian Pediatr* 1998; 35(1):63–65.
11. Green C, Yohannan MD: Umbilical arterial and venous catheters: placement, use and complications. *Neonatal Netw* 1998; 17(6):23–28.
12. Chang LY, Horng YC, Chou YH, et al: Umbilical venous line related pericardial effusion in a premature neonate: report of a case. *J Formosa Med Assoc* 1995; 94(6):355–357.
13. Carey BE, Zeilinger TC: Hypoglycemia due to high positioning of umbilical artery catheters. *J Perinatol* 1989; 9(4):407–410.
14. Omene JA, Odita JC, Diakparomre MA: The risks of umbilical vessel catheterization in a neonatal intensive care unit. *Afr J Med Sci* 1979; 8(3–4):115–123.
15. Diamond DA, Ford C: Neonatal bladder rupture: a complication of umbilical artery catheterization. *J Urol* 1989; 142(6):1543–1544.
16. Mogbo KI, Wang DC: Biliary venous fistula from umbilical catheter placement. *Pediatr Radiol* 1997; 27(4):333–335.

Chapter 46
ARTERIAL PUNCTURE AND CANNULATION

Susan Stroud
Robert Rodriguez

INTRODUCTION

Arterial blood gas sampling is an essential component of the care of many Emergency Department patients. It provides key information regarding a patient's oxygenation and acid-base status. Arterial cannulation allows for continuous and accurate blood pressure monitoring and frequent blood gas sampling in the care of the critically ill patient.

ANATOMY AND PATHOPHYSIOLOGY

Knowledge of the arterial anatomy is a key factor in the success of arterial puncture and cannulation. It is important to recognize that nerves and veins are located in close proximity to the desired arteries in order to avoid complications. The anatomy and positioning for radial, brachial, and femoral arterial access is described below.

RADIAL ARTERY

The radial artery is the preferred site for arterial puncture and cannulation. One reason is the comparative ease of identifying the anatomical location of this artery. A second reason is the collateral nature of the arterial blood supply to the hand provided by the radial and ulnar arteries. Terminal branches of these two arteries meet in the palm of the hand to form the deep and superficial palmar arterial arches (Figure 46-1).

The radial artery can be found just medial and proximal to the radial styloid process on the ventrolateral side of the wrist (Figure 46-1). Dorsiflexing the wrist approximately 60 degrees can aid in palpating the arterial pulse. Another notable landmark is the flexor carpi radialis tendon that runs immediately medial to the radial artery. The recommended point of needle or catheter insertion is at the proximal flexor crease of the wrist.

A modified Allen test should be performed to assess the adequacy of the collateral circulation to the hand prior to radial artery puncture or cannulation (Figure 46-2).[1,2] Ask the patient to close their hand tightly into a fist to force blood out of the fingers (Figure 46-2A). Manually occlude the radial and ulnar arteries (Figure 46-2A). Ask the patient to open the hand. The fingers should be blanched due to the occlusion of the arterial inflow. Release the finger occluding the ulnar artery (Figure 46-2B). Measure the time it takes for blushing of the palm to occur. It is considered normal if it is < 7 seconds, equivocal at 8 to 14 seconds, and abnormal if > 14 seconds.[1]

An alternative method of evaluating the collateral circulation involves the use of a pulse oximeter with a visual pulse waveform display.[3] This is useful in unconscious or uncooperative patients. Place the pulse oximeter sensor on the patient's thumb. Occlude the radial artery and examine the waveform on the monitor. An ulnar dominant system with adequate collateral circulation is likely if the waveform remains unchanged during radial artery occlusion.[3]

The performance of an Allen test to confirm adequate collateral circulation to the hand is generally advocated before radial artery puncture or cannulation. There is concern that radial artery occlusion from an intraluminal clot or an external hematoma can result in hand ischemia if the ulnar artery cannot provide adequate collateral blood flow. Some authors have questioned the utility of performing an Allen test.[1,2,4] The relative safety of radial artery cannulation without the Allen test has been demonstrated in a large case series of patients without major peripheral vascular disease.[4] Although an abnormal Allen test may not preclude radial artery puncture or cannulation, it may indicate a greater need for caution and alert the physician to potential problems after the procedure is performed.[2]

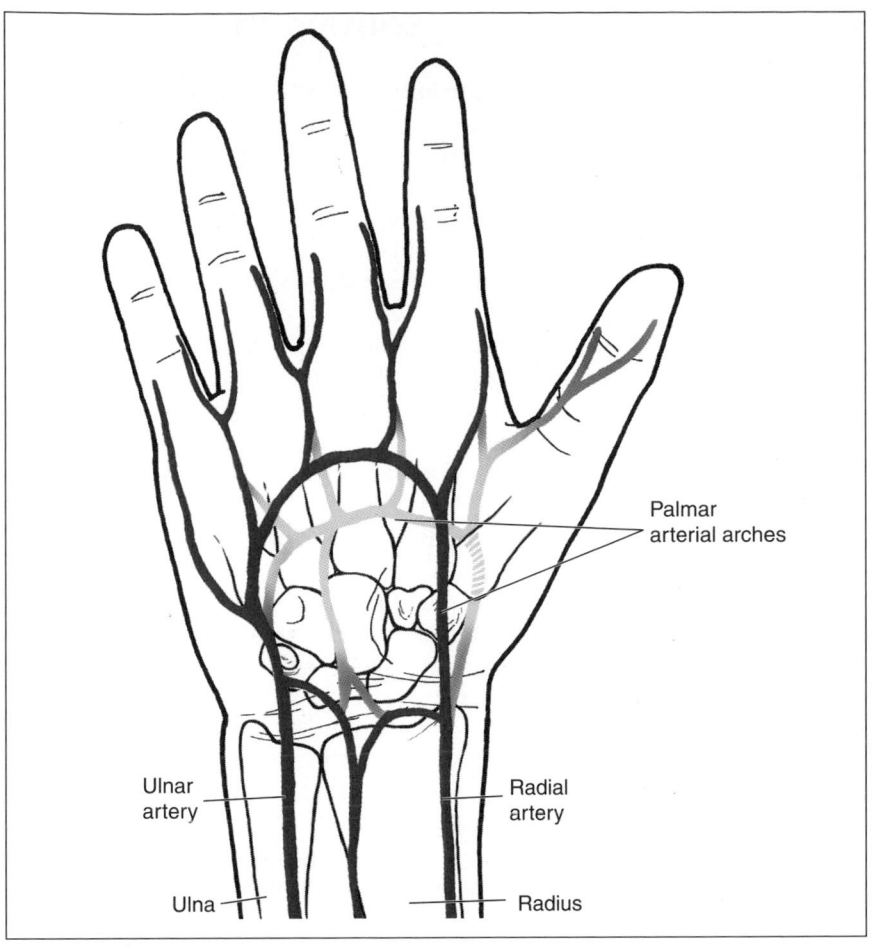

FIGURE 46-1 Anatomical location of the radial and ulnar arteries. Collateral circulation is provided by the superficial and deep palmar arches.

Palmar arterial arches

Ulnar artery

Radial artery

Ulna

Radius

BRACHIAL ARTERY

The brachial artery courses along the medial side of the antecubital fossa just lateral to the median nerve (Figure 46-3). The brachial artery divides at the level of the neck of the radius to become the ulnar and radial arteries. In the antecubital fossa, the brachial artery is located lateral to the medial epicondyle of the humerus and medial to the biceps brachii muscle. The brachial artery is more easily identified when the elbow is fully extended. In order to locate the artery, start by palpating the medial epicondyle of the humerus. Move laterally until the medial edge of the biceps muscle is palpated. The brachial artery pulse should be palpable just medial to the biceps muscle. The arterial pulsation is most easily identified at the level of the proximal flexor crease of the antecubital fossa. The preferred location for puncture or cannulation of the brachial artery is in, or just proximal to, the antecubital fossa. If the artery is to be cannulated, the arm should remain in extension while the cannula is in place.

FEMORAL ARTERY

The bony anatomical landmarks for the femoral artery are the anterior superior iliac spine and the tubercle of the pubic symphysis. The artery lies approximately midway between these two points after it courses under the inguinal ligament to enter the thigh (Figure 46-4). The femoral nerve and vein are found running in parallel and adjacent to the artery. The vein lies just medial to the artery and the nerve just lateral. The femoral artery is larger than other arteries commonly cannulated and lies deeper than the radial or brachial arteries. This makes it necessary to use a longer cannula and, depending on the patient's body habitus, may require a longer needle for a simple arterial puncture to be successful. Extension and slight abduction of the hip maximizes access to the femoral triangle, improves the ability to palpate the artery, and provides a maximal work area for the procedure.

INDICATIONS

The principal indications for arterial blood sampling include the determination of carbon dioxide (CO_2) content, oxygen (O_2) content, and acid-base status.[5,6] The need for arterial blood gas (ABG) sampling for determination of oxygenation has decreased substantially with the advent of pulse oximetry. Pulse oximetry may poorly reflect oxygenation in the settings of severe hypoxia or severe hypotension. Therefore, ABG analysis persists as the true measure of arterial oxygenation.[7] End-tidal CO_2 (E_TCO_2) monitoring has decreased the utilization of ABG samples for CO_2 measurement. In patients who have large dead space ventilation or low cardiac output, E_TCO_2 measurement may grossly underestimate the true CO_2 content of the blood.[8] Arterial blood gas samples are useful for accurate pH monitoring of patients with shock, obstructive lung disease, and other pulmonary disorders. Possibly the most important indication for ABG sampling in the critically ill patient is the determination of the patient's acid-base status. Venous sampling may occasionally suffice for monitoring of pH in a few illnesses such as diabetic ketoacidosis.[9] The measurement of venous blood pH is much less reliable as a surrogate for arterial pH in patients with shock and other critical illnesses.[10] Arterial blood samples are still used for the measurement of carboxyhemoglobin and methemoglobin levels. One study found that venous and arterial co-oximetry carboxyhemoglobin values are closely correlated and may be used to screen patients thought to have been exposed to carbon monoxide.[11]

The two principal indications for arterial catheter placement are the need for continuous monitoring of arterial blood pressure and the need for frequent ABG sampling. Cycled oscillometric blood pressure measurement may be insufficient to gauge rapid hemodynamic changes in critically ill hypertensive or hypotensive patients. Continuous blood pressure monitoring facilitates titration of rapid-acting vasodilators and vasopressors. The accuracy of auscultated or oscillometric blood pressure readings under conditions of severe shock or malperfusion are suspect.[1,2] Centrally measured aortic pressure is the true gold standard.[1,2] However, given the impracticality of measurement of aortic pressure, peripheral arterial pressure measured with an intraarterial catheter connected to a pressure transducer is the next best gauge.

CONTRAINDICATIONS

Contraindications to arterial puncture and catheter placement relate primarily to abnormalities at the insertion sites. Avoid skin and arteries that are already compromised by trauma, burns, infection, severe dermatitis, or severe peripheral vascular disease.[1,5] Puncture or cannulation of synthetic vascular grafts is also relatively contraindicated. **Do not puncture where the artery "should be" if the arterial pulsation cannot be palpated.** Attempts at cannulation of nonpalpable arteries are generally fruitless and sometimes hazardous. Arterial puncture or catheterization is relatively contraindicated in patients with bleeding diatheses and those who have received, or may receive, thrombolytic therapy.

EQUIPMENT

Arterial Puncture for Single ABG Sample

Povidone iodine or alcohol solution
Dorsal wrist extensor splint or small rolled up towel
1% lidocaine, 1 mL in a tuberculin syringe
5 mL syringe for blood collection with cap retained
Prepackaged blood gas syringe with lyophilized heparin pellet
20 to 22 gauge needle for arterial puncture
1 to 2 mL of heparin (1000 U/mL)
Gauze pads
Adhesive tape
Specimen collection bag or cup with 2 to 3 inches of ice

Arterial (Brachial, Radial, Dorsalis Pedis) Cannulation

Povidone iodine or chlorhexidine solution
Dorsal wrist extensor splint or small rolled up towel
1% lidocaine, 1 mL in a tuberculin syringe
4×4 gauze squares
Adhesive tape
Nylon suture, 3–0 or 4–0
20 gauge 1¾ inch polyurethane catheter over a 22 gauge introducer needle
0.45 mm diameter, 5¼ inch spring wire guide compatible with catheter in previous line

Femoral Artery Cannulation

Povidone iodine or chlorhexidine solution
1% lidocaine, 3 mL in a syringe armed with a 25 gauge needle
4×4 gauze squares
#11 scalpel blade
Nylon suture, 3–0 or 4–0
Femoral artery needle, approximately 18 gauge, 2⅞ inches
4 French single lumen catheter, at least 15 cm in length
30 cm guidewire compatible with above needle and catheter

If a syringe that has not been designed specifically for ABG sampling is used, and it has not been pretreated with heparin or does not contain a lyophilized heparin pellet, it is necessary to prepare the syringe using heparin solution. Draw up 1 to 2 mL of heparin solution into the syringe and then expel the heparin, leaving only the heparin remaining in the dead space of the syringe and the needle. This amount of heparin is sufficient to prevent clotting of the sample.[5] It is important to remove all but the necessary amount of heparin as excess heparin has been found to falsely lower the PCO_2 measurement and may elevate the PO_2 measurement.[12] Commercially

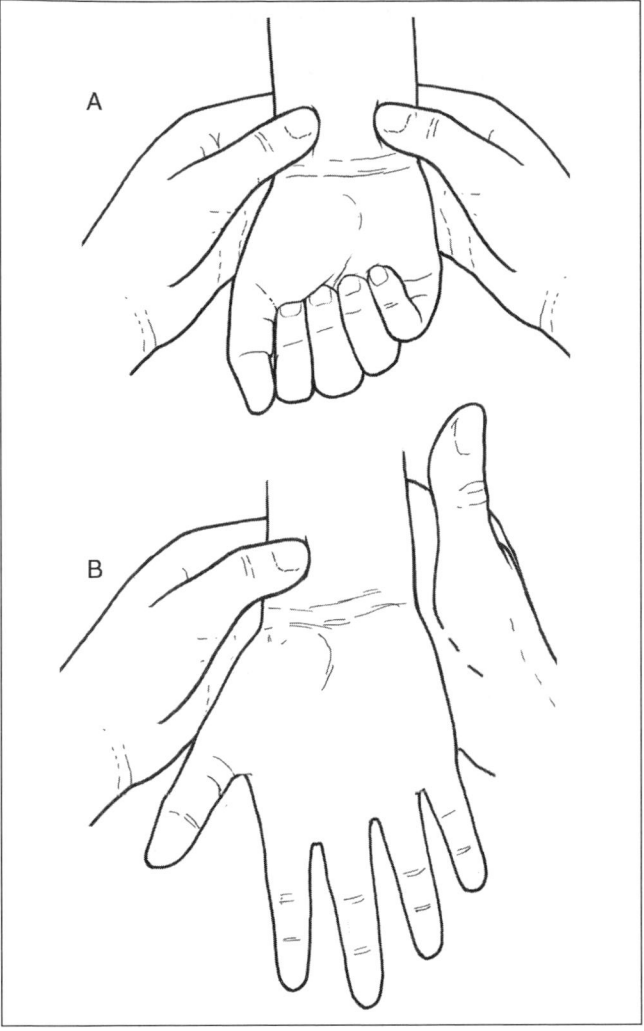

FIGURE 46-2 The modified Allen test. *A.* The distal radial and ulnar arteries are occluded. *B.* The radial artery remains occluded while determining if the ulnar artery can supply adequate blood flow to the hand.

available prepackaged kits are available for arterial puncture and arterial cannulation. These kits are complete and contain all the required equipment. Also available are individually packaged heparinized ABG syringes and arterial line catheters in various sizes.

PATIENT PREPARATION

Explain the procedure, its risks, and benefits to the patient and/or their representative. Obtain an informed consent unless the procedure is being performed emergently or the patient is unable to give consent. Identify by palpation the arterial pulse at the intended skin puncture site. Clean the skin of any dirt and debris. Cleanse the skin with an antiseptic (alcohol, chlorhexidine, or povidone iodine solution).

The use of a local anesthetic agent may greatly aid in the process of arterial puncture or cannulation. Infiltrate 1 mL of local anesthetic solution subcutaneously over the brachial artery, dorsalis pedis artery, or radial artery skin puncture site. Infiltrate 2 to 3 mL of local anesthetic solution subcutaneously over the femoral artery skin puncture site and into the subcutaneous tissues. Aspirate before infiltrating the local anesthetic solution to prevent inadvertent intravascular injection.

Descriptions of the anatomy for arterial puncture or cannulation sites are described in detail earlier in this chapter. The preferred site for the initial attempt at arterial puncture or cannulation is the radial artery.[1] Begin distally where the pulse is most palpable near the proximal wrist flexor crease. If the first attempt at needle or catheter introduction is unsuccessful, and the pulse is still palpable, reattempt the procedure more proximally along this same artery. The radial artery on the contralateral wrist is also a satisfactory second site for attempted access. Other acceptable second-attempt sites of access include the femoral, dorsalis pedis, and brachial arteries. **An attempt at ipsilateral ulnar artery catheterization is not advisable as both limbs of the hand's circulation may be compromised.** The discussion below focuses on puncture or cannulation of the radial and femoral arteries as over 90 percent of arterial punctures or cannulations occur at these sites.[1] The use of other sites generally follows the techniques described below for the radial artery with the exception of the regional anatomic differences. Other useable sites include the dorsal pedis, brachial, posterior tibial, and superficial temporal arteries.

TECHNIQUES

ARTERIAL PUNCTURE FOR A SINGLE SAMPLE

Position the patient to maximize exposure of the skin surface overlying the chosen artery. For the radial artery, this is best accomplished by dorsiflexing the wrist and supporting this position with a small towel rolled up under the dorsal wrist surface (Figure 46-5). For brachial and femoral artery puncture, ensure that the elbow or hip is extended fully. These positions provide maximum exposure and working area for the procedure. Locate the chosen artery, prep the overlying skin, and infiltrate local anesthetic solution subcutaneously.

Reidentify the pulse by palpation with the digits of the nondominant hand (Figure 46-6*A*). Grasp the heparinized syringe with the dominant hand. Withdraw the plunger of the syringe so that 1 to 3 mL of air space is available in the syringe. This will allow for easier assessment of arterial blood return. Insert the needle at a 30 to 45 degree angle to the skin and just above the arterial pulse (Figures 46-5 and 46-6). Advance the needle

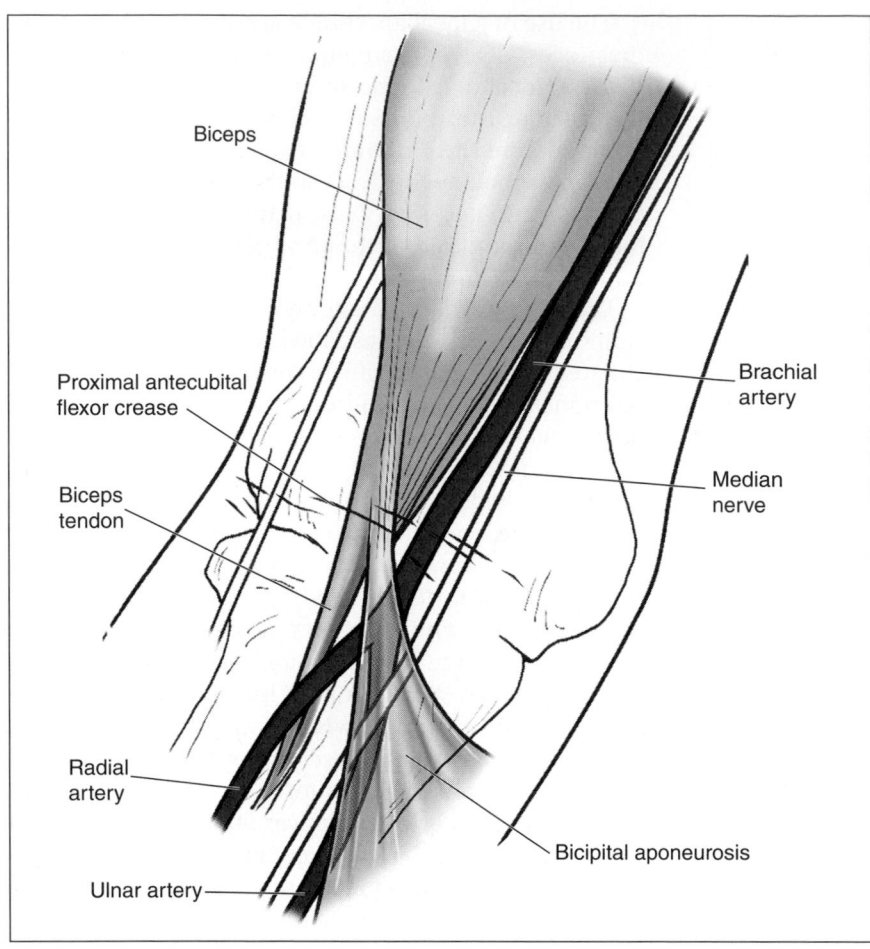

FIGURE 46-3 Anatomical location of the brachial artery. Note the median nerve running just medial to the artery and the biceps brachii muscle just lateral to the artery.

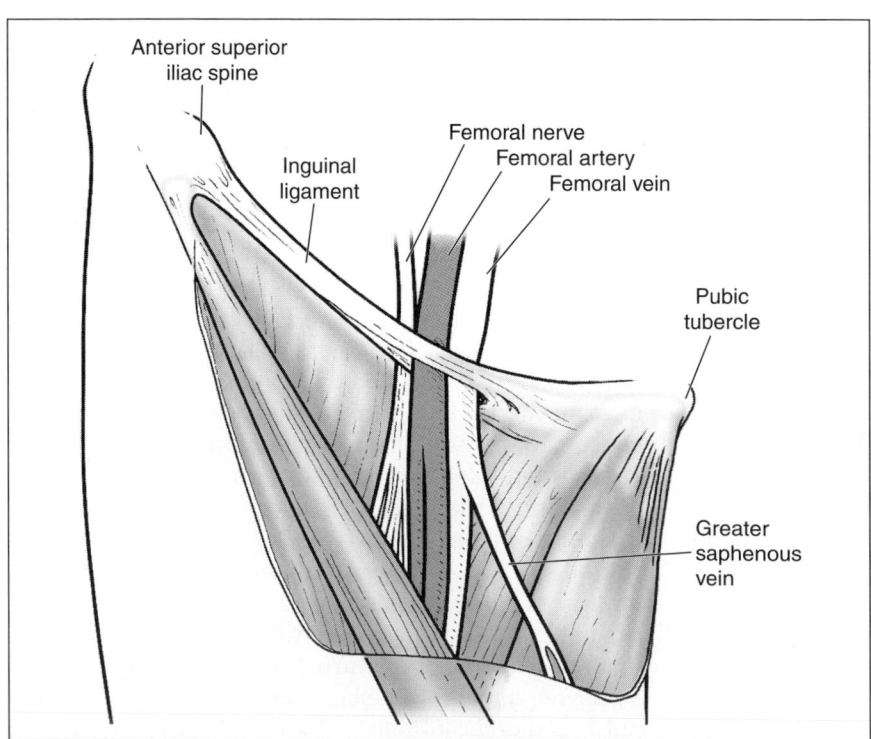

FIGURE 46-4 Anatomical location of the femoral artery. Note the proximity to the femoral nerve and vein.

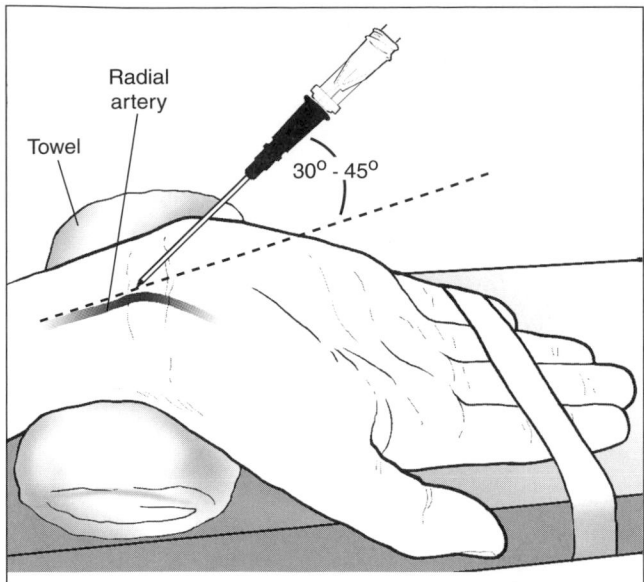

FIGURE 46-5 Correct positioning for radial artery puncture and cannulation. Dorsiflexing the wrist and supporting it with a small towel facilitates palpation of the artery and provides the maximum working space. The needle or catheter-over-the-needle is aimed toward the oncoming blood flow and at a 30 to 45 degree angle to the skin.

through the skin until blood enters the syringe (Figure 46-6B). The blood return will generally fill the syringe without necessitating withdrawal of the plunger in patients with a brisk pulse. If no blood return occurs, slowly withdraw the needle and watch for blood flow into the syringe. **If it is necessary to redirect the needle, it is imperative to first withdraw the needle until the tip is just below the skin surface before changing the angle in order to avoid lacerating the artery or adjacent structures.** To minimize the possibility of error due to the presence of heparin, it is necessary to collect at least 1 mL of blood in a prepackaged syringe or 3 mL of blood if preparing your own syringe with heparin.[5]

Withdraw the needle after the arterial sample has been collected. Apply pressure to the puncture site for 3 to 5 minutes followed by a bandage or gauze dressing applied over the wound. Carefully remove the needle from the syringe. Evacuate any air from the syringe and apply a cap on the syringe. Place the syringe on ice for immediate transportation to the laboratory. Recheck the skin puncture site in 5 to 10 minutes to assess for the formation of a hematoma and/or vascular compromise to the distal extremity.

RADIAL ARTERY CANNULATION: CATHETER-OVER-THE-NEEDLE TECHNIQUE

The most basic method, yet possibly the one associated with the lowest rate of successful cannulation, is direct introduction of the catheter-over-the-needle in a manner similar to that of inserting an intravenous

catheter (Figure 46-7).[13] Clean, prep, and identify the radial artery as described previously. Insert the catheter-over-the-needle at a 30 to 45 degree angle to the skin and directly over the arterial pulse. Advance the catheter-over-the-needle into the artery (Figure 46-7A). Bright red blood in the hub of the needle indicates that the tip of the needle is within the artery. Advance the catheter-over-the-needle another 1 to 2 mm to ensure that the catheter tip is within the arterial lumen. Securely hold the hub of the needle. Advance the catheter over the needle until its hub is against the skin (Figure 46-7B). Remove the needle and confirm pulsatile arterial flow from the hub of the catheter. Free-flowing, pulsatile blood confirms proper catheter placement within the artery. Apply a stopcock or intravenous extension tubing to the hub of the catheter. Secure the catheter to the skin. Apply a dressing to the skin puncture site.

RADIAL ARTERY CANNULATION: SELDINGER-TYPE, SINGLE ARTERIAL WALL PUNCTURE

The second technique for arterial cannulation is a Seldinger-type technique (catheter-over-the-wire) utilizing one of a number of prepackaged commercially available kits. A commercially available one-piece catheter-over-the-needle kit is very popular (Figure 46-8). Open the package, remove the unit, and remove the protective cover over the needle. Advance and retract the guidewire to confirm it moves smoothly and does not get caught on the needle. Retract the guidewire as far back as possible. Identify the arterial pulse with the nondominant hand. Insert the catheter-over-the-needle through the skin and into the artery using a slow and continuous forward motion (Figure 46-8A). A flash of blood in the hub of the needle confirms successful entry through the arterial wall and into the vessel lumen. Stabilize the catheter-over-the-needle.

Advance the guidewire through the needle by pushing the actuating lever as far as possible toward the needle (Figure 46-8B). **Immediately stop if resistance is encountered while advancing the guidewire. The guidewire may be within the artery wall or through the artery wall and into the perivascular tissue. Do not try to force the guidewire into the vessel. Do not retract the guidewire. Withdraw the entire unit and apply pressure to the puncture site to prevent a hematoma.** Obtain a new kit and repeat the procedure.

Once advanced, the guidewire is successfully within the arterial lumen. Firmly grasp the clear hub of the needle and advance the catheter over the guidewire and into the artery (Figure 46-8C). **A rotating motion of the catheter is often helpful to advance it if difficulty is encountered.** Securely hold the catheter at the level of the skin. While firmly holding the catheter hub, remove the guidewire, needle, and feed tube assembly as a unit. Free-flowing, pulsatile blood confirms proper catheter place-

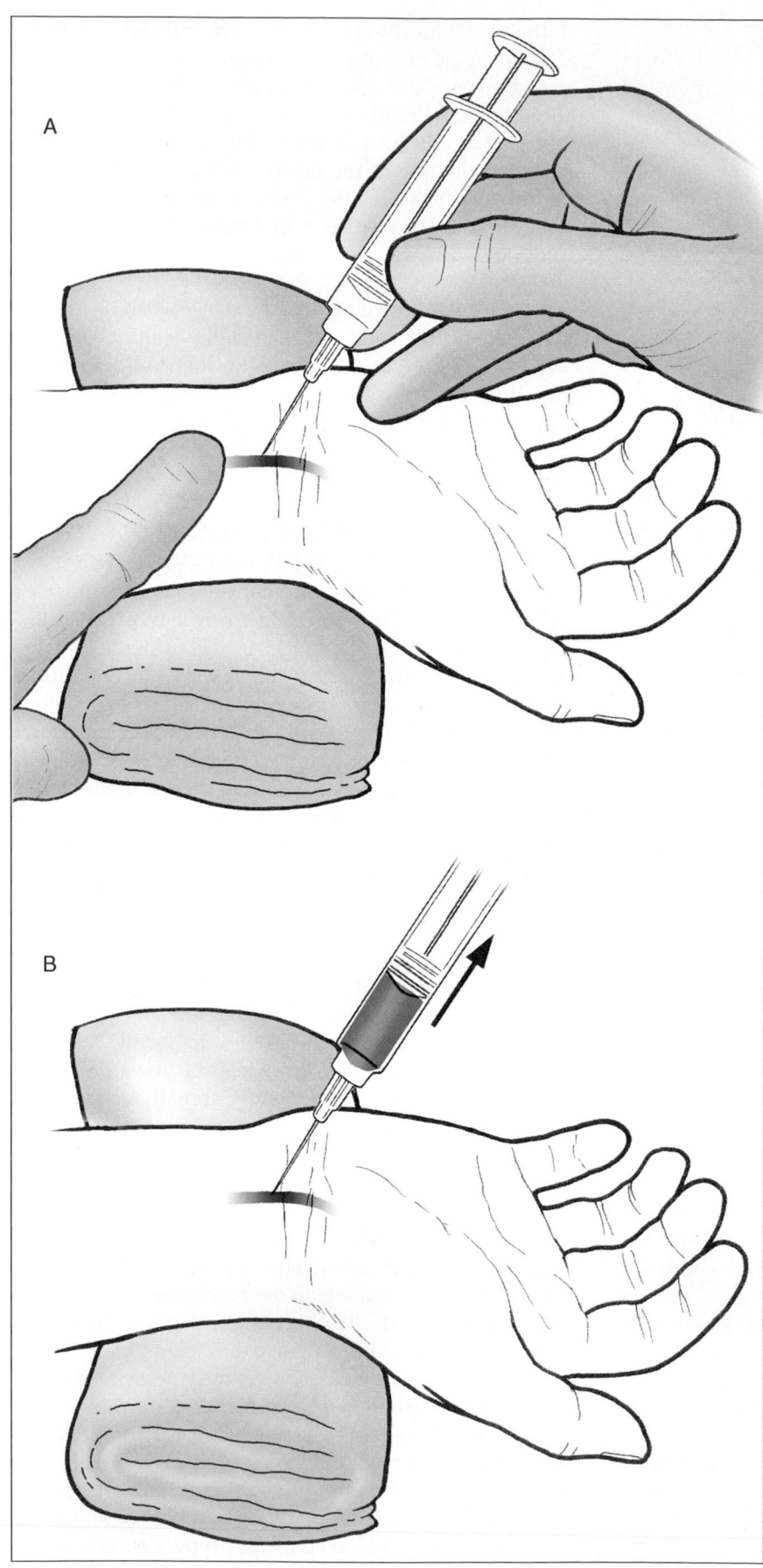

FIGURE 46-6 Radial artery puncture for an ABG sample. *A.* The pulse is palpated with the nondominant hand. The heparinized syringe is inserted at a 30 to 45 degree angle to the skin surface. *B.* Arterial blood fills the syringe.

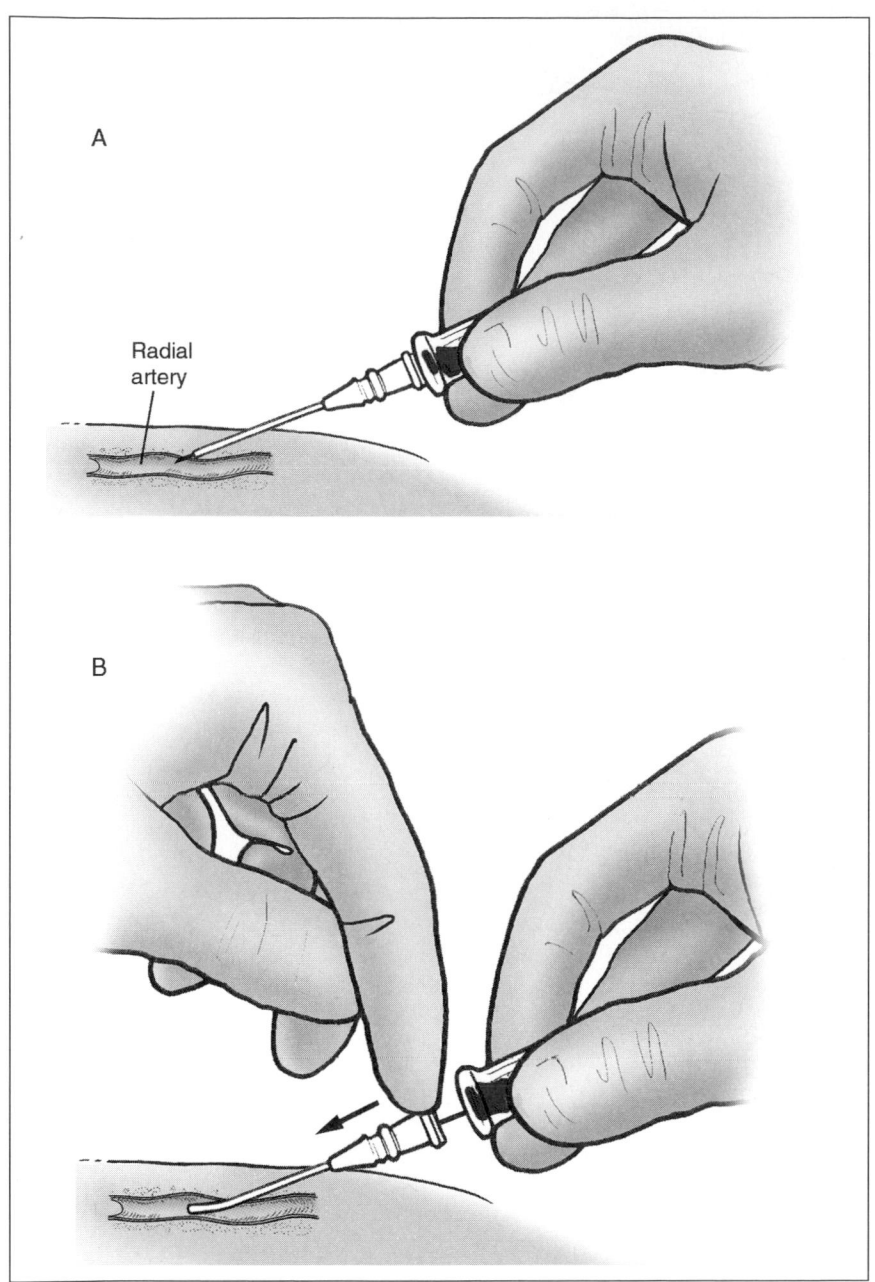

FIGURE 46-7 The catheter-over-the-needle technique for arterial cannulation. *A.* The unit is held at a 30 to 45 degree angle to the skin and advanced into the artery. *B.* The catheter is advanced over the needle and into the artery.

ment within the artery. Apply a stopcock or intravenous extension tubing to the hub of the catheter. Secure the catheter by suturing it to the skin. Apply a dressing to the skin puncture site.

A commercially available Seldinger-type catheter-over-the-needle kit is an alternative to the one-piece unit (Figure 46-9). Open the package and review the equipment it contains. Place the finder needle on the syringe. Withdraw the plunger 1 cm to break the bead of the syringe. Identify the arterial pulse. Insert the needle through the skin and into the artery using a slow and continuous forward motion (Figure 46-9*A*). A flash of blood in the syringe confirms successful entry through

the arterial wall and into the vessel lumen. Stabilize the needle and remove the syringe. Advance the guidewire through the needle (Figure 46-9*B*). The guidewire should advance without resistance. **Immediately stop if resistance is encountered while advancing the guidewire. The guidewire may be within the artery wall or through the artery wall and into the perivascular tissue. Do not try to force the guidewire into the vessel. Do not retract the guidewire. Withdraw the entire unit and apply pressure to the site to prevent a hematoma.** Obtain a new kit and repeat the procedure.

After the guidewire is inserted, withdraw the needle while leaving the guidewire in place (Figure 46-9*C*). **Do**

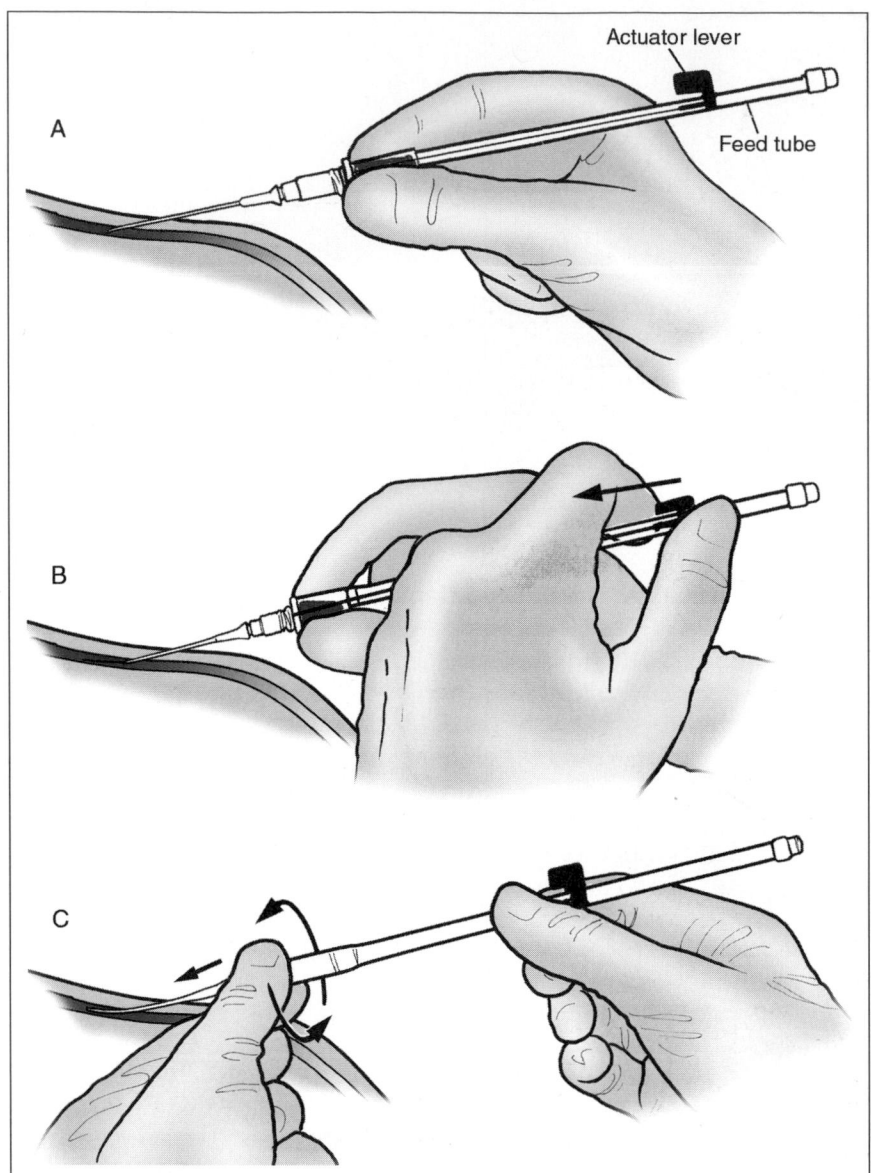

FIGURE 46-8 Catheter-over-the-needle technique using a commercially available one-piece unit. *A.* The catheter-over-the-needle is inserted into the artery. *B.* The guidewire is advanced through the needle and into the artery. *C.* The catheter is advanced over the guidewire and into the artery with a twisting motion.

not readvance the needle as it can shear off the guidewire. Make a 3 mm puncture wound next to the puncture site of the guidewire using a #11 scalpel blade to facilitate inserting the catheter (Figure 46-9*D*). **Use care to not cut the guidewire.** Thread the catheter over the guidewire. Advance the catheter over the guidewire until the hub of the catheter is against the skin (Figure 46-9*E*). **A rotating motion of the catheter is often helpful to advance it if difficulty is encountered.** Securely hold the catheter at the level of the skin. Remove the guidewire while firmly holding the catheter hub. Free-flowing, pulsatile blood confirms proper catheter placement within the artery. Apply a stopcock or intravenous extension tubing to the hub of the catheter. Secure the catheter by suturing it to the skin. Apply a dressing to the site.

RADIAL ARTERY CANNULATION: SELDINGER-TYPE, DOUBLE ARTERIAL WALL PUNCTURE

While localization and needle puncture of the artery is identical in all three techniques, commonly encountered difficulties include threading of the catheter with the first technique and threading of the guidewire into the true vessel lumen with the second technique. If the needle orifice is merely at the vessel edge, blood may enter and rise up through the needle. However, when trying to advance the catheter, it may get hung up outside the lumen with the catheter-over-the-needle technique.[14] The guidewire may not easily pass or may dissect into the vessel wall creating a false lumen when using the Seldinger-type single arterial wall puncture technique. Since pulsatile flow is more easily confirmed prior to the passage of the guidewire, this third tech-

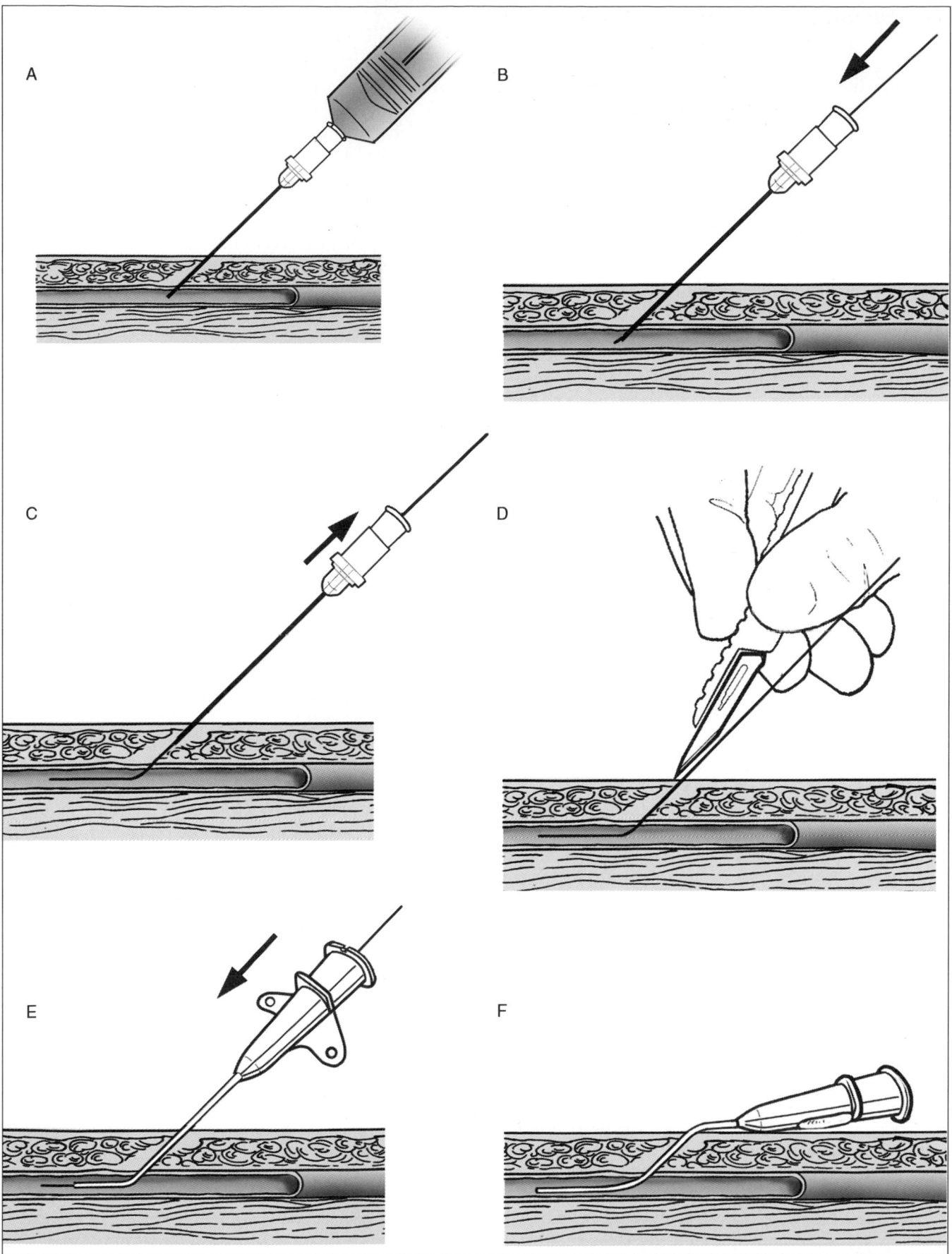

FIGURE 46-9 The Seldinger technique for arterial catheterization. *A.* The needle is inserted into the artery. *B.* The syringe has been removed from the needle. The guidewire is advanced through the needle and into the artery. *C.* The needle is removed while leaving the guidewire in place. *D.* The skin is punctured with a #11 scalpel blade to allow easy insertion of the catheter. *E.* The catheter is advanced over the guidewire and into the artery. *F.* The guidewire is removed.

nique in which both walls of the radial artery are punctured may offer an advantage in passing the guidewire and catheter into the true arterial lumen.

It is imperative that the physician assumes a position out of the trajectory line of the catheter to avoid being sprayed with blood when using this technique. This method is also a Seldinger-type technique that utilizes a guidewire separate from the catheter-over-the-needle. Locate the arterial pulse and insert the catheter-over-the-needle into the artery. Immediately advance the catheter-over-the-needle through the posterior wall of the artery as confirmed by no blood exiting the needle hub. Withdraw the needle leaving the catheter in place through the artery. Flatten the angle of the catheter to the skin to less than 30 degrees. Hold the tip of the guidewire poised at the hub of the catheter. Slowly withdraw the catheter with the nondominant hand. Promptly insert the guidewire through the catheter and into the artery when pulsatile blood flow is noted from the hub of the catheter. Advance the catheter over the guidewire and into the lumen of the artery. Withdraw the guidewire and apply a stopcock or intravenous extension tubing.

This double-puncture technique for cannulation theoretically may be associated with greater vascular damage. The technique should be reserved for instances in which the prior two arterial cannulation techniques have been unsuccessful. However, in an analysis of the complications associated with various techniques of peripheral artery cannulation, investigators found no difference in complications when using this technique.[13]

FEMORAL ARTERY CANNULATION

The femoral artery may be cannulated if the radial artery is inaccessible or attempts at cannulation are unsuccessful. Slightly abduct the leg and identify the femoral artery pulse. Prep, drape, and anesthetize the skin and subcutaneous tissues. Maintain the fingers of the nondominant hand on the arterial pulse. Insert the needle or the catheter-over-the-needle at a 45 degree angle to the skin with the needle bevel pointing superiorly. The remainder of the technique is as described previously.

ALTERNATIVE TECHNIQUE

A cutdown technique may be performed to cannulate an artery. This technique is primarily used for the brachial or radial arteries but may be used to access other peripheral arteries. Clean, prep, anesthetize, and drape the skin overlying the chosen artery. Make a 1.5 to 2.0 cm transverse skin incision centered over the artery. **Do not cut into the subcutaneous tissue so that blood vessels, nerves, and tendons are not transected.** Spread the subcutaneous tissues parallel to the artery with a mosquito hemostat. Expose 1.0 cm of the length of the

artery. Pass a silk suture under the proximal end of the exposed artery. Insert a catheter-over-the-needle through the skin just distal to the incision and advance it into the incision. Elevate the suture to control the artery and occlude distal blood flow. Advance the catheter-over-the-needle into the artery. Release the suture and advance the catheter into the artery. The remainder of the procedure is as described previously. Apply pressure over the incision site for 5 to 10 minutes to prevent the formation of a hematoma or seroma.

AFTERCARE

Apply direct pressure for 3 to 5 minutes to the skin puncture site after an arterial puncture or removal of an arterial catheter. Direct pressure should be applied for 10 minutes or more if the patient has a bleeding diathesis or has received thrombolytic therapy. Apply a bandage or gauze dressing to the skin puncture site. Reassess the skin puncture site in 15 minutes for continued bleeding or hematoma formation.

An arterial catheter must be secured to the skin to prevent inadvertent dislodgement, hematoma formation, and exsanguination. Sew the hub of the catheter to the skin using 3–0 or 4–0 nylon sutures. Apply a protective dressing over the site. A splinting device should be used to secure the limb in the desired position for optimal monitoring if the catheter is in the wrist, arm, or foot. The site should be monitored regularly to assess for signs of bleeding, infection, hematoma, arterial thrombosis, or catheter dislodgement. It is also important to assess the extremity distal to the catheter for evidence of ischemia. The dressing should be replaced regularly in accordance with individual institutional guidelines.

COMPLICATIONS

Arterial puncture and catheterization are generally safe procedures with an incidence of clinically significant complications under 5 percent.[1] The primary complications of arterial catheterization are infection, bleeding, and arterial injury/thrombosis.[2,18–27] While secondary bacteremia and septic emboli may occur, infection is usually limited to the site of catheterization. The risk of catheter site infection is linearly related to the length of time the catheter is in place.[2] Nerve injury from direct puncture of the nerve has been reported in connection with arterial puncture or cannulation.[15] Multiple cases of neuropathy have occurred as a result of a hematoma formation and subsequent nerve compression.[16] In order to minimize hematoma formation after arterial puncture or arterial catheter removal, apply at least 3 minutes of direct pressure to radial, brachial, and dorsalis pedis puncture sites and 5 to 10 minutes of pressure to the femoral site.[15,17] Although small hematomas are common after arterial puncture, major bleeding is unusual and generally occurs only in the concealed retroperitoneum after femoral artery puncture or cannulation. Angiographically demonstrable thrombosis is common (25 to 40 percent) after prolonged arterial catheterization.[2] This rarely results in clinically significant morbidity. Secondary limb ischemia and necrosis requiring amputation occurs in less than 1:2000 arterial catheterizations.[2] Other rare complications include the formation of a pseudoaneurysm or arteriovenous fistula.

SUMMARY

Arterial puncture and cannulation are quick, safe, and simple to perform. Arterial blood sampling may aid in determining the ventilatory and acid-base status of critically ill patients. An arterial catheter is appropriate in patients who need continuous monitoring of arterial blood pressure or frequent ABGs. Arterial puncture and cannulation should be avoided in skin areas with evidence of burn, trauma, infection, severe dermatitis, or severe peripheral vascular disease. Palpation of the arterial pulse and correct anatomical positioning are necessary before these procedures are attempted. It is necessary to monitor the cannulated site for signs of bleeding, hematoma, thrombosis, or infection. After an arterial puncture or removal of an arterial catheter, it is necessary to apply direct pressure to the skin puncture site.

REFERENCES

1. Lodato RF: Arterial pressure monitoring, in Tobin MJ (ed): *Principles and Practice of Intensive Care Monitoring.* New York: McGraw-Hill, 1998:733–747.

2. Schlichtig RI: Arterial catheterization: complications, in Tobin MJ (ed): *Principles and Practice of Intensive Care Monitoring.* New York: McGraw-Hill, 1998:751–756.

3. Pillow K, Herrick IA: Pulse oximetry compared with Doppler ultrasound for assessment of collateral blood flow to the hand. *Anaesthesia* 1991; 46:388–390.

4. Slogoff S, Keats A, Arlund C: On the safety of radial artery cannulation. *Anesthesiology* 1983; 59(1):42–47.

5. AARC Clinical Practice Guidelines: Sampling for arterial blood gas analysis. *Respir Care* 1992; 37(8):913–917.

6. National Committee for Clinical Laboratory Standards: *Procedures for the Collection of Diagnostic Blood Specimens by Skin Puncture*, 3rd ed. Pennsylvania: NCCLS, 1992.

7. Gravenstein N, Good ML, Banner TE: Assessment of cardiopulmonary function, in Vobryys ZKZ, Ysupt TE, Zkitny TT (eds): *Critical Care*, 3rd ed. Philadelphia: Lippincott-Raven, 1997:867–898.

8. Rodriguez RM, Light R: Capnography in the ICU; when and how to monitor carbon dioxide levels noninvasively. *J Crit Illness* 1998; 13(6):372–378.

9. Brandenburg MA, Dire DJ: Comparison of arterial and venous blood gas values in the initial emergency department evaluation of patients with diabetic ketoacidosis. *Ann Emerg Med* 1998; 31:459–465.

10. Markowitz, DH, Irwin RS: Evaluating acid-base disorders: is venous blood gas testing sufficient? *J Crit Illness* 1999; 14(7):403–406.

11. Touger M, Gallagher EJ, Tyrell J: Relationship between venous and arterial carboxyhemoglobin levels in patients with suspected carbon monoxide poisoning. *Ann Emerg Med* 1995; 25(4):481–483.

12. Goodwin NM, Schreiber MT: Effects of anticoagulants on acid-base and blood gas estimations. *Crit Care Med* 1979; 7:473.

13. Jones RM, Hill AB, Nahrwold ML, et al: The effect of method of radial artery cannulation on postcannulation blood flow and thrombus formation. *Anesthesiology* 1981; 55(1):76–78.

14. Beards SC, Doedens L, Jackson A, et al: A comparison of arterial lines and insertion techniques in critically ill patients. *Anaesthesia* 1994; 49:968–973.

15. Okeson GC, Wulbrecht PH: The safety of brachial artery puncture for arterial blood sampling. *Chest* 1998; 114(3):748–751.

16. Nevasier RJ, Adams JP, May GI: Complications of arterial puncture in anticoagulated patients. *J Bone Joint Surg Am* 1976; 35:1118–1123.

17. Chen HE, Foster CL: Arterial and venous access, in Chen HE, Sola JE, Lillemoe KD (eds): *Manual of Common Bedside Surgical Procedures.* Baltimore: Williams & Wilkins, 1996:30–76.

18. Sladen A: Complications of invasive hemodynamic monitoring in the intensive care unit. *Curr Probl Surg* 1988; 25:69–145.

19. Johnson FE, Sumner DS, Strandness DE Jr: Extremity necrosis caused by indwelling arterial catheters. *Am J Surg* 1976; 131(3):375–379.

20. Frezza EE, Mezghebe H: Indications and complications of arterial catheter use in surgical or medical intensive care units: analysis of 4932 patients. *Am Surg* 1998; 64(2):127–131.

21. Clarke SL: Arterial lines: an analysis of good practice. *J Child Health Care* 1999; 3(1):23–27.

22. Downs JB, Rackstein AD, Klein EF: Hazards of radial-artery catheterization. *Anesthesiology* 1973; 38(3):283–286.

23. Clark VL, Kruse JA: Arterial catheterization. *Crit Care Clin* 1992; 8(4):687–697.

24. Fuhrman TM, Reilley TE, Pippin WD: Comparison of digital blood pressure, plethysmography, and the modified Allen's test as means of evaluating the collateral circulation to the hand. *Anaesthesia* 1992; 47:959–961.

25. Spittell JA Jr, Juergens JL, Fairbairn JF II: Radial artery puncture and the Allen test. *Ann Intern Med* 1987; 106(5):771–772.

26. Bedford RF, Wollman H: Complications of percutaneous radial-artery cannulation: an objective prospective study in man. *Anesthesiology* 1973; 38(3):228–236.

27. Barker WJ: Arterial puncture and cannulation, in Roberts JR, Hedges JR (eds): *Clinical Procedures in Emergency Medicine*, 3rd ed. Philadelphia: Saunders, 1998:308–322.

Section Four

GASTROINTESTINAL PROCEDURES

Chapter 47
NASOGASTRIC
INTUBATION

Robert R. Leschke

INTRODUCTION

Nasogastric intubation is one of the common procedures performed in Emergency Departments in the United States.[1] Its use as a conduit into the stomach was first popularized in the early twentieth century mainly through the efforts of Levin. Since then, clinicians have studied its use and have proposed methods to improve the ease with which the tube is inserted as well as ways to diminish the incidence of potentially lethal complications. A nasogastric tube is often placed in patients who have a bowel obstruction, intractable nausea and vomiting, intoxication, significant trauma, and upper gastrointestinal bleeding. The procedure is rapid, simple, and straightforward.

ANATOMY AND PATHOPHYSIOLOGY

The nasal cavity is lined by the very vascular nasal mucosa. The medial wall of the nasal cavity is composed of the septum. The lateral wall of the nasal cavity is covered by the turbinates. The posterior nasal cavities are continuous with the nasopharynx that develops into the posterior oropharynx as you move caudally (Figure 47-1). The oropharynx continues inferiorly as the esophagus that enters the stomach below the diaphragm.[2]

The placement of a nasogastric tube in children is often difficult. Their large tonsils and adenoids may hinder the passage of the nasogastric tube. These tissues are soft, easily injured, and may bleed as the nasogastric tube is passed. The tongue, large by comparison with adults, may push into the oropharynx and impede passage of the nasogastric tube. Their nostrils and nasal passage are quite small and limit the size of nasogastric tube that may be passed.

INDICATIONS

Nasogastric intubation may be performed for diagnostic or therapeutic indications. A nasogastric tube may be inserted to instill air into the stomach to assess for an intraperitoneal perforation. It is used to evaluate the presence, rapidity, and volume of an upper gastrointestinal hemorrhage. Gastric fluid and contents may be aspirated for laboratory analysis. It may also be placed to visualize the stomach on chest radiography to assess for a diaphragmatic hernia. A nasogastric tube is placed in patients for medication administration, relief of a bowel obstruction, treatment of recurrent vomiting, and to perform gastric lavage. They are placed preoperatively, postintubation, prior to a diagnostic peritoneal lavage, or prior to a pericardiocentesis to decompress the stomach.

CONTRAINDICATIONS

Absolute contraindications do not exist for nasogastric tube placement. The relative contraindications are geared toward predicting which patients are more likely to experience complications and which patients are likely to have misplaced tubes. Insertion of a nasogastric tube should be avoided, unless necessary, in the patient with midface trauma. Intubation through the nasal cavity can result in the nasogastric tube being misdirected blindly into the respiratory tract or the rare perforation through the thin cribriform plate of the ethmoid bone and into the brain. Patients with facial trauma are best served with orogastric intubation.[3] Patients with esophageal varices pose potential problems. Placement of a semi-rigid tube into the esophagus or stomach has the potential to cause rupture of the

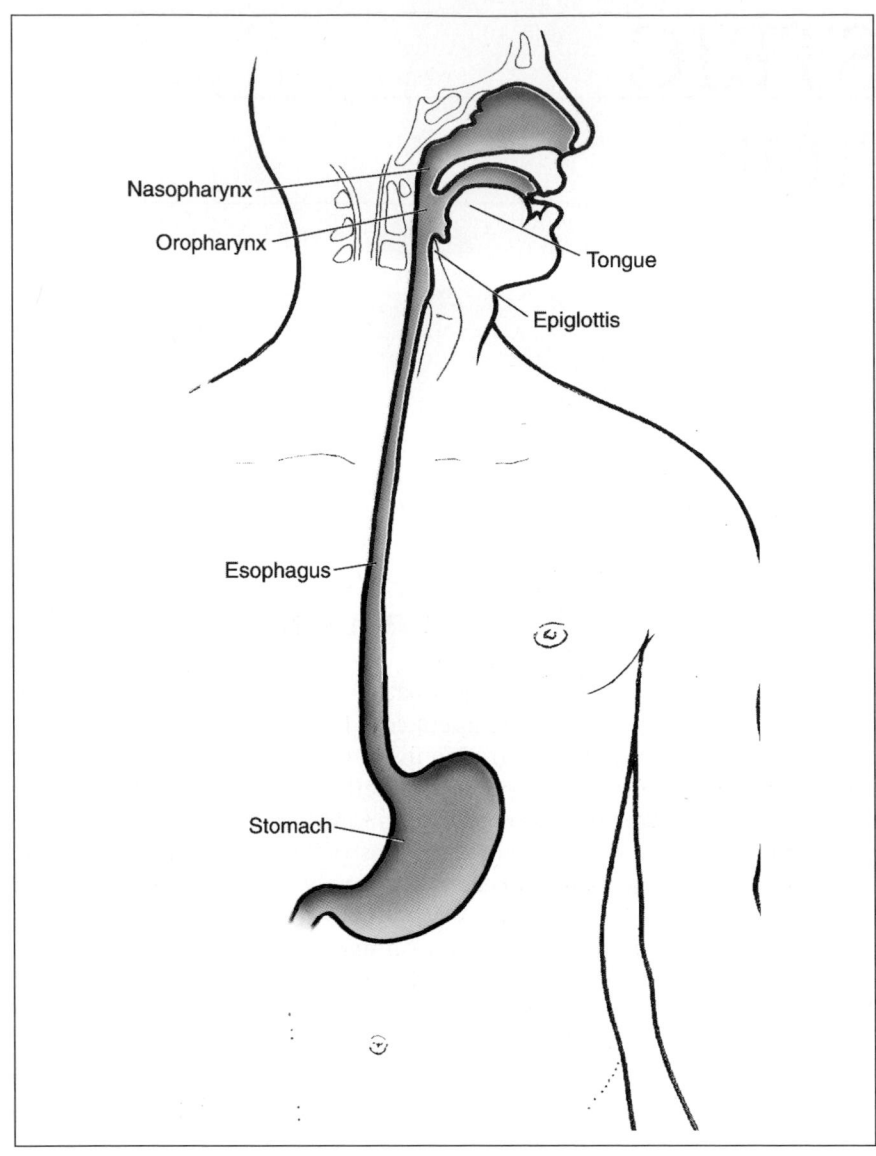

FIGURE 47-1   Basic anatomy of the path of the nasogastric tube.

varices and uncontrollable hemorrhage. Other relative contraindications include patients with coagulopathies, esophageal strictures, ingestions of alkaline substances, nasal obstruction, or recent nasal surgery.

EQUIPMENT

Topical anesthetic (benzocaine spray, cocaine, viscous lidocaine)
Topical vasoconstrictor (phenylephrine, oxymetazoline, cocaine)
Glass of water with straw
Emesis basin
Water-based lubricant
Nasogastric tube
60 mL syringe
Wall suction, set to low intermittent suction
Suction tubing
Benzoin spray
1 inch adhesive tape

Choose a size of nasogastric tube that is appropriate for the patient. A size 16 to 18 French is typically used for an adolescent or adult patient. A formula ([age in years + 16] ÷ 2) may be used to choose the proper size nasogastric tube for children. Typical sizes include 8 French for infants, 10 to 12 French for small children, and 12 to 14 French for older children.

Nasogastric tubes are usually made of clear polypropylene. They are somewhat rigid and single patient use devices. Typically used are the Levin tube and the Salem Sump tube. They both have multiple distal sideports. The Levin tube is a single-lumen tube that is easy to insert. It is simple to use for the aspiration of gastric contents, the instillation of fluids and/or medications, and the application of low intermittent suction. The tube is nonradiopaque. Unfortunately, the amount of suction is difficult to control with the Levin tube. The distal sideports often become occluded with the gastric mucosa, and damage this tissue, when the tube is attached to suction. The Salem Sump tube is a double-lumen, radiopaque tube. It has a smaller suction lumen than the Levin tube. The second lumen allows a constant inward airflow to prevent the sideports from becoming occluded by the gastric mucosa.

PATIENT PREPARATION

The most beneficial factor in the successful placement of a nasogastric tube is a patient who is informed of the procedure and can cooperate with the instructions. Take the patient through each step prior to the start of the procedure to ensure maximal cooperation. Drape the patient to protect them and the bedding from soilage if there is emesis. A glass of water and a straw should be within reach, as should an emesis basin.

Place the patient seated upright in the Fowler's or semi-Fowler's position. Examine the patient for nasal septal deviation or other anatomic abnormalities that may hinder the passage of the nasogastric tube. Ask the patient to breathe through one nostril while the other nostril is occluded to determine which nostril is the most patent.[4] A recent study suggests that the application of topical lidocaine and phenylephrine to the nose and benzocaine spray to the throat resulted in significantly less pain and discomfort than the use of lubricant alone.[5] The patient should be screened for allergies and contraindications, such as hypertension, if these adjuncts are to be used. A sample protocol would include the instillation of 0.5% phenylephrine nasal spray followed by viscous lidocaine. Cetacaine spray can be used to anesthetize the nose and the throat.[4]

Estimate the length of the nasogastric tube to be inserted (Figure 47-2). Place the tip of the nasogastric tube on the patient's xiphoid process and extend it to the tip of the nose and over the earlobe (Figure 47-2A). Mark this distance with a piece of tape.[4] Alternatively, place the tip of the nasogastric tube on the tip of the nose or lip and extend it over the left ear and to just below the left costal margin (Figure 47-2B). Mark this distance with a piece of tape.[4]

TECHNIQUE

Lubricate the first 4 inches (10 cm) of the nasogastric tube with water-soluble lubricant. Position the patient. Place the neck in slight flexion. Gently introduce the nasogastric tube along the floor of the nostril (Figure

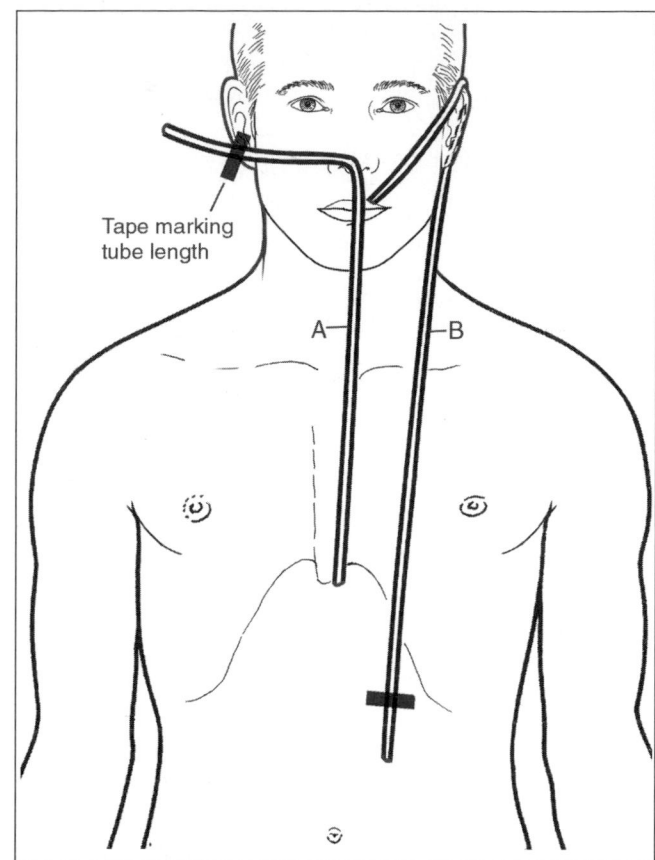

FIGURE 47-2 Determining the proper length of nasogastric tube to insert. *A.* The length is determined by the distance from the xiphoid process to the tip of the nose to the earlobe. *B.* The length is determined by the distance from the tip of the nose or lip to around the left ear and to just below the left costal margin. A piece of tape should be used to mark the distance on the nasogastric tube.

47-3A). Advance the nasogastric tube parallel to the nasal floor until it reaches the nasopharynx as indicated by mild resistance (Figure 47-3A). Do not insert and advance the nasogastric tube in an upward or lateral direction to prevent impingement and damage to the turbinates. Instruct the patient to swallow. This may be assisted by having the patient sip water through a straw. Advance the nasogastric tube (Figure 47-3B). Advancement may be aided by rotating the nasogastric tube medially. **Withdraw the nasogastric tube if at any time resistance, respiratory distress, the inability to speak, or significant nasal hemorrhage occurs.**[5]

Advance the nasogastric tube until the distance previously measured with the tape is at the nostril (Figure 47-4). Verify proper placement by aspirating stomach contents, by auscultating a rush of air over the stomach while 60 mL of air is insufflated through the nasogastric tube, or by radiographically demonstrating the tip of the nasogastric tube in the stomach and below the diaphragm. The latter is the most reliable and should be

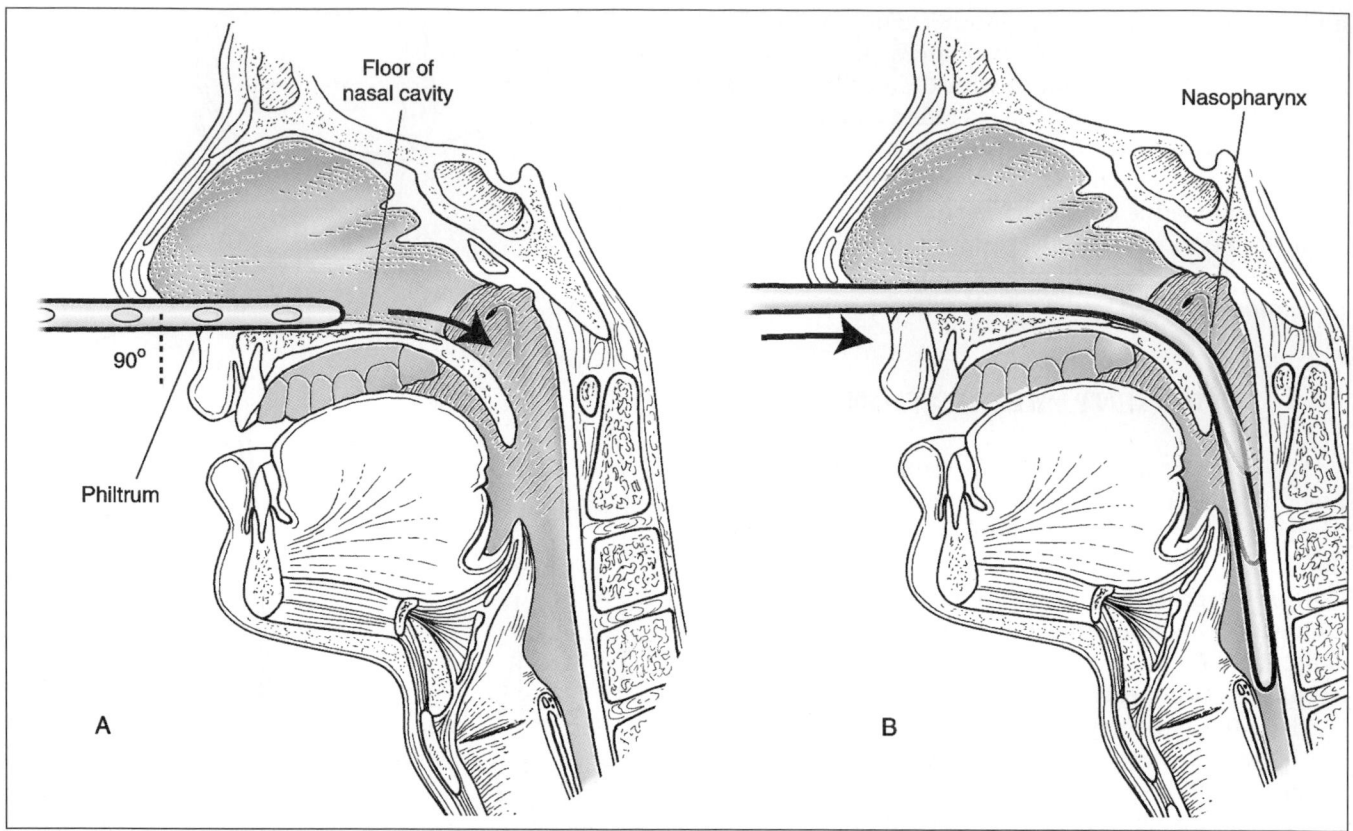

FIGURE 47-3   Insertion of the nasogastric tube. *A.* The nasogastric tube is inserted parallel to the floor of the nasal cavity and at a 90 degree angle to the philtrum. *B.* The tube is advanced along the floor of the nasal cavity, through the nasopharynx and oropharynx, and into the esophagus. The tube is further advanced until the tape mark is at the philtrum.

strongly considered when the nasogastric tube is to be used for medication administration or alimentation.[6] Infusion of substances through a misplaced nasogastric tube could be disastrous. Apply benzoin to the patient's nose. Apply tape to the nose and around the nasogastric tube to secure it in place (Figure 47-5). Attach the nasogastric tube to wall suction.

HELPFUL HINTS

One study attempted to improve the success rate of nasogastric tube placement by providing external and medially directed pressure on the ipsilateral neck at the level of the thyrohyoid membrane.[7] This maneuver will collapse the piriform sinus and eliminate it as a potential site for impaction. This maneuver was successful for difficult nasogastric intubation in 85 percent of patients.

The nasogastric tube may coil in the oropharynx, mouth, or hypopharynx. Cool the tube in cold tap water or ice water for 5 minutes to make the tube stiffer and then reinsert it. A larger bore tube may be inserted and may not coil. A final option is to place several fingers through the patient's mouth and into the oropharynx. The fingers can be used to guide the tube against the posterior oropharyngeal wall and into the hypopharynx.

Do not attempt this unless the patient is unconscious or paralyzed to prevent them from biting the fingers.

The nasogastric tube may easily pass into the hypopharynx but not be able to be passed into the stomach. The tip of the tube may be caught at the level of the cricopharyngeus muscle, behind the left mainstem bronchus, or at the lower esophageal sphincter. Attempt to pass a nasogastric tube that has been cooled with ice water. Grasp the thyroid cartilage and lift it anterior and upward to open the esophagus and allow passage of the nasogastric tube through the upper esophagus.

An orotracheally intubated patient requires a nasogastric tube to decompress the stomach. Unfortunately, one cannot always be passed into the stomach. Remove the respiratory adapter from the proximal end of a second endotracheal tube. Liberally lubricate the endotracheal tube and insert it through the patient's mouth and into the esophagus. Insert a well-lubricated nasogastric tube through the endotracheal tube and into the stomach. Confirm the proper position of the nasogastric tube. Carefully withdraw the endotracheal tube over the nasogastric tube.

The risk for tube misplacement is greater in the intubated patient who is unable to assist with nasogastric in-

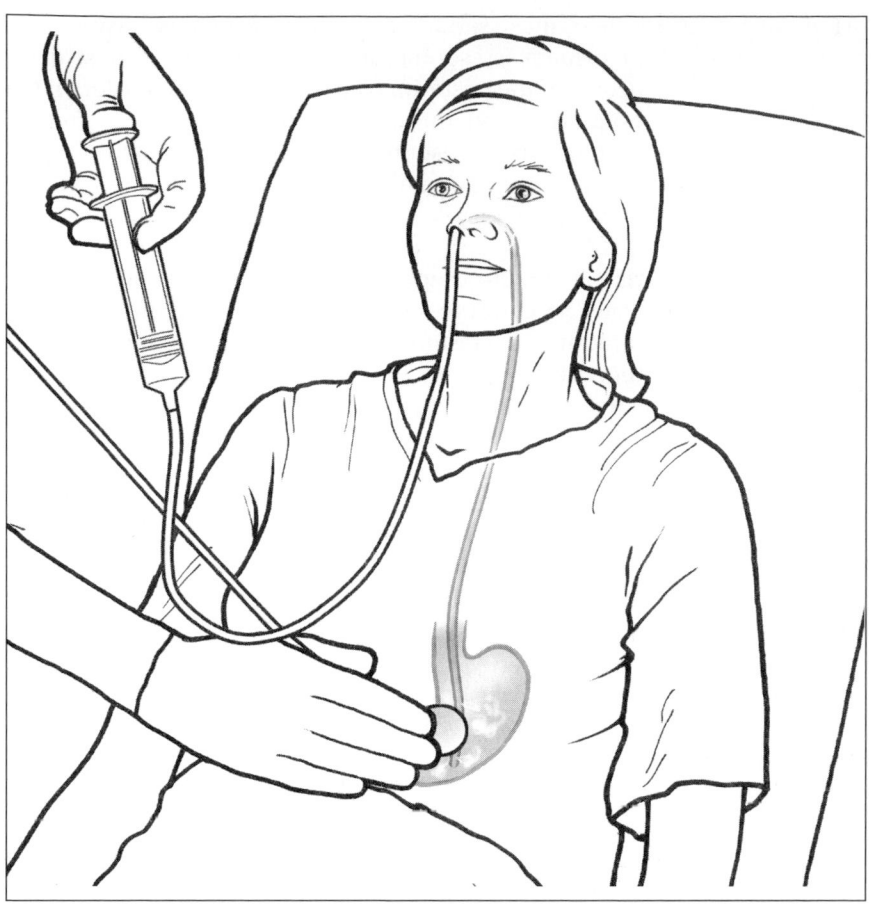

FIGURE 47-4 Proper placement of the nasogastric tube. The tip of the tube resides within the stomach. To confirm proper placement, inject air through the nasogastric tube while simultaneously auscultating over the stomach.

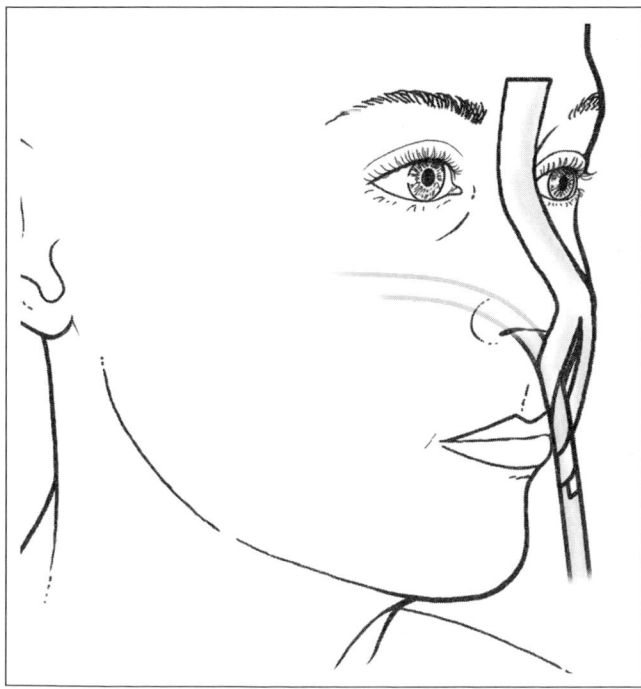

FIGURE 47-5 Securing the nasogastric tube. Apply tincture of benzoin to the bridge of the nose. A piece of tape is attached to the nose with the distal end split into two and intertwined over the tube.

tubation. Observe that the nasogastric tube does not come out of the patient's mouth and that there are no changes in the patient's oxygen saturation when inserting the nasogastric tube. It is very easy for the nasogastric tube to pass by the cuff of an endotracheal tube without much resistance.[7] **It is paramount that correct placement of the nasogastric tube is verified before it is used to instill any fluid or medication.** This may be done radiographically.

ASSESSMENT

The patient should be able to speak without respiratory distress immediately after placement of the nasogastric tube. Observe the patient for complaints of neck pain, substernal chest pain, dysphagia, drooling, trismus, fever, or subcutaneous and mediastinal air. These would be signs of esophageal perforation or errant placement of the nasogastric tube.[6] Although auscultation of air in the stomach has been classically used to determine correct placement, air insufflated into the pleural space or the esophagus after misplacement of the tube can be just as easily heard over the upper abdomen.[6] Gastric contents should be able to be aspirated through the nasogastric tube. Testing the pH of the gastric contents can help predict the placement of the nasogastric tube. The pH of the aspirated fluid will be ≥ 7 in 99 percent of patients if the nasogastric tube is in the respiratory tree.[8] The pH of the aspirated fluid will be ≤ 5 in 70 percent of the patients if the tube was correctly placed in the stomach. The use of H_2 blockers makes the assessment of gastric pH difficult. Radiographic demonstration of the tube in the antral or fundal portion of the stomach is the preferred method of confirmation.[9]

NASOGASTRIC TUBE REMOVAL

Explain to the patient the procedure and what they will experience as the nasogastric tube is removed. Place the patient in the Fowler's or semi-Fowler's position. Place towels or pads over the patient's neck and chest. Have an emesis basin and tissues immediately available. Disconnect the nasogastric tube from suction. Fold over the proximal end of the nasogastric tube and hold it tightly. Ask the patient to slightly flex their neck, breath in, and hold it. Place a drape around the nasogastric tube as it is exiting the patient's nose. Briskly withdraw the nasogastric tube through the drape. Discard the nasogastric tube and the drape.

COMPLICATIONS

The most common complication of nasogastric intubation is discomfort in the nasopharynx and oropharynx. Placement in the nares can result in epistaxis if the nasal mucosa is irritated, abraded, or ulcerated. These complications can be reduced or avoided with generous lubrication of the nasogastric tube and the instillation of topical anesthetics and vasoconstrictors. Sinusitis may occur from the nasogastric tube obstructing the sinus ostia. These complications are usually of no clinical significance.

A more serious consequence of nasogastric intubation is misplacement into the respiratory tree. This is estimated to occur in up to 15 percent of cases.[10] The incidence increases in frequency with the patient who has a diminished gag reflex or a decreased level of consciousness. **The presence of a cuffed endotracheal tube does not preclude passage into the respiratory tree.** The nasogastric tube will pass the cuff of the endotracheal tube without significant resistance. Advancing the tube into the airway can result in perforation of a bronchus or the lung and result in a pneumothorax, hydropneumothorax, pulmonary hemorrhage, empyema, or bronchopulmonary fistula.[10] These complications are increased if medication or alimentation is infused into the respiratory tree.

The most serious complication of nasogastric tube placement is esophageal perforation. This most often occurs in the posterior wall of the cervical portion of the esophagus and through the cricopharyngeus muscle. Risk factors for esophageal perforation include a preexisting esophageal abnormality, altered mental status, cervical osteophytes, cardiomegaly, tracheal intubation, a stiff nasogastric tube, and multiple attempts.[6] Other risk factors for esophageal perforation include esophageal cancer or the ingestion of alkaline substances. Perforation often results in mediastinitis with a subsequent mortality rate of up to 30 percent.[6] Prompt recognition, surgical repair, and parenteral antibiotics can reduce the mortality rate to less than 10 percent. The use of softer and smaller nasogastric tubes with generous lubrication can reduce the risk of esophageal perforation.

Use caution when inserting a nasogastric tube in patients who have suffered trauma to the face and/or skull. Fractures of the base of the skull, cribriform plate, maxilla, nasal walls, orbital floors, and palate may allow a nasally inserted tube to exit the nasal cavity and cause further injury.

SUMMARY

Nasogastric intubation is a widely used procedure in the Emergency Department. It is primarily used to evacuate air and stomach contents in the poisoned, intubated, or obstructed patient. Placement is generally considered easy, though it can be uncomfortable. Recent studies suggest that topical anesthetics and vasoconstrictors, along with generous lubrication, can diminish the discomfort and reduce the chance of misplacement.

Placement of the nasogastric tube into the airway or coiled in the esophagus can result in serious complications. Although auscultation of air has been classically used to determine correct placement, radiographic confirmation of gastric placement is considered the gold standard. Postintubation patients should be carefully observed for signs of esophageal perforation.

REFERENCES

1. McGaig LF, Stussman BJ: *National Hospital Ambulatory Medical Care Survey: 1996 Emergency Department Summary. Advanced Data from Vital Health Statistics; No. 293.* Rockville, MD: National Center for Health Statistics, 1997; DHSS publication no. (PHS) 98-250.
2. Clemente CD: *Anatomy: A Regional Atlas of the Human Body.* Philadelphia: Lea & Febiger, 1975: Figure 537.

ies to be safer and as efficacious when compared with emetics or lavage as a single modality of decontamination. A large randomized controlled trial compared gastric emptying procedures with either ipecac-induced emesis, gastric lavage and activated charcoal, or activated charcoal alone in patients with drug overdoses.[5] No significant difference in mortality, length of hospital stay, or clinical deterioration among the treatment groups was found. These clinical outcomes findings confirm those found in prior studies.[6,7]

Tenenbein et al compared ipecac-induced emesis, activated charcoal, and gastric lavage administered 1 hour after the ingestion of ampicillin to prevent its absorption.[8] They found activated charcoal to be superior in lowering blood ampicillin levels and to decrease absorption by 57 percent. Gastric lavage decreased absorption by 32 percent and emesis decreased it by 38 percent. This study used subtoxic doses of ampicillin on volunteers and is flawed by the small sample size. The authors concluded that activated charcoal without a gastric emptying procedure may be the preferred method of gastrointestinal decontamination.

None of the studies showing the efficacy of activated charcoal have administered it later than 1 hour after the ingestion.[9] This does not mean that charcoal should not be given if the patient presents later than 1 hour after ingestion. It simply means this has not been studied. The American Academy of Clinical Toxicology has noted that there is insufficient evidence to support or exclude the use of activated charcoal more than 1 hour after a toxic ingestion.[10] They also note there is no evidence that the use of activated charcoal improves clinical outcome.

CONTRAINDICATIONS

The only absolute contraindication to the use of activated charcoal is in the patient with an unprotected airway. The patient must be able to maintain an intact gag reflex or should be endotracheally intubated to protect against aspiration. Patients with absent bowel sounds, evidence of gastrointestinal obstruction, or recent gastrointestinal surgery should not receive charcoal secondary to the risk of bezoar formation or perforation and leakage of charcoal into the abdominal cavity.

Activated charcoal is not effective against toxins such as lithium, iron, acids, alkalis, heavy metals, cyanide, boric acid, and alcohols. It is ineffective against petroleum distillates and pesticides. Caustic ingestions are a relative contraindication. Charcoal is minimally effective in adsorption of these corrosives, and endoscopic visualization becomes technically difficult with charcoal in the lumen of the gut. However, a dose of activated charcoal should be given in a mixed ingestion with a toxin that charcoal can absorb. Charcoal combined with

cathartics is contraindicated in children less than one year of age and should be used with caution in renally impaired patients.[11]

EQUIPMENT

Several charcoal preparations are available.[12] These include capsules, tablets, powder, oral suspension, and charcoal with sorbitol suspension. Powder, premixed oral suspensions, and suspensions with sorbitol are the only preparations indicated for use in an acute poisoning. Powder is available in doses from 15 to 500 gm that must be mixed with water to make a slurry. The premixed suspension is available in strengths of 12.5 gm/60 mL to 50 gm/240 mL. Charcoal suspensions with sorbitol are available containing 25 to 50 gm of activated charcoal and 25 to 96 gm of sorbitol in a volume of 120 to 150 mL.

PATIENT PREPARATION

A cuffed endotracheal tube should be placed prior to the administration of activated charcoal in patients who are comatose, drowsy, obtunded, unconscious, or have an absent or impaired gag reflex. Endotracheal intubation should be strongly considered in any patient who has ingested a central nervous system depressant, tricyclic antidepressants, a sympathomimetic or other agent that may result in seizures, or any substances that can cause an altered mental status. A patient may become nauseous and vomit due to the ingested substances, the nasogastric tube, or the activated charcoal slurry. This can be controlled with the intravenous administration of an antiemetic medication.

Thoroughly mix the charcoal slurry prior to opening the container. Some preparations settle with the charcoal in the bottom of the container. Activated charcoal suspensions are gritty and unpleasant to swallow but have no taste. Some newer charcoal preparations dissolve completely when added to water to form a solution that is not gritty (Paddock Laboratories, Minneapolis, MN). The addition of sorbitol causes the suspension to be less gritty and have a sweet taste. This may enhance the palatability of the charcoal. Some manufacturers supply cherry or other flavorings to make the charcoal more palatable.

TECHNIQUE

Charcoal should be administered as early as possible and typically within the first hour after an ingestion as its efficacy is reduced beyond this time frame. An aqueous slurry should be used rather than tablets or powder. The recommended dose is 5 to 10 times the amount of toxin ingested, although standard practice is to give 50 to 100 gm to an adult or 1 gm/kg (maximum 50 gm) to a child.[12] Sorbitol can be premixed with the charcoal. The sorbitol will decrease gastrointestinal transit time and protect against bezoar formation. However, it may increase nausea and the risk of aspiration. An alert patient typically tolerates drinking the slurry well.

Place a nasogastric tube if the patient refuses to drink the charcoal. The nasogastric tube should be at least a size 16 French.[13] **Correct placement of the nasogastric tube in the gastrointestinal tract is essential prior to charcoal administration.** Confirmation of gastric placement can be done radiographically by demonstrating the tube below the diaphragm in the stomach, by auscultation of insufflated air into the stomach over the epigastrium, and by the aspiration of stomach contents through the nasogastric tube. Please refer to Chapter 47 for the details regarding the placement of a nasogastric tube. Attempts should be made to minimize gastric pressures as overly aggressive administration can increase the risk of aspiration. Prior to extubation, charcoal should be held for 4 hours.[13]

Many toxins are transported and metabolized via the enterohepatic circulation. This results in a recycling of the toxin and more available free toxin for absorption. The metabolism of these toxins tend to result in longer half-lives. Multiple doses of activated charcoal can be utilized to bind the recycled toxin and therefore decrease the toxin's half-life and potential toxic effects. Substances shown to respond well to multiple doses of activated charcoal include phenobarbital, theophylline, dapsone, diazepam, amitriptyline, carbamazepine, phenytoin, quinine, salicylates, piroxicam, digoxin, doxepin, quinine, tricyclic antidepressants, and meprobamate. This is evidenced by a significant decrease in their half-lives when multiple-dose charcoal is given. The optimum dose of multiple-dose charcoal is unknown. Typical initial dosing is 50 to 100 grams of activated charcoal with sorbitol, followed every 4 to 6 hours with a dose of 25 to 50 gm of activated charcoal alternating with and without a cathartic.[14]

COMPLICATIONS

The most feared complication of activated charcoal use is aspiration. Activated charcoal can cause severe pneumonitis that can lead to respiratory failure, prolonged ventilatory support, and death. In addition to a pneumonitis, an empyema and bronchiolitis obliterans can occur. Avoiding aspiration is paramount when delivering charcoal. The patient must be awake and have an intact gag reflex in order to protect against aspiration.

The patient should otherwise be intubated and a nasogastric or orogastric tube utilized. Errant placement of nasogastric tubes has been implicated in case reports of aspiration, even in the intubated patient. Nasogastric tubes can and have been inserted past the inflated cuffs of properly placed endotracheal tubes or in the proximal esophagus.[11] **The proper placement of nasogastric tubes must be confirmed prior to their use to instill activated charcoal.**

Intestinal obstruction is a rare complication but carries significant morbidity. Case reports of obstruction and perforation requiring laparotomy have been documented. Charcoal bezoars are the usual culprits. Bezoars can form when intestinal motility is compromised allowing continued absorption of water from the intestinal contents. Once sufficient water has been absorbed, bonds form between charcoal particles and the mass continues to harden. Patients with ingestions of anticholinergic substances, antiperistaltic coingestions, or medications administered during the hospital course are also implicated. Caution should therefore be used when giving these patients narcotic or anticholinergic medications. Typically, patients receiving multiple-dose activated charcoal therapy or activated charcoal without cathartics are at the greater risk. Constipation is a milder form of this complication and is uncommon and rarely of clinical significance.[11]

Charcoal administered with sorbitol or magnesium decreases the risk of intestinal obstruction and constipation. Yet, it can induce its own set of problems. Electrolyte disturbances can result despite the benefits of decreasing transit time throughout the gut and the concomitant decrease in absorption of toxin. Cathartic induced hypernatremia, typically a complication of the very young, can lead to serious central nervous system damage, brain swelling, long-term morbidity, and death. Sorbitol dosing in children is not clearly established, and the typical premixed preparations are not appropriate in the pediatric population. Hypermagnesemia is seen in the adult population when a magnesium-containing cathartic is given in a patient with gastrointestinal abnormalities or renal compromise. Dehydration is a problem encountered in the elderly and young. Osmotic volume loss from the gastrointestinal tract can cause these brittle populations to decompensate.[11]

SUMMARY

Activated charcoal has become a mainstay in the decontamination of the gastrointestinal tract when a susceptible toxin is ingested. Administration of charcoal is relatively easy, especially given today's newer premixed preparations, and is generally well tolerated orally. The usual dose of activated charcoal is 50 to

100 gm in an adult and 1 gm/kg in a child. A cathartic such as sorbitol can be used with the first dose unless contraindicated. The most significant complications occur as a result of aspiration and can be minimized by paying close attention to the patients at risk (those with a decreased level of consciousness or a weakened gag reflex) and by checking placement of the nasogastric tube prior to administration of charcoal. When dealing with toxins that undergo enterohepatic recycling or with long half-lives, the risks and benefits of multiple dosing must be weighed. The evidence favors the administration of activated charcoal for an overdose despite the lack of good randomized controlled studies.

REFERENCES

1. Cooney DO: *Activated Charcoal in Medicinal Applications.* New York: Marcel Decker, 1995.
2. Fountain JS, Beasley DM: Activated charcoal supersedes ipecac as gastric decontaminant. *N Z Med J* 1998; 111(1076):402–404.
3. Levy G: Gastrointestinal clearance of drugs with activated charcoal. *N Engl J Med* 1982; 307:676–678.
4. Bradberry SM, Vale JA: Multiple-dose activated charcoal: a review of relevant clinical studies. *J Toxicol Clin Toxicol* 1995; 33(5):407–416.
5. Pond SM, Lewis-Driver DJ, Williams GM, et al: Gastric emptying in acute overdose: a prospective randomized controlled trial. *Med J Aust* 1995; 163:345–349.
6. Kulig K, Bar-Or D, Cantril SV, et al: Management of acutely poisoned patients without gastric emptying. *Ann Emerg Med* 1985; 14:562–567.
7. Merigian KS, Woodard M, Hedges JR, et al: Prospective evaluation of gastric emptying in the self-poisoned patient. *Am J Emerg Med* 1990; 8:479–483.
8. Tenenbein M, Cohen S, Sitar DS: Efficacy of ipecac-induced emesis, orogastric lavage and activated charcoal for acute drug overdose. *Ann Emerg Med* 1987; 16:838–841.
9. Manoguerra AS: Gastrointestinal decontamination after poisoning. Where is the science? *Crit Care Clin* 1997; 13(4):709–725.
10. Chyka PA, Seger D (for the American Academy of Clinical Toxicology; European Association of Poisons Centres and Clinical Toxicologists): Position statement: single-dose activated charcoal. *J Toxicol Clin Toxicol* 1997; 35(7):721–741.
11. Mauro LS, Nawarskas JJ, Mauro VF: Misadventures with activated charcoal and recommendations for safe use. *Ann Pharmacotherapy* 1994; 28(7–8):915–924.
12. USP DI: *Drug Information for the Healthcare Professional*, 16th ed. Taunton, MA: Rand McNally, 1996: 793–796.
13. Kulig K: General management principles, in Rosen P, Barkin R, Danzl DF, et al (eds): *Emergency Medicine: Concepts and Clinical Practice*, 4th ed. St Louis: Mosby, 1998:1244–1250.
14. Chyka PA: Multiple-dose activated charcoal and enhancement of systemic drug clearance: summary of studies in animals and human volunteers. *J Toxicol Clin Toxicol* 1995; 33(5):399–405.

Chapter 49
GASTRIC LAVAGE

David D. Gummin

INTRODUCTION

Gastric lavage is a method of gastrointestinal decontamination, performed in the setting of an ingested overdose or acute poisoning, to decrease the absorption of substances in the stomach. This technique was first described in 1812 and has been used for nearly 200 years.[1] It was repopularized in the 1950s and 1960s and thrived during the heyday of the "tricyclic era" of the 1970s. Gastric lavage has had a diminishing role in modern toxicology for several reasons. Most notable is the trend toward evidence-based medicine and the growing body of data pointing to the limited efficacy of gastric lavage. The increasing use of other modalities for gut decontamination (e.g., activated charcoal, whole bowel irrigation) has further limited the role of gastric lavage.[1,2]

ANATOMY AND PATHOPHYSIOLOGY

Gastric lavage remains the decontamination modality of choice in a few particular situations. This includes highly toxic or potentially lethal ingestions that present acutely and where no antidotal or other therapies are available. If timed and performed appropriately, this technique can significantly reduce the amount of ingestant available for absorption and thus effectively decrease the total dose absorbed.[2] Gastric lavage has shown greatest benefit if performed promptly and within 1 to 2 hours of an oral ingestion. Efficacy appears greatest in the highest-risk ingestions.

The optimal timing of gastric lavage is controversial. All authors agree that the sooner it is instituted, the better. In volunteer and overdose studies, the range of recovered ingestant is broad at each time point following an ingestion. The trend for mean removal of ingestants is 90 percent recovery at 5 minutes postingestion, 45 percent recovery at 10 minutes, 30 percent recovery at 19 minutes, and as little as 8 percent recovery at 60 minutes.[2]

Undoubtedly, the efficacy of gastric lavage diminishes rapidly over time. Some toxicants or coingestants may cause delayed gastric emptying, while others may form masses or concretions in the stomach. Removal of only a small percentage of the ingested dose may be lifesaving or may avoid permanent sequelae in some cases. A reasonable approach is to consider gastric lavage in the acutely poisoned patient when it can be performed within 1 to 2 hours of a toxic or hazardous ingestion. The decision should be made with consideration to the specifics of the ingestion. Delayed gastric lavage may be indicated in a severely toxic poisoning or where delayed gastric emptying is suspected (e.g., anticholinergic or opioid coingestant). It may be useful to consult a poison control center or a medical toxicologist in borderline or difficult cases.

Nasogastric placement of a gastric lavage tube is generally not indicated. The orogastric route should be used to avoid injury to the nasal mucosa, nasal turbinates, and nasal septum. The use of a small-bore nasogastric tube is discouraged if the objective is gastric emptying. If an appropriately sized nasogastric tube is placed for other reasons and if the ingestant is in liquid form, aspiration of gastric contents can be attempted through a nasogastric tube. Lavage fluid can be instilled through a nasogastric tube with the expectation that the return of gastric contents may be inadequate. Lavage fluid that does not return through the nasogastric tube will pass through the pyloric sphincter and could potentially allow increased absorption of the toxicant.[3] Sustained-release tablets or capsules are particularly large in size and unlikely to be removed through a nasogastric tube or even through a 40 French orogastric lavage tube (Figure 49-1).

Placement of gastric lavage tubes in infants and children can be precarious and may result in complications[4]

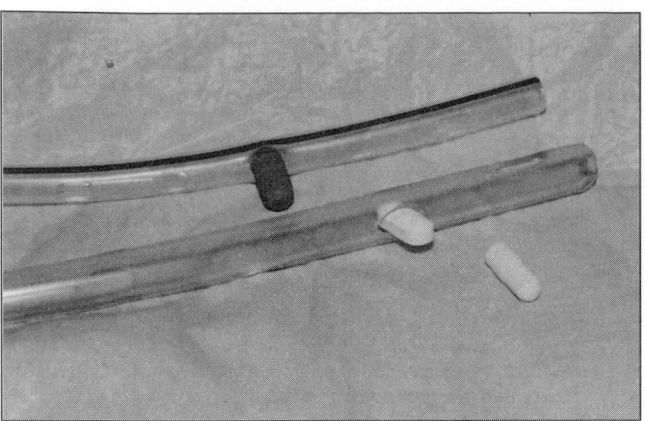

FIGURE 49-1 Orogastric lavage tubes demonstrating sideport size. A 36 French tube with a Stresstab™ 600 multivitamin in the sideport (*top*). A 40 French tube with a 450 mg sustained-release theophylline tablet in the side port (*middle*). A generic 250 mg ampicillin tablet (*bottom*). (Courtesy of F.P. Paloucek, PharmD.)

(Figure 49-2). A formula for the depth of insertion has been prospectively evaluated to ensure adequate placement in this population and is depicted graphically in Figure 49-3.[4,5] Moreover, the size of the oropharyngeal aperture and esophagus are proportional to the size of the individual. Appropriate tube diameter is essential to minimizing complications and is discussed below.

INDICATIONS

Gastric lavage is indicated to empty the stomach immediately, within 1 to 2 hours after an orally ingested overdose or poisoning and when not contraindicated. Consideration should first be given to other less invasive modalities of gastrointestinal decontamination such as activated charcoal or whole bowel irrigation. Consideration should be given to the toxicant, the ingested dose, and the risk versus benefit of performing the procedure. **Gastric lavage should be considered where there is evidence or risk of significant toxicity or imminent fatality and where antidotal or other supportive modalities are inadequate (Table 49-1).** It may be indicated beyond 2 hours in patients with known or suspected delayed gastric motility (e.g., in the setting of anticholinergic or opioid ingestion) or where the evidence of a durable mass (concretion) of pill fragments is a concern.

CONTRAINDICATIONS

The contraindications to performing a gastric lavage are summarized in Table 49-2. **An absolute contraindication to gastric lavage is a deteriorating level of con-**

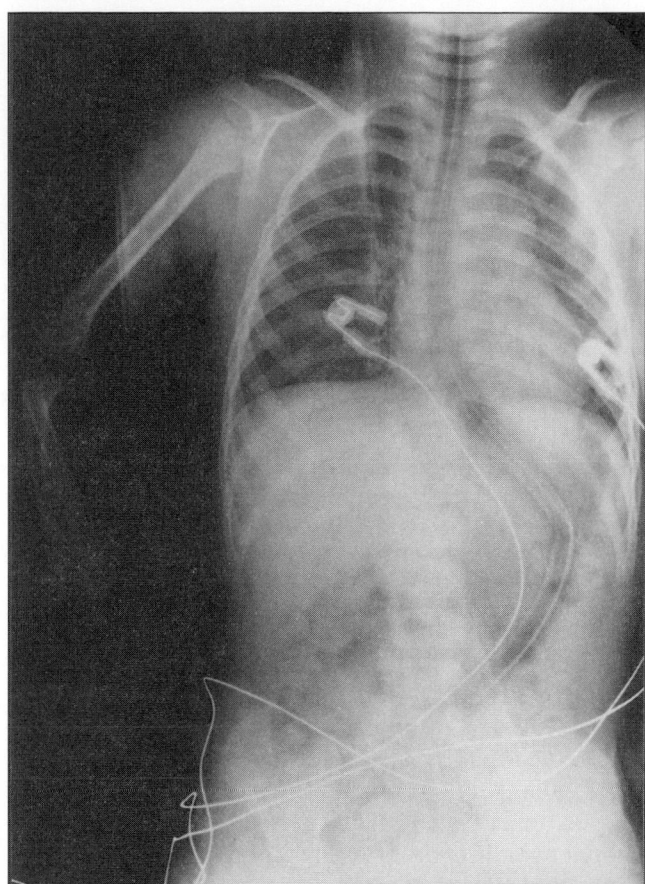

FIGURE 49-2 Malposition of an orogastric tube placed for gastric lavage in a pediatric patient. (Courtesy of Ann E. Klasner, MD, MPH.)

sciousness with loss of protective reflexes or an unprotected airway. In this setting the airway must first be secured by endotracheal intubation. Gastric lavage can then be performed once the airway is protected.[2] Gastric lavage is contraindicated in caustic ingestions. Local mucosal damage amplifies the risk for traumatic perforation. Gastric lavage should not be performed to retrieve large pills, large foreign bodies, or sharp foreign bodies. It is relatively contraindicated in hydrocarbon ingestions, where pulmonary aspiration is a primary concern. This may, however, not be the case when a highly toxic hydrocarbon is ingested (e.g., benzene, *N*-hexane, pesticides). Significantly abnormal upper airway or upper gastrointestinal anatomy (anomaly, stricture, fresh interposition graft) may restrict the use of gastric lavage in rare circumstances.

Vomiting is common after many overdoses and may be protective. Multiple episodes of emesis may clear the majority of a toxicant from the stomach and obviate the need for further intervention. Attempts at gastric intubation in the setting of an actively vomiting patient are likely to be met with minimal success and may cause injury.[6] Gastric lavage is contraindicated unless the vomiting can

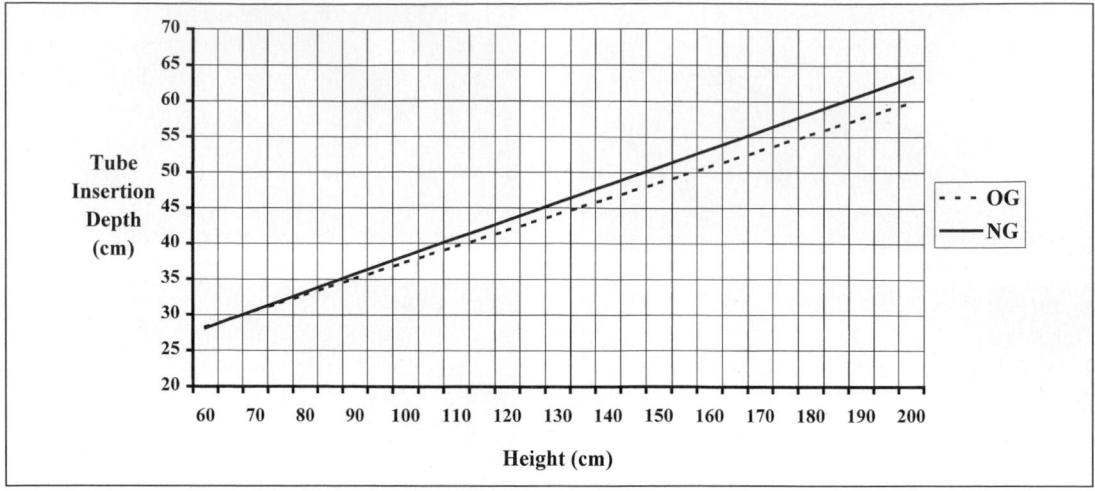

FIGURE 49-3 Estimated lavage tube insertion depth in children based on their height. The lengths for both nasogastric (NG) and orogastric (OG) tubes are represented on the graph. (Reprinted from Scalzo et al,[4] with permission from Elsevier Science.)

be brought under control. Moreover, it is unlikely to be beneficial in this setting.

Gastric lavage is unlikely to change the outcome of a nontoxic or minimally toxic ingestion. It must be ascertained that significant toxicity or death may result if the patient is not lavaged. Otherwise, the risk-benefit ratio is unacceptably high. This is not to say that the patient must manifest toxicity at the time of initial evaluation. The determination of whether to perform a gas-

tric lavage must be individualized and rests upon the evaluating clinician. Consult a toxicologist or poison control center in questionable cases.

EQUIPMENT

Pulse oximeter
Cardiac monitor
Noninvasive blood pressure monitor
Protective clothing
Bite block
Oral airway
Emesis basin
Suction source
Yankauer suction catheter
Suction tubing
Funnel or large (50 to 100 mL) syringe
Tap water or saline
Bulb suction device or large syringe
Water-soluble lubricant
Orogastric lavage tube
Resuscitative equipment readily available

TABLE 49-1. INDICATIONS FOR PERFORMING A GASTRIC LAVAGE

Acute presentation (within 1–2 hours) and:

1. Evident or high risk of morbidity or mortality:

Beta-blockers	Heterocyclic antidepressants
Calcium channel blockers	Iron
Chloroquine	Paraquat
Colchicine	Salicylates
Cyanide	Selenious acid
Heavy metals	

2. Poor absorption by activated charcoal
   Heavy metals
   Iron
   Lithium
   Toxic alcohols

3. Evidence of formed concretion
   Enteric-coated preparations
   Iron
   Phenothiazines
   Salicylates

4. Ineffective or no antidotal therapy available
   Calcium channel blockers
   Colchicine
   Paraquat
   Selenious acid

TABLE 49-2. CONTRAINDICATIONS TO PERFORMING A GASTRIC LAVAGE

Abnormal or absent pharyngeal/upper gastrointestinal anatomy
Active or substantial antecedent vomiting
Caustic ingestion
Coagulopathy
Decreased mental status
Inactive or diminished airway reflexes
Large pills
Large or sharp foreign body
Nontoxic or minimally toxic ingestion
Significant aspiration risk (e.g., hydrocarbon ingestion)

All required instrumentation should be gathered at the bedside prior to initiating the procedure. A variety of orogastric lavage tubes are available. Most have a distal port and at least one sideport. A semirigid tube is preferable to soft rubber or polyvinyl chloride collapsible tubes. Several additional ports should be cut in the sides of the tube near the tip to maximize the return of pill fragments if the tube has only a single sideport. Examples of rigid tubing are shown in Figures 49-1 and 49-4. A larger tube diameter provides less flexibility, so that the tube is less likely to kink, collapse, or curl back on itself. Larger-diameter tubes are more likely to facilitate retrieval of larger pill fragments. A 30 to 50 French lavage tube is preferred in an adult. A 30 to 34 French tube is adequate for an adolescent. Small children can generally accommodate 24 French tubes. Gastric lavage is generally contraindicated in neonates and infants.

There are numerous types of gastric lavage systems. Open systems are less expensive, messy, and time-consuming to use. A passive open system uses gravity to instill and drain the lavage fluid. An active open system uses a large syringe to inject and aspirate lavage fluid through the orogastric tube. The syringe must be removed from the orogastric tube to be filled with fresh lavage fluid, and used lavage fluid must be discarded after each lavage cycle. Closed systems are commercially available, single-patient use devices, self-contained, easy to use, and do not cause a mess (Figure 49-4). The practitioner should be familiar with the type of system available at their institution.

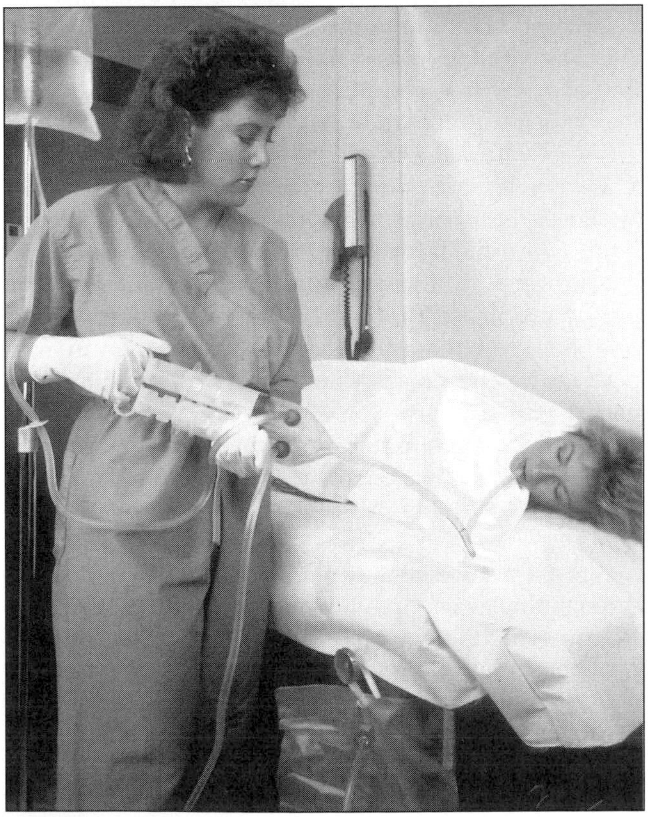

Gastric lavage solution typically consists of tap water or normal saline. **Do not use tap water in small children, as this can result in electrolyte abnormalities.** Specialized lavage solutions may be indicated if the ingested substance is fluoride, formaldehyde, iodine, iron, or oxalic acid. Fluoride ingestions may be lavaged with 15 to 30 gm/L of calcium gluconate to produce an insoluble calcium fluoride. Formaldehyde ingestions may be lavaged with 10 mg/L of ammonium acetate to produce the nontoxic substance methenamine. Iodine ingestions may be lavaged with 75 gm of cornstarch in 1 L of water. Iron ingestions may be lavaged with 2% sodium bicarbonate (50 mEq in 150 mL of normal saline) to produce the insoluble ferrous carbonate. Oxalic acid ingestions may be lavaged with 15 to 30 gm/L of calcium gluconate to form the insoluble calcium oxalate. **These specialized lavage solutions should be used only in consultation with a toxicologist or poison control center.**

FIGURE 49-4 Example of a closed lavage pump system. (Courtesy of Kimberly-Clark Corporation.)

PATIENT PREPARATION

The indications, details of the procedure, risks and benefits, and alternative modalities should be discussed with the patient and/or their representative. Informed consent should be obtained or may be presumed in the setting of a suicidal overdose.

Place the patient in the left lateral decubitus position and in 15 to 20 degrees of Trendelenburg. This position is intended to maximize gastric emptying.[7] However, the removal of ingestants by gastric lavage in the overdose setting is modest, and other circumstances may intervene, such as an uncooperative patient or technical factors.[2] A patient may require chemical restraint, physical restraint, and/or paralysis prior to this procedure. The supine and lateral decubitus positions are associated with a higher risk of pulmonary aspiration in comatose and mechanically ventilated patients.[8–11] It is assumed that this positioning risk is similarly increased in patients not mechanically ventilated and undergoing gastric lavage. Most gastric lavages can be performed safely and effectively with the conscious patient placed in the semi-upright position. The use of a topical anesthetic spray into the oropharynx may decrease the patient's gag reflex and allow easier passage of the orogastric tube. Unfortunately, this can also increase the risk of aspiration.

It is not required but recommended to place the patient on the cardiac monitor, noninvasive blood pressure cuff, and pulse oximeter prior to performing a gastric lavage. This equipment may also be required based upon the patient's physiologic status, the nature of the ingestant or toxin, and/or other underlying problems.

TECHNIQUE

Measure the length of the orogastric tube to be inserted (Figure 49-5). The length should be marked with a permanent marker or a piece of surgical tape. Liberally lubricate the tip of the lavage tube. Place a bite block into the patient's mouth if they are conscious. A bite block or oral airway may preclude biting of the tube by an uncooperative or stuporous patient.[12]

Gently insert the lavage tube into the patient's mouth and direct it into the hypopharynx. Flexion of the patient's neck may facilitate passage of the tube into the

esophagus and avoid endotracheal insertion. Conscious and cooperative patients may be asked to swallow water through a straw or their saliva to facilitate passage of the tube. Stridor, cough, or cyanosis indicates that the lavage tube is in the airway and should prompt removal of the tube. If significant resistance is met in the hypopharynx, applying gentle pressure to the tube while instructing the patient to swallow should allow passage through the upper esophageal sphincter. **The tube should not be forced, as misplacement may damage the larynx or perforate the pyriform sinus.** Slowly advance the tube to the premeasured depth.

Confirmation of intragastric tube placement must precede instillation of any fluid through the tube. Proper placement should be confirmed by aspiration of gastric contents, auscultation of insufflated air over the epigastrium (from a 50 mL Toomey syringe), and/or by radiography. Gastric irrigation should be preceded by aspiration of available gastric contents. The initial aspirate may be sent for toxicologic assay.

Perform the gastric lavage. Instill normal saline or tap water through the orogastric tube. The lavage fluid should ideally be warmed to body temperature. This is often not practical, and room temperature lavage fluid is satisfactory. Instill aliquots of 10 to 15 mL/kg to a maximum of 300 mL of the irrigant solution. Instillation of larger volumes may result in vomiting, with pulmonary aspiration and the passage of gastric contents past the pyloric sphincter where subsequent absorption may occur.[2] Lavage aliquots may be instilled by either placing a funnel in the free end of the lavage tube and allowing gravity instillation or they may be infused with a Toomey syringe. Remove the lavage fluid after a brief (1 to 2 minutes) equilibration period by either gravity drainage into an emesis basin or aspiration with a syringe or suction bulb. Repeat the lavage process until 2 to 3 L of irrigant has been used in the adult or the lavage fluid is free of particulate matter and pill fragments. Some authors have suggested that agitation of the stomach by manual massage of the epigastrium during the equilibration period will ensure mixing of the gastric contents.[12] No substantive data support this approach. Alternatively, closed systems are available for both instilling and suctioning lavage fluids through a common tube (Figure 49-4).

Activated charcoal may be administered, if indicated, through the lavage tube before it is removed. A dose of 1 gm/kg of body weight is typically recommended, either in a premixed slurry or diluted in normal saline or tap water (30 gm charcoal per 240 mL of diluent). Refer to Chapter 48 regarding the details of administering activated charcoal. Remove the orogastric tube. Further gastric access, when needed, should be provided by the subsequent placement of a smaller-bore nasogastric tube.

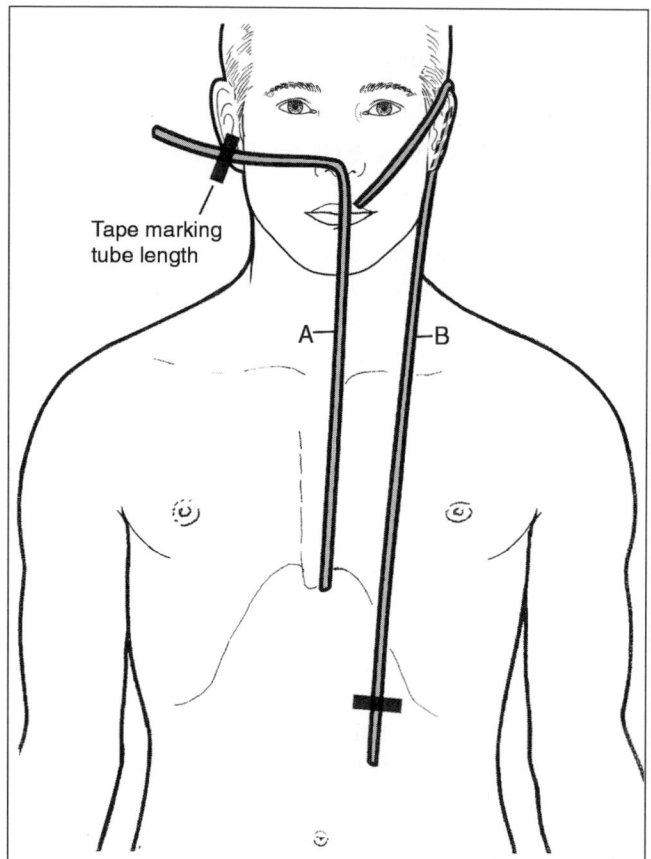

Tape marking tube length

A   B

FIGURE 49-5 Determining the proper length of orogastric tube to insert. *A.* The length is determined by the distance from the xiphoid process to the tip of the nose to the earlobe. *B.* The length is determined by the distance from the tip of the nose or lip, around the left ear, and to just below the left costal margin. A piece of tape is used to mark the distance on the orogastric tube.

ALTERNATIVE TECHNIQUES

Because of concern over toxicants passing through the pyloric valve during the gastric lavage procedure, an alternative sequence could be considered. Administer activated charcoal after the initial aspiration of gastric contents through the lavage tube. Perform the gastric lavage anticipating that a significant amount of activated charcoal will be removed along with the ingestant. Infuse a second dose of activated charcoal through the lavage tube before removal of the tube. The rationale here is an attempt to make charcoal available to adsorb toxicant from any gastric contents pushed into the small bowel during the lavage procedure.[1] While no human data support this technique, it is reasonable to consider.

ASSESSMENT

The patient should be continuously monitored and reassessed throughout the procedure so as to avoid complications. Strict adherence to the procedures noted will minimize the risk of complications. Prompt removal of the lavage tube at the end of the procedure will avoid the risk of delayed complications.

AFTERCARE

Most patients who require gastric lavage for an overdose or poisoning will require inpatient monitoring for complications of the ingestion. A situation wherein a patient requires gastric lavage and is then sent home is conceivable though unlikely. An observation period of 6 to 8 hours for the immediate complications of gastric lavage is probably appropriate (Table 49-3). Delayed complications related to the perforation of the upper gastrointestinal tract may occur.[13]

COMPLICATIONS

The complications associated with gastric lavage are rare and can be avoided by careful patient selection and technique[6] (Table 49-3). Placement of the lavage tube can result in mucosal injury, bleeding, esophageal perforation, gastric perforation, or endotracheal placement. The patient should be monitored, as the procedure may result in cardiac arrhythmias, hypoxemia, and tachycardia.[1,6] Avoid using more than 10 mL/kg or 300 mL aliquots of lavage fluid to prevent vomiting, aspiration, or pushing of gastric contents into the small bowel. The impaction of a lavage tube may prevent its removal.[1,6,13] **Do not use force to remove the lavage tube, as this may injure or rupture the stomach or esophagus.** Evaluate

TABLE 49-3. COMPLICATIONS ASSOCIATED WITH GASTRIC LAVAGE

Cardiac dysrhythmias
Electrolyte abnormalities
Empyema
Esophageal tear or perforation
Gastric perforation
Hypothermia
Laryngospasm
Nasal, oral, or pharyngeal injury
Pneumothorax
Pulmonary aspiration
Pyriform sinus perforation
Tracheal placement
Tube impaction

the tube using fluoroscopy or plain radiographs. A lavage tube that is kinked or knotted will require endoscopically aided or surgical removal.

Gastric lavage with large volumes of cold fluid can result in hypothermia. Warmed lavage fluid should be used if available, although this is somewhat controversial. Warm lavage fluid may dissolve more of the intoxicant and allow rapid access of gastric contents past the pylorus, to be absorbed into the systemic circulation. Electrolyte abnormalities may result, especially in children, if the lavage fluid is hypotonic (i.e., tap water). The use of normal saline for lavage is recommended.

SUMMARY

Gastric lavage is a time-honored procedure to decontaminate the stomach of patients following an ingested overdose or poisoning. While the indications for gastric lavage are diminishing, it remains a safe and effective procedure for specific toxicologic scenarios. Complications are infrequent if the procedure is performed cautiously. Maximal efficacy can be expected if it is performed within 1 to 2 hours following an ingestion. Gastric lavage is not indicated in the setting of a nontoxic or minimally toxic ingestion or where specific and less invasive antidotes are readily available. Consultation with a toxicologist or poison control center may provide valuable information regarding the indications, contraindications, complications, and techniques associated with gastric lavage.

REFERENCES

1. Perrone J, Hoffman RS, Goldfrank LR: Special considerations in gastrointestinal decontamination. *Emerg Med Clin North Am* 1994; 12(2):285–299.
2. Vale JA: Position statement: gastric lavage. *J Toxicol Clin Toxicol* 1997; 35(7):711–719.

3. Saetta JP, March S, Gaunt ME, et al: Gastric emptying procedures in the self-poisoned patient: are we forcing gastric content beyond the pylorus? *J R Soc Med* 1991; 84(5):274–276.

4. Scalzo AJ, Tominack RL, Thompson MW: Malposition of pediatric gastric lavage tubes demonstrated radiographically. *J Emerg Med* 1992; 10(5):581–586.

5. Klasner A, Scalzo A: Pediatric lavage and gastric decompression tubes: a new formula evaluated. *J Toxicol Clin Toxicol* 1999; 37(5):660.

6. Smilkstein MJ: Techniques used to prevent gastrointestinal absorption of toxic compounds, in Goldfrank LR, Floenbaum NE, Lewin NA, et al (eds): *Goldfrank's Toxicologic Emergencies*, 6th ed. Stamford, CT: Appleton & Lange, 1998:35–51.

7. Burke M: Gastric lavage and emesis in the treatment of ingested poisons: a review and a clinical study of lavage in ten adults. *Resuscitation* 1972; 1(2):91–105.

8. Adnet F, Borron SW, Finot MA, et al: Relation of body position at the time of discovery with suspected aspiration pneumonia in poisoned comatose patients. *Crit Care Med* 1999; 27(4):745–748.

9. Drakulovic MB, Torres A, Bauer TT, et al: Supine body position as a risk factor for nosocomial pneumonia in mechanically ventilated patients: a randomised trial. *Lancet* 1999; 354(9193):1851–1858.

10. Orozco-Levi M, Torres A, Ferrer M, et al: Semirecumbent position protects from pulmonary aspiration but not completely from gastroesophageal reflux in mechanically ventilated patients. *Am J Respir Crit Care Med* 1995; 152(4 Pt 1):1387–1390.

11. Torres A, Serra-Batlles J, Ros E, et al: Pulmonary aspiration of gastric contents in patients receiving mechanical ventilation: the effect of body position. *Ann Intern Med* 1992; 116(7):540–543.

12. Tandberg D, Troutman WG: Gastric lavage in the poisoned patient, in Roberts JR, Hedges JR (eds): *Clinical Procedures in Emergency Medicine*, 2nd ed. Philadelphia: Saunders, 1991:655–662.

13. Mariani PJ, Pook N: Gastrointestinal tract perforation with charcoal peritoneum complicating orogastric intubation and lavage. *Ann Emerg Med* 1993; 22(3):606–609.

Chapter 50
WHOLE BOWEL IRRIGATION

David D. Gummin
Steven E. Aks

INTRODUCTION

Whole bowel irrigation is the infusion of polyethylene glycol electrolyte lavage solution into the stomach at flow rates higher than are otherwise commonly used. This is a relatively new technique used to decontaminate the gastrointestinal tract after an acute toxic ingestion or overdose. Most of the literature supporting its use is in the form of case reports or case series.[1] While available reports are compelling, the indications for whole bowel irrigation will likely evolve as more extensive data becomes available. To date, the demonstrated role of whole bowel irrigation remains limited.

ANATOMY AND PATHOPHYSIOLOGY

Current methods of gastrointestinal decontamination (emesis, gastric lavage, activated charcoal administration) focus primarily on decontaminating the stomach. Absorption of most toxicants occurs principally in the proximal small bowel. Sustained- or delayed-release preparations continue to liberate drug during intestinal transit that is then available for absorption throughout the bowel. Infusion of polyethylene glycol electrolyte lavage solution decreases the enteric transit time, attenuating the contact time of a toxicant with the gastrointestinal mucosa. This reduces absorption of the drug or toxin throughout the gastrointestinal tract. The 3500 dalton molecular weight polyethylene glycol solution is specifically designed to prevent electrolyte and fluid shifts.

INDICATIONS

Whole bowel irrigation is indicated for acute ingestions where severe or potentially fatal toxicity is anticipated (Table 50-1). Other decontamination methods, such as activated charcoal, should be employed if they are known to be effective rather than whole bowel irrigation. Whole bowel irrigation may be indicated in situations where activated charcoal is known to be ineffective. Whole bowel irrigation has been effectively utilized to decrease bioavailability of ingested iron, lithium, and heavy metals.[2–6] Whole bowel irrigation is effective at flushing the gastrointestinal tract free of toxicant before absorption can be affected by sustained-release preparations.[7] Whole bowel irrigation may speed gastrointestinal transit of ingested packets or vials of illicit drugs ingested by a "body packer" or "body stuffer."[8] While the indications are limited, additional settings may be envisioned where whole bowel irrigation might be useful. Unfortunately, there is not yet data to support broader indications.

CONTRAINDICATIONS

There are few contraindications to performing whole bowel irrigation (Table 50-2). The infusion of polyethylene glycol into a patient with a potentially compromised or unprotected airway could result in pulmonary aspiration.[1] Significant vomiting may hinder the ability to perform whole bowel irrigation until the vomiting can be brought under control. Theoretical contraindications include abnormal upper airway or upper gastrointestinal anatomy (anomaly, stricture, fresh interposition graft). Ingestion of toxic substances that markedly slow gastrointestinal motility (e.g., anticholinergics, opioids) may cause an ileus, diminishing the ability to perform whole bowel irrigation effectively. The administration of polyethylene glycol in a patient with a bowel obstruction will result in vomiting with the potential for aspiration. This solution should not be used in patients with an actual or suspected perforated bowel. The risk of whole bowel irrigation is quite small but the procedure is not without effort, expense, and risk of complications. In this light, the risk-benefit ratio would be high if whole bowel irrigation were used to treat a nontoxic ingestion.

TABLE 50-1. CONDITIONS IN WHICH WHOLE BOWEL IRRIGATION SHOULD BE CONSIDERED

1. Acute, life-threatening, or serious ingestion
2. Any of the following:
   Delayed or enteric-coated preparation
   Heavy metals
   Ingested packets of illicit drug
   Iron
   Lithium
   Toxin or toxicant poorly adsorbed by activated charcoal

TABLE 50-2. CONTRAINDICATIONS TO PERFORMING WHOLE BOWEL IRRIGATION

Bowel obstruction or perforation
Ileus
Intractable vomiting
Nontoxic ingestion
Potentially compromised or unprotected airway
Significant gastrointestinal bleeding

EQUIPMENT

Nasogastric or enteral feeding tube, size 10 to 12 French
Water-soluble lubricant
Nasal decongestant and anesthetic
Enteral feeding reservoir and tubing
Polyethylene glycol electrolyte lavage solution (packets or reconstituted)
Emesis basin
Stethoscope
Toomey syringe
Intravenous extension tubing

The equipment required for whole bowel irrigation is readily available in most Emergency Departments. A small-bore, 10 to 12 French, nasogastric tube is sufficient for an adult or adolescent. An enteral feeding tube can be substituted if a sufficient flow rate can be ensured. A smaller tube is required in infants or very small children. Infants will tolerate an 8 French tube and a 10 to 12 French tube is adequate beyond the first year.[9,10]

Standard enteral feeding reservoirs and tubing are typically available as packaged kits. An enteral feeding or an enema bag with enteral feed tubing may be substituted. Enteral feeding pumps, however, are not useful, as the flow rate through the pump is typically inadequate to perform whole bowel irrigation effectively. Alternatively, an empty 1 L intravenous fluid bag with intravenous extension tubing can be used for the procedure.

PATIENT PREPARATION

Where possible, explain the procedure, risks, benefits, and alternatives to the patient and/or their representative. Informed consent should be obtained. Informed consent can be assumed in the case of suicidal ingestions. Inspect the nasal passage and oropharynx to rule out anatomic abnormalities or obstruction that would preclude the passage of a nasogastric tube.

Place the patient in the upright or semi-upright position (Figure 50-1).[10] The supine and lateral decubitus positions are associated with a higher risk of pulmonary aspiration in comatose and mechanically ventilated patients.[11–14] It can be assumed that this positioning risk is similarly increased in patients undergoing whole bowel irrigation.

Choose the smallest diameter nasogastric or feeding tube that will allow adequate flow of polyethylene glycol electrolyte lavage solution into the stomach. All necessary equipment should be placed at the bedside and assembled prior to beginning the procedure.

A cuffed endotracheal tube should be placed prior to performing whole bowel irrigation in patients who are comatose, drowsy, obtunded, unconscious, or have an absent or impaired gag reflex. Endotracheal intubation should be strongly considered in any patient who has ingested a central nervous system depressant, tricyclic antidepressants, a sympathomimetic or other agent that may result in seizures, or any substances that can cause an altered mental status.

TECHNIQUE

Insert a nasogastric tube. Refer to Chapter 47 for the complete details regarding nasogastric tube placement. Measure the length of the nasogastric tube to be inserted. Place the tip of the nasogastric tube over the xiphoid process. Extend the tube over the anterior chest, lateral neck, behind the angle of the mandible, and to the tip of the nose. Mark this length with a permanent marker or a piece of surgical tape. Liberally lubricate the tip of the nasogastric tube. The application of a nasal anesthetic and decongestant is optional but can facilitate the passage of the nasogastric tube.

Gently insert the nasogastric tube into the naris. Advance it posteriorly along the nasal floor into the nasopharynx and through to the hypopharynx. Flexion of the neck may facilitate passage of the tube into the esophagus and avoid endotracheal insertion. The conscious and cooperative patient may be asked to swallow water through a straw or to swallow their saliva to facilitate passage of the tube. Stridor, cough, or cyanosis may indicate endotracheal passage and should prompt removal of the tube. Gentle pressure and patient swallowing should allow passage through the upper esophageal sphincter if significant resistance is met in the hy-

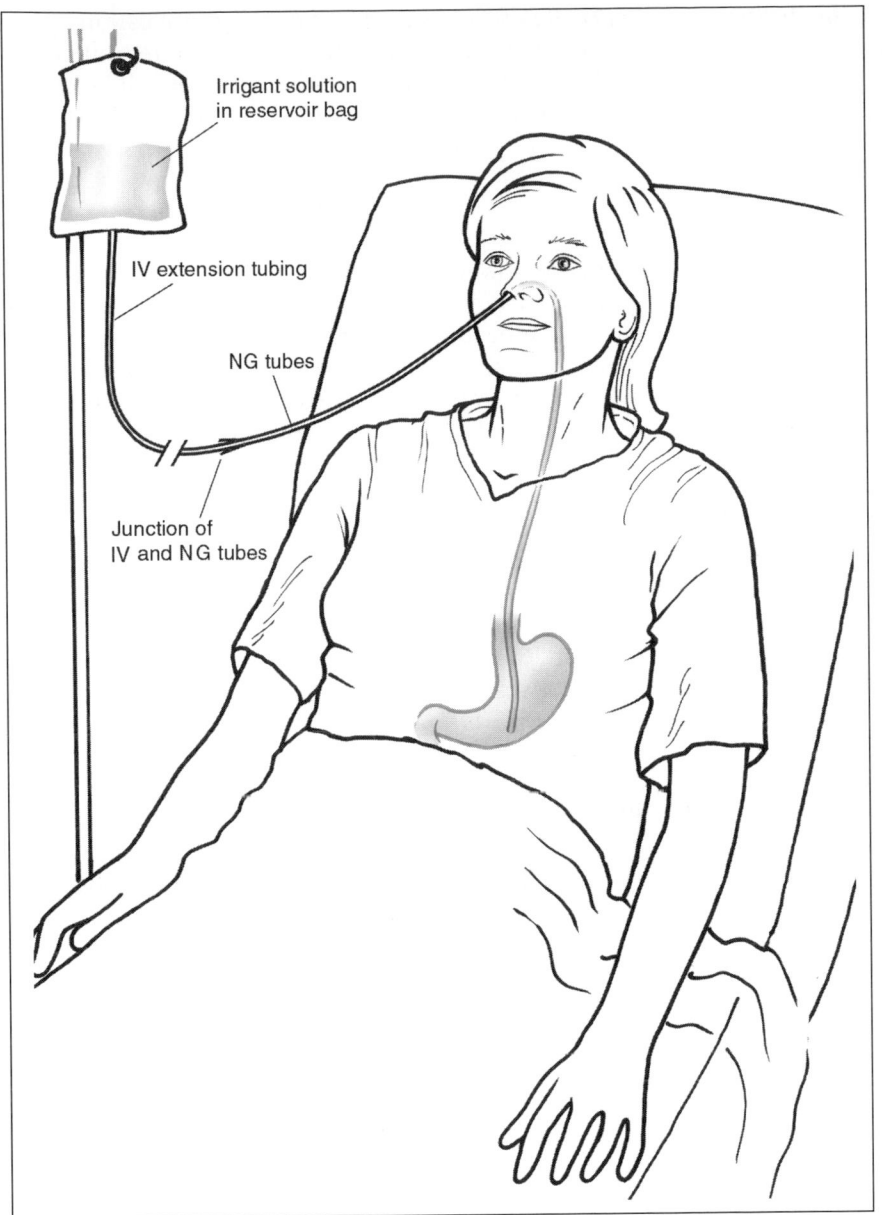

FIGURE 50-1 Setup required to perform whole bowel irrigation.

popharynx. **Do not force the nasogastric tube as misplacement may damage the larynx or perforate the pyriform sinus.** Advance the nasogastric tube to the marked level. Confirm proper placement by the aspiration of gastric contents, by auscultation of insufflated air over the epigastrium (from a 50 mL syringe), and/or by radiography. **Confirmation of intragastric placement must precede administration of any fluids through the nasogastric tube.**

Instill the polyethylene glycol electrolyte lavage solution through a setup such as that shown in Figure 50-1. Flow rates are dependent upon the size of the patient. Begin instillation at an initial rate of 25 to 30 mL of polyethylene glycol electrolyte lavage solution per kilogram per hour. Adults may tolerate more than 3 L of solution per hour. The rate may be adjusted somewhat to accommodate patient tolerance (e.g., vomiting, abdominal distension). Irrigation should be continued until the patient passes the ingestant in the stool or until clear liquid rectal effluent is passed. Liquid stools will continue to be passed after discontinuing whole bowel irrigation. Irrigation should be stopped if the patient vomits, develops an ileus, or if gastrointestinal perforation is suspected.

ALTERNATIVE TECHNIQUES

Some providers may attempt whole bowel irrigation by offering the patient polyethylene glycol electrolyte lavage solution to drink. This is rarely successful. Experience shows that whole bowel irrigation is ineffectively performed if a nasogastric tube is not placed. Even the most cooperative patient is unlikely to drink the solution at the required administration rate.

ASSESSMENT

Patient assessment must be continuous throughout the process of whole bowel irrigation. Abdominal distension, gassiness, and mild discomfort are common side effects in at least 50 percent of patients and do not mandate discontinuation of whole bowel irrigation.[15] Providers must be vigilant in monitoring the patient's bowel sounds. If bowel sounds cease or significant abdominal distension is noted, the irrigation should be held for 30 to 90 minutes and the patient reassessed. Resume the irrigation at a reduced rate if bowel sounds return, if the clinical status improves, and if the patient then tolerates the infusion. Significant electrolyte or osmotic shifts do not occur solely from whole bowel irrigation. Electrolytes may be monitored if otherwise indicated for the type of ingestion or for overall patient status. Of greater concern is vomiting with the risk of aspiration. The patient's posture should be maintained in the upright sitting or the semi-upright position to facilitate passage of irrigant solution into the small bowel and to protect against aspiration.

AFTERCARE

Patients who undergo whole bowel irrigation must all be admitted to the hospital for ongoing assessment of the intervention and the underlying intoxication. In most cases, intensive care or step-down monitoring will be required to ensure adequacy of the intervention and to monitor for complications of the ingestion or overdose. Delayed complications are unlikely once the procedure is completed.

COMPLICATIONS

To date, no serious complications have been attributed to whole bowel irrigation. Theoretical complications include pulmonary aspiration of the irrigant solution and/or ingestant. This would be especially concerning in the patient with an unprotected and potentially compromised airway. Osmotic and electrolyte abnormalities will not occur with the standard preparations of high molecular weight (c. 3500 daltons) polyethylene glycol electrolyte lavage solutions (e.g., Colyte, GoLYTELY, NuLYTELY). Complications of nasogastric tube placement are well described and theoretically can

occur. Refer to Chapter 47 for the complications associated with nasogastric tubes. These are unlikely if proper technique is employed and can be minimized by use of the smallest effective diameter nasogastric tube.

SUMMARY

Whole bowel irrigation is a technique performed to speed gastrointestinal transit and decontaminate the gut after an acute toxic ingestion. Available reports are convincing and show that whole bowel irrigation can decrease bioavailability of toxicants by two thirds.[3,10] It appears useful where activated charcoal is not expected to adequately bind ingestants (e.g., iron, lithium). Efficacy appears greatest in the setting of sustained- or delayed-release preparations. Whole bowel irrigation is not the method of choice, however, when more effective methods of gastrointestinal decontamination are possible (e.g., repetitive-dose activated charcoal for sustained-release theophylline). Until further data emerge, whole bowel irrigation's role in managing the toxic ingestion remains limited.

REFERENCES

1. Tenenbein M: Position statement: whole bowel irrigation. *J Toxicol Clin Toxicol* 1997; 35(7):753–762.
2. Everson GW, Bertaccini EJ, O'Leary J: Use of whole bowel irrigation in an infant following iron overdose. *Am J Emerg Med* 1991; 9:366–369.
3. Smith SW, Ling LJ, Halstenson CE: Whole bowel irrigation as a treatment for acute lithium overdose. *Ann Emerg Med* 1991; 20(5):536–539.
4. Burkhart KK, Kulig KW, Rumack B: Whole bowel irrigation as treatment for zinc sulfate overdose. *Ann Emerg Med* 1990; 19(10):1167–1170.
5. Lee DC, Roberts JR, Kelly JJ, et al: Whole bowel irrigation as an adjunct in the treatment of radiopaque arsenic. *Am J Emerg Med* 1995; 13:244–245.
6. Roberge RJ, Martin TG: Whole bowel irrigation in an acute oral lead intoxication. *Am J Emerg Med* 1992; 10(6):577–583.
7. Buckley N, Dawson AH, Howarth D, et al: Slow-release verapamil poisoning. Use of polyethylene glycol whole-bowel lavage and high-dose calcium. *Med J Aust* 1993; 158(3):202–204.
8. Hoffman RS, Smilkstein MJ, Goldfrank LR: Whole bowel irrigation and the cocaine body-packer: a new approach to a common problem. *Am J Emerg Med* 1990; 8(6):523–527.
9. Carlson DW, DiGuilio GA, Gewitz MH, et al: Nasogastric tube placement, in Fleisher GR, Ludwig S, Henretig FM, et al (eds): *Textbook of Pediatric Emer-*

gency Medicine, 3rd ed. Philadelphia: Williams & Wilkins, 1993:1633.

10. Tenenbein M: Whole bowel irrigation, in Henretig FM, King C, Joffe MD, et al (eds): *Textbook of Pediatric Emergency Procedures.* Philadelphia: Williams & Wilkins, 1997:1309–1312.

11. Adnet F, Borron SW, Finot MA, et al: Relation of body position at the time of discovery with suspected aspiration pneumonia in poisoned comatose patients. *Crit Care Med* 1999; 27(4):745–748.

12. Drakulovic MB, Torres A, Bauer TT, et al: Supine body position as a risk factor for nosocomial pneumonia in mechanically ventilated patients: a ran-

domised trial. *Lancet* 1999; 27;354(9193):1851–1858.

13. Orozco-Levi M, Torres A, Ferrer M, et al: Semirecumbent position protects from pulmonary aspiration but not completely from gastroesophageal reflux in mechanically ventilated patients. *Am J Respir Crit Care Med* 1995; 152(4 Pt 1):1387–1390.

14. Torres A, Serra-Batlles J, Ros E, et al: Pulmonary aspiration of gastric contents in patients receiving mechanical ventilation: the effect of body position. *Ann Intern Med* 1992; 116(7):540–543.

15. Anonymous: *Physician's Desk Reference,* 53rd ed. Montvale, NJ: Medical Economics, 1999:766, 2897.

Chapter 51
ESOPHAGEAL FOREIGN BODY REMOVAL

Bashar M. Attar

INTRODUCTION

Most foreign bodies (90 percent) that are ingested enter the gastrointestinal tract while 10 percent enter the tracheobronchial tree.[1] Approximately 1500 people die annually in the United States from ingested foreign bodies in the upper gastrointestinal tract.[2] Most objects (80 to 90 percent) usually pass spontaneously but about 10 to 20 percent must be removed endoscopically. Approximately 1 percent require surgical removal.[3] Most (80 percent) esophageal foreign bodies occur in children followed by edentulous adults, prisoners, and psychiatric patients.[4] Recurrent episodes of foreign body ingestion occur in 5 to 10 percent of patients, especially prisoners and psychiatric patients.[1]

The presentations are best divided according to accidental and deliberate ingestors.[1-5] The accidental ingestor is usually cooperative and has a single foreign body. Conversely, the deliberate ingestor is often uncooperative and the foreign bodies are multiple and unusual. It is important to identify such individuals at their initial presentation since foreign body removal is usually performed under conscious sedation or general anesthesia.

The patient's history is the most important part of the diagnostic evaluation.[3] The identity of the object ingested is usually known to the patient. Persistent odynophagia, dysphagia, or foreign body sensation may indicate the presence of an esophageal foreign body despite negative radiographic results. A high index of suspicion must be maintained in younger children and mentally retarded adults.

The physical examination is most likely negative unless complications are present. Stridor, wheezing, signs of consolidation, and the absence of breath sounds should be sought. Subcutaneous emphysema in the neck or chest indicates perforation of the esophagus or the stomach. The most common sites for a foreign body to get trapped are where the esophagus is narrow: at the cricopharyngeus muscle, where the aortic arch crosses the esophagus, and at the gastroesophageal junction.

Radiographic evaluation is often helpful in the evaluation of an esophageal foreign body.[3-6] Obtain plain radiographs of the neck and chest in the posteroanterior and lateral positions. Evaluate the radiographs for the presence of a foreign body in all planes. Air in the subcutaneous tissues, mediastinum, and/or beneath the diaphragm is indicative of a perforation. Barium studies are undesirable in patients with a food bolus impaction and obscure endoscopic visualization. Esophagrams performed using a minimal amount of thin barium may be necessary in situations where the foreign body is made of wood, thin metals, aluminum can tops, and plastics. Meglumine diatrizoate (Gastrografin) is contraindicated in food bolus impactions because it is highly hypertonic and can lead to severe chemical pneumonitis if aspirated into the lungs.[5] Computerized tomography may be useful, especially in cases where the foreign body could not be detected as it may have become embedded in or penetrated the esophageal wall.[6]

Endoscopy is important for both the diagnosis and possible removal of an esophageal foreign body. Extraction with the flexible endoscope is successful in 84 to 98 percent of cases with no associated complications.[12,13] Success is more likely and complications are minimized with proper patient preparation.

INDICATIONS

Esophageal foreign body extraction is required in a minority of patients, as most foreign bodies will pass spontaneously into the stomach. The indications for removal depend upon the type of foreign body and whether it impacts in the esophagus.

Meat boluses are commonly impacted in the esophagus. Patients will swallow large pieces that may or may not be well chewed. Impaction of a meat bolus, or another foreign body, at or just below the cricopharyngeus muscle with tracheal compression and resultant respiratory obstruction is a true emergency. The Heimlich maneuver may be lifesaving in this situation.[7] The patient should be immediately orotracheally intubated or a cricothyroidotomy performed if the Heimlich maneuver is unsuccessful. Early removal of meat bolus impactions is recommended, even when the bolus is located in the distal third of the esophagus. Delays in extraction allow the food to soften, making extraction more difficult.

Blunt and round objects may become impacted in the esophagus. Earlier removal is necessary if a blunt object is impacted higher in the esophagus with associated sialorrhea and the potential for pulmonary aspiration. Esophageal obstruction at lower levels requires prompt, but not emergent, treatment. Most rounded objects in the lower third of the esophagus will pass spontaneously into the stomach. Therefore, a 12 hour period of observation is permissible in this situation.[8] It is common for sharp, pointed, and elongated objects to become impacted in the esophagus. Toothpicks, open safety pins, nails, and chicken bones are associated with up to a 35 percent incidence of esophageal perforation and should be removed.[9,10] Toothpicks should be removed promptly from the esophagus or stomach even if they are not impacted because they are particularly prone to penetration of the gastrointestinal wall. Toothpicks may migrate into surrounding structures, leading to vascular and other serious complications.[9]

Numerous other objects can also become impacted in the esophagus. Elongated, narrow foreign bodies such as stiff wires are prone to penetration and perforation of the esophageal wall. They should be removed even if they passed through the esophagus and into the stomach. These objects may become trapped by the retroperitoneally fixed angles of the duodenum and eventually result in perforation. Plastic bag clips, although not sharp and pointed, should be removed before they pass from the esophagus into the stomach and through the pylorus. They have claws that can attach to the small bowel mucosa leading to ulceration, stricture formation, and bleeding.[11] Toxic foreign bodies such as button batteries that become impacted in the esophagus should be removed promptly to prevent perforation and systemic toxicity.

CONTRAINDICATIONS

There are no absolute contraindications to the removal of an esophageal foreign body. Serious, life- and limb-threatening injuries should be treated prior to esophageal foreign body removal. The patient's airway, breathing, and circulation should be evaluated and supported as necessary prior to removing the foreign body.

EQUIPMENT

Flexible upper gastrointestinal endoscope
Rigid gastroscope
Through-the-scope-balloon
Steigmann-Goff friction-fit adaptor of the esophageal variceal rubber banding ligating kit
Glucagon
44 French Maloney rubber dilator
Lubricant gel
Endoscopic overtube, for use with sharp or pointed foreign bodies
Soft latex protector hood for the flexible scope
Laryngoscope
Laryngoscope blades, Miller and Macintosh of various sizes
Curved clamp
Medications for providing conscious sedation
Cardiac monitoring
Pulse oximetry
Supplemental oxygen
Foley catheters, 14 to 16 French
Topical anesthetic spray
Water-soluble contrast material
5 mL syringe
Fluoroscopy machine, optional

PATIENT PREPARATION

If possible, obtain a duplicate sample of the ingested foreign body. Manipulate the duplicate object with available foreign body forceps and snares. Determine which instrument is best suited to grasping the foreign body. Instruments that are most useful include alligator and rat-toothed forceps, polypectomy snares, and Dormia baskets.

Explain the risks, benefits, and aftercare of the procedure to the patient and/or their representative. Obtain an informed consent for the procedure. Place the patient supine. Obtain intravenous access. Apply the cardiac monitor, pulse oximeter, and supplemental oxygen to the patient. Administer intravenous sedation or conscious sedation as necessary.

TECHNIQUES

GENERAL PRINCIPLES

The flexible upper gastrointestinal endoscope should be inserted under direct visualization to avoid inadvertently striking an object and further impacting

it or causing it to penetrate the esophageal wall. Blunt foreign bodies such as coins can be securely grasped with a forceps or a snare. **A firm grasp on the foreign body is required before withdrawal is attempted.** Otherwise, the foreign body may become dislodged at points of anatomic narrowing such as the hypopharynx and the cricopharyngeus muscle. This can result in aspiration of the foreign body. An overtube should be used if multiple insertions and withdrawals of the endoscope are needed. Pointed foreign bodies should be withdrawn with the point trailing to avoid perforating any structures. Objects with sharp edges, such as razor blades, should be extracted through an overtube to prevent secondary injury. Elongated foreign bodies such as wires or pens should be grasped with a snare close to the cephalad end of the object so it can align itself with the long axis of the esophagus during withdrawal. Foreign bodies that penetrate the mucosa can be safely extracted with the endoscope if frank perforation or vascular penetration has not occurred.

FOOD IMPACTIONS

Endoscopy: Food impactions are more likely to occur in the distal esophagus. If the patient is symptomatic, there is no need for barium studies because it will obscure visualization during endoscopy. **Endoscopic intervention should be carried out immediately to prevent aspiration if the patient is salivating and unable to handle oral secretions. The impacted food bolus should not remain in the esophagus for more than 12 hours. Thereafter, the risk of complications increases significantly.**

Underlying esophageal disease is found in 65 to 97 percent of adults presenting with esophageal food impaction.[13,14] **Endoscopic removal is the procedure of choice if a meat bolus does not pass spontaneously or after an unsuccessful trial of gas-forming agents, glucagon, nifedipine, or nitroglycerine.** The entire bolus could be removed slowly with a polypectomy snare or Dormia basket under direct visualization. When the endoscope is just below the cricopharyngeus muscle, snugly pull the snare with the food bolus against the tip of the endoscope. Extend the patient's head and quickly remove the endoscope.[15]

If the food bolus is soft, a piecemeal approach can be accomplished with several passages of the endoscope through an overtube.[16] The overtube will facilitate reinsertion of the endoscope. Insert a Maloney rubber dilator (44 French) into the esophagus and proximal to the foreign body. Pass the overtube, lubricated internally and externally, over the Maloney dilator. Remove the Maloney dilator. Introduce the flexible endoscope through the overtube.

Another method, the push technique, has been useful in dealing with an impacted food bolus.[13] A small-caliber flexible endoscope may be used to bypass the food bolus and evaluate the area distal to the obstruction. If the endoscope is able to pass into the stomach successfully, pull it back until it is just proximal to the food bolus. Use the endoscope to gently push the food bolus into the stomach. It is preferable to push from the right side of the food bolus rather than straight, especially in patients with a hiatal hernia, since the gastroesophageal junction usually takes a left turn as it enters the hernia. The presence of a bone spicule should always be considered, whether the meat bolus is being extracted or pushed into the stomach.

A newer technique is accomplished by attaching the Steigmann-Goff friction-fit adaptor of the esophageal variceal rubber banding ligating kit to the tip of the endoscope.[17] The tip of the endoscope is replaced with a screw-on drum from the variceal ligation kit. After placing an esophageal overtube proximal to the food bolus, the endoscope is passed through the overtube.[18–21] To avoid the risk of dropping the food in the trachea, a Roth retrieval net may be passed through the endoscope to retrieve food from the esophagus.[22,23]

A last resort approach is the use of Nd:YAG laser to burn an opening in the center of an impacted meat bolus. This method is expensive and carries a high risk of complications.[24] Finally, if a food impaction of the esophagus cannot successfully be removed using the flexible endoscope, rigid endoscopy under general anesthesia should be considered.[25]

Gas-forming agents: Gas-forming agents can be used to relieve a distal esophageal food impaction. They are occasionally used in an attempt to relieve a food impaction in the proximal and middle thirds of the esophagus. These agents produce carbon dioxide gas that distends the esophagus, relaxes the lower esophageal sphincter, and "pushes" the food bolus through the gastroesophageal junction with the aid of esophageal peristalsis. Gas-forming agents may be used in conjunction with glucagon, nifedipine, or nitroglycerine to help relieve the impacted food bolus. Complications associated with gas-forming agents include aspiration, vomiting, forceful vomiting, and esophageal perforation due to distention and/or vomiting. Many physicians do not use these agents due to the risk of perforation.

Three classes of gas-forming agents have been used. Commonly used are commercially available agents that are used by Radiologists for upper gastrointestinal contrast studies. A mixture of tartaric acid (1.5 to 3.0 gm in 15 mL H_2O) immediately followed by sodium bicarbonate (1.5 to 3.0 gm in 15 mL H_2O) has been successfully used. A final agent is carbonated soda pop.

Glucagon: A trial of intravenous glucagon before endoscopic therapy is a reasonable approach. It may disimpact a food bolus in the distal esophagus and allow it to pass into the stomach. Glucagon relaxes the smooth muscle of the lower esophagus and decreases lower-esophageal sphincter tone. It relaxes the esophageal smooth muscle within 1 minute of intravenous injection, and its effects last approximately 20 to 25 minutes. Glucagon has no effect on the proximal third of the esophagus that is composed of skeletal muscle. It has a minimal effect on the middle third of the esophagus that is composed of both skeletal and smooth muscle. Glucagon has an overall success rate of ≤ 50 percent. Glucagon has been also combined with gas-forming agents to enhance esophageal clearance.

The dose of glucagon is 0.03 to 0.1 mg/kg intravenously with a maximum dose of 1 mg in children and 2 mg in adults. It should be administered over 1 to 2 minutes. **It is recommended to give a test dose (1/10 of the dose) and observe the patient for 5 minutes for signs of hypersensitivity or hypotension before giving the full dose.** Have the patient take 1 to 2 sips of water after the administration of glucagon to stimulate lower esophageal peristalsis. Administer a second dose of glucagon if the food bolus impaction is not relieved within 10 to 20 minutes.

Glucagon is a relatively safe medication. It should not be administered to patients with known hypersensitivity to glucagon, esophageal fibrosis, esophageal rings, esophageal strictures, insulinomas, pheochromocytomas, sharp or irregular foreign bodies, or Zollinger-Ellison syndrome. Exogenous glucagon stimulates the release of catecholamines. It can stimulate a pheochromocytoma to release catecholamines resulting in marked hypertension and tachycardia. The hypertension can be controlled using 5 to 10 mg of intravenous phentolamine. Glucagon's hyperglycemic effect can cause an insulinoma to release insulin and cause subsequent hypoglycemia. Common complications associated with glucagon include nausea, vomiting, transient hyperglycemia, allergic reactions, tachycardia, and hypertension. Glucagon is a polypeptide hormone synthesized in nonpathogenic *Escherichia coli* that have been genetically altered. This is the basis of the allergic/hypersensitivity reactions. A transient rise in blood pressure and heart rate is often seen after administration of glucagon. Patients taking beta-blockers may be more susceptible to transient hypertension and tachycardia. These side effects are short-lived as the half-life of glucagon is 8 to 18 minutes.

Nifedipine: Nifedipine is a calcium channel blocker that decreases lower esophageal sphincter tone. It has been administered to allow an impacted food bolus to pass into the stomach. It should not be administered if the patient has an allergy to calcium channel blockers, has hypotension, or ingested a sharp or irregular shaped

foreign body. With a single dose, nifedipine has few side effects. These are usually minimal (dizziness, flushing, headache, hypotension, lightheadedness, muscle cramps, nausea, nervousness, and palpitations) and do not preclude its use. **The most significant effect of nifedipine is hypotension that may last 6 to 8 hours.** Some patients will have a significant hypotensive response to nifedipine and there is no way to predict which patients will be affected. For these reasons, many physicians will not use nifedipine in the elderly or in patients with a history of cardiac disease, coronary artery disease, or stroke or who are concurrently taking antihypertensive medications. The typical dose is 10 mg of oral nifedipine. The medication may be chewed then held in the mouth and subsequently swallowed. Alternatively, open the capsule, place the medicine sublingually, and have the patient hold it in their mouth and then swallow the nifedipine. Attempt another technique if the food bolus does not pass with one dose of nifedipine.

Nitroglycerine: Sublingual nitroglycerine (0.3, 0.4, or 0.5 mg) relaxes vascular smooth muscle and the smooth muscle contained within the middle and distal thirds of the esophagus. The use of sublingual nitroglycerine may allow the esophagus to dilate enough so that a food bolus can pass into the stomach. **Nitroglycerine should not be administered if the patient is hypotensive or has ingested a sharp or irregular shaped foreign body.** The onset of action is within 1 to 3 minutes with a maximum effect by 4 to 5 minutes. The major side effect of nitroglycerine is hypotension, but that is short-lived. Administer one pill sublingually and allow 4 to 5 minutes for an effect. The dose may be repeated a second time. Attempt another technique if the food bolus does not pass after two doses of nitroglycerine.

Papain: Papain is a proteolytic enzyme that has been used to dissolve an impacted food bolus. It is available in markets as meat tenderizer and in health food stores as a digestive supplement. It will dissolve the esophageal mucosa and continue to work its way through the esophageal wall and into the mediastinum if it does not first dissolve the food bolus. The use of papain to dissolve an impacted food bolus may be associated with fatal esophageal perforation and, if aspirated, hemorrhagic pulmonary edema. **Papain should never be used to dissolve an impacted food bolus.**

SHARP AND POINTED FOREIGN BODIES

Removal of sharp and pointed objects requires extreme caution due to potential life-threatening complications, higher morbidity, and higher mortality. An experienced Endoscopist should manage these cases. It may be safer, in some cases, to consider surgical intervention. Toothpicks and bones are the most common foreign bodies requiring surgical removal.[26–28] Nails, needles, razor blades, safety pins, and dental prostheses may be removed endoscopically.[26–28] It is important to remember that "advancing points puncture while trailing points do not."[29] Objects longer than 5 cm and wider than 2 cm will rarely pass through the pylorus.[30] Intravenous glucagon (0.4 to 0.6 mg in adults) may be used to facilitate extraction from the stomach and duodenum.

An alligator forceps or snares are needed to grasp the object over the feeding tube. A plastic overtube should be considered for the removal of any sharp object.[18,31] The overtube should be at least 60 cm long to remove a sharp object from the stomach. This will limit objects for endoscopic removal to those smaller than 11 to 15 mm in diameter that fit within the overtube.[32] A soft latex protector hood may be used for the removal of large objects.

Razor blade ingestions may be managed with the flexible esophagoscope in adults. An alligator forceps, a snare, and an overtube will be needed. A razor blade that has passed the pylorus will often traverse through the intestinal tract without difficulty.

Safety pins and toothpicks pose additional risks due to their sharp ends that may perforate the esophagus. An open safety pin in the esophagus, with the open end proximal, should be pushed into the stomach with the flexible endoscope. Once in the stomach, the object is turned and the hinged end is grasped and pulled out first. A closed safety pin in the stomach will often pass without difficulty. Grasp a toothpick with an alligator forceps or snare very close to the tip so that the longitudinal axis of the toothpick is parallel to the scope as it is withdrawn into the overtube.[15]

Numerous other sharp objects are often encountered in the esophagus. Pens, pencils, thermometers, and wires are extracted in a fashion similar to a toothpick with a snare grasping the end of the object.[14] Glass may be withdrawn similarly or by using an end-hood attachment.[31,33]

Attempts should be made to remove all sharp and pointed foreign bodies before they pass from the stomach. Approximately 15 to 35 percent of sharp or pointed foreign bodies will cause intestinal perforation, especially in the area of the ileocecal valve.[34,35]

BUTTON BATTERIES

Most button batteries ingested (96 percent) are small and 7.9 to 11.6 mm in diameter.[36] The majority of them contain manganese dioxide, silver oxide, mercuric oxide, zinc air, mercuric oxide, or lithium. Obtain anteroposterior and lateral abdominal and chest radiographs to distinguish between coins and button batteries. A double density shadow is suggestive of batteries. The coin has a much sharper edge.

A button battery lodged in the esophagus is a true emergency and immediate removal is indicated to avoid the rapid corrosive action of the alkaline substance on the mucosa and subsequent complications.[36,37] Endotracheal intubation is usually necessary to protect the airway prior to endoscopic removal. The battery is removed from the esophagus under direct viewing using a through-the-scope balloon. A biopsy forceps may be needed to free the edge of the battery prior to removal. Alternatively, the battery may be pushed to the stomach and then removed using a polypectomy snare or a Dormia basket. **Do not use a Foley catheter or a magnet to remove a button battery without the aid of endotracheal intubation and general anesthesia due to the possibility of the button battery falling into the airway.** The patient should be admitted to the intensive care unit and monitored for signs of perforation and sepsis if they suffered severe esophageal injury when evaluated by endoscopy after removal of the button battery. If the injury is localized to the anterior wall of the esophagus, bronchoscopy may be performed to evaluate the extent of injury.

Generally, a button battery in the stomach need not be removed unless the patient is symptomatic with abdominal pain, tenderness, or gastrointestinal bleeding. Asymptomatic patients with button batteries less than 15 mm in diameter in their stomachs need follow-up abdominal radiographs every 24 hours to document progress until it is expelled. In a child less than 6 years old, the battery should be endoscopically removed if it is larger in size and has not passed within 48 hours.[36,38] Patients may be placed on H_2 blockers and/or proton pump inhibitors to decrease the acid in the stomach and therefore decrease the battery reaction. If mercury poisoning is expected, serum and urine mercury levels should be obtained and monitored.

FOLEY CATHETER TECHNIQUE

A Foley catheter has been successfully used to remove recently ingested smooth and blunt foreign bodies that are radiographically opaque from the esophagus. This technique is inexpensive, has a high success rate, does not require hospitalization, and avoids the complications associated with endotracheal intubation and general anesthesia. Coins are the foreign bodies primarily removed with a Foley catheter. The technique has also been used to remove button batteries, food boluses, and other smooth foreign bodies.

This technique cannot be used on all patients with an esophageal foreign body. This technique should not be attempted in patients who are confused or uncooperative. Patients with an altered mental status, airway compromise, or potential airway compromise should be endotracheally intubated prior to Foley catheter removal of the foreign body. Sharp or irregular shaped objects can lacerate or perforate the esophagus upon removal. Known or suspected esophageal perforation is a contraindication to this technique. Patients with complete esophageal obstruction, as demonstrated by an esophageal air-fluid level on radiographs, are not candidates. Esophageal fibrosis, esophageal tumors, anatomic anomalies, or a history of prior esophageal surgery are also contraindications.

The equipment required for the technique is minimal. This includes topical anesthetic spray, a bite block, and a size 12 to 16 Foley catheter with a 5 to 10 mL balloon. The technique may be performed ideally in a fluoroscopy suite or blindly in the Emergency Department. A water-soluble contrast agent is required if using fluoroscopy. **The most dangerous and immediate complication of this technique is airway obstruction. Airway and emergency equipment must be available if this technique is to be performed.**

Explain the procedure to the patient, including the sensations they will experience. The use of a topical anesthetic spray for the oropharynx is beneficial but optional. Its use may increase the risk of aspiration. The use of physical restraints, conscious sedation, and/or intubation may be required as needed on a case-by-case basis. Preinflate the Foley catheter balloon with 5 to 10 mL of water-soluble contrast material. Inspect the integrity of the balloon. Withdraw the contrast material back into the syringe to deflate the balloon. The small amount of contrast material left in the balloon will facilitate identification under fluoroscopy. Place the patient prone in 10 to 20 degrees of Trendelenburg or in the left lateral decubitus position in 10 to 20 degrees of Trendelenburg. The fluoroscopy technique and then the blind technique are described in the following paragraphs.

Insert the Foley catheter. Some physicians insert a bite block and place the Foley catheter through the mouth (Figure 51-1). Others use the nasal route. The oral route avoids the potential problem of lodging the foreign body in the nasopharynx with subsequent aspiration. Advance the Foley catheter under fluoroscopy until the balloon is just distal to the foreign body (Figure 51-1*A*). Slowly inflate the balloon with 5 mL of contrast material (Figure 51-1*B*). Stop inflating the balloon if the patient complains of pain; deflate the balloon, then reposition the catheter before reinflating. Withdraw the catheter with moderate and steady traction until it exits the mouth (Figures 51-1*C* and *D*). **Stop withdrawing the catheter if resistance is met to prevent an esophageal tear or perforation.** The balloon may occasionally slide past the foreign body as the catheter is being withdrawn. Reinsert the catheter and inflate the balloon with 7 to 8 mL of contrast material and then withdraw the catheter. **Do not overinflate the balloon as it can rupture the esophagus.** Do not attempt this technique more than twice. The balloon will pull the foreign body ahead of it into the hypopharynx and then the mouth. Tell the patient to spit out the foreign body; or you can grasp it with fingers, forceps, or a hemostat.

This technique may also be used "blindly" if fluoroscopy is not available. Estimate the distance, on the radiographs, from the mouth or nose to the foreign body. Place the Foley catheter over the radiograph with the balloon just distal to the foreign body. Mark the distance with tape on the catheter as it exits the mouth or nose. The catheter will then be inserted into the patient until the tape is positioned at their mouth or nose. Use saline rather than contrast material to inflate the balloon. Obtain repeat radiographs if the foreign body is not expelled with the catheter as it may have been pushed into the stomach. The remainder of the technique is the same as described for removal under fluoroscopy.

Complications with the technique are uncommon but do occur. This technique may not be able to remove the foreign body. Insertion of the catheter can cause laryngospasm or vomiting. The Foley catheter may enter the airway, resulting in coughing and laryngospasm. The esophagus may be lacerated or perforated if the foreign body is large, completely impacted, sharp, irregular, or has been in place for over 12 to 24 hours. Overinflation of the balloon can rupture the esophagus. Removal through the nose may result in epistaxis or impaction of the foreign body in the nasopharynx or nasal cavity. The most feared complication is complete or partial airway obstruction if the foreign body falls into the larynx.

BOUGIENAGE

The use of a Bougie dilator to push an esophageal foreign body into the stomach has been used in children.[39–41] The technique has been successfully used in asymptomatic children who have radiographs documenting a coin in the esophagus, no history of esophageal disease, and less than 24 hours has passed from the time of ingestion. The advantages of this technique are that it is quick, simple to perform, does not require sedation, and does not require intravenous access.

Apply a topical anesthetic spray to the child's oropharynx. Select an appropriate size Bougie dilator. Physically restrain the patient while they are sitting upright or standing on the bed. Place the tip of the Bougie dilator at the mouth and run the rest of the dilator to the earlobe and to just below the left costal margin. Place a piece of tape on the Bougie dilator 3 to 4 cm below the costal margin. Insert the Bougie dilator through the mouth and advance it in one smooth motion until the tape is at the mouth. Remove the Bougie dilator. Obtain a repeat radiograph to confirm that the coin is now in the stomach.

Complications can occur and are avoided with proper patient selection. Esophageal perforation may occur if the patient has known esophageal disease, prior esophageal surgery or manipulation, a sharp foreign body, or an irregular shaped foreign body. A foreign

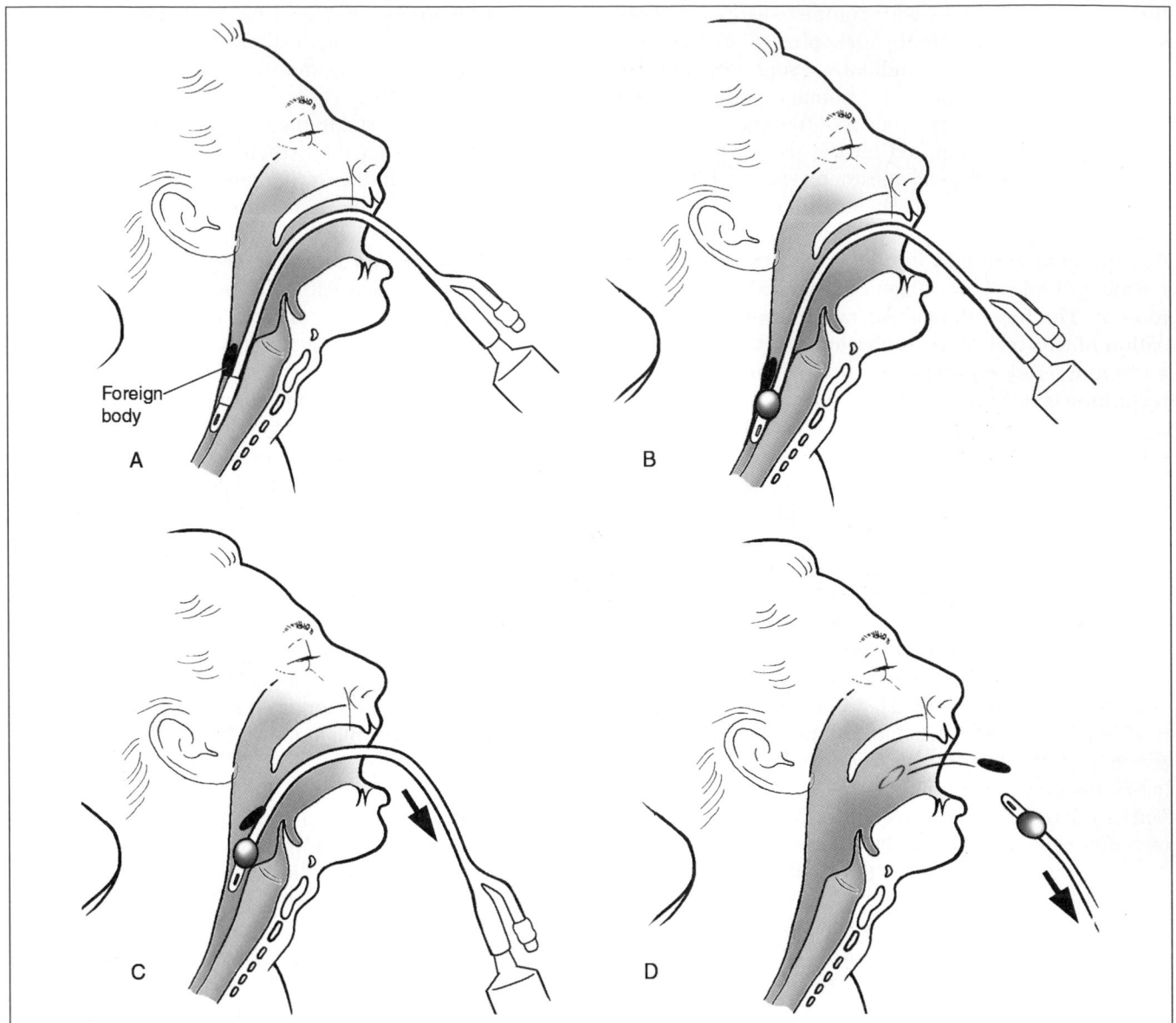

FIGURE 51-1 The Foley catheter technique to remove an esophageal foreign body. This illustration demonstrates the oral route for catheter insertion. The nasal route may also be utilized. *A.* The catheter is inserted and advanced until the balloon is just distal to the foreign body. *B.* The balloon is inflated. *C.* The catheter is withdrawn and pulls the foreign body into the hypopharynx. *D.* Completely withdrawing the catheter will pull the foreign body into and out the mouth. Steps *C* and *D* are performed in one smooth motion.

body present for more than 24 hours can cause pressure-necrosis to the esophagus and increase the risk of perforation.

OROGASTRIC TUBE MAGNET

The orogastric tube magnet (OGTM) is an orogastric tube that has a magnet sealed within the distal end. It may be used to retrieve smooth, metallic foreign bodies from the esophagus and stomach under fluoroscopy. Place the patient in the lateral decubitus position. Apply a topical anesthetic spray to the oropharynx. Insert the OGTM through the mouth. Advance the OGTM under

flouroscopy into the esophagus and directed toward the foreign body until it makes contact. Withdraw the OGTM and the foreign body out the mouth. This is a rarely used technique.

ALTERNATIVE TECHNIQUES

Numerous other methods for the removal of esophageal foreign bodies have been tried and reported in the literature. Surgical removal is rarely indicated except when complications such as perforation or vascular penetration have occurred. **Do not blindly push food boluses into the stomach.** This is hazardous because many patients have underlying esophageal disease. **Blind maneuvers can result in esophageal perforation.**

PEDIATRIC CONSIDERATIONS

Children less than 4 years of age are predisposed to occasionally have an esophageal foreign body. They explore objects with their mouth, have a high curiosity level, lack molars to chew food, and have poor motor and sensory coordination. Common esophageal foreign bodies include balls, button batteries, buttons, candies, coins, gumballs, jacks, marbles, partially chewed food, and pen caps. A high index of suspicion must be maintained as a history of an ingestion may not be obtained.

Children may present asymptomatically or with cough, drooling, dysphagia, respiratory distress, unwillingness to eat, or vomiting. An asymptomatic child with an esophageal coin or round object, except button batteries, can be admitted to the hospital and watched for 24 hours to see if the object will spontaneously pass into the stomach. The object should be removed with a Bougie dilator, a Foley catheter, or an endoscope if the child is or becomes symptomatic, or if the object does not pass within 24 hours. Foreign bodies in a mainstem bronchus require removal by an Otolaryngologist in the operating room with a rigid bronchoscope. Turning the child upside down or performing the Heimlich maneuver may move the foreign body into the trachea or larynx and cause a complete airway obstruction.

ASSESSMENT

The patient should be observed until the effects of the sedation have resolved. This includes monitoring the vital signs as per protocol of the hospital. The patients should be given a trial of liquids to swallow prior to discharge. The patient may be safely discharged after they tolerate oral fluids, are awake and oriented, and are able to ambulate without difficulty. The patient should be driven home by another person if sedation was used to extract the foreign body.

Admission is required in a few instances. The inability to tolerate oral fluids is a contraindication to discharge. Foreign bodies that are not retrievable must be removed. These patients should be admitted for observation, further endoscopy, or operative removal. Any patient with evidence of esophageal perforation should be admitted, observed, and evaluated by a Surgeon.

The esophagus should be endoscopically examined after removal of most foreign bodies. A Gastroenterologist should be consulted on anyone with an esophageal foreign body. All patients discharged from the Emergency Department should follow up with a Gastroenterologist in 24 to 48 hours. The presence of any lacerations, perforations, or erosions should be noted and may require repair. Any strictures will require dilation in the future. Some recommend a second endoscopic follow-up in 3 to 6 weeks for reevaluation of the esophagus. This is Endoscopist-specific.

AFTERCARE

The patient should be instructed to only ingest liquids for the first 12 to 18 hours. A soft diet should begin after this trial period of liquid and advanced to a general diet over 24 hours. The patient should be instructed to take small bites of food and completely chew any food before swallowing. They should immediately return to the Emergency Department if they experience abdominal pain, chest pain, dysphagia, hematemesis, hemoptysis, melena, or odynophagia, or if they have any concerns.

COMPLICATIONS

Esophageal perforation can occur due to the foreign body or the extraction procedure. The patient may present with fever, tachycardia, shortness of breath, chest pain, abdominal pain, and crepitation in the neck. An immediate chest radiograph and/or a radiographic contrast study should be performed if the extraction of the foreign body has been difficult.[1–3] An aortoesophageal fistula can form due to sharp foreign bodies in the esophagus that erode through the esophageal wall. This should be considered when the patient presents with dysphagia and significant hematemesis.[13,32] A latency period between the ingestion of the foreign body and hematemesis is usually 1 to 3 weeks, though it can occur years later.[14] Tracheoesophageal fistulas can occur more than a year after ingestion of the foreign body.[3]

Other life-threatening cardiopulmonary emergencies include mediastinitis, lung abscess, pericarditis, cardiac tamponade, pneumothorax, and pneumomediastinum. These complications mostly result from a delay in recognizing an esophageal perforation.[12–14] The remaining complications are discussed with each of the individual techniques of foreign body removal.

SUMMARY

Foreign body ingestion and food bolus impaction in the upper gastrointestinal tract are relatively common problems seen in the Emergency Department. Several studies have shown that 80 to 90 percent of foreign bodies in the GI tract will pass spontaneously. Approximately 10 to 20 percent will require nonoperative intervention while 1 percent will require surgical removal.[3,42] The most common presenting symptoms are chest or pharyngeal pain, odynophagia, dysphagia, foreign body sensation, and sialorrhea.[42] Despite performing emergent upper endoscopy, no foreign body could be found in almost half of patients.[43] The urgency for the endoscopic examination depends on the potential risk of aspiration or perforation, the type and size of the foreign body, the degree of obstruction, and the inability to manage secretions.[13] The presence of dysphagia and the immediate onset of symptoms would increase the probability of a positive foreign body finding on endoscopy.

Numerous techniques may be used to remove an esophageal foreign body. The technique of choice depends upon the level of patient cooperation, the type of foreign body, the time since ingestion, physician experience and comfort, Gastroenterology consultation, and presenting symptoms. Complications can be minimized by the proper selection of the removal technique and the appropriate patient for the technique.

REFERENCES

1. Webb WA, Taylor MB: Foreign bodies of the upper gastrointestinal tract, in Taylor MB, Gollan JL, Steer ML, et al (eds): *Gastrointestinal Emergencies*, 2nd ed. Baltimore: Lippincott Williams & Wilkins, 1997:3–18.

2. Schwartz GF, Polsky HS: Ingested foreign bodies of the gastrointestinal tract. *Am Surg* 1976; 42:236–238.

3. American Society for Gastrointestinal Endoscopy: Guideline for the management of ingested foreign bodies. *Gastrointest Endosc* 1995; 42(6):622–625.

4. Barros JL, Caballero A Jr, Rueda JC, et al: Foreign body ingestion: management of 167 cases. *World J Surg* 1991; 15(6):783–788.

5. Gelfand DW: Complications of gastrointestinal radiographic procedures: 1. Complications of routine fluoroscopic procedures. *Gastrointest Radiol* 1980; 5:293–315.

6. Gamba JL, Heaston DK, Korobkin M: CT diagnosis of an esophageal foreign body. *Am J Radiol* 1983; 140:289–290.

7. Haugen RK: The café coronary: sudden death in restaurants. *JAMA* 1963; 186(2):142–143.

8. Spitz L: Management of ingested foreign bodies in childhood. *Br Med J* 1971; 4:469–472.

9. Cockerill FR III, Wilson WR, Van Scoy RE: Travelling toothpicks. *Mayo Clin Proc* 1983; 58:613–616.

10. Rosch W, Classen M: Fiber endoscopic foreign body removal from the upper gastrointestinal tract. *Endoscopy* 1972; 4:193–197.

11. Guindi MM, Troster MM, Walley VM: Three cases of an usual foreign body in small bowel. *Gastrointest Radiol* 1987; 12:240–242.

12. Vizcarrondo FJ, Brady PG, Nord HJ: Foreign bodies in the upper gastrointestinal tract. *Gastrointest Endosc* 1983; 29(3):208–210.

13. Webb WA: Management of foreign bodies of the upper gastrointestinal tract. *Gastroenterology* 1988; 94(1):204–216.

14. Brady P: Esophageal foreign bodies. *Gastroenterol Clin North Am* 1991; 20(4):691–701.

15. Yoshida C, Peura D: Foreign bodies in the esophagus, in Castell D, Richter JE (eds): *The Esophagus.* Boston: Little, Brown, 1995:379–394.

16. Rogers BGH, Kot C, Meiri S, et al: An overtube for the flexible fiberoptic esophagogastroduodenoscope. *Gastrointest Endosc* 1982; 28(4):256–257.

17. Saeed ZA, Michaletz PA, Feiner SD, et al: A new endoscopic method for managing food impaction in the esophagus. *Endoscopy* 1990; 22:226–228.

18. Pouagare M, Brady PG: New techniques for the endoscopic removal of foreign bodies, in Barkin JS, O'Phelan CA (eds): *Advanced Therapeutic Endoscopy*, 2nd ed. New York: Raven Press, 1994:165–174.

19. Pezzi J, Shiau YF: A method for removing meat impactions from the esophagus. *Gastrointest Endosc* 1994; 40(5):634–636.

20. Mamel JJ, Weiss D, Pouagare M, et al: Endoscopic suction removal of food boluses from the upper gastrointestinal tract using Stiegmann-Goff friction-fit adaptor: an improved method for removal of food impactions. *Gastrointest Endosc* 1995; 41(6):593–596.

21. Ramirez FC: Endoscopic removal of esophageal meat impaction. *Gastrointest Endosc* 1995; 41(6):617.

22. Neustater B, Barkin JS: Extraction of an esophageal food impaction with a Roth retrieval net. *Gastrointest Endosc* 1996; 43(1):66–67.

23. Faigel DO, Stotland BR, Kochman ML, et al: Device choice and experience level in endoscopic foreign object retrieval: an in vivo study. *Gastrointest Endosc* 1997; 45(6):490–492.

24. Klein I: Resourceful management of esophageal food impaction. *Gastrointest Endosc* 1990; 36:80.

25. Berggreen PJ, Harrison E, Sanowski RA, et al: Techniques and complications of esophageal foreign body extraction in children and adults. *Gastrointest Endosc* 1993; 39(5):626–630.

26. Schwartz JT, Graham DY: Toothpick perforation of the intestines. *Ann Surg* 1977; 185(1):64–66.

27. Budnick LD: Toothpick-related injuries in the United States, 1979 through 1982. *JAMA* 1984; 252(6):796–797.

28. Guber MD, Suarez CA, Greve J: Toothpick perforation of the intestine diagnosed by a small bowel series. *Am J Gastroenterol* 1996; 91(4):789–791.

29. Jackson C, Jackson CL: *Disease of the Air and Food Passages of Foreign Body Origin.* Philadelphia: Saunders, 1937.

30. Koch H: Operative endoscopy. *Gastrointest Endosc* 1977; 24(2):65–68.

31. Macon N: Overtubes and foreign bodies. *Can J Gastroenterol* 1990; 4:599–602.

32. Bertoni G, Pacchione D, Gonigliaro R, et al: Endoscopic protector hood for safe removal of sharp-pointed gastroesophageal foreign bodies. *Surg Endosc* 1992; 6:255–258.

33. Tuen HH, Lai ECS, Fan ST: Endoscopic retrieval of ingested broken glass in the esophagus and stomach by end-hood and suction technique. *Gastrointest Endosc* 1989; 35(4):357–358.

34. Macmanus JE: Perforation of the intestine by ingested foreign bodies. Report of two cases and re-view of the literature. *Am J Surg* 1941; 53(3):393–400.

35. Maleki M, Evans WE: Foreign body perforation of the intestinal tract. *Arch Surg* 1970; 101:475–477.

36. Sheikh A: Button battery ingestion in children. *Pediatr Emerg Care* 1993; 9(4):224–229.

37. Blatnik BS, Toohill RJ, Lehman RH: Fatal complications from an alkaline battery foreign body in the esophagus. *Ann Otol Rhinol Laryngol* 1977; 86: 611–615.

38. Litovitz T, Schmitz BF: Ingestion of cylindrical and button batteries: an analysis of 2,382 cases. *Pediatrics* 1992; 89(4):747–757.

39. Bonadio WA, Jona JZ, Glicklich M, et al: Esophageal bougienage technique for coin ingestion in children. *J Pediatr Surg* 1988; 23:917–918.

40. Jona JZ, Glicklich M, Cohen RD: The contraindications for blind esophageal bougienage for coin ingestion in children. *J Pediatr Surg* 1988; 23:328–330.

41. Kelley JE, Leech MH, Carr MG: A safe and cost-effective protocol for the management of esophageal coins in children. *J Pediatr Surg* 1993; 28:898–900.

42. Ginsberg GG: Management of ingested foreign objects and food bolus impactions. *Gastrointest Endosc* 1994; 41(1):33–38.

43. Ciriza C, Garcia L, Suarez P, et al: What predictive parameters best indicate the need for emergent gastrointestinal endoscopy after foreign body ingestion? *J Clin Gastroenterol* 2000; 31(1):23–28.

Chapter 52

BALLOON TAMPONADE OF GASTROINTESTINAL BLEEDING

Bashar M. Attar

INTRODUCTION

Gastroesophageal varices are among the most dangerous complications associated with cirrhosis. They are present in 50 to 60 percent of cirrhotic patients, and about 30 percent of them will experience an episode of variceal hemorrhage within 2 years of the diagnosis of varices.[1] The major factors that determine the risk of bleeding in cirrhotics are variceal size and the degree of liver dysfunction.[1-3] While variceal bleeding stops spontaneously in 20 to 30 percent of cases, it recurs in 70 percent within 1 year of the initial episode.[1-4] Mortality is as high as 50 percent in the first year.[5] Variceal bleeding accounts for almost one-third of deaths in cirrhotic patients. Variceal hemorrhage has a poor prognosis if it is associated with coexisting or subsequent complications including rebleeding, infection, hepatic dysfunction, and portal pressure ≥ 12 mmHg.[6-7] Splanchnic vasoconstrictors can reduce portal pressure by reducing portal venous inflow, while venodilators reduce portal pressure by reducing resistance to portal flow.[7,8]

Doctors Sengstaken and Blakemore developed the concept of balloon tamponade to control bleeding esophageal and gastric varices in 1950. They developed a triple-lumen and double-balloon system that bears their names. The Sengstaken-Blakemore (SB) tube is used as a temporizing measure to stop variceal bleeding until more definitive means are available. A variant of the SB tube is the Minnesota tube. It is a quadruple-lumen, double-balloon system. These tubes are rarely used today due to the significant complications and the widespread availability of endoscopy. Emergency Physicians should become familiar with the SB and Minnesota tubes, as they can be potentially lifesaving in an emergent setting.

ANATOMY AND PATHOPHYSIOLOGY

Cirrhosis results in portal venous hypertension and a decrease in blood flow through the portal system. Collateral circulation develops, so that the blood in the portal vein can find an alternative route to the inferior vena cava. Large collateral systems include the esophageal, gastric, paraumbilical, and rectal veins. The left gastric and esophageal veins form one of the larger collateral circulation channels due to the pressure generated from the portal venous system and the large volume of blood flow through them. The collateral veins distend from the pressure and large volume of blood flow, resulting in weakening of the walls of the vein. Ulceration and rupture of these veins can result in large amounts of blood entering the esophagus and stomach. Patients may present with bright red blood per rectum, hematemesis, hemorrhagic shock, hypotension, or complications associated with hypotension and hemorrhage (e.g., cerebrovascular accidents and myocardial infarction).

INDICATIONS

Balloon tamponade should be considered in patients with acute bleeding from esophageal and/or gastric varices if medical therapy (e.g., somatostatin, octreotide, vasopressin) or emergent endoscopic therapy (banding or sclerotherapy) is not available, contraindicated, or unsuccessful.

CONTRAINDICATIONS

Absolute contraindications to balloon tamponade of variceal bleeding include a history of esophageal stricture, a history of recent surgery involving the gastro-

446

esophageal junction, or if the bleeding has terminated based upon nasogastric lavage and aspiration.

There are numerous relative contraindications to balloon tamponade of variceal bleeding. The procedure should not be performed if the equipment required is defective or missing components. Untrained support staff make the procedure as well as the aftercare more difficult. Significant active medical problems (respiratory failure, congestive heart failure, and cardiac arrhythmias) preclude the use of balloon devices. Incomplete gastric lavage leaving particulates in the stomach can cause retching and elevated intraabdominal pressure. The balloons will not properly position and may perforate the esophagus if the patient has a hiatal hernia. Esophageal ulcerations preclude the use of the esophageal balloon (a gastric balloon may be used). The device is not helpful if a variceal source of bleeding cannot be demonstrated by examination, history, and/or nasogastric aspiration. Patients with altered mental status, confusion, diminished gag reflexes, hypoxemia, or who are uncooperative should have their airway secured by endotracheal intubation prior to this procedure. Recurrent bleeding after the initial successful tamponade should be followed by endoscopic or operative intervention.

EQUIPMENT

SB tube (or Minnesota tube)
Topical anesthetic spray
Tongue blades
Lidocaine or water-soluble jelly
60 mL syringe
Catheter tips for the syringe
Two wall-suction setups with plastic connectors and
    suction tubing
Adhesive tape
Rubber shod clamps, hemostats, or plugs
Scissors
Y-adapter or 3-way stopcock
Intravenous extension tubing
Pressure bulb
Mercury manometer or handheld manometer
Bite block
Nasogastric tube
Football helmet, catcher's mask, or endotracheal tube
    holder

The SB tube is a triple-lumen and double-balloon system (Figures 52-1 and 52-2). It is available in a variety of sizes, including pediatric sizes. The proximal end contains three ports. A syringe attaches to the esophageal balloon inflation port to inflate the esophageal balloon. A syringe attaches to the gastric balloon inflation port to inflate the gastric balloon. The gastric aspiration port may be used to aspirate gastric contents, instill fluid into the stomach, or lavage the stomach. The ports may be opened and closed by the application of rubber shod clamps, hemostats, or plugs. The tube is made of a soft rubber and is extremely flexible. The proximal or esophageal balloon is elongated. The distal or gastric balloon is round. The maximum volume to inflate each balloon is manufacturer- and size-specific. Numerous perforations in the distal end of the tube allow for gastric aspiration and lavage.

The Minnesota tube is a quadruple-lumen and double-balloon system (Figure 52-3). It is similar to the SB tube with the exception of an additional port and lumen. The esophageal aspiration port allows saliva and esophageal secretions to be aspirated from a perforation just above the esophageal balloon. The only advantage of this tube over the SB tube is that the SB tube requires a nasal or oral tube to be passed into the esophagus to aspirate secretions.

PATIENT PREPARATION

Explain the risks and benefits of the procedure to the patient and/or their representative. An informed consent should be obtained for the procedure. Thoroughly assess the patient's airway and breathing. Have a low threshold to protect the airway by endotracheal intubation. Endotracheal intubation is required before performing the procedure if the patient has altered mental status, airway compromise, or the potential for airway compromise. Patients are often ill and require intubation anyway. The procedure and the tube are not well tolerated, and intubation makes it easier. Endotracheal intubation reduces the risk of aspiration. The patient should be resuscitated, including blood transfusion, to stabilize them hemodynamically.

Place the patient sitting upright to semi-upright by elevating the head of the bed at least 45 degrees. This is the ideal position. The procedure can be performed with the patient in the left lateral decubitus position if he or she cannot sit upright. The procedure can be performed with the patient supine if he or she is endotracheally intubated. Apply topical anesthetic spray to the nostrils and pharynx. Insert a nasogastric tube or Ewald tube. Aspirate the stomach contents. Evacuate the stomach with tap-water lavage through the nasogastric tube (or Ewald tube), then remove the nasogastric tube. The patient should have intravenous access established with at least two large-bore catheters. Cardiac monitoring, continuous pulse oximetry, and supplemental oxygen should be applied to the patient. The patient may require the judicious use of intravenous sedatives and soft restraints during the insertion and inflation of the tube.

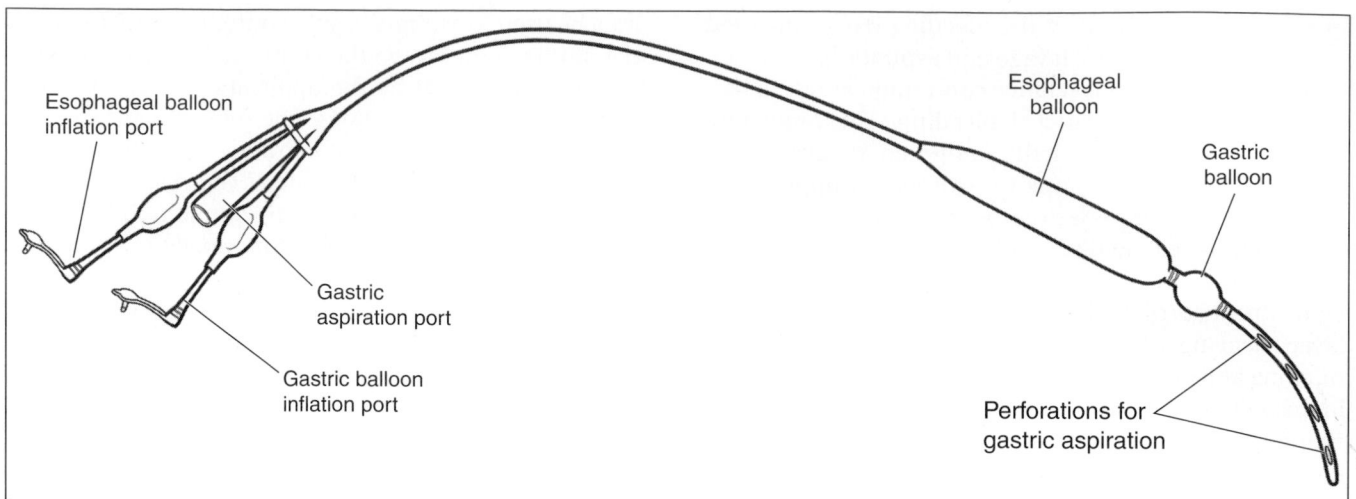

FIGURE 52-1 Schematic illustration of the Sengstaken-Blakemore tube.

Prepare the equipment. Flush the aspiration ports with air to ensure their patency. Inflate the balloons with the maximum recommended volume of air and check for leaks. It is advisable to inflate the balloons under water to look for small leaks. Connect the mercury manometer to the balloon ports and inflate the balloons to the recommended pressures and check for leaks.

Completely deflate the balloons. Record the manometric pressure of each balloon when it is deflated. Insert the plastic plugs in the balloon inflation ports or loosely clamp each port with a hemostat or rubber shod clamp.[9–11] Lubricate the SB tube with a water-soluble lubricant. Place the SB tube on a table. Position a nasogastric tube next to the SB tube so that the tip of the

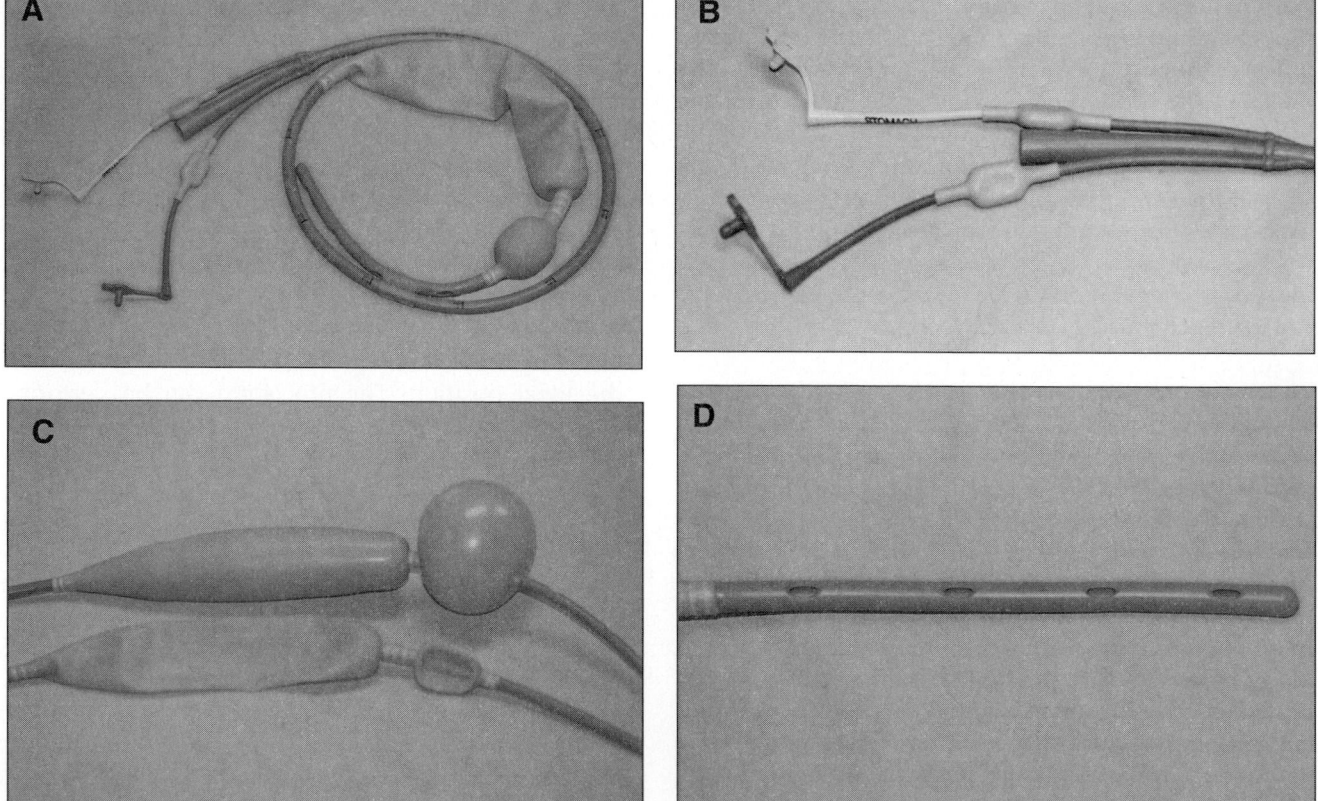

FIGURE 52-2 The Sengstaken-Blakemore tube. *A.* Overall view of the SB tube. *B.* The proximal ports. *C.* The esophageal and gastric balloons in the inflated and deflated states. *D.* The distal end.

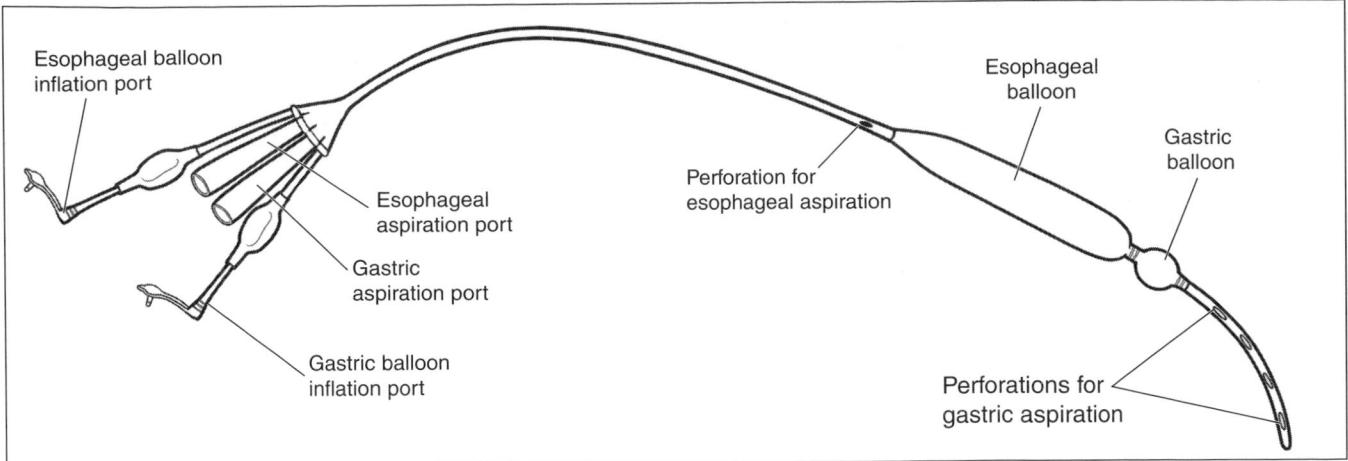

FIGURE 52-3 Schematic illustration of the Minnesota tube.

nasogastric tube is just above the esophageal balloon (Figure 52-4). Place a piece of tape on both tubes to mark a common point, proximal to the 50 cm mark of the SB tube, that will be outside of the patient. The nasogastric tube will be inserted after the SB tube is placed. Alternatively, position the tubes as above and tape both tubes together at two or three sites. This allows the nasogastric tube to be inserted simultaneously with the SB tube.

The SB tube may be inserted through the nose or through the mouth. The nasal route is more difficult to use and may be associated with a higher rate of complications. Despite this, many physicians recommend this route in the awake patient. The oral route is the preferred route of insertion by some physicians, especially if the patient is intubated. Apply topical anesthetic spray into the nasal cavity and oropharynx if the SB tube will be placed nasogastrically. Apply topical anesthetic spray

into the oropharynx if the SB tube will be placed orogastrically. Place a bite block in the patient's mouth if the SB tube will be placed orogastrically to prevent the patient from biting the SB tube.

TECHNIQUE

Insert the lubricated SB tube until the 50 cm mark is located just outside the nares, or outside the teeth if inserted through the mouth. Flush the gastric aspiration port with air while auscultating over the epigastrium (Figure 52-5). A rush of air should be heard to ensure that the distal end of the SB tube is properly positioned within the stomach. If possible, confirm the position of the SB tube with portable plain radiographs or fluoroscopy. **It is imperative to know that the gastric bal-**

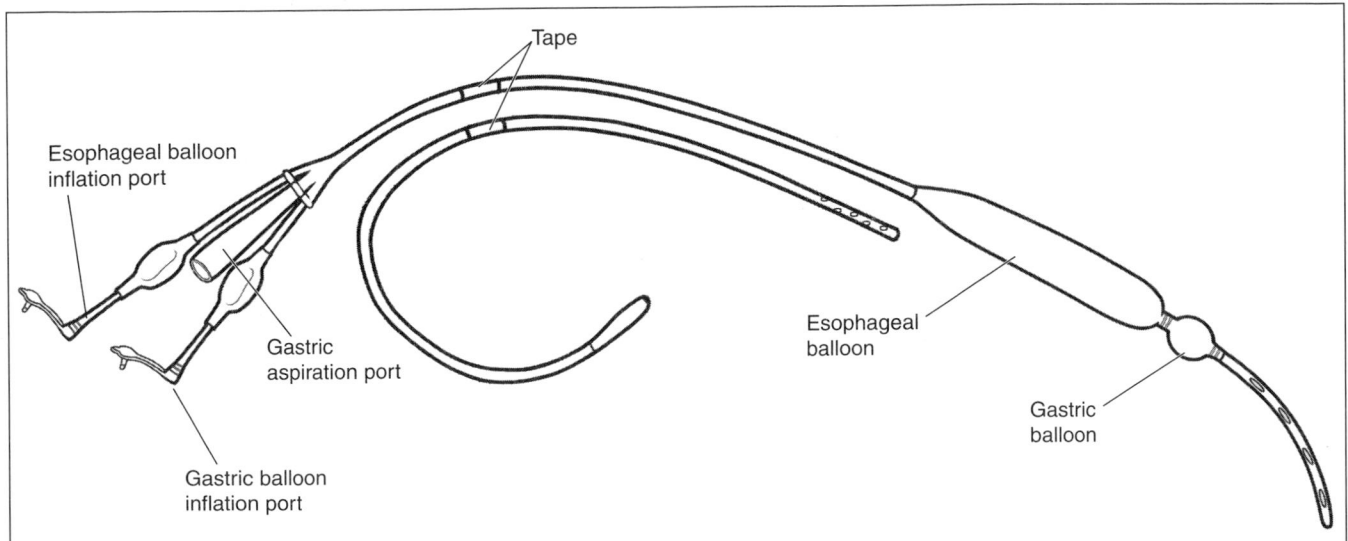

FIGURE 52-4 Preparing the nasogastric tube. Place the nasogastric tube alongside of the SB tube with the tip just above the esophageal balloon. Place tape on both tubes to mark a common point proximal to the 50 cm mark on the SB tube.

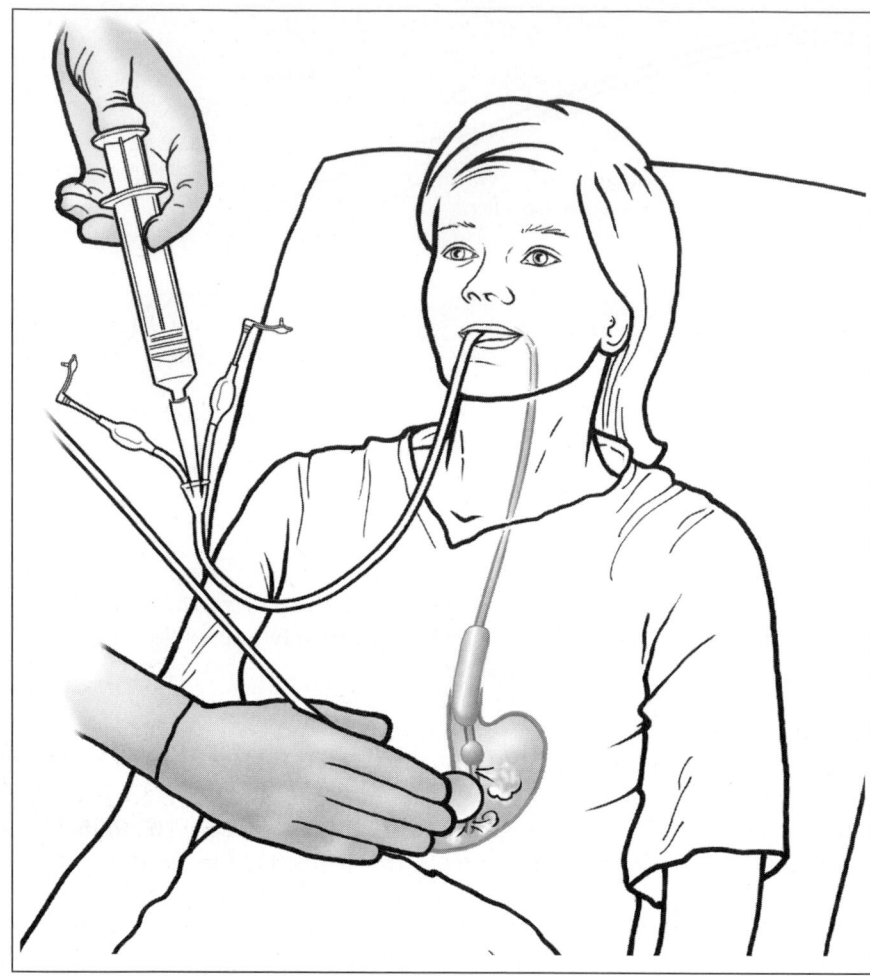

FIGURE 52-5 The SB tube has been inserted until the 50 cm mark is just outside the teeth. Inject 50 mL of air while auscultating over the epigastric area. A rush of air should be heard if the distal end of the SB tube is within the stomach.

loon is within the stomach before it is inflated. Apply suction to the gastric and esophageal aspiration ports.

Remove the rubber shod clamp and plastic plug from the gastric balloon inflation port. Connect the Y-adapter with a handheld or mercury manometer and a pressure bulb or a 50 mL syringe with a catheter tip to the gastric balloon inflation port (Figure 52-6). Measure the intragastric balloon pressure. **If the intragastric balloon pressure after intubation is 15 mm Hg greater than that prior to the intubation, deflate the balloon, as it may be located within the esophagus.** Inflate the gastric balloon in increments with 50 to 100 mL boluses of air (Figure 52-7). **Deflate the balloon immediately if the patient experiences chest pain. This signifies that the gastric balloon is in the esophagus.** Clamp the gastric balloon inflation port when the gastric balloon is inflated with 250 to 300 mL of air. Gently pull the SB tube back until resistance is felt as the gastric balloon lodges against the gastroesophageal junction (Figure 52-8).

Apply slight tension to the SB tube to occlude the veins at the gastroesophageal junction. This tension must be maintained by one of several methods. Fix the upper end of the SB tube as it exits from the mouth or nose to the crossbar of a football helmet or a catcher's mask (Figure 52-9). Apply over-the-bed traction with a one pound weight. Alternatively, fix the upper end of the SB tube, if it emerges from the nostril, by a cuff of sponge rubber held in place by an adhesive tape band. Insert the nasogastric tube until the tape is at the level of the tape on the SB tube (Figure 52-10).

Connect the gastric aspiration port and the nasogastric tube to the suction source (Figure 52-11). Place the gastric aspiration port and the nasogastric tube on low intermittent suction. Unclamp the esophageal balloon port clamp. Attach the Y tubing, manometer, and pressure bulb (or 50 mL syringe) to the esophageal balloon port. Inflate the esophageal balloon to a pressure of 25 mmHg if bleeding continues through the gastric aspiration port or the nasogastric tube. If bleeding continues to persist, increase the esophageal balloon pressure in 5 mmHg increments until 45 mmHg is achieved or the bleeding stops. Double clamp the SB tube to prevent accidental deflation of the balloons.

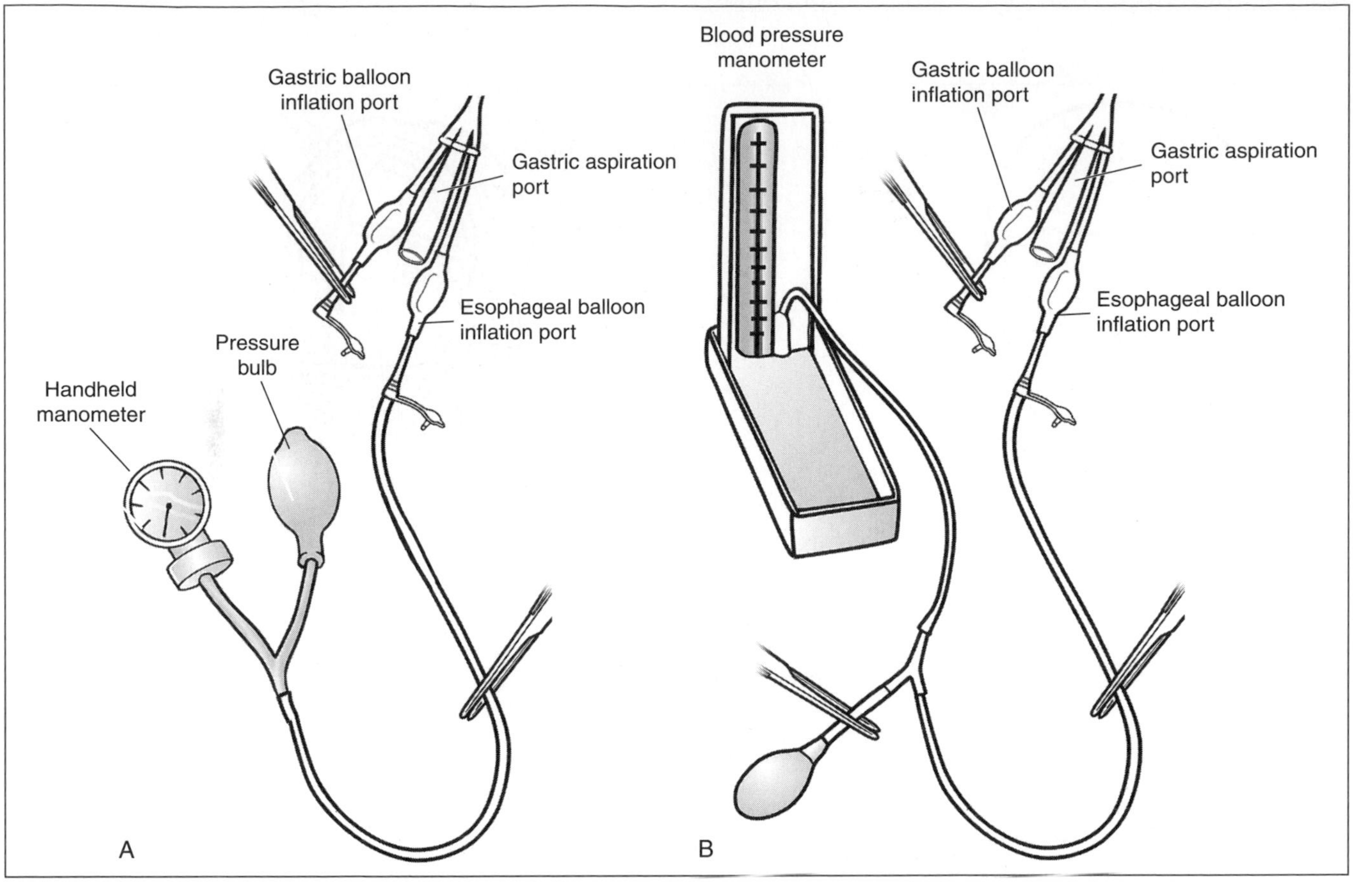

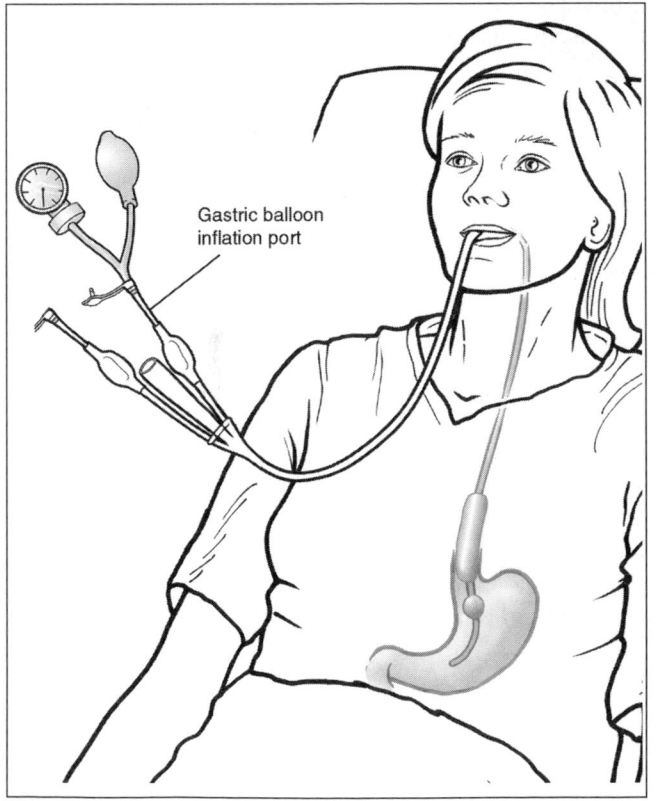

FIGURE 52-6 Connecting the handheld manometer (*A*) or mercury manometer (*B*) to the gastric aspiration port. A 50 mL syringe may be used if a handheld pressure bulb is not available.

Gastric balloon inflation port

Gastric balloon inflation port

Gastric aspiration port

Gastric aspiration port

Esophageal balloon inflation port

Esophageal balloon inflation port

Pressure bulb

Handheld manometer

Blood pressure manometer

A

B

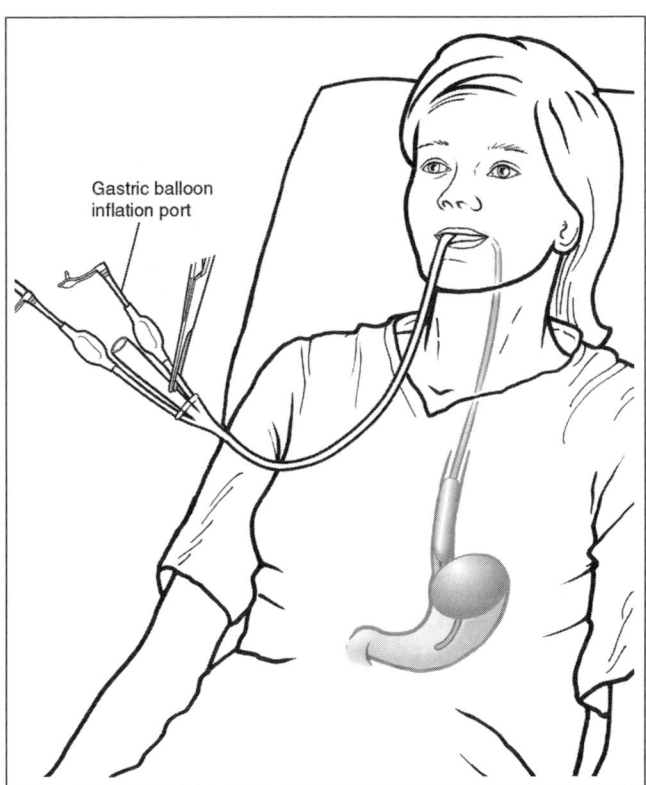

Gastric balloon inflation port

Gastric balloon inflation port

FIGURE 52-7 The gastric balloon is inflated with 50 to 100 mL increments of air to a volume of 250 to 300 mL.

FIGURE 52-8 Tension is applied to the SB tube to lodge the gastric balloon against the gastroesophageal junction.

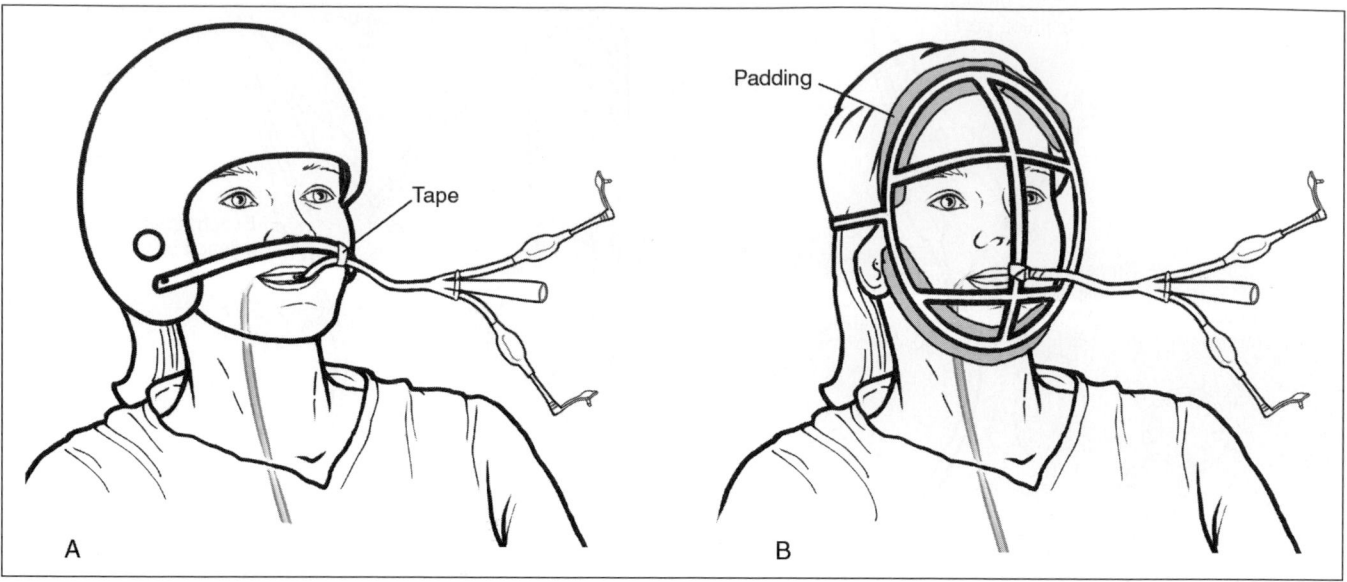

FIGURE 52-9 The SB tube is commonly secured to the faceguard of a football helmet (*A*) or to a catcher's mask (*B*).

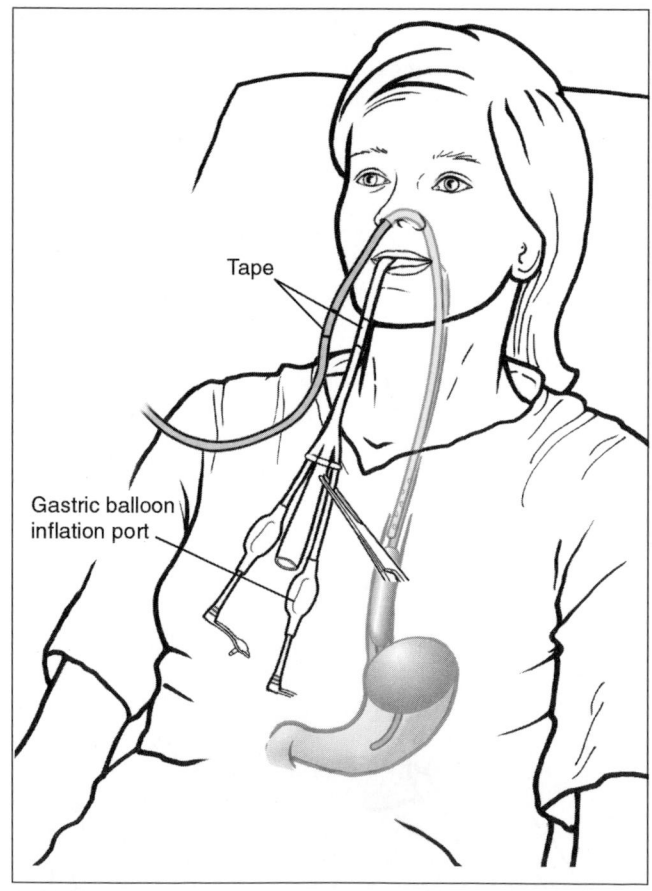

FIGURE 52-10 The nasogastric tube is inserted until the tape mark lines up with the tape mark on the SB tube. The football helmet/catcher's mask is omitted from this illustration for the sake of clarity.

ALTERNATIVE TECHNIQUE

The above technique is also applicable to the four-lumen esophagogastric tamponade tube (Minnesota tube). This tube is a modification of the triple-lumen Sengstaken-Blakemore tube that incorporates a separate esophageal suction port to the existing gastric suction port.[12,13] The design of the Minnesota tube may help prevent aspiration of esophageal contents.[14] Always check the manufacturer characteristics regarding the maximum inflation volume of both the gastric and esophageal balloons, as these are dependent upon the tube manufacturers.

Recently proposed is an effective methodology for placement of the SB tube endoscopically.[15] This method will avoid the need to obtain radiologic confirmation of the gastric balloon within the stomach.[15] Delay in treatment while waiting for a radiologic confirmation may put patients at risk, as they are almost always in critical condition and require immediate attention.[4–6] If endoscopic intervention is not successful, pass an SB tube and confirm the position of the gastric balloon under direct visualization through the endoscope. The balloon is inflated and secured in the usual fashion.[15]

ASSESSMENT

Check the pressure in the balloons periodically with the mercury manometer or keep the manometer attached for constant monitoring. Obtain a portable radio-

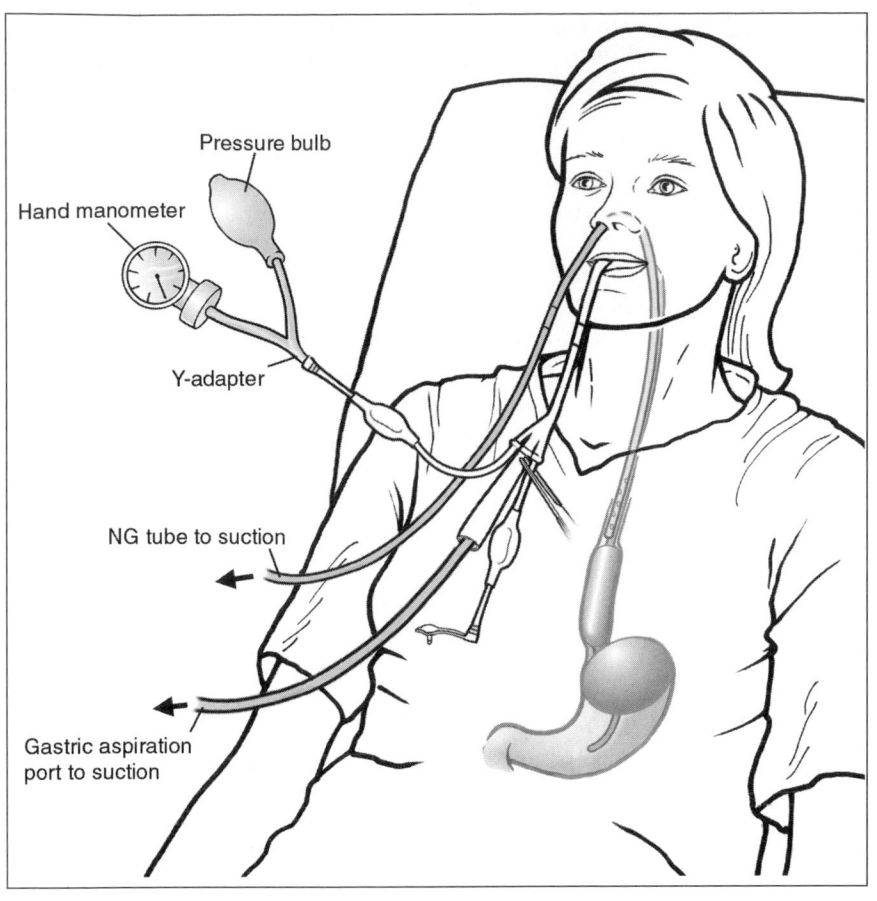

FIGURE 52-11 The esophageal balloon is inflated after the gastric aspiration port and the nasogastric tube have been attached to a suction source. The football helmet/catcher's mask is omitted from this illustration for the sake of clarity.

graph to confirm proper placement of the SB tube and the inflated balloons. The patient may be reclined, but always maintain at least 6 to 10 inches of head elevation on the bed to prevent aspiration in the awake patient. Tape a scissors to the head of the bed for quick access in case the balloon requires emergent deflation (Figure 52-12).

AFTERCARE

If the bleeding is controlled, reduce the esophageal balloon pressure by 5 mmHg every 3 hours until 25 mmHg is reached without bleeding from the nasogastric tube in the esophagus or the gastric aspiration port. Deflate the esophageal balloon for 5 minutes every 6 hours to avoid esophageal pressure necrosis. Give the patient nothing by mouth. Oral medications, if required, may be administered through the gastric aspiration port. Check the tension on the SB tube every 3 hours and adjust it as necessary. Verify patency of the SB and nasogastric tubes by checking the gastric and esophageal return regularly and periodically flushing both lumens.

Monitor the patient continuously for signs of chest pain, respiratory distress, and aspiration. Migration of the esophageal balloon into the hypopharynx of an awake patient will result in respiratory distress. **This situation is a true emergency and the tube should be removed immediately.** Cut the SB tube between the ports and the patient with a scissors (Figure 52-12). The balloons will immediately deflate and allow the removal of the SB tube.

The esophageal balloon should not remain inflated for more than 24 hours to avoid mucosal necrosis. The SB tube is usually left in place with the gastric or gastric and esophageal balloons inflated for 24 hours if variceal bleeding is controlled. If there is no bleeding after 24 hours, deflate the esophageal balloon and leave the gastric balloon inflated for an additional 24 hours. The SB tube may be left in place for an additional 24 hours after both balloons are deflated. If variceal hemorrhage recurs, the appropriate balloons should be reinflated while alternative therapy to control bleeding is sought. Patients who rebleed have a higher mortality rate. Therefore other therapeutic interventions—such as rubber banding, sclerotherapy, transjugular intrahepatic portocaval shunt, or surgery—should be considered. Remove the SB tube if hemostasis persists for 24 hours after deflation of both balloons. Control of esophageal variceal bleeding can be achieved by balloon tamponade in 50 to 94 percent of patients.[17,19–21] However, rebleeding occurs in 38 percent.

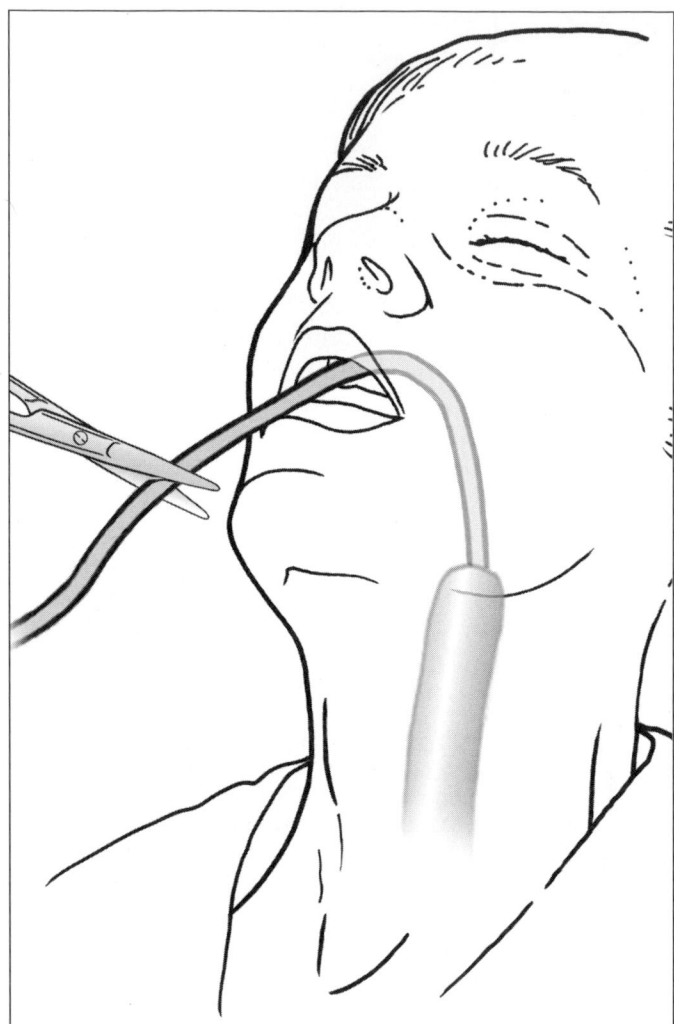

FIGURE 52-12 Emergent removal of the SB tube. Cut the SB tube between the ports and the patient to deflate both balloons rapidly.

COMPLICATIONS

Major complications occur in 0 to 15 percent of patients. Lethal complications have been described in 0 to 6.5 percent of patients.[17,19–21] **Complications associated with the SB tube are often life-threatening.** The airway may become occluded due to proximal migration of the esophageal balloon into the hypopharynx of the awake patient from traction on the SB tube.[16] The patient will begin choking and gagging if not intubated. Cut the SB tube distal to the ports to immediately deflate the balloons and allow the SB tube to be removed. Pulmonary aspiration, and subsequent pneumonia, may occur during SB tube insertion. Airway protection by endotracheal intubation should be considered in all patients prior to insertion of the SB tube.[17] Excessive balloon pressure or prolonged balloon inflation may lead to pressure necrosis and ulcerations of the esophagus, gastroesophageal junction, and/or stomach. Periodic deflation of the

esophageal balloon every 6 hours will help prevent this. Rupture or lacerations of the esophagus, stomach, or small intestine may occur.[18] Esophageal rupture can result in mediastinitis, abscess formation, and sepsis. These can be prevented by adhering to proper balloon inflation techniques with pressure monitoring. Cardiac arrhythmias and pulmonary edema can occur and require continuous monitoring in the setting of an intensive care unit. Pulmonary edema is often due to pressure from the esophageal balloon on mediastinal structures.

Numerous other complications are associated with the use of the SB or Minnesota tube. Unintentional deflation of the balloons can be prevented by the application of rubber shod clamps or hemostats to the balloon inflation ports after the balloons are inflated. Cut the SB tube distal to the ports if the balloons will not deflate. The patient may become agitated from the discomfort of the tube, migration of the tube into the hypopharynx resulting in hypoxemia and asphyxiation, or as chest and back pain is experienced from a misplaced or overdistended balloon. Hiccoughs are due to pressure on the diaphragm by the balloons. Excessive traction on the tube can result in epistaxis or pressure necrosis of the lips, nose, or tongue. Use air and not a liquid to inflate the balloons. Liquid in the balloons causes them to be heavy, increases the risk of pressure necrosis, and makes them hard to deflate.

SUMMARY

Balloon tamponade of variceal bleeding is an uncommonly performed procedure in the Emergency Department. The SB tube plays an important role in the temporary control of hemorrhage from esophageal or gastric varices.[19–21] It is used in cases of variceal bleeding, usually documented by endoscopy, that continues despite aggressive medical management including lavage, correction of blood clotting abnormalities, intravenous somatostatin or vasopressin infusion, rubber banding, and emergent sclerotherapy.[15,22–24] The SB tube can also be placed if these methods are contraindicated or unavailable. Despite the initial success of balloon tamponade in the control of variceal hemorrhage, sustained control of bleeding occurs in only 40 to 50 percent of patients.[25] Balloon tamponade has been shown to be as effective as intravenous vasopressin in controlling esophageal variceal bleeding. Only 25 percent of patients with ascites, jaundice, and encephalopathy achieve lasting hemostasis with balloon tamponade. Long-term efficacy in terms of rebleeding depends in part on the patient's underlying liver disease.[15] Maintain a low threshold to intubate the patient endotracheally in order to prevent aspiration, protect the airway, and prevent airway occlusion from migration of the esophageal balloon.

REFERENCES

1. Pagliaro L: Portal hypertension in cirrhosis: natural history, in Bosch J, Groszmann RJ (eds): *Portal Hypertension, Pathophysiology and Treatment.* Oxford, England: Blackwell, 1994:190.

2. North Italian Endoscopic Club for the Study and Treatment of Esophageal Varices: Prediction of the first variceal hemorrhage in patients with cirrhosis of the liver and esophageal varices: a prospective multicenter study. *N Engl J Med* 1988; 319(15):983–989.

3. Goff JS: Gastroesophageal varices: pathogenesis and therapy of acute bleeding. *Gastroenterol Clin North Am* 1993; 22(4):779–800.

4. Navarro VJ, Garcia-Tsao G: Variceal hemorrhage. *Crit Care Clin* 1995; 11(2):391–414.

5. Graham DY, Smith JL: The course of patients after variceal hemorrhage. *Gastroenterology* 1981; 80(4):800–809.

6. Smith JL, Graham DY: Variceal hemorrhage: a critical evaluation of survival analysis. *Gastroenterology* 1982; 82(5 pt 1):968–973.

7. Groszmann RJ: Reassessing portal venous pressure measurements. *Gastroenterology* 1984; 86(6):1611–1614.

8. Angelico M, Carli L, Piat C, et al: Isosorbide-5-mononitrate versus propranolol in the prevention of the first bleeding in cirrhosis. *Gastroenterology* 1993; 104(5):1460–1465.

9. Kashiwagi H, Shikano S, Yamamoto O, et al: Technique for positioning the Sengstaken-Blakemore tube as comfortably as possible. *Surg Gynecol Obstet* 1991; 172:63.

10. Isacs KL, Levinson SL: Insertion of the Minnesota tube, in Drossman DA (ed): *Manual of Gastroenterology Procedures,* 3rd ed. New York: Raven Press, 1993:27–35.

11. Pasquale MD, Cerra FB: Sengstaken-Blakemore tube placement: use of balloon tamponade to control bleeding varices. *Crit Care Clin* 1992; 8(4):743–753.

12. Edlich RF, Landé AJ, Goodale RL, et al: Prevention of aspiration pneumonia by continuous esophageal aspiration during esophagogastric tamponade and gastric cooling. *Surgery* 1968; 64(2):405–408.

13. Boyce MHW: Modification of the Sengstaken-Blakemore balloon tube. *N Engl J Med* 1962; 267(4):195–196.

14. Mitchell K, Silk DBA, Williams R: Prospective comparison of two Sengstaken tubes in the management of patients with variceal hemorrhage. *Gut* 1980; 21:570–573.

15. Lin TC, Bilir BM, Powis ME: Endoscopic placement of Sengstaken-Blakemore tube. *J Clin Gastroenterol* 2000; 31(1):29–32.

16. Pitcher JL: Safety and effectiveness of the modified Sengstaken-Blakemore tube: a prospective study. *Gastroenterology* 1976; 61(3):291–298.

17. Panes J, Teres J, Bosch J, et al: Efficacy of balloon tamponade in treatment of bleeding gastric and esophageal varices: results in 151 consecutive episodes. *Dig Dis Sci* 1988; 33(4):454–459.

18. Goff JS, Thompson JS, Pratt CF, et al: Jejunal rupture caused by a Sengstaken-Blakemore tube. *Gastroenterology* 1982; 82(3):573–575.

19. Chojkier M, Conn HO: Esophageal tamponade in the treatment of bleeding varices. A decadal progress report. *Dig Dis Sci* 1980; 25(4):267–272.

20. Hunt PS, Korman MG, Hansky J, et al: An 8-year prospective experience with balloon tamponade in emergency control of bleeding esophageal varices. *Dig Dis Sci* 1982; 27(5):413–416.

21. Haddock G, Garden OJ, McKee RF, et al: Esophageal tamponade in the management of acute variceal hemorrhage. *Dig Dis Sci* 1989; 34(6):913–918.

22. Teres J, Planas R, Panes J, et al: Vasopressin/nitroglycerin infusion vs esophageal tamponade in the treatment of acute variceal bleeding: a randomized controlled trial. *Hepatology* 1990; 11(6):964–968.

23. Correia JP, Alves MM, Alexandrino P, et al: Controlled trial of vasopressin and balloon tamponade in bleeding esophageal varices. *Hepatology* 1984; 4(5):885–888.

24. Lo GH, Lai KH, Ng WW, et al: Injection sclerotherapy preceded by esophageal tamponade versus immediate sclerotherapy in arresting active variceal bleeding: a prospective randomized trial. *Gastrointest Endosc* 1992; 38(4):421–424.

25. Pinto-Correia J, Alves MM, Alexandrino P, et al: Controlled trial of vasopressin and balloon tamponade in acute hemorrhage from esophagogastric varices: a prospective controlled randomized trial. *Hepatology* 1984; 4(5):580–583.

Chapter 53
GASTROSTOMY TUBE REPLACEMENT

Karen S. Cosby

INTRODUCTION

Gastrostomy tubes are used to provide prolonged enteral support in patients who are unable to obtain sufficient nutrition orally. They are an adjunct to the supportive care of many chronically ill patients. A few of the indications for feeding tubes include nervous system disorders (stroke, spinal cord injury, dementia, coma), swallowing dysfunction (neuromuscular diseases), obstructive lesions (esophageal cancer, oropharyngeal trauma), and chronic debilitating disorders (severe malnutrition, advanced cancer, respiratory failure). Simplified techniques for their placement and improved materials have made gastrostomies commonplace in acute and chronic health care settings. Repair and replacement of problematic gastrostomy tubes are best handled in an expedient manner. Primary Care and Emergency Physicians fill a valuable role in solving gastrostomy tube problems. This chapter reviews the methods and materials used in gastrostomies and the approaches to replacing displaced or malfunctioning gastrostomy tubes.

ANATOMY AND PATHOPHYSIOLOGY

There are many different procedures that may be used to place feeding gastrostomies and dozens of commercially available gastrostomy tubes. Familiarity with the basic techniques used to create gastrostomies and the characteristics of common gastrostomy tubes is helpful in solving problems with their function and selecting appropriate replacement tubes.

PLACEMENT OF GASTROSTOMY TUBES

Formal surgical techniques for the placement of feeding tubes have been used for more than a century. Sedillot is given credit for having performed the first open human gastrostomy in 1845.[1] However, the first postoperative gastrostomy survival was not reported until 30 years later.[2] The evolution of techniques in surgical gastrostomy has a colorful history, with many contributors.[1-3] Three main procedures that remain in use today are the Stamm (described in 1894), the Witzel (described in 1891), and the Dupage and Janeway (described in 1913)[1-6] (Figure 53-1). Operative gastrostomies require a laparotomy and general anesthesia. They all share the common goal of providing long-term access to the stomach for feedings or decompression while attempting to minimize the potential for gastric leakage.

Each of the techniques attempts to create a leakproof interface between the stomach, the feeding tube, and the anterior abdominal wall. The Stamm gastrostomy secures the stomach to a feeding tube using a double purse-string suture to invaginate the stomach about the feeding tube (Figure 53-1A). The Witzel technique places the feeding tube through a seromuscular tunnel in the stomach wall (Figure 53-1B). The Janeway technique creates a formal tunnel from a gastric flap to envelop the feeding tube and form a gastrocutaneous stoma (Figure 53-1C). These surgical gastrostomies are considered long-term, semipermanent stomas.

Modern endoscopic techniques have provided a simpler option for the placement of percutaneous feeding tubes, also known as gastrostomy tubes, percutaneous endoscopic gastrostomies, or PEGs.[7] Endoscopic gastrostomies have become competitive with the more formal surgical gastrostomies due to their relative ease of placement, avoidance of a laparotomy, avoidance of general anesthesia, and a lower morbidity rate.[2,8] The first endoscopic gastrostomy techniques to gain wide acceptance were described by Gauderer and Ponsky in 1980.[7] Several popular endoscopic techniques in use

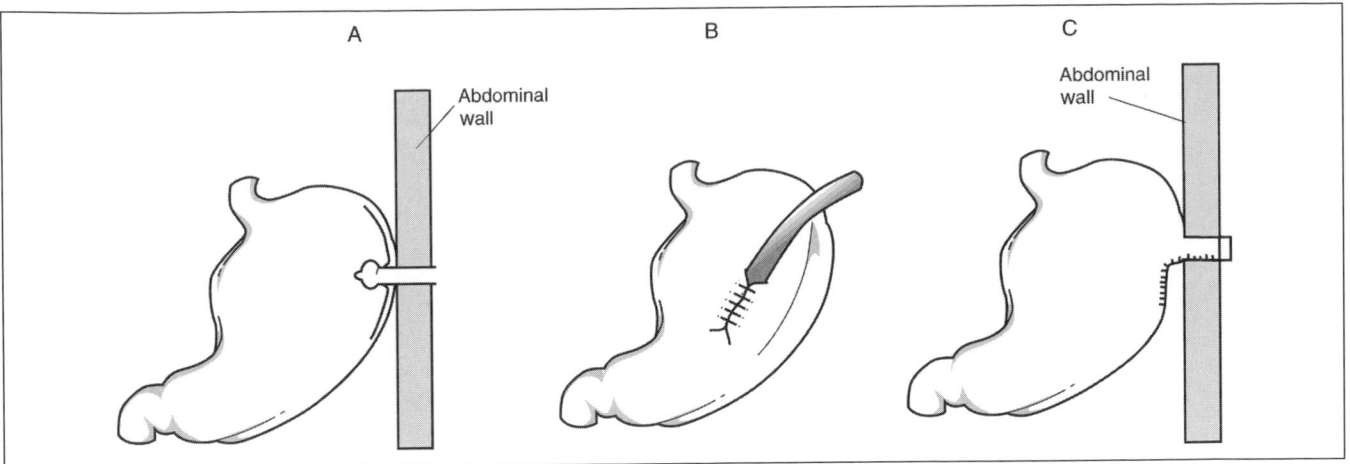

FIGURE 53-1 Surgical gastrostomies. *A.* The Stamm technique. A double purse-string suture invaginates the stomach about the feeding tube. *B.* The Witzel technique. The feeding tube is directed away from the gastric puncture through a sero-muscular tunnel. *C.* The Janeway technique. A full-thickness tube fashioned from the greater curvature of the stomach envelops the feeding tube.

today require two persons—an endoscopist and an operator at skin level.

An endoscope is first advanced into the stomach (Figure 53-2*A*). The stomach is then insufflated with air to displace adjacent loops of bowel and appose the stomach wall to the anterior abdominal wall (Figure 53-2*B*). The operator then visualizes the light of the endoscope as it transilluminates the abdominal wall. The operator then pierces the anterior abdominal wall with a cannula or needle, depending upon the elected procedure (Figure 53-2*C*). The endoscopist confirms placement of the device into the gastric lumen (Figure 53-2*C*).

The gastrostomy tube is then placed. A suture or guidewire is fed into the stomach, grasped with a snare, and pulled out of the patient's mouth. The "Ponsky pull" procedure uses a suture placed through a cannula that is grasped by the endoscopist's snare and pulled through the patient's mouth. The suture is secured around a feeding tube and pulled retrogradely from the mouth to the exit site on the anterior abdominal wall (Figure 53-3*A*). The alternate "Ponsky push" technique substitutes a guidewire for the suture. Instead of pulling the gastrostomy tube, it is pushed down the guidewire toward the gastrostomy site[9] (Figure 53-3*B*). A third technique popularized by Russell eliminates the need to direct the feeding tube through the mouth.[10] Under direct visualization, a dilator is used to enlarge the puncture site. An introducer and peel-away sheath are then used to place the feeding tube directly through the anterior abdominal wall (Figure 53-3*C*). Regardless of which technique is used to establish the gastrostomy, a fibrous tract eventually forms between the anterior abdominal wall and the stomach. The maturation of this tract is an important consideration in assessing gastrostomy tubes.

TYPES OF GASTROSTOMY TUBES

A vast array of feeding tubes have been developed and marketed commercially as the spectrum and versatility of endoscopic techniques has expanded. While few physicians will be experienced with all gastrostomy tubes, a basic understanding of their components is useful. Familiarity with the characteristics of gastrostomy tubes is helpful in assessing tube function and determining appropriate replacements.

The gastrostomy tube, reduced to its most basic form, is simply a conduit for enteral feedings. The essential features of the modern gastrostomy tube include four components: the tube itself, an internal bolster, an external fixation (bolster or retention) device, and the ports (Figure 53-4). The main body of the gastrostomy tube is made of silicone or polyurethane. It is designed to minimize tissue reactions and optimize patient comfort. Gastrostomy tubes come in a variety of sizes ranging from 12 to 24 French. Some are reinforced with an inner steel wire. Many come with external identification marks to denote caliber, commercial brand name, centimeter markings to aid in positioning, and radiopaque lines to aid in radiographic identification (Figure 53-4). Some tubes note if external traction can be used to remove the tube.

The internal bolster fixes the gastrostomy tube within the lumen of the stomach and creates a seal to discourage leaking (Figure 53-4). Commercially available PEG catheters come with a variety of choices for internal bolsters including balloons, crossbars, T-bars, flanges, round disks, three-leaf retainers, soft domes, and others (Figure 53-5). The most basic tubes use a balloon as an internal bolster. Surgical gastrostomies commonly use Foley balloon catheters, mushroom-tip de Pezzer

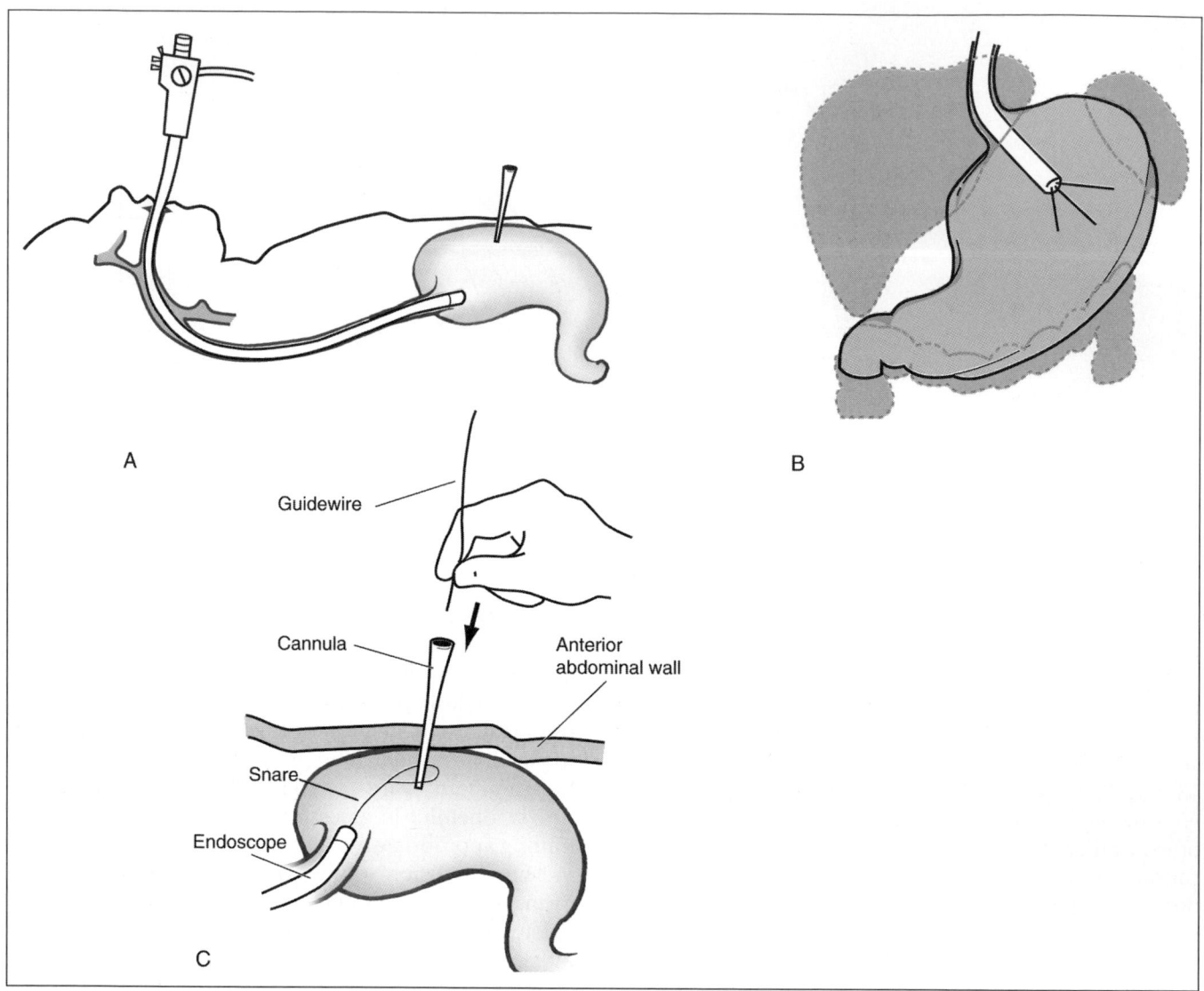

FIGURE 53-2 Endoscopic gastrostomy tube placement. *A.* The endoscope is inserted. *B.* The stomach is inflated with air and transilluminated. *C.* The anterior abdominal wall is pierced with a cannula or needle under endoscopic guidance. A suture or guidewire is then introduced into the gastric lumen and grasped with a snare.

catheters, or Malecot catheters. Some internal bolsters are deformable and allow removal with gentle traction on the external tube. Others are not intended to give way with traction and require more invasive techniques for removal. The nature of the internal bolster will determine if a gastrostomy tube can be removed at the bedside or requires endoscopic removal.

External bolsters are devices at the exit site that secure the gastrostomy tube to the abdominal wall and prevent inward migration (Figure 53-4). Surgical gastrostomies frequently rely on only a silk suture. PEGs typically use a T-bar or retention disk. The external bolster has little impact on the function of the gastrostomy tube or the technique used to place it. The external bolster may cause the gastrostomy tube to kink, fracture, or clog if it is too tight. The gastrostomy tube may migrate inward with peristalsis if the external bolster is too loose.

Inappropriate care of the external bolster may lead to problems that contribute to the need for replacement, although it does not affect the ability to remove the gastrostomy tube. Identification and correction of problems with the external bolster can prevent unnecessary damage to the gastrostomy tube.

The distal end of the gastrostomy tube contains the port(s) to access the lumen(s). Many tubes have a Y port, with one port for enteral feedings and a pop-off valve port to access a balloon (Figure 53-4). Some tubes have multiple ports to access each separate lumen that is designated for a specific purpose, such as medication administration. Others have a suction port for gastric suctioning and a port for distal feeding.

In an effort to improve patient comfort and acceptance, some manufacturers now supply skin-level devices. These are also referred to as low-profile systems or

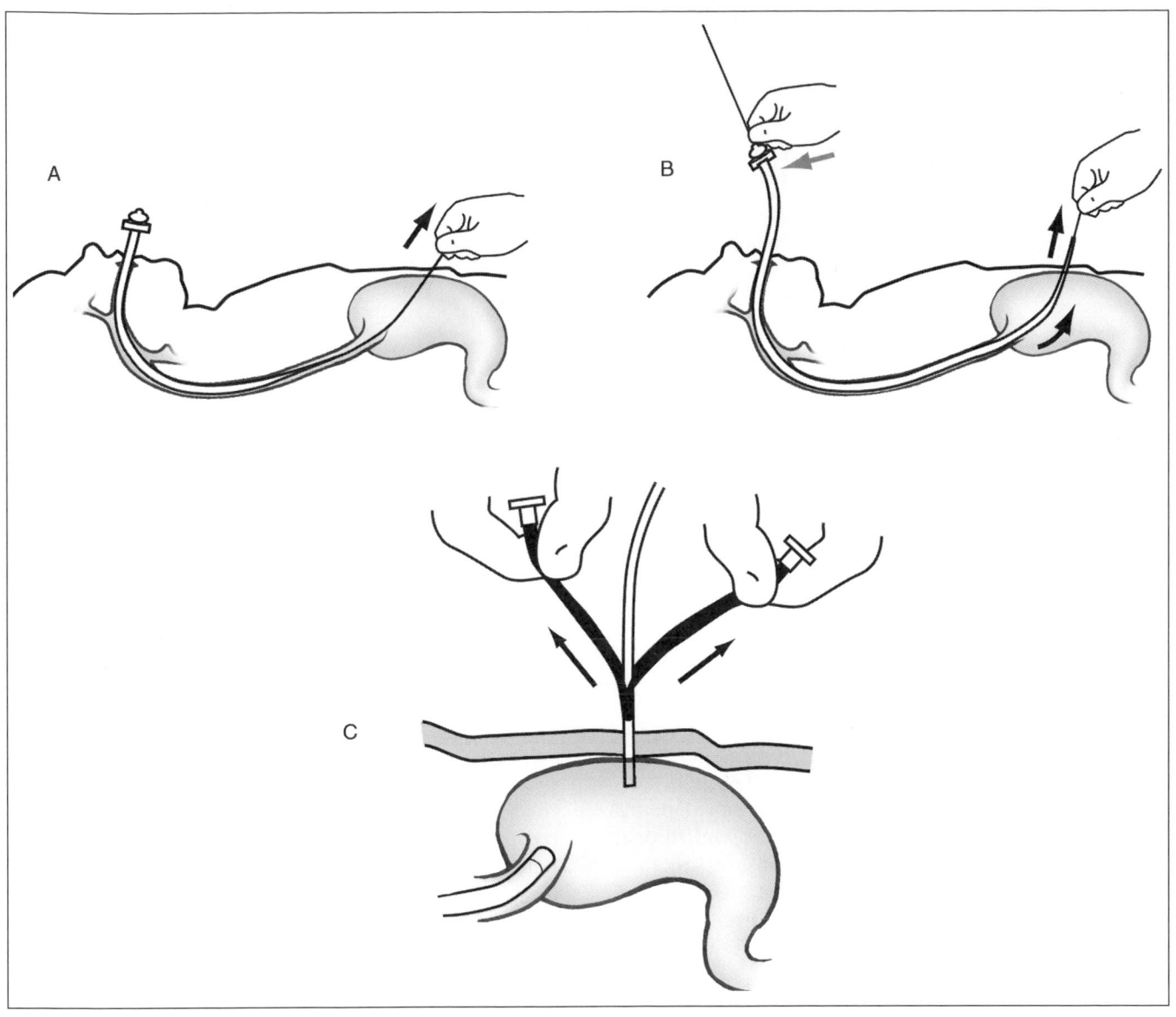

FIGURE 53-3 Endoscopic gastrostomy tube placement. *A.* The "Ponsky pull." A suture is attached to a modified gastrostomy tube and pulled in a retrograde direction through the anterior abdominal wall. *B.* The "Ponsky push." A guidewire serves as a trolley for the gastrostomy tube to be pushed over. *C.* The "Russell poke." The gastrostomy tube is inserted through a peel-away sheath.

buttons. These tubes combine the distal access port and the external bolster to give a more cosmetically appealing look without a dangling tube.

INDICATIONS

There is no need for routine removal or replacement of gastrostomy tubes. The most common reason for replacement is accidental removal. Occasionally, tubes require replacement because they wear out, kink, or fracture. They should be replaced if the lumen becomes clogged with precipitate. Most of these problems can be avoided with diligent care of the gastrostomy tube. Feedings should never be forced—a common error that can weaken the tube. The feeding tube should be flushed with water after each use. Medications should never be mixed with enteral feeding solutions. Proper care of the gastrostomy tube should prevent premature loss. Family members and health care providers should receive detailed instructions regarding gastrostomy tube management so as to avoid common problems.

CONTRAINDICATIONS

A damaged, malfunctioning, or displaced gastrostomy tube should be replaced as soon as possible, with a few exceptions. The existing tube should be left in place if the tract is immature. Premature removal of a tube in

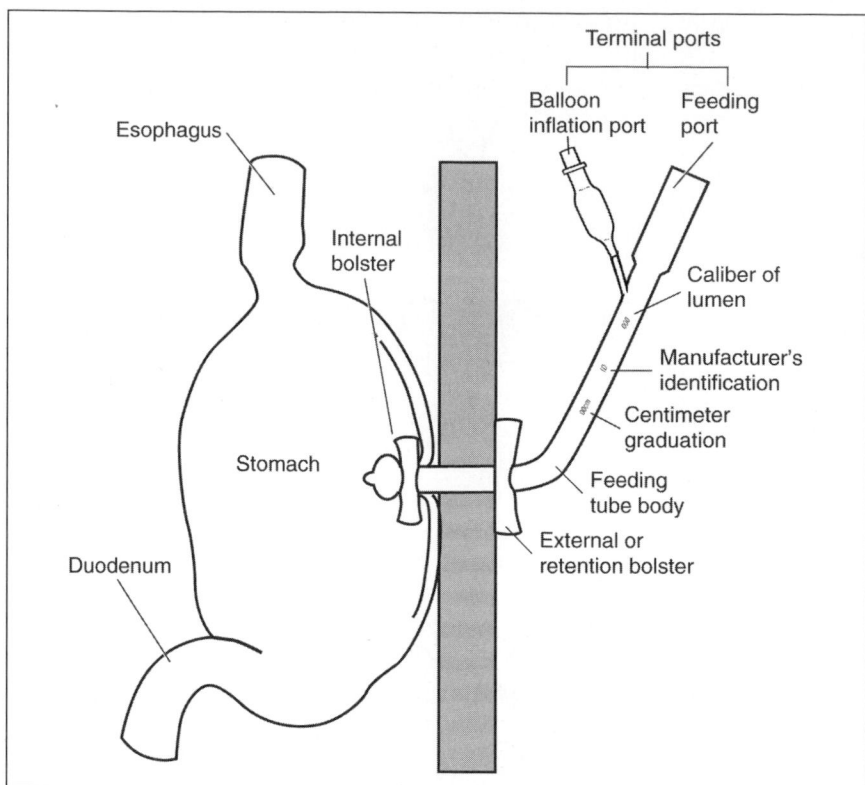

FIGURE 53-4 The basic gastrostomy or percutaneous endoscopic gastrostomy (PEG) tube.

an immature tract can lead to gastric spillage and peritonitis. The exact time for a tract to mature depends upon the procedure used and the patient's nutritional status. A conservative approach is to consider any tract less than 4 weeks old to be immature. The specialist who performed the original procedure should be consulted prior to any manipulation of the immature tract. The tract should be left alone and a Surgeon consulted if a patient has peritonitis at the time of presentation. If the patient has acute abdominal pain after manipulation of a gastrostomy site, feedings should be withheld until an investigation determines the source of the problem. Do

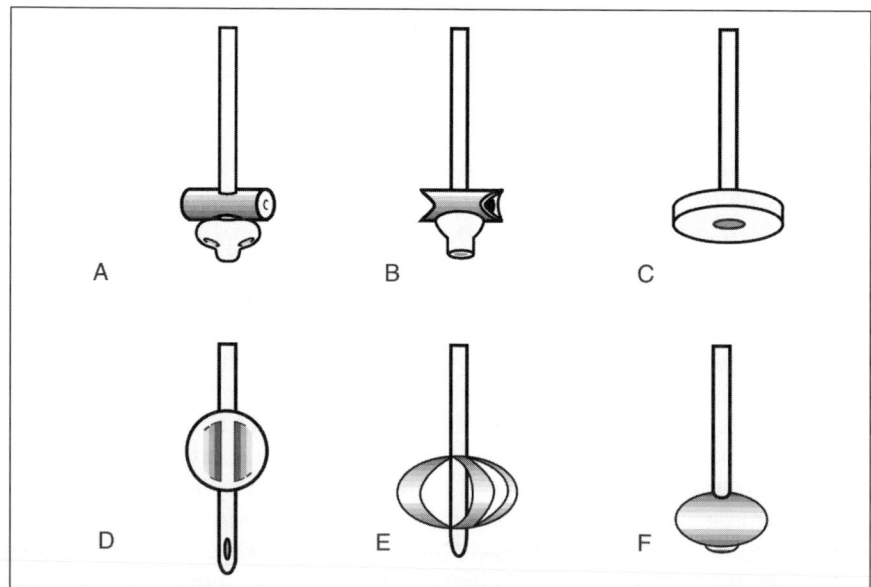

FIGURE 53-5 Examples of internal bolsters used in PEGs. *A.* Mushroom tip with de Pezzer flange. *B.* Crossbar. *C.* Round disk. *D.* Balloon tip. *E.* Malecot. *F.* Soft dome.

not manipulate or change the gastrostomy tube if the patient has pain at the skin entry site or with movement of the tube. This may alert the clinician to an underlying abscess, infection, or intraabdominal pathology.

EQUIPMENT

Povidone iodine solution or other skin antiseptic
Commercial replacement gastrostomy tube kits
Foley catheter of a similar caliber as the original tube
20 mL syringe with saline to fill the Foley balloon
Water-soluble lubricant
Toomey syringe or bulb syringe to aspirate gastric
    contents
Some form of external bolster (see text below)
Adapter to cap off Foley catheter or attach it to feeding
    assembly
Gloves

PATIENT PREPARATION

Explain the procedure to the patient and/or their representative. Gastrostomy tube replacement can usually be accomplished with little preparation or anesthesia. Place the patient supine. Clean the skin surrounding the entry site of any dirt and debris. Apply povidone iodine and allow it to dry. Anesthesia should not be necessary, as the gastrostomy site should not be tender. Significant pain at the site should alert the clinician to an infection, abscess, or intraabdominal pathology. **If anything more than minor discomfort occurs, the gastrostomy should not be manipulated.** Small children or anxious patients may benefit from mild sedation.

TECHNIQUES

The technique for replacing a gastrostomy tube will depend upon the original procedure used to place the tube, the maturity of the tract, and the nature of the internal bolster. Seek as much information as possible about the age and nature of the existing tube. The following discussion reviews the procedure for replacing gastrostomy tubes in mature tracts, factors to consider prior to removing an existing but dysfunctional tube, and techniques to employ in fashioning replacement systems.

REPLACING A DISLODGED GASTROSTOMY TUBE

Every effort should be made to replace a dislodged gastrostomy tube as soon as possible. Gastrostomies begin to close as soon as the tube is removed. The tract will close within hours to days depending on the age,

maturation, and size of the tube. If the original tube is in good condition, it can simply be reinserted to stent the tract until a permanent replacement is found. A commercially available replacement that is compatible with the original tube may be used. Foley catheters are simple to use, are widely available, and function well as temporary replacements.[8,11-13] Select a tube of similar caliber to the patient's gastrostomy tube. A decision regarding the choice of external fixation should be made and the tube adapted appropriately prior to its insertion (see discussion below). Lubricate the replacement tube liberally. Gently insert the replacement tube through the tract. **Do not advance the tube against any significant resistance. Advancement against more than mild resistance can result in complications.** Aspirate gastric contents to confirm proper placement. Inflate the Foley balloon with saline. Pull the catheter snug to lodge the balloon immediately behind the anterior abdominal wall. **The entire process should be painless and should not require dissection or force.**

A few types of feeding tubes merit special attention. While many gastrostomies have a short, direct route to the stomach, the Witzel uses a more circuitous tunnel and a smaller tube. The tract may be difficult to maneuver. A guidewire is sometimes helpful. The procedure should be aborted if any difficulty occurs with this approach.

Not all feeding tubes terminate in the stomach. In some cases, the feeding tube enters the stomach and then feeds through a distal lumen into the jejunum. If a patient is known to have a jejunostomy (sometimes referred to as a percutaneous endoscopic jejunostomy, or PEJ), the tract may be stented with a replacement gastrostomy tube. More information should be obtained prior to resuming feedings.

Some catheters are not intended to be replaceable. Small needle jejunostomies may use 5 to 7 French catheters. Should such a catheter become disrupted or occluded, there is little one can do to correct it. Consult with the patient's primary care provider to discuss the variable options for management and follow-up.

PLACING AN EXTERNAL BOLSTER

Attention should be directed toward the skin exit site after the successful insertion of a replacement tube. The tube should be kept at 90 degrees relative to the skin and fixed in some way to prevent migration into the distal bowel. A short-term solution is to dress the site with 4×4 gauze squares, building them up along the exit site to create a pyramid-shaped dressing several inches high. Alternatively, a strip of urethane foam can be used to bolster the tube[14] (Figure 53-6A). Brummer and Cheng describe an alternate technique using a 3 cm section of latex tubing wrapped about the base of the gastrostomy tube and secured with a plastic cable tie[15] (Figure

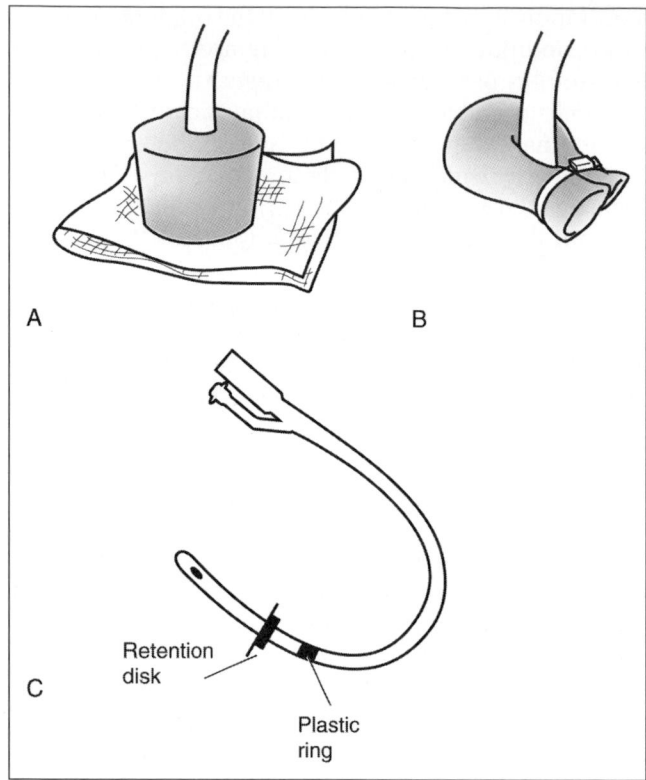

FIGURE 53-6 Types of external bolsters. *A.* Urethane foam dressing. *B.* Latex tubing wrapped about the base of the tube and secured with a plastic cable tie. *C.* A Foley catheter modified with a retention disk and plastic ring.

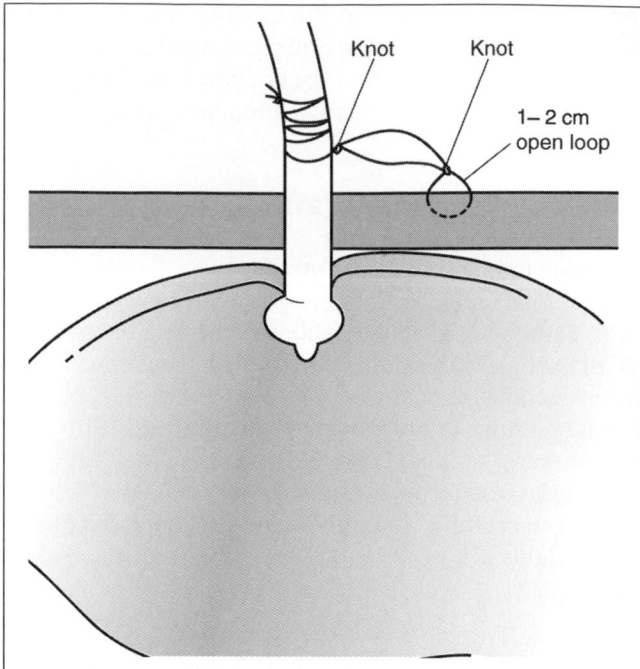

FIGURE 53-7 Simple external fixation using a silk suture laddered up the gastrostomy tube.

53-6*B*). Kadakia has described a modification to a Foley catheter that uses a retention disk and a plastic ring from a nasogastric tube[13] (Figure 53-6*C*).

Another option is to secure and bolster the tube with a suture (Figure 53-7). Place a suture using a large bite of tissue near the skin exit site. This serves as a retention suture. Leave an open loop of 1 to 2 cm between the skin and the knot to avoid unnecessary traction on the skin. Wrap the ends of the suture up the gastrostomy tube in a laddered fashion and tie them securely. This method allows some room for the gastrostomy tube to move while preventing inward migration as the patient changes position.

These techniques are adequate for short-term use, but a more permanent form of external fixation is desirable. A number of external bolsters have been described that can be fashioned from materials available in most health care facilities. A T-bar external bolster can be made by cutting a 3 cm piece of tubing from a latex or silicone Foley catheter or feeding tube[11] (Figure 53-8). Fold the piece of tubing in half. Make two diamond-shaped cuts placed on the sides of the fold and opposite each other (Figure 53-8*A*). Insert a hemostat through the holes and grasp the replacement gastrostomy tube

(Figure 53-8*B*). Slide the latex T-bar along the catheter (Figures 53-8*C* and *D*). In order to function satisfactorily, the latex T-bar must be snug enough to prevent migration but not so snug as to compress the gastrostomy tube lumen. After placement of the gastrostomy tube, position the latex T-bar so that it is about 0.5 to 1.0 cm from the skin surface.

There are several commercially available products designed specifically for replacement gastrostomies. They are convenient. Unfortunately, they are expensive, may not be compatible with the original tube, and may not be on hand at the moment they are needed.

Once the replacement tube's position is confirmed and secured, the end of the tube should be clamped or fitted with an appropriate feeding adapter.

NONFUNCTIONING GASTROSTOMY TUBES

A patient may present with a clogged, leaking, or fractured gastrostomy tube. A number of factors should be considered prior to removing any existing tube. Is the tract mature? Is replacement actually necessary or can other measures remedy the problem? What is the type of internal bolster and can it be removed by external traction? **The most important factor is the age and maturity of the tract. Premature removal of the gastrostomy tube from a fresh tract may lead to peritoneal contamination with gastric contents and peritonitis. A new gastrostomy site should not be manipulated without consultation with the specialist who placed the original tube. A malfunctioning tube may have to remain in**

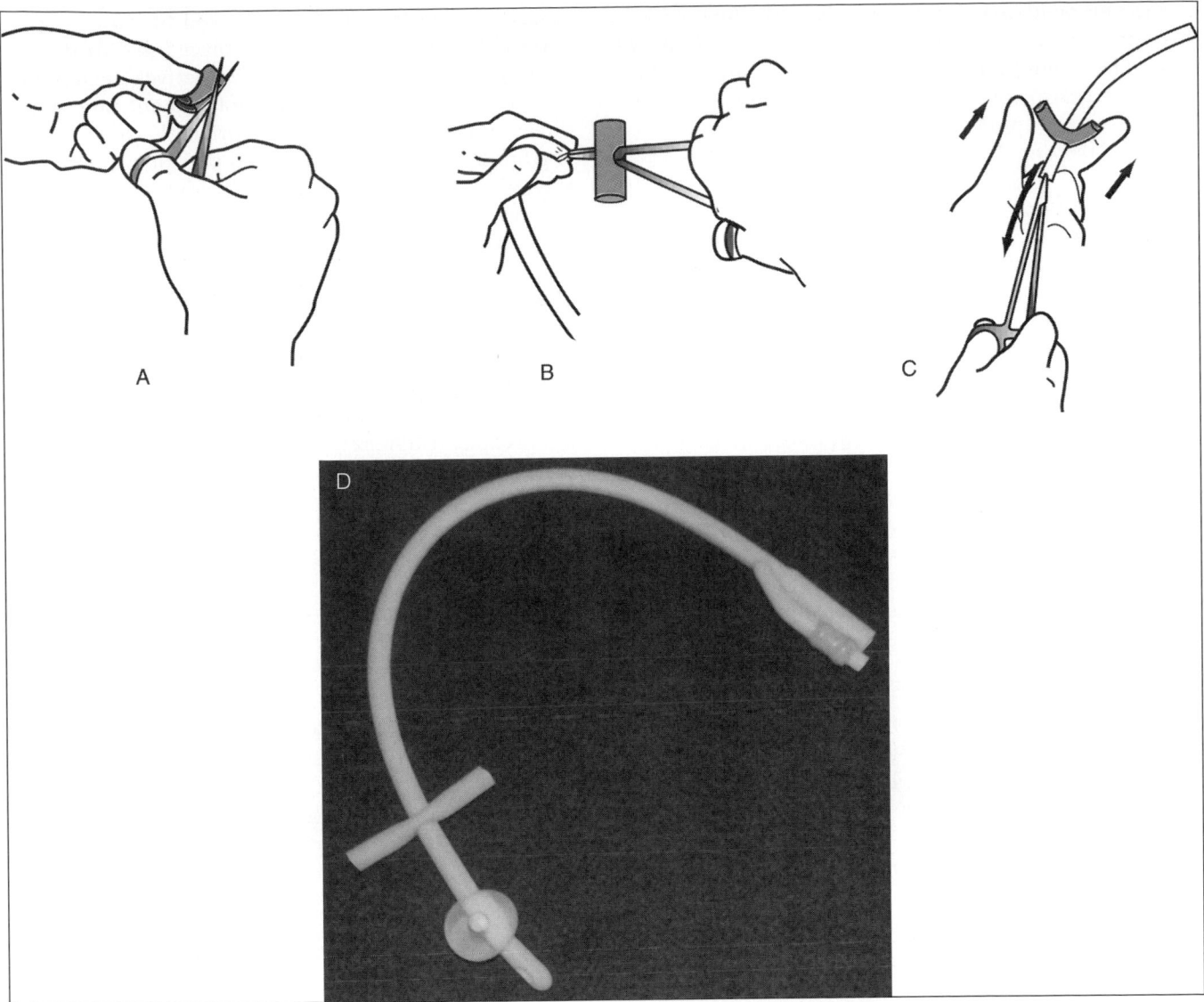

FIGURE 53-8 Fashioning an external bolster from a latex tube and a Foley catheter. *A.* The 3 cm piece of latex tube is folded and cut. *B.* A hemostat is inserted through the latex T-bar and grasps the distal end of the Foley catheter. *C.* The latex tube T-bar is advanced onto the catheter and pulled into position. *D.* The modified Foley catheter with a latex T-bar.

place to stent a fresh tract while alternative methods of nutritional support are provided to the patient.

The underlying problem with a nonfunctioning gastrostomy tube should be investigated prior to its removal and replacement. A fractured tube or a tube with a ruptured balloon will need replacement. A kinked tube may only need revision of the external bolster. A clogged tube should first be irrigated with tap water or saline in an attempt to open the lumen. **Do not force the irrigation fluid into the gastrostomy tube, as it may then rupture and injure the patient.** A variety of other options may be tried to open a clogged gastrostomy tube. These include the instillation of enzymes or attempts to break up or dislodge the clog with an endoscopic snare, biopsy for-

ceps, or Fogarty catheter.[16,17] The latter methods are usually performed by a consultant and not the Emergency Physician.

Once the decision has been made to replace a gastrostomy tube, information should be obtained regarding the type of tube in place. Many are removable by gentle external traction. **Never apply more than gentle traction when removing a gastrostomy tube.** If the internal bolster is a balloon, simply deflating the balloon will allow the tube to be removed. Other bolsters such as soft domes and T-bars may deform easily with gentle constant traction. If gentle traction is not sufficient to remove the gastrostomy tube, either the internal bolster is not intended to be removed externally or it may have become embedded within the gastric wall. When a gastrostomy tube fails to withdraw with ease, it will likely have to be removed using endoscopic techniques. Difficulty with gastrostomy tube removal sometimes occurs. The most likely problems and alternate solutions are discussed below.

The Balloon Does Not Deflate

The balloon may not deflate if the balloon inflation port is clogged or damaged. There are four options to remedy this situation. Simply cutting the gastrostomy tube may allow the balloon to deflate on its own. Cut the gastrostomy tube close to the ports. Maintain a firm hold, manually or with a hemostat, so that the cut tube does not migrate inside the patient and require endoscopic removal. The gastrostomy tube can be pulled taut to the skin and a needle advanced into the tract to puncture the balloon.[18–20] Alternatively, a guidewire may be advanced through the balloon port to puncture and deflate the balloon.[21] If these fail, the balloon may have to be ruptured internally with an endoscopic snare.

The Tube Does Not Withdraw with Ease

One may simply cut the feeding tube at the skin level and push the remaining tube through the tract and into the stomach. This will allow the internal components to pass through the patient's gastrointestinal tract. Retained gastrostomy tube components have been known to cause bowel obstructions and perforations; however, the majority pass without incident.[22] This procedure works for many types of gastrostomy tubes, but it is not clear that this is a safe option for balloon bolsters that have not been deflated. **This option should be used only if a Primary Care Provider agrees with that choice and is available to follow the patient until the contents have passed.** Radiopaque components can be followed by plain radiographs at 48 hour intervals. The gastrostomy "hardware" may have to be retrieved endoscopically or surgically if it fails to pass within 2 to 3 weeks or the patient experiences obstructive symptoms. This option is not recommended for small children under the age of 6 years or weighing less than 20 kilograms.[23] These patients have a greater risk for complications.[23]

Inadvertent Removal of the Tube from a Fresh or Immature Tract

Whenever a fresh tract is disrupted, there is the possibility of gastric spillage and peritonitis. In such an event, all enteral feedings should be discontinued and the patient observed for the development of peritonitis. A number of replacement options have been described. The tract may be allowed to close spontaneously and a replacement PEG placed in 7 to 10 days if the patient remains well.[24] Alternatively, endoscopy can attempt to reintroduce a replacement tube under direct visualization through the original tract.[25] A General Surgeon should be consulted and laparotomy considered if peritonitis develops. Under these circumstances, the Surgeon may choose to place a surgical gastrostomy.

The Tract Is Closed

A gastrostomy tract that is not stented will begin to close within hours. A lost tract may require a repeat procedure. This problem requires consultation with an Endoscopist. Dilation of a closing gastrostomy site has been described using filiform catheters and followers, a procedure adapted from urology.[26] This procedure should be reserved for the subspecialist, as it can result in numerous complications.

Early Balloon Rupture in an Intact Tube in an Immature Tract

In this instance, the tract is stented but there is the risk of gastric leakage about a deflated balloon. Esker and Hall report successful replacement using a guidewire to exchange the gastrostomy tube.[27] This technique is performed using endoscopic guidance to snare the guidewire and withdraw the original gastrostomy tube.

ASSESSMENT

The replacement gastrostomy tube should be placed to gravity drainage or the stomach contents should be aspirated. Use of the gastrostomy tube can be resumed if there is free flow of gastric contents. If there was any difficulty with placement of the gastrostomy tube or if the return is equivocal, its position should be confirmed radiographically. A small amount of water-soluble radiopaque contrast should be administered through the gastrostomy tube and a flat plate of the abdomen obtained. Normal gastrostomy tube placement will show intraluminal contrast. Any extravasation of contrast is abnormal and requires enteral feedings to be withheld and a General Surgeon to be consulted. In most instances, the patient will require hospitalization for parenteral antibiotics, observation, and bowel rest until the tract heals. Some physicians elect to evaluate all replaced gastrostomy tubes radiographically prior to their use. While doing so is harmless to the patient and causes no complications, this process cannot be routinely recommended, as it is time-consuming and expensive.

AFTERCARE

Routine maintenance can resume after successful replacement of the gastrostomy tube. Any factors that contributed to the malfunction should be addressed to prevent a recurrence. The patient and/or their caregivers should be taught the proper care and maintenance of a gastrostomy tube. The patient should follow up with their primary physician in 24 to 48 hours for evaluation, removal of the temporary tube, and placement of a gastrostomy tube. Instruct the patient to immediately return to the Emergency Department if they develop a fever, abdominal pain, nausea, or vomiting.

COMPLICATIONS

A variety of complications may accompany the initial insertion of a feeding gastrostomy.[2,6] However, replacement at a mature site should be relatively free of problems. Excessive force during replacement can disrupt the tract. A misdirected tube may end in a blind pouch or the peritoneal cavity if the stomach separates from the anterior abdominal wall. Installation of enteral feedings will cause a chemical peritonitis. This should be suspected if there is poor return from the replaced gastrostomy tube, there is difficulty installing feedings, or the patient develops pain or fever after the procedure. Peritonitis is preventable if proper positioning is confirmed prior to using the replacement tube.[28]

A replacement gastrostomy tube must be sufficiently secured externally so that the effect of peristalsis does not carry it distally. This is particularly true of balloon-tipped tubes. Once the tube migrates past the pylorus, it can cause bowel obstructions and perforations.[2,6] This can be avoided by carefully securing the replacement gastrostomy tube with an external device or suturing it securely to the skin.

Always advance the Foley catheter into the stomach before carefully and slowly inflating the balloon. Inflation of the balloon within the gastrocutaneous tract can result in hemorrhage, pain, and rupture of the tract. Overinsertion of the catheter can cause the balloon to enter the esophagus, duodenum, or gastroesophageal junction. These structures can rupture when the balloon is inflated. These complications can be avoided by inserting the Foley catheter 8 to 10 cm, slowly inflating the balloon, and not inflating the balloon to its maximal volume.

A mature gastrostomy tract begins to close as soon as the tube is removed. The tract narrows without the presence of the gastrostomy tube to keep it patent. Replace the gastrostomy tube as soon as possible. **Never force a tube through the tract.** This can result in bleeding, gastric perforation, intraperitoneal penetration, pain, and

the formation of a false passage. Pass a smaller-size tube if necessary to reestablish the tract and maintain its patency.

An indwelling or replacement gastrostomy tube may result in a gastric outlet obstruction. The patient usually presents with distention of the stomach and vomiting. Immediately and gently, pull back on the gastrostomy tube until it is snug against the abdominal wall. Secure the gastrostomy tube with an external bolster. Observe the patient for resolution of their symptoms and any complications.

The skin exit site may become edematous, erythematous, and tender. A simple cellulitis should be managed with oral antibiotics and local wound care. A dermatitis can result from leakage of gastric contents around the gastrostomy tube. Ensure that the internal bolster is secured against the anterior abdominal wall. If the leakage persists, replace the gastrostomy tube with a larger one that occludes the tract. Local wound care is all that is necessary once the problem with the gastrostomy tube is corrected. Occasionally, hypersensitivity to the adhesive, cleansing solutions, or the gastrostomy tube itself may develop. The use of different materials and topical corticosteroids will correct this problem. A yeast infection (*Candida albicans*) appears erythematous and moist, with satellite lesions. Topical antifungal creams and local wound care will alleviate the yeast infection. Granulation tissue around the stoma can be eliminated by coagulation with silver nitrate sticks. The patient should follow up with their primary physician in 24 to 48 hours for a reevaluation of all these clinical entities.

SUMMARY

There are a variety of techniques and supplies for establishing a gastrostomy. Despite their differences, they all result in a simple fibrous tract connecting a feeding tube to the stomach. A mature tract can be safely and easily manipulated. An immature tract should prompt further questioning and possibly consultation. Techniques for the basic maintenance and repair of gastrostomy tubes are straightforward. Familiarity with the procedures and equipment used to establish modern gastrostomies will help the clinician solve common gastrostomy tube problems and intervene in an appropriate and timely manner.

REFERENCES

1. Cunha F: Gastrostomy, its inception and evolution. *Am J Surg* 1946; 72(4):610–634.
2. Gauderer MWL, Stellato TA: Gastrostomies: evolution, techniques, indications, and complications. *Curr Probl Surg* 1986; 23:661–719.

3. Engel S: Gastrostomy. *Surg Clin North Am* 1969; 49(6):1289–1295.

4. Stamm M: Gastrostomy by a new method. *Med News* 1894; 65:324–326.

5. Janeway HH: Eine neue gastrostomiemethode. *Muench Med Wochnschr* 1913; 60:1705–1707.

6. O'Keefe KP: Complications of percutaneous feeding tubes. *Emerg Med Clin North Am* 1994; 12(3):815–826.

7. Gauderer MWL, Ponsky JL, Izant RJ: Gastrostomy without laparotomy: a percutaneous endoscopic technique. *J Pediatr Surg* 1980; 15(6):872–875.

8. Graneto JW: Gastrostomy tube replacement, in Henretig FM, King C (eds): *Textbook of Pediatric Emergency Procedures.* Baltimore: Williams & Wilkins, 1997:915–920.

9. Ponsky JL: Percutaneous endoscopic stomas. *Surg Clin North Am* 1989; 69(6):1227–1236.

10. Russell TR, Brotman M, Norris F: Percutaneous gastrostomy: a new simplified and cost-effective technique. *Am J Surg* 1984; 148:132–137.

11. Samuels L: Feeding tubes: removal, replacement, and unclogging, in Roberts JR, Hedges JR (eds): *Clinical Procedures in Emergency Medicine,* 2nd ed. Philadelphia: Saunders, 1991:662–674.

12. Kadakia SC, Cassaday M, Shaffer RT: Prospective evaluation of Foley catheter as a replacement gastrostomy tube. *Am J Gastroenterol* 1992; 87(11):1594–1597.

13. Kadakia SC, Cassaday M, Shaffer RT: Comparison of Foley catheter as a replacement gastrostomy tube with commercial replacement gastrostomy tube: a prospective randomized trial. *Gastrointest Endosc* 1994; 40(2):188–193.

14. Beck AR, Allen JE: An improved gastrostomy dressing. *Arch Surg* 1967; 94:904–906.

15. Brummer B, Cheng EH: Simple external retention device for Foley replacement gastrostomy tubes. *J Clin Gastroenterol* 1995; 20(4):337–338.

16. Simon T, Fink AS: Current management of endoscopic feeding tube dysfunction. *Surg Endosc* 1999;13:403–405.

17. Persaud M: Unclogging percutaneous endoscopic gastrostomy tubes. *Gastrointest Endosc* 1990; 36(6):640.

18. Dobrota JS: Deflating replacement gastroscopy tubes. *Gastrointest Endosc* 1994; 40(6):778.

19. Rogers JJ: Failure to deflate the balloon of replacement gastroscopy tubes. *Gastrointest Endosc* 1994; 40(5):649.

20. Waldstreicher S: Replacement of gastrostomy tube. *Am J Gastroenterol* 1999; 92(4):728.

21. Kadakia SC, Parker A, Angueira C, et al: Failure to deflate the balloon of replacement gastrostomy tubes. *Gastrointest Endosc* 1993; 39(4):576–578.

22. Korula J, Harma C: A simple and inexpensive method of removal or replacement of gastrostomy tubes. *JAMA* 1991; 265(11):1426–1428.

23. Yaseen M, Steele MI, Grunow JE: Nonendoscopic removal of percutaneous endoscopic gastrostomy tubes: morbidity and mortality in children. *Gastrointest Endosc* 1996; 44(3):235–238.

24. Marshall JB, Bodnarchuk G, Barthel JS: Early accidental dislodgement of PEG tubes. *J Clin Gastroenterol* 1994; 18(3):210–212.

25. Galat SA, Gerig KD, Porter JA, et al: Management of premature removal of the percutaneous gastrostomy. *Am Surg* 1990; 56(11):733–736.

26. Benson M, Slater G: Technique for the replacement of a feeding gastrostomy tube. *Am J Surg* 1979; 138(5):732.

27. Esker AH, Hall CH: Replacement of the damaged percutaneous endoscopic gastrostomy feeding tube in the immature tract. *Gastrointest Endosc* 1990; 36(4):389–391.

28. Fox VL, Abel SD, Malas S, et al: Complications following percutaneous endoscopic gastrostomy and subsequent catheter replacement in children and young adults. *Gastrointest Endosc* 1997; 45(1):64–71.

Chapter 54
PARACENTESIS

Susan B. Promes

INTRODUCTION

Ascites (also called abdominal or peritoneal dropsy, hydroperitonia, and hydrops abdominis) is defined as an abnormal accumulation of fluid in the abdominal cavity. The word *ascites* is derived from the Greek *askos,* meaning "bag" or "sac." The presence of ascites has important implications diagnostically, therapeutically, and prognostically. Cirrhosis of the liver is usually related to alcoholism, which accounts for 75 percent of cases of ascites; malignancy accounts for an additional 10 to 12 percent, and cardiac failure for another 5 percent. The remaining cases have a variety of etiologies.[1] Unfortunately, the physical examination is not very reliable when it comes to detecting ascites, making paracentesis an important clinical tool.[2]

Peritoneal aspiration of ascitic fluid or paracentesis was first described by Saloman in the early twentieth century.[3] With the introduction of diuretics as well as a fear of procedure-related complications, paracentesis fell out of favor in the 1950s, being replaced by medical management. At that time, large-bore needles were being used and complication rates were significant. Clinical studies published in the late 1980s demonstrated that performing a paracentesis was, in fact, a safe procedure.[4,5] Nowadays, the procedure is commonplace in Emergency Departments.

Paracentesis is an important diagnostic tool for patients with new-onset ascites to determine its etiology and in those patients with long-standing ascites to detect the presence of infection. Spontaneous bacterial peritonitis can be a very subtle disease. It is well known that some patients with spontaneous bacterial peritonitis are asymptomatic, making peritoneal fluid aspiration and cultures imperative.[6] In addition to the diagnostic usefulness of paracentesis, large volumes of ascitic fluid can be removed therapeutically by this procedure in order to improve a patient's respiratory status and comfort level from tense ascites. This often occurs in patients with end-stage liver disease as well as in some cases of malignancy. Malignant ascites may occur with carcinoma of the ovary, pancreas, stomach, colon, breast, testes, and a variety of sarcomas and lymphomas.

ANATOMY AND PATHOPHYSIOLOGY

The gross anatomy of the abdomen is well known to practitioners and is important to review in preparing for a paracentesis. The abdominal cavity is lined by the peritoneum and is protected from the environment by the abdominal wall musculature, fat, and skin. The right and left rectus muscles, which are nourished by the epigastric vessels, meet in the midline at the avascular linea alba. The umbilicus is located along the lower portion of the linea alba. The layers of the anterior abdominal wall structures vary above and below the level of the anterosuperior iliac spine (Figure 54-1).

The liver sits in the upper right quadrant; when enlarged, it can be palpated in the lower right quadrant. The spleen is normally contained in the upper left quadrant, but when it is enlarged, it can extend into the left lower quadrant of the abdomen. The intestines occupy most of the abdominal cavity and are not rigidly adherent, allowing them to move about in the abdominal cavity. The bladder sits in the pelvis but can enter the abdominal cavity when it is distended with urine.

The abdominal cavity is divided into compartments according to mesenteric attachments. Ascitic fluid can be found anywhere in the peritoneal cavity. The location of the ascitic fluid depends primarily upon the amount of fluid present and the patient's position. Fluid follows the law of gravity. Small amounts of fluid generally accumulate in the cul-de-sac and pericolic gutters. Large amounts of fluid can be found bathing the intestines. There can also be distinct pockets of fluid in areas of

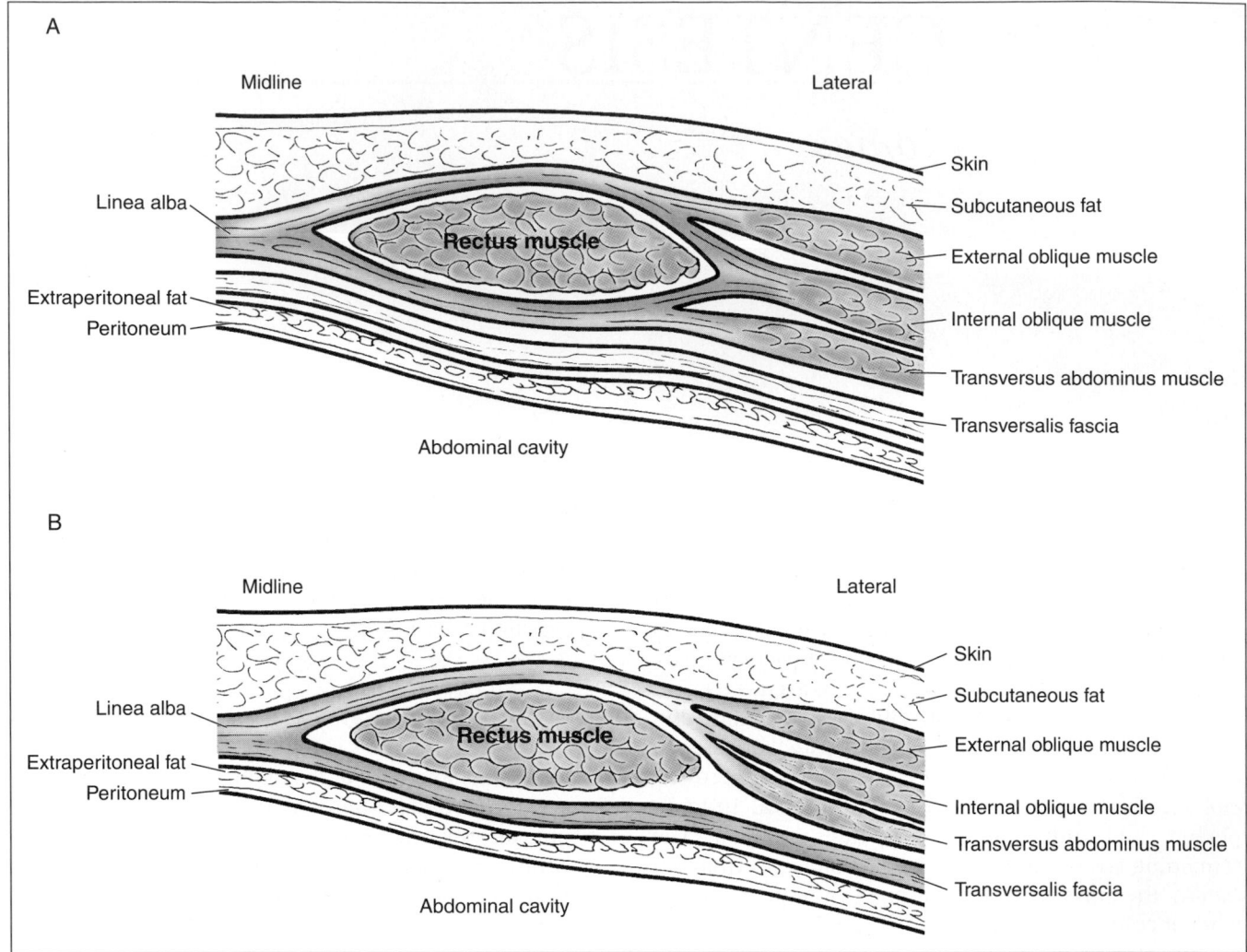

FIGURE 54-1 The layers of the anterior abdominal wall vary above (*A*) and below (*B*) the level of the anterosuperior iliac spine.

bowel adhesions or scarring. These localized areas of fluid are typically found in those patients who have had previous surgery, trauma, or infection. Ultrasound can be helpful in identifying, localizing, and quantifying ascitic fluid (Figure 54-2).

INDICATIONS

A paracentesis can be performed for diagnostic or therapeutic reasons. A paracentesis or "abdominal tap" is warranted in a patient with new-onset ascites to establish the etiology of the fluid. On the other hand, a patient with a history of ascites may or may not need the procedure, depending upon whether or not other associated signs and symptoms such as fever, dyspnea, or pain are present. A paracentesis can be performed therapeutically for patients in whom medical management

with diuretics has not been successful. It is most commonly performed when an intraperitoneal infection is suspected. Some clinicians now advocate that patients with ascites admitted to the hospital, whether or not they have symptoms of spontaneous bacterial peritonitis, should undergo a paracentesis.[7] Paracentesis has been used to aid in the diagnosis of ruptured ectopic pregnancy, bowel perforation, and hemoperitoneum due to trauma; more accurate diagnostic procedures are available and should be used rather than a paracentesis for these conditions.

CONTRAINDICATIONS

There are no absolute contraindications to performing a paracentesis. The relative contraindications include pregnant patients or patients who have a history

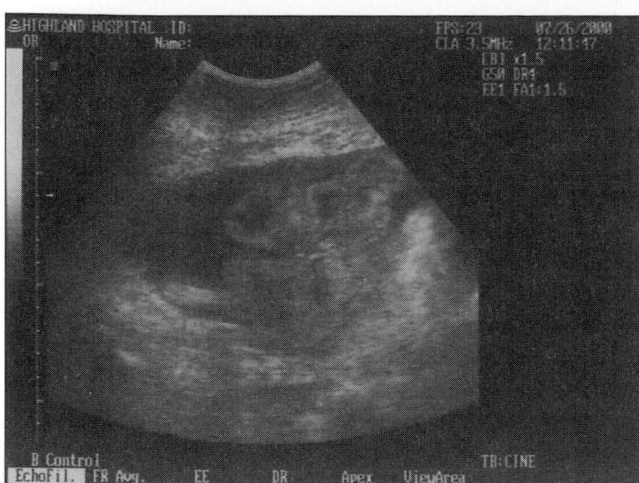

FIGURE 54-2 Ultrasound of the abdomen demonstrating loops of bowel floating in ascitic fluid (*black*).

of abdominal surgery, a current bowel obstruction, or a coagulopathy. Pregnancy is listed because the gravid uterus may fill the space where the procedure is normally performed. The paracentesis should be performed superior to the uterine fundus. It is important to avoid sites of previous surgical incisions, because adhesions may fix the bowel wall to the abdominal wall, thus increasing the possibility of perforation. Many patients who are subjected to a paracentesis have underlying liver disease and resultant coagulopathies. Some advocate that patients with thrombocytopenia or an abnormal international normalized ratio (INR) should have platelet transfusions or factor replacement prior to performing a paracentesis. This practice is controversial and there are no controlled data to support these contentions. Many, however, would suggest using an infraumbilical midline, also known as a linea alba, approach in coagulopathic patients. This area is free of vasculature, thus reducing the possibility of bleeding complications.

EQUIPMENT

Protective eyewear
Sterile gloves
Sterile gown, hat, and mask
Povidone iodine solution
Sterile 4×4 gauze
Sterile drape
Local anesthetic solution with epinephrine
25 gauge needle
10 mL syringe
18 gauge needle, 3½ inch needle or spinal needle
Seldinger-type guidewire kit

Catheter-through-the-needle
Catheter-over-the-needle
60 mL syringe for fluid collection
Intravenous tubing or blood collection tubing if vacuum bottles are used
Collection bottles (vacuum) or collection bag
Bandage
3-way stopcock
Blood collection tubes, purple and red tops
Blood culture bottles
Sterile specimen container for cytology (optional)

PATIENT PREPARATION

Explain the procedure, its risks, and its benefits to the patient and/or their representative. Obtain an informed consent for the procedure. The patient's bladder should be empty. Place a Foley catheter to decompress the bladder if the patient is unable to urinate voluntarily. Placement of a nasogastric tube is recommended prior to proceeding, thus making an iatrogenic gastric perforation less likely, especially if a concomitant bowel obstruction is present.

There are two recommended areas of entry for the paracentesis needle (Figure 54-3). The primary site is in the midline and 2 cm below the umbilicus. Alternatively, the site 4 to 5 cm superior and just medial to the anterosuperior iliac spine in one of the lower quadrants may be used. Some physicians choose the right lower quadrant to avoid the sigmoid colon and spleen. Others choose the left lower quadrant to avoid the cecum and liver. Neither of these recommendations is supported by scientific data. Remember to exercise caution in the region of a scar, prominent veins, caput medusa, or over an area of inflamed or infected skin to minimize complications. Ultrasound may be helpful to identify fluid in complicated cases.

Place the patient sitting upright for a midline or linea alba approach, lying in the right lateral decubitus position for a right lower quadrant approach, or lying in the left lateral decubitus position for a left lower quadrant approach. Another position one might consider is having the patient assume a hand-knee or "crawling" position. This position, however, is awkward for the physician performing the procedure. Remember that the fluid will pool in dependent areas and the bowel will float on top of it (barring any adhesions or masses).

Prepare the patient. Clean the skin around the chosen puncture site of any dirt and debris. Apply povidone iodine solution and allow it to dry. Apply sterile drapes to delineate a sterile field. Inject 2 to 5 mL of local anesthetic solution subcutaneously and along the needle insertion tract. Allow 3 to 5 minutes for the local anesthetic to take effect.

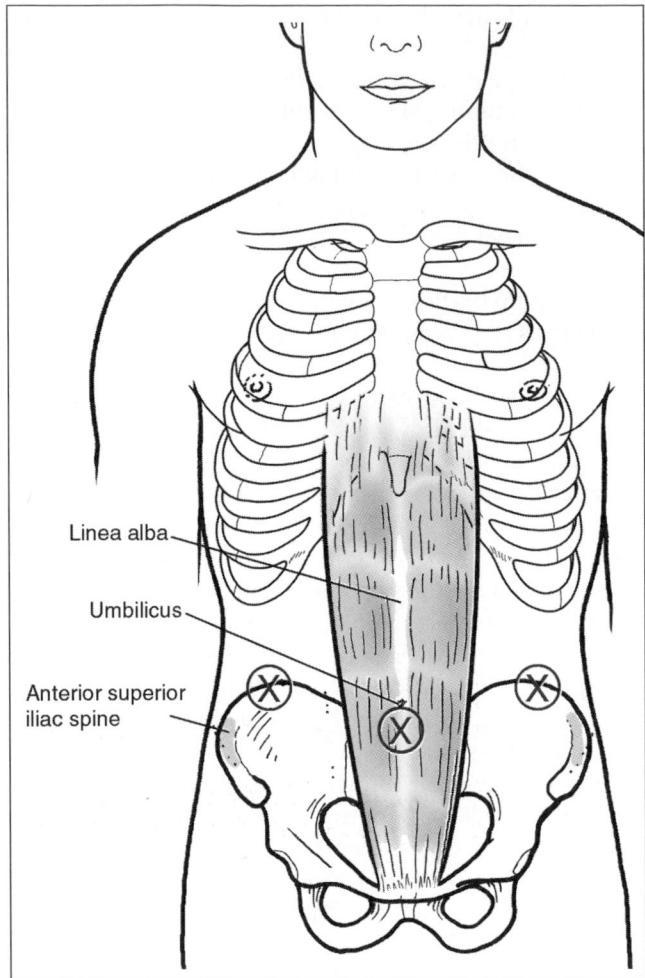

FIGURE 54-3 Needle insertion sites to perform a paracentesis (indicated by a red ⊗). The preferred site is in the midline and 2 cm below the umbilicus. Alternative sites are just medial and 4 to 5 cm above the anterosuperior iliac spines.

Linea alba

Umbilicus

Anterior superior iliac spine

TECHNIQUES

Z-TRACT TECHNIQUE

A "Z-tract" is used to decrease the possibility of an ascitic fluid leak, especially in patients with tense ascites (Figure 54-4). This is the preferred method for inserting the needle. This technique should also be followed in using the techniques described below. Apply traction on the skin cephalad or caudad to the needle insertion site so that the skin is pulled taut when the needle enters the peritoneum (Figures 54-4A and B). The idea is that when the skin tension is released, the skin returns to its normal position and seals off the pathway of the paracentesis needle.

Apply an 18 gauge, 3½ inch needle or spinal needle onto a 60 mL syringe. Slowly insert and advance the needle perpendicular to the skin (Figure 54-4A) or at 45 degrees to the skin and aimed caudally (Figure 54-4B). Ap-

ply negative pressure to the syringe as it is being advanced. A loss of resistance should be felt as the needle enters the peritoneal cavity. Stop advancing the needle when ascitic fluid enters the syringe. Continue to aspirate until the syringe is one-half to three-fourths filled with fluid.

The omentum or a loop of bowel may be occluding the needle if ascitic fluid suddenly stops flowing into the syringe. Release the plunger of the syringe. Reattempt to aspirate. If fluid still will not flow, inject 1 to 2 mL of ascitic fluid, then reattempt to aspirate. Reposition the needle if ascitic fluid still does not flow into the syringe. **Never reposition the needle while the tip is within the peritoneal cavity. The needle can lacerate the bowel, the omentum, or a blood vessel.** Withdraw the needle to the dermis, reposition it, then readvance it into the peritoneal cavity.

Note the color and clarity of the ascitic fluid. Aspirate 30 to 50 mL if the procedure is being performed for diagnostic purposes. Withdraw the needle after obtaining the fluid. Immediately place the fluid into the red-top, purple-top, and culture tubes.[8] If the reason for the paracentesis is therapeutic and there is a large collection of fluid that must be drained, hold the needle securely and remove the syringe. An assistant can place the sample into laboratory containers. Connect the needle to intravenous tubing. Connect the other end of the intravenous tubing to a suction bottle or bag in order to drain off the desired amount of ascitic fluid. Remove the needle once the procedure has been completed. Removal of the needle results in the formation of the Z-tract, so that ascitic fluid will not leak from the skin (Figure 54-4C). Apply a bandage to the skin puncture site.

SELDINGER TECHNIQUE

First described by Seldinger in 1953, this technique allows for the placement of a catheter over a wire (Figure 54-5). The wire used must be longer than the catheter. The needle used to insert the wire can be short and of a smaller gauge than the catheter. Materials needed for catheter insertion are commercially available in a prefabricated kit. The Seldinger technique is most commonly used for central venous catheter insertion.

Choose the puncture site and prepare the patient for the procedure. Insert the thin-walled introducer needle in a Z-tract manner while applying negative pressure to the syringe (Figure 54-5A). The introducer needle has a tapered hub on the proximal end to guide the wire into the needle lumen. Avoid using a standard hypodermic needle, as it will not allow for the passage of the guidewire. A flash of fluid in the needle hub signifies that the tip of the needle is within the peritoneal cavity (Figure 54-5A). Advance the needle an additional 1 to 2 mm. Hold the needle in place securely and remove the syringe.

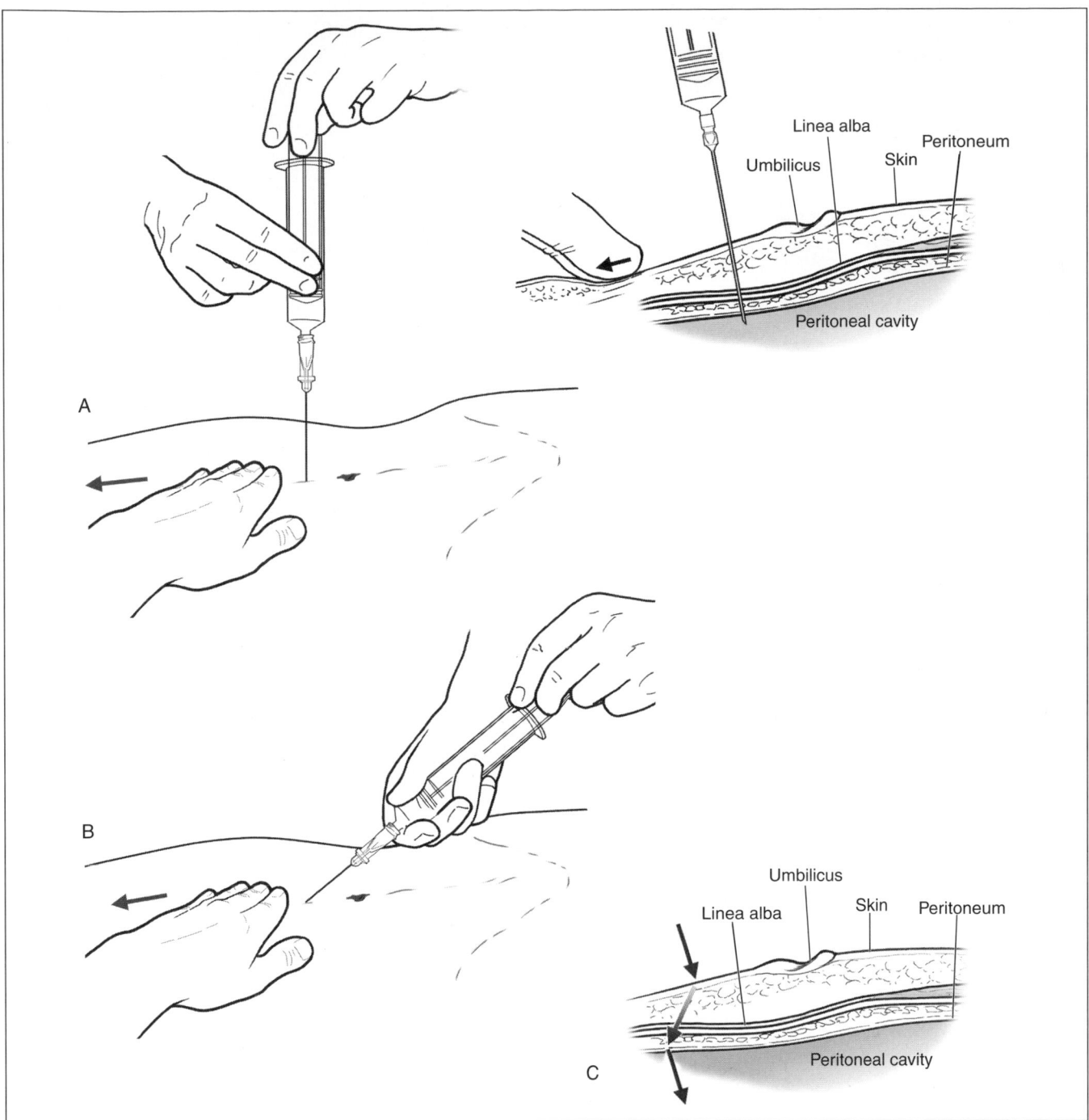

FIGURE 54-4 The Z-tract. *A.* The needle is inserted perpendicular to the skin while the skin is pulled taut. *B.* Alternatively, the needle can be inserted at 45 degrees to the skin and aimed caudally. *C.* The resultant Z-tract (*arrows*).

Occlude the needle hub with a sterile gloved finger. This will prevent air from entering and ascitic fluid from exiting. Insert the guidewire through the hub of the needle (Figure 54-5*B*). Advance the guidewire to the desired depth, ensuring that it is at least several centimeters beyond the beveled end of the needle. **Never let go of the guidewire with both hands at the same time, in order to prevent loss of the wire into the peritoneal cavity.**

Hold the guidewire securely in place. Remove the needle over the guidewire (Figure 54-5*C*). Make a small nick in the skin adjacent to the guidewire with a #11 scalpel blade (Figure 54-5*D*). **Direct the sharp edge of the scalpel blade away from the guidewire to avoid nicking the guidewire.**

Place the dilator through the sheath to form a unit. Advance the dilator and sheath unit over the guidewire

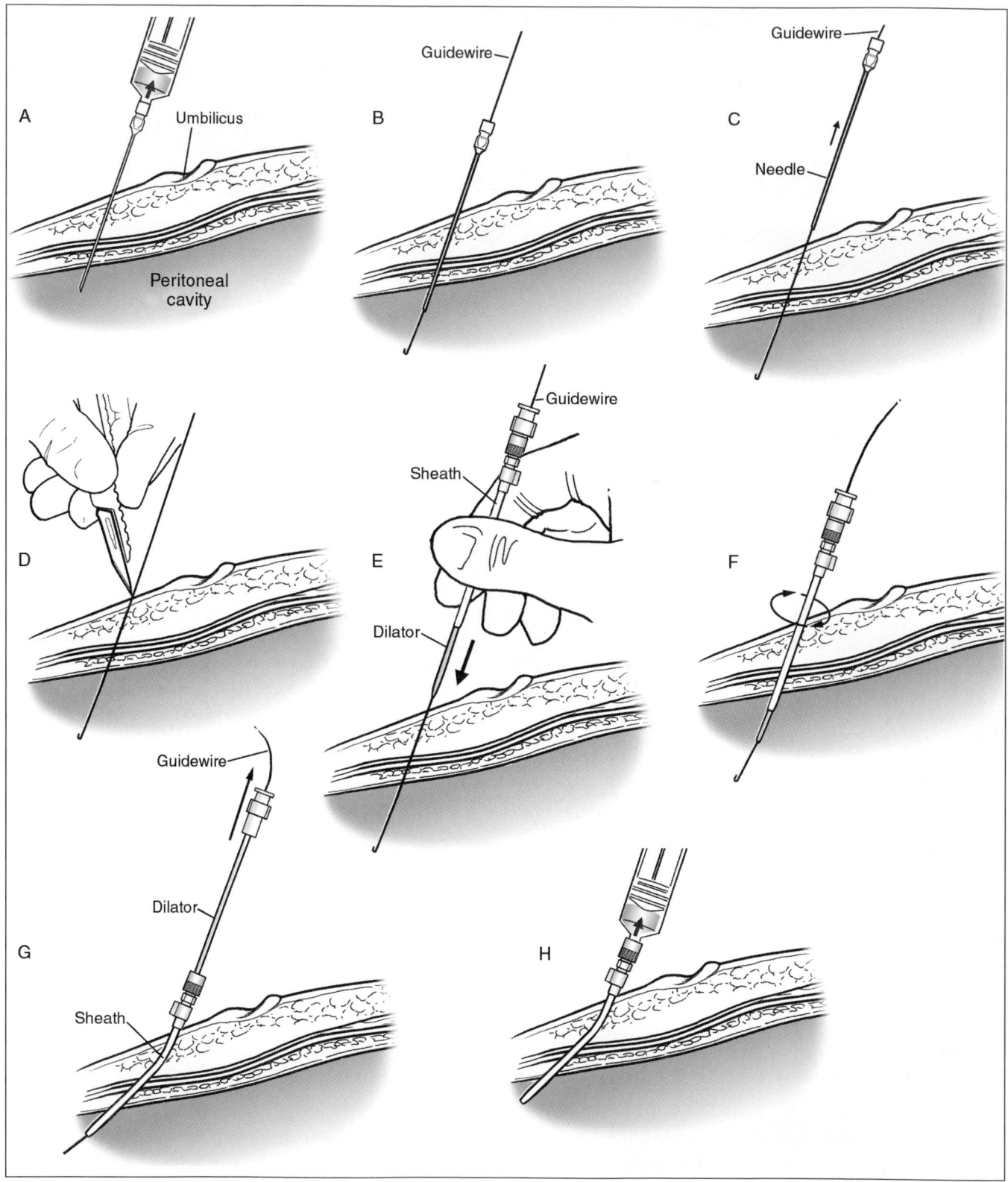

FIGURE 54-5 The Seldinger technique. *A.* The needle is advanced into the peritoneal cavity. *B.* The syringe is removed and a guidewire is inserted through the needle and into the peritoneal cavity. *C.* The needle is removed, leaving the guidewire in place. *D.* An incision is made where the guidewire enters the skin. *E.* The dilator and sheath are advanced as a unit over the guidewire. *F.* The dilator and sheath are advanced into the peritoneal cavity with a twisting motion. *G.* The guidewire and dilator are removed as a unit, leaving the catheter in place. *H.* A syringe is attached to the catheter. The aspiration of ascitic fluid confirms proper intraperitoneal placement of the catheter.

(Figure 54-5*E*). Continue to advance the dilator and sheath unit over the guidewire and into the peritoneal cavity (Figure 54-5*F*). A twisting motion may aid in its advancement through the skin and into the peritoneal cavity (Figure 54-5*F*). Advance the unit until the hub of the catheter is against the skin. Hold the hub of the catheter securely. Remove the guidewire and dilator as a unit (Figure 54-5*G*). Attach a syringe to the hub of the catheter (Figure 54-5*H*).

Aspirate fluid from the catheter to confirm intraperitoneal placement. Hold the hub of the catheter securely and remove the syringe. Pass the syringe to an assistant to place the sample into laboratory containers. Connect the catheter to intravenous tubing. Connect the other end of the intravenous tubing to a suction bottle or bag in order to drain off the desired amount of fluid. An alternative is to attach a 3-way stopcock to the distal end of the intravenous tubing. A syringe may then be attached to the stopcock to withdraw laboratory samples or "pump out" the ascitic fluid into a nonsterile container. Remove the catheter once the procedure is completed. Apply a bandage to the skin puncture site. While this technique seems complicated at first glance, it is easy to learn and can be performed in a few minutes by an experienced physician.

CATHETER-THROUGH-THE-NEEDLE TECHNIQUE

This system is used most commonly for central venous access. Select a catheter size that is appropriate for the patient and the site of entry. Packaged with each catheter is a needle and a needle guard. The needle will have an inner diameter that is slightly larger than the outer diameter of the catheter. The needle guard has a beveled channel in which the needle can reside. The needle guard hinges closed over the needle to hold it securely and prevent the needle from shearing the catheter.

Choose the puncture site and prepare the patient for the procedure. Place the needle on a tuberculin syringe. Insert the needle through the skin in a Z-tract manner and into the peritoneal cavity while applying negative pressure to the syringe (Figure 54-6*A*). A flash of fluid in the syringe confirms that the tip of the needle is within the peritoneal cavity. Advance the needle an additional 2 or 3 mm to ensure that the tip of the needle is completely within the peritoneal cavity. Securely grasp and hold the needle with the nondominant hand. Remove the syringe with the dominant hand. Immediately place the nondominant thumb over the needle hub to prevent air from entering and fluid from exiting.

Insert the catheter through the hub of the needle (Figure 54-6*B*). Advance the catheter through the needle until the desired length of catheter is within the peritoneal cavity. **If the catheter will not advance, remove the catheter and needle as a unit. Never withdraw the catheter through the needle. The sharp bevel of the needle may cut the catheter as it is being withdrawn and result in a catheter embolism in the peritoneal cavity.**

Withdraw the needle over the catheter (Figure 54-6*C*). **Do not allow the catheter to be withdrawn through the needle.** Continue to withdraw the needle until the tip is completely outside the skin. Apply the needle guard over the needle (Figure 54-6*D*). Attach a syringe onto the hub of the catheter. Aspirate fluid from the catheter to confirm intraperitoneal placement. Hold the hub of the catheter securely and remove the syringe. Pass the syringe to an assistant to place the sample into laboratory containers. Connect the catheter to intravenous tubing. Connect the other end of the tubing to a suction bottle or bag in order to drain off the desired amount of fluid. An alternative is to attach a 3-way stopcock to the distal end of the tubing. A syringe may then be attached to the stopcock to withdraw laboratory samples or "pump out" the ascitic fluid into a nonsterile container. Remove the catheter once the procedure is completed. Apply a bandage to the skin puncture site.

The main disadvantage of this technique is the possibility of the needle tip shearing off the catheter and resulting in a catheter embolism. **This can be prevented by not withdrawing the catheter through the needle and applying the needle guard immediately after the needle is withdrawn from the skin.** Another disadvantage is that the contaminated needle must be handled to some extent, creating a potential risk for needle-stick injuries.

CATHETER-OVER-THE-NEEDLE TECHNIQUE

The catheter-over-the-needle systems are the most commonly used for peripheral venous access. The infusion catheter fits closely over a hypodermic needle. The needle and the catheter are advanced as a unit into the peritoneal cavity. They are inexpensive (about $1 to $4 each), come in a variety of diameters (12 to 24 gauge) and lengths, and are widely available. Versions designed to minimize accidental needle-stick injuries are available, and their use is encouraged (Figure 36-7*B*). Placement of these catheters is usually quick and simple.

Choose the puncture site and prepare the patient for the procedure. Insert the catheter-over-the-needle through the skin in a Z-tract manner and into the peritoneal cavity (Figure 54-7*A*). A flash of fluid in the hub of the needle confirms that the tip of the needle is within the peritoneal cavity. Advance the catheter-over-the-needle an additional 2 or 3 mm to ensure that the catheter is within the peritoneal cavity. Hold the hub of the needle securely. Advance the catheter over the needle until its hub is against the skin (Figure 54-7*B*). Withdraw the needle. Attach a syringe onto the hub of the

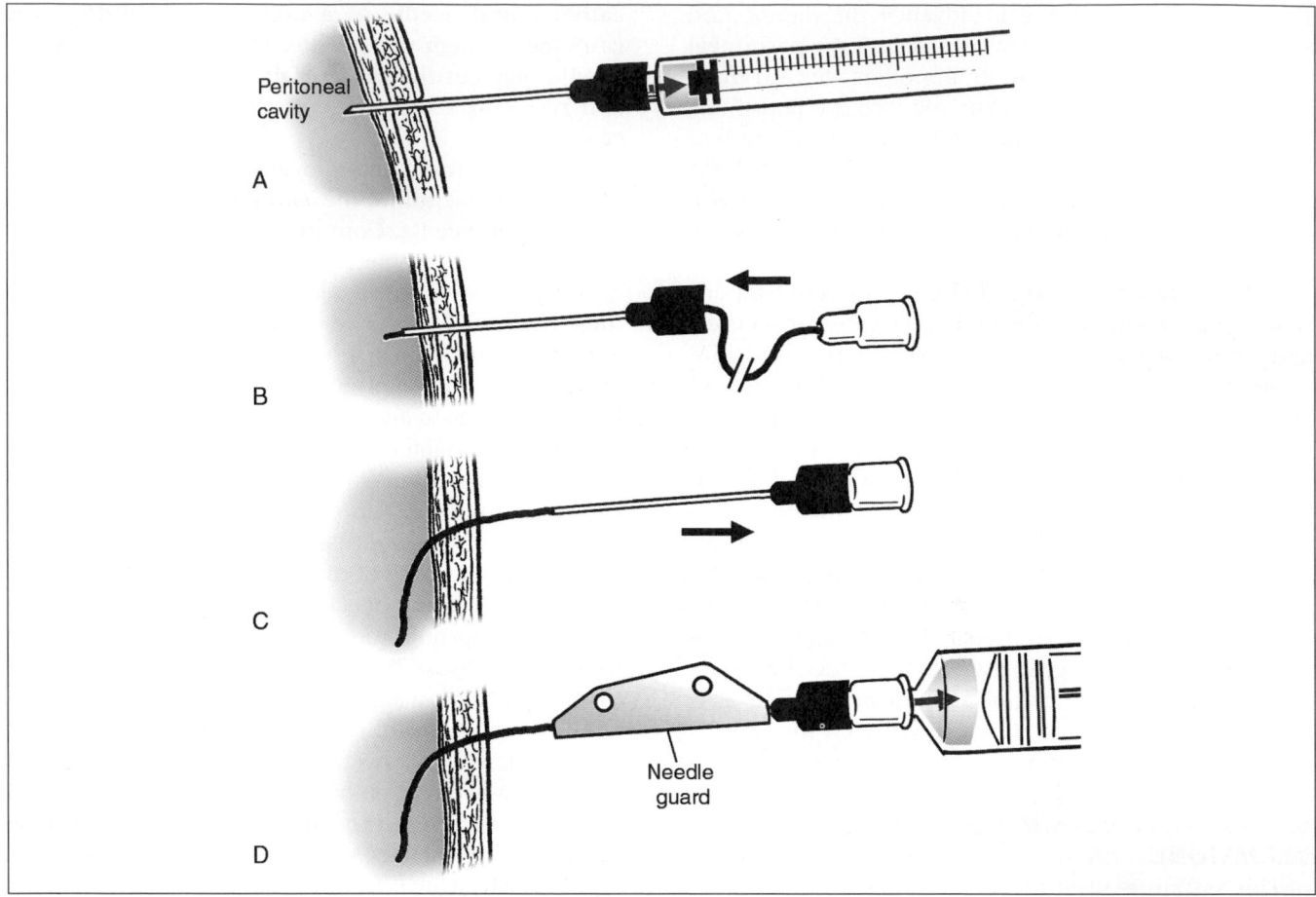

FIGURE 54-6 The catheter-through-the-needle technique. *A.* The needle is advanced into the peritoneal cavity while maintaining negative pressure on the syringe. *B.* The syringe has been removed. The catheter is inserted through the needle. *C.* The needle is withdrawn and the catheter is left within the peritoneal cavity. *D.* A syringe is attached to the catheter. The aspiration of ascitic fluid confirms proper intraperitoneal placement of the catheter.

catheter (Figure 54-7*C*). Aspirate fluid from the catheter to confirm intraperitoneal placement. Hold the hub of the catheter securely and remove the syringe. Pass the syringe to an assistant to place the sample into laboratory containers. Connect the catheter to intravenous tubing. Connect the other end of the tubing to a suction bottle or bag in order to drain off the desired amount of fluid. An alternative is to attach a 3-way stopcock to the distal end of the tubing. A syringe may then be attached to the stopcock to withdraw laboratory samples or "pump out" the ascitic fluid into a nonsterile container. Remove the catheter once the procedure is completed. Apply a bandage to the skin puncture site.

AFTERCARE

Once the procedure is completed, the paracentesis puncture site should be bandaged. The site will occasionally ooze fluid in patients with tense ascites. These patients should be directed to change their dressings regularly. Occlusive tape is helpful to prevent the fluid from leaking onto the patient's clothing and bedding. At times, a simple suture is necessary to control the drainage. The patient may be discharged home if the purpose of the paracentesis was to relieve tense ascites and no signs or symptoms of spontaneous bacterial peritonitis exist. The patient should immediately return to the Emergency Department if they develop abdominal pain, nausea, vomiting, abdominal distention, or a fever.

The patient requires hospitalization and intravenous antibiotics if spontaneous bacterial peritonitis is suspected or diagnosed. Empiric antibiotics that cover gram-negative enterics (of which *Escherichia coli* is the most likely) and streptococcal species (including *Enterococcus*) should be administered in the Emergency Department. A third-generation cephalosporin, such as cefotaxime, that covers 98 percent of the causative agents in this disorder should be administered. Ampicillin may

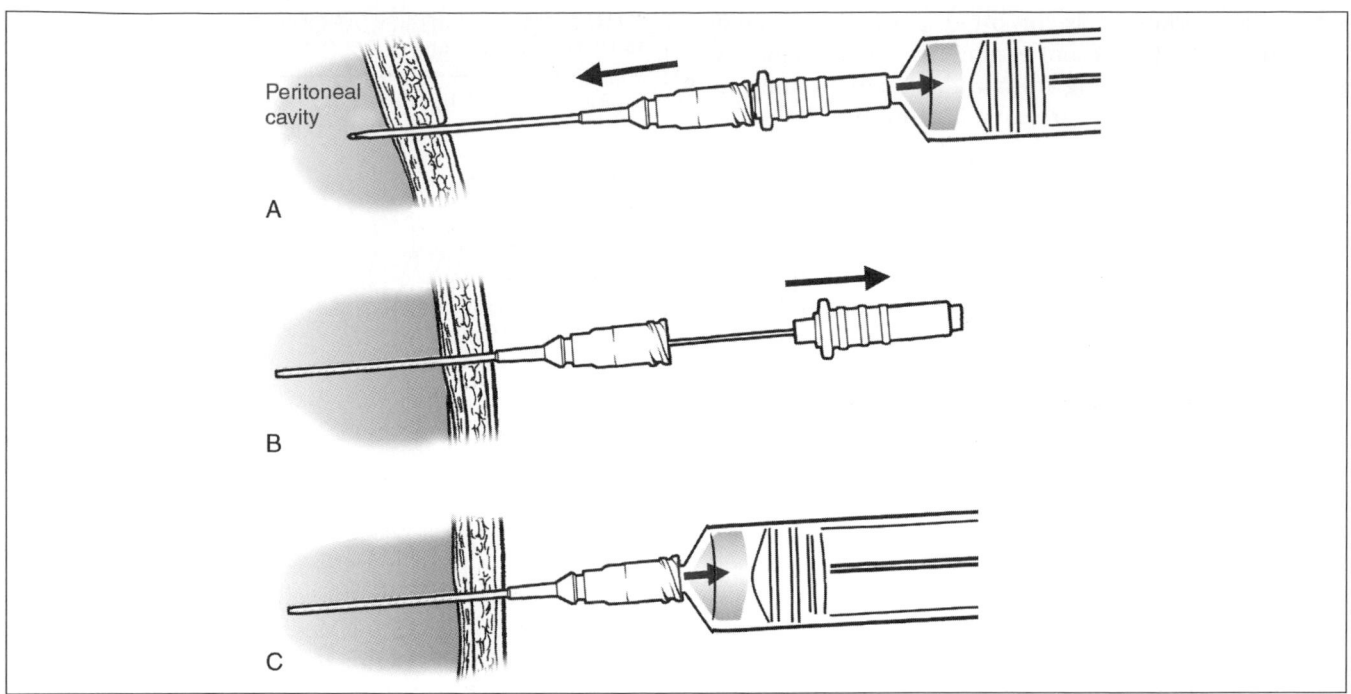

FIGURE 54-7 The catheter-over-the-needle technique. *A.* The catheter-over-the-needle is inserted into the peritoneal cavity while maintaining negative pressure on the syringe. *B.* The needle is removed. *C.* A syringe is attached to the catheter. The aspiration of ascitic fluid confirms proper intraperitoneal placement of the catheter.

be added if *Enterococcus* is suspected. Check previous culture results for antibiotic sensitivities if the patient has a history of spontaneous bacterial peritonitis.

COMPLICATIONS

Complications from abdominal paracentesis are infrequent and rarely serious. However, known complications include shearing of the peritoneal catheter, abdominal wall hematoma, hemoperitoneum, bowel perforation, infection, persistent ascitic fluid leak, and systemic hemodynamic compromise.

Although bleeding is a potential complication of paracentesis, administration of prophylactic blood products such as fresh frozen plasma does not appear to be warranted.[9] Spontaneous hemoperitoneum secondary to mesenteric variceal bleeding has been reported to occur in patients receiving large-volume (> 4000 mL) paracentesis.[10] Patients who developed this complication have had advanced cirrhosis with refractory ascites, previous large-volume paracentesis, and hemorrhagic shock without evidence of gastrointestinal bleeding. Mortality for this complication is exceedingly high. An additional vascular complication of an inferior epigastric artery pseudoaneurysm has been described as a complication of therapeutic paracentesis.[11]

Perforation of the bowel during paracentesis is rare. Additionally, most of these injuries are self-sealing and develop no further problems. Generalized peritonitis and abdominal wall abscesses have also been reported and are exceedingly rare. Do not move the needle when it is within the peritoneal cavity in order to avoid lacerating the bowel wall.

Ascitic fluid may continue to leak from the site of paracentesis. A simple suture at the site will correct the problem. Patients with persistent leaks should also be evaluated for peritonitis.

Rapid removal of significant amounts of ascitic fluid has been found to cause hemodynamic compromise. Initially, removal of large amounts of ascites causes improvement in circulatory function, likely related to both mechanical (improved cardiac venous return) and neurohumoral factors. However, total paracentesis in cirrhotic patients may cause delayed (> 12 to 24 hours post-procedure) effective hypovolemia by accentuation of baseline arteriolar vasodilation through neurohumeral mechanisms.[12] The literature suggests that some of the post-paracentesis circulatory dysfunction may be avoided by pretreating patients with an intravenous colloid such as albumin.[13] This is not a universally accepted practice.

ASCITIC FLUID ANALYSIS

Normal ascitic fluid should appear clear with a yellow color. Increased turbidity may suggest infection, elevated triglyceride levels, or other particulate matter. Sanguinous fluid is present in patients with malignancy, intraperitoneal bleeding from the intraabdominal organs (spontaneous or iatrogenically introduced), or tuberculous peritonitis.

The specific analytical tests ordered on ascitic fluid should reflect the physician's clinical suspicion (Table 54-1). Simple analysis of fluid with a cell count and differential, routine cultures, and albumin concentration are all that is necessary in patients with uncomplicated cirrhosis. These initial tests can be supplemented depending upon clinical suspicion. Total protein, glucose, LDH, amylase, triglyceride, and bilirubin levels are not helpful except in select circumstances and are not warranted on a routine basis. The serum-ascites albumin gradient is approximately 97 percent accurate in indicating portal hypertension.[4,14] The gradient is calculated by subtracting the ascitic fluid albumin concentration from the simultaneously measured serum albumin concentration. A gradient of $\geq$ 1.1 gm/dL suggests portal hypertension as the etiology of the ascites (Table 54-2). A gradient of < 1.1 gm/dL suggests that the patient does not have portal hypertension and that the ascites has some other etiology (Table 54-2).

Peritoneal carcinomatosis should be suspected and cytology ordered in those patients with a history of breast cancer, colon cancer, gastric cancer, pancreatic cancer, or the suspicion of undiagnosed malignancy and ascites. Cultures for mycobacteria are approximately 50 percent sensitive. They should be ordered when the suspicion for tuberculous peritonitis is high, as in patients who have immigrated from endemic areas or have an immunocompromised status.

Patients with uncomplicated ascites secondary to cirrhosis should have an ascitic white blood cell (WBC) count < 500 cells/mm^3. The cells should be predominantly lymphocytes and there should be no clinical evidence of peritonitis. If an infection is suspected, a WBC count of > 250 cells/mm^3 with greater than 50 percent polymorphonuclear leukocytes confirms spontaneous bacterial peritonitis. A Gram's stain is usually not helpful other than in the case of spontaneous bowel rupture. Otherwise, the concentration of bacteria is too low to justify utilization of a Gram's stain. All potentially infected ascitic fluid should be cultured by directly inoculating blood culture bottles at the bedside.[8]

TABLE 54-1. LABORATORY TESTS FOR ASCITIC FLUID

Mandatory	Optional	Unusual
Cell count	Total protein	Acid-fast smear and culture
Albumin	Glucose	Cytology
Cultures	LDH	Triglycerides
	Amylase	
	Gram's stain	

TABLE 54-2. CLASSIFICATION OF ASCITES BY THE SERUM-ASCITES ALBUMIN CONCENTRATION GRADIENT

High gradient ($\geq$ 1.1 gm/dL)	Low gradient (< 1.1 gm/dL)
Cirrhosis	Peritoneal carcinomatosis
Alcoholic hepatitis	Tuberculous peritonitis
Cardiac ascites	Pancreatic ascites
Massive liver metastases	Nephrotic syndrome
Fulminant hepatic failure	Serositis in connective tissue
Budd-Chiari syndrome	diseases
Portal vein thrombosis	
Venoocclusive disease	
Fatty liver of pregnancy	
Myxedema	
Mixed ascites	

SUMMARY

Paracentesis is a safe procedure that is common in the practice of Emergency Medicine. There are few contraindications to its performance. It is most commonly performed diagnostically to detect spontaneous bacterial peritonitis. It can also be performed therapeutically for symptomatic relief in patients with tense ascites. Complications, although they do occur, are rare.

REFERENCES

1. Rocco VK, Ware AJ: Cirrhotic ascites: pathophysiology, diagnosis and management. *Ann Intern Med* 1986; 105(4):573–585.
2. Cattau E Jr, Benjamin SB, Knuff TE, et al: The accuracy of the physical examination in the diagnosis of suspected ascites. *JAMA* 1982; 247(8):1164–1166.
3. Saloman H: Die diagnostische punction des bausches. *Berl Klin Wochenschr* 1906; 43:45.
4. Runyon B: Paracentesis of ascitic fluid: a safe procedure. *Arch Intern Med* 1986; 146:2259–2261.
5. Pinto PC, American J, Reynolds TB: Large-volume paracentesis in the nonedematous patient with tense ascites: its effect on intravascular volume. *Hepatology* 1988; 8(2):207–210.
6. Pinzello G, Simonetti RG, Craxi A, et al: Spontaneous bacterial peritonitis: a prospective investigation in predominately nonalcoholic cirrhotic patients. *Hepatology* 1983; 3(4):545–549.
7. Runyon BA: Care of patients with ascites. *N Engl J Med* 1994; 330(5):337–341.
8. Runyon BA, Canawati HN, Arkriviadis EA: Optimization of ascitic fluid culture technique. *Gastroenterology* 1988; 95(5):1351–1355.
9. Runyon BA: Management of adult patients with ascites caused by cirrhosis. *Hepatology* 1998; 27(1):264–272.

10. Arnold C, Klaus H, Blum HE, et al: Acute hemoperitoneum after large-volume paracentesis. *Gastroenterology* 1997; 113(3):978–982.

11. Lam EY, McLafferty RB, Taylor LM, et al: Inferior epigastric artery pseudoaneurysm: a complication of paracentesis. *J Vasc Surg* 1998; 28(3):566–569.

12. Vila MC, Sola R, Molina L, et al: Hemodynamic changes in patients developing effective hypovolemia after total paracentesis. *J Hepatol* 1998; 28:639–645.

13. Gines A, Fernandez-Esparrach G, Monescillo A, et al: Randomized trial comparing albumin, dextran-70, and polygeline as plasma expanders in cirrhotic patients with ascites treated by total paracentesis. *Gastroenterology* 1996; 111(4):1002–1010.

14. Runyon BA, Montano AA, Akriviadis EA, et al: The serum-ascites albumin gradient is superior to the exudate-transudate concept in the differential diagnosis of ascites. *Ann Intern Med* 1992; 117(3):215–220.

Chapter 55
DIAGNOSTIC PERITONEAL LAVAGE

Kimberly Nagy

INTRODUCTION

Diagnostic peritoneal lavage (DPL) is a useful test to determine which patients require a laparotomy based upon the presence of a hemoperitoneum. The physical examination may be misleading in up to 45 percent of patients with blunt abdominal trauma. It is helpful to use the DPL to diagnose the need for a laparotomy sooner and with greater accuracy.[1,2]

The technique of DPL was first described in 1964 by Dr. Root in an attempt to improve the identification of the patient with blunt abdominal trauma who required a laparotomy.[3] His description of the DPL represented an improvement upon the use of paracentesis to identify a hemoperitoneum as described by Salomon in 1906.[4] Root's initial description of DPL utilized a trocar placed into the peritoneal cavity to instill fluid. The fluid was visually inspected upon removal and the patient then underwent a laparotomy if it appeared bloody.

DPL has undergone several modifications since its initial description. The trocar technique was abandoned first in favor of the open technique and later the Seldinger or closed technique.[5,6] While the DPL was first described for blunt trauma, it has found an indication in the patient with penetrating trauma as well.[2] Initial attempts to quantify the effluent based on its appearance have been replaced by the red blood cell count, the white blood cell count, and the measurement of various enzymes.[7–9] The debate still rages in the literature as to which criterion best determines the need for laparotomy.

ANATOMY AND PATHOPHYSIOLOGY

The gross anatomy of the abdomen is well known to practitioners and is important to review when preparing for a DPL. The abdominal cavity is lined by the peritoneum and is protected from the environment by the abdominal wall musculature, fat, and skin. The right and left rectus muscles, which are nourished by the epigastric vessels, meet in the midline at the avascular linea alba. The umbilicus is located along the lower portion of the linea alba. The layers of the anterior abdominal wall structures vary above and below the level of the anterior superior iliac spine (Figure 55-1).

DPL, unlike a paracentesis, is always performed in the anterior midline of the abdomen (Figure 55-2). The linea alba is an avascular location through which the peritoneal cavity may be entered using either an open technique or a closed Seldinger type technique. This midline location minimizes the number of false positive lavages that occur due to bleeding from the abdominal wall muscles or blood vessels. This also allows the Surgeon to perform a midline laparotomy, if necessary, through the lavage site and avoid the formation of an avascular skin bridge.

Most DPLs may be safely performed 1 to 2 cm below the umbilicus (Figures 55-2 *A* and *B*). This location allows the DPL catheter to be directed into the pelvis, minimizes the occurrence of inadvertent vascular injury, and increases the likelihood that fluid will be sampled from a dependent portion of the abdomen. It is more difficult to retrieve fluid if the DPL is performed above the umbilicus due to interference from the omentum. All closed and semi-open DPLs, as well as many open DPLs, are performed below the umbilicus.

The resultant retroperitoneal hematoma in patients with a pelvic fracture may extend anteriorly to the level of the linea semilunaris. **Therefore, it is important to perform the DPL in patients with a pelvic fracture using an open technique above the umbilicus** (Figure 55-2*C*). This will avoid a false positive DPL and the inadvertent decompression of the hematoma.[10]

Another special situation occurs in the pregnant patient. **The DPL should be performed using an open**

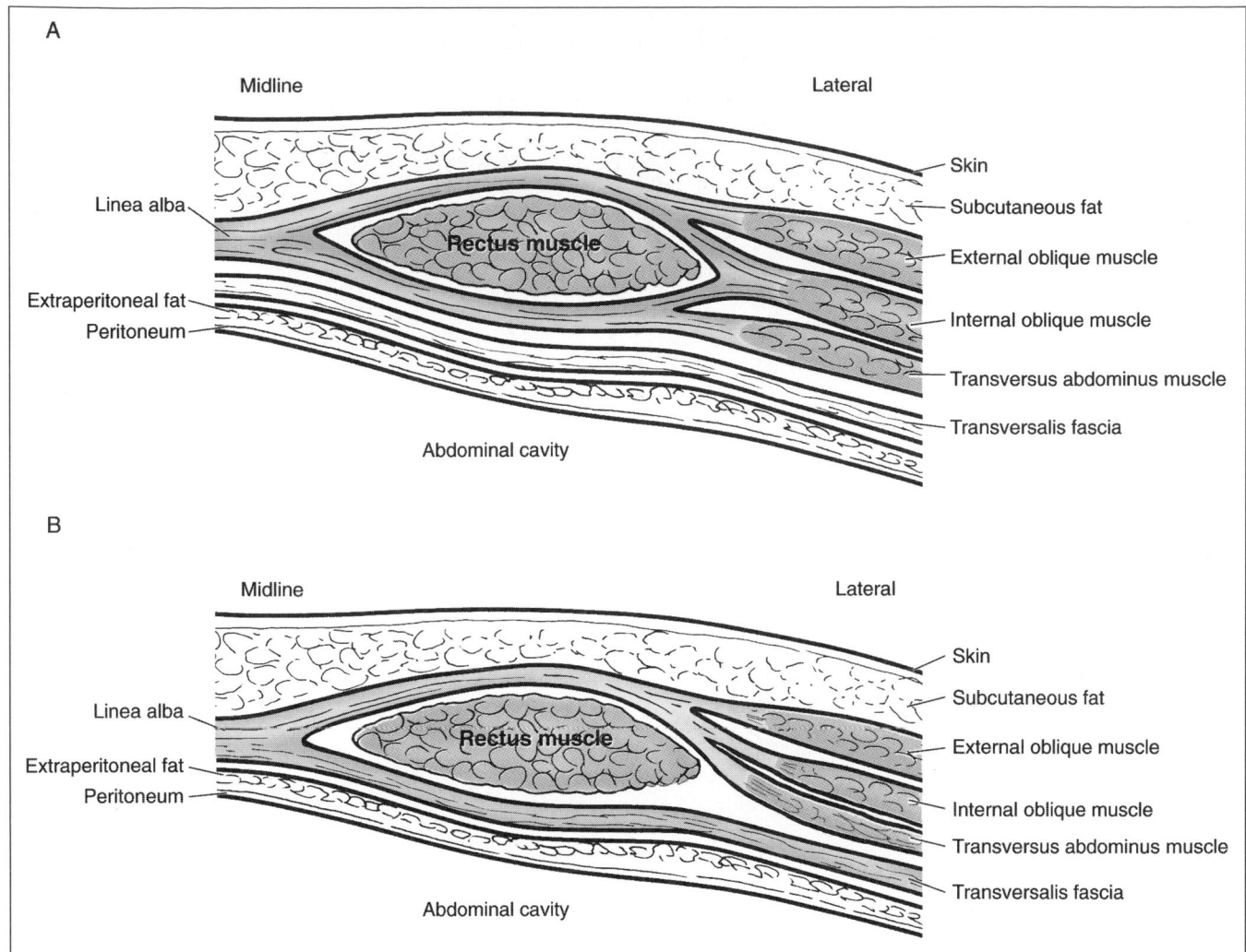

FIGURE 55-1 The layers of the anterior abdominal wall vary above (*A*) and below (*B*) the level of the anterior superior iliac spine.

technique superior to the uterine fundus.[5] The DPL may be performed below the umbilicus if the patient is in an early stage of pregnancy. The DPL should be performed more cephalad as the pregnancy progresses to minimize the chance of injuring the gravid uterus.

The third situation that may necessitate a change in the location to perform the DPL is in the patient with previous abdominal surgery. These patients must be individualized based upon the location of their scar. The DPL should be performed supraumbilically if the patient has a lower abdominal scar. The DPL should be performed infraumbilically if the patient has an upper abdominal scar.[1,7] In all cases of previous surgery, the DPL should be performed using an open technique to avoid any adhesions and minimize complications.[11]

INDICATIONS

DPL is indicated in any patient with suspected abdominal trauma, blunt or penetrating, that does not have an obvious indication for a laparotomy and in whom serial physical examinations are not practical. It can be performed quickly, will reliably exclude significant intraabdominal trauma, and allow the diagnosis and treatment of associated injuries. It does not require transfer of the patient out of the monitored environment of the Emergency Department, as does a computed tomogram (CT scan). It likewise does not require sophisticated equipment and extensive training comparable to those required to perform abdominal ultrasonography.

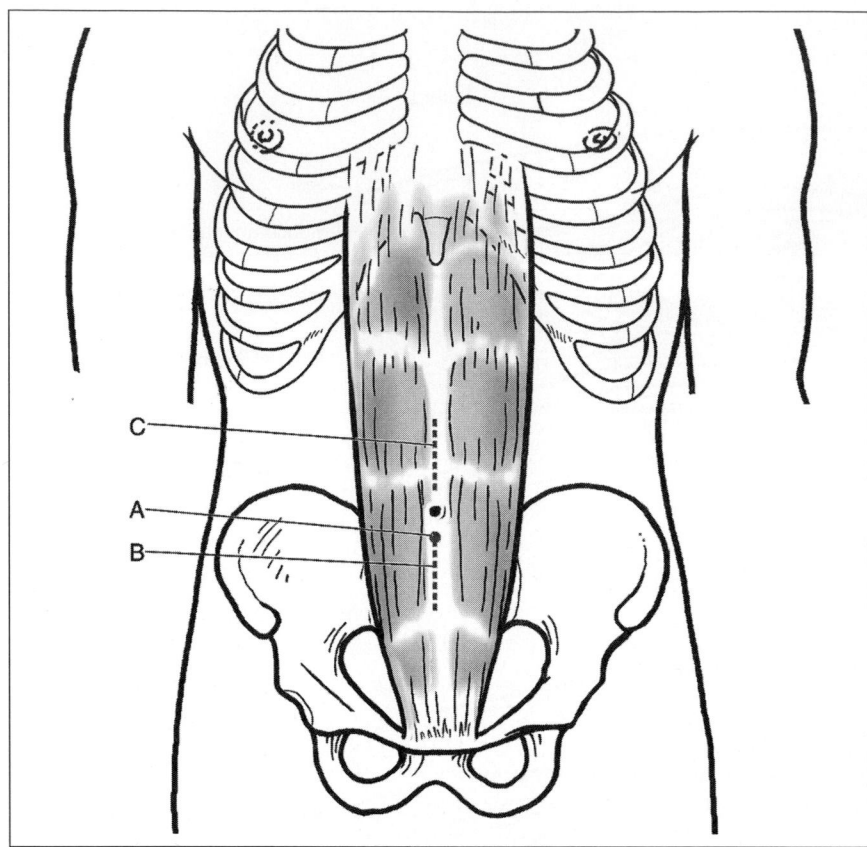

FIGURE 55-2 The preferred sites to perform a DPL. *A.* The midline and approximately 1 to 2 cm below the umbilicus is the location for a closed DPL. *B.* A midline incision beginning 1 to 2 cm below the umbilicus and extending inferiorly for 5 to 6 cm is the location for semi-open and select open DPLs. *C.* A midline incision beginning 2 cm above the umbilicus and extending superiorly for 5 to 6 cm is the location for most open DPLs.

It is especially useful in patients with an unreliable abdominal examination, or an equivocal examination, and those who will be unavailable for serial examination. The patient with an altered mental status (e.g., alcohol, drugs, head injury, etc.) or with abnormal sensation due to a spinal cord injury is considered to have an unreliable physical examination.[5,9,12] Patients may have an equivocal examination due to tenderness from surrounding fractures of the ribs, spine, or pelvis.[9,11] They may also have tenderness of the wound or area of injury that is difficult to distinguish from peritonitis. The third group of patients are those who undergo surgery for another injury such as a neurosurgical or orthopedic procedure.[12] These patients are unavailable for serial examinations while in the operating room. Their examination is altered postoperatively as well due to the analgesics that they receive.

DPL may be useful in the occasional circumstance when the patient presents in shock with other potential sources of hemorrhage, such as intrathoracic or retroperitoneal bleeding. DPL may rule out or confirm the abdomen as the source of the patient's bleeding and shock.[5] **It is important to remember that an injury confined to the retroperitoneum will not result in a positive DPL.**[13]

CONTRAINDICATIONS

The only absolute contraindication to performing a DPL is if the patient has an obvious indication for a laparotomy. Patients who present following abdominal trauma who are in shock, have peritonitis, pneumoperitoneum on chest radiography, evisceration, blood per orifice, or a retained stabbing implement have obvious indications for a laparotomy.

Several relative contraindications to DPL exist. These actually represent contraindications to performing the closed technique. Patients with a pelvic fracture may have a large retroperitoneal hematoma that extends anteriorly to the linea semilunares. The DPL may be performed using the open technique above the umbilicus to avoid decompression of the hematoma.[10] Pregnant patients should not have a closed DPL performed because of the risk of injury to the uterus. It is safe, however, to perform an open DPL above the uterine fundus.[5] Patients with evidence of previous abdominal surgery may have adhesions of the viscera to the abdominal wall that make intraabdominal injury more likely to result when a closed DPL is performed.[1,7] Open DPL may be performed in a location away from the scar.[11] One must recognize, however, that compartmentalization of the abdomen may have occurred due to intraperitoneal adhesions, thus making it more likely to have a falsely negative DPL result.

The DPL should be performed using the open technique in patients who are unable to have a Foley catheter placed due to urethral injury or stricture. This minimizes the chance of inadvertent injury to the bladder. Morbid obesity is a relative contraindication to closed DPL. This represents a difficulty in technically performing the DPL when the abdominal wall is thicker than the 2.5 inch long locator needle. It is useful to perform the DPL in these patients using a semi-open technique.[14]

EQUIPMENT

Closed Technique

Povidone iodine
Face mask
Sterile gloves
Sterile gown
4×4 gauze squares
Local anesthetic solution
Purple top blood collection tube
5 mL syringes
18 gauge needles
25 gauge needles
Nasogastric tube
Foley catheter
1 L of IV fluid to infuse, 0.9% NaCl or lactated Ringer solution
Commercial Peritoneal Lavage Kit (e.g., Arrow AK-0900)

Semi-Open or Open Technique

All items listed above
Razor
#10 scalpel blade on a handle
Abdominal skin retractors, Weitlaner or skin rakes
2 tissue forceps
2 Allis clamps
4 hemostats
Needle driver
Suture for vessel ligation (4–0 Vicryl, 4–0 Dexon, or 4–0 chromic)
Suture for fascial closure (0 Vicryl, 0 Dexon, 0 Maxon, or 0 Prolene)
4–0 nylon suture or skin stapler for skin closure
Suture scissors

A commercially available, disposable, and single-patient use peritoneal lavage kit is available from numerous manufacturers. The kit includes all the material required to perform a closed DPL except lavage fluid. An example is the Arrow kit (Arrow International, Reading, PA). It contains 10% povidone iodine swabs, gauze squares, fenestrated drape, IV fluid administration tubing, 1% lidocaine, 5 mL syringes, 22 and 25 gauge needles, an 18 gauge × 2.5 inch introducer needle, an 0.89 mm × 45 cm J-tipped guidewire, an 8 French lavage catheter, and a #11 scalpel blade on a handle.

PATIENT PREPARATION

Explain the procedure, its risks, and benefits to the patient and/or their representative. This should include the possible complications. Informed consent should be obtained from the patient. Informed consent should be obtained from the family, if possible, if the patient is unable to consent due to age or mental status. **The consent process should not unduly delay the performance of the DPL in an unstable patient.**

The patient is probably in the supine position already. If not, place the patient supine. A distended stomach or bladder may be inadvertently perforated during the procedure. These organs require decompression prior to performing a DPL (Figure 55-3). Decompress the stomach using a nasogastric or orogastric tube.[12,15] Refer to Chapter 47 regarding the details of nasogastric tube insertion. Decompress the bladder using a Foley catheter once a urethral injury has been ruled out.[5,6,12,15] Refer to Chapters 121 and 124 regarding the details of urethral catheterization and evaluation of a urethral injury.

Prepare the abdomen.[12] Shave the area surrounding the incision site if an open or semi-open DPL is to be performed. Clean the skin of any dirt, debris, and blood. Apply povidone iodine and allow it to dry. Apply sterile drapes to delineate a sterile field. Each health care provider who is involved in the procedure should don a face mask, a sterile gown, and sterile gloves.[12]

TECHNIQUES

PERCUTANEOUS (CLOSED) TECHNIQUE

The closed technique is the preferred method to perform a DPL unless contraindications exist (Figure 55-4). The closed DPL can be performed in significantly shorter time than the open DPL.[16,17] There is no difference in the amount of fluid retrieved from the abdomen, the diagnostic accuracy, or the complication rate between the closed and open techniques.[16]

The closed DPL is performed in the midline and approximately 1 to 2 cm below the umbilicus (Figure 55-2A).[15] Prepare the patient as described previously. Infiltrate the skin, subcutaneous tissue, and fascia with local anesthetic solution to provide anesthesia. Place the 2.5 inch introducer needle onto a 5 mL syringe. Insert the needle in the midline and 1 to 2 cm below the umbilicus. Advance the needle at a 45 degree angle and directed

Continue the procedure. Pass the proximal end of the IV tubing to a nonsterile assistant to insert into a bag of IV fluid (0.9% NaCl or Ringer lactate) and prime the tubing. Warmed IV fluid is preferable to room temperature fluid, if available. Attach the distal end of the IV tubing to the lavage catheter (Figure 55-5A). Open the clamp on the IV tubing and allow the lavage fluid to flow freely into the peritoneal cavity (Figure 55-5A). The lavage catheter may not be within the peritoneal cavity if the lavage fluid does not flow quickly but seems to drip in slowly. Reassess the catheter position. If necessary, remove and reinsert the lavage catheter. Infuse 1 L in the adult patient and 10 to 20 mL/kg (maximum 1 L) in the pediatric patient.[6,11] Stabilize the catheter with one hand during the infusion of the lavage fluid.

After the lavage fluid has been instilled, place the IV bag on the floor to allow the fluid to flow out from the peritoneal cavity (Figure 55-5B). There should be a steady rate of flow. Diminution of flow usually results from the omentum blocking the side holes of the lavage catheter. Firm palpation of the patient's abdomen may increase the flow rate if it seems to drop off. The lavage catheter may need to be withdrawn slightly and reinserted. These maneuvers may help to dislodge the omentum. If manipulation of the catheter does not improve flow, a second liter of fluid may be infused (additional 10 mL/kg in children). If this becomes necessary, the threshold for a positive DPL must be halved (i.e., down from 100,000 to 50,000 RBC/mm^3 in blunt trauma); as twice the fluid is infused and results in a halving of the red blood cell count.

At least 200 to 250 mL of lavage fluid should be returned from the peritoneal cavity to result in a reliable cell count.[17-19] This fluid is referred to as the effluent. Place a new lavage catheter if less than 200 to 250 mL of effluent is obtained after the manipulations described above.[6] Remove the existing lavage catheter while maintaining the sterility of the distal end of the IV tubing. Place a second lavage catheter 1 cm inferior to the site of the first lavage catheter. Reconnect the IV tubing and place the IV bag to gravity drainage to obtain the effluent.

Remove the lavage catheter after obtaining as much effluent as possible from the peritoneal cavity. Place a small gauze dressing over the skin puncture site and remove the drapes. Transfer a small aliquot of the lavage effluent to a purple top blood collection tube. Transport the tube to the laboratory for a cell count. The remainder of the lavage effluent may be discarded.

OPEN TECHNIQUE

Prepare the patient as described previously. Infiltrate the skin, subcutaneous tissue, and fascia with local anesthetic solution in the area where the incision is to be made. The incision should begin 2 cm below the umbilicus and extend 5 to 6 cm inferiorly in patients who have an upper abdominal scar (Figure 55-2B). The incision should begin 2 cm above the umbilicus and extend 5 to 6 cm superiorly in patients with a pelvic fracture or lower abdominal scar (Figure 55-2C). The incision should be made in the midline above the uterine fundus in patients who are pregnant.

Incise the skin and subcutaneous tissue longitudinally for a distance of 5 to 6 cm in the midline (Figure 55-6A). The incision may need to be longer in an obese patient. Clamp and ligate any small vessels that are bleeding with absorbable suture prior to incising the fascia. This will minimize the incidence of false positive lavage results. Retract the skin and subcutaneous tissues with a Weitlaner retractor or skin rakes to aid in viewing the fascia (Figure 55-6B). The fascial midline may be identified by the interdigitation of its fibers (Figure 55-6B). Incise the fascia longitudinally along the length of the previous skin incision (Figure 55-6C). Identify the peritoneum. Any preperitoneal fat that is present can be gently moved aside by an assistant using either a forceps or gauze. Grasp and elevate the peritoneum using two Allis clamps (Figure 55-6D). **Use extreme care to ensure that no bowel is included in the clamps.**

Make a small (< 5 mm) incision in the peritoneum. Insert the lavage catheter through the incision and directed caudally into the pelvis (Figure 55-6E).[5] The remainder of the procedure is as described above in the percutaneous (closed) technique. It may be necessary to gently retract the peritoneum upward with the Allis clamps to prevent leakage of the lavage fluid around the catheter.

Remove the lavage catheter and Allis clamps after obtaining as much effluent as possible from the peritoneal cavity. It is not necessary to suture the peritoneum. Close the fascia with # 0 Maxon, Prolene, Vicryl, or Dexon suture in a running fashion. Inspect the edges of the incision for any bleeding blood vessels. Obtain hemostasis of the subcutaneous tissue by ligating small vessels with absorbable suture. Close the skin with interrupted 4-0 nylon sutures or skin staples. Place a gauze dressing over the incision site. Remove the drapes.

SEMI-OPEN TECHNIQUE

This technique is used primarily for patients in whom there is no contraindication to performance of a closed lavage, however their abdominal wall is thicker (> 2.5 inches) than the length of the introducer needle. The procedure often begins as a closed technique and is converted to a semi-open technique once it is realized that the introducer needle is not long enough to enter the peritoneal cavity. It is a modification of both the closed and open techniques.[14]

Prepare the patient and begin the procedure as if performing the open technique. Make the midline incision

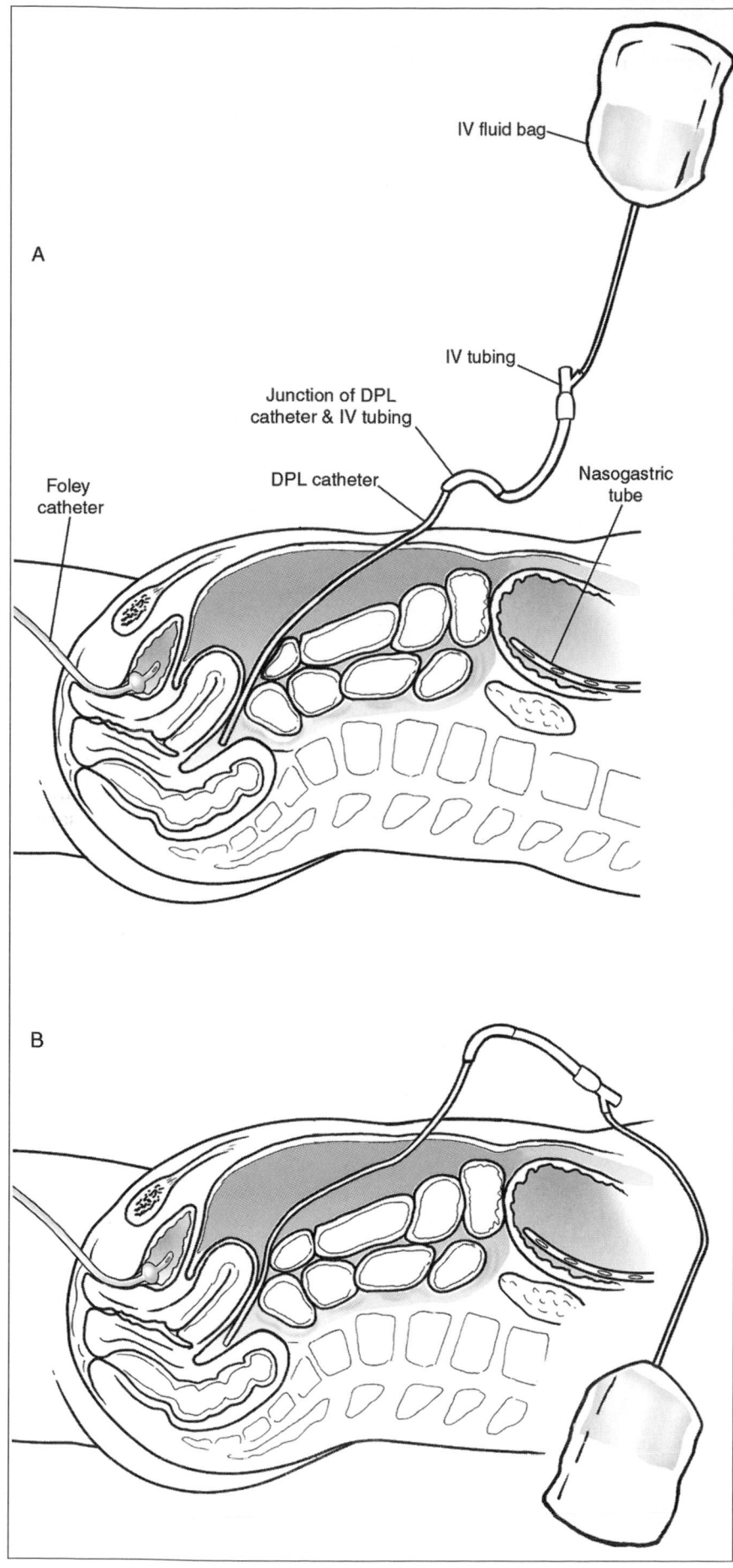

FIGURE 55-5 The instillation and removal of lavage fluid. *A.* The bag of IV fluid is attached to the lavage catheter using IV tubing. The bag of fluid is then suspended in the air and allowed to infuse into the peritoneal cavity. *B.* The IV bag is placed on the floor to allow the lavage fluid to exit the peritoneal cavity and flow back into the bag.

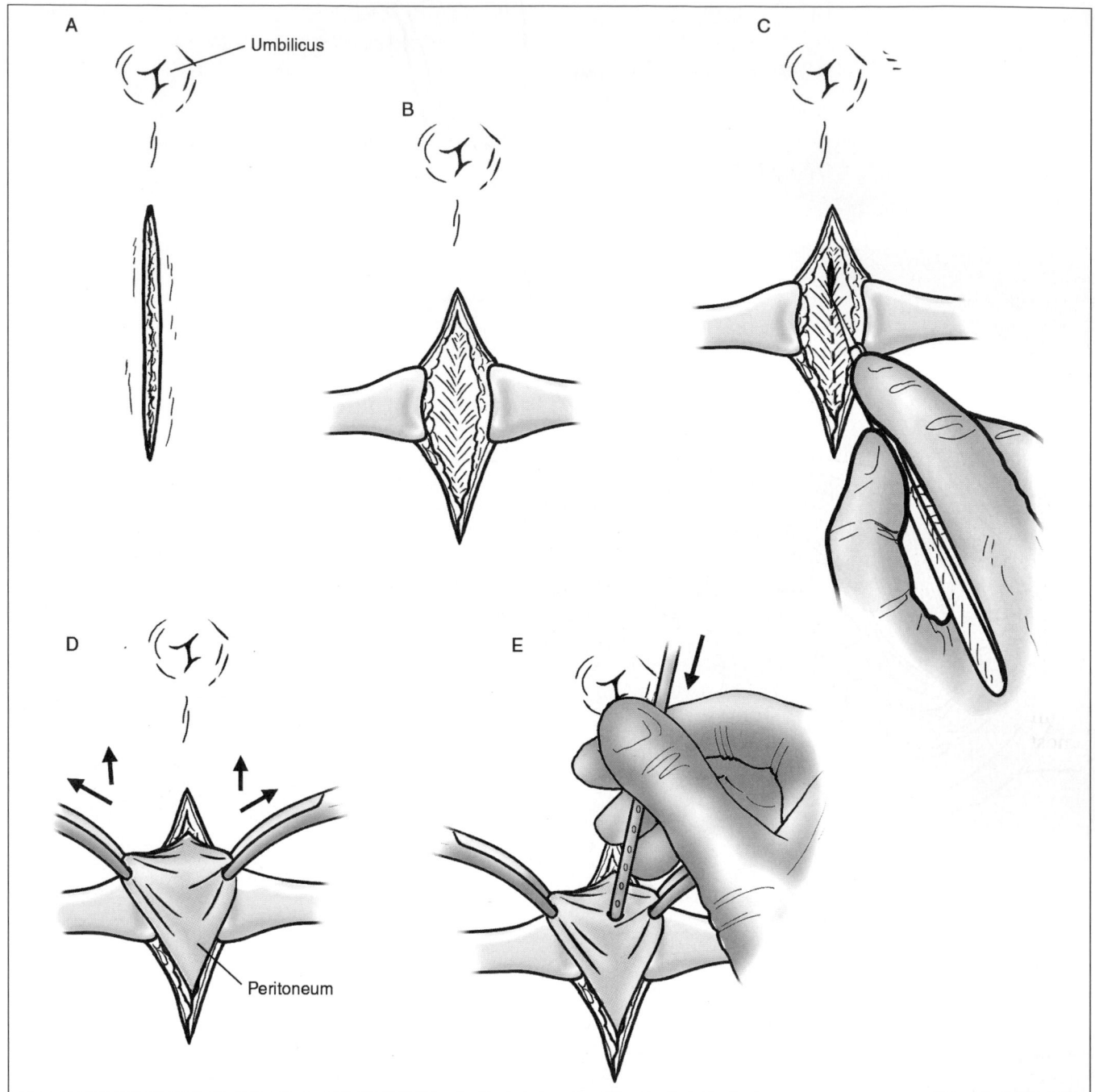

FIGURE 55-6 The open DPL. *A.* An incision is made in the skin and subcutaneous tissues. *B.* The skin and subcutaneous tissues are retracted. Note the interdigitation of the fibers of the fascia in the midline. *C.* An incision is made in the fascia. *D.* The peritoneum is grasped and elevated with Allis clamps. *E.* The lavage catheter is inserted through a small incision (< 5 mm) in the peritoneum.

and retract the tissues (Figures 55-6*A* and *B*). Identify the interdigitations of the fascia in the midline. Place the introducer needle on a 5 mL syringe. Insert the introducer needle through the midline and at a 45 degree angle directed toward the pelvis (Figure 55-4*A*). Apply negative pressure to the syringe while advancing the needle. A pop will be felt as the introducer needle penetrates the

peritoneum. The remainder of the procedure is as described above under the percutaneous or closed technique.

Remove the lavage catheter after obtaining as much lavage fluid as possible from the peritoneal cavity. Inspect the edges of the incision for any bleeding blood vessels. Obtain hemostasis of the subcutaneous tissue by ligating small vessels with absorbable suture. Close the skin using interrupted 4–0 nylon sutures or skin staples. Place a gauze dressing over the skin incision site. Remove the drapes.

ANALYSIS OF PERITONEAL LAVAGE FLUID

There are several laboratory evaluations that can be performed on the lavage effluent to determine whether the patient requires a laparotomy. Gross evidence of injury exists when there is a positive peritoneal tap (gross blood obtained through the introducer needle or gross blood noted upon opening the peritoneum during the open DPL), bile stained peritoneal fluid is noted, or enteric contents are seen in the effluent.[7,20] The most commonly used laboratory determination is that of the erythrocyte or red blood cell (RBC) count. Other determinations include the leukocyte count and the presence of amylase in the lavage effluent.

Peritoneal lavage was first described as utilizing visual inspection of fluid for the presence of blood.[1,3,7] This has been subsequently shown to be very inaccurate, even when performed by experienced physicians.[21] A much better method of quantification of the presence of blood utilizes the counting of erythrocytes, done either manually or with an automated cell counter.

In blunt abdominal trauma, 100,000 RBCs/mm^3 is the most commonly used threshold for a laparotomy.[5,9,20] This corresponds roughly to the presence of 20 mL of blood in the peritoneal cavity. Using the count of 100,000 RBCs/mm^3 to determine the presence of a hemoperitoneum provides a sensitivity of 97 percent, a specificity of 99.6 percent, and an accuracy of 99 percent.[9] The false positives that occur are usually the result of bleeding from the lavage site. False negative DPLs usually result in red blood cell counts in the mid-10,000s, what some authors refer to as indeterminate.[5] The injuries that are missed by a count of 100,000 RBCs/mm^3 are injuries to hollow viscera and the diaphragm; in other words, organs that may not bleed enough to result in a positive lavage.

Penetrating trauma, on the other hand, has no universally agreed upon threshold for a laparotomy. Documentation of penetration of the peritoneal cavity is felt to be an indication for laparotomy in all gunshot wounds and most stab wounds to the abdomen. Penetration of the peritoneum by a gunshot wound results in a significant intraperitoneal injury in 98 percent of cases.[22] Therefore, DPL to prove abdominal penetration is useful in cases of potentially tangential gunshot wounds.[13,23] Likewise, penetration into the peritoneal cavity from a thoracoabdominal wound results, by definition, in a diaphragmatic injury that should be repaired.[13,24] Penetration through the retroperitoneum,

from the back or flank, will cause a significant injury in 73 percent of cases.[15,25] Therefore, DPL is useful in these wounds as well. Penetration of the peritoneal cavity may not bleed enough to result in a 100,000 RBCs/mm^3 count. Most authors believe that a lower red blood cell count should be used. Unfortunately, there is little consensus as to what that count should be.

The red blood cell count varies from 1,000 to 50,000 RBCs/mm^3 as a threshold for laparotomy in penetrating trauma.[9,13,17,25–27] The higher the count that is used, the more likely there will be a missed injury with an increased false negative rate.[9,12,15] The lower the count that is used, the more likely that a negative laparotomy will result with an increased false positive rate.[9,12,15] At our institution, we feel that a threshold of 10,000 RBCs/mm^3 provides the most acceptable balance between false negative and false positive results.[15,23,24] This threshold results in a sensitivity of 88 to 99 percent, a specificity of 97 to 98 percent, and an accuracy of 95 to 98 percent.[12,15,24]

A special case of penetrating abdominal trauma exists when there is a stab wound to the anterior abdomen. We know that only two-thirds of these wounds will penetrate the peritoneum and, of those that penetrate, less than 50 percent will cause an injury that requires repair.[13] Therefore, using a lower threshold for DPL to determine penetration will result in a greater than 50 percent negative laparotomy rate. For this reason, wounds to the anterior abdomen are lavaged with the standard red blood cell count of 100,000 RBCs/mm^3 to determine injury and not penetration as the threshold for an operation.[28]

Many laboratories will routinely report the white blood cell (WBC) count on the lavage effluent. The presence of over 500 WBCs/mm^3 is often quoted as a standard indication for laparotomy.[20] Unfortunately, the presence of an elevated lavage white blood cell count by itself has poor predictive value in the trauma patient.[18] Most commonly, there is an associated elevation in the red blood cell count that will trigger a laparotomy. A recently described "cell count ratio" may help to diagnose the presence of a hollow viscus injury by comparing the WBC/RBC ratio in the lavage effluent to the WBC/RBC ratio in the blood.[29] If the lavage ratio is greater than that of blood, there is a high likelihood of hollow viscus injury. This ratio has only recently been described and is not universally accepted.

While the quantification of red blood cells, and occasionally white blood cells, in the DPL effluent is the most common test, other laboratory tests may be utilized in indeterminate cases. The most commonly used is the determination of amylase.[2,5,7] Amylase may be elevated in the presence of an injury to the gastrointestinal tract. Unfortunately, the amylase level is neither sensitive nor specific.[8] We do not routinely analyze the lavage effluent for amylase at our institution.

AFTERCARE

The patient should be observed in hospital for up to 24 hours after performance of a negative DPL. The Foley catheter and nasogastric tube may be removed if they are no longer needed for other indications. Reexamine the patient periodically during this observation period for the development of peritonitis that may result from a false negative lavage or a complication of the lavage procedure. The performance of the lavage should not alter the patient's examination, although there may be localized wound tenderness if the lavage was performed using the open or semi-open technique.[1] The patient should receive analgesics as needed after an open or semi-open DPL. Keep the patient NPO during the initial portion of their observation. They can be fed near the end of the 24 hours to insure that they tolerate oral intake prior to discharge.

Discharge instructions given to the patients should instruct them to return for the development of a fever, increasing abdominal pain, nausea, vomiting, worsening wound pain, or wound drainage. After undergoing an open or semi-open DPL, the patient should be seen in 7 to 10 days for removal of the skin sutures or staples.

COMPLICATIONS

The complication rate for diagnostic peritoneal lavage is relatively low. The complication rate varies between 0.6 to 2.3 percent of all DPLs.[11,30] There is no difference in complication rates between the three techniques.[17] The complications may be classified as wound-related or puncture-related.

Wound-related complications occur primarily with open or semi-open lavage techniques. Inadequate hemostasis during performance of the DPL may result in bleeding and a hematoma formation at the wound site.[5,11,30] As with any surgical procedure, there is a risk of wound infection at the lavage site.[5] This infection is usually due to skin flora and may be treated simply by opening the wound and performing wet-to-dry dressing changes.

Puncture-related complications may occur after any DPL technique. Virtually any organ within the abdominal cavity may be punctured by the introducer needle, the guidewire, or the catheter. Puncture of the bladder and stomach may be avoided by placing a Foley catheter and nasogastric tube prior to performing the DPL.[12,15] A punctured bladder is usually noted by obtaining urine during syringe aspiration or by lavage fluid exiting through the Foley catheter. Removing the lavage catheter and continuing Foley catheter drainage for 24 to 48 hours will treat this complication.[7] Puncture of the small bowel, colon, and their mesenteries may also oc-

cur.[5,11,12,23,30] Likewise, puncture of blood vessels ranging from mesenteric vessels to iliac vessels has been described.[1] These latter complications will usually result in a positive DPL based on bleeding or return of enteric contents and are repaired at laparotomy.

Occasionally, the lavage fluid may be instilled into the abdominal wall or the retroperitoneum.[1,12] This may result in a false positive lavage, a false negative lavage, or more commonly an inadequate fluid return. This complication requires no specific treatment other than recognition. The body will reabsorb the fluid over time.

SUMMARY

The diagnostic peritoneal lavage is a well-described procedure for determining the need for a laparotomy after trauma. It has undergone several modifications since its initial description over 35 years ago. The procedure may be performed using a closed, semi-open, or open technique depending upon the patient's history and associated injuries. All three techniques are safe, accurate, and easily performed. Several criteria may indicate a positive result, and knowledge of these criteria is important in the evaluation of the DPL effluent.

Because this is an invasive procedure, it is important that it be performed after informed consent (if feasible) and using aseptic technique. There is a small risk of complications as well as missed injuries necessitating the close observation of the patient with a negative DPL.

The DPL remains one of the most useful tests in the patient with abdominal trauma. Despite advances in imaging technology, the DPL remains the test of choice in the patient with penetrating abdominal trauma and in select patients with blunt abdominal trauma.

REFERENCES

1. Olsen WR, Hildreth DH: Abdominal paracentesis and peritoneal lavage in blunt abdominal trauma. *J Trauma* 1971; 11(10):824–829.
2. Danto LA, Thomas CW, Gorenbein S, et al: Penetrating torso injuries: the role of paracentesis and lavage. *Am Surg* 1977; 43:164–170.
3. Root HD, Hauser CW, McKinley CR, et al: Diagnostic peritoneal lavage. *Surgery* 1965; 57(5):633–637.
4. Salomon H: Die diagnostische punktion des bauches. *Berl Klin Wochensch* 1906; 45:45–46.
5. Fischer RP, Beverlin BC, Engrav LH, et al: Diagnostic peritoneal lavage: fourteen years and 2,586 patients later. *Am J Surg* 1978; 136:701–704.
6. Lazarus HM, Nelson JA: A technique for peritoneal lavage without risk or complication. *Surg Gynecol Obstet* 1979; 149:889–892.

7. Olsen WR, Redman HC, Hildreth DH: Quantitative peritoneal lavage in blunt abdominal trauma. *Arch Surg* 1972; 104:536–543.

8. Root HD, Keizer PJ, Perry JF: Peritoneal trauma, experimental and clinical studies. *Surgery* 1967; 62(4):679–685.

9. Alyono D, Morrow CE, Perry JF: Reappraisal of diagnostic peritoneal lavage criteria for operation in penetrating and blunt trauma. *Surgery* 1982; 92(4):751–757.

10. Mendez C, Gubler KD, Maier RV: Diagnostic accuracy of peritoneal lavage in patients with pelvic fractures. *Arch Surg* 1994; 129:477–482.

11. Henneman PL, Marx JA, Moore EE, et al: Diagnostic peritoneal lavage: accuracy in predicting necessary laparotomy following blunt and penetrating trauma. *J Trauma* 1990; 30(11):1345–1355.

12. Nagy KK, Fildes JJ, Sloan EP, et al: Aspiration of free blood from the peritoneal cavity does not mandate immediate laparotomy. *Am Surg* 1995; 61(9):790–795.

13. Thompson JS, Moore EE: Peritoneal lavage in the evaluation of penetrating abdominal trauma. *Surg Gynecol Obstet* 1981; 153:861–863.

14. Ochsner MG, Herr D, Drucker W, et al: A modified Seldinger technique for peritoneal lavage in trauma patients who are obese. *Surg Gynecol Obstet* 1991; 173:158–160.

15. Merlotti GJ, Marcet E, Sheaff CM, et al: Use of peritoneal lavage to evaluate abdominal penetration. *J Trauma* 1985; 25(3):228–231.

16. Cue JI, Miller FB, Cryer HM, et al: A prospective, randomized comparison between open and closed peritoneal lavage techniques. *J Trauma* 1990; 30(7):880–883.

17. Velmahos GC, Demetriades D, Stewart M, et al: Open versus closed diagnostic peritoneal lavage: a comparison on safety, rapidity, efficacy. *J R Coll Surg Edinb* 1998; 43:235–238.

18. Soyka JM, Martin M, Sloan EP, et al: Diagnostic peritoneal lavage: is an isolated WBC count $\geq 500/\text{mm}^3$ predictive of intra-abdominal injury requiring celiotomy in blunt trauma patients? *J Trauma* 1990; 30(7):874–879.

19. Sweeney JR, Albrink MH, Bischof E, et al: Diagnostic peritoneal lavage: volume of lavage effluent needed for accurate determination of a negative lavage. *Injury* 1994; 25(10):659–661.

20. *Advanced Trauma Life Support*, 6th ed. Chicago, IL: American College of Surgeons, 1997.

21. Bellows DR, Salomone JP, Nakamura SK, et al: What's black and white and red (read) all over? The bedside interpretation of diagnostic peritoneal lavage fluid. *Am Surg* 1998; 64(2):112–118.

22. Lowe RJ, Saletta JD, Read DR, et al: Should laparotomy be mandatory of selective gunshot wounds of the abdomen? *J Trauma* 1977; 17(10):903–907.

23. Nagy KK, Krosner SM, Joseph KT, et al: A method of determining peritoneal penetration in gunshot wounds to the abdomen. *J Trauma* 1997; 43(2):242–246.

24. Merlotti GJ, Dillon BC, Lange DA, et al: Peritoneal lavage in penetrating thoracoabdominal trauma. *J Trauma* 1988; 28(1):17–23.

25. Boyle EM, Maier RV, Salazar JD, et al: Diagnosis of injuries after stab wounds to the back and flank. *J Trauma* 1997; 42(2):260–265.

26. Kelemen JJ, Martin RR, Obney JA, et al: Evaluation of diagnostic peritoneal lavage in stable patients with gunshot wounds to the abdomen. *Arch Surg* 1997; 132:909–913.

27. Moore GP, Alden AW, Rodman GH: Is closed diagnostic peritoneal lavage contraindicated in patients with previous abdominal surgery? *Acad Emerg Med* 1997; 4(4):287–290.

28. Feliciano DV, Bitondo CG, Steed G, et al: Five hundred open taps or lavages in patients with abdominal stab wounds. *Am J Surg* 1984; 148:772–777.

29. Fang JF, Chen RJ, Lin BC: Cell count ratio: new criterion of diagnostic peritoneal lavage for detection of hollow organ perforation. *J Trauma* 1998; 45(3):540–544.

30. Falcone RE, Thomas B, Hrutkay L: Safety and efficacy of diagnostic peritoneal lavage performed by supervised surgical and emergency medicine residents. *Eur J Emerg Med* 1997; 4(3):150–155.

Chapter 56
ANAL FISSURE MANAGEMENT

Julia H. Sone

INTRODUCTION

An anal fissure, or fissure-in-ano, is one of the most common anal disorders seen by physicians. It is a linear tear or crack that extends into the anoderm from the mucocutaneous junction to the dentate line (Figure 56-1). An anal fissure usually results from the passage of hard stool that traumatizes and tears the anoderm. Frequent bowel movements with diarrhea can cause similar "cracks" that eventually result in fissures. A fissure may be acute or chronic, occur at any age, and affect both genders equally. It is the most common cause of rectal bleeding in infants. Fissures occur primarily (90 percent) in the posterior midline. The remaining 10 percent are found in the anterior area. There is a slight gender difference with 1 to 7 percent of anal fissures found anteriorly in men and up to 12 percent anteriorly in women.[1] Atypical locations (e.g., lateral) suggest the presence of an underlying disease such as Crohn's disease, anal cancer, previous anal surgery, leukemia, syphilis, tuberculosis, and other infections.

ANATOMY AND PATHOPHYSIOLOGY

The anal canal begins at the level of the anorectal ring and extends distally for 4 cm to the anal verge. The internal anal sphincter and external anal sphincter muscles surround the anal canal. The internal anal sphincter muscle is a continuation of the involuntary layer of circular smooth muscle of the rectum that begins at the anorectal ring. It is contracted at rest so that the lower margin can be palpated 1 to 2 cm below the dentate line in the intersphincteric groove. The internal anal sphincter muscle supplies up to 60 percent of the resting tone of the anus.[2] The external anal sphincter muscle is an elliptical cylinder of voluntary striated muscle tethered to the coccyx and surrounding the anal canal. Columnar

epithelium lines the upper anal canal while the lower anal canal is lined by squamous epithelium. The transitional zone lies between the two different types of mucosa. The anoderm is a thin layer of stratified squamous epithelium around the anus, distal to the dentate or pectinate line, that lacks sweat glands and hair follicles. This area is richly endowed with cutaneous sensory nerve endings.

It is hypothesized that anal fissures usually occur in the posterior midline secondary to a decreased vascular supply causing ischemia or a decreased number of external sphincter muscle fibers predisposing the posterior area to a weakness.[3] Constipation or a hard bowel movement causes a tear in the anoderm that causes pain. Spasm of the internal anal sphincter muscle occurs, which results in a tighter anal canal that causes more pain with subsequent bowel movements. A vicious cycle results and may lead to a chronic anal fissure.

A tight anal sphincter is another hypothesis for the etiology of a fissure. Anal manometry in patients with fissures reveals an elevation of the resting anal canal pressures and infrequent spontaneous relaxation of the internal anal sphincter muscle.[4] These high pressures can impede blood flow. The·anodermal blood supply passes through the internal anal sphincter muscle and increased resting pressure may result in an ischemic ulcer or fissure.

An acute anal fissure has the appearance of a clean longitudinal tear in the anoderm with minimal inflammation (Figure 56-1). A chronic anal fissure is deeper, and exposed internal anal sphincter muscle fibers may be seen at its base. A skin tag or sentinel pile is usually seen externally and a hypertrophied anal papilla may be found at its upper aspect. Patients with a chronic anal fissure may also complain of anal discharge, pruritus, or "a lump". Many people complaining to their physicians of bright red blood per rectum and anal pain think they are suffering from "hemorrhoids." A good history and

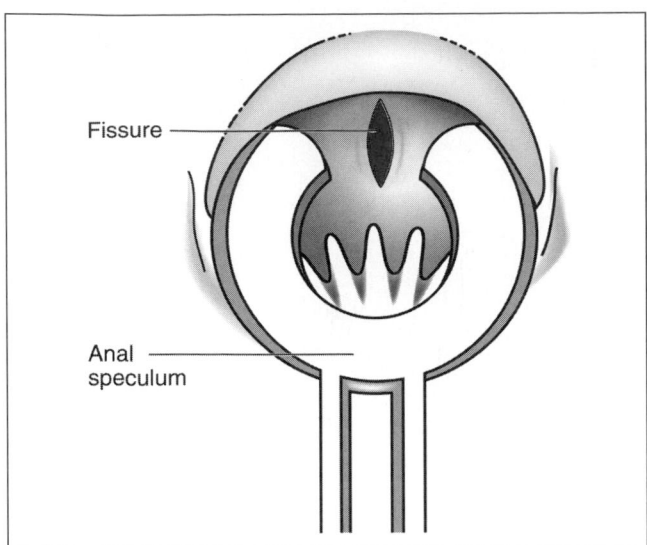

FIGURE 56-1 The anal fissure.

physical examination can confirm the diagnosis of an anal fissure. These patients will typically describe a sharp, burning, or shearing pain with defecation that lasts for a few moments up to an hour afterwards. Some people will complain of a chronic ache that is exacerbated with a bowel movement. The prolonged pain is usually attributed to internal anal sphincter muscle spasm. Bright red blood is usually seen on the stool or toilet paper. Occasionally, a few drops of blood will fall into the toilet bowel.

Patients can usually describe the initial event that triggered the fissure as either an episode of constipation with a hard bowel movement or diarrhea. Most patients with a painful anal fissure will not tolerate a digital rectal examination or anoscopy. A close inspection of the anus can be performed after reassuring the patient and gently pulling the buttocks apart. An anal fissure with a sentinel pile, an abscess, or a thrombosed external hemorrhoid may also be seen. Anesthetic jelly may be needed to examine the patient with an acute, painful anal fissure. Palpating the anal fissure with a cotton swab will reproduce the patient's pain.

INDICATIONS

Anal fissures are extremely painful and uncomfortable for the patient. They can cause poor job attendance or performance. All anal fissures should be treated when they are identified. Initial therapy is conservative (as described in the "Techniques" section), then followed by topical medications and injection therapy. Surgical treatment is warranted for patients for whom nonoperative therapy fails or who experience se-

vere anal pain. The mainstay of operative therapy is a lateral internal sphincterotomy. This technique is curative in 95 percent of patients. Unfortunately, approximately 15 percent of patients will be left with some form of minor incontinence. The technique divides the internal anal sphincter muscle between the dentate line and the anal verge. A meta-analysis of 2727 patients undergoing operative techniques for anal fissures revealed no significant difference between open versus closed lateral internal sphincterotomy for persistence of fissure or incontinence.[5] However, significant differences were found when anal stretch was compared to all forms of sphincterotomy.

CONTRAINDICATIONS

A patient with perianal Crohn's disease or ulcerative colitis is a relative contraindication to performing a lateral internal sphincterotomy. Medical management is advocated to initially treat these fissures associated with inflammatory bowel disease followed by the judicious use of an internal sphincterotomy.[6] A patient who has had multiple fistulotomies in the past or a sphincteroplasty should have their anal sphincter evaluated by anal ultrasound or manometry. The patient may have marginal sphincter function and an internal sphincterotomy can render them completely incontinent. Thus, a sphincterotomy should be performed only by a Colorectal Surgeon in these difficult patients.

EQUIPMENT

Anal Anesthesia

Povidone iodine
10 mL syringe
27 gauge needle, 2 inches long
Local anesthetic solution with epinephrine
4×4 gauze squares
Sodium bicarbonate solution

Lateral Internal Sphincterotomy

Anal speculum
#15 scalpel blade on a handle
Metzenbaum scissors
Forceps
4–0 chromic gut sutures

Dressing

4×4 gauze squares
Gelfoam
2 inch adhesive tape

PATIENT PREPARATION

Explain to the patient and/or their representative the risks, benefits, complications, and the options for treatment. The following discussion applies to the injection or surgical treatment of an anal fissure. Explain the postoperative care if a surgical technique is to be performed. Obtain an informed consent for the procedure. Undress the patient from the waist down. Place the patient prone or in the prone jackknife position (Figure 56-2). Tape the buttocks apart and to the procedure table to gain better exposure of the anus (Figure 56-3). Clean any dirt and debris from around the anus. Apply povidone iodine and allow it to dry. Place drapes to delineate a sterile field.

Perform an anal block. Mix 10 mL of local anesthetic solution with epinephrine in a syringe with 1 mL of sodium bicarbonate. This will decrease the burning sensation upon injection of the anesthetic solution. Inject the anesthetic solution into the subcutaneous tissue circumferentially around the anus, under the fissure, and laterally to anesthetize the pudendal nerves. The use of conscious sedation is recommended but not required.

Gently insert a well-lubricated anoscope into the anal canal. Test for adequate anesthesia. Inspect the lateral areas for an avascular area, usually on the right side between the right posterior and right anterior hemorrhoid complexes. Palpate the intersphincteric groove in the avascular area. It is a palpable depression between the caudal ends of the internal and external anal sphincter muscles.

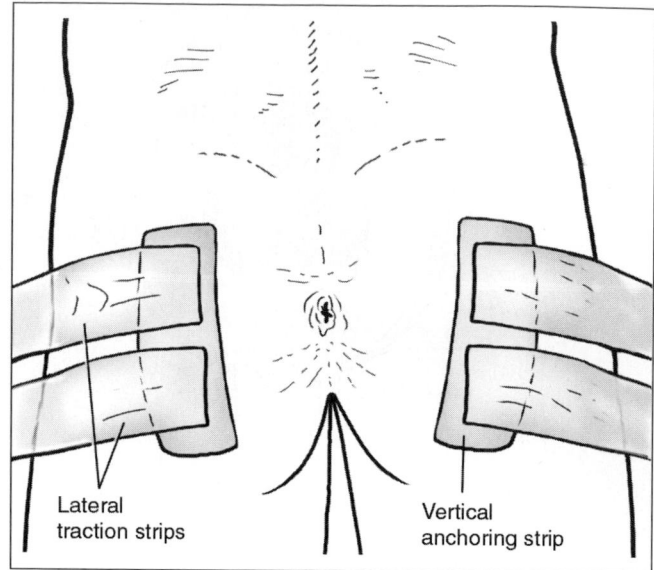

FIGURE 56-3 Taping the buttocks open in the prone patient allows for unobstructed access. The lateral traction strips are taped to the examination table or gurney.

TECHNIQUES

Management of an anal fissure begins conservatively. If unsuccessful, the next steps include topical preparations and injection therapy. A surgical sphincterotomy is the procedure of choice in refractory cases and has a 95 percent success rate.

FOUR-FINGER ANAL STRETCH

In the past, a four-finger anal stretch technique was performed. This involved putting the index and long fingers of both hands into the patient's anal canal and pulling the anal canal forcibly open. This would often cause an uncontrolled tear in the internal anal sphincter muscle. Although patients had relief of their symptoms, 40 percent developed a recurrence of the fissure and a significant proportion had some level of incontinence. **This technique is no longer recommended and should never be performed.**

CONSERVATIVE MANAGEMENT

Most remedies for an anal fissure aim to alleviate internal sphincter hypertonia and anal pain. A trial of conservative treatment is employed for acute fissures and chronic fissures with mild to moderate symptoms. This consists of bulk fiber supplements, a high-fiber diet, increased oral intake of water, sitz baths, and topical anesthetics. The large, soft, bulky stools that result gently dilate the sphincter. The topical anesthetics and sitz baths in warm water alleviate the anal pain and internal anal sphincter muscle spasm. Suppositories are not recom-

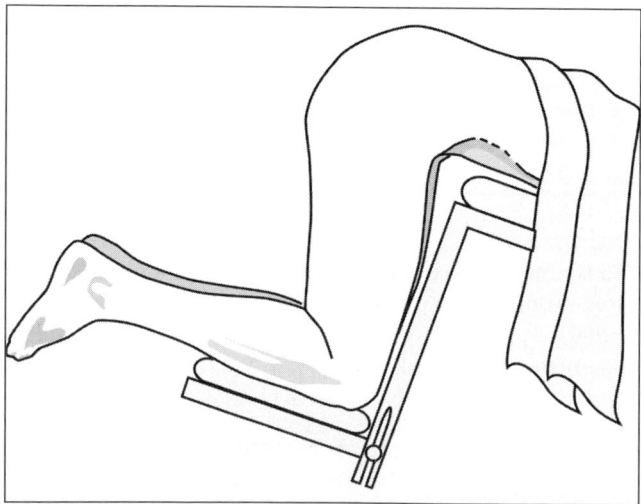

FIGURE 56-2 The prone jackknife position. Note that the lower abdomen is not touching the edge of the table.

mended because they ascend to the rectal ampulla and don't effectively treat the problem within the anal canal. If an initial trial of conservative therapy for 4 weeks fails, the patient can either undergo pharmacological therapy, injection therapy, or operative treatment.

TOPICAL TREATMENT

Nitric oxide has been identified as a chemical messenger mediating relaxation of the internal anal sphincter muscle. Patients treated with 0.2% glyceryl trinitrate ointment to their lower anal canal (near the fissure) twice daily exhibited relief of their anal pain, reduced maximal anal resting pressure, and increased anodermal blood flow (measured by laser Doppler flowmetry).[7] After 8 weeks, 68 percent of patients treated with glyceryl trinitrate had healed their fissures. However, up to 75 percent of patients will have an adverse reaction, mainly a headache unresponsive to mild pain relievers, or develop tolerance to the nitrate.[8] Up to 33 percent of patients will have a recurrence of an anal fissure after the initial anal fissure has healed with nitroglycerin treatment.[9] Topical nifedipine gel in a concentration of 0.2% used every 12 hours for 3 weeks has been successfully used to decrease anal sphincter pressures and help heal fissures.[10] No systemic side effects or significant anorectal bleeding was observed in 141 patients treated with topical nifedipine.[10]

BOTULINUM TOXIN

Botulin toxin is another pharmacological approach to the treatment of a chronic anal fissure. Injection of 20 units of botulinum toxin A (Botox, Allergan, Irvine, CA)

or 0.4 mL (50 U/mL) into the internal anal sphincter muscle on either side of the fissure using a 27 gauge needle can alleviate anal pain, decrease anal sphincter pressure, and promote healing.[11] Unfortunately, this can result in some form of temporary incontinence.

CLOSED LATERAL INTERNAL SPHINCTEROTOMY

The closed lateral internal sphincterotomy technique is preferred by some physicians (Figure 56-4). Its advantage is that a smaller wound is created. Unfortunately, this is a blind procedure and can result in injury to the patient and the physician.

Prepare the patient as described previously. Place a well-lubricated anal speculum into the anal canal. Open the speculum to provide a slight stretch to the anal sphincter muscles. Expose and view the left or right posterolateral quadrant of the anal canal. Place a gloved finger into the anal canal and palpate the internal aspect of the internal anal sphincter muscle. Perform the remainder of this procedure while carefully palpating the course of the scalpel blade with the gloved finger in the anus.

Insert a #11 scalpel blade horizontally through the skin and into the intersphincteric groove (Figure 56-4A). Advance the scalpel blade into the plane between the internal and external anal sphincter muscles and up to the level of the dentate line (Figure 56-4A). Direct the scalpel blade medially by turning it 90 degrees (Figure 56-4B). Slowly divide the full thickness of the internal anal sphincter muscle while withdrawing the scalpel blade. **Do not cut the anoderm.** Withdraw the scalpel from the anal canal. Remove the anal speculum. Close the inci-

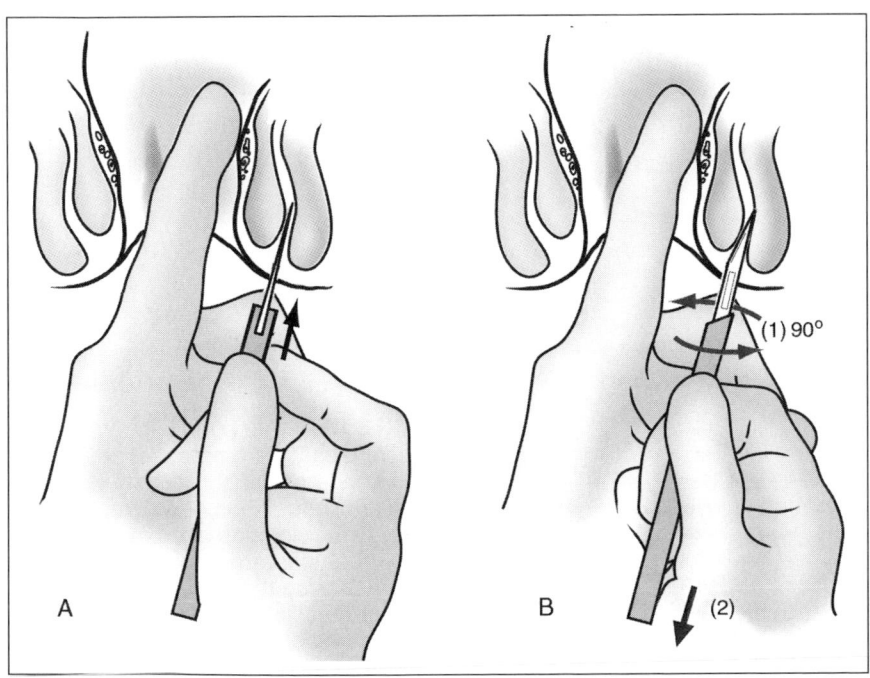

FIGURE 56-4 The closed lateral internal sphincterotomy. *A.* The #11 scalpel blade is inserted horizontally between the internal and external anal sphincter muscles. *B.* The scalpel blade is turned 90 degrees (*1*) then withdrawn (*2*) to transect the internal anal sphincter muscle.

sion site with 1 or 2 chromic gut interrupted sutures. Pack the anal canal with 4×4 gauze squares for 10 to 15 minutes to aid hemostasis and prevent the formation of a hematoma.

OPEN LATERAL INTERNAL SPHINCTEROTOMY

The open technique provides a clear exposure to the anatomy of the region. This is especially important for those less experienced with the procedure. It avoids the potential for injury to the physician when compared to the closed technique.

Prepare the patient as described previously. Place a well-lubricated anal speculum into the anal canal. Open the speculum to provide a slight stretch to the anal sphincters and view the fissure (Figure 56-5A). Rotate the speculum 90 degrees to expose and view the left or right posterolateral quadrant of the anal canal (Figure 56-5B). Place a gloved finger into the anal canal and palpate the internal aspect of the internal anal sphincter muscle.

Make a 1 cm longitudinal incision through the skin and subcutaneous tissue, between the dentate line and the anal verge (Figure 56-5B). This will center the edge of the internal anal sphincter muscle in the middle of the incision. Slide a scissors submucosally along the white internal anal sphincter muscle until the tips are at the level of the fissure, but not beyond the dentate line. Spread the arms of the scissors once to open the jaws of the scissors. Repeat this process on the other (deep) side of the internal sphincter muscle. Grasp and elevate the

internal anal sphincter muscle with a forceps. Use a scissors to make a cut in the internal sphincter muscle the same length as the length of the anal fissure (Figure 56-5C).[12] **Do not completely transect the internal anal sphincter muscle. Preserve at least one-third of the proximal internal sphincter muscle intact.**[12] Pack the anal canal with 4×4 gauze squares to apply pressure to the area for 10 to 15 minutes to aid in hemostasis and to prevent the formation of a hematoma. Suture the incision closed with interrupted chromic gut (Figure 56-5D). Place a small piece of Gelfoam over the wound. Remove the anal speculum. Dress the incision site with 4×4 gauze squares.

AFTERCARE

Instruct the patient to remove the dressing in 12 to 24 hours or before a bowel movement. Warm sitz baths 4 times a day will keep the area clean and alleviate any pain. Prescribe a high-fiber diet with oral stool softener supplements to keep the stools soft and bulky. Oral analgesics such as acetaminophen or nonsteroidal anti-inflammatory medications with supplementary narcotic analgesics will often ease the postoperative pain. The patient should follow-up in 1 to 2 weeks for reevaluation. The patient should immediately return to the Emergency Department if a fever, severe pain, or bleeding from the incision site develops.

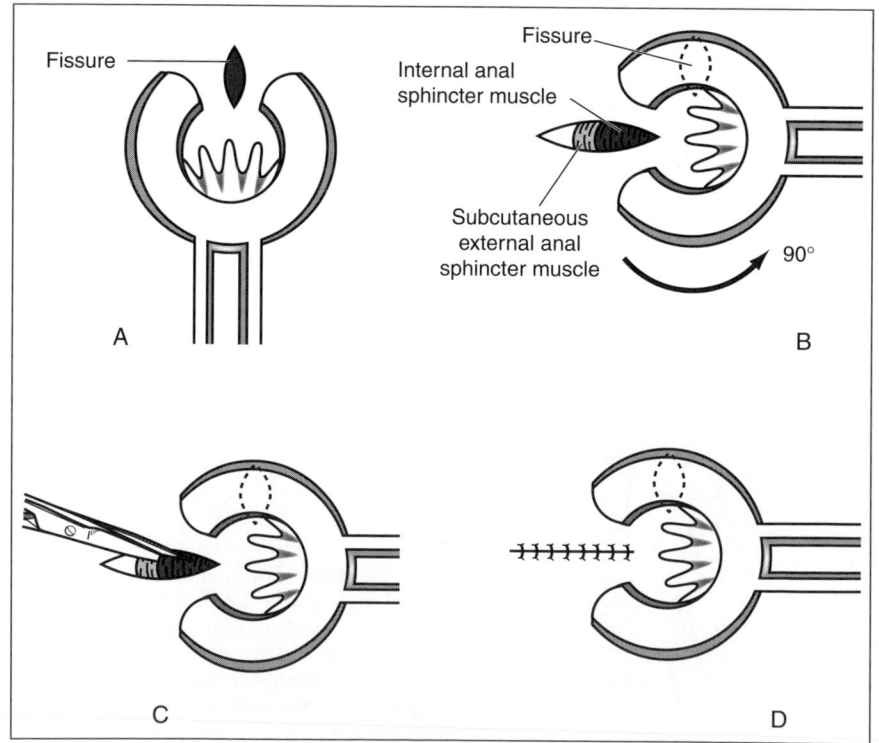

FIGURE 56-5 The open lateral internal sphincterotomy. *A.* The anoscope is inserted so that the anal fissure is visible. *B.* The anoscope has been rotated 90 degrees. An incision has been made through the anoderm and subcutaneous tissue to expose the underlying anal sphincter muscles. *C.* The internal anal sphincter muscle is partially transected with a scissors. *D.* Closure of the incision.

COMPLICATIONS

Many complications have been associated with a lateral sphincterotomy. Itching, burning, bleeding, delayed wound healing, and constipation are minor problems. The patient may complain of mucus drainage or fecal soiling during the healing phase. Bulking agents or a high-fiber diet may help decrease the drainage. Recurrent fissures occur in about 8 percent of patients, 66 percent of which heal with conservative treatment. Up to 45 percent of patients may experience some degree of incontinence, but only 3 percent of patients may have their life affected.[13] A fecal impaction, abscess, or hemorrhage can become significant. Enemas are useful for the constipated patient. An abscess should be incised and drained, preferably in the Operating Room for adequate anesthesia to completely explore the wound and debride any necrotic tissue. A subcutaneous fistula can develop if the anoderm is violated during the sphincterotomy and not recognized. This is easily taken care of by doing a fistulotomy of this superficial skin bridge. The physician may be injured while performing the closed technique. This technique should be reserved for those with experience and a patient that is sedated to decrease the chances of injury.

SUMMARY

Anal pain with bleeding due to a fissure-in-ano is initially treated conservatively with a high-fiber diet, stool softeners, and warm sitz baths. Most patients will respond to these measures. A few will fail conservative therapy and need pharmacological or operative therapy. The goal of all the different regimens is to decrease anal pain, reduce anal sphincter spasm, and heal the fissure.

REFERENCES

1. Hananel N, Gordon PH: Re-examination of clinical manifestations and response to therapy of fissure-in-ano. *Dis Colon Rectum* 1997; 40(2):229–233.

2. Penninckx R, Lestar B, Kerremans R: The internal anal sphincter: mechanisms of control and its role in maintaining anal continence. *Baillieres Clin Gastroenterol* 1992; 6(1):193–214.

3. Lund JN, Binch C, McGrath J, et al: Topographical distribution of blood supply to the anal canal. *Br J Surg* 1999; 86(4):496–498.

4. Keck JO, Staniunas RJ, Coller JA, et al: Computer-generated profiles of the anal canal in patients with anal fissure. *Dis Colon Rectum* 1995; 38(1):72–79.

5. Nelson RL: Meta-analysis of operative techniques for fissure-in-ano. *Dis Colon Rectum* 1999; 42(11):1424–1428.

6. Fleshner PR, Schoetz DJ Jr, Roberts PL, et al: Anal fissure in Crohn's disease: a plea for aggressive management. *Dis Colon Rectum* 1995; 38(11):1137–1143.

7. Lund JN, Scholefield JH: A randomised, prospective, double-blind, placebo-controlled trial of glyceryl trinitrate ointment in treatment of anal fissure. *Lancet* 1997; 349(9044):11–14.

8. Hyman NH, Cataldo PA: Nitroglycerine ointment for anal fissures: effective treatment or just a headache? *Dis Colon Rectum* 1999; 42(3):383–385.

9. Carapeti EA, Kamm MA, McDonald PJ, et al: Randomised controlled trial shows that glyceryl trinitrate heals anal fissures, higher doses are not more effective, and there is a high recurrence rate. *Gut* 1999; 44(5):727–730.

10. Antropoli C, Perrotti P, Rubino M, et al: Nifedipine for local use in conservative treatment of anal fissures: preliminary results of a multicenter study. *Dis Colon Rectum* 1999; 42(8):1011–1015.

11. Maria G, Cassetta E, Gui D, et al: A comparison of botulinum toxin and saline for the treatment of chronic anal fissure. *N Engl J Med* 1998; 338(4):217–220.

12. Littlejohn DR, Newstead GL: Tailored lateral sphincterotomy for anal fissure. *Dis Colon Rectum* 1997; 40(12):1439–1442.

13. Nyam DC, Pemberton JH: Long-term results of lateral internal sphincterotomy for chronic anal fissure with particular reference to incidence of fecal incontinence. *Dis Colon Rectum* 1999; 42(10):1306–1310.

Chapter 57
EXTERNAL HEMORRHOID MANAGEMENT

Charles Orsay

INTRODUCTION

The primary disease process affecting external hemorrhoids is thrombosis. The mainstay of treatment is excision. It is important to remember that the excision is to alleviate or palliate the pain. The natural history of an untreated thrombosed external hemorrhoid is to rupture and spontaneously evacuate the clot or to resorb the clot over time. Therefore, treatment should give the maximum amount of pain relief with the least chance of complications. To make this decision it will be important to obtain a good history of the length of the pain, how severe it is, and whether there has been improvement. It is important to perform a physical examination to rule out prolapsed grade IV internal hemorrhoids, perianal abscesses, and other perianal masses.

ANATOMY AND PATHOPHYSIOLOGY

External hemorrhoids fall into three main groups: left lateral, right anterior, and right posterior (Figure 57-1). They are covered with anoderm and visible on the outside of the anal canal. They are composed of a venous plexus mixed with connective tissue. They drain into the middle and inferior rectal veins that terminate into the internal iliac and femoral veins, respectively. External hemorrhoids do not prolapse like internal hemorrhoids. They engorge and thrombose. It will not benefit the patient to try to reduce an external hemorrhoid since their normal location is mostly outside the anal canal and reduction will not remove the clot. External hemorrhoids are never covered with mucosa. The overlying skin may appear to look shiny, swollen, gangrenous, or like an orange peel mimicking the look of mucosa.

The patient usually complains of a history of the sudden onset of pain and swelling. The exact cause of thrombosed external hemorrhoids is unknown. It is probably related more to straining with lifting, jogging, or bicycling than chronic constipation. This explains why this problem occurs more often than internal hemorrhoidal disease in a younger age group.

External hemorrhoids can be diagnosed when a patient complains of a sudden onset of pain and swelling, usually with no bleeding. The physical examination will reveal a tensely swollen area covered with anoderm. The swelling will be visible by gently spreading the buttocks and inspecting the area near the anal canal. They have a bluish coloration, especially in patients with little skin pigmentation, and almost no redness. The swelling is abrupt, like placing a marble under a sheet and tucking in the edges. This differentiates the appearance of a thrombosed external hemorrhoid from the appearance of an abscess that would have erythema and gently sloping sides from edema.

INDICATIONS

The primary indication for the excision of a thrombosed external hemorrhoid is pain. The excision should occur as soon as possible from the onset of pain and not after the fourth day.[1] The pain should become tolerable in the normal course of events after the fourth day. The clot is already being absorbed at this time and the chance of having problems with bleeding increases and medical management is indicated. Improving pain suggests that medical management is the more appropriate method of care. There is, however, a small subgroup of patients who do not seem to improve with medical management and will require excision, even late in the course of the disease. The thrombosis to be excised should involve one or at most two hemorrhoids. Very large or circumferential thrombosed external hemorrhoids require regional anesthesia and electrocautery or suture ligation to control hemorrhage. These very large

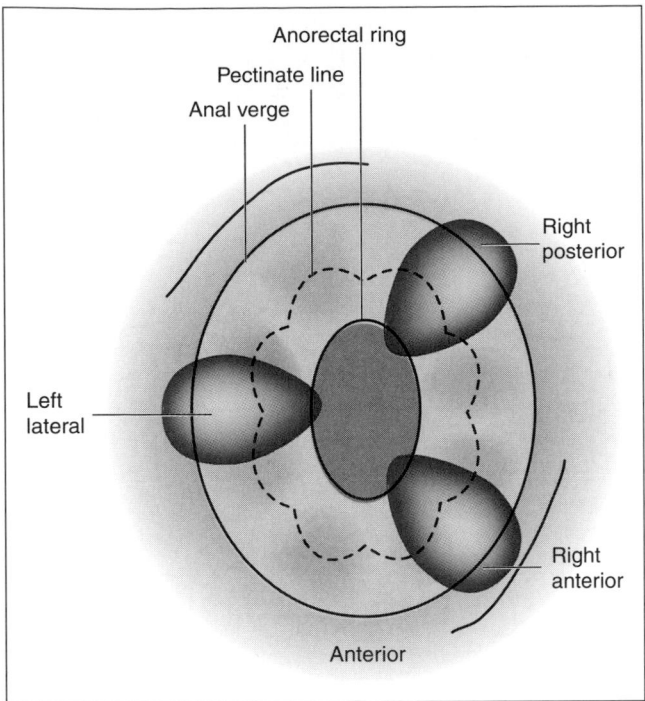

Anorectal ring

Pectinate line

Anal verge

Right posterior

Left lateral

Right anterior

Anterior

FIGURE 57-1 The position of the three main groups of external hemorrhoids.

or circumferential thrombosed external hemorrhoids are best managed in the Operating Room. The remainder of patients with acute pain should have their external hemorrhoid excised to palliate the pain.

CONTRAINDICATIONS

There are several contraindications to the Emergency Department incision and drainage of a thrombosed external hemorrhoid. Grade IV internal hemorrhoids with thrombosed external hemorrhoids or very large thrombosed external hemorrhoids should be managed by a Surgeon in the Operating Room. Patients taking anticoagulants require meticulous care and possible reversal of the coagulopathy. An allergy to local anesthetic agents will require a trip to the Operating Room to excise the hemorrhoid. Painless masses are never thrombosed external hemorrhoids and require evaluation by a Surgeon. Draining external hemorrhoids should be followed-up in 24 hours by a Surgeon. Patients who are unable to cooperate with the procedure may require conscious sedation or general anesthesia. A Surgeon should manage patients who have thrombosed external hemorrhoids and also have inflammatory bowel disease, anorectal fissures, perianal infections, portal hypertension, rectal prolapse, or anorectal tumors or who are immunocompromised. Patients with external hemorrhoids that are not thrombosed should be referred to a Gastroenterologist, General Surgeon, or Colorectal Sur-

geon for management (rubber band ligation, infrared coagulation, direct current, bipolar electrocoagulation, or sclerotherapy).

EQUIPMENT

Povidone iodine
Local anesthetic solution with epinephrine
5 mL syringe
25 gauge needle
18 gauge needle
#11 scalpel blade on a handle
4×4 gauze squares
2–0 absorbable sutures (Vicryl, Dexon, chromic gut, or plain gut)
3–0 absorbable sutures (Vicryl, Dexon, chromic gut, or plain gut)
Small dissecting scissors
Small grasping forceps
2 inch adhesive tape
Tincture of benzoin
Silver nitrate applicator sticks
Moisture resistant drapes

PATIENT PREPARATION

The risks, benefits, and potential complications of the procedures should be explained to the patient and/or their representative. It is also important to explain to the patient what to expect after the procedure. Obtain an informed consent for the procedure.

It is crucial to position the patient so that the anus is clearly visible and the Physician can work with both hands. Place the patient in the prone or prone jackknife position with their hips flexed (Figure 57-2). Tape the buttocks to the procedure table (Figure 57-3). Apply tincture of benzoin to the buttocks and allow it to dry. Place strips of 2 inch adhesive tape on the left and right cheeks of the buttocks and perpendicular to the anus. Apply lateral and slightly cranial traction with adhesive tape to get the proper exposure. Attach the distal ends of the tape to the procedure table or stretcher to maintain exposure during the procedure. This positioning works best in the Operating Room with spinal anesthesia where the patient is unlikely to move. Explain to patients that they must relax and refrain from squeezing their buttocks shut. If the patient is poorly positioned and there is difficulty with hemorrhage in the middle of the procedure, it is very difficult to stop and reposition the patient to place a suture for control. Apply drapes to protect the patient and clothing from spills. Clean the anus and surrounding area of any dirt and debris. Apply povidone iodine and allow it to dry.

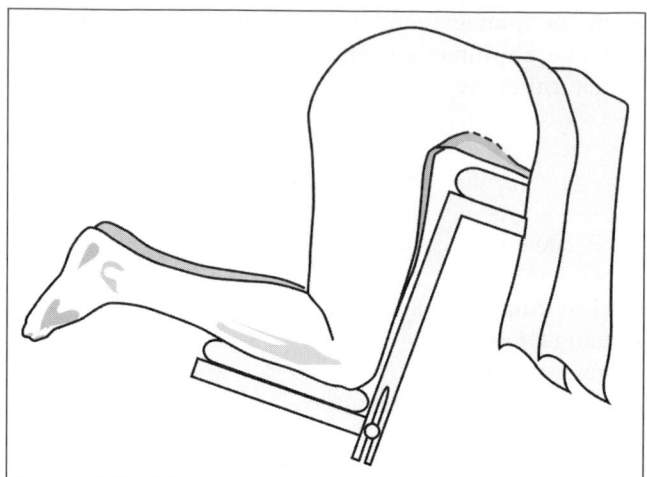

FIGURE 57-2 The prone jackknife position. Note that the lower abdomen is not touching the edge of the table.

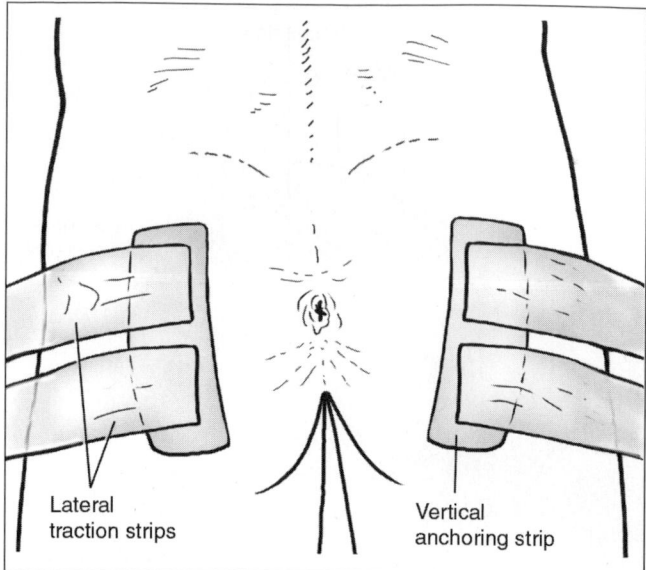

FIGURE 57-3 Taping the buttocks open in the prone patient allows for unobstructed access. The lateral traction strips are taped to the examination table or gurney.

The patient usually is in significant pain. The injection of local anesthetic solution can be excruciating. Consider the use of intravenous analgesics, sedatives, or procedural sedation. This will be greatly appreciated by the patient.

TECHNIQUE

Determine the area of the incision. **The best pain relief will be achieved if the thrombosis is excised rather than incised.** If the hemorrhoid is very large, one-third or greater of the anal circumference, it is best to excise the middle third of the hemorrhoid leaving as much anoderm as possible to prevent the wound healing with a stricture. Excision can be achieved with two radial incisions starting near the center of the anus and enclosing an ellipse of skin that will be removed with the thrombosis (Figure 57-4*A*).

Once the placement of the incision is decided, inject local anesthetic solution containing epinephrine starting laterally and injecting medially to and beyond the thrombosed hemorrhoid (Figure 57-4*B*).[1] The injection should include both lines of the planned incision and, if possible, the area medial to the thrombosis. The local anesthetic agent should also cross the midline anteriorly and posteriorly to include nerve fibers crossing over from the opposite side of the anus. Allow 5 minutes for the local anesthetic to take effect. The degree of local anesthesia can be checked by pinprick or by pinching with forceps.

Make the incisions with a #11 scalpel blade when satisfactory local anesthesia has been achieved. Dissect the ellipse of skin and the underlying clot from lateral to medial with a scissors (Figure 57-4*C*). **Do not cut the anal sphincter at the base of the wound (Figure 57-4*D*). It is important to remove the entire clot since the purpose**

of the excision is only to palliate the patient's pain. Small clots in or between the sphincter muscles may still cause considerable pain. These can be grasped with a fine forceps and removed.

Examine the wound carefully for hemostasis. Localized areas of bleeding can often be controlled with the application of silver nitrate to cauterize the wound. It is my personal belief that there is less discomfort if silver nitrate is used for hemostasis than if one is forced to use suture ligature. However, if there is continued bleeding, a 3–0 absorbable suture can be used in a figure-of-eight formation over the area of bleeding. I prefer plain catgut because the suture will dissolve very quickly. A suture that remains in place for several weeks in this area can sometimes be very uncomfortable for the patient. Dress the wound with 3 or 4 gauze squares folded in half and one piece of tape across the buttocks to hold the dressing in place.

AFTERCARE

The patient should leave the dressing in place until the next day or the next bowel movement. It is best to remove the dressing in the sitz bath and replace it with dry 4×4 gauze placed between the buttocks to collect any moisture. Frequently, tape is not necessary. The patient should be encouraged to take 3 or 4 sitz baths per day and after every bowel movement. The water should be warm, not hot, and the bath should be for 20 minutes. The sitz bath serves two functions. It keeps the wound clean and helps relax the internal anal sphincter muscle

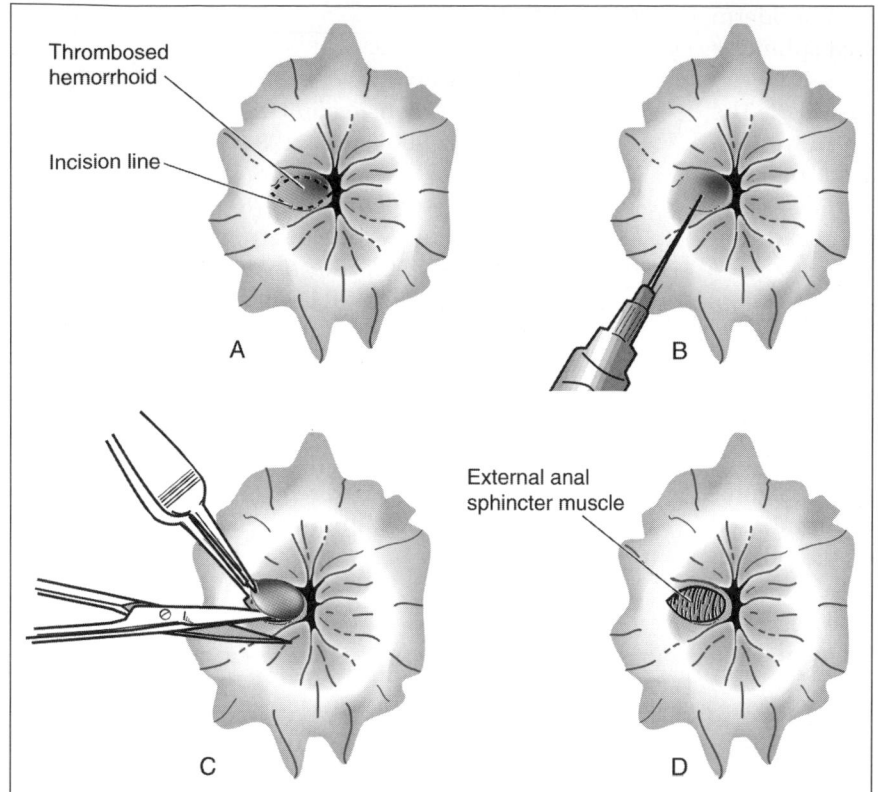

FIGURE 57-4 Excision of the thrombosed external hemorrhoid. *A.* The dotted line represents the incision lines to remove the skin and underlying thrombosis. *B.* Injection of local anesthetic solution. *C.* The skin incision has already been performed. The skin and underlying thrombosis are dissected free with a scissors. *D.* The ellipse of skin and the underlying thrombosis have been removed. The fibers of the underlying external anal sphincter muscle are visible.

spasm, which helps relieve the pain. The sitz baths and dressing changes should continue until the wound is healed.

Fiber supplements and stool softeners should be continued for at least 6 weeks. Prescribe one tablespoon of psyllium products (Metamucil) with water twice a day to soften and bulk the stool. The goal is to achieve an atraumatic stool that gently dilates the anus as it passes. If the patient is unable to tolerate psyllium, 100 mg of docusate once or twice a day can be used to soften the stool but will not give the bulk.

The patient should feel much less pain after the thrombosed hemorrhoid is excised. The remaining pain can frequently be controlled with the sitz baths. Some form of oral analgesia is required. Acetaminophen or ibuprofen is usually adequate. The use of codeine or opiates has a pronounced constipating effect that could result in painful bowel movements. Do not prescribe narcotic analgesics for more than 24 hours. The patient should return to the Emergency Department if the pain is not improved, if bleeding continues, or if they develop a fever. The wound must be watched for infection, which fortunately is very rare.

COMPLICATIONS

The rate of complications for excision of thrombosed external hemorrhoids is not well reported.[1–6] Reported complication rates for more major anal surgery show bleeding occurs in 1.5 to 4.0 percent of patients and infection occurs in 2 percent of patients.[1–3] Considering the persistent fecal contamination at the anus, this is a very low rate of infection. I would estimate the complication rate for the excision of a thrombosed external hemorrhoid would be even less.

Any post-hemorrhoidectomy bleeding that is minimal can be managed by the application of local pressure. Moderate to severe bleeding will require the insertion of a commercially available post-hemorrhoidectomy pack.[6] This is an accordion-like pack that is inserted through the anoscope and into the anal canal. Pulling the two strings of the pack accordions the pack down into the anal canal to tamponade the bleeding. A Foley catheter may be substituted if the packs are not available. These patients require intravenous analgesics, intravenous sedation, and hospitalization.

The treatment for a patient with an infection in the perianal area who has not had surgery is to open the abscess and place the patient on sitz baths. Infection is very unlikely since the wound is already open from the excision procedure and the patient is taking sitz baths. Broad-spectrum antibiotics for aerobic and anaerobic bacteria should be given to any patient with a postprocedural infection and the wound examined under general anesthesia to rule out any underlying pathology.

Long-term theoretical complications include stricture and incontinence. These are exceedingly rare and can be prevented by not removing too much anoderm and not injuring the underlying external anal sphincter muscle.

The use of a linear incision should be avoided. The stretched skin will close and create a pocket in which a hematoma or abscess can form. Removal of clots through a linear incision (rather than an elliptical incision) is often difficult, inadequate, and may lead to a higher incidence of recurrence.

SUMMARY

External hemorrhoids may thrombose and cause the patient considerable pain. The natural history of this disease is for the clot to drain or resorb without significant long-term morbidity. Excision of the thrombosed external hemorrhoid will provide considerable relief if the patient presents acutely. It is important to achieve good hemostasis and not damage the underlying external anal sphincter muscle or remove too much anoderm to avoid problems with continence or stricture formation. Fiber supplements and sitz baths should be prescribed rather than surgical excision if the patient presents later in the course of the disease.

REFERENCES

1. Gordon PH, Nivatvongs S: *Principles and Practice of Surgery for the Colon, Rectum and Anus*. St. Louis: Quality Medical Publishing, 1992:192–193.
2. Corman ML: *Colon and Rectal Surgery*, 3rd ed. Philadelphia: Lippincott, 1993:78–79.
3. Buls JG, Goldberg SMM: Modern management of hemorrhoids. *Surg Clin North Am* 1978; 58:469–478.
4. Ganchrow MI, Mazier WP, Friend WG, et al: Hemorrhoidectomy revisited—a computer analysis of 2038 cases. *Dis Colon Rectum* 1971; 14:128–133.
5. Walker WA, Rothenberger DA, Goldberg SM: Morbidity of internal sphincterotomy for anal fissure and stenosis. *Dis Colon Rectum* 1985; 28:832–835.
6. Simon RR, Brenner BE: *Emergency Procedures and Techniques*, 3rd ed. Baltimore: Williams & Wilkins, 1994:22–25.

Chapter 58
PROLAPSED RECTUM REDUCTION

Jamil D. Bayram
Eric F. Reichman

INTRODUCTION

Rectal prolapse is an uncommon condition. It was first described in the Bible (2 Chronicles 21). "You yourself will be very ill with a lingering disease of the bowels, until the disease causes your bowels to come out. . . . After all this, the Lord afflicted Jehoram with an incurable disease of the bowels. In the course of time, at the end of the second year, his bowels came out because of the disease, and he died in great pain." The pathophysiology of a rectal prolapse has been evolving since 1543 when Vesalius described the detailed anatomy of the anorectum. Today, three types of rectal prolapse are recognized and they represent three stages of a continuum.[1]

Rectal prolapse usually affects people at the extremes of age. It is most common in the very young and the elderly. The condition usually manifests itself in children within the first 4 years of life, with the highest incidence occurring in the first year.[2] The gender incidence is equal or slightly weighted toward males.[1] The peak incidence in the elderly is approximately between 60 and 70 years of age. It affects primarily women, with a 6:1 ratio of females to males.[3]

ANATOMY AND PATHOPHYSIOLOGY

A rectal prolapse is classified into one of three stages (Figure 58-1). An internal prolapse is the prolapse of the upper rectum and sigmoid colon into the rectal ampulla (Figure 58-1A). It is also known as a hidden or occult prolapse. This type of prolapse does not emerge through the anus. Mucosal prolapse is more common in children. It results from the loose attachment of the mucosa to the submucosal layers and an associated weakness of the anal sphincter. A mucosal prolapse is diagnosed by the presence of radial folds and the absence of muscular wall.[3]

If the condition progresses, it leads to the protrusion of part or all layers of the rectum through the anal orifice. If only the mucosa is prolapsed, it is classified as an incomplete prolapse (Figures 58-1B and C). Synonyms include mucosal prolapse and partial prolapse. A complete rectal prolapse occurs when all bowel layers, including the muscular wall, are involved (Figures 58-1D and E). This condition is also known as a procidentia. The complete rectal prolapse is more common in the elderly. It results from generalized weakening of the pelvic floor and anal sphincter muscles. A complete rectal prolapse is characterized by the presence of concentric folds. A double thickness muscular wall will be felt upon palpation.[4]

Numerous risk factors are associated with a rectal prolapse.[4-10] These include malnutrition, chronic constipation, excessive straining, and diarrheal disorders such as amoebiasis, giardiasis, and other parasitic infections. Rectal prolapse in children is often idiopathic. However, there is an association with paraplegia, meningomyelocele, and pinworms. Anatomic variations such as a vertical course of the rectum, flat sacrum and coccyx, and lack of levator ani support can also result in a rectal prolapse. Children placed on adult toilet seats for prolonged periods of time may develop a rectal prolapse. One of the most serious risk factors for a rectal prolapse in children is cystic fibrosis.[6] Patients with cystic fibrosis have an 18 percent incidence of rectal prolapse. Children with no apparent cause for a rectal prolapse should be considered for a sweat chloride test. In the elderly, rectal prolapse is associated with collagen vascular diseases, pelvic floor weakness, mental retardation, organic brain syndrome, stroke, chronic psychiatric conditions, and chronic neurologic conditions (tabes dorsalis, cauda equina, and multiple sclerosis).[5] It is important to note that patients with rectal prolapse often present with no apparent causes. The physician should maintain a high index of suspicion for the risk factors mentioned above.

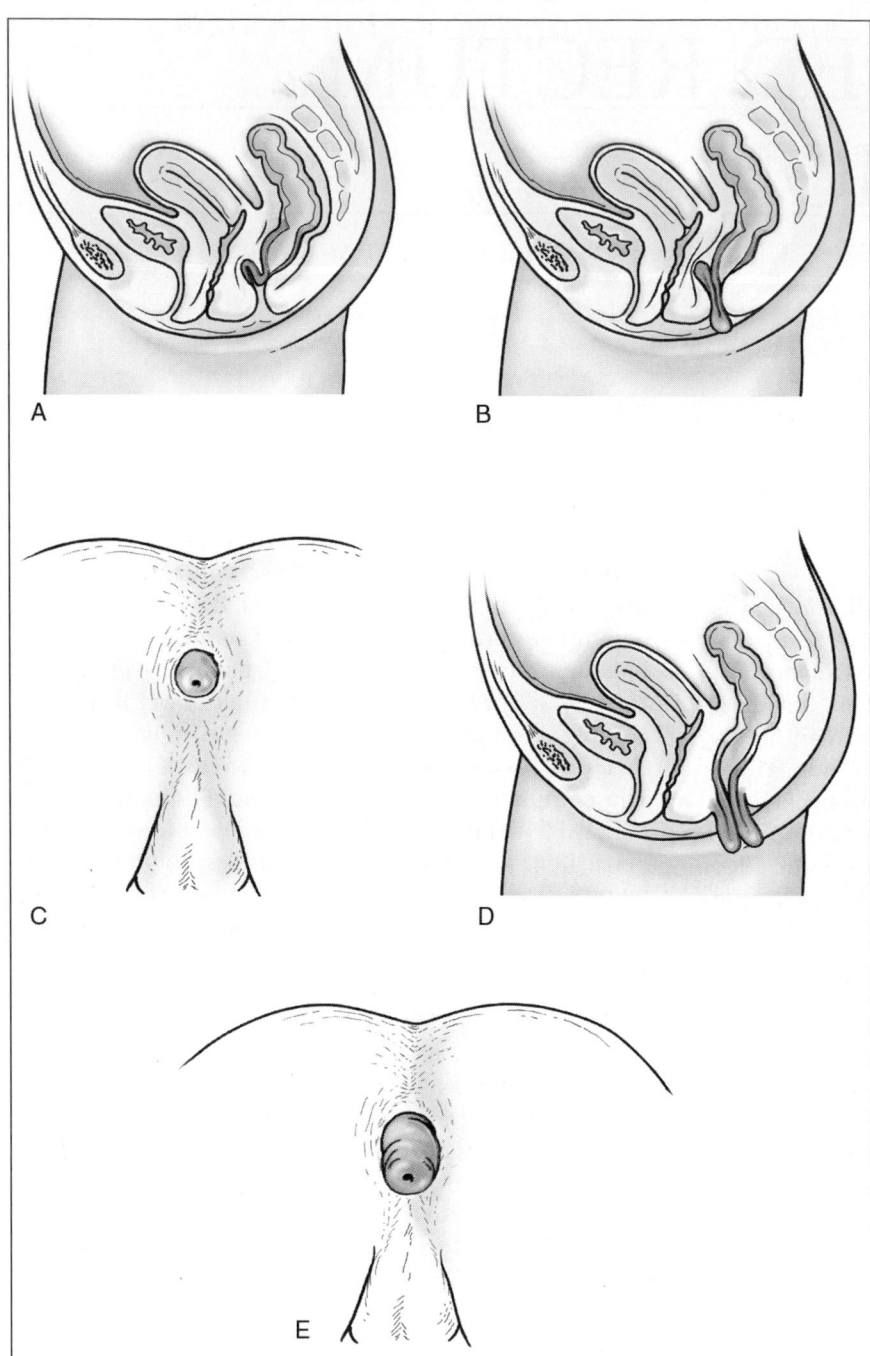

FIGURE 58-1 Types of rectal prolapse. *A.* Midsagittal view of the internal, hidden, or occult prolapse. *B.* Midsagittal view of the incomplete, mucosal, or partial prolapse. *C.* Posterior view of the incomplete, mucosal, or partial prolapse. *D.* Midsagittal view of the complete prolapse or procidentia. *E.* Posterior view of the complete prolapse or procidentia.

The diagnosis can be difficult in the early stages when the prolapse remains in the upper canal (internal or hidden prolapse). The patient may complain of anorectal pain, back pain, discomfort during defecation, difficulty initiating a bowel movement, feeling of incomplete evacuation, tenesmus, pelvic fullness or pain, bloody discharge, or mucoid discharge. At this stage, asking the patient to strain may provoke the prolapse.

The diagnosis becomes easier in a partial or complete prolapse because it protrudes through the anus (Figures 58-1*C* and *E*). These patients may complain of an anal mass when they sit, stand, or walk.[1,5] It is usually the parent who notes the anal mass during defecation in the pediatric patient. The physician should consider the mass described by the parents to be a rectal prolapse if the physical examination is negative.[2] Spontaneous reduction will often occur in this age group. It might also be noted as an incidental finding by a physician.

The differential diagnosis of a rectal prolapse includes anal warts, hemorrhoids, intussusception, prolapsed rectal polyp, or a prolapsed rectal tumor. **Mistaking an intussusception for a rectal prolapse may result in significant morbidity and mortality.** An intussusception, although rare, may result in bowel strangulation and gangrene if not reduced early. **Differentiating features of intussusception include the ability to pass the finger between the prolapsed bowel and the anal sphincter (Figure 58-2). This is in contrast to patients with a rectal prolapse in which the protruding mucosa is continuous with the perianal skin and the examiner's finger will not pass that junction (Figure 58-1D).**[1,2,7] Patients with an intussusception usually appear ill whereas those with a rectal prolapse appear well.[2] Prolapsing hemorrhoids are more often seen in adolescents and adults, are usually purple in color, have deep grooves between the areas of prolapsing tissue, and lack radial or concentric folds. A prolapsed polyp or tumor is plum-colored, does not involve the entire anal circumference, is movable, and is usually palpable as a small growth on a stalk.[2,8]

INDICATIONS

Reduction should be attempted on all patients with a visible rectal prolapse as soon as possible to avoid vascular compromise of the bowel. It is easier to reduce before edema occurs from prolonged prolapse. Early reduction may avoid complications and stretch damage to the pelvic floor ligaments, the pelvic floor muscles, and the anal sphincter muscles.

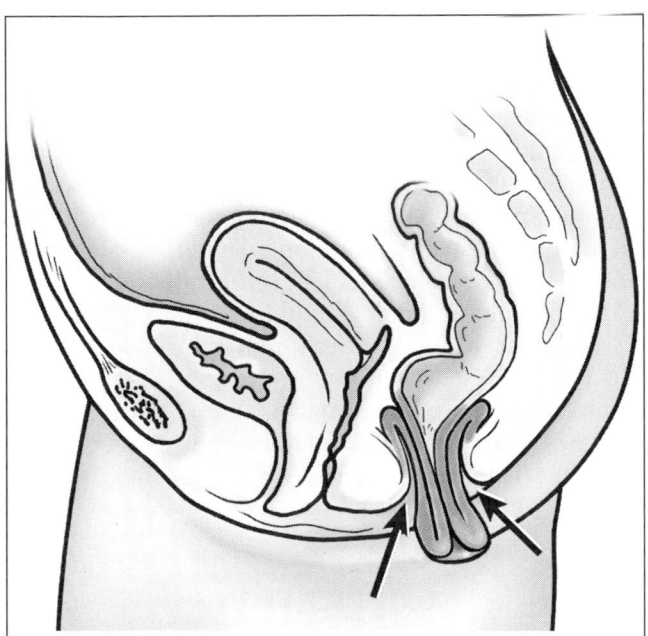

FIGURE 58-2 An intussusception. Note the junction where the finger can be passed (arrows).

CONTRAINDICATIONS

There are few absolute contraindications to the reduction of a rectal prolapse. Gangrene, necrosis, or ulceration of the mucosa are signs of vascular compromise or ischemia and require an emergent consultation by a General Surgeon or Colorectal Surgeon. **Do not reduce ischemic tissue as it may precipitate peritonitis or cause a perforation of the rectum. If the Surgeon's arrival is delayed, prompt gentle reduction should be attempted only after discussions with the Surgeon.** Do not reduce an intussusception. Consult a Surgeon for further evaluation and management of an intussusception.

EQUIPMENT

Gloves
Water-soluble lubricant
4×4 gauze squares
2 inch wide adhesive tape
Benzoin spray or swabs
Petrolatum gauze
Sedation as necessary

PATIENT PREPARATION

Explain the reduction procedure to the patient and/or their representative. Reduction is most likely successful in a relaxed and nonstraining patient. Sedation may sometimes be required in adults. Sedation is more often needed in pediatric patients. Children tend to be more anxious, crying, fighting, or straining, which will increase the intraabdominal pressure and make reduction more difficult. The sedation may be administered intramuscularly, intravenously, orally, or subcutaneously.

Position the patient.[8,9] Place the child in the prone knee-chest position on the parent's lap or on the examination table (Figure 58-3). Place the adult patient in the prone position on an examination table. Large buttocks or tense buttocks may interfere with the reduction of a prolapsed rectum. In these cases, apply benzoin to the buttocks and allow it to dry. Tape the buttocks open for better access (Figure 58-4). Alternatively, in both age groups, the patient can be placed in the lateral decubitus position.

TECHNIQUE

Position the patient. Liberally apply water-soluble lubricant onto the prolapsed rectum. Apply gauze squares onto the prolapsed tissue at the 3 o'clock and 9 o'clock

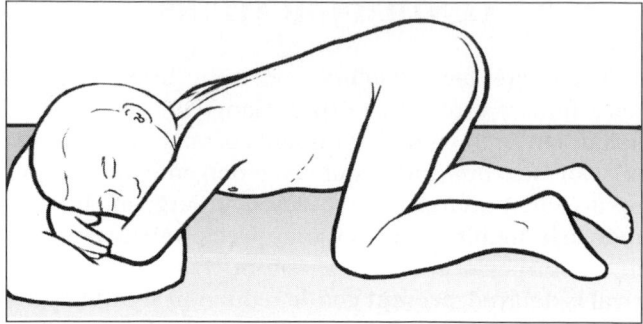

FIGURE 58-3 The prone knee-chest position for children.

positions (Figure 58-5). The bowel wall is quite slippery after lubrication and the gauze will improve the grip on the mucosa. Place both thumbs near the bowel lumen with the hands stabilized on the buttocks (Figure 58-5A). Apply steady, gentle thumb pressure to gently roll the prolapsed rectum back through the anus. Alternatively, the index and the middle fingers can be used to reduce the prolapsed rectum (Figure 58-5B). Regardless of the method used, constant and steady pressure must be applied to the prolapse. It may take up to 15 minutes to reduce a prolapsed rectum.

The rectum will become edematous, and swelling will be noted, if the rectal mucosa has been prolapsed for a prolonged period of time. Wrap a gauze square around the prolapsed rectum and apply manual compression for 3 to 5 minutes before attempting the reduction. If the first effort is unsuccessful without sedation, a second at-

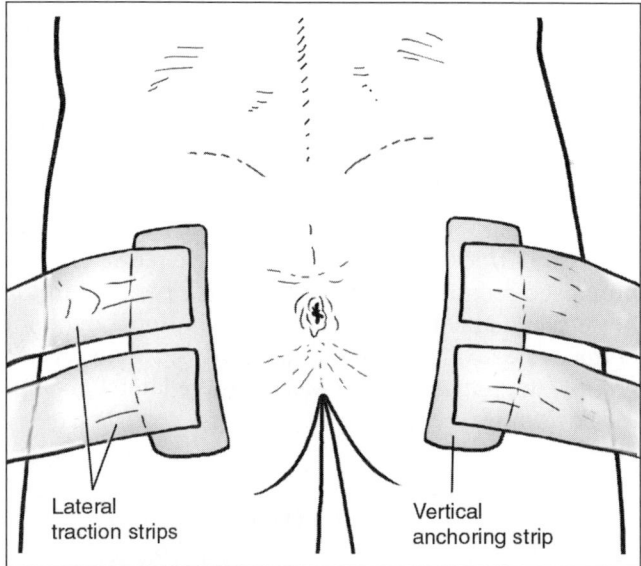

Lateral
traction strips

Vertical
anchoring strip

FIGURE 58-4 Taping the buttocks open in the prone patient allows for unobstructed access. The lateral traction strips are taped to the gurney or examination table.

tempt at reduction after administering sedation is appropriate. If the prolapse rectum will not reduce (i.e., incarcerated), consult a General Surgeon or Colorectal Surgeon for reduction under general anesthesia and possible surgical repair.

ASSESSMENT

Perform a digital rectal examination to ensure that the reduction is complete.[8] If not, apply pressure with the examination finger to completely reduce the prolapse.

AFTERCARE

The application of a bulky pressure dressing will prevent an acute recurrence of the prolapse. Apply petrolatum gauze over the anus. Apply several gauze squares over the petrolatum gauze and into the gluteal cleft. Tape the buttocks together. **The patient and the family must be informed that reduction might be temporary and the prolapse could recur.** Training cooperative parents to reduce the prolapse is warranted in cases of recurrent rectal prolapse in the pediatric age group. Be sure to send them home with gauze squares, gloves, and lubricant.

The underlying cause of the rectal prolapse should be treated. A prophylactic regimen of laxatives and stool softeners should be started if the patient is constipated. Instruct the patient on proper eating habits including fruits, vegetables, and roughage. In cases of diarrhea, treatment should target the underlying causes. Seating children on a child's potty-chair or on an adult toilet seat with a small hole may prevent future episodes of rectal prolapse. Discourage excessive squatting and straining.[3]

All patients who have undergone successful reduction should be referred for further evaluation. Children should be followed up to rule out serious etiologies such as cystic fibrosis. As the child grows, the supporting tissue around the rectum develops. Therefore rectal prolapse in this age group is usually self-limited and surgery is rarely required. Adults should be referred for proctosigmoidoscopy to rule out a tumor. Conservative management in the elderly is rarely successful and most patients eventually require surgical repair. Early referral to a Surgeon can avoid complications and stretch damage to the pelvic floor ligaments, pelvic floor muscles, and the anal sphincter muscles.

COMPLICATIONS

The complications of the procedure are often minimal. The reduction itself may lead to minimal mucosal

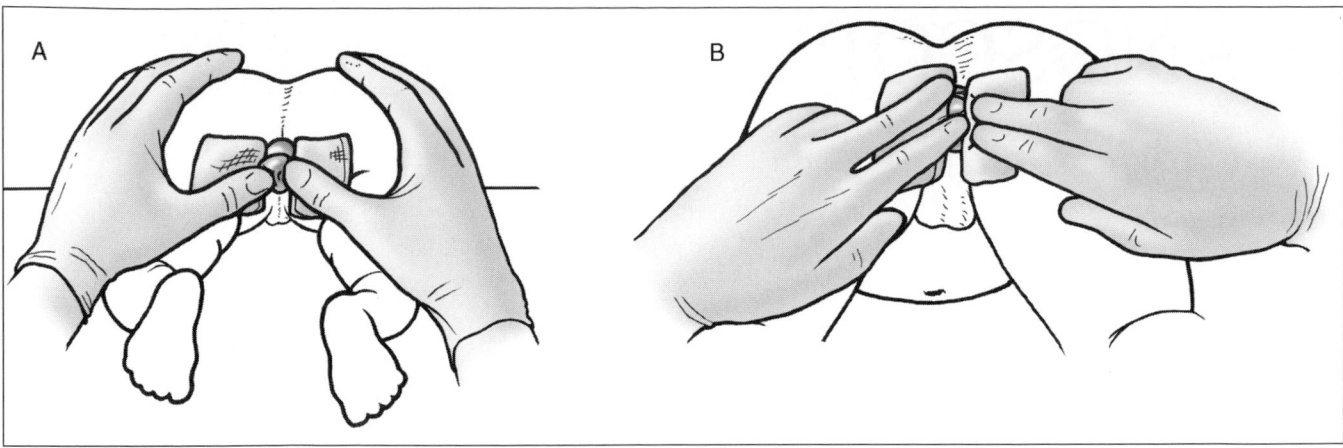

FIGURE 58-5 Rectal prolapse reduction techniques. *A.* Thumb method. *B.* Finger method.

bleeding that is self-limited. The patients may experience a slight discomfort in the anus (pain in the butt) for up to 24 hours after the reduction. This can be managed with oral acetaminophen or nonsteroidal anti-inflammatory drugs.

The inability to reduce a rectal prolapse is an indication for surgical consultation in the Emergency Department. An incarcerated rectal prolapse can lead to vascular compromise. Signs of vascular compromise include mucosal gangrene, necrosis, and ulceration. These patients require admission to the hospital with emergency surgical consultation, even if the reduction is felt to be successful, due to the risk of reducing ischemic bowel that could perforate. Very rarely, the rupture of an incarcerated rectal prolapse with small bowel herniation through the tear has been reported during attempted reduction.[10] Fecal and urinary incontinence may also occur as a result of a long-standing prolapse. This is due to the entrapment and stretching of the pudendal or perineal nerve resulting in neurovascular dysfunction and not a complication of the reduction procedure.

SUMMARY

Rectal prolapse is an uncommon condition affecting the very young and the elderly. Reduction can usually be performed in the Emergency Department. It is important to differentiate a prolapsed rectum from an intussusception. The reduction procedure is quick and simple. The application of constant, firm, and gentle pressure to the rectum in a relaxed and nonstraining patient will reduce most rectal prolapses. All patients with a prolapsed rectum should be referred for further evaluation to rule out underlying pathologic causes for the prolapse.

REFERENCES

1. Heine JA, Wong WD: Rectal prolapse, in Mazier WP (ed): *Surgery of the Colon, Rectum, and Anus.* Philadelphia: Saunders, 1995:515–537.
2. Siafakas C, Vottler TP, Andersen JM: Rectal prolapse in pediatrics. *Clin Pediatr* 1999; 38(2):63–72.
3. Andrews NJ, Jones DJ: Rectal prolapse and associated conditions. *BMJ* 1992; 305:243–246.
4. Yamada T, Alpers DH, Laine L, et al: *Textbook of Gastroenterology,* 3rd ed. Vol 2. Philadelphia: Lippincott Williams & Wilkins, 1999:2091–2092.
5. Keighley MRB, Williams NS: *Surgery of the Anus, Rectum, and Colon.* Vol 1. London: Saunders, 1993:675–715.
6. Stern RC, Inzant R J Jr, Boat IF, et al: Treatment and prognosis of rectal prolapse in cystic fibrosis. *Gastroenterology* 1982; 82(4):707–710.
7. Walter I, Allan W: *Pediatric Gastrointestinal Disease,* 2nd ed. Vol 1. St. Louis: Mosby, 1996:581–582.
8. Alessandrini EA: Reduction of rectal prolapse, in Dieckmann RA, Fiser DH, Selbst SM (eds): *Pediatric Emergency and Critical Care Procedures.* St. Louis: Mosby, 1997:375–376.
9. Schwartz G: Reducing a rectal prolapse, in Hentrig F, King C, Joffe MD, et al (eds): *Textbook of Pediatric Emergency Procedures.* Baltimore: Williams & Wilkins, 1997:947–950.
10. Hovey MA, Metcalf AM: Incarcerated rectal prolapse—rupture and ileal evisceration after failed reduction: report of a case. *Dis Colon Rectum* 1997; 40(10):1254–1257.

Chapter 59
ANOSCOPY

Charles Orsay

INTRODUCTION

Examination of the anal canal is important to evaluate several common patient complaints relating to the anus including itching, pain, and bleeding. While it is possible to examine parts of this area with flexible instruments or a rigid rectosigmoidoscope, the only method that will give a consistent clear view of the anal canal is anoscopy.[1] To properly perform this examination it is necessary to thoroughly understand the anatomy, be aware of the possible causes of the symptoms you are evaluating, use the appropriate equipment, and position the patient correctly.

ANATOMY AND PATHOPHYSIOLOGY

It is necessary to understand the anatomy of the anal canal in order to evaluate the patient's signs and symptoms properly. The anatomy can be divided into topical anatomy and major supporting structures.[2] The topical anatomy is depicted in Figure 59-1.

Perineal skin covers the perineum, is fully innervated, and includes both hair follicles and apocrine glands. It can be grossly distinguished from the anoderm surrounding the anal canal by the visible hair. The anoderm is specialized squamous epithelium that lines the majority of the anal canal. It is fully innervated but does not have apocrine glands or hair follicles. This epithelium is very thin, elastic, and if destroyed by surgery or infection may relate to stricture formation during healing.

Looking into the anal canal, the anoderm can be seen to end in an irregular line called the dentate line. This is a demarcation of anoderm to transition zone mucosa. Proximal to the dentate line there is no longer cutaneous sensation. This allows minor therapeutic procedures like banding or suture ligation to be done without an anesthetic agent. It is also the reason internal hemorrhoids

do not routinely cause pain. The transition zone continues proximally for a variable length of 6 to 12 mm before it becomes the rectal mucosa. The junction of the transitional zone with the rectal mucosa is not visible to the naked eye. The rectal mucosa decreases in diameter in the area of the transitional zone. The mucosa appears to be bunched together in columns called the Columns of Morgagni at the level of the dentate line. Crypts are formed between the columns as the transitional zone becomes the dentate line. Under the anoderm in the crypts are multiple anal glands. Blockage of the anal glands by foreign material leads to infection. This or primary infection of the glands causes the majority of abscesses that arise around the anus. The crypts also are areas to look for foreign bodies such as fish or chicken bones.

External hemorrhoids are located in the left-lateral, right-posterior, and right-anterior portions of the distal anal canal and are covered with anoderm. Their normal position is outside the anal canal and they can be examined by gently spreading the buttocks. The internal hemorrhoids also are located at the left-lateral, right-posterior, and right-anterior positions. They are normally located in the distal rectum and are covered with transitional epithelium and rectal mucosa. They can best be examined with an anoscope if they are not prolapsed. It is possible to see them with a retroflexed sigmoidoscope or colonoscope but the increased air pressure tends to flatten them out giving a false impression as to their size.

The anoscope is used to examine the closed portion of the anal canal. It dilates the anal sphincter and allows one to examine the underlying canal through an opening cut out from the side of the anoscope called a fenestration. It is important to understand the anatomy and functions of the anal sphincter musculature to properly perform this examination (Figure 59-2). Immediately below the anoderm is the internal anal sphincter muscle.

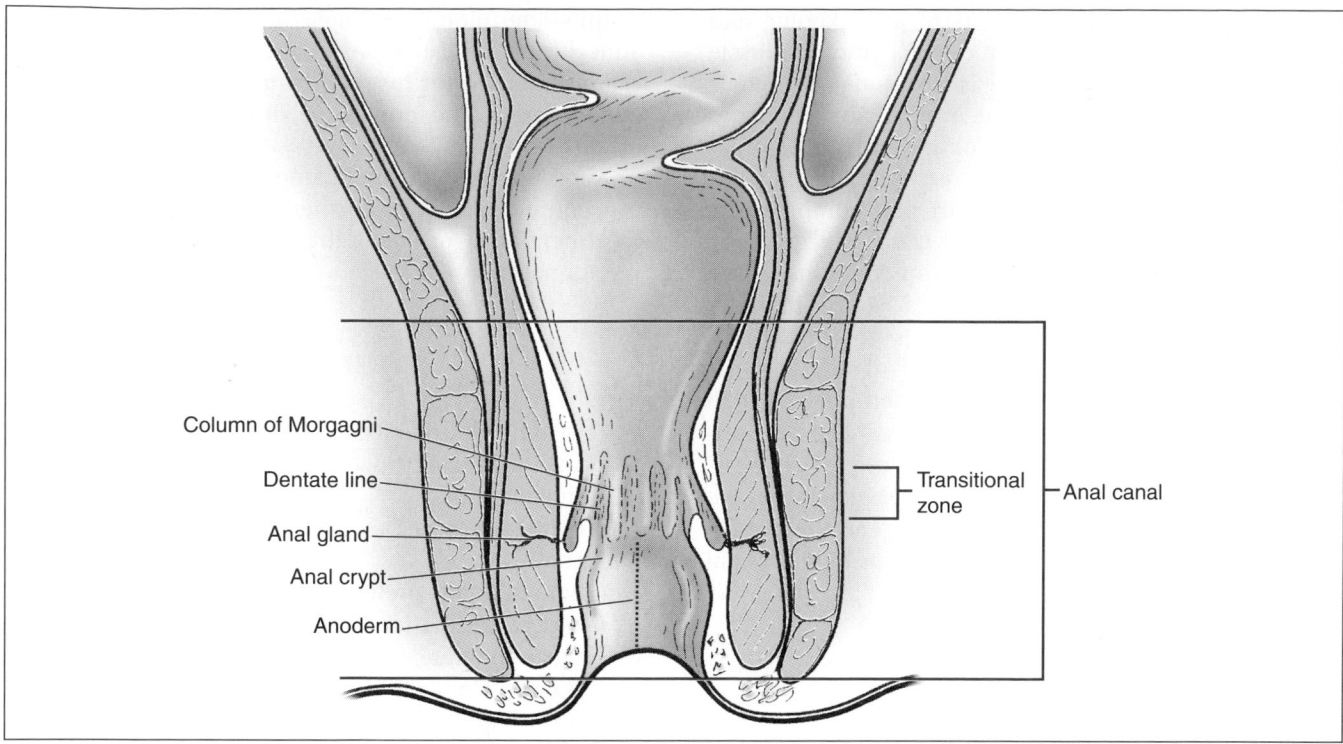

FIGURE 59-1 The topical anatomy of the anal canal.

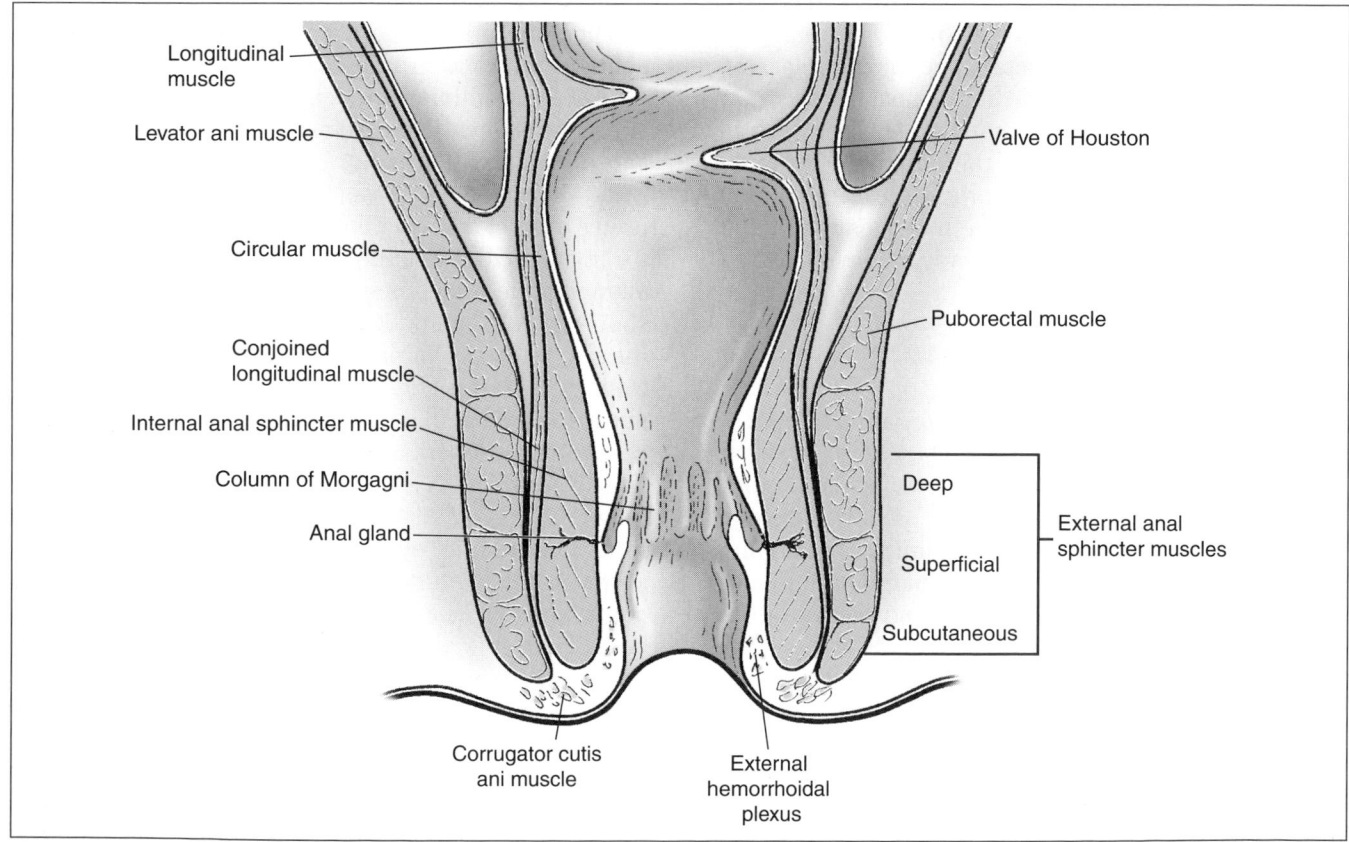

FIGURE 59-2 The major supporting structures of the anal canal.

It is circumferential and consists of a thickening and rounding of the continuation of circular smooth muscle from the rectum. This muscle is not under conscious control. The first response of the internal anal sphincter muscle to a rectal examination or anoscopy is contraction. It is necessary to pause and use slow gentle dilatation to prevent patient discomfort and complete the examination. The axis of the anal canal will normally follow an imaginary line drawn from the anus to the umbilicus. Surrounding the internal anal sphincter muscle is the external anal sphincter muscle. This is comprised of three external sphincters of striated muscle that are more loop-like than circumferential. Deep to these muscles and at the top of the anal canal is the puborectalis muscle. This forms a sling, pulling the anus anterior. It is connected to both the anal sphincters and the levator ani group of muscles. The puborectalis muscle can be felt as funnel-shaped during the digital rectal examination.

INDICATIONS

Anoscopy is indicated in the evaluation of most anal symptoms.[1–6] There are numerous common complaints and conditions where an anoscope, in conjunction with visualization and a digital rectal examination, would be used for evaluation or therapy.[3–5] Anoscopy can be used diagnostically to evaluate rectal bleeding, anal pain, pain with defecation, perirectal infections, fistulas, foreign bodies, internal hemorrhoids, anal masses, and abnormal digital rectal examinations. Anoscopy can be used therapeutically to open the anus and allow the application of medications, procedures to be performed, or for observation in the management of anal fissures, intraanal condylomata, and hemorrhoids.

CONTRAINDICATIONS

Most contraindications to anoscopy are relative. The amount of discomfort a patient will undergo relates to their tolerance. Minor discomfort associated with topical skin excoriations can be treated with 2% lidocaine jelly used as a lubricant and the examination can then continue. Moderate pain can be managed with the application of intravenous sedation and analgesics. Severe pain associated with anal fissures or anal abscesses can best be managed in the Operating Room under general anesthesia.

Strictures can occur from postsurgical changes, inflammatory bowel disease, chronic diarrhea, and other disease processes. Anoscopy should not be performed if the patient has anal strictures, a partially imperforate anus, or a completely imperforate anus. The physician should determine if the anoscope will pass through the anus during the visual examination and the digital rectal examination. **Never insert the anoscope if resistance is encountered. The anoscope should not be used to dilate the anus.**

Anoscopy is contraindicated if any recent surgical procedure has been performed on the anus. The possible exception is for that of the physician who performed the surgical procedure.

EQUIPMENT

Water-soluble lubricant
Lidocaine jelly, can be used as lubricant for patients with pain
Anoscope or Vernon-David rectal speculum
Drapes
Examination table, preferably a proctoscopy table
Nonsterile examination gloves
4×4 gauze squares
Large cotton-tipped applicators
4–0 chromic gut suture
Suction, optional
Bright directional light source
Tincture of benzoin
2 inch adhesive tape

There are many different types of anoscopes available. The type of instrument chosen is largely the preference of the examining physician. The Vernon-David type anoscope is often preferred as it has a wide fenestration and a diameter that is not too large for most patients while allowing the best view. The Ives anoscope may be used if a larger diameter instrument is required. Some of the metal reusable and plastic disposable anoscopes allow for the attachment of a fiberoptic light source. Unfortunately, many of these anoscopes do not allow the same view as a Vernon-David anoscope. Some physicians use a glass test tube as a substitute for an anoscope. This is to be discouraged as the test tube can break and cause serious complications.

The anoscope is a two-piece device (Figure 59-3). It ranges from 7 to 25 cm in length. It can be manufactured from clear plastic, opaque plastic, or metal. The anoscope may have a handle that allows the operator to control its movements. The proximal end is funnel-like and tapers into the cylindrical shaft that is approximately 2.5 cm in diameter. The distal end of the anoscope is tapered on one side and known as the fenestration. The fenestration allows the mucosa to be viewed within the anoscope. It is also where procedures are performed through the anoscope. Some anoscopes have a site proximally to attach a light source. The obturator is smooth tipped, fits within the anoscope, and oc-

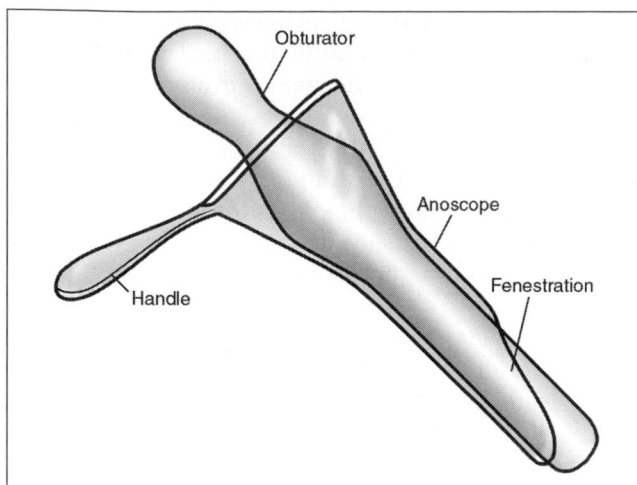

FIGURE 59-3 An example of an anoscope.

cludes the anoscope. Its distal end protrudes from the anoscope. The obturator is used each time the anoscope is inserted to prevent trauma to the anal mucosa. It is removed after the anoscope is inserted to allow viewing through the anoscope.

PATIENT PREPARATION

The area being examined is within the anal canal and requires no special preparation to view correctly. The patient should be given an opportunity to voluntarily evacuate their bowels prior to the examination. It is necessary to have the patient remove their clothes from the waist down and provide protective barriers to protect the patient, the patient's clothing, and the surrounding area from spills. It is usually wise to avoid enema prepa-

rations, as liquid stool is much more difficult to contain than solid stool.

Explain the risks, benefits, and potential complications of the procedure to the patient and/or their representative. Explain to the patient what to expect. Discuss the order of examination, the importance of relaxing, the reason for multiple insertions and withdrawals of the anoscope, and what you are looking for or expect to find.

Anoscopy can be performed with the patient in one of many positions. The position that allows the best observation in most patients is the knee-chest or prone position (Figure 59-4). This allows the buttocks to be to either side and places the anus at the proper angle. Examination of the anus in this position is easiest on a proctoscopy table, but can also be performed on an examination table. The lateral decubitus position with the knees drawn up and the buttocks protruding partly off the table is acceptable for limited diagnostic examinations. Large buttocks may prevent the examination. Apply tincture of benzoin to the buttocks and allow it to dry. Apply 2 inch adhesive tape to the buttocks and tape them to the examination table to spread the buttocks apart (Figure 58-4). Place a Mayo stand or bedside examination table next to the patient's buttocks.

Carefully inspect the entire perineum and anal verge. Many types of pathology such as fissures, fistulas, hemorrhoids, condylomata, and dermatologic conditions can be seen at this time. **A digital rectal examination with a well-lubricated gloved finger prior to anoscopy is mandatory.** The digital rectal examination has many advantages. It allows one to find pathology that is better palpated than viewed. It gives the examiner the size and angle of the anal canal. It will allow the examiner to identify if the patient has tenderness that would preclude anoscopy. Any strictures will be identified, allowing

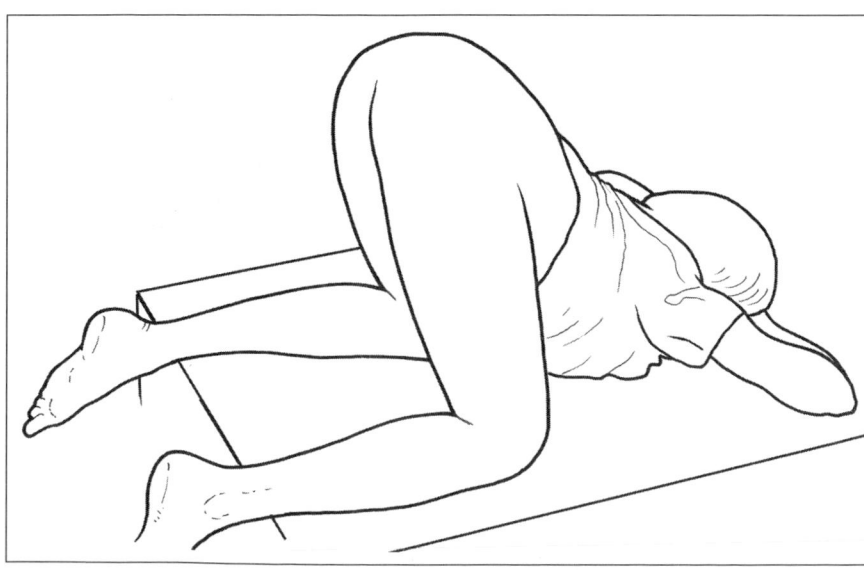

FIGURE 59-4 The knee-chest position.

the examiner to prevent the anoscope from advancing through these strictures and lacerating the tissues. It may identify pathology, so that the examiner can focus the anoscopy in a specific area. It prelubricates the anal canal, making insertion of the anoscope easier. Lidocaine jelly can be used as a lubricant and as an anesthetic if the patient has pain from excoriation. The use of intravenous analgesics, intravenous sedatives, procedural sedation, or general anesthesia may be occasionally required if the patient has significant pain.

TECHNIQUE

The technique of anoscopy is rather simple.[6] Look closely at the anoscope and be sure it is intact and correctly assembled. Liberally lubricate the obturator and anoscope. Ensure that the obturator is easily removed and replaced from within the anoscope. Grasp the anoscope in one hand with the obturator secured in place with the thumb of that hand (Figure 59-5A).

Use the nondominant hand to spread the anus (Figure 59-5A). Place the obturator at the center of the anus. Slowly insert the anoscope, giving time for the internal anal sphincter muscle to relax. Direct the tip of the obturator towards the patient's umbilicus (Figure 59-5A). Insert the anoscope to its fullest depth to start the examination with the area of fenestration pointed towards the area you wish to view first (Figures 59-5B and C). Slowly remove the obturator and place it on a Mayo stand or a bedside table where it can easily be retrieved. Adjust the directional light for the best illumination.

The usual starting place for the examination is the posterior midline (Figures 59-5B and C). Slowly withdraw the anoscope under direct observation to evaluate the entire depth of the anal canal exposed by the fenestration. Remove any fecal material with a cotton-tipped applicator. Note the appearance of the dentate line, the mucosa, and the anoderm. Note the presence and location of any blood, hemorrhoids, masses, mucus, purulence, or other abnormalities. If the anoscope does not fully dilate the columns of mucosa, a cotton-tipped applicator can be used to gently move the mucosa to view between the columns. Continue to withdraw the anoscope as the mucosa is viewed.

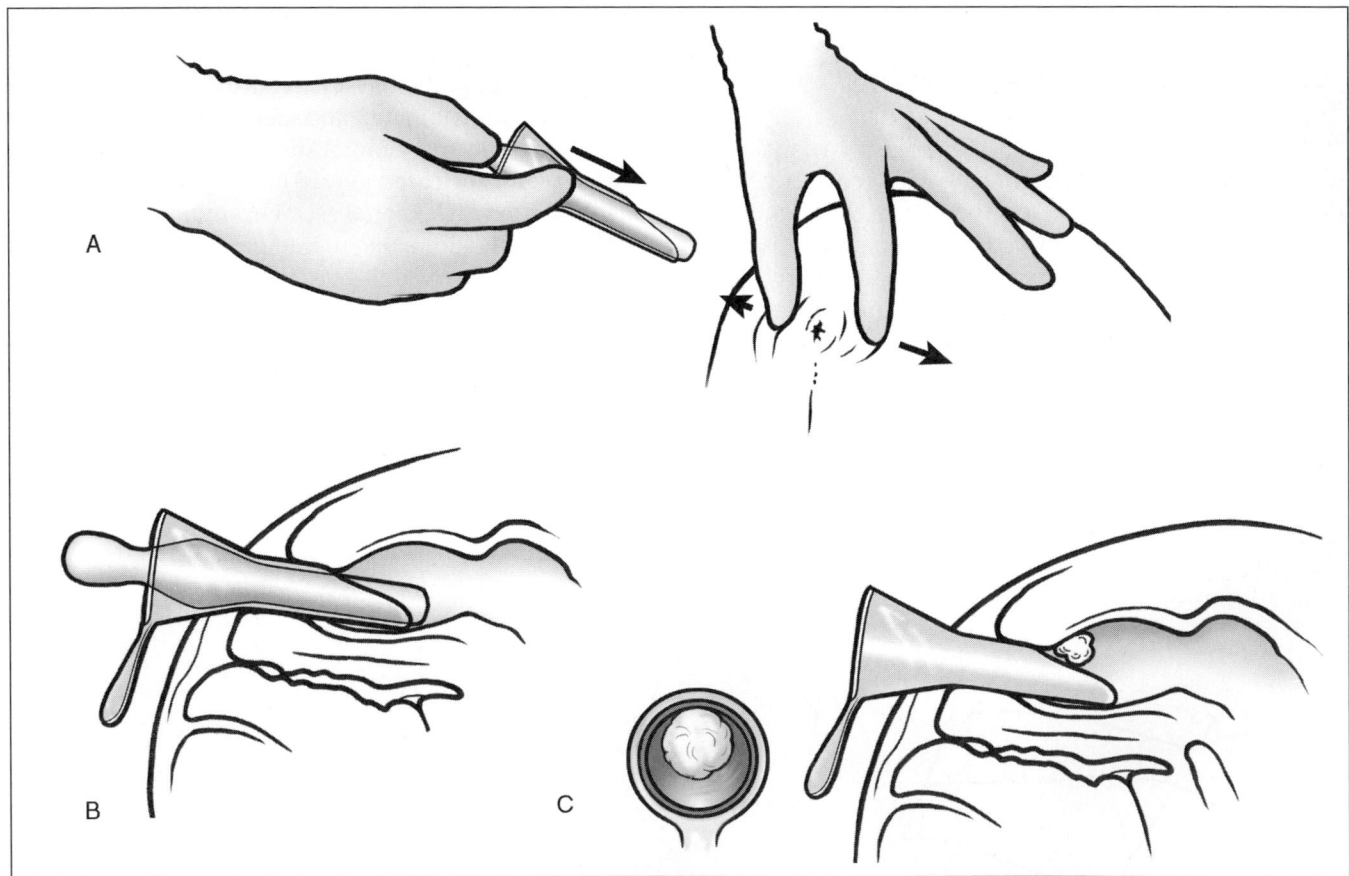

FIGURE 59-5 Placement of the anoscope. *A.* The nondominant hand is used to spread the anus. The anoscope is inserted at an angle and aimed towards the umbilicus. Note that the dominant thumb is used to secure the obturator within the anoscope. The anoscope is completely inserted with the fenestration pointed towards the posterior midline (*B*) or the area of interest (*C*).

Replace the obturator when the anoscope is fully removed from the patient. Rotate the anoscope 30 to 40 degrees and reinsert it into the anal canal. It often takes four or five repeated insertions to evaluate the entire circumference of the anal canal. Some physicians prefer to replace the obturator and rotate the anoscope while it is still within the anal canal. This method is discouraged as it may pinch the tissue of the anus between the obturator and the viewing tube and does not allow the examiner to see the entire depth of the anal canal.

It is helpful to ask the patient to bear down when examining the left-lateral, right-posterior, and right-anterior sections of the anal canal when evaluating the internal hemorrhoids. It is often possible to reproduce the prolapsing of internal hemorrhoids to evaluate the grade of the hemorrhoids. Bearing down is particularly important if bleeding is the symptom. It is possible to identify the area of bleeding.

ANOSCOPY IN CHILDREN

Anoscopy may be performed in children for the same indications as an adult. An anoscope of 8 to 10 cm in length and 1 cm in diameter is appropriate for a neonate and young infant. An anoscope of over 12 cm in length and 1.5 cm in diameter is appropriate for an older infant and child. An adult anoscope is appropriate for an older child and adolescent. Position the young child supine with their buttocks at the edge of the examination table. Have an assistant grasp, abduct, and flex the child's thighs so they touch the abdomen without compressing the abdominal wall. The remainder of the procedure is as described above.

COMPLICATIONS

Examination of the anal canal with an anoscope should have minimal or no complications. It is possible to cause abrasions or lacerate the very thin anoderm. This is normally avoidable with adequate lubrication, the use of the obturator when inserting the anoscope, and gentle technique. Minimal bleeding from mucosal irritation is common and self-limited. Dislodgement of a clot may result in hemorrhoidal bleeding that can be controlled with direct pressure, packing the anal canal with gauze squares, or a 4–0 chromic gut figure-of-eight suture. The most common complication is pain. This is avoidable by allowing enough time for the anus to relax while gently inserting the anoscope. The presence of an anal fissure may preclude the examination. The use of a topical anesthetic will usually allow the examination to proceed.

SUMMARY

Anoscopy is a commonly performed procedure in the Emergency Department. The anal canal is a cylindrical structure surrounded by sensitive anoderm and contracting anal sphincter muscles. The best way to examine this area is with a side-viewing fenestrated anoscope. Anoscopy allows direct viewing of the anal canal to best evaluate anal and perianal complaints. Anoscopy will give the most information with minimal discomfort when properly performed. Always perform a digital rectal examination prior to anoscopy.

REFERENCES

1. Corman ML: *Colon and Rectal Surgery,* 3rd ed. Philadelphia: Lippincott, 1993:5–6.
2. Gordon PH, Nivatvongs S: *Principles and Practice of Surgery for the Colon, Rectum and Anus.* St. Louis: Quality Medical Publishing, 1992:11–12.
3. Hyman NH: Anorectal disease: how to relieve pain and improve other symptoms. *Geriatrics* 1997; 52(4):75–76, 85–88, 91.
4. Rompalo AM: Diagnosis and treatment of sexually acquired proctitis and proctocolitis: an update. *Clin Infect Dis* 1999; 28(Suppl 1):84–90.
5. Segal WN, Greenberg PD, Rockey DC, et al: The outpatient evaluation of hematochezia. *Am J Gastroenterol* 1998; 93(2):179–182.
6. Pearl RK: *Gastrointestinal Endoscopy for Surgeons.* Boston: Little, Brown, 1984:165–179.

Chapter 60
RIGID
RECTOSIGMOIDOSCOPY

Charles Orsay

INTRODUCTION

Rigid rectosigmoidoscopy has largely been replaced by the flexible sigmoidoscope for routine elective screening and diagnostic workups. The rigid rectosigmoidoscope is superior to the flexible sigmoidoscope in measuring distances accurately, examining an unprepared patient, and when trying to work within the bowel lumen, for example when removing foreign bodies. The larger lumen of the rigid rectosigmoidoscope allows for a larger biopsy of lesions where pathology is in question. The cost associated with this examination is less than that for flexible sigmoidoscopy. The rigid rectosigmoidoscope can be purchased in a disposable model that performs well. It is important for a physician who evaluates and treats problems related to the colon, rectum, and anus to be familiar with rigid rectosigmoidoscopy.

ANATOMY AND PATHOPHYSIOLOGY

The significant anatomy of the anal canal that is necessary to understand and to perform rigid rectosigmoidoscopy is covered in Chapter 59 describing the anatomy for anoscopy (Figures 59-1 and 59-2). The gross anatomy of the colon is reviewed in Figure 60-1A. It is important to be aware of the large folds that impinge on the lumen of the colon called the valves of Houston (Figure 60-1B). These folds must be gently flattened to advance the rigid rectosigmoidoscope and clearly see the proximal side of the valve when looking for pathology. It is also necessary to understand the three-dimensional path followed by the distal colon, rectum, and anus. The direction to follow will be towards the patient's umbilicus for 3 to 5 cm initially. The anus then turns posteriorly as it becomes the rectum and follows the curve of the sacrum. The rectosigmoid junction is reached at 10 to 15 cm, at which point the lumen sharply angulates anteriorly and to the left. Because the scope is rigid and straight, it is necessary to angle the tip of the rigid rectosigmoidoscope towards the lumen of the bowel and then gently flatten the haustra or move the patient's colon so that the lumen is in a straight line.

INDICATIONS

Many of the indications for rigid rectosigmoidoscopy are the same as those for performing flexible sigmoidoscopy. The rigid scope is more useful when the bowel is not properly prepared, if a bigger biopsy is needed, or if a larger instrument needs to be passed to the last 25 centimeters. The following is a list of such indications.

The rigid rectosigmoidoscope may be used to evaluate the rectum and sigmoid colon in the office or the Emergency Department. Rectal bleeding can be evaluated in the unprepared patient. It is particularly helpful to determine if stool is mixed with blood when evaluating hematochezia and determining if colonoscopy is indicated. Foreign bodies in the rectum or sigmoid colon can be removed. The rigid rectosigmoidoscope will allow a much larger biopsy and grasping forceps to assist in removing foreign bodies. Traumatic injuries can be assessed. Since the rectum is seldom prepared in the evaluation of a traumatic injury and flexible instruments are unable to clear solid or thick stool, the rigid rectosigmoidoscope is superior in this instance. A sigmoid volvulus can be decompressed using the rigid rectosigmoidoscope to pass a tube to splint the volvulus. It is much easier to suction out a large volume of obstructed material in the colon and leave a large tube with the rigid rectosigmoidoscope. It can be used for surveillance of colon or rectal cancer after subtotal colectomy. It can be used to accurately measure the distance to rectal lesions from the anus prior to surgery.

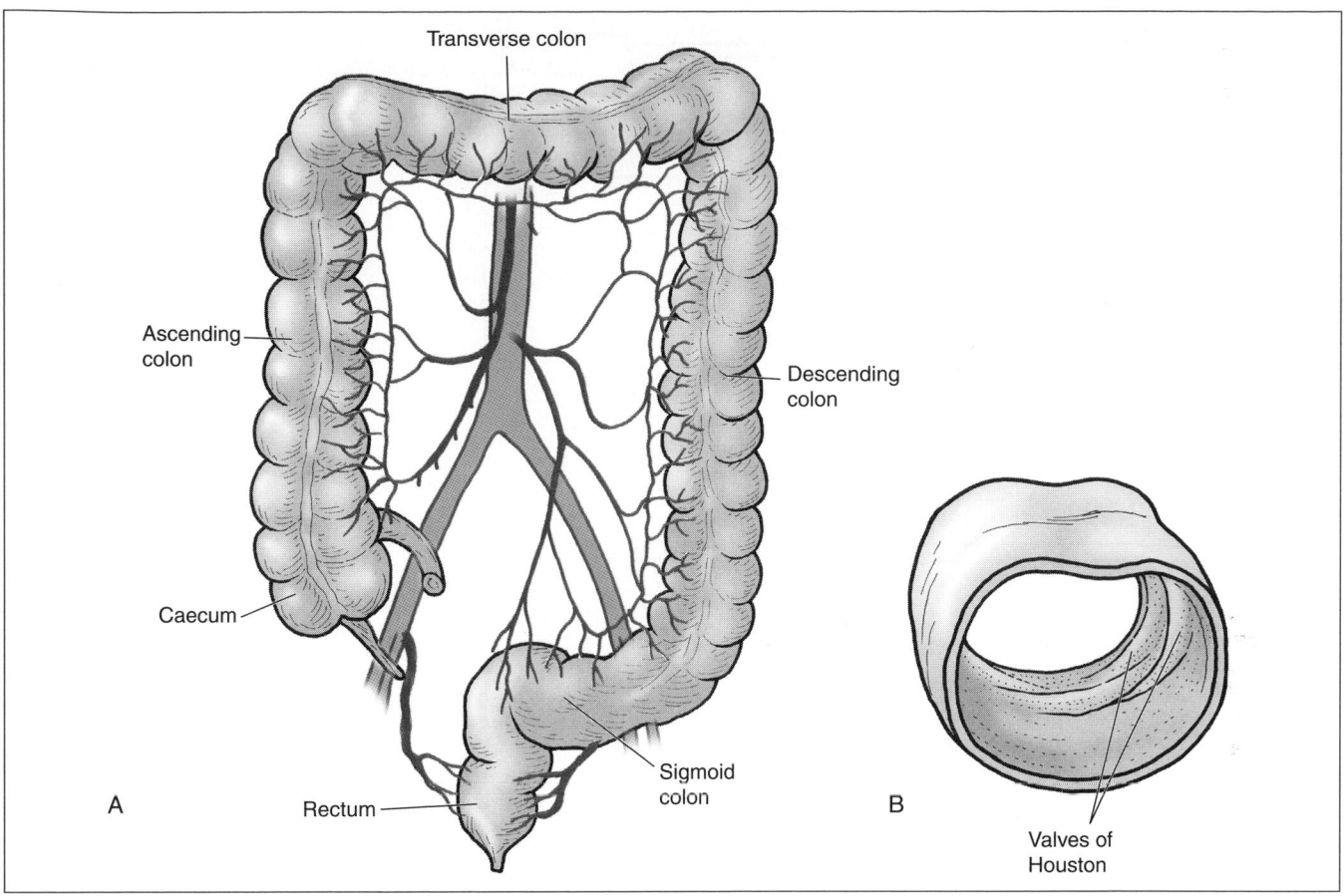

FIGURE 60-1 Anatomy of the colon. *A.* The gross anatomy. *B.* Cross-section through the colon demonstrating the valves of Houston.

CONTRAINDICATIONS

There are no absolute contraindications to rigid rectosigmoidoscopy.[1] Relative contraindications include severe anal pain that may require general anesthesia, recent surgical anastomosis in the distal 25 cm of the colon and rectum, severe stenosis of the anus or rectum, and peritonitis. This procedure should not be performed by anyone unfamiliar with the equipment and technique as significant complications can occur.

EQUIPMENT

Phosphate soda enemas
Rigid rectosigmoidoscope with obturator, air insufflator, eyepiece, and light source
Suction catheter
Suction machine or wall suction
Biopsy forceps
Long cotton-tipped applicator with a silver nitrate applicator on the opposite end
Proctoscopy table or examination table
Protective drape with exam fenestration
4×4 gauze squares
Water-soluble lubricant
Exam gloves
Impermeable gown
Instrument stand
Anoscope, should be available to examine the anal canal if indicated

The rigid rectosigmoidoscope and other required instruments are available in preassembled sterile trays. The tray usually contains the rigid scope, an obturator, a suction catheter, polypectomy snare, and biopsy forceps (Figure 60-2). These trays are available from the Operating Room, hospital central supply, or the surgical clinics. The trays may contain disposable single-use instruments or multiuse instruments depending upon the institution. The remainder of the equipment must be gathered from around the Emergency Department.

The rigid rectosigmoidoscope is a simple instrument (Figures 60-2*A* and *B*). The shaft is approximately 30 to 40 cm in length and has 1 cm increments marked on the outside. Attached to the proximal end are an eyepiece, a

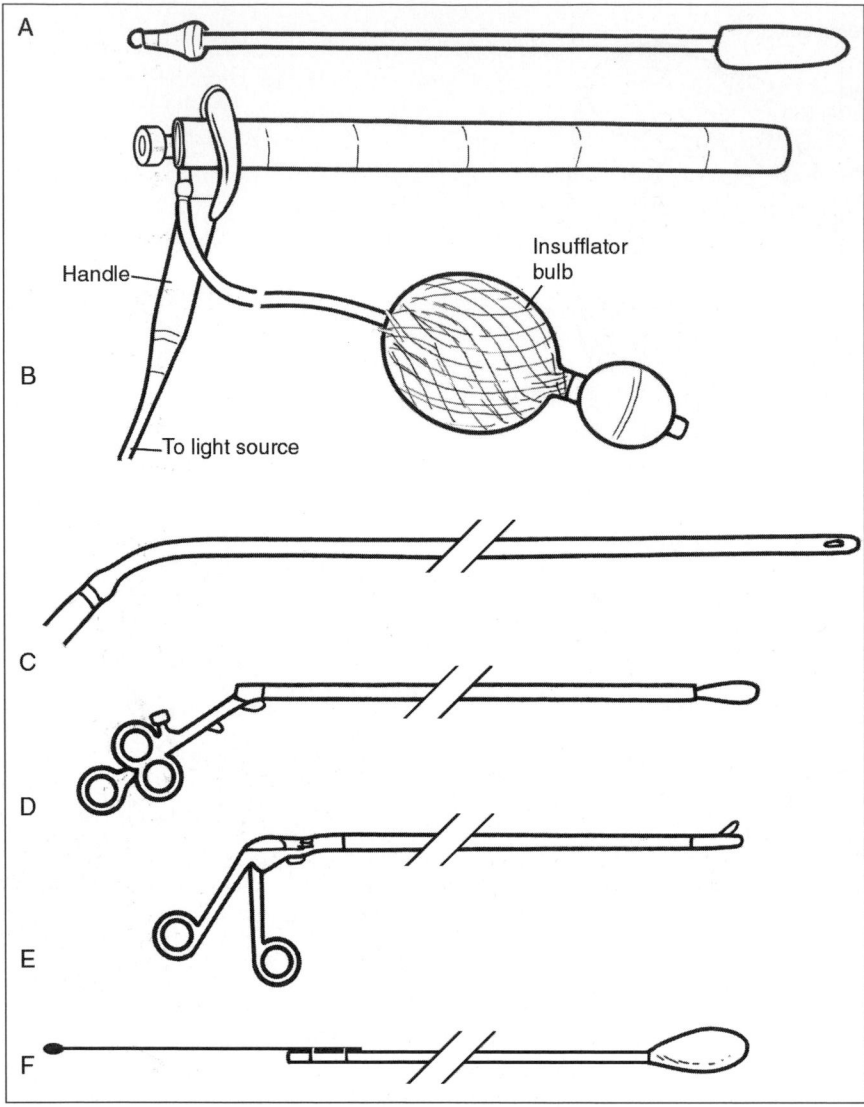

FIGURE 60-2 The instruments required to perform rigid rectosigmoidoscopy. *A.* Obturator. *B.* Rigid rectosigmoidoscope. *C.* Suction catheter. *D.* Polypectomy snare. *E.* Biopsy forceps. *F.* Cotton-tipped applicator with silver nitrate matchstick taped to the opposite side.

handle, and an inflation port. The eyepiece swings to open and close over the proximal shaft of the scope. The handle is used to direct and move the scope. Inside the handle is a fiberoptic light source that transmits into the shaft. The insufflator bulb and tubing attach to the inflation port. These are used to insufflate air through the scope and into the colon. The obturator fits within the shaft of the scope. The distal end of the obturator is smooth, occludes the shaft of the scope, and projects 1 to 2 cm distal to the scope.

PATIENT PREPARATION

Explain the risks, benefits, and potential complications of the procedure to the patient and/or their representative. It is also important to explain to the patient what to expect. Discuss the order of examination, the importance of relaxing, the reason for multiple inser-

tions and withdrawals of the rigid rectosigmoidoscope, and what you expect to find. It is important to explain the reason for insufflating air and how this may produce discomfort. Explain that the procedure should not require procedural sedation and that the patient should inform the physician of any discomfort. Assure the patient that the complaint of pain will stop the examination. Perforations are unlikely with a relaxed, cooperative patient.Obtain a signed informed consent for this procedure.

While it is possible to perform a rigid rectosigmoidoscopy with this instrument on an unprepared rectum, more information about the mucosa will be obtained if the bowel has been prepared. Two 4 ounce phosphate soda enemas given at 2 and 1 hours before the examination will give an adequate preparation in most patients. The use of high-volume PEG preparations, saline, or mannitol should be reserved for colonoscopy. There is no need to clean the entire colon. The preparations used for colonoscopy are expensive, involve too much preparation, and cause patient discomfort for the extent of this examination. The judicious use of intravenous sedation may be required in some patients who are anxious.

Disrobe the patient from the waist down. Place the patient in the prone jackknife position on a proctoscopy table if one is available (Figure 60-3A). If the patient is unable to get in this position, or only a routine examination table or stretcher is available, place the patient in the left lateral decubitus or Sims position (Figure 60-3B). The examiner should be prepared with an impermeable gown and one glove on the left hand and two on the right hand (if right handed). If possible, it is helpful to have someone assist with the remainder of this procedure. Place the fenestrated drape over the patient so that the buttocks are completely exposed (Figure 60-3). Place a Mayo stand or bedside procedure table within reach of the patient's buttocks.

As in anoscopy, it is important to carefully inspect the entire perineum and anal verge prior to the examination. Many types of pathology such as fissures, fistulas, hemorrhoids, condylomata, and dermatologic conditions may be seen at this time.

Digital rectal examination prior to the procedure with a well-lubricated, gloved finger is mandatory. It gives the following advantages. It allows the examiner to find pathology that is better palpated than viewed. It gives the examiner the size and angle of the anal canal. It will allow the examiner to identify if the patient has tenderness that would preclude the examination. It may identify pathology so that the examiner can focus in a specific area. It prelubricates the anal canal, making insertion of the rigid rectosigmoidoscope easier. If the patient has pain from excoriation, 2% lidocaine jelly can be

used as a lubricant and will provide some local anesthesia. This examination is usually performed with the right hand. Remove the extra glove from the dominant hand before picking up the rigid sigmoidoscope. This prevents the contaminated glove from holding the scope near the examiner's face.

It is important to check the equipment prior to its insertion into the patient. Open the tray and place the instruments and supplies on the Mayo stand. The eyepiece on the proximal end of the scope should open easily, close easily, and seal against the rigid rectosigmoidoscope. Open the eyepiece and insert the obturator completely within the rigid sigmoidoscope. The handle, including the light source, must be firmly attached. Turn on the light source. The light must be seen coming from the end of the scope. The bulb of the insufflator must pump air into the rigid rectosigmoidoscope and should reinflate after the bulb is released. Liberally lubricate the distal 5 cm of the rigid rectosigmoidoscope and the obturator. Reinsert the obturator into the rigid rectosigmoidoscope.

TECHNIQUE

Stand to the left side of or directly behind the patient. Place the left, or nondominant, hand on the patient's buttocks (Figure 60-4A). Grasp the handle of the rigid rectosigmoidoscope with the right, or dominant, hand. Place the right thumb on the obturator to keep it properly seated (Figure 60-4B). Spread the buttocks with the left hand (Figure 60-4). Insert the rigid rectosigmoidoscope into the anus and aimed towards the patient's umbilicus. Advance it to the 5 cm mark (Figure 60-6A).

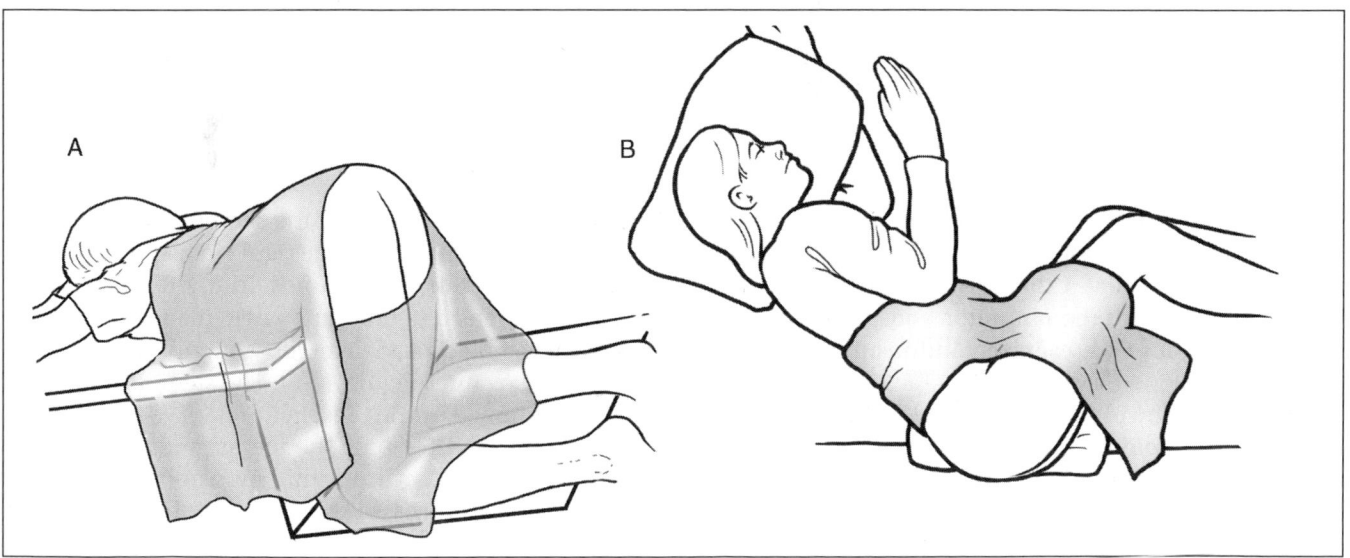

FIGURE 60-3 Patient positioning. *A.* The prone jackknife position on a proctoscopy table. *B.* The left lateral decubitus position on an examination table with the buttocks extended over the edge of the table. Note that the drape is placed so that the buttocks are completely exposed.

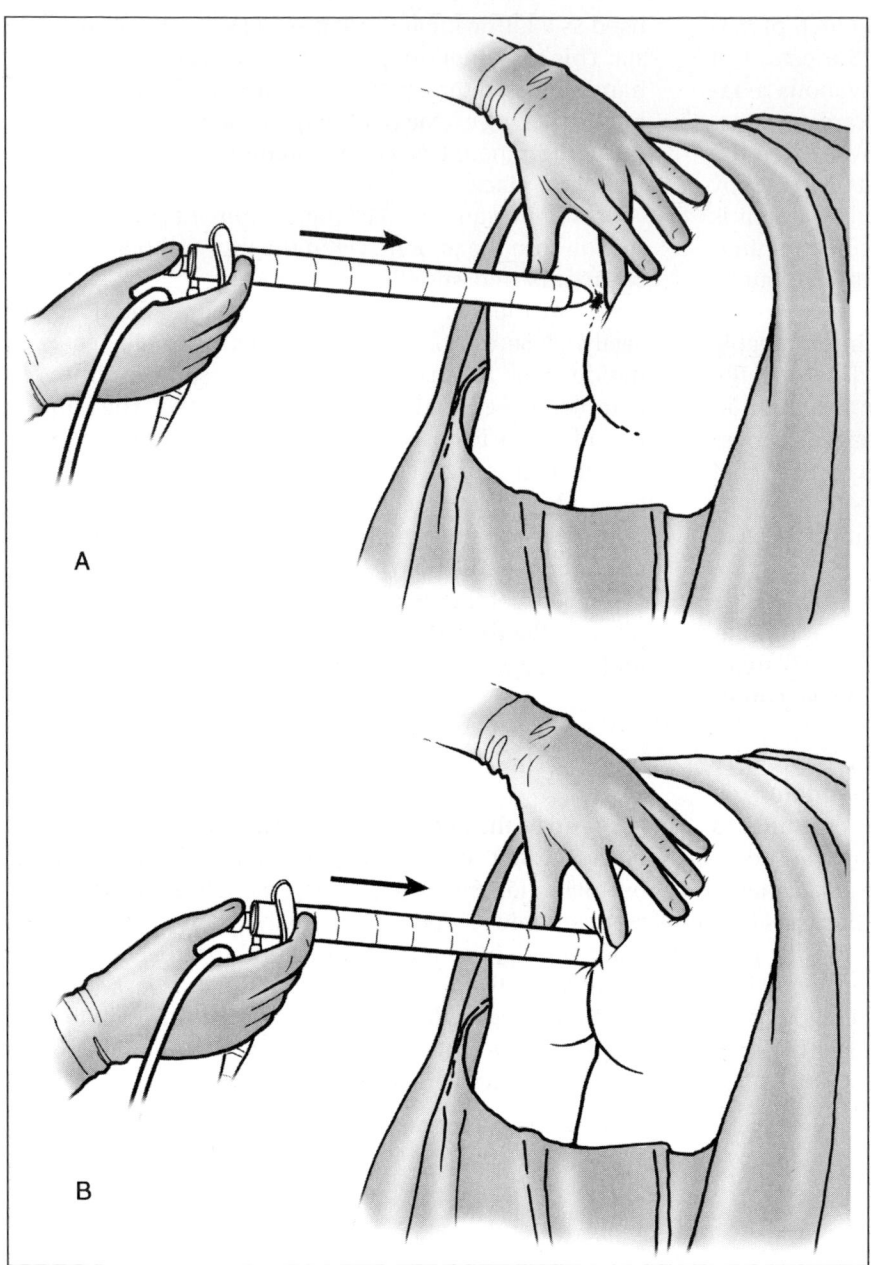

FIGURE 60-4 Insertion of the rigid rectosigmoidoscope. *A*. The left (nondominant) hand is placed on the buttocks and used to spread the buttocks. *B*. The right (dominant) hand is used to insert and advance the scope while the thumb keeps the obturator properly seated.

Support the rigid rectosigmoidoscope at the anus with the left hand (Figure 60-5*A*). This is necessary so that if the patient moves, the instrument will move with the patient. Remove the obturator and place it on the Mayo stand. Close the eyepiece and insufflate air into the rectum.

One must control the insertion and direction of the rigid rectosigmoidoscope with the right hand while stabilizing it with the left hand (Figure 60-5*A*). Continue to slowly advance the rigid rectosigmoidoscope under direct viewing while simultaneously insufflating air to distend the walls of the colon (Figure 60-5*A*). The anal canal is approximately 4 to 5 cm in length (Figure 60-6). The rectum will be seen to turn somewhat posteri-

orly and follow the hollow of the sacrum (Figure 60-5*B*). Moving the right hand and the rigid rectosigmoidoscope anteriorly will direct the tip posteriorly (Figure 60-6*B*). Use the left hand as a fulcrum to help maneuver the distal tip of the rigid rectosigmoidoscope to follow the lumen of the rectum (Figure 60-6). The sigmoid colon can also be identified by the presence of transverse folds that are lacking in the rectum. The rectosigmoid junction is approximately 16 cm from the anus and can be seen when the lumen turns anteriorly and to the right (Figure 60-6*C*). It is necessary to use the rigid rectosigmoidoscope to gently straighten the colon while completely inserting the instrument to a depth of 25 centimeters. **It is important to view the bowel lumen at all times. Never**

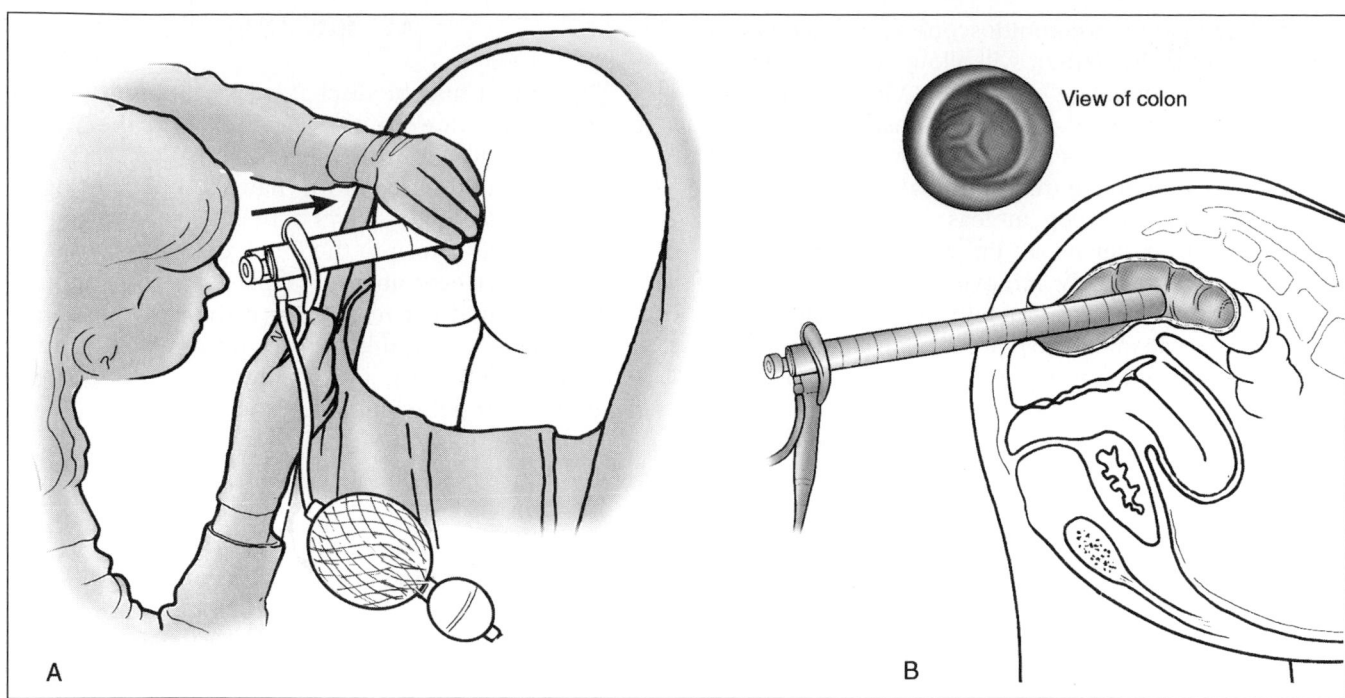

FIGURE 60-5 Advancement of the rigid rectosigmoidoscope. *A.* The nondominant hand stabilizes the scope while the dominant hand advances it under direct visualization. *B.* The rectum begins as the anal canal turns posteriorly towards the sacrum.

advance the instrument blindly as this may cause a perforation.

Maintain communication with the patient, inform them of what is happening, and elicit the status of their comfort. Open the eyepiece if it becomes clouded with moisture and wipe it with dry gauze so the view is kept clear. Do not keep your face near the eyepiece when opening the eyepiece. The insufflated air may forcefully expel stool and secretions. The bowel must be reinflated when the eyepiece is reclosed.

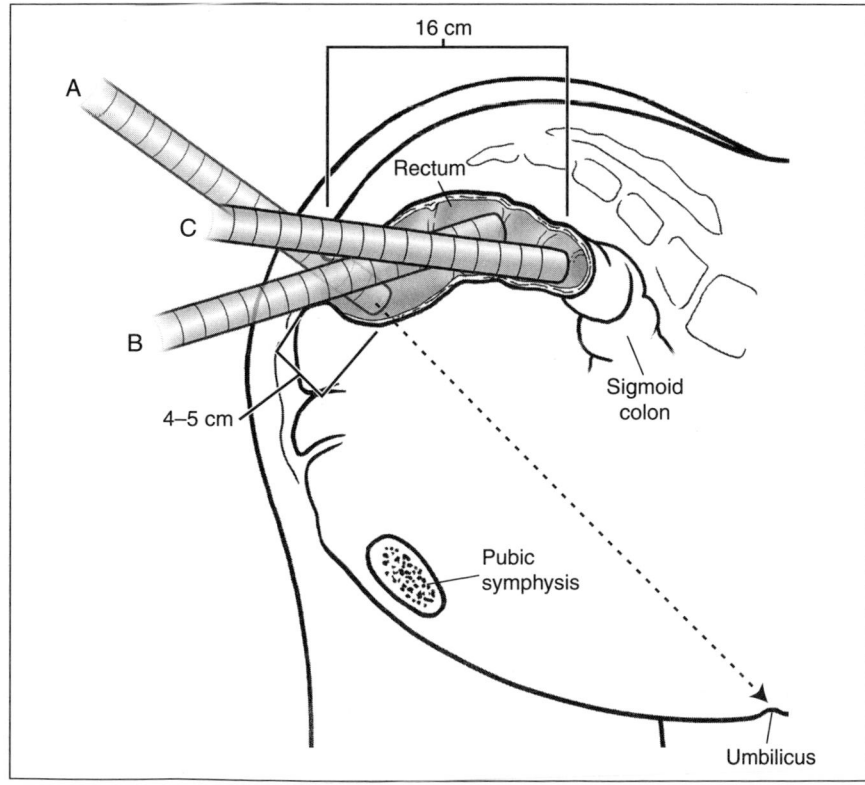

FIGURE 60-6 Insertion and advancement of the rigid rectosigmoidoscope. *A.* The scope is inserted and aimed towards the umbilicus. *B.* Moving the handle anteriorly will direct the tip of the scope posteriorly. *C.* The rectosigmoid junction is located approximately 16 cm from the anus, where the rectal lumen turns anteriorly and to the right.

After the rigid rectosigmoidoscope is advanced to 25 cm, or as far as the patient will allow, slowly remove it with a circular motion (Figure 60-7). View the mucosa while removing the rigid rectosigmoidoscope in a circular motion. This flattens out the haustra and valves of Houston so that the entire mucosal surface can be viewed. Attempt to keep at least 50 percent of the colonic lumen in view at all times. Open the eyepiece just prior to completely removing the rigid rectosigmoidoscope to release as much of the insufflated air as possible. This will make the patient more comfortable.

The viewing window, which seals in the air, must be opened if it is necessary to biopsy or to grasp something. This will result in the collapse of the rectum and loss of view. It is important to place the tip of the rigid rectosigmoidoscope over the area in question so it will stay in the examiner's view. The obturator should be reinserted if it is necessary to reinsert or readvance the rigid rectosigmoidoscope.

ASSESSMENT

Completely and carefully inspect the colonic mucosa. Note the presence, location (anterior, posterior, left, right), and depth of any bleeding, diverticulum, fistulas, hemorrhoids, lesions, masses, mucosal irregularities, and/or polyps. Document any findings in the medical record.

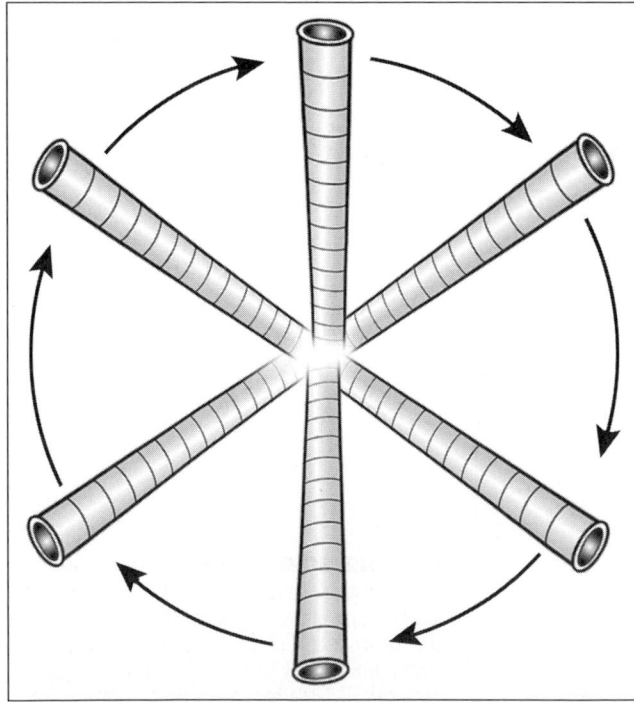

FIGURE 60-7 The rigid rectosigmoidoscope is rotated in a circular motion while simultaneously withdrawing the scope and visualizing the mucosa.

AFTERCARE

The patient may be discharged home after the procedure if there are no complications and there is no other reason to admit them to the hospital. They may experience mild discomfort, flatus, and spotting of blood in the stool for several hours. Instruct the patient to immediately return to the Emergency Department if they develop a fever, abdominal pain, nausea, vomiting, bright red blood per rectum, or if they have any concerns. Follow-up should be arranged with a Family Practitioner, Internist, Gastroenterologist, or Surgeon depending upon the findings of the examination.

COMPLICATIONS

The primary complication of rigid rectosigmoidoscopy is perforation of the rectum or sigmoid colon. Air insufflation may cause an existing perforation, such as may be associated with diverticulitis, to burst, and is the reason one should not perform this examination if the patient has existing peritonitis. Perforation can occur with forceful insertion of the instrument without viewing the colonic lumen or if the patient moves suddenly and the scope is not supported with the left hand. Perforation may also occur with instrumentation in related procedures, such as a biopsy. Perforation should be almost nonexistent if one supports the scope well, views the colonic lumen while advancing the scope, and listens to the patient about complaints of pain.

Minor complications may occur. Trauma to the mucosa from the rigid rectosigmoidoscope or instrumentation in related procedures, such as a biopsy, can result in minor bleeding that is usually self-limited. Brisk bleeding can be controlled by the judicious use of a silver nitrate matchstick. Bacteremia may occur in up to 10 percent of patients. Antibiotic prophylaxis for endocarditis should be administered, if indicated, prior to the procedure. Mild abdominal discomfort and flatus can last a few hours.

SUMMARY

Rigid rectosigmoidoscopy is inexpensive, easy to perform, and useful in bowels with poor preparation or where a wider access is needed. These characteristics make the instrument useful in many indications. With proper training and understanding of the anatomy, this examination is well tolerated by the patient and will be useful to diagnose and treat many colonic and rectal problems.

REFERENCES

1. Pearl RK: *Gastrointestinal Endoscopy for Surgeons.* Boston: Little, Brown, 1984.

Chapter 61
RECTAL FOREIGN BODY EXTRACTION

Charles Orsay

INTRODUCTION

Foreign bodies within the rectum are the result of an ingestion from above or are placed into the anus from below.[1] Fortunately, the majority of items ingested from above that pass the pylorus and ileocecal valve also pass the anal sphincter. The most frequent types of items found in the anus from above are undigested fish or chicken bones. Foreign bodies that are placed into the rectum from the anus are placed iatrogenically (enema tips and thermometers), inserted by the patient in an attempt to remove impacted stool, inserted by the patient or their partner as a form of anorectal auto-eroticism, forcibly placed in the anus during a rape, or placed in the rectum to smuggle objects across a border illegally.

The items placed into the rectum from the anus seem to be limitless and represent all the shapes and sizes imaginable.[2] This makes their removal more difficult. **It is important to attempt to identify the characteristics of the foreign body in order to devise the safest way of removal.** As an example, consider the typical electric lightbulb. The glue that attaches the metal base to the glass loosens with moisture and time. Pulling off the metal base exposes a thin, sharp glass edge. The glass globe is very thin and breaks very easily. If the glass breaks, it may take a long time to remove the fragments and cause considerable damage to the surrounding rectal mucosa or the examining finger. The idea is to remove the foreign body without causing further damage to the rectum or the anal sphincter muscle. The more knowledge the physician has about the foreign body and how it was inserted, the more likely it is that it will be removed safely.

ANATOMY AND PATHOPHYSIOLOGY

The significant anatomy of the anal canal is discussed in Chapter 59, describing the anatomy for anoscopy. Important anatomic considerations in removing rectal foreign bodies include the axis of the lumen of the anus. The anus is pointed toward the patient's umbilicus, while the curve of the sacrum forms a posterior arc. If the length of the foreign body is longer than the curve of the sacrum, such as a long vibrator or dildo, the sacral promontory causes the distal end of the foreign body to be directed toward the tip of the sacrum or coccyx. When the object is being removed by bringing the distal end anteriorly, the middle portion may push anteriorly (into the prostate, uterus, or bladder) and cause considerable discomfort.

The important physiologic considerations include the anal sphincter muscles, edema, and the creation of a vacuum. The anal sphincter is a complex group of muscles. The external anal sphincter muscle is made up of voluntary muscle fibers. The internal anal sphincter muscle is made of smooth muscle fibers. The reflex response to dilatation of the rectum is contraction of the external anal sphincter muscle. The normal tone of the anal sphincter comes from the internal anal sphincter, which can go into spasm with manipulation. Therefore it is very important to try to remove foreign bodies with slow and steady traction. Maintain constant pressure and wait for the sphincter muscle to fatigue. The technique is not too dissimilar to the methods used to relocate a shoulder. The slow and constant traction will also help with the edema that forms around rectal foreign bodies that have remained in the rectum for a prolonged period of time. Finally, it is important to consider the formation of a vacuum, which may result from pulling a large, smooth foreign body such as a bottle or lightbulb. It is sometimes necessary to place one or more soft catheters above the foreign body so that air may get around the object as it is removed. This will prevent the formation of a vacuum and allow the foreign body to be removed. Large Foley catheters with the balloon inflated can be used for air insertion to prevent the vacuum and traction to bring the object further down into the rectum.

INDICATIONS

The indication to remove a foreign body from the rectum is the identification of a foreign body in the rectum. The majority of patients with this problem have already tried to pass the item with a bowel movement. They may also have already tried oral laxatives. It is impossible to estimate the number of rectal foreign bodies that are removed at home. It is estimated that very few objects inserted through the anus will pass spontaneously. Waiting is detrimental for the vast majority of items. Sharp foreign bodies may already have begun to perforate the rectum. Large foreign bodies will continue to cause irritation and edema, making removal more difficult with the passage of time.

CONTRAINDICATIONS

There are a few absolute contraindications to removing a rectal foreign body in the Emergency Department. However, the removal of a rectal foreign body that has not perforated is not an emergency. Time taken to plan the removal and obtain adequate anesthesia and relaxation of the anal sphincter muscles is well spent if the object is not easily retrieved. The patient's general condition must be taken into account. Patients with peritonitis require operative removal and exploration. The time taken to remove the object is wasted and identification of the perforation is easier in the Operating Room with the item in place. Patients with lower abdominal pain and fever may have a perforation below the peritoneum that can be confirmed with a water-soluble contrast enema. Foreign bodies that are large, irregularly shaped, or have sharp edges should be extracted in the Operating Room. In patients who have been assaulted, a complete assessment of all the patient's injuries is mandatory. It usually is better to leave the object in place to help identify all the possible associated injuries that may have occurred. The foreign body should be removed in the Operating Room if it is not palpable, not visible upon dilating the anus, or removal of the object may cause injury to the patient. Packets containing illicit

drugs should be extracted with a rigid rectosigmoidoscope or in the Operating Room. Rupture of the packets can result in significant morbidity and mortality.

EQUIPMENT

Local anesthetic solution with epinephrine (1% lidocaine or 0.5% bupivacaine)
25 gauge needle, 2 inches long
10 mL syringe
Anoscope
Ring forceps
Tenaculum
Park retractor
Hill-Ferguson retractor
Large spoons
Foley catheters
Endotracheal tubes
Endoscopic snare
Rigid rectosigmoidoscope
Vacuum extractor (optional)

PATIENT PREPARATION

The patient must undergo a complete history and physical examination. It is important to ascertain the overall health of the patient in case it is necessary to go to the Operating Room to extract the foreign body. **Attempt to identify patients with rectal perforations as they need to go to Operating Room quickly.** Biplane plain radiographs with an upright are useful to determine the number, shape, and location of the foreign bodies as well as the presence of free air under the diaphragm. It is necessary to look at both the anteroposterior view as well as the lateral view to completely appreciate the object in three dimensions.[1] It is important to inform the patient in advance that while 90 percent of the objects can be removed from below, some may require general anesthesia or even an operation and a temporary colostomy. Explain the local anesthesia and the extraction procedures to the patient and/or their representative. Obtain an informed consent for the extraction of the foreign body.

Ascertain the type and number of objects in the rectum. It is possible to remove one foreign body and miss others that the physician was not aware were present. Unfortunately, it is common to find that the patient is unsure of this part of the history; this is why plain radiographs can be so helpful. It is also important to identify the technique of insertion. Patients with objects that were inserted forcefully should undergo a traumaoriented workup, and sexual abuse must be considered. Determine the length of time since insertion. Edema formation will be significant if the object has been present more than 24 hours. This will make it more likely that an anesthetic will be needed or that it will be necessary to use catheters to break the vacuum that forms during extraction.

The parts of the physical examination that are most helpful are the abdominal and rectal examinations. The abdominal examination should focus on the presence or absence of tenderness, peritonitis, and the palpation of a mass. Many objects are long enough to be palpated in the left lower quadrant. It may be useful to apply pressure on the lower portion of the abdomen to help remove the object. The rectal examination should include a careful external examination looking for evidence of trauma. The digital portion of the examination should roughly quantify the sphincter tone and squeeze pressure.

The remainder of the examination should consist of careful palpation of the foreign body to determine its location, texture, and mobility and to identify possible areas to grasp. Examples would include the open end of a bottle or the narrow end of a lightbulb. Determining if the object is hard, soft rubber, or plastic will help determine which tool would be best suited to grasp the object. One exception to performing the digital rectal examination would be determining, on radiographs or by history, whether the object is sharp (such as a knife blade) or consists of broken glass. Some physicians recommend postponing the digital rectal examination, especially in prisoners and psychiatric patients, until a radiograph rules out a sharp foreign body. If the examiner is not able to palpate the foreign body, a rigid rectosigmoidoscope should be used to identify and remove the object. The technique of rigid rectosigmoidoscopy is described in Chapter 60.

ANESTHESIA

The second general consideration is to have a relaxed anal sphincter. The use of intravenous or procedural sedation will relax the patient and relieve any discomfort associated with the procedure. It may be necessary to inject the anus with local anesthetic solution if the patient experiences pain or if slow steady traction will not overcome the tone of the anal sphincter.[3,4] Anesthesia of the sphincter muscles will provide for patient comfort and allow dilation of the sphincter muscles. Place the patient in the lithotomy position (Figure 61-1A). Inject local anesthetic solution subcutaneously and circumferentially around the anus (Figure 61-1A). Inject 1 to 1.5 mL of local anesthetic solution into the anal sphincter muscles at the 12, 3, 6, and 9 o'clock positions (Figure 61-1B).

An alternative is a pudendal nerve block. Determine if the ischial spines are palpable through the rectum. Insert the needle through the skin and towards the ischial spine. Use the finger inside the rectum to palpate and guide the needle to the ischial spine. Inject 3 to 5 mL of local anesthetic solution just medial to the ischial spine. Repeat this procedure on the other side. The main disadvantage of the pudendal nerve block is that it is a blind procedure and has the potential for a needle stick. If these are not successful, it will be necessary to take the patient to the Operating Room for regional or general anesthesia.

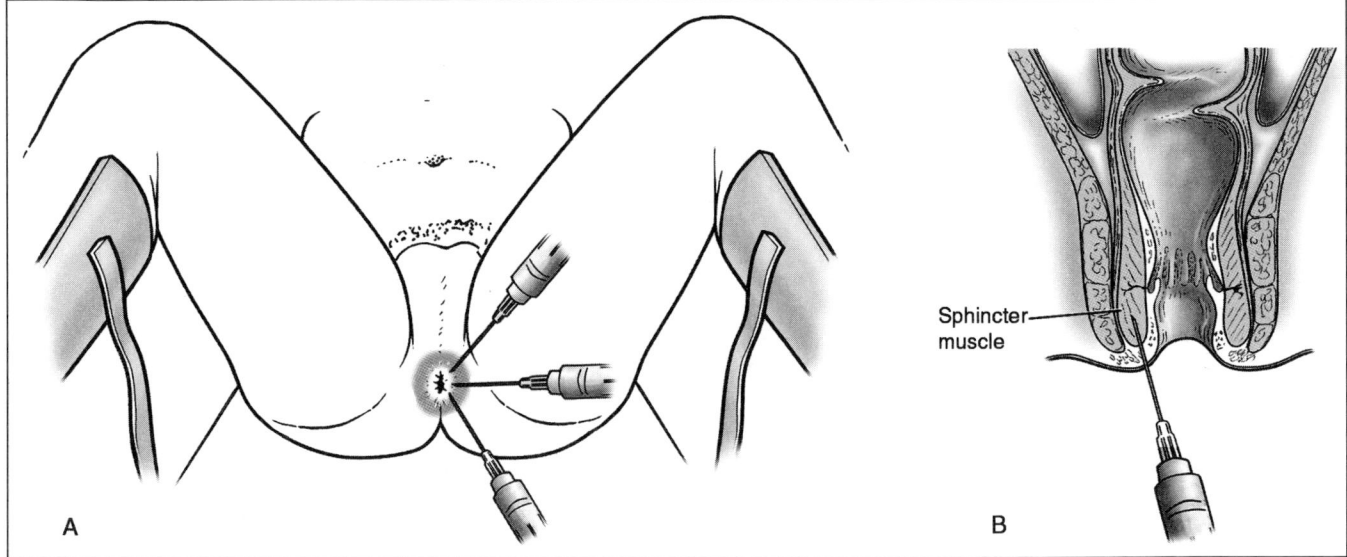

FIGURE 61-1 Anesthesia of the anal region. *A.* Local anesthetic solution is infiltrated subcutaneously and circumferentially around the anus. *B.* Injection of local anesthetic solution into the anal sphincter muscles.

The patient may remain in the lithotomy position for the extraction of the foreign body (Figure 61-2A). Other positions include the modified Lloyd Davies position (Figure 61-2B) and the Sims position (Figure 61-2C). The choice of positions is physician dependent and limited by patient comfort.

TECHNIQUES

It is important to understand that since the types of foreign bodies found in the rectum are so variable, it is impossible to give exact instructions on how to remove them. There are some general considerations to remember. The first is to visualize the foreign body. Gentle suprapubic pressure will often push the foreign body into the distal rectum. The distal end of the foreign body may get caught along the curve of the sacrum. Place a finger in the rectum to redirect the orientation of the foreign body. The second consideration is to grasp the object. Sometimes an object is low-lying and may be grasped with gloved fingers. The object can then be removed by gentle continuous traction. Low-lying objects may be soft enough to be grasped with an instrument. **It is necessary to do this under direct vi-**

sion so that the rectum will not be damaged in the attempt to grasp the foreign body. Hard, low-lying objects made of metal or plastic may be grasped with a tenaculum.

Insert two well-lubricated fingers into the anesthetized anus and gently dilate the anal sphincter muscles. The anus can be maintained in the open position by the insertion of a Park retractor (Figure 61-3A) or a Hill-Ferguson retractor (Figure 61-3B). An anoscope or vaginal speculum may be used if these retractors are not readily available in the Emergency Department. View the distal end of the foreign body. **Never insert instruments unless the foreign body is visualized. Blind insertion of instruments may push the foreign body more proximally. Never grasp a foreign body blindly. This can cause injury to the rectum upon removal of the instrument if the rectal mucosa is entrapped between the instrument and the foreign body.**

DIGITAL EXTRACTION TECHNIQUE

Foreign bodies within reach may be grasped with the fingers and extracted. This often proves very difficult as the foreign body will be coated with lubricant, mucus, and/or stool. Instruct the patient to bear down as if having a bowel movement. The intraabdominal pres-

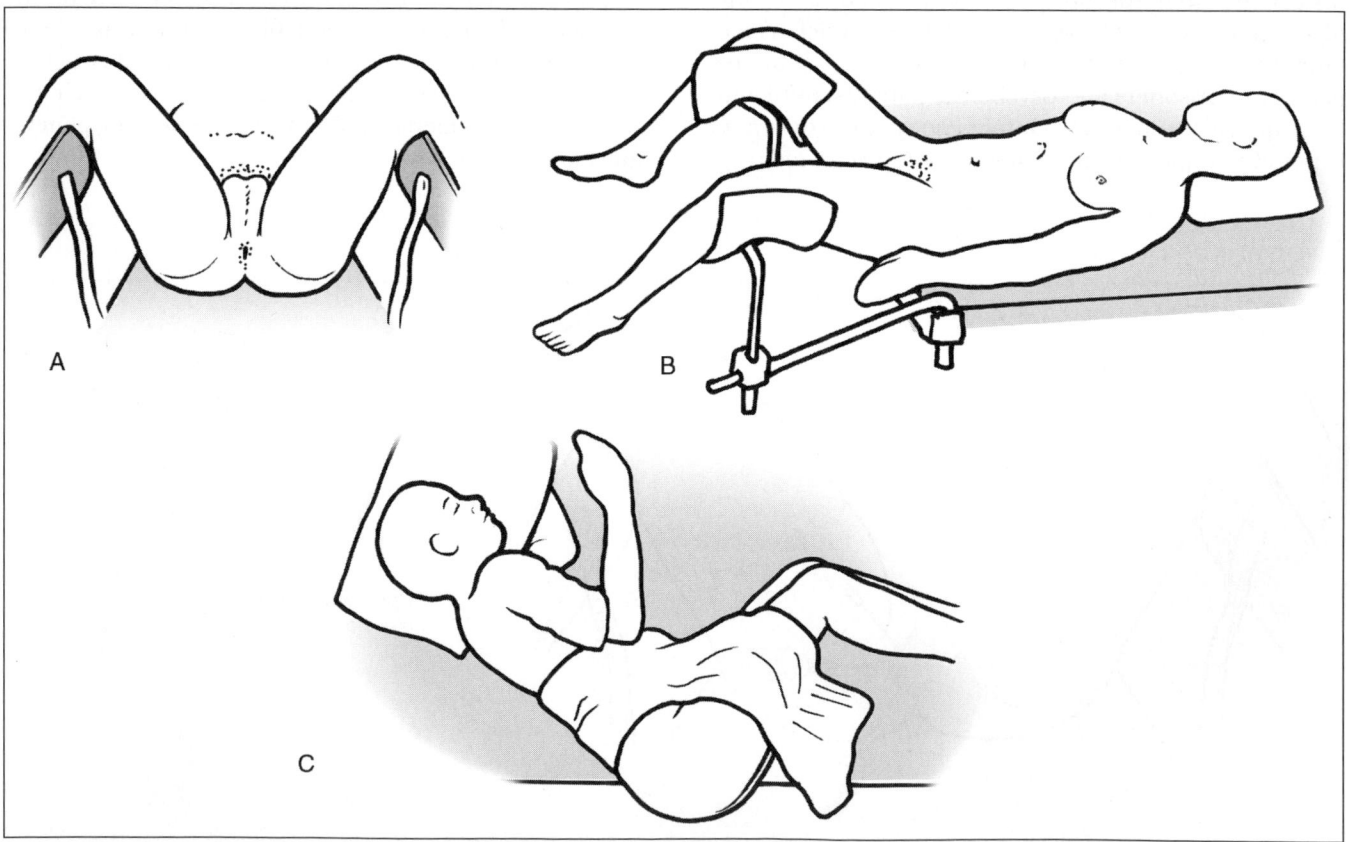

FIGURE 61-2 Patient positioning for removal of rectal foreign bodies. *A.* Lithotomy position. *B.* Modified Lloyd Davies position. *C.* Sims or lateral decubitus position.

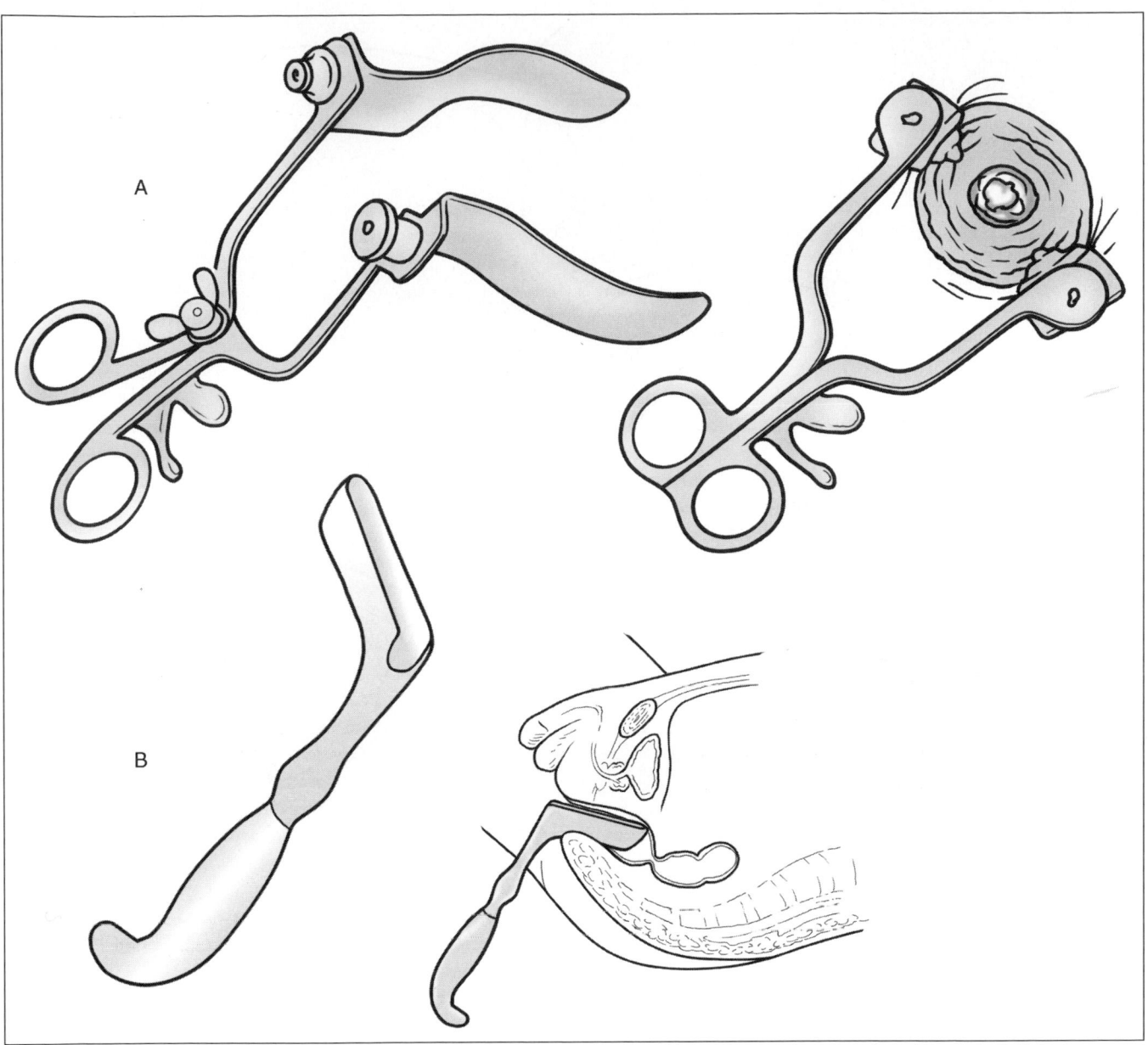

FIGURE 61-3 Retractors placed in the anus allow for better exposure and easier extraction of the foreign body. *A.* The Park retractor. *B.* The Hill-Ferguson retractor.

sure generated in this way may expel the foreign body. The foreign body may become entrapped against the sacrum. Insert a finger into the rectum to dislodge the foreign body from against the sacrum as the patient continues to bear down. Attempt one of the techniques described below if digital extraction is ineffective.

FOLEY CATHETER TECHNIQUE

A Foley catheter has been successfully used to aid in the extraction of rectal foreign bodies.[5–7] This is especially helpful if the foreign body is made of glass, an inverted bottle or can, large, or present for more than 12 to 24 hours. Pulling these types of foreign bodies can result in the formation of a vacuum proximally and inhibit their extraction.

Liberally lubricate a Foley catheter. Insert the Foley catheter between the foreign body and the rectal mucosa. Advance the catheter until the balloon is proximal to the foreign body (Figure 61-4*A*). Inflate the balloon with 30 mL of saline or water. Inject air with a syringe through the Foley catheter to break the vacuum proximal to the foreign body. Remove the syringe so that air can move freely through the Foley catheter and prevent a vacuum from becoming reestablished. Apply constant, gentle, and steady traction to the Foley catheter. This will prevent the foreign body from migrating proximally. It

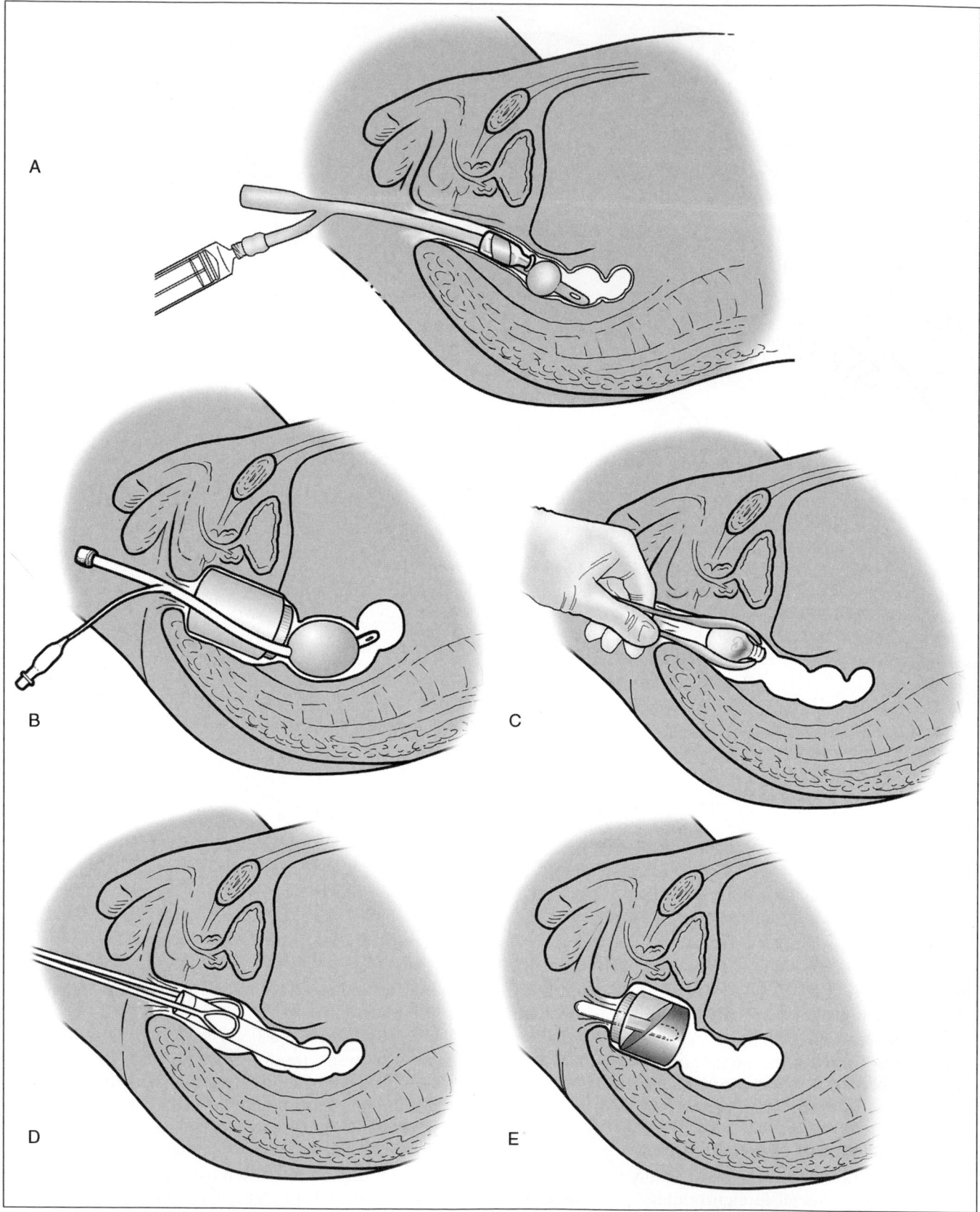

FIGURE 61-4 A sampling of methods to remove rectal foreign bodies. *A*. Foley catheter technique. *B*. Endotracheal tube technique. *C*. Spoons to remove a fragile object. *D*. Ring forceps technique. *E*. Plaster and a tongue depressor are placed in a jar. After the plaster cures, the tongue depressor can be used as a handle to remove the jar.

may also move the foreign body distally so that it can be grasped and extracted with fingers or an instrument. The use of two to four circumferentially placed Foley catheters may apply evenly distributed traction to extract the foreign body more easily.

ENDOTRACHEAL TUBE TECHNIQUE

An endotracheal tube has been used in place of a Foley catheter by some physicians (Figure 61-4*B*). The advantage of using an endotracheal tube is that it is relatively stiff and can apply more traction than a Foley catheter to help remove the foreign body. Unfortunately, there are also disadvantages. The endotracheal tube is larger and less flexible than a Foley catheter. This may result in difficulty advancing it past the foreign body. The larger and stiffer endotracheal tube can more easily lacerate the rectal mucosa and perforate the rectum. For these reasons, the use of an endotracheal tube cannot be recommended.

SPOON TECHNIQUE

The removal of smooth, round, fragile, or glass foreign bodies can be problematic. This can include lightbulbs, balls, fruits, and vegetables. These foreign bodies can be extracted with a pair of large spoons. Liberally lubricate the posterior surface of a pair of spoons. Insert a Foley catheter to eliminate the vacuum proximal to the foreign body. Insert the spoons until they are cupping the foreign body (Figure 61-4*C*). Grasp and gently squeeze the handles of the spoons so that they hold the foreign body. Withdraw the spoons and the foreign body.

A more readily available alternative to large spoons are obstetric forceps. These have also been successfully used to extract a rectal foreign body. **The use of obstetric forceps cannot be recommended due to their large size, unfamiliarity to most physicians, and the potential to perforate the rectum.**

RING FORCEPS OR TENACULUM TECHNIQUE

Rectal foreign bodies that are not fragile may be grasped with a ring forceps or tenaculum and then extracted. Insert a Foley catheter to eliminate the vacuum proximal to the foreign body. Firmly grasp the foreign body with a ring forceps or a tenaculum (Figure 61-4*D*). **This must be performed under direct visualization to ensure that the rectal mucosa is not entrapped between the instrument and the foreign body.** Apply gentle, firm traction to extract the foreign body.

VACUUM EXTRACTION TECHNIQUE

A vacuum dart or obstetrical vacuum extractor may be used to extract a rectal foreign body.[6,8] Emergency Physicians are usually not trained in the proper use of a vacuum extraction device. It may be beneficial to have an Obstetrician, Gynecologist, Family Practitioner with obstetric experience, or a Nurse Midwife to assist with this technique. Insert a Foley catheter to eliminate the vacuum proximal to the foreign body. Place the vacuum cup of the device onto the foreign body. **Ensure that none of the rectal mucosa is entrapped between the rim of the suction cup and the foreign body.** Apply the suction to seal the cup against the foreign body. **Recheck to ensure that none of the rectal mucosa has become entrapped.** Apply steady traction to extract the foreign body.

MISCELLANEOUS TECHNIQUES

Numerous other techniques have been devised to remove a rectal foreign body.[9–12] These include the use of proctoscopes and snares, de Pezzer catheters, cyanoacrylate glue, clamps covered with rubber tubing, a tonsil snare, Sengstaken-Blakemore tubes, and plaster of Paris. Cyanoacrylate glue can be used to attach a handle to the foreign body. The foreign body can be extracted by withdrawing the handle after the glue has dried. A Sengstaken-Blakemore tube can be inserted into a foreign body with a small opening (glass bottle, soda can, etc.). Inflate the balloons and apply traction to extract the foreign body. Plaster of Paris can be used to fill a hollow object and allowed to harden around a tongue blade (Figure 61-4*E*). This is analogous to making a popsicle on a stick. The major disadvantage of using plaster of Paris is that it generates heat as it hardens. This heat may damage the rectal mucosa or shatter a glass bottle. The technique used and the choice of devices are limited only by one's imagination.

ASSESSMENT

Examine the rectum with a rigid rectosigmoidoscope to assess the mucosa for tears or perforations after the foreign body is extracted. Some physicians believe that this examination is not necessary if the patient is asymptomatic, the foreign body is smooth, it was extracted atraumatically, and no complications arose from the extraction procedure. These patients may be discharged with follow-up as an outpatient for rectosigmoidoscopy. If obvious damage to the mucosa exists, the patients should remain in the hospital for observation. The patient should remain NPO and be prepared for possible surgery. Other indications for admissions include abdominal pain, significant bleeding, or the suspicion of a rectal perforation. Broad-spectrum intravenous antibiotics should be administered if a rectal perforation is suspected.

Perform a digital rectal examination to document the presence and quality of anal sphincter tone after the procedure. This should be delayed until the effects of any general, local, or regional anesthesia have dissipated. Rectal tone that is decreased or diminished from the initial (preprocedural) digital rectal examination requires the consultation of a General or Colorectal Surgeon.

AFTERCARE

Patients may be discharged home after the extraction procedure if they are asymptomatic, have normal rectal tone, and have no complications demonstrated on rigid rectosigmoidoscopy. They should be instructed to return to the Emergency Department immediately if they develop abdominal pain, pelvic pain, bright red blood per rectum, or a fever.

COMPLICATIONS

The major complications include rectal bleeding, rectal perforation, and damage to the anal sphincter. **Since the patient may very well have presented with these complications, it is important to document them or their absence on the initial (preprocedural) examination.** Rectal bleeding is common after a difficult extraction. It is important to rule out a perforation. This can be performed with the rigid rectosigmoidoscope after the extraction. Most perforations occur at the rectosigmoid junction, approximately 15 to 16 cm from the anus. Perforation above the peritoneal reflection will result in peritonitis and free air noted under the diaphragm on upright plain radiographs. Perforation below the peritoneal reflection may take several days to manifest pelvic pain, signs of a pelvic abscess, or sepsis. If there is no evidence of perforation or significant mucosal damage, the patient may still be discharged. However, large amounts of bleeding or significant mucosal damage require observation at the least. A Gastrografin enema without the use of the balloon may be used to identify a perforation if there is significant concern that it exists. Patients with perforation of an unprepared rectum require surgical intervention and broad-spectrum intravenous antibiotics. Any evidence of acute sphincter damage requires a surgical evaluation for possible debridement. The majority of these lesions are observed, allowed to heal secondarily, and then repaired surgically.

SUMMARY

The majority of rectal foreign bodies can undergo transanal extraction. Removal of rectal foreign bodies should include an appropriate history and physical;

biplane abdominal radiographs; relaxation of the anal sphincter; firm attachment to the foreign body and slow, firm traction extraction; and postextraction rectosigmoidoscopy. Inpatient observation is indicated if the rectal mucosa is traumatized. The patient should be taken to the Operating Room if the foreign body cannot be removed in the Emergency Department, for pain control, if a perforation is suspected, or if removal may result in secondary injury.

REFERENCES

1. Kingsley AN, Abcarian H: Colorectal foreign bodies: management update. *Dis Colon Rectum* 1985; 28(12):941–944.
2. Busch DB, Starling JR: Rectal foreign bodies: case reports and a comprehensive review of the world's literature. *Surgery* 1986; 100(3):512–519.
3. Sohn N, Weinstein M: Office removal of foreign bodies in the rectum. *Surg Gynecol Obstet* 1978; 146(2):209–210.
4. Schecter WP, Albo RJ: Removal of rectal foreign bodies, in Nyhus LM, Baker RJ, Fischer JE (eds): *Mastery of Surgery,* 3rd ed. Boston: Little, Brown, 1997:1555–1559.
5. Simon RR, Brenner BE: *Emergency Procedures and Techniques,* 3rd ed. Baltimore: Williams & Wilkins, 1994:27–28.
6. Diwan V: Removal of 100-watt electric bulb from rectum. *Ann Emerg Med* 1982; 11(11):643–644.
7. Garber H, Rubin R, Eisenstat T: Removal of a glass foreign body from the rectum. *Dis Colon Rectum* 1981; 24(4):323.
8. Mackinnon RP: Removing rectal foreign bodies: is the ventouse gender specific? *Med J Aust* 1998; 169:670–671.
9. Kantarian JC, Riether RD, Sheets JA, et al: Endoscopic retrieval of foreign bodies from the rectum. *Dis Colon Rectum* 1987; 30(11):902–904.
10. Siroospour D, Dragstedt L: A large foreign body removed intact through the anus: report of a case. *Dis Colon Rectum* 1975; 18(7):616–619.
11. Steven K, Lykke, J, Hansen T: A simple suction device for removing foreign bodies in the rectum. *Br J Surg* 1979; 66(6):418.
12. Hughes J, Marice H, Gathwright J: Method of removing a hollow object from the rectum. *Dis Colon Rectum* 1976; 19(1):44–45.

Section Five

ORTHOPEDIC AND MUSCULOSKELETAL PROCEDURES

Chapter 62
BURSITIS AND TENDONITIS THERAPY

Teresita M. Hogan
Dedra R. Tolson

INTRODUCTION

Musculoskeletal complaints are frequently lumped into the wastebasket diagnoses of bursitis and tendonitis. Patients are often begun on nonsteroidal anti-inflammatory drugs with orthopedic follow-up in a few days. However, joint and soft tissue injections are diagnostically and therapeutically powerful interventions that are effective for patients with musculoskeletal complaints. These injections are a critical component of a multifaceted treatment regimen that should be in the arsenal of the trained Emergency Physician.

The techniques of aspiration and injection are easily mastered. These injections are both safe and effective if appropriate guidelines are followed.[1] The effectiveness of injection therapy is dependent upon "hitting the target structure," followed by a comprehensive rehabilitation program. In selected patients, the Emergency Physician may begin definitive care by administration of a steroid injection. The clinical response to injectable corticosteroids is generally quite positive.[2–5]

ANATOMY AND PATHOPHYSIOLOGY

Bursae are round, flat, pad-like sacs or cavities in connective tissue. They are usually found in the vicinity of joints, at areas of friction, or in areas of possible impingement. Bursae are lined with a synovial membrane and contain synovial fluid. They act to reduce friction. There are approximately 160 bursae in the body. Tendons are fibrous connective tissue bands attaching muscles to bones. A synovial sheath containing synovial fluid surrounds most tendons.

Tendonitis and bursitis are inflammations of these respective structures. They are grouped together because the patient's history, symptomatology, physical examination findings, and the treatment for these two inflammatory processes often overlap.

Corticosteroid injections serve to decrease inflammation, provide pain control, and promote healing. The goal of injection into joints, tendon sheaths, and bursae is to attain concentrated synovial fluid steroid levels to maximize the local anti-inflammatory effect while minimizing systemic effects.

INDICATIONS

Injections of corticosteroids should be performed for an inflammatory bursitis or synovitis when systemic therapy is contraindicated (renal failure, cardiac failure, hypertension, or diabetes) and as an adjunct to physical therapy or systemic therapy. Many conditions, including articular and nonarticular processes, are improved with local corticosteroid injection therapy.[1,6,7] The articular processes that are helped by injection therapy include rheumatoid arthritis, spondyloarthropathy, ankylosing spondylitis, osteoarthritis, gout, and pseudogout. Joint injection in patients with these conditions should usually be deferred to the patient's Family Practitioner, Internist, or Rheumatologist. The nonarticular processes that are helped by injection therapy include bursitis, periarthritis, adhesive capsulitis, tenosynovitis, tendonitis, lateral and medial epicondylitis, plantar fasciitis, and neuritis.

CONTRAINDICATIONS

There are absolute and relative contraindications to corticosteroid injection therapy. The absolute contraindications include overlying cellulitis, septic arthritis, bacteremia, unstable joints, and joints containing prostheses. The relative contraindications include inaccessibility of the joint, joints requiring radiographic guidance to ensure proper needle placement, meniscal or labral tears as a cause of symptoms, joints with loose bodies as a cause of symptoms, coagulopathy, anticoagulant therapy, or more than three injections annually into a weight-bearing joint.

EQUIPMENT

Povidone iodine solution or swabs
Sterile gloves
Sterile drapes
18 gauge needles, 2 inches long
22 gauge needles, 2 inches long
23 gauge needles, 2 inches long
25 gauge needles, 2 inches long
Syringes (1 mL, 5 mL, 10 mL)
Injectable steroidal preparation (Table 62-1)
Lidocaine (1%) without epinephrine
Bupivacaine (0.25%) without epinephrine
Mepivacaine (1%) without epinephrine
Adhesive bandages

PATIENT PREPARATION

Explain the procedure, its risks, and its benefits to the patient and/or their representative. Obtain an informed consent to perform the procedure. Position the patient so that they are comfortable and the injection site is easily accessible. Identify the injection site according to anatomic landmarks. It may be necessary to outline structures with a black or red skin pencil when landmarks are difficult to palpate. Clean any dirt and debris from the skin. Apply povidone iodine solution over the injection site and surrounding skin. Allow it to dry. Sterile drapes and gloves are not considered necessary, especially once greater skill has been acquired. A no-touch technique is indicated if a sterile field is not created. It is suggested that the novice use sterile drapes and gloves to enhance aseptic technique.[8]

TECHNIQUES

Dosing in joint injections is influenced by the joint size, the presence or absence of synovial fluid, the presence or absence of edema, the severity of synovitis, and the steroid preparation selected. Table 62-1 summarizes the characteristics of commonly available corticosteroid preparations. Duration of action is chiefly dependent on the solubility of the preparation. A dose of 20 to 30 mg of methylprednisolone acetate or equivalent is appropriate for large spaces such as the subacromial, olecranon, and trochanteric bursae. This can be increased to a 30 to 40 mg dose if a large amount of joint fluid is present. A dose of 10 to 20 mg is appropriate for intermediate-size bursae, wrists, knees, and heels. A dose of 5 to 15 mg is appropriate for tendon sheaths. Triamcinolone hexacetonide and acetonide are the least soluble and therefore the most potent preparations available. The local effects of these preparations may last weeks or months. More soluble preparations such as hydrocortisone acetate have effects that last a few days. Many physicians prefer triamcinolone due to its prolonged duration of action. Corticosteroids are often mixed with a local anesthetic solution prior to injection. The local anesthetic solution provides immediate pain relief for the patient. It also confirms for the physician that the injection was placed at the appropriate anatomic site.

SUBACROMIAL BURSITIS

The subacromial bursa lies between the rotator cuff muscles inferiorly (supraspinatus, infraspinatus, teres

TABLE 62-1. CORTICOSTEROID PREPARATIONS AVAILABLE FOR INJECTION

Generic name	Trade name	Strength (mg/mL)	Relative potency	Dose range (mg)	Biological half-life (h)
Hydrocortisone acetate	Cortef Solu-Cortef	25	1	12.5–100	8–12
Triamcinolone acetonide	Kenalog –10 Kenalog – 40	10 40	2.5 10.0	4.0–40	18–36
Triamcinolone hexacetonide	Aristospan	20	8	4.0–25	18–36
Dexamethasone acetate	Decadron, Hexadrol, Dexone	4, 8	20–30	0.8–4.0	36–54
Betamethasone sodium phosphate	Celestone	6	20–30	1.5–6.0	36–54
Methylprednisolone acetate	Medrol, Depo-Medrol, Solu-Medrol	20, 40, 80	5, 10, 20	4.0–30	18–36

minor, and subscapularis muscles) and the overlying acromion, teres major muscle, and deltoid muscle. The subacromial space contains the long head of the biceps, the rotator cuff tendons, and the subacromial bursa. The syndromes of calcific tendonitis, supraspinatus tendonitis, and subacromial bursitis are so similar that the signs of each are difficult to distinguish. Anatomic proximity may cause secondary irritative inflammation of adjacent structures, so that these conditions overlap and coexist. Pain from these syndromes is elicited by shoulder abduction.

Patients often present holding the affected arm in a protective fashion against the chest wall. The classic sign of subacromial bursitis is tenderness over the greater trochanter that disappears with arm adduction. The "subacromial painful arc" is painful active abduction of the shoulder with maximal pain occurring during 60 to 120 degrees of abduction. Acromioclavicular joint inflammation results in a painful arc from 120 to 180 degrees of shoulder abduction.

Three techniques are described to inject the subacromial bursa: the lateral approach, the anterior approach, and the posterior approach. The lateral approach is the one preferred by the editors. Some prefer the anterior (or subcoracoid) approach provided that the practitioner has good familiarity with the landmarks. However, the anterior approach is far more difficult for the less experienced.

Place the patient seated upright or supine on a gurney. Palpate the indentation under the acromion process of the scapula for the lateral approach. This indentation is located between the acromion process and the greater tuberosity of the humerus. Arm a syringe containing 1 mL of local anesthetic solution and 1 mL of dexamethasone with a 22 to 25 gauge needle. Insert the needle into the indentation and direct it superomedially. Advance the needle until the tip touches the inferior surface of the acromion (Figure 62-1). Inject the steroid-anesthetic mixture. Withdraw the needle and apply a bandage.

Alternative approaches include the anterior and posterior approaches. Position the patient as above for the anterior approach. Insert the needle 1.5 cm lateral to the coracoid process. Direct the needle horizontally and posteriorly. Advance the needle approximately 2.5 cm to gain direct access to the subacromial space.

The posterior approach may also be used. The distance from the coracoacromial ligamentous arch in this approach is great and may limit efficacy. Place the patient sitting upright with the affected forearm resting in their lap. Palpate the most lateral point of the acromion process posteriorly. Insert the needle at this landmark. Aim the needle toward the center of the humeral head and at an upward angle of 10 degrees (Figure 62-2). Advance the needle 3 to 5 cm until the bursa is entered.

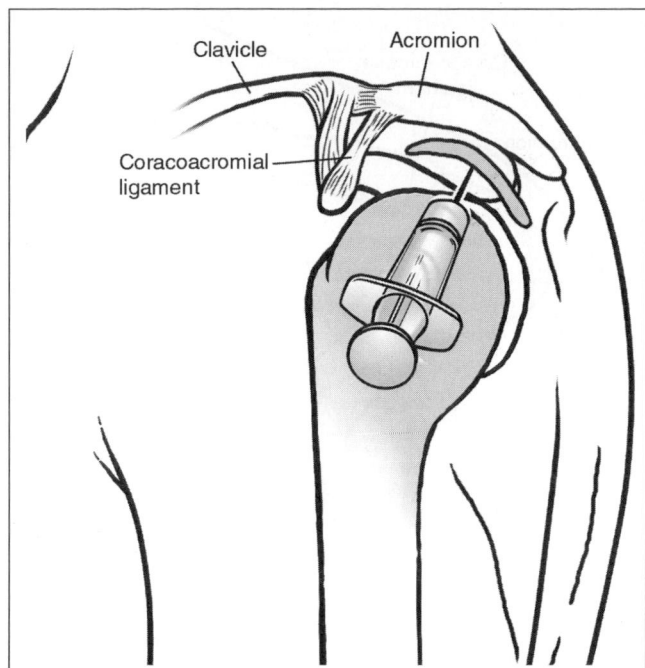

FIGURE 62-1 Lateral approach for subacromial bursitis.

SHOULDER IMPINGEMENT SYNDROME

Impingement syndrome results from rotator cuff, particularly supraspinatous, compression between the humerus and the coracoacromial arch. This is part of a pathophysiologic continuum with an endpoint of complete rotator cuff rupture in some cases. A history of overhead activities such as painting a ceiling is common. The clinical hallmark is a painful arch of abduction from 60 to 120 degrees. Pain typically begins at 60 to 70 degrees of abduction and is maximal from 100 to 120 degrees. Tenderness at the tendon insertion site over the greater tuberosity may be present.

The impingement injection test may separate the pain of impingement from other causes of shoulder pain. First, the examiner prevents scapular rotation by holding the scapula against the rib cage. Extend the patient's affected arm in forced forward elevation. Pain with this movement may signify a number of inflammatory shoulder conditions. Repeat this maneuver after injecting 10 mL of local anesthetic solution beneath the anterior acromion process. The absence of pain after anesthetic injection defines an impingement syndrome.

Place the patient sitting upright or supine on a gurney. Identify the coracoacromial ligament, which is found by palpating the coracoid process and the tip of the acromion process. The coracoacromial ligament connects these two bony points. This ligament is a thick, dense, fibrous band. Arm a syringe containing 80 mg of triamcinolone and 2 mL of bupivacaine or mepivacaine with a 22 to 25 gauge needle.[8] Insert the needle under the coracoacromial arch and inject the steroid-

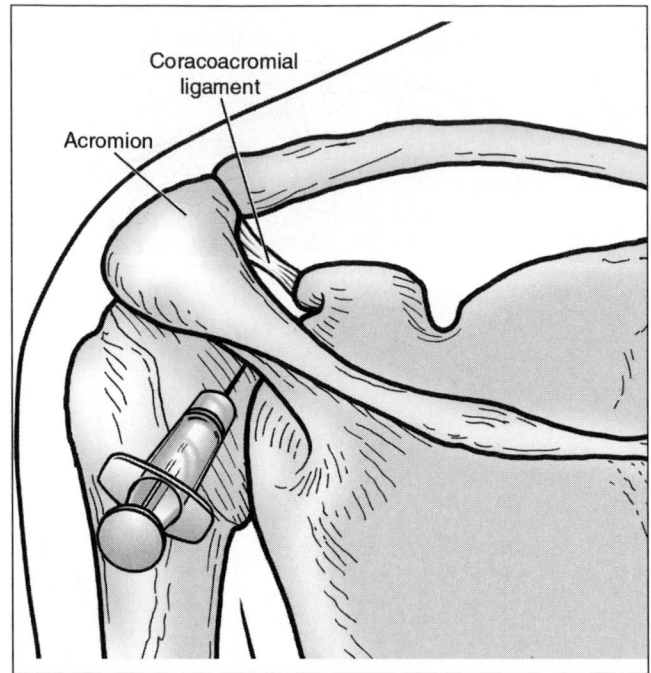

FIGURE 62-2 Posterior approach for subacromial bursitis.

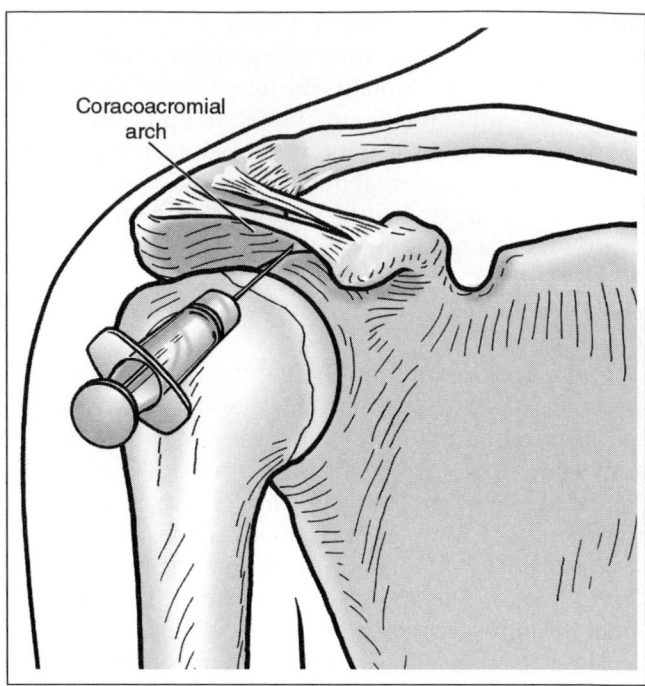

FIGURE 62-3 Injection for painful arch (impingement) syndrome.

anesthetic mixture (Figure 62-3). **The plunger should depress easily and without resistance. Forceful injection indicates that the tip of the needle is within the rotator cuff tendons.** Advance the needle another 0.5 cm and reattempt the injection, seeking minimal resistance. Withdraw the needle and apply a bandage.

BICIPITAL TENDONITIS

The long head of the biceps tendon passes through the bicipital groove of the humerus (Figure 62-4). In this condition, the inflamed tendon is tender to palpation along the anterior humerus. Yergason's test is a clinical indicator of bicipital tendonitis. Flex the patient's elbow 90 degrees. Grasp the patient's affected arm as if shaking hands. A positive test is the elicitation of pain in the biceps muscle while the examiner provides resisted supination to the patient's hand. Lipman's test is another clinical indicator of bicipital tendonitis. Tenderness of the bicipital tendon as it is rolled or plucked within the grove is considered a positive test. In general, pain causes restricted motion. Shoulder elevation will aggravate the patient's symptoms.

Place the patient seated with the arm affected externally rotated 20 degrees. The bicipital groove and tendon are now pointing directly anterior. Arm a syringe containing 10 to 15 mg of triamcinolone and 2 mL of local anesthetic solution with a 22 to 25 gauge needle. Palpate the bicipital tendon and identify the point of maximal tenderness. Insert and direct the needle into the tendon sheath and aimed toward one border of the bicipital

groove at the site of maximal tenderness (Figure 62-4). Inject one-third of the dose into the peritendinous space. **Confirmation of needle placement within the tendon sheath is made by free flow of the steroid-anesthetic mixture with minimal resistance. Difficulty depressing the plunger indicates that the tip of the needle is within the tendon.** If resistance to injection occurs, withdraw the needle slightly and aim more parallel to the tendon to allow penetration of the sheath and not the tendon substance. Withdraw the needle to just under the skin and redirect it 2.5 cm inferiorly, touching the border of the bicipital groove, and inject another one-third of the dose. The final one-third of the dose is deposited by again withdrawing the needle to the subcutaneous area and redirecting the tip 2.5 cm superiorly to the first injection site and touching the border of the bicipital groove. Withdraw the needle and apply a bandage.

LATERAL EPICONDYLITIS (TENNIS ELBOW)

Lateral epicondylitis, or tennis elbow, is pain at the origin of the wrist and finger extensor muscles. Pain is elicited on palpation of the lateral epicondyle of the humerus. It is also elicited during resisted wrist extension. A history of playing racquet sports or doing manual labor is common.

Locate the injection site by palpating the base of the lateral epicondyle with the elbow flexed 90 degrees. Arm a syringe containing 1 mL of local anesthetic solution,

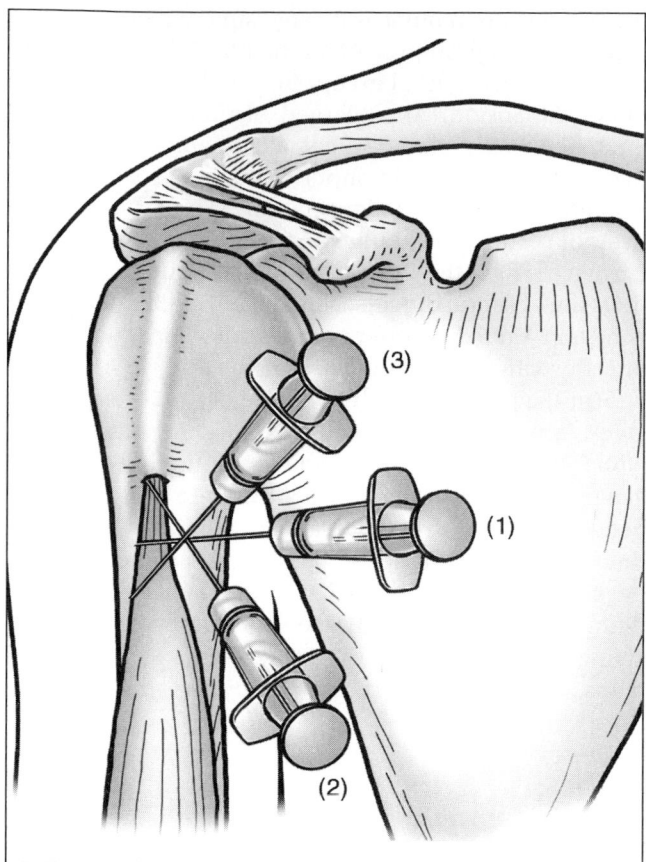

FIGURE 62-4 Injection for bicipital tendonitis.

1 mL of methylprednisolone, and 0.5 mL of dexamethasone with a 22 to 25 gauge needle. Alternatively, mix the local anesthetic with 40 mg of triamcinolone. A total volume of 2 mL is required. Insert the needle in the indentation between the lateral epicondyle and the radial head, beginning at the radial head (Figure 62-5A). Slowly advance the needle toward the lateral epicondyle. **The radial nerve runs in this area, and care must be taken not to penetrate and inject the nerve.** Paresthesias and pain will be felt if the needle enters the nerve.

Inject 0.5 mL of the steroid-anesthetic mixture into the tenoperiosteum at the base of the lateral epicondyle. Withdraw the needle until the tip is at the level of the radial head while simultaneously infiltrating with 0.25 mL of the steroid-anesthetic mixture. Infiltrate 0.5 mL of the steroid-anesthetic mixture when the tip of the needle reaches the level of the radial head. Redirect the needle over the extensor muscle bellies (Figure 62-5B). Inject the remaining steroid-anesthetic mixture in a fan-like pattern over the extensor muscle bellies (Figure 62-5B). Withdraw the needle and apply a bandage.

MEDIAL EPICONDYLITIS (GOLFER'S ELBOW)

Patients affected with medial epicondylitis, or golfer's elbow, are most commonly Little League pitchers, golfers, and bowlers. Pain is felt in the medial aspect of the elbow upon flexion and supination of the wrist. Tenderness is elicited on palpation just distal to the medial epicondyle. It is important to exclude an avulsion of the medial epicondyle or compression fracture of the sub-

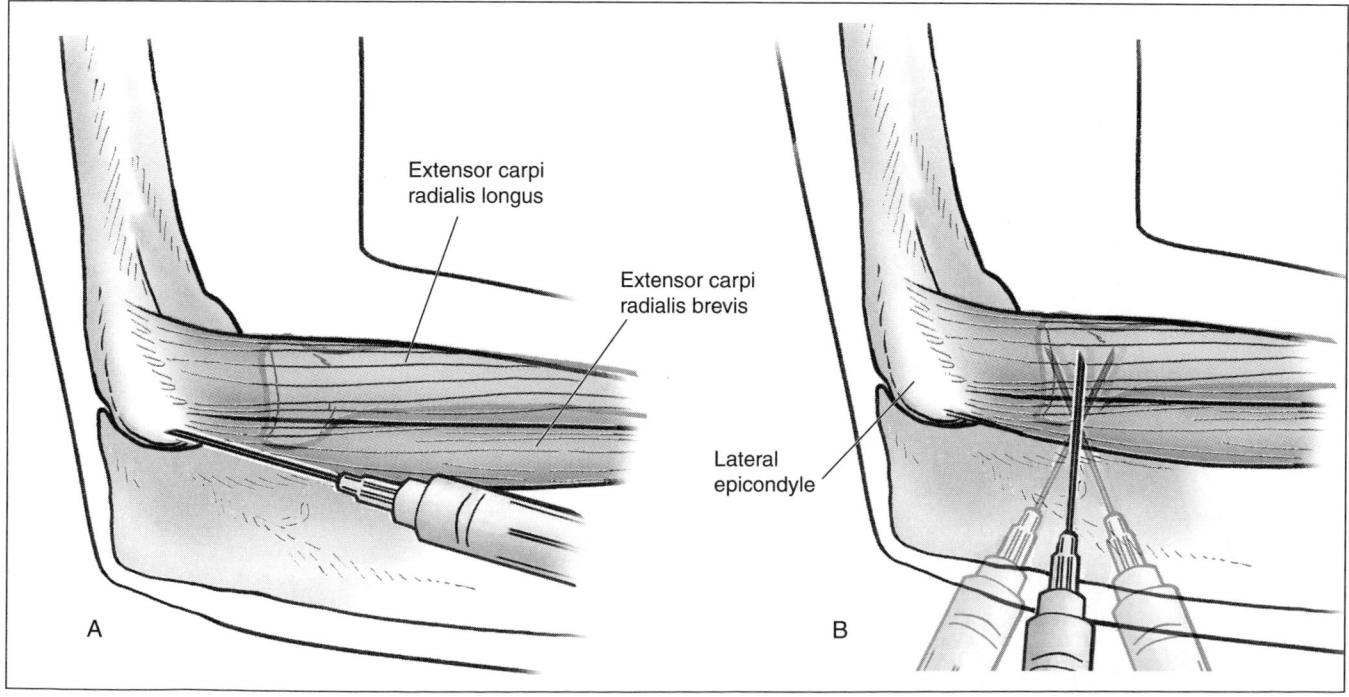

Extensor carpi
radialis longus

Extensor carpi
radialis brevis

Lateral
epicondyle

A

B

FIGURE 62-5 Injection for lateral epicondylitis. *A.* The needle is inserted at the level of the radial head and advanced to the base of the lateral epicondyle. *B.* The needle is redirected in a fan-like pattern over the muscle bellies.

chondral bone of the lateral condyle or radial head in children with nonfused epiphyses. Radiographs are suggested to exclude these causes.

Place the patient supine on a gurney. Place the arm in 90 degrees of external rotation and abducted 90 degrees. Flex the elbow 90 degrees. Prepare a steroid-anesthetic mixture similar to that used for lateral epicondylitis. Identify by palpation the volar surface of the medial epicondyle. Insert the needle 2 cm proximal to the medial epicondyle and advance it distally to the tenoperiosteal region (Figure 62-6). The ulnar nerve is better protected than the radial nerve, as it runs posterior to the epicondyle. Proximal needle insertion prevents striking the ulnar nerve. Paresthesias and pain are indicators of nerve penetration. Inject 1.5 mL of the steroid-anesthetic mixture over the medial epicondyle while withdrawing the needle. Apply a bandage after withdrawing the needle.

OLECRANON BURSITIS

Olecranon bursitis is usually sterile even though the olecranon bursa is the most frequent site of septic bursi-tis. The olecranon bursa is located subcutaneously overlying the olecranon process of the ulna. Olecranon bursitis is not very painful except for the discomfort due to bursal expansion. An enlarged olecranon bursa may limit elbow extension. Studies have demonstrated corticosteroid injection is superior to oral regimens for resolution of bursal inflammation.[9] Simple aspiration without corticosteroid injection is often followed by recurrence. Since the olecranon bursa is the most common site of septic bursitis, aspiration with fluid analysis is recommended before corticosteroid injection unless infection can be ruled out clinically.

Seat the patient upright with the elbow flexed 90 degrees. Arm a syringe containing 30 to 40 mg of triamcinolone and 1 mL of local anesthetic solution. Insert an 18 gauge needle on an empty syringe into the most dependent aspect of the bursal sac. Aspirate the bursal fluid to drain it completely. The bursa may be "milked" by palpation and compression of the tissues toward the draining needle. Hold the needle securely. Remove the syringe while the tip of the needle remains within the bursa. Attach the syringe containing the steroid-

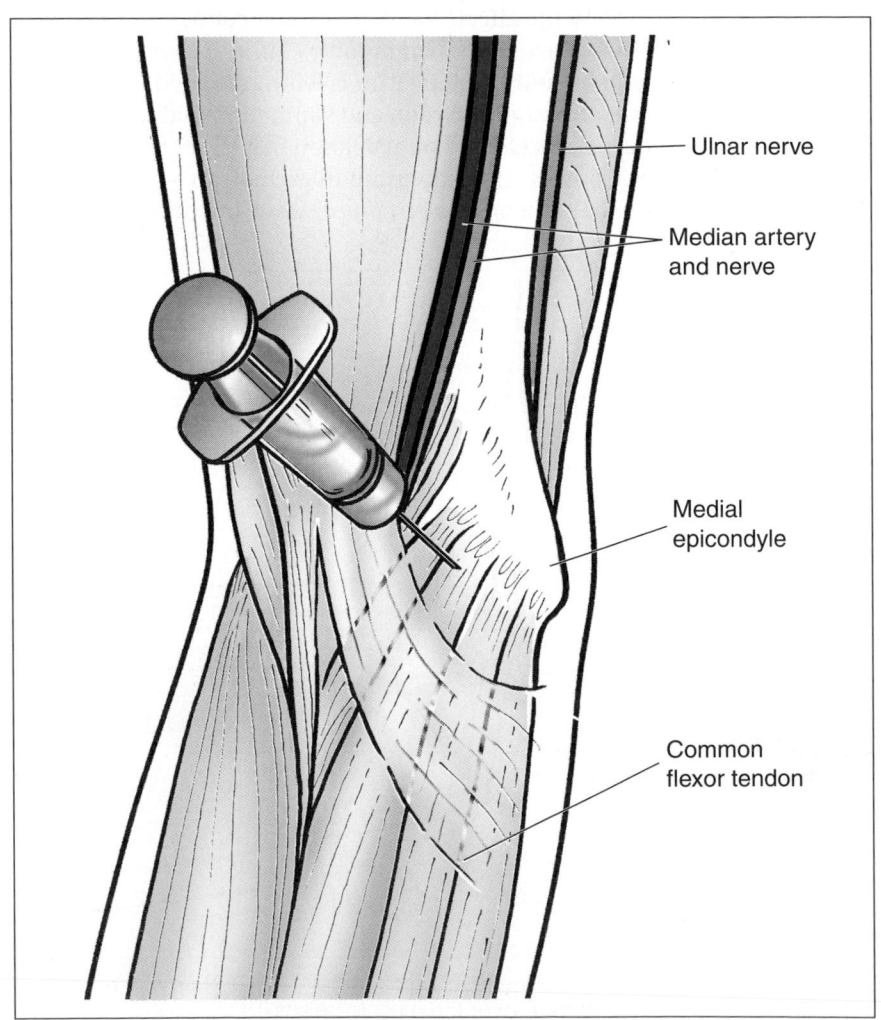

Ulnar nerve

Median artery and nerve

Medial epicondyle

Common flexor tendon

FIGURE 62-6 Injection for medial epicondylitis.

anesthetic mixture. Inject the steroid-anesthetic mixture. Withdraw the needle and apply a bandage. Wrap the elbow region with an elastic compression bandage (Jones compression dressing) for 7 to 10 days. Instruct the patient to limit movement for 7 to 10 days to prevent reaccumulation of the fluid.[18]

DEQUERVAIN'S TENOSYNOVITIS

DeQuervain's tenosynovitis is an inflammation of the tendon sheaths of the abductor pollicis longus and extensor pollicis brevis muscles as they cross the wrist (Figure 62-7A). Pain is elicited by the classic Finkelstein test, in which the patient deviates the wrist ulnarly while holding the thumb between the palm and fingers (Figure 62-7B). Palpation along the course of the tendons will also cause pain.

Arm a syringe containing 40 mg of triamcinolone and 1 to 2 mL of mepivacaine or bupivacaine with a 25 gauge needle. Introduce the needle through the skin overlying the point of maximal tenderness, usually just distal to the radial styloid process (Figure 62-8). The editor (RRS) has found that bending the needle approximately 30 degrees makes it easier to negotiate the area and insert the needle alongside the tendon. Inject the

steroid-anesthetic mixture into the tendon sheath. **Resistance to injection signifies that the tip of the needle is within the tendon.** Withdraw the needle slightly and reinject, feeling for the loss of resistance. Withdraw the needle and apply a bandage. Apply a light thumb splint for approximately 10 days. The splint is especially useful at night or when there is significant activity.

TROCHANTERIC BURSITIS

Trochanteric bursitis typically affects women in the fourth to sixth decades of life. It also occurs in runners, ballet dancers, and as a form of overuse or trauma to the hip. Hip pain often prevents the patient from sleeping on the affected side. Pain is also severe with walking, especially up stairs. The deep trochanteric bursa lies between the tendon of the gluteus maximus and the greater trochanter. Another lies between the gluteus medius and the greater trochanter (Figure 62-9). Pain is elicited upon palpation of the greater trochanter of the femur. Pain can be reproduced by hip adduction in superficial bursitis or on resisted active abduction in deep bursitis.

The principal bursa lies between the gluteus maximus and the posterolateral prominence of the greater trochanter. Pain may radiate from the greater trochanter down the lateral or posterior thigh, mimicking sciatica or hip joint disease. In contrast to these syndromes, passive range of motion of the hip is nearly painless in trochanteric bursitis. However, active abduction of the affected hip while the patient is lying on the unaffected side increases symptoms. Pain is also elicited by abduction and external rotation of the hip.

Place the patient prone on a gurney. Arm a syringe containing 80 mg of triamcinolone and 3 to 10 mL of local

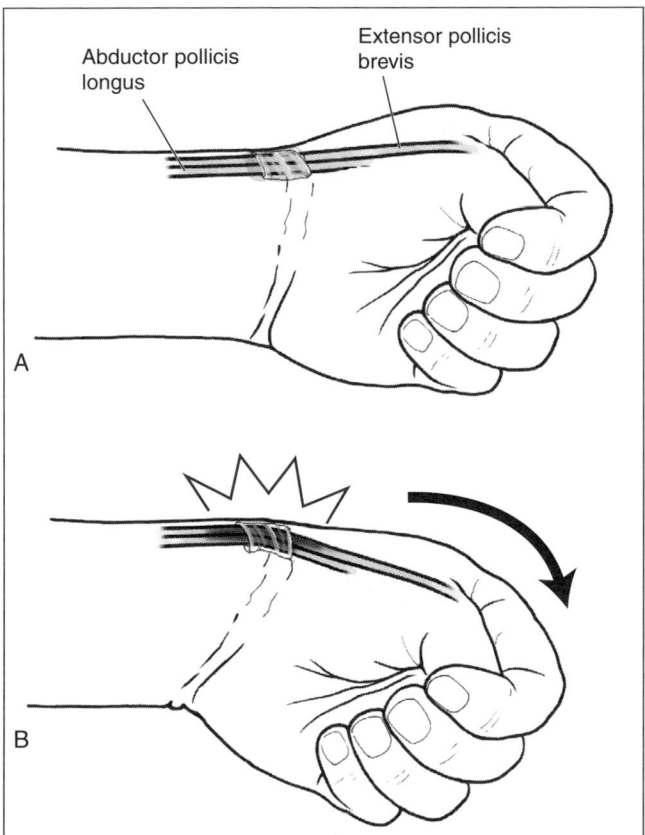

FIGURE 62-7 DeQuervain's tenosynovitis. *A.* Anatomy. *B.* Finkelstein test.

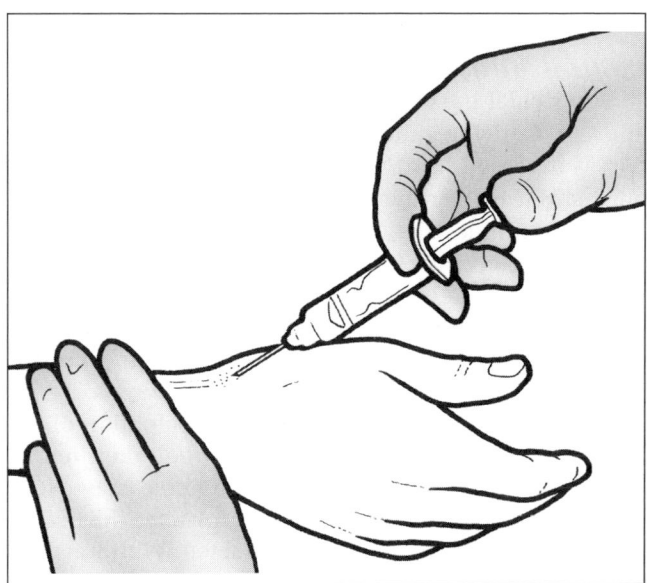

FIGURE 62-8 Injection for DeQuervain's tenosynovitis.

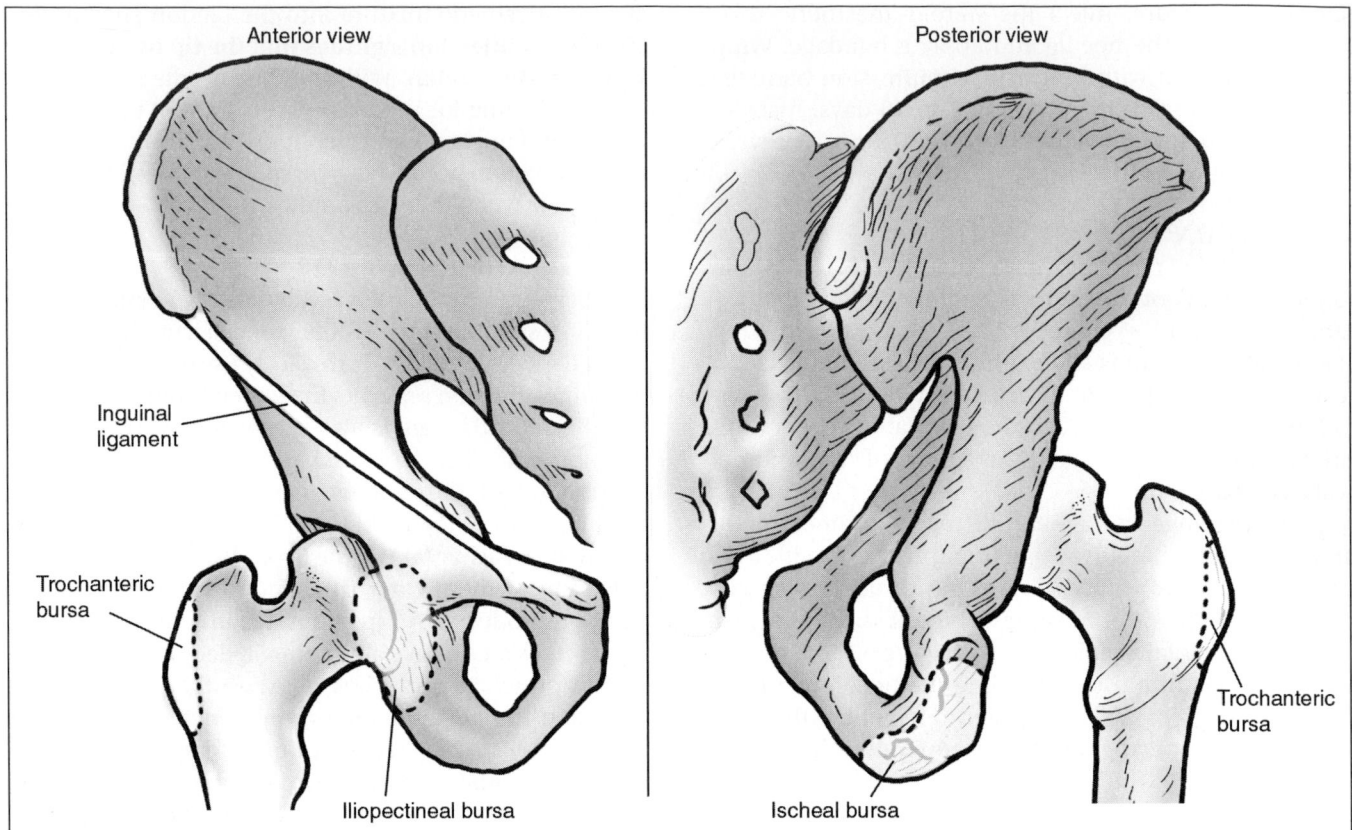

FIGURE 62-9 Selected bursa of the hip region.

anesthetic solution with a 22 to 23 gauge needle. Insert the needle at the point of maximal tenderness. Advance the needle until the tip strikes the greater trochanter. Withdraw the needle 1 to 2 mm and inject the steroid-anesthetic mixture. Withdraw the needle and apply a bandage.

ISCHIAL BURSITIS

The ischial bursa lies between the ischial tuberosity and the overlying gluteus maximus (Figure 62-9). It becomes inflamed from trauma or prolonged sitting on a hard surface. Pain may radiate down the back of the thigh and mimic sciatica. Pain can be elicited by applying pressure over the ischial tuberosity.

Place the patient prone on a gurney. Arm a syringe containing 30 to 40 mg of triamcinolone and 5 to 10 mL of local anesthetic solution with a 22 to 23 gauge needle. Insert the needle over the most prominent section of the ischium. Hip flexion may facilitate palpation of the ischium in obese patients. **Care must be taken not to injure the sciatic nerve.** Striking the nerve may cause paresthesias of the buttocks and leg. Advance the needle until the ischial tuberosity is contacted. Withdraw the needle 2 to 3 mm and inject the steroid-anesthetic mixture. Withdraw the needle and apply a bandage.

ILIOTIBIAL BAND SYNDROME

Patients with iliotibial band syndrome present with lateral knee pain. This condition is commonly seen in cyclists, dancers, long-distance runners or walkers, and football players. These patients have a painful limp that is exacerbated with walking or running. Climbing stairs or walking up an incline will increase their pain. Tenderness is elicited with the patient lying supine and knee flexed 90 degrees. Instruct the patient to extend their knee as you press over the lateral femoral condyle. Pain will be localized to the lateral femoral condyle. The patient will have pain at 30 degrees of flexion as the iliotibial band slides over the condyle. A positive Renne test occurs when the patient stands with their weight on the affected leg and flexes the knee. Pain at 30 degrees of flexion is considered a positive test.

Place the patient supine on a gurney. Arm a syringe containing 80 mg of triamcinolone and 2 mL of local anesthetic solution with a 22 to 25 gauge needle. Typically, at 30 degrees of flexion, the iliotibial band is at the midpoint of the lateral femoral condyle (Figure 62-10). Support the patient's leg in this position to bring the tendon to its most superficial point. Identify the point of maximal tenderness as the patient flexes the knee. Insert the needle perpendicular to the skin and 1 cm caudad to

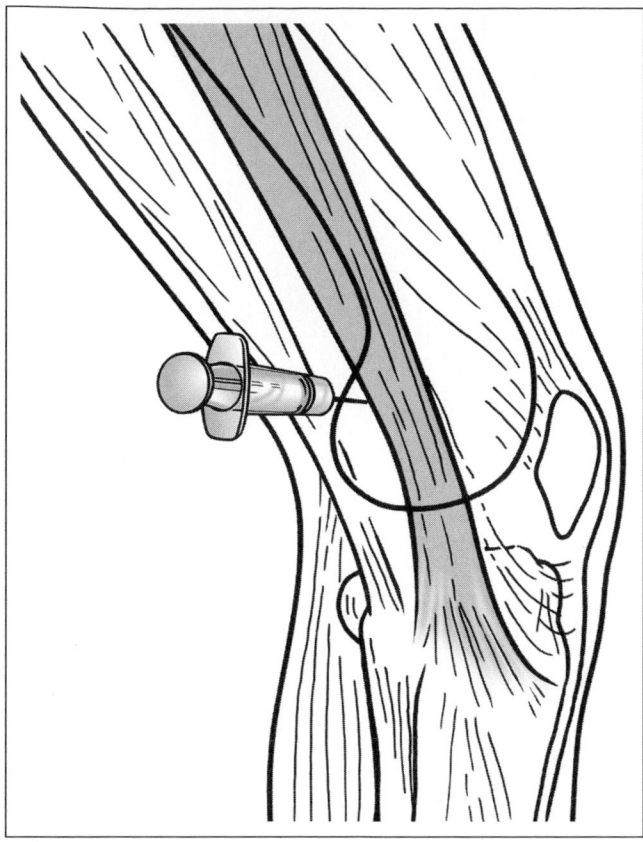

FIGURE 62-10 Injection for iliotibial band syndrome. The knee is flexed 30 degrees to bring the tendon to its most superficial position overlying the midportion of the lateral femoral condyle.

the point of maximal tenderness. Angle the needle cephalad. Inject the steroid-anesthetic mixture in an arc from anterior to posterior. The goal is to deposit corticosteroid in the tendon sheath and the surrounding inflamed tissues. **Resistance to injection indicates that the tip of the needle is within the tendon.** Withdraw the needle slightly and reinject, feeling for the loss of resistance. Withdraw the needle and apply a bandage.

ANSERINE BURSITIS

Anserine or pes anserine bursitis is an inflammation of the bursa located 5 cm below the medial joint line of the knee at the tibial insertion of the gracilis, sartorius, and semitendinosus muscles (Figure 62-11). The anserine bursa is superficial to the tibial insertion of the medial collateral ligament. This syndrome occurs predominately in overweight women with osteoarthritis of the knees. It may also be found in equestrians and was previously known as Cavalryman's disease. The anserine bursa will be tender to palpation.

Place the patient supine with the affected leg externally rotated. Identify the anteromedial joint line of the knee. The bursa is located inferior to the joint line at the insertion of the sartorius, gracilis, and semitendinosus

tendons (Figure 62-11). Palpate the area of maximal tenderness at this site. Arm a syringe containing 40 mg of triamcinolone and 2 to 4 mL of local anesthetic solution with a 23 to 25 gauge needle. Insert the needle and direct its tip into the bursa at the point of maximal tenderness. Inject the steroid-anesthetic mixture into the bursa. Withdraw the needle and apply a bandage.

PREPATELLAR BURSITIS

Prepatellar bursitis is caused by direct pressure, as when a person is kneeling on a firm surface. It is also known as nun's, rug cutter's, or housemaid's knee. Tenderness is elicited by direct palpation overlying the patella. Extreme knee flexion causes pain. There is often a fluctuant, well-circumscribed, warm bursal pouch overlying the patella. Crepitus may be found upon palpation. The prepatellar space is a common site for septic bursitis. Aspiration with fluid analysis is recommended to rule out an infection before any corticosteroid injection is considered.

Place the patient supine on a gurney with the knee slightly flexed. Note that the bursa is very superficial and may be entered by passing the needle just through the skin and subcuticular tissues (Figure 62-11). Arm a syringe containing 30 to 40 mg triamcinolone and 1 to 2 mL of local anesthetic solution with a 23 to 25 gauge needle.[18] Insert the needle into the bursa at the point of maximal fluctuance. Instill the steroid-anesthetic mixture into the bursa. Withdraw the needle and apply a bandage.

INFRAPATELLAR BURSITIS

The infrapatellar bursa has two components (Figure 62-11). The superficial infrapatellar bursa lies between the patellar ligament and the skin. The deep infrapatellar bursa lies between the patellar ligament and the anterior tibia. Inflammation of the superficial bursa occurs due to friction from the overlying skin. Clinically, there is no pain with passive flexion. Active knee flexion and extension causes pain in the deep infrapatellar bursa. Edema and tenderness may be found on both sides of the patellar tendon.

Place the patient supine on a gurney with the leg and knee extended. Palpate the patellar tendon. Identify the superficial inflamed bursa. Arm a syringe containing 20 mg of triamcinolone and 1 mL of local anesthetic solution with a 23 to 25 gauge needle. Insert the needle into the superficial bursa and inject the steroid-anesthetic mixture. Withdraw the needle and apply a bandage.

Patients with deep infrapatellar bursitis have maximal tenderness and swelling both medially and laterally to the patellar tendon. Arm a syringe containing 30 mg of triamcinolone and 1 to 2 mL of local anesthetic solution with a 23 to 25 gauge needle. Insert the needle into the infrapatellar bursa, either medially or laterally to the

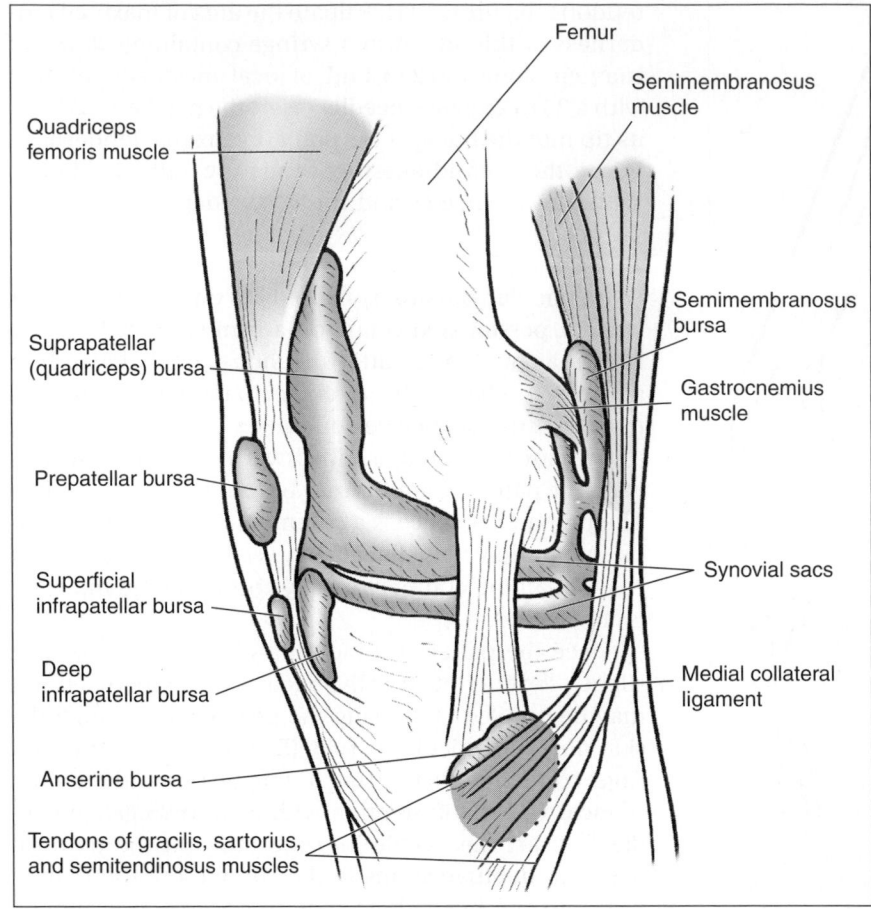

FIGURE 62-11 Bursae of the knee.

patellar tendon. Attempt to aspirate, although fluid accumulation is minimal and usually no return will be found. Inject the steroid-anesthetic mixture. Withdraw the needle and apply a bandage.

ACHILLES TENDONITIS

Achilles tendonitis causes tightness and pain in the heel region upon first awaking. This discomfort improves with ambulation. The Achilles tendon will be tender to palpation and may be visibly swollen. Corticosteroid injection around the Achilles tendon has been associated with tendon rupture.[16] This injection is reserved for the Podiatrist or the Orthopedic Surgeon.[16]

PLANTAR FASCIITIS

Plantar fasciitis is a common problem presenting to the Emergency Department and the primary care physician. Patients complain of medial heel pain, particularly after standing for a long period of time. These patients have minimal to no swelling but feel acute tenderness to palpation over the calcaneal insertion of the plantar fascia. Maximum tenderness is palpated just beneath the

spring ligament at the site of insertion of the plantar fascia on the calcaneous. Radiographs may demonstrate a calcaneal spur. However, the presence of a spur does not correlate with plantar fasciitis. Patients may have plantar fasciitis with or without a calcaneal spur. The optimal therapy for these patients is to elevate the heel with a felt heel pad inserted in the shoe. In addition, they may begin stretching exercises that are designed to stretch the plantar fascia. This often relieves the condition without an injection. In significant cases where conservative therapy is unsuccessful, injection of the calcaneal insertion of the plantar fascia with a steroid-lidocaine mixture is advocated.

Place the patient supine on a gurney with the leg externally rotated. Arm a syringe containing 20 mg of triamcinolone and 1 mL of local anesthetic solution with a 25 gauge needle. Insert the needle into the medial aspect of the foot and aimed just anterior to the base of the calcaneous (Figure 62-12). Advance the needle 1.5 cm and inject the steroid-anesthetic mixture. Withdraw the needle and apply a bandage. The patient should avoid weight bearing for 3 to 4 days and begin oral nonsteroidal anti-inflammatory drugs.

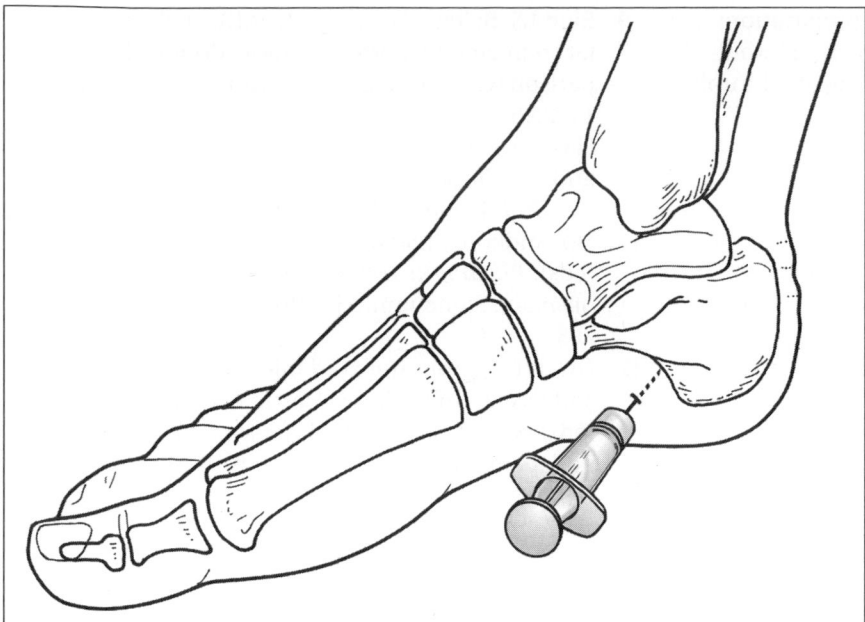

FIGURE 62-12 Injection for plantar fasciitis.

ASSESSMENT

Observe the patient for several minutes after the injection. Reexamine the patient to compare pre- and postinjection tenderness and mobility. The patient's symptoms will abate within a few minutes if a local anesthetic has been used. Lack of relief indicates deposition of the steroid-anesthetic mixture away from the target structure. In these cases, a second attempt may be performed if the injection site can be properly identified. Otherwise, refer the patient to their primary care physician or an Orthopedic Surgeon.

AFTERCARE

Instruct the patient to limit movement and/or weight bearing of the affected area after a corticosteroid injection. The duration of rest is dependent on the injection site. Larger and weight-bearing joints may require up to 2 to 3 weeks of rest, with range-of-motion exercises encouraged. Immobilization with splints or bandages may be necessary to prevent weight bearing. A rehabilitation program including range-of-motion exercises, stretching, and strengthening may be recommended depending upon the chronicity and severity of the presenting condition.

COMPLICATIONS

Local infection is rare after corticosteroid joint injection and occurs from 1 in 17,000 to 50,000 injec-

tions.[1,10–12] A local reaction consisting of heat, swelling, and tenderness may occur a few hours postinjection and last up to 2 days. This is known as the "postinjection flare" or "steroid flare."[11] It is not to be confused with an infection, is self-limited, and responds to ice packs and nonsteroidal anti-inflammatory drugs. It is attributed to preservatives in the suspension inducing a local synovitis. Steroid flares occur in approximately 2 percent of patients injected with corticosteroids.[1]

Tendon rupture is a theoretical complication thought to be due to corticosteroids weakening the collagen matrix. Tendon ruptures after corticosteroid injections have been reported, but direct causality has not been established.[13–17] Rupture is more likely if the injection is made into the tendon matrix rather than the synovial sheath, if the patient does not rest the tendon appropriately after the injection, or with multiple repeat injections.

Subcutaneous atrophy of the overlying skin may develop if the steroid is injected less than 5 mm beneath the skin surface. A depigmentation in darker-skinned individuals may also occur due to superficial steroid injections. This depigmentation typically resolves over a period of 6 months to 1 year.

SUMMARY

Local corticosteroid injections are useful diagnostic and therapeutic adjuncts for the Emergency Physician. Many patients with an inflammatory bursitis or tendonitis will benefit greatly from these simple and effective injections. Mastery of the techniques is simple. They require a familiarity with the indications, the local anatomy, and the injectable corticosteroid preparations. Complications associated with the injection of a steroid-anesthetic mixture are minimal if it is not injected into an infected space.

REFERENCES

1. Pfenninger JL: Injections of joints and soft tissue: part I. General guidelines. *Am Fam Physician* 1991; 44(4):1196–1202.
2. Scott WA: Injection techniques and use in the treatment of sports injuries. *Sports Med* 1996; 22(6):406–416.
3. Holt MA, Keene JS, Graf BK: Treatment of osteitis pubis in athletes. *Am J Sports Med* 1995; 23(5):601–695.
4. Campbell RB, Cannistra LM, Fadale PD, et al: The effects of local corticosteroid injection on the healing of rat medial collateral ligaments. *Trans Orthop Res Soc* 1991; 16:112.
5. Wiggins ME, Fadale PD, Barrach H, et al: Healing characteristics of a type 1 collagenous structure treated with corticosteroids. *Am J Sports Med* 1994; 22(2):279–288.
6. Smith DL, McAfee JH, Lucas LM, et al: Treatment of nonseptic olecranon bursitis: a controlled, blinded prospective trial. *Arch Intern Med* 1989; 149:2527–2530.
7. Anderson B, Kaye S: Treatment of flexor tenosynovitis of the hand ("trigger finger") with corticosteroids: a prospective study of the response to local injection. *Arch Intern Med* 1991; 151:153–156.
8. Zuckerman JD, Meislin RJ, Rothberg M: Injection for joint and soft tissue disorders: when and how to use them. *Geriatrics* 1990; 45(4):45–55.
9. Bain LS, Baleh HW, Wetherly JMR, et al: Intraarticular triamcinolone hexacetonide: double–blind comparison with methylprednisolone. *Br J Clin Pract* 1972; 26:559–561.
10. Haslock I, MacFarlane D, Speed C: Intra-articular and soft tissue injections: a survey of current practice. *Br J Rheumatol* 1995; 34:449–452.
11. Hollander JL: Injection therapy, in Riggs GK, Gall E (eds): *Rheumatic Diseases Rehabilitation and Management.* Stoneham, MA: Butterworth, 1984:199–203.
12. Owen DS: Aspiration and injection of joints and soft tissues, in Ruddy S, Harris ED, Sledge CB, et al (eds): *Kelley's Textbook of Rheumatology,* 6th ed. Philadelphia: Saunders, 2001:583–604.
13. Smith AG, Kosygan K, Newman RJ: Common extensor tendon rupture following corticosteroid injection for lateral tendinosis of the elbow. *Br J Sports Med* 1999; 33(6):423–424.
14. Karpman RR, McComb JE, Volz RG: Tendon rupture following local steroid injection: report of four cases. *Postgrad Med* 1980; 68(1):169–174.
15. Kleinman M, Gross AE: Achilles tendon rupture following steroid injection. Report of three cases. *J Bone Joint Surg Am* 1983; 65(9):1345–1347.
16. Shrier I, Matheson GO, Kohl HW: Achilles tendonitis: are corticosteroid injections useful or harmful? *Clin J Sports Med* 1996; (4):245–250.
17. Lambert MI, Gibson ASC, Noakes TD: Rupture of the triceps tendon associated with steroid injection (letter). *Am J Sports Med* 1995; 23(6):778.
18. Simon RR, Koenigsknecht SJ: *Emergency Orthopedics: The Extremities,* 4th ed. New York: McGraw-Hill, 2001.

Chapter 63
COMPARTMENT PRESSURE MEASUREMENT

Amy M. Hutson
David Rovinsky

INTRODUCTION

The ability to diagnose a compartment syndrome is a critical skill for the Emergency Physician. Early identification of a compartment syndrome can enable the appropriate treatment and may facilitate limb salvage. A compartment syndrome begins when an imbalance of volume and pressure within a myofascial compartment results in diminished blood flow.[1] A compartment syndrome has been classically described in the early literature as a Volkmann ischemic contracture following vascular insufficiency in the forearm.[3]

A compartment syndrome can occur in almost any muscle group that is contained within a confined fascial space. Common locations include the leg, forearm, and gluteal area. There are many causes of a compartment syndrome. These include protracted muscle ischemia (secondary to necrosis from a contusion), swelling (secondary to volume overload states or a fracture), or a thrombus in a vessel that traverses the compartment. In the Emergency Department, a compartment syndrome is most commonly associated with long bone fractures or blunt trauma.[2] Other etiologies for a compartment syndrome include complications from a coagulopathy, dialysis, surgery, or states of obtundation.[4–6]

Identifying a compartment syndrome in a timely fashion can be challenging. **The hallmark symptom is persistent and progressive pain that is disproportionate to the underlying cause.** The pain typically increases with passive motion. **A catastrophic mistake is to attribute the etiology of the patient's pain solely to the underlying problem, such as the fracture.**[7,8] Other signs and symptoms associated with a compartment syndrome occur late in the course and include paresthesias of the involved nerve, paralysis of the involved muscle group, pallor of the skin, and diminished pulses.[9] Waiting for the development of all the clinical signs and symptoms is an invitation for permanent and dangerous sequelae, including muscle necrosis and possible loss of a limb. Measurement of elevated tissue pressure within the muscle compartment is currently the most common objective means of diagnosing this syndrome. The compartment pressure must be released by performing an emergent fasciotomy of the involved compartments once a compartment syndrome is identified.

ANATOMY AND PATHOPHYSIOLOGY

The anatomy of a compartment syndrome is variable, as it can occur in any enclosed muscle group. Any muscle tissue that is confined in space by fascia, skin, or any external forces (e.g., casting material) is a potential site for the development of a compartment syndrome. The muscles, nerves, and vasculature within the affected muscle group are all potentially compromised by a prolonged ischemic state followed by swelling.

The initial imbalance of a compartment syndrome occurs between the volume and pressure within the myofascial compartment. The arterial inflow and venous outflow diminish as either intracompartmental volume or pressure increases. The blood begins to be shunted via capillaries into the muscle tissue. This compensatory shunting of blood further disturbs the volume-pressure balance, resulting in impaired tissue oxygenation.[2,9,10]

The extent of the tissue damage is determined by the duration of ischemia. Numerous experimental studies have documented a lack of muscle viability after 6 to 8 hours of total ischemia and a lack of nerve viability after 8 hours of total ischemia.[11,12] Thus, reversing the ischemia well before this time period is crucial to restoring tissue function. The definitive factor in the development of a compartment syndrome is the alteration of the pressure gradient between arterial and venous flow. Measurement of the intracompartmental pressures is used to determine the extent of ischemia.

The pressure of a healthy muscle compartment ranges between 0 and 8 mmHg.[13] The absolute value of the pressure that determines the presence of a compartment syndrome varies depending upon the source. Some texts refer to an absolute value of 30 to 35 mmHg as the cutoff point for performing a fasciotomy.[9,14,15] Although this value is referred to commonly, several studies confirm that a compartment syndrome does not develop definitively at or above this pressure threshold.[16,17] Other studies use a compartmental pressure that is within 10 to 30 mmHg of the patient's diastolic pressure as one of the indications for a fasciotomy.[2,11] Finally, a measurement that is within 10 to 30 mmHg of the patient's mean arterial pressure is also suggested as an indication for a fasciotomy.[18] **Nonetheless, if the compartmental pressure is 30 mmHg or greater, one must consider the development of a compartment syndrome.**

A compartment syndrome can occur in any muscle group. This includes the hand, foot, thigh, arm, and intercostal spaces, to name a few. This chapter reviews the anatomy of the two most common sites of a compartment syndrome, the leg and the forearm.

LOWER EXTREMITY: LEG

The lower leg consists of four distinct muscle compartments: anterior, lateral, deep posterior, and superficial posterior (Figure 63-1). A general understanding of the components of each compartment is important.[19,20]

The anterior compartment contains the four extensor muscles of the leg. These muscles function together to dorsiflex the foot. The deep peroneal nerve travels through this compartment to innervate the extensors and provide sensory innervation to the web space between the first and second toes. The anterior tibial artery travels through this compartment.

The lateral compartment consists of the peroneus longus and brevis muscles. Their chief function is to evert the foot, with some consequent abduction and plantarflexion of the foot. The superficial peroneal nerve travels in the lateral compartment to supply sensory innervation to the lower leg and foot.

A fascial layer divides the posterior muscle group into superficial and deep compartments. The superficial posterior compartment contains the muscles of plantarflexion (gastrocnemius, soleus, and plantaris tendons). No major nerves or blood vessels travel in the superficial compartment. The deep posterior compartment contains the four deep flexor muscles (flexor digitorum longus, flexor hallucis longus, tibialis posterior, and popliteus). This group of muscles contributes to inverting and adducting the foot in addition to flexing the toes and foot. The primary sensory innervation is from the tibial nerve, which courses through the deep posterior compartment. The posterior tibial artery and the peroneal artery are also contained within this compartment.

Although any of these compartments can suffer from ischemia, **the deep posterior compartment and the**

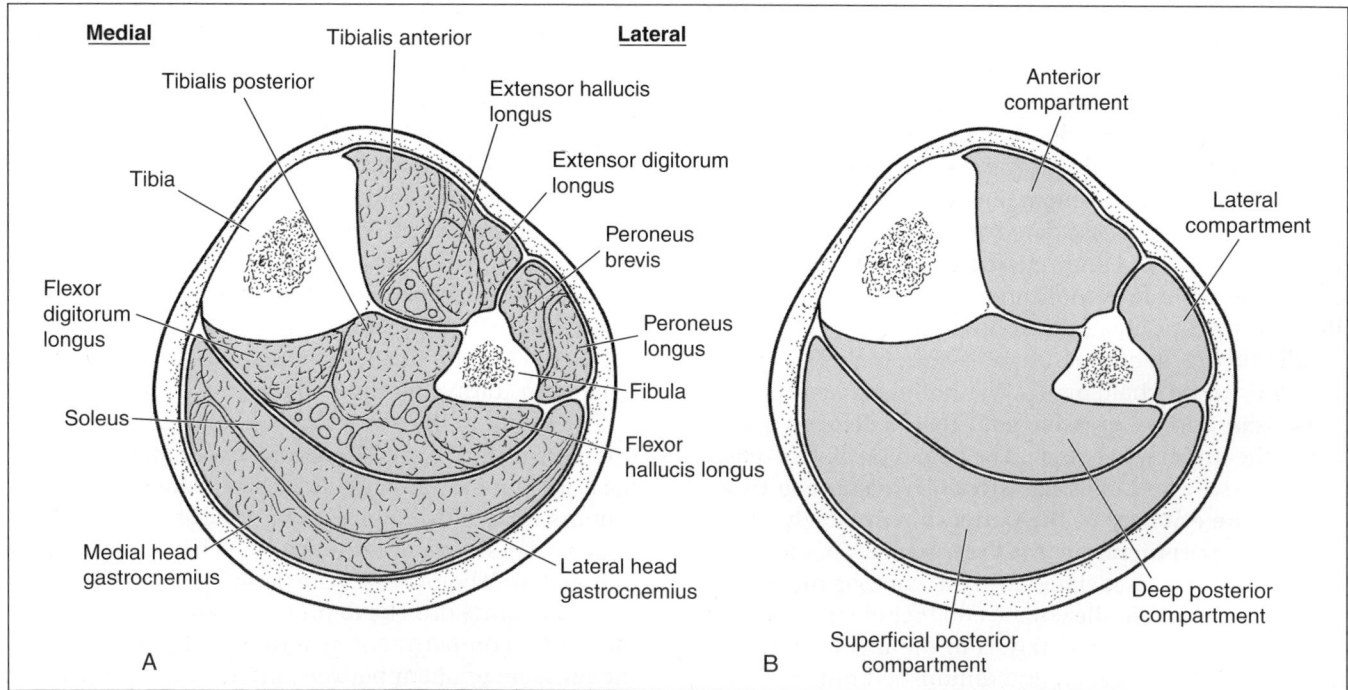

FIGURE 63-1 Cross-section through the middle of the right leg demonstrating the four compartments. The size and proportion of the compartments change as one travels proximally or distally from this middle section.

anterior compartment have the highest incidence of developing a compartment syndrome.[17] It is difficult to simply observe the patient in the face of a normal compartmental pressure when they clinically present with increasing pain and the features suggestive of a compartment syndrome. **Thus, multiple compartmental syndrome readings must be taken when the suspicion is high and the compartmental pressures are normal.**

UPPER EXTREMITY: FOREARM

The forearm consists of three compartments that are interconnected at various levels.[20,21] This interconnection is significant because release of the pressure in one compartment will reduce some of the pressure in the adjacent compartments. **The volar compartment is most at risk for development of a compartment syndrome in traumatic injuries of the forearm.**

The forearm includes the volar, dorsal, and mobile wad compartments (Figure 63-2). The volar compartment contains all of the hand and forearm flexor muscles. The median and ulnar nerves course through the volar compartment. The vascular contents of this compartment include the radial, ulnar, and common interosseous arteries. The mobile wad contains the brachioradialis, the extensor carpi radialis brevis, and the extensor carpi radialis longus muscles. No major arteries or nerves are contained within this compartment. The radial artery and a branch of the radial nerve may sometimes lie between the mobile wad and the volar com-

partment. The dorsal compartment consists of the hand and forearm extensor muscles. The dorsal compartment contains the posterior interosseous artery and nerve.

INDICATIONS

The earliest and most reliable indication for measuring compartment pressures is the development of increasing pain in a tense and swollen muscle group.[2] This pain tends to be disproportionate to the underlying cause (fracture, soft tissue contusion, thrombus, etc.). Pain that increases with passive motion of the affected muscles is also an indication for compartmental pressure measurement. Sensory deficits and paresis of the affected muscles are two late findings for the development of compartment syndrome.[9] **It is important to remember that the presence of palpable pulses and capillary refill do not rule out an evolving acute compartment syndrome.** The absence of pulses may suggest arterial injury or hypovolemia. One must measure and monitor all compartments at risk if the patient is obtunded or unreliable. This usually refers to the forearm and lower leg compartments in the multiple trauma patient.

Have a very low threshold for measuring pressures within a muscle compartment. Compartmental pressures must be measured if a compartment syndrome is considered as a diagnosis. Do not rely solely on the compartmental pressure measurements to make a

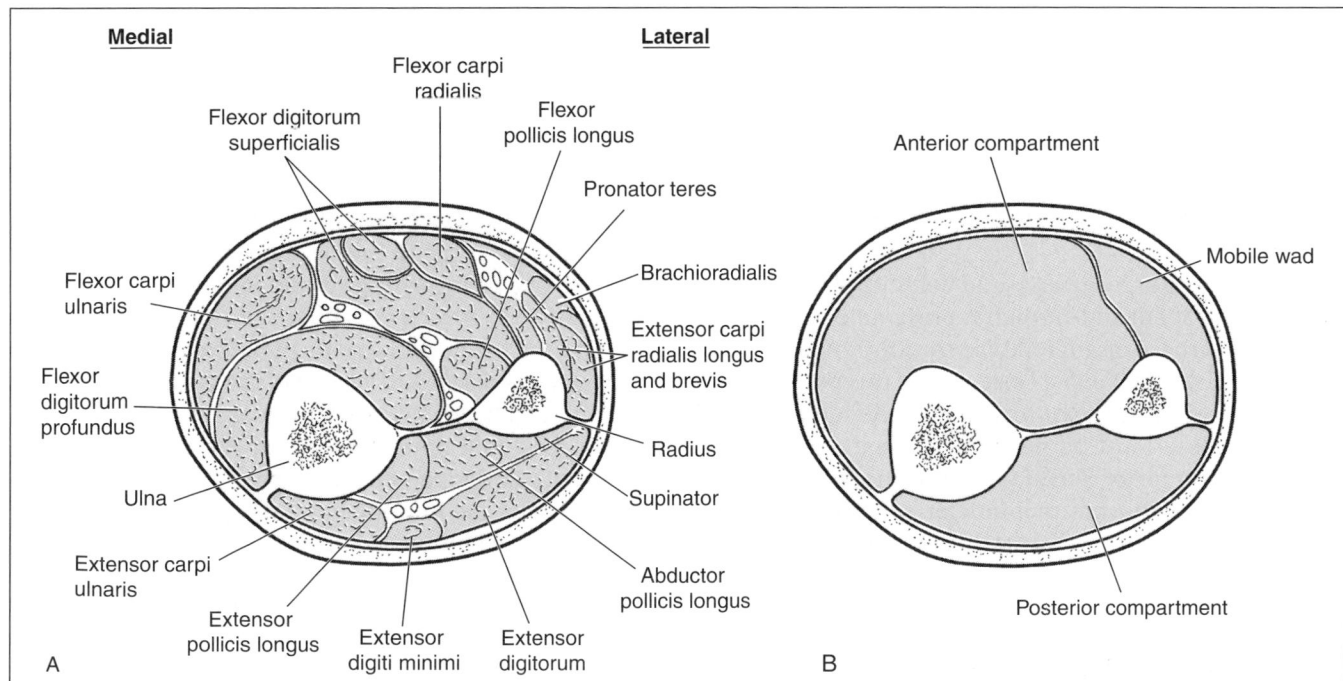

FIGURE 63-2 Cross-section through the middle of the right forearm demonstrating the dorsal and volar compartments separated by the line of the radius, the ulna, and the interosseous membrane. The mobile wad forms a distinct muscle compartment coursing along the radius.

decision regarding the need for fasciotomy. A compartment syndrome is primarily a clinical diagnosis.

CONTRAINDICATIONS

There are no absolute contraindications for measuring compartmental pressures. The physician can still assess the compartmental pressures even though the patient may be undergoing other invasive and/or surgical procedures. **Time is of the essence. Postponing compartmental pressure measurements or a fasciotomy may lead to irreversible damage to the affected extremity.**

EQUIPMENT

General Supplies

Povidone iodine solution
4×4 gauze squares
Sterile drapes or towels

Needle Manometer Technique

Intravenous extension tubing
18 gauge needles, 1.5 inches long
20 mL syringe
Four-way stopcock
Sterile saline
Mercury manometer or electronic arterial pressure
   monitor

Stryker Monitor System

Stryker pressure monitor
Quick pressure monitor set

PATIENT PREPARATION

Explain the purpose, risks, and benefits of this procedure to the patient and/or their representative. Obtain a written or verbal consent for this procedure. A note must be written as to the medical exigency of this procedure if the patient is obtunded or has an altered mental status. This procedure must be performed using sterile technique. Determine the site(s) for needle insertion prior to setting up the pressure manometer system. Clean the skin of any dirt and debris. Apply povidone iodine solution and allow it to dry. Apply sterile drapes to delineate a sterile field.

TECHNIQUES

Many techniques for measuring compartmental pressures have been developed. Some use isolated intracompartmental pressure measurements while others monitor pressure continuously. Obtaining isolated intracompartmental pressure measurements is most important in the Emergency Department. The needle manometer technique modified by Whitesides et al[22] and the modern electronic system developed by Stryker[23] are described below. Similar systems that introduce a wick or slit catheter into the tissue have been shown to be equally effective. For simplicity's sake, explanations of these techniques have been omitted, as they are rarely performed. The needle manometer system can be easily assembled using readily available supplies. The Stryker system is available for the Emergency Physician's use in most hospitals.

The exact location at which to measure the intracompartmental pressures is not clearly defined. There were no clearly established guidelines for determining the appropriate location for compartmental pressure measurements in patients with fractures prior to the recent study of Heckman and Whitesides.[24] The results of their study suggest that measurements must be performed at the level of the fracture "as well as locations proximal and distal to the zone of the fracture." A 5 cm distance was used from the fracture site to the proximal and distal needle insertion sites. **The authors recommend using the highest measured intracompartmental pressure in making the decision for further intervention.**

Clinical judgment is important if the patient does not have a fracture-induced compartment syndrome. The needle should be inserted where the examining physician feels maximal tightness. **Again, multiple measurements at multiple sites are recommended in this scenario.** The needle insertion sites for the leg are demonstrated in Figure 63-3A and described in Table 63-1. The needle insertion sites for the forearm are demonstrated in Figure 63-3B and described in Table 63-2.

NEEDLE MANOMETER TECHNIQUE

Begin by setting up the system (Figure 63-4A). Attach the hub of a 20 mL syringe to the middle port of a three-way stopcock. Attach one end of the intravenous extension tubing to one of the ports of the stopcock. Attach an 18 gauge needle to the free end of the intravenous extension tubing. Insert a second 18 gauge needle into a container of sterile normal saline to release the vacuum. Insert the 18 gauge needle attached to the intravenous extension tubing into the normal saline so that the needle port is well immersed. Open the stopcock ports only to the syringe and the extension tubing. Aspirate the saline to fill one-half of the length of the intravenous extension tubing. **Make sure that no bubbles enter the system.** Turn the stopcock valve so that the port to the saline is closed.

Attach a second piece of intravenous extension tubing to the last port of the stopcock (Figure 63-4B). Attach the free end of this tubing to a manometer or arterial-

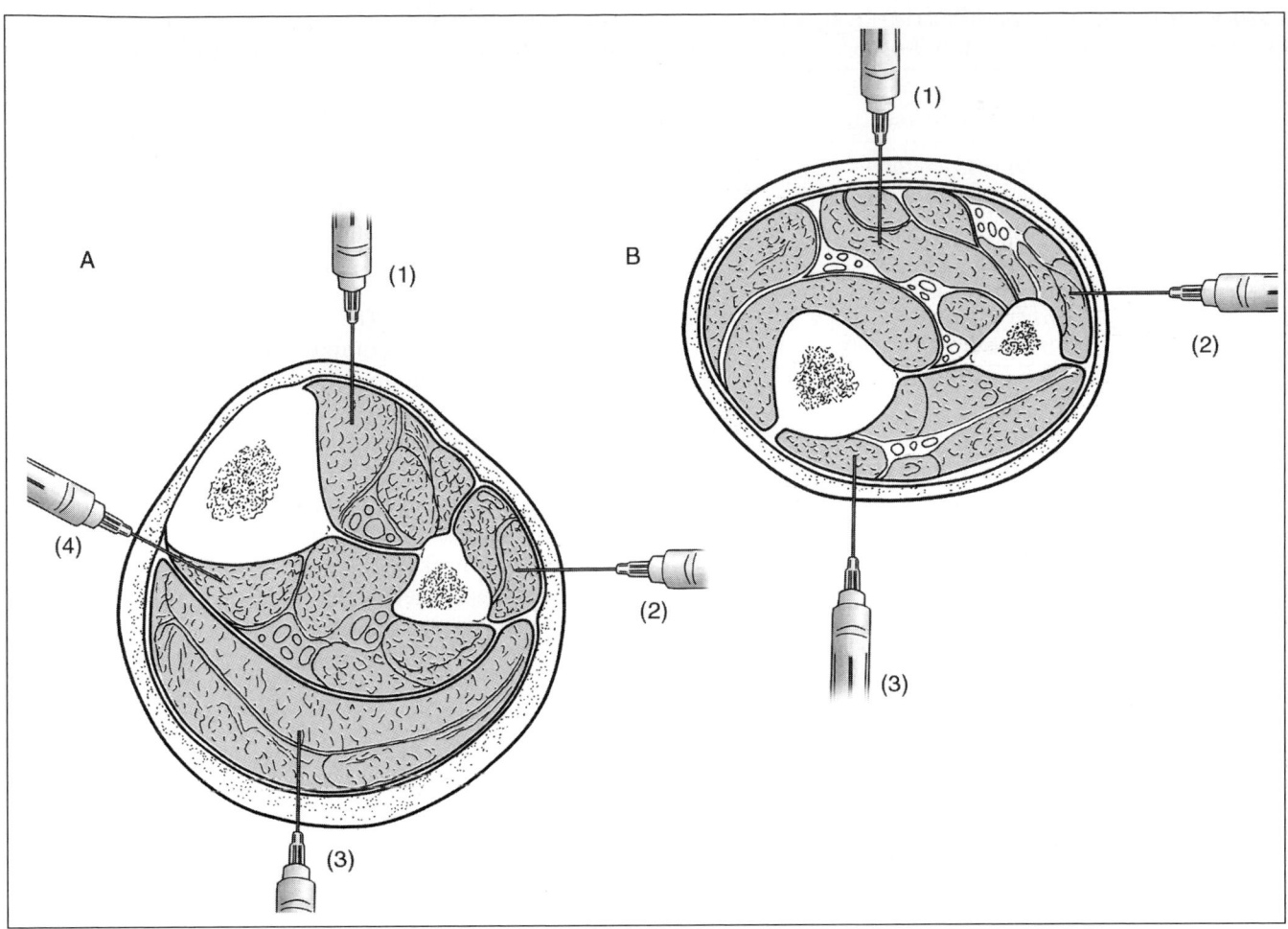

FIGURE 63-3 Needle insertion sites to measure intracompartmental pressures. *A.* The leg compartments: anterior (1), lateral (2), superficial posterior (3), and deep posterior (4). *B.* The forearm compartments: anterior (1), mobile wad (2), and posterior (3).

TABLE 63-1. NEEDLE INSERTION SITES FOR THE COMPARTMENTS OF THE LEG

Compartment	Needle insertion site	Insertion depth (cm)
Anterior	1 cm lateral to the anterior tibial ridge and directed perpendicular to the long axis of the leg	1.0–3.0
Lateral	Just anterior to the posterior border of the fibula and directed toward the fibula	1.0–1.5
Superficial posterior	3 cm medial or lateral to a vertical line drawn through the midcalf	2.0–4.0
Deep posterior	Just posterior to the medial border of the tibia, directed posterolaterally and toward the posterior border of the fibula	2.0–4.0

pressure monitor. Remove the 20 mL syringe from the system and aspirate 15 mL of air into the syringe. Reattach the syringe to the stopcock. Remove the extension tubing with the 18 gauge needle from the saline container.

Insert the 18 gauge needle into the affected muscle compartment (Figure 63-4*B*). Turn the stopcock valve so that all three ports are open. Position the intravenous extension tubing with the normal saline so that the meniscus of the saline-air interface is exactly level with the tip of the needle inserted into the patient's tissue. **The position of the saline-air interface in relation to the tip of the needle is important for an accurate intracompartmental pressure measurement.**

The saline-air interface will form a meniscus when the needle is in the patient. The meniscus will be convex-shaped away from the patient when the tissue pressure is greater than the pressure within the system (Figure 63-5*A*). Depress the plunger of the syringe gradually and delicately to increase the pressure within the system. The shape of the meniscus begins to flatten as the plunger is depressed. **The point where the meniscus is**

TABLE 63-2. NEEDLE INSERTION SITES FOR THE COMPARTMENTS OF THE FOREARM

Compartment	Needle insertion site	Insertion depth (cm)
Anterior	1.5 cm medial to a vertical line drawn through the middle of the forearm	1.0–2.0
Mobile wad	Perpendicular to the long axis of the radius and into the muscles lateral to the radius	1.0–1.5
Posterior	1–2 cm lateral to the posterior aspect of the ulna	1.0–2.0

flat and the saline column begins to move equals the pressure within the compartment (Figure 63-5B). Note and document the pressure on the manometer.

It is important to equilibrate the system between measurements. With the needle still positioned in the tissue, pull back on the syringe plunger until the manometer reads 0 mmHg. Withdraw the needle from the tissue. This will prevent any saline from being deposited in the tissue. The same needle can be reinserted in another location to obtain additional pressure measurements if sterile technique was used throughout the procedure.

The needle puncture sites will bleed. It is important to complete the procedure by properly dressing these puncture wounds. Apply gauze over the puncture sites and tape it in place.

STRYKER TECHNIQUE

The Stryker intracompartmental pressure monitor system is a self-contained device that is convenient, accurate, and relatively easy to use (Figure 63-6). The unit should be kept in a secure place, as it is often misplaced or "borrowed" from the Emergency Department. The pressure monitor is a battery operated, nondisposable unit with a digital display (Figure 63-6A). The quick pressure monitor pack is a disposable, single-patient-use kit that contains a needle, the diaphragm chamber, and a saline-filled syringe (Figure 63-6B).

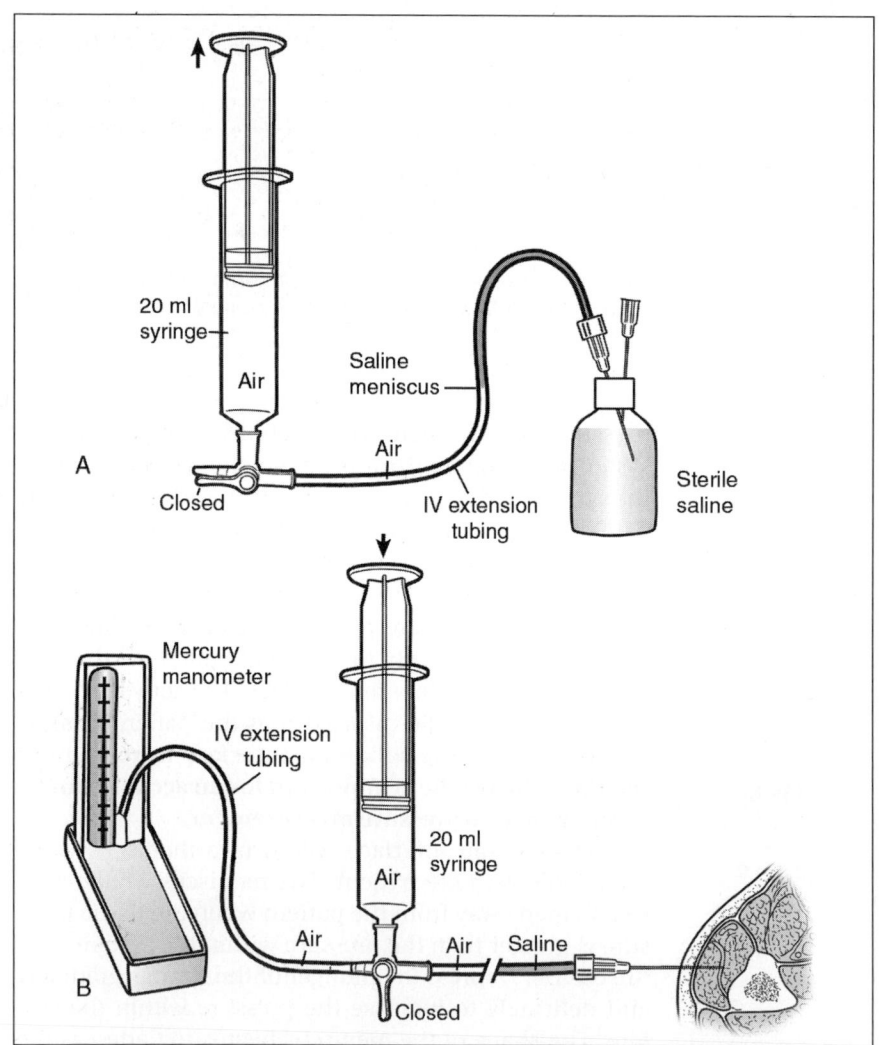

FIGURE 63-4 The needle manometer technique. *A.* The initial system setup. *B.* The final system should form a closed system of space from the manometer through the tissue space.

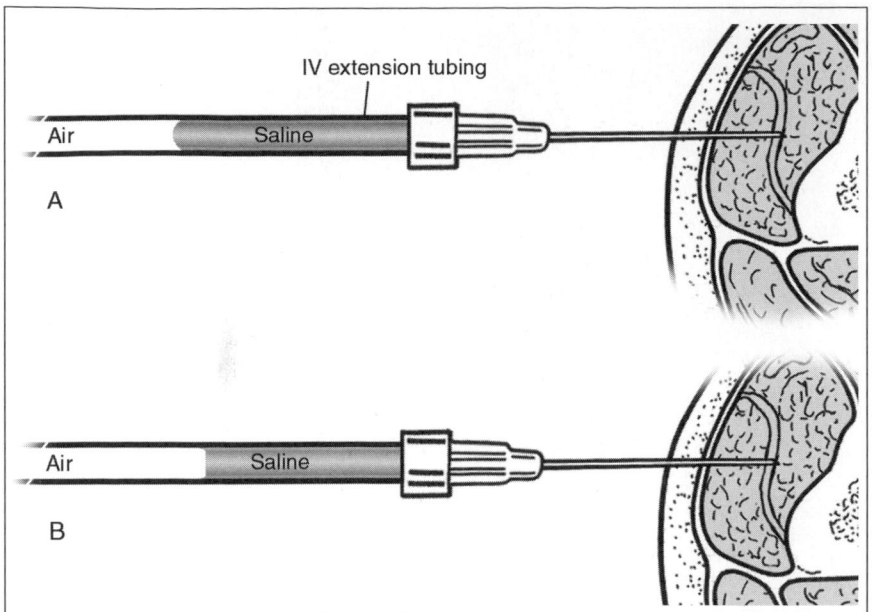

IV extension tubing

Air   Saline

A

Air   Saline

B

FIGURE 63-5 The air-saline interface. *A.* The air-saline meniscus will form a convex shape away from the patient when the tissue pressure is greater than the pressure of the system. *B.* The meniscus will flatten out when the pressure within the system equals that of the patient's tissue.

Turn the pressure monitor unit on. The digital display should read 0 to 9 mmHg. The steps for setting up the system must be performed using sterile technique. Take the diaphragm chamber from the quick pressure monitor pack. This chamber ensures sterility between the system and the patient. Place the 18 gauge, 2.5 inch side-ported needle firmly on the tapered stem of the diaphragm chamber (Figure 63-7*A*). **This needle must remain sterile.** Uncap the 3 mL syringe filled with sterile normal saline and screw it onto the stem of the diaphragm chamber (Figure 63-7*A*). Open the clear plastic lid of the monitor unit. Place the needle-diaphragm chamber-syringe unit on the monitor such that the chamber diaphragm sits in the well (Figure 63-7*B*). Push down gently so that the diaphragm is firmly and evenly positioned on the monitor. Close the cover so that a snap is heard at the latch site.

Hold the monitor unit so that the needle is at a 45 degree angle from the horizontal. Depress the plunger of the syringe to pass saline through the diaphragm chamber and needle and to make sure that no air remains within the system. Position the needle next to the skin at the angle needed for insertion (Figure 63-7*C*). Press the "zero" button on the pressure monitor. The display should read "00" after a few seconds. **Insert the needle into the desired compartment at the same angle used during the zeroing process.** Slowly inject 0.3 mL of saline into the compartment. This volume of fluid is used to equilibrate with the interstitial fluids. Wait a few seconds as the system is measuring the compartmental pressure. The final compartmental pressure measurement will be displayed on the digital screen. Remove the needle from the patient.

Reset the system to zero before taking additional measurements. This is accomplished by positioning the needle at a new site and desired angle of insertion and pressing the zero button. This must be repeated between each measurement. Apply bandages over the skin puncture sites.

An optional indwelling slit catheter set is also available for use on the Stryker pressure monitor. This set substitutes a slit catheter, breakaway needle, and extension tubing for the side-ported needle. The slit catheter is intended to be left within the patient so that multiple sequential intracompartmental pressure measurements may be obtained. This is not intended for use in the Emergency Department.

COMPLICATIONS

There should be no complications for the patient if sterile technique is maintained throughout this procedure. Inserting a needle into a tissue compartment introduces the theoretical risk of infection or damage to the nerves or vessels. No study has shown this to be a significant complication.

A realistic complication of the procedure is obtaining erroneous values. The greatest risk to the patient is if an artificially low pressure is obtained and the needed fasciotomy is not performed. Although false high-pressure readings may also be obtained, the consequences of receiving an unnecessary fasciotomy are less disastrous.

It is important to understand how the mechanics of the needle-manometer system can alter the pressure readings. Injection of normal saline into the tissue will

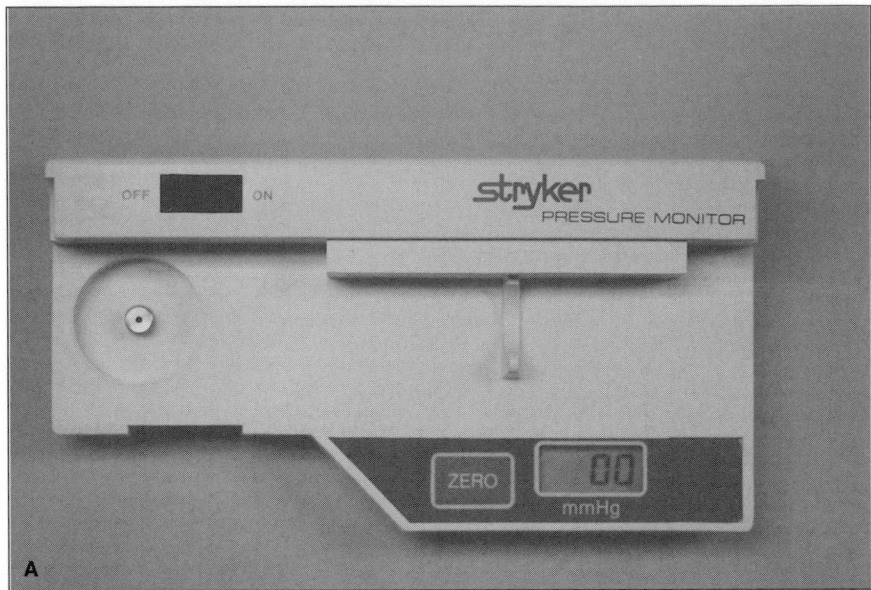

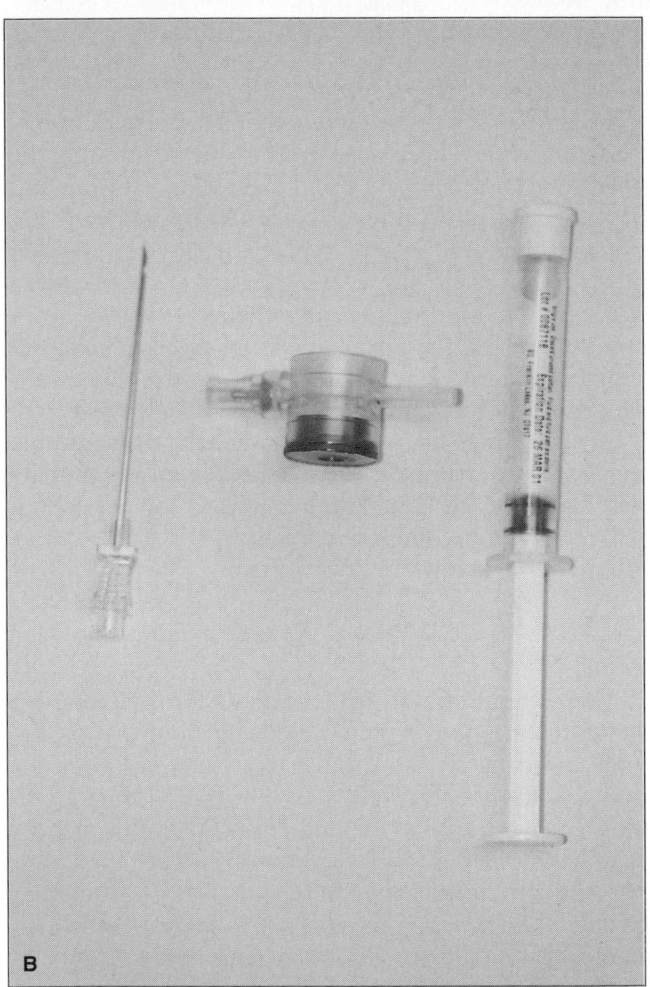

FIGURE 63-6 The Stryker intracompartmental pressure monitor system. *A.* The monitoring unit. *B.* The quick pressure monitor pack contains (*from left to right*): an 18 gauge 2.5 inch side-ported needle, the diaphragm chamber, and a 3 mL syringe filled with sterile saline.

the needle and lead to erroneous pressure measurements. Failing to match up the saline-air meniscus with the level of the needle in the tissue can produce false pressure measurements as well.

One must take multiple pressure measurements around the injury site. To decide whether or not to perform a fasciotomy on an isolated pressure reading is to proceed without all the necessary data. It becomes difficult to simply observe the patient when they clinically present with increasing pain and features suggestive of a compartment syndrome when the compartmental pressure measurement is normal. Thus, multiple readings must be taken when suspicion is high and the compartment pressures are read as normal.

SUMMARY

A compartment syndrome is a well-documented phenomenon. The clinical presentation is variable and changes over time. Determining the pressure within a compartment is a fundamental and essential tool to aid in this diagnosis. Many methods exist for the measurement of compartment pressures. Use of the traditional needle manometer system and the Stryker pressure monitor kit are two established techniques that can easily be performed in the Emergency Department. These two techniques represent the standard of practice in most Emergency Departments. Other methods using noninfusing catheter tips and emission tomography are under investigation as potentially noninvasive procedures.[25,26] Any concern for a compartment syndrome should be followed-up with an orthopedic or surgical consultation, as continuous observation and repeated measurements are often indicated.

raise the pressure reading. The manometer reading will not accurately reflect the pressure of the compartment if the needle is inserted into a tendon rather than the muscle. A piece of tissue from the compartment can obstruct

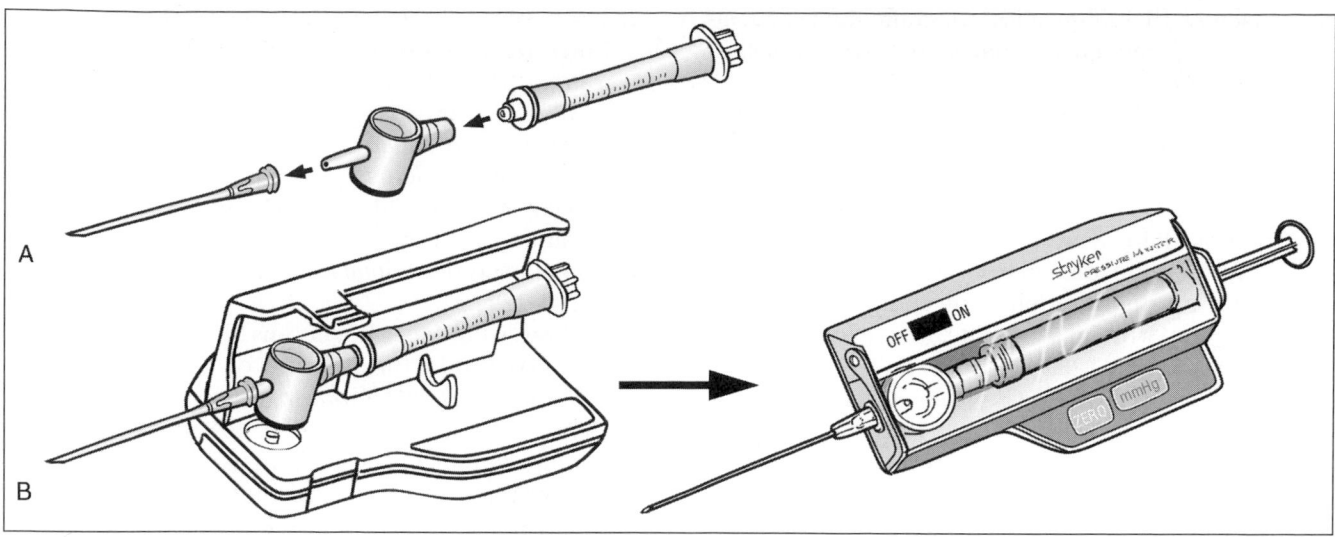

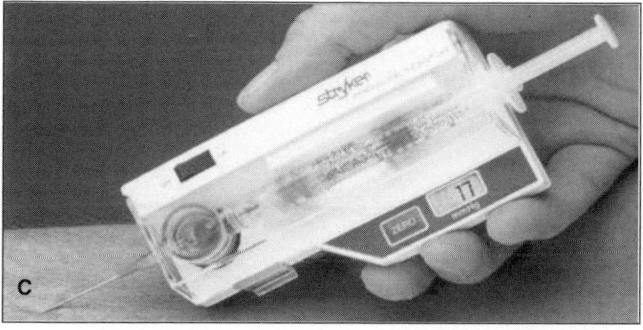

FIGURE 63-7 Measuring intracompartmental pressure with the Stryker system. *A.* The contents of the quick pressure monitor pack are assembled. *B.* The assembled needle-diaphragm-syringe is placed onto the monitor. *C.* The needle is positioned at a 45 degree angle, zeroed, and then advanced into the tissue.

REFERENCES

1. Matsen FA III: Compartment syndrome: a unified concept. *Clin Orthop* 1975; 113:8–14.
2. Whitesides TE, Heckman MH: Acute compartment syndrome: update on diagnosis and treatment. *J Am Acad Orthop Surg* 1996; 4(4):209–218.
3. Volkman R: Die ischaemuschen Muskellahmungen und Kontrakturen. *Zentrabl Chirurg* 1881; 8:801.
4. Christensen KS, Klaerke M: Volkman's ischemic contracture due to limb compression in drug-induced coma. *Injury* 1985; 16:543–545.
5. Heim M, Martinowitz U, Horoszowski H: The short foot syndrome—an unfortunate consequence of neglected raised intracompartment pressure in a severe hemophiliac child. A case report. *Angiology* 1986; 37:128–131.
6. Kunkel JM: Thigh and leg compartment syndrome in the absence of lower extremity trauma following mast application. *Am J Emerg Med* 1987; 5:118–120.
7. Gelberman RH, Garfin SR, Hergenroeder PT, et al: Compartment syndrome of the forearm. Diagnosis and treatment. *Clin Orthop* 1981; 161:252–261.
8. Lee BY, Brancato RF, Park IH, et al: Management of compartment syndrome. Diagnosis and surgical considerations. *Am J Surg* 1984; 148:383–388.
9. Browner BD, Jupiter JB, Levine AM, et al: *Skeletal Trauma.* Philadelphia: Harcourt Brace, 1992: 285–309.
10. Rorabeck CH, Clarke KM: The pathophysiology of the anterior tibia compartment syndrome: an experimental investigation. *J Trauma* 1978; 18:299–306.
11. Whitesides TE, Harada H, Morimoto K: Compartment syndromes and role of fasciotomy: its parameters and techniques. *Instr Course Lect* 1977; 26:179–196.
12. Matara MJ, Whitesides TE, Seiler JG, et al: Determination of the compartment pressure threshold of muscle ischemia in a canine model. *J Trauma* 1994; 37:50–58.
13. Seiler JG III, Womack S, De L'Aune WR, et al: Intracompartmental pressure measurements in the normal forearm. *J Orthop Trauma* 1993; 7:414–416.
14. Geiderman JM: Orthopedics injuries: management principles, in Rosen P, Barkin R, Danzl DF, et al (eds): *Emergency Medicine Concepts and Clinical Practice,* 4th ed. St. Louis: Mosby, 1998:611–613.
15. Mubarak SJ, Owen CA, Hargens AR, et al: Acute compartment syndrome: diagnosis and treatment with the aid of the wick catheter. *J Bone Joint Surg Am* 1978; 60(8):1091–1095.

16. Matsen FA III, Winquist RA, Krugmire RB: Diagnosis and management of compartmental syndromes. *J Bone Joint Surg* 1980; 62(A):286–291.

17. Heckman MM, Whitesides TE, Grewe SR, et al: Compartment pressure in association with closed tibial fractures. *J Bone Joint Surg Am* 1994; 76(9):1285–1292.

18. Heppenstall RB, Scott R, Sapega A, et al: A comparative study of the tolerance of skeletal muscle to ischemia: tourniquet application compared with acute compartment syndrome. *J Bone Joint Surg Am* 1986; 68:820–828.

19. Hollinshead WH, Rosse C: *Textbook of Anatomy,* 4th ed. Philadelphia: Harper & Row, 1985:231–260.

20. Netter FH, Colacino S: *Atlas of Human Anatomy.* Summit, NJ: Ciba-Geigy, 1990.

21. Hollinshead WH, Rosse C: *Textbook of Anatomy,* 4th ed. Philadelphia: Harper & Row, 1985:413–434.

22. Whitesides TE, Hanet TC, Hirada H, et al: A simple method for tissue pressure determination. *Arch Surg* 1975; 110:1311.

23. *STRYKER Intra-compartmental Pressure Monitor System: Instructional Manual.* Kalamazoo, MI: Stryker Instruments.

24. Heckman MM, Whitesides TE, Grewe SR, et al: Compartment pressure in association with closed tibial fractures. *J Bone Joint Surg Am* 1994; 76(9):1285–1292.

25. Edwards PD, Miles KA, Owens SJ, et al: A new noninvasive test for the detection of compartment syndromes. *Nucl Med Commun* 1999; 20(3):215–218.

26. Willy C, Gerngross H, Sterk J: Measurement of intra-compartmental pressure with use of a new electronic transducer-tipped catheter system. *J Bone Joint Surg Am* 1999: 81(2):158–168.

Chapter 64
EXTENSOR TENDON REPAIR

Amy M. Hutson
David Rovinsky

INTRODUCTION

The Emergency Physician commonly encounters lacerations or trauma to the hand. In examining these patients, one must examine the hand and explore the wound for extensor tendon lacerations. The extensor mechanism of the hand and forearm is typically disrupted in association with penetrating trauma. Blunt trauma, such as sudden forced flexion, can also result in injury to the extensor tendons. Performing extensor tendon repair is an important skill in the Emergency Physician's surgical armamentarium.

Although it is important that any deficit in the extensor tendon mechanism be identified at the initial examination, the timing of tendon repair is not a critical aspect of its management. Successful repair of extensor tendons can be accomplished either acutely or within a 7 day window following injury.[1] One should also be aware that at some anatomic sites, splint immobilization of the damaged tendon can produce the same optimal outcome as surgical reapproximation. This is most evident in conservative management of a mallet finger injury.

Repair of an extensor tendon in the Emergency Department requires that the physician be familiar with the anatomy of the region and skilled in the surgical technique. Although complications of tendon repair are more frequently associated with flexor tendons, follow-up studies of extensor tendon repairs reveal similar pitfalls and problems.[2] Adhesion, loss of length, and diminished flexion can all complicate the repair of an extensor tendon.[3]

The anatomy of the extensor mechanism is such that following a laceration or partial disruption, the tendons seldom retract far from the site of injury.[4] This is mostly due to the tethering of tendons by multiple interconnections as the tendons cross the dorsum of the hand. Additionally, the tendons over the dorsum of the hand are ensheathed in a paratenon layer of tissue. This covering is extrasynovial, thus exposing the tendons but containing them in a layer that prevents their wide separation. The physician can proceed safely with the surgical repair if both ends of a lacerated extensor tendon are identified.

The surgical technique for repairing extensor tendons originates in studies of flexor tendon repairs. The goal of the repair is to restore tendon continuity and function while minimizing interference from the repair itself. The suture techniques of Kessler and Bunnell are two of the methods traditionally used in this repair. Modifications of these original methods have resulted in the greatest outcome measurements of tendon strength.[5] Facility with these two suture techniques is essential in repairing any extensor tendon in the Emergency Department.

ANATOMY AND PATHOPHYSIOLOGY

The extensor tendon mechanism is an intricate system of pulleys and levers coursing along the dorsum of the forearm, wrist, and hand.[6,7] The function of these tendons is to extend the fingers and wrist from a flexed position. This function is complemented in the fingers by the actions of the intrinsic muscle groups (lumbricals and interossei).

The elegant anatomy of the hand extensor mechanism is best appreciated in diagrammatic representation (Figure 64-1). The forearm tendons pass through the extensor retinaculum of the wrist to travel unprotected across the dorsum of the hand to each of the fingers. The extensor tendons are reinforced in the fingers by the lateral bands of the intrinsic muscles to form a complex tendon that inserts into the distal phalanx (Figure 64-2).

Knowledge of the anatomy of the extensor mechanism reveals certain salient points. The extensor retinaculum of the wrist is a complicated structure of fibrous canals through which the tendons pass and whose repair necessitates a Hand Surgeon's intervention. The paucity of soft tissue covering the dorsum of the hand makes the tendons quite vulnerable to penetrating trauma. The exten-

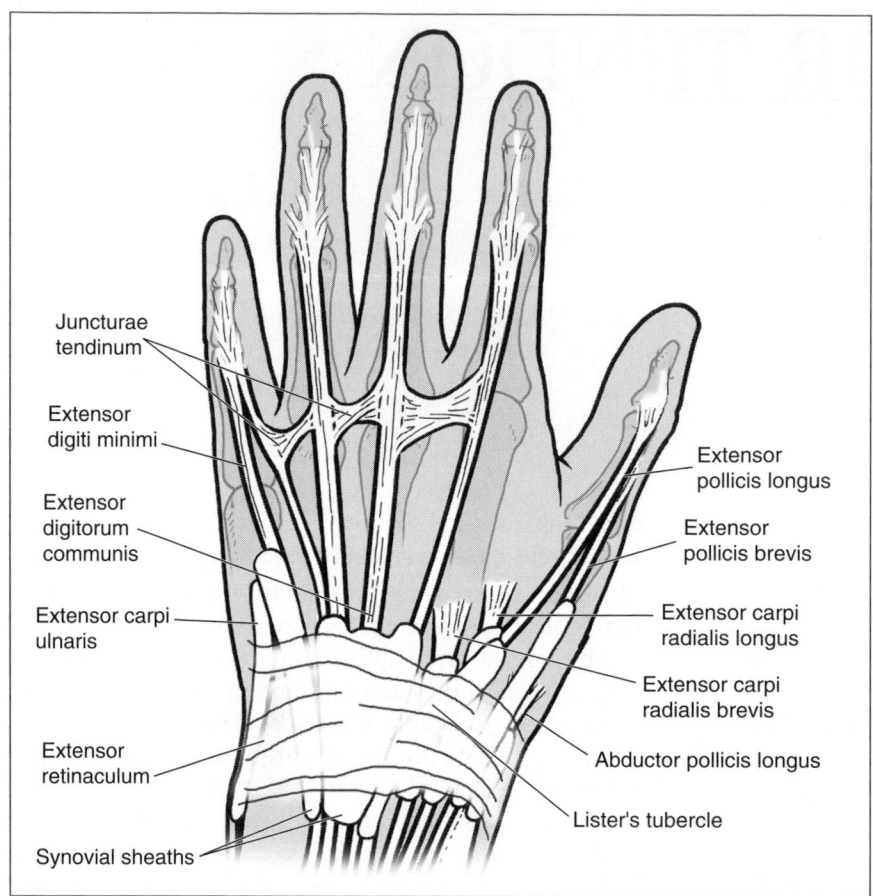

Juncturae
tendinum

Extensor
digiti minimi

Extensor
digitorum
communis

Extensor carpi
ulnaris

Extensor
retinaculum

Synovial sheaths

Extensor
pollicis longus

Extensor
pollicis brevis

Extensor carpi
radialis longus

Extensor carpi
radialis brevis

Abductor pollicis longus

Lister's tubercle

FIGURE 64-1 The extensor tendons of the hand begin just proximal to the extensor retinaculum. After exiting from under this encasing sheath, the tendons form an interconnected network as they cross the dorsum of the hand.

sor tendons of the fingers are interconnected across the dorsum of the hand. An isolated tear of the extensor tendon (like the digiti minimi) will usually not result in lack of function because of the contributing band from the extensor digitorum communis (Figure 64-3). This interconnection of tendons, called the juncturae tendinum, distributes the work of extension among the involved fingers. It is important to realize that there is great anatomic variability in the detailed distribution of these tendons.

The location of an extensor tendon injury is important in determining whether tendon repair in the acute setting is feasible. A range of eight zones defines the location of an extensor tendon injury. The zone chart first described by Kleinert and Verdan helps to classify and organize the modes of repair.[8] The odd-numbered zones refer to areas over the joints, while the even-numbered zones refer to the bony areas (Figure 64-4). Although any zone can undergo injury and repair, the outcome is variable, depending upon the suture technique and the mode of rehabilitation.

INDICATIONS

The decision to surgically repair a lacerated extensor tendon is multifactorial. One must consider the extent of the tendon laceration, the involvement of other tis-

sues (bone or joint space), and the location of the tendon injury. Studies that define a minimum laceration width that requires tendon repair have not been performed. **It is generally accepted that a laceration greater than 50 percent of the tendon width requires surgical repair.**[1] A tendon that has a laceration less than 50 percent of its width will usually heal with conservative management. **One must put the finger through its entire range of motion to confirm normal function and movement of the affected tendon prior to making the decision as to whether conservative management is appropriate.** A lacerated tendon that is associated with significant overlying skin loss, joint space penetration, or a bony fracture will need repair. This repair should not occur in the Emergency Department. Consult an Orthopedic or Hand Surgeon for surgical repair.

Defining the location of the tendon injury according to the Kleinert zone system guides one in deciding which tendons can safely be repaired in the Emergency Department. Although there are no published guidelines on where these procedures should be performed, a thorough understanding of the extensor tendon's anatomy and a good dose of common sense are imperative. The following zones and types of injury represent sites where extensor tendon repair in the Emergency Department is feasible with minimal complications. The thickness of

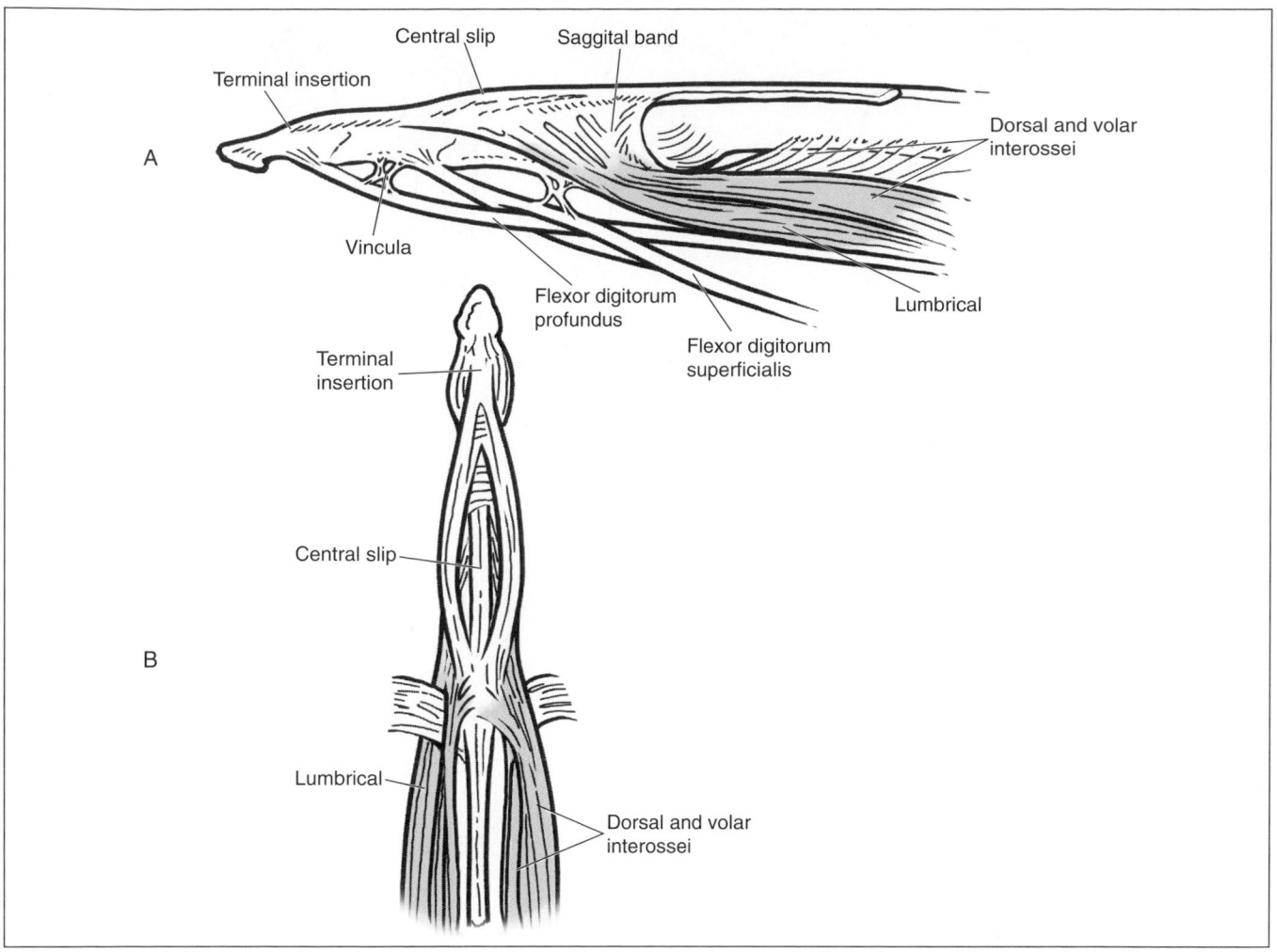

FIGURE 64-2 The central extensor tendons of the digits are reinforced and aided by the lateral bands of the interosseous and lumbrical muscles. The extensor tendon is tethered to the joint surface by a sagittal band, which forms a protective hood. *A.* Lateral view. *B.* Superior view.

the extensor pollicis longus allows for a core-type suture in zone 2 of the thumb. The broad configuration of the extensor tendon allows for a core-type suture in zone 4 of all digits. Isolated involvement of the extensor tendon allows for a core-type suture unless the joint is involved (rare) in zone 5 of the fingers. Isolated involvement of the extensor tendon allows for a core-type suture and good prognosis in zone 6 of the hand.

CONTRAINDICATIONS

There are definite contraindications to repairing an extensor tendon in the Emergency Department. First and foremost, the lack of skill on the part of the physician performing this repair may result in loss of function or may further compromise the patient's hand. Loosely close the skin over the wound, splint the hand, and refer the patient for delayed repair of the extensor tendon if a skilled physician is not available to perform this procedure. Sur-

gical repair of the tendon is not recommended if less than 50 percent of the tendon is lacerated and the finger functions as well as the corresponding finger on the unaffected opposite hand. The presence of a bony fracture, an open joint space, or the lack of adequate soft tissue or skin covering are contraindications to repairing an extensor tendon in the Emergency Department. A tendon laceration as a result of a human bite wound is an absolute contraindication to closure and repair of the injury. The management and rehabilitation of these wounds necessitate consultation with the appropriate surgical specialist.

The Kleinert zone chart can be used to help determine the suitability of repairing an extensor tendon in the Emergency Department. The following zones on the arm and hand represent areas where wound care, skin closure, and splinting are highly recommended until an Orthopedic or Hand Surgeon can perform the definitive surgical repair. Extensor tendon remnants may be too short in zone 1 of all digits. Except in the thumb, extensor tendons of the fingers that are very thin in zone 2 should not be repaired.

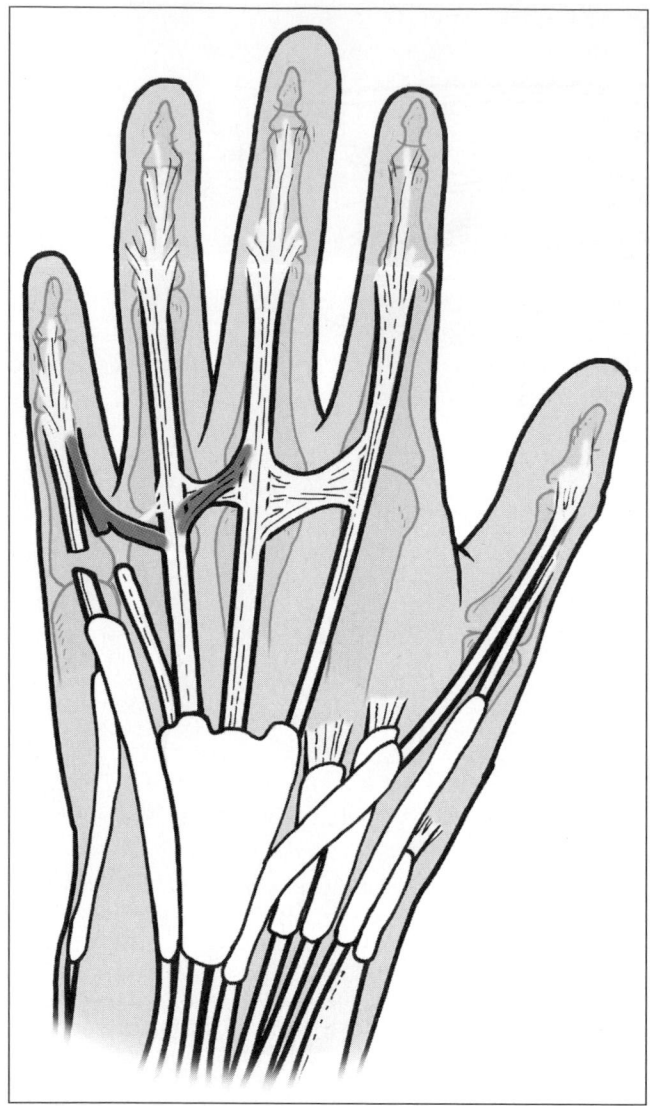

FIGURE 64-3 Division of an extensor tendon in the dorsum of the hand may still allow for full finger extension because of the communicating juncturae tendinum.

Actual or potential joint or lateral band involvement in zone 3 of all digits should not be repaired. Actual or potential joint or sagittal band involvement in zone 5 of all digits should not be repaired. Actual or potential extensor retinaculum involvement in zone 7 should not be repaired. The actual or potential need for tendon transfer in zone 8 requires an Orthopedic or Hand Surgeon.

EQUIPMENT

Digital or Hand Anesthesia

Povidone iodine solution
10 mL syringe
25 to 27 gauge needle, 2 inches long
Local anesthetic solution without epinephrine

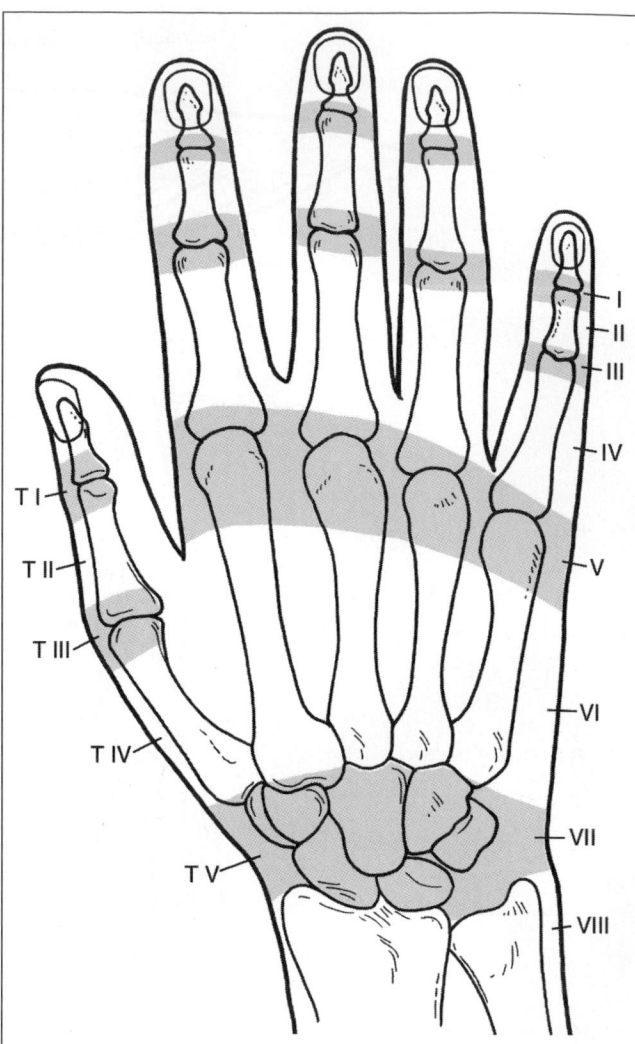

FIGURE 64-4 The extensor tendons of the hand are easily classified by the Kleinert zone system. The odd numbers represent joint spaces. The even numbers represent long bones. Note that the thumb zones are distinct from the other digits.

Extensor Wound Irrigation and Preparation

250 to 500 mL of sterile saline or Ringer's lactate
    solution
Irrigation set
60 mL syringe
16 gauge angiocatheter
Intravenous tubing
Protective facial shield
Blood pressure cuff, preferably automatic
Overhead lamp or source of intense lighting

Extensor Tendon and Skin Repair

Sterile surgical towels
4×4 gauze squares

Forceps
Needle driver
Nonabsorbable, synthetic, and braided suture (4–0, 5–0, and 6–0 Ethibond or Mersilene)
Nylon suture (4–0 and 5–0) for skin closure

Wound Dressing and Splint

Topical antibiotic ointment
Gauze squares
Elastic gauze bandage
Splint material

PATIENT PREPARATION

Explain the risks, benefits, and complications of the procedure to the patient and/or their representative. Additionally, alternative forms of therapy should be discussed. Upon receiving verbal or written consent, the physician may proceed with prepping and positioning the patient.

Place the patient in a supine and comfortable position to minimize movement during the course of the procedure. Place the involved hand on a bedside procedure table at body or heart level so that the patient's arm is resting comfortably. Temporarily diminish arterial blood flow with either a digital tourniquet or a blood pressure cuff applied to the arm if vascular bleeding is active and obscures the site of repair. The maximum time for tourniquet application is generally 2 hours.[8] Any surgical procedure that takes this long should not be performed in the Emergency Department.

Anesthesia to the affected area can be best accomplished with either a digital or wrist block. The choice of procedures depends upon the location and extent of the injury. Descriptions of these procedures can be found in Chapter 106. Once the patient has adequate anesthesia, the wound can be debrided and copiously irrigated with 250 to 500 mL of sterile saline (if no open joint is involved). Following irrigation, the wound is considered sterile; all techniques must be aseptic from this point forward. Apply sterile drapes or towels to delineate a sterile field. Place a sterile drape over the bedside procedure table. Lay out the required instruments and suture material on the bedside procedure table.

TECHNIQUE

Many techniques are used to repair lacerated tendons. All of the original techniques were described with reference to flexor tendons. The application of these techniques, with some modifications, has been extended to include the repair of the extensor tendons. Four com-
mon suture techniques used for a "core" repair of the extensor tendon include the mattress stitch, the figure-of-eight stitch, the modified Bunnell stitch, and the modified Kessler stitch (Figure 64-5). No study has determined the optimal stitch for repair of each zone of injury. However, evidence does exist that the modified Kessler and modified Bunnell stitches produce the greatest strength for a core-type tendon repair.[5] The modified Bunnell and Kessler are equally effective suture techniques for zone 4.[5] The modified Bunnell technique produces the optimal outcome for zone 6.[10] While the literature supports the use of the modified Bunnell and Kessler suture techniques, it has been the editors' experience that these suture techniques are not as useful in the Emergency Department for extensor tendon injuries in zone 4 or zone 6. The reason for this is that the tendon tends to be so thin in this area that it makes the use of these techniques quite difficult. The Bunnell and Kessler techniques are more useful in round, thicker tendons such as the flexor tendons or selected extensor tendons.

MODIFIED KESSLER STITCH

This "core" stitch is designed to place the direction of force perpendicular to the longitudinal axis of the tendon (Figure 64-5C). If the force of the suture is placed in the tendon's longitudinal axis there is a tendency for the suture to pull through and shred the tendon.

Identify the two ends of the lacerated extensor tendon. **Handle the cut ends with maximal care. Blindly or bluntly grabbing the ends traumatizes the tendons and compromises the repair.** A retracted tendon can be held in place with a needle piercing it perpendicularly. Carefully debride the tendon ends if they are jagged or dirty. **Do not remove too much length from the tendon.** Place the affected digit in maximum extension to facilitate approximation of the tendon ends.

Hold one end of the tendon gently with your fingers or a stitch. Introduce the needle into the cut end of the tendon (Figure 64-5C-1). The entrance point should be about one-third of the diameter of the tendon, beginning on either its ulnar or radial side. For simplicity, we begin on the radial side. Pass the suture approximately 1 cm through the length of the tendon and exit dorsally (Figure 64-5C-2). Wrap the suture around the tendon (Figure 64-5C-3). Reenter the radial side of the tendon perpendicularly and 1 to 2 mm closer to the tendon end (Figure 64-5C-3). Pull the suture straight through the tendon to exit on its ulnar side (Figure 64-5C-4). Wrap the suture around the tendon (Figure 64-5C-5). Enter the dorsal aspect of the ulnar half of the tendon (Figure 64-5C-5). This entrance stitch must line up with the first dorsal stitch (Figure 64-5C-2). Pass the needle through the length of the tendon to exit the end of the tendon (Figure 64-5C-6). The needle must exit on the ulnar one-third of the tendon.

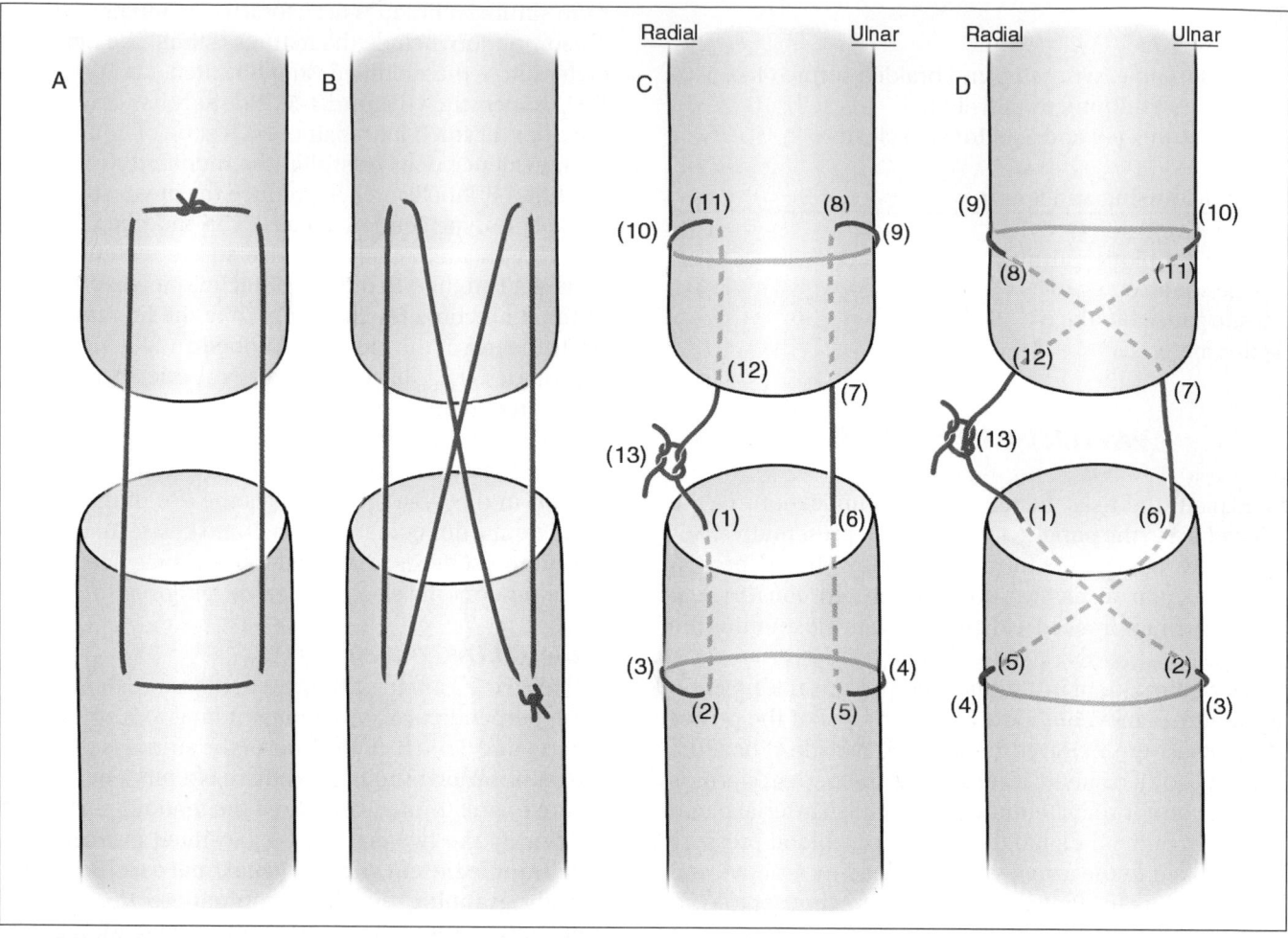

FIGURE 64-5 Suture techniques for extensor tendon repair. *A.* Mattress stitch. *B.* Figure-of-eight stitch. *C.* The modified Kessler stitch. The numbers represent the sequence of steps. *D.* The modified Bunnell stitch. The numbers represent the sequence of steps.

Repeat the same stitch on the opposing piece of the tendon. Pass the needle into the ulnar one-third of the tendon (Figure 64-5C-7). Pass the suture approximately 1 cm through the length of the tendon and exit dorsally (Figure 64-5C-8). Wrap the suture around the tendon (Figure 64-5C-9). Reenter the ulnar side of the tendon perpendicularly and 1 to 2 mm closer to the tendon end (Figure 64-5C-9). Pull the suture straight through the tendon to exit its radial side (Figure 64-5C-10). Reenter the dorsal aspect of the radial half of the tendon (Figure 64-5C-11). The stitch must line up with the previous dorsal stitch (Figure 64-5C-8). Pass the needle through the length of the tendon to exit the end of the tendon (Figure 64-5C-12). The needle must exit on the radial one-third of the tendon.

The two free ends of the suture should be on the radial side of the tendon. Apply tension to the two free ends of the suture to gently approximate the ends of the lacerated tendon. **Do not apply so much force that the ends buckle up.** Secure the stitch with a knot that will remain buried between the tendon ends (Figure 64-5C-13).

MODIFIED BUNNELL STITCH

This stitch follows the same principle as the Kessler stitch. It incorporates a crossing of the suture in its pathway (Figure 64-5D). Remember to minimize the handling of the tendon in performing this stitch. **Instrumentation of the tissue is detrimental to its nutritional supply and can lead to adhesions.** Ideally, one should immobilize the tendon ends with one's fingers or a single suture.

Enter the tendon end on the radial half and at approximately one-third of the diameter of the tendon (Figure 64-5D-1). Pass the needle diagonally through the tendon and exit on the ulnar side (Figure 64-5D-2). Wrap the suture around the tendon (Figure 64-5D-3). Reenter the tendon on its dorsal half (Figure 64-5D-3). Pass the needle directly through the tendon to exit the dorsal surface of the radial aspect of the tendon (Figure 64-5D-4). Enter the radial side of the tendon (Figure 64-5D-5). Cross the suture diagonally through the tendon to exit its ulnar end (Figure 64-5D-6). The needle must exit through the ulnar one-third of the tendon end.

Repeat the same stitch on the opposing piece of the tendon. Pass the needle into the ulnar one-third of the tendon (Figure 64-5D-7). Pass the needle diagonally through the tendon and exit on the radial side (Figure 64-5D-8). Wrap the suture around the tendon (Figure 64-5D-9). Reenter the tendon on its dorsal half (Figure 64-5D-9). Pass the needle directly through the tendon to exit the dorsal surface of the ulnar aspect of the tendon (Figure 64-5D-10). Wrap the suture around the tendon (Figure 64-5D-11). Enter the ulnar side of the tendon (Figure 64-5D-11). Cross the suture diagonally through the tendon to exit the radial end of the tendon (Figure 64-5D-12). The needle must exit through the ulnar one-third of the tendon end.

The two free ends of the suture should be on the radial side of the tendon. Pull gently on the suture ends to approximate the ends of the lacerated tendon. **Do not apply so much force that the ends buckle up.** Secure the stitch with a knot, which will remain buried within the tendon ends (Figure 64-5D-13).

AFTERCARE

Close the overlying skin with nylon suture. Apply topical antibiotic ointment. Apply 4×4 gauze squares to cover the wound. Apply an elastic bandage for protection. Splint the extremity to immobilize the repaired tendon and its associated muscle belly.

The patient may be discharged home with follow-up arranged within 24 to 48 hours with an Orthopedic or Hand Surgeon. Instruct the patient to elevate the extremity. They should return to the Emergency Department immediately if there is increased pain, numbness or tingling in the digits, if the digits become cold or blue, or if a fever develops. Pain can be controlled by the use of nonsteroidal anti-inflammatory drugs supplemented with an occasional narcotic analgesic.

Static immobilization may not be the optimal postoperative management for extensor tendon repairs. The affected tendon may benefit from early mobilization exercises or dynamic splinting depending upon the zone of injury. Dynamic extension splinting may produce fewer complications and less postoperative adhesions.[11-13] Tendon injuries in zones 1 to 4 can be temporarily immobilized in extension until follow-up by an Orthopedic Surgeon determines the definitive splinting management. Tendon injuries in zones 5 to 8 can be placed in a temporary static splint with the wrist in 30 degrees of extension, the MCP joints in 15 degrees of flexion, and the interphalangeal joints in full extension.

The aftercare of extensor tendon lacerations necessitates close follow-up by an Orthopedic or Hand Surgeon for wound evaluation and rehabilitation strategy. **Proper aftercare and hand rehabilitation is crucial to ensure successful results of a tendon repair.**

COMPLICATIONS

Surgical repair of any open wound or tendon laceration can result in unforeseen infections. Careful instructions for wound care and follow-up evaluations are important for early detection and treatment of tissue infection.

Failure of the tendon repair can be due to several etiologies. Disruption of the surgical repair, the formation of adhesions, and joint stiffness can produce an inadequate outcome.[9] It is rare to encounter these complications in the Emergency Department. Nonetheless, they are real complications that both the physician and patient must discuss before proceeding with the repair procedure.

SUMMARY

The repair of an extensor tendon laceration can and does occur in the Emergency Department. While the literature and authors have found that the use of the Bunnell and Kessler stitches for the repair of extensor tendon injuries produce good results, it has been the editors' experience that the mattress technique and figure-of-eight stitch are more useful in the thinner extensor tendons. Even if the tendon repair does not occur in the Emergency Department, the wound must be irrigated, explored, and closed for delayed surgical repair. Postoperative rehabilitation is crucial to ensure an optimal outcome. Splinting in the emergency setting should be only a temporizing immobilization procedure until rehabilitation therapy occurs.

REFERENCES

1. Newport ML: Extensor tendon injuries in the hand. *J Am Acad Orthop Surg* 1997; 5(2):59–66.
2. Newport ML, Blair WF, Steyers CM Jr: Long-term results of extensor tendon repair. *J Hand Surg (Am)* 1990; 15:961–966.
3. Klutz JE, Bennet DL: *Methods and Concepts in Hand Surgery: Tendon Injuries.* London: Butterworths, 1986.
4. McFarlane RM, Hampole MK: The treatment of extensor tendon injuries of the hand. *Can J Surg* 1973; 16:366–375.

5. Newport ML, Pollack GR, Williams CD: Biomechanical characteristics of suture techniques in extensor zone IV. *J Hand Surg* 1995; 20A:650–656.

6. Netter FH, Colacino S: *Atlas of Human Anatomy.* Summit, NJ: Ciba-Geigy, 1990.

7. Hollinshead WH, Rosse C: *Textbook of Anatomy,* 4th ed. Philadelphia: Harper & Row, 1985.

8. Kleinert HE, Verdan C: Report of the committee on tendon injures. *J Hand Surg* 1983; 8:794–798.

9. Green DP, Hotchkiss RN, Pederson WC: *Green's Operative Hand Surgery,* 4th ed. Philadelphia: Churchill Livingstone, 1999.

10. Newport ML, Williams CD: Biomechanical characteristics of extensor tendon suture techniques. *J Hand Surg (Am)* 1992; 17:1117–1123.

11. Evans RB, Thompson DE: An analysis of factors that support early active short arc motion of the repaired central slip. *J Hand Ther* 1992; 5:187–202.

12. Feehan LM, Beauchene JG: Early tensile properties of healing chicken flexor tendons: early controlled passive motion versus postoperative immobilization. *J Hand Surg (Am)* 1990; 15:63–68.

13. Hung LK, Chan A, Chang J, et al: Early controlled active mobilization with dynamic splintage for treatment of extensor tendon injuries. *J Hand Surg (Am)* 1991;16:1145–1150.

Chapter 65
ARTHROCENTESIS

Eric F. Reichman
Richard Waddell

INTRODUCTION

Arthrocentesis is the removal of synovial fluid from a joint cavity. Fluid can be aspirated from almost any joint. Arthrocentesis is used to diagnose and make treatment decisions regarding a joint. Obtaining synovial fluid is safe, simple, relatively pain free, inexpensive, and extremely beneficial to the patient.

Arthrocentesis may be diagnostic or therapeutic. Diagnostically, it is performed to identify the cause of an acute arthritis, to identify an intraarticular fracture, to identify the causes of an effusion, or to give a therapeutic trial of pharmaceuticals. It can also be therapeutic by relieving pain from elevated intraarticular pressure, to drain septic or crystal-laden fluid, or to inject pharmaceuticals.

Synovial fluid analysis will provide unique and valuable information about the affected joint. It is the only method to definitively diagnose or rule out a septic arthritis. The fluid should be analyzed for the presence of crystals. A white blood cell count and differential may help identify the causes of an effusion. A Gram's stain can be quickly performed to identify bacteria in the synovial fluid. A culture of the synovial fluid should be performed to definitively identify any microbiologic pathogen in the joint.

There are several general principles that should be followed when performing an arthrocentesis (Table 65-1). The physician must know the anatomical relationships around the joint. The needle should go around and not through any tendons. Avoid piercing the articular cartilage, which is avascular and may not heal. Do not bounce the needle off the bone, as this is extremely painful for the patient. Insert the needle through the extensor surface of the joint. The synovial cavity is closest to the skin over the extensor surface of the joint. The extensor surface has fewer tendons and ligaments than the flexor surface. Most of the blood vessels and nerves are located on the flexor surface of the joint. Using the extensor surface of the joint for the procedure will avoid potential injury to these structures. Place the joint in slight flexion to maximize the size of the joint cavity. Apply distal in-line traction to the small joints of the wrists, hands, and feet to enlarge the joint cavity. This allows the needle to more easily enter the small joint spaces. Compression of large joints will mobilize peripheral fluid. This is helpful when the volume of synovial fluid is small. Compression may be applied manually or with an elastic bandage.

It is critical to use sterile technique to prevent the infection of a nonseptic joint as well as to ensure the joint fluid is uncontaminated for microbiological cultures. Sterile drapes, sterile gloves, and face masks are not needed to perform the procedure.[1-3] It is necessary to wear gloves to prevent transmission of blood-borne diseases to the physician.[1,4] The skin should be cleansed and prepped in the usual manner. The needle may then be grasped, with clean gloves, at the hub and inserted. As long as the skin and needle are not handled, sterile gloves are not required. This is sometimes difficult to master when the physician has little practice with the technique of arthrocentesis. It may be better to err on the side of conservatism and use sterile gloves and drapes; particularly with inexperienced physicians and in training situations.

TABLE 65-1. GENERAL PRINCIPLES FOR ARTHROCENTESIS

Know the anatomical relationships
Use sterile technique
Provide adequate analgesia
Place the joint in slight flexion
Apply distal traction to small joints
Apply compression to large joints
Enter the extensor surface

INDICATIONS

Arthrocentesis is indicated to evaluate the cause of an arthritis or a joint effusion (Table 65-2).[4-7] All patients presenting with an acute monoarthritis or an acute nontraumatic effusion should undergo arthrocentesis when the diagnosis is not clear based upon the history and physical examination. Analysis of the synovial fluid is essential to help differentiate inflammatory from noninflammatory causes of joint disease. **Arthrocentesis is the only reliable method to confirm the presence of an infectious agent as the cause of an arthritis.** The presence of crystals within the synovial fluid can diagnose gout or pseudogout from other crystal-induced arthritides. Always keep in mind that two or more types of arthritis can coexist in a patient or in a single joint.[4]

Arthrocentesis may be therapeutic.[8] A large effusion, regardless of the cause, stretches the joint capsule, causing pain and limiting range of motion. Removal of the fluid will decrease pain and increase the joint's range of motion. An effusion caused by inflammation or sepsis contains numerous mediators of inflammation. Removal of this synovial fluid will help to relieve the patient's discomfort. The removal of purulent fluid will decrease the number of organisms in the joint cavity and, theoretically, may limit further joint destruction.

Injection of therapeutic agents into nonseptic joints is commonly performed in the Emergency Department. Local anesthetic solutions may be injected to relieve pain. A joint examination after trauma may be limited secondary to pain. Injection of local anesthetic solutions

TABLE 65-2. THE INDICATIONS FOR PERFORMING AN ARTHROCENTESIS

To evaluate a monoarticular arthritis
To diagnose and treat a traumatic arthritis
To diagnose an intraarticular fracture
To diagnose an intraarticular ligamentous disruption
To relieve pain
To diagnose inflammatory versus noninflammatory disorders
To identify the cause of an effusion
To rule out an infection
To identify a crystal-induced arthritis
To inject therapeutic agents

can relieve pain and allow an examination for ligamentous and joint instability. Corticosteroids are injected into joints to control inflammation and arthritis pain. Sometimes, corticosteroids and local anesthetic solutions are combined into one syringe and injected intraarticularly. The local anesthetic provides immediate pain relief and assures the physician of proper needle placement.

Arthrocentesis can be used to diagnose and treat traumatic arthritides. The traumatic event is usually acute, obvious, and followed by joint pain and swelling. Occasionally, the trauma is minimal or remote and not recalled by the patient. A traumatic effusion can be grossly bloody and, if acute, may contain a large amount of red blood cells. The bloody synovial fluid represents an intraarticular fracture or a disruption of intraarticular structures. An intraarticular fracture may be suspected based on mechanism of injury and yet radiographic findings may be negative. The synovial fluid may then be evaluated for fat globules, which are released from the marrow cavity of the fractured bone, which confirm the presence of an intraarticular fracture.

CONTRAINDICATIONS

There are no absolute contraindications to arthrocentesis. All contraindications are relative. The risks and benefits of the procedure should be evaluated and a decision made with the informed consent of the patient. **If a septic joint is suspected, it should be aspirated despite the presence of any relative contraindication. The benefit of the procedure outweighs any relative contraindication when compared to the morbidity of an undiagnosed septic arthritis.**

The presence of a suspected or known skin cellulitis, or other infection overlying the joint, are relative contraindications. A dermatitis or skin lesion overlying the joint should also be avoided. The skin or subcutaneous tissue can harbor organisms that may contaminate the joint when the needle passes through the dermatitis or skin lesion. Often, an alternative site can be found to perform the arthrocentesis and avoid the above obstacles. If the needle is inserted into the joint through any potential or obvious source of infection, antibiotic treatment is required due to the theoretical risk of introducing an infection into the joint cavity.[5] In these cases, patients should be admitted for 23 hours of intravenous antibiotics whose spectrum covers skin flora.

Infections after arthrocentesis, in previously sterile joints, have been reported in bacteremic patients.[5] It is not clear whether the source of the septic arthritis was from the arthrocentesis or bacteremia coincidentally seeding the joint. It is recommended to avoid arthrocentesis in any patients with bacteremia or sepsis except to rule out a septic arthritis.

Patients may be coagulopathic due to heparin or Coumadin therapy, factor deficiencies, liver dysfunction, or many other causes. When possible, the coagulopathy should be reversed prior to arthrocentesis. Unfortunately, this is not always possible or practical. An experienced physician can safely perform the procedure without reversing the coagulopathy. Use the smallest needle gauge possible (22 or 23 gauge) to aspirate the joint fluid. Avoid injury to the articular cartilage by identifying the anatomic landmarks prior to the procedure. Do not bounce the needle off any bony surfaces.

The procedure may be difficult in some patients. In the morbidly obese, it may be difficult to identify anatomic landmarks. The standard needle may be too short to enter the joint cavity. A spinal needle may be required to perform an arthrocentesis in an obese patient. Uncooperative patients require sedation and/or restraint prior to performing the procedure.

A prosthetic joint increases the risk of a septic arthritis. Arthrocentesis is technically more difficult secondary to scar formation and alteration of the normal anatomic relationships. **Joints that contain a prosthesis should be aspirated only to rule out a septic arthritis. Arthrocentesis for other reasons, including joint injection, should be referred to a consultant.**

Corticosteroids are instilled into joints for a variety of conditions. If the patient has no response to the injection within a few weeks, it may be repeated. If multiple injections cause no improvement, an alternative form of therapy should be explored.[9] Multiple injections into a joint increase the risk of complications.

EQUIPMENT

Clean gloves
Gauze squares
Povidone iodine solution
Local anesthetic (injectable, vapor coolant, or ice)
25 to 27 gauge needle
3 mL syringe
Needles to aspirate fluid (18/20/22 gauge)
Syringes to aspirate fluid (1/3/5/10/20/30/60 mL)
Hemostat
Specimen tubes
Culturettes or culture tubes

Arthrocentesis should be performed with a needle of sufficient bore to allow the aspiration of thick fluid, fluid with debris, or purulent fluid. An 18 to 20 gauge needle is recommended for large joints (shoulder, elbow, ankle, knee, hip). A 22 to 23 gauge needle is recommended for all other joints. Using too small a needle makes the procedure technically more difficult and more painful for the patient.

PATIENT PREPARATION

A complete history and physical examination should be performed prior to the arthrocentesis. The affected joint should be thoroughly assessed. Inspect the skin overlying the joint for breaks, infection, old scars, prior incisions, superficial lesions, or any wounds. Palpate the joint to identify any warmth, tenderness, or effusion. Evaluate the joint for any crepitation, deformity, ligamentous instability, or limitations in motion.

As with any nonemergent procedure, consent should be obtained from the patient or their representative. Ideally, the consent should be documented in the medical record and signed by the patient. Some prefer to note on the patient's chart "indications, risks, and benefits were discussed with the patient" rather than having the patient sign a consent form.[4,10] The following is a sample consent for performing an arthrocentesis (which may be written on the medical record and signed by the patient):

Arthrocentesis involves inserting a small needle into your _____ joint. The skin is anesthetized prior to the procedure. Ordinarily, the procedure has no significant complications. Occasionally, a patient may experience bleeding into the joint, infection of the joint or skin, pain, bruising, nerve injury, or an allergic reaction to the medications administered. These complications are minimized due to the use of sterile technique and proper techniques.

Position the patient based on the specific joint to be aspirated and the approach to be used. Expose the joint and surrounding areas. Identify the anatomic landmarks required for proper needle placement. The landmarks may be difficult to identify on a swollen and tender joint. Compare the "affected" joint to the "normal" joint on the opposite side of the body. Identify the joint and a landmark on the normal joint and transfer this to the affected joint. Clean any dirt and debris from the skin. Scrub the needle insertion site with povidone iodine solution and allow it to dry.

Apply anesthesia to the skin and subcutaneous tissue using 1% lidocaine, topical vapor spray, or ice.[11] The administration of some form of local anesthesia is recommended but not required.[4,12] The most common local anesthetic used is a short-acting injectable anesthetic solution of 1% lidocaine. **Do not inject the local anesthetic solution deeper than the subcutaneous tissues.** Deep injections may instill anesthetic solution into the joint cavity, which may interfere with the synovial fluid analysis. There is disagreement if the additional needle stick to administer the anesthesia causes as much discomfort as aspiration without any anesthesia. This decision is specific to each physician.

Alternative methods of anesthesia include ice and topical vapor coolants. A sterile drape may be placed over the prepped skin and a bag of ice water placed over the drape. Remove the ice water bag and drape after 5 minutes and perform the procedure. Ethinyl chloride topical vapor coolant may be used as an anesthetic. Spray the solution onto the area of skin in which the needle will be inserted. Apply the spray from 6 inches above the skin. Spray until the skin turns white and frosty. This usually takes 5 to 10 seconds. Immediately perform the procedure, as the anesthesia lasts only 30 to 60 seconds.

TECHNIQUES

THE BASIC TECHNIQUE

The general procedure preferred by one of the authors and editors (EFR) will be described. The other editor (RRS) prefers to insert the needle into the joint space and then attach the syringe. Specifics will be addressed with each individual joint.

Apply the needle to the syringe and break the resistance. This avoids any sudden and painful movements of the needle within the joint cavity. Stretch the skin over the site where the needle will be inserted. Penetrate the skin briskly with the needle and enter the joint cavity. Gently aspirate synovial fluid. If bone is encountered, slightly withdraw the needle and readvance it in a different direction. If no fluid is obtained, reevaluate the joint to determine if an effusion is present, if another site is more appropriate for the procedure, or if another physician may offer a different perspective. For diagnostic aspirations, it is not necessary to aspirate all of the fluid from the joint. Synovial fluid analysis can usually be performed on 1 to 5 mL of fluid.

If additional fluid is to be removed after the original syringe is filled, or if pharmaceuticals are to be injected into the joint, do not remove the needle from the joint cavity. Grasp the hub of the needle with a hemostat. Remove the syringe and attach the second syringe. Continue to aspirate fluid or inject the desired pharmaceutical. Remove the needle when the procedure has been completed. Apply a bandage to the skin. Transfer the synovial fluid into appropriately labeled tubes or containers. Document the procedure in the medical record. A sample procedure note is described below:

After informed consent, the skin overlying the _____ joint was cleaned and prepped with povidone iodine solution. The skin was anesthetized with (_____ mL of _____ % lidocaine, ethyl chloride vapor coolant, ice for _____ minutes). Using sterile technique, a _____ gauge needle was inserted on the (supero-/infero-, medial/lateral/inferior/superior) surface of the joint. It was directed (supero-/infero-, medially/laterally/inferiorly/superiorly). _____ mL of fluid was obtained. It was (thin, thick, yellow, clear, straw-colored, bloody, purulent, with debris, without debris). No complications were noted.

The joint was injected with _____ mL of _____ % (name of local anesthetic) and/or _____ mL of _____ % _____ (name of corticosteroid). No complications were noted.

STERNOCLAVICULAR JOINT ARTHROCENTESIS

Landmarks: The sternal end of the clavicle and the suprasternal notch are the landmarks for this joint (Figure 65-1). The joint can be palpated just medial to the sternal end of the clavicle and just lateral to the suprasternal notch.

Patient positioning: Place the patient supine on a stretcher with the arm hanging over the edge of the table (Figure 65-1A). Abduct the arm 90 degrees. Externally rotate the arm so that the palm faces upward. This position maximally opens the sternoclavicular joint to allow easy access.

Needle insertion and direction: Insert a 23 gauge needle through the anterior joint surface and perpendicular to the skin (Figure 65-1B). Advance the needle to a depth of 2 to 5 mm.

Remarks: This joint is often involved with degenerative arthritis. Septic arthritis is commonly seen in intravenous drug abusers who inject drugs into the great vessels; also known as "pocket shooting." This joint may only contain 0.25 to 0.50 mL of fluid.

Joint injection: A maximum volume of 1 mL may be instilled into this joint. A maximum dose of 10 mg of corticosteroids may be instilled into this joint.

ACROMIOCLAVICULAR JOINT ARTHROCENTESIS

Landmarks: The acromioclavicular (AC) joint is very superficial (Figure 65-2). Palpate the clavicle and move laterally until a prominence is felt. This is the AC joint. Have the patient move their arm to confirm the joint location.

Patient positioning: Place the patient sitting upright on a stretcher with the affected arm hanging by their side. A weight may be placed in the patient's hand to distract and open the joint space.

Needle insertion and direction: Insert a 22 gauge needle through the superior surface of the AC joint and perpendicular to the skin (Figure 65-2). Advance the needle to a depth of 3 to 5 mm.

Remarks: The acromioclavicular joint is very superficial. It has a dense, thick capsule anteriorly that is lacking on its superior surface. The joint may contain only 0.25 to 0.50 mL of fluid.

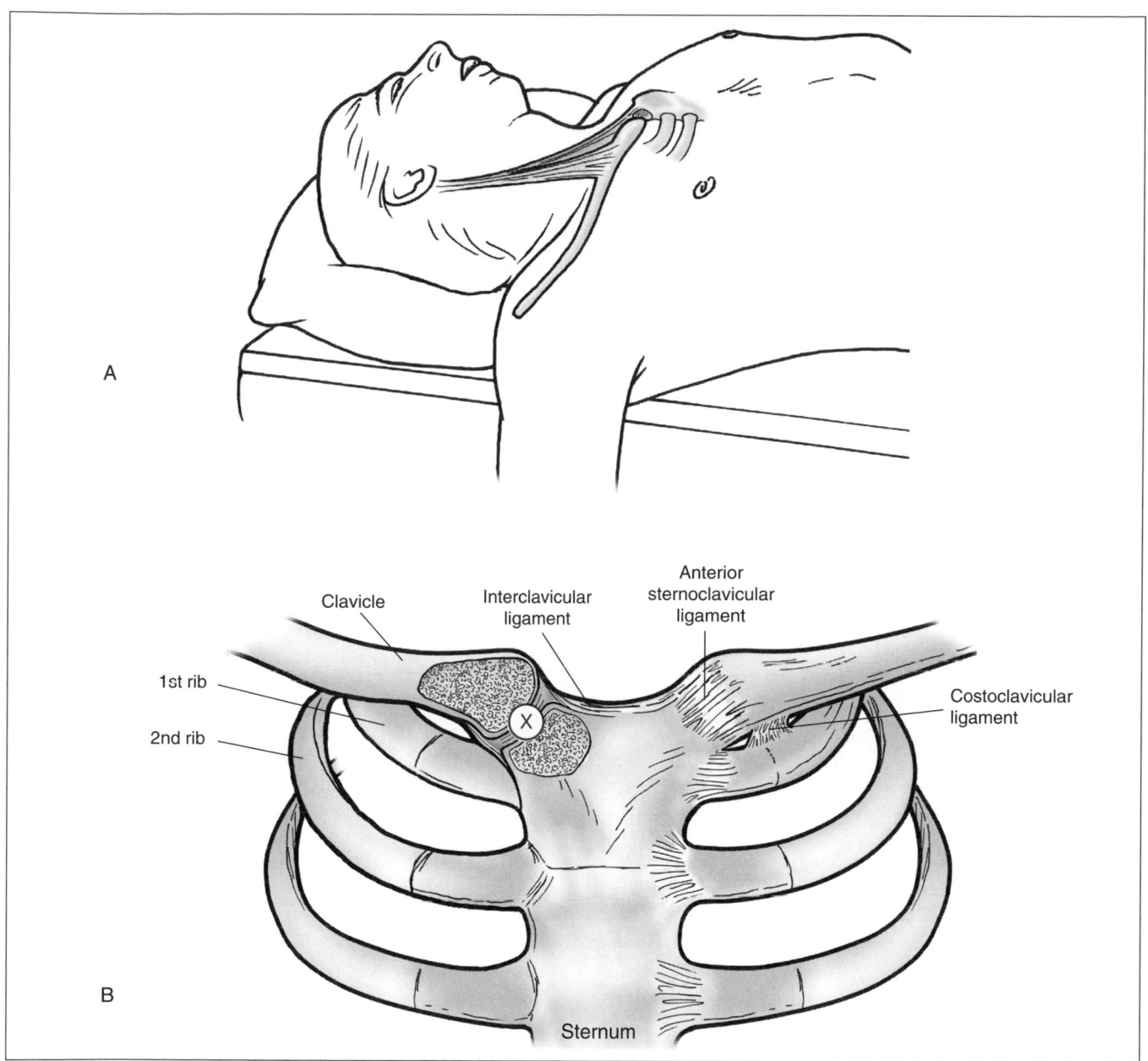

FIGURE 65-1 Sternoclavicular joint arthrocentesis. *A*. Patient positioning. *B*. Anatomy and needle insertion. The site of needle insertion is represented by an ⊗.

Joint injection: A maximum volume of 1.5 mL may be instilled into this joint. A maximum dose of 10 mg of corticosteroids may be instilled into this joint.

GLENOHUMERAL JOINT (SHOULDER) ARTHROCENTESIS, ANTERIOR APPROACH

Landmarks: Palpate the coracoid process of the scapula (Figure 65-3). It will be found below the lateral third of the clavicle. Internally rotate and adduct the humerus. Palpate the groove between the coracoid

process and the humeral head. This groove is the landmark for introduction of the needle.

Patient positioning: Place the patient sitting upright or supine on a stretcher. Flex the elbow 90 degrees. Internally rotate and adduct the arm. In the proper position, the forearm is resting against the patient's abdomen.

Needle insertion and direction: Insert an 18 gauge needle perpendicular to the skin and into the groove just lateral to the coracoid process (Figure 65-3*B*). Aim the

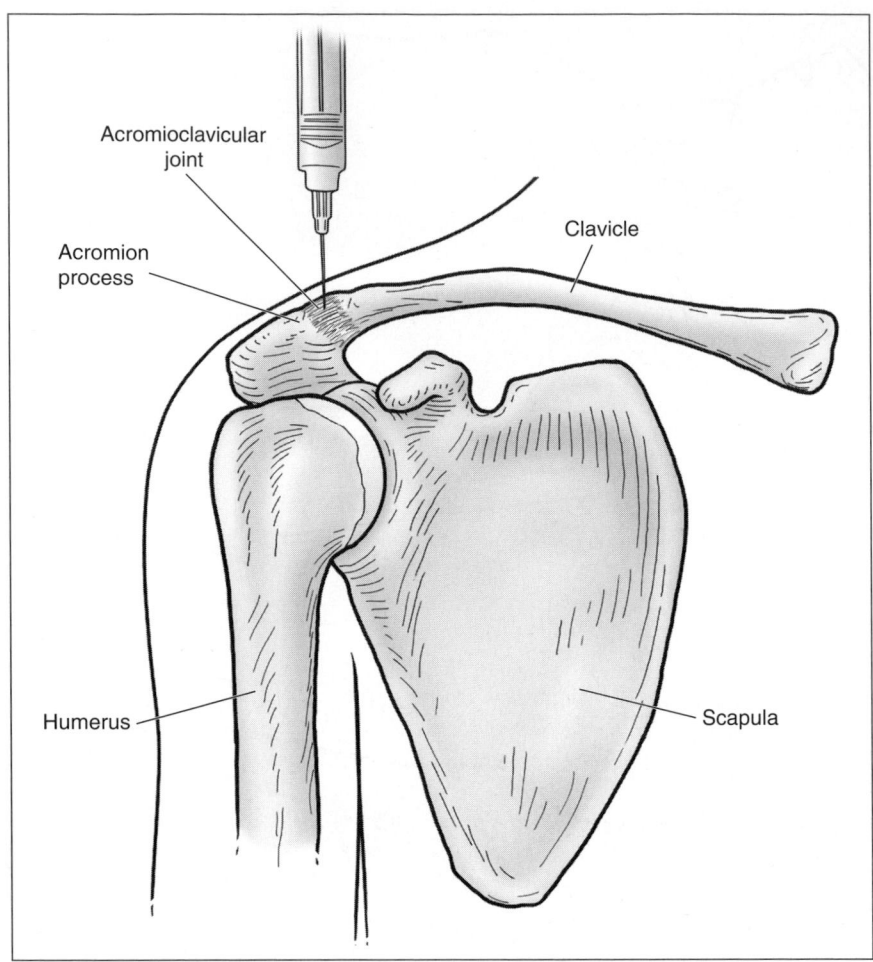

FIGURE 65-2 Acromioclavicular joint arthrocentesis.

needle directly posterior. Advance the needle until a loss of resistance is felt as the joint cavity is entered.

Remarks: This approach is the simplest yet most painful of the three approaches. The needle must penetrate the tendons of the coracobrachialis, subscapularis, biceps, and pectoralis major muscles in addition to the very tough anterior joint capsule. The major disadvantage of this approach is the possible (but rare) penetration of the brachial plexus or the axillary vessels with the needle. The patient can view the large needle as it approaches the skin and this may increase their anxiety level.

Joint injection: A maximum volume of 15 mL may be instilled into this joint. A maximum dose of 30 mg of corticosteroids may be instilled into this joint.

GLENOHUMERAL JOINT (SHOULDER) ARTHROCENTESIS, LATERAL APPROACH

Landmarks: Identify the acromion process of the scapula (Figure 65-3). A groove can be found just inferior to the lateral surface of the acromion and above the greater tubercle of the humerus.

Patient positioning: Place the patient sitting upright on a stretcher with the affected arm hanging by their side. A weight may be placed in the patient's hand to distract and open the joint cavity.

Needle insertion and direction: Insert an 18 gauge needle into the midpoint of the groove (Figure 65-3*A*). Direct the needle medially and slightly posterior. Advance the needle to a depth of 2.5 to 3 cm.

Remarks: Immediately below the deltoid muscle is the subacromial bursa. This bursa does not communicate with the shoulder joint. The needle must be inserted 2.5 to 3 cm to ensure the needle is in the shoulder joint and not in the subacromial bursa. The anterior or posterior approach to shoulder arthrocentesis avoids this potential problem.

Joint injection: A maximum volume of 15 mL may be instilled into this joint. A maximum dose of 30 mg of corticosteroids may be instilled into this joint.

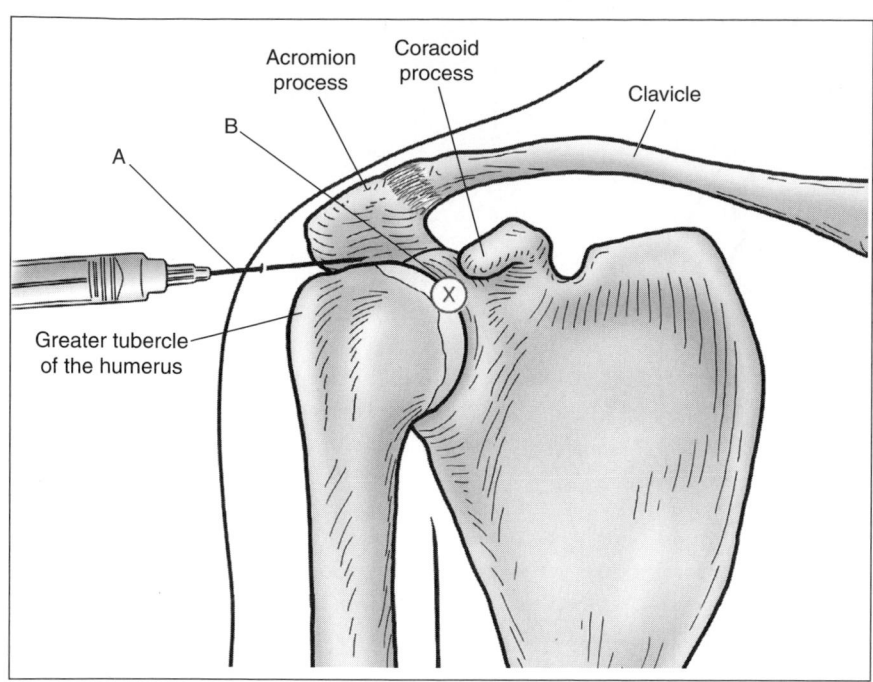

FIGURE 65-3 Shoulder joint arthrocentesis. *A.* Lateral approach. *B.* Anterior approach. The site of needle insertion is represented by an ⊗.

GLENOHUMERAL JOINT (SHOULDER) ARTHROCENTESIS, POSTERIOR APPROACH

Landmarks: Identify the spine of the scapula (Figure 65-4). Follow the spine laterally until it turns anterior to become the acromion process. This posterior border of the acromion process is the landmark for this technique. Locate the coracoid process of the scapula, just inferior to the lateral third of the clavicle.

Patient positioning: Place the patient sitting upright on a stretcher. Place the palm of the hand of the affected shoulder on the anterior surface of the opposite shoulder. The arm and forearm should be held against the chest. This position maximally opens the posterior joint space.

Needle insertion and direction: Place the nondominant thumb on the posterior border of the acromion process. Place the nondominant index finger on the coracoid process. Insert an 18 gauge needle 1 to 2 cm below the thumb and parallel to the floor (Figure 65-4). Aim the needle towards the tip of the index finger, approximately 30 degrees medially. Advance the needle to a depth of 2 to 3 cm.

Remarks: This is felt by some physicians to be the preferred approach to shoulder arthrocentesis. The needle will pierce the deltoid and infraspinatus muscles and avoid the tendons of the rotator cuff. This approach avoids the anxiety associated with the patient observing the large needle and syringe used for the procedure during the anterior or lateral approach. The posterior joint capsule is much thinner and more easily penetrated than the anterior joint capsule. There are no significant neurovascular structures that may be injured from this approach.

Joint injection: A maximum volume of 15 mL may be instilled into this joint. A maximum dose of 30 mg of corticosteroids may be instilled into this joint.

HUMERORADIOULNAR JOINT (ELBOW) ARTHROCENTESIS, LATERAL APPROACH

Landmarks: The lateral epicondyle of the humerus, the radial head, and the tip of the olecranon process of the ulna are the landmarks for this joint (Figure 65-5*A*). Flex the elbow 45 degrees and pronate the hand. Pronation of the hand stretches the radial collateral ligament, moves the radial nerve out of the needle's path, and widens the synovial cavity. Identify the depression between the landmarks. The depression is located proximal to the radial head in the area where no bony structures are palpated.

Patient positioning: Place the patient sitting upright or supine on a stretcher. Flex the elbow 45 degrees and pronate the hand. This position widens the joint cavity and avoids any neurovascular structures.

Needle insertion and direction: Insert a 22 gauge needle perpendicular to the skin and into the depression just proximal to the radial head (Figure 65-5*A*). Advance the needle to a depth of 0.75 to 2.0 cm.

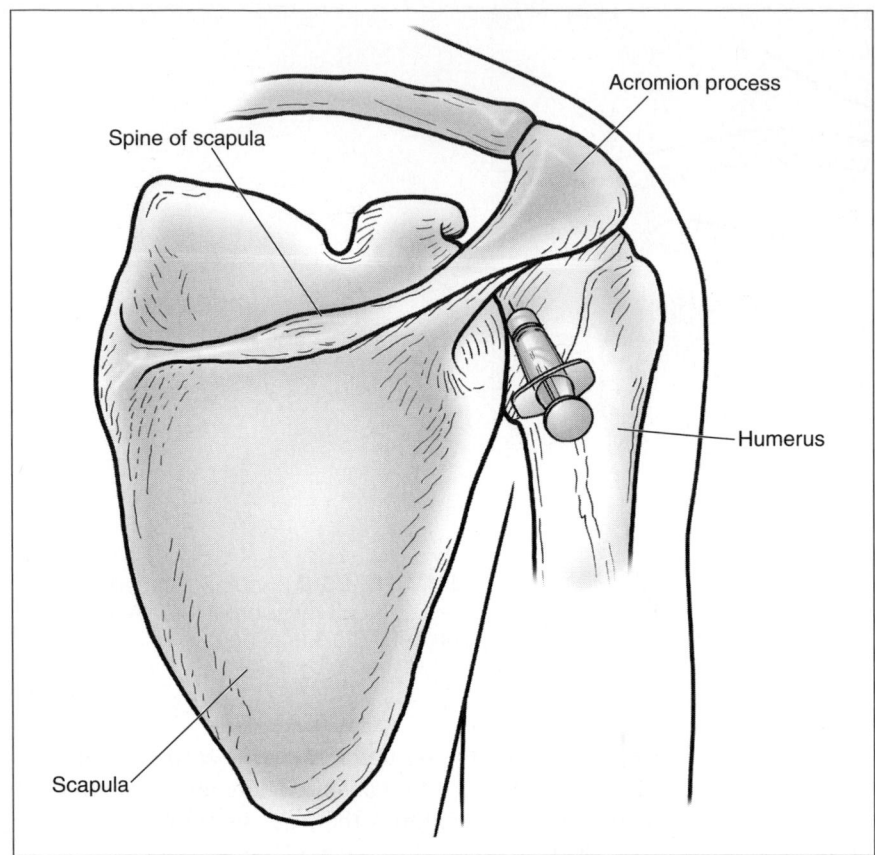

FIGURE 65-4 Posterior approach for shoulder joint arthrocentesis.

Remarks: This is the preferred approach for elbow arthrocentesis. It avoids tendons and neurovascular structures, thereby reducing the risk of complications.[13]

Joint injection: A maximum volume of 5 mL may be instilled into this joint. A maximum dose of 20 mg of corticosteroids may be instilled into this joint.

HUMERORADIOULNAR JOINT (ELBOW) ARTHROCENTESIS, POSTERIOR APPROACH

Landmarks: Identify the top of the olecranon process of the ulna and the triceps muscle insertion into the olecranon process (Figure 65-5B). Find the point just proximal to the top of the olecranon and just lateral to the triceps insertion. This point is the landmark for insertion of the needle.

Patient positioning: Place the patient sitting upright on a stretcher. Flex the elbow 90 degrees with the hand supinated. The forearm and hand should be resting on a tabletop or on the patient's leg.

Needle insertion and direction: Approach the joint from the posterolateral surface with the needle parallel to the radial shaft. Insert a 22 gauge needle perpendicu-

lar to the skin at the landmark (Figure 65-5B). Advance the needle to a depth of 1 cm.

Remarks: Potential complications include needle penetration of the triceps tendon or the radial nerve. This approach is reserved for patients in whom the lateral approach is contraindicated.

Joint injection: A maximum volume of 5 mL may be instilled into this joint. A maximum dose of 20 mg of corticosteroids may be instilled into this joint.

HUMERORADIOULNAR JOINT (ELBOW) ARTHROCENTESIS, POSTEROLATERAL APPROACH

Landmarks: Identify the lateral surface of the olecranon process of the ulna and the lateral epicondyle of the humerus (Figure 65-5C). Find the indentation just lateral to the olecranon and just distal to the lateral epicondyle. This point is the landmark for the insertion of the needle.

Patient positioning: Place the patient sitting upright on a stretcher. Flex the elbow 90 degrees with the hand supinated. The forearm and hand should be resting on a tabletop or on the patient's leg.

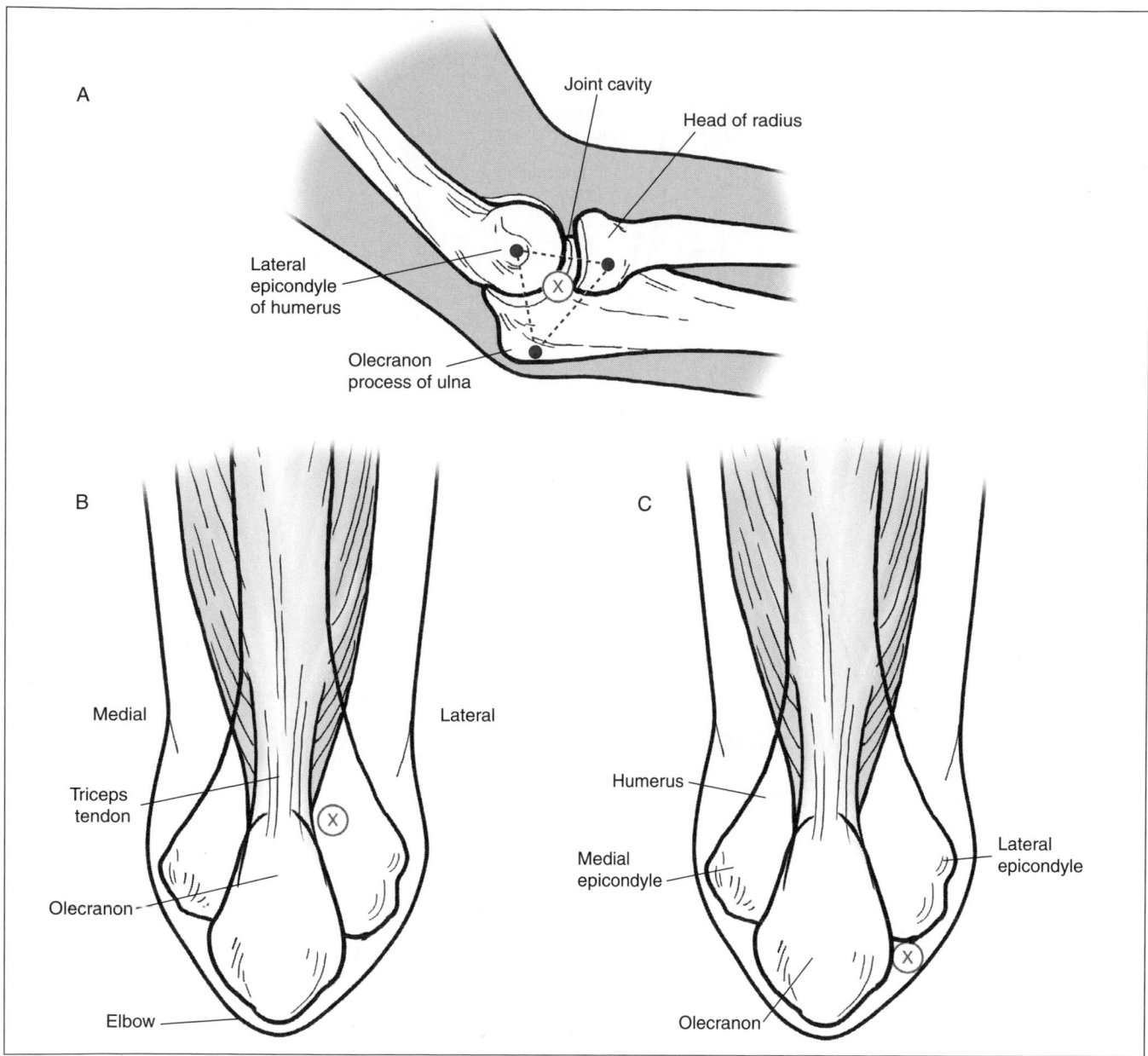

FIGURE 65-5 Elbow joint arthrocentesis. The site of needle insertion is represented by an ⊗. *A.* Lateral approach. *B.* Posterior approach. *C.* Posterolateral approach.

Needle insertion and direction: Approach the joint from the posterolateral surface with the needle parallel to the radial shaft. Insert a 22 gauge needle perpendicular to the skin at the landmark (Figure 65-5*C*). Advance the needle to a depth of 1 cm.

Remarks: This approach is an alternative when the lateral approach is contraindicated.

Joint injection: A maximum volume of 5 mL may be instilled into this joint. A maximum dose of 20 mg of corticosteroids may be instilled into this joint.

RADIOCARPAL JOINT (WRIST) ARTHROCENTESIS

Landmarks: Identify the lunate bone (Figure 65-6). Palpate the middle (third) metacarpal and follow it proximally until a rounded bean-like elevation is felt (Figure 65-6*A*). This is the lunate. Palpate the indentations proximal and distal to the lunate. The indentation proximal to the lunate is the landmark for needle insertion.

Alternatively, identify Lister's tubercle and the extensor pollicis longus (EPL) tendon (Figure 65-6*B*). Lister's

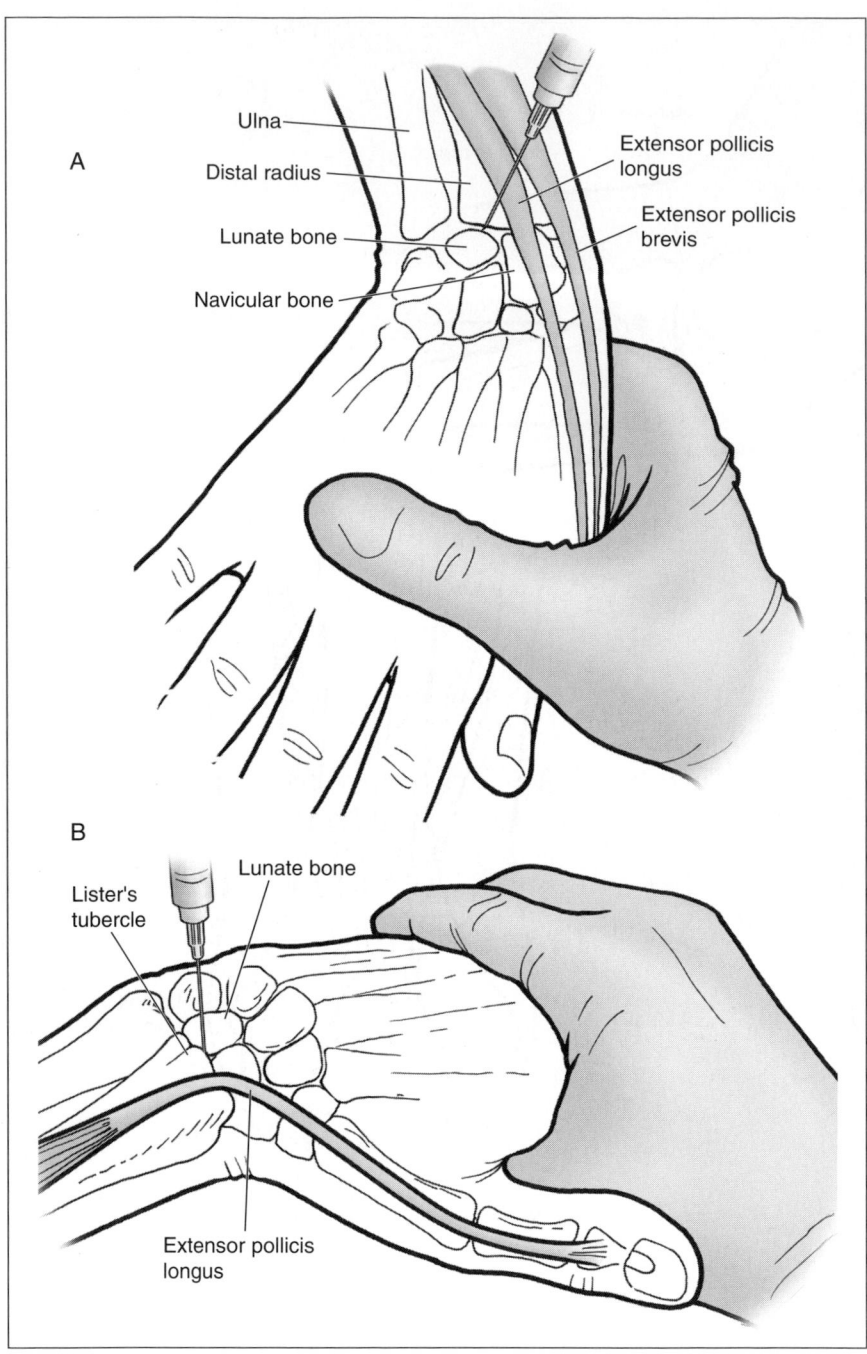

FIGURE 65-6 Radiocarpal joint arthrocentesis.

tubercle is a bony prominence in the center of the dorsal aspect of the distal radius. The EPL tendon can be found lateral (radial) to Lister's tubercle. If the EPL tendon is difficult to find, extend the hand and thumb against resistance and it will become prominent. The lunate is the bony prominence distal to Lister's tubercle. The indentation proximal to the lunate is the landmark for needle insertion.

Patient positioning: Place the patient sitting upright or supine on a stretcher. Pronate the hand with the wrist in slight (20 to 50 degrees) flexion and ulnar deviation (Figure 65-6*A*). The palm of the physician's nondominant hand should be holding the patient's palm. Reidentify the lunate with the nondominant thumb.

Needle insertion and direction: Insert a 22 gauge needle perpendicular to the skin in the indentation proximal to the lunate (Figure 65-6*A*). Advance the needle to a depth of 0.75 to 1.25 cm. Alternatively, insert the needle in the indentation just distal to Lister's tubercle and ulnar to the EPL tendon (Figure 65-6*B*).

Remarks: The preferred, and easiest, method is to identify the lunate and then insert the needle in the indentation just proximal to the lunate.

Joint injection: A maximum volume of 2 mL may be instilled into this joint. A maximum dose of 20 mg of corticosteroids may be instilled into this joint.

INTERCARPAL JOINT ARTHROCENTESIS

Landmarks: Identify the lunate bone (Figure 65-6). Palpate the middle (third) metacarpal and follow it proximally until a rounded bean-like elevation is felt (Figure 65-6A). This is the lunate. Palpate an indentation distal to the lunate and proximal to the base of the third metacarpal. This indentation is the landmark for insertion of the needle.

Patient positioning: Place the patient sitting upright or supine on a stretcher. Pronate the hand with the wrist in slight (20 to 50 degrees) flexion and ulnar deviation (Figure 65-6A). The palm of the physician's nondominant hand should be holding the patient's palm. Reidentify the landmarks with the nondominant thumb.

Needle insertion and direction: Insert a 22 gauge needle perpendicular to the skin in the indentation distal to the lunate. Advance the needle to a depth of 0.5 to 1.0 cm.

Remarks: The joints between the carpal bones are all connected to each other (Figure 65-7). Fluid aspirated from one of these joints is representative of all the joints. Likewise, injection of one joint allows the pharmaceutical to be distributed to all the joints.

Joint injection: A maximum volume of 1.5 mL may be instilled into this joint. A maximum dose of 15 mg of corticosteroids may be instilled into this joint.

CARPOMETACARPAL JOINT OF THE THUMB ARTHROCENTESIS

Landmarks: The base of the first metacarpal and the abductor pollicis longus (APL) tendon are the landmarks for this joint (Figure 65-8). Identify the radial aspect of the base of the first metacarpal. Have the patient rotate the affected thumb to help identify the joint. Identify the APL tendon by extending the patient's thumb against resistance.

Patient positioning: Place the patient sitting upright or supine on a stretcher. Flex the thumb into the palm with the tip of the thumb touching the fifth metacarpal head. Clench the remaining fingers into a fist (Figure 65-8A).

Needle insertion and direction: Insert a 22 gauge needle into the joint space at the radial aspect of the base of the first metacarpal and just lateral (radial) to the APL tendon (Figure 65-8A). Direct the tip of the needle towards the base of the fourth metacarpal. Advance the needle to a depth of 0.5 to 1.0 cm.

Remarks: If difficulty is encountered when inserting the needle, try an alternative thumb position (Figure 65-8B). Flex the first carpometacarpal joint 45 degrees and apply traction to the distal thumb. This in-line traction will enlarge the joint cavity and allow easier access.

Joint injection: A maximum volume of 1.5 mL may be instilled into this joint. A maximum dose of 10 mg of corticosteroids may be instilled into this joint.

METACARPOPHALANGEAL JOINT ARTHROCENTESIS

Landmarks: Identify the metacarpophalangeal (MCP) joint and the extensor digitorum tendon (Figure 65-9A). The MCP joint can be located just proximal to the prominence at the base of the proximal phalanx of the finger. Identify the extensor tendon by having the patient extend the finger against resistance.

Patient positioning: Place the patient sitting upright or supine on a stretcher. Pronate the hand and abduct the fingers. Grasp the finger and apply distal traction.

Needle insertion and direction: Insert a 22 gauge needle into the dorsal joint space just medial or lateral to the extensor tendon (Figure 65-9B). Direct the tip of the needle towards the center of the joint. Advance the needle to a depth of 0.3 to 0.5 cm.

Remarks: The application of distal traction often causes a depression to appear on both sides of the extensor tendon (Figure 65-9B). These depressions can be used as landmarks for the site of needle insertion into the joint cavity.

Joint injection: A maximum volume of 1 mL may be instilled into this joint. A maximum dose of 5 mg of corticosteroids may be instilled into this joint.

INTERPHALANGEAL JOINT OF THE FINGER ARTHROCENTESIS

Landmarks: Identify the interphalangeal (IP) joint and the extensor tendon (Figure 65-9A). The IP joint can be located just proximal to the prominence at the base of the middle or distal phalanx of the finger. Identify the extensor tendon by having the patient extend the finger against resistance.

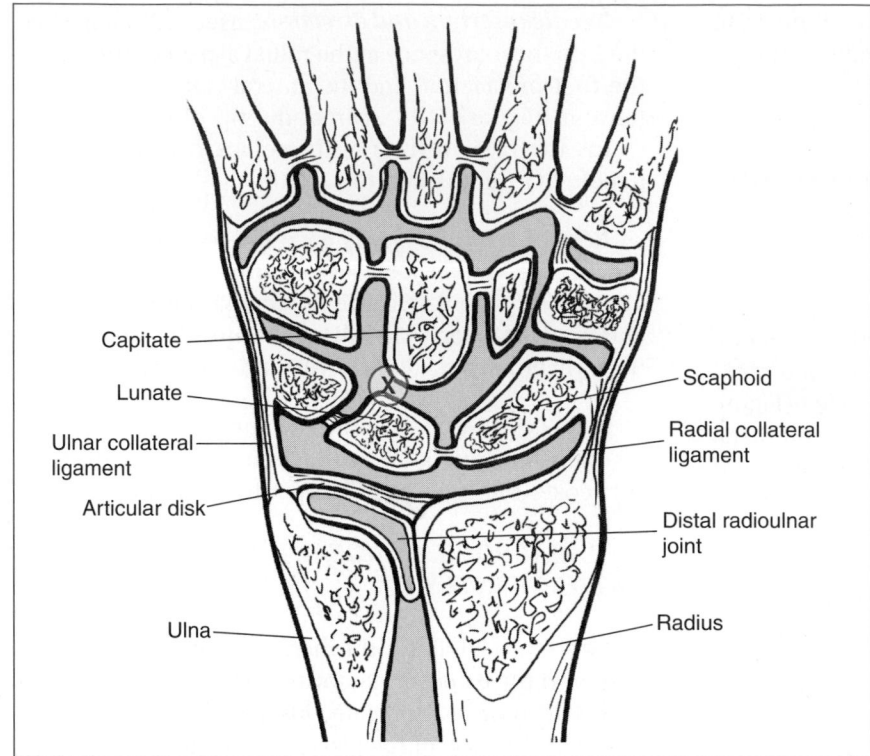

Capitate

Lunate

Ulnar collateral
ligament

Articular disk

Ulna

Scaphoid

Radial collateral
ligament

Distal radioulnar
joint

Radius

FIGURE 65-7 Intercarpal joint arthrocentesis. Coronal section through the wrist and hand demonstrating that the joints between the carpal bones are all interconnected. The site of needle insertion is represented by an ⊗.

Patient positioning: Place the patient sitting upright or supine on a stretcher. Pronate the hand and abduct the fingers. Grasp the finger and apply distal traction.

Needle insertion and direction: Insert a 22 gauge needle into the dorsal joint space just medial or lateral to the extensor tendon (Figure 65-9*B*). Direct the tip of the needle towards the center of the joint. Advance the needle to a depth of 0.3 to 0.5 cm.

Remarks: The application of distal traction often causes a depression to appear on both sides of the extensor tendon (Figure 65-9*B*). These depressions can be used as landmarks for the site of needle insertion into the joint cavity. The joints are small and normally contain almost no synovial fluid. When inflamed or infected, the joint cavity may contain up to 2 mL of synovial fluid.

Joint injection: A maximum volume of 1 mL may be instilled into this joint. A maximum dose of 5 mg of corticosteroids may be instilled into this joint.

HIP JOINT ARTHROCENTESIS, ANTERIOR APPROACH

Landmarks: Identify the anterior superior iliac spine (ASIS) and the femoral pulse (Figure 65-10). The landmark for insertion of the needle is 2 to 3 cm below the ASIS and 2 to 3 cm lateral to the femoral artery pulse.

Patient positioning: Place the patient supine on a stretcher with the affected leg internally rotated.

Needle insertion and direction: Insert a 3.5 inch, 18 gauge needle at the landmark (Figure 65-10). Direct the tip of the needle posteromedially. Insert the needle at a 60 degree angle to the skin of the thigh. Advance the needle until bone is encountered. Slightly withdraw the needle and begin aspirating the synovial fluid.

Remarks: This approach is technically easier and recommended by many authors. A long spinal needle is usually required for this procedure. Use caution as the needle may injure the articular cartilage. This procedure should be performed by an Orthopedist, a Rheumatologist, or a Radiologist under fluoroscopic guidance.

Joint injection: A maximum volume of 10 mL may be instilled into this joint. A maximum dose of 40 mg of corticosteroids may be instilled into this joint.

HIP JOINT ARTHROCENTESIS, LATERAL APPROACH

Landmarks: The greater trochanter is the landmark for this technique (Figure 65-11). Place the patient supine with the affected leg internally rotated. Palpate the greater trochanter.

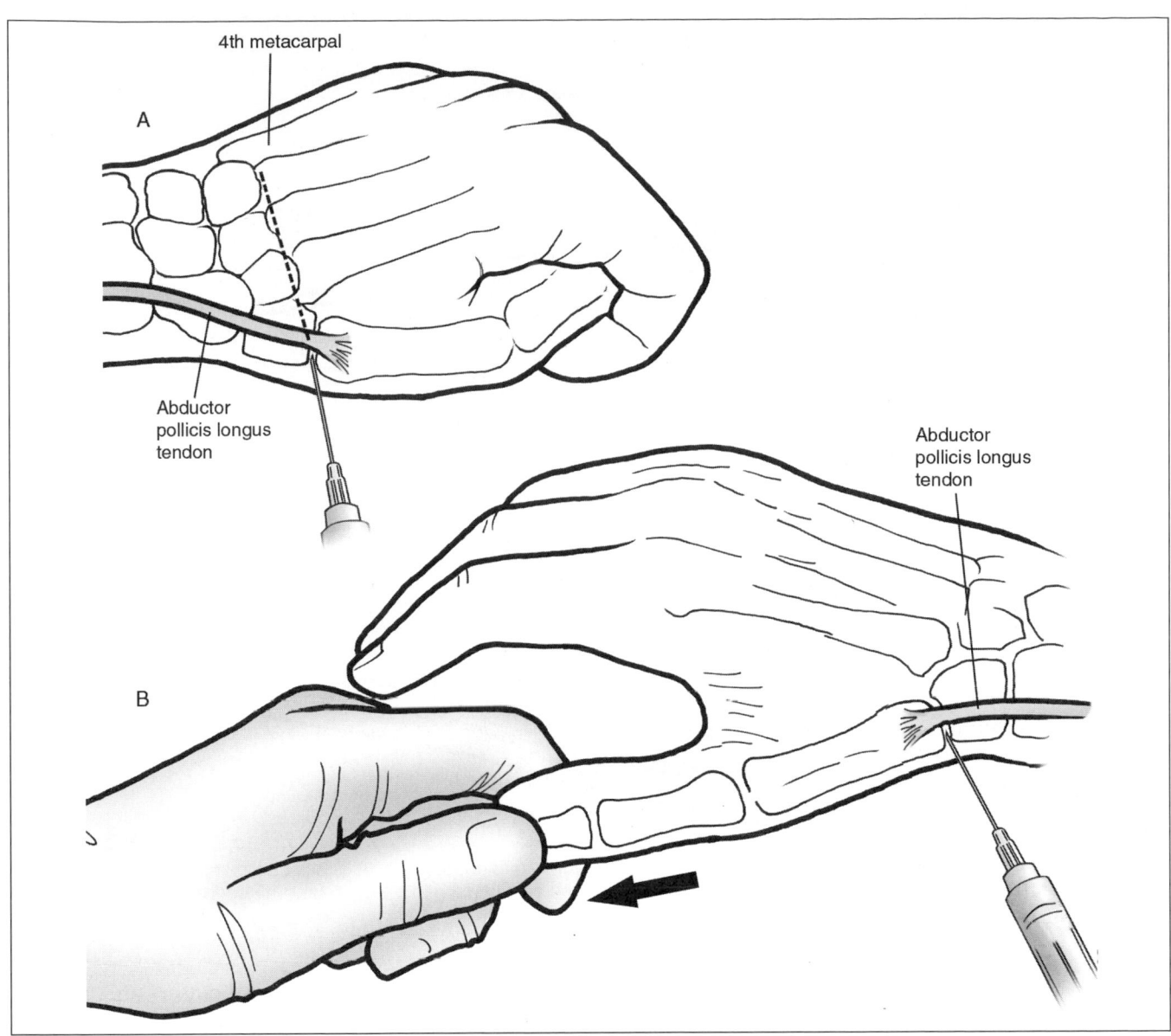

FIGURE 65-8 Carpometacarpal joint of the thumb arthrocentesis. *A.* Recommended approach. The dotted line represents the proper direction for needle insertion, towards the base of the fourth metacarpal. *B.* An alternative technique. The arrow represents the application of distal traction.

Patient positioning: Place the patient supine on a stretcher with the affected leg internally rotated (Figure 65-11*A*). Identify the greater trochanter and hold it between the thumb and index finger. A second patient position may be used for the alternative approach (Figure 65-11*B*). Place the patient lying on the unaffected side. Flex the unaffected, lower, leg 90 degrees. Fully extend the upper, affected, leg with a pillow supporting the ankle.

Needle insertion and direction: Insert a 3.5 inch, 18 gauge needle just superior to the superior margin of the greater trochanter (Figure 65-11*A*). Advance the needle horizontally, parallel to the stretcher, until it contacts the femoral neck. Withdraw the needle 2 to 4 mm and redirect it slightly cephalad. Advance the needle while applying negative pressure to the syringe until synovial fluid enters the syringe. Stop advancing the needle and continue to aspirate the synovial fluid. The alternative technique requires the insertion of the needle perpendicular to the skin and 1 cm proximal to the greater trochanter (Figure 65-11*B*). Advance the needle until the femoral neck is contacted. Withdraw the needle 2 mm and begin aspirating synovial fluid.

Remarks: In the morbidly obese, the greater trochanter may not be palpable. This approach is technically more difficult than the anterior approach. The ad-

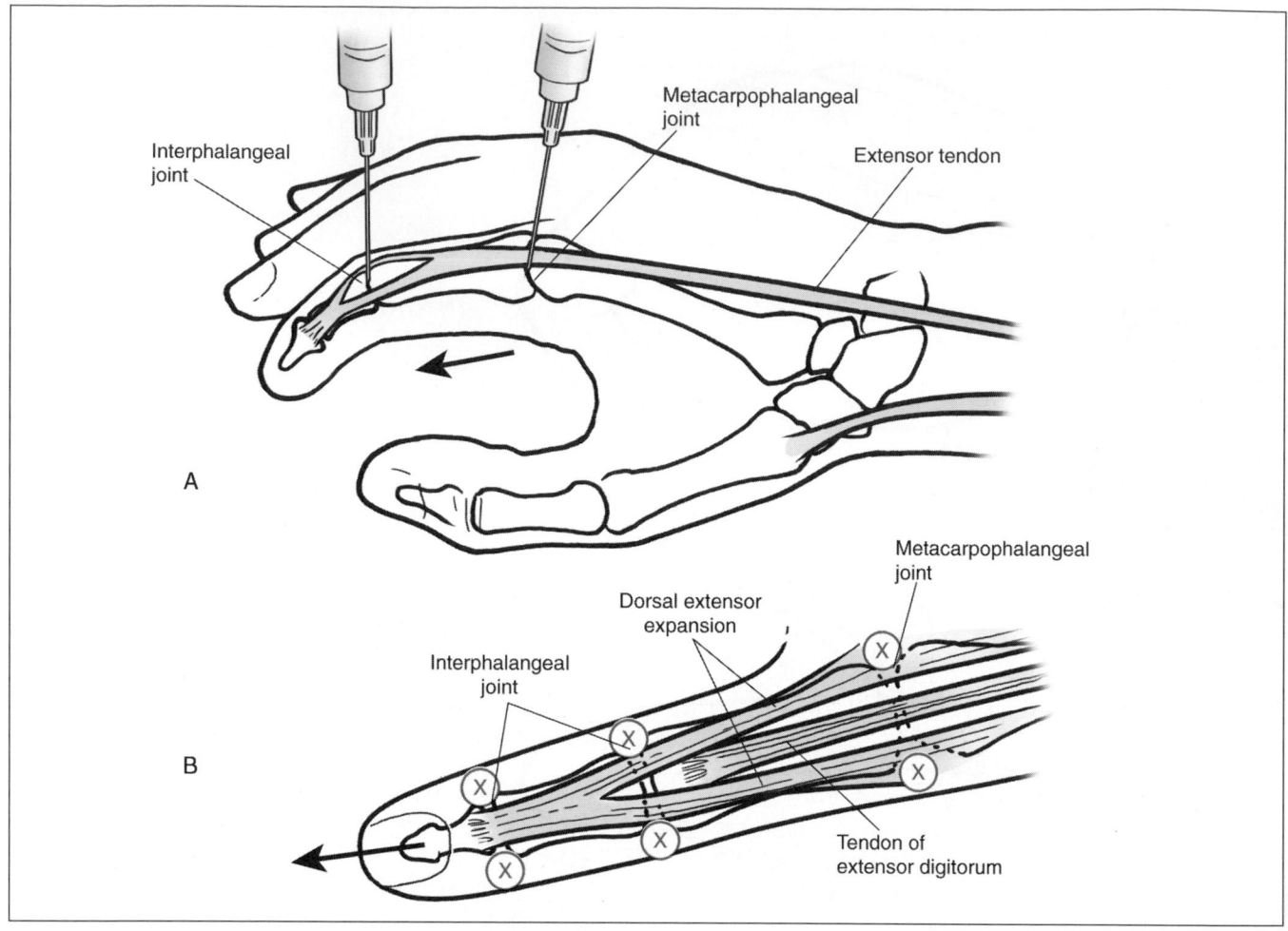

FIGURE 65-9 Arthrocentesis of the metacarpophalangeal and interphalangeal joints. *A.* Proper needle placement. *B.* Distal traction will cause dimpling of the skin noted by the ⊗. These areas of skin dimpling are the landmarks for needle insertion. The arrow represents the application of distal traction.

vantage of this approach is that the articular cartilage will not be in the needle's path and so avoids injury. This procedure should be performed by an Orthopedist, a Rheumatologist, or a Radiologist under fluoroscopic guidance.

Joint injection: A maximum volume of 10 mL may be instilled into this joint. A maximum dose of 40 mg of corticosteroids may be instilled into this joint.

PATELLOFEMOROTIBIAL JOINT (KNEE) ARTHROCENTESIS, SUPRAPATELLAR APPROACH

Landmarks: Identify the midpoint of the superolateral or superomedial border of the patella (Figure 65-12*A*). Either of these landmarks may be used as the site for needle insertion.

Patient positioning: Place the patient supine on a stretcher with the affected knee fully extended.

Needle insertion and direction: Insert an 18 gauge needle through the midpoint of the superolateral or superomedial border of the patella (Figure 65-12*A*). Direct the tip of the needle towards the intercondylar notch of the femur. Advance the needle to a depth of 1.5 to 3.0 cm.

Remarks: The needle enters the suprapatellar bursa and avoids any potential damage to the articular cartilage. The bursa is a direct continuation of the synovial cavity. There are no neurovascular structures of significance to injure with this approach. If the knee effusion is minimal, synovial fluid may not be able to be aspirated from this approach. Approximately 10 percent of the population has a plica completely separating the suprapatellar bursa from the knee joint. If this variation exists in the patient, the bursa fluid will not represent synovial fluid.

Joint injection: A maximum volume of 10 mL may be instilled into this joint. A maximum dose of 40 mg of corticosteroids may be instilled into this joint.

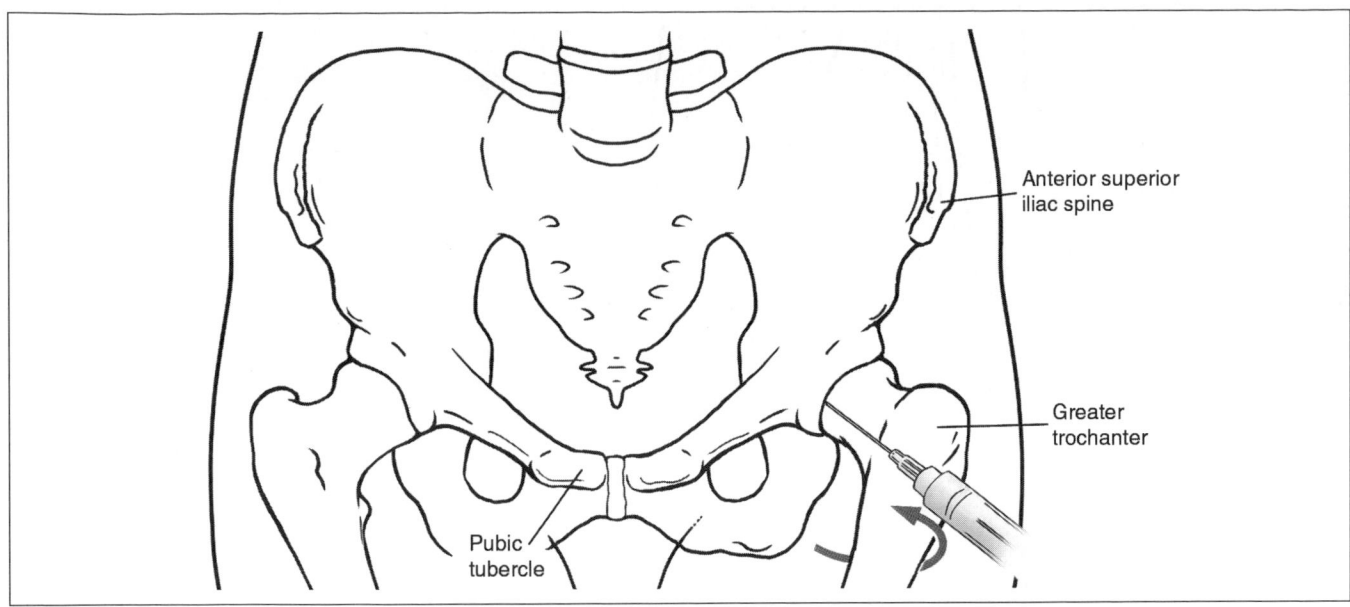

FIGURE 65-10 Anterior approach for hip joint arthrocentesis. The curved arrow represents internal rotation of the femur.

PATELLOFEMOROTIBIAL JOINT (KNEE) ARTHROCENTESIS, PARAPATELLAR APPROACH

Landmarks: Identify the midpoint of the lateral or medial border of the patella (Figure 65-12*B*). Either of these landmarks may be used as the site for needle insertion.

Patient positioning: Place the patient supine on a stretcher with the affected knee fully extended.

Needle insertion and direction: Insert an 18 gauge needle just below the midpoint of the lateral or medial border of the patella (Figure 65-12*B*). Direct the needle

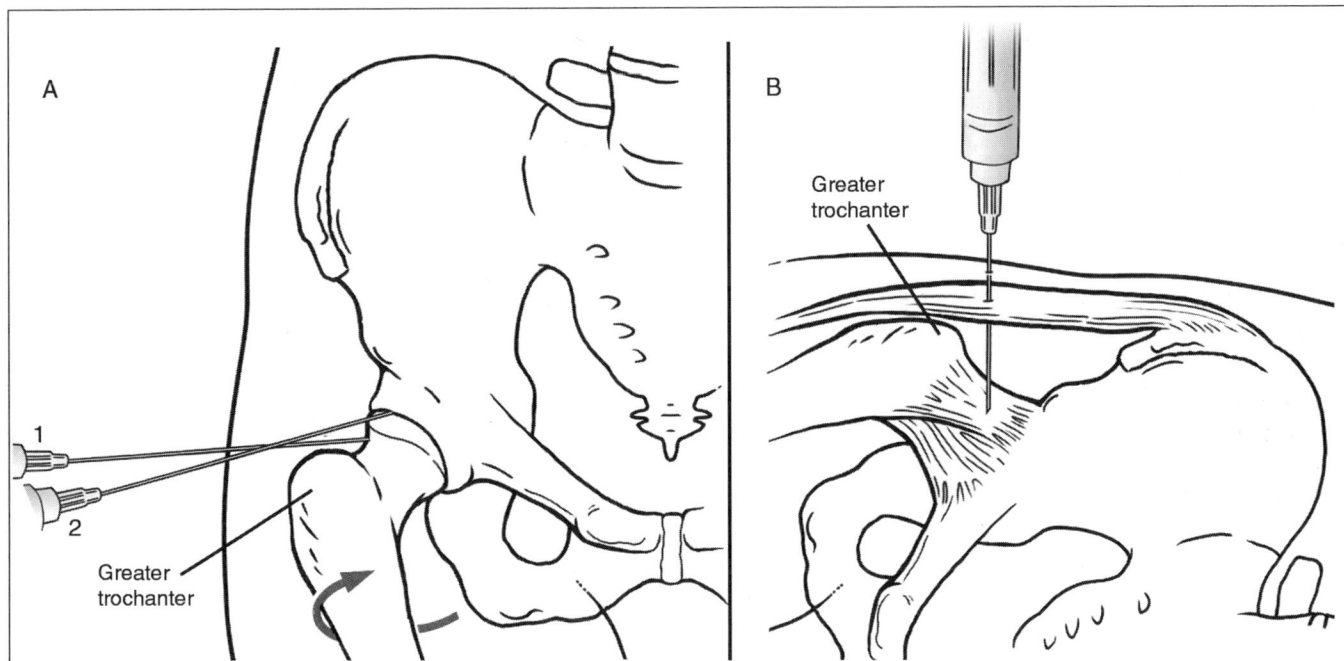

FIGURE 65-11 Lateral approach for hip joint arthrocentesis. *A.* The patient is supine with the leg internally rotated (*curved arrow*). A needle is inserted above the greater trochanter and advanced until the femoral neck is encountered (*1*). The needle has been withdrawn slightly, redirected cephalad, then readvanced into the joint cavity (*2*). *B.* An alternative approach.

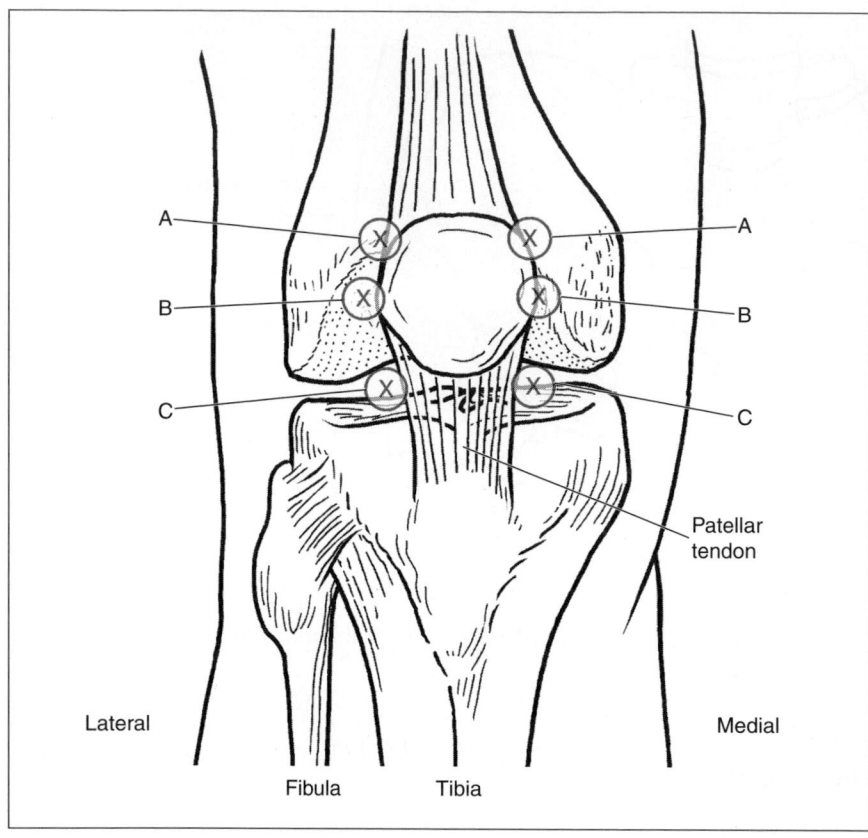

FIGURE 65-12 Knee joint arthrocentesis. The site of needle insertion is represented by an ⊗. *A.* Medial and lateral suprapatellar approach. *B.* Medial and lateral parapatellar approach. *C.* Medial and lateral infrapatellar approach.

perpendicular to the long axis of the leg and aimed towards the intercondylar notch of the femur. Advance the needle to a depth of 1 to 2 cm.

Remarks: The easiest site for arthrocentesis is the medial parapatellar region. There are no disadvantages to using the medial parapatellar site.

Joint injection: A maximum volume of 10 mL may be instilled into this joint. A maximum dose of 40 mg of corticosteroids may be instilled into this joint.

PATELLOFEMOROTIBIAL JOINT (KNEE) ARTHROCENTESIS, INFRAPATELLAR APPROACH

Landmarks: Identify the inferior border of the patella and the patellar tendon (Figure 65-12*C*). The tendon is a thick band that passes from the inferior border of the patella to the tibial tuberosity.

Patient positioning: Place the patient sitting upright on a stretcher with the affected knee bent 90 degrees over the edge of the bed and the leg hanging freely and unsupported.

Needle insertion and direction: Insert an 18 gauge needle 0.5 cm below the inferior border of the patella at the level of the joint line and just medial or lateral to the

patellar tendon (Figure 65-12*C*). Direct the needle perpendicular to the long axis of the leg and aimed towards the intercondylar notch of the femur. Advance the needle to a depth of 1.5 to 2.0 cm.

Remarks: The weight of the leg helps to open the joint cavity. The risk of injury to the articular cartilage is minimal. This approach was popular in the past but is not often used today. Do not pierce the patellar tendon with the needle.

Joint injection: A maximum volume of 10 mL may be instilled into this joint. A maximum dose of 40 mg of corticosteroids may be instilled into this joint.

TIBIOTALAR JOINT (ANKLE) ARTHROCENTESIS, ANTEROLATERAL APPROACH

Landmarks: Identify the joint cavity, the lateral malleolus, and the extensor digitorum longus (EDL) tendons (Figure 65-13). The joint cavity is located below the distal edge of the fibula and between the bases of the malleoli. Extend the toes against resistance to identify the EDL tendons. Palpate the base of the lateral malleolus.

Patient positioning: Place the patient sitting upright or supine on a stretcher. The patient can also be placed

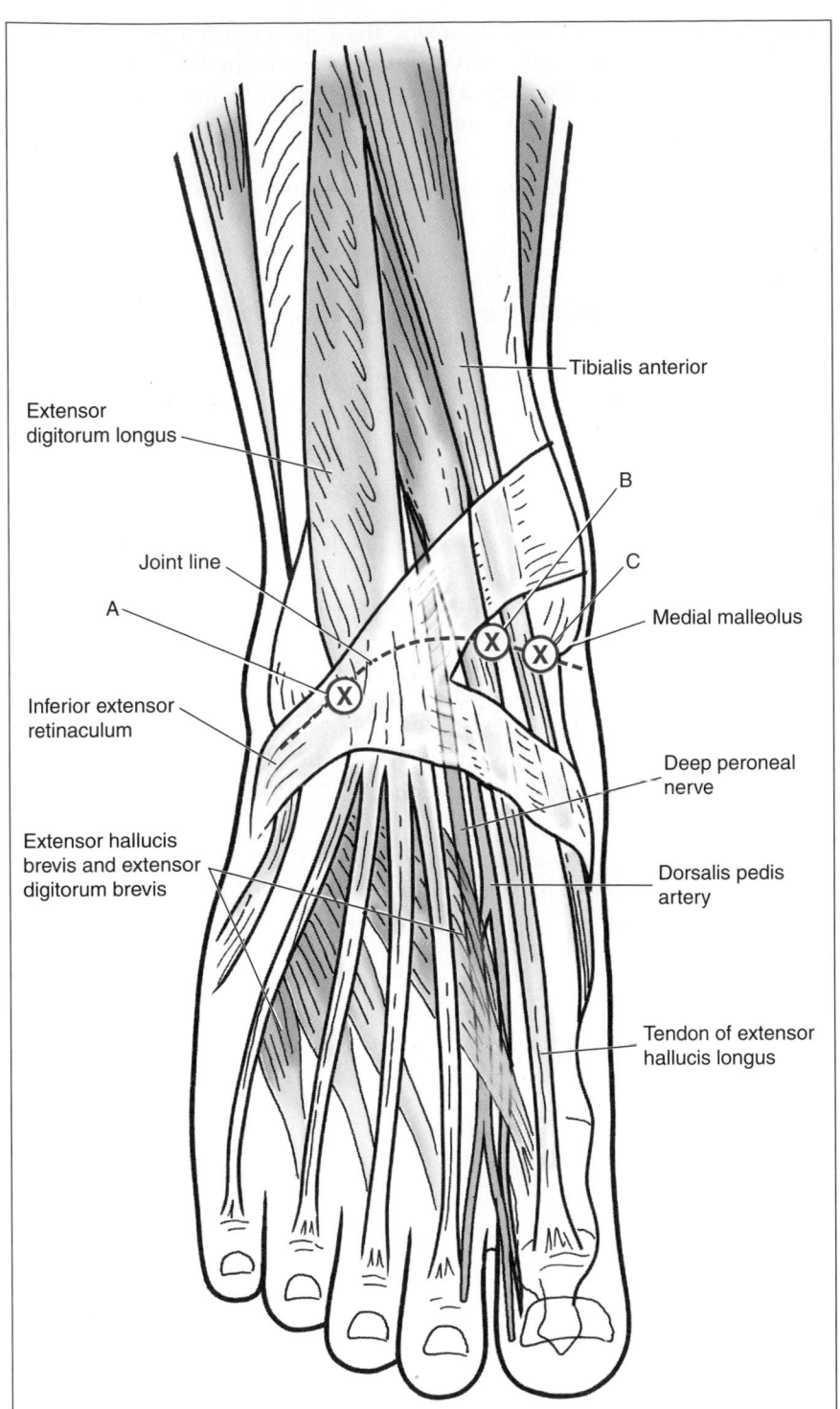

Extensor
digitorum longus

Tibialis anterior

Joint line

B

C

A

Medial malleolus

Inferior extensor
retinaculum

Deep peroneal
nerve

Extensor hallucis
brevis and extensor
digitorum brevis

Dorsalis pedis
artery

Tendon of extensor
hallucis longus

FIGURE 65-13 Arthrocentesis of the ankle joint. The site of needle insertion is represented by an ⊗. *A.* Anterolateral approach. *B.* Anteromedial approach. *C.* An alternative technique for the antero-medial approach.

sitting upright on a stretcher with affected knee bent 90 degrees over the edge of the bed and the foot hanging freely and unsupported. Plantar flex the ankle.

Needle insertion and direction: Insert a 22 gauge needle perpendicular to the fibular shaft at the level of the base of the lateral malleolus; midway between the malleolus and the lateral border of the EDL tendon

(Figure 65-13*A*). Advance the needle to a depth of 0.5 to 1.0 cm.

Remarks: This approach avoids potential injury to the dorsalis pedis vessels and the deep peroneal nerve.

Joint injection: A maximum volume of 3 mL may be instilled into this joint. A maximum dose of 20 mg of corticosteroids may be instilled into this joint.

TIBIOTALAR JOINT (ANKLE) ARTHROCENTESIS, ANTEROMEDIAL APPROACH

Landmarks: Identify the joint cavity, the medial malleolus, and the tendons of the tibialis anterior (TA) and the extensor hallucis longus (EHL) muscles (Figure 65-13). The joint cavity is located below the distal edge of the tibia and between the bases of the malleoli. Extend the great toe against resistance to identify the EHL tendon. Plantar flex the ankle against resistance to identify the TA tendon. Palpate the base of the medial malleolus.

Patient positioning: Place the patient sitting upright or supine on a stretcher. The patient can also be placed sitting upright on a stretcher with the affected knee bent 90 degrees over the edge of the bed and the foot hanging freely and unsupported. Plantar flex the ankle to use the EHL tendon as the landmark for the procedure. Alternatively, plantar flex the ankle and invert the subtalar joint to use the TA tendon as the landmark for the procedure.

Needle insertion and direction: Insert a 22 gauge needle perpendicular to the tibial shaft at the level of the base of the malleolus and medial to the EHL tendon (Figure 65-13B). Alternatively, insert the needle medial to the TA tendon (Figure 65-13C).

Remarks: If using the EHL tendon as the landmark, use caution to avoid the dorsalis pedis vessels and the deep peroneal nerve that usually lie immediately lateral to the EHL tendon.

Joint injection: A maximum volume of 3 mL may be instilled into this joint. A maximum dose of 20 mg of corticosteroids may be instilled into this joint.

SUBTALAR JOINT ARTHROCENTESIS

Landmarks: Identify the tip of the medial malleolus. Palpate the sustentaculum tali of the calcaneus (Figure 65-14). It is approximately 1.5 to 2.0 cm below the tip of the medial malleolus.

Patient positioning: Place the patient supine on a stretcher with the foot held at a right angle to the leg. Externally rotate the hip until the medial malleolus is pointing upward.

Needle insertion and direction: Insert a 22 gauge needle immediately above and slightly posterior to the sustentaculum tali (Figure 65-14). Advance the needle to a depth of 1.5 to 2.0 cm.

Remarks: This is a difficult procedure because the joint space is very small. Fluoroscopy may be required to

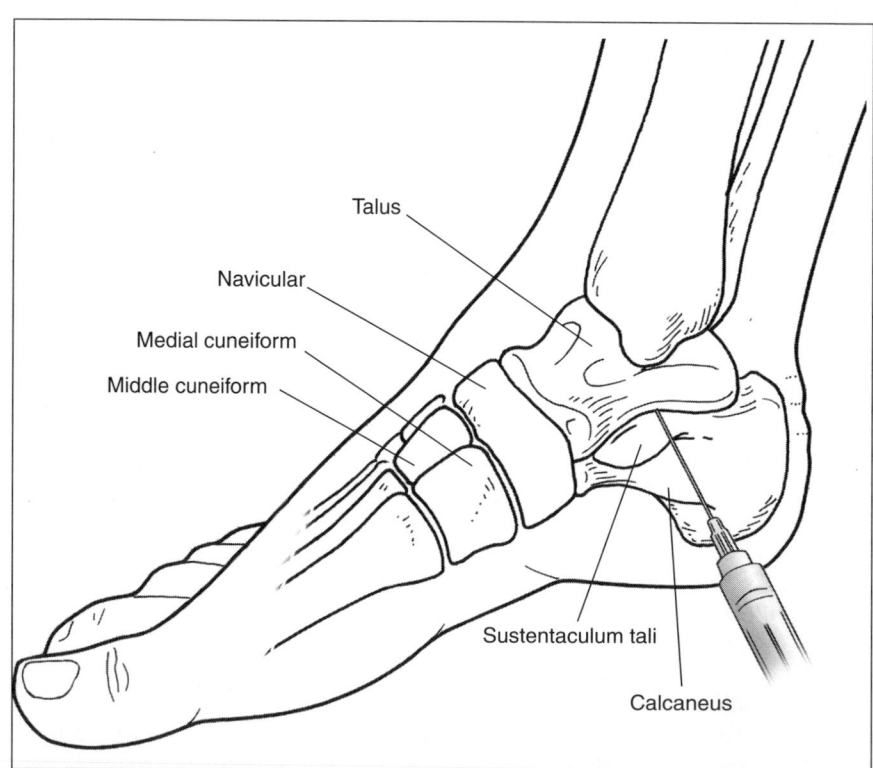

Talus

Navicular

Medial cuneiform

Middle cuneiform

Sustentaculum tali

Calcaneus

FIGURE 65-14 Subtalar joint arthrocentesis.

gain entry into the joint cavity. This procedure is seldom performed in the Emergency Department.

Joint injection: A maximum volume of 1.5 mL may be instilled into this joint. A maximum dose of 20 mg of corticosteroids may be instilled into this joint.

INTERTARSAL JOINT ARTHROCENTESIS

There are no specific landmarks for the many intertarsal joints. Radiographs are required to identify the location of a specific joint. Plain radiographs are often not helpful and fluoroscopic guidance is required. For these reasons, arthrocentesis of these joints is not routinely performed in the Emergency Department. Some authors recommend probing the general area of the joint with a needle until it enters the joint cavity. This is extremely painful for the patient and risks injury to the articular cartilage. Therefore, this technique cannot be recommended.

METATARSOPHALANGEAL JOINT ARTHROCENTESIS

Landmarks: Identify the metatarsophalangeal (MTP) joint and the extensor tendon. The MTP joint can be located just proximal to the prominence at the base of the proximal phalanx of the toe. Identify the extensor tendon by having the patient extend the toe against resistance.

Patient positioning: Place the patient sitting upright or supine on a stretcher. Plantar flex the foot. Grasp and plantar flex the toe 15 to 20 degrees and apply distal traction (Figure 65-15A).

Needle insertion and direction: Insert a 22 gauge needle into the dorsal joint space and just medial or lateral to the extensor tendon (Figure 65-15B). Direct the tip of the needle towards the center of the MTP joint. Advance the needle to a depth of 0.3 to 0.5 cm.

Remarks: The application of distal traction often causes a depression to appear on both sides of the extensor tendon. These depressions can be used as landmarks for the site of needle insertion into the joint cavity.

Joint injection: A maximum volume of 1.5 mL may be instilled into this joint. A maximum dose of 10 mg of corticosteroids may be instilled into this joint.

INTERPHALANGEAL JOINT OF THE TOE ARTHROCENTESIS

Landmarks: Identify the interphalangeal (IP) joint and the extensor tendon. The IP joint can be located just proximal to the prominence at the base of the mid-dle or distal phalanx of the toe. Identify the extensor tendon by having the patient extend their toes against resistance.

Patient positioning: Place the patient sitting upright or supine on a stretcher. Plantar flex the foot. Grasp and plantar flex the toe 15 to 20 degrees and apply distal traction (Figure 65-15A).

Needle insertion and direction: Insert a 23 gauge needle into the dorsal joint space and just medial or lateral to the extensor tendon (Figure 65-15B). The needle should be aimed toward the center of the joint. Advance the needle to a depth of 0.3 to 0.5 cm.

Remarks: The application of distal traction often causes a depression to appear on both sides of the extensor tendon. These depressions can be used as landmarks for the site of needle insertion into the joint cavity. These joints are small and normally contain almost no synovial fluid. When inflamed or infected, the joint cavity may contain up to 1.5 mL of synovial fluid.

Joint injection: A maximum volume of 1 mL may be instilled into this joint. A maximum dose of 5 mg of corticosteroids may be instilled into this joint.

JOINT INJECTION TECHNIQUE

A joint may be injected with corticosteroids and/or local anesthetic solution to relieve pain and inflammation. Identify the anatomic landmarks, prepare the patient, and insert the needle as if performing an arthrocentesis. Inject the pharmaceutical(s), remove the needle, and apply a bandage.

Occasionally, synovial fluid may be required for analysis prior to injection of pharmaceuticals. Identify the anatomic landmarks, prepare the patient, and insert the needle as if performing an arthrocentesis. Aspirate the synovial fluid into the syringe. With the needle still in the joint, grasp the hub of the needle with a hemostat. Remove the original syringe containing the aspirated synovial fluid. Attach a second syringe containing the pharmaceutical(s) to be injected into the synovial cavity. Reaspirate to confirm that the needle tip remained within the synovial cavity. Inject the pharmaceutical(s). While injecting, no resistance should be felt. If resistance is encountered, the needle may have dislodged from the joint cavity. Remove the needle, reinsert it into the synovial cavity, aspirate to confirm proper positioning, and then inject the pharmaceutical(s). After injection, remove the needle and apply a bandage.

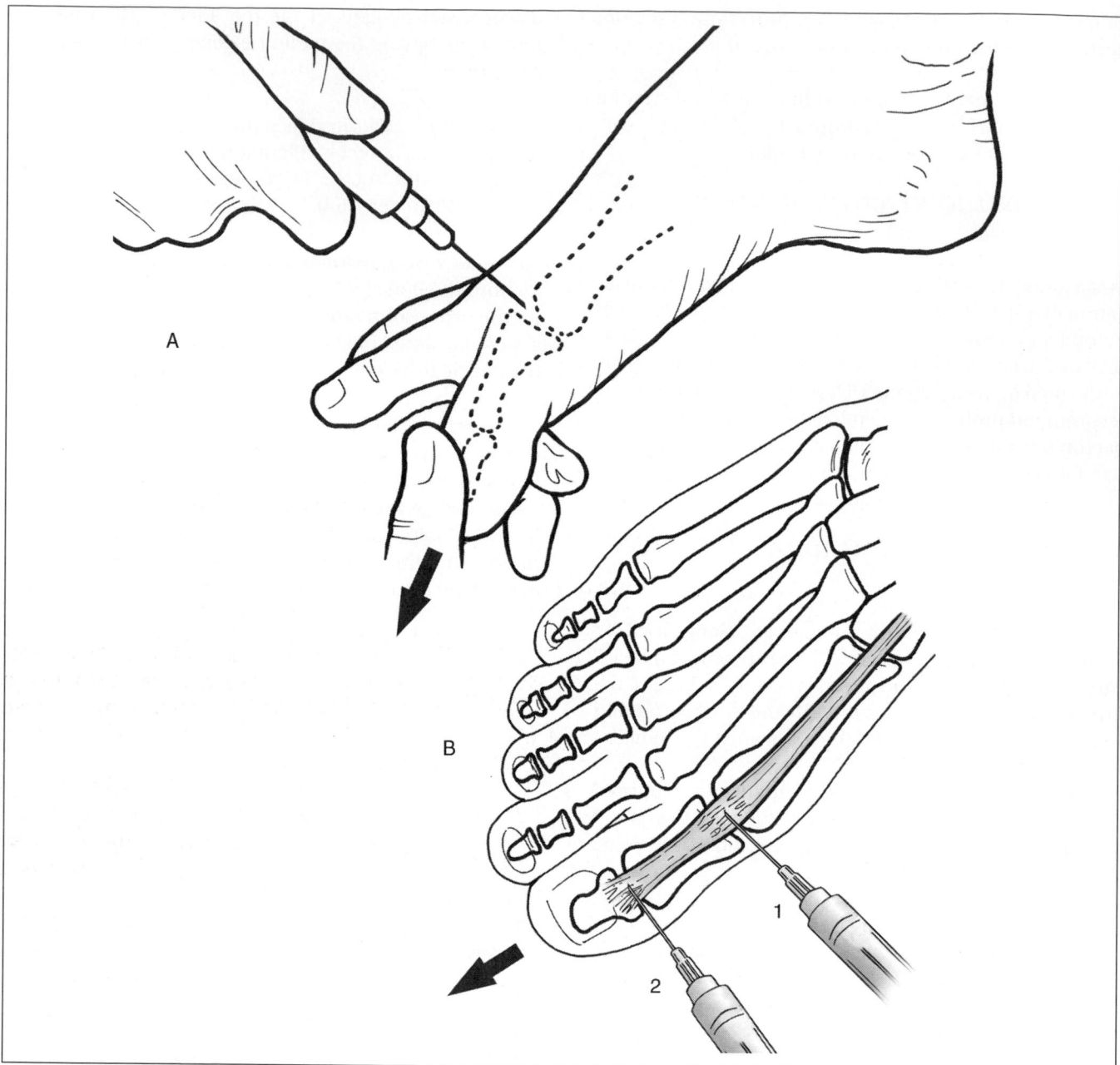

FIGURE 65-15 Arthrocentesis of the metatarsophalangeal and interphalangeal joints of the foot. *A.* The ankle is plantar flexed. The affected toe is flexed 15 to 20 degrees at the metatarsophalangeal joint and distal traction is applied (*arrow*). *B.* The needle is inserted just medial or lateral to the extensor tendon at the level of the metatarsophalangeal joint (*1*) or the interphalangeal joint (*2*).

AFTERCARE

There is no special care or precautions required after performing an arthrocentesis. Pain can be relieved with the use of ice, elevation, and nonsteroidal anti-inflammatory drugs. Joint injection, on the other hand, often requires some precautions. Some recommend limiting joint activity for 4 to 8 hours if an anesthetic solution is injected into a joint. An anesthetized joint, especially weight-bearing joints, may be susceptible to further injury. Injection of corticosteroids into a joint

cavity often requires a period of immobilization. This discussion is beyond the scope of this chapter. The readers should refer to a rheumatology or orthopedic textbook, or the medical literature, for this information.

COMPLICATIONS

Complications can occur with joint aspiration and/or injection (Table 65-3). Most of the complications are minor. Significant complications are rare; but they do occur.

TABLE 65-3. COMPLICATIONS ASSOCIATED WITH THE ASPIRATION AND/OR INFECTION OF JOINTS

Allergic reactions
Bleeding
Cartilage injury
Dry tap
Infection
Joint instability
Needle-associated complications
Corticosteroid-induced complications
Vasovagal reactions

ALLERGIC REACTIONS

Allergic reactions can occur from hypersensitivity to the local anesthetic solution. Symptoms can range from mild itching and urticaria to circulatory collapse and death. Severe allergic reactions are extremely rare but may occur. Taking a thorough history can prevent many allergic reactions. The preservative in the local anesthetic solution is often the cause of the allergic reaction. Local anesthetic solutions containing no preservatives are an alternative. Some authors believe local anesthesia is not required, as the pain of anesthetic injection is equal to performing the procedure without injectable anesthesia.[4,12] If one is concerned about a potential allergic reaction associated with local anesthetic solutions, topical ice or vapor coolant is an acceptable alternative to nothing. A solution of 1 to 2% diphenhydramine can also be used as an injectable local anesthetic agent.

CARTILAGE INJURY

The articular cartilage can be damaged from improper needle insertion or needle movement within the joint cavity. The actual incidence of cartilage injury is unknown. The cartilage is avascular and injuries do not heal. Damaged cartilage can lead to focal degenerative changes and be a nidus for future infection. Injury to the articular cartilage can be prevented with a few simple steps. Select a site for the procedure and a needle path that avoids the articular cartilage. Aspirate as you slowly enter the joint cavity and stop inserting the needle when synovial fluid enters the syringe. There is no advantage to plunging the needle into the middle of the joint cavity. Avoid needle movement once the joint cavity has been entered. Finally, do not try to completely aspirate all the fluid within the joint cavity.

DRY TAP

A needle inserted into a joint does not always guarantee fluid will be aspirated.[14] A dry tap can occur due to improper needle placement, small or absent effusion, mechanical obstruction, or chronic inflammation.

A dry tap can result from improper needle placement. If the needle is not within the joint cavity, no fluid will be aspirated. Slightly withdraw the needle and reinsert it at a different angle. Alternatively, remove the needle, re-identify the anatomic landmarks, and then reinsert the needle.

One of the most common reasons for a dry tap is the lack of an effusion or a small effusion. It may be difficult on physical examination to determine if an effusion is present. This is especially true if the patient is obese or if a large amount of subcutaneous edema is present. Try using the non–syringe-bearing hand to "milk" fluid towards the needle while aspirating. Alternatively, if a small effusion is suspected, inject a small amount of sterile saline into the joint cavity. Allow the saline to remain for 30 to 60 seconds, then aspirate the fluid.

Synovial fluid may be loculated or inaccessible by the chosen site of needle entry if the joint has been previously injured. Choose an alternate approach or site to enter the joint cavity. This may facilitate synovial fluid aspiration.

Mechanical obstruction can result in a dry tap. Gently move the needle tip to determine if it can move freely. If it doesn't, it may be caught or embedded in cartilage, periosteum, or synovium. Withdraw the needle 1 to 2 mm and reaspirate. The needle may also be within the intraarticular fat pad. Slightly withdraw the needle and reaspirate. A plica may be obstructing the lumen of the needle. Rotate the needle and reaspirate. If no fluid is aspirated, slightly advance the needle and reaspirate.

The synovial fluid itself may be the cause of a dry tap. The presence of purulent fluid or fluid with debris may clog the needle. Remove the needle and repeat the procedure with a larger gauge needle. If the needle clogs during the aspiration, try reinjecting a small amount of the synovial fluid to dislodge the obstruction and then reaspirate. A larger gauge needle may be required to complete the procedure.

Aspiration of synovial fluid from a chronically inflamed joint may be problematic. The synovium may undergo fatty replacement known as lipoma arborescens. Long-standing inflammatory fluid may be resorbed, leaving a thick gelatinous material that is difficult to aspirate. In these cases, arthrocentesis should be referred to the experienced clinician or a consultant.

HEMORRHAGE

Significant bleeding is extremely rare. External hemorrhage can be controlled with direct pressure over the puncture site. Hemarthroses are small, self-limited, and only require observation.

Arthrocentesis can be safely performed in patients who are anticoagulated or have a bleeding disorder. If a significant hemarthrosis or external hemorrhage occurs, treatment may be required to reverse the anticoagulant or replace clotting factors. The readers should refer to another source for management of these complications, as a detailed discussion is beyond the scope of this chapter.

INFECTION

Infection of a sterile joint can occur when the needle penetrates unclean skin, cellulitic skin, or infected subcutaneous tissues. If proper aseptic technique is used, the risk of infecting a sterile joint occurs in less than 1:10,000 arthrocenteses.[4] The risk of infection is negligible when the skin is properly cleansed, aseptic technique is used, and the skin is not punctured through an obvious infection or through a skin lesion that may harbor micro-organisms.

HYPODERMIC NEEDLE-ASSOCIATED COMPLICATIONS

The hypodermic needle can be the source of complications in rare circumstances. The needle may separate from the hub during the procedure and require a minor surgical procedure to recover it.[15] The needle tip may be advanced too deep and become embedded in the bony skeleton surrounding the joint. Upon withdrawing the syringe, the needle tip may break off and remain embedded in the bone or the needle may separate from the hub.

CORTICOSTEROID-INDUCED COMPLICATIONS

Corticosteroid-induced complications can be acute or chronic.[3,4,16-18] The most severe acute complication is injection of corticosteroids into an infected joint. **A septic arthritis must be ruled out prior to instillation of corticosteroids into a joint cavity.** Other local complications include steroid arthropathy, Charcot arthropathy, osteonecrosis, aseptic necrosis, tissue atrophy, tendon rupture, fat necrosis, formation of calcifications, joint instability, intraneural injection, and postinjection flare. Systemic complications include flushing, pancreatitis, posterior subcapsular cataracts, and hyperglycemia. Due to the potential for complications, many clinicians defer corticosteroid injections to the Orthopedist, Rheumatologist, or Sports Medicine consultant.

VASOVAGAL REACTIONS

The patient may experience an increase in vagal tone from apprehension, needle phobias, and/or pain. Vasovagal reactions are relatively common and may be associated with light-headedness and/or fainting. To prevent secondary injury to the patient, arthrocentesis should be performed with the patient on a stretcher or in a chair that reclines. These vasovagal reactions are self-limited and only require reassurance.

SYNOVIAL FLUID ANALYSIS

Hailed as the most valuable test in rheumatology, synovial fluid analysis provides essential diagnostic information for the appropriate management and treatment of urgent and emergent arthritic conditions.[4] It has been established as a fundamental component to the complete and appropriate work-up of arthritic diseases. With the possibility of potential joint destruction and chronic disability, **the role of synovial fluid analysis in the expedient diagnosis and treatment of acute joint disease cannot be overemphasized.**

Controversy exists concerning what constitutes the appropriate guidelines for a "routine" synovial fluid analysis.[4,19–21,23,24] This controversy arises from multiple issues that include the clinical scenario, physician competency with appropriate arthrocentesis techniques, the sensitivity and specificity of individual tests, the availability and proficiency of laboratories, and cost. Classification schemes have been established based upon gross, microscopic, biochemical, and microbiological analyses. The most traditional and cited classification for synovial fluid is normal, noninflammatory, inflammatory, septic, or hemorrhagic (Table 65-4).[4,19,20,24] Despite the controversy that exists with guidelines and classification schemes, **it is critical to differentiate between an inflammatory and noninflammatory process, with the intent of expediting the diagnosis and treatment of a possible infectious etiology.**[4]

A detailed discussion of synovial fluid analysis is beyond the scope of this book. A brief discussion of the most essential components that can be performed in the Emergency Department will be presented.

PATHOPHYSIOLOGY OF SYNOVIAL FLUID

Synovium refers to the 1 to 3 cell thick structure that lines the joint space and terminates at the articular cartilage margin.[19] This structure overlies a highly vascularized subsynovium, both of which are supported by the dense fibrous joint capsule.[19] The synovium produces synovia, an ultrafiltrate of plasma that includes hyaluronate. The synovia serves to lubricate, nourish, and clear the metabolic waste of the avascular articular cartilage.[20]

The synovium has been described as a double barrier in which molecules must pass through the endothelial microvasculature as well as the synovium and its matrix.[20] This double barrier is responsible for the retention of plasma protein. In the presence of an inflammatory process, the barrier is disrupted and protein can leak through the synovium. Difficulty arises in the diagnostic interpretation of protein and smaller molecules (i.e., sodium, chloride, urea, urate, lactate) found in synovial fluid secondary to the effects of damaged endothelial permeability and variable lymphatic drainage.[20,23,24]

GROSS ANALYSIS OF SYNOVIAL FLUID

The color of synovial fluid varies depending on the amount of protein, blood, and breakdown products of hemoglobin. Normal synovial fluid usually appears clear

TABLE 65-4. SYNOVIAL FLUID ANALYSIS

	Normal	Noninflammatory	Inflammatory	Septic	Hemorrhagic
Gross analysis					
color	clear/yellow/ straw	straw/xanthochromic	xanthochromic/ cloudy/white	white/variable	red
clarity	transparent	transparent	translucent/opaque	opaque	opaque
viscosity	very high	high	low	very low/variable	
mucin clot	good/firm	fair-to-good/firm	fair-to-poor/friable	poor/friable	
Microscopic analysis					
total leukocyte count (WBC/mm^3)	< 150	< 3000	3000–50,000	> 50,000	
polymorphonuclear leukocytes (%)	< 25	< 25	> 70	> 90	
Biochemical analysis					
glucose (mg/dL)†	normal	normal	70–90	> 90	
protein (mg/dL)‡	1.3–1.8	3–3.5	> 4.0	> 4.0	
Microbiological analysis					
Gram's stain	negative	negative	negative	positive•	negative
culture	negative	negative	negative	positive•	negative
Differential diagnosis					
		osteoarthritis	rheumatoid arthritis	bacterial infections	trauma
		traumatic arthritis	acute crystal synovitis		coagulopathy
		early rheumatoid arthritis	viral arthritis		anticoagulant therapy
		avascular necrosis	psoriatic arthritis		tumor
		crystal synovitis~	Reiter's syndrome		Charcot's arthropathy
		osteochondritis dissecans	arthritis of IBD°		hemangioma
		SLE	SLE		A-V malformation
		polyarteritis	polyarteritis		sickle cell disease
		scleroderma	scleroderma		postsurgical
		amyloidosis	amyloidosis		joint prosthesis

WBC = white blood cells; † and ‡ variable interpretation (refer to text); • variable results depending on organism (refer to text); ~ chronic or subsiding; SLE = systemic lupus erythematosus; ° IBD = inflammatory bowel disease.

to a straw or yellow color. Inflammatory and purulent synovial fluid may appear xanthochromic to white. Hemorrhagic synovial fluid is red and must be distinguished from a traumatic arthrocentesis. A traumatic aspiration usually clots and is more than often nonhomogenous.[19,20] A hematocrit may be sent on a bloody aspirate to distinguish between a traumatic tap and hemorrhagic fluid. A vein was pierced by the needle (traumatic tap) if the synovial fluid hematocrit is equal to the serum hematocrit.[20]

The clarity of synovial fluid refers to the amount and type of particles within the fluid. Normal synovial fluid is usually transparent and newspaper print can be easily read through a glass tube containing this fluid.[19] Inflammatory and purulent synovial fluid is translucent to opaque secondary to the presence of leukocytes. Opaque fluid can also represent crystals and other particulate matter. Infected synovial fluid cannot be differentiated from noninfected synovial fluid based on gross appearance alone.[4]

Synovial fluid viscosity is determined by the intactness and concentration of hyaluronate. Viscosity can grossly be assessed by observing a drop of fluid fall from the tip of the needle. The "string" formed will normally be 5 to 10 cm in length.[22] In inflammatory and septic synovial fluid, the hyaluronidase is depolymerized and degraded.[20] The string formed in these conditions is shorter, or not formed at all, and the fluid falls as a drop. Processes resulting in a significant effusion without inflammation may also dilute hyaluronate without degrading it and result in decreased viscosity. Clotted white blood cells may enhance viscosity in the presence of inflammation.[20] Clinicians must be cautious with their interpretations of viscosity because even quantitative measures often fail to distinguish between inflammatory and noninflammatory states.[4]

The mucin clot test evaluates the degree of polymerization of hyaluronate.[4,19] The mucin clot test is performed by one of two methods. The first method involves mixing the supernatant of a centrifuged specimen with a few drops of glacial acetic acid. The second method involves mixing 1 mL of synovial fluid to 4 mL of 2% acetic acid. A "good" clot consists of a dense white precipitant that indicates a high degree of polymerization and a high viscosity.[19] A "poor" clot consists of little to no precipitate and suggests an inflammatory process that has depolymerized the hyaluronate. Controversy exists concerning the subjectiveness of the clot's endpoint.[4]

MICROSCOPIC ANALYSIS OF SYNOVIAL FLUID

The total leukocyte count, more than any other test, aids in distinguishing between an inflammatory, noninflammatory, and septic process.[20] Although a significant overlap may exist, the total leukocyte count can be used to identify synovial fluid as normal, noninflammatory, inflammatory, or septic (Table 65-4). Using this classification scheme, a total leukocyte count of less than 3000 cells/μL is considered noninflammatory. A count between 3000 and 20,000 cells/μL is considered inflammatory. The range of 20,000 to 50,000 cells/μL may be inflammatory or septic. A count greater than 50,000 cells/μL is considered septic until proven otherwise. **The overlap between categories is considerable and clinicians must be cautious of basing a diagnosis solely on the total leukocyte count.** Depending on the acuteness of the inflammation, several arthritic conditions such as gout, pseudogout, and rheumatoid arthritis may yield a significantly elevated total leukocyte count approaching 100,000 cells/μL.[21] Immunocompromised hosts and some infectious diseases, such as tuberculosis and *Neisseria gonorrhoeae*, may have lower absolute counts than expected.[4]

The differential leukocyte count may further aid in distinguishing between inflammatory, noninflammatory, and septic synovial fluid. Inflammatory processes generally have greater than 70 percent neutrophils while septic synovial fluid has greater than 90 percent neutrophils.[19] Again, the overlap can be significant depending on the arthritic process and its acuteness. Crystal-induced processes may present with high neutrophil counts, while immunocompromised hosts, fungal infections, and tuberculosis may present with lower neutrophil counts.[4,21] **In general, a synovial fluid containing greater than 90 percent neutrophils in the presence of an elevated total leukocyte count should be highly suspicious of a septic process.** High eosinophil counts may suggest parasitic infection, allergic reactions, tumor, or Lyme disease.[20,23] High monocyte counts may suggest viral infection (e.g., rubella and hepatitis B) or serum sickness.[22]

Crystal identification is an essential component of synovial fluid analysis. Crystal identification requires the use of a polarized light microscope with higher-powered lenses and oil immersion capabilities. Crystals can be identified based on their shape, size, and birefringence. Birefringence is defined as the crystals' ability to bend the light passing through it into two distinct directions, negative or positive. The light's ability to bend negatively or positively is transformed into a specific color (yellow or blue) under the polarized microscope.[19,20] Caution must be taken as artifact and tissue debris can often imitate birefringent material.

Crystal analysis requires an experienced technician and is rarely if ever performed in the Emergency Department. Monosodium urate crystals are commonly seen in gout. These crystals are needle-shaped, 2 to 25 μm in length, and have strong negative birefringence. They may clump together in sheets.[22,25] Local anesthetic has the ability to dissolve monosodium urate crystals. Therefore, the joint cavity should not be penetrated with the needle when anesthetizing the skin and subcutaneous tissue.[21] Calcium pyrophosphate dihydrate crystals are seen in pseudogout. These crystals are rhomboidal or rectangular, 2 to 10 μm in length, and have weak positive birefringence.[22,25] These crystals may be more difficult to detect than monosodium urate crystals because of the weaker birefringence. Cholesterol crystals may present in multiple forms and sizes. They are typically flat rhomboidal plates, 5 to 50 μm in length, and have both negative and positive birefringence.[22] Artifact "crystals" can be produced by a variety of substances. Corticosteroids can be detected weeks after injection and have variable shapes but no regular geometric form. Maltese crosses are strong birefringent particles that are secondary to multiple compounds such as talc powder, lipids, calcium oxalate, and dust.[22]

BIOCHEMICAL ANALYSIS OF SYNOVIAL FLUID

As discussed previously under the pathophysiology section, difficulty arises with the interpretation of total protein secondary to the effects of damaged endothelial permeability and variable lymphatic drainage.[20] In theory, the damage caused by an inflammatory process should increase the permeability of proteins into the synovial fluid. Multiple studies have shown that protein samples were only able to classify synovial fluid into an inflammatory or noninflammatory process in approximately 50 percent of the cases.[23] Furthermore, the total protein count was unable to differentiate among various groups of arthritides, including rheumatoid arthritis and osteoarthritis.[4]

Theoretically, inflammatory and infectious processes consume glucose and thus lower the level present in synovial fluid. One study has shown that glucose levels were able to classify synovial fluid into an inflammatory or noninflammatory process in less than 50 percent of cases.[23] In 50 percent of the septic joints analyzed, the glucose level was not significantly decreased. Another study by Shmerling reports glucose analysis having a sensitivity of 20 percent and specificity of 84 percent in detecting inflammatory joint disease.[24] Synovial fluid glucose levels can vary from serum glucose levels when taken less than 6 hours after oral intake.[24] These studies are just a few of many that confirm synovial fluid glucose levels are not reliable to diagnose or rule out a septic joint.

Other biochemical markers have been studied to elicit a marker to differentiate a septic from a nonseptic joint. These include lactate, lactic dehydrogenase, and numerous immunologic and inflammatory mediators. These biochemical markers, at present, are not sensitive or specific to rule out a septic joint. They are not recommended for routine synovial fluid analysis.

MICROBIOLOGICAL ANALYSIS OF SYNOVIAL FLUID

The Gram's stain is an easily performed test that yields rapid results and can lead to the expedient diagnosis and treatment of a septic joint. The Gram's stain has a sensitivity of 50 to 70 percent for nongonococcal infections and less than 10 percent for gonococcal joint infections.[24] Although the sensitivity of this test is low, the specificity of the Gram's stain approaches 100 percent. This makes it an essential component of routine synovial analysis. *Neisseria gonorrhoeae* is identified as a gram-negative intracellular diplococci. *Staphylococcus aureus* and *Streptococcus* are responsible for approximately 70 percent of nongonococcal septic arthritis and can be identified as gram-positive cocci in clusters and gram-positive cocci in chains, respectively.[27]

Bacterial identification is essential when confronted with the possibility of a septic joint. Synovial fluid cultures have a sensitivity of 75 to 95 percent for nongonococcal bacteria and 10 to 50 percent for gonococcal bacteria in the absence of previous antibiotic treatment. Difficulty arises from the low sensitivity of cultures for some organisms, culture methods, specimen preparation, and the length of time for some bacteria to grow.[24] Recent advances with the use of polymerase chain reaction techniques have shown increased sensitivity and specificity for detecting *Neisseria gonorrhoeae*.[19,26]

SPECIMEN COLLECTION

Minimal quantities of synovial fluid can yield valuable information. Analysis can be performed with as little as two drops of synovial fluid.[21] The total leukocyte count, differential leukocyte count, crystal analysis, and Gram's stain can be obtained from the first drop while the second drop can be sent for cultures.[21] Unfortunately, few institutions or laboratories can perform synovial fluid analysis with only two drops of fluid.

The specimen may be transported for analysis by one of two methods. First, the syringe with the synovial fluid may be capped and sent to the laboratory. The laboratory technicians will then divide the specimen for analysis. Alternatively, the synovial fluid may be placed into tubes. A new sterile needle, different from the arthrocentesis needle, should be used to place fluid in the test tubes. A needle used for steroid injection should never be used secondary to the formation of a crystal-like substance.[4] Synovial fluid for microscopic analysis should be collected in test tubes with and without preservatives. Fluid should be placed in a Culturette or culture bottle for microbiological analysis. Synovial fluid for crystal analysis should be sent in a test tube with liquid heparin (green-topped tube) because EDTA and powdered anticoagulants interfere with crystal identification.[21] A red-topped tube containing no preservatives should be used to test for chemistries, serology, and viscosity. A tube with an anticoagulant (purple-topped tube) is used for the cell count, cell differential, and cytology.

SUMMARY

Arthrocentesis is used to diagnose and make treatment decisions regarding a joint. It is a safe, easy, and simple procedure. Arthrocentesis is relatively painless and extremely beneficial to the patient. It may be performed for diagnostic information and/or therapeutic treatment. Analysis of the synovial fluid provides unique and valuable information about a joint. It is the only method to accurately and definitively diagnose or rule out a septic arthritis. Arthrocentesis is indicated to evaluate the cause of an arthritis or a joint effusion. All patients presenting with an acute monoarthritis or an acute, nontraumatic effusion should undergo arthrocentesis when the diagnosis is not clear based upon the history and physical examination.

REFERENCES

1. Council on Rheumatologic Care, American College of Rheumatology: *Safety Guidelines for Performing Arthrocentesis.* 1999. http://www.rheumatology. org/Position/safetyguide.html.
2. Hazleman BL: Principles of joint aspiration and steroid injection, in Doherty M, Hazleman BL, Hutton CW, et al (eds): *Rheumatology Examination and Injection Techniques.* London: Saunders, 1992:121–123.

3. Pfenninger JL: Injections of joints and soft tissue: part I. General guidelines. *Am Fam Physician* 1991; 44(4):1196–1202.

4. Hasselbacher P: Arthrocentesis, synovial fluid analysis, and synovial biopsy, in Schumaker HR Jr, Klippel JH, Koopman WJ (eds): *Primer on Rheumatic Diseases,* 10th ed. Atlanta: Arthritis Foundation, 1993:67–72.

5. Schumacher HR Jr: Arthrocentesis of the knee. *Hosp Med* 1997; 33(7):60–64.

6. Benjamin GC: Arthrocentesis, in Roberts JR, Hedges HR (eds): *Clinical Procedures in Emergency Medicine,* 3rd ed. Philadelphia: Saunders, 1998:919–932.

7. Schaffter TC: Joint and soft tissue arthrocentesis. *Primary Care* 1993; 20:757–770.

8. Holdsworth BJ, Clement DA, Rothwell PNR: Fractures of the radial head—the benefit of aspiration: a prospective controlled trial. *Injury* 1987; 18(1): 44–47.

9. Zuckerman JD, Meislin RJ, Rothberg M: Injections for joint and soft tissue disorders: when and how to use them. *Geriatrics* 1990; 45(4):45–55.

10. Hedges JR: Pearls for the teaching of procedural skills at the bedside. *Acad Emerg Med* 1994; 1(4):401–404.

11. Samuelson CO Jr, Cannon GW, Ward JR: Arthrocentesis. *J Fam Pract* 1985; 20(2):179–184.

12. Pfenninger JL: Injections of joints and soft tissue: part II. Guidelines for specific joints. *Am Fam Physician* 1991; 44(4):1690–1701.

13. Quigley TB: Aspiration of the elbow joint in the treatment of fractures of the head of the radius. *N Engl J Med* 1949; 240:915.

14. Roberts WN, Hayes CW, Breitbach SA, Owens DS Jr: Dry taps and what to do about them: a pictorial essay on failed arthrocenteses of the knee. *Am J Med* 1996; 100:461–464.

15. Gottlieb NL: Hypodermic needle separation during arthrocentesis. *Arthritis Rheum* 1981; 24:1593–1594.

16. Gottlieb NL, Riskin WG: Complication of local corticosteroid injections. *JAMA* 1980; 243:1547–1548.

17. McCarty DJ: Treatment of rheumatoid joint inflammation with triamcinolone hexacetonide. *Arthritis Rheum* 1992; 15:157–173.

18. Gray RG, Gottlieb NL: Intra-articular corticosteroids, an updated assessment. *Clin Orthop* 1983; 177:235–263.

19. McCarty DJ: Synovial fluid, in Koopman WJ: *Arthritis and Allied Conditions.* Baltimore: Williams & Wilkins, 1997:81–102.

20. Gatter RA, Schumacher HR: *A Practical Handbook of Joint Fluid Analysis.* Philadelphia: Lea & Febiger, 1991:1–35.

21. Kolba KS: The approach to the acute joint and synovial fluid examination. *Primary Care* 1984; 11: 211–218.

22. Doherty M: Examination of synovial fluid, in Doherty M, Hazleman BL, Hutton CW, et al (eds): *Rheumatology Examination and Injection Techniques.* London: Saunders, 1992:124–127.

23. Shmerling RH, Delbanco TL, Tosteson ANA, et al: Synovial fluid tests. What should be ordered? *JAMA* 1990; 264:1009–1014.

24. Shmerling RH: Synovial fluid analysis. A critical reappraisal. *Rheum Dis Clin North Am* 1994; 20:503–512.

25. Barland P, Gibofsky A, Lipstein E: Crystal-induced arthritis: an overview. *Am J Med* 1996; 100(2A):46S–52S.

26. Angulo JM, Espinoza LR: Gonococcal arthritis. *Comprehens Ther* 1999; 25:155–162.

27. Sack K: Monarthritis: differential diagnosis. *Am J Med* 1997; 102(1A):30S–34S.

Chapter 66
STERNOCLAVICULAR JOINT DISLOCATION REDUCTION

Shawn Janes
Eric F. Reichman

INTRODUCTION

Sternoclavicular dislocations are uncommon injuries and account for less than 3 percent of shoulder girdle dislocations.[1] The medial clavicle may be displaced anteriorly or posteriorly. Anterior dislocations are more common by a ratio of 3:1 to 20:1.[2,3] Case reports of the less common posterior dislocations are more common in the literature due to the higher incidence of associated complications. Posterior sternoclavicular joint dislocations are often seen in younger individuals.[2,4]

Sternoclavicular dislocations are the result of direct trauma to the sternoclavicular joint or to the glenohumeral joint with the force directed toward the sternoclavicular joint. **This injury is usually associated with a tremendous force.** The most commonly reported mechanisms of injury are motor vehicle collisions and contact sports.[2,5] Anterior dislocations are often due to indirect forces transmitted through the anteromedial shoulder. As the shoulder is externally compressed and rolled backward, the lateral clavicle is pulled back and down beyond its limit of motion. The first rib acts as a fulcrum to spring the sternal end of the clavicle anteriorly from its articulation.[2,6]

Posterior dislocations may be due to direct or indirect forces.[3,4,7–13] With indirect trauma, the shoulder is externally compressed and rolled forward from a posterolaterally applied force to the shoulder. The costoclavicular ligament acts as a fulcrum that produces displacement of the sternal end of the clavicle posteriorly from its articulation.[4,9,11,13] Less commonly, a posterior dislocation may be due to a direct blow to the anteromedial clavicle.

There are reports of spontaneous and nontraumatic sternoclavicular subluxations and dislocations.[14] These are usually seen in females less than 20 years of age with sternoclavicular joint laxity. The clavicle dislocates anteriorly during abduction or flexion of the arm to the overhead position. The clavicle reduces spontaneously when the arm is returned to the side. This condition is usually associated with laxity in numerous other joints.

ANATOMY AND PATHOPHYSIOLOGY

The sternoclavicular joint is a diarthrodial joint with both surfaces covered by fibrocartilage (Figure 66-1). The intraarticular disk ligament divides the joint into two separate compartments, each of which is lined with synovium.[15] This joint is freely movable and functions almost like a ball-and-socket joint in that it has motion, including rotation, in almost all planes.[3,6,16] This includes 30 to 35 degrees of upward elevation, 35 degrees of combined forward/backward movement, and 40 to 45 degrees of rotation about its long axis.[3,6,16] Less than half of the medial clavicle articulates with the upper angle of the sternum. This gives the sternoclavicular joint the distinction of having the least amount of bony stability of any of the major joints.[3] Given this amount of joint incongruity, it is surprising that sternoclavicular joint dislocations are uncommon. However, its stability comes from strong surrounding ligaments (Figure 66-1). These ligaments include the intraarticular disk ligament, the extraarticular costoclavicular ligament (rhomboid ligament), the anterior and posterior sternoclavicular ligaments, and the interclavicular ligament.[15]

The region that lies directly posterior to the sternoclavicular joint contains numerous vital structures (Figure 66-2). Within the confines of the thoracic inlet are the trachea, esophagus, lungs, and great vessels. This proximity, and the small size of the thoracic inlet, accounts for the injuries that may occur to these structures with posterior sternoclavicular joint dislocations.

The medial clavicular epiphysis is the last epiphysis of the long bones to appear. It usually ossifies by the age

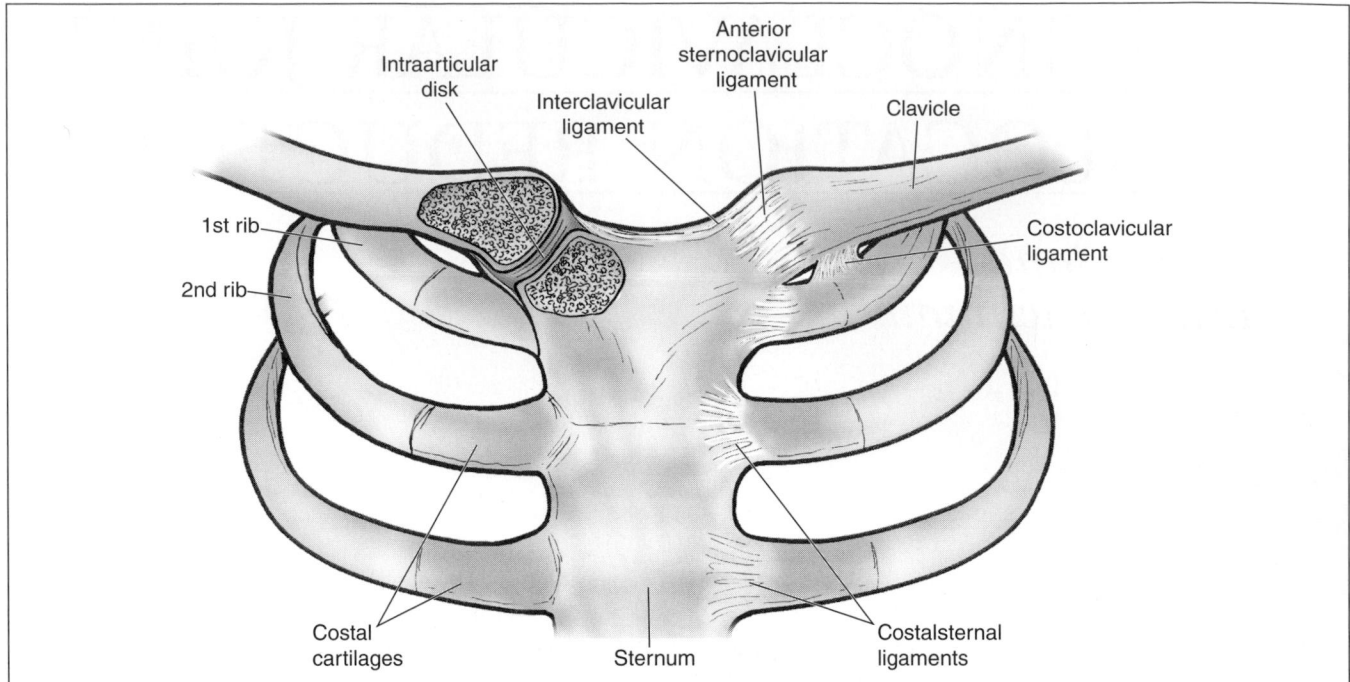

FIGURE 66-1 Anatomy of the sternoclavicular joint and surrounding structures.

of 18 to 20 and occasionally not until the age of 25.[3,17] It is also the last to fuse.[3,17] This epiphysis is difficult to see on plain radiographs. Many injuries in patients under 25 years of age that are initially felt to be sternoclavicular joint dislocations are actually Salter I or II epiphyseal injuries.[3,10,18–23]

The diagnosis of a traumatic sternoclavicular joint dislocation may be difficult and delayed. This is particularly true in the patient with multiple injuries.[7,24,25] Symptoms include severe pain that increases with movement of the ipsilateral arm. Physical signs include edema and ecchymosis over the region of the sternoclavicular joint. The patient usually holds the injured arm adducted across the trunk. Their head may be tilted toward the affected side to relieve the pain caused by traction of the sternocleidomastoid muscle on the medial clavicle. With anterior dislocations, the medial end of the clavicle may be palpated anterior to the sternum. It may also be fixed or mobile. A visible depression may be noted or a hollow palpated at the location of the sternoclavicular joint with posterior sternoclavicular joint dislocations. However, accompanying edema may obscure these physical findings. The shoulder may be held forward. When the patient is supine, the affected shoulder does not lie flat against the bed.

Additional signs and symptoms associated with a posterior sternoclavicular joint dislocation may also be due to injury or compression of mediastinal structures.[3,4,7,9,11–13,18,25–32] **It is extremely important to perform a careful and complete physical examination, as associated injuries are common.** Compression of the trachea or esophagus may result in cyanosis, dyspnea, or dysphagia. Circulation to the ipsilateral arm may be reduced if the subclavian artery is compressed. Venous congestion of the upper extremity or neck can result from compression of the subclavian or jugular veins. The patient may present in shock due to compression or injury to the retrosternal great vessels. Paresthesias of the upper extremity are due to a brachial plexus injury. Voice changes are due to compression of the recurrent laryngeal nerve. Tracheal or lung injuries can result in pneumothoraces.

The clinician cannot always rely on the clinical findings of observation and palpation to distinguish between anterior and posterior sternoclavicular joint dislocations.[3] Documentation with appropriate radiologic studies is recommended prior to the decision to treat. Routine radiographs of the sternoclavicular joint are often difficult to interpret due to overlapping structures. Several different radiographic projections have been reported to improve the ability to demonstrate asymmetry of the joints.[3,8,9,33] Computed tomography (CT) is the preferred imaging modality to study the sternoclavicular joint. It should always be performed if the diagnosis is uncertain.[9,10] The use of ultrasound to aid in the diagnosis has also been reported.[12,34]

With posterior sternoclavicular joint dislocations, the physician should also consider appropriate studies to rule out associated injuries to neighboring structures. This could include a chest radiograph, which may

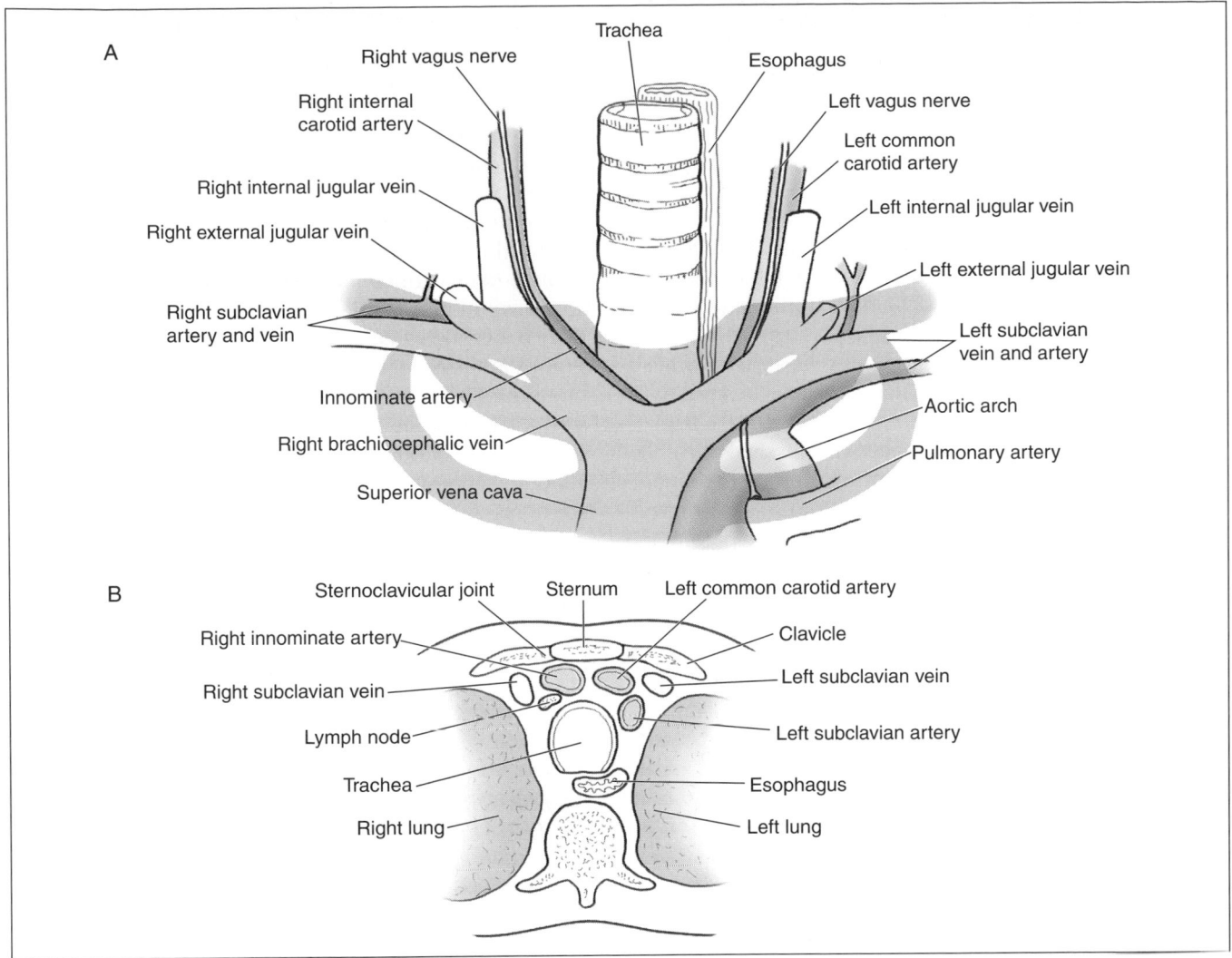

FIGURE 66-2 Anatomic relationships of structures to the sternoclavicular joint. *A.* Anteroposterior view. *B.* Cross-section through the level of the sternoclavicular joint.

reveal mediastinal widening, a pneumomediastinum, or a pneumothorax. CT will reveal the relationship of the clavicle to the great vessels, esophagus, and trachea. It may also demonstrate compression of these structures, a mediastinal hematoma, or mediastinal emphysema. Angiography, venography, and Doppler studies may be considered to investigate potential vascular injury. Esophagoscopy and/or an esophagram may be employed to evaluate the esophagus. Bronchoscopy is indicated if a tracheal or bronchial injury is suspected.

INDICATIONS

It is generally held that closed reduction should be attempted on all acute traumatic anterior and posterior sternoclavicular joint dislocations.[3,10,27] Anterior sterno-clavicular joint dislocations have been reduced via closed techniques up to 10 days postinjury.[9] Successful closed reduction of posterior sternoclavicular joint dislocations has been reported up to 5 days postinjury.[12,27] Posterior sternoclavicular joint dislocations are uncommon injuries. Early consultation with an Orthopedic Surgeon is recommended. Careful evaluation of the patient's airway, breathing, and circulation should be performed prior to the reduction. It is recommended that the reduction be performed where staff and facilities are immediately available to intervene should any thoracic emergency develop.[25] **The dislocation should be reduced emergently if neurologic or vascular compromise exists in the affected extremity.**

Many of these injuries are in fact Salter-Harris I or II epiphyseal injuries in patients less than 25 years of age.[3,10,18–23] Closed reduction should still be attempted after consultation with an Orthopedic Surgeon.

CONTRAINDICATIONS

Reduction may be postponed to attend to more serious injuries unless a posterior sternoclavicular joint dislocation is present and is compromising adjacent structures. Open reduction of posterior sternoclavicular joint dislocations may be preferred if surgery is planned for associated injuries.

Attempted reduction of chronic traumatic anterior dislocations or spontaneous anterior dislocations is not indicated. These patients usually have minimal discomfort, normal range of motion, and can return to normal activity.[3,14] Patients do well without treatment other than nonsteroidal anti-inflammatory drugs, the application of heat, and rest.[2,14,35] The results of operative treatment of such injuries have not been impressive.[3,14]

There is controversy regarding the necessity of reducing chronic posterior sternoclavicular joint dislocations. Some feel that all should be reduced due to the potential compression of adjacent structures or erosion into them.[3,28,36,37] However, there have been reports of patients who have chronic dislocations without sequelae.[6] Treatment decisions for such injuries should be made in consultation with an Orthopedic Surgeon. Reduction would require general anesthesia and operative intervention.[35]

EQUIPMENT

Sandbags or folded towels
Povidone iodine solution
Sterile towel clamps
Sterile gloves
Local anesthetic solution
18 gauge needles
25 gauge needles
10 mL syringe

PATIENT PREPARATION

Explain the risks, benefits, potential complications, and aftercare of the procedure to the patient and/or their representative. Obtain a signed consent to perform the reduction.

Place the patient supine with the affected side near the edge of the gurney. Place sandbags or towels between the patient's scapulae. They should be thick enough to raise the patient 5 cm off the gurney.[4]

A form of anesthesia and analgesia is required to reduce a sternoclavicular joint dislocation. Closed reduction of anterior sternoclavicular joint dislocations may be performed with local anesthetic solution infiltrated about the medial clavicle and sternoclavicular joint. Consider the administration of supplementary intravenous sedation or procedural sedation. Posterior sternoclavicular joint dislocations have also been reduced using local anesthesia. However, procedural sedation or general anesthesia is recommended. Infiltrate local anesthetic solution about the medial clavicle and sternoclavicular joint if procedural sedation will be performed.

TECHNIQUES

ANTERIOR STERNOCLAVICULAR JOINT DISLOCATION REDUCTION

Position the patient as mentioned above. The patient's arms should be at their sides (Figure 66-3A). Apply analgesia and sedation. Instruct an assistant to apply downward pressure to the anterior surface of both shoulders (Figure 66-3B). Pushing the shoulders posteriorly pulls the clavicles laterally and distracts the dislocated medial clavicle. Push the medial clavicle posteriorly and into anatomic position (Figure 66-3C). Relocation of the clavicle usually occurs promptly. Carefully sit the pa-

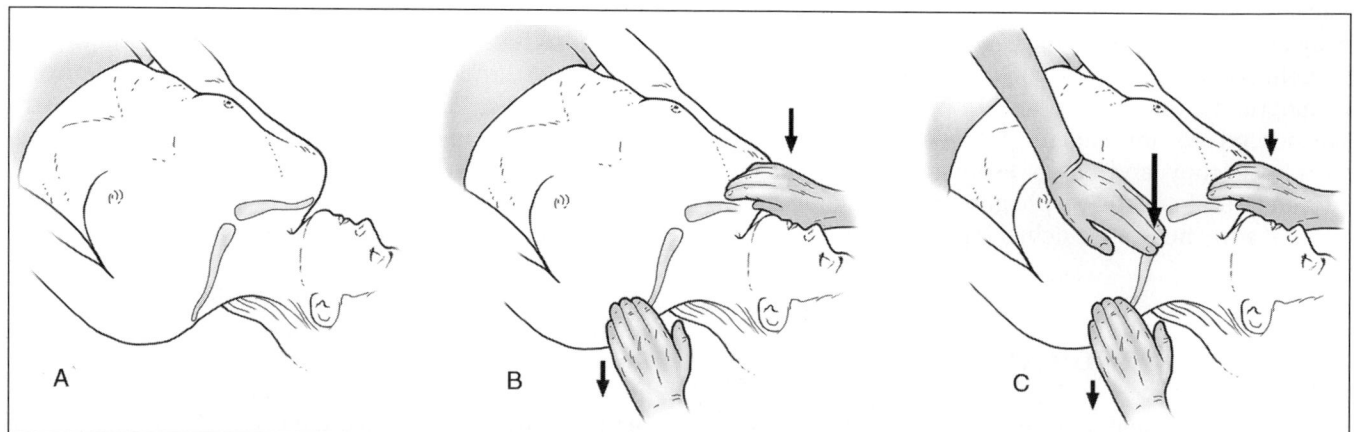

FIGURE 66-3 Reduction of an anterior sternoclavicular joint dislocation. *A.* Patient positioning. *B.* An assistant applies anterior pressure to both shoulders. *C.* The medial clavicle is pushed posteriorly.

tient upright while the assistant maintains the shoulders in a posterior position. Apply a figure-of-eight splint (Figure 75-3*C*).

POSTERIOR STERNOCLAVICULAR JOINT DISLOCATION REDUCTION

Position the patient as mentioned previously. Apply analgesia and sedation. Abduct the affected extremity 90 degrees and extend it 20 degrees in line with the clavicle (Figure 66-4*A*). Spontaneous reduction may occur at this point. If not, instruct an assistant to apply distal in-line traction to the extremity (Figure 66-4*B*). This may be aided by wrapping a sheet about the patient's upper torso to provide countertraction. The clavicle may reduce under traction. Keep the patient's arm abducted, extended, and under traction if the sternoclavicular joint does not reduce. Manually manipulate the clavicle into position. Grasp the medial clavicle and pull it upward into anatomic position (Figure 66-4*C*).

It may be difficult at times to achieve a secure grasp on the medial clavicle. In such cases, clean the skin surrounding the medial clavicle of any dirt and debris. Apply povidone iodine solution and allow it to dry. Grasp through the skin and around (not through) the shaft of the medial clavicle with a towel clamp (Figure 66-4*D*). The thick cortical bone often prevents purchase of the towel clamp into the clavicle. Elevate the medial clavicle into anatomic position while the assistant is maintaining traction on the abducted and extended extremity (Figure 66-4*D*).

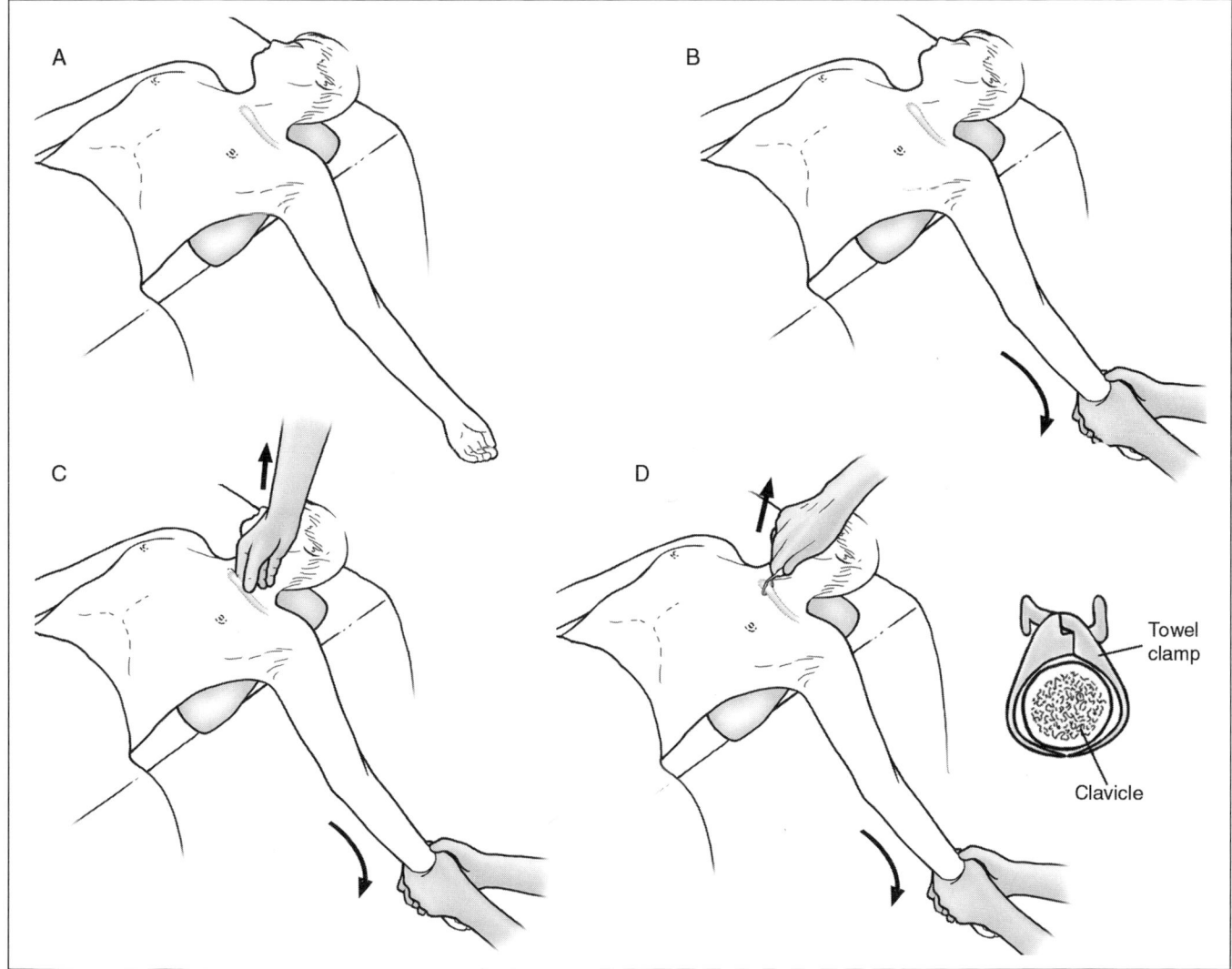

FIGURE 66-4 Reduction of a posterior sternoclavicular joint dislocation. *A.* Patient positioning. *B.* An assistant applies distal in-line traction. *C.* The medial clavicle is grasped and elevated while maintaining distal traction on the extremity. *D.* An alternative technique. A towel clamp is placed around the medial clavicle. The clamp is used to elevate the medial clavicle while maintaining distal traction on the extremity.

ALTERNATIVE TECHNIQUES

An alternative technique may be applied to reduce a posterior sternoclavicular joint dislocation.[4] It uses the first rib as a lever and has been reported to be successful when the previous technique has failed. Position the patient with their arms adducted (Figure 66-5A). Apply analgesia and sedation. Instruct an assistant to apply distal in-line traction to the adducted arm (Figure 66-5B). This will lever the medial clavicle over the first rib and above the superior sternum (Figure 66-5B, inset). Apply downward pressure to the anterior shoulder, forcing it into retraction (Figure 66-5C). This will lever the medial clavicle anteriorly and laterally into anatomic position (Figure 66-5C, inset). Reduction may occur at this point. If not, elevate the medial clavicle either by manual grasp or using a towel clamp, as described previously. It is postulated that this technique requires less force than the prior technique. A variation of this technique involves applying lateral traction to the upper humerus using a sheet looped around the upper arm.[38]

Other methods of closed reduction for a posterior sternoclavicular joint dislocation have been described but are not often performed. Successful reduction has been described using 4.5 kg (10 pounds) of lateral skin traction on the abducted arm for 30 minutes.[39] Reduction has also been achieved by simple forced retraction of the lateral clavicle.[8] Reduction has also been reported in a sedated patient who was placed, for 8 hours on rolled towels between the scapulae.[13]

ASSESSMENT

Assess all patients, both initially and following any reduction attempts, for neurologic and vascular integrity of the upper extremity. Obtain post-reduction radiographs to confirm proper bony positioning. The

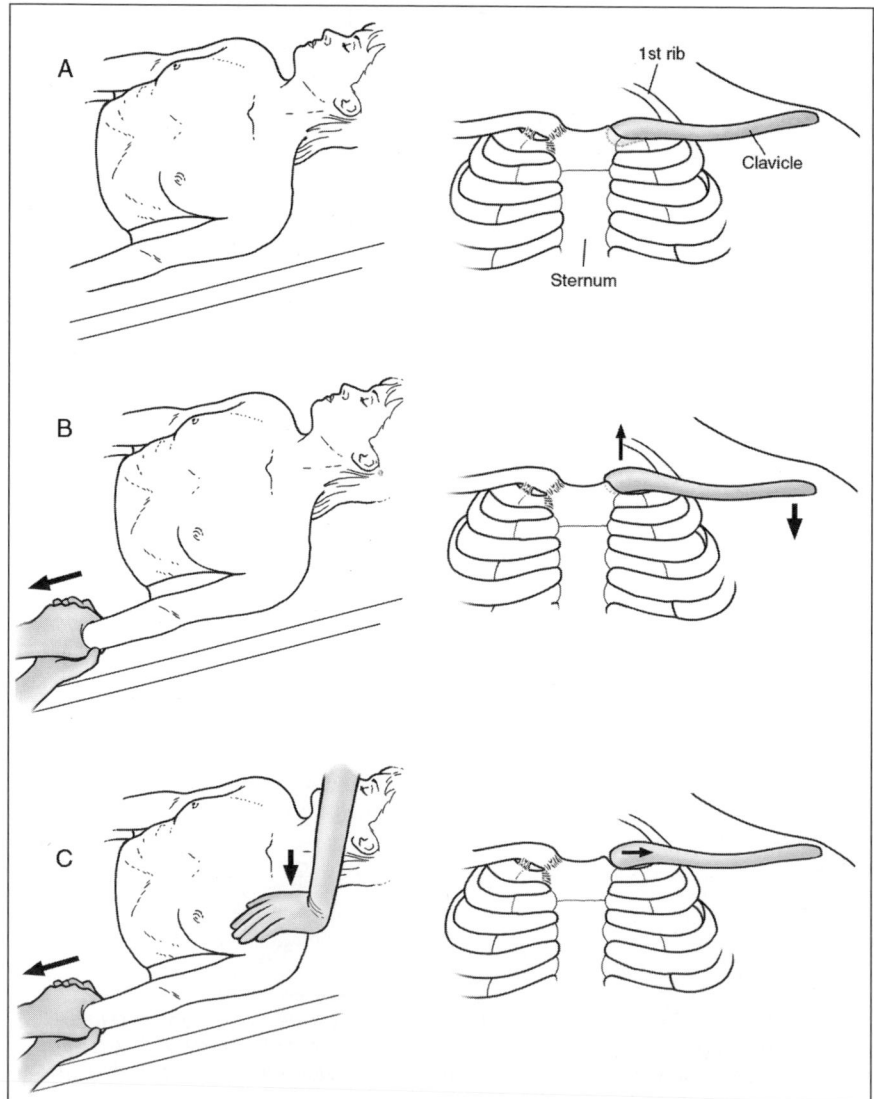

FIGURE 66-5 An alternative technique for reducing a posterior sternoclavicular joint dislocation. (Modified from Buckerfield and Castle.[4]) *A.* Patient positioning. *B.* An assistant applies distal in-line traction (*large arrow*). The medial clavicle will be elevated above the sternum (*small arrow*). *C.* A posteriorly directed force is applied to the shoulder to draw the medial clavicle anteriorly and laterally into its normal anatomic position.

procedure may be repeated if the radiographs show incomplete reduction. **Positioning is not critical if the reduction was performed for neurologic or vascular compromise. The primary consideration is the relief of the compromised nerve and/or artery.** The Orthopedic Surgeon can later reduce the defect that remains.

AFTERCARE

The general principles of orthopedic care should be applied. These include rest, ice, nonsteroidal anti-inflammatory drugs, and supplemental narcotic analgesics.

ANTERIOR STERNOCLAVICULAR JOINT DISLOCATIONS

The sternoclavicular joint is often unstable following reduction. These injuries require splinting to maintain the normal anatomic relationships and allow ligamentous healing. This is best accomplished with a figure-of-eight splint (Figure 75-3*C*). Unfortunately, patients do not often tolerate this splint. Alternatives include a sling, sling and swath, or a sling and Velpeau dressing (Figures 75-3*A* and *B*). Apply one of the above splints if the medial clavicle will not remain reduced. Orthopedic follow-up should be scheduled within 5 to 7 days of the reduction.

POSTERIOR STERNOCLAVICULAR JOINT DISLOCATIONS

The sternoclavicular joint is usually stable following reduction. The splinting and follow-up are the same as with an anterior sternoclavicular joint dislocation.

COMPLICATIONS

ANTERIOR STERNOCLAVICULAR JOINT DISLOCATIONS

Complications of the reduction are relatively minor. The sternoclavicular joint is usually unstable post-reduction and often dislocates spontaneously. This should be explained to the patient prior to attempted reduction. A "cosmetic bump" can remain if reduction is not maintained. Occasionally, these patients will continue to have persistent pain.[3]

POSTERIOR STERNOCLAVICULAR JOINT DISLOCATIONS

Most complications result from the original injury and are due to compression or injury of neighboring structures. The incidence of associated injuries is reported to be 25 percent.[25] Death secondary to these complications has been reported.[31,40]

Complications of the reduction include pain, incomplete reduction, subclavian vessel injury, and brachial plexus injury. A higher incidence of injury to the subclavian vessels may be seen if a towel clamp is used in the reduction.

SUMMARY

Sternoclavicular joint dislocations are uncommon injuries. They are usually due to high-impact forces from motor vehicle collisions or contact sports. Anterior sternoclavicular joint dislocations are easily reduced but often do not maintain reduction. However, patients tend to do well with persistent dislocations. Posterior sternoclavicular joint dislocations are even less common. The practitioner should be aware of the high incidence of associated injuries. These dislocations tend to be stable after reduction.

REFERENCES

1. Rowe CR: Shoulder girdle injuries, in Cave EF, Burke JF, Boyd RJ (eds): *Trauma Management.* Chicago: Year Book, 1974:399–453.
2. Nettles JL, Linscheid RL: Sternoclavicular dislocations. *J Trauma* 1968; 8(2):158–164.
3. Rockwood CA Jr, Wirth MA: Injuries to the sternoclavicular joint, in Rockwood CA Jr, Green DP, Bucholtz RW, et al (eds): *Rockwood and Green's Fractures in Adults,* 4th ed. Philadelphia: Lippincott-Raven, 1996:1415–1471.
4. Buckerfield CT, Castle ME: Acute retrosternal dislocation of the clavicle. *J Bone Joint Surg* 1984; 66A(3):379–385.
5. Omer GE Jr: Osteotomy of the clavicle in surgical reduction of anterior sternoclavicular dislocation. *J Trauma* 1967; 7(4):584–590.
6. Savastano AA: Traumatic sternoclavicular dislocation. *Int Surg* 1978; 63(1):10–13.
7. Mehta JC, Sachdev A, Collins JJ: Retrosternal dislocation of the clavicle. *Injury* 1973; 5:79–83.
8. Heinig CF: Retrosternal dislocation of the clavicle: early recognition, x-ray diagnosis, and management. *J Bone Joint Surg* 1968; 50A:830.
9. Cope R: Dislocations of the sternoclavicular joint. *Skel Radiol* 1993; 22:233–238.
10. Selesnick FH, Jablon M, Frank C, et al: Retrosternal dislocation of the clavicle. *J Bone Joint Surg* 1984; 66A(2):287–291.
11. Gazak S, Davidson SJ: Posterior sternoclavicular dislocations: two case reports. *J Trauma* 1984; 24(1):80–82.

12. Benson LS, Donaldson JS, Carroll NC: Use of ultrasound in management of posterior sternoclavicular dislocation. *J Ultrasound Med* 1991; 10:115–118.

13. Elting JJ: Retrosternal dislocation of the clavicle. *Arch Surg* 1972; 104:35–37.

14. Rockwood CA Jr, Odor JM: Spontaneous atraumatic anterior subluxation of the sternoclavicular joint. *J Bone Joint Surg* 1989; 71A(9):1280–1288.

15. Gray H: *Anatomy of the Human Body*, 30th ed. Philadelphia: Lea & Febiger, 1985:366–368.

16. Lucas DB: Biomechanics of the shoulder joint. *Arch Surg* 1973; 107:425–432.

17. Owings-Webb PA, Meyers-Suchey J: Epiphyseal union of the anterior iliac crest and medial clavicle in a modern multiracial sample of American males and females. *Am J Phys Anthropol* 1985; 68:457–466.

18. Winter J, Sterner S, Maurer D, et al: Retrosternal epiphyseal disruption of medial clavicle: case and review in children. *J Emerg Med* 1989; 7:9–13.

19. Zaslav KR, Ray S, Neer CS: Conservative management of a displaced medial clavicular physeal injury in an adolescent athlete. *Am J Sports Med* 1989; 17(6):833–836.

20. Leighton D, Oudjhane K, Mohammed HB: The sternoclavicular joint in trauma: retrosternal dislocation versus epiphyseal fracture. *Pediatr Radiol* 1989; 20:126–127.

21. Brooks AL, Henning GD: Injury to the proximal clavicular epiphysis. *J Bone Joint Surg* 1972; 54A: 1347–1348.

22. Lewonowski K, Bassett GS: Complete posterior epiphyseal separation. *Clin Orthop* 1992; 281:84–88.

23. Denham RH Jr, Dingley AF Jr: Epiphyseal separation of the medial end of the clavicle. *J Bone Joint Surg* 1967; 49A(6):1179–1183.

24. Worrell J, Fernandez GN: Retrosternal dislocation of the clavicle: an important injury easily missed. *Arch Emerg Med* 1986; 3:133–135.

25. Worman LW, Leagus C: Intrathoracic injury following retrosternal dislocation of the clavicle. *J Trauma* 1967; 7(3):416–422.

26. Kennedy JC: Retrosternal dislocation of the clavicle. *J Bone Joint Surg* 1949; 31B(1):74–75.

27. Leighton RK, Buhr AJ, Sinclair AM: Posterior sternoclavicular dislocations. *Can J Surg* 1986; 29(2):104–106.

28. Stankler L: Posterior dislocation of the clavicle. *Br J Surg* 1962; 50:164–168.

29. Derkson EJ, Eykelhoff JA, Schenk KE, et al: Retrosternal dislocation of the clavicle. *Acta Orthop Belg* 1992; 58(3):297–300.

30. Jougon JB, Lepront DJ, Dromer CEH: Posterior dislocation of the sternoclavicular joint leading to mediastinal compression. *Ann Thorac Surg* 1996; 61:711–713.

31. Gardner MAH, Bidstrup BP: Intrathoracic great vessel injury resulting from blunt chest trauma associated with posterior dislocation of the sternoclavicular joint. *Aust N Z J Surg* 1983; 53:427–430.

32. Nettles JL, Linscheid RL: Sternoclavicular dislocations (discussion). *J Trauma* 1968; 8(2):158–164.

33. Hobbs DW: Sternoclavicular joint: a new radiographic view. *Radiology* 1968; 90:801.

34. Pollock RC, Bankes MJK, Emery RJH: Diagnosis of retrosternal dislocations of the clavicle with ultrasound. *Injury* 1996; 27(9):670–671.

35. Wirth MA, Rockwood CA Jr: Chronic conditions of the acromioclavicular and sternoclavicular joints, in Chapman MW (ed): *Operative Orthopedics*, 2nd ed. Philadelphia: Lippincott, 1993:1683–1693.

36. Gangahar DM, Flogaites T: Retrosternal dislocation of the clavicle producing thoracic outlet syndrome. *J Trauma* 1978; 18(5):369–372.

37. Rayan GM: Compression brachial plexopathy caused by chronic posterior dislocation of the sternoclavicular joint. *J Okla State Med Assoc* 1994; 87:7–9.

38. Butterworth RD, Kirk AA: Fracture dislocation sternoclavicular joint—case report. *Va Med Monthly* 1952; 79:98–100.

39. Stein AH: Retrosternal dislocation of the clavicle. *J Bone Joint Surg* 1957; 39A(3):656–660.

40. Wasylenko MJ, Busse EF: Posterior dislocation of the clavicle causing fatal tracheoesophageal fistula. *Can J Surg* 1981; 24(6):626–627.

Chapter 67

SHOULDER JOINT DISLOCATION REDUCTION

Sanford Scot Sineff
Eric F. Reichman

INTRODUCTION

The shoulder joint is the most commonly dislocated of all joints.[1-4] Shoulder dislocations were depicted in Egyptian murals as early as 3000 B.C.[1] Despite 5000 years of medical advancements, shoulder dislocations continue to be a major cause of Emergency Department visits. They account for more than 50 percent of all joint complications treated by Emergency Physicians.[2]

The human shoulder is remarkable for its degree of motion. The anatomic features that contribute to this mobility also contribute to its instability.[3] The shallow glenohumeral joint allows the shoulder to be dislocated anteriorly, posteriorly, or inferiorly. The anterior shoulder dislocation is the most common and accounts for 95 percent of all shoulder dislocations.[1-4] The overall incidence of shoulder dislocations is 17 per 100,000. There is a bimodal age distribution.[1,4] It occurs in males from 20 to 30 years of age most commonly related to athletics and trauma. The other large group is women from 60 to 80 years of age, primarily due to falls.

ANATOMY AND PATHOPHYSIOLOGY

The shoulder (glenohumeral) joint is a multiaxial ball-and-socket type of synovial joint that permits a wide range of motion. Unfortunately, the range of motion is at the expense of stability.[5] The shoulder has greater than 180 degrees of motion in both the sagittal and coronal planes as well as 180 degrees of rotary movement.[6] The spheroidal head of the humerus articulates with the shallow glenoid fossa of the scapula. The glenoid fossa accommodates roughly one-third of the humeral head. The bony landmarks surrounding the shoulder joint are the coracoid and acromion processes of the scapula. A loose, thin fibrous capsule encloses the glenohumeral joint. The muscular component of the shoulder is a fu-

sion of four separate muscles (supraspinatus, infraspinatus, teres minor, and subscapularis) that together form the rotator cuff. These muscles have a tendency to be torn and injured in shoulder dislocations, especially posterior and inferior dislocations.[7] The shoulder receives its blood supply from the anterior and posterior circumflex humeral arteries. These arteries are branches of the axillary artery. Innervation of the shoulder is from branches of the suprascapular, axillary, and lateral pectoral nerves. The axillary nerve lies at the level of the humeral neck. When it is dislocated anteriorly, the humeral head is displaced into the quadrangular space where it may compress and damage the axillary nerve. This can result in neuropraxia or paralysis of the deltoid muscle and sensory loss to the skin over the shoulder.

Shoulder dislocations can occur anteriorly, posteriorly, or inferiorly depending on the mechanism of injury. Anterior shoulder dislocations are by far the most common and account for 95 percent of all dislocations. An anterior dislocation usually results from direct or indirect forces causing abduction, extension, and external rotation of the limb. Anterior dislocations are classified based on the location of the humeral head into subcoracoid, subglenoid, subclavicular, and intrathoracic. Subcoracoid dislocations account for 75 percent of all anterior shoulder dislocations. The dislocated humeral head can shift between the first three positions but generally remains in one anatomic location.[2] In younger patients, the injury is usually linked to athletics, such as spiking a volleyball or blocking a basketball shot. Older patients may sustain anterior shoulder dislocations from falling on an outstretched arm or from a direct blow on the posterior shoulder.[4] The patient will present in obvious distress, holding the affected arm in slight abduction and internal rotation. Typically, the elbow is flexed and supported by the unaffected arm. The shoulder will have the typical "squared off" appearance, with loss of the normal deltoid contour. The humeral head may be palpable anteriorly.[1]

Posterior shoulder dislocations account for 4 percent of all shoulder dislocations.[1-4] They have a tendency to be missed, even by experienced physicians. Delayed diagnoses have been made up to a year after the initial injury.[8] The mechanism of injury is usually indirect, with a combination of internal rotation, adduction, and flexion. The most common precipitating mechanism is a seizure. Other etiologies include electrocution, direct trauma, and falls.[3] Direct trauma, such as a head-on motor vehicle collision in which the patient braces their hands against the dashboard, can result in bilateral posterior shoulder dislocations in rare instances. Posterior shoulder dislocations are classified based on the location of the humeral head into subacromial, subglenoid, or subspinous. Subacromial dislocations account for 98 percent of posterior shoulder dislocations.[2,8] The patient usually presents with the arm held in adduction and internal rotation.[9] The shoulder will appear flat anteriorly. The coracoid process of the scapula will be visually prominent and palpable.[1]

Inferior shoulder dislocations are the least common type.[1-4] They represent less than 0.5 percent of all shoulder dislocations. The inferior shoulder dislocation is also known as luxatio erecta, because the dislocated extremity is extended upward. Inferior shoulder dislocations are usually sustained from indirect forces with the arm hyperabducted, causing the rotator cuff to tear and the arm to rotate 180 degrees externally.[7] Alternatively, a direct axial force applied to the arm above the head, as in a fall or Olympic-style weight lifting, will drive the humeral head inferiorly.[10] The patient will present with the affected arm shortened and fixed above his or her head, with the hand rotated as if asking a question.[7] The humeral head may be palpable along the lateral chest wall. Inferior shoulder dislocations are often associated with fractures.[1] The fractures can involve the acromion process, coracoid process, clavicle, greater tuberosity, humeral head, and/or glenoid rim.[1,2,6,11] Complete disruption of the rotator cuff often occurs with inferior shoulder dislocations.[1,2,6,11] Dislocations can cause capsular and rotator cuff tears, compression or tears of the axillary artery and its branches, and injury to the subclavian vein. Because of their anatomic proximity, damage to the brachial plexus, suprascapular nerve, and the axillary nerve occur at a rate of 21 to 36 percent due to traction and compression of these nerves.[8] Prompt reduction of the dislocation may alleviate compression injuries and enable a more thorough examination and evaluation of all components of the shoulder.

Radiographs are required to classify the type of dislocation and diagnose fractures. Associated fractures are detected in up to 24 percent of anterior shoulder dislocations.[3] They include fractures of the greater tuberosity, humeral head, coracoid process, acromion process, clavicle, and glenoid. Anecdotal evidence suggests that clinically obvious dislocations without a high-energy mechanism can be reduced without prior radiographs. The current literature recommends that all patients have at least two-view pre-reduction plain radiographs of the affected joint.[12] Post-reduction films should be obtained both to document the reduction of the joint and any injury induced by the reduction technique as well as to document bony abnormalities (Hill-Sachs lesions, Bankart lesion) or previously hidden fractures that were not visible on the initial radiographs. There is some evidence that post-reduction radiographs may be unnecessary, but further study is required before this can be made the standard of care.[13,14]

The anteroposterior (AP) view will clearly demonstrate anterior dislocations, inferior dislocations, and humeral fractures. In evaluating radiographs of anterior shoulder dislocations, look for an impaction fracture defect in the posterolateral portion of the humeral head, called a Hill-Sachs deformity. These are found in up to 50 percent of all anterior shoulder dislocations.[2] A Bankart lesion is an avulsed fragment of the glenoid labrum with contiguous bone.[6] Both lesions tend to get worse the longer the humeral head remains dislocated.

In patients with posterior shoulder dislocations, however, the AP view often shows a "normal" picture, which accounts for the high incidence of missed dislocations. There are three features that suggest a posterior dislocation on AP films. First is the loss of the normal elliptical pattern produced by overlap of the humeral head and the posterior glenoid rim. Second, the distance between the anterior glenoid rim and the articular surface of the humeral head will be increased. This is also known as the "rim sign." Finally, internal rotation of the greater tuberosity makes the humerus take on a "lightbulb" or "ice cream cone" appearance.[2,4] If there is any question, a lateral view (either the Y view or an axillary view) will help delineate the posterior position of the humeral head behind the glenoid fossa.[1] One study showed that up to 50 percent of posterior shoulder dislocations were missed using only the AP view, whereas lateral views increased the diagnostic accuracy to 100 percent.[15] An isolated fracture of the lesser tuberosity on the AP view is suggestive of a posterior shoulder dislocation until proven otherwise.[2]

INDICATIONS

Shoulder dislocations, whether first-time or recurrent, are typically very painful and distressing for the patient. **All attempts should be made to reduce the joint as quickly as possible once the diagnosis is made.** In general, uncomplicated joint dislocations should be reduced within 20 to 30 minutes to alleviate further injury to surrounding neurologic and vascular structures. **A patient with a neurologic deficit or a compromised distal** pulse in the setting of a shoulder dislocation should undergo immediate reduction.

CONTRAINDICATIONS

There are no absolute contraindications to reducing a dislocated shoulder. The patient's airway, breathing, and circulation should be assessed and managed prior to reducing the dislocated shoulder. Any life- or limb-threatening injuries should be managed before the shoulder reduction is attempted.

An Orthopedic Surgeon should be consulted prior to the reduction of a shoulder dislocation in patients with posterior and inferior dislocations. They are relatively rare, there is a high incidence of complications requiring operative management, dislocations associated with fractures may make the reduction difficult, and other indications for surgical management may exist. The indications for surgical intervention in anterior shoulder dislocations include complete rotator cuff tears, fracture of the greater tuberosity with displacement of more than 1 cm, or fractures of the glenoid rim that are displaced more than 5 millimeters.[2] Posterior shoulder dislocations with major displacement of a fractured lesser tuberosity or an impression defect greater than 20 percent of the articular surface necessitate surgical intervention or open reduction.[2,3] Open dislocations require operative management but may be reduced in the Emergency Department if there is a delay in getting the patient to the Operating Room. Surgical reduction is indicated in patients with evidence of hemorrhagic shock from a suspected axillary artery injury sustained during a shoulder dislocation.

An Orthopedic Surgeon should be consulted before reducing a dislocated shoulder that presents greater than 7 to 10 days after the acute injury. There is a higher risk of vascular injury when an "old" dislocation is mistaken for an acute injury and subsequently reduced. The axillary artery, which is bound down by the pectoralis major muscle and anterior pericapsular scarring, becomes brittle and may not withstand the traction required to reduce an "old" dislocation. This is especially true in the elderly. A 1941 study reported a 50 percent hemorrhage-related mortality in patients who had shoulder reductions performed several weeks after initial injury.[11]

Shoulder dislocations in children present unique problems. Pediatric patients whose ossification centers have not yet fused tend to have Salter-Harris type fractures of the epiphyseal plate. **An Orthopedic Surgeon should be consulted prior to reduction of a pediatric shoulder dislocation unless neurologic or vascular compromise is present in the affected extremity.** Otherwise, the same techniques for reduction can be applied to both adult and pediatric patients.

EQUIPMENT

General Supplies

Equipment and supplies for procedural sedation
   (Chapter 109)
Assistants
Sheets
10 to 15 pounds of weights
Sling and swath or shoulder immobilizer
Splinting material (plaster, fiberglass, prepackaged
   casting material)

Intraarticular Analgesia

Povidone iodine solution
20 mL syringe
25 gauge, 2.5 inch needle
Local anesthetic solution (carbocaine, lidocaine,
   bupivacaine)

PATIENT PREPARATION

The risks, benefits, potential complications, and aftercare of the procedure should be explained to the patient and/or their representative. Obtain an informed consent for the reduction procedure. An informed consent should be obtained for procedural sedation and/or an intraarticular injection if they are performed in addition to the reduction procedure.

Place the patient in a position of maximal comfort with the affected extremity supported and its motion limited. Placing the patient supine or prone is difficult, painful, and often requires analgesia before being attempted. The patient presenting in spinal immobilization should remain supine. If the spine cannot be cleared, shoulder reduction can be performed without changing the patient's position. Intravenous access should be obtained if indicated. Pain should be addressed quickly and aggressively.

ANALGESIA

There are several methods to control pain for patient comfort before and during the joint reduction procedure. Intravenous or intramuscular narcotics should not be withheld pending prolonged radiographic studies. Commonly administered medications include morphine, meperidine, hydromorphone, and fentanyl.

An alternative to intramuscular or intravenous narcotics is the intraarticular instillation of local anesthetic solution.[16] This was formally introduced in 1991 as an effective method of analgesia for anterior shoulder dislocations. It is often used in addition to procedural sedation. It can also be used as the only method of analgesia when procedural sedation is contraindicated. Clean the anterolateral shoulder of any dirt and debris. Apply povidone iodine solution to the shoulder area and allow it to dry. Identify the hollow 2 cm inferior to the lateral border of the acromion process (Figure 67-1). Using sterile technique, insert a 25 gauge needle perpendicular to the skin and into the hollow to a depth of 2 cm (Figure 67-1). Inject 10 to 20 mL of a 50:50 mixture of sterile saline and local anesthetic solution. This technique is effective in controlling muscle spasm and pain. The editor and one of the authors (EFR) believe this should be performed on every dislocated shoulder before attempts at reduction.

Several sources suggest that patients with an anterior shoulder dislocation without a significant trauma history may actually accept some degree of discomfort as a trade-off for the prompt resolution of pain by reduction without anesthesia.[17–19] Patient comfort should not be sacrificed for expediency. Anterior shoulder dislocations may require procedural sedation prior to reduction, depending on the patient's level of discomfort and the reduction method chosen. Posterior and inferior shoulder dislocations require procedural sedation prior to reduction.

ANTERIOR SHOULDER DISLOCATION REDUCTION TECHNIQUES

The methods for treating a closed shoulder dislocation depend on overcoming muscular spasm to relocate the humeral head into the glenoid fossa. Reduction techniques are classified into traction techniques, leverage techniques, scapular manipulation, and combinations of the three previous techniques. A study evaluating the various reduction techniques found similar success rates of 70 to 90 percent regardless of the technique.[20] However, postreduction complications rates are variable.[20] The major considerations in deciding which technique to use are physician experience, familiarity with the technique, availability of time, and the presence or absence of an assistant.[20]

HENNIPEN TECHNIQUE

The Hennipen technique, popularized at Hennipen County Medical Center, is often the preferred method to reduce anterior shoulder dislocations (Figure 67-2). This technique can be accomplished with no anesthesia or with the intraarticular instillation of local anesthetic so-

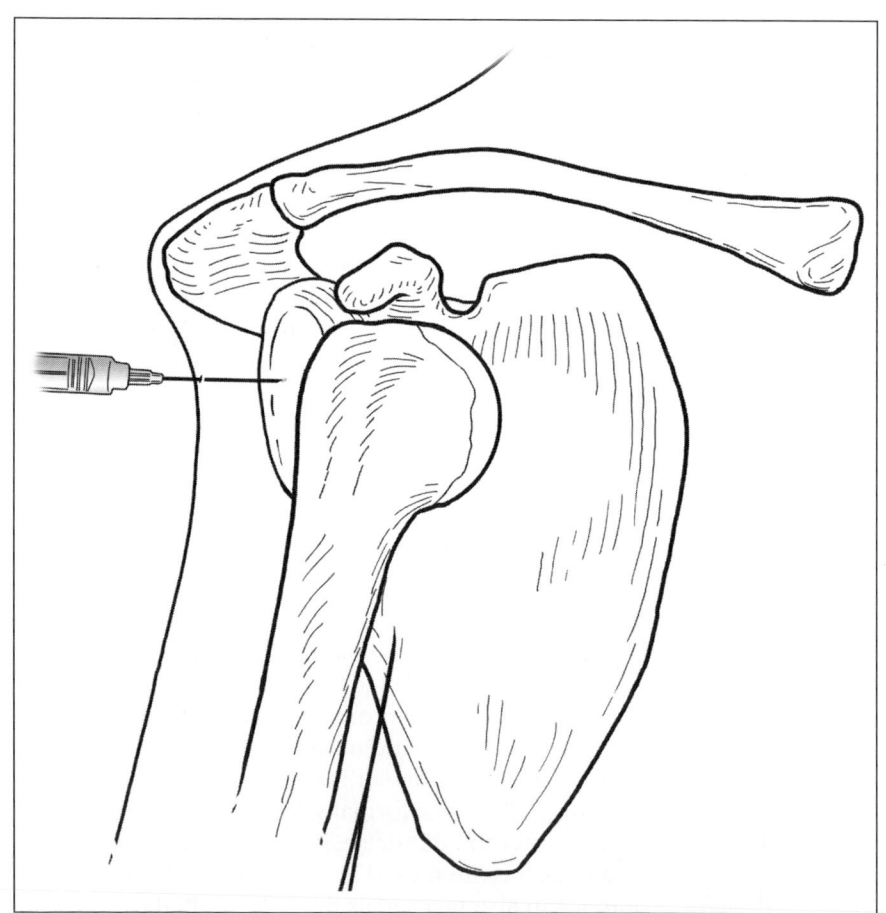

FIGURE 67-1 Local anesthesia for a shoulder dislocation. The needle is introduced in the hollow under the lateral surface of the acromion process.

lution. Procedural sedation is not required but may be used if the patient has severe pain and muscle spasms.

Place the patient seated, supine, or reclined 45 degrees on a gurney (Figure 67-2A). Place the affected arm in adduction. Flex the elbow 90 degrees. Support the patient's flexed elbow against their torso with the nondominant hand. Grasp the patient's forearm with the dominant hand. Slowly rotate the arm externally. **If pain becomes severe, typically as a result of rotator cuff spasm, stop the motion and wait until the spasm subsides. Do not release the arm or return it to its original position.** Continue to rotate the arm externally until the humeral head reduces or the arm reaches the coronal plane (90 degrees of external rotation). This can take up to 10 minutes to accomplish. If the humeral head is still dislocated, slowly abduct the arm until the humeral head reduces or full abduction is obtained[2] (Figure 67-2B). Full abduction occurs when the patient's hand crosses over their head and is able to touch the contralateral ear. Adduct the arm until it is against the patient's torso. Another technique should be attempted if the humeral head is still dislocated.

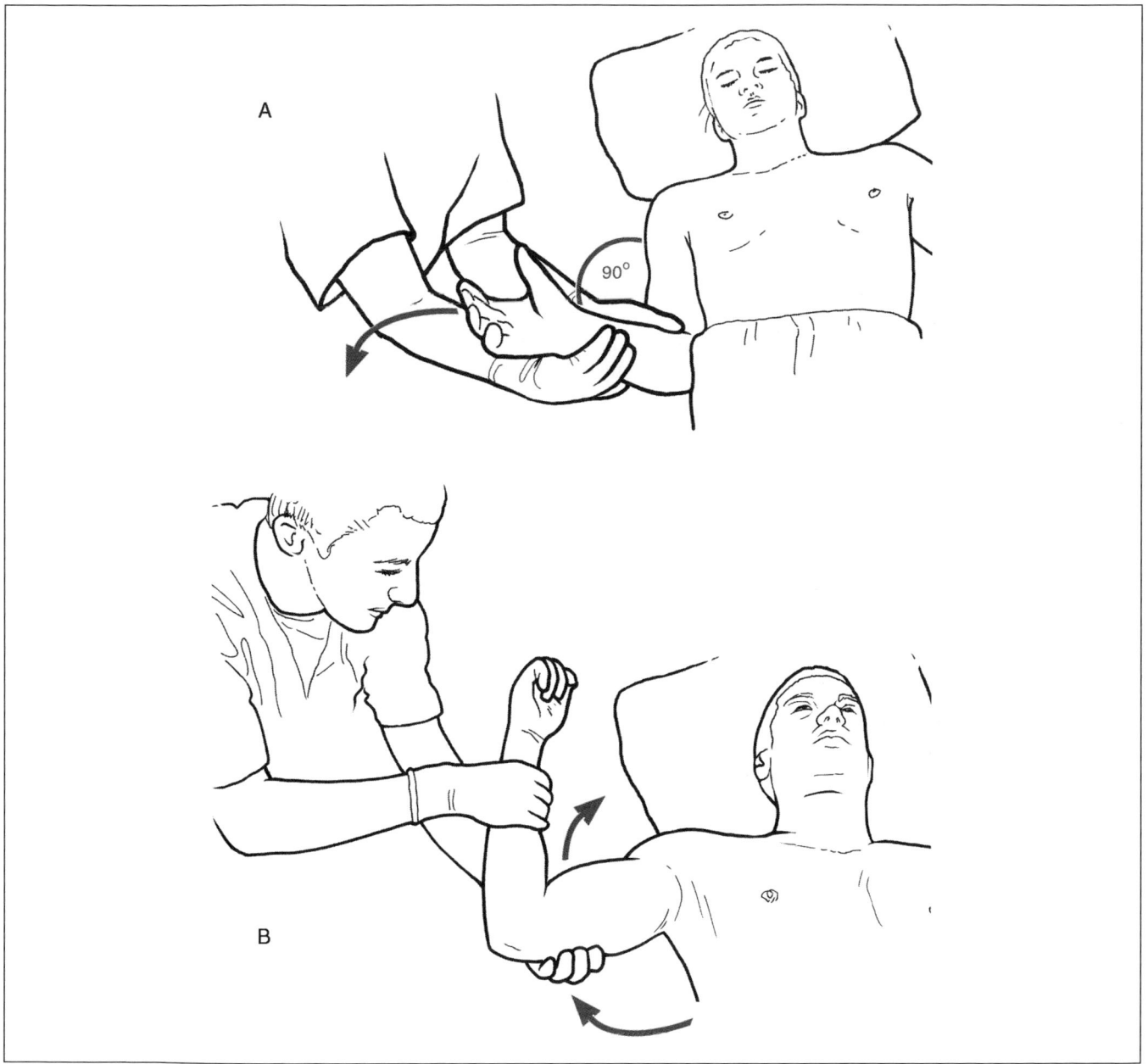

FIGURE 67-2 The Hennepin technique to reduce an anterior shoulder dislocation. *A.* Patient positioning and external rotation of the humerus. *B.* Abduction of the arm with the elbow flexed 90 degrees.

The advantages of this technique include little to no patient manipulation or positioning, the relative ease of reduction, minimal equipment, the requirement of only a single operator, and the ability to perform the reduction without analgesia. The success rate when performed by Emergency Physicians is approximately 80 percent, with 36 percent of patients not requiring analgesia.[3] The major disadvantage is that patients are often too apprehensive and experiencing too much discomfort to relax their arms sufficiently to allow for reduction to occur. This problem can be eliminated by the intraarticular instillation of local anesthetic solution. Occasionally, patients will require procedural sedation.

EXTERNAL ROTATION TECHNIQUE

This is a modified version of the Hennipen technique.[21–24] The technique is identical to the Hennipen technique except that the procedure is terminated when the arm reaches 90 degrees of external rotation. The step of abduction is not performed. The advantages and disadvantages are as listed for the Hennipen technique.

STIMSON TECHNIQUE

The Stimson technique is a safe first-line technique that uses gravity and weights to overcome muscle spasm and reduce the dislocated shoulder[25–28] (Figure 67-3). Instill intraarticular local anesthetic solution into the shoulder joint prior to attempting the reduction. Procedural sedation is usually not necessary. The patient must be under constant observation to monitor pulse oximetry and respiratory status if procedural sedation is used because of the patient's prone positioning.

Place the patient prone with the dislocated arm hanging over the side of the gurney (Figure 67-3). Flex the shoulder 90 degees. A pillow or folded sheets may be placed beneath the affected shoulder for patient comfort. Tie a sheet around the patient's hips and the gurney to prevent them from falling off the bed (Figure 67-3). Apply 10 to 15 pounds of weight to the wrist or forearm. The weights can be attached by a commercially available device, hung off a padded wrist restraint, or hung off gauze wrapped circumferentially around the wrist. Raise the gurney so that the weights are suspended off the ground (Figure 67-3). The weights will provide traction in a position of forward flexion and are usually sufficient for reduction to take place within 15 to 30 minutes.[4] If the reduction is unsuccessful after 30 minutes, grasp the patient's forearm and twist it to gently rotate the humerus externally and then internally while the patient is prone and the arm is maintained under traction. This maneuver will often reduce the dislocation if the weights alone are unsuccessful.

An alternative method is to have the patient grip a bucket approximately half full of water. This will provide the necessary traction weight to reduce the joint. The disadvantage of the bucket technique is that the patient will have to grip the bucket for a considerable length of time without releasing it.

The advantage of the Stimson technique is that it is safe and does not require the presence of an assistant. A 96 percent success rate has been reported with this technique.[3] The disadvantage of the procedure is that the patient must be placed in a prone position that may be painful, uncomfortable, or impossible because of other injuries. There is a small risk of the patient slipping off the elevated gurney. A strap or sheet tied around the patient and the gurney is recommended in order to prevent this. Procedural sedation is not recommended due to the prolonged prone positioning required, which may interfere with the patient's respiration. Additionally, procedural sedation for 15 to 30 minutes is relatively contraindicated and difficult to maintain without potential complications.

SCAPULAR MANIPULATION TECHNIQUE

Scapular manipulation accomplishes reduction by repositioning the glenoid fossa rather than manipulating the humeral head[4,29–33] (Figure 67-4). This is a popular technique due to its low complication rate and high patient satisfaction. This technique can be accomplished with no anesthesia or with the intraarticular instillation of local anesthetic solution. Procedural sedation is not required.

Place the patient prone with the dislocated extremity hanging over the side of the gurney (Figures 67-4A and B). Flex the shoulder 90 degrees. A pillow or folded sheets may be placed below the affected shoulder for patient comfort. Place 5 to 15 pounds of weights suspended from the patient's wrist or in their hand. If weights are not available, an assistant may apply downward traction on the extremity (Figure 67-4B). The weights or the assistant will provide in-line traction to the arm.

Identify the scapula and its borders. The scapular tip will "wing" laterally. Stabilize the superior portion of the scapula with one hand (Figure 67-4A). Place the thumb of the stabilization hand along the superolateral border of the scapula. Apply constant and firm medial and upward pressure to the inferior tip of the scapula using the other hand or thumb. The thumb of the stabilizing hand can also be used to apply medially directed pressure to the tip of the scapula. Push the tip of the scapula as far medially as possible. The shoulder should reduce within 1 to 3 minutes. A small degree of dorsal displacement of the scapular tip has also been recommended.[3,33] If the reduction is unsuccessful, slight external rotation of the humerus (by an assistant) while the scapula is being manipulated and the arm is under traction may facilitate reduction (Figure 67-4B). This maneuver releases

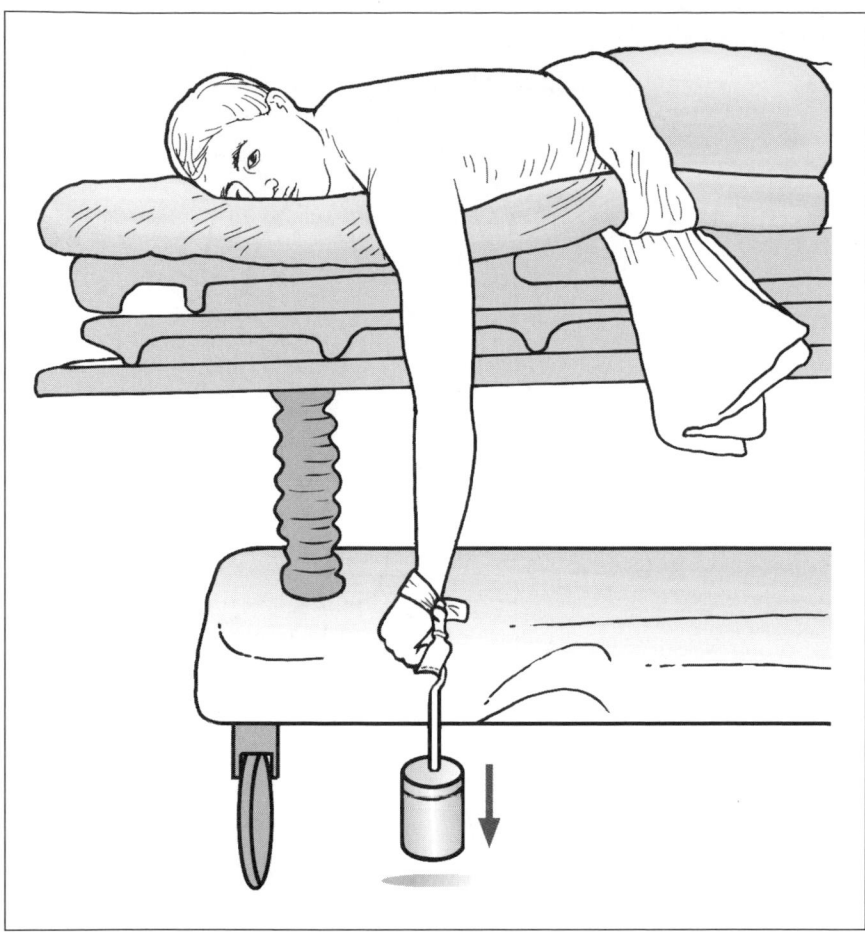

FIGURE 67-3 The Stimson technique to reduce an anterior shoulder dislocation.

the superior glenohumeral ligament and presents a favorable profile of the humeral head to the glenoid fossa.[31,33]

The scapular manipulation technique may be performed with the patient supine (Figure 67-4C). This is particularly helpful when other injuries or conditions preclude using the prone position. Flex the affected shoulder 90 degrees. Instruct an assistant to grasp the forearm and apply upward traction to elevate the shoulder off the bed. Apply your hands to stabilize and manipulate the scapula as described in the previous paragraph.

This technique may also be performed with the patient sitting (Figure 67-4D). This is particularly helpful when other injuries or conditions preclude using the prone or the supine position. Flex the affected shoulder 90 degrees. Instruct an assistant to grasp the forearm and apply horizontal traction. Apply your hands to stabilize and manipulate the scapula as described in the previous paragraphs. This method is technically a more difficult version of the scapular manipulation technique because the patient's torso is not stabilized and moves during the traction and scapular manipulation.[3,31,33]

The reduction of an anterior shoulder dislocation by the scapular manipulation technique is usually quite subtle and may be missed by both the patient and the physician. In a few rare cases, the act of lying prone will be sufficient to relocate the shoulder. Success rates of over 90 percent have been reported with this technique.[3,30–33] The procedure is well tolerated.[3,29–33] In addition, there is a very low incidence of complications with this procedure and it can be performed without analgesia and monitoring. Disadvantages include the prone position and the need for an assistant to apply traction on the arm.

TRACTION-COUNTERTRACTION TECHNIQUE

The traction-countertraction technique is commonly performed in the Emergency Department, mostly out of tradition (Figure 67-5). It may be used as a first-line technique or a backup for patients who have failed the Stimson technique.[2] This technique requires anesthesia and analgesia. Instill local anesthetic solution intraarticularly. This may be sufficient, but most patients will require procedural sedation. This technique can cause significant patient discomfort.

Place the patient supine. Pass a sheet around the chest and axilla of the affected arm (Figure 67-5A). Abduct the affected arm 45 degrees. Instruct an assistant to grasp the loose ends of the sheet firmly. Grasp the patient's wrist

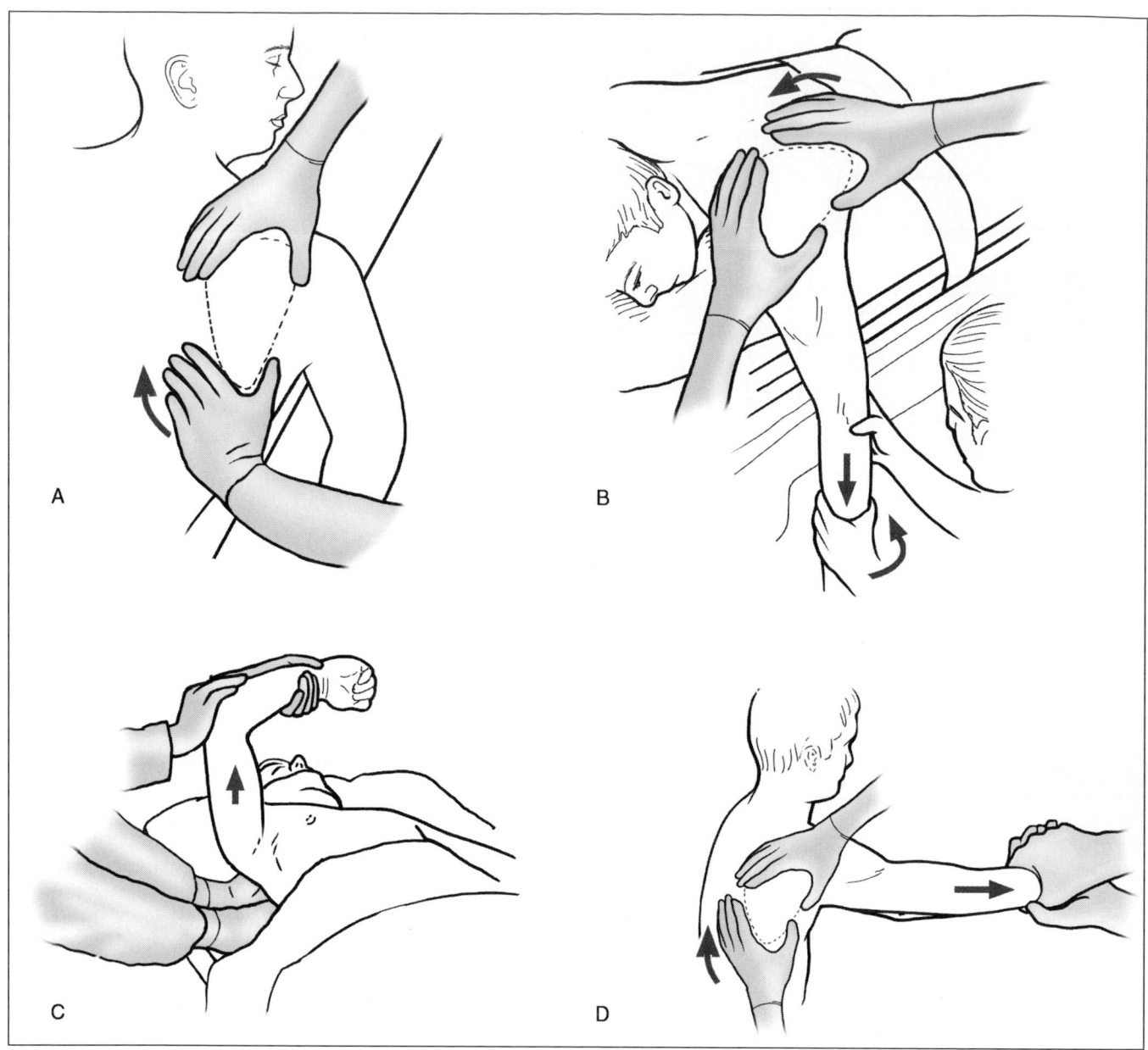

FIGURE 67-4 The scapular manipulation technique to reduce an anterior shoulder dislocation. *A.* Proper hand positioning. The upper hand stabilizes the base of the scapula while the lower hand applies medial and upward pressure on the tip of the scapula (*curved arrow*). *B.* Reduction with the patient prone. Traction is applied by an assistant (*straight arrow*). Occasionally, external rotation is also required (*curved arrow*). *C.* Reduction with the patient supine. Traction is applied on the humerus to elevate the shoulder off the bed (*arrow*). *D.* Reduction with the patient sitting. Traction is applied on the humerus (*arrow*).

and apply slow and steady traction. Instruct the assistant to apply countertraction. The assistant and physician should be exerting equal and opposite forces. **If pain becomes severe, typically as a result of rotator cuff spasm, stop the motion and wait until the spasm subsides. Do not release the arm or return it to its original position.** After the spasm subsides, continue applying traction and countertraction until the shoulder reduces.

Direct traction on the extended arm may result in rapid operator fatigue. This is especially true if the physi-

cian is creating most of the force of traction through contraction of their biceps (Figure 67-5*A*). A less strenuous alternative is available and preferred (Figure 67-5*B*). Position the patient as above. Flex the elbow of the affected arm 90 degrees. Place a looped sheet over the proximal forearm and the physician's hips. Do not loop the sheet around the physician's back, as this can cause low back strain. This method allows the physician to lean back slowly and use their body weight to supply the traction force. The physician's arms should be extended

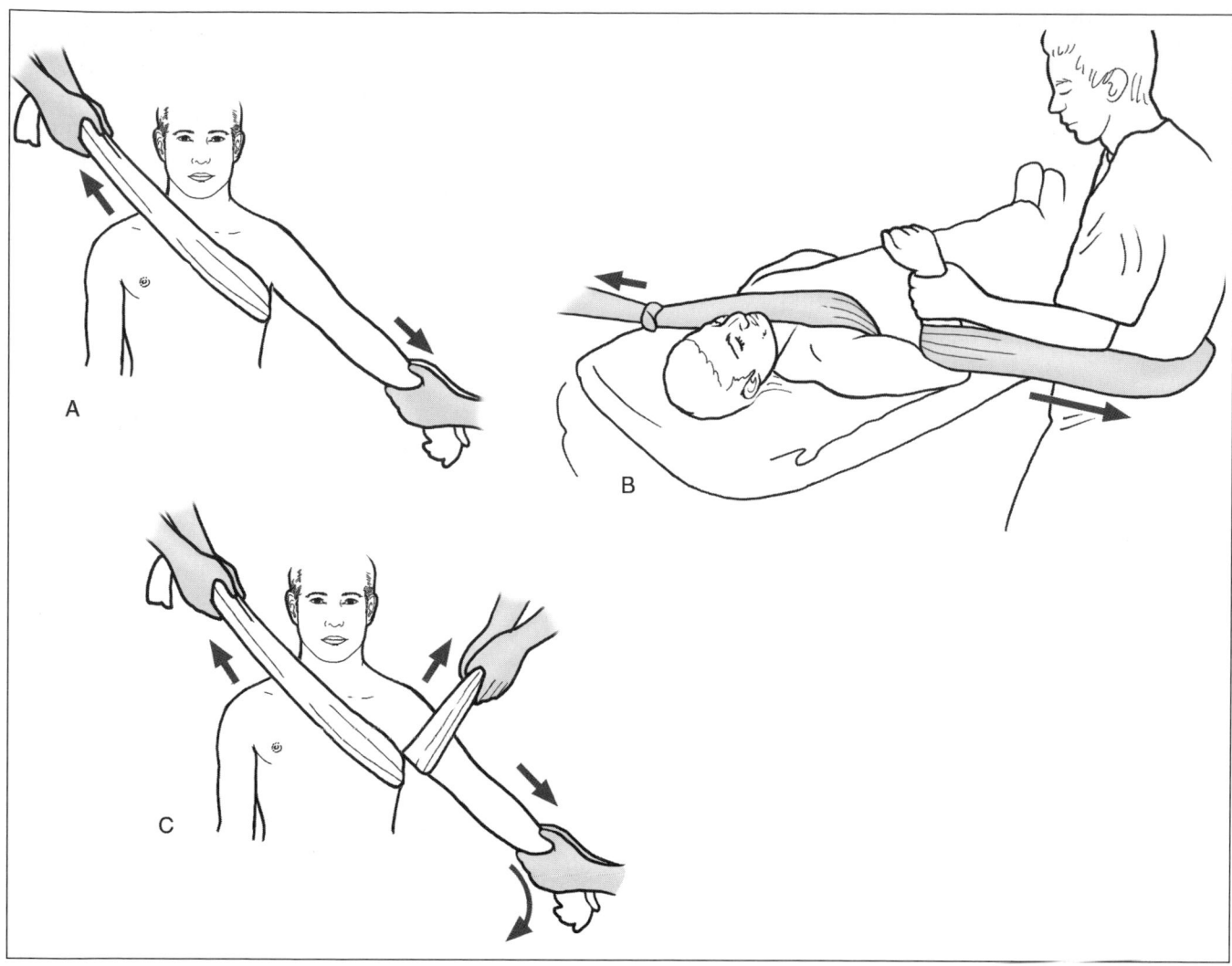

FIGURE 67-5 The traction-countertraction technique to reduce an anterior or posterior shoulder dislocation. *A.* In-line traction is applied to the affected extremity after it is abducted 45 degrees. An assistant provides equal and opposite countertraction with a sheet. *B.* An alternative method. A sheet is looped around the flexed forearm and the physician's hips. The physician leans back (*arrow*) to allow their body to do the work of reduction. *C.* An additional assistant is applying traction 90 degrees to the traction-countertraction axis with a sheet in the axilla. Simultaneous adduction (*curved arrow*) and in-line traction by the physician may aid in the reduction.

with the hands grasping the patient's distal forearm. When leaning back to apply traction, the hands should maintain the patient's forearm upright with the elbow flexed 90 degrees.

Traction may have to be applied for several minutes. The application of gentle and limited external rotation to the affected arm while under traction may speed up the reduction. Alternatively, a second assistant can apply lateral pressure (lateral traction) on the humeral head with their hands. A variation of this technique involves a second assistant with a looped sheet placed high in the patient's axilla and around the assistant's hips (Figure 67-5*C*). This second assistant is used to create lateral traction at the proximal humerus that is perpendicular (90 degrees) to the traction-countertraction

axis.[2] As lateral traction is applied, the physician continues in-line traction and can simultaneously adduct the patient's arm to maneuver the humeral head back into position (Figure 67-5*C*). The second assistant may also be used with the technique demonstrated in Figures 67-5*A* or *B*.

Successful reduction is noted by a lengthening of the arm, a noticeable "clunk," and/or a brief fasciculation of the deltoid muscle. Disadvantages of the traction-countertraction technique include the need for more than one operator, the significant degree of force required, the prolonged time and endurance required of the operator, and the need for procedural sedation. **This technique should not be used to reduce shoulder dislocations associated with significant fractures. The force**

required for this technique can displace fracture fragments, necessitating an open reduction or operative management of the displaced fragments.

SNOWBIRD TECHNIQUE

The Snowbird technique was named after a ski area in Utah where this technique originated.[34] It was developed in order to reduce the large number of ski-related glenohumeral dislocations quickly while also conserving time and resources. This is an effective alternative reduction technique as compared with the more traditional methods. While this technique can be accomplished with no anesthesia, the intraarticular instillation of local anesthetic solution is highly recommended. Procedural sedation is not required for this reduction technique.

Place the patient in a sitting position on a chair with a back (Figure 67-6). Completely adduct the affected arm. Flex the elbow to greater than 90 degrees. Support the affected arm with the other arm or a pillow. Make a 3 foot long loop of 4 inch wide cast stockinette. Place the stockinette around the proximal forearm. Instruct the patient to sit as straight as possible. Instruct an assistant to maintain the patient in an upright position by standing adjacent to the unaffected shoulder and clasping their hands around the chest, in the axilla, of the affected shoulder. The physician then places one foot in the stockinette loop and applies firm downward trac-

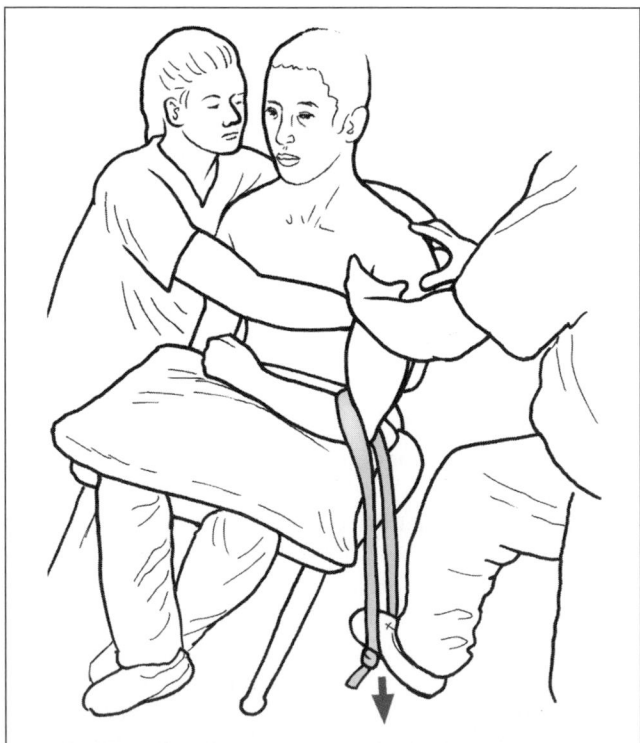

FIGURE 67-6 The Snowbird technique to reduce an anterior shoulder dislocation.

tion with the foot while the patient tries to keep the shoulder relaxed and the affected elbow flexed. Instruct the assistant to provide countertraction to keep the patient from moving. The shoulder may reduce. If not, with continued downward traction on the stockinette, the physician will have both hands free to apply gentle rotation and pressure on the humeral head until the shoulder is reduced.[34]

The Snowbird physicians had a 97 percent success rate and were able to reduce 93 percent of anterior shoulder dislocations without any form of analgesia.[34] The advantages of this technique include the relative ease of setup, the rapid nature of the technique, limited use of analgesia, and limited patient positioning. Potential disadvantages include the use of an assistant and the fact that this technique was used and developed on a limited patient population (young, healthy skiers).

MILCH TECHNIQUE

Milch, in describing this technique, wrote that a fully abducted arm is in a natural and neutral position in which there is little tension on the muscles of the shoulder girdle.[35–37] Accordingly, the technique that Milch developed relies on gentle manipulation through abduction, external rotation, and traction on the arm.[19,35–40] The patient's affected arm moves in a gradual arc, assisted by the physician, to reduce the dislocation without extensive or forceful manipulation (Figure 67-7). While this technique can be accomplished with no anesthesia, the intraarticular instillation of local anesthetic solution is highly recommended. Procedural sedation is not required for this reduction technique.

Place the patient supine. Position one hand with the thumb under the dislocated humeral head (Figure 67-7*A*). Slowly abduct the affected arm 180 degrees to an overhead position (Figure 67-7*B*). This can be accomplished by having the patient lift the affected arm. Many patients are unable to do this due to pain, muscle spasm, or apprehension. Gently grip the elbow or wrist and slowly abduct the arm to 180 degrees (Figure 67-7*B*). Once the arm is fully abducted, grasp the patient's distal arm or proximal forearm with one hand. Apply gentle longitudinal traction with slight external rotation to the arm (Figure 67-7*C*). The humeral head may reduce. If not, while maintaining traction with external rotation, apply upward pressure under the humeral head with the other hand to guide it into the glenoid fossa (Figure 67-7*C*).

Successful reduction is attained in 70 to 90 percent of the cases with no requirement for assistance, other equipment, or medications.[19,35–40] Advantages of the Milch technique include its gentleness, high success rate, limited complications, and good patient tolerance. Disadvantages include positioning the arm in full abduction with or without analgesia, as many patients cannot attain the optimal position due to severe pain, muscle spasm, and/or apprehension.

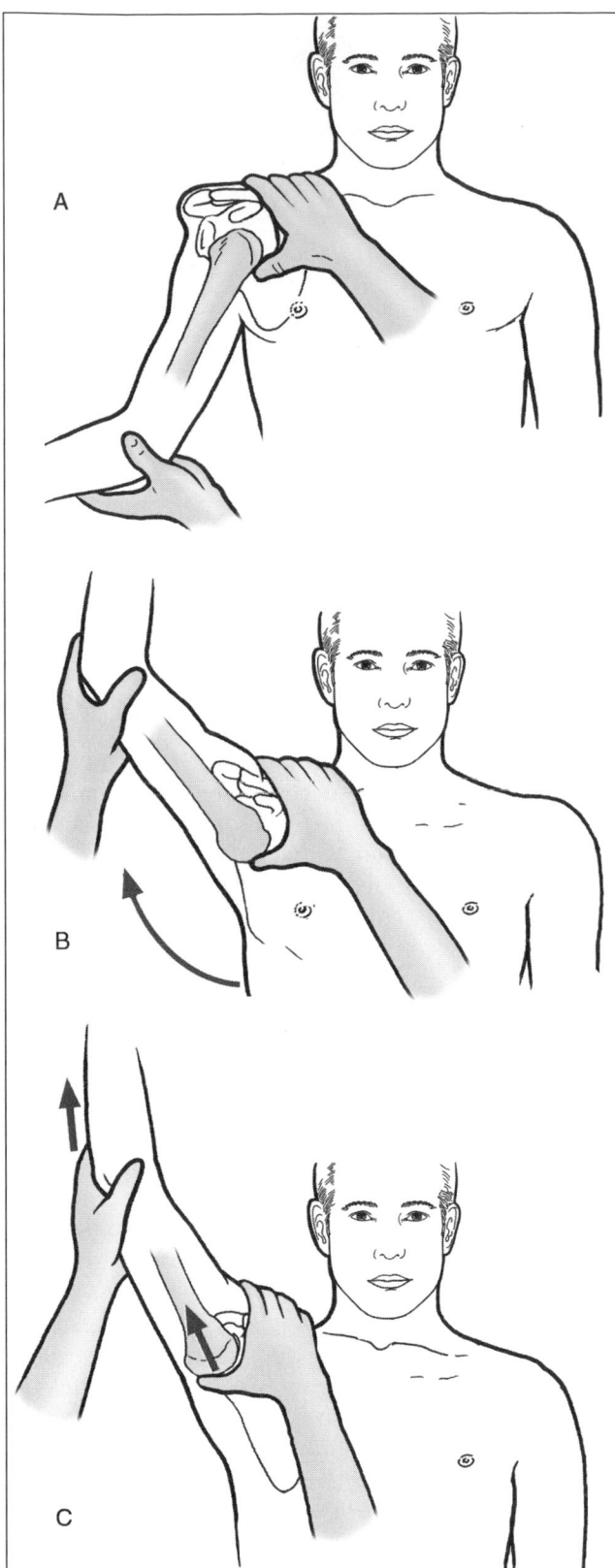

FIGURE 67-7 The Milch technique to reduce an anterior shoulder dislocation. *A.* The distal humerus is grasped with one hand while the thumb of the other hand is placed under the dislocated humeral head. *B.* The arm is abducted to 180 degrees. *C.* In-line traction is applied to the humerus while the thumb pushes the humeral head into the glenoid fossa.

ALTERNATIVE ANTERIOR SHOULDER DISLOCATION REDUCTION TECHNIQUES

Numerous alternative and less commonly used techniques are available to reduce an anterior shoulder dislocation. Some of these are modifications of existing methods. Others are original techniques that had too many associated complications and were modified with time and experience. Some are well known and effective techniques that have been used for many years. **None of these techniques are advocated as first-line treatments for the reduction of shoulder dislocations. Their inclusion here is for the sake of completeness; it does not constitute an endorsement for their use.** Only a select few of these techniques are discussed.

HIPPOCRATIC TECHNIQUE

The Hippocratic technique is the original traction-countertraction technique[41] (Figure 67-8). It is one of the oldest documented techniques to reduce a shoulder dislocation.[2,11, 26,41] This technique has the advantage that it can be performed by a single operator in any setting. It is not recommended due to the great force required to achieve reduction. Common complications of the technique include fractures, brachial plexus injury, vascular injury, and poor patient tolerability.[2,6,11]

The patient is placed supine (Figure 67-8). The wrist of the affected arm is grasped and the arm abducted 20 to 30 degrees. The physician places one foot into the axilla of the affected arm. With a firm grasp of the patient's wrist, the physician applies traction to the arm while the foot in the axilla is extended to provide countertraction.

KOCHER TECHNIQUE

The Kocher technique was first recorded on an Egyptian mural dated 1200 B.C.[42] It is another traditional method that has come into disfavor. This maneuver relies upon leverage and humeral manipulation to reduce the shoulder (Figure 67-9). The humeral head is levered on the anterior glenoid while the humeral shaft is levered against the anterior thoracic wall until reduction is achieved.[11,42,43] A substantial amount of force must be applied while adducting and externally rotating the arm in order to reduce the joint.

The patient is placed sitting at a 45 degree incline or supine. The affected arm is abducted 45 degrees and the elbow flexed 90 degrees (Figure 67-9A). The physician grasps the patient's distal humerus with the dominant hand and the patient's wrist with the nondominant hand (Figure 67-9A). In-line traction is applied to the distal humerus. The arm is then rotated externally to its maximal extent while in-line traction is maintained (Figure 67-9B). The patient's elbow is brought across their chest and to the midline while traction is maintained (Figure 67-9C), with the elbow held tightly against the patient's chest. Finally, the arm is rotated internally until

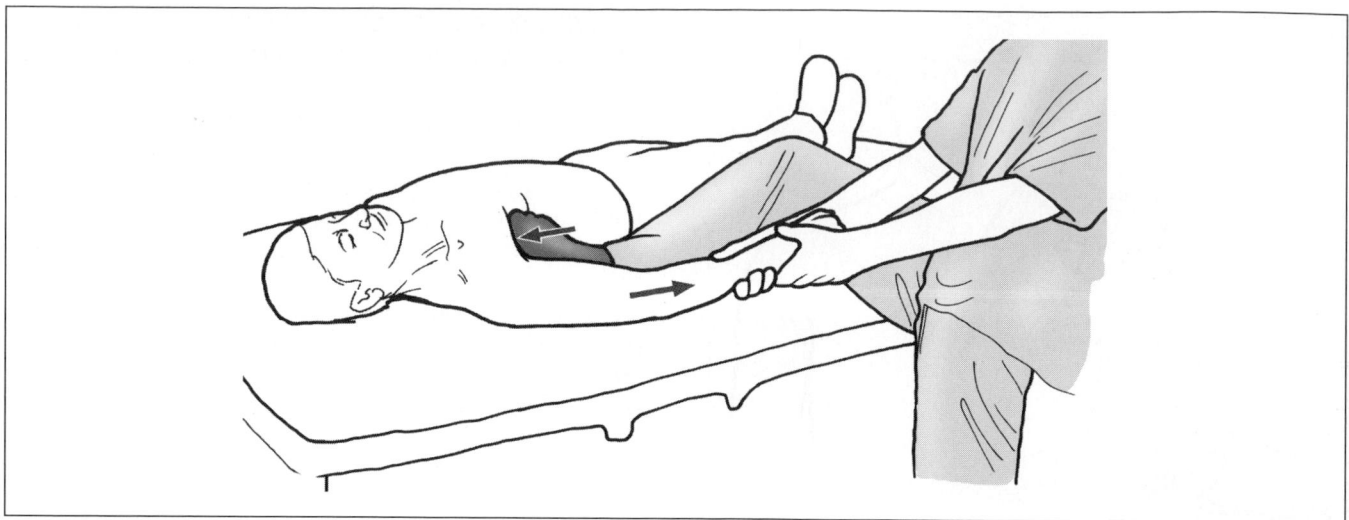

FIGURE 67-8 The Hippocratic technique to reduce an anterior shoulder dislocation.

the patient's hand touches their opposite shoulder (Figure 67-9D).

The main advantage of this method is that it is a single-operator technique that has withstood the test of time. However, studies have shown that the forces generated are sufficient to cause fractures of the humeral neck, spiral humeral fractures, vascular trauma, and brachial plexus injury.[11]

ESKIMO TECHNIQUE

The Eskimo technique uses the patient's body weight and gravity as a traction mechanism to reduce an anterior shoulder dislocation.[44] It can be performed in the field, where access to a health care facility may be limited. Disadvantages of this technique include the strength and stamina required to lift the patient, physician injury due to heavy lifting, poor patient tolerability, and increased stress on the brachial plexus and axillary vessels.

The patient is placed on the floor and lying on the unaffected side (Figure 67-10). The affected arm is placed tightly adducted, with the elbow flexed 45 degrees (Figure 67-10A). The physician grasps the injured arm and slowly lifts the patient 6 to 12 inches off the ground (Figure 67-10A) so that the patient's body weight produces enough traction to reduce the joint. Poulsen initially described this technique and reported a 74 percent success rate.[44] Alternatively, the patient can be positioned on the unaffected side with the affected arm abducted 90 degrees (Figure 67-10B). One or two people can then grasp the patient's wrist and forearm and lift the patient 6 to 12 inches off the ground (Figure 67-10B).

CHAIR TECHNIQUE

The chair technique is a simple method to reduce an anterior shoulder dislocation.[45–47] It is a variation of

the traction-countertraction technique. The patient is placed sitting sideways or backwards in a chair with the affected arm draped over the back rest (Figure 67-11). The physician supinates the patient's wrist and applies downward traction while the patient attempts to stand and provide countertraction (Figure 67-11). This technique has a 72 percent success rate.[3] The advantages include the simplicity of the technique and the fact that analgesia is not required. Unfortunately, a large amount of force is required to reduce the shoulder. These forces can cause injury to the brachial plexus and axillary vessels as the axilla is impinged on the back of the chair.

WRESTLING TECHNIQUE

Zahiri recently described a new technique based on optimal anatomic positioning with limited complications.[48] The patient is placed supine with the elbow of the affected shoulder flexed 120 degrees. With one hand, the physician grasps the dislocated arm just above the humeral condyles and applies distal traction to the arm. The physician grasps the distal forearm overhanded with the opposite hand and moves the hand from the condyles through the acute angle of the arm, grasping the wrist of the hand holding the forearm. The wrestling hold is now established (Figure 67-12). With the hold in place, the patient's forearm will be used as a fulcrum. The patient's shoulder is abducted 45 degrees while constant traction is maintained. The arm is then rotated externally in a slow, smooth motion. While maintaining traction and external rotation, the physician brings the patient's arm over the chest wall and rotates it internally.[1] The shoulder should then reduce.

This technique has the advantages of requiring no equipment, no analgesia, and no assistants. It may be used in the field where a health care facility is not read-

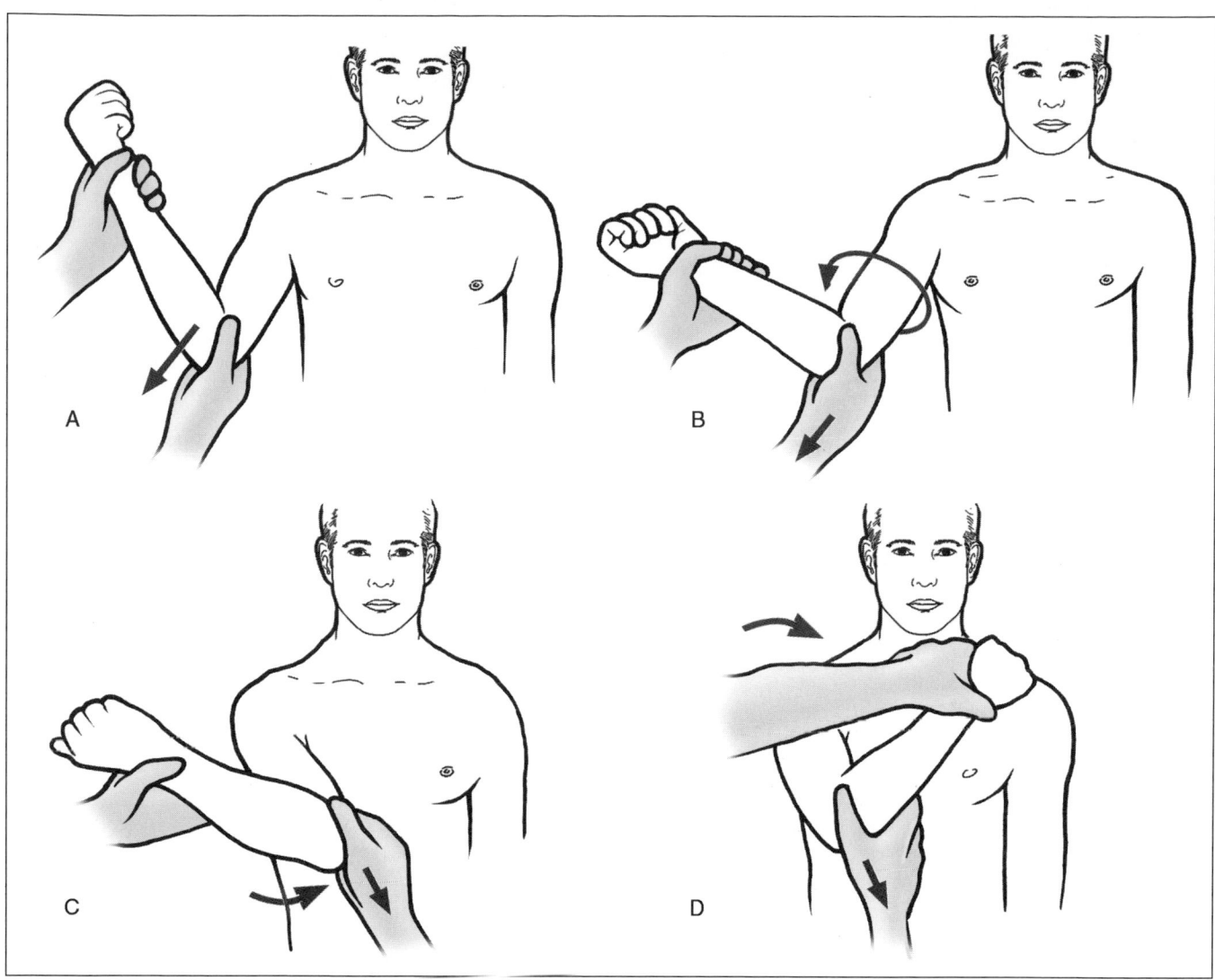

FIGURE 67-9 The Kocher technique to reduce an anterior shoulder dislocation. *A.* The arm is abducted 45 degrees with the elbow flexed 90 degrees. In-line traction is applied to the humerus (*arrow*). *B.* The arm is rotated externally (*curved arrow*) while traction is maintained (*straight arrow*). *C.* The elbow is brought across the chest to the midline while the arm is still rotated externally and traction on the arm is maintained (*straight arrow*). *D.* The arm is rotated internally until the patient's hand touches their opposite shoulder.

ily available. The main disadvantage is the amount of force applied to the shoulder and surrounding structures. The twisting of the forearm as a lever can displace fracture fragments or cause fractures. This technique also requires the physician to have a significant amount of upper body strength and arms long enough to accomplish the wrestling hold, especially if the patient has large arms. The series of movements is difficult to accomplish while always maintaining distal traction.

PNEUMATIC STRETCHER TECHNIQUE

This technique was developed to reduce a shoulder dislocation when assistants were not available or if the physician did not have the physical strength required to

use other techniques.[49] It is a modification of the traction-countertraction technique. **This technique should never be used to reduce a shoulder dislocation.** It will cause stretching and possible rupture of the brachial plexus, ligaments of the shoulder region, muscles and tendons crossing the shoulder, nerves of the upper extremity, vascular structures of the upper extremity, and injury to other joints. Tremendous forces are applied to the extremity with this technique.

The patient is placed prone, with the affected arm hanging off the gurney (Figure 67-13). A sheet is wrapped around the patient's waist and hips and the gurney to hold the patient in position. The ends of the sheet are tied into a knot or held by an assistant. The patient's wrist is wrapped with gauze and then tied to the base or

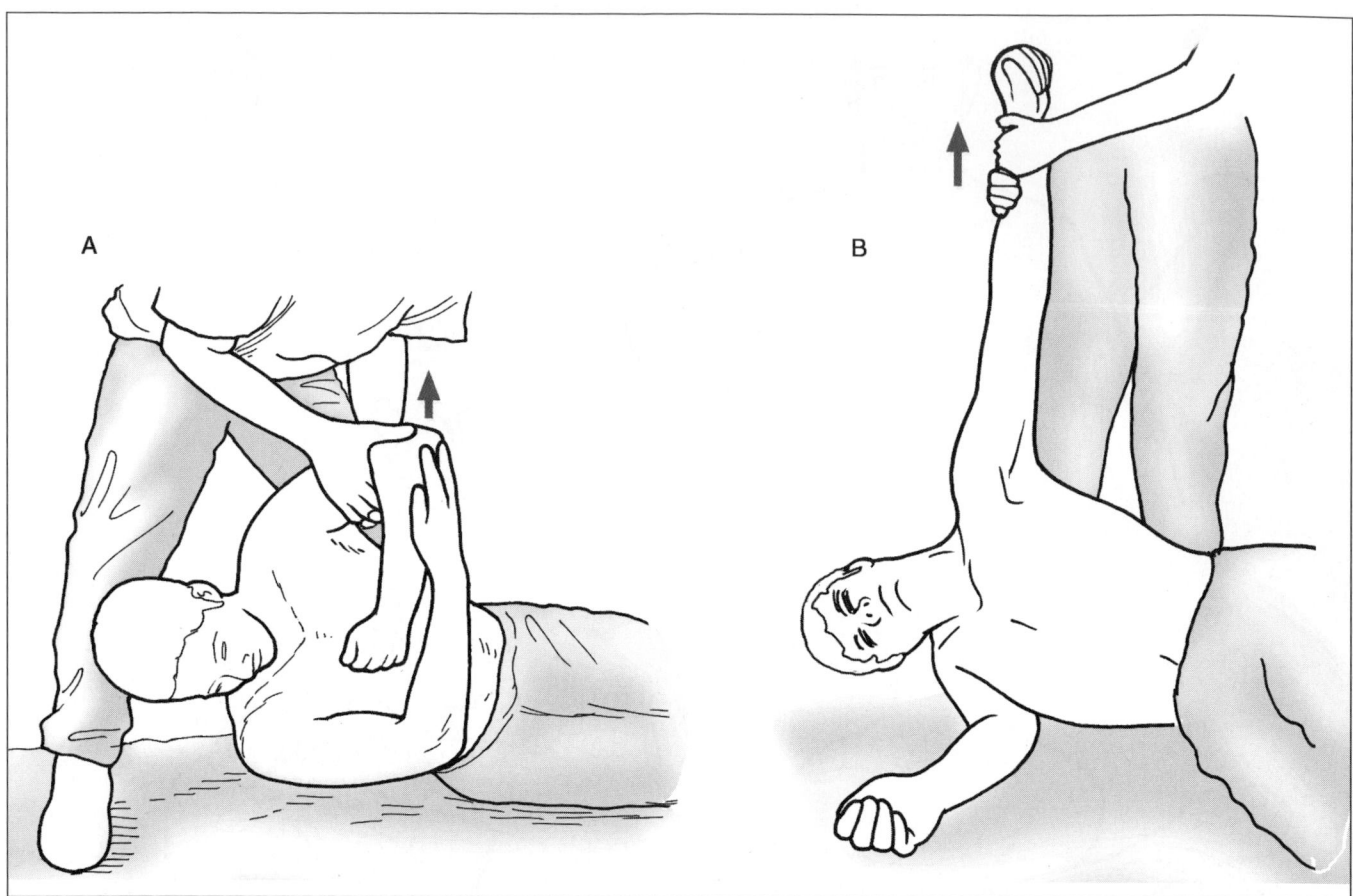

FIGURE 67-10 The Eskimo technique to reduce an anterior shoulder dislocation. The patient is lying on the floor on the unaffected side. *A.* The patient is lifted off the ground by grasping the adducted arm. *B.* The patient is lifted off the ground by grasping the distal forearm of the affected arm.

wheel of the gurney, which is then elevated until the dislocation is reduced.

POSTERIOR SHOULDER DISLOCATION REDUCTION TECHNIQUE

An Orthopedic Surgeon should be consulted before attempting to reduce the shoulder due to the rarity of posterior shoulder dislocations, the difficulty of reduction, the high incidence of associated injuries, and the need to operate to repair the associated injuries.[2,4,8,11] **The only exception is when the affected extremity has signs of neurologic or vascular compromise and the Orthopedic Surgeon is not immediately available to reduce the shoulder.** The patient will require intraarticular instillation of local anesthetic solution and procedural sedation for the performance of this technique.

Place the patient supine. Perform procedural sedation. Pass a sheet around the axilla and torso of the af-

fected arm in the same manner as in the traction-countertraction technique (Figure 67-5A). Grasp the distal forearm. Apply axial traction in-line with the humerus. Instruct an assistant to apply countertraction on the sheet looped around the patient's torso. The traction and countertraction should be equal in force and in opposite directions. While maintaining traction, gently internally rotate and adduct the arm. The shoulder may reduce. If not, instruct a second assistant to apply simultaneous lateral pressure on the humeral head.[3] While continuing to exert pressure on the humeral head, in trying to work it over the glenoid rim, the arm may need to be gently rotated externally. If this fails to reduce the shoulder, apply lateral traction, with a second assistant using a sheet looped around the proximal humerus, and repeat the process (Figure 67-5C). If the shoulder will still not reduce, this is an indication for general anesthesia and an open or closed reduction in the Operating Room.[4,9] The shoulder joint is usually unstable and may not remain articulated once it is reduced.

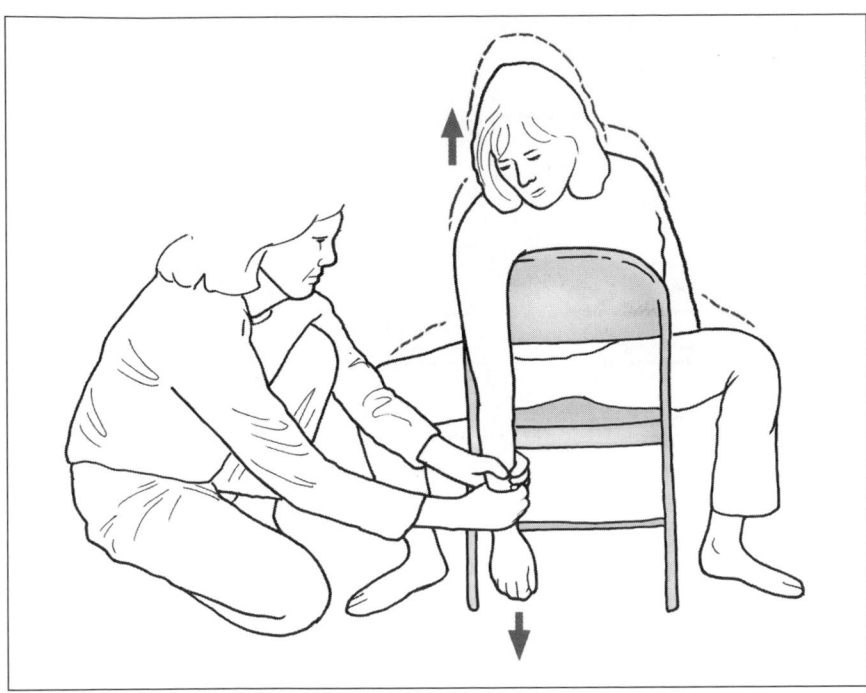

FIGURE 67-11 The chair technique to reduce an anterior shoulder dislocation.

An alternative to grasping the forearm is to apply a padded wrist restraint. Tie the loose ends of the restraint straps to create a loop around the physician's hips. A second alternative is to loop a sheet around the patient's flexed forearm and the physician's hips as in the traction-countertraction technique (Figure 67-5*B*). These two alternatives are preferred, as they allow the physician's body to reduce the shoulder rather than depending on biceps strength.

INFERIOR SHOULDER DISLOCATION REDUCTION TECHNIQUE

Like posterior shoulder dislocations, **inferior shoulder dislocations require an Orthopedic Surgeon to be consulted before attempting closed reduction unless neurologic or vascular compromise is present in the affected extremity.** Consultation is required because of the rarity of inferior shoulder dislocations, the difficulty

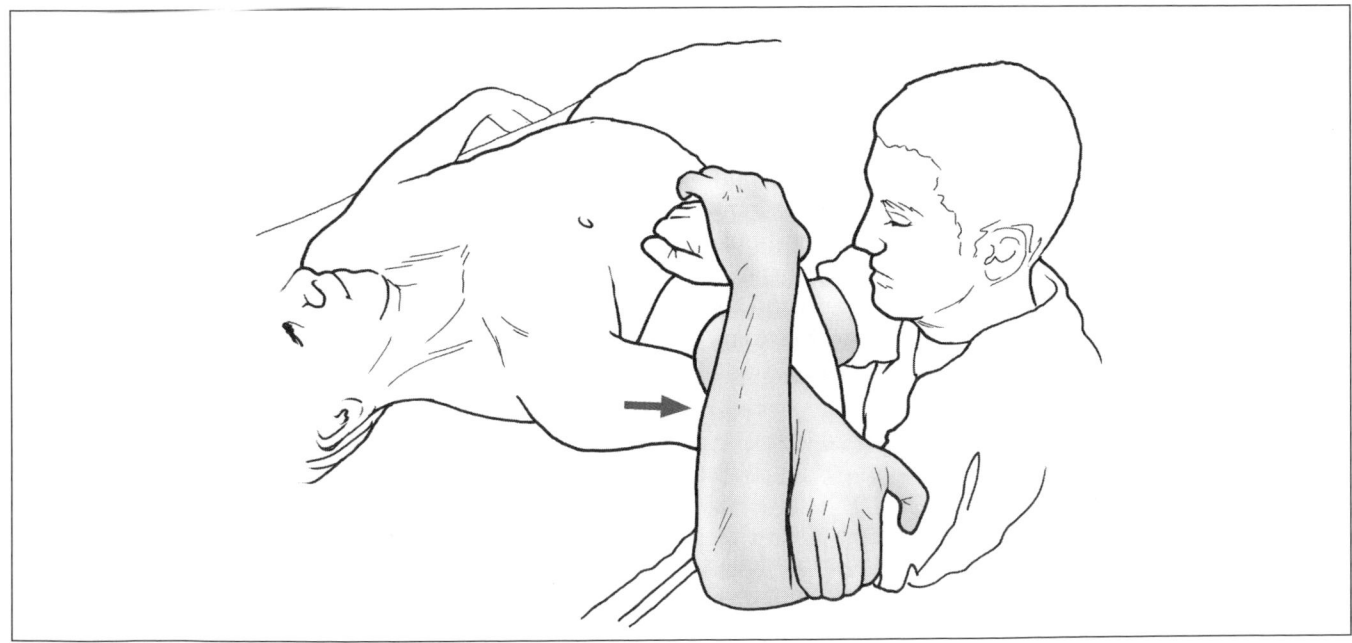

FIGURE 67-12 The wrestling technique to reduce an anterior shoulder dislocation.

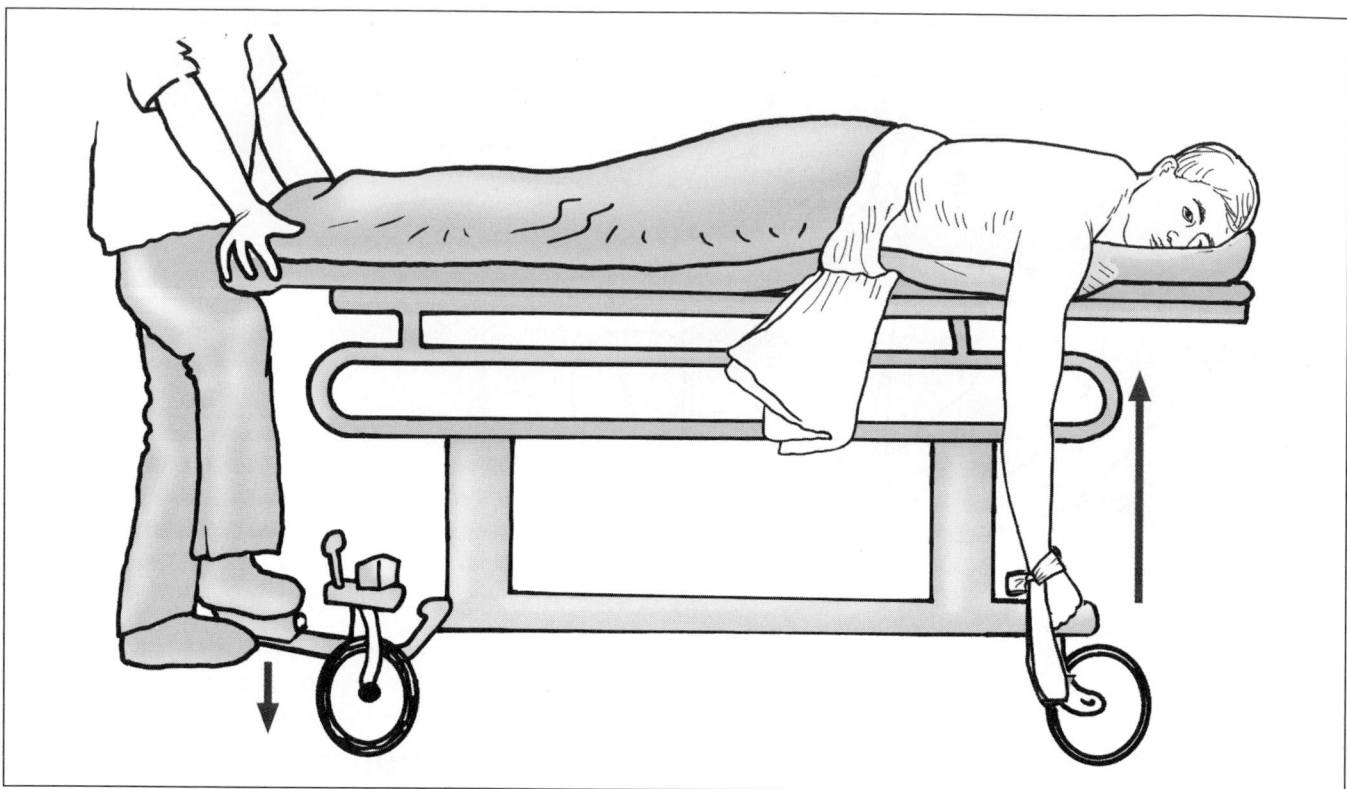

FIGURE 67-13 The pneumatic stretcher technique to reduce an anterior shoulder dislocation.

of reduction, the high incidence of associated injuries, and the need to operate to repair the associated injuries.[2–4,10,50–52] The patient will require intraarticular instillation of local anesthetic solution and procedural sedation for the performance of this technique.[4]

Place the patient supine. Loop a sheet over the clavicle of the affected shoulder with the loose ends of the sheet at the opposite hip (Figure 67-14). Stand above the patient's head and grasp the distal forearm. Apply axial traction to the arm. Instruct an assistant to apply equal countertraction on the sheet. While maintaining axial traction on the humerus, gently adduct the arm in a full arc from the patient's head to their side (Figure 67-14). The shoulder should reduce. The shoulder joint is usually unstable and may not remain articulated once reduced. In rare instances, buttonholing of the joint capsule will prevent closed reduction and require an open reduction.[2]

ASSESSMENT

The post-procedural care of the dislocated shoulder is as important as the initial reduction. Successful shoulder reduction is usually sensed by the operator as a shift or "clunk" in the shoulder joint. Sometimes this can be a very subtle sign. Generally, the normal contour of the shoulder is restored and patients often report marked improvement in their pain. A simple test to evaluate the success of the reduced joint, especially in anterior and posterior dislocations, is to have the patient touch their nose or contralateral shoulder with the hand of the affected limb.[3] The ability to do so usually signifies a relocated shoulder joint. **The patient should have a thorough examination to evaluate the extremity for vascular and/or neurologic compromise.** Any compromise requires immediate consultation with an Orthopedist.

It is important to prevent further external rotation or abduction of the reduced shoulder. Place the affected extremity in a shoulder immobilizer (Figure 67-15A) or a conventional sling with a swath (Figure 67-15B).[1,2,11,20,53,54] The shoulder should be immobilized in external rotation in a spica cast if a successful reduction is unstable[3] (Figure 67-15C). Post-reduction films are indicated after immobilization to confirm the reduction of the joint, to rule out missed fractures on the original radiographs, to rule out a fracture from the reduction procedure, and to evaluate for displacement of fracture fragments. There is some evidence that post-reduction radiographs may be unnecessary, but further study is warranted before this can be routinely recommended.[13,14]

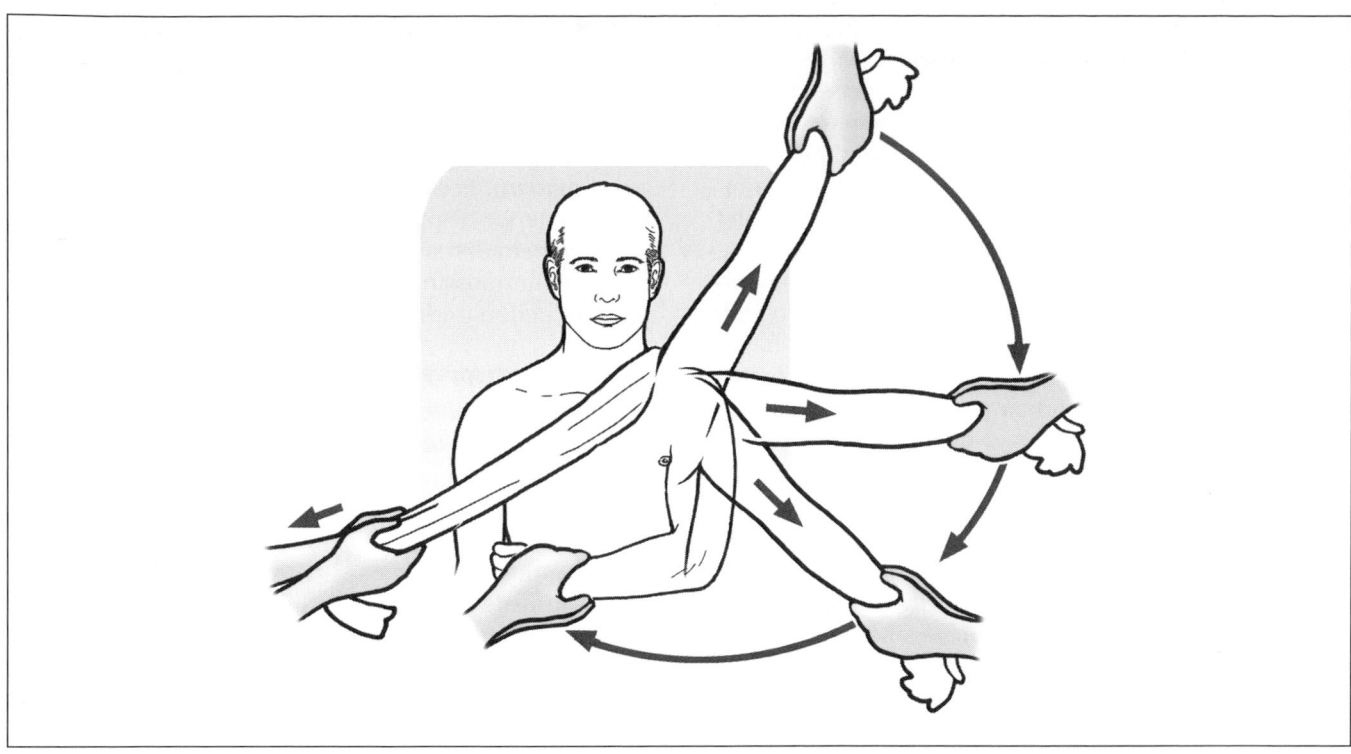

FIGURE 67-14 Reduction of an inferior shoulder dislocation (luxatio erecta). Axial traction (*straight arrows*) is applied and maintained on the dislocated extremity while it is simultaneously hyperadducted (*curved arrows*).

AFTERCARE

Following procedural sedation, the patient will need to be observed before being discharged home in the care of friends or family. It is necessary to have the patient awake, alert, oriented, and to have the pain adequately controlled before discharge. The patient should be discharged with adequate pain control and follow-up care by an Orthopedic Surgeon. Generally, oral nonsteroidal anti-inflammatory drugs are sufficient to control pain. Oral narcotics may be given as needed for 2 to 3 days to aid with pain during the acute inflammatory response period. Orthopedic follow-up should be arranged within 24 hours for anterior shoulder dislocations complicated by fractures or soft tissue injuries beyond ligamentous strain. Orthopedic follow-up within 5 to 7 days is generally sufficient for uncomplicated anterior shoulder reductions.

The duration of immobilization depends on the patient's age.[2,11,20] The only large-scale prospective study of first-time anterior shoulder dislocations followed patients over a 10 year period. It found that the duration

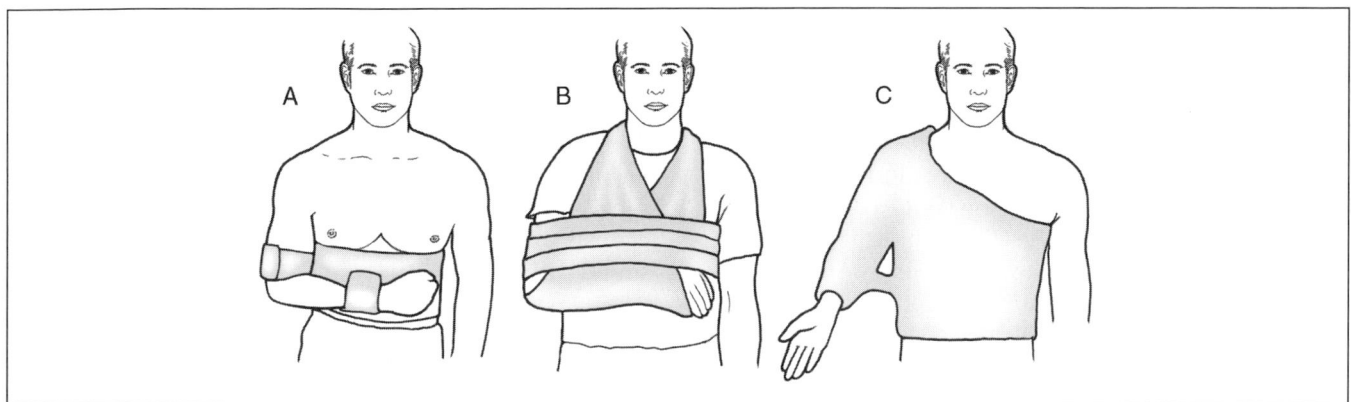

FIGURE 67-15 Methods of shoulder immobilization after reduction of a dislocation. *A.* Shoulder immobilizer. *B.* Velpeau dressing. *C.* Spica cast.

of immobilization had no effect on the incidence of recurrence. Age was the only prognostic factor for recurrence. Patients under 20 years of age should be immobilized for 3 weeks and then begin active range-of-motion exercises. Patients aged 20 to 40 years should be immobilized for 1 to 2 weeks and begin active range-of-motion exercises 5 days post-reduction. Patients older than 60 years of age should have minimal immobilization—less than 1 week—and begin active range-of-motion exercises within 72 hours post-reduction to limit subsequent shoulder stiffness.[2,11] Patients should be instructed to avoid external rotation and abduction activities, such as combing their hair, to avoid a recurrent dislocation.[1]

Range-of-motion exercises should include dangling-arm rotation.[2,11] While supporting the torso with the other arm, the patient makes a small circular motion with the injured arm against the force of gravity. For anterior dislocations, strengthening the subscapularis muscle by doing internal rotation against a resistance band with the elbow flexed 90 degrees is advocated.[2]

COMPLICATIONS

Complications of shoulder dislocations can occur as a result of the initial injury, the reduction technique, or a combination of both. Complications are discussed with respect to both the initial injury and the reduction. They include fractures, displacement of fracture fragments, rotator cuff tears, vascular injury, neurologic injury, recurrence of dislocation, hemarthroses, and the inability to reduce the shoulder.

FRACTURES

Most fractures are caused during the dislocation and rarely during the reduction procedure if the proper techniques are used.[2,4,8,11,50] Pre-reduction radiographs will identify most fractures. Post-reduction radiographs are required to identify fractures initially missed or new ones associated with the reduction. Fractures of the humerus and coracoid process are rare and almost always associated with traumatic anterior shoulder dislocations.[1,2,8] These fractures make closed reduction very difficult and should generally be treated under general anesthesia by an Orthopedic Surgeon or by open reduction.

More common bony injuries include the Hill-Sachs deformity and the Bankart lesion, both caused during and from the dislocation. The Hill-Sachs lesion occurs in up to 50 percent of shoulder dislocations.[1,2] More significant fractures can occur during reduction in rare situations in which the humeral head is dislocated anteriorly with impaction on the glenoid rim.[1,2,8,11] The Bankart lesion is more commonly seen in recurrent dislocations and is associated with rupture of the joint capsule, but it spares the rotator cuff.[1,2,8,11]

DISPLACEMENT OF FRACTURE FRAGMENTS

Pre-reduction radiographs should be obtained on all shoulder dislocations. They will identify most fractures and any associated displacement. Many of the reduction techniques use significant force and may displace a fracture fragment. Post-reduction radiographs are required to evaluate for displacement of fracture fragments. The displacement of fracture fragments may make reduction difficult or impossible, in some cases necessitating operative reduction under general anesthesia.

ROTATOR CUFF TEARS

Rotator cuff injury is most commonly seen in inferior dislocations and in patients greater than 60 years of age.[11,51,52] Overall, 38 percent of shoulder dislocations will have associated rotator cuff tears at the time of injury. This injury is not typically seen as a complication of the reduction technique.[3,11] Rotator cuff tears generally do not impede reduction, as they are often missed during the initial evaluation. One study showed that 86 percent of shoulder dislocations had rotator cuff tears diagnosed by arthroscopy an average of 7 months after the dislocation.[1,4] Rotator cuff injuries complicate restoration of normal shoulder function and may require surgical correction.

VASCULAR INJURY

Vascular injuries are seen in the arteries and veins of the shoulder region in association with shoulder dislocations.[1,8,11,50,55,56] **An evaluation for the signs of an axillary artery injury should be sought before and after any reduction attempt.** The most common vessel injured, during both dislocation and forceful reduction, is the axillary artery. Such an injury is usually seen in older patients who have brittle vessels that have lost some elasticity. Inferior dislocations have the highest association with vascular injuries.[11] The second and third parts of the axillary artery are deep to the pectoralis major muscle and sustain the most damage.[8] These injuries include decreased radial pulse, an axillary mass, an axillary bruit, or lateral chest wall bruising.[1] An angiogram is indicated if a vascular injury is suspected.

The subclavian vein is rarely injured. Direct injuries to venous vessels are atypical. The most common injury is a venous thrombosis. Physical signs include extremity edema and occasionally paresthesias. However, these signs are typically seen days after the reduction. The diagnostic test of choice for venous evaluation is an ultrasound with Doppler study.[8]

NEUROLOGIC INJURY

Neurologic injury is seen in 5 to 12 percent of all shoulder dislocations.[8,11,50,56–59] **An evaluation for the signs of any neurologic injury should be sought before and after any reduction attempt.** Anterior shoulder dislocations with humeral fractures have a 45 percent incidence of nerve injury, with the axillary nerve being injured in up to 36 percent of cases.[8] Older patients tend to be more prone to nerve injury from the dislocation and the reduction techniques.[8] Of the techniques described, those that cause significant downward traction typically cause more reduction-induced neurologic injuries. Fortunately, most neurologic injuries are neuropraxias and will completely resolve within 2 to 5 months.[11] A small percentage of axillary nerve injuries that do not resolve may require nerve grafting. Brachial plexus injuries are much more common in posterior and inferior shoulder dislocations. Because the brachial plexus surrounds the axillary artery, injuries to the artery should raise the suspicion for a brachial plexus injury.

DISLOCATION RECURRENCE

The incidence of recurrence is variable, age-dependent, and gender-dependent.[54,60] Among patients under the age of 20 years, 90 percent will dislocate again, while only 14 percent of those over the age of 40 will redislocate.[1] Recurrences are much more common in men, with a ratio of 4:1 to 6:1 as compared to women.[11] Recurrent shoulder dislocations have other associated morbidities. A triad of lesions—including a detached labrum and anterior capsule, a Hill-Sachs deformity, and erosion of the anterior glenoid—develops in 85 percent of recurrent shoulder dislocations.[4] The methods for reduction are not different from those of a first-time shoulder dislocation. Patients who have had multiple shoulder dislocations are generally easier to reduce using nonanalgesic manipulation techniques. The orthopedic literature suggests that three shoulder dislocations in a single extremity indicate the need for surgical repair.[11]

HEMARTHROSIS

Blood collections in the shoulder joint are rare complications and are seen almost exclusively in traumatic shoulder dislocations associated with fractures. Typically, older patients (greater than 60 years of age) will return to the Emergency Department within 24 to 48 hours with a tense, swollen, painful shoulder. The shoulder joint should be aspirated. Refer to Chapter 65 for the complete details regarding shoulder arthrocentesis. Aspiration is usually sufficient to relieve pain and restore function.

INABILITY TO REDUCE

There are a few reasons for the inability to reduce a dislocated shoulder completely. The most common is inadequate medication and sedation to overcome muscle spasm and pain. Occasionally, the humeral head may be "buttonholed" through the joint capsule.[11] A fracture fragment may be impinged or interposed between the humeral head and the glenoid cavity. Significant or complete disruption of ligamentous structures, as in an inferior or posterior dislocation, will not allow the humeral head to remain in the glenoid cavity. The inability to reduce a shoulder dislocation is an indication for reduction, open or closed, under general anesthesia.

SUMMARY

Shoulder dislocations are common due to the inherent instability of the glenohumeral joint. There are three different types of dislocation, each of which has different mechanisms of injury and incidences of associated injuries. The vast majority are anterior shoulder dislocations. The diagnosis of a shoulder dislocation is generally uncomplicated given the history and patient presentation. The physician must be expeditious in reducing the dislocated joint once the patient is stabilized, other injuries have been ruled out, pain control has been addressed, and radiographs have been obtained to confirm the type of dislocation along with associated injuries.

Orthopedic Surgeons may need to be involved with the acute care of a dislocated shoulder. They should be involved in the initial reduction care of all posterior and inferior dislocations because of the rarity of these shoulder dislocations, the difficulty of reduction, the high incidence of associated injuries, and the need to operate to repair the associated injuries.

Multiple closed reduction techniques are available. They have similar success rates. The method chosen, as well as the decision to use analgesia, is individualized to the physician and the patient. Certain traditional techniques (Hippocratic and Kocher) have been demonstrated to have a higher incidence of complications and should be avoided. Patients should be thoroughly evaluated before and after any closed reduction attempt for neurologic, vascular, soft tissue, or bony injury. The shoulder should be immobilized after it is reduced.

Patients should be instructed on proper aftercare and should be provided with adequate oral analgesia. This can be accomplished with nonsteroidal anti-inflammatory drugs supplemented with narcotics. All patients discharged from the Emergency Department should follow-up with an Orthopedic Surgeon within 24 hours to 5 days based on associated injuries and age.

REFERENCES

1. Price DD, Wilson SR: *Shoulder Dislocations.* 1999: 1–11. http://www.E-medicine.com.
2. Simon R, Koenisknecht S: *Emergency Orthopedics: The Extremities,* 3rd ed. Stamford, CT: Appleton & Lange, 1996:388–400.

3. McNamara R: Management of common dislocations, in Roberts JR, Hedges JR (eds): *Clinical Procedures in Emergency Medicine,* 3rd ed. Philadelphia: Saunders, 1998:818–830.

4. Daya M: Shoulder, in Rosen P, Barkin R, Danzl DF, et al (eds): *Emergency Medicine: Concepts and Clinical Practice,* 4th ed. St. Louis: Mosby, 1998:726–732.

5. Moore K: *Clinically Oriented Anatomy,* 3rd ed. Baltimore: Williams & Wilkins, 1992:611–615.

6. Blake R, Hoffman J: Emergency department evaluation and treatment of the shoulder and humerus. *Emerg Med Clin North Am* 1999; 17(4):859–870.

7. Bruno RG, Carter W: Shoulder dislocation, in Rosen P, Barkin RM, Hayden SR, et al (eds): *The 5 Minute Emergency Medicine Consult.* Philadelphia: Lippincott, Williams & Wilkins, 1999:1032–1033.

8. Beeson M: Complications of shoulder dislocations. *Am J Emerg Med* 1999; 17(3):288–295.

9. Neviaser JS: Posterior dislocations of the shoulder, diagnosis and treatment. *Surg Clin North Am* 1963; 43(6):1623–1630.

10. Brady WJ, Knuth CJ, Pirrallo RG: Bilateral inferior glenohumeral dislocation: luxatio erecta, an unusual presentation of a rare disorder. *J Emerg Med* 1995; 13(1):37–42.

11. Rockwood CA Jr, Wirth MA: Subluxations and dislocations about the glenohumeral joint, in Rockwood CA Jr, Green DP, Bucholz RW, et al (eds): *Rockwood and Green's Fractures in Adults,* 4th ed. Philadelphia: Lippincott-Raven, 1996:1193–1340.

12. Ferkel RD, Hedley AK, Eckardt JJ: Anterior fracture-dislocations of the shoulder: pitfalls in treatment. *J Trauma* 1984; 24(4):363–367.

13. Harvey RA, Trabulsy ME, Roe L: Are postreduction anteroposterior and scapular Y views useful in anterior shoulder dislocations? *Am J Emerg Med* 1992; 19(2):149–151.

14. Hendey G, Kinlaw K: Clinically significant abnormalities in postreduction radiographs after anterior shoulder dislocation. *Ann Emerg Med* 1996; 28(4):299–402.

15. Elberger S, Brody G: Bilateral posterior shoulder dislocations. *Am J Emerg Med* 1995; 13(3):331–332.

16. Matthews DE, Roberts T: Intraarticular lidocaine versus intravenous analgesic for reduction of acute anterior shoulder dislocations. *Am J Sports Med* 1995; 23(1):54–59.

17. Kolb JC, Krupnick J: Shoulder reduction without anesthesia. *Ann Emerg Med* 1996; 28(5):581–582.

18. Parvin RW: Closed reduction of common shoulder and elbow dislocations without anesthesia. *AMA Arch Surg* 1957; 75:972–975.

19. Garnavos C: Technical note: modifications and improvement of the Milch technique for the reduction of anterior dislocation of the shoulder without premedication. *J Trauma* 1992; 32(6):801–803.

20. Wen DY: Current concepts in the treatment of anterior shoulder dislocation. *Am J Emerg Med* 1999; 17(4):401–407.

21. Liedelmeyer R: Reduced! A shoulder, subtly and painlessly. *Emerg Med* 1977; 9:233–234.

22. Mirick MJ, Clinton JE, Ruiz E: External rotation method of shoulder dislocation reduction. *JACEP* 1979; 8(12):528–531.

23. Plummer D, Clinton J: The external rotation method for reduction of acute anterior shoulder dislocation. *Emerg Med Clin North Am* 1989; 7(1):165–175.

24. Danzl DF, Vicario SJ, Gleis GL, et al: Closed reduction of anterior subcoracoid shoulder dislocation, evaluation of an external rotation method. *Orthop Rev* 1986; 15(5):311–315.

25. Stimson LA: An easy method of reducing dislocations of the shoulder and hip. *Med Rec* 1900; 57(9):356–357.

26. Riebel GD, McCabe JB: Anterior shoulder dislocation: a review of reduction techniques. *Am J Emerg Med* 1991; 9(2):180–188.

27. Lippert FG: A modification of the gravity method of reducing anterior shoulder dislocations. *Clin Orthop Rel Res* 1982; 165:259–260.

28. Rollinson PD: Reduction of shoulder dislocations by the hanging method. *S Afr Med J* 1988; 73:106–107.

29. Doyle WL, Ragar T: Use of the scapular manipulation method to reduce an anterior shoulder dislocation in the supine position. *Ann Emerg Med* 1996; 27(1):92–94.

30. Anderson D, Zvirbulis R, Ciullo J: Scapular manipulation for reduction of anterior shoulder dislocations. *Clin Orthop Rel Res* 1982; 164:181–183.

31. Kothari RU, Dronen SC: The scapular manipulation technique for the reduction of acute anterior shoulder dislocations. *J Emerg Med* 1990; 8:625–628.

32. Kothari RU, Dronen SC: Prospective evaluation of the scapular manipulation technique in reducing anterior shoulder dislocations. *Ann Emerg Med* 1992; 21(11):1349–1352.

33. McNamara RM: Reduction of anterior shoulder dislocations by scapular manipulation. *Ann Emerg Med* 1993; 22(7):1140–1144.

34. Westin CD, Gill EA, Noyes ME, et al: Anterior shoulder dislocation: a simple and rapid method for reduction. *Am J Sports Med* 1995; 23(3):369–371.

35. Milch H: The treatment of recent dislocations and fractures-dislocations of the shoulder. *J Bone Jt Surg* 1949; 31A(1):173–180.

36. Milch H: Treatment of dislocation of the shoulder. *Surgery* 1938; 3:732–740.

37. Milch H: Pulsion-traction in the reduction of dislocations or fracture dislocations of the humerus. *Bull Hosp Jt Dis* 1963; 24:147–152.

38. Lacey T II, Crawford HB: Reduction of anterior dislocations of the shoulder by means of the Milch abduction technique. *J Bone Joint Surg* 1952; 34A(1): 108–109.

39. Russell JA, Holmes EM III, Keller DJ, et al: Reduction of acute anterior shoulder dislocations using the Milch technique: a study of ski injuries. *J Trauma* 1981; 21(9):802–804.

40. Janecki CJ, Shahcheragh GH: The forward elevation maneuver for reduction of anterior dislocations of the shoulder. *Clin Orthop Rel Res* 1982; 164:177–180.

41. Hippocrates: Injuries of the shoulder, dislocations (Tsemanis VS, trans). *Clin Orthop Rel Res* 1989; 246:4–7.

42. Hussein MK: Kocher's method is 3,000 years old. *J Bone Joint Surg* 1968; 50B(3):669–671.

43. Thakur AJ, Narayan R: Painless reduction of shoulder dislocation by Kocher's method. *J Bone Joint Surg* 1990; 72(3):524.

44. Poulsen SR: Reduction of acute shoulder dislocations using the Eskimo technique: a study of 23 consecutive cases. *J Trauma* 1988; 2B(9):1382–1383.

45. Parisien VM: Shoulder dislocation, an easier method of reduction. *J Maine Med Assoc* 1979; 70(3):102.

46. White ADN: Dislocated shoulder—a simple method of reduction. *Med J Aust* 1976; 2:726–727.

47. Noordeen MHH, Bacarese–Hamilton IH, Belham GJ, et al: Anterior dislocation of the shoulder: a simple method of reduction. *Injury* 1992; 23(7):479–480.

48. Zahiri CA, Zahiri H, Tehrany F: Anterior shoulder dislocation reduction technique revisited. *Orthopedics* 1997; 20:515–521.

49. Shackelford HL: Hydraulic stretcher reduction technique for anterior dislocation of the shoulder. *W Va Med J* 1982; 78(1):9.

50. Davids JR, Talbott RD: Luxatio erecta humeri: a case report. *Clin Orthop Rel Res* 1990; 252:144–149.

51. Pirrallo RG, Bridges TP: Luxatio erecta: a missed diagnosis. *Am J Emerg Med* 1990; 8(4):315–317.

52. Saxena K, Stravas J: Inferior glenohumeral dislocation. *Ann Emerg Med* 1983; 12(11):718–720.

53. Pick RY: Treatment of dislocated shoulder. *Clin Orthop Rel Res* 1977; 123:76–77.

54. Relovszky K: Prognosis of primary dislocation of the shoulder. *Acta Orthop Scand* 1969; 40:216–224.

55. Kirker JR: Dislocation of the shoulder complicated by rupture of the axillary vessels: a case report. *J Bone Joint Surg* 1952; 34B(1):72–73.

56. Curley SA, Osler T, Demarest GB: Traumatic disruption of the subclavian artery and brachial plexus in a patient with Ehlers-Danlos syndrome. *Ann Emerg Med* 1988; 17(8):850–852.

57. DeLaat EAT, Visser CPJ, Coene LNJEM, et al: Nerve lesions in primary shoulder dislocations and humeral neck fractures: a prospective clinical and emg study. *J Bone Joint Surg* 1994; 76B(3):381–383.

58. Toolanen G, Hildingsson C, Hedlund T, et al: Early complications after anterior dislocation of the shoulder in patients over 40 years: an ultrasonographic and electromyographic study. *Acta Orthop Scand* 1993; 64(5):549–552.

59. Travlos J, Goldberg I, Boome RS: Brachial plexus lesions associated with dislocated shoulders. *J Bone Joint Surg* 1990; 72B(1):68–71.

60. Hoelen MA, Burgers AMJ, Rozing PM: Prognosis of primary anterior shoulder dislocation in young adults. *Arch Orthop Trauma Surg* 1990; 110:51–54.

Chapter 68
ELBOW JOINT DISLOCATION REDUCTION

Angelique S. Kelly Campen

INTRODUCTION

The elbow is inherently subjected to dislocations because of its mechanical structure.[1] Elbow dislocations are one of the more common joint dislocations in the body, second only to dislocations of the shoulders and fingers.[2] Injuries to the elbow have a high potential for complications and residual disability.[3] Timely reduction is imperative to relieve pain and reduce the possibility of neurovascular sequelae.[3] Closed reduction of the elbow is unlikely to be successful if not performed promptly.[4]

The most common mechanism for a dislocation is a fall onto an extended and abducted arm. The patient usually presents with a swollen and painful arm that is held in flexion. Elbow dislocations require a significant amount of force. Up to 20 percent of elbow dislocations are associated with fractures.[2] Simple elbow dislocations have a better prognosis and are less likely to require surgical intervention than complex ones (fracture-dislocations). This chapter deals with the closed reduction of simple elbow dislocations.

One particular type of dislocation pertains primarily to the pediatric population. Subluxation of the radial head, often referred to as a "nursemaid's elbow," occurs commonly in preschool children. It is rarely seen after age 7 and represents 20 percent of upper extremity injuries in children.[5] It occurs after sudden traction on the radius with an extended elbow, as when an adult pulls a child up into a standing position by one arm. The annular ligament slips between the capitellum and the head of the radius, impeding supination of the arm. The patient will present with the arm held in slight flexion and pronation, usually in not much distress, and not using the affected arm. The simple reduction of this dislocation is also addressed.

ANATOMY AND PATHOPHYSIOLOGY

The elbow is a hinge joint comprising articulations between the humerus, the ulna, and the radius (Figure 68-1). The distal humerus consists of the extraarticular medial and lateral epicondyles, which are diverging columns separated by the intraarticular trochlea and capitellum. The trochlea articulates with the proximal ulna. The articular surfaces of the trochlea extend from the coronoid fossa anteriorly to the olecranon fossa posteriorly. The anterior and posterior fossae provide space for the coronoid and olecranon, respectively, at the extremes of motion. The capitellum is a spherical structure that articulates with the concave radial head.

Numerous neurovascular structures cross the elbow (Figure 68-2). The prominent medial epicondyle protects the ulnar nerve, which travels in its posterior sulcus. The radial nerve travels just anterior to the lateral epicondyle. The median nerve travels with the brachial artery through the antecubital fossa.

There are four ligamentous structures of importance in considering injuries to the elbow: the radial collateral ligament, the ulnar collateral ligament, the annular ligament, and the anterior capsule (Figure 68-3). The annular ligament and radial collateral ligament hold the radial head in position. The annular ligament allows the radial head to rotate under it during pronation and supination.

The relationship of the radius and ulna to the humerus is used to classify elbow dislocations into posterior, anterior, medial, lateral, and divergent. The majority of elbow dislocations are posterior in direction.[6] The other types of elbow dislocations are uncommon.[6] The radius and ulna are held tightly together by the annular ligament and the interosseous membrane (Figure 68-3). Posterior elbow dislocations result in the radius and ulna projecting posterior to the humerus (Figures 68-4A and B). The radius and ulna may be slightly lateral or medial in posterior elbow dislocations in addition to being posteriorly displaced. This does not affect the management or prognosis. The presence of a fracture of the radial head or coronoid process may frequently render any attempt at reduction unstable and will usually require an open reduction.[7] Anterior elbow dislocations occur from traction of the forearm with the elbow extended or a blow to the posterior aspect of the flexed elbow. Anterior elbow dislocations result in the radius and

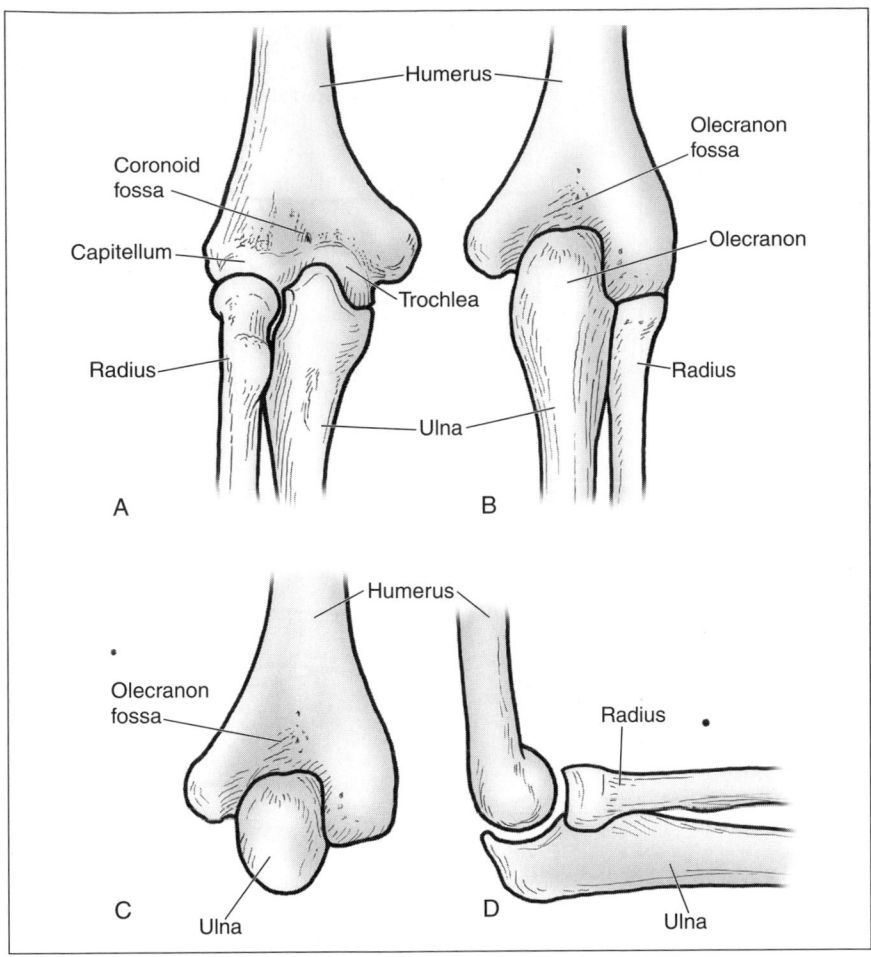

FIGURE 68-1 Bony anatomy of the elbow region. The right arm is demonstrated in these illustrations. *A.* Anterior view. *B.* Posterior view. *C.* Posterior view of the elbow in 90 degrees of flexion. *D.* Lateral view of the elbow in 90 degrees of flexion.

ulna projecting anterior to the humerus (Figure 68-4*C*). Medial and lateral dislocations are rare injuries with poorer prognoses. Divergent dislocations are rare injuries that are distinct from the other types of elbow dislocations because there is dissociation of the radius and ulna. The annular ligament and interosseous membrane must be torn for a divergent dislocation to occur.

The patient usually presents with pain and swelling of the elbow. All elbow dislocations are characterized by loss of the normal relationship of the humeral epicondyles to the tip of the olecranon. The bony landmarks may be identified if the patient is seen immediately after the injury. However, the swelling and hemarthrosis that develop over time make it difficult to palpate these landmarks. Posterior dislocations are further apparent by a shortening of the forearm and the elbow being fixed in flexion.

INDICATIONS

All elbow dislocations require reduction. Early reduction of a dislocation, by open or closed means, is of para-

mount importance if good functional results are to be obtained. Closed reduction is unlikely to be successful if attempted later than 14 days after the injury.[4] The more promptly the reduction is attempted, the more likely it is to be successful.

The vascular status of the extremity also dictates the need for emergent relocation. **Emergent and immediate relocation is necessary when there is neurologic or vascular compromise of the distal extremity.** Relocation can await titration of sedation and analgesia when the extremity is neurovascularly intact.

CONTRAINDICATIONS

There are no absolute contraindications to the closed reduction of an elbow dislocation. A relative contraindication to the procedure is when there is uncertainty, before radiographic evaluation, if the injury is a dislocation or a fracture. Closed reduction is not indicated if there is an interposed osteochondral fragment preventing concentric reduction or when there is a concomitant displaced fracture of the radial head or neck. Elbows that

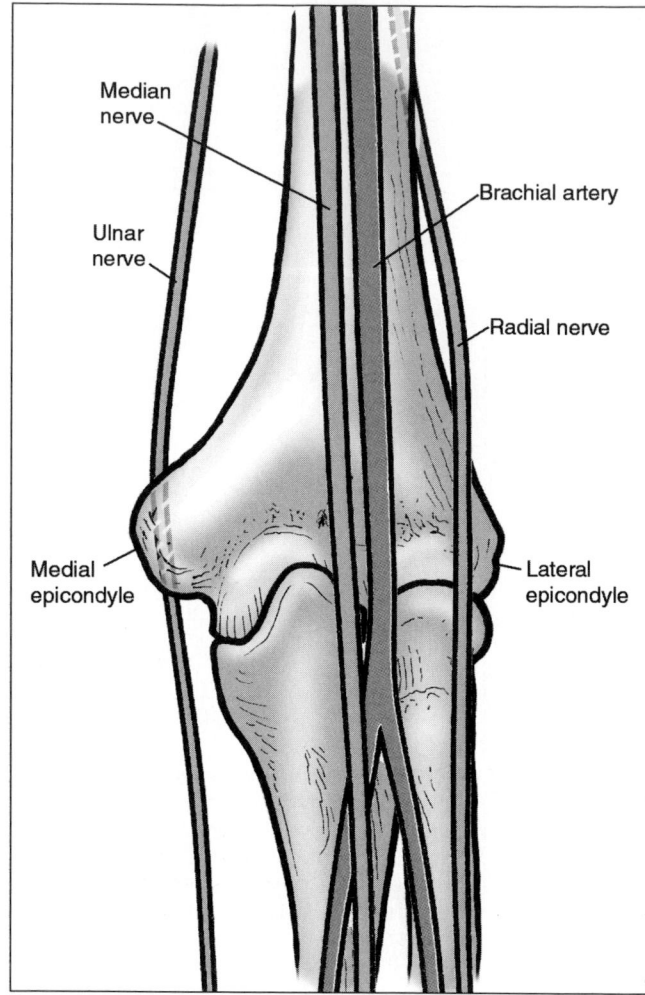

FIGURE 68-2 Major neurovascular structures that cross the elbow.

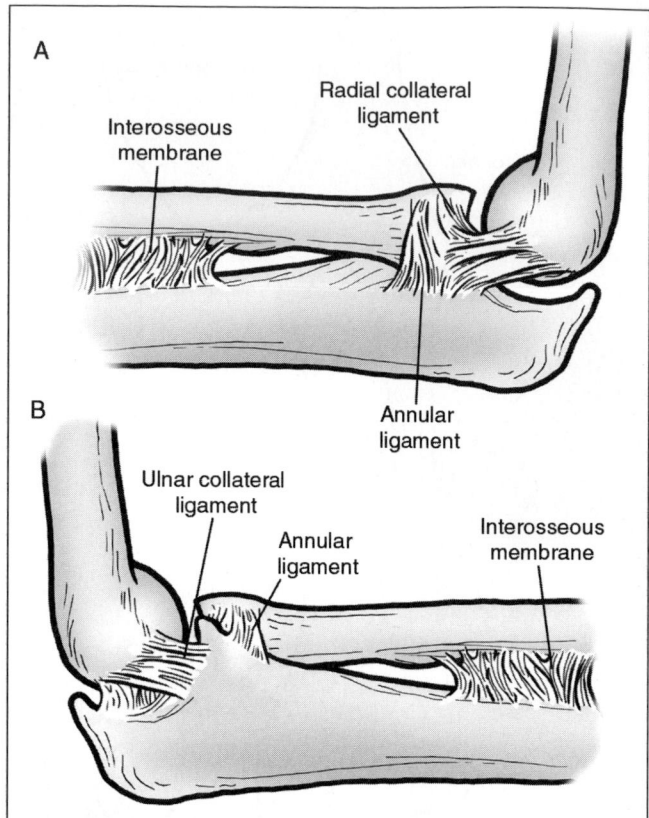

FIGURE 68-3 Major ligamentous structures of the elbow. *A.* Lateral view. *B.* Medial view.

have been dislocated for a prolonged period of time may have closed reduction attempted but will most likely require an open procedure.

EQUIPMENT

Towel or sheet to aid in applying traction
Splinting materials
Weight (sandbag, bucket with water, or any other weight)
Procedural sedation supplies (see Chapter 109)

PATIENT PREPARATION

Explain the risks, benefits, and potential complications to the patient and/or their representative. The post-procedural care should also be discussed. Obtain an informed consent for the reduction procedure.

Carefully assess and document the pre-procedural neurologic (median, radial, and ulnar nerves) and vascular (brachial, radial, and ulnar arteries) status of the extremity. Splint and/or sling the affected extremity until radiographs are obtained and a closed reduction can be performed. Obtain anteroposterior and lateral radiographs to confirm the diagnosis of an elbow dislocation. Oblique views may be helpful to further define the relationship between the distal humerus, radius, and ulna. **The only case for which a pre-procedure radiograph is not indicated is when neurologic or vascular compromise exists in the distal extremity and an expeditious reduction is required.**

Closed reduction of elbow dislocations requires adequate analgesia and muscle relaxation. In most cases, procedural sedation is useful. Regional anesthesia (axillary nerve or Bier blocks) are useful if procedural sedation is contraindicated. Refer to Chapters 106 and 107 for details regarding regional anesthesia of the upper extremity. General anesthesia with fluoroscopy is rarely necessary unless the dislocation is associated with an undisplaced fracture of the radial head or neck.

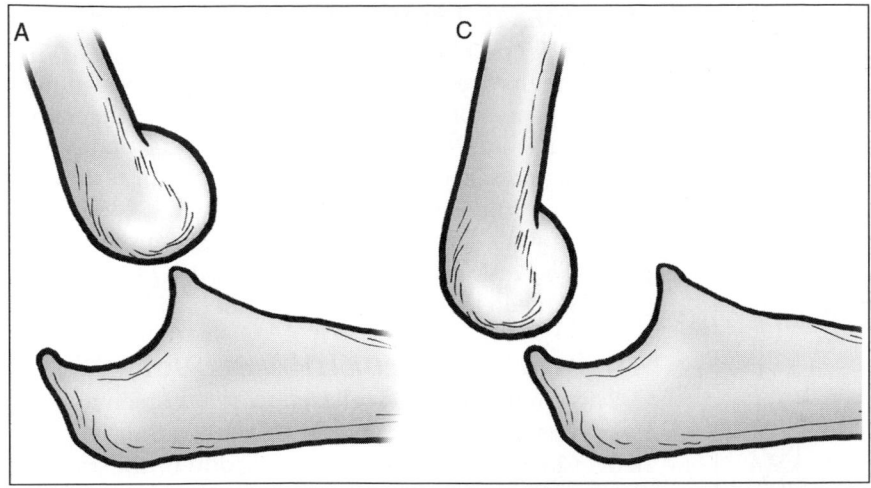

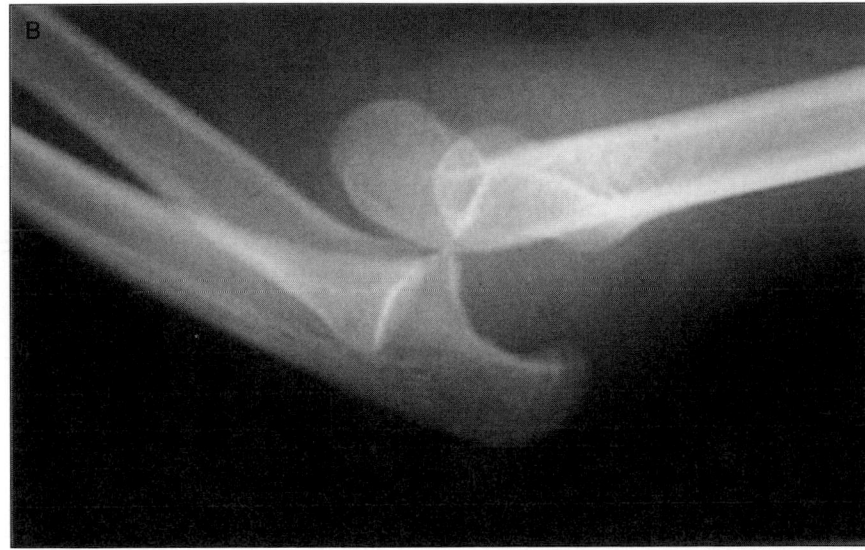

FIGURE 68-4 Elbow dislocations.
A. The posterior elbow dislocation. *B.* Radiograph of a posterior elbow dislocation.
C. The anterior elbow dislocation.

TECHNIQUES

POSTERIOR ELBOW DISLOCATION REDUCTION TECHNIQUES

Stimson Technique

The goal of closed reduction is to distract the radius and ulna, allowing them to relocate. The preferred technique that provides the least complications is a modification of the Stimson technique used for shoulder dislocations.[8] Place the patient prone with the affected arm hanging off the gurney (Figure 68-5). Place padding anteriorly in front of the arm and shoulder so that the arm does not drag along the side of the gurney. Care must be taken that the patient does not fall from the gurney. Tie a sheet circumferentially around the patient's hips and the gurney. **Ensure that the patient does not have any respiratory difficulty while in the prone position.** Suspend a weight from the patient's wrist to apply traction to the arm (Figure 68-5). The weight should be approximately 5 pounds and may go up to 15 pounds, depending on the patient's musculature and weight. Allow the arm to dangle over the edge of the gurney for 10 minutes. If the elbow dislocation will not reduce, attempt the traction-countertraction technique.

Traction-Countertraction Technique

The traction-countertraction technique can be performed but is not the optimal approach. Place the patient's arm in slight flexion. Grasp the patient's mid-humerus with the nondominant hand and the patient's wrist with the dominant hand (Figure 68-6). Alternatively, an assistant can grasp the humerus while the physician uses both hands to grasp the patient's wrist. Stabilize the patient's humerus. Apply steady and constant traction to the patient's wrist to distract the coro-

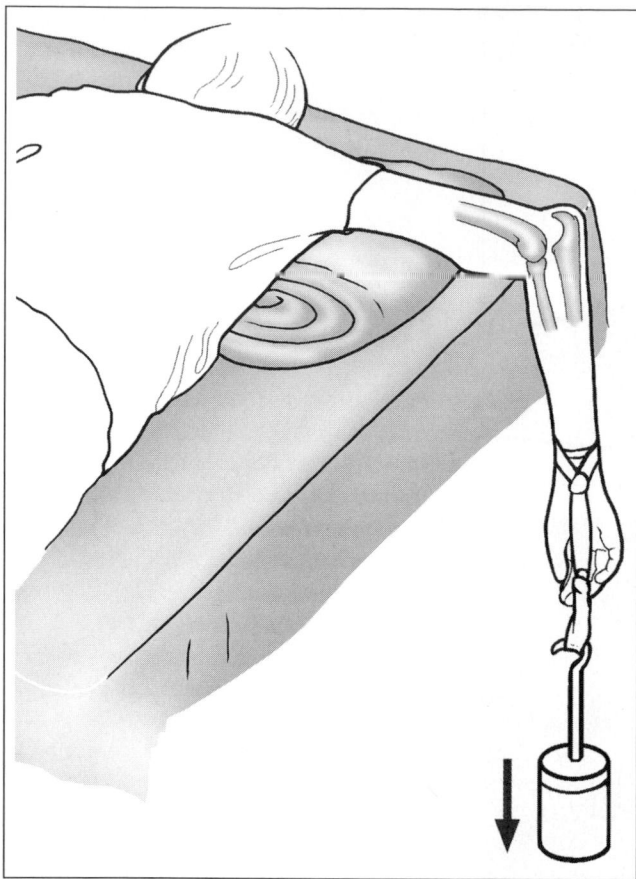

FIGURE 68-5 The modified Stimson technique for reducing posterior elbow dislocations.

noid process and allow it to slip past the humerus and back into anatomic position.

MEDIAL AND LATERAL ELBOW DISLOCATION REDUCTION TECHNIQUE

Medial and lateral dislocations of the elbow are extraordinarily uncommon. They are usually associated with a posterior elbow dislocation. These dislocations can be reduced in a similar manner to that of the posterior elbow dislocation. Emergency Physicians should not reduce a medial or lateral elbow dislocation. They are uncommon, may be associated with neurovascular complications, have severe ligamentous tears, and should be reduced by an Orthopedic Surgeon.

ANTERIOR ELBOW DISLOCATION REDUCTION TECHNIQUE

Anterior elbow dislocations are uncommon. They are often associated with intimal injuries to the brachial artery, from being stretched during the injury. Anterior elbow dislocations should be reduced by an Orthopedic Surgeon in the Operating Room for the same reasons as a medial or lateral elbow dislocation.

DIVERGENT ELBOW DISLOCATION REDUCTION TECHNIQUE

Fortunately, divergent dislocations are exceedingly rare. They are commonly associated with severe articular damage, interosseous ligamentous tears, neurologic injuries, and vascular injuries. The reduction technique is complex; the elbow is reduced as a two-part dislocation and often requires fixation to be stabilized. Divergent elbow dislocations should be reduced by an Orthopedic Surgeon in the Operating Room.

RADIAL HEAD SUBLUXATION REDUCTION

This condition is also referred to as a "nursemaid's elbow." Reduction of a radial head subluxation is a maneuver involving supination and flexion of the affected forearm. The forearm is quickly supinated and the elbow flexed completely in one smooth motion. A pop or click is sometimes heard or felt by the physician as the subluxation is reduced. Most patients are asymptomatic within 5 to 10 minutes and 90 percent within 30 minutes.[9] The physician should leave the room for 5 to 10 minutes after the procedure. Ask the parents to distract the child to see if he or she begins to move the arm. A fearful child will often not use a successfully reduced arm in fear of pain. Place a toy (car keys, popsicle, or other object the child may want) within grasp of the reduced extremity to encourage the child to use the extremity. Refer to Chapter 69 for the complete details regarding the reduction of a radial head subluxation.

ASSESSMENT

After a reduction, gently move the joint through the entire range of motion to ensure smooth movement and proper joint placement. This also tests for joint stability and whether or not the joint will easily redislocate. The joint may need to be repaired operatively if it dislocates during this examination. **The neurovascular status of the extremity must again be evaluated and documented.** The integrity of the median, ulnar, and radial nerves as well as the brachial artery must be evaluated and documented. All reductions except radial head subluxations should have post-procedural radiographs to ensure proper bony alignment and the lack of a fracture. If full and smooth passive range of motion is not possible, which is especially common in children, post-reduction radiographs should be examined for entrapment of the medial epicondyle.

AFTERCARE

Place the reduced extremity in a posterior long arm splint, from the midhumerus to the base of the fingers,

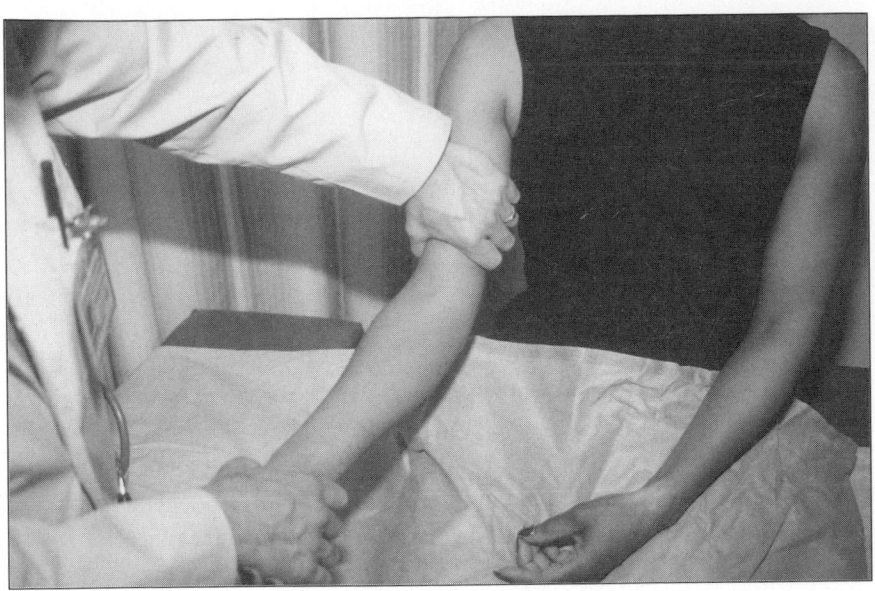

FIGURE 68-6 The traction-countertraction technique to reduce a posterior elbow dislocation. The physician stabilizes the humerus with one hand and distracts the forearm with the other hand.

with the elbow in 90 degrees of flexion. Do not apply a circumferential cast due to the subsequent swelling and edema. Suspend the arm with a sling to aid in elevating the extremity. The patient should be carefully observed for 12 to 36 hours for vascular impairment. Instruct the patient to return to the Emergency Department if they develop weakness, numbness, paresthesias, cold fingers, or cyanotic fingers. The patient should be admitted for observation if there is any question of neurovascular compromise. Gentle range-of-motion exercises can be started as early as 3 to 5 days post-reduction if the elbow is stable.[10] Orthopedic follow-up should be scheduled for 3 to 4 days post-reduction to test for joint stability. Prescribe nonsteroidal anti-inflammatory drugs supplemented with narcotic analgesics to control pain.

No immobilization is necessary for a radial head subluxation that is reduced. Immobilization in a sling with follow-up by an Orthopedic Surgeon is recommended if this is a recurrent radial head subluxation.

COMPLICATIONS

Several serious complications exist with elbow dislocations. The most serious and first to happen are ischemic complications. Damage to and obstruction of the brachial artery can occur with any of the elbow dislocations. Brachial artery injury occurs in 5 to 13 percent of patients with an elbow dislocation.[11] It is a serious complication that can occur even without an associated fracture.[11] **The presence of a distal pulse is not proof that there is no vascular injury.** Any suspicion of a brachial artery injury necessitates prompt angiography.[12]

The second serious complication resulting from an elbow dislocation is nerve injury from traction or entrapment. Loss of median nerve function post-reduction should prompt an immediate consultation with an Orthopedic Surgeon. The ulnar nerve is most commonly injured; this is seen in 8 to 20 percent of patients with posterior elbow dislocations.[13]

Fractures commonly occur with elbow dislocations. **Radiographs should always be obtained before and after any attempt at reduction. The only exception to obtaining pre-reduction radiographs is if the extremity has signs of distal neurovascular compromise and obtaining radiographs will delay the reduction.** A fractured coronoid process can sometimes become entrapped in the joint, requiring an open reduction. Fractures of the coronoid process are commonly associated injuries and will usually come into near-normal opposition once reduction occurs (Figure 68-7). Large fragments that are displaced may require operative fixation.

Late complications of elbow dislocations include posttraumatic stiffness, posterolateral joint instability, ectopic ossification, and occult distal radioulnar joint disruption.[14]

SUMMARY

Elbow dislocations are the second most common large joint dislocations that occur in adults. The majority of dislocations are posterior elbow dislocations, although the radius and ulna can dislocate into just about any other position. Relocation involves distracting the forearm while stabilizing the humerus and putting pressure counter to the direction of the dislocation.

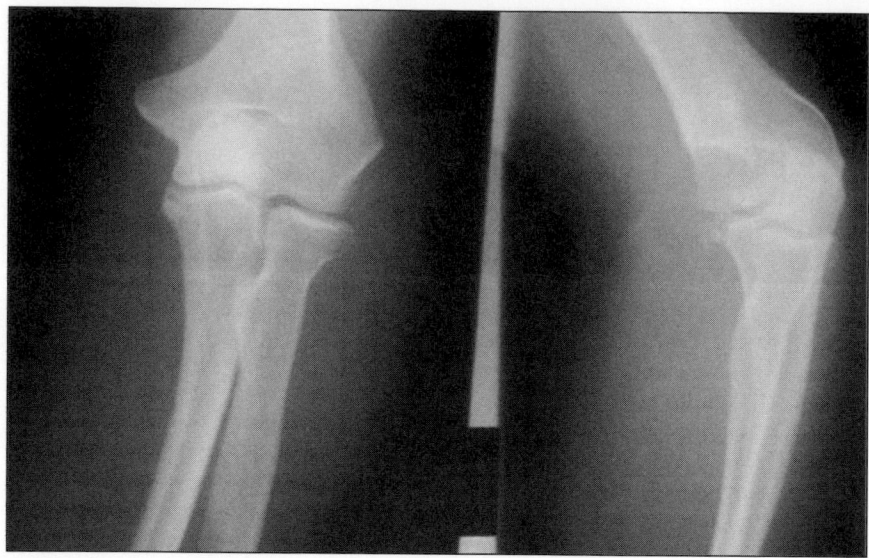

FIGURE 68-7 Post-reduction radiograph demonstrating a fracture of the coronoid process.

It is not uncommon to have associated fractures, so radiographic studies are imperative. The neurovascular status of the extremity must be carefully monitored and documented both before and after any attempts at reduction. Splint the elbow in flexion post-reduction. Orthopedic follow-up and early range-of-motion exercises are recommended to ensure proper joint function.

REFERENCES

1. Royle SG: Posterior dislocation of the elbow. Clin Orthop 1991; 269:201–204.
2. Hildebrand KA, Patterson SD, King GJ: Acute elbow dislocations: simple and complex. *Orthop Clin North Am* 1999; 30(1):63–79.
3. Perry MO, Thal ER, Shires GT: Management of arterial injuries. *Ann Surg* 1971; 173(3):403–408.
4. Bruce C, Laing P, Dorgan J, et al: Unreduced dislocation of the elbow: case report and review of the literature. *J Trauma* 1993; 35(6):962–965.
5. Quan L, Marcuse EK: The epidemiology and treatment of radial head subluxation. *Am J Dis Child* 1985; 139(12):1194.
6. Geiderman J, Magnusson A: Humerus and elbow, in Rosen P, Barkin R, Danzl D, et al (eds): *Emergency Medicine: Concepts and Clinical Practice,* 4th ed. St. Louis: Mosby, 1998:690–708.
7. Kennedy J, Blaisdell F: *Extremity Trauma.* New York: Thieme, 1992:146–148.
8. Simon RR, Koenigsknecht SJ: *Emerency Orthopedics—The Extremities,* 4th ed. Stamford, CT: Appleton & Lange, 1995:378–380.
9. Schunk JE: Radial head subluxation: epidemiology and treatment of 87 episodes. *Ann Emerg Med* 1990; 19(9):1019.
10. Schippinger G, Seibert FJ, Steinbock J, et al: Management of simple elbow dislocations. Does the period of immobilization affect the eventual results? *Langenbecks Arch Surg* 1999; 384(3):294–297.
11. Platz A, Heinzalmann M, Ertel W, et al: Posterior elbow dislocation with associated vascular injury after blunt trauma. *J Trauma* 1999; 46(5):948–950.
12. Endean ED, Veldenz HC, Schwarcz TH, et al: Recognition of arterial injury in elbow dislocation. *J Vasc Surg* 1992; 16(3):402–406.
13. Galbraith KA, McCullough CJ: Acute nerve injury as a complication of closed fractures or dislocation of the elbow. *Injury* 1979; 11(2):159–164.
14. Cohen MS, Hastngs H: Acute elbow dislocation: evaluation and management. *J Am Acad Orthop Surg* 1998; 6(1):15–23.

Chapter 69
RADIAL HEAD SUBLUXATION ("NURSEMAID'S ELBOW") REDUCTION

Mark P. Kling
Eric F. Reichman

INTRODUCTION

Subluxation of the radial head is one of the most common pediatric orthopedic injuries. This can occur in children whose age ranges from less than 6 months to the preteens. The majority of radial head subluxations occur between 1 and 3 years of age.[1] It is a rare injury before 1 year of age and after 8 years of age.

ANATOMY AND PATHOPHYSIOLOGY

Historically, the classic mechanism involves axial or longitudinal traction on an extended elbow with the forearm pronated. This often occurs while someone is holding onto the child by the hand or wrist. While being held, the child is then pulled or the child falls and is suspended by the arm. The subluxation is seen more often in the left arm than the right. This is due to more people being right-handed and holding the child's left hand or wrist while walking. It is not uncommon, however, for the child to present with a history of a fall or rolling over in bed.[1]

This orthopedic injury involves the region of the elbow (Figure 69-1). The annular ligament is a thick band that wraps around the upper radial neck and radial head (Figure 69-1A). It guides the radial head as the forearm moves through pronation and supination. The injury causes the radial head to become partially dislocated from its articulation with the ulna and the capitellum of the humerus while the forearm is in a pronated state.

The annular ligament then slips proximally and its lateral end becomes entrapped between the radial head and the capitellum (Figure 69-1B). The forearm becomes locked in pronation due to the entrapped annular ligament. This condition is painless as long as the forearm is held in pronation. Supination of the forearm causes pain, so the child holds the extremity in pronation. The act of supination would also spontaneously return the annular ligament to its anatomic position and reduce the subluxation.

Children will present in no apparent distress.[2] They are usually resting comfortably and have some reservation in using the affected extremity. The arm will be held with slight flexion of the elbow and pronation of the forearm (Figure 69-2A). The child may point to an area of pain, but this is not often the case. A child may be much more comfortable with the parent examining and questioning areas of tenderness as opposed to the unknown and sometimes intimidating physician.

Radiographs are not required unless other trauma or diagnoses are suspected. If radiographs are obtained, the child often returns from the radiology suite using the affected extremity. Radial head subluxations often reduce spontaneously during positioning for radiographs.

INDICATIONS

Any child presenting with the inability to utilize the partially flexed elbow, the forearm pronated and adducted, and a mechanism for a radial head subluxation

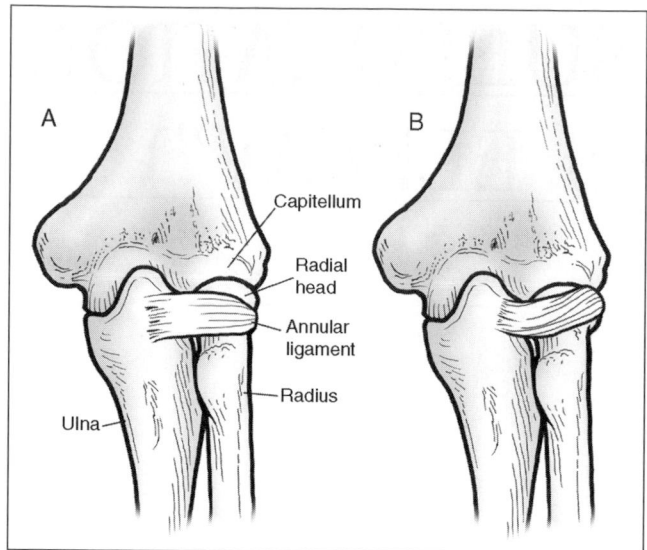

FIGURE 69-1 Anatomy of the elbow region. *A.* Normal anatomy. *B.* A radial head subluxation. Note the entrapped annular ligament.

should be reduced. Many physicians may be hesitant to repeat the procedure multiple times if a child was not utilizing the arm normally within 15 to 30 minutes after a clinically successful reduction. However, if the radiographs appear normal and a repeat history and physical examination are consistent with the original diagnosis, a decision to repeat the reduction should be considered.

CONTRAINDICATIONS

The presence of edema, ecchymoses, tenderness other than over the radial head, suspicion of a fracture, or a mechanism of injury not consistent with a radial head subluxation should first be evaluated radiographically. The presence of any distal neurologic or vascular compromise excludes the diagnosis of a radial head subluxation.

EQUIPMENT

No equipment is required for the reduction of a radial head subluxation.

PATIENT PREPARATION

Explain the procedure to the patient and caregiver. Obtain an informed consent to perform the procedure. Place the patient sitting in the parent's lap or supine on an examination table or gurney. No premedication is required.

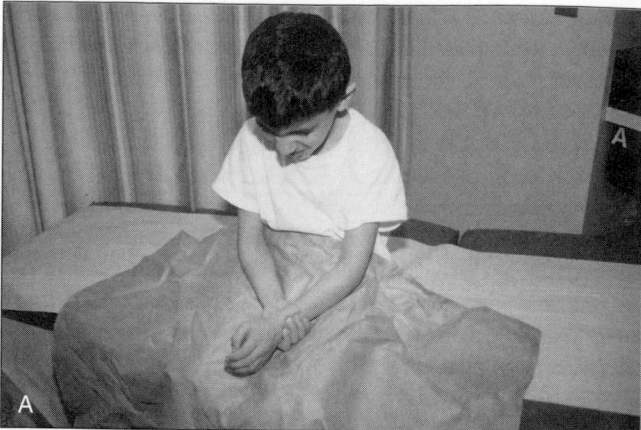

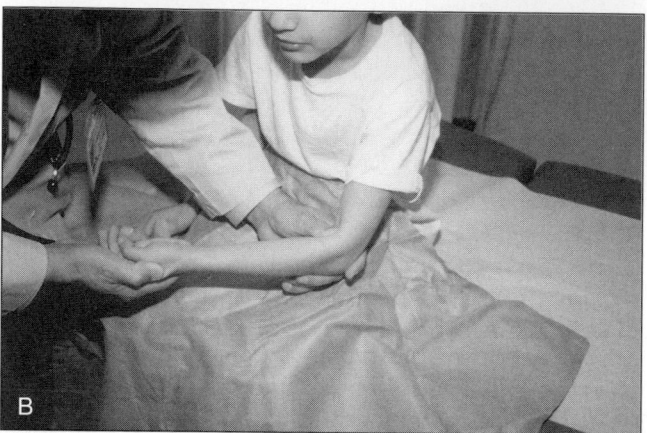

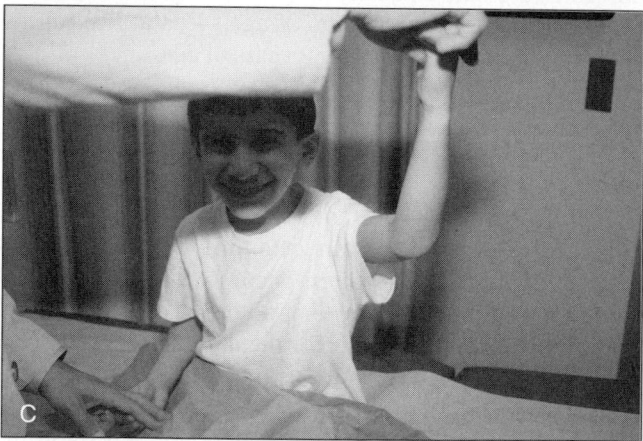

FIGURE 69-2 A child with a radial head subluxation. *A.* The subluxed right forearm is held flexed, pronated, and adducted. *B.* Reduction technique. *C.* Post-reduction. The forearm is freely mobile with normal extension and abduction.

TECHNIQUE

Place the nondominant hand on the child's elbow with the thumb over the radial head (Figure 69-3*A*). This will aid in palpation of the traditional "click" of reduction. Gently grasp the child's wrist with the dominant hand

(Figure 69-3A). Perform the following maneuvers in one smooth motion to reduce the subluxation. Apply distal traction while supinating the forearm (Figure 69-3B), followed by flexion of the elbow (Figure 69-3C). A click may be felt as the radial head is reduced.[1,4] If not, flex the forearm until the hand is upright. Other methods of reduction are often compared to this method.[3,5]

If you feel the traditional click or feel satisfied with the attempted reduction, allow 5 to 15 minutes to pass and return for a repeat examination. Children may cry at the end of the procedure but will generally only do so for a moment. As the child feels more comfortable, they will proceed to use the arm (Figure 69-2C). This freedom of use can be accelerated by the caregiver or physician stimulating the patient to use the arm with an incentive (e.g., by offering candy, a pen, or a popsicle for the child to grab).

ASSESSMENT

The child should have uninhibited use of the forearm within 30 minutes. If not, reconsider the diagnosis. Alternative diagnoses include clavicular fractures, distal humeral fractures, osteomyelitis, radial head fractures, septic arthritis, and stress fractures. Reevaluate the elbow joint for signs of trauma. Obtain plain radiographs if not done previously. Full recovery may take 24 to 48 hours if the reduction is delayed for more than 8 hours from the time of injury.

AFTERCARE

Radiographs, immobilization, splinting, analgesics, and orthopedic follow-up are not necessary if the subluxation is reduced and the child is using their arm. Educate the caregiver regarding the mechanism of injury and prevention of future subluxations.

Phone consultation with an Orthopedic Surgeon is recommended if the reduction is unsuccessful. It is not unusual to have a spontaneous reduction on repeat examination and follow-up. Immobilize the arm until the child is evaluated by an Orthopedic Surgeon. Immobilization will aid in pain relief. Consider the use of nonsteroidal anti-inflammatory drugs.

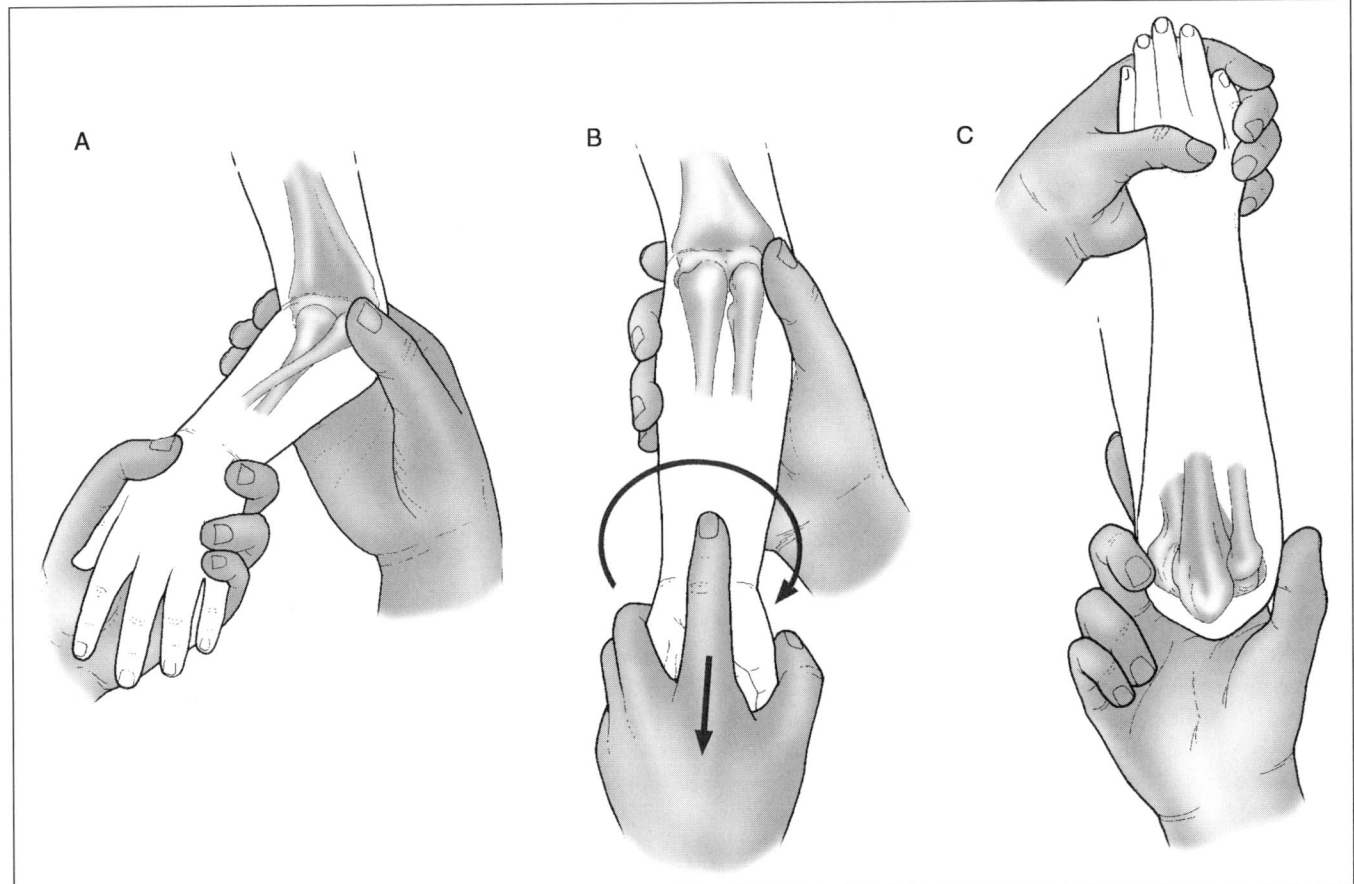

FIGURE 69-3 Reduction of a radial head subluxation. *A.* Positioning of the physician's hands. *B.* Distal traction is applied (*straight arrow*) while supinating the forearm (*curved arrow*). *C.* The forearm is maximally flexed.

COMPLICATIONS

There are no complications associated with the reduction of a radial head subluxation.

SUMMARY

A radial head subluxation is one of the more common orthopedic injuries of childhood. Children present with the inability to utilize the affected upper extremity. They hold the forearm flexed, pronated, and adducted. The reduction technique is quick and simple. It is important to educate the caregivers regarding the mechanism of injury and prevention of future subluxations.

REFERENCES

1. Schunk JE: Radial head subluxation: epidemiology and treatment of 87 episodes. *Ann Emerg Med* 1990; 19(9):1019–1023.

2. Quan L, Marcuse EK: The epidemiology and treatment of radial head subluxation. *Am J Dis Child* 1985; 139:1194–1197.

3. McDonald J, Whitelaw C, Goldsmith LJ: Radial head subluxation: comparing two methods of reduction. *Acad Emerg Med* 1999; 6(7):715–718.

4. McNamara R: Management of common dislocations, in Roberts JR, Hedges JR (eds): *Clinical Procedures in Emergency Medicine*, 3rd ed. Philadelphia: Saunders, 1998:834–836.

5. Macias CG, Bothner J, Wiebe R: A comparison of supination/flexion to hyperpronation in reduction of radial head subluxations. *Pediatrics* 1998; 102(1):133.

6. Teach SJ, Schutzman SA: Prospective study of recurrent radial head subluxation. *Arch Pediatr Adolesc Med* 1996; 150(2):164–166.

7. Jongschaap HC, Youngson GG, Beattie TF: The epidemiology of radial head subluxation ("pulled elbow") in the Aberdeen city area. *Health Bull (Edinb)* 1990; 48(2):58–61.

8. Gotrell CB: Radiologic findings in radial head subluxation. *Am J Dis Child* 1986; 140(4):856.

Chapter 70
INTERPHALANGEAL JOINT DISLOCATION REDUCTION

Geraldine L. Stratton
Ritu Malik

INTRODUCTION

Closed hand injuries, including dislocations of the interphalangeal (IP) joints of the fingers, are among the most common injuries encountered in the Emergency Department.[1-3] Many finger dislocations are secondary to sports-related events. The proximal interphalangeal (PIP) joint is especially vulnerable in ball-handling activities.[2,4] IP dislocations are second only to shoulder dislocations in incidence and are generally easy to reduce.[4] IP joint dislocations may lead to chronic pain, swelling, stiffness, deformity, or early degenerative arthritis if not properly treated.[1,5,6] Emergency Physicians must be capable diagnosing and managing IP joint dislocations.

ANATOMY AND PATHOPHYSIOLOGY

The PIP joint is a hinge joint with a bicondylar formation (Figure 70-1). It allows only for flexion and extension from 0 degrees to approximately 120 degrees.[1,7,8] The convex proximal phalangeal head articulates with the concave base of the middle phalanx.[4] This configuration provides the inherent static stability of the joint. Further stability, both static and dynamic, is provided by the surrounding ligaments and tendons that essentially form a box complex around the joint (Figure 70-2). The box complex supporting the articular surface is composed of the volar plate, the lateral and collateral accessory ligaments, and the extensor tendon. The volar plate is attached to the middle phalanx distally, where it is made of a dense, fibrous connective tissue. The volar plate thins proximally into a membranous portion that becomes continuous with the synovial reflection, allowing for folding with flexion of the digit. This configuration provides resistance against dorsal displacement of the middle phalanx.[4] The extensor mechanism is composed of three slips: the central slip and two lateral slips (or bands) on the radial and ulnar sides (Figures 70-3 and 70-4). These slips provide dorsal support against dislocation of the joint. The lateral collateral ligaments bridge across the PIP joint on either side and stabilize it against lateral stress.[3]

The distal interphalangeal (DIP) joint is a broad-based hinge joint that allows approximately 90 degrees of flexion.[3] Like the PIP joint, the DIP joint permits very little lateral or rotatory motion.[3] The distal phalanx is attached firmly to the skin and subcutaneous tissue by osteocutaneous fibers. This firm attachment to the overlying soft tissue explains why DIP joint dislocations are almost always open.

The IP joint of the thumb is similar in structure to the DIP joint of the other fingers. Thumb IP joint dislocations tend to be open, similar to DIP dislocations. Thumb dislocations are uncommon despite the fact that it is the most mobile joint of the hand and provides 50 percent of the hand's function.

PATTERNS OF INJURY

Dislocations of the PIP joint are the most common and may be classified as dorsal, volar, and lateral (Figure 70-5).[1,4] Each type of dislocation results from a different mechanism of injury and has specific associated complications.

Dorsal (or posterior) dislocations are the most common type of PIP joint dislocation (Figures 70-5A and 70-6). They usually result from hyperextension injuries.[4,7,8] A dorsal dislocation occurs when the middle phalanx is displaced dorsally from the proximal phalanx. These dislocations involve injury to the volar plate and may be associated with an avulsion fracture of the base of the middle phalanx. Avulsion fractures involving greater than 30 percent of the articular surface are considered unstable and require immediate referral to an Orthopedic Surgeon[4] (Figure 70-5B).

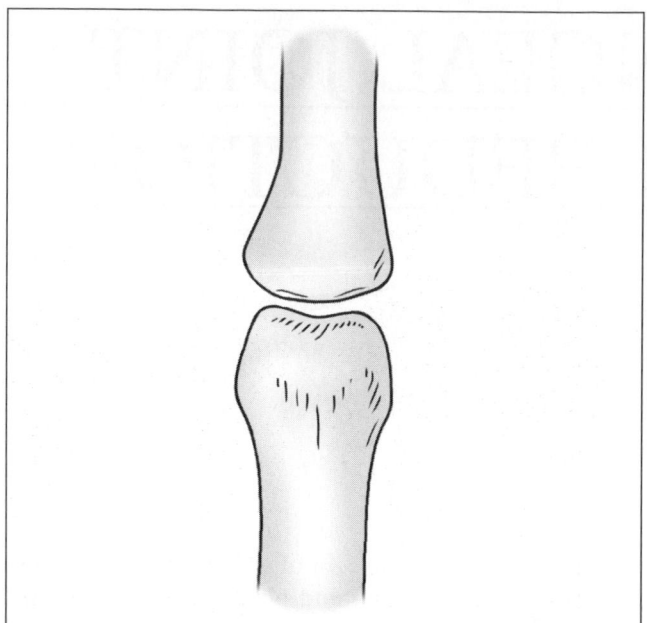

FIGURE 70-1 The bicondylar IP joint.

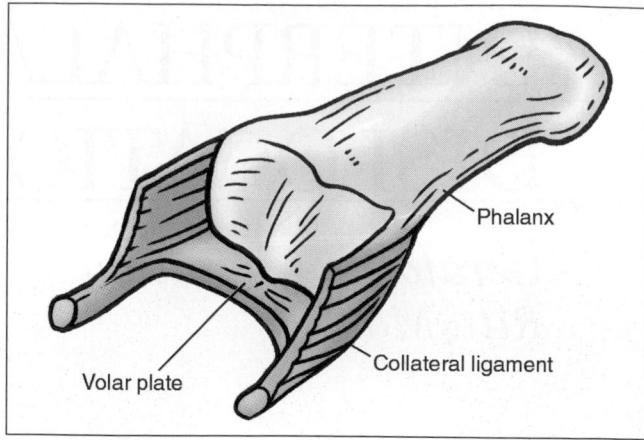

FIGURE 70-2 A schematic drawing of the box complex surrounding the PIP joint.

Volar (or anterior) PIP joint dislocations are far less common and are more severe than dorsal PIP joint dislocations (Figure 70-5C). They occur from a simultaneous axial load and a rotational force on the IP joint. Volar PIP joint dislocations are associated with rupture of the collateral ligament and disruption of the central slip of the extensor tendon mechanism. These injuries may preclude closed reduction.[4] If left untreated, volar PIP joint dislocations may result in a boutonniere deformity.[1]

Lateral PIP joint dislocations are uncommon.[3] They result from a pure radial or ulnar force on the joint with either partial or complete rupture of the collateral ligament (Figure 70-5D). Lateral PIP joint dislocations are often reducible by closed methods.

Distal IP joint dislocations and IP joint dislocations of the thumb (Figure 70-7) are rare. They are often due to a direct blow to the distal portion of the digit.[7] They are most often dorsally dislocated and frequently open due to the firm attachment of the distal phalanx to the subcutaneous tissue and skin. All open dislocations require immediate orthopedic consultation.

IP joint dislocations of the toes are primarily dorsal. They occur secondary to an axial compression load to the digit, such as kicking a toe against a wall. IP joint dislocations of the toe are reduced similarly to dorsal IP dislocations of the finger.

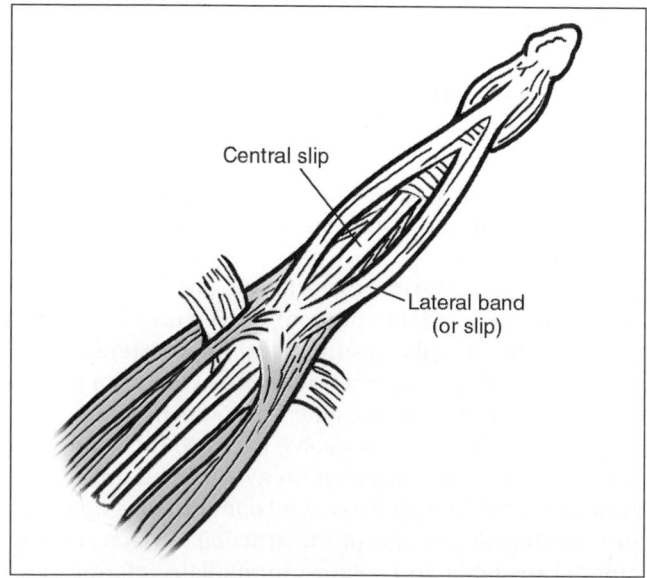

FIGURE 70-3 Dorsal view of the extensor mechanism.

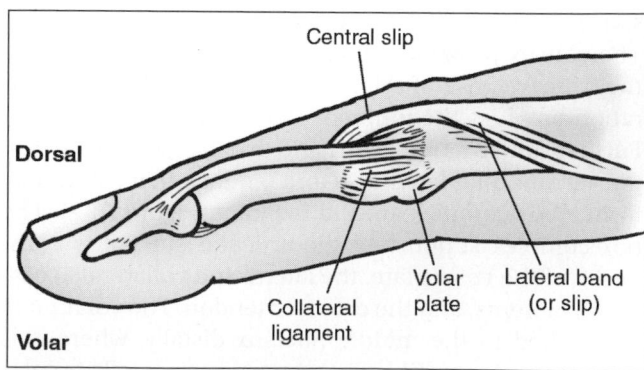

FIGURE 70-4 Lateral view of the digit, demonstrating the anatomy and supporting structures. This support consists of the collateral ligaments and the volar plate, forming a box complex around the volar and lateral aspects of the joint. The extensor mechanism consists of the central and the lateral slips on the dorsal aspect of the digit.

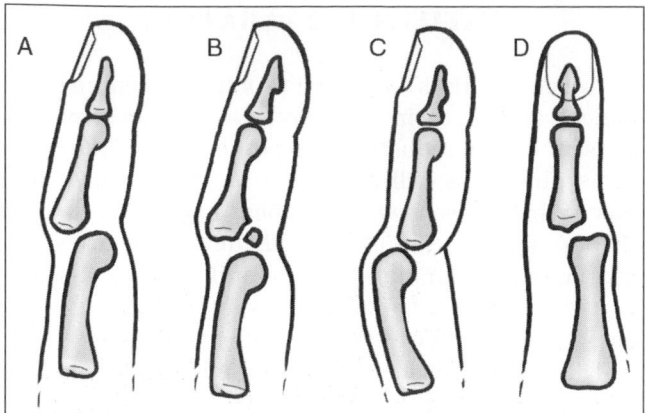

FIGURE 70-5 Dislocations of the proximal interphalangeal joint. *A.* Dorsal dislocation. This is the most common type of dislocation. The middle phalanx is displaced posteriorly in relation to the proximal phalanx. *B.* Fracture-dislocation. A complicated dislocation with a fracture involving greater than 30 percent of the articular surface. *C.* Volar dislocation. The middle phalanx is displaced anteriorly in relation to the proximal phalanx. *D.* Lateral dislocation. The middle phalanx is displaced laterally in relation to the proximal phalanx.

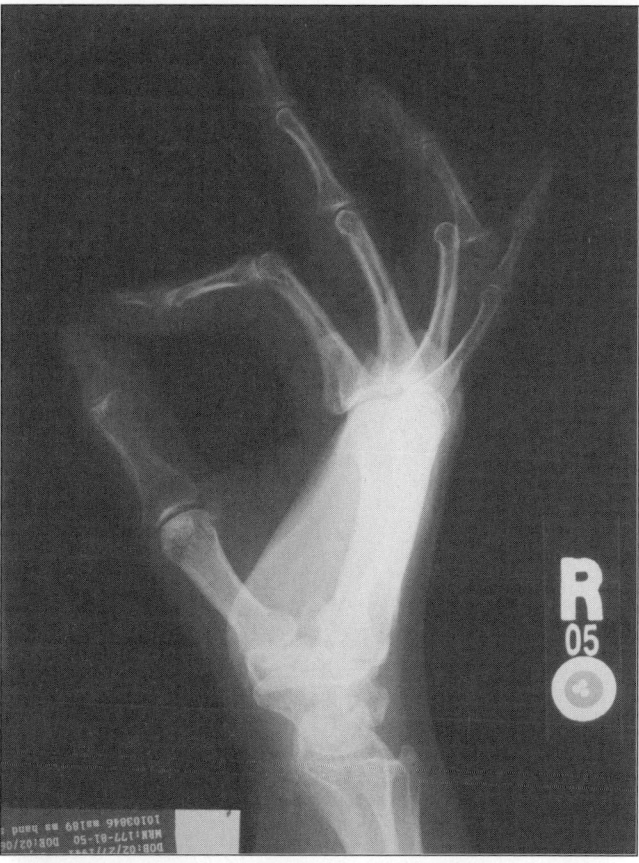

FIGURE 70-6 Radiograph of a dorsal dislocation of the PIP joint of the fourth finger.

INDICATIONS

The two principal indications for closed reduction of dislocated IP joints are the potential for joint stability after the reduction and the proximity to the date of injury. Joint stability is determined by a physical examination in which there is no displacement during active range of motion or gentle passive stressing of the joint after reduction. Administering a digital block may facilitate the physical examination.[4] Joint dislocations that are usually stable after reduction include dorsal and lateral dislocations, dislocations with small avulsion fractures involving less than 30 percent of the articular surface, and dislocations with incomplete tears of surrounding ligaments. Anteroposterior and lateral radiographs should be obtained prior to the reduction to evaluate the digit completely. The lateral film will aid in picking up subtle dislocations and avulsion fractures. Acute IP dislocations presenting fewer than 3 weeks from the time of injury can be safely reduced in the Emergency Department.[6]

The acute volar dislocation is a rare injury and its management is controversial. Some experts feel that at least one attempt should be made at closed reduction, while others feel that these injuries should be managed by surgical reduction.[8] The authors believe that these injuries should be immediately evaluated by an Orthopedic Surgeon.

CONTRAINDICATIONS

Certain dislocations require immediate evaluation by an Orthopedic Surgeon for repair and reduction. Closed reduction should not be attempted in the Emergency Department for unstable, chronic, complex, and open injuries. Instability in a joint through active range of motion indicates complete and multiple ligament disruption requiring surgical repair.[3,8] A fracture-dislocation involving greater than 30 percent of the articular surface represents an unstable joint.[3] Chronic injuries greater than 3 weeks old generally necessitate surgical repair.[7] Occasionally, ligaments and/or tendons may become trapped by bony and soft tissue structures in and around the IP joint that will resist traction and reduction. These complex or irreducible dislocations require surgical release of the interposed soft tissue.[1,7,9,10] Open IP joint dislocations require immediate referral to an Orthopedic Surgeon for reduction after initiation of antibiotics in the Emergency Department.

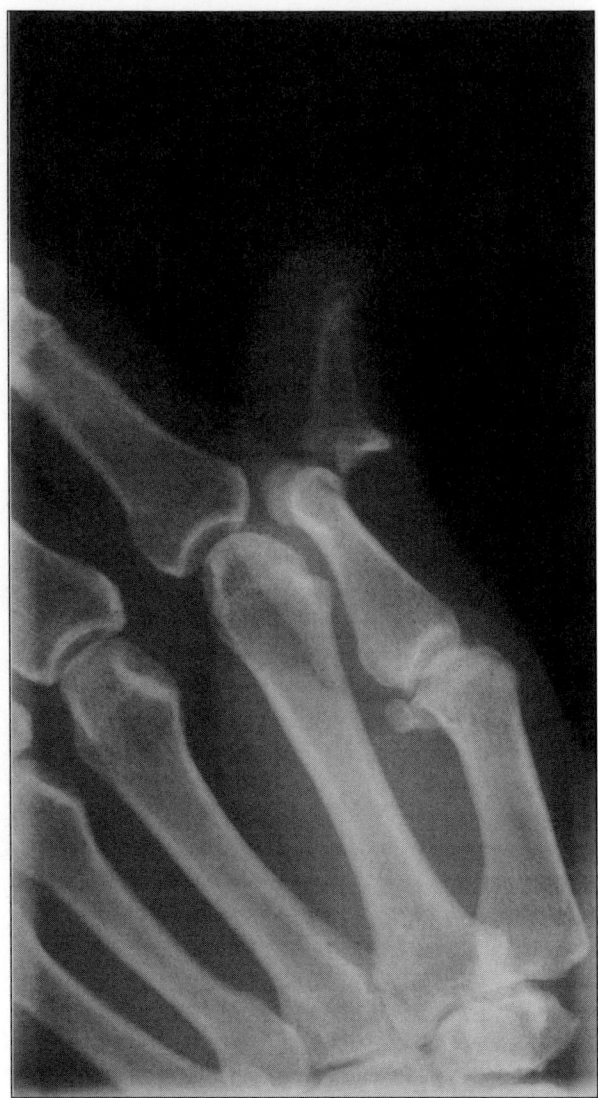

FIGURE 70-7 Radiograph of a dorsal dislocation of the IP joint of the thumb.

EQUIPMENT

Digital Block

Povidone iodine solution
27 gauge needle, 2 inches long
5 mL syringe
Alcohol swab
Local anesthetic solution without epinephrine, 1% lidocaine or 0.25 to 0.5% bupivacaine

Post-Reduction Splint

Adhesive tape, ½ inch
Gauze padding
Aluminum finger splint with foam padding
Scissors

PATIENT PREPARATION

Explain the risks and benefits of the procedure to the patient and/or their representative. Obtain a written consent for the reduction procedure. As an alternative, some physicians will document in the patient's chart that verbal consent was obtained. Inform the patient that up to 30 percent of PIP and DIP joint injuries may remain swollen for many months and will likely result in permanent joint enlargement. Loss of motion and residual soreness may last several months.[1,6]

The use of local anesthesia is based on physician and patient preference. Many physicians and patients believe that the pain of reduction is less than that of a digital block and more tolerable. For this reason, many physicians will reduce an IP joint dislocation without the use of local anesthesia.

Clean the finger of any dirt and debris. Apply povidone iodine solution and allow it to dry. Insert a 27 gauge needle into the lateral aspect of the base of the proximal phalanx. Inject 0.5 mL of local anesthetic solution. Redirect the needle dorsally while depositing 1 mL of local anesthetic solution. Withdraw the needle and redirect it volarly while depositing 1 mL of local anesthetic solution. Repeat the procedure on the medial aspect of the base of the proximal phalanx. Refer to Chapter 106 for a more detailed description of the methods to anesthetize a finger.

TECHNIQUES

DORSAL DISLOCATION OF THE PIP JOINT

A dorsal dislocation of the PIP joint involves a partial or complete disruption of the volar plate. Most dorsal dislocations of the PIP joint are easily reduced (Figure 70-8). Firmly grasp the affected finger with the dominant hand. Grasp the base of the proximal phalanx with the nondominant hand. Hyperextend the PIP joint and apply longitudinal traction to separate the articular surfaces (Figure 70-8B). The nondominant hand is used to stabilize the proximal phalanx and apply countertraction. Flex the PIP joint while maintaining traction and apply dorsal pressure on the base of the middle phalanx (Figure 70-8C). This should restore the proper alignment of the proximal and middle phalanx.

Immobilize the reduced PIP joint in 30 degrees of flexion for approximately 3 weeks (Figure 70-8D). Alternatively, tape the injured finger to an adjacent unaffected finger ("buddy taping"). Gauze padding must be placed between the fingers before buddy taping to prevent skin breakdown. During immobilization, it is important to avoid hyperextension if the finger is buddy taped, as this may lead to further injury of the volar plate. The presence of an avulsion fracture involving less

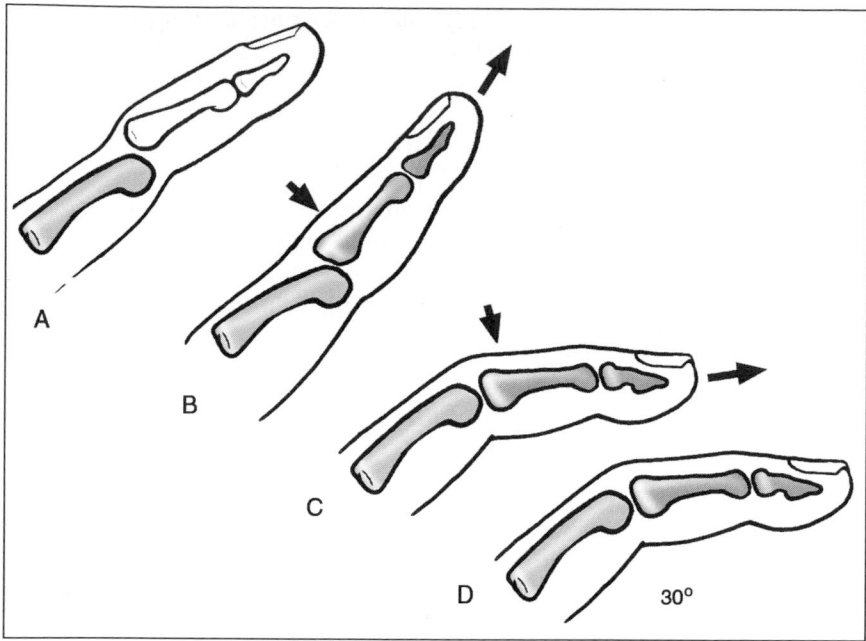

FIGURE 70-8 Reduction of a dislocation. *A.* Dorsal dislocation of the PIP joint. *B.* The deformity is exaggerated by hyperextending the distal phalanx and applying longitudinal (distal) traction to the digit. *C.* The PIP joint is flexed while placing dorsally applied pressure on the base of the middle phalanx and maintaining distal traction. *D.* The PIP joint is placed in 30 degrees of flexion prior to immobilization.

than 30 percent of the articular surface does not alter this management plan.

Rarely, a dorsal dislocation can be irreducible due to interposed soft tissue or impingement of the proximal phalangeal head between the central slip and the lateral bands.[9] This type of dislocation is referred to as "complex." Failure of two or three attempts at closed reduction should raise the suspicion of an irreducible joint and an Orthopedic Surgeon should be consulted.

VOLAR DISLOCATION OF THE PIP JOINT

Volar dislocations of the PIP joint are almost always accompanied by an injury to the central slip of the extensor tendon, causing an inability to extend the PIP joint (Figure 70-9). These dislocations are generally irreducible and need early consultation with an Orthopedic Surgeon for operative repair due to the extensive soft tissue damage. Although controversial, some authors recommend a single attempt at closed reduction by applying a longitudinal (distal) force, hyperextending the joint, and applying dorsal pressure to the base of the middle phalanx. During this procedure, the metacarpophalangeal and DIP joints should be flexed and the wrist extended to relax the anteriorly displaced lateral bands and extensor mechanism. Splint the joint in extension and arrange for early follow-up with an Orthopedic Surgeon if closed reduction is achieved. **It is important to note that splinting in even mild flexion or "buddy taping" may lead to a boutonniere deformity (Figure 70-9).**

LATERAL DISLOCATION OF THE PIP JOINT

Lateral dislocations of the PIP joint involve a partial or complete rupture of the radial and ulnar collateral ligaments. There is a 6:1 ratio of radial to ulnar collateral ligament tears with the digit being displaced in the opposite direction of the ligament rupture.[3] Generally, reduction is easy and the joint is stable after the procedure. Recreate the injury and apply longitudinal (distal) traction to the finger. Bring (move) the distal phalanx in line with the proximal phalanx.

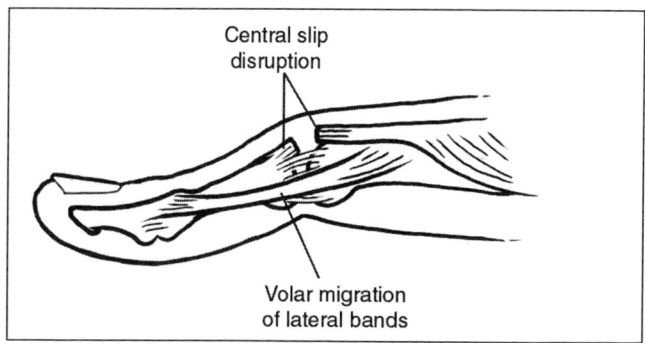

Central slip
disruption

Volar migration
of lateral bands

FIGURE 70-9 The boutonniere deformity of the finger is a potential complication of a volar dislocation of the PIP joint. This results from a disruption of the central slip of the extensor tendon over the PIP joint on the dorsal aspect of the finger. A central slip disruption should be suspected in patients with pain primarily over the PIP joint and the inability to extend the middle phalanx fully against active resistance. Radiographic findings are usually unremarkable.

After reduction, determine by physical examination if the collateral ligaments are partially or completely torn. Buddy tape the finger to the adjacent finger for 3 weeks for incomplete collateral ligament tears. Early active motion of the finger is encouraged after this time. Complete collateral ligament tears are repaired operatively and require early consultation by an Orthopedic Surgeon.

INTERPHALANGEAL JOINT OF THE THUMB DISLOCATION

Dislocations of the IP joint of the thumb are rare. The injury is usually dorsal and open. If the dislocation is closed, the joint can be reduced in the same manner as PIP dislocations of the fingers.[11] Splint the reduced joint in slight flexion and arrange for early follow-up by an Orthopedic Surgeon.

DISTAL INTERPHALANGEAL JOINT DISLOCATION

DIP joint dislocations are rare, usually dorsal, and open. They are easily reduced in a similar manner to other IP joint dislocations and are generally stable after reduction.[12] Reduction is accomplished by application of longitudinal (distal) traction, hyperextension of the distal phalanx, and the application of dorsal pressure on the base of the distal phalanx. Immobilize only the DIP joint with a dorsal splint in 5 to 10 degrees of flexion. Arrange for follow-up with an Orthopedic Surgeon.

The DIP joint may be irreducible if there is an avulsion and entrapment of the volar plate in the joint, entrapment of the long flexor tendon in the joint, or entrapment of a bony fragment. Immediate consultation with an Orthopedic Surgeon should be sought if the DIP joint is irreducible.

ASSESSMENT

Obtain post-reduction radiographs of the digit to identify an avulsion injury or an incomplete reduction. Test the joint for functional stability by having the patient actively move the injured finger through a full range of motion. Stability of the joint is maintained if the collateral ligaments and volar plate are intact. Test the collateral ligaments by applying radially and ulnarly directed stresses with the joint in 20 degrees of flexion. Test the integrity of the volar plate by having the patient hyperextend the joint and comparing the range of motion to that of the other fingers. The joint is considered stable if there is no displacement during active range of motion and passive stressing of the joint. If stable, place the joint in an appropriate splint and refer the patient to an Orthopedic Surgeon for follow-up. Immediately consult an Orthopedic Surgeon if the joint is not easily reduced or if it is not stable after the reduction. All open dislocations require immediate evaluation by an Orthopedic Surgeon for irrigation, reduction, and closure.

AFTERCARE

Splinting of any finger injury should provide adequate immobilization and protection while allowing maximal range of motion of the unaffected joints. The method of splinting for each specific dislocation is discussed in the "Technique" section for each type of dislocation.

COMPLICATIONS

Most complications of IP joint dislocations are secondary to the injury itself rather than the reduction procedure. Even seemingly minor injuries can have complications such as prolonged swelling, pain, and stiffness. A thorough evaluation of the digit, prompt diagnosis, and proper treatment will help minimize these complications.

Complications of the reduction procedure are primarily related to failure of reduction. Entrapment of soft tissues should be suspected in cases with multiple failed attempts at reduction. Numerous attempts at reduction may lead to trauma at the articular surface, predisposing to the development of premature degenerative arthritis. Irreducible or complex IP joint dislocations require an immediate evaluation by an Orthopedic Surgeon.

Prolonged or improper splinting of a joint can lead to chronic complications. Extended splinting and immobilization can lead to permanent joint stiffness. In general, IP joints should not be immobilized for greater than 3 weeks. Inappropriate splinting of a volar dislocation in even mild flexion may lead to long-term complications such as the boutonniere deformity (Figure 70-9).

SUMMARY

Injuries to the IP joints of the hand are commonly encountered in the Emergency Department and may be associated with significant morbidity. The most common injury encountered is a dorsal IP joint dislocation. Other dislocations include volar and lateral IP joint dislocations. A thorough understanding of the anatomy and function of the IP joint is essential to diagnose and treat these common injuries appropriately. A detailed physical examination of the soft tissues, bones, and neurovascular structures is necessary. Radiographic evaluation is required for all potential injuries, including an anteroposterior and a lateral view of the affected digit. Acute stable dislocations can be reduced immediately in the Emergency Department. An Orthopedic Surgeon should evaluate any unstable, chronic, open, or complex dislocation. Joints reduced in the Emergency Department must be splinted and appropriate follow-up arranged with an Orthopedic Surgeon.

REFERENCES

1. Frieberg A, Pollard BA, Macdonald MR, et al: Management of proximal interphalangeal joint injuries. *J Trauma* 1999; 46(3):523–528.
2. Mastey RD, Weiss AP, Akelman E: Primary care of hand and wrist athletic injuries. *Clin Sports Med* 1997; 16(4):705–724.
3. Hossfeld GE, Uehara DT: Acute joint injuries of the hand. *Emerg Med Clin North Am* 1993; 11(3):781–795.
4. Bailie DS, Benson LS, Marymont JV: Proximal interphalangeal joint injuries of the hand: Part 1. Anatomy and diagnosis. *Am J Orthop* 1996; 25(7):474–477.
5. Kiefhaber TR, Stern PJ: Fracture dislocations of the proximal interphalangeal joint. *J Hand Surg (Am)* 1998; 23(3):368–380.
6. Benson LS, Bailie DS: Proximal interphalangeal joint injuries of the hand: Part 2. Treatment and complications. *Am J Orthop* 1996; 25(8):527–530.
7. Green DP, Butler TE: Fractures and dislocations in the hand, in Rockwood CA, Green DP, Bucholz RW, et al (eds): *Rockwood and Green's Fractures in Adults,* 2nd ed. Philadelphia: Lippincott, 1996:607–744.
8. McNamara R: Management of common dislocations, in Roberts RR, Hedges JR (eds): *Clinical Procedures in Emergency Medicine,* 3rd ed. Philadelphia: Saunders, 1998; 836–843.
9. Hoffman DF, Schaffer TC: Management of common finger injuries. *Am Fam Physician* 1991; 43(5):1594–1607.
10. Stiles BM, Drake DB, Gear AJ, et al: Metacarpophalangeal joint dislocation: indications for open surgical reduction. *J Emerg Med* 1997; 15(5):669–671.
11. Nakae H, Endo S, Hoshi S: Two cases of closed dislocation of the interphalangeal joint of the thumb. *Arch Orthop Trauma Surg* 1996; 115(3–4):236–237.
12. Abouzahr MK, Poblete JV: Irreducible dorsal dislocation of the distal interphalangeal joint: case report and literature review. *J Trauma* 1997; 42(4): 743–745.

Chapter 71
HIP JOINT DISLOCATION REDUCTION

Teresita M. Hogan

INTRODUCTION

Hip dislocations are true orthopedic emergencies. The Emergency Physician must be capable of reducing a dislocated hip. Neurovascular damage to the hip and leg is a consequence of a hip dislocation. The complication of avascular necrosis is time-dependent. **The longer a hip is dislocated, the higher the incidence of avascular necrosis.** Dislocation of a hip for more than 6 hours almost universally results in this devastating complication.

The main etiologies of a hip dislocation are traumatic dislocations of a normal hip, mechanical dislocations of a prosthetic hip, spontaneous dislocations, and pathologic dislocations. Less impressive mechanisms may result in hip dislocations in the young and the elderly. A simple fall from standing may dislocate a geriatric hip. Dislocations may occur with minor force in children, as during athletic activities.

Many techniques have been described to reduce dislocated hips.[1-7] The Emergency Physician must be familiar with some of these methods and how to apply them appropriately to optimize patient management and outcome. Dislocations of both normal and prosthetic hips are seen in the Emergency Department. Dislocations of prosthetic hips are now more common than those of normal hips.[8] While these are not associated with avascular necrosis, the pressure from the dislocated prosthetic head may result in other neurovascular complications.

ANATOMY AND PATHOPHYSIOLOGY

Ball-and-socket joints are inherently stable. The strong muscles, ligaments, and fibrous joint capsule of the hip reinforce this innate stability. Consequently, in the average adult, a great deal of force must be transmitted to dislocate the hip. This is significant, as the patient with a hip dislocation may have other life-threatening injuries that take precedence over the management of the hip dislocation. The mortality associated with a hip dislocation results from associated injuries of the head, thorax, or pelvis.

Hip dislocations are classified into anterior, posterior, and central based upon the relationship of the dislocated femoral head to the acetabulum. Anterior hip dislocations occur with the leg in a neutral or abducted position. The femoral head is pushed anterior to the coronal plane of the acetabulum. These patients present in extreme pain with the hip and knee flexed 90 degrees. The leg will be held in external rotation. A slight shortening of the leg may be noted, but this is difficult to detect with the knee in flexion. There are three subtypes of an anterior hip dislocation: anterior obturator, anterior iliac, and anterior pubic. The femoral head displaces medially and lies in the obturator canal in anterior obturator dislocations. The femoral head moves superiorly and lies over the iliac wing in anterior iliac dislocations. The femoral head moves inferiorly over the pubic ramus in anterior pubic dislocations.

Posterior hip dislocations are the most common type. They account for nearly 90 percent of all hip dislocations. This is because the posterolateral half of the femoral neck lies outside the joint capsule and the weaker posterior support of the hip. Posterior dislocations result from force transmitted along the femoral shaft with the leg adducted. The most common mechanism of injury is a motor vehicle collision where the knees strike the dashboard and the femoral head is pushed posterior to the coronal plane of the acetabulum. The presentation of a posterior dislocation is of a patient in extreme pain. The leg will be internally rotated with marked knee flexion and adduction of the thigh. The femoral head is rarely visible but may be palpable in the buttock region. Posterior hip dislocations are further categorized into posterior ischial and posterior iliac subtypes. The femoral head is displaced inferiorly and lies over the ischium in posterior ischial dislocations. The femoral head is displaced superiorly and lies over the iliac wing in posterior iliac dislocations.

Central hip dislocations are the rarest form. The femoral head remains on the same coronal plane as the acetabulum in central dislocations. However, it is displaced superiorly. Most central hip dislocations are associated with acetabular fractures.

INDICATIONS

All hip dislocations must be reduced. **Emergent hip reduction is indicated when distal neurologic or vascular deficits are present or if the Orthopedic Surgeon is not immediately available.** The incidence of avascular necrosis is time-dependent and necessitates reduction as soon as possible to limit this complication.

CONTRAINDICATIONS

Any life-threatening conditions must be treated before the hip is reduced. Closed reduction is contraindicated if a surgical indication for repair exists. Surgical exploration is required for hip dislocations associated with femoral head fractures, femoral shaft fractures, or the finding of sciatic nerve dysfunction. Surgery is also indicated for an irreducible dislocation, persistent instability of the joint after closed reduction, and for any postreduction neurovascular deficits.

EQUIPMENT

Procedural sedation equipment and supplies
   (Chapter 109)
Assistants
Sheets

PATIENT PREPARATION

The patient must be appropriately stabilized with prioritization of the ABCs (airway, breathing, and circulation). Life-threatening associated injuries and comorbid conditions must be adequately addressed. Obtain plain radiographs to define the anatomic dislocation pattern, to rule out any associated fractures, and to guide relocation attempts.

Explain the risks, benefits, complications, and aftercare of the reduction procedure and obtain an informed consent from the patient and/or their representative.

The patient must be sedated to achieve optimal muscle relaxation and pain control. Perform procedural sedation after obtaining a separate informed consent for this procedure.

TECHNIQUES

Hip reduction techniques have been described with the patient in every imaginable position.[1-9] The relative success rates for each technique have not been reliably reported.[8] Therefore physicians typically use the technique that was demonstrated to them during their residency training. **The editors recommend the use of the Allis maneuver as the treatment of choice for the reduction of posterior hip dislocations.** The other techniques are described in the text primarily for historical information, to give the reader full information regarding procedures that have been used and described for the reduction of this common problem, and as alternative techniques if the Allis maneuver is not successful in reducing the hip.

ALLIS MANEUVER
This is the most common hip reduction method (Figure 71-1A). It was described by Allis in 1893.[1] The technique has been improved by the addition of procedural sedation. Place the patient supine and perform procedural sedation. Instruct an assistant to stabilize the pelvis to the gurney by pressing down on the anterior superior iliac spines. It may be necessary for the assistant to use both hands on the side of the pelvis associated with the hip dislocation to stabilize the pelvis. Flex the affected knee and hip 90 degrees. Grasp the affected knee in both hands. Apply axial traction to the thigh with incrementally increasing force. Simultaneously rotate the femur laterally and medially until the hip relocates.

If relocation is not easily accomplished, instruct a second assistant to apply lateral traction to the inner thigh of the affected proximal femur (Figure 71-1B). Repeat the entire procedure with the addition of lateral traction to reduce the dislocation.

MODIFIED ALLIS MANEUVER
This technique incorporates all of the maneuvers described above. Additionally, place the hip in maximum adduction. Apply longitudinal traction to the femur while an assistant presses down on the pelvis with one hand and pushes the head of the affected femur toward the acetabulum with the other hand.

GRAVITY METHOD OF STIMSON
Place the patient prone on the gurney. Perform procedural sedation. Monitoring may be more difficult due to the prone positioning. **Extra attention must be paid to**

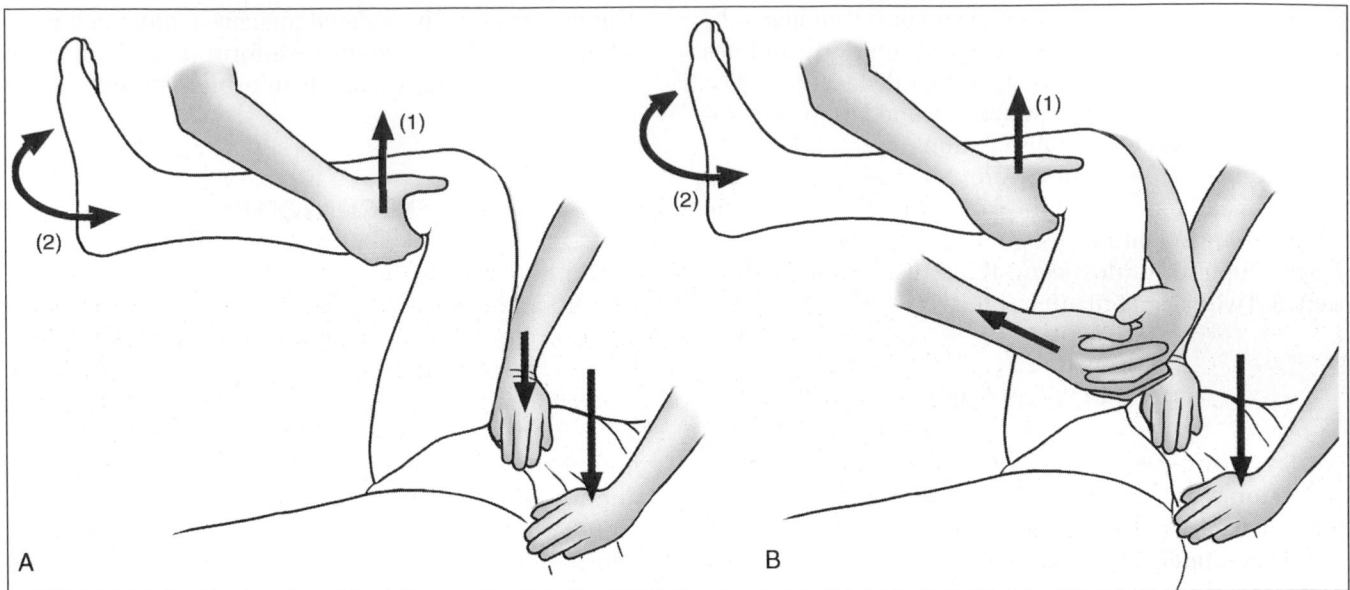

FIGURE 71-1 The Allis maneuver. *A.* An assistant stabilizes the pelvis. The physician simultaneously distracts the femur and rocks it medial to lateral (*curved arrow*). *B.* The same maneuver with the addition of a second assistant to apply lateral traction to the thigh.

the patient's airway and breathing when placed prone. Associated injuries may preclude prone positioning of the patient.

Place the affected leg hanging over the side of the gurney with the knee and hip each flexed 90 degrees. Alternatively, hang both legs off the distal edge of the gurney with the knees and hips flexed 90 degrees (Figure 71-2*A*). Instruct an assistant to hold the patient down on the gurney by applying downward pressure on the anterior superior iliac spines.

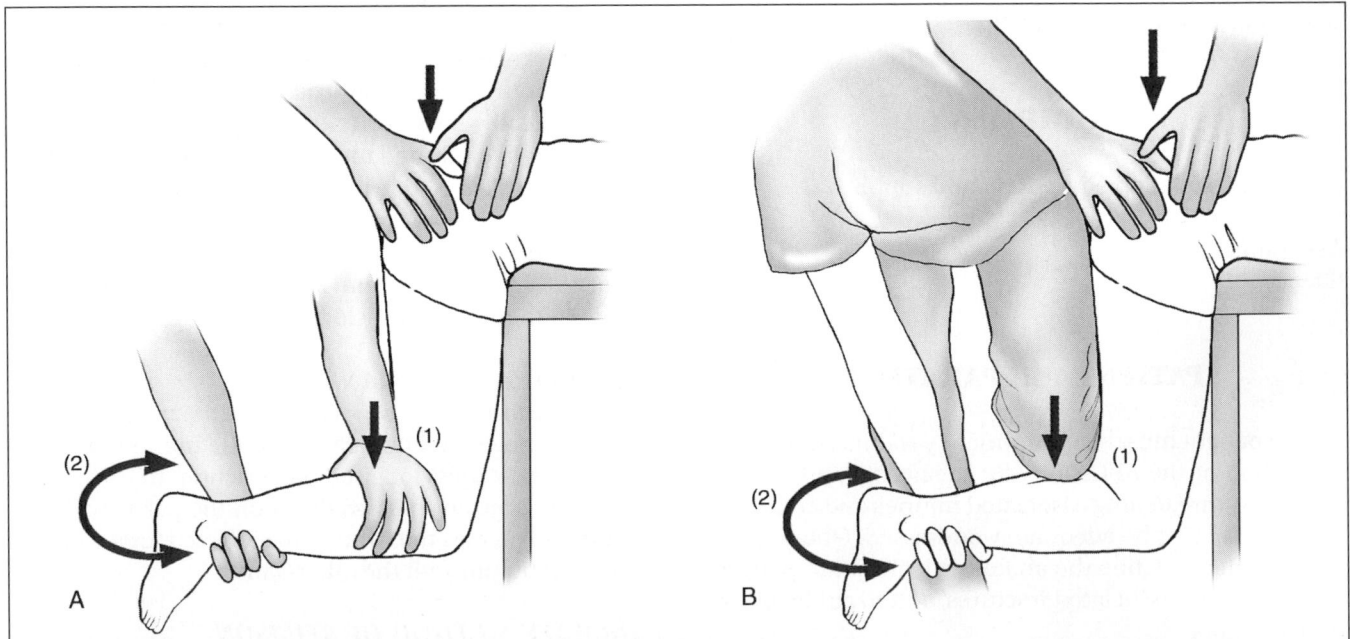

FIGURE 71-2 The gravity method of Stimson. *A.* An assistant stabilizes the pelvis. The physician applies downward pressure on the calf (*straight arrow*) while applying subtle and external rotation to the femur (*curved arrow*). *B.* An alternative method.

Grasp the ankle in one hand to support the limb and to be able to apply internal and external rotation to the extremity (Figure 71-2A). Place the other hand on the proximal posterior calf. Exert gradual longitudinal traction on the femur by placing pressure on the affected calf until the hip is felt to pop into place. A subtle internal and external rotary motion may help to move the femoral head over the acetabular rim. **Care must be taken not to compress the structures in the popliteal fossa with excessive pressure behind the knee.**

A much greater degree of force can be applied to the hip if the physician, instead of generating traction with their arm, places a knee in the affected popliteal fossa (Figure 71-2B). Pull the affected ankle upward while simultaneously exerting downward force on the calf to reduce the dislocation.

WHISTLER / ROCHESTER / TULSA TECHNIQUE

This technique was described at three separate sites (Figure 71-3). Whistler Health Care Center in Vancouver, Canada, described it in 1997.[10] The Orthopedic Associates of Rochester described it in 1999. Vosburgh described it in 1995 as the "Tulsa method."[11] It is reported as being easier to implement than the other techniques and appropriate for use in the Emergency Department.[10,11] Another advantage is that it can be performed without the aid of an assistant. Pelvic stabilization is provided by a counterforce on the uninjured knee. The force and counterforce occur through the same fulcrum and are therefore exactly equivalent.[9]

Place the patient supine. Perform procedural sedation. Stand to the side of the injured leg. Flex the unaffected knee 130 degrees. Place an elbow under the affected knee, allowing the injured leg to dangle over the forearm. Reach to grasp the flexed unaffected knee with the palm. Grasp the affected ankle with the other hand in order to flex the knee and rotate the hip. The hold is now established (Figure 71-3).

Elevate the affected knee by raising your shoulder and using your arm as a lever. Simultaneously apply a longitudinal force by progressively flexing the patient's knee over your arm. This applies traction to the femoral head, moving it anteriorly and around the acetabular rim. Once the acetabular rim is cleared, externally rotate the leg to allow the femoral head to reduce. External rotation is achieved by swinging the ankle laterally. A pop should be felt as the femoral head falls into the acetabulum. Reduction can be verified by internal and external rotation of the hip. An assistant may occasionally be required to stabilize the pelvis.

FULCRUM TECHNIQUE

Lefkowitz described this technique in 1993 and Bergman described it in 1994.[6] The advantage of this technique is that leverage allows greater reduction forces to be applied to the hip with less strength and effort on the part of the physician (Figure 71-4). A steady and constant force can easily be applied that reduces the risk of fractures and nerve injuries. This constant traction is superior to the sudden jerks that are inevitable in some of the other reduction techniques.[6]

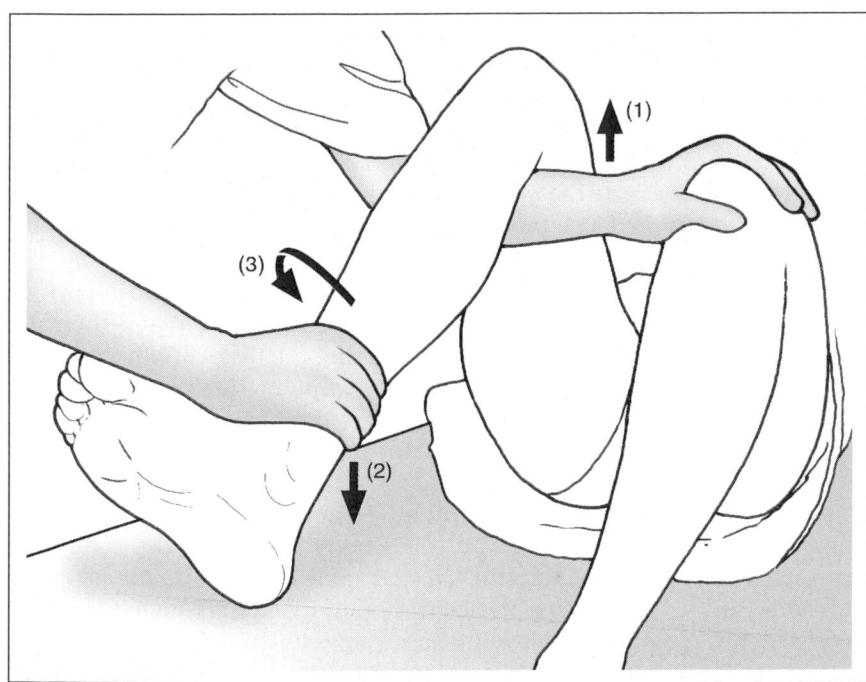

FIGURE 71-3 The Whistler (or Rochester, or Tulsa) technique. Elevation of the physician's shoulder while simultaneously flexing the patient's knee moves the femoral head anteriorly and around the acetabular rim. Externally rotating the patient's leg (*curved arrow*) by swinging the ankle laterally allows the femoral head to reduce.

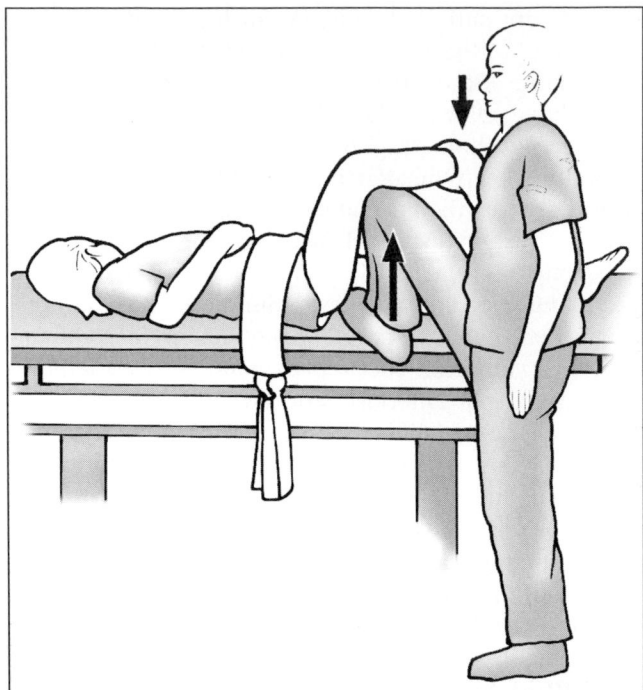

FIGURE 71-4 The fulcrum technique. The physician applies downward pressure on the patient's ankle while simultaneously plantarflexing the patient's foot to move the femoral head around the acetabular rim and reduce the hip.

Place the patient supine and perform procedural sedation. Lower the bed, preferably to within 2 to 3 feet of the floor. Stand on the side of the affected hip. Place one foot on the edge of the bed at the level of the patient's hip. A platform or footstool may be used to gain a mechanical advantage if the level of the bed is too high or you are too short.

Flex the affected knee 90 degrees over your knee (Figure 71-4). Grasp and hold the affected ankle. Apply steady, gentle downward traction on the ankle to flex the knee while simultaneously plantarflexing your foot on the gurney. This will cause the knee to exert an upward force on the patient's knee, raising the femoral head around the edge of the acetabulum and reducing the hip. It may be necessary to gently rotate the affected foot internally and externally if the hip does not reduce easily.

SIMPLE LONGITUDINAL TRACTION

This technique is similar to the reduction of a shoulder dislocation (Figure 71-5). Place the patient supine and perform procedural sedation. Extend the affected lower extremity at the hip and knee. Wrap a sheet around the affected proximal thigh. Grasp the patient's ankle with both hands. **Do not grasp the foot, as this can result in secondary injury.** Instruct an assistant to apply lateral traction to the sheet and proximal thigh to move

the femoral head over the acetabular rim while simultaneously exerting longitudinal traction to the leg by pulling on the patient's ankle to reduce the hip (Figure 71-5).

One of the editors (EFR) prefers to use a padded leather restraint around the affected ankle. Wrap the two ties of the restraint around your hips and secure them with a knot. You can then slowly lean backward to allow your body weight to reduce the hip. This method is especially useful if you are small in stature or do not have significant upper body strength. Do not wrap the ties around your waist, as this can cause low back strain.

BIGELOW MANEUVER

Bigelow described this technique in the literature in 1870 (Figure 71-6). It was the first documented hip reduction technique. Perform procedural sedation. Place the patient supine with the affected hip and knee flexed 90 degrees (Figure 71-6A). Hold the affected knee in the crook of the flexed elbow with the patient's foot in the opposite hand. Instruct an assistant to stabilize the pelvis by applying downward pressure to the anterior superior iliac spines. Lift the shoulder and arm supporting the patient's knee to apply distal traction to the femur (Figure 71-6A). Externally rotate and extend the hip while distracting the femur to reduce the hip (Figure 71-6B).

This is considered the "classic" reduction technique. Its disadvantages are that it requires great strength on the part of the physician to reduce the hip. The force applied is often jerking and inconsistent. The aid of a strong assistant is required to stabilize the pelvis.

LATERAL REDUCTION TECHNIQUE

This technique was described in 1986 by Skoff.[8,12] It gives a mechanical advantage to the physician, as most of the force exerted is by the physician's own body weight (Figure 71-7). It also capitalizes on the principle of recreating the position of injury in order to exactly reverse the forces of the injury to produce the reduction.

Place the patient in the lateral decubitus position lying on the unaffected extremity. Perform procedural sedation. Flex the affected hip 100 degrees and allow it to gravitate to adduction. This position recreates the typical position of the hip during the dislocation. Internally rotate the hip 45 degrees while maintaining 45 degrees of adduction to exaggerate the hip dislocation. Place a looped sheet around the patient's hips and an assistant's hips. Place a second looped sheet around the patient's knee and your own hips. The use of sheets allows optimal leverage by using body weight as the reduction force. Grasp the affected ankle to maintain the patient's knee flexed 90 degrees. Apply distal traction to the femur by slowly leaning backward while the assistant simultaneously applies posteriorly directed counterpressure to

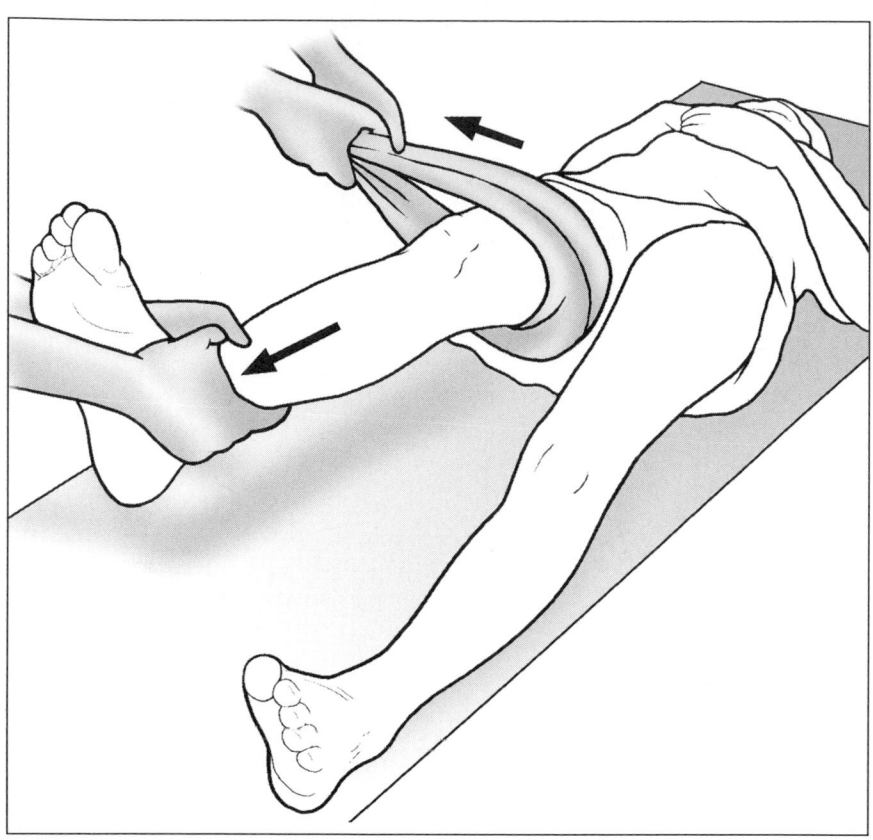

FIGURE 71-5 The simple longitudinal traction technique. An assistant applies lateral traction to the thigh while the physician simultaneously applies in-line traction to the leg.

the femoral head. The assistant can use their hands to apply a distally directed force to the femoral head to assist in the reduction.

ASSESSMENT

The appropriate evaluation of any dislocation requires a thorough pre- and post-reduction neurologic and vascular examination of the distal extremity. Any neurologic or vascular deficits require immediate evaluation by an Orthopedic Surgeon. Obtain a post-reduction radiograph to confirm the reduction and rule out any fractures missed on the initial radiographs or as a result of the reduction procedure. Monitor the patient until they recover from the procedural sedation. A computed tomography scan may help identify any acetabular or osteochondral fractures.

AFTERCARE

All patients with a hip dislocation require an evaluation by an Orthopedic Surgeon. All native hip dislocations and most prosthetic hip dislocations require hospitalization and traction after reduction.[13]

COMPLICATIONS

The complications of a hip dislocation itself are fractures, avascular necrosis of the femoral head, injury to the sciatic and femoral nerve, and injury to the femoral artery. Posttraumatic arthritis, recurrent dislocation, and myositis ossificans can also occur.[13] Complications may occur despite the most expedient treatment, and prosthetic hip replacement may become necessary.

The complication of avascular necrosis is time-dependent. Reductions delayed over 6 hours are at an extreme risk for avascular necrosis. The risk of avascular necrosis increases as the time of the dislocation increases. Reductions that apply steady, nonjerking force to the limb have a lower incidence of associated fractures as well as fewer neurovascular complications.

SUMMARY

Multiple techniques exist to reduce hip dislocations. The Emergency Physician should master one or two methods in order to provide essential care to these patients, limit complications, and enhance outcomes. The sooner a dislocated hip is reduced, the fewer the potential complications.

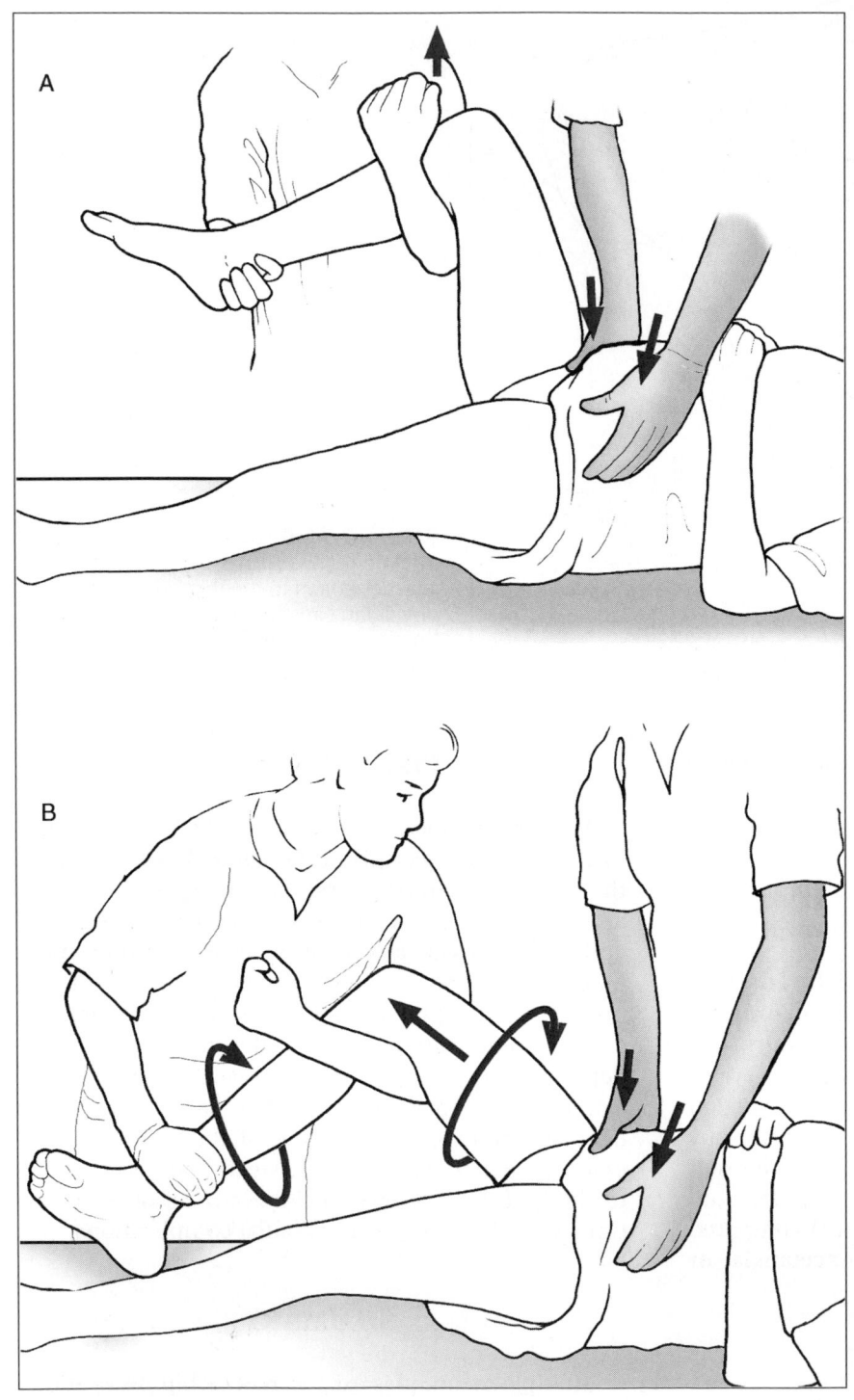

FIGURE 71-6 The Bigelow maneuver. *A.* The physician applies upward traction on the femur while an assistant stabilizes the pelvis. *B.* The hip is externally rotated and extended while the femur is distracted.

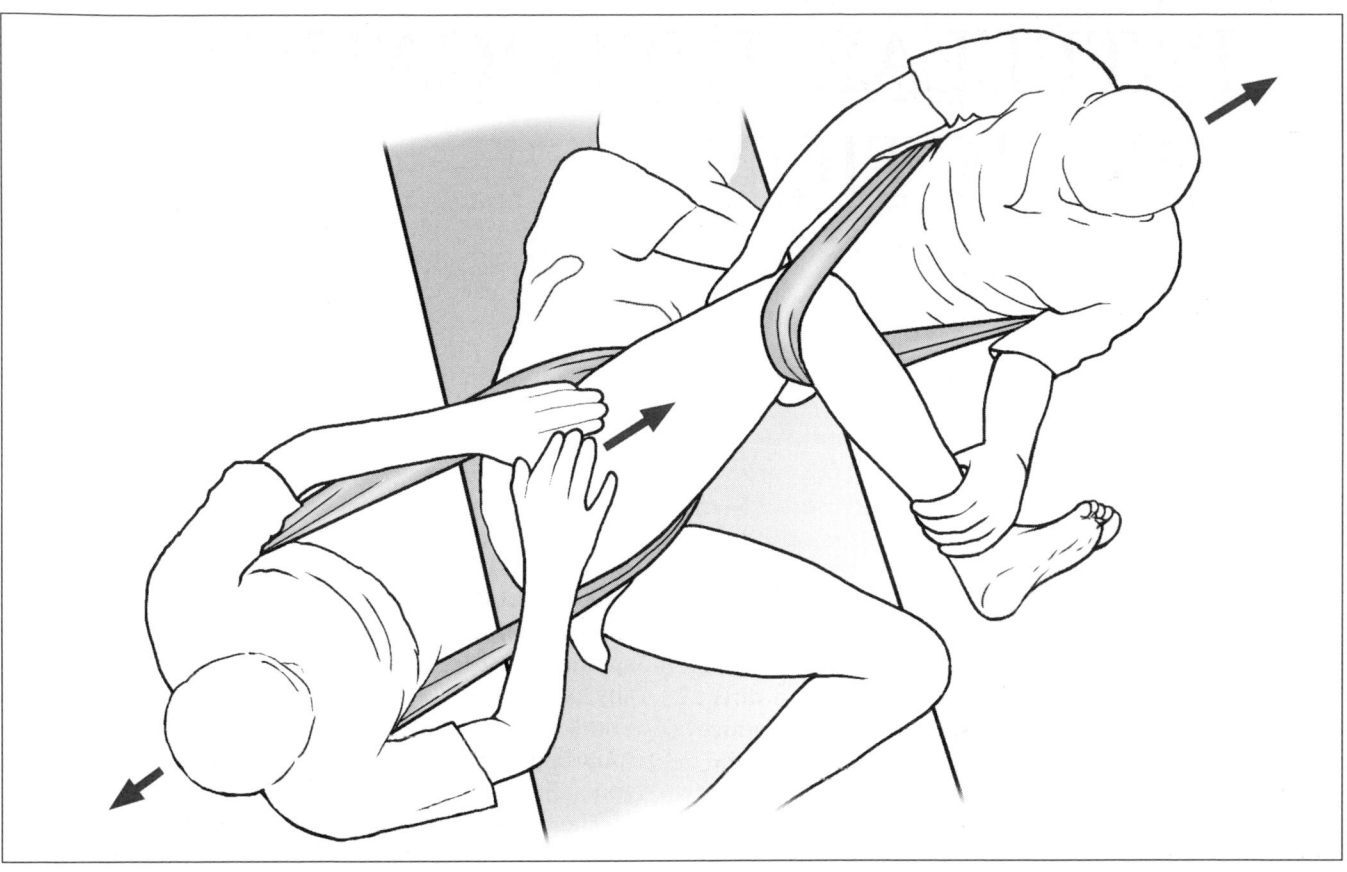

FIGURE 71-7 The lateral reduction technique. The hip is flexed 100 degrees, adducted 45 degrees, and rotated internally 45 degrees. The physician applies traction to the femur. The assistant applies counterpressure to the femoral head while applying distal traction with their hands.

REFERENCES

1. Allis OH: *The Hip*. Philadelphia: Dorman, 1893:14–16.
2. Bergman NJ: Reduction of posterior dislocation of the hip. *Tropic Doc* 1994; 24:134–135.
3. Brav EA: Traumatic dislocation of the hip. *J Bone Joint Surg* 1962; 44A:1115–1134.
4. Epstein HC: Posterior fracture-dislocation of the hip. *J Bone Joint Surg* 1974; 56A:1103–1127.
5. Howard CB: A gentle method of reducing traumatic dislocation of the hip. *Injury Br J Accid Surg* 1992; 23:481–482.
6. Lefkowitz M: A new method for reduction of traumatic dislocations. *Orthop Rev* 1993; 2:253–256.
7. Skoff HD: Posterior hip dislocation: a new technique for reduction. *Orthop Rev* 1986; 15:405–409.
8. Nordt WE: Maneuvers for reducing dislocated hips. A new technique and a literature review. *Clin Orthop Rel Res* 1999; 360:260–264.
9. Stefanich RJ: Closed reduction of posterior hip dislocation: the Rochester method. *Am J Orthop* 1999; 28:64–65.
10. Walden PD, Hamer JR: Whistler technique used to reduce traumatic dislocation of the hip in the emergency department setting. *J Emerg Med* 1999; 17(3):441–444.
11. Vosburgh CL, Vosburgh JB: Closed reduction for total hip arthroplasty reduction. The Tulsa technique. *J Arthrop* 1995; 10(5):693–696.
12. Dahners LE, Hundley JD: Reduction of posterior hip dislocations in the lateral position using traction-countertraction: safer for the surgeon? *J Orthop Trauma* 1999; 13(5):373–374.
13. Hogan TH: Hip and femur, in Hart RG, Rittenberry TJ, Uehara DT (eds): *Handbook of Orthopaedic Emergencies*. Philadelphia: Lippincott–Raven, 1999:309–315.

Chapter 72
PATELLAR DISLOCATION REDUCTION

Mark P. Kling

INTRODUCTION

Dislocation of the patella generally results from a traumatic event. It is most commonly due to a direct blow to the flexed knee. Many patients may not notice the dislocation as it may spontaneously reduce immediately after the injury. There are numerous theories as to the predisposition, if any, to a patellar dislocation.[1,2] This condition is most common in adolescents and females.

ANATOMY AND PATHOPHYSIOLOGY

The knee consists of the patellofemoral and the tibiofemoral joints. The patellofemoral joint is a gliding joint. The patella is an oval-shaped sesamoid bone that develops in the tendon of the quadriceps muscle. It is attached to the quadriceps superiorly and the tibial tuberosity inferiorly. The patella articulates between the femoral condyles. It is held in place by the vastus medialis muscle, the medial retinaculum, the medial and lateral patellofemoral ligaments, and the patellotibial ligament.

The patella may dislocate in numerous directions (Figure 72-1). Lateral dislocations are the most common type (Figure 72-2). The patella usually dislocates laterally due to its asymmetrical shape and the normal upward and lateral pull of the quadriceps muscle. The patella may also dislocate superiorly, medially, and intraarticularly in rare instances.[3,4]

The clinical determination of a lateral patellar dislocation is usually simple and quite obvious (Figure 72-3). The knee is held in partial flexion. The patella can be seen and palpated on the lateral surface of the knee. This may be accompanied by edema and/or ecchymoses over the anterolateral knee.

Pain over the parapatellar ligaments may be the only clinical sign in patients whose patellar dislocation has spontaneously reduced. The physical examination usually reveals mild edema in the parapatellar recesses. There is often laxity in the tendons and ligaments surrounding the patella. A patellar apprehension test is generally positive. The knee joint is usually stable.

The pathophysiology of this dislocation may include abnormalities secondary to malalignment, laxity, and hyper-elasticity of the joint. Osteochondral fractures are common but seen only on arthroscopy.[1,2,5] Magnetic resonance imaging, bone scans, and arthroscopy are considerations for further evaluation and diagnosis of the patellofemoral joint by the Orthopedic Surgeon.

Pre-reduction radiographs should be obtained to document patellar fractures or other bony abnormalities prior to the reduction. Radiographs may also be used to identify a foreign body if abrasions or lacerations are present over the knee. The patella often reduces spontaneously in the radiology suite as the leg is extended to obtain the radiographs.

INDICATIONS

Any medial or lateral patellar dislocation that does not reduce spontaneously should be reduced manually.

CONTRAINDICATIONS

As with any traumatic injury, the evaluation and management of the patient's airway, breathing, circulation, and other significant injuries takes priority over the reduction of a patellar dislocation. There are a few relative contraindications to the reduction of a patellar dislocation. An Orthopedic Surgeon should be consulted

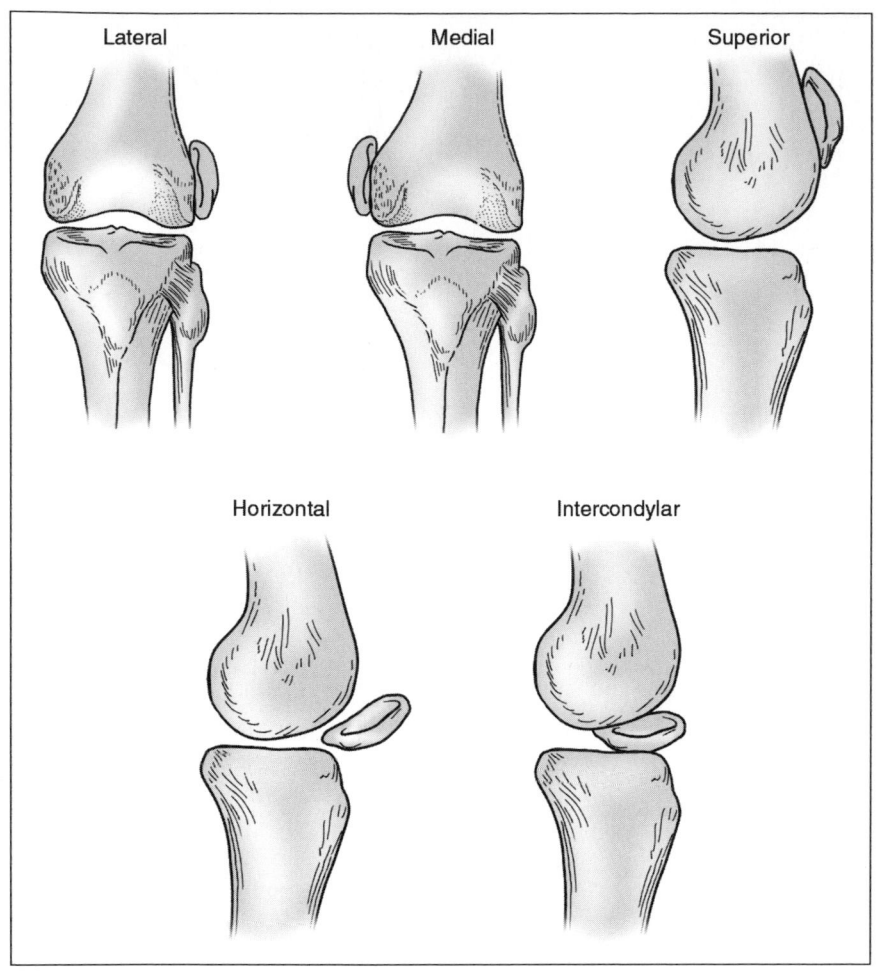

FIGURE 72-1 Types of patellar dislocations.

for the evaluation and reduction if the dislocation is superior, horizontal, intercondylar, or associated with fractures of the distal femur or proximal tibia. **The only exception to this is if there is neurologic and/or vascular compromise of the distal extremity**. This requires immediate reduction by the Emergency Physician if, after phone consultation, the Orthopedic Surgeon is not immediately available to perform the reduction.

EQUIPMENT

No special equipment is required for the reduction of the dislocation. A knee immobilizer or splinting material (plaster, fiberglass, prepackaged splints) should be available to temporarily splint the patella after the reduction.

PATIENT PREPARATION

Patient preparation is minimal in the case of a lateral or medial patellar dislocation. Explain the risks, benefits, complications, and aftercare to the patient and/or their representative. Obtain an informed consent prior to performing the procedure. Verbal consent is usually sufficient, since the reduction of a patellar dislocation is relatively simple, with infrequent complications. Place the patient supine on a gurney. No premedication or sedation is required for this procedure.

TECHNIQUES

The technique for the reduction of a lateral patellar dislocation is rather simple (Figure 72-4). Flex the patient's hip to release the tension on the quadriceps muscles. Slowly and gently extend the knee (Figure 72-4A). The patella may relocate spontaneously by simply extending the knee. If it is still dislocated, apply gentle and medially directed pressure to the lateral surface of the patella (Figure 72-4B). This will allow the patella to move into its normal anatomic position in the intercondylar fossa of the femur. The technique to reduce a medially dislocated patella is similar with the exception of the application of a laterally directed force on the patella.

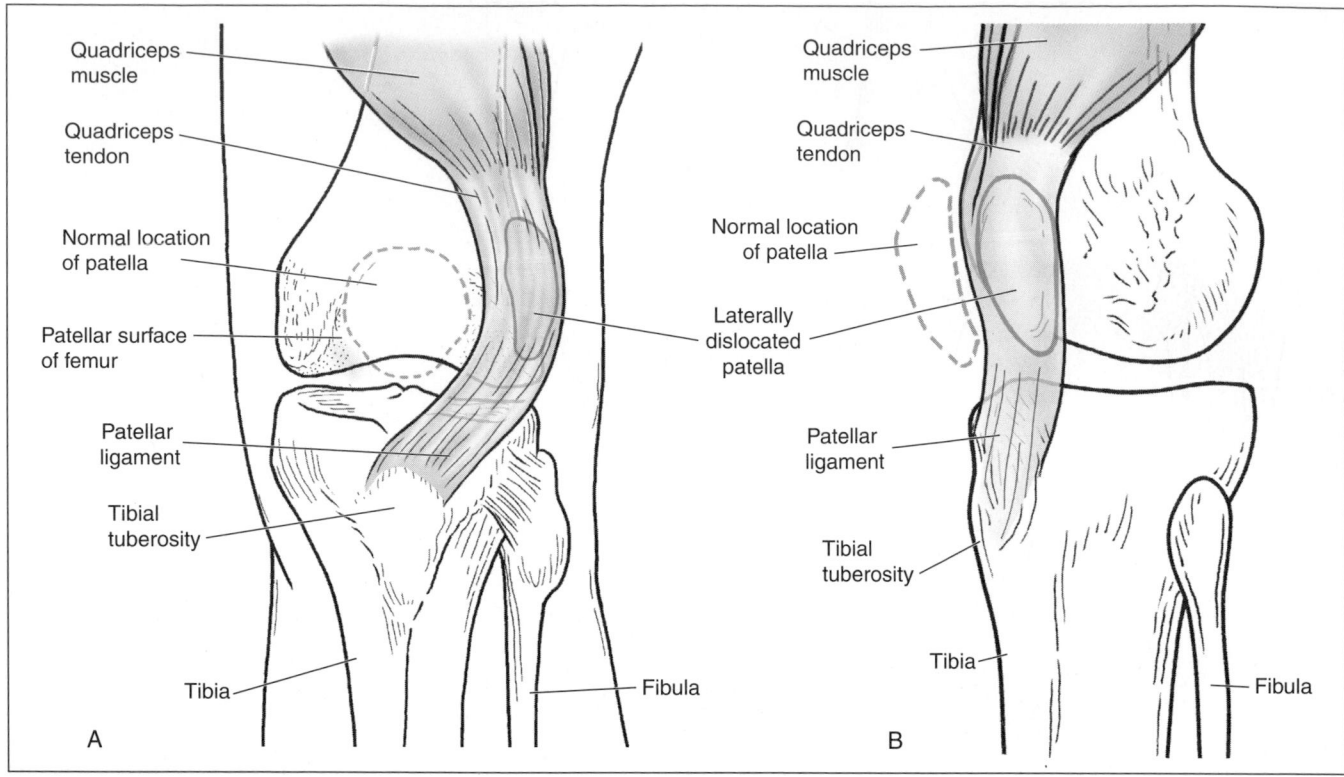

FIGURE 72-2 Anatomy of a lateral patellar dislocation. *A.* Anteroposterior view. *B.* Lateral view.

Intraarticular and horizontal patellar dislocations are sometimes reduced by closed manipulation, although most require open reduction. Superior patellar dislocations require operative reduction. These dislocations should not be reduced in the Emergency Department. Patients with these types of patellar dislocations require

urgent consultation with an Orthopedic Surgeon and hospital admission for reduction.

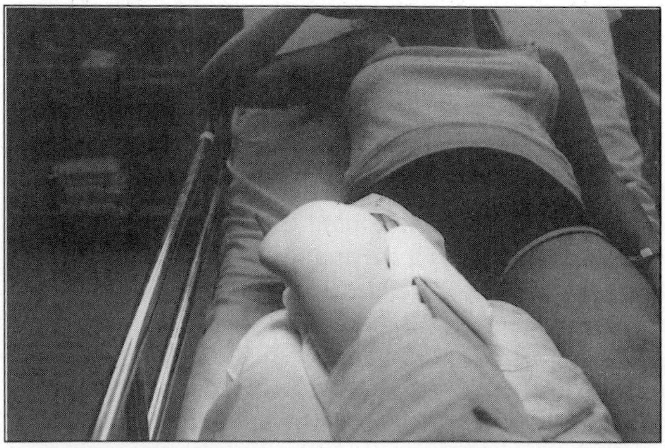

AFTERCARE

Obtain a post-reduction radiograph to rule out any osteochondral fractures that were not diagnosed initially and to ensure proper positioning of the patella. Maintain the knee in extension by immobilization with a splint, cast, or knee immobilizer. Many Orthopedic Surgeons will elect a conservative approach with the leg in a long leg cast and the knee in full extension for 6 weeks.[6] Some Orthopedic Surgeons believe that all first-time dislocations should be repaired surgically. Thus, phone consultation with an Orthopedic Surgeon is recommended before the patient is discharged home.

The general principles of orthopedic care can be applied. These include rest, ice, elevation, and non-steroidal anti-inflammatory drugs. Narcotic analgesics are not necessary or required in most cases. The patient should follow-up with an Orthopedic Surgeon in 5 to 7 days. The patient will most likely need physical therapy. The instability and resultant tracking abnormalities will require strength, proprioceptive, and isometric rehabilitation.[7] Patients who are placed in splints or casts

FIGURE 72-3 The lateral patellar dislocation. The presentation is often clinically dramatic. (Photograph courtesy of Dr. Robert R. Simon.)

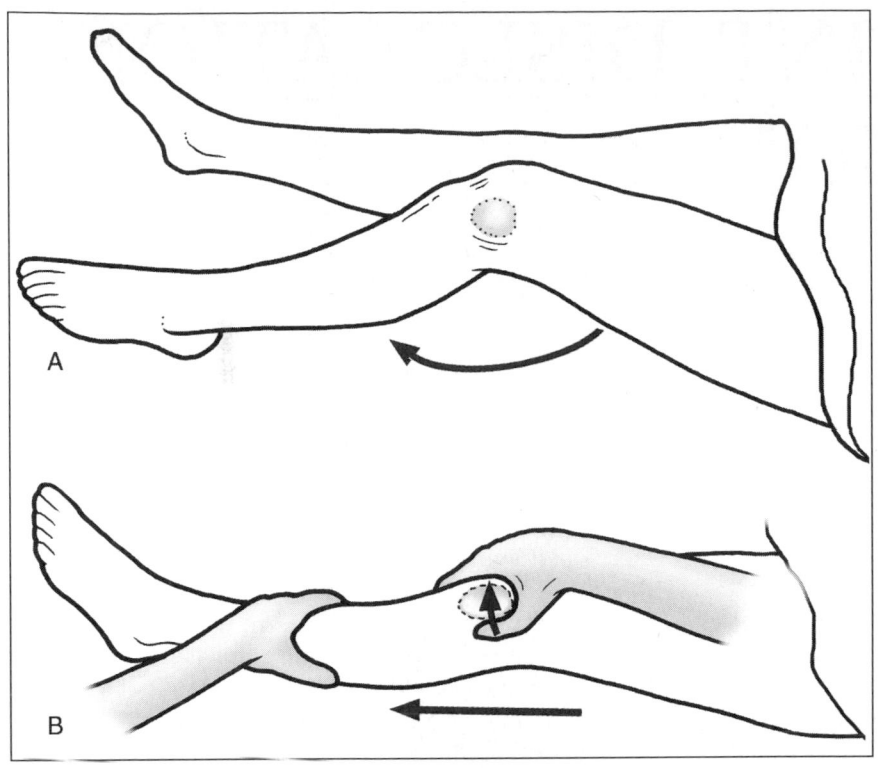

FIGURE 72-4 Reduction of a lateral patellar dislocation. *A.* Manipulation of the knee begins with gradual extension. *B.* Medially directed pressure applied to the patella reduces the dislocation.

should use crutches and not bear weight on the affected extremity. Crutches may be of use to those placed in a knee immobilizer.

COMPLICATIONS

Patellar dislocations are subject to degenerative arthritis, osteochondral fractures (which may be difficult to diagnose initially), and recurrent dislocations or subluxations. No complications are associated with the reduction procedure.

SUMMARY

Patellar dislocations are common. The reduction of a lateral or medial patellar dislocation is a safe, simple, and gratifying procedure. Education of the patient and follow-up with an Orthopedic Surgeon is a requirement for successful rehabilitation.

REFERENCES

1. Hawkins RJ, Bell RH, Anisette G: Acute patellar dislocations: the natural history. *Am J Sports Med* 1986; 14(2):117–120.
2. Burks RT, Desio SM, Bachus KN, et al: Biomechanical evaluation of lateral patellar dislocations. *Am J Knee Surg* 1998; 11(1):24–31.
3. Harries M, Williams C, Stanish W: *Oxford Textbook of Sports Medicine,* 2nd ed. Oxford, England: Oxford Medical Publications, 1998:407–414.
4. Dimentberg RA: Intra-articular dislocation of the patella: case report and literature review. *Clin J Sport Med* 1997; 7(2):126–128.
5. Apostolaki E, Cassar-Pullicino VN, Tyrrell PNM, et al: MRI appearances of infrapatellar fat pad in occult traumatic patellar dislocation. *Clin Radiol* 1999; 54(11):743–747.
6. Maenpaa H, Lehto MUK: Patellar dislocation. The long-term results of non-operative management in 100 patients. *Am J Sports Med* 1997; 25(2):213–217.
7. Holmes SW Jr, Clancy WG: Clinical classification of patellofemoral pain and dysfunction. *J Orthop Sports Phys Ther* 1998; 28(5):299–306.

Chapter 73
KNEE JOINT DISLOCATION REDUCTION

Sharad Pandit
Zach Kassutto

INTRODUCTION

Dislocations of the knee are rare. They are true orthopedic emergencies and have a significant association with soft tissue injuries and neurovascular compromise. A dislocated knee occurs most commonly after a major force is applied to the knee joint from motor vehicle trauma, pedestrian-vehicle collisions, bicycle collisions, or motorcycle collisions. The forces necessary to cause a dislocation of the knee joint often fracture the bones of the leg.

Complete dislocation of the knee joint results in a gross deformity that is confirmed by plain radiographs. Reduction by the Emergency Physician may be reasonable if the Orthopedic Surgeon is not immediately available and/or if the injured extremity shows signs of distal neurologic or vascular compromise.

A careful examination of the distal extremity must be performed and documented. **It must include an assessment of the capillary refill, the dorsalis pedis pulse, the posterior tibial pulse, peroneal nerve function, and tibial nerve function.**

ANATOMY AND PATHOPHYSIOLOGY

A knee dislocation is the displacement of the tibiofemoral articulation. It involves the rupture of the anterior cruciate ligament, the posterior cruciate ligament, the joint capsule, and/or the collateral ligaments of the knee. Anterior knee dislocations are the most common type of knee dislocation. This injury is defined as anterior displacement of the tibia relative to the femur. It results from an acute hyperextension injury to the knee joint that ruptures the anterior cruciate ligament completely, the posterior cruciate ligament partially, and the posterior joint capsule, allowing for anterior tibiofemoral displacement. The collateral ligaments usually remain in-

tact. Tibial spine fractures, osteochondral fractures of the tibia or femur, and meniscal injuries are avulsion-type fractures resulting from the rupture of the anterior cruciate ligament. Distal femoral epiphyseal separation, rather than complete dislocation, as a result of a hyperextension injury is more common in children.

An anterior knee dislocation is associated with a popliteal artery injury in 30 to 40 percent of patients.[1] The popliteal artery is at particular risk for injury because it is anchored proximally at the adductor hiatus and distally at the soleus arch. The collateral circulation around the knee joint is relatively poor. Therefore disruption of the popliteal artery may result in distal ischemia and limb loss if the reduction is delayed. **It is important to note that the presence of distal peripheral pulses and capillary refill does not preclude an arterial injury.**

A posterior knee dislocation is defined as the posterior displacement of the tibia relative to the femur. It occurs less commonly than an anterior knee dislocation. It results from a direct force applied to the anterior tibia with the knee slightly flexed, which ruptures the posterior joint capsule and both cruciate ligaments. The collateral ligaments usually remain intact. It is associated with popliteal artery damage and disruption of the extensor mechanism of the knee joint.

A posterolateral knee dislocation is a rare type of knee dislocation that is associated with peroneal nerve injury in 35 percent of patients.[2-4] These patients must be examined for peroneal nerve dysfunction (i.e., anesthesia or paresthesia on the lateral aspect of the leg and impaired dorsiflexion of the foot).

Anteroposterior and lateral radiographs of the knee will confirm the diagnosis of a knee dislocation. Post-reduction films in two planes will detect any occult fractures of the tibial spine, the distal femoral physis, or the proximal tibial physis. Obtain post-reduction stress views if damage to the collateral ligaments is suspected.

Radiographs of the pelvis and hip should also be considered to rule out any associated injuries.

Medial, lateral, and rotary dislocations of the knee joint are less common than anterior or posterior knee dislocations. Medial knee dislocations result from an adduction force on the tibia that ruptures the lateral collateral ligament, the posterior joint capsule, and both cruciates. Damage to the peroneal nerve is common, while injury to the popliteal artery is not. Lateral knee dislocations result from an abduction force on the tibia that ruptures the medial collateral ligament, the posteromedial joint capsule, and both cruciates. Neurovascular injuries are uncommon with a lateral knee dislocation.

Rotary dislocations are subdivided into posterolateral and posteromedial types. Posterolateral rotary dislocations result from an anteromedial force on the tibia that ruptures the posterior and medial joint capsule, partially avulses the gastrocnemius, damages the menisci, and has an associated chondral fracture. Posteromedial rotary dislocations result from an anterolateral force on the tibia that ruptures both cruciates, the medial collateral ligament, the posteromedial joint capsule, partially avulses the gastrocnemius, damages the menisci, and has an associated chondral fracture. Both of these rotary dislocations are associated with peroneal nerve and popliteal artery injuries.

Medial, lateral, and rotary dislocations of the knee are uncommon injuries that should be managed by an Orthopedic Surgeon. The reduction technique for these dislocations is quite similar to that for the reduction of anterior or posterior knee dislocations.

INDICATIONS

Any dislocation of the knee joint requires prompt reduction in order to reestablish the normal anatomy of the knee joint. The reduction should ideally be accomplished within 6 to 8 hours after the injury. The incidence of limb loss is greater than 85 percent if the knee is dislocated longer than 6 to 8 hours.[5] **Knee dislocations associated with distal neurologic or vascular insufficiency require immediate and emergent reduction.**

CONTRAINDICATIONS

There are no absolute contraindications to the reduction of a dislocated knee joint. Reduction of the knee joint may be performed intraoperatively if the patient requires surgery for other reasons. An Orthopedic Surgeon should reduce the knee if it is dislocated medially, laterally, or rotatorily; if it is associated with fractures of the extremity; or if the joint is open. **Emergent reduction by the Emergency Physician is indicated if the**

Orthopedic Surgeon is not immediately available and/or if there is evidence of distal neurologic or vascular compromise.

EQUIPMENT

Procedural sedation equipment and supplies
    (Chapter 109)
Assistants
Compressive cotton wrap (Webril)
Splinting material
Elastic bandage

PATIENT PREPARATION

Explain the risks, benefits, and potential complications of the procedure to the patient and/or their representative. The necessary post-procedural care should also be discussed. Obtain an informed consent for the reduction procedure as well as for the procedural sedation. Place the patient supine on a gurney. Apply procedural sedation. The key to performing this procedure is to have the patient adequately sedated and their muscles relaxed.

TECHNIQUES

ANTERIOR KNEE DISLOCATION REDUCTION

Reduction of an anterior knee dislocation is usually performed without difficulty. Instruct an assistant to grasp the tibia and apply in-line traction while a second assistant grasps the thigh and applies countertraction (Figure 73-1). **It is extremely important to avoid putting pressure over the popliteal fossa as this could injure the structures traversing that space.** The physician then pushes the proximal tibia posteriorly while simultaneously lifting the distal femur anteriorly into anatomic position (Figure 73-1). **Do not allow the knee to become hyperextended.**

Some physicians feel that the reduction procedure may be easier to perform if the patient is in the prone position. Performing the procedure in the prone position is quite cumbersome, it is a difficult position to attain if other injuries are present, and it makes monitoring patients undergoing procedural sedation difficult. Therefore placing the patient in the prone position is not recommended.

POSTERIOR KNEE DISLOCATION REDUCTION

Reduction of a posterior knee dislocation is similar to that of an anterior knee dislocation. The two assistants provide in-line traction and countertraction while the

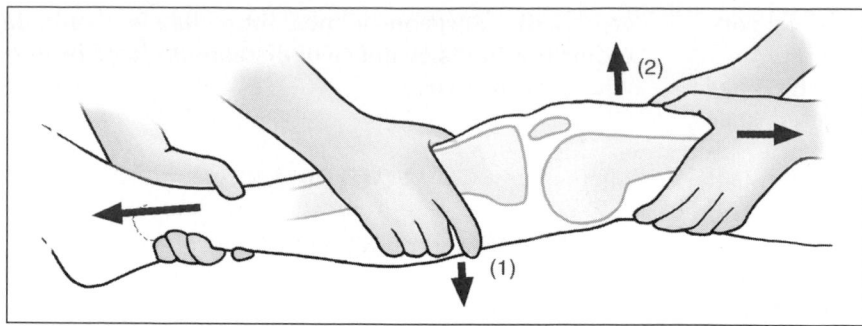

FIGURE 73-1 Reduction of an anterior knee dislocation. An assistant applies in-line traction to the tibia while a second assistant applies countertraction to the femur. The physician then pushes the proximal tibia posteriorly (*1*) and pulls the distal femur anteriorly (*2*) to reduce the dislocation.

physician grasps the proximal tibia and pulls it anteriorly into anatomic position (Figure 73-2).

MEDIAL KNEE DISLOCATION REDUCTION

Reduction of a medial knee dislocation is similar to that of the anterior knee dislocation. The two assistants provide in-line traction and countertraction while the physician grasps the proximal tibia and pulls it laterally into anatomic position.

LATERAL KNEE DISLOCATION REDUCTION

Reduction of a lateral knee dislocation is similar to that of the anterior knee dislocation. The two assistants provide in-line traction and countertraction while the physician grasps the proximal tibia and pulls it medially into anatomic position.

ROTARY KNEE DISLOCATION REDUCTION

Reduction of a posteromedial knee dislocation is similar to that of the anterior knee dislocation. The two assistants provide in-line traction and countertraction while the physician grasps the proximal tibia and simultaneously externally rotates and lifts it upward into anatomic position.

Reduction of a posterolateral knee dislocation should be performed in the Operating Room. These dislocations are irreducible using closed reduction techniques. The medial femoral condyle evaginates through the medial joint capsule in a process known as "buttonholing."

This dislocation requires open reduction under general anesthesia.

ASSESSMENT

Immediately evaluate and document the neurologic and vascular status of the distal extremity after any attempts at reduction. Any diminished or absent sensation, motor deficits, and/or pulses require immediate angiography and operative intervention. Obtain post-reduction radiographs to confirm proper anatomic reduction, to rule out any fractures not evident on the pre-reduction radiographs, and to rule out the displacement of any fracture fragments. Stress radiographs are recommended if injury to the collateral ligaments is suspected.

AFTERCARE

The post-procedural care of the knee joint is as important as the initial reduction. Immobilize the extremity in a posterior long leg splint with the knee in 15 degrees of flexion. Administer intravenous and/or oral analgesics as necessary to control the patient's pain.

All patients require admission to the hospital for observation and monitoring of the distal neurovascular status of the extremity. Arteriography should be ob-

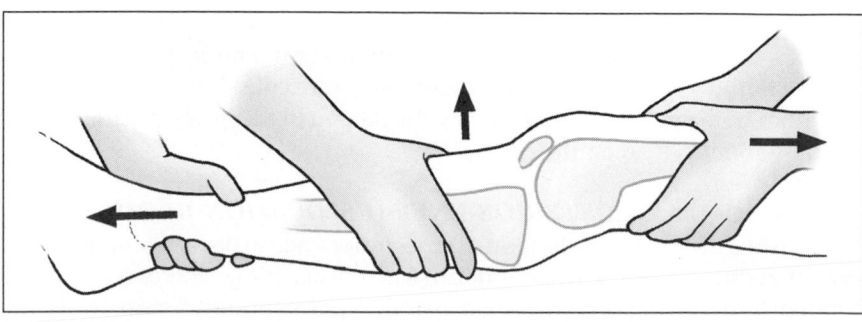

FIGURE 73-2 Reduction of a posterior knee dislocation. An assistant applies in-line traction to the tibia while a second assistant applies countertraction to the femur. The physician then pulls the proximal tibia anteriorly to reduce the dislocation.

tained to exclude injury to the popliteal artery, especially if there is any irregularity in the dorsalis pedis or posterior tibial pulse before or after the reduction. Arteriography may not be necessary if the distal pulses are normal before and after the reduction; however, the vascular status should be closely monitored for 48 to 72 hours after the reduction.[6]

An inpatient magnetic resonance imaging (MRI) scan of the knee joint should be obtained to evaluate ligamentous injury. The patient may require reconstructive surgery on the knee joint. This is especially true if they are young, physically active, and well motivated to cooperate with rehabilitation therapy.[7]

COMPLICATIONS

The complications are primarily related to injuries of the neurovascular structures crossing the popliteal fossa. **These injuries and any associated fractures should not be missed. Pressure to the popliteal fossa during the reduction and hyperextension of the knee postreduction must be avoided to prevent neurovascular damage.** Injuries to neurologic and vascular structures can occur during the reduction. These include lacerations, traction injuries, and entrapment between the tibial plateau and the femoral condyles.

Irreducible dislocations may be secondary to interposed soft tissue, ligamentous instability, buttonhole tears in the medial joint capsule, or entrapment of the medial femoral condyle. These patients require operative reduction under general anesthesia by an Orthopedic Surgeon.

SUMMARY

Knee dislocations occur after significant trauma to the knee joint. Fortunately, knee dislocations are rare events. They are associated with significant morbidity and require prompt reduction to restore the normal alignment of the bony structures. Arteriography to rule out damage to the popliteal artery and an MRI scan to rule out soft tissue injuries should be performed after the knee joint has been reduced and adequately splinted. All patients require admission for observation and eventual reconstructive surgery. Frequent neurovascular evaluation is extremely important during the hospitalization. Evidence of ischemia requires immediate vascular exploration.

REFERENCES

1. Beaty JH: Fractures and dislocations of the knee: knee injuries, knee dislocations, in Rockwood CA, Wilkins KE, and King RE (eds): *Fractures in Children*, 3rd ed. Philadelphia: Lippincott, 1991:1254–1255.
2. Manaster BJ, Andrews CL: Fractures and dislocations of the knee and proximal tibia and fibula. *Semin Roentgenol* 1994; 29(2):113–133.
3. Schenck RC Jr: The dislocated knee. *Instr Course Lect* 1994; 43:127–136.
4. Scuderi GR, Scott WN, Insall JN: Injuries of the knee, in Rockwood CA, Green DP, Bucholz RW, et al (eds): *Rockwood and Green's Fractures in Adults*, 3rd ed. Philadelphia: Lippincott, 1996:2001–2126.
5. Ogden JA: Knee, in Ogden JA (ed): *Skeletal Injury in the Child*, 2nd ed. Philadelphia: Saunders, 1990:745–786.
6. Merrill KD: Knee dislocations with vascular injuries. *Orthop Clin North Am* 1994; 25(4):707–713.
7. Gustilo RB, Cabatan DM: Traumatic dislocation of the knee, in Gustilo RB, Kyle RF, Templeman DC (eds): *Fractures and Dislocations*. St. Louis: Mosby, 1993:885–895.

Chapter 74
ANKLE JOINT DISLOCATION REDUCTION

Jim Comes

INTRODUCTION

The foot and the ankle are the most frequently injured parts of the body. Fractures of the ankle associated with dislocations of the ankle joint (fracture-dislocations) are serious injuries that can lead to long-term morbidity. They occur most commonly in young people who participate in sports, in those suffering from falls, or in those involved in motor vehicle collisions. The ankle mortise and surrounding ligaments make the ankle joint strong and stable. As a result, isolated ankle dislocations are rare. Ankle dislocations are usually associated with malleolar fractures or a fracture of the tip of the tibia. They are open 25 percent of the time. While there are limited data on the mechanism of injury, most ankle dislocations lead to posterior or posteromedial displacement and occur from a force against a plantarflexed foot. Fracture-dislocations are often treated definitively in the Operating Room. Despite this, patients benefit from early analgesia and prompt reduction.

Ankle dislocations can be successfully reduced in the Emergency Department with the use of procedural sedation and longitudinal traction-countertraction.[1] Postreduction management invariably involves leg immobilization and admission to the hospital after consultation with an Orthopedic Surgeon. Some closed ankle dislocations may be managed nonoperatively with good long-term results from a closed reduction and casting for 6 to 9 weeks.[2–5]

ANATOMY AND PATHOPHYSIOLOGY

The ankle joint is composed of the talus, tibia, and fibula. The inferior articular surface of the tibia is concave in both the coronal and sagittal planes. The articular surface of the talus is broader anteriorly and longer on its medial and lateral aspects.[6] The ankle mortise lim-

its rotation of the talus, making the ankle joint inherently stable.

There are three groups of ligaments that provide added stability to the ankle joint. It is stabilized laterally by the anterior talofibular, the calcaneofibular, and the posterior talofibular ligaments (Figure 74-1). It is stabilized medially by the deltoid ligament, which comprises a group of four adjoining ligaments: the anterior and posterior tibiotalar, the tibionavicular, and the tibiocalcaneal ligaments (Figure 74-2). The third group of ligaments stabilizes the tibia to the fibula and forms the tibiofibular syndesmosis. This includes the anterior and posterior tibiofibular ligaments.

Almost all ankle dislocations are associated with ligamentous ruptures, either partial or complete (Figure 74-3). Approximately 25 percent of ankle dislocations are open. Posterior or posteromedial ankle dislocations are the most common dislocations of the ankle joint[4,7] (Figures 74-3A and 74-4). While this is what is documented in the literature, by far the most common ankle dislocations seen by the editors are lateral ankle dislocations (Figure 74-3B). Posterior and lateral ankle dislocations are commonly associated with malleolar fractures and distal fibular fractures. Posterior ankle dislocations are associated with posterior marginal fractures of the tibia. An anterior ankle dislocation is even more rare and frequently is associated with a fracture of the anterior margin of the tibia (Figure 74-3C). The talus may also dislocate laterally or medially if the tibiofibular ligaments are disrupted or a fracture of one or both malleoli occurs. The medial and lateral ligamentous complexes are usually stronger than the malleoli. This results in one or both malleoli fracturing, rather than the ligaments tearing, with a lateral fracture-dislocation.[8]

Due to the low incidence of reported ankle dislocations without fractures, data on the mechanism of injury are incomplete.[9] A posteromedial ankle dislocation occurs when a force is applied against the posterior distal

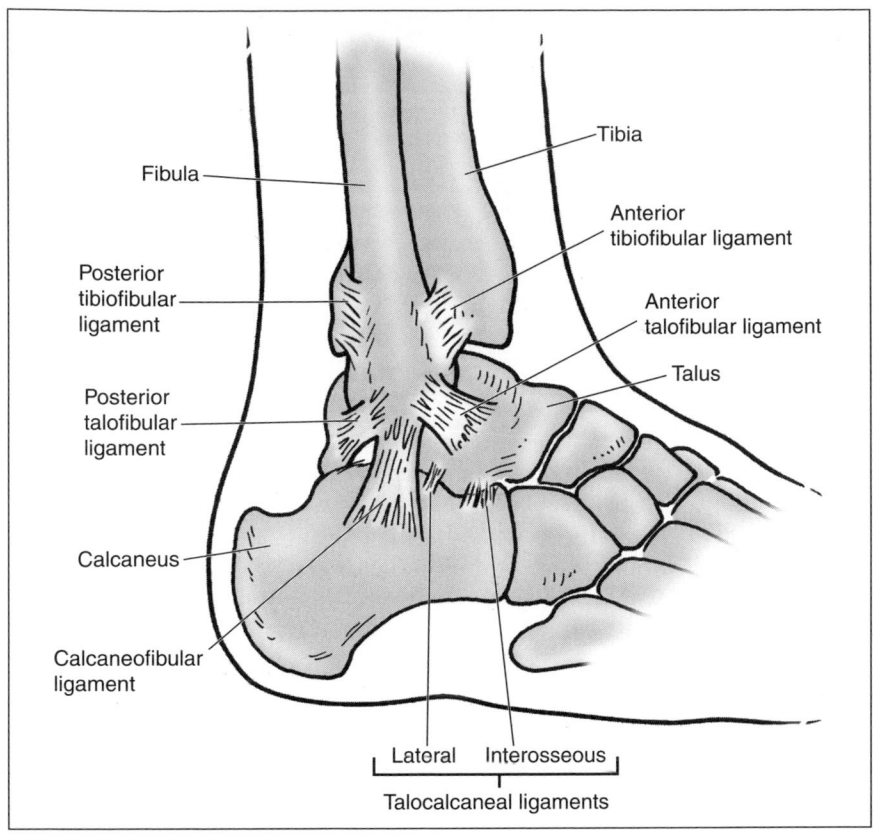

FIGURE 74-1 The bony and ligamentous structures of the lateral ankle.

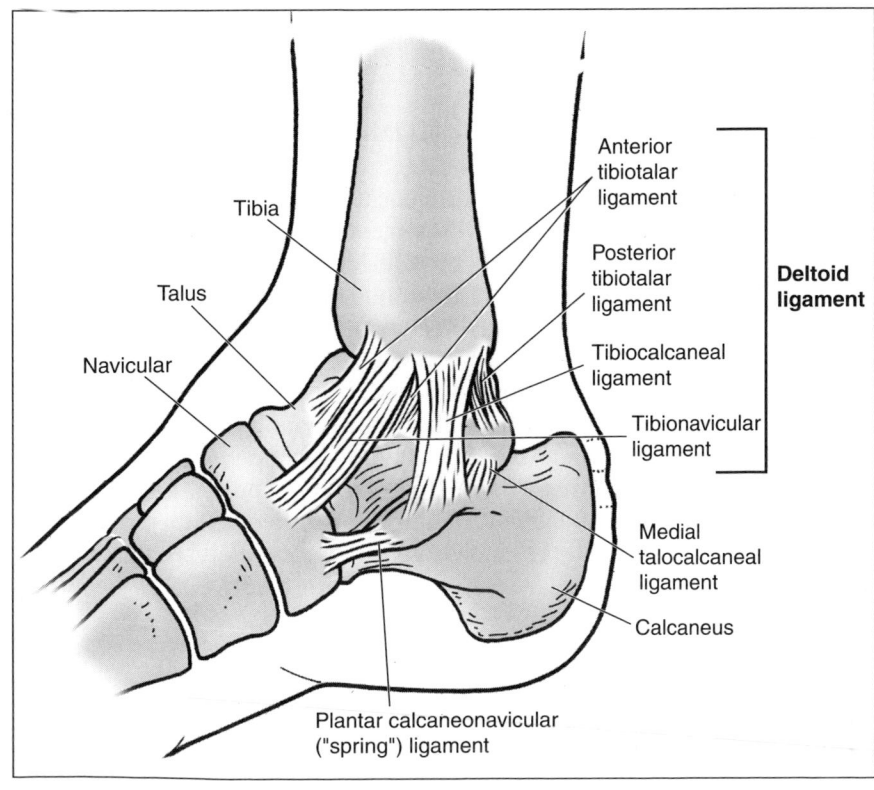

FIGURE 74-2 The bony and ligamentous structures of the medial ankle.

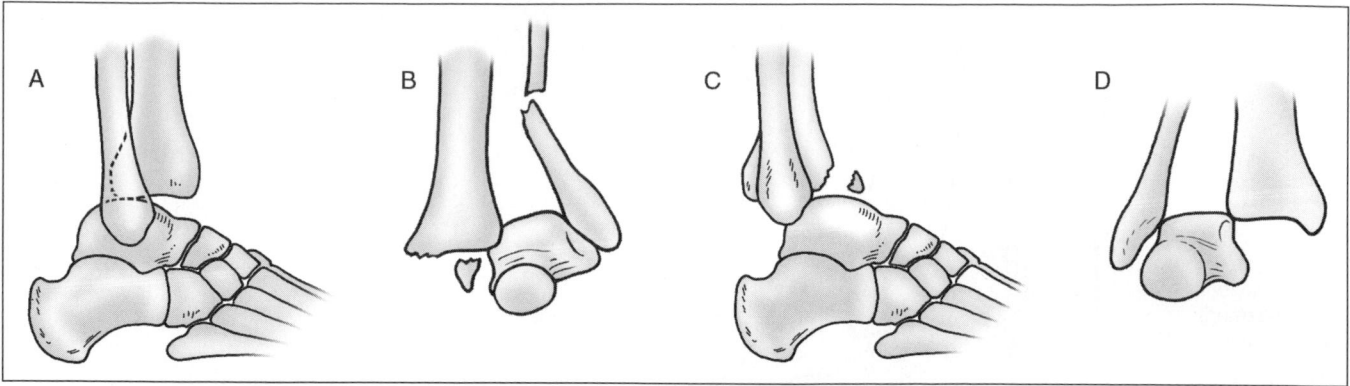

FIGURE 74-3 Types of ankle dislocations. *A.* Posterior. *B.* Lateral. *C.* Anterior. *D.* Superior.

tibia with the foot plantarflexed. Anterior ankle dislocations occur from a forcible dorsiflexion of the foot (fall on the heel with the foot dorsiflexed) or from a force applied to the distal anterior tibia while the foot is fixed. Injury to the tibiofibular joint is variable, and the fibula may be dislocated posteriorly or anteriorly. Diastasis of the tibiofibular syndesmosis is uncommon. Lateral ankle dislocations are always associated with fractures of the malleoli. They occur from a force on the distal fibula with the foot fixed to the ground. Superior ankle dislocations are uncommon (Figure 74-3*D*). They occur when a force from above is driven through the leg and to the ankle (e.g., a fall from a height).

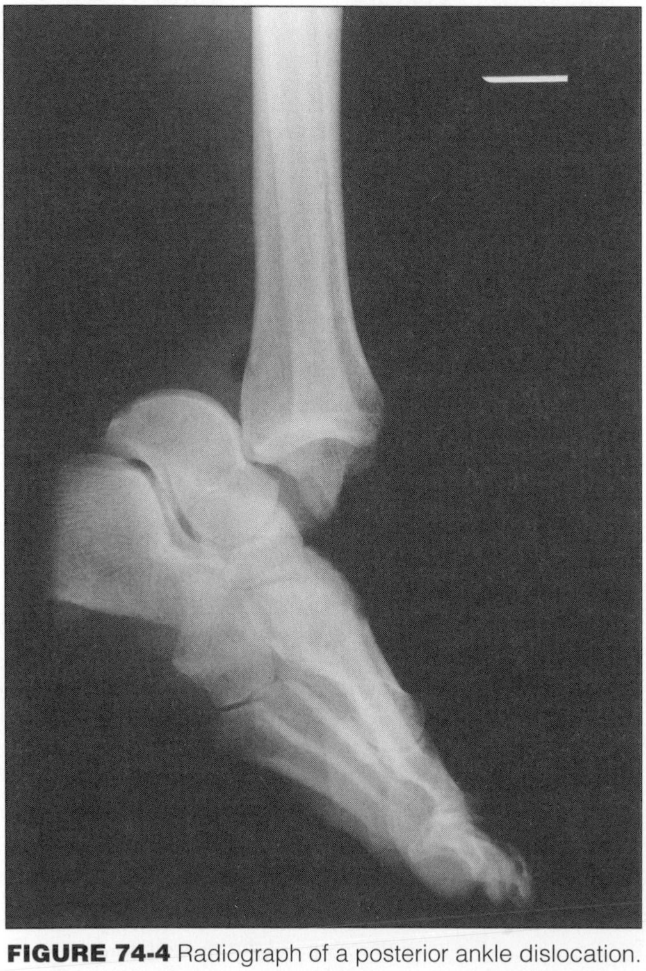

Physical examination often reveals the type of ankle dislocation. Prominence of the talus and a change in the length of the foot are common. Neurovascular injury is uncommon, although there is a higher incidence of this in open dislocations. Ankle dislocations are associated with a risk of vascular injury and the development of a compartment syndrome from severe swelling.[7] Most vascular injuries are to the dorsalis pedis or posterior tibial vessels and may be accompanied by damage to the adjacent superficial peroneal nerve or sural nerve, respectively.[1,6] Tibiotalar dislocations rarely result in avascular necrosis.

INDICATIONS

All closed ankle dislocations should be reduced emergently. Some authors recommend reduction even prior to radiography.[10] **Any dislocation, open or closed, that has evidence of distal neurologic or vascular compromise must be reduced emergently.** Extreme lateral deviation may compromise the dorsalis pedis artery and requires prompt reduction.[10] All open dislocations require intravenous antibiotics, irrigation, surgical debridement, and reduction by an Orthopedic Surgeon in the Operating Room. However, reduction should occur in the Emergency Department if the Orthopedic Surgeon or the Operating Room is not immediately available.[3]

CONTRAINDICATIONS

There are no absolute contraindications to reducing a dislocated ankle. Some authors would not recommend Emergency Department reduction of an open fracture-

FIGURE 74-4 Radiograph of a posterior ankle dislocation.

dislocation without evidence of neurovascular compromise or in a setting where immediate orthopedic and operative intervention was available.

EQUIPMENT

Local anesthetic solution
18 gauge needle
22 gauge needle, 2 inches long
Equipment and supplies for procedural sedation
  (Chapter 109)
Stockinette
Compressive wrap (Webril)
Plaster, fiberglass, or commercially prepared splinting
  material
Elastic bandage

PATIENT PREPARATION

Explain the risks, benefits, and potential complications of the reduction procedure and the procedural sedation to the patient and/or their representative. Obtain an informed consent for both procedures. Place the patient supine with the affected foot at the edge of the gurney. Patients should be premedicated with an opioid analgesic prior to the procedure and ideally prior to radiography. The editors have found that the use of procedural sedation provides excellent analgesia, muscle relaxation, and sedation, allowing the reduction procedure to be more tolerable for both the patient and the physician. A Bier block (Chapter 107) or the intraarticular instillation of local anesthetic solution (Chapter 65) are reasonable alternatives if procedural sedation is contraindicated.

TECHNIQUES

The techniques described below to reduce ankle dislocations have three things in common. The hip and knee are flexed to relieve the tension on the gastrocnemius and soleus muscles. The foot is flexed (plantarflexed or dorsiflexed) to unlock or disengage the talus. Finally, the talus is maneuvered into its proper anatomic position.

LATERAL ANKLE DISLOCATIONS
Flex the patient's hip and knee by placing a pillow behind their knee. Grasp the calcaneus with one hand and the forefoot with the other hand (Figure 74-5A). Instruct an assistant to grasp the patient's calf. Apply distal traction to the heel while the assistant provides countertraction to the leg (Figure 74-5A). The next step is to rotate

the foot medially so that the great toe is in alignment with the anterior tibia while simultaneously dorsiflexing the foot and distracting the heel (Figure 74-5B). The talus will reduce easily with a palpable and audible "clunk."

POSTERIOR ANKLE DISLOCATIONS
Flex the patient's hip and knee by placing a pillow behind their knee. Grasp the calcaneus with one hand and the forefoot with the other hand (Figure 74-6A). Instruct an assistant to grasp the patient's calf. Simultaneously apply distal traction to the heel and plantarflex the foot while the assistant provides countertraction to the leg (Figure 74-6A). The next step is to dorsiflex the foot while distracting the heel and a second assistant provides posteriorly directed pressure on the distal leg (Figure 74-6B). The talus will reduce with a palpable and audible "clunk."

ANTERIOR ANKLE DISLOCATIONS
Flex the patient's hip and knee by placing a pillow behind their knee. Grasp the calcaneus with one hand and the forefoot with the other hand (Figure 74-7A). Instruct an assistant to grasp the patient's calf. Simultaneously apply distal traction to the heel and dorsiflex the foot until the toes point upright while the assistant provides countertraction to the leg (Figure 74-7A). The next step is to push the foot posteriorly while distracting the heel and a second assistant provides anteriorly directed pressure on the distal leg (Figure 74-7B). The talus will reduce with a palpable and audible "clunk."

SUPERIOR ANKLE DISLOCATIONS
Superior ankle dislocations are associated with significant soft tissue and articular damage. Neurovascular injury is uncommon with these dislocations. Superior ankle dislocations should be splinted and managed by an Orthopedic Surgeon.

OPEN ANKLE DISLOCATIONS
The Emergency Physician occasionally reduces open ankle dislocations if neurologic and/or vascular compromise of the foot is present and an Orthopedic Surgeon is not immediately available. Copiously irrigate the wound with sterile saline before attempting the reduction. The technique to reduce an open ankle dislocation is the same as that for a closed ankle dislocation.

ASSESSMENT

Verify and document the neurologic and vascular status of the foot before and after any attempts at reduction. Any diminution or absence of neurologic or

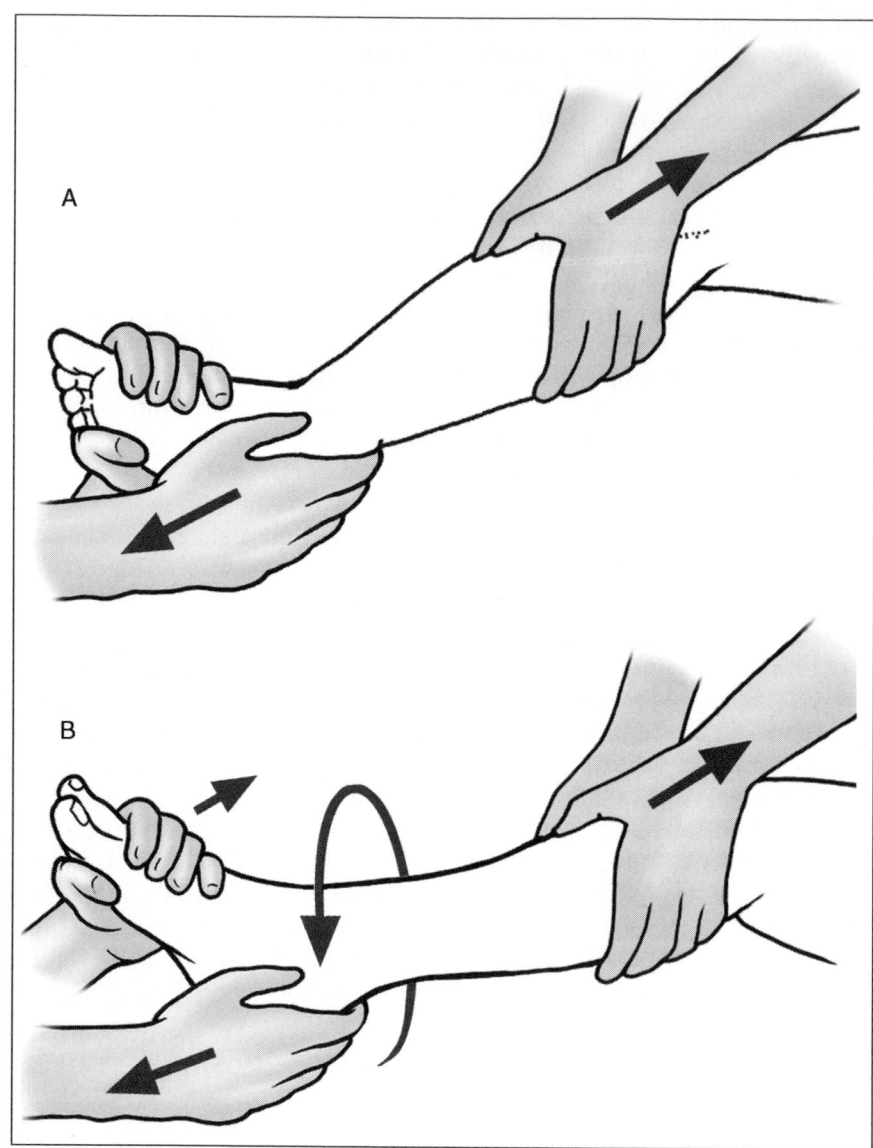

FIGURE 74-5 Closed reduction of a lateral ankle dislocation. *A.* The heel is distracted while an assistant provides countertraction. *B.* Simultaneously, medially rotate and dorsiflex the foot while distracting the heel.

vascular signs requires emergent consultation with an Orthopedic Surgeon.

AFTERCARE

Splint the extremity. Apply a three-sided short leg splint or bivalved cast from the base of the toes to just below the knee for posterior, lateral, and superior ankle dislocations that have been reduced. Immobilize the ankle in 90 degrees of flexion and in a neutral position with respect to inversion and eversion.[7] A short leg splint is preferred to a bivalved cast, due to the likelihood of increasing swelling, for anterior ankle dislocations that have been reduced. Immobilize the reduced anterior ankle dislocation with the ankle in slight plantarflexion. All patients with ankle dislocations require admission to the hospital. The limb should be elevated and not bear weight; it should have frequent neurologic and vascular checks and have frequent assessments for the development of the signs associated with a compartment syndrome.[7]

COMPLICATIONS

Most complications occur as a result of the fracture-dislocation and not the reduction procedure. This includes neurologic damage, vascular damage, and compartment syndromes. A posttraumatic peroneal tendon dislocation can occur and may be initially unrecognized. The patient usually becomes symptomatic after the acute stage, when the tendon subluxes and dislocates. There is a low rate of subsequently developing avascular necrosis and degenerative joint disease with isolated ankle dislocations.

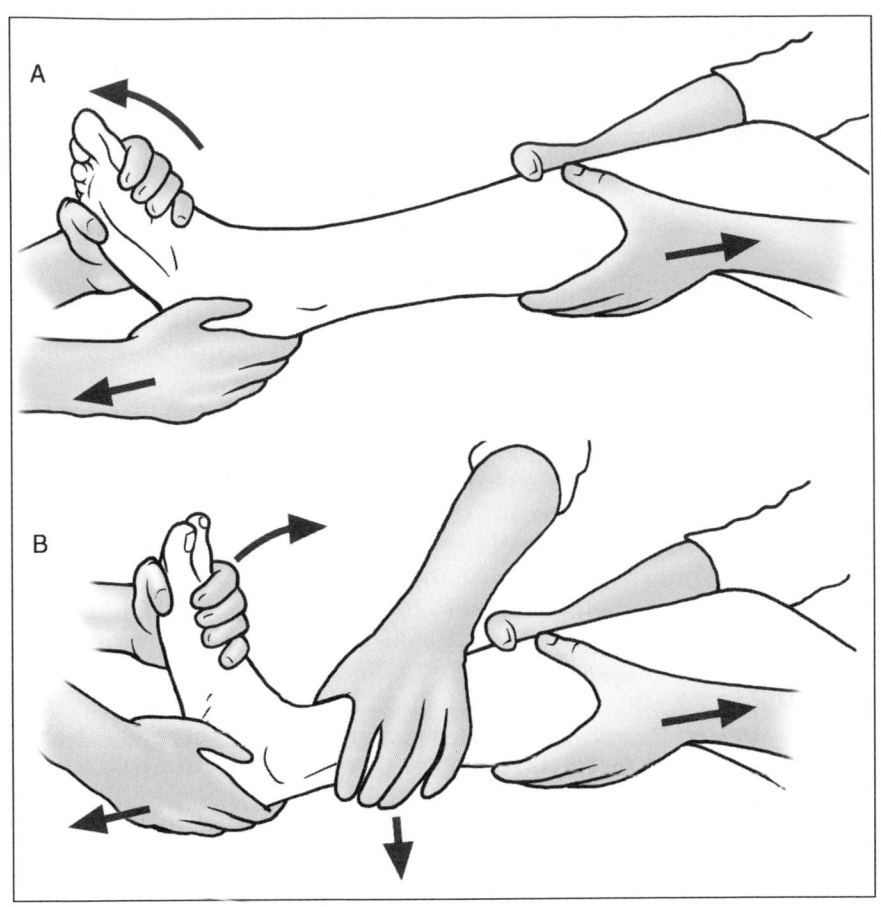

FIGURE 74-6 Closed reduction of a posterior ankle dislocation. *A.* The heel is distracted and the foot is plantarflexed while an assistant provides countertraction. *B.* The foot is dorsiflexed while the heel is distracted and a second assistant applies posterior traction on the distal leg.

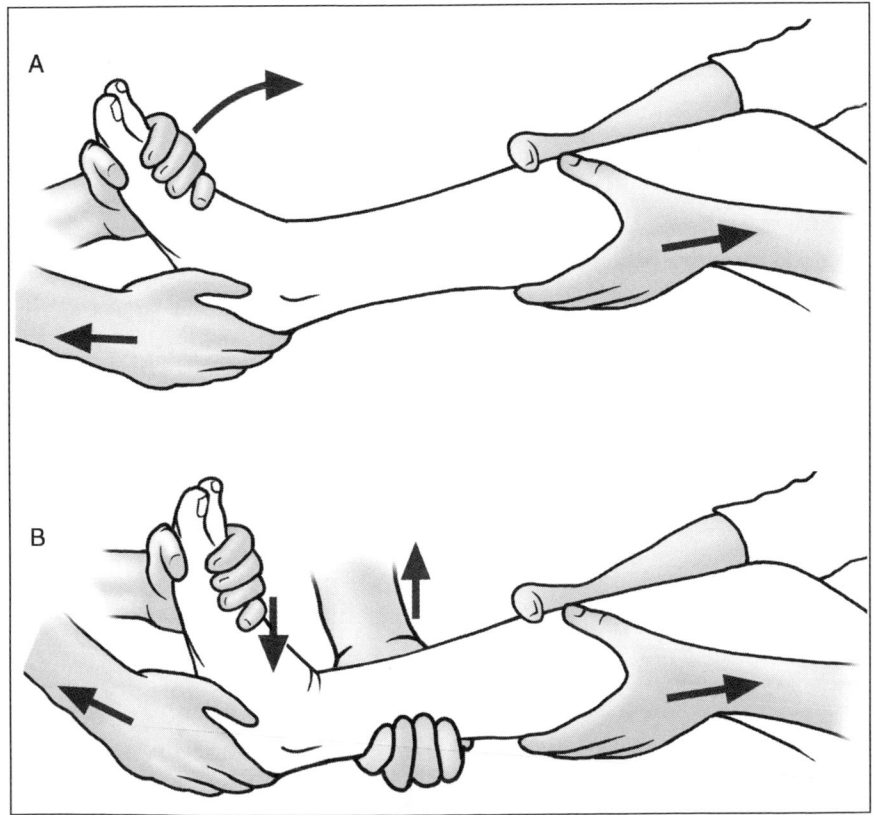

FIGURE 74-7 Closed reduction of an anterior ankle dislocation. *A.* The heel is distracted and the foot is dorsiflexed until the toes are upright, while an assistant provides countertraction. *B.* The foot is pushed posteriorly while the heel is distracted and a second assistant applies anterior traction on the distal leg.

Complications associated with the reduction procedure, if they occur at all, are usually neurologic and vascular injuries. These structures may become impinged, or trapped, in the relocated joint or on a fracture fragment. **Emergently consult an Orthopedic Surgeon if there is any diminished or absent function of any nerve or artery.**

SUMMARY

Ankle dislocations without fractures are uncommon yet serious injuries. Closed ankle dislocations can be reduced emergently and successfully with the use of procedural sedation. Open ankle dislocations should be irrigated in the Emergency Department and reduced rapidly after consultation with an Orthopedic Surgeon. Reduction, irrigation, and debridement are all likely to occur in the Operating Room if an Orthopedic Surgeon is immediately available. Any ankle dislocation with evidence of distal neurovascular compromise should be reduced immediately. All patients with ankle dislocations should have an Orthopedic Surgeon consulted, the ankle immobilized and elevated, and be admitted to the hospital. The majority of closed ankle dislocations are managed nonoperatively with good long-term results.

REFERENCES

1. Geissler WB, Tsao AK, Hughes JL: Fractures and injuries of the ankle, in Rockwood CA, Green DP, Bucholz RW, et al (eds): *Rockwood and Green's Fractures in Adults,* 4th ed. Philadelphia: Lippincott-Raven, 1996:2250–2251.

2. Colville MR, Coville JM, Manoli A: Posteromedial dislocation of the ankle without fracture. *J Bone Joint Surg* 1987; 69A(5):706–711.

3. Segal D, Wasilewski S: Total dislocation of the talus. *J Bone Joint Surg* 1980; 62A(8):1370–1372.

4. Wilson AB, Toriello EA: Lateral rotatory dislocation of the ankle without fracture. *J Orthop Trauma* 1991; 5(1):93–95.

5. Wroble RR, Nepola JV, Marvitz TA: Ankle dislocation without fracture. *Foot Ankle* 1988; 9(2):64–74.

6. Toohey JS, Worsing RA: A long-term follow-up study of tibiotalar dislocations without associated fractures. *Clin Orthop Rel Res* 1989; 239:207–210.

7. Connolly JF: *Fractures and Dislocations: Closed Management.* Philadelphia: Saunders, 1995:898–901.

8. Conwell HE, Alldredge RH: Complete compound dislocation of the ankle joint without fracture with primary healing. *JAMA* 1937; 108(24):2035–2036.

9. Moehring HD, Tan RT, Marder RA, et al: Ankle dislocation. *J Orthop Trauma* 1994; 8(2):167–172.

10. Watson JAS, Hollingdale JP: Early management of displaced ankle fractures. *Injury* 1992; 23(2):87–88.

Chapter 75
COMMON FRACTURE REDUCTION

Mark E. Johnson
Eric F. Reichman

INTRODUCTION

Extremity fractures are a common reason for Emergency Department visits. If there is no neurologic or vascular compromise, most closed fractures can be managed conservatively in the Emergency Department with splinting and Orthopedic Surgeon follow-up. This chapter addresses four common fractures of the upper extremity that may require reduction by the Emergency Physician. These include clavicular fractures, Colles fractures, displaced surgical neck fractures of the humerus, and supracondylar fractures of the humerus. **The reduction of fractures in the Emergency Department should involve consultation with an Orthopedic Surgeon prior to performing the procedure. The only exception to this is if neurologic or vascular compromise exists in the extremity.**

CLAVICULAR FRACTURES

INTRODUCTION

Clavicular fractures are common and represent approximately 5 percent of all fractures.[1-3] Most of these occur at the junction of the middle and distal third of the clavicle, just medial to the coracoclavicular ligament. The clavicular fracture is the most common fracture encountered in childhood and occurs most often as a result of a fall. These fractures are usually detectable clinically, with plain radiographs helping to confirm the diagnosis. Although these fractures are relatively common, there is a small but definite risk of associated complications.

ANATOMY AND PATHOPHYSIOLOGY

The clavicle is the only bony attachment of the upper extremity to the axial skeleton. It serves as a strut to support the shoulder girdle. It provides support and stabi-

lization of the upper limb while allowing a broad range of movements. The clavicle is securely attached at both the acromioclavicular and sternoclavicular joints by ligaments (Figure 75-1). The great vessels of the upper extremity and nerves of the brachial plexus pass posteriorly to the clavicle at its midportion where it overlies the first rib. The proximity of these neurovascular structures, as well as the underlying lung, accounts for most of the potential complications of clavicular fractures.

The most commonly used classification for clavicular fractures was proposed by Allman.[4] This simple classification is useful clinically and mechanistically to the Emergency Physician. Group I fractures are midclavicular and account for approximately 80 percent of clavicular fractures. These most often result from a shearing force applied to the lateral aspect of the shoulder. Group II fractures involve the distal third of the clavicle and account for approximately 15 percent of all clavicular fractures. These most often result from a direct blow to the top of the shoulder. Several additional subclassifications have been proposed for these fractures based on the location of the fracture and associated ligamentous injury. Operative repair is suggested for some of these subtypes. All distal clavicular fractures should therefore be referred for follow-up within 24 hours to an Orthopedic Surgeon.[1,2] Group III fractures represent about 5 percent of clavicular fractures and involve the proximal third of the clavicle. They often result from a direct blow to the chest.

Patients with clavicular fractures are easily identified clinically. The clavicle is almost entirely subcutaneous, allowing most fractures to be palpated. Presenting signs and symptoms include localized pain, ecchymoses, and edema. Physical examination findings include upward and backward displacement of the proximal portion of the clavicle due to traction from the sternocleidomastoid muscle (Figure 75-2). The shoulder is often displaced inferiorly by the weight of the upper extremity

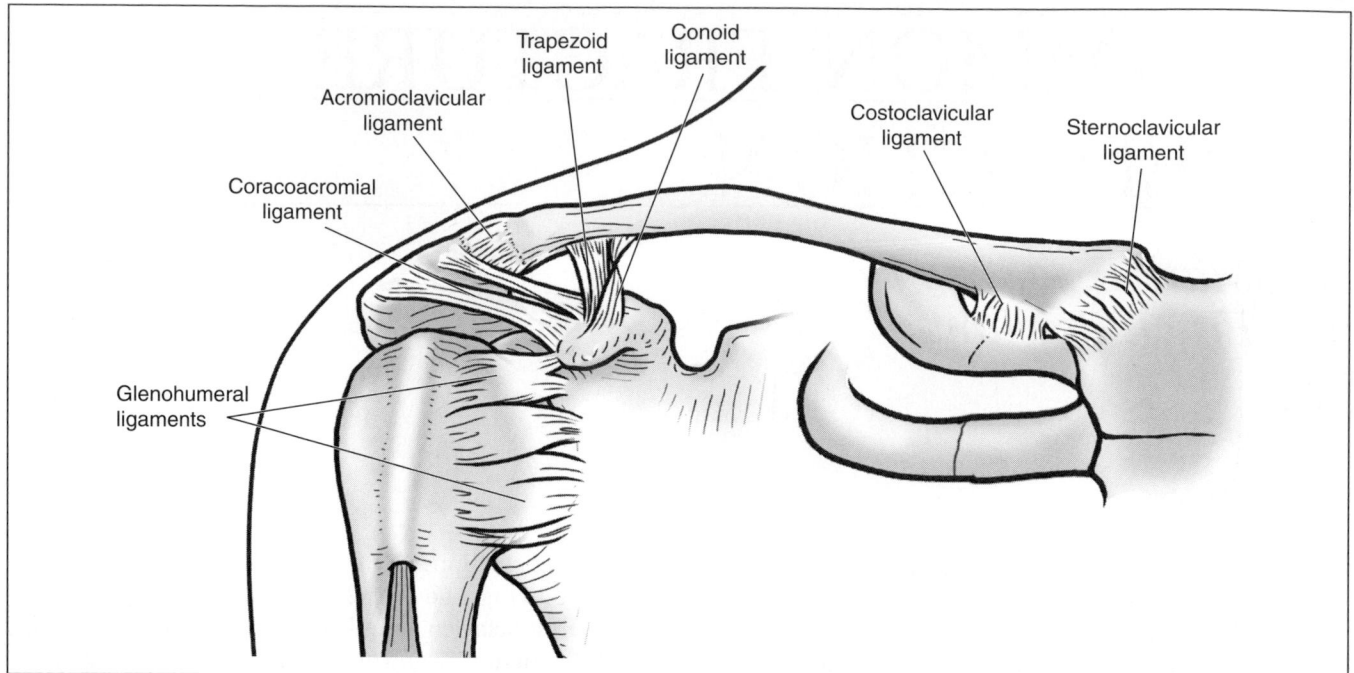

FIGURE 75-1 The clavicle serves as a strut between the torso and upper extremity; it is held firmly by the acromioclavicular and sternoclavicular ligaments. The brachial plexus and great vessels pass behind the middle third of the clavicle.

and the force of gravity. Medial displacement of the shoulder may be seen due to traction from the pectoral and the latissimus dorsi muscles.

Most fractures are readily identifiable on standard anteroposterior radiographs. Some group II and III fractures may not be readily identifiable.[1] Additional views at a 45 degree angle cephalad (apical lordotic view) may be useful to assess displacement.[1,3] Special views (cone views, tomograms, and upper rib films) may be required and are best determined in consultation with an Orthopedic Surgeon.

Clavicular injury and pain in children present two concerns. First, nondisplaced greenstick fractures to the clavicle may not be radiographically visible for 7 to 10 days.[2,3] Clinical suspicion of a clavicular fracture with a negative radiograph should prompt conservative management. Follow-up should be arranged for 7 to 10 days after the injury to obtain repeat radiographs. Second, it may be unclear if the epiphyses are involved in some group II and III fractures.[2,3] **Any fracture through the epiphysis, or possibly through the epiphyses, requires an urgent referral to an Orthopedic Surgeon.**

INDICATIONS

Reduction of most clavicular fractures is not usually necessary in either the pediatric or adult patient.[1,2] A sling for simple arm support provides results comparable to the figure-of-eight reduction without the risk of brachial plexus injury or patient discomfort.[1–3]

The sling may be additionally supported by a swath (Figure 75-3*A*) or a Velpeau wrap (Figure 75-3*B*). However, many physicians still prefer the use of a figure-of-eight strap (Figures 75-3*C* and *D*). The figure-of-eight splint still represents the treatment of choice in patients over the age of 10 years in the presence of greatly displaced fragments.[2,3] Despite this, there is no evidence that the figure-of-eight splint offers any advantage over a simple sling for midclavicular fractures.

Reduction of clavicular fractures is necessary in a few circumstances. **It is required if neurologic and/or vascular compromise is present in the affected extremity.** Consider patients who are actively involved in athletics or have jobs that require overhead use of their arms (e.g., painters) for operative reduction by an Orthopedic Surgeon. Distal clavicular fractures that are displaced should be reduced. Otherwise, reduction is optional and at the discretion of the treating physician.

CONTRAINDICATIONS

Contraindications to the reduction of a clavicular fracture include other injuries that represent a threat to life or limb. The patient's airway, breathing, and circulation must first be addressed and stabilized. Patients with open clavicular fractures require emergent consultation by an Orthopedic Surgeon, intravenous antibiotics, and hospital admission for possible open reduction and internal fixation. Reduction is also contraindicated if an expanding hematoma, indicative of a vascular injury, is

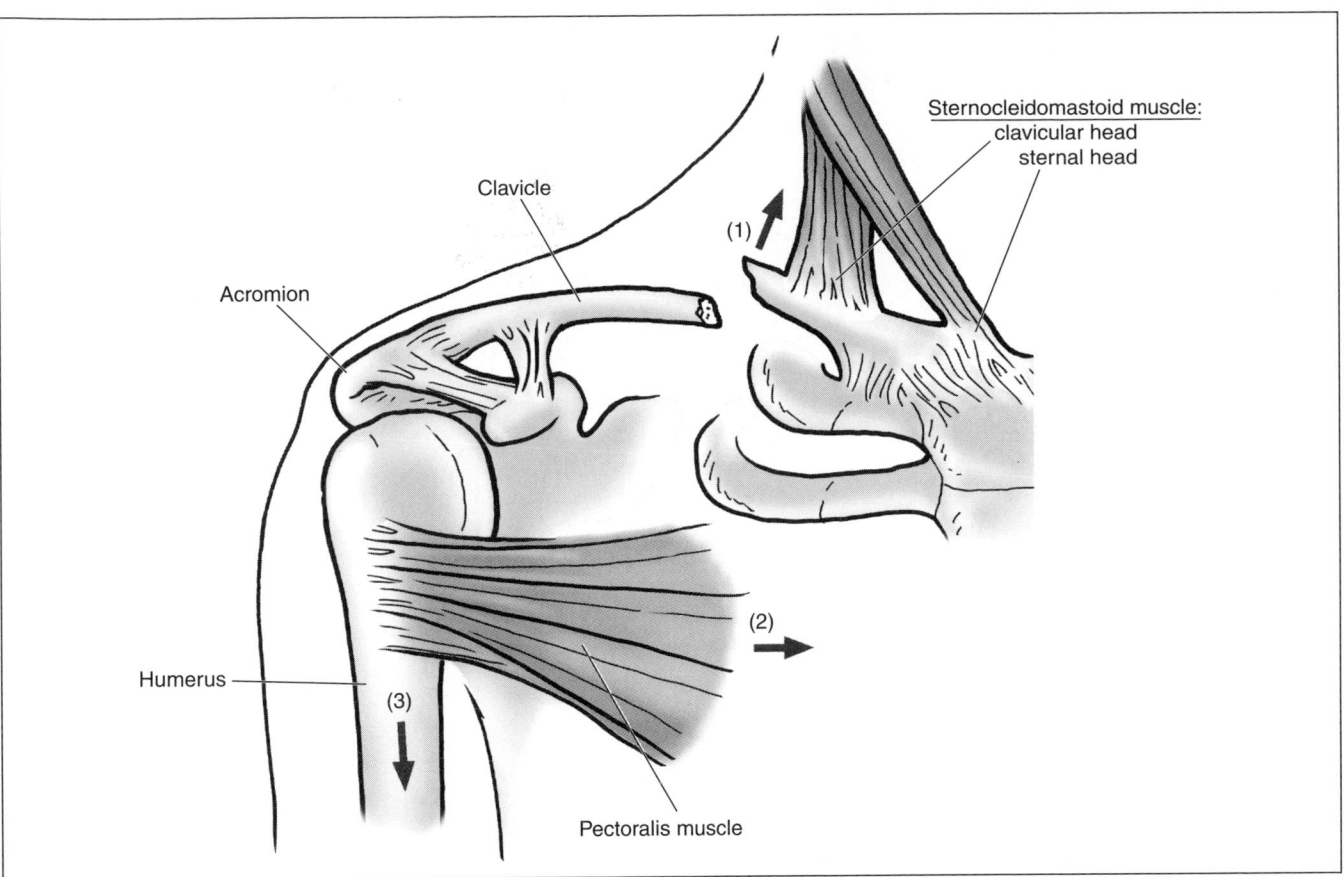

FIGURE 75-2 Displacement of the clavicle and shoulder after a clavicular fracture. The clavicular head of the sternocleido-mastoid muscle displaces the proximal clavicular fragment superiorly and posteriorly (*1*). The pectoralis major and latissimus dorsi muscles pull the shoulder medially (*2*). The force of gravity displaces the distal clavicle and shoulder inferiorly (*3*).

observed. Finally, unfamiliarity with technique is a relative contraindication.

EQUIPMENT

Figure-of-eight splint strap (commercially available)
Sling
Kerlix rolls
Elastic bandage

PATIENT PREPARATION

Explain the reduction technique and aftercare to the patient and/or their representative. As with any procedure, informed consent should be obtained. Consider the administration of oral, intramuscular, or intravenous analgesics for patient comfort during the procedure. Procedural sedation is not needed or required for this fracture reduction.

TECHNIQUE

Sit the patient upright on the side of the stretcher with their feet on the floor. Alternatively, the patient may be standing upright. Stand behind the patient. Grasp

and pull both of the patient's shoulders backward as if the patient were standing at attention. Instruct an assistant to apply the figure-of-eight splint while the patient is in this position. Apply the splint like a backpack and tighten the straps (Figure 75-3). Reassess the neurologic and vascular integrity of the affected extremity after application of the splint.

ASSESSMENT

The neurologic and vascular integrity of the upper extremity should be assessed for all patients both initially, following any reduction attempts, and after the application of a figure-of-eight splint. Any neurologic and/or vascular compromise requires an emergent consultation with an Orthopedic Surgeon.

AFTERCARE

Patients with uncomplicated fractures should be referred to an Orthopedic Surgeon in 7 to 10 days. Patients with group II distal fractures and any fracture in a child potentially involving the epiphysis should have an urgent consultation with an Orthopedic Surgeon within 24

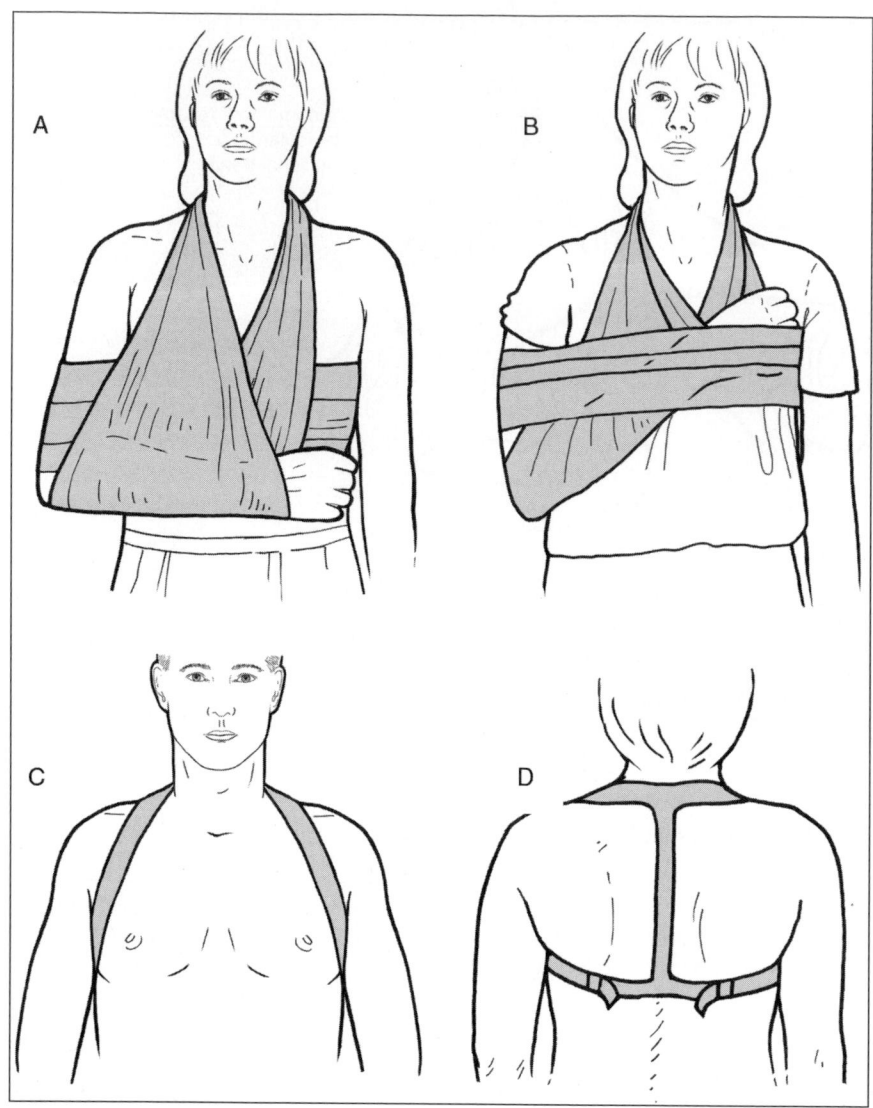

FIGURE 75-3 Treatment of clavicular fractures. *A.* Sling-over-swath immobilization. *B.* Velpeau sling immobilization. *C.* Anterior view of the figure-of-eight splint *D.* Posterior view of the figure-of-eight splint.

to 48 hours. Any patient with neurologic or vascular compromise, a pneumothorax, or signs of vascular injury should be admitted to the hospital after an emergent consultation by an Orthopedic Surgeon.

General principles of orthopedic care are recommended. These include the application of ice, rest, nonsteroidal anti-inflammatory drugs, and narcotic analgesics as needed. Most patients find the figure-of-eight splint extremely uncomfortable and remove it shortly after its application. If the patient tolerates the splint, it should be tightened daily. The figure-of-eight strap should be worn until there is evidence of clinical union and the arm can be abducted without pain. This generally requires 3 to 5 weeks in children and 6 or more weeks in adults.[1,2] It may be more advantageous to apply a sling and swath or a sling and Velpeau wrap for patient

comfort and compliance (Figures 75-3*A* and *B*). Alternatively, apply a shoulder immobilizer.

The sling is used to immobilize and elevate the elbow, forearm, and hand. It is also used to support the upper extremity. Slings are often used to support casts or splints of the upper extremity. These devices are simple, inexpensive, and effective. **It is imperative that the sling not be too short to allow the wrist and hand to hang over the sling.** This can result in an ulnar nerve neuropraxia.

The addition of a swath to a sling is used to immobilize dislocated shoulders that have been reduced and proximal humeral fractures (Figure 75-3*A*). The swath immobilizes the humerus against the torso to limit motion at the shoulder. A shoulder immobilizer may be substituted for a sling and swath.

The Velpeau wrap is a sling-and-swath technique that positions the forearm diagonally rather than horizontally (Figure 75-3B). The Velpeau wrap has no practical advantages over a sling and swath.

The figure-of-eight strap is difficult to apply, uncomfortable for the patient, and often removed after the patient leaves the Emergency Department. Its use has no advantage over a sling or a sling and swath.

COMPLICATIONS

Complications of the reduction procedure include injuries to the brachial plexus and to the subclavian artery and vein.[1,2] These are more commonly the result of the injury and not the reduction procedure. **It is imperative to perform a neurologic and vascular examination prior to and after any attempt at reducing a clavicular fracture.**

SUMMARY

Clavicular fractures are common, easily diagnosed, and often treated in the Emergency Department. Fractures of the distal or medial third may be more challenging. Although the incidence of complications is low, a thorough search for resultant or concomitant injury is required. Any evidence of neurologic or vascular compromise requires an emergent consultation with an Orthopedic Surgeon.

COLLES FRACTURE

INTRODUCTION

A Colles fracture is a transverse fracture of the distal radial metaphysis with dorsal displacement and angulation of the distal fragment. The fracture usually occurs 2 cm from the distal end of the radius (Figure 75-4). The most common mechanism producing a Colles fracture is a fall on an outstretched hand.[5,6] The majority of fractures occur in patients 50 years of age and older.[5,6] This fracture is more commonly seen in women than in men.

The Colles fracture is the most common fracture of the wrist.[5,6] Familiarity with its presentation, indications for reduction, and method of reduction are essential for the Emergency Physician. Consult an Orthopedic Surgeon for the reduction of most fractures, due to the high incidence of long-term complications that may result, even when these fractures are appropriately managed and reduced.[5,6]

ANATOMY AND PATHOPHYSIOLOGY

The distal radius is involved in two important articulations. First is the distal radioulnar joint, which is responsible for pronation and supination of the forearm. The second is the wrist articulation. The distal radius normally displays approximately 15 to 30 degrees of angulation relative to the ulna. It also has a volar tilt of up

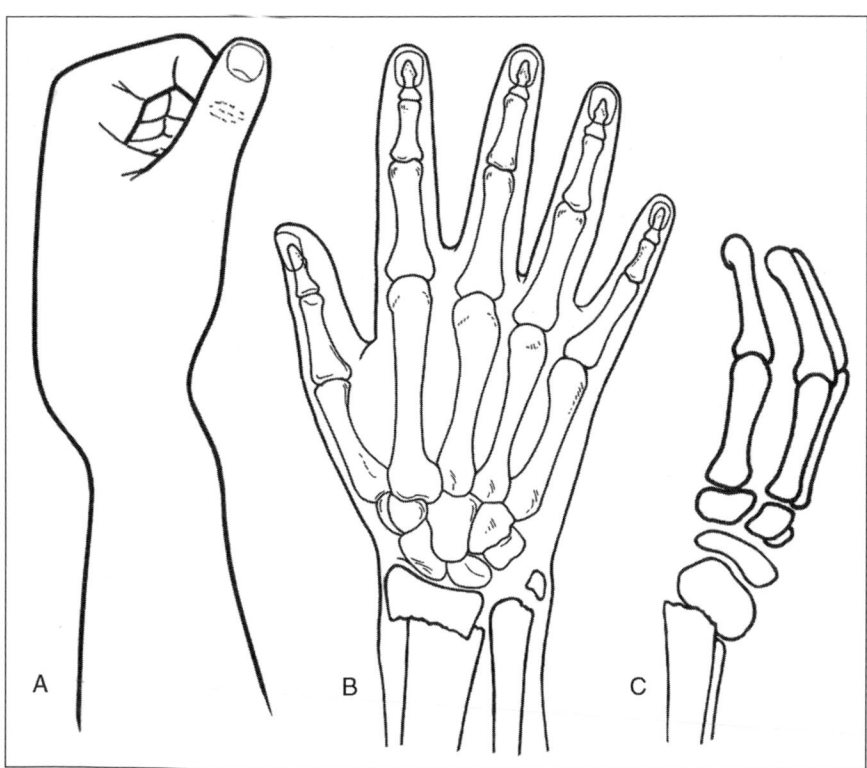

FIGURE 75-4 The Colles fracture. *A.* The dinner fork deformity, which is often seen. *B.* Anteroposterior view. *C.* Lateral view.

660 SECTION FIVE / ORTHOPEDIC AND MUSCULOSKELETAL PROCEDURES

to 23 degrees. It is important to maintain this anatomic position of the distal radius with the reduction of a Colles fracture so that the patient retains good function of the wrist and distal radioulnar joints.[6]

The Colles fracture can be associated with several other significant injuries. Up to 60 percent of patients have a fracture of the ulnar styloid process.[5,6] Other injuries include carpal fractures, distal radioulnar joint subluxations, flexor tendon injuries, median nerve injuries, ulnar neck fractures, and ulnar nerve injuries. A thorough physical examination and evaluation of the radiographs will uncover these injuries.

Standard radiographs include the anteroposterior and lateral views of the wrist. The Colles fracture is classically described as a "dinner fork" deformity when seen on lateral view (Figure 75-4A). Intraarticular involvement with the fracture is rare and should prompt an emergent consultation with an Orthopedic Surgeon in the Emergency Department for reduction.[6]

A variation of the Colles fracture is the Smith fracture (reversed Colles). The Smith fracture is similar to the Colles fracture except that the distal fracture fragment is displaced in a volar direction. This fracture most often results from a direct blow to the wrist while the hand is flexed. It is more commonly seen in young males. The management of these fractures is similar to that of the Colles fracture.

INDICATIONS

Nondisplaced Colles fractures can be placed in a splint or cast and the patient follow-up with an Orthopedic Surgeon on an outpatient basis. Displaced fractures should be reduced in the Emergency Department.[5,6] Simple Colles fractures may be reduced after consultation with an Orthopedic Surgeon. Many Orthopedic Surgeons prefer to reduce these fractures themselves, often prior to open reduction and internal fixation. **It is necessary to emergently reduce the fracture if the patient has neurologic and/or vascular compromise.** The Emergency Physician should reduce the fracture if the Orthopedic Surgeon is not immediately available. The goal is to relieve the neurologic and/or vascular compromise. Ideal positioning is not required. The Orthopedic Surgeon can later reduce the bony defect.

CONTRAINDICATIONS

Contraindications to the reduction of a Colles fracture include other injuries that represent a threat to life or limb. Airway, breathing, and circulation must first be addressed and stabilized. An Orthopedic Surgeon should reduce any fractures that involve the radioulnar or wrist joint. Complex, comminuted, or open fractures also require reduction by an Orthopedic Surgeon. Unfamiliarity with the reduction technique is a relative contraindication.

Any patient presenting with a Colles fracture should be evaluated for the presence of a compartment syndrome. **Any suspicion of a compartment syndrome necessitates having intracompartmental pressures measured. Elevated compartmental pressures require emergent consultation with an Orthopedic Surgeon or General Surgeon.** Reduction and fasciotomies should be performed in the Operating Room. Refer to Chapter 63 for the details regarding a compartment syndrome.

EQUIPMENT

Povidone iodine solution
Local anesthetic solution, 1 to 2% lidocaine
10 mL syringe
18 gauge needle
Chinese finger trap
Compressive cotton bandage (Webril)
Elastic wrap
8 to 10 pounds of weights
Casting material (plaster, fiberglass, prepackaged splints)

PATIENT PREPARATION

Obtain an informed consent for reduction of the fracture after explaining to the patient and/or their representative the indications, anticipated outcome, risks, benefits, and potential complications.

The patient should be given adequate anesthesia for the procedure. This can often be accomplished with a hematoma block. Clean the skin overlying the fracture of any dirt and debris. Apply povidone iodine solution to the skin and allow it to dry. Place a subcutaneous wheal of local anesthetic solution over the area of the hematoma. Insert an 18 gauge needle through the anesthetized skin and into the hematoma. Aspirate blood from the hematoma site to confirm proper needle placement. Inject 5 to 10 mL of the local anesthetic solution into the hematoma surrounding the fracture. Although a hematoma block will provide adequate anesthesia in most patients, it may be incomplete. Adjunctive or alternative anesthesia includes intramuscular analgesics, intravenous analgesics, regional nerve blocks (Chapter 106), Bier blocks (Chapter 107), and procedural sedation (Chapter 109).

TECHNIQUE

Place the patient supine on a stretcher. Perform a hematoma block as described above. Provide supplemental analgesia to the patient if required. Position the patient as in Figure 75-5A. Abduct the arm 90 degrees and allow it to hang over the edge of the bed. Flex the elbow 90 degrees with the hand pointing upright. Insert the thumb, index finger, and long finger into the Chinese finger trap (Figure 75-5B). Suspend 8 to 10 pounds of weights from the elbow (Figure 75-5C). Allow the pa-

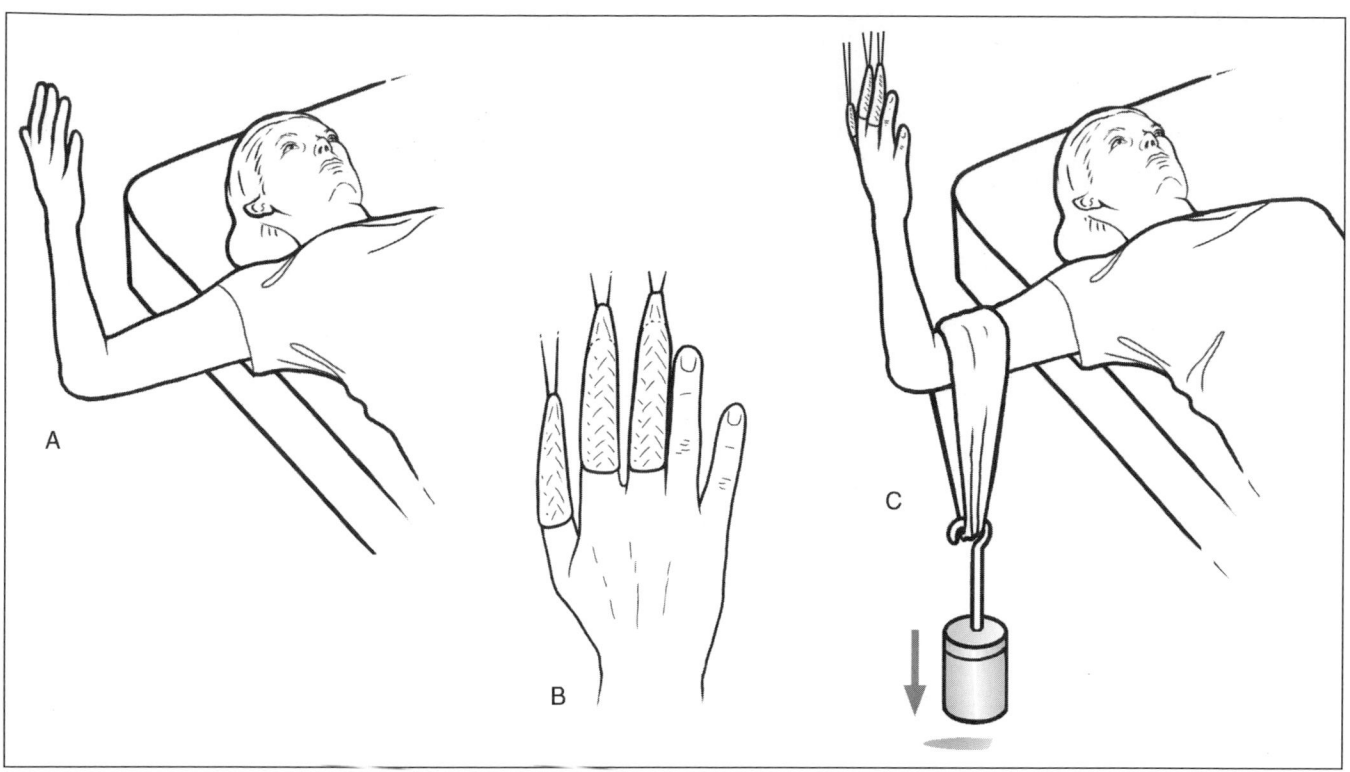

FIGURE 75-5 Positioning for the reduction of a Colles fracture. *A*. The arm is abducted 90 degrees and the elbow is flexed 90 degrees. *B*. The thumb, index finger, and long finger are placed in the Chinese finger trap. *C*. Weights are suspended from the elbow.

tient to remain in this position for 5 to 10 minutes to distract and disimpact the fracture fragments.

The fracture reduction involves traction followed by manipulation of the distal radial fragment to reverse the action that resulted in the fracture (Figure 75-6). Place both hands around the patient's wrist with the thumbs at the base of the fracture site (Figure 75-6*A*). Displace the fracture fragment distally with the thumbs while maintaining traction with the Chinese finger trap and the weights (Figure 75-6*A*). This maneuver allows the distal fragment to become free from any contacts with the proximal radius, which may prevent its movement. Continue to manipulate the fragment distally while simultaneously manipulating it in a volar direction until the fragment assumes the proper anatomic position. Slight ulnar deviation of the fragment is often necessary (Figure 75-6*B*). Remove the weights. Palpation of a smooth surface at the radial and dorsal aspects of the radius indicates an appropriate reduction. Remove the Chinese finger trap and the weights.

Immobilize the forearm with a sugar tong splint. Place the forearm in a neutral position, halfway between pronation and supination. Place the wrist in 15 to 20 degrees of flexion and 20 degrees of ulnar deviation. Unstable fractures are best splinted immediately after the reduction while the hand is still maintained in the Chinese

finger trap for traction (Figure 75-6*C*). If a long arm cast is applied, be sure to bivalve it to prevent complications. A short arm splint or cast may be used if the fracture is stable and impacted or is stable in an elderly person who needs to maintain mobility of the elbow.

ASSESSMENT

All patients should be assessed both initially and following any reduction attempts for neurologic and vascular integrity of the extremity. Post-reduction radiographs should be obtained to confirm proper bony positioning. The procedure may be repeated if the radiographs show incomplete reduction. The goal is the restoration of the normal relationships and angles of the radius with congruity of the radiocarpal and radio-ulnar joints. The lateral radiograph should reveal a 23 degree angle of the radiocarpal joint in a palmar direction with no dorsal angulation. The anteroposterior radiograph should reveal a radioulnar joint angle of 15 to 30 degrees with the ulna in relation to the radiocarpal joint.

Positioning is not critical if the reduction was performed for neurologic and/or vascular compromise. The primary consideration is the relief of the compromised nerve and/or artery. The Orthopedic Surgeon can later reduce the bony defect that remains.

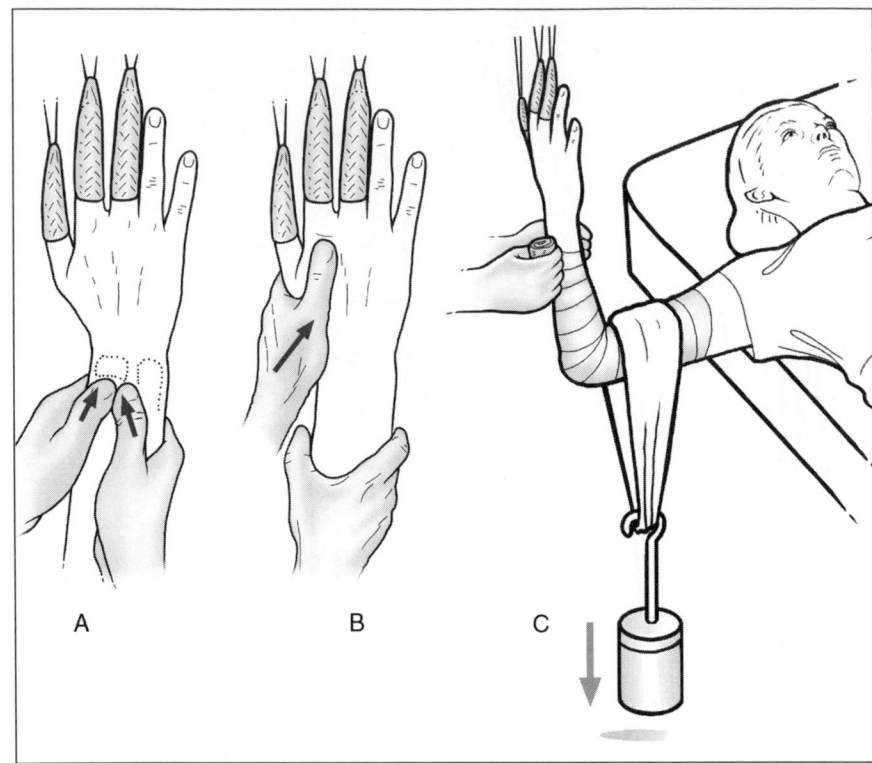

FIGURE 75-6 Reduction of a Colles fracture. *A.* Proper positioning of the physician's hands. The arrows represent the application of a distally directed force. *B.* Application of an ulnar-directed force to reduce the radial deviation. *C.* The application of a splint.

AFTERCARE

Patients with uncomplicated or nondisplaced fractures should be referred to an Orthopedic Surgeon in 24 to 48 hours. Patients with unstable fractures should be evaluated within 24 hours. **All patients should be given written instructions regarding the signs and symptoms of the splint or cast being too tight or a potential compartment syndrome.** Any patient with an open fracture, evidence of neurologic and/or vascular compromise, or suspicion of a compartment syndrome should be admitted to the hospital after an emergent consultation with an Orthopedic Surgeon.

General principles of orthopedic care are recommended. These include rest, elevation of the arm, nonsteroidal anti-inflammatory drugs, and narcotic analgesics as needed. The patient should be instructed to exercise the fingers and shoulder to prevent weakness, muscular atrophy, and the ligaments surrounding these joints from becoming taut.

COMPLICATIONS

Complications of the reduction procedure include post-reduction edema and bleeding into the forearm. These may contribute to the development of a compartment syndrome. Although infrequent, a neuropraxia of the median nerve is possible. Most complications result from the injury that produced the fracture and underlie

the need for a good neurologic and vascular examination prior to attempts at reduction. Any diminished or absent neurologic or vascular function requires an emergent consultation with an Orthopedic Surgeon. Incomplete reduction can result in future morbidity (pain, decreased range of motion, and deformity).

SUMMARY

The Colles fracture is the most common fracture of the wrist. Familiarity with its presentation and method of reduction are essential for the Emergency Physician. Many Orthopedic Surgeons prefer to reduce these fractures. Consultation is advised prior to reduction unless the extremity has evidence of neurologic or vascular compromise. These fractures have a high incidence of long-term complications, even when appropriately managed and reduced.[5,6]

DISPLACED SURGICAL NECK FRACTURE OF THE HUMERUS

INTRODUCTION

Proximal humeral fractures are relatively common. Most patients presenting to the Emergency Department with a proximal humeral fracture are elderly and usually have osteoporosis. The most common mechanism of injury involves a fall on an outstretched hand with the elbow extended.[3,7] The Emergency Physician can manage most of these fractures conservatively. However, the Emergency Physician must have a basic knowledge of the types of proximal humeral fractures, those that should be managed by the Orthopedic Surgeon, and the indications for emergent reduction.

ANATOMY AND PATHOPHYSIOLOGY

The proximal humerus is composed of the articular segment, the greater and lesser tuberosities, and the proximal humeral shaft. This anatomic division is based on the epiphyseal lines and the development of the humerus.[2,3,7] The commonly used Neer classification utilizes the observation that proximal humeral fractures separate primarily along these epiphyseal lines.[2,3,7] Using this classification, it is the displacement of fragments, not the total number of fracture lines, that is important. Significant displacement is considered to be a separation of greater than 1 cm or angulation of more than 45 degrees.[3,7] The classification separates fractures into one- to four-part fractures. The vast majority, approximately 80 percent, of proximal humeral fractures are one-part or minimally displaced fractures.[3,7] These fractures can be managed conservatively. Multiple-part fractures often require surgical intervention by an Orthopedic Surgeon. **A surgical neck fracture of the humerus is the only proximal humeral fracture that should be reduced by the Emergency Physician.**

INDICATIONS

Surgical neck fractures of the humerus may be reduced in the Emergency Department after consultation with an Orthopedic Surgeon. **If the patient has neurologic and/or vascular compromise, the reduction should be undertaken emergently after consultation with the Orthopedic Surgeon.**

CONTRAINDICATIONS

Contraindications to the reduction of humeral fractures include other injuries that represent a threat to life or limb. Airway, breathing, and circulation must first be addressed and stabilized. An Orthopedic Surgeon should manage any open fracture, complex comminuted fracture, or multiple-part fracture as the patient often requires operative repair and reduction.[2,3,7] Unfamiliarity with the reduction technique is a relative contraindication. Children presenting with separation of the proximal humeral epiphyses require meticulous realignment; their fractures should be reduced by an Orthopedic Surgeon.[2]

EQUIPMENT

Supplies and equipment for procedural sedation
  (Chapter 109)

Compressive cotton bandage (Webril)
Casting material (plaster, fiberglass, prepackaged
  splints)
Sling
Elastic wrap

PATIENT PREPARATION

Obtain an informed consent for reduction of the fractures after explaining to the patient and/or their representative the indications, anticipated outcome, risks, benefits, and potential complications of the procedure. Adequate anesthesia for this procedure is best accomplished with procedural sedation. Obtain an informed consent for the procedural sedation procedure. Refer to Chapter 109 for complete details regarding procedural sedation.

TECHNIQUE

Place the patient supine. Apply procedural sedation. Completely flex the patient's elbow. Apply a distractive force along the long axis of the humerus by applying traction on the patient's elbow (Figure 75-7A). Simultaneously slightly adduct the arm across the chest (to allow relaxation of the pectoralis muscle), slightly flex the arm, and apply lateral pressure to the fracture site while distracting the humerus (Figure 75-7B). Slowly release the traction on the elbow as the fragments come into good reduction.

Apply a sugar tong splint from over the deltoid muscle, under the elbow, and up into the axilla (Figure 75-8A). Secure the splint in the usual manner with an elastic wrap. Apply a sling (Figure 75-8B). Place the arm slightly across the chest and apply a sling and swath in the event of an unstable proximal humeral fracture (Figure 75-3A). This can help to limit the pull of the pectoralis muscle on the fracture site.

ASSESSMENT

All patients should be assessed both initially and following any reduction attempts for neurologic and vascular integrity of the extremity. Post-reduction radiographs should be obtained to confirm proper bony positioning. The procedure may be repeated if the radiographs show incomplete reduction.

Positioning is not critical if the reduction was performed for neurologic or vascular compromise. The primary consideration is the relief of the compromised nerve and/or artery. The Orthopedic Surgeon can later reduce the bony defect that remains.

AFTERCARE

Patients with uncomplicated or nondisplaced fractures should be referred to an Orthopedic Surgeon in 24 to 48 hours. **All patients should receive written instructions on the signs and symptoms of the splint being too**

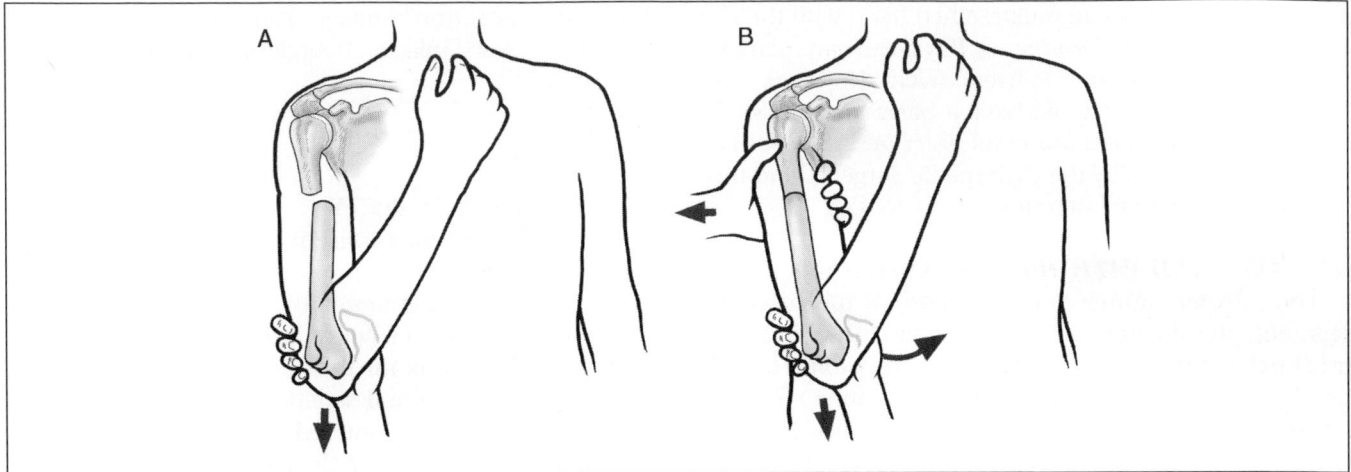

FIGURE 75-7 Reduction of a displaced surgical neck fracture of the humerus. *A.* The application of distal traction to the elbow. *B.* Lateral pressure is applied to reduce the fracture while maintaining distal traction, adducting the elbow, and slightly flexing the arm.

tight or a potential compartment syndrome. Patients with unstable fractures should be evaluated within 24 hours. Any patient with an open fracture, evidence of neurologic and/or vascular compromise, or suspicion of a compartment syndrome should be admitted to the hospital after an emergent consultation with an Orthopedic Surgeon.

COMPLICATIONS

Complications of the reduction procedure include primarily neurologic and/or vascular compromise. However, most complications result from the injury that pro-

duced the fracture; this underlies the need for a good neurovascular examination prior to reduction.

SUMMARY

Proximal humeral fractures are common. The Emergency Physician can manage most of these appropriately. A displaced surgical neck fracture is the only proximal humeral fracture that should be reduced in the Emergency Department. Reduction is often reserved for patients who have evidence of neurologic and/or vascular compromise. Most of these injuries require open reduction and internal fixation in the Operating Room by

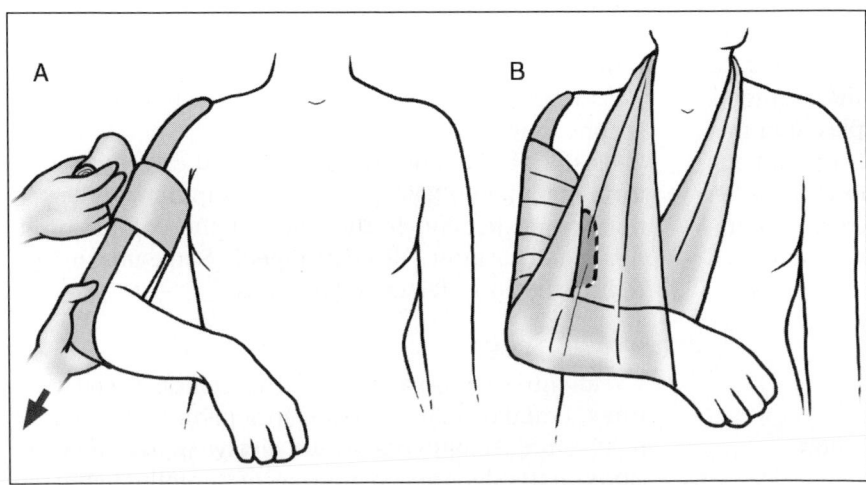

FIGURE 75-8 Immobilization of the reduced surgical neck fracture of the humerus. *A.* Application of a sugar tong splint. *B.* A sling is applied after padding is placed between the upper arm and the thorax.

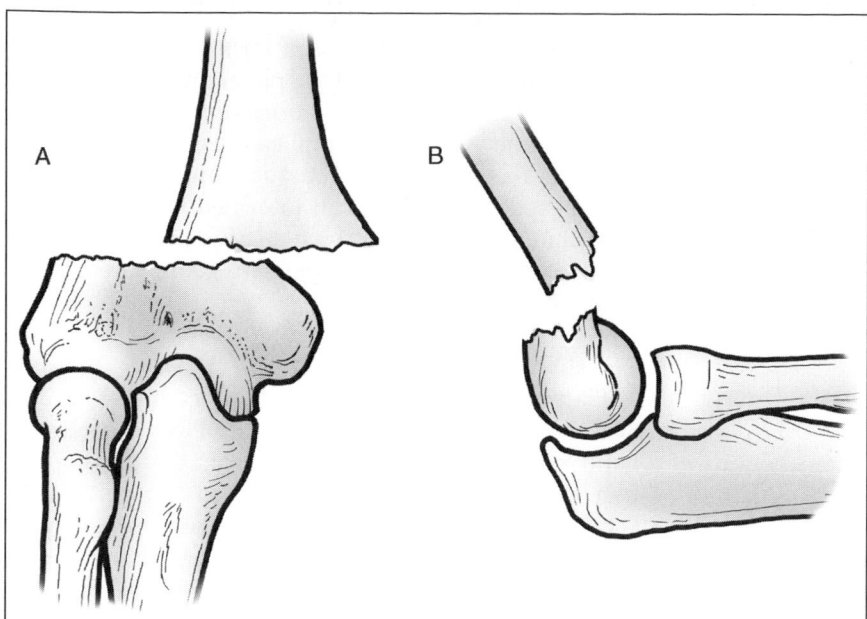

FIGURE 75-9 Supracondylar fracture of the humerus. *A.* Anteroposterior view. *B.* Lateral view.

an Orthopedic Surgeon. Close follow-up should be arranged for any patient discharged from the Emergency Department.

SUPRACONDYLAR FRACTURE OF THE HUMERUS

INTRODUCTION

Distal fractures of the humerus that are located just proximal to the epicondyles are known as supracondylar fractures (Figure 75-9). Supracondylar fractures are classified as extension and flexion fractures.[8–10] These fractures are common in children under the age of 15 and are rare in people over the age of 20.[8–10] The most common mechanism of injury involves a fall onto an outstretched hand with the elbow locked in extension.[8–10] The same mechanism of injury in an adult often results in a posterior elbow dislocation. The bones of an adult are much stronger than those of a child, so that the ligaments rupture rather than the bone fracturing.[8,9] **These injuries have a significant incidence of associated neurologic and/or vascular injury. There is a significant incidence of a subsequent compartment syndrome.** All supracondylar fractures should be referred to an Orthopedic Surgeon for follow-up care.

ANATOMY AND PATHOPHYSIOLOGY

On presentation, the child will be holding the affected extremity with the elbow flexed 90 degrees and the arm adducted.[8,10] Localized tenderness and swelling will be found upon examination. Extension fractures have posterior displacement of the distal fragment of the humerus that is aggravated by the pull of the triceps muscle.[8,10] The olecranon will be displaced posteriorly due to traction from the triceps muscle. The posterior displacement of the olecranon may mimic a posterior elbow dislocation. **Anterior angulation of the sharp proximal fragment (Figure 75-9*B*) may injure the brachial artery or median nerve (Figure 75-10). A thorough neurovascular examination is essential.** There will be loss of the normal olecranon prominence with flexion injuries. These fractures are frequently open and vascular injury is less frequent.[8,10]

Radiologic evaluation of supracondylar fractures is best appreciated on the lateral view. One-quarter of these fractures in children are of the greenstick variety.[8,10] The posterior fat pad sign and anterior humeral line should be closely examined. Even without any radiologic signs, a child with localized tenderness in the supracondylar area should be treated conservatively with splinting and referral to an Orthopedic Surgeon.[8,10] The anteroposterior view allows an assessment of any displacement. Displaced fractures should be emergently referred to and reduced by an Orthopedic Surgeon.

INDICATIONS

The only indication for reducing a supracondylar fracture of the humerus emergently is neurologic and/or vascular compromise of the extremity distal to the fracture.

CONTRAINDICATIONS

Contraindications to the reduction of a supracondylar fracture include other injuries that represent a threat to life or limb. The patient's airway, breathing, and circu-

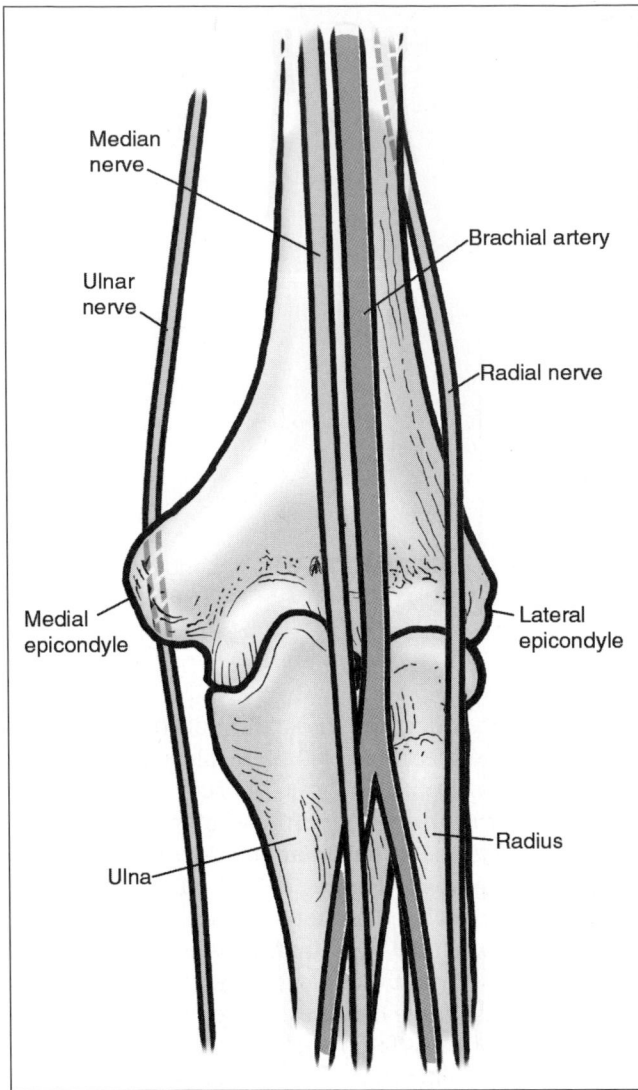

FIGURE 75-10 Major neurologic and vascular structures crossing the elbow.

lation must first be addressed and stabilized. An Orthopedic Surgeon should manage any open or displaced fractures. Unfamiliarity with the reduction technique is a relative contraindication. If the physician is uncomfortable with the reduction procedure, simple traction on the extended elbow may be sufficient to restore neurologic and/or vascular integrity.

EQUIPMENT

Supplies and equipment for procedural sedation (Chapter 109)
Compressive cotton bandage (Webril)
Elastic wraps
Casting material (plaster, fiberglass, prepackaged splints)
Prepackaged splinting sheets
Sling

PATIENT PREPARATION

Obtain an informed consent for the reduction of the fracture after explaining to the patient and/or their representative the indications, anticipated outcome, risks, benefits, and potential complications. Adequate anesthesia for this procedure is best accomplished with procedural sedation. Obtain an informed consent for this procedure in addition to the reduction procedure. Refer to Chapter 109 for complete details regarding procedural sedation.

TECHNIQUE

Place the patient supine. Apply procedural sedation. Slightly abduct the affected extremity. Place the patient's hand in the midposition between pronation and supination with the thumb pointing upward (Figure 75-11*A*). Grasp the patient's elbow region with the dominant hand and grasp the wrist with the nondominant hand (Figure 75-11*A*). Instruct an assistant to stabilize the proximal humerus (Figure 75-11*A*). Apply distal traction in line with the long axis of the arm by pulling on the wrist while simultaneously correcting any medial or lateral displacement at the elbow (Figure 75-11*A*). Supinate the patient's arm and correct any remaining medial or lateral displacement at the elbow while simultaneously distracting the wrist (Figure 75-11*B*). Place the thumb of the dominant hand across the joint line of the elbow with the fingers behind the olecranon process and slowly flex the elbow to just beyond 90 degrees while distracting the wrist (Figure 75-11*C*). Splint the arm in this position.

ASSESSMENT

All patients should be assessed both initially and following any reduction attempts for neurologic and vascular integrity of the extremity. Post-procedural swelling is common. Post-reduction radiographs should be obtained to confirm proper bony positioning. The procedure may be repeated if the radiographs show incomplete reduction.

Positioning is not critical if the reduction was performed for neurologic or vascular compromise. The primary consideration is the relief of the compromised nerve and/or artery. The Orthopedic Surgeon can later reduce the bony defect that remains.

AFTERCARE

Patients with supracondylar fractures should be admitted to the hospital to be monitored for a delayed compartment syndrome, neurologic compromise, or vascular compromise. Any patient with an open fracture, evidence of neurologic or vascular compromise, or suspicion of a compartment syndrome should be admitted to the hospital after an emergent consultation with an Orthopedic Surgeon.

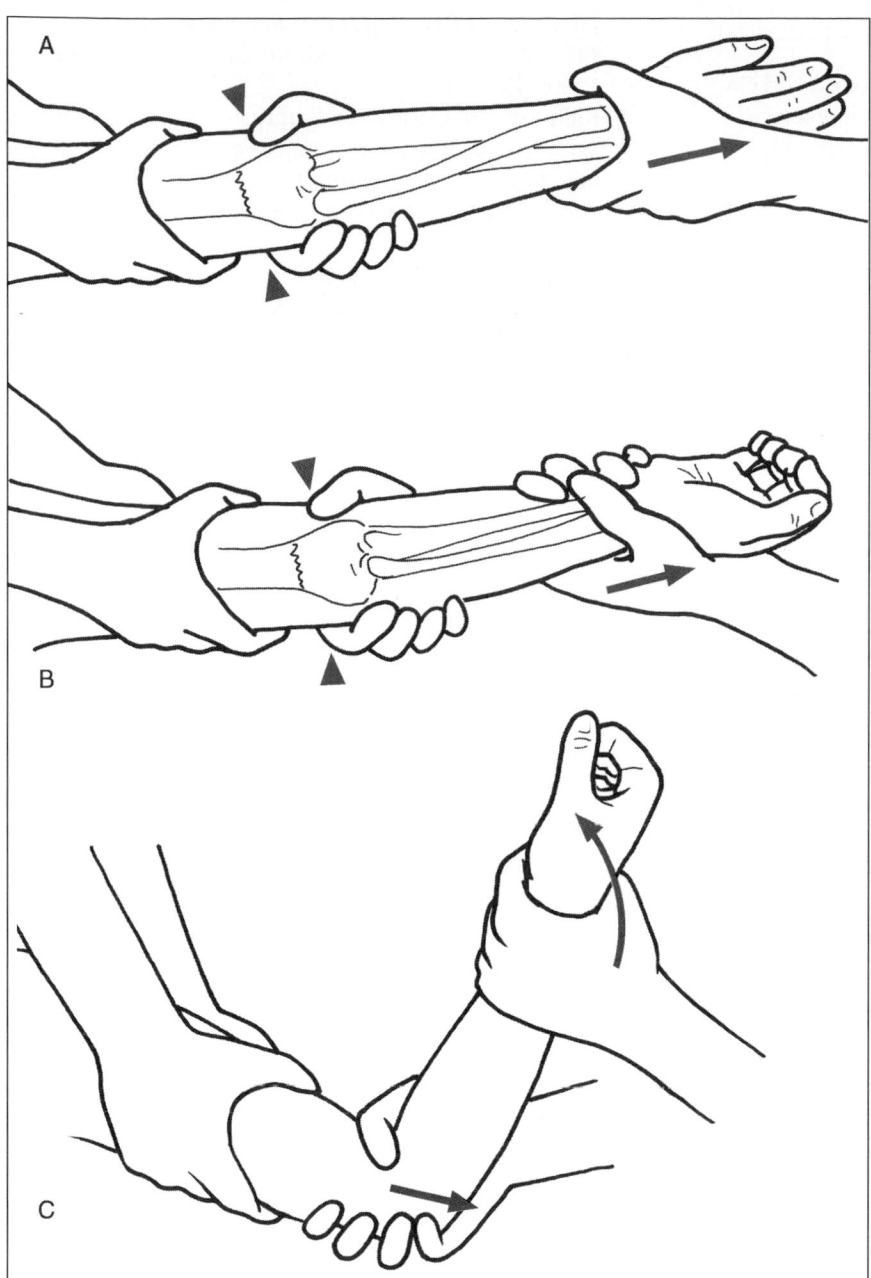

FIGURE 75-11 Reduction of a supracondylar fracture. *A.* Positioning of the hands of the physician and the assistant. Distal traction is applied (*arrow*) while reducing the medial or lateral displacement (*arrowheads*). *B.* The patient's hand is supinated while maintaining distal traction (*arrow*). Any remaining medial or lateral displacement is also corrected (*arrowheads*). *C.* The patient's elbow is flexed (*curved arrow*) just beyond 90 degrees while maintaining distal traction (*straight arrow*).

COMPLICATIONS

Most complications result from the injury that produced the fracture and not the reduction. Complications of the reduction procedure include primarily neurologic and vascular compromise. This is most often a neuropraxia and may involve any of the three nerves crossing the fracture. The neurovascular structures crossing the fracture may become lacerated or entrapped during the reduction. **The necessity of an accurate and complete neurovascular examination prior to and after reduction cannot be overemphasized.**

SUMMARY

Supracondylar fractures of the humerus are common in children under the age of 15 and rare over the age of 20. The most common mechanism of injury involves a fall onto an outstretched hand with the elbow locked in extension. These injuries have a significant incidence of associated neurologic injury, vascular injury, and the subsequent development of a compartment syndrome. The only indication for the reduction of a supracondylar fracture of the humerus by the Emergency Physician is neurologic and/or vascular compromise distal to the fracture.

REFERENCES

1. Craig EV: Fractures of the clavicle, in Rockwood CA, Green DP, Bucholz RW, et al (eds): *Rockwood and Green's Fractures in Adults,* 4th ed. New York: Lippincott, 1996:1109–1162.
2. Sanders JO, Rockwood CA, Curtis RJ: Fractures and dislocations of the humeral shaft and shoulder, in Rockwood CA, Green DP (eds): *Fractures in Children,* 4th ed. New York: Lippincott, 1996:905–1022.
3. Daya M: Shoulder, in Rosen P, Barkin R (eds*): Emergency Medicine: Concepts and Clinical Practice,* 3rd ed. St. Louis: Mosby, 1992:626–658.
4. Allman FL: Fractures and ligamentous injuries of the clavicle and its articulation. *J Bone Joint Surg Am* 1967; 49A:774–784.
5. Chin HW, Propp DA, Orban DJ: Forearm and wrist, in Rosen P, Barkin R (eds): *Emergency Medicine: Concepts and Clinical Practice,* 3rd ed. St. Louis: Mosby, 1992:626–658.
6. Cooney WP, Linscheid RL, Dobyns JH: Fractures and dislocations of the wrist, in Rockwood CA, Green DP, Bucholz RW, et al (eds): *Rockwood and Green's Fractures in Adults,* 4th ed. New York: Lippincott, 1996:745–868.
7. Richards RR, Corley FG: Fractures of the proximal humerus, in Rockwood CA, Green DP, Bucholz RW, et al (eds): *Rockwood and Green's Fractures in Adults,* 4th ed. New York: Lippincott, 1996:1055–1108.
8. Magnusson AR: Humerus and elbow, in Rosen P, Barkin R (eds): *Emergency Medicine: Concepts and Clinical Practice,* 3rd ed. St. Louis: Mosby, 1992:609–626.
9. Hotchkiss RN: Fractures and dislocations of the elbow, in Rockwood CA, Green DP, Bucholz RW, et al (eds): *Rockwood and Green's Fractures in Adults,* 4th ed. New York: Lippincott, 1996:929–1024.
10. Wilkins KE: Supracondylar fractures of the distal humerus, in Rockwood CA, Green DP (eds): *Fractures in Children,* 4th ed. New York: Lippincott, 1996:669–750.

Chapter 76
CASTS AND SPLINTS

Amy M. Hutson
David Rovinsky

INTRODUCTION

External immobilization of the extremities is one of the oldest forms of fracture treatment. References to plaster use and immobilization techniques are scattered throughout historical records. The use of plaster of paris (plaster) in fracture management dates back to the eighteenth-century Turkish Empire. Plaster bandages became commercially available in 1931. Despite the development of plastic casting products, the plaster bandage persists as the most economical and versatile material for immobilization techniques.[1]

Immobilization of an injured extremity begins at the scene of the accident. According to Advanced Trauma Life Support guidelines, the injured extremity must be aligned and immobilized after the appropriate management of life-threatening problems.[2] Prehospital immobilization of fractures is invaluable for pain control, prevention of soft tissue injury, and management of edema. External immobilization with splinting or casting is often the definitive management of injured extremities in the Emergency Department. Knowledge of and expertise in this therapeutic procedure is essential for any Emergency Physician.

Splints are commonly used for the immobilization of upper and lower extremity injuries. A splint is a hard bandage that is not circumferential and prevents movement of the injured extremity. Splinting may be the definitive management of certain injuries. Splints have the distinct advantage of being quick and easy to apply. They are designed to accommodate postinjury swelling. The major disadvantage of splints is that they provide slightly less rigid immobilization than casting.

Casts, which are generally circumferential, are better suited for the definitive treatment of fractures and ligamentous injuries. Casts provide superb immobilization and allow for the maintenance of a reduced fracture. The rigidity of a cast limits the amount of swelling and soft tissue edema and is therefore associated with an increased risk of developing a compartment syndrome. **Casts should be used with caution in the management of acute fractures. They are often split (bivalved) to allow swelling and prevent the development of a compartment syndrome before the patient is discharged from the Emergency Department.**

ANATOMY AND PATHOPHYSIOLOGY

Casts and splints rely on the principle of a three-point mold to maintain fracture reduction (Figure 76-1). **When applying a cast or splint, the application of directed force to the underlying bones should be uppermost in one's mind.** To obtain a three-point mold, place one point of contact over the convex side of the fracture site. The other two points of force are aimed in an opposite direction, proximal and distal to the fracture on the concave side. This is the classic teaching of Sir John Charnley, who noted that "a curved plaster is necessary in order to make a straight limb."[3] A skin-tight cast that closely follows the contours of the extremity will not maintain the fracture in alignment, as it does not apply appropriate pressure to the underlying bones.

Casts and splints also rely on hydraulic force to maintain limb length and alignment. One may think of the soft tissues surrounding the broken bones as constituting a flexible cylinder that contains the underlying fracture hematoma and edema. Axial loading of the bones will cause the soft tissue to expand and allow the limb to shorten. A well-applied cast or splint will resist the outward expansion from axial loading and provide additional support for the limb.[4]

Plaster is made of finely ground calcium sulfate that has been dehydrated by heat. The calcium sulfate is impregnated into muslin sheets containing dextrose or starch. The addition of various chemicals (alum, alu-

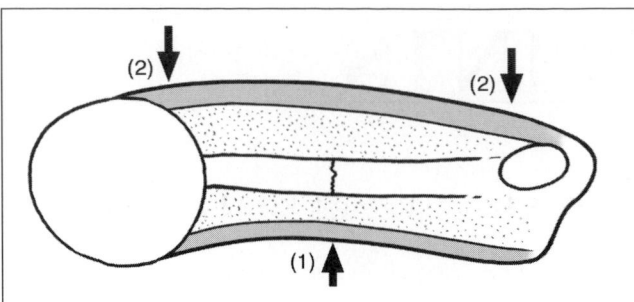

FIGURE 76-1 Three points of force are acting on the injured extremity in a well-applied cast or splint. One force is applied to the convex side of the fracture site (*1*). Two opposing forces are applied at sites proximal and distal to the fracture and on the concave side of the fracture (*2*).

minum, copper, iron, magnesium, salicylic acid, or zinc) to the calcium sulfate alters the rate of hardening after the addition of water. Plaster grades include fast-setting and extra-fast-setting plaster, which are useful for different applications. Long cylindrical crystals form and interlock as the cast sets to give strength to the cast. For this reason, plaster should not be moved once it begins to set, as these crystals may fracture, causing the plaster to lose strength. Careful lamination of the plaster while it is still wet will add strength by enabling the formation of longer crystals.

Crystal formation during the setting of plaster is an exothermic process that is initiated by the addition of water to the plaster. Using warm water will accelerate the chemical reaction and decrease the setting time. Unfortunately, the use of very warm or hot water will also increase heat production while the plaster sets. The use of very thick splints or fast-setting plaster will also increase the heat produced during setting. Using cold water to activate the plaster will increase the setting time and decrease the heat produced during setting. **Great care should be taken if warm water is used in applying a cast or splint to an anesthetized patient or an insensate limb, as the setting plaster may burn the skin.** Rubbing and working with the plaster will also accelerate the setting process.[5] These same principles apply to the use of fiberglass, which consists of cloth impregnated with resin and a water-activated catalyst.

INDICATIONS

SPLINTS

An injured extremity should be splinted as soon as possible after the injury. Reduction of pain, reduction of edema, and the prevention of further soft tissue injury are all achieved by splinting.[6] Any available material can be used to immobilize or realign the affected extremity

in the prehospital setting. **A thorough neurologic and vascular examination of the extremity should be performed and documented, followed by temporary splinting of the extremity before the patient undergoes radiographic studies.** Immobilize an extremity in the appropriate splint after diagnosing and stabilizing the fracture.

An extremity fracture is the most common reason for placement of a splint. A splint is also indicated following the reduction of a dislocated joint. The patient with ligamentous sprains or muscle strains will also receive great relief with splint immobilization. Splints are placed following orthopedic or soft tissue surgery of the extremities.

CASTS

There are few reasons to immobilize an acutely injured extremity with a cast in the Emergency Department. Most injuries can be initially stabilized with a splint. Following reduction of certain fractures, placement of a cast will secure the bones in their proper alignment and allow for a primary union (e.g., distal radius, tibial shaft).[6,7] **Placement of a cast instead of a splint should be performed only if the patient has access to close follow-up or can return to the Emergency Department for a cast check.**

Patients with casts may present to the Emergency Department with various cast-associated problems. The cast may have become wet and lost its strength and integrity. It may no longer fit properly if the affected extremity has decreased in size from reduction of swelling. The cast must be removed and the affected area examined if the patient complains of persistent pain.[6,7] All these patients may safely be placed in a cast. They may also be placed in an appropriate splint and follow-up arranged with an Orthopedic Surgeon for casting.

CONTRAINDICATIONS

SPLINTS

There are no absolute contraindications for the placement of a splint. Relative contraindications include soft tissue injuries or wounds that need regular care and evaluation. In this setting, the wounds should be appropriately dressed and padded and the splint constructed so that it can easily be removed and replaced. The splint should not place pressure over the wound.

CASTS

Do not cast an extremity that may develop a compartment syndrome. An injured extremity with significant edema or soft tissue injuries should not be constrained by a cast. Similarly, infections of joint spaces or soft tissues must remain exposed for frequent evaluations. Any fracture that is not adequately reduced by closed manipulation should not be placed in a cast.[3,7] A cast should not be applied by someone unfamiliar with the technique and unable to manage the associated complications.

EQUIPMENT

Bucket to hold water
Source of cool or tepid water
Cotton cast padding (Webril), various sizes
Plaster strips or rolls, various sizes
Bias stockinette, various sizes
Cloth tape, 1 inch wide
Sling

The width of the cotton cast padding, plaster, and bias stockinette required will vary by the site of application. In general, 3 to 4 inch wide material can be used for the upper extremity and 5 to 6 inch wide material can be used for the lower extremity. Alternative materials include fiberglass strips and rolls instead of plaster strips. Elastic bandages (Ace wraps) can be substituted for bias stockinette. Prefabricated splinting material is also available, with the padding and fiberglass (or plaster) already assembled and covered with cotton material (e.g., Orthoglass).

PATIENT PREPARATION

Whether reducing a fracture or simply manipulating the extremity to place a cast or splint, make sure that the patient has appropriate analgesia. Conduct a thorough examination of the skin overlying the site of injury. **It is inexcusable to miss the diagnosis of an open fracture. All skin wounds must be inspected and explored.** Exploration of the wound is undertaken cautiously with a sterile probe or gloved finger according to wound size. Fractures may puncture the skin from the "inside-out," resulting in an innocuous appearing pinhole in the skin. These are grade I open fractures and carry with them a 5 percent risk of infection.[8] Cover any open fractures with sterile saline-soaked gauze until formal irrigation and debridement can be undertaken in the Operating Room. Do not examine open wounds repeatedly due to the risk of increased contamination.

Document a thorough neurologic and vascular examination of the injured extremity before and after splinting or casting. Change in the neurovascular status of an extremity may be the result of the fracture reduction, the splint or cast application, or a compartment syndrome. The fracture may have to be reduced and held in position while a splint or a cast is applied. If no

reduction is needed, splint the affected extremity in a position of stability. Techniques for achieving and maintaining fracture reduction are beyond the scope of this chapter.

GENERAL SPLINTING CONSIDERATIONS

The general considerations and techniques common to the application of all splints are discussed in this section. It describes the techniques for splints utilizing cotton cast padding, plaster, and bias stockinette. Many alternative materials are available and may be substituted, such as fiberglass for plaster or elastic wraps for stockinette. Prefabricated splint materials that incorporate padding may also be used. The techniques described in these chapters are applicable for all splinting materials. Where alterations in technique are required, they are so noted.

Splints are constructed of cotton padding overlaid by strips of plaster and subsequently held in position by an overwrap of bias stockinette. Splint padding should be thick enough to provide protection for the skin from the plaster. **The splint or cast will be unable to provide sufficient immobilization of the fracture to maintain a reduction if the padding is too thick.** One to two layers of cotton cast padding are sufficient over the fracture site. Three to four layers of cotton cast padding are required at the proximal and distal extents of the splint to distribute the stresses. Thinner padding can be used when maintenance of fracture reduction is a priority (e.g., with a fracture of the distal radius).

Plaster strips are available in precut slabs measuring either 4 by 15 or 5 by 30 inches. The precut strips have the advantage of speed and ease of application. Alternatively, plaster is available in rolls of various widths ranging from 2 to 8 inches. The plaster may be rolled out to the precise length desired and torn appropriately. The plaster rolls are useful for splints requiring long strips of plaster, such as coaptation splints. **The ideal thickness for most upper extremity splints is 10 sheets or layers of plaster. The use of 15 sheets or layers of plaster is preferable for lower extremity splints.** The strength of the plaster splint depends on the number of sheets as well as the lamination of the plaster sheets during their application.

A piece of cotton cast padding may be used as a template for the length of the plaster strips. Roll a piece of cotton cast padding over the desired location of the splint to determine the length of the plaster strips required (Figure 76-2A). Roll out the plaster strips to the appropriate lengths and tear them slightly shorter than the template. Prepare strips of cotton cast padding. **The strips of cotton cast padding should always be longer and wider than the plaster.** This prevents the plaster

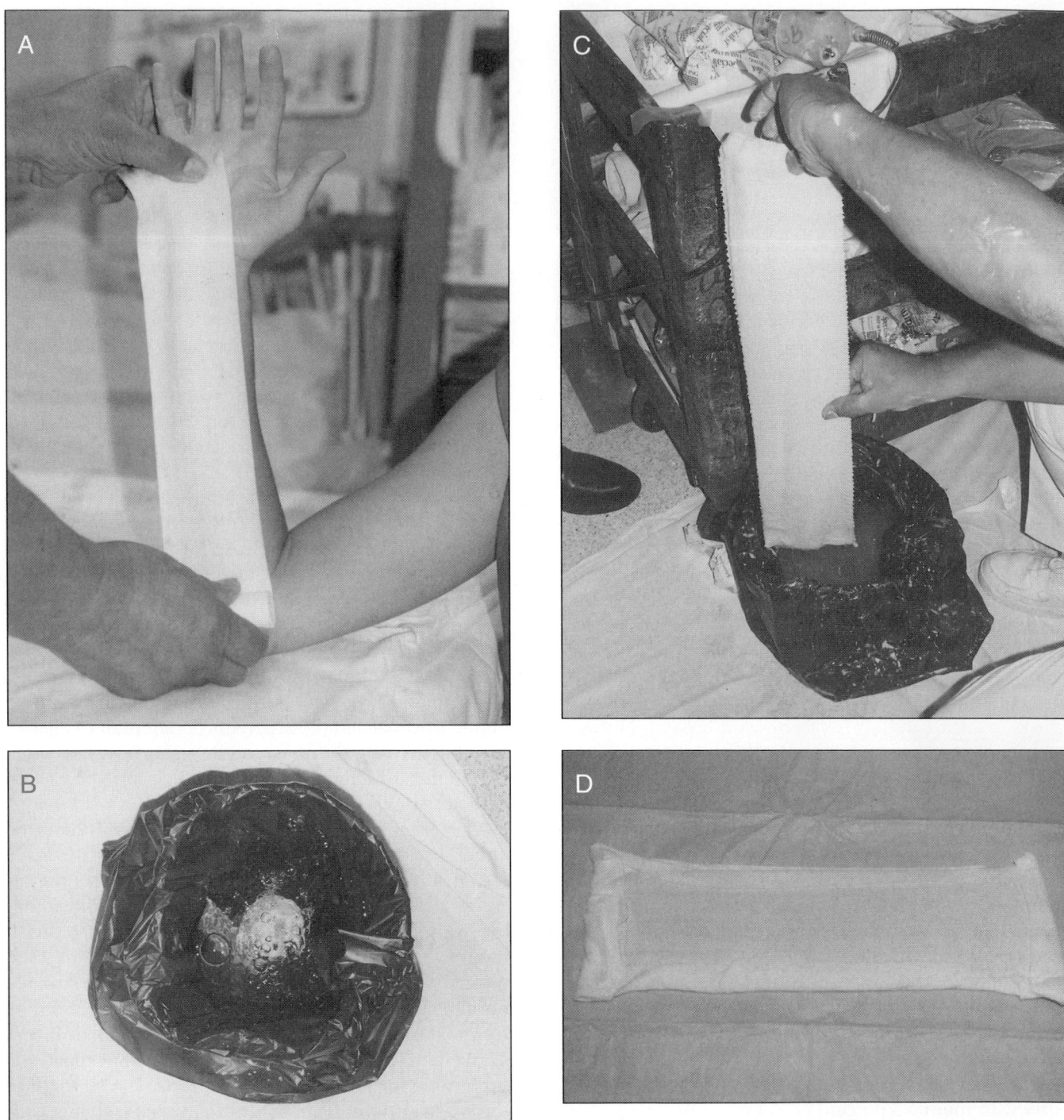

FIGURE 76-2 Preparing the splint. *A.* The use of cotton cast padding to measure the length of material needed for proper extremity immobilization before cutting the plaster lengths. *B.* The plaster is submersed in tepid water. It is ready to use once all the air bubbles have stopped rising from it. *C.* Suspend the lengths of wet plaster over the bucket. Use the lengths of your fingers to squeeze out the excess water. This should take only two or three passes along the length of the plaster. *D.* Place the plaster sheets on the cotton cast padding. Fold the cotton padding over all the edges to protect the skin from the plaster.

from touching the skin and causing a pressure sore, an abrasion, or a burn. Padding is especially important at the proximal and distal edges, as this is where significant pressure originates. Apply additional padding over pressure points and bony prominences (e.g., the olecranon) as needed. Alternatively, cotton cast padding may be applied directly by wrapping it circumferentially around the extremity (as is done in cast application).

Begin applying the splint once the padding and plaster have been cut to the appropriate lengths. Be sure that all required materials have been collected before dipping the plaster in water. Only a limited amount of time, less than 10 minutes, is available for splint application and molding once the plaster is wet. Completely immerse all of the plaster strips in a bucket of tepid, clean tap water. Keep the plaster submersed until no more bubbles arise from the plaster under water (Figure 76-2*B*). At this point the plaster can absorb no more water. Suspend the plaster strips over the bucket and lightly squeeze out the excess water by running your fingers down its length (Figure 76-2*C*). **It should only take two or three passes of the fingers to remove the excess water. Do not wring the plaster strips like a dish rag, as that will cause loss of plaster into the bucket!** Lay the plaster strips on a clean flat surface. Run your hands over the plaster to laminate the individual plaster strips into one slab. Laminating the plaster strips together adds significant strength. Lay the plaster onto the cotton cast padding. Fold the edges of the cotton cast padding over the plaster to cover all the plaster edges completely (Figure 76-2*D*). Apply the splint to the extremity.

An alternative method that is preferred by many is to apply the cotton cast padding over the extremity, overlapping each layer by 50 percent, and then applying the plaster sheets. In this fashion, the plaster will "stick" to the cotton cast padding. **Smooth the plaster sheets with the broad aspect of your hand and not your fingers to help minimize irregular indentations.**

The cotton cast padding should be facing the patient and no plaster should directly contact the skin regardless of the method used. Secure the splint with a wrap of bias stockinette. The wrap must be applied under minimal tension when you are using an elastic wrap to affix the splint. The elastic may cause increasing pressure over time. Apply three strips of tape to the end of the wrap to secure the bias stockinette or the elastic wrap.

The plaster may be molded at this point to achieve greater conformity to the extremity or better reduction of the fracture. **All molding must stop once the plaster begins to harden.** The plaster is quite fragile, and cracks that weaken the splint may be propagated. Apply 1 inch wide tape in a spiral fashion to secure the bias (or elastic wrap after the plaster has hardened). **Tape should never be applied circumferentially, as this can impede expansion of the splint due to underlying swelling and create a tourniquet effect. Application of the spiral tape before the splint is completely hard will cause indentations in the plaster and result in pressure points on the underlying skin.**

Fiberglass rolls must be cut to the appropriate length with scissors, because the fibers are too strong to be torn by hand. Gloves should always be worn when handling fiberglass because the resin will stick to hands and is exceedingly difficult to remove.[4–6] Otherwise, the same principles described above apply to fiberglass.

GENERAL CASTING CONSIDERATIONS

The general considerations and techniques common to the application of all casts are discussed in this section.[3,5,6,10] Casting requires careful circumferential turns of material instead of longitudinal layers of material, as for splints. Plaster casts are constructed of cotton cast padding overlaid with plaster bandages. Padding, pressure points, plaster application, and molding are four areas that require particular attention and are discussed in this section.

Begin by organizing the equipment. Cast application requires the same material as that used in splinting (cotton cast padding, stockinette, and plaster). The width of the padding and plaster depends on the size of the extremity. Generally, the 6 inch wide plaster rolls are used for lower extremity casts while 3 or 4 inch wide plaster rolls are used for the upper extremity. **Use the widest plaster available and possible in order to limit the number of turns of the plaster roll over joints or other curved surfaces.** Place all materials on a tray near the bedside, including a bucket of tepid water. An assistant designated to dip and drain the plaster is immensely helpful.

Prepare the patient. Position the extremity and the patient appropriately for cast placement. The patient is frequently able to assist in the process. Cover the patient with gowns or towels to keep plaster off their clothes.

Apply tubular stockinette to the extremity (Figure 76-3*A*). The stockinette is not a necessary component of casting, but many physicians use it as a first layer.[5] It provides a smooth covering over the skin that wraps neatly over both ends of the cast. Roll up the stockinette. Place it over the distal extremity as if you were putting on a sock (Figure 76-3*A*). Unroll the stockinette up the leg (Figure 76-3*B*). Care must be taken to apply the stockinette gently. **Do not create tension in the stockinette by pulling it tightly. Eliminate any creases or redundancy of material by trimming any overlapping folds with a scissors.**

The primary layer of padding is provided by the cotton cast padding. **Casts and cast padding should be applied from distal to proximal.** Begin wrapping the cotton cast padding at a point that will be distal to the start of the plaster (Figure 76-3*B*). This initial band of padding is essential for protection against the cast edge. Keep the roll of padding in contact with the skin so that the material conforms easily to the contours of the extremity as it unrolls. Unroll the padding in a circumferential manner

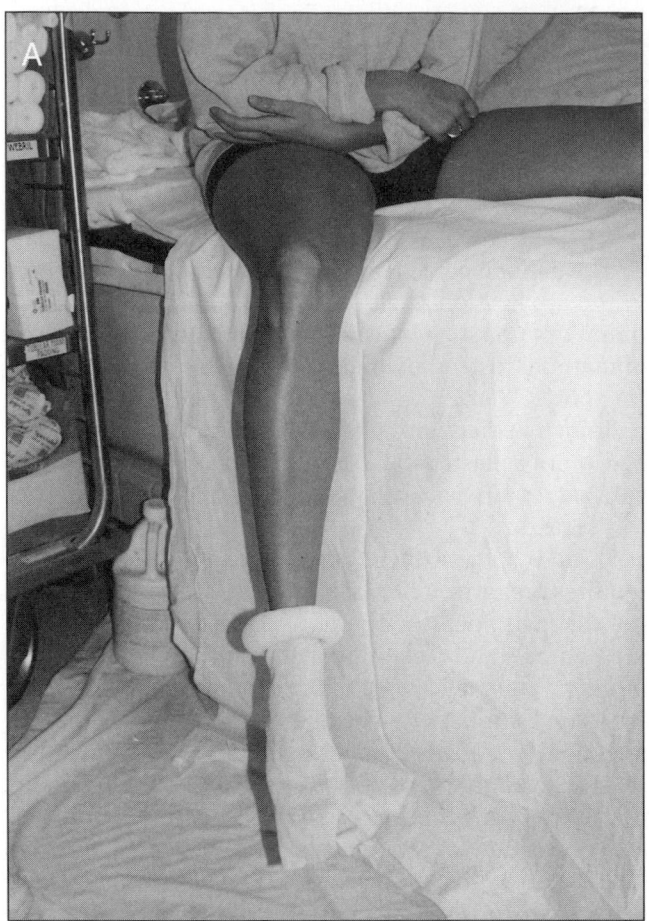
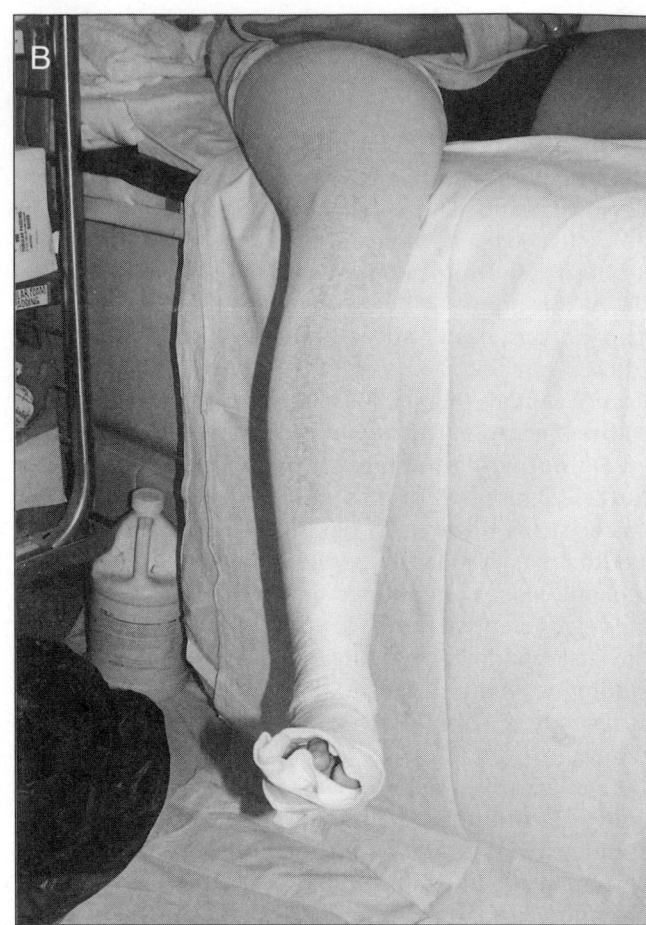

FIGURE 76-3 Preparing to place a cast. *A.* Apply an initial layer of tubular stockinette. *B.* The stockinette has been unrolled over the extremity. Begin and end the layering of the cotton cast padding at a site distal and proximal to where the plaster material will end. This ensures protection at the cast edges. Excess length can easily be torn away after the plaster is applied.

around the extremity (Figure 76-3*C*). **The cotton cast padding must be laid down neatly and cleanly with no kinks or creases.** Each turn should overlap one-third to one-half of the previous turn. Tear off the extra cotton cast padding to eliminate excess material as you turn angles (ankle, heel, elbow, or thumb). **Lay the torn edges down by rubbing the padding smoothly.** Continue applying the padding, ensuring that it extends beyond the proximal end of where the cast edge will be. Typically, two layers of cotton cast padding are adequate for protection between the skin and the casting material.

Pressure points occur over bony prominences or where excess padding has created an unnatural prominence. Palpate the obvious bony prominences to get a sense of whether or not there is adequate padding after the application of the two layers of padding. If the area feels vulnerable, place torn off pieces of cotton cast padding onto the exposed areas (Figure 76-3*D*). **Do not over-pad bony prominences, as excess layering can also lead to excess pressure.** Rub the torn edges of the padding so that they fuse smoothly to the underlying padding.

Place the rolls of plaster material in a bucket of tepid water so that they are standing on end. Let the plaster remain submersed as long as air bubbles rise out from the center of the roll (Figure 76-2*B*). Remove the rolls of plaster when all bubbles stop rising. Hold the plaster roll in both hands and squeeze some of the water out (Figure 76-4). **Do not wring the roll. Do not eliminate all the water from the plaster roll.** The remaining water in the roll of plaster is necessary for smoothing and molding the plaster into one solid unit. In general, casts should be applied with "wetter" plaster and splints with "drier" plaster.

Apply the plaster (Figure 76-5). Place the roll of plaster on the extremity (Figure 76-5*A*). Unroll the plaster in a circumferential fashion around the extremity. **Never lift the plaster roll off the extremity!** Continue each consecutive wrap around the extremity by overlapping the plaster by 50 percent. The free border of the plaster will have excess material in it as the extremity changes in size. Grasp this excess plaster with the thumb and index finger of the nondominant hand (Figure 76-5*B*). Pull it outward to create a tuck or a fold. Wrap this fold around the

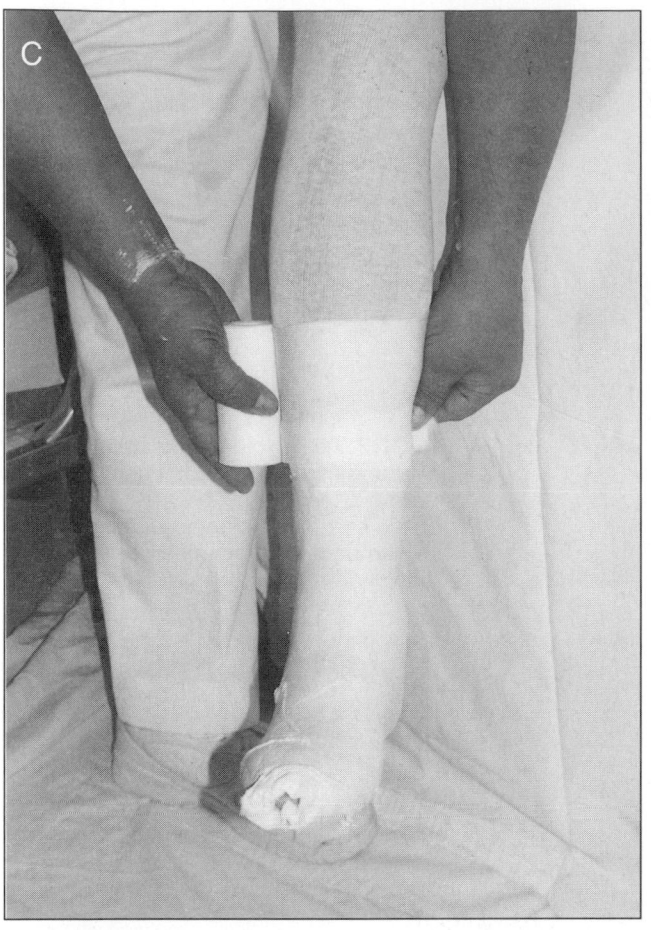
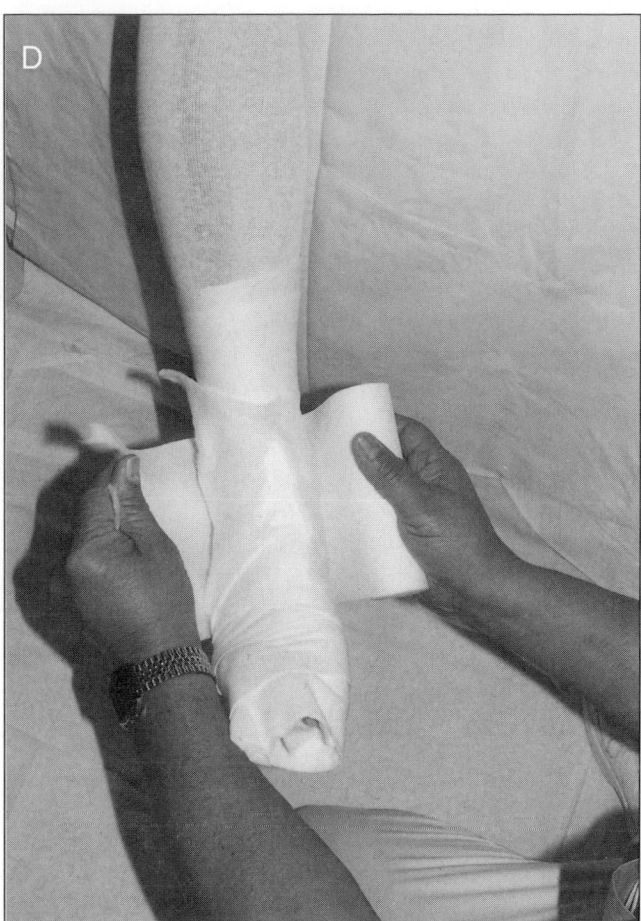

FIGURE 76-3 *(continued) C.* Unroll the plaster in a circumferential manner, covering each preceding layer by one-third to one-half of its width. *D.* The cotton cast padding tears easily to provide additional layers of padding over bony prominences.

extremity (Figure 76 5*C*) and smooth the fold down against the plaster. This fold will barely be noticeable in the final product. As one roll of plaster ends, another should begin with a small amount of end-to-end overlap.

Continuously mold and smooth the plaster with wet hands as each layer is applied. **This action ensures continuity of plaster material throughout the cast and forms a smooth cast that conforms to the contours of the extremity. Use the palmar surface of the hands and proximal digits (Figure 76-5D). Excess use of the fingertips will produce irregular indentations and pressure points.** Molding around irregular bony areas is best accomplished with two hands simultaneously rubbing the plaster. **Do not allow excess time to pass between each layering of plaster, as lamination between layers may not occur. This will weaken the cast considerably.**

A cast thickness of 1/4 inch is felt to be adequate. This usually requires four to five layers of plaster. Allow the cast to set and dry with no further manipulations. The time for drying is variable depending upon the casting material used, the water temperature, and the thickness of the cast. Typically, one should let the casting material

set over a period of 10 to 15 minutes. Fold the free ends of the cotton cast padding and the stockinette over the edges of the cast as it sets (Figure 76-6). This prevents the rough edges of the plaster from irritating and abrading the skin. Secure the edges of the cotton cast padding neatly with tape or thin strips of plaster.

It is a common practice to bivalve the cast with a saw if increased swelling of the extremity is a concern (Figure 76-7). Cut completely through the length of the cast in two spots 180 degrees apart (i.e., medial and lateral or anterior and posterior). This simple maneuver provides some room for edema without compromising the integrity of the reduction or the strength of the cast. **The underlying cast padding must also be split. Splitting the plaster alone will not reduce the pressure sufficiently.**

UPPER EXTREMITY CASTS AND SPLINTS

COAPTATION SPLINT

A coaptation ("to bring together") splint is used primarily in the acute setting for humeral shaft fractures

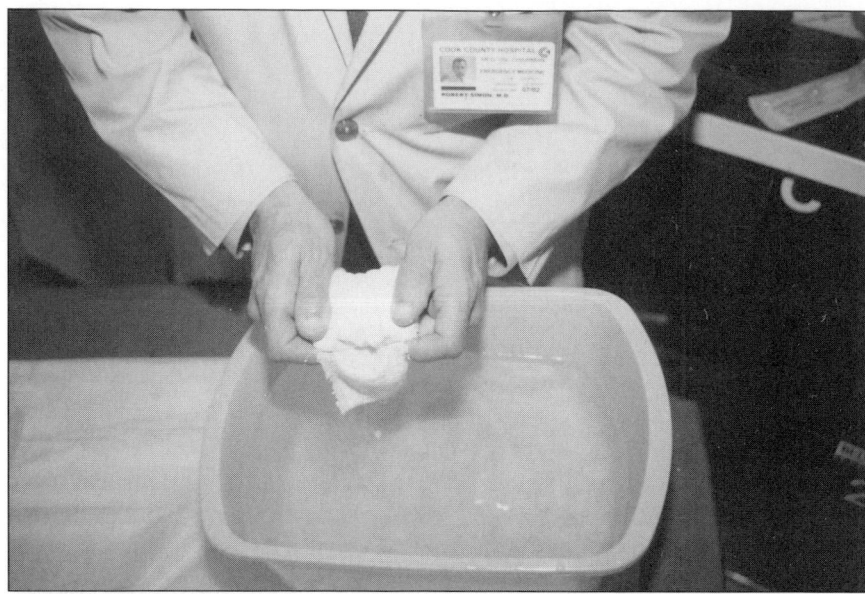

FIGURE 76-4 Hold the plaster roll in both hands and gently twist each end to squeeze out the excess water. Keeping the free end of the plaster folded over will facilitate access after it has been removed from the water.

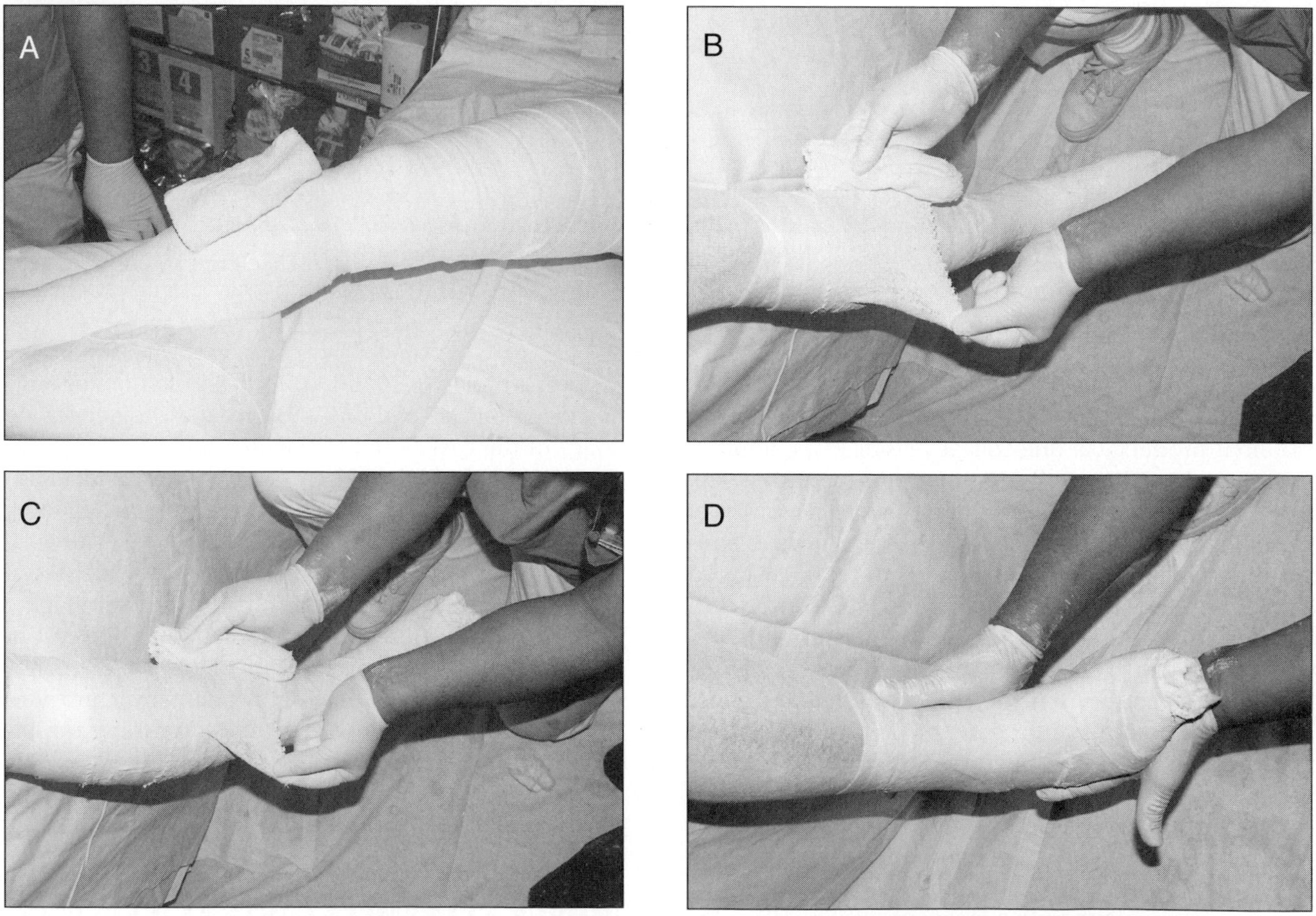

FIGURE 76-5 Applying a plaster cast. *A.* Lay the plaster on the extremity and unroll it. Never lift and pull the plaster around the extremity. *B.* As the limb changes in girth, there will be excess plaster. Use the nondominant hand to pull on the excess material. *C.* Fold the excess material back onto the plaster in a neat tuck. Each tuck should be laid down smoothly with a molding of the hand. *D.* The plaster is laminated smoothly with a continuous motion of the palmar surface of the hand and the proximal fingers.

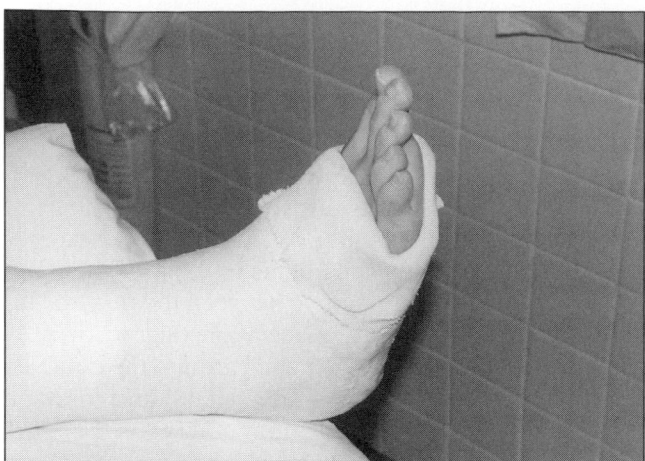

FIGURE 76-6 Fold the free ends of the cotton cast padding and the stockinette over the edges of the plaster to finish the cast.

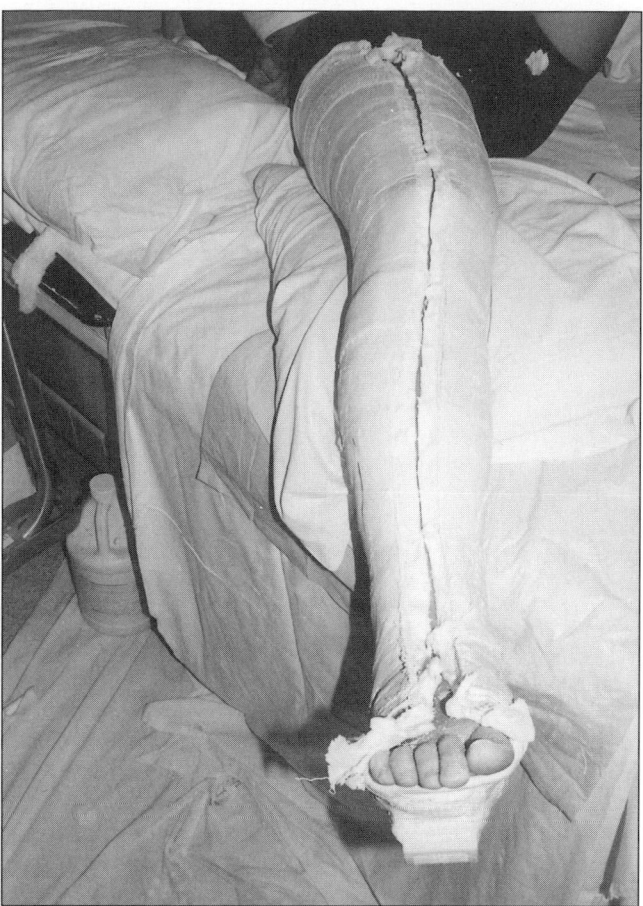

FIGURE 76-7 Splitting of the cast can be achieved with a cast saw that cuts through the thickness of the plaster. Cut the underlying protective material with a scissors. Cotton cast padding or stockinette that is left intact exerts excess pressure on the limb.

that are nondisplaced or minimally displaced. This splinting technique allows for motion of the hand and wrist while limiting shoulder and elbow mobility. The length of the plaster extends from the axilla, around the 90 degree flexed elbow, along the outer arm, over the deltoid muscle, and over the acromion process (Figure 76-8). **It is critical that the plaster extend over the deltoid muscle and the acromion process.** The shoulder portion can be held down by applying 3 inch wide tape over the portion of the splint that covers the acromion. The major pitfall is making the splint too short and having it fall off! Always leave plenty of length over the shoulder. Padding is required to minimize axillary irritation. The disadvantages of this splint include the possibility of fracture displacement and extremity shortening. The splint should be replaced with a functional brace or cast after a short period of immobilization for pain control.[4]

SUGAR TONG SPLINT

Sugar tong splints may be used for mid- and distal forearm fractures. They are most commonly recommended for minimally displaced and distal ulnar and radial fractures (Colles, Smith). This splint immobilizes the elbow and wrist joints to prevent supination and pronation of the forearm (Figure 76-9). The splint begins at the palm, just proximal to the metacarpophalangeal (MCP) joints. Measure the required length of plaster along the volar surface of the hand (starting just proximal to the MCP joints) and forearm, around the elbow, and back on the dorsal surface of the forearm ending just proximal to the MCP joints (Figure 76-9*A*). **The MCP joints should be left completely free to prevent stiffness.** Early mobilization of the fingers will help to reduce swelling. Apply cotton cast padding from the MCP joints to just proximal to the elbow (Figure 76-9*B*). The ulnar styloid and olecranon are two bony prominences

that need extra padding for comfort and prevention of pressure sores. The ends of the splint also need added protection to minimize hand discomfort. Apply the splint. **Mold the plaster with great caution to prevent closure of the sides of the splint, thus forming a closed cast.** Fold and cut the dorsal aspect to ensure that the MCP joints are freely mobile (Figure 76-9*C*).

POSTERIOR LONG ARM SPLINT

Distal humeral fractures and proximal forearm fractures can be immobilized in a posterior long arm splint (Figure 76-10). It is also useful for fractures of the radial head and neck, olecranon fractures, and severe ligamentous injuries to the elbow. The posterior long arm splint extends from the axillary crease area, behind the elbow, then traveling distally to incorporate the wrist joint (Figure 76-10). This splint immobilizes the elbow in a range of 45 to 90 degrees with the forearm in supination, pronation, or neutral positioning depending upon the type of injury. The wrist can also be in a flexed, extended,

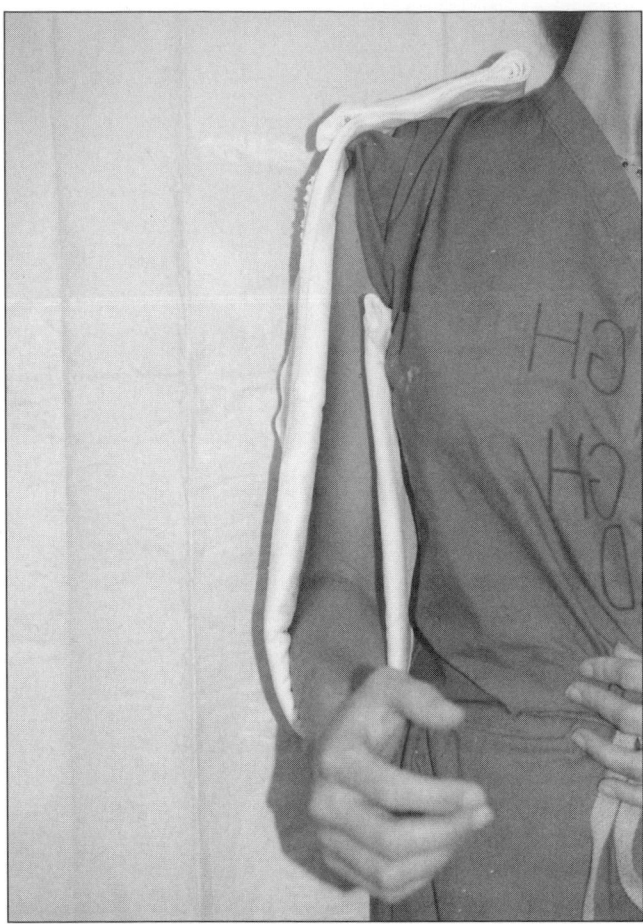

FIGURE 76-8 The coaptation splint. Adequate splint length is needed to extend over the deltoid muscle and acromion process. Care is taken at the axilla to ensure adequate padding and protection. The padding and overwrap have been omitted for easier visualization of the splint.

or neutral position. **The metacarpals should not be immobilized in this splint.** Despite the many possibilities, the posterior long arm splint is usually applied with the elbow flexed 90 degrees, the forearm neutral, and the wrist neutral (Figure 76-10).

RADIAL GUTTER SPLINT

The radial gutter splint is used for the treatment of stable phalangeal and metacarpal fractures of the index or middle fingers. The plaster extends from the pulp of the distal fingers to the proximal forearm (Figure 76-11). It is helpful to measure and cut a hole in the middle of the plaster to allow for the insertion of the thumb prior to wetting the plaster. Place cotton cast padding between the index and middle fingers to prevent skin maceration. Mold the width of the plaster around the radial aspect of the hand and forearm to create a stabilizing force. The ulnar aspect of the hand and forearm is left entirely free. The hand is immobilized in what is considered a "safe" position with the wrist dorsiflexed 20 de-

grees, the MCP joints flexed 60 to 90 degrees, and the interphalangeal (IP) joints extended or slightly flexed at 10 degrees[9] (Figure 76-11).

ULNAR GUTTER SPLINT

This splint is used for the treatment of stable metacarpal and phalangeal fractures of the ring and small fingers (Figure 76-12). The long axis of the plaster extends from the pulp of the distal fingers to the proximal forearm. Place cotton cast padding between the ring and little fingers to prevent any maceration (Figure 76-12A). The width of the plaster must wrap around the ulnar aspect of the hand and forearm. The radial side of the hand is left entirely free. The hand is immobilized in the "safe" position with the wrist dorsiflexed 20 degrees, the MCP joints flexed 60 to 70 degrees, and the IP joints extended or slightly flexed at 10 degrees[9] (Figure 76-12B).

VOLAR SPLINT

The volar splint can be used for the treatment of radial styloid fractures, ulnar styloid fractures, metacarpal fractures, middle phalangeal fractures, and proximal phalangeal fractures. This splint remains only on the volar surface of the hand and forearm, as the name suggests. The splint begins at the proximal forearm and ends just proximal to the MCP joints (Figure 76-13). The splint can be extended to include the fingers for phalangeal fractures with the wrist dorsiflexed 20 degrees, the MCP joints flexed 60 to 90 degrees, and the IP joints extended or slightly flexed at 10 degrees.

DORSAL ("CLAM DIGGER") SPLINT

The dorsal splint can be used in place of a volar splint for injuries of the distal forearm, wrist, or hand. The splint runs along the dorsal surface of the forearm and hand, from the proximal forearm to the ends of the digits. As with the volar splint, the wrist is extended 15 to 20 degrees, the MCP joints are flexed 60 to 90 degrees, and the IP joints are extended or slightly flexed to a maximum of 10 degrees.

The dorsal splint maintains better control of the MCP and IP joints, assuring that the hand remains in the "safe position," when compared to the volar splint. Pad the splint adequately to prevent pressure sores, since the dorsal surface of the hand lacks the intrinsic fat pads of the palm.

THUMB SPICA SPLINT

Scaphoid injuries, carpometacarpal subluxations of the thumb, and collateral ligament injuries of the thumb can all be immobilized in a thumb spica splint (Figure 76-14). This splint can extend to the proximal forearm or it can include the elbow joint. It is positioned on the forearm, like a radial gutter splint, but only the thumb is immobilized. There are several methods to forming a

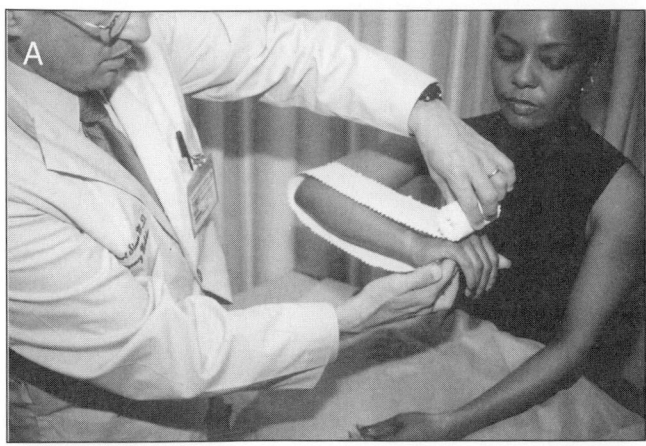
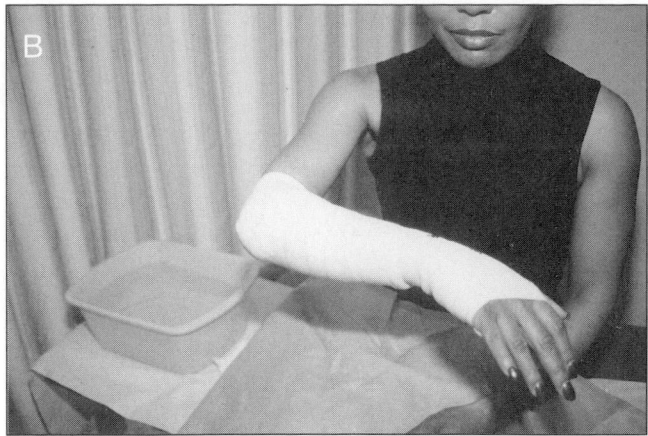
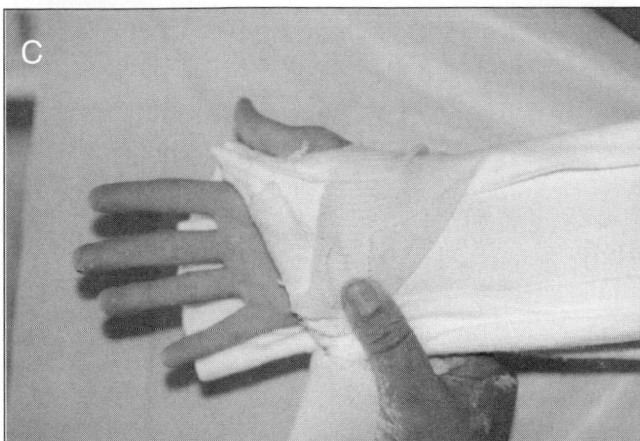
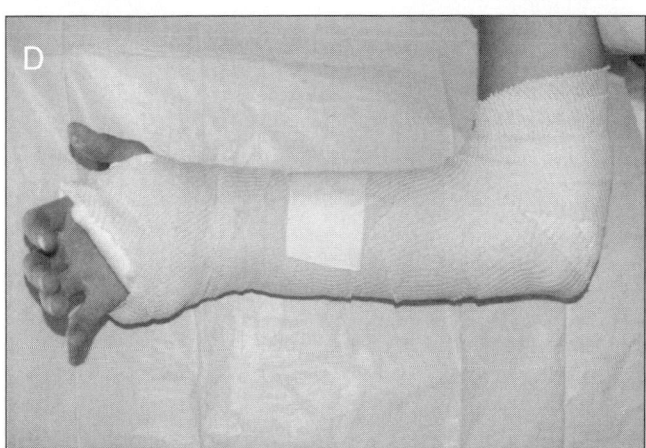

FIGURE 76-9 The sugar tong splint. *A.* The lengths of plaster for the sugar tong splint should leave the metacarpal joints free for flexion and extension. *B.* Cotton cast padding is applied from the metacarpophalangeal (MCP) joints to just above the elbow. *C.* The dorsal aspect is cut and folded back to free the MCP joints. *D.* The final product with the elbow immobilized at 90 degrees.

thumb spica splint. One can simply lay the plaster over the radial aspect of the forearm and thumb. It is useful to cut one side of the splint into a shape that conforms to the thumb to facilitate the placement of the splint material around the thumb (Figure 76-14*A*). Cutting a wedge

out of one side of the plaster will allow for easier splinting of the thumb without excess material collecting in the first web space (Figure 76-14*B*). Position the thumb as if a glass were being held in the hand with the wrist in 20 degrees of dorsiflexion (Figure 76-14*C*).

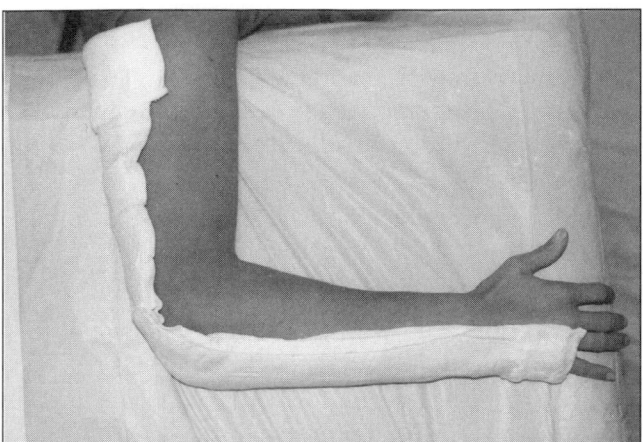

FIGURE 76-10 The posterior long arm splint secures the elbow at 90 degrees. The forearm and wrist are shown in a neutral position.

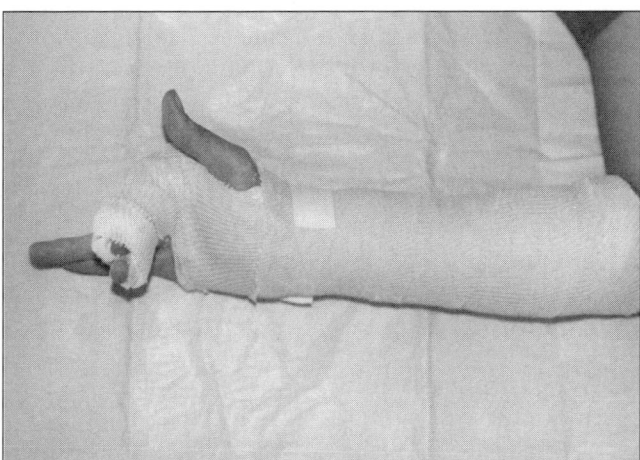

FIGURE 76-11 The radial gutter splint with the hand in the "safe" position.[9]

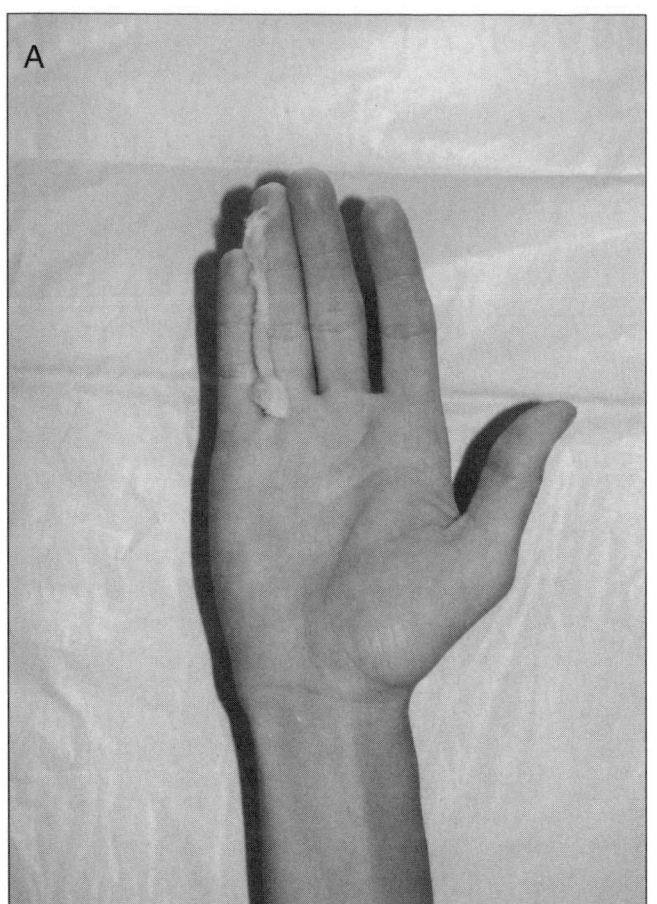
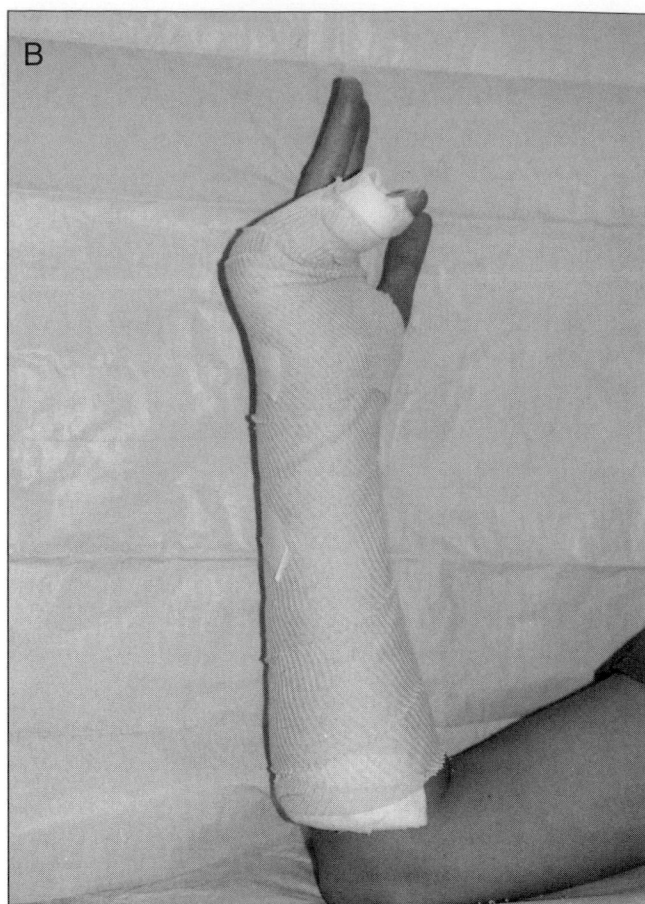

FIGURE 76-12 The ulnar gutter splint. *A.* Padding is necessary between any fingers that are immobilized together. *B.* The final product with the hand in the "safe" position.[9]

FINGER SPLINTS

Immobilization of the finger lends itself to great creativity in the field of splinting. Finger splints may be adequate for immobilization of stable finger fractures, dislocated joints, or ligamentous strains. Splint the finger in full extension if it involves an extraarticular fracture of the distal phalanx. Splint the finger in slight flexion if it involves the strain of a joint or ligament. The finger can be splinted in isolation, or it can be immobilized with the adjacent finger for additional stability. Plaster is rarely used for finger splints in the modern hospital setting. The creation of foam-padded metal or plastic splints has facilitated immobilization of the affected digit. Nonetheless, small strips of cut plaster can still be used to stabilize any finger injuries. **The juxtaposition of the affected finger with its neighboring finger requires padding between the digits to prevent skin maceration and breakdown.**

SHORT ARM CAST

The short arm cast is used for stable fractures of the metacarpals, the carpal bones, the distal radius, and the radial or ulnar styloid process (Figure 76-15). The short arm cast begins at the proximal forearm and extends to include the palm and the dorsum of the hand. The metacarpophalangeal and elbow joints are left exposed to allow for full motion at these joints. Flex the patient's elbow 90 degrees (Figure 76-15*A*). Place the wrist in the desired position. The extent of flexion and ulnar-radial deviation of the wrist is determined by the underlying injury. The forearm can be in a neutral, pronated, or supinated position. Apply bias stockinette (Figure 76-15*B*). Apply cotton cast padding (Figure 76-15*C*). Ensure that extra padding is applied to the bony prominences of the base of the thumb and the ulnar styloid.

Apply the plaster. Roll the plaster over the padding from the hand to the forearm. A quick trim of the material will allow for a better fit as the plaster passes around the thumb (Figure 76-15*D*). **Provide adequate space for the thumb so that its motion is not limited.** The application of additional layers to the anteromedial surface will strengthen the cast (Figure 76-15*E*). Mold the cast with an anterior–posterior force applied to the forearm (Figure 76-15*F*). Trim the plaster while it is still wet to even out the thumb opening and the cast ends (Figure 76-15*G*). Ensure that all protective padding is pulled out from under the plaster material to protect the skin from

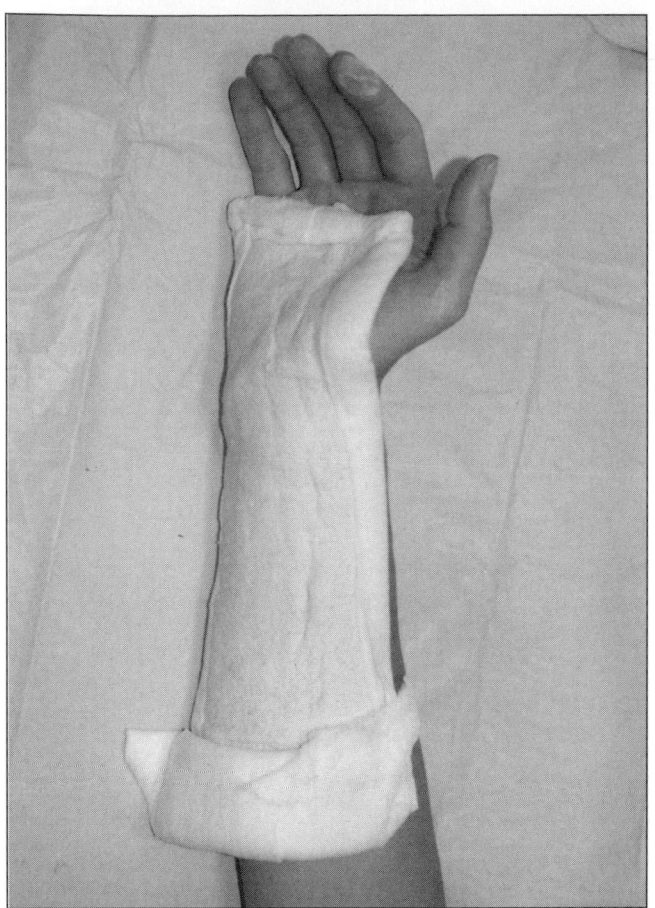

FIGURE 76-13 The volar splint.

the sharp edges (Figure 76-15*G*). The patient should be able to touch the tips of the thumb and index fingers when the cast is properly applied (Figure 76-15*H*).

LONG ARM CAST

A short arm cast can easily be extended into a long arm cast if needed. Simply extend the cast proximally with the elbow in 90 degrees of flexion. Extend the padding and the plaster to the proximal humerus, ending two or three finger breadths distal to the axilla (Figure 76-16). Be careful to provide adequate padding around the axilla or the patient will complain about the sharp cast edge.

LOWER EXTREMITY SPLINTS AND CASTS

LONG LEG SPLINT

This splint is commonly used for knee and tibial injuries prior to and after surgical fixation. Posterior, medial, and lateral lengths of plaster are used to stabilize the leg while the anterior aspect of the leg is left exposed. The application of medial and lateral plaster begins at the upper thigh and travels down the knee, calf, and an-

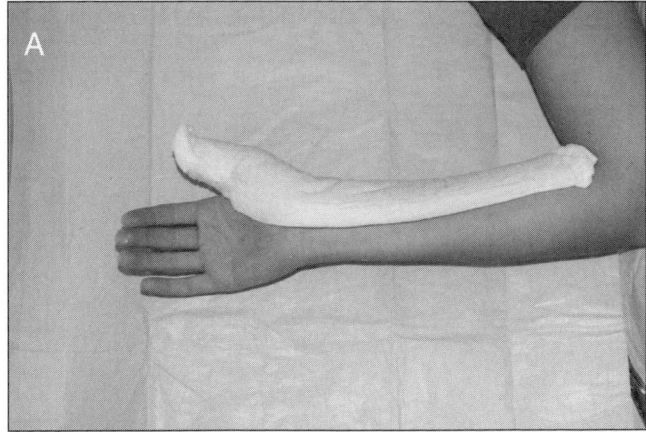

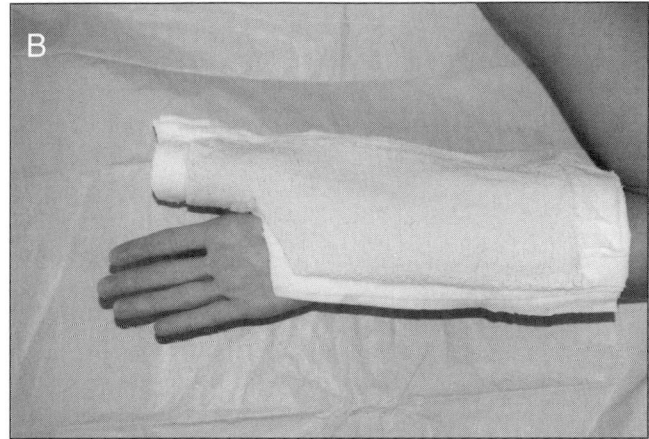

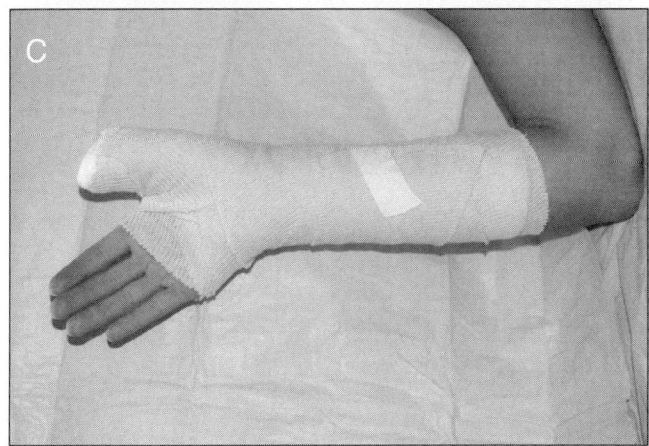

FIGURE 76-14 The thumb spica splint. *A.* One technique of thumb spica application with the plaster cut to conform to the thumb. *B.* Cutting the plaster facilitates this different technique of thumb spica application. *C.* The final product with the wrist dorsiflexed 20 degrees and the thumb positioned as if a glass were being held in the hand.

kle. The posterior portion of plaster begins at this same level and travels down the posterior aspect of the leg, behind the knee, curving around the heel, and ending just beyond the ends of the toes. Place the foot 90 degrees to the tibia and flex the knee 10 to 20 degrees.

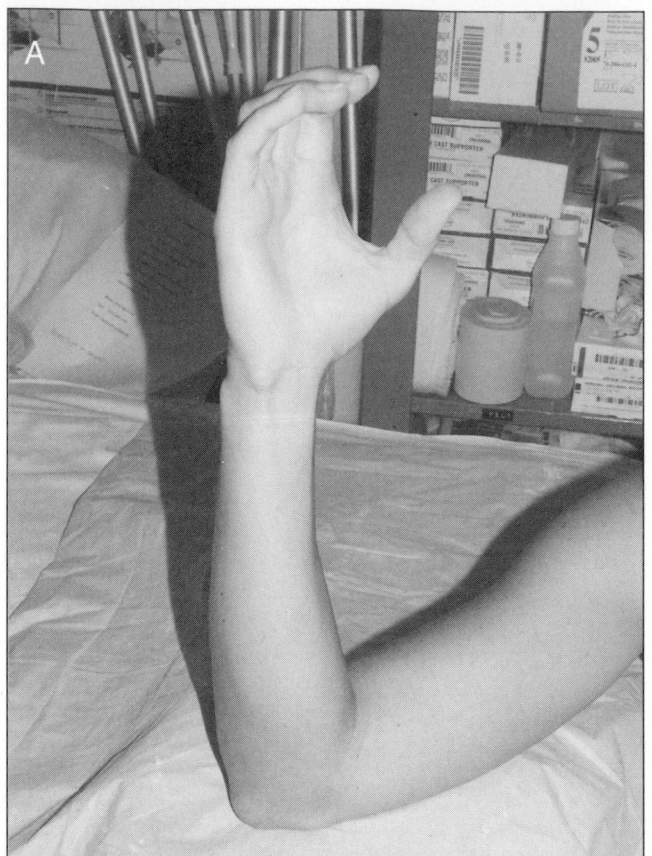
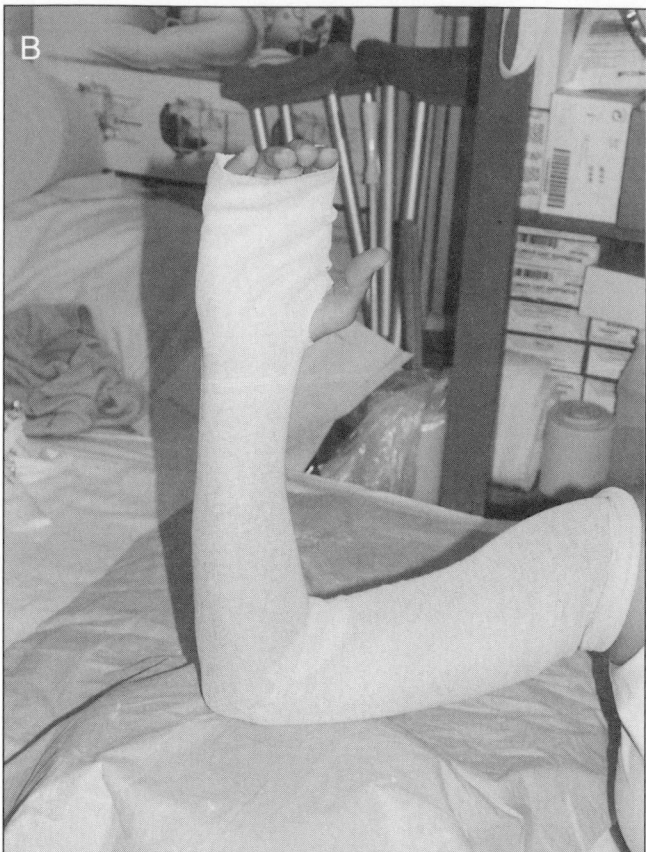
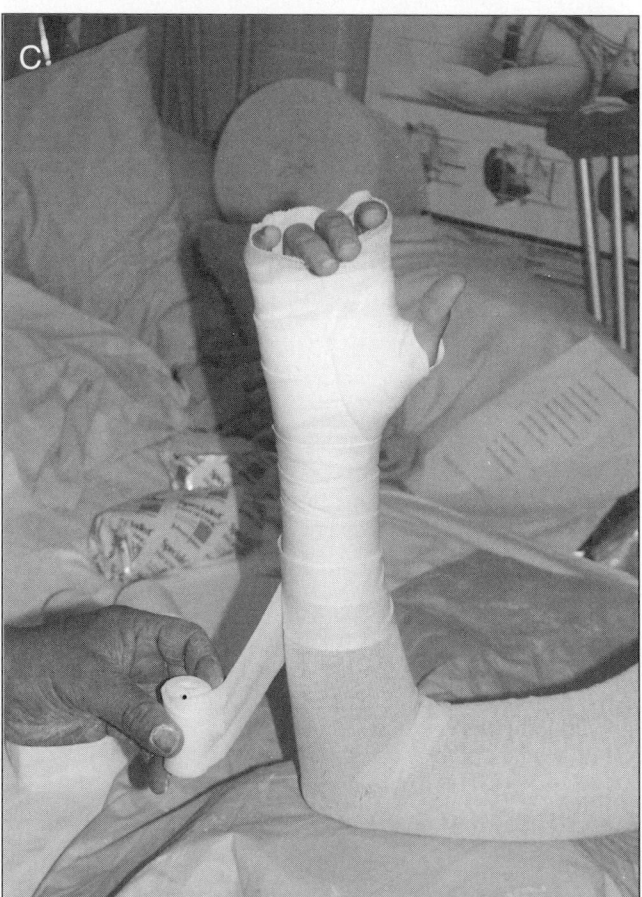
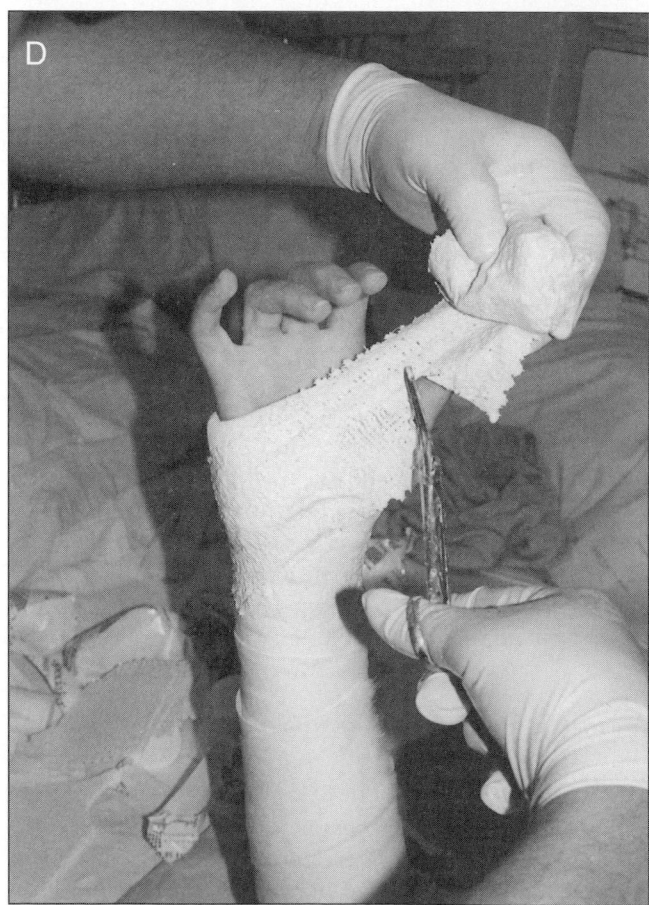

FIGURE 76-15 The short arm cast. *A.* Flex the elbow 90 degrees. The patient can help position the wrist and fingers in a position of function. *B.* Tubular stockinette is applied to the entire arm in anticipation of a long arm cast. *C.* Cotton cast padding is applied to the forearm. Adequate padding is also needed at the thumb, as it will remain exposed and mobile. *D.* Cut one side of the plaster as it is wrapped around the thumb. Less bunching of excess material occurs with quick cuts of the plaster. *(continued)*

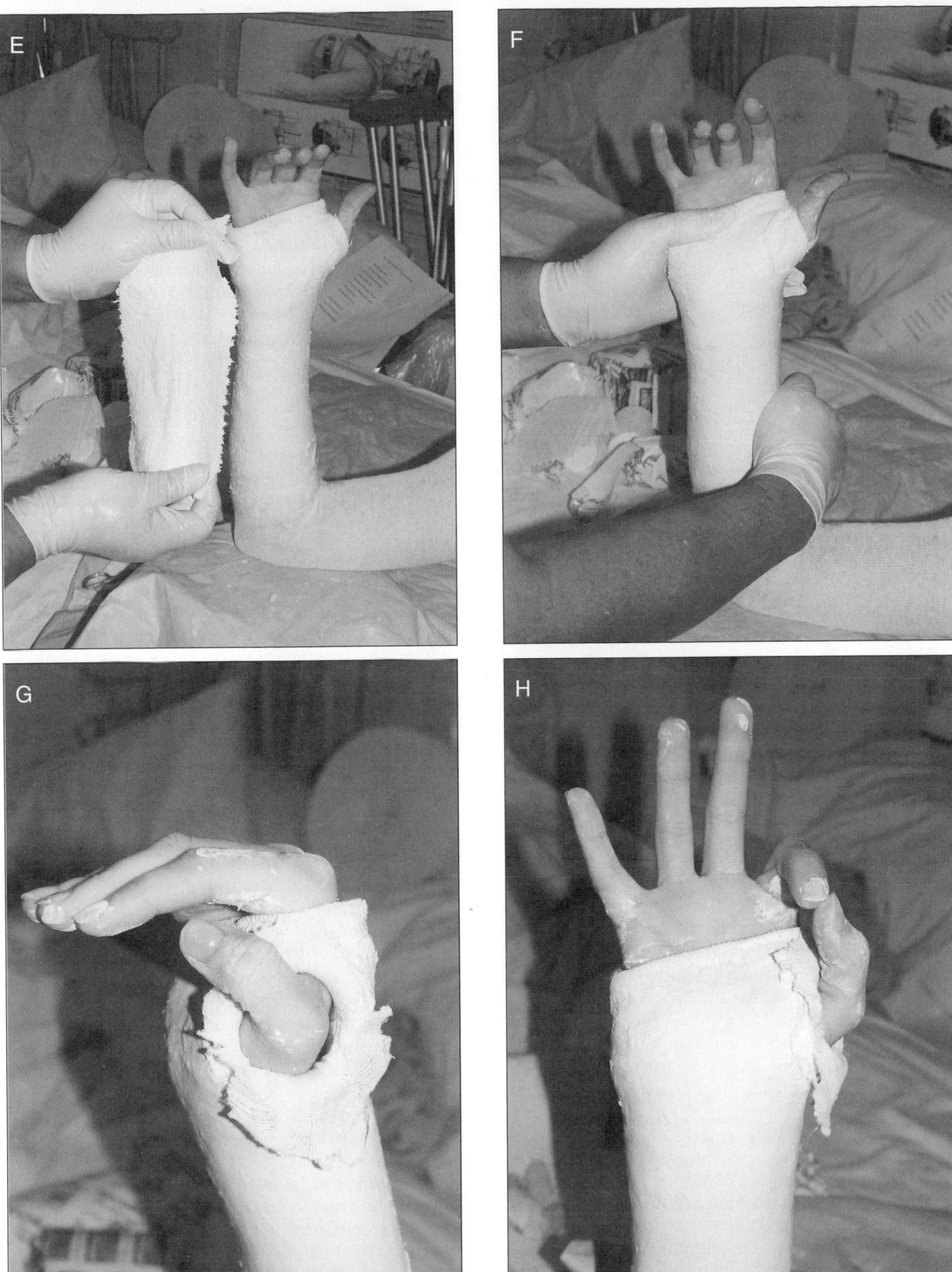

FIGURE 76-15 *(continued)* *E.* An additional length of plaster material (five layers) can be applied along the ulnar length of the cast. This serves as reinforcement if additional strength is necessary. *F.* Mold the cast with the palmar aspect of the hands using smooth, rapid, and repetitive motions. The motion does not consist of simple up-and-down strokes. *G.* The wet plaster and underlying padding are cut and folded back to fully expose the thumb. *H.* The "okay" sign of a properly exposed thumb.

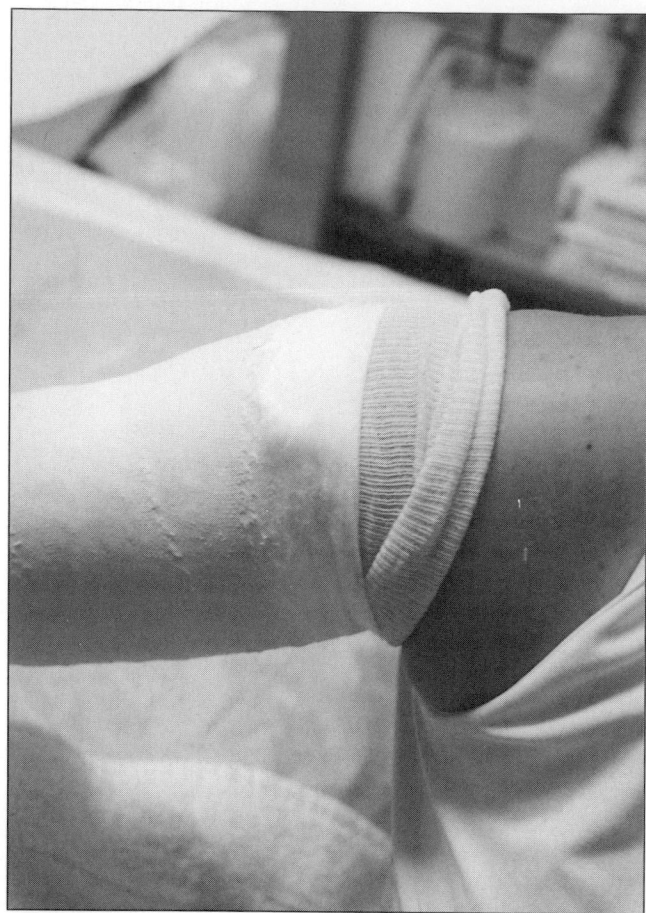

FIGURE 76-16 The short arm cast is extended into a long arm cast. The axilla needs adequate padding for protection of its sensitive skin.

ANKLE SPLINT

The ankle splint helps to immobilize isolated ankle injuries with the joint at a 90 degree angle (Figure 76-17). This splint is commonly used for ankle fractures and sprains. It can also be helpful for certain stable fractures of the foot. This splint can be applied as a posterior splint or a lateral to medial stirrup splint.[13] Combining the two techniques can provide additional support for the ankle. The first part (posterior splint) provides posterior support to the foot and ankle. The second part creates a medial-to-lateral stirrup-like splint around the sides of the ankle.

Place the patient prone with their knee flexed 90 degrees and the foot pointing upward (Figure 76-17A). Place the posterior support of plaster from the proximal posterior calf to pass under the heel and along the plantar surface of the foot (Figure 76-17B). The plaster should extend under the toes to provide protection. Place the foot 90 degrees to the tibia and in neutral rotation.

For a "stirrup" support of the ankle, begin by applying plaster to the length of the medial aspect of the proximal calf, over the medial malleolus, under the heel, and up the lateral aspect of the ankle and calf (Figure 76-17C). Fold and smooth the edges of the stirrup around the heel (Figure 76-17D). Keep the ankle flexed 90 degrees with the foot neutral while the plaster sets (Figure 76-17E).

SPLINT FOR ACHILLES TENDON RUPTURE

Rupture of the Achilles tendon can be managed surgically or conservatively with immobilization. Surgery is often delayed and the patient will require immobilization. Position the patient as if placing an ankle splint or have the patient sit up with the affected extremity hanging over the table's edge. Position the foot in 20 to 30 degrees of plantarflexion (Figure 76-18). This is a position that the foot will naturally relax into. Place a posterior splint on the lower extremity extending from the proximal calf to the distal aspect of the toes. Cut out wedges of plaster in order to minimize buckling at the malleoli as the splint material wraps around the heel.

SHORT LEG CAST

The short leg cast is used for stable ankle fractures and stable fractures of the hindfoot, midfoot, and forefoot (Figure 76-19). Place the patient either supine or sitting on the edge of the gurney. Place a padded block under the distal thigh if the patient is supine. Instruct an assistant to hold the patient's toes to help keep the lower extremity in a good position. Holding the leg by the toes may allow the force of gravity to disrupt fracture alignment. Care must be taken to prevent this outcome. The patient can sit upright on the edge of the gurney with the affected leg hanging down freely if no assistant is available.

The short leg cast begins at the proximal calf, below the knee, and extends down to the toes (Figure 76-19). The knee is left entirely free to allow for full flexion and extension. The toes can be left entirely exposed or the cast can provide a hard sole of support and protection beneath the toes. Apply cotton cast padding with extra attention to the areas of bony prominence such as the fibular head, the lateral malleolus, and the medial malleolus. Apply the plaster from the calf to the toes as if applying a short arm cast. Mold the plaster around the Achilles tendon, away from the malleoli and to conform to the plantar arch. Cut the wet plaster under the metatarsal heads to expose the toes or leave it long to support the entire toes.

Converting a short leg non-weight bearing cast to a walking cast requires small adjustments to the existing cast. Supplement the arched foot of the short leg cast with additional plaster to form a flat surface. **Apply a preformed heel after the cast has completely dried to prevent any indentation.** Place the walking heel in the midsagittal plane of the foot with the center aspect lining up with the anterior calf. Secure the heel in place

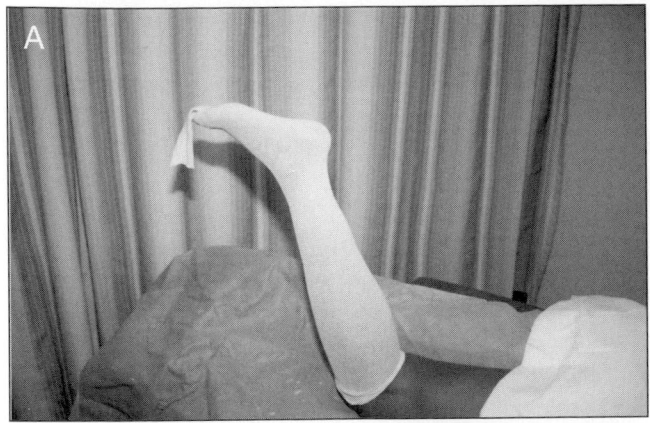
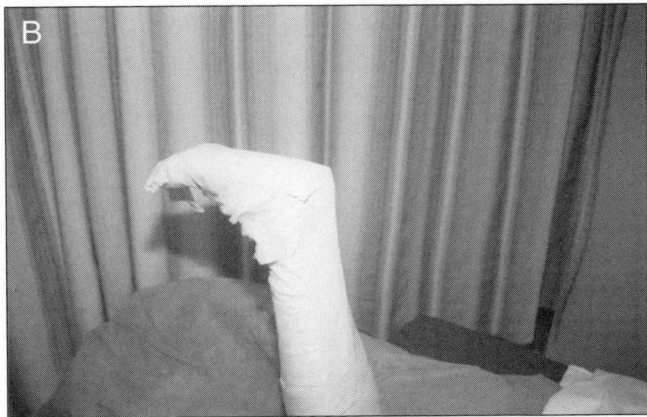
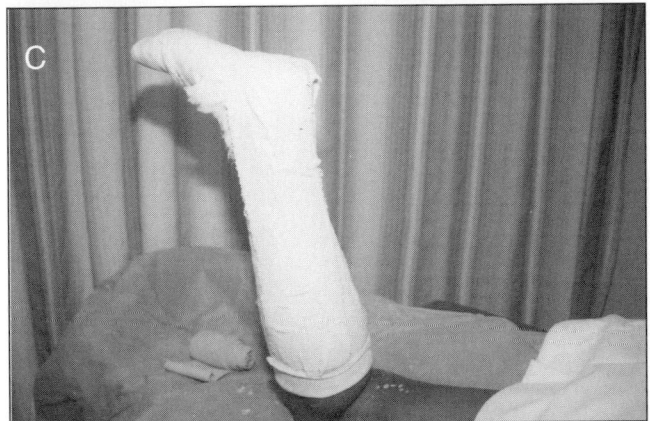
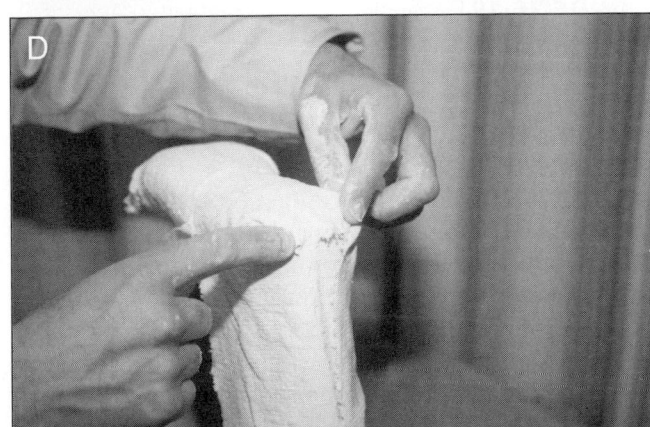
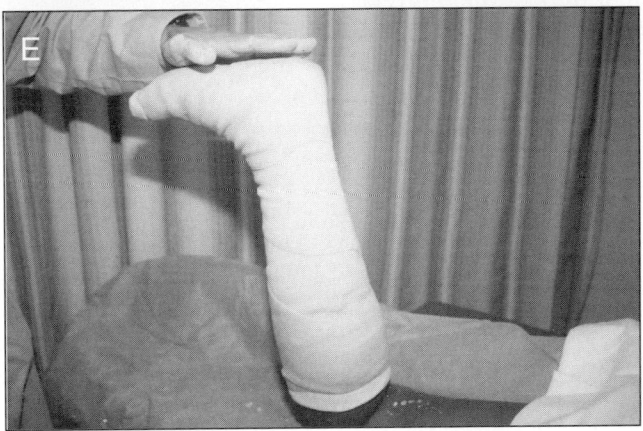

FIGURE 76-17 The ankle splint. *A.* Stockinette is applied and the leg is positioned. *B.* The plaster splint is applied posteriorly. *C.* A stirrup plaster splint is applied around the medial to lateral ankle and over the posterior splint. *D.* Fold the corners and smooth out the splint. *E.* An elastic wrap is applied over the splint after folding back the stockinette. The foot is maintained in this position until the plaster sets.

with copious plaster wrapped around the foot and ankle (Figure 76-20).

LONG LEG CAST

The long leg cast can be used for immobilization of distal femoral or proximal tibial fractures (Figure 76-21). The cast extends from the metatarsal heads to several finger breadths below the groin. The leg is immobilized with the knee in slight flexion and the foot 90 degrees to the tibia with no inward or external rotation (Figure 76-21*A*). Extending the short leg cast up to the groin is a safe, stepwise technique of forming a long leg cast. Be sure to provide sufficient overlap of plaster at the junction between the two casts. Inadequate overlap will weaken the integrity of the cast. Support the knee in slight flexion while the plaster sets (Figure 76-21*B*). Make sure that there is adequate padding around the proximal free edge of the cast to protect the groin (Figure 76-21*C*).

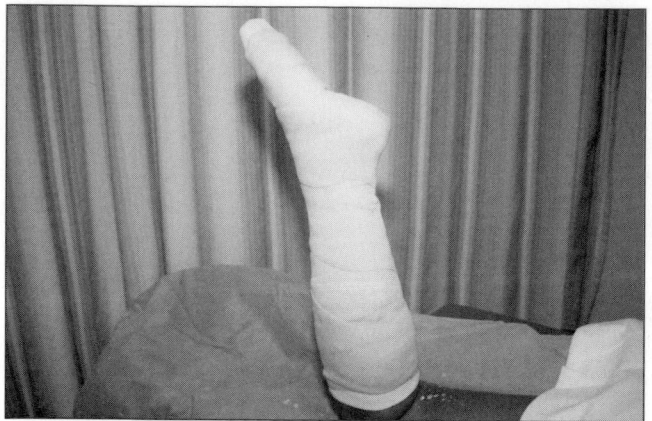

FIGURE 76-18 Positioning of the patient for an Achilles tendon splint.

AFTERCARE

The most feared complication of a splint or cast application is the development of a compartment syndrome. Aftercare is geared toward edema reduction and patient education. Instruct the patient regarding the early signs of a compartment syndrome. This includes increased pain, pain with passive motion, paresthesias, pallor, decreased or altered sensation, as well as delayed capillary refill. The patient should return to the Emergency Department immediately if they develop any of these symptoms, if the digits become cold or blue, or if the patient has other concerns. The extremity should be maintained above the level of the heart for the first 48 to 72 hours after the injury. Ice should be applied to the surface of the cast or splint for at least 15 minutes three times a day. The cold therapy will be transmitted through the plaster and result in significant reduction of edema. Active motion of the fingers and toes should be encouraged to help reduce edema in the extremity. **The**

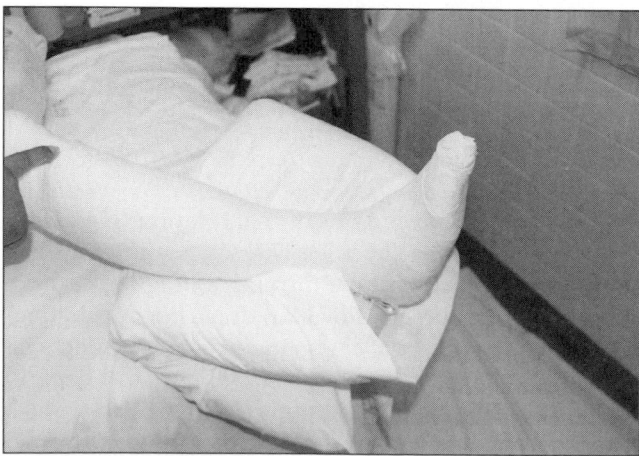

FIGURE 76-19 The short leg cast leaves the knee and tibial tuberosity exposed.

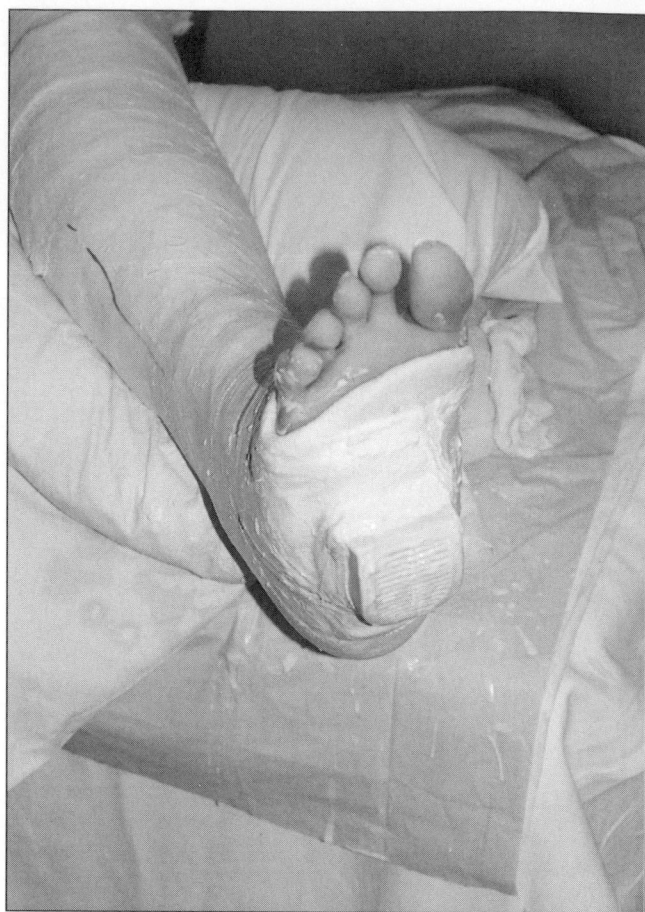

FIGURE 76-20 Converting the short leg cast into a walking cast. A walking heel is secured with an additional plaster foundation and overwrappings of plaster.

cast or splint must be kept completely dry. Should bathing be desired, instruct the patient to place two plastic bags over the extremity and tape the proximal edge to the skin of the extremity. Sufficient pain medication should be supplied to last the patient until the follow-up visit. This should include nonsteroidal anti-inflammatory drugs supplemented with narcotic analgesics. A sling may facilitate mobilization for some upper extremity injuries.

COMPLICATIONS

The most common complications associated with the application of a cast or splint include plaster sores, compartment syndrome, joint stiffness, thermal injury, infection, and allergic reactions. The following section focuses on the prevention of these complications.[4,6,10]

PLASTER SORES

Plaster sores result from ischemic necrosis of the skin underneath a cast or splint. The skin begins to exhibit necrosis after only 2 hours of continuous pressure. **Great**

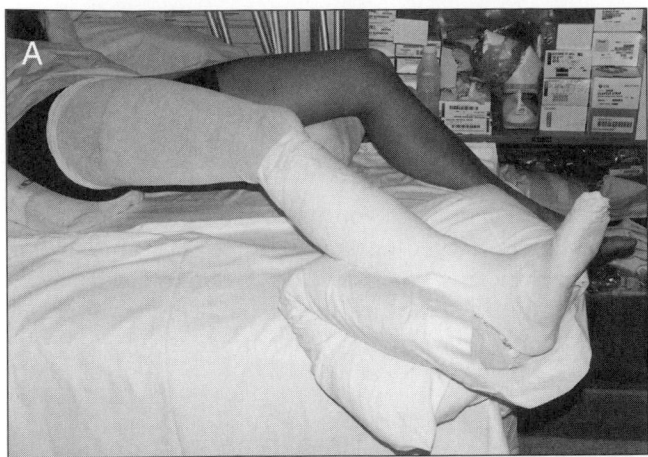

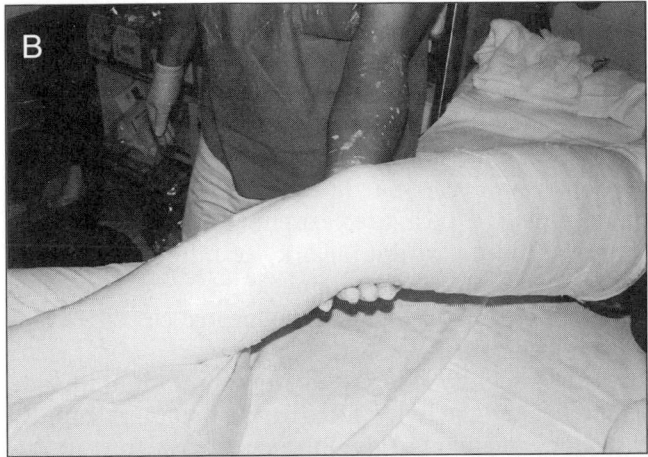

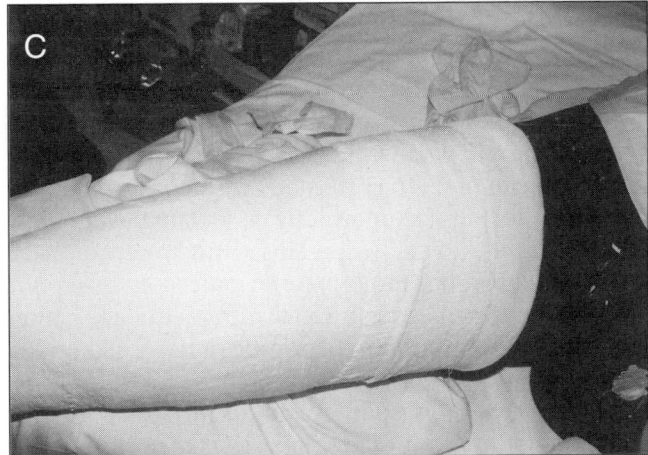

FIGURE 76-21 The long leg cast. *A.* Positioning the patient for a long leg cast. Place a bump under the patient's hip to facilitate extending a short leg cast into a long leg cast. *B.* Support the leg as the cast hardens to ensure proper positioning. *C.* Adequate padding at the groin area will add to patient comfort and cast longevity.

care should be taken in applying a cast or splint to mold the plaster with the broad surfaces of the hands. Molding with the fingers can result in indentations of the plaster and localized areas of pressure. The cast or splint should never be allowed to rest on a hard or

pointed surface until it is completely dry. Points of contact on the hard surfaces may cause impressions that result in increased pressure. Extra padding over bony prominences may decrease the incidence of plaster sores.

Complaints of pain should be taken very seriously. The cast or splint should be split or removed immediately and the skin examined. If the pressure point is not addressed rapidly, the pain will often subside as the skin becomes necrotic. This oversight often results in a foul smelling pressure sore under the cast when the patient returns for follow-up. Cast and splint treatment may be rife with complications for patients with limited sensation from underlying medical conditions (i.e., diabetes, paraplegia, myelomeningocele). Great care should be taken and extra padding used when casting or splinting these individuals.

Common areas of pressure necrosis also include the proximal and distal extent of the cast or splint. These are areas of stress concentration. Great care should be taken in padding the ends of the cast or splint during the application. No plaster should ever touch the skin directly. If the edges of the splint are sharp or too long, they should be folded out and away from the patient.

COMPARTMENT SYNDROME

A compartment syndrome is a significant complication from the application of a cast or, less commonly, a splint. The rigid immobilization of the cast prevents soft tissue expansion from edema and decreases the amount of fluid needed to raise compartment pressures.[11] In cases of acute fractures, casts should be used with caution and always split in the direction perpendicular to the force needed to maintain the reduction. For example, after casting a distal radial fracture where a dorsal mold is needed to maintain the reduction, split the cast longitudinally on the volar and dorsal surfaces (bivalved) to allow for mediolateral spread of the plaster.

It is not sufficient to split only the plaster. The plaster and underlying cotton cast padding must be split to visualize the skin underneath. Making a single longitudinal cut (univalving) in the cast can also decrease the compartment pressure. Univalving the cast can decrease intracompartmental pressures by 30 percent.[12] Spreading the cast 1 cm after cutting it can lower the pressure 60 percent.[12] Splitting the cotton cast padding will decrease the pressure by 70 percent.[12]

JOINT STIFFNESS

Joint stiffness is a significant complication of joint immobilization with casts and splints. Sometimes the immobilization is unavoidable, as the incorporation of the ankle and the knee in a long leg cast. Every effort should be made to decrease adjacent joint immobilization as soon as it is safe and practical. For example, by converting a long leg cast into a short leg cast.

Immobilize the extremity in a position of function as long as this does not interfere with the maintenance of fracture reduction. For example, take great care not to immobilize the ankle in plantarflexion when applying a lower extremity splint or cast. This mistake is commonly seen when a long leg cast is placed. This pitfall may be avoided by the stepwise application of the cast. First apply the cast to the foot and ankle with the ankle held 90 degrees to the tibia. Second, extend the cast proximally to become a short leg cast and mold the reduction. Finally, extend the cast up the thigh as needed. An additional benefit is the reduction of anterior compartment pressures of the leg when the foot is held in 0 to 37 degrees of dorsiflexion.

Great care should also be taken in splinting the upper extremity. **Every effort should be made to leave the fingers mobile at the metacarpophalangeal joints.** Immobilization of the metacarpophalangeal joints in extension results in shortening of the collateral ligaments and limitation of flexion. **Immobilize the metacarpophalangeal joints in 90 degrees of flexion if they must be immobilized.** This position keeps the collateral ligaments in a lengthened position and allows a rapid return to function.

THERMAL INJURY

Thermal injury may result from the exothermic reaction of plaster as it sets (dries). The heat generated during the setting of the plaster increases as the number of layers (thickness) of plaster increases as well as the temperature of the water increases. Also important is the ability to dissipate the heat generated by the drying plaster. Placing a cast or splint on a plastic pillow as it dries will result in reflection of the heat and increased temperature within the cast. The use of cloth pillows or towels under the cast material allows for some dissipation of the heat. Optimal heat dissipation occurs by exposing the cast to circulating air.

Sufficient cotton cast padding must be used to protect the skin. Plaster must never touch the skin directly. The incidence of thermal injury can be decreased by using cool water and as thin a layer of plaster as possible to accomplish stable immobilization of the extremity. Great care should be used in the application of plaster to anesthetized patients, insensate limbs, or confused patients.

INFECTION

Infection secondary to a cast or splint is uncommon and is usually related to open wounds or exposed surgical pins underneath the plaster. Fresh water should be used to wet the plaster. Do not use standing or previously used water, as it is an excellent culture medium. All wounds should be dressed with sterile gauze and cotton cast padding prior to applying the cast or splint. Windows can be created over wound sites to allow for regular care and evaluation. Patients should be instructed to keep casts and splints clean and dry so as to prevent skin maceration.

ALLERGIC REACTIONS

Allergic reactions to cotton or plaster have been reported but are exceedingly rare. Orthopedists and orthopedic technicians may develop a contact dermatitis from continued exposure to plaster over many years. Gloves should be worn for plaster application.

SUMMARY

The initial management of orthopedic trauma is a fundamental aspect of Emergency Medicine. Fractures and dislocations of the extremities are routinely handled in the Emergency Department with prompt Orthopedic follow-up or consultation. The application of external immobilization can be the definitive or temporizing management of the injured extremity. The application of splints accounts for the majority of immobilization of injured extremities. Cast application plays a role in maintaining bony alignment following closed reductions of fractures.

Clear benefits of external immobilization include pain relief and the reduction of further soft tissue injury from bony fragments. Immobilization of the fracture decreases motion and traction on the nerve-rich periosteum.[4,7] The immobilization of fracture ends protects adjacent neurovascular structures from injury and helps prevent bony fragments from penetrating the skin. External immobilization also reduces the area available for hemorrhage and decreases bone bleeding.[4] Early immobilization leading to fracture stabilization is also important in reducing the morbidity associated with long bone fractures.[12] Finally, the closed treatment of fractures facilitates the body's natural processes of repair. External periosteal and internal intramedullary callus formation is optimized in the setting of bony alignment that has been secured by casting or splinting.

The application of splints is an essential skill for any Emergency Physician. The application of a cast in the Emergency Department is appropriate in some select situations. The casting or splinting of an extremity is simple, easy to perform, and relatively quick.

REFERENCES

1. Stewart JDM, Hallett JP: *Traction and Orthopaedic Appliances.* Edinburgh: Churchill Livingstone, 1983:195–210.

2. Alexander RH, Proctor HJ: *Advanced Trauma Life Support. Course for Physicians.* Chicago: American College of Surgeons, 1993:221–239.

3. Charnley J: *The Closed Treatment of Common Fractures.* Baltimore: Williams & Wilkins, 1972, chaps 1, 2, and 5.

4. Browner BD, Jupiter JB, Levine AM, et al: *Skeletal Trauma: Fractures, Dislocations, Ligamentous Injuries.* Philadelphia: Saunders, 1992, chaps 9 and 38.

5. Department of the Army: *Orthopedic Specialist, Department of the Army and Air Force Technical Manual.* Washington, DC: U.S. Government Printing Office, 1967:103–149.

6. Lewis RC: *Handbook of Traction, Casting and Splinting Techniques.* Philadelphia: Lippincott, 1977, chaps 3, 4, and 6.

7. Harkess JW, Ramsey WC, Harkess JW: Principles of fractures and dislocations, in Rockwood CA, Green DP, Bucholz RW, et al (eds): *Rockwood & Green's Fractures in Adults,* 4th ed. Philadelphia: Lippincott-Raven, 1996:3–121.

8. Gustilo RB, Anderson JT: Prevention of infection in the treatment of 1025 open fractures of long bones: retrospective and prospective analyses. *J Bone Joint Surg Am* 1976; 58(4):453–458.

9. James JIP: The assessment and management of the injured hand. *Hand* 1970; 2(2):97–105.

10. Schneider FR: *Handbook for the Orthopaedic Assistant.* St. Louis: Mosby, 1976: 95–125.

11. Bingold AC: On splitting plasters. A useful analogy. *J Bone Joint Surg Br* 1979; 61(3):294–295.

12. Garfin SR, Mubarak SJ, Evans KL, et al: Quantification of intracompartmental pressure and volume under plaster casts. *J Bone Joint Surg Am* 1981; 63(4):449–453.

13. Bone LB, Johnson KD, Weigelt J, et al: Early versus delayed stabilization of femoral fractures: a prospective randomized study. *J Bone Joint Surg Am* 1989; 71(3):336–340.

14. Simon RR, Koenigsnecht S: *Emergency Orthopedics: The Extremities,* 4th ed. New York: McGraw-Hill, 2000.

Acknowledgment: We wish to thank Frank Anguiano, cast technician at San Francisco General Hospital, for his tremendous help in preparing the figures for this manuscript.

Section Six

SKIN AND SOFT TISSUE PROCEDURES

Chapter 77
GENERAL PRINCIPLES OF WOUND MANAGEMENT

Ardena L. Flippin

INTRODUCTION

An acute wound can be defined as an unplanned disruption in the integrity of the skin, including the epidermis and dermis. The goals of wound management are to restore tissue continuity and function, minimize infection, repair with minimal cosmetic deformity, and be able to distinguish wounds that require special care. The principles of wound management should be emphasized over the repair technique. Appropriate wound management prior to approximating the wound will allow it to heal with minimal complications. This includes wound cleansing, debridement of the wound edges, wound approximation, and prevention of secondary injury.

HEALING OF WOUNDED TISSUE

PHASES OF WOUND HEALING

The response of tissue to an injury is described in three phases. The first phase is coagulation and inflammation. The second phase is the proliferative phase. The final phase is the reepithelialization or remodeling phase.

Phase I consists of coagulation and inflammation. It occurs in the first 5 days. This phase is also known as the vascular phase. A fibrin clot forms a transitional matrix that allows for the migration of cells into the wound site over a period of 72 hours. Inflammatory cells (i.e., neutrophils, monocytes, and macrophages) kill microbes, prevent microbial colonization, break down soluble wound debris, and secrete cytokines. The cytokines signal synthetic cells, such as fibroblasts, to initiate phase II.

Phase II is the proliferative phase. It occurs during days 5 to 14 after the injury. Fibroblasts proliferate and synthesize a new connective tissue matrix that replaces the transitional fibrin matrix. Granulation tissue consisting of fibroblasts, immature connective tissue, epi-dermal cells that have migrated, and abundant capillaries forms within the wound. Fibroblasts release collagen, a protein substance that is the chief constituent of connective tissue. **At 5 days, the tensile strength of the wound itself is 5 percent that of normal skin. Collagen formation peaks at day 7.**

Phase III is known as the remodeling, reepithelialization, or maturation phase. It occurs from day 14 and lasts until there is complete healing of the wound. The new granulation tissue is being converted into a scar. The scar consists of a rich matrix with decreasing cell density, decreasing vascular density, and increasing thickness of collagen fiber bundles packed in parallel arrays.[1] **The wound will have 15 to 20 percent of its full strength at 3 weeks and 60 percent of its full strength at 4 months.** Tensile strength continues to increase up to 1 year after wounding. The skin will eventually regain 70 to 90 percent of its original tensile strength.

FACTORS AFFECTING NORMAL REPAIR

The most common causes of improper wound healing are tension on the wound edges, necrosis and/or ischemia of the tissues from local conditions (crushes and contusions decrease blood flow and lymphatic drainage, which alters local defense mechanisms), or shock. Hypovolemia is the major deterrent to wound healing in patients with hemorrhage and shock, hemorrhage from inadequate hemostasis, infection, or retention of foreign bodies. Systemic conditions including malnutrition, immunosuppression, shock, diabetes secondary to microangiopathy, decreased oxygen and nutrient delivery to the wound, renal insufficiency, cytotoxic drugs, vitamin deficiency, trace metal deficiency, and collagen vascular disease can result in poor wound healing. Polymorphonuclear leukocyte function is known to be impaired from hyperglycemia, jaundice, uremia, cancer, or chronic infections.

Drugs and medications can contribute to good wound healing or affect it adversely. Malnutrition, lack of protein, and lack of vitamins (e.g., vitamins A and C) may inhibit or prolong healing. Zinc deficiency, which is reversible, may play a role in retarding the healing process.[3] Anti-inflammatory drugs (e.g., colchicine, aspirin, and glucocorticoids) disrupt macrophage function, collagen synthesis, and polymorphonuclear neutrophil concentrations. Pretreatment or early introduction of glucocorticoids results in retarded wound repair by slowing cell proliferation.[4]

SCAR FORMATION

Some 6 to 12 months are required to form a mature scar. This explains why scars should not be revised until 12 months have passed. A wider scar, inadequate wound closure, or a wound dehiscence may occur in areas with increased skin tension or if the wound is an area of excessive motion (e.g., over joints). **Adequate immobilization of the approximated wound (but not necessarily the entire anatomic part) is mandatory after wound closure for efficient healing and minimal scar formation.** Contractures can develop when a scar crosses perpendicular to a joint crease. These patients may require physical therapy to prevent the loss of range of motion secondary to contractures.

Hypertrophic scars result from full-thickness injuries. **Hypertrophic scars are characterized by a thick and raised scar that remains within the boundaries of the original injury.** They must often be corrected by surgical intervention.[1]

Keloids are raised scars that exceed the boundaries of the initial injury. They can develop from superficial injuries and appear to have a genetic basis. Surgical intervention rarely resolves keloids. They may be prevented or minimized by the local application of pressure dressings, Silastic dressings, glucocorticoids, and calcium channel blockers.[1]

The repair procedure may result in more scar tissue. Absorbable suture materials contribute to the formation of suture marks because of their increased reactivity, whereas nonabsorbable materials do not. Wounds that are approximated too tightly can result in tissue ischemia and more scar tissue formation.

WOUND CLOSURE TECHNIQUES

PRIMARY INTENTION

Primary intention involves surgically approximating the wound edges shortly after the time of injury. The skin's greatest strength is in the dermal layer. The best repair results when the entire depth of the dermis is accurately approximated to the entire depth of the opposite dermis. **Accurate approximation of the epidermis gives a cosmetically appealing effect to the repair but does not contribute to its strength. Wound eversion and the use of buried sutures can greatly improve healing by primary intention.**

SECONDARY INTENTION

Secondary intention involves allowing the wound to heal without any surgical intervention. The wound is left open and allowed to heal from the inner layer to the outer surface. It is a more complicated and prolonged healing process than primary intention. Infection, excessive trauma, tissue loss, or imprecise approximation of tissue can result due to healing by secondary intention. Wound contraction by granulation tissue containing myofibroblasts is the major influence on this type of healing. Wound contraction becomes more significant when the dermis is lost.

Concave skin wounds heal with the best results. These areas often heal better by secondary intention than by primary intention. Such concave areas include the inner ear, the nasal alar crease, the nasolabial fold, the temple, and the concave areas of the pinna. Flat surfaces can also heal well by secondary intention, although surgical intervention may be best. Some examples include the forehead, the side of the nose, and periorbital areas. Wounds on convex surfaces are not optimal for healing by secondary intention. Convex surfaces include the malar cheek, the tip of the nose, and the vermilion border of the lip.[2]

TERTIARY INTENTION

Tertiary intention, or delayed primary closure, can often decrease infection rates. Wound closure by tertiary intention is accomplished 3 to 5 days following the initial injury. It is a combination of allowing the wound to heal secondarily for 3 to 5 days and then primarily closing the wound. It is the safest method of repair for wounds that are contaminated, dirty, infected, traumatic, associated with extensive tissue loss, at high risk for infection, and for wounds that are "too old" to close. The ultimate cosmetic result is the same as that of primary wound closure.

WOUND INFECTION

Wound infections occur as a result of the patient's resident flora and the environment. It is related to wound age, the amount of devitalized tissue, and the tissue concentration of pyogenic bacteria. A wound infection exists when there are bacterial densities of more than 10,000 organisms per gram of tissue.[5] Bacteria slow wound healing by secreting proteases that directly injure the tissue in the wound.[2] They also secrete other factors that lead to excess inflammatory cells in the wound, which also injures the tissue.[2]

PATIENT EVALUATION AND ASSESSMENT

HOST HISTORY

A thorough and accurate history and physical examination are essential for optimum wound management. Documentation of the patient's age, prior tetanus immunization history, systemic illnesses, medications, allergies, and the circumstances of the injury are essential to good wound management. These principles are emphasized because the presence of disease processes (such as diabetes mellitus, chronic malnutrition, alcoholism, hepatic or renal insufficiency, asplenism, malignancies, and extremes of age) may impair host defenses or complicate wound healing.[6,7] **Second, the wound itself is often less important than an associated injury to an adjacent structure or cavity. Associated injuries can easily be missed without a specific directed search for their presence.**

TETANUS PROPHYLAXIS

A thorough history must be obtained concerning the patient's tetanus immunization status. Important factors to consider in assessing the risk of developing tetanus include prior immunization history, the type of wound, the degree of wound contamination, the time from injury to treatment, and the presence of underlying medical disease.

Wounds may or may not be prone to tetanus (Table 77-1). The administration of tetanus prophylaxis is based upon the patient's immunization history and the risk of developing tetanus (Table 77-2). Current guidelines state that tetanus toxoid (Td) may be deferred in patients with "clean, minor" wounds who have completed a primary series or received a booster dose (Td 0.5 mL IM) within 10 years. Consider tetanus immune globulin (TIG 250 to 500 U IM) in addition to Td for patients at risk of developing tetanus. Elderly patients without documentation of a primary series, patients from nonindustrialized nations, and those from rural or inner-city areas may never have received tetanus immunization and should be considered for TIG.

MECHANISM OF INJURY

Severity of injury as well as associated injuries can be anticipated by determining the precise mechanism of injury. This will often indicate additional soft tissue injury, the presence of a foreign body, or the amount of contamination present.

Soft tissue injuries are rarely surgical emergencies. The patient's general condition should be attended to, with priority given to observing the ABCs (airway, breathing, and circulation) of Emergency Medicine. The skin margins of a laceration can be tacked together with well-placed atraumatic sutures and the wound covered with a moist pressure dressing until the time is more opportune for definitive repair.

Important questions and answers that must be documented are exactly how the injury occurred, when and where the injury occurred, and what contaminants were present or involved. If the injury involves the hand, what position was the hand in at the time of the injury, what kind of work does the patient do, and which is the patient's dominant hand?

CLASSIFICATION OF WOUNDS

Wounds are described and classified based upon their cause and the type of injury. Abrasions are the result of grinding or abrading forces on the skin. The epidermis and/or dermis is disrupted but not removed in its entirety. Crush injuries are due to compressive forces. The patient sustains a large amount of kinetic energy that results in microvascular disruption, edema, and devitalized tissue. Crush wounds are 100-fold more likely to become infected than lacerations because of the much lower bacterial loads required for infection.[8]

Lacerations are wounds that are caused by shear forces that result in a tearing of the tissue. They are subclassified as avulsion, shear, or tension lacerations. Avulsion lacerations are injuries where there is sharp trauma at an angle that removes the epidermal and possibly also the dermal layer of skin. The injury creates a skin flap. Shear lacerations are produced by a sharp force, usually

TABLE 77-1. CHARACTERISTICS OF TETANUS-PRONE AND NON-TETANUS-PRONE WOUNDS

Clinical feature	Tetanus-prone wounds	Non-tetanus-prone wounds
Contaminants (feces, foreign body saliva, soil)	Present	Absent
Devitalized tissue	Present	Absent
Infection	Present	Absent
Ischemic or denervated tissue	Present	Absent
Mechanism of injury	Burn, crush, bullet	Sharp and smooth (knife or glass)
Wound age	> 6 hours	< 6 hours
Wound depth	> 1 cm	< 1 cm
Wound type	Abrasion, avulsion, crush, irregular, stellate	Linear or straight

TABLE 77-2. TETANUS PROPHYLAXIS

Immunization history	Tetanus-prone wounds	Non-tetanus-prone wounds
History of adsorbed Td	Td and TIG	Td and TIG
Unknown or less than three doses	Td, TIG, and complete the series	Td and complete the series
Fully immunized, > 5 years and < 10 years since last dose	Td	None needed
Fully immunized; ≤ 5 years since last dose	None needed	None needed
Fully immunized; ≥ 10 years since last dose	Td and TIG	Td

Td, tetanus and diphtheria toxoids; TIG, tetanus immune globulin.

perpendicular to the skin surface, that results in a tidy or clean wound. These wounds are usually caused by knives, glass, or sharp metal objects. There is little tissue damage, and this type of wound is not prone to infection. Tension or tensile lacerations are injuries with jagged or contused edges that are created by a compressive force. These wounds pose a greater risk for infection.[8]

Punctures result in a wound that is deeper than it is wide. The skin opening is small and the depth of the wound is often unknown. Such wounds are made by discrete and thin objects, and they carry a high risk for infection. Irrigation is mandatory for puncture wounds; however, the pressure must not be so high as to drive contaminants deeper into the wound.

The wound may also be clinically classified based upon an estimate of microbial contamination and the subsequent risk of infection. Clean wounds are those that occur under aseptic technique. These are usually surgical incisions that are elective in nature and preceded by a thorough skin cleansing and decontamination process. Clean-contaminated wounds are those associated with the usual and normal flora of the region. There is no contamination from foreign bodies or pus. Contaminated wounds are those that are traumatic (e.g., lacerations, open fractures), less than 12 hours old, or associated with a break in aseptic technique. Most wounds seen in the Emergency Department are of the contaminated type. They may be associated with the introduction of "dirt" or foreign bodies into the wound. Dirty wounds are those that are heavily contaminated (e.g., soil or feces), occur through infected tissue, are over 12 hours old, are associated with retained foreign bodies, or associated with devitalized tissue.

TIME OF INJURY

This is probably the most pertinent factor of the history. After 3 to 6 hours, the bacterial count in a wound increases dramatically. Few studies have been conducted to determine the maximal time in which lacerations can be closed without resulting in infectious complications. One study performed in an underdeveloped country indicated that wounds might be closed up to 18 hours postinjury.[9] Lacerations of the face and scalp that are reasonably clean may be closed primarily up to 12 to 24 (or even 48) hours postinjury with little risk of infection because of the excellent circulation in these areas. Other lacerations may generally be closed primarily if they are less than 6 to 12 hours old provided that they are not heavily contaminated or located in high-risk areas (i.e., hand or foot). The infection rate rises rapidly after 12 hours.

WOUND ASSESSMENT

A complete examination and documentation of the laceration is necessary. This includes noting the location and depth of the laceration, the presence of any gross contamination, the presence of an obvious foreign body, and any associated injuries.

Assessment of soft tissue wounds involves an examination of the surrounding tendons as well as the vascular and neurologic structures; bony injuries and foreign bodies should also be looked for. Emergency Physicians must possess a working knowledge of functional anatomy, particularly of the face and distal upper extremity.

Hemostasis can be achieved by direct pressure with a gauze sponge or gloved finger for simple lacerations. Suturing the wound best controls bleeding of the scalp. Extremity wounds, particularly of the wrist and hand, should have a pneumatic tourniquet applied after the extremity is elevated for 1 minute to promote venous drainage. Inflate the cuff 20 to 30 mmHg above the patient's systolic blood pressure. A blood pressure cuff may be substituted if a pneumatic tourniquet is not available. **Vascular structures (with the exception of small arterioles, small venules, and vessels within muscles) should not be clamped and may require special techniques for hemostasis.**

Wounds may cross tissue planes, opening them and creating potential pockets or dead spaces. Elimination of the dead space has been advocated in the past to decrease the probability of this area becoming a nidus for infection. This once traditional practice of obliteration of dead space to avoid infection of a nonvascularized space or to prevent hematoma formation is now considered controversial. Studies in animal models have found the incidence of infected wounds to be consistently proportional to the number of suture layers.[10,11] Leaving dead space open resulted in lower rates of infection than obliterating it with sutures.[10,11] Studies in 1995 and 1996 concluded that buried absorbable sutures increase the infection rate and the degree of inflammation in contaminated wounds and do not significantly increase the degree of inflammation in noncontaminated wounds.[12] Sutures placed in fat contribute no strength to the repair and fail to prevent hematoma formation and infection. **Deep absorbable sutures may be placed to repair the periosteum, muscles, or fascia or to minimize tension on skin sutures. Use only enough subcutaneous sutures to restore anatomic and functional integrity.** In most wounds, however, leaving potential space may be preferable to attempting to obliterate it.

It is important to explore the deep structures through a full range of motion in order to detect partial tendon lacerations or joint capsule disruption. **Tendons can be evaluated by inspection, but individual muscles must also be tested for full range of motion and full strength.**

A distal neurologic and vascular examination should be performed on extremity injuries. Capillary refill should be checked distally and take less than 2 seconds. Neurologic assessment involves checking distal muscle strength and sensation. **Check two-point discrimination prior to the administration of anesthesia for hand and finger lacerations.** Two-point discrimination at 5 mm on the radial and ulnar aspects of the finger pads is the most efficient method of assessing median and ulnar nerve function. Two-point discrimination should be less than 1 cm at the fingertips. A crush injury may be associated with decreased two-point discrimination and may take several months for recovery. Numbness may also be the first sign of a developing compartment syndrome. Nerve lacerations can be repaired immediately or the wound can be loosely approximated and repair of the lacerated nerve delayed.

Obvious as well as questionable fractures should receive a radiograph of the area. Bone injuries require checking the overlying skin to exclude an open fracture. An open fracture is an indication for surgical debridement and repair except in the case of a distal phalanx fracture, which can be treated with copious irrigation, oral antibiotics, and detailed discharge instructions.

WOUND FOREIGN BODIES

Foreign bodies and foreign matter greatly enhance the infectivity of a given bacterial inoculum.[13] Retained foreign bodies are a common complication of simple wound repair. **Perform a thorough inspection to attempt to diagnose the presence of a foreign body.** Missed foreign bodies are the second leading cause (14

percent) of lawsuits brought against Emergency Physicians.[14] Some foreign bodies cause an inflammatory reaction (wood, thorns, splinters, cloth, teeth, and rubber from shoes or foam insoles), while others do not (metal, glass, most plastics, and pencil graphite).

Wound exploration, irrigation, and radiography may be needed when the clinical setting suggests a possible foreign body. **Spread the tissue during exploration. Do not cut tissue and risk neurovascular injury.** Puncture wounds have not been proven to benefit by coring or probing to determine the depth of the wound. Imaging may be required to detect retained foreign bodies. Retained wood, thorns, and plastic are often detectable only by wound exploration and may not be visible on plain radiographs. Radiographs will identify retained metallic fragments and more than 90 percent of glass foreign bodies if the glass does not have a low lead content and the fragments are at least 2 mm long.[15,16] Wound markers can be used during radiography. Radiographs obtained in two planes can help localize the object for recovery. Glass may penetrate at an angle and be buried deeper than it appears. The use of ultrasound is controversial because of its lack of specificity, lack of sensitivity, and operator dependency.

Foreign bodies that do not cause an inflammatory reaction are often not removed from lacerations. This is especially true if there are multiple fragments or if excessive tissue disruption will result with attempted removal. **The patient should be made aware of any retained foreign bodies at the time of discharge, their benign presence, why removal was not attempted, the possibility of later infection, and the fact that they may eventually self-extrude. This must also be documented in the medical record.** If the wound is in a complex area, such as the palm, it may be necessary to gain consultation for immediate or delayed removal. The wound can be approximated loosely and immobilized for comfort and to avoid further tissue disruption, antibiotics can be prescribed, and arrangements made for appropriate follow-up.

Soils have varied levels of contamination potential. Sandy soils present a low risk of wound contamination. Clay-containing soils are pyogenic because they impair host defense mechanisms and promote inflammation. Organic soils contain *Clostridium tetani* and a more concentrated bacterial inocula. Soil contaminants, when present, can be removed by copious irrigation. These contaminated wounds should be left open and allowed to heal by secondary or tertiary intention.

HIGH-RISK WOUNDS

Many wounds require special consideration in deciding upon the method of closure, the type of suture to use, and the use of antibiotic prophylaxis. These include wounds contaminated by saliva, feces, vaginal secretions, soil, and organic material. **Wounds in immunocompromised patients or patients taking immunosuppressive drugs may require antibiotics and longer times for the sutures to remain before removal.** Hand wounds, including bite wounds, and foot wounds require special care. Wounds greater than 6 to 12 hours old, other than wounds on the face, may require delayed closure. Puncture wounds may require radiographs, incision and exploration, and antibiotic prophylaxis. Wounds accompanied by excessive tissue damage and devitalization or crush injuries are prone to infection. Wounds with retained foreign bodies may require radiographs, exploration, and removal. Major tissue defects may be closed with advanced wound closure techniques. Wounds overlying sites of active infection require antibiotics and delayed closure. These topics are covered further on in this chapter and in other chapters of this book (see Chapters 79 and 80 for details).

SKIN AND WOUND PREPARATION

SKIN CLEANSING

Meticulous preparation of the skin surrounding the wound and the actual wound, irrigation, and wound debridement are tantamount to good wound healing. The goal is to remove bacteria, foreign matter, and tissue debris. Wounds should be adequately anesthetized prior to cleansing and/or local exploration. Adequate light, anesthesia, and equipment are a must in order to avoid inadequate debridement, a retained foreign body, or a wound hematoma that can result in a necrotizing soft tissue infection.

Disinfecting the intact skin surrounding the wound and ridding it of foreign bodies, debris, and particulate matter is the initial step in wound preparation. This technique can be accomplished by scrubbing the skin with either povidone iodine (Betadine) or poloxamer 188 (Shur Clens) skin-prep solutions, being careful not to expose the wound to these solutions. Povidone iodine solution is bactericidal and works as it dries. Its toxicity to wound tissue is controversial. Shur Clens has no tissue toxicity but also has no antibacterial activity. A wide area surrounding the wound should be prepped with an antimicrobial agent, preferably povidone iodine solution.

HAIR REMOVAL

Hair removal is often unnecessary prior to closing wounds and can be embarrassing for the patient after repair. Shaving can cause minimal soft tissue trauma and wound infections.[17] **Eyebrows should never be shaved, as they can grow back unpredictably or not at**

all. Simple scalp lacerations can be exposed by using antibiotic ointment (or lubricating gel) to plaster the hair down at the wound margins.

WOUND IRRIGATION

Wound cleansing and preparation have been proven to be the foundations of proper wound management and the prevention of wound infections. Irrigation removes contaminants, reduces infection, and improves visualization. There are two concerns regarding wound irrigation: the pressure required for adequate cleansing of the wound and the means to irrigate the wound safely while protecting the health care worker from the threat of human immunodeficiency virus and hepatitis B [by contamination of their own skin surfaces, mucosal surfaces (eyes, nose, or mouth), or minor open skin wounds].

Irrigation pressures of 8 to 12 pounds per square inch (psi) are felt to be adequate to cleanse a wound that is not heavily contaminated. This surface pressure can be generated by the combination of a 35 mL syringe and a 19 gauge angiocatheter held 2 cm from the wound surface.[18] Unfortunately, this process can be quite messy (Figure 77-1). High-pressure irrigation, which generates peak pressures of 25 to 40 psi, has been a controversial issue in the recent Emergency Medicine literature. The theory is that high pressures may cause tissue disruption and increase infection rates. High-pressure irrigation should be reserved for highly contaminated wounds. High-pressure irrigation may drive contaminants deeper into puncture wounds and should be avoided.

Though there are a variety of irrigation fluids, the optimal type is unknown. Normal saline and a 1% povidone iodine solution (a 1:9 dilution of the stock 10% solution) have both been recommended, but neither is superior to the other in the prevention of infec-

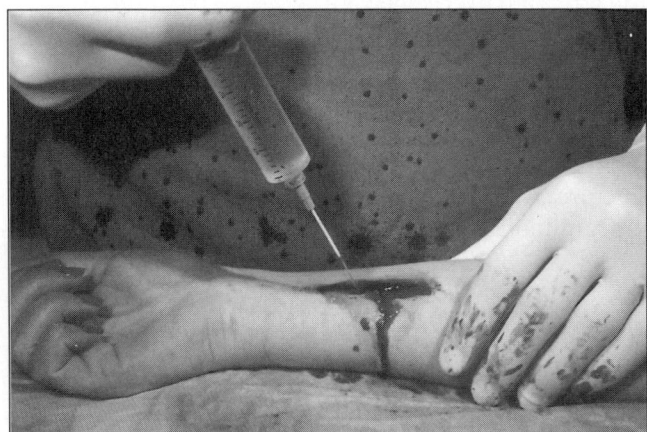

FIGURE 77-1 Wound irrigation with an angiocatheter on a syringe. This process is quite messy and can result in an occupational exposure. (Photo courtesy of Zerowet Incorporated.)

tion. The volume of irrigation fluid to be used has not been well established. The use of 100 to 300 mL has been suggested in the literature. Heavily contaminated wounds require larger amounts of irrigant. Anecdotal recommendations suggest using 50 mL/cm for clean wounds and 100 mL/cm for dirty wounds. Heavily contaminated wounds may have to be scrubbed (after adequate anesthesia) with fine-mesh gauze or a micropore sponge using a 1% solution of povidone iodine or poloxamer 188. Soaking of wounds is discouraged as a poor substitute for the preparation of contaminated or clean wounds.

Numerous commercially available devices are available to irrigate a wound (Figure 77-2). The Combiport (Ethox Corp., Buffalo, NY) is a wound irrigation device that inserts directly into the port of an intravenous fluid bag (Figure 77-2A). Squeeze the bag of saline and direct the stream of fluid through the device and into the wound. Wound Wash Saline (Blairex Laboratories Inc., Columbus, IN) is sterile normal saline within a pressurized can (Figure 77-2B). Direct the tip of the can toward the wound, press the button, and direct the saline stream into the wound. This is also available at retail stores for patients to use at home for wound care. The company offers a convenient chart that uses wound depth and base characteristics to determine how much saline to use to irrigate the wound. The can controls the pressure (6 to 13 psi), so that tissue is not devitalized during the irrigation.

The operator should use barrier protection to shield their face, eyes, skin, and submucosal surfaces during the irrigation process. There are several barrier devices on the market that decrease the splatter of irrigation fluid[19] (Figure 77-2). Some of these devices are pre-attached to a wound irrigation device. Others can be attached to a wound irrigation device. The Zerowet Splashield (Zerowet Inc., Palos Verdes Peninsula, CA) is a dome-shaped device that attaches to a syringe (Figure 77-2C). The Combiguard Irrigation Splash Guard (Ethox Corp., Buffalo, NY) is similar in function to the Zerowet Splashield and has a slightly different shape. The Combiguard can attach to a syringe or the Combiport Wound

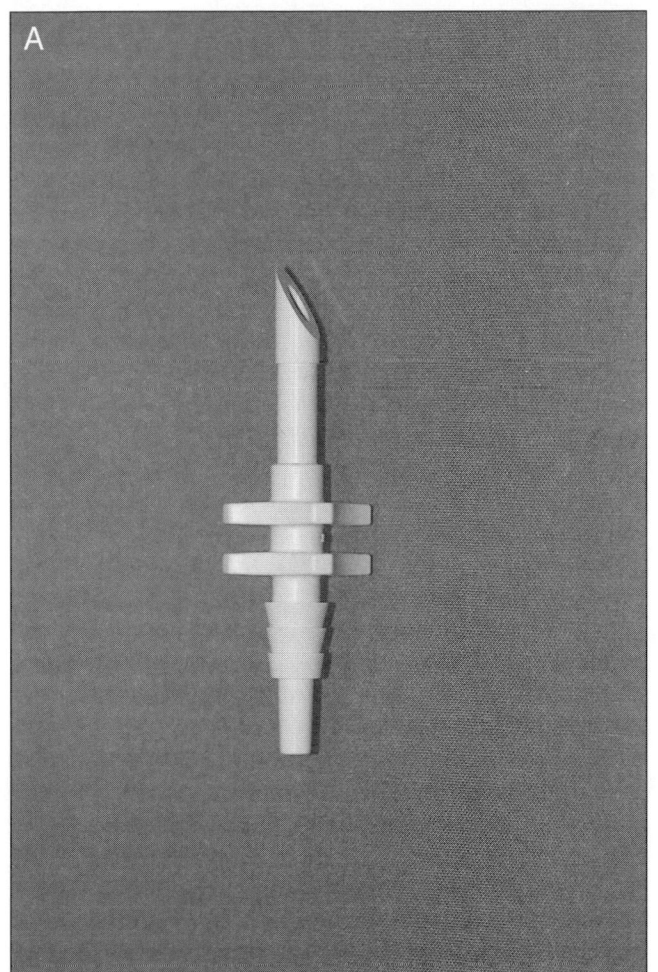
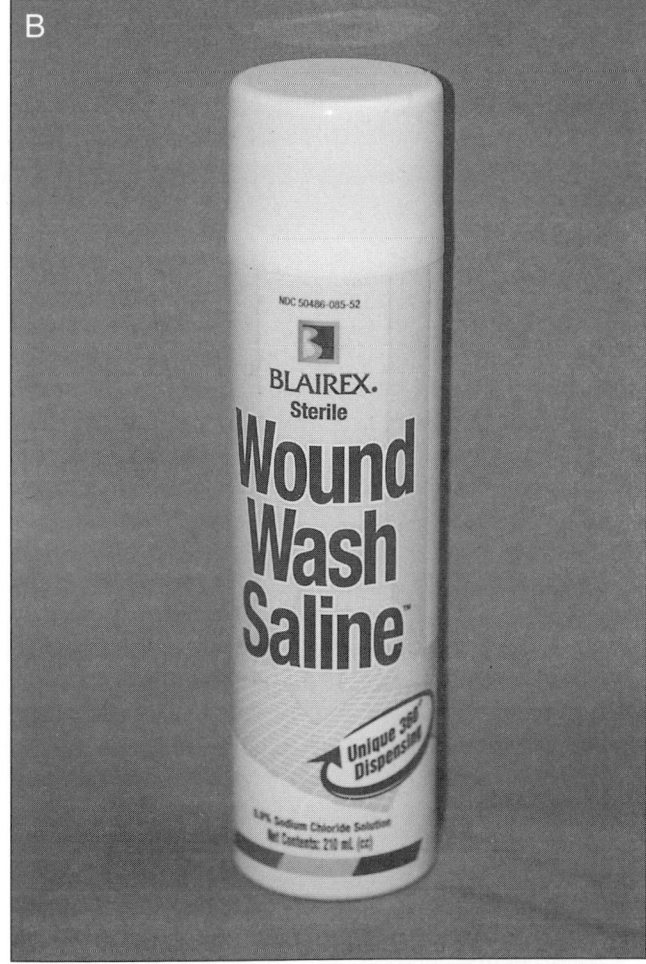

FIGURE 77-2 Commercially available wound irrigation devices. *A.* The Combiport Wound Irrigation Device (Ethox Corp., Buffalo, NY). *B.* Wound Wash Saline (Blairex Laboratories Inc., Columbus, IN). *(continued)*

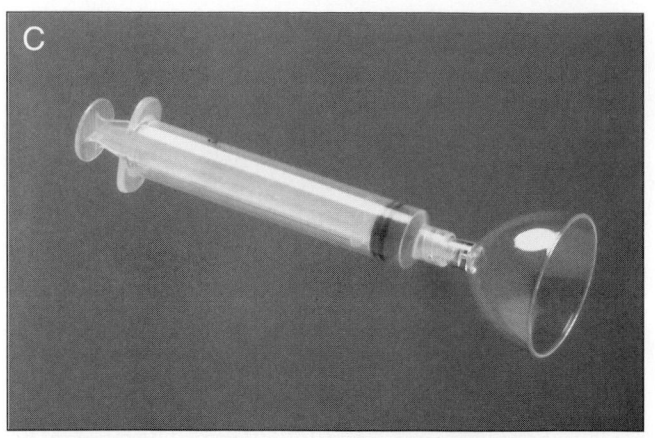

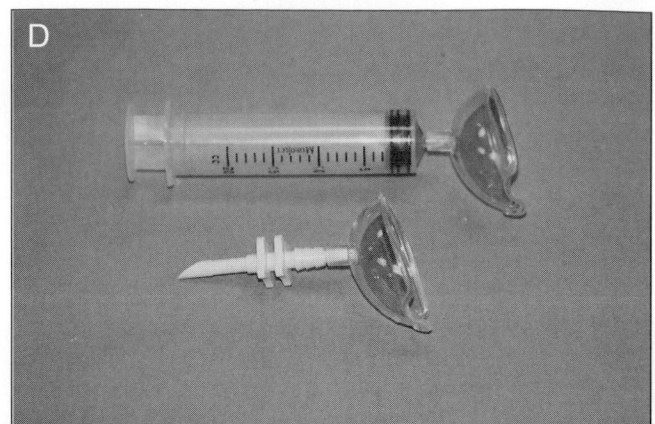

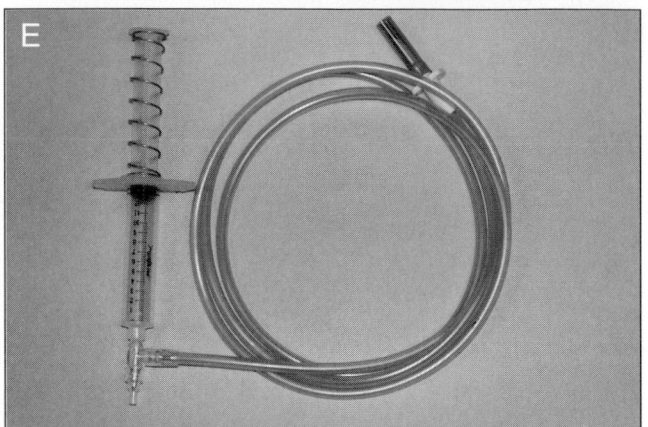

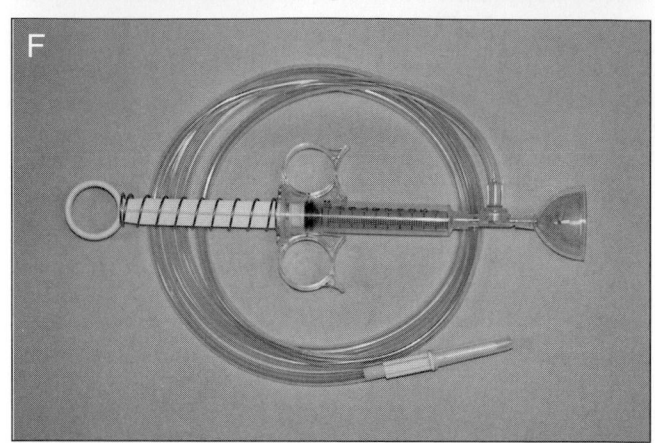

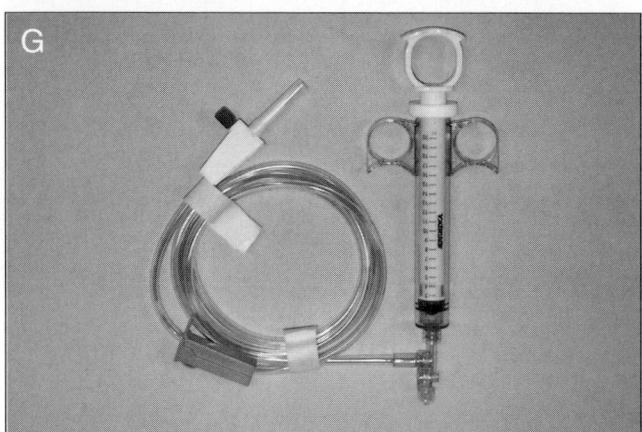

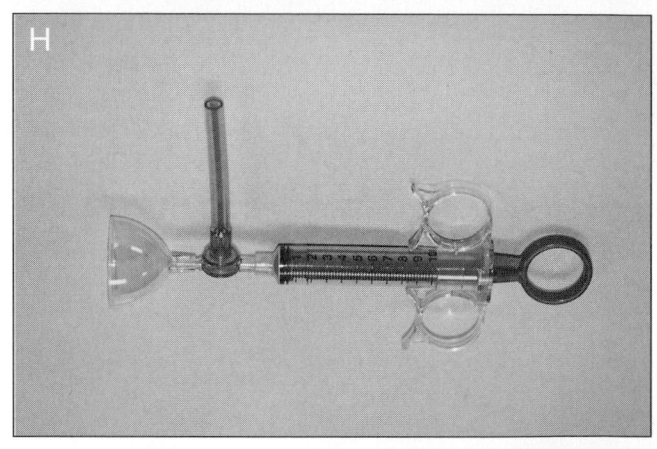

FIGURE 77-2 (continued) *C.* The Zerowet Splashield (Zerowet Inc., Palos Verdes Peninsula, CA). *D.* The Combiguard (Ethox Corp., Buffalo, NY) attaches to the Combiport or a syringe. *E.* The Irrijet (Ackrad Laboratories Inc., Cranford, NJ). *F.* The Canyons Wound Irrigation System (Canyons International Inc., Salt Lake City, UT). *G.* The Squirt Wound Irrigation Kit (Merit Medical Systems Inc., South Jordan, UT). *H.* The Klenzalac (Zerowet Inc., Palos Verdes Peninsula, CA).

Irrigation Device (Figure 77-2*D*). The Igloo Wound Irrigator (Bionix Medical Technologies, Toledo, OH) is a similar device that provides a multiport shower effect to deliver the irrigation solution. The Irrijet (Ackrad Laboratories Inc., Cranford, NJ) is a spring-loaded, self-refilling system that is operated with one hand (Figure 77-2*E*). A Splashield, Splash Guard, or Igloo can be at-

tached to the Irrijet. The Canyons Wound Irrigation System (Canyons International Inc., Salt Lake City, UT) is a similar device with the exception of using the built-in Zerowet Splashield (Figure 77-2*F*). The Squirt Wound Irrigation Kit (Merit Medical Systems Inc., South Jordan, UT) is a manually operated system that may be used alone or attached to the Splashield, Combiguard, Igloo, or an angiocatheter (Figure 77-2*G*). The Klenzalac (Zerowet Inc., Palos Verdes Peninsula, CA) is a similar device with the exception of using the built-in Zerowet Splashield (Figure 77-2*H*).

WOUND DEBRIDEMENT

Debridement creates straight and clean wound edges that are easier to repair by removing tissue that is devitalized, contaminated by bacteria, or contaminated by foreign matter and may impair the ability of the tissue to resist infection. Successful wound closure may require the transformation of a ragged laceration, the removal of devitalized tissue, or the removal of contaminated tissue in order to convert a traumatic wound into a surgical wound. Devitalized and necrotic tissue must be removed in order to remove a nidus for bacterial growth and wound infection.[20]

Close approximation of the wound requires that debridement of jagged edges not be too vigorous in order to avoid widening the scar and making it difficult to close. Wounds of the face or areas that are devoid of redundant tissue require conservative debridement. Debridement to simplify wound closure is not always the answer for a superior cosmetic result in the repair of irregular wound edges. The meticulous repair of complex wound edges can often provide a superior cosmetic result.

Debridement can be accomplished mechanically, hydrodynamically, or with a combination of both methods. Tissue must be removed mechanically with a #11 or #15 scalpel blade or a scissors (Figure 77-3). Superficial debris and contaminants can be removed with a pulsatile stream of normal saline solution during the irrigation process. **Debridement must be performed using aseptic technique. Scrubbing is not a substitute for debridement of heavily contaminated tissue. Wound edges should be handled delicately or gingerly in order to avoid further soft tissue damage and devitalization of injured tissue.**

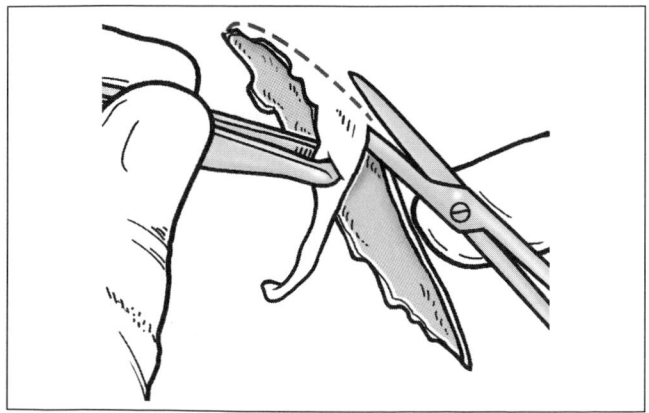

FIGURE 77-3 Wound debridement. Removal of the wound edges with a scissors (or a scalpel).

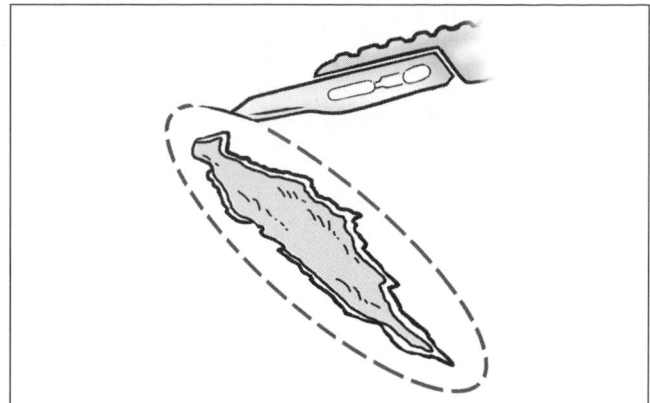

FIGURE 77-4 Wound excision. Removal of an ellipse of tissue that contains the wound results in smooth, clean edges that can be approximated.

WOUND EXCISION

The entire wound may be excised in areas of excess tissue or tissue laxity if no blood vessels, nerves, tendons, or joints lie within or at the base of the wound (Figure 77-4). The excision of a wound creates smooth, clean edges that may be approximated with sutures. This is especially useful in wounds that are heavily contaminated. Most wounds are excised with an elliptical incision (Figure 77-4). Other types of wound excision are discussed in Chapters 79 and 80.

Carefully plan the excision before removing any tissue. Mark the edges of the proposed incision with a marking pen. The long axis of the ellipse should be three to four times as long as the greatest width of the ellipse. Removal of too much tissue will produce a large defect that may not be possible to close primarily. Remove the tissue using aseptic technique, preventing any contamination of the new wound edges.

WOUND UNDERMINING

The undermining of tissue creates a "flap" that involves the separation of the skin and superficial subcutaneous tissue from the deeper subcutaneous tissue and fascia (Figure 77-5). The process of undermining tissue minimizes skin tension, allows for eversion of the approximated skin edges, and relieves the extrinsic tension from sutures. **Undermining is performed when the wound cannot be closed due to a tissue defect or if a wound is under tension.** This procedure requires the physician to be familiar with the local anatomy so that no blood vessels, nerves, or tendons are injured in the process. **Do not undermine contaminated wounds.** Undermining can separate the skin from its underlying blood supply and result in a diminished blood flow that predisposes the area to infection. Undermining may be useful on the forehead, scalp, arm, forearm, thigh, calf, and torso. **Never undermine wounds on the palms, soles, and face.**

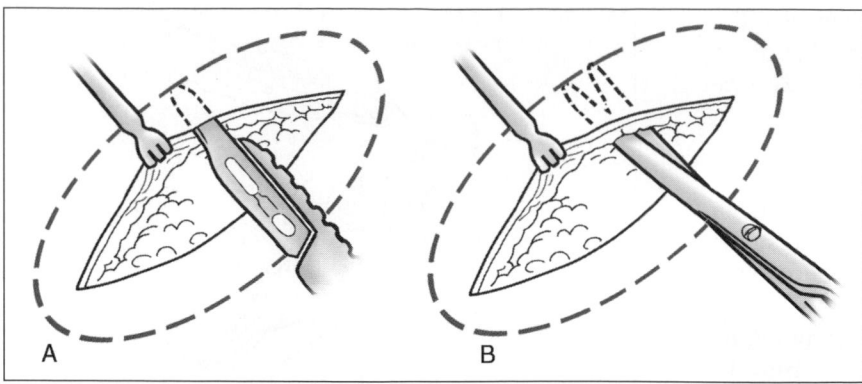

FIGURE 77-5 Wound undermining. *A.* Sharp undermining with a #15 scalpel blade. *B.* Blunt undermining with a Mayo scissors.

Tissue should be undermined at the dermal-epidermal junction or within the subcutaneous adipose tissue. The amount of undermining necessary to close a laceration is approximately double the width of the gap of the laceration at its widest point. A 1 cm wide laceration should be undermined for 1 cm on both sides of the wound, including the ends (Figure 77-5). The use of a Mayo scissors versus a #15 scalpel blade to undermine tissue is based on physician experience and preference. A Mayo scissors is recommended as it may cause less secondary injury, especially in experienced hands.

EMERGENCY DEPARTMENT VERSUS OPERATING ROOM MANAGEMENT OF WOUNDS

Laceration repair may sometimes have to be performed in the Operating Room. Indications for Operating Room repair of lacerations include those associated with open fractures, major or complex wounds involving devitalized tissue, heavily contaminated wounds, associated injuries (visceral, neurovascular, fracture, tendon), perineal wounds, large or complicated soft tissue injuries, compartment syndromes, wounds with extensive amounts of necrotic or ischemic tissue, and high-pressure injection injuries.

ANTIBIOTIC PROPHYLAXIS

Despite the best wound care and management, the rate of infection has been determined to be approximately 1 to 12 percent. Not all wounds result in infection. Most uncomplicated wounds heal without the need for antibiotics. Wounds associated with an increased risk for infection are those of the extremities (especially the lower), complex wounds, or wounds over 3 to 5 cm in length. The use of antibiotics for traumatic wounds is controversial. Prophylactic antibiotics are not indicated for uncomplicated minor wounds with a low chance of becoming infected. It has not been proven that antibiotic administration following injury actually reduces the probability of infection.

It is necessary to identify those patients who may benefit from antibiotics early. Antibiotic therapy should be considered in the following situations: where wounds are heavily contaminated or associated with major soft tissue injury; wounds associated with active infection; when there is a delay in care that results in a prolonged time from debridement or treatment (> 3 hours); when the patient is immunocompromised or has cardiac valvular disease; when there are bites to the hand or face, deep puncture wounds, or lacerations to lymphedematous tissue; or when the patient has prosthetic joints.

ANESTHESIA

Wounds must be anesthetized with either local or regional techniques prior to cleansing and repair. Local anesthesia distorts wound edges; therefore regional nerve blocks should be used where appropriate (e.g., the hand, face, ear, nasal cartilage, palm, sole). Refer to Chapters 105 to 109 for a complete discussion of local anesthetic agents, nerve blocks, nitrous oxide anesthesia, and procedural sedation.

One-percent lidocaine (Xylocaine) in a dose not to exceed 5 to 7 mg/kg is an effective and standard agent. Lidocaine anesthesia lasts approximately 60 minutes. If a longer period of anesthesia is required, 0.75% bupivacaine (Marcaine or Sensorcaine), which lasts approximately 90 to 120 minutes, may be used. A 1 : 100,000 dilution of epinephrine can be added to prolong the duration of anesthesia, promote hemostasis, and reduce systemic absorption of locally infiltrated lidocaine. Epinephrine is a potent vasoconstrictor and should not be used near end organs such as the fingers or toes. It may decrease blood flow and induce ischemia. Epinephrine should also be avoided near the nasal tip, the ear, and the penis.

Animal model studies have consistently shown that epinephrine increases the incidence of infection in contaminated wounds. This may be due to vasospasm induced local ischemia. Epinephrine should not be used to enhance anesthesia in contaminated wounds.

The use of a 27 or 30 gauge needle, slower and deeper infiltration (into the dermis), and the addition of bicarbonate to lidocaine (9 mL lidocaine to 1 mL of bicarbonate) may decrease the pain of anesthetic injection.[21–26] Other strategies involve anesthetizing as much tissue as possible through a single site and starting proximally on extremities and moving distally.

Most "allergic" reactions are actually vasovagal or other adverse responses. Allergies to "caines" are attributed to what is often a vasovagal or other side effect. True allergies to local anesthetics are rare and are generally seen only with esters. If an allergy to lidocaine (an amide class of local anesthetic) is suspected, the use of an ester class of local anesthetic is suggested. An alternative is the use of cardiac lidocaine, which contains no preservative. It is felt that the preservative in lidocaine is responsible for the allergic effect. Another alternative is to use a 1% to 2% solution of diphenhydramine (Benadryl). This provides adequate but not ideal anesthesia. The most common complication of local anesthesia infiltration is hypotension and bradycardia as a result of a vasovagal reaction.

Topical anesthesia is an attractive alternative to injection, particularly in the management of pediatric patients with simple wounds. Lidocaine/epinephrine/tetracaine (LET) gel or tetracaine/adrenaline/cocaine (TAC) are two agents that can be used as effective local anesthesia.[27] Both of these agents contain epinephrine and should not be used on areas involving an end artery or contaminated wounds.

TAC involves expense and incorporates problems with the use and maintenance of a controlled substance. TAC should also concern physicians because of its potential for toxicity, especially with application to mucosal surfaces. EMLA (eutectic mixture of local anesthetics) cream, also used for local anesthesia, has been found to provide effective anesthesia for extremity lacerations. EMLA is a combination of 2.5% lidocaine and 2.5% prilocaine suspended in an oil-in-water emulsion. Studies have found that it takes longer to obtain optimal anesthesia with EMLA than with TAC.[28]

SUTURES

SUTURE TYPES

Proper size suture material can be summarized as the smallest suture needed to approximate the edges of a wound. This will reduce tissue damage caused by the suture, and the resulting scar will be minimized. The tensile strength of the suture should never exceed the tensile strength of the tissue, or it can pull through and damage the tissue. The sutures should be at least as strong as the normal tissue through which they are being placed.

The size of the suture material is related to the diameter of the suture. As the number of 0's in the suture size increases, the diameter of the strand decreases. For example, size 5–0, or 00000, is smaller in diameter than size 4–0, or 0000. The smaller the size, the less tensile strength the suture will have.

Suture description entails numerous characteristics. Sutures can be classified into two major groups based upon the number of strands of which they are composed. Monofilament sutures are made of a single strand of material. They encounter less resistance passing through tissue and resist harboring organisms that may cause suture-line infections. Multifilament sutures consist of several filaments, or strands, that are twisted or braided together. This affords greater tensile strength, pliability, and flexibility. Unfortunately, bacteria can migrate between the filaments and into the wound.

Another classification is based on the ability of the body to break down and absorb the suture material. Absorbable sutures are digested by body enzymes or hydrolyzed in body tissue. Nonabsorbable sutures are not digested by body enzymes or hydrolyzed.

Absorbable suture can be made of natural or synthetic material. Natural absorbable suture is classified as surgical gut (plain or chromic). Plain surgical gut is composed of collagen from bovine or sheep intestine. It is rapidly absorbed, maintaining its tensile strength for only 7 to 10 days and is completely absorbed within 70 days. Chromic gut is treated with a chromium salt solution to resist body enzymes. It retains its tensile strength for 10 to 14 days and is absorbed over 90 days.

Synthetic absorbable sutures include polyglactin 910 (Vicryl, Ethicon) and polyglycolic acid (Dexon). They were developed because of the tissue reaction, suture antigenicity, and unpredictable rates of absorption of natural absorbable sutures. These sutures are braided synthetic materials that retain 50 percent of their initial strength at 4 weeks. The synthetic absorbable sutures retain their tensile strength long enough to ensure the security of the subcutaneous layers after the removal of percutaneous sutures.

Nonabsorbable sutures are made of silk, nylon, polypropylene, cotton, linen, or metal. They can be monofilament or multifilament in construction. Nylon is the most commonly used suture in the Emergency Department. It is used to approximate lacerations at the skin surface. Silk may occasionally be used in the mouth. It causes significant tissue reactions that result in inflammation and granuloma formation as the body "fights off" this natural fiber. The other types of nonabsorbable sutures are generally not utilized in the Emergency Department.

Several factors must be considered in choosing suture material. Choose sutures that match the healing properties of the tissues. Approximate slow-healing tissues (fascia and tendons) with nonabsorbable sutures or a long-lasting absorbable suture. Foreign bodies in potentially contaminated tissues may result in an infection. Multifilament sutures can act as a foreign body and may convert a contaminated wound into an infected one. Multifilament sutures should generally be avoided. Use monofilament sutures or absorbable sutures that resist harboring infection. Use the smallest inert monofilament suture materials (such as nylon or polypropylene), avoid using skin sutures alone (use subcuticular closure whenever possible), and use sterile skin closure strips for apposition when possible.

NEEDLES

Needles are generally of two types, tapered and cutting (Figure 77-6). Cutting needles have sharp ends and sharp edges that act as a cutting instrument (Figure 77-6A). The cutting needle is commonly used for tougher tissues such as subcutaneous, intradermal, and cutaneous (skin) closure. In addition to the two cutting edges, conventional cutting needles have a third cutting edge on the inside concave curvature of the needle. This needle type may be prone to "cutout" of tissue because the inside cutting edge cuts toward the edges of the incision or wound.

Reverse cutting needles are as sharp as the conventional cutting needle except that the third cutting edge is located on the outer convex curvature of the needle (Figure 77-6B). Reverse cutting needles have more strength than similar-sized conventional cutting needles. The danger of tissue "cutout" is greatly reduced. The hole left by the needle leaves a wide wall of tissue against which the suture is to be tied.

Taper point needles have a pointed end (Figure 77-6C). The rest of the needle is a smooth, rounded tube with no cutting edges. This type of needle is commonly used in surgery to close tissues with minimal trauma. It is used for all tissues except skin.

Two other types of needles are often available but not used in the Emergency Department. The blunt point needle has a smooth tip and tapered body (Figure 77-6D). It is used for suturing friable tissue and blunt dissection. The taper cut needle has a cutting tip and a tapered body (Figure 77-6E). It is a combination of the tapered point and cutting needle. It is used to place sutures through tough tissues. Numerous other needles are available, as are modifications of the five basic needle types. These needles are used by surgeons for specialized tissues.

Always keep some general principles in mind when suturing. **Needles should be pulled through tissue using a needle driver and never a hemostat.** A hemostat or other clamp can damage the needle. Avoid injury to yourself and others. **Keep all open needles in a place so that they will not injure you or your assistant.** Account for and discard all suture needles in a "sharps" container. Following these two steps will dramatically decrease the chance for a needle-stick injury.

HANDLING SUTURES

Always use a needle driver when suturing. The use of a hemostat or other type of "clamp" can damage the needle and cause it to bend or break in the tissue. Needle drivers are generally made of steel with a jaw designed to hold the needle securely without damaging it. They come in numerous sizes and shapes. Choose a needle driver that is an appropriate size for the needle that is to be grasped. Grasp and remove a clean needle from its package with your hands (forceps or a needle driver may also be used). Securely grasp the proximal one-third to one-

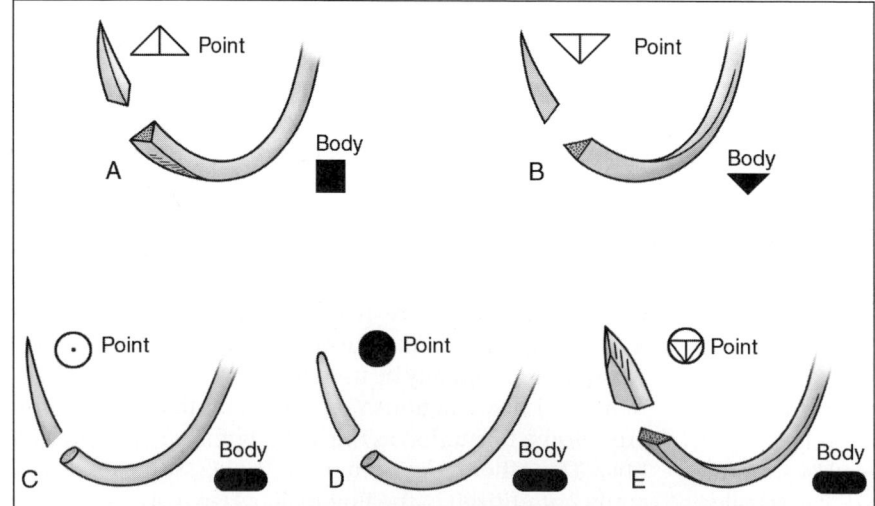

FIGURE 77-6 Common types of suture needles. *A.* The cutting needle. *B.* The reverse cutting needle. *C.* The taper point needle. *D.* The blunt point needle. *E.* The taper cut needle.

half of the needle with the needle driver (Figure 77-7*A*). **Do not grasp the distal one-third of the needle.** This can damage its cutting surfaces. **Always use the tips of the needle driver to grasp the needle** (Figure 77-7*B*). Grasping a needle with the base of the jaws may damage the needle.

Use the needle driver when pushing the needle through the tissue to place a suture (Figure 77-7*C*). **Apply the force in a direction following the curve of the needle. Do not twist or force the needle to push the point through the tissue and out the other side.** Use a larger needle if the first one is too short or too small. **Do not use a needle that has become dull and difficult to pass through the tissue.** Obtain a new needle and continue the procedure. Grasp the distal tip of the needle with a needle driver when it emerges from the tissues (Figure 77-7*D*). **Always grasp the needle proximal to its distal third to prevent damage to the cutting edges.**

Always use caution when handing a needle driver armed with a needle to another person. Grasp the needle driver between the thumb, index, and middle fingers (Figure 77-7*E*). Hand the base of the needle driver to another person. **Do not blindly pass the needle driver. Do not pass the needle driver over a third party without their knowledge of the transfer. Never grasp the distal end of an armed needle driver.**

WOUND CLOSURE

The goal of wound closure is approximation of the skin under minimal tension while achieving eversion of the wound edges (Chapter 78). Wound eversion slightly raises the wound edges to keep the epidermal cells from migrating into the dermal layers, therefore leaving a flat scar (Figure 77-8). The time from the injury to the presentation and the mechanism of injury will indicate whether the laceration mandates delayed closure instead of primary closure and whether tetanus prophylaxis is required. With the exception of patients who are immunocompromised or taking immunosuppressive therapy, those with high-risk wounds should be considered for delayed closure.

SINGLE-LAYER VERSUS MULTILAYER CLOSURE

The greatest strength of the skin (and of the wound) is contained within the dermis. The better the coaptation of the dermal edges, the narrower the scar will be. The best results occur when the entire depth of the dermis is accurately approximated to the entire depth of the opposite dermis. Dermal closure is best performed with synthetic monofilament absorbable suture that requires enzymatic degradation. Chromic or plain catgut suture dissolves much more rapidly by means of hydrolysis.

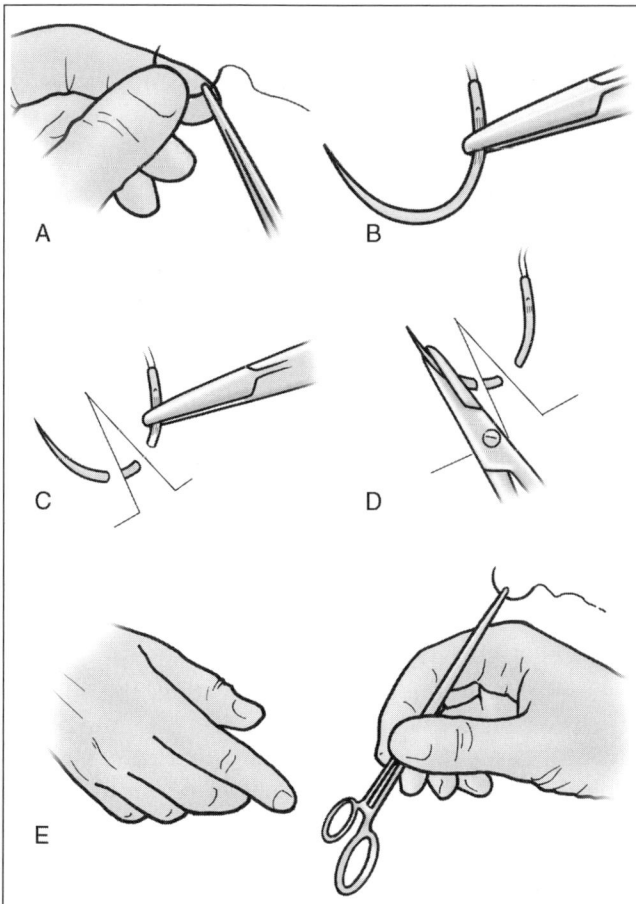

FIGURE 77-7 Using a needle driver. *A.* Grasp the proximal one-third to one-half of the needle. *B.* Always use the tips of the jaws to grasp the needle. *C.* Drive the needle through the tissue following the natural curve of the needle. *D.* Grasp the distal needle proximal to the cutting edges. *E.* Correct method to pass a needle driver armed with a needle.

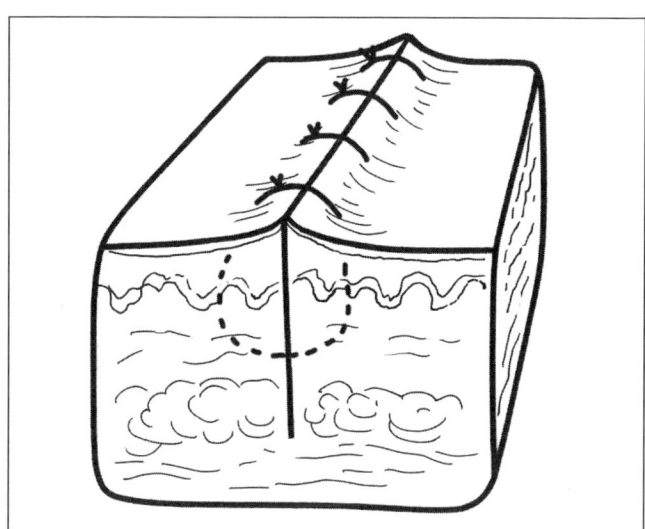

FIGURE 77-8 Eversion of the wound edge signifies proper suture placement and knot tension.

Close the wound in multiple layers if the goal is cosmesis. Close the wound with a minimal number of sutures in a single layer if the goal is a functional result. Do not suture through fat and muscle. Fat has no tensile strength. Sutures placed tightly in fat can cause ischemia and necrosis in the wound and increase the risk of a wound infection. Muscle fibers do not support sutures. Muscle is best treated by repair of the overlying fascia and immobilization to prevent motion and to allow coaptation of the muscle fibers.

WOUND CLOSURE PROCEDURE

Clean any dirt and debris from the skin. Scrub the area surrounding the wound with antiseptic skin cleanser. Anesthetize the wound with a 27 to 30 gauge hypodermic needle and local anesthetic solution. Irrigate the wound with normal saline. Use a mask with a face shield to prevent exposure to the patient's blood and tissue fluid. Debride and undermine the wound as necessary. Irrigate the wound again to remove exposed debris and devitalized tissue. Repair the wound with sutures or pack it with saline-soaked fine-mesh gauze for delayed closure. Clean the repaired wound with normal saline and apply a dressing for comfort and protection. Consider the application of a splint for wounds covering joints or muscle lacerations.

Write a procedure note describing the sterile preparation of the wound, the type and volume of anesthesia administered, the type of suture(s) used in the repair, the layers repaired, the type of repair (interrupted versus continuous), and how the procedure was tolerated by the patient. Any complications should also be noted.

AFTERCARE

Wound care has become a specialty involving sophisticated research in many areas, including dressings and the environment in which wounds heal best. Clean the area surrounding the repaired wound with normal saline to remove any antimicrobial agents and blood. It has been demonstrated that optimal growth of fibroblasts in tissue culture occurs at low partial pressures of oxygen (5 to 10 mmHg). Epidermal cell growth is inhibited at oxygen levels higher than that in surrounding air. It has been shown clinically that hydrocolloid dressings are capable of maintaining low oxygen tension independent of the underlying disease process.[29] The application of an occlusive dressing has been shown to increase the rate of wound healing by approximately 40 percent, as well as preventing environmental trauma and keeping bacteria out of the wound.

Dressings, regardless of the type used, should produce a moist but not macerated wound that is free of infection, toxic chemicals, and foreign material while maintaining an optimum temperature and pH. Layered dressings of nonadherent gauze, such as Xeroform, covered with dry gauze can be used for large sutured lacerations and abrasions. This dressing draws exudate into a layer that can be replaced without disturbing the underlying wound. Shear wounds or hematomas may require gauze that is fluffed and formed into a pressure dressing. Dressings of antibiotic ointment with a standard adhesive bandage (e.g., Band-Aid) provide adequate healing and protection for smaller repaired lacerations. The topical application of antibiotics to the suture line after wound closure helps to protect against exogenous bacterial contamination. The use of paper gauze and Telfa pads is not advisable.

DISCHARGE INSTRUCTIONS

High-risk wounds such as animal and/or human bites, hand wounds, heavily contaminated wounds, and wounds that require prophylactic antibiotic coverage should be reevaluated within 24 hours.

Patients should be made aware, orally and in writing, that up to one in ten persons develops a wound infection that can be treated with an oral antibiotic. Puncture wounds are considered high-risk injuries that can result in bone infections. Patients should immediately return to the Emergency Department or their primary physician if a wound becomes red or has a discharge, if redness or red streaks are emanating from the wound, or if they develop a fever.

Explain briefly the progression of healing. The new scar's appearance is usually worst at 3 to 5 weeks. Most scars remodel within 6 to 12 months. Any revision of the wound should be postponed for approximately 6 to 12 months from the time of injury.

SUTURE REMOVAL

The length of time that the sutures remain in place depends upon the location of the wound, the amount of tension on the wound, and the healing time of the involved tissue. Some general guidelines are listed in Table 77-3. Appropriate and timely removal of sutures minimizes scarring. Leaving sutures in too long results in epithelialization of the suture tracts, larger scars, and possibly infections. Suture removal kits are commercially available (Figure 77-9). They typically contain a forceps, a scissors, and gauze squares. These kits are inexpensive, disposable, and intended for single-patient use.

Sutures should be removed using aseptic and sterile technique. Clean the wound with saline. Apply hydro-

TABLE 77-3. SUTURE REMOVAL RECOMMENDATIONS

Location	Days
Face	3–4 (child), 3–5 (adult)
Neck	2–3 (child), 3–4 (adult)
Upper extremity	7–10
Hand	10–14
Chest	7–10
Back	10–14
Buttocks	10–14
Legs	8–10
Foot	10–14
Delayed closure	8–12
Retention sutures	14–30
Overlying joints	10–14

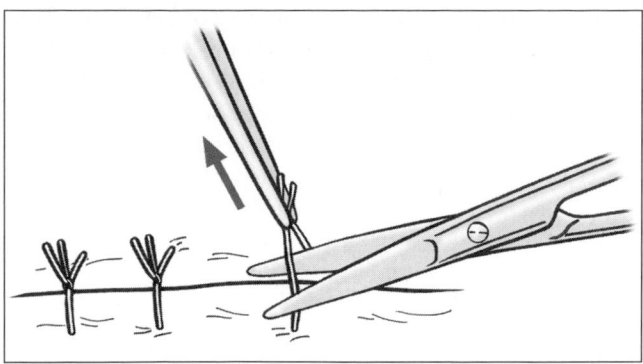

FIGURE 77-10 Suture removal.

gen peroxide to remove any dried blood and serum encrusted around the sutures. Grasp the suture at the knot with forceps (Figure 77-10). Lift the knot off the skin. Cut the suture as close to the skin as possible with a scissors and where the suture enters the skin (Figure 77-10). This will avoid drawing contaminated suture through the depth of the wound. Sutures that are close together, small, or tight may require a #11 scalpel blade to cut them rather than a scissors. Gently pull the suture strand out of the tissue with the forceps and across the wound. Pulling a suture out away from the wound may result in the wound edges opening (dehiscing). Remove one to three sutures and ensure that the wound edges do not dehisce. Remove the remaining sutures. Apply skin adhesive strips (Steri-strips) across the wound to provide support.

Full-thickness sutures can be left in place for 2 or more weeks without risk of suture-track formation in areas where sebaceous glands and other adnexal structures are not present, such as the plantar and palmar surfaces.

MANAGEMENT OF PUNCTURE WOUNDS

Puncture wounds are considered to be at higher risk for infection than simple lacerations. They should be allowed to heal by delayed intention, particularly if they penetrate into the subcutaneous tissues. Local cleansing is the initial step in management. High-pressure irrigation, coring, and probing are generally not recommended.

Infection is most frequently due to *Staphylococcus aureus, Staphylococcus epidermidis,* or streptococcal species. Treatment should be reserved for compromised hosts, dirty wounds, or actual infected wounds.[30] Puncture wounds of the foot are of special concern due to the risk of *Pseudomonas aeruginosa* infection, particularly with wounds through athletic shoes. A tender wound that is not infected usually indicates that there is a retained foreign body. Persistent infection from a plantar wound suggests an underlying osteomyelitis that requires radiographs and treatment with a fluoroquinolone.[31]

PEDIATRIC ISSUES OF WOUND HEALING

Pediatric patients less than 15 years of age experience infection rates of less than 1 percent for clean surgical wounds.[7] This is less than that seen in adults. Young chil-

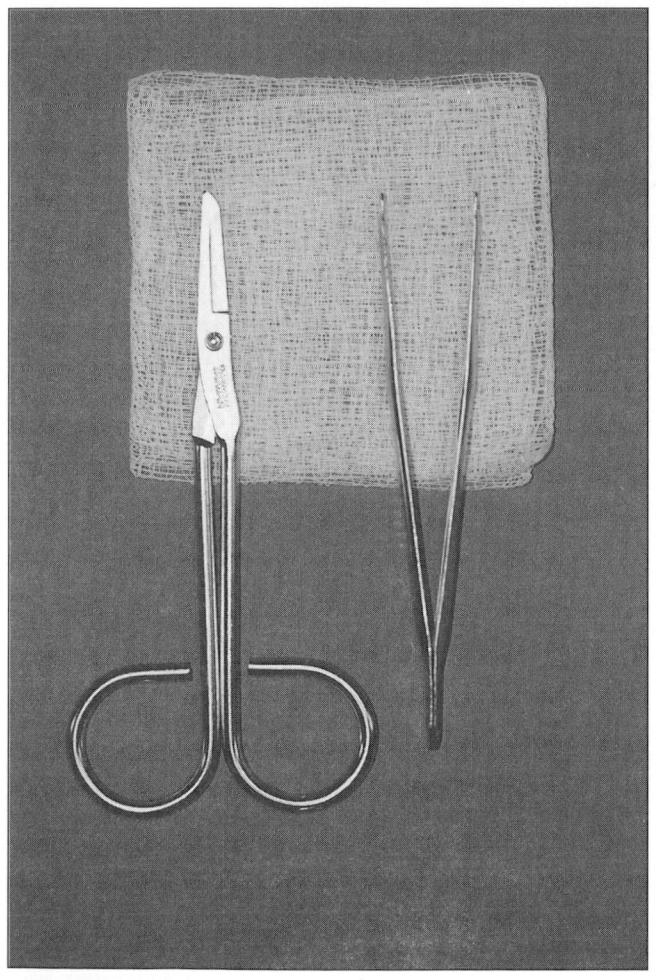

FIGURE 77-9 Contents of a commercially available suture removal kit.

dren, despite the ultimate in the way of gentle reassurance, will sometimes require sedation in order to make painful or difficult procedures possible. Safe and effective sedation for patient comfort or cooperation to facilitate or expedite medical care is described in Chapter 109. Undermining is not useful in most pediatric wounds as they do not usually require advancement of skin over a significant tissue defect. Scalp lacerations account for 30 percent of pediatric lacerations. Scalp lacerations are well suited for single-layer repair with staples. Cosmetic results are comparable with those of sutured repairs, with no differences in complication and infection rates. Staples are six times faster, less expensive in cost of supplies and physician time than standard sutures, and can be implanted rapidly and accurately, even in a moving child.

ALTERNATIVE CLOSURES

Alternative methods of wound closure include skin closure tapes, tissue adhesives, and staples. These are mentioned briefly below. A more complete discussion can be found in Chapter 78.

SKIN CLOSURE TAPES

Skin closure tapes are adhesive strips that are used when skin tension and wound contamination are not concerning factors. Adhesive-backed long and narrow strips are used for approximating the edges of lacerations (with or without staples or sutures) and for closing the skin following many operative procedures. The most common type is the Steri-strip. Skin closure tapes are felt to develop and increase wound tensile strength faster than sutured wounds because uniformly orienting collagen fibers apply equal stress across the wound. Skin closure tapes are porous, which allows for good air inflow and the escape of water vapor from the wound during the healing process.

TISSUE ADHESIVES

Tissue adhesives such as the older and weaker butyl cyanoacrylates focused on small linear lacerations. A newer and stronger medical-grade octyl cyanoacrylate formulation has recently been approved by the U.S. Food and Drug Administration. It has been clinically proven that there is no difference 1 year after treatment in the cosmetic outcome of wounds repaired with suture versus those closed with octyl cyanoacrylate tissue adhesive.[32]

STAPLES

Staple closure is time-efficient compared to the suture repair of lacerations.[33] It is primarily used for large wounds that are not on the face. Stapling is especially useful for closure of incisions in hair-bearing skin (scalp) areas as well as the trunk and extremities. The wound edges require manual eversion with forceps prior to placing the staples.

SUMMARY

Expert wound management consists of attention to the details surrounding the wound, gleaning important information concerning the host's history, as well as meticulous wound preparation. Aggressive attention to the presence of foreign bodies, underlying injury to anatomic structures of significance, and the possibility of subsequent wound infection should be kept in mind at all times. An effort should be made to educate the patient about the possible outcomes of wounds and lacerations and to encourage expedited follow-up.

REFERENCES

1. Ehrlich HP: The physiology of wound healing. A summary of normal and abnormal wound healing processes. *Adv Wound Care* 1998; 11(7):326–328.
2. Moy LS: Management of acute wounds. *Dermatol Clin* 1993; 11(4):759–766.
3. Pollack SV: Wound healing: a review. III. Nutritional factors affecting wound healing. *J Enterostom Ther* 1982; 9(2):28–33.
4. Pollack SV: Wound healing: a review. IV. Systemic medications affecting wound healing. *J Dermatol Surg Oncol* 1982; 8(8):667–672.
5. Robson MC: Disturbances of wound healing. *Ann Emerg Med* 1988; 17(12):1274–1278.
6. Berk WA, Welch RD, Bock BF: Controversial issues in clinical management of the simple wound. *Ann Emerg Med* 1992; 21(1):72–80.
7. Cruse PJ, Foord R: A five-year prospective study of 23,649 surgical wounds. *Arch Surg* 1973; 107(2):206–210.
8. Cardany CR, Rodeheaver G, Thacker J, et al: The crush injury: a high risk wound. *J Am Coll Emerg Physicians* 1976; 5(12):965–970.
9. Berk WA, Osbourne DD, Taylor DD: Evaluation of the 'golden period' for wound repair: 204 cases from a third world emergency department. *Ann Emerg Med* 1988; 17(5):496–500.
10. Condie JD FD: Experimental wound infections: contamination versus surgical technique. *Surgery* 1961; 50:367–371.
11. De Holl D, Rodeheaver G, Edgerton MT, et al: Potentiation of infection by suture closure of dead space. *Am J Surg* 1974; 127(6):716–720.
12. Mehta PH, Dunn KA, Bradfield JF, et al: Contaminated wounds: infection rates with subcutaneous sutures. *Ann Emerg Med* 1996; 27(1):43–48.

13. Lammers RL: Soft tissue foreign bodies. *Ann Emerg Med* 1988; 17(12):1336–1347.
14. Schlager D: Ultrasound detection of foreign bodies and procedure guidance. *Emerg Med Clin North Am* 1997; 15(4):895–912.
15. Tandberg D: Glass in the hand and foot: will an x-ray film show it? *JAMA* 1982; 248(15):1872–1874.
16. Courter BJ: Radiographic screening for glass foreign bodies—what does a "negative" foreign body series really mean? *Ann Emerg Med* 1990; 19(9):997–1000.
17. Alexander JW, Fischer JE, Boyajian M, et al: The influence of hair-removal methods on wound infections. *Arch Surg* 1983; 118(3):347–352.
18. Singer AJ, Hollander JE, Subramanian S, et al: Pressure dynamics of various irrigation techniques commonly used in the emergency department. *Ann Emerg Med* 1994; 24(1):36–40.
19. Pigman EC, Karch DB, Scott JL: Splatter during jet irrigation cleansing of a wound model: a comparison of three inexpensive devices. *Ann Emerg Med* 1993; 22(10):1563–1567.
20. Haury B, Rodeheaver G, Vensko J, et al: Debridement: an essential component of traumatic wound care. *Am J Surg* 1978; 135(2):238–242.
21. Palmon SC, Lloyd AT, Kirsch JR: The effect of needle gauge and lidocaine pH on pain during intradermal injection. *Anesth Analg* 1998; 86(2):379–381.
22. Scarfone RJ, Jasani M, Gracely EJ: Pain of local anesthetics: rate of administration and buffering. *Ann Emerg Med* 1998; 31(1):36–40.
23. Christoph RA, Buchanan L, Begalla K, et al: Pain reduction in local anesthetic administration through pH buffering. *Ann Emerg Med* 1988; 17(2):117–120.
24. Bartfield JM, Homer PJ, Ford DT, et al: Buffered lidocaine as a local anesthetic: an investigation of shelf life. *Ann Emerg Med* 1992; 21(1):16–19.
25. Bartfield JM, Ford DT, Homer PJ: Buffered versus plain lidocaine for digital nerve blocks. *Ann Emerg Med* 1993; 22(2):216–219.
26. Bartfield JM, Gennis P, Barbera J, et al: Buffered versus plain lidocaine as a local anesthetic for simple laceration repair. *Ann Emerg Med* 1990; 19(12):1387–1389.
27. Schilling CG, Bank DE, Borchert BA, et al: Tetracaine, epinephrine (adrenalin), and cocaine (TAC) versus lidocaine, epinephrine, and tetracaine (LET) for anesthesia of lacerations in children. *Ann Emerg Med* 1995; 25(2):203–208.
28. Zempsky WT, Karasic RB: EMLA versus TAC for topical anesthesia of extremity wounds in children. *Ann Emerg Med* 1997; 30(2):163–166.
29. Varghese MC, Balin AK, Carter DM, et al: Local environment of chronic wounds under synthetic dressings. *Arch Dermatol* 1986; 122(1):52–57.
30. Dire DJ: *Emergency Medicine*, 2nd ed. Philadelphia: Lippincott-Raven, 1998.
31. Eron LJ: Targeting lurking pathogens in acute traumatic and chronic wounds. *J Emerg Med* 1999; 17(1):189–195.
32. Quinn JV, Drzewiecki A, Li MM, et al: A randomized, controlled trial comparing a tissue adhesive with suturing in the repair of pediatric facial lacerations. *Ann Emerg Med* 1993; 22(7):1130–1135.
33. Orlinsky M, Goldberg RM, Chan L, et al: Cost analysis of stapling versus suturing for skin closure. *Am J Emerg Med* 1995; 13(1):77–81.

Chapter 78
BASIC WOUND CLOSURE TECHNIQUES

Ardena L. Flippin
Hazel Cebrun
Eric F. Reichman

INTRODUCTION

Wound management is crucial to the practice of Emergency Medicine. Emergency Physicians routinely care for wounds ranging from simple lacerations to complex injuries in the trauma patient. Wound repair is always secondary to the evaluation and stabilization of any life-threatening emergencies. However, patients are often legitimately concerned about the outcome of wounds and lacerations. There are several basic suture principles that will help to provide optimal wound healing and ensure a more than acceptable cosmetic result. The previous chapter outlines the essential principles of wound closure. This chapter describes the basic methods used to close wounds.

SUTURES

The choice of suture materials is important in wound closure. Sutures are made of a wide variety of materials, both natural and synthetic. Natural substances include gut (sheep and beef), cotton, and silk. **Natural substance sutures cause more tissue reactions and scarring, which limits their use.** Cotton sutures are not discussed, as they are no longer used in clinical practice. Synthetic sutures can be made of nylon, Dacron, polyglactin, polypropylene, polyglycolic acid, and metal. Metal sutures are used in the Operating Room and not in the Emergency Department as they are difficult to handle and prone to breakage. Synthetic sutures tend to have a problem with "memory." That is, they tend to retain the shape of their packaging. This can make it difficult to manipulate the suture during wound closure.

Sutures are constructed as monofilaments or polyfilaments. Polyfilament fibers consist of multiple filaments braided together to form one suture. They are easier to handle than monofilament sutures, as they tend to be more pliable. Polyfilament sutures have better knot security and therefore reduce the incidence of knot slippage. However, they can be associated with a higher incidence of infection than monofilament sutures. They allow bacteria to migrate (or wick) between the strands of the suture located at the skin surface and into the wound.

Select the smallest diameter suture that can adequately hold the tissue edges together in order to reduce tissue damage and scarring. The largest suture material available is size #5. The suture sizes decrease to zero (#4, #3, #2, #1, #0) and then are followed by #00 (2–0), #000 (3–0), and #0000 (4–0), in decreasing size. The smallest suture commonly used in the Emergency Department is 6–0 for facial lacerations, hand lacerations, as well as lacerations in other cosmetically sensitive areas. The tensile strength of sutures is related to their size. The tensile strength of suture increases as the size increases. For example, 4–0 is stronger than 5–0.

The other main category of suture classification is absorbable versus nonabsorbable. Absorbable sutures are primarily used to close the subcutaneous layers of a wound. Nonabsorbable sutures are primarily used for skin closure.

ABSORBABLE SUTURE MATERIALS

Absorbable sutures are degraded by the body and do not require removal. They usually do not maintain their tensile strength for longer than 60 days. Body enzymes dissolve the absorbable sutures with the aid of an inflammatory reaction. The rate of absorption of the sutures varies based upon the tissue where it is placed and the size of the suture. Absorbable sutures placed in mucous membranes absorb faster than those placed in muscle tissue or fascia. Smaller sizes of suture dissolve faster than larger sizes.

There are several types of absorbable sutures, both natural and synthetic (Table 78-1). The most commonly used absorbable sutures in the Emergency Department are plain gut, chromic gut, polyglycolic acid (Dexon),

TABLE 78-1. ABSORBABLE SUTURE MATERIALS

Suture type	Source	Tensile strength	Tissue reaction	Knot security	Absorption
Plain surgical gut	Beef or sheep collagen	Poor	Moderate	Poor	1–2 weeks
Chromic surgical gut	Beef or sheep collagen	Poor	Moderate	Fair	2–3 weeks
Monocryl	Polylicaprone 25	20% remains by 3 weeks	Minimal	Good	3 months
Coated Vicryl	Polyglycolic 910, polyglactin 370, and calcium stearate	65% remains at 2 weeks; 40% at 3 weeks	Minimal	Fair	3–6 months
PDS polydioxanone	Polyester polymer	70% remains at 2 weeks; 50% at 4 weeks	Slight	Poor	6 months

and polyglactin (Vicryl). Plain gut and chromic gut are both natural forms of absorbable sutures. They are made from the intestines of sheep and cattle. Gut is a tissue irritant and can cause a substantial tissue reaction while it is being absorbed and degraded by the body. Chromic gut is plain gut that has been soaked in chromic acid salts. This process helps to extend the half-life of the suture and allows it to maintain its tensile strength longer than plain gut. Chromic gut may retain its tensile strength for 2 to 3 weeks, while plain gut retains its tensile strength for 1 to 2 weeks. Both types of gut are packaged wet in order to keep them from drying out and becoming stiff.

Synthetic absorbable sutures, such as Dexon and Vicryl, are typically used more often than natural absorbable sutures in the Emergency Department. They are degraded by the body more slowly than natural fibers and can therefore help maintain the strength of the wound longer. Vicryl and Dexon maintain their tensile strength at 80 days and 120 days, respectively. They cause less reaction in the tissues as they break down when compared to natural absorbable sutures.

NONABSORBABLE SUTURE MATERIALS

Nonabsorbable sutures are not degraded by the body and must be removed. They maintain their tensile strength for longer than 60 days. They are composed of monofilament or polyfilament strands of organic, synthetic, or metal fibers (Table 78-2). Nonabsorbable sutures generally have greater tensile strength and lower tissue reactivity than absorbable sutures. They are used in a variety of applications including skin closure. Nonabsorbable sutures can be used within a body cavity and subcutaneously, where they will become encapsulated in connective tissue.

Nonabsorbable sutures can be classified as organic, synthetic, and wire. Organic sutures include those made of cotton or silk. Cotton is the oldest of the nonabsorbable sutures. It is not discussed here as cotton sutures are no longer used in general medical practice. Silk is a polyfilament suture that has limited use in the practice of Emergency Medicine. There are several advantages to silk suture material. Its pliability makes it very easy to handle. It holds knots better than other types of suture. However, as with all natural and/or polyfilament sutures, it has a greater tendency to cause wound infections. The polyfilament braids can provide a place for bacteria to lodge. Silk suture may actually protect the bacteria from attack by the body's defenses if the wound becomes infected. The primary use of silk sutures is for the repair of lip, oral cavity, and tongue lacerations.

Synthetic sutures are available in monofilament and polyfilament forms. Commonly used synthetic sutures include nylon, polypropylene, polybutester, and Dacron.

TABLE 78-2. NONABSORBABLE SUTURE MATERIALS

Suture type	Source	Tensile strength	Tissue reaction	Knot security	Absorption
Silk (braided)	Organic protein	Gradual loss by progressive degradation	High	Good	Gradual encapsulation by connective tissue
Ethilon	Polyamide (nylon)	Progressive hydrolysis may result in gradual loss of tensile strength	Minimal	Fair	Gradual encapsulation by connective tissue
Nurolon	Polyamide (nylon)	Progressive hydrolysis may result in gradual loss of tensile strength	Minimal	Fair	Gradual encapsulation by connective tissue
Prolene	Polyamide (nylon)	Not subject to degradation	Minimal	Poor	Nonabsorbable
Mersilene	Polyester	No significant change occurs	Minimal	Good	Gradual encapsulation by connective tissue
Ethibond	Coated polyester	No significant change occurs	Minimal	Good	Gradual encapsulation by connective tissue
Stainless steel	Stainless steel	Indefinite	Minimal	Good	Nonabsorbable

Nylon, polypropylene, and polybutester are monofilament synthetic sutures. Dacron is a polyfilament synthetic suture. The synthetic nonabsorbable sutures have several advantages over the natural nonabsorbable sutures. They are less reactive in tissues, generally stronger than the natural sutures, and retain their tensile strength over many years.

Nylon (Ethilon, Dermalon) is the most common nonabsorbable suture used in the Emergency Department. It is a monofilament suture, it is inert, and it does not tend to harbor bacteria. It is primarily used for skin closure. Nylon has good tensile strength and minimal tissue reactivity. However, nylon is difficult to handle and difficult to tie. It requires more knots to achieve good knot security than other types of suture. This is primarily due to the tendency of the suture to return to its packaged shape. This tendency is also known as "memory." Because the knot can unravel or slip, it is important to place at least four or five knots when using nylon suture.

Polypropylene and polybutester are less commonly used synthetic nonabsorbable sutures. Polypropylene (Prolene) is stronger but more difficult to work with than nylon because it has greater memory. Polybutester (Novafil) is a newer suture in this category. It is stronger than the other monofilaments and does not have significant memory. Therefore, it is easier to work with than the other monofilament synthetic sutures.

EQUIPMENT

Needle drivers, 4.5 and 6.0 inch
Skin hooks
Scalpel blades (#10, #11, #15)
Scalpel handles
Iris scissors, straight 4 inch and curved 4 inch
Suture scissors, 6 inch
Forceps, toothed Adson
Metzenbaum scissors, curved 6 inch
Hemostats, straight 6 inch, and curved mosquitoes
Suture material
Skin closure tapes
Benzoin solution, swabs or spray
Tissue adhesive
Tissue adhesive forceps
Gauze, 4×4 squares

The above equipment can be purchased in single-use, sterile, and disposable kits from several commercial manufacturers (Figure 78-1A). These kits tend to be expensive and occasionally have a limited amount of equipment. Many hospitals package and sterilize their own wound repair kits (Figure 78-1B). This decreases the cost, as the equipment can be repeatedly sterilized and

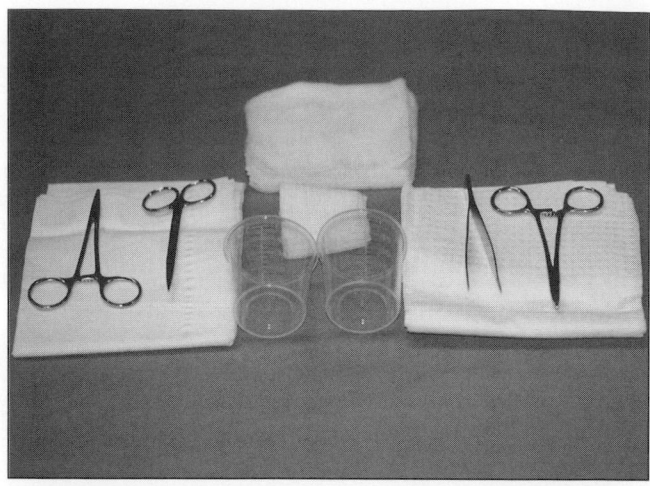

A

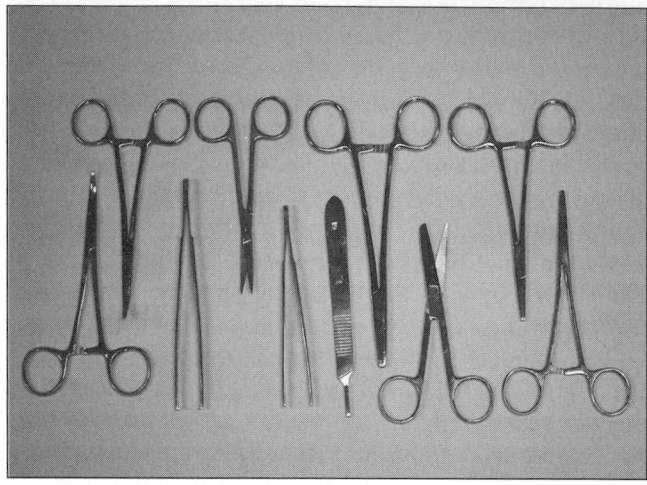

B

FIGURE 78-1 The equipment required for basic wound closure techniques. *A.* The contents of a disposable and commercially available wound closure kit (Clinipad Corp., Guilford, CT). *B.* A hospital packaged kit with reusable instruments.

reused. It also allows the kits to contain a wide variety of instruments for multiple situations (minor laceration, large laceration, plastics closure).

Needle drivers come in a variety of sizes. A 4.5 inch needle driver can be used comfortably with most types of needles. A 6 inch needle driver may be required if large needles are used to close a wound. Hold the needle driver with the fingertips to provide greater flexibility. The fingers can also be placed through the finger holes, but this is not as efficient when closing a wound. Grasp the needle one-third of the way from the swag (distal) end with the tip of the needle driver.

The skin must be grasped and manipulated during wound repair to allow for proper suture placement. Forceps are most commonly used to grasp and manipulate the skin. **Smooth (nontoothed) forceps should never be used to grasp skin.** They require the application of a large amount of force to grasp the tissue. This can crush tissue very easily. An Adson forceps is the forceps of choice. It has fine teeth that grasp tissue securely with minimal force.

A skin hook is a sharp, pointed instrument that is inserted into the wound edge and grasps the tissue from the undersurface. It produces a small puncture wound in the subcutaneous tissues and does not penetrate the skin surface. Skin hooks are preferable to forceps, as they do not crush tissues. A skin hook is awkward to use at first. With proper instruction and experience, the physician will most certainly prefer a skin hook to forceps.

Several types of scissors are required for proper wound closure. Iris scissors have sharp, delicate tips for making precise cuts in tissue. They should not be used to cut suture material, as this rapidly dulls and nicks the blades. Suture scissors have one blunt tip and one pointed tip. Both blades of the suture scissors are sharp. Suture scissors are used to cut adhesive tape, gauze, rubber drains, and suture material. Metzenbaum scissors should be used to debride heavy tissue, bluntly dissect tissue, and undermine tissue.

Hemostats are used to clamp small vessels that are bleeding, to explore a wound, and to grasp fascia. Hemostats are available in a variety of sizes and styles. A straight 6 inch hemostat is used for most purposes during wound repair. A curved 5 inch mosquito hemostat can be used for small wounds or delicate tissues.

Three different scalpel blades should be available when a wound is being repaired. A #11 blade is used to make stab incisions. It is often used for the incision and drainage of abscesses, cricothyroidotomies, and the removal of small or tight sutures. A #10 blade is used to make straight cuts in the skin and debride wound edges. It is rarely used in laceration repair. A #15 blade is small and curved to allow precise incisions. It is used for excising foreign bodies and wound debridement.

SUTURE TECHNIQUES

Proper wound closure requires an understanding of certain basic principles. **The needle should enter and exit the skin at a 90 degree angle and perpendicular to the wound edges.** By doing so, when the suture loop is closed, the wound edges will be everted. **Sutures should be placed as close to the wound edge as possible (2 to 3 mm) in order to avoid excessive tension on the wound.** More force will be required to close the wound if the sutures are placed too far from the wound edge. Edema develops in a wound in the first 48 hours after closure. Sutures placed too far from the wound edge can result in large scars when the edema subsides. **The layers of the wound should be matched evenly and each layer should be closed separately.** If a wound involves the deeper layers of skin, fascia should be matched to fascia, dermis should be matched to dermis, and epidermis should be matched to epidermis. **The proper matching of layers avoids an uneven closure, helps to prevent an unnecessarily large scar, and eliminates dead space.**

The epidermal edges of the wound must be everted to allow for proper healing. Scars contract with time. They will flatten and heal with a better cosmetic result if the wound edge is everted and slightly elevated. The wound edges will contract into a "pit" below the plane of the skin, will be more noticeable, and the final result will be less appealing cosmetically if the wound edges are not everted.

Handle the tissues gently and do not squeeze or twist them too tightly with the instruments. This helps to avoid strangulation, which can result in tissue necrosis. **The sutures should be placed carefully and with the proper amount of tension to help promote healing.** Sutures should be snug. Attempts should be made to avoid excessive tension on the wound edges in order to prevent wound dehiscence. The use of the smallest suture size necessary to approximate the wound edges will reduce tissue damage and minimize scarring. Table 78-3 lists the appropriate suture types and sizes for each body region.

If there will be a temporary delay in the closure of a laceration because of other injuries that may be life-threatening or of greater importance, cover the wound with a saline-soaked gauze in order to keep the tissues from drying.

PRINCIPLE OF HALVING

Large wounds gape open and are difficult to approximate. Closure of the deeper layers will often bring the skin edges into apposition. If not, the principle of halving may be used to approximate the wound (Figure 78-2). Identify the midpoint of the laceration. Place the first suture at the midpoint (Figure 78-2A). This stitch is known as the central suture. The next sutures are placed in halves on each side of the central suture (Figures 78-2B and C). Continue the process by placing sutures halfway between previous sutures until the wound is approximated. This results in even closure of the wound edge. This principle can be used for closure of both the deep layers and the skin.

TWO-HANDED SQUARE KNOT

This is the easiest and most reliable method of tying most suture materials. It involves the classic "right-over-left and left-over-right" tie (Figure 78-3). The incorrect "right-over-left and right-over-left" is a granny knot which will slip if it is tied in this manner. This square knot is quick and simple to perform. However, it does take significant practice to master this technique.

TABLE 78-3. TYPICAL SUTURE CHOICES FOR EACH BODY SITE

Anatomic site	Deep-layer suture size	Deep-layer suture material	Skin-layer suture size	Skin-layer closure material
Scalp	2–0, 3–0, or 4–0	Absorbable	4–0 or 5–0	Nylon, polypropylene, or staples
Eyelid	5–0, 6–0, or 7–0	Absorbable	6–0 or 7–0	Nylon or polypropylene
Face	4–0 or 5–0	Absorbable	5–0 or 6–0	Nylon or polypropylene
Neck	4–0 or 5–0	Absorbable	4–0 or 5–0	Nylon or polypropylene
Trunk	3–0 or 4–0	Absorbable	3–0 or 4–0	Nylon, polypropylene, or staples
Extremities	3–0 or 4–0	Absorbable	3–0, 4–0, or 5–0	Nylon, polypropylene, or staples
Hands and feet	Not advisable	Not applicable	4–0 or 5–0	Nylon or polypropylene
Sole of foot	3–0 or 4–0	Absorbable	3–0 or 4–0	Nylon or polypropylene

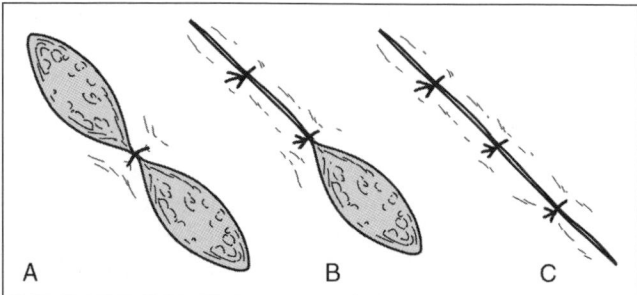

FIGURE 78-2 The principle of halving. *A.* The first suture is placed in the middle of the laceration. *B.* The second suture is placed halfway between the first suture and the upper end of the laceration. *C.* The third suture is placed halfway between the first suture and the lower end of the laceration.

Place a suture through the skin on both sides of the laceration (Figure 78-3*A*). Pull the suture through the wound until half is on each side of the laceration. Grasp the right half of the suture with the right thumb and index finger (Figure 78-3*A*). Grasp the left half of the suture with the left third through fifth fingers and the suture draped over the thumb (Figure 78-3*A*). Cross the right hand toward the left hand (Figure 78-3*B*). Continue to move the right hand until the suture is between the left thumb and index finger (Figure 78-3*C*). Close the left thumb and index finger to entrap the right half of the suture in the pads of the fingers (Figure 78-3*D*). Pull the right hand down and to the left so that the two halves of the suture form an X over the left thumb (Figure 78-3*E*). Flex the left wrist to slide the X off the left thumb and onto the left index finger (Figure 78-3*F*). Lift the left thumb backward and upward so that the X overlies the tip of the left index finger (Figure 78-3*G*). Reapply the left thumb over the left index finger to entrap the X (Figure 78-3*H*). Extend the left wrist to push the left thumb and the X through the loop (Figure 78-3*I*). Release the suture held with the right hand (Figure 78-3*J*). Regrasp the suture with the right hand after it passes through the loop (Figure 78-3*K*). Pull the suture completely through the loop with the right hand. Simultaneously move the left hand toward the left and move the right hand toward the right (Figure 78-3*L*). Cross the hands so that the left

hand goes toward the right side and the right hand goes toward the left side (Figure 78-3*M*). Continue to pull both sides of the suture until the knot lies flat and the skin edges are apposed (Figure 78-3*M*). The first half of the knot is now complete.

Make the second half of the knot to complete the square knot. Raise both hands upward and uncross them until an X is formed over the left index finger (Figure 78-3*N*). Close the left thumb and index finger to entrap the suture being held with the right hand (Figure 78-3*O*). Extend the left wrist to push the left thumb through the loop (Figure 78-3*P*). Lift the left index finger upward (Figure 78-3*Q*). Move the right hand away from you until the suture it holds drapes over the left thumb (Figure 78-3*R*). Reapply the left index finger onto the thumb to entrap the suture held with the right hand (Figure 78-3*S*). Release the suture held with the right hand (Figure 78-3*T*). Flex the left wrist to push the left index finger and suture through the loop (Figure 78-3*U*). Regrasp the free suture with the right hand after it passes through the loop (Figure 78-3*V*). Move the right hand upward and to the right to complete the second half of the knot overlying the left index finger (Figure 78-3*W*). Simultaneously move the left hand towards the left and move the right hand towards the right (Figure 78-3*X*). Continue to pull both halves of the suture until both halves of the knot come into contact (Figure 78-3*Y*). Pull both halves of the suture to secure the knot. The square knot is now complete. Continue the process to add additional knots onto the suture. Cut off excess suture on both sides of the knots.

SURGEON'S KNOT

The physician may choose to use a surgeon's knot instead of a square knot (Figure 78-4). The square knot has one loop in the first throw and one loop in the second throw (Figure 78-4*A*). The surgeon's knot has two loops in the first throw and one loop in the second throw (Figure 78-4*B*). The only difference between these two knots is the two loops in the first throw. The second throw and subsequent knots are exactly the same for both knots. The advantage of the surgeon's knot is that the two loops are more secure and stay in place while the second throw

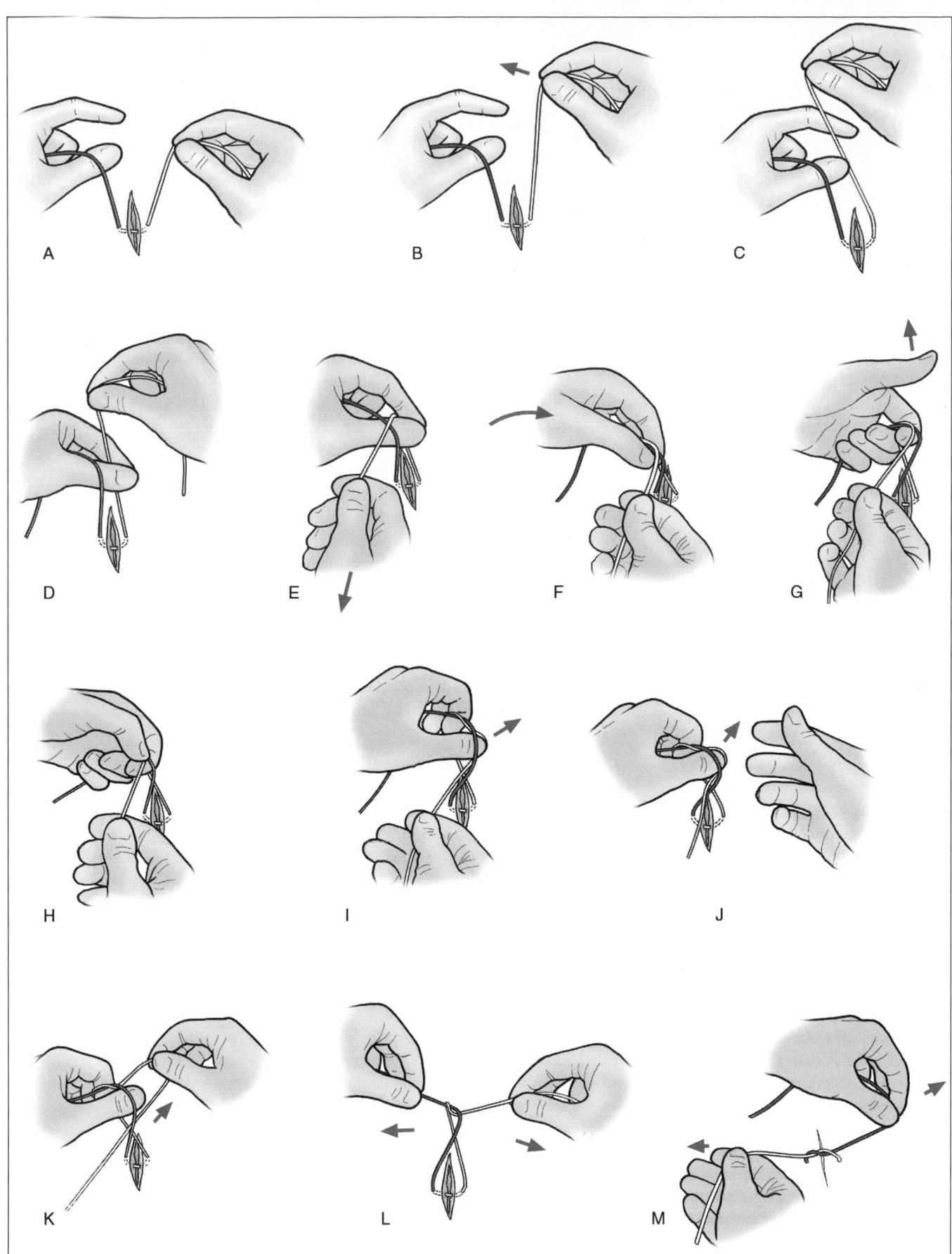

FIGURE 78-3 The two-handed square knot. *(continued)*

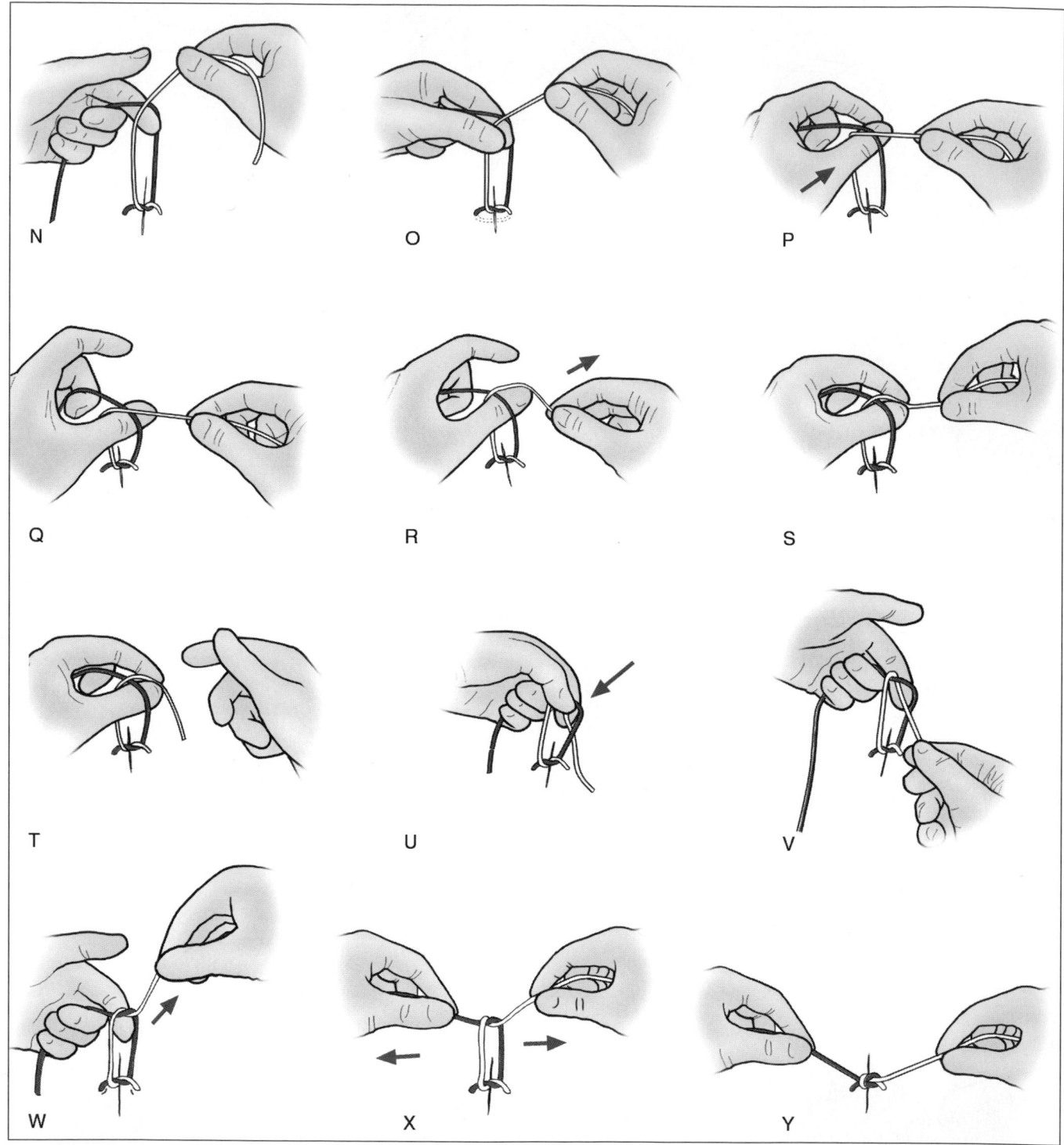

FIGURE 78-3 *Continued.*

is being tied. The choice to use either knot is dependent on the experience and the training of the physician.

INSTRUMENT TIE

The instrument tie is the most efficient method to complete a simple interrupted suture (Figure 78-5). It is the tie that is most commonly used in the Emergency Department. An instrument tie is often quicker, requires less dexterity, and is easier to perform than the two-handed method. It may be used with the square knot or the surgeon's knot.

Place a suture through the skin on both sides of the laceration (Figure 78-5A). Carefully grasp the needle in its midportion and pull it through the laceration (Figure

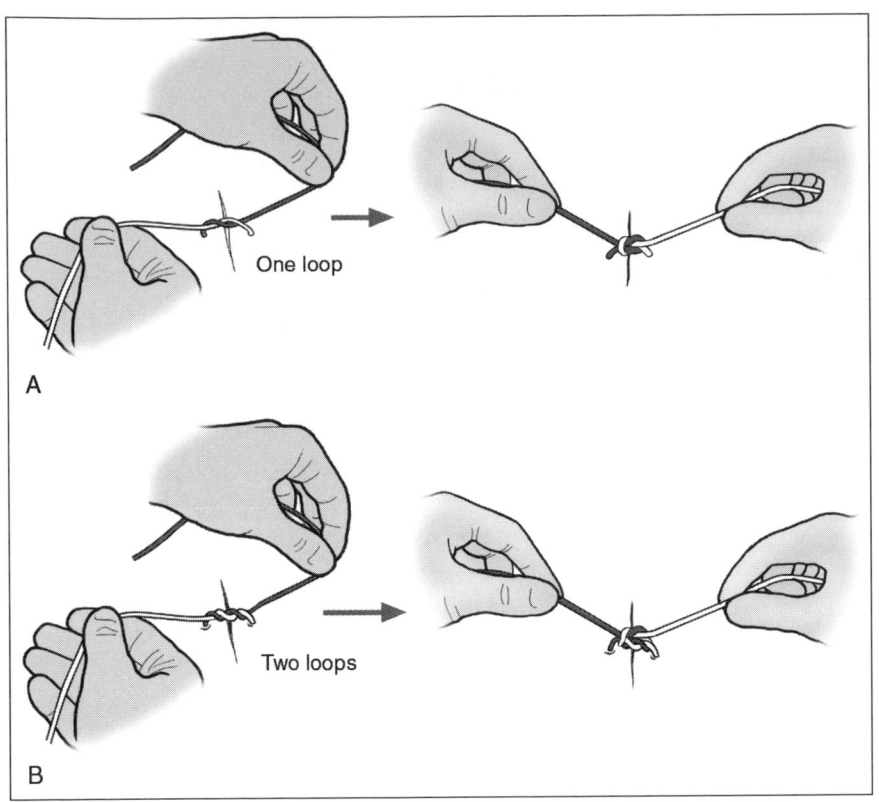

One loop

A

Two loops

B

FIGURE 78-4 The square knot (*A*) versus the surgeon's knot (*B*). The first throw of the square knot has one loop (*A*), while that of the surgeon's knot has two loops (*B*). The second throw of both knots are a simple loop.

78-5*B*). Continue to pull the needle until approximately 1 to 2 cm of suture on the tail end remains outside the laceration (Figure 78-5*C*). A large amount of suture will be wasted if the tail is left too long, as it will be later cut off and discarded. On first learning the instrument tie, it may be best to leave a tail of 3 to 4 cm until one is proficient with this technique.

Place the needle driver over the laceration but not touching it (Figure 78-5*C*). Loosely loop the needle end of the suture over (Figure 78-5*D*) and around (Figure 78-5*E*) the needle driver. Loosely loop the needle end of the suture over and around the needle driver a second time (Figures 78-5*F* and *G*). This will eventually result in the first half of a surgeon's knot. Looping the suture once around the needle driver will result in a square knot. Move the tip of the needle driver toward the tail of the suture without letting the loops fall off the needle driver (Figure 78-5*H*). Grasp the tail of the suture with the needle driver (Figure 78-5*I*). Pull the tail of the suture through the loop (Figure 78-5*J*). Pull the tail completely through the loops (Figure 78-5*K*). Simultaneously move the left hand toward the right and the right hand/needle driver toward the left (Figure 78-5*L*). Continue to pull both sides of the suture until the hands are opposite each other, the knot lies flat, and the skin edges are apposed (Figure 78-5*M*). The first half of the knot is now complete.

Make the second half of the knot. Continue to hold the needle and release the tail of the suture from the

needle driver (Figure 78-5*N*). Place the needle driver over the laceration but not touching it (Figure 78-5*N*). Loosely loop the needle end of the suture over (Figure 78-5*O*) and around (Figure 78-5*P*) the needle driver. Move the tip of the needle driver toward the tail of the suture without letting the loop fall off the needle driver (Figure 78-5*Q*). Grasp the tail of the suture with the needle driver (Figure 78-5*R*). Pull the tail of the suture completely through the loop (Figure 78-5*S*). Simultaneously move the left hand toward the left and the right hand/needle driver toward the right (Figure 78-5*T*). Continue to pull both sides of the suture until both halves of the knot come into contact. Pull both sides of the suture to secure the knot. The knot is now complete. Continue this process three or four more times, each in alternative directions, to place additional knots. Cut off the excess suture on both sides of the knots.

SIMPLE INTERRUPTED STITCH

The simple interrupted stitch is the most commonly used suture technique and is useful in many situations (Figure 78-6). One major advantage is that each stitch is placed independent of the others. Therefore tension on each stitch can be adjusted separately. Additionally, the entire repair is not compromised if one suture should happen to come out. The other sutures will remain in place to help assure proper wound healing. **The needle must enter and exit the skin at a 90 degree angle to help evert the wound edges. Take equal volumes of skin**

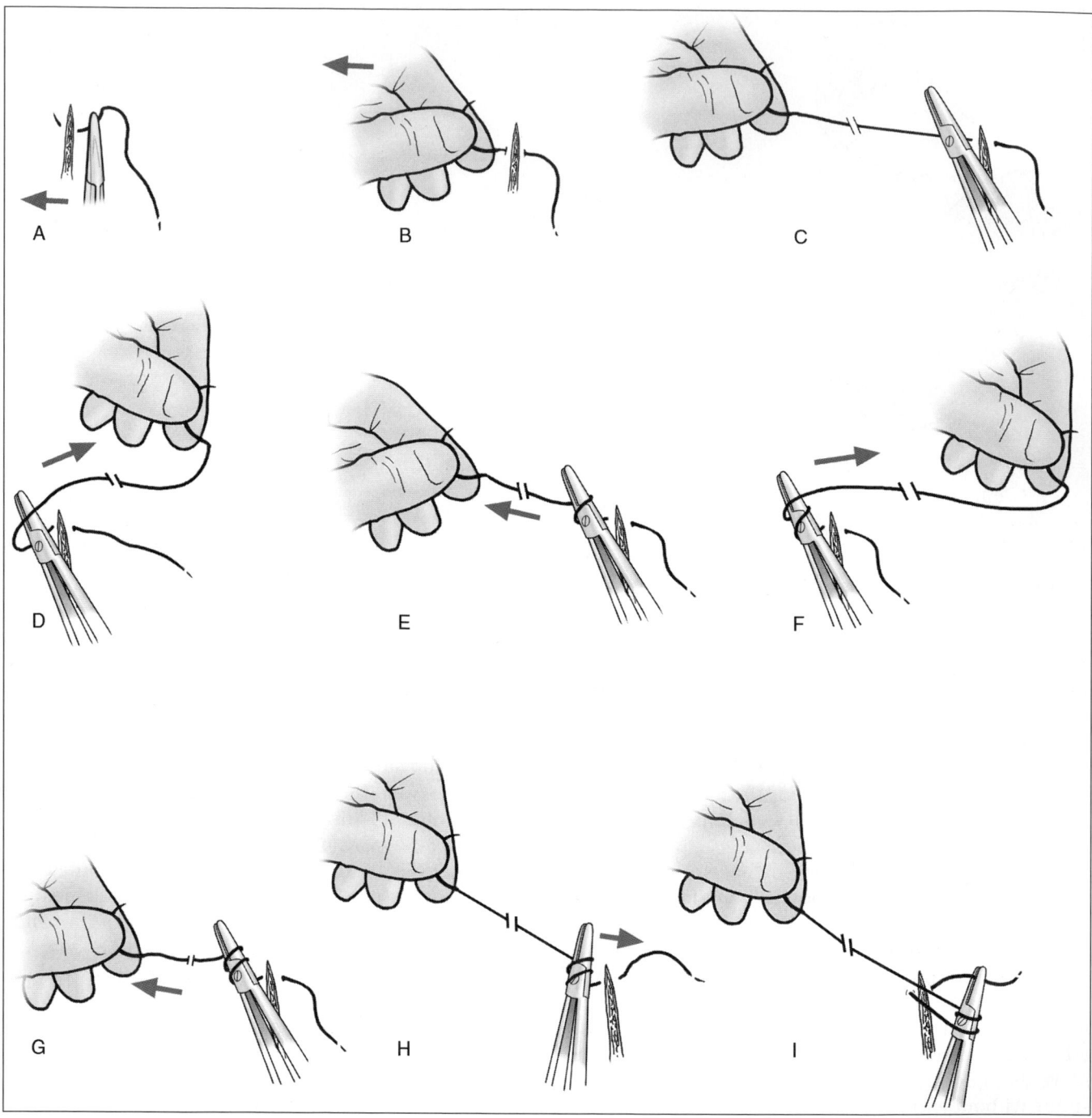

FIGURE 78-5 The instrument tie. *(continued)*

from each side of the area being sutured. Drive the needle equidistantly into and out of the wound edges and incorporate the base of the wound.

Insert the needle at a 90 degree angle to the skin (Figure 78-6A). Drive the needle through the tissue until the tip exits the skin (Figure 78-6B). Grasp the needle behind the tip and pull it through the wound (Figure 78-6C). **The suture should enter and exit the skin equidistant from the wound edges (Figure 78-6D). If it does not, pull the suture out and repeat the stitch so that it is equidistant from the wound edges.** Make a loop in the

suture with the two-handed tie or the instrument tie. Pull the suture to appose the wound edges and cinch down the knot (Figure 78-6E). The tissue at the base of the wound will come into apposition before the tissue at the skin surface and thus evert the wound edge. Complete the knot to one side of the laceration (Figure 78-6F). Just prior to cinching the second throw onto the first, quickly pull the ends so that the knot is not directly over the wound and the edges of the wound remain in apposition. Apply additional sutures equidistant from each other until the wound is closed (Figure 78-6G).

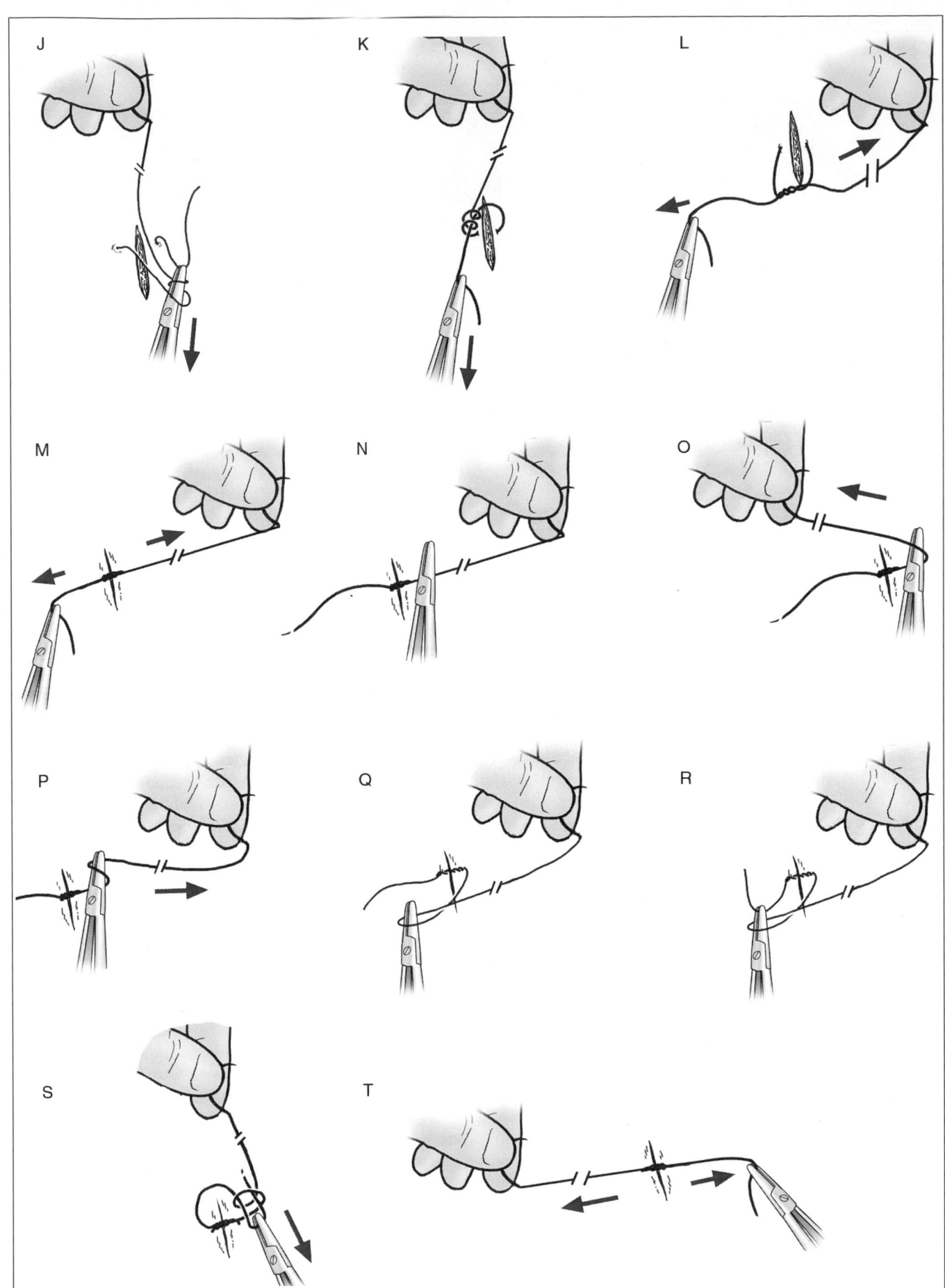

FIGURE 78-5 *Continued.*

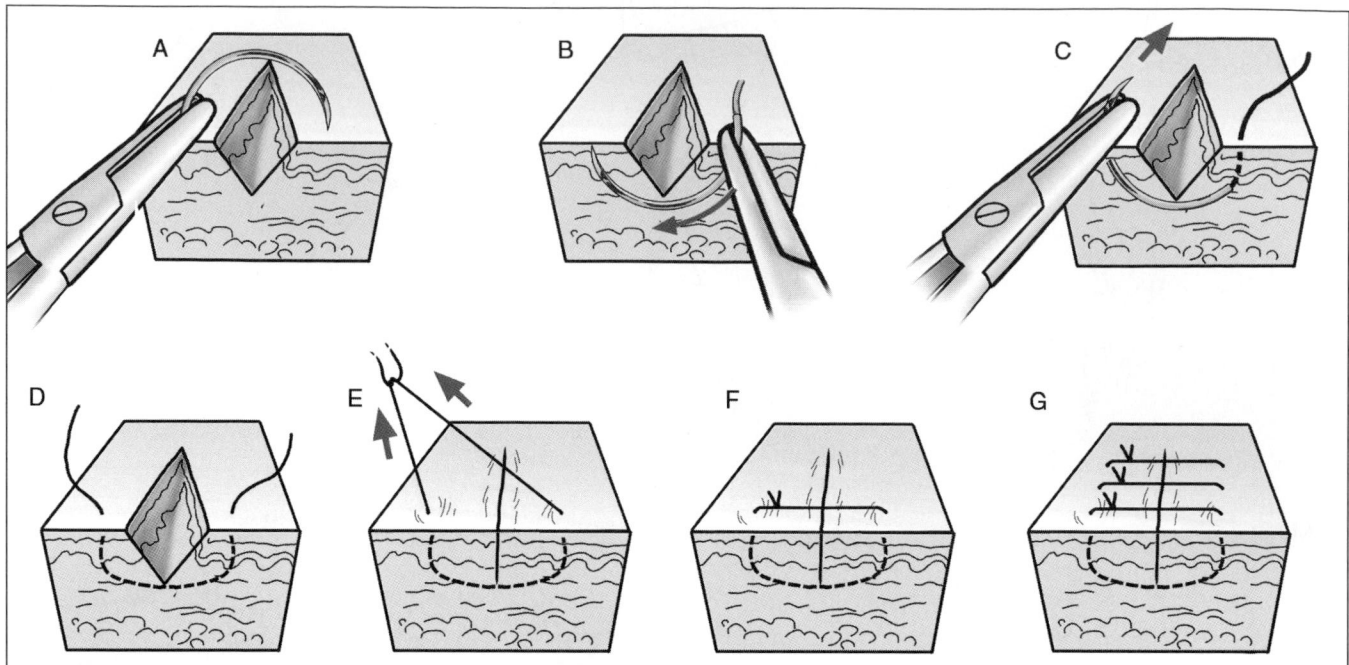

FIGURE 78-6 The simple interrupted stitch.

OPEN-LOOP SIMPLE INTERRUPTED STITCH

The open-loop simple interrupted stitch is a variation of the simple interrupted stitch (Figure 78-7). The same basic technique is used except that the knot is tied differently. The tie involves laying down the first throw with an instrument tie. However, the second throw placed on the suture is not pulled all the way through. Pull the second knot through only until it starts to deform the first knot (Figure 78-7A). In other words, the second knot is loosely tied, leaving a loop between the first and second knots. Place a third throw as a single throw knot square to the second knot (Figure 78-7B). Cinch the third knot tightly to the second knot. This "locks" the second knot onto the third knot.

This knot is indicated when there is the possibility of edema forming at the suture site. If edema forms, the first knot will have room to open as it slides toward the second knot. This stitch avoids excessive tension on the wound and prevents the suture from cutting into the skin. This stitch facilitates suture removal when numerous small stitches are placed next to a wound edge. Cutting the open loop unravels the knot and allows for easy removal of the suture. This stitch should not be used in areas where the skin is thin or if there is little subcutaneous tissue (e.g., dorsal hand and foot). In these areas, the wound edges often become unopposed while the knot is being secured.

INTERLOCKING SLIP KNOT

This technique can be used in patients who will be traveling, camping, or otherwise away from their primary source of medical care (Figure 78-8). The patient can easily remove the sutures without having to find an unfamiliar or foreign health care provider for routine suture removal. The interlocking slip knot can be removed by hand without the use of a scissors or a scalpel. This can be useful for suture removal in pediatric patients, who may find it hard to sit still for suture removal.

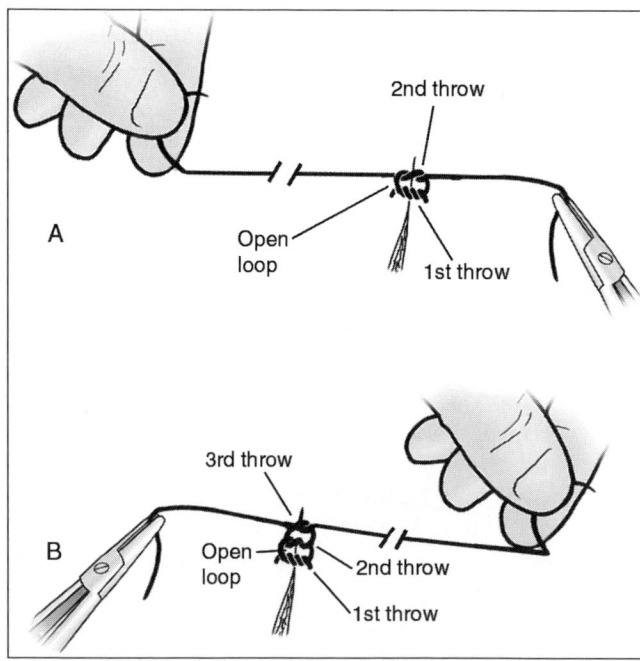

FIGURE 78-7 The open-loop simple interrupted stitch.

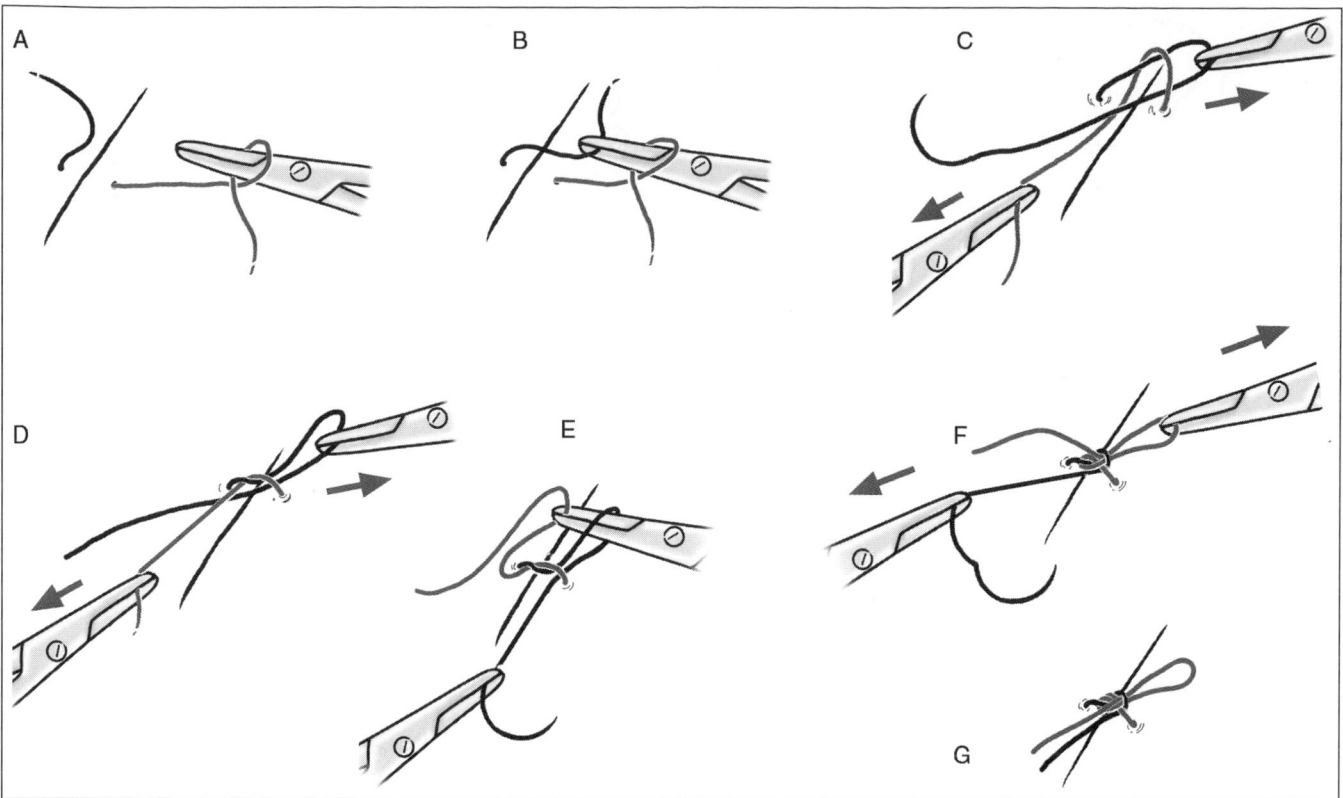

FIGURE 78-8 The interlocking slip knot.

Place a suture through the skin on both sides of the laceration (Figure 78-8*A*). Loop the tail end of the suture around the tip of the needle driver (Figure 78-8*A*). Grasp the needle end of the suture with the needle driver (Figure 78-8*B*). Pull the needle end of the suture through the loop while simultaneously pulling on the tail end of the suture with a second needle driver (Figure 78-8*C*). Continue to pull both suture halves in opposite directions until a knot is formed against the skin and the wound edges are apposed (Figure 78-8*D*). Release the needle driver holding the now formed loop. Insert the needle driver through the loop and grasp the tail end of the suture (Figure 78-8*E*). Grasp the needle end of the suture with the second needle driver (Figure 78-8*E*). Pull the needle drivers in opposite directions to lock and secure the knot (Figure 78-8*F*). The knot is now complete (Figure 78-8*G*). To remove the stitch, pull the free end of the suture to unlock the knot. Continue to pull the suture until it is free from the skin.

CONTINUOUS OVER-AND-OVER STITCH (SIMPLE RUNNING STITCH)

Continuous (simple running) sutures minimize the time required for laceration repair. Stitches can be placed very quickly, since each individual stitch does not have to be tied. This stitch provides strength and applies equal tension on all sutures in the repair. This stitch can be used to achieve hemostasis. The wound must be long and straight. Simple running stitches can effectively be used in partial-thickness lacerations and wounds under minimal tension.

However, there are several disadvantages to this stitch. It can be associated with significant epithelialization of the suture track. This is especially true if the suture is not removed early and remains for a prolonged period of time. Inclusion cysts may form within a few weeks after removal of the sutures. **Simple running stitches should not be used on any wound under tension.** If one suture breaks, the entire wound may open. **This stitch should not be used when closing a wound where there is a risk of subsequent hematoma formation.** Hematoma formation would require the removal of all of the sutures in order to drain the hematoma. Although this suture is not commonly used in the Emergency Department, it can be very helpful for closing bleeding scalp wounds, as the injury will be covered with hair and cosmesis is a secondary concern.

Place the initial stitch as a simple interrupted stitch (Figures 78-9*A*). Do not cut the suture after the knots are securely tied. Place a second stitch 3 to 5 mm from the first stitch as if placing another simple interrupted stitch (Figures 78-9*B* and *C*). Place a third stitch 3 to 5 mm from the second stitch (Figures 78-9*D* and *E*). Continue to

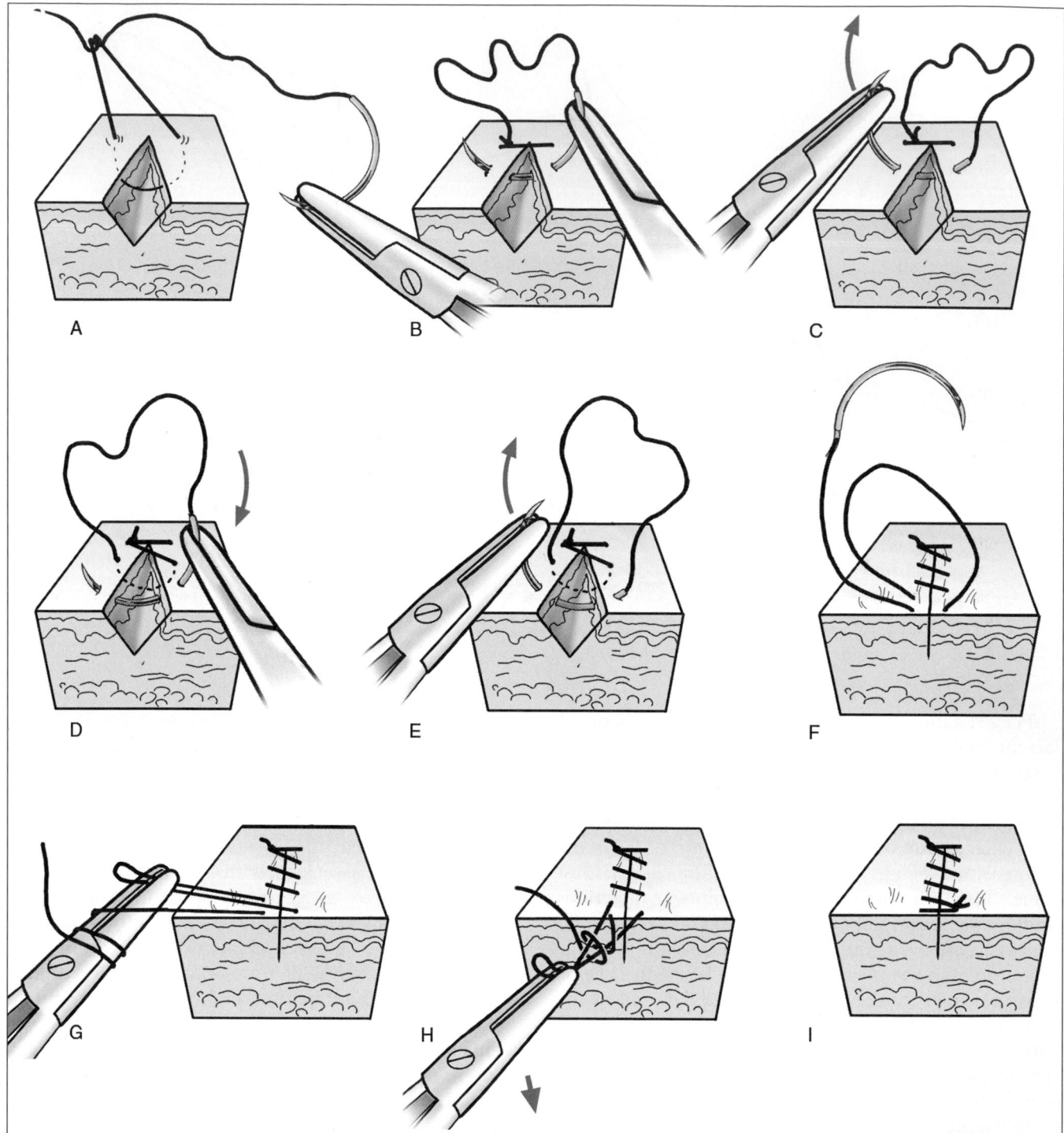

FIGURE 78-9 The continuous over-and-over or simple running stitch.

place additional stitches until the end of the laceration is reached. Do not pull the last throw taut against the skin (Figure 78-9F). The loop will act as the tail end of the suture for knot tying. Loop the needle end of the suture twice around the tip of the needle driver (Figure 78-9G). Grasp the last throw with the tips of the needle driver (Figure 78-9G). Pull the last throw through the loops until the knot is against the skin (Figure 78-9H). Perform

three to five more instrument ties to secure the knot, then cut off the excess suture (Figure 78-9I).

CONTINUOUS SINGLE-LOCKED STITCH (RUNNING-LOCKED CLOSURE)

This stitch may promote less epithelialization of the suture track than the continuous over-and-over stitch. It maintains the advantages of a continuous suture. This variation of the simple running closure locks each stitch after it is placed (Figure 78-10). It provides a secure apposition of the wound edges while each subsequent stitch is placed. The main disadvantage of this stitch is the time it takes compared to a continuous over-and-over stitch.

Place the initial stitch as a simple interrupted stitch (Figure 78-10A). Do not cut the suture after the knots are securely tied. Loop the tail end of the suture over the nondominant fifth finger (Figure 78-10B). Apply slight tension on the tail end of the suture while placing the second stitch (Figures 78-10C and D). As the needle exits the skin, move the nondominant hand to bring the suture loop down and over the needle (Figure 78-10E). Grasp the front of the needle with the needle driver. Simultaneously pull the needle and suture through the laceration while releasing the loop from the fifth finger (Figure 78-10F). Repeat this procedure until the laceration is closed (Figure 78-10G). **Do not pull the last throw taut against the skin.** The loop will act as the tail end of the suture for knot tying. Loop the needle end of the suture twice around the tip of the needle driver (Figure 78-10H). Grasp the last throw with the tips of the needle driver. Pull the last throw through the loops until the knot is against the skin (Figure 78-10I). Perform three to five more instrument ties to secure the knot; then cut off the excess suture (Figure 78-10J).

VERTICAL MATTRESS STITCH

The vertical mattress stitch is a double stitch that provides for excellent wound eversion (Figure 78-11). It optimizes wound closure of single layers under tension. This stitch is useful in areas where the skin is very lax, such as the elbow and the dorsum of the hand. This stitch provides for both superficial as well as deep closure of lacerations. **This stitch is contraindicated in lacerations involving the volar aspect of the hands and feet or the face, as it requires the blind placement of a deep suture.** The main disadvantage of the vertical mattress closure is the time it takes to place it.

Place the first throw much like a simple interrupted stitch with a few noted differences. The needle should enter and exit the skin 1.0 to 1.5 cm from the wound edge. The needle should traverse the base of the wound and grasp a large amount of tissue (Figures 78-11A and B). Reverse the needle. The second throw should enter and exit the skin approximately 2 to 3 mm from the wound edge (Figures 78-11C and D). **The first and second throws must be directly over each other and parallel.** Tie the suture to approximate the wound edges (Figures 78-11E). The first throw will close the wound base and relieve the tension at the skin surface. The second throw approximates and everts the skin edges.

The newer version of the classic vertical mattress is referred to as the "shorthand" vertical mattress stitch (Figure 78-12). It provides wound eversion in half the time as the traditional method. Place the first throw close to the lacerated wound edge to approximate the skin edges (Figures 78-12A and B). Grasp and pull the suture to elevate the wound edges (Figure 78-12C). This allows the needle to more easily take a large bite of tissue on the second throw. Place the second throw 1.0 to 1.5 cm from the wound edge (Figures 78-12C and D). Release the suture. Tie the suture to approximate the wound edges and evert the skin surface (Figure 78-12E). The final product looks exactly the same as the traditional vertical mattress suture (Figure 78-12F).

LOCKED VERTICAL MATTRESS STITCH

The locked vertical mattress stitch is useful in areas that are widely separated and where deep sutures must be avoided (Figure 78-13). This stitch helps to reduce the amount of tension needed to close a wound. It helps to avoid the pain and scarring that can result if too much tension is applied to a laceration. It does not put an excessive amount of tension on the deep throw, as does the vertical mattress stitch.

This is a modification of the vertical mattress stitch (Figures 78-11 and 78-12). Place the first two throws as if placing a vertical mattress stitch (Figure 78-13A). Leave the suture lax with a loop above the wound surface. Pass the needle end of the suture through the open loop (Figure 78-13B). This step will form the locked portion of the stitch. Pull the needle end of the suture taut to appose the wound edges (Figure 78-13C). Tie and secure the suture in the standard manner.

HORIZONTAL MATTRESS STITCH

The horizontal mattress stitch is placed along the axis of the wound and helps to eliminate tension on the wound (Figure 78-14). It is a good closure technique for wounds with relatively poor circulation to the wound edges because, theoretically, no suture is placed through the wound edges. This helps to avoid tension on the wound edges from the suture and subsequent local necrosis. This stitch is placed more rapidly than the vertical mattress stitch. It requires fewer stitches to close a wound with horizontal rather than vertical mattress stitches. The throws are side by side rather than on top of each other, as with the vertical mattress, and each stitch closes more tissue. This closure may be used on the volar surfaces of the hands and fingers, as these delicate skin areas may swell and be cut by simple interrupted sutures. The main disadvantage of the horizontal mattress stitch is that it takes more experience to properly place this stitch to achieve wound eversion than with the vertical mattress stitch.

Place the first throw much like a simple interrupted stitch with a few noted differences. The needle should enter and exit the skin 0.5 to 1.0 cm from the wound edge. The needle should traverse the base of the wound

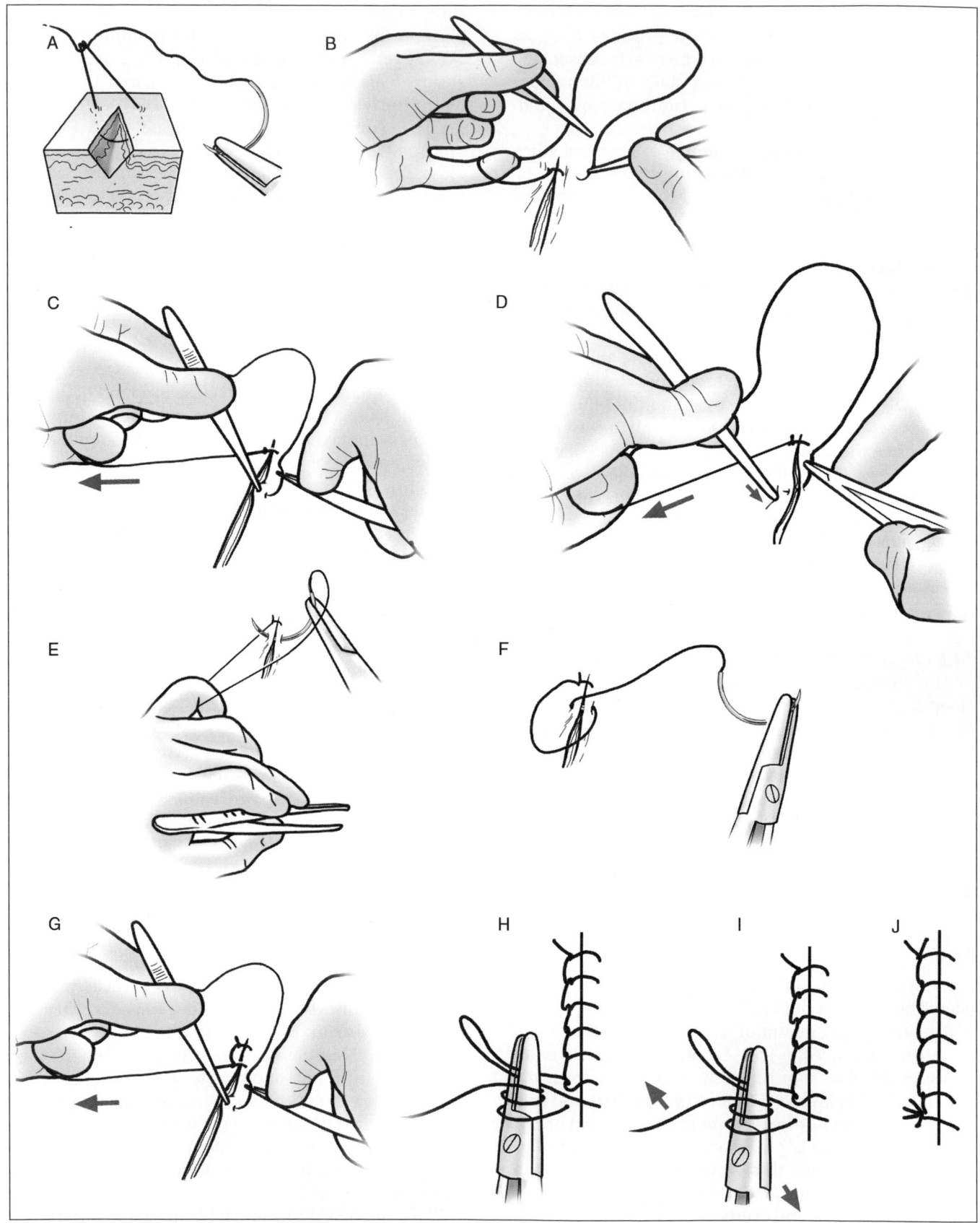

FIGURE 78-10 The continuous single-locked or running-locked stitch.

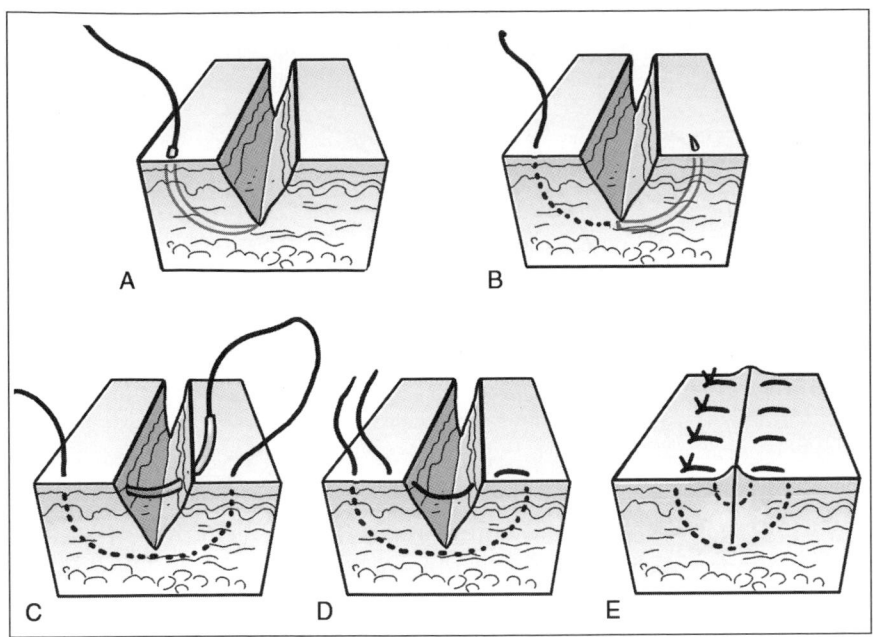

FIGURE 78-11 The vertical mattress stitch.

(Figures 78-14*A* and *B*). Reverse the needle and make a second throw 0.5 cm from the first (Figure 78-14*C*). **The needle must enter and exit the skin and the wound edges so that the first and second throws are parallel to** **each other** (Figures 78-14*C* and *D*). Pull the free ends of the suture taut to appose and evert the wound edges (Figures 78-14*E* and *F*). Tie and secure the suture in the standard manner.

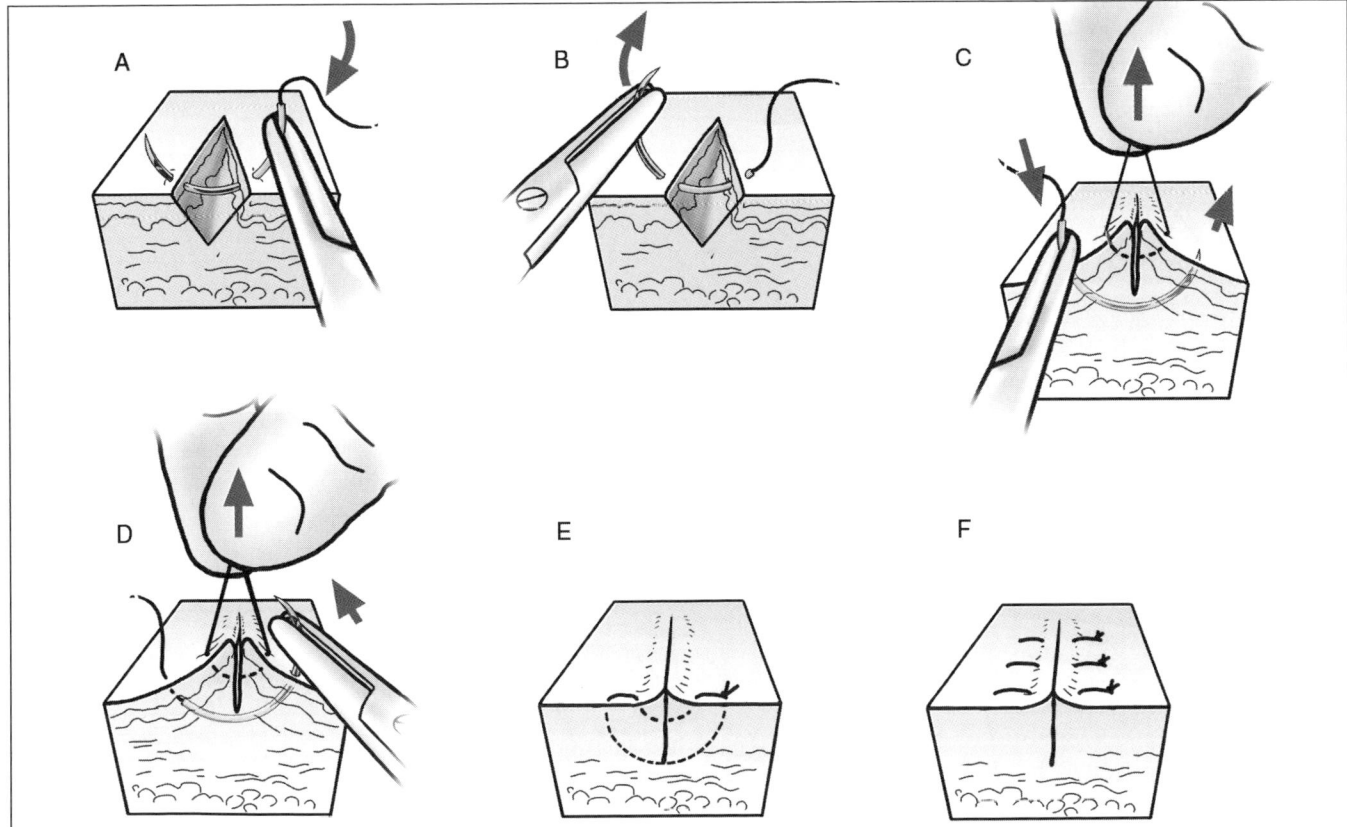

FIGURE 78-12 The "shortcut" vertical mattress stitch. An alternative method to place the vertical mattress stitch.

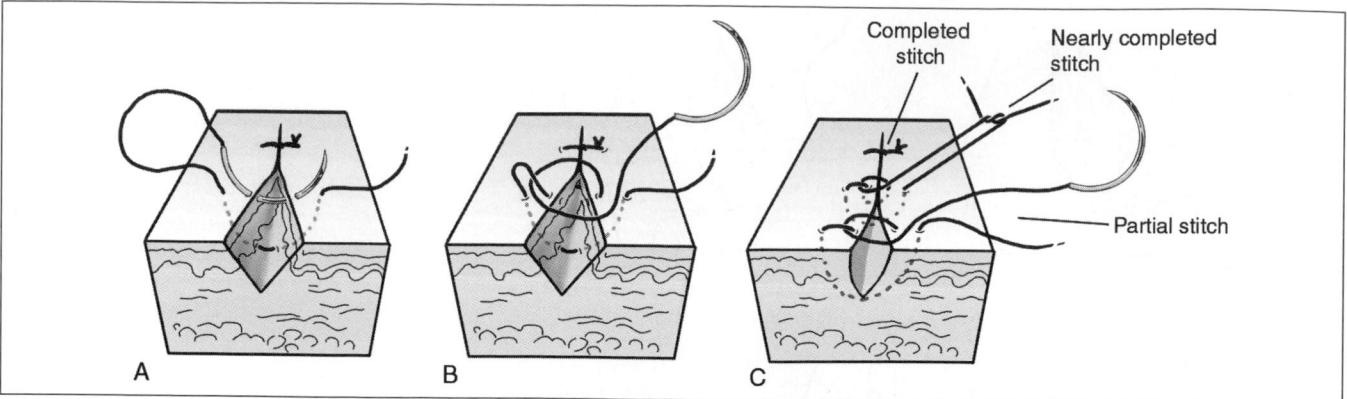

FIGURE 78-13 The locked vertical mattress stitch.

HALF-BURIED HORIZONTAL MATTRESS STITCH

This is the stitch of choice to close complex wounds with multiple flaps in a single-layer closure. This stitch is ideal to close stellate, Y-shaped, V-shaped, and T-shaped lacerations. The half-buried horizontal mattress stitch allows a tissue flap to be reapproximated without tension on the edges of the flap. The vascular supply to a flap is derived from its base. The flaps sometimes have a limited or poor vascular supply. This stitch may be used to approximate a flap-like laceration in which the corner has limited vascularity and/or viability.

The key to this stitch is that the needle and suture pass through the dermis of the flap and not the epidermis (Figure 78-15). Begin by placing the first stitch per-

cutaneously through the skin adjacent to the tip of the flap (Figure 78-15*A*). Advance the needle through the dermal layer of the flap, the dermal layer of the skin adjacent to the tip of the flap, and out the skin adjacent to the tip of the flap opposite to where the stitch began (Figure 78-15*A*). **The needle must traverse the dermis of the flap and adjacent tissue at the same level of the dermis to properly approximate the wound edges.** Gently pull on the free ends of the suture to approximate the flap against the adjacent skin edges. Tie and secure the suture in the usual manner. Secure the edges of the flap with half-buried horizontal mattress stitches (Figure 78-15*A*), simple interrupted stitches, vertical mattress stitches, or horizontal mattress stitches.

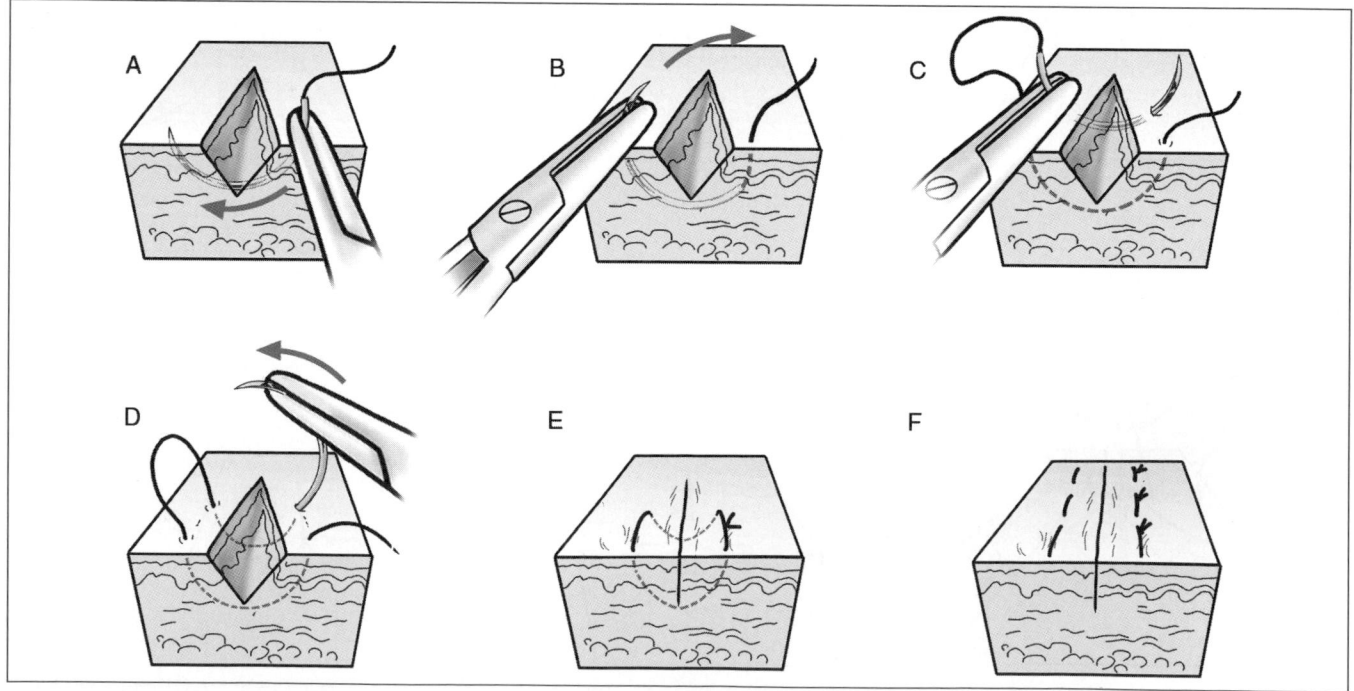

FIGURE 78-14 The horizontal mattress stitch.

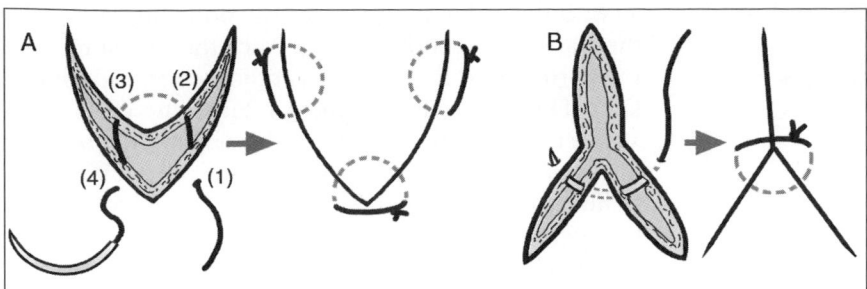

FIGURE 78-15 The half-buried horizontal mattress stitch is used to approximate a star-shaped (stellate) laceration (*A*) and a Y-shaped laceration (*B*).

Stellate lacerations are often seen in the Emergency Department. They occur due to bursting of the skin from crush injuries. These lacerations are often encountered on the extremities, forehead, and scalp. Begin by inserting the needle through the skin of the largest flap. Advance the needle so that its tip exits the dermis. Continue to advance the needle through the dermis of each flap. The half-buried horizontal mattress stitch should encompass the tips of all the flaps (Figure 78-15*B*). The remainder of the procedure is as described above.

CONTINUOUS (RUNNING) HORIZONTAL MATTRESS STITCH

The running horizontal mattress stitch is indicated in areas of the body where there is loose skin that tends to overlap or invert, such as the skin of the upper eyelids or the dorsum of the hand. This stitch can also be used as the surface closure in a multiple-layer closure if there is a tendency for wound inversion. Like the traditional horizontal mattress stitch, it provides good apposition and can be placed rapidly. The running horizontal mattress stitch is contraindicated in wounds under tension if the goal of wound closure is optimal cosmesis.

This stitch begins with a simple interrupted stitch at one end of a laceration (Figure 78-16). The needle is then run along the length of the wound while placing horizontal mattress stitches. The difference between this and the standard horizontal mattress stitch is that the suture is not tied and cut after each individual stitch.

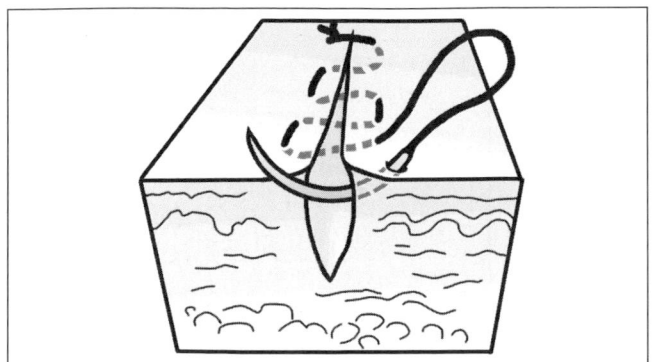

FIGURE 78-16 The continuous or running horizontal mattress stitch.

Rather, the stitch is continued (running) the length of the laceration. At the end of the laceration, the stitch is tied and secured in the same way as the simple running stitch (Figure 78-9).

CONTINUOUS SUBCUTICULAR STITCH

This closure is ideal for lacerations of the face and neck. It provides excellent cosmesis, leaves no suture marks on the skin, and causes minimal scarring. It requires more time and skill to place than other types of stitches. It may be performed for the temporary (pull-out) or permanent placement of subcutaneous sutures. Polypropylene or nylon sutures must be used for this stitch. Polypropylene is preferred as it is stiffer, stronger, and easier to remove than nylon.

The use of this stitch is limited to lacerations that are clean, straight, have sharp edges, and are less than 6 cm in length. It may be extremely difficult to remove the suture material for the pull-out technique if the laceration is greater than 6 cm in length. The laceration can be longer if the permanent placement of absorbable sutures is being used. The dermis and subcutaneous tissue must be apposed before proceeding with this stitch. If necessary, apply buried absorbable sutures to appose the dermis before applying this stitch. **The superficial wound surface must be tension-free, as this stitch is for cosmesis and not strength.** The wound may require undermining to release the tension from the wound edges. Refer to Chapter 77 for details regarding wound undermining.

The pull-out technique allows the subcuticular stitch to be removed after the laceration heals (Figure 78-17). The subcuticular suture should enter the intact skin 3 to 4 mm from one end of the laceration and burrow through the dermal-epidermal junction to emerge through the skin at the other end of the laceration (Figure 78-17*A*). The suture will continuously pass through the subcuticular layer on alternate sides of the laceration. **The point of entry of each stitch should be directly across from or slightly behind the exit point of the previous stitch. It is very important to keep the needle at the same level of depth throughout the wound. The tension on the suture should be adjusted to ensure that there is no puckering of the skin.** Tape the free

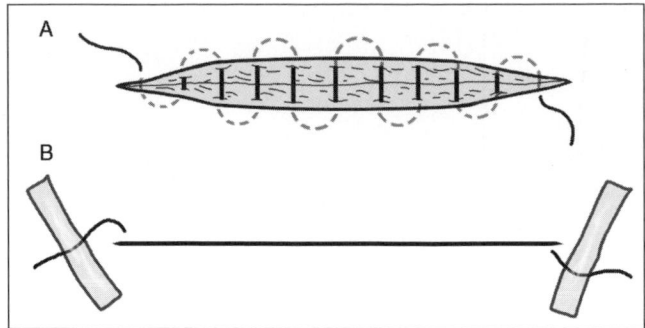

FIGURE 78-17 The continuous subcuticular pull-out stitch.

suture at both ends of the laceration to the skin (Figure 78-17*B*). Place wound tape (e.g., Steri-strips) across the laceration to help maintain the apposition of the epidermis. This stitch is easily removed. Remove the tape and pull one end of the suture with a needle driver.

As an alternative, the continuous stitch may be placed using absorbable suture material to provide longer-lasting strength to the wound (Figure 78-18). Suture material of choice includes Dexon, PDS, or Vicryl. The same indications, preparation, and stitch are used

as with the pullout technique. The only difference is in the starting and ending stitch. Place the first stitch into the dermis, just inside the laceration edge, as a buried knot (Figures 78-18*A*, *B*, and *C*). Place the continuous suture until the opposite end of the laceration is reached (Figure 78-18*D*). The final throw should be left lax with a trailing loop of suture (Figure 78-18*E*). The loop should be used as the "tail end" to perform an instrument tie (Figure 78-18*F*). Tie three or four knots in the suture. Lift the free ends of the suture and cut them just above the knot. Apply wound tape across the laceration to help maintain the apposition of the wound.

BURIED (SUBCUTANEOUS) KNOT STITCH

This stitch helps to decrease potential dead space underneath a laceration and gives tensile support for up to 4 to 6 weeks, while the wound is still weak. The loop is constructed so that the knot lies at the bottom of the wound base (Figure 78-19). This helps to keep the skin surface smooth and flat. The buried knot stitch is most useful in closing subcutaneous tissue just under the skin surface.

This stitch requires practice to master. Insert the needle into one side of the base of the wound (Figure 78-19*A*).

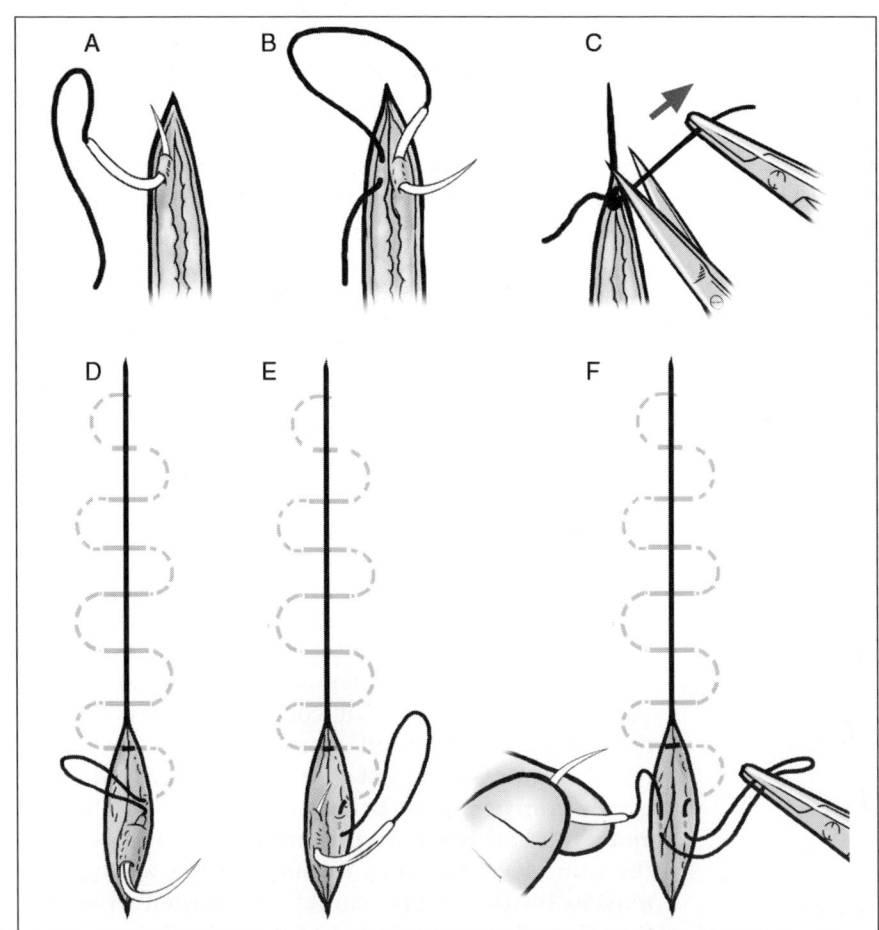

FIGURE 78-18 The continuous subcuticular permanent stitch.

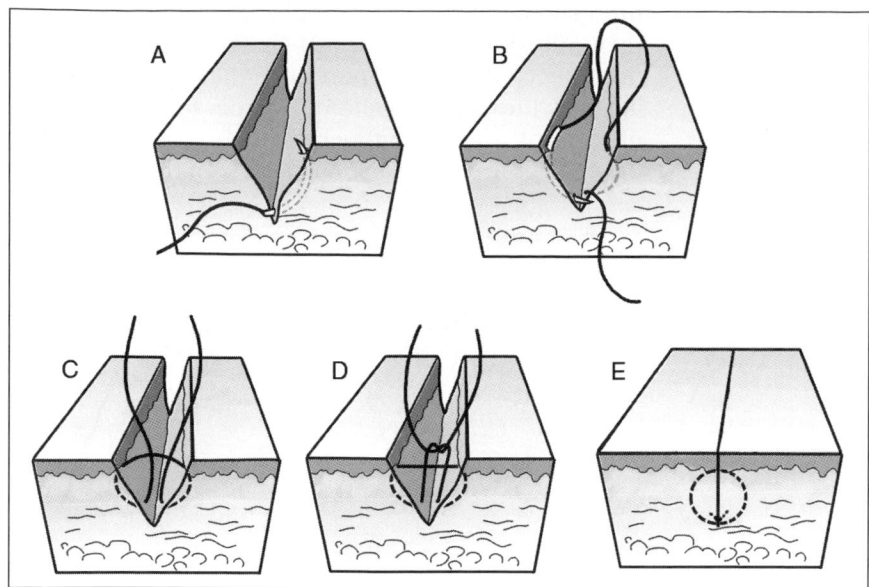

FIGURE 78-19 The buried (subcutaneous) knot stitch.

Drive the needle from deep to superficial and exiting at the dermal-epidermal junction (Figure 78-19*A*). Insert the needle through the dermal-epidermal junction on the opposite side of the wound and drive it through the base of the wound (Figure 78-19*B*). **The suture should exit the base of the wound across from and level with the entrance site of the first throw.** Pull both free ends of the suture up and out through the laceration (Figure 78-19*C*). Tie a knot in the suture (Figure 78-19*D*). Pull both free ends of the suture to lower the knot to the base of the wound and appose the tissue (Figure 78-19*E*). Tie two additional knots to secure the suture. Cut off any excess suture.

REINFORCING (RETENTION) SUTURES FOR WOUNDS UNDER TENSION

Reinforcing (retention) sutures are particularly useful for wounds in which the edges are widely separated or where the skin is too atrophic to approximate without the suture cutting through the skin. The reinforcing sutures help to decrease the tension on the wound by providing more support for the wound edges. Reinforcing sutures can be placed using sterile buttons or rubber tubing (Figure 78-20). Heavy sizes of nonabsorbable suture materials are used for reinforcing sutures. This is not for strength but to avoid the finer suture from cutting through the tissue.

Ideally, a double-swaged (needle) suture should be used to place suture from the inside of the wound toward the outside skin to avoid pulling potentially contaminated epithelial cells through the wound. The stitch is placed like the horizontal mattress stitch and sterile buttons or rubber tubing is used to achieve approximation to a point where the wound edges can be closed without significant tension (Figures 78-20*A* and *B*). **Do not attempt to appose the wound edges when using retention sutures.** Appose the remaining skin edges with simple interrupted, vertical mattress, or horizontal mattress stitches. The reinforcing sutures should remain in place after the skin sutures are removed. The reinforcing sutures should be removed after the wound has healed and gained significant tensile strength.

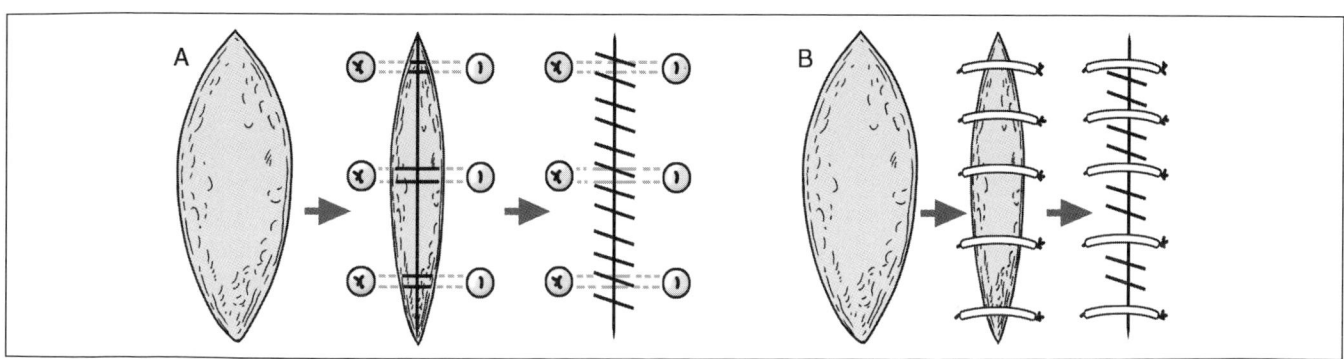

FIGURE 78-20 Reinforcing sutures for wounds under tension. Sterile buttons (*A*) or pieces of sterile rubber tubing (*B*) can be used to secure the suture and prevent injury to the soft tissues.

SUTURE REMOVAL TECHNIQUES

Remove sutures as soon as possible to avoid the possibility of infection and prevent the formation of suture marks. However, if they are removed too early, wound dehiscence may occur. Simple interrupted su-

tures should be cut at the end away from the knot and then pulled out (Figure 78-21*A*). This helps to prevent the outer contaminated portion of the suture from passing back through the wound. In order to remove a running simple or running-locked stitch, grasp the knot at the end of the closure and cut each loop (Figures 78-21*B*

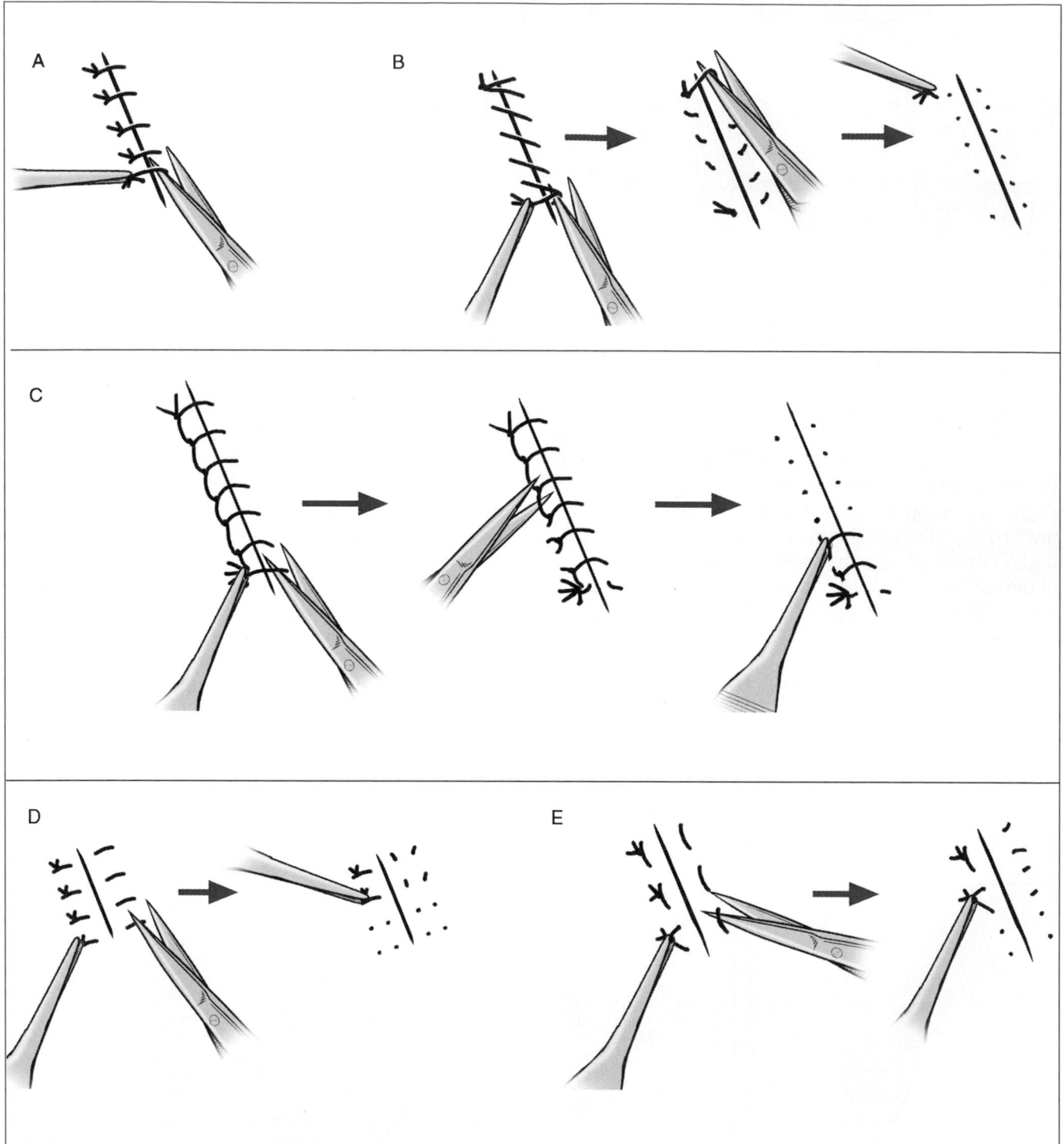

FIGURE 78-21 Suture removal techniques. *A.* Simple interrupted stitch. *B.* Simple running stitch. *C.* Running-locked stitch. *D.* Vertical mattress stitch. *E.* Horizontal mattress stitch.

and *C*). Pull out each individual suture piece. Vertical and horizontal mattress sutures can be removed in much the same way as the simple interrupted stitch (Figures 78-21*D* and *E*).

SKIN ADHESIVE CLOSURE (CYANOACRYLATES)

Skin adhesives (skin glues) are best used to close low-tension, small, straight-edged, and superficial wounds (Figure 78-22). They should not be used for lacerations that are bleeding, lacerations over joints, or lacerations under tension. There must be adequate hemostasis and the tissue must be as dry as possible. The major advantage to the use of tissue adhesives is speed. Wounds can be repaired quickly and without anesthesia. Other contraindications to this type of closure are angled or beveled wounds. Petroleum-based ointments or similar products will dissolve the tissue adhesive and should be avoided on this type of closure.

Crush the glass ampule containing the adhesive with finger pressure (Figure 78-22*A*). Allow the adhesive to moisten the cotton tip of the applicator. Approximate the wound edges with forceps. Commercially available, disposable, single-patient-use tissue forceps can be used (Bionix Development Corp., Toledo, OH). These are specifically designed to approximate the wound edges prior to using cyanoacrylates (Figure 78-22*B*). Apply the adhesive in two or three layers along the wound edge (Figure 78-22*C*). The adhesive may also be applied in spots over the laceration (Figure 78-22*D*) or across the laceration, like wound tape (Figure 78-22*E*). Droplets or lines should be placed 0.5 cm from each other. Support the wound for 30 to 60 seconds while the adhesive polymerizes.

SKIN CLOSURE TAPES

Skin closure tapes are used to close very low tension wounds that are tidy and small. They can be used as the primary closure technique for superficial wounds (Figure 78-23) or they can provide reinforcement after su-

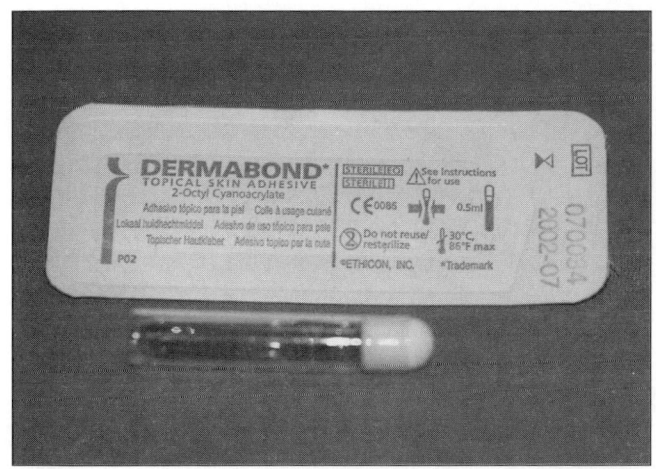

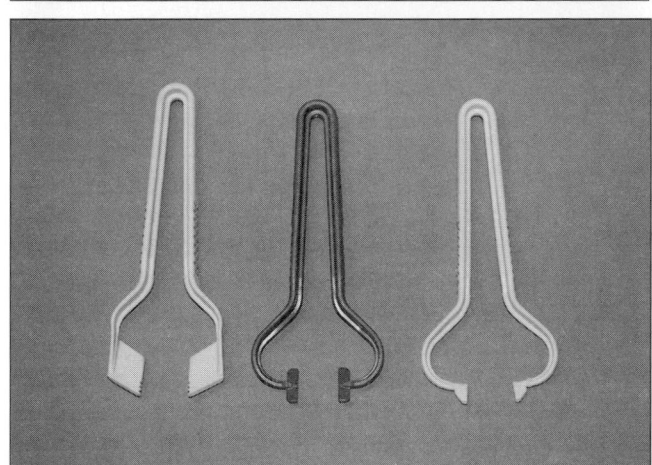

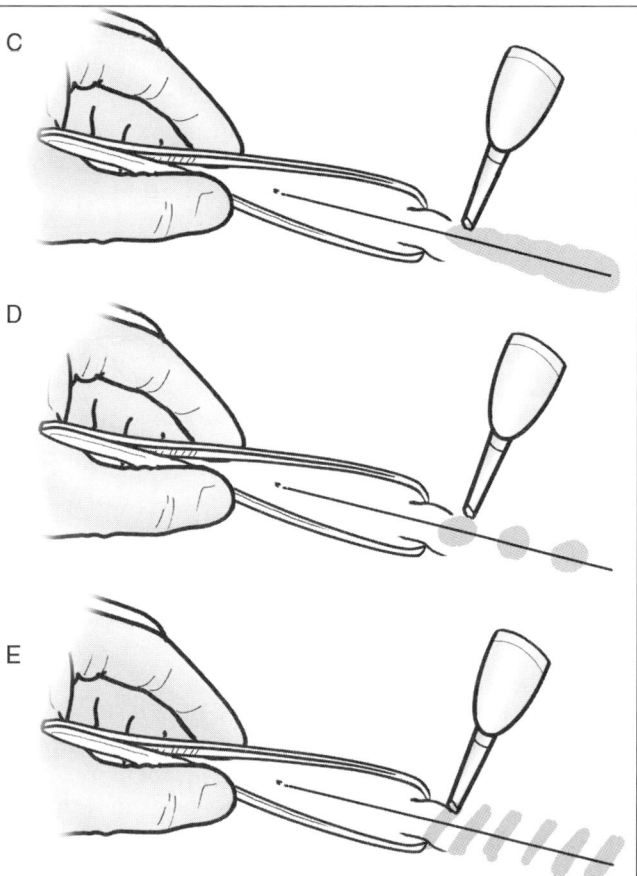

FIGURE 78-22 Laceration repair with cyanoacrylate skin adhesive. *A.* The skin adhesive. *B.* Commercially available wound forceps (Bionix Development Corp., Toledo, OH). *C.* Wound adhesive applied continuously over the laceration. *D.* Wound adhesive applied in spots over the laceration. *E.* Wound adhesive applied across the laceration.

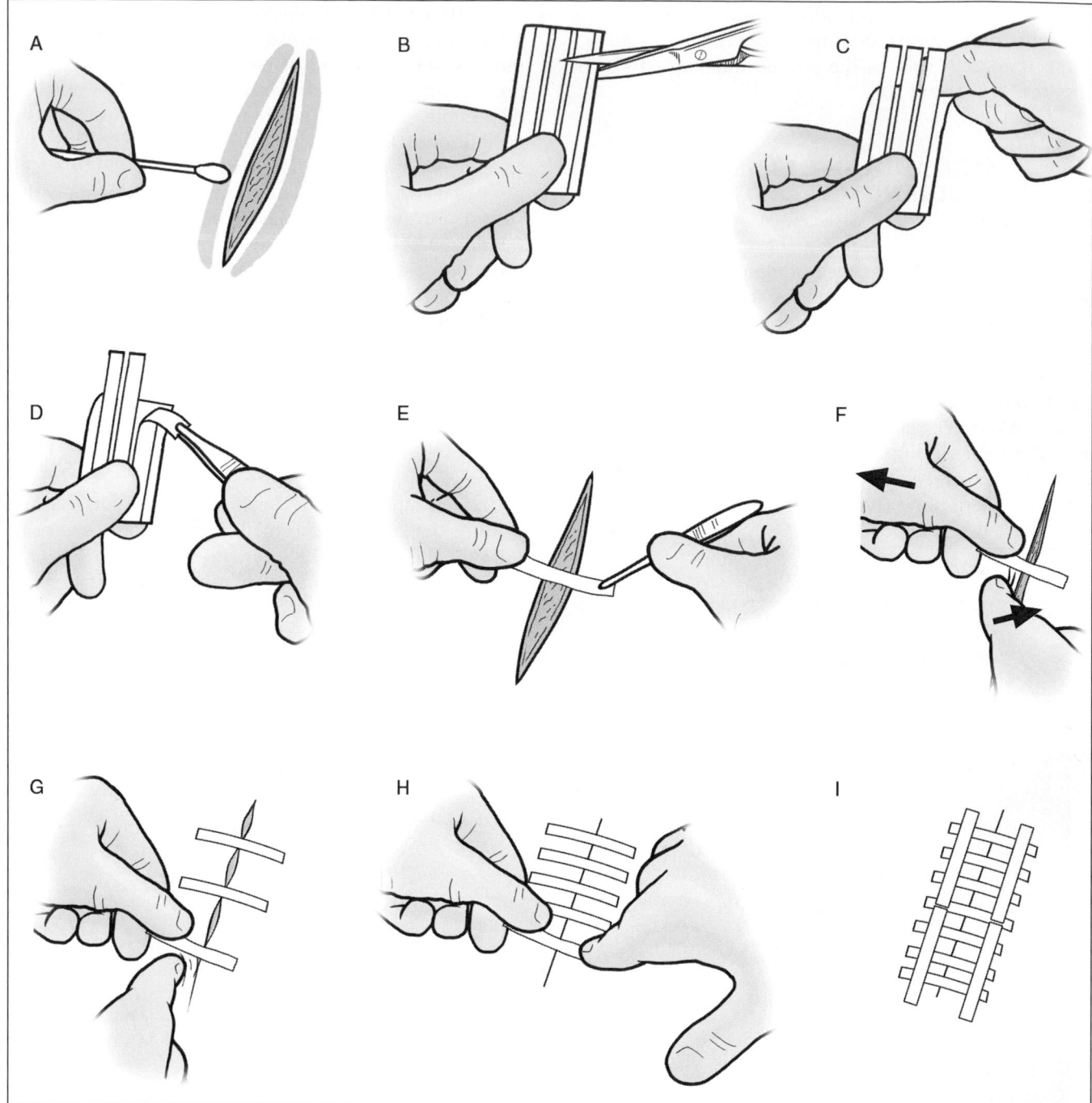

FIGURE 78-23 Skin closure tapes to close a laceration primarily.

tures have been placed (Figure 78-24). Skin tapes are easy to use and can be placed relatively quickly. They do not leave suture marks and have no skin reactivity.

Skin closure tapes should not be used in wounds where the edges are widely separated or on parts of the body where there is a lot of movement or moisture. This technique does not work well on irregularly shaped wounds or wounds where there will be a propensity for swelling of the wound edges. Care should be taken in us-

ing these tapes in a child. If they are not secured properly, the child may remove them prematurely.

After the initial cleansing of the skin, clean the skin surface with acetone or alcohol to remove any surface oils. Allow the skin to dry. Apply benzoin solution to the skin on both sides of the wound with a cotton applicator (Figure 78-23A). Cut the skin closure tapes to the proper length (Figure 78-23B). Gently tear the end-tab off the back of the card to prevent the strips from deforming

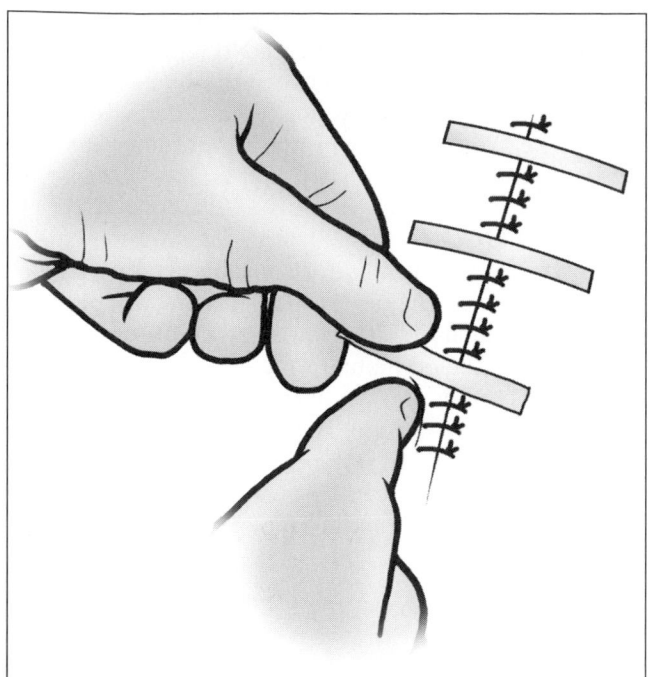

FIGURE 78-24 Skin closure tapes can be used to provide reinforcement for sutures.

(Figure 78-23*C*). Remove a strip from the card (Figure 78-23*D*). Firmly secure the tape to one side of the wound (Figure 78-23*E*). Use the nondominant hand to appose the wound edges as the tape is brought over and secured to the skin on the opposite wound edge (Figure 78-23*F*). Place additional tapes at 2 to 3 mm intervals until the wound edges are apposed (Figures 78-23*G* and *H*). Place pieces of tape across the tape edges to prevent premature removal and skin blistering from the tape ends (Figure 78-23*I*).

Skin closure tapes may be placed over a sutured laceration (Figure 78-24). The tapes will provide additional support to the wound edge and help to prevent dehiscence. This technique is especially useful in areas of cosmetic concern, such as the face.

The skin closure tapes should remain in place for at least as long as the sutures. They must be kept dry to prevent them from coming off and the wound from dehiscing. The wound should be observed daily for signs of infection.

Skin closure tapes may be placed across a wound when sutures or staples are removed. The tapes will maintain the apposition of the epidermis as the wound matures. Apply benzoin solution to the skin before removing the sutures or staples. Remove several sutures or staples and apply the skin closure tapes. Continue this process until all the sutures or staples have been removed and the wound is covered with skin closure tapes. Alternatively, remove all of the sutures or staples and then apply the skin closure tapes.

STAPLE CLOSURE

Stapling is a rapid closure technique that is useful for superficial scalp lacerations and linear lacerations of the trunk and extremities. Staples should not be used on the face, neck, hands, or feet. These areas have little subcutaneous tissue and the staples can damage underlying structures. Staples should also be avoided in any area of the body that will be exposed to computed tomography (CT) or magnetic resonance imaging (MRI). The staples are made of an inert material, which helps to decrease tissue reactivity.

The skin stapler is a simple device (Figure 78-25). It is a single-patient-use, sterile, disposable unit that is preloaded with staples. It is grasped and held with one hand. When the handle is squeezed, a staple is inserted into the tissue. The stapler automatically loads the next

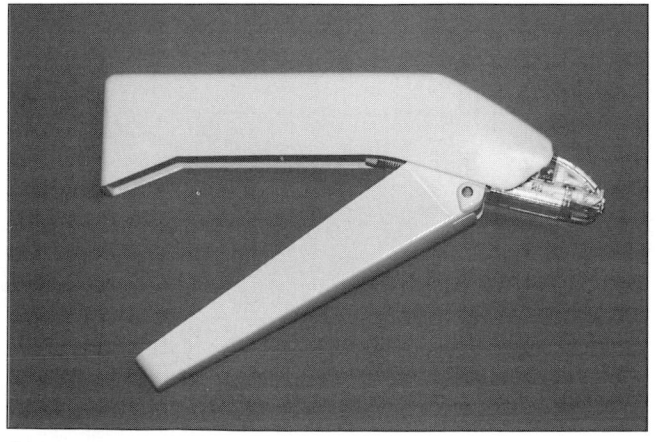

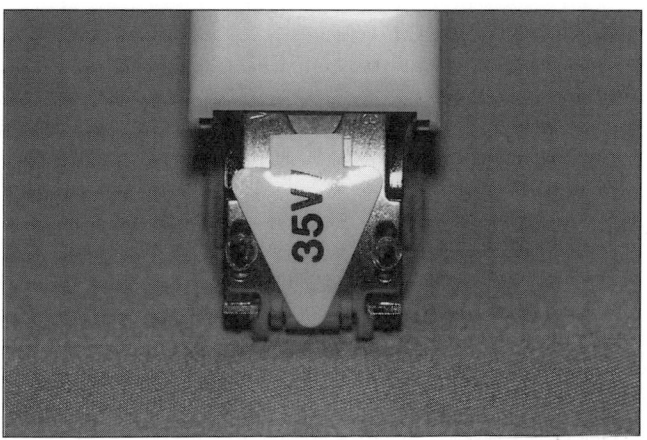

A   B

FIGURE 78-25 The skin stapler. *A.* Overview of the wound stapler. *B.* The distal end of the wound stapler.

staple after one staple is discharged. Skin staplers typically have 10 or 35 preloaded staples.

Prepare the wound for stapling. Place deep sutures to close the subcutaneous tissue and, if the wound is gaping, bring the wound edges into apposition. Approximate the skin edges with the dominant hand (Figure 78-26A). Evert the wound edges with a forceps held in the nondominant hand (Figure 78-26A). Grasp the stapler with the dominant hand. Gently place the skin stapler over the laceration (Figure 78-26B). **Do not indent the skin with the stapler, as this will cause the staples to be placed too deep.** Align the arrow on the front of the stapler over the laceration (Figure 78-26C). Squeeze the handle of the stapler. A plunger will advance a staple into the wound margins (Figure 78-26D). An anvil will bend the staple into a square or rectangular shape to secure the staple (Figure 78-26E). Continue to evert the wound edges and apply staples every 3 to 5 mm until the wound is approximated (Figure 78-26F). A small space will be visible between the skin surface and the staple if it is properly positioned. If the staple is against the skin, it has been placed too deep. Remove the staple and replace it.

STAPLE REMOVAL

The staple remover is a disposable, sterile, single-patient-use device (Figure 78-27A). It is made of metal or plastic with metal tips. The lower jaw of the stapler has two upwardly angled metal prongs (Figure 78-27B). The upper jaw of the stapler is a flat piece of metal. Insert the prongs of the lower jaw of the staple remover between the staple and the skin (Figure 78-28A). Close the handles of the staple remover. This will cause the upper jaw to compress the center of the staple and the arms of the

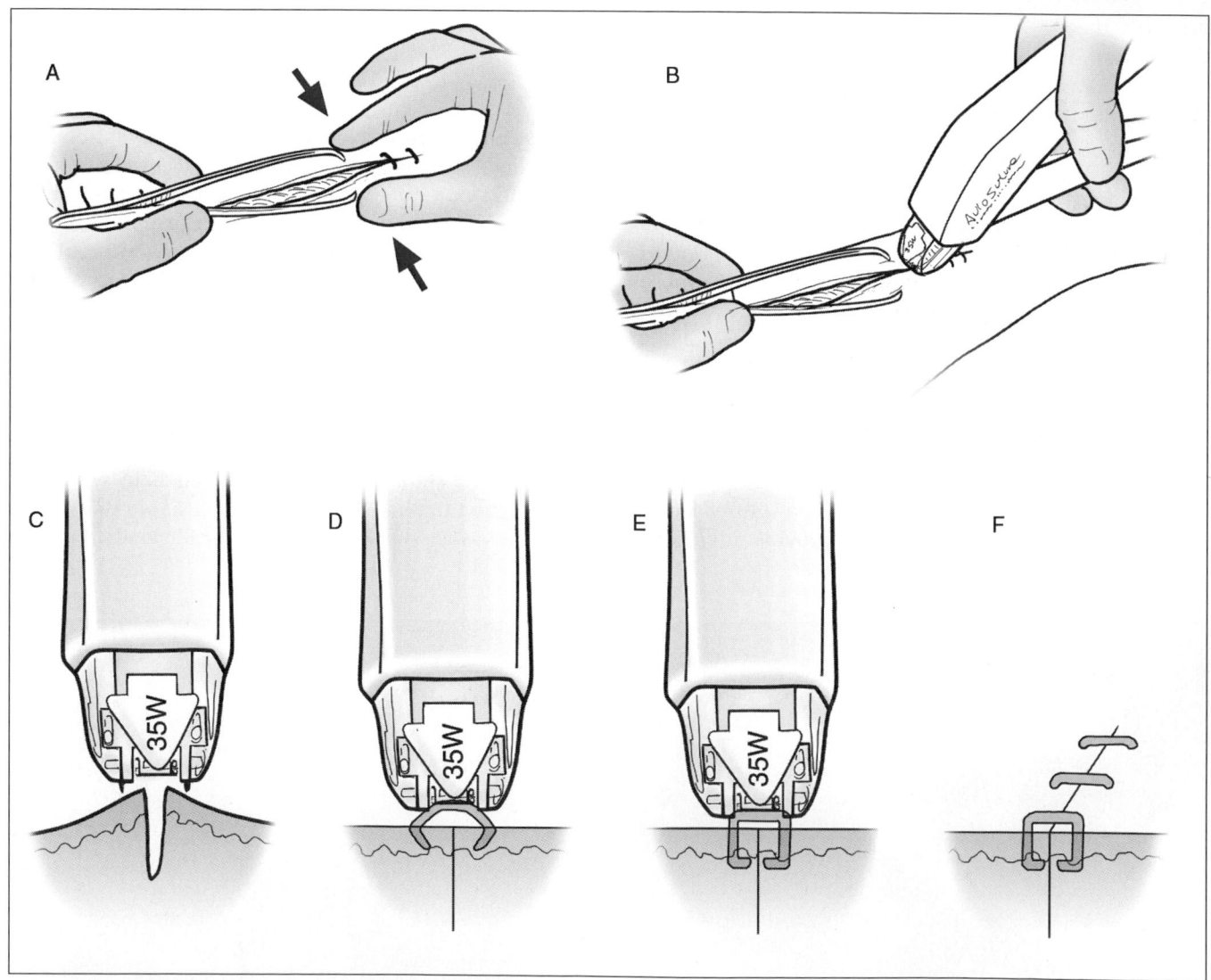

FIGURE 78-26 Laceration repair with staple closure. *A.* The wound edges are apposed and everted. *B.* The stapler is applied over the laceration. *C.* The stapler is applied over the everted wound edges. *D.* The plunger advances the staple into the wound margins. *E.* The anvil bends the staple into shape. *F.* The final product.

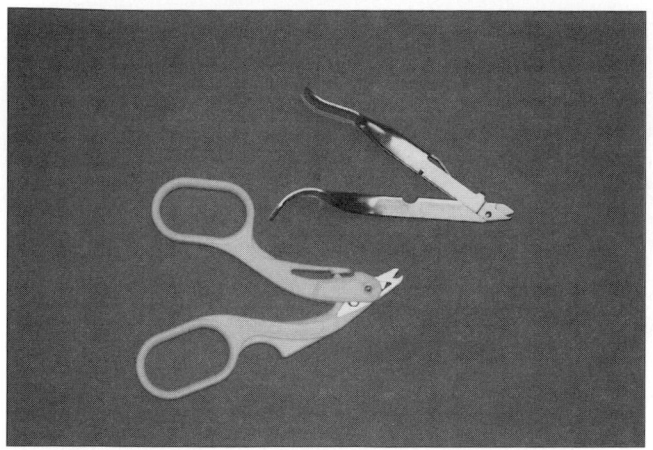

A

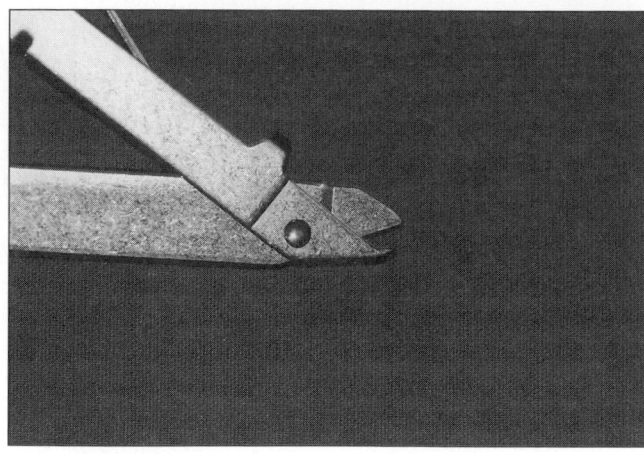

B

FIGURE 78-27 The staple remover. *A.* Overview. *B.* The tip with the jaws open.

staple to withdraw from the skin (Figure 78-28*B*). Lift the staple remover and staple off of the skin. Discard the staple and continue the process until all the staples have been removed.

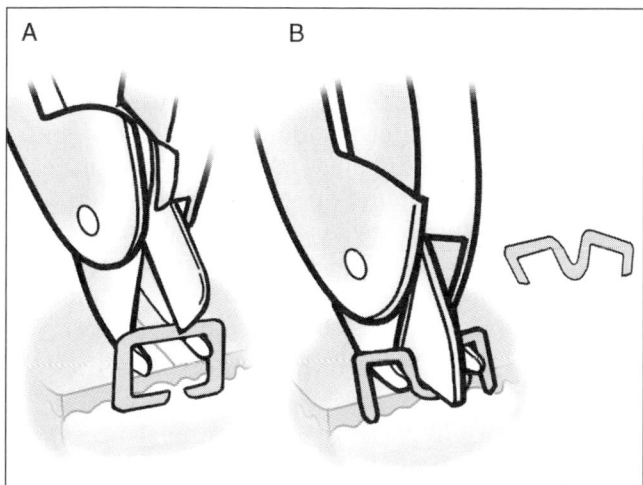

FIGURE 78-28 Staple removal. *A.* The lower jaw of the staple remover is placed under the staple. *B.* The upper jaw compresses the center of the staple and allows the staple arms to exit the skin.

SUMMARY

There are multiple techniques available for basic wound closure. The principles discussed above will help to provide the most appropriate closure for the various types of wounds that are seen in the practice of Emergency Medicine. Care should be taken to provide the best closure possible to provide good cosmesis and avoid complications.

REFERENCES

1. Simon RR, Brenner BE: *Emergency Procedures and Techniques,* 3rd ed. Baltimore: Williams & Wilkins, 1994:286–325.
2. Ethicon: *Wound Closure Manual.* Somerville, NJ: Ethicon, Inc., 1999.
3. Sherris DA, Kern EG: *Basic Surgical Skills.* Rochester: Mayo Clinic Scientific Press, 1999.
4. Roberts JR, Hedges JR: *Clinical Procedures in Emergency Medicine.* Philadelphia: Saunders, 1998.
5. Trott A: *Wounds and Lacerations.* St. Louis: Mosby-Yearbook, 1997.

Chapter 79
ADVANCED WOUND CLOSURE TECHNIQUES

Eric F. Reichman
Lukas Kolm

INTRODUCTION

Traumatic wounds or skin lacerations are among the most common injuries, occurring in people of all ages, that require evaluation and treatment in the Emergency Department. The result of many if not all wound closures is scar formation. Although most wounds heal with a surprisingly pleasing cosmetic transformation from their initial presentations, it is not uncommon for some wounds to present complications during the healing period as well as to produce an undesirable scar. A systematic approach to wound management serves to help in deciding how to close complicated wounds, reduce the risk for infection, and minimize less favorable outcomes.

Wound management in the Emergency Department includes an assessment of the mechanism and conditions that were present at the time of injury. Initially, one must address the concerns of the patient, family members, or friends with a concise explanation of how the wound will be treated and what can be anticipated for aftercare. Many lawsuits and concerns of poor care evolve from poor cosmetic outcomes. **It is recommended that verbal wound care instructions be offered once wound closure is completed, in addition to giving the patient written discharge instructions.**[1]

Regardless of the severity of the wound or possible inherent complications associated with the injury, many patients are primarily concerned with the potential for scarring or disfigurement. Most patients expect cosmetic and functional perfection as an ultimate result after their wounds are treated and the healing process is completed. These expectations are often not clearly expressed during the evaluation and treatment in the Emergency Department. **The Emergency Physician must openly explain and discuss the fact that virtually no wound heals without a scar following wound closure.**[1,2] A clear understanding of this is not to be used as an explanation for a poor outcome but to counter any misconception that a wound will heal to look exactly like the previously intact skin. Treatment is rendered to offer the best possible functional and esthetic outcome while reducing the risk of potential soft tissue infection.

An overall plan of wound site preparation and closure will be needed to provide the greatest likelihood of a pleasing cosmetic result.[1] The mechanism of injury, severity of the wound, location of the wound, and the presence or risk of necrotic tissue can all influence the risk of infection. Additionally, the decision of how to approach wound closure will be affected by the patient's skin type, age, gender, occupation, and hobbies.

Wound healing ultimately takes place over at least 6 to 9 months. Any wound presenting with concerns for a poor outcome or an obvious likelihood of wound revision in the future should be evaluated and treated by a Plastic Surgeon when possible.[1,2] All other wounds requiring complex closures should be properly assessed and treated by the Emergency Physician.

ANATOMY AND PATHOPHYSIOLOGY

In order to have a better understanding of scar tissue formation and the antecedent techniques of wound closure, the Emergency Physician should have knowledge of specific physiologic conditions and anatomic areas that may increase the chances of unfavorable scarring following wound repair.[2,3] The age of the patient and appearance of the patient's intact skin should be taken into consideration. The younger patient tends to heal more rapidly, while the older patient tends to have a more favorable cosmetic outcome with wound closure. Older patients have less overall elastic and subcutaneous tissue and more wrinkling, thus decreasing the tension on the healing wound and making scarring less noticeable.[2,3] Wrinkling, or lines of minimal tension, makes wound repair more technically challenging.

Suturing of asymmetrical, deep, or large wounds requires particular attention to the preexisting lines of minimal tension or lines of facial expression. Without properly addressing such preexistent anomalies, the cosmesis of wound repair can be grossly affected.[2,3] Scars from wounds closed perpendicular to preexisting functionally anatomic lines undergo repetitive physical stress and may result in hypertrophic scar tissue. With markedly less skin elasticity and subcutaneous fat, older patients will often experience more favorable cosmetic results from less complex wound closures. However, younger patients will benefit from more advanced wound closure techniques to properly close large or complicated wounds. Rotational and advancement flaps are frequently performed to make scarring less obvious when suturing across lines of tension.[3]

The type of skin, regardless of age, will affect scar formation.[3,4] Oily or hyperpigmented skin more frequently has poor scar tissue formation, resulting in scars that are hypertrophic, deep, and asymmetrical. Consideration of wound outcome should be given to areas of the skin that are rich in sebaceous glands or simply hyperpigmented (from environmental exposure or ethnicity). Patients with underlying connective disease disorders or conditions with a high likelihood of concomitant vitamin deficiencies should also be scrutinized, as wound closure and healing may be compromised in such cases, resulting in highly variable and less predictable outcomes.

The mechanism of injury, including environmental exposure to underlying tissue, should not be overlooked, so that adequate debridement and preparation may be done prior to a complex wound closure. This allows the physician to better visualize the anatomic layers of the skin. It can be difficult to determine a clear delineation between the anatomic layers of the skin when the wound was a result of a crush injury, shredding mechanism, or any circumstance resulting in uneven or macerated wound edges. Delineate the pigmented epidermis from the thicker underlying dermis, especially when multilayer wound closures are required, as suturing may then become unnecessarily complicated and affect the overall integrity of the wound closure.

It should be noted that the literature supports a significant underutilization of multilayer closures, though these are often necessary. Single-layer closures and excessively large suture materials are the greatest causes of residual scar tissue.[1] It is recommended to prepare the wound edges by creating a bevel or undercutting of the wound margin to allow subtle epidermal eversion, thus augmenting the natural process of scar formation.[1,2] This allows the natural flattening and depression of the forming scar to occur without excessive depression from the wound margins.[2] This will also help to reduce the thickness of the scar tissue and decrease the refraction of light from the scar, making it less noticeable.

Depending on the presentation of the tissue defect, more than one wound closure technique may be used to adequately close a wound. Utilizing more than one technique will help remove underlying tension and allow better approximation of the epidermis. With the help of specific camouflage techniques used in closing the epidermis, irregularly shaped wounds can heal with less obtrusive scarring. Familiarity with a few of these techniques and their application will allow the Emergency Physician to comfortably close the more challenging wounds encountered, with expectantly more favorable cosmetic prognoses.

INDICATIONS

Advanced wound closure techniques are indicated for closing wounds with irregularly shaped defects. They can be used to close circular, square, elliptical, or asymmetrical skin defects. Advanced wound closure techniques are beneficial when there is a need to reduce skin tension and contracture, which are likely to result in hypertrophic scar formation.[3,4] Rotational and advancement flap techniques are useful in areas where tissue loss must be avoided and the undermining of wound edges must be minimized. This is often encountered with facial wounds in proximity to the eyelids, eyebrows, canthi, nasolabial folds, or lip borders. These techniques allow the initial shape of the wound to be altered such that there is reduced tension on the wound edges, which may then be closed simply.

CONTRAINDICATIONS

Specific wound closure techniques should take into account the potential for scar formation to occur in an undesirable location. This can happen when a wound must be elongated to create parallel lines and to decrease the tension on the wound edges. Elongation of a wound may bring it into proximity of other anatomic positions or landmarks, thus further complicating the healing process. If not planned well, excessively large defects may result, making it more likely that the scar will require later revision. More obvious conditions may exist that compromise complex wound closures. Particular attention must be given to crush injuries with devitalized or contaminated tissues. Severely contaminated wounds, including those with prolonged exposure, generally are at greater risk of infection with multilayer closures. Careful wound assessment may result in a decision to use simple approximation of the wound edges with close follow-up for ongoing wound care. Contraindications to complex wound closures will at times be reliant on temporal factors, such as the need to close a wound prior to the patient receiving surgical intervention for more life threatening injuries. There must be a commonsense approach in deciding how to close more challenging wounds in the Emergency Department.

PATIENT PREPARATION

Explain the risks, benefits, and complications of the wound closure to the patient and/or their representative. Discuss the presence of a visible scar after the repair, which may require subsequent revision. Explain the aftercare and follow-up. Obtained a signed informed consent for the procedure.

Place the patient in a position of comfort that is equally comfortable for the physician. This should allow for appropriate stretcher or seat height, lighting, and maneuverability so that physical obstacles are not a complicating variable during the wound repair. Clean the wound and surrounding skin of any dirt and debris. Flush the wound with normal saline. Apply povidone iodine solution to the surrounding skin, not the wound, and allow it to dry. Anesthetize the area using local or regional anesthesia (refer to Chapters 105 through 109).

Examine the wound for obvious foreign bodies or contaminants. Remove these with pressure irrigation using sterile saline. Apply sterile drapes to demarcate a sterile field. Apply the drapes so that the wound may be approached easily from different angles and without the risk of contaminating the site or any of the materials being used. There can be a great degree of variability in sterile techniques; therefore it is important to note that the best way to avoid wound infections is to employ and maintain consistency with sterile procedures throughout the wound repair.

TECHNIQUES

Z-PLASTY

It can be challenging to change the axis of orientation of a wound. **The reason for changing the orientation of a wound is to create a more functionally and cosmetically pleasing scar.** The Z-plasty has been described as a basic technique for scar revision, though its application also proves useful to lengthen and reorient wounds.[5] Wound lengthening reduces the formation of contractures, which often occur when the wound crosses areas of flexion. The Z-plasty should not be used for wounds from burn injuries where normal skin is not present. It also breaks up a linear scar into an accordion-like scar that has some degree of elasticity.

The Z-plasty is generally described to redirect a wound occurring across a flexion crease, over a joint, or on the face. It requires two incisions that create two triangular flaps with approximately 60 degrees of separation between the flaps, though the angle may vary between 30 and 90 degrees (Figure 79-1).[5] The greater the angle, the greater the gain in wound length. Sharper angles increase the risk of necrosis in the tip of the flap. Broader angles result in difficulty in rotating the flaps. Angles of 60 degrees increase the wound length by 75 percent. Angles of 45 degrees increase the wound length by 50 percent. Angles of 30 degrees increase the wound length by 25 percent. **The length of both arms of the incision must be the same length as the wound.** The undermining and separation of the two triangular flaps lengthens the wound and allows it to be reoriented perpendicularly to the original location. Additionally, small Z-plasties may be used in sequence to offset the appearance of straight wounds crossing lines of flexion or where contractures are likely to occur, so that the wound site then becomes parallel to the lines of flexion, further reducing occurrence of contracture formation.[3,4]

Clean, prep, and anesthetize the wound and surrounding skin. If the wound edges are irregular, sharply debride them using a #15 scalpel blade to form straight edges (Figure 79-1A). Measure and draw 60 degree angles from the ends of the laceration (Figure 79-1B). Draw the arms of the Z on the patient's skin with a skin-marking pen. **The arms must be the same length as the original laceration.** Incise the arms of the Z using a #15 scalpel blade (Figure 79-1C). Undermine the flaps of the Z and the surrounding skin. Elevate the flaps of the Z (Figure 79-1D). Transpose the flaps so that the wound is reoriented (Figure 79-1E). Place simple interrupted sutures to approximate the wound edges (Figure 79-1F).

APPROXIMATING THE EDGES OF A LACERATION WITH GROSSLY UNEQUAL LENGTHS

Creating an equilateral triangle from the midpoint of the longest wound edge allows wound edges of unequal length to be closed easily (Figure 79-2).[3-5] Determine the widest point between the two wound edges. Determine which of the two wound edges is longer. Mark the middle of the longest wound edge (Figure 79-2A). Draw an equilateral triangle centered at this mark (Figure 79-2B). **The sides and base of the triangle must all be of equal length and the same length as the widest part of the original wound.** Incise the arms of the equilateral triangle with a #15 scalpel blade and remove the tissue (Figure 79-2B). Undermine the wound edges. Close the wound and the perpendicular incision from the triangle with simple interrupted or running sutures (Figure 79-2C). Closure of the two wounds results in a clean linear wound with a short perpendicular

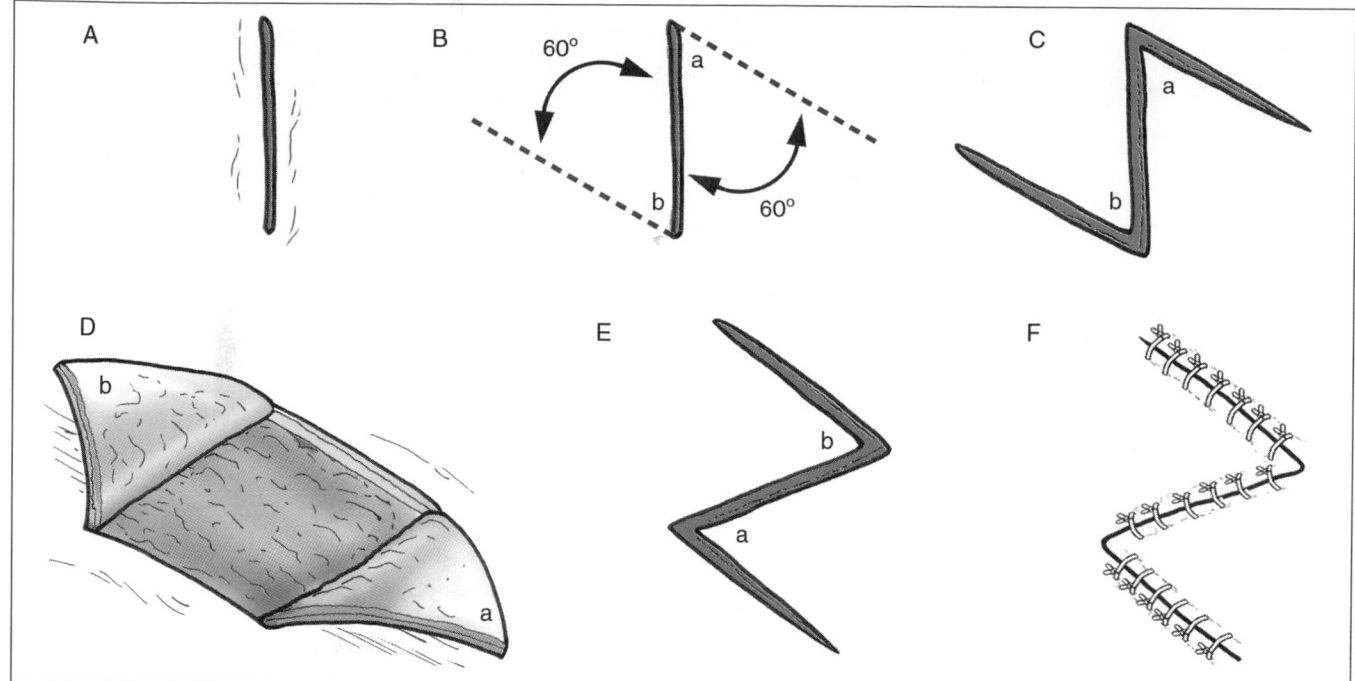

FIGURE 79-1 The Z-plasty. *A.* The original laceration. *B.* Draw the arms of the Z at a 60 degree angle from the ends of the lacerations. The arms must be the same length as the laceration. *C.* The skin has been incised to form the Z. *D.* Undermine and elevate the flaps. *E.* Transpose the flaps to reorient the wound. *F.* Approximate the wound edges with simple interrupted sutures.

linear wound offsetting the previously unequal edges (Figure 79-2*C*).

CLOSING A SQUARE-SHAPED DEFECT

Wounds are rarely square-shaped after an injury (Figure 79-3*A*). Debride the wound to make a square-shaped defect (Figure 79-3*B*). Square-shaped defects can be difficult to close and require a single pedicle advancement flap.[3] Elongating two sides of the square allows small and moderate-sized defects to be closed primarily (Figure 79-3*C*). Draw lines to extend two parallel edges of the square by twice their length (Figure 79-3*C*). Draw Burow's triangles on the ends of the extended lines (Figure 79-3*C*). These triangles will be removed, allowing the flap to be transposed into the wound and creating a more symmetrical flap.[3–5] Draw the Burow's

triangles as equilateral triangles whose sides are half the length of the square defect (Figure 79-3*C*).

Incise along the extended lines and Burow's triangles with a #15 scalpel blade. Remove the tissue of the Burow's triangles. Undermine the rectangular flap and the area surrounding the base of the flap. **Do not undermine the area lateral to the extended lines**. Advance the tissue flap to close the defect (Figure 79-3*D*). Place a simple interrupted suture in the center of the short edge of the flap to hold it in position. Place half-buried horizontal mattress sutures to secure the corners of the flap. Approximate the wound edges with simple interrupted sutures along the long arms. Approximate the corner of the Burow's triangles with half-buried horizontal mattress stitches and the rest of the triangle with simple interrupted sutures.[3–5]

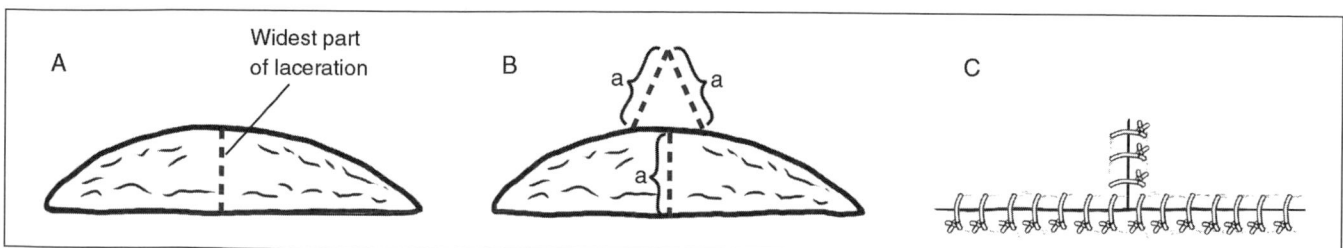

FIGURE 79-2 Approximating edges of grossly unequal lengths in repairing a laceration. *A.* The laceration. *B.* Draw an equilateral triangle along the longest side and centered about the widest part of the laceration. The sides of the triangle must be equal to the length of the widest part of the original laceration. *C.* Approximate the wound edges with simple interrupted sutures.

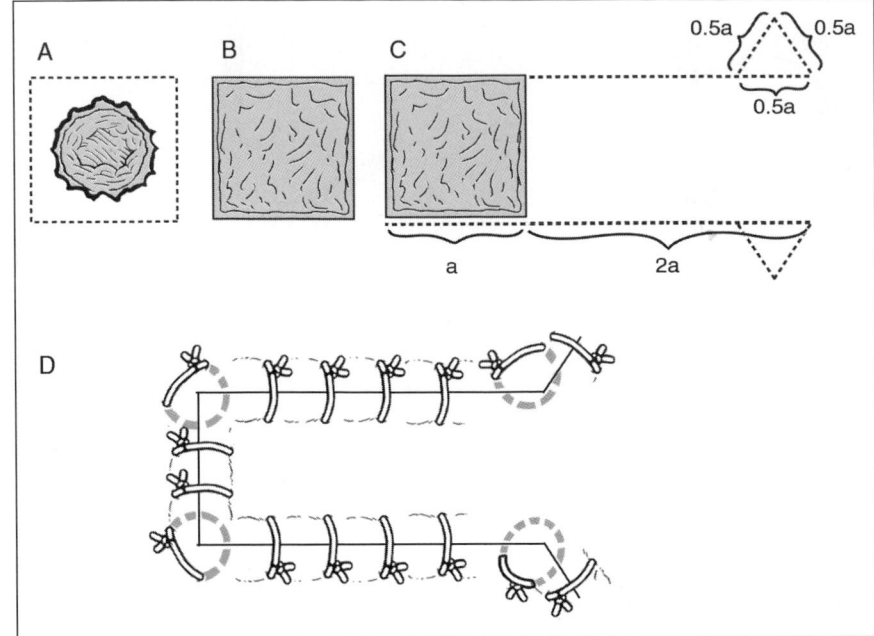

FIGURE 79-3 Closure of a square-shaped defect. *A.* The original tissue defect. Draw lines around the defect to form a square. *B.* The skin has been incised and the original defect removed to create a square-shaped defect. *C.* Draw lines to extend two sides of the square into a rectangle. Draw Burow's triangles at the ends of the rectangular lines. *D.* Advance the flap and approximate the wound edges.

CLOSURE OF A DIAMOND-SHAPED DEFECT

Diamond- or rhomboid-shaped defects require the rotation of a flap referred to as a Limberg flap. **The Limberg flap is a transposition flap suitable only for closing a diamond- or rhomboid-shaped defect. It requires the formation of two adjacent angles of the rhomboid that must be 60 and 120 degrees for an optimal flap.**

Wounds are rarely diamond-shaped after an injury (Figure 79-4A). Debride the wound to make a diamond-shaped defect (Figure 79-4A). Draw a line to extend the distance of the short diagonal of the defect to double its total length (Figure 79-4B). Draw a line from the extended line and parallel (back cut) to the adjacent wound edge that is equal to the length of the extended line (Figure 79-4B). Incise along the extended lines with a #15 scalpel blade. Undermine the flap and adjacent skin. Rotate the flap into the diamond-shaped defect (Figure 79-4C). Approximate the wound edges with simple interrupted sutures along the linear edges and half-buried horizontal mattress sutures at the intersection or angles of the wound edges (Figure 79-4D).[3–5] Depending on the location of loose tissue and adjacent structures, one of four Limberg flaps can be created to close the defect (Figure 79-4E).

CLOSURE OF AN ELLIPTICAL DEFECT

Wounds are often irregular and elliptical (Figure 79-5A). Creating an ellipse from a wound allows more even closure of asymmetrical wounds. This is also referred to as an S-plasty. This technique may be used when there is concern of significant scarring and contracture formation from an associated thermal burn injury and Z-plasties are not recommended.[4] The less acute and more rounded edges of the ellipse tend to result in less tissue necrosis.[3,4]

Draw lines to debride the wound and form an S-shaped defect (Figure 79-5A). Incise the extended lines with a #15 scalpel blade to form the S-shaped defect and excise the wound (Figure 79-5B). Undermine the wound edges. Place buried sutures to close the wound and prevent tension on the wound edges. Approximate the wound edges by placing simple interrupted sutures alternating at each end of the S-shaped defect and ending in the middle (Figure 79-5C). Suturing from the ends and moving inward reduces the tension on the wound edges.[3,4]

CLOSURE OF A V-Y ADVANCEMENT FLAP

The V-Y flap is not a rotational flap but rather a V-shaped flap created away from the wound site, which then allows the skin to be advanced into the defect (Figure 79-6).[3–6] These advancement flaps may be used to avoid defects from lacerations of the fingertips, lips, or face.

Wounds may be oval and elliptical (Figure 79-6A). Creating an oval from a wound allows more even closure of asymmetrical wounds. Draw lines to debride the wound and form an oval-shaped defect (Figure 79-6A). Incise along the lines with a #15 scalpel blade to form the oval-shaped defect and excise the wound (Figure 79-6B). Draw a V-shaped line adjacent to the oval-shaped defect (Figure 79-6C). **The line should be the length of the oval-shaped defect and approximately the width of the original wound away from the defect along its entire length.** Although the two sites do

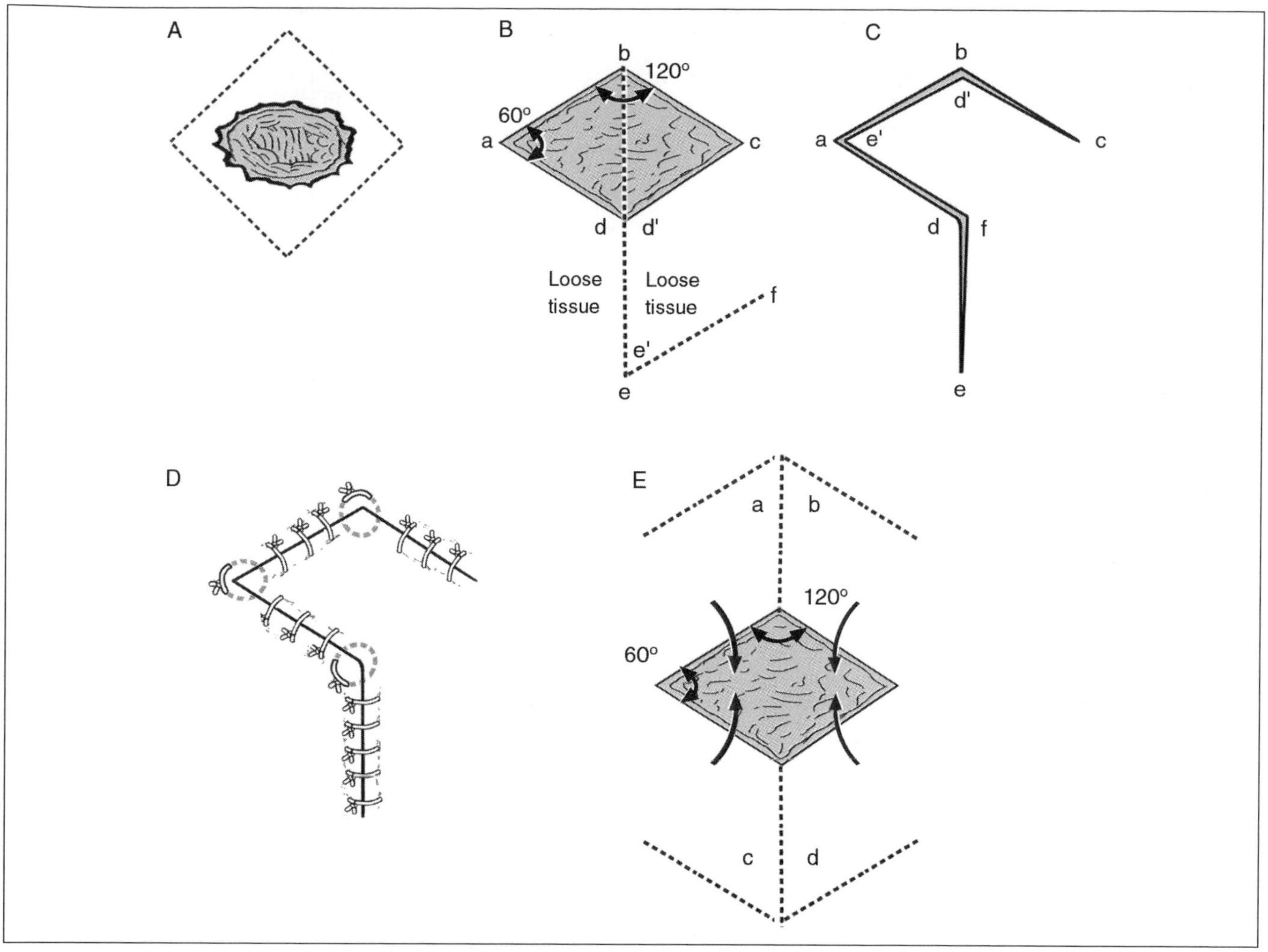

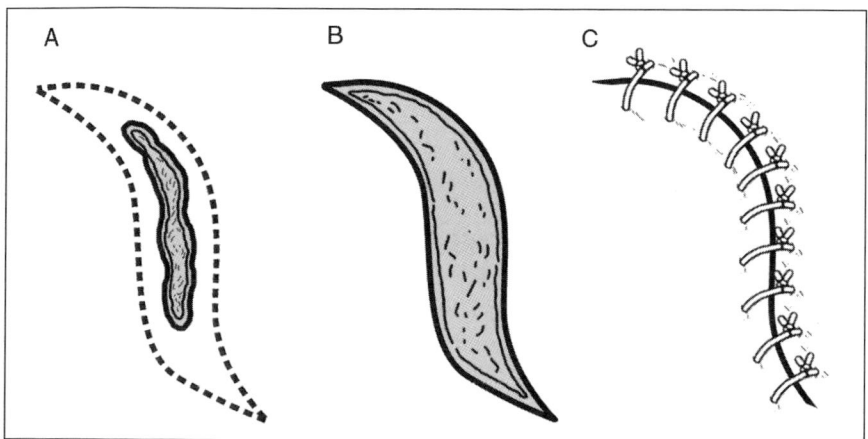

FIGURE 79-4 Closure of a diamond- or rhomboid-shaped defect. *A.* The original tissue defect. Draw lines around the defect to form a diamond or rhomboid. *B.* The skin has been incised to create a diamond-shaped defect. Draw lines to form the flap. Extend the short diagonal (BD) by one times its length to form line DE. Draw line EF parallel to line CD and the same length as line CD. *C.* Transpose the flap to close the defect. *D.* Approximate the wound edges. *E.* The four available Limberg flaps that can be created to fill the defect.

FIGURE 79-5 Closure of an elliptical defect. *A.* The original tissue defect. Draw lines around the defect to form an S-shaped defect. *B.* The skin has been incised and the original defect removed to create an S-shaped defect. *C.* Approximation of the wound edges with simple interrupted sutures.

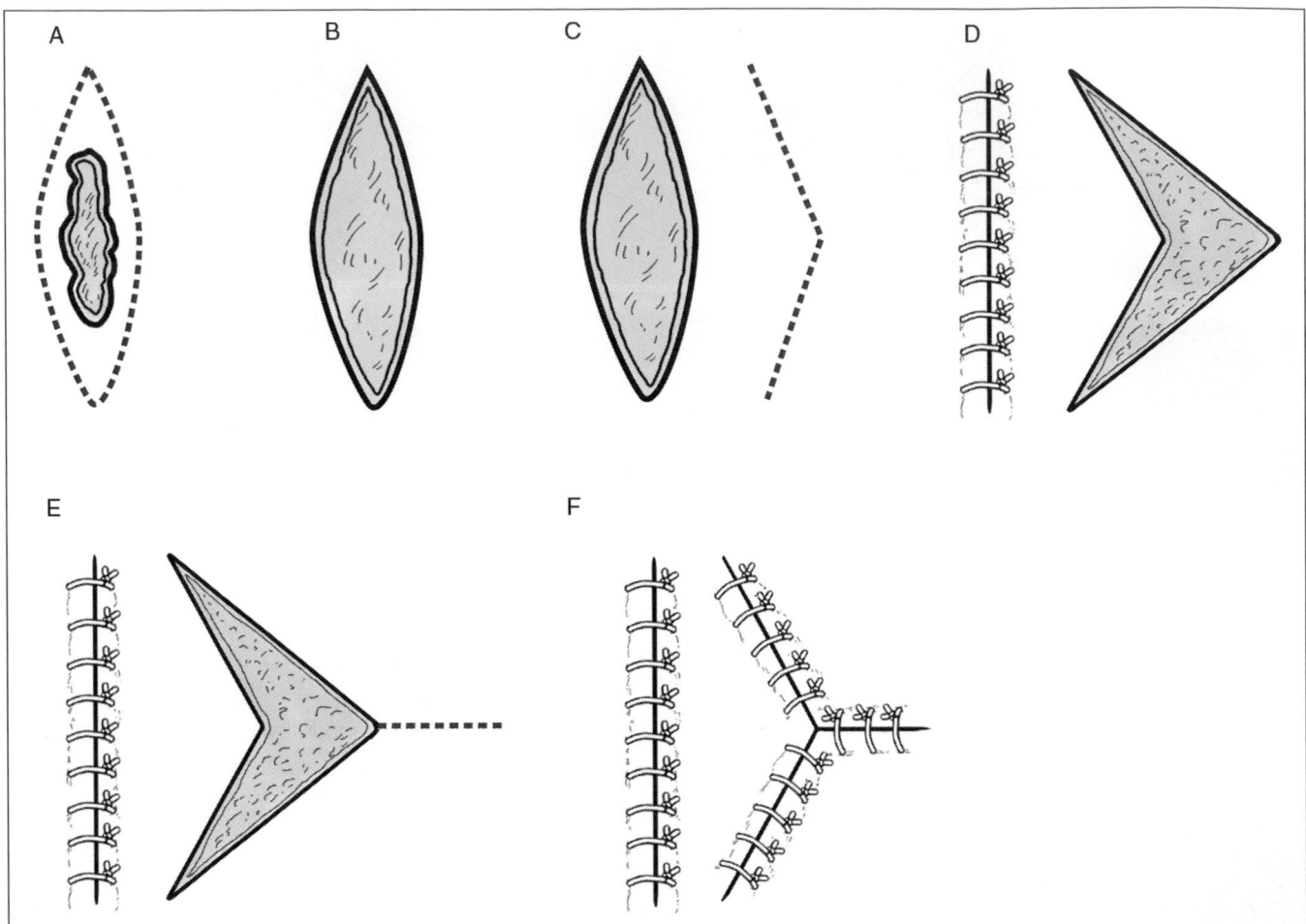

FIGURE 79-6 Closure of a V-Y advancement flap. *A.* The original tissue defect. Draw lines around the defect to form an oval. *B.* The skin has been incised and the original defect removed to form an oval-shaped defect. *C.* Draw a V-shaped line adjacent to the oval defect. It should be positioned the maximum width of the oval defect from the wound edge. *D.* Incise the V and undermine the skin edges. Approximate the oval-shaped defect with buried sutures and simple interrupted sutures. *E.* Draw and incise a line perpendicular to the apex of the V and equal to the maximum width of the V-shaped defect. This forms the V into a Y. *F.* Approximation of the Y-shaped defect.

not directly communicate with each other, the V-shaped incision allows the original wound to be closed primarily and without tension. Undermine the wound and the V-shaped incision. Approximate the oval-shaped defect with buried sutures, if necessary, and simple interrupted sutures (Figure 79-6*D*). This will result in an opening of the V-shaped defect (Figure 79-6*D*). Draw and incise a line perpendicular to the apex of the V-shaped defect with a #15 scalpel blade (Figure 79-6*E*). The line should be as long as the width of the V-shaped defect. Approximate the arms of the defect with simple interrupted sutures to form a Y (Figure 79-6*F*).

An alternative V-Y advancement flap can be used to close the injury without making a second wound (Figure 79-7). Draw lines to debride the wound and form a V-shaped defect (Figure 79-7*A*). Incise along the lines with a #15 scalpel blade to form the V-shaped defect and excise the wound (Figure 79-7*B*). Draw and incise a line

perpendicular to the apex of the V-shaped defect with a #15 scalpel blade (Figure 79-7*C*). The line should be as long as the width of the V-shaped defect. Undermine the V-shaped defect and the perpendicular line. Place a half-buried horizontal mattress suture to close the center of the Y (Figure 79-7*D*). Approximate the edges of the defect with simple interrupted stitches (Figure 79-7*D*).

CLOSURE OF A RECTANGULAR DEFECT

Wounds may be in the form of an ellipse or oblong (Figure 79-8*A*). These can be converted into a rectangular defect to allow primary closure.[3] Draw lines to debride the wound and form a rectangular defect (Figure 79-8*A*). Incise along the lines with a #15 scalpel blade to form the rectangular defect and excise the wound (Figure 79-8*B*). Draw lines to convert the short ends of the rectangle into triangles (Figure 79-8*C*). **The width of the rectangle should serve as the measurement to**

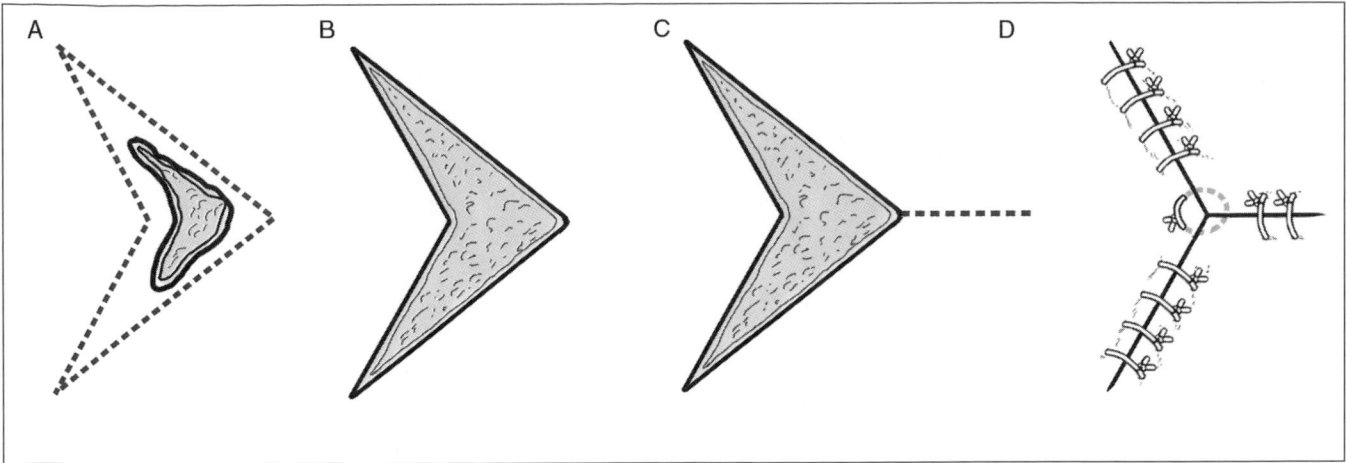

FIGURE 79-7 An alternative V-Y advancement flap closure. *A.* The original tissue defect. Draw lines around the defect to form a V. *B.* The skin has been incised and the original defect removed to form a V-shaped defect. *C.* Draw and incise a line perpendicular to the apex of the V and equal to the maximum width of the V-shaped incision. *D.* Approximate the center of the Y with a half-buried horizontal mattress suture. Approximate the arms of the Y with simple interrupted sutures.

create an equal distance between the base and the apex of the triangle. Excising triangles from the ends of the rectangular defect reconfigures the ends of the wound. Incise along the lines with a #15 scalpel blade and remove the triangles (Figure 79-8*D*). Undermine the skin surrounding the defect. Approximate the wound edges with simple interrupted sutures to form a straight line (Figure 79-8*E*).

CLOSURE OF A TRIANGULAR DEFECT (ROTATION FLAP)

Closing of a triangular defect can be accomplished with the use of a rotational flap (Figure 79-9). These flaps can be turned on a pivot point. **The flap must be planned carefully so that the direction of rotation co-**

incides with the geometry of the defect.[3-5] **Always plan and draw the arch of the flap carefully to visualize the pivot point and direction of rotation prior to making the incision. The creation of a rotation flap is a significant procedure. It can result in a vascular disaster and leave a deformity greater than the original defect it was supposed to correct. Do not create a rotation flap unless you have experience with this technique and know that the flap has an adequate vascular supply.**

Wounds are often irregular and elliptical (Figure 79-9*A*). Draw lines to debride the wound and form an isosceles triangular defect. Incise along the lines with a #15 scalpel blade to form the triangular defect and excise the wound (Figure 79-9*B*). **Draw the rotation flap very carefully.** The edge of the flap is an arch from the base of the trian-

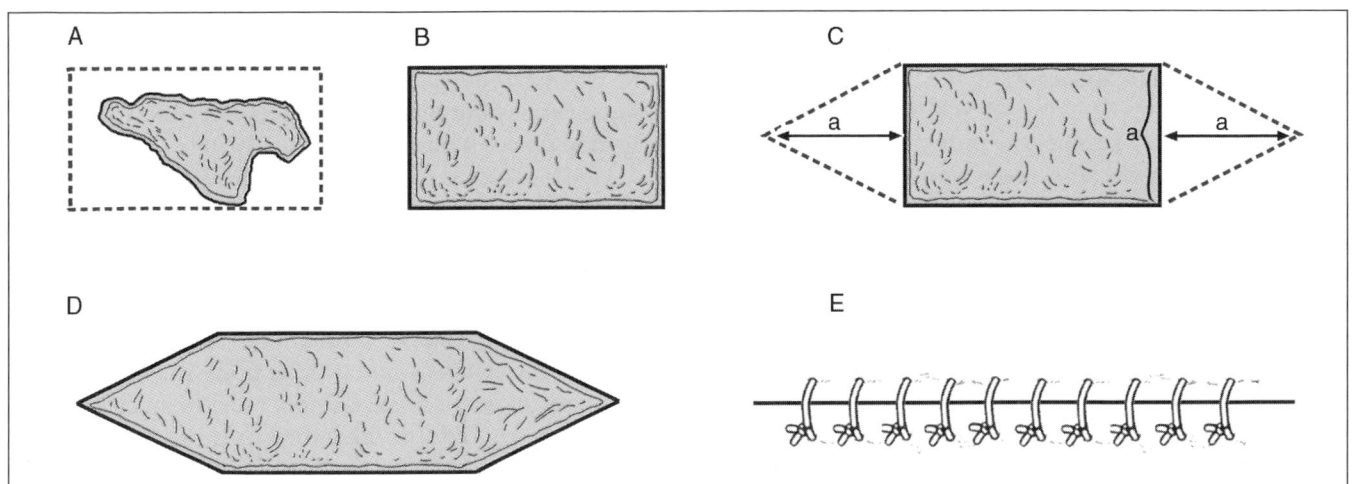

FIGURE 79-8 Closure of a rectangular defect. *A.* The original defect. Draw lines around the defect to form a rectangle. *B.* The skin has been incised and the original defect removed to form a rectangle. *C.* Draw triangles along the short sides of the rectangle. The length from the apex to the base of the triangle must be equal to the width of the rectangle. *D.* The resulting defect after incising and removing the triangles. *E.* Approximation of the wound edges to form a linear scar.

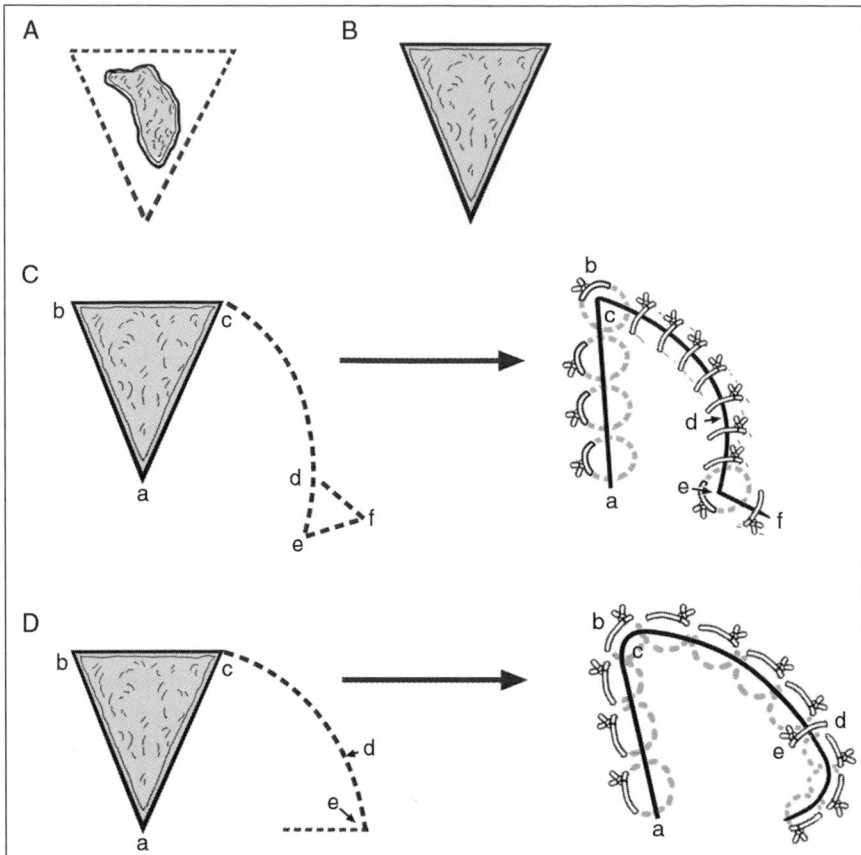

FIGURE 79-9 Closure of a triangular defect. *A.* The original defect. Draw lines around the defect to form a triangle. *B.* The skin has been incised and the original defect removed to form a triangle. *C.* Draw a line to extend the base of the triangle in a wide arc that is three to four times the length of the base of the triangle. Make sure that the arc is drawn beyond the line from point a to point d. Draw a Burow's triangle at the end of the arc. The base of the Burow's triangle should be half the length of the base of the triangular defect. Approximate the triangular defect and any corners with half-buried horizontal mattress sutures. *D.* An alternative technique. Draw a wide arc from the base of the triangle similar to that in *C* but which ends opposite the apex of the triangle (point a). Draw a line to make a back-cut that is three-fourths the length of the base of the triangular defect. Approximate the entire wound edge with half-buried horizontal mattress sutures.

gle and three to four times longer than the actual base of the triangle (Figures 79-9*C* and *D*).[3] Draw a second triangle as a Burow's triangle in the area next to the pivot point of the flap (Figure 79-9*C*).[3–5] **The base of the Burow's triangle should be half the length of the base of the triangular defect, with one corner of the base formed by the end of the arch.** Incise along the lines with a #15 scalpel blade. Remove the Burow's triangle. Undermine the rotation flap and the surrounding skin. Rotate the flap to close the defect and approximate the wound edges with interrupted sutures (Figure 79-9*C*). Place half-buried horizontal mattress sutures to approximate the triangular defect and any corners. Place simple interrupted sutures to approximate the remaining wound edges.

A triangular defect may be closed with a modification to the above technique when there is minimal room to form and excise the Burow's triangle or if lines of skin tension limit the location of the pivot point.[3] **This modified technique should be considered only when necessary, which may occur from poor planning of the initial flap or in areas where fascia can be separated from the subcutaneous layer (scalp wounds and areas involving the trunk).[3–5]** Form the triangle to debride the wound and draw the arch as described previously. **Do not draw the area beyond the point perpendicular to the apex of the triangle (Figure 79-9*D*).** Rather than drawing a

Burow's triangle for excision, draw a line to make a back-cut from the pivot point (the end of the arc) and along the base of the flap (Figure 79-9*D*).[3,5] **This line should be three-fourths the length of the base of the triangular defect.** Incise along the lines with a #15 scalpel blade. Undermine the defect and the rotation flap. Rotate the flap to close the defect and approximate the entire wound edge with half-buried horizontal mattress sutures (Figure 79-9*D*). Suture the back-cut prior to closing the triangular defect or the arch.[3] **This alternative technique carries the risk of having a poor blood supply to the flap due to its small base.**

CLOSURE OF AN OVAL DEFECT

Oval defects can be closed by creating a rotational or interpolation flap from the intact adjacent tissue (Figure 79-10).[3] Wounds are often irregular and elliptical (Figure 79-10*A*). Choose a side of the oval defect to form the flap. The adjacent skin used to make the flap must be vascularly intact to avoid the risk of tissue necrosis once the flap is sutured into position. Draw lines to debride the wound and form an oval defect (Figure 79-10*A*). Incise along the lines with a #15 scalpel blade to form the oval defect and excise the wound (Figure 79-10*B*). **Draw the rotation flap very carefully. Draw a mirror image of the defect abutting the original wound (Figure 79-10*C*).**

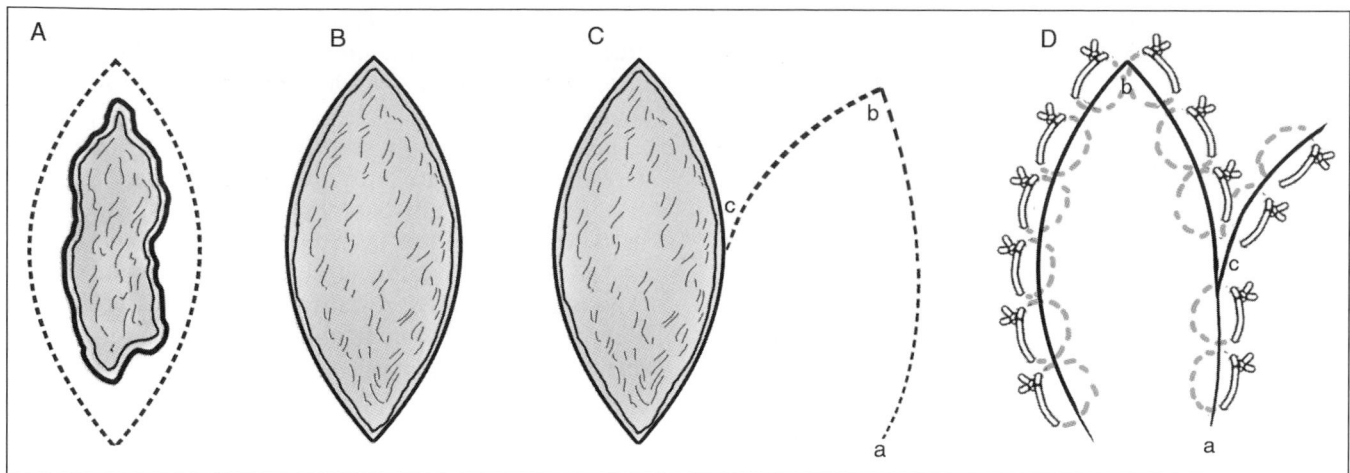

FIGURE 79-10 Closure of an oval-shaped defect. *A.* The original defect. Draw lines around the defect to form a rectangle. *B.* The skin has been incised and the original defect removed to form an oval. *C.* Draw a mirror image of the defect so that it is abutting the defect. *D.* The flap has been rotated and the wound margins approximated with half-buried horizontal mattress sutures.

Incise only along the lines noted with a #15 scalpel blade. Undermine the rotation flap and surrounding skin. Rotate the flap to close the defect (Figure 79-10*D*). Approximate the edges of the flap with half-buried horizontal mattress sutures (Figure 79-10*D*). Approximate the wound from where thc flap originated with simple interrupted sutures, if it is not excessively large or under tension, or with half-buried horizontal mattress sutures.

CLOSURE OF A CIRCULAR DEFECT

Some defects can be closed primarily. Examples include circular defects or triangular defects that are con-

verted to ellipses (Figure 79-11). Excise the tissue defect to form a circle. Excise a surrounding ellipse of tissue centered about the circle (Figure 79-11*A*). **The ellipse must be 2½ to 3 times as long as its greatest width.** Undermine the edges of the ellipse. Close the resulting defect with deep suturcs if required and cutaneous sutures (Figure 79-11*B*).

Larger defects require the use of a double V-Y closure (Figure 79-12). Create two sliding pedicle flaps with a #15 scalpel blade. **Incise the skin and dermis but not the underlying subcutaneous tissue**, to form an ellipse centered about the tissue defect (Figure 79-12*A*). Remove

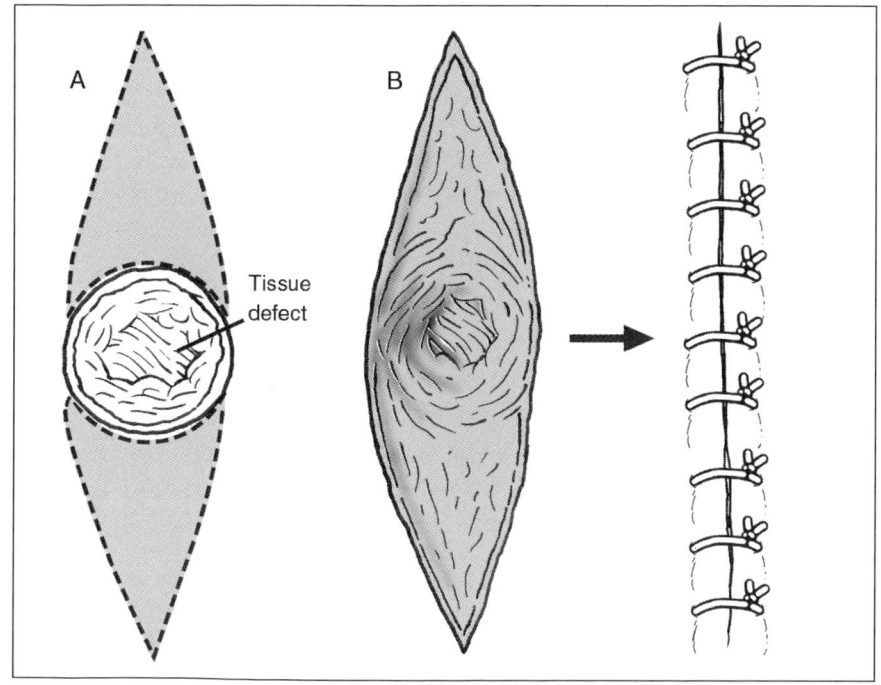

FIGURE 79-11 Closure of a circular tissue defect. *A.* Excise the defect and a surrounding ellipse. *B.* Approximation of the wound edges with deep and cutaneous sutures.

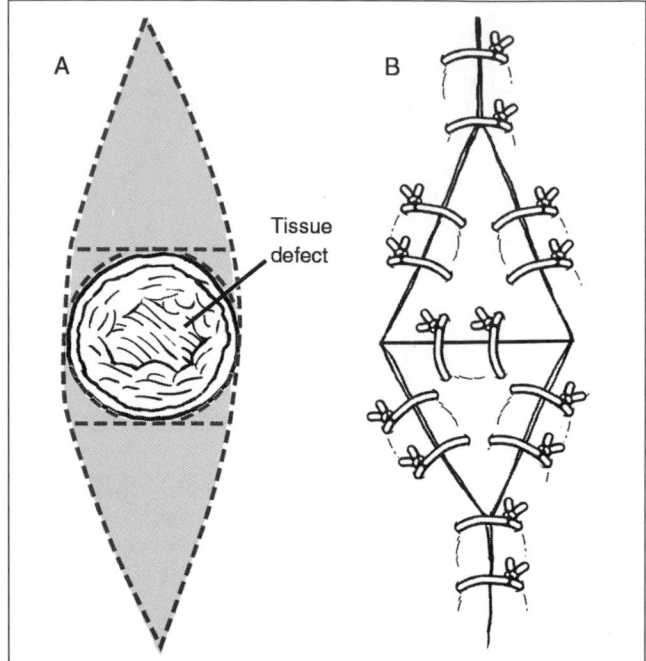

FIGURE 79-12 The double V-Y closure to repair a tissue defect. *A.* Create an ellipse centered about the tissue defect. Remove the tissue defect and form straight edges at the bases of the triangular flaps. *B.* Approximate the bases of the triangular flaps, followed by the arms and bases of the "Y's," using simple interrupted sutures.

the tissue defect and debride the tissues at the base of the flaps to form two straight edges (Figure 79-12*A*). Gently undermine the edges of the ellipse. **Do not undermine the triangular tissue flaps, so that their vascular supply is preserved.** Slide (advance) the flaps on their subcutaneous pedicles until the bases are touching. Approximate the base of one flap to the other using simple interrupted sutures (Figure 79-12*B*). Approximate the arms and bases of the Y's using simple interrupted sutures.

ASSESSMENT

Inspect the wound edges carefully for adequate approximation. Observe the wound for a period of time to make sure that it remains viable and is not compromised due to a poor blood supply or tight sutures. **A nonviable repair requires immediate removal of the sutures and consultation with a Plastic Surgeon.**

AFTERCARE

Pull the suture knots lying directly over the wound margin to one side so that all the knots lie on the same side. Wipe off any residual povidone iodine solution with sterile saline. Apply a topical antibiotic ointment to the wound, followed by sterile gauze or a nonadherent dressing. Arrange follow-up in 24 hours with the patient's Primary Care Provider, a Plastic Surgeon, or the Emergency Department.

Instruct the patient and/or their representative regarding wound care and dressing changes. Provide clear instructions of what to look for regarding possible signs of early infection, both localized around the wound site as well as systemic symptoms. Any patient who experiences excessive swelling, erythema, a purulent or foul smelling discharge, significant pain from the wound site, or fever should return to the Emergency Department immediately.

COMPLICATIONS

A brief discussion of the complications of wound closure is presented below. Refer to Chapter 77 for a more complete discussion. The complications of any wound can be greatly affected by the preparation of the wound prior to wound closure. The maintenance of sterile technique throughout wound closure and adequate irrigation of the wound will limit the risk of infection. It is unrealistic to expect any wound site to be bacteria-free.

Wounds may show poor scar formation or delayed healing due to several factors. Poor aftercare without adequate dressing changes or neglect (including premature exposure to environmental irritants such as dirty water, direct and excessive sun exposure, or chemicals) will likely result in a less favorable and unpredictable healing process. The wound site should be protected from excessive contact or use during the initial healing period. Mechanical trauma or overuse can increase the chance of edema or hematoma formation, leading to wound dehiscence or atypical scar formation.

Proper follow-up should be arranged and stressed within the initial 24 to 48 hours following the treatment and thereafter as may be warranted. Awareness that wound healing takes place in sequential physiologic steps is needed to properly direct patients, so that the risk of complications or the need for antibiotics will be minimal.

SUMMARY

Patients present to the Emergency Department with a wide variety of wound types. The use of local flap techniques allows the Emergency Physician to close difficult and complex wounds. If primary closure is not possible, these techniques decrease the tension on a wound and allow for appropriate cosmesis. They require close follow-up and appropriate patient selection if complications are to be prevented.

REFERENCES

1. Farrior RT: Management of lacerations and scars. *Laryngoscope* 1977; 87(6):917–933.
2. Rudolph R, Schneider G: Scar revision, in Georgiade GS, Riefkohl R, Levin SL (eds): *Georgiade Plastic, Maxillofacial, and Reconstructive Surgery,* 3rd ed. Baltimore: Williams & Wilkins, 1997:115–121.
3. McGregor AD, McGregor IA: *Fundamental Techniques of Plastic Surgery and Their Surgical Application.* London: Churchill Livingstone, 2000.
4. McCarthy JG: Introduction to plastic surgery, in McCarthy JG, May JW, Littler W (eds): *Plastic Surgery,* 3rd ed. Philadelphia: Saunders, 1990:1–68.
5. Place MJ, Herber SC, Hardesty RA: Basic techniques and principles in plastic surgery, in Aston SJ, Beasley RW, Thorne CHM, et al (eds): *Grabb and Smith's Plastic Surgery,* 5th ed. Philadelphia: Lippincott-Raven, 1997:13–25.
6. Ulusoy MG, Akan IM, Sensoz O, et al: Bilateral extended V-Y advancement flap. *Ann Plast Surg* 2001; 46(1):5–8.

Chapter 80

MANAGEMENT OF SPECIFIC SOFT TISSUE INJURIES

David A. Harter
Shayle Miller

INTRODUCTION

Blunt and penetrating trauma can lead to a myriad of soft tissue injuries. The management of the majority of these injuries is discussed elsewhere in this text. Some soft tissue injuries require detailed explanations for their repair. These injuries are discussed below.

WOUNDS OF UNEQUAL THICKNESS

Wounds of unequal thickness are not suited for repair with simple interrupted sutures. Unequal tissue loss on each edge of a wound creates a thick edge–thin edge wound. **The depressed edge must be elevated to the level of the nondepressed edge in order to attain proper wound apposition and cosmesis.**

There are two techniques to repair wounds with edges of unequal thickness. One technique utilizes a half-buried horizontal mattress suture (Figure 80-1).[1] Place the suture through the thick edge of the wound, across the wound and buried into the subcutaneous tissue of the thin edge, and back out the skin of the thick edge (Figure 80-1A). Apply traction to the suture and tie it to approximate the wound (Figure 80-1B). Apply an ointment-based compressive dressing.

The second technique requires undermining both wound edges at the same depth in the subcutaneous tissue plane (Figure 80-2).[2] Make an incision in the subcutaneous tissues of both wound edges and at the same level (Figure 80-2A). Undermine the area to free the tissue flaps (Figure 80-2B). Grasp the subcutaneous tissue flap from the thicker side and insert it under the thinner side beneath the undermined area (Figures 80-2B and C). Place a buried horizontal mattress suture to maintain the flaps in position. This "flap" elevates the depressed wound edge and facilitates appropriate wound approximation (Figure 80-2).[2] Place interrupted sutures to approximate the wound edges (Figure 80-2C).

Tangential flap lacerations over thin skin, such as the dorsum of the hand or the pretibial area, where there is very little subcutaneous tissue can be approximated with a specially placed simple interrupted suture. Insert the needle through the tip of the thin edge, across the wound, into the dermis of the thick edge, and out the skin of the thick edge. Apply traction to the suture to pull the thick edge up to meet the thin edge, producing good approximation rather than overlap of the edges. Apply an ointment-based compressive dressing.

MULTIPLE FOREHEAD LACERATIONS

Forehead lacerations are common in all age groups. Their visibility requires meticulous attention to detail. Knowledge of the principles regarding their repair allows for good cosmesis. The repair of forehead lacerations differs from that of other soft tissue injuries due to the role of skin tension lines, the lack of extra tissue, and scarring promoted by too many deep dermal sutures.[3–5] Forehead injury repair is governed by three principles: (1) skin tension lines run parallel to the skin creases and play a major role in the outcome of any forehead laceration; (2) lacerations running perpendicular to skin tension lines are more likely to result in a noticeable scar[3,4]; and (3) there is little excess tissue on the forehead to allow later wound revisions. **Resist the temptation to excise ragged wounds.**[5] This leaves enough tissue for the Surgeon to work with if further revision is required. **Place as few deep sutures as possible.** Deep sutures tend to promote more tissue reaction and more noticeable scar formation.[4]

All forehead lacerations require repair in order to promote cosmesis and provide hemostasis. Perform primary repair at any time up to 24 hours after the initial insult. This allows referral to a consultant if there is any question about one's ability to achieve satisfactory cosmesis or if the wounds are so extensive as to take the

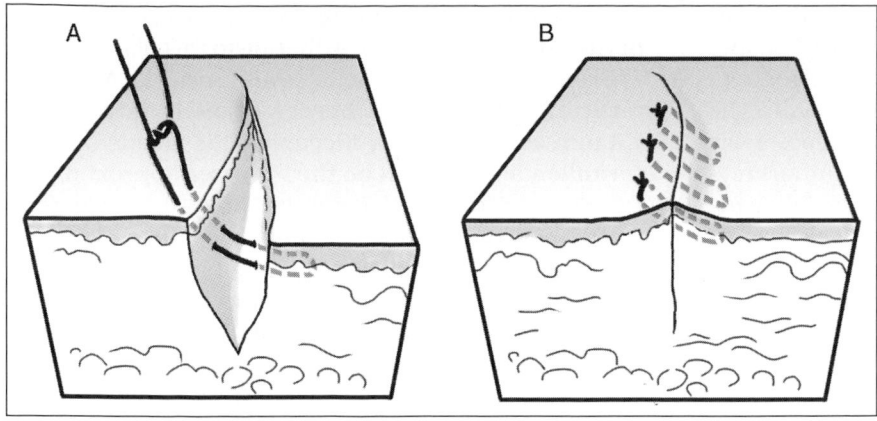

FIGURE 80-1 Closing a wound with edges of unequal thickness using half-buried horizontal mattress sutures.

Emergency Physician away from their departmental responsibilities for an unacceptably long time regardless of the level of complexity.

Laceration repair is dependent on the type of laceration. Close small and uncomplicated lacerations with simple interrupted 6–0 nylon sutures. Close flaps smaller than 5 mm using simple interrupted 6–0 nylon sutures. Close larger flaps using the half-buried horizontal mattress stitch. Allow partial-thickness abrasions and gouges less than 1 cm wide and 2 mm deep to heal by secondary intention.[3,6,7] Bunched-up, small flap lacerations can be excised together and the resulting defect repaired primarily.[7] This technique is described under "Multiple Small Skin Flaps" in this chapter.

TONGUE LACERATIONS

The majority of tongue lacerations heal well without intervention. Lacerations that do not require repair are generally small, linear, and superficial lacerations located in the central tongue region or small flaps on the edge of the tongue that can be excised. The tongue's generous blood supply allows these wounds to heal well. Some wounds require closure and can be very challenging to repair.[8–11] These include large lacerations (> 1 cm), gaping wounds, actively bleeding lacerations, U-shaped lacerations, wounds that bisect the tongue, and large flaps on the tongue edge. The main problem is not the repair itself but achieving control of the area to facilitate the repair.

Anesthetize the tongue via local wound infiltration or a lingual nerve block for the anterior two-thirds of the tongue (Chapter 154). These can be supplemented with procedural sedation techniques (Chapter 109). Instruct an assistant to gain control of the tongue. Grasp the anesthetized tip of the tongue with a towel clip, a suture through the tip of the tongue, or a gauze square. Consider inserting a bite block to further protect the patient and the physician from injury during the repair process. Thoroughly irrigate the wound. Close the laceration using absorbable 4–0 plain gut or chromic gut sutures. Take large bites that include the mucosal and muscular layers of the tongue. Buried sutures are not required in repairing tongue lacerations.

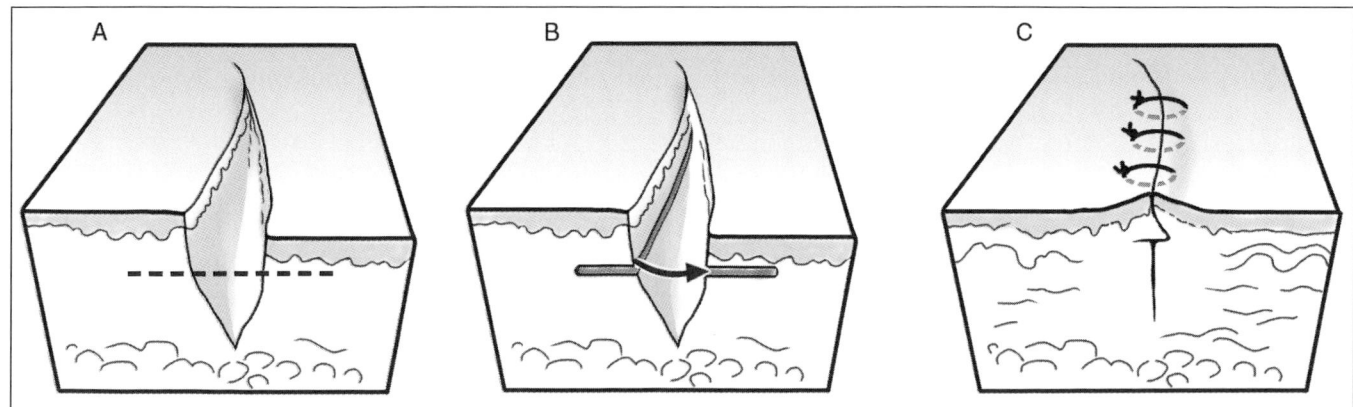

FIGURE 80-2 An alternative technique to close a wound with edges of unequal thickness. *A.* Make an incision in the subcutaneous tissue of both wound edges. *B.* Undermine the edges. Transpose the subcutaneous tissue of the thicker side into the undermined area of the thinner side (*arrow*). *C.* Approximate the wound edges using interrupted sutures.

Instruct the patient to follow the same aftercare instructions as for other laceration repairs with a few specific additions. A diet of soft foods and liquids is recommended for the first 2 to 3 days after the repair. The mouth should be rinsed gently two or three times a day and after meals with Peridex solution. Some authors recommend the use of prophylactic antibiotics following tongue laceration repair, although this is controversial.[12]

GINGIVAL LACERATIONS

Gingival lacerations differ from other lacerations in that there is often no subcutaneous tissue available to anchor the flap. Small gingival lacerations tend to heal well without intervention because of the extensive blood supply in this area. Repair wounds that are large, actively bleeding, gaping open, or that fall onto the occlusive surface of the teeth.

Flap lacerations exposing the alveolar ridge and tooth roots pose a special problem, as there is no subcutaneous support to anchor the mucosa. The technique requires the placement of a circumferential suture that is absorbable (plain gut or chromic gut) and tied posteriorly to the tooth (Figure 80-3). Place the suture 2 to 3 mm proximal to the gingival margin (Figure 80-3A). Place the suture through the gingiva so that it passes circumferentially around the tooth to secure the flap (Figure 80-3B). Loosely tie the suture on the inner aspect of the tooth so that the knot does not irritate the lip or strangulate the tissues (Figure 80-3B). The aftercare is the same as described under "Tongue Lacerations" in this chapter.

LIP LACERATIONS

Attention to detail is essential for attaining a good cosmetic result in repairing lip lacerations, as they can result in devastating cosmetic defects if not repaired properly. Anesthetize the lip using a nerve block to avoid tissue distortion and allow proper tissue apposition (Chapters 106 and 154). **Always close the vermilion border followed by the orbicularis muscle, the mucosal border and then the skin.** Adhering to this plan of attack will allow the best cosmetic result possible. **Misalignment of the vermilion border by as little as 0.5 to 1.0 mm will be easily noticeable. This means that the vermilion border must be the first area approximated.** Other anatomic areas that require careful approximation to attain good cosmesis include the mucosal border (separating the intraoral and extraoral portions of the lip) and the orbicularis oris muscle. Through-and-through lip lacerations often violate all three of these structures.

The first step in any lip laceration repair is to approximate the vermilion border or "white line" (the transition between the oral mucosa and the skin) using 6–0 nylon sutures (Figure 80-4A). Repair the orbicularis muscle with 5–0 plain gut or chromic gut suture (Figure 80-4B). Approximate the mucosa with the same type of suture. Take care to meticulously line up the muscle and the mucosal border. Close the skin with interrupted 6–0 nylon sutures (Figure 80-4C).

The aftercare for a sutured lip laceration is much the same as for a tongue laceration. Instruct the patient to avoid bringing excessive pressure to bear on the suture line. Remove the skin sutures in 4 to 5 days to avoid scarring.

DEBRIDEMENT OF GUNSHOT WOUNDS

The lack of primary literature on this subject makes it a controversial area. Wounds created by low-velocity bullets tend to cause damage only along the bullet track. Debridement is unnecessary for wounds created by bullets with muzzle energy of less than 400 foot-pounds, as many consider bullets to be sterile.[13] Devitalized and contaminated tissue is more likely to result from shotgun wounds and high-velocity bullets.[14] The shock wave created by the bullet damages tissue distant from the track of the bullet.[14] Consider these wounds for debridement.

Not all gunshot wounds require debridement. Consider debriding shotgun wounds and wounds from high-

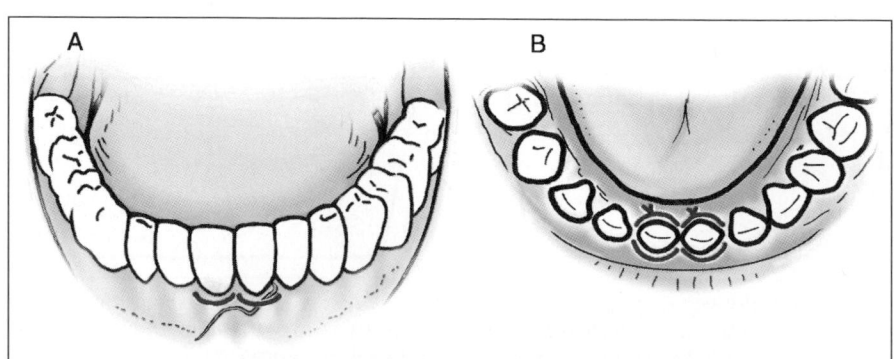

FIGURE 80-3 Gingival laceration repair. *A.* Place the suture 2 to 3 mm proximal to the gingival margin. *B.* Place the suture through the gingiva and circumferentially around a tooth to secure the flap.

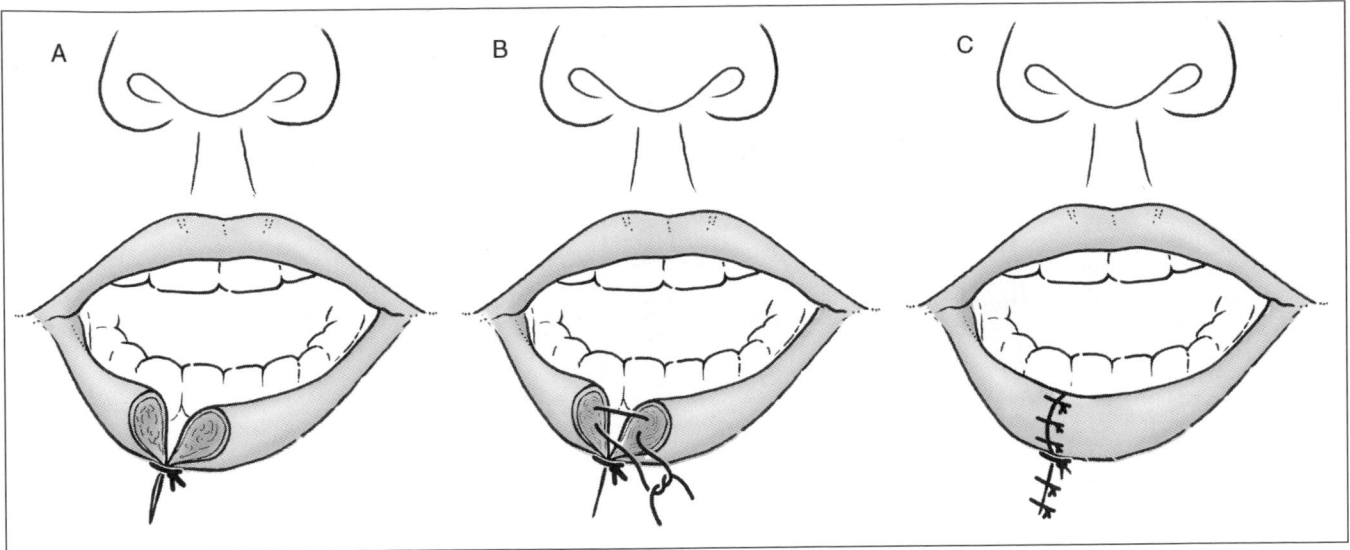

FIGURE 80-4 Lip laceration repair. *A.* Always approximate the vermillion border first. *B.* Approximation of the orbicularis oris muscle. *C.* Approximation of the mucosal surface and the skin.

velocity weapons.[14] These wounds are more often associated with tissue destruction and contamination.[14] The debridement of gunshot wounds requires exposure of the entire bullet track and treatment as a delayed closure, followed by referral for skin grafting if needed.

Clean, prep, and anesthetize the skin overlying the path of the bullet (or shotgun blast). Incise the wound with a #11 scalpel blade to expose the area. Sharply debride any devitalized and contaminated tissue. Treat the area with delayed closure techniques. Large areas of tissue destruction may require a skin graft for adequate closure.

AVULSION INJURIES

The treatment of tissue avulsion injuries varies depending on the amount of tissue lost and its depth. Allow full-thickness defects less than 1 to 2 cm^2 to heal by secondary intention after debridement. Full-thickness defects greater than 2 cm^2 require a different approach utilizing skin grafts, flaps, or converting the wound to one that can be closed primarily. Treat avulsed tissue as an "amputated part" that may be used in the repair process. Consider consulting a Plastic Surgeon for a large avulsion that cannot be closed primarily or to convert it into a wound that can be closed primarily.

Some defects can be closed primarily. Examples include circular defects or triangular defects that are converted to ellipses (Figure 80-5).[15] Excise the tissue defect to form a circle. Excise a surrounding ellipse of tissue centered about the circle (Figure 80-5A). The ellipse must be 2½ to 3 times as long as its greatest width. Undermine the edges of the ellipse. Approximate the

center of the resulting defect using a locked vertical mattress stitch, which allows approximation of the remainder of the wound with minimal extrinsic tension. Approximate the remainder of the resulting defect with deep sutures, if required, and cutaneous sutures (Figure 80-5B).

Larger defects require the use of a double V-Y closure (Figure 80-6).[15] Create two sliding pedicle flaps with a #15 scalpel blade. **Incise the skin and dermis, but not the underling subcutaneous tissue,** to form an ellipse centered about the tissue defect (Figure 80-6A). Remove the tissue defect and debride the tissues at the base of the flaps to form two straight edges (Figure 80-6A). Gently undermine the edges of the ellipse. **Do not undermine the triangular tissue flaps, so that their vascular supply is preserved.** Slide (advance) the flaps on their subcutaneous pedicles until the bases are touching. Approximate the base of one flap to the other using simple interrupted nylon sutures (Figure 80-6B). Approximate the arms and bases of the Y's using interrupted nylon suture.

EAR LACERATIONS

Ear lacerations can result from blunt or sharp trauma to the auricle. The primary goals are to preserve the normal contours of the auricle and prevent chondritis.[16] The skin of the ear is extremely vascular. The underlying auricular cartilage is avascular and receives its nourishment from the overlying skin. **Minimize any debridement of the auricular soft tissues to ensure that the repair covers all exposed cartilage.** Auricular laceration repair follows the same principles as other laceration repair techniques. Differences to be appreciated include

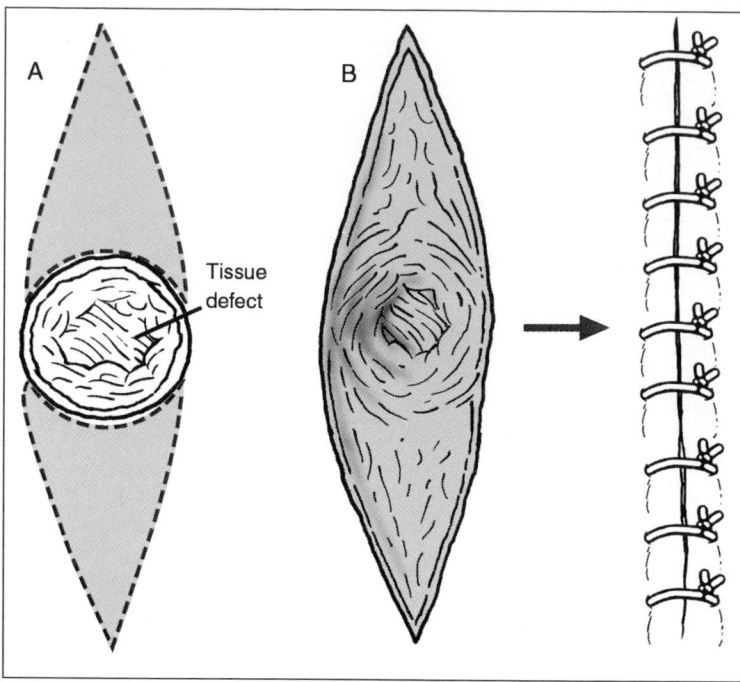

FIGURE 80-5 Closure of a tissue defect. *A.* Excise the defect and a surrounding ellipse. *B.* Approximation of the wound edges with deep and cutaneous sutures.

the importance of debriding as little soft tissue as possible, always covering exposed cartilage, splinting the ear appropriately after the repair, and realizing the indications for consulting a Plastic Surgeon (cartilage defects

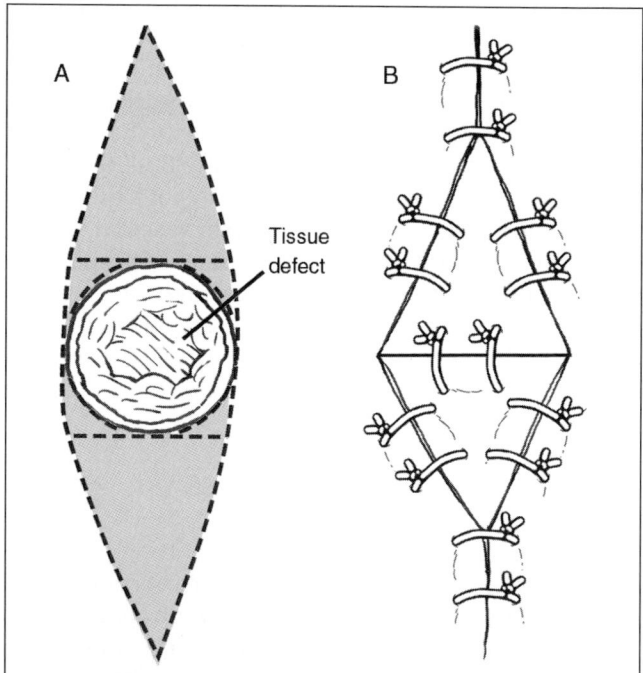

FIGURE 80-6 The double V-Y closure to repair a tissue defect. *A.* Create an ellipse centered about the tissue defect. Remove the tissue defect and form straight edges at the bases of the triangular flaps. *B.* Approximate the bases of the triangular flaps followed by the arms and bases of the Y's, using interrupted sutures.

> 5 mm, inability to cover exposed cartilage, and amputation injuries).

Clean, prepare, and anesthetize the auricle. Refer to Chapter 144 regarding the techniques of auricular anesthesia. Consider local infiltration for small, isolated wounds without cartilage involvement or an auricular block for complicated or extensive lesions. Use only a local anesthetic agent without epinephrine to prevent potential complications. Close simple lacerations primarily with interrupted 6–0 nylon suture.

Close wounds involving soft tissue and cartilage loss of less than 5 mm with a wedge excision and repair technique (Figure 80-7). The auricular skin does not stretch to allow coverage of defects. The wedge excision technique allows a primary closure that would otherwise have been difficult to achieve without distortion or buckling the anatomy of the auricle due to the underlying cartilage.

Excise a full-thickness triangle of tissue in the antihelix with a #15 scalpel blade (Figure 80-7*A*). Approximate the skin on the anterolateral surface followed by the posterior surface with interrupted 6–0 nylon sutures. **Carefully approximate the ridges and valleys to minimize the cosmetic defect. Place the sutures through the skin and perichondrium, not the cartilage.** The skin and underlying cartilage are so adherent to each other that it is not necessary to close the cartilage separately. A preferred technique by some, who believe that the cartilage fragments will be drawn together and heal much better, is to place numerous interrupted sutures through the skin and perichondrium on either side of the wound (Figure 80-7*B*) and then approximate the wound edges (Figure 80-7*C*).

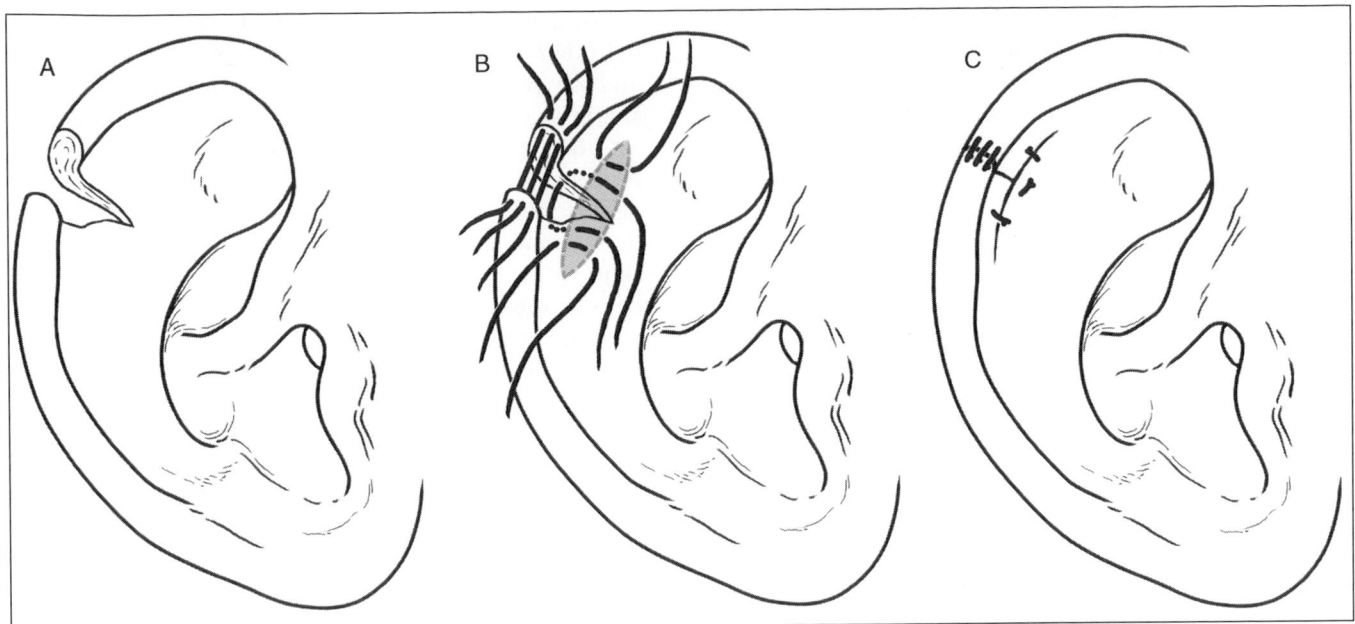

FIGURE 80-7 The wedge excision and repair technique for auricular lacerations. *A.* Excise a full-thickness triangle of tissue. *B.* Place interrupted nylon sutures through the skin and perichondrium. *C.* Approximate the wound edges by tying the sutures.

Auricular lacerations can involve one or all layers without any loss of tissue. The cartilage may protrude into the wound further than the overlying skin (Figure 80-8*A*). This type of wound is difficult to close primarily without debridement as the skin does not stretch to cover the cartilage. Use a #15 scalpel blade to carefully trim the cartilage back to the level of the skin or so that the skin overhangs the cartilage by 1 mm (Figure 80-8*B*). This allows the skin edges to be everted when closed. Approximate the skin and perichondrium with interrupted 6–0 nylon sutures.

Extensive lacerations of the auricle are managed in a similar manner. Trim any protruding cartilage as described above. Place interrupted 6–0 Vicryl or 6–0 Dexon sutures through the perichondrium to approximate the cartilage at important landmarks and remove tension from the wound edges. Approximate the skin and perichondrium with interrupted 6–0 nylon sutures.

Lacerations of the external auditory canal require repair only if the underlying cartilage is exposed. This is done in an attempt to prevent chondritis. Otherwise, pack the external auditory canal with a nonabsorbent wick (petrolatum gauze wrapped around a cotton ball) to approximate the wound edges and speed the healing process.

Consult a Plastic Surgeon for wounds with tissue loss of greater than 5 mm, wounds with exposed cartilage that cannot be covered without sacrificing greater than 5 mm of cartilage, complete or almost complete ear avulsion injuries, and injuries with obvious devitalization of the auricle. **Care for the avulsed auricle as an "amputated part" to preserve viability should the consultant desire to pursue reimplantation.**

Uncomplicated wounds not involving the auricular cartilage require local wound care and suture removal in 4 to 5 days. Larger wounds and those involving the auricular cartilage require oral antibiotics to cover skin flora and a dressing that conforms to the anatomic configuration of the auricle. The dressing will provide support and prevent an auricular hematoma from forming. Refer to Chapter 144 regarding the details of placing this dressing.

The complications following ear laceration repair are similar to those occurring after all wound repairs. Specific problems include the development of a chondritis, which is much more likely if the auricular carti-

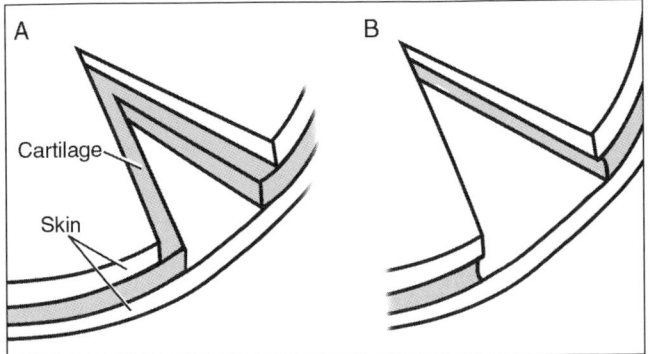

FIGURE 80-8 Repair of an auricular laceration. *A.* The skin has retracted and the cartilage protrudes into the wound. *B.* Trim the cartilage so that it is level with the skin or so that skin overhangs the cartilage by 1 millimeter.

lage is left exposed. Deformities can be due to the injury itself, poor repair techniques, or the development of an auricular hematoma secondary to poor ear splinting. Refer to Chapter 144 for a complete discussion of these complications.

FLAP LACERATIONS

Flap lacerations occur when shearing forces to the skin tear the dermis from the underlying subcutaneous tissues. This type of laceration is problematic. The flap is now separated from its blood supply except for the blood entering through the base. This low-flow state makes the flap susceptible to necrosis and infection. As a general rule, a flap will remain viable if the base of the flap is three times its length.[17] Flaps with a ratio of less than 3:1 are less likely to survive intact; therefore alternative methods of closure should be entertained.

Flap lacerations are unique in their tendency to necrose or become infected if the ratio of the base to the length is less than 3:1. Techniques such as debriding the fatty tissue from the flap before a primary repair or converting the flap to a different shape (V to Y closure or an ellipse) prior to the repair can increase the chances of successful primary closure. Healing by secondary intention or referral for skin grafting are other options in cases where the former techniques are unlikely to succeed.

A flap can easily be repaired primarily if it has viable edges and meets or exceeds the 3:1 ratio of base to length. Anesthetize, clean, and prepare the area. Trim the excess fatty tissue from the underside of the flap. This will improve the chances of healing. Place a half-buried horizontal mattress suture as the first stitch to close the corner or the tip of the flap. Approximate the sides of the flap with interrupted sutures or half-buried mattress sutures.

Some viable flaps have nonviable edges that must be debrided prior to closure to ensure proper cosmesis and survival of the tissue. Debride the nonviable edges sharply with a #15 scalpel blade or an iris scissors (Figures 80-9A and B). Place a half-buried horizontal mattress suture as the first stitch to close the corner. This is necessary to close the flap, as the debridement has left the flap too small to close the wound. Approximate the sides of the flap with simple interrupted sutures, mattress sutures, or half-buried mattress sutures.

Some flaps may be too small after debridement or be under too much tension to stretch across the wound. Close the flap by forming a Y closure instead of a V closure (Figure 80-9C). Place a half-buried horizontal mattress suture to close the tip of the flap. Approximate the base and arms of the Y with interrupted sutures.

A flap laceration may present difficulties. It may not be possible to revise and repair it or it may obviously be nonviable. It is often possible to "ellipse" the flap (Figure 80-5). Excise the flap and create a soft tissue defect three times longer than it is wide. Close the ellipse primarily with nonabsorbable interrupted sutures. In some cases, there is simply not enough tissue to cover the defect, no matter what technique is attempted. These wounds may be left to heal by secondary intention if small or referred to a Plastic Surgeon for skin grafting. The only complication unique to the repair of flap lacerations is the possibility that the flap may not survive, requiring referral and revision or skin grafting.

DISTAL FINGERTIP AMPUTATIONS

Amputations of the distal fingertip are defined as loss of the tissues distal to the insertions of the extrinsic flexor and extensor tendons on the distal phalanx. This may include skin, pulp, bone, the nail matrix, or the nail

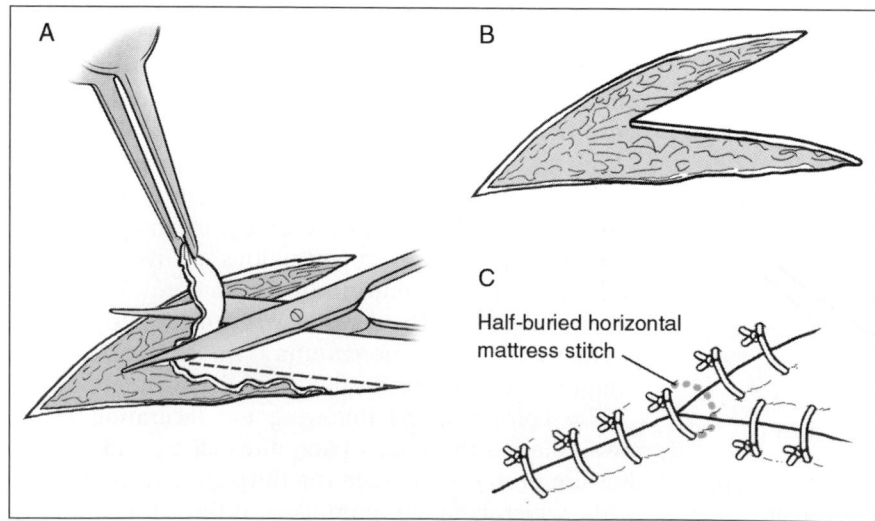

FIGURE 80-9 Repair of a flap laceration. *A.* Sharply debride the edges. *B.* The resultant defect. *C.* Approximation of the wound edges. First place a half-buried horizontal mattress suture to close the tip of the flap. Approximate the remaining wound edges with interrupted sutures.

plate. Treatment options have evolved remarkably over the past 30 years, though change in clinical practice has lagged. Multiple treatment modalities exist and depend on whether the amputated part was retrieved, its condition, the character of the injury, the patient's preference and underlying health status, as well as the availability and sophistication of consultants.

The long-held doctrine regarding the limitation of the extent of an amputation (< 1 cm^2) that can be treated nonoperatively and by secondary intention (conservative management) has evolved.[18–20] If the amputated part is unavailable or terminalization is preferred, conservative nonsurgical management with serial dressing changes of nonadherent gauze is appropriate treatment for distal fingertip amputations, both with and without bone exposure. Nonoperative open management has been shown to be as efficacious or more so than primary closure, local and distant tissue-transfer flap procedures, and grafts.[20–27] Anatomic classification schemes for the level of injury are multiple and make literature comparisons problematic. Therefore it is best to describe injuries related to anatomic landmarks.

No single method is applicable to all amputations. The literature supports the use of conservative therapy (healing by secondary intention), unless reimplantation is being considered, for amputations distal to the lunula.[20–27] Amputations proximal to the lunula are less common. Those who address the issue specifically recommend shortening and primary closure without discussion or data. These injuries require emergent consultation for possible replantation. Injuries from the flexor digitorum profundus insertion to approximately the level of the mid-nail can be replanted if the amputated part is available.[28–30] The purpose of replantation is the restoration of cosmesis and function. The patient's perception may be that replantation will restore functional and cosmetic normality. Inform the patient that this is doubtful.

Conservative therapy usually provides acceptable preservation of contour and better salvage of two-point discrimination than grafts, is cheaper than replantation, is associated with a virtual absence of postsurgical infections, and limits joint stiffness. It is equivalent to other techniques for time off work, preservation of length, and functional use. Moreover, eventual patient satisfaction may be even greater than with surgical techniques. Patients may have to be convinced that closure by secondary intention is both rational and, in fact, optimal. A set of photographs demonstrating this is often helpful.

Anesthetize, clean, and prepare the finger. Fingertip amputations tend to bleed profusely. Hemostasis can be achieved in some wounds with direct pressure using a nonadherent dressing while the hand is raised above heart level for several minutes. Do not remove the dressing if this is successful. Consider the application of Gelfoam covered with a nonadherent dressing and the application of pressure if the bleeding continues. Attempts at cauterizing bleeders are usually unsuccessful because of the tissue's vascularity. Apply a sterile Penrose drain as a tourniquet, without excessive constriction, to provide a dry field if debridement of devitalized tissue is required.

The presence of protruding bone poses several treatment options. Some physicians rongeur any significantly protruding bone until it is flush with the wound surface and thereafter continue open treatment. There is no published evidence supporting rongeuring of protruding bone in adults. Anecdotal statements supporting this technique exist in texts.[21,27] Published reports support not shortening protruding bone in children under the age of 12.[25,31] Consider trimming the nail bed back to the bone margin if a remnant overhangs or is not supported by adequate bone.

Dress the wound with either a bulky hand dressing or tube gauze and a four-pronged disposable (metal or plastic) splint. There is no documented benefit for the use of topical antibiotic ointment. The literature is inconsistent regarding the use of oral antibiotic prophylaxis, and there is no documented benefit. Some prescribe antibiotic prophylaxis only to grossly contaminated wounds, others use none (even with bone exposure), and still others use antibiotics in all patients. Refer all patients to a Hand Surgeon or Primary Care Provider in 24 to 48 hours.

Inform all patients of the 30 to 50 percent incidence of sensory impairment (diminished sensation, cold intolerance, dysesthesia), impaired function, or cosmetic deformity.[20,22,26,27,32] Document this in the medical record. The possibility of a wound infection is very small with conservative treatment.[24] Healing may be prolonged if protruding bone is not debrided or if it is debrided at a later time.

EYELID LACERATIONS

The objective of eyelid repair is the restoration of normal alignment and anatomic function. Eyelid lacerations are classified as marginal if they cross the eyelid margin or extramarginal if they do not cross the eyelid margin.[33] **A careful history and a thorough physical examination looking for concealed injury or foreign bodies is imperative.** The examination must specifically address and eliminate canthal injuries, lacrimal apparatus (most commonly canalicular) injuries, and/or deep structure injuries. Injuries medial to the lacrimal punctum must explicitly address the possibility of a lacrimal apparatus (canalicular) injury. Consult an Ophthalmologist for a probe evaluation of the lacrimal apparatus. Failure to identify canalicular interruptions can compromise outcome, as canalicular repair delayed beyond several days is less successful than primary repair. A delay of 2 to 3 days may be advantageous, as the cut medial ends may become edematous, whitened, and easier to locate.[34,35]

Recognition and management of injuries to deep structures—including the lacrimal apparatus, orbicularis oculi muscle, levator palpebrae muscle, tarsal plates, and medial or lateral canthal tendons—is necessary to prevent dysfunctional tearing, lid misalignment, ptosis, functional abnormalities, and cosmetic defects.

Awareness of the eyelid's anatomy is essential to the proper recognition and repair of less evident impairment due to injury. The eyelid's anatomy is complex. Certain key features are reviewed here as they are necessary to prevent overlooked injury and understand proper repair.

The eyelid's skin is the thinnest in the body, with that of the upper eyelid being thinner than that of the lower eyelid. The skin moves freely over the deeper tissues and can be easily mobilized with forceps. Surface landmarks include—from posterior (nearest the globe) to anterior (nearest the skin)—the mucocutaneous junction, the orifices of the meibomian glands, the gray line, and the lash line. The gray line is a key landmark. It consists of an isolated strip of pretarsal orbicularis oculi muscle just anterior to the tarsus (Riolan's muscle). There are three or four irregular rows containing approximately 100 lashes on the upper eyelid and two or three rows of approximately 50 lashes on the lower eyelid.

The levator palpebrae muscle arises from the roof of the orbit. It inserts into the midtarsus and overlying skin, intimately associating with the orbicularis oculi muscle. Suspect levator injuries with any horizontal laceration of the upper eyelid. Improper repair or failure to repair a laceration may result in ptosis or a deformity of the supratarsal fold.

Canthal injuries must be actively sought. Determine whether the medial or lateral canthal tendon is injured. Apply lateral traction on the eyelid. Displacement of the punctum laterally may be due to a disruption of the medial canthal tendon. Such a disruption is likely to be associated with nasal fractures, orbital fractures, ethmoid fractures, and canalicular injuries.[36] Apply medial traction on the eyelid. Displacement of the lateral canthus medially is due to a disruption of the lateral canthal tendon.

Evidence of a canalicular injury must be specifically sought after any injury medial to the punctum. Inspection and/or probing through the wound may confirm canalicular interruption. Secondary repair is less successful than primary repair within 2 to 3 days. Consult an Ophthalmologist, as meticulous repair is mandatory to avoid damaging the lacrimal apparatus.

The orbicularis oculi muscle closes the eyelids tightly. Failure to properly repair the levator muscle, the tarsal fascia, or the orbicularis muscle in a deep upper eyelid laceration may result in ptosis. Consult an Ophthalmologist for all deep upper eyelid lacerations.

There are at least six published variations on the techniques described for repair of the eyelid margin with less than one-third of tissue loss measured horizontally; there is no literature comparing outcomes.[33,36–42] The experience and skill of the practitioner are vital. Each minor variation aims for precise apposition to avoid misalignment or notching of the eyelid margin. Each technique varies the sequence, number, or type of margin sutures or the order of margin sutures (final or temporary) versus tarsal suture placement and closure (if required).

A recently published edition of a major emergency medicine text maintains that only Ophthalmologists or Oculoplastic Surgeons should close marginal lacerations. Consult an Ophthalmologist prior to repairing any marginal lacerations. Repair requires considerable experience, the use of magnification, and the placement of deep sutures.

Eyelid lacerations without marginal involvement are considered "superficial." Approximate these lacerations with interrupted 6–0 sutures. The skin and orbicularis muscle may be closed in one layer. Consult an Ophthalmologist or Oculoplastic Surgeon for lacerations involving the tarsal plates.

Eyelid lacerations with tissue loss require individualization.[34,36] Wound edge loss of less than 25 percent of the horizontal length of the eyelid can often be closed primarily. Approximate the wound edges with a toothed forceps to evaluate wound tension. Freshen ragged edges without loss of tissue. Avoid penetration to the conjunctival surface to avoid contact with the cornea. Accurate repair of the tarsus is vital because it forms the skeleton of the lid. Remove sutures in 5 days. Tissue loss of greater than 25 percent may require a canthotomy, cantholysis, or a tissue flap. Refer these injuries to an Ophthalmologist or Oculoplastic Surgeon. Older patients with skin laxity may be able to tolerate a greater than 25 percent loss with adequate cosmesis.[34,36]

Some eyelid lacerations without eyelid margin involvement may involve the levator muscle. Evaluate horizontal lacerations of the upper eyelid for levator interruption. Visible fat indicates orbital septum penetration and raises the suspicion of levator involvement. Ptosis related to swelling may simulate levator injury.[36] **An eyelid crease and/or minimal levator function will suggest an intact levator.**[36]

The orbital septum lies deep to the orbicularis oculi muscle. The levator palpebrae lies deep to the orbital septum. The septum is rigidly attached to the orbit and does not move on traction with a forceps. Grasp the levator muscle with a forceps and instruct the patient to look up. A brief pull will be felt as the muscle contracts. It is crucial to distinguish between the levator apparatus and the orbital septum. **The septum must not be included in a repair of the levator, as it will restrict movement of the levator.** Consult an Ophthalmologist or Oculoplastic Surgeon for deep extramarginal lacerations with suspected levator or tarsoorbital fascia/septal involvement.[43]

Complications associated with eyelid repair include misalignment, missed canalicular lacerations with attendant tearing dysfunction, missed foreign bodies, corneal abrasions, missed globe injury, missed canthal interruption, and missed fractures with entrapment. Unless the practitioner has adequate familiarity with the techniques, referral to an Ophthalmologist or Oculoplastic Surgeon is recommended.

ANIMAL BITES

Animal bites must be carefully explored to rule out underlying fractures, retained teeth, penetrated joints, tendon injuries, nerve injuries, and/or blood vessel injuries. Not all animal bites require antibiotic therapy. Some bite wounds may be closed primarily and others require delayed closure. **Adequate debridement and proper irrigation are imperative to a good outcome.**

Infections following a bite wound are polymicrobial. The most frequent bacteria isolated from infected dog and cat bites are *Pasteurella,* staphylococci, streptococci, and anaerobes. Human bites result in infections due mainly to anaerobes and less commonly staphylococci, streptococci, and *Eikenella corrodens.*[44,45]

Any bites to the hand, especially a clenched-fist injury human bite, are the most likely to be complicated by infection. Human bites in other locations do not have higher rates of infection than other types of lacerations.

E. corrodens is isolated from a significant percent of clenched-fist injury human bites, may cause a septic arthritis or osteomyelitis, and can be resistant to several commonly prescribed antibiotics (clindamycin and penicillinase-resistant penicillin). Severe infections occasionally develop after bite wounds.[45] Consider the presence of *Capnocytophaga canimorsus* infection in dog bites, *E. corrodens* in human bites, and *Bartonella henselae* in cat bites with persistent lymphadenopathy and/or drainage.

There are no prospective studies confirming the indications for repairing bite wounds. Primary closure with subsequent antibiotic therapy of head and neck wounds from dogs, cats, and humans have low infection rates in studies of a small number of patients. Suturing head and neck lacerations within 6 hours of a dog bite, following a meticulous debridement and irrigation protocol, was successful without subsequent antibiotic use.[46] Therefore, some bite wounds can be safely closed primarily while others are left open for delayed primary closure (Table 80-1). The issue of closure applies only to wounds of cosmetic significance. Allow wounds without notable cosmetic significance to be left open for delayed primary closure or healing by secondary intention. Do not primarily close puncture wounds, hand wounds, human bites, extremity wounds, wounds less than 2 cm in size, facial wounds more than 12 to 24 hours old, or nonfacial wounds more than 6 to 12 hours old. **Limit the use of buried sutures, as they can increase the infection rate of a repaired bite wound.**

Preparation of the wound for closure is of the utmost importance. Obtain radiographs of the bite wound if there is the possibility of a fracture, a retained tooth, or penetration of a joint. Debride any devitalized tissue, compromised tissue, or dirty wounds. Gently scrub the

TABLE 80-1. THE REPAIR OF LACERATION-TYPE BITE WOUNDS

Location	Dog bites	Cat bites	Human bites
Face	PC	PC	PC
Scalp	PC	PC	PC
Neck	PC	PC	PC
Trunk	PC if > 2 cm DPC if < 2 cm	PC if > 2 cm DPC if < 2 cm	PC or DPC
Arm	PC if > 2 cm DPC if < 2 cm	PC if > 2 cm DPC if < 2 cm	PC if > 2 cm DPC if < 2 cm
Hand with foreign body, extensor tendon injury, joint capsule injury, or bone involvement	Hand Surgeon consultation, exploration, and intravenous antibiotics	Hand Surgeon consultation, exploration, and intravenous antibiotics	Hand Surgeon consultation, exploration, and intravenous antibiotics
Hand with only soft tissues involved	DPC or secondary closure	DPC or secondary closure	DPC or secondary closure
Leg	PC if > 2 cm DPC if < 2 cm	PC if > 2 cm DPC if < 2 cm	PC if > 2 cm DPC if < 2 cm
Foot	DPC	DPC	DPC

KEY: PC, primary closure; DPC, delayed primary closure.

surrounding skin, and not the wound, with povidone iodine solution or soap and water. Copiously irrigate the wound. **Antibiotic coverage is no substitute for meticulous wound cleansing.** Refer to Chapter 77 for a complete discussion of wound irrigation principles and techniques. Some studies report lower infection rates when wounds have been irrigated with a topical antibiotic.[47] This cannot be recommended as standard practice at this time.

Bites to the hand require radiographs to rule out a fracture, retained tooth, or air in the joint cavity. Bite wounds, especially human bite wounds, involving a joint cavity or tendon require operative debridement and parenteral antibiotics. Bite wounds not involving a joint or tendon can be cleaned, debrided, splinted, watched expectantly on an outpatient basis, and treated with oral antibiotics.[48] Instruct the patient to keep the hand elevated and return in 12 to 24 hours for a reevaluation.

The use of antibiotics for an infected bite wound is beneficial. However, there is little concurrence regarding the routine use of prophylactic antibiotics. Data demonstrating effectiveness are limited. Differences in wound care, antibiotic regimens, and the severity of wounds makes comparison of studies problematic. Prophylactic treatment should ideally allow infection rates to be less than 5 percent.[49] There is a trend toward benefit for the prophylactic treatment of hand wounds and bites presenting more than 8 hours after the injury.[45,48,50]

High-risk wounds include puncture wounds (as opposed to laceration-type wounds), cat bites, bites to the hands, severe crush injuries, wounds in immunocompromised patients, and bites requiring surgical repair. The relative risk of infection can be reduced with prophylactic antibiotics (Table 80-2). Dog bites have the lowest associated infection rate of all bite wounds.[45,48,50] Higher rates of infection in cat bites may be due to the fact that a greater proportion of cat bites are puncture-type wounds that are especially vulnerable to infection.

TABLE 80-2. INDICATIONS FOR PROPHYLACTIC ANTIBIOTIC THERAPY FOR BITE WOUNDS

	Dog bites	Cat bites	Human bites
Puncture wound	Yes	Yes	Yes
Hand bites	Yes	Yes	Yes
Facial bites	No	Consider	No
Non-hand-laceration-type bites	No	Consider	No
Immunocompromised patients*	Yes	Yes	Yes
Surgical closure	Yes	Yes	Yes
Severe crush	Yes	Yes	Yes

*Immunocompromised includes age > 50, diabetics, alcoholics, asplenics, and patients with any other illness associated with an impaired immune status.

It is unclear whether all cat bites require prophylactic antibiotic treatment. It may eventually be proven that superficial laceration- type cat bites may not require treatment beyond irrigation and debridement.[51] Recommended treatment regimens for prophylaxis are 5 to 7 days for all bites with a beta lactam-beta lactamase inhibitor antibiotic (amoxicillin/clavulanate) or clindamycin and a fluoroquinolone for penicillin-allergic patients.[52]

Immunoprophylaxis may be required. Administer tetanus immune globulin and tetanus toxoid as indicated. With any animal bite, consider rabies postexposure prophylaxis. In North America, bites from bats, raccoons, skunks, and foxes carry a special risk. Consult the local public health department for guidelines and the incidence of rabies in your community.

The discharge instructions are just as important as the Emergency Department management. Provide the patient with a written copy of a wound care sheet, regardless of whether the wound was closed primarily. Instruct the patient to elevate any involved extremity, even with antibiotic treatment.[53] Arrange follow-up within 24 to 48 hours for a reevaluation of the wound. Physical therapy following a hand infection may be required and initiated 3 to 5 days after the infection resolves.[45]

INCOMPLETE LACERATIONS

Lacerations involving the epidermal and superficial papillary layers of the skin but sparing the deep papillary layer are referred to as incomplete lacerations. Excise the loose epidermal pieces of skin, then cover the wound with petrolatum gauze and a pressure dressing.

MULTIPLE SMALL SKIN FLAPS

Numerous small skin flaps that are bunched up, as commonly seen following a forehead versus a windshield accident, are difficult to repair individually. Excise them as a group to form a single laceration that can be repaired primarily (Figure 80-10). Larger and more "spread out" groups of flap lacerations can be repaired in a manner similar to that described under "Multiple Forehead Lacerations," above.

SUTURING THROUGH HAIR

It is inadvisable to shave hair bordering the edges of a laceration, as this only serves to increase the likelihood of a wound infection.[54] Instead of shaving the hair, brush it aside or mat it down using petroleum jelly or antibiotic ointment prior to wound repair. **It is of par-**

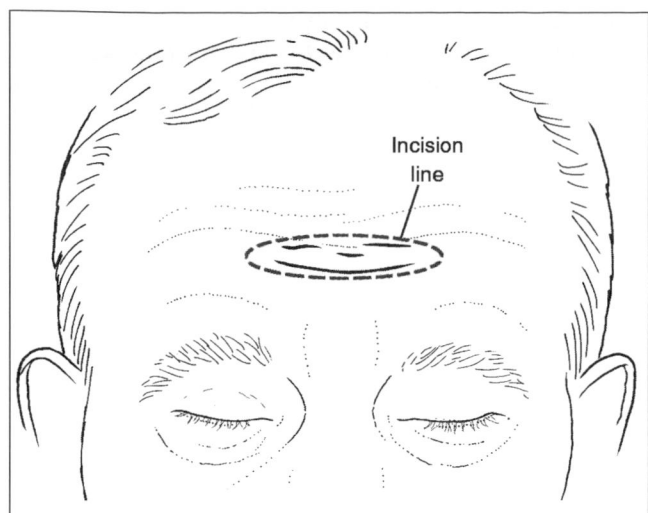

FIGURE 80-10 Repair of multiple small lacerations. Excise the lacerations as a group to form a single wound that can be closed primarily.

ticular importance never to shave eyebrows or eyelashes, as they will take months to grow back if they grow back at all. Always debride an eyebrow laceration oblique to the hair follicles and not perpendicular to the skin edge (Figure 80-11). This will reduce the loss of hair follicles.

ABRASIONS

An abrasion is a skin wound created by tangential trauma to the epidermis and dermis. The skin is forced against an abrasive surface in a rubbing fashion and the resultant injury resembles a thermal burn. The goals of managing an abrasion include the prevention of infection, promotion of healing, and prevention of "tattooing" with retained foreign bodies. Large and heavily contaminated abrasions are best managed in the Oper-

ating Room, as the volume of local anesthetic required to achieve anesthesia would likely exceed toxic limits.

Prepare the wound. Anesthesia may be required prior to wound management. Perform a field block or regional nerve block (Chapter 106) as appropriate. Large abrasions may be anesthetized by applying 5% lidocaine gel topically for 5 to 10 minutes. Remove any dirt, debris, and foreign bodies using a sterile scrub brush and surgical soap (or saline). Use the tip of a #11 scalpel blade to remove deeply embedded and larger particles from the wound. Apply Vaseline or Neosporin to remove embedded tar.[55] Apply an antibacterial ointment to the wound.

Instruct the patient to cleanse the wound three to four times a day. The wound may also be covered with petrolatum gauze and sterile gauze. Instruct the patient on how to properly cleanse the wound and reapply the bandage. Provide the patient with wound care supplies prior to discharge from the Emergency Department.

ORAL MUCOSAL LACERATIONS

Lacerations of the oral mucosa generally heal without intervention. Wounds requiring repair are those large enough to trap food particles (greater than 2 to 3 cm) and wounds with a tissue flap that falls between the occlusive surfaces of the teeth. Approximate lacerations with interrupted dissolvable sutures (plain gut or chromic gut). The sutures will dissolve and fall out on their own. Some physicians prefer to place silk sutures, as they are not irritating to the patient and do not tempt the patient to "play" with them with their tongue. The disadvantage of silk sutures is that they require a return visit for removal. The choice of using gut or silk is physician-dependent. Tissue flaps that fall between the occlusal surfaces of the teeth may be approximated or excised. Of more importance in the management of oral mucosal lacerations is the aftercare, as described under "Tongue Lacerations," above.

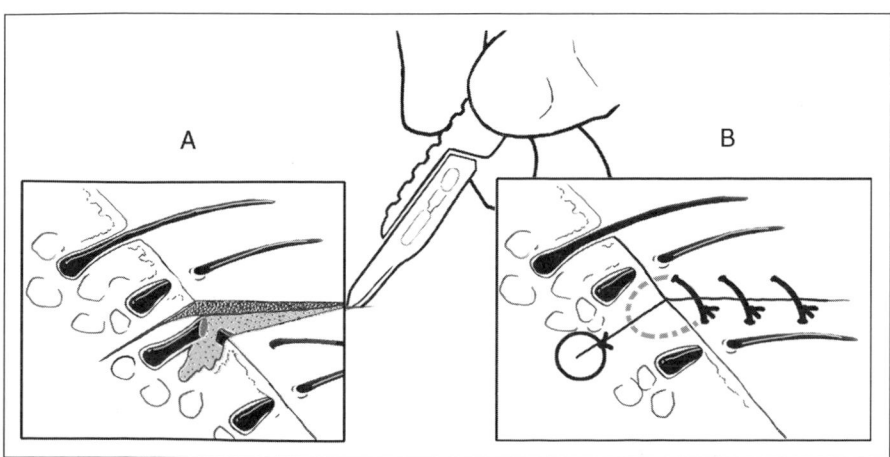

FIGURE 80-11 Repair of eyebrow lacerations. *A.* Debride the wound edges obliquely and parallel to the hair follicles and not perpendicular to the wound edges. *B.* Approximate the wound edges.

NASAL LACERATIONS

Important points to note in dealing with nasal lacerations are the extent of the laceration and the structures involved. Cartilage involvement increases the likelihood of developing a subsequent infection. Lacerations are difficult to close because the skin is inflexible and lacks redundancy. Associated injuries, such as nasal fractures and septal hematomas, must also be managed.

The repair of nasal lacerations requires local anesthesia, which can be achieved using an infraorbital nerve block (Chapter 106), a nose block (Chapter 146), or direct infiltration of local anesthetic solution without epinephrine. The nasal mucosa can be anesthetized using cocaine soaked pledgets (Chapter 146).

Lacerations limited to the outer aspect of the nose (i.e., skin lacerations and not through-and-through lacerations) can be repaired as simple lacerations. Minimize any debridement, as the lack of redundancy of nasal skin can result in disfiguring scarring.[56]

Lacerations involving the nasal cartilages require a thorough cleansing, minimal if any debridement, and a multilayered closure. **Do not place stitches through the avascular nasal cartilages, as this increases the chances of a postrepair infection.** Approximation of the nasal mucosa, subcutaneous tissues, and skin will appose the cartilage edges. The repair proceeds from inside outward. Approximate the nasal mucosa with interrupted 5–0 or 6–0 Vicryl sutures. Approximate the subcutaneous tissues with interrupted 5–0 or 6–0 Vicryl sutures. Approximate the skin with 5–0 or 6–0 nylon sutures. **Pay careful attention to the alignment of the tissues in order to avoid the postrepair complication known as "notching."**

MUSCLE LACERATIONS

The repair of muscle lacerations begins with a careful assessment of the extent of injury and the level of contamination prior to repair. Large and/or grossly contaminated muscle injuries require operative management. All other muscle injuries can be managed in the Emergency Department.

Lacerations of the fascia surrounding a muscle are common. Thoroughly cleanse the area and debride any devitalized tissue. Approximate small violations of the muscle fascia with interrupted 3–0 or 4–0 Vicryl (or other long absorbable) sutures. Closing small rents will prevent symptomatic herniation of muscle tissue through them in the future. Do not repair large violations of the muscle fascia. Anecdotal reports of muscle compression and compartment syndromes after such repairs abound.

Lacerations through the muscle require a thorough cleansing and debridement of any devitalized tissue.

Repair the laceration with 3–0 or 4–0 Vicryl suture. **Place horizontal mattress stitches to close the laceration.** Interrupted sutures are not effective, as they tend to pull through the muscle fibers and not hold.

REFERENCES

1. Trott AT: *Wounds and Lacerations,* 2nd ed. St. Louis: Mosby–Year Book, 1997:174–176.
2. Simon RR, Brenner BE: *Emergency Procedures and Techniques,* 3rd ed. Baltimore: Williams & Wilkins, 1994:332–333.
3. Lammers RL: Principles of wound management, in Roberts JR, Hedges JR (eds): *Clinical Procedures in Emergency Medicine,* 2nd ed. Philadelphia: Saunders, 1991:547.
4. Trott AT: *Wounds and Lacerations,* 2nd ed. St. Louis: Mosby–Year Book, 1997:183.
5. Duschoff IM: About face. *Emerg Med* 1974; 11:25–77.
6. Trott AT: *Wounds and Lacerations,* 2nd ed. St. Louis: Mosby–Year Book, 1997:183–186.
7. Simon RR, Brenner BE: *Emergency Procedures and Techniques,* 3rd ed. Baltimore: Williams & Wilkins, 1994:338.
8. Simon RR, Brenner BE: *Emergency Procedures and Techniques,* 3rd ed. Baltimore: Williams & Wilkins, 1994:90.
9. Trott AT: *Wounds and Lacerations,* 2nd ed. St. Louis: Mosby–Year Book, 1997:203.
10. Quinn PD, Loiselle J: Management of soft tissue injuries of the mouth, in Henretig FM, King C, Joffe MD, et al (eds): *Textbook of Pediatric Emergency Procedures.* Baltimore: Williams & Wilkins, 1996:741–749.
11. Lammers RL: Principles of wound management, in Roberts JR, Hedges JR (eds): *Clinical Procedures in Emergency Medicine,* 2nd ed. Philadelphia: Saunders, 1991:549.
12. Steele MT, Sainsbury CR, Robinson WA, et al: Prophylactic penicillin for intraoral wounds. *Ann Emerg Med* 1989; 18(8)847–852.
13. Hampton OP: The indications for debridement of gunshot (bullet) wounds of the extremities in civilian practice. *J Trauma* 1961; 1:368.
14. Tejani F, Aufses AH: A new technique for skin closure. *Surg Gynecol Obstet* 1976; 142(3):406–407.
15. Trott AT: *Wounds and Lacerations,* 2nd ed. St. Louis: Mosby–Year Book, 1997:171–172.
16. Liston SL, Cortez EA, McNabrey WK: External ear injuries. *J Am Coll Emerg Physicians* 1978; 7(6): 233–236.
17. Grabb WC: Introduction to the clinical aspects of flap repair, in Grabb WC, Myers MB (eds): *Skin Flaps.* Boston: Little, Brown, 1975.

18. Fox, JW, Golden GT, Rodeheaver G, et al: Nonoperative management of fingertip pulp amputation by occlusive dressings. *Am J Surg* 1977; 133:255–256.
19. Chow SP, Ho E: Open treatment of fingertip injuries in adults. *J Hand Surg* 1982; 7(5):470–476.
20. Louis DS: Open treatment, in Neviaser RJ (ed): *Controversies in Hand Surgery.* New York: Churchill Livingstone, 1990:21–26.
21. Söderberg T, Nyström A, Hallmans G, et al: Treatment of fingertip amputations with bone exposure. *Scand J Plast Reconstr Surg* 1983; 17:147–152.
22. Holm A, Zachariae L: Fingertip lesions. An evaluation of conservative treatment versus free skin grafting. *Acta Orthop Scand* 1974; 45:382–392.
23. Bossley CJ: Conservative treatment of digit amputations. *NZ Med J* 1975; 82:379–380.
24. Lamon P: Open treatment of fingertip amputations. *Ann Emerg Med* 1983; 12(6):358–360.
25. Illingworth CM: Trapped fingers and amputated finger-tips in children. *J Pediatr Surg* 1974; 9(6):853–858.
26. Louis DS, Palmer AK, Burney RE: Open treatment of digital tip injuries. *JAMA* 1980; 244(7):697–698.
27. Louis DS, Jebson PJ, Graham TJ: Amputations, in Green DP, Hotchkiss RN, Pederson WC, et al (eds): *Green's Operative Hand Surgery,* 4th ed. New York: Churchill Livingstone, 1999:48–89.
28. Goldner RD, Urbaniak JR: Replantation, in Green DP, Hotchkiss RN, Pederson WC, et al (eds): *Green's Operative Hand Surgery,* 4th ed. New York: Churchill Livingstone, 1999:1139–1157.
29. Shaw Wilgas EF: Replantation, in Neviaser RJ (ed): *Controversies in Hand Surgery.* New York: Churchill Livingstone, 1990:3–7.
30. Foucher G, Norris RW: Distal and very distal digital replantations. *Br J Plast Surg* 1992; 45:199–203.
31. Douglas BS: Conservative management of guillotine amputation of the finger in children. *Aust Paediatr J* 1972; 8:86–89.
32. Bojsen-Moller J, Pers M, Schmidt A: Finger-tip injuries: late results. *Acta Chir Scand* 1961; 122:177–183.
33. Simon RR, Brenner BE: *Emergency Procedures and Techniques,* 3rd ed. Baltimore: Williams & Wilkins, 1994:286–362.
34. Baker S, Hurwitz JJ: Management of orbital and ocular adnexal trauma. *Ophthalmol Clin North Am* 1999; 12(3):451–452.
35. Lemke BN, Della Rocca RC: *Surgery of the Eyelids and Orbit—An Anatomic Approach.* Stamford, CT: Appleton & Lange, 1990:108.
36. Rocca RD, Weiner W, Maher E: Lid laceration and avulsions, in Roy FH, Media PA (eds): *Master Techniques in Ophthalmic Surgery.* Baltimore: Williams & Wilkins, 1995:422–428.
37. Coates W: Lacerations to the face and scalp, in Tintanelli, Krone, Ruiz (eds): *Emergency Medicine—A Comprehensive Study Guide,* 5th ed. New York: McGraw Hill, 2000:303–309.
38. Lemke BN, Della Rocca RC: *Surgery of the Eyelids and Orbit—An Anatomic Approach.* Stamford, CT: Appleton & Lange, 1990:212.
39. Smith BC, Cherubini: Transmarginal lacerations—suturing techniques, in Smith BC (ed): *Oculoplastic Surgery: A Compendium of Principles and Techniques.* St. Louis: Mosby, 1970:9–10.
40. Reeh MJ: *Practical Ophthalmic Plastic and Reconstructive Surgery.* London: Henry Kimpton, 1976:44–45.
41. Beyer-Machule CK: Operations on the eyelids, the lacrimal apparatus, and the orbit, in Naumann HH, Helms J, Herberhold C, et al (eds): *Head and Neck Surgery,* 2nd ed. New York: Thieme, 1998:169–181.
42. Lemke BN, Della Rocca RC: *Surgery of the Eyelids and Orbit—An Anatomic Approach.* Stamford, DT: Appleton & Lange, 1990:211–212.
43. Marrone AC: Eyelid and canalicular trauma, in Roy FH (ed): *Master Techniques in Ophthalmic Surgery.* Baltimore: Williams & Wilkins, 1995:83–96.
44. Talan, DA, Citron, DM, Abrahamian FM, et al: Bacteriologic analysis of infected dog and cat bites. *N Engl J Med* 1999; 340:85–92.
45. Smith PF: Treating mamalian bite wounds. *J Clin Pharm Ther* 2000; 25(2):85–99.
46. Guy RJ, Zook EG: Successful treatment of acute head and neck dog bite wounds without antibiotics. *Ann Plast Surg* 1986; 17(1):45–48.
47. Sabiston: *Textbook of Surgery,* 15th ed. Philadelphia: Saunders, 1997:289–290.
48. Zubowicz VN, Gravier M: Management of early human bites of the hand: a prospective randomized study. *Plast Reconstr Surg* 1991; 88(1):111–114.
49. Fleisher GR: The management of bite wounds. *N Engl J Med* 1999; 340(2):138–140.
50. Dire DJ: Management of animal bites. *Acad Emerg Med* 1994; 1(2):178–179.
51. Dire DJ: Cat bite wounds: risk factors for infection. *Ann Emerg Med* 1991; 20(9):973–979.
52. Talan DA: New concepts in antimicrobial therapy for emergency department infections. *Ann Emerg Med* 1999; 34(4):503–516.
53. Goldstein EJC: Bite wounds and infection. *Clin Infect Dis* 1992; 14:633–640.
54. Seropian R, Reynolds BM: Wound infections after preoperative depilatory versus razor preparation. *Am J Surg* 1971; 121(3):251–254.
55. Demling RH, Buerstatte WR, Perea A: Management of hot tar burns. *J Trauma* 1980; 20(3):242.
56. Spira M, Gerow FJ, Hardy SB: Windshield injuries of the face. *J Trauma* 1968; 8(4):513–526.

Chapter 81

SUBCUTANEOUS FOREIGN BODY IDENTIFICATION AND REMOVAL

Samuel J. Gutman

INTRODUCTION

Wounds with retained foreign bodies are a frequent presenting complaint to Emergency Departments. Up to 38 percent of embedded objects are missed on the initial assessment.[1] Identification and removal of debris and foreign bodies promotes optimal healing of traumatic wounds. **The presence of an unrecognized foreign body can lead to complications that include infection, pain, loss of function, joint injury, tenosynovitis, tendon rupture, and osteomyelitis.[2–5] Patients presenting with chronic, recurrent, or delayed skin infections should be assessed for the presence of an unrecognized foreign body.** Failure to diagnose and treat a foreign body is a common cause of litigation against Emergency Physicians. The presence of a foreign body may not be obvious. A high index of suspicion and careful methodical examination, including appropriate imaging, must be undertaken to identify a foreign body.

It is important to be familiar with the characteristics of different types of foreign bodies and the interactions they may have with a host patient. This information is crucial in determining the urgency or necessity of removal (not all implanted objects require removal), the appropriate imaging techniques, the approach to removal, and whether specialty referral is required. The removal of foreign bodies from subcutaneous tissue can be a frustrating and time-consuming endeavor when it is ill conceived. **The successful removal of a foreign body requires a directed history and physical examination, appropriate imaging, adequate light, anesthesia, exposure, hemostasis, patient cooperation, an uninterrupted time period for attempted removal, appropriate wound care, and assured post-procedural follow-up.**

ANATOMY AND PATHOPHYSIOLOGY

Only a small percentage of wounds actually contain concealed foreign bodies.[6] The mechanism of injury may give some idea of the likelihood of a retained object.[1] Crush wounds and puncture wounds, especially those involving the sole of the foot, as well as wounds deeper than 5 mm involving adipose tissue are associated with a higher incidence of foreign bodies that are often difficult to find.[6] Wounds caused by objects that shatter, splinter, or break in the process of causing injury have a higher risk of having a retained foreign body.[7] Lip or facial lacerations associated with dental fractures must be explored for pieces of teeth. Thorns, spines, or slivers tend to penetrate deeply and break. Broken-off needles are common foreign bodies in injection drug users. Objects greater than 4.5 mm in diameter that penetrate the skin may push fragments of epidermis deep into the wound producing an epidermal inclusion cyst, which can act as a foreign body.[8]

Depending upon the type of material retained and the physical form of the foreign object, excess inflammation may result. This can delay healing or destroy surrounding soft tissues. Retained organic foreign bodies trigger the most severe inflammatory reactions and can lead to chronic granulomatous reactions, periosteal reactions, osteolytic lesions, or severe infections such as fatal necrotizing fasciitis.[8–10] The presence of soil in wounds markedly lowers the concentration of bacteria required to cause an infection by its interaction and interference with white blood cells.[11] Wounds tend to be resistant to antibiotics when a foreign body is present.[2,3,12] It may be impossible to eradicate the infection until the foreign body is removed.[2,3,12] Metals that oxidize may cause mild to moderate inflammation. Some retained foreign bodies, like lead, have the potential to produce systemic effects, especially when in contact with pleural, peritoneal, cerebrospinal, or joint fluid.[13] Inert objects with smooth, nonporous surfaces like glass or plastic elicit a minimal tissue reaction. Retained foreign bodies that are not dissolved or extruded by the body's defenses become encapsulated, after which the inflammation will subside.[3]

HISTORICAL AND PHYSICAL ASSESSMENT

Patients presenting after an injury require a focused history including the details of the incident, the wounding agent, and the mechanism of injury. This information may suggest the presence of a retained foreign body and direct which imaging study may be required.[14,15] Historical features that may signal unusual circumstances or difficult wound healing and management include diabetes, renal failure, immunosuppression, lymphedema, or peripheral vascular disease.[16] Past anesthetic history and the potential for aspiration should be assessed if procedural sedation is to be considered.[17] Medications and allergies should be queried. Tetanus status must be confirmed and booster doses provided as required (Table 77-2).

A directed physical examination should begin with a brief inspection and documentation of the distal neurovascular status and function. An injured extremity must be carefully examined through a full range of motion to ensure the integrity of the tendons. Discoloration of the skin may suggest a foreign body.[8] Palpation may reveal superficial foreign bodies. Sharp localized pain with palpation over a puncture wound may suggest a retained foreign body. Adequate anesthesia, lighting, and good hemostasis are required to allow a thorough examination of the wound. **The examiner must avoid probing only superficially since the subcutaneous tissue can reapproximate and give the appearance of a superficial wound.** The wound edges should be extended with a scalpel to facilitate inspection if there is concern regarding a retained foreign body and direct visualization is difficult.

A retained foreign body can be ruled out with a negative predictive value of 96 percent for wounds less than 5 mm deep if the bottom of the wound is visible.[6] A gloved finger can carefully probe the cavity, being careful to avoid injury to the operator from sharp foreign bodies. Gentle blind probing with a hemostat is an acceptable and preferred alternative. A grating sensation that can be appreciated by the examiner is produced if the probe strikes a metallic or glass foreign body. Direct visualization is preferable when examining wounds of the face, feet, or hands. **Blind grasping within a wound using a hemostat should be avoided.**

RADIOLOGIC ASSESSMENT

Imaging is indicated in most cases where a retained foreign body is suspected but not found during wound exploration, when thorough exploration of the entire wound cavity is not possible, or if the patient feels that there is a retained foreign body.

PLAIN RADIOGRAPHY

Most foreign bodies missed during the initial clinical examination can be seen on plain radiographs.[14] Plain radiographs are readily available. Some authors suggest radiographic evaluation of nearly any penetrating wound involving an extremity.[1,4,18] Standard anteroposterior and lateral radiographs should be performed using an underpenetrated "soft-tissue technique" to increase the contrast between the foreign body and the surrounding tissue.[3] Visibility of foreign material in soft tissues is dependent upon its composition, relative density, configuration, size, and orientation.[19,20] Oblique and other views can be added to avoid superimposition of the object over bony structures. Even radiopaque foreign bodies may be invisible if they are projected over bone or impacted in bone.[21] Metal, bone, teeth, pencil graphite, certain plastics, gravel, sand, and aluminum are all visible on plain radiographs.[3,20,22] Glass fragments have been thought to require lead or heavy metal content to be visible. However, glass fragments as small as 0.5 mm appear on two-view plain radiographs if not obscured by bone fragments; and glass fragments as small as 2 mm appear in the presence of overlaying bone regardless of lead content.[23,24]

Organic materials and plastics are not reliably detected on plain radiographs. They may be indirectly shown as a radiolucent filling defect when the object is less dense than the surrounding tissue, making plain radiography worthwhile even in cases of suspected radiolucent foreign bodies.[25,26]

It is important to examine the entire radiograph for the appearance and location of an unexpected foreign body.[27] The evaluation can be terminated after adequate wound exploration and plain radiographs for a known radiopaque foreign body, if nothing is found. Other imaging modalities are required if there is a strong suspicion for a retained foreign body of the type that is not usually demonstrated on plain radiographs.

The advantages of plain radiographs include their universal availability, low cost, and familiarity to most physicians. The disadvantages include the inability to resolve objects with densities similar to body tissues. Plain films do not demonstrate anatomic structures that may be intervening between the skin and foreign body along the planned surgical approach. It may be difficult to accurately judge the depth of a foreign body using two-dimensional radiographs.[8] Despite these drawbacks, standard radiographs remain the most clinically practical means of screening for foreign bodies.[19]

COMPUTED TOMOGRAPHY (CT) SCAN

CT scanning can be obtained to rule out objects not routinely visible on plain radiography. CT is the modality of choice because it is more sensitive in differentiating densities and thus is capable of detecting more types of foreign bodies.[14,28–31] Subtle density differences can be distinguished with a narrow radiographic density window adjustment, particularly if a computer workstation is used to vary the gain and contrast.[29,32] CT images can be created in multiple planes and can demonstrate the relationship of a foreign body to important anatomic structures.[28,33] CT-guided percutaneous placement of a catheter or needle can guide surgical dissection to a foreign body, aiding in the subsequent removal.[28,33] The disadvantages of CT scanning include its higher cost, radiation dosage, the need for patient cooperation, and variable availability.

ULTRASOUND

High-resolution real-time ultrasound using a 7.5 MHz or greater linear array head, in the hands of a skilled operator, can detect nonradiopaque superficial foreign bodies with a similar radiographic density as the surrounding tissue.[8,34–38] This can include wood, small glass fragments, fish bones, sea urchin spines, and other vegetative material.[8,34–38] The scanning beam must be oriented parallel to the long axis of a hemostat, which can be directed toward the long axis of the foreign body.[35] Ultrasound also has the ability to localize a foreign body within three dimensions, thus helping to establish its relation to adjacent bone, muscle, tendons, and tendon sheaths.[36] Additionally, there is no radiation exposure. Preoperative ultrasound results in less damage to the surrounding tissues, reduced operative time, and reduced postoperative morbidity.[36,39]

The disadvantages of ultrasound include the level of physician skill required for its use in diagnosing musculoskeletal foreign bodies.[37–41] Studies assessing the accuracy of ultrasound have shown a sensitivity of 30 to 100 percent and a specificity of 70 to 90 percent.[41] These values have been mostly demonstrated in referred patients studied by Radiologists and certified technicians.[42,43] Usage of ultrasound by Emergency Physicians has a specificity of only 59 percent under conditions that replicate a typical Emergency Department situation.[43] Another disadvantage is that false positives can occur with tendons, old scar tissue, small bones, calcifications, fresh bleeding, sutures, or air in wounds.[8,38] Ultrasound appears to be less reliable than other methods for confirming the presence or absence of nonradiopaque foreign bodies. Lack of universal availability and the time required to find foreign bodies make it difficult to generalize a definitive role for ultrasound in routine clinical practice. Perhaps the best usage of ultrasound is in place of fluoroscopy to guide removal of objects located by plain film or CT scanning.[36]

MRI

MRI appears to be more accurate than any other modality for identifying wood, glass, plastic, spines, and thorns.[14,28] It is superior to CT scanning in detecting the presence and extent of edema, hemorrhage, and infection surrounding foreign bodies.[14,28] MRI's other advantages include the high resolution and contrast between adjacent tissues. It allows the precise localization of foreign bodies in three dimensions to aid in surgical planning and assessment of the need for advanced exploration, debridement, and irrigation. It does not expose the patient to radiation.[44]

The disadvantages of MRI include its lack of availability and high cost. Patients must be assessed to rule out a magnetic foreign body due to the risk of movement of the foreign body during MRI scanning.[45] Prior history of an ocular or other metallic foreign bodies must also be sought prior to MRI scanning to prevent iatrogenic injury. This often requires a thorough screening history and plain radiographs prior to MRI scanning. Gravel and ferromagnetic substances produce severe artifact.[14]

XERORADIOGRAPHY

Xeroradiography has been used to localize and identify foreign bodies. It is sometimes advantageous over plain radiography because of its ability to increase contrast between the edges of a foreign body and the surrounding soft tissue.[37,46] The disadvantages of this technique include the lack of availability and its high radiation dose compared to standard radiographs. Imaging of nonradiopaque objects, like wood or plastic, with xeroradiography does not reveal any detail that could not be seen on standard radiographs.[14,19] In general, other modalities provide comparable or superior information.

INDICATIONS

Every effort should be made to identify foreign bodies, even if they are not likely to be removed. It must be decided whether a foreign body needs to be removed immediately, electively, or at all once identified. Factors that influence the decision to proceed with attempted removal include the size and reactivity of the foreign body, its proximity to vital structures, and associated injuries. These must be weighed against the potential for further tissue damage and contaminating the wound.

A foreign body requires immediate removal if it is likely to provoke significant tissue inflammation or

injury.[3,47,48] Contaminated objects such as teeth, soil, or foreign bodies located in the presence of an established infection should be immediately removed.[3,11] Allergenic foreign bodies, toxic foreign bodies, or those causing hemorrhage or ischemia should be immediately removed.[3,48] Foreign bodies interfering with sensory or motor function, or having the potential for migration, should be urgently removed.[3] Foreign bodies in the hands and feet usually require removal as they may cause persistent pain and can sever nerves or tendons much later.[5] The foreign body may require removal for cosmetic or psychological reasons only in some cases.[1]

CONTRAINDICATIONS

The foreign body should be urgently removed under ideal conditions by an appropriate Surgeon when it is associated with a neurovascular injury or is located near tendons, nerves, or blood vessels.[1,3] Deep exploration of the hands should be avoided to prevent injuring the intricate structures. Large, deep, and impaled foreign bodies are assumed to be tamponading hemorrhage, should initially be left in place, and urgently removed in the Operating Room.[27] Foreign bodies associated with fractures or located within a joint require prompt surgical debridement to prevent osteomyelitis.[48] Urgent surgical intervention is required for all high-pressure injection accidents. These injuries may initially appear innocuous but often cause extensive damage and carry a significantly high risk of complications.[48] Consider referral based on one's own experience, anticipated problems related to the foreign body's location or depth of penetration, the duration of retention, or other patient factors likely to complicate the procedure or follow-up.

A deeply embedded, inert object not near vital structures can be left alone. The difficulty of removal is usually not worth the potential tissue damage. These patients can be referred for elective removal, if necessary.[1,48] **If the decision is made not to remove a foreign body, the patient must be informed and the issues discussed including the potential for migration and infection.**

EQUIPMENT

18 gauge needles
27 gauge needles
10 mL Syringes
Povidone iodine or chlorhexidine solution
Lidocaine (1%) with and without epinephrine
Depilatory wax, rubber cement, or hardening facial gel

#11 scalpel blade
#15 scalpel blade
Scalpel handle
Nylon suture, 1–0 or 2–0
Methylene blue
Paper clips
Wire grid
Eye magnet
Hemoclips
Hemoclip applier
Fluoroscopy unit
Hemostats, two sizes
Forceps
22 gauge needles for foreign-body localization
Magnification eye loupes
Normal saline
19 gauge blunt-tip needle or angiocatheter
35 mL syringe
Blood pressure cuff or Penrose drains
4×4 gauze squares
Adhesive tape

PATIENT PREPARATION

Foreign body removal can be frustrating and time consuming, even when performed under ideal conditions. It is appropriate to set a time limit that is reasonable based upon the staffing and volume of the Emergency Department. Approximately 10 to 30 minutes is appropriate to find and remove an embedded foreign body. Inform the patient of the planned time limit at the outset. The search should be discontinued and the patient referred to a Surgeon after expiration of the predetermined time.

Apply povidone iodine or chlorhexidine to the skin site surrounding the wound. Avoid spilling the solution into the wound cavity as both are toxic to wound defenses and may increase the incidence of a subsequent wound infection.[12] Obtain a bloodless field for the examination. Place a blood pressure cuff proximal to the injury. Elevate the extremity for at least one minute and then inflate the cuff to a pressure greater than the patient's systolic blood pressure. Although it will cause some discomfort, this is safe for up to 2 hours.[49] A local vasoconstrictor can be used with the anesthetic to control localized capillary bleeding if no contraindications exist. A 0.25 to 0.50 inch Penrose drain can be wrapped tightly around a finger or toe and secured in place with a clamp as a tourniquet.

Adequate anesthesia is crucial to the procedure. A field block or regional nerve block, depending upon the location of the foreign body, best accomplishes anesthesia without distorting the wound further by local infiltration.[50] The techniques of regional anesthesia are described in Chapter 106. Procedural sedation (Chapter

109) or general anesthesia may be required, especially in children where cooperation may not be otherwise possible.

TECHNIQUES

SUPERFICIAL WOOD OR ORGANIC SPLINTER REMOVAL

Very fine foreign bodies can be difficult to visualize. One method to help localize them is to spread soft soap very lightly over the skin.[51] Only superficial organic splinters and foreign bodies should be pulled out with forceps as they often come apart leaving a fragment that is more difficult to remove.[3,52] Occasionally, cactus spines or wood splinters lie superficial and parallel to the skin surface. Make an incision parallel to the long axis of the foreign body and then lift it out of the wound. Enlarge the skin entrance wound with a scalpel so that the foreign body can be grasped and withdrawn with a hemostat under direct visualization if it is lodged in the subcutaneous tissue.

Small cactus spines may be difficult to locate and remove directly. Application of a depilatory wax, rubber cement, or a water-soluble facial gel with a brush can successfully aid in the removal of small fine spines.[47] Apply the wax, rubber cement, or facial gel over the skin containing the protruding spines. Apply a layer of gauze over the wet substance. Allow the substance to dry onto the skin and the gauze. Remove the gauze to lift off the dried substance and attached spines. Repeat this process as required to remove the remaining spines.

PUNCTURE WOUNDS

Puncture wounds of the foot are commonly seen in Emergency Departments. Punctures often drive pieces of clothing, shoes, or other debris deep into the wound resulting in an infection rate of approximately 10 percent.[53,54] Although often difficult, puncture wounds in the distal foot may profit from debridement and irrigation.

Puncture wounds can be trimmed or ellipsed to remove contaminated and/or embedded foreign bodies (Figure 81-1).[3] This technique also works well for foreign bodies that are difficult to localize. Make an ellipse in the skin surrounding the foreign body with a #15 scalpel blade (Figure 81-1A). Lift up the ellipse of skin and separate it from the underlying dermis (Figure 81-1B). The foreign body may be visible. Grasp it with a hemostat or forceps and remove it from the tissue.

If unable to exactly localize the object, the foreign body and the ellipsed puncture wound can both be extracted in a block of tissue (Figure 81-1B, dotted line).[50] **First ensure that no nerves, blood vessels, or tendons will be injured.** Alternatively, make the skin ellipse and extract the block of tissue containing the foreign body without dissecting the skin from the subcutaneous tissue (Figure 81-1C). Both techniques allow for the removal of foreign bodies and better cleaning of the wound. Puncture wounds of the foot require careful follow-up due to the risk of infection.

There are several alternative techniques if removing an ellipse of skin and/or tissue is contraindicated or if the physician is not comfortable with this technique (Figures 81-2 and 81-3). A foreign body may be embedded perpendicular to the skin (Figure 81-2A). Make a linear incision that passes 1 mm to the side of the puncture wound with a #15 scalpel blade (Figures 81-2A and B). Spread the incision open. Visualize the foreign body, grasp it with a hemostat, and remove it.

The final technique of removing a foreign body from a puncture wound involves making a superficial skin inci-

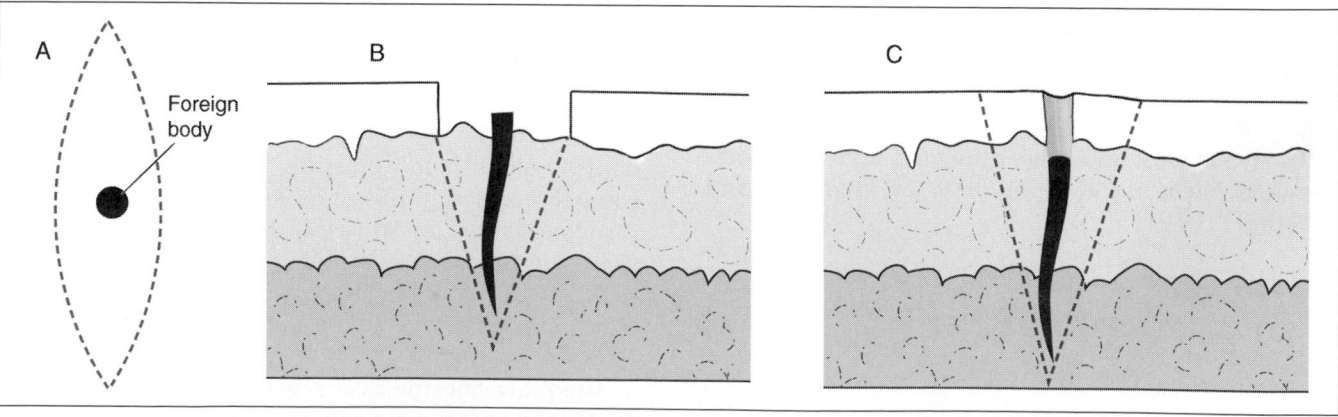

FIGURE 81-1 Creating an ellipse to remove a contaminated or embedded foreign body. *A.* An ellipse is made in the skin surrounding the foreign body. *B.* The epidermis is removed to expose the foreign body. A block of subcutaneous tissue (dotted line) can be removed if the foreign body is difficult to visualize. *C.* The skin, the subcutaneous tissue, and the foreign body can be removed *en bloc.*

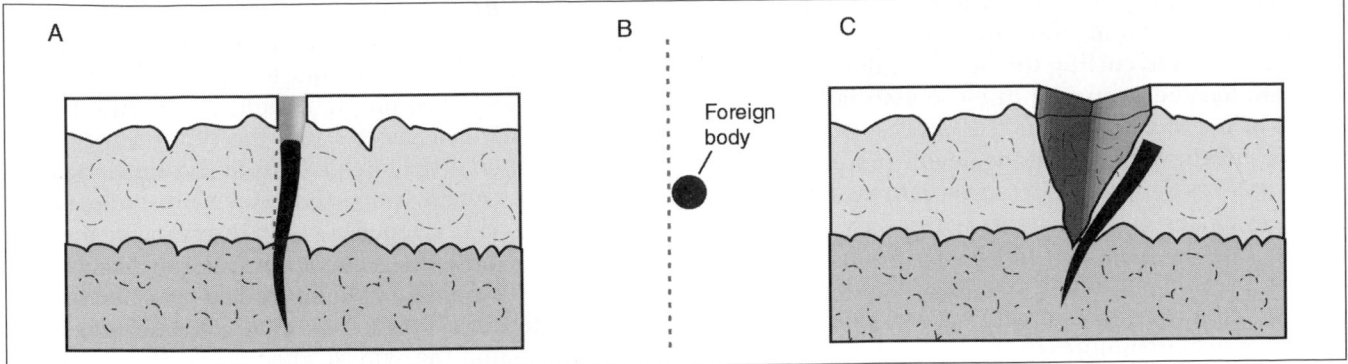

FIGURE 81-2 Removal of a foreign body embedded perpendicular to the skin. *A.* The embedded foreign body. The dotted line represents the proposed incision line. *B.* A linear incision is made 1 mm lateral to the foreign body. *C.* The incision is spread open to visualize and remove the foreign body.

sion and manually expressing the foreign body (Figure 81-3). Make an elliptical incision surrounding the foreign body or a linear incision over the foreign body (Figure 81-3*A*). Remove the ellipse of skin or spread the linear incision. Undermine the subcutaneous tissues surrounding the foreign body (Figure 81-3*B*). Apply digital pressure over the undermined areas to displace the foreign body into the center of the wound and upward (Figure 81-3*B*). Grasp the foreign body with a hemostat and remove it.

NYLON SUTURE TECHNIQUE

One technique described for use in fresh wounds involves the localization of a foreign body by marking its entry tract with a nylon suture.[55] Grasp a piece of 1–0 or 2–0 nylon suture between the thumb and index finger. Rotate the suture while pushing it into the wound so that it follows the tract made by the foreign body. It is reported that the foreign body is easily felt when the nylon contacts the foreign body.[55] Leave the suture in the wound tract. Open the wound tract by cutting alongside the nylon suture until the foreign body is reached, at

which time it is removed. A 92 percent success rate up to 48 hours after the time of injury has been reported with this technique.[55]

GEOMETRIC APPROACH FOR A NEEDLE IN THE FOOT

A technique that is useful for the removal of a needle in the plantar surface of the foot involves the use of standard anterior, posterior, and lateral radiographs to identify the cutaneous site corresponding to the location of the needle.[56] The incision site is determined by bisecting the midpoint of the needle, as seen in each projection, by a line drawn at right angles to the long axis of the needle. The ideal plane of dissection is perpendicular to the needle's midpoint, which is correlated with the surface anatomy of the foot.

Prepare and anesthetize the skin after determining the dissection plane. Make a 0.5 to 1.0 cm skin incision in the plane perpendicular to the needle in its midpoint. Advance an iris scissors into the incision and along the dissection plane with the blades slightly open. Advance the scissors 1 to 2 mm and close the blades. Withdraw

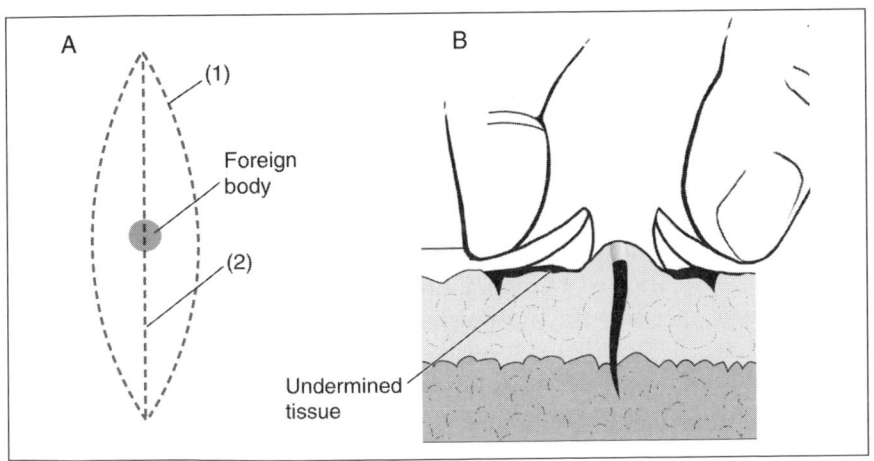

FIGURE 81-3 An alternative technique to remove a foreign body from a puncture wound. *A.* Incise and remove an ellipse of epidermis (*1*). Alternatively, make a linear incision centered over the foreign body (*2*). *B.* Undermine the subcutaneous tissue surrounding the foreign body. Apply digital pressure to visualize and express the foreign body.

the scissors slightly. Open the blades of the scissors, advance them 1 to 2 mm, and close the blades. **Care must be taken to avoid cutting the flexor tendons, although they are located deep and in close association to the bones of the foot.** Continue this process of advancing and closing the blades until the needle prevents closure of the scissors. Advance a hemostat into the wound and over the blades of the scissors. Grasp and secure the needle. Pull the hemostat out of the wound to simply back the needle out of its entry tract. This procedure is reported to have a 100 percent success rate and takes approximately 10 minutes.[56]

DYE TECHNIQUE FOR LOCALIZING A NEEDLE

Methylene blue may be used to track the location of a foreign body.[57] Identify the presence of a needle on plain radiographs. Clean and prepare the skin. Sterilely inject 0.1 to 0.2 mL of methylene blue very gently through the entrance wound of the foreign body. The dye will travel along the path of least resistance, that is, the path of the foreign body. Make an *A-, U-, V-,* or *Y*-shaped incision from the point of entry and raise a flap of tissue. The blue dot of dye serves as a guide to the location of the foreign body. This procedure is often complicated by seepage of dye and is therefore of limited value.

PAPER CLIP X-RAY LOCALIZATION

Simple paper clips may be used to locate a foreign body.[58,59] Obtain plain radiographs to demonstrate the presence of a radiopaque foreign body. Bend two or more paperclips into different shapes. Place the ends over the wound entry site. Secure the paper clips in position with tape. Obtain two plain radiographs taken at right angles to each other. Examine the radiographs to determine the cutaneous location of the foreign body in relation to the paper clips and note its depth from the skin surface. Mark the exact cutaneous location of the foreign body on the patient's skin with a permanent ink pen. Remove the paper clips. Clean, prepare, and anesthetize the skin. Make a stab incision at a 90 degree angle to the middle of the foreign body, taking the shortest distance between the skin and the foreign body, and following the method discussed for the geometric approach for a needle in the foot. Insert a small hemostat in the incision. Advance the hemostat allowing localization of the object with minimal probing. Grasp and remove the foreign body.

WIRE GRID LOCALIZATION

This technique follows a similar approach to the paper clip method.[60] Place a wire grid over the skin. Obtain radiographs in two planes to locate the object within the grid system. Mark the skin and remove the grid. Remove the foreign body as discussed for the paper clip technique.

NEEDLE GRID LOCALIZATION

The grid principle may also be used to remove superficial and nonlinear radiopaque foreign bodies after they have been identified on plain radiographs. Insert three 25 gauge, 1.5 inch needles into the skin near the estimated location of the foreign body and at right angles to each other. Obtain two orthogonal plain radiographs. This process can be repeated, each time moving the needles slightly until one is superimposed on the foreign body. Determine the cutaneous position of the foreign body by noting its position within the needle grid. Mark this position on the skin. It must be remembered that this technique does not provide a true three-dimensional image since divergence and parallax distortion of images occurs on the radiographs.[3]

The operator must recall that tendons and other structures may block the planned path to the object.[7] Make a 0.5 to 1.0 cm incision in a plane perpendicular to the long axis of the foreign body to an appropriate depth or dissect along the path of the closest needle.[27] Identify and remove the foreign body. A drawback of this technique is the potential for dislodging of the needles with attendant repeated trips to the Radiology Department. The use of a portable fluoroscopy unit will prevent this problem.

Another similar technique involves the placement of 3 to 4 needles of different gauges at 90 degrees to each other in the anesthetized subject.[61] Obtain repeat radiographs to identify which needle is closest to the object. Remove all but the closest needle. Make an incision down to the estimated depth where the foreign body is located. Identify and remove the foreign body.

EYE MAGNET

Another technique reported to have a good success rate in removing metallic foreign bodies utilizes a handheld eye magnet.[62] Confirm the presence of a radiopaque foreign body with plain radiographs. Prepare, drape, and anesthetize the area. Slightly enlarge the entry wound to permit entrance of the magnet tip. Gently probe the wound track with the magnet until a "click" is appreciated. Withdraw the magnet with the foreign body attached to the magnet. Perform further and more directed wound exploration with the magnet if resistance is met.

TAGGED HEMOCLIPS

It can be difficult to find foreign bodies once the dissection actually begins since the tissues may be distorted by retraction, edema, or local anesthesia; even with the most elaborate marking system using grids or needles. The tagged Hemoclip method was developed to address this problem.[63] It requires a skin incision and dissection down to where the operator believes the foreign body to be, based as observed on plain radiographs.

Prepare two or three Hemoclips with a long silk suture attached to each one. Place them into the Hemoclip applier. Dissect down to where the foreign body is believed to be located. Place two or three Hemoclips into the depths of the wound. Obtain repeat radiographs to show the relationship of the foreign body to the Hemoclips. Remove all but the closest Hemoclip. Dissect towards the Hemoclip and the foreign body. Identify and remove the foreign body. Remove the Hemoclip. If the foreign body is not readily found, repeat the procedure after placing two or three additional Hemoclips. Follow the trail of Hemoclips to the foreign body.

FLUOROSCOPIC TECHNIQUES

Fluoroscopy offers an excellent aid in the removal of radiopaque foreign bodies.[64] Make an incision over the foreign body as judged from plain radiographs. Localize the foreign body under fluoroscopy. Guide a curved hemostat to the foreign body with brief intermittent exposures of the fluoroscopy unit.[65] Grasp and remove the foreign body. This procedure exposes the operator's hands to radiation and may risk damaging structures in the wound by blind manipulation of the hemostat.[66]

The grid and needle localization techniques described previously can be applied under fluoroscopy. Rotate the site of injury under the fluoroscope to visualize the foreign body between the markers. This may improve the ability to judge the location of the foreign body in three dimensions and aid in its removal. Intermittent exposure with a fluoroscope can allow repositioning of the needles until the foreign body is localized between two needles or at the tip of a single needle. Make a small incision carried down to the foreign body and remove it.[66,67]

Additional techniques using fluoroscopy and neurosurgical stereotactic devices have been described.[3] The cost, availability, and practicality makes these approaches unattractive in the Emergency Department and are therefore not discussed further.

AFTERCARE

It is often prudent to take post-extraction radiographs to ensure complete removal of the foreign body, especially if multiple objects are involved or if there is concern about the object fragmenting.[61] Carefully irrigate and debride the wound of all epidermal fragments.[3] The most effective form of wound cleansing is jet lavage irrigation with normal saline to decrease the number of bacteria and the incidence of infection.[68] This can be obtained with a 35 mL syringe and a 19 gauge angiocatheter or needle.[12] The quality of mechanical cleaning is important to wound prognosis.[1] Clean, thoroughly irrigated, and debrided wounds with a good blood supply do not require antibiotics and may be sutured closed af-

ter removal of the foreign body. Patients should be followed up in 5 to 7 days for suture removal.

If complete cleansing of the wound is not assured or if the wound is at significant risk for infection for other reasons, delayed primary closure or healing by second intention should be considered.[12,69] Delayed primary closure involves packing the wound open for 4 to 5 days, after which it is reassessed and closed primarily if the edema has resolved, no infection is present, and exudate has been removed. This technique results in minimal tissue damage. It is especially useful in clean contaminated and contaminated wounds, achieving a 90 percent success rate in appropriate patients. Antibiotic therapy may be considered in those with wounds that are at significant risk for infection, **but antibiotics are not a replacement for proper wound care.** Close follow-up is especially important in these patients. Prophylaxis for endocarditis is not recommended unless foreign body removal is undertaken through an area of an established infection.[70] Splint the involved extremity if the foreign body is near a joint, a highly mobile region, or a vital structure to prevent injury and/or migration of the foreign body if the patient is referred for delayed removal.[8]

A more complete discussion on wound cleansing, wound irrigation, and the general principles of wound management can be found in Chapter 77. The techniques to approximate a wound can be found in Chapters 77, 78, 79, and 80.

TETANUS PROPHYLAXIS

Wounds with foreign bodies must be considered for tetanus prophylaxis (Table 77-2).[71] Wounds contaminated with feces, soil, or saliva; puncture wounds; avulsions; and wounds resulting from missiles, crushing, burns, and frostbite are classified as tetanus prone. If the most recent tetanus toxoid booster in a patient who has previously received a full primary series is more than 5 years, a booster dose of Td (0.5 mL IM) should be given if the wound is tetanus prone. A booster is not indicated until 10 years have elapsed since the last dose of toxoid if it is a minor wound in a previously fully vaccinated patient. Patients who have not completed a primary series require tetanus toxoid and passive immunization at the time of wound cleaning and debridement, and follow-up to complete a primary series. Refer to Chapter 77 for more complete details regarding tetanus prophylaxis.

COMPLICATIONS

The removal of embedded foreign bodies is relatively free of complications if properly conceived. **Care must be taken to document the functional and neurovascular status prior to and after any significant manipula-**

tions. Appropriate referral of complicated cases, including those with foreign bodies located deep in the hands, the feet, or near vital structures, will lessen the risk of unfavorable outcomes. Infection remains the most common complication of a retained foreign body, even when the object itself is not contaminated. Aseptic technique and avoidance of excessively prolonged manipulation and searching for embedded foreign bodies is important to prevent introducing infection into a previously sterile area. In cases where the foreign body cannot be found, it may be necessary, although less than ideal, to wait for an abscess formation in order to pinpoint the location of an object at a later time.[3] Referral for additional imaging and removal may be appropriate. The patient must be advised in detail of the likely course, and follow-up must be assured and documented.

SUMMARY

Nearly all embedded subcutaneous foreign bodies should be identified and located with rigorous assessment of each and every traumatic wound and a high index of suspicion. The history and physical examination should guide the search for retained foreign bodies and the approach to locating them. The majority of foreign bodies are visible on plain radiographs. Wounds for which a radiopaque foreign body may be retained should be imaged with standard radiographs utilizing a soft tissue technique. A decision must be made regarding the necessity of immediate or urgent removal in the Emergency Department or by referral to a specialist. Additional imaging with CT, ultrasound, or MRI may be indicated if the suspected foreign body is likely to be radiolucent. Once identified and located, several techniques are available to aid in localization and removal. Inert foreign bodies that are unlikely to cause long-term complications may be left in situ with information provided to the patient explaining the reasoning behind this conservative approach. Appropriate wound care is crucial to satisfactory healing, and post-procedure follow-up must be assured.

REFERENCES

1. Anderson MA, Newmeyer WL III, Kilgore ES: Diagnosis and treatment of retained foreign bodies in the hand. *Am J Surg* 1982; 144(1):63–67.
2. Zimmereli W, Zak O, Vosbeck K: Experimental hematogenous infection of subcutaneously implanted foreign bodies. *Scand J Infect Dis* 1985; 17:303–310.
3. Lammers RL: Soft tissue foreign bodies. *Ann Emerg Med* 1988; 17(12):1336–1347.
4. Merrell JC, Russell RC, Zook EG: Nonsuppurative tenosynovitis secondary to foreign body migration. *J Hand Surg* 1983; 8(3):340–341.
5. Jablon M, Rabin SI: Late flexor pollicis longus tendon rupture due to retained glass fragments. *J Hand Surg* 1988; 13A(5):713–715.
6. Avner JR, Baker MD: Lacerations involving glass: the role of routine roentgenograms. *Am J Dis Child* 1992; 146(1):600–602.
7. Lamers RL: Soft tissue foreign bodies, in Tintinalli JE, Kelen GD, Stapczynski JS (eds): *Emergency Medicine: A Comprehensive Study Guide*, 5th ed. New York: McGraw-Hill, 1999:323–330.
8. Lammers RL, Magill T: Detection and management of foreign bodies in soft tissue. *Emerg Med Clin North Am* 1992; 10(4):767–781.
9. Cracchiolo A III: Wooden foreign bodies in the foot. *Am J Surg* 1980; 140:585–587.
10. Gilad J, Borer A, Weksler N, et al: Fatal necrotizing fasciitis caused by a toothpick injury. *Scand J Infect Dis* 1998; 30(2):189–190.
11. Haury BB, Rodeheaver GT, Pettry D, et al: Inhibition of nonspecific defenses by soil infection potentiating factors. *Surg Gynecol Obstet* 1977; 144:19–24.
12. Edlich RF, Rodheaver GT, Morgan RF, et al: Principles of emergency wound management. *Ann Emerg Med* 1988; 17(12):55–73.
13. Farrell SE, Vandevander P, Schoffstall JM, et al: Blood lead levels in emergency department patients with retained lead bullets and shrapnel. *Acad Emerg Med* 1999; 6(3):208–212.
14. Russell RC, Williamson DA, Sullivan JW, et al: Detection of foreign bodies in the hand. *J Hand Surg* 1991; 16A(1):2–11.
15. Marquis GP: Radiolucent foreign bodies in the hand: case report. *J Trauma* 1989; 29(3):403–404.
16. Colin JF, Elliot P, Ellis H: The effect of uraemia on wound healing: an experimental study. *Br J Surg* 1979; 66:793–797.
17. American College of Emergency Physicians: Clinical policy for procedural sedation and analgesia in the emergency department. *Ann Emerg Med* 1998; 31:663–677.
18. Edlich RF, Kenney JG, Morgan RF, et al: Antimicrobial treatment of minor soft tissue lacerations: a critical review. *Emerg Med Clin North Am* 1986; 4(3):561–580.
19. Charney DB, Manzi JA, Turlik M, et al: Non-metallic foreign bodies in the foot: radiography versus xeroradiography. *J Foot Surg* 1986; 25(1):44–49.
20. Chisholm CD, Wood CO, Chua G, et al: Radiographic detection of gravel in soft tissue. *Ann Emerg Med* 1997; 29(6):725–730.
21. Roobottom CA, Weston MJ: The detection of foreign bodies in soft tissue—comparison of conventional

and digital radiography. *Clin Radiol* 1994; 49:330–332.

22. Ellis G: Are aluminum foreign bodies detectable radiographically? *Am J Emerg Med* 1993; 11:12–13.

23. Tandberg D: Glass in the hand and foot. Will an x-ray film show it? *JAMA* 1982; 248(15):1872–1874.

24. Courter BJ: Radiographic screening for glass foreign bodies: what does a "negative" foreign body series really mean? *Ann Emerg Med* 1990; 19(9):997–1000.

25. DeLacey G, Evans R, Sandin B: Penetrating injuries: how easy is it to see glass and plastic on radiographs? *Br J Radiol* 1985; 58(685):27–30.

26. Mucci B, Stenhouse G: Soft tissue radiography for wooden foreign bodies—a worthwhile exercise? *Injury* 1985; 16(6):402–404.

27. Rusnak RA: Removal of foreign bodies from the skin, in Schwartz G, Cayten CG, Mangelsen MA, et al (eds): *Principles and Practice of Emergency Medicine*, 3rd ed. Philadelphia: Lea & Febiger, 1890–1897:1992.

28. Bodne D, Quinn SF, Cochran CF: Imaging foreign glass and wooden bodies of the extremities with CT and MR. *J Comput Assist Tomog* 1988; 12(4):608–611.

29. Bauer AR, Yutani D: Computed tomographic localization of wooden foreign bodies in children's extremities. *Arch Surg* 1983; 118:1084–1086.

30. Kuhns LR, Borlaza GS, Seigel RS, et al: An in vitro comparison of computed tomography, xeroradiography, and radiology in the detection of soft-tissue foreign bodies. *Radiology* 1979; 132:218–219.

31. Rhoades CE, Soye I, Levine E, et al: Detection of a wooden foreign body in the hand using computed tomography—case report. *J Hand Surg* 1982; 7(3):306–307.

32. Reiner B, Siegel E, McLaurin T, et al: Evaluation of soft-tissue foreign bodies: comparing conventional plain film radiography, computed radiography printed on film, and computed radiography displayed on a computer workstation. *Am J Roentgenol* 1996; 167:141–144.

33. Haaga JR, Stewart BH, Alfidi RJ: Foreign body localization and removal utilizing computerized axial tomography. *Urology* 1978; 11(3):306–307.

34. Ginsburg MJ, Ellis GL, Flom LL: Detection of soft-tissue foreign bodies by plain radiography, xerography, computed tomography an ultrasonography. *Ann Emerg Med* 1990; 19(6):701–703.

35. Turner J, Wilde CH, Hughes KC, et al: Ultrasound-guided retrieval of small foreign objects in subcutaneous tissue. *Ann Emerg Med* 1997; 29(6):731–734.

36. Fornage BD, Schernberg FL: Sonographic diagnosis of foreign bodies of the distal extremities. *Am J Roentgenol* 1986; 147:567–569.

37. De Flaviis L, Scaglione P, Del Bo P, et al: Detection of foreign bodies in soft tissue: experimental comparison of ultrasonography and xeroradiography. *J Trauma* 1988; 28(3):400–404.

38. Gilbert FJ, Campbell RSD, Bayliss AP: The role of ultrasound in the detection of non-radiopaque foreign bodies. *Clin Radiol* 1990; 41:109–112.

39. Crawford R, Matheson AB: Clinical value of ultrasonography in the detection and removal of radiolucent foreign bodies. *Injury* 1989; 20:341–343.

40. Storrow AB, Manthey DE: Ultrasound retrieval of foreign bodies. *Ann Emerg Med* 1997; 29(6):779–780.

41. Schlager D, Sanders AB, Wiggins D, et al: Ultrasound for the detection of foreign bodies. *Ann Emerg Med* 1991; 20:189–191.

42. Manthey DE, Storrow AB, Milbourn JM, et al: Ultrasound versus radiography in the detection of soft-tissue foreign bodies. *Ann Emerg Med* 1996; 28(1):7–9.

43. Hill R, Conron R, Greissinger P, et al: Ultrasound for the detection of foreign bodies in human tissue. *Ann Emerg Med* 1997; 29(3):353–356.

44. Nelson EW, DeHart MM, Christensen AW, et al: Magnetic resonance imaging characteristics of a lead pencil foreign body in the hand. *J Hand Surg* 1996; 21A(1):100–103.

45. Lewis TT, Case A, Troughton A, et al: Metallic foreign body localization with magnetic resonance imaging. *Radiography Today* 1991; 57(644):16–17.

46. Carneiro RS, Okunski WJ, Hefferman AW: Detection of a relatively radiolucent foreign body in the hand by xerography. *Plast Reconstr Surg* 1977; 59(6):862–863.

47. Lindsey D, Lindsey WE: Cactus spine injuries. *Am J Emerg Med* 1988; 6(4):362–369.

48. Smoot EC, Robson MC: Acute management of foreign injuries of the hand. *Ann Emerg Med* 1983; 12(7):434–437.

49. Simon B, Hern HG Jr: Wound management principles, in Rosen P, Barkin RM, Braen RC, et al (eds): *Emergency Medicine: Concepts and Clinical Practice*, 5th ed. St. Louis: Mosby-Year Book, 2001:737–752.

50. Rees CE: The removal of foreign bodies: a modified incision. *JAMA* 1939; 113:35–36.

51. Sutcliffe H: Detecting fine skin splinters—the soft soap method. *Aust Fam Physician* 1994; 23(3):493.

52. Stein F: Foreign body injuries of the hand. *Emerg Med Clin North Am* 1985; 3(2):383–390.

53. Patzakis MJ: Wound site as a predictor of complications following deep nail punctures to the foot. *West J Med* 1989; 150(5):545–547.

54. Joseph WS, LeFrock JL: Infections complicating puncture wounds of the foot. *J Foot Surg* 1987; 26(1 suppl):S30–S33.

55. Lannigan S: Finding and removing small foreign bodies: a new technique for A & E. *J Accident Emerg Med* 1996; 13(2):151.

56. Gilsdorf JR: A needle in the sole of the foot. *Surg Gynecol Obstet* 1984; 163:573–574.

57. Bhavsar MS: Technique of finding a metallic foreign body. *J Surg* 1981; 141:305.

58. Gahhos F, Arons MS: Soft tissue foreign body removal: management and presentation of a new technique. *J Trauma* 1984; 24(4):340–341.

59. Leidelmeyer R: The embedded broken-off needle. *J Am Coll Emerg Physicians* 1976; 5(5):362–363.

60. Weinstock RE: Noninvasive technique for the localization of radiopaque foreign bodies. *J Foot Surg* 1981; 20(2):73–75.

61. Rickoff SE, Bauder T, Kerman BL: Foreign body localization and retrieval in the foot. *J Foot Surg* 1981; 20(1):30–34.

62. Bocka JJ, Godfrey J: Emergency department use of an eye magnet for the removal of soft tissue foreign bodies. *Ann Emerg Med* 1994; 23(2):350–351.

63. Mladick RA: Easy location of foreign body with "tagged hemo-clips." *Plast Reconstr Surg* 1978; 61:459–460.

64. Cohen DM, Garcia CT, Dietrich AM, et al: Miniature c-arm imaging: an in vitro study of detecting foreign bodies in the emergency department. *Pediatr Emerg Care* 1997; 13(4):247–249.

65. Wayne R, Carnazzo AJ: Needle in the foot. *Am J Surg* 1975; 129(6):599–600.

66. Ariyan S: A simple stereotactic method to isolate and remove foreign bodies. *Arch Surg* 1977; 112:857–859.

67. Simon RR, Brenner BE: *Emergency Procedures and Techniques,* 3rd ed. Baltimore: Williams & Wilkins, 1994:360–365.

68. Rodheaver GT, Pettry D, Thacker JG, et al: Wound cleansing by high-pressure irrigation. *Surg Gynecol Obstet* 1975; 141:357–362.

69. Dimick AR: Delayed wound closure indications and techniques. *Ann Emerg Med* 1988; 17(12):1303–1304.

70. Dajani AS, Taubert KA, Wilson W, et al: Prevention of bacterial endocarditis: recommendations by the American Heart Association. http://www.american heart.org/Scientific/statements/1997/079701.html

71. Center for Disease Control: Diphtheria, tetanus, pertussis: recommendations for vaccine use and other preventive measures: recommendation of the immunization practices advisory committee (ACIP). *MMWR Morb Mortal Wkly Rep* 1991; 40(RR-10):1–28.

Chapter 82
TICK REMOVAL

Jeffrey Gordon

INTRODUCTION

Ticks are blood-feeding external parasites (Figure 82-1). Ticks are a significant infectious disease problem in the United States as well as worldwide. They have been implicated as vectors in the transmission of a large number of diseases including Lyme disease, ehrlichiosis, babesiosis, Rocky Mountain spotted fever, tularemia, and tick borne relapsing fever. Disease transmission is postulated to occur when stomach contents and saliva from the tick are introduced into the host during the blood-feeding process. There is significance in how long a tick has been attached and how quickly a feeding tick can be removed. Early removal is felt to greatly limit the transmission of disease. Current entomological thinking suggests that the tick must be attached for at least 24 hours in order to transmit *B. burgdorferri,* the spirochete responsible for Lyme disease.[1]

ANATOMY AND PATHOPHYSIOLOGY

There are two main families of ticks.[2] Hard body ticks belong to the Ixodidae family. Soft body ticks belong to the Argasidae family. Hard body ticks are responsible for the transmission of the majority of human diseases and will be the focus of this chapter. Hard ticks pass through four life cycle stages from birth (egg, larva, nymph, and adult). They require a blood meal in order to progress into the next stage of their development.

The bite of a tick is painless and often not noticed until the tick is seen attached to the skin. Ticks are often encountered in the late spring, summer, and early fall. Ticks are more prevalent in rural and wooded areas. They like to feed in dark (covered) and moist areas of the body such as the axilla, groin, or scalp.

Ticks have specialized mouthparts that make their removal difficult (Figure 82-2).[2] They screw their mouthparts into the skin in a clockwise direction. Mouthparts include the palps, the chelicerae, and the hypostome.

The chelicerae are used to cut through the epidermis and allow passage of the hypostome, through which the feeding takes place. Ticks attach themselves to their host by inserting the rod-like hypostome into the skin. The hypostome has many backward pointing sharp projections on it that prevent it from being pulled out. The tick secretes a cement-like material around the hypostome to secure its attachment to the host while it feeds. The tick releases its mouthparts from the host after the meal is complete. It can take hours to days for a tick to finish its blood meal.

INDICATIONS

Any tick found attached to the skin should be removed. Transmission of bacteria, spirochetes, viruses, or other infectious agents is directly related to length of time of attachment. It is felt that ticks attached less than 24 hours are very low risk for transmission of disease.[3]

CONTRAINDICATIONS

There are no absolute or relative contraindications to the removal of a tick.

EQUIPMENT

Povidone iodine or isopropyl alcohol swabs
Gloves
Mosquito hemostat or fine forceps
Magnifying headlamp
Local anesthetic solution
3 mL syringe armed with a 27 gauge needle
Skin biopsy punches
#15 surgical scalpel blade on a handle
5–0 nylon suture
Specimen container with isopropyl alcohol

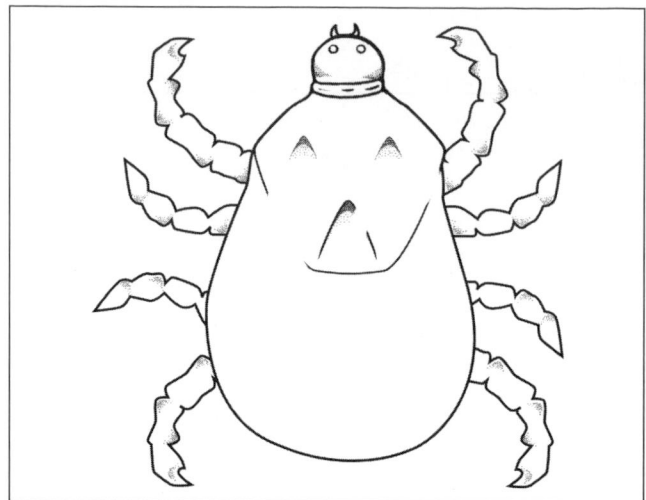

FIGURE 82-1 The tick.

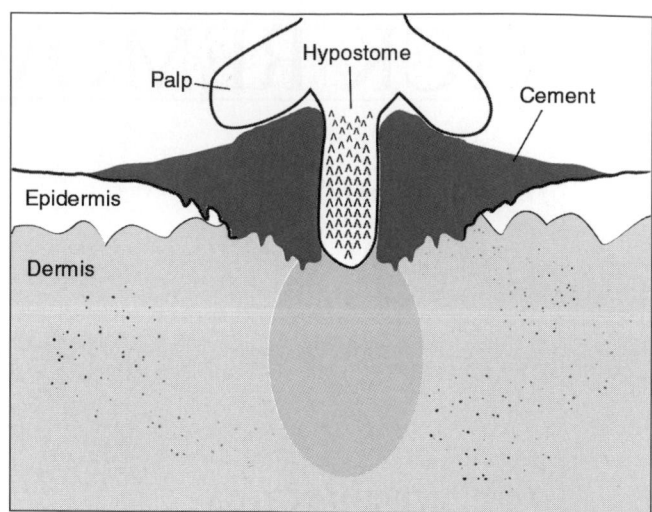

FIGURE 82-2 The specialized mouthparts of the tick.

PATIENT PREPARATION

Explain the risks and benefits of the procedure to the patient and/or their representative. Risks include failure to remove all tick parts and infection. Obtain an informed consent for the procedure. Clean any dirt and debris from the skin. Apply an alcohol swab or another antiseptic solution to the skin surrounding the tick.

TECHNIQUE

Direct mechanical removal of the tick is the only recommended technique. Grasp the tick tightly with a fine forceps or mosquito hemostat as close to the patient's skin as possible. Firmly pull the tick upward. **Do not crush, puncture, squeeze, or tear the ticks' abdomen.** A rotary counterclockwise movement combined with the firm pull may be more effective.[4] A technique has been described of first rotating the tick two complete revolutions around its axis to loosen its attachment prior to pulling it away from the skin.[5] **Care must be taken not to leave pieces of the tick's mouthparts embedded in the skin after removal of the body.**

ALTERNATIVE TECHNIQUES

Some physicians prefer a surgical technique to remove the tick and its attachment to the skin to ensure that no fragments of the tick mouthparts remain within the patient. Inject 0.25 to 0.50 mL of local anesthetic solution subcutaneously immediately underneath the tick's mouthparts. Apply povidone iodine to the skin and allow it to dry. Stretch the skin on each side of the tick with the nondominant hand. Apply the skin biopsy punch per-

pendicular to the skin. Make sure that the tick is centered within the skin biopsy punch. Advance the skin biopsy punch downward using a twisting (clockwise-counterclockwise) motion until a loss of resistance is felt. The loss of resistance indicates that the skin biopsy punch is through the epidermis and at the level of the dermis. Remove the skin biopsy punch. Lift the punched skin with forceps. Cut the skin at the dermal-epidermal junction with an iris scissors or a #15 scalpel blade. Alternatively, remove the tick and skin with a #15 surgical scalpel blade. The skin site may be closed with a single interrupted 5–0 nylon suture or left open to granulate.

Many other alternate techniques have been described in the literature. Techniques that involve coating the tick with some type of noxious stimulant (kerosene, lidocaine, nail polish) to cause the tick to voluntarily withdraw its attachment have not been shown to be successful.[4,6] Techniques that involve suffocating the tick with petroleum jelly are also not felt to be useful due to the low respiratory rate of 3 to 10 breaths per hour in a feeding tick.[5] The use of a heated object, e.g., a match tip or piece of metal, applied to the abdominal surface of the tick has not been shown to effect rapid tick detachment and presents a risk of burning the patient. Subcutaneous injection of local anesthetic solution at the attachment site was studied and also found not to stimulate tick detachment.[7] There are specific devices that are commercially available and advertised to aid in manual tick removal. Some of these devices have been tested and are not felt to offer any advantage over forceps removal.[8,9]

ASSESSMENT

Inspect the area to ensure no foreign material has been retained. The tick can be discarded unless further serologic testing is desired. The tick can be stored in iso-propyl alcohol until testing can be performed by a laboratory or the local public health department.

AFTERCARE

Cleanse the area with a mild disinfectant or soap and water. Administer tetanus prophylaxis if the immunization history is not up-to-date. The appearance of any rash or the occurrence of any febrile illness 2 to 12 days after a documented tick exposure should prompt further medical follow-up. The patient should inspect the site twice a day for signs of an infection. Patients should return to the Emergency Department or their Primary Physician if they develop redness, tenderness, swelling, or a discharge at the bite site. Please consult the current medical literature or an Infectious Disease Physician regarding the use of prophylactic antibiotics against tick-borne diseases. The use of antistaphylococcal antibiotics is not routinely recommended.

Patients should be educated about ticks and preventative measures. Prevention is the best protection. Unfortunately, avoiding the outdoors and its associated activities is not practical. Patients should be advised to wear clothes to cover the arms, legs, and torso; tuck the cuffs of pants into boots; apply a repellent to clothes and exposed skin; and physically check for the presence of a tick at the end of the activity or the end of the day.

COMPLICATIONS

The major complication of the direct removal technique is the separation of the tick body from the embedded head. Leaving foreign material in the wound can become a site for future infection.[5] Any remaining pieces of the tick should be removed using an 18 gauge needle, a skin biopsy punch, or sharp dissection with a #15 scalpel blade.

Inadvertent crushing of the tick may allow stomach contents or saliva from the tick to enter the wound. It is theorized that grasping the tick too distal to its head, across its thorax/abdomen, could induce regurgitation of stomach contents into the wound and increases the risk of disease transmission.[5]

SUMMARY

Ticks are a vector for numerous serious diseases and should be removed from the skin as soon as they are identified. Disease transmission is felt unlikely if the tick has been attached less than 24 hours. The only recommended technique for tick removal is manual detachment using forceps.

REFERENCES

1. Zung JL, Lewengrub S, Rudzinska MA, et al: Fine structural evidence for the penetration of the Lyme disease spirochete *Borrelia burgdorferi* through the gut and salivary tissues of *Ixodes dammini. Can J Zool* 1989; 67:1737–1748.
2. Story K: Biology and control of ticks. *Pest Control Tech* 1989; June:54–56.
3. De Boer R, Van Den Bogaard AEJM: Removal of attached nymphs and adults of *Ixodes ricinus. J Med Entomol* 1993; 30(4):748–752.
4. Needham GR: Evaluation of five popular methods for tick removal. *Pediatrics* 1985; 75(6):997–1002.
5. Schultheis L: A novel technique to remove the common dog tick. *Am Fam Physician* 1998; 58(2):354–357.
6. Dolan DL, McKinsey JJ: Removing a tick. *N C Med J* 1985; 46:471.
7. Lee MD, Sonenshine DE, Counselman FL: Evaluation of subcutaneous injection of local anesthetic agents as a method of tick removal. *Am J Emerg Med* 1995; 13(1):14–16.
8. Karras DJ: Tick removal. *Ann Emerg Med* 1998; 32(4):519.
9. Bowles DE, McHugh CP, Spradling SL: Evaluation of devices for removing attached *Rhipicephalus sanguineus* (acari: Ixodidae). *J Med Entomol* 1992; 29(5):901–902.

Chapter 83
FISHHOOK REMOVAL

Alfred E. Tober
Eric F. Reichman

INTRODUCTION

Depending on practice location and season of the year, the presentation of a fishhook embedded in the subcutaneous tissue can be common. Often, the patient or a well-meaning bystander will have already attempted removal that was prevented by the hook's barb. Removal can be difficult as a fishhook is designed not to pull out of a fish's mouth. Several methods of removal have been described.[1–5] The method chosen depends on the type and size of the hook, the depth of penetration, and the anatomical location of injury.

ANATOMY AND PATHOPHYSIOLOGY

Most fishhooks become embedded in the skin and subcutaneous soft tissue. The anatomy of a fishhook is simple (Figure 83-1). The long, straight section is known as the shaft. The proximal end of the shaft has a closed circle, the eyelet, where the fishing wire attaches. The distal end of the shaft curves in a semicircle known as the belly of the fishhook. The belly tapers into a sharp point with a barb. The barb is usually located on the inner surface of the hook, pointing away from the tip. The barb, once pierced through the skin, becomes embedded within the tissue and prevents removal of the fishhook. Additional barbs may be located along the shaft of the fishhook.

INDICATIONS

Any embedded fishhook must be removed from the body. There is no reason a fishhook should not be removed by the primary physician or Emergentologist if no contraindication exists.

CONTRAINDICATIONS

There are no absolute contraindications to fishhook removal. Occasionally, the procedure should be referred to a consultant. Globe perforation or laceration requires emergent consultation with an Opthalmologist. Place the patient supine with a shield, not a patch, over the eye. Please see Chapter 138 for the complete details regarding eye patching and eye shields. **Penetration of, or near, vital structures (e.g., the neck, groin, or major neurovascular structures) should be given consideration for the appropriate surgical consultation prior to removal of the fishhook.**

EQUIPMENT

Povidone iodine
Local anesthetic solution without epinephrine
3 mL syringe armed with a 25 gauge needle
Wire cutter
Needle driver
Hemostat
18 gauge needle
#11 scalpel blade on a handle
String, fishing line, or a strong silk tie, at least 50 cm in length
Safety glasses/goggles

PATIENT PREPARATION

Explain the risks and benefits of the procedure to the patient and/or their representative. Obtain a signed consent form prior to beginning the procedure. Cleanse the skin of any dirt and debris. Apply povidone iodine to the skin surrounding the embedded fishhook and allow it to dry.

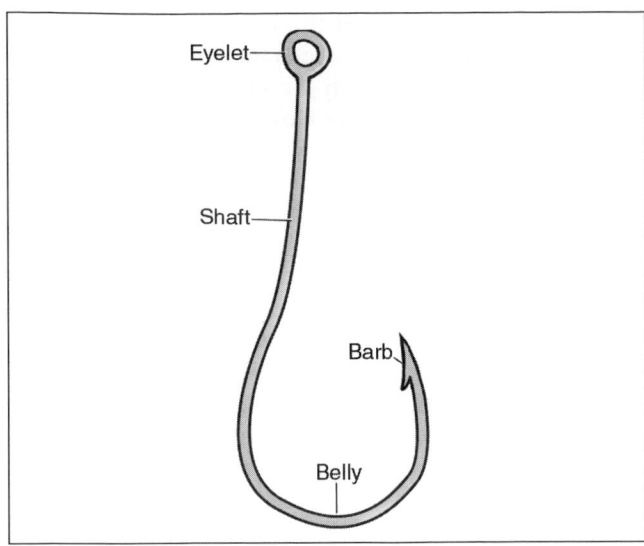

FIGURE 83-1 Anatomy of a fishhook.

TECHNIQUES

PULL-THROUGH TECHNIQUE

This is the traditional method that is used for larger sized hooks embedded in the soft tissue with the barb near the skin surface. This is the preferred technique for fishhooks embedded in the ear, a joint, or in the nasal cartilages. Experienced fishermen often perform this technique in the field, as they would hate to lose prime fishing time to go to the hospital.

Identify the barbed end of the fishhook, located under the skin surface. Inject 0.5 to 1.0 mL of local anesthetic solution into the subcutaneous tissue overlying the barbed end of the fishhook to raise a skin wheal (Figure 83-2*A*). Allow 3 to 4 minutes for the local anesthetic solution to take effect. Grasp the shaft of the fishhook with a needle driver (Figure 83-2*B*). Advance the fishhook until the barbed end protrudes through the anes-

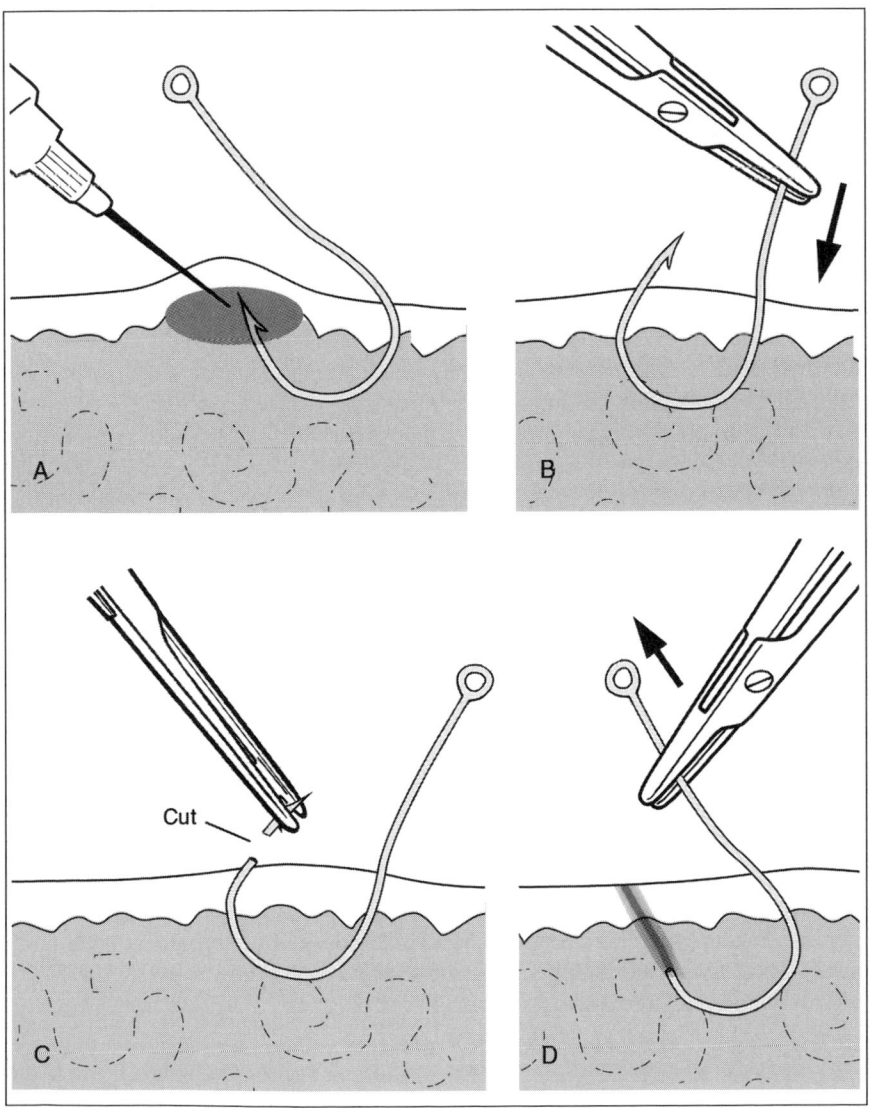

FIGURE 83-2 The pull-through technique for fishhook removal. *A*. Subcutaneous anesthetic is placed over the barb. *B*. The fishhook is advanced until the barb protrudes from the skin. *C*. A hemostat is placed over the barb before it is cut off with wire cutters. *D*. The fishhook is removed.

thetized skin (Figure 83-2*B*). **Securely clamp a hemostat over the barb.** This will prevent it from becoming a projectile when cut and injuring someone. Cut the belly of the fishhook just proximal to the barbed end with a wire cutter (Figure 83-2*C*). Grasp the shaft of the fishhook with the needle driver and withdraw it along its direction of entry (Figure 83-2*D*).

Occasionally, fishhooks may have additional barbs on the shaft or the belly (Figure 83-3). Inject 0.5 to 1.0 mL of local anesthetic solution into the subcutaneous tissue overlying the barbed end of the fishhook (Figure 83-3*A*). Allow 3 to 4 minutes for the local anesthetic solution to take effect. Grasp the shaft of the fishhook with a needle driver (Figure 83-3*B*). Advance the fishhook until the barbed end protrudes through the anesthetized skin (Figure 83-3*B*). Continue to advance the fishhook until all the barbs on the belly and shaft are below the skin surface (Figure 83-3*B*). Securely clamp a hemostat over the proximal shaft of the fishhook (Figure 83-3*C*). Cut

the shaft of the fishhook at the level of the skin with a wire cutter (Figure 83-3*C*). Grasp the fishhook just proximal to the barbed end with the needle driver and pull the remainder of the fishhook out of the subcutaneous tissues (Figure 83-3*D*).

BARB-SHEATH TECHNIQUE

This method is reserved for small fishhooks embedded near the skin surface. This technique should not be used for fishhooks in the ear, nose, or a joint cavity. Inject 0.5 to 1.0 mL of local anesthetic solution to form a wheal subcutaneously around the area where the fishhook enters the skin. Insert an 18 gauge needle along the entrance wound and aimed towards the barb (Figure 83-4*A*). The bevel of the needle should face the barb with the goal being to engage and cover the barb. Advance the needle and engage the barb in the core of the needle (Figure 83-4*B*). Gently twist and pull the hook back through the entrance wound while the needle covers the barb (Figure 83-4*C*).

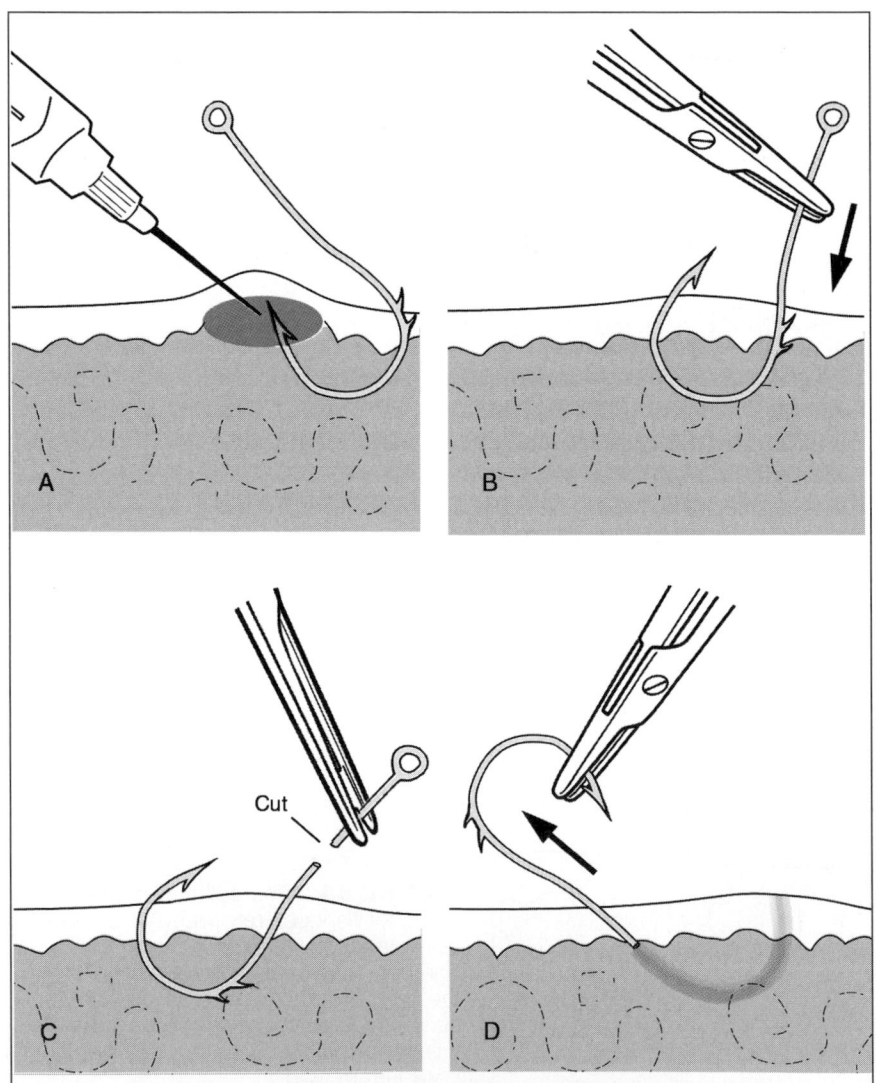

FIGURE 83-3 An alternative pull-through technique for the removal of a multibarbed fishhook. *A.* Subcutaneous anesthetic is placed over the barb. *B.* The fishhook is advanced until all of the proximal barbs are under the skin. *C.* The shaft is cut. *D.* The fishhook is removed.

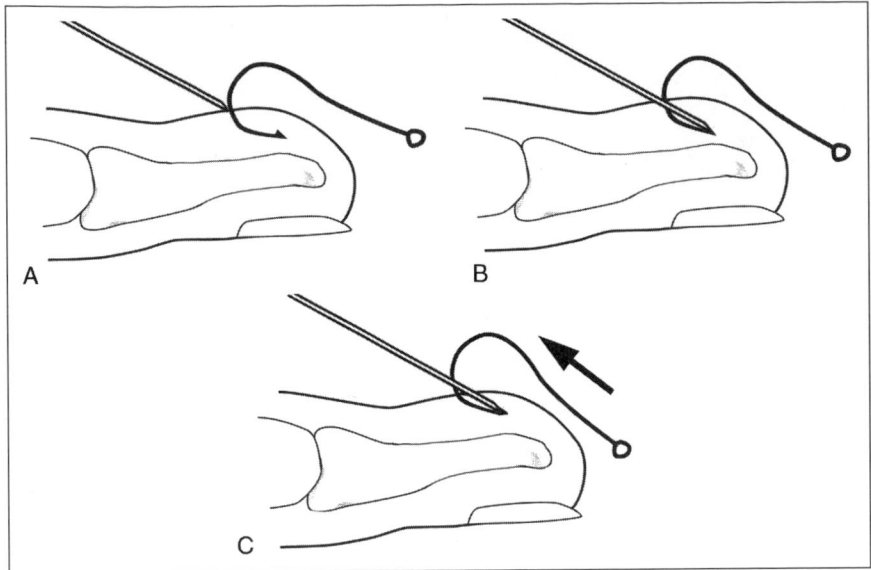

FIGURE 83-4 The barb-sheath technique for fishhook removal. *A.* Insert the needle through the entrance wound and aimed toward the barb. *B.* Advance the needle through the entry site to catch the barb in the core of the needle. *C.* The needle and fishhook are removed as a unit.

An alternative method is to insert a #11 scalpel blade parallel to the shaft of the fishhook at the site it enters the skin. Advance the scalpel blade until it is adjacent to the barb. Withdraw the fishhook and scalpel through the tract. The barb will be resting against the scalpel blade and not get embedded in the subcutaneous tissues. This method is not recommended due to the blind insertion of a scalpel blade into the soft tissues and the potential for secondary injury.

STRING-YANK TECHNIQUE

This method has been extensively described and is often performed by experienced fishermen in the field. It is rapid, effective, easy to perform, and relatively painless. This technique should not be used for fishhooks in the ear, nose, or a joint cavity. **The care providers should take caution for themselves, the patient, and bystanders. The hook often forcibly flies out of the patient. Ensure the suspected path of the fishhook is clear. Eye protection is recommended with this technique for the physician and the patient.**

Place the body part that the fishhook entered firmly on a flat surface. Local anesthetic solution can be infiltrated, at the care provider's discretion, into the area where the fishhook enters the skin. Wrap the midpoint of a string around the belly of the fishhook at the site it enters the skin (Figure 83-5*A*). The string ends should be firmly wrapped around and secured to the index and middle fingers of the physician's dominant hand. Using the nondominant thumb and index finger, firmly depress the shaft of the fishhook against the skin, until slight resistance is met (Figure 83-5*B*). The shaft should be parallel to the skin and touching the skin. This will disengage the barb from the soft tissues. Quickly and

firmly jerk the string (Figure 83-5*C*). This maneuver will release the fishhook from the subcutaneous tissues and pull it out through the entry wound.

AFTERCARE

The wound should be cleaned of any blood and a dry dressing applied. Administer tetanus prophylaxis if the immunization history is not up-to-date. A radiograph is indicated if there is any suspicion of a retained foreign body. Antistaphylococcal antibiotic prophylaxis remains controversial.[1,2] The use of antibiotics is left to the discretion of the care provider and should include consideration for the anatomic site of injury, depth of penetration, and evidence of gross contamination. Nonsteroidal anti-inflammatory drugs will provide any required analgesia.

The patient should be instructed to clean the area with warm soapy water 3 times a day and to keep the wound covered until healed. Instruct the patient as to the signs of infection. They should return to the Emergency Department, or their physician, if signs of an infection develop. Follow-up is arranged at the discretion of the care provider but is often not required.

COMPLICATIONS

Complications include infection or damage to the surrounding tissue. Infection is often due to either the contaminated fishhook inoculating the tissues or the fishhook penetrating contaminated skin. Using proper removal techniques will minimize, but not eliminate, any damage to the soft tissues.

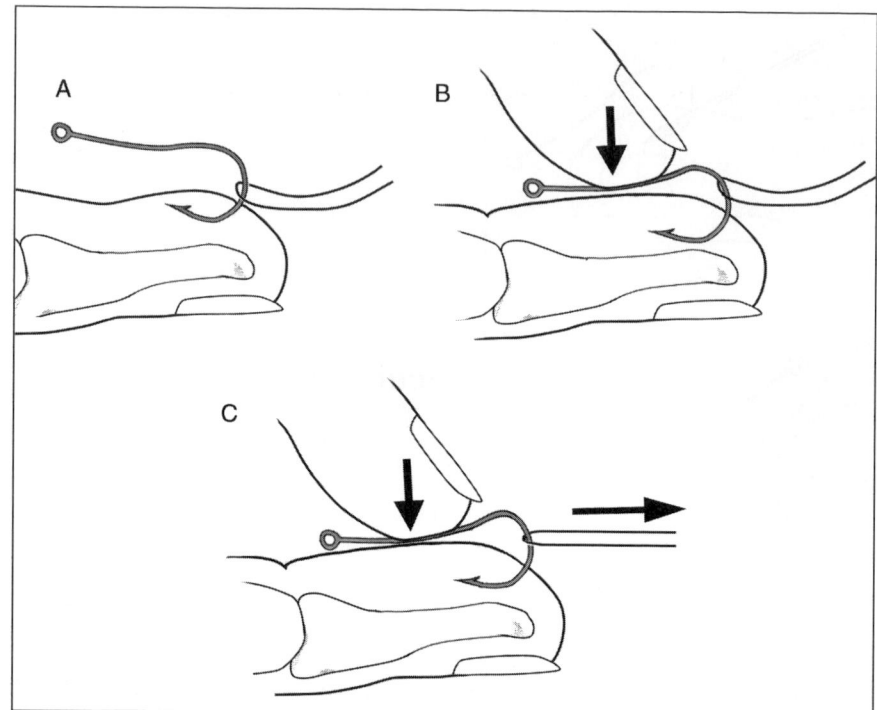

FIGURE 83-5 The string-yank technique for fishhook removal. *A.* A string is wrapped around the belly of the fishhook. *B.* The shaft of the fishhook is depressed until resistance is encountered. The shaft should be parallel to the skin and touching the skin. *C.* A quick tug on the string will remove the fishhook.

Use caution when extracting fishhooks to avoid secondary injury to bystanders, the patient, or the care provider. Protective eyewear should be worn with all three techniques of fishhook extraction. Ocular injury has been reported to occur during this procedure.[2] When using the pull-through technique, clamping a hemostat to the exposed portion of the fishhook that is to be cut off will prevent flying shrapnel.

SUMMARY

Fishhook removal can be accomplished by one of several simple techniques. It can be performed in the Emergency Department, the office, or the field with minimal supplies. Almost painless removal is possible in most cases. This procedure is gratifying both for the patient and the care provider.

REFERENCES

1. Diekema DS, Quan L: Fishhook removal, in Henretig FM, King C (eds): *Textbook of Pediatric Emergency Procedures.* Baltimore: Williams & Wilkins, 1997: 1223–1227.
2. Dunmire SM, Paris PM: *Atlas of Emergency Procedures.* Philadelphia: Saunders, 1994:110–112.
3. Freidenberg S: How to remove an embedded fishhook in five seconds without really trying. *N Engl J Med* 1971; 284:733–734.
4. Haynes JH III: Fishhook removal, in Pfenninger JL, Fowler GC (eds): *Procedures for Primary Care Physicians.* St. Louis: Mosby, 1994:128–132.
5. Rudnitsky GS, Barnett RC: Soft tissue foreign body removal, in Roberts JR, Hedges JR (eds): *Clinical Procedures in Emergency Medicine,* 3rd ed. Philadelphia: Saunders, 1998: 623–624.

Chapter 84
RING REMOVAL

Steven H. Bowman

INTRODUCTION

The need to remove rings is not uncommon in the Emergency Department. Patients may present with an initial primary complaint that they are no longer able to remove a ring or that a ring has become painful. A variety of conditions may necessitate the urgent removal of a ring, including swelling from extremity trauma, infections or burns, increases in total volume status, and allergic reactions. Swelling of the digit can rapidly progress, causing the ring to become a constricting band. Patients who are critically ill and being admitted to intensive care settings or undergoing emergency surgery may need to have rings removed urgently. The information in this chapter applies to rings on the fingers and toes.

ANATOMY AND PATHOPHYSIOLOGY

The second through fourth digits receive their blood supply through four vessels: the palmar radial digital arteries, the palmar ulnar digital arteries, the dorsal radial digital arteries, and the dorsal ulnar digital arteries. The thumb receives its blood supply from the dorsalis pollicis and princeps pollicis arteries. Blood returns from the digits via the dorsal digital veins. When the digit is compressed for prolonged periods by a tight-fitting ring, which acts as a tourniquet, venous return is impeded and swelling ensues. The swelling results in greater compression and further propagation of this cycle. In theory, the increased swelling will eventually impede the arterial supply to the digit.

The greatest circumference of the finger is at the proximal interphalangeal (PIP) joint. Rings usually become entrapped proximal to the PIP joint. Skin breakdown and tissue necrosis occur if the constricting ring is not removed. If left untreated, the digit is at risk for infections such as cellulitis, tenosynovitis, and osteomyelitis.

In severe cases, the digit's viability may be threatened. There have been several case reports of rings that have become embedded in the soft tissue of the digits.[1-5]

Most patients will experience pain and seek medical attention prior to the development of severe complications. Patients with an altered mental status, psychiatric illness, peripheral neuropathies, peripheral vascular disease, or other chronic disability may present later with complications.[1,2,4,5]

INDICATIONS

Rings are removed to prevent ischemia of a digit. Rings should be removed whenever patients complain that a ring is causing pain. Generally, even a tight-fitting ring will not be painful. Rings must be removed from any injured digit where edema is a possible consequence: sprains, contusions, fractures, lacerations, crush injuries, and burns. Rings should be removed from all digits on the involved side for any hand or foot injury where edema is a possible consequence. Other nontraumatic conditions that may necessitate emergent ring removal include infections of the upper or lower extremity, acute increases in volume status, and allergic reactions. Urgent ring removal should be considered in patients with markedly decreased levels of consciousness and in all critically ill patients, particularly those being admitted to intensive care settings or undergoing emergent surgery.

CONTRAINDICATIONS

There are no absolute contraindications to removing a ring. It is important to note that certain techniques may be more applicable than others, depending on the individual patient. The practitioner's goal is to remove the ring in a timely manner and not cause additional injury.

EQUIPMENT

Metacarpal Block

Povidone iodine or isopropyl alcohol swab solution
3 mL syringe
25 or 27 gauge needle, 1 inch long
3 to 5 mL local anesthetic solution without epinephrine

Lubricant Technique

Lubricant (K-Y jelly, Surgilube, petrolatum, mineral oil, or liquid soap)

String Technique

String (1–0 silk suture, cotton umbilical string, tracheal tape, Penrose drain, or intravenous tourniquet)
Mosquito hemostat

Rubber Band Technique

3 to 4 mm wide rubber band
Lubricant (K-Y jelly, Surgilube, petrolatum, mineral oil, or liquid soap)
Mosquito hemostat

Glove Technique

Latex rubber gloves
Lubricant (K-Y jelly, Surgilube, petrolatum, mineral oil, or liquid soap)
Mosquito hemostat
Scissors

Ring Cutter Technique

Ring cutter, manually operated or battery-powered
Steinman pin cutter if ring cutter not available
Two large hemostats or needle drivers
Pliers (optional)

PATIENT PREPARATION

Place the patient sitting upright or in a semirecumbent position. Explain the procedure to the patient and/or their representative. A signed informed consent is not required for the removal of a ring. Analgesia should be provided in the form of a metacarpal block for patients who are complaining of pain. Refer to Chapter 106 for the complete details regarding a metacarpal block.

The removal of a tight ring should be considered a two-step process: first reduce the edema in the finger,

then remove the ring.[6] The patient's involved hand should be elevated to reduce edema prior to any attempts at manipulation. A Penrose drain, piece of tape, gauze, or elastic bandage may be wrapped around the finger, from distal to proximal, to further reduce swelling.

The simplest and most effective way to remove a ring from a finger is simply to cut the ring using a ring cutter. Reassure the patient that cut rings can be repaired by a jeweler. However, patients may still be reluctant to have expensive rings or rings with sentimental value removed in such a way. The practitioner must consider time, the individual circumstances regarding the entrapment, and which alternative techniques may be effective.

TECHNIQUES

LUBRICANT TECHNIQUE

This technique works for mild cases of ring entrapment with minimal swelling and without significant trauma. Many patients will attempt to remove the ring using some type of lubricant at home prior to presenting to the Emergency Department. Despite this, the same technique may also be tried in the Emergency Department prior to attempting other techniques. Liberally apply a lubricant (K-Y jelly, Surgilube, petrolatum, mineral oil, or liquid soap) to the digit and beneath the ring. Advance the ring over the PIP joint with steady traction.

STRING TECHNIQUE

Several authors have extensively described the string technique and its modifications[5–7] (Figure 84-1). This technique consists of using a "string" to compress the edematous tissue, exsanguinate the digit, and then facilitate the passage of the ring over the PIP joint. This technique should be avoided if the patient has a laceration, a fracture, or an embedded ring.[7,8]

Pass a length of 1–0 silk suture underneath the ring (Figure 84-1A). Avoid monofilament sutures and smaller-size sutures as they may break or inadvertently cut the patient if wound too tightly. Passage of the string or suture may be facilitated with the use of a mosquito hemostat.[7–9] Wind the distal portion of the suture tightly around the digit in a closed spiral (Figure 84-1B). **There should be no interposition of skin between the turns of the suture material so as to ensure even compression of the skin and soft tissue.** Continue the spiral distally to just beyond the PIP joint. Grasp the proximal end of the suture. Unwind the suture while maintaining traction in the distal direction (Figure 84-1C). The ring will be pushed distally as the suture unwinds. The ring is easily removed once it clears the PIP joint (Figure 84-1D).

Other materials—such as umbilical tape, cotton gauze, rubber intravenous tourniquets, or Penrose drains—have also been used.[6,10,11] These materials have certain practical advantages. Since they are wider than sutures, shorter lengths and fewer turns are required to encircle the finger. It is easier to wind these materials around the digit without interposition of the skin between the turns. The umbilical tape method is the author's preferred method of ring removal (Figure 84-2).

Insert the umbilical tape under the ring, from distal to proximal, with the aid of a mosquito hemostat (Figure 84-2*A*). Pull 6 to 7 cm of the umbilical tape proximal to the ring (Figure 84-2*B*). Wind the distal portion of the umbilical tape tightly around the digit in a closed spiral (Figure 84-2*C*). There should be no interposition of skin between the turns of the umbilical tape. Continue to spiral distally to just beyond the PIP joint (Figure 84-2*C*).

Grasp the proximal end of the umbilical tape. Unwind the proximal end of the umbilical tape while maintaining traction in a distal direction (Figure 84-2*D*). Continue to unwind the umbilical tape until the ring passes the PIP joint (Figure 84-2*E*). The ring is easily removed once it clears the PIP joint (Figure 84-2*F*).

RUBBER BAND TECHNIQUE

This technique utilizes a 3 to 4 mm wide rubber band, which is used to apply traction on the ring to facilitate its passage over the PIP joint[9] (Figure 84-3). Though success has been reported using rubber bands, this technique should be reserved for less severe ring entrapments. This technique should be avoided if the patient has a laceration, a fracture, or an embedded ring.

Lubricate the finger liberally, as described above. Pass the rubber band beneath the ring using a mosquito

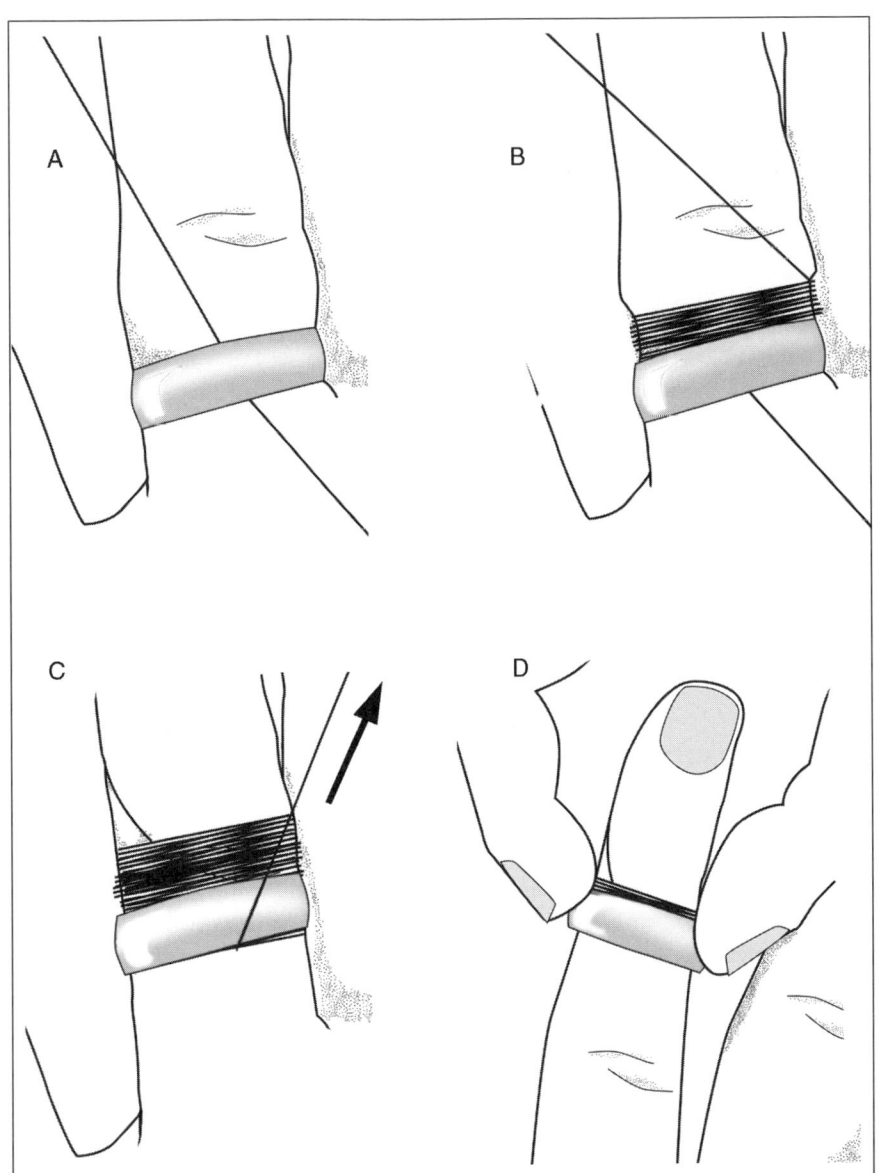

FIGURE 84-1 The string technique. *A.* A string is passed between the ring and the finger. *B.* The string distal to the ring is wound tightly around the finger and continued distally to the level just below the PIP joint. *C.* The string proximal to the ring is slowly unwound and moves the ring distally. *D.* When the ring passes the PIP joint, it usually comes off without effort.

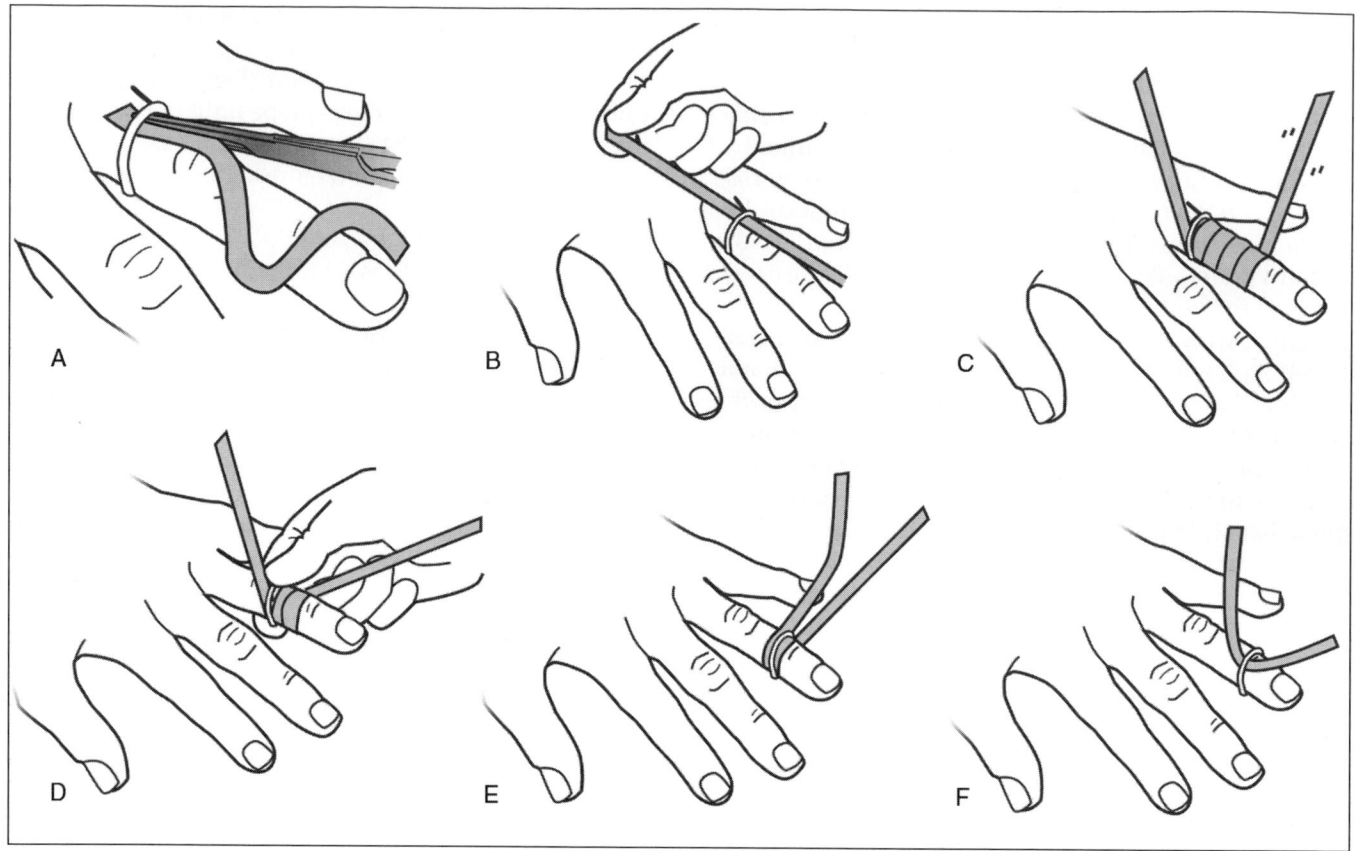

FIGURE 84-2 The string technique with umbilical tape. *A.* The umbilical tape is inserted under the ring with a hemostat. *B.* The umbilical tape is pulled through to the other side of the ring. *C.* The umbilical tape distal to the ring is wound tightly around the finger to the level just below the PIP joint. *D.* The umbilical tape proximal to the ring is slowly unwound and moves the ring distally. *E.* The ring passes the PIP joint. *F.* The ring is free and usually comes off without effort.

hemostat (Figures 84-3*A* and *B*). Position the rubber band so that equal lengths are on each side of the ring (Figure 84-3*C*). Insert a finger through both loops of the rubber band (Figure 84-3*D*). Pull the loops of the rubber band distally while simultaneously moving them circumferentially (Figure 84-3*D*). Continue the motion until the ring is removed (Figure 84-3*E*).

GLOVE TECHNIQUE

This technique has been advocated for use in patients with underlying soft tissue injury to the finger.[12,13] Its success is anecdotal. The glove technique uses a finger cut from an appropriately sized latex glove (Figure 84-4). The latex finger provides mild compression, acts as a barrier to protect damaged soft tissue, and provides a "leading edge" to guide the ring over the damaged tissues. Despite these theoretical advantages, the glove technique may be no more effective than any other in cases of severe finger edema.

Choose a glove that fits the patient snugly. Use the patient's other hand to aid in choosing the right size glove. Cut the finger from a latex glove to match the finger of the patient (Figure 84-4*A*). Cut off the tip of the finger of the glove to create a latex cylinder (Figure 84-4*A*). Slide the latex cylinder onto the patient's finger. Advance the proximal portion of the latex cylinder beneath the ring using a mosquito hemostat (Figure 84-4*B*). Lubricate the latex cylinder and the ring with K-Y jelly, Surgilube, petrolatum, mineral oil, or liquid soap. Pull the proximal edges of the latex cylinder, with your fingers or mosquito hemostats, to advance the ring distally (Figure 84-4*C*). Continue to pull on the proximal latex cylinder until the ring moves past the PIP joint and falls off the finger.

RING CUTTER TECHNIQUE

The definitive method for ring removal is cutting the ring. The ring should be cut if the patient presents with an underlying injury, severe swelling, an embedded ring, or entrapment with nonjewelry items. Cutting a ring is generally rapid and safe.

Many devices will cut rings. The standard rotary ring cutter should be available in every Emergency Department (Figure 84-5). The ring cutter's blade should be periodically inspected and it should be sharp. Battery-powered ring cuttesrs are also available (W.M. Mooney & Co., Ashland, OR). The advantage of the powered ring

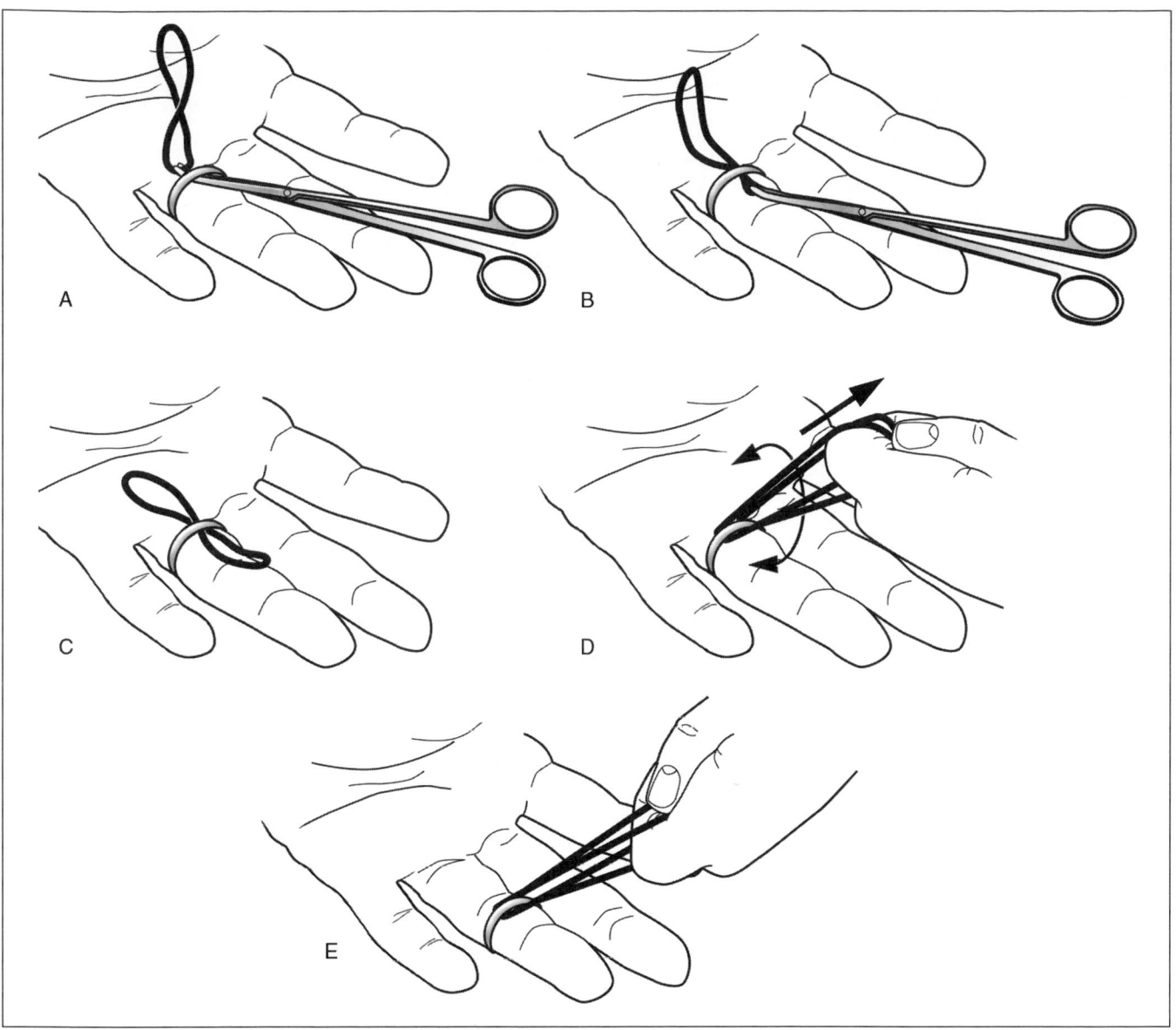

FIGURE 84-3 The rubber band technique. *A.* A mosquito hemostat is passed below the ring and grasps the rubber band. *B.* The rubber band is pulled beneath the ring and out the other side. *C.* The rubber band is positioned with equal lengths of loop on each side of the ring. *D.* Both loops of the rubber band are grasped and pulled distally while it is simultaneously rotated circumferentially. *E.* When the ring passes the PIP joint, it usually comes off without effort.

cutters is that they are easy to use, lightweight, fast, powerful, can easily cut nonjewelry items, and do not rely on the strength of the care provider to use them. In the absence of a ring cutter, another medical device that has been used successfully to cut rings is the Steinman pin cutter.[14] Our Emergency Department also maintains a sharp pair of diagonal pliers that are effective at removing small rings.

Pass the finger guard between the ring and the digit at the thinnest part of the ring (Figure 84-6). Care should be taken to place the ring cutter correctly and avoid additional injury. The ring may be squeezed using a heavy needle driver, hemostat, or pliers to change its shape from round to oval to facilitate passage of the

finger guard (Figure 84-7). This additional distortion of the ring will not further exacerbate the entrapment.[14] Lower the cutting blade onto the ring. Turn the turn key to rotate the blade while maintaining pressure on the ring. Pry apart the ring with hemostats or a needle driver once it is completely cut through.

If an open wound is present, it should be irrigated with normal saline to remove any small metal fragments that may result from the cutting process. There has been a case report of a foreign body granuloma caused by metal particles left in a finger wound in a patient following ring removal.[15]

Patients may rarely present with other heavy circular objects on their digits such as steel rings, nuts, or washers

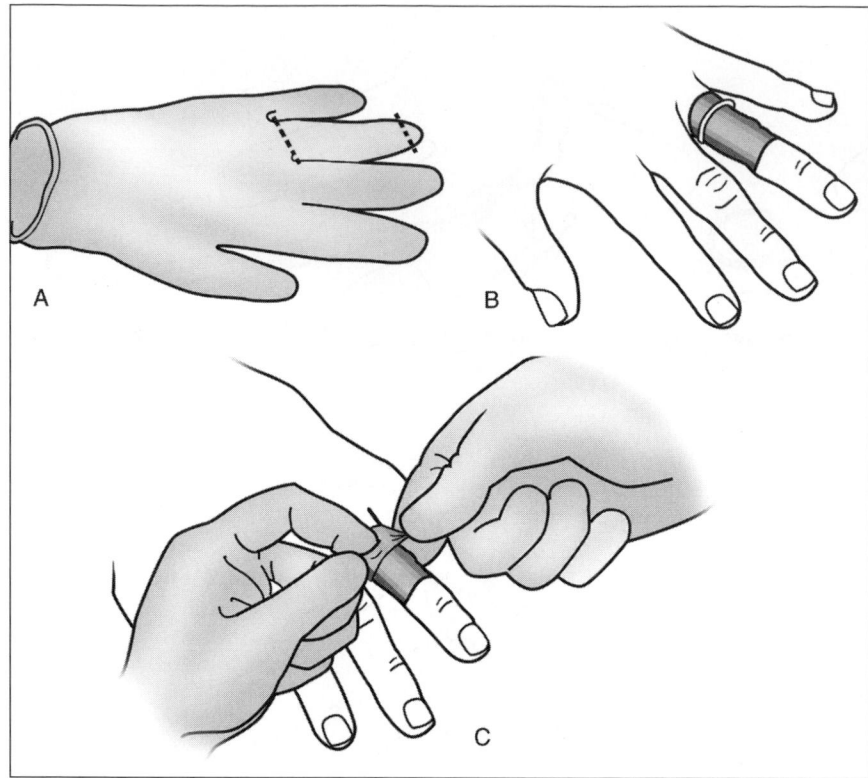

FIGURE 84-4 The latex glove technique. *A.* The finger matching the one on which the ring is lodged is cut from an examination glove. *B.* The latex cylinder is put on the finger. The proximal edges of the cylinder are pulled under and proximal to the ring using a mosquito hemostat. *C.* The proximal edges of the latex cylinder are slowly pulled distally to roll the ring off the finger.

that cannot be removed using a manually operated ring cutter. Powered cutting tools such as heavy-duty saws and bolt cutters may be needed to remove these objects. Battery-powered ring cutters may be ideal in these situations. Power saws with carbon blades have been used to successfully remove hardened steel rings from a patient's fingers.[5] If it becomes necessary to use a powered metal cutting device, additional care should be taken to protect the patient from secondary injury from the cutting element and the heat these powered devices may generate.

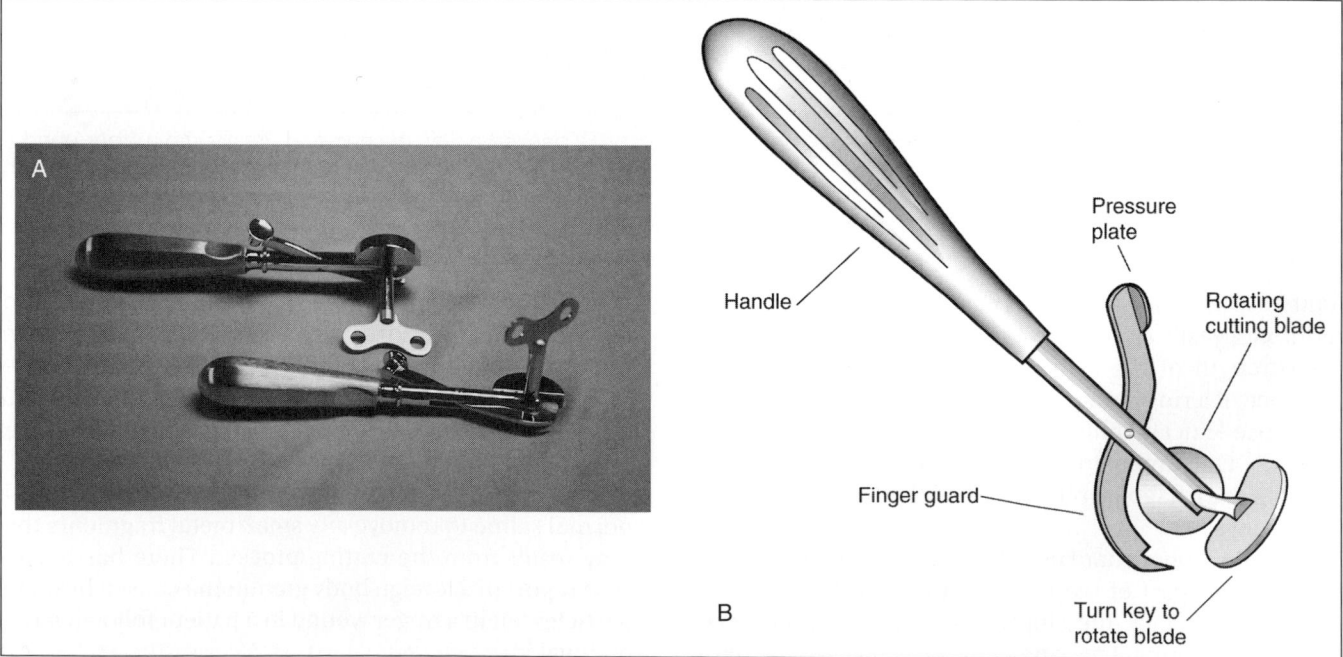

FIGURE 84-5 Manually operated ring cutters. *A.* Examples of manually operated ring cutters. *B.* The anatomy of a ring cutter.

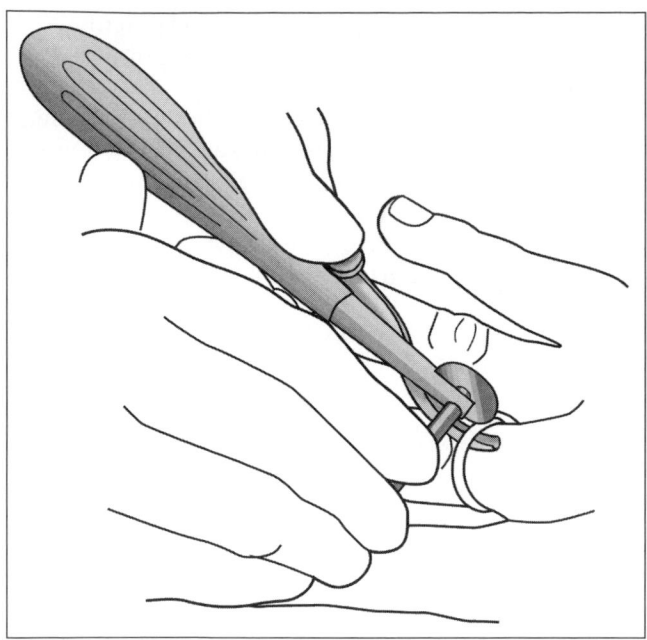

FIGURE 84-6 Ring removal using a ring cutter.

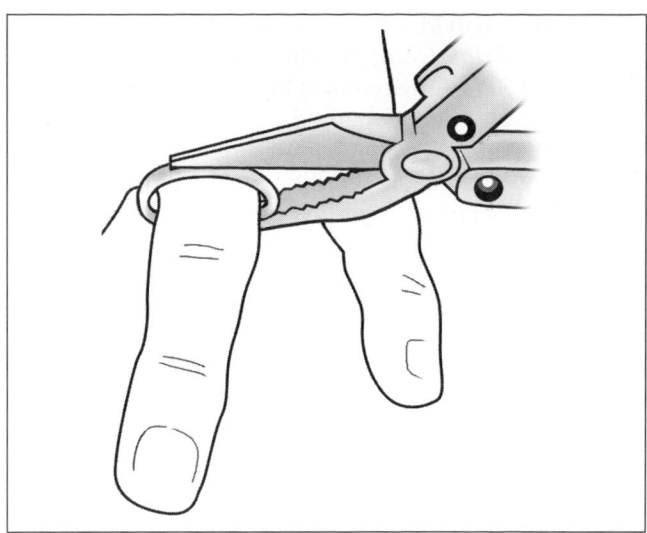

FIGURE 84-7 A pair of pliers is used to make the ring "oval" in shape. This may facilitate the use of a ring cutter.

ASSESSMENT

The finger should be thoroughly examined for any injuries after the ring is removed. Reassess perfusion to the digit by noting the capillary refill time, the color, and the pulse oximeter reading on the digit compared to adjacent fingers.

AFTERCARE

No specific aftercare is required following the ring removal process. Elevation, nonsteroidal anti-inflammatory agents, and local wound care are all that is necessary. Consultation with a Hand Surgeon, Orthopedic Surgeon, Plastic Surgeon, or Podiatrist is recommended in severe cases that include embedded rings, infections, vascular compromise, and/or neurologic compromise. The aftercare is based on any lacerations and/or fractures of the digit. The patient's tetanus immune status should be ascertained and, if the skin is broken, the appropriate tetanus prophylaxis administered. Instruct the patient not to place any rings on the digit until the edema has completely resolved.

COMPLICATIONS

The direct complications are minor compared to the complications that may occur from failure to remove a ring. Direct complications include secondary injury to soft tissues, vascular structures, and nerves and granuloma formation.

SUMMARY

Ring removal is a relatively straightforward and simple procedure. In situations in which the ring is extremely difficult to remove, a variety of potential approaches may assure success. Use of the ring cutter is the most reliable and quickest technique. The decision to use a ring cutter should be based upon the urgency with which the ring must be removed and not upon the monetary or sentimental value of the ring.

REFERENCES

1. Drake DA, Lewis F, Newmeyer WL, et al: An unusual ring injury. *J Hand Surg* 1977; 2(2):111–112.
2. Kuscher SH, Gellman H, Hume M: Embedded ring injuries. *Clin Orthop Rel Res* 1992; 276:192–193.
3. Shafiroff BB: Easy removal of a partially embedded ring from a finger. *Plast Reconstr Surg* 1979; 63(6):841–842.
4. Woodhouse C: Ulceration of a ring into a phalanx. *Hand* 1976; 8(2):186–188.
5. Rubman MH, Taylor K: A rapid method for emergency ring removal. *Am J Orthop* 1996; 25(1):42–44.
6. Cresap CR: Removal of a hardened steel ring from an extremely swollen finger. *Am J Emerg Med* 1995; 13(3):318–320.
7. Mizrahi S, Lunski I: A simplified method for ring removal from an edematous finger. *Am J Surg* 1986; 151(3):412–413.
8. Belliappa PP: A technique for removal of a tight ring. *J Hand Surg [Br]* 1989; 14(1):127.
9. McElfresh EC, Peterson-Elijah RC: Removal of a tight ring by the rubber band. *J Hand Surg [Br]* 1991; 16(2):225–226.

10. Thilagarajah M: An improved method of ring removal. *J Hand Surg [Br]* 1999; 24(1):118–119.

11. Mullet STH: Ring removal from an oedematous finger, an alternative method. *J Hand Surg [Br]* 1995; 20(4):496.

12. Clarke AC, Spencer RF: Ring removal from the injured or swollen finger. *J R Coll Surg Edinb* 1991; 36(2):59.

13. Inoue S: Another simple method for ring removal. *Anesthesiology* 1995; 83(5):1133–1134.

14. Wee JTK, Chandra D: A rapid method of removal of rings impacted in fingers. *J Hand Surg [Br]* 1989; 14(1):126–127.

15. Fasano FJ Jr, Hansen RH: Foreign body granuloma and synovitis of the finger: a hazard of ring removal by the sawing technique. *J Hand Surg [Am]* 1987; 12(4):621–623.

16. Rubio PA: A simplified method for ring removal from an edematous finger. *Am J Surg* 1987; 153(1):A42.

Chapter 85
SUBUNGUAL HEMATOMA EVACUATION

Steven H. Bowman

INTRODUCTION

Fingertips are sensitive, mobile, and prone to injury. Blunt trauma to the tip of the finger or toe may result in a variety of injuries including fractures, avulsions to the nail and nail apparatus, contusions, lacerations, and amputations. The most common injuries to the distal fingers and toes are crush injuries. The most common mechanism of injury is closure of some type of door (car, house, etc.) on the finger. Dropped objects, hand tools, and power tools constitute the majority of the remaining mechanisms of injury.

Subungual hematomas very commonly develop following blunt trauma to the distal finger or toe.[1–3] They result from the accumulation of blood between the nail and the nail bed. Treatment of a subungual hematoma is relatively straightforward, yet in some cases it is still controversial. It is important to understand the structure of the distal finger or toe, to determine whether simple drainage will be sufficient management, and to consider how initial management may affect outcome.

ANATOMY AND PATHOPHYSIOLOGY

The distal digits of the fingers and toes and the nail apparatus are complex structures (Figure 85-1). The perionychium is composed of the nail bed and the surrounding soft tissue. The hyponychium is the junction of the nail bed at the sterile matrix and the fingertip skin beneath the distal margin of the nail. The eponychium is the distal portion of the nail fold where it attaches to the proximal surface of the nail. The lunule is the white arc seen in the proximal portion of the nail. The nail bed consists of the germinal matrix on the proximal ventral floor of the nail fold and the sterile matrix, which extends from the lunule to the hyponychium. The germinal matrix is primarily responsible for the growth of the nail, with a significant contribution from the sterile matrix.[4,5]

The nail bed must be smooth for normal nail growth. A nail matrix that has not been well approximated to minimize scar formation may develop a deformed nail.[1,3–8]

The nail bed receives its blood supply from the two terminal branches of the volar digital artery, which communicate to form blood sinuses. Venous drainage begins at the proximal portion of the nail bed and the skin proximal to the nail fold.[4]

Force applied to the fingertip disrupts the vascular structures in the nail bed. Trauma causes the capillaries of the nail bed to be compressed between the nail and the distal phalanx. Blood collects between the nail bed and the nail, forming a subungual hematoma (Figure 85-2). The patient's pain is directly related to the injury itself and the increased pressure from the hematoma. The hematoma is a black-and-blue or black-and-purple area under the nail that is extremely tender to palpation.

Nail bed injuries may be classified as simple lacerations, stellate lacerations, severe crush injuries, and avulsions.[1] It is important to understand that each of these types of nail bed injuries may result in a subungual hematoma.

The management of subungual hematomas is still somewhat controversial. The approach to management was initially very aggressive, since subungual hematomas are often seen with fractures of the distal phalanx, damage to the nail, and damage to the nail apparatus.[1,2,4–8] The surgical literature generally recommends removal of the nail, inspection of the nail bed, and repair of any nail bed injury if the subungual hematoma involves 25 percent or more of the nail surface.[1,2,4–9] This practice has been questioned recently by newer controlled studies that demonstrated excellent outcomes in patients with large (greater than 25 percent) subungual hematomas treated by trephination alone, regardless of the presence of fractures.[11,12] Larger hematomas involving over 50 percent of the nail surface may be treated successfully with trephination. Many authors still advocate the removal of the nail to thoroughly inspect the nail bed

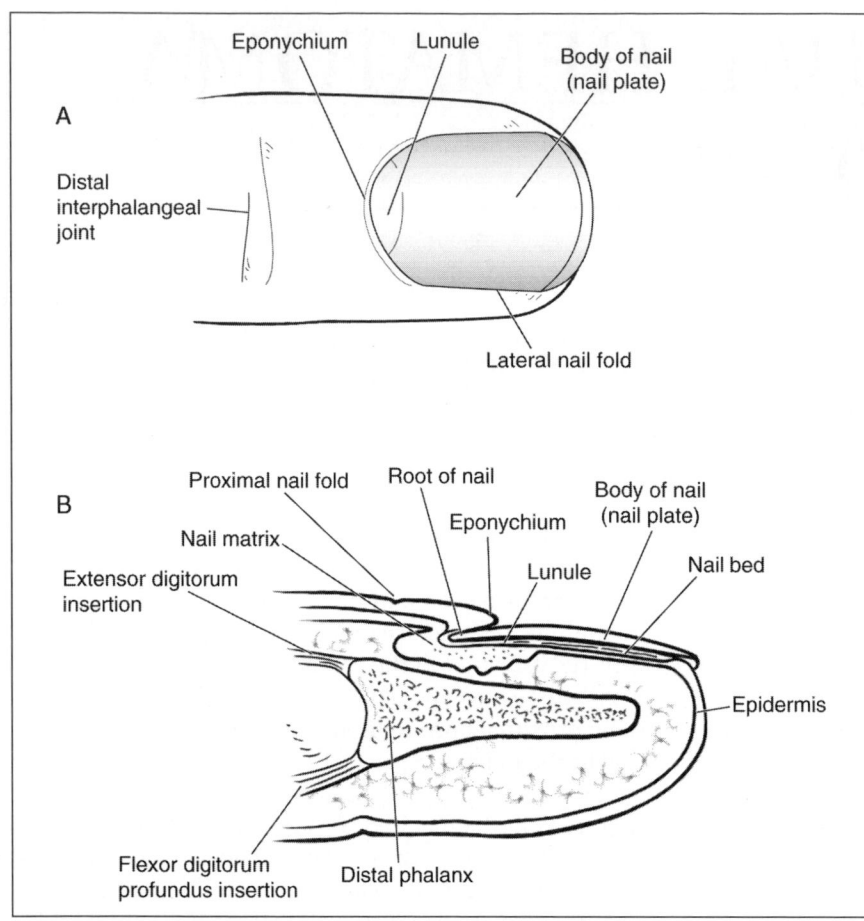

FIGURE 85-1 The anatomy of the distal fingertip and nail bed. *A.* Surface anatomy. *B.* Midsagittal view.

and effect repair in all patients who present with a subungual hematoma. Though this aproach is time-honored, more recent studies have demonstrated that it is not necessary if the patient's nail is still attached to the matrix, even in the presence of a distal phalanx fracture.[11,12]

INDICATIONS

Patients who present to the Emergency Department after sustaining an injury with a resultant subungual

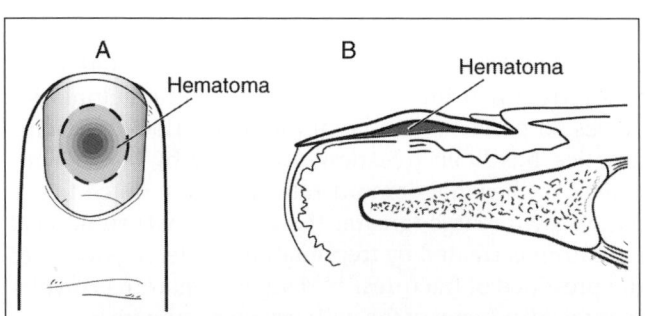

FIGURE 85-2 The subungual hematoma. *A.* Surface view. *B.* Sagittal view.

hematoma will generally complain of severe pain. Trephination, the process of making a small hole in the nail to allow the collected blood to escape, will provide significant relief for most patients.[2,9] **The trephination procedures described below should be utilized when patients present with a subungual hematoma and an intact (not fractured or avulsed) nail that is still attached to the matrix. If the nail is partially or completely avulsed from the matrix, simple evacuation of the hematoma may not constitute adequate therapy.[9,11,13]**

CONTRAINDICATIONS

Simple trephination is reserved for patients with intact nails. **Patients who present with nail fractures, avulsions of the nail, or partial amputations may require more extensive therapy with removal of the nail and repair of the nail bed.** A description of these techniques is provided in Chapters 80 and 87. Trephination using heat-based methods should be avoided in patients wearing artificial nails due to the potential for igniting the nail or nail adhesive.[13]

EQUIPMENT

Digital/Metacarpal Block

Povidone iodine or isopropyl alcohol pads
3 mL syringe
25 or 27 gauge needle, 1 inch long
Local anesthetic solution without epinephrine

Electrocautery

Povidone iodine or isopropyl alcohol pads
Battery-powered electrocautery device

Paper Clip Technique

Povidone iodine or isopropyl alcohol pads
Heat source (open flame)
Paper clip
Hemostat

Drill Technique

Povidone iodine or isopropyl alcohol pads
18 gauge needle
Cotton-tipped applicators

PATIENT PREPARATION

Explain the procedure to the patient and emphasize that pain relief rapidly follows nail trephination. Obtain a consent to perform the procedure. Place the patient supine or seated on a gurney. The practitioner should sit facing the patient. Place the hand with the injured digit palm side down on a flat surface such as a procedure table. Cleanse the injured digit of any dirt and debris. Apply povidone iodine solution and allow it to dry. A digital block is generally not needed in using heat-based methods to penetrate the nail.[2,5,9,13] The nail is not innervated and the hematoma prevents contact with the nail bed. A digital block may be required if the patient is excessively anxious, if additional injury is present, or if a drill technique is to be performed. Refer to Chapter 106 for the complete details regarding digital and metacarpal blocks. The techniques described below may be used on fingernails and toenails.

TECHNIQUES

ELECTROCAUTERY TECHNIQUE

Electrocautery is the preferred technique to drain a subungual hematoma. Battery-operated microcautery devices are generally available in the Emergency Depart-

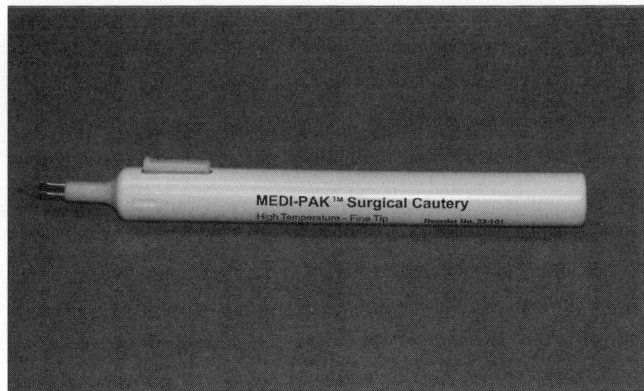

FIGURE 85-3 The battery-operated electrocautery device.

ment (Figure 85-3). Assure the patient that he or she will not be burned. Stabilize the injured digit proximally with the nondominant hand. Grasp the cautery unit like a pencil with the dominant hand. Press the button on the cautery unit to heat the tip. Place the hot tip on the nail plate, centered over the hematoma (Figure 85-4). The cautery will penetrate the nail easily. The tips of some microcautery devices are shaped in such a way that they will not make a hole that is wide enough to allow adequate drainage. Slightly rotate the cautery unit as it traverses the nail plate to ensure an adequate sized drainage hole.

Darkened blood will flow out of the hole as the hematoma space is entered. The nail will regain its normal color after the hematoma is drained. Apply slight digital pressure to the nail plate to ensure complete drainage of the hematoma. The patient will usually begin to feel pain relief at this point. Some physicians prefer to make one or two additional holes in the nail plate to ensure drainage if the first hole should become occluded.

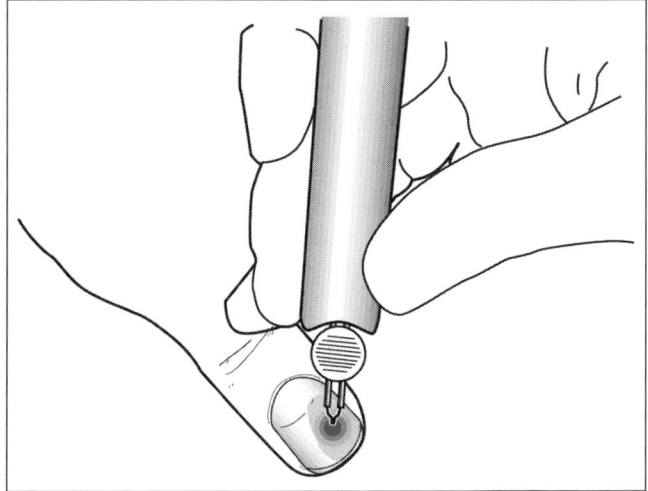

FIGURE 85-4 The electrocautery technique. The hot tip of the unit is centered over the subungual hematoma and allowed to penetrate the nail plate.

PAPER CLIP TECHNIQUE

This technique is similar to that using the electrocautery unit. Unfold and heat the tip of a paper clip with a flame from a lighter or alcohol lamp. Place the heated tip of the paper clip against the nail plate, centered over the subungual hematoma (Figure 85-5). Apply slight downward pressure to allow the paper clip to perforate the nail plate. A drop of blood will be seen as the paper clip enters the hematoma.

The paper clip will not get as hot as a cautery device. More than one attempt may be necessary to penetrate a thick nail. Another disadvantage of this technique is the possibility of introducing carbonaceous material into the hole. In some settings, it may be difficult and potentially more dangerous to use an open flame.

DRILL TECHNIQUE

This technique uses a needle as a small drill to penetrate the nail plate (Figure 85-6). Small electric nail drills are available that greatly simplify this procedure, though they may not be readily available in the Emergency Department. Drilling through the nail plate may require a digital block. This is particularly true if there is a fracture, another associated injury, or the nail plate is very thick. Grasp an 18 gauge needle by its hub with the thumb and forefinger (Figure 85-6A). Place the tip of the needle over the nail plate, centered over the subungual hematoma. Spin the needle back and forth while applying gentle downward pressure. Small shavings will appear as the needle begins to drill through the nail plate. A loss of resistance will be felt as the hematoma is entered and darkened blood will flow out of the hole.

One of the editors uses a modified version of this technique (Reichman, personal communication). A cotton-tipped applicator may be wedged into the needle hub to facilitate the drilling (Figure 85-6B). This method makes the drilling more efficient, as the cotton-tipped applicator is easier to hold and offers a mechanical advantage. The drill technique is useful in the absence of a cautery device or flame and paper clip.

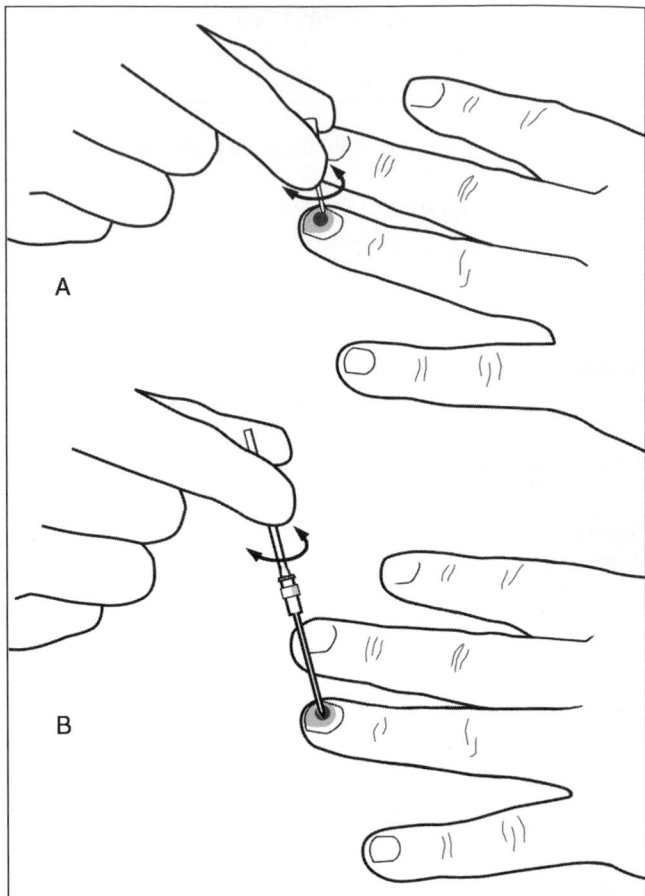

FIGURE 85-6 Drill techniques. *A.* Grasping the 18 gauge needle with the thumb and index finger, a twisting motion is used to penetrate the nail plate. *B.* A cotton-tipped applicator has been inserted into the hub of the needle. The applicator is grasped with the thumb and index finger. A twisting motion is used to penetrate the nail plate.

ASSESSMENT

Squeeze the nail plate to evacuate the hematoma. Any underlying injury should be evaluated and managed.

AFTERCARE

The patient should keep the wound clean and monitor drainage. The nail may be covered with a nonadherent dressing. The hematoma may continue to drain for several hours. If there is a reaccumulation, denoted by the reappearance of darkened blood beneath the nail, the nail can be soaked in warm water and pressure applied to express the hematoma. A splint should be applied if a distal phalanx fracture is present. No studies have demonstrated that prophylactic antibiotics are beneficial in the management of a subungual hematoma.[9,14] The patient should immediately return to the Emergency Depart-

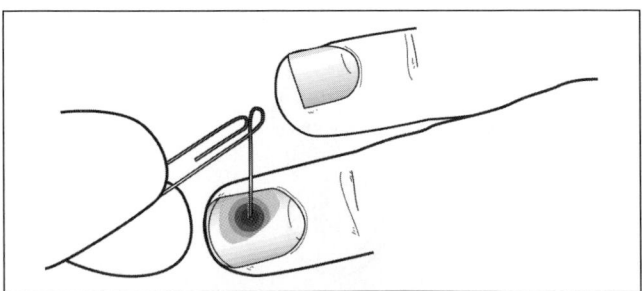

FIGURE 85-5 The paper clip technique. The hot tip of the paper clip is centered over the subungual hematoma and allowed to penetrate the nail plate.

ment or their primary physician if a fever develops or if there is increased pain, a purulent or foul-smelling drainage from the nail, or reddening of the digit.

COMPLICATIONS

Direct complications from nail trephination are rare.[11–13] Complications will more likely result from the original injury and include nail loss, nail deformity, cosmetic changes, and infection. Patients should be warned that as the nail grows out, loss of the nail is a possibility. The hematoma may reaccumulate if the hole in the nail is too small and becomes occluded. Reaccumulation can be prevented by making a large hole or multiple holes in the nail plate.

SUMMARY

Fingertip injuries are common. Patients will often present to the Emergency Department with a subungual hematoma and a complaint of pain. Rapid relief of pain and good outcomes can be obtained in the majority of cases by simply performing a nail trephination. It is important to distinguish when trephination alone will not be adequate therapy. Patients presenting with nail fractures, avulsions of the nail, or partial finger amputations will require removal of the nail and repair of the nail bed.

REFERENCES

1. Zook EG, Guy RJ, Russell RC: A study of nail bed injuries: causes, treatment, and prognosis. *J Hand Surg [Am]* 1984; 9A(2):247–252.
2. Newmeyer WL, Kilgore ES: Common injuries of the fingernail and nail bed. *Am Fam Physician* 1977; 16(4):93–95.
3. Guy RJ: The etiologies and mechanisms of nail bed injuries. *Hand Clin* 1990; 6(1):9–19.
4. Zook EG, Brown RE: The perionychium, in Green DP, Hotchkiss RN, Pederson WC (eds): *Green's Operative Hand Surgery,* 4th ed. New York: Churchill Livingstone, 1999:1353–1380.
5. Hart RG, Kleinert HE: Fingertip and nailbed injuries. *Emerg Med Clin North Am* 1993; 11(3):755–765.
6. Melone CP Jr, Grad JB: Primary care of fingernail injuries. *Emerg Med Clin North Am* 1985; 3(2):255–261.
7. Van Beek AL, Kassan MA, Adson MH, et al: Management of acute fingernail injuries. *Hand Clin* 1990; 6(1):23–35.
8. Russell RC, Casas LA: Management of fingertip injuries. *Clin Plast Surg* 1989; 16(3):405–425.
9. Blumstein H: Incision and drainage, in Roberts JR, Hedges JR (eds): *Clinical Procedures in Emergency Medicine,* 3rd ed. Philadelphia: Saunders, 1998:634–659.
10. Simon RR, Wolgin M: Subungual hematoma: association with occult laceration requiring repair. *Am J Emerg Med* 1987; 5(4):302–304.
11. Seaberg DC, Angelos WJ, Paris PM: Treatment of subungual hematomas with nail trephination: a prospective study. *Am J Emerg Med* 1991; 9(3):209–210.
12. Roser SE, Gellman H: Comparison of nail bed repair versus nail trephination for subungual hematomas in children. *J Hand Surg [Am]* 1999; 24(6):1166–1170.
13. Chudnofsky CR, Sebastian S: Special wounds: nail bed, plantar puncture, and cartilage. *Emerg Med Clin North Am* 1992; 10(4):801–822.
14. Lammers RL, Trott AT: Methods of wound closure, in Roberts JR, Hedges JR (eds): *Clinical Procedures in Emergency Medicine,* 3rd ed. Philadelphia: Saunders, 1998:560–599.

Chapter 86
SUBUNGUAL FOREIGN BODY REMOVAL

Steven H. Bowman

INTRODUCTION

Subungual foreign bodies are often difficult to treat. Foreign bodies such as wood or metal splinters, pencil lead, thorns, spines, or hair may become lodged beneath the fingernail.[1-3] Tradesmen such as carpenters, landscapers, auto mechanics, and individuals who work without hand protection with materials that produce small splinters are at risk for this type of injury. Subungual foreign bodies may also present less commonly under the toenails.

Patients generally present for medical intervention complaining of pain after unsuccessfully attempting to remove the foreign body. Prior removal attempts often result in breakage of the foreign body or pushing it further beneath the nail; both of which complicate the next extraction attempt. Left untreated, retained subungual foreign bodies will often become infected or cause tissue reactions and granuloma formation. These injuries may be treated rapidly with complete removal of the foreign body and without causing additional patient discomfort.

ANATOMY AND PATHOPHYSIOLOGY

The distal fingertip and nail apparatus are complex structures (Figure 86-1). The perionychium is composed of the nail bed and the surrounding soft tissue. The hyponychium is the junction of the nail bed at the sterile matrix and the fingertip skin beneath the distal margin of the nail plate. The eponychium is the distal portion of the nail fold where it attaches to the proximal surface of the nail plate. The lunule is the white arc seen on the proximal portion of the nail plate. The nail bed consists of the germinal matrix on the proximal ventral floor of the nail fold and the sterile matrix that extends from the lunule to the hyponychium. The germinal matrix is primarily responsible for the growth of the nail. The subungual space is the area immediately beneath the nail plate.

Foreign bodies may enter the subungual space at the distal fingertip beneath the nail, or may penetrate the nail plate directly (Figure 86-2). In either event, separation of the nail from the nail bed results in severe pain.

Patients generally immediately attempt to remove the foreign body because of this intense pain. Infection or foreign body reaction is likely to ensue if the foreign body is not removed in its entirety.

INDICATIONS

Subungual foreign bodies should be removed to prevent the complications of infection, foreign body reaction, and possible nail deformity. Deeply embedded foreign bodies, splintered foreign bodies, those that traverse the nail plate, or contaminated foreign bodies may require the removal of the nail plate to extract the foreign body. Refer to Chapter 87 regarding the details of removing the nail plate. A Hand Surgeon should be consulted if the foreign body cannot be removed, if the site is infected, or if significant injury to the digit is present.

CONTRAINDICATIONS

There are no absolute contraindications to the removal of a subungual foreign body.

EQUIPMENT

General Supplies

Povidone iodine
Sterile saline solution
Topical antibiotic ointment
Nonadherent dressing (e.g., petrolatum gauze)
4×4 gauze squares
Adhesive tape

Digital / Metacarpal Block

3 mL syringe
25 or 27 gauge needle, 1 inch long
3 to 5 mL local anesthetic solution without epinephrine

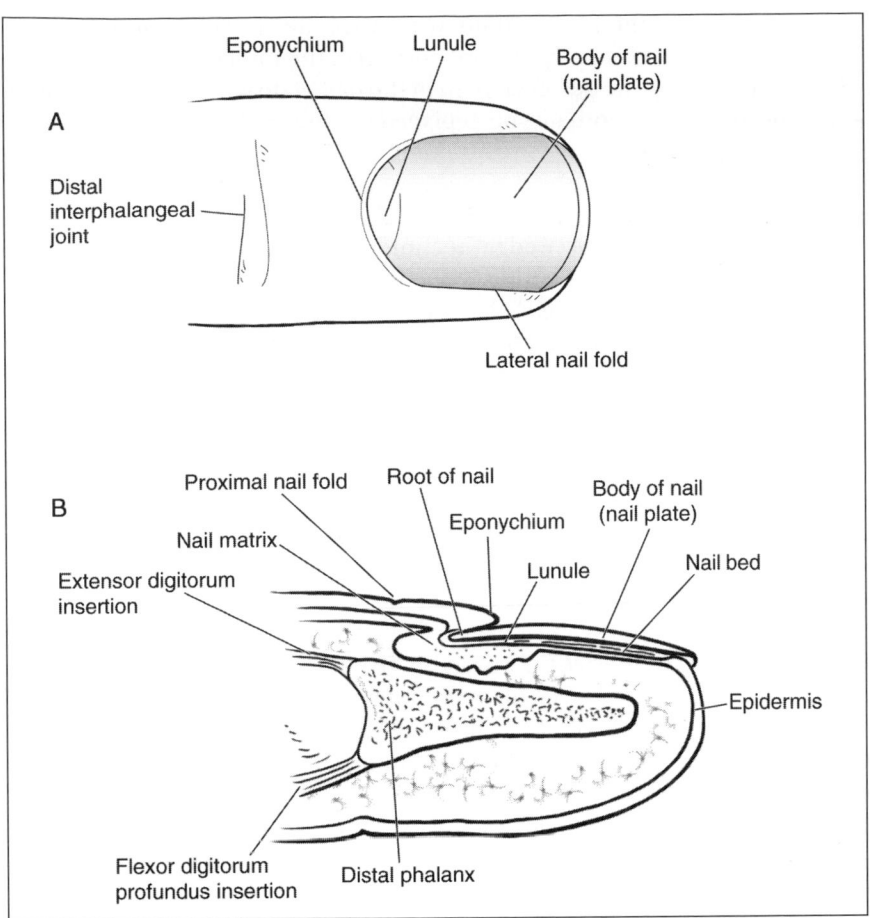

FIGURE 86-1 The anatomy of the distal fingertip and nail bed. *A.* Surface anatomy. *B.* Midsagittal view.

Scrape Technique

Splinter forceps
#11 or #15 scalpel blade on a handle

Wedge Technique

Splinter forceps
Tissue scissors or nail clippers

Needle Technique

Needles, 19 and 25 to 27 gauges
Splinter forceps
Hemostat

PATIENT PREPARATION

Explain the risks and benefits of the procedure to the patient and/or their representative. Obtain an informed consent for the procedure. Ascertain the patient's tetanus immune status and administer the appropriate tetanus prophylaxis. The practitioner should attempt to gain the patient's cooperation. Place the patient on a gurney with the hand on a bedside procedure table. Clean any dirt and debris from the affected finger. Apply povidone iodine and allow it to dry. Any manipulation of the nailbed will result in additional patient discomfort. Determine the need for a digital or metacarpal block depending on the type and extent of the foreign body and the removal technique. Please refer to Chapter 106 for the complete details regarding anesthesia of the finger or toe.

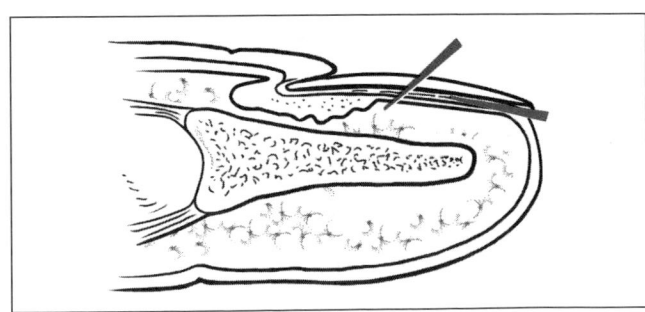

FIGURE 86-2 Subungual foreign bodies can enter from under the distal nail plate or through the nail plate.

TECHNIQUES

Foreign bodies protruding through or from underneath the nail plate may be grasped with a forceps and removed. A scalpel blade or 18 gauge needle may be used to entrap a small protruding tip of the foreign body against the nail plate and draw it out. Superficially located subungual foreign bodies may be removed by one of the following techniques.

SCRAPE TECHNIQUE

This technique has been described anecdotally.[4,5] It appears promising as it does not require the administration of a digital block and causes less trauma to the nail and the nail bed compared to other techniques. This technique works well for subungual foreign bodies that either traverse the nail plate or are lodged beneath the distal or middle portion of the nail.

Support the patient's hand on a procedure table. The practitioner should sit facing the patient. Place a #11 or #15 scalpel blade on the nail plate and directly over the foreign body (Figure 86-3A). Hold the blade perpendicular to the surface of the nail plate. Draw the scalpel blade from proximal to distal using short strokes and gentle pressure over the foreign body (Figure 86-3A). A small shaving of the nail plate is removed with each stroke of the scalpel blade. The finger may be soaked in lukewarm water for 15 to 20 minutes to soften the nail plate if it is difficult to shave the nail plate. Removing successive slivers of the nail plate will eventually create a U-shaped defect and expose the foreign body (Figure 86-3B). Grasp the foreign body with a splinter forceps and remove it once a significant portion of the foreign body is exposed. The defect created in the nail plate will move distally and eventually be replaced as the nail plate continues to grow.

WEDGE TECHNIQUE

The wedge technique works well for subungual foreign bodies lodged beneath the distal portion of the nail plate.[1,6] Patients will require a digital or metacarpal block prior to attempting this technique since it involves manipulation of the nail bed.

The practitioner should sit facing the patient. Cut a triangular wedge from the distal portion of the nail plate overlying the foreign body with a small pair of tissue scissors or nail clippers (Figure 86-4A). Remove the wedge of nail. This will provide enough exposure to grasp and remove the foreign body with splinter forceps (Figure 86-4B).

NEEDLE TECHNIQUES

The needle technique works well for subungual foreign bodies located beneath the distal portion of the nail plate.[1] Patients will require a digital or metacarpal block prior to attempting this technique. Insertion of a needle into the nail bed is extremely painful. The major drawback of this technique is the potential for leaving fragments of the foreign body beneath the nail plate.

The practitioner should sit facing the patient. Introduce a 19 gauge needle beneath the nail plate and along the track of the foreign body (Figure 86-5A). Tease out

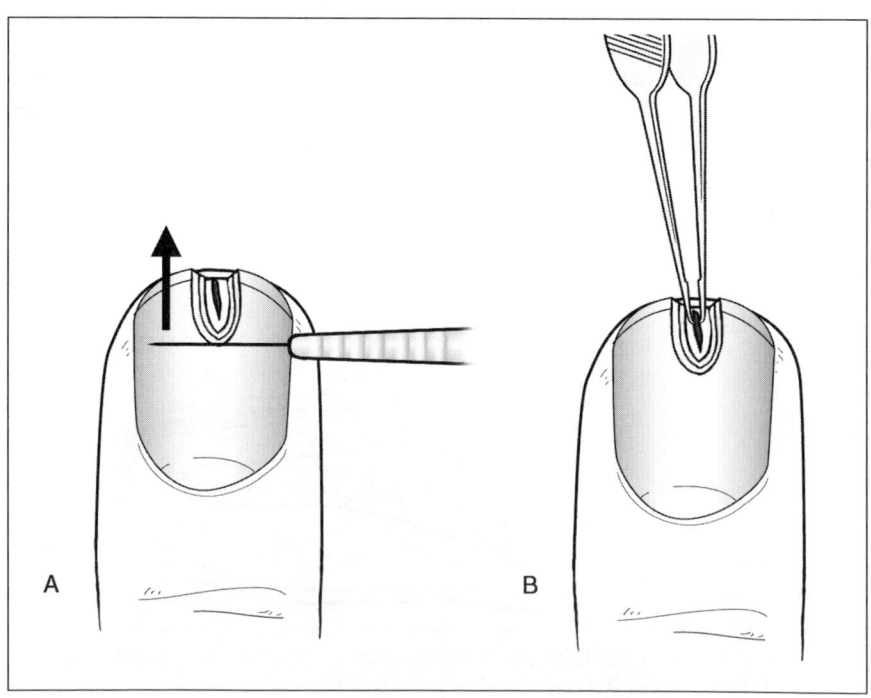

FIGURE 86-3 The scrape technique. *A.* With the scalpel blade held 90 degrees to the nailbed, strokes are made in a proximal to distal direction. A U-shaped defect will be created to expose the foreign body. *B.* The foreign body is removed with a forceps.

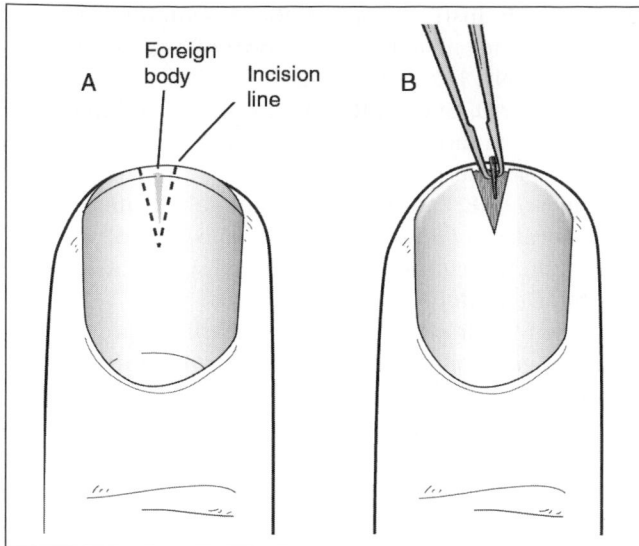

FIGURE 86-4 The wedge technique. *A.* A triangular incision is made in the nail plate overlying the foreign body. *B.* The cut section of the nail plate has been removed. The foreign body is grasped with a forceps and removed.

and move the foreign body distally so that it may be grasped with a splinter forceps.

Two alternate techniques have also been described for the needle extraction of a subungual foreign body.[7,8] The first is a modification of the needle technique.[7] Place a hook in the distal end of a 25 to 27 gauge needle with a hemostat or needle driver (Figure 86-5*B*). Pass the needle along the foreign body tract to tease out and move the foreign body distally so that it may be grasped with a splinter forceps. A third technique involves the excision of a small portion of the nail place overlying the foreign body with an 18 gauge needle.[8] This is similar to the shave technique with the exception of an 18 gauge needle being used instead of a scalpel blade.

ASSESSMENT

The subungual area should be inspected for any remaining fragments of the foreign body that may have broken off in the nail bed. **Any remaining fragments of the foreign body must be removed.** Refer the patient to a specialist if the foreign body fragments cannot be removed.

AFTERCARE

In most cases, local wound care and the application of a topical antibiotic are all that is required. Irrigate the foreign body tract and excision site with sterile saline. Apply topical antibiotic ointment to the area. Apply a nonadherent dressing over the nail. Follow-up with a

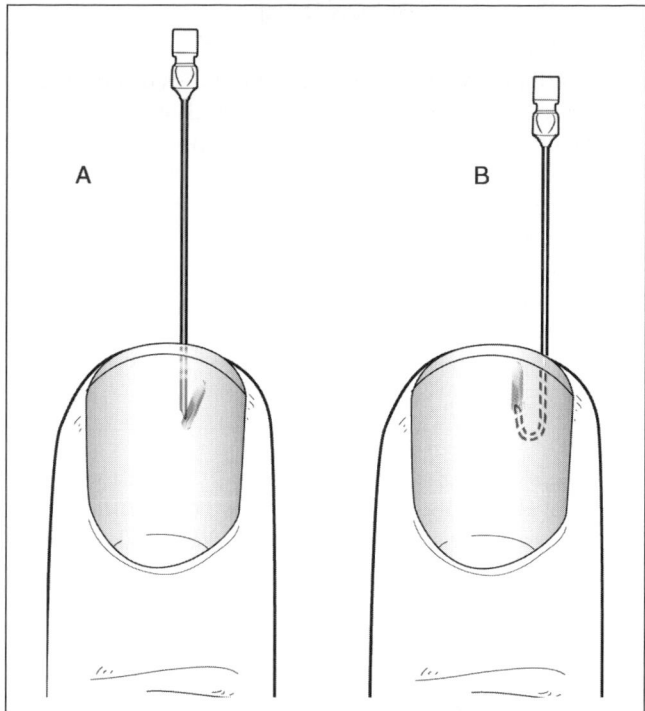

FIGURE 86-5 Needle techniques. *A.* A 19 gauge needle is inserted along the tract of the foreign body. The tip is used to tease the foreign body out of the tissues. *B.* The tip of a 25 to 27 gauge needle has been formed into a hook with the aid of a hemostat. The needle is inserted along the tract of the foreign body. The tip is used to grasp the foreign body and pull it out of the tissues.

hand specialist and systemic antibiotics may be necessary in severe cases, such as the presence of a nail deformity or chronic foreign bodies with infection. Postprocedural pain can be managed with acetaminophen or nonsteroidal anti-inflammatory drugs. The use of prophylactic antibiotics is not recommended unless the foreign body was contaminated or had deeply penetrated into the digit. The patient should immediately return to the Emergency Department for pus in the wound, increased tenderness of the digit, redness of the nail bed or digit, or fever.

COMPLICATIONS

There are a few potential complications from subungual foreign body removal. Damage to the nail bed can result in a residual nail deformity. Failure to completely remove a subungual foreign body may result in a nail deformity, infection (usually a paronychia), or a foreign body reaction with granuloma formation. An infection can result if sterile technique is not followed.

Significant pain during the procedure can be avoided by first performing a digital or metacarpal block.

SUMMARY

Patients with subungual foreign bodies often present in severe pain after prior unsuccessful attempts at removal or after complications develop. Though sometimes challenging, it is important that the practitioner completely remove the foreign material in the subungual space to prevent further complications. Providing adequate anesthesia and using the appropriate instruments and technique will allow the successful removal of most subungual foreign bodies.

REFERENCES

1. Rudinsky GS, Barnett RC: Soft tissue foreign-body removal, in Roberts JR, Hedges JR (eds): *Clinical Procedures in Emergency Medicine,* 3rd ed. Philadelphia: Saunders, 1998:623.

2. Haneke E, Tosti A, Piraccini BM: Sea urchin granuloma of the nail apparatus: report of 2 cases. *Dermatology* 1996; 192(2):140–142.

3. de Berker D, Dawber R, Wojnarowska F: Subungual hair implantation in hairdressers. *Br J Dermatol* 1994; 130(3):400–401.

4. Schwartz GR, Schwen SA: Subungual splinter removal. *Am J Emerg Med* 1997; 15(3):330–331.

5. Epstein E: Treatment of subungual splinters. *J Am Acad Dermatol* 1996; 35 (3 Pt 1):491.

6. Miller MA, Brodell RT: Surgical pearl: treatment of subungual splinters. *J Am Acad Dermatol* 1995; 33(4):667–668.

7. Davis LJ: Removal of subungual foreign bodies. *J Fam Pract* 1980; 11(5):714.

8. Andrus CH: Instrument and technique for removal of subungual foreign bodies. *Am J Surg* 1980; 140(4): 588.

Chapter 87
NAIL BED REPAIR

Brian C. Sullivan

INTRODUCTION

The fingernail plays an important functional role in the mechanism of pinch and grasp.[1,2] It increases the sensitivity of the fingertip.[2] The fingernails are frequently injured due to their anatomic location and their functional role. Immediate primary repair is the ideal management when these injuries involve the nail bed and surrounding skin fold structures.[2,3] Careful repair is necessary to avoid functional impairment and cosmetic derangement of the nail plate.[4] The following discussion will refer primarily to the fingernail. The toenail has less importance, both cosmetically and functionally, as grasp and pinch are not needed. However, all the principles and recommendations made also apply to the toenail.[5]

ANATOMY AND PATHOPHYSIOLOGY

The nail plate enhances the sensibility of the fingertip by applying a counterforce to the pulp space nerve endings.[2] The digital tip and the nail plate also function in unison to smoothly coordinate normal pinch and grasp, which are important for picking up fine objects such as coins and pins.[1,2]

The nail plate is comprised of compacted, flattened, and elongated anucleated cells that originate from cornified epithelial cells.[6] There are three atomic sites where these cells exist.[1,3] The nail bed contains two of the sites: the sterile matrix and the germinal matrix.[1] The other location is the dorsal roof matrix (Figure 87-1A). Of these, the germinal matrix is the most important for normal nail growth.[3] The germinal matrix is responsible for approximately 90 percent of the nail plate by volume.[1] The sterile matrix is responsible for a small percent of the nail plate by volume and varies from individual to individual. This cell production accounts for the nail plate being thicker at its distal tip compared to its proximal origin.[1] The nail cells from the dorsal roof matrix are small in number and form a very thin layer on the surface of the nail plate. These cells are responsible for the shine of the nail. If the dorsal roof is destroyed, the nail will lose its shine and become dull.

Skin overlies the nail plate proximally and laterally (Figure 87-1B).[6] The proximal skin fold is referred to as the eponychium. The eponychium protects the germinal matrix located in the proximal nail bed and is the home of the dorsal roof matrix. The skin immediately over the dorsal roof is called the nail wall.[1] The lateral skin folds, the adjacent cutaneous areas, and the adjacent nail bed (germinal matrix and sterile matrix) are collectively referred to as the perionychium (Figure 87-1B).[1,4,6] The lunule is the pale arc just distal to the eponychium and roughly corresponds to the location of the germinal matrix.[1,6]

The nail bed is comprised of the germinal matrix proximally and the sterile matrix distally. The borders of the nail bed are the proximal nail fold, the lateral nail folds, and the hyponychium distally. The hyponychium is the thick layer of cells at the junction of the distal nail bed (sterile matrix) and the fingertip skin.[1] It is located just under the distal free margin of the nail plate (Figure 87-1A). The hyponychium serves as a barrier preventing the delicate nail bed from exposure to bacteria and fungi.[1]

The rate of nail growth varies from finger to finger as well as from individual to individual.[1,2] Progression of the distal nail occurs at a rate of 0.1 mm/day or 0.5 to 1 mm/week.[2,6] This rate varies and is usually faster in fingers than in toes, and faster in the summer months.[2] The pressure of new cells being formed leads to the flattening and elongation of the older cells as well as their progression distally.[1]

The sterile matrix is more adherent to the nail plate than to the adjacent germinal matrix. Therefore, avulsions involving nail bed tissue are more likely to occur at the sterile matrix.[1,7,8] Conversely, the nail plate is loosely held to the germinal matrix. This accounts for the pecu-

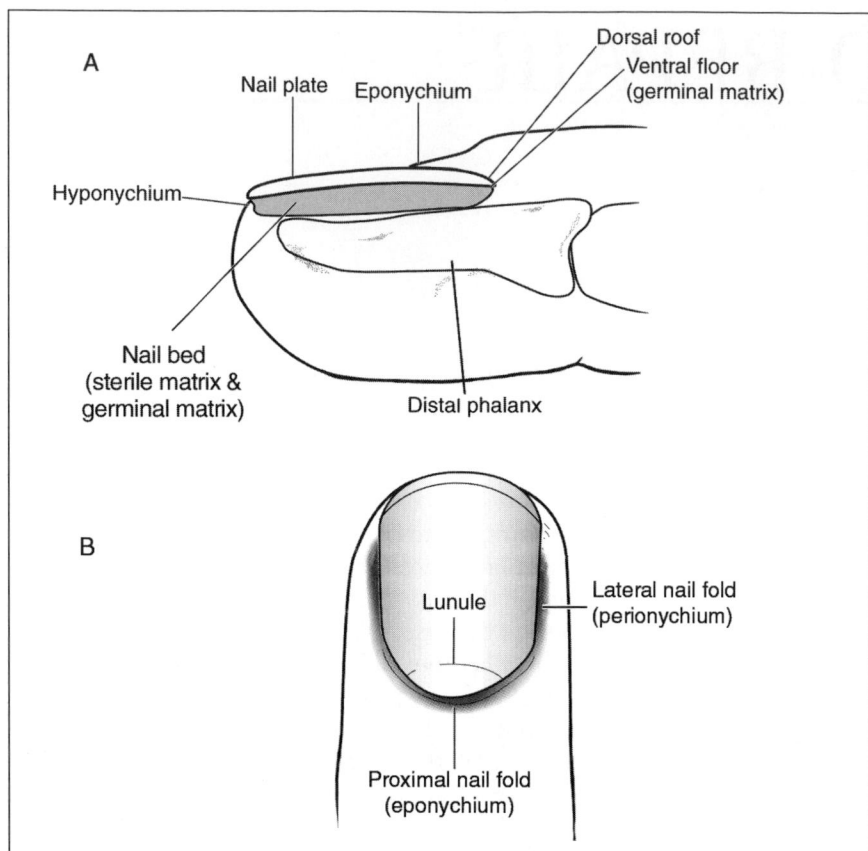

FIGURE 87-1 Anatomy of the fingernail. *A.* Lateral view. *B.* Top view. The colored area represents the perionychium.

liar injury of avulsions of the proximal nail plate from the proximal nail fold while the distal nail plate remains attached (Figure 87-2).

The extensor tendon inserts onto the epiphysis of the distal phalanx at a location just proximal to the germinal matrix.[1,8] The sterile matrix closely adheres to the dorsal periosteum of the distal phalanx.[1] Fractures of the distal phalanx may cause disruption of the nail bed and lead to the appearance of a subungual hematoma.[4] A subungual hematoma is a collection of blood between the nail bed and the nail plate. Although a large subungual hematoma may require repair of the underlying nail bed, this is controversial. Physicians must consider in each case whether there exists enough damage to require surgical repair. It is important to note that significant force is required to break, penetrate, or avulse the nail plate.[4] Therefore, the fragile nail bed is most likely disrupted if the nail plate is disrupted.

INDICATIONS

The indications to repair nail beds are functional and cosmetic. The most important consideration is functional.[6] Normal nail growth after injury requires a smooth nail bed. Therefore, nail bed injuries must be repaired to prevent cosmetic deformities and functional

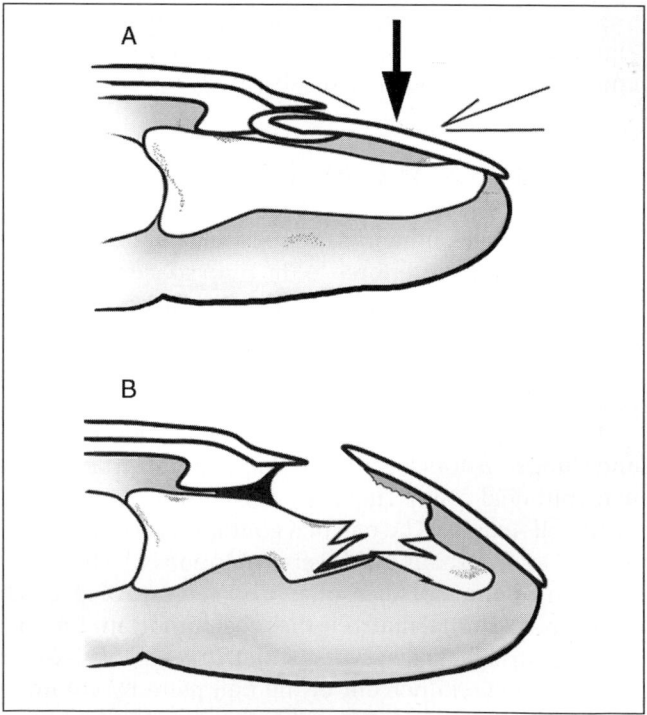

FIGURE 87-2 A crush injury to the distal fingertip. *A.* Proximal nail bed avulsion. *B.* A more severe crush injury can result in a proximal nail bed avulsion and fracture of the distal phalanx. Note that the distal nail plate remains attached to the sterile matrix in both of these injuries.

impairment.[6–8] Scar tissue may form between the wound edges if the nail bed is not accurately approximated. This scar tissue will not form the intermediate nail cells responsible for nail adherence.[1] Furthermore, loss of the germinal matrix alone will result in permanent loss of the nail plate.[3,9] The skin folds surrounding the nail margins must also be preserved.[3,8] Failure to do so will result in the painful complication of adhesion formation between the skin fold and the nail bed.[3,8] Secondary repair of these spaces, or of the nail bed, requires more complex procedures and are usually associated with a poor outcome.[7] **Therefore, every effort should be made to primarily repair all significant nail bed injuries.**

CONTRAINDICATIONS

No absolute contraindications exist for primary nail bed repair.

EQUIPMENT

Povidone iodine or antiseptic cleansing solution
Restraining device, as necessary
10 mL syringe armed with a 27 gauge needle
Local anesthetic solution without epinephrine, 1% lidocaine or 0.25% bupivacaine
Digital tourniquet, Penrose drain, or other device
#15 scalpel blade on a handle
Magnification device
Sterile prefabricated nail, if available
Nonadherent petrolatum gauze
6–0 or 7–0 chromic gut on a p-3 cutting needle
6–0 monofilament nylon sutures
Needle driver
Curved hemostat
Fine scissors
Forceps
Sterile towels or drapes
Sterile gloves
Dry gauze/tube gauze
Splinting material
Battery powered electrocautery device

PATIENT PREPARATION

All significant injuries to the fingertip should be evaluated radiographically for fractures. The management of fingertip injuries may differ in the presence of a fracture. Thoroughly evaluate and document a complete neurovascular examination, tendon function and intactness, and ligamentous stability of the joints. Ascertain the patient's tetanus immune status and administer prophylaxis if required.

It is important to explain both the risks of doing the procedure and of not doing the procedure. Document this conversation and obtain an informed consent. Place the patient on a gurney with the hand on a bedside procedure table in a well-lit area. Be prepared to use age-appropriate sedation or to apply appropriate restraints for children.[8] Apply a type of magnification device if available. This may consist of a head-strap device, a swing arm device, magnification glasses, or loupe magnification glasses.

Anesthetize the injured digit(s). Anesthesia may be achieved with a digital block or a metacarpal block when only a single digit is involved.[4] Multiple metacarpal blocks or an axillary nerve block may be performed if multiple digits are involved.[4] Please refer to Chapter 106 for the details regarding regional nerve blocks.

Thoroughly clean the hand of any dirt and debris. Apply povidone iodine and allow it to dry. Irrigate the wound with sterile saline. If the nail plate has been avulsed, irrigate it with a dilute povidone iodine solution followed by a gentle rinse with sterile saline. **It is important not to scrub the undersurface of the avulsed nail plate because adherent squamous tissue may be destroyed.[4]**

A bloodless field is desired and, in many cases, necessary. Apply a digital tourniquet.[4] This tourniquet usually consists of a sterile Penrose drain wrapped around the base of the finger and secured with a hemostat (Figure 87-3). Alternatively, cut a finger from a sterile glove as a substitute for the Penrose drain. A commercially available finger tourniquet may also be used. If available, a pneumatic tourniquet may be placed on the arm instead of using the digital tourniquet. The pneumatic tourniquet is especially helpful when the patient has fractures or lacerations of the proximal digit that preclude the use of a digital tourniquet. Avoid using a blood pressure cuff, as these tend to deflate during use. **As with all tourniquets, limit the amount of time in which**

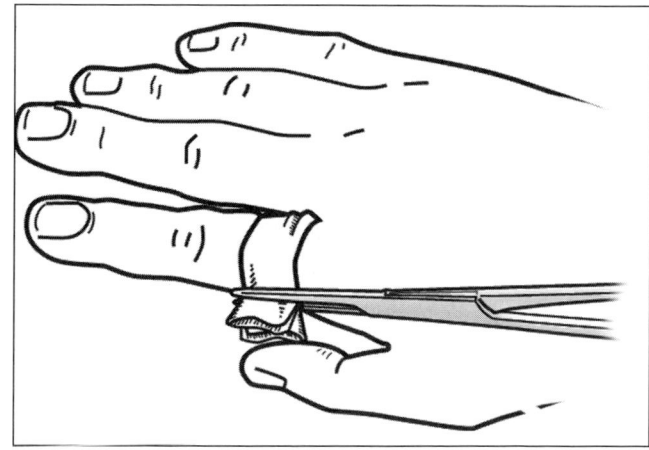

FIGURE 87-3 A sterile Penrose drain used as a digital tourniquet.

the tourniquet is in place. Create a sterile field by applying sterile towels.

TECHNIQUES

Adhering to certain principles will improve the outcome when repairing nail beds. Avoid or severely limit the amount of debridement.[3] The germinal matrix must be meticulously repaired and the proximal nail fold preserved or that space is obliterated within a few days.[3] Thoroughly clean and replace the nail plate whenever possible. This will preserve the nail folds surrounding the nail bed, allow the nail plate to serve as a splint for fractures, and act as a protective cover for the healing nail bed.[4]

The technique of nail bed repair depends upon the type of injury as well as which structures are involved. Nail bed injuries are classified as simple lacerations, crushing lacerations, avulsion-lacerations, lacerations with associated fractures, lacerations with loss of skin and pulp, and fingertip amputations.[9]

NAIL PLATE REMOVAL

Remove the nail plate to repair nail bed injuries or to inspect the nail bed for potential injuries (Figure 87-4). Insert the closed tips of a fine scissors between the nail bed and the nail plate. Hold the scissors parallel to the long axis of the finger. Slightly angle the tips of the scissors towards the nail plate to prevent any damage to the nail bed.[8] Advance the tips of the scissors 1 to 2 millimeters. Open the blades of the scissors to separate the nail bed from the nail plate. Close the blades of the scissors. Continue to advance the tips of the scissors in 1 to 2 mm increments and separate the nail bed from the nail plate. Stop advancing the scissors when the tips of the blades are at the level of the eponychium. Grasp the nail plate with a hemostat. Pull the nail plate parallel to the long axis of the finger to completely remove it from the finger.

SIMPLE LACERATIONS

Carefully approximate simple nail bed lacerations using fine (6–0 or 7–0) chromic gut sutures.[4] Repair any skin lacerations adjacent to the nail bed using 6–0 or 5–0 monofilament nylon sutures.[3] Nail fold lacerations may require repair in layers in order to preserve these spaces.[6]

CRUSHING LACERATIONS

The second type of injury is a crush injury with resultant lacerations. Crushing injuries may result in stellate lacerations and fragmentation of the nail bed (Figure 87-5A). Attempt to meticulously repair the fragmented nail bed using 6–0 or 7–0 chromic gut sutures to achieve the smoothest result possible (Figure 87-5B).[4]

AVULSION-LACERATIONS

The third type of nail bed injury is the avulsion-laceration (Figure 87-6A). Distal nail bed avulsions simply require petrolatum gauze to be placed over the injury followed by sterile gauze. Suture the petrolatum gauze and sterile gauze in place using 6–0 nylon suture (Figure 87-6B).[3] Avulsion-laceration injuries may require consultation with a Hand Surgeon depending on the amount of tissue involved and whether the germinal matrix is involved.[4,8,9] More severely damaged nail beds

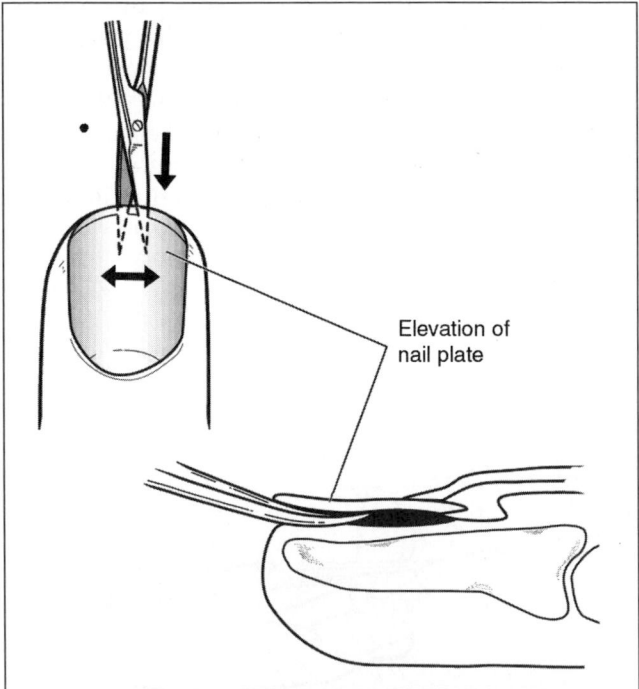

Elevation of nail plate

FIGURE 87-4 Removal of the nail plate. Dissect along the plane between the nail plate and the nail bed using a pair of fine scissors.

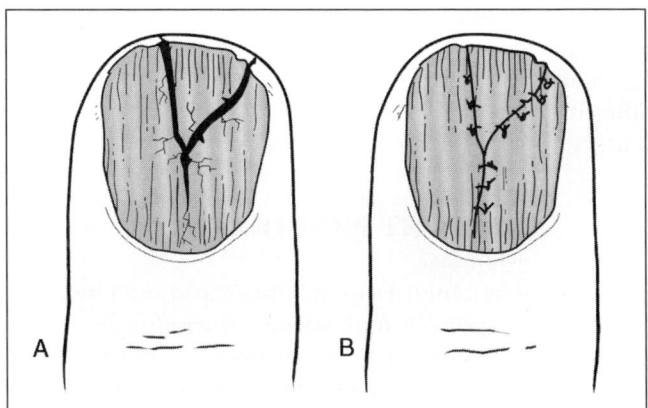

FIGURE 87-5 Crushing lacerations to the nail bed. *A.* Stellate or complex lacerations of the nail bed can occur after a crush injury. *B.* Approximation of the nail bed with fine absorbable sutures.

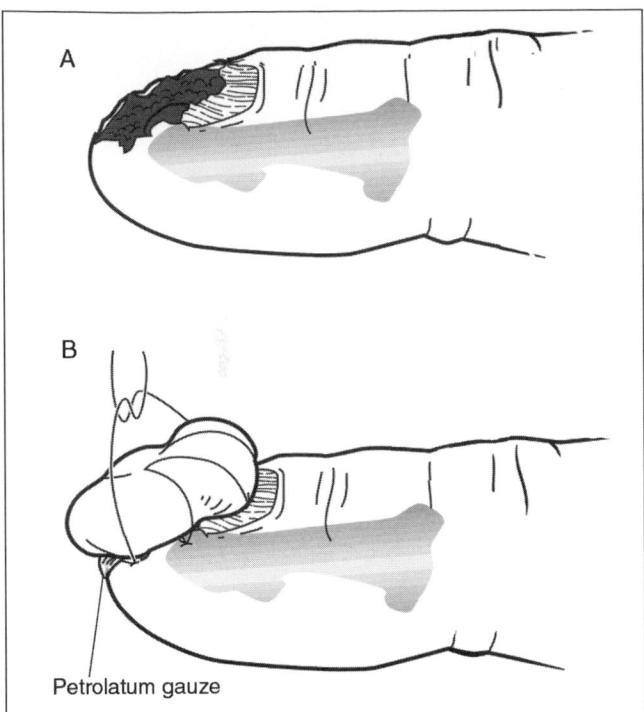

FIGURE 87-6 Avulsion-lacerations of the nail bed. *A.* The dorsal aspect of the fingertip is avulsed with the nail plate. *B.* Petrolatum gauze is placed over the injury. This is subsequently covered with sterile gauze and sutured into place for 10 days.

with a large amount of avulsed tissue usually require dermal grafts or split-thickness matrix grafts.[4]

Small fragments of avulsed nail bed may remain attached to the nail plate. These may be simply treated by carefully replacing the nail plate in its anatomic position.[10] Larger segments of avulsed nail bed that remain attached to the nail plate should be repaired (Figures 87-7*A* and *B*). Gently shave away the nail bed from the nail plate with a #15 scalpel blade (Figure 87-7*C*). Replace the avulsed nail bed and suture it in place with 5–0 or 6–0 chromic gut (Figure 87-7*D*).[7,10] Apply a petrolatum gauze dressing and replace the nail plate.

A special type of avulsion injury occurs when there is a crush to the distal fingernail. This results in an avulsion of the proximal nail plate with or without involvement of the germinal matrix (Figure 87-2). Remove the nail plate if the proximal nail plate is avulsed without involvement of the germinal matrix. Clean the nail plate and nail bed with sterile saline. Replace the nail plate. More often with these injuries, the germinal matrix is avulsed as well. In these cases, the germinal matrix should be replaced by a series, usually three, of 6–0 nylon simple interrupted or horizontal mattress sutures (Figure 87-8).[3,4,7] Place all three sutures before returning the nail bed to its proper location. Making two linear incisions

with a scalpel at 90 degrees from the eponychial edge will allow exposure to the germinal matrix for repair (Figure 87-9).[5] This allows the eponychium to be folded back and therefore increase exposure of the germinal matrix. Place a piece of petrolatum gauze between the eponychium and the germinal matrix after the repair (Figure 87-8*B*). Larger germinal matrix avulsions require consultation with a Hand Surgeon.[4,8]

LACERATIONS WITH ASSOCIATED FRACTURES

The fourth type of nail bed injury is lacerations associated with fracture(s). The nail bed laceration should be repaired as previously described and the fracture addressed as a separate entity.[3] It is important to remember that the sterile matrix is closely adherent to the dorsal periosteum of the distal phalanx. Therefore, fractures require precise anatomic reduction in order for normal nail bed healing to take place.[4,7,9] Replacing the nail plate and splinting the finger after repair of the nail bed laceration is often enough to reduce these fractures. Occasionally, fixation may be employed by a Hand Surgeon using Kirschner wires.[4]

LACERATIONS WITH SKIN LOSS AND FINGERTIP AMPUTATIONS

The final two classifications are lacerations with loss of skin and pulp, and fingertip amputations. They can be further classified according to zones based upon the functional anatomy of the fingertip (Figure 87-10).[2] Zone I injuries occur distal to the bony phalanx. These do not result in the loss of function and rarely result in a cosmetic deformity. Management consists of cleansing, placing topical antibiotic ointment over the injured area, and then applying a layer of petrolatum gauze. This should be followed by a sterile dressing and a splint.

Zone II injuries occur distal to the lunule and over the bony phalanx. These injuries often have exposed bone. Zone III injuries occur proximal to the distal end of the lunule. Zone II and Zone III injuries should be managed in consultation with a Hand Surgeon. Either type of injury may require reconstruction with a pedicle flap and/or skin grafting.[2]

TREPHINATION

The management of subungual hematomas is discussed separately because these injuries are typically minor and are treated by simple trephination. A complete discussion of the management of subungual hematomas can be found in Chapter 85. A subungual hematoma is a collection of blood under the nail plate caused by blunt trauma to the fingertip. The nail bed is usually crushed or lacerated with resultant extravasation of blood into the plane between the nail plate and the nail bed.[8] As pressure builds up, compression of nail bed nerves occurs

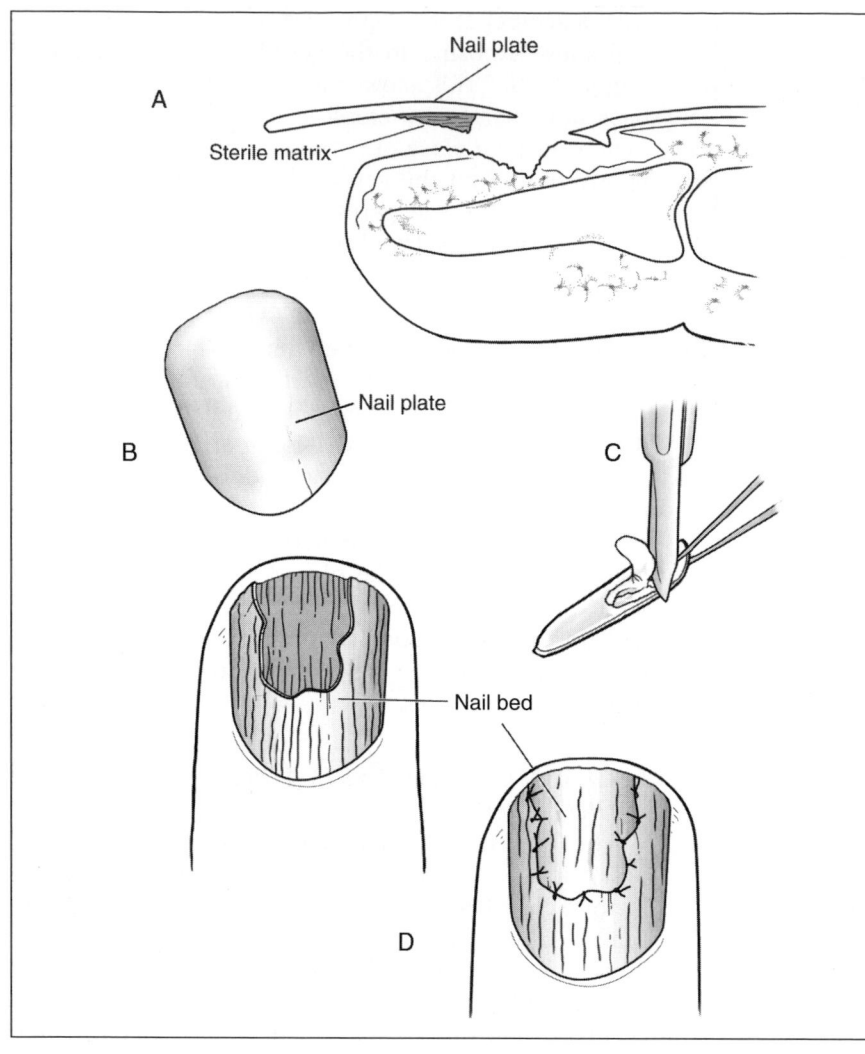

FIGURE 87-7 Large avulsion of the nail bed that is adherent to the nail plate. *A.* Lateral view of injury. *B.* Top view of injury. *C.* Gently shave away the avulsed segment. *D.* Repair the nail bed using the avulsed segment and chromic gut sutures.

and often causes significant pain. Usually this pain is what causes the patient to seek medical attention.

The following discussion applies to simple subungual hematomas. The nail plate should be removed and the nail bed and margins repaired, as previously discussed, if there is any disruption of the nail plate or of the nail margins.

It is generally accepted that smaller subungual hematomas (< 25 to 50 percent) may be drained by simple trephination (puncture) of the nail plate.[3,4,8,11,12] This allows for drainage of blood and immediate pain relief. No anesthesia is necessary for this procedure. Ideally, this is accomplished with the use of an electrocautery device creating a 3 to 4 mm hole in the nail plate overlying the hematoma. The nail plate should be clean and dry for this procedure. If an electrocautery device is not available, a heated paperclip may be used.[5]

Some controversy exists over the management of larger subungual hematomas (> 25 to 50 percent). The concern is that a larger hematoma may hide an occult laceration that requires repair in order to avoid the complication of step-off with subsequent ridging as the new nail grows back. Some authors feel that it is impossible to accurately assess the amount of damage beneath a subungual hematoma unless the nail plate is removed to directly inspect the nail bed.[4] These authors noted that subungual hematomas that have separated greater than 50 percent usually have lacerations that require repair. Another study found that a subungual hematoma with more than 50 percent separation had a 60 percent incidence of having a nail bed laceration that required repair and up to a 95 percent incidence when there was an associated phalanx fracture.[12] In contrast to these studies, a prospective study found no complications at 6 months follow-up for subungual hematomas treated by electrocautery trephination alone.[11] This was regardless of the size of the subungual hematoma or the presence of a fracture. These authors feel that removing the nail plate and attempting repair may actually cause further trauma to the nail bed.[11]

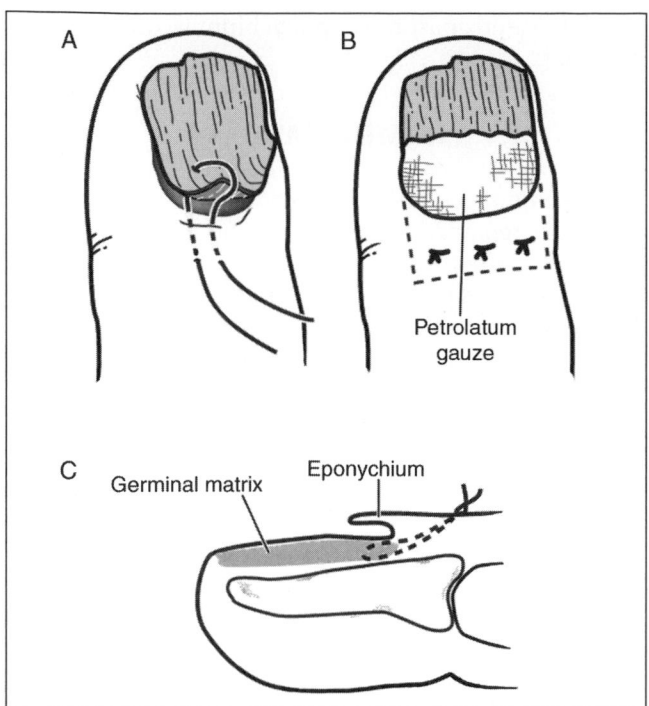

FIGURE 87-8 Repair of the germinal matrix after an avulsion. *A.* A series of horizontal mattress sutures are placed. *B.* The nail bed is returned to its proper location and the sutures tied. *C.* Lateral view of the repair.

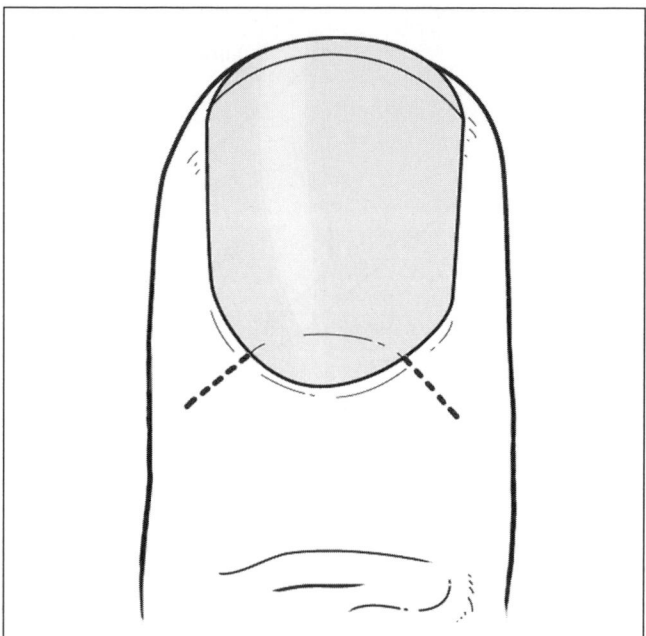

FIGURE 87-9 Incisions can be made at 90 degrees to the corners of the eponychium for better exposure of the germinal matrix.

In summary, most subungual hematomas may be treated by simple nail trephination using an electrocautery device. This procedure will lead to beneficial drainage only if done before 36 to 48 hours from the time of the injury.[8] The clinical benefit of nail bed repair with larger subungual hematomas is controversial. **It may be prudent to maintain a lower threshold for nail bed repair with a larger subungual hematoma, particularly if an ideal cosmetic outcome is desired.**

AFTERCARE

Whenever possible, the nail plate should be replaced after repairing any of the above mentioned injuries. The nail plate covers the sensitive nail bed and protects it from injury, maintains the proximal nail fold (eponychium) to allow for growth of a new nail, and splints the nail bed. In order to accomplish the best outcome, place a hole in the center of the nail plate to allow for drainage.[8] Suture the nail plate in place using 6–0 nylon sutures through the lateral skin folds (Figure 87-11).[4,7,8] These sutures should remain in place for 7 days. An artificial nail may be used if the original nail plate is not available. The potential problem with sterile prefabricated nails is that there exists an increased risk for infection and a risk of erosion into the nail bed or nail folds.[4] We recommend petrolatum gauze be used to maintain

the nail fold structures when the original nail plate is not available or significantly damaged (Figure 87-12).

After repair of the nail bed, the digit(s) involved will need to be bandaged in order to protect it from infection, moisture, and trauma. Place petrolatum gauze over the nail bed to avoid adherence from secretions. Apply a tube gauze dressing followed by a digital aluminum splint.[2] Movement of the distal interphalangeal joint should be restricted for 7 to 10 days with a splint.[4] For infants and young children, the entire hand should be dressed. If petrolatum gauze was used to keep the proximal nail fold (eponychium) open, it should be removed in 5 to 10 days.[4] Petrolatum gauze used to keep open the

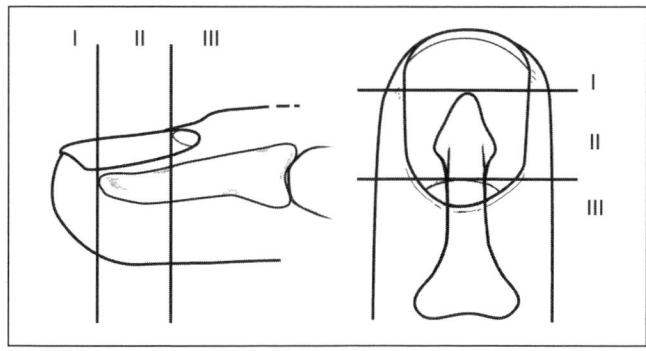

FIGURE 87-10 Classification of fingertip injuries. Zone I is distal to the bony phalanx. Zone II is distal to the lunule and over the bony phalanx. Zone III is proximal to the distal end of the lunule.

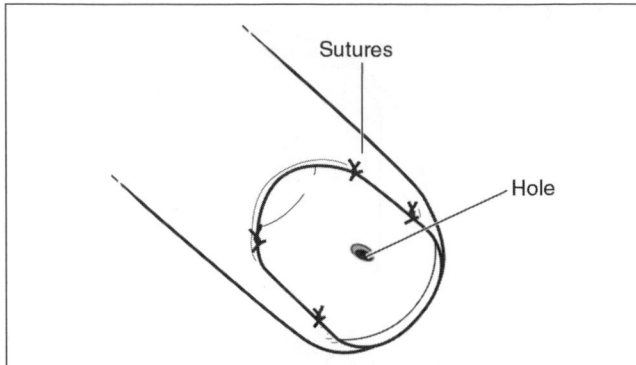

FIGURE 87-11 A hole should be placed in the nail plate before it is sutured in place after repair of the nail bed.

lateral nail folds (perionychium) should remain in place for 10 days.[3] Any sutures placed in the skin structures or nail folds should be removed in 7 days.[3]

Prophylactic antibiotics are not routinely required. They are recommended for large avulsions, amputations, and associated fractures when there is contamination with organic material.[4] Topical antibiotics may be applied to Zone I fingertip amputations. All injuries require a wound check in 24 to 72 hours.[2–4] A tetanus booster should be administered if the patient has not received one in the past 5 years. The hand should be elevated whenever possible. Narcotic analgesics may be prescribed as needed for pain control.

It is important to explain to the patient that regeneration of a new nail may take up to 6 to 12 months.[4] Warn the patient that as the new nail forms, it may look irregular and snag on cloth or string objects.[4] The patient should trim and file the leading edge of the new nail once it extends past the hyponychium in order to avoid snagging.

COMPLICATIONS

The complications associated with failure to repair or improper repair of a nail bed can be either functional, cosmetic, or both. The more serious complications are those which impair function or cause pain. There are basically seven complications that may arise. These exclude the infectious complications (abscess formation, cellulitis, and lymphangitis) that are inherent to all wounds. The occurrence of osteomyelitis from these injuries is rare, even with open fractures. The seven complications are loss of nail, split nail, nonadherent nail, ingrown nail, malaligned nail, wide nails, and narrow nails.[9]

The complete loss of a nail could result in significant functional impairment to the fingertip as well as an abnormal looking fingertip. Complete nail loss occurs when there is complete disruption of the germinal matrix, either by significant avulsion of the matrix or amputation. Remember that if the germinal or roof matrices are not repaired, the pouch deep to the proximal skin fold (eponychium) is obliterated within a few days.[11]

A split nail occurs when the germinal matrix is improperly approximated.[3,4,9] A wide scar will result that will not form a new nail. Subsequently, a split nail develops. This can be avoided by the careful approximation of the nail bed with sutures.

A nonadherent nail occurs when the nail bed is not repaired and granulation tissue forms secondarily. The nail plate will not adhere at the site of the granulation tissue and distal to the granulation tissue as well.[9] The

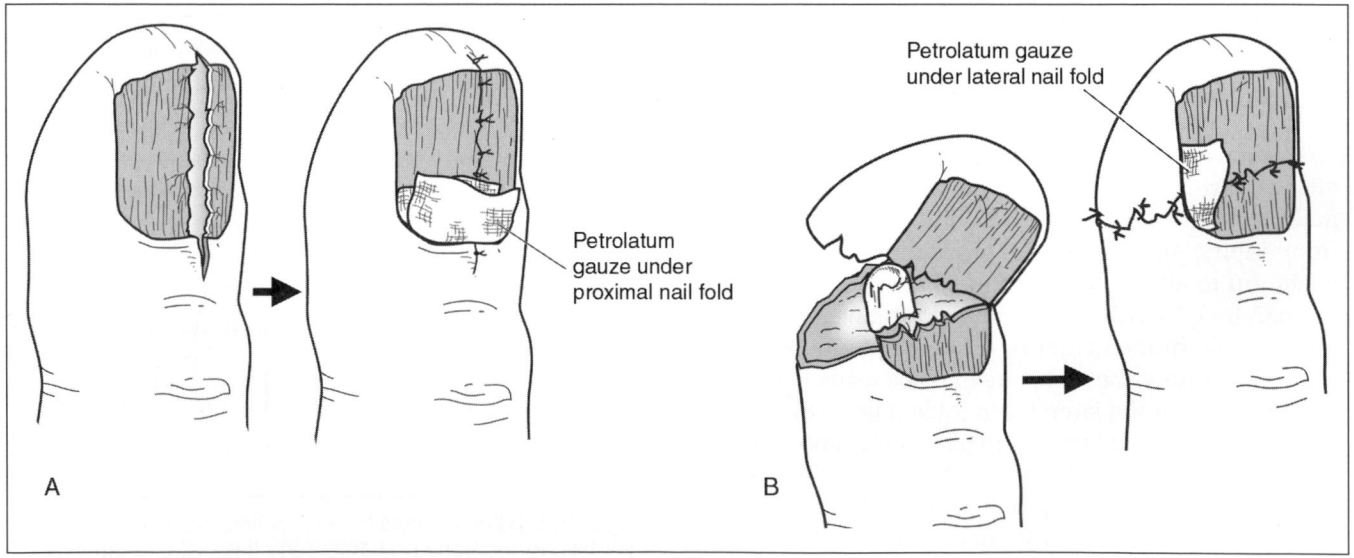

FIGURE 87-12 Petrolatum gauze may be placed between the dorsal roof and germinal matrix (*A*) or between the lateral skin fold and nail bed (*B*) to preserve the skin fold spaces.

nail can snag and be exposed to repeated tears once the nail plate loses adhesion to the nail bed.

The nail plate may ingrow if the lateral skin folds or sulci are not maintained and kept open.[9] Adhesions that form between the skin and nail bed can be very painful when the new nail tries to grow through that space.[3] Ingrown nails also have the long-term problem of a higher rate of infections (paronychia). This can be avoided by the replacement of the nail plate or the placement of petrolatum gauze to elevate the lateral nail fold from the nail bed.

The nail plate will grow in a malaligned direction if the matrix is displaced or repaired in such a manner that it is improperly aligned.[9] Functional impairment and cosmetic deformity may ensue depending upon the degree of this misdirected growth.

Wide nails often result from a crush injury with a tuft fracture.[9] Separated bony fragments leave the nail bed flatter and wider. Narrow nails occur when a central avulsion-laceration is not repaired. Scar tissue forms in the center and allows the intact lateral portions to contract towards each other.[9] The new nail subsequently becomes narrow and thick.

SUMMARY

Nail bed injuries are common and may result in a cosmetically deformed or functionally impaired fingertip. Complications may occur even with precise repair. The treatment of choice is immediate primary repair of the nail bed and surrounding structures. Remember to minimize any debridement and to replace the nail plate whenever possible. Injuries with associated fractures and simple subungual hematomas are managed separately from the nail bed injury. Always be thorough and meticulous when repairing nail bed injuries to provide the best possible outcome. Finally, know when to consult with a Hand Surgeon.

REFERENCES

1. Zook EG: Anatomy and physiology of the perionychium. *Hand Clin* 1990; 6(1):1–7.
2. Rosenthal EA: Treatment of fingertip and nail bed injuries. *Orthop Clin North Am* 1983; 14(4):675–697.
3. Simon RR, Brenner BE: *Emergency Procedures and Techniques,* 3rd ed. Baltimore: Williams & Wilkins, 1994:351–353.
4. VanBeek AL, Kassan MA, Adson MH, et al: Management of acute fingernail injuries. *Hand Clin* 1990; 6(1):25–35.
5. Zook EG: Discussion of "Management of acute fingernail injuries." *Hand Clin* 1990; 6(1):37–38.
6. Lammers RC, Freemyer BC: Hand, in Rosen P, Barkin R (eds): *Emergency Medicine: Concepts and Clinical Practice,* 3rd ed. St. Louis: Mosby, 1992:544–588.
7. Shepard GH: Management of acute nail bed avulsions. *Hand Clin* 1990; 6(1):39–56.
8. Eberlein R: Hand and finger injuries, in Henritig FM, King C (eds): *Textbook of Pediatric Emergency Procedures.* Baltimore: Williams & Wilkins, 1997:1047–1061.
9. Ashbell TS, Kleinhert HE, Putcha SM, et al: The deformed finger nail, a frequent result of failure to repair nail bed injuries. *J Trauma* 1967; 7(2):177–189.
10. Zook EG: Discussion of "Management of acute nail bed avulsions." *Hand Clin* 1990; 6(1):57–58.
11. Seaberg DC, Angelos WJ, Paris PM: Treatment of subungual hematomas with nail trephination: a prospective study. *Am J Emerg Med* 1991; 9(3):209–210.
12. Simon RR, Wolgin M: Subungual hematoma: association with occult laceration requiring repair. *Am J Emerg Med* 1987; 5:302–304.

Chapter 88
GANGLION CYST ASPIRATION AND INJECTION

Thomas P. Graham

INTRODUCTION

Ganglion cysts, also known as synovial cysts or ganglia, are the most common soft tissue tumors of the wrist and hand.[1] They are a common reason for patients to present to the Emergency Department. Their chief complaint is usually a mild pain or ache exacerbated by movement and localized to a 1 to 2 cm mass on the wrist or hand. Patients may also present with concern about a painless "lump." Acute trauma prior to presentation is uncommon, though patients often give a history of repetitive motion at the site. The mass usually increases in size progressively over time or, occasionally, may grow rapidly over a short period. Patients presenting to the Emergency Department with ganglia may have already attempted one of several popular home remedies, including homeopathic medications or striking the cyst firmly with a large book or hammer.

Ganglion cyst aspiration is a relatively simple procedure that may be performed by the Emergency Physician. However, cysts recur in many cases. There are reports of up to and even greater than 50 percent recurrence postaspiration.[2,3] The practice of Emergency Department aspiration has been challenged because of the high recurrence rate.[4] However, the procedure usually alleviates presenting symptoms, is occasionally curative, and is more cost-effective than referring all patients for surgical treatment.[5]

ANATOMY AND PATHOPHYSIOLOGY

Ganglia are benign synovial cysts that arise from a joint capsule or tendon sheath. It is unclear whether they are formed by herniation of the tendon sheath, myxomatous degeneration of connective tissue, or some other mechanism. Contained within the cyst is a viscous, jelly-like fluid. Ganglia often connect with the underlying synovial cavity or tendon sheath by a stalk.

Hyaluronic acid makes up all or part of the mucoid fluid.[6]

Ganglia are usually encountered on the dorsum of the wrist, in particular over the scapholunate ligament (Figure 88-1). They may also be found on the palmar surface of the wrist, the lateral surface of the wrist, or on the hand itself. Ganglia of the foot and ankle, while less common, are also seen.[7] Ganglia are occasionally encountered in other areas such as the shoulder, hip, elbow, knee (including the anterior cruciate ligament), the lumbar spine, temporomandibular joint, or even the odontoid process of the cervical spine.[8–10]

Ganglia present as fixed or slightly movable masses that are usually solitary. Frequently characterized as smooth and "rubbery," cysts may become more noticeable with wrist flexion. They vary in size from barely palpable to 3 cm in diameter (smaller than 1.5 cm being the norm). Tenderness is sometimes but not invariably present. Ganglion cysts will transilluminate, as they are fluid-filled.

Diagnosing a ganglion is usually not difficult. However, ganglia of the foot, in particular, and those occurring in other uncommon locations may be difficult to palpate despite causing significant discomfort. The differential diagnosis of ganglia includes joint capsulitis, neuromas, and other soft-tissue neoplasms such as sarcomas and chondrosarcomas. Ganglia themselves have no malignant potential. Radiographs and laboratory tests are not helpful in making the Emergency Department diagnosis. However, MRI and ultrasound are sometimes employed on an outpatient basis to aid in the diagnosis of occult ganglia or ganglia presenting atypically.[8]

INDICATIONS

The most common indication for ganglion aspiration is worsening pain and swelling, in particular when normal range of motion is restricted or occupational disabil-

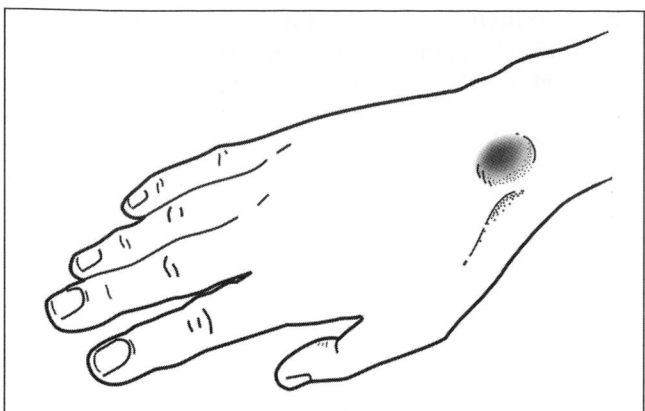

FIGURE 88-1 Oblique view of the wrist demonstrating a ganglion cyst overlying the scapholunate joint.

ity is present. Failure of conservative measures such as rest, splinting, and the use of nonsteroidal anti-inflammatory medications to resolve symptoms may also prompt ganglion aspiration in the Emergency Department.

CONTRAINDICATIONS

There are few contraindications to ganglion cyst aspiration. Introducing a needle through an area of cellulitis should be avoided. However, cellulitis overlying a ganglion is uncommon and should raise suspicion for an alternate diagnosis such as a skin abscess. The procedure can be safely deferred, with the patient being given a referral to a Hand Surgeon, if the diagnosis of a ganglion is uncertain.

The location of a ganglion is not a contraindication to aspiration. The procedure should be deferred if there is a concern that the aspirating needle could damage an adjacent structure and cause neurologic or vascular injury. Aspiration of lower extremity ganglia may be performed in a similar fashion to hand and wrist lesions, with similar results.[7,11] Some literature suggests that volar wrist ganglion cysts recur at an even higher rate than those of the dorsal wrist and lower extremity; leading some authors to recommend surgical excision, and not aspiration, as the primary therapy for this subset of ganglia.[12]

EQUIPMENT

Sterile gloves
Povidone iodine solution
Local anesthetic solution without epinephrine, lidocaine or bupivacaine

25 or 27 gauge needle on a 3 mL syringe for local anesthesia
16 or 18 gauge needle on a 5 or 10 mL syringe for aspiration
10 to 15 mg methylprednisolone acetate (20 mg/mL) or prednisolone tebutate (20 mg/mL)

PATIENT PREPARATION

Explain the risks and benefits of the procedure to the patient and/or their representative. Obtain an informed consent, either signed or verbal, with adequate documentation to support the latter method. Place the patient on a gurney with the hand on a bedside procedure table. Clean the skin of any dirt and debris. Apply povidone iodine and allow it to dry. The use of local anesthesia is optional. The cyst can be aspirated and/or injected without the use of local anesthesia. It is recommended to provide local anesthesia for patient comfort. Place a subcutaneous wheal of local anesthetic solution immediately over or adjacent to the periphery of the ganglion.

TECHNIQUE

Manipulate the wrist (or other affected extremity) to expose more of the cyst and facilitate needle entry into the cavity. Insert a 16 or 18 gauge needle on a 5 or 10 mL syringe through the anesthetized tissue and into the ganglion cyst cavity (Figure 88-2). Apply negative pressure to the syringe to aspirate the cyst contents once the tip of the needle is within the cyst cavity. The contents

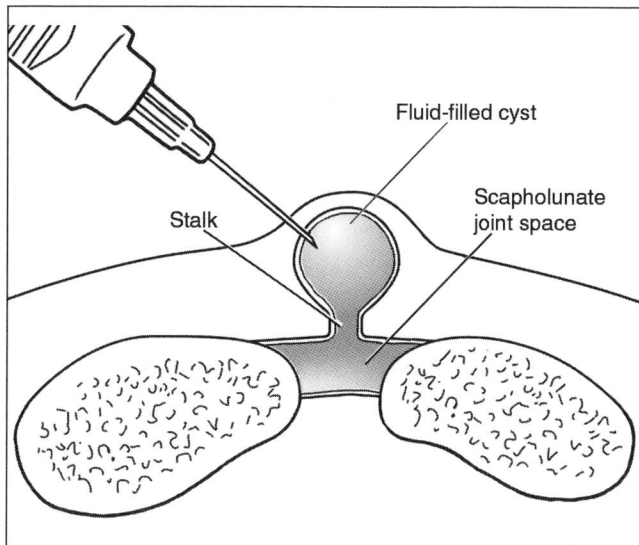

Fluid-filled cyst

Scapholunate joint space

Stalk

FIGURE 88-2 Cross-section through the scapholunate joint demonstrating a ganglion cyst. The needle is inserted into the cyst cavity to aspirate its contents.

may be difficult to aspirate, as the mucinous contents of the cyst are quite viscous. The cyst can be manipulated and compressed to express more of the contents into the syringe once the very viscous, clear or yellow material begins to flow into the syringe. Generally, 1 to 2 mL of fluid can be aspirated from a typical ganglion. Withdraw the needle when fluid can no longer be expressed. Apply a simple dressing. A pressure dressing may also be temporarily applied, taking care not to compromise neurologic or vascular function.

ALTERNATIVE TECHNIQUES

The infiltration of glucocorticoids into a ganglion cyst immediately after aspiration is commonly recommended. However, the literature has not shown a clear benefit to steroid use over aspiration alone.[13] If a steroid injection is desired, securely hold the aspirating needle in place after the cyst contents have been withdrawn and remove the syringe. Place a second syringe containing the glucocorticoid solution onto the needle. Inject the contents into the cyst cavity. Withdraw the needle and apply a dressing.

Other variations of ganglion cyst aspiration have been described in the literature. Puncturing the ganglion wall at multiple separate locations has been advocated.[14] This technique has not been proven to decrease the recurrence rate when compared to aspiration at a single point alone.[14] The injection of hyaluronidase into the cyst, with or without corticosteroids, has been studied with some favorable results.[15,16] Further study is necessary before this technique can be recommended for widespread use in the Emergency Department.

ASSESSMENT

Patients usually report total or near-total relief of their symptoms immediately after aspiration. Obtaining highly viscous, clear or yellow fluid from the cyst virtually confirms the diagnosis. Obtaining purulent fluid suggests a skin abscess and not a ganglion cyst. Failure to obtain fluid does not rule out the diagnosis of a ganglion, but should prompt an evaluation for alternative diagnoses.

AFTERCARE

Patients should be reassured that ganglia are not malignant tumors. Immobilization of the affected limb may be performed temporarily for patient comfort. However, splinting limits the ability of patients to function normally and does not appear to affect recurrence rates.[17] Aftercare instructions should direct patients to return to the Emergency Department for any significant increase

in pain, erythema at the site or up the extremity, swelling beyond the ganglion's original size, purulent discharge, continued bleeding, or the development of a fever. Patients should also be directed to elevate the extremity, avoid strenuous activity of the affected limb, and rewrap the pressure dressing (if one is applied) to make it snug but not uncomfortable. Acetaminophen or nonsteroidal anti-inflammatory medications may be recommended for relief of mild post-procedure pain. Oral corticosteroids have not been demonstrated to play a role in ganglion therapy.

All patients with ganglion cysts aspirated in the Emergency Department should be informed of the potential for recurrence and the possibility of definitive ganglion treatment by surgical excision. Referral to a Hand Surgeon should be provided, if desired by the patient. Although reports of postsurgical recurrence rates vary widely, currently the most effective therapy for ganglion cysts involves open excision. During this procedure, a Hand Surgeon removes the cyst and, if possible, the stalk or pedicle that connects it to the normal synovium. Arthroscopic removal of wrist ganglia has also been described and performed successfully in a number of patients.[18]

COMPLICATIONS

Complications of ganglion cyst aspiration are uncommon. They include bleeding and infection. Bleeding is self-limited and easily controlled with manual pressure. The use of sterile technique will prevent any infectious complications (abscess, cellulitis, or septic arthritis). Rare complications of corticosteroid injection include localized depigmentation that is due to injection outside of the cyst capsule or leakage out of the cyst capsule through the needle tract.[19]

SUMMARY

Ganglion cysts are common growths of the wrist and hand. They frequently progress to cause pain to the point of disability. Contraindications to the aspiration of a ganglion cyst in the Emergency Department are few. The procedure is often warranted due to debilitating pain, deformity, or inability on the patient's part to promptly seek the care of a surgical specialist. The procedure is simple, quick, and only slightly uncomfortable if performed correctly. Although the injection of steroids into the cyst is commonly advocated to prevent recurrence, the efficacy of this procedure has not been conclusively demonstrated. Ganglia recurrence is very common after aspiration and may occur even after surgical excision. This fact must be clearly relayed to the patient. All patients should be offered referral to a Hand Surgeon on a nonemergent basis to discuss further intervention.

REFERENCES

1. Diao E, Moy OJ: Common tumors. *Orthop Clin North Am* 1992; 1:187–196.
2. Oni JA: Treatment of ganglia by aspiration alone. *J Hand Surg [Br]* 1992; 17B(6):660.
3. Thornburg LE: Ganglions of the hand and wrist. *J Am Acad Orthop Surg* 1999; 7(4):231–238.
4. Razemon JP: Surgical treatment of ganglions of the wrist by partial excision of the joint capsule. Report on 303 cases. *Ann Chir Main* 1983; 2(3):230–243.
5. Zubowicz VN: Management of ganglion cysts of the hand by simple aspiration. *J Hand Surg [Am]* 1987; 12A(4):618.
6. Hernandez-Lugo AM, Dominguez-Cherit J, Vega-Memije ME: Digital mucoid cyst: the ganglion type. *Int J Dermatol* 1999; 38:533–535.
7. Rozbruch SR, Chang V, Bohne WH, et al: Ganglion cysts of the lower extremity: an analysis of 54 cases and review of the literature. *Orthopedics* 1998; 21(2):141–148.
8. Treadwell EL: Synovial cysts and ganglia: the value of magnetic resonance imaging. *Semin Arthritis Rheum* 1994; 24(1):61–70.
9. Ferrick MR, Marzo JM: Suprascapular entrapment neuropathy and ganglion cysts about the shoulder. *Orthopedics* 1999; 22(4):430–434.
10. Campagnolo MD, Davis BA, Blacksin MF, et al: Computed tomography-guided aspiration of a ganglion cyst of the anterior cruciate ligament: a case report. *Arch Phys Med Rehabil* 1996; 77:732–733.
11. Pontius J, Good J, Maxian SH: Ganglions of the foot and ankle. A retrospective analysis of 63 procedures. *J Am Podiatr Med Assoc* 1999; 89(4):163–168.
12. Wright TW, Cooney WP, Ilstrup DM: Anterior wrist ganglion. *J Hand Surg [Am]* 1994; 19(6):954–958.
13. Varley GW, Needoff M, Davis TR, et al: Conservative management of wrist ganglia: aspiration versus steroid infiltration. *J Hand Surg [Br]* 1997; 22(5):636.
14. Stephen AB, Lyons AR, Davis TR: A prospective study of two conservative treatments for ganglia of the wrist. *J Hand Surg [Br]* 1999; 24(1):104–105.
15. Paul AS, Sochart DH: Improving the results of ganglion aspiration by the use of hyaluronidase. *J Hand Surg [Br]* 1997; 22(2):219–221.
16. Otu AA: Wrist and hand ganglion treatment with hyaluronidase injection and fine-needle aspiration: a tropical African perspective. *J R Coll Surg Edinb* 1992; 37(6):405–407.
17. Korman J, Pearl R, Hentz VR: Efficacy of immobilization following aspiration of carpal and digital ganglions. *J Hand Surg [Am]* 1992; 17(6):1097–1099.
18. Osterman AL, Raphael J: Arthroscopic resection of dorsal ganglion of the wrist. *Hand Clin* 1995; 11(1):7–12.
19. Stapczynski JS: Localized depigmentation after steroid injection of a ganglion cyst on the hand. *Ann Emerg Med* 1991; 20(7):807–809.

Chapter 89

SUBCUTANEOUS ABSCESS INCISION AND DRAINAGE

Samuel J. Gutman

INTRODUCTION

Subcutaneous abscesses are common in the Emergency Department. Approximately 1 to 2.5 percent of patients present with this chief complaint.[1–3] Abscesses occur in numerous anatomical areas with varied etiology and bacteriology. Classically, an abscess is a tender and fluctuant mass located in the dermal or subdermal tissue. It demonstrates the classic inflammatory responses of rubor, tumor, dolor, and calor. Although the abscess is usually tender, the surrounding and underlying tissue should not be tender.[4,5] There is minimal surrounding erythema in a mature abscess.

Incision and drainage is the definitive treatment of a soft tissue abscess.[6] This procedure results in significant improvement in symptoms and a rapid resolution of the infection in uncomplicated cases.[7] However, premature incision before localization of pus will not be curative and may be deleterious. In cases of immature abscesses or cellulitis, oral antibiotics and warm compresses may be of value in helping the infection to coalesce. These methods are not a substitute for incision and drainage and should not be continued for more than 24 to 36 hours without reassessment of the patient.

ANATOMY AND PATHOPHYSIOLOGY

PATHOGENESIS

An abscess is a localized collection of pus caused by suppuration buried in a tissue, organ, or confined space.[8] Intact skin is very resistant to bacterial invasion. Localized pyogenic infections are usually initiated by a breakdown in the normal epithelial defense mechanisms in the normal host. Plugging of the ducts of a superficial exocrine gland, such as apocrine and sebaceous glands or a congenital cyst or sinus, may initiate the process. Occlusion prevents desquamation and provides a moist environment for organisms to proliferate.

The combination of a high concentration of organisms, the presence of nutrients, and sufficient damage to the corneal layer to allow organisms to penetrate the skin defenses results in abscess formation.[1,9]

Abscesses may begin as a cellulitis with organisms that cause necrosis, liquefaction, and accumulation of leukocytes and debris. Early stages appear as an area of hyperemia and tender inflammation that later becomes fluctuant as an exudate of leukocytes, necrotic material, and cellular debris accumulates. This is followed by loculation and walling off of the pus. As the process progresses, the area of liquefaction increases until it "points" and eventually ruptures into the area of least resistance.[5]

The body area involved depends upon host factors such as drug use, employment-related exposures, or minor trauma.[9,10] Areas with a compromised blood supply will be more prone to infection as normal host cell mediated immunity is not as available.[9] The frequency of occurrence in different areas includes the buttocks and perirectal area in 25 percent of cases, the head and neck in 20 percent, the extremities in 18 percent, the axilla in 16 percent, and the inguinal area in 15 percent.[1]

BACTERIOLOGY

The majority of abscesses are polymicrobial with the isolated organisms usually representing the normal resident flora associated with the body area on which the abscess is found.[1,11] Nonresident bacteria are found in abscesses that occur as a result of direct inoculation of extraneous organisms such as those following human bite wounds, intravenous drug use, or bacterial seeding of embedded foreign bodies.[12] In normal hosts, aerobic *Staphylococcus* and group A *Streptococcus* are the most common organisms isolated from abscesses of the head, neck, extremities, and trunk.[11,13] Anaerobes are found in all areas of the body but predominate in abscesses of the buttocks and perirectal regions.[11,13] *Staphylococcus aureus* occurs in 24 to 60 percent of abscesses and in pure cultures is the only organism in 21 to 72 percent of cases.[1,13–16]

Abscesses occur with increased frequency in intravenous drug abusers (IVDAs) and are often atypical in location and the isolated organisms.[10,17] The cause of this difference is multifactorial and includes intrinsic immune deficiencies, increased carriage of *Staphylococcus*, frequent breaking of the skin defense integrity by needle punctures under nonsterile conditions, licking of needles, inadvertent subcutaneous injection, deposition of foreign bodies such as talc, and broken needles.[18–21] These patients are at increased risk of severe necrotizing soft tissue infections.[22] Abscesses in IVDAs often occur at common sites of injection such as the extremities, breasts, and lateral buttocks.[18,21] In one series, 63 percent of abscesses in this population were polymicrobial, including 67 percent growing anaerobes and only 19 percent growing *Staphylococcus aureus*.[23] In another series, the most common organisms were gram-negative and oral flora.[18] In other studies of IVDAs, the most common gram-positives were *Streptococcus* species with variable isolation of *Staphylococcus*.[10,18] Abscesses in IVDAs in Ireland were found to contain *Staphylococcus aureus* in 64 percent of cases and *Streptococcus* species were isolated in 90 percent of abscesses that were polymicrobial.[21] It is thought that the particular bacteriology of an abscess in any given IVDA will vary based on individual lifestyle, drug use practices, the specific flora in that particular addict, and geographic location.[18]

Immunocompromised patients (such as those with diabetes, acute leukemia, renal failure, HIV, or transplant recipients) have an increased frequency for abscess formation. They are susceptible to much more severe and progressive infections. These hosts are also predisposed to infections with unusual organisms (such as fungi, nocardia, or parasites) and may respond poorly to standard treatment.[23,24] These patients should be considered for early intravenous antibiotic therapy, surgical consultation, and very close follow-up.

Up to 17 percent of abscesses are sterile.[1,7,13] Nearly 40 percent of these are secondary to drug abuse and most likely result from injection of necrotizing chemical irritants.[3] Viruses (e.g., herpes), autoimmune mechanisms, or systemic illnesses including metastatic tumors, benign tumors, and granulomatous disease may also cause sterile abscesses.[4,25] These atypical etiologies may present with the absence of local symptoms and only with an exacerbation of the underlying disease process.

SPECIFIC CLINICAL ENTITIES

Furuncles, or boils, are acute circumscribed abscesses of the skin and subcutaneous tissue that most commonly occur on the face, neck, buttocks, thigh, perineum, breast, or axilla. Carbuncles are aggregates of interconnected furuncles that frequently occur on the back of the neck where the thick skin causes lateral extension of the infection rather than pointing towards the skin surface. These occur with a high frequency in diabetics. They can be large and cause systemic symptoms and complications. Carbuncles often require surgical consultation and treatment in the Operating Room.

Hidradenitis suppurativa is a chronic relapsing inflammatory disease process affecting the apocrine glands primarily in the axilla, the inguinal region, or both.[26] Initially, this process will appear like any other abscess and is only identifiable in its chronic scarring phase when there are multiple lesions with tender areas of induration and inflammation in various stages of healing. The chronic process leads to draining fistulous tracts that require ongoing surgical management. Emergency Department management involves the usual incision and drainage procedure of any area of fluctuance. Patients should be informed that the intervention is not curative and that the problem is chronic. Referral to a General Surgeon, Dermatologist, or Plastic Surgeon for long-term follow-up should be arranged.

Up to 80 percent of breast abscesses occur in nonlactating women.[4] Peripheral and superficial lesions are similar to abscesses elsewhere on the body and respond to conservative incision and drainage with an incision that radiates out (centripetally) from the nipple.[27] Deeper and periareolar abscesses are often complex, require surgical referral, and general anesthesia to properly treat. Postpartum mastitis is common and precipitated by milk stasis and bacterial invasion through a cracked nipple. The offending organism is commonly *Staphylococcus aureus* or *Streptococcus* species. Treatment includes the application of heat, oral antibiotics, and continued breast emptying with a breast pump or feeding the baby. The process may evolve into an abscess and is often associated with systemic symptoms. Appropriate antibiotic therapy and follow-up in 24 to 48 hours is required.

Sebaceous cysts are a common cause of a subcutaneous abscess. They can persist for long periods as nontender subcutaneous swellings before becoming infected. They appear like most other abscesses. Sebaceous cysts can be identified by a small punctate sinus tract near the center of the fluctuant area. The initial treatment is incision and drainage. The contents are usually thick cheesy material that needs to be manually expressed. A sebaceous cyst has a definite shiny white capsule that must be excised, preferably at the time of incision and drainage or at the first follow-up visit, to prevent recurrence. The area is then treated as any other healing abscess cavity.

The recurrence of an abscess that has been previously drained should suggest the possibility of underlying osteomyelitis, a retained foreign body, or the presence of unusual organisms such as mycobacteria or fungi. Recurrent abscesses should prompt further investigation including an assessment of the patient's immune status.

SPECIAL CONSIDERATIONS

The precise risk for endocarditis associated with subcutaneous abscesses is unknown. Up to 5 percent of patients with abscesses have bacteremia at the time of presentation.[4,16] Incision and drainage of cutaneous abscesses not uncommonly results in transient bacteremia with the same organism causing the abscess.[7,14,28] More recently, the clinical relevance of this bacteremia has become controversial.[16] At this time, patients at high and moderate risk for endocarditis are recommended to receive antimicrobial prophylaxis before incision and drainage (Table 89-1).[29] IVDAs as a group have a high incidence of undiagnosed endocarditis and thus prophylaxis should be considered prior to incision and drainage. Some authors suggest that IVDAs with a fever require admission, parenteral antibiotics, and blood cultures until a firm diagnosis can be identified as physicians are unable to accurately predict who will ultimately have endocarditis.[19]

TABLE 89-1. CARDIAC CONDITIONS AT RISK FOR ENDOCARDITIS THAT REQUIRE ANTIBIOTIC PROPHYLAXIS[29]

Endocarditis prophylaxis recommended
High-risk categories
  Prosthetic cardiac valves, including bioprosthetic and homograft valves
  Previous bacterial endocarditis
  Complex cyanotic congenital heart disease (e.g., single ventricle states, transposition of the great arteries, tetralogy of Fallot)
  Surgically constructed systemic pulmonary shunts or conduits
Moderate-risk categories
  Most other congenital cardiac malformations (other than above and below)
  Acquired valvar dysfunction (e.g., rheumatic heart disease)
  Hypertrophic cardiomyopathy
  Mitral valve prolapse with valvar regurgitation and/or thickened leaflets

Endocarditis prophylaxis not recommended
Negligible-risk categories (no greater risk than the general population)
  Isolated secundum atrial septal defect
  Surgical repair of atrial septal defect, ventricular septal defect, or patent ductus arteriosus (without residua beyond 6 mo)
  Previous coronary artery bypass graft surgery
  Mitral valve prolapse without valvar regurgitation
  Physiologic, functional, or innocent heart murmurs
  Previous Kawasaki disease without valvar dysfunction
  Previous rheumatic fever without valvar dysfunction
  Cardiac pacemakers (intravascular and epicardial) and implanted defibrillators

Bacterial endocarditis prophylaxis should be directed at the most likely pathogen causing the infection. An antistaphylococcal penicillin or a first generation cephalosporin is an appropriate choice for most soft tissue infections (Table 89-2). Clindamycin is an acceptable alternative for patients allergic to penicillin. Vancomycin is the regimen of choice for those unable to take oral antibiotics or who are known to have methicillin-resistant *Staphylococcus aureus* bacteremia.[29] Oral prophylactic regimens should be administered 1 hour prior to the procedure. Parenteral prophylactic regimens should be administered within 30 minutes of the procedure.

Patients with immunodeficiency and localized soft tissue abscesses may be at higher risk for developing septicemia secondary to bacteremia induced by incision and drainage, but it is unclear if they are at higher risk of complications and death.[30,31] These patients probably benefit from prophylactic antibiotics prior to incision and drainage, but only indirect evidence and no controlled studies are available.[32]

PATIENT ASSESSMENT

Prior to the treatment of an abscess, a directed history should be taken assessing for trauma, intravenous drug abuse, history of fevers, and past medical history (specifically: diabetes, renal failure, steroid use or other immune suppression, peripheral vascular disease, or valvular heart disease). Past anesthetic history and the potential for aspiration should be assessed if procedural sedation is to be considered.[33] Medications and allergies should be queried. Tetanus status must be confirmed and booster doses provided as required.

A brief physical examination documenting function and intact distal neurovascular status of extremities involved is required. Evidence of pain on passive or active movement of fingers may suggest a deep space infection.[4] A high index of suspicion is required, especially in IVDAs, to identify those simple cutaneous abscesses that unpredictably evolve into extensive necrotizing soft tissue infections.[22] General assessment of the airway and cardiopulmonary system, vital signs, and mental status is indicated if procedural sedation is to be employed.[33]

Routine laboratory studies are not indicated in otherwise healthy individuals. In immunocompromised patients, a CBC looking for leukopenia or toxic granulations should be considered. Diabetics should have electrolytes, BUN, creatinine, and glucose assessed. Elevated potassium in diabetics possibly indicates myonecrosis.[34] A urinalysis for myoglobinuria can be considered.

Cultures of an abscess are of little value since incision and drainage is nearly always curative and antibiotic therapy has not been shown to affect the course when

TABLE 89-2. PROPHYLACTIC REGIMENS FOR DENTAL, ORAL, RESPIRATORY TRACT, OR ESOPHAGEAL PROCEDURES[29]

Clinical situation	Agent	Dose*	Timing
Standard general prophylaxis	Amoxicillin	Adults: 2.0 gm Children: 50 mg/kg	Orally, 1 hour prior to the procedure
Unable to take oral medications	Ampicillin	Adults: 2.0 gm Children: 50 mg/kg	Intravenously or intramuscularly, 30 minutes prior to the procedure
Allergic to penicillin	Clindamycin	Adults: 600 mg Children: 20 mg/kg	Orally, 1 hour prior to the procedure
Allergic to penicillin	Cephalexin** or cefadroxil**	Adults: 2.0 gm Children: 50 mg/kg	Orally, 1 hour prior to the procedure
Allergic to penicillin	Azithromycin or clarithromycin	Adults: 500 mg Children: 15 mg/kg	Orally, 1 hour prior to the procedure
Allergic to penicillin and unable to take oral medications	Clindamycin	Adults: 600 mg Children: 20 mg/kg	Intravenously 30 minutes prior to the procedure
Allergic to penicillin and unable to take oral medications	Cefazolin**	Adults: 1.0 gm Children: 25 mg/kg	Intravenously or intramuscularly, 30 minutes prior to the procedure

*Total child dose should not exceed adult dose.
**Cephalosporins should not be used in patients with immediate-type hypersensitivity reactions (urticaria, angioedema, or anaphylaxis) to penicillin.

given after the procedure in normal patients.[1,2] Gram's stain and cultures for both aerobic and anaerobic bacteria may be helpful in those patients who are febrile, systemically unwell, immunocompromised, or who present atypically.

Consider obtaining radiographs of the affected areas if there is a history of trauma, drug abuse, or evidence of deep infection. Foreign bodies and fractures may not be easily identifiable because of the edema and tenderness caused by the infection. Gas or osteolytic lesions on plain radiographs may indicate severe deeper infection, the need for urgent surgical consultation, and prompt antibiotic therapy.[23] CT scanning or ultrasound can differentiate abscesses from cellulitis, although this is rarely required.

INDICATIONS

The presence of a fluctuant mass in an area of induration, erythema, and tenderness is clinical evidence that an abscess exists. These require incision and drainage. Examination alone may not definitively indicate an abscess, especially if it is deep. If the diagnosis is unclear, needle aspiration can confirm the presence of an abscess.[4] Obtaining pus on aspiration is an indication for incision and drainage.[4] If no pus is aspirated, oral antibiotics, warm compresses, and follow-up in 24 hours must be arranged for reassessment.

CONTRAINDICATIONS

The only absolute contraindication to incision and drainage of an abscess in the Emergency Department is the possible association with a mycotic aneurysm.[10,34] Commonly, abscesses overlie large vessels including those in the anterior triangle of the neck, the supraclavicular fossa, the deep space of the axilla, the antecubital fossa, the groin, and the popliteal space.[35] In these locations, or if the abscess is pulsatile, fine needle aspiration for blood and/or angiography is indicated prior to incision and drainage.

Relative contraindications to incision and drainage include an inability to achieve adequate anesthesia. An abscess associated with a deep foreign body that requires additional real-time imaging such as a fluoroscopy or ultrasound may require surgical referral.[36,37] Proximity of a lesion to important neurovascular or tendinous structures may require specialty consultation and magnification under Operating Room conditions. Deep space infections or involvement of any joint requires admission for parenteral antibiotic therapy and possible operative debridement. Patients presenting with soft tissue infections exhibiting pain out of proportion to physical examination findings or deep anesthesia of the involved or distal area should raise the possibility of deeper infections such as necrotizing fasciitis or myonecrosis.[23] Perirectal and periurethral abscesses are often larger and deeper than they appear and may be complicated by sinus tracts that require exploration under general anesthesia. Manipulation of abscesses in the "danger triangle" of the face (corners of the mouth to glabella) can lead to septic thrombosis of the cavernous sinus. Periorbital or orbital abscesses require ophthalmologic assessment and treatment.

EQUIPMENT

Anesthesia

18 and 27 gauge needles, 1½ inches long
10 mL syringes
Povidone iodine or chlorhexidine solution
Local anesthetic solution with epinephrine
Local anesthetic solution without epinephrine if abscess is near an end arteriolar system
Ethyl chloride spray
Ice pack

Procedure

#11 and #15 scalpel blades on a handle
2 hemostats, in two sizes for breaking up loculations and probing the cavity
Scissors
Normal saline
10 or 20 mL syringe with a 20 or 22 gauge angiocatheter
Suction source, tubing, and catheter for larger abscesses
4×4 gauze squares
Iodoform gauze packing
Adhesive tape

PATIENT PREPARATION

Explain the procedure, its risks, and benefits to the patient and/or their representative. Patients should be warned of potential cosmetic complications prior to proceeding. Obtain an informed consent to perform the procedure. Clean the skin of any dirt and debris. Apply povidone iodine to the skin and allow it to dry. Alternatively, prep the skin with chlorhexidine solution. Apply drapes to delineate a sterile field. Many physicians regard this last step optional, as the procedure is not considered sterile but clean.

The value of antibiotics prior to incision and drainage of a mature abscess is somewhat controversial, with many arguing that the antibiotic levels in the abscess cavity are low and therefore not of value.[7,38] Others suggest that decreased healing times may occur when antibiotics are administered.[2,14] Antibiotics are not indicated in an uncomplicated abscess in an otherwise healthy patient without significant systemic involvement or local erythema and lymphangitis.[16] If endocarditis prophy-

laxis is indicated, oral regimens should be given 1 hour prior to the procedure and parenteral regimens within 30 minutes of the procedure.

ANESTHESIA

It is usually possible to achieve adequate anesthesia for the skin incision but any addition manipulation may be painful. Local anesthetic infiltration is often less effective than in other procedures. The pH of infected tissue is often low and retards the diffusion of the local anesthetic solution into nerve axons (Figure 89-1A).[39] A regional field block can be instituted by injecting a ring of 1% lidocaine or 0.5% bupivacaine subcutaneously approximately 1 cm away from the perimeter of the erythematous border of the abscess. The onset of anesthesia occurs in about 5 minutes. A small amount of local anesthetic solution can be injected intradermally into the roof of the abscess in a linear fashion along the line of the planned incision (Figure 89-1A).[4] Be careful during this portion of the procedure as the abscess may be under pressure. The inadvertent injection of local anesthetic solution into the abscess cavity may cause fluid to be forcibly ejected toward the operator. Appropriate universal precautions should be employed including mask and eye protection.

In superficial abscesses or furuncles, which are unlikely to require significant exploration, topical ethyl chloride spray can be used to provide anesthesia. Invert the bottle and compress the spray nozzle to begin the flow of fluid. Direct the spray towards the planned site of incision. The pain relief from ethyl chloride is variable and fleeting and it is highly flammable.[5] The application of an ice pack secured with an elastic bandage for 15 minutes can also be effective. This may be especially useful for children, those with severe needle phobias, or in cases of true anesthetic allergy.

Nitrous oxide is safe and was previously thought to be effective as an adjunct to the incision and drainage of abscesses.[40] More recently, it has been shown to cause no significant reduction in pain and to only be marginally effective as an anxiolytic.[41] Procedural sedation with agents such as fentanyl and midazolam can be useful in deep abscesses that require extensive probing since it is difficult to obtain adequate pain control, even with a well-performed field block. A dissociative agent such as ketamine may be a good choice in IVDAs. It may be difficult to achieve adequate pain control and sedation with narcotics and benzodiazepines in these patients.

TECHNIQUES

ASPIRATION

Aspiration is performed as a diagnostic procedure in cases of soft tissue infections where the presence of an

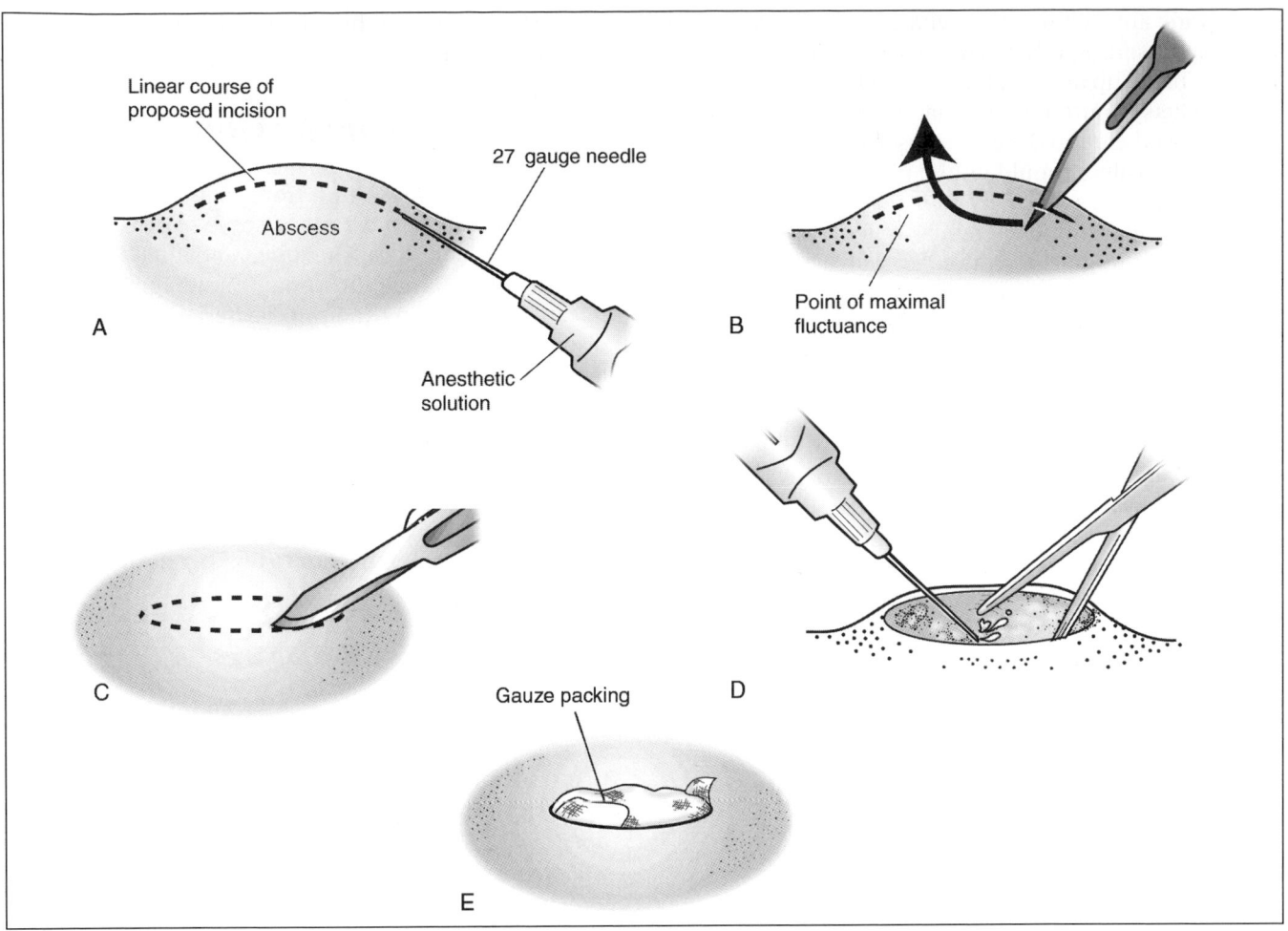

FIGURE 89-1 Incision and drainage of a subcutaneous abscess. *A.* Infiltration of local anesthetic solution over the abscess. *B.* A straight incision to drain the abscess. *C.* An elliptical incision to drain the abscess. *D.* The wound is irrigated with sterile saline. Any pockets of pus are opened by blunt dissection with the hemostat. *E.* The wound is packed open.

abscess is unclear, a mycotic aneurysm must be ruled out, or samples for Gram's stain and culture are required. **Aspiration is not a therapeutic procedure in and of itself.** Insert an 18 gauge needle attached to a 10 mL syringe into the skin. Apply negative pressure to the syringe. Advance the needle into the area where pus or blood is presumed to be loculated. The procedure should be terminated and incision and drainage to follow immediately if pus is obtained. Anaerobic and aerobic culture bottles should be inoculated directly from the syringe if cultures are indicated. Simple swabbing of the purulent material after incision and drainage is inadequate for growth of anaerobic organisms. If blood is aspirated, the procedure should be terminated and firm pressure applied to the area to prevent a hematoma from forming. Angiography with surgical consultation should immediately follow. If no pus or blood is aspirated, redirect the needle in several directions to confirm the absence of an abscess. Discharge the patient with oral antibiotics, warm compresses, and follow-up in 24 hours to reassess the situation.

INCISION AND DRAINAGE

Make an incision spanning the entire area of fluctuance and parallel to the relaxed skin tension lines to reduce scarring.[34] A straight incision with a #11 scalpel blade is usually performed (Figure 89-1B). An elliptical incision with a #15 scalpel blade is an alternative and often results in a similar appearing final scar (Figure 89-1C). The purpose of the elliptical incision is to remove a full thickness wedge of tissue so that the wound will remain open. This type of incision should not be made in cosmetically sensitive areas (face, neck, or breasts) or in areas with minimal subcutaneous tissue (hands and feet). **It is important to ensure a large enough incision to promote adequate drainage with the exception of cosmetically sensitive areas where a stab incision may be initially attempted to limit scar formation.[5]**

Debride any necrotic or devitalized tissue. Probe the cavity by inserting a hemostat. Gently spread the jaws open to break up any loculations and to release any further pockets of purulent material (Figure 89-1D).[6] Rotate the hemostat around the entire abscess to break any loculations. A scalpel should not be used for the blunt dissection of an abscess cavity as it may cause additional tissue damage and bacteremia.[14] Remove the tough shiny capsule by grasping the edges with a hemostat and applying firm traction if the abscess is due to an infected sebaceous cyst. The capsule can often by removed intact in this manner.

Irrigate the abscess cavity with an 18 gauge angiocatheter attached to a 10 mL syringe containing sterile saline (Figure 89-1D). This will flush away all loosened purulent and necrotic material. Loosely pack iodoform gauze into the abscess cavity (Figure 89-1E). Leave 1 to 2 cm of gauze exiting from the cavity to prevent the incision from sealing over and ensure an adequate drainage tract for the cavity. The value of antiseptic impregnated gauze over plain gauze is uncertain. Overly packing the abscess cavity may interfere with the inflammatory hyperemia necessary for healing or retard drainage and reproduce "abscess-like" conditions.[6] Apply an absorbent dressing of 4×4 gauze over the wound. Splinting and elevation of the affected area may be beneficial.

AFTERCARE

Antibiotics after incision and drainage of uncomplicated abscesses are of no benefit.[1,2,4,15] Abscesses that are surrounded by lymphangitis or cellulitis, or that have signs of a more extensive infection should be considered for treatment with parenteral antibiotics. Patients with signs and symptoms of a systemic infection should be considered for 23-hour admission and parenteral antibiotics.

Diabetics or others with impaired healing capacities may require admission for more frequent wound care, packing changes, and early reassessment within 24 hours.[5] Wounds at high risk for complications, such as human bites, hand wounds, or face wounds, require close follow-up. It is often preferable to have follow-up done by the same physician who performed the procedure.

Follow-up in 24 to 48 hours to remove the packing and assess the response to therapy should be arranged. The cavity should be repacked about every 48 hours until granulation tissue is developing throughout the wound and the drainage tract is well established if a large amount of drainage continues.[15,42] At that time, the remaining packing is removed and the patient is instructed to soak the area in warm water three to four times per day.[3] Healing occurs in 5 to 9 days in most cases.[4,6,15] The patient may be discharged from medical care when all signs of infection (erythema, drainage, pain and induration) have resolved.

COMPLICATIONS

Complications resulting from incision and drainage are uncommon. In most cases, some scarring will result from the deliberate packing open and intended secondary intention granulation of the wound. Infectious complications, including inciting bacterial endocarditis as discussed earlier, are possible. **Endocarditis can be avoided with appropriate screening of patients and the application of prophylactic antibiotic therapy.** Precipitation of septicemia because of transient bacteremia in an immunodeficient patient must be considered prior to the procedure. **Incision and drainage of a mycotic aneurysm simply should not occur if an appropriate assessment is completed prior to making the incision.**

SUMMARY

Simple incision and drainage under local or regional anesthesia in the Emergency Department can effectively treat most subcutaneous abscesses. Adjunctive procedural sedation may be required to adequately probe a deep cavity. A directed history and physical examination will identify those who may require additional lab work, imaging, or specialty consultation and follow-up. The majority of patients will not require antibiotics. Attention must be paid to requirements for endocarditis prophylaxis and consideration given to the possible effects of inducing bacteremia in any given patient.

REFERENCES

1. Meislin HW, Lerner SA, Graves MH, et al: Cutaneous abscesses: anaerobic and aerobic bacteriology and outpatient management. *Ann Intern Med* 1977; 87(2):145–149.
2. Llera JL, Levy RC: Treatment of cutaneous abscesses: a double-blind clinical study. *Ann Emerg Med* 1985; 14(1):15–19.
3. Meislin HW, McGhee MD, Rosen P: Management and microbiology of cutaneous abscesses. *JACEP* 1978; 7(5):186–191.
4. Burney RE: Incision and drainage procedures: soft tissue abscesses in the emergency service. *Emerg Med Clin North Am* 1986; 4(3):527–542.
5. Warden TM, Fourre MW: Incision and drainage of cutaneous abscesses and soft tissue infections, in Roberts JR, Hedges JR (eds): *Clinical Procedures in Emergency Medicine*, 2nd ed. Philadelphia: Saunders, 1991:591–609.

6. Simms MH, Curran F, Johnson RA, et al: Treatment of acute abscesses in the casualty department. *Br Med J* 1982; 284:1827–1829.

7. Ghoneim ATM, McGoldrick J, Blick PWH, et al: Aerobic and anaerobic bacteriology of subcutaneous abscesses. *Br J Surg* 1981; 68:498–500.

8. Robbins SL, Cotran RS, Kumar V: *Pathologic Basis of Disease,* 3rd ed. Philadelphia: Saunders, 1984:63–64.

9. Simms RL: Life-threatening soft tissue infections, in Peterson PK, Sabath LD, Caleron JE, et al (eds): *The Management of Infectious Diseases in Clinical Practice.* New York: Academic Press, 1982:211–228.

10. Biderman P, Hiatt JR: Management of soft-tissue infection of the upper extremity in parenteral drug abusers. *Am J Surg* 1987; 154(5):526–528.

11. Brook I, Frazier EH: Aerobic and anaerobic bacteriology of wounds and cutaneous abscesses. *Arch Surg* 1990; 125:1445–1451.

12. Zimmereli W, Zak O, Vosbeck K: Experimental hematogenous infection of subcutaneously implanted foreign bodies. *Scand J Infect Dis* 1985; 17:303–310.

13. Brook I, Finegold SM: Aerobic and anaerobic bacteriology of cutaneous abscesses in children. *Pediatrics* 1981; 67(6):891–895.

14. Blick PWH, Flowers MW, Marsden AK, et al: Antibiotics in the surgical treatment of acute abscesses. *Br Med J* 1980; 281:111–112.

15. MacFie J, Harvey J: Treatment of acute superficial abscesses: a prospective clinical trial. *Br J Surg* 1977; 64:264–266.

16. Bobrow BJ, Pollack Jr CV, Gamble S, et al: Incision and drainage of cutaneous abscesses is not associated with bacteremia in afebrile adults. *Ann Emerg Med* 1997; 29(3):404–408.

17. Podzamczer D, Ribera MD, Gudiol F: Skin abscesses caused by *Candida albicans* in heroin abusers. *J Am Acad Dermatol* 1987; 16(2 Pt 1):386–387.

18. Orangio GR, Silvio D, Pitlick MD, et al: Soft tissue infections in parenteral drug abusers. *Ann Surg* 1984; 199(1):97–100.

19. Marantz PR, Linzer M, Feiner CJ, et al: Inability to predict diagnosis in febrile intravenous drug abusers. *Ann Intern Med* 1987; 106:823–828.

20. Gonzales MH, Garst J, Nourbash P, et al: Abscesses of the upper extremity from drug abuse by injection. *J Hand Surg* 1993; 18A(5):868–870.

21. O'Sullivan M, Beattie T, Keane CT: A review of drug addict abscesses. *Ir Med J* 1984; 77:68–70.

22. Callahan TE, Schecter WP, Horn JK: Necrotizing soft tissue infections masquerading as cutaneous abscess following illicit drug injection. *Arch Surg* 1998; 133:812–819.

23. Webb D, Thadepalli H: Skin and soft tissue polymicrobial infections from intravenous abuse of drugs. *West J Med* 1979; 130(3):200–204.

24. Boudreau S, Hines HC, Hood AF: Dermal abscesses with *Staphylococcus aureus,* cytomegalovirus and acid-fast bacilli in a patient with acquired immunodeficiency syndrome (AIDS). *J Cutan Pathol* 1988; 15(1):53–57.

25. Manji N, Hulyalkar AR, Keroack MA, et al: Cutaneous pseudo abscesses: an unusual presentation of severe pancreatitis. *Am J Gastroenterol* 1988; 83(2):177–179.

26. Paletta C, Jurkiewicz MJ: Hidradenitis suppurativa. *Clin Plast Surg* 1987; 14(2):383–390.

27. Scholefield JH, Duncan JL, Rogers K: Review of hospital experience of breast abscesses. *Br J Surg* 1987; 74(6):469–470.

28. Fine BC, Sheckman PR, Bartlett JC: Incision and drainage of soft-tissue abscesses and bacteremia. *Ann Intern Med* 1985; 103(4):645.

29. Dajani AS, Taubert KA, Wilson W, et al: Prevention of bacterial endocarditis: recommendations by the American Heart Association, http://www.americanheart.org/Scientific/statements/1997/079701.html.

30. Roca B, Vilar C, Perez EV, et al: Breast abscess with lethal septicemia due to *Pseudomonas aeruginosa* in a patient with AIDS. *Presse Med* 1996; 25(17): 803–804.

31. Fichtenbaum C, Dunagan WC, Powderly WG: The incidence and outcome of bacteremia in HIV-infected patients. *Int Conf AIDS* 1993; 9(1):318.

32. Styrt BA, Chaisson RE, Moore RD: Prior antimicrobials and staphylococcal bacteremia in HIV-infected patients. *AIDS* 1997; 11(10):1243–1248.

33. American College of Emergency Physicians: Clinical policy for procedural sedation and analgesia in the emergency department. *Ann Emerg Med* 1998; 31(5):663–677.

34. Connell P, Ellis JI: Cutaneous abscesses and gas gangrene, in Schwartz G, Cayten CG, Mangelsen MA, et al (eds): *Principles and Practice of Emergency Medicine.* Philadelphia: Lea & Febiger, 1992:1890–1897.

35. Simon RR, Brenner BE: *Emergency Procedures and Techniques,* 3rd ed. Baltimore: Williams & Wilkins, 1994:357–360.

36. Cohen DM, Garcia CT, Dietrich AM, et al: Miniature c-arm imaging: an in vitro study of detecting foreign bodies in the emergency department. *Pediatr Emerg Care* 1997; 13(4):247–249.

37. Fornage BD, Schernberg FL: Sonographic diagnosis of foreign bodies of the distal extremities. *AJR Am J Roentgenol* 1986; 147:567–569.

38. Joiner KA, Lowe BR, Dzink JL, et al: Antibiotic levels in infected and sterile subcutaneous abscesses in mice. *J Infect Dis* 1981; 143(3):487–490.

39. Meislin HW: Soft tissue infections, in Rosen P, Barkin RM, Braen RC, et al (eds): *Emergency Medicine: Concepts and Clinical Practice,* 3rd ed. St. Louis: Mosby Year-Book, 1992:850–861.

40. Flomenbaum N, Gallagher EJ, Eagen K, et al: Self-administered nitrous oxide: an adjunct analgesic. *JACEP* 1979; 8(3):95–97.

41. Leeson Payne CG, Edbrooke DL, Davies GK: Minor procedures in the accident and emergency department: can entonox help. *Arch Emerg Med* 1991; 24:24–32.

42. Dimick AR: Delayed wound closure indications and techniques. *Ann Emerg Med* 1988; 17(12):1303–1304.

Chapter 90
PARONYCHIA OR EPONYCHIA INCISION AND DRAINAGE

Lisa R. Palivos

INTRODUCTION

A paronychia is an infection or abscess of the tissues around the base and along the sides of the nail plate. It is the most common infection in the hand.[1] A paronychia can be located on the fingers or the toes. It occurs in all age groups. It can cause significant pain and discomfort leading to a visit to the Emergency Department.

A paronychia initially presents with redness, swelling, and tenderness along the edges of the nail plate. This can progress to an abscess that requires drainage. An infection that extends to the overlying proximal cuticle is termed an eponychia. In this chapter, we will discuss different treatments that vary with the extent of the infection.

ANATOMY AND PATHOPHYSIOLOGY

The dorsal aspect of the distal digit consists of the nail plate, the nail bed (matrix), and the perionychium (Figure 90-1). The nail bed is situated beneath the nail plate and is responsible for growth of the nail. The perionychium consists of the soft tissue surrounding the nail plate (eponychium and lateral nail folds).

A paronychia is usually the result of frequent trauma, aggressive manicures, hangnails, or nail biting.[2] A disruption of the seal between the nail plate and nail fold allows bacteria to enter, leading to pus formation in the eponychial space (Figure 90-1). It begins as a swelling and erythema in the dorsolateral corner of the nail fold that can progress to an abscess. The most common organism to cause a paronychia is *Staphylococcus aureus*.[3] In chil-

dren, paronychia are often caused by anaerobes secondary to finger sucking or nail biting.[4] Gram-negative organisms should be considered in immunocompromised hosts. Chronic paronychia are usually caused by *Candida albicans*.[5]

INDICATIONS

An early paronychia with signs of cellulitis may be treated nonsurgically with frequent warm soaks, immobilization, elevation, oral antibiotics, and follow-up in 24 hours.[2,6] A progression of the infection results in fluctuance and the formation of an abscess. The presence of an abscess, fluctuance, or pus beneath the nail plate requires an incision and drainage procedure.

CONTRAINDICATIONS

A herpetic whitlow is a herpes simplex virus infection of the distal phalanx that can be confused with an early paronychia or felon. The presence of multiple clear vesicles that coalesce suggests a herpetic whitlow. The herpetic whitlow is a nonsurgical and self-limited infection. Treatment consists of a dry dressing to the affected finger in order to prevent autoinoculation and transmission of the infection, oral antiviral agents, and analgesics. Incision and drainage is not recommended, will prolong the recovery, and lead to secondary bacterial infection.[7] A chronic paronychia should be referred to a Hand Surgeon or Dermatologist for treatment.

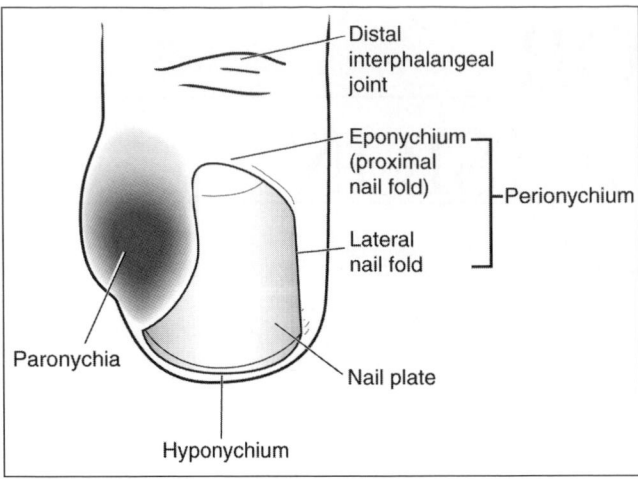

FIGURE 90-1 The distal finger illustrating a paronychia and the surface anatomy.

EQUIPMENT

Povidone iodine
Sterile gloves
11 scalpel blade or an 18 gauge needle
Local anesthetic solution without epinephrine
18 and 27 gauge needles
5 to 10 mL syringe
Forceps
Mosquito hemostat
Ribbon gauze packing, ½ inch wide
Scissors
4×4 gauze squares
18 gauge angiocatheter
20 mL syringe
Sterile saline
Adhesive tape

PATIENT PREPARATION

Explain the procedure, its risks, and benefits to the patient and/or their representative. Obtain an informed consent for the procedure. Place the patient on a gurney with the extremity on a bedside procedure table in a well-lit room. Soak the digit in warm water for 5 minutes to soften the skin. Perform a digital nerve block if the patient is apprehensive, has significant tenderness, or if it is not a simple paronychia or eponychia. Refer to Chapter 106 for the complete details regarding anesthesia techniques. Apply povidone iodine and allow it to dry. The digit can be secured to a sterile tongue depressor for better control, especially in uncooperative children.

TECHNIQUES

SIMPLE PARONYCHIA OR EPONYCHIA

There is no need for a skin incision in an uncomplicated paronychia or eponychia. Simply lifting the eponychium off the nail at the point of maximal tenderness and/or fluctuance is usually curative. Slide the tip of a #11 scalpel blade (or an 18 gauge needle) under the paronychia, or eponychia, at the site of maximal fluctuance (Figure 90-2). Advance the scalpel blade to lift the soft tissue from the nail plate until there is an efflux of purulent fluid. Apply digital pressure to the area to express the pus. Gently place a hemostat under the soft tissue to break any loculations. Irrigate the pocket with an angiocatheter on a syringe containing sterile saline.

Packing a paronychia is controversial and physician-dependent. To pack, place a small piece of ribbon gauze under the elevated soft tissue followed by a dressing. If packing is not necessary, most physicians apply an antibiotic ointment followed by a bandage. Oral antibiotics are usually not recommended in an uncomplicated paronychia or eponychia.

PARONYCHIA WITH EXTENSION UNDER THE LATERAL NAIL PLATE

A more extensive incision and drainage is required when pus accumulates laterally and beneath the nail plate. Remove the lateral nail plate to allow adequate drainage (Figure 90-3A). Use scissors to cut the nail plate longitudinally. Remove the lateral nail plate with a hemostat. A small (2 to 3 mm) incision may be required in the corner of the nail fold to remove the nail plate (Figure 90-3A). This will result in the egress of pus. Irrigate the area with saline. Insert a small piece of petrolatum gauze under the nail fold (Figure 90-3B). This will prevent the nail fold from fusing to the nail bed.

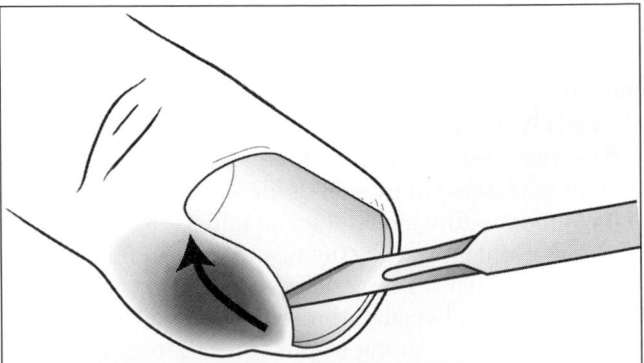

FIGURE 90-2 Drainage of a simple paronychia or eponychia. The eponychial fold is elevated from the nail plate with a # 11 scalpel blade. Note that the blade is parallel to the nail plate, thereby avoiding injury to the matrix.

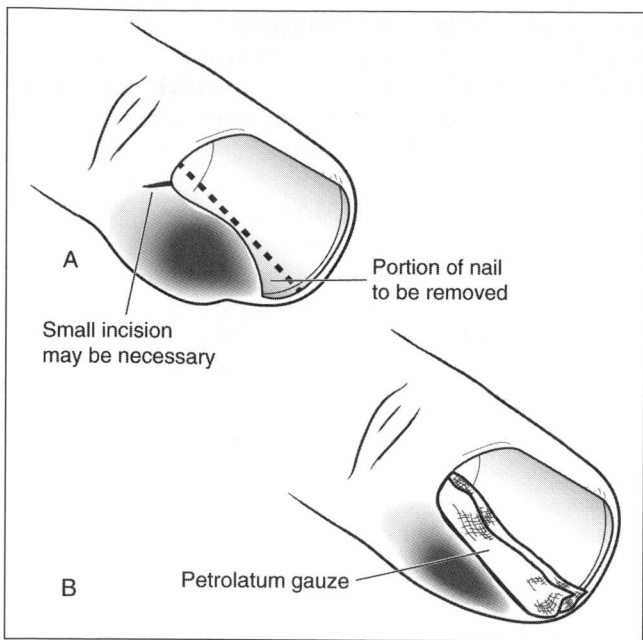

FIGURE 90-3 Removal of the lateral nail plate is required when pus extends laterally below the nail plate. *A.* The dotted line over the nail represents the incision required to remove the nail plate. An additional incision may be required on the eponychium. *B.* The lateral portion of the nail plate has been removed and gauze packing has been inserted to keep the nail fold elevated from the nail bed.

PARONYCHIA WITH EXTENSION UNDER THE PROXIMAL NAIL PLATE

A paronychia with extension under the proximal nail plate also requires the removal of a portion of the nail plate (Figure 90-4). Make two 3 to 4 mm long incisions at the corners of the nail folds (Figure 90-4*A*). Cut the proximal one-third of the nail plate with scissors (Figure 90-4*B*). Grasp and remove the proximal segment of the nail plate with a hemostat. This will result in the egress of pus. Irrigate the area with saline. Insert a piece of petrolatum gauze under the nail fold to prevent it from fusing to the nail bed (Figure 90-4*C*).

Removal of the entire nail is rarely necessary except in cases of extensive subungual abscesses. An alternative to nail removal is trephination with a heated paper clip or a microcautery unit.[8] A large opening or multiple holes are required with this technique in order to eliminate the pus. Refer to Chapter 85 for the complete details regarding trephination.

CHRONIC PARONYCHIA

A chronic paronychia occurs from recurrent episodes of inflammation or from neglected infections. It is much more difficult to treat and eradicate than an acute infection. A chronic paronychia is seen frequently in immunosuppressed patients, such as those with diabetes

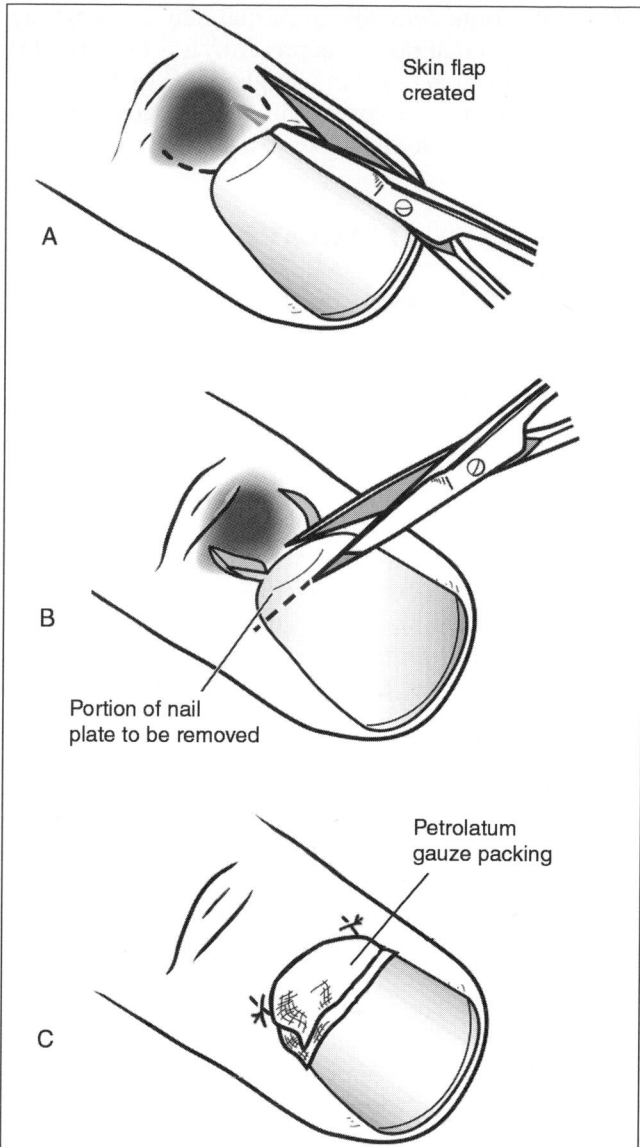

FIGURE 90-4 Removal of the proximal nail plate is required when pus extends proximally below the nail plate. *A.* Two incisions are required through the eponychium, represented by dotted lines. *B.* The dotted line over the nail plate represents the incision required to remove the nail plate. *C.* The proximal portion of the nail plate has been removed and gauze packing has been inserted to keep the nail fold elevated from the nail bed.

or cancer. A chronic paronychia is also common in people who wash their hands often, such as dishwashers and health care providers. The most frequently isolated organism is *Candida albicans* that commonly coexists with *Staphylococcus aureus*.[5,6] Treatment for a chronic paronychia is eponychial marsupialization. This involves removal of a crescent shaped piece of skin proximal to the nail fold and parallel to the eponychium, extending from the radial to ulnar borders. In addition to marsupialization, complete or partial nail removal may be necessary if nail ridging is present.[9] It is best to refer chronic paronychia to a Hand Surgeon due to the higher rate of recurrence, the complexity in management, and where follow-up care can be more consistent.

AFTERCARE

Immobilize and elevate the digit. Remind the patient to avoid nail biting or sucking. Any discomfort can be treated with acetaminophen or nonsteroidal anti-inflammatory medications. Follow-up care in 24 hours is important. Packing of a simple paronychia should be removed in 24 hours. Warms soaks can begin immediately if packing is not placed. Otherwise, warm soaks should be delayed until the packing is removed in 24 hours. Oral antibiotics are not necessary unless the nail bed is involved, there is apparent cellulitis of the surrounding tissue, or if there are systemic signs of infections such as lymphangitis and fever.[6] Patients should return to the Emergency Department if they develop a fever, reaccumulation of pus, redness extending up the finger and hand, or increased tenderness to the digit.

Most simple paronychias resolve within a few days. If they persist longer or are recurrent, a Hand Surgeon should be consulted for more aggressive therapy, such as eponychial marsupialization and nail plate removal.

Paronychia or eponychia that extend under the nail plate require follow-up in 24 hours. The packing must be maintained between the nail fold and the nail bed for at least 5 to 7 days. The nail fold will fuse to the nail bed if the packing is removed too soon and a new nail plate will not form. These infections require a 5 to 7 day course of oral antistaphylococcal antibiotics. Nonsteroidal anti-inflammatory medications supplemented with occasional narcotic analgesics will provide adequate pain control for these patients.

COMPLICATIONS

Complications, even in a properly drained paronychia, include osteomyelitis of the distal phalanx. Superinfection with *Candida albicans* or other fungi can also

occur. Care must be taken if the proximal nail plate is removed to avoid damaging the underlying matrix so that a nail deformity does not result. Fusion of the nail fold to the nail bed will result in a new nail not being formed.

SUMMARY

A paronychia is one of the most common hand infections. The treatment depends on the extent of the infection. The procedures are quick, simple, and easy to perform. Simple paronychias require elevation of the nail fold with no incision. A more extensive incision and drainage is required along with nail excision when pus accumulates below the nail plate. Follow-up is critical as complications may occur, even when treatment is optimal. Complications should be referred to a Hand Surgeon.

REFERENCES

1. Neviaser RJ: Infections, in Green DP (ed): *Operative Hand Surgery*, 3rd ed. New York: Churchill Livingstone, 1993:1021–1038.
2. Siegel DB, Gelberman RH: Infections of the hand. *Orthop Clin North Am* 1988; 19(4):779–789.
3. Canales FL, Newmeyer WL, Kilgore ES: The treatment of felons and paronychias. *Hand Clin* 1989; 5(4):515–523.
4. Brook I: Bacteriologic study of paronychia in children. *Am J Surg* 1981; 141:703–705.
5. Barlow AJ, Chattaway FW, Holgate MC, et al: Chronic paronychia. *Br J Dermatol* 1970; 82:448–453.
6. Moran GJ, Talan DA: Hand infections. *Emerg Med Clin North Am* 1993; 11(3):601–619.
7. Louis DS, Silva Jr J: Herpetic whitlow: herpetic infections of the digits. *J Hand Surg [Am]* 1979; 4(1):90–94.
8. Blumstein H: Incision and drainage, in Roberts JR, Hedges JR (eds): *Clinical Procedures in Emergency Medicine*, 3rd ed. Philadelphia: Saunders, 1998:634–659.
9. Bednar MS, Lane LB: Eponychial marsupialization and nail removal for surgical treatment of chronic paronychia. *J Hand Surg [Am]* 1991; 16A(2):314–317.

Chapter 91
FELON INCISION AND DRAINAGE

Lisa R. Palivos

INTRODUCTION

A felon is a subcutaneous infection or abscess in the pulp space on the volar aspect surface of the distal phalanx. It is usually caused by penetrating trauma, an abrasion, or a minor cut with invasion of bacteria. A felon can also develop in the presence of a foreign body, such as a wood splinter or a thorn.[1] It can be iatrogenic from multiple fingersticks for glucose determination.[2] The offending organism is usually *Staphylococcus aureus.* Mixed infections and gram-negative infections may occur in the immunocompromised patient. A felon can less commonly occur on the toes. The information in this chapter can be applied to a felon of the finger or the toe.

ANATOMY AND PATHOPHYSIOLOGY

Felons initially present with a gradual onset of pain and erythema in the distal finger. Intense throbbing pain, warmth, and swelling develop with the formation of an abscess as the infection progresses. **The proper treatment for a felon is incision and drainage.** There are multiple techniques to incise and drain a felon. The patient requires digital elevation, immobilization, oral antistaphylococcal antibiotics, oral analgesics, and close follow-up to prevent complications following the incision and drainage.[3-7]

The distal finger consists of a closed compartment that is bound by the nail plate dorsally, by the skin ventrally and distally, and by the flexion crease proximally (Figure 91-1). This pulp region is divided by multiple vertical septa.[8] These septa extend from the volar surface of the fat pad to the periosteum of the distal phalanx. They divide and compartmentalize the pulp area. When an abscess occurs, it is confined by the septa. They also limit the proximal spread of an infection. Unfortunately, they also inhibit the abscess from reaching the surface and inhibit drainage after the incision and drainage pro-

cedure. Blood is supplied by branches of the digital arteries that run parallel and lateral to the phalanx and terminate in the pulp region. The terminal branches of the digital nerves lie palmer and superficial to the arteries. The flexor digitorum profundus tendon inserts on the volar surface of the proximal distal phalanx.

INDICATIONS

All felons that are fluctuant should be incised and drained.

CONTRAINDICATIONS

Felons that are not yet fluctuant, as in an early infection, may be treated with warm soaks, elevation, oral antibiotics, and follow-up in 24 hours.[6,7] A herpetic whitlow can sometimes be confused with a felon.[5,9] A herpetic whitlow can be clinically distinguished by the presence of multiple vesicles and a history of recurrence or simultaneous genital or oral lesions. Treatment of a herpetic whitlow is nonsurgical and consists of a protective dry dressing, oral antiviral agents, and analgesics. Incision and drainage of a herpetic whitlow may spread the virus and predispose the patient to secondary bacterial infection.[9]

EQUIPMENT

Povidone iodine
Sterile gloves
#11 scalpel blade on a handle
Local anesthetic solution without epinephrine
18 and 27 gauge needles
5 or 10 mL syringe

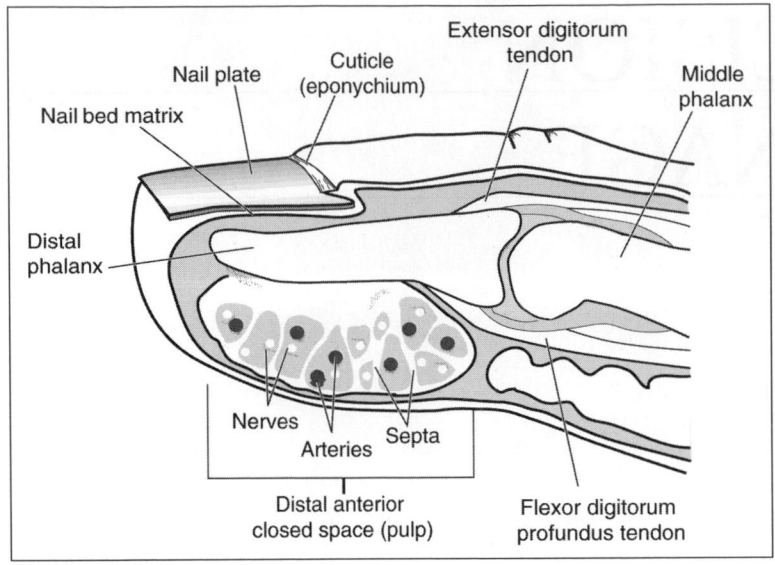

FIGURE 91-1 Midsagittal section demonstrating the anatomy of the distal finger.

20 mL syringe
Sterile saline
18 gauge angiocatheter
Mosquito hemostat
Iodophor gauze, ½ inch wide ribbon
Bandage material
Digital splint (plaster, preformed, or tongue depressor)
Sling
Digital tourniquet, optional

PATIENT PREPARATION

Explain the procedure, its risks, and benefits to the patient and/or their representative. Obtain an informed consent for the procedure. Some physicians prefer to obtain anteroposterior and lateral radiographs of the digit to rule out an osteomyelitis prior to performing the procedure. A positive radiograph for osteomyelitis will alter the time course for antibiotic therapy and require follow-up with a Hand Surgeon. Radiographs should be obtained if there is a suspicion for a foreign body.

Place the patient on a gurney with the extremity on a bedside procedure table in a well-lit room. Soak the digit in warm water for 5 minutes to soften the skin. Perform a digital or metacarpal nerve block. Refer to Chapter 106 for the complete details regarding anesthesia techniques. Apply povidone iodine and allow it to dry. Apply sterile drapes to delineate a sterile field. The digit can be secured to a sterile tongue depressor for better control, especially in uncooperative children. The application of a digital tourniquet to create a bloodless field is optional.

TECHNIQUES

Multiple incisions can be employed. Make an incision in the area of greatest fluctuance or tenderness with a #11 scalpel blade.[3–6] Make a longitudinal incision if the maximal tenderness is in the center of the pulp of the distal fingertip (Figure 91-2A). **The incision should not cross the crease of the distal interphalangeal joint, as this can lead to flexor tenosynovitis and flexion contractures.**[7] Make the incision along the lateral surface of the finger if the felon has maximal tenderness on the radial or ulnar aspect of the finger (Figure 91-2B). Purulent and/or bloody pink fluid will exit from the incision. Gently probe the loculations with a mosquito hemostat. Irrigate the wound with an 18 gauge angiocatheter on a

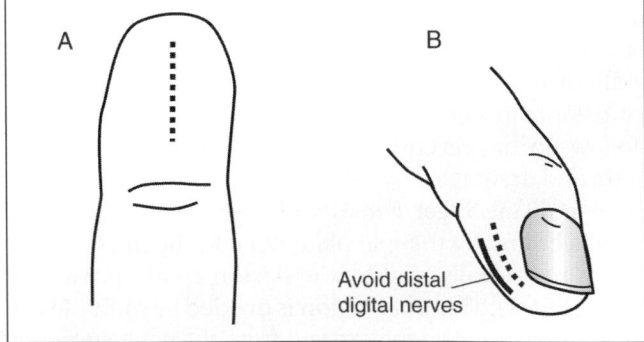

FIGURE 91-2 Recommended incisions for the incision and drainage of a felon. A felon should be incised and drained in the area of maximal fluctance. *A.* The longitudinal fat pad incision over the area of maximum fluctance. *B.* The unilateral longitudinal incision is high, lateral, and just below the level of the nail.

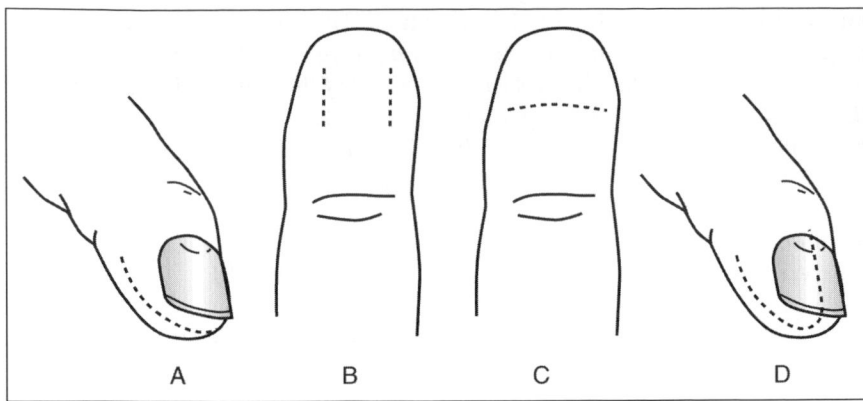

FIGURE 91-3 Incisions not recommended for the drainage of a felon. *A.* The hockey stick incision. *B.* The through-and-through or bilateral longitudinal incision. *C.* The transverse palmar incision. *D.* The fishmouth incision.

5 or 10 mL syringe containing sterile saline. Place a piece of iodophor gauze into the wound. Apply a dry bulky dressing.

ALTERNATIVE TECHNIQUES

Alternative incisions have been advocated but are not recommended because they have higher complication rates (Figure 91-3). These incisions can result in neurovascular injury, painful scars, and altered fingertip sensation. The hockey stick incision can result in digital nerve injury and produce numbness to the fingertip (Figure 91-3*A*).[5] The through-and-through or bilateral longitudinal incision can result in bilateral digital nerve injury and complete anesthesia of the fingertip (Figure 91-3*B*).[6] The transverse palmar incision may transect the digital neurovascular bundles (Figure 91-3*C*). The fishmouth or horseshoe incision is very extensive, can take a long time to heal, produces a large scar, and an unstable pulp (Figure 91-3*D*).[5]

AFTERCARE

Splint the involved digit. Give the patient a sling to keep the hand elevated. Oral antistaphylococcal antibiotics such as penicillinase-resistant penicillins (dicloxacillin) or first-generation cephalosporins (cephalexin) should be prescribed for 5 to 7 days.[10] Nonsteroidal anti-inflammatory medications supplemented with narcotic analgesics will control any post-procedural pain. The patient should be reevaluated in 24 to 48 hours for removal of the gauze and inspection of the digit.

Remove the iodoform gauze during the follow-up visit. Perform a digital or metacarpal block. Irrigate the wound with sterile saline and break up any further loculations, if needed. Replace the gauze for another 24 to 48 hours if there is continued drainage. Instruct the patient to soak the digit in warm water several times a day to speed healing. Patients should immediately return to the Emergency Department if they experience fever, increased pain, difficulty using the finger, redness of the finger or hand or arm, or a discharge from the wound.

COMPLICATIONS

Untreated or mistreated felons may cause skin necrosis, osteitis or osteomyelitis of the distal phalanx, septic arthritis of the distal interphalangeal joint, extension of the infection into the palm and adjacent fingers, suppurative tenosynovitis, and lymphangitis. Flexor tenosynovitis can occur if the incision is extended too far proximally and too deep. Improperly placed incisions can result in mobility of the pad of the finger, neurologic compromise, and/or vascular compromise. The lack of improvement within 24 to 48 hours requires consultation with a Hand Surgeon.

SUMMARY

Felons require incision and drainage. The procedure is quick, simple, and easy to perform. The incision should be made at the point of maximal fluctuance while avoiding injury to the digital arteries, digital nerves, the flexor digitorum profundus tendon, and the distal interphalangeal joint. Close follow-up is mandatory to prevent any complications. Consult a Hand Surgeon for any complications associated with the felon.

REFERENCES

1. Hausman MR, Lisser SP: Hand infections. *Orthop Clin North Am* 1992; 23(1):171–185.
2. Perry AW, Gottlieb LJ, Zachary LS, et al: Fingerstick felons. *Ann Plast Surg* 1988; 20(3):249–251.
3. Canales FL, Newmeyer WL, Kilgore ES: The treatment of felons and paronychias. *Hand Clin* 1989; 5(4):515–523.

4. Jebson PJL: Infections of the fingertip paronychias and felons. *Hand Clin* 1998; 14(4):547–555.

5. Blumstein H: Incision and drainage, in Roberts JR, Hedges JR (eds): *Clinical Procedures in Emergency Medicine*, 3rd ed. Philadelphia: Saunders, 1998:634–659.

6. Bethel CA: Incision and drainage of a felon, in Henretig FM, King C, Joffe MD, et al (eds): *Textbook of Pediatric Emergency Procedures*. Baltimore: Williams & Wilkins, 1997:1211–1215.

7. Kilgore ES, Brown LG, Newmeyer WL, et al: Treatment of felons. *Am J Surg* 1975; 130:194–198.

8. Kanavel AB: *Infections of the Hand*, 4th ed. Philadelphia: Lea & Febiger, 1921.

9. Louis DS, Silva J Jr: Herpetic whitlow: herpetic infections of the digits. *J Hand Surg Am* 1979; 4(1):90–94.

10. Moran MD, Talan MD: Hand infections. *Emerg Med Clin North Am* 1993: 11(3):601–619.

Chapter 92
PILONIDAL ABSCESS OR CYST INCISION AND DRAINAGE

Paula L. Ward

INTRODUCTION

Pilonidal disease was first described in 1880 by Hodges.[1] He used the term "pilonidal sinus" to describe a chronic infection that contained hair and was usually found between the buttocks. "Pilonidal" comes from "pilus" or hair and "nidus" or nest. It literally means "nest of hair." The condition did not receive much attention until it became a significant problem in the armed services around the time of World War II. In 1940, in the United States Navy, the number of sick days caused by pilonidal disease and its complications exceeded those of either syphilis or hernias.[2] The term "jeep disease" was coined by Buie in 1944.[3] It related the condition to drivers and passengers of jeeps.

Pilonidal sinus disease primarily affects Caucasian males. Blacks are infrequently affected. The condition is rare in Asians and Indians. Males are affected three times as frequently as females. The condition is prevalent from the onset of puberty to young adulthood. It is unusual after the age of forty. The peak age of incidence is 21 years. The increased incidence in adolescents and young adults is attributed to hormonal effects of increased hair on the torso, increased activity of sebaceous and sweat glands, fat deposition on the buttocks, and deepening of the gluteal cleft. Other risk factors may include hirsutism, obesity, and poor personal hygiene. Repeated trauma to the area may also contribute to the formation of pilonidal disease. There is an increased prevalence in drivers and others with occupations requiring long periods of sitting.[4,5]

Patients with pilonidal sinus disease may present with mild discomfort and a chronically draining sinus in the upper gluteal region. Others may note sinuses or pits that are asymptomatic. Approximately 50 percent of patients with symptomatic pilonidal disease will present acutely with severe pain and disability indicative of a pilonidal abscess that necessitates incision and drainage.[6,7] Inspection will reveal one or more midline sinus tract openings, often with protruding tufts of hair. The area will be tender, erythematous, and indurated when an abscess is present. Fluctuance and swelling may not be readily appreciated. The sinuses may be quite extensive depending upon the chronicity of the disease process prior to presentation.

ANATOMY AND PATHOPHYSIOLOGY

A pilonidal sinus consists of a characteristic midline opening, or series of openings, in the upper aspect of the gluteal cleft and approximately 4–5 cm from the anus (Figure 92-1). The skin enters the sinus giving the opening a smooth edge. This primary tract leads into a subcutaneous cavity that contains granulation tissue and often a nest of hairs (Figure 92-2). The hairs may be seen projecting through the skin opening. Many sinuses have lateral or secondary openings (fistulas) extending from the pilonidal abscess (Figure 92-2).

There have been various opinions as to the etiology of the condition since the first description of the disease. In the first half of the twentieth century, it was generally attributed to a congenital lesion. Some authors believed that the pilonidal sinus originated from a remnant of the medullary canal that subsequently became infected. However, pilonidal disease can form in other areas of the body that lack hair, as some barbers have experienced in interdigital spaces.[8,9] Piloidal disease is often recurrent despite excising the affected area of skin.[8,9]

It is now generally believed that the condition is acquired. Loose hairs from the adjacent gluteal region are thought to form a bristly tuft and penetrate into the skin, perhaps in an area of skin irregularity. This process may be aided by pressure on the region in persons with occupations that require long hours of driving or sitting. The hairs may also be pulled in by a suction effect between

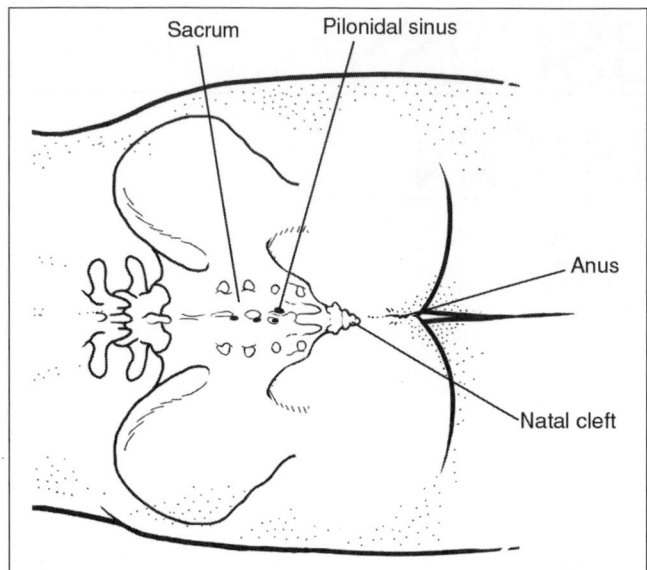

FIGURE 92-1 Pilonidal sinuses occur in the midline, approximately 4 to 5 cm above the anus and in the natal cleft.

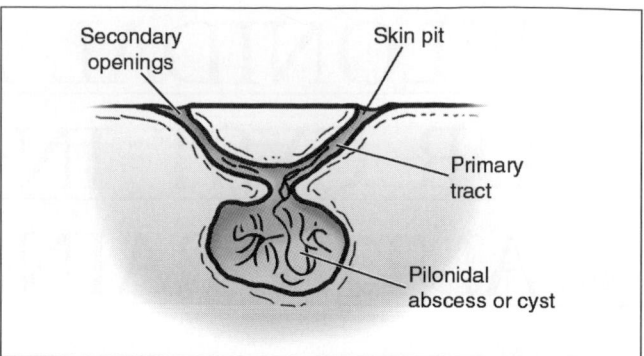

FIGURE 92-2 Cross-section through a pilonidal abscess and sinus. A primary tract and skin pit leads to the subcutaneous abscess. There may be secondary or lateral openings (fistulas).

the moving buttocks. The hair penetrates the skin and causes a foreign body reaction and secondary inflammation with the potential for infection and abscess formation. The sinuses spread cranially and laterally. They rarely approach the anus and generally remain superficial to the presacral fascia.[7,8,10]

INDICATIONS

Incision and drainage is indicated whenever a patient presents with a pilonidal abscess. The procedure will relieve the patient's pain. Antibiotics alone are ineffective in treating pilonidal abscesses. Rarely, systemic signs and symptoms may ensue. There are reported cases of necrotizing fasciitis from neglected pilonidal sinus disease. Thus it is preferable to treat pilonidal abscesses expeditiously.

CONTRAINDICATIONS

The great majority of pilonidal abscesses may be drained in the Emergency Department. Patients occasionally present with fever or toxicity. They should be admitted to the hospital for parenteral antibiotics, incision and drainage, and observation. This is particularly true if the patient has diabetes or is immunocompromised. Consult a Surgeon to manage these patients. Extensive abscesses should be incised and drained in the Operating Room under general anesthesia. Patients who are asymptomatic do not require an incision and drainage and can be referred to a Surgeon for removal.

EQUIPMENT

Benzoin solution
Povidone iodine solution
Skin razor
10 mL syringe
25 to 30 gauge needle, 2 inches long
Local anesthetic solution with epinephrine, lidocaine, or bupivacaine
#11 scalpel blade on a handle
#15 scalpel blade on a handle
Curved hemostat
4×4 gauze squares
Ribbon gauze, plain or iodoform
Adhesive tape

PATIENT PREPARATION

Explain the risks, benefits, and potential complications of the procedure to the patient and/or their representative. The post-procedure care should be explained as well. Document the discussion of the risks and benefits of the procedure. Obtain an informed consent for the procedure.

The best visualization of the sacral region, particularly in obese patients, occurs with the use of a proctoscopic examination table, if available (Figure 92-3A). Place the patient prone on a gurney or on the proctoscopy table. Alternatively, place the patient in the lateral knee-chest position to expose the affected area (Figure 92-3B). Apply benzoin solution to the buttocks and allow it to dry. Apply adhesive tape to the buttocks and tape them open (Figure 92-4). Clean any dirt and debris from the skin overlying the abscess or cyst. Apply povidone iodine and allow it to dry. However, this is probably not necessary because by definition the drainage of an abscess is not a sterile procedure. Shaving the

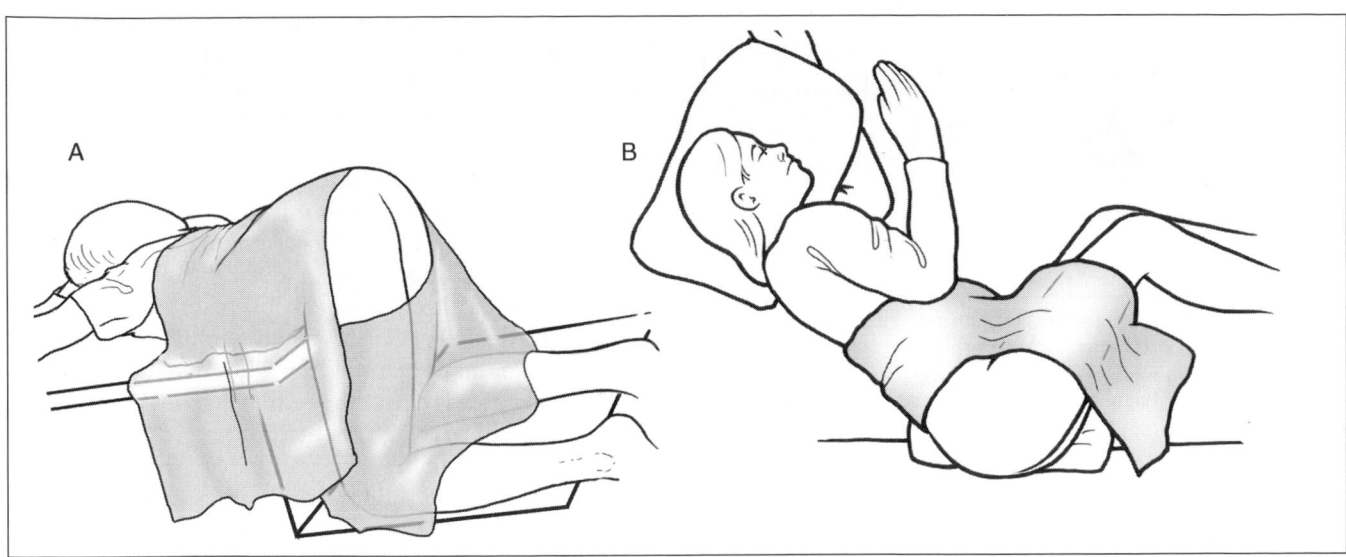

FIGURE 92-3 Patient placement. *A.* Place the patient prone on a proctoscopy table. The patient may also be placed prone on a gurney. *B.* The lateral knee-chest position.

surrounding area, if the patient is hirsute, will aid the application of the dressing after the procedure. Some authors advocate shaving the sacral region to prevent recurrence as well, although this has not been proven to be effective.

ANESTHESIA

Local anesthesia should be administered, recognizing that it is often difficult to obtain complete anesthesia by direct infiltration of an abscess. Local anesthetics are weak acids and are less effective in the acidic environment of an abscess. The skin over the abscess cavity usually becomes insensate, but anesthesia of the abscess

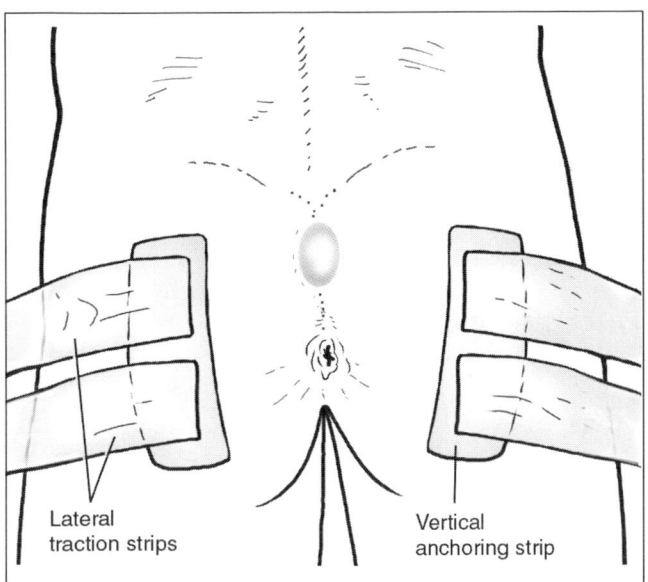

Lateral traction strips

Vertical anchoring strip

FIGURE 92-4 Exposure of the abscess.

cavity itself is not possible. The pain caused by injection of the local anesthetic solution is related to the rate that the anesthetic is injected and the force necessary to inject it. **Inject the local anesthetic solution slowly through a small-bore needle (25 to 30 gauge) as the needle is withdrawn through the dermis.** The needle bore will create a passage through the subcutaneous tissue as it is inserted that enables the local anesthetic solution to be infiltrated slowly and with less discomfort.

Hold the syringe horizontal in reference to the skin surface. Inject 3 to 4 mL of local anesthetic solution intradermally over the dome of the abscess (Figure 92-5). The skin will blanch if the injection is given properly. **Do not inject the local anesthetic solution into the abscess cavity.** The increased pressure within the cavity will cause more discomfort to the patient and may cause the solution to be forcefully expelled if there is an opening in the skin.

Additional anesthesia is accomplished by performing a field block (Figure 92-6).[11] Inject local anesthetic solution subcutaneously around the periphery of the abscess (Figure 92-6A). Inject local anesthetic solution deep to the abscess in a fan-like pattern (Figure 92-6B).

Systemic analgesia (i.e., procedural sedation) is usually required since it is quite difficult to obtain adequate anesthesia of an abscess locally. Refer to Chapter 109 regarding the details of procedural sedation. Self-administered nitrous oxide is an alternative. Nitrous oxide may be supplemented with an opiate, such as morphine or meperidine, although this must be tailored to the individual. Refer to Chapter 108 regarding the details of nitrous oxide anesthesia. Obtain an additional informed consent for the procedural sedation or nitrous oxide procedure. **The procedure should be conducted**

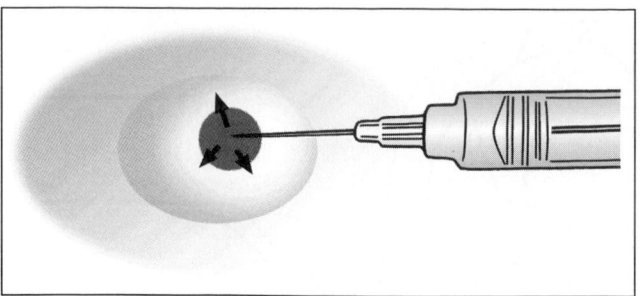

FIGURE 92-5 Subcutaneous infiltration of local anesthetic solution. The needle and syringe are held parallel to the skin. The needle is inserted into the subcutaneous tissue overlying the pilonidal abscess. Infiltrate the local anesthetic solution as the needle is withdrawn. The skin should blanch (shaded area) if injected properly.

under general anesthesia in the Operating Room if adequate anesthesia cannot be obtained and pain limits the procedure.

TECHNIQUE

Incise the skin over the area of maximum fluctuance with a scalpel blade. A 10 percent recurrence rate after drainage of chronic abscesses through a vertical incision lateral to the midline has been reported.[12] This may be due to better healing of wounds that are off the midline. Thus, some authors and Colorectal Surgeons recommend that the incision for an acute abscess be off the midline if the abscess can be drained adequately through the incision (Figure 92-7A). Extend the incision the length of the abscess to allow for proper drainage. A thin ellipse of skin can be removed to prevent premature closure of the skin edges. Approximately 40 percent of pilonidal abscesses will be cured from simple incision and drainage alone.[13] It is not necessary to perform more radical excision procedures in the Emergency Department.

It is important that loculations be lysed and the area thoroughly drained to minimize recurrence. Several methods can be used to lyse adhesions within the cavity. A gloved finger may be used to bluntly break up the adhesions. Hemostats can be inserted and spread within the abscess cavity. A useful technique employs a gauze 4×4 square clamped in a hemostat and swirled inside the abscess cavity to break adhesions and remove debris (Figure 92-7B). This technique aids in removing hair and the infected lining of the cyst. Irrigation of the cavity with normal saline is optional and used by some physicians.

Loosely pack the cavity with ribbon gauze. Packing the cavity too tightly may cause ischemia to the surrounding tissue, delays healing, and is uncomfortable for the patient. The purpose of the packing is to keep the skin edges from adhering before the cavity closes. Cover the incision with gauze and adhesive tape. A thick layer of absorbent gauze will soak up any continued drainage.

AFTERCARE

Antibiotics are generally unnecessary to treat a simple abscess when there is no cellulitis surrounding the wound.[14] No data could be found on the optimal duration of antibiotic treatment if the overlying skin is cellulitic. The conventional 7 to 10 day course of antibiotics is probably adequate. Likewise, no studies could be

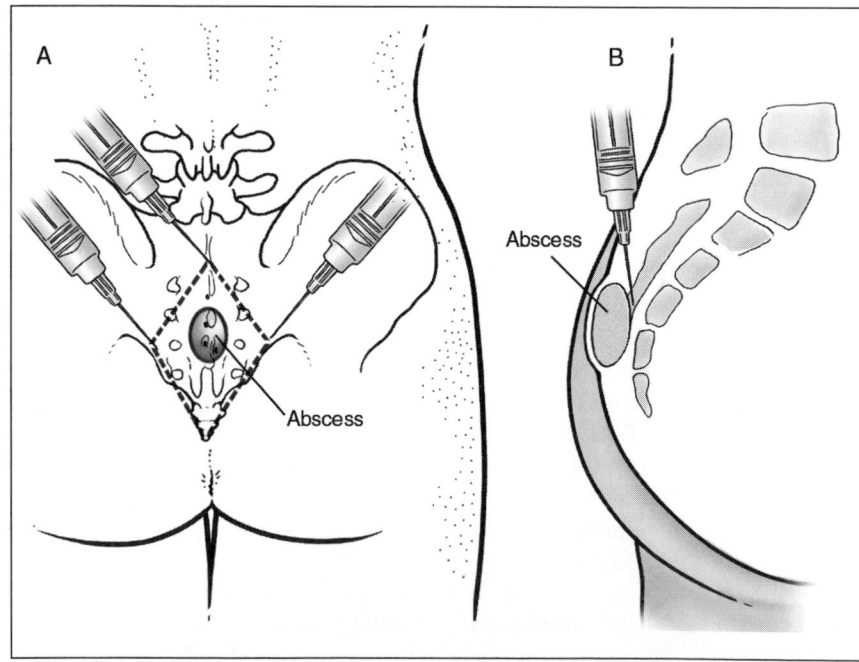

FIGURE 92-6 Field block anesthesia for a pilonidal abscess. *A.* Local anesthetic solution is infiltrated subcutaneously on all four sides of the abscess. *B.* The local anesthetic solution is infiltrated deep to the abscess cavity in a fan-like pattern.

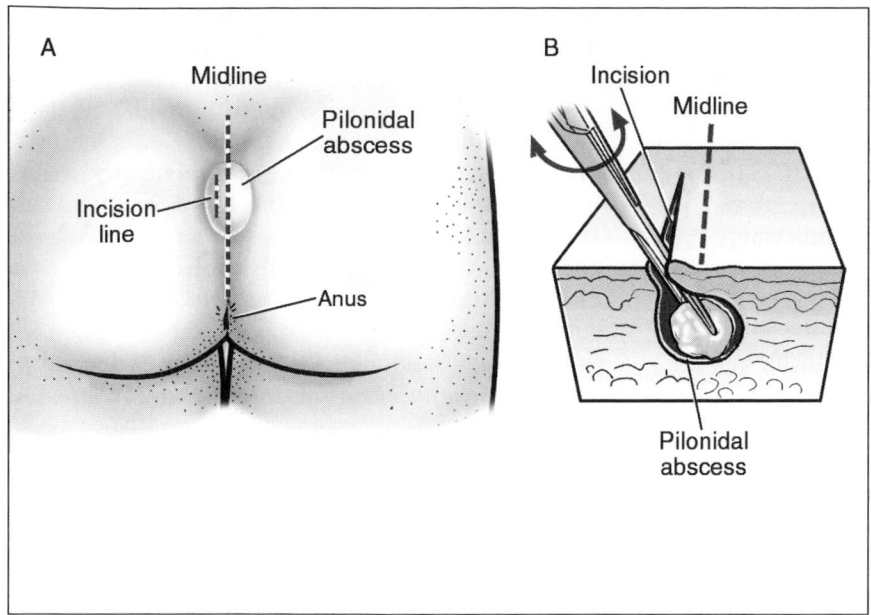

FIGURE 92-7 Incision and drainage of a pilonidal abscess. *A.* An incision is made lateral to the midline and overlying the abscess cavity. *B.* A hemostat with gauze clamped in the jaws is inserted into the abscess cavity and rotated to break loculations and remove debris.

found regarding treating patients with diabetes, cardiac valve disease, those who have hardware in their body, or those who are immunocompromised and have a pilonidal abscess. These patients are at risk for infectious complications and it is advised that they be treated with antibiotics.

There is a disparity in the literature regarding the bacteriology of pilonidal abscesses. *Staphylococcus aureus* is the most commonly found bacteria and, surprisingly, *Escherichia coli* is rarely found.[15] A report in children recovered primarily anaerobes from pilonidal cysts.[16] *Escherichia coli* was the most common aerobe cultured from this series. In light of these conflicting results, and in the event that antibiotics are deemed necessary, coverage for skin flora as well as aerobes and gram-negative organisms would be advised. A combination of a first generation cephalosporin or penicillinase-resistant penicillin along with metronidazole or clindamycin is recommended.

Instruct the patient to change the gauze dressing as often as necessary to keep the outside of the dressing dry. The patient should return for follow-up in 48 hours for a wound check and removal of the packing. If the wound is large, reinsert the packing upon follow-up. Incisions that remain open or that removed an ellipse of skin do not require packing. The patient is advised to have the packing changed every 24 to 48 hours, depending upon the amount of drainage. Decrease the amount of packing each time to allow the wound to heal from the base outward. The patient should thoroughly wash the wound with soap and water in the shower or take a sitz bath each time the packing is removed. It is helpful to let the stream of shower water run inside the wound to aid in wound irrigation. Discontinue the packing once the wound is well granulated and there is no concern that the skin edges will ad-

here to each other. The patient must continue to clean the wound thoroughly every day until it is fully healed. Healing may take several weeks depending upon the size of the abscess cavity. Instruct the patient that they must return to the Emergency Department if they develop a fever, increased pain, or increased redness of the skin surrounding the abscess. Patients often have pain in the first 2 to 3 days after the incision and drainage. This can be controlled with nonsteroidal anti-inflammatory drugs supplemented with narcotic analgesics.

Inform the patient that incision and drainage in the acute care setting is not definitive treatment and that the condition may recur. Definitive treatment of a chronic pilonidal abscess or sinus includes various excisional options under general anesthesia. Arrange follow-up with a physician who can provide wound care as well as definitive therapy if surgery is required.

Educate the patient about their role in the prevention of a recurrence. Recurrence may be prevented with meticulous hygiene and periodic shaving of the area.[8,11] Instruct the patient on the need for meticulous hygiene in the area, even after the wound has healed. Repeated trauma to the area should be avoided. This includes exercises such as sit-ups and leg lifts, and prolonged periods of sitting.

COMPLICATIONS

Pilonidal disease may return, even with radical and extensive surgical excision procedures. Thus, recurrence is to be expected and the patient alerted of this possibility. Rarely, pilonidal lesions progress to necrotizing fasciitis. Proceed cautiously with patients who are diabetic or otherwise immunocompromised as they are at risk for widespread infections. Those with systemic signs and symptoms are best admitted for treatment. Necrotizing fasciitis is a surgical emergency and requires extensive operative debridement, systemic antibiotics, and intensive supportive care.

Rarely, a nonhealing pilonidal infection may be a pilonidal sinus malignancy.[17] Squamous cell carcinoma has been described to arise from chronic sinus tracts. This emphasizes the importance of follow-up for all patients with pilonidal sinus disease.

Other complications include infection and tissue injury. The incision and drainage procedure can result in a subsequent cellulitis, endocarditis, fasciitis, meningitis, myositis, sacrococcygeal osteomyelitis, or septicemia. The sharp and blunt dissection can injure underlying or adjacent structures including the blood vessels, the coccyx, muscles, nerves, and tendons.

SUMMARY

Pilonidal disease is common in the young adult population. It is probably an acquired condition caused by hair that penetrates an irregular area of skin in the sacral area. Pits occur in the skin that in turn lead to cysts in the subcutaneous tissue. Patients may present with asymptomatic pits noted incidentally, as chronically draining sinuses, or an acute painful abscess. No treatment is necessary for asymptomatic patients. Nontender sinuses may be referred for surgical treatment. Abscesses should be drained expeditiously under adequate analgesia and anesthesia. Antibiotics are not indicated unless the patient has surrounding cellulitis or is immunocompromised. Recurrences are common and patients must be referred for follow-up with a physician who can provide wound care as well as surgical treatment for chronic cases.

REFERENCES

1. Hodges RM: Pilonidal sinus. *Boston Med Surg J* 1880; 103:485.
2. Lane WZ: Pilonidal cysts and sinuses in the Navy. *US Navy Med Bull* 1943; 41:1284–1295.
3. Buie LA: Jeep disease (pilonidal disease of mechanized warfare). *South Med J* 1944; 37(2):103–109.
4. Sebastian MW: Pilonidal cysts and sinuses, in Sabiston, DC (ed): *Textbook of Surgery,* 15th ed. Philadelphia: Saunders, 1997:1332–1333.
5. Clothier PR, Haywood IR: The natural history of the post anal (pilonidal) sinus. *Ann R Coll Surg Engl* 1984; 66(3):201–203.
6. Eftaiha M, Abcarian H: The dilemma of pilonidal disease: surgical treatment. *Dis Colon Rectum* 1977; 20(4):279–286.
7. Golz A, Argov S, Barzilai A: Pilonidal sinus disease: comparison among various methods of treatment and a survey of 160 patients. *Curr Surg* 1980; 37(2):77–85.
8. Stephens FO, Stephens RBH: Pilonidal sinus: management objectives. *Aust N Z J Surg* 1995; 65:558–560.
9. Chamberlain JW, Vawter GF: The congenital origin of pilonidal sinus. *J Pediatr Surg* 1974; 9(4):441–444.
10. Lord PH: Anorectal problems: etiology of pilonidal sinus. *Dis Colon Rectum* 1975; 18(8):661–664.
11. Hanley PH: Acute pilonidal abscess. *Surg Gyn Obstet* 1980; 150(1):9–11.
12. Bascom J: Pilonidal disease: origin from follicles of hairs and results of follicle removal as treatment. *Surgery* 1980; 87(5):567–572.
13. Jensen SL, Harling H: Prognosis after simple incision and drainage for a first-episode acute pilonidal abscess. *Br J Surg* 1988; 75:60–61.
14. Llera JL, Levy RC: Treatment of cutaneous abscess: a double-blind clinical study. *Ann Emerg Med* 1985; 14(1):15–19.
15. Shons AR, Mountjoy JR: Pilonidal disease: the case for excision with primary closure. *Dis Colon Rectum* 1971; 14(5):353–355.
16. Brook I, Anderson KD, Controni G, et al: Aerobic and anaerobic bacteriology of pilonidal cyst abscess in children. *Am J Dis Child* 1980; 134:679–680.
17. Davis KA, Mock CN, Versaci A, et al: Malignant degeneration of pilonidal cysts. *Am Surg* 1994; 60(3):200–204.

Chapter 93
PERIANAL ABSCESS INCISION AND DRAINAGE

Paula L. Ward

INTRODUCTION

Anorectal infections are common but vary widely in their presentation. An understanding of the anorectal anatomy is essential to make a diagnosis and plan proper treatment. Failure to diagnose and treat an extensive abscess may be life threatening. It is imperative to obtain a surgical consultation if one is unsure of the extent of an abscess.

The peak age of incidence of anorectal infections is in the third or fourth decade of life. Perianal abscesses are two to three times more common in men than women.[1] Male predominance is even more pronounced in the pediatric population.[2] In one series, all patients under 2 years of age were males, while 60 percent of the children greater than 2 years were males.[2] The increased incidence of perianal infection in males may be related to androgen conversion in the anal glands.[3] In infants, deep anal crypts are associated with perianal abscesses.[4]

Abscesses may completely resolve after the incision and drainage procedure. However, 50 percent recur or develop a chronic epithelialized tract or fistula-in-ano. Abscesses and fistulas are different sequelae of the same process.[5]

ANATOMY AND PATHOPHYSIOLOGY

Knowledge of the anatomy of the region is important to understand the pathophysiology of anorectal infections (Figures 93-1 and 93-2). Columnar epithelium transitions to squamous epithelium where there are vertical folds of tissue called the columns of Morgagni at the level of the dentate line. Semilunar folds of epithelium called anal valves connect the inferior borders of the anal columns. At the base of each anal valve is an anal crypt, into which opens the ducts of the anal glands. The anal glands secrete mucous to aid in evacuation of feces. The anal glands are located in the space between the internal and external anal sphincter muscles. Most anorectal infections begin in this intersphincteric space due to blockage and resultant infection of the anal glands.[6]

The spread of an infection is determined by the anatomy of the anorectal region. There are five anatomic spaces into which an infection can spread (Figure 93-3).[5] The perianal space is located at the area of the anal verge. The ischiorectal space, which is continuous with the perianal space, extends from the levator ani muscle to the perineum. The intersphincteric space lies between the internal and external anal sphincter muscles. It connects inferiorly with the perianal space and superiorly with the rectal wall. The supralevator (or pelvirectal) space is located superior to the levator ani muscle and is bounded superiorly by the peritoneum. The rectum forms its medial border and the pelvic wall forms the lateral boundary. The deep postanal space is located between the tip of the coccyx and the anus. It courses through the superficial external anal sphincter and the levator ani. The superficial postanal space lies posterior to the anal verge and is subcutaneous. The retrorectal space is high in the pelvis. It occupies the area between the distal rectum and the sacrum.

Most anorectal infections begin in the intersphincteric space. Natural barriers are broken down by formation of an abscess and the infection can spread to contiguous spaces. Abscesses are classified according to their location. Perianal abscesses are common, ischiorectal abscesses occur less frequently, and supralevator abscesses are least common.[7] Bilateral involvement may occur when an infection spreads circumferentially via the deep postanal space, resulting in a horseshoe abscess.

Patients with anorectal abscesses present with buttock pain and swelling. There is, occasionally, spontaneous drainage from the abscess site. Symptoms depend upon the location of the abscess. Patients with perianal infections have anal pain that increases with defecation or sitting. Pain associated with deeper infections may be

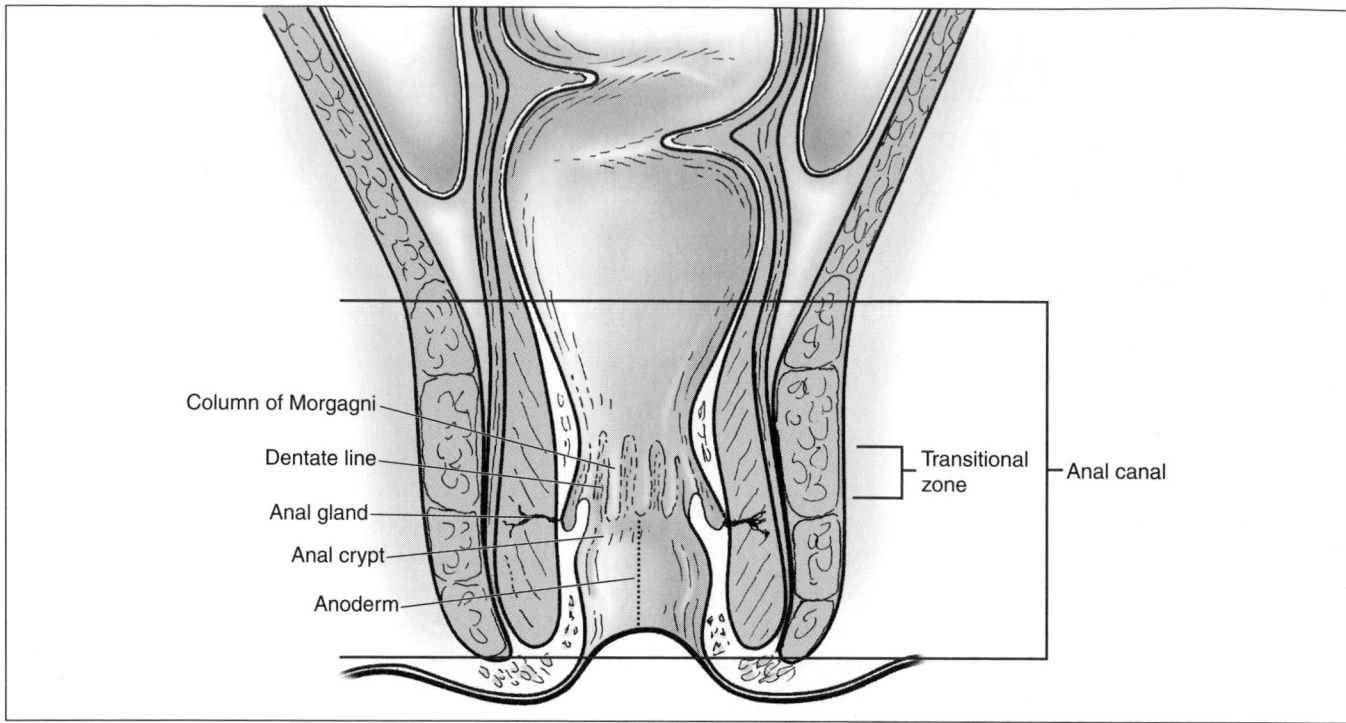

FIGURE 93-1 The topical anatomy of the anal canal.

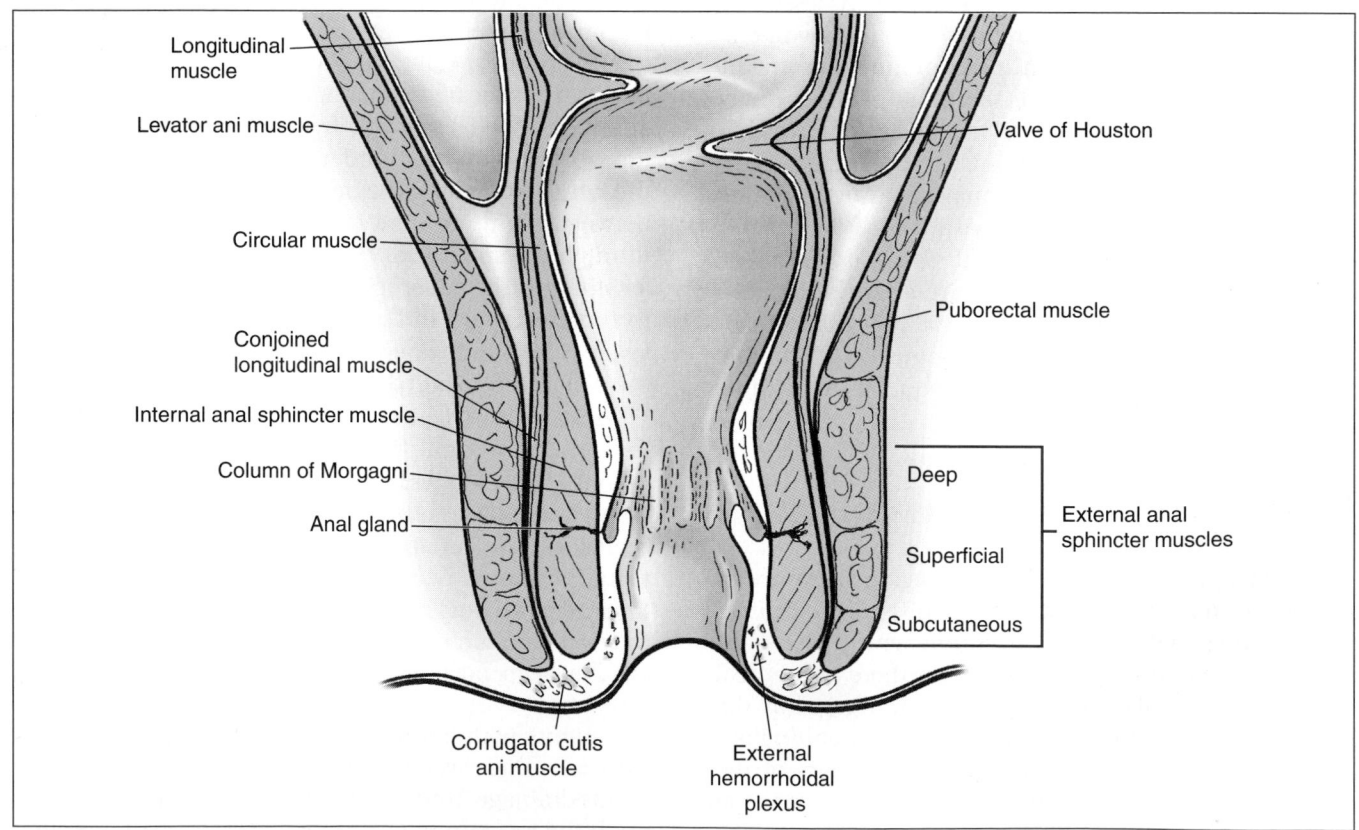

FIGURE 93-2 The major supporting structures of the anal canal.

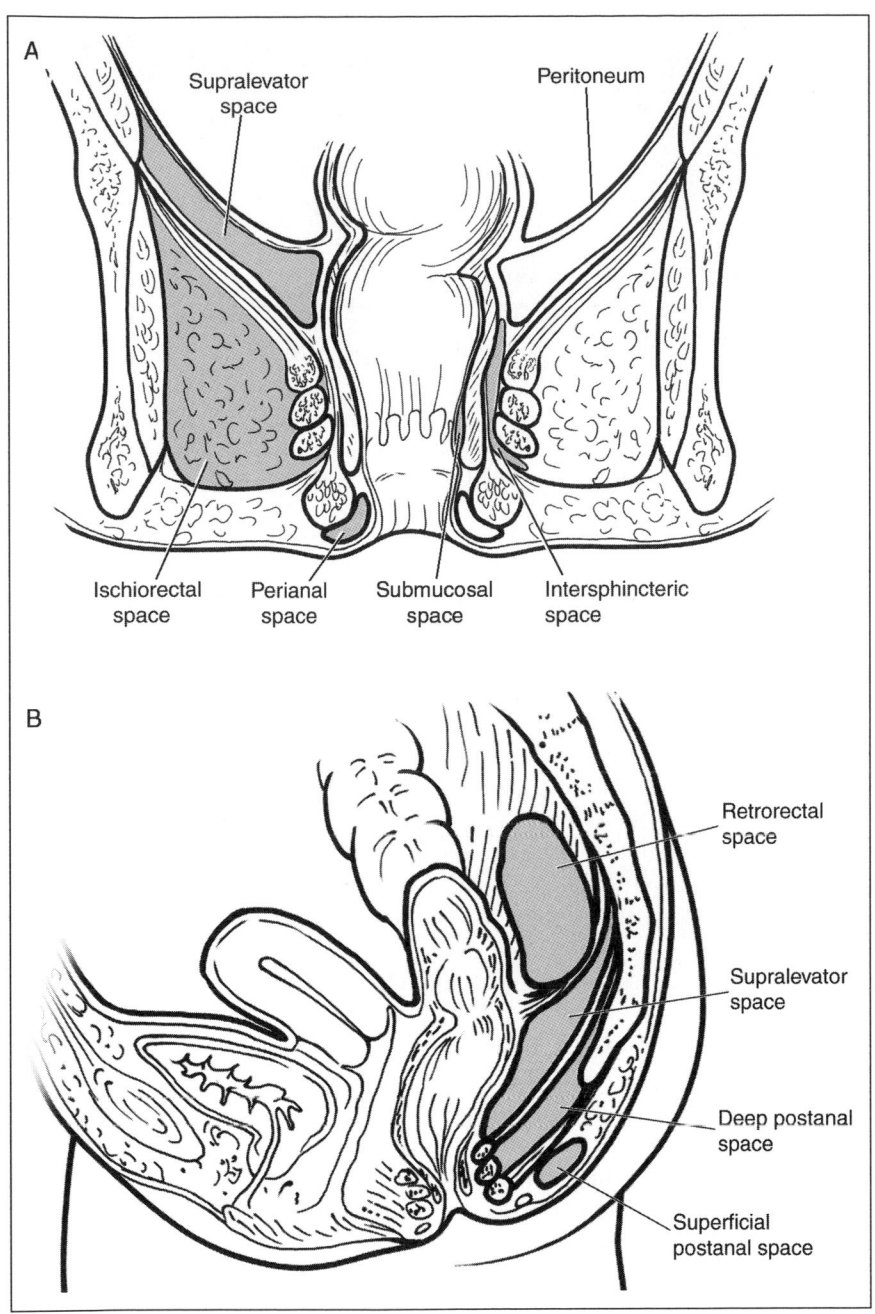

FIGURE 93-3 The anorectal spaces.
A. Coronal section through the pelvis.
B. Sagittal section through the pelvis.

atypical. Patients with supralevator abscesses may have deep rectal pain, gluteal pain, dysuria, or other urinary symptoms.

Erythema, swelling, and fluctuance are often present at the abscess site. The location of the swelling and fluctuance of a perianal abscess is at the anal verge. Ischiorectal space infections track farther from the anus onto the buttock. Supralevator and intersphincteric abscesses may have minimal or no external signs.[8] **The diagnosis of perianal cellulitis is highly suspect. These patients have either an anorectal abscess or Fournier's Gangrene until proven otherwise. Patients with gluteal**

pain and a small amount of erythema in the perianal area have a deep-seated abscess until proven otherwise.

Intersphincteric, deep postanal, and submucosal abscesses can be found only on a digital rectal examination. **A superficial digital examination of the anal canal alone is inadequate for detection of some abscesses. The gloved finger must extend into the rectum seeking tenderness and a mass.** Unfortunately, some deep abscesses may not be detected with a digital rectal examination because of patient discomfort. Seek surgical consultation for an examination under anesthesia or obtain a CT scan of the pelvis if a deep abscess is suspected. The

CT scan should be ordered in consultation with the Surgeon when possible.

A fistula-in-ano represents the chronic phase of an unhealed perianal abscess. Fistulas may form due to persistent obstruction of the anal gland or inadequate drainage of an abscess. The tract eventually becomes epithelialized with glandular tissue. Fistulas may also form as a result of epithelialization by cells derived from the transitional zone of the anal canal and thus may be unrelated to persistent anal gland disease.[9] Patients with a fistula-in-ano will often give a history of a previous abscess in the same area that was either drained surgically or spontaneously. Patients may complain of chronic drainage from the site or subacute pain.

Physical examination of a fistula-in-ano reveals an external opening with scant drainage and visible surrounding granulation tissue. Digital rectal examination may reveal an indurated cord-like structure beneath the skin within the anal canal. The internal opening may be palpable along the dentate line. Pus may be expressed externally or from within the anus upon palpation of the fistulous tract.

The greater the distance from the anus that the external opening is located, the more complex is the fistulous tract. Goodsall's rule describes the likelihood of the location of fistulous tracts and internal opening based upon the location of the external opening (Figure 93-4). Anterior external openings tend to communicate in a linear fashion with the internal opening in the anal canal. Fistulas with posterior external openings tend to communicate in a curvilinear fashion with the internal opening.

Patients with multiple or recurrent fistulas require evaluation of the bowel for Crohn's disease. This is particularly true if associated with chronic diarrhea or cramping which suggests inflammatory bowel disease. Recurrent fistulas may be indicative of tuberculosis or a sexually transmitted disease such as lymphogranuloma venereum. **It is imperative that these patients be referred to a Surgeon who is experienced in managing anorectal disease.**

INDICATIONS

Incision and drainage is the treatment for an anorectal abscess. Perianal abscesses and submucosal abscesses may be drained in the Emergency Department. Use caution in draining ischiorectal abscesses in the Emergency Department, especially if they are large. The ischiorectal space is quite large, particularly in the obese patient, and adequacy of drainage is not assured except under general anesthesia. It is not uncommon for an abscess to have a small erythematous and swollen area on the buttock overlying an extensive and deep abscess. Attempts at drainage in the Emergency Department may be inadequate.

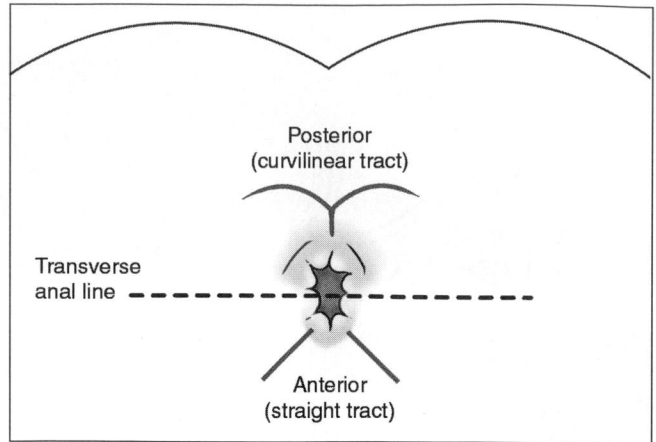

FIGURE 93-4 Goodsall's rule.

Perianal disease is commonly encountered in the HIV-infected patient. Complication rates were noted to be high in the past and a hands-off approach was espoused. However, more recent data suggest that those patients with a relatively preserved immune system may safely undergo standard surgical drainage. Small perianal abscesses may be drained in the outpatient setting. Consult a General or Colorectal Surgeon for those patients with late-stage HIV disease. Infections are more likely to be extensive and anorectal sepsis is more common because these patients have poor wound healing.[10]

CONTRAINDICATIONS

Most small perianal and submucosal abscesses can be drained in the Emergency Department. **A General or Colorectal Surgeon should drain all other types of anorectal abscesses. Caution is urged when an abscess is on the buttock for it may manifest an ischiorectal abscess.** Consult a Surgeon if the infection is extensive or if the extent of the abscess cannot be determined. Surgical consultation is also necessary for patients with purulent drainage from inside the anus. Internal findings may indicate that the patient has an intersphincteric or a supralevator abscess; the full extent of which can be determined only under general anesthesia.

Patients with fever or toxicity should be admitted to the hospital for parenteral antibiotics, incision and drainage in the Operating Room, and observation. Anorectal infections occasionally progress to necrotizing fasciitis, a true surgical emergency. Physical examination findings in such cases may initially be minimal except for systemic signs or symptoms. Patients with late-stage HIV infection should be referred to an experienced Surgeon due to the higher complication rate and increased risk of extensive infection.

Chronically draining fistulas without an acute infection should be referred to a General or Colorectal Surgeon for care. Patients with purulent drainage from the anus, even if there is no significant tenderness, should be examined under general anesthesia as they may still have an internal abscess along with a fistulous tract.

EQUIPMENT

Povidone iodine solution
10 mL syringe
25 to 30 gauge needle, 2 inches long
Local anesthetic solution with epinephrine, lidocaine, or bupivacaine
#11 scalpel blade on a handle
#15 scalpel blade on a handle
Curved hemostat
4×4 gauze squares
10 to 16 French mushroom (de Pezzer) catheter, optional
Adhesive tape
Feminine napkin, optional
Normal saline
18 gauge angiocatheter
20 mL syringe

PATIENT PREPARATION

Explain the risks, benefits, and potential complications of the procedure to the patient and/or their representative. The post-procedure care should be explained as well. Document the discussion of the risks and benefits of the procedure. Obtain an informed consent for the procedure.

The best visualization of the sacral region, particularly in obese patients, occurs with the use of a procto-scopic examination table, if available (Figure 93-5A). Place the patient prone on a gurney or on the proctoscopy table. Alternatively, place the patient in the lateral knee-chest position to expose the affected area (Figure 93-5B). Apply benzoin solution to the buttocks and allow it to dry. Apply adhesive tape to the buttocks and tape them open (Figure 93-6). Clean any dirt and debris from the skin overlying the abscess or cyst. Apply povidone iodine and allow it to dry. However, this is probably not necessary since by definition the drainage of an abscess is not a sterile procedure. Shaving the surrounding area, if the patient is hirsute, will aid the application of the dressing after the procedure.

ANESTHESIA

Local anesthesia should be administered, recognizing that it is often difficult to obtain complete anesthesia by direct infiltration of an abscess. Local anesthetics are weak acids and are less effective in the acidic environment of an abscess. The skin over the abscess cavity usually becomes insensate, but anesthesia of the abscess cavity itself is not possible. The pain caused by injection of the local anesthetic solution is related to the rate that the anesthetic is injected and the force necessary to inject it. **Inject the local anesthetic solution slowly through a small-bore needle (25 to 30 gauge) as the needle is withdrawn through the dermis.** The needle bore will create a passage through the subcutaneous tissue as it is inserted that enables the local anesthetic solution to be infiltrated slowly and with less discomfort.

Hold the syringe horizontal in reference to the skin surface. Inject 3 to 4 mL of local anesthetic solution intradermally over the dome of the abscess (Figure 93-7). The skin will blanch if the injection is given properly. **Do not inject the local anesthetic solution into the abscess cavity.** The increased pressure within the cavity will

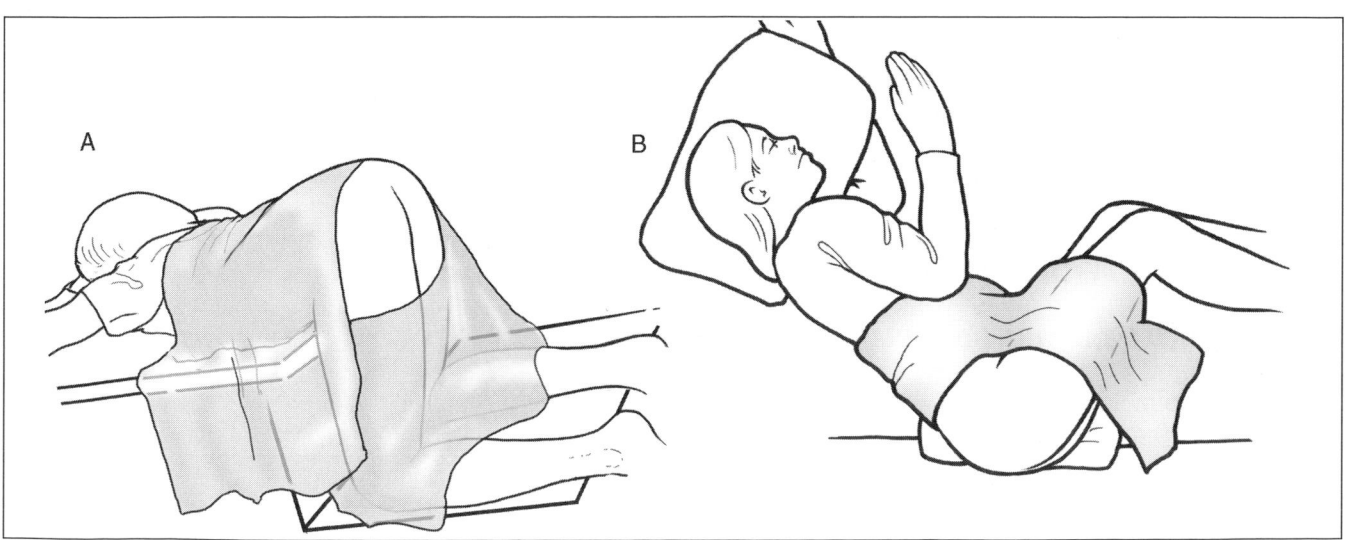

FIGURE 93-5 Patient placement. *A.* Place the patient prone on a proctoscopy table. The patient may also be placed prone on a gurney. *B.* The lateral knee-chest position.

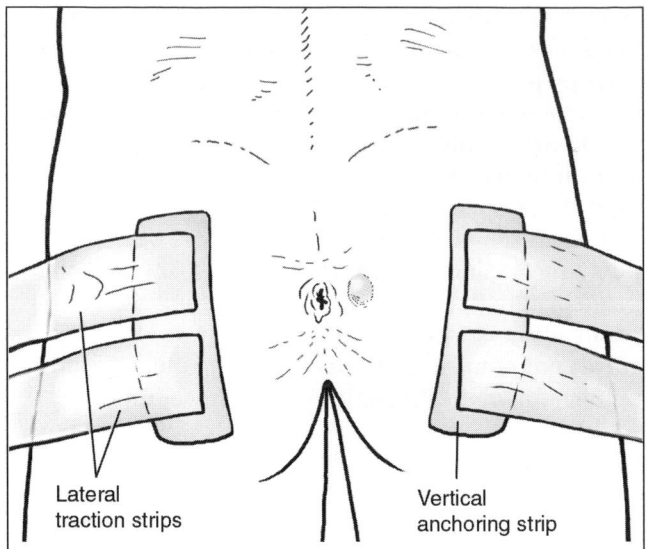

FIGURE 93-6 Exposure of the abscess.

Lateral traction strips

Vertical anchoring strip

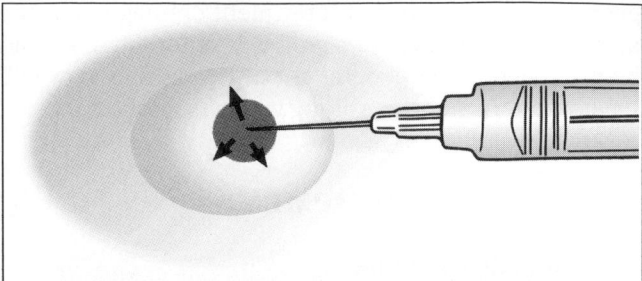

FIGURE 93-7 Subcutaneous infiltration of local anesthetic solution. The needle and syringe are held parallel to the skin. The needle is inserted into the subcutaneous tissue overlying the abscess. Infiltrate the local anesthetic solution as the needle is withdrawn. The skin should blanch (shaded area) if injected properly.

cause more discomfort to the patient and may cause the solution to be forcefully expelled if there is an opening in the skin.

Additional anesthesia is accomplished by performing a field block (Figure 93-8). Inject local anesthetic solution subcutaneously around the periphery of the abscess (Figure 93-8A).[11] Inject local anesthetic solution deep to the abscess in a fan-like pattern (Figure 93-8B).

Systemic analgesia (i.e., procedural sedation) is usually required since it is quite difficult to obtain adequate anesthesia of an abscess locally. Refer to Chapter 109 regarding the details of procedural sedation. Self-administered nitrous oxide is an alternative. Nitrous oxide may be supplemented with an opiate, such as morphine or meperidine, although this must be tailored to the individual. Refer to Chapter 108 regarding the details of nitrous oxide anesthesia. Obtain an additional informed consent for the procedural sedation or nitrous oxide procedure. **The procedure should be conducted under general anesthesia in the Operating Room if adequate anesthesia cannot be obtained and pain limits the procedure.**

TECHNIQUES

INCISION AND DRAINAGE OF PERIANAL ABSCESSES

Make a stab incision with a #11 scalpel blade in the skin overlying the area of fluctuance to decompress the abscess. **Make the incision as close to the anus as possible so that if a fistula forms, its size will be limited.** This maneuver will minimize the length of a fistulotomy, should it become necessary, in the future. Extend the

incision with the #11 scalpel blade or a #15 scalpel blade. Continue the excision in an elliptical pattern (Figure 93-9A). Remove the ellipse of skin (Figure 93-9B). An ellipse of skin is excised to prevent premature closure of the skin edges. Alternatively, make a cruciate incision over the abscess and excise the edges (Figure 93-10).[5] Both of these techniques delay cutaneous healing while the abscess is decompressing and allow it to drain freely without the need for packing.

It is important that loculations be lysed and the area thoroughly drained to minimize recurrence. Several methods can be used to lyse adhesions within the abscess cavity. A gloved finger may be used to bluntly break up the adhesions. Hemostats can be inserted and spread within the cavity. A useful technique employs a gauze square clamped in a hemostat and swirled inside the ab-

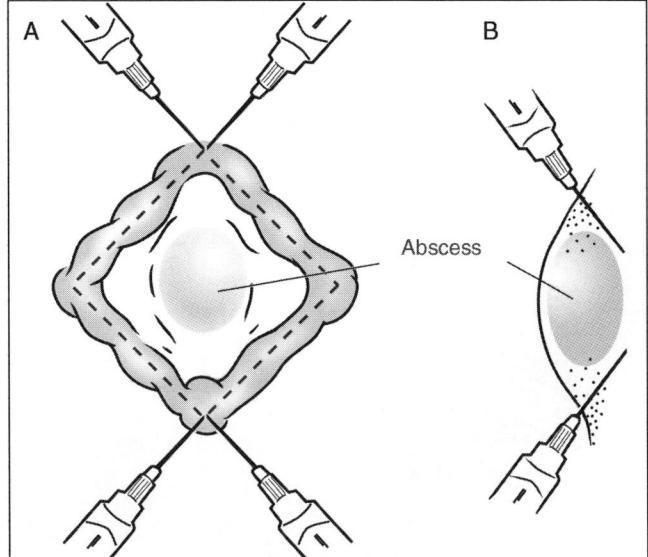

FIGURE 93-8 Field block anesthesia. *A.* Local anesthetic solution is infiltrated subcutaneously on all four sides of the abscess. *B.* The local anesthetic solution is infiltrated deep to the abscess cavity in a fan-like pattern.

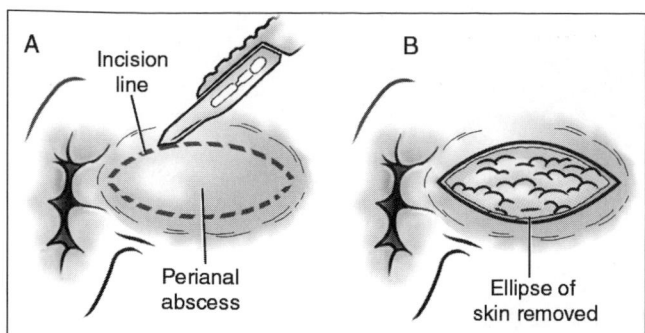

FIGURE 93-9 Drainage of a perianal abscess. *A.* An elliptical incision is made in the skin. *B.* The ellipse of skin is removed to prevent premature closure of the skin edges.

scess cavity to break adhesions and remove debris. Irrigation of the cavity with normal saline is optional and used by some physicians.

It is not necessary to pack an incised and drained perianal abscess. Cover the wound with a thick layer of absorbent gauze to soak up continued drainage. A feminine napkin may also be used to absorb drainage and obviates the need for taping the dressing in place.

CATHETER DRAINAGE OF PERIANAL ABSCESSES

Another method used to drain perianal abscesses, and preferred by some Colorectal Surgeons, is catheter drainage. The mushroom or de Pezzer catheter has a tunnel through a solid mushroom-shaped tip (Figure 93-11*A*).[12] Make a stab incision with a #11 scalpel blade over the anal side of the area of fluctuance (Figure 93-11*B*). Insert a hemostat into the abscess cavity. Open and close the jaws of the hemostat to lyse any adhesions and express the pus. Flush the abscess cavity with normal saline using an 18 gauge angiocatheter on a 20 mL syringe.

Insert a 10 to 16 French latex mushroom catheter using a hemostat to stretch the tip so that it will fit through the incision. Place the tip of the hemostat through the hole in the mushroom catheter. With one hand holding the hemostat, use the other hand to pull on the tubing to stretch the mushroom tip and enable it to fit into the abscess cavity (Figure 93-11*C*). Release the traction on the hemostat once the catheter tip is within the abscess cavity and the mushroom shape will be restored (Figure 93-11*D*). Remove the hemostat from the abscess cavity. Cut the catheter so that it protrudes only 2 to 3 cm from the incision (Figure 93-11*E*). Suture the catheter in place. Apply a dressing of gauze squares or a feminine napkin.

Many Colorectal Surgeons prefer the catheter method. On subsequent visits they can assess the wound for the presence of a fistula without removing the catheter. Hydrogen peroxide can be infused through the catheter. Bubbles seen escaping from an opening within the anal canal are diagnostic for a fistula. Hydrogen peroxide is also used to produce an ultrasound interface that facilitates the definition of a fistulous tract and the internal opening.[5]

SUBMUCOSAL ABSCESSES

The majority of submucosal abscesses may be drained in the Emergency Department. The procedure requires the use of an anoscope to visualize the abscess. Refer to Chapter 59 for the complete details regarding the use of an anoscope. Make a superficial stab incision in the abscess with a #11 scalpel blade. Gently insert a hemostat and lyse any adhesions. Remove a small ellipse of the mucosa to allow the abscess to drain. Arrange follow-up with a Colorectal Surgeon within 24 hours.

AFTERCARE

Antibiotics are generally unnecessary to treat a simple abscess when there is no cellulitis surrounding the wound.[13] No data could be found on the optimal duration of antibiotic treatment if the overlying skin is cellulitic. The conventional 7 to 10 day course of antibiotics

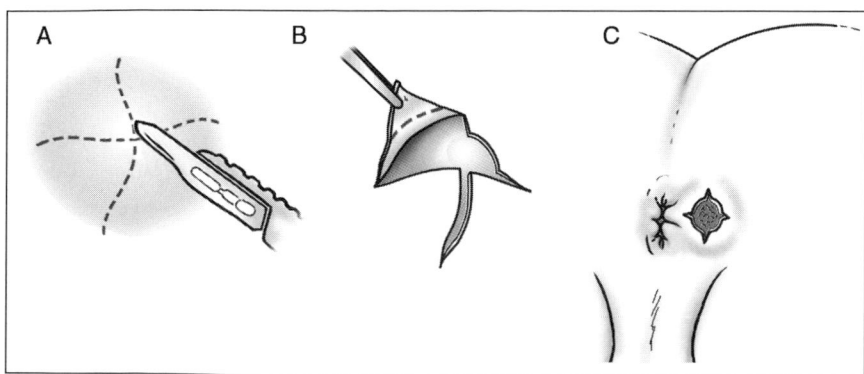

FIGURE 93-10 Drainage of perianal abscess employing a cruciate incision. *A.* The cruciate incision is made over the abscess. *B.* Excision of the skin flap edges. *C.* The final appearance.

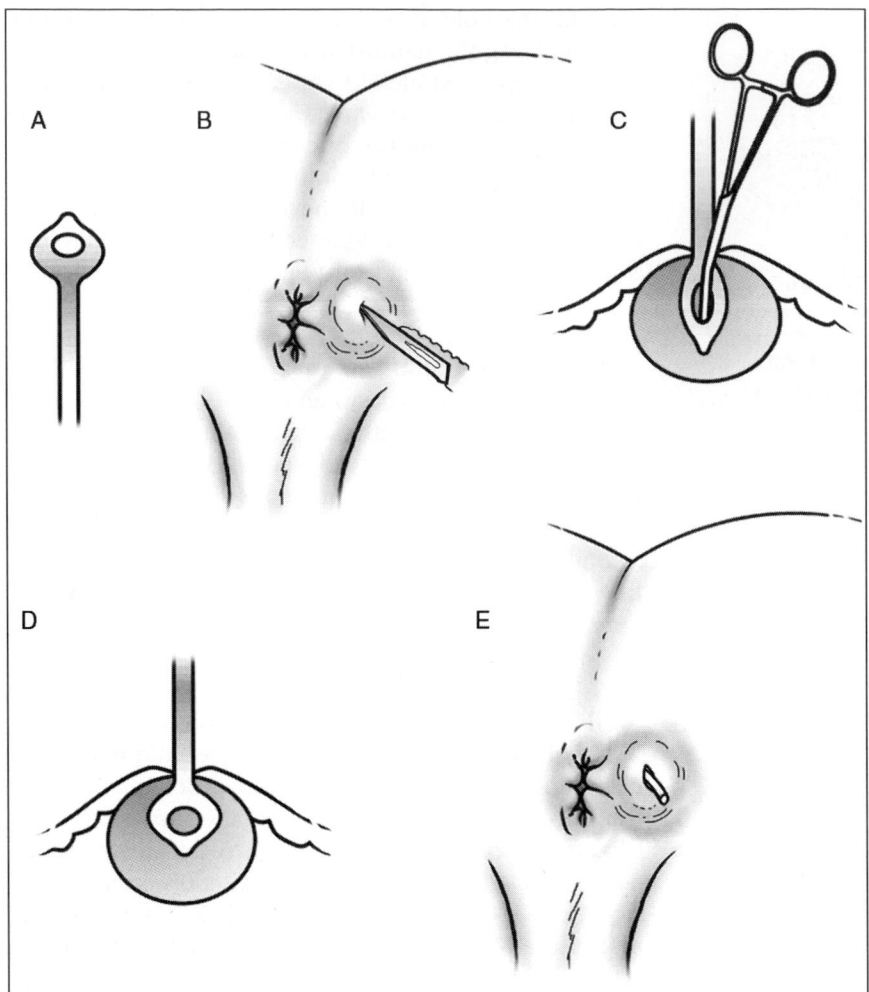

FIGURE 93-11 Catheter drainage of an abscess. *A.* The mushroom (de Pezzer) catheter. *B.* A stab incision is made over the area of maximal fluctuance. *C.* Place the tip of the hemostat through the side hole to stretch the tip of the catheter. Insert the stretched catheter through the stab incision. *D.* Remove the hemostat to expand the head of the catheter so that it remains within the abscess cavity. *E.* The catheter is cut so that it protrudes 2 to 3 cm from the skin incision.

is likely adequate. Likewise, there is no data in the literature regarding the treatment of patients with diabetes, cardiac valve disease, those who have hardware in their body, or those who are immunocompromised with antibiotics for a perianal abscess. These patients are at risk for infectious complications. It is advised that they be treated with antibiotics. Bacteriology of anorectal abscesses usually reveals a mixed infection, with coliforms and anaerobes predominating.[14] Recommended antibiotics include an extended spectrum β-lactam, a second- or third-generation cephalosporin with metronidazole or clindamycin, or a newer fluoroquinolone with metronidazole or clindamycin.

The patient may change the gauze dressing as often as necessary to keep the outside of the dressing dry. Instruct the patient to return for follow-up in 48 hours for a wound check. The patient may begin sitz baths or showers 24 hours after the procedure. They should thoroughly clean the wound with soap and water at least once a day until the wound is fully healed. It is helpful to let the stream of shower water run inside the wound to

aid in irrigation. Healing may take a few weeks depending upon the size of the abscess. Additional measures to aid in healing and comfort include stool bulking agents and stool softeners. Pain can be controlled with nonsteroidal anti-inflammatory drugs supplemented with occasional narcotics analgesics.

Advise the patient that the condition is likely to recur. They must be referred to a General or Colorectal Surgeon who is experienced in the management of anorectal infections. Inform the patient that they may require an operation to prevent future recurrences. Instruct the patient to immediately return to the Emergency Department if they develop a fever or increased pain.

COMPLICATIONS

Perianal abscesses may recur or a fistula may form. Recurrence is more likely if the patient has had abscesses in the same location in the past. Occasionally, anorectal infections progress to necrotizing fasciitis. Patients with any systemic signs and symptoms require surgical consultation, hospital admission, parenteral antibiotics, and a drainage procedure.

SUMMARY

Anorectal infections are commonly seen in the Emergency Department. They are thought to be due to obstruction and subsequent infection of the anal glands that in turn form an abscess. Small perianal abscesses and submucosal abscesses can safely be drained in the Emergency Department. A digital rectal examination may aid in determining the extent of an abscess. A General or Colorectal Surgeon should manage patients with fever, signs of toxicity, evidence of an infection beyond the perianal area, or who are immunocompromised. Be alert that abscesses with maximum fluctuance on the buttock are more likely to have ischiorectal extension, are more complex, and greater in size. Perianal abscesses must be drained expeditiously to prevent their spread. Approximately 50 percent of anorectal abscesses will develop a fistulous tract. Patients require referral for follow-up with a General or Colorectal Surgeon who can provide wound care as well as manage chronic cases.

REFERENCES

1. Doberneck RC: Perianal suppuration: results of treatment. *Am Surg* 1987; 53(10):569–572.
2. Piazza DJ, Radhakrishnan J: Perianal abscess and fistula-in-ano in children. *Dis Colon Rectum* 1990; 33(12):1014–1016.
3. Lunniss PJ, Jenkins PJ, Besser GM, et al: Gender differences in incidence of idiopathic fistula-in-ano are not explained by circulating sex hormones. *Int J Colorectal Dis* 1995; 10(1):25–28.
4. Shafer AD, McGlone TP, Flanagan RA: Abnormal crypts of Morgagni: the cause of perianal abscess and fistula-in-ano. *J Pediatr Surg* 1987; 22(3):203–204.
5. Vasilevsky CA: Fistula-in-ano and abscess, in Beck D, Wexher S (eds): *Fundamentals of Anorectal Surgery,* 2nd ed. Philadelphia: Saunders, 1998:153–173.
6. Parks AG: Pathogenesis and treatment of fistula-in-ano. *Br Med J* 1961; 1:463–469.
7. Read DR, Abcarian H: A prospective survey of 474 patients with anorectal abscess. *Dis Colon Rectum* 1979; 22(8):566–568.
8. Parks AG: Intersphincteric abscess. *Br Med J* 1973; 2:537–539.
9. Lunniss PJ, Sheffield JP, Talbot IC, et al: Persistence of idiopathic anal fistula may be related to epithelialization. *Br J Surg* 1995; 82(1):32–33.
10. Weiss EG, Wexner SD: Surgery for anal lesions in HIV-infected patients. *Ann Med* 1995; 27:467–475.
11. Hanley PH: Acute pilonidal abscess. *Surg Gynecol Obstet* 1980; 150(1):9–11.
12. Philip RS: A simplified method for the incision and drainage of abscesses. *Am J Surg* 1978; 135(5):721.
13. Llera JL, Levy RC: Treatment of cutaneous abscess: a double blind clinical study. *Ann Emerg Med* 1985; 14(1):15–19.
14. Seow-Choen F, Hay AJ, Heard S, et al: Bacteriology of anal fistula. *Br J Surg* 1992; 79(1):27–28.

Chapter 94
SEBACEOUS CYST INCISION AND DRAINAGE

Paula L. Ward

INTRODUCTION

Sebaceous cysts are common, may be located anywhere on the body, and frequently become infected. Patients will often present complaining of pain. The Emergency Physician must be acquainted with the principles involved in treating abscesses, particularly if they are located on cosmetically important areas such as the face.

ANATOMY AND PATHOPHYSIOLOGY

Sebaceous cysts are the result of obstruction of sebaceous gland ducts. They are freely mobile, round, and located in the subcutaneous tissues. The cysts are made of a thin white capsule filled with a thick, cheesy, and keratinous material. They frequently become infected and subsequently form an abscess. Sebaceous cysts may be present for many years before infection occurs. Physical examination often reveals a subcutaneous mass that is fluctuant and tender. The overlying skin may appear normal or erythematous.

The initial treatment of an infected sebaceous cyst is incision and drainage. **The sebaceous material is too thick to allow for spontaneous drainage and it must be expressed.** The sebaceous cyst will likely recur, however, unless the capsule of the cyst is removed. Patients may have the initial incision and drainage performed in the Emergency Department with follow-up at some later date to remove the cyst capsule. Alternatively, the cyst capsule may be removed at the time of the initial incision and drainage.

INDICATIONS

Incision and drainage is indicated whenever a patient presents with a tender sebaceous cyst consistent with abscess formation. The procedure will relieve the patient's pain. Antibiotics alone are ineffective in treating abscesses.[1] The vast majority of infected sebaceous cysts may be drained in the Emergency Department, clinic, or office setting. A noninfected sebaceous cyst may be removed electively and for cosmetic purposes in the clinic or office setting by the Primary Care Provider or a Surgeon.

CONTRAINDICATIONS

There are no absolute contraindications to the incision and drainage or removal of an infected sebaceous cyst. Incision and drainage is preferred if the overlying skin is cellulitic. The capsule can be removed at a later time. Extremely large abscesses or those in which adequate anesthesia is not possible should be managed in the Operating Room by a General Surgeon or Plastic Surgeon. Refer patients with noninfected sebaceous cysts to their Primary Care Provider or a Surgeon for removal.

EQUIPMENT

Povidone iodine solution
10 mL syringe
25 to 30 gauge needle, 2 inches long
Local anesthetic solution, with or without epinephrine
#11 scalpel blade on a handle
#15 scalpel blade on a handle
Curved hemostat
Iris scissors
Ribbon gauze, plain or iodinated
4×4 gauze squares
Adhesive tape
Sterile saline
Nylon sutures for skin closure, various sizes

PATIENT PREPARATION

Explain the risks, benefits, and potential complications of the procedure to the patient and/or their representative. The post-procedure care should be explained as well. Document the discussion of the risks and benefits of the procedure. Obtain an informed consent for the procedure.

ANESTHESIA

Local anesthesia should be administered, recognizing that it is often difficult to obtain complete anesthesia by direct infiltration of an abscess. Local anesthetics are weak acids and less effective in the acidic environment of an abscess. The skin over the abscess cavity usually becomes insensate, but anesthesia of the abscess cavity itself is not possible. The pain caused by injection of the local anesthetic solution is related to the rate that the anesthetic is injected and the force necessary to inject it. **Inject the local anesthetic solution slowly through a small-bore needle (25 to 30 gauge) as the needle is withdrawn through the dermis.** The needle bore will create a passage through the subcutaneous tissue as it is inserted that enables the local anesthetic solution to be infiltrated slowly and with less discomfort.

Hold the syringe horizontally in reference to the skin surface. Inject 3 to 4 mL of local anesthetic solution intradermally over the dome of the abscess (Figure 94-1). The skin will blanch if the injection is given properly. **Do not inject the local anesthetic solution into the abscess cavity.** The increased pressure within the cavity will cause more discomfort to the patient and may cause the solution to be forcefully expelled if there is an opening in the skin.

Additional anesthesia is accomplished by performing a field block (Figure 94-2).[2] Inject local anesthetic solution subcutaneously around the periphery of the abscess (Figure 94-2A). Inject local anesthetic solution deep to the abscess in a fan-like pattern (Figure 94-2B).

Systemic analgesia (i.e., procedural sedation) may occasionally be required because it is quite difficult to obtain adequate anesthesia of an abscess locally. Refer to Chapter 109 regarding the details of procedural sedation. Self-administered nitrous oxide is an alternative. Nitrous oxide may be supplemented with an opiate, such as morphine or meperidine, although this must be tailored to the individual. Refer to Chapter 108 regarding the details of nitrous oxide anesthesia. Obtain an additional informed consent for the procedural sedation or nitrous oxide procedure. **The procedure should be conducted under general anesthesia in the Operating Room if adequate anesthesia cannot be obtained and pain limits the procedure.**

TECHNIQUES

INCISION AND DRAINAGE

Make a stab incision with a #11 scalpel blade in the skin overlying the area of fluctuance (Figure 94-3A). The incision should be parallel to any lines of tension to produce the least conspicuous scar, particularly in cosmetically important areas such as the face. Extend the incision the length of the fluctuant area with a #11 or #15 scalpel blade unless the abscess is in a cosmetically important area. A linear incision is adequate, although some advocate a cruciate incision (Figure 93-10). The cruciate incision results in greater scarring, however, and probably is not necessary. An elliptical incision can be performed in non-cosmetically important areas (Figure 94-3B). The purpose of the elliptical incision is to remove a full thickness wedge of tissue so that the wound will remain open. **Limit the length of the incision on cosmetically important areas to 3 to 4 mm.** This is just large enough to drain the abscess.

Express the thick sebaceous material. It is too thick to drain spontaneously. It is important that loculations be lysed and the area thoroughly drained to minimize recurrence. Insert a hemostat and spread the jaws within the cavity (Figure 94-3C). A useful technique employs a gauze square clamped in the jaws of a hemostat and

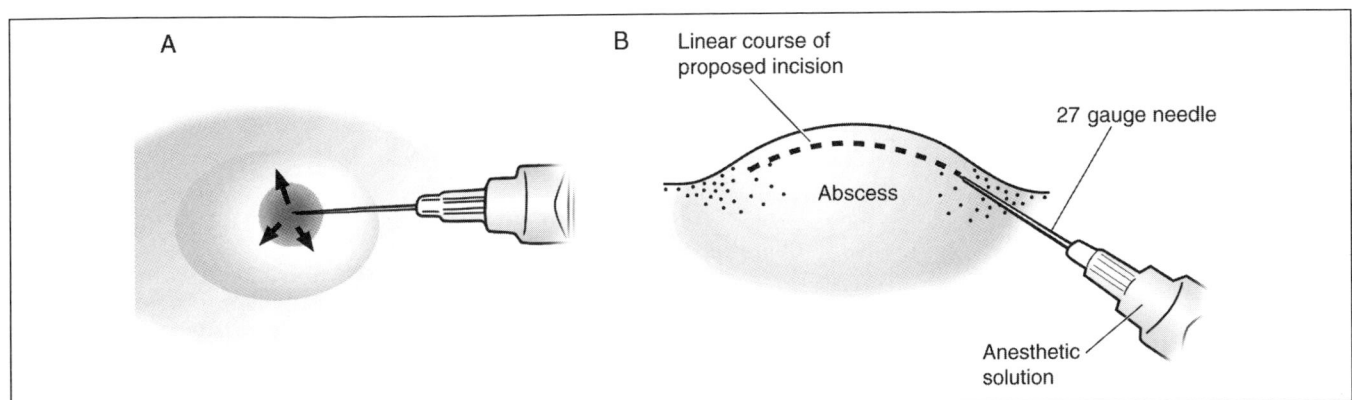

FIGURE 94-1 Subcutaneous infiltration of local anesthetic solution. The needle and syringe are held parallel to the skin. The needle is inserted into the subcutaneous tissue overlying the infected sebaceous cyst. Infiltrate the local anesthetic solution as the needle is withdrawn. The skin should blanch (shaded area) if injected properly. *A.* Superior view. *B.* Lateral view.

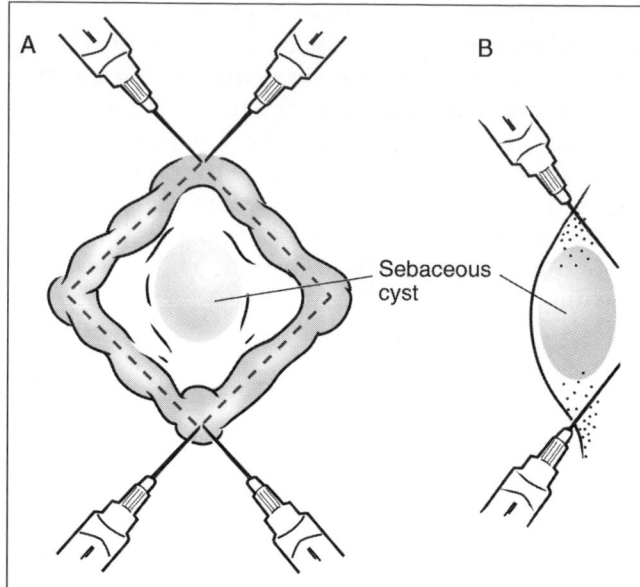

FIGURE 94-2 Field block anesthesia. *A.* Local anesthetic solution is infiltrated subcutaneously on all four sides of the infected sebaceous cyst. *B.* Local anesthetic solution is infiltrated deep to the infected sebaceous cyst in a fan-like pattern.

swirled inside the abscess cavity to break adhesions and remove debris. Irrigation of the cavity with normal saline is optional and used by some physicians (Figure 94-3C).

Loosely pack the wound with ribbon gauze or gauze squares to prevent the skin edges from closing prema-

turely if a linear incision was made (Figure 94-3D). Cruciate and elliptical incisions do not require packing of the wound. Cover the wound with a bulky gauze dressing to soak up continued drainage.

INCISION AND DRAINAGE WITH PRIMARY CYST REMOVAL

The entire sebaceous cyst, including the capsule, can be removed at the time of the incision and drainage.[3] Make an incision in the skin overlying the center of the sebaceous cyst. Extend the incision to be slightly longer than the diameter of the sebaceous cyst. **Do not cut into the dermis or subcutaneous tissues.** Sharply dissect the sebaceous cyst free of the surrounding subcutaneous tissues with an iris scissors. The delineation between the thin, shiny, white capsule and the surrounding tissues is very obvious. **Do not puncture the capsule of the sebaceous cyst.** Doing so and spilling some of the contents sets up a nidus for subsequent infection or reformation of the sebaceous cyst. Carefully grasp the cyst with a forceps and remove it from the subcutaneous tissue. Irrigate the wound with at least 200 mL of normal saline solution. Approximate the skin edges with nylon sutures.

This technique results in fewer days to heal, less pain for the patient, and less scarring than with incision and drainage alone.[3] This was not a blinded study and no other studies could be found to verify their results. The researchers noted that primary resection

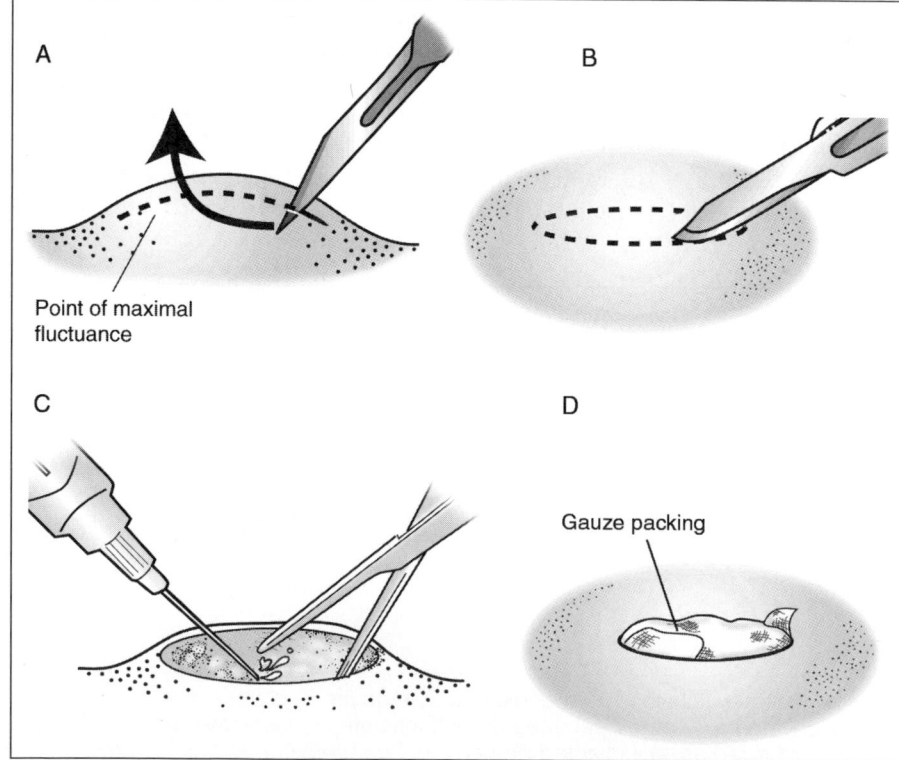

FIGURE 94-3 Incision and drainage of an infected sebaceous cyst. *A.* A straight incision to drain the abscess. *B.* An elliptical incision to drain the abscess. *C.* The wound is irrigated with sterile saline. Any pockets of pus are opened by blunt dissection with the hemostat. *D.* The wound is packed open.

(average of 50 minutes) takes longer than simple incision and drainage (average of 10 minutes). This may limit its use in the Emergency Department.

AFTERCARE

Antibiotics are generally unnecessary to treat a simple abscess unless there is cellulitis of the skin surrounding the wound.[1] No data could be found regarding patients with an abscess who are diabetic, have cardiac valve disease, who have hardware in their body, or who are immunocompromised. These patients are at risk for infectious complications. It is advised to cover these patients with antibiotics. Likewise, there is no data on the optimal duration of antibiotic treatment. The conventional 7 to 10 day course of antibiotic coverage is probably adequate.

Bacteriology of cutaneous abscesses remote from the rectum usually show aerobic skin flora, with *Staphylococcus* and *Streptococcus* being the most common etiologies.[4] Antibiotics recommended are a first-generation cephalosporin, a penicillinase-resistant penicillin, or a newer fluoroquinolone.

Instruct the patient to change the gauze dressing as often as necessary to keep the outside of the dressing dry. Patients should return for follow-up in 48 hours for a wound check and removal of the packing. The packing should be removed in 24 hours if the wound is on the face. If the wound is large, reinsert the packing upon follow-up. Incisions that remain open or that have an elliptical or cruciate incision do not require packing. Advise the patient to change the packing every 24 to 48 hours, depending on the amount of drainage. Decrease the amount of packing each time to allow the wound to heal from the base outward. The patient should thoroughly wash the wound with soap and water in the shower each time the packing is removed. It is helpful to let the stream of shower water run inside the wound to aid in wound irrigation. Discontinue the packing once the wound is well granulated and there is no concern that the skin edges will adhere to each other. The patient must continue to clean the wound thoroughly every day until it is fully healed.

Healing may take one to several weeks depending upon the size of the abscess cavity. Instruct the patient to return to the Emergency Department immediately if they develop a fever, increased pain, or increased redness of the skin surrounding the abscess. Pain relief can be provided with nonsteroidal anti-inflammatory drugs.

Occasionally, narcotic analgesics may be required in the first 24 hours after the procedure.

Inform the patient that incision and drainage in the acute care setting is not definitive treatment and that the condition is likely to recur unless the cyst is removed. Refer the patient to a physician who can provide wound care as well as remove the cyst capsule.

COMPLICATIONS

Sebaceous cyst infections may spread if the wound is inadequately drained. Attention must be paid to underlying anatomical structures, such as cranial nerve VII when draining facial abscesses, to avoid complications caused by inadvertently incising these structures. Incomplete removal of the cyst wall or spillage of the cyst contents sets up a nidus for future infection and/or recurrence of the sebaceous cyst.

SUMMARY

Infected sebaceous cysts are commonly seen in the Emergency Department. They are thought to be due to blockage of the ducts of sebaceous glands that subsequently become infected and form an abscess. Most cutaneous abscesses can be drained in the Emergency Department. Obtain surgical consultation for those patients with large abscesses who require drainage in the Operating Room. Patients with signs of fever or toxicity should be admitted for parenteral antibiotics, incision and drainage, and observation. Refer patients to a physician who can provide wound care as well as definitive excision of the sebaceous cyst.

REFERENCES

1. Llera JL, Levy RC: Treatment of cutaneous abscess: a double-blind clinical study. *Ann Emerg Med* 1985; 14(1):119.
2. Hanley PH: Acute pilonidal abscess. *Surg Gynecol Obstet* 1980; 150(1):9–11.
3. Kitamura K, Takahashi T, Toshiharu Y, et al: Primary resection of infectious epidermal cyst. *J Am Coll Surg* 1994; 179:607.
4. Meislin HW, Lerner SA, Graves MH, et al: Cutaneous abscesses: anaerobic and aerobic bacteriology and outpatient management. *Ann Intern Med* 1977; 87(2):145–149.

Chapter 95
HEMORRHAGE CONTROL

Karen S. Cosby

INTRODUCTION

Control of external hemorrhage from an injury is a priority of basic first aid, beginning with the first responder in the prehospital setting and continuing with Emergency and Trauma Physicians in the resuscitation suite. Bleeding from extremity wounds is common. Most extremity bleeding is a minor inconvenience for the busy Emergency Physician in the crowded Emergency Department, prolonging wound closure and complicating wound healing. However, major exsanguinating extremity hemorrhage can be a life threat. Hemorrhage from extremity injuries was a leading cause of death in the Vietnam War and Operation Desert Storm.[1,2] Methods for rapid and effective control of bleeding are essential in managing traumatic injuries and optimizing wound management.

ANATOMY AND PATHOPHYSIOLOGY

Hemostasis is the first biological response to injury.[3–5] Hemostatic platelet plugs form at the ends of transected vessels within seconds of traumatic disruption of the skin. Fibrin fibers gather about the platelet plug within minutes. This fibrin mesh becomes part of an early matrix that initiates wound healing.[3]

Hemostasis is also the first priority in wound management for the physician caring for traumatic wounds. **Control of bleeding is necessary to establish hemodynamic stability and prevent further blood loss.** Hemostasis is the first step in preparing for wound closure. Inadequate hemostasis with hematoma formation impairs wound healing, increases the risk of wound infection, leads to tissue ischemia, and results in hypertrophic scars.[6,7] Large hematomas may cause delayed wound dehiscence.

Bleeding from wounds may be superficial or deep. Superficial wounds, such as abrasions, avulsions, or simple lacerations, involve damage to the epidermis, dermis, and subcutaneous tissue. Bleeding from most superficial wounds is predominantly from capillaries, small veins, or arterioles. Wounds deep to the fascia involve larger vessels and are typical of deep puncture wounds, gunshot wounds, or major crush injuries. The approach to the bleeding wound will depend upon the nature of bleeding (large vessel versus small, discrete source versus diffuse), the site of injury, and its association with other major organ injury.

INDICATIONS

The immediate control of excessive bleeding is always a priority and should occur during the first contact with the patient. The timing and selection of specific measures to isolate and treat the bleeding source will depend upon the management priorities of each patient. A simple compressive dressing or tourniquet may be used as a first-line measure to control bleeding in a multiple trauma patient. Measures that are more definitive may be taken early to identify and treat the specific injury if it is isolated.

CONTRAINDICATIONS

There are no absolute contraindications to any particular technique to control bleeding. The physician should choose the technique best suited to the individual situation. An impressive wound should not distract or divert attention away from other injuries that may be less dramatic but more immediate life threats. **The simplest and most effective techniques should be used to control hemorrhage when faced with multiple injuries.**

EQUIPMENT

Pressure Control

Blood pressure cuff
Sterile 4×4 gauze pads
Elastic bandage

Wound Manipulation

Hemostats
Needle driver
Assorted suture
Scissors
Sterile saline
20 mL syringes
10 mL syringes
18 gauge needles
27 gauge needles

Anesthetic

Lidocaine, with and without epinephrine
Bupivacaine, with and without epinephrine
18 gauge needles
27 gauge needles
10 mL syringes

Wound Cautery

Silver nitrate (AgNO$_3$)
Electrocautery unit

Vasoconstrictors

Epinephrine, 1:1000
Cocaine, 1% to 4%
Tetracaine, epinephrine, and cocaine (TEC) solution

Local Hemostatic Agents

Gelfoam
Surgicel

Miscellaneous Supplies

Penrose drain
Finger tourniquet
Hemoclips
Hemoclip applicator
Bone wax

PATIENT PREPARATION

Control of hemorrhage is the priority. Attention to wound preparation should not delay definitive action to control bleeding. Obtain intravenous access and a type and crossmatch for blood products in any patient with active bleeding and hemodynamic compromise while applying direct pressure to the bleeding site. Explain the procedures to the patient while preparing for and performing the procedures. A local anesthetic can

be administered prior to significant wound manipulation if the injury is minor and the patient is stable. Contaminated wounds should be irrigated free of foreign bodies and debris and the surrounding area cleaned with an antiseptic solution.

TECHNIQUES

DIRECT PRESSURE

The quickest and easiest method to stop bleeding is the application of direct pressure to the bleeding site.[8–10] Poor lighting may prevent the exposure and visualization necessary to identify discrete bleeding sites in the prehospital setting. A compressive dressing may be the best option to control bleeding. Unfortunately, most compressive bandages apply too little pressure over too wide an area and act more like a sponge than a pressure dressing. Significant blood loss can be hidden within a bulky dressing.

Explore a bleeding wound as soon as lighting is sufficient and circumstances allow. Even brisk bleeding frequently has a few discrete sources that can be easily managed once identified. Direct pressure over bleeding vessels allows time for a platelet plug to form and gives a chance for the body's natural mechanisms of hemostasis to take place. Apply pressure over arterial wounds for 10 to 15 minutes to control most bleeding. Apply pressure to a proximal artery to impede arterial inflow and control, or slow, the bleeding when wound exploration is not practical.[11,12]

TOURNIQUETS

The use of tourniquets for extremity hemorrhage has received a great deal of attention throughout history. In reality, tourniquets are seldom necessary to control hemorrhage, even in major crush wounds, amputations, and in wilderness settings.[13] Direct pressure is more effective and causes less tissue ischemia. Tourniquets may be required to control bleeding and free rescue personnel to attend to other concerns if there is significant bleeding in a mass casualty disaster. Tourniquets should be used as a last resort when other methods fail and the patient's life is in jeopardy.[11,13]

SUTURE LIGATION

Thoroughly inspect briskly bleeding wounds. Place a blood pressure cuff proximally and inflate it until a dry bloodless field is obtained. Large vessel bleeding will first become apparent as the cuff pressure is slowly dropped. Large and intermediate sized vessels will need to be ligated or oversewn for effective control. Familiarity with the vascular supply to the extremities will help the clinician anticipate major arterial injuries and look for likely bleeding sources. **Whenever a transected ves-**

sel is seen, the other end should be searched for. A retracted artery in spasm will likely bleed later and should be actively sought and ligated.

Bleeding vessels that can be visualized should be ligated with suture (Figure 95-1). Grasp the cut end of the bleeding vessel with a hemostat (Figure 95-1A). Pass an appropriate sized suture around the vessel (Figure 95-1B). Use absorbable sutures that do not lose their tensile strength too soon (e.g., Vicryl, Monocryl, and PDS). Tie and secure the suture around the base of the bleeding vessel (Figure 95-1C). Gently release the hemostat from the blood vessel.

Cut blood vessels, especially arteries and arterioles, often retract into the tissue and are difficult to visualize. A suture can be used to control the bleeding (Figure 95-2). Place a figure-of-eight stitch (Figure 95-2A) or a pursestring stitch (Figure 95-2B) to encompass the blood vessel. These sutures are simple, quick, and easy to place.

CAUTERY

Smaller bleeders will be identified as the cuff pressure is gradually reduced. The next most likely source of significant bleeding is from veins and dermal arterioles. Venous bleeding usually stops with direct pressure alone. Dermal arterioles tend to resist pressure and cause persistent oozing from the wound edges. Blood vessels are best identified by picking up the wound edges and inspecting the dermis. These bleeding vessels are effectively treated with electrocautery or chemical cauterization.

Electrocautery is surprisingly easy and effective against aggressive bleeding from small vessels less than 2 mm in diameter.[9] Handheld battery-driven electrocautery units use a heated electrode to deliver a thermal burn to the tissue and char the ends of vessels. They are simple, inexpensive, and stocked in most Emergency Departments. More versatile electrosurgical units, such as the Bovie and Hyfrecator, are extremely effective coagulators.[14] Unfortunately, they are not routinely available in most Emergency Departments.

Chemical cauterization with silver nitrate ($AgNO_3$) is an effective alternative. The silver nitrate is a dark material that is provided on the end of a wooden applicator stick, resembling a large matchstick. Rub the silver nitrate over the bleeding vessel. It forms an insoluble precipitate with tissue protein to form an artificial clot that occludes vessel lumens.

Apply the electrocautery or chemical cautery directly to the bleeding source. More liberal use to the surrounding tissue will leave unnecessary damage and impair wound healing. Neither technique will work well unless the field is dry. This can be achieved with the use of suction, or the wound can be dabbed dry with gauze or cotton-tipped applicators.

VASOCONSTRICTORS

Smaller bleeding vessels will usually constrict and eventually stop on their own once major vessels have been treated. If not, the use of local vasoconstrictors and topical hemostatic agents is effective.[15] Epinephrine is a convenient and effective vasoconstrictor.[16] It can be injected into the wound edges with local anesthetic or placed directly into the wound. Spray 1 to 2 mL of 1:1000 epinephrine over the wound surface with a 25 gauge needle and cover the wound with a sterile saline-soaked gauze for 2 to 4 minutes.[17]

A more dilute epinephrine solution can be used in larger wounds to minimize potential side effects. Solutions as dilute as 1:100,000 to 1:1,000,000 are used to control the brisk bleeding that accompanies tangential burn wound excision and graft donor sites.[18] Topical cocaine (1 to 4 percent) is a potent vasoconstrictor commonly used on mucous membranes. Combinations of

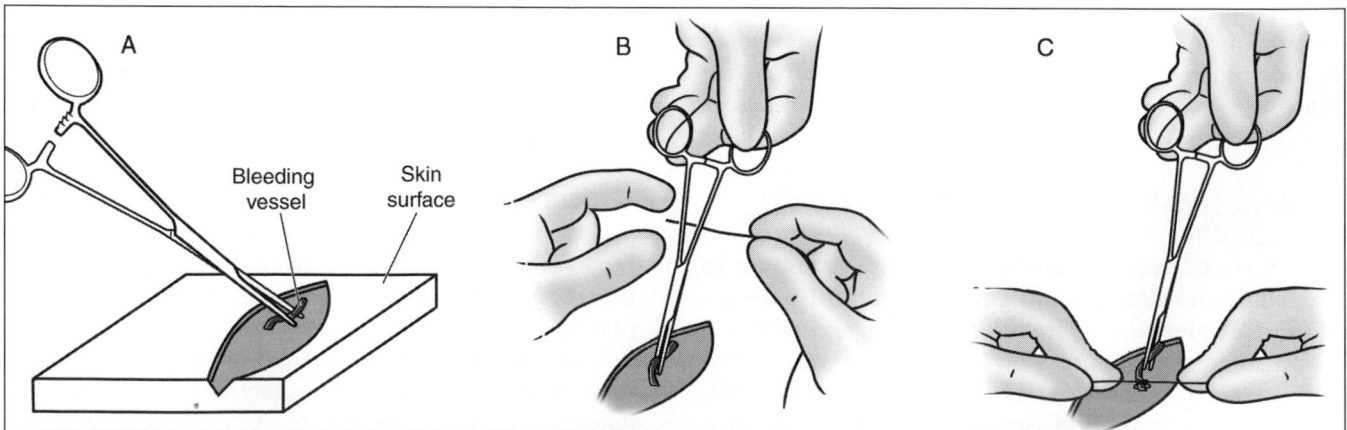

FIGURE 95-1 Control of the bleeding vessel that is visualized. *A.* Clamp the cut end of the vessel with a hemostat. *B.* Wrap a suture ligature about the base of the vessel. *C.* Tie and secure the suture around the base of the bleeding vessel.

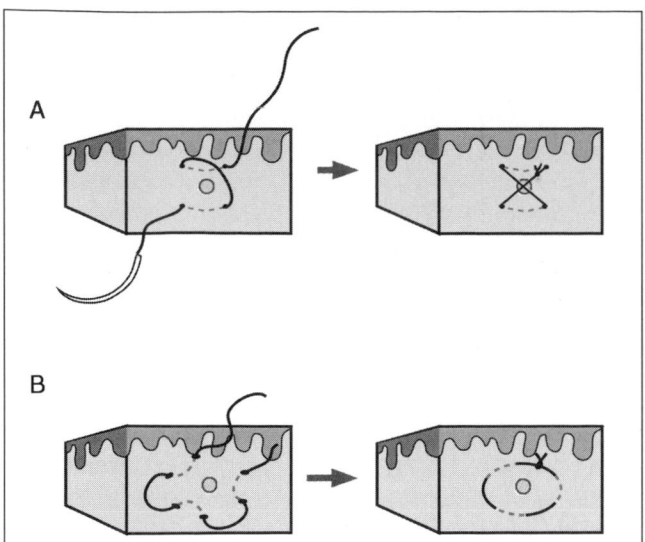

FIGURE 95-2 Control of a bleeding vessel deep in tissue. *A*. The figure-of-eight stitch. *B*. The pursestring stitch. Note that both of these stitches are not tied tightly for the sake of clarity. In real use, both of these stitches will be tied tightly to seal the bleeding vessel.

0.5 percent tetracaine, 1:2000 epinephrine (adrenalin), and 11.8 percent cocaine (TAC) are used for topical anesthesia and hemostasis in pediatric wounds.[19] Apply 1 to 2 mL of these solutions directly into the wound followed by an occlusive dressing.

TOPICAL HEMOSTATIC AGENTS

Occasionally, diffuse oozing persists after obvious blood vessels have been ligated. This seldom poses a hemodynamic risk but may be a problem in small wounds where even a small amount of blood impedes wound closure and jeopardizes a cosmetic outcome. The application of oxidized cellulose (Surgicel) or dry gelatin (Gelfoam) can provide a matrix for platelet deposition and aid hemostasis.[6,15] Troublesome wounds can be treated with these agents and covered with a pressure dressing. After a few minutes, the dry field can be approximated with sutures. Another option is to simply leave the hemostatic agent in the wound, close the wound, and apply a pressure dressing. These techniques will be effective for many wounds.

Bleeding may persist because of recent aspirin or anticoagulant use. The bleeding may actually worsen as attempts at wound repair are made. Topical thrombin or microfibrillar collagen (Avitene) may be useful hemostatic agents in these problematic cases.[15] Apply topical thrombin in powder form or diluted with saline and sprayed on the wound. Concentrations of 100 units/mL are usually effective. Concentrations of 1000 to 2000 units/mL can be used if the bleeding is severe. Alternatively, microfibrillar collagen can be used to encourage platelet aggregation. Both thrombin and microfibrillar collagen are expensive and are not usually supplied outside the Operating Room. Their use should be restricted to the unusual patient with a coagulopathy or severe bleeding unresponsive to other measures.

Hemostatic dressings may be available in the future to manage serious hemorrhage in the field. The United States Military and the American Red Cross have jointly worked on the development of a dry fibrin sealant bandage.[20] This gauze mesh is impregnated with fibrinogen and thrombin, which activate when exposed to fresh blood. Wrapped about a hemorrhaging extremity, it can provide hemostasis in prehospital settings. Fibrin glues and sealants are already in use in Europe but technical factors have slowed their acceptance in the United States. These products may eventually prove beneficial in the early phase of trauma management.

WOUND CLOSURE VERSUS PACKING

The wound can be approximated, a pressure dressing applied, and the limb elevated when oozing cannot be controlled by any other method. Alternatively, the wound can be packed until better control is achieved. A coagulation profile should be checked in anyone with persistent diffuse bleeding. If a correctable coagulopathy is identified, the wound can be approximated after the defect is corrected.

ALTERNATIVE TECHNIQUES

The general techniques discussed above apply to bleeding from most sites. There are a number of techniques applicable to specific anatomic sites.

THE HAND

Hand injuries pose special problems. Strict hemostasis is necessary to examine the wound and identify any associated damage to tendons, nerves, and joint capsules. A tourniquet can be placed to exsanguinate the extremity and facilitate wound inspection. Elevate the limb and wrap it with an elastic bandage to milk the venous return toward the heart. Apply a blood pressure cuff and inflate it above the systolic blood pressure. This prevents arterial inflow while minimizing the backflow from venous engorgement to reliably provide a bloodless field.

A digital tourniquet may expedite the examination if the injury is confined to a single digit.[21,22] A number of methods are effective (Figure 95-3). A Penrose drain can be wrapped about the base of the finger and secured with a hemostat (Figure 95-3*A*). Mark a 0.25 inch Penrose drain with two lines placed 26 mm apart. Stretch the Penrose drain about the base of an average adult finger until the lines meet. Clamp the Penrose drain with a hemostat to generate a sufficient but safe pressure.[21] An

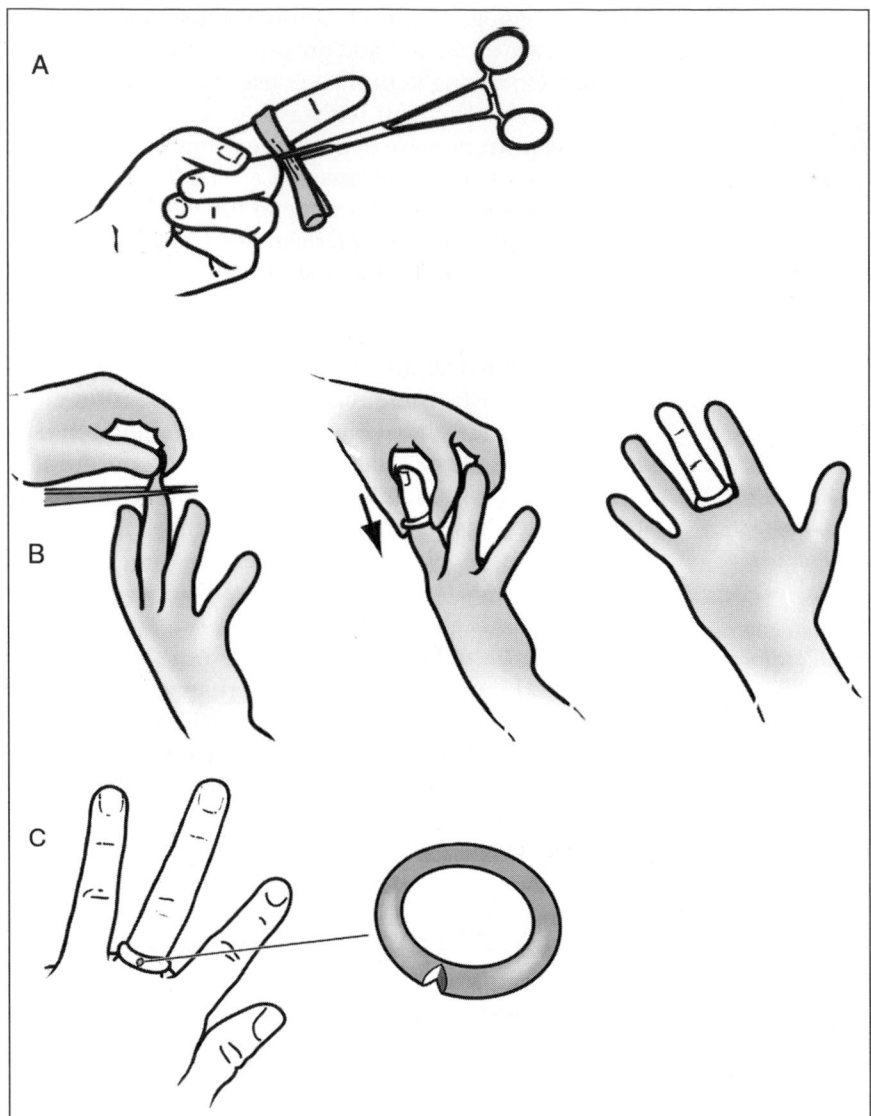

FIGURE 95-3 Finger tourniquets. *A.* A Penrose drain wrapped about the base of the finger provides effective hemostasis. *B.* A finger of a surgical glove has been cut and rolled down the finger. *C.* A commercial finger tourniquet.

alternative is to use a surgical glove with the fingertip cut off and rolled down the finger to leave a tight band at the base of the digit (Figure 95-3*B*). Use a glove size larger than what would typically fit the patient for general use to avoid generating excessive pressure.[21] Disposable, preformed, rubber digital tourniquets are commercially available and may be useful (Mar-Med Co., Grand Rapids, Michigan).[23] These digital tourniquets are available in numerous sizes. Roll the digital tourniquet over the finger until it is at the base of the digit (Figure 95-3*C*). This will exsanguinate the digit and prevent arterial inflow. **Tourniquets should be used for no more than 20 minutes to avoid injury to the digital nerves.**

Although hemostasis is important, it should not be pursued without regard to the surrounding tissues. **Hand wounds should not be explored or probed deep to surface structures. Blind exploration or clamping is never advised. Vasoconstrictors, such as epinephrine, should not be used on the digits.** Consult a Hand Surgeon if wounds require deep exploration.

THE SCALP

Scalp wounds frequently occur in association with other major intracranial, spinal, thoracic, and intra-abdominal injuries. Control of scalp bleeding is frequently not the first priority in the multiple trauma patient, although continued brisk bleeding from the scalp can contribute to hemorrhagic shock.[24] Techniques for vascular control of the damaged scalp should be simple and fast, and should not interfere with the ongoing assessment and treatment of other injuries.

A few techniques can help gain rapid control of bleeding with a minimal investment of time or personnel (Figures 95-4). The fastest and most effective method is the application of Raney scalp clips (Figure 95-4*A*). These

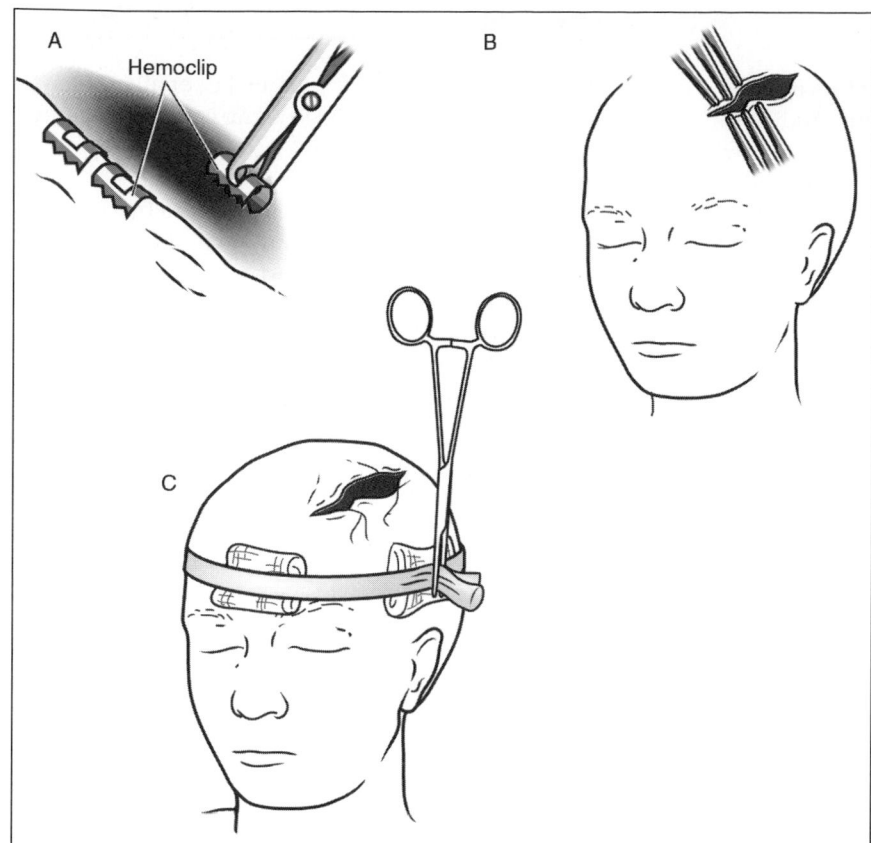

FIGURE 95-4 Hemorrhage from scalp wounds can easily be controlled. *A.* Hemostatic Raney scalp clips seal the wound edge. *B.* Hemostats applied about the edge of the wound. *C.* A Penrose drain wrapped about the head.

have been used for years by Neurosurgeons performing craniotomies.[25] If these are not available, apply hemostats at the wound edges where the bleeding is brisk (Figure 95-4*B*). Inject local anesthetic solution with epinephrine into the wound edges to constrict smaller vessels. A Penrose drain can be wrapped about the head as a temporary tourniquet (Figure 95-4*C*).[11] A time-honored method is to place figure-of-eight, simple running, or mattress sutures to temporarily close the wounds. A more definitive closure can be performed after the patient has been stabilized.

MAJOR EXTREMITY INJURY

Amputations, major crush wounds, soft tissue avulsions, and fractures of the extremity may present with active bleeding. Diffuse bleeding from muscle and soft tissue may be difficult to localize and treat. Immobilize the extremity and apply direct pressure if discrete bleeding sites cannot be identified. Reduction of long bone fractures and immobilization of soft tissue injuries can stabilize the damaged tissue and minimize blood loss. The application of a MAST suit or air splint may stabilize bony fragments and tamponade active bleeding.[26] These conservative and simple measures can dramatically reduce ongoing blood loss.

EXPOSED BONE

Exposed bone will tend to ooze. This can be especially troublesome in amputations and crush wounds. Bone wax can tamponade these sites and temporarily halt the bleeding until more definitive action can be taken. Open a sterile package of bone wax and hold it in a sterile-gloved hand to warm it up and make it more pliable. Remove a piece of the bone wax and mold it over the end of the broken bone. Firmly push the bone wax into the bone to seal the edges. Use care to prevent lacerating your glove and finger, resulting in a significant exposure.

ARTERIAL INJURIES

Puncture wounds and deep lacerations may be complicated by arterial injuries. These may be obvious if they present with dramatic pulsatile bleeding. However, the elastic recoil of arteries frequently causes the damaged vessel to retract deep within the wound, only to rebleed after wound closure. Recurrent pulsatile bleeding and deep hematoma formation are characteristics of unrecognized arterial injuries. This is particularly true of puncture wounds where the damage may be deep and not visible to the examiner's eye. These wounds may require angiography, embolization, or wound exploration to identify the source if they rebleed despite local measures.

ASSESSMENT

The ideal goal in wound care is to achieve a dry bloodless field without compromising the vitality of the tissue. Simply controlling the hemorrhage and preserving life is the goal in major trauma victims. Expediting wound closure and preventing hematoma formation is a more modest goal for minor injuries.

AFTERCARE

A healthy wound is proof of adequate hemostasis. Routine wound care should verify a healthy incision line and the absence of a hematoma or an infection. Refer to Chapters 77 through 80 regarding the details of wound care and repair.

COMPLICATIONS

The techniques in this chapter are all safe and effective when used as described. Complications occur when they are used in excess or in the wrong setting. There is a risk of limb ischemia and eventual limb loss any time a tourniquet is used. Tourniquet use should be restricted to 20 to 30 minutes. The tourniquet should be released periodically and the extremity reassessed. Use the minimal tourniquet pressure necessary to maintain hemostasis. Overzealous use of electrocautery and chemical cautery can cause unnecessary tissue necrosis and increase the risk of infection. Hand wounds should not be probed and bleeding vessels should never be clamped to avoid damage to small nerves and other structures. Epinephrine and other vasoconstrictors should not be used in a finger, toe, ear, nose, or penis where ischemia may cause tissue loss. Scalp clips should only be used on the thick skin of the scalp. Use elsewhere can crush and devitalize thin skin or damage subcutaneous structures. Injudicious reliance on hemostatic agents should not replace a methodical approach to wound care and a meticulous search for bleeding vessels. Topical vasoconstrictors should be used with diligent attention to the total dose administered to avoid systemic side effects such as hypertension, tachycardia, and seizures.

SUMMARY

There are a number of techniques available for the control of hemorrhage. A methodical approach to the bleeding wound will optimize the outcome. Simple measures should be used first and progressive systematic steps taken until hemostasis is achieved. All bleeding eventually stops! The goal is to halt the bleeding before irreparable harm occurs.

REFERENCES

1. McCaughey BG, Garrick J, Carey LC, et al: Naval support activity hospital Da Nang combat casualty deaths January to June 1968. *Mil Med* 1987; 152(6):284–289.
2. Carey ME: Analysis of wounds incurred by U.S. Army Seventh Corps personnel treated in corps hospitals during Operation Desert Storm, February 20 to March 10, 1991. *J Trauma* 1996; 40(3):S165–S169.
3. Wester J, Sixma JJ, Geuze JJ, et al: Morphology of the early hemostasis in human skin wounds. Influence of acetylsalicylic acid. *Lab Invest* 1978; 39(3):298–311.
4. Lawrence WT: Physiology of the acute wound. *Clin Plast Surg* 1998; 25(3):321–340.
5. Hotter A: The physiology and clinical implications of wound healing. Part I. Wound healing physiology. *Plast Surg Nurs* 1984; 4(1):4–13.
6. Parker RK, Dinehart SM: Hints for hemostasis. *Dermatol Clin* 1994; 12(3):601–606.
7. Salasche SJ: Acute surgical complications: cause, prevention, and treatment. *J Am Acad Dermatol* 1986; 15(6):1163–1185.
8. Borja AR, Lansing AM: Immediate control of intermediate vascular bleeding. *Surg Gynecol Obstet* 1971; 132(3):494–496.
9. Lammers RL: Principles of wound management, in Roberts JR, Hedges JR (eds): *Clinical Procedures in Emergency Medicine*, 3rd ed. Philadelphia: Saunders, 1998:533–559.
10. Breitenbach KL, Bergera JJ: Principles and techniques of primary wound closure. *Prim Care* 1986; 13(3):411–431.
11. Kelly JJ: Control of exsanguinating external hemorrhage, in Henretig FM, King C (eds): *Textbook of Pediatric Emergency Procedures*. Baltimore: Wiliams & Wilkins, 1997:367–376.
12. Simon RR, Brenner BE: *Emergency Procedures and Techniques*, 3rd ed. Baltimore: Williams & Wilkins, 1994:308.
13. Morris JA, Swiontkowski MF, Herrman HJ: Wilderness trauma emergencies, in Auerbach PS, Geehr EC (eds): *Management of Wilderness and Environmental Emergencies*, 2nd ed. St. Louis: Mosby, 1989:223–265.
14. Sebben JE: The status of electrosurgery in dermatologic practice. *Dermatol Surg* 1988; 19(3):542–549.
15. Larson PO: Topical hemostatic agents for dermatologic surgery. *J Dermatol Surg Oncol* 1988; 14(6):623–632.
16. Munchow OB, Denson JS: The effect of various vasoconstrictors on the blood vessels of human skin. A pilot study with a new method. *Surgery* 1964; 56(5):989–992.

17. Glasson DW: Topical Adrenalin as a hemostatic agent. *Plast Reconstr Surg* 1984; 74(3):451–452.

18. Snelling CFT, Shaw K: The effect of topical epinephrine hydrochloride in saline on blood loss following tangential excision of burn wounds. *Plast Reconstr Surg* 1983; 72(6):830–836.

19. Shafi S, Gilbert JC: Minor pediatric injuries. *Pediatr Clin North Am* 1998; 45(4):831–851.

20. Holcomb JB, Pusateri AE, Hess JR, et al: Implications of new dry fibrin sealant technology for trauma surgery. *Surg Clin North Am* 1997; 77(4):943–952.

21. Lubahn JD, Koeneman J, Kosar K: The digital tourniquet: how safe is it? *J Hand Surg [Am]* 1985; 10A(5):664–669.

22. Rohrer TET, Lewlie B, Grande DJ: Dermatologic surgery of the hand. *J Dermatol Surg Oncol* 1994; 20:19–34.

23. Trott AT: *Wounds and Lacerations: Emergency Care and Closure,* 2nd ed. St. Louis: Mosby, 1997.

24. Lemos MJ, Clark DE: Scalp lacerations resulting in hemorrhagic shock: case reports and recommended management. *J Emerg Med* 1988; 6:377–379.

25. Coleman RJ, Rocko JM: Rapid control of hemorrhage of the scalp in the patient with trauma. *Surg Gynecol Obstet* 1988; 166:165–166.

26. Kaback KR, Sanders AB, Meislin HW: MAST suit update. *JAMA* 1984; 252(18):2598–2603.

Section Seven

NEUROLOGIC AND NEUROSURGICAL PROCEDURES

Chapter 96
LUMBAR PUNCTURE

Brian Fong
Jeffrey M. VanBendegom

INTRODUCTION

Meningitis and subarachnoid hemorrhage are serious life-threatening conditions. They require prompt and accurate diagnosis in the Emergency Department due to their significant morbidity and mortality. There are many diagnostic modalities available to the Emergency Physician to assist in the diagnosis. However, lumbar puncture (LP) is still considered the gold standard. Lumbar puncture is a procedure that is often performed in the Emergency Department to obtain information about the cerebrospinal fluid (CSF) to aid in the diagnosis of a variety of medical conditions. Knowledge about the proper indications, contraindications, various techniques, equipment, and recognition and treatment of its complications is vital to any physician that performs this procedure. **A lumbar puncture should be performed after a thorough neurological exam. Significant morbidity and mortality can result if the procedure is performed on the wrong patient.**

ANATOMY AND PATHOPHYSIOLOGY

While the entire cavity of the brain and spinal cord has a volume of approximately 1650 mL, CSF occupies approximately 150 mL of this volume. The brain literally floats in the CSF because the specific gravity of the CSF and brain are approximately the same. Approximately 500 mL (0.35 mL/min) of CSF is produced each day. Most (over two-thirds) of the CSF is produced by the choroid plexus within the lateral ventricles. Small amounts of choroid plexus can also be found in the third and fourth ventricles. Small amounts of CSF are secreted by the ependymal surfaces of the ventricles. A minimal volume of CSF is produced by the brain through the small perivascular spaces that surround the blood vessels entering the brain substance.

The flow of CSF through the ventricular system is rather simple (Figure 96-1). CSF produced in the lateral ventricles flows through the foramina of Monro into the midline third ventricle. It then passes through the Aqueduct of Sylvius into the fourth ventricle. From the fourth ventricle, the CSF flows into the cisterna magna via two lateral openings (foramina of Luschka) and one midline opening (foramen of Magendie). The cisterna magna is located beneath the medulla and cerebellum and is continuous with the subarachnoid space that surrounds the brain and spinal cord. The CSF then flows through the subarachnoid space to bathe the brain and spinal cord. The CSF is absorbed back into the venous system by way of arachnoid villi.

CSF pressure should average 130 mmH$_2$O when measured in the lateral decubitus position. It can range from 70 to 180 mmH$_2$O in a normal person. Since the CSF production rate is constant, the pressure is regulated by the rate of CSF absorption by the arachnoid villi that act as one-way valves into the venous blood of the dural sinuses. Certain disease states may impede reabsorption and lead to increased intracranial pressure.[1]

Familiarity with the anatomy of the spinal column is important when performing a lumbar puncture. The anatomy will be briefly reviewed from superficial to deep as the spinal needle traverses the midline structures. The skin and subcutaneous tissue are the first layers encountered. These are followed by the supraspinous and intraspinous ligaments, located between the spinous processes of adjacent vertebrae. Deep to these ligaments is the thick ligamentum flavum that accounts for the characteristic "pop" that is described when performing a lumbar puncture. The next layers encountered are the epidural fat in the epidural space followed by the dura mater and finally the subarachnoid space.

When considering the lateral approach, there are subtle anatomic differences. The layers include skin and subcutaneous tissue followed by the paraspinal ligaments.

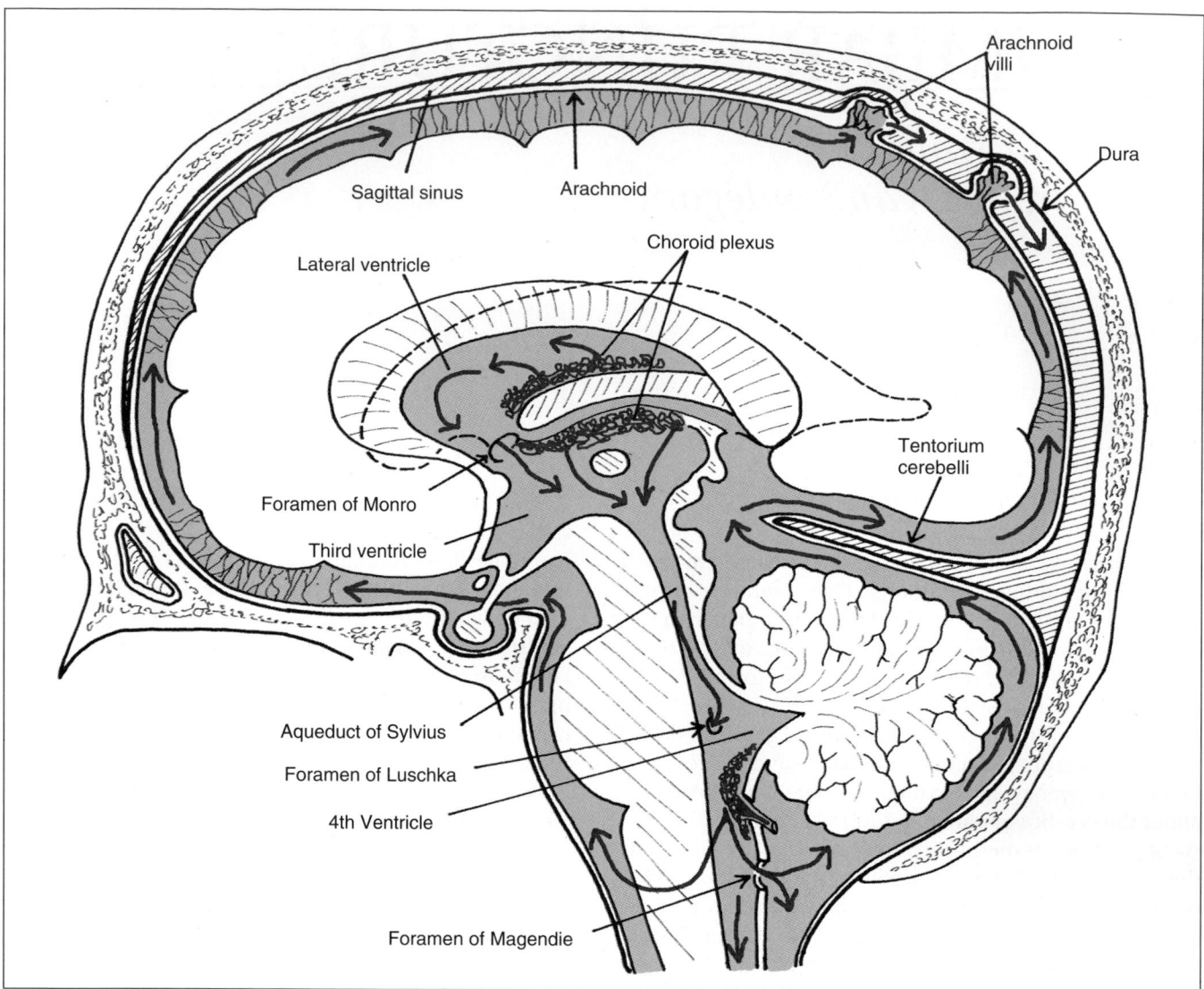

FIGURE 96-1 CSF circulation around the brain and upper spinal cord.

The intraspinous ligament is less likely to be encountered with an extreme lateral approach, as this is a midline structure. The ligamentum flavum and deeper structures should be encountered in the same fashion regardless of the approach.

INDICATIONS

There are many indications for performing a lumbar puncture. The primary indications to perform a lumbar puncture are the suspicion for a central nervous system infection, such as meningitis, or for a subarachnoid hemorrhage. It may also be performed to relieve CSF pressure and confirm the diagnosis of pseudotumor cerebri. Other indications include CSF evaluation (Guillain-Barré, multiple sclerosis, systemic lupus erythematosus), to con-

firm demyelinating or inflammatory diseases, to administer antibiotics or chemotherapeutic agents, to aid in radiologic imaging procedures (cysternography or myelography), and to diagnose meningeal carcinomatosis.

SUSPICION OF MENINGITIS IN ADULTS

A lumbar puncture should be performed in adults when there is a clinical suspicion of a central nervous system (CNS) infection. While a fever is often present (most sources consider a fever > (100.4° F or 38° C), it is not a dependable sign. Meningeal signs include nuchal rigidity, Kernig's sign, and Brudzinski's sign. Other signs of a possible CNS infection include a severe headache, photophobia, or a petechial rash. Unfortunately these signs may or may not be present. This is especially true in the elderly, the young, or the immunocompromised patient. **A lumbar puncture should be a routine proce-**

dure in febrile adults with an altered mental status and no source of fever.

The most commonly looked-for signs of meningitis include the Kernig's sign and the Brudzinski's sign (Figure 96-2). Place the patient supine to test for these physical examination signs. Passively flex the patient's head until their chin touches the sternum. Flexion of the patient's hips and knees in response to the head flexion is known as the Brudzinski's sign (Figure 96-2A). The patient may also experience neck pain and resistance to flexion if meningitis is present. Passively flex one of the patient's legs to 90 degrees at the hip and to 90 degrees at the knee (Figure 96-2B). Passively extend the knee. Pain in the lower back or resistance to knee extension is known as the Kernig's sign.[2]

SUSPICION OF MENINGITIS IN CHILDREN

When evaluating the febrile infant, the decision of whether to perform a lumbar puncture will be based on the clinical suspicion of meningitis, the age and appearance of the child, and whether an identifiable source of fever is present. The physician will often be faced with a well-appearing febrile infant with no obvious source

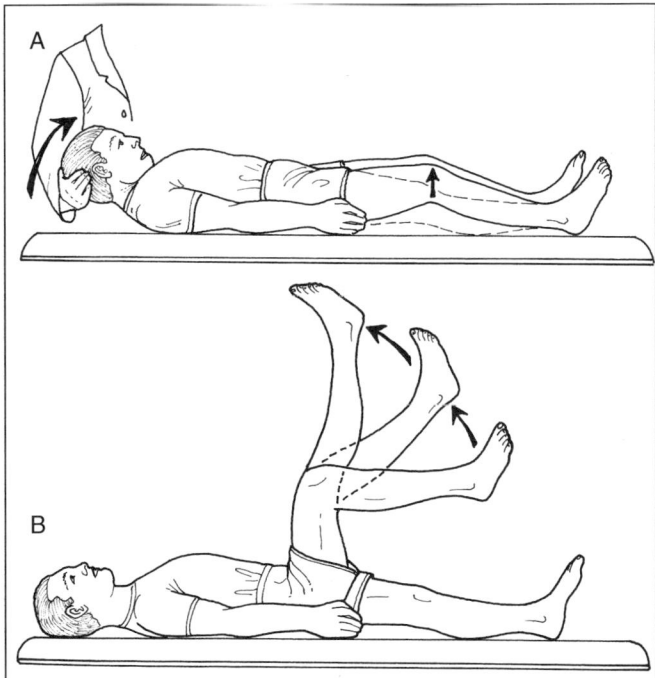

FIGURE 96-2 Physical examination of meningeal signs. *A.* Brudzinski's sign. Upon passive elevation of the head by the examiner, the patient complains of neck and low back pain, and may have involuntary flexion of the knees and hips suggesting meningeal irritation. *B.* Kernig's sign. Begin with the patient starting in a supine position with their hips and knees flexed 90 degrees. Gradually extending the knee causes the patient to complain of neck or lower back pain.

of fever. Until recently, many institutions managed all febrile infants less than three months old with a full sepsis workup (including LP) and admission to the hospital.

More recent guidelines, based on an extensive literature review and meta-analysis by an expert panel, identify patients at low risk for serious bacterial infection (SBI), where lumbar puncture and hospitalization may or may not be indicated.[3] Examples of serious bacterial infections include meningitis, sepsis, osteomyelitis, septic arthritis, urinary tract infections, pneumonia, and enteritis. Since clinical evaluation alone is inadequate to exclude serious bacterial infections in infants, it must be combined with laboratory studies that can define low-risk criteria. These criteria apply to nontoxic-appearing infants with reliable parents and prearranged follow-up: previously healthy infant, absence of focal bacterial infection on physical examination (except otitis media), and a negative laboratory screening panel. This includes a white blood cell (WBC) count of 5000 to 15,000/mm^3 with less than 1500 bands/mm^3, a normal urinalysis, and a stool white blood cell count of < 5 per high-power field when diarrhea is present. Although these criteria pertain to infants from 0 to 90 days of age, many institutions hospitalize all febrile infants less than 30 days old and administer parenteral antibiotics until meningitis is ruled out. A more detailed discussion regarding the evaluation of the child with a fever is beyond the scope of this chapter.

It should be noted that any febrile child, regardless of age, who appears "toxic" should have a lumbar puncture as an integral part of the sepsis workup. Certain bacterial infections have a high propensity for dissemination and systemic bacteremia. Examples include epiglottitis, buccal cellulitis, periorbital cellulitis, and septic arthritis. These children should also be considered for a lumbar puncture in their evaluation and work-up.

IS LUMBAR PUNCTURE INDICATED FOR THE FIRST FEBRILE SEIZURE?

The Emergency Physician will be faced with the decision of whether to perform a lumbar puncture when evaluating infants and children with a first febrile seizure. The American Academy of Pediatrics recommends that a lumbar puncture be "strongly considered in infants less than 12 months of age" and "considered in children 12 to 18 months of age."[4] This is based on the lack of clinical signs and symptoms often associated with meningitis in this age group. For children over 18 months of age, a lumbar puncture should only be performed if there is a clinical suggestion of meningitis. Clinical signs and symptoms that have been shown to correlate with the presence of meningitis include petechiae, nuchal rigidity, coma, persistent drowsiness, Kernig's or Brudzinski's sign, status epilepticus, and paralysis.[5]

Benign febrile seizures are those that occur in children 3 months to 5 years of age, are associated with a fever at the onset of an illness, have a single generalized seizure lasting less than 15 minutes in a child with normal psychomotor development, have no history of prior febrile seizures with this current illness, and have no evidence of an intracranial infection or acute neurological illness. These children generally appear well except for the fever and generally do not require a lumbar puncture. This is based upon the level of physician comfort in a nontoxic-appearing child.

Complex febrile seizures are those that do not meet the criteria of a benign febrile seizure. These children require a complete septic work-up including a lumbar puncture. Criteria include seizures that begin focally, seizures lasting over 15 minutes, children with a prolonged postictal period, suspicious findings on physical examination, children less than 12 months of age, children already receiving antibiotics, children who have seen a physician for an illness in the preceding 24 hours, or those who have had multiple seizures during a single period of illness. Seizures not associated with the onset of an illness have an increased risk of being due to meningitis or bacteremia. Children seizing upon presentation to the Emergency Department are considered to be seizing over 15 minutes or to have recurrent seizures. Suspicious findings on physical examination that suggest a complex seizure include rashes, petechiae, cyanosis, hypotension, abnormal respirations, increased or floppy tone, stiff neck, difficult to console, deviated eyes, doll's eyes, nystagmus, ataxia, photophobia, bulging or tense fontanelles, unable to fix and follow, or children that do not respond to voice or painful stimuli.

SUBARACHNOID HEMORRHAGE

A suspected subarachnoid hemorrhage (SAH) is the other common indication for a lumbar puncture. The classic description of a subarachnoid hemorrhage is the sudden onset of an excruciating headache ("thunderclap") during exertion that may or may not be associated with syncope, nausea, vomiting, diaphoresis, or meningeal signs. Physical examination findings may include nuchal rigidity, an altered level of consciousness, papilledema, retinal hemorrhage, third-nerve palsy, sixth-nerve palsy, bilateral lower leg weakness, nystagmus, ataxia, aphasia, or hemiparesis. Additional risk factors for a SAH include cigarette smoking, hypertension, alcohol abuse, a family history of subarachnoid hemorrhage, polycystic kidney disease, connective tissue disorders, or sickle cell anemia.

It is estimated that 20 to 50 percent of patients with a subarachnoid hemorrhage may have sentinel bleeds or small leaks that precede the major bleeding event. **It is important to diagnose a sentinel bleed because early management and intervention can improve the overall outcome for the patient. A sentinel bleed may precede a major SAH by hours, days, weeks, or months.**[6,7]

A CT scan of the head is often the first study used to investigate a patient complaining of the sudden-onset headache. The sensitivity of CT scan for SAH can range from 92 to 98 percent when performed within 24 hours of the onset of symptoms.[8,9] The sensitivity decreases markedly (about 76 percent) when performed 48 to 72 hours after onset of symptoms.[10,11] The head CT is often negative in patients with a sentinel bleed.

A lumbar puncture must be performed if the CT scan is negative and a subarachnoid hemorrhage is still suspected. The presence of xanthochromia or red blood cells in the CSF will confirm the presence of bleeding. While the CSF will usually confirm a SAH, it is possible that the lumbar puncture may be negative despite a recent subarachnoid hemorrhage if there has not been sufficient time for the red blood cells to migrate to the lumbar spine area. In this case, despite a negative head CT or lumbar puncture, a cerebral angiogram or follow-up lumbar puncture in 12 to 18 hours should be performed.

CONTRAINDICATIONS

Knowledge of the contraindications to performing a lumbar puncture is important because the physician will often have to weigh the potential risks of performing the procedure with the benefits of obtaining the CSF. The decision must be made whether the procedure should be performed immediately or can be delayed until further studies are completed. Absolute contraindications to performing a lumbar puncture include a cellulitis or abscess at the skin puncture site or increased intracranial pressure. The lumbar puncture should be delayed in patients with an unstable airway, hypotension, shock, or status epilepticus until the patient has been stabilized. Hypoxemia, clinical deterioration, apnea, and cardiopulmonary arrest are reported complications of lumbar puncture in unstable patients. Relative contraindications to performing a lumbar puncture include the presence of a brain abscess, epidural or subdural fluid collection, brain tumors, and spinal cord tumors.

Note that antibiotics should not be delayed if meningitis is suspected and the LP must be delayed. If meningitis is highly suspected but the patient is unstable, treatment should be initiated with parenteral antibiotics and the lumbar puncture delayed until the patient's condition is stabilized.

INCREASED INTRACRANIAL PRESSURE

Lumbar puncture is relatively contraindicated in the presence of increased intracranial pressure. This includes patients with space-occupying lesions (tumor or abscess), lateralizing signs such as hemiparesis on the physical examination, or when signs of uncal herniation are present (unilateral third-nerve palsy). Brain herniation or coning has also been reported in patients with meningitis and increased intracranial pressure. The sudden drop in intracranial pressure induced by a lumbar puncture may precipitate a pressure cone or herniation.

BRAIN ABSCESS

Patients with brain abscess are at high risk for herniation.[12,13] Brain abscesses may present with a progressively worsening headache, low-grade fever, and the development of focal neurological signs (hemiparesis, papilledema, visual field deficits, mild obtundation). Suspect a brain abscess in patients with a history of otic or paranasal sinus infection, orbital cellulitis, chronic pulmonary or abdominal infection, endocarditis, congenital heart disease, recent dental procedures, dental abscesses, recent neurosurgery, craniofacial trauma, open skull fractures, or recent meningitis.

WHEN IS A CT SCAN INDICATED BEFORE LUMBAR PUNCTURE?

It should be emphasized that increased intracranial pressure by itself is not necessarily a contraindication to lumbar puncture. Intracranial pressure is usually mildly elevated in patients with meningitis.[14] A CT scan does not need to be routinely performed in straightforward cases of suspected meningitis in patients with a normal neurological examination.[15–19] The inability to visualize the optic discs does not constitute a focal finding and, by itself, is not an indication for a head CT prior to the lumbar puncture.[17]

Most literature suggests that CT scans be performed prior to lumbar puncture when patients are comatose or altered, have focal neurological signs, are HIV positive, have a progressively worsening headache, or have papilledema.[17–19] **The lack of papilledema is not always a reliable sign of normal intracranial pressure, as it often takes greater than 48 hours to develop papilledema.[15]** Papilledema may be absent in up to 15 percent of adults and up to 50 percent of children with early increased intracranial hypertension.

The CT scan should be evaluated for mass lesions, shift of midline structures, or hydrocephalus due to obstructing masses, cisternal obstruction, and cerebral edema.[19] There are three findings that may predispose a patient to herniation if a lumbar puncture is performed.[20] The first finding is midline shift. This suggests unequal pressures across the midline. The second finding is a loss of the suprachiasmatic and basilar cisterns. This suggests unequal pressures between the supratentorial and infratentorial compartments. The third finding is any evidence of a posterior fossa mass, obliteration of the superior cerebellar cistern, or obliteration of the quadrigem-

inal plate cistern caudal to the midbrain. These findings all suggest the presence of increased infratentorial pressure.

Do not delay the initiation of antibiotics if meningitis is suspected and a CT scan is indicated before performing the lumbar puncture. Administer the antibiotics before the patient undergoes CT scanning. Several studies have shown that delays in the initiation of antibiotics are common in the Emergency Department. These delays are usually physician generated and result from the need for a CT scan prior to lumbar puncture, waiting for lumbar puncture results before administering antibiotics, and not giving antibiotics before a patient is transferred to the ward.[21–24]

COAGULATION DEFECTS

Lumbar puncture is relatively contraindicated in patients with a coagulopathy. This includes hemophiliacs, those on anticoagulants, and patients with thrombocytopenia. Lumbar puncture can result in a spinal epidural or subdural hematoma with subsequent spinal cord compression. Appropriate replacement of platelets and/or clotting factors should be undertaken prior to attempting the lumbar puncture if the procedure can be delayed.[25] **The most experienced physician should perform the procedure with a small gauge needle when immediate lumbar puncture is indicated in these patients.**

BACTEREMIA

Some sources list bacteremia as a contraindication to lumbar puncture, especially in children. While there is some suggestion that there may be an association between performing a lumbar puncture in a bacteremic patient and the later development of meningitis, the risk of this is low. **Lumbar puncture should not be withheld for fear of inducing meningitis.** The risk of delaying the diagnosis of meningitis clearly outweighs the small chance of causing meningitis with a lumbar puncture.[26]

EQUIPMENT

Most of the equipment necessary for performing a lumbar puncture is available in prepackaged commercial kits (Figure 96-3). These kits usually contain a 20 gauge Quincke spinal needle, syringes, needles (25 gauge and 22 gauge) for local anesthesia, manometer with stopcock, sterile drapes, specimen tubes, gauze, brushes for prepping the skin, and bandages. Some kits provide povidone iodine swab sticks whereas other kits have a small basin that needs to be filled. The physician should become familiar with the kit used at their institution.

Additional supplies may be needed to perform the procedure without interruption. For example, some physicians prefer a smaller gauge Quincke needle or a nontraumatic needle such as a Sprotte or Whitacre that are not

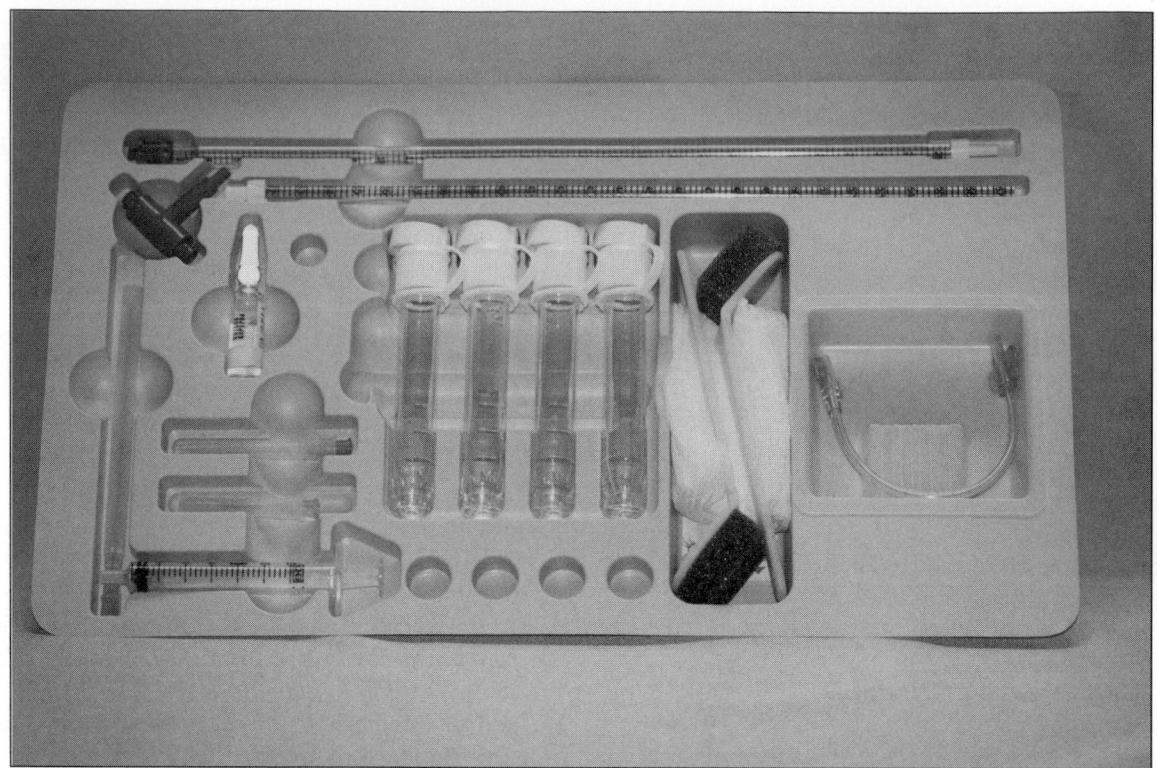

FIGURE 96-3 A commercially available lumbar puncture kit.

often provided in the commercial kits (Figure 96-4). The use of a 25 gauge spinal needle is recommended as it causes a smaller puncture hole and less post-procedural headaches.[27] In general, it is a good idea to have extra spinal needles, lidocaine, gauze, and povidone iodine when performing the procedure.

There are subtle differences among the spinal needles commonly available (Figure 96-4). The standard Quincke needle has a sharp tip with a broad bevel at the end. The Whitaker and Sprotte needles have smaller tips with smaller diameter bevels. The bevel of the Sprotte needle is broader with a rounded tip so as to separate fibers of the dura as opposed to cutting through them. **Always remember to keep the bevel oriented superiorly when performing a lumbar puncture regardless of needle style.**

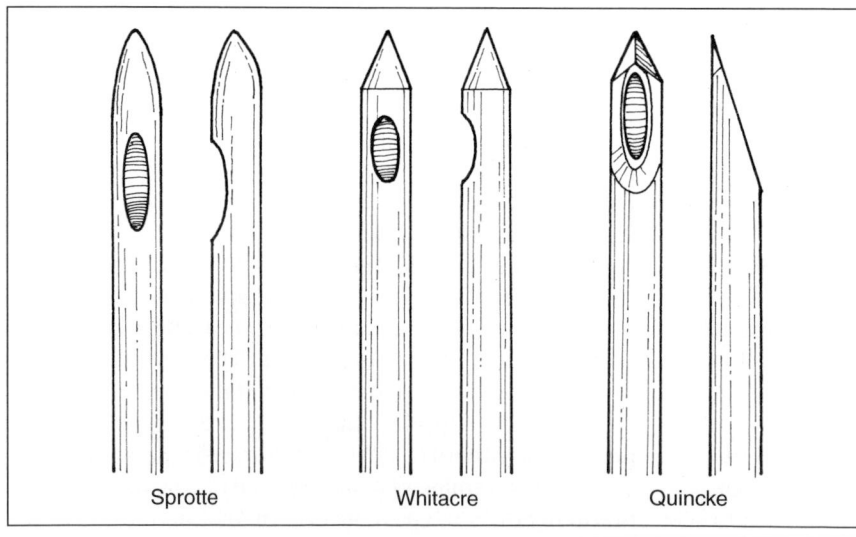

Sprotte   Whitacre   Quincke

FIGURE 96-4 The three types of spinal needle tips. The standard Quincke needle has a sharp, beveled end. The Whitacre and Sprotte needles are designed to spread atraumatically, rather than cut dural fibers.

PATIENT PREPARATION

Explain the risks, benefits, and complications of the procedure to the patient and/or their representative. Obtain a signed informed consent for the procedure. If the patient is a child or minor, ask the parents or caregivers whether or not they would like to be present for the lumbar puncture.

There are a variety of different patient positions that can be used to perform the lumbar puncture (Figure 96-5).[27–29] Knowledge and proficiency in more than one approach will be useful for the physician, especially when encountering a difficult tap. The position of the patient will be chosen based upon the patient's body habitus, their ability to assume a position, their level of cooperativeness, and physician preference.

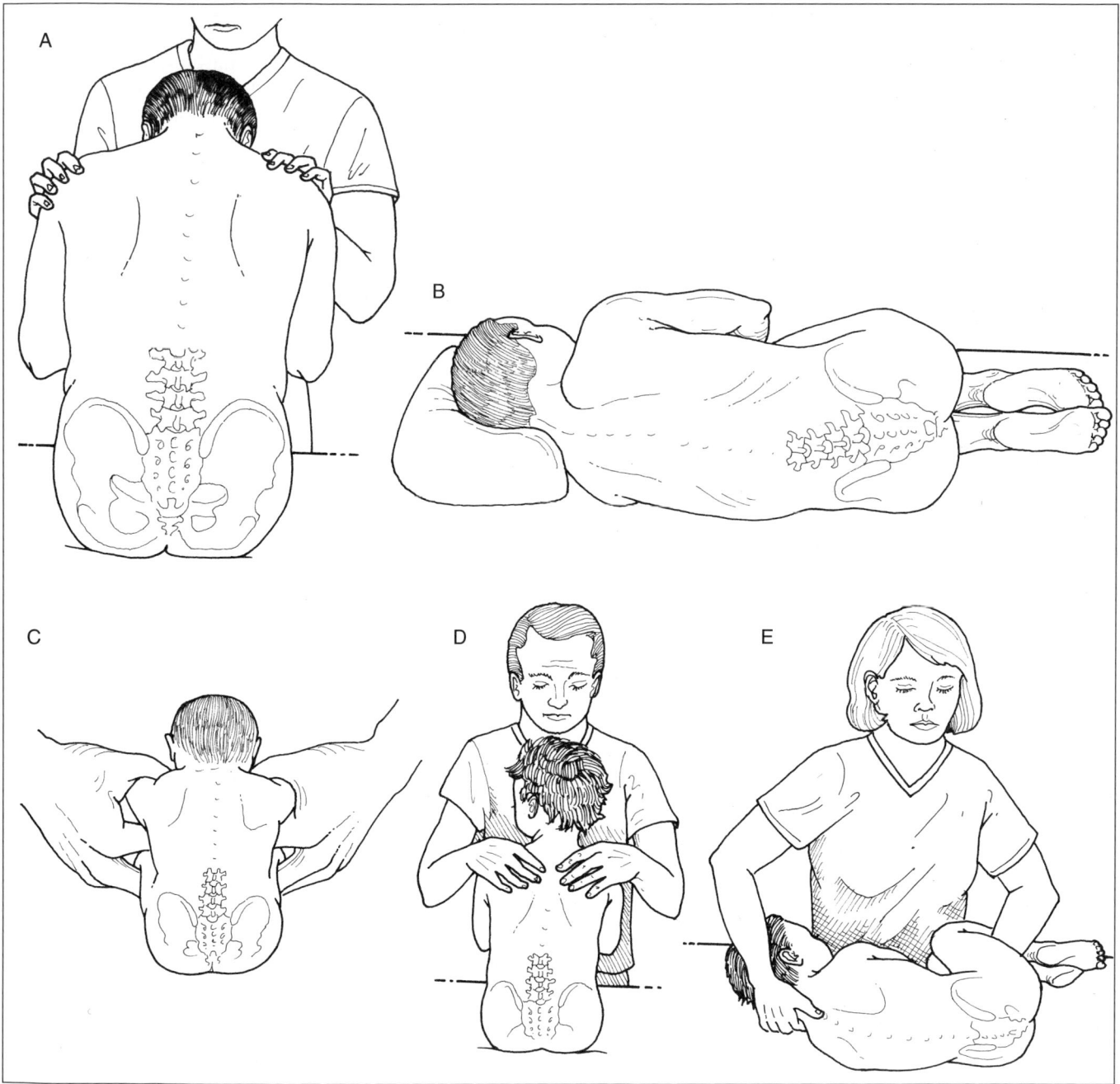

FIGURE 96-5 Patient positioning for a lumbar puncture. *A.* An adult in the sitting position. *B.* An adult in the lateral decubitus position. *C.* An infant restrained in the sitting position. *D.* A child restrained in the sitting position. *E.* A child restrained in the lateral decubitus position.

The sitting position is more commonly used in adults than the lateral decubitus position. It is easier to identify the midline and palpate the spinous processes with the patient sitting (Figure 96-5A). The sitting position is particularly useful when patients are obese. While the lumbar puncture can still be performed in the lateral decubitus position for obese patients, palpating the spinous processes and identifying the midline can be difficult. The measurement of hydrostatic pressure in the CSF is not accurate with the patient sitting. It gives a falsely elevated pressure reading.

The lateral decubitus position is often the most comfortable position for the patient (Figure 96-5B). Place the patient with their knees flexed, the upper back arched to spread the interlaminar spaces, and the neck slightly flexed. Ensure that the patient's shoulders, back, and hips are exactly perpendicular to the stretcher and floor. This will increase the chances of keeping the needle in the midline as it is introduced parallel to the surface of the stretcher. This is particularly important in infants and children where an assistant may be called upon to hold the patient in position. Severe neck flexion is not necessary and can lead to airway obstruction or lack of CSF flow.

Children can be placed in the sitting or lateral decubitus position. An assistant can easily maintain neonates and infants in the sitting position (Figure 96-5C). Toddlers and school-aged children can also often be maintained in the sitting position (Figure 96-5D). The lateral decubitus position can be used for any child (Figure 96-5E). **It is important to assess the child visually and with pulse oximetry during the procedure. These positions may cause respiratory difficulty resulting in oxygen desaturation and hypoxemia.**

The subarachnoid space must be entered below the termination of the spinal cord that is situated at the lower level of L1 or the body of L2 (Figure 96-6). Identify by palpation the vertebral spinous processes in the midline and the posterior superior iliac spines. An imaginary line connecting the posterior superior iliac spines should intersect the midline at approximately the L4 spinous process or the L3-L4 interspace. One can select any of the spaces between L2-L3 to L5-S1 to perform the lumbar puncture. Palpate the intended interspace before prepping the area. Some physicians mark the site lightly with a pen or make a small indentation with the hub of a needle. Adjust the bed height so that you can sit in a comfortable position while performing the procedure.

Prepare the lumbar puncture kit. Open the kit using sterile technique and place it on a bedside table. Place povidone iodine solution into the basin provided with the kit. Place any additional needles or supplies onto the sterile field. Apply sterile gloves and prepare the stopcock and manometer. The manometer is usually in two pieces that slide together. Insert the manometer into the vertical port of the stopcock. Turn the handle toward the outflow side of the stopcock. In general, the stopcock handle will occlude the port that it points to.

Prepare the patient's back. Clean the skin of any dirt and debris. Apply povidone iodine using a circular motion from the intended site of entry outward. Prepare an area of at least 10 cm in diameter. Most kits include a solid drape and a fenestrated drape. Place the solid drape between the patient's hip and the bed. Place the fenestrated drape with the adhesive side towards the patient's back and the opening centered at the desired level for the procedure.

Reidentify the anatomic landmarks. Place a finger over the desired interspace to use for the procedure. Place a skin wheal of local anesthetic solution subcutaneously over the desired interspace using a 25 gauge needle. Infiltrate and anesthetize the deeper tissue of the interspace along the projected needle track using the 22 gauge needle.

Alternatively, a field block can easily be performed to produce anesthesia of the skin, interspinous ligaments and muscles, and the periosteum. The interspinous ligament and the periosteum are supplied by the recurrent spinal nerves branching off the nerve roots exiting the spinal canal at the same level. Inject local anesthetic solution into the interspinous ligaments, between the spinous processes superior and inferior to the intended puncture site, and on either side of the interspinous space (Figure 96-7).[27] A topical anesthetic (e.g., EMLA cream) may be applied over the interspace for 30 to 60 minutes prior to performing the lumbar puncture if the patient is awaiting a CT scan of the head and antibiotics have been administered. Unfortunately, this only anesthetizes the skin and superficial subcutaneous structures. The patient will still require an anesthetic injection.

TECHNIQUES

LATERAL DECUBITUS POSITION AND MIDLINE APPROACH

Palpate the intended interspace. Introduce the needle in the middle of the interspace and parallel to the bed. **Orient the bevel parallel to the longitudinal dural fibers to increase the chances that the fibers will be separated rather than cut by the tip of the needle.** This has been shown to decrease the incidence of postdural puncture headache.[30–32] The bevel should point up or down with the patient in the lateral decubitus position. Angle the needle 10 degrees cephalad, or towards the umbilicus, and advance it slowly. The needle can be held between both index fingers and advanced with the thumbs (Figure 96-8A). Alternatively, it can be guided with a thumb and forefinger near the puncture site while

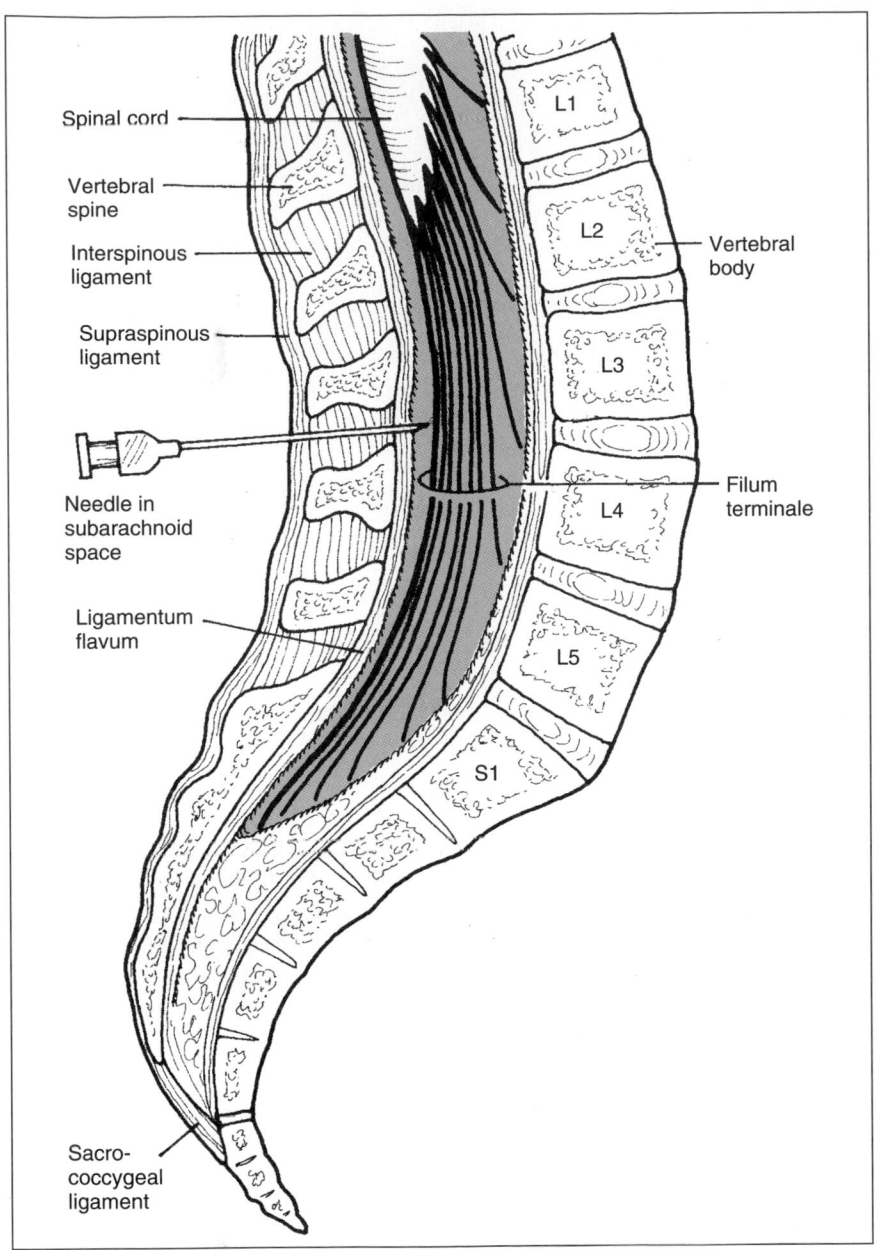

FIGURE 96-6 Midsagittal section of the lumbosacral region with a spinal needle in the L3-L4 interspace. The needle has penetrated the supraspinal ligament, the interspinous ligament, the ligamentum flavum, the dura mater, and the arachnoid mater.

the other hand holds the hub of the needle and advances it (Figure 96-8*B*).

Resistance will be felt as the needle penetrates the interspinous ligaments. Stop advancing the needle and remove the stylet frequently to check for the presence of CSF. Many describe a characteristic "pop" that is felt when the needle enters the subarachnoid space. The commonly used Quincke needles often decrease or eliminate this sensation. If bone is encountered, withdraw the needle to the subcutaneous tissue, confirm your landmarks, and readvance the needle in the midline. If bone is still encountered, redirect the needle slightly more cephalad and readvance it. Perform the procedure at a different level if still unsuccessful.

CSF should flow freely once the subarachnoid space is entered. Attach the stopcock and manometer directly to the needle. Alternatively, use the short extension tubing provided in most kits to connect the needle to the manometer. **Hold the hub of the needle firmly between the thumb and index finger and brace your hand against the patient's back when attaching or removing anything from the spinal needle.** This will prevent the needle from advancing or withdrawing. The stopcock handle should point posteriorly and CSF will begin to fill the manometer. **Ensure that the manometer hub remains at the level of the needle in order to get an accurate reading if using the extension tubing.** Phasic changes with respirations should be noted as the

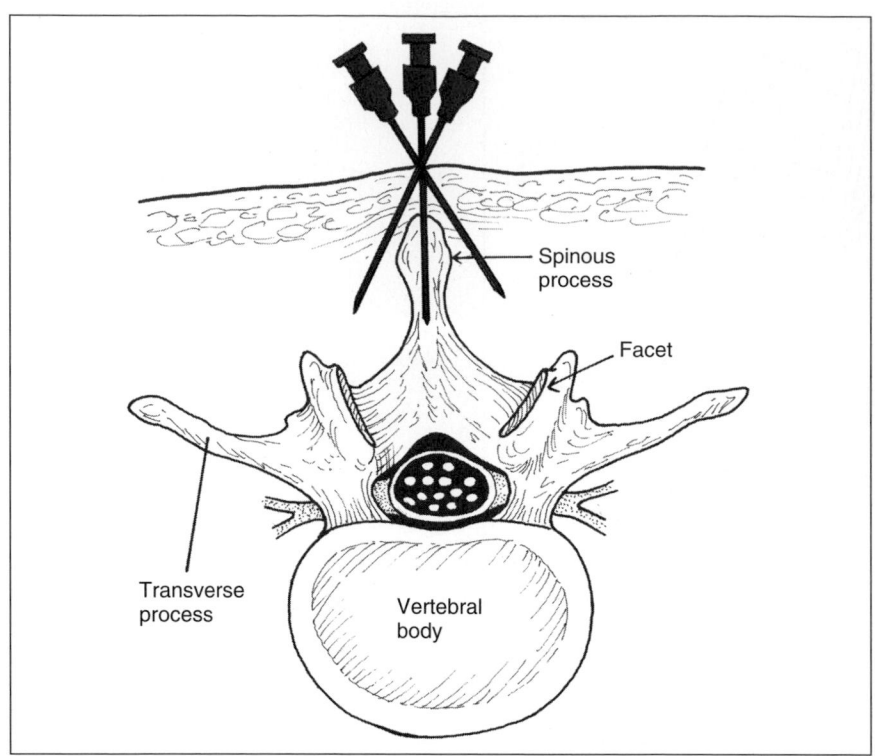

FIGURE 96-7 Field block for lumbar puncture anesthesia.

manometer fills. Instruct the patient, or an assistant, to gently extend the patient's legs to decrease intraabdominal pressure and lower the reading. Normal opening pressure is 70 to 180 mmH$_2$O. Obtain the pressure reading once the CSF flow stops. Turn the stopcock handle towards the needle hub (or patient) to empty the contents of the manometer into the first tube for collection. To continue collection, remove the stopcock or simply remove the manometer and continue collection through the stopcock by pointing the handle towards the manometer port.

In general, 1.0 mL of CSF in each of the four tubes should be adequate to perform the CSF analysis. Collect 2 mL in each tube if cytology or antigen testing is necessary. When the samples have been collected, replace the stylet and remove the needle.

SITTING POSITION AND MIDLINE APPROACH

Place the patient sitting on the edge of the bed. Ask the patient to flex the lower back and lean forward onto some support, such as an assistant or bedside stand, in order to open the interlaminar spaces in the lumbar area. Orient the bevel of the needle laterally (to the left or right). The remainder of the procedure is the same as previously described.

LATERAL APPROACH

The lateral approach may be useful in avoiding the calcified supraspinous and interspinous ligaments often encountered in elderly patients. This approach may be performed with the patient in the lateral decubitus position or the sitting position. Though it is less commonly used than the midline approach, it is a good idea for the Emergency Physician to become familiar with this technique as an alternate approach if the midline approach has failed. This may prove easier in the patient who has had multiple previous midline lumbar punctures.

Position the patient and select an appropriate interspace. Cleanse, drape, and anesthetize the area as previously described. Insert the spinal needle 1.5 to 2.0 cm lateral to the midline. The needle can approach from either side (left or right) if the procedure is being performed in the sitting position. Approach from the inferior side if performing the LP in the lateral decubitus position (Figure 96-9A). Direct the needle 10 degrees cephalad and approximately 20 degrees to the midline. This angle will direct the needle through the erector spinae muscles and lateral to the supraspinous and interspinous ligaments. The needle will penetrate the ligamentum flavum, the dura, and then the subarachnoid space (Figure 96-9B). If bone is encountered, partially withdraw the needle and redirect it at the same angle towards the midline but slightly more cephalad. The remainder of the procedure is as described previously.

LUMBAR PUNCTURE IN INFANTS AND CHILDREN

Performing a lumbar puncture in an infant or child is similar to that of an adult. Place the patient in the lateral

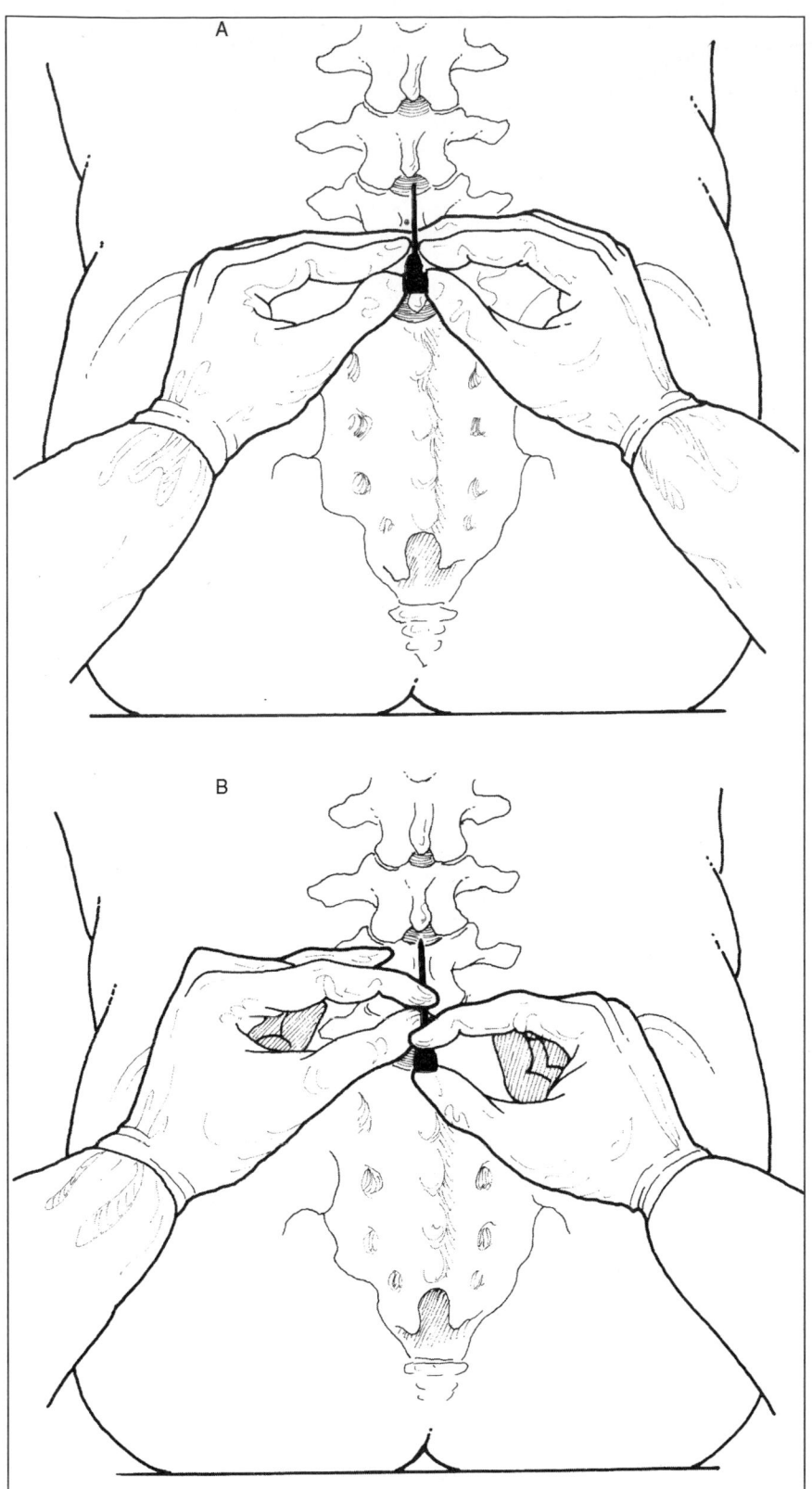

FIGURE 96-8 Two-handed techniques for spinal needle insertion. *A.* The index fingers guide the tip while the thumbs advance the needle. *B.* An alternative technique. One hand is placed at the needle tip and the other is at the base of the needle.

decubitus position or the sitting position. Place the neck in midflexion in the lateral decubitus position. Severe flexion of the neck does not facilitate the procedure and can result in the lack of CSF flow or airway obstruction.

Hypoxemia has been reported during lumbar puncture in infants. The increased intraabdominal pressure caused by flexing the knees into the abdomen may lead to compression of the diaphragm, ventilation-perfusion

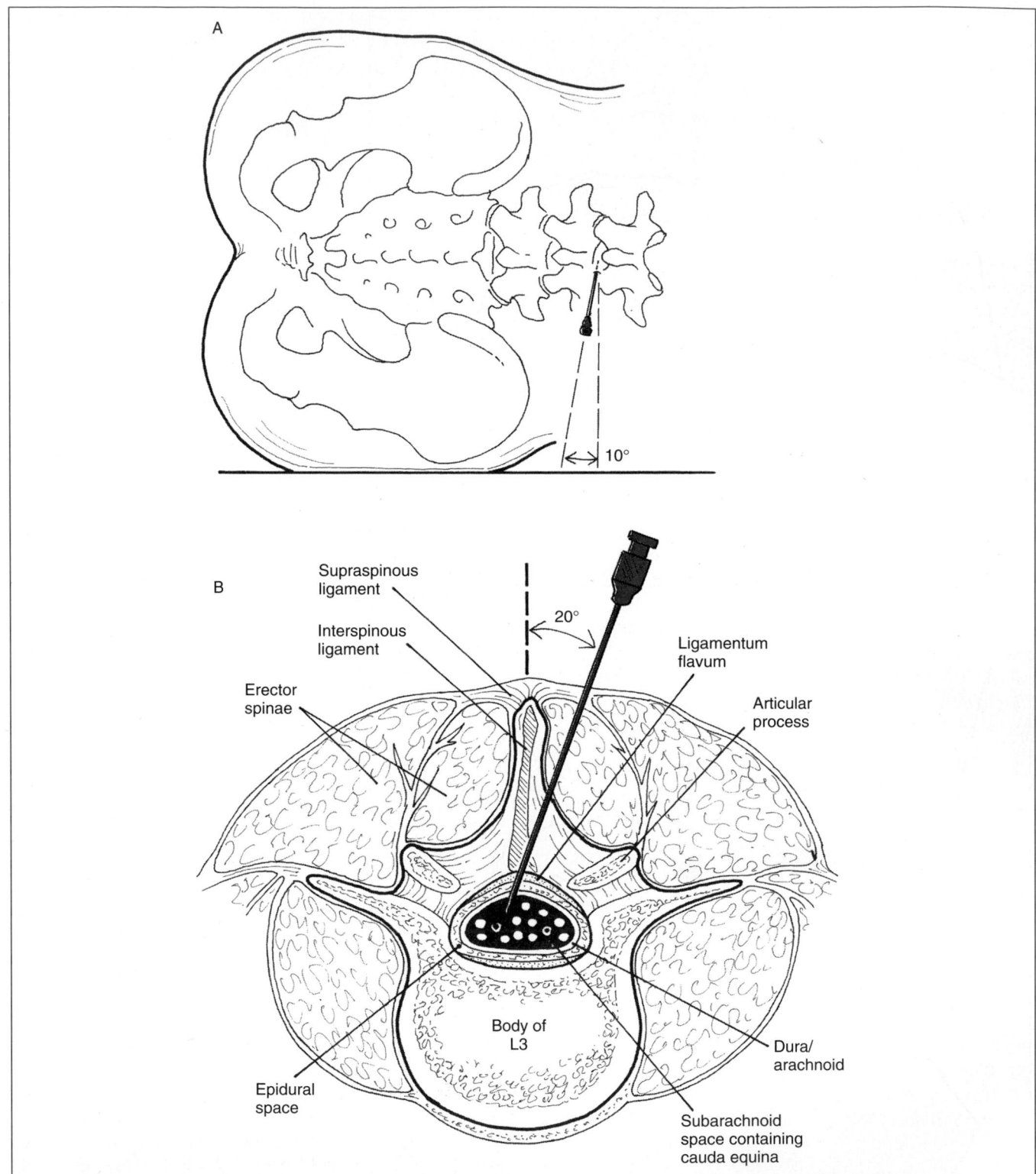

FIGURE 96-9 The lateral approach. *A.* If the patient is in the lateral decubitus position, insert the spinal needle approximately 2 cm below the midline and directed approximately 20 degrees towards the midline, and 10 degrees cephalad. *B.* Cross-section of the spinal column showing the path of the spinal needle during the lateral approach. Notice that it avoids the calcified supraspinal and interspinal ligaments.

mismatch, and hypoxemia.[33] For this reason, the sitting position or modified lateral decubitus position (hips only flexed to 90 degrees) is preferred.[34] Preoxygenation with 100 percent oxygen via face mask for 2 to 5 minutes may prevent hypoxemia.[35] **Consider the use of continuous pulse oximetry in infants and young children undergoing a lumbar puncture.**

Some authors advocate the use of a butterfly needle and using the tubing as a manometer to get a general idea of the opening pressure. The use of nonstyletted needles, however, may occasionally result in the implantation of cells and a subsequent epidermoid tumor. In some low intracranial pressure syndromes, CSF may fail to flow during the procedure and gentle suction with a 1 mL syringe can be used.

Local anesthesia should be used in all patients, even in neonates. There is evidence that pain perception is present even in premature neonates.[36] The use of local anesthetic is often omitted in the neonate and young infant, possibly in fear of obscuring anatomical landmarks. Pinheiro et al studied the success rate of lumbar puncture in neonates given local anesthetic, the amount of struggling during lidocaine injection, and the amount of struggling during spinal needle insertion.[37] They found that local anesthesia did not alter the success rate of the procedure and led to a decreased amount of struggling during spinal needle insertion.

The use of a eutectic mixture of local anesthetics (EMLA) cream or similar topical anesthetic is common and effective for venipuncture in children. It also can be used successfully before lumbar puncture in children and adults.[38,39] EMLA has been shown in some studies on adults to be more effective than lidocaine infiltration.[40,41] The major disadvantage of EMLA cream is that it requires application for a minimum of 30 minutes before the procedure is performed. In general, it is more effective if it stays on longer. It also does not anesthetize the deeper tissues and local infiltration is still required.

Procedural sedation is usually reserved for those children getting routine lumbar punctures for intrathecal chemotherapy. If absolutely necessary, procedural sedation can be used while performing a diagnostic lumbar puncture. Procedural sedation should not be used unless the child has a normal mental status and is hemodynamically stable. The decision regarding procedural sedation must be considered on a case-by-case basis.

AFTERCARE

Clean the excess povidone iodine from the patient's back and apply a dressing or bandage to the puncture site. Immediately place the patient supine to decrease the potential for postdural puncture headache and decrease the risk of local bleeding. Recumbent positioning will decrease the postural headache that sometimes follows lumbar puncture, but it has not been shown to decrease the incidence of postdural puncture headache.

COMPLICATIONS

The use of proper technique is essential when performing a lumbar puncture. It is also important that the physician is aware of potential complications, how to recognize them, and how to manage the complications that can result from a lumbar puncture. Refer to the article by Evans for a complete review of the recent literature on lumbar puncture complications.[42] Postdural puncture headache is the most common complication and cerebral herniation is the most immediately life-threatening. Localized cellulitis, dural abscesses, discitis, and localized bleeding are also potential problems.

CEREBRAL HERNIATION

The most serious complication that may result from a lumbar puncture is brain herniation or coning. Theoretically, if a large pressure gradient exists between the cranial and lumbar compartments, herniation across the tentorial incisura or foramen magnum may occur after removal of CSF from the lumbar area. Patients with increased intracranial pressure secondary to intracranial mass lesions, cerebral edema, and acute hydrocephalus are at greater risk for cerebral herniation or coning. Herniation has also been known to occur in patients with meningitis. For many years, the role of lumbar puncture in precipitating brain herniation has been the subject of debate. Several studies suggest that lumbar puncture is relatively safe in the patient with increased intracranial pressure.[43–45] However, each individual patient's risks and benefits must be considered before proceeding.

Herniation has resulted from lumbar puncture in patients with meningitis and subarachnoid hemorrhage.[46–48] The actual role that lumbar puncture has in precipitating or facilitating the process of herniation is not known.[46] **Patients with decorticate or decerebrate posture, focal neurologic signs, or no response to pain should receive antibiotics but not a lumbar puncture; this is true even in the face of a normal CT in suspected cases of meningitis.**[46,48] Deterioration after lumbar puncture has been reported in patients with a subarachnoid hemorrhage. Fortunately, it is a rare outcome as a result of lumbar puncture. **A CT scan should be obtained before performing a lumbar puncture if there is a suspicion for subarachnoid hemorrhage.**[49,50]

POSTDURAL PUNCTURE HEADACHE (PDPH)

PDPH is the most common complication of a lumbar puncture. It is thought to be the result of continued CSF leakage at the puncture site. The reason why this causes a headache is unclear. It is thought that the lower CSF pressure induced by the leakage causes the brain to "sag." This leads to traction on pain-sensitive structures in the brain such as the dura, nerves, and bridging veins. Intracranial venous dilation and increased brain volume may lead to a neurohumoral response identified as pain.

The headache begins within 24 hours of the procedure in 65 percent of cases and within 48 hours in 90 percent of cases. Delayed development of a PDPH 5 to 14 days after the procedure has been reported. The headache typically resolves within 7 days. It has been reported to last several months in rare individuals. The headache is usually located in the frontal or occipital area. It may vary in intensity. The PDPH is usually described as bilateral pressure that is throbbing or achy and improves with supine positioning. Associated symptoms may include nausea, vomiting, neck stiffness, auditory symptoms, and vestibular symptoms.[51]

The incidence of PDPH has been reported to be anywhere from 1 to 70 percent. The wide range is most likely due to the fact there are several identifiable risk factors that influence its development. Age and gender play a significant role.[51–53] The highest incidence occurs in the 18 to 30 year old range. There seems to be a decreased incidence after the age of 60, the reason for which is unknown.

The type of needle and its diameter also influence the development of PDPH. This is based upon the amount of trauma and the size of the rent it makes in the dura. Smaller diameter needles and atraumatic needles lower the incidence of PDPH. However, a 22 or larger gauge needle must be used to determine the opening pressure and to collect samples in a timely fashion when performing a diagnostic lumbar puncture.[54] The bevel orientation should be parallel to the longitudinal dural fibers when using a Quincke needle. This significantly reduces the incidence of PDPH.[55,56,32] The use of an atraumatic needle may also decrease the incidence of PDPH.[57,58] These needles are designed to separate rather than shear the dural fibers. Replacement of the stylet before removing the spinal needle has been shown to decrease the incidence of PDPH.[59] Repeated dural punctures have been associated with an increase in the incidence of PDPH.[60]

Other nonproven risk factors for a PDPH include psychogenic factors, the rapidity of CSF withdrawal, race, patient positioning, and hydration status. Bed rest for 24 hours is still widely recommended. However, it has not been shown to decrease the incidence of PDPH.[61–63] Other studies have shown bed rest to increase the risk of PDPH.[64,65] Dehydration was once felt to impair the patient's ability to produce CSF to compensate for the leaking CSF. Dieterich and Brandt found that the incidence of PDPH was independent of daily fluid intake.[66] They

postulated that it is the closure of the dural defect and not the CSF loss that is the critical factor in the termination of the PDPH.

Supine positioning can provide some symptomatic relief for initial or mild PDPHs. A single 300 mg dose of oral caffeine may provide transient relief.[67] While offering no advantage over caffeine, an oral dose of theophylline can also be given. Administer 500 mg of intravenous caffeine, or 5 to 6 mg/kg of intravenous aminophylline, for more severe headaches. In the only study to date describing the use of intravenous caffeine, Sechzer and Abel reported an approximately 70 percent success rate in treating PDPH.[68] A more recent study suggests that intravenous caffeine administered prophylactically may minimize the incidence of PDPH.[69] There is some promise in the use of sumatriptan.[70] These authors reported initial relief of the PDPH in six of six cases. The headache recurred in two of the patients, one of which was relieved by a second injection.

A more definitive but invasive treatment for the PDPH is the epidural blood patch. This procedure is to be performed by an Anesthesiologist. It involves injecting 10 to 20 mL of autologous blood into the epidural space at the level of the previous lumbar puncture. The blood acts to tamponade any further CSF leakage and allows healing of the dural rent. Epidural blood patching is successful in 85 percent of patients after one injection and about 98 percent of patients if a second blood patch is required.[71–73] Epidural blood patching should be performed no sooner than 24 hours after the lumbar puncture. Complications of the blood patch include back pain, paresthesias, radiculopathies, and weakness; all of which are transient. A rare complication is the spinal subdural hematoma.[74] Other modalities for PDPH relief that have been used but not widely studied are epidural saline injections, dextrose injections, gelatin injections, and epidural morphine.

INFECTIONS

Local infections including cellulitis, abscesses (lumbar epidural or spinal cord), and discitis can result from a lumbar puncture. Performing a lumbar puncture through an area with a local infection, such as a cellulitis or an abscess, can introduce bacteria into the CSF and lead to meningitis. Contamination of the needle by airborne pathogens can also occur. Always wear a mask while performing a lumbar puncture.

It was once thought that a lumbar puncture could induce meningitis in a bacteremic patient. Further studies have shown this idea to be unfounded.[75–77] **Bacteremia is not a contraindication to performing a lumbar puncture.** Proper cleaning and disinfecting of the skin, avoiding infected areas with the spinal needle, and using sterile technique will minimize any risk of infection.

HEMORRHAGE

Traumatic lumbar puncture is a common occurrence. Up to 72 percent of lumbar punctures have anywhere from 1 to over 50 red blood cells.[78] This is a common and usually uncomplicated occurrence in patients with normal coagulation. Traumatic lumbar puncture can result in a spinal epidural or spinal subdural hematoma in patients with coagulation abnormalities. Epidural hematomas most likely result from needle trauma to the internal vertebral plexus or radicular vessels (Figure 96-10).[78] The radicular vessels course down the length of each nerve root. It has been suggested that the bevel of the spinal needle can induce trauma and bleeding to these vessels much like they produce paresthesias when touching the nerve roots.

Subdural or subarachnoid hemorrhage is a rare but catastrophic complication in patients with a coagulopathy. Edelson et al recommend that the procedure be performed only if absolutely necessary in patient's with thrombocytopenia.[79] Platelets should be transfused prior to lumbar puncture in patients with platelet counts less than 20,000 or if platelet counts are dropping rapidly. The most skilled physician should perform the lumbar puncture using a 22 gauge (or smaller) needle.[79] Patients should be observed after the procedure for the development of neurological signs suggesting a hematoma. Such signs include paraplegia, lower extremity weakness, sensory deficits, or incontinence.

Another rare bleeding complication is an intracranial subdural hematoma.[80,81] This may result from the same mechanism causing PDPH, namely downward displacement of the brain from decreased CSF volume and persistent leakage after lumbar puncture. This may occasionally cause tearing of the bridging veins and lead to a unilateral or bilateral subdural hematoma. Suspect this diagnosis when a headache sounding like a PDPH lasts

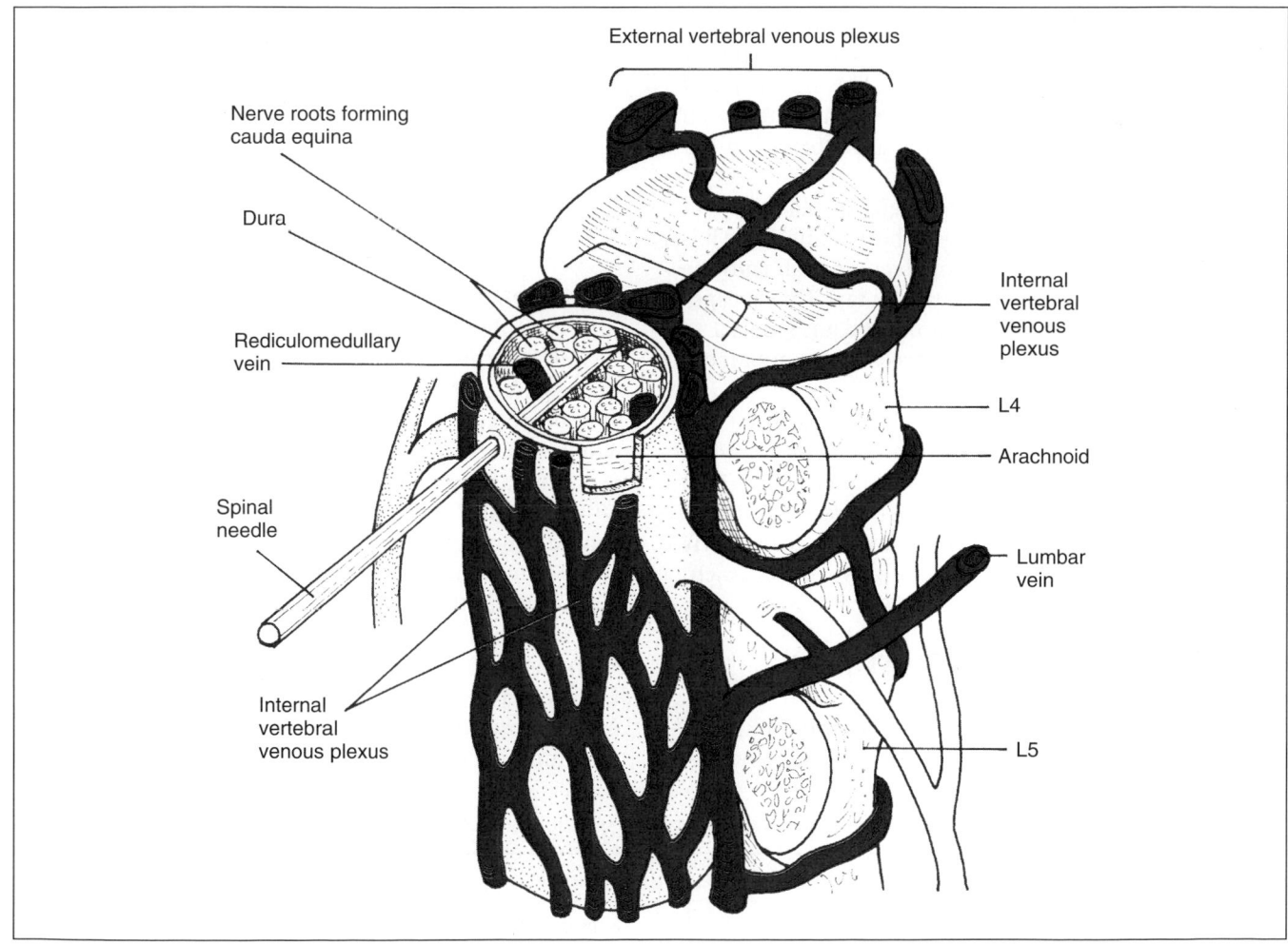

FIGURE 96-10 Illustration of the spinal cord and the potential sources of needle-induced bleeding. In patients with coagulation abnormalities or thrombocytopenia, needle-induced injury to the internal vertebral plexus could lead to spinal epidural hematomas. Note, however, that the correct path of the needle should usually avoid the internal vertebral venous plexus. The needle may lacerate the small radicular vessels that accompany each nerve root of the cauda equina when it enters the subarachnoid space. This is the most likely source of most needle-induced bleeding. This can lead to spinal subdural hematomas in patients with coagulation defects or thrombocytopenia.

for more than a week, is no longer postural in nature, or returns after initially improving.[82]

MISCELLANEOUS COMPLICATIONS

Neuropathies involving cranial nerves III, IV, V, VI, VII, and VIII have been reported. They most likely result from traction on the nerves caused by low intracranial pressure after the lumbar puncture. Typical complaints may include visual and auditory symptoms.

Mild low back pain is a common complaint that results from the local trauma of the needle tract. Transient dysesthesias are fairly common, resulting from needle contact with the nerve roots. A needle that passes beyond the subarachnoid space into the annulus fibrosis can cause disc herniation. This can also result in discitis and vertebral collapse.[83]

Intraspinal epidermoid tumors are composed of well-differentiated stratified squamous epithelium surrounding a mass of caseous substance formed by the desquamation of epidermal tissue. They are often congenital but may result from the introduction of epidermal fragments into the spinal canal. This may occur if the stylet of the needle is not used. Spinal epidermoid tumors may present months to years after a lumbar puncture.[84,85]

A dry tap is often the result of lateral displacement of the needle. Maintain the needle in the midline while it is being advanced. Not penetrating deep enough with the spinal needle can also result in a dry tap. This is especially true in obese patients that may require long, 7 to 10 inch, spinal needles to gain access to the subarachnoid space.

Prevent secondary injury by always inserting the stylet into the spinal needle before removing it. Withdrawing the spinal needle without the stylet can result in the aspiration of a lumbar nerve root or arachnoid tissue into the epidural space. If this occurs, the patient will require a laminectomy to replace the nerve root or arachnoid tissue.

CSF INTERPRETATION

Proper interpretation of the CSF is an important skill for the physician who performs the lumbar puncture.

Table 96-1 and Table 96-2 list the normal CSF values and the CSF values in a variety of different medical conditions.[86,87]

CSF PRESSURE

Normal CSF pressure ranges from 70 to 180 mmH_2O in adults and from 50 to 80 mmH_2O in infants and children. Note that many manometer kits use cmH_2O on the demarcations whereas results are commonly interpreted in mmH_2O. Elevated CSF pressure may be seen in bacterial meningitis, viral meningitis, brain abscesses, tuberculous meningitis, fungal meningitis, encephalitis, meningeal carcinomatosis, subarachnoid hemorrhage, pseudotumor cerebri, and Guillain-Barré syndrome. It may be falsely elevated when the patient is tense or creating a lot of intraabdominal pressure by flexing their knees into the abdomen. The pressure will also be falsely elevated if the patient is in a sitting position. Although CSF pressure is not routinely recorded in infants and children (most likely because they are often crying, struggling, or difficult to hold), it should be recorded whenever possible. Low CSF pressure may be the result of a spinal root obstructing the flow of CSF into the needle or obstruction of flow from a spinal mass.

CELL COUNTS AND DIFFERENTIAL

A variable amount of white blood cells (WBCs) may be normally present in the CSF depending upon the age of the patient. Neonates may have up to 32 WBCs/mm³ with 60 percent polymorphonuclear leukocytes. Infants 4 to 8 weeks of age may have up to 22 WBCs/mm³. However, most sources consider anything greater than 8 to 10 WBCs/mm³ to be abnormal.[88,89] Normal adult CSF should contain no more than 5 WBCs/mm³ with a differential of mononuclear cells or lymphocytes. The presence of more than one polymorphonuclear cell should be considered abnormal.

In cases of bacterial meningitis, cell counts are usually greater than 500 WBCs/mm³ with a predominance of polymorphonuclear cells; though lymphocytosis can uncommonly occur.[90] The CSF will usually contain less

TABLE 96-1. NORMAL CSF VALUES. ADAPTED FROM REFERENCE 86

	Preterm infant	Term infant	Child	Adult
White blood cell count (WBC/mm³)	9 (range 0–32) 57% PMNs	8 (range 0–22) 61% PMNs	0–7 0% PMNs	0–5 0% PMNs
Glucose (mg/dL)	24–63 (mean 50)	34–119 (mean 52)	40–80	50–80
CSF/blood glucose ratio				
Normal ratio	55–105%	44–128%	50%	60–70%
Abnormal ratio	< 0.5–0.6	< 0.5–0.6	< 0.4–0.5	< 0.4–0.5
Protein (mg/dL)	65–150 (mean 115)	20–170 (mean 90)	5–40	15–45

TABLE 96-2. CSF VALUES IN VARIOUS NEUROLOGICAL CONDITIONS. ADAPTED FROM REFERENCE 87

Condition	Appearance	Pressure	Cell count (mm³)	Glucose (mg/dL)	Protein (mg/dL)
Bacterial meningitis	Clear, cloudy, or purulent	Elevated	500–10,000+ cells with 90–95% PMNs	0–40	>50
Partially treated bacterial meningitis	Possibly cloudy	Normal or elevated	1–500 cells, lymphs or monos may predominate	Low or normal	>50 and <500
Brain abscess	Clear, cloudy, or purulent	Elevated	Possibly >100,000 cells if abscess ruptures. PMNs predominate.	Normal	<200
Tuberculous meningitis	Clear, opalescent, or ground glass	Elevated	25–500 WBCs, PMNs early but usually lymphs predominate	10–40	50–500
Fungal meningitis	Clear or cloudy	Elevated	10–500 WBCs, lymphs predominate. PMNs early.	<40	<600
Viral meningitis or encephalitis	Clear, may have faint opalescence	Normal or elevated	6–1000 cells, predominance of lymphs. PMNs early.	Normal but may be low with herpes or mumps	<200
Acute syphilitic meningitis and leptospirosis	Clear or turbid	Elevated	100–500 WBCs, usually lymphs	Normal or decreased	<200
Meningeal carcinomatosis	Clear or mucinous	Elevated	10–500 WBCs, lymphs predominate	<40	<500
Subarachnoid hemorrhage	Bloody, xanthochromia, clear	Elevated	1000–3.5 × 10⁶ RBCs	Normal, but can be decreased in 10–15% of cases	Increased
Multiple sclerosis	Clear	Normal	0–20 lymphocytes, >50 rare	Normal	45–75
Progressive multifocal leukoencephalopathy	Clear	Normal	<10 monos	Normal	Normal
Guillain-Barré syndrome	Clear or xanthochromic	Normal or elevated	Normal, but 10–200 WBCs, predominantly lymphs	Normal	May be as high as 1000
Pseudotumor cerebri	Clear	Elevated	Normal	Normal	Normal
Subacute sclerosing panencephalitis	Clear	Normal	Usually normal	Normal	Increased, check CSF measles titers & CSF gamma-globulin
Neuro-Behçet's syndrome	Clear	Normal or elevated	Up to 3000 WBCs, PMNs predominate	Normal	Increased

than 1000 WBCs/mm^3 in patients with viral meningitis and have a differential of 100 percent lymphocytes. Early in the course of viral meningitis (< 48 hours), 20 to 75 percent of patients will have a predominance of polymorphonuclear cells in the CSF, making it difficult to distinguish it from bacterial meningitis.[91] Within 8 to 12 hours, approximately 90 percent of patients will show a switch to a mononuclear pleocytosis on repeat lumbar puncture.[92]

Normal cell counts and differentials do not always exclude meningitis. Approximately 95 percent of the population does not normally have any polymorphonuclear leukocytes (PMNs) in their CSF. The presence of one PMN could represent an abnormality. One polymorphonuclear leukocyte may be seen in approximately 5 percent of normal children. Bonadio and colleagues reviewed 424 lumbar punctures of which 106 had PMNs but no pleocytosis.[93] All 106 patients had negative Gram's stains and cultures. The authors concluded that the older child without pleocytosis or abnormal CSF chemistries can be considered at very low risk for meningitis. If meningitis is suspected and the CSF is normal or has PMNs, close clinical observation and hospitalization for treatment and repeat lumbar puncture should be considered until CSF culture results are negative.

A traumatic lumbar puncture can often make the interpretation of the CSF difficult as peripheral WBCs can be introduced into the CSF. Clearing of the red hue of the CSF from the first to last tube suggests that the tap was traumatic. However, this is not always a reliable sign. Traditionally, the ratio of the RBCs to the WBCs in the blood is compared to the ratio in the CSF. This is based upon the assumption that when blood is introduced into the CSF, the ratio of RBCs to WBCs should stay the same. Some physicians use a set RBC to WBC ratio of 750:1 or 500:1. This is not always accurate as a peripheral leukocytosis may often be present. By comparing the ratios, a predicted WBC count for the CSF can be obtained (predicted CSF WBC = CSF RBC × blood WBC ÷ blood RBC). The actual WBC count will then be the predicted WBC subtracted from the observed or measured WBC (actual CSF WBC = observed CSF WBC − predicted CSF WBC).

Most studies on patients with traumatic taps that did not have meningitis have shown that these formulae are often inaccurate. Oftentimes, the observed CSF WBC count is less that the predicted CSF WBC count. This raises concerns that in the presence of meningitis, the diagnosis could be missed. Mayefsky and Roghmann studied the use of the formula in patients that had meningitis and found that it led to a lot of false-positive and false-negative results.[94] They investigated the value of an O:P ratio (observed CSF WBC/predicted CSF WBC) in predicting the presence of meningitis. They found that a ratio greater than 10 had a sensitivity of 88 percent and a specificity of 90 percent in predicting culture posi-

tive meningitis. They concluded, along with others, that pleocytosis in bacterial meningitis is rarely masked by a traumatic tap.[94,95]

GLUCOSE

Normal values for CSF glucose are listed in Table 96-1. Compare the ratio of CSF glucose to simultaneously determined blood glucose levels to determine if low CSF glucose (hypoglycorrhachia) exists. The ratio is abnormal in preterm infants if it is lower than 0.5 to 0.6. A ratio of less than 0.4 to 0.5 in children and adults is abnormal. Approximately 58 percent of patients with bacterial meningitis will have a glucose of < 40 mg/dL. The sensitivity for detecting bacterial meningitis increases to about 70 percent if a CSF-to-serum glucose ratio of < 0.31 is used.[96] The normal steady state of 0.6 tends to decrease as serum glucose increases. Ratios of less than 0.3 should be considered abnormal in cases of severe hyperglycemia. The CSF-to-serum glucose ratio is less accurate when there are rapid changes in the serum glucose. **A low CSF-to-serum glucose ratio should always raise the concern of bacterial or fungal meningitis.** Other conditions such as tuberculous or syphilitic meningitis, meningeal carcinomatosis, or subarachnoid hemorrhage can also be the etiology. Approximately 15 to 20 percent of patients with a subarachnoid hemorrhage will have hypoglycorrhachia.[97,98] Normal CSF-to-serum glucose ratios are usually seen with aseptic meningitis, encephalitis, brain abscesses, and subdural empyemas.

PROTEIN

The normal CSF protein levels are listed in Table 96-1. Elevated CSF protein levels, often greater than 150 mg/dL, are seen in acute bacterial meningitis. Others causes of increased CSF protein include any type of meningitis, encephalitis, CNS tumors, subarachnoid hemorrhage, demyelinating syndromes, and traumatic lumbar puncture.[99] Correct the CSF protein by subtracting 1 mg/dL of protein for each 1000 RBCs in traumatic lumbar punctures.

GRAM'S STAIN

The Gram's stain is a very reliable test when performed by properly trained individuals. In general, it is positive in identifying approximately 80 percent of bacterial CNS infections.[100] The probability of detecting bacteria on a Gram's stain depends upon the number of bacteria present in the CSF.[101] Approximately 25 percent of smears are positive with ≤ 10^3 colony-forming units (CFU)/mL, 60 percent with 10^3 to 10^5 CFU/mL, and 97 percent with > 10^5 CFU/mL. False negatives can result from partially treated meningitis where the sensitivity decreases to about 60 percent.[102] False positives can result from the use of contaminated lumbar puncture trays or reagents, or the use of an unoccluded spinal needle.[103]

CSF CULTURES

CSF cultures should be obtained in all patients suspected of having meningitis. Positive cultures are assumed to be 100 percent specific but may only occur in 80 percent of patients thought to have bacterial meningitis.[104] Transport the CSF specimens to the laboratory promptly, as *H. influenza* and meningococcus will not survive storage or variations in temperature. In general, antibiotics given prior to lumbar puncture can sterilize the CSF. However, depending upon the amount of bacteria in the CSF and the elapsed time from initiation of antibiotics, there is probably a window of about 2 to 3 hours where antibiotics do not affect the culture results. The percentage of positive CSF cultures decreases from 33 percent to 4 percent and Gram's stains from 41 percent to 7 percent when antibiotics are given prior to lumbar puncture.[105] Blazer et al studied the effect of full intravenous antibiotic treatment on CSF cultures by performing an initial lumbar puncture and then a repeat lumbar puncture in 44 to 66 hours.[106] All but one of the cultures became negative whereas the cytology and biochemistry were not affected. They concluded that partial treatment with antibiotics may alter the culture results but does not distort the other characteristics of a "bacterial" CSF.

SUBARACHNOID HEMORRHAGE

It is imperative to interpret the CSF results correctly when a lumbar puncture is performed after a negative head CT to rule out the possibility of a subarachnoid hemorrhage. Most sources agree that the presence of xanthochromia, which results from lysis of red blood cells, confirms the presence of intracranial bleeding.[107,108] Xanthochromia, when measured by spectrophotometry, has a sensitivity that approaches 100 percent when performed between 12 hours and 2 weeks from the initial subarachnoid hemorrhage. Others have suggested that the presence of erythrocytes alone may suggest a subarachnoid hemorrhage.

So how should patients that present within 12 hours of their symptom onset be managed? Delaying a lumbar puncture for 12 hours would require holding patients in an Emergency Department or admitting everyone who required a lumbar puncture for evaluation. This presents a legitimate logistical problem. Edlow et al suggest that patients that have a negative CT should undergo immediate lumbar puncture.[109] If the CSF is persistently bloody without xanthochromia, and clinical suspicion is high, vascular imaging should be the next step.

SUMMARY

Most lumbar punctures will be performed in suspected cases of meningitis or for subarachnoid hemorrhage after a negative head CT. The risks of performing a lumbar puncture need to be weighed against the potential benefits of diagnosing these two potentially life-threatening illnesses promptly. Knowledge of the proper indications, contraindications, technique, and interpretation of the CSF findings will undoubtedly help the physician to minimize the complications that can be associated with the procedure. Although most complications are rare, awareness of their existence, presentation, and proper treatment is imperative for any physician that performs this procedure.

REFERENCES

1. Guyton AC: *Textbook of Medical Physiology,* 7th ed. Philadelphia: Saunders, 1986:373–377.
2. Reilly BM: *Practical Strategies in Outpatient Medicine,* 2nd ed. Philadelphia: Saunders, 1991:95–100.
3. Baraff LJ, Bass JW, Fleisher GR, et al: Practice guidelines of infants and children 0 to 36 months of age with fever without source. *Pediatrics* 1997; 92(1):1–12.
4. Duffner PK, Baumann RJ: A synopsis of the American Academy of Pediatrics' practice parameters on the evaluation and treatment of children with febrile seizures. *Pediatr Rev* 1999; 20(8):285–287.
5. Offringa M, Beishuizen A, Derksen-Lubsen G, et al: Seizures and fever: can we rule out meningitis on clinical grounds alone? *Clin Pediatr* 1992; 31(9):514–522.
6. LeBlanc R: The minor leak preceding subarachnoid hemorrhage. *J Neurosurg* 1987; 66:35–39.
7. Juvela S: Minor leak before rupture of an intracranial aneurysm and subarachnoid hemorrhage of unknown etiology. *Neurosurgery* 1992; 30:7–11.
8. Van der Wee N, Rinkel GJ, Hasan D, et al: Detection of subarachnoid haemorrhage on early CT: is lumbar puncture still needed after a negative scan? *J Neurol Neurosurg Psychiatry* 1995; 58:357–359.
9. Sidman R, Connolly E, Lemke T: Subarachnoid hemorrhage diagnosis: lumbar puncture is still needed when the computed tomography scan is normal. *Acad Emerg Med* 1996; 3:827–831.
10. Kassel NF, Torner JC, Haley EC, et al: The international cooperative study on the timing of aneurysm surgery. 1. Overall management results. *J Neurosurgery* 1990; 73:18–36.
11. Adams HO, Kassell NF, Torner JC, et al: CT and clinical correlations in recent aneurysmal subarachnoid hemorrhage: a preliminary report of the cooperative aneurysm study. *Neurology* 1983; 33:981–988.
12. Brewer NS, MacCarty CS, Wellman WE: Brain abscess: a review of recent literature. *Ann Intern Med* 1975; 82:571–576.

13. Samson DS, Clark K: A current review of brain abscess. *Am J Med* 1973; 54:201–210.

14. Minns RA, Engleman HM, Stirling H: Cerebrospinal fluid pressure in pyogenic meningitis. *Arch Dis Child* 1989; 64:814–820.

15. Haslan RHA: Role of CT in management of bacterial meningitis. *J Pediatr* 1991; 119(1):157–159.

16. Cabral DA, Flodmark O, Farrell K, et al: Prospective study of computed tomography in acute bacterial meningitis. *J Pedriatr* 1987; 111:201–205.

17. Archer BD: Computed tomography before lumbar puncture in acute meningitis: a review of the risks and benefits. *CMAJ* 1993; 148(6):961–965.

18. Gopal AK, Whitehouse JD, Simel DL, et al: Cranial computed tomography before lumbar puncture. A prospective clinical evaluation. *Arch Intern Med* 1999; 159:2681–2685.

19. Baker ND, Kharazi H, Laurent L, et al: The efficacy of routine head computed tomography (CT scan) prior to lumbar puncture in the emergency department. *J Emerg Med* 1994; 12(5):597–601.

20. Gower DJ, Baker AL, Bell WO, et al: Contraindications to lumbar puncture as defined by computed cranial tomography. *J Neurol Neurosurg Psychiatry* 1987; 50:1071–1074.

21. Talan DA, Guterman JJ, Overturf GD, et al: Analysis of emergency department management of suspected bacterial meningitis. *Ann Emerg Med* 1989; 18:856–862.

22. Bryan CS, Reynolds KL, Crout L: Promptness of antibiotic therapy in acute bacterial meningitis. *Ann Emerg Med* 1986; 15:544–547.

23. Meadow WL, Lantos J, Tanz RR, et al: Ought "standard care" be the "standard of care"? *Am J Dis Child* 1993; 147(1):40–44.

24. Talan DA, Zibulewsky J: Relationship of clinical presentation to time of antibiotics for the emergency department management of suspected meningitis. *Ann Emerg Med* 1993; 22(11):1733–1738.

25. Silverman R, Kwiatkowski T, Bernstein S, et al: Safety of lumbar puncture in patients with hemophilia. *Ann Emerg Med* 1993; 22(11):1739–1742.

26. McLellan D, Giebink GS: Perspectives on occult bacteremia in children. *J Pediatr* 1986; 109(1):1–7.

27. Simon RR, Brenner BE: *Emergency Procedures and Techniques,* 3rd ed. Baltimore: Williams & Wilkins, 1994:167–175.

28. Levinson G: Spinal anesthesia, in Benumof JL (ed): *Clinical Procedures in Anesthesia and Intensive Care.* Philadelphia: Lippincott, 1992:645–661.

29. Kooiker JC: Spinal puncture and cerebrospinal fluid examination, in Roberts JR, Hedges JR (eds): *Clinical Procedures in Emergency Medicine,* 3rd ed. Philadelphia: Saunders, 1998:1054–1077.

30. Norris MC, Leighton BL, DeSimone CA: Needle bevel direction and headache after inadvertent dural puncture. *Anesthesiology* 1989; 70:729–731.

31. Mihic DN: Postspinal headache and relationship of needle bevel to longitudinal fibers. *Reg Anesth* 1985; 110:76–81.

32. Flaaten H, Thorsen T, Askeland B, et al: Puncture technique and postural postdural puncture headache. A randomized, double-blind study comparing transverse and parallel puncture. *Acta Anesthesiol Scand* 1998; 42:1209–1214.

33. Gleason CA, Martin RJ, Anderson JV, et al: Optimal position for a spinal tap in preterm infants. *Pediatrics* 1983; 71:31–35.

34. Weisman LE, Merenstein GB, Steenbarger JR: The effect of lumbar puncture position in sick neonates. *Am J Dis Child* 1983; 137:1077–1079.

35. Fiser DH, Gober GA, Smith CE, et al: Prevention of hypoxemia during lumbar puncture in infancy with preoxygenation. *Pediatr Emerg Care* 1993; 9(2):81–83.

36. Anand KJ, Hickey PR: Pain and its effects in the human neonate and fetus. *N Engl J Med* 1983; 317:1321–1329.

37. Pinheiro JMB, Furdon S, Ocho LF: Role of local anesthesia during lumbar puncture in neonates. *Pediatrics* 1991; 91:379–382.

38. Halperin DL, Koren G, Solh H, et al: Topical skin anesthesia for venous, subcutaneous drug reservoir and lumbar punctures in children. *Pediatrics* 1989; 84:281–284.

39. Ralston SJ, Head-Rapson AG: Use of EMLA cream for skin anesthesia prior to extradural insertion in labour. *Anaesthesia* 1993; 48:65–67.

40. Sharma SK, Garaj NM, Sidawi JE, et al: EMLA cream effectively reduces the pain of spinal needle insertion. *Reg Anesth* 1996; 21:561–564.

41. Koscielniak-Nielsen Z, Hesselbjerg L, Brushoj, et al: EMLA patch for spinal puncture. A comparison of EMLA patch with lidocaine infiltration and placebo patch. *Anaesthesia* 1998; 53:1209–1227.

42. Evans RW: Complications of lumbar puncture. *Neurol Clin* 1998; 16(1):83–105.

43. Lubic LG, Marotta JT: Brain tumor and lumbar puncture. *Arch Neurol Psychiatry* 1954; 72:568–572.

44. Korein J, Craviato H, Leicach: Reevaluation of lumbar puncture. *Neurology* 1959; 9:290–297.

45. Zisfrein J, Tuchman AJ: Risks of lumbar puncture in the presence of intracranial mass lesions. *Mt Sinai J Med* 1988; 55:283–287.

46. Horwitz SJ, Boxerbaum B, O'Beill J: Cerebral herniation in bacterial meningitis in childhood. *Ann Neurol* 7; 5:524–528.

47. Durand ML, Calderwood SB, Weber DJ, et al: Acute bacterial meningitis in adults. A review of 493 episodes. *N Eng J Med* 1993; 328(1):21–28.

48. Rennick G, Shann F, de Campo J: Cerebral herniation during bacterial meningitis in children. *BMJ* 1998; 306:953–955.

49. Duffy GP: Lumbar puncture in spontaneous subarachnoid hemorrhage. *Br Med J* 1982; 285:1163–1164.

50. Hillman J: Should computed tomography scanning replace lumbar puncture in the diagnostic process in suspected subarachnoid hemorrhage? *Surg Neurol* 1986; 26:547–550.

51. Leibold RA, Yealy DM, Coppola M, et al: Post-dural puncture headache: characteristics, management, and prevention. *Ann Emerg Med* 1993; 22:1863–1870.

52. Lybecker H, Djernes M, Schmidt JF: Postdural puncture headache (PDPH): onset, duration, severity, and associated symptoms. An analysis of 75 consecutive patients with PDPH. *Acta Anaesthesiol Scand* 1995; 39:605–612.

53. Ramamoorthy C, Geiduschek JM, Braton SL, et al: Postdural puncture headache in pediatric oncology patients. *Clin Pedriatr* 1998; 37:247–252.

54. Carson D, Serpell M: Choosing the best needle for diagnostic lumbar puncture. *Neurology* 1996; 47:33–37.

55. Norris MC, Leighton BL, DeSimone CA: Needle bevel direction and headache after inadvertent dural puncture. *Anesthesiology* 1989; 70:729–731.

56. Mihic DN: Postspinal headache and relationship of needle bevel to longitudinal fibers. *Reg Anesth* 1985; 110:76–81.

57. Engelhardt A, Ohelm S, Neundorfer B: Post-lumbar puncture headache: experiences with Sprotte's atraumatic needle. *Cephalalgia* 1992; 12(4):259.

58. Braune HJ, Huffman G: A prospective double blind clinical trial comparing the sharp Quincke needle (22G) with an "atraumatic" needle (22G) in the induction of post-lumbar puncture headache. *Acta Neurol Scand* 1992; 86:50–54.

59. Strupp M, Brandt T, Muller A: Incidence of post-lumbar puncture syndrome reduced by reinserting the stylet: a randomized prospective study of 600 patients. *J Neurol* 1998; 245:589–592.

60. Seeberger MD, Kaufmann M, Staender S, et al: Repeated dural punctures increase the incidence of postdural puncture headache. *Anesth Analg* 1996; 82:302–305.

61. Dieterich M, Brandt T: Is obligatory bed rest after lumbar puncture obsolete? *Eur Arch Psychiatry Neurol Sci* 1985; 235:71–75.

62. Carbaat PAT, van Crevel H: Lumbar puncture headache: controlled study on the preventative effect of 24 hours bed rest. *Lancet* 1981; 2:1133–1135.

63. Cook PT, Davies MJ, Beavis RE: Bed rest and postlumbar puncture headache: the effectiveness of 24 hours' recumbency in reducing the incidence of postlumbar puncture headache. *Anaesthesia* 1989; 445:389–391.

64. Vilming ST, Schrader H, Monstad I: Post-lumbar-puncture headache: the significance of body posture: a controlled study of 300 patients. *Cephalalgia* 1988; 8:75–78.

65. Kuntz KM, Kokmen E, Stevens JC, et al: Post-lumbar puncture headaches: experience in 501 consecutive patients. *Neurology* 1992; 42:1884–1887.

66. Dieterich M, Brandt T: Incidence of post-lumbar puncture headache is independent of daily fluid intake. *Eur Arch Psychiatry Neurol Sci* 1988; 237:194–195.

67. Camann WR, Murray RS, Mushlin PS, et al: Effects of oral caffeine on postdural puncture headache: a double-blind, placebo-controlled trial. *Anesth Analg* 1990; 70:181–184.

68. Sechzer PH, Abel L: Post-spinal anesthesia headache treated with caffeine: evaluation with demand method. Part 1. *Curr Ther Res* 1978; 24:307–331.

69. Yücel A, Özyalçin S, Talu G, et al: Intravenous administration of caffeine sodium benzoate for postdural puncture headache. *Reg Anesth Pain Med* 1999; 24:51–54.

70. Carp H, Singh PJ, Vadhera R, et al: Effects of the serotonin-receptor agonist sumatriptan on postdural puncture headache: report of six cases. *Anesth Analg* 1994; 79:180–182.

71. Tarkkila PJ, Miralles JA, Palomaki EA: The subjective complications and efficiency of the epidural blood patch in the treatment of post-dural puncture headache. *Reg Anesth* 1989; 14:247–250.

72. Abouleish E, de la Vega S, Blendinger, et al: Long-term follow-up of the epidural blood patch. *Anesth Analg* 1975; 54:459–463.

73. McGruder JM, Cooke JE, Conroy JM, et al: Epidural blood patch in the treatment of post dural puncture headache. *South Med J* 1988; 81:1249–1252.

74. Olsen KS: Epidural blood patch in the treatment of post-lumbar puncture headache. *Pain* 1987; 30:293–301.

75. Eng RHK, Seligman SJ: Lumbar puncture-induced meningitis. *JAMA* 1981; 245(14):1456–1459.

76. Shapiro ED, Aaron NH, Wald ER, et al: Risk factors for development of bacterial meningitis among children with occult bacteremia. *J Pediatr* 1986; 109:15–19.

77. Krishna V, Liu V, Singleton AF: Should lumbar puncture be routinely performed in patients with suspected bacteremia? *J Natl Med Assoc* 1983; 75(12):1153–1157.

78. Breuer AC, Tyler HR, Marzewski DJ, et al: Radicular vessels are the most probable source of needle induced blood in lumbar puncture. Significance for the thrombocytopenic cancer patient. *Cancer* 1982; 49:2168–2172.

79. Edelson RN, Chernik NL, Posner JB, et al: Spinal subdural hematomas complicating lumbar puncture. Occurrence in thrombocytopenic patients. *Arch Neurol* 1974; 31:134–137.

80. Hart IK, Bone I, Hadley DM: Development of neurological problems after lumbar puncture. *BMJ* 1988; 296:51–52.

81. Edelman JD, Wingard DW: Subdural haematomas after lumbar puncture. *Anesthesiology* 1980; 52:166–167.

82. Vos PE, de Boer WA, Wurzer JAL, et al: Subdural hematoma after lumbar puncture: two case reports and review of the literature. *Clin Neurol Neurosurg* 1991; 93(2):127–131.

83. Bhatoe HS, Gill HS, Kumar N, et al: Post lumbar puncture discitis and vertebral collapse. *Postgrad Med J* 1994; 70:882–884.

84. Potgieter S, Dimin S, Lagae L, et al: Epidermoid tumours associated with lumbar punctures performed in early neonatal life. *Dev Med Child Neurol* 1997; 39:266–269.

85. McDonald JV, Klump TE: Intraspinal epidermoid tumors caused by lumbar puncture. *Arch Neurol* 1986; 43:936–939.

86. Oski FA: *Principles and Practice of Pediatrics,* 2nd ed. Philadelphia: Lippincott, 1994.

87. Gorelick PB, Biller J: Lumbar puncture: technique, indications, and complications. *Postgrad Med* 1986; 79(8):257–268.

88. Bonadio WA, Stanco L, Bruce R, et al: Reference values of normal cerebrospinal fluid composition in infants ages 0–8 weeks. *Pediatr Infect Dis J* 1992; 11(7):589–591.

89. Klein JO, Feigin RD, McCracken GH Jr: Report of the task force on the diagnosis and management of meningitis. *Pediatrics* 1986; 78(5pt2):959–982.

90. Powers WJ: Cerebrospinal fluid lymphocytosis in acute bacterial meningitis. *Am J Med* 1985; 79:216–220.

91. Ratzan KR: Viral meningitis. *Med Clin North Am* 1985; 69(2):399–413.

92. Feigen RD, Shakelford PG: Value of repeat lumbar puncture in the differential diagnosis of meningitis. *N Engl J Med* 1973; 289:571–574.

93. Bonadio W: Bacterial meningitis in children whose cerebrospinal fluid contains polymorphonuclear leukocytes without pleocytosis. *Clin Pediatr* 1988; 27:4198–4200.

94. Mayefsky JH, Roghmann KJ: Determination of leukocytosis in traumatic spinal tap specimens. *Am J Med* 1987; 82:1175–1181.

95. Bonadio WA, Smith DS, Goddard S, et al: Distinguishing cerebrospinal fluid abnormalities in children with bacterial meningitis and traumatic lumbar puncture. *J Infect Dis* 1990; 162:251–253.

96. Powers WJ: Cerebrospinal fluid to serum glucose ratios in diabetes mellitus and bacterial meningitis. *Am J Med* 1981; 71:217–220.

97. Marton KI, Gean AD: The spinal tap: a new look at an old test. *Ann Intern Med* 1986; 104:840–848.

98. Conly JM, Ronald AR: Cerebrospinal fluid as a diagnostic body fluid. *Am J Med* 1983; 75:102–108.

99. Lavoie FW: Meningitis, encephalitis, and central nervous system abscess, in Rosen P, Barkin R: *Emergency Medicine Concepts and Clinical Practice,* 4th ed. St. Louis: Mosby-Year Book, 1998:2198–2211.

100. Karandanis D, Shulman JA: Recent survey of infectious meningitis in adults: review of laboratory findings in bacterial, tuberculous, and aseptic meningitis. *South Med J* 1976; 69(4):449–457.

101. LaScolea JL: Connotation of bacteria in cerebrospinal fluid in blood of children with meningitis and its diagnostic significance. *J Clin Microbiol* 1984; 19:187.

102. Jarvis CW, Saxena KM: Does prior antibiotic treatment hamper the diagnosis of acute bacterial meningitis. *Clin Pediatr* 1972; 11(4):201–204.

103. Bolan G, Barza M: Acute bacterial meningitis in children and adults. A perspective. *Med Clin North Am* 1985; 69(2):231–241.

104. Wiebe RA, Crast FW, Hall RA, et al: Clinical factors relating to prognosis of bacterial meningitis. *South Med J* 1972; 65(3):257–264.

105. Talan DA, Hoffman JR, Yoshikawa TT, et al: Role of empiric parenteral antibiotics prior to lumbar puncture in suspected bacterial meningitis: state of the art. *Rev Infect Dis* 1988; 10:365–376.

106. Blazer S, Berant M, Alon U: Effect of antibiotic treatment on cerebrospinal fluid. *Am J Neurosurg Psychiatry* 1988; 51:342–344.

107. Vermeulen M: Subarachnoid haemorrhage: diagnosis and treatment. *J Neurol* 1996; 243:496–501.

108. Vermeulen M, Hasan D, Blijenberg BG, et al: Xanthochromia after subarachnoid haemorrhage needs no revisitation. *J Neurol Neurosurg Psychiatry* 1989; 52:826–828.

109. Edlow JA, Caplan LR: Avoiding pitfalls in the diagnosis of subarachnoid hemorrhage. *N Engl J Med* 2000; 342(1):29–36.

Chapter 97
BURR HOLES

Yogesh Ghandhi
Don W. Penney

INTRODUCTION

Burr holes in the Emergency Department setting are uncommonly performed for diagnostic and therapeutic purposes. Diagnosis and treatment of increased intracranial pressure (ICP) in a timely fashion can be a lifesaving measure. Increased ICP can be the result of trauma, tumors, hemorrhage, or infections. There has been less need to make exploratory burr holes in head injured patients since CT scanning has become widely available.

Burr holes can be lifesaving on rare occasions when the patient is worsening neurologically or has blown a pupil and CT scan is unavailable. Suspect a space-occupying lesion when there is clinical evidence of tentorial herniation or upper brain stem dysfunction. This includes pupillary dilation with a decreased or absent light reflex, progressive deterioration in the patient's level of consciousness, and/or hemiparesis including posturing (decerebrate/decorticate) or flaccidity. The placement of a temporal burr hole on the side of the mydriatic pupil can be lifesaving. Up to 70 percent of patients with evidence of brain stem dysfunction soon after head trauma have significant intracranial mass lesions, most of which are extra-axial blood collections.[1]

ANATOMY AND PATHOPHYSIOLOGY

Sixty percent of patients with fatal head injuries die before reaching the hospital. The cause of death is usually a result of an expanding intracranial hemorrhage, extensive basilar skull fractures with associated injury to the venous sinuses, intracranial carotid artery laceration, and/or major cortical vessel laceration. Skull fractures are present in up to 90 percent of adults who develop an intracranial hematoma. Children are less likely to suffer a skull fracture after head trauma than adults.

The middle meningeal artery is a branch of the maxillary artery and enters the cranium via the foramen spinosum. It is usually located between the periosteal and meningeal layers of the dura mater. Shortly after entering the skull it divides into anterior and posterior branches. The larger branches of the middle meningeal artery lie within the dura and are accompanied by veins. Their superficial location in the dura produces grooves on the interior of the cranium. This location makes them vulnerable to injury, especially from fractures of the temporal bone. The bony vault of the skull is fairly thick, approximately 5 mm in thickness, and shows considerable individual and regional variation. The temporal bone, in particular the squamous temporal bone, is much thinner than other areas of the skull. This renders it vulnerable to fracture with associated injury to the middle meningeal vessels.

Posttraumatic epidural hematomas usually develop in the temporal or temporoparietal location as a result of an injury to the middle meningeal vessels (Figures 97-1*A* and *B*). Epidural hematomas occur laterally over the cerebral hemispheres with the epicenter at the pterion in approximately 70 percent of patients (Figure 97-2). The remaining epidural hematomas are distributed in the frontal area, occipitoparietal area, and the posterior fossa. Other sources of epidural hematomas include a torn venous sinus or an injury to the carotid artery before it enters the intracranial dural mater. More than 50 percent of all epidural hematomas result from an injury to the middle meningeal artery itself.

Subdural hematomas are collections of blood between the dura mater and the brain (Figures 97-1*C* and *D*). They usually are the result of blunt trauma to the cranium.[1] These result from the tearing of a bridging vein as the brain forcefully moves within the skull. The patient will present with an abnormal neurological examination minutes to hours after the acute injury.

Pupillary changes are not an early sign of an intracranial hematoma. However, when they do occur, they signify cerebral compression and transtentorial herniation. Other causes of acute pupillary changes need to be ruled out. Hematomas are usually found ipsilateral to the pupillary change in up to 85 percent of cases.

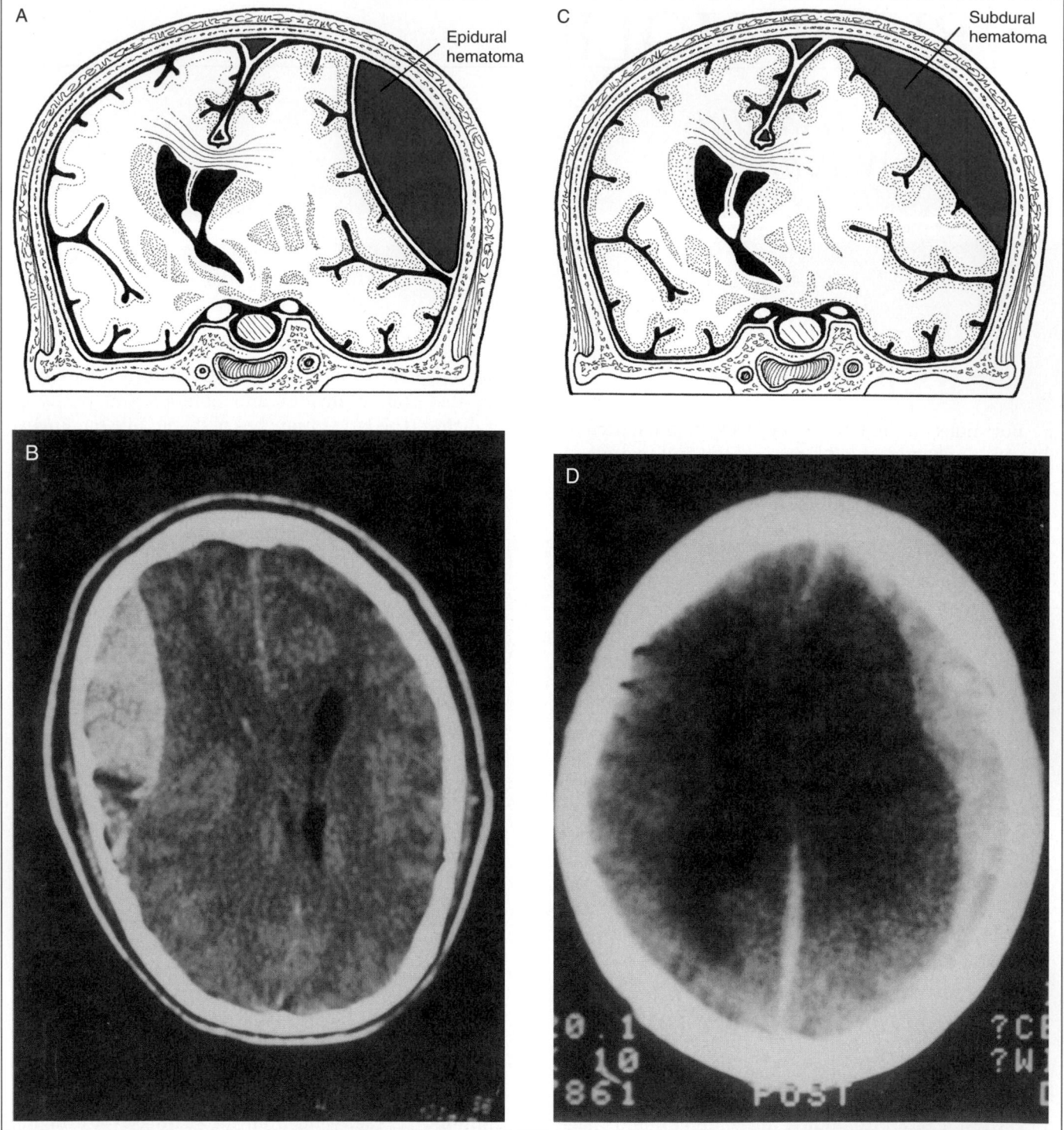

FIGURE 97-1 Hematomas requiring drainage through a burr hole. *A*. Illustration of an epidural hematoma. *B*. CT scan of an epidural hematoma. *C*. Illustration of a subdural hematoma. *D*. CT scan of a subdural hematoma.

INDICATIONS

There are a few indications to emergently place a burr hole in the Emergency Department. These include monitoring of intracranial pressure, the emergent drainage of an intracranial hematoma, and the emergent cannulation of the ventricular system. This procedure may be performed by trained Emergency Physicians if a Neurosurgeon has been consulted and is not immediately available.

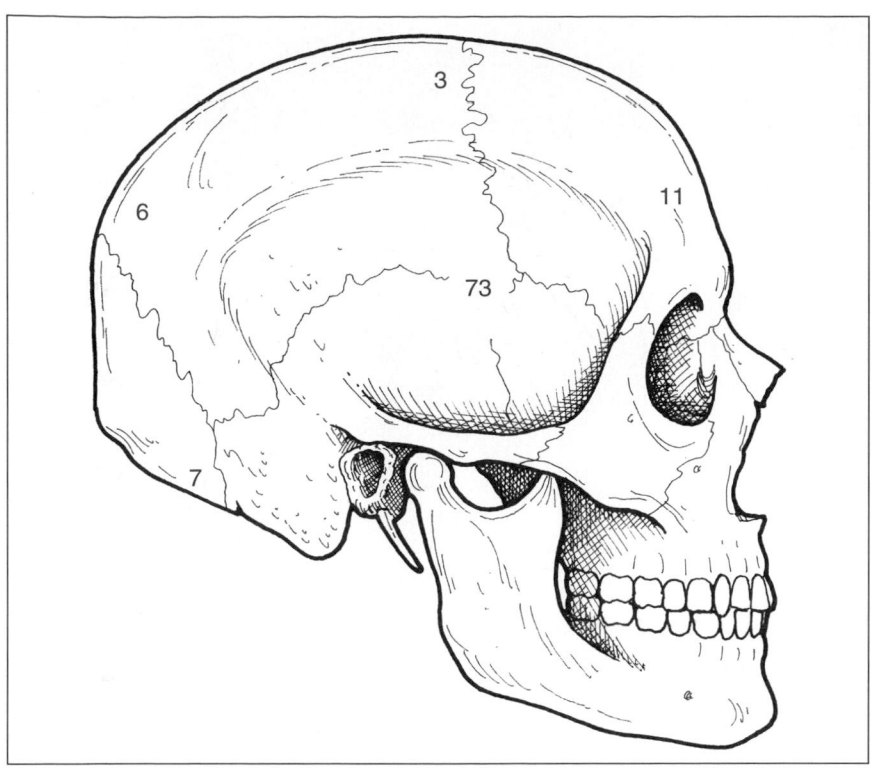

FIGURE 97-2 Percentages of epidural hematomas by anatomic location.

CONTRAINDICATIONS

The only absolute contraindication is a patient who is coagulopathic. Otherwise, the available physician with the most skill and experience in performing this technique should be the one to place the burr hole. This procedure should not be performed by anyone not properly trained.

EQUIPMENT

Sterile prep kit
Povidone iodine solution
Sterile drapes
Local anesthetic solution containing epinephrine
22 gauge needles
5 mL syringe
#10 scalpel blades
#11 scalpel blades
#3 scalpel handle
Bipolar cautery, optional
Self-retaining mastoid retractors
Hudson brace drill
Skull perforator bits
Conical burr bits
Small hook
Bone wax
Thrombin-soaked Gelfoam
Periosteal elevator
Suction catheter kit
Head covers, masks, and sterile gowns
Ventriculostomy catheter (optional)
Bone rongeur
Mayo scissors
4–0 nylon suture
Potts scissors

The required equipment is all contained within a prepared sterile tray that can be obtained from the Operating Room or hospital central supply (Figure 97-3). A completely disposable single patient use instrument set is also available (Spectrum Surgical Instruments Corp., Stow, Ohio). The Hudson brace drill is a handheld device (Figure 97-4). It has a stabilizing handle in series with a handle that rotates in circles. The distal end has a snap lock chuck that slides to allow easy insertion and removal of the bits. The bits come in a variety of shapes and sizes (Figure 97-5). The perforator bits have a sharp point. The tip of the perforator bit is designed to penetrate the inner table of the skull and lock without allowing it to puncture the dura or the brain (Figure 97-6). **However, exercise extreme caution as the bit may occasionally not lock.** The burr bits are rounded. They are used to enlarge the hole in the skull made by the perforator bit (Figure 97-6).

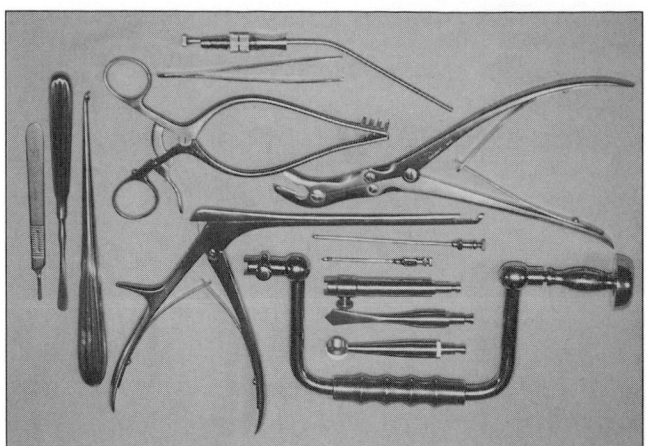

FIGURE 97-3 The contents of the hospital-prepared burr hole tray.

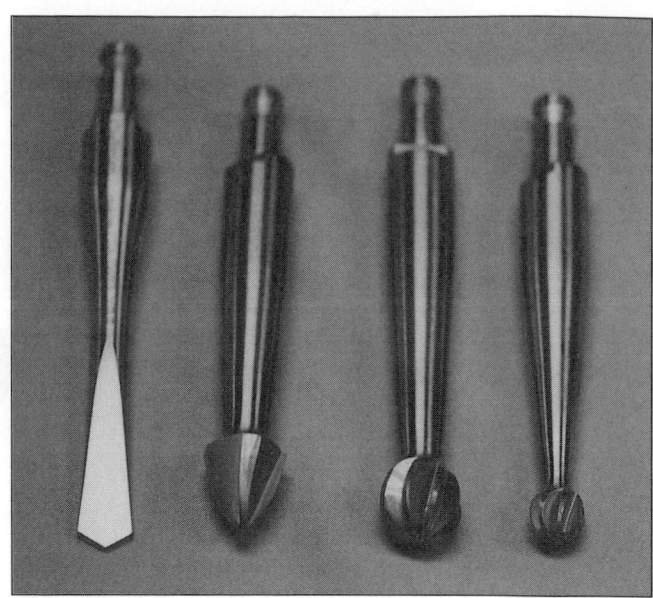

FIGURE 97-5 Examples of perforator bits (left) and burr bits (right).

PATIENT PREPARATION

Explain the risks, benefits, and complications of the procedure to the patient and/or their representative. Obtain an informed consent. However, in the patient who is deteriorating neurologically with tentorial herniation, consciousness is usually lost and time is of the essence.

Determine the site for the skin incision and the burr hole (Figure 97-7). A frontal or anterior burr hole is made just anterior to the coronal suture and 3 cm lateral to the midline, approximately along the midpupillary line (Figure 97-7A). The coronal suture is often palpable. If not, draw a perpendicular line midway between the lateral canthus of the orbit and the external auditory meatus. The frontal burr hole can be used to drain an intracranial hematoma or to perform a ventriculostomy. The temporal burr hole is made two finger breadths above the zygomatic arch and two finger breadths anterior to the external auditory meatus (Figure 97-7B). The parietal or posterior burr hole is made two finger breadths behind the external auditory meatus and three finger breadths above the mastoid process (Figure 97-7B).

Prepare the patient. Orotracheally intubate the patient to protect and secure the airway. Insert a nasogastric tube to decompress the stomach. Shave the scalp at least 5 cm in all directions from the proposed skin incision. Clean the skin of any dirt or debris. Cleanse the skin first using 70 percent alcohol followed by povidone iodine prep solution. Allow the povidone iodine to dry. Isolate the surgical field by using sterile drapes. Prophylactic intravenous antibiotic coverage is recommended if time permits. Administer a broad-spectrum antibiotic that

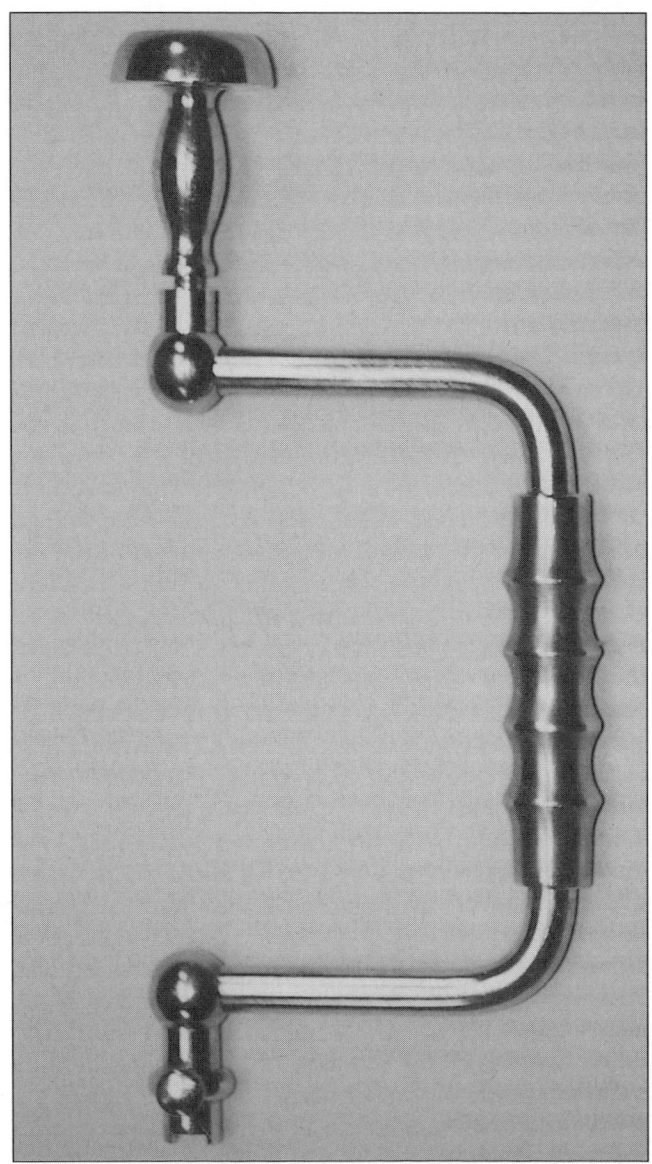

FIGURE 97-4 The Hudson brace drill.

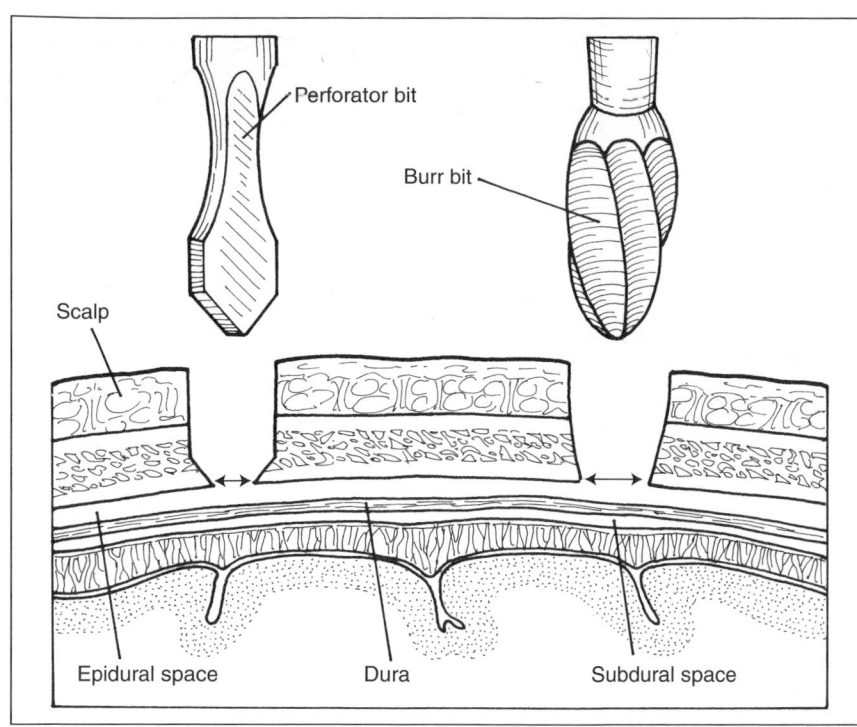

FIGURE 97-6 The perforator bit is used to make a hole through the skull and just penetrate the inner table of bone. The burr bit is used to enlarge the hole.

covers gram-positive skin flora. Position the patient so that the proposed incision site is visible and easily accessible. Place the patient supine with a folded blanket or towel under the ipsilateral shoulder. Turn the head to the contralateral side if the cervical spine has been cleared. Instruct an assistant to hold and steady the head.

TECHNIQUES

BURR HOLES

Identify the site to make the burr hole. Infiltrate 5 mL of local anesthetic solution containing epinephrine along the proposed incision site. This will result in analgesia and vasoconstriction that may aid in hemostasis. Make a 2 cm long skin incision centered about the site to make the burr hole. Carry the incision down to the bone of the skull. The incision must traverse all layers of the scalp including the skin, the subcutaneous tissue, the temporalis muscle (if present), and the periosteum. Remove the periosteum overlying the skull with a periosteal elevator. The periosteum will otherwise get caught in the perforator bit and make it difficult to turn. Insert a small self-retaining retractor into the wound (Figure 97-8A). Hemostasis can often be obtained with the use of the retractor. However, having cautery available can be helpful. Small bleeding vessels may be tied off with absorbable suture.

Fit the Hudson brace with a perforator bit. Grasp the stabilizing handle of the Hudson brace with the non-dominant hand. Grasp the rotating handle with the dominant hand. Place the tip of the perforator bit against the skull (Figure 97-8B). Turn the rotating handle clockwise with the dominant hand in a smooth and slow motion. **Always maintain the drill perpendicular to the skull. Maintain controlled pressure on the Hudson brace.** Watch as the perforator bit cuts through the skull. Frequently remove the perforator bit to examine the hole. Irrigate the area. Use suction to remove the bone fragments and the irrigation fluid. Gently probe the hole to determine if the inner table has been penetrated. Continue to drill until the inner table has been penetrated or the perforator bit locks (Figure 97-8C). **Do not apply too much downward pressure on the brace to prevent it from plunging into the brain. Exercise extreme caution as the bit does not always lock when the inner table is perforated.**

Remove the perforator bit from the Hudson brace. Place the burr bit on the Hudson brace. Place the burr bit into the hole in the skull. Hold the Hudson brace as described above. Rotate the handle clockwise to enlarge the hole in the skull (Figure 97-8D). Frequently remove the burr bit to examine the hole. Irrigate the area. Use suction to remove the bone fragments and the irrigation fluid. Continue to drill until the hole in the inner table is enlarged enough to accept the tip of the bone rongeur. **Do not apply too much downward pressure on the Hudson brace to prevent it from plunging into the brain.**

Control bleeding from the bone with bone wax and from the epidural space with Gelfoam. The clot of an epidural hematoma will be obvious as it separates the inner table of the skull from the dura. This clot will

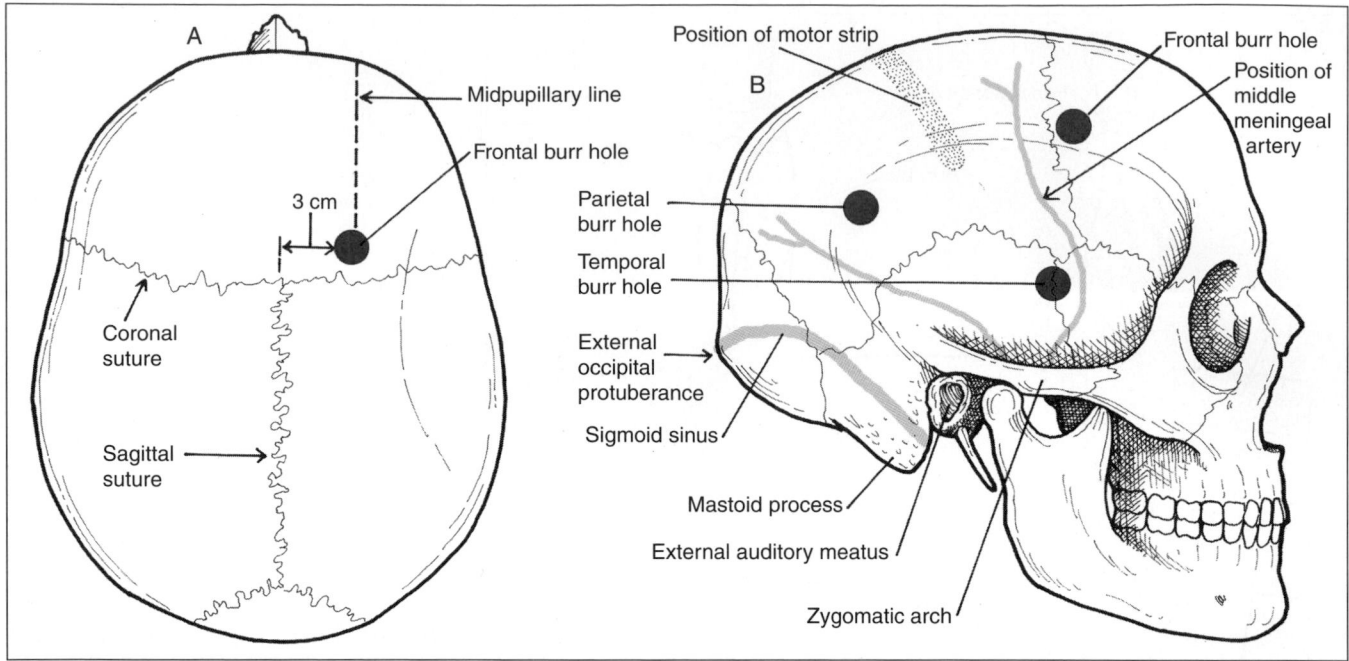

FIGURE 97-7 Typical locations for burr holes. *A.* Superior view of the skull. *B.* Lateral view of the skull.

be gelatinous in consistency and drainage through a single burr hole can be difficult. Free the underlying dura from the bone edge with a Penfield elevator. **Gently insert the elevator between the inner table of the skull and the dura. Gently separate the dura from the skull.** Enlarge the burr hole in order to facilitate aspiration of the blood clot. Insert a bone rongeur into the hole. Take small bites of the skull to enlarge the hole. Do not concern yourself with making the hole smooth or symmetric. The Neurological Surgeon will later trim and repair the bony defect.

HEMATOMA DRAINAGE

An epidural hematoma is aspirated by gentle suction and irrigation with normal saline through an adequate bone opening (Figure 97-8*E*). **Pay close attention to the temperature of the irrigation solution. It should ideally be body temperature.** Use wall suction with a #9 or #11 French aspirator.

Epidural and subdural hemorrhages are usually clotted in the acute stages. In the event that an epidural hematoma is not identified after placement of the burr hole, inspect the underlying dura for a possible subdural hematoma. The presence of a subdural hematoma causes the dura to have a bluish hue or tinge (Figure 97-9*A*). Carefully place a traction suture using 4–0 nylon through the outer layer of the dura (Figure 97-9*B*). Apply traction on the suture to elevate the dura. Incise the dura with a fine Mayo scissors or a #11 scalpel blade (Figure 97-9*B*). **Exercising extreme caution during the maneuver is mandatory to prevent lacerating the brain.** Open the dura in a cruciate fashion. Drain the subdural clot

using suction and gentle irrigation. **At no time should any pressure be placed on the brain. Care should be taken not to irrigate with any force directly against the brain surface.**

VENTRICULOSTOMY

The burr hole can be made in order to place a ventriculostomy catheter. Incise the dural edges with a #11 scalpel blade. Cauterize the edges of the dura. Cauterize the pia and cortical surface with bipolar cautery, if available. Perform a ventriculostomy using an appropriate ventricular catheter. Anatomical landmarks suggestive for placement of the catheter within the ventricular system are to insert the catheter perpendicular to the skull and directed towards the ipsilateral inner canthus.[2] Advance the catheter to a depth of approximately 5 to 6 cm. If unsuccessful after three attempts, place the parenchymal monitor or a subarachnoid bolt. Refer to Chapter 99 for the complete details of performing a ventriculostomy.

ASSESSMENT

Assessment and stabilization of the head injury victim prior to placement of the burr hole, during the procedure, and post-procedurally requires attention to securing the patient's airway, adequate and aggressive treatment of hemodynamic instability and shock, stabilization of the cervical and thoracolumbar spine, and concomitant treatment of any extracranial injuries. **Aggressive management of hypoxia and hypotension cannot be overemphasized. Hyperventilation in the**

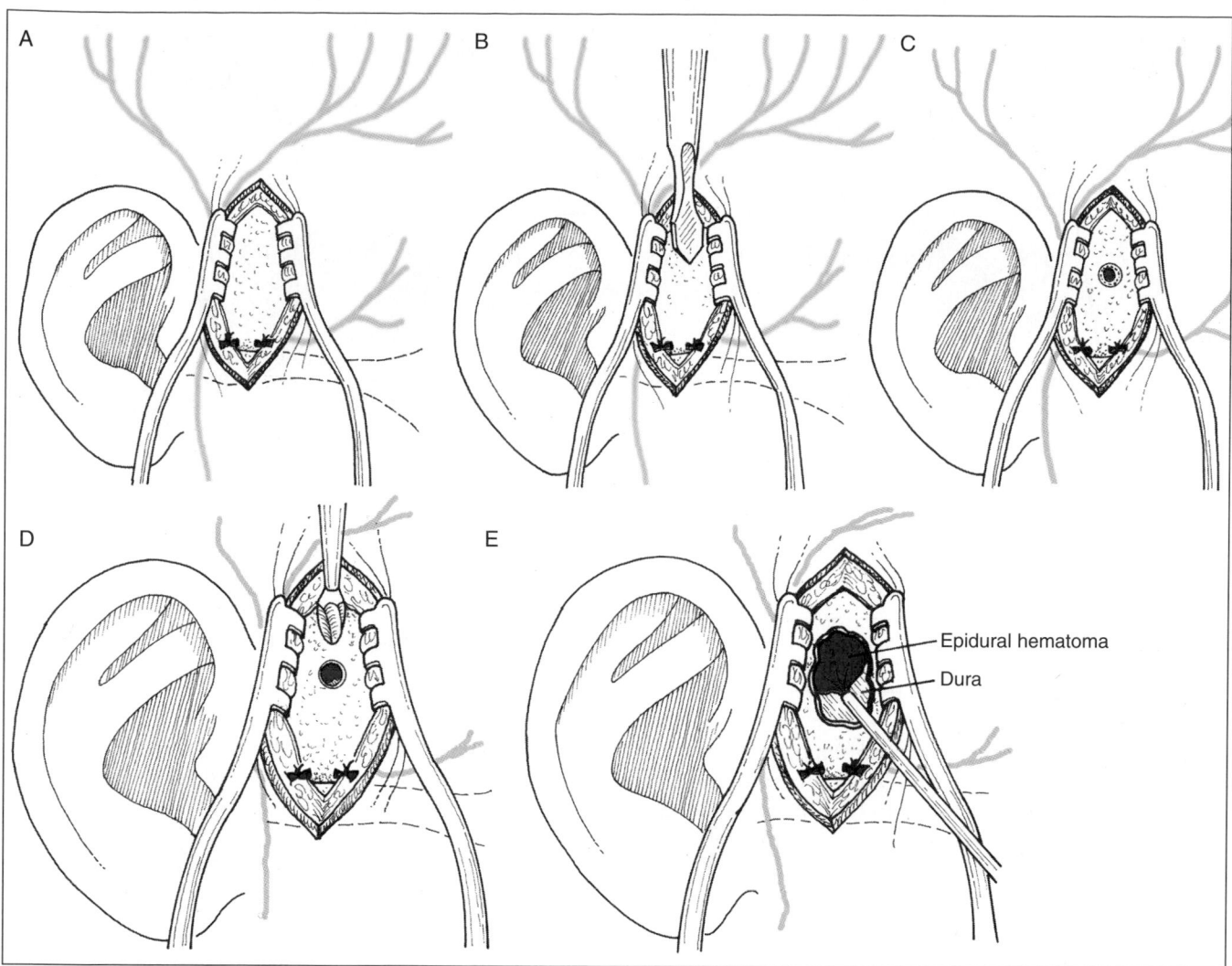

FIGURE 97-8 Drainage of an epidural hematoma. *A.* An incision is made through the skin, subcutaneous tissue, temporalis muscle, and galea aponeurotica. The incision is held open with a self-retaining mastoid retractor. *B.* A Hudson brace fitted with a perforator bit is used to penetrate the skull to the inner table. *C.* A hole has been made with the perforator bit. *D.* The hole is opened with a burr bit on the Hudson brace. *E.* The bone edges have been removed with a rongeur to expose the epidural hematoma. The hematoma is gently removed by suction.

first 24 hours after severe head injury should be avoided as it can reduce cerebral blood flow. The assessment should include hemodynamic parameters, Glasgow Coma Score, and frequent neurological examinations. The neurological examination should include pupillary size and reaction, extraocular muscle function, and motor movements of the extremities. Intubation utilizing rapid sequence technique antecedes burr hole placement in the patient with severe head injury. This precludes a detailed neurological examination as most patients will have received neuromuscular blockade.

Reduction in pupillary size can be appreciated postevacuation of the hematoma in patients who have had pupillary changes anteceding the burr hole placement. Repeat the hemodynamic and neurological assessments often, every five minutes, and document this in the pa-

tient's record. Obtain a post-procedural CT scan of the head as early as possible to check the status of the hematoma. CT scanning also verifies catheter location and reduction in ventricular size in patients in which trephination has been completed for ventricular catheter placement.

AFTERCARE

Patients who have had burr hole placement because of neurological deterioration require further definitive management by a Neurological Surgeon. A craniotomy is indicated for a more thorough evaluation, irrigation of the epidural or subdural space, and for hemostasis. Post-procedural CT scanning should not be performed if

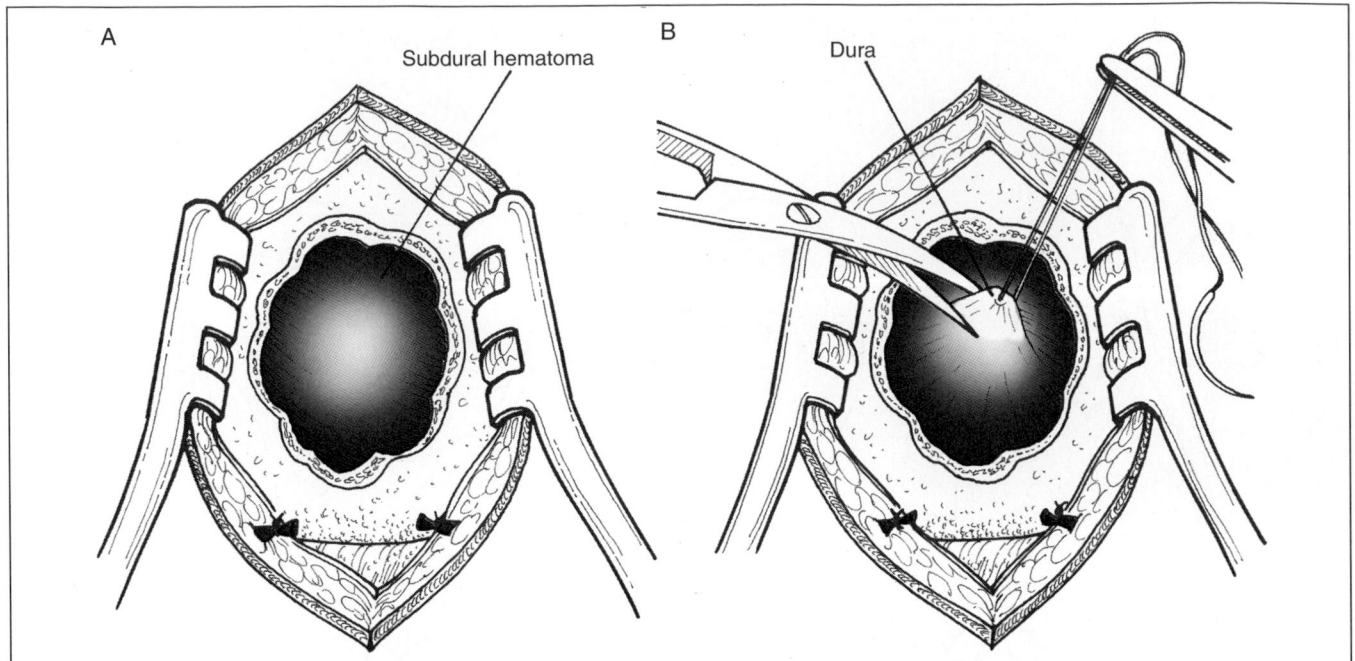

FIGURE 97-9 Drainage of a subdural hematoma. *A.* The dura is exposed and a hematoma is visible below it. *B.* Traction is placed on a suture that has been placed through the center of the exposed dura. The tented dura is carefully opened with a scissors or scalpel to expose the underlying hematoma.

definitive management by a Neurological Surgeon is available. It is an unnecessary waste of time and the patient should proceed directly to the Operating Room. Cranioplasty is often not completed initially after burr hole placement in order to minimize the infectious risk. Post-procedural treatment often requires airway protection with continued endotracheal intubation, adequate fluid resuscitation, management of hypoxia, management of hypotension, management of seizures, and management of any coagulopathy. Secondary injuries can evolve, even after adequate hematoma evacuation. They need to be anticipated, recognized, and treated aggressively.

A two-layer closure is recommended in the event a craniotomy is not to follow or will be delayed. The dura is usually not closed. Cover the dura with a small piece of thrombin-soaked Gelfoam. Close the galea with 3–0 absorbable suture. Close the scalp/skin with 3–0 nylon suture. Apply a dry dressing to the scalp wound. Alternatively, apply sterile saline soaked gauze over the wound and cover this with a dry dressing.

COMPLICATIONS

Wound infections, abscesses, and postoperative hematomas are major complications. These can be avoided by using sterile precautions, antibiotic prophylaxis, and fine surgical technique. Other complications include plunging with the perforator bit or the burr bit resulting in a penetrating injury to the brain, cortical lacerations, cortical contusions, and seizures. Blunt or penetrating brain injuries can result in delayed stroke and hemorrhage. At times, this can be produced by a post-traumatic aneurysm or arteriovenous fistula. In the severely head injured patient, a multitude of coagulopathic abnormalities can occur including hypercoagulable and fibrinolytic states as well as disseminated intravascular coagulation (DIC).

Significant bleeding complications can occur from this procedure. Penetration of the sagittal sinus can result in significant hemorrhage and possible exsanguination. Prevent this by staying at least 2 cm from the midline and properly identifying the landmarks before drilling into the skull. Avoid lacerating the middle meningeal artery or its branches. Prevent injuries to these arteries by not drilling beyond the inner table and carefully separating the dura from the skull before using the bone rongeur. Another option is to obtain a lateral plain radiograph of the skull. Note the position of the grooves in relation to the external auditory meatus. Avoid these grooves, and thus the branches of the middle meningeal artery, when determining the exact site to place the burr hole.

SUMMARY

The prognosis for the severely head injured patient with clinical evidence of tentorial herniation and brainstem compression is poor. Rapid evacuation of an intra-cranial mass lesion may help to improve the outcome. Ideally, these patients are resuscitated and a CT scan of the head is completed in order to determine the presence of a mass lesion. Patients may at times undergo rapid neurological deterioration prior to CT scanning or CT scanning may not be readily available. Diagnostic burr hole exploration and evacuation of an extra-axial hematoma can be a lifesaving measure. The authors do not wish to suggest that exploratory surgery should replace CT scanning in the management of all patients with severe head injury. The CT scan is invaluable in assessing and identifying accurately the location of any mass lesion intracranially. Burr hole evacuation in a trauma setting should be considered only in the presence of rapid neurological deterioration with evidence of herniation and brainstem compression and the unavailability of a Neurological Surgeon to perform the procedure.

REFERENCES

1. Stone JL, Rifai MHS, Sugar O, et al: Subdural hematomas: I. Acute subdural hematoma: progress in definition, clinical pathology, and therapy. *Surg Neurol* 1983; 19:216–231.
2. Ghajar JBG: A guide for ventricular catheter placement: technical note. *J Neurosurg* 1985; 63:985–986.

Chapter 98
LATERAL CERVICAL PUNCTURE

Yogesh Ghandhi
Don W. Penney

INTRODUCTION

The safest procedure to obtain cerebrospinal fluid is lumbar puncture. However, there are situations where lumbar puncture is either contraindicated or technically not feasible. This includes infections in the lumbar area, obesity, previous spinal surgery, previous spinal fusion, previous arachnoiditis, and the previous injection of chemotherapeutics. The usual and safe alternative method is a lateral cervical puncture under such circumstances. Cisternal puncture describes the suboccipital access to cisterna magna, a cerebral spinal fluid (CSF) containing space. It is a less frequently used procedure due to the high incidence of complications. As a result, cisternal puncture should be performed by a Neurological Surgeon for patients whose CSF cannot be accessed by lumbar puncture or lateral cervical puncture.[1]

Dr. Mullan introduced a method for performing a percutaneous cordotomy using a lateral cervical puncture in the early 1960s.[2] He introduced a strontium-90 needle through the C1-C2 interspace and entered the subarachnoid space under fluoroscopic guidance. He then directed the needle anteriorly towards the anterior dura mater to interrupt the spinal thalamic fibers in an attempt to control intractable pain. The lateral cervical puncture is a direct derivative of this technique.

ANATOMY AND PATHOPHYSIOLOGY

Lateral cervical puncture involves the placement of a spinal needle into the C1-C2 interspace, posterior and inferior to the vertebral artery. The vertebral artery ascends through the foramina in the transverse processes of the cervical vertebrae beginning at the sixth cervical vertebra. It winds behind the lateral mass of the atlas (C1) to enter the skull through the foramen magnum (Figure 98-1). Inserting the needle 1 cm inferior to the tip of the mastoid process and 1 cm posterior from that point will avoid puncturing the vertebral artery (Figure 98-2).

The spinal canal is formed by sequential vertebral foramina and is triangular in shape. Its lateral width is greater than the anteroposterior width. The spinal canal is more spacious in the upper cervical spine allowing for safe placement of a needle into the C1-C2 interspace. The sagittal diameter of the spinal canal is approximately 23 mm at C1 and 20 mm at C2. The cross-sectional area of the cervical spinal canal is greatest at C2 and progressively decreases. It is smallest at the level of C7. The vertebral canal is narrower in women than in men. The spinal canal at the level of C1-C2 can be divided into three parts. The anterior third is occupied by the odontoid process. The middle third is occupied by the spinal cord itself. The posterior third is occupied by the subarachnoid space. The spinal cord is suspended and cushioned within the subarachnoid space by cerebral spinal fluid. The anterior boundary of the spinal canal is formed by the posterior aspect of the vertebral bodies and the intervertebral disks. The lateral wall of the spinal canal is formed by the pedicles and the intervertebral foramen. The posterior wall of the spinal canal is formed by the lamina, the ligamentum flavum, and the lateral masses or articular processes.

The morphology of the spinal cord demonstrates considerable individual variation in size and shape. The spinal cord changes in morphology throughout the entire spinal canal. It is cylindrical in shape and larger in transverse diameter than anteroposterior diameter. The spinal cord is largest from C3 to C6, obtaining approximately 13 to 14 mm in maximal transverse diameter. The average sagittal diameter of the cervical spinal cord is approximately 11 mm at C1 and 10 mm at C2.

The cervical nerve roots usually occupy the inferior one-third of the neural foramen. The first cervical spinal nerve root exits between the occiput and C1. The C2

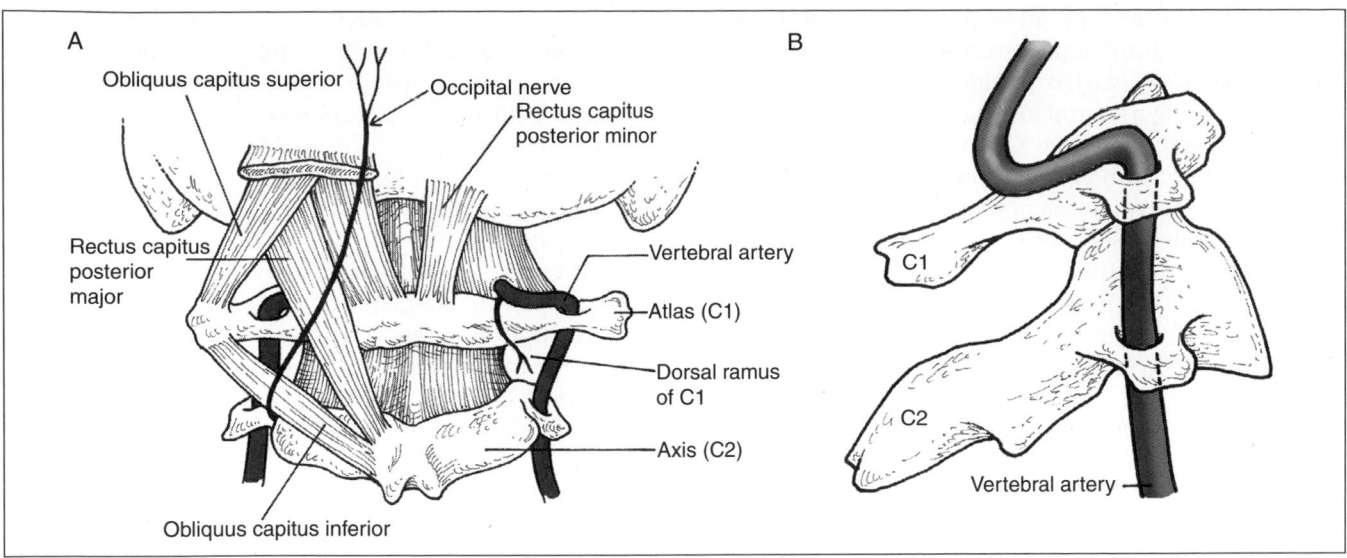

FIGURE 98-1 The course of the vertebral artery at the level of C1-C2. *A.* Posterior view. *B.* Lateral view.

through C7 spinal nerves exit above their corresponding numbered vertebra. Each nerve root innervates a specific dermatome and myotome, with considerable anatomical variation and overlap. The C1-C2 interspace is guarded laterally by the ligamentum flavum. The ligamentum flavum is composed of a yellow elastic tissue, the fibers of which are almost perpendicular in direction. It is attached to the lower part of the anterior surface of the lamina above and the posterior surface of the upper margin of the lamina below.

INDICATIONS

Lateral cervical puncture is an alternative method for obtaining CSF when lumbar puncture is not feasible or successful. Conditions that make lumbar puncture difficult are considered contraindications such as lumbar arachnoiditis, marked obesity, infections in the lumbar area, prior lumbar spine surgery, prior administration of lumbar intrathecal chemotherapeutics, and known congenital anomalies of the lumbar area (meningocele and

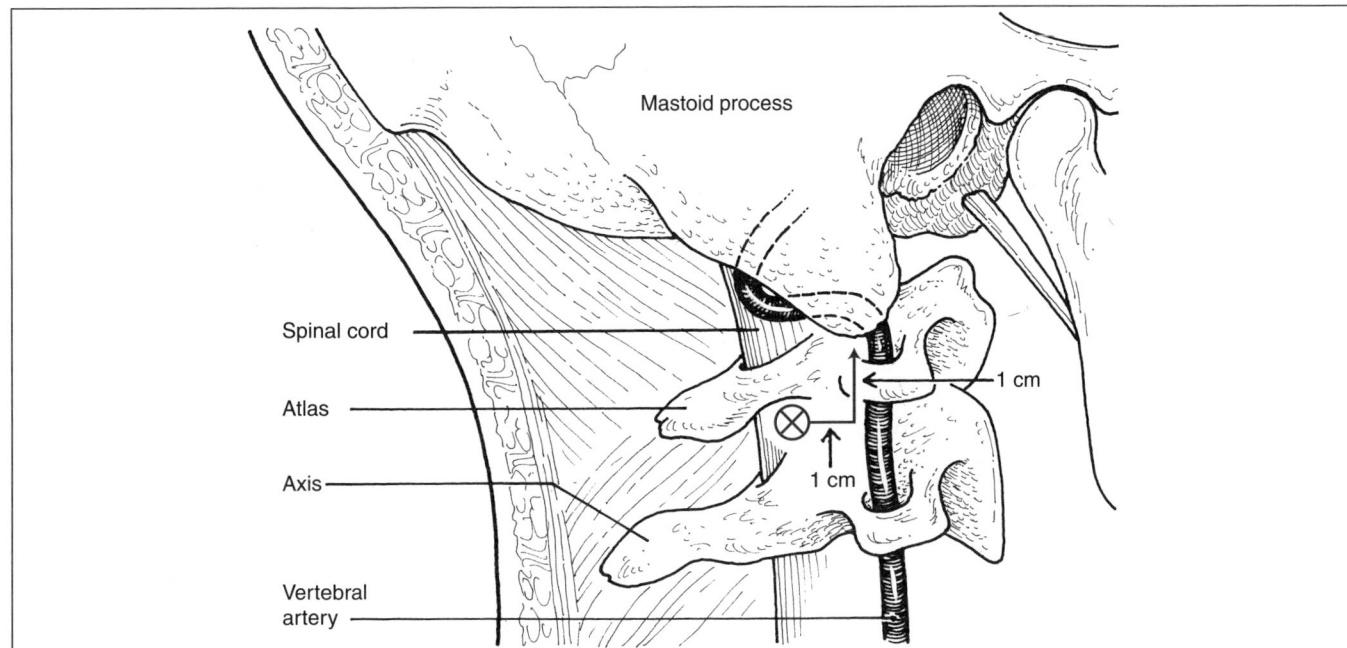

FIGURE 98-2 Anatomic landmarks for cisternal puncture. The site for insertion of the needle is represented by an ⊗.

myelomeningocele). The lateral cervical puncture is performed, like the lumbar puncture, in order to obtain CSF for analysis. CSF analysis is indicated in patients suspected of having a central nervous system infection or a subarachnoid hemorrhage. Other indications for lateral cervical puncture include the installation of antineoplastic or antimicrobial agents. Lateral cervical puncture may also be necessary for the introduction of dye for radiographic evaluation.

CONTRAINDICATIONS

Contraindications for lateral cervical puncture include local infections, coagulopathy, inflammatory adhesions, increased intracranial pressure, posterior fossa tumors, brain abscesses, and posterior fossa abscesses. Arnold-Chiari malformations and other congenital abnormalities in the region of the foramen magnum are also a relative contraindication. These include achondroplasia, basilar impression, Dandy-Walker malformation, Klippel-Feil syndrome, and syringomyelia.

EQUIPMENT

20 gauge spinal needle with a stylette
23 gauge spinal needle with a stylette
3 mL syringe
20 gauge needles
22 gauge needles
3-way stopcock
Manometer
Extension tubing, optional
4 specimen vials with caps
Gauze pads
Povidone iodine swab sticks
Sterile towels
Fenestrated sterile drape
Lidocaine hydrochloride, 1%
Sterile gloves
Povidone iodine solution
Fluoroscopy unit, optional

All the required equipment is contained within commercially available lumbar puncture kits (Figure 96-3). Refer to Chapter 96 for details of the lumbar puncture kit.

PATIENT PREPARATION

Explain the procedure, its risks, and benefits to the patient and/or their representative. Explain the postprocedural care. Obtain an informed consent for the procedure. Place the patient supine on the gurney, without a pillow, and the neck as straight as possible. Limit any head rotation from the true supine position. The landmark for needle insertion is 1 cm caudal and 1 cm posterior to the tip of the mastoid process (Figure 98-2).

Clean the skin of any dirt and debris. Swab the area with alcohol pads. Shave the area so that the mastoid tip is contained within the sterile field. Apply povidone iodine to the skin and allow it to dry. Apply sterile towels and drapes to delineate a sterile field. Consider the administration of intravenous diazepam or midazolam, if not contraindicated, to relax the patient. Inject local anesthetic solution subcutaneously at the above identified landmark.

TECHNIQUE

Maintain the patient in the supine position with absolutely no head movement. An assistant may be required to stabilize the head. Introduce a 21 or 22 gauge needle perfectly horizontal, parallel to the plane of the bed, and perpendicular to the neck (Figure 98-3). The needle will cross a number of tissue planes including the skin, subcutaneous tissue, trapezius muscle, suboccipital muscles, and the meninges. Advance the needle slowly and in 2 to 3 mm increments. Remove the stylette frequently to check for CSF. The subarachnoid space is approximately 6 cm from the skin surface in most adults. Puncture of the dura is often felt as a "pop" or loss of resistance. Frequent checks for CSF prevent excessive penetration of the needle through subarachnoid space, overshooting the spinal canal, or inadvertent puncture of the spinal cord or vertebral artery. **Immediately remove the spinal needle if the patient develops any neurological symptoms.**

CSF flow through the needle signifies that the tip is within the subarachnoid space. If CSF is not draining after puncture of the dura and removal of the stylet, rotate the needle 30 degrees. The use of a portable fluoroscopic unit can confirm the needle's trajectory and exact position. Carefully apply the 3-way stopcock and manometer to the spinal needle to measure the pressure of the CSF. Carefully remove the stopcock and the manometer from the spinal needle. **Do not allow the spinal needle to move while applying and removing the stopcock and manometer. Keep in mind that the needle is not very well supported by the soft tissue as in the lumbar puncture. Hence, the needle must be supported more carefully.** Collect 1 to 2 mL of CSF in each tube. Insert the stylet into the needle. Remove the needle and stylet as a unit. Apply a bandage to the skin puncture site.

Encountering arterial blood from the needle usually indicates that it was pointing too far anteriorly and that the vertebral artery was penetrated. The venous plexus

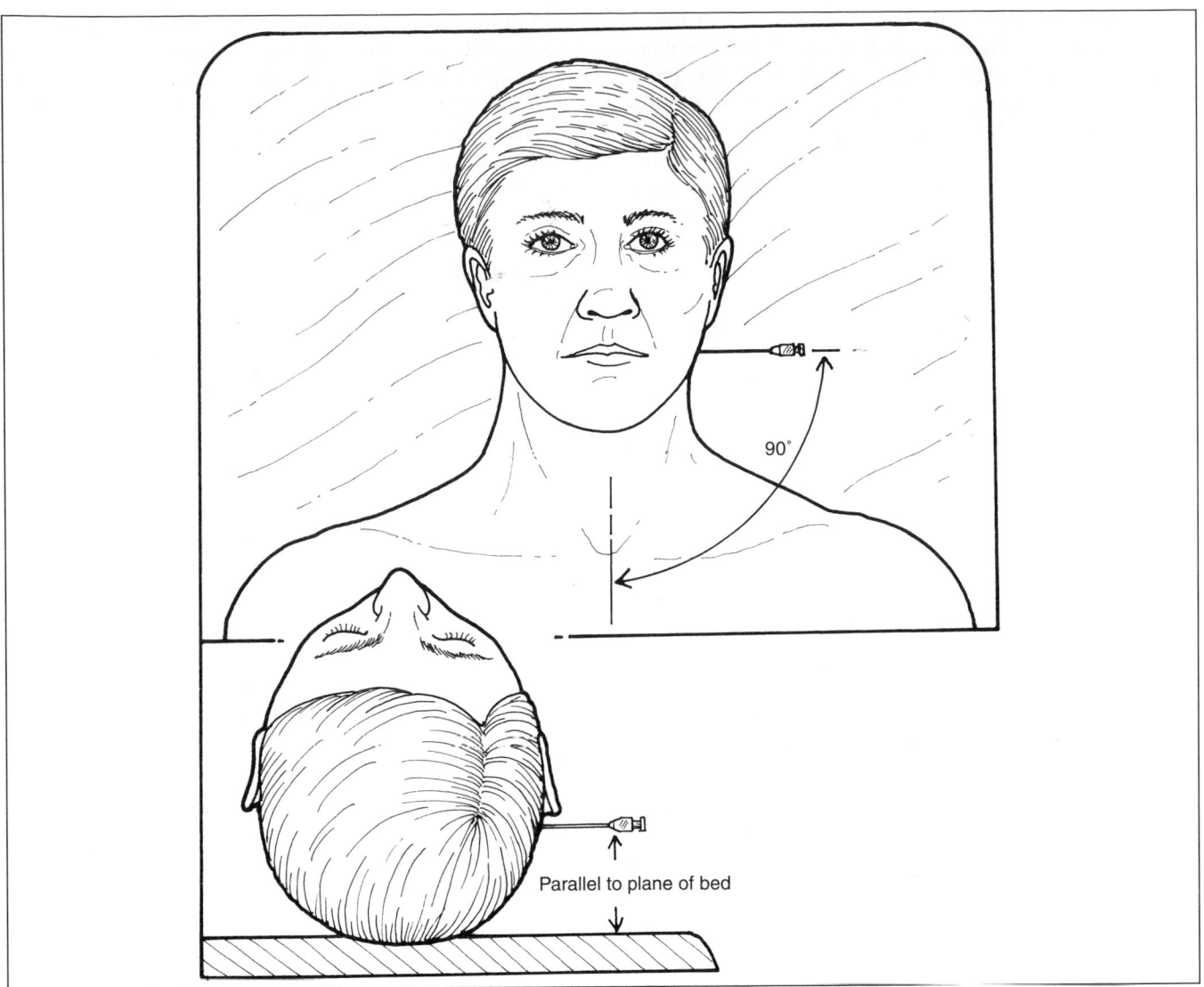

FIGURE 98-3 Proper needle trajectory for a cisternal puncture.

surrounding the vertebral artery may also be penetrated. Remove the needle and apply manual pressure if the vertebral artery is inadvertently entered. Reattempt the procedure with the tip of the needle directed slightly more posteriorly. Directing the needle too far posteriorly causes it to enter the spinal musculature and miss the spinal canal. In the event that bone is encountered, meaning that either the lateral arch of C1 or C2 is encountered, redirect the needle slightly rostrally or caudally and advance it into the subarachnoid space.

AFTERCARE

Maintain the patient in a supine position after the procedure. A small bandage is usually sufficient to control any soft tissue bleeding or continued CSF leakage.

Postdural puncture headaches can be minimized by utilizing a small gauged spinal needle inserted with the bevel parallel to the fibers of the dura. Resting in the supine position for 24 hours also reduces the incidence of postdural puncture headaches. Monitor the patient's neurological status. Any change in patient's baseline neurological examination requires a CT scan of the posterior fossa and occipital-cervical junction in order to rule out an epidural or intradural hemorrhage.

COMPLICATIONS

The complications associated with lumbar puncture are also possible during the lateral cervical puncture. Specific complications from lateral cervical puncture include penetration of the vertebral artery with subsequent hematoma formation and puncture of the spinal cord with resultant neurological deficits. Minimize complications by utilizing a small gauge spinal needle. These complications should result in no serious consequences if unilateral and recognized.[3] Approximately 0.4 percent of the population has an anomalously positioned vertebral artery. There has been a single case report of a death from a subdural hematoma due to puncture of this vessel.[4] A nerve root may be irritated with passage of the needle resulting in local pain or possibly a headache. Other complications include infection, herniation syndromes, neck pain, and headache. The incidence of postdural puncture headache is less with the lateral cervical puncture than with a lumbar puncture. Refer to Chapter 96 for the complete details regarding the complications associated with a lumbar puncture.

SUMMARY

A lumbar puncture is still the preferred technique to obtain cerebrospinal fluid for analysis as well as for injection of contrast material. Lateral cervical puncture is a safe alternative method. One can avoid the complications of puncturing the vertebral artery or the spinal cord by observing maximum attention to detail. Lateral cervical puncture can be performed at the bedside. However, the availability of a portable fluoroscopy unit facilitates the procedure.

REFERENCES

1. Ward E, Orrison W, Watridge C: Anatomic evaluation of cisternal puncture. *Neurosurgery* 1989; 25(3):412–415.
2. Mullan S, Harper PV, Hekmatpnah J, et al: Percutaneous interruption of spinal-pain tracts by means of a strontium 90 needle. *J Neurosurg* 1963; 20:931–939.
3. Zivin J: Lateral cervical puncture: an alternative to lumbar puncture. *Neurology* 1978; 28:616–618.
4. Rogers LA: Acute subdural hematoma and death following lateral cervical puncture. *J Neurosurg* 1983; 58:284–286.

Chapter 99
VENTRICULOSTOMY

Lauren S. Grossman

INTRODUCTION

Performing an emergent ventriculostomy may be lifesaving when faced with a patient who is deteriorating rapidly from a neurologic perspective and all other therapeutic options have been employed.[1] This chapter will discuss some of the situations when this procedure may be considered, other therapeutic options, and an explanation of how to perform an emergent ventriculostomy.

ANATOMY AND PATHOPHYSIOLOGY

The cranium is a fixed space after infancy that has little capacity for added volume or mass. Pathologic conditions such as tumors, intracranial hemorrhage, infection, massive infarctions, and edema can exert direct pressure on the brain or interrupt flow of the cerebrospinal fluid (CSF). These processes result in fluid accumulation and increased intracranial pressure (ICP).

The patient with increased ICP may display the classic clinical signs of headache, vomiting, and papilledema.[1] Vomiting is particularly associated with acute increases in ICP. Other signs include an abducens nerve palsy (cranial nerve VI) that causes diplopia, decreased consciousness, and an elevated blood pressure with bradycardia (Cushing's phenomenon). An increase in ICP may eventually progress to brain herniation.

Herniation occurs when there exists a force in part of the brain great enough to push other parts of the brain into different compartments. The cranial contents are divided into compartments by invaginations of the dura mater (Figure 99-1).[2] The supratentorial space is separated from the infratentorial space by the tentorium cerebelli. The right and left hemispheres are separated by the falx cerebri.

When a unilateral supratentorial mass exerts enough force, the ipsilateral cerebral hemisphere is pushed medially toward the opposite hemisphere (Figure 99-2A).

The medial aspect of the temporal lobe is pushed down towards the brainstem and over the edge of the tentorium cerebelli (Figure 99-2B). This process is known as tentorial herniation. Symptoms of tentorial herniation include a worsening of any headache with vomiting, progressively decreasing consciousness, anisocoria, hemiparesis, and Parinaud's syndrome (an upward gaze paresis). Compression of the oculomotor nerve results in a sluggish and dilated pupil, usually on the same side as the mass lesion. A progression to a fixed and dilated pupil, with decerebrate rigidity (extensor posturing), is an ominous sign of increased ICP.

Mass effect in the infratentorial compartment of the skull may produce downward pressure of the cerebellum into the foramen magnum (Figure 99-3A) or upward pressure of the midbrain into the supratentorial compartment (Figure 99-3B), the former being more common. The downward pressure is known as tonsillar or cerebellar herniation and the terminal events surrounding this condition may occur more urgently and fatally than a supratentorial herniation (Figure 99-3A). For example, an acute respiratory arrest may occur from compression of the medulla. Other important signs of tonsillar herniation include profuse vomiting, irregular respirations (ataxic breathing), neck pain, and neck stiffness. The patient may not necessarily lose consciousness or have pupillary changes prior to the terminal events of tonsillar herniation. Upward herniation forces the cerebellum and upper brainstem through the tentorial notch (Figure 99-3B). The patient is usually obtunded or comatose with small or anisocoric pupils that may, at first, be reactive. There may be an associated paresis of the extremities which progresses to decorticate posturing.

Any patient with these potentially life-threatening neurologic findings should be considered unstable and worked up accordingly. An emergent head CT scan, if available, is the diagnostic test of choice after the patient's airway, breathing, and circulation have been stabilized. Signs of herniation on the head CT include an

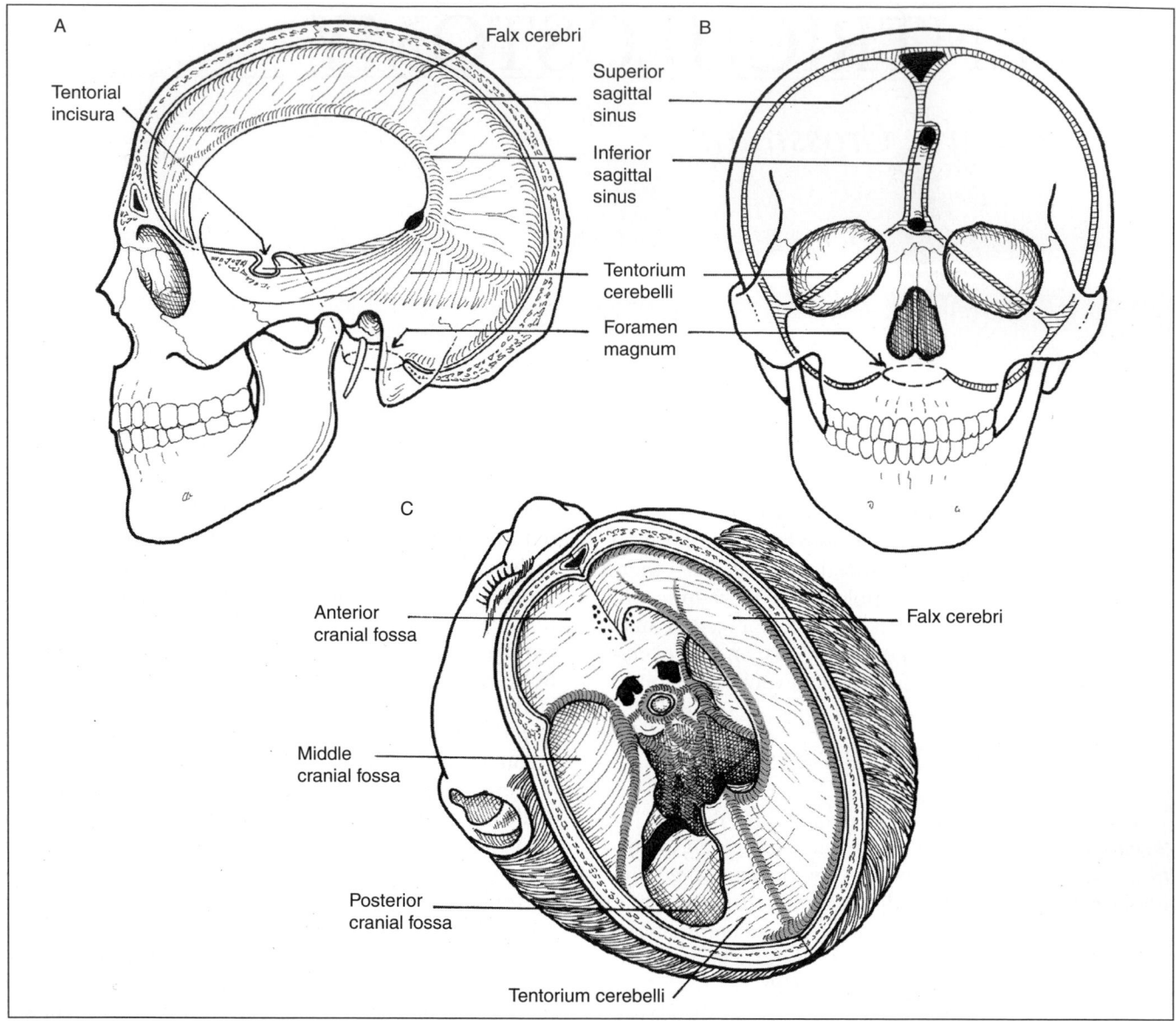

FIGURE 99-1 The falx cerebri and tentorium cerebelli divide the skull into compartments. *A.* Sagittal view. *B.* Coronal view. *C.* Top of the skull removed with a section of tentorium cerebelli also removed.

anterior midline shift with brain tissue from one side pushed under the falx and into the opposite side of the brain (subfalcial herniation; Figure 99-2*A*). Other signs include generalized cerebral edema with effacement of the sulci, the ventricles, the basilar cisterns, and the fourth ventricle.

There are several clinical interventions that should be implemented immediately once increased ICP, hydrocephalus, or herniation is suspected and the patient's condition is declining. The airway must be stabilized and rapid-sequence intubation is the procedure of choice. Pretreatment with lidocaine is useful in diminishing the elevation in ICP that occurs during direct laryngoscopy. Thiopental, etomidate, and propofol are the induction agents of choice as they decrease the ICP.

Neuromuscular blockade is accomplished with succinylcholine after administering a defasciculating dose of a nondepolarizing neuromuscular blocking agent. Paralytics may only be necessary for a brief period during intubation. **It is preferable to avoid paralysis for any length of time when the patient's neurologic status needs to be followed closely.** However, the need to follow the patient's neurologic course should be balanced by the need to reduce elevated ICP that may be accomplished, in part, with sedatives and paralytics. The potential for succinylcholine increasing ICP is most prevalent in patients with neoplasms of the central nervous system and may not be significant for acute trauma or bleeds.[3] Maintain the patient's oxygen saturation at 100 percent. Elevate the head of the bed to 30 degrees.

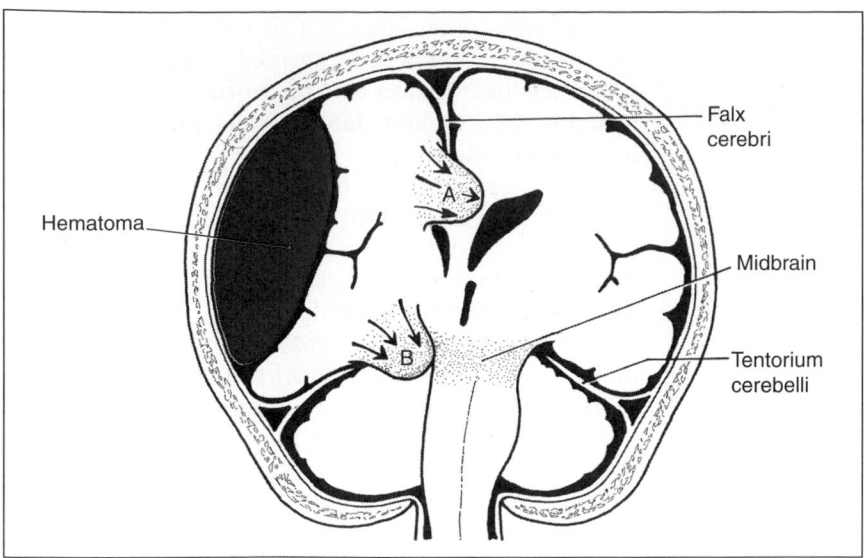

FIGURE 99-2 Supratentorial herniation of the brain. *A.* Tentorial herniation. *B.* Subfalcial herniation.

Place the patient in the reverse Trendelenburg position if a cervical spine injury is suspected.

It is desirable for the mean arterial pressure to be 90 mmHg or higher in order to maintain an adequate cerebral perfusion pressure and diminish the risk of cerebral ischemia. The commonly employed modalities of hyperventilation and osmotic diuresis are still used in the acutely deteriorating patient but their value is limited because of the ischemic and metabolic complications related to their use. Reducing the pCO_2 to 25 mmHg via hyperventilation can reduce the ICP in the acute resuscitation phase. The pCO_2 should not be maintained below 35 mmHg during the immediate postresuscitation period. The use of osmotic diuretics, such as mannitol, can also reduce ICP quickly. Unfortunately, any extended duration of use of osmotic diuretics places the patient at an increased risk for cerebral ischemia. Other methods to consider include the use of dexamethasone in patients with edema surrounding a neoplastic mass or abscess. Pentobarbital can be used to induce a coma that will reduce the ICP but also cause hypotension. An ICP monitoring device must be put into place since the ability to do sequential neurological checks is lost.

INDICATIONS

The aforementioned procedures are temporizing measures only. It is preferable to treat an identifiable pathologic process as soon as possible. This usually requires intervention by a Neurosurgeon. The Neurosurgeon may be able to take the patient to the Operating

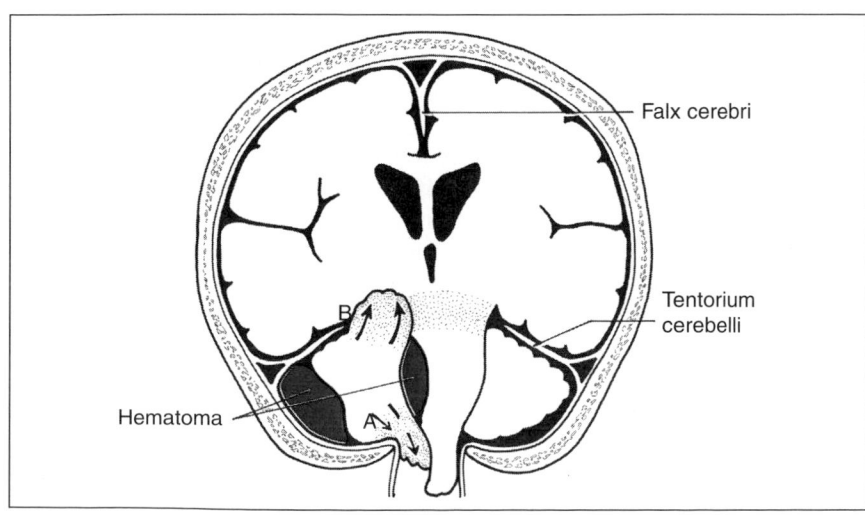

FIGURE 99-3 Infratentorial herniation of the brain. *A.* Downward tonsillar herniation through the foramen magnum. *B.* Upward herniation into the supratentorial compartment.

Room to place an indwelling ventricular shunt system in an expedited fashion. The ICP can be reduced by draining CSF via a ventriculostomy if the patient continues to deteriorate and a definitive procedure cannot be immediately arranged.

CONTRAINDICATIONS

Performing a ventriculostomy could precipitate or worsen herniation and hasten the patient's mortality if an infratentorial mass has been identified and it appears to be inducing upward pressure into the supratentorial compartment. Any coagulopathic conditions make a ventriculostomy dangerous to perform.

EQUIPMENT

Skin razor
Skin prep kit
Povidone iodine solution
Skin marker
Ventricular catheter with stylet
Drainage tubing and collection system
Measuring implement
Scalpel handle
#15 scalpel blade
Sterile surgical gloves
10 mL syringe
25 gauge needle
Lidocaine with epinephrine, 1%
Twist drill with a ¼ inch bit
Sterile towels
Bipolar cautery
Needle driver
3–0 nylon suture
Suction source
Suction tubing
Suction catheters
Headlight, optional
Curette, optional
3-way stopcock, optional

It is most useful to have either a commercially available ventriculostomy kit or assemble one to have available in the resuscitation area. Complete, disposable, and single-patient use kits are convenient and cost-effective (Integra Neurocare LLC, San Diego, California).

PATIENT PREPARATION

This procedure is often performed emergently. Explain the procedure, its risks, and benefits to the patient and/or their representative. If it will not unduly delay the treatment, obtain an informed consent to perform the procedure. **Always test for normal blood clotting function (PT, PTT, and platelet levels) prior to performing this procedure.**

Place the patient supine on a gurney with the head elevated 30 degrees. Identify the burr hole entry site. This is located 3 cm to the right of midline and 10 cm behind the glabella in the midpupillary line or 1 cm anterior to the coronal suture in the midpupillary line (Figure 99-4). Shave the right side of the head, the nondominant side in most people, for 4 to 5 cm surrounding the burr hole entry point. The hair from the entire frontal area back to the ear may be shaved, but it is probably unnecessary to do so. Clean the scalp of any dirt and debris. Apply povidone iodine solution and allow it to dry. Denote the landmark on the skin with a sterile skin marker. Apply sterile drapes to the head so that the medial canthus of the right eye can be visualized. Note the premade markings on the ventricular catheter or mark 4, 5, and 7 cm on the catheter prior to insertion.

TECHNIQUE

Infiltrate the marked area with 3 to 5 mL of local anesthetic solution containing epinephrine. Make a 1 to 2 cm incision with a #15 scalpel blade. Carry the incision down to and through the periosteum. Tie off or cauterize any bleeding vessels. Insert the self-retaining retractor into the incision to provide adequate exposure.

Prepare the drill. Choose the appropriate drill bit and insert it into the drill. Adjust the safety stop on the drill bit to the estimated skull thickness. Secure the safety stop on the drill bit firmly with an Allen wrench. Drill through the outer and inner tables of the skull. **Take care not to penetrate the dura. Do not apply too much force against the drill to prevent plunging the drill bit into the brain. Stop drilling when a loss of resistance is felt.** Flush the hole with warm sterile saline to remove any debris. Make an opening in the dura with an 18 gauge needle or a #11 scalpel blade.

A simple ventricular catheter or a fiberoptic catheter with a screw-in mechanism should be available. Apply gentle pressure while inserting the catheter into the brain matter and aiming for the medial canthus of the ipsilateral eye (Figure 99-4A). A loss of resistance or a "give" will often be felt as the catheter enters the ventricle. There should be a return of CSF at a depth of 4 to 5 cm. Withdraw the stylet and advance the catheter 1 cm farther. **Do not insert the catheter more than 7 cm deep.** If no CSF is obtained, withdraw the catheter and reinsert it while aiming slightly more medially and posteriorly; as the position of the ventricles may be distorted by the underlying pathologic process.

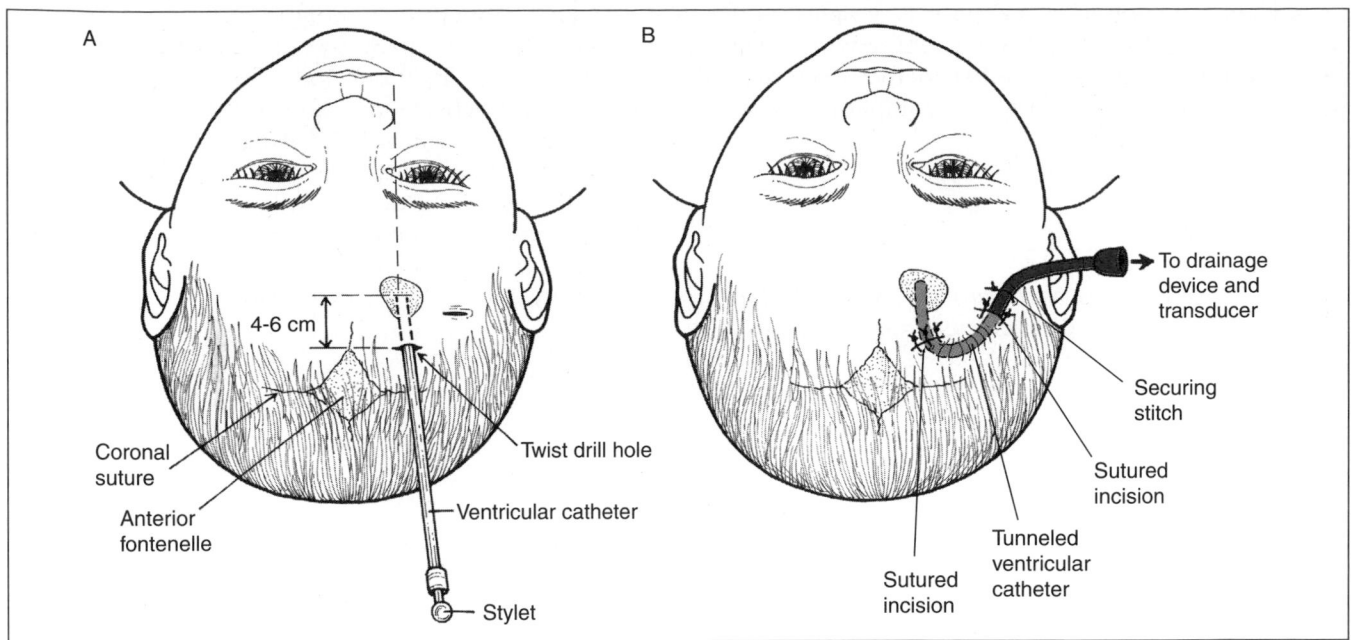

FIGURE 99-4 Placement of a ventriculostomy catheter. *A.* Insertion of the ventricular catheter. *B.* The catheter is tunneled and the skin closed.

It is desirable to tunnel the drainage tubing subcutaneously for several centimeters to reduce the risk of infection (Figure 99-4*B*).[1,4] Suture the ventricular catheter and tubing to the skin so that it remains in place (Figure 99-4*B*). Close the skin around the ventricular catheter. If a pressure transducer is being utilized, obtain a measurement prior to allowing any quantity of CSF to drain. Attach the sterile fluid collection system. If a simple drainage bag is being used, ensure that it is kept at the level of the ventricle to avoid overdrainage. Recheck the patient's neurologic status frequently.

COMPLICATIONS

The most common complication of placement of an emergent ventriculostomy is a CSF infection. The risk of infection increases the longer the drain is left in place. Fortunately, infections are rare for those in place for fewer than 4 days. Tunneling the drainage tubing, adhering to strict aseptic technique, and administering prophylactic antibiotics can reduce the incidence of infection. The usual infecting organisms are *Staphylococcus epidermidis* and *Staphylococcus aureus*. Appropriate antibiotic coverage includes third-generation cephalosporins and penicillinase-resistant penicillins. It is useful to send a baseline sample of CSF for culture, cell count, chemistry, and cytology (if applicable) after ventriculostomy placement.

Ventricular puncture can result in an acute bleed in the subdural, intraparenchymal, or ventricular spaces. This can occur from direct trauma to the vascular system or excessive CSF drainage that shrinks the brain and tears the bridging vessels to the subdural space. **An emergent head CT is indicated if the patient's condition deteriorates further after ventriculostomy placement. Patients should always be tested for normal blood clotting function prior to performing a ventriculostomy.**

The most feared complication of this procedure is plunging with the drill bit uncontrollably into the brain substance. This procedure should not be performed by those unfamiliar and untrained in the technique. Apply the minimal amount of pressure to the drill so that the bit penetrates the bone. Never use a twist drill without the safety stop.

SUMMARY

The patient who presents with a rapidly deteriorating neurologic status may have increased ICP or be in the process of brain herniation. There are several tools, in addition to emergent ventriculostomy placement, that can temporarily stabilize the patient's changing neurological status. This includes intubation, hyperventilation, osmotic diuresis, maintenance of cerebral perfusion pressure, dexamethasone administration, and barbiturate coma. While the ultimate goal is to treat the primary pathologic condition, this chapter was designed to describe the use of CSF drainage via ventriculostomy and its use in the context of the other methods commonly used to reverse the life-threatening complications of an acutely increasing ICP.

REFERENCES

1. Black PM, Rossitch E: *Neurosurgery, An Introductory Text.* New York: Oxford University Press, 1995:99–100.

2. Sugiura K, Robinson G, Stuart D: *Illustrated Guide to the Central Nervous System.* St. Louis: Ishiyaku EuroAmerica, 1989:144–150.

3. Danzl D: Tracheal intubation and mechanical ventilation, in Tintinalli J, Kelen G, Stapczynski (eds): *Emergency Medicine: A Comprehensive Study Guide,* 4th ed. New York: McGraw-Hill, 2000:85–97.

4. Mapstone T, Ratcheson R: Techniques of ventricular puncture, in Wilkins R, Rengachary S (eds): *Neurosurgery,* 2nd ed. New York: McGraw-Hill, 1996:179–183.

Chapter 100
VENTRICULAR SHUNT EVALUATION AND ASPIRATION

Lauren S. Grossman

INTRODUCTION

Pediatric and adult patients with ventricular shunts frequently seek medical attention in acute care settings with complaints that may or may not be caused by a malfunction and/or infection of these indwelling devices. The challenge for the clinician is to determine if the shunt system is functioning properly and if it is a direct cause of the patient's acute problem. This chapter will discuss the complications of ventricular shunt malfunction including infection.

Complications in children with ventricular shunts are common whereas those in adults occur less frequently. Approximately 30 percent of infants will experience shunt complications during their first year following shunt placement.[1] Children who had shunts placed as infants will require two shunt revisions secondary to obstruction within their first 10 years.[1] The overall shunt infection rate is 10 to 20 percent.[1–3] Approximately 90 percent of these infections will present within 3 months of the shunt placement.[1] These statistics apply to the population with conventionally treated hydrocephalus using indwelling ventricular shunt devices. It is significant to note that with the wide application and development of neuroendoscopic techniques, many of the complications discussed in this chapter will be eliminated or significantly reduced.

Complications resulting from ventricular shunts take many forms. These include proximal obstruction (most common), distal obstruction, disconnection, wound and cerebrospinal fluid (CSF) infections, seizures, epidural hygromas, subdural hematomas, low (overdrainage) and high pressure (slit ventricle) syndromes, and cranial deformities. There are other unique complications experienced by the smaller number of patients who have ventriculoatrial (V-A) and ventriculopleural shunt systems and these will be discussed separately. Unless stated otherwise, the reader should assume that reference is being made to the more common ventriculoperitoneal (V-P) shunt device.

Patients with shunts may present with clinical entities as benign as a viral upper respiratory infection or with a life threat like hydrocephalus; the wide range of possibilities is a challenge to the practitioner's diligence and clinical acumen. Common presenting symptoms include headache, fever, vomiting, decreased alertness, neck stiffness, visual changes, malaise, abdominal pain, abdominal distension, and surgical site problems.

ANATOMY AND PATHOPHYSIOLOGY

Hydrocephalus, a condition defined by an excessive quantity of CSF, is the condition most frequently associated with the initial need for a ventricular shunt or a shunt revision if it malfunctions. Most abnormal accumulations of CSF are identified in the ventricles, although it may also occur in the subarachnoid or subdural spaces. Several types of hydrocephalus are cited in the literature.

Communicating hydrocephalus occurs when there is unobstructed flow of CSF between the ventricular system of the brain and the spinal cord. It frequently occurs in patients who have had a hemorrhage or infectious process whereby particulate matter interferes with the normal circulation and absorption of CSF. A congenital problem such as aqueductal stenosis or a mass lesion in the posterior fossa may obstruct the flow of CSF between the brain and spinal cord causing obstructive hydrocephalus or noncommunicating hydrocephalus. Normal pressure hydrocephalus is usually a diagnosis made in older people who present with the clinical triad of dementia, ataxic gait, and urinary incontinence. The CSF is found to flow within a normal pressure range, but the patient accumulates excess CSF due to decreased absorption. Hydrocephalus ex vacuo is the result of excessive CSF and ventricular enlargement due to brain atrophy. It presents a challenge to the acute care practitioner who may need to decide if a patient with large ventricles on head CT has a pathologic condition or has so much brain atrophy that the fluid filled spaces appear excessively large.[4]

The clinical presentation of hydrocephalus will vary depending upon its acuity and the age of the patient. The individual who experiences shunt failure may present in the same way as one who is presenting with hydrocephalus initially. Infants may have an enlarged head circumference, a bulging anterior fontanel, separation of the cranial sutures, bilateral or unilateral palsy of the abducens nerve (medial eye deviation), or Parinaud's syndrome.[5] Parinaud's syndrome is a paralysis of upward gaze (also known as "sunset eyes" or the setting sun sign), unequal pupils, and the loss of convergence.[5]

Within hours of an acute cause of hydrocephalus, the patient (past infancy) will commonly experience a headache with nausea and vomiting secondary to the quick increase in intracranial pressure (ICP). The patient may less commonly have a focal neurological deficit due to the pressure exerted by the brainstem from a dilated third ventricle. There may also be visual changes that include Parinaud's syndrome. A change in mental status may occur as the increase in ICP persists. Finally, signs of herniation signify a terminal event. It will be observed with, for example, decorticate or decerebrate posturing, a third cranial nerve palsy, and the Cushing reflex (elevated blood pressure accompanied by bradycardia). The process of herniation is nearly completely reversible with immediate ventricular drainage through emergent revision of a malfunctioning shunt or the de novo placement of a ventricular drain.

Chronic hydrocephalus can present with a variety of signs and symptoms. The patient may complain of an isolated bifrontal headache, a generalized headache, vomiting, a change in behavior, a change in mentation, or a change in cognition. Ocular findings include papilledema, a unilateral or bilateral abducens nerve palsy, Parinaud's syndrome, or even a bitemporal hemianopsia. The extremities may be involved with spasticity in the legs that is more pronounced than that found in the arms.

Once the diagnosis of hydrocephalus is made, the Neurosurgeon will be responsible for treating the primary causes (e.g., tumor, bleed, congenital abnormality) along with placement of an indwelling ventricular shunt. The components of a standard shunt system include a ventricular catheter, a one-way valve, and distal tubing that enters the cavity into which the fluid is being shunted (Figure 100-1). It is standard practice to enter the right lateral ventricle and tunnel the valve system and distal tubing subcutaneously along the right temporoparietal region of the skull, the lateral neck, the

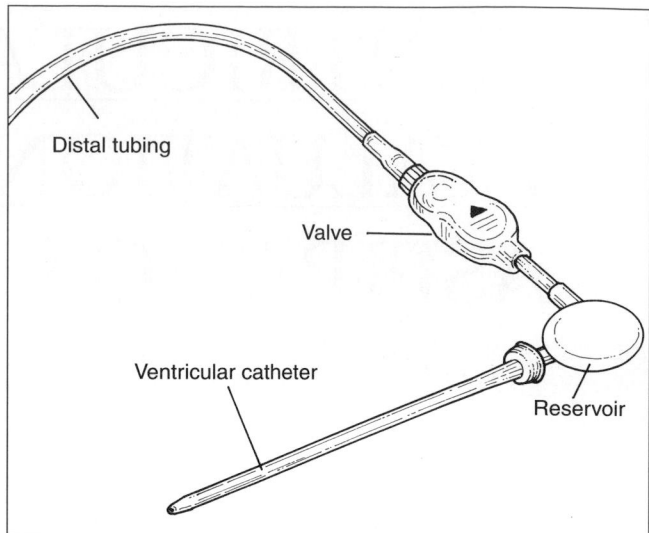

FIGURE 100-1 The components of a ventricular shunt.

anterolateral chest wall, and finally into the peritoneal space just superior or lateral (right side) to the umbilicus (Figure 100-2). The shunt system may occasionally be found on the left side in some patients.

Much of the shunt pathway is palpable on physical examination (Figure 100-2). The entire system may be visualized on plain radiographs. The system is impregnated with radiopaque material either entirely or with intermittent markings.

The ventricular catheter is inserted through a burr hole and into the lateral ventricle. The distal end of the ventricular catheter is connected to one of many different types of valves currently available. Functionally, there are two main types. The differential pressure valve allows the Surgeon to select a low, medium, or high pressure system whereby the CSF will flow out of the ventricle through a one-way system when the CSF pressure or CSF flow rate builds to a specified level. A variable resistance constant flow valve keeps CSF rates constant and, therefore, provides a more physiologic system by varying the resistance in the valve as the individual changes position. Some of these valves, although palpable on physical examination, do not allow access to the CSF for aspiration nor do they allow for any non-invasive assessment of CSF flow. A bubble-like reservoir (may be single or two bubbles in tandem) for the draining of CSF is a common addition to the standard three-part shunt system. While they can be inserted anywhere in the system, they are most frequently located adjacent to the valve mechanism on the lateral aspect of the skull (Figure 100-2).

The distal tubing is made of a flexible and soft synthetic rubber material that is attached to the reservoir/valve system and tunneled subcutaneously through

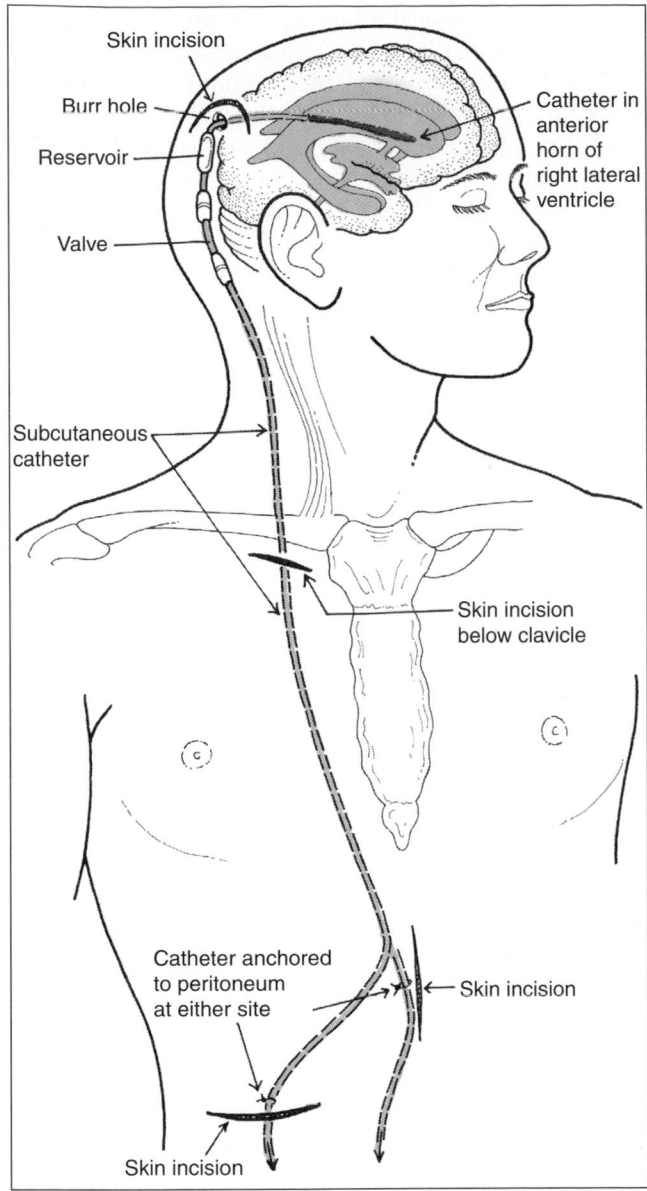

FIGURE 100-2 The anatomical pathway of a ventriculoperitoneal shunt.

the lateral neck, chest, and abdominal wall. A small incision is made in the skin and the peritoneum where the tubing is brought from the subcutaneous tissue into the peritoneal cavity. After securing the tubing to the peritoneum, a generous portion of tubing is left free floating inside the peritoneal cavity. This allows for the distal end to lengthen as the patient grows and lends further stability to its place within the abdominal cavity.

The distal tubing in ventriculoatrial and ventriculopleural shunt systems will terminate in the right atria and right pleural cavity, respectively. However, these configurations are not used frequently. One may also come across a patient with a lumboperitoneal shunt that avoids any invasive procedures to the brain directly. This system is inserted into the lumbar subarachnoid space with the valve/reservoir system located above the iliac crest and the distal tubing tunneled subcutaneously in the abdominal wall and into the abdominal cavity.

The patient is subject to a host of complications due to mechanical malfunctioning that can occur anywhere along the path of the system. There is the risk of infection, as is the case with any indwelling medical device. The remainder of this chapter will guide the reader through the process of identifying the various types of shunt problems.

INDICATIONS

The clinician is obliged to assess the patency, placement, and integrity of the shunt system when a patient presents with any symptoms even remotely related to hydrocephalus. The presence of systemic signs or local signs of infection is a reason to consider aspirating CSF from the system. This includes fever, warmth, tenderness, bogginess, or redness along the shunt tract. That is not to say that every child with an upper respiratory infection requires that the shunt be tapped. It is not uncommon to have overlapping findings in that an infection may obstruct the system and therefore require both mechanical and infectious complications to be addressed. The withdrawal of CSF from the shunt can be lifesaving and sustain the patient who is herniating, in extremis, or deteriorating neurologically until a Neurosurgeon can repair the shunt.

CONTRAINDICATIONS

There are no contraindications to performing a thorough physical examination of the shunt system, obtaining a head CT, and obtaining plain radiographs to assess its integrity. There is some controversy, however, that surrounds the tapping of a shunt by personnel other than a Neurosurgeon. It is possible to disrupt the pressure and valve mechanism by the manipulation of the needle that is required to perform the tap. The reservoir may develop a leak if the correct technique is not employed or if the shunt is tapped too frequently. There is the risk that bacteria will be introduced into the system. Many patients have had multiple complications related to both a primary disease and the shunt, with some already having undergone a number of shunt revisions. **It is prudent to assume a conservative approach with each of these patients and consult a Neurosurgeon prior to tapping the shunt.**

SHUNT ASSESSMENT

The technique of shunt evaluation begins with taking a complete history and performing a thorough physical examination. Palpate the entire system starting with the cranium. Examine the surrounding scalp carefully for any bogginess (indicating that CSF may have extravasated from the system), redness, tenderness, or warmth. The suture line should be examined as well if the shunt has been placed recently. Examine the scalp on the right side for a burr hole. This is where you may palpate a shunt reservoir that is placed subcutaneously. The reservoir feels like a firm fluid-filled bubble. Compress the bubble gently to assess if there is brisk refilling of the CSF. Quick filling of the reservoir is an indication that the proximal portion of the system may be patent, but this is by no means a perfect test. Resistance to compression indicates a distal malfunction. **Avoid pumping the reservoir repeatedly.**

A double bubble (reservoir system) may be occasionally palpated. Compress the proximal reservoir to empty it and fill the distal reservoir. While still compressing the proximal reservoir, compress the distal reservoir. Any resistance to compression indicates a distal malfunction. With both reservoirs compressed, release the proximal reservoir. It should refill very quickly. Any delay in filling of the proximal reservoir indicates a proximal malfunction.

Move down and palpate the temporal region of the scalp and the neck. Note any gaps in the system that could indicate a disconnection. The individual components of the shunt system are commonly joined by small connectors that may come apart. Continue to palpate the tubing along the neck and chest until you reach the abdomen. Perform a thorough abdominal examination, specifically noting the presence of any tenderness, masses, distension, or erythema of the abdominal wall.

The distal end of the shunt may not function for several reasons. The tip may have withdrawn out of the peritoneal cavity and into the preperitoneal fat or subcutaneous tissue of the abdominal wall where the CSF cannot be resorbed. This may have occurred simply because the patient had grown and used up the extra length of catheter that was originally left in the peritoneal cavity just for this reason. Intraperitoneal infections, particularly those caused by anaerobic organisms, may cause loculations around the catheter tip forming a pseudocyst. It is important to note that these patients may not have any signs of a systemic infection. Additional causes of distal catheter obstruction include kinking of the intraabdominal tubing, debris collection around the tube openings, and compression secondary to pregnancy or other processes that increase the intraabdominal pressure.

After completing the history and physical examination, including an assessment of the shunt system, the differential diagnoses will help initiate an appropriate work-up. One or more of the following studies may be indicated: plain radiograph shunt series, computerized tomography (CT) of the head, shunt aspiration of CSF, or a radioisotope shunt scan. **Stabilize the patient and arrange for an emergent head CT if any life-threatening signs of neurologic dysfunction appear.**

There are several important points to note. Findings consistent with hydrocephalus include enlargement or effacement of the ventricles, particularly looking for fullness of the temporal horns of the lateral ventricles (Figure 100-3). It can be difficult to determine if there is a change in the ventricular system because congenital or chronic abnormalities can give the CT scan an abnormal

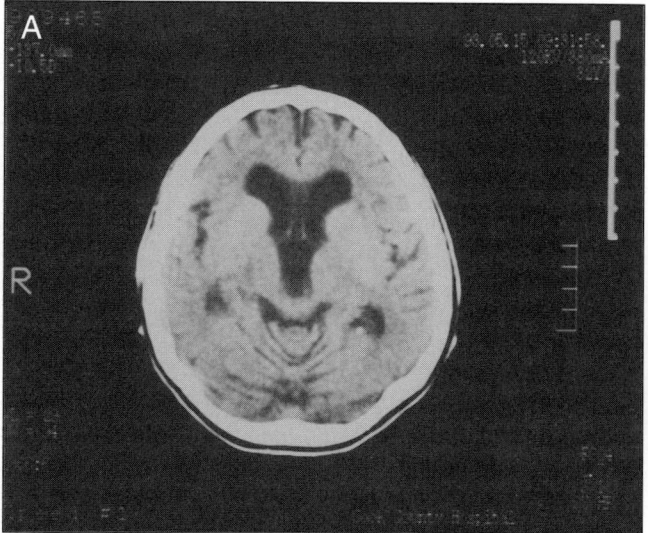

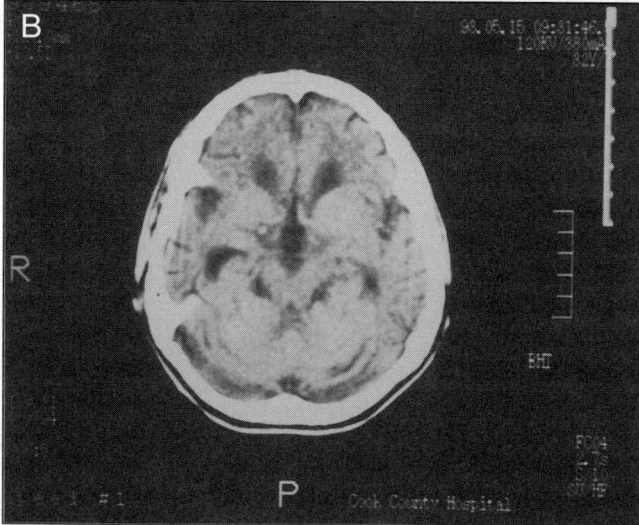

FIGURE 100-3 Head CT of a patient with hydrocephalus. *A.* The ventricles are enlarged with effacement. *B.* Pronounced temporal horns.

appearance. The best way to approach this situation is to compare the current scan to a previous one, preferably by comparing the two scans side by side. Brain atrophy causes the ventricles to appear abnormally full when, in fact, they appear large because of the relative loss of brain tissue.

Impending herniation may be a concern if the brain appears to be under increased pressure with a loss of the sulcal markings, loss of the differentiation between the gray and white matter, or an inability to visualize the fourth ventricle. The ventricles can appear unusually small which may be an indication of a shunt system that is draining CSF too vigorously. Overdrainage may be the problem if the patient complains of a positional headache that is worse in the upright position and less severe when supine. **If this is the case, it is important to carefully examine the CT scan for any subdural hematomas that can result from the brain shrinking away from the dura and tearing a bridging vein secondary to overdrainage of CSF.** The patient's scan may reveal small ventricles accompanied by signs of increased ICP in the slit ventricle syndrome. While the slit ventricle syndrome is poorly understood, it is theorized that ventricles with poor compliance (common in those with chronic hydrocephalus) will respond to small increases in CSF pressure with large increases in ICP.

Obtain a plain radiograph shunt series if there is the slightest suspicion of a shunt malfunction or infection. This study consists of anteroposterior and lateral plain radiographs of the skull, neck, chest, and abdomen. These films are useful for assessing placement and integrity of the connections within the shunt system. Shunt materials are impregnated with a radiopaque substance either completely or in regularly placed markings so that the entire device can be visualized on plain radiographs. **It is important to obtain and review the lateral abdominal film as this view is frequently overlooked.** It is impossible to determine if the shunt tubing lies within the peritoneal cavity or not if the lateral abdominal film is excluded. The entire path of the shunt system should be visualized. Particular findings to note on this study include placement of the ventricular catheter inside of the ventricle, the integrity of the connections around the valve and/or reservoir, and the identification of the distal catheter within the peritoneal cavity. Examine the chest radiographs closely for a pleural effusion or a pneumothorax in a patient with a ventriculopleural shunt.

SHUNT ASPIRATION

Tapping the ventricular shunt should be considered whenever there are signs of localized infection, systemic infection, or in some cases of suspected obstruction without an identifiable cause. It should also be per-

formed if the patient is in extremis, deteriorating neurologically, or has signs of herniation on the CT scan. This can temporarily restore cerebral perfusion and sustain the patient until a Neurosurgeon can repair the shunt. **It is recommended that a Neurosurgeon be consulted and given the first option to perform the procedure.** The Neurosurgeon may have already manipulated the hardware multiple times and will ultimately be responsible for any shunt revisions and follow-up. Patients with ventriculoatrial shunts are a particular concern when there are any signs of an infection. The distal catheter sits at the intersection of the right atrium and the superior vena cava. This puts the patient at risk for life threats such as endocarditis and septic emboli.

Tapping a ventricular shunt is a quick and simple procedure. Palpate the lateral aspect of the skull (usually the right side of the patient) for the reservoir. Plain radiographs may be helpful if it is difficult to identify upon palpation. Prepare for the procedure by having the following equipment available: four sterile fluid specimen tubes with tight fitting tops (those supplied in the standard lumbar puncture kit are ideal), a 23 to 25 gauge butterfly needle, a 5 to 10 mL syringe, a shave-prep set, an antibacterial cleansing preparation (povidone iodine), a fenestrated drape, and sterile gloves.

Local anesthetic is not required for this procedure. Place the patient in whatever position is mutually comfortable. Shave a small patch of hair overlying the reservoir. Clean the skin of any dirt and debris. Apply povidone iodine and allow it to dry. Place the drape over the patient's head so that the fenestration overlies the reservoir and prepped skin.

Insert the needle at approximately 45 degrees from the vertex of the reservoir bubble with the tip pointed toward the center of the reservoir (Figure 100-4). This is where the greatest amount of CSF is located. **Avoid inserting the needle into any of the connections or internal pressure mechanisms that may be at either end of the reservoir.** Allow the CSF to passively drain from the butterfly tubing into sterile tubes. It may be necessary to very gently aspirate 4 to 5 mL of CSF. The ventricular end of the shunt is obstructed if CSF cannot be aspirated. Withdraw the needle from the shunt reservoir. Transport the tubes of CSF to the laboratory for a cell count and differential, Gram's stain, culture, and chemistry (protein and glucose). Obtain a sample of the patient's serum glucose at the same time so as to more accurately determine what level of glucose in the CSF to call abnormal. A normal level of CSF glucose should not be any lower than 50 to 66 percent of the serum level.

It is possible to attach the end of the butterfly tubing to a manometer so that an opening pressure can be measured. This must be done, however, with the patient in the lateral decubitus position, reservoir side up, and the head level with the heart.

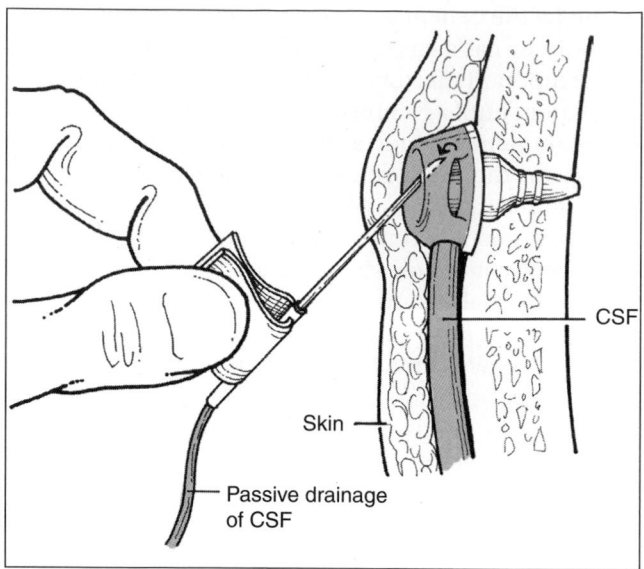

FIGURE 100-4 Tapping the shunt reservoir.

Obtain a nuclear medicine test ("shunt-o-gram") if CSF cannot be aspirated to determine proximal patency of the system. A radioactive isotope (technetium) is injected into the reservoir after manually occluding the distal shunt tubing. The flow, or lack thereof, of the radioactive isotope is then imaged.[3] **A lumbar puncture should never be performed in lieu of tapping the shunt. Obstruction of the shunt system can result in obstructive hydrocephalus. Lumbar puncture in a patient with obstructive hydrocephalus can cause a significant pressure differential and precipitate brain herniation.**

CSF ASSESSMENT

The CSF obtained from the shunt is interpreted in the same way as CSF from a lumbar puncture. A high white cell count with a large number of polymorphonuclear leukocytes, low glucose, and a high protein level indicates a high likelihood of bacterial infection. However, the positive Gram stain and culture make the definitive diagnosis. Unfortunately, there is no standard for the number of white cells that definitively indicates an infection. Some patients with indwelling shunts may have a chronically elevated CSF white blood cell count, albeit with more lymphocytes or eosinophils than polymorphonuclear leukocytes.[2] Refer to Chapter 96 for a more detailed discussion regarding the evaluation of CSF. Antibiotic coverage should be initiated if a shunt is being tapped. *Staphylococcus epidermidis* causes the vast majority of infections with *Staphylococcus aureus* and gram-negative bacilli following in frequency. Empiric therapy includes vancomycin with either cefotaxime or ceftriaxone for children and vancomycin with rifampin for adults.[6]

COMPLICATIONS

There are a few complications associated with the aspiration of a ventricular shunt. The introduction of bacteria into the reservoir can result in meningitis, peritonitis, brain abscesses, shunt occlusion, or infection anywhere along the course of the shunt tubing. It is of the utmost importance to maintain strict sterile technique. The needle can damage the reservoir and result in a permanent hole necessitating its removal and replacement. A misplaced needle can damage the connections or valves of the shunt system.

SUMMARY

Patients with indwelling ventricular shunt devices are subject to many complications throughout their lives. This most commonly includes obstruction, infection, and malfunction secondary to loss of placement or connection. Clinicians will see patients of all ages with shunts and who present with headache, fever, nausea, vomiting, seizures, irritability, or a change in mental status. The challenge, frequently a formidable one, will be to determine whether or not the patient's complaint is related to the shunt. This chapter discussed some of the common shunt complications and an approach to their diagnosis. The head CT, the plain film shunt series, and the shunt tap will prove most useful. Of course, a careful history and a skilled physical examination will set the clinician on a path towards a good outcome for the patient. A Neurosurgeon should be consulted if available. A conservative approach to diagnosis, management, and patient disposition is strongly recommended due to the life-threatening nature of shunt complications.

REFERENCES

1. Pople I: Management of shunt complications, in Palmer JP (ed): *Neurosurgery 96: Manual of Neurosurgery.* New York: Churchill Livingstone, 1996:590–592.
2. Scott RM: Shunt complications, in Wilkins R, Rengachary S (eds): *Neurosurgery,* 2nd ed. New York: McGraw-Hill, 1996:3655–3664.
3. Muhonen M, Wellman J: Hydrocephalus and benign intracranial cysts, in Grossman R, Loftus C (eds): *Principles of Neurosurgery,* 2nd ed. Philadelphia: Lippincott-Raven, 1999:93–114.

4. *Stedman's Illustrated Medical Dictionary,* 27th ed. Baltimore: Williams & Wilkins, 2000.

5. Netter FH: *The CIBA Collection of Medical Illustrations, Volume I, Nervous System, Part II Neurologic and Neuromuscular Disorders.* Summit, NJ: CIBA, 1986:8–9.

6. Gilbert DN, Moellering RC, Sande MA: *The Sanford Guide to Antimicrobial Therapy 2001,* 31st ed. Hyde Park, VT: Antimicrobial Therapy, 2001:5.

7. Black PML, Ojemann RG: Hydrocephalus in adults, in Youmans JR (ed): *Neurological Surgery,* 3rd ed. Philadelphia: Saunders, 1990:1277–1298.

Chapter 101
SUBDURAL HEMATOMA ASPIRATION IN THE INFANT

Yogesh Ghandhi
Don W. Penney

INTRODUCTION

Extra-axial fluid collections in children are classified as symptomatic and asymptomatic. Symptomatic, chronic extra-axial fluid collections have been variously classified as hematomas, effusions, or hygromas with differing definitions associated with each. It has been proposed that they all be classified together as extra-axial fluid collections because their appearance on CT scan and treatment is identical.[1] Symptomatic, chronic extra-axial fluid collections usually show ventricular compression and flattening or obliteration of the cerebral sulci on CT scans. Benign subdural fluid collections usually appear as a hypodensity over the frontal lobes with dilatation of the interhemispheric fissure, cortical sulci, and Sylvian fissure. The ventricles are usually normal or slightly enlarged with no evidence of transependymal flow.

Seizures, a large head, vomiting, irritability, and lethargy are common presenting symptoms of symptomatic extra-axial fluid collections. Physical examination reveals a full fontanel, macrocephaly, fever, lethargy, hemiparesis, retinal hemorrhages, generalized increased tone, or gaze paresis. Markwalder has done an excellent review of the pathophysiology and experimental studies of chronic subdural hematomas.[2]

The majority of extra-axial fluid collections result from head trauma. Other causes include bacterial meningitis (postinfectious) and the placement of a ventriculoperitoneal shunt. Chronic subdural fluid collections are common problems during infancy. Males are affected more commonly than females. **A clear history of injury or trauma should be sought in cases of acute or chronic subdural hematomas.** If a history of injury is not forthcoming, every opportunity should be seized to investigate the child and the social setting to screen for child abuse. **It is incumbent upon the medical team to rule out abuse.** This may require a period of observation, social services consultation, a radi-ological skeletal survey, a bone scan, and possibly an ophthalmological assessment. **The presence of retinal hemorrhages in association with a subdural fluid collection is highly suspicious for child abuse.** Admission to the hospital for further observation is warranted if child abuse cannot be ruled out. The presence of congenital anomalies may predispose the child to subdural hematoma formation.

Percutaneous removal of the subdural fluid is useful in diagnosing active infection and rapidly lowering intracranial pressure in patients who are symptomatic. Repeated removal of the fluid by percutaneous aspirations has been advocated by some Neurosurgeons for definitive treatment of chronic extra-axial fluid collections.[3,4] Subdural fluid collections in infants have a tendency to increase in size, are often bilateral, can be difficult to diagnose, and are most often seen in children under the age of two years. The combination of CT and MRI imaging is usually diagnostic.

ANATOMY AND PATHOPHYSIOLOGY

A subdural aspiration (or tap) is usually performed by puncturing the anterior fontanel. However, it can also be approached through the coronal suture as well as through the soft cranium. The diamond-shaped anterior fontanel is formed by the junction of the sagittal, coronal, and frontal sutures (Figure 101-1). It measures approximately 4 cm in the anteroposterior plane and 2.5 cm in the transverse plane. The bones of the infant calvarium are separated by connective tissue bands referred to as sutures. The fontanels are readily palpable clinically. Other fontanels are present in the infant's head in addition to the anterior and posterior fontanel. Six of the fontanels are located at each of the corners of the two parietal bones. Two of these, the anterior and posterior fontanels, are in the midline. The anterior fontanel, the largest of the neonatal fontanels, is utilized

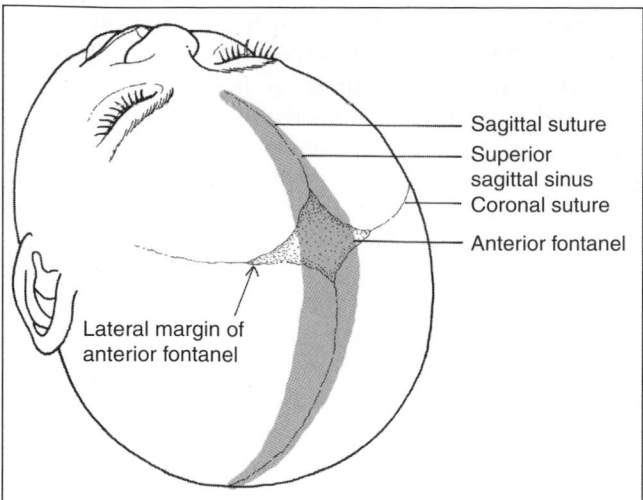

FIGURE 101-1 Surface anatomy of the infant skull. The red line represents the underlying superior sagittal sinus.

TABLE 101-1. THE ETIOLOGIES FOR INTRACRANIAL AND EXTRA-AXIAL FLUID COLLECTIONS

Coagulopathy
Infection
Masqueraders
  Craniocerebral disproportion
  Extracerebral space is enlarged and filled with CSF-like fluid as a result of the head being too large for the enclosed brain
  External hydrocephalus in a child with ventriculomegaly and extracerebral fluid
Neoplastic
  Metastatic
  Primary
Spontaneous
Vascular
  Aneurysm
  Vascular malformation

for percutaneous subdural aspiration. The anterior fontanel is located at the junction of the coronal and sagittal sutures. The posterior fontanel is at the junction of the lamboidal and sagittal sutures. In general, the anterior fontanel has usually closed by 18 months of age but can be patent up to the age of 2 years. The posterior fontanel usually closes earlier in life and is usually complete by 6 weeks of age.

The anterior fontanel is composed of connective tissue and easily perforated with a spinal needle. Continued penetration with the needle would then perforate the underlying dura allowing the needle to rest within the subdural space. Traversing the dura is usually associated with a definite change in resistance as the subdural space is entered. Successful entry into the subdural clot can be confirmed by removal of the stylet and observing spontaneous drainage from the needle hub. The anterior fontanel is readily palpable and bulging in cases of symptomatic chronic extra-axial fluid collections. The lateral extent of the anterior fontanel is continuous with the coronal suture (Figure 101-1).

INDICATIONS

A subdural tap is performed for diagnostic purposes as well as for rapid decompression of subdural fluid collections. The etiology of intracranial hemorrhage and extra-axial fluid collections are quite varied (Table 101-1). Aspiration of extra-axial fluid collections can reduce the intracranial pressure dramatically. Subdural aspiration of fluid allows for culture and sensitivity, identification of microorganisms, and aids in the selection of bacterial specific antimicrobial agents if an infectious etiology is considered to be the cause of the extra-axial fluid collection.

CONTRAINDICATIONS

The main contraindications to performing a subdural aspiration include localized infections of the scalp, patients who are coagulopathic, children over the age of two, children who have an absence of the anterior fontanel as a result of premature closure, a solid clot that is not liquefied, and children with congenital anomalies of the skull or brain. This procedure should not be performed by those unfamiliar with the technique and its complications.

EQUIPMENT

Sterile prep kit
Povidone iodine solution
Sterile drapes
Local anesthetic solution with epinephrine
20 or 21 gauge short spinal needle
Tincture of benzoin
Cotton swab
Bandage
Bundling blanket
Syringe for aspirating fluid
IV extension tubing, optional

All of this equipment can be found in commercially available pediatric lumbar puncture kits.

PATIENT PREPARATION

Explain the procedure to the parents and/or guardian of the child if time permits. Obtain an informed consent to perform the procedure. Place the patient supine on a stretcher. The child may need to be restrained to prevent moving during the procedure. Bundling an infant in a blanket and placing their head close to the edge of the bed facilitates aspiration. The aid of an assistant to hold the child's body with the head straight and upright is recommended if the child is restless. Some children may require the administration of parenteral sedatives.

Shave the frontal and parietal regions of the child's head. Clean any dirt and debris from the scalp. Identify by palpation the anterior fontanel, the coronal suture, and the lateral margin of the coronal suture. Apply povidone iodine solution to the skin and allow it to dry. Ensure that the solution is not allowed to drain onto the baby's face or eyes as it can cause burns. Apply sterile drapes leaving the frontal and parietal regions of the skull exposed. A local anesthetic agent is usually not required but may be used at the physician's discretion. If used, place a skin wheal using 0.25 to 0.50 mL of local anesthetic solution at the site the needle will enter the scalp.

TECHNIQUE

Form a Z-tract by gently sliding the scalp skin laterally. Insert a 22 gauge spinal needle into the lateral margin of the anterior fontanel, about 3 cm off the midline (Figure 101-2). Advance the spinal needle beneath the frontal bone at a 45 degree angle to the skin surface until the subdural space is penetrated. A loss of resistance is usually appreciated as the dura is penetrated and the subdural space is entered. **Do not ad-**

vance the needle any further. Securely hold the spinal needle so that it does not move (Figure 101-3). Remove the stylet. Spontaneous drainage is often appreciated. This fluid may appear hemorrhagic. However, it is not uncommon, especially in patients who require multiple taps, to drain xanthrochromic fluid.

The initial subdural tap usually results in spontaneous drainage through the spinal needle. Apply a syringe to the spinal needle and gently aspirate the fluid if it does not spontaneously drain. **Use minimal negative pressure to just aspirate the fluid collection and prevent pulling the brain or any bridging veins into the needle.** Alternatively, apply digital pressure to the anterior fontanelle to increase the flow through the spinal needle. However, subsequent taps may require gentle aspiration with a syringe. Some physicians apply intravenous extension tubing to the spinal needle to allow the subdural fluid to drain away from the patient and into tubes. This is left to physician preference. Observe the gradual flattening of the anterior fontanel to determine the endpoint for the procedure. Generally, on any one occasion, no more than 25 to 30 mL of subdural fluid should be aspirated. Remove the spinal needle and apply a bandage.

ALTERNATIVE TECHNIQUES

Consult a Neurological Surgeon to evaluate and manage the patient. There are numerous alternatives to the aspiration of the fluid collection. These include observation, burr hole drainage, drainage through an

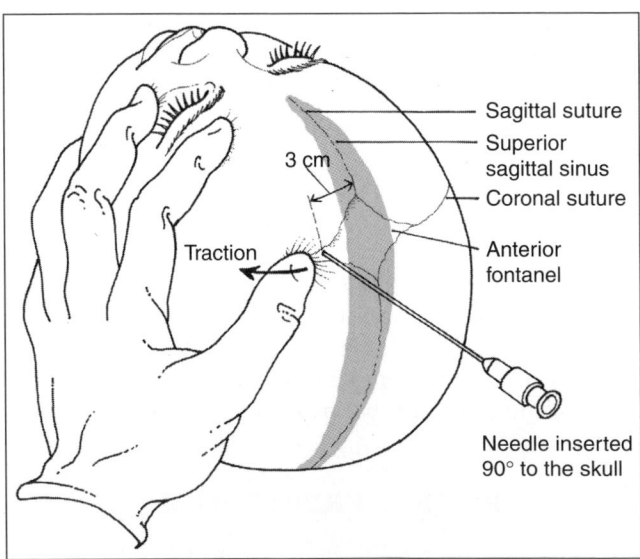

FIGURE 101-2 Subdural fluid aspiration. The needle is inserted at the lateral border of the coronal suture and at 90 degrees to the skull.

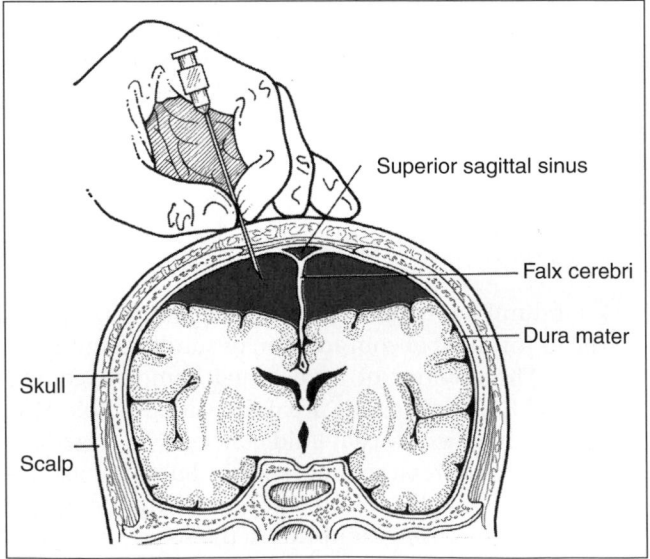

FIGURE 101-3 Coronal section through the skull at the level of the coronal suture. The needle is visible along its trajectory.

external collecting system, placement of a subdural-to-peritoneal shunt, and a craniotomy. A craniotomy should be performed in patients with a symptomatic nonliquefied clot or extensive membrane development precluding aspiration.

Some physicians prefer to use an intravenous catheter rather than the spinal needle. Removal of the metal needle leaves a soft Teflon catheter in place that minimizes the risk of injury to the brain or intracranial vascular structures. The use of an intravenous catheter set rather than a spinal needle is left to the discretion of the physician.

ASSESSMENT

Monitor the child for a change in their level of functioning after subdural aspiration. Comparison to the child's baseline neurological examination is essential. It is mandatory to document serial neurological examinations in the patient's chart. The clinical examination is age-related. It is often prudent to observe the infant in the arms of a parent or health care worker while monitoring their level of alertness, facial expression, extraocular movement, pupillary response, and limb movement. Obtain daily head circumference measurements and plot them on a head circumference chart. Note the size and feel of the anterior fontanel. Infection can be prevented with careful attention to aseptic technique.

A simple bandage placed over the puncture site is usually sufficient and can be removed 48 to 72 hours after the procedure. Continued spontaneous drainage through the puncture site should be monitored carefully as it poses an infectious risk. This complication can be prevented by tunneling the needle under the scalp prior to penetrating the lateral margin of the anterior fontanel (Figure 101-4).

AFTERCARE

Perform an ultrasound or CT scan of the head to determine if the fluid collection has been adequately drained. Bedside ultrasonography is an effective tool in neonates and young children. Any changes in the child's neurological examination requires an emergent head CT scan or ultrasonography to determine if the subdural fluid collection has reaccumulated.

COMPLICATIONS

Injury to the superior sagittal sinus or draining veins is best avoided by inserting the spinal needle 3 cm lat-

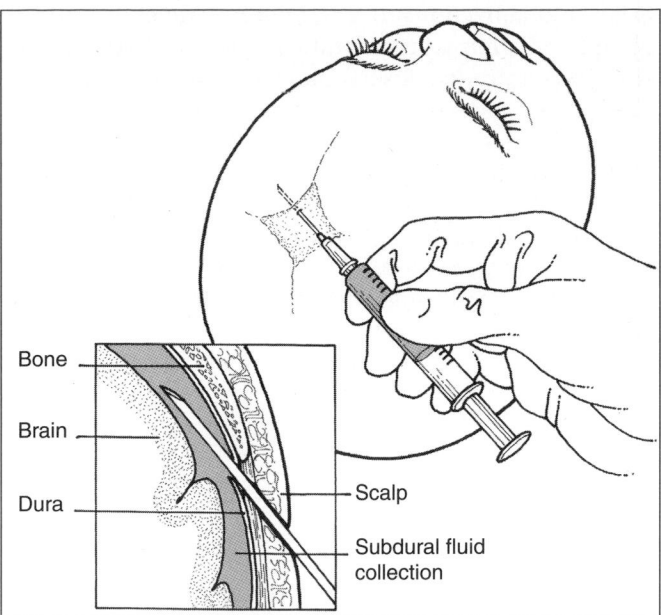

FIGURE 101-4 An alternative method for subdural fluid aspiration. The inset shows the oblique trajectory of the needle into the subdural space.

eral to the midline. **At no time should the trajectory of the needle be in the midline or parasagittal in location.** Overpenetration of the spinal needle can result in intracerebral hemorrhage. Have an assistant immobilize the child to prevent them from moving and the needle lacerating the brain or a blood vessel. Persistent leakage of subdural fluid from the puncture site can be the result of insufficient fluid aspiration or failure to use a Z-tract. This leakage can usually be controlled with local pressure, head elevation, and rarely by using cotton soaked with tincture of benzoin. Placement of a single suture at the puncture site will usually control continued leakage if less invasive methods fail. Introducing infection into the subdural space has also been reported following a subdural tap.[5] This is best avoided by maintaining strict sterile technique.

SUMMARY

Chronic subdural fluid collections are common problems during infancy. They are regarded as posttraumatic lesions in the great majority of cases. Birth trauma is sometimes implicated but uncommon. It appears that minor injuries during infancy or even more violent injuries such as infant shaking and/or cranial impact are the inciting events. It is incumbent upon the practitioner to rule out any possibility of child abuse! Report actual or suspected abuse to the appropriate state agency as required by law. Aspiration of chronic extra-axial fluid collections in the symptomatic child can be completed safely with very little risk to the child. Admission and continued observation are mandatory.

REFERENCES

1. Litofsky NS, Raffel C, McComb JG: Management of symptomatic extra-axial fluid collections in pediatric patients. *Neurosurgery* 1992; 31(3):445–450.

2. Markwalder T: Chronic subdural hematomas: a review. *J Neurosurg* 1981; 54:637–645.
3. Aoki N: Chronic subdural hematoma in infancy. *J Neurosurg* 1971; 73:201–205.
4. McLaurin RL, Isaacs E, Lewis HP: Results of nonoperative treatment in 15 cases of infantile subdural hematoma. *J Neurosurg* 1971; 34:753–759.
5. Cohle D, Hinds D, Yawn DH: Propionibacterium acnes infection following subdural tap. *Am J Clin Pathol* 1981; 75(3):430–431.

Chapter 102

SKELETAL TRACTION (GARDNER-WELLS TONGS) FOR CERVICAL SPINE DISLOCATIONS AND FRACTURES

Yogesh Ghandhi
Don W. Penney

INTRODUCTION

Traumatic injuries to the cervical spine result from forces acting on the head and neck. The incidence of spinal cord injury in the United States is approximately 5 per 100,000 population. Approximately 60 to 80 percent of spinal cord injuries involve the cervical spine. Motor vehicle collisions are the cause of one-third of cervical spine injuries. The second one-third of cervical spine injuries result from falls. Penetrating wounds and other types of injuries account for the remaining one-third.

The primary aim of therapy in the treatment of the person with an acute spinal cord injury is to minimize secondary injury to the spinal cord, to realign the spine, to improve neurological recovery, to maintain spinal stability, and to obtain an early functional recovery. This is achieved by decompression of the neural tissue either by restoring the normal sagittal diameter of the spinal canal or by removing a compressive lesion surgically. This is particularly important in patients who have sustained an incomplete spinal cord lesion and are found to have a progressing neurological deficit. Restoring the normal anatomic position also provides for relief of pain.

Early operative intervention is currently being investigated in the treatment of acute cervical fractures to achieve decompression and restore normal alignment. The use of skeletal traction in the acute spinal cord injury patient remains a very safe and straightforward me-thod of reducing fractures and maintaining the spinal canal in anatomical alignment.

Fabricius Hildanus utilized forceps in treating fractures or dislocations of the cervical spine as early as 1646. Crutchfield developed a pair of self-tightening tongs in 1933 that allowed him to apply traction to the cranium in a patient with a cervical spine fracture.[1] These tongs were subsequently modified and have essentially been replaced by the Gardner-Wells tongs.[2]

ANATOMY AND PATHOPHYSIOLOGY

Cervical spinal cord injuries can be divided into the upper (occiput to C3) and lower (C3 to C7) injuries. Numerous classification systems exist. These are based upon the morphology and the mechanism of injury. Included in this chapter is the classification proposed by the Orthopedic Trauma Association (Table 102-1).[3] No classification is ideal. However, critical to all cervical classifications is the determination of stability of a fracture or dislocation. Stability of the vertebral column is dependent upon the integrity of the vertebra, the intervertebral disk, the facet joints, and most importantly the ligamentous structures.

Clinical stability of the cervical spine is determined by the ability of the spine under physiological loads to maintain its normal anatomical relationship so that there is no damage to the spinal cord or nerve roots. It has been proposed that spinal instability be separated

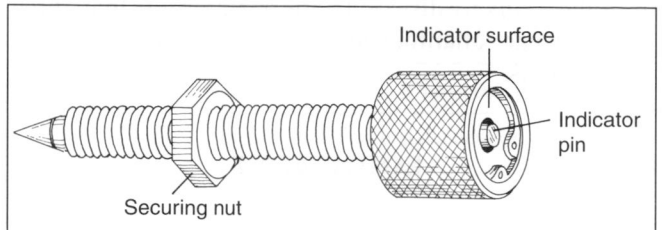

FIGURE 102-2 The calibration pin of the Gardner-Wells tongs.

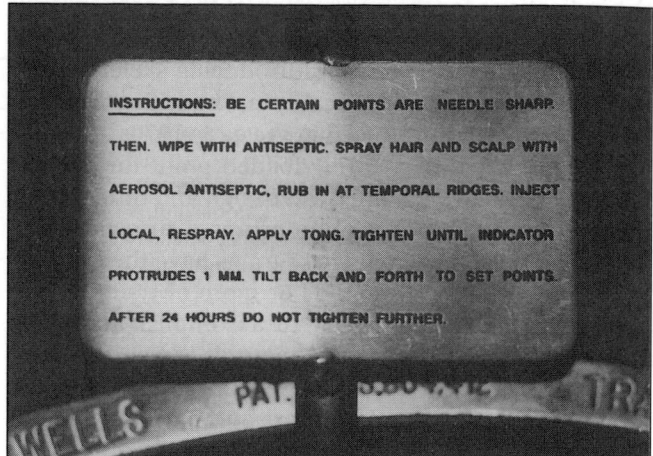

FIGURE 102-3 Instructions for the use of the Gardner-Wells tongs.

PATIENT PREPARATION

Explain the procedure, its risks, and benefits to the patient and/or their representative. Obtain an informed consent to apply the Gardner-Wells tongs. Signed consent may be omitted in cases where the patient is immobilized or has an altered mental status. Document the reason for the lack of a signed consent in the medical record. Intravenous sedation may be required in certain cases, at the discretion of the treating physician.

Identify the anatomic landmarks required to place the Gardner-Wells tongs. The pins are introduced in the temporal region, 2 to 3 finger-breadths (3 to 4 cm) above the pinna of the ear (Figure 102-5). Place them directly above the external auditory meatus for neutral distraction, 2 to 3 cm posterior to the external auditory meatus for flexion distraction, and 2 to 3 cm anterior to the external auditory meatus for extension distraction. A helpful landmark is the squamosal line where the temporalis muscle inserts into the skull. Tong placement should be below this line to allow adequate traction. Another useful landmark is to observe for the widest biparietal diameter of the patient's skull. This usually corresponds to the landmark just inferior to the squamosal line.

Shave the hair around the proposed pin sites. Clean the skin of any dirt and debris. Apply povidone iodine to the skin and allow it to dry. Infiltrate 1 mL of local anesthetic solution into each of the two proposed pin sites. Infiltrate subcutaneously and down to the level of the periosteum of the skull.

TECHNIQUE

Assemble the Gardner-Wells tongs by inserting the pins into the threaded holes. Place the pins of the Gardner-Wells tongs over the proposed pin sites. **The instructions on the S-hook must be facing upward and readable. If not, the tongs are upside down.** Screw in the pins equally on both sides of the tongs (Figure 102-5*B*). Note that a small spring loaded indicator pin is observed on one side of the tongs when adequate tension is applied. Recommendations by the manufacturer suggest that the pins should be tightened until there is a 1 mm protrusion of the indicator pin beyond the flat surface (Figure 102-6). Tighten the securing nuts to prevent the tongs from loosening.

The points of the pins will not pull out when properly applied. The depth of penetration of the pins is self-limited by a gradual lessening of the spring tension and an increase in the surface area of contact between the tips of the pins and the skull. The pressure exerted by each pin is exactly the same, regardless if one pin has been advanced farther than the other. The curve of the rigid rod allows the traction loop to find its proper position.

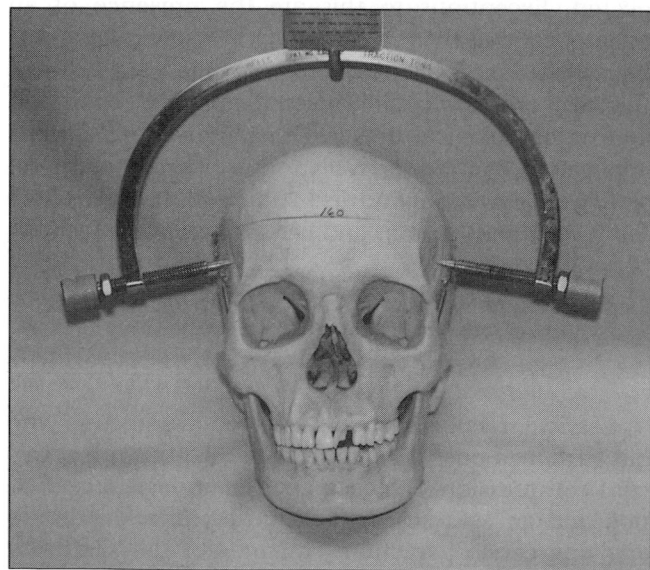

FIGURE 102-4 Application of the Gardner-Wells tongs to a human skull.

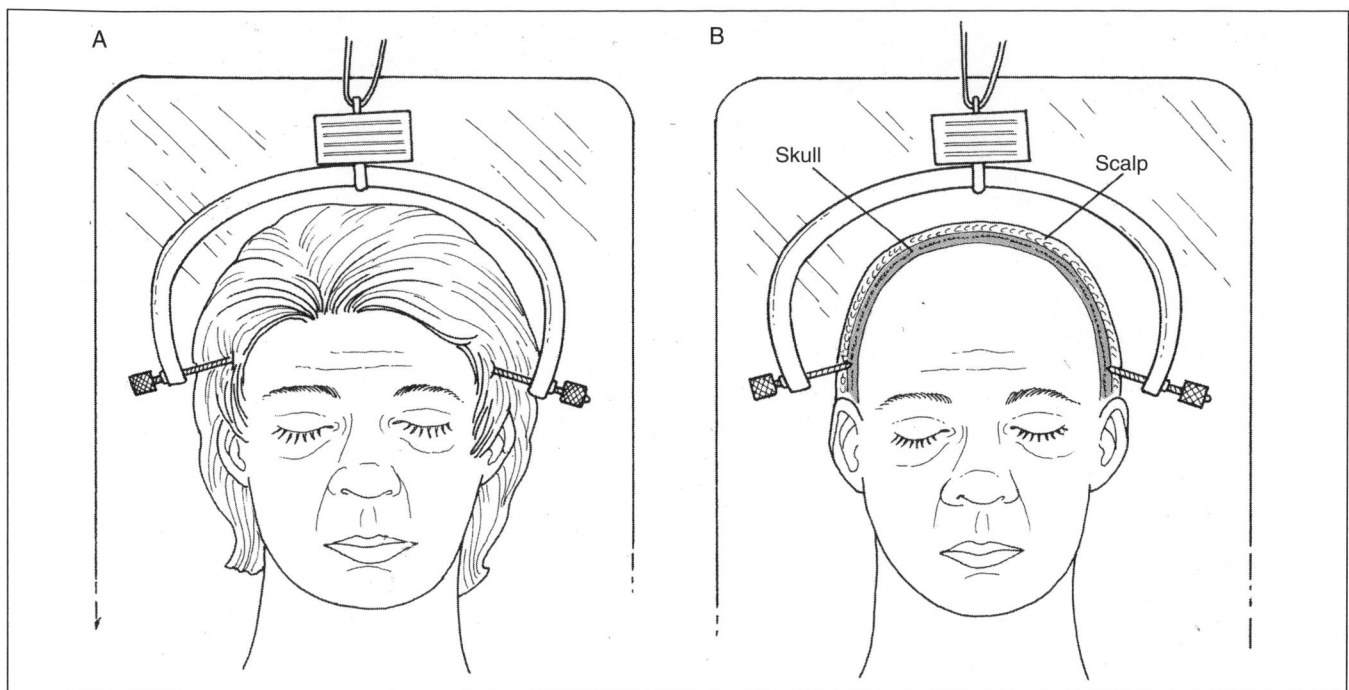

FIGURE 102-5 Application of the Gardner-Wells tongs. *A.* It can be positioned and applied without shaving the patient's entire head. *B.* Schematic demonstrating the pin position into the skull.

ASSESSMENT

Gently rock the Gardner-Wells tongs to assure that the pins are properly seated within the outer table of the skull (Figure 102-7). Place the patient in the reverse Trendelenburg position (Figure 102-8). Tie a rope to the S-shaped hook. Feed the other end of the rope through a pulley at the head of the bed and apply weights. Proper attention to the head position and the axis of distraction are important elements in achieving closed reduction. The initial weight to apply is 10 pounds for the head and 5 pounds for each vertebral segment above the level of the injury. Obtain a lateral cervical spine radiograph. Increase the weight in 3 to 5 pound increments. Obtain repeat lateral cervical spine radiographs each time weight is added. Stop adding weights when the radiographs demonstrate appropriate alignment of the cervical spine. **Careful assessment and documentation of the patient's neurological function is mandatory throughout the application of skeletal traction.**

AFTERCARE

Clean the pin sites every shift with povidone iodine or hydrogen peroxide solution followed by iodine ointment. Obtain daily cervical spine radiographs to follow the spinal alignment. Reduce the weight by 50 percent to maintain the alignment if spinal realignment is obtained with traction.

The points of the pins tend to penetrate the outer table of the skull due to the continuous pressure exerted by the springs on a very small area. Readjust the pins in 24 hours, again setting the indicator pin so that it protrudes approximately 1 mm from the flat surface. Further adjustment of the Gardner-Wells tongs is not necessary and is not recommended as it can result in erosion of the pin point through the skull.

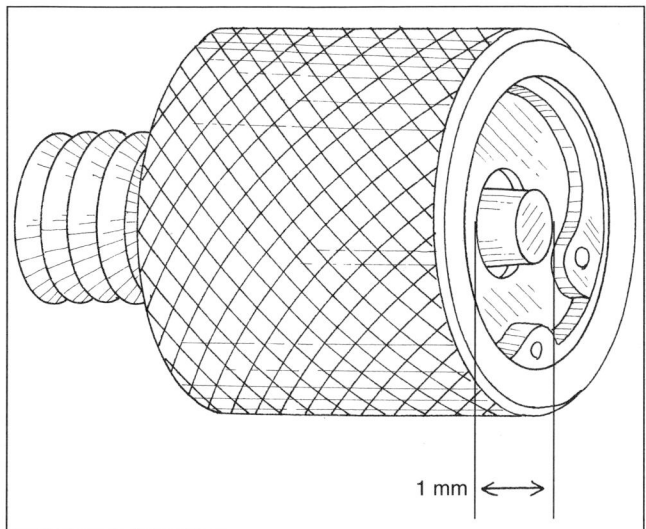

FIGURE 102-6 The calibration pin indicator is at 1 mm when the pins are properly seated in the skull.

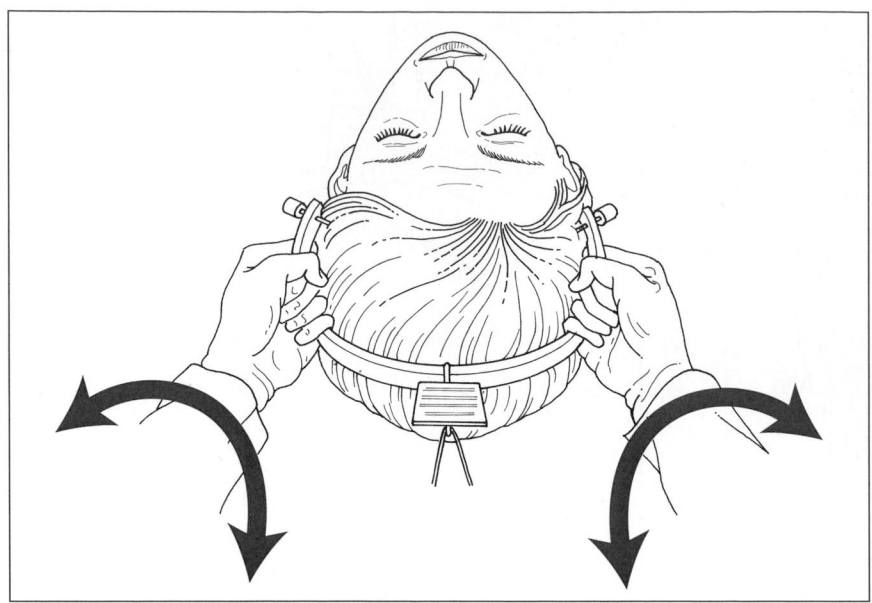

FIGURE 102-7 The Gardner-Wells tongs have been applied. The arms are grasped and gently twisted to confirm proper seating of the pins.

COMPLICATIONS

Skull penetration from placing the pins too low in the temporal region where the skull is thinnest can lead to dural tears, epidural hematomas, and possibly intracranial injury. Pins located in the temporal fossa pierce the temporalis muscle and can cause painful mastication. Overdistraction can lead to iatrogenic injury. This is best prevented by the initial use of a minimal amount of weight necessary to distract or reduce the cervical spine injury. Pin site infections are prevented by close attention to surgical technique and daily hygiene. Other complications reported include intracranial aneurysms, CSF leaks, and osteomyelitis of the skull.

SUMMARY

The application of skeletal traction in the form of Gardner-Wells tongs is a safe, simple, and quick procedure when there is evidence of clinical or radiological cervical spine instability. It requires only local anesthesia and antiseptic preparation of the skin. Careful attention to the application technique utilizing the suggested anatomical landmarks will reduce the chances of complications. Monitoring realignment and/or reduction procedures with frequent cervical spine radiographs is prudent. Gardner-Wells tongs are not recommended as a long-term immobilization technique. Definitive management of cervical spine instability can require surgical stabilization and/or halo bracing.

REFERENCES

1. Crutchfield WG: Redesigned Crutchfield skull tongs, technical note describing the combined "squeeze" and "hook" principle. *J Neurosurg* 1966; 25:656–657.
2. Gardner WJ: The principle of spring-loaded points for cervical traction, technical note. *J Neurosurg* 1973; 39:543–544.
3. Orthopedic Trauma Association: Comprehensive classification of fractures. *J Orthop Trauma* 1995; 9(suppl):129–140.
4. Maiman DJ, Barolat G, Larson SJ: Management of bilateral locked facets of the cervical spine. *Neurosurgery* 1986; 18(5):542–547.
5. Wolf A, Levi L, Mirvis S, et al: Operative management of bilateral facet dislocation. *J Neurosurg* 1991; 75:883–890.

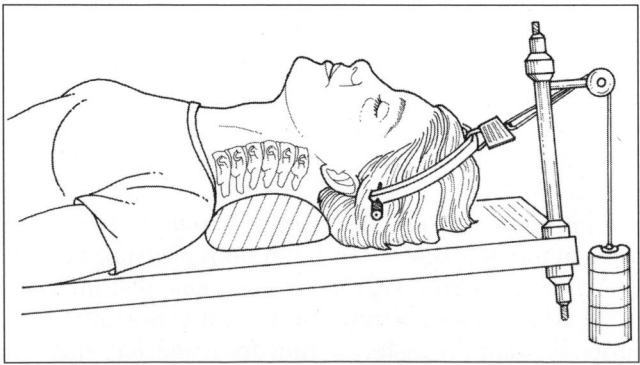

FIGURE 102-8 The patient is placed in reverse Trendelenburg and traction is applied.

Chapter 103

REFLEX EYE MOVEMENTS (CALORIC TESTING AND DOLL'S EYES)

Atilla B. Üner

INTRODUCTION

A central nervous system induced coma is either the result of bilateral diffuse impairment of the hemispheres or impairment of the paramedian reticular formation in the high pons of the brainstem. Examination of the pupils and reflex horizontal eye movements (vestibulo-ocular reflex and oculocephalic reflex) in the Emergency Department will aid in determining the location of the lesion responsible for the comatose state to either the brainstem, the hemispheres, or both.[1,2] **This testing is considered to be part of a thorough and complete neurological examination in the comatose patient.**

ANATOMY AND PATHOPHYSIOLOGY

EXAMINATION OF THE PUPILS

It is imperative to first assess the pupillary reflex to light and the presence of spontaneous eye movements in the comatose supine patient. The pupillary light reflex involves the pretectal nucleus in the upper midbrain of the brainstem.[3] Damage to areas of the brainstem can result in characteristic abnormalities of the pupils.[1] Pontine lesions can produce pinpoint pupils with preserved reaction to light upon close examination. Midbrain tegmental lesions can result in midrange pupils that may be irregular, unequal, and unreactive to light. Midbrain pretectum lesions may cause midrange fixed pupils that do respond to accommodation.

Impaired brainstem function may be seen in patients who are in a toxic or metabolic coma. This can present with impaired eye movements or even a complete ophthalmoplegia. However, pupillary function is preserved in these cases. **Preserved pupillary function in a comatose patient suggests decreased brainstem function** likely caused by a toxic or metabolic disorder and not structural damage to the brainstem.[1]

Spontaneous roving eye movements in the comatose patient are typically slow and horizontal indicating bilateral hemispheric disease with a relatively intact brainstem, particularly the pons and the midbrain.[1,2] Ocular dipping describes the slow downward movement of the eyes with rapid return to a neutral position with preserved spontaneous roving horizontal eye movements and suggests global hypoxic encephalopathy.[1] Ocular bobbing describes an intermittent rapid downward movement of the eyes with delayed return to a neutral position in the absence of horizontal eye movements and suggests severe damage to the pons, including the "locked-in syndrome".[1]

Spontaneous full roving eye movements or impaired eye movements with preserved pupillary reaction to light permit adequate localization of the cause of coma. Further testing of reflex eye movements is only indicated if spontaneous lateral eye movements are limited or absent.[1,2]

OCULOCEPHALIC REFLEX (DOLL'S EYES)

The brainstem is comprised of the medulla, the pons and the midbrain. It contains all three nuclei involved in the oculocephalic reflex. **Hence an intact oculocephalic reflex response suggests intact brainstem function.[2]** The lateral semicircular canals, the vestibulocochlear nerve, the abducens nerve, the oculomotor nerve, and the medial and lateral ocular rectus muscles must also be intact for a physiologic response to occur. Note that the optic nerve is not involved and vision or light perception is not required for this reflex to function.

A simplified model of the physiological oculocephalic reflex is described in this paragraph. Neural stimulation of the lateral semicircular canal is mediated by the inertia of the endolymph fluid resulting in a deflection of the cupula that is directly proportional to instantaneous head velocity.[4] Fairly rapid movements are thus necessary to elicit a response. Neural excitation from the lateral semicircular canal travels via the ipsilateral vestibulocochlear nerve to the ipsilateral medial vestibular nucleus in the medulla. It continues from there to the contralateral abducens nucleus in the pons and results in abduction of the contralateral eye via the abducens nerve and the lateral rectus muscle. The contralateral medial longitudinal fasciculus then excites the ipsilateral oculomotor nucleus in the ipsilateral midbrain resulting in ipsilateral eye adduction via the oculomotor nerve and the medial rectus muscle (Figure 103-1).[1]

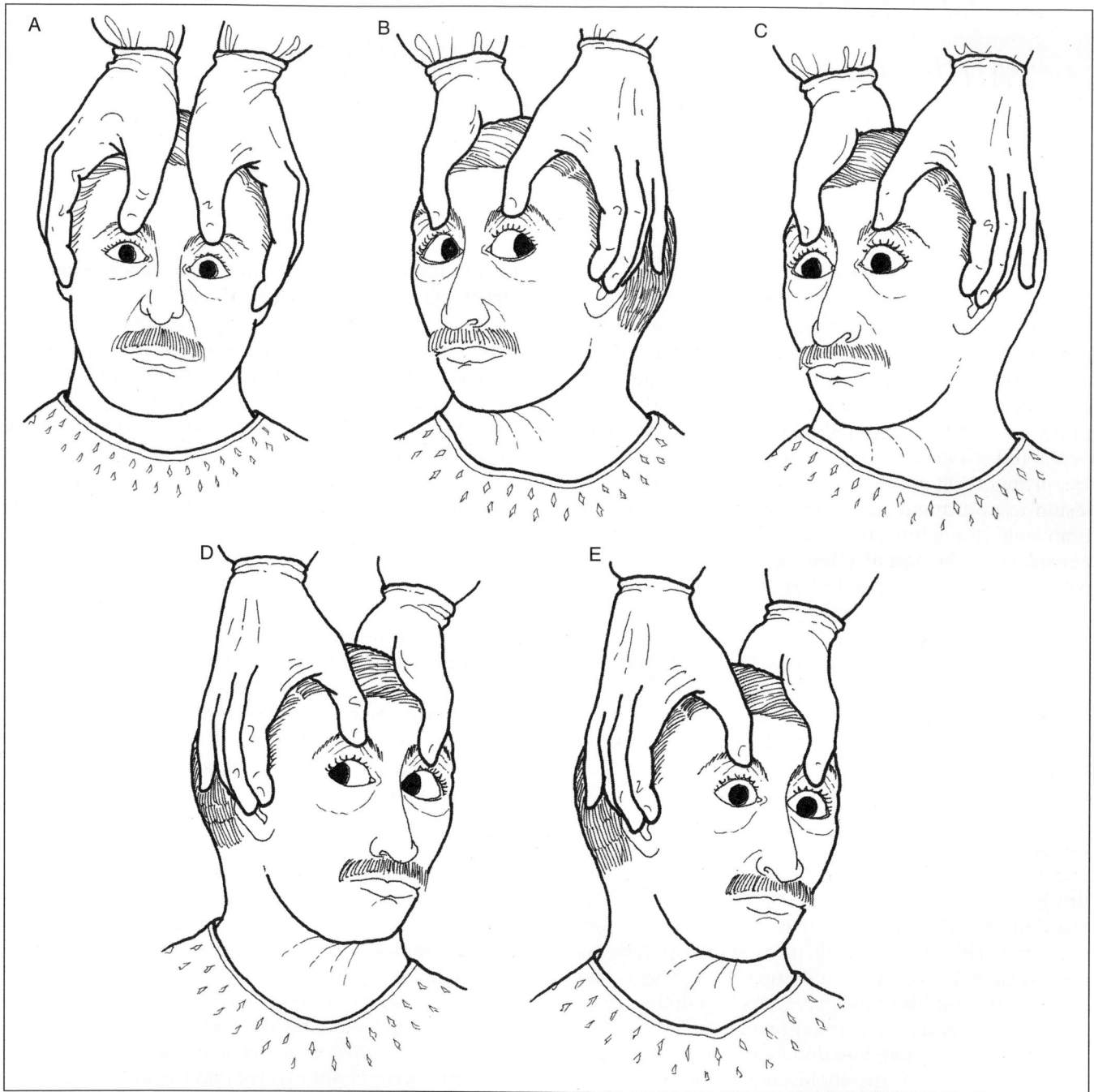

FIGURE 103-1 The oculocephalic (doll's eyes) reflex in a patient with an intact brainstem. *A.* The head is facing upright and grasped. *B.* The head is rotated 90 degrees to the right and the eyes deviate to the left (opposite side). *C.* The eyes spontaneously return to the midline. *D.* The head is rotated 180 degrees to the left and the eyes deviate to the right (opposite side). *E.* The eyes spontaneously return to the midline.

Turning the head to one side will cause an increase in the resting neuronal discharge rate of the lateral semicircular canal on that side. **Turning the head to the right will result in abduction of the left eye and adduction of the right eye in a comatose patient whose brainstem function is intact (Figures 103-1A, and B). The eyes then spontaneously return to the midline (Figure 103-1C). Turning the head to the left will result in abduction of the right eye and adduction of the left eye in a comatose patient whose brainstem function is intact (Figure 103-1D). The eyes then spontaneously return to the midline (Figure 103-1E). The result is conjugate ("parallel") eye movement contralateral to the direction of head deviation.** It will appear as though the patient is compensating for the passive head motion by moving both eyes to the other side and "maintaining visual fixation of a stationary target" when the head is turned. This indicates intact brainstem function and is termed a positive oculocephalic reflex (doll's eyes). A negative oculocephalic reflex ensues if the patient's eyes remain fixed in the orbits in a neutral position and do not move in response to passive turning of the head, implying impaired brainstem function. A partial response may be caused by impaired brainstem function, oculomotor nerve palsy, or abducens nerve palsy.[2]

A vertical oculocephalic response can similarly be tested by moving the patient's head up and down. This should result in "compensatory" vertical eye movements. This test will only be useful if the horizontal oculocephalic reflex is negative. A positive (intact) vertical oculocephalic reflex with a negative horizontal oculocephalic reflex suggests a pontine lesion. However, the vertical oculocephalic reflex is often negative in normal elderly patients and is only helpful if positive.[1]

VESTIBULO-OCULAR REFLEX

Ice and warm water caloric testing of the vestibulo-ocular reflex involves the same structures as the oculocephalic reflex (Figure 103-2). This test needs only be performed when the oculocephalic reflex is negative or cannot be performed.[2] Instilling ice water into the external auditory canal generates a temperature gradient that causes movement of the endolymph of the lateral semicircular canal.[5] This results in an ampullifugal deflection of the cupula in the supine patient leading to a decrease in the lateral semicircular canal resting neuron discharge rate on the ipsilateral side and an active increase of the resting neuron discharge rate of the medial vestibular nucleus on the contralateral side. This leads to an activation of the contralateral medial vestibular nucleus of the medulla resulting in conjugate eye deviation to the ipsilateral side (towards the ice water irrigated side) if all involved brainstem structures are intact.[1,2]

Irrigation of the external auditory canal with warm water will cause an increase in the resting neuron discharge rate of the ipsilateral lateral semicircular canal and conjugate eye deviation to the contralateral side (away from the warm water irrigated side). The results are reverse if the patient is prone.[1,2,6]

Density changes caused by temperature changes of the endolymph demonstrate the greatest effect when the lateral semicircular canals are in the vertical planes for maximum gravity effect. This is achieved by elevation of the supine patient's upper body to 30 degrees above the horizontal.[5,6] The observable oculomotor response is terminated after about 100 seconds by neural adaptation, although the residual thermal stimulation of the lateral semicircular canal can last up to 10 minutes.[5]

Unilateral vestibulo-ocular testing in an awake patient with ice water results in slow eye movements (slow phase nystagmus) ipsilateral to (toward) the irrigated side and rapid eye movements (fast phase nystagmus) contralateral to (away from) the irrigated side (Figure 103-2). Warm water testing in an awake patient results in slow eye movements (slow phase nystagmus) contralateral to (away from) the irrigated side and rapid eye movements (fast phase nystagmus) ipsilateral to (toward) the irrigated side. This quick phase, if present, indicates alertness of the pontine or midbrain reticular formation.[1] The direction of nystagmus is named after the direction of the quick phase, giving rise to confusion.

Bilateral vestibulo-ocular testing in an awake patient can be used to test vertical eye movements (Figure 103-2). Bilateral cold water irrigation results in slow eye movements (slow phase nystagmus) downward and rapid eye movements (fast phase nystagmus) upward. Bilateral warm water irrigation results in slow eye movements (slow phase nystagmus) upward and rapid eye movements (fast phase nystagmus) downward.

The presence of nystagmus indicates a noncomatose state. Typical examples of noncomatose states include catatonia, conversion reactions, malingering, psychiatric illness, or schizophrenia. Hypoactive responses are often due to neurologic and vestibular disorders. Hyperactive responses are often due to mastoid disease or a perforated tympanic membrane.

Rapid phase nystagmus is absent in the patient with an acute coma. The quick phase may return with persistent vegetative states. **It is important to note that you are searching for the slow, full eye deviation in response to caloric stimulation when assessing the comatose patient and not nystagmus.**[1,2]

INDICATIONS

Reflex eye movement testing is indicated when information is needed regarding the brainstem function of a

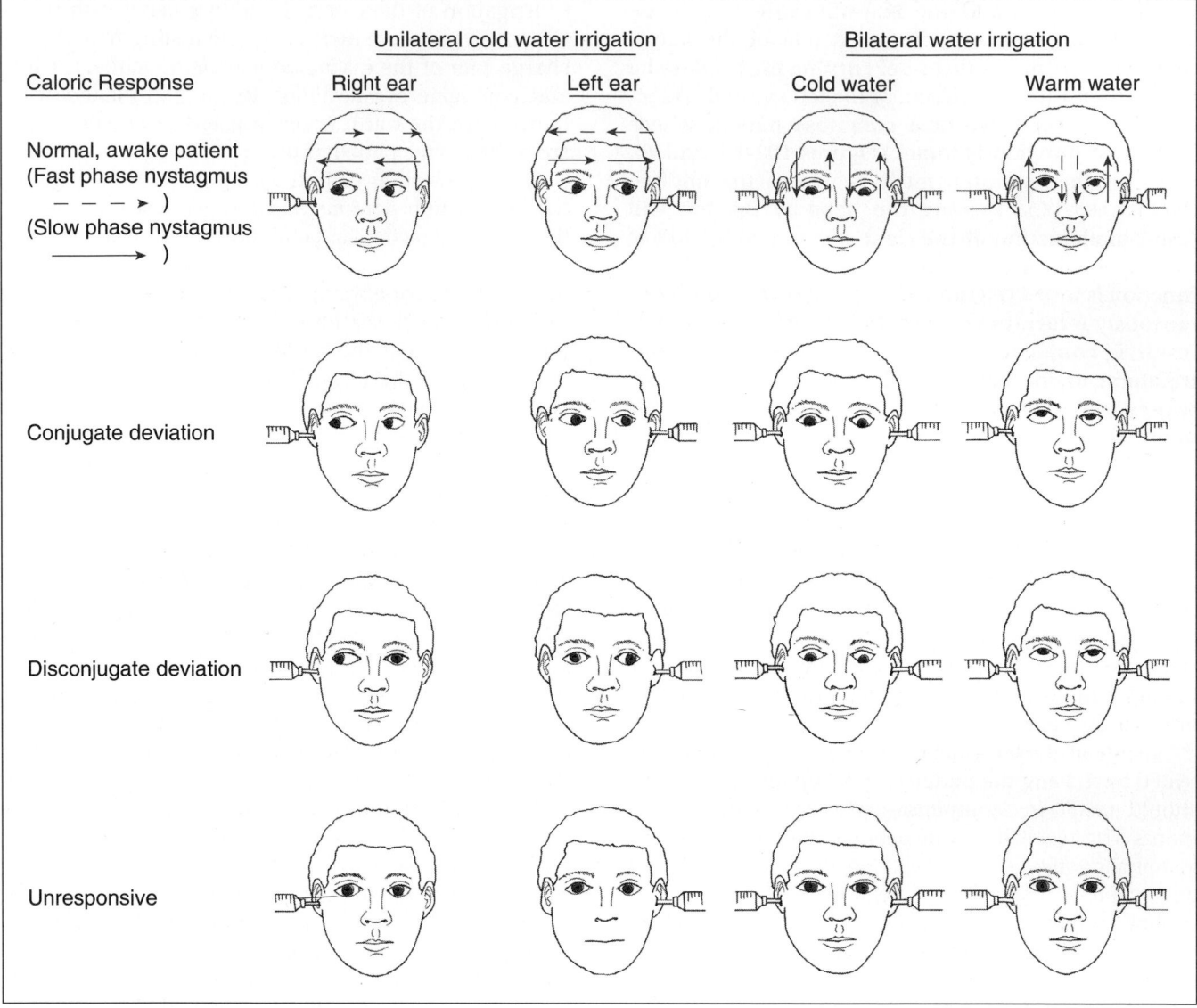

FIGURE 103-2 The vestibulo-ocular reflexes associated with unilateral cold water irrigation, bilateral cold water irrigation, and bilateral warm water irrigation.

comatose patient. Oculocephalic reflex (doll's eyes) testing is indicated in any comatose patient if both spontaneous roving horizontal eye movements and pupillary reactions to light are limited or absent. Vestibulo-ocular reflex testing is indicated in any comatose patient if the oculocephalic reflex assessment is abnormal or cannot be performed.[1]

CONTRAINDICATIONS

Any suspicion of an occult cervical spine injury or basilar skull fracture is an absolute contraindication to oculocephalic reflex (doll's eyes) testing. It cannot be performed if the patient's cervical spine is immobilized. A history of rheumatoid arthritis increases the risk of atlantoaxial subluxation with resulting spinal cord compression. Osteoporosis and cervical spine ankylosis increase the risk of injury to the cervical spine with manipulation. These are relative contraindications to oculocephalic reflex testing.

Contraindications to vestibulo-ocular reflex testing include perforation of the tympanic membrane, the presence of tympanostomy tubes, any suspicion of CSF otorrhea, and basilar skull fractures. There is a significant risk of introducing bacteria into the central nervous system through a tear in the dura mater.

EQUIPMENT

Otoscope
Warm water
Ice water
16 to 18 gauge angiocatheter
60 mL syringe
Emesis basin
Towels or chux

PATIENT PREPARATION

Explain the procedure, its utility, and potential outcomes to the patient's representatives. Place the patient supine for testing. The cervical spine must be cleared radiographically and clinically to rule out any fractures, dislocations, or ligamentous instability before oculocephalic reflex (doll's eyes) testing.

The external auditory canals and tympanic membranes must be visualized by otoscopy before performing vestibulo-ocular reflex testing. The absence of blood, cerebrospinal fluid, tympanostomy tubes, and tympanic membrane perforation must be ascertained before performing this test. Remove any cerumen from the external auditory canal so that the irrigation fluid can reach the tympanic membrane. Place towels and an emesis basin under the ear to be irrigated to catch the draining fluid.

TECHNIQUE

OCULOCEPHALIC REFLEX TESTING

Stand above the head of the bed and grasp the patient's head with both hands (Figure 103-1A). Use the thumbs of both hands to open the patient's eyelids. Rapidly move the patient's head to one side while simultaneously observing for presence or absence of horizontal eye movements (Figures 103-1B and C). Observe the eyes for several seconds. Repeat the test by rotating the patient's head towards the other side (Figures 103-1D and E). Document the presence or absence of horizontal eye movements.

VESTIBULO-OCULAR REFLEX TESTING

Elevate the head of the bed to 30 degrees. Remove the plastic angiocatheter from the needle. Discard the needle. Place the catheter on a 60 mL syringe. Draw ice water into the syringe. Place the catheter into the external auditory canal. Irrigate the external auditory canal over 30 seconds with the water. Simultaneously observe the patient's eyes for the presence, or absence, and direction of horizontal eye movements.[1] The water should freely enter and exit the external auditory canal.[6] The stimulus is dependent upon the water temperature and not water pressure. Therefore slow irrigation will suffice. Reflex horizontal eye movements may be delayed for up to one minute after irrigation of the external auditory canal.[1] It may be easier for the physician to observe the patient's eye movements while an assistant irrigates the external auditory canals.

At least 5 to 10 minutes should elapse before testing the contralateral side.[1] The same external auditory canal can also be irrigated with warm water at 44°C (111.2°F) if, for any reason, the contralateral side cannot be tested. Warm water testing may be performed if there is no response to cold testing. Some physicians also perform simultaneous bilateral external auditory canal irrigation and observe for vertical eye movements. This requires the simultaneous irrigation of both external auditory canals with equal volumes of water.

ASSESSMENT

OCULOCEPHALIC REFLEX TESTING

Head movement to the right should result in conjugate eye movement to the left and return to midline whereas head movement to the left should result in conjugate eye movement to the right and return to midline (Figure 103-1). **This is a positive oculocephalic reflex and indicates a functionally intact brainstem in the comatose patient. Incomplete or absent horizontal eye movements in response to head movement (eyes remain in the midline) is called a negative oculocephalic reflex. This indicates impairment of the brainstem and vestibulo-ocular reflex testing should be performed if not contraindicated.**

VESTIBULO-OCULAR REFLEX TESTING

Full horizontal eye movements indicate that the etiology of the patient's coma is located in the cerebral hemispheres and not in the brainstem. This is true whether the eye movements are noted spontaneously, upon oculocephalic reflex testing, or upon vestibulo-ocular reflex testing. Unilateral ice water irrigation of the external auditory canal resulting in ipsilateral conjugated full eye deviation (towards the irrigated ear) followed slowly by a returning to midline is a positive response. Unilateral warm water irrigation of the external auditory canal resulting in contralateral full eye deviation (away from the irrigated ear) followed slowly by a returning to midline is a positive response. **A positive response indicates intact brainstem function. Impaired or absent reflex horizontal eye movements indicates impaired brainstem function at or below the level of the oculomotor nucleus.** This may or may not be the sole cause of the patient's coma.[1,2]

Full vertical eye movements indicate that the etiology of the patient's coma is located in the cerebral hemispheres and not in the brainstem. Bilateral ice water irrigation of the external auditory canals resulting in downward movement of the pupils followed slowly by a return to midline is considered a positive response. Bilateral warm water irrigation of the external auditory canals resulting in upward movement of the pupils followed slowly by a return to midline is considered a positive response. **A positive response indicates intact brainstem function. Impaired or absent reflex vertical eye movements indicates impaired brainstem function at or below the level of the oculomotor nucleus.**

Absent bilateral vestibulo-ocular reflexes in a comatose patient may be due to a variety of reasons. Inadequate irrigation can be due to cerumen impaction, low irrigation volumes, or poor technique. These causes are obvious and easily corrected. The patient may have other causes for the coma, including toxin-induced and metabolic. The patient may also have a preexisting dysfunction of their vestibular apparatus.

AFTERCARE

Dry the patient off to prevent skin maceration from moisture if vestibulo-ocular reflex testing was performed. Examine the tympanic membranes and external auditory canals to assess for any injury related to the testing.

COMPLICATIONS

No significant complications are to be expected if patients with contraindications are excluded. Injury to the tympanic membrane and external auditory canal can occur from the angiocatheter or forceful irrigation. Never use a sharp or metal object to irrigate the external auditory canals. Other potential complications from vestibulo-ocular reflex testing include meningitis, otitis media, and vomiting.

SUMMARY

Central nervous system induced coma can occur only in the presence of bilateral (or diffuse) hemispheric lesions, brainstem lesions, or a combination of both. Spontaneous roving eye movements are seen in bilateral hemispheric disease with a relatively intact brainstem. Perform oculocephalic reflex testing if spontaneous roving eye movements in the comatose patient are impaired or absent. The brainstem function is intact if passive turning of the patient's head results in conjugate contralateral eye deviation.

Vestibulo-ocular reflex testing needs only to be performed when oculocephalic reflex testing is abnormal or cannot be performed. Irrigation of the ear canal with ice water will result in eye deviation towards the irrigated ear in the comatose patient with intact brainstem function. Intact full reflex horizontal eye movement indicates that the lesion or lesions causing the coma lies in the cerebral hemispheres and not in the infratentorial brainstem. Incomplete or absent horizontal eye movements suggest a lesion in the brainstem, that may or may not be the sole cause of coma.

REFERENCES

1. Lewis SL, Topel JL: Coma, in Weiner WJ, Shulman LM (eds): *Emergent and Urgent Neurology,* 2nd ed. Baltimore: Lippincott Williams & Wilkins, 1999:1–22.
2. Fisher CM: The neurological exam of the comatose patient. *Acta Neurol Scand* 1969; 45 (suppl 36):1–56.
3. Duus P: *Topical Diagnosis in Neurology,* 3rd ed. New York: Thieme Medical, 1998.
4. O'Neill G: The caloric stimulus: mechanisms of heat transfer. *Br J Audiol* 1995; 29:87–94.
5. Barnes G: Adaptation in the oculomotor response to caloric irrigation and the merits of bithermal stimulation. *Br J Audiol* 1995; 29:95–106.
6. Halmagyi GM, Yavor RA, McGarvie LA: Testing the vestibulo-ocular reflex. *Adv Otorhinolaryngol* 1997; 53:132–154.

Chapter 104

EDROPHONIUM (TENSILON) TESTING

Austen Chai
Eric F. Reichman

INTRODUCTION

Myasthenia gravis is an autoimmune disorder that occurs when polyclonal antibodies bind to a significant number of postsynaptic acetylcholine receptors at the neuromuscular junction leading to inadequate neuromuscular transmission. It most commonly affects 10 to 30 year old females and 70 to 90 year old males. Multiple tests are available to diagnose myasthenia gravis. These include the use of curare, edrophonium chloride (Tensilon), electromyography, ice packs, neostigmine, nerve stimulation, and serologic testing for acetylcholinesterase receptor antibodies or striational antibodies. Many of these techniques are seldom used and not feasible to perform in the Emergency Department. For these reasons only the edrophonium test and the ice pack test will be described in this chapter.

ANATOMY AND PATHOPHYSIOLOGY

Acetylcholine is a neurotransmitter of the neuromuscular junction that is released by the presynaptic nerve terminals when stimulated. An electrical potential is produced at the myoneural end plate when sufficient numbers of the postsynaptic receptors at the neuromuscular junction are bound by the released acetylcholine. This electric potential then propagates and ultimately leads to muscle contraction. Simultaneously, acetylcholinesterase rapidly terminates the neurotransmission by metabolizing the acetylcholine in the synaptic cleft of the neuromuscular junction.

Myasthenia gravis is an autoimmune disorder that occurs when polyclonal antibodies bind to postsynaptic acetylcholine receptors at the neuromuscular junction. This leads to inactivation of the receptors and inadequate neuromuscular transmission. Myasthenia gravis is characterized clinically by muscle weakness that develops after repetitive muscle contraction.

Patients are divided into two clinical groups. The first are patients that present with ocular complaints. Patients most commonly present with some degree of ocular muscle involvement. Diplopia is the most common patient complaint. Ptosis is the most visible sign noted on the physical examination. Diplopia with disconjugate gaze can be elicited by having the patient maintain a vertical gaze for approximately 3 minutes. Ptosis can also be made to worsen by having the patient maintain an upward gaze for the same duration of time. These patients may or may not have associated weakness of the pharyngeal and facial muscles that present with the complaints of dysarthria and dysphagia. These symptoms can often be elicited by having the patient count backwards from 100.

The second group are patients with proximal muscle weakness. Weakness of the limbs usually involves the proximal muscles and may be asymmetric. Weakness of the muscles can be elicited by having the patient perform repetitive exercises involving the muscle groups in question. **Involvement of respiratory and pharyngeal muscles should be taken very seriously as it may lead to respiratory failure or aspiration.**[2–5]

Edrophonium chloride is a short-acting acetylcholinesterase inhibitor (anticholinesterase) used in the diagnosis of myasthenia gravis. Its onset of action is rapid (within 1 to 2 minutes) and the duration of action is brief (2 to 5 minutes). These characteristics make it ideal to use in the Emergency Department.

Edrophonium given intravenously to patients with myasthenia gravis briefly inhibits the actions of the acetylcholinesterase, thus prolonging the interaction between the acetylcholine and the postsynaptic receptors. This results in a temporary but noticeable improvement in muscle contraction.[1,4] Edrophonium can rapidly, and temporarily, reverse the signs of myasthenia gravis.

INDICATIONS

Testing is indicated when the patient's condition is suggestive of myasthenia gravis. Edrophonium chloride is reserved for patients presenting with diplopia, facial muscle weakness, appendicular muscle weakness, or ptosis suggestive of myasthenia gravis. The ice pack test can be used to evaluate patients presenting with ptosis.

CONTRAINDICATIONS

Edrophonium testing is relatively contraindicated in patients with known myasthenia gravis that are taking oral pyridostigmine (Mestinon) and present with increasing weakness. The weakness may be due to insufficient drug treatment (myasthenic crisis) or too much drug treatment (cholinergic crisis). The patient will improve with edrophonium testing if the etiology of the weakness is a myasthenic crisis. The symptoms will worsen with edrophonium testing if the etiology of the weakness is a cholinergic crisis. Consult a Neurologist, for these reasons, prior to performing an edrophonium test on a patient with myasthenia gravis who is already taking oral medications.

A patient with known myasthenia gravis complaining of respiratory distress should be assessed and managed similar to any other patient with respiratory compromise. An edrophonium test is contraindicated if it is being used to improve a patient's respiratory distress.

The use of edrophonium is contraindicated in pregnancy. It may induce the patient into preterm labor. A neostigmine test is safer if testing is required. Testing should be performed only after consultation with an Obstetrician and a Neurologist.

Edrophonium testing is relatively contraindicated in patients with asthma, bronchospastic disease, cardiac dysrhythmias, or if a group of muscles that are weak are not easily observable. Edrophonium testing should be deferred in favor of neurological consultation and consideration of other testing methods.

EQUIPMENT

10 mg edrophonium chloride (Tensilon)
Tuberculin syringe
10 mL syringe containing 9 mL of sterile normal saline
Intravenous access with normal saline solution
    attached to the IV catheter
Cardiac monitor
Pulse oximeter
Noninvasive blood pressure monitor
Supplemental nasal oxygen
Resuscitative equipment and medications
Polaroid camera with instant film

PATIENT PREPARATION

Explain the risks, benefits, and potential complications to the patient and/or their representative. Obtain a signed consent for the procedure. Place the patient sitting upright or supine in a bed. Obtain intravenous access. Apply supplemental oxygen, pulse oximetry, cardiac monitoring, and noninvasive blood pressure monitoring. **Resuscitative equipment and medication must be immediately available if required**.

Identify a group of muscles that can easily be observed and monitored for improvement of function. If possible, the muscle group to be tested should be fatigued. For example, have the patient look upward for 3 minutes to accentuate ptosis. Muscle groups of the extremities can be exercised for several minutes until the patient experiences fatigue. Take a picture of the muscle group to be observed after it has been fatigued. This is the "before" photograph.

TECHNIQUE

Prepare the edrophonium chloride. It is supplied in a concentration of 10 mg/mL. Place 10 mg (1 mL of 10 mg/mL) of edrophonium into a syringe containing 9 mL of normal saline. The resulting solution will contain 1 mg of edrophonium chloride per mL of fluid. Administer the edrophonium soon after the weakened muscle is identified, carefully noted, and fatigued. Ideally, one person should administer the medication while another person observes the patient for the effects of the edrophonium chloride.

Administer the edrophonium chloride. **It may be administered in increasing doses up to a total of 10 mg.** Inject 1 mg (1 mL) of edrophonium chloride intravenously followed by a saline flush. Physical improvement in the observed muscle group should be seen within 30 seconds to 2 minutes if the edrophonium is effective. Muscle improvements will revert to their original state after 2 to 3 minutes. **The test is concluded if there is a positive response to the edrophonium in the observed muscle group.** Inject 3 mg (3 mL) of edrophonium chloride intravenously followed by a saline flush if there is no improvement after the first dose. **The test is concluded if improvement is seen in the muscle group.** Inject the remaining 6 mg (6 mL) of the edrophonium chloride intravenously followed by a saline flush if there is no response within 2 to 3 minutes after the second dose. **The test is considered negative and concluded if there is no response to the third dose of edrophonium (total of 10 mg). A negative test argues against myasthenia gravis, but does not completely exclude the diagnosis.**[3,5]

Some Neurologists prefer to give the entire 10 mg (10 mL) dose of edrophonium chloride as a single intravenous bolus and observe the muscle group for improvement. **This has the potential to cause significant bradycardia and is not recommended.**

The total dose of edrophonium to administer to children is 0.15 mg/kg, not to exceed 10 mg of edrophonium. An initial dose of 1 mg is appropriate for children with subsequent doses of 1 to 2 mg to a maximum of 0.15 mg/kg or 10 mg of edrophonium.

ALTERNATIVE TECHNIQUE

ICE PACK TEST FOR OCULAR MYASTHENIA GRAVIS

The ice pack test can be used to diagnose patients with ocular signs of myasthenia gravis. This test is reserved for the patient presenting with ptosis and/or diplopia suggestive of myasthenia gravis. The basis of this test is the finding that patients with myasthenia gravis have symptoms that worsen in warm weather and that improve in cold weather. Based on this clinical observation, studies have shown that placement of a bag of ice directly over the eyes of myasthenia patients with ptosis actually relieved the symptoms and signs of ocular myasthenia gravis.[6,7] This test is quick, simple, inexpensive, and easy to perform in the Emergency Department. It has none of the potential complications associated with the intravenous administration of edrophonium chloride. There are no contraindications to performing in this test.

Place a bag of ice directly over the eye with ptosis and/or diplopia for 2 minutes or until the patient is no longer able to tolerate the cold. An alternative to an ice pack is ice cubes placed in a glove or instant cold packs that are activated by compression. Remove the ice pack from the eye and observe the patient for any improvement in the ptosis or diplopia. **A clear improvement of the ptosis indicates a positive test.** This test may be limited by the patient's intolerance to the ice pack.

ASSESSMENT

These tests can be positive and confirm the diagnosis of myasthenia gravis. **Objective findings of improved muscle function must be observed to identify the test as positive.** It is very common to observe fasciculations of the facial muscles or tongue after the intravenous administration of edrophonium chloride. **Muscle fasciculations are not considered a positive test.** The patient having the subjective feeling of "feeling better" without objective evidence of improved muscle function is also not considered a positive test. Document improvement by taking a photograph. This is the "after" photograph. Place both the "before" and "after" photographs in the patient's medical record.

AFTERCARE

The patient may be safely discharged if they are ambulatory and without respiratory distress. All patients with suspected or proven myasthenia gravis should be referred to their Primary Care Physician and a Neurologist for further evaluation and management.

COMPLICATIONS

Muscarinic side effects can be seen due to the prolonged cholinergic stimulation in patients hypersensitive to edrophonium chloride. These effects include increased salivation, increased lacrimation, and miosis. Some patients may experience bradycardia due to the increased vagal effects of the prolonged acetylcholine stimulation of the heart. Older patients may experience a resultant postural syncope. **These effects are usually transient and self-limited. Intravenous atropine in low doses (0.5 mg) is effective to counteract any of the above symptomatology.**

There are no complications associated with the proper use of the ice pack test. Leaving the ice pack on the eyelids too long can result in a frostbite injury.

SUMMARY

Myasthenia gravis is an autoimmune disease that results in muscle weakness. The edrophonium test allows for a rapid, simple, and safe way to diagnose myasthenia gravis in the Emergency Department. The ice pack test for ocular myasthenia gravis offers a simple alternative to diagnose myasthenia gravis. Obtain prompt Neurological consultation for all patients presenting with signs and symptoms suggestive of myasthenia gravis.

REFERENCES

1. Rowland LP: Diseases of chemical transmission at the nerve-muscle synapse: myasthenia gravis, in Kandel ER, Schwartz JH, Jessell TM (eds): *The Principles of Neural Science,* 4th ed. New York: McGraw-Hill, 2000:298–309.

2. Drachman DB: Myasthenia gravis. *N Engl J Med* 1994; 330(25):1797–1810.

3. Seybold ME: Myasthenia gravis: diagnosis and therapeutic perspectives in the 1990's. *Neurologist* 1995; 1:345–360.

4. Wald JJ, Albers JW: Neuromuscular disorders, in Shah SM, Kelly KM, Wigenstein JG (eds): *Emergency Neurology: Principles and Practice.* Cambridge: Cambridge University Press, 1999:253–272.

5. Gilchrist JM: Myasthenia gravis, in Feldmann E, Feldman E (eds): *Current Diagnosis in Neurology.* St. Louis: Mosby-Year Book, 1994:350–352.

6. Golnik KC, Pena R, Lee AG, et al: An ice test for the diagnosis of myasthenia gravis. *Ophthalmology* 1999; 106(7):1282–1286.

7. Sethi KD, Rivner MH, Swift TR: Ice pack test for myasthenia gravis. *Neurology* 1987; 37(8):1383–1385.

Section Eight
ANESTHESIA AND ANALGESIA

Chapter 105
LOCAL ANESTHESIA

Michael J. Armstrong

INTRODUCTION

Cocaine appeared in the first published reports of an effective local anesthetic agent in 1884 and 1885.[1] Halstead's experiments with cocaine demonstrated its effectiveness in more than 1000 minor surgical cases.[1] Modern local anesthetic agents have supplanted cocaine as the agent of choice as they are more efficacious and safer to use.[2] They are all synthetic derivatives of cocaine. The Emergency Physician will routinely be confronted with acute wounds, abscesses, and other injuries requiring local anesthesia. An expert knowledge of local anesthesia is a required piece of our armamentarium. One must know the agents available, the techniques for optimum pain relief, and the methods to avoid and treat adverse reactions.

PHARMACOLOGY AND PATHOPHYSIOLOGY

The molecule that comprises the structure of any commercially available local anesthetic agent has three major components. They consist of a lipophilic aromatic chain joined by either an amide or an ester linkage to a hydrophilic tertiary amide.[3] Local anesthetics are classified according to their intermediate chain as either esters or amides. Procaine was the first available injectable ester local anesthetic agent and was synthesized in 1905.[4] Lidocaine was the first amide anesthetic agent and was first produced in 1945.[4] Researchers have produced agents with varied anesthetic properties based upon potency, onset, and duration of action by making substitutions at different sites on the basic molecule.[4] An appreciation of these different properties permits the Emergency Physician to make logical choices regarding the optimal use of these agents.

Neural depolarization results from a rapid influx of sodium ions through special sodium channels within the nerve cell membrane.[3,5,6] Local anesthetic agents function by reversibly binding to specific protein receptors within these sodium channels.[3,5,6] The local anesthetic agent impedes sodium influx and blocks depolarization.[4,5,7,8] Local anesthetic agents with longer protein binding to the sodium channel results in a longer duration of blockade and anesthesia. Small diameter nerve fibers responsible for pain and temperature sensation are blocked preferentially before fibers that propagate touch, motor function, and proprioception.[3,6,9]

Local anesthetic potency is determined by the lipid solubility of the agent.[8,10] Highly lipid-soluble agents more readily traverse the lipoprotein nerve cell membrane and are more effective at inducing blockade.

The primary determinant of a local anesthetic's onset of action is its pKa.[11] The pKa is the pH at which a given drug exists in equal proportions as ionized and unionized molecules. The unionized molecules more readily cross the nerve cell membrane. A portion of the molecule becomes charged once inside the neuron. It is this ionized portion that binds most completely to receptor proteins within the sodium channels.[3,10] Commercially available local anesthetic agents are weak bases with pKa's of 7.6 to 8.9.[3] Agents with a lower pKa at physiologic pH (7.4) will have relatively more uncharged molecules free to cross the nerve cell membrane (i.e., faster onset) than agents with a higher pKa.[6,10] Low tissue pH, such as seen in abscess cavities, results in so little local anesthetic in the uncharged form that the agent is ineffective.[6] The onset of action also depends upon the total dose of local anesthetic agent administered. Larger doses provide more molecules for access to the cell membrane and diffusion into the neuron.[4,7] The rate at which a local anesthetic agent diffuses through surrounding nonneuronal tissues also appears to be an important variable.[5,7]

The degree of protein binding influences the duration of action.[4,6,7,10] Agents with greater protein binding are less rapidly washed out and have a longer duration of action.[4,10] All of the available injectable local anesthetic agents cause local vasodilatation at common doses. The more vasodilatory agents, such as lidocaine, result in an increased absorption from the injection site and a decrease in their duration of action.[4,5,10] Increasing the total anesthetic dose or adding a vasoconstriction agent, such as epinephrine, to counter vasodilatation prolongs the anesthetic effect.[3,12]

The two classes of local anesthetic agents undergo metabolism via different mechanisms.[4,5,13–15] Esters are metabolized rapidly by plasma pseudocholinesterase to the major metabolite para-aminobenzoic acid or PABA.[4,5,13] PABA is allergenic and likely responsible for the infrequent allergic reactions to ester agents.[4,5,14] Patients with atypical pseudocholinesterase are at increased risk for systemic toxicity from ester anesthetic agents.[14,15] Amide anesthetic agents are metabolized more slowly by the liver to a variety of metabolites that are unrelated to PABA. Patients with impaired liver function are at increased risk for systemic toxicity from amide anesthetic agents.[14,15]

INDICATIONS

Local anesthetic agents are used in the Emergency Department for local infiltration, regional nerve blockade, peripheral nerve blockade, and topical application. General principles concerning their use will be discussed here. A complete review of specific techniques and procedures are available elsewhere in this text.

CONTRAINDICATIONS

The primary and most important contraindication to the use of a local anesthetic agent is a history of an allergic reaction. Less than 1 percent of all adverse reactions from local anesthetic agents are due to true IgE mediated allergic phenomena.[16] Ester agents are responsible for the majority of such cases, whereas allergic reactions to amide anesthetics are exceptionally rare.[4,13,17–19] The allergic potential of an ester anesthetic agent is related to PABA, its primary metabolite. Methylparaben is a close analog of PABA and a preservative commonly used in multidose preparations of amide agents. It may account for the rare occurrence of an apparent allergic reaction to the amide class of local anesthetic agents.[4,13,14,19–21]

An agent from the opposite class may be chosen if a history of a prior allergic reaction to a particular agent is obtained from a patient requiring local anesthesia. There is no cross reactivity between esters and amides.[4] A preservative-free preparation should be chosen, however, to avoid possible reaction from this source.[20] Solutions intended for single use or intravenous use tend to be free of preservatives.

Topical anesthetic agents are contraindicated on mucous membranes, the eye, denuded skin, or burned skin as they are rapidly absorbed through these tissues. Such absorption can produce severe systemic toxicity and death. Eye contact can produce corneal injury. Topical agents containing cocaine and epinephrine are contraindicated in regions of end artery flow because they can result in intense vasoconstriction.[23]

Infiltration of a wound with 1% diphenhydramine is clinically effective as an alternative agent in the rare circumstance that a patient has a true IgE mediated allergy to the local anesthetic agents.[24] Diphenhydramine is more painful to inject than the local anesthetics. It was less effective at attaining adequate anesthesia when compared to local anesthetic agents. **Reserve the use of diphenhydramine for the rare instance of a patient with an actual local anesthetic allergy.**[24] Dilute the 5% parenteral formulation of diphenhydramine to 1% to make a solution for local infiltration (add 1 mL of diphenhydramine to 4 mL of normal saline).

EQUIPMENT

Universal precautions are of utmost importance in performing any procedure using a local anesthetic agent. It is vital to wear gloves when administering topical anesthetic agents to protect the fingers and to prevent introduction of bacteria into the wound. Wear a mask with a face shield or goggles to prevent accidental mucous membrane exposure if the local anesthetic solution shoots out of the wound margins.

One of the most important determinants of pain response during administration of a local anesthetic agent is needle size. Use a 25 gauge or smaller needle for infiltration to minimize pain. A long needle decreases the number of times tissues must be punctured, but should not be inserted more than two-thirds of its length to prevent inadvertent breakage within the tissues.[11] Another important factor is the rate of infiltration. A slow steady method minimizes the pain response.

Most Emergency Departments have a small tray or basket containing the necessary equipment for providing local anesthesia. Such a kit may include the following items. Needles in sizes from 18 to 30 gauge, 1 to 2 cm long, and 4 cm long. Syringes ranging from 1 mL (tuberculin) through 10 mL. Cotton-tipped applicators for the application of topical agents. Local anesthetic agents such as 1% and 2% lidocaine, 0.25% and 0.5% bupivacaine, and lidocaine with 1:200,000 epinephrine. Sodium bicarbonate may be used for buffering the local anesthetic agent. Alcohol and povidone iodine swabs are required for cleansing the skin. Nonsterile and sterile examination gloves are required for the infiltration of the local anesthetic agent and performing the procedure.

PATIENT PREPARATION

Discuss the procedure with the patient. The most common adverse reaction to a local anesthetic agent is a vasovagal reaction.[11] **The physician must take precautions to alleviate secondary injury to the pa-**

tient. **Place the patient lying in a bed with side rails up to prevent injury no matter how minor the procedure.** Friends and family members observing the procedure should be asked to sit or leave the room. Sedation can minimize the response to treatment while maintaining stable vital signs and spontaneous respirations when the patient exhibits considerable anxiety. Refer to Chapter 109 regarding the details of procedural sedation.

LOCAL INFILTRATION AND PERIPHERAL NERVE BLOCKADE

LOCAL ANESTHETIC DOSING

It is important to keep in mind the maximal recommended doses for the chosen local anesthetic agent to avoid systemic toxicity (Table 105-1). The disadvantages of local infiltration is that a large amount of local anesthetic must be used for a small area. Extensive wounds may require toxic doses of local anesthetic agents. A lower concentration or the addition of epinephrine will allow a larger volume of local anesthetic to be used. Local infiltration may distort the wound edges and com-plicate the repair.

The maximal recommended dose of a local anesthetic agent is the same for local infiltration or regional nerve blockade. **It is important to properly calculate the amount of local anesthetic agent administered to a patient.** Local anesthetic solutions are supplied with the concentration denoted as a percentage (e.g., 1% lidocaine, 0.25% bupivacaine, 4% cocaine). This percentage must be converted to mg/mL. A 1% local anesthetic solution is prepared by dissolving 1 gm of the local anesthetic agent in 100 mL of diluent. This results in a concentration of 10 mg/mL (1 gm/100 mL = 1000 mg/ 100 mL = 10 mg/mL). **A simple method to calculate the strength of a local anesthetic solution is to move the decimal point one place to the right** (e.g., 0.25% = 2.5 mg/mL, 2% = 20 mg/mL, 4% = 40 mg/mL).

EPINEPHRINE CONTAINING AGENTS

Epinephrine can be added to a local anesthetic solution to prolong its duration of action, to assist with hemostasis by local vasoconstriction, and to slow the absorption of the local anesthetic agent. It can be combined with the local anesthetic solution in a dilution of 1:100,000 or 1:200,000. Begin by obtaining 1:1000 epinephrine that is usually administered to patients for severe allergic reactions or bronchospasm. This solution of 1:1000 contains 1 mg/mL of epinephrine. Place 0.1 mL of 1:1000 epinephrine into 10 mL of local anesthetic solution to make a dilution of 1:100,000 (or 0.010 mg/mL). Place 0.1 mL of 1:1000 epinephrine into 20 mL (or 0.05 mL in 10 mL) of local anesthetic solution to make a dilution of 1:200,000 (or 0.005 mg/mL). Local anesthetic agents containing epinephrine are also commercially available and do not have to be made.

REDUCING THE PAIN OF INFILTRATION

Local anesthetic agents are weak bases. They are packaged, however, as hydrochloride salts with a pH of 4 to 6 to increase their solubility and shelf life. This acid pH causes much of the pain associated with the injection of local anesthetic agents.[3,6] **Buffering lidocaine, mepivacaine, or bupivacaine with sodium bicarbonate has been shown to reduce the pain of injection significantly.**[23,25,26] Raising the pH of the agent increases the percentage of local anesthetic molecules in the uncharged diffusible state.[26] This may allow nearly instantaneous penetration of the nerve cell membrane by the anesthetic molecules and block the pain of infiltration.[26] Buffering local anesthetic agents does not appear to affect the duration or degree of anesthesia. There does not appear to be an increase in serum levels or toxicity of buffered anesthetic agents.

Caution must be exercised when buffering highly lipophilic and less soluble anesthetic agents, like bupivacaine, because precipitation can occur.[3] Add 1 mL of 8.4% (1 meq/mL) sodium bicarbonate to 10 mL of 1% lidocaine or 1% mepivacaine, with or without epinephrine, to achieve buffering.[26] Add 0.05–0.10 mL of 8.4% (1 meq/mL) sodium bicarbonate to each 10 mL of 0.5% bupivacaine.[25]

The use of warm lidocaine [37 °C (98.6 °F) to 42 °C (107.6 °F)] decreases the pain of infiltration. The exact etiology of this is unknown. It is hypothesized that warm lidocaine does not stimulate cold receptors and it dif-

TABLE 105-1 PROPERTIES AND DOSAGES FOR INJECTABLE LOCAL ANESTHETIC AGENTS[7,10,20,33]

Anesthetic agent	Relative potency	Relative onset of action	Duration of action (minutes)*	Maximum dose with epinephrine (mg/kg)	Maximum dose without epinephrine (mg/kg)
Procaine (ester)	1	Slow	60–90	7.0	9.0
Lidocaine (amide)	2	Rapid	90–200	4.5	7.0
Mepivacaine (amide)	2	Rapid	120–240	7.0	8.0
Bupivacaine (amide)	8	Moderate	180–600	2.0	3.0

* Longer times represent the addition of epinephrine to the local anesthetic solution.

fuses into tissues faster. Warm the local anesthetic agent by placing it in a blanket warmer or a water bath.

The pain upon injection of local anesthetic agents can be reduced by following a few simple suggestions. Warm and/or buffer the local anesthetic agent as discussed previously. Inject the local anesthetic agent slowly. Inject open wounds through the wound edges and not through intact skin. An exception to this is grossly contaminated wounds. Infiltrate subdermally to minimize pain and tissue distention. Insert and advance the needle to create a tract and inject as the needle is withdrawn to minimize tissue distention. Do not totally withdraw the needle after infiltration. Leave the tip of the needle within the skin and redirect the needle to prevent excessive skin punctures.

COMBINING LOCAL ANESTHETIC AGENTS

Physicians have for some time combined various local anesthetic agents in an attempt to achieve both rapid onset of action and prolonged duration. Lidocaine, with its rapid onset, can be safely mixed in a 1:1 ratio with longer acting bupivacaine or mepivacaine. The value of such an approach is questionable. It is important to realize that the toxic effects in an overdose situation are additive, even if an amide and ester are combined. **It is also difficult to determine the maximum dose if two local anesthetic agents are mixed together.** The combination of local anesthetic agents can therefore not be recommended. Use lidocaine containing epinephrine to prolong the anesthetic effect rather than combining it with a second local anesthetic agent.

TOPICAL ANESTHESIA

Topical agents offer several advantages over local infiltration anesthesia. They are less painful to apply, cause less distortion of wound margins, and decrease the need for sedation in the pediatric population.[27] The major limitation of topical anesthesia has been the lack of adequate analgesia in many clinical situations and the time required to achieve anesthesia. The exact components of topical anesthetic agents vary depending upon your hospital. It is important for the physician to become familiar with the agent used in their department to know specifics in regard to allergic tendency and toxicity.[28]

TAC

Many Emergency Departments use a combination of 0.5% tetracaine, 1:2000 or 0.05% epinephrine, and 11.8% cocaine (also known as TAC) for topical anesthesia. Pharmacists compound these for application in individual use vials. The degree of anesthesia achieved with TAC is comparable to that of local infiltration with lidocaine for wounds on the face and scalp.[28] The effects are less profound for wounds of the trunk and extremities.[28] Use in these areas should be limited, if at all.

Dose recommendations generally call for 5 mL of TAC for lacerations smaller than 3 cm in length and 10 mL for lacerations greater than 3 cm in length.[28] Apply the chosen volume to 2×2 inch gauze pads or cotton balls. Apply these within the wound margins for 5 to 15 minutes or until visible skin blanching occurs. The gauze pad can be held in place by the patient, a parent, a responsible adult, or tape. **Blanching tends to signal the presence of adequate analgesia.**[29] **Always wear gloves when handling TAC to prevent percutaneous absorption and avoid the introduction of more bacteria into the wound. TAC should never be placed on tissues with end arteriole supply.**

LET

There are numerous combinations of anesthetic agents to use topically on wounds. The two most commonly used are TAC [0.5% tetracaine, 0.05% adrenalin (1:2000 epinephrine), 11.8% cocaine] and LET [4% lidocaine, 0.1 (1:1000) epinephrine, 0.5% tetracaine]. **LET is safer, more practical, and more cost effective to use than TAC.** LET is not a controlled substance and has no potential for abuse. It does not require the documentation and monitoring associated with a controlled substance. The systemic absorption of cocaine (in TAC) has resulted in respiratory arrest, seizures, and death in children. LET is just as effective as TAC and costs significantly less. LET can be applied by dripping it into the wound or taping a LET soaked cotton ball over the wound. The addition of methylcellulose to LET makes a gel that can be painted on wounds. The gel form will not drip or run into mucous membranes. The maximum allowable dose of LET is 5 mL. It should not be placed on the digits, ear, nose, penis, or other areas that are supplied by end arteries.

EMLA CREAM

The use of EMLA (eutectic mixture of local anesthetics) cream has gained significant popularity. It is an emulsion of 2.5% lidocaine and 2.5% prilocaine in a 1:1 ratio by weight. Each gram of EMLA contains 25 mg of lidocaine and 25 mg of prilocaine. EMLA is dosed in terms of milligrams of cream and not milligrams of the local anesthetic agent. **Apply EMLA to intact skin and not open wounds.** It is nonsterile and preservative free. It is now also available in prepackaged transdermal disks.

EMLA is indicated prior to performing arterial punctures, accessing indwelling ports and reservoirs, lumbar puncture, minor skin procedures, regional nerve blockade, and venipuncture. Apply EMLA to intact skin and cover it with an occlusive dressing (e.g., Tegaderm) or apply a transdermal disk. Allow at least 1 hour for the EMLA to work. Analgesia is usually satisfactory after 1 hour, peaks at 2 hours, and persists for about 1 hour after removed from the skin. The prolonged time required for anesthesia to take effect limits its use in the Emergency Department. EMLA should not be applied to infants less than 3 months of age due to the theoretical risk of methemoglobinemia.

REFRIGERANT SPRAYS

Refrigerant sprays (ethyl chloride and fluori-methane) are sterile liquids that vaporize upon contact with the skin. They are commercially available in containers with a tip that directs a precise stream of liquid when compressed. The liquid lowers the skin temperature in the area of contact to $-20\,°C$ ($-4\,°F$) as it vaporizes. The skin becomes temporarily frozen. Refrigerant sprays are convenient, effective, provide immediate anesthesia, and provide a "needle-less" form of anesthesia. They may be used prior to accessing indwelling ports and reservoirs, arterial puncture, intramuscular injections, local anesthetic injection, lumbar puncture, and minor skin procedures (incision and drainage of an abscess, or venipuncture).

Clean and prep the skin prior to using a refrigerant spray. Hold the inverted container of refrigerant spray 10 to 20 cm above the skin. Spray the liquid onto the skin until a white frost appears and the skin turns white. Immediately perform the procedure as the anesthesia only lasts 30 to 60 seconds. These sprays only provide superficial anesthesia.

Avoid spraying for prolonged periods as it may result in frostbite. Do not use refrigerant sprays on mucous membranes. These agents are highly volatile and must be used in well-ventilated areas. Never spray around open flames or an electrocautery unit as the refrigerant sprays are highly flammable. Do not use refrigerant sprays on open wounds as it may delay wound healing.

ABRADED SKIN

Paint denuded regions of the skin with 2% lidocaine jelly and cover the area with a gauze square for 5 to 10 minutes before any manipulations to provide adequate anesthesia. Five percent lidocaine cream has been shown to reduce the pain of partial thickness burns significantly when applied at a dose of $1\,mg/cm^2$, up to a maximum dose of 2 grams.[11] This dose resulted in no toxicity or adverse effects on wound healing in a study of burn patients greater than 12 years of age. **Caution must be taken when using topical anesthesia on large wounds. The total dose should be calculated carefully to avoid toxicity.**

MUCOUS MEMBRANE ANESTHESIA

Numerous agents may be used to provide anesthesia to mucous membranes. This includes benzocaine, cocaine, lidocaine, and tetracaine. These local anesthetic agents produce only superficial anesthesia. They do not provide for any pain relief that originates submucosally or deeper. **The total dose applied should be one-third to one-half the dose used for infiltration. The systemic absorption from mucous membranes is much more rapid than infiltration and results in higher blood levels of the local anesthetic agent. Use the agents cautiously as they can suppress the gag reflex and increase the risk for aspiration.**

Benzocaine is a commonly used mucous membrane anesthetic. It is available in spray, liquid, and gel form in a concentration of 14 to 20% (Cetacaine, Hurricaine, Americaine). It is nontoxic when applied to intact mucous membranes due to its poor water solubility. It provides brief analgesia. **Use benzocaine sparingly as it has the potential to produce methemoglobinemia.**

Cocaine is supplied in solution at concentrations of 4% and 10%. It is an extremely effectively mucous membrane anesthetic with significant vasoconstrictive properties. Enhanced systemic absorption occurs when it is applied to inflamed mucous membranes. The maximum dose is 3 mg/kg. This dose still has the potential to result in toxicity and serious complications. Do not use cocaine in patients with hypertension, cardiomyopathy, known or suspected coronary artery disease, or patients sensitive to exogenous catecholamines.

Lidocaine is available in jelly and liquid form with a concentration of 2% to 10%. The 2% to 4% viscous solution is often used in the Emergency Department. Instruct the patient to swish the solution in their mouth for 30 to 60 seconds then spit it out. It can result in significant systemic absorption if swallowed. The maximal dose is 300 mg in adults (15 mL of 2% or 7.5 mL of 4%) and 3 mg/kg in children. **Use extreme caution when sending patients home with viscous lidocaine for intraoral use.** Frequent use and swallowing can both result in elevated blood levels of the parent drug and its metabolites, both of which can result in potential toxic effects.

Tetracaine is available in liquid and aerosol form with a concentration of 0.25% to 1.0%. It is significantly cardiotoxic and not often used in the Emergency Department.

ASSESSMENT

It is important to wait long enough after the local anesthetic agent is administered to allow the onset of adequate anesthesia before the planned procedure is started. A period of 5 to 10 minutes is adequate for subcutaneous local infiltration. A period of 15 to 30 minutes is required for peripheral nerve blocks. A simple examination of the area being anesthetized with fine touch and pinprick is important to insure adequate anesthesia prior to the procedure. It may be necessary to inject additional agent in areas of continued sensitivity, keeping in mind the total dose injected to avoid toxicity.

AFTERCARE

The Emergency Physician should observe the patient for a minimum of 15 minutes following the use of local anesthesia to insure no evidence of an adverse reaction. The length of time analgesia is maintained depends upon the agent used for the procedure (Table 105-1). The patient need not wait in the Emergency Department for normal sensation to return prior to discharge. They should be instructed to return to the Emergency Department if normal sensation has not returned within 12 to 24 hours.

COMPLICATIONS

Toxic reactions to local anesthetics agents are far more common than allergic sequelae.[11,15] The propensity for toxicity is directly proportional to the potency of the drug.[4,8,10] Table 105-1 lists the recommended maximal doses for commonly used local anesthetic agents. **These are only estimates and in certain circumstances the toxic dose might be considerably less.[4,18] Infiltration into highly vascular areas, inadvertent intravascular injection, or application to mucous membranes may cause toxicity at accepted standard doses.[4]**

It is unlikely that toxic serum concentrations of local anesthetic agents will be reached in most clinical situations in the Emergency Department. For example, the maximum dose of 1% lidocaine without epinephrine in a 70 kg patient would be approximately 31.5 mL, a volume more than adequate for most wounds. **It is important to be vigilant of the total dose administered, especially in patients with large or multiple lacerations in whom higher doses of local anesthetics may be required.** A less concentrated form of the local anesthetic agent (e.g., 0.5% lidocaine as opposed to 1%) may be used when the maximum dose could be exceeded. General anesthesia may be required to repair larger wounds.

The major manifestations of local anesthetic toxicity occur in the central nervous system (CNS) and the cardiovascular system.[6,8,11,13] Initial signs and symptoms are of CNS excitation. This occurs as a result of the suppression of inhibitory cortical neurons that permits unopposed functioning of facilitory pathways. Signs and symptoms include lightheadedness, dizziness, nystagmus, sensory disturbances (e.g., visual difficulties, tinnitus, perioral tingling, metallic taste in the mouth), restlessness, disorientation, and psychosis. Slurred speech, muscle twitching, and/or tremors may immediately precede seizures. There may also be augmentation of medullary and sympathetic activity with resultant tachypnea, hyperpnea, hypertension, and tachycardia. Generalized depression of the entire CNS can occur and is manifested as drowsiness, coma, and respiratory arrest.[8,13]

The cardiovascular system is relatively resistant to local anesthetic toxicity in comparison with the CNS.[15,22] The cardiovascular system does not exhibit toxicity until much higher blood levels are reached.[15,22] Complications are the result of negative inotropism, peripheral vasodilatation, and slowing of the myocardial conduction system.[8,13] The end results are hypotension, bradycardia, prolonged electrocardiographic intervals, and cardiac arrest.[8,10,13] Vasopressors with positive inotropic effects, such as dopamine, will treat profound cardiovascular depression.[4]

Management of CNS toxicity should begin with an assessment of the patient's airway, breathing, and circulation. Hypoxia and acidosis enhance CNS and myocardial absorption of local anesthetic agents and must be addressed aggressively. Hypocapnia raises the seizure threshold (to prevent convulsions) by inducing cerebral vasoconstriction and by decreasing the delivery of the local anesthetic agent to the CNS.[4,30] An alert and cooperative patient may be instructed to hyperventilate if early signs of toxicity are present.[6,18,31] Manage seizures with intravenous benzodiazepines as they raise the CNS threshold to local anesthesia-induced convulsions. The metabolism of local anesthetics is short enough that loading patients with long-acting antiseizure agents, such as phenytoin, is generally not required. Administer short-acting neuromuscular blocking agents, such as succinylcholine or vecuronium, until serum levels of the local anesthetic agent decline if the seizures fail to respond to benzodiazepines.[4] Succinylcholine, however, is metabolized by pseudocholinesterase. This is the same plasma enzyme that metabolizes ester anesthetic agents. Therefore, avoid succinylcholine in ester-induced seizures.[4,6,18]

Adding epinephrine to a local anesthetic agent increases both the amount of drug that can be administered and the duration of action.[3,12] It also decreases bleeding into the surgical field. There are, however, significant drawbacks to the use of epinephrine. This includes increased pain of infiltration, increased wound inflammation, increased wound infection rates, uncomfortable side effects in susceptible patients (e.g., palpitations, tremors, syncope), and the potential for severe tissue ischemia if used in the digits, the tip of the nose, the pinna, or the penis.[11] Prolonged vasospasm and ischemia in these areas can be reversed with the subcutaneous infiltration of 1.5 to 5.0 mg of phentolamine diluted with saline in a 1:1 mixture. Caution must be used when administering epinephrine to patients who are elderly, taking beta-blockers, or with a history of coronary artery disease, hypertension, hyperthyroidism, or pheochromocytoma.[6,11] Inadvertent intravascular injection of epinephrine can have fatal consequences.[32,33]

True allergic reactions are rare adverse events to the local anesthetic class of medications. Effective management of an allergic reaction depends upon its severity and may include the use of epinephrine, antihistamines, steroids, and vasopressors. A complete review of the management of allergic reactions and anaphylaxis can be found in standard Emergency Medicine textbooks.

Injection of local anesthetic agents can cause complications in the area of the infiltration. These agents have not been shown to increase the incidence of wound infections. Do not inject local anesthetic agents into a joint prior to obtaining synovial fluid. They can result in false-negative culture results, false-negative crystal analysis, and false-positive (anesthetic crystals) crystal analysis. Needle punctures of arteries, nerves, and veins are usually a temporary inconvenience with no long-lasting consequences. Intraneural injection can result in temporary or permanent nerve injury. Never inject local anesthetic agents if the patient experiences paresthesias (indicating intraneural needle placement). Withdraw the needle 1 to 2 mm and allow the paresthesias to resolve before infiltrating with the local anesthetic solution. Never redirect the needle when more than the tip is subcutaneous to prevent needle breakage.

SUMMARY

Emergency Physicians often rely on local anesthetic agents to relieve patient discomfort and provide wound care. These agents have been found to be safe and effective in daily clinical practice. An expertise in the use of these agents plays an important role in our practice of the art of medicine. For hundreds of years physicians have sought to relive the pain and suffering of our patients. These agents allow us to come closer to attaining that goal.

REFERENCES

1. Halstead WS: Practical comments on the use and abuse of cocaine; suggested by its invariably successful employment in more than a thousand minor surgical operations. *N Y Med J* 1885; 42:294–295.

2. Green SM: What is the role of diphenhydramine in local anesthesia? *Acad Emerg Med* 1996; 3(3): 198–200.

3. Akerman B: On the chemistry and pharmacology of local anesthetic agents, in Loftstrom JB, Sjostrand U (eds): *Monographs in Anesthesiology. Local Anesthesia and Regional Blockade: Pharmacology, Physiology and Clinical Effects,* vol 15. New York: Elsevier Science Publishers, 1988:1–22.

4. Covino BG: *Local Anesthetics: Mechanisms of Action and Clinical Use.* New York: Grune and Stratton, 1976.

5. Covino BG: New developments in the field of local anesthetics and the scientific basis for their clinical use. *Acta Anaesth Scand* 1982; 26:242–249.

6. McLeskey CH: Rational use of local anesthetic drugs. *N C Med J* 1982; 43(7):496–500.

7. Covino BG: Pharmacology of local anesthetic agents. *Br J Anaesth* 1986; 58:701–716.

8. Covino BG: Pharmacology of local anesthetics. *Res Staff Phys* 1982; 28:60–70.

9. Strichartz G: Molecular mechanisms of nerve block by local anesthetics. *Anesthesiology* 1976; 45(4):421–441.

10. Covino BG: Local anesthetic agents for peripheral nerve blocks. *Reg Anesth* 1980; 3:33–37.

11. Stewart RD: Local anesthesia, in Paris PM, Stewart RD (eds): *Pain Management in Emergency Medicine.* Norwalk, CT: Appleton & Lange, 1988:33–50.

12. Albæert J, Löfström B: Effects of epinephrine in solutions of local anesthetic agents. *Acta Anaesth Scand* 1965; 16:71–77.

13. Covino BG: Local anesthesia (first of two parts). *N Engl J Med* 1972; 286(18):975–983.

14. Glinert RJ, Zachary CB: Local anesthetic allergy: its recognition and avoidance. *J Dermatol Surg Oncol* 1991; 17:491–496.

15. Savarese JJ, Covino BG: Basic and clinical pharmacology of local anesthetic drugs, in Miller RD (ed): *Anesthesia,* 2nd ed. New York: Churchill Livingstone, 1986:985–1013.

16. Giovannitti JA, Bennett CR: Assessment of allergy to local anesthetics. *J Am Dent Assoc* 1979; 98:701–706.

17. Brown DT, Beamish D, Wildsmith JAW: Allergic reaction to an amide local anesthetic. *Br J Anaesth* 1981; 53:435–437.

18. DeJong RH: Toxic effects of local anesthetics. *JAMA* 1978; 239(12):1166–1168.

19. McLeskey CH: Allergic reaction to an amide local anesthetic. *Br J Anaesth* 1981; 53:1105–1106.

20. Murphy MF: Local anesthetic agents. *Emerg Med Clin North Am* 1988; 6(4):769–776.

21. Johnson WT, DeStigter T: Hypersensitivity to procaine, tetracaine, mepivacaine, and methylparaben: report of a case. *J Am Dent Assoc* 1983; 106:53–56.

22. Reynolds F: Adverse effects of local anesthetics. *Br J Anaesth* 1987; 59:78–95.

23. Dronen SC: Complications of TAC. *Ann Emerg Med* 1983; 12(5):333.

24. Berk WA, Welch TCD, Bock BF: Controversial issues in clinical management of the simple wound. *Ann Emerg Med* 1992; 21(1):72–80.

25. Cheney PR, Molzen G, Tandberg D: The effect of pH buffering on reducing the pain associated with sub-cutaneous infiltration of bupivacaine. *Am J Emerg Med* 1991; 9(2):147–148.

26. Christoph RA, Buchanan L, Begalla K, et al: Pain reduction in local anesthetic administration through pH buffering. *Ann Emerg Med* 1988; 17(2): 117–120.

27. Hegenbarth MA, Altieri MF, Hawk WH, et al: Comparison of topical tetracaine, adrenaline and cocaine with lidocaine infiltration for repair of lacerations in children. *Ann Emerg Med* 1990; 19(1): 63–67.

28. Cannon CR, Chouteau S, Hutchinson K: Topically applied tetracaine, adrenaline and cocaine in the repair of traumatic wounds of the head and neck. *Otolaryngol Head Neck Surg* 1989; 100(1):78–79.

29. Moore DC, Bonica JJ: Convulsions and ventricular tachycardia from bupivacaine with epinephrine: successful resuscitation—congratulations! *Anesth Analg* 1985; 64:(8)844–846.

30. Englesson S, Matousek M: Central nervous system effects of local anesthetic agents. *Br J Anaesth* 1975; 47(suppl):241–246.

31. Mallampati SR, Liu PL, Knapp RM: Convulsions and ventricular tachycardia from bupivacaine with epinephrine: successful resuscitation. *Anesth Analg* 1984; 63:856–859.

32. Ernst AA, Marvez-Valls E, Nick TG, et al: Comparison trial of four injectable anesthetics for laceration repair. *Acad Emerg Med* 1996; 3(3):228–233.

33. Pedersen H, Finster M: Selection and use of local anesthetics. *Clin Obstet Gynecol* 1987; 30(3):505–514.

Chapter 106

REGIONAL NERVE BLOCKS (REGIONAL ANESTHESIA)

Eric F. Reichman
Dedra R. Tolson

INTRODUCTION

Regional anesthesia or regional nerve blocks are defined as infiltration of a peripheral nerve with local anesthetic agents to attenuate motor output and sensory input.[1,2] It provides anesthesia to allow problems to be treated efficiently and with minimal discomfort. Patients typically tolerate nerve blocks better than direct wound infiltration. Nerve blocks often require less local anesthetic solution than does infiltration of large wounds.

Regional anesthesia provides sensory blockade of a region without altering the normal anatomic features of the area to be repaired. It may be considered for use in the repair of extensive wounds, incision and drainage of abscesses, foreign body removal, wound exploration, burn care, fracture reduction, or pain control. Once familiar with the body's sensory innervation, the physician can easily employ regional anesthesia techniques within the Emergency Department.

Locating and anesthetizing a peripheral nerve is accomplished in one of three ways. First is to identify the general location of the nerve using anatomy and landmarks. Infiltrate local anesthetic solution at that site and allow it to diffuse over the area. The second is to locate a nerve by using the injecting needle to elicit paresthesias. Once paresthesias are elicited, slightly withdraw the needle and allow the paresthesias to resolve before injecting the local anesthetic solution. Finally, a nerve stimulator can be used to accurately locate peripheral nerves with motor fiber components. Use of a nerve stimulator does not require cooperation on the part of the patient. However, due to its complexity, a physician skilled in its use is required. Nerve stimulaters are rarely available in Emergency Departments.

Cocaine was the first local anesthetic agent used in medical practice. In the 1880s, Halsted demonstrated that cocaine can be used to block nerve conduction.[3–5] There are two main classes of local anesthetics agents in use today: the esters and the amides.[5,6] They stabilize the nerve cell membrane by inhibiting the ionic fluxes required for initiation and conduction of nerve impulses.[6–9] Ester anesthetics include cocaine, procaine, benzocaine, and tetracaine.[8] The amide agents include the most commonly used anesthetics: lidocaine and bupivacaine. Other amide agents include etidocaine, mepivacaine, prilocaine, and ropivacaine.[9] **Ester agents can be substituted for amide agents if a patient has had a prior allergic reaction to an amide and vice versa.**

Adding epinephrine to local anesthetic agents increases their duration of action; however, it can result in significant vasoconstriction. **Use epinephrine-containing agents only in areas of good perfusion.**[10] Avoid epinephrine-containing agents in and around the fingers, toes, penis, ears, and nose. Avoid using these agents in crushed or damaged tissue with poor perfusion.

The addition of buffering agents to the local anesthetic solution results in less pain upon injection than nonbuffered agents.[3,11] The addition of bicarbonate to a local anesthetic agent can significantly decrease the pain of injection and improve the ease of performing a nerve block. Add 1 mL of sodium bicarbonate (44 meq per 50 mL) to 9 mL of lidocaine, for a total of 10 mL, to buffer the local anesthetic solution.[6,11,16,24] Buffering the agent does not compromise the efficacy of the anesthetic.

It is common to encounter children complaining of pain in the Emergency Department. Regional anesthesia is frequently overlooked in children. Its use is increasing and serves as an excellent opportunity to minimize pain in the pediatric population.[1,2,12] It can be administered safely and effectively in these patients. A child may require intravenous or intramuscular sedation in conjunction with nerve blockade in more complicated cases.

The use of nitrous oxide with pediatric patients in the Emergency Department has been found to be successful when used for forearm fracture manipulation.[13] It can also be used for other procedures. Refer to Chapter 108 regarding the use of nitrous oxide as a supplement or to perform the regional nerve block. The disadvantages of regional nerve blocks in children include the extra time required to perform the block, mandatory technical dexterity, and assistant support because the child may not remain still for the procedure.

This chapter covers regional anesthetic blocks of the head, neck, upper extremity, lower extremity, and two of the many torso blocks (Table 106-1). Dental blocks are discussed in Chapter 154. Refer to Chapter 105 for a more complete discussion on the properties of local anesthetic agents.

ANATOMY AND PATHOPHYSIOLOGY

There is a topographic arrangement of axons within peripheral nerves[1,6,14] (Figure 106-1*A*). Axons located in the outer or mantle layer innervate proximal structures. Axons in the center of the nerve or core layer innervate distal structures. Local anesthetic solution injected near a nerve diffuses from the mantle layer to the core layers. **This explains why anesthesia slowly spreads along the nerve distribution in a proximal to distal direction.**

Avoid intraneural injection when performing peripheral nerve blocks. The nerve has a tough, fibrous outer sheath that acts as a physical barrier to trap intraneural fluid (Figure 106-1*B*). Injection of local anesthetic agents into the nerve bundle will compress the fragile axons and their capillary blood supply.[7,15,16] This can result in axonal necrosis and permanent nerve damage. **Paresthesias elicited upon needle insertion indicate that the tip of the needle is within the nerve bundle. Withdraw the needle 1 to 2 mm and allow the pares-**

thesias to resolve, usually within 15 to 30 seconds. The anesthetic agent can be safely injected when the paresthesias resolve.

Cutaneous innervation is referenced to a segment known as a dermatome.[1,6] This is defined as an area of skin supplied by a single spinal or segmental nerve. This type of innervation is best represented in worms, where each body segment has its own nervous supply. The pattern of segmental innervation still holds true with some minor modifications as one moves up the phylogenetic tree. The truncal dermatomes in humans are represented as simple bands while the extremity dermatomes are serpiginous and follow the embryonic rotation of the limb buds. The most commonly used dermatomal chart is that developed by Keegan and Garrett[14] (Figure 106-2). Their model of the extremity dermatomes is in strips of innervation, all originating from the limb base and extending distally. This system is used in clinical medicine today.

INDICATIONS

Regional anesthesia produces profound analgesia with minimal physiologic or anatomic alteration. These techniques are especially useful in large or extensive lacerations that would otherwise require infiltration of large amounts of local anesthetic agent. Nerve blocks can avoid a patient being taken to the Operating Room because the volume of local anesthetic required for extensive wound repair may require toxic doses. These techniques are also useful in cosmetic repairs where local infiltration may cause distortion of tissues or loss of anatomic landmarks making approximation and repair difficult. The necessity to palpate deep tissue for excision is also an indication for regional anesthesia.[17,18] Regional nerve blocks can be performed prior to burn care, dislocation or fracture reduction, foreign body re-

TABLE 106-1. NERVES AND ANATOMICAL AREAS THAT CAN BE ANESTHETIZED IN THE EMERGENCY DEPARTMENT USING A REGIONAL BLOCK

Head and neck	Lower extremity	Upper extremity	Torso
Supraorbital nerve block	Femoral nerve block	Brachial plexus block	Intercostal block
Supratrochlear nerve block	Saphenous nerve block	Median nerve block	Penile nerve block
Infraorbital nerve block	Lateral femoral cutaneous nerve block	Ulnar nerve block	
Mental nerve block	Obturator nerve block	Radial nerve block	
Greater occipital nerve block	Sciatic nerve block	Wrist block	
Lesser occipital nerve block	Popliteal fossa block	Digital nerve block	
Greater auricular nerve block	Common peroneal nerve block		
Scalp block	Superficial peroneal nerve block		
External ear block	Deep peroneal nerve block		
External auditory canal block	Sural nerve block		
Cervical plexus block	Posterior tibial nerve block		
	Ankle block		
	Digital nerve block		

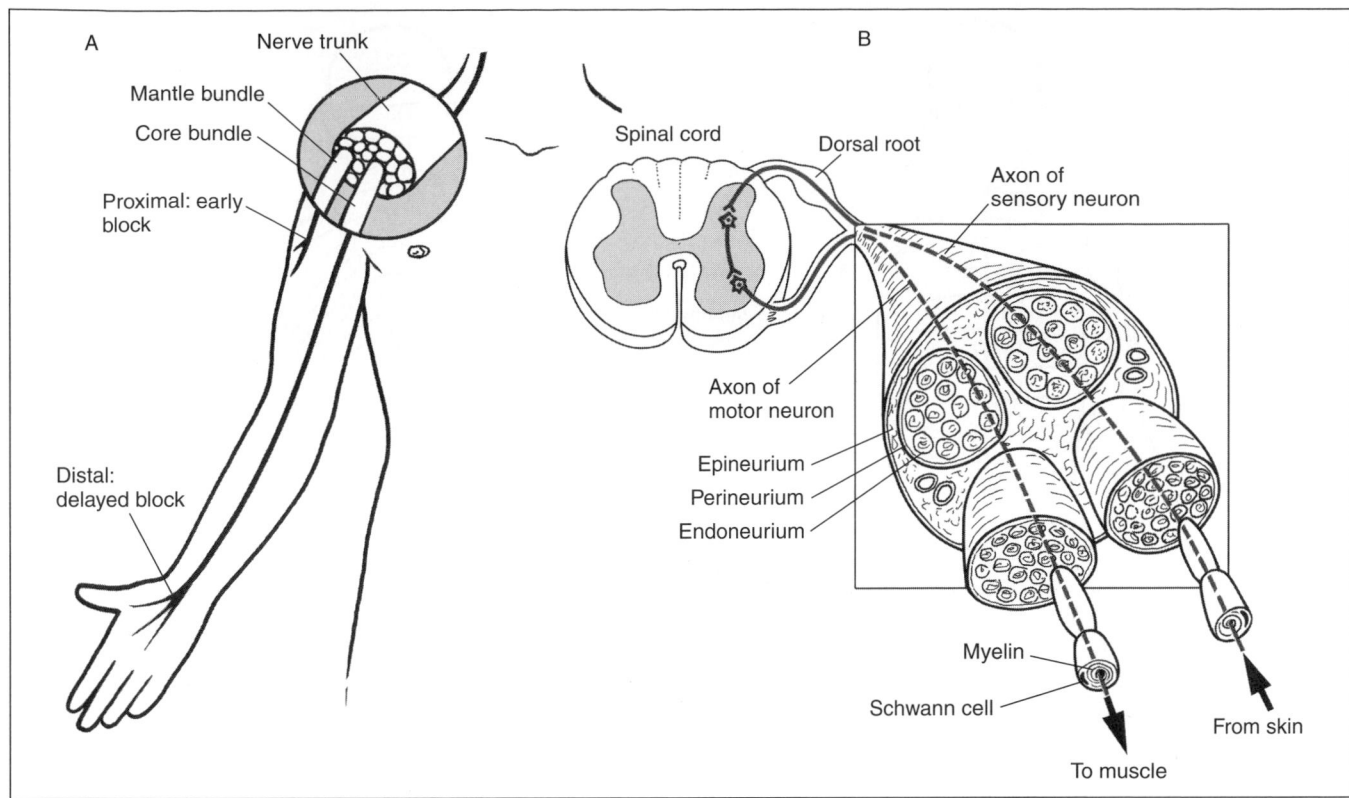

FIGURE 106-1 The anatomy and topographic arrangement of axons in a peripheral nerve. *A.* The gross anatomy of a peripheral nerve. *B.* The microscopic anatomy of a peripheral nerve.

moval, incision and drainage of abscesses, pain control, and wound care.

CONTRAINDICATIONS

There are few contraindications to regional anesthesia.[5,6,10] Absolute contraindications include injection through infected tissue, history of a bleeding disorder or a coagulopathy, or an allergy to the anesthetic agent. Relative contraindications include preexisting neurologic damage prior to the procedure. This should carefully be documented before any anesthetic injection. Additionally, patient uncooperativeness can make the procedure technically more difficult. Therefore, procedural sedation may be a necessary adjunct.[3,12] This is particularly true of the pediatric population and those with altered mental status.[19]

EQUIPMENT

Sterile gloves
Sterile drapes
Povidone iodine solution
Alcohol swabs
Local anesthetic solution (Table 106-2 and Chapter 105)
18 gauge needle to draw up local anesthetic solution
20 to 30 gauge needles for injection, 2 inches long
22 to 24 gauge spinal needles
1, 3, 5, 10, and 60 mL syringes
Intravenous extension tubing

All of the required equipment is available in any Emergency Department.[20] Some have a preprepared tray containing all the equipment.

PATIENT PREPARATION

Explain the procedure, its risks, and benefits to the patient and/or their representative. Emphasize that there are few complications with this procedure. However, all possible complications should be discussed beforehand. Inform the patient of the possibility of paresthesias during the procedure and of the expected duration of action of the local anesthetic agent (Table 106-2). Obtain an informed consent for the regional nerve block in addition to the procedure for which it is performed. Ideally, the consent should be docu-

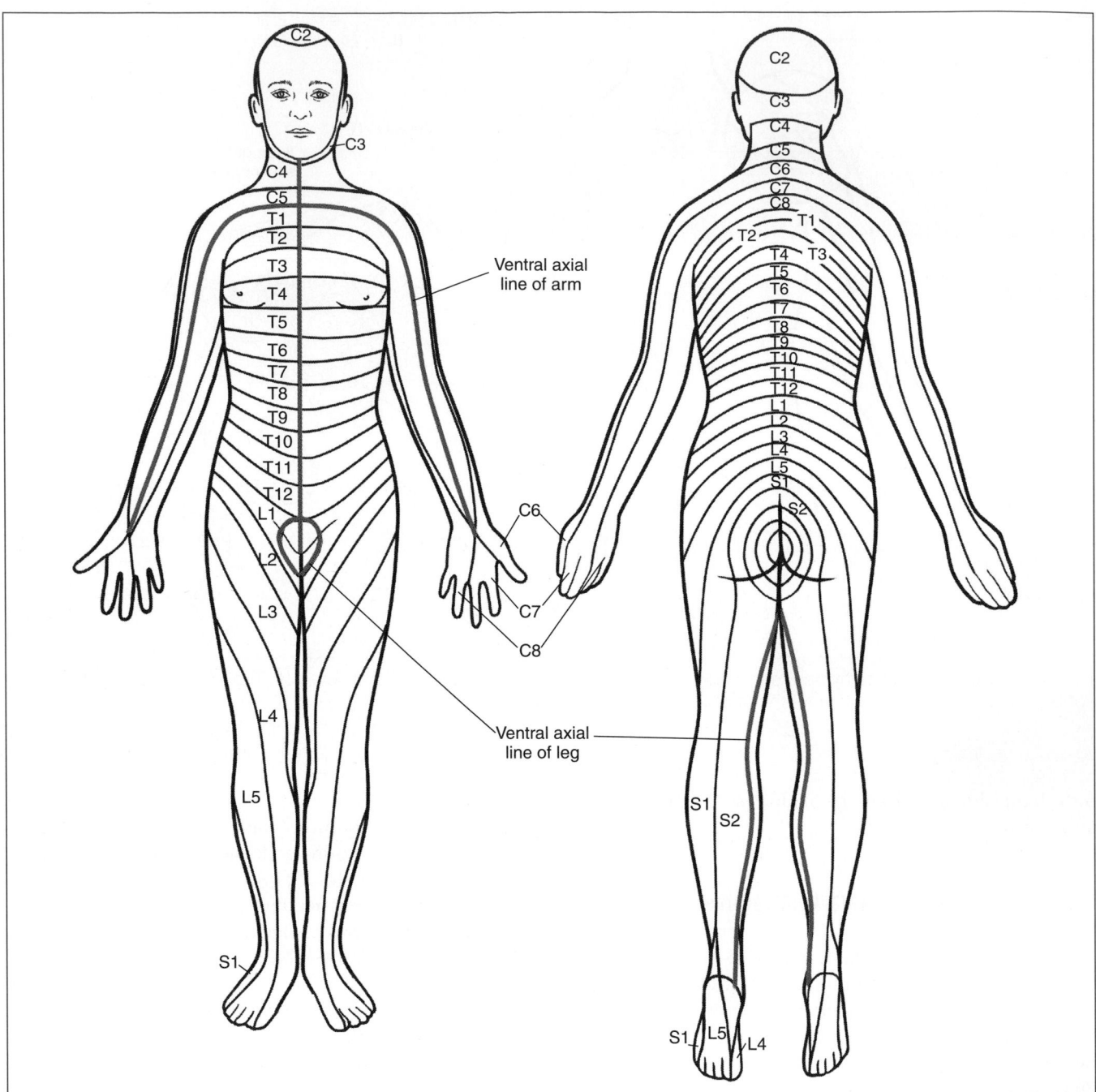

FIGURE 106-2 The dermatomal chart of the human body.

mented in the medical record and signed by the patient. Some physicians prefer to note on the patient's chart "indications, risks, and benefits were discussed with the patient" rather than having the patient sign a consent form.[21]

Perform and document a neurological examination of the area to be anesthetized before performing regional anesthesia.[21,23] Include a description of any neurological deficit in the document of informed consent

for the procedure. Have the patient sign an agreement that the defect was present prior to the administration of the local anesthetic agent.

Position the patient based upon the specific regional block to be performed. Place the patient supine on a gurney or procedure table prior to the procedure in most cases. If the patient must sit upright, place the patient on an adjustable bed. The patient's comfort should be optimized to prevent unexpected complications such as

TABLE 106-2. MAXIMUM DOSES OF LOCAL ANESTHETIC AGENTS

Anesthetic agent	Maximum dose (mg/kg)	Duration of action (min)
Procaine (2%)	6	15–30
Procaine (2%) with epinephrine	8	30–90
Tetracaine (0.25%)	1	120–140
Tetracaine (0.25%) with epinephrine	2	240–280
Chloroprocaine (2%)	8	15–30
Chloroprocaine (2%) with epinephrine	10	30–90
Lidocaine (1%)	3	30–120
Lidocaine (1%) with epinephrine	5	60–400
Etidocaine (0.5%)	3	30–120
Etidocaine (0.5%) with epinephrine	4	60–200
Mepivacaine (1%)	3	30–120
Mepivacaine (1%) with epinephrine	5	60–400
Bupivacaine (0.25%)	1.75	120–240
Bupivacaine (0.25%) with epinephrine	2.25	240–480
Prilocaine (4%)	5	30–60
Prilocaine (4%) with epinephrine	6	120–300

vasovagal syncope.[4,6,22] Expose the area of the injection and identify the anatomic landmarks required for proper needle placement. Clean all dirt and debris from the skin. Scrub the needle insertion site with povidone iodine solution and allow it to dry.

TECHNIQUE

The general procedure will first be described and specifics will be addressed with each individual nerve block.

Identify the nerve or nerves to be blocked and their associated anatomic landmarks. Carefully clean and prepare the skin over the injection site in a sterile fashion. Draw up the local anesthetic agent to be used. The amount will vary based upon the specific block. Always keep in mind the maximum allowable dose of local anesthetic (Table 106-2). Reidentify the anatomic landmarks. Insert the needle into the site. Withdraw the plunger to ensure that the tip of the needle is not within a blood vessel, thus avoiding intravascular injection. If paresthesias are elicited, withdraw the needle 1 mm and allow them to resolve. Inject the local anesthetic solution. Apply an appropriate bandage to the site. Allow 5 to 15 minutes for the block to take effect. Confirm that anesthesia has been achieved with pinprick prior to performing a procedure. Document the anesthesia procedure, the procedure for which regional anesthesia was performed, and any complications in the medical record.[23–26] A sample regional anesthesia procedure note is described in Table 106-3.

TABLE 106-3. A SAMPLE REGIONAL ANESTHESIA PROCEDURE NOTE

After informed consent and identification of the necessary landmarks, the skin overlying _____ (location) was cleaned and prepped with povidone iodine solution. Using sterile technique, a skin wheal of local anesthetic solution was placed. A _____ gauge needle was used to anesthesize the _____ nerve with _____ mL of ___ % _____ (lidocaine, marcaine, procaine, etc.). Anesthesia was confirmed with needle pinprick testing. No complications were noted.

REGIONAL ANESTHESIA TECHNIQUES FOR THE HEAD AND NECK

SUPRAORBITAL NERVE BLOCK

Anatomy: The supraorbital foramen lies on the supraorbital ridge along a line drawn through the pupil in the midposition (Figures 106-3 and 106-4). The supraorbital foramen may be palpable as an indentation. The supraorbital nerve is a branch of the ophthalmic division of the trigeminal nerve (Figure 106-4A). It emerges through the supraorbital foramen, or notch, at the midline of the superior orbital ridge. Its area of innervation includes the forehead, beginning at the superior orbital ridge and extending superiorly to the vertex of the scalp. It is blocked simultaneously with the supratrochlear nerve, as there is considerable overlap in their areas of innervation.[17,27,28]

Patient positioning: Place the patient supine, or sitting, and facing the operator.

Landmarks: Identify, under the eyebrow, the superior orbital rim and the supraorbital foramen by palpation.

Needle insertion and direction: Place a skin wheal of local anesthetic solution over the midline of the forehead at the level of the eyebrow. Insert a 25 or 27 gauge needle through the skin wheal and aimed laterally (Figure 106-4B). Advance the needle while infiltrating subcutaneously with 3 to 5 mL of local anesthetic solution. Always maintain the needle just above the supraorbital ridge while advancing it (Figure 106-4B). Stop infiltrating when the needle passes the midline of the bony orbit.

Remarks: This technique will anesthetize both the supraorbital and supratrochlear nerves. Infiltrate 2 mL of local anesthetic solution directly over the supraorbital foramen, or notch, if it is palpable rather than subcutaneously infiltrating above the supraorbital ridge.

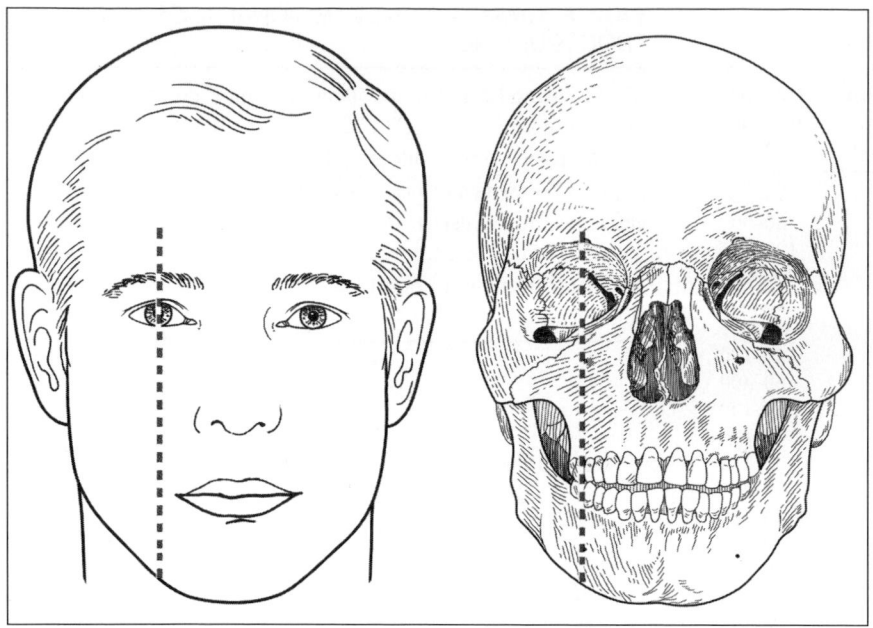

FIGURE 106-3 The supraorbital foramen, the infraorbital foramen, and the mental foramen all lie along a straight line drawn through the pupil in the midposition.

SUPRATROCHLEAR NERVE BLOCK

Anatomy: The supratrochlear nerve is a branch of the ophthalmic division of the trigeminal nerve. It emerges through the trochlea at the supermedial aspect of the bony orbit (Figure 106-4*A*). It provides innervation to the middle of the forehead beginning at the superior orbital ridge and extending superiorly to the vertex of the scalp. It is often blocked simultaneously with the supraorbital nerve, because there is considerable overlap in their areas of innervation.[17,27,28]

Patient positioning: Place the patient supine, or sitting, and facing the operator.

Landmarks: Identify, under the eyebrow, the superior orbital rim by palpation.

Needle insertion and direction: Place a skin wheal of local anesthetic solution over the midline of the forehead at the level of the eyebrows. Insert a 25 or 27 gauge needle through the skin wheal, aimed laterally (Figure 106-4*B*). Advance the needle while infiltrating subcu-

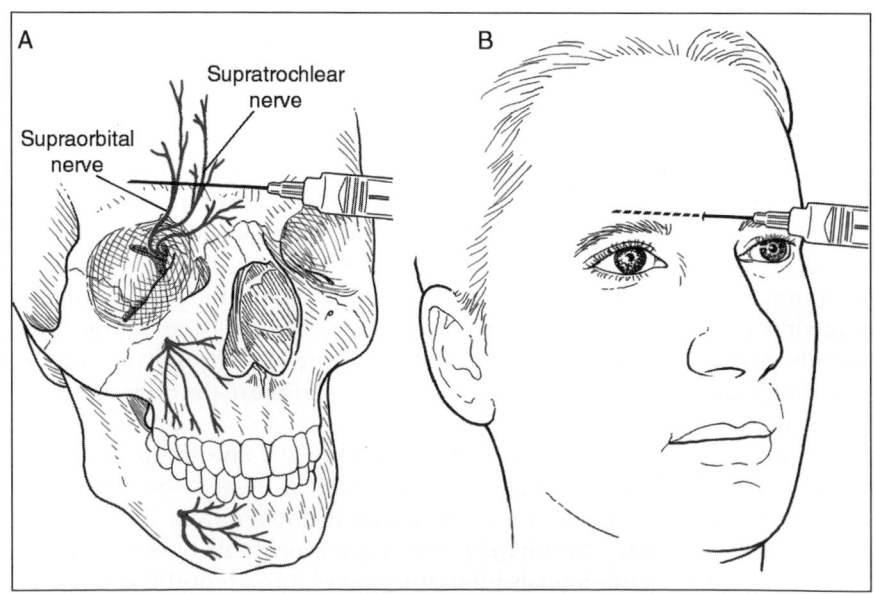

FIGURE 106-4 The supraorbital and supratrochlear nerve block. *A.* The location of the nerves. *B.* Insertion of the needle.

taneously with 3 to 5 mL of local anesthetic solution. Always maintain the needle just above the supraorbital ridge while advancing it (Figure 106-4*B*). Stop infiltrating when the needle passes the midline of the bony orbit.

Remarks: Stop infiltrating 1.5 cm from the skin wheal so as to block only the supratrochlear nerve.

INFRAORBITAL NERVE BLOCK, EXTRAORAL APPROACH

Anatomy: The infraorbital nerve is a branch of the maxillary division of the trigeminal nerve. It emerges through the infraorbital foramen, 1 cm below the middle to medial third of the inferior orbital ridge (Figure 106-5*A*). It lies in the same plane as the supraorbital foramen and pupil that is in the midposition (Figures 106-3 and 106-5). The nerve exits the infraorbital foramen and travels inferiorly and medially. It provides sensory innervation to the medial cheek, nasal ala, upper lip, and the skin between the upper lip and nose.[2,27,28] The infraorbital nerve terminates as the anterior and middle superior alveolar nerves. They provide sensory innervation to the maxillary incisors, canine, and premolar teeth, as well as their bony support and surrounding soft tissues.

Patient positioning: Place the patient supine, or sitting, and facing the operator.

Landmarks: Identify the infraorbital foramen by palpation. Significant tenderness will be elicited when the infraorbital nerve is palpated as it exits the infraorbital foramen.

Needle insertion and direction: Insert a 25 or 27 gauge needle just above the infraorbital foramen (Figure 106-5*B*). Advance the needle until the maxilla is contacted. Inject 1 to 2 mL of local anesthetic solution.

Remarks: The infraorbital nerve can be blocked intraorally.[17,28] The intraoral route results in the patient experiencing less pain than the extraoral route.

INFRAORBITAL NERVE BLOCK, INTRAORAL APPROACH

Anatomy: The anatomy and innervation of the infraorbital nerve is described in the previous section.

Patient positioning: Place the patient supine, or sitting, and facing the operator.

Landmarks: Identify the infraorbital foramen by palpation. It lies in a plane with the supraorbital foramen and the pupil in the midposition (Figures 106-3 and 106-6*A*).

Needle insertion and direction: Place the index finger of the nondominant hand over the infraorbital foramen (Figure 106-6*B*). Use the nondominant thumb to retract the upper lip.

Insert a 2.5 to 4.0 cm, 25 or 27 gauge needle through the mucous membranes, directed at the index finger. Ad-

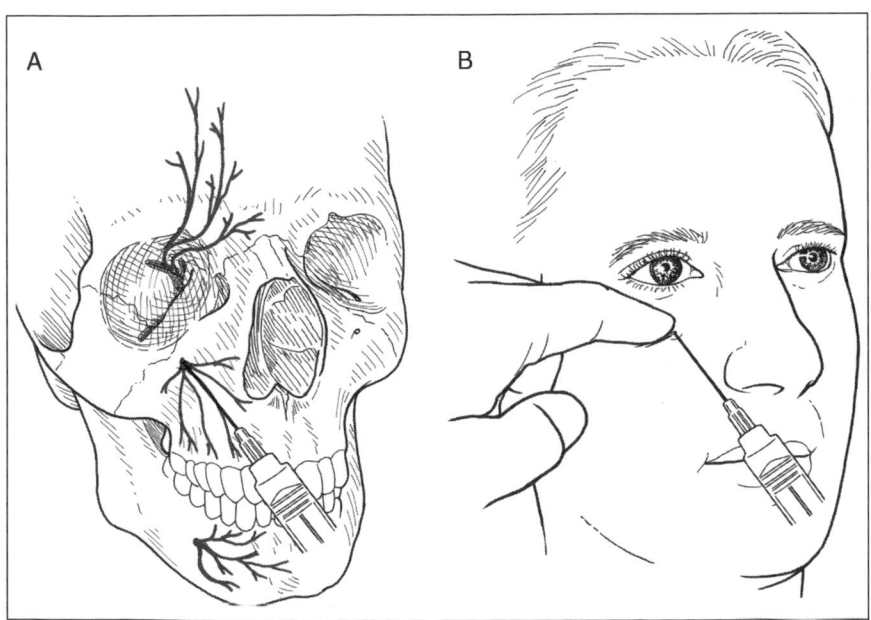

FIGURE 106-5 The extraoral approach to the infraorbital nerve block. *A*. Location of the nerve. *B*. Insertion of the needle.

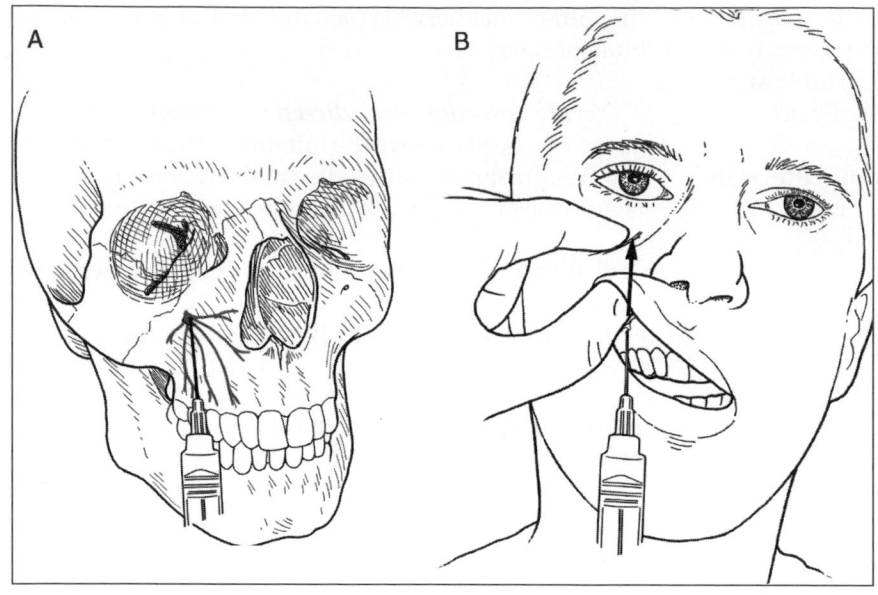

FIGURE 106-6 The intraoral approach to the infraorbital nerve block. *A.* Location of the nerve. *B.* Insertion of the needle.

vance the needle until its tip is palpable at the infraorbital foramen by the index finger. The estimated depth of needle penetration is 1.0 to 1.5 cm. Inject 2 mL of local anesthetic solution.

Remarks: This is the preferred route to block the infraorbital nerve. It can also be blocked extraorally.[17,28]

MENTAL NERVE BLOCK, EXTRAORAL APPROACH

Anatomy: The mental nerve is a branch of the mandibular division of the trigeminal nerve. It emerges from the mental foramen. The foramen lies in a vertical plane with the supraorbital foramen, the infraorbital foramen, and the pupil that is midposition (Figures 106-3 and 106-7). The nerve travels inferiorly and anteriorly to provide sensory innervation to the skin of the lower lip and chin.[2,27,28]

Patient positioning: Place the patient supine, or sitting, and facing the operator.

Landmarks: Identify the vertical plane consisting of the supraorbital foramen, the infraorbital foramen, and the midposition pupil. Identify the point where the

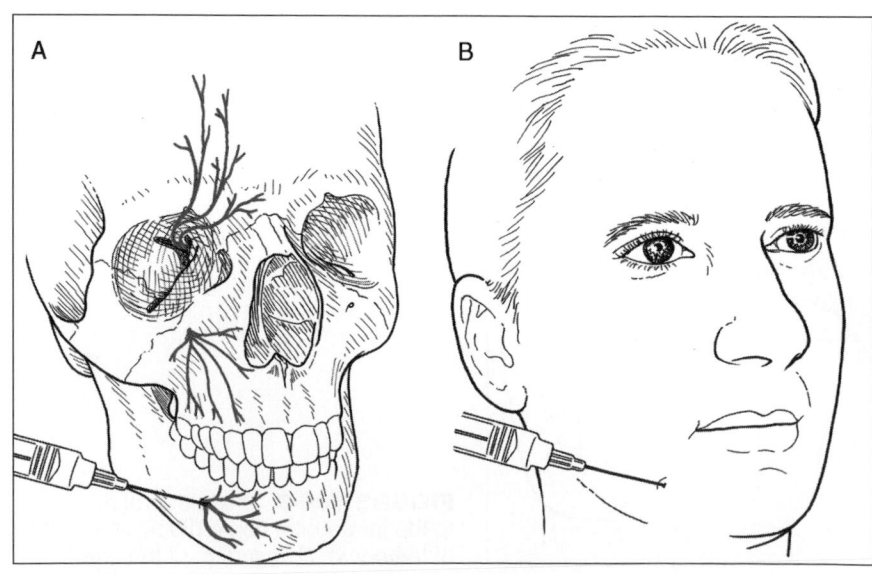

FIGURE 106-7 The extraoral approach to the mental nerve block. *A.* Location of the nerve. *B.* Insertion of the needle.

vertical plane crosses the middle of the body of the mandible (Figure 106-7A). This is where the mental nerve exits the mental foramen.

Needle insertion and direction: Insert a 25 or 27 gauge needle at the above identified landmark (Figure 106-7B). Place a skin wheal of local anesthetic solution at this intersection. Advance the needle through the skin wheal until the mandible is contacted. Inject 1 to 2 mL of local anesthetic solution.

Remarks: This nerve can also be blocked intraorally.

MENTAL NERVE BLOCK, INTRAORAL APPROACH

Anatomy: The anatomy and innervation of the mental nerve is described in the previous section.

Patient positioning: Place the patient supine, or sitting, and facing the operator.

Landmarks: Retract the lower lip and identify the junction of the first and second premolars. The patient's mouth may be open or closed.

Needle insertion and direction: Insert a 25 or 27 gauge needle directed inferiorly and posteriorly through the gingival mucosa at the junction of the first and second premolars (Figure 106-8). Advance the needle one-third the depth of the mandible and contact the mandible. Inject 1 to 2 mL of local anesthetic solution.

Remarks: This is the preferred approach to block the mental nerve. The intraoral route results in the patient experiencing less pain than the extraoral route.

GREATER OCCIPITAL NERVE BLOCK

Anatomy: The greater occipital nerve is a branch of the dorsal ramus of the second cervical nerve.[17,27,28] It provides sensory innervation to the posterior neck, extending superiorly to the vertex of the scalp (Figure 106-9). It emerges on the posterosuperior neck, just below the line connecting the external occipital protuberance and the mastoid process (Figure 106-10). The posterior occipital artery accompanies the greater occipital nerve.

Patient positioning: Place the patient prone.

Landmarks: Identify the external occipital protuberance and mastoid process by palpation (Figure 106-10A). Connect these landmarks with a line. Identify the occipital artery by its palpable pulse, approximately one-third the distance from the external occipital protuberance.

Needle insertion and direction: Place a skin wheal of local anesthetic solution over the pulse of the occipital artery. Insert a 25 gauge needle 1 to 2 mm to the left of the occipital artery pulse. Inject 1 mL of local anesthetic solution. Redirect the needle 1 to 2 mm to the right of the pulse and inject 1 mL of local anesthetic solution.

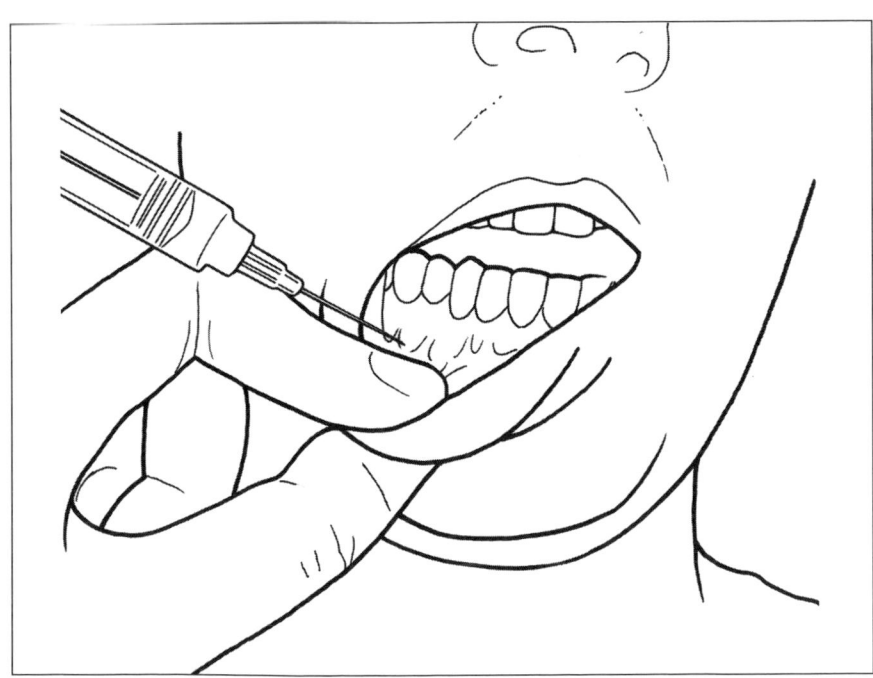

FIGURE 106-8 The intraoral approach to the mental nerve block.

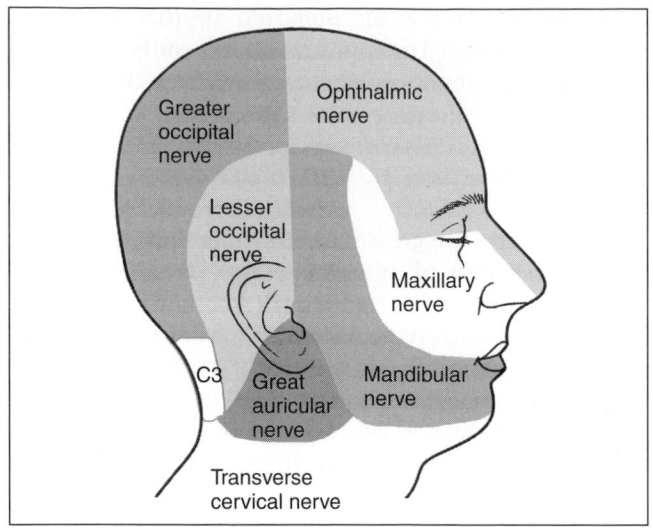

FIGURE 106-9 The cutaneous nerve supply to the face, scalp, and upper neck.

Remarks: This block is useful for laceration repair as well as relief of occipital muscular or tension headaches.[27,28] If the pulse of the posterior occipital artery is not palpable, divide the line between the external occipital protuberance and the mastoid process into thirds. Infiltrate the middle third subcutaneously with 5 to 8 mL of local anesthetic solution (Figure 106-10*A*). This technique will also anesthetize the great occipital nerve.

LESSER OCCIPITAL NERVE BLOCK

Anatomy: The lesser occipital nerve is a branch of the cervical plexus. It provides sensory innervation to the skin and scalp between the ear and the mastoid process (Figure 106-9). It emerges at the middle third of the posterior border of the sternocleidomastoid muscle and travels superiorly toward the mastoid process (Figure 106-10).

Patient positioning: Place the patient supine or sitting with their head turned toward the side opposite that being anesthetized.

Landmarks: Identify the mastoid process by palpation.

Needle insertion and direction: Place a skin wheal of local anesthetic solution just posterior to the mastoid process. Insert a 25 gauge needle directed anteriorly through the skin wheal. Advance the needle while infiltrating local anesthetic solution subcutaneously until the

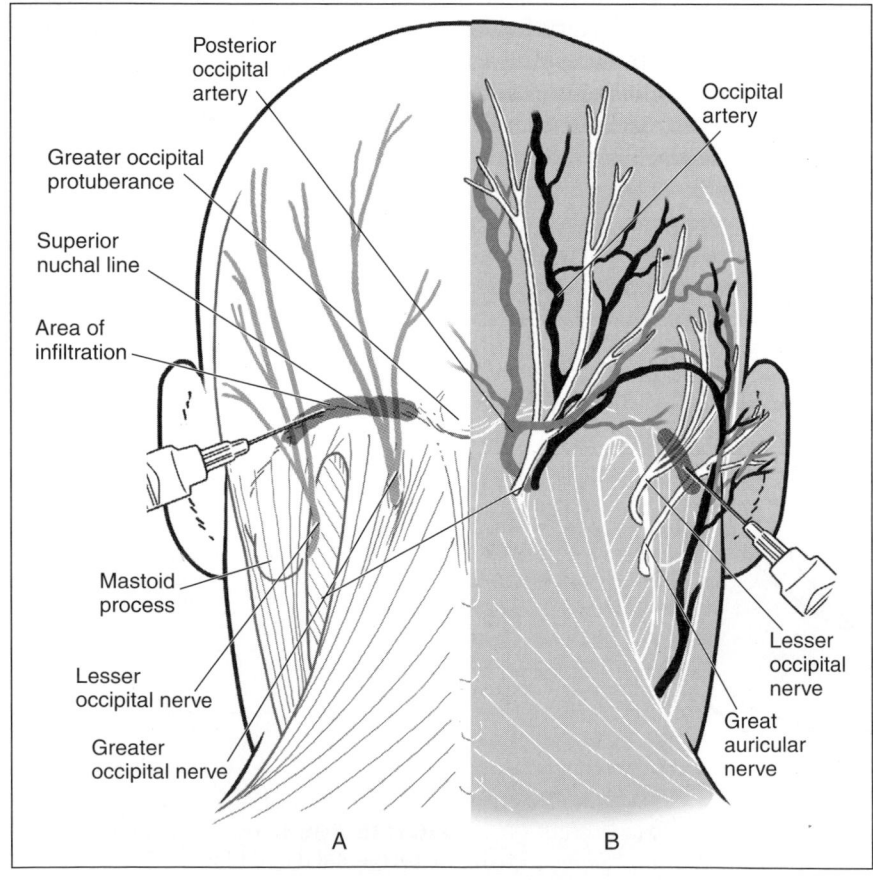

FIGURE 106-10 Regional anesthesia of the posterolateral scalp. *A.* The greater occipital nerve block. *B.* The lesser occipital and great auricular nerve blocks.

posterior ear is contacted (Figure 106-10*B*). This requires 3 to 7 mL of local anesthetic solution.

Remarks: The lesser occipital nerve can be blocked at the level of the cervical plexus. Refer to the section on cervical plexus blockade below.

GREAT AURICULAR NERVE BLOCK

Anatomy: The great auricular nerve is a branch of the cervical plexus. It emerges at the middle third of the posterior border of the sternocleidomastoid muscle and travels superiorly with the external jugular vein (Figure 106-10*B*). This nerve provides sensory innervation to the skin and scalp behind the ear, the posterior ear, and the lobule (Figure 106-9).

Patient positioning: Place the patient supine with their head turned toward the side opposite that being anesthetized.

Landmarks: Identify the lobule of the ear, the mastoid process, and the sulcus behind the ear.

Needle insertion and direction: Place a skin wheal of local anesthetic solution just posterior to the mastoid process. Insert a 25 gauge needle directed anteriorly

through the skin wheal. Advance the needle while infiltrating local anesthetic solution subcutaneously until the posterior ear is contacted (Figure 106-10*B*). This requires 3 to 7 mL of local anesthetic solution. Complete and successful anesthesia occurs within 10 minutes.[2,27]

Remarks: The great auricular nerve block is indicated for lacerations of the auricle, debridement, and hematoma evacuations. It is rarely performed without simultaneous blockade of the auriculotemporal nerve.[27] The great auricular nerve can be blocked at the level of the cervical plexus. Refer to the section on cervical plexus blockade below.

SCALP BLOCK

Anatomy: The scalp receives its sensory innervation from branches of the trigeminal nerve anteriorly and the cervical plexus posteriorly (Figure 106-11). The scalp may be anesthetized anywhere along the anterior midline to the posterior midline. This involves blocking the supratrochlear, supraorbital, auriculotemporal, lesser occipital, great auricular, and greater occipital nerves.[1,2,27]

Patient positioning: Place the patient supine with their head turned toward the side opposite that being anesthetized.

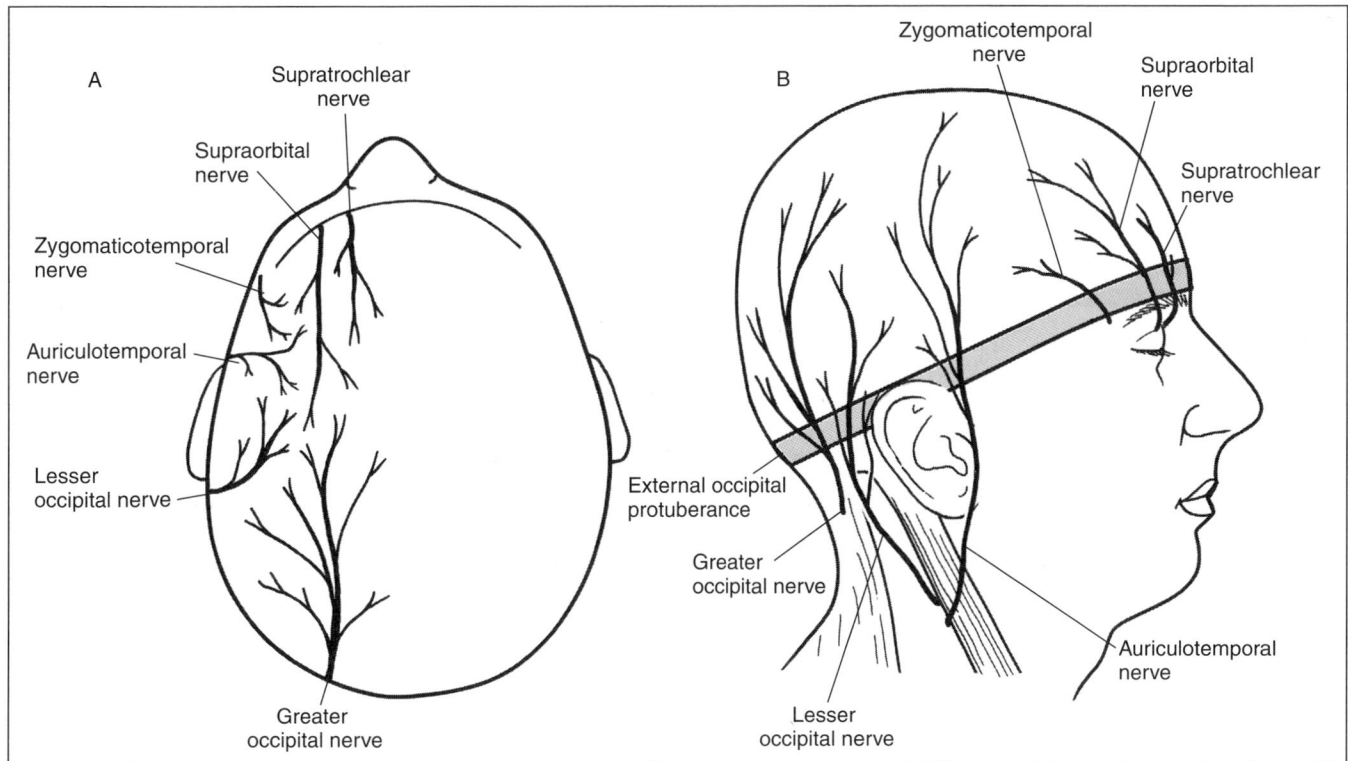

FIGURE 106-11 The scalp block. *A.* The sensory innervation of the scalp. *B.* Local anesthetic solution is injected subcutaneously along the base of the scalp.

Landmarks: Identify the glabella and the external occipital protuberance by palpation.

Needle insertion and direction: Place a skin wheal of local anesthetic solution over the glabella. Insert a 25 gauge needle through the skin wheal. Infiltrate a continuous line of local anesthetic solution subcutaneously between the glabella and the external occipital protuberance (Figure 106-11*B*). This requires 15 to 30 mL of local anesthetic solution.

Remarks: Infiltrate the local anesthetic solution subcutaneously along the scalp base inferior to the area in which the procedures will be performed to block only a portion of the scalp. It is useful to add epinephrine (1:200,000) to the local anesthetic solution to cause vasoconstriction and prevent excessive blood loss. Significant systemic absorption of the local anesthetic agent does not occur despite the extensive vascularity of the scalp.[27] Scalp blocks provide anesthesia for laceration repair, drainage of superficial abscesses, and the exploration of scalp wounds. Complications are fairly rare. There is a case report of a temporary facial nerve palsy after a scalp block.[29]

EXTERNAL EAR BLOCK

Anatomy: The ear is a difficult structure to anesthetize. It is innervated by a large number of sensory fibers that originate from the cervical plexus, the trigeminal nerve, and the vagus nerve. The external ear, or pinna, is innervated by the cervical plexus and the auriculotemporal branch of the trigeminal nerve[1,2,28] (Figures 106-9 and 106-11).

Patient positioning: Place the patient supine or sitting upright with their head turned toward the side opposite that being anesthetized.

Landmarks: Identify the angle of the mandible by palpation.

Needle insertion and direction: Place a skin wheal of local anesthetic solution over the angle of the mandible. Insert a 25 gauge needle through the skin wheal. Infiltrate local anesthetic solution subcutaneously in an anterior and superior direction, from the angle of the mandible to the superior surface of the ear, to block the auriculotemporal nerve (Figure 106-12*A*). Infiltrate local anesthetic solution subcutaneously in a posterior and superior direction, from the angle of the mandible to the superior surface of the ear, to block the great auricular and lesser occipital nerves (Figure 106-12*A*). This requires a total of 8 to 15 mL of local anesthetic solution.

Remarks: Some physicians prefer to anesthetize the auriculotemporal nerve trunk by injecting local anesthetic solution just above the posterior aspect of the zygomatic arch (Figure 106-12*B*). It requires less local anesthetic solution and hurts less than subcutaneous infiltration. An alternative technique is to circumferentially infiltrate local anesthetic solution subcutaneously around the ear (Figure 106-12*C*).

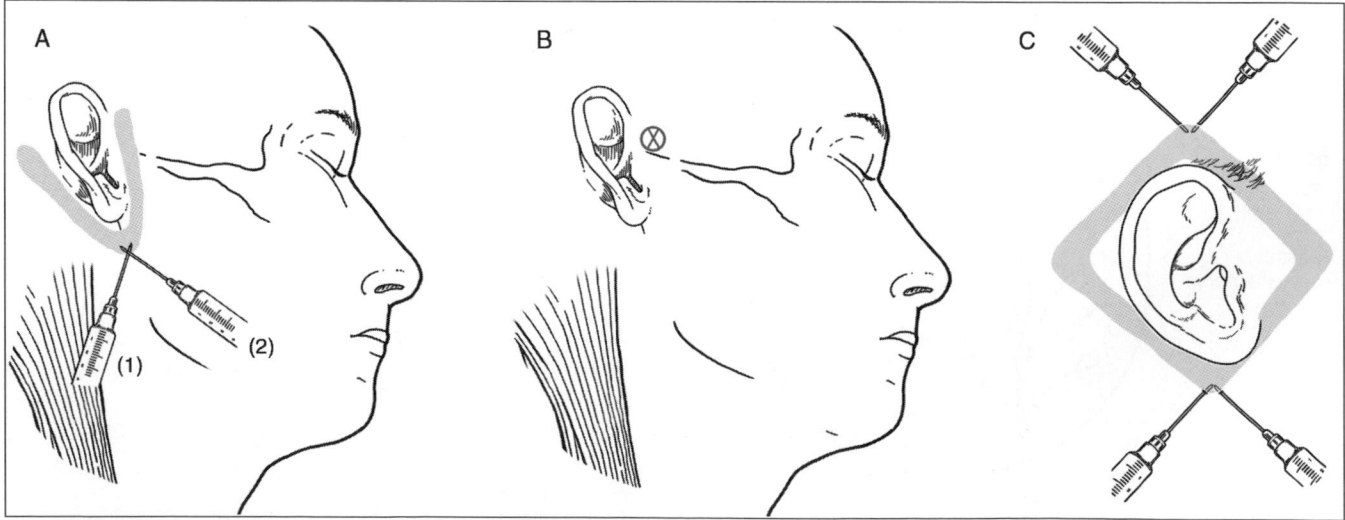

FIGURE 106-12 The external ear block. *A.* Infiltration of local anesthetic solution from the angle of the mandible to the anterior (*1*) and posterior (*2*) superior surfaces of the ear. *B.* The site for anesthetizing the trunk of the auriculotemporal nerve. *C.* An alternative method.

EXTERNAL AUDITORY CANAL BLOCK

Anatomy: The external auditory canal (and the tympanic membrane) receives its innervation from the auriculotemporal nerve and the vagus nerve.

Patient positioning: Place the patient sitting upright or supine with their head turned toward the side opposite that being anesthetized.

Landmarks: Identify the helix, the tragus, and the lobule of the ear to be anesthetized (Figure 106-13).

Needle insertion and direction: Anesthetize the external auditory canal using a four-quadrant block (Figure 106-13). Insert a 25 gauge needle, advance it 0.5 to 0.75 cm, and inject 1 mL of local anesthetic solution at each of the four landmarks identified in Figure 106-13.

Remarks: This block can be quite painful for the patient. The authors recommend to first anesthetize the external ear before anesthetizing the external auditory canal. This block also anesthetizes the tympanic membrane.[2]

CERVICAL PLEXUS BLOCK

Anatomy: The cervical plexus originates from the anterior rami of cervical nerves two through four. These

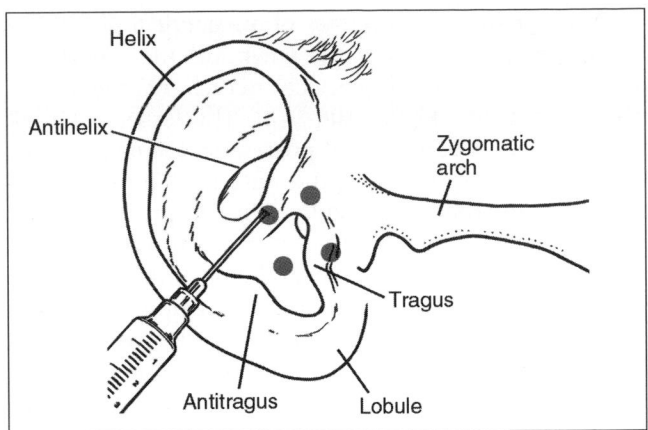

FIGURE 106-13 External auditory canal block. Inject local anesthetic solution at each of the four landmarks. This block also anesthetizes the tympanic membrane.

rami form numerous loops that anastomose to form nerves that provide sensory innervation to the anterolateral neck, the scalp, the ear, and the infraclavicular area. The four nerves of the cervical plexus become superficial at the midportion of the posterior border of the sternocleidomastoid muscle and then distribute to their respective sensory areas (Figure 106-14A). The cervical plexus provides motor innervation to the strap muscles of the neck.[1,2]

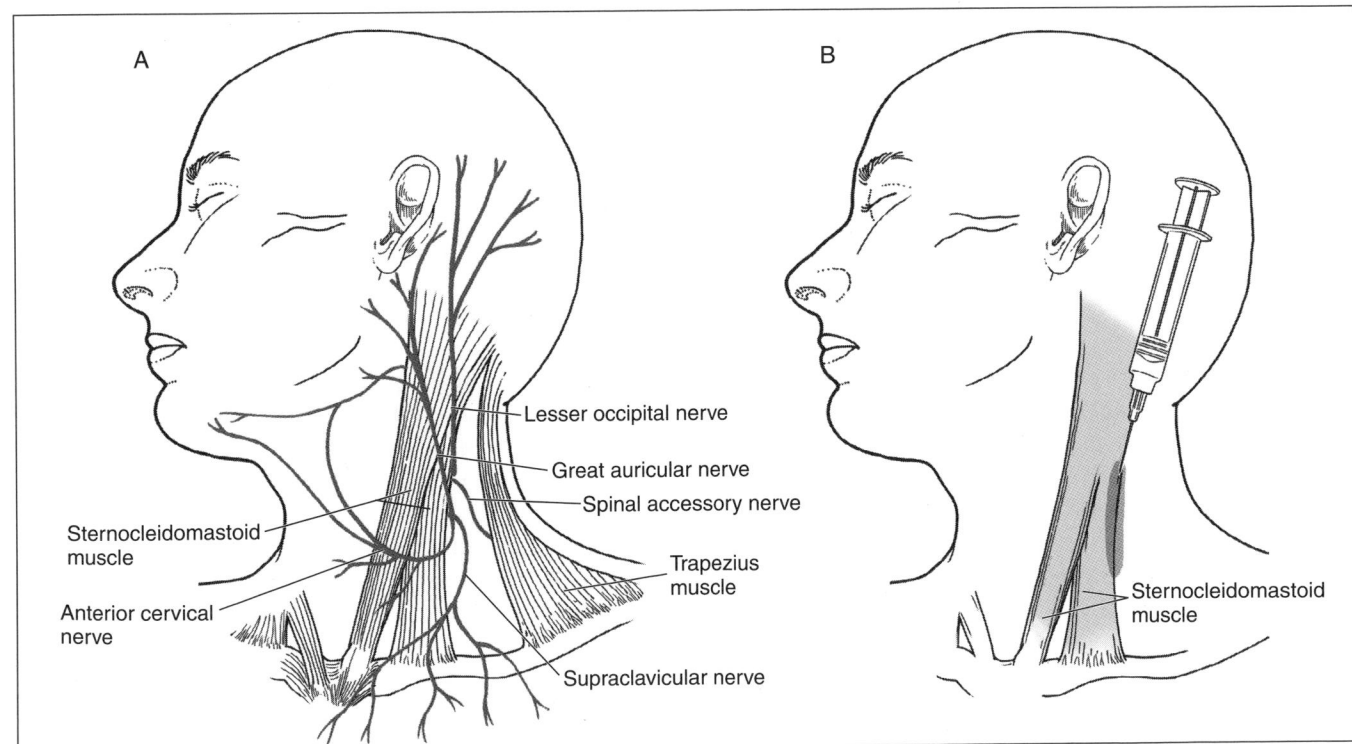

FIGURE 106-14 The cervical plexus block. *A.* The cutaneous nerves of the cervical plexus. *B.* Injection of local anesthetic solution posterior to the middle third of the sternocleidomastoid muscle.

The four superficial nerves of the cervical plexus are the lesser occipital nerve, the great auricular nerve, the anterior (or transverse) cervical nerve, and the supraclavicular nerve (Figure 106-14*A*). The lesser occipital nerve travels superiorly and posteriorly to provide sensory innervation to part of the posterior surface of the upper ear and the postauricular skin. The great auricular nerve travels superiorly and anteriorly to provide sensory innervation to the skin over the posterior surface of the ear, the anterior lower half of the ear, and over the angle of the mandible. The anterior, or transverse, cervical nerve of the neck travels anteriorly to provide sensory innervation to the skin of the neck, from the inferior border of the mandible to the sternum. The supraclavicular nerves travel inferiorly to provide sensory innervation to the skin over the clavicle down to the second rib.

Patient positioning: Place the patient supine with their head turned toward the side opposite of that being anesthetized.

Landmarks: Identify the posterior border of the sternocleidomastoid muscle by palpation. Divide this border into thirds.

Needle insertion and direction: Place a skin wheal of local anesthetic solution over the middle third of the posterior border of the sternocleidomastoid muscle. Insert a needle through the skin wheal. Infiltrate 5 to 10 mL of local anesthetic solution subcutaneously over the middle third of the posterior border of the sternocleidomastoid muscle (Figure 106-14*B*).

Remarks: This block is useful when managing burns or suturing lacerations on the anterolateral neck.

REGIONAL ANESTHESIA TECHNIQUES FOR THE UPPER EXTREMITY

BRACHIAL PLEXUS BLOCK

The brachial plexus innervates the entire upper extremity. Blockade of the brachial plexus can be performed to repair tendons or extensive lacerations, to reduce fractures and dislocations, or to provide anesthesia for burn care, to name a few uses.[2,30] Protect the arm from injury if this procedure is to be performed by properly supporting the arm, padding the ulnar nerve and pressure points, and not extending or displacing the arm posteriorly.[31]

The brachial plexus may be blocked from the supraclavicular, interscalene, infraclavicular, or axillary approach. The preferred method for the Emergency Physician is the axillary block, which will be described in detail.

The other blocks will be mentioned for the sake of knowledge only because they require the use of a nerve stimulator and have a high risk of associated complications.

BRACHIAL PLEXUS BLOCK, SUPRACLAVICULAR APPROACH

Anatomy: The brachial plexus arises from the C5 to T1 nerve roots (Figure 106-15). The nerve roots fuse to form three trunks. Each trunk divides into an anterior and posterior division that then redistributes to form the lateral, medial, and posterior cords. These cords divide in the region of the axilla to form the musculocutaneous nerve, the median nerve, the ulnar nerve, the axillary nerve, the radial nerve, and several cutaneous nerves. The brachial plexus crosses the midclavicle to enter the axilla (Figure 106-16*A*). This approach blocks the brachial plexus at the level of the trunks, where it is most compactly arranged.[32]

Patient positioning: Place the patient supine with the ipsilateral arm in any position of comfort for the patient.

Landmarks: The subclavian artery is the main landmark. Palpate the subclavian artery immediately lateral to the clavicular head of the sternocleidomastoid muscle in the interscalene groove. Identify the midpoint of the clavicle.

Needle insertion and direction: Place a skin wheal of local anesthetic solution 2 cm above the midclavicle. Insert a 25 gauge needle directed caudally through the skin wheal (Figures 106-16*B* and *C*). Advance the needle until the patient experiences paresthesias. Withdraw the needle 1 mm and allow the paresthesias to resolve. Aspirate to ensure that the tip of the needle is not within a blood vessel. Inject 40 mL of local anesthetic solution.

Remarks: This block is characterized by a quick onset of anesthesia and a complete block. A high volume of anesthetic is required with a quick onset of anesthesia. There is no chance of missing peripheral or proximal nerve branches because of failure of the local anesthetic solution to spread along the sheath of the brachial plexus.[30,31] Unfortunately, this technique is difficult to teach and to master without considerable experience. This technique has a high incidence of pneumothorax, reportedly up to 6 percent.[31] Other complications include blockade of the phrenic nerve, arterial puncture, and Horner's syndrome. Unintentional intravascular injection can result in high blood levels of the local anesthetic agent.

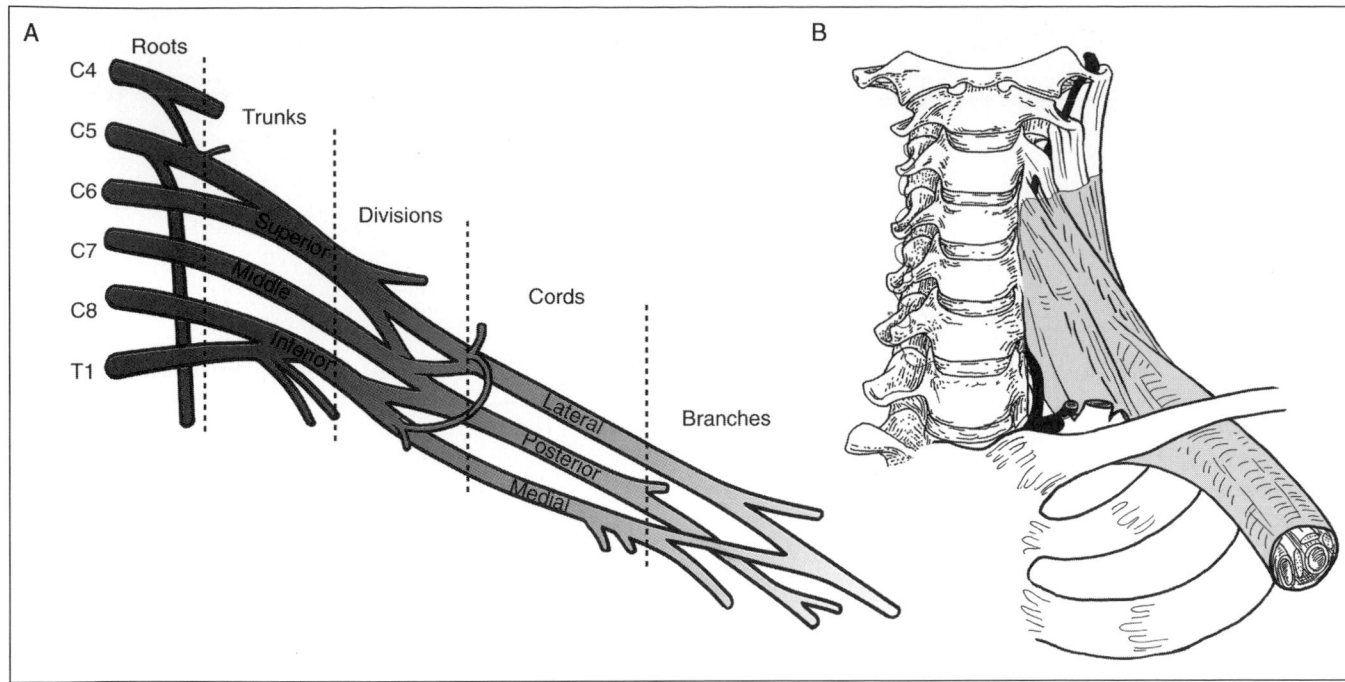

FIGURE 106-15 The brachial plexus. *A.* The anatomy of the brachial plexus. *B.* The brachial plexus is contained within a sheath. The subclavian artery and vein enter the sheath at the level of the clavicle.

BRACHIAL PLEXUS BLOCK, INTERSCALENE APPROACH

Anatomy: The anatomy of the brachial plexus is described above. This approach blocks the brachial plexus at the level of the trunks (Figure 106-17*A*).

Patient positioning: Place the patient supine with their head turned 45 degrees from midline and toward the side opposite that being anesthetized. Place the ipsilateral arm in any position of comfort.

Landmarks: Identify the posterior border of the clavicular head of the sternocleidomastoid muscle by palpation. Move the palpating finger laterally until it rolls into the interscalene groove between the anterior and middle scalene muscles, at the level of the cricoid cartilage (Figure 106-17*B*).

Needle insertion and direction: Place a skin wheal of local anesthetic solution in the interscalene groove, at the level of the cricoid cartilage. Slowly insert a 25 gauge needle through the skin wheal in a dorsal, medial, and caudal direction (Figure 106-17*B*). Advance the needle until the patient experiences paresthesias. Withdraw the needle 1 mm and allow the paresthesias to resolve. Aspirate to ensure that the tip of the needle is not within a blood vessel. Inject 40 mL of local anesthetic solution.

Remarks: The advantages and disadvantages are similar to those of the supraclavicular approach with the exception of possibly not achieving anesthesia of the lower trunk.[30,31] This may require supplementary blockade of the median and ulnar nerves.

BRACHIAL PLEXUS BLOCK, AXILLARY APPROACH

Anatomy: The anatomy of the axillary nerve block is rather simple. The neurovascular bundle is easily found at the anterior axillary fold by palpating for the pulsations of the axillary artery. The neurovascular bundle is surrounded by the fibrous axillary sheath (Figure 106-18*A*). The axillary sheath is bound medially by skin and connective tissue, anteriorly by the biceps and coracobrachialis muscles, inferiorly by the triceps muscle, and laterally by the neck of the humerus. The axillary artery is the central reference structure within the neurovascular bundle. Within the axillary sheath, the median nerve is anterior, the radial nerve is posterolateral, and the ulnar nerve is posterior to the axillary artery; the axillary vein is medial to the artery; and the medial antebrachial cutaneous nerve and the medial brachial cutaneous nerve are medial to the artery (Figure 106-18*A*). The only sensory nerve outside the neurovascular bundle is the musculocutaneous nerve. This nerve exits the axillary sheath as it crosses the clavicle.

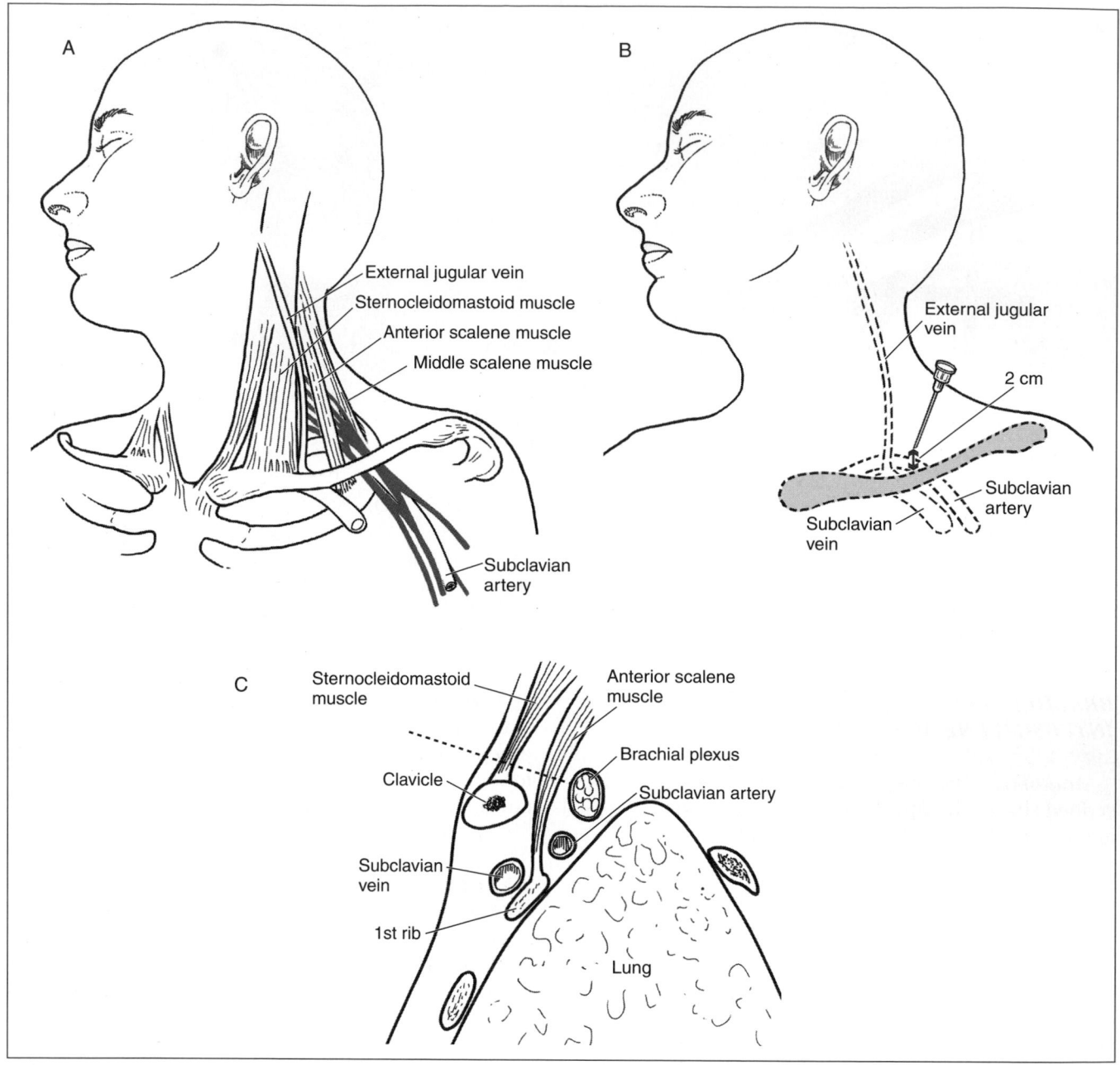

FIGURE 106-16 The supraclavicular approach to the brachial plexus block. *A.* The course of the brachial plexus. *B.* The needle is inserted perpendicular to the skin and 2 cm superior to the middle of the clavicle. *C.* Sagittal section demonstrating the trajectory of the needle (dotted line).

Patient positioning: Place the patient supine with their head turned toward the side opposite that being anesthetized (Figure 106-18*B*). Abduct the arm 90 degrees. Flex the elbow 90 degrees so that the forearm is parallel to the long axis of the body and the palm is facing upward.

Landmarks: Identify the brachial artery by its palpable pulse. Trace it proximally to the anterior axillary fold, formed by the pectoralis major muscle. Use the index and middle fingers of the nondominant hand to secure the neurovascular bundle (identified by the pulse) against the humerus (Figure 106-18*B*).

Needle insertion and direction: Place the skin wheal of local anesthetic solution overlying the axillary artery pulse, just posterior to the anterior axillary fold. Insert a 22 gauge spinal needle just above the fingertip on the axillary pulse, directed toward the apex of the axilla and in the direction of the neurovascular bundle

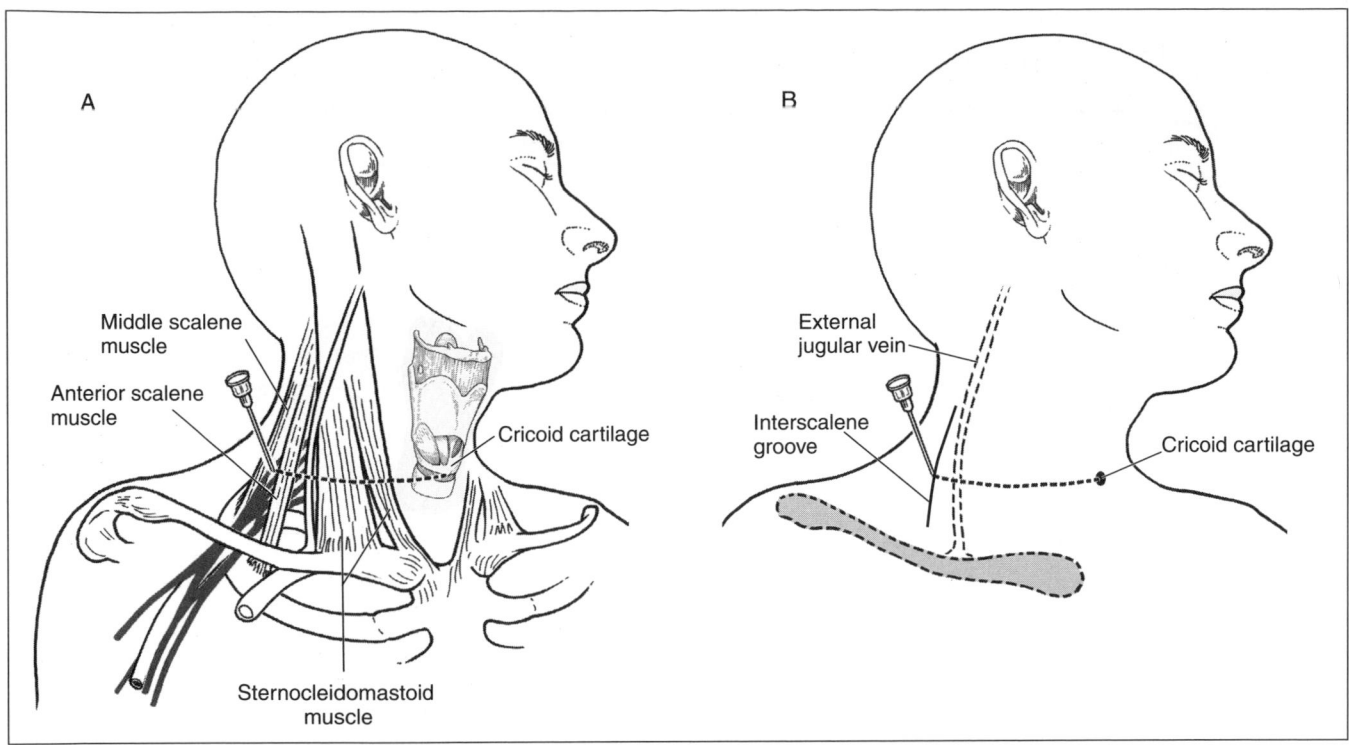

FIGURE 106-17 The interscalene approach to the brachial plexus block. *A.* The anatomy of the region. *B.* The needle is inserted into the interscalene groove at the level of the cricoid cartilage.

(Figure 106-18*B*). Advance the needle. A "pop" will be felt as the axillary sheath is penetrated. The correct needle position is confirmed by eliciting paresthesias, observing blood flow in the needle, or observing pulsations of the needle that match the pulse. Instruct an assistant to attach the distal end of intravenous extension tubing to the hub of the needle, and the proximal end to a 60 mL syringe containing local anesthetic solution. The physician must always maintain pressure against the neurovascular bundle with the nondominant hand while stabilizing the needle with the dominant hand. Instruct the assistant to aspirate to ensure that the tip of the needle is not within a blood vessel. Withdraw the needle 2 mm if blood flow or paresthesias are elicited.

Apply digital pressure to the neurovascular bundle just distal to the tip of the needle with the nondominant fingers. This prevents the local anesthetic solution from flowing distally. Inject the local anesthetic solution into the axillary sheath after the paresthesias have resolved and a negative aspiration has been achieved. Instruct the assistant to inject a volume of approximately 40 mL in the adult patient. This volume has been shown to consistently block the entire brachial plexus. Reduce the volume based upon the patient's body size and the maximal allowable dose to prevent toxicity.[31] **Continue to apply digital pressure to the neurovascu-**

lar bundle just distal to the needle during and after injection of the local anesthetic.

Withdraw the needle while the assistant simultaneously injects 3 to 5 mL of local anesthetic solution into the subcutaneous tissue. This blocks the medial brachial cutaneous nerve and the intercostobrachial nerve. Abduct the patient's arm 30 degrees to 45 degrees after the needle is withdrawn. Maintain this position, while continuing to apply digital pressure to the neurovascular bundle just distal to the needle insertion site, for 2 to 3 minutes.

Remarks: The axillary approach to the brachial plexus is the most commonly used and preferred technique. The procedure is easily mastered, has no major complications, and is easily performed in the obese patient. The disadvantages of this technique include insufficient anesthesia of the shoulder and upper arm. The musculocutaneous nerve provides sensory innervation to the radial aspect of the forearm and may be missed by the local anesthetic agent. The subcutaneous infiltration of local anesthetic solution usually blocks the musculocutaneous nerve. **Proximal flow of the local anesthetic solution is required to ensure adequate anesthesia.** Abduction of the arm while maintaining pressure on the neurovascular bundle allows proximal flow of the local anesthetic solution. It also prevents the humeral head

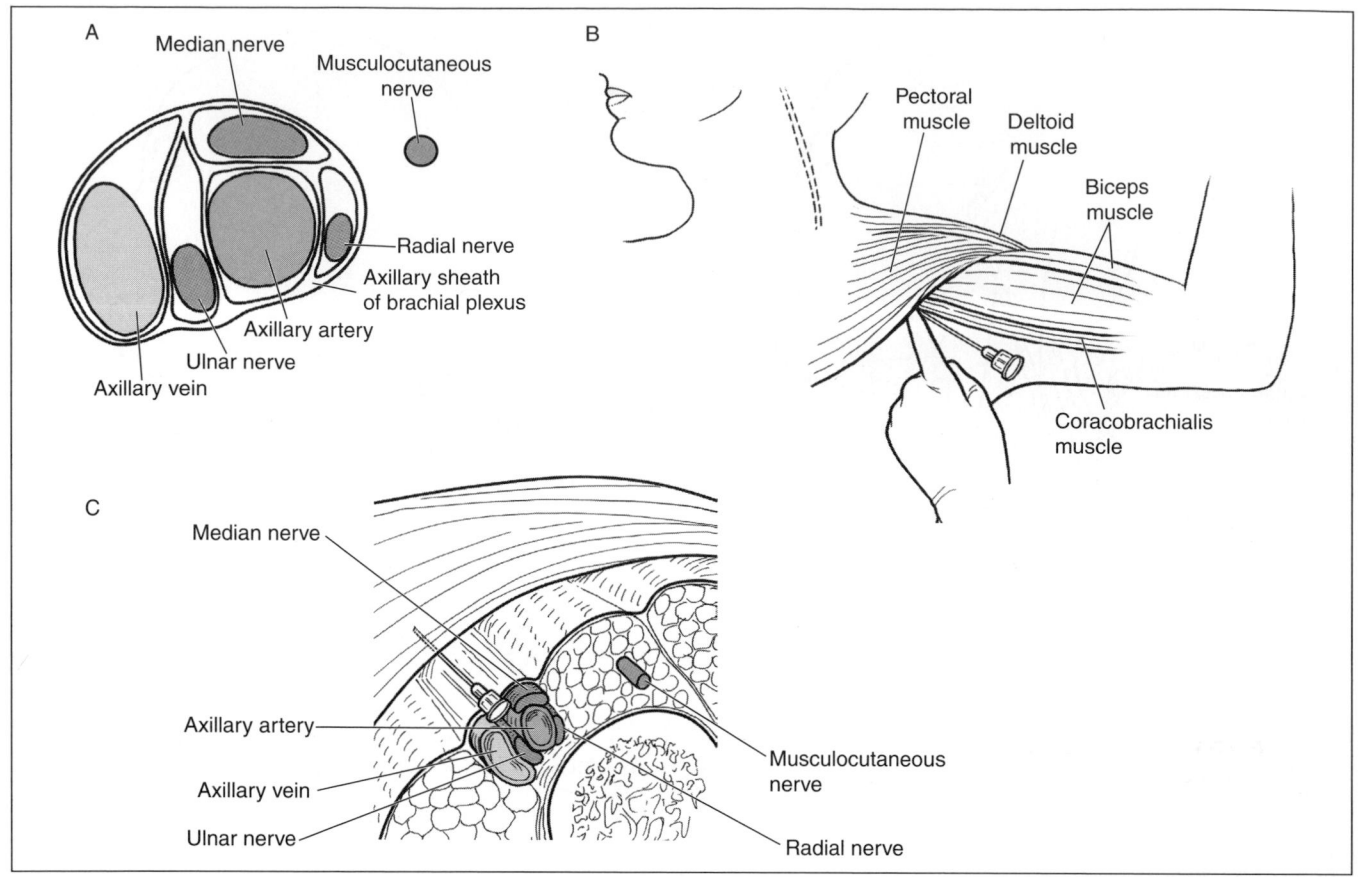

FIGURE 106-18 The axillary approach to the brachial plexus block. *A.* The topographical arrangement of the contents of the axillary sheath at the level of the blockade. *B.* The patient is positioned and the axillary artery pulse is palpated with one finger. The needle is inserted above the pulse and along the course of the axillary sheath. *C.* The needle may travel above the sheath and enter it at a higher level.

from limiting proximal spread due to compression of the brachial plexus.

BRACHIAL PLEXUS BLOCK, INFRACLAVICULAR APPROACH

This approach to the brachial plexus has many advantages and few serious complications. Unfortunately, this technique requires considerable experience on the part of the operator and a nerve stimulator to locate the brachial plexus (Figure 106-19). For these reasons, it will not be described.

MEDIAN NERVE BLOCK, AT THE ELBOW

Anatomy: The median nerve innervates all the muscles of the anterior forearm except the flexor digitorum profundus to the ring and little fingers and the flexor carpi ulnaris.[2,18,33] It innervates the thenar muscles and the lumbrical muscles to the index and middle fingers in

the hand. It provides sensory innervation to the palmar aspect of the thumb, index finger, middle finger, radial portion of the ring finger, and the lateral half of the palm (Figure 106-20*A*). The median nerve provides a variable amount of sensory innervation to the dorsal distal surfaces of the lateral three and one-half fingers.[1,2,18]

Patient positioning: Place the patient supine with their arm abducted 45 degrees, the elbow in full extension, and the hand supinated (Figure 106-21*A*).

Landmarks: Identify the medial and lateral epicondyle of the humerus by palpation. Connect the epicondyles with a straight line (Figure 106-21*A*). Identify the brachial artery by palpating for its pulse just medial to the biceps tendon and over the line just drawn. Mark the site of the palpable pulse with a marker.

Needle insertion and direction: Place a skin wheal of local anesthetic solution just medial to the pulse, at the level of the intercondylar line. Insert a 25 gauge nee-

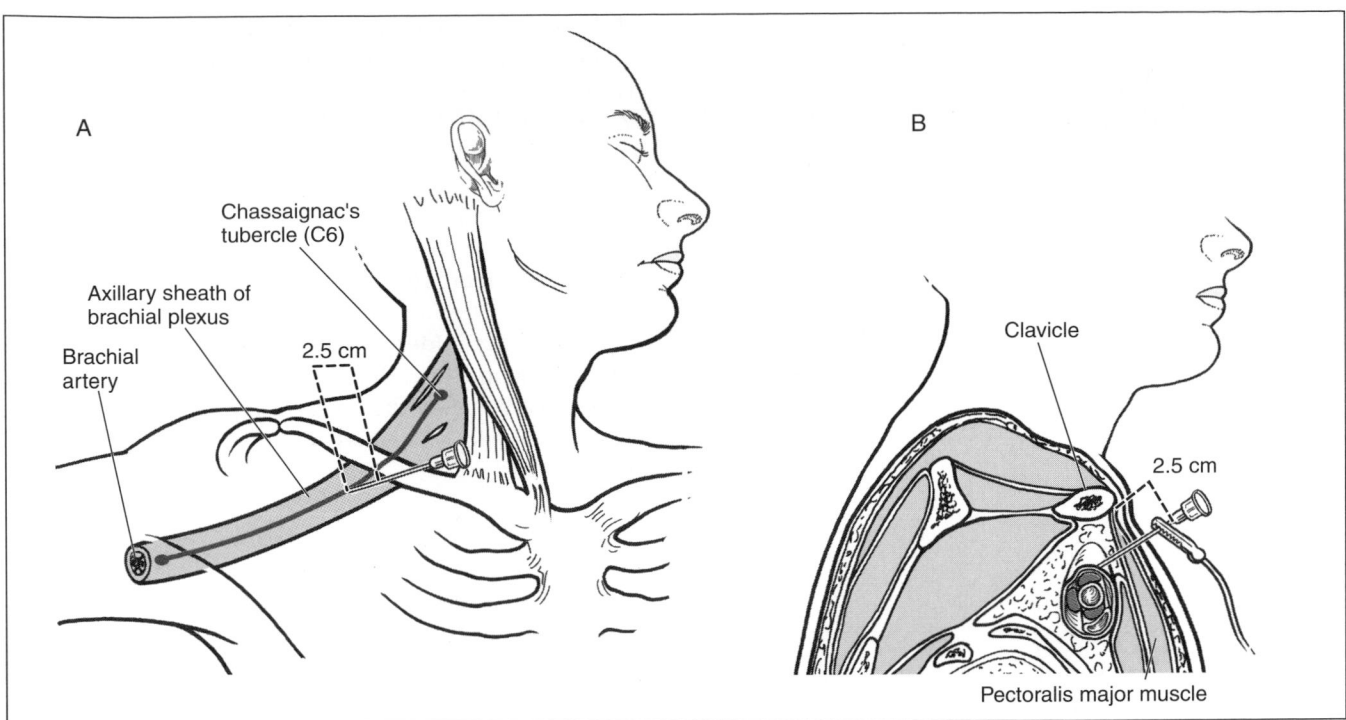

FIGURE 106-19 The infraclavicular approach to the brachial plexus block *A*. Needle insertion and direction. *B*. Sagittal section demonstrating needle insertion into the neurovascular bundle. The alligator clip is attached to a nerve stimulator.

dle perpendicular to the skin and slowly advance it. If paresthesias are elicited, withdraw the needle 1 to 2 mm and allow the paresthesias to resolve. Inject 3 to 5 mL of local anesthetic solution. If paresthesias are not elicited, slowly move the needle in a fan-like pattern to elicit paresthesias. Withdraw the needle 1 to 2 mm, allow the paresthesias to resolve, and inject 3 to 5 mL of local anesthetic solution.

Remarks: The median nerve has no sensory branches in the forearm. Therefore, there is no advantage to blocking the median nerve at the elbow. Inserting the needle to elicit paresthesias can be quite painful for the patient. Blockade at the wrist is usually easier to perform, especially in obese patients.[2,15]

MEDIAN NERVE BLOCK, AT THE WRIST

Anatomy: The median nerve lies in the carpal tunnel on the volar aspect of the wrist. It is located between the tendons of the flexor carpi radialis and palmaris longus muscles (Figure 106-21). The innervation of the median nerve is described in the previous section.

Patient positioning: Place the patient supine with their arm abducted 45 degrees, the elbow in full extension, and the hand fully supinated (Figure 106-21*A*).

Landmarks: Identify the palmaris longus tendon by flexing the patient's clenched hand against resistance. Mark the radial border of the palmaris longus tendon. Note the position of the proximal and distal wrist creases.

Needle insertion and direction: Place a skin wheal of local anesthetic solution along the radial border of the palmaris longus tendon, between the proximal and distal wrist creases. Insert a 25 gauge needle perpendicular to the skin wheal and advance it slowly (Figure 106-21*B*). If paresthesias are elicited, withdraw the needle 1 to 2 mm and allow them to resolve. Inject 3 to 5 mL of local anesthetic solution. If paresthesias are not elicited, inject 5 to 10 mL of local anesthetic solution. Injection of the local anesthetic solution should not raise a skin wheal and should flow effortlessly if the needle is within the carpal tunnel.[1,18]

Remarks: A small percentage of the population (10 to 15 percent) does not have a palmaris longus tendon. Identify the flexor carpi radialis tendon by the same method as identifying the palmaris longus tendon. Inject the local anesthetic solution 1 cm medial to the ulnar edge of the flexor carpi radialis tendon, between the proximal and distal wrist creases. The technique is otherwise as noted above.

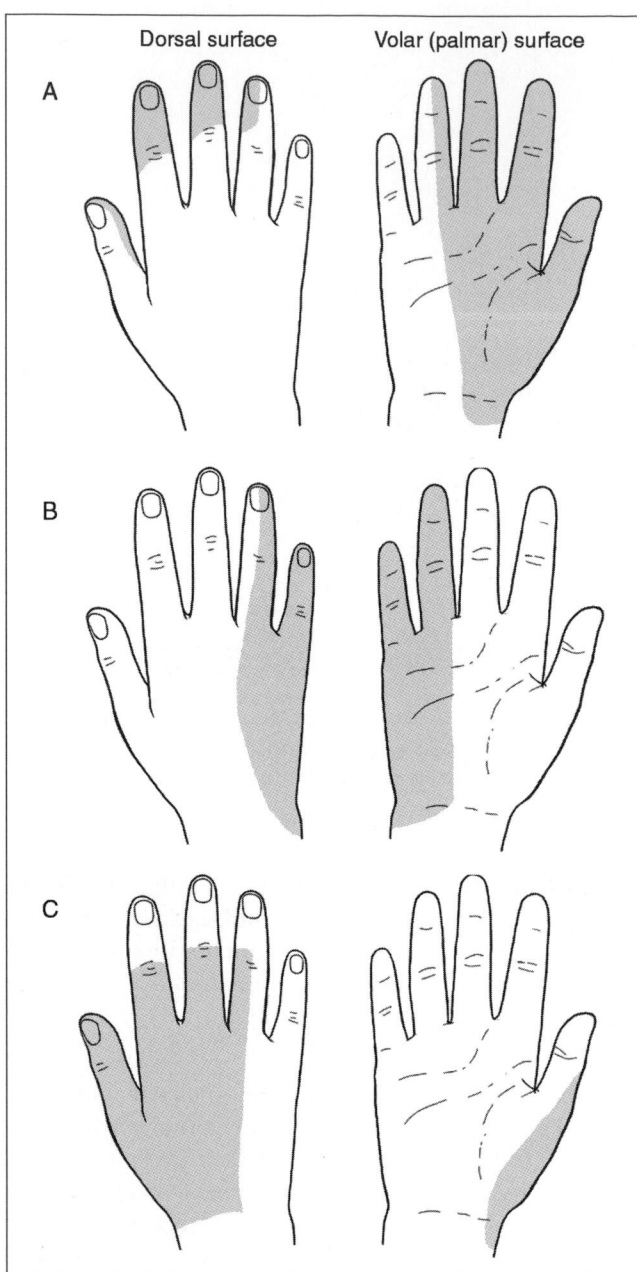

FIGURE 106-20 The sensory innervation of the hand. *A.* The median nerve. *B.* The ulnar nerve. *C.* The radial nerve.

ULNAR NERVE BLOCK, AT THE ELBOW

Anatomy: The ulnar nerve lies in the ulnar groove of the humerus at the elbow, between the olecranon process and medial condyle of the humerus (Figure 106-22*A*). It provides motor innervation to the flexor carpi ulnaris, the ring and little finger portion of the flexor digitorum profundus, the palmaris brevis, the hypothenar muscles, the third and fourth lumbricals, the interossei, and the adductor pollicis muscles. It provides sensory innervation to the medial one-third to one-half of the palm, the palmar aspect of the ulnar half of the ring finger, and the entire little finger (Figure 106-20*B*). The ulnar nerve provides sensory innervation to the dorsomedial half of the hand, the little finger, and the ulnar half of the ring finger on the dorsal surface of the hand.[34]

Patient positioning: Place the patient supine with their elbow flexed 90 degrees and the shoulder flexed 45 degrees (Figure 106-22*A*).

Landmarks: Identify the olecranon process and the medial epicondyle of the humerus by palpation. Palpate the groove between the olecranon process and the medial epicondyle. The ulnar nerve is located within this groove.

Needle insertion and direction: Place a skin wheal of local anesthetic solution 1 to 2 cm proximal to the ulnar groove. Insert a 25 gauge needle through the skin wheal and directed towards the ulnar groove. Aim the needle parallel to the ulnar groove and the course of the nerve (Figure 106-22*A*). Advance the needle into the ulnar groove and inject 5 to 7 mL of local anesthetic solution. If paresthesias are elicited, withdraw the needle 1 mm and allow them to resolve before injecting the local anesthetic solution.

Remarks: The ulnar nerve has no sensory branches in the forearm and thus may be blocked at the wrist or at the elbow. Blockade of the ulnar nerve at the elbow is not recommended. A fibrous sheath surrounds the ulnar nerve at the elbow requiring intraneural injection for successful blockade. This can lead to residual neuritis and nerve dysfunction. Blocking the ulnar nerve several centimeters above the elbow may prevent these complications. Blockade at the wrist is very reliable and does not have the associated complications as at the elbow.

ULNAR NERVE BLOCK, AT THE WRIST

Anatomy: The ulnar nerve lies between the distal and proximal flexor skin creases of the wrist, lateral (or radial) to the flexor carpi ulnaris tendon and medial (or ulnar) to the ulnar artery (Figure 106-22*B*). The innervation of the ulnar nerve is described in the previous section.

Patient positioning: Place the patient supine with their arm abducted 45 to 90 degrees, the elbow fully extended, and the hand supinated (Figure 106-22*B*).

Landmarks: Identify the flexor carpi ulnaris tendon by flexing the patient's clenched hand against resistance. Mark the medial aspect of the flexor carpi ulnaris ten-

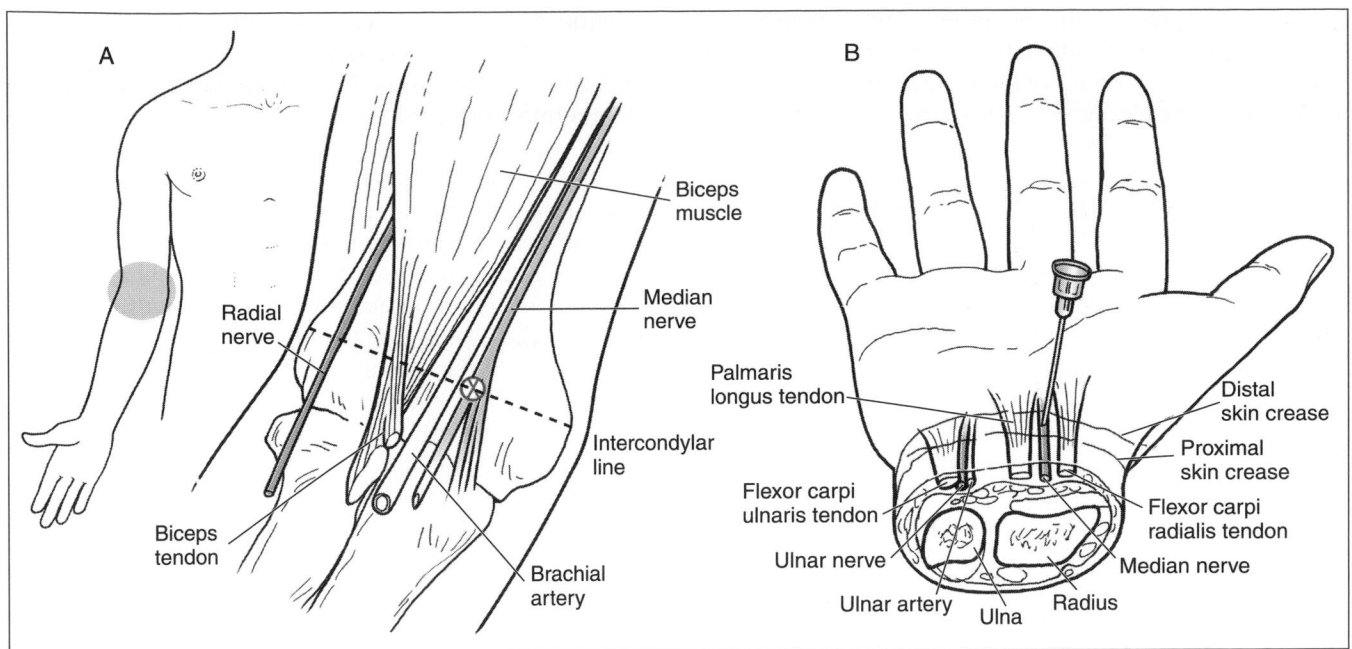

FIGURE 106-21 The median nerve block. *A.* Blockade at the level of the elbow. *B.* Blockade at the level of the wrist.

don. Identify the ulnar artery by its palpable pulsations between the proximal and distal wrist crease. Note the position of the proximal and distal wrist creases.

Needle insertion and direction: Place a skin wheal of local anesthetic solution in the quadrangle defined by the proximal flexor skin crease, the distal flexor skin crease, the lateral aspect of the flexor carpi ulnaris tendon, and medial to the ulnar artery. Insert a 25 gauge needle perpendicular to the skin wheal and slowly advance it 0.5 cm (Figure 106-22*B*). If paresthesias are elicited, withdraw the needle 2 mm and allow them to resolve. Inject 2 mL of local anesthetic solution once the paresthesias resolve. If paresthesias are not elicited, inject 3 to 5 mL of local anesthetic solution.

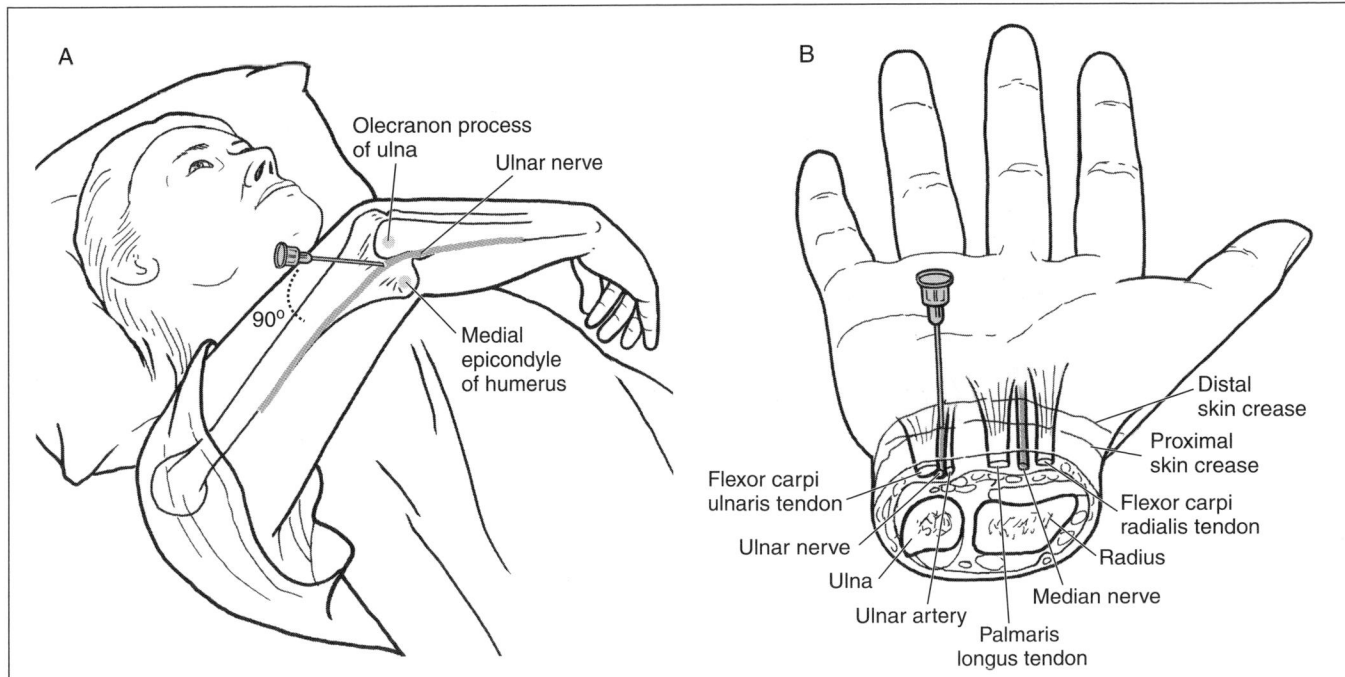

FIGURE 106-22 The ulnar nerve block. *A.* Blockade at the level of the elbow. *B.* Blockade at the level of the wrist.

Remarks: This is the preferred approach to block the ulnar nerve. Blockade of the ulnar nerve at the wrist is very reliable and does not have the associated complications as at the elbow.[35]

RADIAL NERVE BLOCK, AT THE ELBOW

Anatomy: The radial nerve and the sensory branch of the musculocutaneous nerve run together in the sulcus between the biceps and the brachioradialis muscle on the anterolateral aspect of the elbow. The radial nerve provides sensory innervation to portions of the dorsal arm and forearm, the dorsolateral half of the hand, and the dorsal proximal aspects of the thumb, index, middle, and radial half of the ring fingers[18,36] (Figure 106-20). It provides motor innervation to the muscles on the posterior aspect of the arm, forearm, and hand.

Patient positioning: Place the patient supine with their elbow flexed 15 to 30 degrees.

Landmarks: Palpate the tendon of the biceps muscle in the antecubital fossa. Identify the flexion skin crease of the elbow. Palpation of the biceps tendon is greatly facilitated by having the patient flex their elbow 90 degrees then contract and relax their biceps muscle.

Identify the medial and lateral condyles of the humerus. Draw a line between the humeral condyles (Figure 106-23). This line should be located at the level of the antecubital crease.

Needle insertion and direction: Place a skin wheal of local anesthetic solution 2 cm lateral to the biceps tendon and 1 cm proximal to the antecubital crease (Figure 106-23A). Insert a 25 gauge needle through the skin wheal and perpendicular to the skin (Figure 106-23A). Advance the needle 1 to 2 cm. Probe in a fan-like pattern until paresthesias are elicited. Withdraw the needle 1 to 2 mm and allow the paresthesias to resolve. Inject 5 to 7 mL of local anesthetic solution.

Remarks: Blockade of the radial nerve at the elbow is difficult, has limited applications, is painful for the patient, and often results in a large antecubital hematoma. The preferred technique is blockade at the wrist.

RADIAL NERVE BLOCK, AT THE WRIST

Anatomy: The radial nerve at the wrist consists of a trunk and terminal branches that arise in the forearm (Figure 106-23B). The innervation of the radial nerve is described in the previous section.

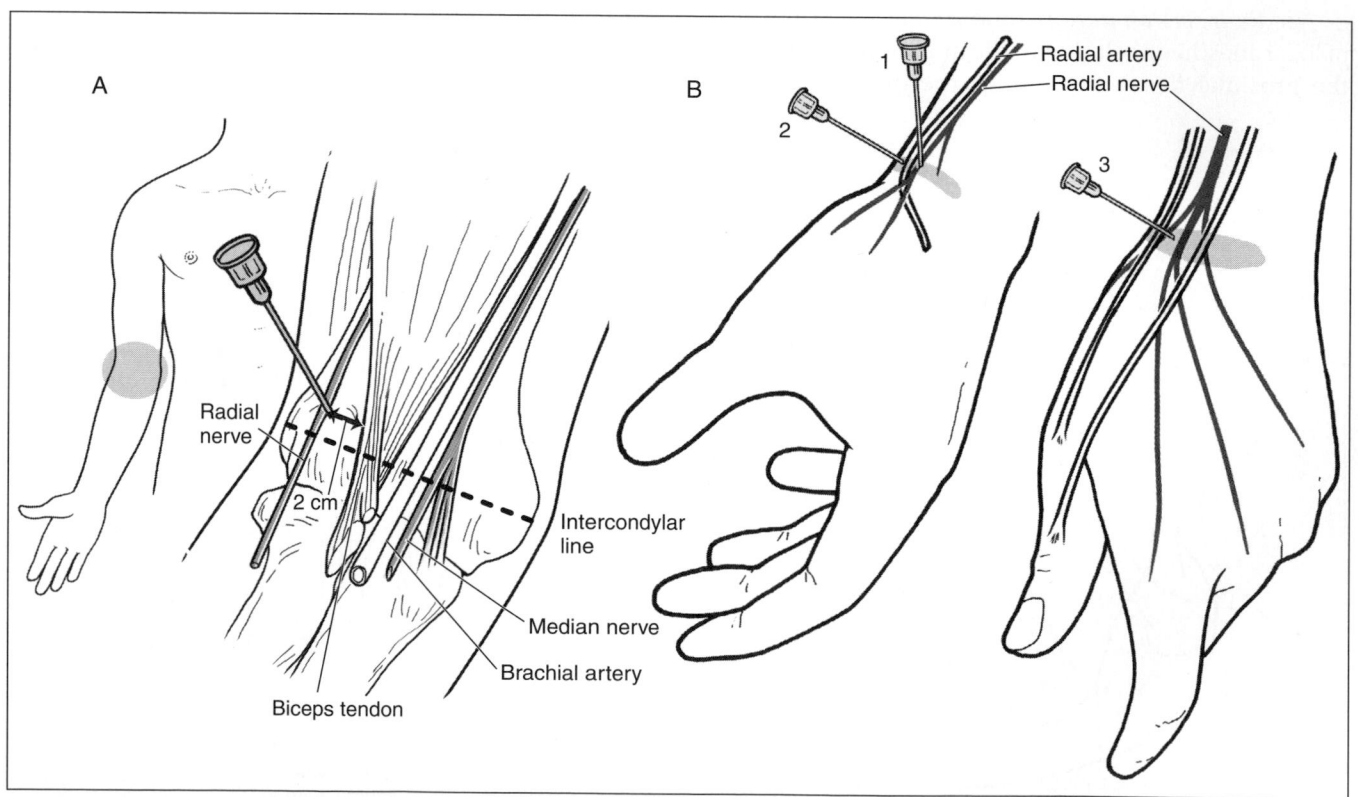

FIGURE 106-23 The radial nerve block. *A.* Blockade at the level of the elbow. *B.* Blockade at the level of the wrist. The numbers represent the three injections required to anesthetize the branches of the radial nerve.

Patient positioning: Place the patient supine with their arm abducted 45 degrees, the elbow fully extended, and the hand midway between supination and pronation (Figure 106-23*B*).

Landmarks: Identify the radial artery by its pulsation at the level of the proximal wrist crease.

Needle insertion and direction: Place a skin wheal of local anesthetic solution 1 mm lateral to the radial pulse. Insert a 25 gauge needle 1 mm lateral to the radial pulse, through the skin wheal, and perpendicular to the skin (Figure 106-23*B*). Advance the needle 0.5 cm. If paresthesias are elicited, withdraw the needle 1 to 2 mm and allow them to resolve. Inject 2 mL of local anesthetic solution. If paresthesias are not elicited, inject 3 to 5 mL of local anesthetic solution. This will anesthetize the terminal trunk of the radial nerve. Infiltrate 5 to 7 mL of local anesthetic solution at the level of the extensor wrist crease, from the lateral aspect of the radius to the base of the fourth metacarpal (Figure 106-23*B*). This will anesthetize the terminal branches that arise in the forearm.

Remarks: This is the preferred technique for blockade of radial nerve.

WRIST BLOCK

Perform the wrist block by blocking the radial, ulnar, and median nerves at the wrist. The technique for each specific nerve block was discussed previously. The wrist block provides complete anesthesia to the hand and is commonly used in hand surgery.[1,3,36] It can be performed in the Emergency Department to provide anesthesia for burn management, foreign body removal, wound exploration, or extensive laceration repair. Wrist blockade is reliable but slow, as it requires extended time to block all three nerves at the wrist.[18,36]

INTERMETACARPAL NERVE BLOCK

Anatomy: The principal nerves supplying the finger are the palmar digital nerves, which originate from the deep volar branches of the ulnar and median nerves in the region of the wrist. These nerves follow the artery along the lateral aspects of the bone and supply sensation to the volar skin, the interphalangeal joints, the distal finger, and the fingertip of all five digits.[36]

Two dorsal and two palmar nerves supply each finger. These nerves run along the phalanxes in the 2, 4, 8, and 10 o'clock positions.[2,3,37] These nerves also supply the dorsal, distal aspect of the finger, including the fingertip and nail bed. The dorsal digital nerves originate from the radial and ulnar nerves that wrap around the dorsum of the hand. They supply the nail bed of the thumb and small finger and the dorsal aspect of all five digits up to the distal interphalangeal joints. The palmar and dorsal nerves need to be blocked in the case of the thumb and fifth finger.[2,36]

Patient positioning: Place the patient sitting upright or supine with their hand pronated on a bedside examination table.

Landmarks: Locate the web spaces and the metacarpal heads on each side of the finger to be blocked.

Needle insertion and direction: Insert a 25 gauge needle into the dorsal aspect of the web space on one side of the digit to be anesthetized (Figure 106-24*A*). Advance the needle approximately 0.5 cm. Inject 1 mL of local anesthetic solution. Repeat the procedure on the other side of the digit to be blocked. When blocking the second and fifth digits, a half-ring block is required on the ulnar aspect of the fifth digit and radial aspect of the second digit. When blocking the thumb, infiltrate the dorsum and sides in a half-ring manner.

An alternative is the metacarpal head block. This technique can be used to anesthetize any of the fingers. Insert a 25 gauge needle perpendicular to the dorsum of the hand and adjacent to the metacarpal head on one side of the finger to be blocked (Figure 106-24*B*). Advance the needle 0.5 cm and inject 1 mL of local anesthetic solution. Repeat the procedure on the other side of the finger to be blocked. Some physicians prefer to perform this block on the volar aspect of the hand (Figure 106-24*C*). This technique is extremely painful and should be avoided.

Remarks: This block produces less swelling than does the ring block.[1,36] Subsequently, there is less risk of vascular compromise. This is a less painful technique than the ring block.

DIGITAL NERVE BLOCK (RING BLOCK) OF THE FINGER

Anatomy: The anatomy and innervation of the digital nerves are described in the previous section.

Patient positioning: Place the patient sitting upright or supine with their hand pronated on a bedside examination table.

Landmarks: Locate the dorsum of the proximal phalanx to be anesthetized.

Needle insertion and direction: Insert a 25 gauge needle on the dorsal surface of the base of the proximal phalanx (Figure 106-24*D-1*). Inject 1 mL of local anes-

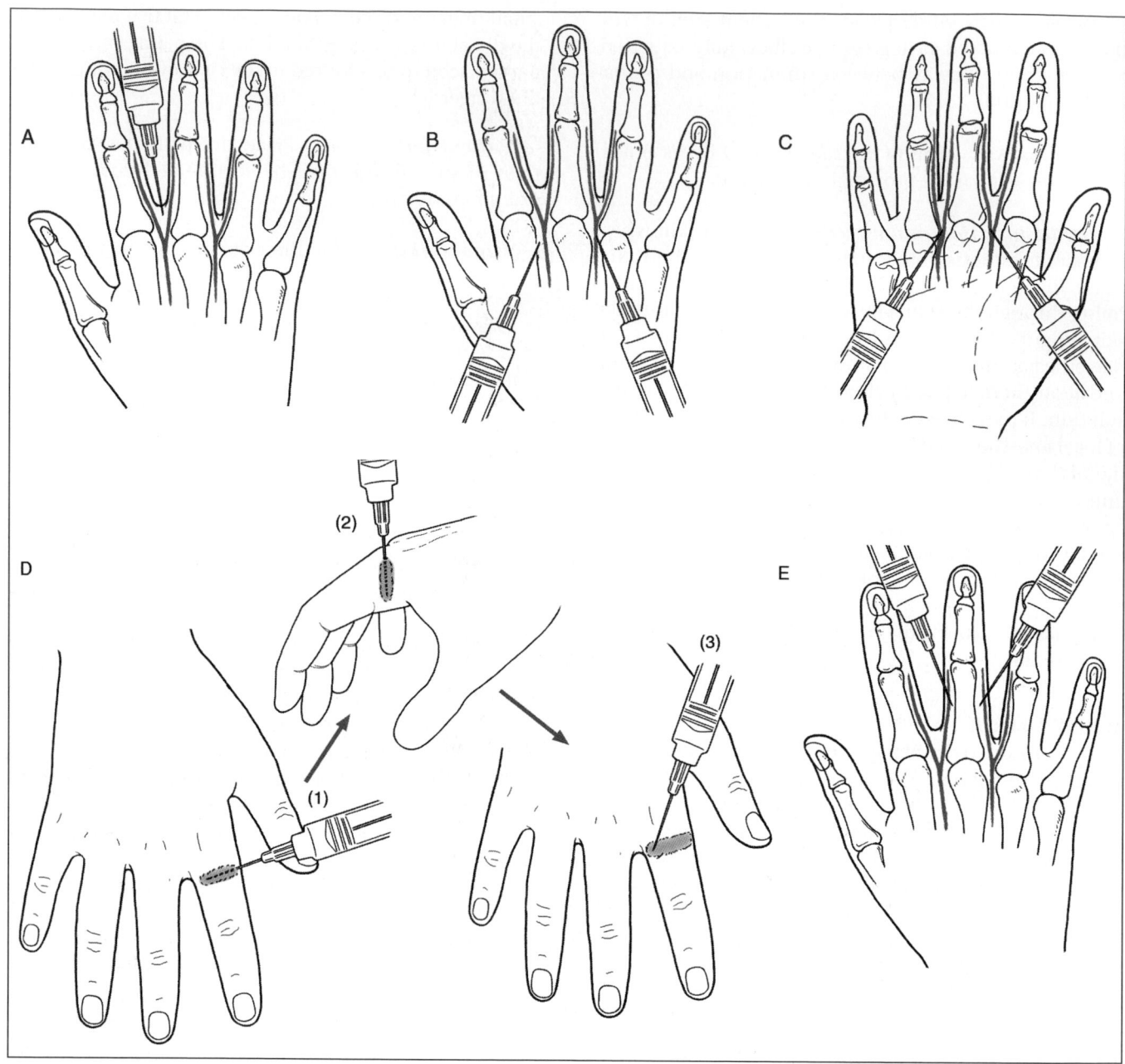

FIGURE 106-24 Techniques to anesthetize the digital nerves of the fingers. *A.* Intermetacarpal nerve block through the web space. *B.* Intermetacarpal nerve block on the dorsal surface of the hand, between the metacarpal heads. *C.* Intermetacarpal nerve block on the ventral surface of the hand, between the metacarpal heads. *D.* The ring block. *E.* The half-ring block.

thetic solution along the dorsal surface of the finger. Remove the needle and reinsert it downward, perpendicular to the phalanx and to a depth just past the base of the phalanx (Figure 106-24*D-2*). Inject 1.0 to 1.5 mL of local anesthetic along the lateral aspect of the finger. Withdraw the needle, reinsert it on the other side of the finger to be blocked, and inject 1.0 to 1.5 mL of local anesthetic solution (Figure 106-24*D-3*).

An alternative is the half-ring block (Figure 106-24*E*). It is a variant of the ring block (Figure 106-24*D*). Inject 1.0 to 1.5 mL of local anesthetic solution on one side of the base of the proximal phalanx to be anesthetized. Repeat this procedure on the other side of the finger. The injection of local anesthetic on one side of the finger is termed the half-ring block. It takes two half-ring blocks to anesthetize a finger.

Remarks: The indications for a digital block include repair of finger lacerations and amputations, reductions of fractures and dislocations, incision and drainage of infections, removal of fingernails, and relief of pain from burns. Do not inject more than 5 mL of local anesthetic solution into a digit.[36] Using local anesthetic agents that contain epinephrine is not recommended because the finger contains end arteries and may experience ischemia from the epinephrine.

REGIONAL ANESTHESIA TECHNIQUES FOR THE TORSO

INTERCOSTAL NERVE BLOCK

Anatomy: The intercostal nerves originate from the thoracic spinal cord and have four major branches[11] (Figure 106-25). The first is the gray rami communicans to the sympathetic ganglion. The second branch is the posterior cutaneous nerve that supplies the paravertebral muscles and overlying skin. The third branch is the lateral cutaneous nerve that arises about the midaxillary line. It divides into an anterior and posterior division to supply most of the chest and the abdominal wall. The final branch is the terminal anterior cutaneous nerve. It supplies the anterior chest and abdominal wall adjacent to the midline. Each intercostal nerve travels within a neurovascular bundle behind the inferior border of each rib (Figure 106-25B). The intercostal nerve lies inferior to the intercostal vein and artery. The intercostal nerve

may be blocked at several sites along its course. The most common site is at the angle of the rib.[1,11] The technique described will be the blockade of the intercostal nerves at the angle of the rib.

Patient positioning: Place the patient prone with a pillow under the midabdomen to straighten the lumbar curve and increase the size of the intercostal spaces posteriorly.

Landmarks: **The most important step is to correctly identify the anatomy of the patient.** Draw a line along the vertebral spines corresponding to the levels to be anesthetized. Palpate laterally from the vertebral spines to the edge of the paraspinal muscles. This is the location where the ribs are most superficial. This distance can vary from 6 to 8 cm from the midline in the average adult. Draw vertical lines parallel to the first line and along the edge of the paraspinal muscles (Figure 106-26A). These lines must angle slightly medially over the upper ribs to avoid the scapula. Palpate and mark the inferior edge of each rib along these two vertical lines (Figure 106-26A).

Needle insertion and direction: **This procedure requires the utmost of care to prevent inducing a pneumothorax.**[38] Inject local anesthetic solution to make a skin wheal at the intersection of the horizontal lines with the vertical paraspinal muscle lines. Use the index finger

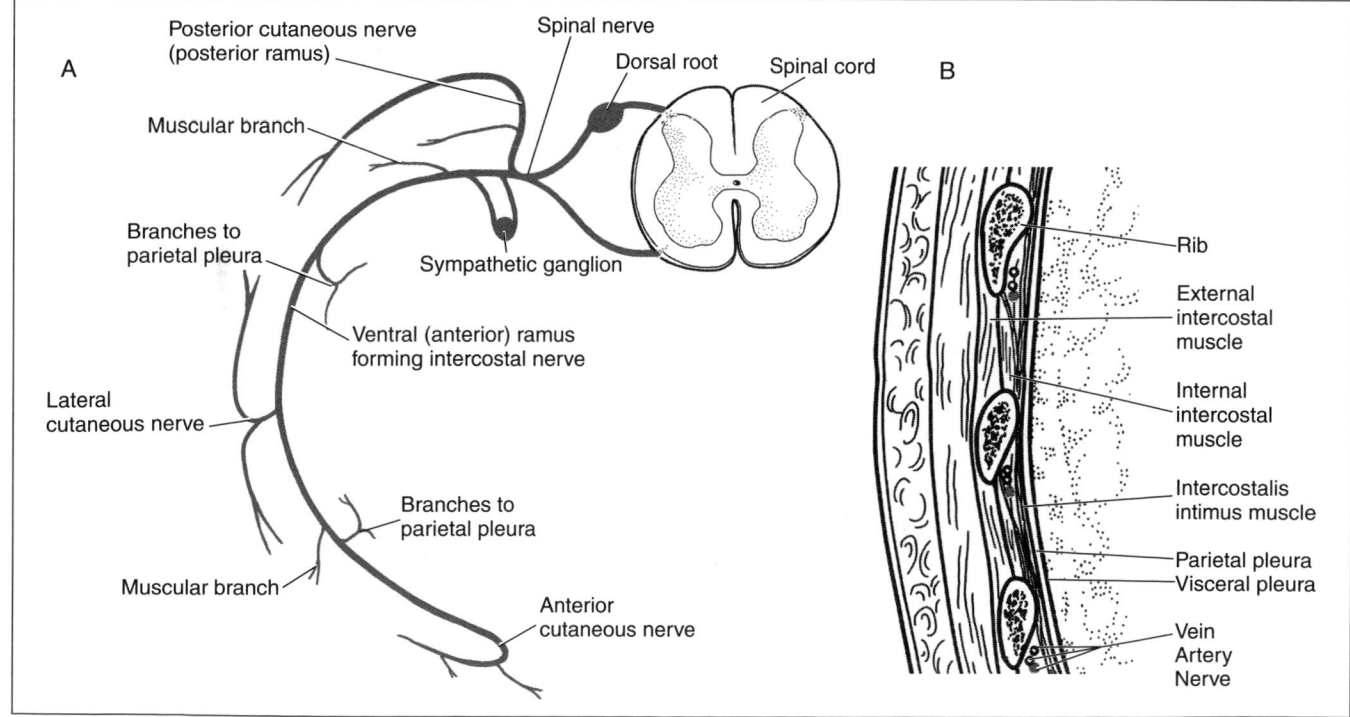

FIGURE 106-25 The intercostal nerve. *A.* The anatomy of a typical thoracic spinal nerve. *B.* Cross-section through the chest wall. The intercostal nerves are contained within a neurovascular bundle that lies behind the inferior border of each rib.

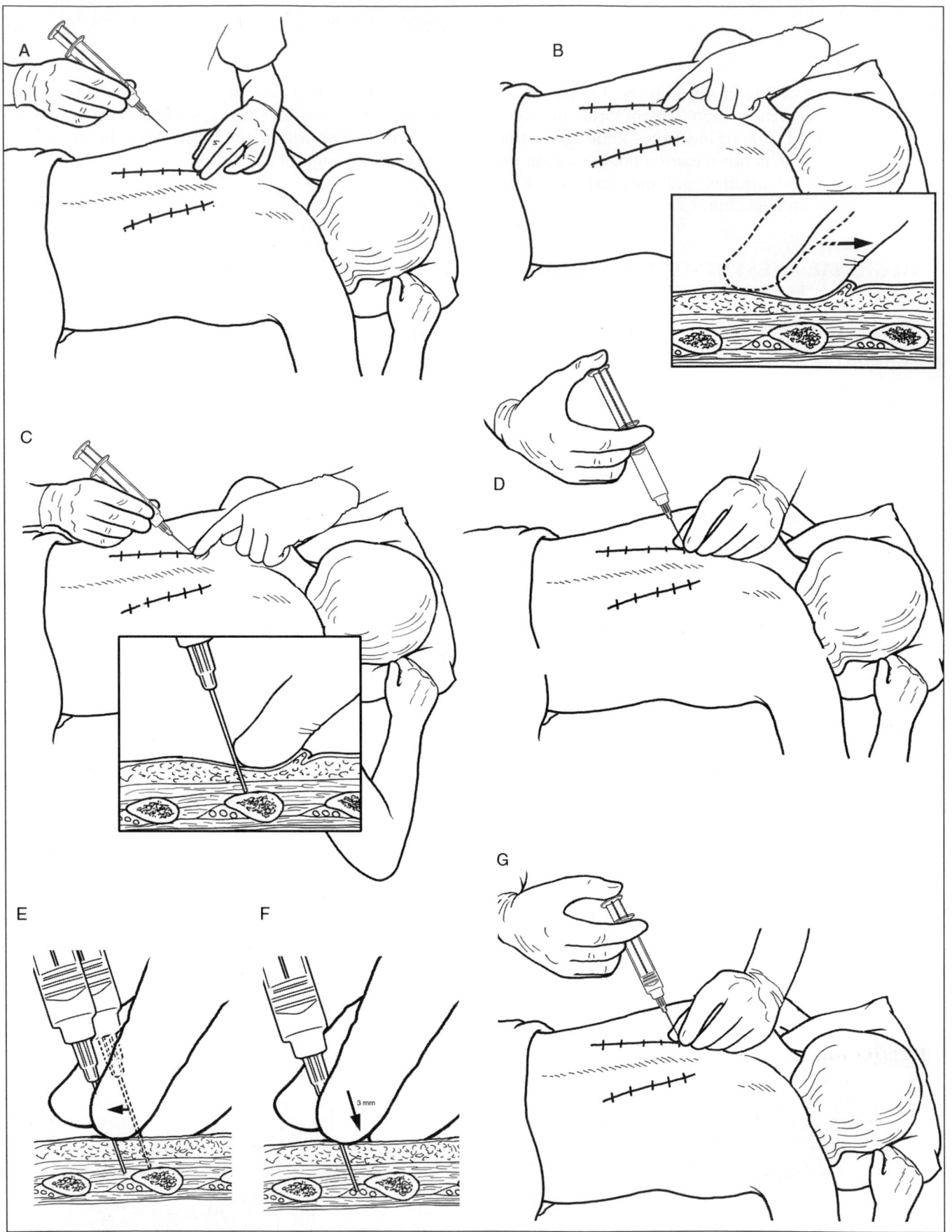

FIGURE 106-26 The intercostal nerve block. *A.* The patient is placed prone. A line is drawn along the lateral border of the paraspinal muscles. Note that the upper end is angled medially to avoid the scapula. Cross-marks are drawn to denote the inferior border of the rib and the location to perform the block. *B.* The index finger of the nondominant hand pulls the skin overlying the inferior border of the rib upward. *C.* The dominant hand is resting against the patient. The needle is inserted at a 60 degree angle to the skin and advanced until the rib is contacted. *D.* The fingers of the nondominant hand grasp and stabilize the needle. *E.* The needle is "walked" off the inferior border of the rib. *F.* The needle is advanced 3 mm so that the tip is within the neurovascular bundle. *G.* Inject 1 to 2 mL of local anesthetic solution while maintaining the needle in a stable position with the dominant hand.

of the nondominant hand to pull the skin at the lower edge of the rib up onto the rib (Figure 106-26*B*). Grasp the syringe in the dominant hand. Insert the 25 gauge needle at a 60 degree angle along the tip of the nondominant index finger while the dominant hand is resting on the patient's back (Figure 106-26*C*). Advance the needle until the rib is contacted (Figure 106-26*C* inset).

Reposition the nondominant hand so that it is resting against the patient's back and holding the needle between the thumb, index, and middle fingers (Figure 106-26*D*). Use the nondominant hand to slowly and carefully "walk" the needle off the inferior rib margin (Figure 106-26*E*). Advance the needle 3 mm with the nondominant hand (Figure 106-26*F*). **It is imperative that the needle not be advanced more than 3 mm after it is "walked" off the inferior border of the rib to prevent a pneumothorax. Aspirate to ensure that the tip of the needle is not within a blood vessel or the lung.** Inject 1 to 2 mL of local anesthetic solution (Figure 106-26*G*). Remove the needle and repeat the procedure at the other desired interspaces.

Remarks: Local anesthetic solution for intercostal blocks should contain 1:200,000 or less of epinephrine.[11] **Obtain a postprocedural chest radiograph to ensure that the patient does not have a pneumothorax.**

PENILE BLOCK

The penis may be anesthetized for the purposes of circumcision, laceration repair, foreign body removal, zipper entrapment, or to perform the release of a phimosis or paraphimosis.[1–3] The dorsal nerves of the penis provide sensory innervation to the penis.[12,39] They emerge from under the pubis, just lateral to the symphysis, and course along the dorsal surface of the penis. These nerves are located approximately 0.5 cm from the dorsal penile midline. These nerves are blocked at the base of the penis. Refer to Chapter 125 for the complete details of the penile block.

REGIONAL ANESTHESIA TECHNIQUES FOR THE LOWER EXTREMITY

The sensory innervation of the lower extremity is illustrated in Figure 106-27. Note that the nerves provide patches of innervation rather than stripes of innervation beginning at the torso and extending to the foot.

FEMORAL NERVE BLOCK

Anatomy: The femoral nerve is formed from the lumbar plexus.[40–42] It travels in the pelvis between the iliacus and psoas major muscles. It enters the thigh below the inguinal ligament, midway between the anterior superior iliac spine and the pubic tubercle (Figure 106-28*A*). The femoral nerve lies anterior to the iliopsoas muscle and lateral to the femoral artery in the proximal thigh. The femoral nerve has both sensory and motor components. It provides motor innervation to the anterior thigh muscles. It provides sensory innervation for the anterior thigh, anteromedial thigh, medial thigh, medial leg, and the medial border of the foot (Figure 106-27).

Patient positioning: Place the patient supine with their hip and knee extended.

Landmarks: Identify the anterior superior iliac spine and the pubic tubercle by palpation. Connect these landmarks with a straight line to roughly approximate the position of the inguinal ligament. Identify the femoral artery by its palpable pulse 1 to 2 cm below the midpoint of the inguinal ligament.

Needle insertion and direction: Place a skin wheal of local anesthetic solution just lateral to the femoral artery pulse. Insert a 25 gauge needle through the skin wheal and perpendicular to the skin (Figure 106-28*B*). Slowly advance the needle while remaining perpendicular to the skin. The femoral nerve is identified once paresthesias are elicited. Withdraw the needle 2 mm and allow the paresthesias to resolve. Inject 15 to 20 mL of local anesthetic solution.

Remarks: The femoral nerve is contained within a fibrous sheath that is separate from the other contents (femoral artery and vein) of the femoral triangle (Figure 106-28*B*). **Paresthesias must be elicited to confirm the proper position of the tip of the needle before injecting the local anesthetic solution.** Deposition of the local anesthetic solution outside of the fibrous sheath will not result in any anesthesia except in the area of the injection.

SAPHENOUS NERVE BLOCK, AT THE KNEE

Anatomy: The saphenous nerve is the terminal branch of the femoral nerve.[43,44] It travels across the anterior thigh in a medial direction to become superficial at the medial knee after emerging between the tendons of the gracilis and sartorius muscles (Figure 106-29*A*). It follows the great saphenous vein from above the knee to below the medial malleolus (Figure 106-29*B*). It provides sensory innervation to the anteromedial leg, medial leg, posteromedial leg, and medial

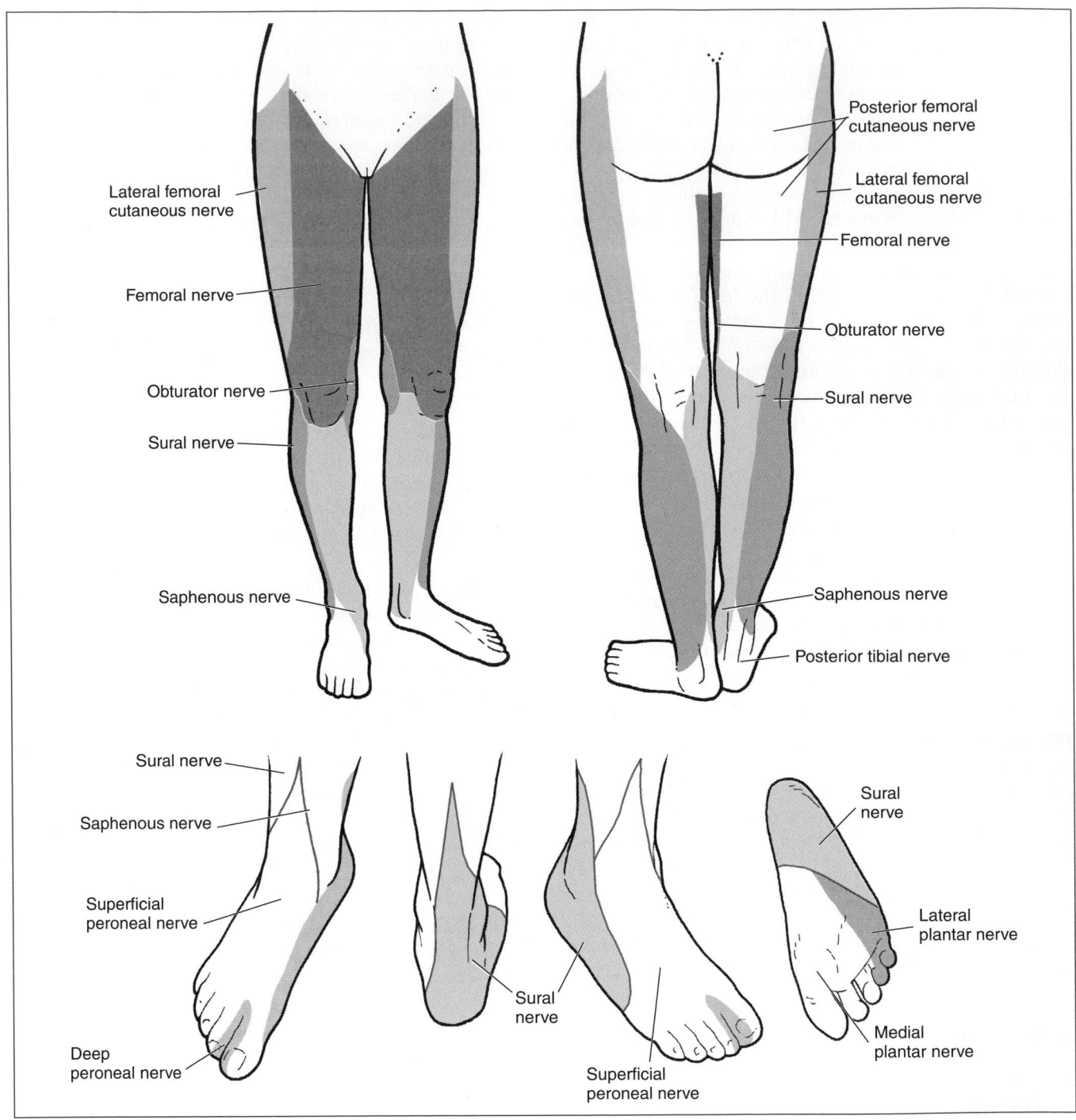

FIGURE 106-27 The sensory distribution of the cutaneous nerves of the lower extremity.

border of the foot to the ball of the great toe (Figure 106-27). It has no motor component.

Patient positioning: Place the patient supine with their ankle supported on a pillow or blanket, the knee extended, and the leg externally rotated.

Landmarks: Identify the femoral condyle above the knee or the tibial condyle below the knee by palpation.

Needle insertion and direction: Place a skin wheal of local anesthetic solution over the posteromedial aspect of either condyle (femoral or tibial). Insert a 25

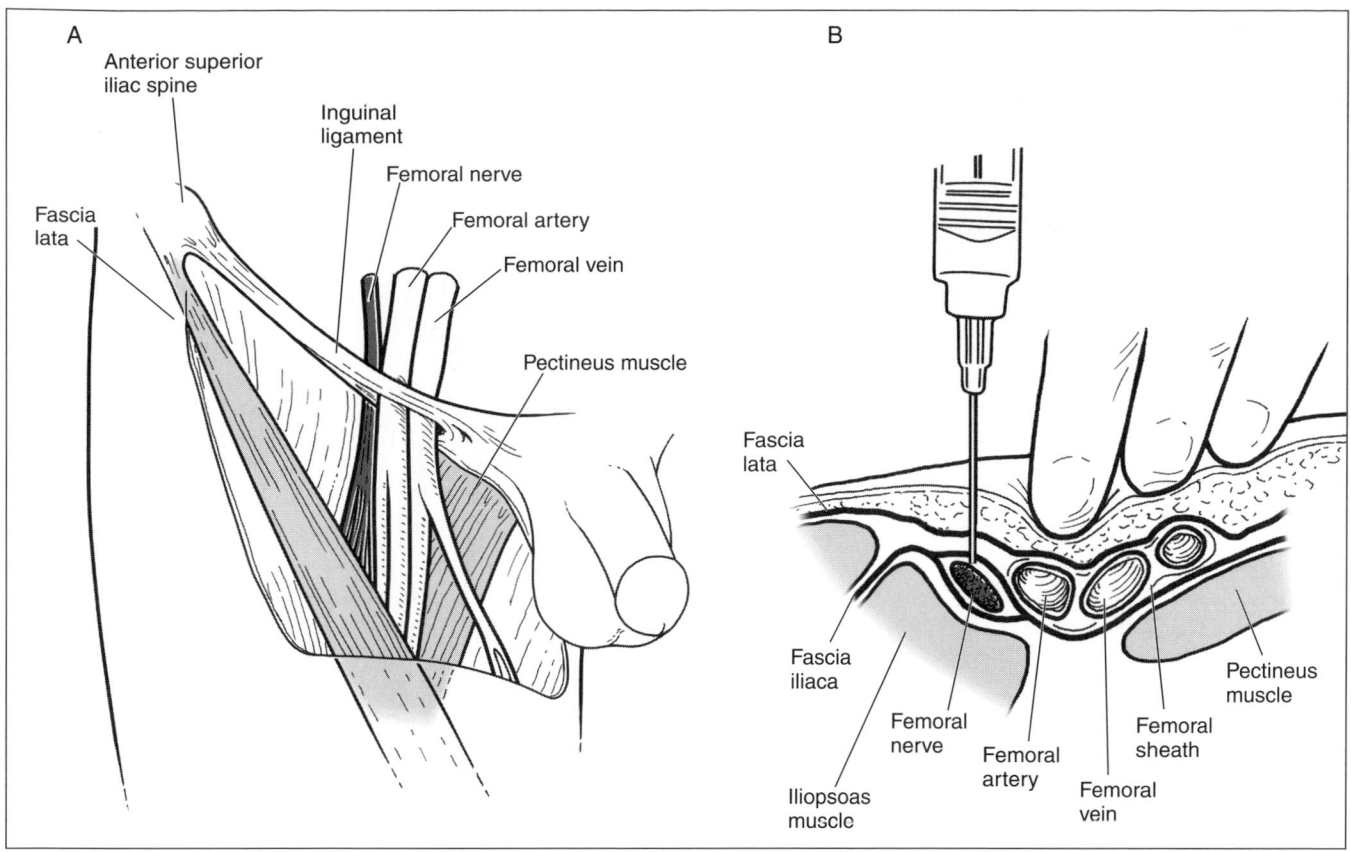

FIGURE 106-28 The femoral nerve block. *A.* The anatomy of the inguinal region. *B.* Blockade of the femoral nerve.

gauge needle through the skin wheal. Infiltrate 7 to 10 mL of local anesthetic solution subcutaneously in a transverse line from the posteromedial to the anteromedial aspect of either condyle (Figure 106-29*C*).

Remarks: The saphenous nerve may be blocked at the ankle if anesthesia of the leg is not required.

SAPHENOUS NERVE BLOCK, AT THE ANKLE

Anatomy: The saphenous nerve divides into numerous terminal branches in the distal leg. These terminal branches travel across the anteromedial ankle (Figure 106-29*B*) to innervate the anteromedial aspect of the ankle and foot (Figure 106-27).

Patient positioning: Place the patient supine with their ankle supported on a pillow or blanket, the knee extended, and the leg externally rotated.

Landmarks: Identify the anterior border of the medial malleolus and the great saphenous vein by palpation.

Needle insertion and direction: Place a skin wheal of local anesthetic 1.5 cm superior and anterior to the medial malleolus. Insert a 25 gauge needle through the skin wheal. Infiltrate 3 to 5 mL of local anesthetic solution subcutaneously in a fan-like pattern around the great saphenous vein.

Remarks: Alternatively, infiltrate 5 to 7 mL of local anesthetic solution subcutaneously in a transverse line from the anterior border of the medial malleolus to the anterior border of the anterior tibial ridge (Figure 106-29*D*).

LATERAL FEMORAL CUTANEOUS NERVE BLOCK

Anatomy: The lateral femoral cutaneous nerve enters the thigh through or below the inguinal ligament, 1 to 2 cm medial to the anterior superior iliac spine[9] (Figure 106-30*A*). It crosses through or over the sartorius muscle to lie on its anterior surface and deep to the fascia lata. This nerve provides sensory innervation to the anterolateral and lateral thigh (Figure 106-27). It has no motor components.

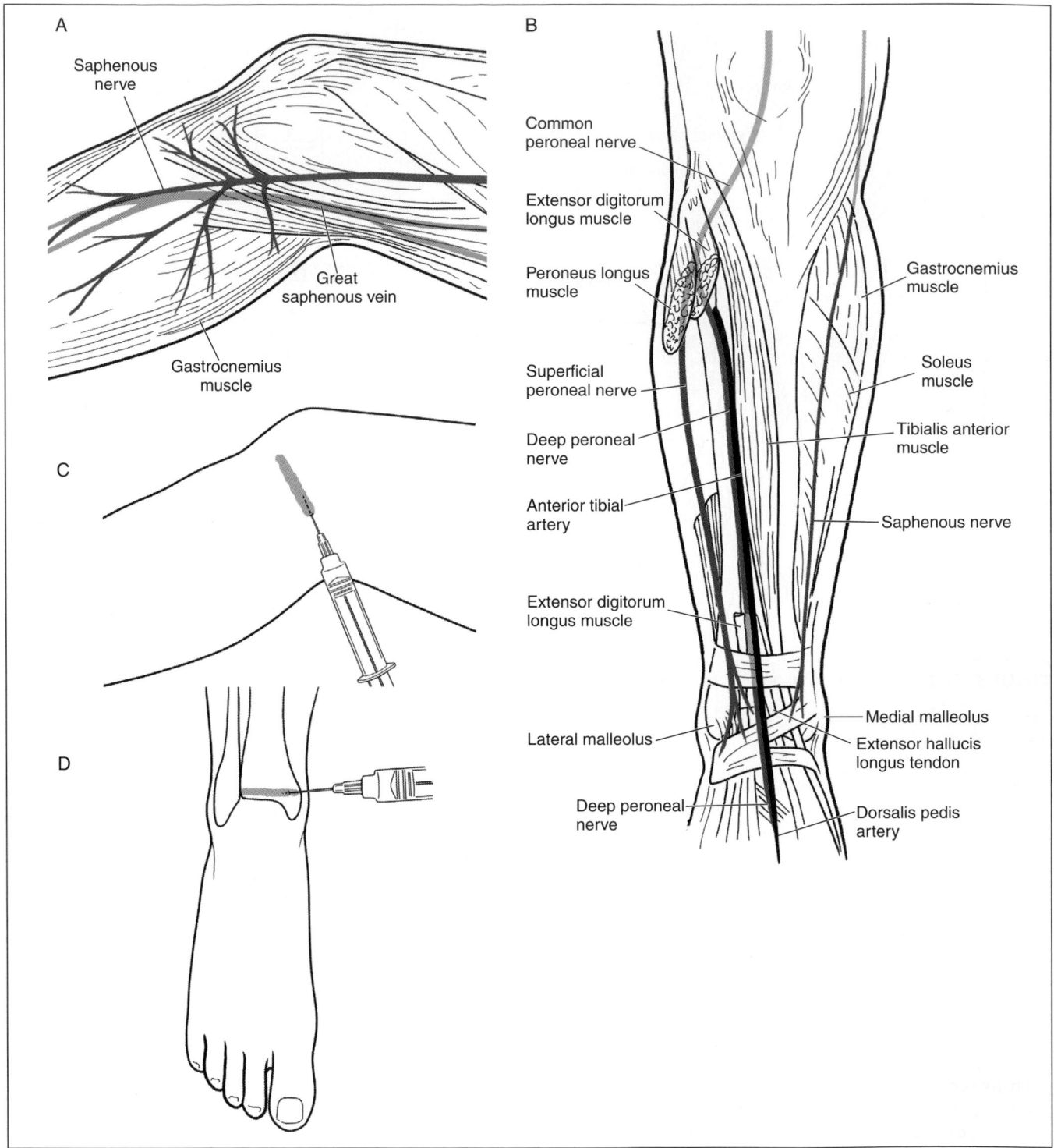

FIGURE 106-29 The saphenous nerve block. *A.* The course of the saphenous nerve at the medial knee. *B.* The course of the saphenous nerve in the leg. *C.* Blockade at the level of the knee. *D.* Blockade at the level of the ankle.

Patient positioning: Place the patient supine with their hip and knee extended.

Landmarks: Identify the anterior superior iliac spine by palpation.

Needle insertion and direction: Place a skin wheal of local anesthetic solution 2 to 3 cm inferior and 2 to 3 cm medial to the anterior superior iliac spine. Insert a 25 gauge needle perpendicular to the skin wheal. Advance the needle through the fascia lata. A "pop" will be

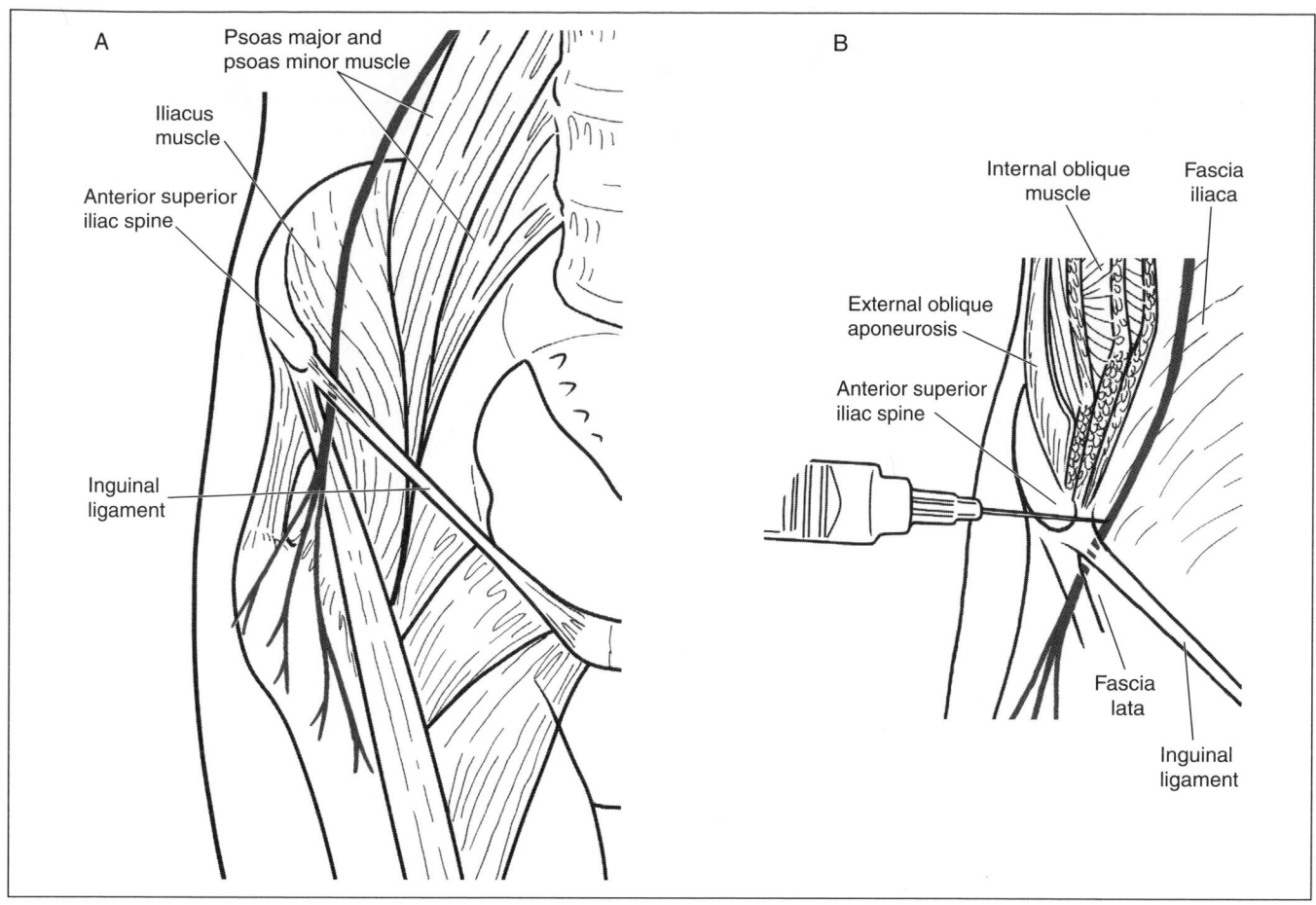

FIGURE 106-30 The lateral femoral cutaneous nerve block. *A.* The course of the lateral femoral cutaneous nerve. *B.* The third or alternative approach to blockade of the nerve.

felt as the needle traverses through the fascia lata.[2,45] Infiltrate 10 mL of local anesthetic solution subcutaneously in a superior to inferior fan-like pattern.

A second approach begins with making the same skin wheal. Insert the needle through the skin wheal, directed laterally and superiorly. Advance the needle to contact the iliac bone just medial and inferior to the anterior superior iliac spine. Infiltrate 10 mL of local anesthetic solution subcutaneously in a fan-like pattern about the iliac bone.

Remarks: A third, or alternative, approach is often used (Figure 106-30*B*). Place a skin wheal of local anesthetic solution just medial to the anterior superior iliac spine. Insert the needle through the skin wheal and perpendicular to the skin. Advance the needle until a "pop" is felt as the needle transverses the aponeurosis of the external oblique muscle. Continue to slowly advance the needle until a second "pop" is felt as the needle transverses through the internal oblique muscle and underlying iliac fascia. Inject 5 to 10 mL of local anesthetic solution. This approach blocks the nerve in its canal as it begins to pass under the inguinal ligament.

OBTURATOR NERVE BLOCK

Anatomy: The obturator nerve originates from the lumbar plexus. It passes through the pelvis and obturator canal to exit the obturator foramen into the thigh with its accompanying artery and vein (Figure 106-31*A*). It divides within the obturator canal into anterior and posterior branches. The anterior branch provides the sensory innervation to the hip and motor innervation to the anterior adductor muscles. There may also be a small and inconsistent area of cutaneous innervation over the medial thigh (Figures 106-27 and 106-31*B*). The posterior branch provides motor innervation to the deep adductor muscles and sensory innervation to the knee joint.[1,2]

Patient positioning: Place the patient supine with their hip and knee extended. Abduct the hip 10 to 20 degrees.

Landmarks: Identify the pubic tubercle by palpation.

Needle insertion and direction: Place a skin wheal of anesthetic solution 1.5 cm inferior and 1.5 cm lateral to

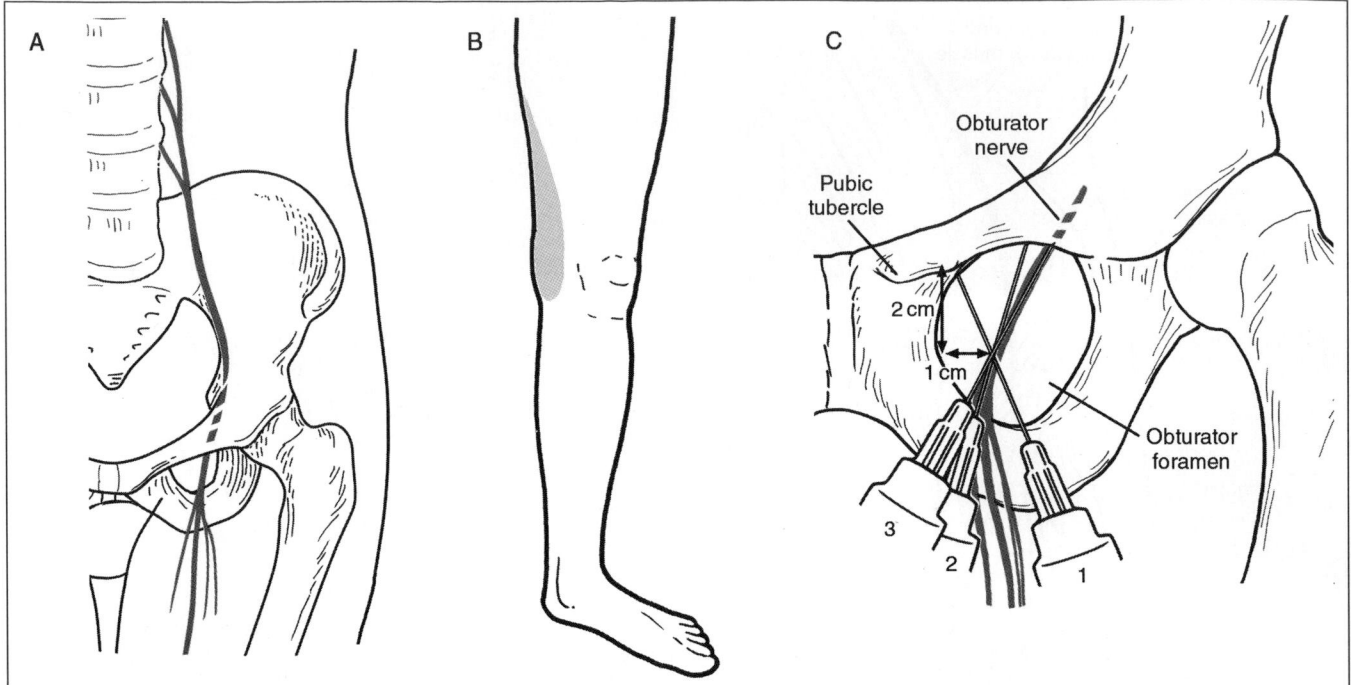

FIGURE 106-31 The obturator nerve block. *A.* The course of the obturator nerve. *B.* The sensory distribution of the obturator nerve. *C.* Blockade of the obturator nerve.

the pubic tubercle. Insert a 7 to 10 cm, 22 to 25 gauge spinal needle directed medially through the skin wheal. Advance the needle until it contacts the horizontal ramus of the pubic bone (Figure 106-31*C-1*). Withdraw the needle slightly (2 to 3 mm) and redirect it 45 degrees superiorly. Advance the needle to identify the superior bony portion of the obturator canal (Figure 106-31*C-2*). Withdraw the needle slightly (2 to 3 mm). Redirect the needle slightly laterally and inferiorly towards the obturator canal. Advance the needle 2 to 3 cm (Figure 106-31*C-3*). Inject 10 to 15 mL of local anesthetic solution.

Remarks: The purpose of this block is to provide analgesia for an acute hip fracture when the administration of intravenous analgesics is contraindicated. The technique requires significant experience and is time-consuming. **The obturator nerve must be anesthetized within the bony canal to prevent the needle from perforating the bladder or vagina.** This block is rarely, if ever, performed in the Emergency Department.

SCIATIC NERVE BLOCK, CLASSIC OR POSTERIOR APPROACH

Anatomy: The sciatic nerve arises from the lumbosacral plexus and leaves the pelvis through the greater sciatic foramen, inferior to the piriformis muscle (Figure 106-32). It is located midway between the ischial tuberosity and the greater trochanter of the femur.[46,47]

The nerve is superficial and accessible at the inferior border of the gluteus maximus muscle. The sciatic nerve provides the motor innervation to the muscles of the posterior thigh, leg, and foot. It provides sensory innervation to the posterior thigh, anterolateral leg, posterolateral leg, lateral leg, and almost the entire foot. There are four techniques for sciatic nerve blockade. These approaches were developed to allow sciatic nerve blockade from a variety of positions, therefore eliminating positioning problems that are encountered in the elderly, the infirm, and the trauma patient.

Patient positioning: Place the patient on the side opposite that to be blocked. Flex the hip and knee of the upper leg until the heel is over the dependent knee (Figure 106-33*A*).

Landmarks: **Identification of the anatomic landmarks is the key to success (Figure 106-33*A*).** Identify the greater trochanter of the femur and the posterior superior iliac spine by palpation. Connect these two landmarks with a straight line. Identify the midpoint of this line and draw a perpendicular bisector downward for 3 cm. This point represents the site of local anesthetic injection. Verify the position for injection with a second line. Reidentify the greater trochanter of the femur and the sacral cornu. Draw a line starting from 1.5 cm below the sacral cornu to the greater trochanter. This line should cross the end of the perpendicular bisector and be directly over the sciatic nerve.

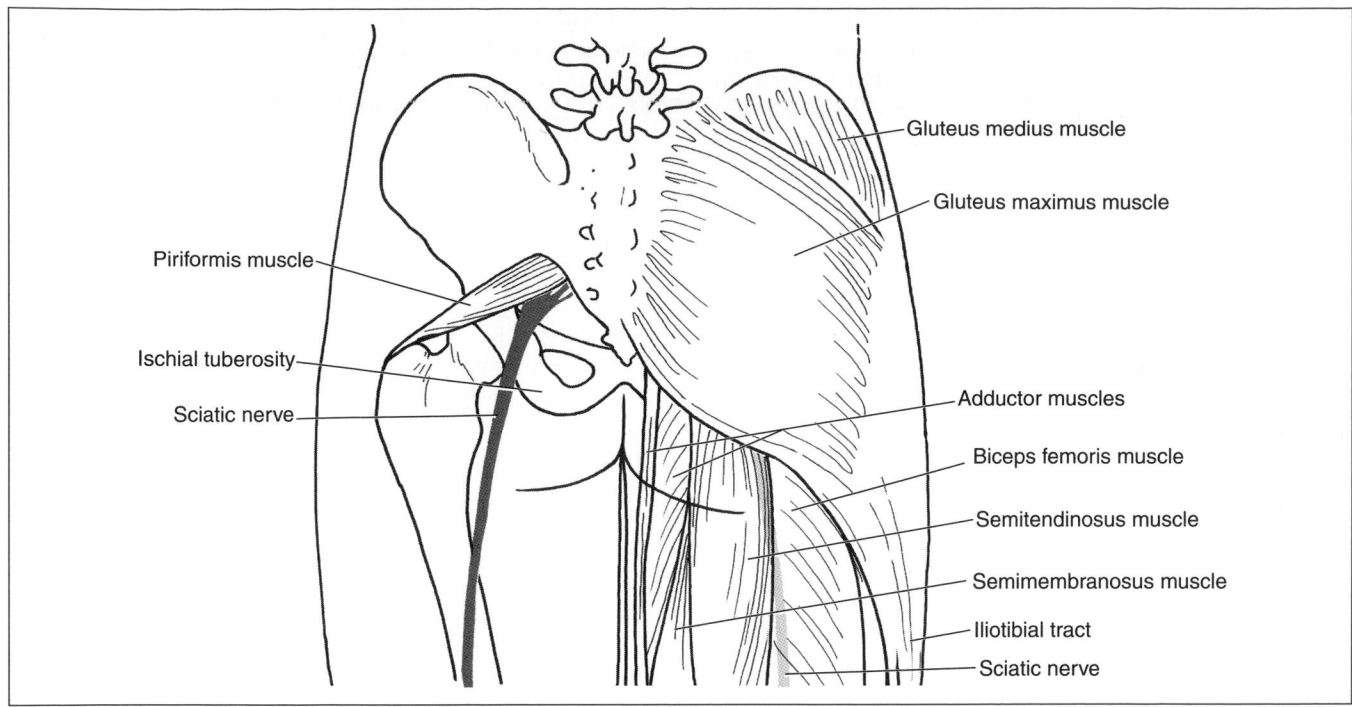

FIGURE 106-32 The course of the sciatic nerve.

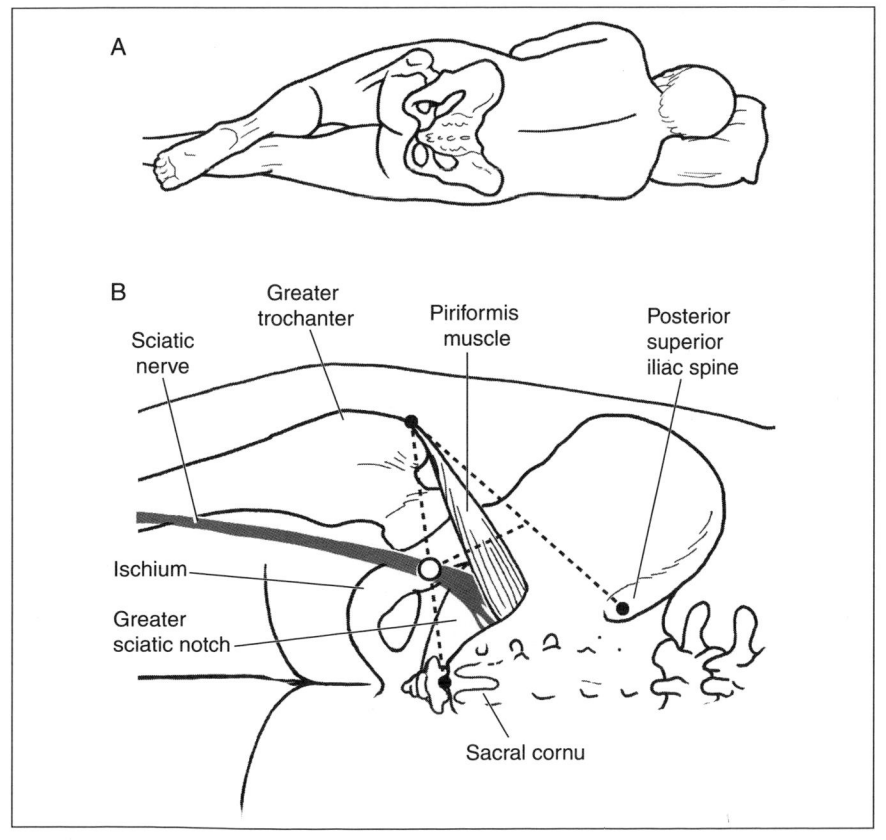

FIGURE 106-33 The classic or posterior approach to the sciatic nerve block. *A*. Patient positioning. *B*. Identification of the landmarks required to perform the block.

Needle insertion and direction: Place a skin wheal of local anesthetic solution at the identified injection site. Insert a 22 gauge needle perpendicular to the skin wheal. Advance the needle until paresthesias are elicited. **If paresthesias are not elicited, redirect the needle to find the sciatic nerve. The nerve must be located prior to infiltration with the local anesthetic solution to achieve proper anesthesia.**[46,48] Withdraw the needle 2 mm and allow the paresthesias to resolve. Inject 20 to 30 mL of local anesthetic solution.

Remarks: Blockade of the sciatic nerve can be used for fracture reduction, extensive laceration repair, incision and drainage of abscesses, wound exploration, or anesthesia from burns or trauma.[1,46,47] The posterior approach is the most commonly performed technique.

SCIATIC NERVE BLOCK, ANTERIOR APPROACH

Anatomy: The anatomy and innervation of the sciatic nerve are described in the previous section. This approach can be used for patients who cannot be turned onto their side.[47]

Patient positioning: Place the patient supine with their hip and knee extended.

Landmarks: **Identification of the anatomic landmarks is the key to success (Figure 106-34A).** Identify the anterior superior iliac spine and the pubic tubercle by palpation. Connect these points with a straight line (Figure 106-34A, Line 1). This line represents the location of the inguinal ligament. Trisect the inguinal ligament line into three equal parts. Draw a line perpendicular from the junction of the medial and middle thirds (Figure 106-34A, Line 2). Identify the tuberosity of the greater trochanter by palpation. Draw a line from the tuberosity medially across the anterior thigh and parallel to the line representing the inguinal ligament (Figure 106-34A, Line 3). The point of intersection of this line (Figure 106-34A, Line 3) with the perpendicular line from the inguinal ligament (Figure 106-34A, Line 2) represents the point of injection.

Needle insertion and direction: Place a skin wheal of local anesthetic solution at the identified injection site. Insert a 10 to 15 cm long, 22 gauge needle perpendicular to the skin and aimed slightly lateral. Advance the needle until the femur is contacted (Figure 106-34B-1). Withdraw the needle 1 cm and redirect it medially. Advance the needle 5 cm past the location where the bone was found (i.e., 6 cm; Figure 106-34B-2). The needle should be within the neurovascular bundle containing the sciatic nerve. The average distance from

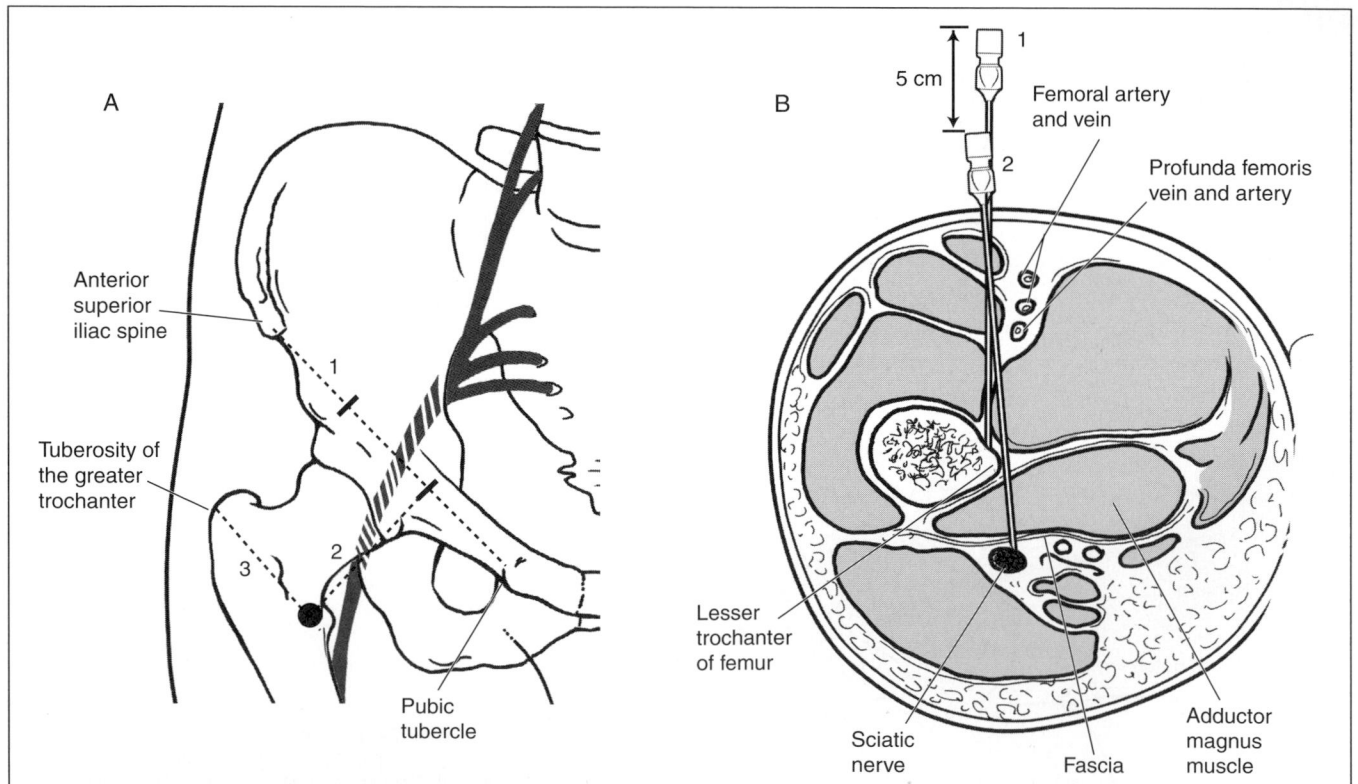

FIGURE 106-34 The anterior approach to the sciatic nerve block. *A.* Identification of the landmarks. *B.* Blockade of the sciatic nerve.

the surface of the femur to the neurovascular bundle is 4.5 to 6.0 cm in adults. **Inject a small test dose of local anesthetic solution to determine the ease of injection. The tip of the needle is within muscle or a fascial plane if significant resistance is encountered.** Advance the needle until resistance to injection is at a minimum. Eliciting paresthesias is extremely helpful in identifying the correct location of the needle. If paresthesias are elicited, withdraw the needle 2 mm and allow them to resolve. Inject 15 to 30 mL of local anesthetic solution.

Remarks: The posterior femoral cutaneous nerve, which accompanies the sciatic nerve, may sometimes be missed with this approach. This technique is extremely painful and not often performed.

SCIATIC NERVE BLOCK, LITHOTOMY APPROACH

Anatomy: The anatomy and innervation of the sciatic nerve are described in the previous section. The sciatic nerve lies anterior to the gluteus maximus muscle when the patient is in the lithotomy position. The nerve is more superficial in this position than in the other approaches.[46,47]

Patient positioning: Place the patient supine. Maximally flex the hip and knee of the extremity to be anesthetized. Use a bed or examination table with foot stirrups if available and not contraindicated.

Landmarks: Identify the ischial tuberosity and the greater trochanter of the femur by palpation. Connect these landmarks with a straight line. Identify the midpoint of this line.

Needle insertion and direction: Place a skin wheal of local anesthetic solution at the midpoint of the line from the ischial tuberosity to the greater trochanter. Insert a 10 to 15 cm long, 22 gauge spinal needle perpendicular to the skin wheal. Slowly advance the needle until paresthesias are elicited. Withdraw the needle 2 mm and allow the paresthesias to resolve. Inject 20 to 25 mL of local anesthetic solution.

Remarks: This approach is more difficult to master than the previous two techniques. It is time-consuming and requires locating the sciatic nerve by eliciting paresthesias prior to injecting the local anesthetic solution.

SCIATIC NERVE BLOCK, LATERAL APPROACH

The lateral approach will not be described. This approach requires considerable experience, a nerve stimulator, and does not provide any advantage over the other approaches.

POPLITEAL FOSSA NERVE BLOCK, ANATOMICAL OR POSTERIOR APPROACH

Anatomy: The popliteal fossa is a diamond-shaped area on the posterior aspect of the knee (Figure 106-35). Its boundaries are the long head of the biceps femoris muscle superolaterally, the semimembranous and semitendinous muscles superomedially, and the medial and lateral heads of the gastrocnemius muscle inferiorly. This space contains the tibial and common peroneal nerves, the popliteal artery and vein, and loose fatty connective tissue (Figure 106-35A). The nerves are superficial to the arteries and veins, midway between the skin and the posterior surface of the femur. The average distance between the skin and the nerves is 1.5 to 2.0 cm in adults.[49] These nerves are responsible for the motor innervation of all the muscles below the knee. They also provide sensory innervation to the entire leg below the knee except the area innervated by the saphenous nerve.

Patient positioning: Place the patient prone with a pillow or blanket under their ankle to position the knee in slight flexion (10 to 20 degrees).

Landmarks: Identify the borders of the popliteal fossa. Divide the fossa into a superior and inferior triangle with a line drawn medial to lateral across the skin fold or crease (Figure 106-35B). Draw a line from the apex to the base of the superior triangle, making two smaller and equal triangles. Identify the spot 5 cm superior and 1 cm lateral to the midline of the upper triangle. This spot represents the landmark for needle insertion.

Needle insertion and direction: Place a skin wheal of local anesthetic solution 5 cm superior and 1 cm lateral to the midline of the upper triangle (Figure 106-35B). Insert a 25 gauge needle through the skin wheal, directed superiorly and at a 45 to 60 degree angle to the skin surface. Advance the needle anteriorly and superiorly until paresthesias are elicited. Withdraw the needle 2 mm and allow the paresthesias to resolve. Infiltrate 35 to 45 mL of local anesthetic solution.

Remarks: This block is difficult to use in patients who cannot lie in the prone position. This includes pregnant patients, the morbidly obese, spinal injury patients, hemodynamically unstable patients, and those on mechanical ventilation.[49]

COMMON PERONEAL NERVE BLOCK

Anatomy: The common peroneal nerve originates in the popliteal fossa as one of the terminal branches of the sciatic nerve[2,11] (Figure 106-36A). It courses posterolater-

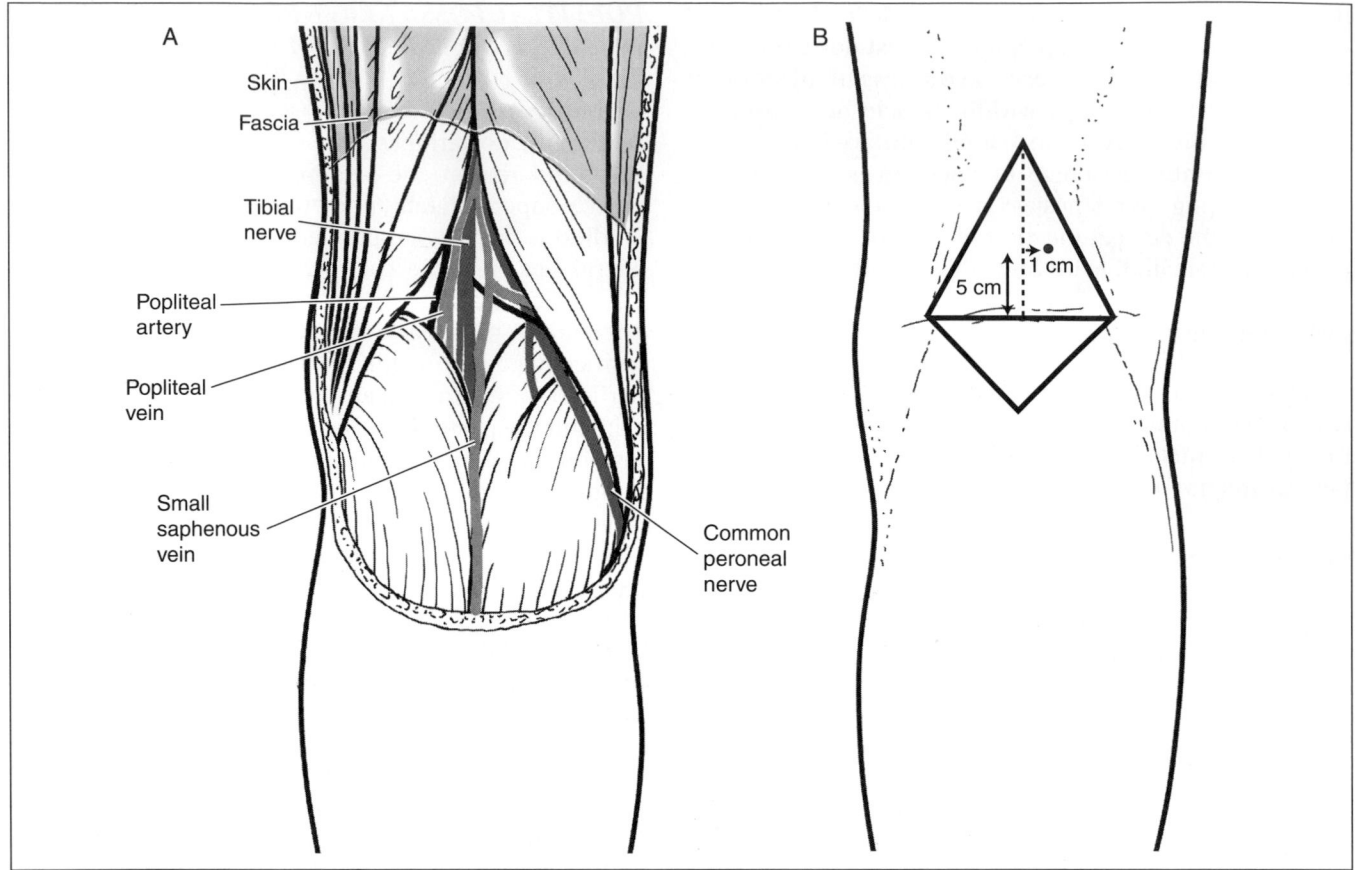

FIGURE 106-35 The anatomical or posterior approach to the popliteal fossa nerve block. *A.* The contents of the popliteal fossa. *B.* Identification of the landmarks required to perform the block.

ally around the neck of the fibula where it can be palpated. It provides motor innervation to the peroneal muscles and the muscles of the anterior leg and foot. It provides sensory innervation to the anterior leg, dorsum of the foot and toes, and to the medial great toe (Figure 106-27).

Patient positioning: Place the patient lying on the side opposite that being anesthetized. Alternatively, place the patient supine with their leg internally rotated.

Landmarks: Identify the head and neck of the fibula and the common peroneal nerve by palpation.

Needle insertion and direction: Place a skin wheal of local anesthetic solution over the neck of the fibula (Figure 106-36*B*). Insert a 25 gauge needle through the skin wheal to elicit paresthesias. Withdraw the needle 2 mm and allow the paresthesias to resolve. Inject 3 to 5 mL of local anesthetic solution. If paresthesias are not elicited, subcutaneously infiltrate the area with 5 to 7 mL of local anesthetic solution.

Remarks: The common peroneal nerve may not always be palpable. Apply digital pressure over the neck of

the fibula. Significant discomfort will be elicited when compressing the nerve against the fibula. This site is the location of the common peroneal nerve.

SUPERFICIAL PERONEAL NERVE BLOCK

Anatomy: The superficial peroneal nerve is one of the terminal branches of the common peroneal nerve[2,50] (Figure 106-37*A*). It perforates the investing fascia of the anterior leg to become subcutaneous in the lower third of the leg. It provides motor innervation to the peroneus longus and brevis muscles. It provides sensory innervation to the anterolateral leg, medial great toe, and dorsum of the foot and toes except the first web space and the area covered by the saphenous and sural nerves (Figure 106-27).

Patient positioning: Place the patient supine with their ankle supported on a pillow or blanket.

Landmarks: Identify the anterior border of the medial and lateral malleolus by palpation.

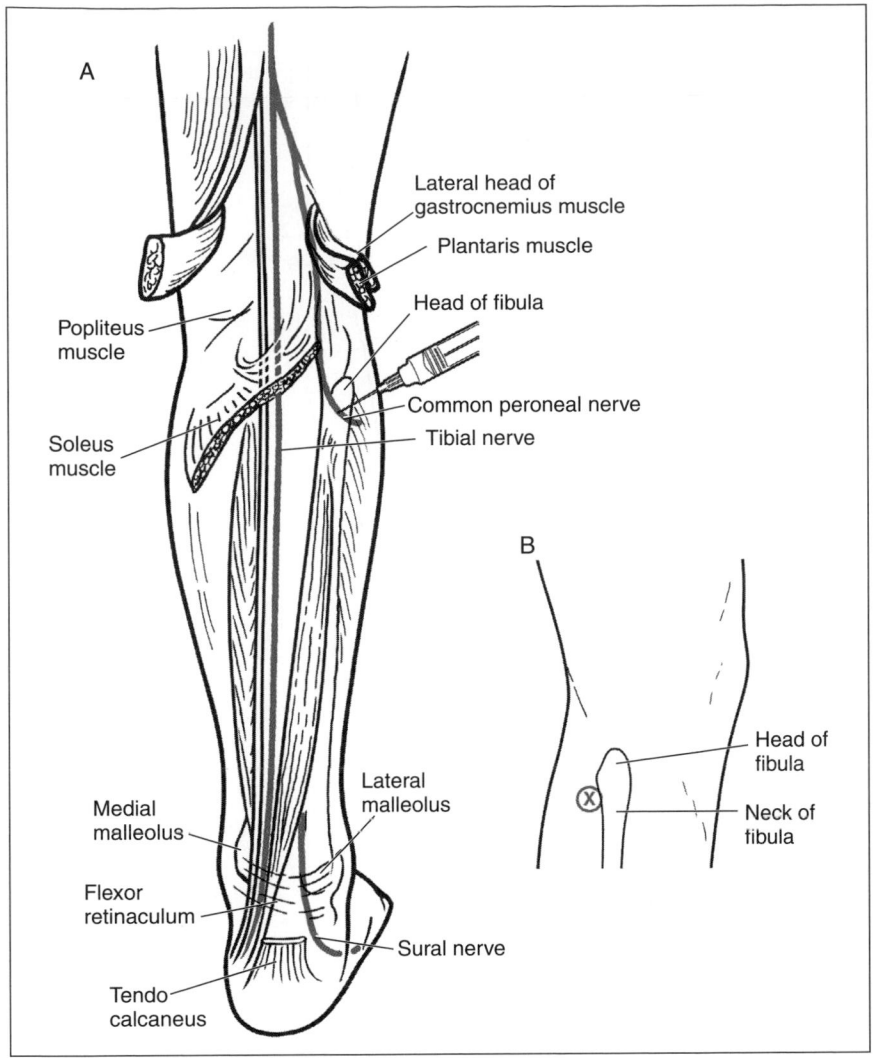

A
Lateral head of gastrocnemius muscle
Plantaris muscle
Head of fibula
Popliteus muscle
Common peroneal nerve
Tibial nerve
Soleus muscle
Medial malleolus
Lateral malleolus
Flexor retinaculum
Sural nerve
Tendo calcaneus

B
Head of fibula
Neck of fibula

FIGURE 106-36 The common peroneal nerve block. *A.* The course of the common peroneal nerve. *B.* The landmark for performing the block.

Needle insertion and direction: Place a skin wheal of local anesthetic solution anterior to the distal aspect of the lateral malleolus. Insert a 25 gauge needle through the skin wheal. Infiltrate 6 to 10 mL of local anesthetic solution subcutaneously in a transverse line to the anterior border of the medial malleolus (Figure 106-37*B*).

Remarks: The superficial peroneal nerve may also be blocked at the level of the ankle. Infiltrate 4 to 8 mL of local anesthetic solution subcutaneously in a transverse line from the anterior border of the lateral malleolus to the anterior tibial ridge.

DEEP PERONEAL NERVE BLOCK

Anatomy: The deep peroneal nerve is one of the terminal branches of the common peroneal nerve.[2,51] It descends over the interosseous membrane into the dorsal foot, lateral to the dorsalis pedis artery (Figure 106-38*A*). It travels between the tendons of the tibialis anterior and extensor hallucis longus muscles at the level of the ankle

joint and above. It travels between the tendons of the extensor digitorum longus and the extensor hallucis longus muscles at the level of the malleoli. It may or may not contribute a motor branch to the peroneus longus muscles. It provides sensory innervation to only the first web space (Figure 106-27).

Patient positioning: Place the patient supine with their ankle supported on a pillow or blanket.

Landmarks: Identify the tendons of the tibialis anterior and the extensor hallucis longus muscles by palpation. Identify the anterior tibial artery by its pulse at the level of the ankle joint.

Needle insertion and direction: Place a skin wheal of local anesthetic solution between the two tendons and just lateral to the anterior tibial artery (Figure 106-38*B*). Insert a 25 gauge needle through the skin wheal and perpendicular to the skin. Advance the needle 3 mm and inject 3 to 5 mL of local anesthetic solution.

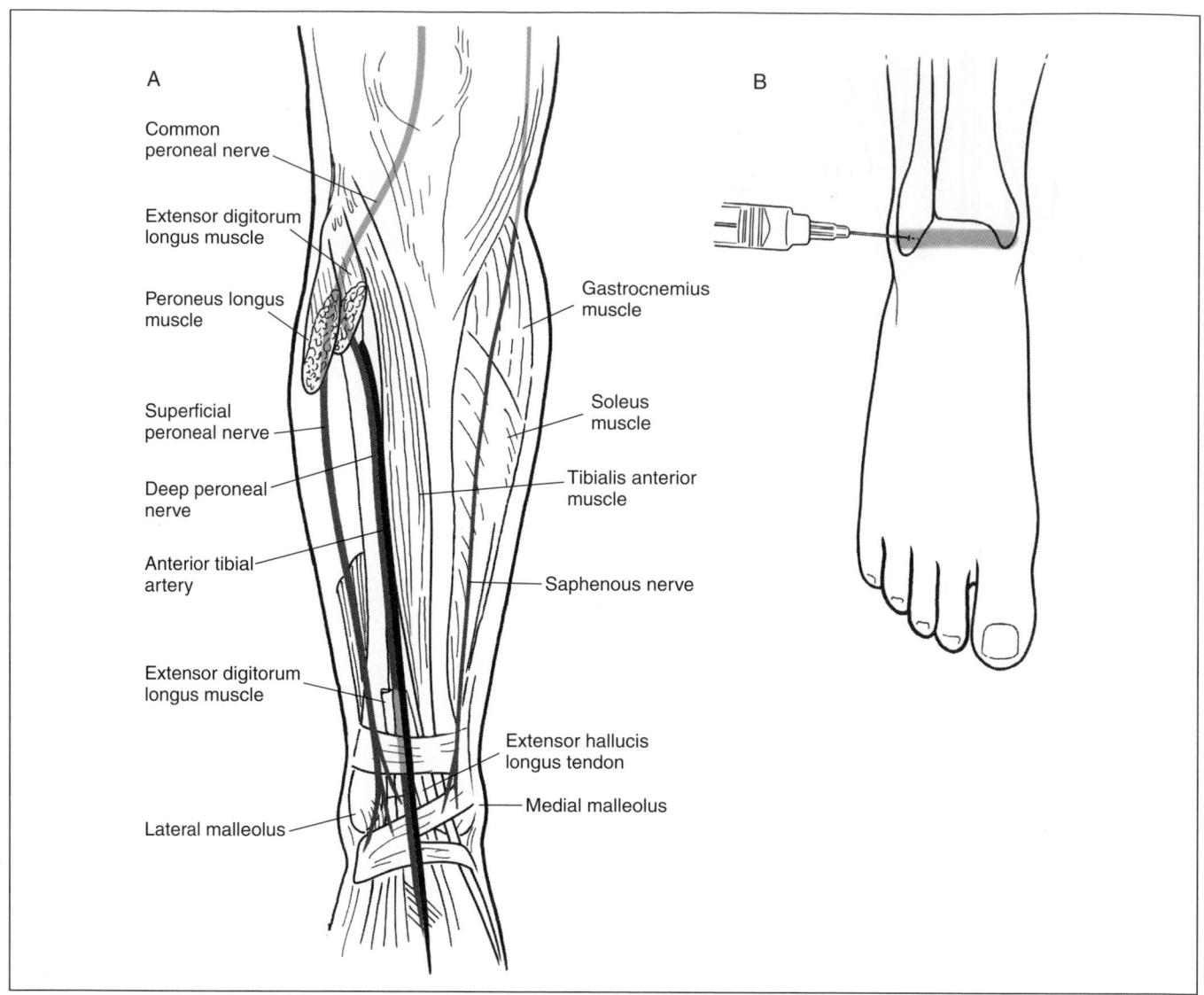

FIGURE 106-37 The superficial peroneal nerve block. *A.* The course of the nerve. *B.* Blockade of the superficial peroneal nerve.

Remarks: The deep peroneal nerve may also be blocked at the level of the malleoli. Identify the tendons of the extensor digitorum longus and extensor hallucis longus muscles by palpation and the dorsalis pedis artery by its pulse at the level of the malleoli. Place a skin wheal of local anesthetic solution between the tendons and lateral to the dorsalis pedis artery. Insert the needle perpendicular to the skin. Advance the needle 3 mm and inject 2 to 4 mL of local anesthetic solution.

SURAL NERVE BLOCK

Anatomy: The sural nerve originates from the tibial nerve and the common peroneal nerve in the popliteal fossa.[52] It is superficial after its orgin and travels on the lateral leg and foot (Figure 106-39). It has already divided at the level of the ankle into numerous superficial branches, all located behind the lateral malleolus. The sural nerve provides sensory innervation to the antero-lateral surface of the foot and little toe (Figure 106-27).

Patient positioning: Place the patient prone with their ankle supported on a pillow or blanket and the leg externally rotated. Alternatively, place the patient supine with their ankle supported on a pillow or blanket and the leg internally rotated.

Landmarks: Identify the posterior border of the lateral malleolus and the Achilles tendon by palpation.

Needle insertion and direction: Place a skin wheal of local anesthetic solution, at the level of the lateral malleolus, just lateral to the Achilles tendon. Insert a 25 gauge needle through the skin wheal and angled toward

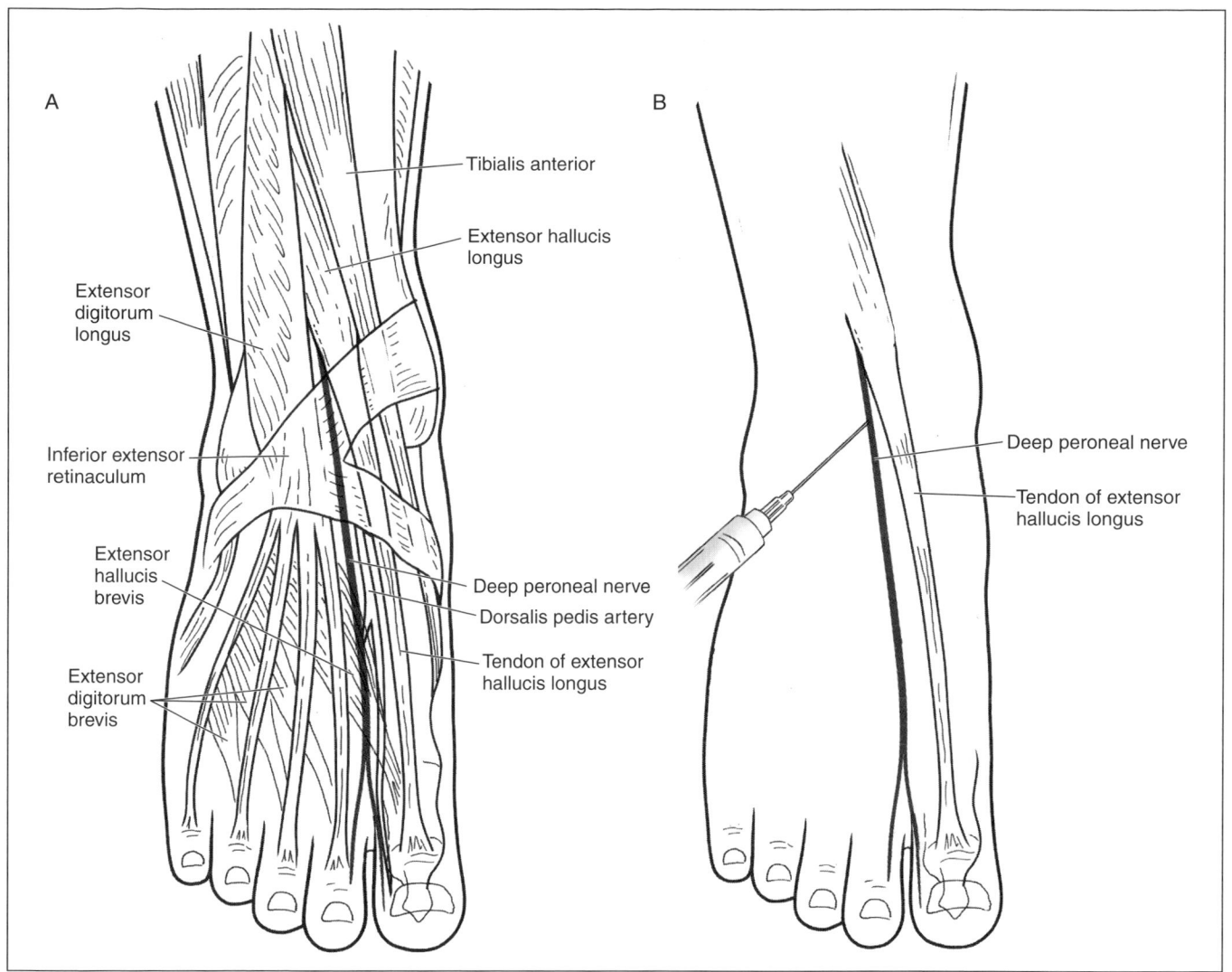

FIGURE 106-38 The deep peroneal nerve block. *A.* The course of the deep peroneal nerve. *B.* Blockade of the deep peroneal nerve.

the lateral malleolus (Figure 106-39). Infiltrate 5 mL of local anesthetic solution subcutaneously in a transverse line to the lateral malleolus.

Remarks: **Ensure that the needle is not within the Achilles tendon before injecting the local anesthetic solution.**

POSTERIOR TIBIAL NERVE BLOCK

Anatomy: The posterior tibial nerve travels in the posterior leg and exists medial to the Achilles tendon, several centimeters above the ankle.[2] It is superficial at the ankle, midway between the medial malleolus and the heel (Figure 106-40). It lies between the tendons of the flexor digitorum longus and flexor hallucis longus muscles. It travels with, and slightly posterior to, the posterior tibial artery. The posterior tibial nerve divides

at the inferior border of the calcaneus to form the medial and lateral plantar nerves. It provides motor innervation to the intrinsic foot muscles. The lateral plantar nerve provides sensory innervation to the lateral one-third of the sole and plantar surface of the lateral one and one-half toes (Figure 106-27). The medial plantar nerve provides sensory innervation to the medial two-thirds of the sole and the plantar surface of the medial three and one-half toes (Figure 106-27).

Patient positioning: Place the patient supine with their ankle supported on a pillow or blanket and the leg externally rotated.

Landmarks: Identify the medial malleolus by palpation and the posterior tibial artery by its pulsation.

Needle insertion and direction: Place a skin wheal of local anesthetic solution, at the level of the upper

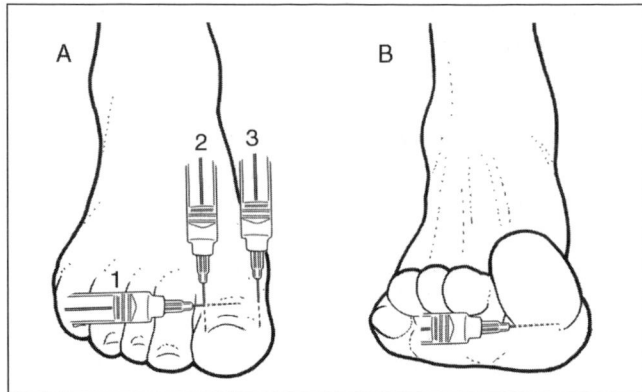

FIGURE 106-42 The digital block of the toe. *A.* The three-sided ring block may be used on any of the toes. *B.* The great toe requires an additional injection to achieve anesthesia.

aspect of the toe while infiltrating with 1.0 to 1.5 mL of local anesthetic solution. Repeat the infiltration on the lateral aspect of the toe. Anesthesia should be complete within 10 minutes. The great toe, due to its unique nerve supply, requires an additional anesthetic injection on the plantar aspect[1–3,55] (Figure 106-42B).

Remarks: This technique is commonly employed in the Emergency Department. The indications include repair of lacerations, incision and drainage of infections, removal of toenails, manipulations of fractures and dislocations, and painful procedures requiring anesthesia. Other techniques to anesthetize the toes are similar to those of anesthetizing the fingers (Figure 106-24).

ASSESSMENT

Allow 5 to 10 minutes for most regional anesthesia blocks to take effect. Up to 20 minutes may be required for blockade of major nerves (axillary, femoral, sciatic, and popliteal fossa). **Incomplete or inadequate anesthesia is the result of not properly identifying the anatomic landmarks or not inserting the needle properly. The procedure may be repeated if the administration of a second dose of local anesthetic solution does not result in the patient receiving a toxic dose of the anesthetic agent** (Table 106-2).

AFTERCARE

Perform frequent neurovascular checks until baseline function has returned. Injury to the anesthetized limb can result if the patient is permitted to use it, to use heat or cold application, or to perform wound care before the anesthesia has worn off.[1,22,26] **If extensive**
or major nerve blockade was performed, discharge the patient home only after the sensation and function have returned to baseline.** The patient may be discharged home immediately after minor blockade, but should be properly cautioned. Avoid compression dressings as they may result in ischemia, which is improperly sensed by the anesthetized area or limb.

COMPLICATIONS

Complications can occur from the injection of local anesthetic solution, most of which are minor. Significant complications are rare; yet, they do occur. Complications generally result from poor technique. General precautions include measures to minimize nerve injury, intravascular injection, and systemic toxicity. The physician must be prepared to institute quick and immediate abortive care, cardiac monitoring, and airway control if complications do arise.

ALLERGIC REACTIONS
Allergic reactions can occur from hypersensitivity to the local anesthetic solution. Symptoms can range from mild itching and urticaria to circulatory collapse and death. Severe allergic reactions are extremely rare but may occur. The preservative in the local anesthetic solution is often the cause of an allergic reaction. Local anesthetic solutions containing no preservatives are an alternative. One example is "cardiac" lidocaine that is used for Advanced Cardiac Life Support (ACLS) protocols. Topical ice or vapor coolant is an acceptable alternative to nothing if one is concerned about a potential allergic reaction from the local anesthetic solutions. A solution of 1% to 2% diphenhydramine can also be used as an injectable local anesthetic.[6,10,26]

HEMORRHAGE
Significant bleeding is extremely rare. Injection of a local anesthetic solution can be performed safely in patients who are anticoagulated or have a bleeding disorder.[6,10,26] A hematoma may commonly develop due to an arterial puncture. The application of direct pressure can be helpful if significant external hemorrhage occurs. However, if bleeding continues, treatment may be required to reverse the anticoagulant or replace clotting factors.

OVERDOSAGE
Central nervous system (CNS) complications primarily result from local anesthetic toxicity.[56,57] These symptoms range from tremors to convulsions. The most severe complication is respiratory compromise resulting in intubation. The maximum dose of local anesthetic solution should not exceed the doses listed in Table 106-2.[2,6,15] Toxicity after intravascular injection requires even less anesthetic than subcutaneous infiltration.

INFECTION

Infection can occur when the needle penetrates unclean skin. The risk of infection is significantly reduced if proper aseptic technique is used. The risk of infection is negligible when the skin is properly cleansed, sterile technique is used, puncture through obviously infected skin is avoided, and penetrating the needle through a skin lesion that may harbor microorganisms is avoided.

VASOVAGAL REACTIONS

The patient may experience an increase in vagal tone from apprehension, needle phobias, and/or pain. Vasovagal reactions are relatively common and may be associated with light-headedness and/or fainting. **Always perform regional anesthesia with the patient on a stretcher or in a chair that reclines to prevent secondary injury.** Vasovagal reactions are self-limited and only require reassurance.[6,26]

NERVE INJURY

Inflammation of the nerve is the most common nerve injury seen after regional anesthesia.[1,26] Neuritis is a rare complication. Patients may complain of paresthesias, motor deficits, and/or sensory deficits. Most cases are transient and resolve completely, requiring only supportive care and close follow-up. Nerve damage results from direct needle trauma, ischemia due to intraneural injection, and chemical irritation from the anesthetic solution.[1,26,56] Proper needle style, positioning, and manipulation can minimize direct nerve damage. Intraneural injection can cause nerve ischemia with resultant injury. **Elicitation of paresthesias or severe pain indicates that the needle has made contact with the nerve. Withdraw the needle slightly and allow the paresthesias to resolve before injecting the local anesthetic solution.** Concentrated anesthetics can produce chemical irritation of the nerve.[56,57]

INTRAVASCULAR INJECTION

Intravascular injection results in both systemic and limb toxicity. Inadvertent intravascular injection produces high blood levels of the anesthetic agent and resultant toxicity. Particular care must be taken when administering large amounts of local anesthetic solution in close proximity to large blood vessels.

Intraarterial injection of local anesthetic solution containing epinephrine may cause peripheral vasospasm and subsequent ischemia that further compromises injured tissue. The local anesthetic solution is not toxic to the limb itself, although it may produce transient blanching of the skin by displacing blood from the vascular tree. α-Adrenergic antagonists have been used with success in relieving arterial vasospasm secondary to intraarterial injection of local anesthetics.[58,59]

SUMMARY

Regional anesthesia can serve as a valuable adjunct to the Emergency Physician's armamentarium. It is used for wound anesthesia prior to exploration, irrigation, debridement, and repair. Regional anesthesia may also be used to reduce the pain of procedures such as reduction of fractures and dislocations. Nerve blocks are especially useful when pain-sensitive structures such as fingers, toes, hands, and feet are involved. The application of regional anesthesia is frequently overlooked and underutilized in the emergency care of not only adults but even more so in the case of children. The use of regional nerve blocks is simple, safe, and effective for providing analgesia in the Emergency Department.

REFERENCES

1. Moy JG, Pfenninger JL: Peripheral nerve blocks and field blocks, in Pfenninger JL, Fowler GC (eds): *Procedures for Primary Care Physicians.* St. Louis: Mosby, 1994:145–155.
2. Dunmire SM, Paris PM: *Atlas of Emergency Procedures,* 2nd ed. Philadelphia: Saunders, 1994:35–54.
3. Walton SA, Hodge D: Regional anesthesia, in Dieckmann RA, Fiser DH, Selbst SM (eds): *Illustrated Textbook of Pediatric Emergency and Critical Care Procedures.* St. Louis: Mosby, 1997:87–92.
4. Yentis SM, Vlassakov KV: Vassily von Anrep, forgotten pioneer of regional anesthesia. *Anesthesiology* 1999; 90(3):890–895.
5. MacKenzie TA, Young ER: Local anesthetic update. *Anesth Prog* 1993; 40:29–34.
6. Norris RL: Local anesthetics. *Emerg Med Clin North Am* 1992; 10(4):707–718.
7. Cleveland Clinic Foundation Department of General Anesthesiology: Local anesthetic properties and determinants of blockade. 1999. http://www.anes.ccf.org:8080/pilot/ortho/la_prop.htm.
8. Cleveland Clinic Foundation Department of General Anesthesiology: Preparation for regional anesthesia. 1999. http://www.anes.ccf.org:8080/pilot/ortho/prep4reg.htm.
9. Cleveland Clinic Foundation Department of General Anesthesiology: Amino ester local anesthetics. 1999. http://www.anes.ccf.org:8080/pilot/ortho/laester.htm.
10. Cleveland Clinic Foundation Department of General Anesthesiology: Contraindications to regional anesthesia. 1999. http://www.anes.ccf.org:8080/pilot/ortho/contra.htm.
11. Dean E, Orlinsky M: Nerve blocks of the thorax and extremities, in Roberts JR, Hedges JR (eds): *Clinical Procedures in Emergency Medicine,* 3rd ed. Philadelphia: Saunders, 1998:473–496.

12. Lewis L, Stephan M: Local and regional anesthesia, in Henretig FM, King C (eds): *Textbook of Pediatric Emergency Procedures,* 3rd ed. Baltimore: Williams & Wilkins, 1997:465–496.

13. Gregory PR, Sullivan MD, Sullivan JA: Nitrous oxide compared with intravenous regional anesthesia in pediatric forearm fracture manipulation. *J Pediatr Orthop* 1996; 16(2):188–191.

14. Keegan JJ, Garrett FD: The segmental distribution of the cutaneous nerves in the limbs of man. *Anat Rec* 1948; 102:409–437.

15. Baker JD, Blackman BB: Local anesthesia. *Clin Plast Surg* 1985; 12(1):25–31.

16. Tuckley JM: The pharmacology of local anesthetic agents. 1999. http://www.nda.ox.ac.uk/wfsa/html/u04/u04_014.htm.

17. Kretzschmar JL, Peters JE: Nerve blocks for regional anesthesia of the face. *Am Fam Physician* 1997; 55(5):1701–1704.

18. Earle AS, Blanchard JM: Regional anesthesia in the upper extremity. *Clin Plast Surg* 1985; 12(1):97–114.

19. Yaster M, Maxwell LG: Pediatric regional anesthesia. *Anesthesiology* 1989; 70:324–338.

20. Cleveland Clinic Foundation Department of General Anesthesiology: Equipment for regional anesthesia. 1999. http://www.anes.ccf.org:8080/pilot/ortho/equip.htm.

21. Cleveland Clinic Foundation Department of General Anesthesiology: Patient selection and informed consent. 1999. http://www.anes.ccf.org:8080/pilot/ortho/prepare.htm.

22. Auroy Y, Narchi P, Messiah A, et al: Serious complications related to regional anesthesia. *Anesthesiology* 1997; 87(3):479–486.

23. Cleveland Clinic Foundation Department of General Anesthesiology: Preparation for regional anesthesia. 1999. http://www.anes.ccf.org:8080/pilot/ortho/prep4reg.htm.

24. Cleveland Clinic Foundation Department of General Anesthesiology: Choosing a local anesthetic. 1999. http://www.anes.ccf.org:8080/pilot/ortho/chooseL.A.htm.

25. Cleveland Clinic Foundation Department of General Anesthesiology: Sedation for regional anesthesiology. 1999. http://www.anes.ccf.org:8080/pilot/ortho/sedation.htm.

26. Cleveland Clinic Foundation Department of General Anesthesiology: Complications of regional anesthesia. 1999. http://www.anes.ccf.org:8080/pilot/ortho/complica.htm.

27. Giannoni CM: Local and regional anesthesia in the head and neck. 1993. http://www.bcm.tmc.edu/oto/grand/52793.html.

28. Giannoni CM: Local and regional anesthesia in the head and neck. 1993. http://www.bcm.tmc.edu/oto/grand/52793.html.

29. Harbers JB, Beems T, Hoen MB, et al: A case of temporary facial nerve palsy after regional anesthesia of the scalp. *Anesth Analg* 1998; 87(6):1375–1376.

30. Cleveland Clinic Foundation Department of General Anesthesiology: Axillary brachial plexus block. 1999. http://www.anes.ccf.org:8080/pilot/ortho/axillary.htm.

31. Dannemiller Memorial Educational Foundation: Regional anesthesia for shoulder and elbow surgery. 1998. http://www.pain.com/regional/racme_jan98_shoulderelbow.cfm.

32. University of Washington: Brachial plexus anatomy. 1999. http://www.weber.u.washington.edu/ael/regionalplexus/brachialplexusanatomy.html.

33. Blasier RD, White R: Intravenous regional anesthesia for management of children's extremity fractures in the emergency department. *Pediatr Emerg Care* 1996; 12(6):404–406.

34. Philip BK: Supplemental medication for ambulatory procedures under regional anesthesia. *Anesth Analg* 1985; 64:1117–1125.

35. Baker JD, Blackman BB: Local anesthesia. *Clin Plast Surg* 1985; 12(1):25–31.

36. University of Washington: Ulnar nerve block. 1999. http://www.weber.u.washington.edu/ael/regional/ulnarnerve/ulnarnerveblock.html.

37. Carter PR: Regional anesthesia of the injured hand, in Carter PR (ed): *Common Hand Injuries and Infections—A Practical Approach to Early Treatment.* Philadelphia: Saunders, 1983:67–73.

38. Ferrera PC, Chandler R: Anesthesia in the emergency setting: Part I. Hand and foot injuries. *Am Fam Physician* 1994; 50(3):569–573.

39. Holzer A, Kapral S, Heilwagner K, et al: Severe pneumothorax after intercostal blockade: a case report. *Acta Anaesth Scand* 1998; 42(9)1124–1126.

40. Holman JR, Stuessi KA: Adult circumcision. *Am Fam Physician* 1999; 59(6):1514–1518.

41. Cleveland Clinic Foundation Department of General Anesthesiology: Femoral nerve block. 1999. http://www.anes.ccf.org:8080/pilot/ortho/femnerve.htm.

42. Dannemiller Memorial Educational Foundation: Femoral nerve block. 1998. http://www.pain.com/regional/racmejan98/rajan98femoral.cfm.

43. University of Washington: Femoral nerve block. 1999. http://www.weber.u.washington.edu/ael/regional/femoral/femoraltext.html.

44. Cappellino A, Jokl P, Ruwe PA: Regional anesthesia in knee arthroscopy: a new technique involving femoral and sciatic nerve blocks in knee arthroscopy. *Arthroscopy* 1996; 12(1):120–123.

45. Cleveland Clinic Foundation Department of General Anesthesiology: Saphenous nerve block. 1999. http://www.anes.ccf.org:8080/pilot/ortho/saph.htm.

46. Cleveland Clinic Foundation Department of General Anesthesiology: Lateral femoral cutaneous nerve block. 1999. http://www.anes.ccf.org:8080/pilot/ortho/lfe.htm.

47. Cleveland Clinic Foundation Department of General Anesthesiology: Sciatic nerve block. 1999. http://www.anes.ccf.org:8080/pilot/ortho/sciatic. htm.

48. University of Washington: Sciatic nerve block. 1999. http://www.weber.u.washington.edu/ael/regional/sciatic/sciatictext.html.

49. Hadzie A, Vloka JD: A comparison of the posterior versus lateral approaches to the block of the sciatic nerve in the popliteal fossa. *Anesthesiology* 1998; 88:1480–1486.

50. Cleveland Clinic Foundation Department of General Anesthesiology: Popliteal nerve block. 1999. http://www.anes.ccf.org:8080/pilot/ortho/poplit.htm.

51. Cleveland Clinic Foundation Department of General Anesthesiology: Superficial peroneal nerve block. 1999. http://www.anes.ccf.org:8080/pilot/ortho/superfpn.htm.

52. Cleveland Clinic Foundation Department of General Anesthesiology: Tibial nerve block. 1999. http://www.anes.ccf.org:8080/pilot/ortho/tibil.htm.

53. Cleveland Clinic Foundation Department of General Anesthesiology: Sural nerve. 1999. http://www.anes.ccf.org:8080/pilot/ortho/sural.htm.

54. Cleveland Clinic Foundation Department of General Anesthesiology: Ankle block. 1999. http://www.anes.ccf.org:8080/pilot/ortho/anklanat.htm.

55. Dannemiller Memorial Educational Foundation: Anesthesia for ankle and foot surgery. 1998. http://www.pain.com/regional/racme_jan98/rajan98_anklefoot.cfm.

56. Hess J: A review of regional blocks for the foot. *J Am Assoc Nurse Anesthetists* 1998; 66(1):82–87.

57. Cleveland Clinic Foundation Department of General Anesthesiology: Toxicity of local anesthetics. 1999. http://www.anes.ccf.org:8080/pilot/ortho/la_toxic.htm.

58. Dannemiller Memorial Educational Foundation: Choice of local anesthetic agent: a matter of safety as well as efficacy. 1998. http://www.pain.com/regional/racme_jan98/rajan98_choiceof.cfm.

59. Eisenach JC, De Kock M, Klimscha W: α_2-Adrenergic agonists for regional anesthesia: a clinical review of clonidine (1984–1995). *Anesthesiology* 1996; 85(3):655–674.

Chapter 107
INTRAVENOUS REGIONAL ANESTHESIA

Kenneth D. Candido
Eric L. Pedicini
Alon P. Winnie

INTRODUCTION

The technique of intravenous regional anesthesia (IVRA) was first introduced by August Bier in 1908.[1] IVRA essentially consists of injecting local anesthetic solution into the venous system of an extremity (upper or lower) that has been exsanguinated by compression and/or gravity and isolated from the central circulation by means of a tourniquet. Procaine in concentrations of 0.25% to 0.5% was injected through an intravenous cannula placed between two Esmarch bandages utilized as tourniquets to divide the arm into proximal and distal compartments in Bier's original technique.[2–4] He noted two distinct types of anesthesia. The first was an almost immediate onset of "direct" anesthesia between the two tourniquets. An "indirect" anesthesia distal to the distally placed tourniquet was noted after a delay of 5 to 7 minutes. This technique was eventually renamed the Bier block.

Bier performed dissections of the venous system of the upper extremity in cadavers after injecting methylene blue. He was able to determine that the "direct" anesthesia was the result of the local anesthetic agent bathing bare nerve endings in the tissues. The "indirect" anesthesia was most probably due to the local anesthetic agent being transported into the substance of the nerves via the vasa nervorum, where a typical conduction block is affected. Bier's conclusion was that there were two mechanisms of anesthesia associated with his technique: peripheral infiltration block and conduction block.

The only major modification of Bier's technique in the past 90 years has been the development of the double tourniquet technique in current clinical practice.[5–7] The Bier block is appropriate for brief surgical procedures of the upper or lower extremity. However, the technique has certainly gained its greatest acceptance for use in the former case as tourniquet problems and safety issues seem to arise more frequently when IVRA is undertaken in the leg. The Bier block is a procedure that has found utility as a treatment adjunct for patients suffering from complex regional pain syndromes (CRPS, formerly reflex sympathetic dystrophy or sympathetically maintained pain) as an alternative to repeated sympathetic blocks. Chemical sympathectomy using IVRA with agents such as guanethidine or bretylium may last up to five days, as compared to local anesthetic blocks that typically provide analgesia lasting only hours.

INDICATIONS

Intravenous regional anesthesia is appropriate for procedures, surgeries, and manipulations of the extremities requiring anesthesia of up to one hour in duration. It is most suited for laceration repair, reduction of fractures and dislocations, burn care, and minor soft tissue procedures in the Emergency Department. The necessity of exsanguinating the extremity is a potentially painful maneuver that may preclude certain procedures from being undertaken with this technique. The Bier block is acceptable in the anticoagulated patient, a feature that distinguishes this technique from other regional anesthesia procedures (spinal block, epidural block, or plexus blocks).

CONTRAINDICATIONS

The only absolute contraindication for IVRA is patient refusal. Relative contraindications include crush injuries of an extremity, the inability to obtain peripheral venous access in the affected extremity, local skin infections, cellulitis, and compound fractures. Patients having manifested a previous allergy to local anesthetic agents should probably be excluded from consideration. Patients with severe vascular injuries to the extremity requiring treatment are not suitable candidates for IVRA. Patients with arteriovenous fistulas should be excluded from consideration, as well as anyone in whom a tourniquet is unsuitable (e.g., severe peripheral vascular disease). The feasibility of using a pneumatic tourniquet in a patient with sickle cell disease must be balanced against the need for performing this type of anesthesia. Tourniquet use in sick patients may induce localized stasis of blood flow, acidosis, and hypoxemia with subsequent formation of sickle cells and a pain crisis.

EQUIPMENT

Povidone iodine solution
Alcohol swabs
Gauze 4×4 squares
Local anesthetic solution, 0.25% to 0.50% lidocaine hydrochloride or 0.50% prilocaine
Penrose drain, 12 to 18 inches long and 7/8 inches wide
18 to 20 gauge angiocatheter
500 to 1000 mL bag of intravenous solution connected to an infusion set
Intravenous catheter, crystalloid solution, and infusion set for the contralateral upper extremity
2 pneumatic tourniquets, size appropriate for the extremity
Esmarch bandage, 60 inches long and 4 inches wide
50 mL Luer-lock syringe
100 mL sterile graduated measuring cup, for mixing of solution
Adhesive tape
Cardiac monitor
Noninvasive blood pressure cuff
Pulse oximeter
Resuscitation equipment
Adjuvants to local anesthesia, parenteral analgesics, and sedatives

PATIENT PREPARATION

Explain the procedure, its risks, and benefits to the patient and/or their representative. Discuss the discomfort that may be experienced during the procedure. Obtain an informed consent to perform the procedure. Place the patient supine on a gurney. Alternatively, place the patient in any other position so long as the vein selected for placement is readily accessible. Assemble all of the required equipment (Figure 107-1). Test the pneumatic tourniquets.

Obtain intravenous access in the affected extremity with a saline-locked angiocatheter. The addition of saline-locked intravenous extension tubing to the angiocatheter is optional and preferred by some physicians. Place the angiocatheter in the forearm or antecubital fossa for procedures involving the elbow region. Place the angiocatheter in the dorsum of the hand for procedures involving the hand or forearm. Place the angiocatheter in a foot, ankle, or lower leg vein for lower extremity procedures. Obtain intravenous access in a nonprocedural extremity. Alternatively, central venous access may be secured if required for other reasons.

Place the patient on the cardiac monitor, noninvasive blood pressure cuff, and pulse oximeter. Obtain, record, and assess baseline vital signs. Administer small aliquots of intravenous analgesics (i.e., 1 to 2 µg/kg fentanyl) if the patient is in severe pain to facilitate the exsanguination procedure. **Total patient cooperation is not essential to be successful.** Administer small doses of benzodiazepines (e.g., 15 to 25 µg/kg midazolam) for anxiolysis. An important added benefit to choosing a benzodiazepine is the suppression of the usual convulsant response associated with local anesthetic toxicity, a valid concern in the patient receiving intravenous regional anesthesia. **Check to ensure that resuscitative equipment is present and working properly. The time to look for resuscitative equipment is not when it is needed.**

UPPER EXTREMITY TECHNIQUE

APPLICATION OF THE PNEUMATIC TOURNIQUET

Apply the double pneumatic tourniquet (Figure 107-2). Place one cuff high on the upper arm. Place the second cuff above the angiocatheter and just below the proximal cuff. Elevate the arm. Tightly apply a rubber Esmarch bandage spirally around the arm, starting at the hand and terminating at the distal cuff of the double tourniquet (Figure 107-3). The process of arm elevation followed by the application of an Esmarch bandage exsanguinates the arm. Place the tourniquets about the elbow and proximal forearm for procedures of the hand, wrist, and distal forearm (Figure 107-4).

Apply digital pressure to occlude the axillary artery. Inflate the proximal cuff of the double tourniquet to 50 to 100 mmHg above the patient's systolic blood pressure. **It is important to compress the axillary artery both before and during the inflation of the pneumatic tourniquet.** Venous outflow is prevented before arterial inflow is occluded as the pressure in the tourniquet rises. Exsanguination of the extremity may be incomplete without occlusion of the arterial inflow before the tourniquet is inflated. Remove the Esmarch bandage.

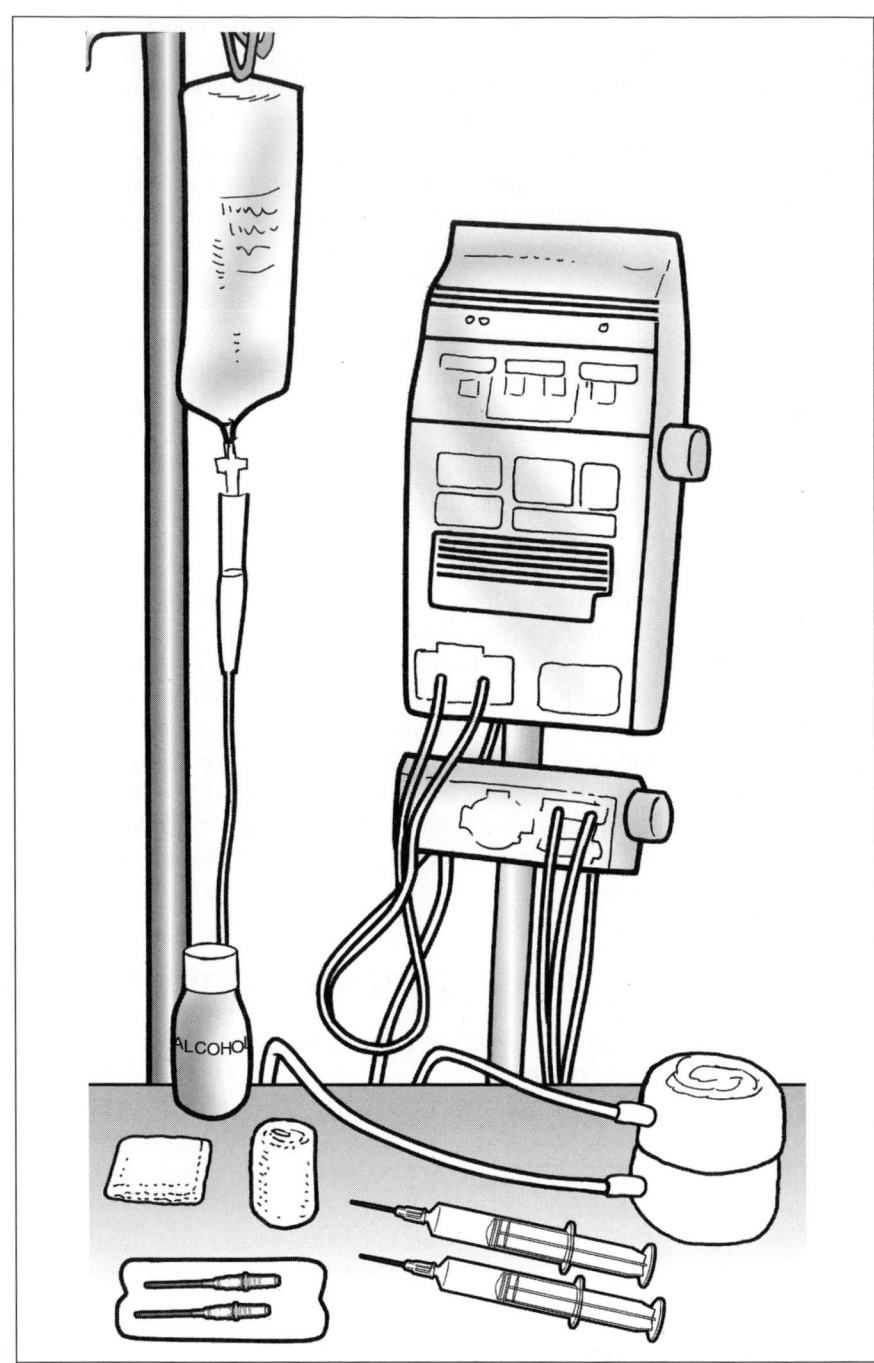

FIGURE 107-1 Essential equipment for IVRA.

INJECTION OF THE LOCAL ANESTHETIC AGENT

Slowly inject 30 to 50 mL, maximum 3 mg/kg, of 0.5% lidocaine hydrochloride. The precise volume depends upon the size of the arm being anesthetized and the maximal anesthetic dose based upon the patient's weight (Table 105-1). **Slow and controlled injection rates are an absolute necessity to avoid the development of elevated venous pressures.** The onset of anesthesia should begin in approximately 5 to 7 minutes. Inflate the distal cuff to 50 to 100 mmHg above the patient's systolic blood pressure approximately 25 to 30 minutes after the onset

of anesthesia. **Slowly deflate the proximal cuff to prevent a rush of local anesthetic solution back into the central circulation.** Deflation of the proximal cuff will minimize the development of tourniquet pain. Begin the procedure for which the IVRA was performed.

The usual dose of lidocaine to administer is approximately 3 mg/kg. This is a relatively large dose in terms of systemic toxicity. Systemic toxic reactions can and do occur due to leakage past the tourniquet, sudden accidental deflation of the tourniquet during the procedure, or intentional deflation following brief surgical proce-

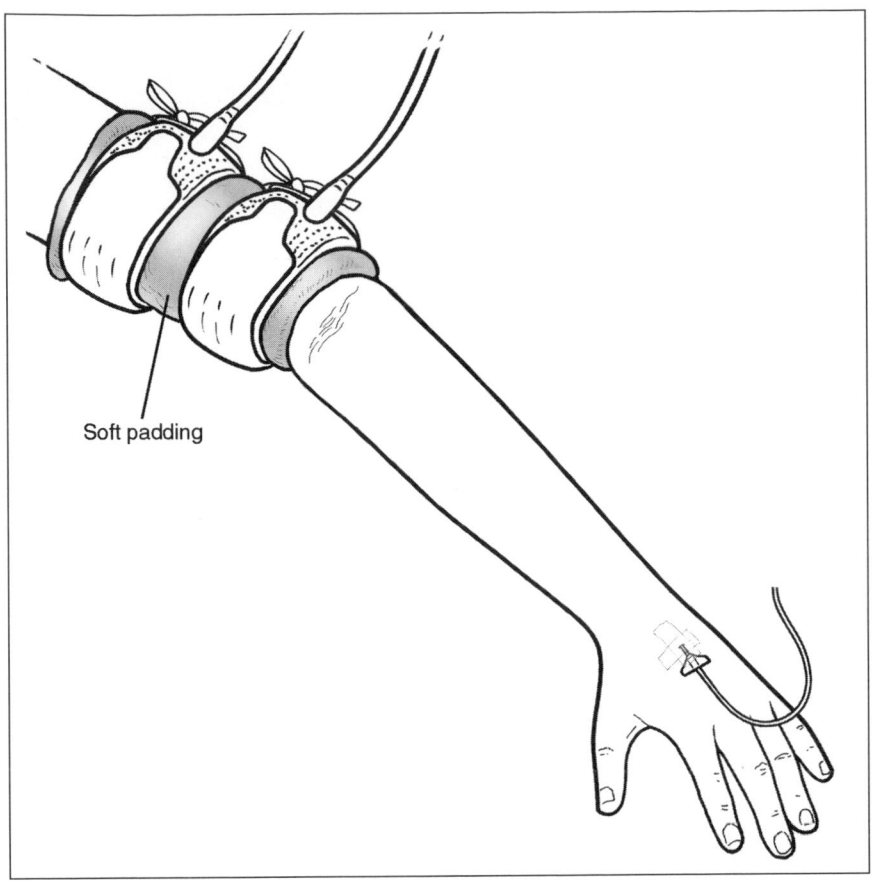

Soft padding

FIGURE 107-2 Preparatory steps. An angiocatheter is inserted into a dorsal hand vein. The double tourniquet is applied to the upper arm after the application of protective padding.

dures.[8,9] Opiate receptors have been discovered in the peripheral nervous system.[10,11] It has been demonstrated that opioids may produce effective, long-lasting analgesia when injected with local anesthetics for brachial plexus blockade.[12–15,33] Several investigators have attempted to decrease the potential for lidocaine toxicity by adding opioids in order to reduce the volume of lidocaine. Although it has not been proven, it appears that the addition of fentanyl to lidocaine for IVRA results in improved analgesia while reducing the risks of lidocaine toxicity.[16,17] Other investigators have found that adding an opioid and a muscle relaxant to 0.25% lidocaine provides the same analgesia and muscular relaxation as 0.5% lidocaine alone and reduces the likelihood of systemic toxicity.

Adjuvants added to 0.25% lidocaine have included 50 μg of fentanyl plus 0.5 mg of pancuronium, fentanyl plus rocuronium, and fentanyl plus D-tubocurarine.[18–21] The authors reported outstanding operating conditions in each of these cases. The lidocaine concentration was reduced in half to 0.25% and the potential for systemic toxicity was also halved. A small dose of any nondepolarizing muscle relaxant may be chosen as an adjunct to the local anesthetic. Avoid using D-tubocurarine as it releases histamine, even in small doses. Other attempts

to improve IVRA have included alkalization by mixing bicarbonate with lidocaine.[22] This has not been demonstrated to hasten the onset or prolong the duration of anesthesia. Adding ketorolac to the lidocaine to suppress tourniquet pain while enhancing postoperative analgesia has shown some efficacy.[23]

Lidocaine is the most commonly utilized local anesthetic agent for IVRA in the United States. Prilocaine (0.5%) is more routinely chosen in Europe. Prilocaine is metabolized to orthotoluidine, an oxidizing compound capable of converting hemoglobin to methemoglobin. This is usually only of concern when the dose of prilocaine is greater than 600 mg, which, even for lower extremity IVRA and volumes as high as 100 mL, should not be attained.

DEFLATION OF THE PNEUMATIC TOURNIQUET

Deflation of the tourniquet, after the procedure was performed, is a critical step to minimizing the possibility of toxicity associated with IVRA. It is absolutely mandatory that the tourniquet not be deflated unless at least 30 minutes have elapsed since the injection of the local anesthetic agent, even if the duration of surgery or manipulation has been very brief. At least one case of cardiac arrest has been reported when the

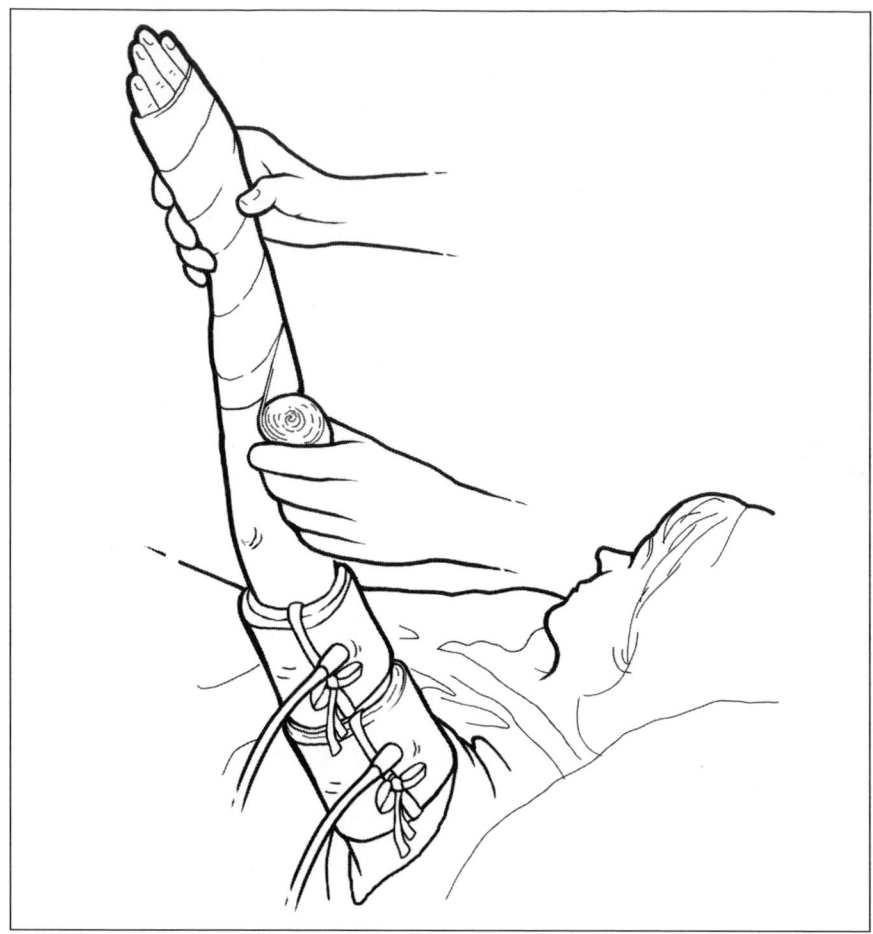

FIGURE 107-3 Exsanguination of the arm. The patient's arm is elevated and an Esmarch bandage is tightly applied.

tourniquet was released soon after the injection of the local anesthetic solution and the duration of surgery was extremely short.[24]

It is absolutely mandatory to deflate the tourniquet in a cyclical fashion. Deflate the cuff and immediately reinflate it to 50 to 100 mmHg above the patient's systolic blood pressure. Observe the patient for 1 minute and question them carefully for the occurrence of symptoms associated with local anesthetic toxicity such as tinnitus, lightheadedness, and a metallic taste in the mouth. Obvious signs of central nervous system stimulation may also represent local anesthetic toxicity. If there are no such signs or symptoms after approximately 1 minute, deflate the cuff and once again immediately reinflate the cuff. Observe the patient for a period of approximately 1 to 2 minutes and question them again for the symptoms associated with local anesthetic toxicity. The tourniquet may be safely deflated and removed if there are no signs and symptoms of local anesthetic toxicity. The safety of the cycled deflation/reinflation allows only a small fraction of the administered (and unbound) local anesthetic agent to enter the systemic circulation.[25] This minimizes

the possibility of a sudden sustained increase in the blood level of the local anesthetic agent.[25]

LOWER EXTREMITY TECHNIQUE

The lower extremity requires double the anesthetic volume for IVRA and is otherwise completely analogous to the upper extremity. Obtain intravenous access in the lower extremity. Place the proximal tourniquet just distal to the femoral pulse. Place the distal tourniquet just above the site of the procedure. Exsanguinate the extremity. Apply digital pressure to the femoral artery while inflating the proximal tourniquet. Inject the local anesthetic agent. Inflate the distal tourniquet and deflate the proximal tourniquet. Perform the procedure for which IVRA was performed. Cyclically deflate the tourniquet.

A modification of the above technique can be performed for procedures about the distal leg, ankle, and foot (Figure 107-5). Place the proximal tourniquet just above the knee joint and the distal tourniquet just below the knee joint. There is one major advantage of this technique. It allows the same volume of local anesthetic

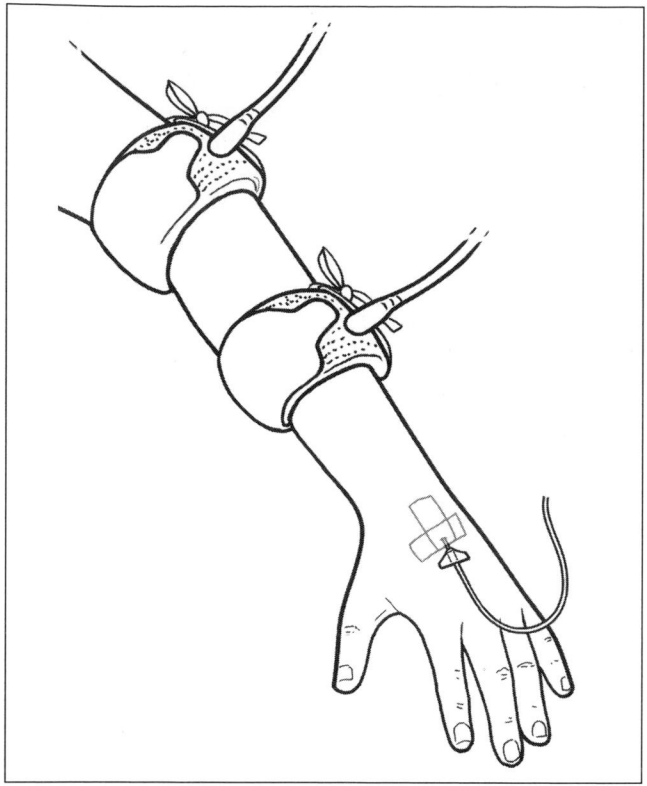

FIGURE 107-4 A modified setup for procedures involving the hand, wrist, and distal forearm.

agent to be used as would be for the upper extremity in the same patient. This is half of the volume required for the entire leg.

ALTERNATIVE TECHNIQUES

Some patients, especially those with painful fractures of the upper or lower extremity, may not be able to tolerate the placement of an Esmarch bandage for exsanguination of the extremity. It may be completely appropriate to forego the Esmarch bandage. Instead, simply elevate the extremity while occluding the axillary artery for a minimum of 5 minutes to effect the requisite venous drainage of the extremity.

Alternatively, exsanguination may be painlessly and effectively accomplished using a zippered pneumatic splint if simply elevating the extremity is not sufficient to effect this process and IVRA is still considered the technique of choice.[26] Apply the double tourniquet. Place the patient's extremity on the open splint and close the zipper. Inflate the splint to a pressure well above the patient's systolic pressure. Inflate the proximal cuff of the tourniquet. Deflate and remove the splint. The gradual inflation of the pneumatic splint is usually more comfortable whereas applying an Esmarch bandage to a painful fracture produces excessive pain. This improves

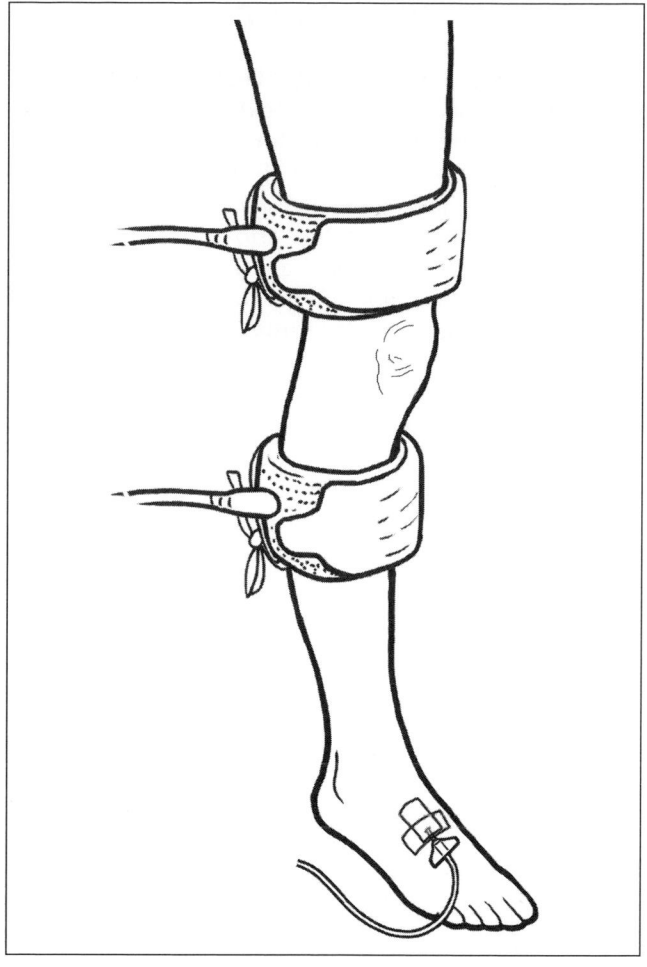

FIGURE 107-5 Placement of the double tourniquet for IVRA of the foot, ankle, and distal leg.

the likelihood of the patient accepting the technique and hence enhances the chance for success with IVRA.

Prilocaine (0.5%) is usually selected for IVRA in countries outside the United States. The addition of opioids to prilocaine has not been shown to improve success with the technique.[27–29] The addition of bicarbonate to prilocaine shortens the onset time of anesthesia and prolongs the duration of anesthesia.[30,31] The addition of clonidine to prilocaine dramatically suppresses tourniquet pain but does not alter postoperative pain following tourniquet deflation.[32]

The addition of long-acting and potent lipophilic opioids with agonist-antagonist activity, such as buprenorphine, to local anesthetics administered for brachial plexus blockade has recently been demonstrated to provide effective anesthesia and long-lasting postblock analgesia. This technique, being a single-shot procedure, may supplant other methods of anesthetizing the upper extremity and perhaps the lower extremity. It offers a method of prolonging pain management long into the recovery period, which IVRA does not.[33]

ASSESSMENT

Patients must be carefully observed for signs and symptoms of local anesthetic toxicity following injection of local anesthetic agents for IVRA. It is mandatory to remain in verbal contact with patients. Continually monitor their vital signs including the electrocardiogram, blood pressure, pulse, and oxygen saturation. Adjuvants added to the local anesthetic agent may result in concomitant side effects or toxicities unrelated to the local anesthetic agent utilized. Muscle relaxants can result in patients developing muscle weakness if the medications gain access directly into the systemic circulation. This may necessitate assisted or controlled ventilation and, occasionally, the establishment of an artificial airway if symptoms are severe. Opioids can result in signs of sedation and respiratory depression. This would be quite rare following the small doses of opioid that would normally be administered as supplementation for IVRA.

Just as important as assessing patients for adverse reactions due to technical or pharmacological methodology in IVRA, it is important to ensure that IVRA has been effective in providing appropriate analgesia for the intended surgery or manipulation to proceed uneventfully. Fortunately, the success rate with IVRA has been reported to be as high as 96 percent in one large series of patients.[41] Supplemental local anesthesia, intravenous sedatives and analgesics, or general anesthesia may be required if IVRA is unsuccessful or only partially effective in preventing nociceptive stimuli from being experienced by the patient.

Patients must be treated following standard basic and advanced cardiac and pulmonary life-support protocols, with oxygen always being the first administered intervention should toxicity or complications develop following IVRA.

The patient assessment does not end after completing the mechanical portion of IVRA. Tourniquet problems may develop during the procedure and result in leakage of local anesthetic and/or adjuvant into the systemic circulation (see section on complications). Release and deflation of the tourniquet may be associated with significant morbidity if strict adherence to the guidelines in this text are not followed.

AFTERCARE

Carefully observe the patient after IVRA has been completed. It is important to keep the extremity relatively quiescent in the immediate post-procedural period. Remove the intravenous cannula and apply a sterile dressing over the injection site. Assess the extremity for signs of venous or arterial insufficiency every 30 minutes, or at more frequent intervals if necessary. Peripheral nerve function will rapidly return following the deflation of the tourniquet, but should nevertheless be examined and documented. Continually monitor vital signs at intervals no greater than every 5 minutes for the first 30 minutes, and as indicated by the patient's clinical status thereafter. Additional intravenous or intramuscular analgesics may be administered at this time if the patient is experiencing pain as IVRA affords no prolongation of antinociception once the tourniquet has been deflated. Patients must be able to bear weight and ambulate (if appropriate) prior to being discharged if the lower extremity was chosen for IVRA. Patients may be discharged into the care of a responsible adult (for outpatients) or back to their respective wards or units (for inpatients) once they meet the established criteria if there have been no untoward effects of the procedure and the IVRA. Instruct the patient regarding the use of the extremity, depending of course upon the nature of the intervention performed upon it.

Perform a detailed follow-up within 24 hours, either by telephone for outpatients or in person for inpatients. Place the emphasis on peripheral sensory, motor, and sympathetic nerve function.

COMPLICATIONS

Local anesthetic agents themselves have relatively narrow therapeutic indices. Systemic toxicity involves primarily the central nervous system and the cardiovascular system. There also may be localized neural and skeletal muscle irritation or allergic phenomena, all supporting the admonition for vigilance following injection for IVRA. Local anesthetic toxicity usually progresses through several well-defined stages unless a gross overdosage has been directly administered systemically. These include numbness of the tongue and lightheadedness followed by visual and auditory disturbances. This progresses to muscular twitching, unconsciousness, convulsions, coma, respiratory depression, cardiovascular depression, and with death ensuing in the absence of treatment.

These events progress along plasma concentrations of about 3 to 24 μg/mL of lidocaine for the most severe signs and symptoms. A correlation exists between the convulsive blood level of various local anesthetic agents and their relative anesthetic potencies. Prilocaine and lidocaine are on the lower, least potent, and least toxic end of that spectrum. However, the rate of injection and the rapidity with which a particular blood level is achieved will influence the toxicity of these agents.

The patient's acid-base status will have a profound influence on the CNS activity of the local anesthetic agent. Convulsive thresholds are inversely related to arterial $PaCO_2$. This further emphasizes the importance of continually assessing patients, both verbally as well as by noninvasive monitors, following injection of the local anesthetic agent. Avoid oversedation as it tends to result in respiratory depression and the concomitant elevation of arterial CO_2.

Lidocaine is well known to depress the maximal rate of cardiac depolarization and cardiac contractility while not significantly altering the resting membrane potential of cardiac muscle. **Continually assess the electrocardiogram during and after the injection of this agent for IVRA.** Blood pressure monitoring is also mandatory, since local anesthetic agents exert a biphasic action on smooth muscle of peripheral blood vessels. Vasoconstriction is seen early followed by vasodilatation if levels continue to rise unabated. Strict adherence to the recommended doses presented in this chapter will essentially prevent most of the dreaded complications due to excessive dosing.

Lidocaine and prilocaine are both amino-amide type local anesthetic agents having pKa's of 7.7 and are between 55 to 65 percent protein bound. They therefore react rather similarly when utilized for IVRA. **Assess the patient for the development of methemoglobinemia if prilocaine is administered for IVRA.** The methemoglobinemia resulting from prilocaine is spontaneously reversible. It can alternatively be corrected by administering intravenous methylene blue. The incidence of allergic phenomena associated with the use of lidocaine and prilocaine is not common because amino-amide agents are not derived from para-aminobenzoic acid. Nevertheless, patients must be monitored for the development of allergic reactions following injection for IVRA.

Complications due to IVRA may be classified either as drug-related or tourniquet-related. Drug-related complications depend both upon the agent being administered directly into the vascular system and the equipment utilized to isolate the vascular space from the systemic circulation. Inadvertent deflation of the cuff, cuff failure, a sudden increase in venous pressure within the occluded tissue to a level higher than cuff pressure, and an intact interosseous circulation may all contribute to drug-related complications when using IVRA.

Lidocaine is the most commonly utilized local anesthetic for IVRA and is therefore the agent about which most complications have been reported. Fortunately, lidocaine does not accumulate to any great extent at sodium channels at therapeutic plasma concentrations.[34,35] Toxic accumulation of the drug at the sodium channels is atypical since it both rapidly binds to and dissociates from the channel.[34,35] Excessive plasma concentrations of lidocaine associated with intravenous boluses of large doses with a faulty tourniquet system result in peripheral vasodilatation and diminished cardiac contrac-

tility that manifests clinically as hypotension. The onset and termination of lidocaine anesthesia is relatively rapid.[36] The usual onset of IVRA using 0.5% lidocaine is about 4.5 ± 0.3 minutes. The termination of anesthesia once the tourniquet has been deflated is about 5.8 ± 0.5 minutes. There are usually no signs or symptoms of cardiovascular or central nervous system toxicity if the tourniquet is deflated at least 5 minutes after the drug is injected into the venous system, although tinnitus has been noted.[37]

Approximately 70 percent of the administered lidocaine dose remains within the tissues of the isolated limb after tourniquet deflation.[35] The remaining 30 percent enters the systemic circulation during the ensuing 45 minutes.[35] **Much more local anesthetic is released from the tissues of the isolated limb into the circulation after tourniquet deflation if the limb is inadvertently exercised. This emphasizes the importance of maintaining the previously anesthetized extremity quiescent for some time immediately following tourniquet deflation.**

The other commonly utilized local anesthetic agent for IVRA, prilocaine, is associated with the formation of methemoglobin in about 4 to 8 hours after administration.[34] Fortunately, significant methemoglobinemia has not been reported when prilocaine has been used for IVRA. Prilocaine administered for IVRA has an onset of analgesia in about 11 ± 6.8 minutes.[38] Termination of analgesia following tourniquet deflation averages 7.2 ± 4.6 minutes.[38] The use of prilocaine for IVRA appears to be extraordinarily safe. There were no serious side effects or deaths reported by using this technique in one survey of 45,000 prilocaine blocks.[39] The effectiveness of prilocaine seems to be equivalent to lidocaine when used for IVRA.

Opioids can be administered in combination with local anesthetic agents for IVRA in an attempt to prolong analgesia following cuff deflation. Occasional side effects typically attributed to opioids given systemically may be noted following cuff deflation. These include nausea, vomiting, and mild sedation.[16,27]

Neuromuscular blocking drugs can be administered in conjunction with local anesthetic agents to improve conditions for patients undergoing fracture reduction. There have been no reports of significant complications due to this adjuvant.

An intact tourniquet system is absolutely essential for the successful performance of IVRA. Unintentional deflation of the tourniquet or the presence of an arteriovenous communication, even with an intact tourniquet, may result in serious sequelae due to IVRA. The tourniquet itself may be a source of complications. It may result in discomfort or ischemic pain. Systemic hypertension can occur from prolonged tourniquet inflation. Equipment misuse or malfunction is an important and avoidable source of complications. An intact and functioning tourniquet may be associated with leakage of local anesthetic agents from a supposedly isolated extremity into the systemic circulation.[40,41] Lower limb IVRA has almost a 100 percent incidence of local anesthetic leakage from beneath the tourniquet versus a 25 percent incidence for the upper extremity.[42] The use of IVRA for lower extremity analgesia has an associated incidence of poor quality block in almost 40 percent of patients in one prospective study.[43] Local anesthetic may leak past an apparently fully functioning cuff due to the interosseous circulation that is not affected by occlusion of muscles and soft tissues. The functional significance of this circulation has been recognized for almost 35 years, yet it does not appear to be a significant factor in the production of complications due to IVRA.[44]

Tourniquet deflation after IVRA is associated with signs and symptoms of systemic local anesthetic toxicity ranging from mild CNS-related events, such as tinnitus and perioral numbness, to devastating cardiovascular collapse. These correlate with the local anesthetic concentrations in arterial blood and not to venous concentrations.[25,45] Intermittent cuff deflation may effectively prolong the time to achieve peak local anesthetic arterial concentrations, but may not be entirely reliable in minimizing toxicity due to release of local anesthetic agents into the circulation.[25] **Just as importantly, the tourniquet should not be deflated until at least 10 minutes, and for greater safety 30 minutes, have elapsed from the time the local anesthetic is injected into the isolated venous system.**

Another complication of IVRA is tourniquet pain that commonly occurs if a double pneumatic tourniquet is not utilized.[41] We recommend the use of such a tourniquet for any procedure performed under IVRA expected to last longer than 30 minutes.

There are very rare and isolated reports of neurological complications associated with IVRA that include damage to the median, ulnar, and musculocutaneous nerves.[46] The etiology of such complications appears to be direct pressure from the tourniquet. These nerves subsequently exhibit histologic changes resembling crush injuries. It is recommended that the tourniquet time not exceed 2 hours duration to reduce the likelihood of capillary and muscle damage secondary to tissue acidosis.[46,47]

A compartment syndrome may rarely occur following IVRA. This is especially true when IVRA is used for reduction of long bone lower extremity fractures. It may be due to the large volume of anesthetic injected to effect analgesia as well as inadequate or incomplete exsanguinations of the limb prior to performing the block.[48,49] A compartment syndrome resulted from the inadvertent injection of hypertonic saline solution instead of local anesthetic solution.[50] One case report of a compartment syndrome resulted in the amputation of an arm in a 28 year old patient who thrombosed her radial and ulnar arteries following IVRA after a relatively brief tourniquet occlusion time.[51] Whether this resulted from unsuspected intraarterial injection of drug, a drug administration error, or perhaps an idiosyncratic drug reaction is purely speculative.

SUMMARY

Intravenous regional anesthesia is a valuable adjunct to the armamentarium of clinicians in any specialty dealing with the acutely injured patient. The simplicity of the technique and the relative safety, if strict adherence to the above listed rules is maintained, make it an attractive alternative to a brachial plexus block, spinal block, or epidural block. Simply being able to identify a peripheral vein, secure intravenous access, and use a pneumatic tourniquet makes this one of the most user-friendly regional anesthetic procedures. One of the only potential downsides to IVRA is the very finite duration of anesthesia and the inability to prolong analgesia into the postoperative or post-procedural period.

REFERENCES

1. Bier A: Uber einen neun weg localanaesthesia an den gliedmassen zu erzeugen. *Arch Klin Chir* 1908; 86:1007–1016.
2. Bier A: On a new method of local anesthesia. *Muench Med Wschir* 1909; 56:589.
3. Bier A: Concerning venous anesthesia. *Berl Klin Wschr* 1909; 46:477–489.
4. Bier A: On local anesthesia with special reference to vein anesthesia. *Edinburgh Med J* 1910; 5:103–123.
5. Morrison JT: Intravenous local anesthesia. *Brit J Surg* 1930–31; 18:641–647.
6. Herreros LG: Regional anesthesia by the intravenous route. *Anesthesiology* 1946; 7:558–560.
7. Holmes CMcK: Intravenous regional analgesia. A useful method of producing analgesia of the limbs. *Lancet* 1963; 1:245–247.
8. Brown EM, McGriff JT, Malinowski RW: Intravenous regional anesthesia (Bier block): a review of 20 years' experience. *Can J Anaesth* 1989; 36(3):307–310.
9. Mazze RI, Dunbar RW: Intravenous regional anesthesia—report of 497 cases with a toxicity study. *Acta Anaesthesiol Scand* 1969; 36:27–34.
10. Fields HL, Emson PC, Leigh BK, et al: Multiple opiate receptor sites on primary afferent fibers. *Nature* 1980; 284:351–353.
11. Young WS, Wamsley JK, Zarbin MA, et al: Opioid receptors undergo axonal flow. *Science* 1980; 210:76–78.

12. Boogaerts JR, Balatoni E, Lafont N, et al: Utilisation des morphiniques dans les blocs nerveux peripheriques. *Congres Ser Ars Medicina* 1985; 3:143–150.

13. Gobeaux D, Landais A: Utilisation de deux morphineiques dans les blocs du plexus brachial. *Can J Anaesth* 1988; 36(6):437–440.

14. Gobeux D, Landais A, Bexon G, et al: Adjonction de fentanyl la lidocaine adrenaline pour le blocage du plexus brachial. *Can J Anaesth* 1987; 35(3):195–199.

15. Viel EJ, Eledjam JJ, de la Coussaye JE, et al: Brachial plexus block with opioids for postoperative pain relief: comparison between buprenorphine and morphine. *Reg Anesth* 1989; 14(6):274–278.

16. Arthur JM, Mian T, Heavner JE, et al: Fentanyl and lidocaine versus lidocaine for Bier block. *Reg Anesth* 1992; 17(4):223–227.

17. Bobart V, Hartmannsgruber MWB, Atanassoff PG, et al: Analgesia/anesthesia after fentanyl + lidocaine vs. plain lidocaine for intravenous regional anesthesia. *Anesth Analg* 1998; 86:S3.

18. Abdulla WY, Fadhil NM: A new approach to intravenous regional anesthesia. *Anesth Analg* 1992; 75:597–601.

19. Sztark F, Thicoipe M, Favarel-Garriques JF, et al: The use of 0.25% lidocaine with fentanyl and pancuronium for intravenous regional anesthesia. *Anesth Analg* 1997; 84:777–779.

20. Subxedar DV, Gevirtz CM, Malik V, et al: Intravenous regional anesthesia: prospective evaluation of 0.25% lidocaine, with fentanyl and rocuronium. *Reg Anesth* 1997; 22:41.

21. Thapar P, Skerman JH: Evaluation of 0.2% lidocaine with fentanyl and D-tubocurarine for intravenous regional anesthesia. *Anesth Analg* 1997; 84:S342.

22. Benlabed M, Hamza J, Jullian P, et al: Alkalization of 0.5% lidocaine for intravenous regional anesthesia. *Reg Anesth* 1990; 15(2):59–60.

23. Reuben SS, Steiberg RB, Kreitzer JM, et al: Intravenous regional anesthesia using lidocaine and ketorolac. *Anesth Analg* 1995; 81:110–113.

24. Kennedy BR, Duthie AM, Parbrook GD, et al: Intravenous regional anesthesia: an appraisal. *Brit Med J* 1965; 1:954–957.

25. Sukhani R, Garcia CJ, Munhall RJ, et al: Lidocaine disposition following intravenous regional anesthesia with different deflation technics. *Anesth Analg* 1989; 68:633–637.

26. Winnie AP, Ramamurthy S: Pneumatic exsanguination for intravenous regional anesthesia. *Anesthesiology* 1970; 33(6):664–665.

27. Armstrong P, Power I, Wildsmith JAW: Addition of fentanyl to prilocaine for intravenous regional anesthesia. *Anaesthesia* 1991; 46:278–280.

28. Gupta A, Bengtsson M, Bjornsson A, et al: Lack of peripheral analgesic effect of low-dose morphine during intravenous regional anesthesia. *Reg Anesth* 1993; 18(4):250–253.

29. Pitkanen MT, Rosenberg PH, Pere PJ, et al: Fentanyl-prilocaine mixture for intravenous regional anesthesia in patients undergoing surgery. *Anaesthesia* 1992; 47:395–398.

30. Armstrong P, Brockway M, Wildsmith JAW: Alkalinization of prilocaine for intravenous regional anesthesia. *Anaesthesia* 1990; 45:11–13.

31. Solak M, Akturk G, Erciyes N, et al: The addition of sodium bicarbonate to prilocaine solution during I.V. regional anesthesia. *Acta Anesthesiol Scand* 1991; 35:572–574.

32. Cucchia G, Chasot-Di Dio V, VanGessei E, et al: Effect of addition of clonidine to local anesthetic during the Bier block on the pre- and postoperative analgesia. *Br J Anaesth* 1997; 78 (suppl 1):78–79.

33. Candido KD, Khan MA, Raja DS, et al: Brachial plexus block with buprenorphine for postoperative pain relief. *Reg Anesth* 2000; 25(2):23.

34. Bader AM, Concepcion M, Hurley RJ, et al: Comparison of lidocaine and prilocaine for intravenous regional anesthesia. *Anesthesiology* 1988; 69(3):409–412.

35. Tucker GT, Boas RA: Pharmacokinetic aspects of intravenous anesthesia. *Anesthesiology* 1971; 34(6):538–548.

36. Ware RJ: Intravenous regional analgesia using bupivacaine. a double blind comparison with lignocaine. *Anaesthesia* 1979; 34:231–235.

37. Smith CA, Steinhaus JE, Haynes CD: The safety and effectiveness of intravenous regional anesthesia. *South Med J* 1968; 61:1057–1060.

38. Pitkanen MT, Suzuki N, Rosenberg PH: Intravenous regional anaesthesia with 0.5% prilocaine or 0.5% chloroprocaine. a double-blind comparison in volunteers. *Anaesthesia* 1992; 47:618–619.

39. Bartholomew K, Sloan JP: Prilocaine for Bier's block: how safe is safe? *Arch Emerg Med* 1990; 7:189–195.

40. Mazze RI, Dunbar RW: Plasma lidocaine concentrations after caudal, lumbar epidural, axillary block, and intravenous regional anesthesia. *Anesthesiology* 1966; 27(5):574–578.

41. Dunbar RW, Mazze RI: Intravenous regional anesthesia: experience with 779 cases. *Anesth Analg* 1967; 46(6):806–811.

42. Davies JA, Walford AJ: Intravenous regional anaesthesia for foot surgery. *Acta Anaesthesiol Scand* 1986; 30:145–147.

43. Kim DD, Shuman C, Sadr B: Intravenous regional anesthesia for outpatient foot and ankle surgery: a prospective study. *Orthopedics* 1993; 16(10): 1109–1112.

44. Cotev S, Robin GC: Experimental studies on intravenous regional anaesthesia using radioactive lignocaine. *Br J Anaesth* 1966; 38:936–940.

45. Hargrove RL, Hoyle JR, Parker JB, et al: Blood lignocaine levels following intravenous regional analgesia. *Anaesthesia* 1966; 21(1):37–41.

46. Larsen UT, Hommelgaard P: Pneumatic tourniquet paralysis following intravenous regional analgesia. *Anaesthesia* 1987; 42:526–528.

47. Shaw-Wilgis EF: Observations on the effects of tourniquet ischemia. *J Bone Jt Surg Br* 1971; 53A(7):1343–1345.

48. Mabee JR, Bostwick TL, Burke MK: Iatrogenic compartment syndrome from hypertonic saline injection in Bier block. *J Emerg Med* 1994; 12(4):473–476.

49. Quigley JT, Popich GA, Lanz UB: Compartment syndrome of the forearm and hand: a case report. *Clin Orthop* 1981; 161:247–251.

50. Hastings H II, Misamore G: Compartment syndrome resulting from intravenous regional anesthesia. *J Hand Surg* 1987; 12A(4):559–562.

51. Luce EA, Mangubat E: Loss of hand and forearm following Bier block: a case report. *J Hand Surg* 1983; 8A(3):280–283.

Chapter 108
NITROUS OXIDE ANESTHESIA

Robert Bilkovski

INTRODUCTION

Joseph Priestly discovered nitrous oxide in 1772, shortly after his discovery of oxygen. Humphry Davy was the first to identify the analgesic and anesthetic effects of nitrous oxide in the late eighteenth century. Oxygen was added to the nitrous oxide mixture in 1868 in order to prevent hypoxia that was commonly seen. The first detailed analysis of nitrous oxide-oxygen mixtures as they apply to pain relief without sedation or hypoxia was published by Stanislav Klikovich in 1881.

Nitrous oxide-oxygen mixtures were first applied in an ambulatory setting in 1955; dentists in Denmark used them for office-based procedures. A 50-50 mixture of nitrous oxide with oxygen (Entonox) has been used by the British Ambulance Service in a self-administered format since 1970.[1] Nitrous oxide-oxygen mixtures became popular in the United States as a sedative/analgesic for use in the Emergency Department during the late 1970s.[2]

ANATOMY AND PATHOPHYSIOLOGY

Nitrous oxide (N_2O) is a colorless gas; it has a sweet odor and is heavier than air. The gas diffuses rapidly across biologic membranes, resulting in a rapid onset and short duration of action. The precise mechanism of action is unknown. However, involvement of the endogenous opioid system has been suggested.[3] **The gas has the five actions of mild sedation, anxiolysis, mild to moderate analgesia, weak anesthesia, and mild dissociative effects.**[4]

Nitrous oxide is 34 times more soluble in plasma than nitrogen. It quickly diffuses across biologic membranes (lung-blood and blood-CNS), which accounts for its rapid onset of action (60 to 90 seconds). The maximal effect occurs within 2 minutes of administration. Its duration of action is 2 to 5 minutes after discontinuation of the administration. **Nitrous oxide does not have significant cardiovascular or respiratory depressant effects.**

It does not result in a loss of the patient's protective airway reflexes. It rapidly depresses all cerebral cortical functions including all five senses. Nitrous oxide rapidly diffuses into pockets of trapped gas (dilated bowel, pneumothorax, pneumoperitoneum). Nitrogen is displaced and replaced by larger amounts of nitrous oxide that results in increased pressure and volume within the confined space. Nitrous oxide is lipid insoluble resulting in minimal uptake in fat, muscle, and solid organs.

Nitrous oxide has been shown to be effective in 85 percent of cases involving mild to moderate pain.[5] The agent is a more potent anxiolytic than an analgesic. Anxiolysis is obtained by inducing a state of euphoria with a concurrent mild sedating effect. The analgesic effect is a result of an increase in the pain threshold. Combination therapy is often required due to its relatively weak analgesic effects, especially for painful procedures. For example, the infiltration of a local anesthetic agent for laceration repair is made more tolerable following the use of nitrous oxide.

Nitrous oxide used in an ambulatory care setting (e.g., Emergency Department, Dentist Office) is mixed with oxygen in a 50:50 mixture. Nitrous oxide becomes a more effective general anesthetic when concentrations exceed this level. Hypoxemia is a concern at general anesthetic doses. The nitrous oxide-oxygen ratio must be adjusted for altitude due to the effects of a lower atmospheric pressure as well as a lower partial pressure of the gas. Nieto showed that a 70:30 ratio of nitrous oxide to oxygen was effective in Denver, with an elevation of 5000 feet.[6] The sex of the patient does not influence the response to nitrous oxide administration.[6]

INDICATIONS

Nitrous oxide-oxygen mixtures have been shown effective in both the Emergency Department and the prehospital setting to alleviate anxiety as well control mild to moderate pain states. The indications for nitrous oxide use are reserved for patients with mild to moderate pain states, who are anxious, or who will undergo a painful procedure. A more detailed outline of the general uses of nitrous oxide is contained in Table 108-1.

CONTRAINDICATIONS

There are few contraindications to the use of nitrous oxide anesthesia (Table 108-2). **Given that the gas is self-administered, normal cognitive function is required for its safe and effective use.** Patients with altered consciousness, head injuries, or the inability to understand instructions for administration should all be excluded. Children who are younger than 4 years of age cannot properly follow the instructions for the use of the system. Hysterical patients, somnolent patients, and those with altered mental status also cannot comprehend and follow the instructions for the proper use of the system. It is important to restate that nitrous oxide is a relatively weak analgesic and commonly requires supplemental analgesic use (e.g., local anesthetic infiltration or intravenous analgesic administration). Nitrous oxide has the ability to rapidly cross membranes and exchange with nitrogen. Patients with risks for a closed nitrogen-containing space injury are not eligible candidates. This includes patients with a pneumothorax, a pneumoperitoneum, or a bowel obstruction. Rapid diffusion of nitrous oxide into a closed gas-containing space, in combination with its inability to leave the space quickly, results in an increased volume of the space and an increased pressure within the space. Patients undergoing decompression sickness should also be excluded.

EQUIPMENT

Nitrous oxide tank
Oxygen tank
Mixing valve
Scavenging device
Demand valve apparatus
Nasal mask
Face mask
Sensor to measure ambient levels of nitrous oxide
Pulse oximeter
Cardiac monitor
Supplemental oxygen source
Intravenous catheters, tubing and fluid
Analgesic agents
Anxiolytic/sedative agents

A typical hospital-based device applicable for Emergency Department use is shown in Figure 108-1. The

TABLE 108-1. INDICATIONS FOR NITROUS OXIDE ADMINISTRATION

Anginal chest pain	Joint dislocation reduction
Biliary colic	Labor pain
Bladder catheter insertion	Laceration repair
Cervical and uterine procedures	Migraine headache
Cluster headache	Pancreatitis
Colonoscopy	Pelvic and physical
Dental procedures	examinations
Dilation and curettage	Renal colic
Foreign body removal	Tube thoracostomy
Fracture reduction	
Incision and drainage of cysts or abscesses	

mixing valve ensures that a 50:50 mixture of both gases is delivered to the patient. The sources for the nitrous oxide-oxygen mixture can be from premixed cylinders, individual cylinders, or wall units. The device has a fail-safe mechanism that prevents gas flow when either tank becomes empty. It is required, in accordance with the National Institute of Occupational Safety and Health (NIOSH), to have a sensor to monitor ambient levels of nitrous oxide within the treatment area. The scavenging device reduces the ambient levels of nitrous oxide within the treatment area. Elevated levels of nitrous oxide have been associated with a decreased fertility rate, an increased rate of spontaneous abortion, and neurologic disturbances among dental assistants.[7] Ambient levels of nitrous oxide were measured and noted to be 500 ppm following 8 minutes of patient administration.[8] The ambient levels in a similarly sized room were 0 when a scavenging device was added.[9]

Portable units are available for use in clinics and ambulances (Figure 108-2). The nitrous oxide levels will vary in an ambulance with the airflow within the patient compartment. Trace levels of the gas are reduced to safe levels, even without the use of a scavenging device, if the air-conditioning or fans are operating and the ambulance is in motion.[10]

A face mask or nasal mask (suited for pediatric patients) connected to a demand valve will help minimize the unwanted release of nitrous oxide into the treatment area. The demand valve allows for the self-

TABLE 108-2. CONTRAINDICATIONS TO THE USE OF NITROUS OXIDE

Acute myocardial infarction	Hypotension
Alcohol intoxication	Inability to follow or understand instructions
Altered consciousness	
Bowel obstruction	Pneumothorax
Congestive heart failure	Pneumoperitoneum
Decompression sickness	Pregnancy
Facial trauma	Pulmonary edema
Head injuries	Shock

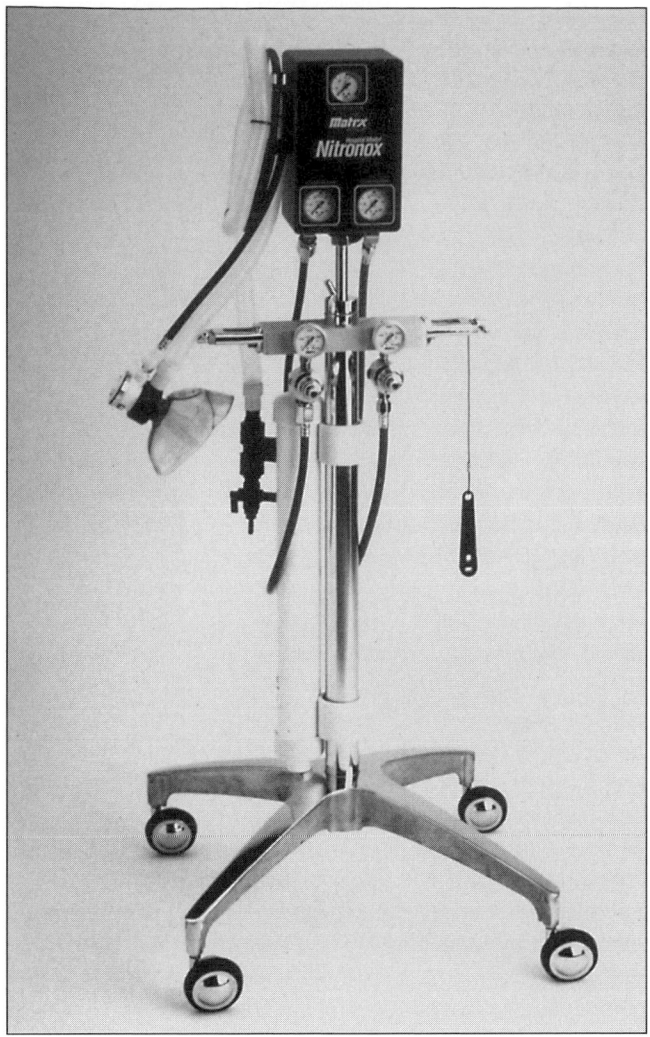

FIGURE 108-1 The free-standing Nitronox machine. Photo courtesy of MDS Matrx, Orchard Park, New York.

administration of the gaseous mixture. A negative inspiratory flow (-1 to -5 cmH$_2$O) must be generated in order to activate the gas flow. An airtight seal is required between the patient's face and the mask in order to achieve a negative inspiratory flow. The demand valve provides for a safe administration of nitrous oxide, minimizes the risk of oversedation, guards against human error, and protects against equipment failure.

PATIENT PREPARATION

Inform the patient and/or their representative of the risks and benefits of nitrous oxide anesthesia. Obtain a signed informed consent for the nitrous oxide anesthesia in addition to the consent for the procedure for which nitrous oxide is administered. Establish intravenous access. Apply cardiac monitoring and pulse ox-

imetry to the patient. Place the patient supine on a gurney or sitting in a procedure (dental) chair that reclines. Preoxygenate the patient for 2 to 3 minutes with 100% oxygen. Encourage the patient to remain calm and breathe in a controlled manner, with special emphasis not to breathe too deeply or rapidly.

TECHNIQUE

The nitrous oxide-oxygen gas mixture can be administered via a nasal mask or a face mask. The nasal mask is used primarily by dentists. It has been shown to be more effective in pediatric patients and patients undergoing procedures around the mouth and chin. The size and positioning of the nasal mask are important for ensuring a snug fit. Encourage the patient to breathe through their nose as opposed to their mouth in a controlled manner (i.e., not too fast or too deep).

The demand valve prevents gas flow unless a negative inspiratory pressure is applied with a self-administered face mask. The patient applies the face mask ensuring an airtight seal that covers both the mouth and nose (Figure 108-3). Do not remove the face mask between breaths unless adverse effects are noted (e.g., dysphoria, headache, nausea, vomiting, lightheadedness, or vertigo). In these circumstances, remove the mask and administer 100% oxygen via a non-rebreather mask for 5 minutes or until the adverse symptoms resolve. The analgesic effects of nitrous oxide are commonly noted within 90 to 120 seconds of the onset of administration.[11] Once the patient becomes mildly sedated (3 to 5 minutes), supplemental analgesics (e.g., wound infiltration of a local anesthetic) may be administered as needed or the procedure can be performed.

The patient cannot overdose on nitrous oxide if the mask is not attached to their face with tape or a strap. The patient will often remove the hand and the mask from their face as a state of analgesia and euphoria develops. The mask will fall off or loosen if the seal is not maintained and the demand valve will not be triggered. **It is extremely important not to secure the mask to the patient's head with straps or tape so that nitrous oxide delivery will cease as the patient falls asleep.** The patient may reapply the mask and self-administer additional nitrous oxide upon awakening or the experience of pain.

Remove the face mask upon completion of the procedure. Administer 100% oxygen for 5 minutes. This increases the rate of elimination of nitrous oxide and minimizes the side effects such as dizziness, lightheadedness, nausea, vomiting, headache, or dysphoria.[12] Record the amount of gas and the duration of time used in the patient's chart. Record this information in the log maintained with the nitrous oxide device. Clean

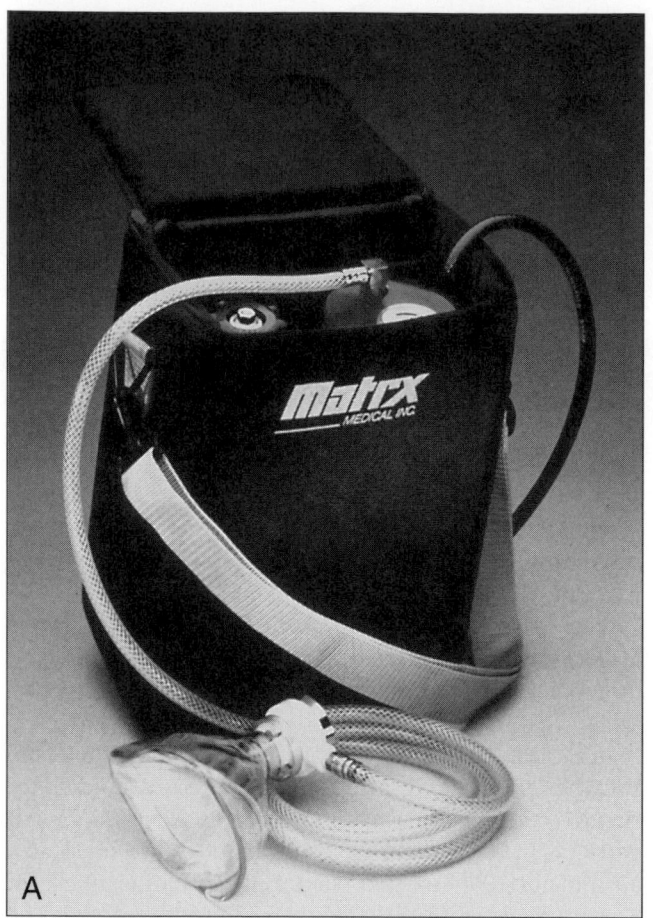
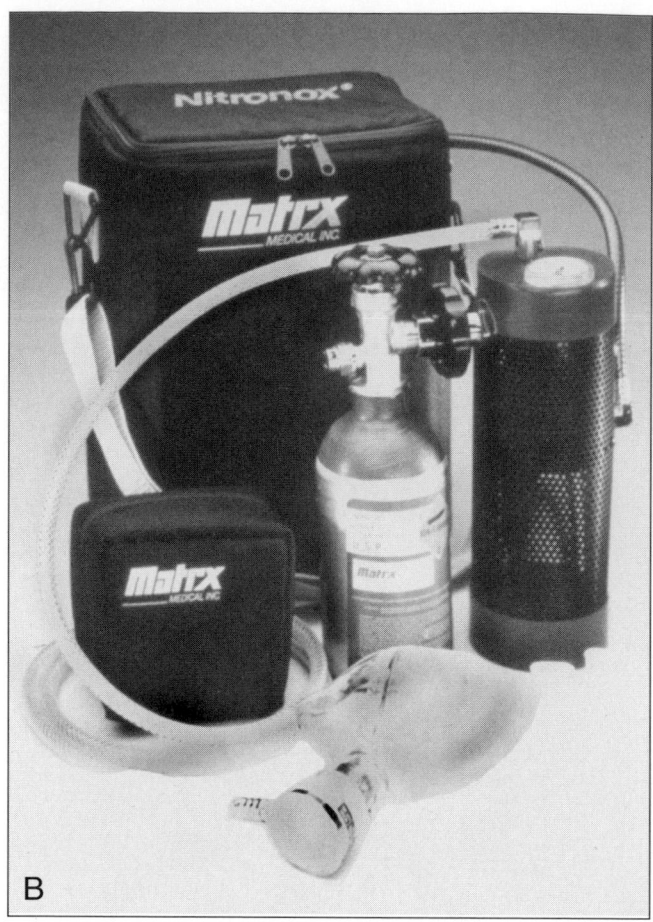

FIGURE 108-2 The portable Nitronox machine. *A.* The unit in a case. *B.* The unit removed from the case. Photos courtesy of MDS Matrx, Orchard Park, New York.

the demand valve apparatus prior to and after each administration.

ASSESSMENT

Ensure that the patient is experiencing adequate analgesia before performing the procedure for which nitrous oxide is administered. Nitrous oxide analgesia is supposed to be the equivalent of administering 10 to 20 mg of morphine. Real use has shown that patients experience a wide range of pain relief (none, mild, moderate, or marked). Nitrous oxide administration may require supplementation with parenteral analgesics, parenteral sedatives, or other anesthetic techniques.

AFTERCARE

There is no aftercare related to the administration of nitrous oxide anesthesia other than 5 minutes of supplemental 100% oxygen via a non-rebreather mask.

COMPLICATIONS

The side effects of a 50:50 nitrous oxide-oxygen mixture are relatively mild. Lightheadedness is most common with the occasional patient complaining of paresthesias or nausea. Donen reported a 19 percent incidence of dizziness, lightheadedness, or vertigo; 4 percent of patients had paresthesias, headache, or amnesia; 5 percent had nausea; and 1 percent had vomiting.[1] There is little to no risk of inducing anesthesia or losing protective reflexes if used in concentrations of 50 percent or less.

The concept of diffusion hypoxia was first described by Fink in 1955.[13] He noted the rapid diffusibility of nitrous oxide could displace oxygen from the alveoli after discontinuation of the gas.[13] This concept has led practitioners to administer 100% oxygen for 5 minutes following discontinuation of nitrous oxide administration. There has been evidence to disprove diffusion hypoxia in low-dose nitrous oxide mixtures (e.g., 50:50 nitrous oxide-oxygen). It is only a legitimate concern at higher concentrations such as that used during general anesthesia. Given the safety of a short course of

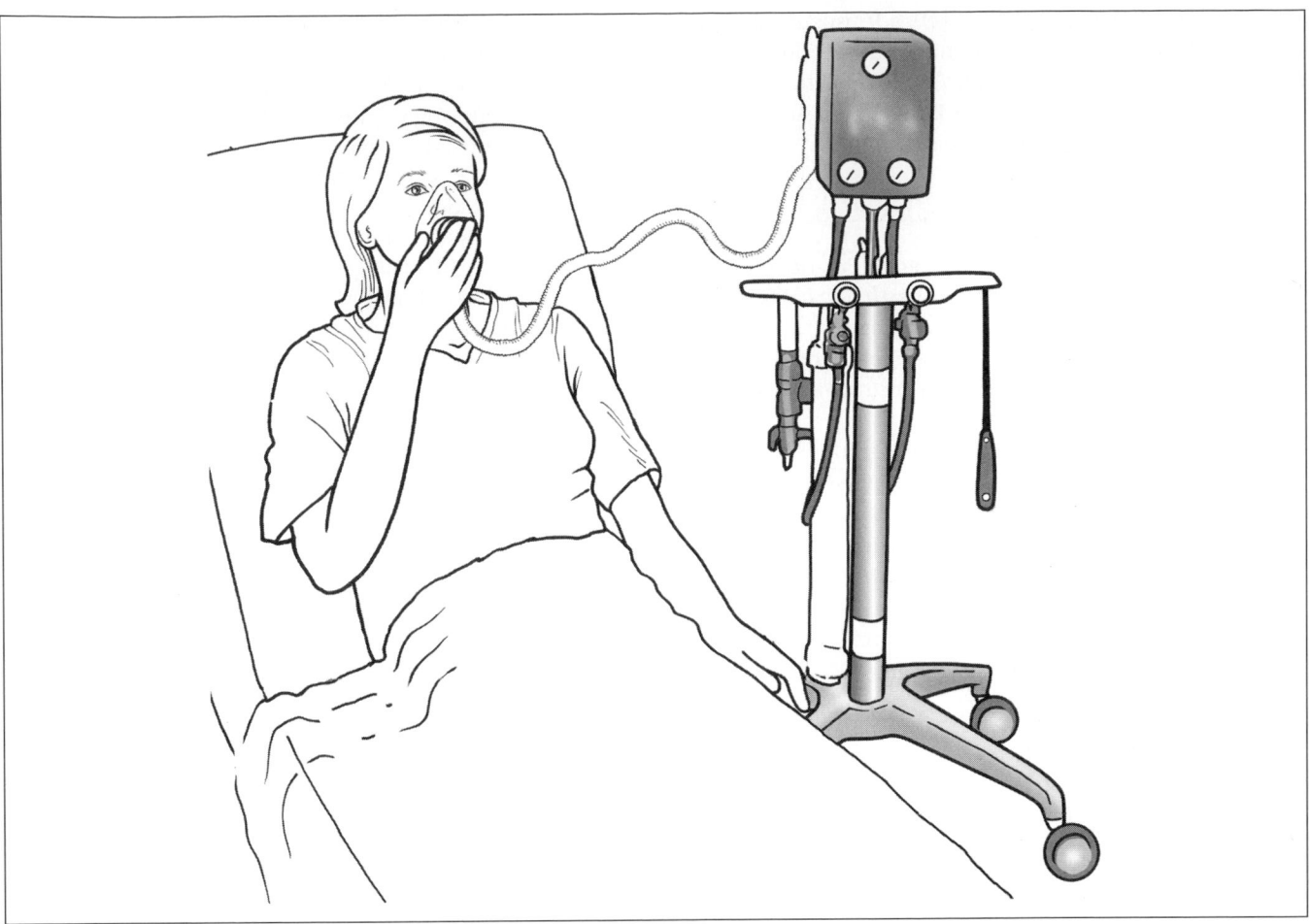

FIGURE 108-3 Use of the Nitronox system by a patient.

100% oxygen, its use following cessation of the nitrous oxide gas is still suggested. The increased oxygen concentration found in the nitrous oxide-oxygen mixture can depress the respiratory drive of patients with COPD, necessitating close monitoring of their ventilatory status.

There has been a growing concern regarding the safety of trace levels of nitrous oxide in the Operating Room, Emergency Department, and dental clinics. There is evidence to show that elevated levels of nitrous oxide are associated with reduced fertility among female dental assistants.[7] Scavenging devices help reduce the ambient levels of nitrous oxide within treatment areas. The demand valve system allows for all exhaled gases to escape into the surrounding environment without a scavenging device. A scavenging device will collect the exhaled gas and remove it from the patient care area.[9] Scavenging devices can maintain ambient levels of nitrous oxide below 1200 ppm according to the guidelines proposed by the National Institute of Occupational Safety and Health (NIOSH).

There has been concern raised about the experimental use of nitrous oxide gas by medical personnel. Prepare a strict protocol on the use of the gas and its associated demand valve apparatus prior to the implementation of nitrous oxide-based procedural sedation in the Emergency Department. Record the volume of gas administered in the patient's chart as well as in a log kept with the nitrous oxide device following each use of nitrous oxide. The demand valve apparatus can be safely secured in the narcotic cabinet or within a Pixis system until it is required for patient use.

SUMMARY

The administration of a nitrous oxide-oxygen mixture has been shown to be safe, effective, and easy to administer in an ambulatory care setting. The gas provides rapid onset of sedation as well as hypnosis. It is a mild anesthetic that helps to facilitate the performance of mildly to moderately painful procedures. The adverse effects are minimal and, given a self-administered application of the gas, concerns of hemodynamic compromise are negligible. The use of nitrous oxide in a closed-space environment should be accompanied by a scavenging device to minimize ambient levels of the gas.

REFERENCES

1. Donen N, Tweed WA, White D, et al: Pre-hospital analgesia with entonox. *Can Anesth Soc J* 1982; 29(3):275–279.

2. Flomenbaum N, Gallagher EJ, Eagen K, et al: Self-administered nitrous oxide: an adjunct analgesic. *JACEP* 1979; 8(3):95–97.

3. Gillman MA: Analgesic (subanesthetic) nitrous oxide interacts with the endogenous opioid system: a review of the evidence. *Life Sci* 1986; 39(14):1209–1221.

4. Pinell MC, Linscott MS: Nitrous oxide in the emergency department. *Am J Emerg Med* 1987; 5(5):395–399.

5. Johnson JC, Atherton GL: Effectiveness of nitrous oxide in a rural EMS system. *J Emerg Med* 1991; 9(1–2):45–53.

6. Nieto JM, Rosen P: Nitrous oxide at higher elevations. *Ann Emerg Med* 1980; 9(12):610–612.

7. Rowland AS, Baird DD, Weinberg CR, et al: Reduced fertility among women employed as dental assistants exposed to high levels of nitrous oxide. *N Engl J Med* 1992; 327(14):993–997.

8. Dula DJ, Skiendzielewski JJ, Royko M: Nitrous oxide levels in the emergency department. *Ann Emerg Med* 1981; 10(11):575–578.

9. Dula DJ, Skiendzielewski JJ, Snover SW: The scavenger device for nitrous oxide administration. *Ann Emerg Med* 1983; 12(12):759–761.

10. Stewart RD: Nitrous oxide, in Paris PM, Stewart RD (eds): *Pain Management in Emergency Medicine.* Norwalk, CT: Appleton and Lange, 1988:221–238.

11. Johnson RAA: Entonox in general practice. *Practitioner* 1979; 222(1331):681–683.

12. Thal ER, Montgomery SJ, Atkins JM, et al: Self-administered analgesia with nitrous oxide: adjunctive aid for emergency medical care systems. *JAMA* 1979; 242(22):2418–2419.

13. Fink BR: Diffusion anoxia. *Anesthesiology* 1955; 16:511–519.

Chapter 109
PROCEDURAL SEDATION AND ANALGESIA (CONSCIOUS SEDATION)

Ronald F. Hayden

INTRODUCTION

Procedural sedation and analgesia techniques are an essential skill for any Emergency Physician. Our daily practice employs painful and anxiety-provoking measures to perform diagnostic testing or therapeutic interventions. These skills not only apply to the operator, but to the individual monitoring the procedure as well. Procedural sedation and analgesia is a skill that may require a credentialing procedure at your respective institution. It probably has evoked a written procedural guide in your respective department, with or without the input from a hospital-wide procedural sedation and analgesia committee or the Department of Anesthesiology. It may require annual competency assessments in the form of a written examination or practical scenarios. It is a technique that probably receives a great deal of attention from the continuous quality improvement committee as a result of the Joint Commission of Accreditation of Hospital Organization's directive. It is a skill that, with proper training and well-designed application principles, will provide your patient and their families with a sense of compassion and caring for their physical and emotional distress. It is a skill that may result in horrific outcomes when performed without appropriate training, knowledge, risk-benefit analysis, and anticipation of complications.

An extensive spectrum of painful and anxiety-provoking clinical presentations arrive in an Emergency Department on any given day. There may be a dislocation reduction, a fracture reduction, a diagnostic lumbar puncture, a sexual assault examination on a child, or neuro-imaging on a combative, head injured patient. Each presentation has a separate subset of variables to consider prior to procedural sedation and analgesia. While Anesthesiologists are still considered the experts in sedation, they are not readily available to the Emergency Department's beck and call. Multiple specialties have developed guidelines for the use of procedural sedation and analgesia to account for these limitations and to ensure that safe, effective care can be rendered to their respective patient populations.[1–3]

The environment of the Emergency Department is unique in many facets of procedural sedation and analgesia due to the fact that situations are nonelective. Procedures are relatively brief, thereby making operating suite time neither timely nor cost effective. Intrinsic to procedural sedation and analgesia is the core training and frequent exposure that Emergency Medicine practitioners have to this particular skill. Who better to handle an untoward cardiopulmonary complication of a procedure than a specialist in the area of airway management and resuscitation?

It will be critical to your techniques and drug selection to take a variety of parameters into consideration before the first medication is administered. The potency and effectiveness of today's newer agents is a double-edged sword. They are invaluable with the correct selection and administration. They are also a recipe for disaster if risks are not appropriately identified and minimized. Monitoring techniques, including pulse oximetry and capnography, are effective adjuncts to procedural monitoring. However, they are no substitute for a trained, dedicated observer.

TERMINOLOGY

Textbooks and review articles use various definitions to define components of procedural sedation and analgesia, formerly known as conscious sedation. Terms such as light and deep sedation are often applied to the extremes of the sedation continuum. **The important thing to realize is that sedation is a continuum.**[2] At the far left of the continuum is the alert and anxious patient. Eye opening, speech, and motor responses diminish as the sedation process proceeds. At the opposite end of the spectrum are CO_2 retention, hypoxia, hypotension, and finally death. These later endpoints are obviously not desirable. Anxiolysis and analgesia are other terms that need definition. The following terminology is representative of current procedural sedation and analgesia jargon.

Analgesia equates to pain relief without alteration in mental status. Analgesia is required in a variety of procedures in which painful manipulation or instrumentation is anticipated. Most potent pain medications will also have a component of sedation, especially the opioids. This sedation component needs to be carefully considered during drug selection and dosing calculations to minimize the risk of overshooting the desired sedation endpoint.

Anxiolysis means to relieve apprehension. Patients may be anxious for any variety of reasons besides the thought of a painful forthcoming procedure. Anxiolysis involves allaying the patient's fears. The agents used for anxiolysis are pure sedatives and no pain relief is implied. Although some degree of sedation is to be expected, it should be minimized with appropriate drug and dosing selection.

Sedation blunts the patient's perception of the surroundings and pain with a depression in the state of wakefulness. Levels of procedural sedation do not follow a discrete stepwise progression. Rather, sedation proceeds along a continuum. This continuum ranges from a mild sedation through deep sedation into general anesthesia. The level is determined by a patient's state of anxiety, wakefulness, and mobility in addition to their ability to retain protective reflexes.

Dissociative sedation implies sedation, analgesia, amnesia, and the induction of a cataleptic state. This state preserves ventilatory drive and maintains protective reflexes while maintaining cardiovascular stability. Ketamine is the primary agent used to induce this state.

Neurolepsis is a reduced motor activity state in which the patient has reduced anxiety and indifference to their surroundings. Neurolepsis is best achieved with major tranquilizers such as haloperidol or droperidol. Its application is best suited to the agitated or violent patient whose behavior places either themself or others at risk for harm.

General anesthesia represents the extreme right of this continuum. The patient has no awareness of the environment and has lost the ability to self-maintain protective reflexes. This is not an endpoint one would desire during procedural sedation and analgesia in the Emergency Department.

Procedural sedation and analgesia is "a technique of administering sedation or dissociative agents with or without analgesics to induce a state that allows the patient to tolerate unpleasant procedures while maintaining cardiorespiratory function. Procedural sedation and analgesia produces a depressed level of consciousness which allows the patient to maintain airway control

independently and continuously. Specifically, the drugs, doses, and techniques used are not likely to produce a loss of protective reflexes" according to the American College of Emergency Physicians Clinical Policy for Procedural Sedation and Analgesia in the Emergency Department.[1]

Standardizing levels of sedation along a continuum has been attempted with various scoring systems.[4] The Ramsey scale was specifically devoted to providing objective determinations of sedation during drug-induced sedation practices. Scoring consists of six sequential scoring levels (Table 109-1).

Another scoring system is the Observer's Assessment of Alertness/Sedation (OAA/S) Scale. It was designed as a research tool for studies incorporating pharmacologic studies with benzodiazepines.[4] The scoring system was based upon the assessment of the patient for responsiveness, speech, facial expressions, and ocular appearance. The OAA/S scale incorporates the patients' responsiveness to the effects of the agents given, in contrast to the similar observational scoring used in the Ramsey scale.

INDICATIONS

A wide variety of clinical presentations and procedures would entail the appropriate use of anxiolysis, sedation, analgesia, or dissociation for case management (Table 109-2). **There are four goals of procedural sedation and analgesia. The first and foremost is to assure patient safety. This is accomplished with a careful risk-benefit assessment and a well-defined clinical procedure to maximize benefit, limit risk, and foresee potential complications. Second is to appropriately assess and deliver adequate analgesia, anxiolysis, sedation, and amnesia as dictated by the patient's needs. Third is to consider the psychological impact of the forthcoming procedure and minimize the impact of these events. Fourth is to provide a fluid transition to the pre-procedural physical and mental status while assuring a safe discharge and post-procedural observation.**

TABLE 109-1. THE RAMSEY SCALE FOR STANDARDIZED LEVELS OF SEDATION[4]

Level	Clinical status	Sedation equivalent
1	Awake, anxious, agitated	None
2	Awake, cooperative, oriented and tranquil	Anxiolysis
3	Awake, responds to commands only	Mild sedation
4	Asleep, responds to brisk stimuli	Moderate sedation
5	Asleep, sluggish response to stimuli	Deep sedation
6	Asleep, no response to stimulation	Anesthesia

TABLE 109-2. THE INDICATIONS FOR PROCEDURAL SEDATION AND ANALGESIA

Anxiolysis/mild sedation (analgesia minimal)
Painless diagnostic studies, i.e., CT scanning
Lumbar puncture
Posterior nasal packing
Pediatric foreign body removal
Pediatric slit lamp examination

Mild sedation and analgesia
Pediatric hand/finger injuries (with local analgesia)
Disimpaction
Vaginal/rectal foreign bodies

Moderate sedation and analgesia
Traction splints for fractures
Burn debridement
Cardioversion
Fracture/joint reduction

Deep sedation and analgesia
I & D perineal/perirectal abscesses
Complex pediatric lacerations
Extensive road rash debridement

Pediatric dissociative sedation
Multiple trauma procedures
Fracture/dislocation reduction
Abscess I & D
Paraphimosis reduction
Complex facial lacerations
Tongue lacerations
Complex hand lacerations
Burn debridement
Sexual assault examination

Adult dissociative sedation
Asthma intubation
Trauma resuscitation
Hemodynamic instability requiring
  sedation
Lengthy and painful procedures

CONTRAINDICATIONS

There are three contraindications to the use of procedural sedation and analgesia. First, known allergy to the individual agent(s) being considered is an absolute contraindication. Ketamine and nitrous oxide have agent specific contraindications. Second is the lack of experienced or credentialed personnel. Procedural sedation and analgesia requires personnel appropriately trained in airway management. Finally, appropriate monitoring capabilities must be available. This includes appropriate equipment monitors as well as personnel to observe the monitors, record procedural flow, and monitor post-procedural recovery.

Issues such as the time of the last oral intake should be considered in the risk-benefit analysis. However, a full stomach does not constitute an absolute contraindication. Concomitant drug or alcohol use is a complicating variable that needs to be recognized and accounted for prior to the procedure. Complicated airway anatomy should also receive particular attention in case emergent airway management is necessary.

EQUIPMENT

Crash cart with resuscitation equipment
Defibrillator
Oxygen source
Oxygen masks
Nasal oxygen cannulas
Oral airways
Nasal airways
Bag-valve-mask device
Continuous pulse oximetry
Capnography, if available
Continuous cardiac monitoring
Intravenous access supplies (catheters, tubing, fluids, etc.)
Suction source
Suction catheters
Pharmaceutical agents
Reversal agents (naloxone, flumazenil)
Succinylcholine

It is imperative that resuscitation equipment be immediately available prior to the onset of procedural sedation and analgesia. Such requirements should be part of the pre-procedural checklist. Age-appropriate equipment must be immediately available. The immediate availability of reversal agents is a prerequisite to the administration of opioids or benzodiazepines. Succinylcholine should be readily available in case of laryngospasm or opioid-induced chest wall tightness.

PATIENT PREPARATION

INFORMED CONSENT

The issue of informed consent is institution specific. Most institutions function under the premise that if a particular procedure has any significant level of risk inherent in its application, informed consent regarding the risks and benefits of the procedure be undertaken with the patient and/or their representative. The benefit to the patient is a careful calculated means at reducing the pain and anxiety associated with a planned diagnostic or therapeutic intervention. The risks are inherent in the medications selected, the patient's current state of physical condition, and complicating conditions (such as time of last meal, recent drug use, or recent alcohol use).

PERSONNEL COMPETENCY/CREDENTIALING

Any physician practicing procedural sedation and analgesia must be competent in airway management and resuscitation. Competency credentialing is institution specific. Physicians may be granted privileges on the basis of their residency training or current practice. Other institutions may mandate a written competency examination or advanced airway/resuscitation training such as ACLS certification.

Nursing personnel must be proficient in medication profiles, medication administration, and patient monitoring. The staff needs to be aware of the department's policies and procedures. Competency testing may be a prerequisite to providing procedural sedation and analgesia. All personnel involved must meet these departmental/institutional requirements prior to initiation of procedural sedation and analgesia.

RISK-BENEFIT ASSESSMENT

Pre-procedural assessment constitutes both a risk assessment and a pre-procedural baseline determination. Assessment requires a determination of the patient's current health and an evaluation of potential risk, adverse reactions, and procedural complications. The old adage "an ounce of prevention is worth a pound of cure" certainly applies with procedural sedation and analgesia. **Thorough preparation is critical to minimize patient risk.** Department procedural flowsheets, complete with pre-procedural assessment checklists, can be a valuable adjunct.

Assign patients an American Society of Anesthesiologists (ASA) Physical Status Classification (Table 109-3). Emergency Department procedural sedation and analgesia would normally be limited to class I or class II patients. Class III or class IV patients are best served in consultation with an Anesthesiologist. Never perform procedural sedation and analgesia on class V patients.

Perform a complete history and physical examination prior to the application of procedural sedation and analgesia. Special emphasis should be directed toward allergies to any analgesic or sedation agent. Previous anesthesia and related complications may be critical to drug selection and/or the involvement of an Anesthesiologist. Conduct a separate assessment of the patient's airway, including dentition. **Age-appropriate**

TABLE 109-3. THE AMERICAN SOCIETY OF ANESTHESIOLOGIST'S (ASA) PHYSICAL STATUS CLASSIFICATION

I.	Healthy patient
II.	Mild systemic disease—no functional limitation
III.	Severe system disease—definite functional limitation
IV.	Severe systemic disease—constant threat to life
V.	Moribund patient—not expected to survive without the operation

airway management equipment must be immediately available in the event airway control becomes necessary. A patient's breathing is an important continuous determinate that needs to be observed and recorded before the procedure, throughout the procedure, and during recovery. Hypoventilation or bronchospasm may be clinically evident with observation before an alteration in heart rate or oximetry is detected. The patient's state of wakefulness and ability to follow commands are markers for sedation. Depending on the procedure, a patient's mental status may be minimally depressed whereby they may respond to environmental stimuli, whereas deep sedation requires moderate stimulation to arouse the patient.

A full meal less than 6 hours, or liquids less than 2 to 3 hours, prior to the procedure places adults at risk for aspiration if sedation inadvertently results in loss of protective airway reflexes. These time requirements are not a contraindication to the use of procedural sedation and analgesia. Agents used to promote gastric emptying or altering gastric pH to minimize the effects of aspiration are typically impractical in the Emergency Department setting due to their delayed onset for effectiveness. These procedures cannot usually be delayed due to the urgency of the matter.

Obtain baseline measurements of the patient's weight, blood pressure, heart rate, oxygen saturation, and capnography (if available). Procedural sedation and analgesia can result in both hypoxia and hypercapnia. The underlying mechanism is opioid/sedative-induced hypoventilation. While pulse oximetry is routinely used, the degree of desaturation does not correlate alone with poor outcomes.[5] It would stand to reason that capnography would provide an earlier warning to a hypoventilatory condition, yet its routine application is rarely practiced. Oxygen application is considered routine, yet its value has not been established. The routine application of oxygen may delay recognition of a profound hypoventilatory state if capnography is not used.

AGENT SELECTION

A patient may present with a number of conditions that may require sedation, analgesia, or a combination of both. The first step is to determine exactly what is needed: anxiety relief and/or pain control. Levels of sedation range from light or minimal depression of mental status to deep or heavy sedation where protective airway reflexes or hemodynamic stability may be compromised. **The goal of procedural sedation and analgesia is to achieve the desired endpoint with minimal risk of cardiorespiratory compromise.**

Light sedation is aimed at blunting the level of awareness to environmental stimuli and painful perceptions. Anxiety is alleviated and the patient maintains responsiveness to verbal and physical stimuli. Protective airway reflexes are maintained. Deep sedation produces profound depression of awareness with the inability to respond to verbal stimuli. Careful monitoring of cardiorespiratory status is essential in this setting as protective airway reflexes may be lost.

Certain agents, themselves or in combination, produce varied results in different patient subgroups. Each patient requires individual consideration. Selecting the appropriate agent requires knowledge of the agent's potency, duration to onset, duration of drug effect, titratability, interaction with other drugs, and adverse effects profile. Increasing dosages of an agent reduces its drug-specific effect in exchange for a nonspecific sedative effect complete with cardiorespiratory compromise. The most common mistake in sedation is choosing the wrong agent for the specific goal. For example, sedating a patient does not relieve pain. Sedation must be accompanied by analgesia if a patient is undergoing a painful procedure. This agent should ideally be titratable. The only reliable and precise means of this is via intravenous administration. Deep sedation should be provided only via the intravenous route. **Intravenous access is required if the patient undergoes deep sedation in case cardiorespiratory support is required or in the event that reversal agents must be administered.** Anxiolysis or mild sedation does not necessarily require intravenous access. Patients may be assessed on an individual basis as to whether intravenous access is deemed appropriate.

Synergistic effects must be considered when choosing a dosing schedule. For example, combining a benzodiazepine with a narcotic analgesic increases the potential effect of either agent alone.[6] **Reduce the initial doses of multiple agents owing to the additive sedative effects. Small and incremental dosing enables a controlled titration to effect. Physicians must have a fundamental knowledge of the pharmacological profiles of these agents. Allow the medications to reach peak effect before administering additional medication. Physicians are best served with a thorough knowledge of a few drugs as opposed to little knowledge over the entire procedural sedation agent spectrum.**

It would behoove a physician to develop and practice four procedural sedation and analgesia drug regimens: sedative plus analgesic, pure sedation, dissociative analgesia and sedation (ketamine), and inhalation anesthesia (nitrous oxide). **Become well versed in the applications of these regimens and do not stray from your routine unless circumstances dictate a different regimen.** At that time, identify your limitations and obtain peer or Anesthesiology backup prior to procedural initiation. Provide adequate analgesia first when performing a painful procedure. Some degree of sedation will have already been established. Provide sedation with a pure sedative to obtain the endpoint of relaxation/sedation required to complete the procedure.

DRUG PROFILES

Table 109-4 provides a summary review of the agents routinely employed during procedural sedation and analgesia. **It is critical that the physician is well versed on both the individual agent and its effect in combination with other medications. Medication routes, dosing parameters, side effects, contraindications, and anticipated complication management must be well known in advance.**

The ideal agent is a single drug that has amnestic, anxiolytic, analgesic, and sedative properties. It should have a predictable and rapid onset of action. It should have a predictable and short duration of action with a rapid recovery. The ideal agent should be inexpensive, easy to administer, and have a wide safety margin to make loss of consciousness extremely unlikely. It should have little or no side effects, especially cardiovascular and respiratory. It must be easily reversible if necessary. There should be no residual effects at the end of the procedure. It is obvious that no agent meets all these criteria. **We hope to minimize side effects, maximize benefit, allow quick recovery and dispositions, and produce reliable effects using small doses of multiple agents.** The most widely used combinations are fentanyl and midazolam or ketamine and midazolam.

BENZODIAZEPINES

Benzodiazepines produce anterograde amnesia, anxiolysis, sedation, and muscle relaxation. They have no analgesic activity and must be used in conjunction with other agents for painful procedures. The use of a benzodiazepine allows less analgesic agent to be administered and may reduce the severity of adverse reactions. The major adverse effects of benzodiazepines are respiratory depression and hypotension. The respiratory depression is usually transient but can be reversed with flumazenil. Prevent hypotension by ensuring that the patient is euvolemic, using the minimum amount of

TABLE 109-4. THE AGENTS CURRENTLY AVAILABLE FOR PROCEDURAL SEDATION AND ANALGESIA

Agent	Route	Pediatric dosing		Adult dosing		Onset (min)	Duration (min)	Adverse reactions	Contraindications
		Initial	Maximum	Initial	Maximum				
Benzodiazepines									
Midazolam (Versed)	IV	0.05 mg/kg	0.15 mg/kg	0.025 mg/kg	0.1 mg/kg	2–3	30–60	Respiratory depression	Hypersensitivity
	IM	0.05 mg/kg	0.20 mg/kg	0.05 mg/kg	0.15 mg/kg	10–20	60–120	Hallucinations	Renal impairment
	PO	0.5 mg/kg	0.7 mg/kg			10–30	60–90	Hypotension	Uncompressed acute illness
	PR	0.25 mg/kg	0.5 mg/kg			10–30	60–90	Excessive sedation	Recent illicit drug use
	Nasal	0.2 mg/kg	0.5 mg/kg (or 6 mg)			10–15	45–60	Headache	Recent alcohol use
								Nausea	
								Vomiting	
								Hiccups	
								Paradoxical reactions	
Opioids									
Fentanyl (Sublimaze)	IV	0.5–1.0 mcg/kg	2–3 mcg/kg	1–2 mcg/kg		1–2	20–30	Respiratory depression	Hypersensitivity
Sufentanil (Sufenta)	Nasal	0.7 mcg/kg (0.7 mcg/kg if given with nasal midazolam)				5–15	60–120	Puritis	Uncompensated acute illness
								Bradycardia	Recent illicit drug use
								Nausea	Recent alcohol use
								Vomiting	Coma
								Chest wall rigidity	< 6 months of age
								Hypotension	
Morphine	IV	0.1 mg/kg	0.2 mg/kg	0.1 mg/kg	0.2 mg/kg	1–5	180–240	Respiratory depression	Hypersensitivity
	IM/SQ	0.1 mg/kg	0.2 mg/kg	0.1 mg/kg	0.2 mg/kg	30	240–300	Hypotension	
								Nausea	
								Vomiting	
								Histamine release	
								Prolonged sedation	
Barbiturates									
Methohexital (Brevital)	IV	0.5 mg/kg	1.0 mg/kg	0.5 mg/kg	1.0 mg/kg	0.75	5–10	Nausea	Temporal lobe epilepsy
	PR	20 mg/kg	25 mg/kg			10–15	60	Vomiting	Acute intermittent porphyria
								Apnea	
								Respiratory depression	
								Paradoxical hyperactivity	
Thiopental (Pentothal)	IV	0.5–1.0 mg/kg	4 mg/kg			0.25–0.3	3–10	Apnea	Hypotension
	PR	20–25 mg/kg				5–8	60	Respiratory depression	Altered mental status
								Hypotension	Cardiac ischemia
								Histamine release	Cardiac conditions
								Decreased myocardial contractility	

Drug	Route	Dose				Onset (min)	Duration (min)	Side effects	Contraindications
Pentobarbital (Nembutal)	IV	2.5 mg/kg	6 mg/kg (additional increments of 1.25 mg/kg q 30 sec) max 100 mg	1.25 mg/kg	2.5 mg/kg	0.5–1.0	15	Nausea Vomiting Apnea Hypotension Hypoxemia Respiratory depression Paradoxical hyperactivity Decreased myocardial contractility	Acute intermittent porphyria
	IM	4 mg/kg	6 mg/kg	1.25 mg/kg	2.5 mg/kg	10–20	60–240		
	PO	1 mg/kg	6 mg/kg (max 100 mg)	2 mg/kg	6 mg/kg	15–60	60–240		
	PR	*< 4 years:* 3 mg/kg	6 mg/kg (max 100 mg)	2 mg/kg	6 mg/kg	15–60	60–240		
		> 4 years: 1.5 mg/kg	3 mg/kg (max 100 mg)						
Hypnotics									
Chloral hydrate	PO	20 mg/kg	1000 mg			15–60	60–120	Paradoxical hyperactivity Delirium Residual sedation Nausea Vomiting	Hepatic impairment Renal impairment Hypersensitivity
	PR	Not recommended				10–20	60–120		
Ketamine (Ketalar)	IV	0.5 mg/kg	1.0 mg/kg	0.75 mg/kg	1.5 mg/kg (additional 5–10 mg doses as required to effect; 0.01–0.02 mg/kg/min infusion)	0.5–1.5	15–45	Increase intractinal pressure Increased intraocular pressure	< 3 months Active respiratory infections Increased ICP, head trauma, hydrocephalus
	IM	1 mg/kg	6 mg/kg (usually 2–4 mg/kg; may repeat q 5–10 min as needed)			4–10	30–60	Stridor Vomiting Hypersalivation Bronchorrhea Hypertonicity Laryngospasm Emergence reactions	Cardiovascular disease Glaucoma Psychoses Potential for airway instability i.e. tracheal stenosis Relative contraindications Oral procedures Thyroid disease Acute intermittent porphyria
	PO	5.0 mg/kg	10.0 mg/kg			10–15			
	PR	50 mg/kg				4–10	30–60		
						10–15	45–75		
Propofol (Diprivan)	IV bolus	0.5–1.0 mg/kg				0.5	0.5	8–10	Respiratory depression
	IV drip	50–75 mcg/kg/min				0.5	8–10 min after stopped	Apnea Hypotension Similar to thiopental	

(continued)

TABLE 109-4. *CONTINUED*

Agent	Route	Pediatric dosing		Adult dosing		Onset (min)	Duration (min)	Adverse reactions	Contraindications
		Initial	Maximum	Initial	Maximum				
Inhalation anesthetics									
Nitrous oxide		50% N_2O–50% O_2 (self-administered by demand valve mask)		50% N_2O–50% O_2 (self-administered by demand valve mask)		0.5–1.0 (peaks in 3–5 min)	3–5 after withdrawal of gas	Nausea, vomiting Disorientation Agitation Air-filled cavity expansion	Altered mental status Intoxication Pregnancy Opioids within past 4 hours Pneumothorax Pneumomediastinum Bowel obstruction Uncooperative patient Facial trauma Relative contraindications Full meal < 1 hour Age < 5 years (cooperation)
Reversing agents									
Naloxone (Narcan)	IV	*< 12months:* 0.1 mg/kg q 2–3 min *> 12 months:* 1–2 mg/kg q 2–3 min	10 mg	Respiratory arrest: 1–2 mg Respiratory depression: (0.4 g in 9 cc) 1 cc q 2 min		1–2	20–40	May precipitate withdrawal in opioid dependent patient	None
	IM, SL, SQ	*< 12months:* 0.1 mg/kg q 2–3 min *> 12months:* 1–2 mg/kg q 2–3 min	10 mg			5–10	60–90		
Flumazenil (Romazicon)	IV	0.02 mg/kg (max 1 mg) (repeat q 1 min to effect)	1 mg total	0.2 mg q 15–45 sec	1 mg/15 min 3 mg/30 min	1–2	20–40	Nausea, vomiting	Concomitant tricyclic antidepressant ingestion Hypersensitivity In patient with chronic benzodiazepine use—may precipitate seizure
	IM	Same as IV				5–10	60–90		

narcotics to produce analgesia, and carefully titrating the benzodiazepine.

MIDAZOLAM (VERSED)

Midazolam is an ultra-short-acting benzodiazepine that is metabolized by the liver and excreted by the kidney. Intravenous midazolam in dose ranges from 0.02 to 0.10 mg/kg will produce sedation within 2 to 3 minutes, redistribute rapidly, and provide a 20 to 30 minute duration of action. Most adults have adequate sedation and anxiolysis by a total dose of 5 to 7 mg; administered in 0.05 mg/kg or 1 to 2 mg increments every 3 to 5 minutes. **It is important to note the 2 minute delay in the peak CNS effect. Allow midazolam time to work before additional dosing.** It is water-soluble and does not cause vascular irritation on injection, as found in its relative diazepam. Midazolam is three to four times more potent than diazepam. It has anxiolytic and anticonvulsive properties. It is a potent amnestic agent that has the added advantage of providing both antegrade and retrograde amnesia. Like all benzodiazepines, midazolam alters the response to pain but does not reduce pain perception. The addition of an analgesic agent is required when midazolam is administered for a painful procedure.

Midazolam is a potent respiratory depressant, like all sedative agents. Midazolam can cause apnea by depressing the sensitivity of the hypothalamus to hypercapnia. It shifts the CO_2 response curve to the right and depresses its slope. **Its respiratory depressant effects are augmented in patients receiving opioids, with underlying lung disease (e.g., COPD), and with concomitant circulating CNS depressants (including opioids, alcohol, and barbiturates).** Patients may become hypoxic, even with normal respiratory rates.

Pulse oximetry is warranted when administering midazolam. Deaths related to the use of midazolam for sedation during endoscopy prompted the FDA to recommend increased monitoring and particular caution with elderly or debilitated patients. There is a particular propensity for apnea when even very small doses of midazolam are given in conjunction with fentanyl.[6] Midazolam may cause hypotension that is related to the dose and to the rate of administration. This effect is more likely to occur in hypovolemic patients or elderly patients.

DIAZEPAM (VALIUM) AND LORAZEPAM (ATIVAN)

Both diazepam and lorazepam have longer half-lives than midazolam. While either agent may be used for procedural sedation and analgesia, they are more difficult to titrate and have a longer duration of action. Neither of these characteristics is well suited to procedural sedation and analgesia. **Midazolam has greater earlier sedation, less recall, less pain upon injection, higher 90 minute alertness scores, and more patients ready for discharge at 90 minutes post-procedure than diazepam.** Diazepam results in more respiratory depression, hypotension, and phlebitis than midazolam. **Diazepam and lorazepam have no advantage over midazolam if the goal is to produce a short, titratable state of anxiolysis and sedation.** These agents are therefore not often used for procedural sedation and analgesia.

OPIOIDS

Opiates provide analgesia with minimal sedation and no anxiolysis. They have a long track record showing a predictable performance. The respiratory and central nervous system depression can be readily reversed with naloxone and nalmefene. Opiates are relatively inexpensive and often used in a balanced approach to procedural sedation and analgesia. Agents in this class include morphine, fentanyl, meperidine, sufentanil, and alfentanil.

While morphine has been the mainstay narcotic analgesic, the use of potent synthetic short-acting opioids for analgesia and sedation has been common practice for procedural sedation and analgesia. These drugs are particularly appealing for their short half-lives, rapid onset of action, limited cardiovascular side effects, ease of controlled administration, and the availability of a rapidly acting reversal agent. The use of these agents requires a thorough familiarity with their pharmacological properties and side effects. A procedural sedation and analgesia repertoire should include one of the potent synthetic narcotics. It is better to master one drug than dabble in the pharmacology and administration of three different drugs with different dosing regimens. These are not the type of agents you have a full decimal point leeway in dosing.

MORPHINE

Morphine is a "good old" potent analgesic with a lot of clinical experience. It is the prototype opioid to which all others are compared. Incremental intravenous dosing of 0.05 to 0.20 mg/kg every 3 to 5 minutes provides a nice range over which to carefully titrate to an individual analgesia requirement. It begins working in 1 to 3 minutes and peaks within 15 to 20 minutes. Morphine has a duration of activity of 3 to 4 hours, thereby providing often-needed pain relief even after the procedure has been completed. It is metabolized by the liver and excreted by the kidney. Morphine, as with all opioids, decreases the medullary response thereby promoting hypercapnia and hypoxia. Histamine release with hypotension, nausea, vomiting, itching, bronchospasm, and loss of vascular tone are all too common side effects of morphine administration. Morphine has steadily lost ground to the newer, designer opioids with better cardiovascular stability such as fentanyl, sufentanil, and alfentanil.

FENTANYL (SUBLIMAZE)

This opioid is highly lipid soluble and 75 to 125 times more potent than morphine. Peak analgesia is achieved in 2 to 3 minutes after intravenous administration. Although its terminal half-life is 130 to 220 minutes, its clinical effectiveness is limited to approximately 30 minutes due to rapid tissue redistribution. Fentanyl is a "20 minute drug for a 20 minute procedure." It is metabolized in the liver with renal and hepatic excretion. Approximately 20 percent is excreted as the unmetabolized parent compound. The major side effect of fentanyl is respiratory depression. Hypotension is less common than with morphine because fentanyl does not induce histamine release.

Administer fentanyl very slowly and in small increments. Patients may experience rigidity of their chest muscles, coined the "rigid chest syndrome," when it is administered too rapidly. This syndrome can severely impact ventilation to the point that the patient must be paralyzed to facilitate adequate ventilation. Administer incremental doses of 0.5 to 1.0 $\mu g/kg$ or 10 to 100 μg boluses slowly intravenously to a total maximum dose of 2 to 3 $\mu g/kg$.

Fentanyl is contraindicated in children less than six months of age. It stimulates the central vagus nucleus in the brainstem. This can result in a prolongation of the refractory period of the atrioventricular (AV) node and significant bradycardia.

The rigid chest syndrome may occur to the point at which the patient may not be ventilating and attempts at assisted ventilation with a bag-valve-mask device are unsuccessful. The patient may then become hypoxic, bradycardic, and eventually expire. This phenomenon has been well documented in children. The rigid chest syndrome is the reason many physicians are reluctant to administer fentanyl. **It occurs during rapid intravenous administration, so give it slowly.** It only occurs at high doses (> 15 $\mu g/kg$) to anesthetic doses (50 to 100 $\mu g/kg$) ranges. **The doses used for procedural sedation and analgesia are safe and do not result in the rigid chest syndrome.** Immediately administer naloxone intravenously if the rigid chest syndrome develops. Unfortunately, naloxone does not often work to overcome the rigid chest syndrome. The patient may require paralysis and orotracheal intubation to overcome the rigid chest syndrome.

SUFENTANIL (SUFENTA)

Sufentanil is an extremely potent narcotic analgesic. It is 5 to 10 times more potent than fentanyl and 500 to 1000 times more potent than morphine. It is metabolized and eliminated more rapidly than fentanyl. There is no significant advantage to using sufentanil over fentanyl for most procedural sedation and analgesia applications.

The one advantage is that its potency and small volume dosing enables it to be delivered intranasally in the pediatric population. ACEP's Guideline to Pediatric Sedation is a proponent of this particular application.[7] Sufentanil has an onset of action in 5 to 15 minutes and a duration of action lasting 1 to 2 hours when administered intranasally. It provides exceptional cardiovascular stability but maintains the profound respiratory depressive effects inherent in the opioid class of agents. Careful patient selection is well advised when considering sufentanil.

ALFENTANIL (ALFENTA)

Alfentanil is less lipid soluble than fentanyl. It is therefore less likely to accumulate if multiple doses are required. It is 10 to 20 times more potent than morphine. It is one-tenth to one-fifth as potent as fentanyl. The duration of analgesia is ultrashort. Its onset of action is within seconds and lasts only 2 minutes. Alfentanil is too short acting to use for procedural sedation and analgesia. Total dosing is 8 to 10 $\mu g/kg$ delivered in small repeated dosing aliquots. Its half-life is only 80 minutes. The adverse effect profile is identical to fentanyl. The rigid chest syndrome may also be seen with alfentanil. Alfentanil is more appropriate to use for the induction of general anesthesia.

MEPERIDINE (DEMEROL)

Meperidine is one-tenth as potent as morphine. It is the most commonly administered opioid agent for pain in the United States. It is not used for procedural sedation and analgesia because it is hard to titrate and takes a long time to reach peak activity.

DISSOCIATIVE AGENTS

KETAMINE (KETALAR)

Ketamine is a unique pharmaceutical agent in that it provides sedation, amnesia, analgesia, and anxiolysis. Its safe and effective use in pediatric sedation/analgesia is well studied.[8] It is the most commonly used anesthetic agent throughout the world. It has the best safety profile in terms of cardiorespiratory complications of any agent. Ketamine is a derivative of PCP that generates a functional and electrophysical dissociation between the cortical and limbic systems. This results in a dissociative state whereby the patient is in a trance-like cataleptic condition in which sensory perceptions and memory are blunted. Although the patient appears awake, they are dissociated from their environment. Random tonic movements will occur and gentle physical restraint may be required.

Ketamine is a positive inotrope. It increases the heart rate, blood pressure, cardiac output, and intracranial pressure. The blood pressure and heart rate may slightly increase with the use of ketamine. The systolic and diastolic blood pressure increase up to 30 mmHg (average 15 mmHg). The heart rate may increase up to 30 beats per minute with an average of 15 beats per minute. These effects are believed due to decreased uptake of catecholamines at neural endplates.

Ketamine's effect on the respiratory status includes bronchodilation, a slight increased respiratory rate, increased secretions, and potential laryngospasm. Ketamine is a potent bronchodilator. It does not depress airway reflexes like narcotics or benzodiazepines. The side effects of increased respiratory secretions can be blocked with atropine or glycopyrrolate. Administer glycopyrrolate before ketamine in a dose of 0.005 mg/kg to a maximum of 0.25 mg. Administer atropine prior to or concurrently with ketamine in a dose of 0.01 mg/kg to a maximum of 0.3 to 0.5 mg.

Ketamine may be administered by several routes. Rapid predictable effects are best seen with parenteral administration. Intravenous dosing (0.5 to 1.0 mg/kg slowly) is approximately one-fourth of the intramuscular dosing (1 to 6 mg/kg, usually 2 to 4 mg/kg). A dissociative state is produced in less than a minute with intravenous administration and 2 to 10 minutes via the intramuscular route. Intramuscular dosing may be repeated at 10 minutes with an additional 2 to 4 mg/kg if adequate sedation has not been achieved. Although ketamine may be given orally (5 to 6 mg/kg) or rectally (5 to 10 mg/kg), its titratability is poor, which makes its effectiveness much less predictable.

Contraindications to the use of ketamine include age less than 3 months, procedures involving pharyngeal stimulation, known cardiovascular disease, concurrent head trauma with altered mental status, airway compromise including previous tracheal surgery/stenosis, known CNS mass lesions, increased intracranial pressure, active upper or lower respiratory disease, and porphyria.

Patients will exhibit a slow emergence from the effects of ketamine over the course of 1 to 2 hours. Ketamine is metabolized and excreted by hepatic mechanisms. Place the patient in a quiet room that is free of excessive external stimuli to minimize the possibility of them becoming hyperactive or overstimulated by their surroundings.

Emergence reactions are hallucinations that occur as the ketamine wears off and the patient awakens. They may be seen in up to 50 percent of adults and up to 10 percent of children given ketamine. The etiology of these emergence reactions is unknown. There is an association of emergence reactions with an age over 10 years, females, rapid intravenous administration, stimulation during the recovery period, and personality disorders. Rarely will a child less than 10 years of age develop an emergence reaction with hallucinations.

The incidence of emergence reactions can be decreased. Administer the ketamine slowly intravenously. Place the patient in a dark, quiet room with minimal sensory stimulation during the recovery period. Treatment with benzodiazepines is indicated if an emergence reaction develops. The concurrent administration of midazolam in a dose of 0.025 to 0.050 mg/kg is currently used to reduce emergence reactions. One study found no advantage of combining midazolam with ketamine in preventing an emergence reaction.[9] The concurrent use of midazolam is physician-dependent, has no serious sequelae, and may reduce emergence reactions.

SEDATIVE HYPNOTICS

The sedative-hypnotics are a diverse category of agents that include thiopental, methohexital, etomidate, and propofol. These agents provide anxiolysis and sedation with various degrees of amnesia. They provide no analgesia.

BARBITURATES

Short-acting barbiturates (thiopental, pentobarbital, and methohexital) are effective procedural sedation and analgesia agents. They provide good titratability with a rapid onset of action. Barbiturates provide sedation, hypnosis, and amnesia. They are highly lipophilic and cross the blood-brain barrier readily, resulting in an onset of action in less than 1 minute. They have short half-lives that promote a rapid recovery and minimize the risks inherent in prolonged sedation. **Their major drawbacks are respiratory depression, apnea, occasional transient hypotension, and lack of a reversing agent. The window between procedural sedation and analgesia, deep sedation, and general anesthesia is extremely narrow.** These agents are rarely used for procedural sedation and analgesia in the Emergency Department.

THIOPENTAL (PENTOTHAL)

Thiopental is one of the more commonly used barbiturates. It has an extremely rapid onset of action (10 to 20 seconds) with a peak activity in 1 minute. Its sedative effect lasts 3 to 10 minutes. Thiopental is titratable in doses of 0.5 to 1.0 mg/kg intravenously. Rarely is more than 2 mg/kg required.

It may be administered rectally (20 to 25 mg/kg) in children who require sedation without intravenous access. Sedation is achieved within 5 to 8 minutes. Rectal administration does not result in apnea or respiratory depression. Thiopental is often administered rectally for laceration repairs in children.

METHOHEXITAL (BREVITAL)

Methohexital has a profile very similar to thiopental with a few noted exceptions. It is twice as potent as thiopental. It has much less of an effect on decreasing myocardial contractility and decreasing vascular tone. A study has convinced most people not to use this drug in the Emergency Department.[10] One hundred and two patients were given methohexital with a mean cumulative dose of 1.6 mg/kg. Three patients developed hypotension. Twenty-two patients developed respiratory depression requiring bag-valve-mask assistance. Five of the 22 patients with respiratory depression developed transient apnea.

Methohexital may be administered as either repeated incremental bolus dosing or via a titratable continuous infusion. Begin with a 0.5 to 1.0 mg/kg bolus followed by an infusion at 50 μg/kg/min. Titrate infusion rates upward to effect, with a maximum rate of 75 μg/kg/min. Bolus dosing is best delivered as 0.5 to 1.0 mg/kg (maximum 20 mg) every 45 to 60 seconds until the desired endpoint is attained. Maximum sedation is achieved at 40 seconds.

Respiratory depression is common and independent of the dose or concomitant administration of a narcotic or benzodiazepine. Patients may require ventilator assistance until the effect of the drug clears. **Respiratory depression is minimized by first administering the analgesic agent to control pain followed by methohexital to effect.** Do not use methohexital in children younger than 12 years of age.

PENTOBARBITAL (NEMBUTAL)

Pentobarbital is a short-acting barbiturate that is effective for pediatric sedation during nonpainful diagnostic procedures such as computed tomography or magnetic resonance imaging. Controlled sedation levels are best achieved with titrated small incremental intravenous dosing. It may also be administered intramuscularly, orally, and rectally. Intravenous administration will induce sleepiness within 30 seconds with a duration of action up to 15 minutes. Other dosing methods take longer to work, with a duration of action ranging from 1 to 4 hours.

It is primarily administered intravenously or rectally. Initial intravenous dosing at 2.5 mg/kg may be sufficient. Subsequent doses of 1.25 mg/kg every 30 seconds to effect will minimize oversedation and limit hypoxia. Other side effects are nausea, vomiting, and paradoxical hyperactivity. A maximum total dose of 6 mg/kg or 100 mg should mark the dosing endpoint. Older children may exceed this limit with due caution. Rectal dosing is age-dependent. Administer 3 to 6 mg/kg (maximum 100 mg) to children younger than 4 years of age and 1.5 to 3 mg/kg (maximum 100 mg) to children older than 4 years of age.

ETOMIDATE (AMIDATE)

Etomidate is an imidazole derivative that is commonly used for the induction of anesthesia or rapid sequence induction. It produces anxiolysis, sedation, and amnesia equal to that of the barbiturates but with fewer hemodynamic affects. It is ultra-short-acting and in a class of its own. It may produce unconscious sedation similar to the barbiturates. This agent is not commonly used for procedural sedation and analgesia. There is little reference for the use of etomidate in the Emergency Department or in the outpatient setting.

PROPOFOL (DIPRIVAN)

Propofol is a highly lipid soluble compound with ultra-short sedative hypnotic properties. It can produce profound sedation, hypnosis, anxiolysis, and amnesia. Propofol has no analgesic properties. It is unrelated to the barbiturate or benzodiazepine classes. The onset of action is rapid (15 to 30 seconds) with a maximal effect seen within 30 to 45 seconds. The duration of effect is typically only 8 to 15 minutes, even after prolonged administration.

Dosing can be delivered intravenously via repeated small 20 mg doses at 2 minute intervals or initial loading of 0.5 to 2.0 mg/kg followed by infusion rates of 25 to 130 μg/kg/min. A continuous infusion of 50 to 70 μg/kg/min can be used to produce a sleep-like state with minimal respiratory depression. Continuous infusions allow the patient to be easily aroused by verbal stimuli and recover within 2 to 3 minutes of stopping the infusion. Effective total doses may range from 20 to 150 mg. Induction dosing or rapid bolus injection can result in profound respiratory depression and hypotension, especially in the hypovolemic patient. Propofol can be coadministered with fentanyl for painful procedures requiring a combination of sedation and analgesia.

MISCELLANEOUS AGENTS

Several agents can be used for the sedation of children in the Emergency Department and outpatient setting. These agents are not used for procedural sedation and analgesia. These agents include chloral hydrate and DPT. Chloral hydrate is not often used in the Emergency Department. **Never use the DPT cocktail in any outpatient setting.**

CHLORAL HYDRATE

Chloral hydrate is a time-tested, effective, and pure sedative hypnotic. It has no analgesic properties. Its primary usage has been for sedation during nonpainful diagnostic testing. The oral dose is 20 to 100 mg/kg (maximum 2000 mg). Most children require 50 to 75 mg/kg to achieve proper sedation. It has an onset of action of 15 to 60 minutes and a duration of effect of 1 to 2 hours. Its effects may persist for up to 24 hours. Rectal dosing is not recommended due to erratic absorption.

Contraindications include renal impairment, hepatic impairment, or hypersensitivity to the agent itself. The wide dosing range and variability of onset and duration make chloral hydrate a far-from-perfect sedative for use in the Emergency Department. Its primary usage has been with outpatient testing.

DPT

DPT, also known as the "lytic cocktail," was popularized for the induction of general anesthesia. Unfortunately, it was expanded to use in the outpatient setting and had many adverse events. It consists of Demerol, Phenergan, and Thorazine in a 2:1:1 or 4:1:1 mixture. It is administered intramuscularly at a dose of 1 mg/kg based upon the Demerol component. Intramuscular absorption is erratic, with up to one-third of children never obtaining moderate to adequate sedation. It produces too deep a level of sedation that is difficult to reverse in the other two-thirds of the children.

Many children have suffered respiratory depression, hypoxemia, and apnea due to this agent. DPT is an agent of the past due to its prolonged action and significant potential for respiratory depression. The DPT agent has no use in the Emergency Department. Agents now exist that are safer, easier to use, and have a more rapid recovery. The mean time to Emergency Department discharge is 5 hours due to the prolonged sedation. The mean time for the child's behavior to return to normal is 19 ± 15 hours.

INHALATION AGENTS

NITROUS OXIDE (NITRONOX)

Nitrous oxide is an anesthetic gas that has been used in the outpatient procedural arena since the 1950s. It produces anxiolysis, sedation, and amnesia with a variable degree of analgesia. It dissociates a patient from pain and their surroundings. Nitrous oxide is self-delivered via a handheld demand valve mask in a 50-50 mixture with oxygen. The risk of oversedation is minimized with this mode of administration. The patient will drop the mask once they are too sedated to coordinate self-administration.

The onset of action of nitrous oxide is 30 to 60 seconds with a peak in 3 to 5 minutes. It has a similar washout period once delivery is ceased. Nitrous oxide is eliminated unchanged via the lungs, thereby minimizing any drug-drug interactions. Nausea and vomiting are common. The feelings of disorientation and agitation are also common.

Contraindications to the use of nitrous oxide include impaired mental status, concomitant intoxication, pregnancy, potential to expand air-filled cavities (e.g., pneumothorax or bowel obstruction), and coadministration

of narcotics within 4 hours (general anesthesia may be induced). Relative contraindications include a full meal within 1 hour of its use and children less than 5 years of age due to delivery system compliance. Refer to Chapter 108 for the complete details regarding nitrous oxide anesthesia.

REVERSAL AGENTS

It should be well recognized that a desired endpoint can be overshot resulting in an apneic and hypotensive patient despite good pre-procedural assessments, appropriate agent selection, appropriate dosing, and titration. There are two reversal agents, namely naloxone and flumazenil, that can be of help in these situations. **Reversal agents are not routinely required following procedural sedation and analgesia. They are reserved for the patient who develops apnea, hypoxia, and/or hypoventilation.**

FLUMAZENIL (ROMAZICON)

Flumazenil is a benzodiazepine antagonist that works by competitive inhibition at the GABA receptor. Intravenous administration will rapidly reverse CNS depression and respiratory depression from benzodiazepines within 2 minutes. Begin by administering a dose of 0.02 mg/kg to a maximum of 0.2 mg over 15 seconds. Administer additional 0.2 mg doses at 1 minute intervals until the desired state of consciousness is achieved. Maximum dosing is 1.0 mg over 15 minutes or 3.0 mg over 60 minutes. **The benzodiazepine metabolites are active longer than the reversal agent. Therefore, a patient receiving flumazenil must be carefully monitored for resedation.** A safe recommendation would require a minimum observation of 2 hours after the last dose is given.

Flumazenil is contraindicated in patients taking benzodiazepines for an extended amount of time or patients with an underlying seizure disorder. These patients are prone to seizure activity with the administration of flumazenil. It is also contraindicated in patients taking tricyclic antidepressants.

NALOXONE (NARCAN)

Naloxone is a pure opioid antagonist that works by competitively inhibiting narcotics at the opioid receptor. Intravenous administration reverses the respiratory depressive effects of opioids within 1 to 2 minutes. Its clinical duration of effect is approximately 30 minutes. Therefore, long-acting narcotics may cause resedation. The drug can be delivered via multiple routes (intravenously, intramuscularly, sublingually, subcutaneously, and endotracheally). The administration of 1 to 2 mg intravenously (0.1 mg/kg in children) will reverse most respiratory arrest situations. Administer additional doses every 2 to 3 minutes to a total of 10 mg. Another etiology of the sedation and respiratory depression, other than narcotics, should be aggressively sought if the respiratory depression is not reversed after 10 mg of naloxone.

Small (40 μg) aliquots titrated to effect may be delivered in a situation where the patient is slightly oversedated and rapid full reversal of the narcotic is not desired. Mix 0.4 mg of naloxone with 9 mL of normal saline to produce a concentration of 40 μg/mL. Administer 1 to 2 mL aliquots every 1 to 3 minutes to alleviate respiratory depression yet maintain the analgesic effect. Use caution as naloxone can result in opioid withdrawal in those with physical dependence or intoxicated with narcotics.

TECHNIQUE

The technique of procedural sedation and analgesia can be quite variable depending upon the institution and the agents chosen to administer. A sample procedural sedation and analgesia protocol can be found in Table 109-5. This requires two persons at a minimum. One person must monitor the patient while the other administers the medication and performs the procedure. **Take the time to do it right!** The right time to perform procedural sedation and analgesia is not when the

TABLE 109-5. A SAMPLE PROCEDURAL SEDATION AND ANALGESIA PROTOCOL

1. Place the patient supine in bed with the rails up.
2. Obtain IV access with a large bore angiocatheter and hang a 1 L bag of normal saline.
3. Apply the cardiac monitor to record pulse, respiratory rate, and blood pressure at start of procedure and every 3–5 minutes during the procedure.
4. The nurse must monitor the patient's level of consciousness at the start of the procedure and every 3–5 minutes during the procedure.
5. Apply continuous pulse oximetry to monitor and maintain the oxygen saturation > 95%, or no less than 3–5% below baseline.
6. Apply supplemental oxygen by nasal cannula at 2–4 L/min.
7. Place the resuscitation cart at the bedside.
8. Set up suction equipment and ensure that it is working properly.
9. Have the required medicines at the bedside and drawn up into labeled syringes.
10. Have the reversal agents (naloxone and flumazenil) at the bedside, not drawn up unless needed.
11. Administer and titrate the medications to effect.
12. Administer local or regional anesthesia if indicated.
13. Perform the procedure for which procedural sedation and analgesia was performed.
14. Administer additional doses of sedatives and analgesics as needed.
15. Closely observe and monitor the patient until they are awake, alert, and back to baseline.

Emergency Department is full to capacity and/or the acuity of other patients is high. The medications must be titrated to effect, which can take up to 15 minutes.

ASSESSMENT

Nursing personnel managing the care of the patient receiving procedural sedation and analgesia must continuously monitor the patient's airway, breathing, circulation, and mental status. It is imperative to observe the rise and fall of the chest wall with the focus upon the work of breathing. **Relying solely on pulse oximetry may give one a false sense of security.** Observation of a progressive slowing in the patient's respiratory effort is a sign of impending hypercapnia or hypoxia that is seen well ahead of any monitoring alerts or cutoffs. Avoid sterile wraps that cover the entire face or chest for this reason. Observe the patient for a decrease in respiratory rate or depth of breathing. Notice any abnormal airway sounds indicative of partial airway obstruction, laryngospasm, bronchospasm, or stridor. Visually monitor the peripheral perfusion of assessments of skin/mucosa color, temperature, and moisture. Assess pulse quality and rate in addition to frequent blood pressure determinations. Blood pressure monitoring may awaken the patient and forgo the ability to complete the diagnostic or therapeutic interventions in cases of mild sedation (e.g., pediatric sedation for neuroimaging). Continually assess the patient's level of consciousness throughout the procedure and recovery period. The aforementioned scoring systems offer one means of determining the level of sedation. Record the patient's responses to verbal stimuli, if applicable.

AFTERCARE

The patient must meet several criteria to ensure their safety before leaving the Emergency Department. Vital signs must be appropriate to the age of the patient and comparable to pre-procedural parameters. The respiratory effort must return to baseline. Mobility must be equal to or better than that before the procedure. The patient must be able to follow commands and discharge instructions. Pre-procedural levels of consciousness and mental status must be present. The patient must be able to tolerate oral fluids. The pain of the procedure for which procedural sedation and analgesia was performed must be controlled. The patient must be discharged in the care of a responsible adult who understands the discharge instructions. All these criteria must be documented in the medical record and timed prior to discharge.

Patients who have received multiple medications or a reversal agent will require a longer recovery period. A

2 hour observation window is prudent. Provide written discharge instructions and explain them to both the patient and the responsible adult who will accompany the patient home. Examples of preprinted pediatric and adult discharge sheets are presented in Tables 109-6 and 109-7.

COMPLICATIONS

Respiratory depression and hypoxia are inherent risks of procedural sedation and analgesia despite efforts to minimize risk with prudent patient risk-benefit assessment, appropriate drug selection, and appropriate dosing. Individual patient responses to hypnotic, sedative, or analgesic agents can be very unpredictable. Part of the preparation included bedside availability of reversal agents in anticipation of these complications.

The first course of action is simply to provide patient stimulation in the event of respiratory depression. Support the patient's ventilation with a bag-valve-mask device while the appropriate reversal agent(s) are being drawn up if stimulation is inadequate. Naloxone will rapidly reverse the respiratory depression if the patient had only received a narcotic. Flumazenil will reverse the impaired respiratory drive if only a benzodiazepine was administered.

There is no way to determine which reversal agent is best suited to reverse the respiratory depression when both a narcotic and benzodiazepine have been administered. A rational approach is to first administer flumazenil. This maintains the needed analgesia while, hopefully, improving the respiratory drive. Administer naloxone if the flumazenil does not reverse the respiratory depression.

Laryngospasm is a real but relatively rare event during procedural sedation and analgesia provided the appropriate patient and drug selection was employed. Ketamine, midazolam, fentanyl, and phenobarbital may all cause laryngospasm. This tends to be a brief and self-limited event that can be supported with the use of positive-pressure ventilation. Administer succinylcholine (1 to 2 mg/kg intravenously or 4 to 5 mg/kg intramuscularly) and support the patient's airway if laryngospasm is severe or persistent.

Virtually all agents can induce nausea and vomiting. Patients with recent oral intake are at a higher level of risk for aspiration. **Always have suction available if required.** Hypotension induced by opiates or benzodiazepines is responsive to fluid management and the corresponding reversal agent. Chest wall rigidity from short-acting opioids that cannot be reversed with naloxone requires succinylcholine and airway management to support ventilation and oxygenation.

TABLE 109-6. PEDIATRIC PROCEDURAL SEDATION AND ANALGESIA DISCHARGE INSTRUCTIONS

In order to best care for your child, they were given medications that can cause drowsiness and clumsiness over the next few hours. While most of the effect has worn off by this time, their coordination and judgment may still be affected. During this time it is very important to directly watch your child's activity to assure their safety.

Diet . . . Do not let them eat or drink for the next two hours. At that time, start with sips of water or juice before giving them solid foods. Children less than one year may start feeding in one hour.

Activity . . . For the next 6–8 hours, do not allow them to participate in any activity where lack of coordination could cause injury. Examples would include biking, climbing, running, playing on swing sets or monkey bars, swimming, or even stair climbing without your assistance. Your direct observation of their activities is very important during this recovery time. You need to directly watch your child if they are bathing, showering, cooking, or using any tool or device where injury could result due to poor judgment or coordination.

Sleep . . . Your child may wish to nap or sleep for the duration of the night. You need to awaken them in two hours. If they should appear as they normally would after being awoken from sleep you can let them finish their nap or sleep through the night.

Contact or return to the Emergency Department immediately if:

1. You notice anything you feel is unusual about your child.
2. You feel your child's breathing is abnormally fast, slow, or shallow.
3. Your child's skin appears pale or grayish in color.
4. You have more difficulty awakening your child.
5. Your child has repeated vomiting (3 or more times).

Phone number: _____

TABLE 109-7. ADULT PROCEDURAL SEDATION AND ANALGESIA DISCHARGE INSTRUCTIONS

To best manage your condition, you were given medications that can cause drowsiness and clumsiness over the next several hours. While most of the effect has worn off by this time, your coordination and judgment may still be affected.

1. You should avoid all activities that could result in injury due to drowsiness or impaired coordination or judgment. Examples would include driving a motorized vehicle, operating machinery, biking, swimming, skating, or any activity at height where a fall could result.
2. The effects of the medications could cause you to feel weak, shaky, or even nauseated. You should rest during this time and wait 1–2 hours before trying small sips of liquids. You can increase to solid foods once you start feeling better.
3. Take additional pain medications as directed by the doctor.
4. For the next 24 hours, avoid taking anything that could make you drowsy. Examples would include alcohol, sleeping pills, and antihistamine medications.

Please call the Emergency Department if you have any questions or feel anything is unusual about your recovery.

Phone number: _____

Allergic reactions can result from the administration of any of the aforementioned procedural agents. Management is similar to other allergic reactions in terms of treatment with epinephrine, diphenhydramine (H_1 antagonist), an H_2 antagonist, and methylprednisolone.

The use of procedural sedation and analgesia in pregnant and lactating patients must be undertaken with great caution. The safety of many of the agents is unknown or of concern (Table 109-8). Consult an Obstetrician, Gynecologist, or Anesthesiologist prior to performing procedural sedation and analgesia on pregnant and lactating women.

SUMMARY

Procedural sedation and analgesia is a necessary part of Emergency Medicine practice. Skillful application in the appropriate clinical scenarios will offer patients a world of anxiety and pain relief. We have the necessary pharmaceuticals to control the patient's pain and anxiety. It is essential that we possess the knowledge and training to understand our patients' needs and satisfy this requirement with a careful risk-benefit assessment and appropriate drug selection. It is essential we maintain the necessary high standards to safely get our patients through these procedures with a minimum of risk and complications. Competency extends beyond the physician and includes nursing and support personnel. They too must be knowledgeable as to the content of procedural sedation and analgesia with an uneventful recovery.

Everyone must know their limitations. Become very comfortable with a limited set of medications that will enable one to address 95 percent of all procedural sedation and analgesia requirements. Secure the assistance of a colleague or backup from an Anesthesiologist in difficult situations. Procedural sedation and analgesia will never be a substitute for a little patience and a soft, gentle mannerism. Reserve its use for the patient who truly needs the intervention.

TABLE 109-8. PREGNANCY CATEGORIES FOR PROCEDURAL SEDATION AND ANALGESIA AGENTS

Agent	Safety in pregnancy	Safety in lactation
Morphine	C	?
Meperidine	C but +	?
Fentanyl	C	?
Sufentanil	C	?
Alfentanil	C	?
Diazepam	D	–
Midazolam	D	–
Ketamine	?	?
Thiopental	C	?
Methohexital	B	?
Etomidate	C	?
Propofol	B	–
Nitrous oxide	–	?
Chloral hydrate	C	?
Naloxone	B	?
Nalmefene	B	?
Flumazenil	C	?
Atropine	C	–
Glycopyrrolate	B	–

Legend:
(A) Safety established in human studies
(B) Presumed safe based on animal studies
(C) Uncertain safety, animal studies show adverse effects, no human studies
(D) Unsafe
(+) Generally accepted as safe
(–) Generally regarded as safe
(?) Safety unknown or controversial

REFERENCES

1. American College of Emergency Physicians: Clinical policy for procedural sedation and analgesia in the emergency department. *Ann Emerg Med* 1998; 31(5):663–677.
2. Innes G, Murphy M, Nijssen-Jordan C, et al: Procedural sedation and analgesia in the emergency department. Canadian consensus guidelines. *J Emerg Med* 1999; 17(1):145–156.
3. American Academy of Pediatrics Committee on Drugs: Guidelines for monitoring and management of pediatric patients during and after sedation for diagnostic and therapeutic procedures. *Pediatrics* 1992; 89(6 pt 1):1110–1115.
4. Avramov MN, White PF: Methods for monitoring the level of sedation. *Crit Care Clin* 1995; 11(4):803–826.
5. American Medical Association Council on Scientific Affairs: The use of pulse oximetry during conscious sedation. *JAMA* 1993; 270(12):1463–1468.
6. Bailey PL, Pace NL, Ashburn MA, et al: Frequent hypoxemia and apnea after sedation with midazolam and fentanyl. *Anesthesiology* 1990; 73(5):826–830.
7. Krauss B, Shannon M, Damian FJ, et al: *Guidelines for Pediatric Procedural Sedation,* 2nd ed. Dallas: American College of Emergency Physicians, 1998.
8. Green SM, Rothrock SG, Lynch EL, et al: Intramuscular ketamine for pediatric sedation in the emergency department: safety profile in 1,022 cases. *Ann Emerg Med* 1998; 31(6):688–697.
9. Sherwin TS, Green SM, Khan A, et al: Does adjunctive midazolam reduce recovery agitation after ketamine sedation for pediatric procedures? A randomized, double-blind, placebo-controlled trial [see comments]. *Ann Emerg Med* 2000; 35(3):229–238.
10. Zink BJ, Darfler K, Salluzzo RF, et al: The efficacy and safety of methohexital in the emergency department. *Ann Emerg Med* 1991; 20(12):1293–1298.

Section Nine

OBSTETRIC AND GYNECOLOGIC PROCEDURES

Chapter 110
NORMAL SPONTANEOUS VAGINAL DELIVERY

Dudley Brown, Jr.
Susan K. Hendricks
Anthony Waechter

INTRODUCTION

The Emergency Physician will, on occasion, be required to handle the delivery of an infant when an Obstetrician or Family Physician is not available. The management of normal labor and delivery requires a basic understanding of the mechanisms of labor, the assessment and treatment of the mother, the safe delivery of the infant, and careful observation of both in the immediate postpartum period.

Labor is defined as repetitive uterine contractions leading to cervical change (dilation and effacement). The mechanisms of labor, also known as the cardinal movements of labor, describe the changes in the position of the fetal head as it travels through the birth canal. The safe delivery of the infant is the ultimate goal of labor.

ANATOMY AND PATHOPHYSIOLOGY

PELVIC ANATOMY

The success of a vaginal delivery depends on the four P's (presentation, position, place of the fetus, and adequacy of the pelvis). The physician must be able to assess the mother in anticipation of potential problems. The most commonly measured planes of the maternal pelvis are the pelvic inlet and the midplane. The two measurements most clinically useful are the diagonal conjugate and the ischial interspinous or bi-ischial diameter (Figure 110-1). The diagonal conjugate refers to the distance from the inferior border of the pubic symphysis to the sacral promontory (Figure 110-1A). Place the tip of the middle finger at the sacral promontory and note the point on the hand that contacts the pubic symphysis (Figure 110-1B). Measure this distance as the diagonal conjugate. The diagonal conjugate is generally 1.5 to 2 cm longer than the obstetric conjugate. The average

measurement of the anteroposterior diameter of the pelvic inlet is 12.5 cm, with the critical distance being 10 centimeters. Therefore, the critical distance to keep in mind when measuring the diagonal conjugate is 8.5 centimeters. Measure the ischial interspinous diameter. Palpate the ischial tuberosities and measure the distance between them (Figure 110-1C). A value greater than 8 cm is considered adequate. Distances less than these represent potential problems that may result in fetal entrapment, shoulder dystocia, or prolonged labor. It is not often feasible to take these measurements in the Emergency Department as the patient is often delivering precipitously.

TRUE LABOR VERSUS FALSE LABOR

False labor is common in late pregnancy. It is characterized by contractions that are brief, occur at irregular intervals, and whose intensity remains the same. These are often referred to as Braxton-Hicks contractions. These contractions primarily cause discomfort in the lower abdomen. Physical examination often reveals the fetus has not descended and the cervix is not dilated. False labor contractions are relieved by hydration and sedation.

True labor is characterized by contractions that are at regular intervals, the intensity gradually increases, and the interval between contractions gradually shortens. These contractions cause discomfort in the back and upper abdomen. Physical examination reveals that the fetus has descended and the cervix is dilating and effacing.

FETAL POSITIONING

Determine the fetal position and presenting part (i.e., vertex or breech) using the Leopold maneuvers (Figure 110-2). Approximately 97 percent of fetuses will present in the vertex position at full term. The Leopold maneuvers will determine the position of the fetus by

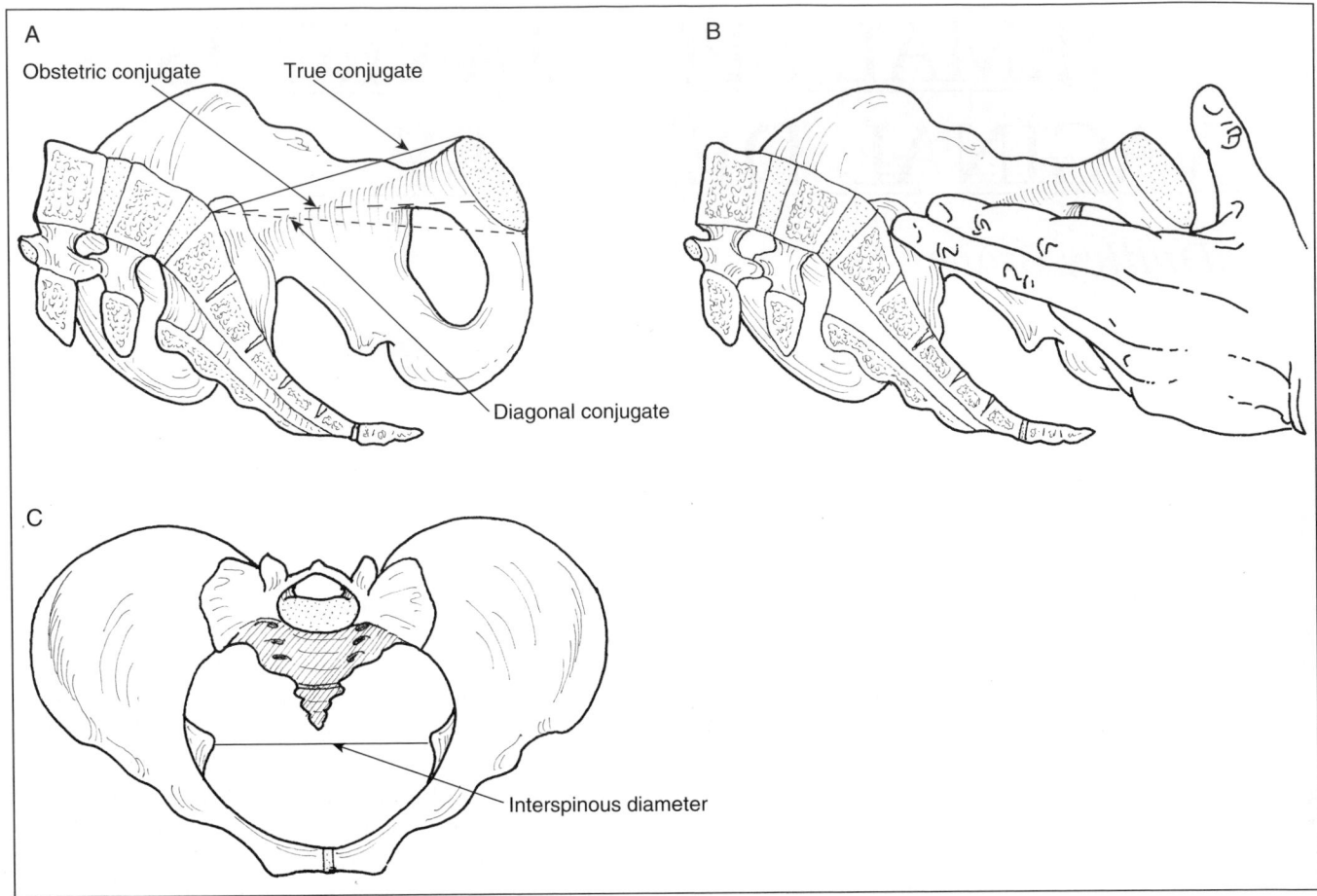

FIGURE 110-1 Measure pelvic distances to determine if there may be difficulties during the delivery. *A.* The pelvic conjugate diameters. *B.* Measuring the diagonal conjugate. *C.* The ischial interspinous distance.

identifying specific fetal landmarks or by revealing a specific relationship between the fetus and the mother (Figure 110-2).

The use of the Leopold maneuvers has been largely replaced by bedside ultrasonography. Nonetheless, they may still be useful when an Emergency Department bedside ultrasound unit is not available. The fetus bends in late pregnancy so that the back is convex while the extremities and neck are sharply flexed, and the fetal arms are crossed across the chest (Figure 110-2A). This posture is assumed so that the growing fetus can fit within the uterine cavity. The lie of the fetus, or its long axis in comparison to the mother, is either longitudinal or transverse. The vast majority of fetuses lie in the longitudinal plane at term. The presentation is the fetal part that is closest to the vagina, as felt through the cervix. The head, buttocks, or feet may be the presenting part if the fetus is in a longitudinal lie. The typical presenting part for a longitudinal lie is the occiput.

Perform the first maneuver. Stand at the patient's side and face her (Figure 110-2A). Gently palpate the mother's abdomen with the fingertips of both hands to determine which fetal part occupies the uterine fundus. The fetal head is palpable as a firm, freely mobile, round, and smooth structure. The fetal buttocks are palpable as an irregular, large, and soft structure in the uterine fundus.

Perform the second maneuver. Stand at the patient's side and face her (Figure 110-2B). Place both hands on either side of the abdomen. Palpate firmly, gently, and deeply to identify the fetal back and the extremities (small parts). Note the lie of the fetus and the position of their back.

Perform the third maneuver. Stand at the patient's side and face her (Figure 110-2C). Place the thumb and middle finger of the dominant hand just above the pubic symphysis. Palpate to determine the presenting part and its relation to the fetal spine. The fetus will be in a vertex or occiput presentation if the cephalic prominence is palpable on the same side as the small parts (i.e., the head is flexed). The fetus will be in a forehead presentation if the cephalic prominence is palpable on the same side as the spine (i.e., the head is extended). The fourth

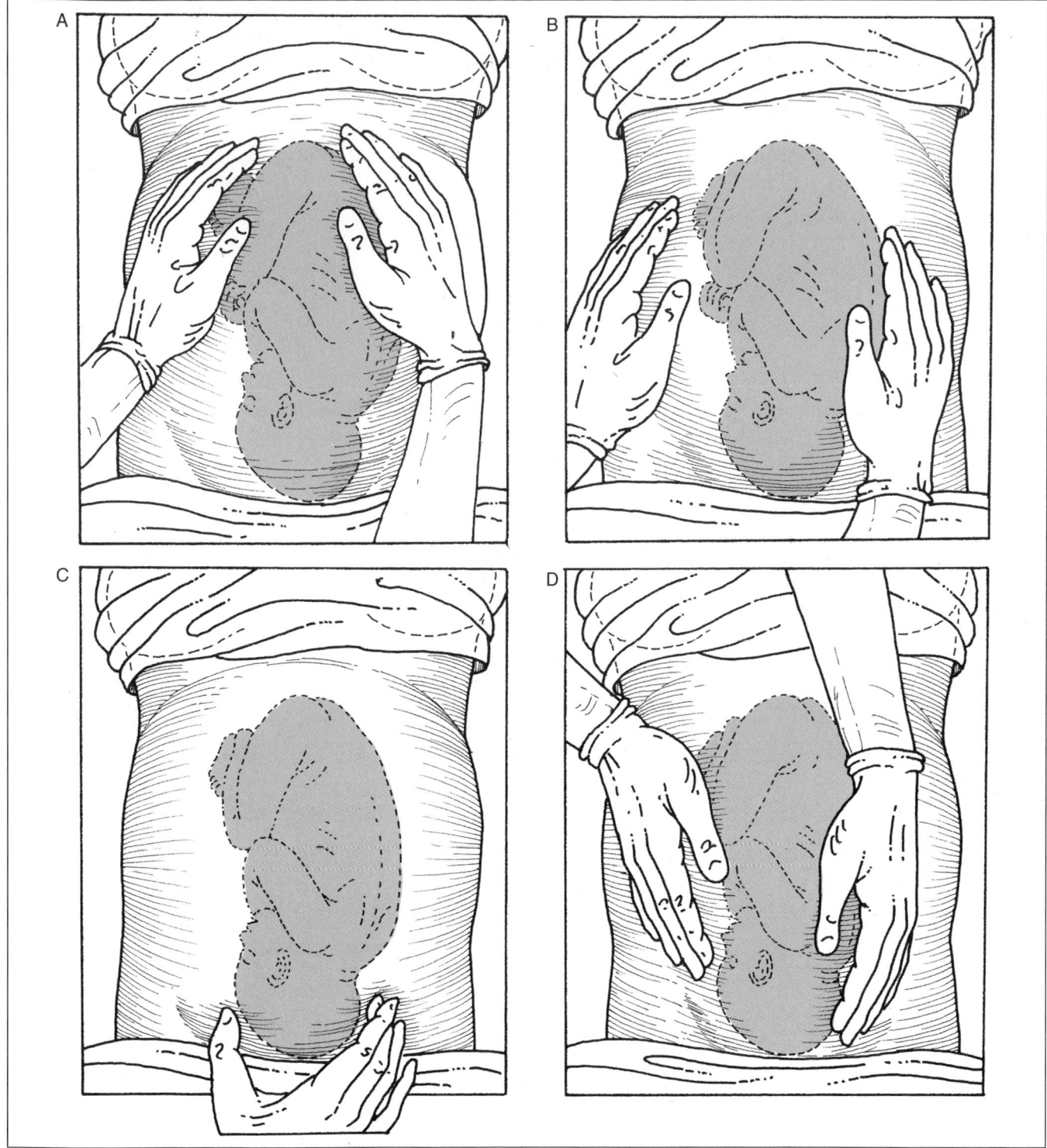

FIGURE 110-2 Leopold's maneuvers. *A.* The first maneuver. *B.* The second maneuver. *C.* The third maneuver. *D.* The fourth maneuver.

maneuver must be performed to determine the presentation if the presenting part is fixed and deep within the pelvis.

Perform the fourth maneuver. Stand at the patient's side and face her feet (Figure 110-2*D*). Place the tips of the thumb, index, and middle fingers over both sides of the lower abdomen. Palpate firmly, gently, and deeply towards the pelvic inlet with both hands. Determine the head position in relation to the fetal spine and small parts.

MECHANISM OF LABOR

Certain movements must occur with the position of the fetal head in relation to the maternal pelvis. These movements are known as the mechanism of labor or the cardinal movements of labor (Figure 110-3). These movements are described as engagement, descent, flexion, internal rotation, extension, external rotation, and expulsion (Figure 110-4).

The fetal head is floating free in the amniotic fluid before it engages the maternal pelvis (Figure 110-4A). Engagement is the mechanism by which the widest diameter of the presenting part of the fetus, the biparietal diameter, passes below the plane of the pelvic inlet (Figure 110-4B). This can be confirmed clinically by palpation of the presenting part, both abdominally and vaginally. Bimanual examination will reveal the presenting

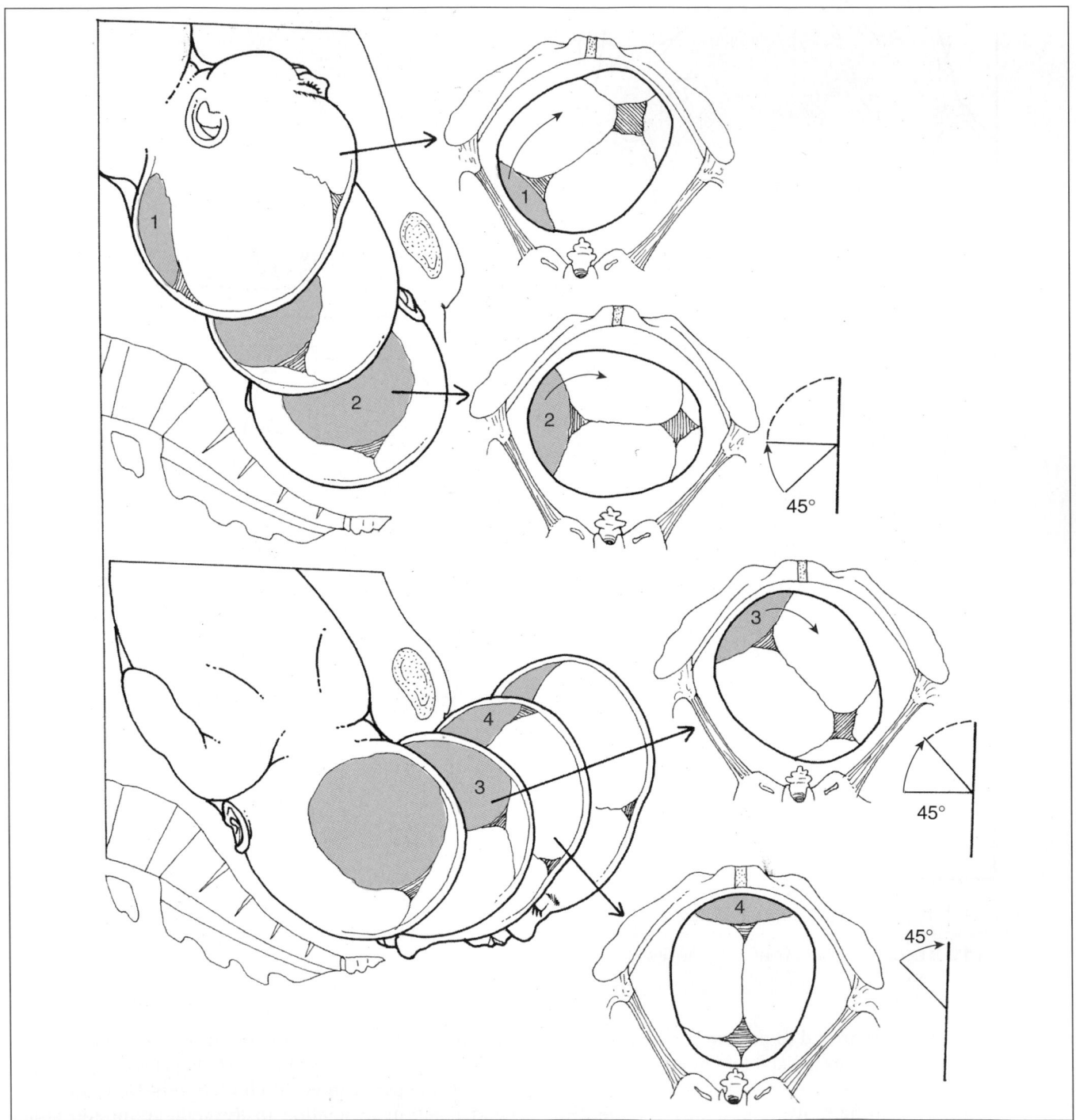

FIGURE 110-3 The mechanism of labor.

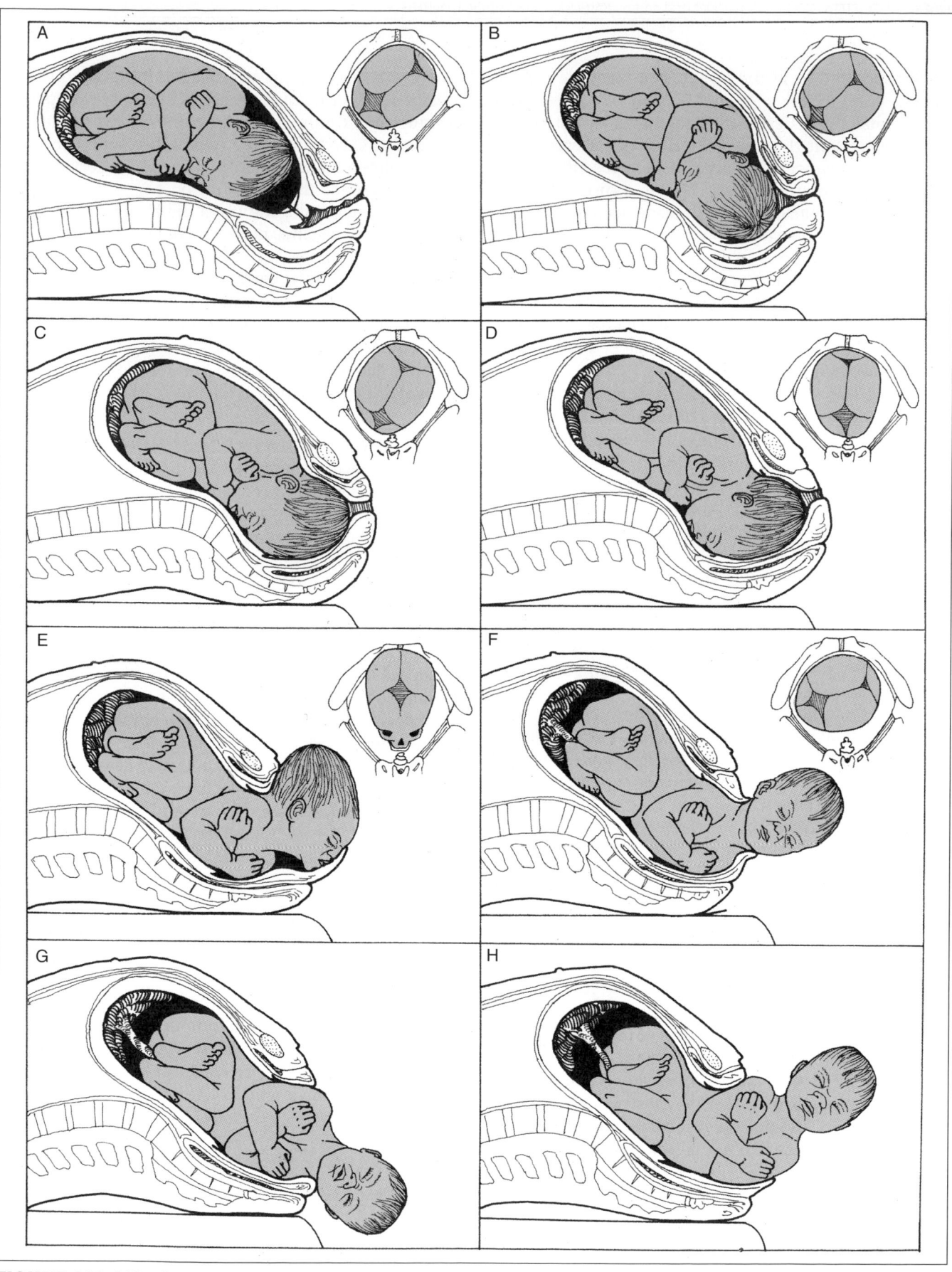

FIGURE 110-4 The fetal movements associated with the mechanism of labor. *A*. The fetal head is floating free. *B*. The head has descended and flexed to engage in the pelvis. *C*. The head descends further and internally rotates. *D*. The head has completely rotated into the direct occiput anterior position. The head begins to extend. *E*. The head completely extends to allow it to be delivered. *F*. External rotation of the head to bring it back to its natural position. *G*. Delivery of the anterior shoulder. *H*. Delivery of the posterior shoulder.

part at station 0 or at the level of the maternal ischial spines.

The fetal head descends into the maternal pelvis after engagement (Figures 110-4*B* and *C*). Descent refers to the downward passage of the presenting part through the maternal pelvis. This is a discontinuous process. The greatest rate of descent occurs near the end of the active phase of labor.

The fetal head flexes as it meets resistance from the cervix, the pelvic wall, and/or the pelvic floor during passage (Figure 110-4*B*). The result of flexion is to present the smallest diameter of the fetal head, the suboccipitobregmatic diameter, for passage through the maternal pelvis. This is a passive movement of the fetal head.

Internal rotation results in the fetal occiput moving anteriorly towards the pubic symphysis to assume the occiput anterior position (Figures 110-4*C* and *D*). It may rotate, less commonly, posteriorly towards the sacral hollow to assume the occiput posterior position. Internal rotation, like flexion, is a passive movement resulting from the contours of the maternal pelvis.

The fetal head begins extension once it descends to the level of the introitus and has completed internal rotation (Figures 110-4*D* and *E*). A combination of the downward force of the contracting uterus and the upward force exerted by the maternal pelvic floor muscles rotates the fetal head in extension around the pubic symphysis. Extension continues until the fetal head is delivered.

External rotation, or restitution, of the fetal head takes place after delivery of the head (Figure 110-4*F*). It brings the occiput and spine back into the same plane with the shoulders. This can occur to either side depending upon the orientation of the fetus.

Expulsion, or delivery of the fetus, occurs after external rotation (Figures 110-4*G* and *H*). The anterior shoulder delivers followed by the posterior shoulder then by delivery of the entire body.

ADMISSION EXAMINATION

Perform a thorough history and physical examination including vital signs, a sterile vaginal examination, and appropriate laboratory analysis on every patient if time permits. Vaginal bleeding in excess of bloody show is a contraindication to a vaginal examination. Appropriate laboratory work-up includes a hematocrit, urine protein, blood type, Rh status, antibody screen, VDRL, and hepatitis screen. The patient's prenatal record should be reviewed, if available. Do not give the patient anything to eat or drink once she enters the Emergency Department as gastric emptying time is delayed in pregnancy. Establish intravenous access.

Examine the cervix for dilatation and effacement. Effacement is said to be 50 percent when the length of the cervix is one-half that of an uneffaced cervix (~ 4 cm). It is said to be completely, or 100 percent, effaced when

the cervix becomes as thin as the lower uterine segment. Dilation is an estimate of the cervical opening expressed in centimeters. The examiner sweeps a finger across the cervix, from one side to the other. The cervix is completely dilated (i.e., 10 cm) when no cervix can be palpated around the presenting part.

Assessment of the station of the fetal head is vital. It measures the distance between fetal vertex and the maternal ischial spines. Zero (0) station is when the lowermost part of the fetal head is at the level of the maternal ischial spines. The system most commonly used for station is the system of thirds. The fetal head above the level of the maternal ischial spines is at a negative station (-1 to -3). The fetal head below the level of the maternal ischial spines is at a positive station ($+1$ to $+3$).

DETECTION OF RUPTURED MEMBRANES

Three specific examinations are performed if rupture of membranes (ROM) is suspected. This includes pooling, the Nitrazine test, and the fern test. First, perform a sterile speculum examination to look for fluid accumulation, or pooling, in the posterior vaginal fornix. Swab the pooled fluid and examine it for ferning and Nitrazine positivity. Any fluid present should also be examined for the presence of meconium.

Amniotic fluid is basic (pH 7.0 to 7.5) whereas the vagina and its secretions are acidic (pH 4.5 to 5.5). Touch a sample of the pooled fluid to pH or Nitrazine paper. The pooled fluid is presumed to be amniotic fluid if the color of the Nitrazine paper changes from yellow to blue. Blood, however, is also basic and may give a false positive result if the sample collected is contaminated.

The third diagnostic test for ruptured membranes, and the most specific, is the ferning test. Place a sample of the pooled fluid on a slide and allow it to air dry. Examine the slide under a microscope. The crystals that make up the amniotic fluid will arborize giving the appearance of fern leaves and thus a positive test.

CLASSIFICATION OF LABOR

Labor is divided into three stages. The first stage of labor is defined as the period from the onset of labor until the cervix is completely dilated. The second stage of labor begins at complete cervical dilation and ends with the delivery of the infant. The third stage of labor is the period from the delivery of the infant until the delivery of the placenta.

FIRST STAGE OF LABOR

The first stage of labor is subdivided into three phases. The first or latent phase is the period between the onset of labor and 3 to 4 cm of cervical dilation. The second phase lasts until cervical dilation is almost complete. The third phase is the final period until maximum cervical dilation.

The average duration of the first stage of labor is approximately 8 hours in nulliparous women and 5 hours in multiparous women. Review all data concerning the patient, including the laboratory data. Reassure the patient if there are no problems detected.

Monitor the fetal heart rate. The American College of Obstetricians and Gynecologists (ACOG) recommends monitoring the fetal heart rate by Doppler immediately following a contraction, every 30 minutes in low-risk pregnancies, and continuously with high-risk pregnancies.[1] Suspect fetal distress if the heart rate following a contraction is repeatedly below 120 beats per minute.[2]

The intensity of a contraction is determined by the degree of firmness that the uterus achieves. Contractions may be palpated or monitored by an external transducer (tocodynamometer) placed upon the mother's abdomen.

Monitor the maternal vital signs during active labor. Obtain a temperature every 2 hours and a blood pressure every 30 minutes.[3] Antibiotic coverage (penicillin) for group B streptococcal infection is recommended if the membranes have been ruptured for greater than 18 hours.[4] This is also known as prolonged rupture of membranes.[2,5]

Perform a vaginal examination immediately after the membranes have ruptured if the fetal head is not engaged. Monitor the fetal heart rate following the next contraction after rupture of the membranes to assess for occult umbilical cord compression.[2]

SECOND STAGE OF LABOR

The second stage of labor lasts approximately 50 minutes in nulliparous women and 20 minutes in multiparous women. It begins with complete dilatation of the cervix and terminates upon delivery of the infant. The recommendation for heart rate monitoring during the second stage of labor is auscultation at least every 15 minutes for low-risk infants and every 5 minutes for those at high risk.[1] Fetal heart rate decelerations may occur with contractions as the head descends.[1] Allow labor to continue if prompt recovery occurs as the contraction diminishes. Decelerations may also occur from progressive compression of an umbilical cord around the fetus, premature placental separation, or reduction in uterine blood flow, which will all lead to fetal compromise.[6] Prolonged fetal heart rate decelerations are an indication for immediate cesarean section.[1–3,5,6]

Bearing down is reflex during the second stage of labor. Coaching may be required for optimal pushing efforts, especially in the presence of epidural anesthesia. Half-flex the patient's legs to increase and improve her pushing efficacy. Encourage the mother to take a deep breath at the onset of a contraction and then push downward or Valsalva. Encourage the mother to rest between contractions, as both the mother and the fetus need to recover from the effects of uterine contractions, breath holding, and the muscular effort.[2]

The perineum will bulge as the fetus descends into the maternal pelvis. Sponge downward any stool that is expelled with a sterile sponge and diluted soap solution. The woman and the fetus are prepared for delivery when the scalp of the fetus becomes visible at the introitus.

INDICATIONS

The indications for the performance of a vaginal delivery in the Emergency Department include a patient in active labor without the ability or time to transfer the patient to a delivery unit; the lack of availability of an Obstetrician, Family Physician, Certified Nurse Midwife, or other obstetric practitioner; fetal distress; or maternal distress.

CONTRAINDICATIONS

There are no contraindications to the emergent delivery of the fetus in the Emergency Department. Delivery is preferred in a well-staffed Obstetrics Department, especially when the delivery is complicated with prematurity, breech delivery, or umbilical cord prolapse.

EQUIPMENT

General Supplies

Electronic fetal monitor
Sterile towels
Povidone iodine
Clock or timer watch
Sterile perineal drapes
Sterile gloves
Needles
Syringes
Chromic suture, 2–0 and 4–0
Vicryl suture, 2–0 and 3–0
Bulb syringe
Local anesthetic solution
Clean towels or blanket for baby
Umbilical cord clamp
Sterile scissors to trim umbilical cord
Infant warmer
Infant resuscitation equipment

Delivery Instrument Pack

Bandage scissors
4 towel clips
2 Allis forceps
4 ring forceps
6 straight Kocher clamps
Straight Mayo scissors
2 suture scissors
Adson forceps, or other forceps with teeth
Russian forceps, 5.5 inches and 8 inches
Gelpe retractor
2 small or medium Richardson retractors
2 Army-Navy retractors
2 needle holders, 6 inches
Placenta basin

PATIENT PREPARATION

The initial step when managing an emergent delivery is to obtain vital signs of the mother and the fetus, if fetal monitoring is available. Explain to the mother the urgency of a delivery in the Emergency Department, including the risks and benefits. Explain what to expect, the procedures that may be performed, and attempt to incorporate maternal cooperation to accomplish a controlled delivery. Obtain intravenous access and send blood to the laboratory to determine maternal Rh status and ABO blood type.

The most commonly used maternal position for delivery is the dorsal lithotomy position. This position increases the diameter of the pelvic outlet. Place the patient supine with her legs in stirrups or leg holders.

Never strap the legs so that quick flexion of the thighs can occur if shoulder dystocia presents. Cleanse the vulvar and perineal area with sterile soap or povidone iodine, if time permits. Apply sterile drapes to only expose the vulvar area (Figure 110-5). Perform a surgical hand scrub and apply a sterile gown and gloves.

Pain relief for a vaginal delivery can be achieved safely and effectively in the form of perineal infiltration with a local anesthetic agent. The pudendal nerve block is a minor regional block that provides adequate analgesia (Figure 110-6A). Palpate the ischial spine through the vagina. Insert a 20 gauge needle between the index and middle finger using a needle guard (Figure 110-6B). Advance the needle and pierce the sacrospinous ligament (Figure 110-6B). Aspirate to ensure that the tip of the needle is not within a blood vessel. Inject 5 to 10 mL of local anesthetic solution. Repeat this procedure on the contralateral side.

A paracervical block can also be used to provide analgesia. However, it can only be used during the first stage of labor. This technique anesthetizes the Frankenhäuser ganglions that contain all the visceral sensory nerve fibers from the uterus, cervix, and upper vagina. Palpate the lateral vaginal fornix (Figure 110-7). Insert a 20 gauge needle along the finger using a needle guard (Figure 110-7). Advance the needle into the submucosa of the lateral vaginal fornix. Aspirate to ensure that the tip of the needle is not within a blood vessel. Inject 5 to 7 mL of local anesthetic solution. Repeat this procedure on the contralateral side. Paracervical block anesthesia has been associated with a relatively high incidence of fetal bradycardia, usually developing 2 to 10 minutes after the block.

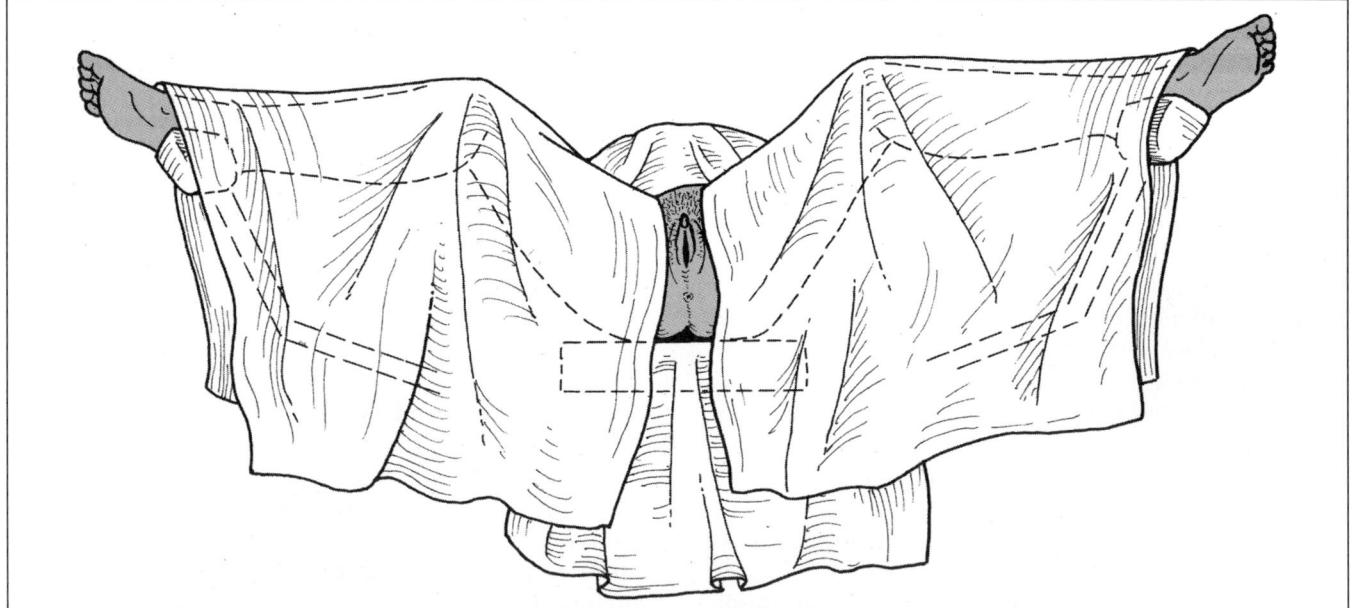

FIGURE 110-5 Patient positioning and sterile drape placement.

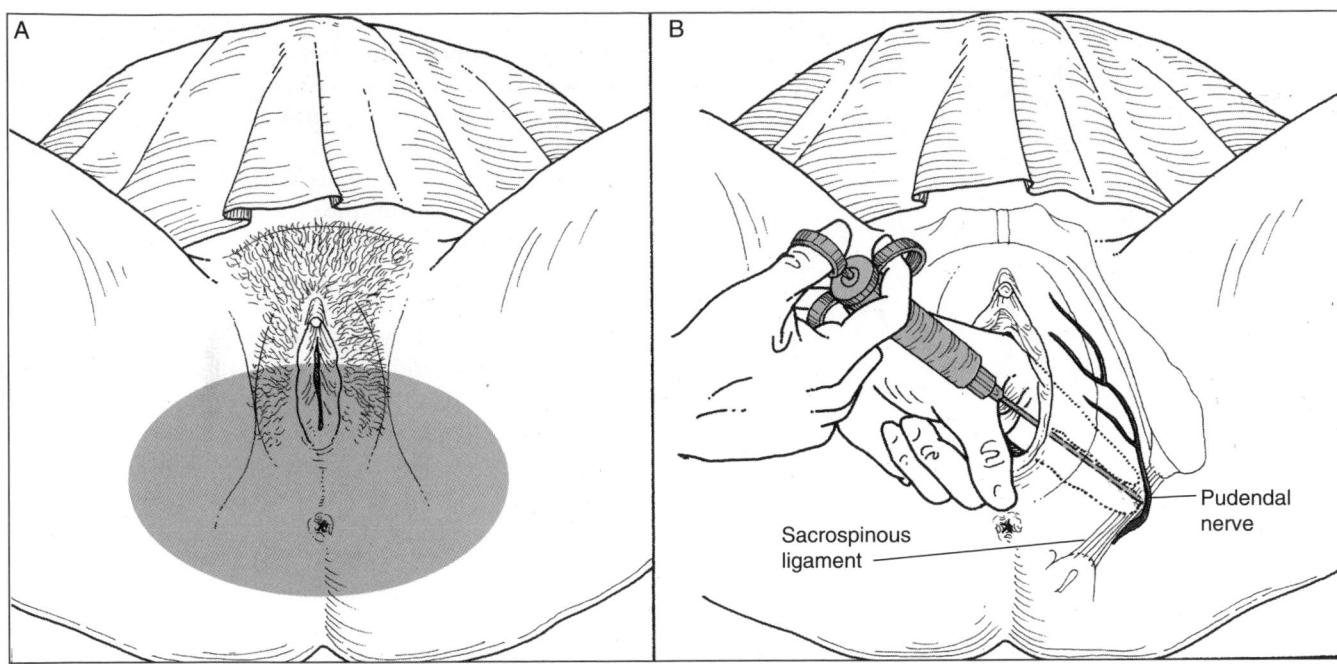

FIGURE 110-6 The pudendal nerve block. *A.* The area of sensory innervation of the pudendal nerve. *B.* Infiltration of local anesthetic solution.

TECHNIQUE

DELIVERY OF THE INFANT

The fetal head becomes increasingly visible at the introitus as labor progresses. It stretches the vaginal outlet and the vulva until they encircle the largest diameter of the fetal head, known as crowning. Gentle digital stretching of the inferior portion of the perineum may aide delivery. The routine use of an episiotomy for delivery has been discouraged due to increases in third-degree and fourth-degree lacerations. However, an episiotomy can be accomplished when the baby is crowning if there appears to be inadequate stretching of the perineum. The most common episiotomy performed is in the midline. Refer to Chapter 111 for the complete details regarding an episiotomy.

Perform the Ritgen maneuver as the head emerges from the introitus (Figure 110-8).[2,5] The Ritgen maneuver applies forward and upward force on the fetal forehead through the perineum, anterior to the coccyx, with a towel-draped hand to protect against fecal contamination. The other hand is placed on the fetal occiput to hold the suboccipital region against the mother's pubic symphysis.

Slowly deliver the fetal head using the Ritgen maneuver. The base of the occiput will rotate towards the posterior aspect of the pubic symphysis while the fetal brow, face, and chin pass over the perineum. **Instruct the**

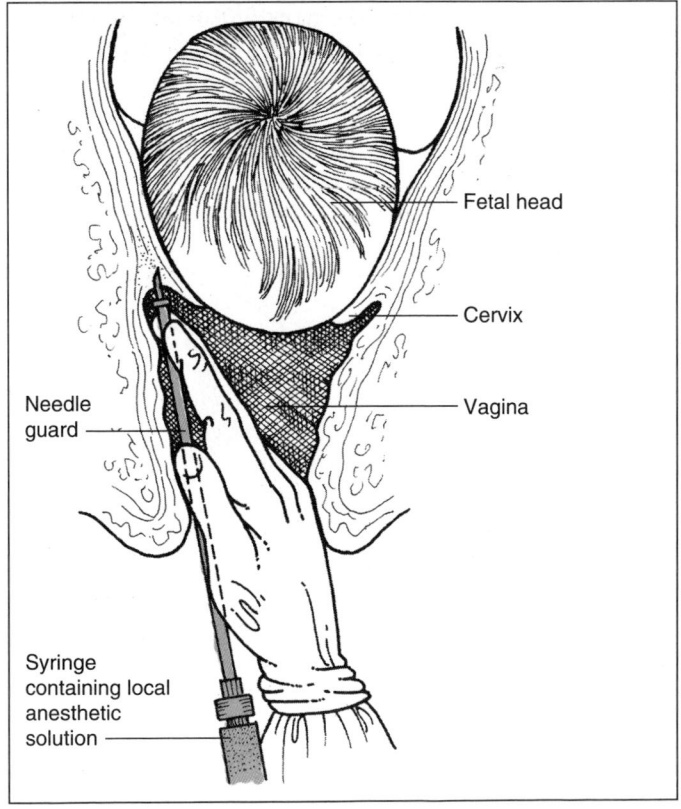

FIGURE 110-7 The paracervical nerve block.

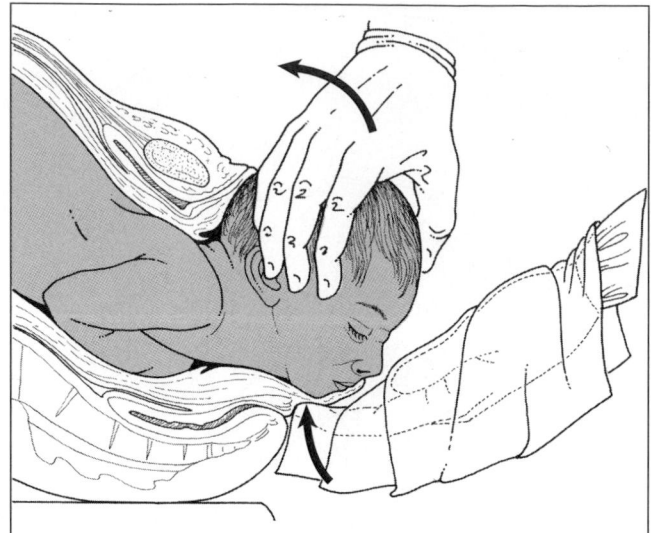

FIGURE 110-8 The Ritgen maneuver. A hand covered with a sterile towel applies moderate upward pressure on the perineum between the anus and the introitus. The other hand extends the fetal head to maintain the suboccipital region against the maternal pubic symphysis. This maneuver assists in the delivery of the fetal head.

mother to stop pushing once the head is delivered. Slightly rotate the infant's head if it does not spontaneously rotate. Suction the nasal cavities and oropharynx (Figure 110-9). This is particularly important if the infant is presenting with meconium.

Pass one hand around the neck of the fetus to check for a nuchal cord.[2,5] **The umbilical cord must be unwound from the fetal neck, if present, prior to continuing with the delivery.**[6] Slip it over the infant's head if possible (Figure 110-10). The umbilical cord can occasionally be wrapped so tight around the fetal neck that it

cannot be slipped over the head. **Carefully grasp and clamp the umbilical cord between two Kocher clamps placed 1 to 2 cm apart. Carefully cut the umbilical cord between the two Kocher clamps with a sterile scissors. Unwind the umbilical cord from around the fetal neck. Immediately deliver the fetus as it no longer can rely on the maternal circulation once the umbilical cord is clamped and cut.**

Deliver the body of the fetus (Figure 110-11). Gently grasp the sides of the fetal head with two hands (Figure 110-11). Apply steady and gentle downward traction until the anterior shoulder appears under the pubic symphysis (Figure 110-11A). The use of gentle traction may avoid brachial plexus injuries. Apply steady and gentle upward pressure until the posterior shoulder is delivered (Figure 110-11B).

The rest of the infant will spontaneously deliver once the shoulders are delivered. **It is still very important to control the delivery of the body to prevent maternal perineal lacerations.** Proper positioning is important during delivery of the body. A combination of amniotic fluid, blood, and vernix makes delivery of the infant very slippery. Position the posterior or left hand underneath the infant's axilla prior to delivering the rest of the body. Use the anterior or right hand to grasp the infant's ankles as they are delivered. This ensures a firm grip on the infant.

Suction the oropharynx and nasal cavities again following delivery of the infant. Place two Kocher clamps on the umbilical cord, approximately 4 to 5 cm from the infant and 1 cm apart. Cut the umbilical cord between the two clamps using a sterile scissors. Instruct an assis-

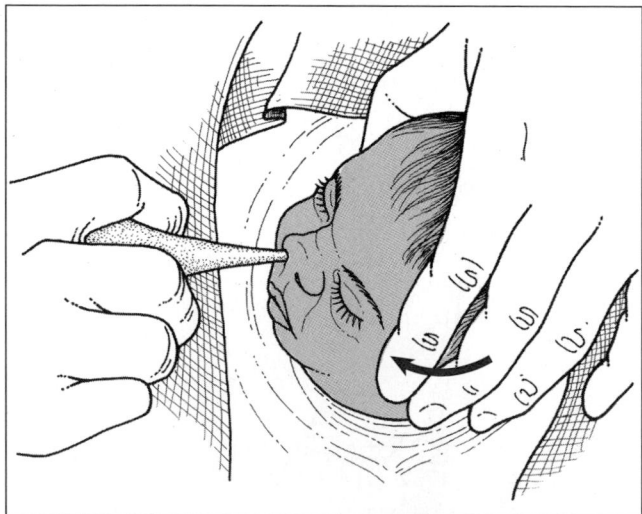

FIGURE 110-9 Slightly rotate the fetal head and suction the nasal cavities and the oropharynx.

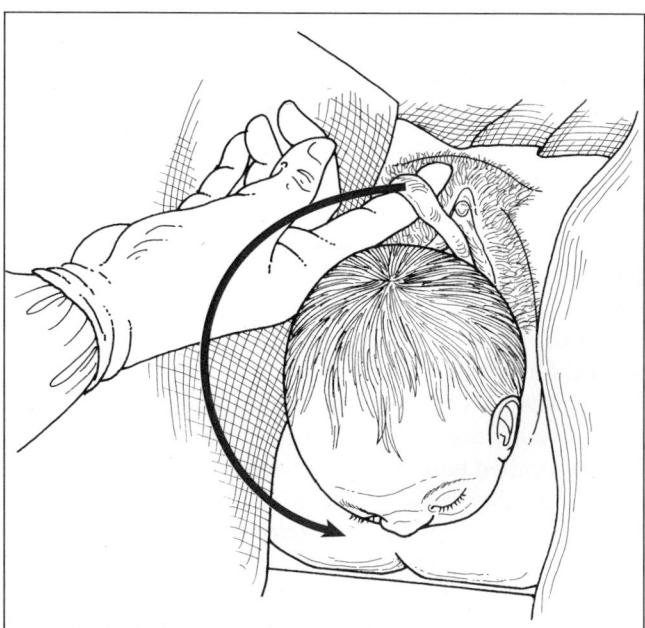

FIGURE 110-10 Slip any loops of umbilical cord that are wrapped around the fetal neck over the head.

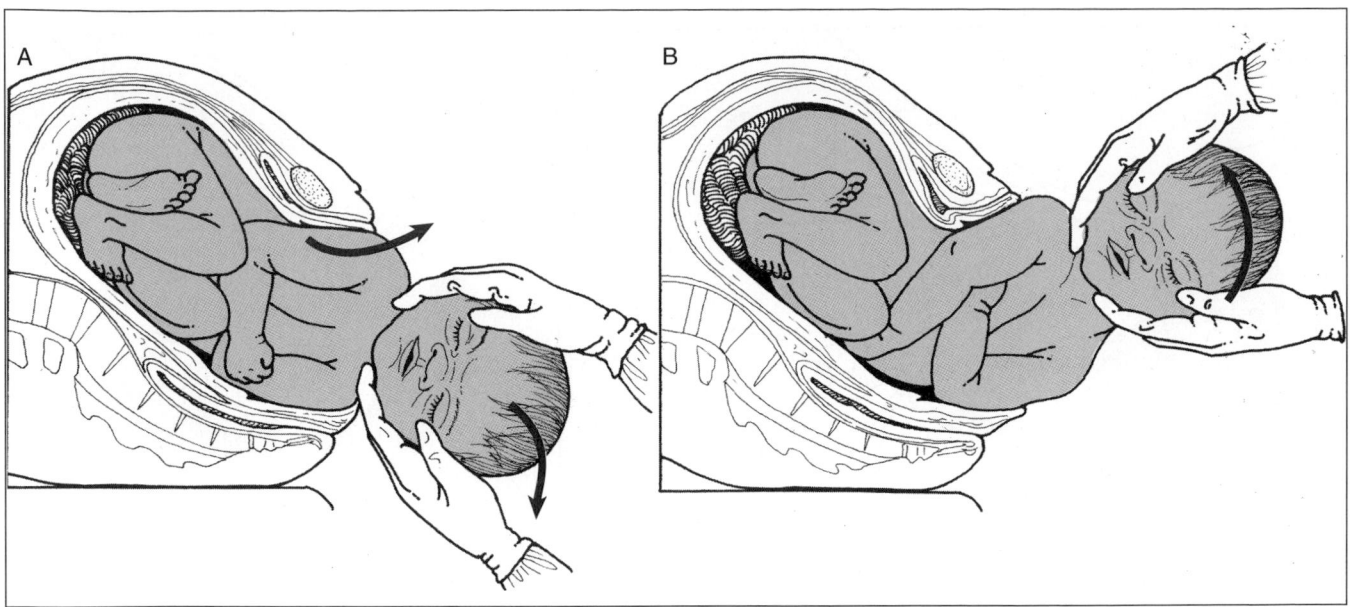

FIGURE 110-11 Delivery of the body. Grasp the head with both hands. *A.* Apply gentle and steady downward traction to deliver the anterior shoulder. *B.* Apply gentle and steady upward traction to deliver the posterior shoulder.

tant to obtain a 10 to 20 mL sample of umbilical cord blood from the placental end for Coombs and VDRL testing.

Dry the infant in a loosely wrapped towel while simultaneously stimulating and assessing it. The mother may immediately hold the infant while the umbilical cord is cut in an uncomplicated birth. The child should respond well to initial stimulation and have an adequately clear airway and good respiratory effort. The infant can be further dried and stimulated in a warm incubator where neonatal resuscitation can occur. Immediately place the infant in the incubator and begin resuscitation in cases where meconium contamination is suspected. Calculate the Apgar scores at 1 minute and 5 minutes after delivery. Scoring involves general color, tone, heart rate, respiratory effort, and reflexes (Table 110-1).

DELIVERY OF THE PLACENTA

Watchful waiting until the placenta separates from the uterus is the usual practice if there is no unusual bleeding after delivery of the infant. The signs of placental separation include a firm and globular uterus, a sudden gush of blood, uterine elevation in the abdomen, and a lengthening of the umbilical cord. These signs are generally present within 5 to 10 minutes after delivery of the infant. Times longer than 30 minutes raise concern regarding a potential retained placenta.

Instruct the patient to bear down when the placenta has separated. This results in increased intraabdominal pressure that aids in expelling the placenta. Apply gentle traction on the umbilical cord to keep it taut without the use of excessive traction (Figure 110-12*A*). **Aggressive traction on the umbilical cord can result in disruption of the placenta, uterine inversion, or tearing of the umbilical cord; all of which can result in excessive bleeding.** Apply suprapubic pressure as the placenta exits the uterus to prevent uterine inversion (Figure 110-12*B*). Deliver the placenta from the uterus (Figure 110-12*C*). Take care to prevent tearing of the placenta and its membranes as it passes through the introitus. Grasp the placenta and membranes with a ring forceps and guide them out the vagina with gentle twisting traction if tearing occurs (Figure 110-12*D*). Gently massage the uterus through the anterior abdominal wall to maintain uterine contraction. **Carefully examine the maternal surface of the placenta for completeness. Any missing pieces represent retained products and must be removed.**

TABLE 110-1. THE APGAR SCORE

Sign	Score = 0	Score = 1	Score = 2
Heart rate	Absent	Slow (< 100)	> 100
Respiratory effort	Absent	Slow or irregular	Good and crying
Muscle tone	Flaccid	Some extremity flexion	Active motion
Reflex irritability	No response	Grimace	Vigorous crying
Color	Blue or pale	Pink body and blue extremities	Completely pink

Sum the scores for each of the five signs to obtain the Apgar score. The maximal possible score is ten.

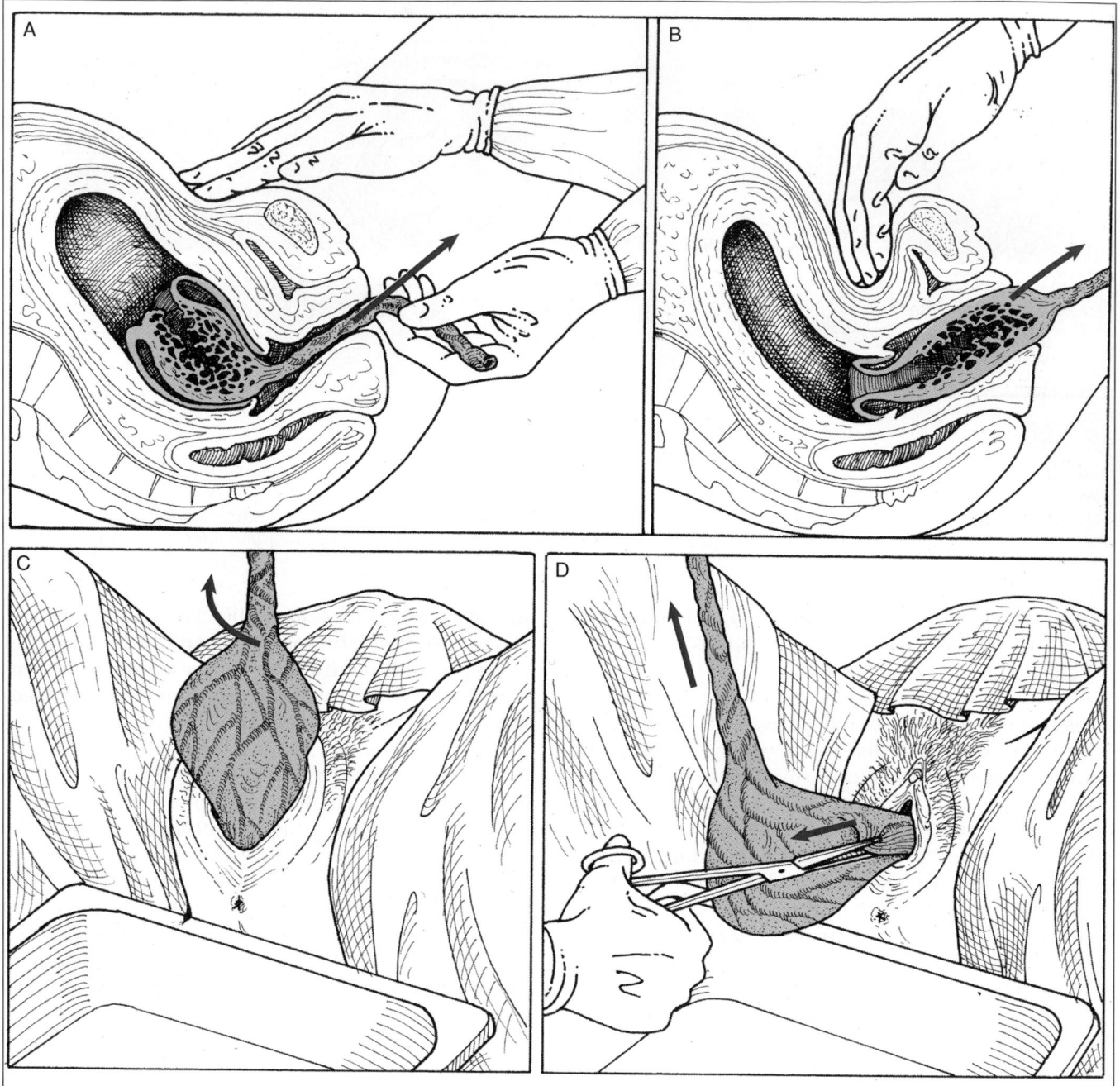

FIGURE 110-12 Delivery of the placenta. *A.* Apply gentle traction on the umbilical cord. *B.* Apply suprapubic pressure to help expel the placenta and prevent inversion of the uterus. *C.* Delivery of the placenta. *D.* Torn membranes or placenta are grasped with a ring forceps and delivered.

ALTERNATIVE TECHNIQUES

Operative vaginal delivery involves the use of forceps or vacuum extractors. This mode of delivery is sometimes controversial, but it can be a safe and effective technique for delivery.[2,5] The use of forceps and vacuums is beyond the scope of this chapter.

ASSESSMENT

Vaginal lacerations are classified as first, second, third, or fourth degree.[2,5] First-degree lacerations involve the fourchette, perineal skin, and vaginal mucous membrane but not the underlying fascia or muscle. Second-degree lacerations involve the above plus the fascia and muscles of the perineal body but not the anal sphincter. Third-degree lacerations involve the anal sphincter, while fourth-degree lacerations extend through the anal mucosa. The repair of vaginal lacerations is beyond the scope of this chapter. Refer to Chapters 111 and 114 for the complete details regarding laceration repair.

AFTERCARE

The hour immediately following delivery is often referred to as the fourth stage of labor. It is a critical time. The mother is at risk for hemorrhage, most commonly the result of uterine atony or lacerations of the birth canal. **Investigate any unusual bleeding immediately**. Administer 20 units of oxytocin, in 1 L of normal saline, intravenously to prevent uterine atony and postpartum hemorrhage. Persistent vaginal bleeding can be managed with additional intravenous oxytocin, 0.2 mg of methyl ergonovine (Methergine) intramuscularly, or 0.2 mg of prostaglandin F-2 alpha (Hemabate) intramuscularly.

COMPLICATIONS

Numerous complications can result during the delivery of an infant. These may affect the infant, the mother, or both the infant and the mother.

UMBILICAL CORD PROLAPSE

The examiner's hand should not be removed if the initial vaginal examination reveals a prolapsed umbilical cord. Elevate the presenting part away from the prolapsed umbilical cord. This reduces compression of the umbilical cord and optimizes blood flow to the fetus. Immediately transport and prep the patient for an emergent cesarean section while keeping the examiner's hand in place.

SHOULDER DYSTOCIA

The shoulders may occasionally impact at the pelvic outlet after delivery of the head. This may occur with delivery of large infants that have larger shoulders compared to their head circumference. Complications of shoulder dystocia include brachial plexus injuries, fetal hypoxia, and compression of the umbilical cord. Suction the infant's nasopharynx and place the mother in the extreme lithotomy position, with her legs sharply flexed up to the abdomen (McRoberts maneuver). An episiotomy may also be made to assist in the delivery. Instruct an assistant to apply suprapubic pressure to help disimpact the anterior shoulder from the pubic symphysis. Refer to Chapter 112 for the complete details regarding the management of shoulder dystocia.

BREECH PRESENTATION

The breech presentation is associated with a higher incidence of fetal distress and umbilical cord prolapse. It usually occurs in premature infants as the final rotation in the uterus may have not yet occurred. The major concern of breech deliveries is entrapment of the head because of an incompletely dilated cervix. **Do not pull on the fetus. This may put additional pressure on the head or further entrap an extremity. Obtain immediate Obstetrical assistance**. Refer to Chapter 113 for the complete details regarding breech deliveries.

PRETERM DELIVERY

Delivery of the preterm fetus must be controlled and slow, reducing the likelihood of trauma to the fragile infant. Immediately dry and warm the preterm infant while making an initial assessment. Resuscitation should occur, even for extreme prematurity, until the determination of viability is made.

POSTPARTUM HEMORRHAGE

Significant bleeding can occur from cervical lacerations, uterine atony, retained products, or first-degree through fourth-degree lacerations. Perform a thorough search for the cause of the postpartum hemorrhage. Refer to Chapter 114 for the complete details regarding the evaluation and management of postpartum hemorrhage.

INJURIES TO THE INFANT

A variety of injuries can occur to the fetus during the process of delivery. These include abrasions, lacerations, bruising, skull fractures, cephalohematomas, intracranial hemorrhage, brachial plexopathies, nerve injuries, clavicle fractures, humerus fractures, femur fractures, spinal cord injuries, and visceral injuries. Most of these can be prevented by using appropriate techniques and care when delivering the infant.

SUMMARY

The Emergency Physician will occasionally be required to perform a delivery of a baby when the Obstetrician is not available or when delivery is imminent. Fortunately, births in the Emergency Department are rare and most proceed with good outcomes. Knowledge of normal labor and delivery mechanics aid in a safe delivery and help identify complications. The Emergency Physician must develop strategies to treat potential complications and must be prepared to intervene.

REFERENCES

1. American College of Obstetricians and Gynecologists: *Technical Bulletin Number 207. Fetal Heart Rate Patterns: Monitoring, Interpretation, and Manage-*

ment. Washington, DC: American College of Obstetricians and Gynecologists, 1995.

2. Cunningham FG, MacDonald PC, Gant NF, et al: *Williams Obstetrics,* 20th ed. Norwalk, CT: Appleton and Lange, 1997.

3. Kjeldsen J: Hemodynamic investigations during labor and delivery. *Acta Obstet Gynecol Scand* 1979; 89(suppl):1–252.

4. American College of Obstetricians and Gynecologists: *Committee Opinion Number 173. Prevention of Early-Onset Group B Streptococcal Disease in Newborns.* Washington, DC: American College of Obstetricians and Gynecologists, 1996.

5. Gabbe SG, Niebyl JR, Simpson JL: *Obstetrics: Normal and Problem Pregnancies.* Philadelphia: Churchill Livingstone, 1996.

6. Hankins GDV, Snyder RR, Hauth JC, et al: Nuchal cords and neonatal outcome. *Obstet Gynecol* 1987; 70:687–691.

Chapter 111
EPISIOTOMY

Arani Forghani
Susan K. Hendricks

INTRODUCTION

An episiotomy or perineotomy is defined as an incision made into the perineal body and vagina to create room for the presenting part of the fetus and facilitate vaginal delivery. It is the most common operation in obstetrics, yet it is highly controversial. It is thought to prevent perineal tearing by substituting a straight surgical incision for a ragged spontaneous laceration that may have a worse outcome after repair. Several studies, however, have shown that the notion of decreased postoperative pain and improved healing with an episiotomy compared to a tear may not be true.

Early studies on episiotomy in the 1940s and 1950s seemed to indicate that an episiotomy was protective of the vagina, urogenital diaphragm, and perineum.[1,2] However, more recent studies have refuted these findings.[3-5] A study of nearly 25,000 deliveries demonstrated that the episiotomy rate from 1980 to 1984 decreased from 73 percent to 45 percent.[6] The incidence of second-degree tears increased from 0.7 percent to 2 percent but the incidence of third-degree lacerations was unchanged at about 5 per 1000.[6] This study further supports the notion that a decreased frequency of episiotomies does not increase the incidence of extended tears.

ANATOMY AND PATHOPHYSIOLOGY

The perineal body is the center of the hub of a wheel that includes the transverse perineal muscles, the capsule of the external anal sphincter muscle, and the bulbospongiosus muscle (Figure 111-1). Connective tissue serves as the insertion site for many of the pelvic floor muscles. The perineal body attaches to the ischial tuberosities and to the inferior pubic rami through the perineal membrane and superficial transverse perineal muscles. The ischiocavernosus muscles attach to the anterior and lateral aspects of the structure. The perineal body is connected to the muscles of the pelvic diaphragm laterally. The perineal body is anchored posteriorly to the coccyx by the anal sphincter. The mediolateral episiotomy transects the superficial muscles of the perineum whereas the midline episiotomy does not.

An episiotomy may be performed in the midline or mediolaterally (Figure 111-2).[7-10] The choice between the two types of episiotomy is largely dependent upon the experience of the practitioner. Factors that influence type of episiotomy include, but are not limited to, the site of prior episiotomies, position of the presenting fetal part, the thickness or rigidity of the patient's perineum, and the obstetric perception of an impending severe laceration that risks a fourth-degree extension. A mediolateral incision may be prudent when an extended episiotomy is required or when the risk of a fourth-degree laceration is significant.[11-13] **Never perform a lateral (Figure 111-2A) or a Schuchardt (Figure 111-2D) episiotomy in the Emergency Department.** These are associated with significant complications.[7]

MIDLINE EPISIOTOMY

The midline episiotomy is a surgical incision made in the midline of the perineal body, starting from the vaginal fourchette to (but not including) the anal sphincter (Figure 111-2B). The incision transects the central tendinous portion of the perineal body. This is the most favored type of episiotomy in the United States. The midline episiotomy is easy to perform and easy to repair.[14,15] A prophylactic episiotomy, though not proven, is thought to prevent pelvic relaxation including cystoceles, rectoceles, and urinary incontinence.[4] The midline episiotomy is associated with quicker healing, less pain (no muscle belly is transected), and less blood loss than the other types of episiotomies. Compared to mediolateral episiotomies, there is an increased risk of third-degree or fourth-degree extensions with midline episiotomies.

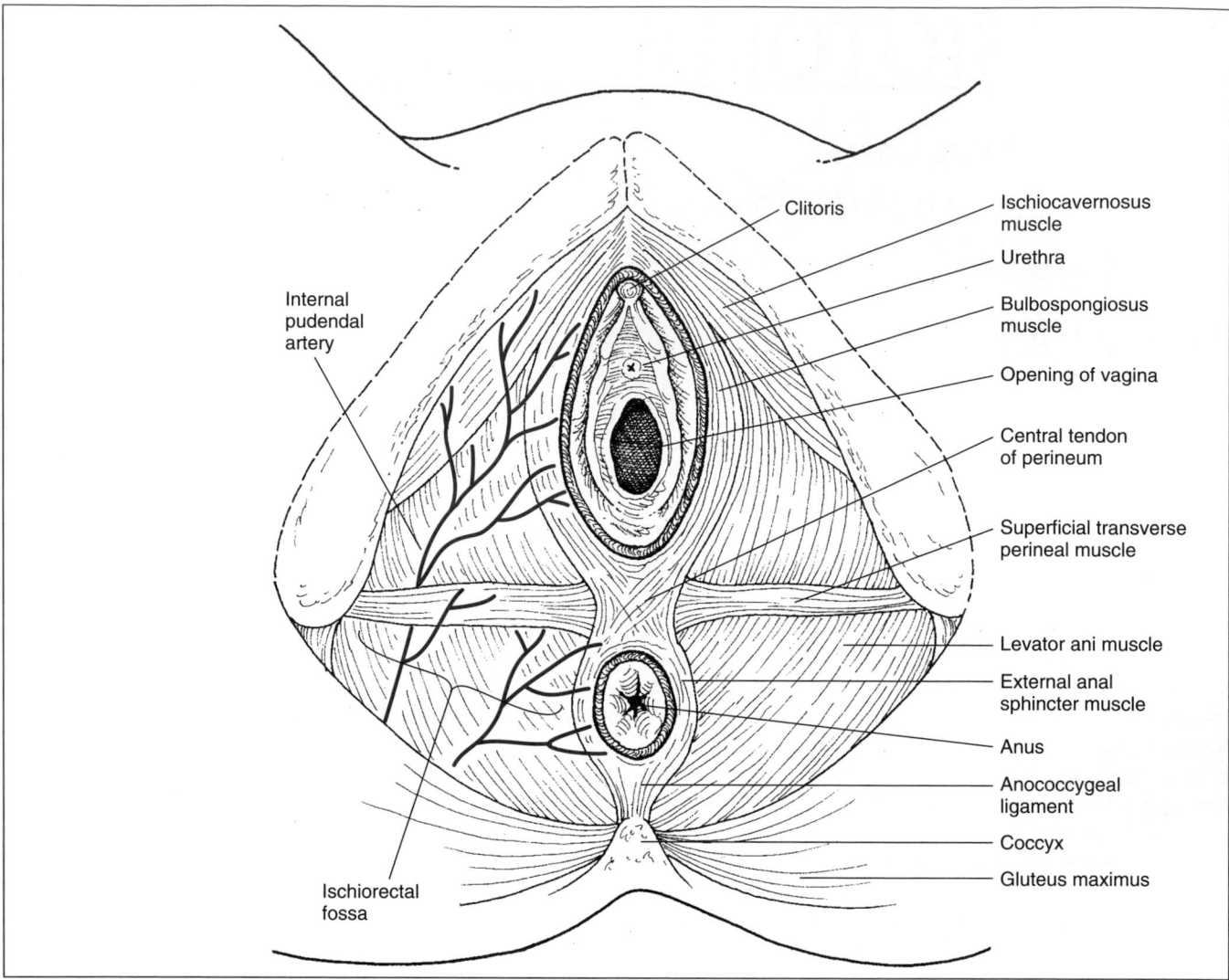

FIGURE 111-1 The anatomy of the perineum. The skin and subcutaneous tissues have been removed.

MEDIOLATERAL EPISIOTOMY

The mediolateral episiotomy is the preferred method in Europe.[18] The mediolateral episiotomy is a surgical incision made from the midline of the posterior vaginal fourchette obliquely towards the ischial tuberosity (Figure 111-2C). The anatomic structures transected are the skin, the subcutaneous tissues, the bulbospongiosus muscle, the superficial transverse perinei muscle, and a portion of the levator ani muscle and fascia.

The midline episiotomy is the preferred technique for many reasons. The mediolateral episiotomy is associated with a decreased risk of third-degree and fourth-degree lacerations, especially when combined with an operative vaginal delivery.[14] It is unfortunately associated with a more painful postpartum course and increased blood loss. It may result in faulty healing, anatomical deformities, and dyspareunia. It also requires a significant familiarity with the anatomy of the perineal body. The mediolateral episiotomy requires a more complicated repair.

INDICATIONS

The rate of episiotomy decreases as one travels the continuum from Obstetrician to Family Practitioner to Certified Nurse Midwife to lay Midwife. Most practitioners consider the performance of an episiotomy to be appropriate in situations of fetal distress or maternal disease requiring urgent delivery. Deliveries necessitating greater space accommodation for effective delivery are also indications for an episiotomy. These situations include shoulder dystocia, breech delivery, forceps or vacuum extractions, occiput posterior positions, and cases of imminent perineal rupture.[17] Other indications include contracted outlet syndrome, face presentations,

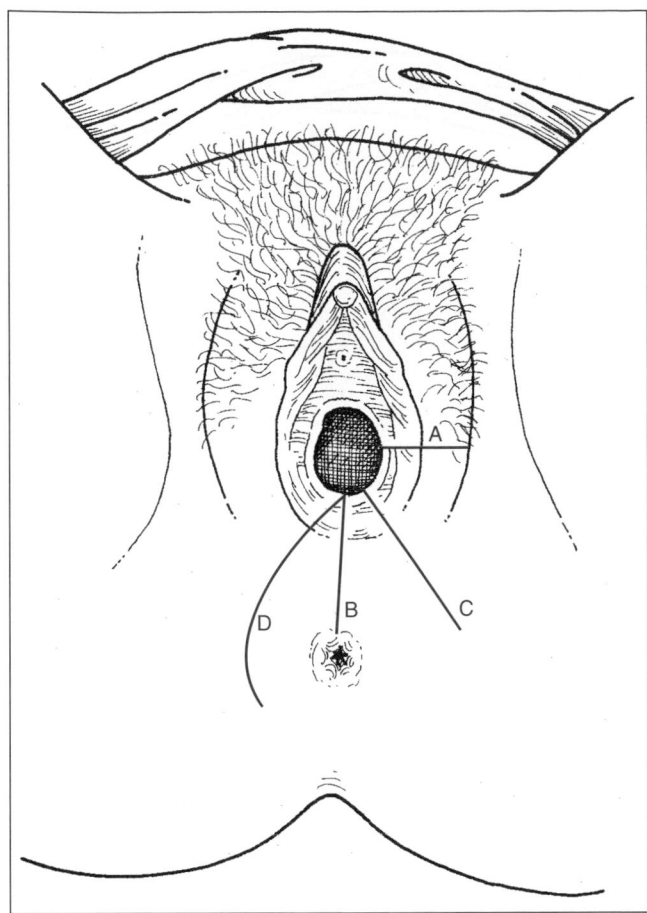

FIGURE 111-2 The types of episiotomies. *A.* Lateral. *B.* Midline. *C.* Mediolateral. *D.* Schuchardt.

and extensive fetal head extension. It is commonly believed that an episiotomy safely aids in shortening the second stage of labor and reduces trauma to the pelvic floor musculature.[4] More perineal and pelvic tissue injury is noted with a precipitous labor; thus a timely episiotomy is critical.[1] A multicenter review of 8647 deliveries demonstrated that the strongest independent predictors of episiotomy were nulliparity and vaginal operative delivery followed by the mother's age at first delivery.[1,2]

CONTRAINDICATIONS

Contraindications to performing an episiotomy include rectal or perineal lesions, prior or concurrent fistulae, inflammatory bowel disease, prior rectal surgery, or prior anal surgery.[16] Maternal diseases that impair healing such as autoimmune disorders (SLE, rheumatoid arthritis), HIV, or pregestational diabetes mellitus are relative contraindications to an episiotomy. Relative contraindications specific to the midline episiotomy are a short perineum, fetal macrosomia, vaginal operative deliveries, and abnormal fetal presentation.

EQUIPMENT

Local anesthetic solution, lidocaine or bupivacaine
Alcohol wipes
16 to 18 gauge needle
10 mL syringe
22 to 25 gauge needle
Straight Mayo scissors
#10 scalpel blade on a handle
Povidone iodine solution
Sterile drapes
Sterile gown and gloves
Chromic or polyglycolic acid suture, 2–0 or 3–0
Vicryl suture, 4–0 and 5–0
Needle driver

PATIENT PREPARATION

Explain the procedure, its risks, and benefits to the patient. Clean the perineum of any dirt, debris, stool, and urine. Apply povidone iodine or apply noniodinated alcohol-based sterilization solutions if the patient is allergic to iodine. Place sterile drapes beneath the buttocks, over the legs, and on the abdomen to prevent contamination from nonsterile areas (Figure 110-5).

Anesthetize the perineal body (Figure 111-3). Infiltrate 10 to 20 mL of local anesthetic solution directly into the perineal body, from the posterior base of the vaginal fourchette to the anus (Figure 111-3*A*). This provides safe and effective anesthesia. It may be performed if the child's head is within the vagina or crowning.

A bilateral pudendal nerve block will also provide excellent pain control (Figure 111-3*B*). It requires more time to perform and cannot be done if the child's head is in the vagina. Place the nondominant index finger in the vagina and palpate the ischial spine. The pudendal nerve and artery lie between the ischial spine and ischial tuberosity. Palpate the ischial tuberosity with the nondominant thumb. Insert a 23 gauge spinal needle just medial to the ischial tuberosity and aimed towards the ischial spine. Carefully advance the needle until the tip is palpable with the nondominant index finger. Infiltrate the area with 4 to 6 mL of local anesthetic solution. Repeat the procedure on the contralateral side.

TECHNIQUES

Place the index and middle fingers of the nondominant hand into the patient's introitus, with the palm of the hand facing outward (Figure 111-4*A*). Pull the perineal body away from the fetal presenting part to protect the fetus from injury. Use a #10 scalpel blade, a #15 scalpel blade, or a straight Mayo scissors to make the

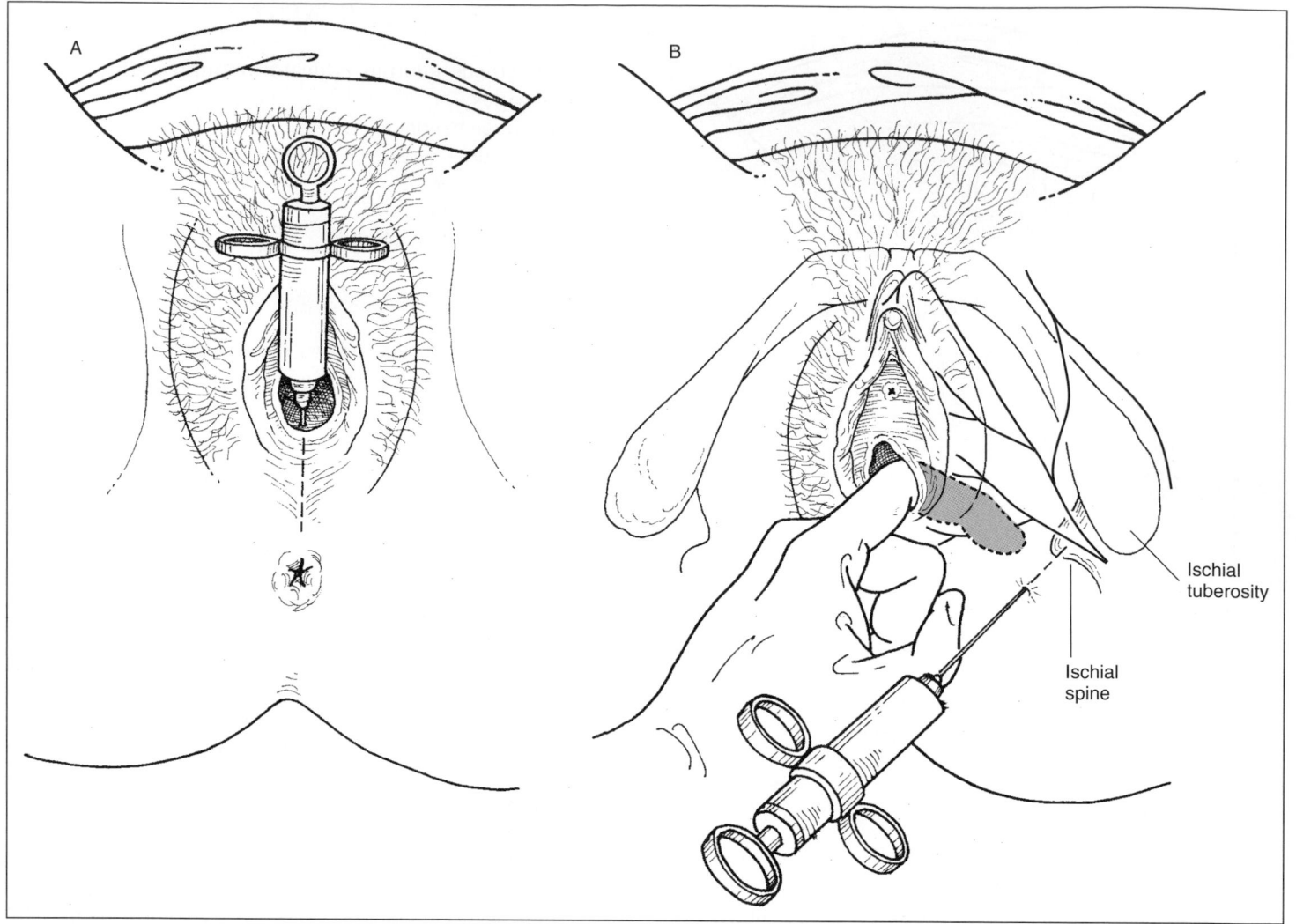

FIGURE 111-3 Anesthesia of the perineum. *A.* Local anesthetic infiltration subcutaneously from the posterior fourchette to the anus. *B.* The pudendal nerve block.

incision. **The editors recommend using only the Mayo scissors. A scalpel can cause significant injury to the fetus, the mother, and/or the physician.**

Insert the Mayo scissors so that one blade lies along the skin and the other is inside the introitus, between the index and middle fingers, and against the vaginal mucosa (Figure 111-4*B*). **Allow the maximum descent of the fetal presenting part and moderate distension of the perineum before making the incision to avoid a third-degree or fourth-degree laceration.** Make the incision when the presenting part has separated the vulva a minimum of 2 to 3 cm, unless early delivery is indicated.[1] Extend the incision 2 to 3 cm vertically up the vaginal mucosa. The introitus will readily open after making the episiotomy (Figure 111-4*C*).

MIDLINE EPISIOTOMY

Make the incision vertically in the midline of the perineal body, from the midpoint of the posterior fourchette to the capsule of the anal sphincter (Figure 111-4). The incision length depends upon the perineal length. **Make it of sufficient length to increase the area of the introitus for successful delivery of the presenting part without compromising the anal sphincter. The incision must include the tendinous central portion of the perineal body.** This involves (in order of progression from anterior to posterior) the muscular attachments of the bulbospongiosus muscle, the superficial transverse perinei muscle, a portion of the levator ani muscle, and the capsule of the anal sphincter muscle. **The most important aspect of the midline episiotomy is extension of the incision upward into the vaginal mucosal and past the hymenal ring.** This releases any constriction and allows maximal room for the presenting part of the fetus.

MEDIOLATERAL EPISIOTOMY

Make an incision at a 45 degree angle to the midline of the posterior fourchette, from the inferior portion of

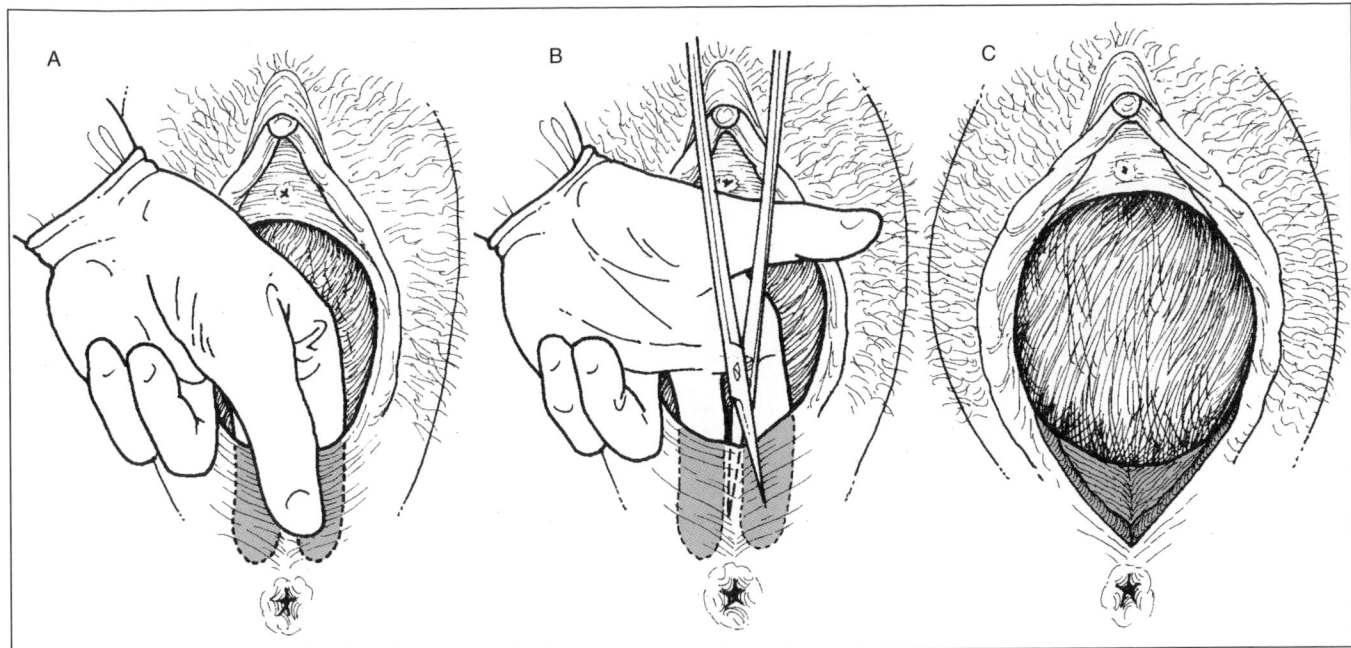

FIGURE 111-4 Performing a midline episiotomy. *A.* Place the nondominant index and middle fingers inside the introitus with the palm facing outward. *B.* Pull the perineal body away from the fetus and insert the straight Mayo scissors. Note that the blades of the Mayo scissors are positioned between the fingers. *C.* The introitus readily opens after making the episiotomy.

the hymenal ring towards the ischial tuberosity (Figure 111-2*C*). The length of the incision is less critical than that for a median episiotomy. Longer incisions require more extensive repair. The side to which the episiotomy is performed is generally the same as the handedness of the operator.[1] Make the incision at approximately 5 o'clock for left-handed dominants or at 7 o'clock for right-handed dominants. The anatomic structures incised and requiring repair (in progression from superficial to deep) are the skin and subcutaneous tissues, the bulbospongiosus muscle, the superficial transverse perinei muscle, and a portion of the levator ani muscle and its fascia.

ASSESSMENT

Carefully examine the vagina, cervix, and lower uterine segment for any signs of injury or laceration immediately following delivery of the infant and placenta. Do not begin repairing the episiotomy until after the delivery of the placenta. The repair may be compromised if manual removal of the placenta or intravaginal procedures must be performed after the episiotomy is reconstructed. Assess the incision for extension (third-degree or fourth-degree). Identify any site of excessive bleeding and immediately control it with a Vicryl ligature. Perform a digital rectal examination to rule out a fourth-degree extension or button-holing (a laceration through to the rectal mucosa which is not contiguous with the episiotomy).

MIDLINE EPISIOTOMY REPAIR TECHNIQUES

The midline episiotomy repair is an easier approximation than the mediolateral episiotomy as the incision is symmetrically situated in the perineal tissue.[14,19,20] The choice of suture is physician-dependent.[20] Chromic gut is associated with an increase in episiotomy breakdown and initial pain because of its shorter tensile strength. Dexon and Vicryl are associated with greater perineal irritation. Use a round needle to close all layers except the capsule and skin to minimize the risk of a subcutaneous hematoma.

VAGINAL MUCOSA REPAIR

Repair the vaginal mucosa first (Figure 111-5). Place the initial suture superior to the apex of the vaginal incision to incorporate any retracted vessels. Tie the suture at the apex of the incision securely. Approximate the wound edges with a running subcuticular stitch (Figure 111-5*A*) or a running simple stitch (Figure 111-5*B*). Place a running locked stitch (Figure 111-5*C*) if there are any concerns about hemostasis. **Do not allow the needle to enter through the rectal mucosa as this can result in the formation of a rectovaginal fistula.**

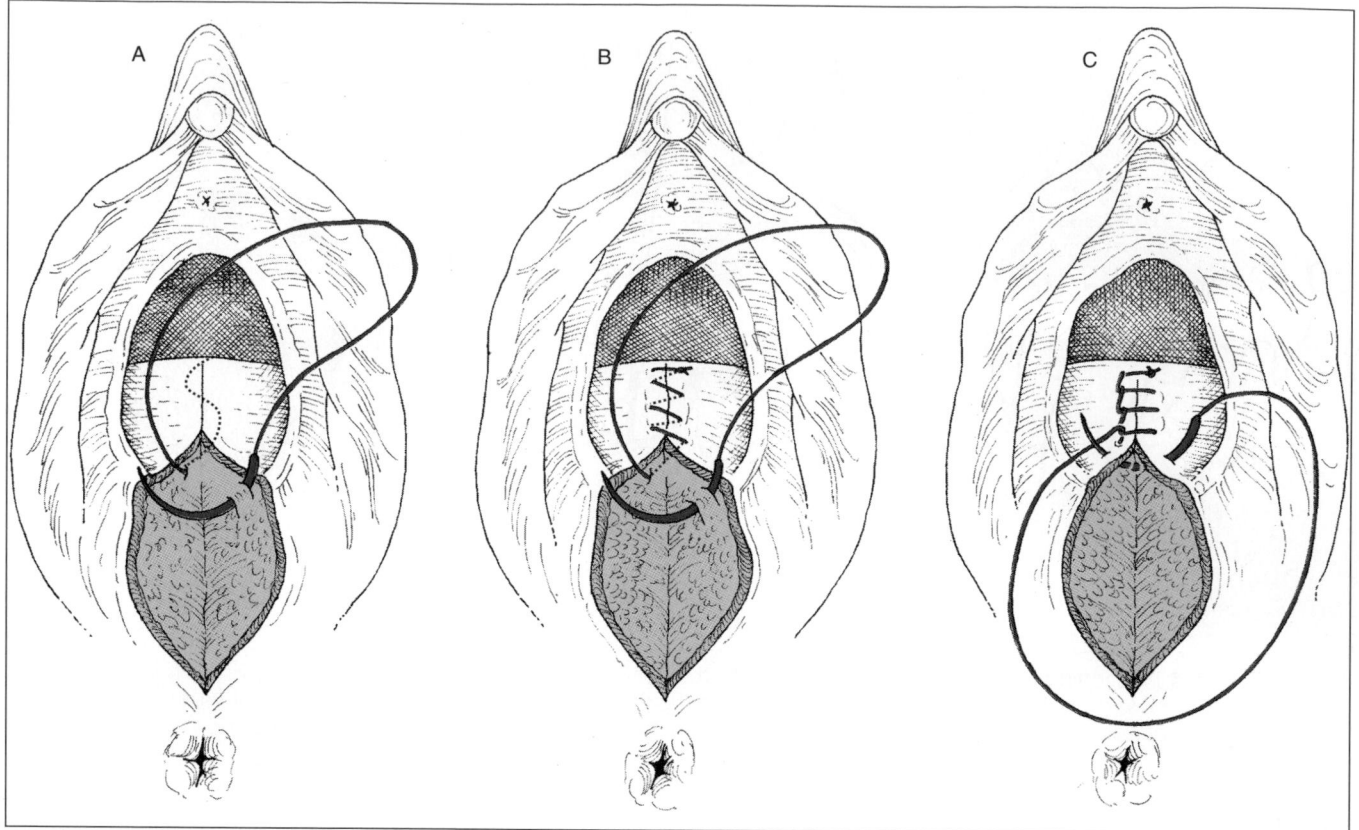

FIGURE 111-5 Methods of closing the vaginal mucosa. *A.* The running subcuticular stitch. *B.* The running simple stitch. *C.* The running locked stitch.

Place each stitch to bring together the mucous membrane of the vagina and the tissue between the vagina and rectum. This method of suturing provides for hemostasis, eliminates dead space, and decreases the risk of subsequent infection. Extend the continuous suture by one to two stitches past the hymenal ring and to the edge of the skin. Place the final suture to incorporate the subcutaneous tissue but not the skin. Finish reapproximating the skin incision with a buried knot.

The second suture is the so-called "crown suture". It is placed at the base of the sutured vaginal wound. Insert the needle into the immediate subcutaneous tissue, perpendicular to the skin, and angled deeply to approximate the edges of the bulbospongiosus muscle and its fascia. Close the remainder of the incision with the one-suture (Figure 111-6) or the two-suture technique (Figure 111-7).

ONE-SUTURE TECHNIQUE

The one-suture technique utilizes one strand of suture to close the entire episiotomy (Figure 111-6). Close the vaginal mucosa, as described previously, with a running stitch (Figure 111-6A). Approximate the hymeneal ring. Continue the running stitch to approximate the

perineal body (Figure 111-6B). Continue the running stitch until the bottom of the episiotomy is reached. Place a running subcuticular stitch from the bottom of the episiotomy to the hymenal ring (Figure 111-6C). Finish approximating the skin incision with a buried knot at the hymenal ring.

TWO-SUTURE TECHNIQUE

This technique utilizes two strands of suture to close the episiotomy (Figure 111-7). Close the vaginal mucosa, as described previously, with a running stitch (Figure 111-7A). Approximate the hymenal ring with this first strand of suture (Figure 111-7B). Close the perineal body using a second strand of suture material. Place running or interrupted stitches (Figure 111-7B). Use the first strand of suture to place a subcuticular running stitch to approximate the skin (Figure 111-7C). Finish approximating the skin incision with a buried knot.

ALTERNATIVE TECHNIQUE

Approximation of an episiotomy with one or two sutures can be time consuming and difficult. An alternative is to close the episiotomy using a simple interrupted

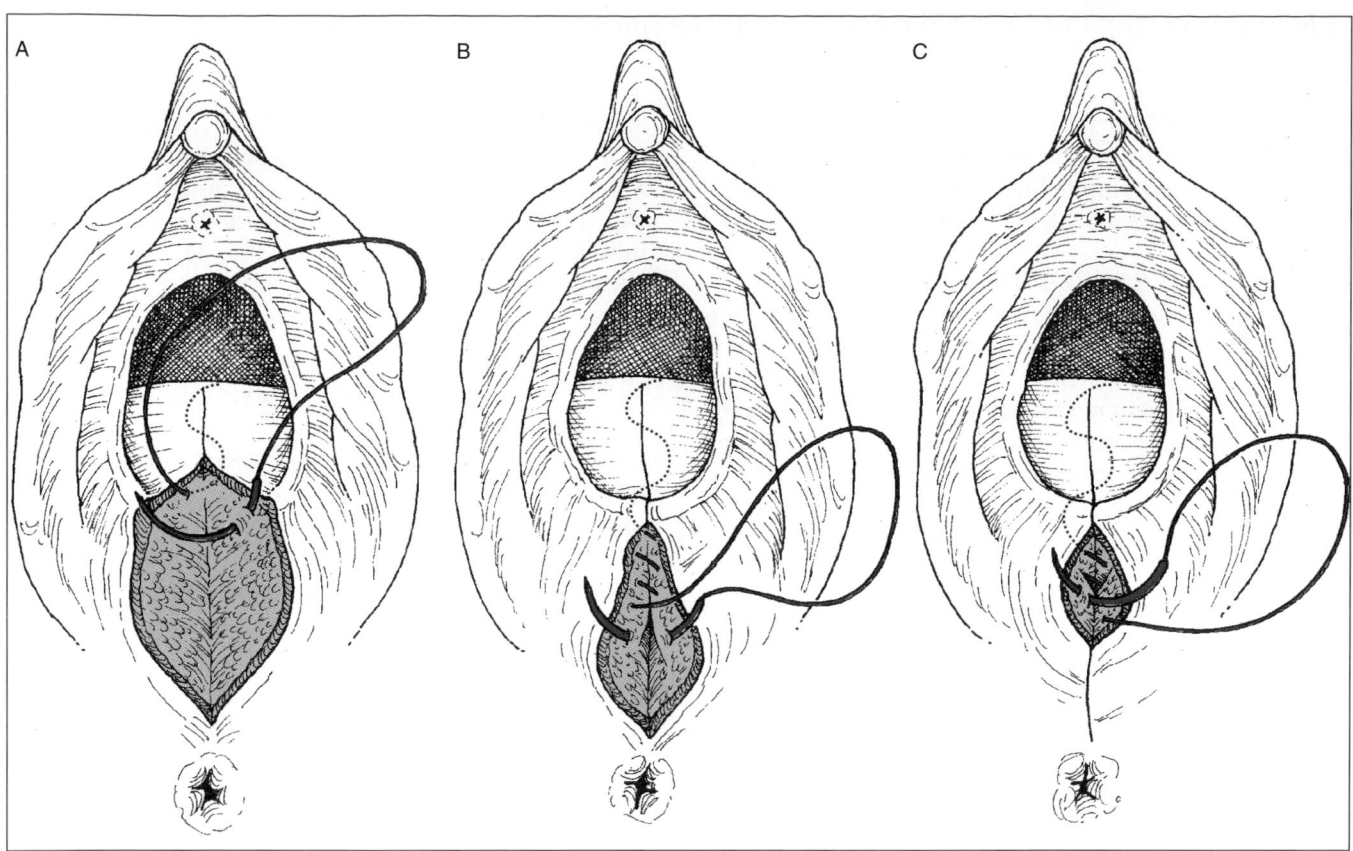

FIGURE 111-6 The one-suture technique to close an episiotomy. *A.* Approximate the vaginal mucosa with a running stitch. *B.* Approximate the hymenal ring followed by a running stitch to approximate the perineal body. *C.* Reverse the suture direction with a running subcuticular stitch to approximate the skin.

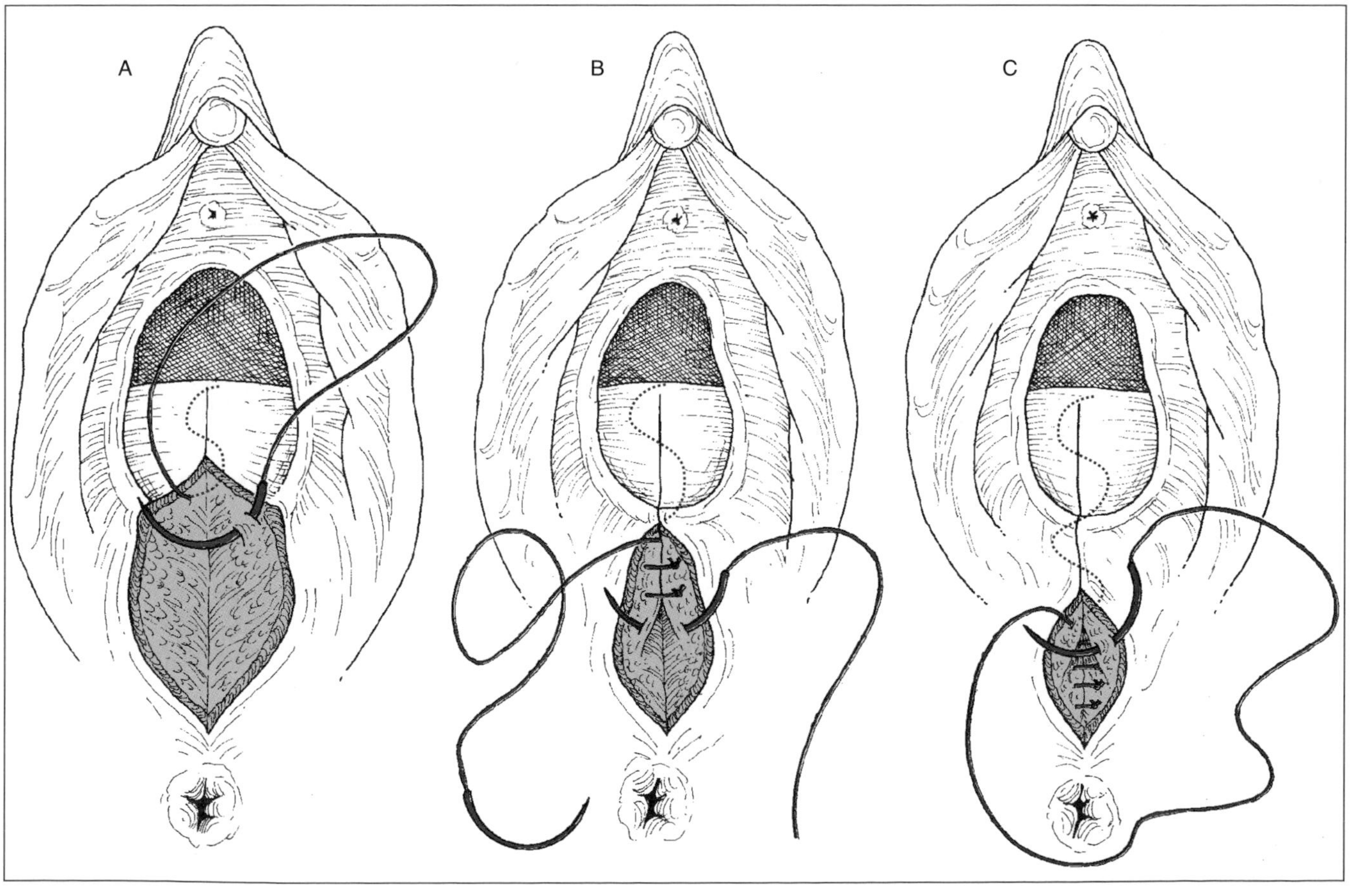

FIGURE 111-7 The two-suture technique to close an episiotomy. *A.* Approximate the vaginal mucosa with a running stitch. *B.* The hymenal ring is approximated with the first suture. The perineal body is approximated with a second suture utilizing an interrupted stitch. *C.* The first suture is continued subcutaneously to approximate the skin.

stitch (Figure 111-8). Take deep bites of tissue with the needle to ensure that the stitches close the subcutaneous tissues and perineal body along with the overlying vaginal mucosa and skin.

THIRD-DEGREE LACERATION REPAIR

A third-degree laceration involves the anal sphincter muscle and spares the anal mucosa. Visually inspect the anal sphincter muscle for partial lacerations. **A patient can have normal anal sphincter tone and a partial anal sphincter muscle laceration.** Repair any anal sphincter muscle lacerations as described in the following section on fourth-degree laceration repair.

FOURTH-DEGREE LACERATION REPAIR

Fourth-degree lacerations may occur as a result of a tearing of the tissues without an episiotomy, an extension of an episiotomy, or from an overvigorous episiotomy. **These lacerations involve the anal sphincter muscle and the anal mucosa. They must be repaired to prevent incontinence.** Approximate the anal mucosa and muscularis with simple interrupted 4–0 or 5–0

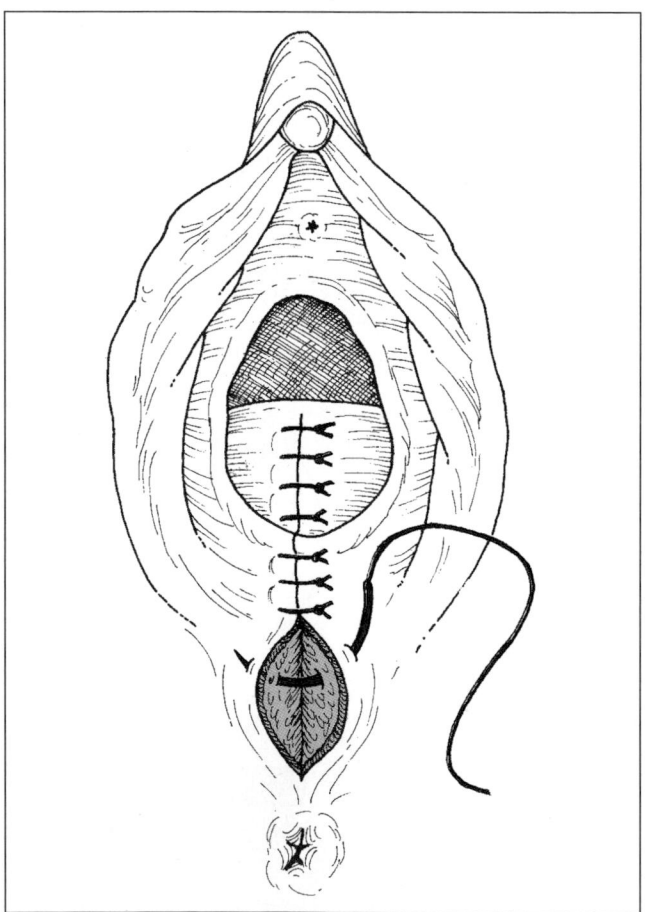

FIGURE 111-8 An alternative technique to close an episiotomy. Place simple interrupted stitches to approximate the mucosa/skin and perineal body.

chromic gut sutures (Figure 111-9A). Find and grasp both transected ends of the anal sphincter muscle with Allis clamps (Figure 111-9A). Place transfixion stitches with 4–0 or 5–0 Vicryl to approximate the anal sphincter muscles (Figure 111-9B). Close the remainder of the episiotomy as previously described.

MEDIOLATERAL EPISIOTOMY REPAIR TECHNIQUE

It is extremely important to locate and repair the transected bulbospongiosus muscle. Find and grasp the transected ends of the bulbospongiosus muscle with Allis clamps. Approximate it using 4–0 and 5–0 Vicryl sutures (Figure 111-10A). Approximate the vagina and deep perineal tissues using the one-suture or the two-suture technique (Figure 111-10B). Approximate the skin of the perineum using a running subcuticular stitch (Figure 111-10C).

AFTERCARE

The aftercare for a perineal incision involves cleanliness and pain control. The use of warm sitz baths three to four times a day in concert with the use of ice packs to the perineum will decrease inflammation and the risk of infection. Routine use of prophylactic antibiotics has never been proven effective to prevent infections after an episiotomy. Prescribe stool softeners to decrease the pain of defecation and the risk of episiotomy disruption, especially if it was associated with a third-degree or fourth-degree extension. Nonsteroidal anti-inflammatory drugs or acetaminophen provide adequate analgesia in most patients. Narcotic analgesics may be required for 24 to 72 hours, especially in cases of mediolateral episiotomies. Many Obstetricians prefer oxycodone or acetaminophen with codeine as they are not as constipating as the other narcotic analgesics. This is especially important in patients with third-degree or fourth-degree lacerations.

COMPLICATIONS

The use of a midline episiotomy may increase the risk of third-degree and fourth-degree lacerations.[21–24] A third-degree laceration is diagnosed when the capsule and/or the muscle of the anal sphincter is interrupted. A fourth-degree laceration involves the anal sphincter and the mucosa of the anus or rectum. Third-degree and fourth-degree lacerations may result in incontinence of feces, incontinence of flatus, and/or rectovaginal fistula formation if not properly repaired. Complications include increased blood loss, especially if the incision is made too early.

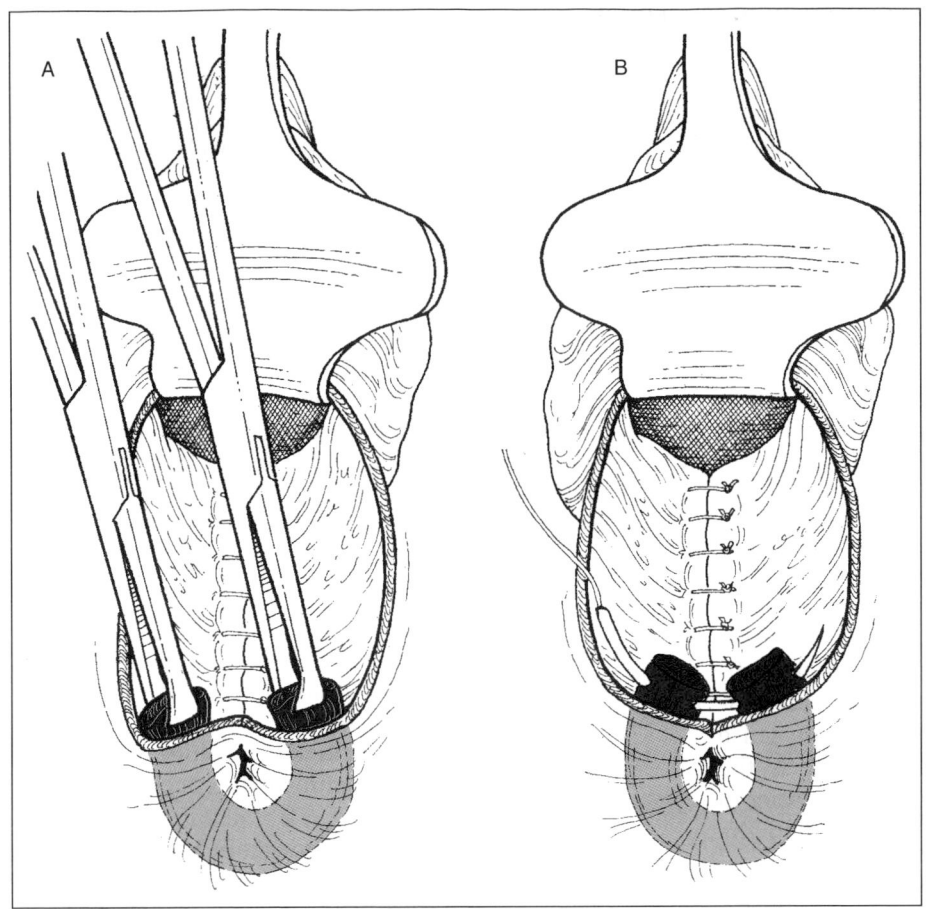

FIGURE 111-9 Repair of a fourth-degree laceration or episiotomy. *A.* Approximate the rectal submucosa and muscularis with simple interrupted sutures. Grasp the cut edges of the anal sphincter muscle with Allis clamps. *B.* Approximate the ends of the anal sphincter muscle with transfixion stitches.

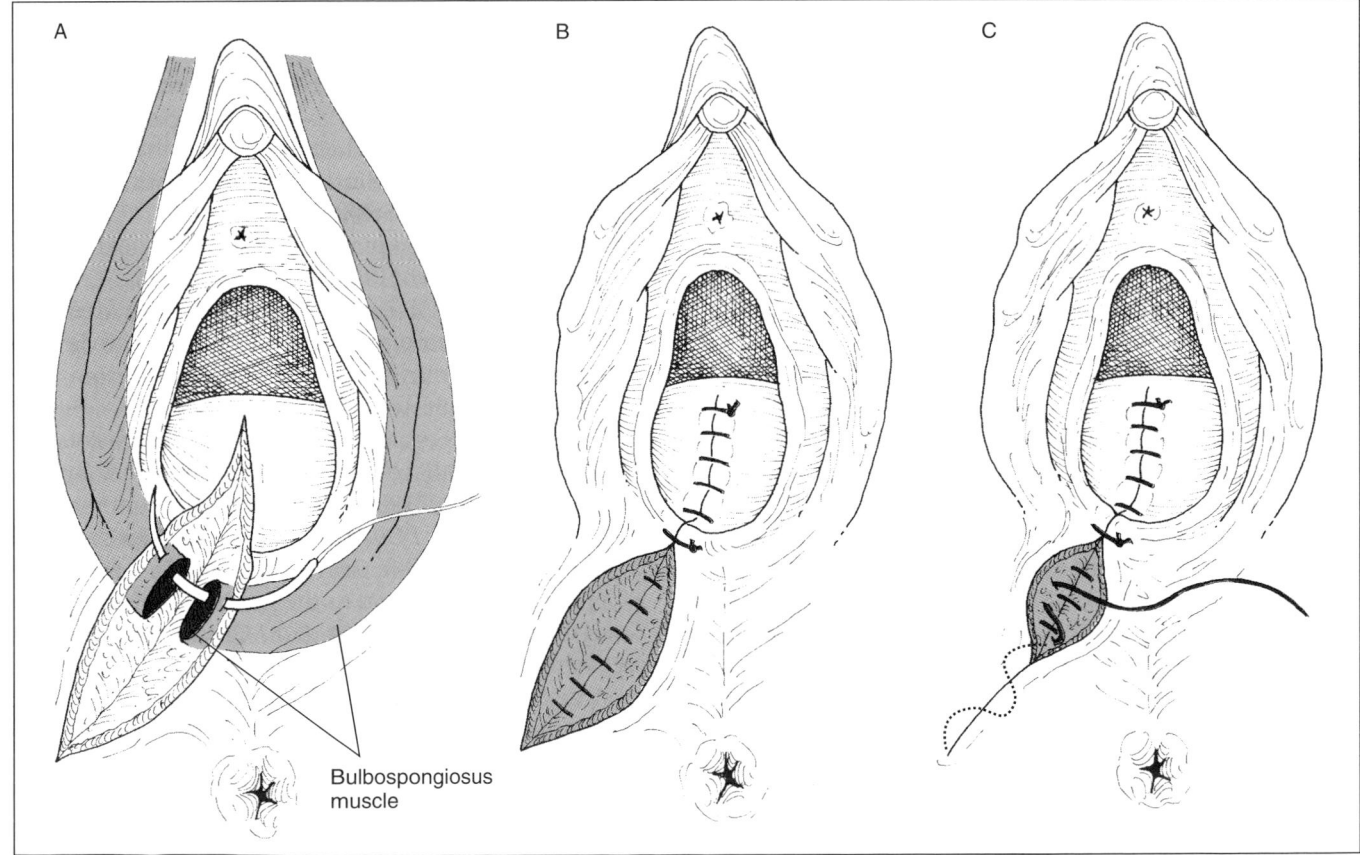

Bulbospongiosus muscle

FIGURE 111-10 Repair of a mediolateral episiotomy. *A.* Find and approximate the ends of the transected bulbospongiosus muscle. *B.* Approximate the vagina and deep peroneal tissues using the one-suture or two-suture technique. *C.* Approximate the skin with running subcuticular stitches.

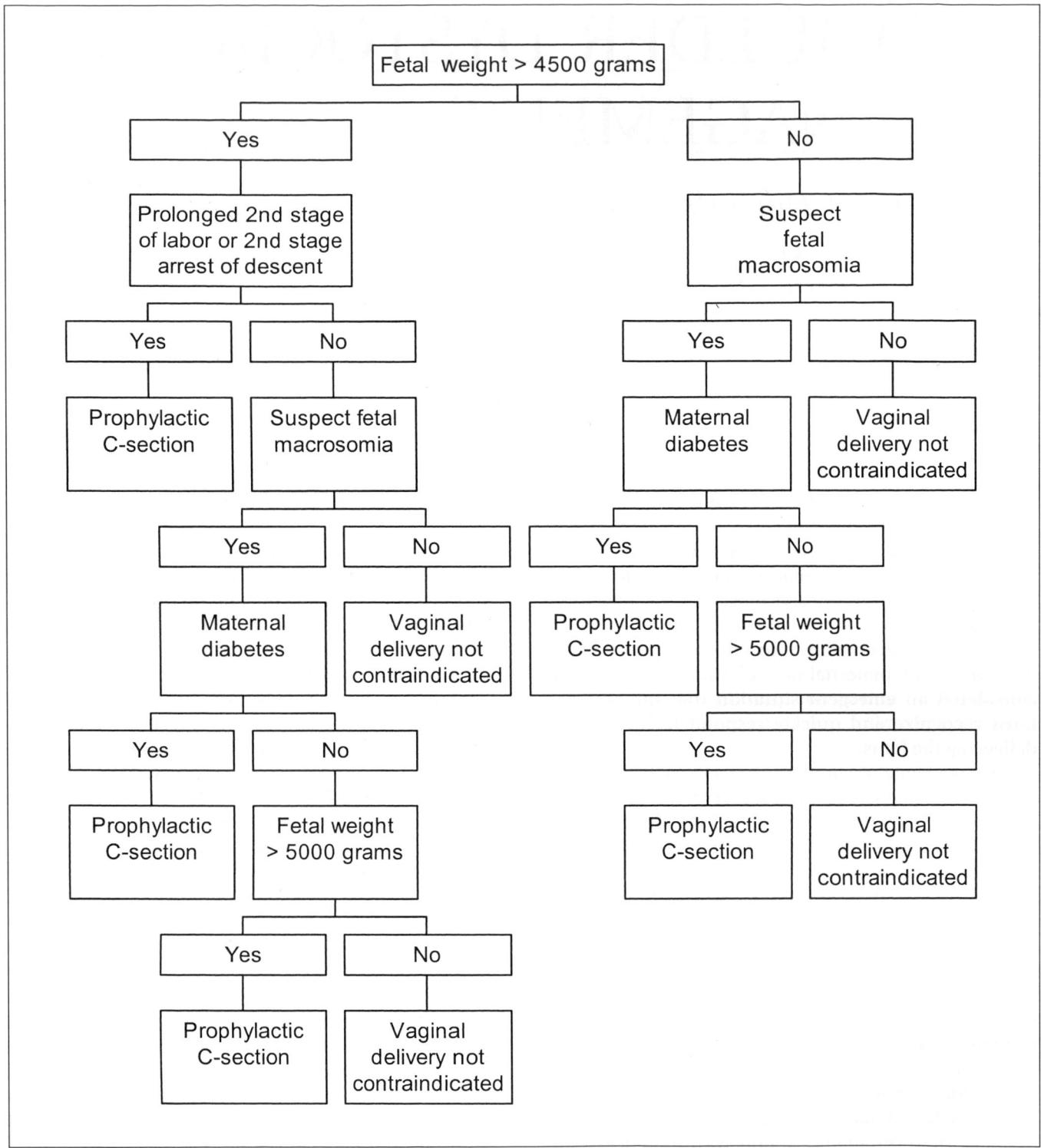

FIGURE 112-1 An algorithm providing a sequence of decisions for evaluation and anticipation of shoulder dystocia.[10]

should be utilized in the approximate order described, from least invasive and easiest to perform to most invasive and difficult to perform.

A symphysiotomy is indicated for shoulder dystocia unresponsive to less invasive techniques and for fetal head entrapment by presumed cephalopelvic disproportion. It is an alternative to the cesarean section when a qualified Obstetrician or Surgeon is unavailable.[10] Refer to Chapter 116 for the complete details regarding a symphysiotomy.

CONTRAINDICATIONS

There are few contraindications to the release maneuvers in an emergent situation of shoulder dystocia and imminent fetal demise. The only absolute contraindication is if the procedure might endanger the mother.

Indications for cesarean delivery are relative contraindications for release maneuvers. Fetal macrosomia has been associated with shoulder dystocia.[10] The American College of Obstetricians and Gynecologists (ACOG) supported the recommendation that planned cesarean delivery may be a reasonable strategy for diabetic pregnant women with estimated fetal weights exceeding 4250 to 4500 grams.[8] ACOG issued guidelines on fetal macrosomia in 2001. The guidelines were based upon limited or inconsistent scientific evidence. ACOG recommended that an estimated fetal weight of more than 4500 gm, a prolonged second stage of labor, or arrest of descent in the second stage of labor are indications for cesarean delivery.[10] ACOG noted that the diagnosis of fetal macrosomia is imprecise and recommended prophylactic cesarean delivery be considered with estimated fetal weights of more than 5000 gm in nondiabetic pregnant women and more than 4500 gm in diabetic pregnant women.[10]

EQUIPMENT

General Supplies

Electronic fetal monitor
Sterile towels
Clock or timer watch
Sterile perineal drapes
Sterile gloves
Chromic suture, 2–0 and 4–0
Vicryl suture, 2–0 and 3–0
Bulb syringe
Clean towels/blanket for baby
Umbilical cord clamp
Sterile scissors to trim umbilical cord
Infant warmer

Delivery Instrument Pack

Bandage scissors
Towel clips
2 Allis forceps
4 ring forceps
6 straight Kocher clamps
Straight Mayo scissors
2 suture scissors
Adson forceps, or other forceps with teeth
Russian forceps, 5½ inches and 8 inches

Gelpi retractor
Richardson retractors, small and medium
Army/Navy retractors
6 inch needle driver

Symphysiotomy

#10 or #15 scalpel blade on a handle
Finger guard
Foley catheter

PATIENT PREPARATION

Pain associated with the first stage of labor can be relieved with a paracervical block (Figure 110-7). Inject 5 mL of local anesthetic solution into the submucosa of the lateral vaginal fornix. Repeat the injection in the contralateral lateral vaginal fornix. Pain transmission is interrupted for all visceral sensory nerve fibers from the uterus, cervix, and upper vagina. The somatosensory fibers from the perineum are not blocked. This technique is effective only during the first stage of labor and before shoulder dystocia occurs.[11,12]

A pudendal nerve block and local perineal infiltration anesthesia are usually administered just before delivery (Figure 111-3).[12] Refer to Chapters 110 and 111 regarding the complete details of these anesthetic techniques. Unfortunately, these techniques must also be performed prior to the occurrence of shoulder dystocia.

The patient should already be in the lithotomy position on a bed with stirrups. Preparation begins with suspicion of fetal macrosomia by clinical examination and/or fetal ultrasonography. Retraction of the fetal head immediately after its delivery and the fetal chin against the maternal thigh (turtle sign) with difficulty suctioning the mouth may signal impending shoulder dystocia (Figure 112-2).

The fetal sagittal suture generally lies oblique to the maternal anteroposterior diameter with the fetal shoulders occupying the opposite oblique diameter after delivery of the fetal head (Figure 112-3). The shoulder may become impacted behind the pubic symphysis and impede delivery if the anterior shoulder descends in the anteroposterior diameter. Apply gentle and downward pressure on the fetal head to move the posterior shoulder into the hollow of the sacrum and deliver the anterior shoulder (Figure 112-4). **Resist applying excessive downward or lateral traction on the fetal head and neck.**

TECHNIQUES

Perform attempts at gentle traction coordinated with maternal expulsive efforts before attempting maneuvers to relieve shoulder dystocia. Initiate a planned sequence of events if delivery is impeded. **Avoid applying fundal**

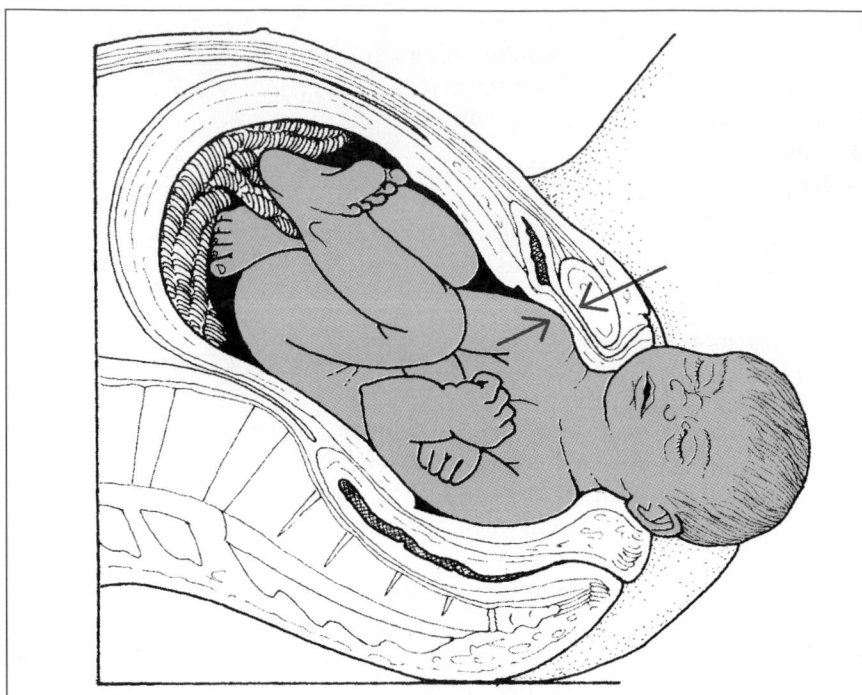

FIGURE 112-2 The head may retract towards the perineum (turtle sign) when delivery of the fetal head is not followed by delivery of the shoulders.

pressure and discontinue maternal pushing efforts until disimpaction has occurred. Contact an Anesthesiologist for pain control. Summon extra personnel for help, with one person designated as a timekeeper. Notify a Neonatologist of the impending delivery. Maneuvers for shoulder dystocia disimpaction will be described in order of ease of implementation and from least invasive to more invasive.

SUPRAPUBIC PRESSURE

This maneuver can be used alone or in combination with the McRoberts maneuver. Apply gentle downward traction to the fetal head while an assistant simultaneously applies moderate suprapubic pressure (Figure 112-5). **Do not apply heavy pressure to prevent injury to the fetus's brachial plexus, neck, and spinal cord.**

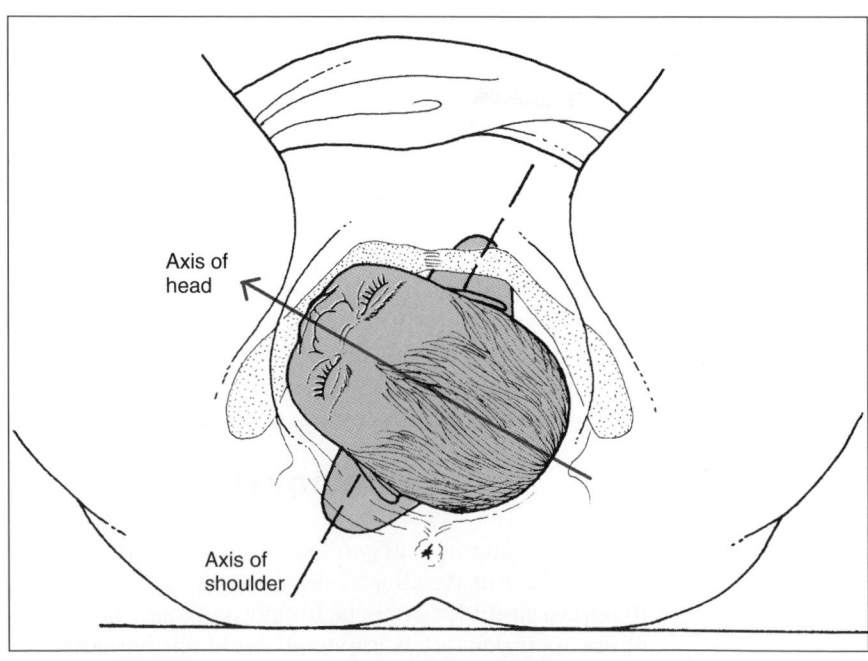

Axis of head

Axis of shoulder

FIGURE 112-3 Restitution (external rotation) of the fetal head normally results in a natural perpendicular relationship of the head to the shoulders.

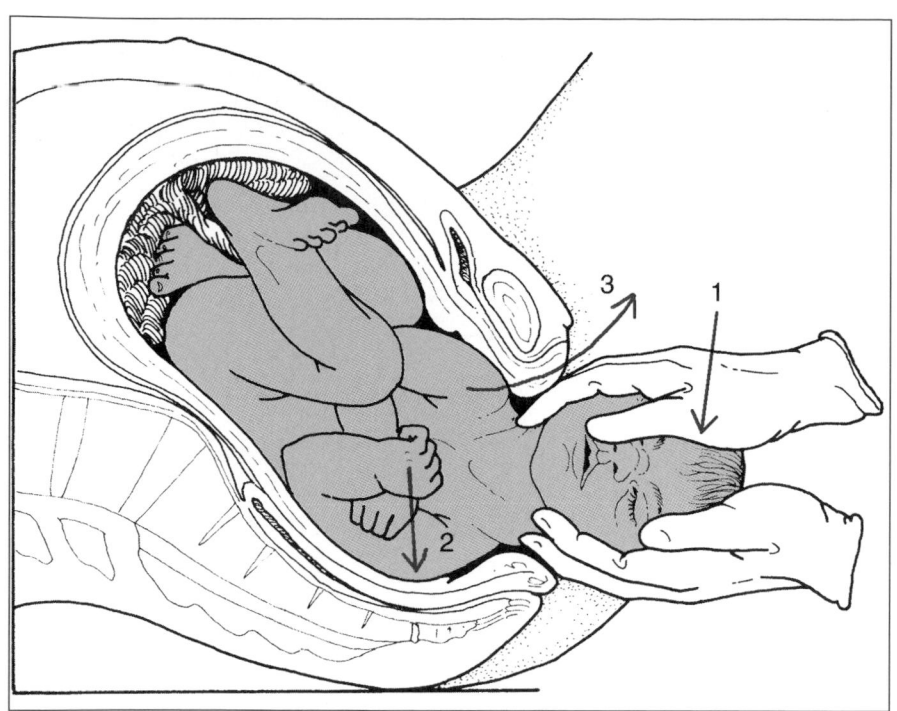

FIGURE 112-4 Apply gentle and downward pressure on the fetal head (1) to move the posterior shoulder into the hollow of the sacrum (2) and deliver the anterior shoulder (3).

McROBERTS MANEUVER

The McRoberts maneuver is easy to perform (Figure 112-6). Place an assistant on each side of the patient. Hyperflex the mother's thighs onto her abdomen (Figure 112-6A). Instruct the assistants to maintain support of the hyperflexion while applying suprapubic pressure (Figure 112-6B). This results in flattening of the maternal lumbosacral curve with rotation of the pubic symphysis

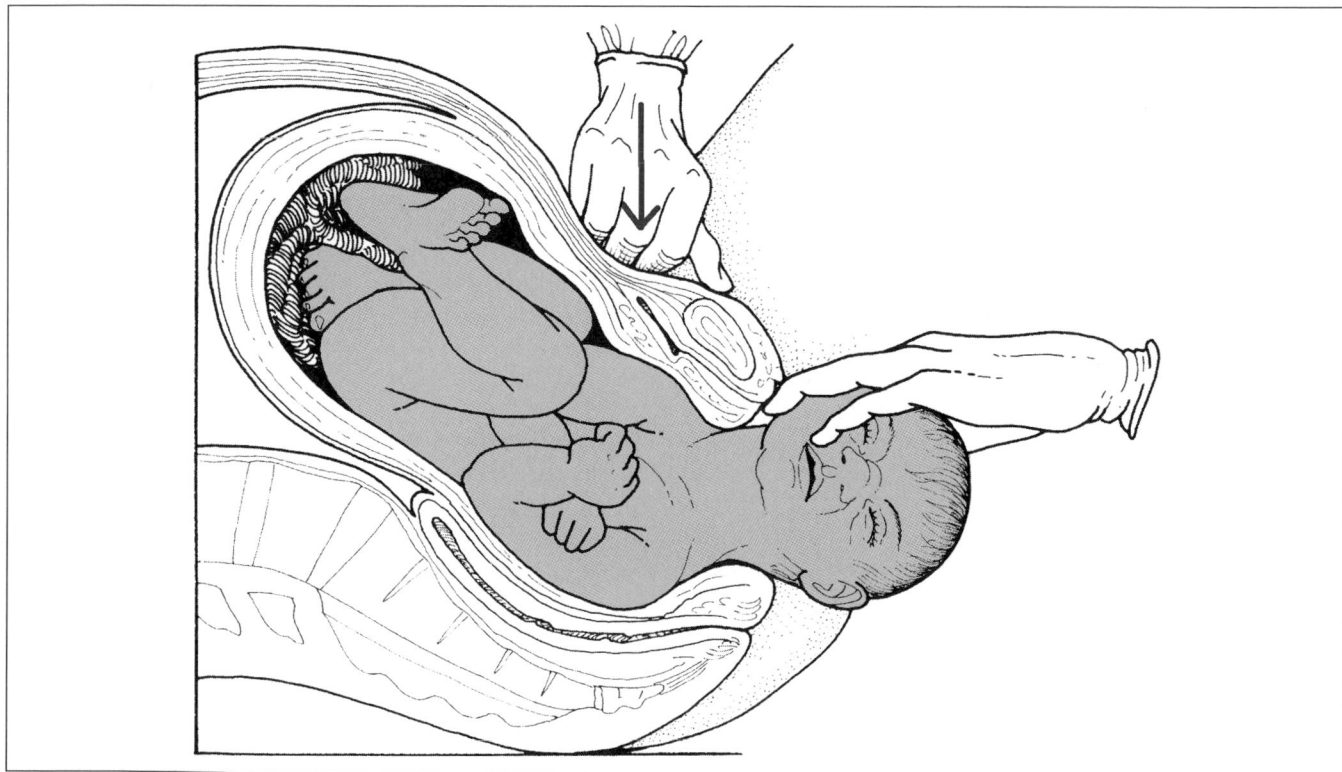

FIGURE 112-5 Moderate suprapubic pressure to disimpact the fetal shoulder.

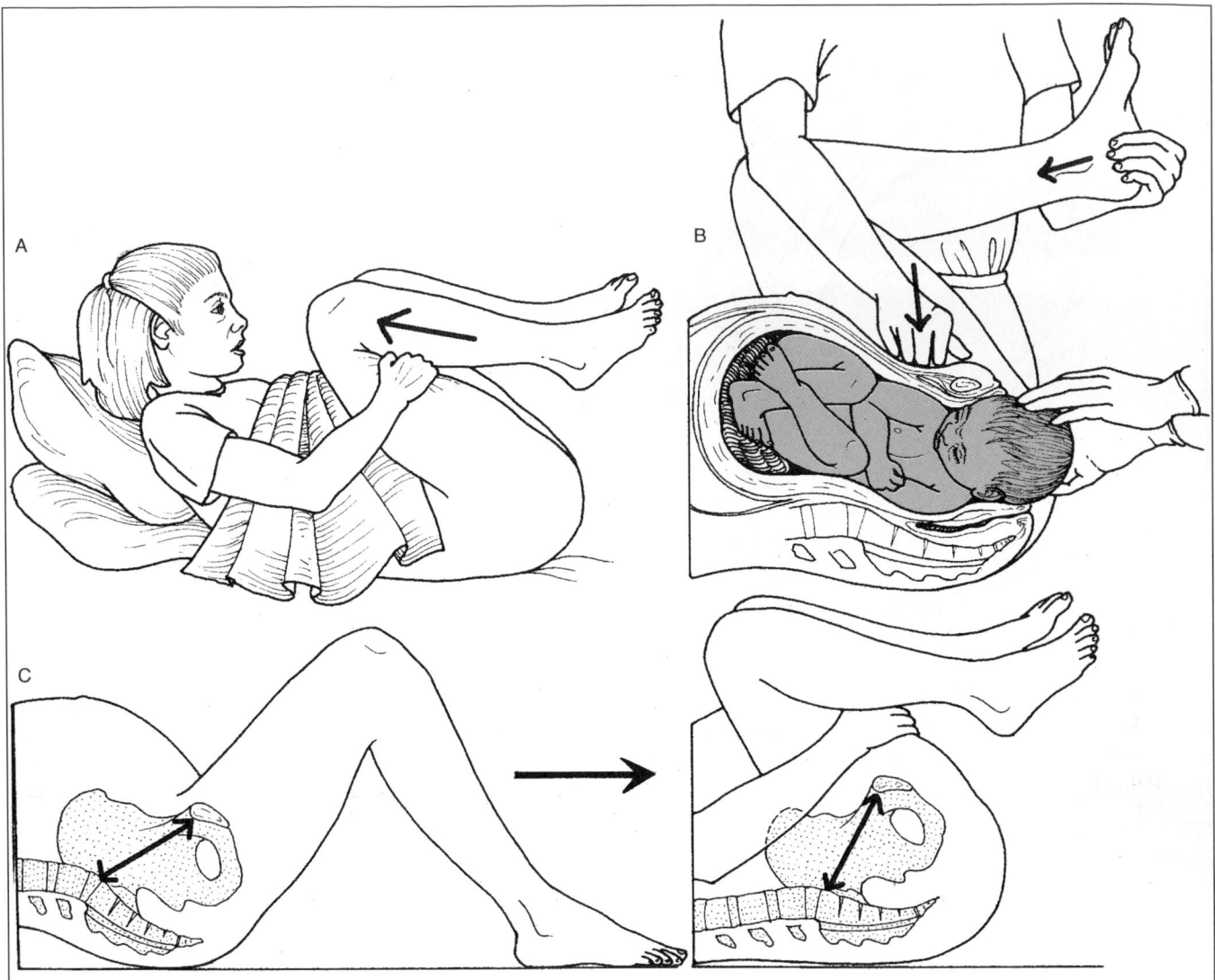

FIGURE 112-6 The McRoberts maneuver. *A.* Hyperflex the maternal thighs upon the abdomen. *B.* An assistant applies suprapubic pressure while maintaining flexion of the legs. *C.* This maneuver results in cephalad rotation of the maternal pelvis and an increase in the size of the pelvic outlet.

cephalad (Figure 112-6*C*). Rotation of the maternal pelvis may free the impacted anterior fetal shoulder.[7,13] This maneuver has the advantages of reducing shoulder extraction forces, brachial plexus stretching, and the incidence of clavicular fractures.[7,13] The McRoberts maneuver is effective in disimpacting the fetal shoulders in 50 to 90 percent of cases of shoulder dystocia.[7,13]

RUBIN MANEUVER

The Rubin maneuver is simple and may lead to the descent and delivery of the anterior fetal shoulder (Figure 112-7). Insert the dominant hand into the vagina. Place the fingers of the hand against the posterior aspect of the anterior fetal shoulder. Rotate the fetal shoulder counterclockwise in a small arc. **The Rubin maneuver compresses and diminishes the size of the fetal shoulder girdle to disimpact the anterior shoulder.** Rotation

in the opposite direction will open the shoulder girdle, increase the size of the shoulder girdle, and further impact the fetus.

WOOD'S CORKSCREW MANEUVER

The Wood's corkscrew maneuver (Figure 112-8) is an alternative to the Rubin maneuver. Insert the dominant hand into the vagina. Place the fingers of the hand against the posterior aspect of the posterior fetal shoulder. Gently rotate the posterior shoulder 180 degrees clockwise (Figure 112-8).[15] This maneuver, like the Rubin maneuver, compresses and diminishes the size of the fetal shoulder girdle to disimpact the anterior shoulder. Rotation in the opposite direction will open the shoulder girdle, increase the size of the shoulder girdle, and further impact the fetus.

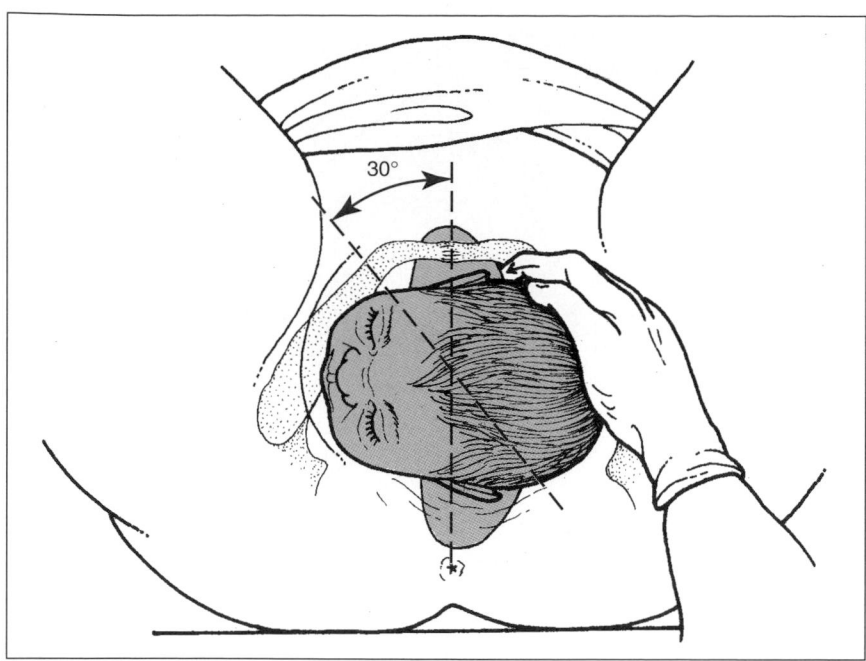

FIGURE 112-7 The Rubin maneuver. Rotation of the anterior shoulder counter-clockwise through a small arc to the oblique position.

DELIVERY OF THE POSTERIOR ARM

Attempt to deliver the posterior arm if the previous maneuvers are unsuccessful (Figure 112-9). Insert the dominant hand into the vagina. Place the fingers of the hand against the posterior fetal humerus (Figure 112-9*A*). Sweep the fetal arm across the chest (Figure 112-9*B*). Palpate for and grasp the fetal hand (Figure 112-9*C*). Gently pull the hand along the side of the face. Continue to gently pull the hand to deliver the posterior arm and shoulder (Figure 112-9*D*). Apply gentle downward traction on the fetal head and arm while an assistant simultaneously applies suprapubic pressure to deliver the anterior

shoulder (Figure 112-9*E*). Rotate the shoulder girdle into the oblique diameter if traction on the fetal head and arm does not deliver the anterior shoulder.[9] This will usually disimpact the anterior shoulder and allow it to be delivered. The major disadvantage of this maneuver is that it may result in a clavicle fracture or a humerus fracture.

DELIBERATE FRACTURE OF THE CLAVICLE

Fracture the fetal clavicle by pressing the anterior clavicle against the maternal pubic symphysis. This will decrease the rigidity and the size of the fetal shoulder girdle. Exert the pressure in a direction away from the

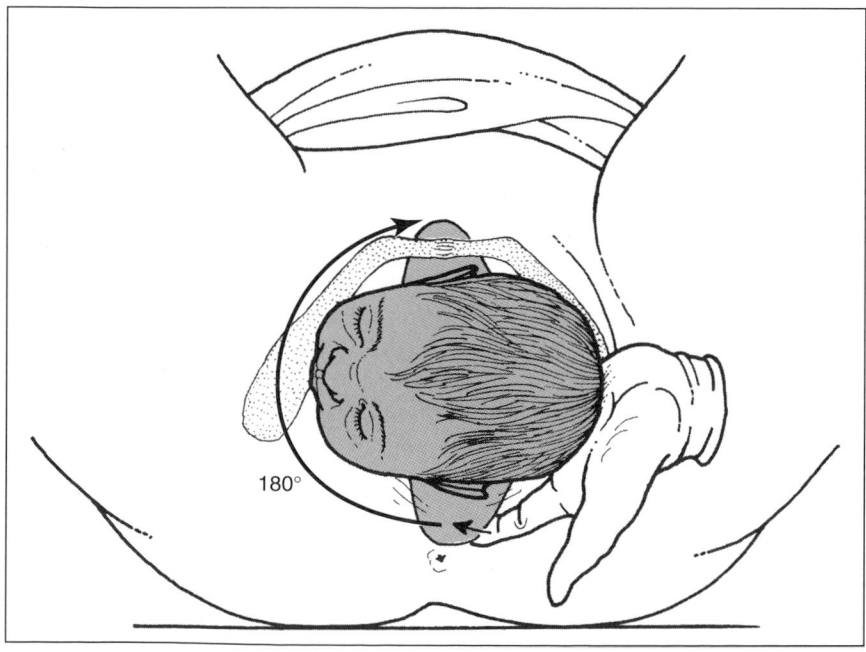

FIGURE 112-8 The Wood's corkscrew maneuver. Rotation of the posterior shoulder through a 180 degree arc.

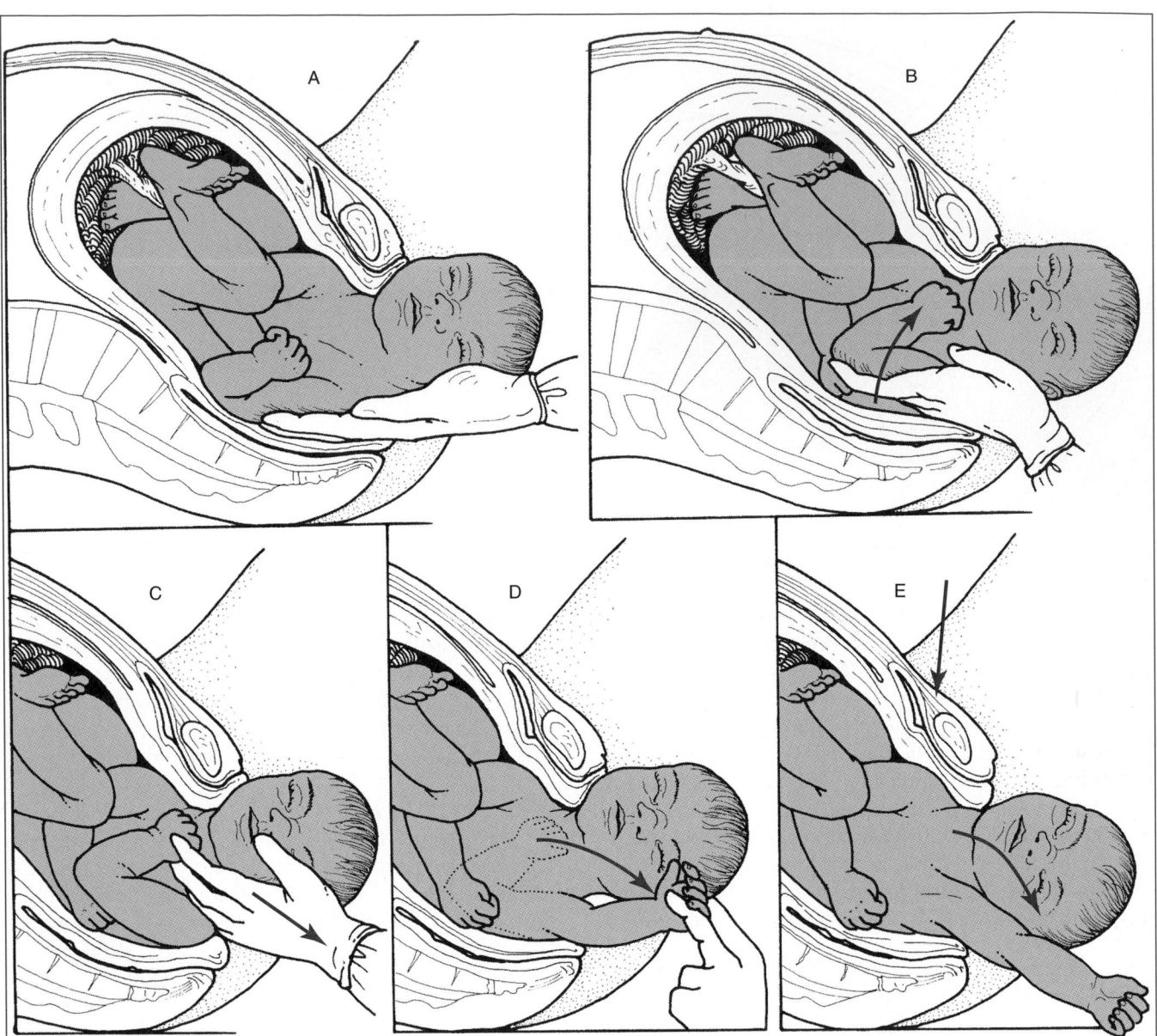

FIGURE 112-9 Delivery of the posterior arm. *A.* Insert a hand into the vagina and along the posterior fetal humerus. *B.* Sweep the fetal arm across the chest. *C.* Grasp the hand and extend the arm along the side of the face. *D.* Deliver the posterior arm and shoulder from the vagina. *E.* Apply gentle downward traction on the fetal head and arm while an assistant simultaneously applies suprapubic pressure to deliver the anterior shoulder.

lungs to avoid a pneumothorax. **Never use an instrument to fracture the clavicle.** It may penetrate into the thoracic cavity, cause a pneumothorax, or result in subsequent osteomyelitis if the skin is punctured.[14] The fracture will heal quickly and is much less serious than a brachial plexus injury, asphyxia, or death. This maneuver is difficult to perform.[15] It is physically and mentally difficult to deliberately fracture the clavicle of a large infant.

ZAVANELLI MANEUVER

The Zavanelli maneuver involves replacement of the fetal head followed by a cesarean section (Figure 112-10).

The expulsed head must undergo two maneuvers to reverse the mechanisms of labor. Manually rotate the fetal head into the prerestitution position (Figure 112-10*A*). This is usually the direct occiput anterior position with full extension of the neck (Figure 112-10*B*). The second maneuver is flexion of the fetal head followed by upward pressure on the head to replace it into the maternal vagina (Figure 112-10*B*). The physician must maintain their hand in the vagina and maintain gentle pressure on the fetal head to prevent re-expulsion.

This series of maneuvers decompresses the fetus. Immediately transport the mother to the Operating Room

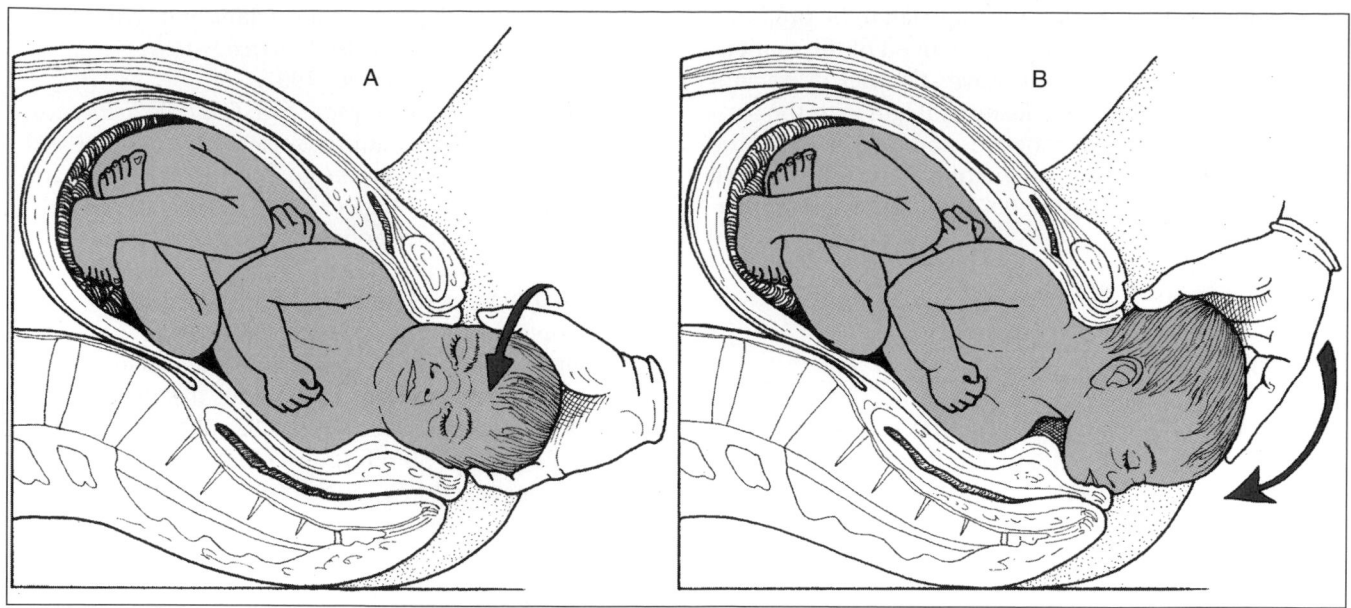

FIGURE 112-10 The Zavanelli maneuver. *A.* Manually return the fetal head to the prerestitution position, if restitution has occurred. This position is usually the direct occiput anterior position. *B.* Flex the fetal head and apply upward pressure to place the fetal head back into the vagina.

for a cesarean section. The Zavanelli maneuver was found to be successful in 84 percent of initial attempts and 91 percent of attempts when uterine relaxing anesthesia or medication was necessary.[16,17] More importantly, it was successful on the first attempt by untrained hands in 69 percent of the cases.

SYMPHYSIOTOMY

A symphysiotomy is an uncommon procedure utilized primarily in two situations. The first is shoulder dystocia unresponsive to less invasive techniques. The second is when the head of a breech delivery is trapped by presumed cephalopelvic disproportion. It serves as an alternative to the more invasive cesarean section. It is especially useful in situations where an Obstetrician or Surgeon is unavailable.[17] Refer to Chapter 116 for the complete details regarding a symphysiotomy.

AFTERCARE

Disimpaction of the shoulder girdle is usually followed by delivery of the infant. Clamp and cut the umbilical cord. Immediately assess and implement any resuscitative measures for the infant without delay. Deliver the placenta. Repair any lacerations, Dührssen's incisions, episiotomy, perineal lacerations, and vaginal lacerations. Refer to Chapter 111 for the complete details regarding episiotomy repair. Refer to Chapter 114 for the complete details regarding postpartum hemorrhage management. Initiate uterine massage and administer intramuscular pitocin following delivery of the

placenta to prevent postpartum hemorrhage. Clearly and completely document the series of events in the medical record.

COMPLICATIONS

Complications can occur for both the mother and the fetus when shoulder dystocia occurs. The most common maternal complications are lower genital tract lacerations, postpartum hemorrhage (secondary to uterine atony or lacerations), and infection.[2,19]

Significant fetal morbidity and mortality is attributable to asphyxia from delayed delivery or trauma sustained during delivery.[9] Perinatal mortality ranges from 2.1 to 29 percent when shoulder dystocia occurs. Neonatal morbidity is immediately apparent in 20 percent of the affected infants.[2] Neonatal trauma may occur in utero secondary to chronic nerve compression from malposition and during delivery.[9] Birth trauma occurring during shoulder dystocia may include brachial plexus injuries or Erb's palsy (6 to 16 percent), Klumpke palsy, clavicular fractures (5 to 13 percent), or humeral fractures.[3,5,6,14,15,19,20]

SUMMARY

The successful management of shoulder dystocia requires considerable judgment by the clinician in a timely fashion. Warning signals such as fetal macrosomia based on clinical estimate, maternal diabetes, and labor disorders should alert the clinician to be prepared for possible shoulder dystocia. Any or all of the maneuvers described will usually resolve shoulder dystocia if performed in a methodical fashion. Begin with the simplest and least invasive maneuver and work towards the more invasive maneuvers. Reduction of the time interval from delivery of the head to delivery of the body is crucial to fetal survival.

REFERENCES

1. Gabbe SG, Niebyl JR, Simpson JL: *Obstetrics: Normal and Problem Pregnancies*, 3rd ed. New York: Churchill Livingstone, 1996:490–494.

2. Benedetti TJ, Gabbe SG: Shoulder dystocia: a complication of fetal macrosomia and prolonged second stage labor with midpelvic delivery. *Obstet Gynecol* 1978; 52(5):526–529.

3. Baskett TF, Allen AC: Perinatal implications of shoulder dystocia. *Obstet Gynecol* 1995; 86:14–17.

4. Gross TL, Sokol RJ, Williams T, et al: Shoulder dystocia: a fetal-physician risk. *Am J Obstet Gynecol* 1987; 156(6):1408–1418.

5. Nocon JJ, McKenzie DK, Thomas LJ, et al: Shoulder dystocia: an analysis of risks and obstetric maneuvers. *Am J Obstet Gynecol* 1993; 168(6):1732–1739.

6. McFarland M, Hod M, Piper JM, et al: Are labor abnormalities more common in shoulder dystocia? *Am J Obstet Gynecol* 1995; 173(4):1211–1214.

7. Gonik B, Allen R, Sorab J: Objective evaluation of the shoulder dystocia phenomenon: effect of maternal pelvic orientation on force reduction. *Obstet Gynecol* 1989; 74(1):44–48.

8. American College of Obstetricians and Gynecologists: *Shoulder Dystocia. Practice Pattern No. 7*. Washington, DC: ACOG, 1997.

9. Creasy RK, Resnik R: *Maternal-Fetal Medicine*, 4th ed. Philadelphia: Saunders, 1999:546–547, 988–989.

10. Chatfield J: ACOG issues guidelines on fetal macrosomia. *Am Fam Physician* 2001; 64(1):169–170.

11. Watterson L: Paracervical block. http://www.manbit.com/oa/c46.htm.

12. Miller RD: *Anesthesia*, 5th ed. Philadelphia: Churchill Livingstone, 2000:2045–2046.

13. Gonik B, Stringer CA, Held B: An alternate maneuver for management of shoulder dystocia. *Am J Obstet Gynecol* 1983; 145(7):882–884.

14. Seigworth GR: Shoulder dystocia—review of 5 years experience. *Obstet Gynecol* 1966; 28(6):764–767.

15. Cunningham FG, MacDonald PC, Gant NF, et al: *Williams Obstetrics*, 20th ed. Norwalk, CT: Appleton & Lange, 1997:509–514.

16. Sandberg EC: The Zavanelli maneuver: a potentially revolutionary method for the resolution of shoulder dystocia. *Am J Obstet Gynecol* 1985; 152(4):479–484.

17. Sandberg EC: The Zavanelli maneuver: 12 years of recorded experience. *Obstet Gynecol* 1999; 93(2):312–317.

18. Hartfield VJ: Symphysiotomy for shoulder dystocia. *Am J Obstet Gynecol* 1986; 155(1):228.

19. Lipscomb KR, Gregory K, Shaw K: The outcome of macrosomic infants weighing at least 4500 grams: Los Angeles County/University of Southern California experience. *Obstet Gynecol* 1995; 85(4):558–564.

20. Acker DB, Sachs BP, Friedman EA: Risk factors for shoulder dystocia. *Obstet Gynecol* 1985; 66(6):762–768.

Chapter 113
BREECH DELIVERY

Susan K. Hendricks
John E. Lewis, Jr.

INTRODUCTION

The breech presentation exists when the cephalic pole of the fetus is positioned in a longitudinal lie and is located within the uterine fundus. The incidence of breech presentation is inversely related to the fetal gestational age.[1] It is greater than 25 percent if the fetal age is less than 27 weeks of gestation and decreases to 3 to 4 percent at term.

Knowledge and preparedness facilitate comfort and promote success in approaching any emergent procedure. The breech delivery is no exception to this rule. Breech delivery is a high-risk obstetric complication generally handled by an Obstetrician. There are situations when a pregnant woman will present to the Emergency Department in active labor with a fetus in the breech position. The preferable method of delivery is a cesarean section if available. Vaginal breech delivery may be the only viable option in the absence of surgical assistance or in the presence of an acute situation such as fetal distress or umbilical cord prolapse.

ANATOMY AND PATHOPHYSIOLOGY

The breech presentation is associated with abnormal fetal conditions that may decrease fetal movement or mobility. An increased incidence of breech or other abnormal presentations is associated with primary neurologic disorders, neuromuscular disorders (myotonic dystrophy), genetic abnormalities (trisomies 13, 18, and 21), prematurity, fetal malformations such as hydrocephalus or a cystic hygroma, and polar placentation.[1] Maternal abnormalities that increase the risk of an abnormal fetal presentation include a small pelvis, small or abnormal pelvic measurements, uterine anomalies, and lower segment leiomyomata.

There are three main types of breech presentation (Figure 113-1). The most common is the frank breech, accounting for 50 to 73 percent of breech presentations. The fetus is flexed at the hips and extended at the knees (Figure 113-1A). The fetus is in the "pike" position. The complete breech is the least common type and accounts for approximately 5 to 11 percent of breech presentations. The fetus is flexed at both the hips and the knees (Figure 113-1B). The footling or incomplete breech accounts for approximately 12 to 38 percent of breech presentations. The fetus is incompletely deflexed at one or both knees or hips (Figure 113-1C). The risks of umbilical cord prolapse and prematurity associated with the breech presentation are listed in Table 113-1.

Breech delivery is divided into three categories. These include unassisted or spontaneous expulsion, partial breech extraction, and total breech extraction. Unassisted or spontaneous expulsion of the fetus occurs when there is no assistance from the provider in the delivery of the infant. This generally occurs only with very premature infants or in precipitous deliveries where the baby delivers so rapidly as not to allow the provider to arrive.

Partial breech extraction is defined as spontaneous delivery of the infant to the level of the umbilicus followed by assistance from the provider. This is the usual manner of breech delivery. **Allowing the fetus to descend naturally into the pelvis avoids an increased incidence of head entrapment, deflexion of the fetal head, nuchal arms, and umbilical cord prolapse.** This is the preferred method of delivery for the Emergency Physician confronted with an actively laboring breech presentation and little hope of obtaining an Obstetrician before delivery.

Total breech extraction occurs when the provider reaches into the uterus and literally pulls or extracts the fetal feet into the vagina and through the vulva, followed by assisted delivery of the remainder of the infant. Total breech extraction is indicated in the absence of an experienced Obstetrician to perform a cesarean section and if performed for the breech presentation of a second twin, acute and profound fetal distress, and/or umbilical cord prolapse.[1]

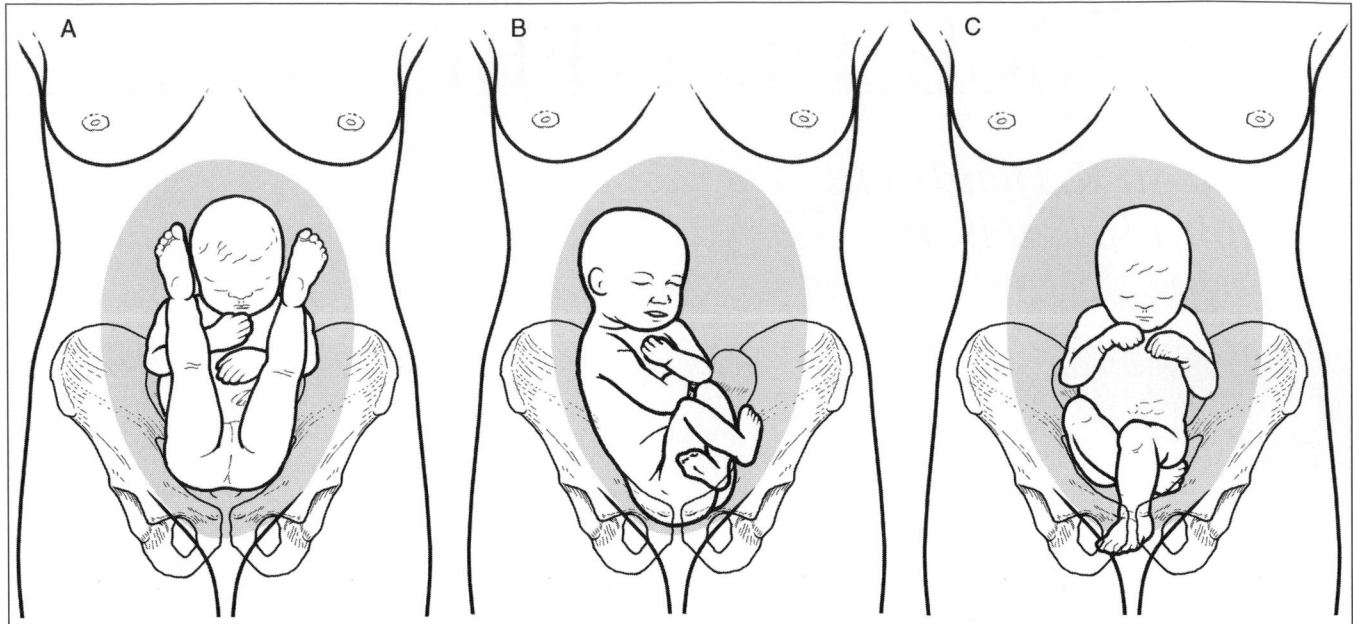

FIGURE 113-1 The main types of breech presentations. *A.* The frank breech. *B.* The complete breech. *C.* The incomplete breech.

The breech presentation alone was accepted for many years as a contraindication for vaginal delivery due to an increased incidence of neonatal morbidity and mortality. However, prospective and retrospective studies over the last two decades are now beginning to refute this practice.[1–14] The perinatal mortality associated with the breech presentation is approximately 9 to 25 percent. This is three to five times greater than that associated with a vertex presentation.

It is difficult to differentiate the primary causation of the increased morbidity and mortality associated with breech presentations. Few randomized controlled studies exist.[1] Many earlier studies reporting a higher incidence of perinatal morbidity and mortality in vaginal breech delivery compared to cesarean section did not utilize fetal monitoring or take into account and control for preexisting maternal and fetal risk factors.[1–10,13,15] Several studies have reported no increase and even lower incidences of maternal and fetal complications in vaginal delivery when these factors are taken into account.[1–4,6,8,10] Maternal morbidity and mortality are higher if an emergency cesarean delivery is performed.

For these reasons, the vaginal delivery of the breech fetus has not yet been rejected by Obstetricians in the United States. The rate of cesarean section for the breech presentation has increased from 10 percent in the late 1960s to greater than 80 percent in the 1990s. No consensus exists concerning the absolute preferred method of breech delivery because of rather conflicting data.[1,9]

Recommendations have been made based upon various studies utilizing factors that increase morbidity and mortality in vaginal and cesarean breech deliveries.[1,3,4,6,7] Maternal risk factors for increased morbidity and mortality with vaginal breech delivery include a small pelvis, pelvic anomalies, uterine masses, uterine malformations, and arrest of labor. Fetal risk factors for increased morbidity and mortality with vaginal breech delivery include extremes of fetal weight, fetal head extension, prematurity, non-frank breech, and a non-reassuring fetal heart rate pattern.

Obstetricians will often perform external cephalic version prior to the delivery dates if a breech presentation is noted.[1,3] This technique is reserved for the experienced Obstetrician, as it can be associated with significant complications. External cephalic version cannot be performed if the mother is in active labor and the fetus is engaged in the maternal pelvis.

TABLE 113-1. BREECH PRESENTATIONS AND ASSOCIATED COMPLICATIONS[1]

Breech presentation	Breech deliveries (%)	Umbilical cord prolapse (%)	Prematurity (%)
Frank	50–73	0.5	38
Complete	5–11	5	12
Incomplete	12–38	14	50

INDICATIONS

Vaginal breech delivery is indicated when the mother is in active labor and an Obstetrician is not available to perform the delivery or a cesarean section.

CONTRAINDICATIONS

There are no agreed upon absolute contraindications to vaginal breech delivery. General consensus recommends that vaginal breech delivery may be contraindicated under certain conditions.[1-10,13,15] These include the absence of provider experience, estimated fetal weight of less than 1500 gm or greater than 4000 gm, nonreassuring fetal heart rate patterns, small maternal pelvis, arrest of progress of labor, a hyperextended fetal head, the footling presentation, or a Zatuchni-Andros score less than four. Many of these conditions are not known in an emergent breech presentation. The Emergency Physician may not have the time or experience to assess these conditions. The Zatuchni-Andros score is based on six factors, including estimated fetal weight and gestational age.[7] Emergent cesarean delivery is indicated if any of the conditions listed above are known and the setting allows for it.

EQUIPMENT

Electronic fetal monitor
Delivery instrument pack (see Chapter 110)
Piper forceps
Towels
Clock or timer watch
Sterile gowns and gloves
Chromic or Vicryl suture, 2–0 or 3–0
Richardson or right-angle retractors
Ring forceps
Straight Mayo scissors
8 inch needle driver
Sterile drapes

Personnel

Two medical practitioners if available
Nursing personnel
Timekeeper
Anesthesiologist or Anesthetist if available
Pediatric or neonatal team if available

PATIENT PREPARATION

Perform an abdominal palpation and cervical examination to assess the fetal position. Apply a fetal monitor and tocodynamometer to the maternal abdomen. Perform ultrasonography if available to confirm the fetal position and to assist in the breech delivery.

Obtain an informed consent for the delivery if possible and time permits. Lumbar epidural anesthesia or a spinal block by an Anesthesiologist is recommended if available and time permits. A pudendal nerve block with local perineal infiltration may be used as an alternative. Refer to Chapter 110 for the details regarding the pudendal nerve block. Place the mother in the lithotomy position. Scrub the perineum with povidone iodine solution or antibacterial soap. The physician should perform a surgical scrub of their hands and arms if time permits. Apply a mask, sterile gown, and sterile gloves. Apply sterile drapes to isolate the patient's perineum.

ASSISTED VAGINAL FRANK BREECH DELIVERY

This method is appropriate for all breech presentations. The fetus enters the maternal pelvis with the bitrochanteric diameter in an oblique position (Figure 113-2A). The sacrum is the point of designation for these presentations. The fetus rotates with labor and descent, so that the bitrochanteric diameter is in the anteroposterior axis and the sacrum is in the transverse axis (Figure 113-2B).

Encourage maternal "pushing" to expel the fetal buttocks (Figure 113-3A). Support the fetal buttocks with a toweled hand. **Do not assist with the delivery of the buttocks as they emerge (Figure 113-4B). Allow the fetus to deliver spontaneously to the level of the umbilicus with only maternal uterine propulsive efforts.** Early extraction of the buttocks increases the risk of head entrapment in a partially dilated cervix, results in deflexion of the fetal head, and increases the risk of nuchal arm entrapment. Perform a midline episiotomy when the buttocks crown. **Do not perform the episiotomy too early, as this may lead to excessive maternal blood loss.** Refer to Chapter 111 for complete details regarding an episiotomy.

Proceed with the delivery of the fetal legs when the umbilicus emerges (Figure 113-4). The legs will likely have delivered themselves by this time if the fetus is in the complete or incomplete breech position. Insert the fingers of the dominant hand along the long axis of the medial fetal thigh (Figure 113-4A). Apply laterally directed pressure on the fetal thigh to flex the knee and externally rotate the leg out and down through the vulva (Figure 113-4A). Simultaneously apply opposite rotation on the fetal hip and pelvis. Deliver the other leg in a similar manner (Figure 113-4B). **Rotation of the hip in a direction opposite the direction of knee flexion facilitates the delivery of the distal extremities. Therefore, rotate the left leg clockwise and the right leg counterclockwise.**

Prepare to deliver the fetal arms (Figure 113-5). Place a sterile towel around the legs and trunk of the fetus for support (Figure 113-5A). Continue to support the fetal body and encourage maternal pushing efforts. **Do not**

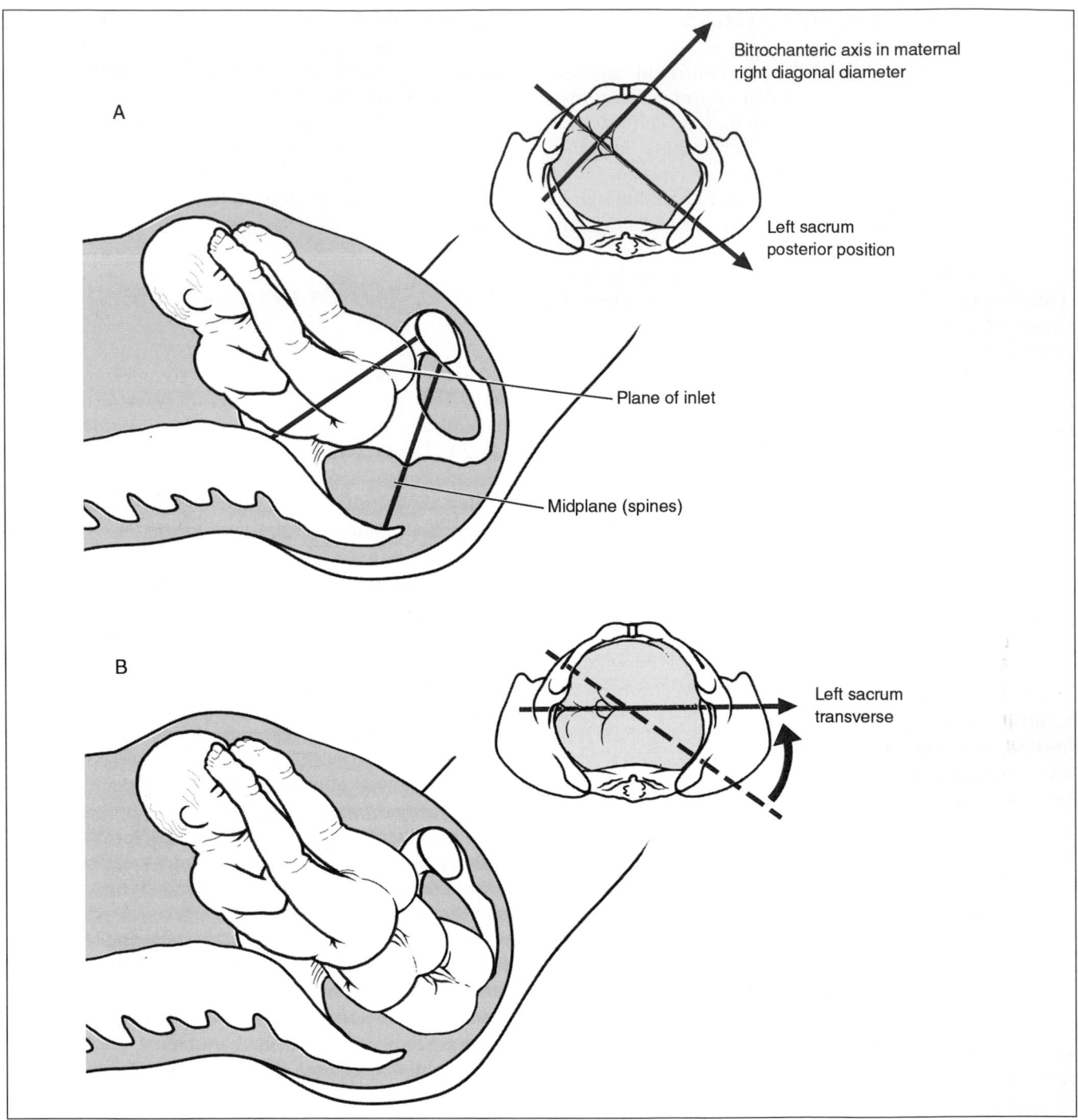

Bitrochanteric axis in maternal
right diagonal diameter

Left sacrum
posterior position

Plane of inlet

Midplane (spines)

Left sacrum
transverse

FIGURE 113-2 Breech engagement of the maternal pelvis. *A.* The bitrochanteric diameter is aligned with one of the diagonal diameters. *B.* Descent causes the bitrochanteric diameter to rotate into the anteroposterior axis and the sacrum to rotate into the transverse axis.

actively assist in the delivery until the fetal scapulae are visible. Aggressive extraction of the fetus following the delivery of the legs may cause deflexion of the vertex or nuchal entrapment of the arms.

Proceed with active delivery of the shoulders and arms as the scapulae emerge from the vagina (Figure 113-5). Rotate the fetal trunk to present the anterior

arm and shoulder (Figure 113-5*A*). Insert the fingers of the dominant hand longitudinally along the humerus of the presenting arm (Figure 113-5*A*). Apply traction to the humerus to flex the elbow. Sweep the arm across the chest and deliver it through the mother's vulva (Figure 113-5*B*). Rotate the fetus in a manner to bring the alternate shoulder into the anterior position (Figure

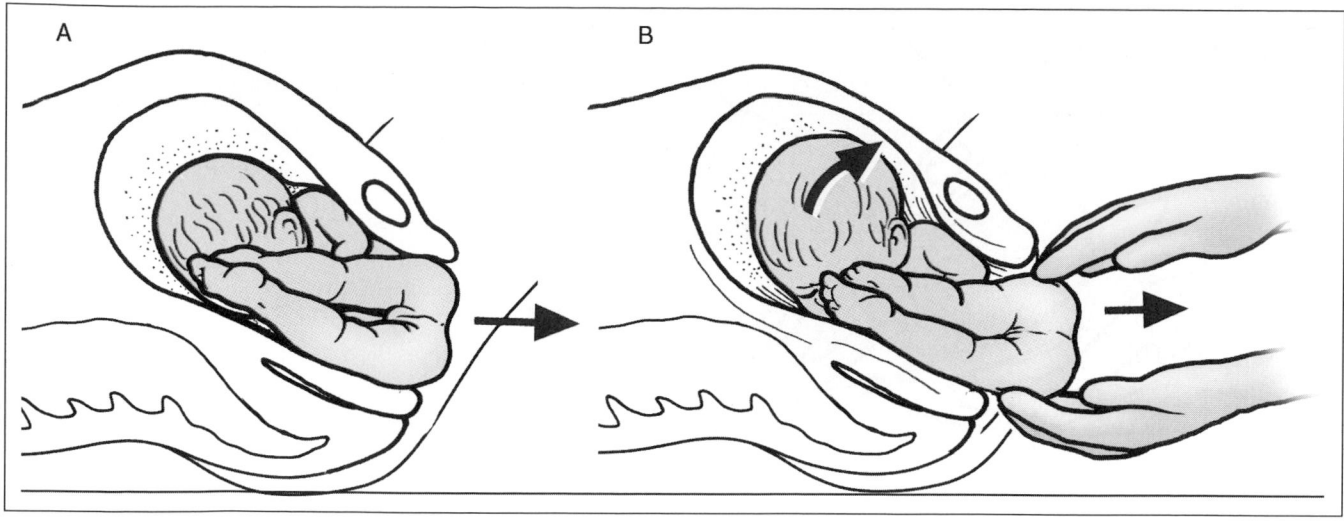

FIGURE 113-3 Delivery of the buttocks. *A.* Uterine contractions result in spontaneous emergence of the buttocks while maintaining cephalic flexion. *B.* Premature traction can result in deflexion of the vertex, head entrapment, or nuchal arms.

113-5*C*). Gently rotate the fetus clockwise to deliver the left arm and counterclockwise to deliver the right arm. This direction of motion prevents the arm from becoming entrapped on the neck. Repeat the procedure to deliver the second arm.

The fetal shoulders and arms may not easily deliver utilizing the above technique. Perform this alternate technique if the arms and shoulders do not deliver. Place the thumbs of both hands over the fetal posterior iliac spines and sacroiliac area. Place the palms and fingers over the fetal hips. **Apply pressure only over the iliac spines. Never grasp the fetal abdomen. The adrenal glands, kidney, liver, and spleen may be injured with excessive pressure during the delivery process.** Elevate the fetal body to deliver the posterior shoulder over the more pliable posterior perineum. Deliver the posterior arm as described above. Lower the fetal trunk. Deliver the anterior shoulder from under the maternal pubic symphysis as described above.

The fetal vertex will generally rotate into the antero-posterior orientation after delivery of the arms and shoulders. The fetal vertex will lie against the maternal

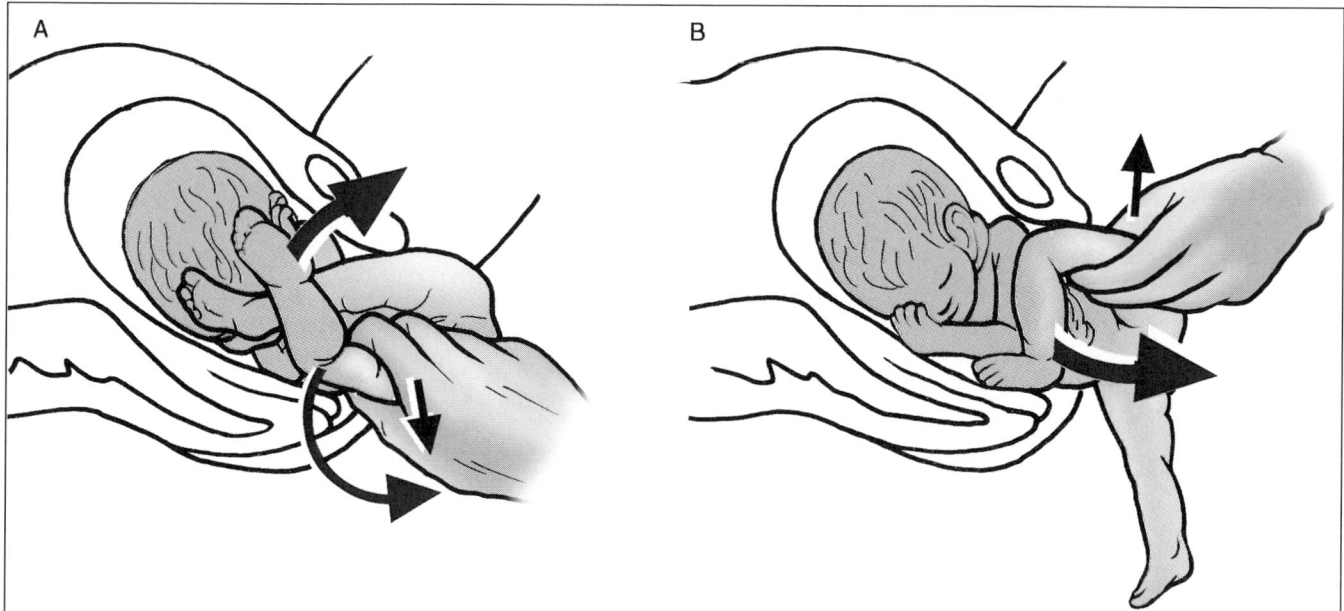

FIGURE 113-4 Delivery of the legs. *A.* Apply laterally directed pressure on the medial thigh with opposite rotation of the pelvis to deliver the leg. *B.* Repeat the procedure to deliver the other leg.

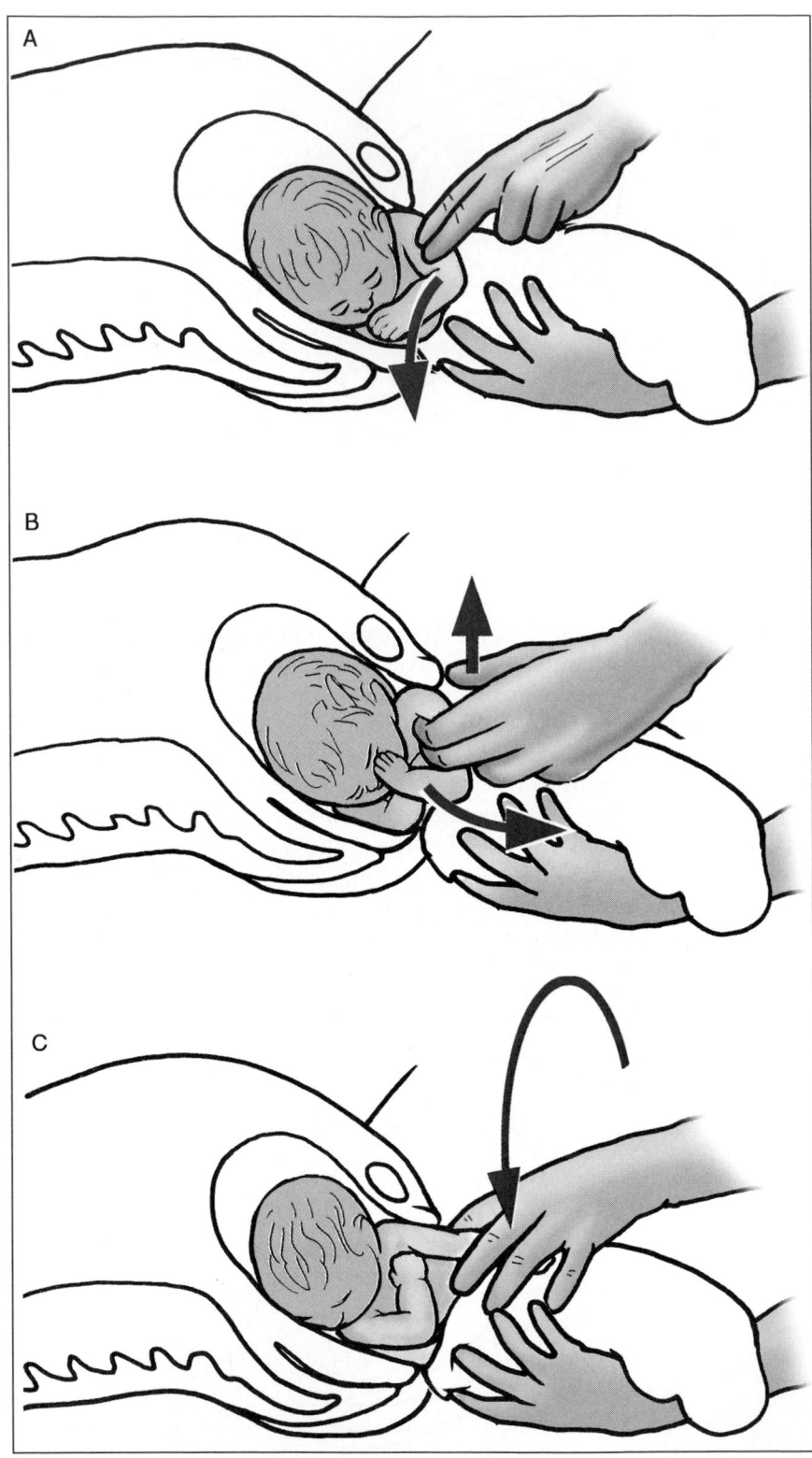

FIGURE 113-5 Delivery of the arms. *A.* Insert the dominant hand along the humerus of the anterior arm. Apply traction (*arrow*) to flex the elbow. *B.* Deliver the arm. *C.* Gently rotate the fetus so that the other arm presents anteriorly.

pubic symphysis. The fetal chin will lie in the posterior aspect of the vagina and/or lower uterine segment. Wrap the fetal arms and trunk in a towel. Encourage maternal pushing efforts. The fetal head may deliver spontaneously. Note when the fetal chin and mouth appear at the posterior perineum. **Instruct the mother to stop pushing.** Suction the fetal mouth. Gently lift the infant upward to deliver the head in a controlled manner (Figure 113-6). **Avoid hyperextending the fetal back.**

Complete the delivery of the infant. Clamp and cut the umbilical cord. Place the infant in the warmer for

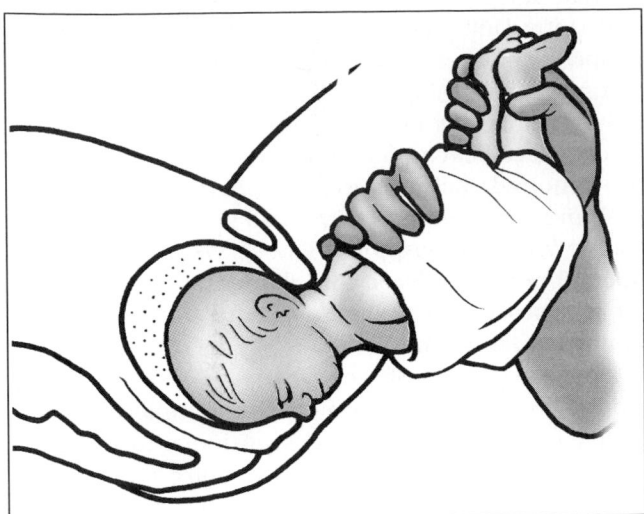

FIGURE 113-6 Delivery of the fetal head.

examination and resuscitation. The Apgar scores for infants delivered from a breech position are generally slightly lower than from a vertex delivery. The infant may show some initial signs of short-term and generally clinically insignificant hypoxia.

DELIVERY OF THE FETAL HEAD

Cervical entrapment (inadequate cervical dilation) is a more common occurrence in the delivery of a fetus in the breech presentation. It is most frequently observed when rapid labor results in the fetal trunk being delivered through a partially dilated cervix or during the delivery of a premature breech when the fetal head is relatively larger than the fetal trunk.

The fetal head often delivers spontaneously with maternal pushing efforts, but it may occasionally fail to do so. Several options exist to aid in the delivery of the fetal head. These include manual extraction, manual extraction with the McRoberts maneuver or the Mauriceau maneuver, forceps-assisted delivery, and Dührssen's incisions.

Adequate anesthesia is vital to the extraction of the fetal head. A pudendal block and peroneal infiltration should have been performed previously. If not, consider the administration of parenteral sedation and analgesia (Chapter 109) and local infiltration. Utilize assistants as needed to offer adequate visualization. Gently place Richardson or Pratt retractors in the vagina to maximize the view.

McROBERTS MANEUVER

Apply the McRoberts maneuver if the fetal head does not deliver. The McRoberts maneuver is easy to perform (Figure 112-6). Place an assistant on each side of the patient. Hyperflex the mother's thighs onto her abdomen (Figure 112-6A). Instruct the assistants to maintain support of the hyperflexion while applying suprapubic pressure (Figure 112-6B). This results in flattening of the lumbosacral curve with rotation of the pubic symphysis cephalad (Figure 112-6C). Perform the manual extraction.

MAURICEAU MANEUVER

Perform the Mauriceau maneuver if the McRoberts maneuver is unsuccessful in the spontaneous delivery of the head (Figure 113-7). Rest the body of the infant on the dominant arm. Place the index and middle finger of the dominant hand on the fetal maxilla. Apply pressure to the maxilla to maintain the fetal head in flexion. **Do not place the fingers on the fetal mandible or in the fetal mouth.** Place the nondominant hand on the posterior aspect of the fetal neck and shoulders. Slightly elevate the fetal body from the horizontal plane.

Exert continued and gentle downward traction with both hands until the occiput moves under the mother's pubic symphysis. **Never hyperextend the fetal trunk. Never apply pressure to the mandible or the fetal mouth during this maneuver. The force applied to the mandible or mouth can dislocate the mandible.** Instruct an assistant to apply firm and gentle suprapubic pressure in conjunction with gentle downward traction by the operator. Continue this process until the head delivers.

FORCEPS-ASSISTED DELIVERY OF THE HEAD

The utilization of forceps may be warranted if none of these maneuvers is successful.[14] The Piper forceps have a minimal pelvic curve, allowing direct application to the fetal head. They are used solely for the delivery of an after-coming head in the breech delivery. **Forceps-assisted delivery can result in significant injury to the fetus and the mother. The use of the Piper forceps is**

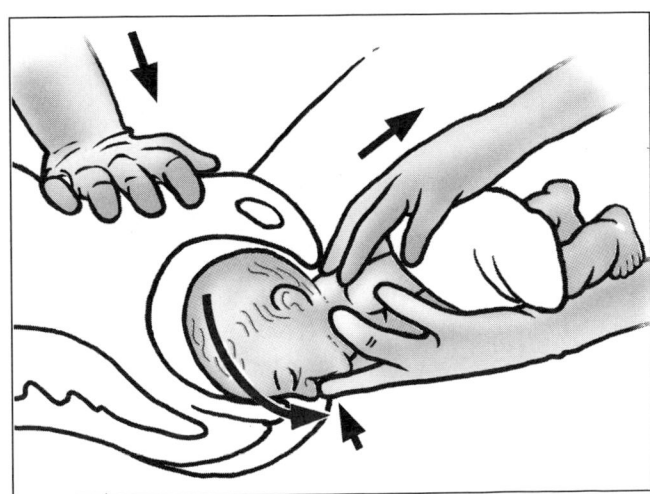

FIGURE 113-7 The Mauriceau maneuver.

not recommended unless the operator has training and experience in their proper use.

Apply the Piper forceps. Instruct an assistant to elevate the fetal trunk slightly above the horizontal plane (Figure 113-8*A*). Kneel below the fetus. Insert the forceps directly into the vagina and along the fetal head. Apply the right forceps blade. Grasp the blade in the left hand. Place the right hand along the left fetal parietal bone, between the fetal head and the right maternal pelvic side wall. Insert and apply the forceps blade. Instruct the assistant to hold the blade in this position. Apply the left forceps blade. Grasp the blade in the right hand. Place the left hand along the right fetal parietal bone, between the fetal head and the left maternal pelvic side wall. Insert and apply the forceps blade. Gently join the forceps handles while avoiding excessive pressure.

Apply gentle downward and outward traction to the forceps blades to deliver the fetal head (Figure 113-8*B*). Slowly elevate the plane of the fetal trunk toward the maternal abdomen as the fetal face delivers. **Do not hyperextend the fetal neck.** Stop the extraction as the mouth appears. Gently suction the fetal mouth. Deliver the head.

DÜHRSSEN'S INCISIONS

Perform Dührssen's incisions if the fetal head is entrapped, if other methods of extraction have failed, and if you are unfamiliar with the use of forceps (Figure 113-9). Dührssen's incisions consist of two to four incisions placed circumferentially around the cervix. **The two required incisions are at the 10 and 2 o'clock positions.** Additional incisions can be made at the 5, 6, and/or 7 o'clock positions. **The cervix must be more than 70 percent effaced and dilated more than 6 cm for the procedure to be successful and to prevent significant hemorrhage.**

Grasp two pairs of ring forceps. Grasp the cervix around the point of the incision. For example, place ring forceps at the 9 and 11 o'clock positions to make the 10 o'clock incision (Figure 113-9*A*). Make the incisions 2 to 3 cm in length with a straight Mayo scissors. Deliver the fetal head.

PERSISTENT FETAL HEAD ENTRAPMENT

The fetal head may become entrapped and unable to be delivered despite the maneuvers described above. True cephalopelvic disproportion must be differentiated from cervical entrapment (inadequate cervical dilation).

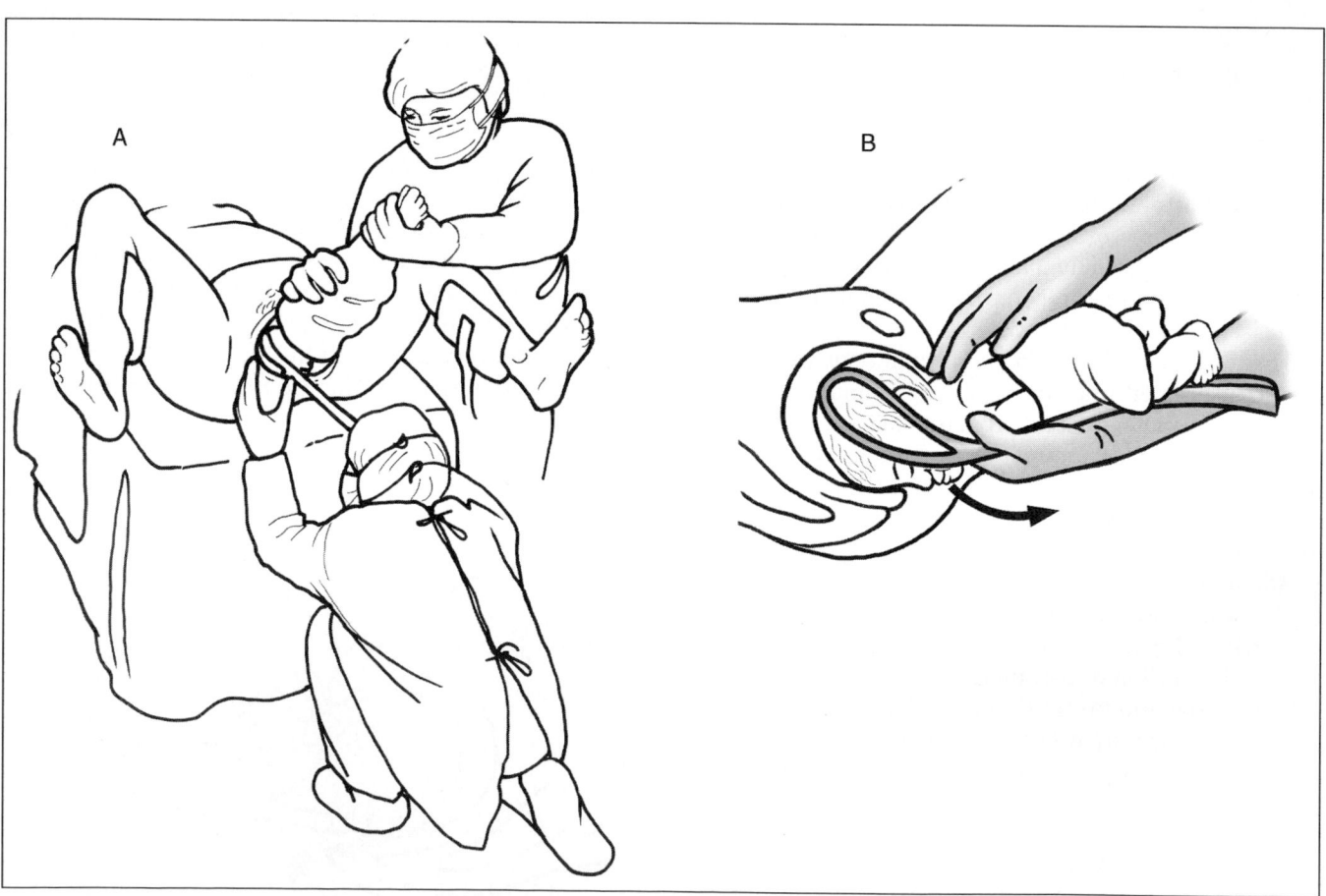

FIGURE 113-8 Forceps-assisted delivery of the head. *A.* Application of the forceps. *B.* Delivery of the fetal head.

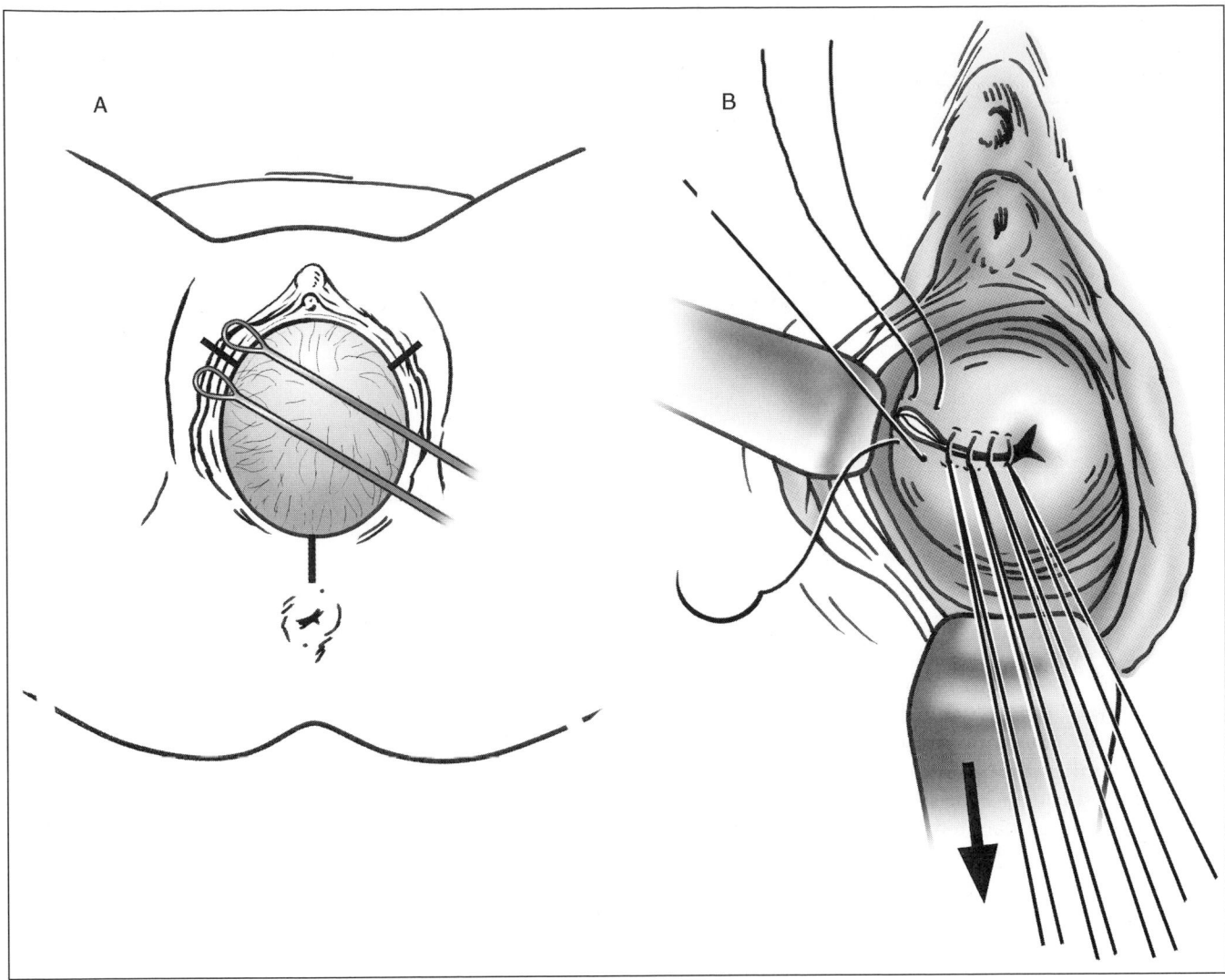

FIGURE 113-9 Dührssen's incisions. *A.* The incisions. *B.* Repair of the incisions.

The options are limited in the rare case of a true cephalopelvic disproportion. The operator can perform a symphysiotomy (Chapter 116), the fetal body can be pushed back into the uterus and a cesarean section performed, or an experienced Obstetrician may perform a destructive procedure if the fetus is nonviable.

BREECH EXTRACTION

Breech extraction is to be performed only in the rare instances of a second twin presenting in a breech position, extreme fetal distress without the capability of performing a cesarean section, and/or umbilical cord prolapse that does not allow time for setup or performance of a cesarean section.[1,11,12,14]

If available, utilize ultrasound to identify the fetal legs and feet. This will ensure you grasp the appropriate extremity. Reach into the lower uterine segment with the dominant hand and firmly grasp the fetal feet. Place the fingers around the fetus's ankles, with the index finger between the two ankles. Apply continuous and firm traction in a downward and outward direction. Deliver the fetal feet and legs through the vaginal opening (Figure 113-10*A*). Continue to apply traction to deliver the fetus to the level of the buttocks (Figure 113-10*B*). Instruct an assistant to support the fetus. Perform a midline episiotomy if necessary. Deliver the fetus to the level of the umbilicus. Grasp the bony sacrum and pelvis. The remainder of the technique is as described above.

COMPLETE AND INCOMPLETE BREECH DELIVERIES

Complete and incomplete breech deliveries may occur in the same fashion as the frank vaginal breech

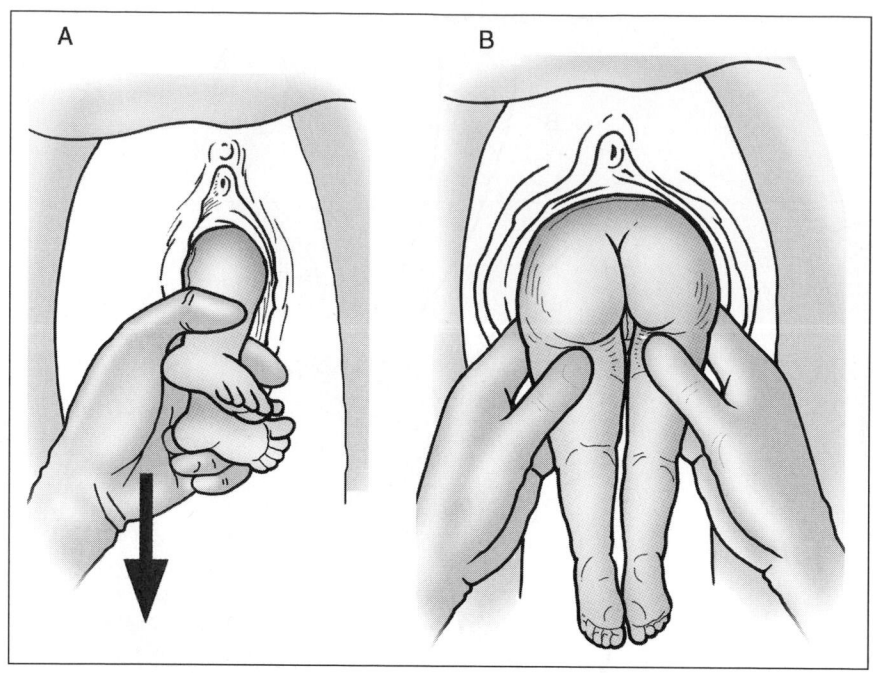

FIGURE 113-10 Breech extraction. Reach into the uterus and grasp the fetal ankles. *A.* Apply traction to deliver the feet and ankles. *B.* Delivery of the buttocks.

delivery. The one exception is that one or both feet may already be extended and not require attention.[1] There is an increased risk of umbilical cord prolapse, umbilical cord entanglement, and entrapment of the after-coming head.[1–3] This is the basis for the recommendation for cesarean delivery in these cases.[1–3] However, one randomized trial reported non-frank vaginal breech delivery to be relatively safe as well.[1,3]

ASSESSMENT

The two patients must now be assessed and treated. If available, a second practitioner or neonatal team can evaluate and resuscitate the infant. Determine the infant's Apgar score. Examine the infant for birth trauma and signs of prematurity (e.g., fusing of eyelids), as both correlate with perinatal morbidity and mortality.

The maternal assessment should occur simultaneously with that of the neonate. Offering reassurance to the mother while delivering the placenta and evaluating for postpartum hemorrhage is of the utmost importance. Deliver the placenta and repair the cervix if there are any lacerations or Dührssen's incisions. An episiotomy, perineal laceration, and/or vaginal laceration must be repaired (Chapters 111 and 114). Initiate uterine massage. Administer pitocin intramuscularly following delivery of the placenta.

AFTERCARE

It is vital that postpartum hemorrhage be managed to prevent maternal morbidity and mortality. Refer to Chapter 114 regarding the details of postpartum hemorrhage management. Grasp the base of each cervical incision or laceration to decrease the bleeding. If the distal angle is difficult to visualize, do not waste time attempting to locate it. Apply traction to the proximal edges of the incision or laceration with ring forceps. Alternatively, place 2–0 chromic, Dexon, or Vicryl sutures along the edges of the cervical incision or laceration that can be visualized. Place progressively proximal interrupted sutures until the base is completely visualized (Figure 113-9*B*). Apply traction to the sutures to better visualize the cervical incision or laceration.

COMPLICATIONS

Maternal complications associated with the performance of a vaginal breech delivery include lacerations (cervical, vaginal, and/or perineal), episiotomy extension, infection, postpartum hemorrhage, and hematomas (vaginal or pelvic). Neonatal complications include hypoxia, anoxia (perinatal asphyxia), umbilical cord prolapse, fractures (cranial, femoral, and clavicular), cerebral hemorrhage, cephalohematomas, lacerations, brachial nerve palsy, cerebral palsy, spinal cord injuries (from head hyperextension), arrest of the after-coming head, and death.[1–10] Recent studies suggest that the occurrence of these complications may be greatly influenced by the urgency of the delivery rather than solely the method of delivery.[1] Thus, an adequately prepared Emergency Physician may not be able to prevent these complications but will less likely contribute to them.

SUMMARY

Perinatal survival is similar for the delivery of a breech infant vaginally or by cesarean section, although controversy still exists.[1,7,8,13] Increased morbidity and mortality may be seen with estimated fetal weights of less than 1500 gm or greater than 4000 gm, single or double footling presentation, a diminished maternal pelvis, cephalic hyperextension, or in the hands of an inexperienced provider. Cesarean section is preferable in these instances if available. The Emergency Physician managing an imminent breech delivery should be well aware of not only the potential complications but also the relative indications for cesarean delivery and the techniques and tools for vaginal delivery in order to lessen the inherent risks to both patients.

REFERENCES

1. Lanni SM, Seeds JW: Malpresentations, in Gabbe SG, Niebyl JR, Simpson JL (eds): *Obstetrics—Normal and Problem Pregnancies*, 4th ed. New York: Churchill Livingstone, 2002:482–493.

2. Collea JV, Chein C, Quilligan EJ: The randomized management of term frank breech presentation: a study of 208 cases. *Am J Obstet Gynecol* 1980; 137(2):235–244.

3. Flanagan TA, Mulchahey KM, Korenbrot CC, et al: Management of the term breech presentation. *Am J Obstet Gynecol* 1987; 156(6):1492–1502.

4. Gimovsky ML, Wallace RL, Schifrin BS, et al: Randomized management of the non-frank breech presentation at term: a preliminary report. *Am J Obstet Gynecol* 1983; 146(1):34–40.

5. Green JE, McLean F, Smith LP, et al: Has an increased cesarean section rate for term breech delivery reduced the incidence of birth asphyxia, trauma, and death? *Am J Obstet Gynecol* 1982; 142(3 pt 1):643–648.

6. Croughan-Minihane MS, Pettiti DB, Gordis L, et al: Morbidity amongst breech infants according to method of delivery. *Obstet Gynecol* 1990; 75(5):821–825.

7. Zatuchni GI, Andros GJ: Prognostic index for vaginal delivery in breech presentation at term. *Am J Obstet Gynecol* 1965; 93(2):237–242.

8. Weissman A, Blazer S, Zimmer EZ, et al: Low birth-weight breech infant: short term and long term outcome by method of delivery. *Am J Perinatol* 1988; 5(3):289–292.

9. Cheng M, Hannah M: Breech delivery at term: a critical review of the literature. *Obstet Gynecol* 1993; 82(4 pt 1):605–618.

10. Bingham P, Lilford RJ: Management of the selected term breech presentation: assessment of the risks of selected vaginal delivery versus cesarean section for all cases. *Obstet Gynecol* 1987; 69(6):965–978.

11. Blickstein I, Schwartz-Shoham Z, Lancet M: Vaginal delivery of the second twin in breech presentation. *Obstet Gynecol* 1987; 69(5):774–776.

12. Fishman A, Grubb DK, Kovacs BW: Vaginal delivery of the nonvertex second twin. *Am J Obstet Gynecol* 1993; 168(3 pt 1):861–864.

13. Danielian PJ, Wang J, Hall MH: Long-term outcome by method of delivery of fetuses in breech presentation at term: population-based follow up. *Br Med J* 1996; 312(7044):1451–1453.

14. Milner RDG: Neonatal mortality of breech deliveries with and without forceps to the aftercoming head. *Br J Obstet Gynaecol* 1975; 82:783–785.

15. Tatum RK, Orr JW, Soong S, et al: Vaginal breech delivery of selected infants weighing more than 2000 grams: a retrospective analysis of 7 years experience. *Am J Obstet Gynecol* 1985; 152(2):145–155.

Chapter 114
POSTPARTUM
HEMORRHAGE
MANAGEMENT

R. Harold Holbrook, Jr.
Susan K. Hendricks
Mark Tanaka

INTRODUCTION

Postpartum hemorrhage, or excessive blood loss following delivery, has been variably defined. It is traditionally defined as blood loss greater than 500 mL after vaginal delivery. The American College of Obstetrics and Gynecology (ACOG) defines postpartum hemorrhage as blood loss that results in a decrease in hematocrit of greater than 10 points or bleeding that requires erythrocyte transfusion. A drop in the hematocrit of 10 points corresponds to the 97th percentile of vaginal and 92nd percentile of cesarean deliveries.[1] Normal blood loss is believed to be 300 to 500 mL following a vaginal delivery and 900 to 1200 mL following a cesarean section.[2] Postpartum hemorrhage can occur at sites within or external to the genitourinary tract (Table 114-1).

The incidence of postpartum hemorrhage ranges from 3.9 to 11 percent of all pregnancies.[1-5] Early postpartum hemorrhage accounts for greater than 90 percent of all cases and occurs within 24 hours of delivery. It is most commonly the result of excessive bleeding from the placental implantation site or trauma to the genital tract. It is associated with a considerable drop in hematocrit and significant maternal complications. Late postpartum hemorrhage occurs more than 24 hours after delivery but before 6 weeks postpartum. It is the result of excessive bleeding from the placental implantation site, endometritis, or a hereditary coagulopathy.[1,5] This chapter reviews the pathophysiology of early postpartum hemorrhage, discusses the diagnosis and assessment of postpartum hemorrhage, and concludes with strategies for treatment.

ANATOMY AND PATHOPHYSIOLOGY

The most common causes of postpartum hemorrhage are uterine atony (70 to 90 percent), lacerations and genital tract injuries (5 to 8 percent), retained products of conception (3 to 5 percent), and hematologic or coagulopathic abnormalities (< 2 percent). Complete and incomplete uterine inversion is a rare cause of postpartum hemorrhage. Risk factors for uterine atony include high parity, advanced maternal age, multiple gestations, polyhydramnios, use of oxytocin or uterine relaxing agents, macrosomia, chorioamnionitis, prolonged third stage of labor, and uterine overdistention.[1] Genital tract injuries include vaginal lacerations, cervical lacerations, lower uterine segment lacerations, vulvar hematomas, vaginal hematomas, uterine rupture, and uterine inversion. Retention of all or part of the placenta can interfere with postpartum uterine contraction and retraction. Hematologic abnormalities include von Willebrand's disease, disseminated intravascular coagulation, and other less common inherited, congenital, or acquired disorders.

Measurement of actual blood loss is difficult. The hypervolemia and increase in plasma volume seen in normal pregnancy may partially compensate for the initial blood loss. Visual estimates of blood loss are inaccurate. **Weigh all pads for an accurate assessment (1 gm = 1 mL of blood).** The signs and symptoms of postpartum hemorrhage include measurable blood loss greater than 500 mL, tachycardia, hypotension, pallor, loss of consciousness, and diaphoresis. Concealed hemorrhage (vaginal hematoma, uterine rupture) must be

TABLE 114-1. ANATOMIC SITES OF POSTPARTUM HEMORRHAGE

Broad ligament
Cervix
Contractile tissue
Lower urinary tract (bladder, urethra)
Lower uterine segment placental implantation site
Noncontractile or poorly contractile tissue
Perineum (perineal body, periurethral area, rectum)
Upper uterine segment placental implantation site
Vagina (fornices, hymen, anomalous septa, side walls)

suspected if the patient is symptomatic in the absence of obvious blood loss.

Patients at risk for postpartum hemorrhage require blood typed and held at the outset. Leading risk factors associated with postpartum hemorrhage in vaginal birth include prolonged third stage of labor, preeclampsia, mediolateral episiotomy, previous postpartum hemorrhage, twins, arrest of descent, and soft tissue lacerations.[3,6] Other risk factors are listed in Table 114-2. Surgical deliveries as compared with vaginal deliveries are invariably associated with increased blood loss. Inhalation anesthesia, especially with halogenated agents, increases the risk for postpartum hemorrhage and should be used sparingly in high-risk cases.[3,7] Other risk factors for postpartum hemorrhage in cesarean deliveries include amnionitis, protracted active phase of labor, and preeclampsia.[2]

INDICATIONS

All postpartum hemorrhage must be controlled as soon as possible to prevent maternal morbidity and mortality. The two foremost causes of postpartum hem-

TABLE 114-2. ETIOLOGIC ASSOCIATIONS FOR POSTPARTUM HEMORRHAGE

Altered maternal anatomy	Operative delivery
Altered uterine contractility	Pitocin use, prolonged
Cesarean section dehiscence or rupture	Placental abruption
	Placenta previa
Chorioamnionitis	Postpartum hemorrhage history
Compound delivery	Precipitous delivery
Dührssen's incisions	Prolonged or tumultuous labor
Endometritis	Retained placental fragments
Fetal scalp electrode injury	Shoulder dystocia
Grand multiparity	Tocolytic use
Infection	Trauma
Intrauterine pressure catheter injury	Uterine anomalies
	Uterine inversion
Myomectomy dehiscence or rupture	Uterine leiomyomata
	Von Willebrand's coagulopathy
Occiput posterior delivery	

orrhage are uterine atony and lower genital tract lacerations. Such lacerations and injuries are most common with difficult deliveries, especially operative vaginal deliveries, and with the use of an episiotomy. Carefully examine the vagina, cervix, and lower uterine segment for injury immediately following delivery of the infant and placenta. If present, these factors should be noted and the possibility of postpartum hemorrhage anticipated.

CONTRAINDICATIONS

There are no absolute contraindications to the management of postpartum hemorrhage. Therapies for postpartum hemorrhage, specifically drug therapy for uterine atony, may have significant side effects. Ergots, such as methylergonovine, are potent vasoconstrictors. They are contraindicated in the presence of cardiac disorders, coronary artery disease, and hypertensive disorders. Prostaglandin F (PGF) is contraindicated in patients with active asthma as it can incite severe bronchospasm in sensitive individuals.[1] It may also result in vasoconstriction of the pulmonary bed.[1]

EQUIPMENT

Physician's gown and gloves
Povidone iodine solution
Sponges
Sponge-tipped applicators
Sterile delivery drapes
Alcohol wipes
16 to 18 gauge needle
10 mL syringe
22 to 25 gauge epidural needle for injection
Weighted vaginal speculum
Six ring forceps
Straight Mayo scissors or sterile scalpel
2–0 or 3–0 suture, chromic gut or polyglycolic acid

Medications

Local anesthetic solution (lidocaine, bupivacaine, or mepivacaine)
Oxytocin (Pitocin)
Methylergonovine maleate (Methergine)
Misoprostol or prostaglandin E-1 (Cytotec)
Carboprost tromethamine or prostaglandin F-2 (Hemabate)

PATIENT PREPARATION

The initial management must be aimed at stabilizing the mother and identifying the bleeding source. Establish intravenous access at two sites with 16 to 18 gauge angiocatheters. Type and crossmatch the patient for any required blood components. Place a Foley catheter for adequate monitoring of urine output. Regulate fluid intake carefully.

Identification of the origin or site of bleeding is critical. Uterine hypotonia is the most frequent source of hemorrhage. Begin with a complete examination of the uterus. Palpation will often exhibit a spongy, boggy, and soft uterus that may be increasing in size due to the accumulation of clots and blood within the endometrial cavity. Continued bleeding from the endometrial cavity through the cervical os is always present. A well-contracted uterus does not bleed significantly in the absence of a severe coagulopathy. Examination of the uterine fundus is performed by palpation of the myometrium and manual exploration of the uterine cavity. Ultrasound may be used to ascertain the presence of placental tissue or clots that may require manual removal and/or curettage.

Continued vaginal hemorrhage with a firm, globular uterus indicates bleeding from another source such as the lower uterine segment, the cervix, or the vagina. **Examine all areas carefully, even after hemorrhage is noted at one site, as there may be more than one source of hemorrhage.** Begin at the most distal aspects of the genital tract and work proximally.

TECHNIQUES

RETAINED PLACENTA

Postpartum hemorrhage, whether early or late, may be caused by retained placental tissue within the uterine cavity. The retained placental tissue may be completely attached, partially separated, or completely separated from the uterine wall. Placental fragments completely attached to the uterine wall may not be removable manually and may require a curettage or laparotomy. Completely or partially separated placental fragments may remain due to a closed cervix entrapping them or inadequate uterine contractions. Manual extraction will remove the retained placental fragments. **Administer adequate anesthesia. A uterine relaxant may be utilized to relax the lower uterine segment in the absence of uterine atony. This must be performed aseptically.**

Insert a sterile gloved hand through the open cervix and into the uterine cavity (Figure 114-1). Place the other hand abdominally and over the fundus of the uterus. Gently and carefully sweep the fingers around the circumference of the uterus to determine if any fragments of placenta remain. Gently remove any placental fragments from the uterine wall by alternately abducting, adducting, and advancing the fingers in a

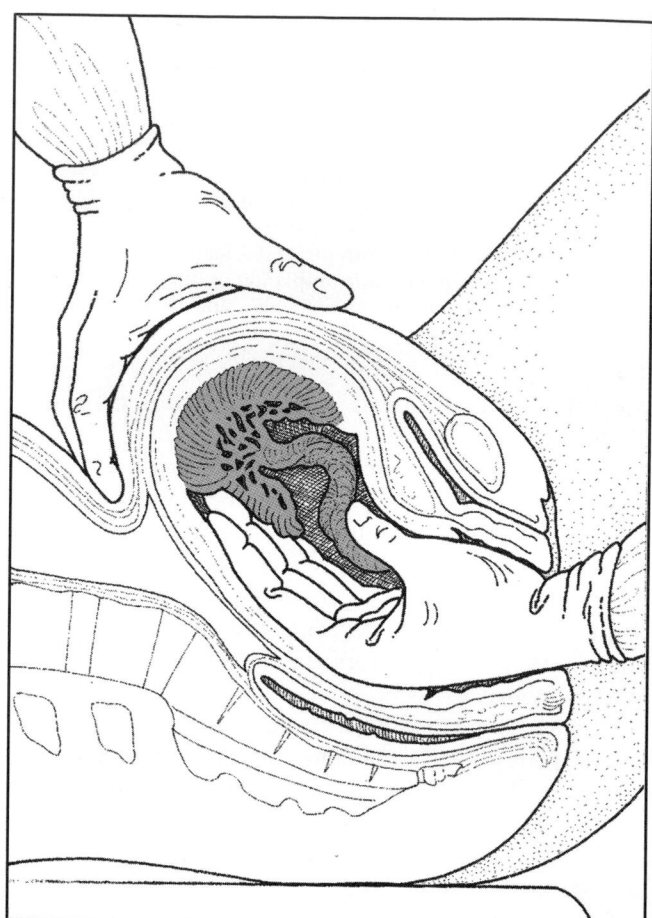

FIGURE 114-1 Manual removal of the placenta. The fingers are abducted, adducted, and advanced continually (in a scissor-like motion) in this sequence of movements until the placenta is completely detached.

scissors-like motion. Grasp and gently remove the placental fragments when separated from the uterine wall. **Ensure that the entire placenta is removed. Reinsert a hand into the uterine cavity and palpate for any remaining placental fragments. Examine the placenta carefully to make sure that no cotyledons are missing.**

Determine if any placental membranes are retained. Reinsert the gloved hand covered with a gauze sponge (Figure 114-2). Wipe the uterine walls with the sponge to collect any retained membranes. Remove the gauze sponge with any adherent membranes.

Identify the edge of the placenta if it has not separated from the uterine wall. Gently place the fingertips under the edge of the placenta, forming a line of cleavage between the uterine wall and the placenta. Alternately abduct, adduct, and advance the fingers in a scissors-like motion until the entire placenta is separated from the fundus[8] (Figure 114-1). Gently remove the placenta from the uterine cavity. **Make sure that the entire placenta is removed. Reinsert a hand into the uterine cavity and palpate for any remaining placental frag-**

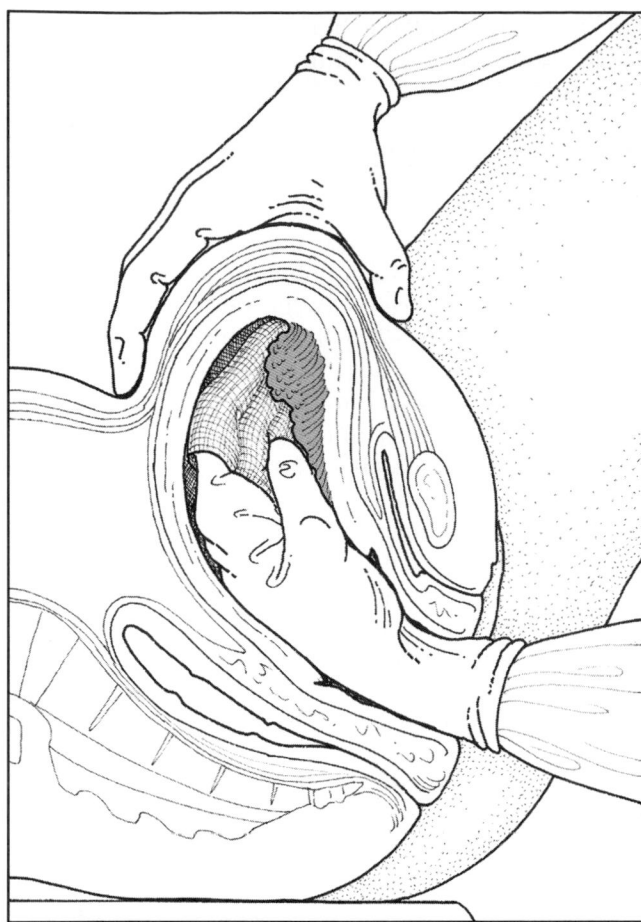

FIGURE 114-2 Manual removal of retained placental membranes.

ments. Examine the placenta carefully to make sure that no cotyledons are missing. Initiate intravenous oxytocin following removal of the placenta.

The placenta is likely embedded into the wall of the uterus if it does not manually separate. This is known as placenta accreta, percreta, or increta, depending on the degree of myometrial penetration. Consult an Obstetrician, as a laparotomy, hysterotomy, and possibly a hysterectomy will be required.

UTERINE ATONY

Uterine atony is identified by palpating a soft and boggy uterus. Begin transabdominal uterine massage to promote uterine muscle contraction. Use one or two hands to palpate the uterus through the abdominal wall and rhythmically press downward. Massage in a firm but gentle manner, without pushing the uterus through the birth canal. **Avoid overvigorous massage, as this can injure the vasculature of the broad ligament.**[8]

Initiate an oxytocin infusion at the same time as transabdominal uterine massage. Inject 20 to 40 U of oxytocin into 1 L of intravenous fluid. Allow this solu-

tion to infuse over 10 minutes. Oxytocin concentrations above 30 to 40 U/L of fluid do not increase the effectiveness of uterine contractions and increase the risk of fluid overload secondary to the ADH-like effects of this hormone.[9] Alternatively, administer 10 U of oxytocin intramuscularly.

Continued bleeding requires the initiation of bimanual uterine compression. Massage the posterior aspect of the uterus with the abdominal hand and the anterior aspect of the uterus through the vagina with the other hand clenched into a fist[8] (Figure 114-3). Use the intravaginal hand to massage the uterus against the external pressure applied by the abdominal hand. This allows for more effective uterine massage. Perform manual uterine exploration if the massage fails to control the hemorrhage. Manual uterine exploration can localize and extract any placental fragments remaining within the uterus.

Begin administering second-line medications to contract the uterus if bimanual massage is ineffective. Administer 0.2 mg of methylergonovine (Methergine) intramuscularly. This is an ergot derivative that causes

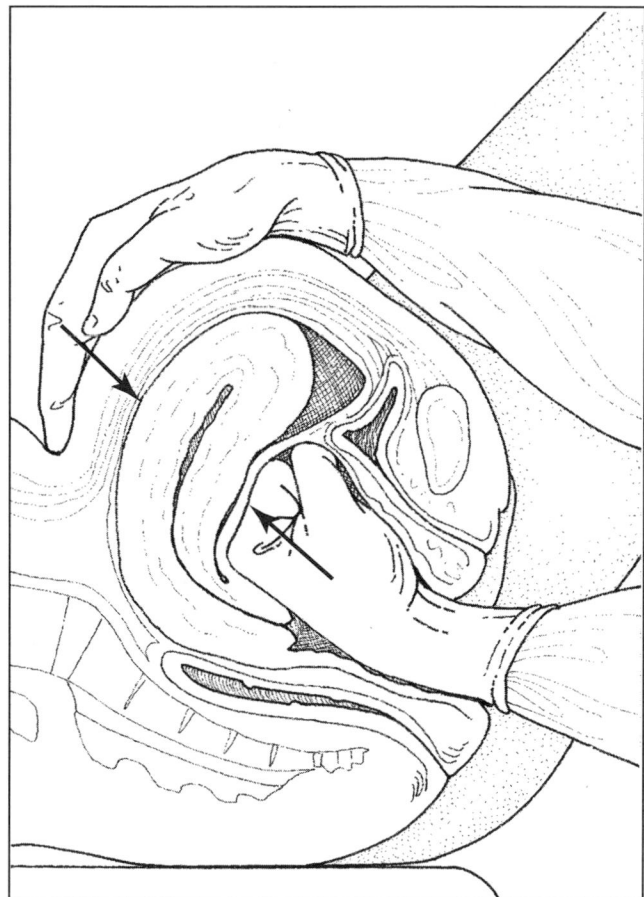

FIGURE 114-3 Bimanual uterine compression for uterine atony.

uterine contraction. Prostaglandin F-2 (Hemabate) is a potent stimulator of uterine contraction.[10] Administer 250 to 500 μg transabdominally into the uterine musculature or intramuscularly. Prostaglandin E-1 or misoprostol (Cytotec) may be utilized intravaginally in the form of 20 mg suppositories, or 25 or 50 mg tablets. Attach the pack string to a hemostat outside the vagina if a vaginal pack is utilized. Continued bleeding requires an Obstetrician for curettage or operative management. A discussion of this technique is beyond the scope of this chapter.

GENITAL TRACT ABNORMALITIES

Bleeding from the lower uterine segment, cervix, or upper vagina is difficult to diagnose and manage. The anatomic locations are awkward and difficult to visualize; excessive bleeding makes visualization even more problematic. It may be almost impossible to see a small laceration or an individual bleeding vessel. The uterotonic medications, such as oxytocin, and the prostaglandins are less effective due to the relative paucity of contractile muscle in these tissues. Management of excessive bleeding from this area may require a laparotomy with uterine artery ligation or a hysterectomy. Discussion of these techniques is beyond the scope of this chapter.

LACERATION REPAIR

All lacerations must be repaired. Always make sure there is adequate exposure and visualization of the laceration. Insert a Foley catheter if the laceration is in proximity to the urethra. This ensures urethral patency and noninclusion in sutures. Scrub the perineum with an iodine-based solution or, if the patient is iodine-allergic, with a noniodinated alcohol-based sterilization solution. Apply sterile drapes beneath the patient's buttocks, on the legs, and on the abdomen to prevent contamination from nonsterile areas. Provide anesthesia with the injection of local anesthetic solution directly into the laceration or with a nerve block. Refer to Chapter 111 for details regarding perineal nerve blocks.

Thorough knowledge of the anatomy and awareness of where sutures are being placed is necessary to avoid perforation of any proximate viscera. Always use absorbable suture. Refer to Chapter 111 for complete details regarding the repair of an episiotomy. A brief description of the repair procedure is given below.

First-Degree Lacerations

First-degree lacerations involve the fourchette, the perineal skin, and the vaginal mucous membrane. They spare the underlying fascia and muscle. Use continuous 2–0 or 3–0 chromic suture to close the vaginal mucosa and submucosa. Interrupted sutures may better approximate the laceration if it is very irregular. Approximate

the cut margins of the hymenal ring with a stitch. Repair skin lacerations with interrupted 3–0 chromic sutures.[11]

Second-Degree Lacerations

Second-degree lacerations involve the perineal skin, vaginal mucous membrane, subcutaneous tissue, fascia, and muscles of the perineum but not the anal sphincter muscle. Repair is essentially the same as for an episiotomy but complicated by the irregularity of the laceration. Begin as in a first-degree laceration by repairing the vaginal mucosa and submucosa. Approximate the hymenal ring. Place interrupted 2–0 or 3–0 chromic gut sutures to close the fascia and muscles of the lacerated perineum. Carry a continuous (running) suture downward to unite the superficial fascia and then upward to close the subcutaneous tissue. Alternatively, place interrupted stitches for better approximation. Close the skin with a running subcuticular stitch. The subcutaneous tissue and skin may be closed together with interrupted 3–0 chromic sutures to minimize the amount of buried suture in the superficial perineal layers.[11]

Third-Degree Lacerations

Third-degree lacerations involve a second-degree laceration that extends into the anal sphincter but not the rectal mucosa. Isolate, approximate, and suture together the cut ends of the anal sphincter with interrupted 2–0 chromic gut or Vicryl sutures. The remainder of the repair is the same as that for second-degree lacerations.[11]

Fourth-Degree Lacerations

Fourth-degree lacerations extend through the rectal mucosa to expose the rectal lumen. Approximate the torn rectal mucosa with interrupted 3–0 or 4–0 chromic gut sutures placed approximately 0.5 cm apart. Cover this muscular layer with a layer of fascia. Proceed as with the repair of third-degree lacerations.[11]

ASSESSMENT

Thoroughly examine the patient to ensure the cessation of bleeding. **Any additional bleeding sites must be found and repaired.** Carefully monitor the patient's vital signs and urinary output. Manage any hypotension with fluid boluses and packed red blood cells as indicated. Follow serial complete blood counts if the patient has lost a significant amount of blood. Persistent hypotension, tachycardia, or a hematocrit less than 21 percent may require a transfusion. Hemodynamically stable patients may be expectantly managed.

AFTERCARE

The aftercare for postpartum hemorrhage is targeted toward the etiology of the bleeding episode. Warm sitz baths alternated with ice packs applied to the perineum three to four times a day will decrease inflammation and the risk of infection in patients with lacerations or episiotomies. Stool softeners will decrease the pain of defecation and the risk of wound dehiscence, especially with third- or fourth-degree lacerations. A high-fiber, low-residue diet may be helpful. Prescribe oral analgesics for pain relief. Nonsteroidal anti-inflammatory drugs or acetaminophen provide adequate analgesia for most patients. Narcotic analgesics, such as oxycodone or acetaminophen with codeine, may be necessary initially. Avoid formulations that increase constipation in patients with third- or fourth-degree lacerations.

Follow complete blood count values until the patient is asymptomatic and stable. Consider a transfusion if the patient's hematocrit is less than 25, the patient is symptomatic from anemia, or is hemodynamically unstable. Prescribe 300 mg of iron sulfate ($FeSO_4$) orally per day.

Follow-up therapy for uterine atony may include the use of oxytocin (10 to 20 U/L of intravenous fluid) for 12 to 24 hours. An alternative is oral Methergine. Initiate therapy after consultation with an Obstetrician.

COMPLICATIONS

Maternal complications resulting from postpartum hemorrhage include the need for blood transfusion, possible complications from the transfusion, the need for surgical intervention (dilatation and curretage or laparotomy) and its associated complications, fatigue, postpartum endomyometritis, or a urinary tract infection. Complications associated with pharmacologic therapy can be avoided by carefully selecting the appropriate patient for each agent (see "Contraindications," above).

SUMMARY

Postpartum hemorrhage is a serious and potentially lethal condition. Early identification of risk factors and a prompt response to the early signs and symptoms of postpartum bleeding will decrease the morbidity and mortality of this situation. Always consult an Obstetrician immediately if the patient experiences postpartum hemorrhage.

REFERENCES

1. Sorokin Y: Obstetrical hemorrhage, in Ransom SB (ed): *Practical Strategies in Obstetrics and Gynecology.* Philadelphia: Saunders, 2000:311–320.
2. Combs CA, Murphy EL, Laros RK: Factors associated with hemorrhage in cesarean deliveries. *Obstet Gynecol* 1991; 77(1):77–82.
3. Combs CA, Murphy EL, Laros RK: Factors associated with postpartum hemorrhage with vaginal birth. *Obstet Gynecol* 1991; 77(1):69–76.
4. Naef RW, Chauhan SP, Chevalier SP, et al: Prediction of hemorrhage at cesarean delivery. *Obstet Gynecol* 1994; 83(6):923–926.
5. Khong TY, Khong TK: Delayed postpartum hemorrhage: a morphologic study of causes and their relation to other pregnancy disorders. *Obstet Gynecol* 1993; 82(1):17–22.
6. Gilbert L, Porter W, Brown VA: Postpartum hemorrhage—a continuing problem. *Br J Obstet Gynecol* 1987; 94:67–71.
7. Gilstrap LC, Hauth JC, Hankins GDV, et al: Effect of type of anesthesia on blood loss at cesarean section. *Obstet Gynecol* 1987; 69(3 pt 1):328–332.
8. Cunningham FG, Gant NF, Leveno, KJ, et al: *Williams Obstetrics,* 21st ed. New York: McGraw-Hill, 2001:619–669.
9. Prendiville W, Ebourne D, Chalmers I: The effects of routine oxytocic administration in the management of the third stage of labour: an overview of the evidence from controlled trials. *Br J Obstet Gynecol* 1988; 95:3–16.
10. Oleen MA, Mariano JP: Controlling refractory atonic postpartum hemorrhage with hemabate sterile solution. *Am J Obstet Gynecol* 1990; 162(1):205–208.
11. Cunningham FG, Gant NF, Leveno, KJ, et al: *Williams Obstetrics,* 21st ed. New York: McGraw-Hill, 2001:309–329.

Chapter 115
PERIMORTEM CESAREAN SECTION

Angela Flippin
Susan K. Hendricks

INTRODUCTION

Trauma is the leading cause of death in women of reproductive age and accounts for 25 to 50 percent of maternal morbidity. Major maternal injury is associated with a 45 to 50 percent fetal loss rate. **The primary goal in the management of the severely injured pregnant patient is maternal assessment and stabilization. Prompt attention to the needs of the gravid patient can save the life of both the fetus and the mother**. Nonetheless, there are occasions when emergent cesarean delivery of the fetus is necessary to save the fetus, and sometimes, the mother. This procedure is best performed by a qualified Surgeon in the Operating Room. However, there are circumstances that may necessitate the performance of this procedure in the Emergency Department. These include the possibility of uterine rupture, placental abruption, fetal distress, and imminent maternal demise.

There are several simple principles to keep in mind. Quickly establish that the mother is deceased or that no further intervention is possible. Quickly open the abdominal wall and uterus with vertical incisions. The use of aseptic technique is not required and only wastes valuable time. Deliver the fetus and begin resuscitation. Manually remove the placenta. Close the uterus and abdominal wall with running sutures.

ANATOMY AND PATHOPHYSIOLOGY

MATERNAL PHYSIOLOGY
The performance of adequate CPR in the gravid patient at or near term is extremely difficult. Adequate CPR produces a cardiac output equivalent to 30 percent of normal under ideal circumstances. The enlarged uterus lies anterior to the inferior vena cava and suppresses venous return in the gravid patient. Place the patient in 15 degrees of left lateral tilt to adequately relieve the obstruction of the inferior vena cava by the uterus. Evacuation of the uterus by cesarean section may save the fetus and, by enabling adequate maternal resuscitation, save the mother as well. The pregnant patient has a decreased tolerance for anoxic brain injury. The fetus can tolerate anoxic injury slightly longer than the mother.

EVALUATION FOR PERIMORTEM CESAREAN SECTION
Quickly determine the fetal age using ultrasonography, the last known menstrual period, the history of term gestation by family members, or fundal height. Perform ultrasonography only if the unit is immediately available and if the operator is experienced in obstetric ultrasound. Note the time of the maternal arrest. Immediately consider performing a perimortem cesarean section in the resuscitation of a pregnant patient with an estimated gestational age of 24 weeks or greater and with cardiac arrest that has not responded to aggressive resuscitation within four minutes from onset. The single most important prognostic factor for neonatal outcome is the time from maternal arrest to delivery. Delivery of the fetus can also maximize maternal resuscitation efforts and minimize the risk of maternal brain injury. Delay the initiation of vasopressor agents until after adequate volume replacement. However, they should not be withheld if needed to resuscitate the patient. Place a wedge under the patient's right flank and hip to displace the uterus laterally.

INDICATIONS

The major indication for perimortem cesarean section is to optimize maternal cardiopulmonary resuscitation. **The rescue of a viable fetus greater than 24 weeks gestation is an important consideration, but such rescue is always secondary to the safety and life of the mother.**

CONTRAINDICATIONS

There are few contraindications to performing a perimortem cesarean delivery. The best fetal outcomes are reported when cesarean delivery occurs within five minutes of maternal arrest. However, perimortem cesarean section should be considered if the time from the maternal arrest to delivery would be no greater than 25 minutes. It is contraindicated if the mother has a serious brain injury but is otherwise hemodynamically stable and the fetus shows no signs of distress. Other contraindications to perimortem cesarean delivery are the inability to adequately resuscitate the infant after delivery or extreme fetal prematurity/immaturity.

Attempt to obtain consent for the procedure. However, there is no documentation of physician liability in these situations. **Do not delay treatment pending consent.** The unanimous consensus in the medical literature and of legal authorities is that a civil suit against a physician for performing a perimortem cesarean delivery, regardless of the outcome, would not result in a judgment against the physician.

EQUIPMENT

10 towel clips
16 Kelly clamps
16 hemostats
10 Peon or Pennington clamps
8 Allis forceps
6 Babcock forceps
6 ring forceps
6 straight Kocher clamps
#10 surgical scalpel blade and handle
#15 surgical scalpel blade and handle
Straight Mayo scissors
Curved Mayo scissors
Metzenbaum scissors
Bandage scissors
2 suture scissors
2 Adson forceps, or other forceps with teeth
2 Russian forceps, 5 1/2 inches and 8 inches
Dressing forceps
Bladder retractor
2 medium Richardson retractors
2 small Richardson retractors
2 malleable retractors
2 Army-Navy retractors
Needle drivers, 8 inches and 6 inches long
2 suction tips
Suction tubing set(s)
Wall suction
Electrocautery unit with disposable tips
Povidone iodine

Sterile drapes
Sterile gloves
2 skin staplers
Chromic, Polysorb, or Vicryl suture (2–0 or 1–0)
Nylon suture, 3–0
Bulb syringe
Clean towels or blanket for baby
Umbilical cord clamp
Sterile scissors to trim umbilical cord
Infant warmer
Neonatal resuscitation equipment

Ideally, all of the equipment should be prepackaged in a sterile cesarean section instrument tray. A pre-prepared sterile instrument tray may not be available because this procedure is rarely performed in the Emergency Department. A standard thoracotomy tray or tube thoracostomy tray will contain all the required equipment except for the bulb syringe and umbilical cord clamp.

PATIENT PREPARATION

Administer adequate anesthesia if the patient is awake and aware of their surroundings. General or epidural/spinal anesthesia is preferred as provided by a qualified Anesthesiologist or Nurse Anesthetist. However, local infiltration of anesthetic solution may be performed in conjunction with procedural sedation. The deceased patient requires no anesthesia.

Surgical preparation in an emergency is minimal. Perform a minimal shave of the lower abdomen and pubic region if time permits. Prepare the abdomen with povidone iodine. Place a Foley catheter to continuously drain the bladder and to decrease the risk of inadvertent entry into the bladder during the procedure. Perform an appropriate surgical scrub if time allows. Apply relevant surgical clothing and covers (hat, mask, booties, sterile gown). Apply sterile surgical drapes over the patient to isolate a surgical field.

The patient will be clinically deceased in most cases if this procedure is performed in the Emergency Department. Patient preparation is not necessary and wastes valuable time when trying to salvage the fetus. The Emergency Physician should follow body fluid precautions (hat, mask, gloves, boots, and sterile gown). Administer broad-spectrum intravenous antibiotics if the mother survives the procedure. Continue CPR until the fetus is delivered.

Every attempt should be made to contact an Obstetrician and Neonatologist if a perimortem cesarean section is anticipated. Consult a General Surgeon if an Obstetrician is not available. Notify the neonatal resuscitation team and Anesthesia (Physician or Nurse Anesthetist) of the impending procedure.

TECHNIQUE

Identify the patient's umbilicus and pubic symphysis. Make a vertical midline skin incision with a #10 scalpel blade beginning 2 to 3 cm above the pubic symphysis and extending to 1 cm below the umbilicus (Figure 115-1*A*). Ignore any subcutaneous bleeding unless it is arterial. Clamp the bleeding artery or use an electrocautery unit to coagulate the vessel if available.

Extend the incision through the subcutaneous fat to the rectus sheath (Figure 115-1*B*). **Do not be overzealous and cut through the rectus sheath, peritoneum, uterus, abdominal organs, or bladder.** Grasp and elevate the rectus sheath using a toothed forceps (Figure 115-1*C*). Make an incision in the rectus sheath with a Mayo scissors. Extend the rectus sheath incision superiorly and inferiorly with a Mayo scissors (Figure 115-1*C*). **Be cautious not to cut any abdominal or pelvic organs.**

Expose the uterus (Figure 115-2). The underlying peritoneal membrane (peritoneum) should be visible (Figure 115-2*A*). It may occasionally be attached to the rectus sheath and opened simultaneously. Insert retractors to fully expose the peritoneal membrane (Figure 115-2*A*). Grasp and elevate the peritoneal membrane with a toothed forceps. Incise the peritoneal membrane with a Mayo or Metzenbaum scissors in a manner similar to that used to open the rectus sheath (Figure 115-2*A*).

Make reasonable attempts to protect the bowel and bladder from injury. Elevate the bowel off the field and cover it with a saline soaked towel. Place a bladder retractor over the pubic symphysis to retract the rectus sheath and bladder (Figure 115-3*A*). This will allow visualization of the uterus and prevent injury to the bladder. Alternatively, grasp and elevate the bladder from the pelvis with a saline soaked gauze or towel (Figure 115-2*B*).

Identify the position of the fetal head by palpating the uterus. Make a 2 to 4 cm midline vertical incision in the uterus (Figure 115-3*A*). The amniotic sac will bulge through the incision if the membranes are intact. **Place a finger into the uterine incision and aimed vertically (Figure 115-3*B*). Insert one blade of a bandage scissors between the finger and the uterine wall (Figure 115-3*B*).** The other blade of the scissors should be outside the uterus. Extend the vertical uterine incision fundally, superior and away from the bladder (Figure 115-3*B*). The finger inside the uterus will protect the fetus

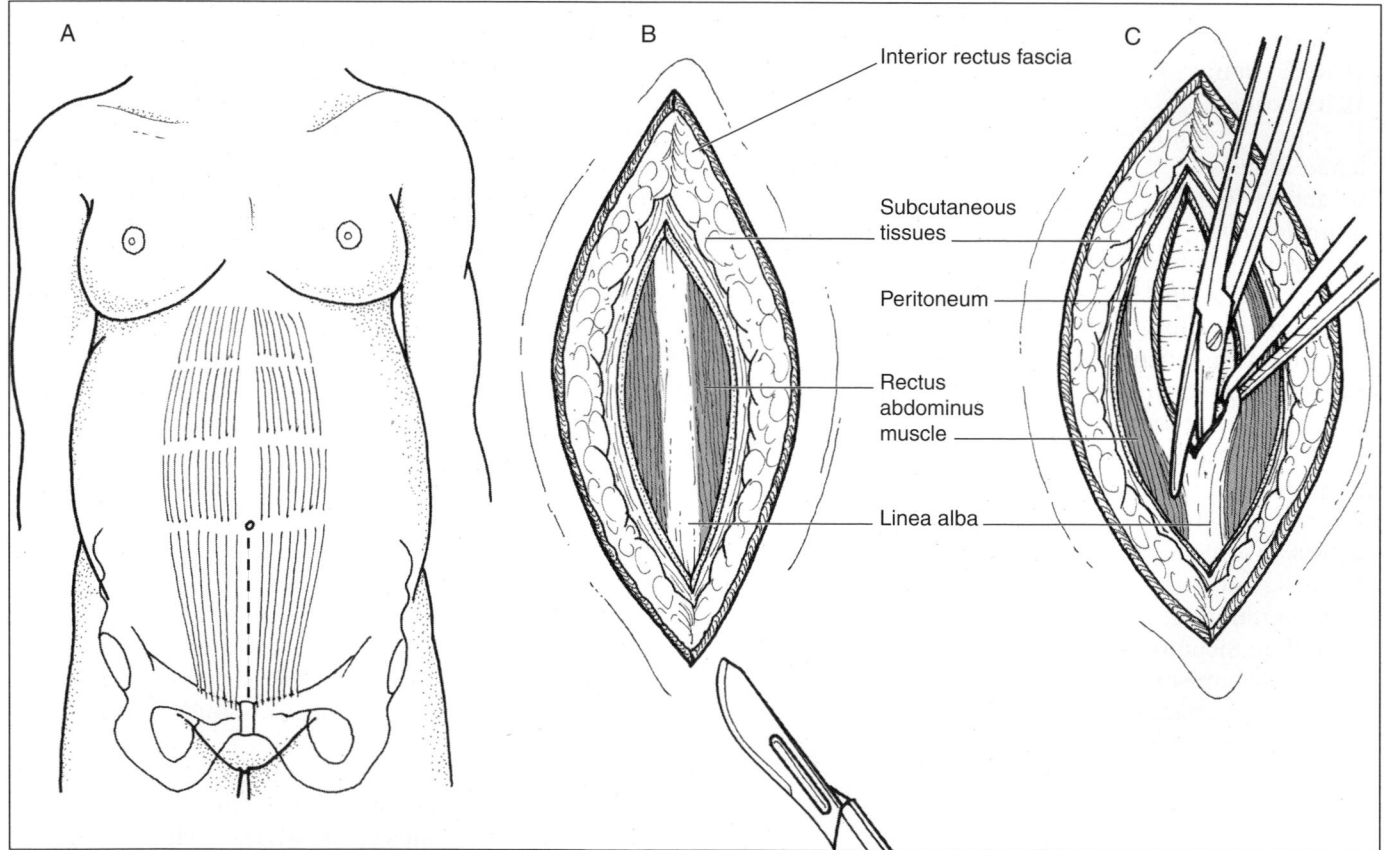

FIGURE 115-1 Accessing the peritoneal cavity. *A.* Make a midline skin incision from just below the umbilicus to just above the pubic symphysis. *B.* Extend the incision through the subcutaneous tissues and down to the linea alba. *C.* Grasp and elevate the rectus abdominis muscle while opening the linea alba with a Mayo scissors.

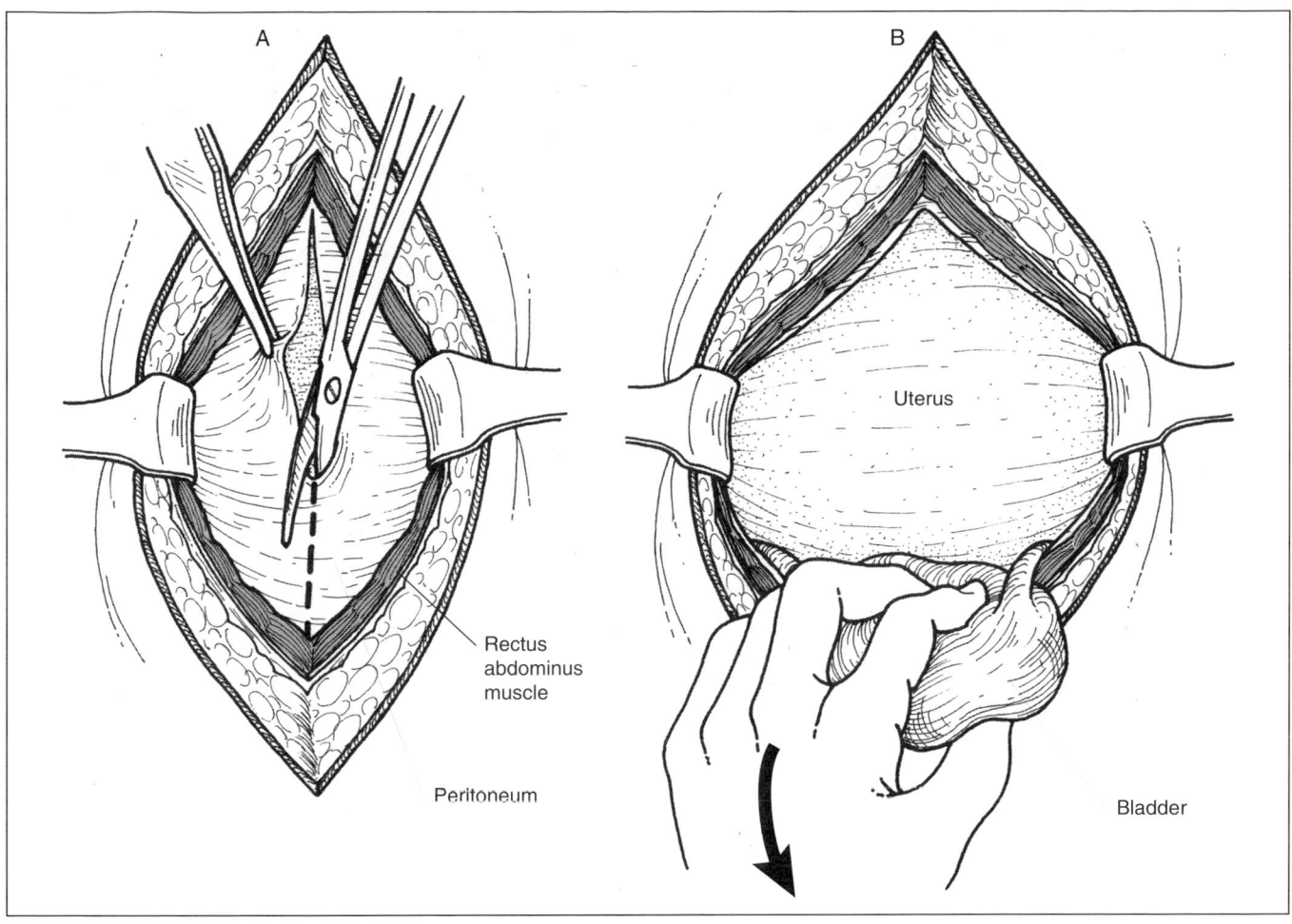

FIGURE 115-2 Exposure of the uterus. *A.* Apply retractors to hold the abdominal wall open. Grasp, elevate, and incise the peritoneal membrane in the midline. *B.* Grasp and elevate the bladder out of the pelvis.

from injury when opening the uterine wall. Repeat this procedure to open the uterine wall inferiorly (Figure 115-3*C*).

Rupture the amniotic membranes with a clamp or other blunt instrument. Carefully transect the placenta if it is anterior to the fetus. **There is an urgency to deliver the fetus and clamp the umbilical cord to prevent significant fetal hemorrhage.** Insert a hand between the pubic symphysis and the fetal occiput (Figure 115-4*A*). Advance the hand to the base of the occiput. Flex the fetal head and apply gentle anteriorly and superiorly directed traction to elevate and deliver the head (Figure 115-4*B*). Deliver the entire fetal head (Figure 115-4*C*). Suction the mouth and nose with a bulb syringe (Figure 115-4*D*). Deliver the shoulders in a manner similar to that of a vaginal delivery (Figure 115-4*E*). Apply gentle upward traction on the head while an assistant applies pressure on the uterine fundus. First deliver the anterior shoulder. Deliver the other shoulder followed by the torso and lower extremities.

Clamp the umbilical cord with a hemostat or umbilical cord clamp approximately 10 to 15 cm from the fetus. Attach a second hemostat or clamp 2 to 3 cm distal to the first. Cut the umbilical cord between the clamps with a Mayo scissors. Hand the neonate to waiting personnel for resuscitation. Resuscitate the neonate yourself if additional help is not available.

AFTERCARE

Deliver the placenta if the patient is still alive or if they regain vital signs (Figure 115-5). Begin an oxytocin infusion of 20 units in 1 liter of normal saline at a rate of 10 mL/hr to help the uterus contract. Apply gentle upward traction on the umbilical cord while holding the uterine wall open (Figure 115-5*A*). Insert the other hand between the placenta and uterine wall (Figure 115-5*B*). Apply gentle pressure to separate the placenta from the uterus.

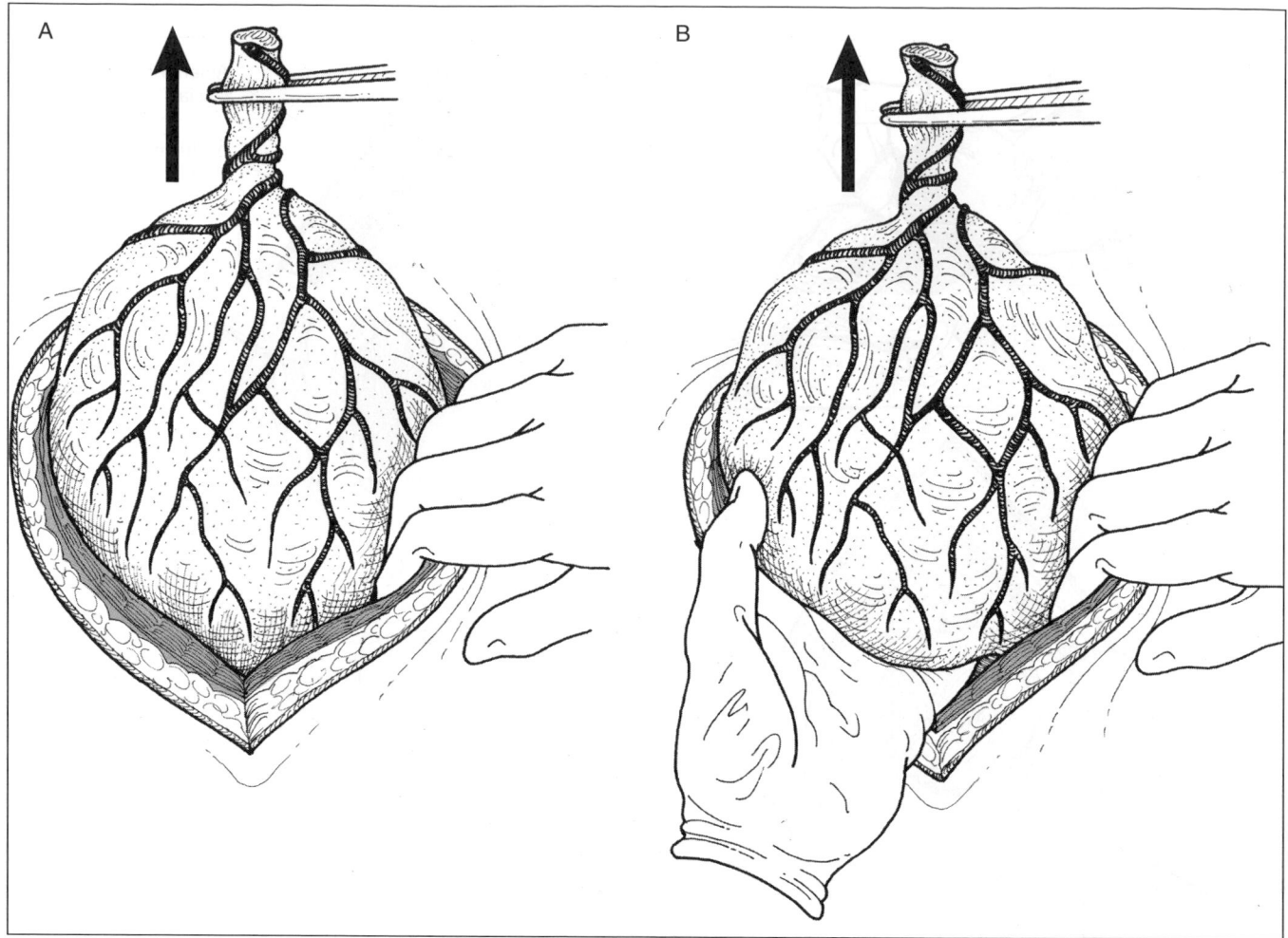

FIGURE 115-5 Delivery of the placenta. *A.* Apply gentle upward traction on the umbilical cord while holding the uterine wall open. *B.* Insert a hand between the placenta and the uterine wall to separate the placenta from the uterus.

Close the patient if they are still alive or if they regain vital signs. Apply ring forceps to the uterine incision. Close the uterus in two layers with 2–0 or 1–0 chromic, Polysorb, or Vicryl suture. Close the first layer in a running locked fashion (Figure 115-6A). This will provide hemostasis. A second running layer may be necessary for hemostasis. Closure of the serosa of the uterus (Figure 115-6B) and the peritoneal membrane (Figure 115-6C) is recommended but not required. Close the serosa and peritoneum with running 2–0 chromic, Polysorb, or Vicryl suture. Identify and grasp the cut ends of the rectus sheath with hemostats. Close the rectus sheath in a running pattern with 2–0 Vicryl suture (Figure 115-6D). Close the skin with running 3–0 nylon (Figure 115-6E) or staples for speed.

The only closure required if the mother will not survive is a minimal closure of the skin. Use either a running baseball stitch closure or skin staples.

COMPLICATIONS

The major associated complications of the procedure include maternal sepsis, maternal visceral injury, maternal hemorrhage, and fetal injury secondary to delivery. The possible benefits of maternal and/or fetal survival should far outweigh these considerations.

SUMMARY

Perimortem cesarean section is a valuable procedure that should be considered in any maternal arrest with an estimated fetal gestational age of greater than 24 weeks. It provides the fetus with a chance for survival in the face of maternal death. In addition to potentially saving the life of the infant, emergent delivery might also aid in the resuscitation of the mother. The medicolegal risks

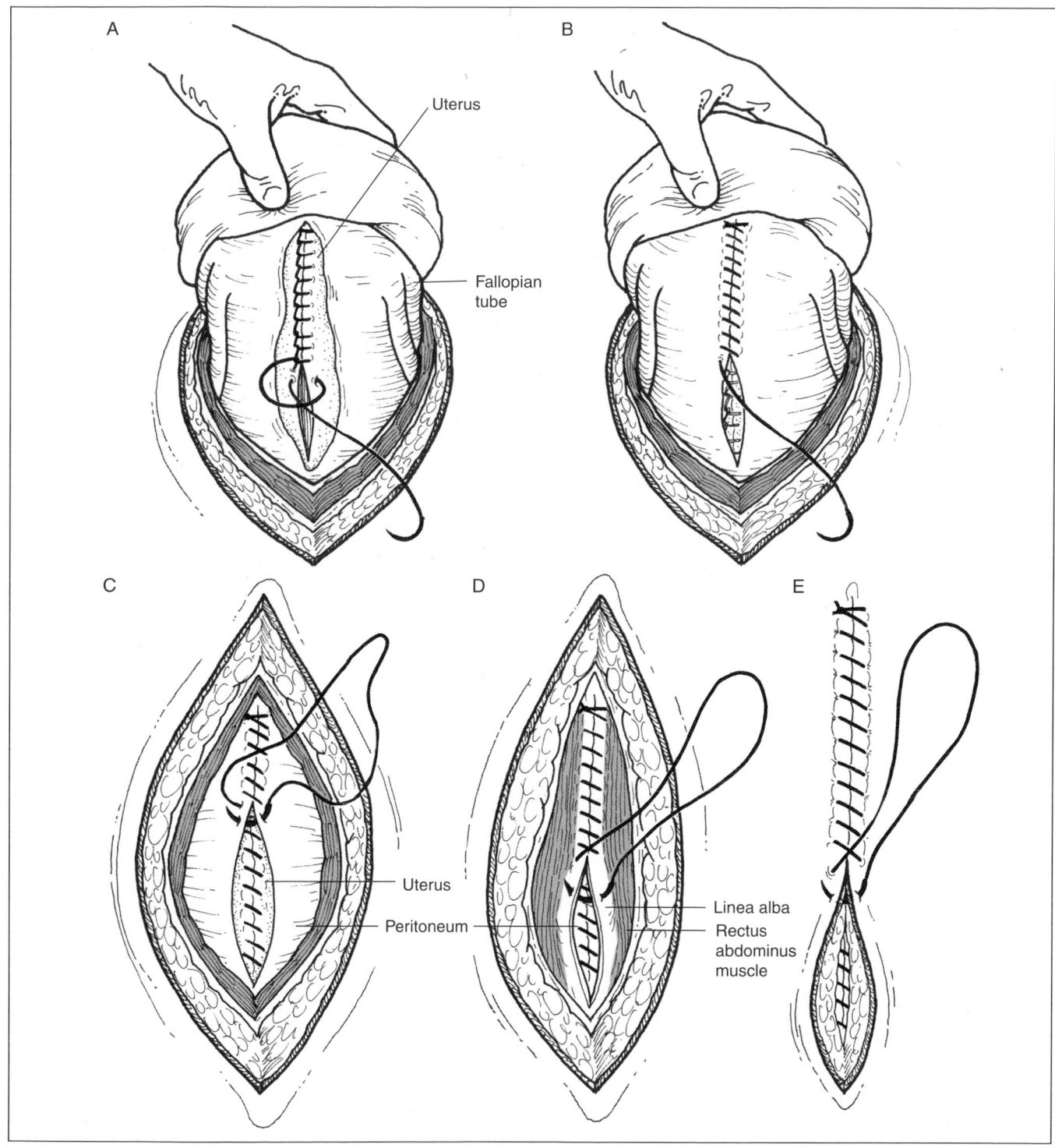

FIGURE 115-6 Closure of the incisions. *A.* Running locked closure of the uterine wall. *B.* Closure of the serosa of the uterus. *C.* Running closure of the peritoneal membrane. *D.* Running closure of the rectus sheath. *E.* Running closure of the skin.

are few. It should be performed within 5 minutes of maternal arrest as this gives the greatest potential for successful fetal, and possibly maternal, resuscitation.

REFERENCES

1. American College of Obstetricians and Gynecologists: *Educational Bulletin Number 251. Obstetric Aspects of Trauma Management.* Washington, DC: American College of Obstetricians and Gynecologists, 1998.

2. Cunningham FG, MacDonald PC, Gant NF, et al: *Williams Obstetrics,* 20th ed. Norwalk, CT: Appleton & Lange, 1997:604.

3. Cunningham FG, MacDonald PC, Gant NF, et al: *Williams Obstetrics,* 20th ed. Norwalk, CT: Appleton & Lange, 1997:1078–1079.

4. Gabbe SG, Niebyl JR, Simpson JL: *Obstetrics: Normal and Problem Pregnancies,* 3rd ed. New York: Churchill Livingstone, 1996:573–578.

5. Gabbe SG, Niebyl JR, Simpson JL: *Obstetrics: Normal and Problem Pregnancies,* 3rd ed. New York: Churchill Livingstone, 1996:585–586.

6. Clark SL, Cotton DB, Hankins GDV, et al (eds): *Critical Care Obstetrics,* 3rd ed. Boston: Blackwell Scientific, 1997.

7. Katz DL, Dotters DJ, Droegemueller W: Perimortem cesarean delivery. *Obstet Gynecol* 1986; 68(4):571–576.

8. Kuhlmann RS, Cruikshank DP: Maternal trauma during pregnancy. *Clin Obstet Gynecol* 1994; 37(2):274–293.

Chapter 116
SYMPHYSIOTOMY

Ikem Ajaelo

INTRODUCTION

Symphysiotomy is the artificial division and separation of the pubic symphysis in order to facilitate vaginal delivery. This is not to be confused with a pubiotomy, or the severance of the pubic bone a few centimeters lateral to the symphysis, for the same purpose. First performed in the seventeenth century, it is indicated in cases of cephalopelvic disproportion and may be a life-saving alternative to cesarean delivery.[1] The reported success rate of this procedure is about 80 percent when performed appropriately.[2]

The procedure itself is well described and can be accomplished under local anesthesia.[2] Early reports of urologic and orthopedic complications led to its decline and lack of acceptance in modern obstetrical practice despite initial successes.[3] Symphysiotomy is performed quite regularly and successfully in developing countries where medical conditions are not as favorable as in the United States.[4]

Indications for a symphysiotomy include breech delivery, cephalopelvic disproportion, and for the relief of shoulder dystocia.[1,5,6] Each of these conditions poses significant potential risks to mother and child, even under optimal conditions. Emergency Physicians should be familiar with the indications and technique of symphysiotomy as expeditious delivery is vital in these scenarios.

ANATOMY AND PATHOPHYSIOLOGY

The pelvis is composed of four bones: the sacrum, the coccyx, and the two innominate bones. Each innominate bone is made up of the fused ischium, ilium, and pubis. The innominate bones are connected at the sacrum by the sacroiliac ligaments and at the pubic symphysis by the superior and arcuate pubic ligaments.[7] Together they determine the size and shape of the pelvis. The fetus assumes positions during labor that are primarily determined by the conformation of the mother's pelvis.[8]

The pelvis is divided into a true pelvis and a false pelvis. They are separated by the linea terminalis, an anatomic boundary formed by the pelvic brim (superior pelvic aperture). The true pelvis lies below the linea terminalis and is the more relevant portion in delivery.[9] Dense ligaments hold the walls of the true pelvis together. The posterior wall is the anterior surface of the sacrum and coccyx. The lateral boundaries are formed by the inner surface of the ischial bones as well as the sacrosciatic notches and ligaments. The ischial spines can be readily palpated during the vaginal or rectal examination. They serve as important landmarks in determining to which level the presenting part has descended into the true pelvis. The true pelvis is bounded anteriorly by the pubic bones, the ascending superior rami of the ischial bones, and the obturator foramina.

The ligaments of the pubic symphysis and the sacroiliac ligaments allow mobility and contribute to the increase in pelvic diameter during pregnancy.[8] The sacral nerves, the coccygeal nerves, and the pelvic portion of the autonomic nervous system innervate the pelvis. The important pudendal nerve arises from the sacral plexus and accompanies the internal pudendal artery. It enters the perineal region via the lesser sciatic foramen and around the sacrospinous ligament to supply the muscles of the perineum.[7] Anesthesia to the perineal region can be accomplished by performing a pudendal nerve block.

INDICATIONS

Symphysiotomy is indicated in any difficult delivery in the presence of fetal distress, when labor is obstructed, and when an Obstetrician is not immediately available. It has traditionally been reserved for complicated breech deliveries or cases of cephalopelvic disproportion in which the fetal head is presenting vertex and at least one-third of the fetal head has entered the pelvic brim and cervical dilatation is no more than 7 centimeters.[1] Symphysiotomy has been advocated more recently for the relief of intractable shoulder dystocia.[5,6]

CONTRAINDICATIONS

There are no absolute contraindications to performing a symphysiotomy. Some authors have recommended limiting symphysiotomy to mothers weighing between 50 to 80 kg and a fetus with an estimated mass of 2700 to 3700 grams.[4,10] Other relative contraindications include the presence of maternal spinal deformities, hip deformities, pelvic deformities, and gross obesity.[10] Symphysiotomy has been performed after a prior cesarean section without added complications despite concerns regarding the safety of symphysiotomy in the presence of a previous cesarean scar.[10]

EQUIPMENT

Local anesthetic solution
Urethral catheter set
Sterile drapes
#10 scalpel blade on a handle
Mayo scissors
Finger guard
Hemostats
Sterile gloves
Neonatal resuscitation equipment
Infant warmer

PATIENT PREPARATION

Explain the risks, benefits, and potential complications to the patient and/or their representative. Obtain an informed consent to perform this procedure if time allows. Place the patient in the lithotomy position with the thighs separated no more than 90 degrees. This position is necessary to prevent undue strain on the sacroiliac joints. Two assistants should be available to assist in proper positioning. Insert a Foley catheter into the bladder. Prep and drape, as time permits, the skin and tissues overlying the pubic symphysis. Shaving is considered optional. Infiltrate the anterior and inferior aspects of the pubic symphysis and the surrounding skin with 5 to 10 mL of local anesthetic solution to anesthetize the pubic symphysis. Leaving the needle in place may be useful in identifying the pubic symphysis joint. Equipment for infant resuscitation should be readily available, as with all deliveries. Notify the pediatric resuscitation team and a Neonatologist of the impending procedure and delivery.

TECHNIQUE

Place the nondominant index finger into the vagina and against the posterior aspect of the pubic symphysis (Figure 116-1). Advance the finger approximately 2 to 3 cm beyond the superior aspect of the pubic symphysis to displace the bladder and urethra. **Do not move this finger until the procedure is complete.**

Grasp the scalpel in the dominant hand with the cutting edge of the blade facing the operator (Figure 116-2). The scalpel blade must be kept in a strict midsagittal plane and perpendicular to the skin overlying the pubic symphysis. Resting the hypothenar eminence of the dominant hand against the patient's pubic ramus will help maintain fine control of hand and finger movements.[2]

Make a midline stab incision 1 cm below the upper edge of the pubic symphysis (Figure 116-3). **Very little resistance should be met as the scalpel blade pierces the hyaline cartilage of the pubic symphysis if the scalpel is in the midline.** Carefully and slowly advance the scalpel blade until the tip is just felt through the anterior vaginal wall. Resistance is usually a result of lateral deviation of the scalpel blade against the pubic bones. Withdraw the scalpel blade 2 to 3 mm and readvance it in the midline. **Use extreme caution so that the scalpel does not lacerate the vagina, the urethra, or the finger.**

Lower the handle of the scalpel blade cephalad, towards the abdomen, using the upper portion of the pubic symphysis as a fulcrum. Cut through the lower half of the pubic symphysis, dividing the cartilage and associated ligaments. Remove the scalpel blade and reinsert it with the cutting edge in the opposite direction and facing the patient. Repeat the same maneuver but with the scalpel handle lowered caudally to divide the upper portion of the pubic symphysis, thereby completing the separation.

Use the nondominant index finger to confirm complete separation of the pubic symphysis. **The symphysiotomy is complete when the index finger pressing through the vaginal wall can fit into the space between the pubic symphysis.** Reinsert the scalpel to complete the division if any ligaments or cartilage remains. A variation of the above technique involves simply dividing the pubic symphysis in a single step by a repeated slow stabbing motion.

Once the symphysiotomy is completed, delivery of the infant should follow. Delivery of the infant usually requires more downward traction than is usually necessary.

AFTERCARE

Carefully return the mother to the supine position with the thighs in normal anatomic position. Close the skin and subcutaneous tissue with simple interrupted 4–0 nylon sutures. Some authors have recommended binding the knees for 12 to 48 hours to prevent inadvertent abduction or external rotation of the hips.[11] Admit the patient to the hospital for observation and monitoring of any potential complications. Leave the Foley catheter in place until any bleeding

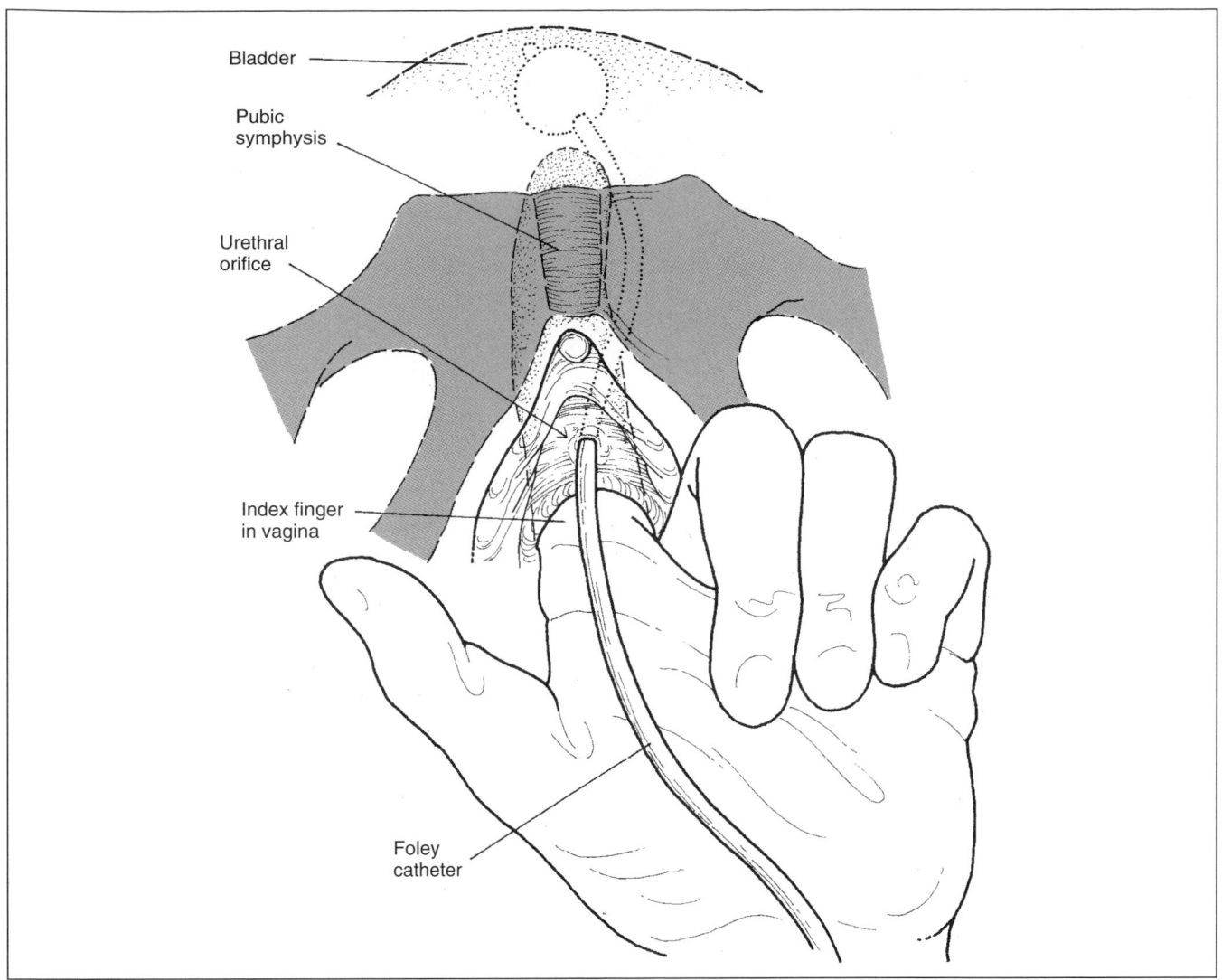

FIGURE 116-1 Frontal view demonstrating the operator's nondominant index finger inserted into the vagina and pushing anteriorly to palpate the pubic symphysis.

resolves or the patient begins to walk. Patients may begin ambulation with assistance between the second and fifth days. They should be warned against any unusual straining or heavy lifting.

COMPLICATIONS

Experience and careful case selection appear to be the most important factors in determining outcome and morbidity associated with this procedure.[2] Immediate complications include bladder lacerations, urethral lacerations, subcutaneous bleeding, and urinary incontinence.[10] Some patients develop gait instability immediately after the operation that tends to be transient and does not appear to affect subsequent pelvic stability.[12]

Lacerations to the operator's fingers are a significant concern.[11,14] Prevent lacerations by using the utmost of care and slowly transect the cartilage and ligaments of the pubic symphysis. The nondominant hand should be double-gloved at a minimum.[11] The use of a Kevlar glove that is resistant to scalpel injury may also be used.[14] A third option is to apply a malleable splint over the palmar aspect of the index finger before double gloving.[11]

Long-term complications include, but are not limited to, stress urinary incontinence, recurrent urinary tract infections, sepsis, and vesicovaginal fistulas.[13] Vaginal fistulas are frequently due to nonplacement of a Foley catheter during the procedure.[3] This important step should never be omitted. The effect of a symphysiotomy on subsequent pregnancies has not been studied in detail. However, the limited data available suggest that a symphysiotomy permanently enlarges the pelvis so that subsequent vaginal deliveries are in fact easier.[12]

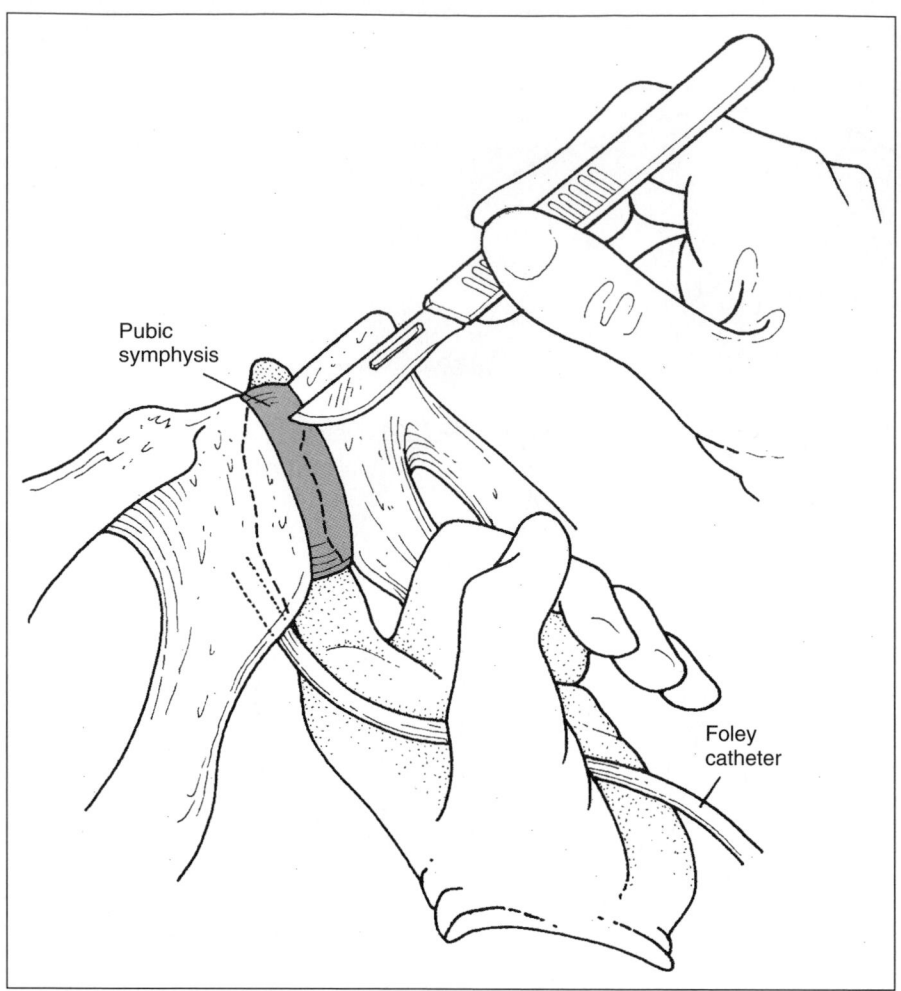

Pubic symphysis

Foley catheter

FIGURE 116-2 Skeletal outline demonstrating the position of the scalpel blade in relation to the pubic symphysis.

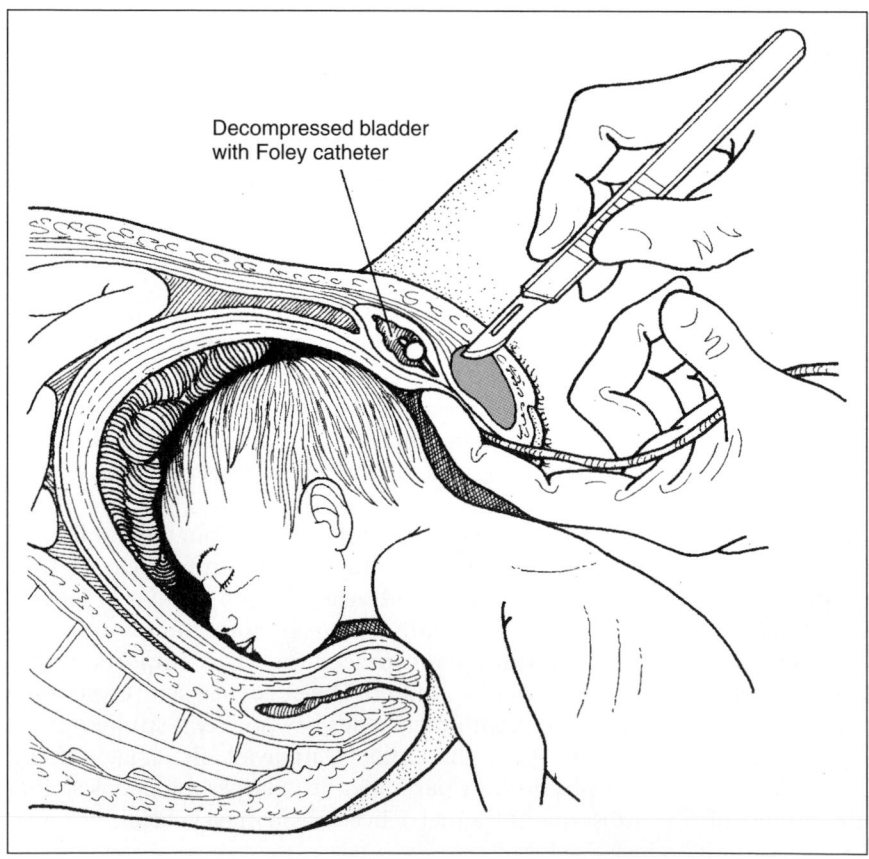

Decompressed bladder with Foley catheter

FIGURE 116-3 Sagittal view of a symphysiotomy using the scalpel blade to divide the pubic symphysis.

SUMMARY

Modern surgical techniques and advances have diminished the practice of symphysiotomy. It still remains a simple and safe method to overcome the common and lethal problems of cephalopelvic disproportion, shoulder dystocia, and breech deliveries. Complications are uncommon when performed correctly. Emergency Physicians can master this procedure.[11] A symphysiotomy is a viable and potentially lifesaving option for those who may be working outside the confines of a well-equipped hospital.

REFERENCES

1. Van Roosmalen J: Symphysiotomy as an alternative to cesarean section. *Int J Gynaecol Obstet* 1987; 25(6):451–458.
2. Menticoglou SM: Symphysiotomy for the trapped aftercoming parts of the breech: a review of the literature and a plea for its use. *Aust N Z J Obstet Gynaecol* 1990; 30(1):1–9.
3. Van Roosmalen J: Safe motherhood: cesarean section or symphysiotomy? *Am J Obstet Gynecol* 1990; 163(1 pt 1):1–4.
4. Norman RJ: Six years' experience of symphysiotomy in a teaching hospital. *S Afr Med J* 1978; 54(27):1121–1125.
5. Goodwin TM, Banks E, Millar LK, et al: Catastrophic shoulder dystocia and emergency symphysiotomy. *Am J Obstet Gynecol* 1997; 177(2):463–464.
6. Toppozada HK: Subcutaneous partial symphysiotomy. *Am J Obstet Gynecol* 1983; 46(3):344.
7. Moore KL: *Clinically Oriented Anatomy*, 3rd ed. Baltimore: Williams and Wilkins, 1992:243–249.
8. Sokol RJ, Brindley BA, Dumbrowski MP: Practical diagnosis and management of abnormal labor, in Scott RJ, DiSaia PJ, Hammond CB, et al (eds): *Danforth's Obstetrics and Gynecology*, 7th ed. Philadelphia: Lippincott, 1994:521–528.
9. Cunningham GF, MacDonald PC, Ganf NF, et al: *Williams' Obstetrics*, 20th ed. Norwalk, CT: Appleton & Lange, 1997:59–67.
10. Armon PJ, Philip M: Symphysiotomy and subsequent pregnancy in the Kilimanjaro region of Tanzania. *East Afr Med J* 1978; 55(7):306–313.
11. Pust RE, Hirschler RA, Lennox CE: Emergency symphysiotomy for the trapped head in breech delivery: indications, limitations and method. *Trop Doct* 1992; 22(2):71–75.
12. Kariuki HC: The place of symphysiotomy in the treatment of disproportion in Uganda. A study of 30 cases. *East Afr Med J* 1975; 52(12):686–693.
13. Hartfield VJ: Late effects of symphysiotomy. *Trop Doct* 1975; 5(2):76–78.
14. Wright JG, McGeer AJ, Chyatte D, et al: Mechanisms of glove tears and sharp injuries among surgical personnel. *JAMA* 1991; 266:1668–1671.

Chapter 117

BARTHOLIN GLAND ABSCESS OR CYST INCISION AND DRAINAGE

Krystaleah Lindsay

INTRODUCTION

Bartholin gland cysts and abscesses are common problems for women of reproductive age with an incidence of 2 percent in this population.[1,2] A Bartholin gland and its duct may enlarge to form a Bartholin cyst or become infected and form a Bartholin abscess. A number of different techniques have been developed for the treatment of both cysts and abscesses.

ANATOMY AND PATHOPHYSIOLOGY

The Bartholin glands were named after Caspar Bartholin, a Danish anatomist.[1,3] It refers to a pair of pea sized vulvovaginal mucous-secreting vestibular glands. They are located in the labia minora beneath the bulbospongiosus muscle, superficial to the deep perineal compartment, and in the 4 and 8 o'clock positions.[4,5] The glands are lined with mucous-secreting epithelium that provides moisture for the vulva but are not necessarily needed for sexual lubrication.[3,6] They drain by a 2.5 cm duct lined proximally with mucous-secreting epithelium and distally with transitional epithelium. The duct exits between the hymenal ring and the labia minora. The distal duct lining becomes squamous epithelium as it terminates.[2,5,7] The Bartholin glands are not normally palpable.

Obstruction of the duct by scar tissue, accumulation of secretions, metaplasia, trauma, or tumor leads to ductal dilation and cyst formation. Cysts may grow as large as 1 to 3 centimeters. Bartholin cysts present as painless unilateral swellings in the labial area. A patient will become symptomatic if they become large enough (some have been documented to be as large as 8 cm) or infected. Patients may complain of vulvar discomfort or pain with activity, sitting, and intercourse.[3,6,8–10] The infected Bartholin gland may be tender, red, hot, and cellulitic.

Carcinoma should be considered in the differential diagnosis of any labial mass. Adenocarcinoma (40 percent), squamous cell carcinoma (40 percent), adenoid cystic carcinoma (15 percent), and transitional cell carcinoma (5 percent) of the Bartholin gland have all been documented.[5,7,11–13] Carcinoma can easily mimic a Bartholin gland cyst or abscess.

The majority of Bartholin gland cysts appear to be sterile or contain bacteria common to the vaginal flora.[14] Studies of Bartholin gland abscesses have shown no bacterial growth in 7, 10, and 30 percent of specimens cultured.[14–16] The causative organisms are multiple in the cultures that do grow bacteria. Brook identified 67 different bacterial isolates from 26 different specimens.[15] The most prevalent organisms isolated were anaerobes, with *Bacteroides* and *Peptostreptococcus* being the most common species. The remainder of the cultures demonstrated either aerobic/facultative isolates with *Escherichia coli* being the most common species or a mixture of both aerobic and anaerobic organisms. *Neisseria gonorrhea* and *Chlamydia trachomatis* have also been implicated as causative agents and have been isolated in 8 to 16 percent of cultures.[14,17]

INDICATIONS

Small and asymptomatic cysts in women less than 40 years of age can be managed expectantly. All others should be treated. Any cyst that becomes large and symptomatic (i.e., painful, interfering with physical or sexual activity) should be treated. Any cyst that appears tender, red, hot, or cellulitic represents a Bartholin abscess and requires treatment.

CONTRAINDICATIONS

There is some controversy about the treatment of Bartholin cysts and abscesses in women over the age of

40. Carcinoma of the Bartholin gland is rare, comprising less than 1 percent of female genital tract neoplasm.[11] It is felt that women over the age of 40 are at an increased risk for having carcinoma of the Bartholin gland, Bartholin duct, or adjacent structures; and thus all of these should be properly biopsied or completely excised and sent to pathology.[1,5,6,7,11,12] Another study reported an incidence of Bartholin gland cancer in postmenopausal women of 0.114 per 100,000 women and suggests that selective biopsy be performed to reduce the number of total excisions.[13] In general, these women should be referral to a Gynecologist for diagnosis and further treatment.

Patients who have had multiple recurrences and previous treatments are best served with a referral to their Gynecologist for more definitive measures.

EQUIPMENT

Simple Incision and Drainage

Sterile prep solution and drapes
Lidocaine, 1 to 2%
3 mL syringe
18 gauge needle
25 gauge needle
2×2 gauze pads
4×4 gauze pads
#11 scalpel blade and scalpel handle
Culture medium for routine bacteria, gonorrhea, and chlamydia
Hemostat
Small wick, 2 inches long

Incision and Insertion of a Word Catheter

Equipment for simple incision and drainage
Word catheter
5 mL sterile saline or water

Marsupialization

Equipment for simple incision and drainage
2 small retractors
Specimen container for excised tissue
Silver nitrate sticks or electrocautery
Vicryl, 3–0 or 4–0 on cutting needle
Scissors
Small toothed forceps

Window Operation

Same as equipment for marsupialization

PATIENT PREPARATION

Explain the risks, benefits, and potential complications of the procedure to the patient and/or their representative. The post-procedural care should also be discussed. Obtain a signed consent for the procedure. Some physicians omit the signed consent and place in the procedure note a statement saying: "the risks, benefits, and complications were described and discussed with the patient. They understood this and gave verbal consent for the procedure."

Place the patient in the lithotomy position. Apply povidone iodine to the labia and allow it to dry. The surface of the labia must be anesthetized. This can be extremely painful. The use of ice packs, topical refrigerant spray (Chapter 105), parenteral sedation, parenteral analgesics, or procedural sedation (Chapter 109) should be considered for patient comfort prior to infiltrating local anesthetic solution. Infiltrate 0.25 to 1.0 mL of local anesthetic solution subcutaneously under the mucosal surface of the labia minora for simple incision and drainage, with or without the use of a Word Catheter. Infiltrate 2 to 3 mL of local anesthetic solution if a marsupialization or window operation will be performed.

TECHNIQUES

A number of different treatments and procedures have been developed to manage a Bartholin cyst or abscess. These are largely influenced by the size, symptoms, the age of the patient, suspected etiology, and previous treatment in the same patient. The techniques include simple incision and drainage, incision and insertion of a Word catheter, marsupialization, a window operation, and complete excision.

SIMPLE INCISION AND DRAINAGE

The standard treatment for most abscesses is simple incision and drainage.[6,8,9,18,19] Simple incision and drainage of a Bartholin cyst or abscess provides immediate pain relief but is often complicated by chronic recurrences. This technique is not recommended but described for the sake of completeness.

Spread open the labia to visualize the area (Figure 117-1). Make a 1 cm vertical incision on the mucosal surface of the labia minora and parallel to the posterior border of the hymenal ring (Figure 117-1). **The incision should ideally be within the hymenal ring, if possible.** Extend the incision into the abscess/cyst cavity. **Do not make incisions along the skin surface of the labia minora.** Skin incisions can lead to the formation of a fistula tract and are fraught with complications. Culture the contents of the sac. Manually express the contents of the sac. Insert a hemostat and break any adhesions. Place a

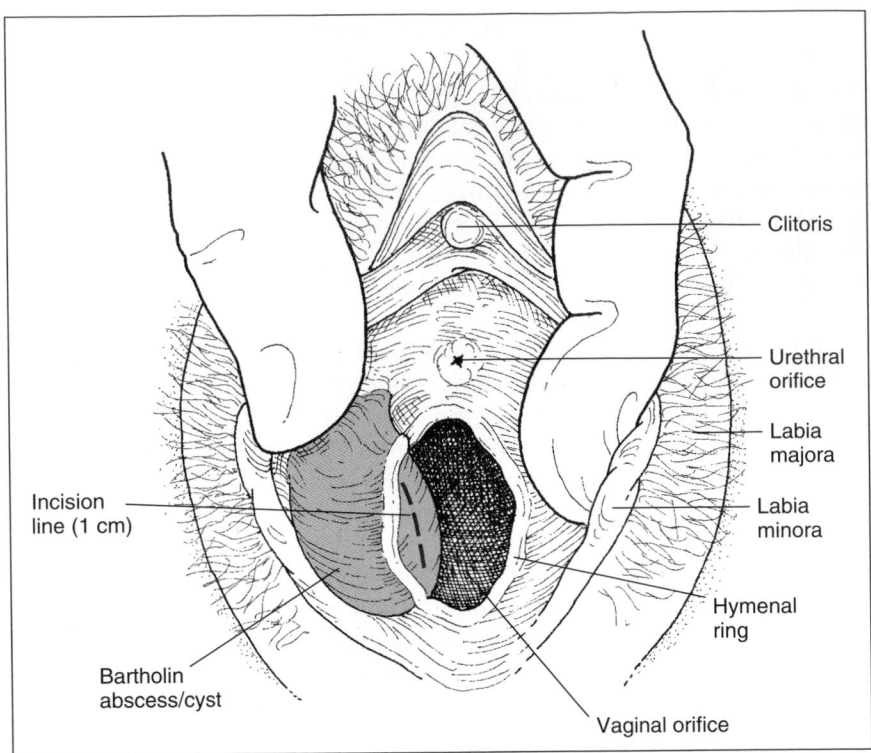

FIGURE 117-1 Simple incision and drainage of a Bartholin cyst or abscess. Spread open the labia to expose the area. The dotted line represents the incision over the cyst or abscess.

small wick within the cavity to allow for complete drainage and prevent premature closure of the skin incision.

INCISION AND INSERTION OF A WORD CATHETER

Dr. B. Word first described this procedure in 1964. It is a relatively simple procedure that can be accomplished in the Emergency Department.[3,6,8,9,20] The catheter is approximately 5 cm long and made of soft pliable latex with a 10 French tip. The tip contains a balloon that inflates up to a volume of 5 mL (Figure 117-2). These catheters cost approximately $17 each (Berkeley Medevices Inc., Berkeley, California).

Spread open the labia to completely visualize the area (Figure 117-3A). Make a 0.5 cm long puncture on the mucosal surface of the labia minora with a #11 scalpel blade into the cyst or abscess cavity (Figure 117-3A). **This puncture should ideally be located just inside the hymenal ring if possible.** Culture the contents of the sac. Manually express the contents of the sac. Insert a small hemostat and break any adhesions.

Insert the tip of the Word catheter deep within the cavity (Figure 117-3B). Inject 2 to 4 mL of sterile saline into the free end of the catheter to inflate the balloon (Figure 117-3C). **Pain upon inflation of the balloon or persistent pain after the procedure indicates overinflation of the balloon. Do not use air to inflate the balloon.** The catheter will stay in place because the in-

flated balloon is larger than the puncture incision. Tuck the free end of the catheter within the vaginal canal. The Word catheter should ideally stay in place for up to 4 weeks. This allows the tract to become epithelialized and prevent a recurrence. The patient should abstain from sexual activity while the catheter is in place.

MARSUPIALIZATION

Marsupialization is the treatment of choice.[1,6,8,9,19,21,22] It is performed once and is curative in 90 percent of cases.[21] Marsupialization can be easily and safely performed in the Emergency Department using local anesthesia. Some Obstetricians prefer to perform this procedure in the Operating Room under general anesthesia.

Make an oval-shaped or elliptical incision approximately 1.5 cm long and 1 cm wide through the vulvar mucosa over the cyst/abscess and just outside the hymenal ring (Figure 117-4A). Remove this piece of mucosa to visualize the anterior wall of the cyst/abscess cavity. Insert a retractor to pull the skin edges open and better visualize the sac (Figure 117-4B). Make a similar incision through the anterior wall of the cyst/abscess cavity (Figure 117-4B). Remove this piece of tissue leaving the cavity exposed. Culture the contents of the sac. Express the contents of the sac. Insert a small hemostat and break any adhesions. Control any bleeding with electrocautery, silver nitrate application, or manual pressure.

Evert the cyst/abscess wall. Approximate the wall of the cyst/abscess to the vestibular mucosa. Sew the wall

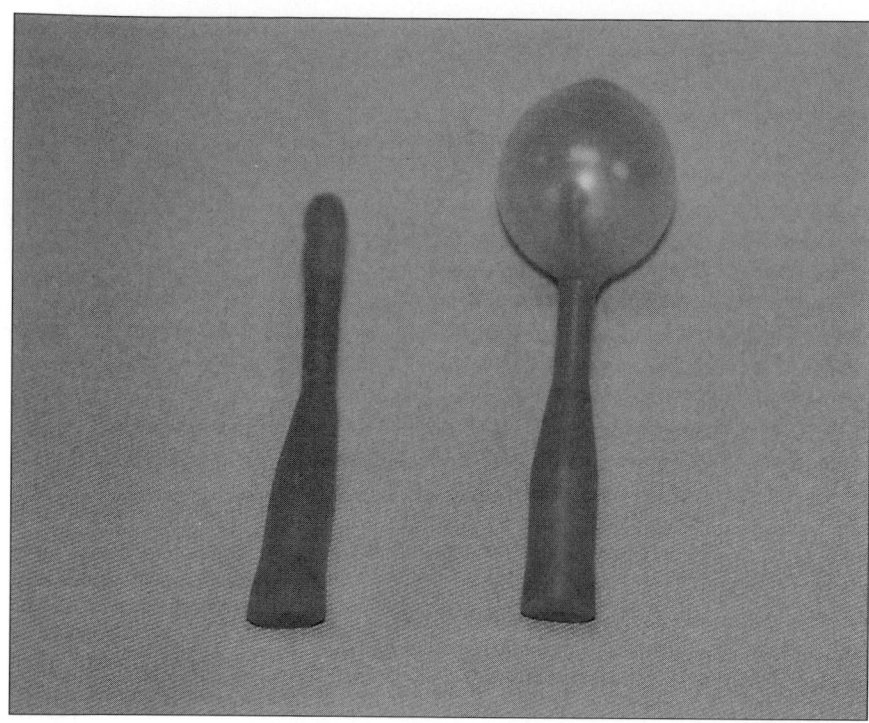

FIGURE 117-2 The Word catheter. The plastic catheter has a port at its proximal end to insert a needle. The distal end contains a balloon that can be inflated.

of the cavity to the mucosa of the labia minora with interrupted 3–0 or 4–0 Vicryl sutures (Figure 117-4C). The orifice will reduce in size, epithelialize, and form a new duct in time. **Send all excised tissue to the Pathology Department to confirm the diagnosis and to rule out neoplasm.**

WINDOW OPERATION

This technique is almost identical to marsupialization.[23] It differs only in the size of the incision. One study claimed this procedure had no long-term complications or recurrences, thus making it a more desirable technique.[23] However, the total patient population was small and the study has not been duplicated and republished. In essence, one follows the exact procedure for marsupialization with the exception of making a larger incision (2 to 3 cm long and 1.5 cm wide). At the completion of the procedure a wide opening is observed. The opening will be approximately one-half its original size at the 1 year follow-up. This much larger and radical incision is not recommended for the Emergency Physician.

COMPLETE EXCISION

This technique is reserved for the treatment of recurrent cysts and abscesses unresponsive to less invasive techniques or those associated with deep infections.[6–10,13,19,23] It is also indicated in patients for whom one suspects carcinoma. Some authors feel that all cysts and abscesses should be completely excised in women over the age of 40. Directly beneath the Bar-

tholin duct is the vestibular bulb that is composed of anastomosing venous channels. Significant bleeding may complicate dissection into this area. This procedure should only be performed by an Obstetrician/Gynecologist in the controlled setting of an Operating Room under general anesthesia.

AFTERCARE

All abscess and cyst contents should be cultured. Initiate the appropriate antibiotics to cover gram-positive, gram-negative, and anaerobic organisms. Cephalexin plus metronidazole may be an appropriate choice if a sexually transmitted disease is suspected. Cefixime plus metronidazole may be considered if gonorrhea is suspected. Azithromycin plus metronidazole may be considered if *Chlamydia* is suspected. The initiation of antibiotics can be delayed pending the culture results, at the discretion of the physician.

All patients should abstain from sexual activity until the inflammation and pain resolves or until the Word catheter is removed. Begin sitz baths in two days. Prescribe appropriate oral analgesics. Nonsteroidal anti-inflammatory drugs will provide most patients with adequate analgesia. Some patients may require a brief course (1 to 3 days) of narcotic analgesics. Give written discharge instructions to each patient explaining the aftercare, the complications, and the actions to take if a complication does arise.

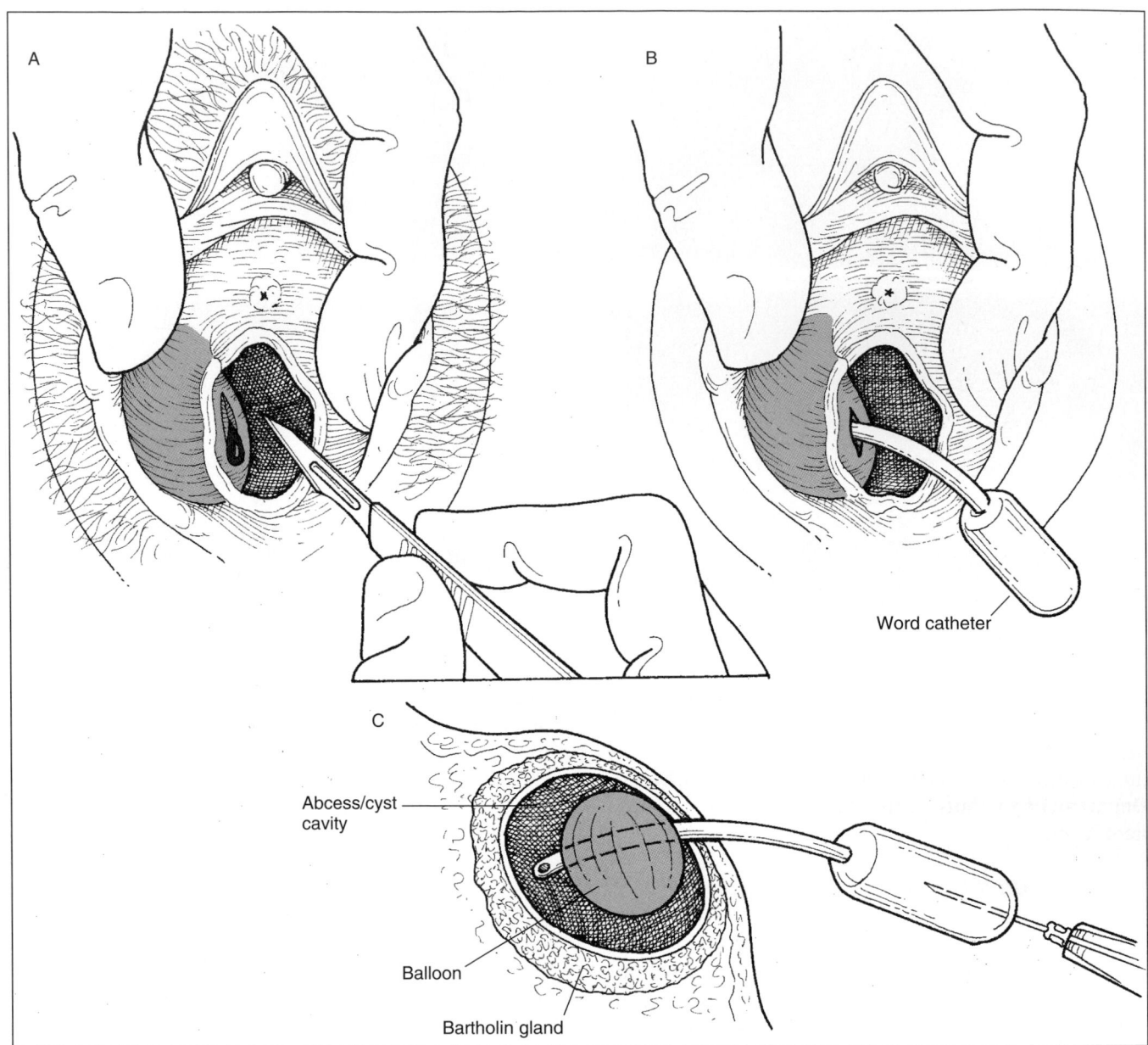

FIGURE 117-3 Incision and insertion of the Word catheter. *A.* Make a 0.5 cm long stab incision on the mucosal surface of the labia minora. *B.* The cavity has been evacuated and the Word catheter inserted. *C.* The balloon is inflated with saline.

COMPLICATIONS

The most common complication with the incision and drainage technique is frequent recurrence. The most common complication of Word catheter insertion is premature loss of the catheter resulting in early incision closure and recurrence. It can also be associated with significant discomfort if the catheter is inserted improperly. Marsupialization has few complications and a recurrence rate of approximately 10 percent. With any of these procedures, one can miss a carcinoma of the

Bartholin duct or Bartholin gland if a biopsy or excision is not performed. Bleeding and progressive infection, including septic shock and toxic shock, are rare but possible complications.[24,25]

The immunocompromised patient (e.g., diabetic, steroid dependent, or HIV positive) needs particular attention paid to sterility during the procedure and afterwards. Though rare, this population is more susceptible to deep-seated infections including necrotizing fascitis, *Clostridia perfringens* gas gangrene, and septic shock.[1] Daily follow-up visits are recommended for these pa-

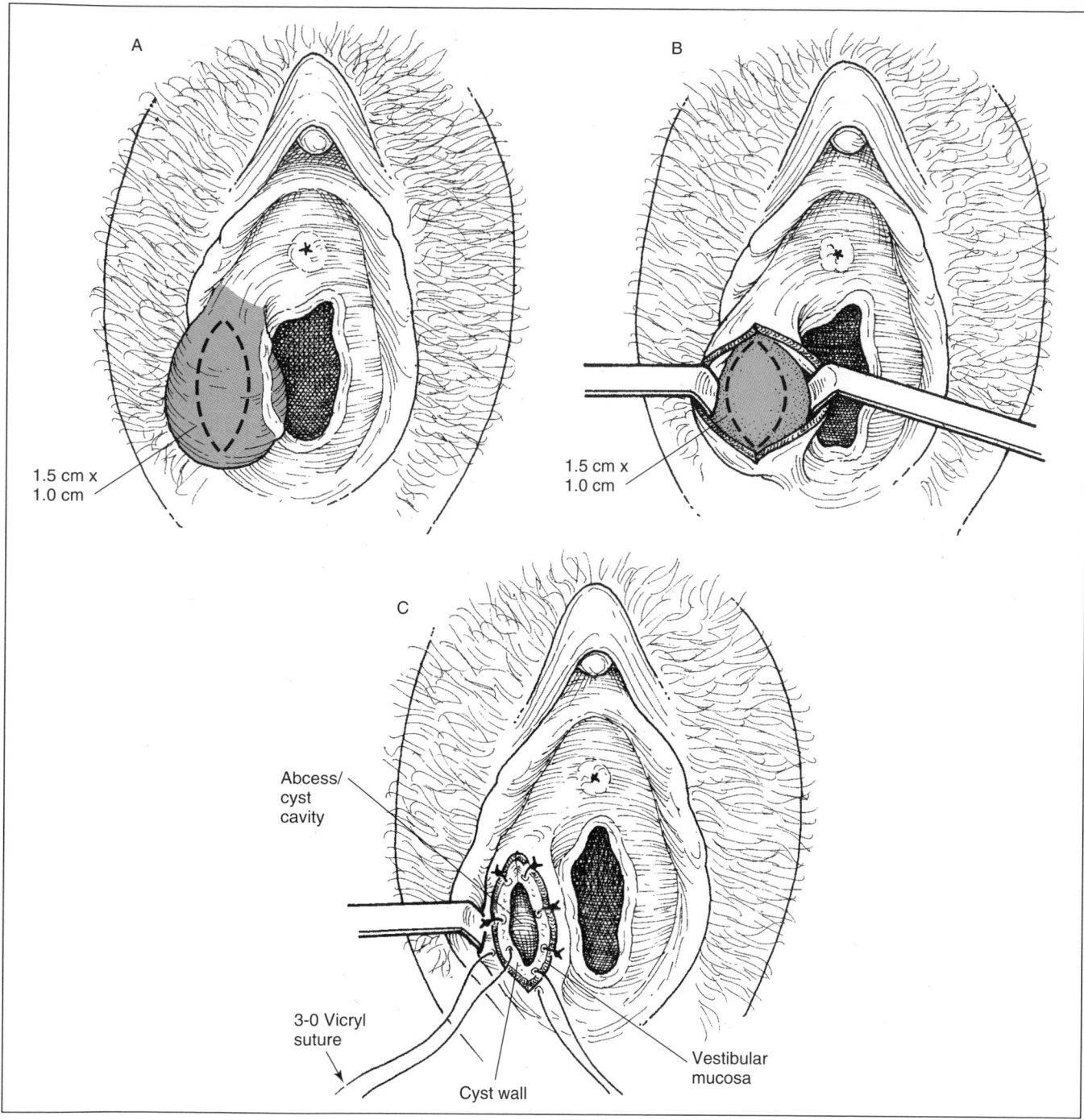

A

1.5 cm x
1.0 cm

B

1.5 cm x
1.0 cm

C

Abcess/
cyst
cavity

3-0 Vicryl
suture

Cyst wall

Vestibular
mucosa

FIGURE 117-4 The marsupialization of a Bartholin cyst or abscess. *A.* An elliptical incision, 1.5 cm in length and 1.0 cm in width, is made through the vulvar mucosa and just outside the hymenal ring. The ellipse of mucosal tissue is then removed. *B.* An elliptical incision (dotted line) is then made through the anterior wall of the cyst or abscess. *C.* Approximation of the cyst or abscess wall to the vestibular mucosa with 3–0 or 4–0 interrupted Vicryl suture.

tients during the initial post-procedural period. Early hospitalization and administration of intravenous antibiotics are warranted if there is any sign of progressive infection.

SUMMARY

Bartholin cysts and abscesses will be encountered by the Emergency Physician and can easily be treated. They present as a painful unilateral swelling of the inferior aspect of the labia. Marsupialization is the procedure of choice, though there are many treatments. Culture all cyst or abscess contents. Treat all abscesses with broad-spectrum antibiotics. Send any tissue removed to the Pathology Department to rule out carcinoma. Refer patients with previously treated cysts or abscesses, those suspicious for carcinoma, and those over the age of 40 to a Gynecologist or Obstetrician for definitive care. Give all patients written discharge instructions at the end of the procedure. All immunocompromised patients require very careful follow-up.

REFERENCES

1. Droegemueller W, Herbst AL, Mishell DR Jr, et al: *Comprehensive Gynecology,* 2nd ed. St. Louis: Mosby, 1992:569–571.

2. Azzan BB: Bartholin's cyst and abscess: a review of treatment of 53 cases. *Br J Clin Pract* 1978; 32: 101–102.

3. Word B: Office treatment of cyst and abscess of Bartholin's gland duct. *South Med J* 1968; 61(5): 514–518.

4. Agur AMR, Lee MJ: *Grant's Atlas of Anatomy,* 9th ed. Baltimore: Williams and Wilkins, 1991:192–196.

5. Wheelock JB, Goplerud DR, Dunn LJ, et al: Primary carcinoma of the Bartholin gland: a report of 10 cases. *Obstet Gynecol* 1984; 63(6):820–824.

6. Hill DA, Lense JJ: Office management of Bartholin gland cysts and abscesses. *Am Fam Physician* 1998; 57(7):1611–1616.

7. Wilkinson EJ: Benign diseases of the vulva, in Kurman RJ (ed): *Blaustein's Pathology of the Female Genital Tract,* 4th ed. New York: Springer-Verlag, 1994:32–34, 50, 63–64, 105, 108–109.

8. Rock JA, Thompson JD: *Te Linde's Operative Gynecology,* 4th ed. Philadelphia: Lippincott, 1997:890–892.

9. Heah J: Methods of treatment for cysts and abscesses of Bartholin's gland. *Br J Obstet Gynaecol* 1998; 95(4):321–322.

10. Scott JR, Di Saia PJ, Hammond CB, et al: *Danforth's Obstetrics and Gynecology,* 6th ed. Philadelphia: Lippincott, 1990:1–15.

11. Copeland LJ, Sneige N, Gershenson DM, et al: Bartholin gland carcinoma. *Obstet Gynecol* 1986; 67(6):794–801.

12. Chamlain DL, Taylor HB: Primary carcinoma of Bartholin's gland: a report of 24 patients. *J Obstet Gynecol* 1972; 39(4):489–494.

13. Visco AG, Del Priore G: Postmenopausal Bartholin gland enlargement: a hospital-based cancer risk assessment. *Obstet Gynecol* 1996; 87(2):786–790.

14. Lee YH, Rankin JS, Alpert S, et al: Microbiological investigation of Bartholin's gland abscesses and cysts. *Am J Obstet Gynecol* 1977; 129(2):150–153.

15. Brook I: Aerobic and anaerobic microbiology of Bartholin's abscess. *Surg Gynecol Obstet* 1989; 169:32–34.

16. Wren MWD: Bacteriological findings in cultures of clinical material from Bartholin's abscess. *J Clin Pathol* 1977; 30:1025–1027.

17. Bleker OP, Smalbraak DJC, Schutte MF: Bartholin's abscess: the role of *Chlamydia trachomatis. Genito-urinary Med* 1990; 66:24–25.

18. Cheetham DR: Bartholin's cyst: marsupialization or aspiration? *Am J Obstet Gynecol* 1985; 152:569–570.

19. Vlasis G: Treatment of Bartholin's cysts. *Am Fam Physician* 1971; 3(6):85–86.

20. Golberg JE: Simplified treatment for disease of Bartholin's gland. *Obstet Gynecol* 1970; 35(1):109–110.

21. Blakey DH, Dewhurst CJ, Tipton RH: The long-term results after marsupialization of Bartholin's cysts and abscesses. *J Obstet Gynaecol Br Cmwlth* 1966; 73:1006–1009.

22. Curtis JM: Marsupialization techniques for Bartholin's cyst. *Aust Fam Physician* 1993; 22:369.

23. Cho JY, Ahn MO, Cha KS: Window operation: an alternative treatment method for Bartholin gland cysts and abscesses. *Obstet Gynecol* 1990; 76:886–888.

24. Shearin RS, Boehlke J, Karanth S: Toxic shock-like syndrome associated with Bartholin's gland abscess: case report. *Am J Obstet Gynecol* 1989; 160(5 pt 1):1073–1074.

25. Lopez-Zeno JA, Ross E, O'Grady JP: Septic shock complicating drainage of a Bartholin gland abscess. *Obstet Gynecol* 1990; 76(5 pt 2):915–916.

Chapter 118
SEXUAL ASSAULT EXAMINATION

David L. Levine

INTRODUCTION

The specific legal definition of sexual assault varies from state to state. Generally, sexual assault is forced sexual contact without consent. Sexual assault occurs along a continuum from unwanted touching and fondling of sex organs to forced penetration (oral, anal, or vaginal). Fingers or objects (such as broomsticks, bottles, or knives) could be used instead of, or in addition to, a penis as a weapon of choice. Drugs such as gamma-hydroxybutyric acid (GHB), Rohypnol (flunitrazepam), or ketamine are known as date rape or club drugs. They can be used to disable the victim prior to a sexual assault. Alcohol has also been used as a date rape drug.

Recent studies show that 13 to 18 percent of women and 3 percent of men have experienced an attempted or completed sexual assault in their lifetime.[1] FBI and crime statistics grossly underestimate the incidence since only 16 percent of sexual assaults are reported to police.[1] Approximately 300,000 to 700,000 adult women are victims of sexual assault annually in the United States, with 40,000 victims treated in Emergency Departments.[1,2]

Sexual assault is not generally a crime among strangers. Most women (78 to 82 percent) are sexually assaulted by someone known to them.[1,3,4] The assailant may include a spouse, boyfriend, family member, co-worker, or neighbor. More than 50 percent of rape victims over the age of 30 are sexually assaulted by an intimate partner.[5] The offender may be someone the victim knows less well, such as a contractor or package delivery person.

There is not a typical profile of a victim, although adolescent girls and young women face particularly high rates of sexual assault.[6] Victims have been reported in all age groups. Sexual assault occurs across all socioeconomic groups, all racial backgrounds, and all ethnic backgrounds. Up to 39 percent of women will be raped more than once during their lifetime.[1]

Some victims will not identify themselves as victims of sexual assault. They may be ashamed or fearful to disclose what happened. They also may be experiencing the rape trauma syndrome, a special category of post-traumatic stress disorder. The use of screening questions, as used for domestic violence, and a high index of suspicion is necessary in identifying these patients. There is a significant increase in the utilization of medical resources after a sexual assault.[7]

The Emergency Department visit of a sexual assault victim plays a vital role in assuring proper medical care, evidence collection, and treatment. The proper follow-up plans and referrals to local rape crisis centers and/or hotlines are crucial to the mental and physical recovery of victims. The initial treatment in the Emergency Department will strongly influence whether the patient will get follow-up care and pursue the case through legal avenues. It is critical to not revictimize the patient and make them feel responsible for the sexual assault.

INDICATIONS

Perform a sexual assault examination, including evidence collection, on all patients who present within 1 week of a sexual assault. Evidence collection has the highest yield if collected within 72 hours after the sexual assault. Proceed with the examination if the victim is unsure of when the assault occurred. A history and physical examination with extra attention to the areas violated should still be performed to evaluate for injuries if the patient presents more than 1 week after the sexual assault. States vary in requirements for evidence collection. **Perform a complete history, as outlined in the technique sections, regardless of when the assault took place. Patients must consent to evidence collections (Figure 118-1).** Evidence collection should proceed if a patient is unable to consent due to a medical condition, with local statutes and hospital policy determining the release of evidence. Minors do not require parental consent for the initial evaluation of life-threatening injuries. Many states require parental permission for the release of evidence.

CONTRAINDICATIONS

Life-threatening injuries and unstable vital signs must be assessed prior to evidence collection. Five percent of sexual assault victims have major nongenital physical injuries.[8] Victims must be able to consent to the examination and evidence collection unless prohibited by a medical condition.

EQUIPMENT

Paper bags for clothing
Paper bag for undergarments
Clean white sheet and large paper sheet to place on floor when patient disrobes
4 sterile cotton-tipped swabs for oropharynx evidence collection
Pharyngeal culturettes for gonorrhea and chlamydia
4 sterile cotton-tipped swabs for vaginal/cervical/penile evidence collection
Culturettes for gonorrhea and chlamydia of the vagina/penis
Slides for vaginal wet mount for trichomonas
4 sterile cotton-tipped swabs for rectal evidence collection
Culturettes for gonorrhea and chlamydia of the rectum
Extra sterile cotton-tipped applicator swabs for miscellaneous stains and bite marks
Comb and a piece of clean white paper for loose pubic hairs
Comb and a piece of clean white paper for loose head hairs
2 sticks for fingernail scrapings
Filter paper for blood collection
Urine or blood collection equipment to test for pregnancy
Equipment for serum collection to test for hepatitis, syphilis, and HIV
Instant camera or forensic photographer
Colposcope, as applicable
Sterile water to moisten speculum and cotton-tipped swabs
Change of clothing for the patient
Separate envelopes to place evidence within for each body site
Tape to seal all evidence

Most states have prepackaged evidence collection kits with most of the necessary equipment included. These kits usually do not contain paper bags for the clothes, culturettes, blood drawing equipment (i.e., needles, Vacutainers), and blood collection tubes; all of which are readily available in any Emergency Department.

PATIENT PREPARATION

Address any life-threatening injuries and unstable vital signs before proceeding to the formal sexual assault examination. Up to 5 percent of rape victims have major nongenital physical injuries.[8] Place a large white sheet on the ground and cover it with a large piece of white paper. Instruct the patient to undress over the large white sheet of paper, if possible. **To best preserve evidence, try not to rip or cut any clothes. Life-threatening interventions always supersede evidence collection, but note on the patient's record if any clothing is cut or torn by medical personnel.**

Conduct the examination in a quiet, private room. It should ideally have the facilities to perform a pelvic examination so that the patient does not have to be moved multiple times. Assign a designated nurse and physician who are trained in the sexual assault protocol and aware of the multiple emotional manifestations that the patient may experience. **Safety and privacy must be ensured.** Notify a community- or hospital-based advocate upon the patient's arrival to the Emergency Department. Advocates can best define their own role. Allow the patient to decide if the advocate should stay for the examination and evidence collection. The number of providers should be kept to a minimum. Contact police per local laws and patient request. Alert hospital security to the possibility that the assailant may come to the hospital.

The patient must give written consent prior to the examination (Figure 118-1). **It is important to let the victim guide the process as much as possible to help them restore control of their life.** Obtaining consent has important legal and psychological implications for the patient. **The sexual assault victim has the right to refuse the sexual assault examination, any medical treatment, and any interviews by advocates or social workers.** Note in the medical record any and all portions of the sexual assault examination and treatment that the patient refuses. **Encourage the patient to have the examination, without the use of the sexual assault kit, so that you can provide proper medical treatment. Encourage the patient to allow the collection of evidence with the sexual assault kit in the event that they later change their mind and decide to prosecute the assailant.**

Discourage the patient from eating, drinking, changing clothes, urinating, or defecating prior to the examination. This is to best preserve evidence, especially if the patient is seen in close time proximity to the sexual assault. Perform examinations specific to the affected area earlier to accommodate the patient if they need to drink or void.

EXAMINATION OF FEMALE PATIENTS

Exact details of the examination will vary depending upon state and local evidence collection requirements. Some states have provisions for special Sexual Assault Nurse Examiners (SANEs) who are specially trained to perform the complete sexual assault examination and testify if the case is prosecuted. The order of the examination may also vary depending upon the patient's needs. The Emergency Department is often the first official system to which the victim reports an assault. **Patients may be reluctant to share their story with personnel in the criminal justice system if they are met with judgmental attitudes or insensitive treatment by emergency medical staff.**[9]

Collect a urine sample early if there is any possibility of the use of a date rape or club drug. The decision to process the urine can be determined later. The window to detect these drugs, such as gamma-hydroxybutyric acid (GHB) or Rohypnol (flunitrazepam), can be as little as 8 hours after ingestion. Most toxicology screens will detect prescription drugs and recreational drugs that the patient may have taken. Some patients may decide not to have their urine tested, as it will pick up other substances they have used.

HISTORY

Proceed with the history and physical examination once the patient is in a private room, has consented to the examination, and an advocate is made available. Obtain a complete history to guide the medical examination and help with possible legal matters (Figure 118-2). **Avoid judgmental questions that may feed into the victim's feeling of self-blame.** Aspects of the history should include the time and place of the assault, the race and number of assailants, and a brief description of the assault including whether there was oral penetration, vaginal penetration, rectal penetration, and/or ejaculation. Elicit any use of force, restraints, foreign bodies, or lubricants. Ask the patient what they have done since the assault, especially things such as changing clothes, douching, bathing, urinating, defecating, or using a tampon as this may change the ability to collect forensic evidence.

The past medical history should emphasize the gynecological history and include last menstrual period, birth control, last consensual intercourse, previous sexually transmitted diseases, previous pregnancies, and previous gynecological surgeries. The time of the last voluntary intercourse is important, as mobile sperm may be found up to 72 hours in the cervix. Address the tetanus immune status. Determine if date rape drugs might have been given, especially if there seems to be a lapse of time.

PHYSICAL EXAMINATION

The physical examination serves to detect injuries and document for future legal prosecution. A complete physical examination must be performed, even if the patient does not want to pursue legal matters. Although up to 70 percent of rape victims reported no physical injuries, 4 to 5 percent sustained serious physical injury and 24 percent sustained minor physical injuries.[1,10] **It is important to help patients guide the examination and allow them to stop at points if they are not ready to proceed. Many patients will need encouragement through the examination.**

Note the patient's general appearance, affect, and emotional status. Instruct the patient to disrobe over a clean paper and sheet if they are wearing the same clothes they wore prior to the assault. Place all clothes in paper bags, with underwear in a separate paper bag. Fold the paper sheet, containing any debris, and place it in a collection envelope. Examine the entire body for abrasions, lacerations, bites, scratches, foreign bodies, and areas of ecchymoses. **Closely examine every laceration to ensure it is not a stab wound.** It is helpful to use a body diagram to document injuries (Figure 118-3). Commonly injured areas besides the vagina include the mouth, throat, wrist, breasts, and thighs.[9] Oral cavity injuries are common and include a torn frenulum and broken teeth. Bite marks on the genitalia and breast are common.[11] Use a Wood's lamp to examine the skin for fluorescent stains that may represent semen. Use an instant camera or a hospital photographer to document any bites, lacerations, scratches, abrasions, or any other injuries. **Photographs are much more informative than body diagrams.**

Collection of forensic evidence usually precedes the gynecological examination unless the patient is bleeding, has severe lower abdominal pain, or has pelvic pain. Most states have set evidence collection kits and the elements required will vary. Evidence is usually helpful up to 5 days after an assault. It is recommended to collect evidence up to a week after an assault as patients may not recall the dates exactly. Most sexual assault kits require fingernail scraping, head hair combing, saliva specimens, and blood type screening. Swab any stain on the patient's body that fluoresces under the Wood's light. Swab all orifices (oral, vaginal, anal), even if not penetrated, as recollection of events may change and a negative examination in a nonpenetrated area helps to validate the patient's story. **Use only sterile water and normal saline to moisten a swab.** Obtain samples of the patient's saliva by having them bite on filter paper in the kit. Obtain a sample of the patient's blood. Place 5 or 6 drops of blood on a piece of filter paper. Use a wooden stick to scrape under all the patient's fingernails. Collect the scrapings over a piece of white paper. **Allow all specimens to air-dry before placing them in envelopes.**

Collect hair samples from the victim. Pluck two or three hairs from the scalp hair and place it in a labeled envelope. Comb the patient's pubic hair over a white piece of paper. Place the comb, paper, and any hair or debris in a labeled envelope. Pluck two or three hairs from the pubic region and place them in a labeled envelope. The process of plucking hairs is painful and somewhat insensitive to the patient. Ask the patient to pluck the hairs for the evidence collection. These can also be obtained later if the case is prosecuted, as the patient's hair samples will not change. **Cutting off pieces of hair is of no value as the roots of the hairs are required for the forensic evidence process.**

Inspect the mouth and perioral structures for any signs of trauma. Carefully inspect the frenulum of the lower lip and tongue for bruising or tears. Examine the tonsils, the tonsillar pillars, and the oropharynx for bruising or lacerations. Swab the oral cavity thoroughly and allow the swabs to air-dry. These will later be tested for sperm acid phosphate and the victim's blood group antigens. Obtain additional swabs for gonorrhea and chlamydia testing in the hospital laboratory. Prepare a wet mount to look for motile spermatozoa.

Thoroughly examine the anorectal area for signs of trauma. This includes abrasions, ecchymoses, and lacerations. Swab the rectum and anal canal. Send one swab to the hospital laboratory for gonorrhea and chlamydia testing. Place the remainder of the swabs in envelopes for later sperm and acid phosphatase testing.

The gynecological examination is usually the most traumatic aspect of the examination for the patient. It may remind them of the assault. **Explain all procedures in simple terms prior to beginning. Allow the patient to help guide the examination.** Do all forensic evidence collection, including combing for pubic hairs and vaginal swabs, at the same time as the gynecological examination. Close attention to the external genitalia is important, as many patients are asymptomatic (Figure 118-4). Eight percent of patients have vulvar trauma.[12] **Only use sterile water to lubricate the speculum. Lubricants interfere with forensic evidence collection.** Examination of the hymen is important, as it is one of the most common areas of injury. A person's previous sexual history helps predict the location of lacerations of the vaginal wall. Lacerations are seen near the introitus in less sexually experienced patients and higher in more sexually experienced patients.

Collect baseline gonorrhea and chlamydia swabs at the time of the pelvic examination from pooled vaginal secretions and the endocervical canal. Obtain additional swabs to test for sperm acid phosphatase and blood group antigens. Colposcopy is used to detect and document more subtle injuries of the cervix and vagina. One study showed that colposcopy increased detection of genital trauma from 6 to 53 percent of victims.[13]

Toluidine blue can be used to identify small lacerations and abrasions that result from traumatic intercourse. It can increase the chances for detection of lacerations in sexual assault victims. Apply the dye with a cotton-tipped applicator to the external genitalia and wipe off the excess. Document and photograph any areas of uptake to toluidine blue. Toluidine blue should be used prior to the speculum examination, as the speculum can result in small lacerations that uptake the dye. Unfortunately, the dye acts as a spermicidal agent and can interfere with wet mount examinations.

EXAMINATION OF MALE PATIENTS

Males should have a complete urogenital examination looking for abrasions, lesions, and bites (Figure 118-4). The same disrobing specimens, and precautions should be observed in male sexual assault victims. Obtain oral, rectal, and urethral swabs for gonorrhea and chlamydia.

EXAMINATION OF CHILDREN

The procedure for a child is similar to that of an adult. Children are often referred to pediatric hospitals or specially trained physicians to perform the sexual assault examination. **Defer the sexual assault examination of a child to a specialist if you do not have experience in this area. The anatomy and examination of a child is different from that of an adult.** Restraining an uncooperative or combative child can result in significant psychological trauma. These children may require an examination under procedural sedation or general anesthesia.

LABORATORY INVESTIGATIONS

Draw blood for tests run at the hospital laboratory including syphilis serology, hepatitis B and C screening, HIV status, and pregnancy status. These are baseline tests and will be repeated in later follow-up testing. Process the gonorrhea and chlamydia probes at the hospital laboratory. Toxicology screens should only be performed at the hospital laboratory if there is a medically necessary reason for the test, such as altered mental status. Individual states have protocols for urine testing, which is done at a crime lab to detect date rape drugs.

CHAIN OF EVIDENCE

The work does not stop after the evidence is collected. All evidence must be properly tagged and secured. Seal all paper bags and evidence with evidence tape. Place your signature across the sealed ends of each bag or envelope and the evidence tape. This will make it easier to determine if they have been opened and tampered with. Clearly label each bag or envelope with the patient's name and hospital identification number, the date of collection, the time of collection, the source of the sample, and the printed and signed name of the nurse or assistant. Secure all the evidence in a locked room or cabinet until it can be turned over to a law enforcement officer. Have the officer sign a form stating the officer's name and badge number, the date and time the evidence was transferred, and the name of the physician or nurse releasing the evidence to the officer (Figure 118-1). Both individuals must sign this form.

AFTERCARE

Referral to a Social Worker or Psychiatrist may be necessary, especially if a patient advocate is not available. Treat any injuries in the standard manner. Be sure to check and update the tetanus status as necessary. Make a written summary of the physical examination findings for the medical record (Figure 118-5). Place any photographs taken in the medical record.

Provide all follow-up instructions in writing (Figure 118-6). Arrange a medical follow-up with a primary care physician in 1 to 2 weeks and again in 2 to 4 months. The follow-up appointment should include an examination for sexually transmitted diseases, HIV testing, and hepatitis immunizations. Give all patients a 24 hour crisis phone number as well as a follow-up in 1 to 2 days with the local rape crisis center, if the community has one. Arrange, with the help of the advocate or Social Worker, a safe place for the patient to stay. This is especially important if the offender is not in custody. Encourage the patient not to stay by themselves. A patient may need to be hospitalized in rare instances for psychiatric issues from the assault or for the patient's safety.

PREGNANCY PROPHYLAXIS

The risk of pregnancy after a sexual assault is estimated to be 2 to 5 percent if the patient is of reproductive age. Offer the patient pregnancy prophylaxis after baseline pregnancy testing is negative. Hormonal therapy within 72 hours of the sexual assault with 100 mcg of ethinyl estradiol immediately and repeated in 12 hours is 74 to 84 percent effective.[14,15] Common preparations include Ovral or Ortho-Novum 1/35. It is best to provide

the patient with the initial dose in the Emergency Department. Promptly refer the patient to a center where she can receive the medication if the hospital has a policy against providing pregnancy prophylaxis. **It must be emphasized that the effectiveness of pregnancy prophylaxis decreases over time. It is not indicated if over 72 hours has passed from the time of the sexual assault.** An intrauterine device (IUD) may be placed if the time of the sexual assault was between 72 hours and 1 week ago. Administer antibiotics prior to IUD placement to decrease the risk of ascending infections.

ANTIMICROBIAL PROPHYLAXIS

Postexposure prophylaxis for sexually transmitted diseases is recommended. The risk of acquiring a sexually transmitted disease is relatively high and the side effects from the medications is relatively low. Risks for acquiring trichomonas is approximately 12 percent, bacterial vaginosis 12 percent, gonorrhea 4 to 12 percent, chlamydia 2 to 14 percent, and syphilis 5 percent.[16–18] The current recommendation is to provide prophylaxis for gonorrhea and chlamydia. The current CDC recommendation is intramuscular ceftriaxone (125 mg) plus oral azithromycin (1000 mg, single dose) or doxycycline (100 mg) twice a day for 10 days.[14] A single dose of oral cefixime (400 mg) may be provided in place of ceftriaxone. Some centers administer 1000 mg of azithromycin to cover for gonorrhea and chlamydia, and increase the dose to 2000 mg if there is fear of resistant strains of gonorrhea.[18] The current guidelines do not recommend prophylaxis for syphilis. The treatment for bacterial vaginosis and trichomonas is a single 2000 mg dose of oral metronidazole. Trichomonas prophylaxis is controversial as ascending infections are rare. The side effects include significant nausea that may interfere or complicate pregnancy prophylaxis.

Administer hepatitis B prophylaxis for high-risk, nonvaccinated patients. High risk is defined as unprotected penetration, contact with the assailant's blood, or contact with the assailant's body fluid. Provide the first dose of the hepatitis B vaccine in the Emergency Department. Boosters are recommended at 1 to 2 months and 4 to 6 months. Immune globulin is not recommended.

There are no solid recommendations for HIV prophylaxis. The risk of HIV transmission from a single sexual assault is estimated at less than 1 percent. The CDC has made no formal recommendations for HIV prophylaxis, although centers are providing prophylaxis to candidates willing to take a full course of medications and who will comply with follow-up testing. Current recommendation is zidovudine (200 mg) three times a day and lamivudine (150 mg) twice a day for 4 weeks.[17] There are significant side effects with this regimen and the patient must be monitored closely.

PLEASE SEE INSIDE BOX COVER

STEP 1

Please print, type or use a patient information stamp.

(patient stamp)

Illinois State Police
Division of Forensic Services

PATIENT CONSENT/AUTHORIZATION TO RELEASE EVIDENCE TO LAW ENFORCEMENT AGENCY

Patient _____

DOB_____ Hospital Patient No. _____

CONSENT

I understand that in addition to consent for medical evaluation and treatment given to the hospital and physician, I also give consent to a medical examination for evidence of sexual assault. I understand that the evidence collected in the State Police Evidence Collection Kit will be sent to the Illinois State Police Forensic Sciences Command for the sole purpose of analysis to determine sexual activity relating to the investigation of sexual assault. I understand that this exam may include reference samples. I also understand that I may withdraw consent at any time for any portion of the exam.

_____
Patient, Parent, Guardian (please circle)

I understand that collection of evidence may include photographing injuries and that these photographs may include the genital area. Knowing this I consent to having photographs taken.

_____
Patient, Parent, Guardian (please circle)

RELEASE

I hereby authorize _____ to release to _____
     (Name of hospital)   (City)   (Law enforcement agency name)

the following information covering treatment given to me on _____.
                  (Month)   (Day)   (Year)

	AUTHORIZED FOR RELEASE	NOT AUTHORIZED FOR RELEASE
	(check those which apply)	
1. Copies of Forensic Laboratory Report Form	☐	☐
2. State Police Evidence Collection Kit	☐	☐
3. Photographs	☐	☐
4. X-rays or copies of x-rays taken in connection with exam	☐	☐
5. Clothing	☐	☐

Authorized for release (list clothing or miscellaneous items)
Article   Description

_____   _____

_____   _____

_____   _____

Signature of person authorizing release of information _____
                     Patient, Parent, Guardian (please circle)

RECEIPT OF INFORMATION

STEP 13

I certify that I have received the following items (check those which apply):

☐ One sealed evidence collection kit   ☐ X-rays   ☐ Photographs   ☐ Swabs/specimens (if no evidence collection kit is used)

☐ Sealed paper clothing bag(s) (if more than one sealed clothing bag, please note)   ☐ Other _____

Signature of person receiving information and/or articles_____ Date_____ Time _____

Officer ID# and rank_____ Representative of _____

Name of hospital representative who is releasing articles _____
                   (Printed name)   (Signature)   ILSP501

(White copy to hospital; yellow copy to law enforcement agency)

FIGURE 118-1 Sample form for patient consent and release of information to a law enforcement agency. It includes the receipt of information form to be signed by the law enforcement officer when the evidence is transferred to their care. Courtesy of Illinois State Police.

STEP 2

FORENSIC LABORATORY REPORT
(4 PAGES)

Illinois State Police
Division of Forensic Services

Please print, type or use a patient information stamp.

(patient stamp)

Patient Name		DOB	Age	
Race	Sex	Arrival Date		Arrival Time
Address		City		
County	State	Zip		Phone
Hospital			ER#	
For Children: Name of Guardian			Relationship	
Person providing history		Relationship to patient		

For children: Avoid multiple interviews. Take time to establish rapport. Avoid leading or yes/no questions. Use direct quotes. Avoid surprise or negative emotions, while still showing concern and support.

1. Chief complaint of person providing history to include physical injuries and methods employed by perpetrator, i.e., weapons, restraint, biting, threats.

2. Chief complaint in child's words to include physical injuries and methods employed by perpetrator, i.e., weapons, restraint, biting, threats.

3. Date of Assault	Time of Assault	4. Location & geographical surroundings of assault

5. Name(s), number, & race of assailant(s) if known.

6. Sexual acts described by patient/historian

Acts Described	Yes	No	Attempted	Unsure	Acts Described	Yes	No	Attempted	Unsure
Penetration of vagina by:					Masturbation:				
penis					of victim by assailant				
finger					of assailant by victim				
foreign object					Did ejaculation occur?				
describe object					inside body orifice				
Penetration of rectum by:					outside body orifice				
penis					If outside body orifice, describe location				
finger					Other sexual acts?				
foreign object					If yes, describe				
describe object					Did assailant use condom?				
Oral copulation of genitals:					Did you bite your assailant?				
of victim by assailant					Were you bitten by your assailant?				
of assailant by victim					Victim was licked/sucked?				

7. Post-assault hygiene/activity   Yes   No
   urinated   ☐   ☐
   defecated   ☐   ☐
   genital wipe/wash   ☐   ☐
   bath/shower   ☐   ☐
   douche   ☐   ☐
   tampon, sponge, diaphragm   ☐   ☐
     removed/inserted (circle)
   oral hygiene/intake/vomit   ☐   ☐
   changed clothes   ☐   ☐

If yes, where_____

Victim licked/sucked assailant?				

If yes, where_____

8. Pertinent medical history
   a. Date of LMP
   b. Sexual activity within 72 hrs. of assault?
      Yes   No
   c. Contraceptive used at time of assault?
   d. Communicable diseases of risk to lab personnel
      (e.g., hepatitis, TB, HIV, lice, etc.)

ILSP502A

(White copy to hospital; yellow copy in kit)

FIGURE 118-2 Sample history form. Courtesy of Illinois State Police.

FORENSIC LABORATORY REPORT — PAGE 2

Please print, type or use a patient information stamp.

(patient stamp)

COMPLETE EVIDENCE COLLECTION STEPS 3, 4, AND 5

GENERAL EXAM

> After STEP 5, obtain appropriate medical specimens from the mouth for clinical lab testing. Patient may rinse out his/her mouth after specimens are obtained. (DO NOT INCLUDE MEDICAL SPECIMENS IN KIT.)

Trauma should be recorded on the diagrams below which may be used in a criminal proceeding. These include: lacerations, scratches, bruises (detail size, shape, color), erythema, bites, patterned injury, burns, fractures and stains/foreign materials on body, swelling, tenderness. Be sure to note even the most minor signs of trauma. In children: include anogenital or behavioral symptoms. Note general appearance.

Note abnormalities in diagram and/or text.

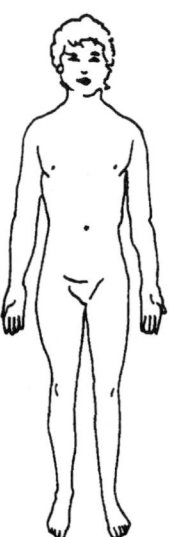 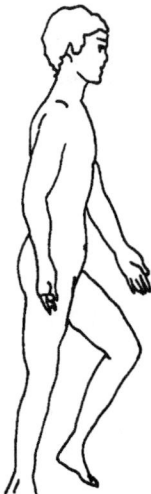 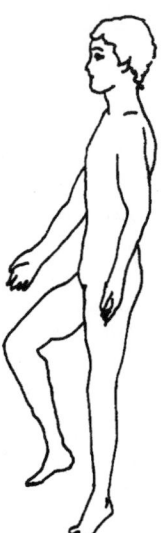 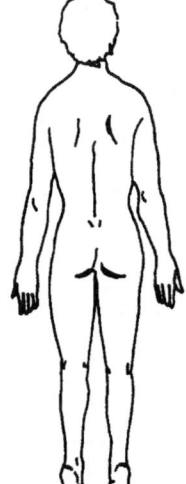 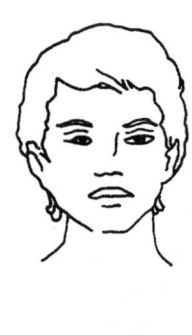

TEXT

GENITAL EXAM

- For children: Take time to establish rapport and proceed slowly. Extent of examination, including physical as well as specimens, must be decided on a case-by-case basis by the attending physician. If the examination would be too physically or emotionally traumatic for the child, then specimens may need to be obtained by gently using a moist swab on the external vaginal and rectal areas, especially with small hymenal openings.

- Note all discharge, stains, and foreign materials. Note any bleeding.

- Draw shape of hymen and anus in diagrams.

- Use sterile, non-bacteriostatic water or saline for lubrication of speculum.

- Record all acute trauma (lacerations, scratches, bruises [detail size, shape and color], erythema, bites, patterned injury, burns, swelling, tenderness) and chronic trauma (scarring, notching, pigmentation changes) on below diagrams.

(White copy to hospital; yellow copy in kit)

ILSP502B

FIGURE 118-3 Sample general physical examination form with body diagrams. Courtesy of Illinois State Police.

FORENSIC LABORATORY REPORT — PAGE 3

Please print, type or use a patient information stamp.

(patient stamp)

EXTERNAL GENITALIA
• Note abnormalities in diagrams and/or text.

Vulva/Hymen

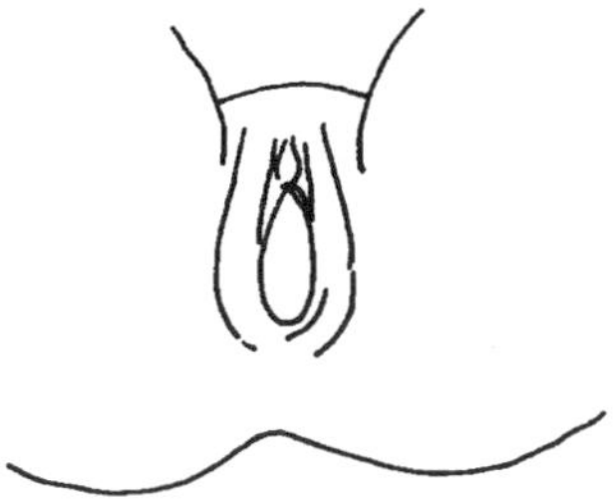

• position during exam	lithotomy	knee chest	supine
• labia majora maneuver?	If yes, outward traction		lateral-down separation
• horizontal hymenal opening (with above position and maneuver)		mm	
• description of hymen			
• draw picture of hymen on diagram			

Penis/Scrotum

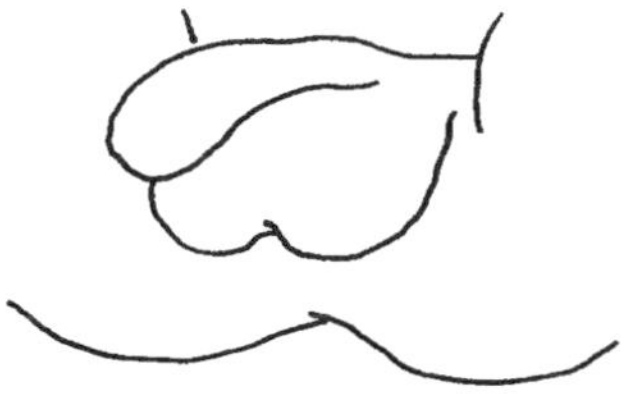

• circumcised?   Yes ☐   No ☐

INTERNAL EXAM
• As noted above, most children require only vaginal introital specimens without speculum or bimanual exams. Please individualize.

Vagina and Cervix

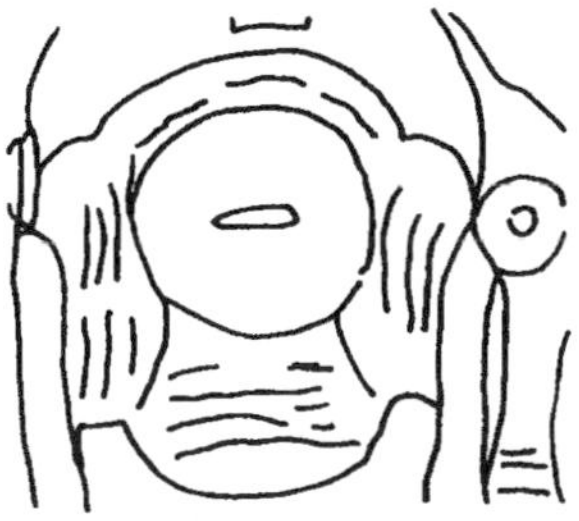

• Note abnormalities in diagram and/or text.

Uterus, Adnexa

• Note abnormalities on bimanual exam, if indicated.

COMPLETE EVIDENCE COLLECTION STEP 6

After Step 6, obtain appropriate medical specimens from the vagina/cervix or male urethra for clinical lab testing. (DO NOT INCLUDE MEDICAL SPECIMENS IN KIT.)

RECTAL EXAM
• Digital or anoscopic exam at discretion of physician.
• Note abnormalities on above diagrams and/or text.

COMPLETE EVIDENCE COLLECTION STEPS 7 - 12

After Step 7, obtain appropriate medical specimens from the rectum for clinical lab testing. (DO NOT INCLUDE MEDICAL SPECIMENS IN KIT.) After Step 11, obtain appropriate blood specimens for clinical lab testing. (DO NOT INCLUDE MEDICAL SPECIMENS IN KIT.)

ILSP502C

(White copy to hospital; yellow copy in kit)

FIGURE 118-4 Sample physical examination form with diagrams for the genital examination. Courtesy of Illinois State Police.

FORENSIC LABORATORY REPORT — PAGE 4

Please print, type or use a patient information stamp.

(patient stamp)

Photographs — may be taken for evidentiary purposes with the written consent of the patient or the patient's guardian if the patient is a minor. If the patient is a minor and the parent/guardian is not immediately available, photographs may be taken but shall be released to law enforcement personnel and state's attorneys only with the written consent of the parent/guardian. If consent is refused, all photographs and negatives shall be given, without charge, to the parent/guardian.

SUMMARY OF FINDINGS

SIGNATURES

| (Attending Physician Signature) | (date) | (Attending Nurse/Assistant Signature) | (date) |

| (Please print) | | (Please print) | |

COMPLETE EVIDENCE COLLECTION STEP 13

FINAL INSTRUCTIONS
1. Make sure all information requested on all sample envelopes and bag labels have been filled out completely.
2. Separate all forms (Steps 1, 2, and 14) and follow distribution requirements on the bottom of each form.
3. With the exception of the large sealed and labeled clothing bags, return all other evidence envelopes/bags to the kit box.
4. Initial and affix red evidence tape on box top.
5. Fill out information required on kit box top.
6. Hand the sealed kit and sealed bags to investigating officer.
NOTE: If officer is not present at this time, place sealed kit and sealed bags in secure area, and hold for pickup by investigating officer.

COMPLETE EVIDENCE COLLECTION STEP 14

(White copy to hospital; yellow copy in kit)

ILSP502D

FIGURE 118-5 Sample form for summary of physical examination findings. Note that the form is signed by the attending physician and the nurse, or assistant, who was present during the examination. Courtesy of Illinois State Police.

Illinois State Police
Division of Forensic Services

STEP 14

Please print, type or use a patient information stamp.

(patient stamp)

PATIENT DISCHARGE MATERIALS

Patient name	DOB/Age
Hospital name/phone	
Date of examination	ER#
Examining physician	

With your consent, a number of specimens were collected from you to provide evidence in court should your attacker be caught and you decide to prosecute.

Additional tests were conducted as follows: ☐ A blood test for syphilis, ☐ A culture for gonorrhea, ☐ Tests for chlamydia, ☐ Other tests_____

_____, and ☐ A pregnancy test to determine pre-existing pregnancy only, not to determine a possible pregnancy as a result of the assault.

VENEREAL DISEASE TREATMENT

☐ You were given an antibiotic to prevent gonorrhea. However, you must return in six weeks following this treatment for another test to be sure you do not have syphilis. Return for this test and possible treatment the week of _____ name of drug _____ dosage _____

☐ You were *not* given treatment to prevent gonorrhea or any other venereal disease because _____

☐ If you wish to obtain follow-up testing or treatment for venereal disease, please visit your local health clinic or contact _____
_____ (name, address, and telephone)

☐ Patient declines

PREGNANCY PREVENTION

☐ You were given medication to prevent pregnancy as a result of the sexual assault. If you should become pregnant despite having been given treatment, you should return immediately to the hospital emergency room or go to your private physician because the drug you were given may cause damage to the fetus.   Name of drug _____   Dosage_____

☐ You were *not* given medication to prevent pregnancy because _____
If you want counseling, referrals and/or follow-up pregnancy testing information, consult the social service department of this hospital or call one of the agencies listed below for assistance.

Agency _____   Agency _____

Address _____   Address _____

Telephone _____   Telephone _____

☐ Patient declines

FOLLOW-UP

☐ An appointment was made for you at this hospital for follow-up *medical* treatment on (date) _____

☐ No appointment was made for follow-up medical treatment because _____

☐ An appointment was made for you at this hospital for follow-up *counseling* on (date) _____

☐ No appointment was made for follow-up counseling because _____

PSYCHOLOGICAL SUPPORT referral to

Was written and verbal information given to patient? ☐ Yes ☐ No

DOCUMENTATION If the patient is less than 18 years of age, was DCFS notified, if appropriate? ☐ Yes ☐ No

Were police notified? ☐ Yes ☐ No   Was Patient Consent and Authorization Form completed? ☐ Yes ☐ No

INFORMATION

I have received the following written information:

☐ Illinois Department of Public Health brochure, "After Sexual Assault"   ☐ Attorney General's Office flyer "Illinois Crime Victims Compensation Act"
☐ Patient Medication information sheets listing anticipated effects and side effects of medicines given to me.

☐ This patient information sheet _____
                          Patient Signature   Date

☐ I do not wish to receive this sheet _____
                          Patient Signature   Date

ILSP514

(White copy to patient; yellow copy to hospital)

FIGURE 118-6 Sample patient discharge instruction form. Courtesy of Illinois State Police.

Treatment for the male sexual assault victim is the same except for trichomonas treatment and pregnancy prophylaxis. These are not necessary in the male patient.

COMPLICATIONS

There are no physical complications to performing the sexual assault examination. **Be aware of potential psychological complications. Treat the patient with the utmost privacy and dignity to help them through this stressful situation and not victimize them. Do not add to the abuse that they have already suffered. Allow the patient to make decisions during the history and physical examination so that they have a voice in the process.**

SUMMARY

The Emergency Department plays a key role in providing quality treatment to the sexual assault victim. Providing compassionate care strongly influences the healing process from being a victim to becoming a survivor. It is important to perform a complete examination for trauma and not just focus on evidence collection. Careful collection and documentation of the elements of the evidence collection kit will impact successful prosecution. Proper follow-up care and a strong link to a local rape crisis center are important.

REFERENCES

1. National Victim Center, Crime Victims Research and Treatment Centers: *Rape in America—A Report to the Nation.* Charleston, SC: Medical University of South Carolina, 1992.
2. Holmes MM, Resnick HS, Kilpatrick DG, et al: Rape-related pregnancy: estimates and characteristics from a national sample of women. *Am J Obstet Gynecol* 1996; 175(2):320–325.
3. Linden JA: Sexual assault. *Emerg Med Clin North Am* 1999; 17(3):685–697.
4. Ullman SE, Siegel JM: Victim-offender relationship and sexual assault. *Violence Vict* 1993; 8(2):121–134.
5. Stark E, Flitcraft A, Zuckerman D, et al: *Wife Abuse in the Medical Setting: An Introduction for Health Personnel.* Rockville, MD: National Clearinghouse on Domestic Violence, 1981.
6. Rennison CM: *Bureau of Justice Statistics. Criminal Victimization 1998: Changes 1997–98 with trends 1993–98.* Washington, DC: US Department of Justice, 1999.
7. Koss MP, Koss PG, Woodruff WJ: Deleterious effects of criminal victimization on women's health and medical utilization. *Arch Intern Med* 1991; 151:342–7.
8. Marchbank PA, Lui KJ, Mercy JA: Risk of injury from resisting rape. *Am J Epidemiol* 1990; 132(3):540–549.
9. Levine DL, Kaufman LE: Rape and sexual violence: the adult and adolescent female victim, in Bernstein E, Bernstein J (eds): *Case Studies in Emergency Medicine and the Health of the Public.* Boston: James & Bartlett, 1996:100–112.
10. Dupre AR, Hampton HL, Morrison H, et al: Sexual assault. *Obstet Gynecol Surv* 1993; 45:640–648.
11. Deming JE, Mittleman RE, Wetli CV: Forensic science aspects of fatal sexual assaults on women. *J Forensic Sci* 1983; 28(3):572–576.
12. Schiff AF: A statistical evaluation of rape. *J Forensic Sci* 1973; 2:339–349.
13. Lenahan LC, Ernst A, Johnson B: Colposcopy in evaluation of the adult sexual assault victim. *Am J Emerg Med* 1998; 16(2):183–184.
14. Centers for Disease Control: Sexual assault and STDs. *MMWR Morb Mortal Wkly Rep* 1998; 47(RR-1):108–115.
15. Yuzpe AA, Smith RP, Rademaker AW: A multicenter clinical investigation employing ethinyl estradiol combined with dl-norgestrel as postcoital contraceptive agent. *Fertil Steril* 1982; 37(4):508–513.
16. Jenny C, Hooton TM, Bowers A, et al: Sexually transmitted disease in victims of rape. *N Engl J Med* 1990; 322(11):713–716.
17. Katz MH, Gerberding JL: The care of persons with recent sexual exposure to HIV. *Ann Intern Med* 1988; 128:306–312.
18. Schwarcz SK, Whittington WL: Sexual assault and sexually transmitted diseases: detection and management in adults and children. *Rev Infect Dis* 1990; 12(6):682–690.

Chapter 119
CULDOCENTESIS

David L. Levine

INTRODUCTION

Culdocentesis is a procedure used to sample peritoneal fluid to help confirm a diagnosis or to obtain a culture. It has mainly been used for diagnosing a ruptured ectopic pregnancy or ruptured ovarian cyst.[1-9] Culdocentesis involves introducing a hollow needle through the posterior vaginal cuff and into the peritoneal space. This is a relatively simple and fast procedure. Ultrasound, with its improved resolution and availability, has virtually replaced culdocentesis as the test of choice.

ANATOMY AND PATHOPHYSIOLOGY

The key anatomy to be familiar with is the vagina and the pouch of Douglas, also known as the rectouterine pouch or the cul-de-sac. The rectouterine pouch is formed by reflections of the peritoneum between the posterior surface of the uterus and the anterior surface of the rectum. It is the most dependent intraperitoneal space in both the upright and supine positions. This allows blood, pus, and other free fluids to pool in this space. The rectouterine pouch separates the upper portion of the rectum from the uterus and the upper portion of the vagina. The small intestine and a small amount of peritoneal fluid often lie within the rectouterine pouch. Sensation of the vagina is greatest near the introitus. There is minimal sensation in the posterior vaginal fornix adjacent to the rectouterine pouch.

INDICATIONS

Culdocentesis has been used in the Emergency Department in the past to diagnose a ruptured viscus, particularly an ectopic pregnancy. The use of culdocentesis has decreased significantly with the emergence of improved serum and urine tests for pregnancy, increased accessibility to ultrasonography, and the increased resolution of ultrasound. Recent studies have clearly shown ultrasonography to be more sensitive and noninvasive in detecting a hemoperitoneum.[1] There still remains three main indications to perform a culdocentesis.

The first indication is a hemodynamically unstable female patient of reproductive age with evidence of peritoneal irritation in the pelvic region. This patient most likely has a ruptured ectopic pregnancy and needs emergent surgery. A diagnostic test is usually not necessary to take the patient directly to the Operating Room if a rapid pregnancy test is positive. An unstable patient cannot be sent to the Radiology Department for an ultrasound. A culdocentesis may be performed if bedside ultrasonography is not available. Approximately 85 to 90 percent of patients with ruptured ectopic pregnancies have a positive culdocentesis.[2]

The second indication for a culdocentesis is a stable pregnant patient with ultrasonographic evidence of free fluid in the pelvis or pouch of Douglas. A culdocentesis can confirm if the fluid is blood. Approximately 65 to 70 percent of patients who have a stable presentation and unruptured ectopic pregnancy have a positive culdocentesis.

A culdocentesis is indicated if ultrasonography or laparoscopy is not readily available. A negative culdocentesis may be used to reassure a physician that following serial quantitative beta-HCG levels can be performed before committing a stable patient to an operative procedure. A positive culdocentesis would indicate intra-abdominal bleeding that requires immediate operative intervention.[3]

Culdocentesis has been used in place of a diagnostic peritoneal lavage to detect a hemoperitoneum since small amounts of blood tend to collect in the rectouterine pouch. Aspiration of clear peritoneal fluid excludes a hemoperitoneum. Ultrasonography and CT scanning have significantly reduced the usefulness of culdocentesis for this indication.

CONTRAINDICATIONS

There are a few contraindications to performing a culdocentesis. A pelvic mass detected on bimanual pelvic examination is a contraindication. A pelvic mass may be a tubo-ovarian abscess, an appendiceal abscess, an ovarian mass, or a pelvic kidney. There is a concern of rupturing an abscess, if present, into the peritoneal cavity with the culdocentesis needle. Other contraindications include a nonmobile uterus and patients with a coagulopathy. The procedure is limited to patients beyond puberty on the basis of anatomy. It is difficult to perform the procedure through a small prepubertal vagina. **A patient with unstable vital signs and a positive bedside pregnancy test should be immediately taken to the Operating Room and does not require a culdocentesis; although they will require fluid and blood resuscitation until the Operating Room and Surgeon is available.**

Culdocentesis may be unsatisfactory in women with previous salpingitis and pelvic peritonitis because the rectouterine pouch may have been obliterated. **The failure to obtain blood does not exclude the diagnosis of a hemoperitoneum and, therefore, cannot exclude an ectopic pregnancy.**[4]

EQUIPMENT

Exam table with stirrups
Water-soluble lubricant
Vaginal speculum
Cervical tenaculum
19 gauge butterfly needle or 18 gauge spinal needle
25 and 27 gauge needles
Ring forceps
20 mL syringe
Povidone iodine
Sterile water
Cotton balls
4×4 gauze squares
Local anesthetic solution with epinephrine
4% cocaine
20% benzocaine
Red top test tube for laboratory analysis
Purple top test tube for laboratory analysis
Culture tubes
Light source

PATIENT PREPARATION

Explain the risks, benefits, potential complications, and alternatives (such as ultrasound or immediate laparoscopy) to culdocentesis to the patient and/or their representative. Obtain a signed consent for the procedure. If verbal consent is obtained, a statement in the chart should state the following: "The risks, benefits, alternatives, and complications were described and discussed in detail. The patient has a clear understanding of these and any questions were answered." A witness should be noted in the record.

Perform a bimanual pelvic examination to rule out a fixed pelvic mass and to assess the position of the uterus prior to the culdocentesis. Place the patient in the lithotomy position with the head of the table slightly elevated (reverse Trendelenburg) so that the intraperitoneal fluid gravitates into the rectouterine pouch. Place the patient's feet in stirrups. Procedural sedation or premedication with intravenous narcotics or sedatives is recommended and may make the procedure more tolerable for the patient. Premedication is not required in an unstable patient.

Some physicians obtain stat upright plain radiographs in stable patients prior to the procedure. These are performed to assess for a pneumoperitoneum. This will also help in determining if a pneumoperitoneum was secondary to the procedure upon obtaining post-procedural radiographs.

TECHNIQUES

Insert a lubricated speculum into the vagina. Open the speculum widely. Grasp the posterior lip of the cervix with the toothed tenaculum or a ring forceps (Figure 119-1A). **Forewarn the patient that grasping of the cervix with a tenaculum may be painful.** Elevate the cervix to elevate a retroverted uterus from the pouch and to stabilize the posterior wall of the uterus during the needle puncture. This also results in a tightening of the vaginal wall adjacent to the rectouterine pouch to expose the puncture site and keep it from moving away from the needle as the vaginal wall is punctured.

Prepare the area. Swab any secretions out of the vagina. Swab the vaginal wall in the area of the rectouterine pouch with povidone iodine followed by sterile water. Some physicians optionally choose to topically anesthetize the area with a cotton ball soaked in 4% cocaine or 20% benzocaine prior to infiltrating with local anesthetic solution. Insert the cocaine or benzocaine soaked cotton ball into the posterior vaginal fornix area and allow it to remain for 3 minutes. The maximum dose of cocaine to apply to the cotton ball is 3 mg/kg. Arm a 5 mL syringe containing local anesthetic solution with epinephrine with a 25 gauge needle. Insert the needle in the midline and 1.0 cm posterior (inferior) to the point at which the posterior vaginal wall joins the cervix (Figure 119-1B). Inject 2 mL of local anesthetic solution containing epinephrine.

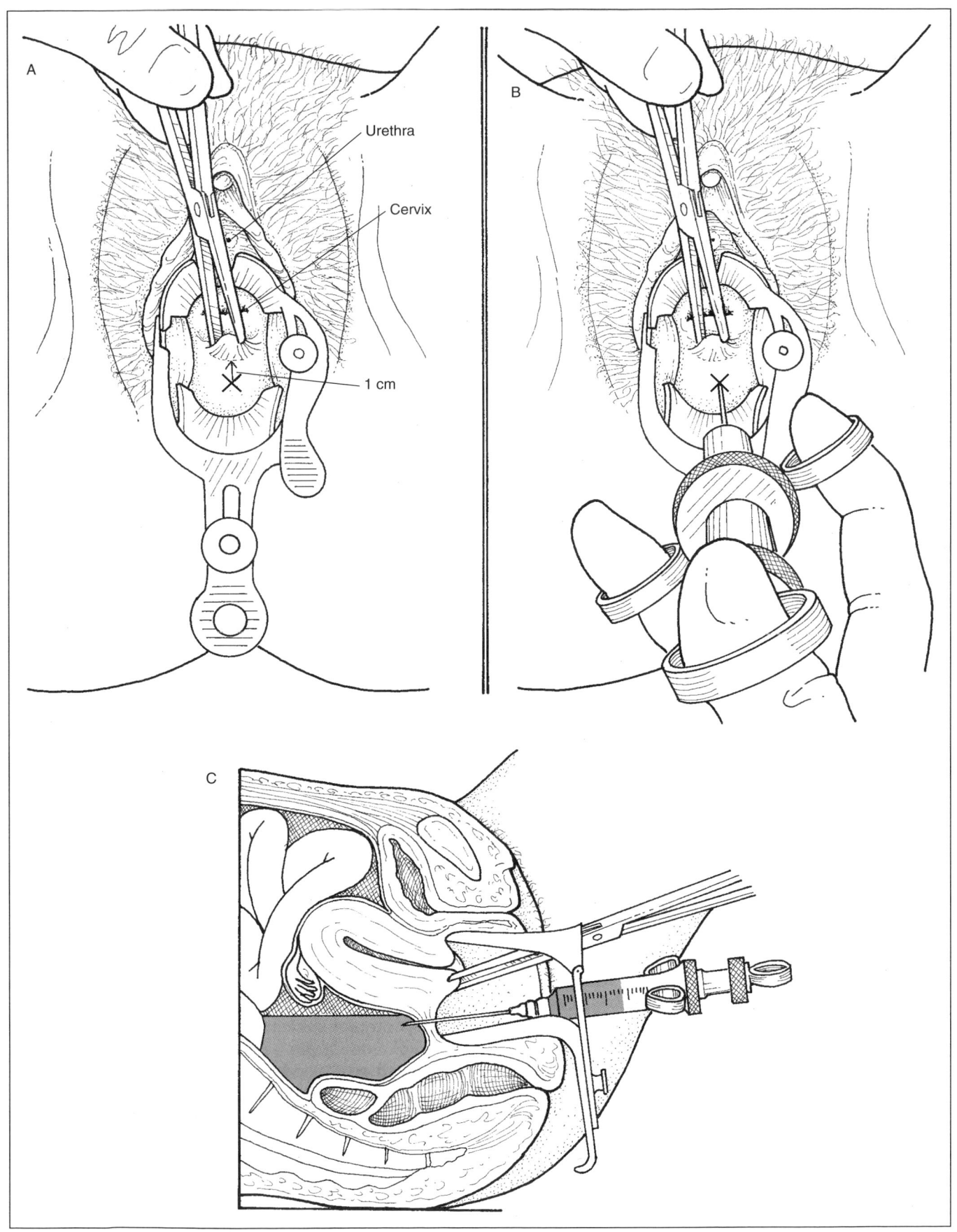

FIGURE 119-1 Culdocentesis. A speculum has been inserted in the vagina and opened. *A.* Grasp the posterior lip of the cervix with a toothed tenaculum and elevate it. The *x* marks a spot 1 cm from the junction of the cervix and posterior vaginal wall where needles will be inserted. *B.* The needles used for anesthesia and culdocentesis are inserted 1 cm from the junction of the cervix and posterior vaginal wall. *C.* Midsagittal section of the female pelvis during a culdocentesis. The needle is inserted and aimed slightly posterior to access the fluid.

6. Cartwright PS, Vaughn B, Tuttle D: Culdocentesis and ectopic pregnancy. *J Reprod Med* 1984; 29(2): 88–91.

7. Wolcott, HD, Stock, RJ, Kaunitz AM: Ectopic pregnancy, in Benrubi GI (ed): *Obstetric and Gynecologic Emergencies.* Philadelphia: Lippincott, 1994:41–50.

8. Cunningham FG, MacDonald PC, Gant NF, et al: *Williams Obstetrics,* 21st ed. New York: McGraw-Hill, 2001:883–910.

9. Brenner PF, Roys S, Mishell DR: Ectopic pregnancy: a study of 300 consecutive surgically treated cases. *JAMA* 1980; 243(7):673–676.

Chapter 120
PROLAPSED UTERUS REDUCTION

Wendy A. Cole
Eric R. Snoey

INTRODUCTION

There is a progressive relaxation of pelvic support for the uterus and vagina with advancing age. This relaxation may in turn lead to symptomatically important uterine prolapse in susceptible women. The quality of life issues associated with prolapse of the uterus have become increasingly more relevant with women living a third of their lives in the susceptible period after menopause. Manual reduction of the prolapsed uterus and placement of a pessary represents a safe, temporizing measure that may be performed in the Emergency Department. Surgical correction may ultimately be necessary. This chapter will address the nonsurgical management of a prolapsed uterus.[1,2]

The structural support of the female pelvis is subject to a number of identifiable stresses that may predispose certain women to uterine prolapse later in life. Multiparity seems to be the most commonly shared trait, suggesting that birth trauma has a primary role to play. Alternative mechanisms include anything that may increase intraabdominal pressure, such as heavy lifting, ascites, obesity, large intraabdominal tumors, or pelvic tumors. Similarly, chronic respiratory disorders (e.g., asthma, bronchitis, or emphysema) may put undue tension on the pelvic floor musculature.[3] Two cases of acute uterine prolapse after restrained motor vehicle collisions were recently described.[4] It was hypothesized that the sudden increase in intraabdominal pressure from the lap belt was the cause of the prolapse. A congenital form of uterine prolapse may be seen in newborns due to vigorous crying.[3] The integrity of the pelvic connective tissues may have a role to play as suggested by the increased incidence of uterine prolapse in women with Marfan syndrome and other connective tissue disorders.[5]

Uterine prolapse is defined as the descent of the uterus and cervix down the vaginal canal towards the vaginal introitus. All forms of genital prolapse are described with reference to the vagina.[6] The degree of uterine prolapse parallels the extent of weakening of the supporting structures.[3] A first-degree or mild prolapse is defined with the cervix palpable as a firm mass in the lower third of the vagina. The patient is usually asymptomatic. Second-degree or moderate prolapse is defined as the cervix being visible and projecting into or through the vaginal introitus. The patient may be experiencing a falling-out sensation or may report the feeling of sitting on a ball. Additional symptoms include heaviness in the pelvis, low backache, lower abdominal discomfort, and inguinal discomfort. Third-degree prolapse, also known as severe prolapse or procidentia, is defined as the cervix and entire uterus projecting through the introitus, completely inverting the vaginal vault (Figure 120-1). The uterine mass frequently has one or more areas of easily bleeding atrophic lesions secondary to exposure and local pressure effects. It may result in leukorrhea, abnormal uterine bleeding, or spontaneous abortions.[3]

ANATOMY AND PATHOPHYSIOLOGY

The pelvic diaphragm, the endopelvic fascia, and the vagina provide the primary support for the pelvic organs. The superficial muscles of the perineum lie below the pelvic diaphragm and indirectly support the pelvic organs by inserting centrally into the perineal body. The perineal body serves to fix the distal vagina and anus. The bony pelvis is the ultimate support of all the soft tissues of the pelvis.[7]

The pelvic diaphragm is made up of a bilaterally paired group of three striated muscles: the pubococcygeus (including the puborectalis), the iliococcygeus, and the coccygeus. The pelvic diaphragm is innervated by fibers originating from sacral segments four and five. The pelvic diaphragm is normally in a state of tonic contraction. It increases its tone reflexively in response to increases in intraabdominal pressure.[7]

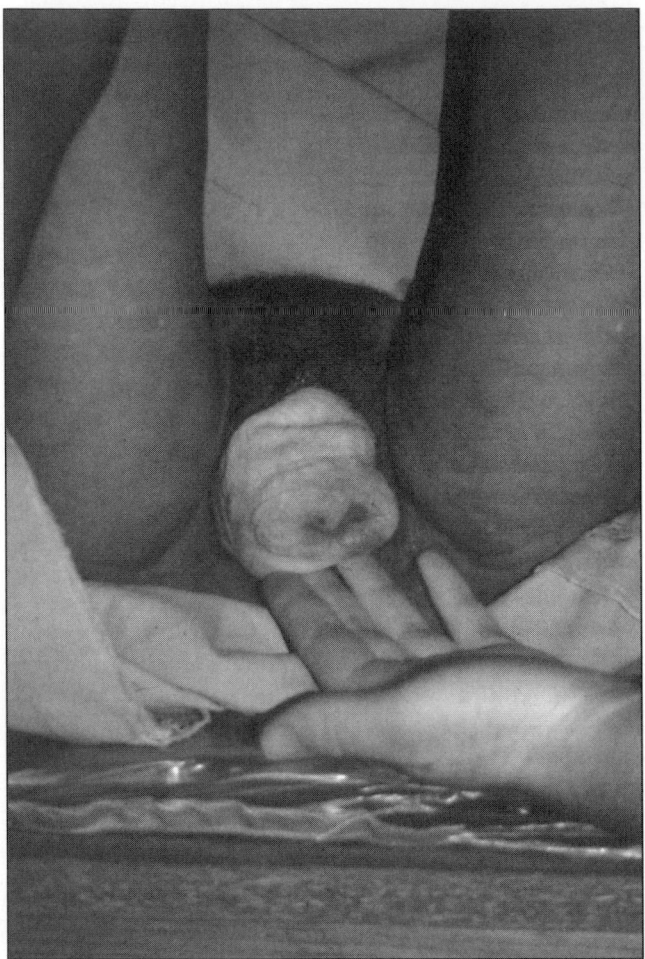

FIGURE 120-1 Uterine procidentia. Photo courtesy of Steve Miller, MD.

The endopelvic fascia is the layer of fibrous connective tissue that envelops all pelvic organs. The endopelvic fascia develops supportive thickenings along lines of tension that are referred to as ligaments (e.g., uterosacral, cardinal). These ligaments provide further support for the pelvic structures. The uterosacral and cardinal ligaments suspend the uterus and are in fact simple extensions of the endopelvic fascia.[7]

The vagina has supportive functions as well. The uterosacral and cardinal ligaments shift the upper one-third of the vagina posteriorly and laterally. This provides support for the cervix. The middle third of the vagina is attached bilaterally to the fascia overlying the pelvic sidewall musculature and supports the bladder. The lower third of the vagina is fused to the tissues about the vaginal outlet.

There are numerous causes that lead to the development of a prolapsed uterus. Prolonged labor can lead to significant pelvic floor damage, suggesting that women who delivered vaginally or who later required cesarean section because of failure to progress are more at risk.[7] As yet, no factor has been identified that allows the iden-

tification of apparently normal individuals in which pelvic floor dysfunction is destined to develop after vaginal delivery.[8] The quantity and quality of collagen appears to deteriorate in women after menopause, likely attributable to the resultant estrogen deficiency.[7,9] It is thought that defective connective tissue contributes significantly to uterine prolapse in the absence of other risk factors. One study of premenopausal women with uterine prolapse found a 25 percent reduction in the collagen content of tissues.[10] Conditions that affect spinal cord pathways and pelvic nerve roots (e.g., muscular dystrophy, trauma, myelodysplasia, meningomyelocele) can result in paralysis of the pelvic floor with the subsequent prolapse of pelvic structures. Spina bifida has been associated with the majority of cases of uterine prolapse in newborn girls and nulliparous women.[7]

Increased intraabdominal pressure is a major factor in the development of pelvic organ prolapse. Obesity contributes to pelvic prolapse by increasing intraabdominal pressure that is, in turn, transmitted to the pelvic organs. Chronic respiratory conditions that are associated with forceful coughing are also thought to predispose to uterine prolapse. Occupational and recreational activities, such as heavy lifting or repeated jumping, result in repeated and prolonged increases in intraabdominal pressure. A review of 1.6 million women found an increase risk of uterine prolapse in a group of nurses whose jobs required heavy lifting.[7] The deterioration in muscle function and connective tissue associated with aging together with gravity, childbirth, neurological deterioration, and hormonal status all combine to lead to a progressive decline in pelvic floor function in older women. This may be compounded by factors that increase intraabdominal pressure leading to the development of symptomatic pelvic floor prolapse.[9]

All aspects of the vaginal support should be carefully surveyed when examining a patient with a uterine prolapse. Examine the patient in the standing position, as well as in the standard dorsal lithotomy position, since the prolapse is almost invariably worse when the patient is upright.[11] It may be necessary to have the patient strain to assess the full extent of the prolapse.[12] Some degree of a cystocele, urethrocele, enterocele, or rectocele may develop or may be associated with a uterine prolapse as the uterus progressively descends. Perform a rectovaginal examination with the patient in the standing position to detect an occult enterocele, suggested by the presence of small bowel easily palpable in the cul-de-sac using the thumb and forefinger.[11]

Asymptomatic uterine prolapse requires no treatment in the Emergency Department. The patient with only intermittent symptoms can prevent against prolapse by simply inserting a tampon or a diaphragm. This additional support is used in anticipation of increased activity or prolonged periods of standing. The patient, however, should be informed that she is losing some aspects of pelvic support and should be referred to a Gynecologist for evaluation of future treatment options.[6] Lifestyle changes can prevent the progression or recurrence of prolapse, precluding the need for future surgical evaluation and complications. Most of these changes focus on decreasing unnecessary increases in intraabdominal pressure like losing weight, removing girdles, avoiding heavy lifting, stopping smoking, and treating allergies or pulmonary disease accordingly.[1] Kegel proposed a series of pelvic muscle exercises for the treatment of urinary incontinence, which can accompany uterine prolapse. These exercises strengthen pelvic muscles but are of limited value in patients with significant prolapse since fascial attachments have been disrupted.[6,13]

Symptomatic women can be treated conservatively or surgically. Pelvic organ prolapse is frequently not recognized until advanced disease because prolapse does not become symptomatic until the descending segment is at or through the introitus.[8] Therapeutic options are variable and relate to the age and health of the patient, the severity of the symptoms, and the degree of prolapse. The options for uterine prolapse include observation, reduction with or without supportive pessary therapy, vaginal hysterectomy with corrective therapy for pelvic relaxation, and some form of colpocleisis.[14]

INDICATIONS

Conservative management of symptomatic uterine prolapse in the Emergency Department involves reduction and subsequent fitting of the patient with a pessary. The pessary is largely used as an alternative to surgery or as a temporizing measure in patients awaiting surgery.[15] Preoperative use of a pessary in advanced degrees of prolapse may aid in decongesting the mucosa, improving circulation, and reestablishing vaginal tonicity. Patients desiring surgical management may be treated conservatively in the Emergency Department and referred to the Gynecologist. Symptomatic women who wish to complete childbearing before having a surgical repair may also be candidates for a vaginal pessary.[1] The gynecologic and obstetric indications for pessary support after reduction of the prolapsed uterus are listed in Table 120-1.[3]

CONTRAINDICATIONS

There are no contraindications to the manual reduction of a prolapsed uterus. Pessaries are contraindicated in patients with acute genital tract infections and in those with adherent retroposition of the uterus.[3] Any vaginal inflammation, ulceration, infection, or atrophy should be treated before pessary fitting to decrease the likelihood of vaginal erosions and granulation tissue.

TABLE 120-1. INDICATIONS FOR THE PLACEMENT OF A PESSARY[3]

Gynecologic indications

Nonsurgical management of uterine prolapse

Aid in the healing of cervical stasis ulceration associated with uterine prolapse

Reduction of cystocele or rectocele

To alleviate the complications of free uterine retroposition and adnexal prolapse

To determine if future hysteroplexy will relieve backache associated with uterine malposition

To facilitate hysteroplexy by holding the uterus in position for operation

To control stress urinary incontinence

To reduce infertility due to cervical retroposition

Obstetric indications

To avoid threatened abortion due to uterine retroposition and chronic passive congestion

To relieve urinary retention and/or pain that can accompany uterine retroposition in pregnancy

To prevent postpartum subinvolution or retroversion of uterus

To prevent and protect against abortion in cervical incompetence

These latter conditions can be mitigated by oral or topical estrogen supplementation. The use of large amounts of lubricants, such as K-Y Jelly, should be encouraged with the pessary in the event that estrogen is absolutely contraindicated.[15]

EQUIPMENT

Pessary

Standard pelvic bed

Vaginal speculum

Water-soluble lubricant

Culture swabs

Biopsy and Pap smear brush, optional

Uterine forceps

Sterile gloves

Sedation, as needed

The vaginal pessary is of ancient lineage. They are now made of plastic, rubber, or silicone that functions to support the uterus, cervical stump, or hernias of the pelvic floor.[3] They are available in numerous sizes and shapes (Figure 120-2). Silicone pessaries have the advantage of being flexible and pliable while causing less vaginal discharge and odor than the rubber pessaries.[14] Pessaries elevate the vagina and maintain normal anatomic relations by supporting prolapsing structures against the perineal body and pubic bone. They thereby reduce vaginal relaxation and increase the tautness of the pelvic floor structures. Usually all that is needed is adequate support anteriorly and a reasonably good perineal body; otherwise, the pessary may slip from behind the symphysis and extrude from the vagina.[3,5] Unfortu-

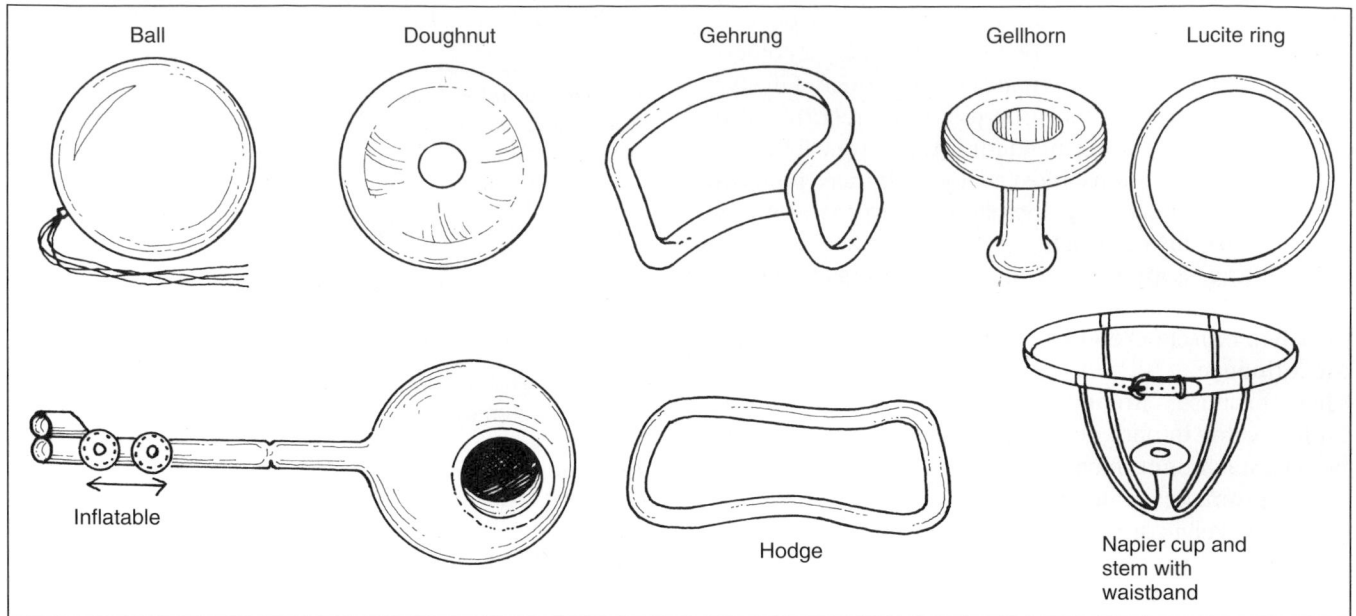

FIGURE 120-2 Examples of different types of pessaries.

nately, the education of physicians is somewhat compromised in the use of pessaries. This is often a trial and error experience for the Emergency Physician as well. Review the accompanying brochures to obtain the most satisfactory results from the pessary.[14]

PATIENT PREPARATION

Explain the procedure, its risks, and complications to the patient and/or their representative. Obtain an informed consent prior to performing the procedure. Place the patient in the lithotomy position with both feet comfortably resting in standard stirrups. One assistant should be available to assist in proper positioning.

TECHNIQUES

The management of uterine prolapse in the Emergency Department depends upon successful replacement of the uterine fundus into the pelvis and subsequent fitting of the appropriate pessary. Surgical management should be appropriately referred. An incarcerated uterus in the pregnant patient is an obstetrical emergency requiring immediate surgical elevation. Other indications include any pregnant patient who develops acute urinary retention or is at risk of aborting.[3]

UTERINE REDUCTION
Insert one gloved and lubricated hand into the vagina with the fingers extended to identify the margins of the cervix. Allow the uterine corpus to rest in the palm of the hand. Apply gentle pressure to elevate the uterine fun-

dus with the gloved hand by pressing against the cervix. Use the fingers on the edges of the uterus closest to the cervix to gently manipulate the uterus in the direction of the umbilicus. Gradually replace the uterus into the pelvis.

If this maneuver is not successful, insert a pessary into the posterior vaginal fornix while the patient is in the lithotomy position. Instruct the patient to sit up and assume the knee-chest position after insertion of the pessary. Instruct the patient to slip slowly into the prone position and then into the lithotomy position. The pessary will maintain the uterus in anteposition. It may be necessary to pack the vagina following manual reduction of a procidentia to maintain the uterine position as a preoperative management decision of an ulcerated, infected prolapse.[3,16] This should be performed in consultation with a Gynecologist.

FITTING OF THE PESSARY
Measure the distance from the introitus to the posterior vaginal vault using uterine forceps after reduction of the uterus. This measurement minus 1 cm is the approximate length of the pessary. To find the width (assuming an ovoid rather than a round pessary is required), place the forceps into the introitus to about the level of the cervix. Separate the handles until the blades touch the walls of the vagina. This represents the greatest diameter of the pessary.[3]

Liberally lubricate the pessary. Insert it with its widest dimension in the oblique diameter of the vagina to avoid painful distension of the introitus. Use the fingers of the nondominant hand to depress the perineum.

Slip the posterior bar behind the cervix using a finger on the dominant hand. The forefinger should pass easily between the sides of the frame and the vaginal wall at any point to ensure adequate fitting. If this is not possible, the pessary is too large.[3]

ASSESSMENT

Ask the patient initially to walk around the examination room to confirm comfort and exclude partial or complete expulsion of the pessary and/or cervix. Replace the pessary with one of a different size or style to prevent any further prolapse.

AFTERCARE

Instruct the patient to remove the pessary each night and clean it with soap and water during the first few weeks of use. Weekly cleanings and overnight removal are adequate after the patient has become comfortable with its use. Apply vaginal cream once a week if the patient is not receiving systemic supplemental estrogen replacement. Warm, low-pressure acetic acid douches or acidic vaginal creams (such as ACI-JEL) may relieve irritation and prevent any discharge caused by the vaginal pessary.[3]

Refer the patient to a Gynecologist. Routine follow-up at 6 to 12 month intervals is recommended after several weeks of a well-managed and appropriately sized pessary. Additional care of these devices includes biannual pelvic examinations and replacement of pessaries every 12 to 18 months.[2] Patients should be counseled on the hazards of leaving the pessary in for prolonged periods of time and the importance of complying with recommended follow-up. It is not uncommon to have to change the pessary size and/or type. Patients are sometimes unable to manage the responsibilities of a pessary. A family member or a nurse trained in the insertion, removal, and care of the pessary is an appropriate alternative.

Advise all patients to return to the Emergency Department for difficulty urinating, defecating, signs of infection, or any problems with insertion and removal of the pessary.

COMPLICATIONS

Attempts at reducing the symptomatic uterine prolapse may be unsuccessful. Review the surgical and medical options with the patient and arrange the appropriate follow-up. Consult a Gynecologist before the patient is discharged from the Emergency Department.

A loose pessary is ineffective and usually will be expelled. The patient may experience pelvic pain, vaginal bleeding, vaginal ulcers, urinary retention, urinary fistulas, bowel fistulas, vaginal discharge, and/or dyspareunia if the pessary is too large. **Therefore, proper fitting is important initially with appropriate follow-up to address these issues.**[14]

Minor complications include ulceration and abrasions of the vaginal mucosa secondary to local pressure effects. Pessaries act as foreign bodies and can become colonized by bacteria and lead to vaginitis. Many patients experience a physiologic watery discharge with pessary use. This should not be confused with an infectious process that usually is accompanied by itching, burning, or odor. Severe vaginitis is more common in the elderly and debilitated patients because of the inability to remove and cleanse the pessary.[17,18] These conditions should be treated accordingly with discontinuation of the pessary until the infection has cleared and local care with estrogen or antibiotic creams.[15]

Serious complications are a result of prolonged, often decades long, uninterrupted use caused by neglect rather than the pessary itself.[15] Case reports described in the literature include vesicovaginal fistulas, rectovaginal fistulas, urosepsis, and malignancy.[19] Cervical and vaginal cancer associated with pessary use is a rare complication and is perhaps related to prolonged irritation or the chemical constituents of some of the older models of pessaries.[19] Pessary-related infections can occasionally develop local complications (e.g., abscess, sinus tract, pelvic cellulitis) or spread to other systems to cause systemic manifestations (e.g., pyelonephritis, peritonitis). Patient counseling and adequate follow-up is important.[15] All of the complications are preventable and point to the need for periodic gynecologic examinations in pessary users.[17]

SUMMARY

Reduction of the prolapsed uterus with subsequent pessary placement is a safe and acceptable mechanism for management of women who present to the Emergency Department with symptomatic prolapse. It is important that Emergency Physicians be familiar with this technique and recognize those women most at risk in order to avoid related complications.

REFERENCES

1. Parker GA, Nichols DH: Genital prolapse, in Altchek A, Deligdisch L (eds): *The Uterus: Pathology, Diagnosis, and Management.* New York: Springer-Verlag, 1991:368–387.
2. Roberge RJ, McCandlish MM, Dorfsman ML: Urosepsis associated with vaginal pessary use. *Ann Emerg Med* 1999; 33(5):581–583.

3. Dor CH III: Relaxation of pelvic supports, in De Cherney AH, Pernoll ML (eds): *Current Obstetric and Gynecologic Diagnosis and Treatment,* 8th ed. Norwalk, CT: Appleton and Lange, 1994:820–829.

4. Mukalian GG: Traumatic uterine prolapse. *J Trauma* 1997; 42(3):553–554.

5. Kistner RW, Berkowitz RS, Barbieri RL (eds): *Kistner's Gynecology: Principles and Practice,* 6th ed. St. Louis: Mosby, 1995:88–95.

6. Videla FLG: Incontinence, prolapse, and disorders of the pelvic floor, in Berek JS, Adashi EY, Hillard PA (eds): *Novak's Gynecology,* 12th ed. Baltimore: Williams and Wilkins, 1996:657–663.

7. Gill EJ, Hurt WG: Pathophysiology of pelvic organ prolapse. *Obstet Gynecol Clin North Am* 1998; 25(4):757–769.

8. Bump RC, Norton PA: Epidemiology and natural history of pelvic floor dysfunction. *Obstet Gynecol Clin North Am* 1998; 25(4):723–746.

9. Bidmead J, Cardozo LD: Pelvic floor changes in the older woman. *Br J Urol* 1998; 82(1):18–25.

10. Jackson SR, Avery NC, Tarlton JF, et al: Changes in metabolism of collagen in genitourinary prolapse. *Lancet* 1996; 347(9016):1658–1661.

11. Mischell DR, Stenchever MA, Droegemueller W, et al: *Comprehensive Gynecology,* 4th ed. St. Louis: Mosby, 1997:547–564.

12. Theofrastous JP, Swift SE: The clinical evaluation of pelvic floor dysfunction. *Obstet Gynecol Clin North Am* 1998; 25(4):783–804.

13. Cundiff GW, Addison WA: Management of pelvic organ prolapse. *Obstet Gynecol Clin North Am* 1998; 25(4):907–921.

14. Morley GW: Treatment of uterine and vaginal prolapse. *Clin Obstet Gynecol* 1996; 39(4):959–969.

15. Sulak PJ: Nonsurgical correction of defects: the use of vaginal support devices, in Rock JA, Thompson JD (eds): *Te Linde's Operative Gynecology,* 8th ed. Philadelphia: Lippincott-Raven, 1997:1077–1084.

16. Doan-Wiggins L: Emergency childbirth, in Roberts JR, Hedges JR (eds): *Clinical Procedures in Emergency Medicine,* 2nd ed. Philadelphia: Saunders, 1991:903–927.

17. Davila GW: Vaginal prolapse: management with nonsurgical techniques. *Postgrad Med* 1996; 99(4):171–185.

18. Zeitlin MP, Lebherz TB: Pessaries in the geriatric patient. *J Am Geriatr Soc* 1992; 40(6):635–639.

19. Schraub S, Sun XS, Maingon P, et al: Cervical and vaginal cancer associated with pessary use. *Cancer* 1992; 69(10):2505–2509.

Section Ten

GENITOURINARY PROCEDURES

Chapter 121
URETHRAL CATHETERIZATION

Sam Stokes, III
Paul S. Ray
Jehangir Meer

INTRODUCTION

Urethral catheterization is the most frequent retrograde manipulation of the urinary tract. It is routinely performed for diagnostic and therapeutic reasons in both urologic and nonurologic diseases.[1–5] Although this is one of the more routinely performed procedures in the Emergency Department, great care must be taken to avoid lower urinary tract injury, reduce the introduction of infection, and minimize patient discomfort. It is important to respect the patient's need for modesty and privacy as much as possible.

ANATOMY AND PATHOPHYSIOLOGY

The genitourinary system is frequently divided into upper and lower urinary tracts. The former refers to the kidneys and ureters or those structures above the bony pelvis. The lower urinary tract includes the bladder and urethra or those structures contained within or below the bony pelvis. Although the entire urinary tract may be catheterized, it is the lower tract, namely the urethra, which will be the focus of this chapter.

Averaging 4 cm in length, the female urethra is rarely a focus of difficulty. Most of the confusion related to urethral catheterization in the female results from poor anatomic knowledge of the external genitalia (Figure 121-1). The clitoris is often mistaken for the urethral meatus. This can result in catheter-related trauma, bleeding, patient discomfort, and frustration. After lateral retraction of the labia minora and exposure of the vaginal vault, the cephalad-most structure is the clitoris. Traveling in a caudal direction, the orifices encountered are the urethra, followed by the vagina, and the anus.

The male urethra is most often the site of catheter-associated difficulty.[3] In contrast to the female, the male urethra may extend upwards of 20 cm in length and follows a tortuous course. The urethra is named based on the anatomic structure it traverses or travels with. The distal-most portion of the male urethra is the meatus, followed by the penile, bulbar, membranous, and prostatic portions (Figure 121-2). Resistance to the advancement of a catheter may occur at any point along the course of the urethra as a result of meatal stenosis, urethral strictures, urethral valves, false urethral passages, enlarged prostates, inflammatory processes, malignant processes, bladder neck contractors, urethral disruptions, and bladder neck disruptions. A careful clinical history and thorough physical examination will, in most cases, uncover these causes. The two most common sites that may be difficult for the catheter to pass are the junction between the bulbar and membranous urethra and the bladder neck.

INDICATIONS

Urinary catheterization can be performed for diagnostic and/or therapeutic reasons.[2,5] Urethral catheterization is often performed in females to collect urine for culture and avoid contamination from skin and vaginal flora. This is usually not necessary in males. Measurement of residual (postvoid) urine, urinary output monitoring, treatment of urinary incontinence, and to allow postsurgical healing are all indications for urethral catheterization. It can be performed to facilitate diagnostic studies, such as retrograde cystography and urodynamics. The main therapeutic indication for urethral catheterization is to relieve acute or chronic urinary retention. Patients with neurogenic bladders are often taught self-catheterization so they may perform this procedure at home.

CONTRAINDICATIONS

The only absolute contraindication to urethral catheterization is in those patients with known or

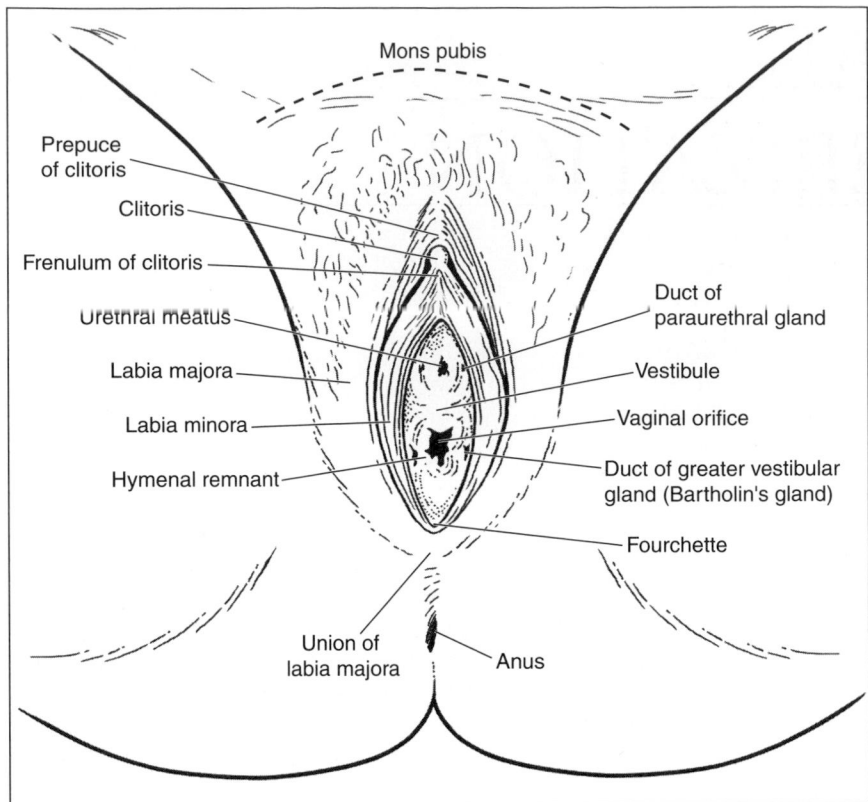

FIGURE 121-1 External anatomy of the female genitourinary tract.

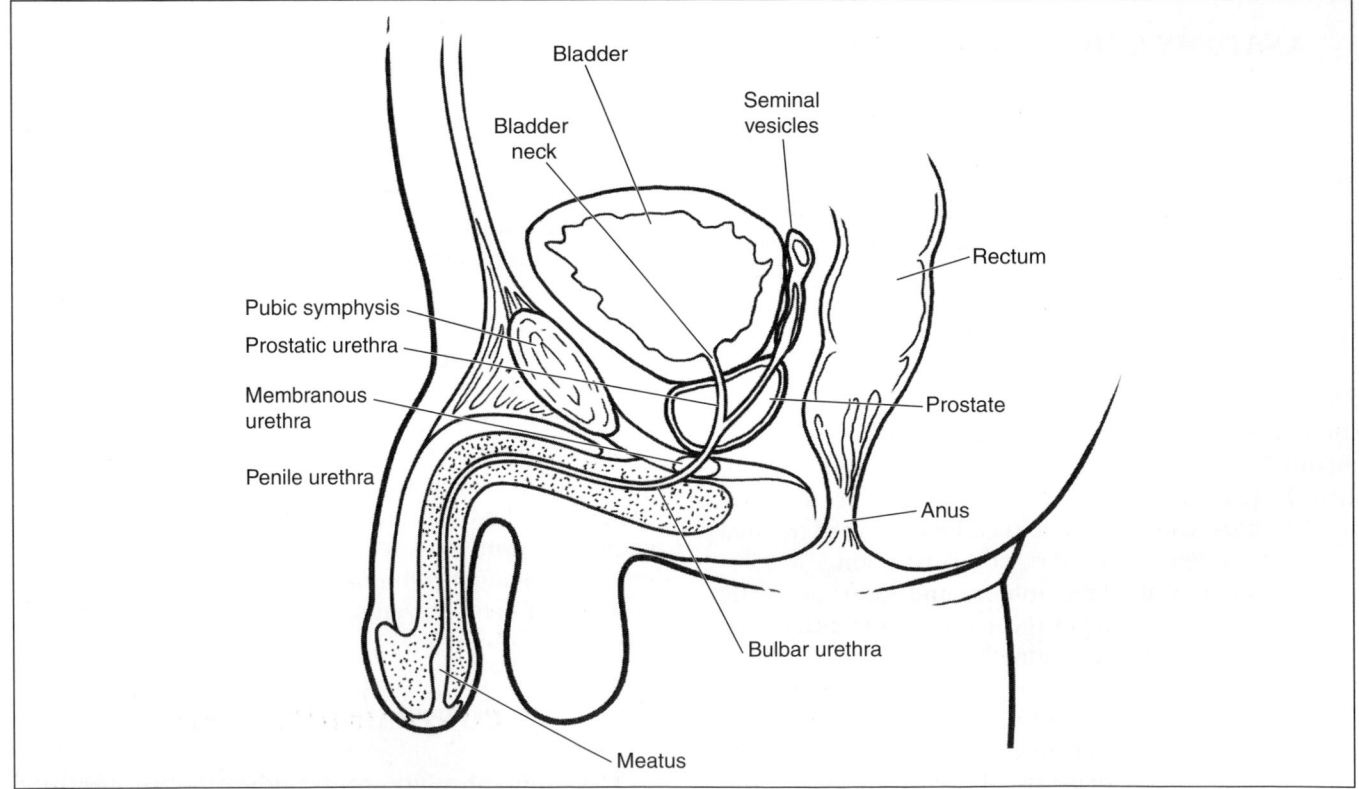

FIGURE 121-2 Anatomy of the male genitourinary tract.

suspected traumatic injury to the lower urinary tract.[2,4,5] They should not undergo urethral catheterization until urethral continuity has been confirmed radiographically. Physical signs on examination that might suggest urethral trauma include blood at the urethral meatus, a perineal hematoma, or a high riding prostate. Attempts at urethral catheterization may convert a partial urethral disruption into a complete disruption. Refer to Chapter 124 for the complete details regarding retrograde urethrography and cystography.

There are a few relative contraindications to urethral catheterization. Microscopic or gross hematuria in the absence of lower urinary tract trauma is not a contraindication to urethral catheterization. Patients with grossly bloody urine are at risk for urinary retention secondary to obstructing clots and require urethral catheterization for bladder irrigation. Although hypocoagulable states are not contraindications to urethral catheterization, great care must be exercised to avoid traumatic injuries and uncontrollable bleeding of the urethra. Prior placement of a penile prosthesis or an artificial urinary sphincter are not contraindications to catheterization. However, vigorous attempts at inserting the catheter are discouraged. Urethral catheterization should not be performed in an uncooperative or combative patient unless they are sedated and/or restrained. A Urologist should be consulted prior to urethral catheterization in patients with known urethral strictures or recent surgery of the urethra or bladder neck.

EQUIPMENT

Povidone iodine
Water-soluble lubrication gel
Lidocaine jelly in penile applicator (i.e., Uro-jet)
Sterile drapes
Sterile gloves
Urethral catheters (Foley, coudé, filiform, and followers)
Christmas tree adapter
Pediatric feeding tubes, sizes 5 to 8 French
Sterile saline
10 mL syringe
Urine meter, if catheter is to be retained
Urine collection system
Urethral catheter leg strap, if catheter is to be retained
1 inch tape
Benzoin solution

PATIENT PREPARATION

Explain the procedure, its risks, and benefits to the patient and/or their representative. Urethral catheterization must be performed using sterile technique. All equipment needed to perform the procedure should be assembled at the bedside prior to beginning the procedure. The preparation for a male patient will be described below. The preparation for a female patient will be described in the techniques section.

Place the male patient in a bed or gurney. In uncircumcised patients, the foreskin must be retracted to expose the glans penis and the urethra. If a phimosis is encountered, it should be approached accordingly. In the pediatric population, male infants and children often have a physiologic phimosis. Attempts at aggressive foreskin retraction should be avoided. Clean any dirt and debris from the penis. Apply povidone iodine solution, with cotton balls or swabs, and allow it to dry. Place sterile drapes around the penis to isolate a sterile field.

Generous lubrication and anesthesia of the male urethra is one of the most important aspects of urethral catheterization. A water-soluble lubricant (e.g., K-Y Jelly) or local anesthetic lubricant (e.g., 2% lidocaine jelly) can be applied to the tip of the urethral catheter before it is inserted. Unfortunately, this provides little-to-no anesthesia. Ideally, commercially packaged blunt-tip syringes of lidocaine jelly (Uro-jet) should be used. Insert the blunt tip of the syringe into the urethral meatus. Firmly squeeze the glans penis to form a seal around the syringe tip. Inject the anesthetic jelly into the urethra. Maintain the syringe tip in the urethral meatus and manual pressure on the glans penis for 10 seconds to prevent egress of the anesthetic jelly.

Prophylactic antibiotic coverage is generally not indicated for urethral catheter placement. Patients with penile prostheses, artificial urinary sphincters, prosthetic heart valves, vascular graphs, and other indwelling foreign bodies may benefit from prophylactic antibiotics. An intravenous dose of a cephalosporin, quinolone, or other antibiotic that covers skin and perineal flora may be administered just prior to inserting the urethral catheter.

MALE CATHETERIZATION TECHNIQUES

FOLEY CATHETER INSERTION

Foley catheters are the most commonly placed urethral catheters. A Foley catheter is a dual lumen tube that contains an inflatable cuff near the distal end (Figure 121-3A). The distal end has two holes for urine to enter the catheter. Urine traverses the large inner lumen of the catheter to exit the proximal port. The second lumen is extremely small and allows air to flow into the inflatable cuff. The proximal end contains two ports. One port allows the egress of urine from the catheter. The second port is an inflation port. An air-filled or saline-filled syringe attaches to this port and is used to inflate the cuff. When inflated, the cuff prevents the distal end of the catheter from slipping out of the bladder.

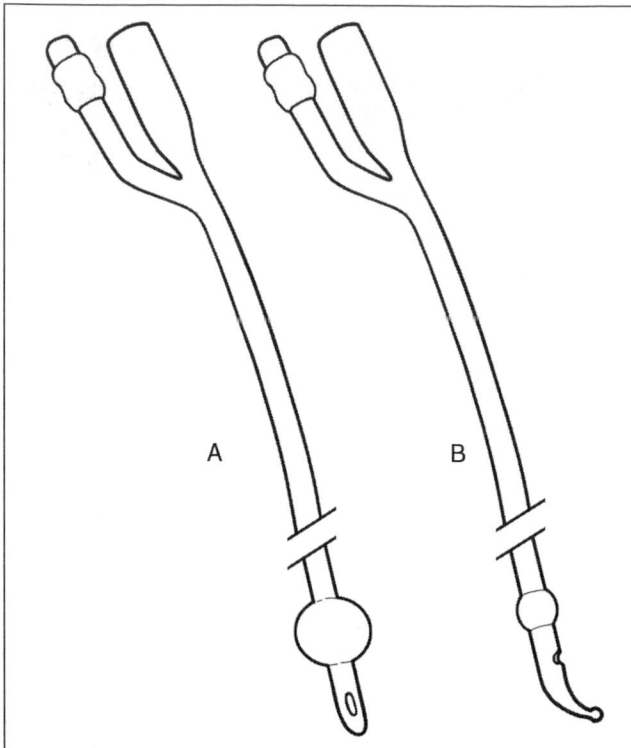

FIGURE 121-3 Urethral catheters. *A.* Foley catheter. *B.* Coudé catheter.

Foley catheters come in a variety of sizes and styles. A 14 or 16 French catheter is the size most commonly used in adolescent or adult patients. The two-way catheter is most commonly used. It is designed for urinary drainage and described in the preceding paragraph. It is a dual lumen tube with a small lumen to inflate the cuff and a large lumen to drain urine from the bladder. Three-way catheters are employed when bladder irrigation, in addition to urinary drainage, is required. These catheters have a small lumen to inflate the cuff, an intermediate sized lumen to instill irrigation solution, and a large lumen to drain urine from the bladder. In the Emergency Department, they are placed in patients with gross hematuria and passage of clots that may or have caused acute urinary retention.

Clean and prep the penis, anesthetize the urethra, and set up a sterile field as mentioned previously. Select an appropriately sized Foley catheter. Inflate the cuff to check its integrity. Deflate the cuff. Grasp the penis with the nondominant hand. Pull the penis taut and upright to straighten out the penile urethra (Figure 121-4*A*). Grasp the Foley catheter with the dominant hand. Dip the tip of the catheter in, or an assistant can apply, water-soluble lubricant or anesthetic jelly (Figure 121-4*A*). Insert the catheter into the penile urethra. Continue to advance the Foley catheter into the urethra until the proximal ports are at the urethral meatus (Figure 121-4*B*).

This ensures that the distal tip of the catheter and the cuff will reside within the bladder (Figure 121-4*C*). **If the distal end of the catheter is not completely within the bladder, inflation of the cuff inside the urethra will result in severe pain, hematuria, and possible urethral rupture.**

Urine should begin to spontaneously flow out of the large port. Insert the proximal end of the catheter into a sterile container to collect the urine. If urine does not spontaneously flow out of the large port, attach a 60 mL syringe to the port and aspirate urine to confirm proper placement of the catheter (Figure 121-4*D*). If no urine is aspirated, remove the catheter from the urethra and reattempt the procedure.

Attach an air-filled or saline-filled syringe to the cuff inflation port (Figure 121-4*E*). Inject the air or saline to inflate the cuff (Figure 121-4*E*). Remove the syringe from the inflation port. Gently withdraw the Foley catheter until resistance is met. This signifies that the cuff is lodged against the bladder neck (Figure 121-4*F*). Attach an adapter and urine collection system to the urine port of the Foley catheter.

Secure the catheter. Wrap tape around the urine port of the Foley catheter and continue it onto the adapter and first 3 to 5 cm of the collection tubing. This will prevent the system from disconnecting. Tape the collection tubing to the patient's thigh to prevent it from pulling out the adapter or the Foley catheter when the patient moves. Some authors also secure the Foley catheter as it exits the penile urethra (Figure 121-5).[5] This is especially important if a red rubber catheter or coudé catheter is used as these catheters do not have a cuff and are not self-retaining. Place three thin strips of tape along the length of the penis and attached to the Foley catheter. Benzoin solution can be applied to the penis to aid in adhesion of the tape. Place a piece of tape circumferentially around the tape ends attached to the catheter. **Never apply tape circumferentially around the penis as it may cause ischemia.**

COUDÉ CATHETER INSERTION

The coudé catheter is similar to a Foley catheter except that the distal end is curved and the tip has a small rounded ball (Figure 121-3*B*). The catheter was designed to bypass the areas of the urethra that a straight catheter could not negotiate. A coudé catheter may be used if a Foley catheter cannot be passed into the bladder. It may also be used if the patient has a known urethral stricture, urethral valve, narrow urethra, or enlarged prostate.

The coudé catheter comes in various sizes and styles. Some models contain a cuff while others do not. The catheter is inserted into the urethra with the elbow on the tip of the catheter facing anteriorly. The procedure for placement of the catheter into the bladder is the same as that for a Foley catheter.

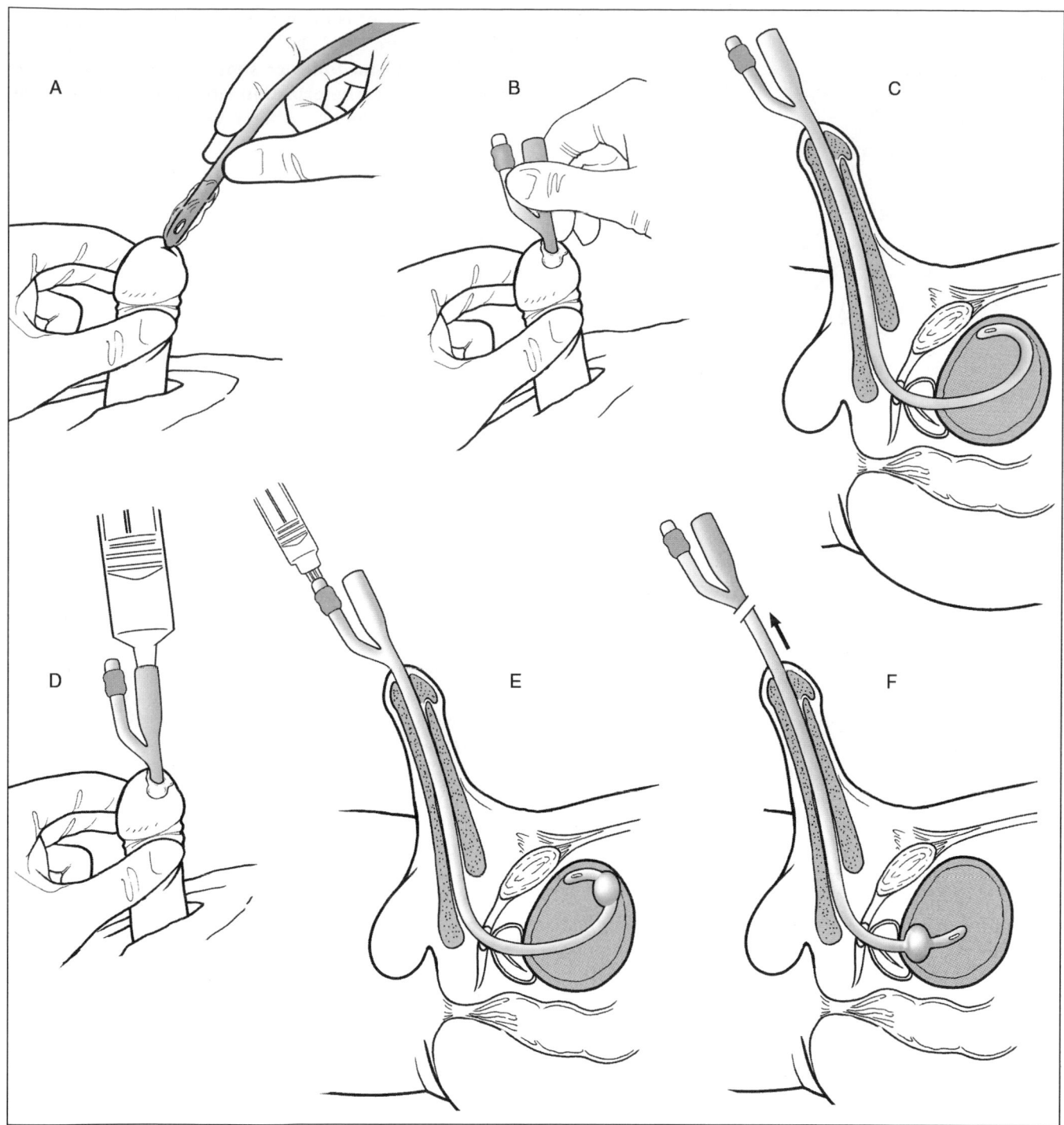

FIGURE 121-4 Foley catheter insertion. *A.* The lubricated catheter is inserted into the urethra. *B.* The catheter is advanced until the ports are at the meatus. *C.* Cross-section of the male pelvis showing the distal catheter and cuff positioned within the bladder. *D.* Urine aspiration confirms proper placement of the catheter. *E.* The cuff at the tip of the catheter is inflated. *F.* The catheter is gently withdrawn to lodge the cuff against the bladder neck.

DIGITAL ASSISTANCE

Occasionally, the Foley or coudé catheter tip will become caught in a posterior fold of the urethra just distal to the urogenital diaphragm (Figure 121-6A). Place the fingers of the nondominant hand on the perineum between the scrotum and anus (Figure 121-6B). Apply upward pressure on the perineum to direct the catheter tip upward while simultaneously advancing the catheter with the dominant hand through the urogenital diaphragm and into the bladder.

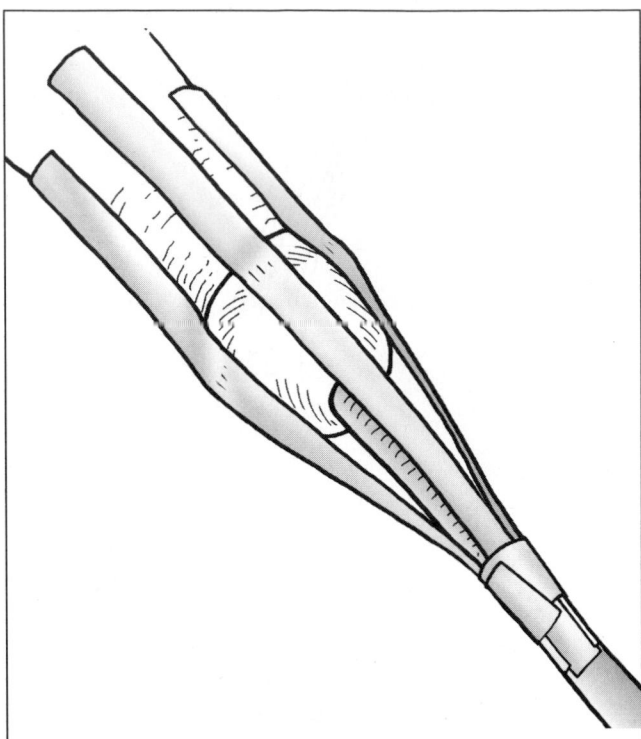

FIGURE 121-5 A method to secure the urethral catheter as it exits the penis.[5]

If the patient has an enlarged prostate, the bladder neck is often elevated superiorly and anteriorly. Digital assistance on the skin of the perineum may be unsuccessful. A finger in the rectum may be used to move the catheter tip anteriorly so that it can be advanced into the bladder.

FILIFORM AND FOLLOWER CATHETERS

In patients with severe urethral strictures or urethral folds, it may be impossible to pass a Foley catheter or a coudé catheter. The next step in the progression to catheterize the bladder is to use filiform and follower catheters. Filiforms are very narrow, flexible, and solid catheters. Their sole function is to successfully negotiate a strictured urethral segment and enter the bladder. The distal end of the filiform catheter may be straight or pig-tailed and are available in a variety of sizes (Figure 121-7A). The proximal end of the filiform catheter is a standard size and contains a metal female connector (Figure 121-7B). The followers are flexible hollow catheters that attach to the filiform catheters. The distal end of the follower catheter contains a metal male connector, to attach to the proximal end of the filiform catheter, and a hole to allow urine to enter the catheter (Figure 121-7C). The follower catheters come in a variety of sizes and allow the physician to dilate the urethra and catheterize the bladder. The proximal end of the

follower catheter is open and accepts a Christmas tree adaptor (Figure 121-7D).

A filiform and follower should be used only after unsuccessful catheterization attempts with a Foley catheter and a coudé catheter. The patient has already been prepped and draped for the prior catheterization attempts. Reinstill anesthetic jelly into the urethra to ensure adequate anesthesia. Numerous sizes and shapes of filiform and follower catheters should be available at the bedside. An assistant will be required to open each sterile packet and hand the filiforms and followers to the physician as needed.

Grasp the penis with the nondominant hand. Pull the penis taut and upright to straighten out the penile urethra (Figure 121-8A). Grasp a filiform catheter and dip the tip in water-soluble lubricant or anesthetic jelly. Gently insert and advance the filiform catheter into the urethra with a twisting motion (Figure 121-8A). Stop advancing the filiform catheter when resistance is met (Figure 121-9A). Insert a second well-lubricated filiform into the urethra with a twisting motion until it meets resistance (Figure 121-9B). Gently attempt to advance the first filiform catheter. If it will not advance, insert a third filiform catheter (Figure 121-9C). Continue to insert filiform catheters and manipulate the previously inserted filiforms (Figure 121-8B). Continue this process until one filiform advances so that its proximal end is 2 cm from the tip of the penis. Remove all the filiform catheters except the one that entered the bladder (Figure 121-9D).

Choose a follower catheter to insert into the bladder. Liberally lubricate the tip of the follower catheter and attach it to the filiform catheter (Figure 121-10A). Gently advance the follower catheter until its proximal end is 3 to 4 cm from the tip of the penis (Figure 121-10B). **If the follower catheter meets resistance during its advancement, do not force it into the urethra.** Instead, withdraw the follower catheter until the tip is 2 to 3 cm outside the penis. Remove the follower catheter from the filiform catheter. Attach a well-lubricated follower catheter onto the filiform catheter that is 1 or 2 French smaller and attempt to advance it into the bladder. Continue this process until a follower catheter can be completely advanced into the bladder. The filiform catheter will be curled up inside the bladder (Figure 121-10B). Urine should spontaneously flow from the follower catheter. If not, attach a 60 mL syringe and Christmas tree adaptor to the follower catheter (Figure 121-10C). Apply negative pressure to the syringe to aspirate urine and confirm the proper placement of the tip of the follower catheter. Attach a urinary collection system to the follower catheter and secure the catheter as described previously.

The patient with urinary obstruction cannot be discharged home with a filiform and follower inserted

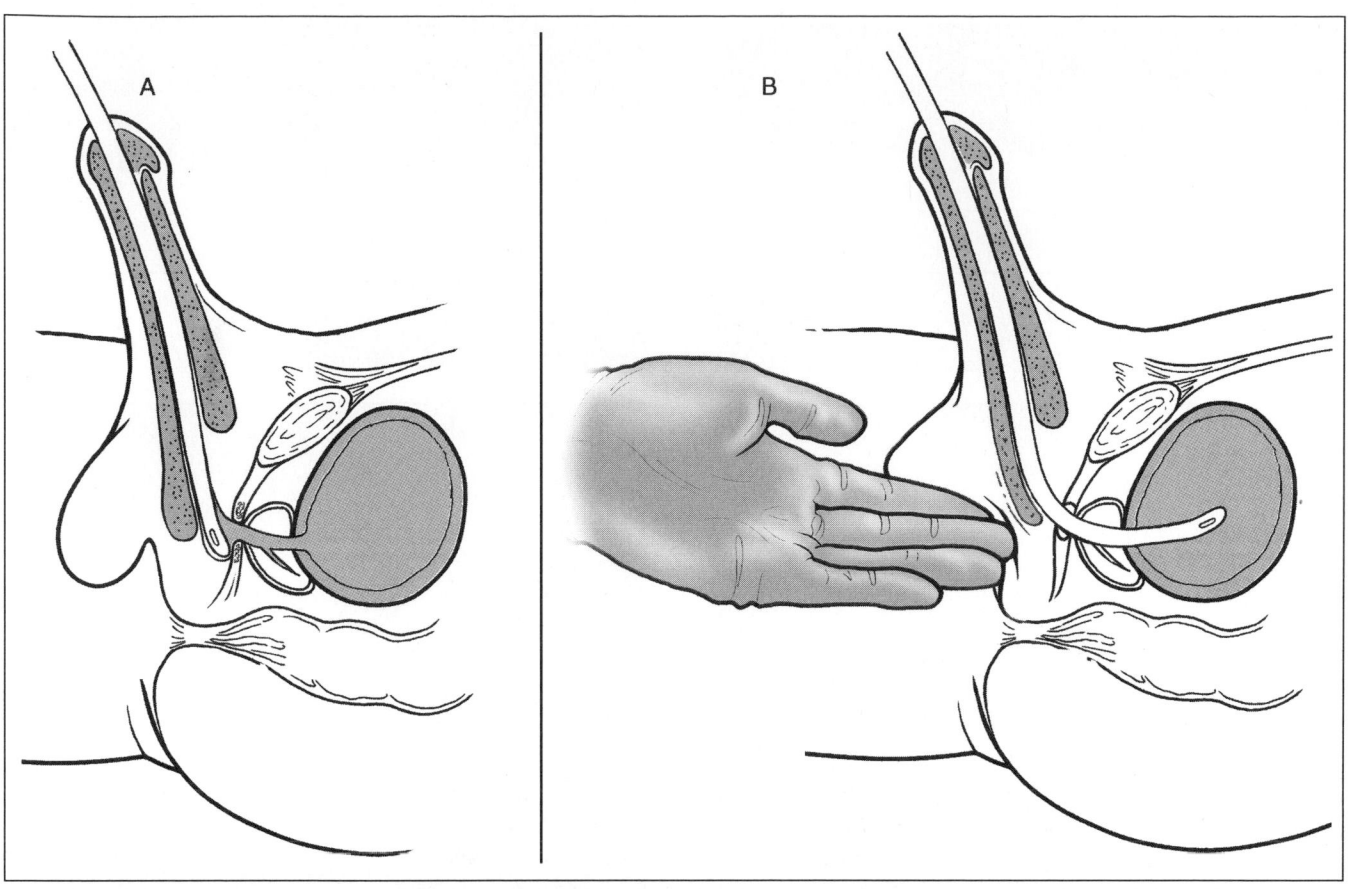

FIGURE 121-6 Digital assistance. *A.* The Foley catheter is caught in a posterior urethral fold. *B.* Digital upward pressure on the perineum will direct the catheter tip upward and through the urogenital diaphragm.

inside the bladder. If the follower catheter is a size 16 or 18 French, completely withdraw it and the filiform catheter and insert a Foley catheter. If the follower catheter is smaller than size 16 French, the urethra must be dilated. Withdraw the follower catheter until the distal tip is 2 to 3 cm outside the penis. Remove the follower catheter from the filiform catheter. Attach a well-lubricated follower catheter onto the filiform catheter that is 1 or 2 French larger than the previous one and gently advance it into the bladder. Continue this process until a follower catheter that is size 16 French easily passes into the bladder. Remove the filiform and follower catheters. Insert a size 16 French Foley catheter. Secure the catheter as described previously.

FEMALE CATHETERIZATION TECHNIQUES

Place the female patient supine in an examination bed. Place the patient in the frog-legged position. If an examination table equipped with stirrups is available, the patient can be placed in the lithotomy position. Sep-arate the labia with the nondominant thumb and index finger to expose the vulva (Figure 121-11). Identify the urethral meatus. Apply povidone iodine solution to the urethral meatus and surrounding vulva. Without moving the nondominant hand, apply sterile drapes to isolate the vulva. A lesser amount of anesthetic jelly is needed to lubricate the female urethra. Place anesthetic jelly on a sterile, cotton-tipped applicator. Insert the cotton-tipped applicator just into the tip of the urethral meatus for 8 to 10 seconds. Remove and discard the cotton-tipped applicator.

Grasp the Foley catheter with the dominant hand. Dip the tip of the catheter in, or an assistant can apply, water-soluble lubricant or anesthetic jelly. Insert the catheter into the urethral meatus (Figure 121-11). Ad-vance the catheter 6 to 8 cm to ensure the distal end and cuff are within the bladder. Urine should sponta-neously begin to flow out of the large port. Insert the proximal end of the catheter into a sterile container to collect urine. If urine does not spontaneously flow out of the large port, attach a 60 mL syringe to the port and aspirate urine to confirm proper placement of the catheter. The remainder of the procedure is exactly the same as previously described for the male patient.

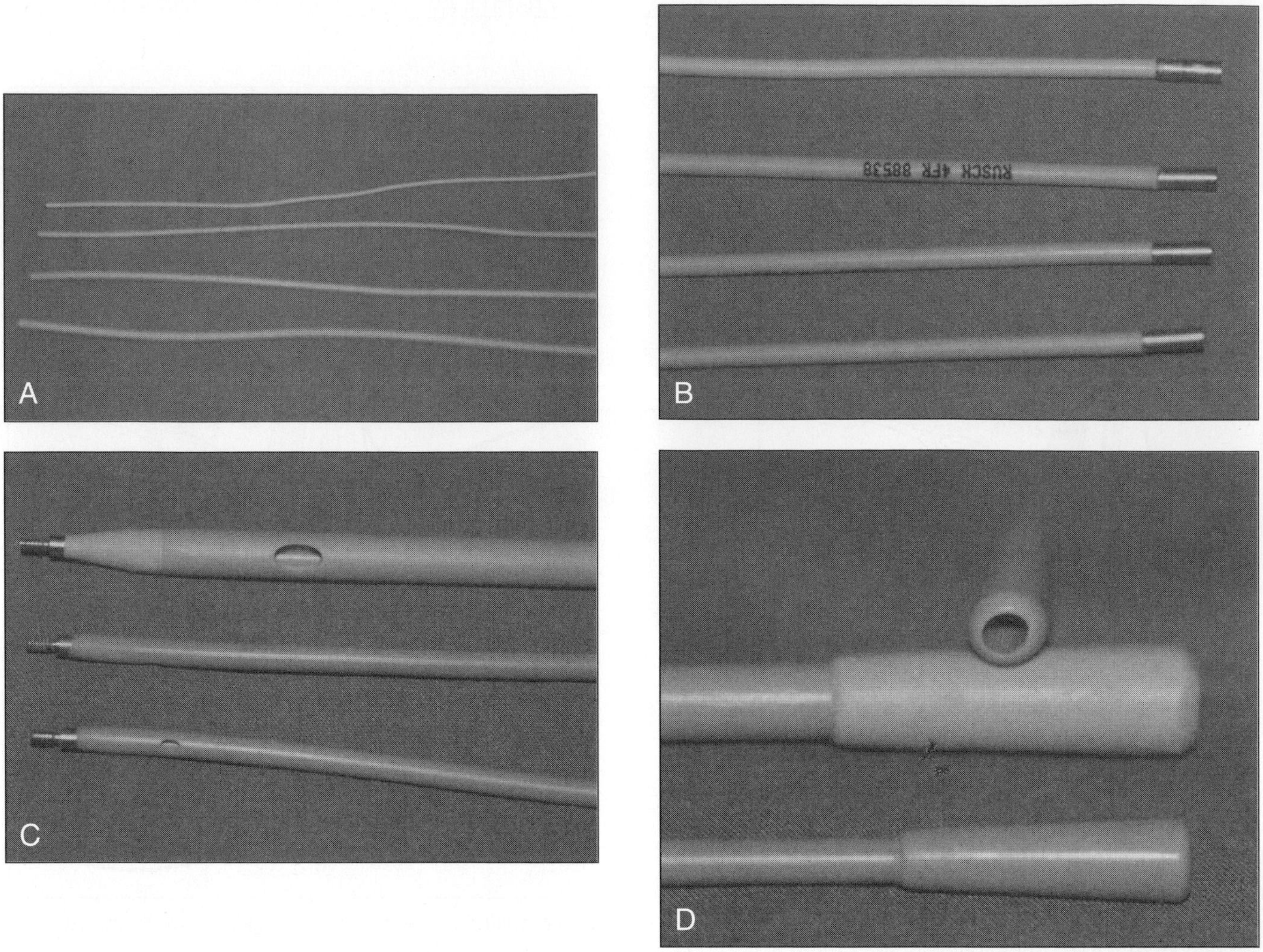

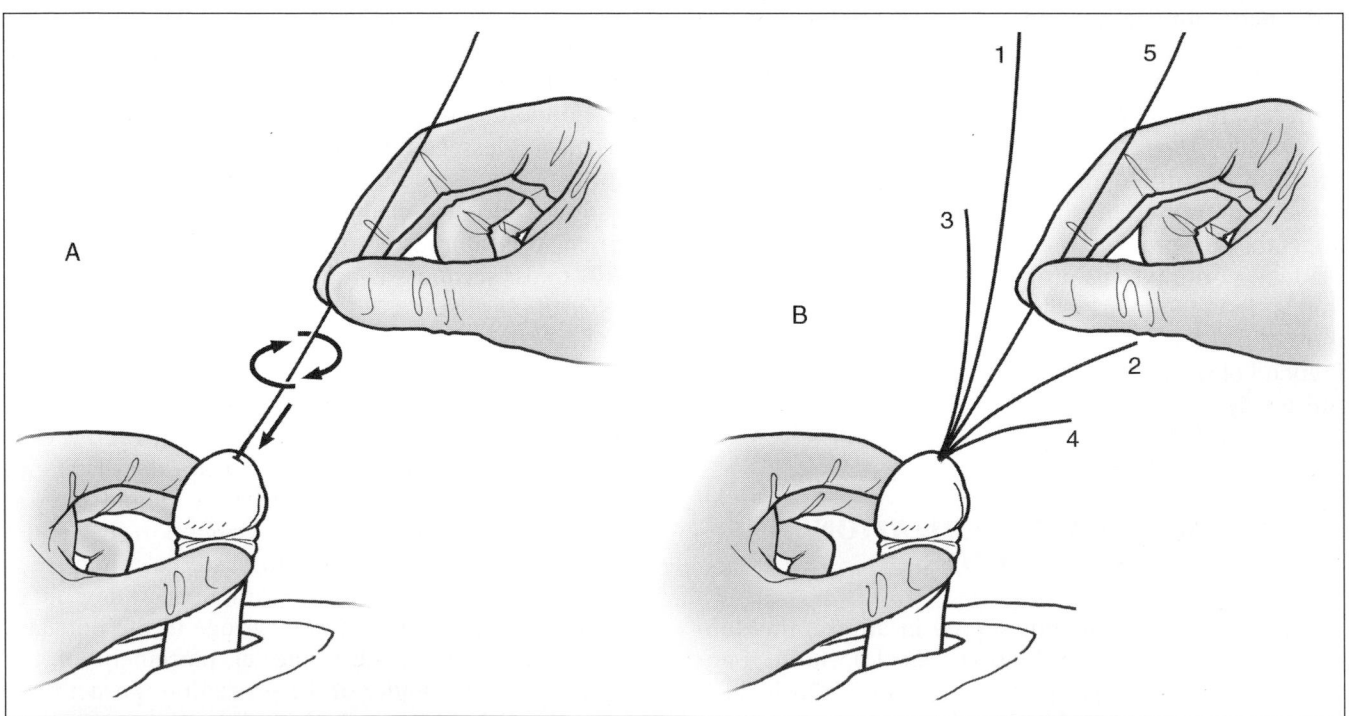

FIGURE 121-7 Photographs of the ends of the filiform and follower catheters. *A.* Distal ends of the filiform catheter. *B.* Proximal ends of the filiform catheter. *C.* Distal ends of the follower catheter. *D.* Proximal ends of the follower catheter.

FIGURE 121-8 Insertion of the filiform catheter. *A.* The catheter is inserted and advanced into the urethra (straight arrow) with a twisting motion (curved arrows). *B.* Additional catheters are inserted until one advances into the bladder. The numbers represent the order of insertion of the filiform catheters.

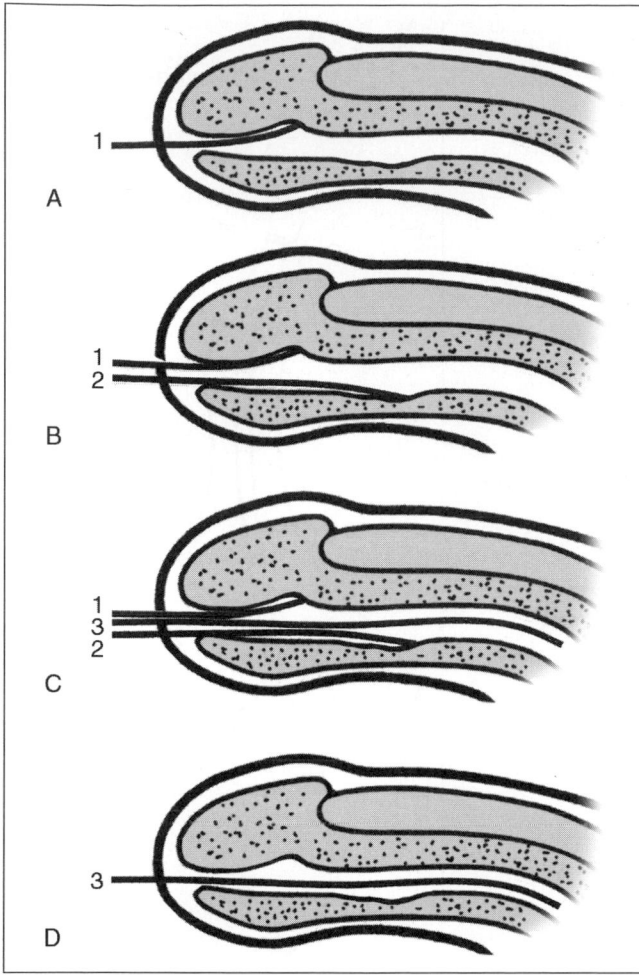

FIGURE 121-9 Midsagittal section of the penis demonstrating insertion of the filiform catheter. *A.* The filiform catheter is inserted until resistance is encountered. *B.* A second filiform catheter is inserted until it encounters resistance. *C.* A third filiform catheter is inserted and advances into the bladder. *D.* Filiform catheters #1 and #2 have been removed.

INFANT AND CHILDREN CATHETERIZATION TECHNIQUES

The indications and contraindications for catheterization of infants and children are the same as for adults. The anatomy of the prepubertal child is similar to the adult, except for the difference in size and lack of secondary sexual characteristics. It is worth noting that the urethral orifice may be difficult to identify in a young female due to abundant hymenal tissue covering the vaginal introitus. This can be circumvented by gentle lateral traction of the labia and downward pressure on the vaginal introital fold with a cotton-tipped applicator. The catheterization of newborns and infants is accomplished with an appropriately sized pediatric feeding tube, usually size 5 to 8 French. Small Foley catheters may be used in large children. The same techniques and cautions followed in the adult patient also apply to the pediatric patient.

ASSESSMENT

Urine drainage is the sign of appropriate catheter placement. Lubricating gel may plug the outflow port of the catheter. If no urine is seen, apply gentle pressure to the suprapubic area to force the flow of urine. If still no urine flows out after this maneuver, irrigate the catheter with sterile saline. The catheter will flush and withdraw fluid with ease if properly positioned in the urinary bladder. Irrigate with an irrigation tray, which includes a 60 mL piston tipped syringe. It may require greater than one fill (i.e., more than 60 mL of saline) to produce two-way flow. The inability to irrigate denotes obstruction or misplacement of catheter. Ensure that the catheter is inserted completely to the hub in males to prevent inadvertent inflation of the cuff in the membranous or prostatic urethra.

AFTERCARE

In uncircumcised males, always remember to reduce the foreskin after catheter placement to avoid the complication of a paraphimosis. Indwelling catheters should be secured to a closed gravity drainage system and attached to the anterior medial thigh. For long-term requirements in males, the catheter should be secured to the anterior abdominal wall to decrease the likelihood of stricture formation.

The patient may be discharged from the Emergency Department with a Foley catheter. Instruct the patient on the proper care and emptying of the leg bag. The patient should immediately return to the Emergency Department if they develop a fever, pain, hematuria, inability to void through the catheter, or abdominal pain.

COMPLICATIONS

Creation of false passages, urethral perforations, bleeding, infection, and catheter misplacement are the complications associated with urethral catheterization. Urethritis is fairly common following catheterization, especially in patients with urethral strictures or prostatic enlargement. Epididymitis, cystitis, and pyelonephritis are uncommon complications and often seen with prolonged catheterization. Bacteremia can occur following the procedure. High-risk patients should receive anti-

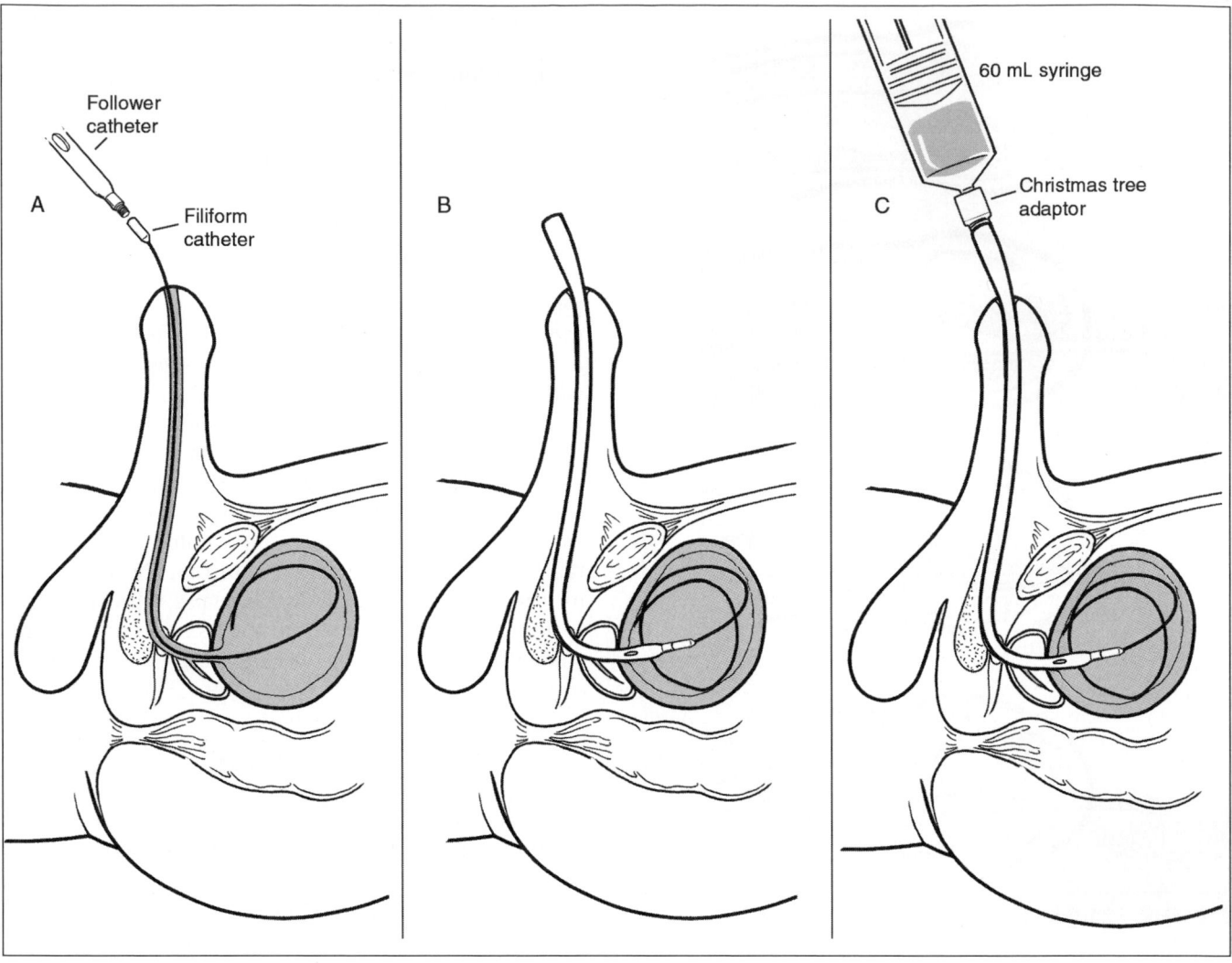

FIGURE 121-10 Insertion of the follower catheter. The filiform catheter has been previously inserted into the bladder. *A.* The follower catheter is screwed into the filiform catheter. *B.* The follower catheter is advanced into the bladder. *C.* Urine aspiration confirms proper placement.

biotic prophylaxis prior to catheterization. Iatrogenic trauma to the urethra can lead to strictures, hemorrhage, and hematuria. Creation of a false passage can occur by inserting the catheter alongside the urethra. Attempts at catheterization in a trauma patient with a urethral injury can convert a partial urethral tear to a complete tear. Failure to reduce the foreskin after catheter placement will result in a paraphimosis.

A less common complication is difficulty removing an indwelling urethral catheter that has an inflated cuff. Inspection of the valve usually reveals the problem. One may attempt to cut proximal to the valve in hopes of evacuating the cuff contents but this is not always successful. Other options include transperineal cuff puncture, transabdominal cuff puncture, or the injection of an organic agent such as ether through the inflation port to dissolve the cuff. Occasionally, a narrow gauge

guidewire may be placed through the cut balloon port to loosen any concretions that may have formed and allow the cuff to deflate. These techniques to reduce the cuff should be performed in consultation with a Urologist.

SUMMARY

Although one of the most routinely performed urologic procedures, urethral catheterization is not a benign process and should be attempted with mindfulness. A working knowledge of genital and perineal anatomy, along with a thorough clinical history and physical examination, is paramount to successful catheter placement and avoidance of complications. Liberal amounts of lubrication should always be used when inserting the catheter. Those patients requiring chronic indwelling

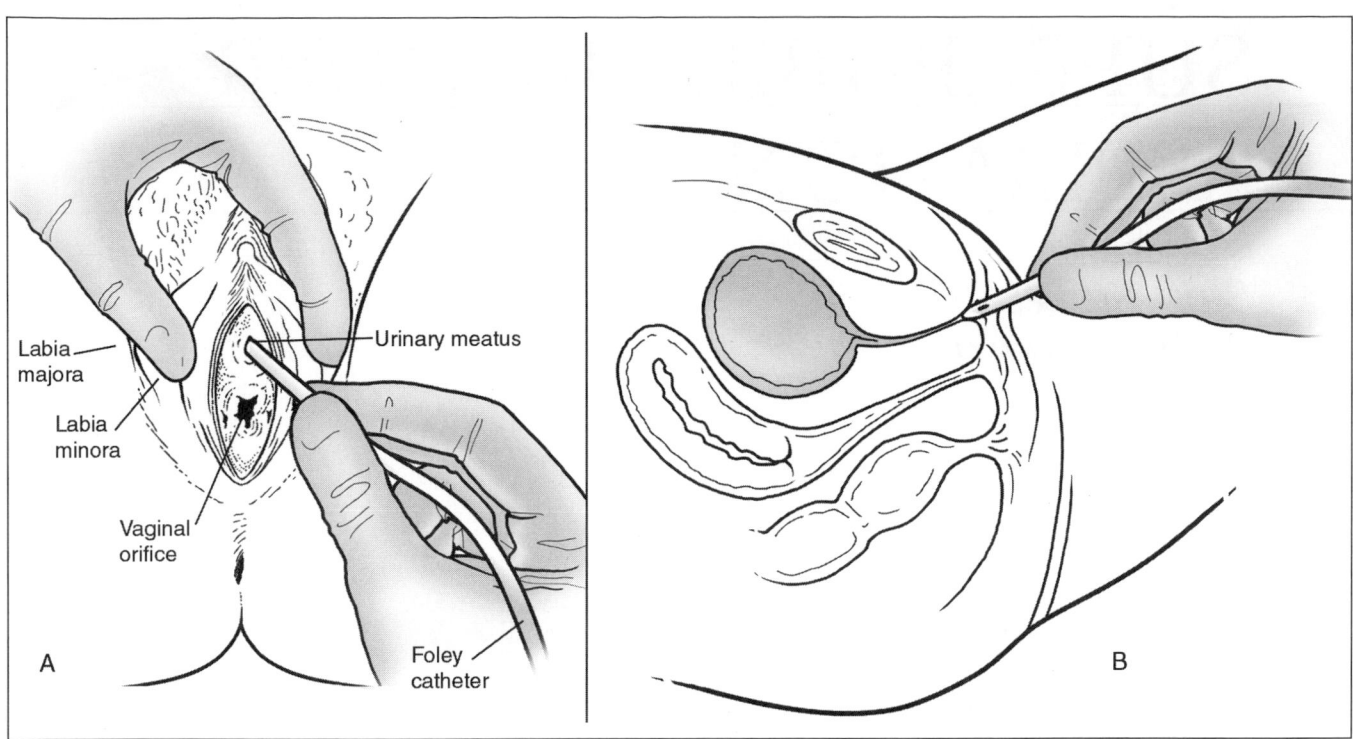

FIGURE 121-11 Female urethral catheterization. *A*. External view of the genitalia. The catheter is inserted into the urethral meatus and advanced. *B*. Midsagittal section of the female pelvis demonstrating catheter insertion.

catheters should be versed in catheter care and have routine medical evaluations for catheter change and follow-up.

REFERENCES

1. Carter HB: Instrumentation and endoscopy, in Walsh PC, Retik AB, Vaughan ED, et al (eds): *Campbell's Urology,* 7th ed. Philadelphia: Saunders, 1998:159–169.

2. McAninch JW: Traumatic injuries of the urethra. *J Trauma* 1981; 21(4):291–297.

3. McCallum RW: The adult male urethra: normal anatomy, pathology, and method of urethrography. *Radiol Clin North Am* 1979; 17:227–244.

4. Wright EJ, Webster GD: Urethral stricture and disruption, in Graham SD Jr, Glenn JF, (eds): *Glenn's Urologic Surgery,* 5th ed. Philadelphia: Lippincott Williams and Wilkins, 1998:425–438.

5. Simon RR, Brenner BE: *Emergency Procedures and Techniques,* 3rd ed. Baltimore: Williams and Wilkins, 1994:366–379.

Chapter 122
SUPRAPUBIC BLADDER ASPIRATION

Sam Stokes, III
Anita Kulkarni

INTRODUCTION

Suprapubic bladder aspiration is the introduction of a needle through the anterior abdominal wall and into the bladder to obtain a urine specimen under strict sterile technique. It is performed primarily to diagnose urinary tract infections.[1–5] It is most commonly performed in children under the age of 2 years as part of the septic work-up. The procedure is quick, simple to perform, safe, and has a low rate of complications. The main advantage of suprapubic bladder aspiration is that it bypasses the urethra and minimizes the risk of obtaining a contaminated urine specimen.

Urinary sampling remains the cornerstone for the diagnosis of many disease processes including metabolic derangements, infectious processes, catabolic states, and neoplastic conditions. In cases when the usual means of voided urine collection or bladder drainage is not possible or preferable, suprapubic bladder aspiration becomes a viable option both therapeutically and diagnostically. If properly performed, this technique can yield an uncontaminated urine sample without urethral or skin flora contamination.

ANATOMY AND PATHOPHYSIOLOGY

The urinary bladder of the neonate and infant begins as an abdominal organ (Figure 122-1A). As the child grows the pelvis enlarges and the bladder migrates down into the pelvis. The bladder eventually assumes its retropubic position that is maintained throughout life (Figure 122-1B).

The anatomic knowledge required to perform this procedure is minimal. The pubic symphysis is in the midline and forms the anterior border of the bony pelvis. The bladder resides posterior and superior to the pubic symphysis in the young child. The needle will pass through the skin and subcutaneous tissue of the lower abdominal wall, the rectus sheath, the peritoneum, and the bladder wall.

The adult urinary bladder resides behind the pubic symphysis and has both retroperitoneal and intraperitoneal attachments (Figure 122-1B). A working knowledge of this anatomy makes percutaneous bladder manipulation both safe and possible. The rectum lies just inferior and posterior to the urinary bladder. This relationship must be kept in mind when attempting percutaneous access. The bladder dome has peritoneal attachments and access in this area carries the potential for bowel injury and intraperitoneal bladder perforation.

Multiple major vascular structures, including the common iliac and hypogastric vessels, reside in the bony pelvis alongside the bladder. These structures are lateral to the bladder and eccentric percutaneous access may result in troublesome hemorrhage.

INDICATIONS

Suprapubic bladder aspiration is the preferred method of urinary sampling and drainage in instances where voided specimens are undesirable or unattainable, and when urethral catheterization is not technically possible or contraindicated.[1–5] It offers the exam-

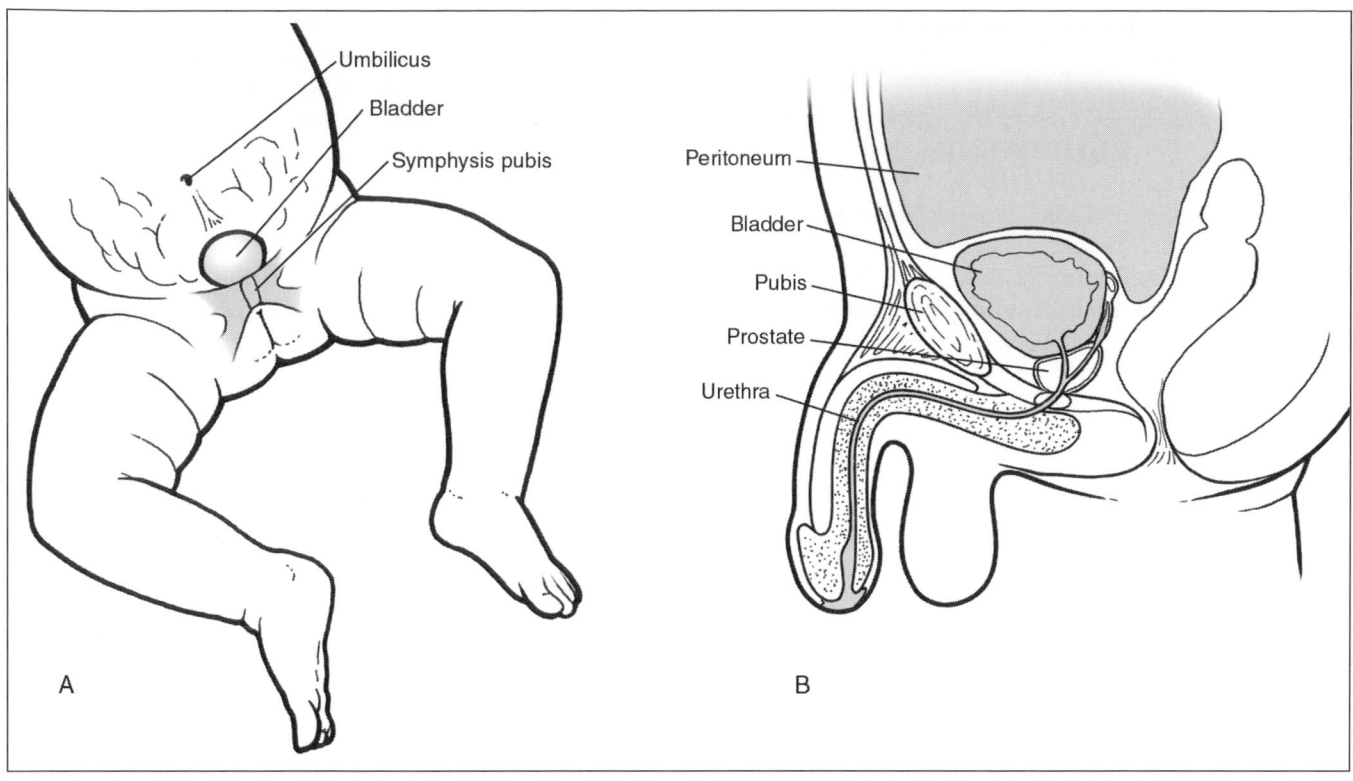

FIGURE 122-1 Position of the bladder. *A.* The bladder is an abdominal organ in the neonate and infant. *B.* The bladder is a pelvic organ in the older child, adolescent, and adult.

iner a viable means of obtaining an uncontaminated urine sample from the bladder. Obtaining a urine sample by urethral catheterization in the neonate or young child may be technically difficult, in which case suprapubic aspiration is a viable alternative. Although urethral catheterization may be an easier method of urine collection in the child or adult, suprapubic aspiration may be required to isolate infravesicular infections, to rule out contamination with asymptomatic bacturia, or in cases of urinary retention from a phimosis. The procedure may be performed to temporarily relieve acute urinary retention.

CONTRAINDICATIONS

The single most important aspect of suprapubic bladder manipulation is the presence of a palpable and distended urinary bladder. Under no circumstances should "blind" percutaneous access be attempted if the bladder is not palpable or visualized with the aid of ultrasonography.

Any physical alteration, spinal deformities, extremity contractures, truncal obesity, or other conditions that would preclude patients from lying supine and inhibiting bladder palpation are contraindications to this procedure. Skin infections overlying the puncture site are a contraindication to bladder aspiration. Abnormalities in genitourinary anatomy or enlargement of pelvic structures (ovarian cysts, uterine fibroids) increase the chance of complications with bladder aspiration. Similarly, distention or enlargement of the abdominal viscera can increase complication rates.

Patients with a coagulopathy are at an increased risk for troublesome hemorrhage from any percutaneous procedure, including suprapubic bladder access. Patients with a bleeding diathesis, anticoagulant therapy, or thrombocytopenia should be corrected prior to performing the procedure. In individuals with prior abdominal surgery, the peritoneal cavity has been violated and the bowel may be displaced more caudal and extend to the level of the urinary bladder. This heightens the risk of inadvertent bowel injury. The procedure should not be performed in patients with abdominal distention or the suspicion of an intestinal obstruction. An uncooperative patient should be sedated and/or restrained for the procedure.

EQUIPMENT

22 to 24 gauge spinal needle, 2 inches and 3 inches
10 mL syringe
Povidone iodine solution
Injectable local anesthetic solution, most commonly 1% lidocaine
4×4 gauze squares
25 gauge needle and 3 mL syringe for anesthetic administration
Sterile towels or drapes
Sterile gloves
Specimen containers for urine analysis and culture
Bandage

PATIENT PREPARATION

Explain the risks, benefits, and alternative procedures to the patient and/or their representative. Obtain an informed consent for the procedure and place this in the medical record. When performing the procedure on a neonate or child, it is advisable to give the parent the option to leave the room or look away as the procedure can be disconcerting to some parents.

It is important to identify the distended bladder by palpation, percussion, or ultrasonography. Transillumination of the full bladder may be conducted in the neonate. Place the patient supine (Figure 122-2). Prepare and drape the abdomen in a sterile fashion from the umbilicus to the pubis. Inject a local anesthetic agent, usually 1% lidocaine, to raise a subcutaneous wheal in the area of the intended skin puncture site. Many consider this step to be optional in the neonate as the amount of discomfort caused by placement of the anesthetic is similar to the actual puncture for bladder aspiration. Slight alterations in technique are required for the suprapubic bladder aspiration of the infant, child, and adult.

TECHNIQUES

INFANTS

Have an assistant place and hold the infant supine in the frog-leg position (Figure 122-2A). Clean any dirt and debris from the abdominal wall. Apply povidone iodine solution to the lower abdomen and allow it to dry. Identify the needle insertion site in the midline and 2 cm cephalad to the pubic symphysis (Figure 122-3). Inject 1 mL of local anesthetic solution subcutaneously and into the abdominal wall musculature at the needle insertion site.

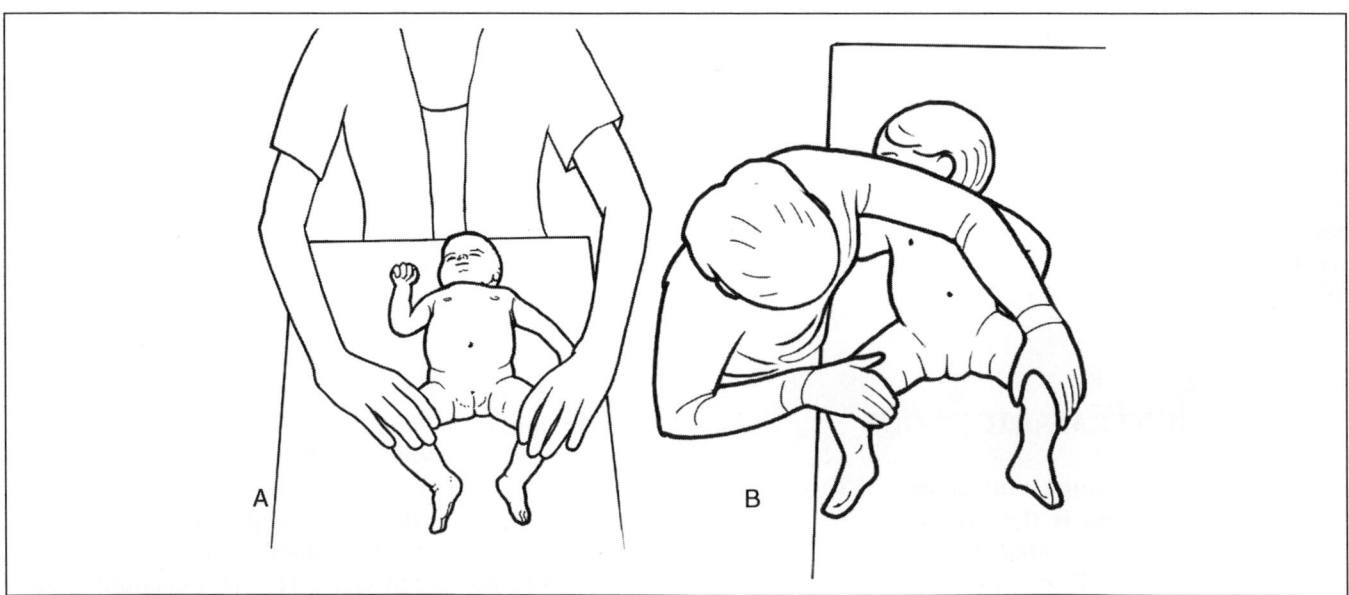

FIGURE 122-2 The frog-leg position. *A.* The infant. *B.* The older child.

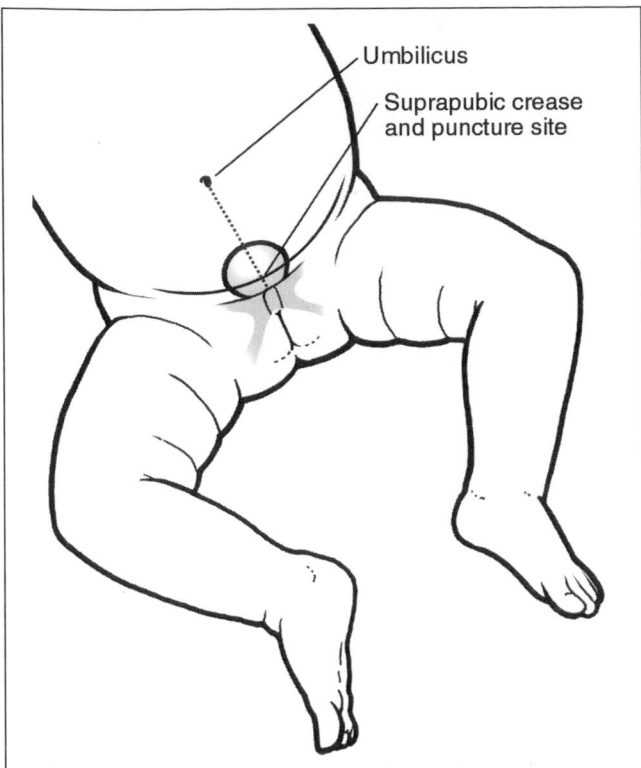

FIGURE 122-3 Anatomical landmarks for suprapubic bladder aspiration in the infant. A line is drawn from the umbilicus to the pubic symphysis (dotted line). The intersection of the line with the suprapubic crease is the landmark for insertion of the needle.

Place a 2 to 3 inch, 24 gauge spinal needle onto a 10 mL syringe. Occlude the urethra to prevent reflexive micturition. Apply manual pressure to the urethral meatus of the female (Figure 122-4A) or the glans penis in the male (Figure 122-4B). Insert the needle through the insertion site and at a 20 degree angle from the true perpendicular to the skin (Figure 122-4). Advance the needle cephalad while applying negative pressure to the syringe. Stop advancing the syringe when urine is aspirated. If no urine is aspirated, withdraw the needle to the subcutaneous tissue and readvance it in a slightly different direction (0 to 10 degrees to the true perpendicular). If the procedure is unsuccessful on the second attempt, delay further attempts until the bladder is more distended, consult a Urologist, or obtain urine through urethral catheterization. After urine is obtained, remove the needle and apply a bandage to the puncture site.

OLDER CHILDREN

The positioning of the older child is similar to that of the neonate or infant (Figure 122-2B). The procedure is similar to that of the infant, although it is more important to identify the location of the distended bladder to assure a successful aspiration. The urinary bladder of the older child may be in the abdomen or may have migrated into the pelvis.

ADULTS

Place the patient supine. Identify the bladder by palpation or ultrasonography. Clean any dirt and debris from the abdominal wall. Apply povidone iodine solution to the lower abdomen and allow it to dry. Apply sterile drapes to delineate a sterile field. Identify the needle insertion site in the midline and 2 to 4 cm cephalad to the pubic symphysis. Inject 1 to 3 mL of local anesthetic solution subcutaneously and into the abdominal wall musculature at the needle insertion site.

Place a 3 inch, 22 to 24 gauge spinal needle onto a 10 mL syringe. Insert the needle through the insertion site and at a 60 degree angle to the skin of the abdominal wall (Figure 122-5). Advance the needle caudally while applying negative pressure to the syringe. Stop advancing the needle when urine is aspirated. If no urine is aspirated, withdraw the needle to the subcutaneous tissue and readvance it in a slightly different direction (50 degrees to the skin of the abdominal wall). After urine is obtained, remove the needle and apply a bandage to the puncture site.

ASSESSMENT

If the first attempt at aspiration is unsuccessful, withdraw the needle to a subcutaneous position and redirect it at a different angle. This should be done only if the bladder is clearly identified. If the procedure is unsuccessful on the second attempt, the procedure should be delayed until the bladder is more distended. A urologic consult may also be necessary.

AFTERCARE

No specific care is required after performing a suprapubic bladder aspiration. **Microscopic hematuria can occur following the procedure although gross hematuria is uncommon.** The patient may complain of mild pain or soreness in the suprapubic area. This can be relieved with acetaminophen or nonsteroidal anti-inflammatory drugs. The patient, if discharged, should be given specific instructions to return immediately if they develop abdominal pain, fever, nausea, vomiting, or infection at the puncture site.

COMPLICATIONS

Numerous complications can be associated with suprapubic bladder aspiration. Fortunately, these are

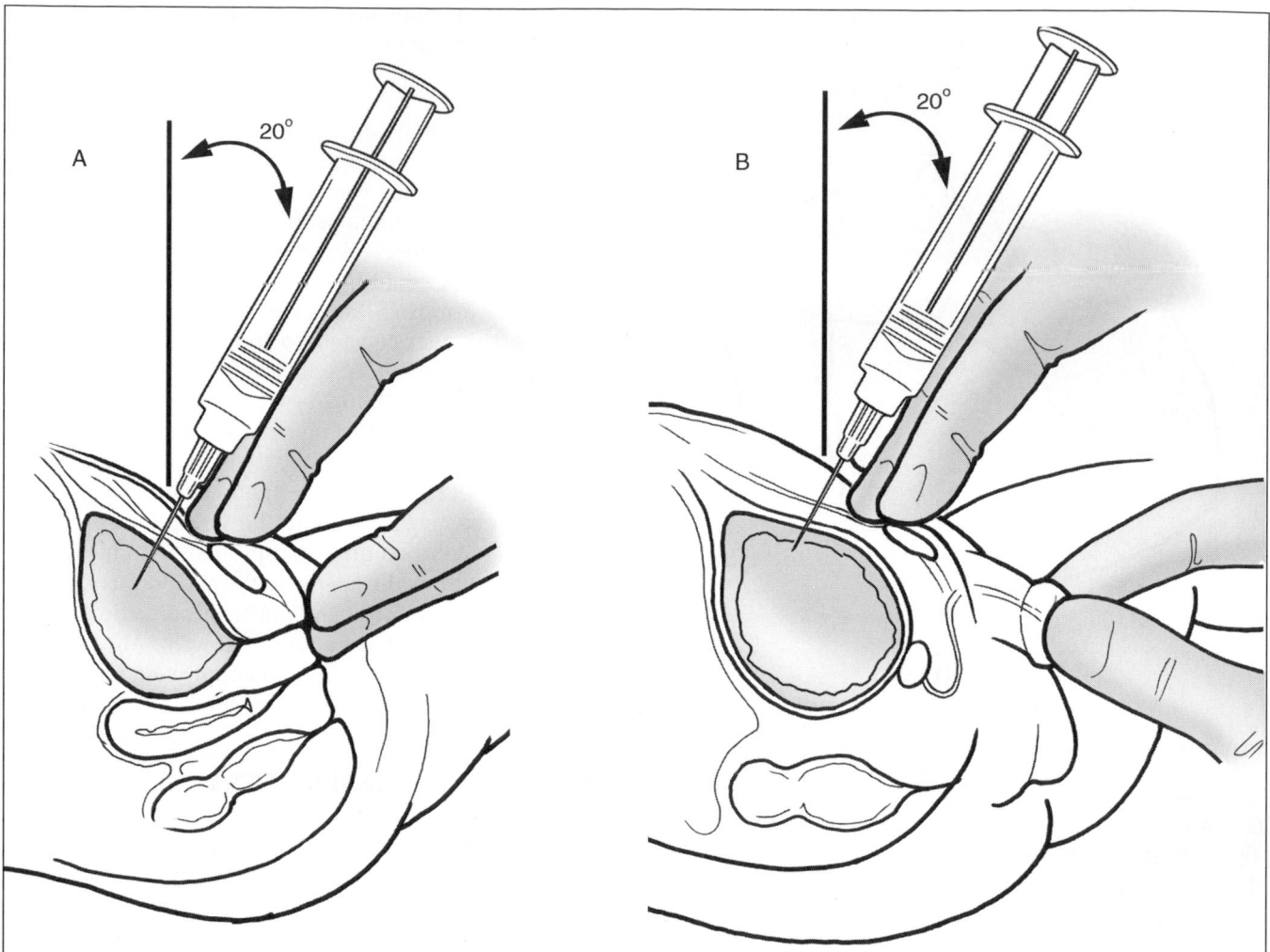

FIGURE 122-4 Suprapubic bladder aspiration in the infant. *A*. Digital pressure on the urethral meatus will prevent micturition in the female. *B*. Digital pressure on the glans penis will prevent micturition in the male.

rare occurrences. Bowel perforation, intraabdominal viscera injury, uncontrolled hemorrhage, and needle misplacement are the major complications of suprapubic bladder aspiration. Infectious complications include abdominal wall cellulitis, abdominal wall abscess, sepsis, and peritonitis. Hematomas of the abdominal wall, bladder wall, and pelvis are usually self-limited and require no treatment.

In the unfortunate situation when bowel contents or continuous blood is aspirated, the appropriate surgical consultant should be contacted. Generally, simple penetration of the bowel is considered harmless and requires no specific treatment. Observe the patient for the development of signs and symptoms of peritonitis.

To avoid complications, it is key that the bladder be clearly identified prior to inserting the spinal needle. The use of strict septic technique should avoid most infectious complications. Delaying the procedure for in-

fants who have urinated within the last hour and the correction of any bleeding diathesis before performing the procedure can help avoid complications.

SUMMARY

In those clinical situations when transurethral urine collection is not desired or possible, suprapubic bladder aspiration is an alternative. A thorough understanding of the pelvic and abdominal anatomy, along with a complete history and physical examination, is necessary to assure patient safety and avoid complications. This procedure is safe and effective to obtain urine as long as the bladder can be properly identified by palpation, percussion, or ultrasonography. Suprapubic bladder aspiration provides urine that is free from urethral contamination.

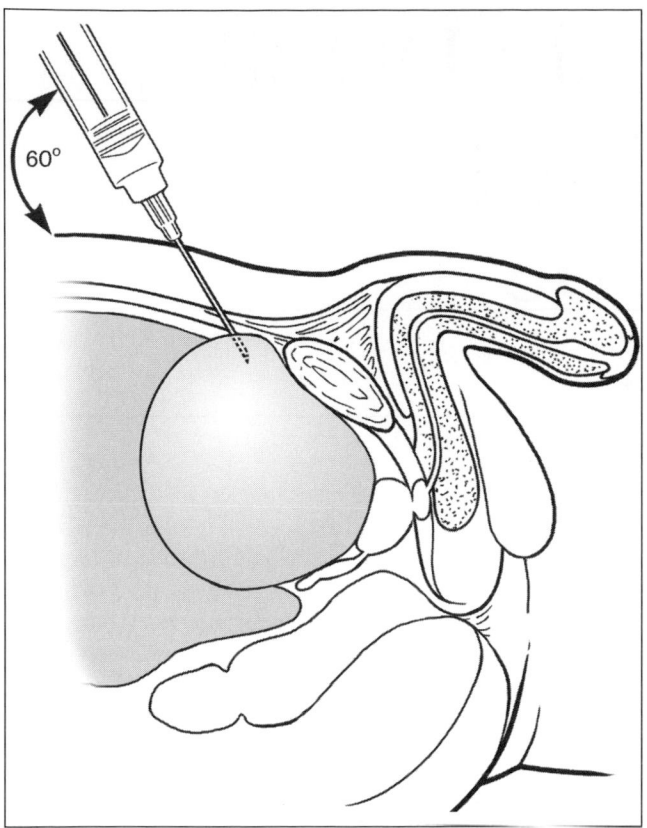

FIGURE 122-5 Suprapubic bladder aspiration in the adult.

REFERENCES

1. Carter HB: Instrumentation and endoscopy, in Walsh PC, Retik AB, Vaughan ED, et al (eds): Campbell's Urology, 7th ed. Philadelphia: Saunders 1998:159–169.
2. Newman CGH, O'Neil P, Parker A: Pyuria in infancy, and the role of suprapubic aspiration of urine in diagnosis of infection of urinary tract. Br Med J 1967; 2:227–279.
3. Schaeffer AJ: Infections of the urinary tract, in Walsh PC, Retik AB, Vaughan ED, et al (eds): Campbell's Urology, 7th ed. Philadelphia: Saunders 1998:533–614.
4. Stamey TA: The prevention of recurrent urinary tract infection. New York: Science and Medicine, 1973.
5. Stoller, ML: Retrograde instrumentation of the urinary tract, in Tanago EA, McAninch JW (eds): Smith's General Urology, 14th ed. Stamford, CT: Simon and Schuster 1995:160–171.

Chapter 123

SUPRAPUBIC BLADDER CATHETERIZATION (PERCUTANEOUS CYSTOSTOMY)

Sam Stokes, III
Daniel Wu

INTRODUCTION

Complaints involving the lower genitourinary system are among the most common urologic problems encountered by the Emergency Physician. The collection and evaluation of urine plays a critical role in the process of diagnosis and treatment. Volitional voiding and transurethral urinary catheterization are the preferred methods of bladder drainage and can be accomplished in most instances. There are situations when the transurethral route is contraindicated or technically not possible and alternate avenues must be explored. A percutaneous approach to urinary bladder drainage and decompression becomes the solution, offering both therapeutic and diagnostic results.[1–6] Suprapubic bladder catheterization has been used for decades as an effective means of accessing the bladder.

Suprapubic bladder catheterization, or percutaneous cystostomy, has become the treatment of choice for the patient with acute urinary retention regardless of the cause. It is commonly performed in the trauma patient with a known or suspected urethral injury. The catheters are well tolerated, easy to care for, and can easily be replaced and/or removed. The placement of a suprapubic catheter into the bladder is fast and may be performed under local anesthesia. It is a relatively safe procedure but does have potential complications that are significant.

ANATOMY AND PATHOPHYSIOLOGY

Residing in the retropubic space approximately 5 cm above the superior margin of the symphysis pubis, the adult urinary bladder has both retroperitoneal and intraperitoneal attachments. A working knowledge of this anatomy makes percutaneous bladder manipulation both safe and possible. The rectum lies just inferior and posterior to the urinary bladder and this relationship must be kept in mind when attempting percutaneous access. The bladder dome has peritoneal attachments and access in this area carries a risk of bowel injury and intraperitoneal bladder perforation.

Multiple vascular structures, including the common iliac and hypogastric vessels, reside in the bony pelvis alongside the bladder. These structures are lateral to the bladder and eccentric percutaneous access may result in troublesome hemorrhage.

INDICATIONS

Suprapubic bladder catheterization is indicated in cases when the transurethral route of bladder drainage or decompression is technically not possible or contraindicated. This includes patients with iatrogenic urethral injuries, obstructing urethral lesions, bladder neck lesions, enlarged prostates (benign hypertrophy or cancer), urethral strictures, urethral scarring, an obstructing phimosis, a urethral foreign body, and a suspected or known traumatic urethral or prostatic disruption. Continuous bladder irrigation can be accomplished via a combined suprapubic and transurethral route.

CONTRAINDICATIONS

The single most important aspect of suprapubic bladder manipulation is the presence of a palpable

and distended urinary bladder and under no circumstances should "blind" percutaneous access be attempted. The bladder must be distended to push the bowel away from the anterosuperior surface of the bladder.

Patients with a coagulopathy are at an increased risk for troublesome hemorrhage from any percutaneous procedure, including suprapubic bladder access. Any coagulopathy, bleeding diathesis, platelet dysfunction, and/or thrombocytopenia should be corrected prior to performing this procedure.

In individuals with prior lower abdominal surgery or traumatic injury, the peritoneal cavity has been violated and the bowel may be displaced more caudal and to the level of the urinary bladder. The bowel may be adhesed to the anterior abdominal wall. This heightens the risk of inadvertent entry into the peritoneal cavity and injury to the bowel.

Relative contraindications to percutaneous bladder catheterization include patients who have a history of pelvic cancer or pelvic radiation therapy, ascites, urinary tract infections, or who are uncooperative. A history of pelvic cancer or irradiation will increase the risk of anatomical distortion, adhesions, and scarring. Attempts at suprapubic cystostomy increase the risk of peritoneal and/or bowel perforation. The return of ascitic fluid may lead the physician to a false sense of security when the catheter is actually intraperitoneal. Urine leakage in patients with a urinary tract infection may result in bacteremia, peritonitis, and/or sepsis. In these circumstances, consult a Urologist for an open suprapubic cystostomy or a Radiologist for a percutaneous cystostomy using fluoroscopic or ultrasonic guidance. An uncooperative patient will require parenteral sedation or procedural sedation prior to performing this procedure.

Any physical alteration, spinal deformities, extremity contractures, truncal obesity, or other conditions that would preclude patients from lying supine and inhibiting bladder palpation are also contraindications to performing a percutaneous cystostomy.

EQUIPMENT

Percutaneous cystostomy catheter kit
Foley catheter, 14 to 16 French
60 mL catheter-tipped syringe
10 mL syringes
24 to 25 gauge spinal needle, 3 inches long
#11 Surgical scalpel blade on a handle
3–0 nylon suture
Needle driver
Povidone iodine solution
Local anesthetic solution, 1% lidocaine

4×4 gauze squares
25 gauge needle, 1 inch long
18 gauge needle
Urine meter or urine leg bag
Sterile towels
Sterile gloves
Sterile drapes
Tincture of benzoin
2 inch tape
Ultrasound machine (optional)

The percutaneous cystostomy catheter kit is commercially available and prepackaged by several manufacturers. One type contains a cystostomy tube, an obturator, and connector tubing (Figures 123-1, 123-2, and 123-4). Another type uses a Seldinger-type kit with a peel-away sheath (Figure 123-3).

A commonly used suprapubic catheter kit is the Rutner Percutaneous Suprapubic Balloon Catheter Set (Cook Urological Inc., Spencer, IN). It consists of a 10 French catheter that is 22 cm long, a needle obturator, a connecting tube, and a 3 mL syringe (Figures 123-1 and 123-2A). The proximal end of the catheter has two ports (Figures 123-1 and 123-2B). One port is for the insertion of the obturator through the catheter. The obturator screws and locks into this port. The other port is an inflation port for the cuff of the catheter. A 3 to 5 mL syringe attaches to this port. The obturator is a hollow tube that tapers to a sharp point distally. When properly inserted and locked into the port, the obturator will project 2.5 mm from the distal end of the catheter (Figures 123-1C and 123-2C). The cuff is donut-shaped and centered 1 cm from the tip of the catheter (Figure 123-2D). The connector tube has a stopcock at its distal end that attaches to the catheter (Figure 123-2E). The proximal end of the connector tube has a flared flange to attach to a urine drainage system.

PATIENT PREPARATION

As with all procedures, the risks and benefits of suprapubic bladder catheterization should be discussed with the patient and/or their representative. Obtain an informed consent and place it in the medical record.

Place the patient supine. Clean any dirt and debris from the abdominal wall. Shave the lower abdomen if the patient is hirsute. Identify the bladder by palpation, percussion, and/or ultrasonography. Apply povidone iodine solution to the lower abdomen, from the umbilicus to the pubis, and allow it to dry. Consider the administration of parenteral analgesics, sedatives, or procedural sedation as this is a painful procedure.

Anesthetize the abdominal wall. Fill a 10 mL syringe with local anesthetic solution. Apply a 24 to 25 gauge spinal needle onto the syringe. Identify the insertion site

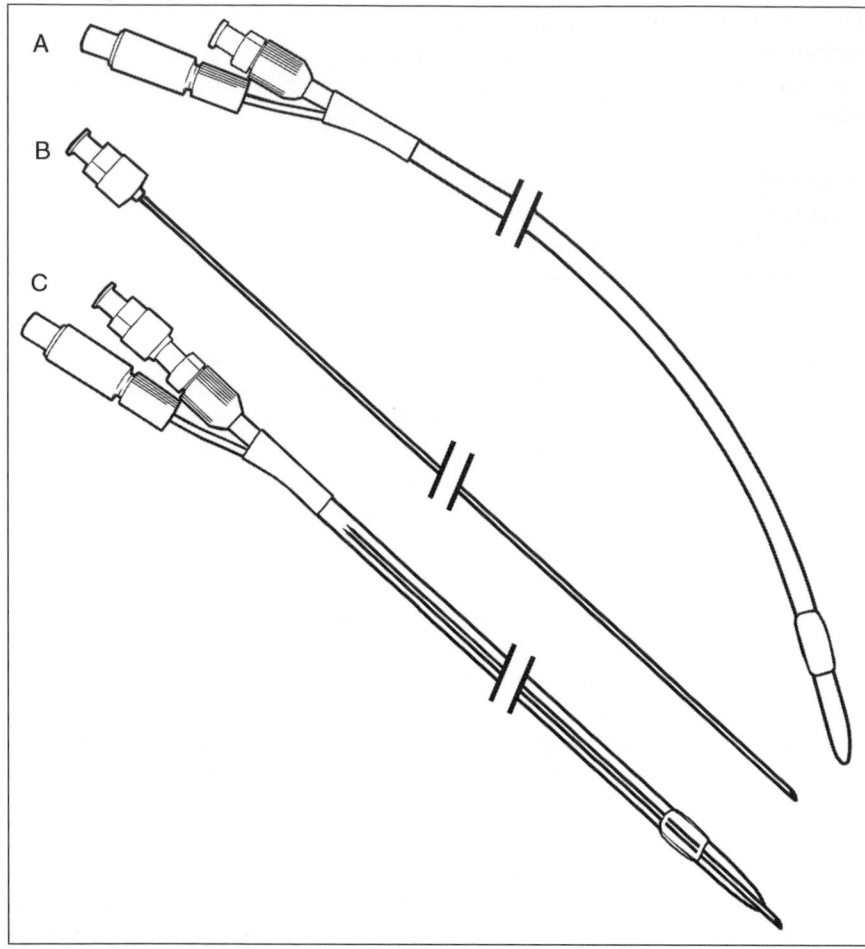

FIGURE 123-1 Schematic of a catheter and obturator system. *A.* The catheter. *B.* The obturator. *C.* The obturator within the catheter.

in the midline and 4 to 5 cm above the pubic symphysis. Make a skin wheal with the local anesthetic solution at the insertion site. Insert the spinal needle at a 20 to 30 degree angle from true vertical and aimed caudally (Figure 123-3*A*). Advance the needle through the subcutaneous tissue, rectus sheath, and retropubic space while simultaneously aspirating and injecting 5 to 10 mL of local anesthetic solution. A loss of resistance will be felt as the spinal needle traverses the rectus sheath and enters the retropubic space. Continue to aspirate while advancing the spinal needle until the bladder is entered and urine fills the syringe. **Note the needle direction and depth of insertion required to enter the bladder.**

TECHNIQUES

SELDINGER TECHNIQUE WITH A PEEL-AWAY SHEATH

This method is similar to that of placing a central venous catheter. The needle is used to locate the bladder. Place the needle on a 10 mL syringe. Insert the needle

through the skin wheal located in the midline and 4 to 5 cm above the pubic symphysis. Direct the needle caudally and at a 20 to 30 degree angle from the true vertical (Figure 123-3*A*). **It is important to ensure that the needle enters, and is advanced, in the midline.** This area is avascular. If the needle is paramedian, it may traverse the rectus muscles and inferior epigastric vessels, and insertion may result in significant hemorrhage. Advance the needle caudally while applying negative pressure with the syringe. Stop advancing the needle when urine is aspirated into the syringe. Advance the needle an additional 2 to 3 cm into the bladder. The aspiration of urine will confirm the proper position of the needle within the bladder.

Firmly hold the needle against the abdominal wall. Carefully remove the syringe from the needle. **Do not allow the needle to move as it may shear the bladder wall.** Advance the guidewire through the needle and into the bladder (Figure 123-3*B*). Withdraw the needle over the guidewire while leaving the guidewire in place. Make a superficial stab incision with the #11 scalpel blade adjacent to the guidewire. This will facilitate passage of the dilator and sheath. Insert the dilator

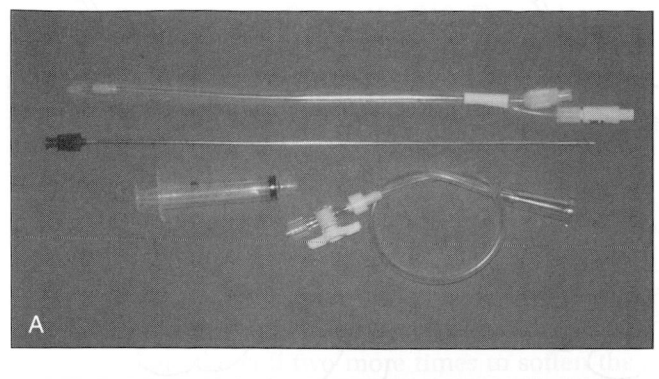
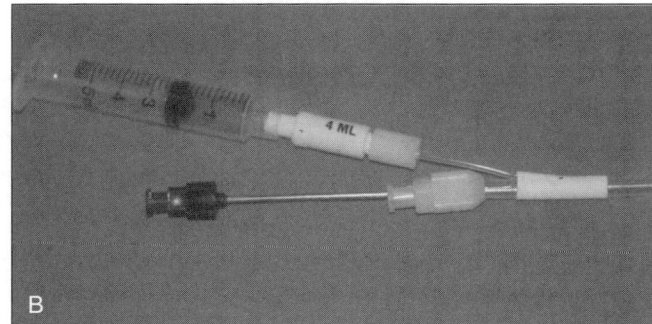
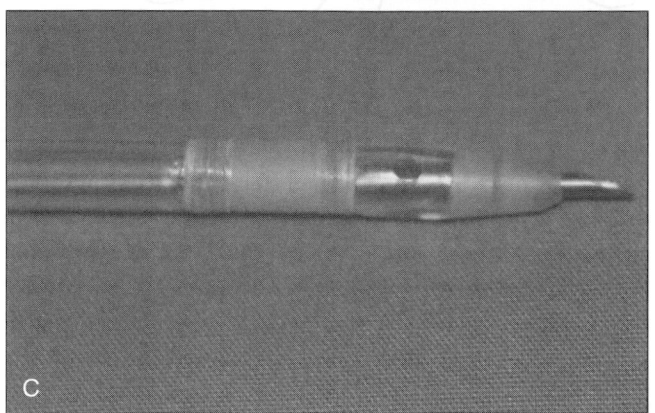
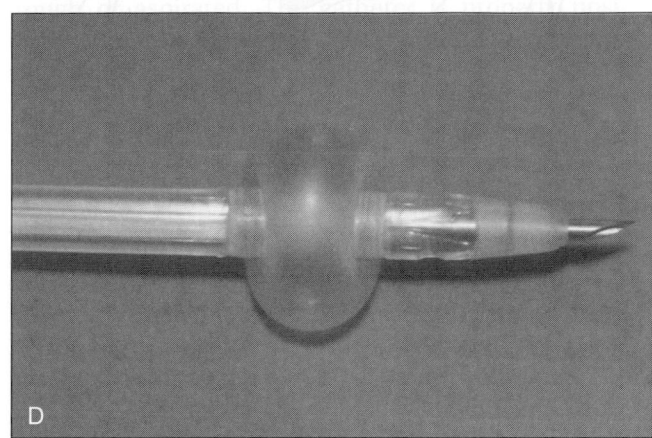
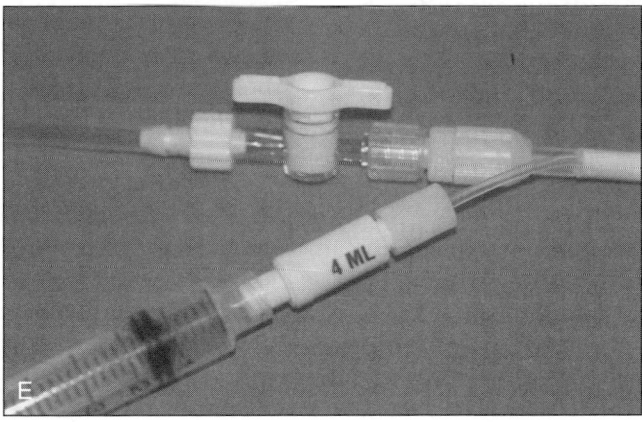

FIGURE 123-2 The Rutner Percutaneous Suprapubic Balloon Catheter Set (COOK Urological Inc., Spencer, IN). *A.* The equipment. *B.* The proximal catheter ports. *C.* The distal end of the catheter with the obturator properly inserted. *D.* The distal end of the catheter with the cuff inflated. *E.* The proximal end of the connector tube contains a stopcock to attach to the catheter. The distal end has a flared flange.

through the peel-away sheath. Advance the dilator and peel-away sheath as a unit over the guidewire and into the bladder (Figure 123-3*C*). Remove the guidewire and dilator as a unit (Figure 123-3*D*), leaving only the peel-away sheath (Figure 123-3*E*).

Insert a Foley catheter through the peel-away sheath and completely into the bladder (Figure 123-3*F*). The Foley catheter should be two sizes (2 French) smaller than the size of the peel-away sheath. Urine should

spontaneously flow from the Foley catheter. If not, insert a 60 mL catheter-tipped syringe into the Foley catheter and aspirate (Figure 123-3*G*). The flow of urine will confirm that the catheter is properly positioned within the bladder. Inflate the cuff of the Foley catheter. Attach a urine collection system to the proximal end of the Foley catheter (Figure 123-3*H*).

Remove the peel-away sheath. Grasp the free ends or arms of the peel-away sheath. Pull the free ends upward

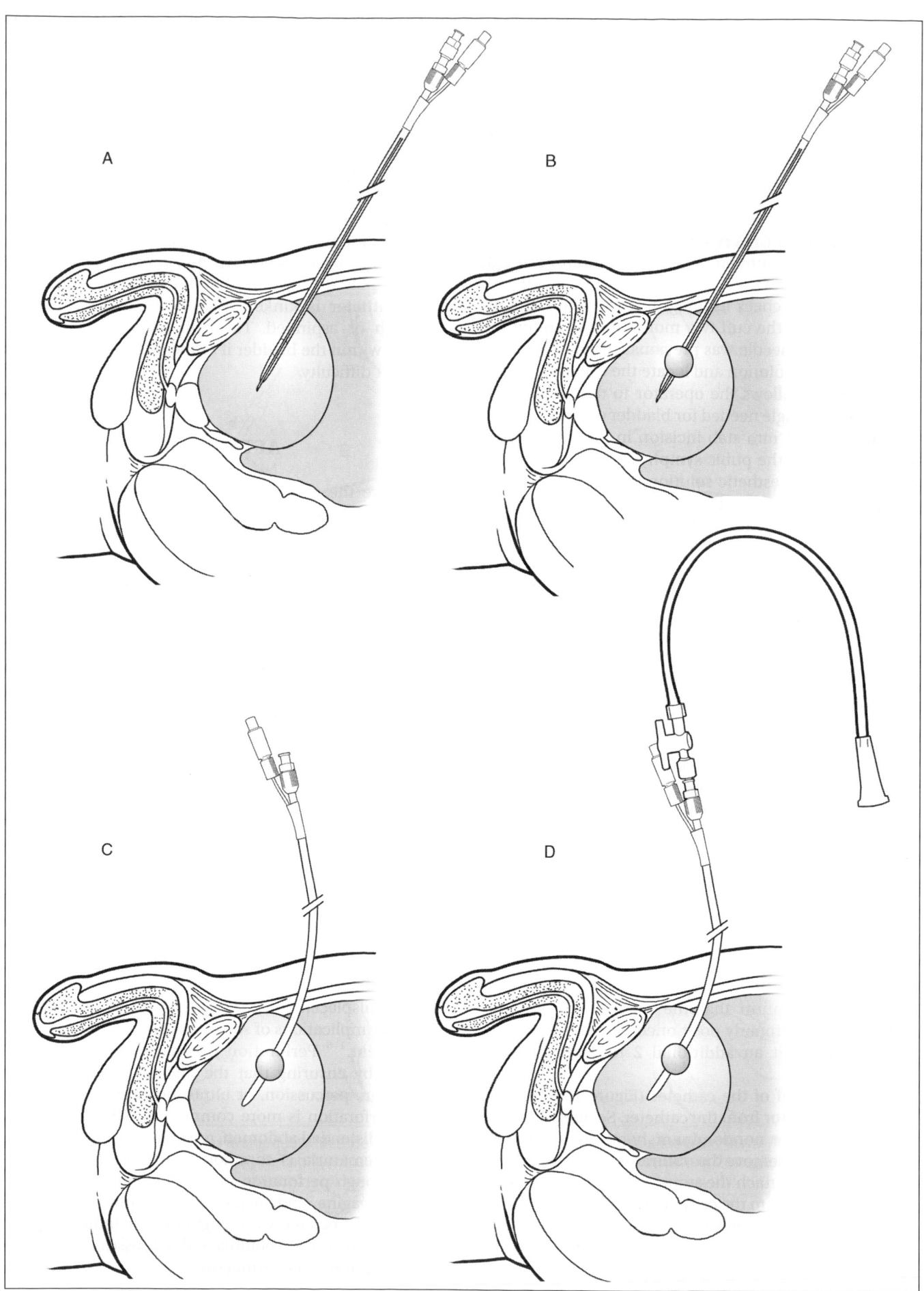

FIGURE 123-4 The obturator technique. *A.* The obturator is within the catheter. The system is inserted 60 degrees to the skin and advanced into the bladder. *B.* The balloon is inflated. *C.* The obturator is removed while the catheter remains within the bladder. *D.* The collecting tube is attached to the catheter.

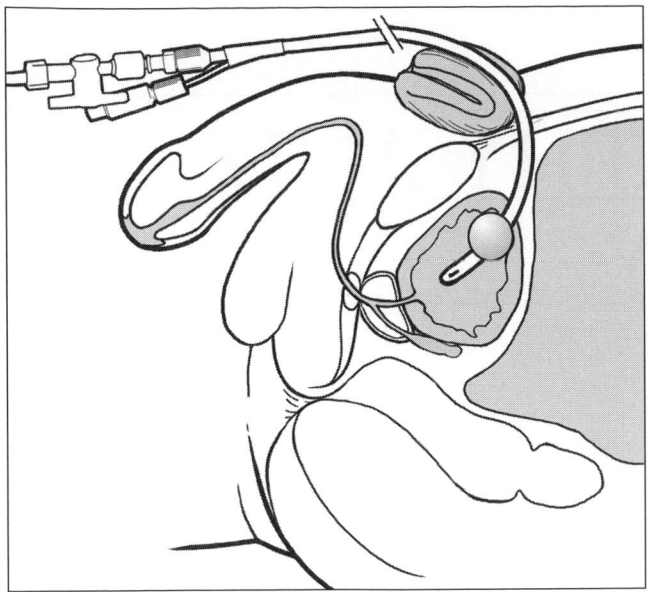

FIGURE 123-5 Secure the catheter. Place gauze squares on the skin to make a gentle curve in the catheter without kinks. Tape the catheter to the abdominal wall.

When catheter placement is in doubt or when a previously draining tube no longer continues to drain, simple flushing and irrigation will usually suffice. However, if concern persists, a gravity cystogram under fluoroscopy is diagnostic. In the unfortunate situation when bowel contents or continuous blood is aspirated or flows from the catheter, the appropriate surgical consultations should be obtained.

SUMMARY

In those clinical situations when transurethral bladder decompression is no longer an option, percutaneous access is the preferred alternative. Although years of experience have demonstrated suprapubic bladder catheterization to be an effective and relatively safe method of accessing the bladder, as with any procedure, a prior understanding of the associated anatomy is paramount in the avoidance of adverse results.

REFERENCES

1. Blocksom BH Jr: Bladder pouch for prolonged tubeless cystostomy. J Urol 1957; 78:398–401.
2. Carter HB: Instrumentation and endoscopy, in Walsh PC, Retik AB, Vaughn ED, et al (eds): Campbell's Urology, 7th ed. Philadelphia: Saunders, 1998:159–169.
3. Papanicolaou N, Pfister RC, Nocks BN: Percutaneous, large-bore, suprapubic cystostomy: techniques and results. AJR Am J Roentgen 1989; 152:303–306.
4. Stroller ML: Retrograde instrumentation of the urinary tract, in Tanago EA, McAninch JW (eds): Smith's General Urology, 14th ed. Stamford, CT: Simon and Schuster, 1995:160–171.
5. Wright EJ, Webster GD: Urethral stricture and disruption, in Graham SD Jr, Glenn J, (eds): Glenn's Urologic Surgery, 5th ed. Philadelphia: Lippincott Williams and Wilkins, 1998:871–878.
6. Zdreic SA, Hanno PM: Suprapubic cystostomy and cutaneous vesicostomy, in Fowler JE (ed): Urologic Surgery. Boston: Little Brown, 1992:235–236.

Chapter 124
RETROGRADE URETHROGRAPHY AND CYSTOGRAPHY

Charles M. Lash
Paul S. Ray
Yanina Purim-Shem-Tov

INTRODUCTION

Urinary tract injuries may result from blunt trauma, penetrating trauma, urologic procedures, or may arise spontaneously. Bladder injuries occur in up to 15 percent of pelvic fractures.[1–3] Associated urethral injuries occur in up to 11 percent of males and up to 6 percent of females.[1–3] The role of retrograde urethrography and cystography in the trauma patient is to rule out a partial urethral rupture, complete urethral rupture, or a bladder rupture. On initial presentation to the Emergency Department there are clear indications for performing these procedures. The importance of proper training in these techniques must be stressed to avoid secondary urologic complications.

The evaluation of a traumatically injured patient should include, if appropriate, an assessment of the bony pelvis and the genitourinary system. The identification of a pelvic fracture must be followed by an examination of the lower genitourinary tract to rule out associated injury. Unfortunately, the lack of a pelvic fracture does not eliminate the possibility of a bladder or urethral injury. The most common signs seen in patients with genitourinary tract injury are gross hematuria (82 percent) and abdominal tenderness (62 percent).[4] Other signs of genitourinary tract injury include blood at the urethral meatus, inability to void, swelling or ecchymosis of the perineum or penis, a boggy prostate, and a high riding prostate. In the presence of any of these signs, an evaluation of the genitourinary tract is indicated. These assessments should be made early and intervention instituted.

ANATOMY AND PATHOPHYSIOLOGY

The lower urinary tract in males consists of the urethra and bladder (Figure 124-1). The urethra is divided into the fossa navicularis, the penile urethra, the bulbar urethra, the membranous urethra, and the prostatic urethra based on its anatomic location. The bladder neck opens into the trigonal canal and funnels into the bladder. The male posterior urethra is 5.0 to 5.5 cm long, fixed to the urogenital diaphragm, and is the area most susceptible to injury.[2,5] The female urethra is short, not rigidly fixed to the pubis or pelvic floor, mobile, and much less susceptible to injury.[3] The female urethra is equivalent to the membranous and prostatic (posterior) urethra in the male.[6]

The periurethral striated sphincter is composed of muscle from the urogenital diaphragm. This muscle layer unites with the distal smooth muscle at the intermuscular incisura. This is frequently seen on the voiding cystourethrogram and may be mistaken for a stricture or posterior urethral valves. The urogenital diaphragm surrounds the membranous urethra and may compress the urethra during voiding or on retrograde flow of contrast.[6]

The verumontanum and urethral crest protrude into the male prostatic urethral lumen and may extend into the membranous urethra. The prostatic gland ducts, prostatic utricle, ejaculatory ducts, and urethral gland ducts usually do not fill on voiding cystourethrogram; and when present, fill usually denotes distal obstruction. These structures, however, may fill during aggressive injection of contrast during the retrograde urethrogram.

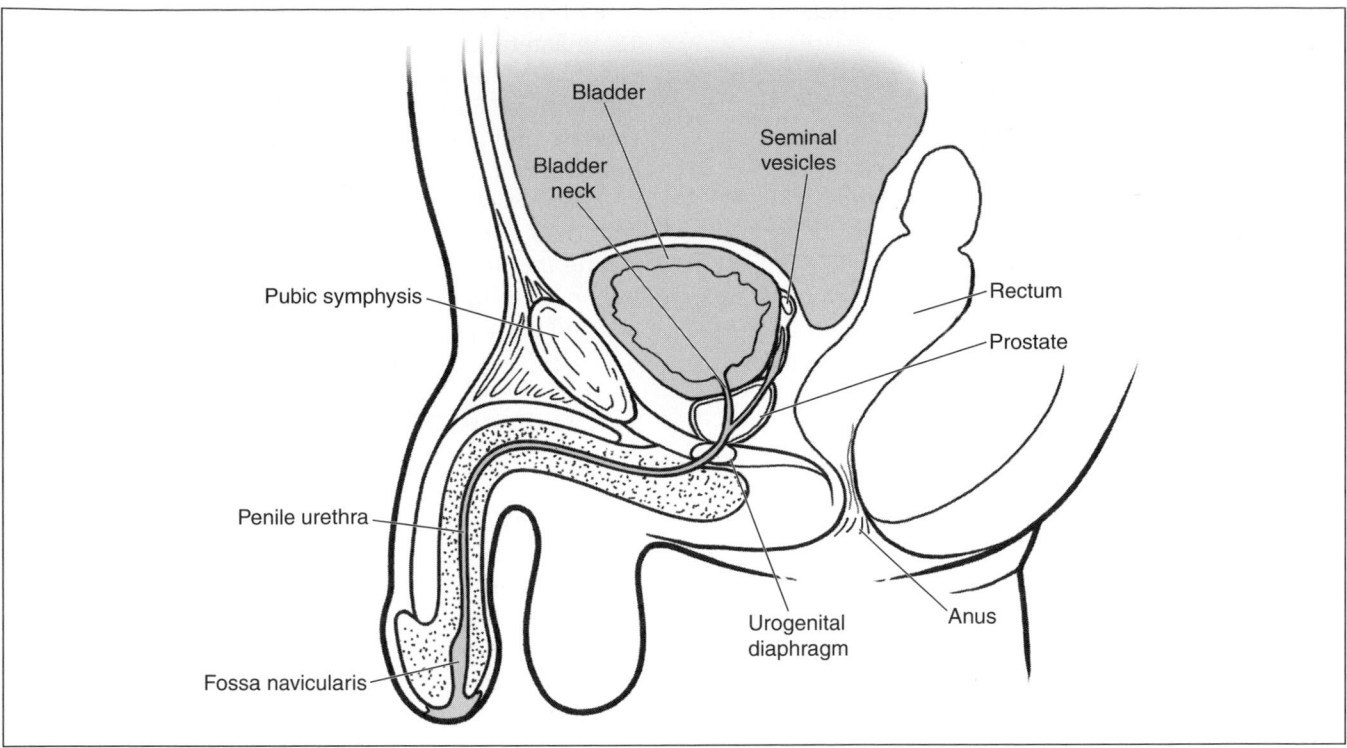

FIGURE 124-1 Anatomy of the male genitourinary tract.

On the lateral view of the bladder, the anterior and posterior baseplate (of which the trigone is part) is seen as a diagonal plane sloping downward from posterior to anterior. The bladder neck is visualized at the junction of the anterior one-third and the posterior two-thirds of the plane. Anteriorly, the pubis abuts the baseplate. The fundus of the bladder becomes more dome-shaped as it fills with fluid. It may be compressed by the uterus or colon in the midline or on either side.[6]

INDICATIONS

The retrograde urethrogram is to be employed in traumatic presentations when there is any indication of a urethral injury. Indications include penetrating injury when involvement of the lower genitourinary tract is suspected, pelvic fractures, perineal or lower abdominal trauma with gross hematuria, inability to void, swelling of the perineum or penis, ecchymosis of the perineum or penis, hematoma of the perineum or penis, a high riding prostate, or a boggy prostate.[7,8] Other indications include urethral strictures and obstructions, congenital abnormalities, periurethral or prostatic abscess, and fistulae or false passages. In females, it may be indicated if urethral diverticula are suspected.

Retrograde cystography should follow retrograde urethrography, especially in patients who recall having a full bladder at the time of trauma and are later unable to void or have small amounts of bloody urine.[9]

CONTRAINDICATIONS

There are few contraindications to retrograde urethrography and cystography. However, the patient's overall condition must be taken into consideration. The lifesaving procedures, such as securing an airway and stabilizing life- and limb-threatening injuries, must take precedence. Because septic shock and irreversible renal damage can occur, a relative contraindication in the setting of acute urethritis exists when the suspicion of genitourinary tract trauma is very low. **A urethral injury identified on the retrograde urethrogram is the only absolute contraindication to transurethral bladder catheterization and retrograde cystography.** A Urologist should be consulted if, in a patient with pelvic trauma, there is any difficulty in passing a urethral catheter into the bladder. **Do not try to advance a catheter against resistance as iatrogenic injury can result.** There is a small risk of allergic reactions to the contrast media. Patients with previous reactions should receive nonionic agents and be premedicated with corticosteroids and antihistamines.

EQUIPMENT

Povidone iodine solution
Sterile drapes
Viscous lidocaine suspension
Foley catheter, 12 to 16 French
Brodney clamp
Contrast material
60 mL catheter tip syringe
Toomey syringe
Christmas tree adaptor
Surgical clamp
Lead apron

A variety of contrast agents are available and may be used to perform retrograde urethrography and cystography. The agents used are specific to each institution. Most commonly used are full strength Hypaque (50% diatrizoate sodium), Renografin-60 (diatrizoate sodium), or Cystografin. Alternatively, the same agents can be diluted with sterile saline in a 1:10 dilution.

PATIENT PREPARATION

Explain the procedure, its risks, and benefits to the patient and/or their representative. While a formal consent is usually not obtained since this is an emergent procedure, document in the medical record that the "risks and benefits were explained to the patient." If not contraindicated, administer parenteral sedation. Place the patient in a 45 degree oblique position with their left side on the bed. Flex the left leg at the knee and abduct the hip. Place a radiolucent wedge or rolled towels under the patient to maintain the oblique position. Completely extend the right leg. This is the ideal patient position. The degree of patient mobility and the medical condition may dictate an alteration of this position.

Prepare the penis and urethra. Clean any dirt and debris from around the penis. Retract the foreskin if the patient is uncircumcised. Apply povidone iodine solution to the penis and allow it to dry. Apply sterile drapes to delineate a sterile field. The retrograde urethrogram must be performed under sterile conditions. **Insert viscous lidocaine into the urethral meatus to anesthetize the urethra. Do not use lidocaine jelly as this may impede the flow of contrast material.** Allow the lidocaine to remain in the urethra for 2 to 4 minutes prior to performing the procedure to provide adequate analgesia.

Obtain a flat plate or KUB (kidney, ureters, and bladder) radiograph. This will be a baseline film for future reference. Carefully examine the radiograph for curva-

ture of the spine, pelvic fractures, fractures of ribs 9 to 12, unilateral or bilateral loss of the normal psoas muscle shadow, or vertebral transverse process fractures. Any of these findings can signify a urinary tract injury. Observe and note any radiopaque material that may be present prior to the injection of contrast material.

The physician should dress appropriately for the procedure. Since the physician must be near the patient during the procedure and while radiographs are taken, put on a lead apron. Dress in a sterile gown and gloves. A cap and mask are not required.

RETROGRADE URETHROGRAPHY TECHNIQUES

FOLEY CATHETER TECHNIQUE

The Foley catheter technique is the preferred method. The Foley catheter causes little or no discomfort, is flexible, and the patient may be able to move if necessary. An advantage to using the Foley catheter is that it can subsequently be advanced into the bladder to perform the cystogram. The newer types of catheters have two cuffs; one at the tip and the other near the hub of the catheter. The proximal cuff will expand when the pressure in the distal cuff exceeds the maximum safe pressure during cuff inflation. This allows the excess pressure to be directed away from the distal cuff and not cause iatrogenic injury. There are some disadvantages to this method. The inflated cuff may conceal an injury of the distal urethra at the fossa navicularis. Air bubbles are difficult to eliminate from the catheter. This may impair the flow of the contrast material or produce artifacts due to air in the urethra. Air bubbles in the Foley catheter will alter the integrity of the study. Prime the tubing with contrast before inserting it into the urethra. Place an x-ray plate under the patient's hips and pelvis.

Insert the catheter into the urethra. Advance it until the cuff is within the fossa navicularis (Figure 124-2A). Inflate the cuff with approximately 3 mL of sterile saline, or to the point that it is snug and does not cause pain to the patient.[10] Gently straighten the urethra by directing the tip of the penis toward the dependent shoulder or nipple and over the thigh. Traction on the penis or catheter is discouraged as it tends to dislodge the catheter. Attach a contrast-filled syringe to the proximal end of the Foley catheter. Gently inject 50 to 60 mL of contrast material over 5 to 10 seconds.

Obtain a radiograph at or near the end of the injection. Have the film developed and review the image. The entire urethra should be visible in a lateral projection. The procedure should be repeated if this is not achieved. Allow the contrast to drain from the urethra through the Foley catheter and into a container. Deflate the cuff and remove the catheter from the urethra. Obtain an additional radiograph of the pelvis as a washout

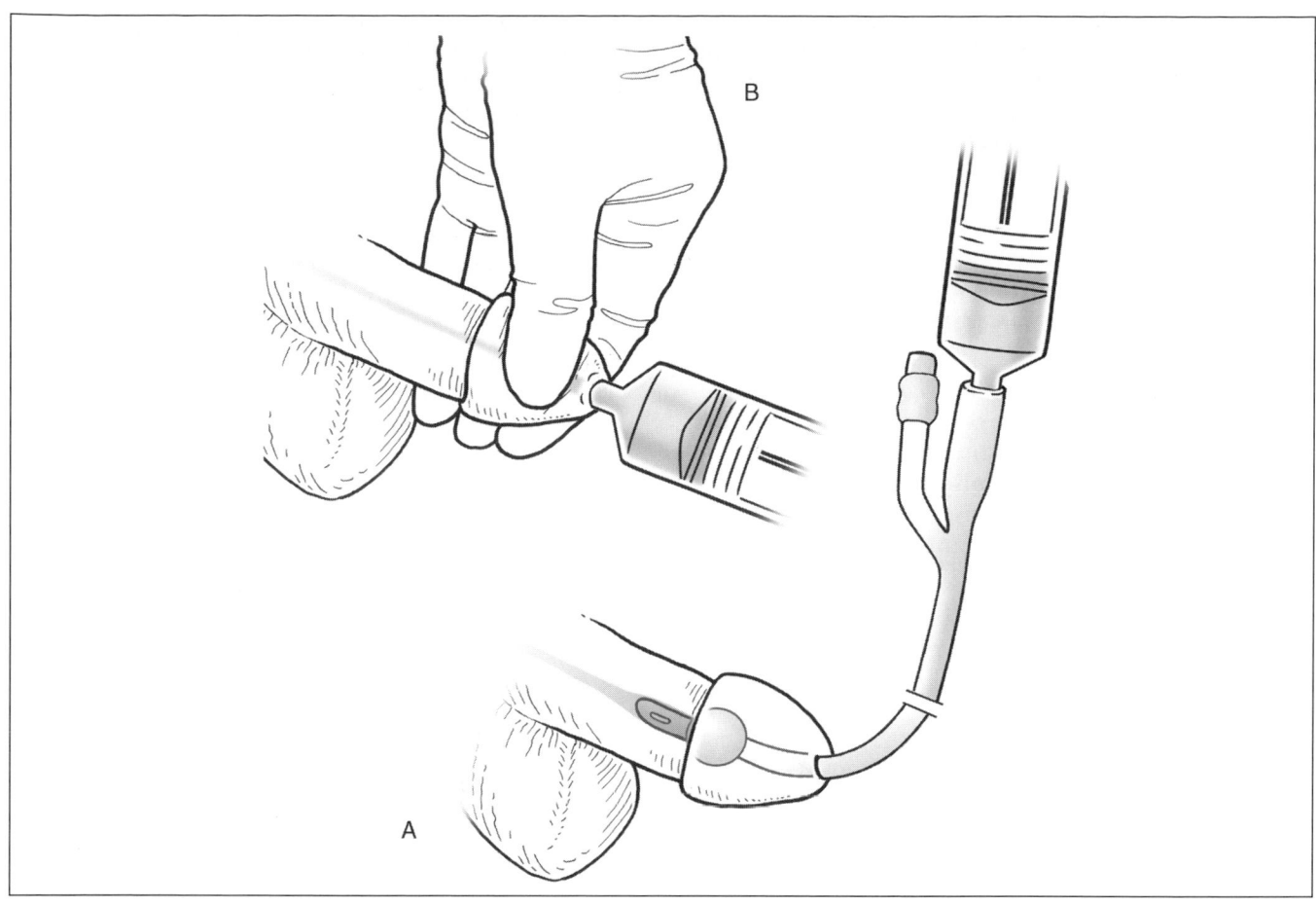

FIGURE 124-2 Retrograde urethrography. *A.* Foley catheter technique. *B.* Syringe technique.

image. Have the film developed and review the image for any abnormalities in the urethra. Although not necessary, fluoroscopy may aid in obtaining an adequate study.[10]

Great care should be taken so as not to allow any contrast to leak out of the catheter or urethra. Any spill of contrast material will cause distortions on the radiographs. The contrast may also cause skin irritation. It should be wiped and rinsed off the skin immediately if this occurs.

SYRINGE TECHNIQUE

If a proximal urethral injury is suspected, the alternative method is to use a 60 mL catheter-tipped Toomey syringe or a 60 mL syringe with a Christmas tree adaptor. Because it is not flexible and cannot be fixed inside the penis, the syringe must be held in place at all times during the procedure. The penile shaft must also be held to secure the tip of the syringe inside the urethra.

Clear, prep, and drape the penis as described previously. Place an x-ray plate under the patient's hips and pelvis. Grasp and cradle the patient's penis with the nondominant hand. Insert the tip of the contrast-filled syringe into the urethra. Firmly squeeze the glans pe-

nis between the thumb and the index and long fingers (Figure 124-2*B*). This will secure the catheter tip within the fossa navicularis. Do not squeeze the shaft of the penis with middle, ring, or little fingers as this will occlude the urethra. Gently straighten the urethra by directing the tip of the penis toward the dependent shoulder or nipple and over the left thigh. The remainder of the procedure is as described above in the Foley catheter section.

BRODNEY CLAMP TECHNIQUE

The Brodney clamp is a cage with rubber feet that clamp behind the corona of the glans.[10] In the center of the device there is a blunt-tipped obturator that inserts into and occludes the urethral meatus. It may be used instead of a Foley catheter or 60 mL syringe for the procedure. The advantage of this device is that both the fossa navicularis and the distal urethra are visible on the radiograph. Air bubbles are easily eliminated from the obturator. The disadvantages of the clamp are that it is not flexible and it is heavy. It must be held during the procedure and fluoroscopy is impossible. If the patient moves, the clamp tends to dislodge. The clamp is difficult to use in boys and in the presence of a phimoses.[10]

Clean, prep, and drape the penis as mentioned previously. Insert the blunt-tipped obturator of the clamp into the urethra. Rotate the feet of the clamp so that they are grasping the coronal sulcus of the penis. These should not be so tight as to occlude the urethra ventrally. The remainder of the technique is as describe in the Foley catheter section.

RETROGRADE CYSTOGRAPHY TECHNIQUE

Any abnormalities in the retrograde urethrogram, such as extravasation of the contrast from the urethra or evidence of strictures, should prompt an urgent urology consult and intervention. If the study is normal, the retrograde cystogram should be performed. Gently advance a Foley catheter into the bladder (Figures 124-3A and B). Inflate the cuff at the tip of the Foley catheter (Figure 124-3B). Gently pull the Foley catheter to lodge the cuff at the bladder neck (Figure 124-3C). Attach a 60 mL catheter-tipped syringe, without the plunger, to the Foley catheter. Pour contrast material into the syringe and let it drain by gravity into the bladder. Continue to allow contrast to fill the bladder until 300 to 350 mL of contrast material is in the bladder of an adult or any child older than 11. In younger children, the instilled volume is estimated by the formula (age in years +2) × 30, or to the point of initiating a bladder contraction.[11] After the contrast is instilled, clamp the Foley catheter with a hemostat.

Obtain two radiographs. These are the anteroposterior (AP) and the oblique, or the lateral, views of the pelvis. Evaluate the radiographs for proper bladder filling with contrast and for extravasation of contrast. Release the hemostat and allow the contrast to drain out of

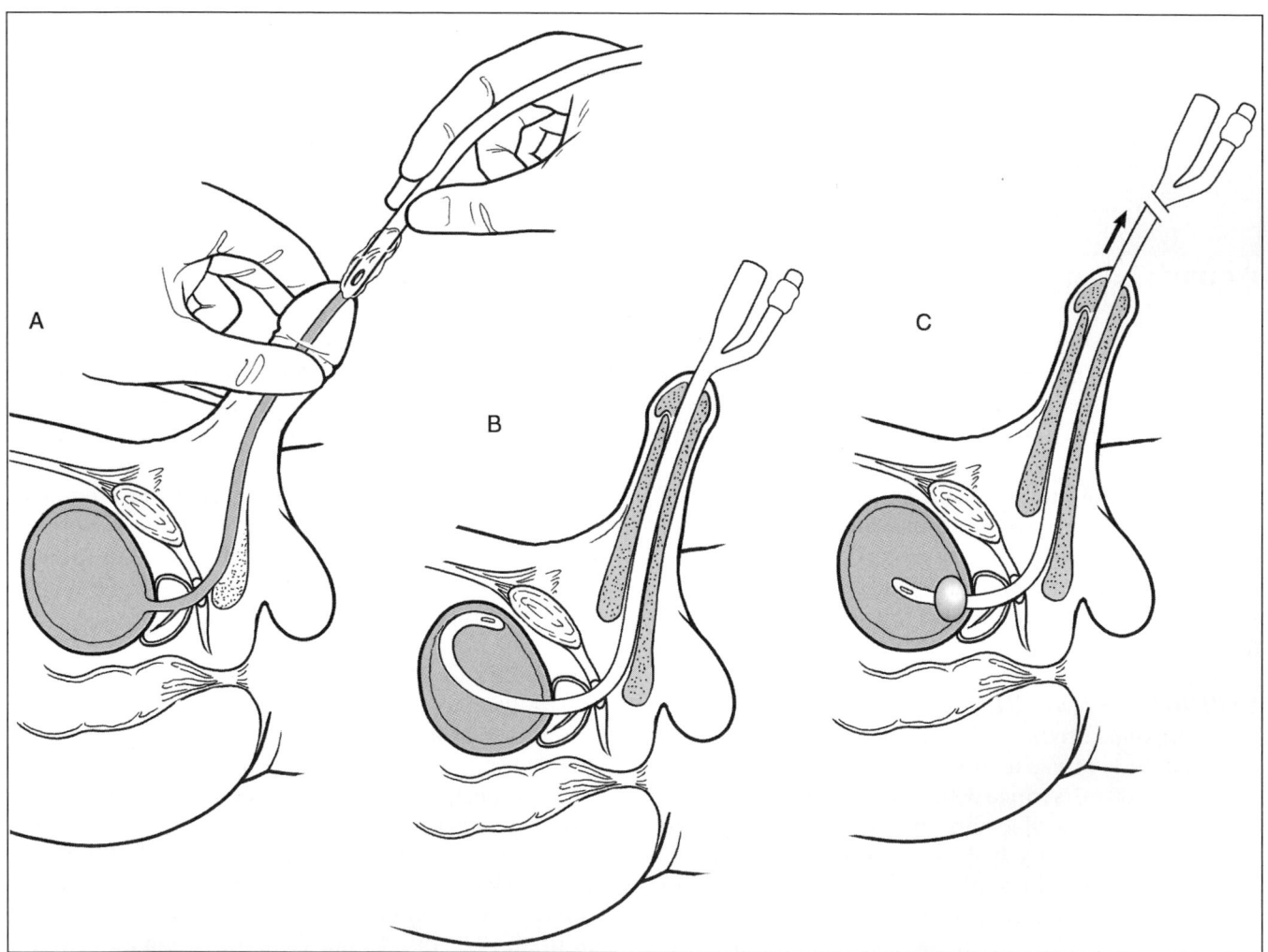

FIGURE 124-3 Retrograde cystography. *A.* The Foley catheter is inserted into the penis. *B.* The Foley catheter is advanced until it is inside the urinary bladder. *C.* The cuff is inflated. The catheter is then pulled until resistance is met to occlude the urethra with the cuff.

the bladder through the Foley catheter and into the container. Obtain another AP radiograph of the pelvis (washout film). This film is often helpful in picking up obscured areas of extravasation not visible on the initial film. In patients with pelvic fractures, all radiographs should be taken with the patient in a supine position. Review the radiographs for intraperitoneal and extraperitoneal bladder rupture.

ASSESSMENT

In a normal retrograde urethrogram, the entire urethra should be visible. Some of the contrast material should also be seen within the bladder. Extravasation of contrast from the urethra will appear as a flame-like density outside the urethra. A partial urethral disruption will show extravasation of contrast as well as contrast within the bladder. In a complete urethral disruption, no contrast material will be visible within the bladder. Occasionally, contrast material may be seen in the venous plexus of the penis due to forceful injection of contrast into the urethra. This is a common phenomenon and should not be mistaken for extravasation. The venous flush will clear spontaneously on a postvoid film.

In the evaluation of the retrograde cystogram, intraperitoneal and extraperitoneal bladder injuries can be differentiated. The extravasation of the contrast material that appears as a flame-like projection confined to the pelvis constitutes the extraperitoneal injury. In patients with intraperitoneal injuries, the contrast tends to outline the intraperitoneal organs. This differentiation is important because each requires a different treatment. All intraperitoneal injuries are managed surgically whereas some extraperitoneal injuries can be managed with Foley catheter drainage or suprapubic cystostomy.[7]

AFTERCARE

Because of the hypertonicity of the contrast material and urethral stretching, patients may experience burning and dysuria. After a normal study, ensure that the patient is well hydrated. The flow of urine will wash the contrast out of the bladder and urethra.

SUMMARY

The retrograde urethrogram should be performed in any male with a pelvic fracture, lower abdominal trauma with gross hematuria, inability to void, hematoma of the perineum, or a high riding or boggy prostate on physical examination. The cystogram should follow to evaluate potential bladder injuries. The cystogram is used to evaluate and differentiate intraperitoneal and extraperitoneal bladder injuries.

Retrograde urethrography and cystography are diagnostic procedures that are easy to perform and have the potential to avoid major complications related to urine leakage. Both of these procedures are safe and simple to perform. With basic equipment, invaluable information can be collected with very little time investment. The early recognition of disruption of the lower genitourinary tract can prevent significant morbidity.

REFERENCES

1. Heare MM, Heare TC, Gillespy T: Diagnostic imaging of the pelvic and chest wall trauma. *Radiol Clin North Am* 1989; 27:873–889.
2. Spirnak JP: Pelvic fracture and injury to the lower urinary tract. *Surg Clin North Am* 1988; 68:1057–1069.
3. Diekmann-Guiroy B, Young DH: Female urethral injury secondary to blunt pelvic trauma. *Ann Emerg Med* 1991; 20:1376–1378.
4. Carroll PR, McAninch JW: Major bladder trauma: mechanisms of injury and a unified method of diagnoses. *J Urol* 1984; 132:254–257.
5. Patterson BM: Pelvic ring injury and associated urologic trauma: an orthopaedic perspective. *Semin Urol* 1995; 13:25–33.
6. Friedland GW, Filly R, Goris ML, et al: Anatomy, in Friedland GW, Filly R, Goris ML, et al (eds): *Uroradiology: An Integrated Approach.* New York: Churchill Livingstone, 1983:118–141.
7. Dixon CM: Diagnosis and acute management of posterior urethral disruptions, in McAninch JW, Carroll PR, Jordan GH (eds): *Traumatic and Reconstructive Urology.* Philadelphia: Saunders, 1996:347–355.
8. Oosterlinck W: Controversies in management of urethral trauma after pelvic fracture in men. *Acta Urol Belg* 1998; 66(2):49–53.
9. Rehm CG, Mure AJ, O'Malley KF, et al: Blunt traumatic bladder rupture: the role of retrograde cystogram. *Ann Emerg Med* 1991; 20(8):845–847.
10. Friedland GW, Goris ML, Gross D: Voiding cystourethrography, retrograde urethrography, and seminal vesiculography, in Friedland GW, Filly R, Goris ML, et al (eds): *Uroradiology: An Integrated Approach.* New York: Churchill Livingstone, 1983:249–264.
11. Schneider RE: Urologic procedures, in Roberts JR, Hedges JR (eds): *Clinical Procedures in Emergency Medicine,* 3rd ed. Philadelphia: Saunders, 1998:947–987.

Chapter 125
ANESTHESIA OF THE PENIS, TESTICLE, AND EPIDIDYMIS

Patricia Vidal
Michael P. Jones

INTRODUCTION

A wide range of urologic procedures are performed using local or regional anesthesia. This includes an orchiectomy, inspection of the painful testis, release of a paraphimosis, dorsal slit, circumcision, and even a hydrocelectomy or varicocelectomy done in the Operating Room. Emergency Physicians can utilize some of the same anesthetic techniques, namely the penile or spermatic cord blocks, to safely and painlessly perform many procedures in the Emergency Department. These techniques are easy to learn, simple to perform, and have a low risk of serious complications.

ANATOMY AND PATHOPHYSIOLOGY

Innervation of the penis arises from the pudendal nerve that is derived from sacral levels 2 to 4. The pudendal nerve divides into the perineal and the inferior rectal nerves. The perineal nerve further divides into the right and left dorsal nerves of the penis. The dorsal nerves of the penis pass under the pubic symphysis to penetrate the suspensory ligament of the penis.[1] They travel under Buck's fascia to supply sensory innervation to the entire penis (Figure 125-1).

The primary nerve supply of the testis and epididymis are from the ilioinguinal and genitofemoral nerves. The ilioinguinal nerve is derived from the first lumbar spinal nerve. It arises slightly inferior and medial to the anterior superior iliac spine and courses toward the pubic tubercle, between the internal and external oblique muscles.[1,2] It enters the inguinal canal on the anterior surface of the spermatic cord. The ilioinguinal nerve provides sensory innervation to the skin of the upper thigh, base of the penis, and the upper scrotum.[3] It also provides sensory innervation to the spermatic cord and testicle. The genitofemoral nerve is derived from the first two lumbar spinal nerves. It divides into the genital branch and the femoral branch. The genital branch enters the inguinal canal at the external inguinal ring and travels with the spermatic cord. It provides sensory innervation to the lower scrotum, cremaster muscle, spermatic cord, and scrotum. The femoral branch supplies the skin of the anteromedial thigh.[3]

INDICATIONS

Emergency Department procedures that are facilitated by local anesthesia of the penis include dorsal slit of the foreskin, release of a phimosis or paraphimosis, repair of penile lacerations, and the release of penile skin entrapped in zippers. Local anesthesia can also be used before performing a circumcision. However, this procedure is usually performed by a Urologist.

Emergency Department indications for a spermatic cord block include the relief of epididymal pain, the facilitation of a manual or ultrasound examination when differentiating between torsion and epididymitis, and to inspect the testis following trauma. Manual detorsion of a testis may be enabled by local anesthesia when a patient cannot tolerate the pain of palpation. However, the risk of compromising the blood supply to the testis and the loss of patient assessment of pain in determining the success of detorsion are often cited as contraindications to spermatic cord blockade when testicular torsion is suspected.

CONTRAINDICATIONS

Local anesthesia is contraindicated in testicular torsion, as there is a risk of compromising the testicular blood supply. The anesthetic effect will also eliminate the patient's assessment of pain that is needed to determine the success of manual detorsion. Agents containing epinephrine are not to be used in or

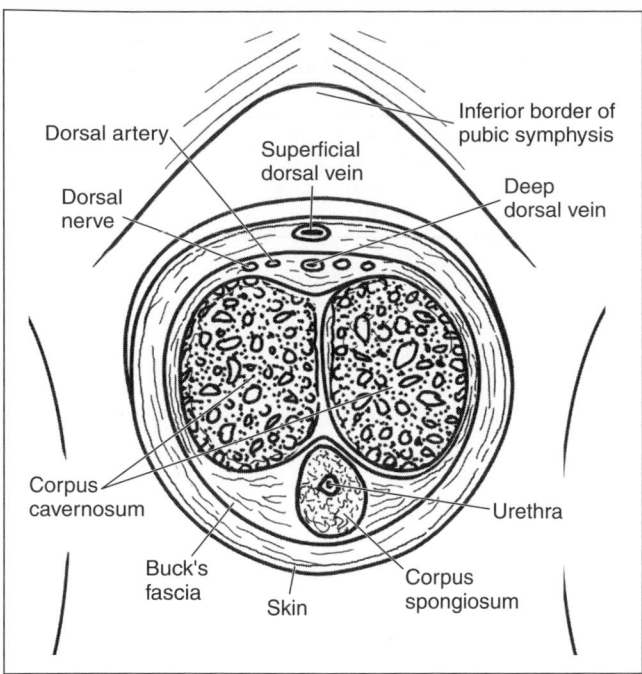

FIGURE 125-1 Transverse section through the base of the penis.

around the phallus.[4] The arteries of the penis are end arteries and vasoconstriction can result in tissue ischemia and sloughing. To minimize the spread of infection, local anesthetic should not be directly injected into an area of local infection.

EQUIPMENT

25 and 27 gauge needles
Syringes (3 mL, 5 mL, 10 mL)
Povidone iodine solution
Alcohol pads
4×4 gauze squares
Local anesthetic solution

Several local anesthetic agents are commonly used for genitourinary anesthesia. These include lidocaine, bupivacaine, mepivacaine, and chloroprocaine (Table 125-1). The anesthetic agent, concentration, and technique must be chosen so that the maximum safe dose is not exceeded. This is especially important when performing anesthesia in children.

PATIENT PREPARATION

The patient must be informed of the procedure, including its risks and benefits. The explanation must include the risks of local anesthetic injection and the possibility that the anesthetic may not effectively eliminate pain. The risks associated with the injection include pain, hematoma formation, and bleeding. Infection is a late risk that can be reduced by prepping the skin and using sterile technique. Obtain an informed consent for the anesthetic procedure and the procedure that will be performed under anesthesia.

The patient's ability to cooperate with the planned procedures must be assessed. Consider oral or parenteral sedation, especially in anxious patients or children. Midazolam (0.02 to 0.04 mg/kg IV) or diazepam (2.5 to 5 mg IV) are often good choices in adults. Children may benefit from midazolam parenterally (0.05 to 0.15 mg/kg IV) or orally (0.5 to 0.7 mg/kg). Ketamine (1.0 to 1.5 mg/kg IV or 2 to 5 mg/kg IM) combined with atropine (0.01 mg/kg) to reduce respiratory secretions is an alternative, especially in children younger than 10.

Clean any dirt and debris from the skin. Identify the anatomic landmarks required to perform the anesthetic injection. Apply povidone iodine solution to the area where the anesthetic is to be injected. The povidone iodine may also be applied to the penis and scrotum if an invasive procedure is subsequently to be performed. Apply sterile drapes to delineate a surgical field. Allow the povidone iodine to dry. Put on sterile gloves and reidentify the anatomic landmarks. Infiltrate with local anesthetic solution using sterile technique.

TECHNIQUES

LOCAL INFILTRATION

Local anesthetic infiltration of the skin of the penis is useful for the repair of superficial lacerations, dorsal slits of the foreskin, or freeing entrapped skin from a zipper. Local infiltration circumferentially around the penis will provide adequate anesthesia distal to the anesthetic injection site. The circumferential subcutaneous injections can be performed directly on the penis or on the abdominal wall and scrotum surrounding the penis. While not contraindicated, some authors avoid direct infiltration of the foreskin as tissue sloughing may result.[2] **Local infiltration of anesthetic agents is often extremely painful for the patient. Consider premedicating the patient with parenteral benzodiazepines and/or narcotic agents.**

Local anesthetic agents can be injected subcutaneously into the penis to provide distal anesthesia. If performing a dorsal slit of the foreskin, raise a skin wheal of local anesthetic solution at the base of the foreskin in the 12 o'clock position (Figure 125-2A). Insert the needle through the skin wheal aimed distally. Inject local anesthetic solution subcutaneously as the needle is advanced to the distal edge of the foreskin. Alternatively, local anesthetic solution can be circumferentially infiltrated

TABLE 125-1. LOCAL ANESTHETIC AGENTS COMMONLY USED FOR GENITOURINARY ANESTHESIA

Anesthetic agent	Strength (%)	Onset of action (minutes)	Duration of action (minutes)	Maximum dose (mg/kg)
Lidocaine	0.5, 1.0, 1.5, 2.0	5–15	45–90	4.5
Bupivacaine	0.25, 0.50	10–15	120–240	2.5
Mepivacaine	1.0, 1.5	10–15	120–240	4.0
Chloroprocaine	2.0, 3.0	10–15	20–40	11.0

around the penis (Figure 125-2*B*). This block usually requires 6 to 10 mL of local anesthetic solution.

PENILE BLOCK

The objective of a penile block is to anesthetize the right and left dorsal nerves of the penis that provide sensation to the penis (Figure 125-1). **The dorsal nerves should be blocked as close to the base of the penis as possible. If the block is performed too distal to the pubic bone, the posterior branches of the dorsal nerves will not be anesthetized and the ventral surface of the penis will retain sensation.**[5,6] Multiple effective techniques will be described to perform a penile block. The technique chosen should depend on the specific procedure to be performed, the level of patient cooperation, and the preference of the physician.

The penis may be anesthetized where it forms along the abdominal wall.[2] This block anesthetizes the nerves to the penis before they reach the penis. Form three skin wheals using local anesthetic solution on the abdominal and scrotal skin, 0.5 to 1.0 cm from the base of the penis, at the 2 o'clock, 6 o'clock, and 10 o'clock positions (Figure 125-3). Infiltrate subcutaneously with local anesthetic solution between the skin wheals to form a triangle of anesthetic that surrounds the base of

the penis. This block usually requires 8 to 12 mL of local anesthetic solution.

The dorsal nerves of the penis can be anesthetized as they course onto the penis. Place a skin wheal of local anesthetic solution at the 2 o'clock and 10 o'clock positions. Slowly insert a 27 gauge needle through the skin wheals until there is a slight loss of resistance indicating penetration of Buck's fascia (Figure 125-4). Aspirate to ensure that the needle is not within a blood vessel. Inject 2 mL of local anesthetic solution at each site.[1]

Another technique blocks the dorsal nerves as they pass through the triangular space bordered by the pubic symphysis, the corpora cavernosa, and Buck's fascia. Place a skin wheal of local anesthetic solution at the dorsal base of the penis. Insert the needle through the skin wheal and to the pubic symphysis. Withdraw the needle slightly and advance it caudally until a loss of resistance is felt, indicating it has penetrated Buck's fascia. Aspirate to ensure that the needle is not within a blood vessel. Inject 10 mL of local anesthetic solution on each side of the suspensory ligament (midline). Alternatively,

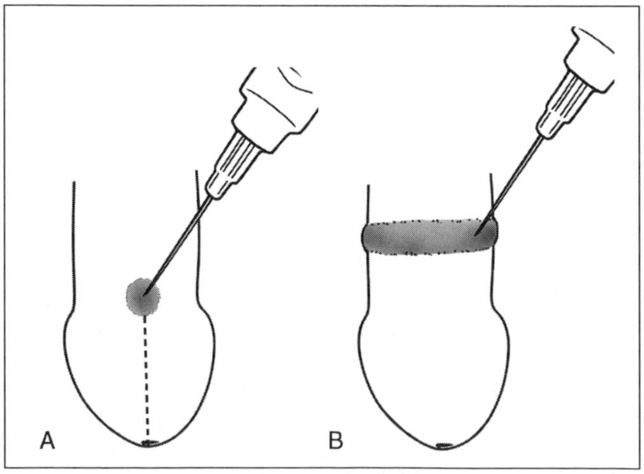

FIGURE 125-2 Local anesthetic infiltration into the penis. *A.* A skin wheal is raised and local anesthetic is injected distally (dotted line). *B.* Circumferential infiltration of local anesthetic solution.

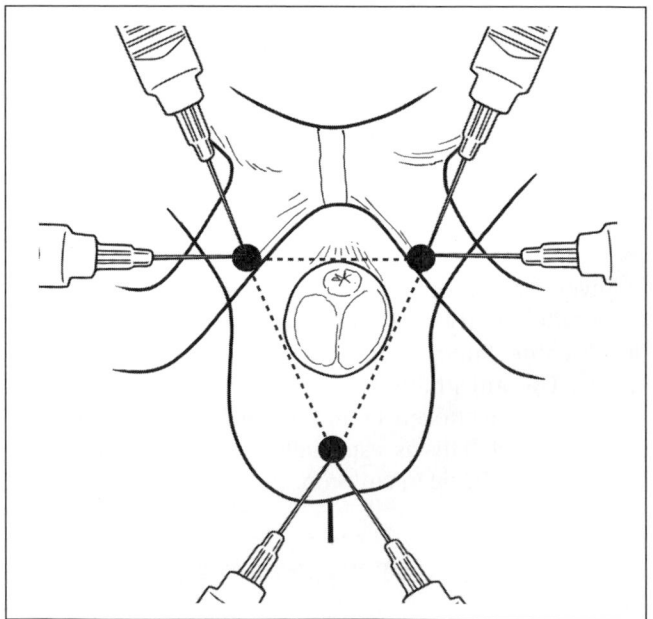

FIGURE 125-3 Local anesthetic infiltration around the base of the penis. Black dots represent the locations of the skin wheals.

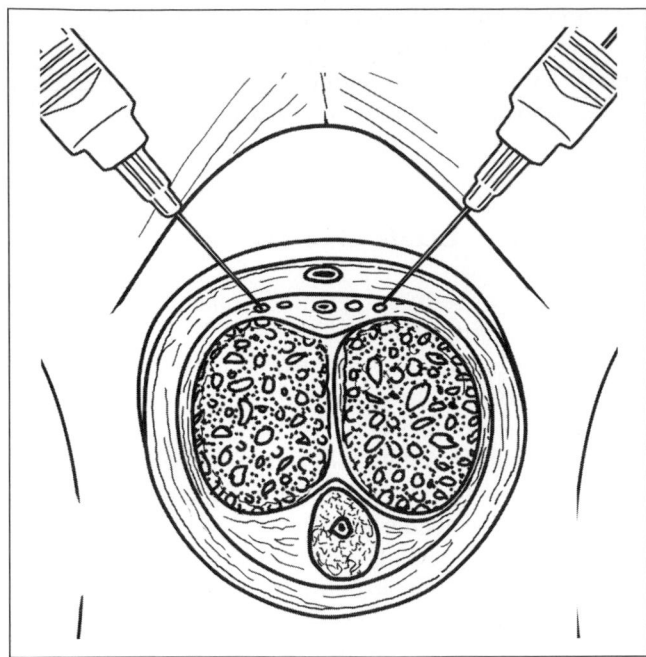

FIGURE 125-4 The penile block anesthetizes the left and right deep dorsal nerves of the penis.

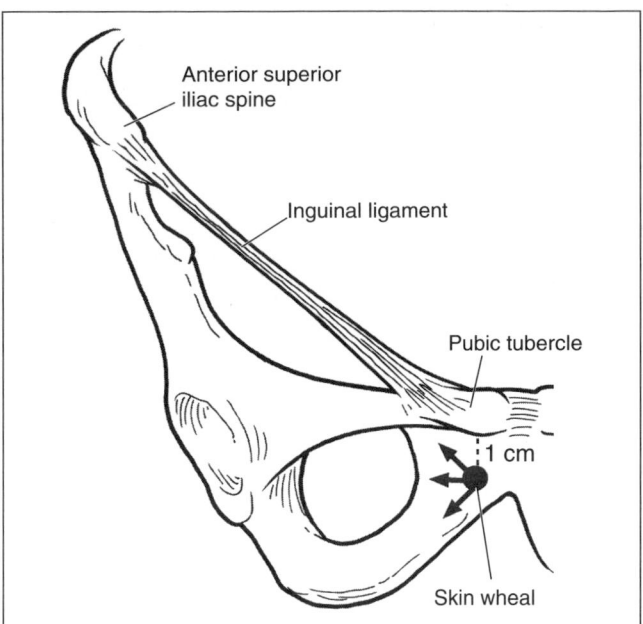

FIGURE 125-5 The spermatic cord can be anesthetized just below the pubic tubercle, if the tubercle is palpable. The arrows represent the three different directions required to inject local anesthetic solution.

the same block can be accomplished with a separate injection on each side of the midline.[1,7]

SPERMATIC CORD BLOCK

As the spermatic cord exits the external inguinal ring, it passes over the pubic tubercle and continues medially towards the scrotum. In this same location, the ilioinguinal nerve travels on the anterior surface of the spermatic cord and the genital branch of the genitofemoral nerve on the posterior surface. These two nerves supply sensation to the spermatic cord, epididymis, and testicle. Anesthesia of the spermatic cord in the region of the pubic tubercle will provide anesthesia to the testis and its covering, the epididymis, and the vas deferens.[6] The spermatic cord block does not provide anesthesia to the skin of the scrotum. Additional subcutaneous infiltration is necessary for an incision of the scrotal skin.

This first spermatic cord block technique is useful in thin patients with a palpable pubic tubercle. Identify the pubic tubercle by palpation. Inject local anesthetic solution to make a skin wheal just medial and 1 cm below the pubic tubercle (Figure 125-5). Gently advance a 25 gauge needle laterally through the skin wheal and spermatic cord until bone is contacted. Aspirate to ensure that the needle is not within a blood vessel. Inject 3 to 4 mL of local anesthetic solution as the needle is slowly withdrawn. Repeat the procedure two more times using the same skin puncture, each time passing through the cord at a slightly different angle. This block requires a total of 10 to 12 mL of local anesthetic solution.[6]

A modified technique is used for the patient in whom the pubic tubercle is difficult to palpate. Grasp the spermatic cord between the nondominant thumb and index finger as it enters the scrotum (Figure 125-6). Place a wheal of local anesthetic solution between the fingers and above the spermatic cord. Insert a 25 gauge needle through the skin wheal. Direct the needle anterior to the spermatic cord. Aspirate to ensure that the needle is not within a blood vessel. Inject 3 to 4 mL of local anesthetic solution. Repeat the process on the medial and lateral side of the spermatic cord.

Alternatively, palpate the spermatic cord as it enters the scrotum.[8] Trace the spermatic cord superiorly to the pubic tubercle where it exits the external inguinal ring. Trap the spermatic cord between the second and third fingers of the nondominant hand and the pubic tubercle. Place a wheal of local anesthetic solution between the fingers and above the spermatic cord. Insert a 25 gauge needle through the skin wheal. Aspirate to ensure that the needle is not within a blood vessel. Inject 3 to 4 mL of local anesthetic solution anteriorly, medially, and laterally as described above. Injection of local anesthetic solution into the spermatic cord as it exits the inguinal canal may be less painful than injection as it enters the scrotum.

ASSESSMENT

Allow 10 to 15 minutes for the local anesthetic solution to take effect for a penile block. Test the level of

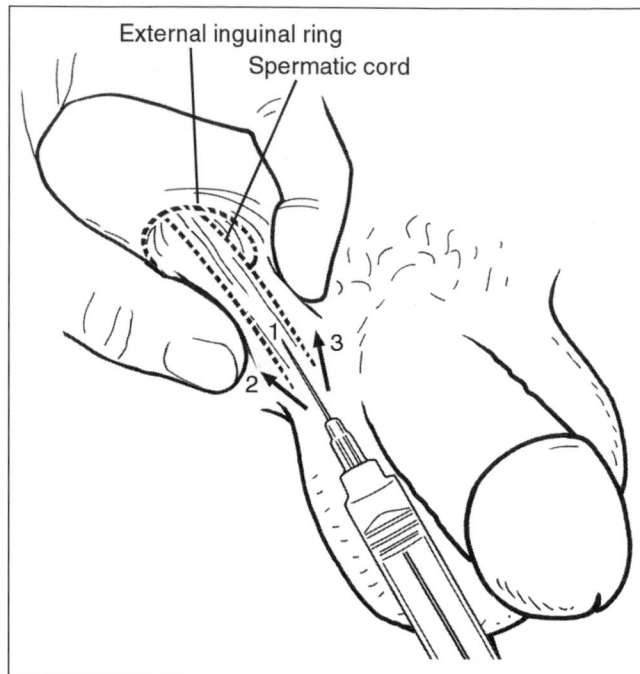

FIGURE 125-6 The spermatic cord block at the base of the scrotum. Local anesthetic solution is injected anteriorly (1), laterally (2), and medially (3) to the spermatic cord.

anesthesia by pinching the skin with a forceps or by pinprick with a needle. The patient may feel a pressure sensation but should not feel pain. If the test stimulus is painful, repeat the block or use additional anesthetic techniques prior to performing the procedure.

Spermatic cord blocks require 10 to 15 minutes for maximal effectiveness. The patient should be warned that, despite an effective block, traction on the spermatic cord might cause nausea and a tugging sensation. These will resolve upon release of the traction.[6] Additional anesthesia must be applied to the scrotal skin for any incisions or procedures as a spermatic cord block does not anesthetize the scrotal skin.

AFTERCARE

Minimal aftercare is required for these local anesthetic techniques. Depending on the agent used, sensation may return in as little as 1 to 2 hours (lidocaine, chloroprocaine) or up to 4 hours (bupivacaine). The skin may reawaken with a pins-and-needles sensation. Patients should use caution when zipping their pants so as not to catch the penis, foreskin, or scrotum as they will not feel the injury. Patients should be warned that the site of a spermatic cord block might remain tender for as long as 10 days.[6] The application of cool compresses to the injection site and oral nonsteroidal anti-inflammatory drugs will provide adequate analgesia for injection site pain. Patients should inspect the injection site and surrounding area three to four times a day for signs of infection. They should return to the Emergency Department immediately if any problems or concerns arise.

COMPLICATIONS

The most procedure-specific complication of a penile block is sloughing of the penile skin. This is more common in the region of the glans. Performing the penile block at the base of the penis and using solutions without epinephrine minimizes this risk.

Hematomas can be quite large in spermatic cord blocks because the venous plexus is usually pierced. The use of a smaller needle and careful application of pressure can help prevent hematomas. Blood loss from puncturing a vascular structure is easily controlled with direct pressure. A Urologist should be consulted urgently in the rare occasion that bleeding does not resolve with pressure.

Local infection at the injection site is possible. Patients should be warned about the signs of infection including fever, erythema, warmth, induration, increased pain, and purulent drainage. Patients should seek immediate medical attention for any of these symptoms.

Toxic levels of anesthetic agents can affect multiple organ systems, most notably the central nervous and cardiovascular systems. Anesthetic agents block the inhibitory neurons of the brain producing a state of neuro-excitation. Initial symptoms may include tinnitus, premolar numbness, disorientation, lightheadedness, or nystagmus. This may progress to seizures that can be accompanied by slow or absent breathing, acidosis, aspiration, and cardiovascular instability. Intravenous diazepam (2.5 to 5 mg) at the first sign of symptoms may stop the cascade.[2] Significantly higher doses of diazepam are required to treat seizures. Very high levels of local anesthetics are cardiotoxic and may result in heart block. Heart block from bupivacaine toxicity is associated with resistance to resuscitative maneuvers. The onset of all local anesthetic toxicities is faster with intravascular injection versus toxic tissue concentrations.

SUMMARY

Local anesthesia allows many painful genitourinary procedures to be performed in the Emergency Department. The techniques are simple and easy to perform with little to no experience. Local anesthetic solutions containing epinephrine should never be used to anesthetize the penis, scrotum, or spermatic cord.

REFERENCES

1. Hinman F: *Atlas of Urologic Surgery,* 1st ed. Philadelphia: Saunders, 1989:958–962.
2. Cassady JF: Regional anesthesia for urologic procedures. *Urol Clin North Am* 1987; 14(1):43–50.
3. Hinman F: *Atlas of Urosurgical Anatomy,* 1st ed. Philadelphia: Saunders, 1993:46–47.
4. Kindscher JD: Operative and postoperative pain management for the urologic patient. AUA Update Series 1007;Vol XVI, Lesson 3:20.
5. Eltherington L, Chase R: Neural blockade for plastic surgery, in Cousins MJ, Bridenbaugh PO (eds): *Neural Blockade in Clinical Anesthesia and Management of Pain,* 2nd ed. Philadelphia: Lippincott, 1999:657–658.
6. Brown TCK, Schultz-Steinberg O: Neural blockade for pediatric surgery, in Cousins MJ, Bridenbaugh PO (eds): *Neural Blockade in Clinical Anesthesia and Management of Pain,* 2nd ed. Philadelphia: Lippincott, 1999:685–688.
7. Kaye KW, Lange PH, Fraley EE: Spermatic cord block in urologic surgery. *J Urol* 1982; 128(4):720–721.
8. Fuchs EF: Cord block anesthesia for scrotal surgery. *J Urol* 1982; 128(4):718–719.

TABLE 126-1. THE ETIOLOGIES OF LOW-FLOW PRIAPISM IN THE ORDER OF INCIDENCE (HIGH TO LOW)

Idiopathic (common)
Hematologic—sickle cell, leukemia (common)
Iatrogenic—intracavernous drug therapy, surgery (common)
Pharmacologic—mainly psychotropic drugs (uncommon)
Traumatic—usually gives high-flow priapism (uncommon)
Neoplastic—metastatic (rare)
Neurogenic—spinal cord problems (rare)
Infectious (rare)

The cause of priapism in metastatic malignancy and leukemia involving the penis is assumed to be local obstruction. Sickle cell hemoglobinopathy has been found in as many as 88 percent of African Americans who present with priapism in one series.[11] Children with sickle cell disease have a high incidence of priapism and multiple episodes are common. The decrease in O_2 tension during erection is thought to predispose the blood to sludging.[12,13] Patients with sickle cell trait or other hemoglobinopathies may develop priapism.[14] The use of injectable vasodilator drugs for the treatment of impotence is becoming a frequent cause of priapism. Drugs are not a common cause but many have been associated with low-flow priapism and the history must review this area. Psychotropic agents with autonomic activity, alpha-adrenergic blockers for hypertension, anticoagulants, cocaine, and other drugs have also been incriminated in priapism.

TREATMENT OF LOW-FLOW PRIAPISM

The successful treatment of low-flow priapism is based on the concept of immediate decompression of the corporal tissue to reverse the ischemia by allowing the inflow of arterial blood (Figure 126-2). Aspiration rarely has to be performed as passive drainage usually is adequate for decompression and is less traumatic. This is followed by the injection of an alpha-adrenergic agonist to initiate smooth muscle contraction and detumescence.[15–17] If done within 12 to 24 hours of the onset of priapism, there is a high rate of success.[1] After 36 hours of low-flow priapism, there is often no significant response of the smooth muscle to alpha-adrenergic simulation and decompression with irrigation is required.[5,18] The success rate of this treatment drops dramatically if the patient presents after 48 hours.[18] A venous shunt procedure should be considered if there is no response to these treatments.

There are some exceptions to these treatments for low-flow priapism. The patient with metastatic cancer involvement of the penis requires only palliative treatment for priapism. The primary treatment of the patient with leukemia has traditionally been chemotherapy. However, decompression and alpha-adrenergic agonist therapy has also been used successfully in a patient with leukemic priapism.[19] Treatment with chemotherapy is still necessary to prevent a recurrence.[20]

The treatment of low-flow priapism in sickle cell hemoglobinopathy has relied on conservative treatment with aggressive hydration, alkalization, analgesics, transfusion, and exchange transfusion.[12,13,21] The goal is

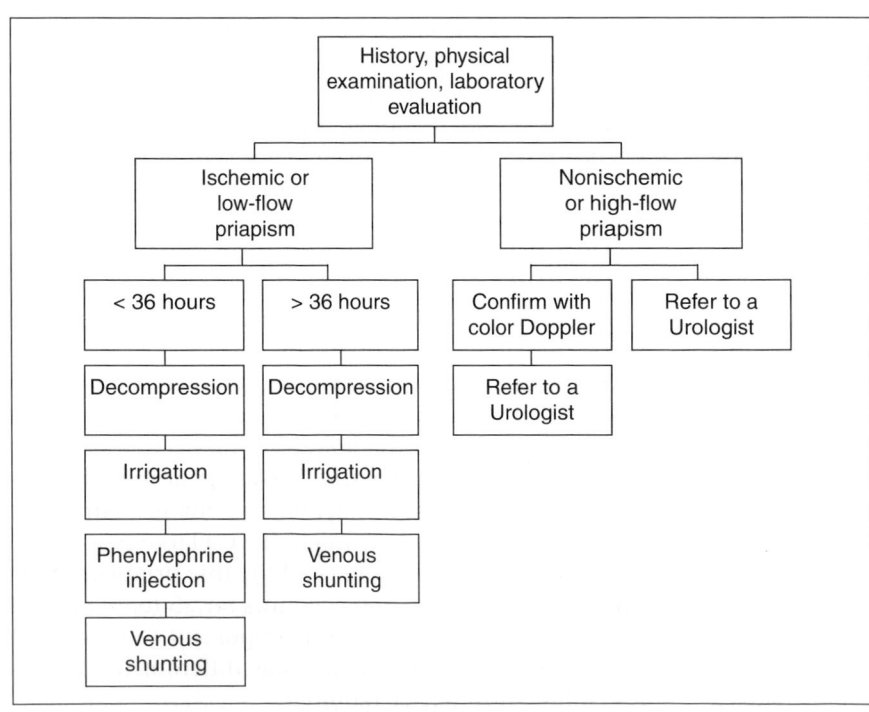

FIGURE 126-2 Management of priapism. Modified from Lue.[1]

to achieve good hydration, correct the corporal acidosis, and lower the hemoglobin S to 30 percent. These measures are intended to restore circulation and oxygenation to the penis that would reverse the red cell sickling. Unfortunately, this treatment is slow at best and erectile dysfunction is common, even if the initial therapy is successful.[22] Serum electrophoresis is not usually available on an emergency basis and the immediate care cannot depend on following hemoglobin S levels.

Traditionally, aspiration and alpha-adrenergic agonist treatment has been initiated after several hours or days of the conservative management described in the previous paragraph. There are no adequate studies that allow a clear recommendation for timing as to when to start aspiration and injection therapy. However, there are authorities who will immediately start treating patients with aspiration and alpha-adrenergic agonist injection therapy along with the conservative medical management instead of waiting 12 to 24 hours for results of the medical therapy.[2] This would include venous shunting if there were no response to the conservative therapy. The basis for this newer approach is that the fundamental requirement in low-flow priapism is to rapidly reverse the ischemia present in the corporal bodies before permanent damage occurs.

Venous shunting for low-flow priapism is a surgical method of decompressing the corpora by creating "fistulas" to the corpus spongiosum or the saphenous vein. It was the first successful form of treatment for priapism. The only indication for venous shunting is for failure of conservative therapy. There are several techniques for shunting. They are usually performed initially in the distal penis (glans) as this area provides the easiest surgical access; proximal procedures should be used only if the distal operation fails.[22–24] The Winter operation using a Tru-Cut biopsy needle to remove pieces of the tip of the corpora through the glans can be performed in the Emergency Department by a Urologist.[25]

TREATMENT OF HIGH-FLOW PRIAPISM

High-flow priapism does not require immediate therapy, since the tissue is not ischemic (Figure 126-2). These patients can frequently present a long period of time after the onset of priapism. Consult a Urologist. The usual treatment is selective arteriography with internal pudendal embolization, although surgical ligation has also been done.[26–28] The need for informing a patient about erectile dysfunction as a consequence of the disease process is also necessary with high-flow priapism.

INDICATIONS

Patients with low-flow priapism should have an expedited work-up and treatment since there is a high failure rate if it is not resolved within 24 hours of the onset.[1] A thorough history and physical examination can frequently determine the cause. A complete blood cell count and urinalysis are performed routinely. A sickle cell prep should be included in appropriate ethnic groups unless there is already a history of sickle cell disease. A serum electrophoresis should be obtained in those patients with a sickling history or if the prep is positive.

If there is doubt with regards to high-flow or low-flow priapism, aspiration of corporal blood with blood gas analysis would determine if the blood is arterial or venous.[1] Usually, looking at the blood is adequate. Duplex ultrasound can confirm the presence of an arterial fistula.

CONTRAINDICATIONS

Medical risks or other priorities making priapism therapy inappropriate will occasionally occur and have to be weighed against the fact that the natural course of priapism is benign. Patients taking monoamine oxidase inhibitors or with significant hypertension should not receive alpha-adrenergic agonists. Patients with unstable angina, arrhythmias, and other high-risk cardiac problems should also not receive alphaadrenergic agonists.

EQUIPMENT

19 gauge butterfly needle or straight needle
21 gauge needles
Syringes (1 mL, 3 mL, 10 mL, 20 mL)
Povidone iodine solution
4×4 gauze squares
Sterile drapes
Sterile basin
3-way stopcock (optional)
Phenylephrine, 10 mg/mL in 1 mL vials
1% lidocaine
Normal saline, 1 liter bottle
Normal saline, 10 mL vial
Blood pressure monitoring equipment
ECG monitoring equipment

PATIENT PREPARATION

Explain to the patient and/or their representative the procedure, its risks and benefits, and the aftercare. Obtain a signed consent and place it in the medical record. Obtain intravenous access. The blood pressure and pulse should be taken before the procedure and at frequent (5 to 10 minute) intervals in all patients. Electrocardiographic monitoring should be performed in patients with a history of hypertension, coronary artery disease, or cardiac dysfunction.

These procedures can be extremely painful. If not contraindicated, perform a penile block (Chapter 125). Alternatively, administer parenteral analgesics, sedatives, and/or procedural sedation. This will be most appreciated by the patient.

Prepare the penis. Clean the penis, scrotum, and surrounding area of any dirt and debris. Apply povidone iodine solution to the penis and allow it to dry. Apply sterile drapes to delineate a sterile field. Some Urologists cleanse and prepare the penis with alcohol rather than povidone iodine. This is not recommended for the Emergency Department unless the patient is allergic to iodine.

TECHNIQUES

Prepare the phenylephrine. It is purchased in sterile 1 mL glass vials with a concentration of 10 mg/mL. Place 10 mg (1 mL) of phenylephrine into a syringe containing 9 mL of normal saline. This provides a solution of 1 mg/mL that allows easy calculation of the doses. Other dilutions can be used, as this is physician-dependent, and the concentration should be clearly marked on the syringe.

Insert a 19 gauge butterfly needle into the lateral midshaft of the penis at the 3 o'clock or 9 o'clock position (Figure 126-3). This will be used for draining or aspirating the penis. The tubing can be capped with a syringe or 3-way stopcock. The 19 gauge needle usually provides free drainage with no aspirating being necessary. **The needle should always be inserted straight in and directed toward the center of the corpora.** If a difficult procedure is anticipated (priapism duration > 24 hours), a 21 gauge butterfly needle can also be inserted in the base of the penis and left in place for either injection or irrigation. **The fewer the injections, the less chance for a hematoma formation.**

Place the catheter end of the butterfly into a sterile basin and allow the blood to drain from the penis. If blood does not spontaneously drain, attach a 10 or 20 mL syringe to the catheter end and aspirate blood from the penis. Cap the butterfly catheter after draining enough blood to significantly soften the penis.

If there is difficulty with the drainage, a 21 gauge butterfly needle should be inserted in the proximal shaft area. Begin gentle irrigation with normal saline through the 21 gauge needle with outflow through the 19 gauge needle. This will help to irrigate out the old blood. **Only normal saline should be used because the endothelium can be damaged if the solution is not isotonic.** Massaging the penis to "milk out" sludge can be helpful. Placement of additional 19 gauge butterfly needles may be used to improve drainage in difficult cases.

Inject 0.25 to 0.5 mL (250 to 500 micrograms) of the phenylephrine solution with an insulin syringe through the butterfly catheter and into the penis. Observe the penis for up to 10 minutes. Repeat the procedure if the erection returns or does not resolve. There is no definite

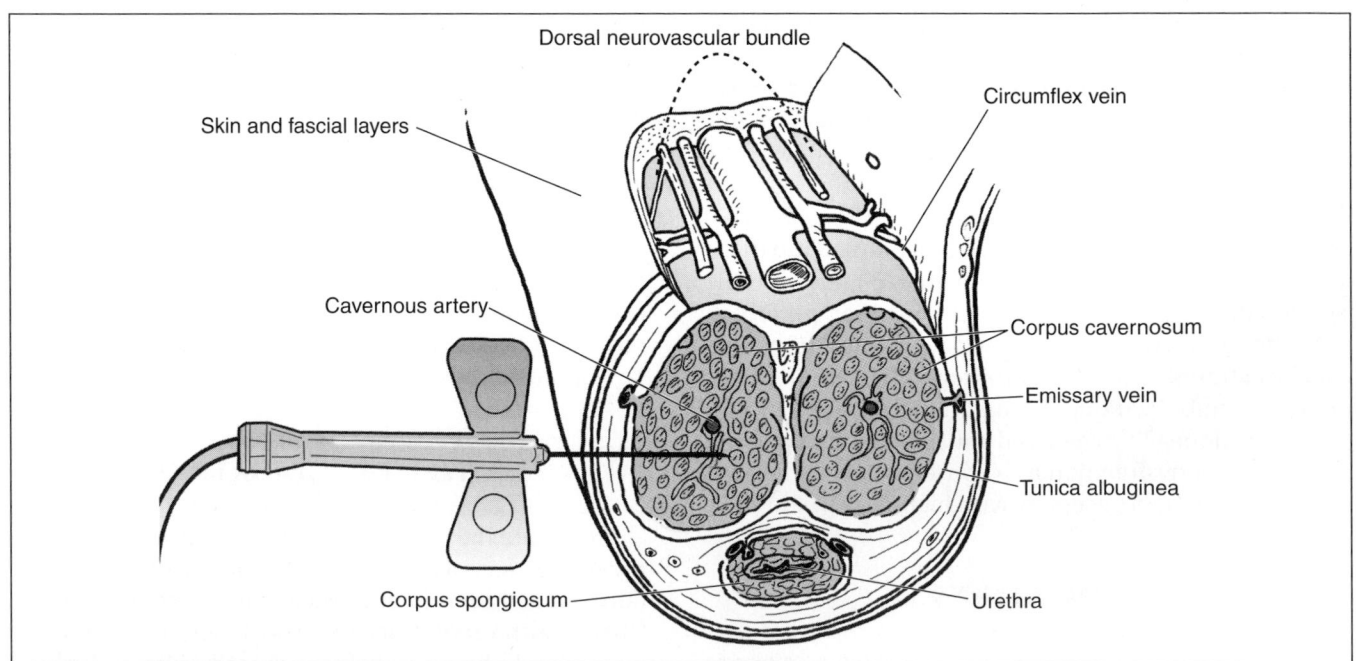

FIGURE 126-3 The technique of penile aspiration.

limit to the amount of phenylephrine used. Most physicians inject up to 1 mg of phenylephrine but up to 2.5 mg has been suggested.

Compression of a puncture site must be done every time a needle is withdrawn from the penis to avoid a hematoma. The penis should resume a soft state. Partial detumescence might occur in some patients. If in doubt and pressure equipment is available, a cavernous pressure below 40 mmHg is considered acceptable. If this has been unsuccessful, venous shunting has to be considered. A Winter procedure using a Tru-Cut biopsy needle through the glans to remove a piece of corporal tissue can be performed in the Emergency Department by a Urologist. Familiarity with this procedure is necessary in order to establish an effective shunt. Other venous types of shunts are performed in the Operating Room to decompress the corpora cavernosa.

AFTERCARE

The patient should be observed for at least 30 minutes before assuming successful detumescence. No dressing should be applied to the penis. Any form of a compression dressing is contraindicated. An oral antibiotic should be prescribed for 24 hours (or longer if there is significant edema or a hematoma). An antibiotic whose spectrum covers skin flora, such as cephalexin, is appropriate. Referral to an appropriate specialist depends on the cause of the priapism. If a medication is a suspected cause, it should be discontinued if possible and the treating physician notified. Follow-up with a Urologist within 24 hours is necessary in all patients.

COMPLICATIONS

The long-term sequelae to unresolved priapism are fibrosis of the corporal tissue and loss of erectile function. Erectile dysfunction may still occur in patients despite successful detumescence. Varying degrees of fibrosis may be found on physical examination at a later date. Treatment by aspiration and irrigation can be associated with hematoma formation, urethral injury, and infection. The use of alpha-adrenergic agonists can have the systemic effects of headache, increased blood pressure, palpitations, and erythema. Deaths have been recorded with agents other than phenylephrine. The use of phenylephrine has not been reported to give rise to serious complications and is the agent of choice.

A prophylactic antibiotic, compression of needle puncture sites, care in alpha-adrenergic agonist dosing, observing the patient, and monitoring the blood pressure and pulse can help prevent untoward outcomes. The patient needs to be fully informed of the long-term risk of sexual dysfunction, even if detumescence is successful. Recurrence of the priapism is common and the patient should be warned to seek immediate care.

SUMMARY

Priapism is either low-flow with ischemia or high-flow, which is nonischemic. Ischemia of the corpora cavernous is associated with permanent damage to the tissue if not treated within 36 hours. Prompt treatment is essential. Although initial care should be suited to the specific cause, the general recommendation for treatment is to establish oxygenation of the tissue as soon as possible by decompressing the corpora, thus allowing arterial inflow with oxygenation of the tissue. If the duration of tumescence is under 36 hours, injection of alpha-adrenergic agonists can be used to further facilitate detumescence. The incidence of erectile dysfunction following low-flow priapism is high. The patient needs to be fully informed and this should be documented in the medical record.

In contrast to ischemic low-flow priapism, high-flow or nonischemic priapism does not require emergency treatment. Patients should have prompt referral to a Urologist for diagnosis and treatment. Sexual dysfunction may less commonly occur in these patients.

REFERENCES

1. Lue TF, Broderick G: Evaluation and nonsurgical management of erectile dysfunction and priapism, in Walsh PC, Retik AB, Vaughan ED Jr, et al (eds): *Campbell's Urology,* 7th ed. Philadelphia: Saunders, 1998:1181–1214.
2. Goldstein I, Lue TF, Mulhall J: Personal communication, October 1999.
3. Chakrabarty A, Upadhyay J, Dhabuwala CB, et al: Priapism associated with hemoglobinopathy in children: long-term effects on potency. *J Urol* 1996; 155(4):1419–1423.
4. Spycher MA, Hauri D: The ultrastructure of the erectile tissue in priapism. *J Urol* 1986; 135(1): 142–146.
5. Kulmala RV, Tamella TLJ: Effects of priapism lasting 24 hours or longer caused by intracavernosal injection of vasoactive drugs. *Int J Impot Res* 1995; 7(2):131–136.
6. Ul-Iltasan M, El-Sakka AI, Lee C, et al: Expression of TGF-B-1 mRNA and ultrastructural alterations in pharmacologically induced prolonged penile erection in a canine model. *J Urol* 1998; 160(6):2263–2266.

7. Jünemann KP, Lue TF, Abozeid M, et al: Blood gas analysis in drug induced penile erection. *Urol Int* 1986; 41:(1)207–211.

8. Lue TF, Hellstrom WJG, McAninch JW, et al: Priapism: a refined approach to diagnosis and treatment. *J Urol* 1986; 136(1):104–108.

9. Sharpsteen R, Powars D, Johnson C, et al: Multisystem damage associated with tricorporal priapism in sickle cell disease. *Am J Med* 1993; 94(1):289–293.

10. Pohl J, Pott B, Kleinhaus G: Priapism: a three-phase concept of management according to etiology and prognosis. *Br J Urol* 1986; 58(1):113–116.

11. Hasen HB, Raines SL: Priapism associated with sickle cell disease. *J Urol* 1962; 88(1):71–75.

12. Tarry CA, Duckett JW Jr, Snyder HMcC III: Urological complications of sickle cell disease in a pediatric population. *J Urol* 1987; 138(2):592–594.

13. Seeler RA: Intensive transfusion therapy for boys with sickle cell anemia. *J Urol* 1973; 110(2):360–361.

14. Hamre MR, Harmon EP, Kirkpatrick DV: Priapism as a complication of sickle cell disease. *J Urol* 1991; 145(1):1–5.

15. Muruve N, Hosking DH: Intracorporal phenylephrine in the treatment of priapism. *J Urol* 1996; 155(1):141–143.

16. Sayer J, Parsons CL: Successful treatment of priapism with intracorporal epinephrine. *J Urol* 1988; 140(3):827–828.

17. Molina L, Bejany D, Lynne CM: Diluted epinephrine solution for the treatment of priapism. *J Urol* 1989; 141(6):1127–1128.

18. Broderick GA, Gordon D, Hypolite, et al: Anoxia and corporal smooth muscle dysfunction: a model for ischemic priapism. *J Urol* 1994; 151(1):259–262.

19. Mulhall J: Personal communication, March 2000.

20. Schreibman SM, Gee TS, Grabstald H: Management of priapism in patients with chronic granulocytic leukemia. *J Urol* 1974; 111(3):786–788.

21. Baron M, Leiter E: The management of priapism in sickle cell anemia. *J Urol* 1978; 119(5):610–611.

22. Emond AM, Holman R, Hayes RJ, et al: Priapism and impotence in sickle cell disease. *Arch Intern Med* 1980; 140(6):1434–1437.

23. Sacher EC, Sayegh E, Fernsilli F, et al: Cavernospongiosum shunt in the treatment of priapism. *J Urol* 1972; 108(1):97–100.

24. Resnick MI, Holland JM, King LR: Priapism in boys: management with cavernosaphenous shunt. *Urology* 1975; 5(4):492–495.

25. Winter CC: Care of idiopathic priapism: new procedure for creating fistula between glans penis and corpora cavernosa. *Urology* 1976; 8(2):389–391.

26. Walker TG, Grant PW, Goldstein I: High-flow priapism: treatment with super-selective transcatheter embolization. *Radiology* 1990; 174(3):1053–1054.

27. Brock G, Breza J, Lue TF: High-flow priapism: a spectrum of disease. *J Urol* 1993; 150(2):968–971.

28. Ercole CJ, Pontes JE, Pierce JM Jr: Changing surgical concepts in the treatment for priapism. *J Urol* 1981; 125(1):210–211.

Chapter 127
PARAPHIMOSIS REDUCTION

Charles M. Lash
Ann Nguyen

INTRODUCTION

A paraphimosis is defined as the inability to reduce a proximally positioned foreskin over the glans penis and back to its normal anatomic position. Some confuse a paraphimosis with a phimosis. The latter is a scarring or narrowing of the foreskin in which it cannot be retracted over the glans of the penis. The most common causes for a paraphimosis are iatrogenic. Following examination or instrumentation of the penis, medical personnel often forget to reduce the foreskin over the glans. This is particularly true of patients who are sedated, confused, demented, delirious, or in a nursing home. Patients may fail to reduce their foreskin after intercourse or urination. In infants and toddlers, the foreskin does not become fully mobile until after three years of age. This predisposes them to a paraphimosis when well-meaning caregivers forcibly retract the foreskin during cleaning. A paraphimosis may also occur when a narrowed (phimotic) foreskin is retracted and unable to be reduced.

A patient with a paraphimosis usually presents with severe pain in the distal penis. The process may have a more indolent presentation in persons with impaired pain sensation, such as the elderly or diabetics. As they are often unable to complain of pain, patients with altered mental status are at risk for complications of a paraphimosis. This includes penile ulceration, infection, gangrene, and partial penile autoamputation.[1] A careful and complete physical examination is mandatory in these patients. Penile edema secondary to a paraphimosis must be differentiated from edema due to infection, trauma, or allergic reactions.

ANATOMY AND PATHOPHYSIOLOGY

The foreskin results from epithelial infolding during the gestational growth of the penis. It is composed of a double layer of epidermis overlying subcutaneous tissue. The foreskin is attached to the skin at the base of the glans penis. It covers the glans to a variable degree and can usually be completely retracted over the glans. The arterial supply to the foreskin is derived from branches of the external pudendal artery that originates from the femoral artery. Once these branches reach the preputial ring, they become tortuous, attenuated, and terminate at the coronal sulcus. These superficial arteries do not communicate with the deep arteries of the penis. The foreskin veins are multiple small branches that drain through the inferior external pudendal vein to the saphenous vein of the thigh.

The glans of the penis is supplied by the paired dorsal arteries of the penis that arise from the penile artery. These dorsal penile arteries course deep to Buck's fascia ventrolaterally to enter the glans at the coronal sulcus. A frenular branch is given off at this point. The blood supply to the glans penis is entirely separate from that of the foreskin.

A retracted foreskin will block lymphatic drainage from the distal penis. As arterial inflow continues, the lack of lymphatic drainage will cause a progressive edema of the penis distal to the retracted foreskin. If the foreskin is not reduced, the edema will eventually obstruct venous outflow. The distal penis will become painful and hyperemic. The edema will progress to eventually obstruct arterial inflow resulting in penile ischemia, necrosis, and gangrene. This series of events, from retraction of the foreskin to arterial inflow obstruction, can occur over a few hours to 1 to 2 days.

A paraphimosis is a simple structural abnormality (Figures 127-1 and 127-2). The foreskin is retracted behind the glans of the penis and becomes edematous. The base of the foreskin is the location of the constricting or phimotic ring. As the foreskin continues to swell, the phimotic ring becomes progressively tighter. To reduce the paraphimosis, the phimotic ring must be advanced (reduced) over the glans of the penis.

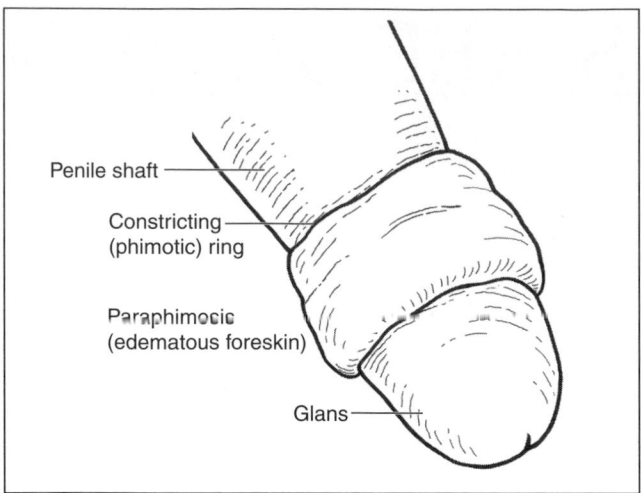

FIGURE 127-1 The anatomy of a paraphimosis.

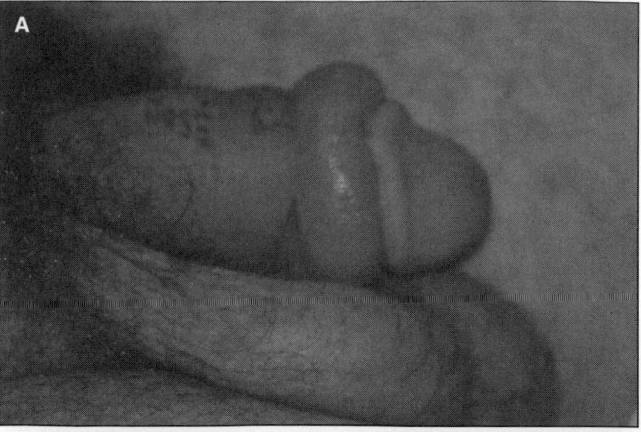

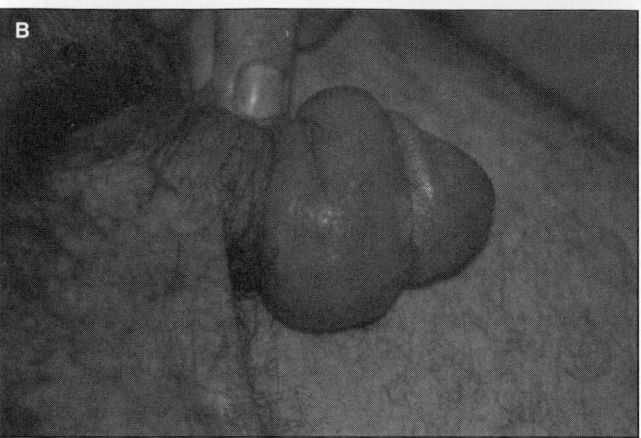

FIGURE 127-2 A paraphimosis. *A.* Superior view. *B.* Inferior view.

INDICATIONS

All paraphimoses require reduction. The earlier a paraphimosis is reduced, the easier it will be to perform the reduction. As the edema progresses, it becomes progressively more difficult to reduce a paraphimosis. **Nonsurgical techniques should be attempted first. If they are unsuccessful or the skin is compromised (infection, ulceration, gangrene), surgical techniques are indicated.**[2]

CONTRAINDICATIONS

There are no absolute contraindications to the reduction of a paraphimosis. Nonsurgical techniques are contraindicated in patients with ulcerated or necrotic foreskins.[2] While all paraphimoses must be reduced, some techniques are contraindicated in certain patient subgroups. Some authors feel that surgical reductions in children should be reserved for Pediatric Urologists.[3,4] **A surgical reduction should not be performed if noninvasive and lesser invasive techniques have not been attempted.** The hyaluronidase technique is contraindicated in penile cancers or infections due to the possibility of spreading infected or malignant cells through the tissue planes.[5]

EQUIPMENT

Povidone iodine solution
Lidocaine jelly
Water-soluble lubricant
Local anesthetic solution (1% lidocaine or 0.5% bupivacaine) without epinephrine
27 gauge needle
10 mL syringe

4×4 gauze squares
Crushed ice
Surgical gloves
Babcock clamps (6 to 8)
2 inch wide roll of elastic bandage (Ace Wrap or Elastoplast)
Sterile drapes
Sterile surgical gloves
Suture scissors
2 straight hemostats
#15 surgical blade with handle
Needle driver
3–0 synthetic absorbable suture or chromic catgut suture
Granulated (table) sugar
Hyaluronidase (Wydase, Wyeth-Ayerst Laboratories, Philadelphia, PA)
Antibiotic ointment, topical
Petrolatum gauze

PATIENT PREPARATION

Reduction of a paraphimosis can be painful and somewhat distressing to patients. Explain to the patient and/or their representative the risks and benefits of the procedure. Also explain that the progression from nonsurgical to surgical techniques may be required. Obtain an informed consent from the patient. If the patient has an indwelling urinary catheter, it should be left in place during the reduction.

While premedication is rarely necessary, some patients may benefit from mild sedation. Procedural sedation and general anesthesia may be required in children.[3,4] Analgesia can sometimes be achieved with the topical application of lidocaine jelly or EMLA cream (2.5% prilocaine and 2.5% lidocaine). If this does not provide adequate patient comfort, a ring block or dorsal penile nerve block can be performed with 0.5% bupivacaine and/or 1% lidocaine.[6] Refer to Chapter 125 for the complete details regarding penile anesthesia.

TECHNIQUES

The techniques described below to reduce a paraphimosis begin with manual compression and progress to incision of the phimotic ring. They should be attempted in a stepwise manner from the least invasive to the most invasive procedure as described below.

MANUAL REDUCTION

This method has been extensively described.[3,7–10] Liberally apply an anesthetic jelly or water-soluble lubricant to the glans and foreskin. Do not coat the penile shaft or else it will be too slippery to facilitate an easy reduction.

Apply manual compression directly to the glans and edematous foreskin by grasping them with the palm of a gloved hand (Figure 127-3). Apply slow and steady pressure for 5 to 10 minutes. Many physicians do not have the time or the strength to apply pressure to a patient's

penis for 5 to 10 minutes. In children, the parent may be asked to provide the manual compression. Compression may also be provided by firmly wrapping a bandage around the penis beginning at the glans and working towards the base of the penis. Apply the bandage so that it places more pressure distally and less proximally. This will mobilize the edematous fluid from distal to proximal. The bandage can be an Ace Wrap or Elastoplast,[10] a gauze sponge soaked in lidocaine jelly, or a gauze sponge soaked in cold water.[7]

Remove the bandage or release manual compression after it has been applied for 5 to 10 minutes. Apply the index and middle fingers of both hands to surround the penile shaft proximal to the phimotic ring (Figure 127-4). Place both thumbs adjacent to the urethral meatus. Push the glans proximally with the thumbs while the fingers simultaneously provide countertraction to pull the phimotic band over the glans. Apply continuous force until the phimotic band moves distal to the glans. This same technique can be applied if the patient has an indwelling urinary catheter (Figure 127-5).

Alternatively, encircle the entire foreskin in one hand and pull distally while simultaneously pushing the glans proximally with the thumb of the opposite hand.[8] It is important to be very deliberate in the first attempt as the patient will become more anxious on subsequent attempts. This same technique can be applied if the patient has an indwelling urinary catheter.

ICED GLOVE TECHNIQUE

This technique combines cold to induce vasoconstriction and compression to reduce swelling.[8] This method uses a glove to provide a circumferential ice

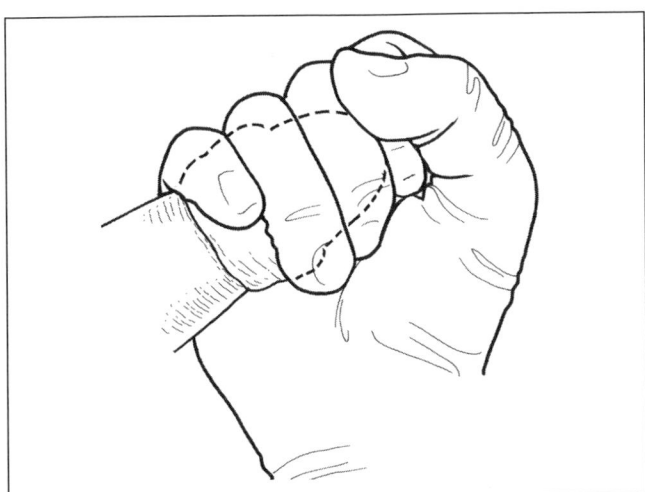

FIGURE 127-3 Manual compression of the glans and foreskin to reduce the edema of the foreskin.

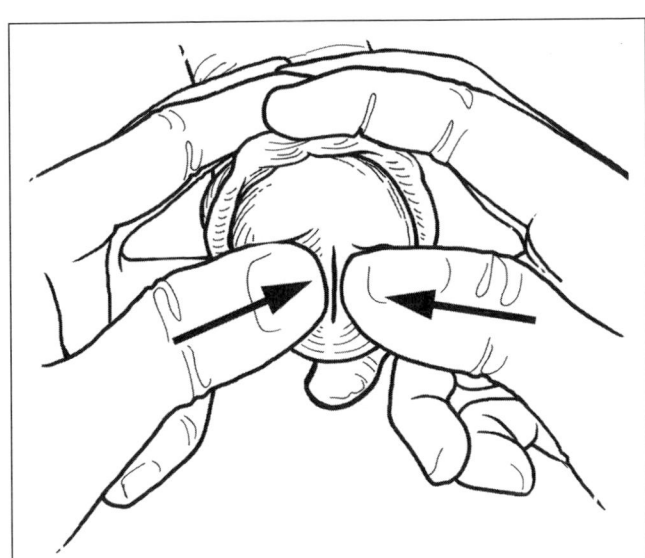

FIGURE 127-4 Manual reduction of a paraphimosis. The thumbs push the glans proximally (arrows) while the fingers provide countertraction to slip the phimotic ring over the glans.

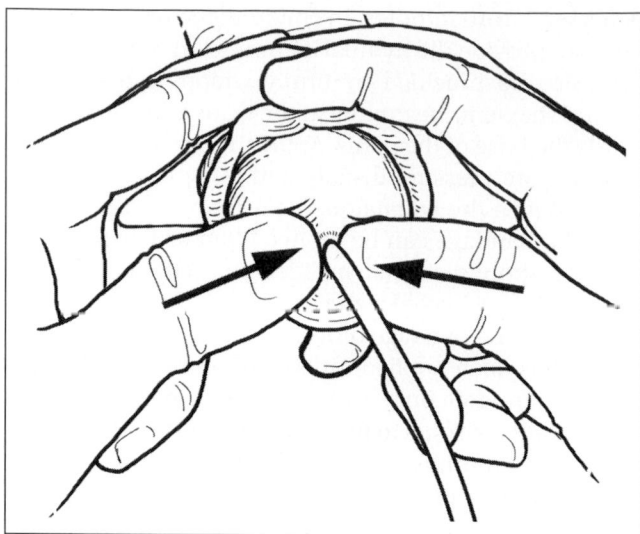

FIGURE 127-5 Manual reduction of a paraphimosis in the patient with an indwelling urinary catheter.

pack to the foreskin to reduce edema. Half-fill a size 8 surgical glove with crushed ice and cold water. Squeeze the air from the glove and tie a knot in the wrist of the glove. Invaginate the thumb into the body of the glove. Liberally lubricate the glans and foreskin. Insert the penis into the invaginated thumb of the glove. Apply manual pressure with a clenched fist or bandage for ten minutes. Attempt manual reduction as described previously.[2,3,4,8]

BABCOCK CLAMP TECHNIQUE

This technique can be used when manual reduction has been unsuccessful. It has a high rate of success in reducing a paraphimosis.[3,8,11,12] It requires penile anesthesia. **Use only Babcock clamps. All other surgical clamps will crush and devitalize tissue.**

Apply 6 to 8 Babcock clamps circumferentially around the phimotic ring (Figure 127-6A). Place one edge of each clamp just proximal to the phimotic ring and the other edge just distal to the phimotic ring. **It is important to grasp a sufficient amount of the constricting ring to avoid tearing the skin once traction is applied.** Space the clamps evenly around the circumference of the penis. Grasp all of the Babcock clamps in one hand. Simultaneously and slowly apply distal traction to pull the phimotic ring over the glans (Figure 127-6B). After reduction, remove the Babcock clamps. Examine the foreskin for any signs of traumatic injury from the clamps.

NEEDLE DECOMPRESSION TECHNIQUE

This technique mechanically expresses fluid from the edematous foreskin via a series of puncture holes in the foreskin.[3,9,13–16] Penile anesthesia is required with this technique. Clean the penis of any dirt or debris. Drape and isolate a sterile field around the penis. Apply povidone iodine solution to the penis and allow it to dry.

Insert a sterile, hollow-bore 18 gauge needle 3 to 5 mm deep into the foreskin. Continue to puncture holes circumferentially around the edematous foreskin (Figure 127-7). An average of 8 to 12 holes are required; different recommendations to use as few as 1 to as many as 20 punctures have been made.[14,15] Wrap a gauze square around the foreskin and glans. Grasp the glans and foreskin in the palm of a gloved hand and apply manual compression. Edema fluid and blood will be expressed from the puncture holes allowing the foreskin

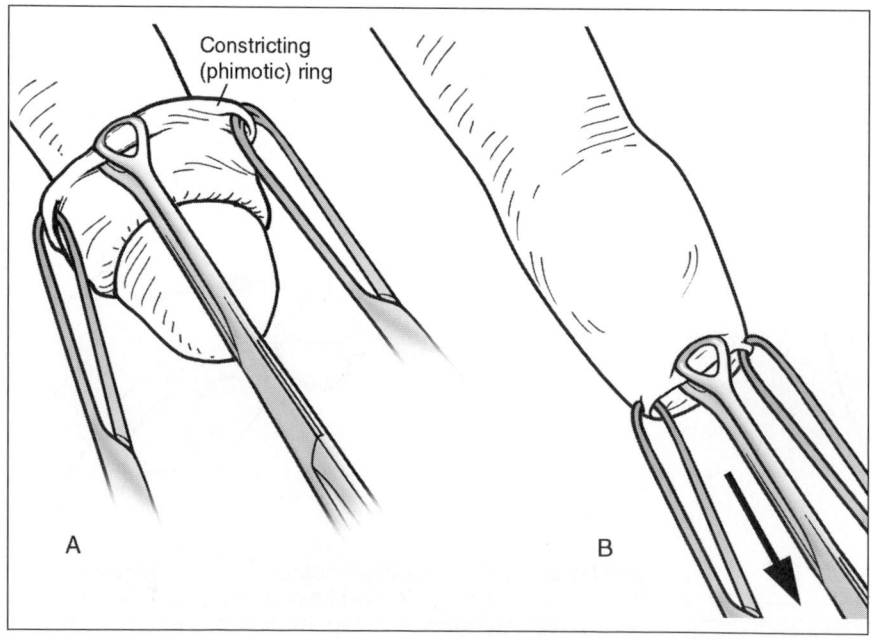

FIGURE 127-6 The Babcock clamp technique. *A.* Place 6 to 8 Babcock clamps along the phimotic ring. Note that only 3 Babcock clamps are seen in the illustration for the sake of clarity. *B.* Traction is simultaneously placed on all the clamps to advance the phimotic ring over the glans.

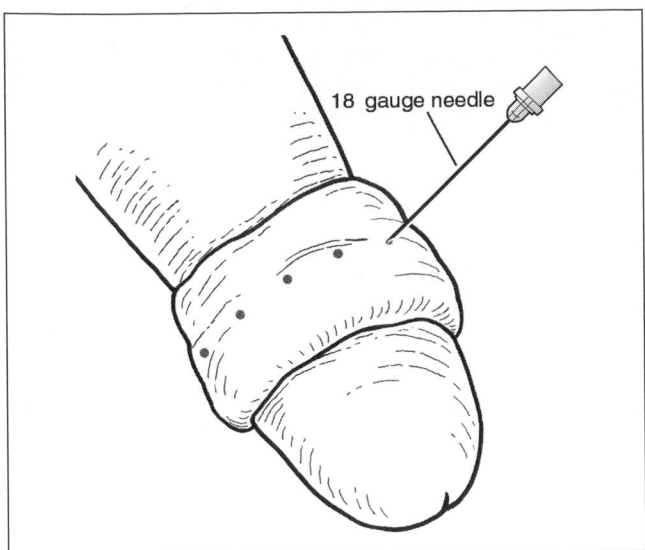

FIGURE 127-7 The needle decompression technique. An 18 gauge needle is used to circumferentially puncture the edematous foreskin 8 to 12 times.

to decompress. The gauze square will allow the physician to maintain a grasp as the penis becomes slippery with blood and edema fluid. After the foreskin is decompressed, reduce it manually or with Babcock clamps.

DORSAL SLIT OF THE FORESKIN

One must always be prepared to perform surgical techniques if nonsurgical reduction is unsuccessful. This technique involves the incision of the phimotic ring under strict sterile technique.[2,6,8] Place the patient supine and anesthetize the penis, if it hasn't been done previously. Apply povidone iodine solution to the penis and let it dry. Apply sterile drapes to isolate a surgical field. Consider the administration of parenteral sedation prior to performing this procedure to alleviate the patient's anxiety.

Clamp a straight-blade hemostat over the foreskin and phimotic ring at the 11 o'clock and 1 o'clock positions. Place one jaw of each hemostat beneath the phimotic ring and the other jaw on top of it. **Be careful not to clamp the skin on the shaft of the penis.** Pull the foreskin taut between the hemostats. Grasp the hemostats with the nondominant hand or have an assistant hold them. Incise the foreskin and phimotic ring at the 12 o'clock position with a scissors or a #15 scalpel blade (Figure 127-8A). **Be careful not to cut the skin on the shaft of the penis.** Remove the hemostats. The incision will open into a pentagonal shape (Figure 127-8B). Reduce the foreskin over the glans. Cover the penis with sterile gauze and allow the edges of the incision to ooze for 10 to 15 minutes.

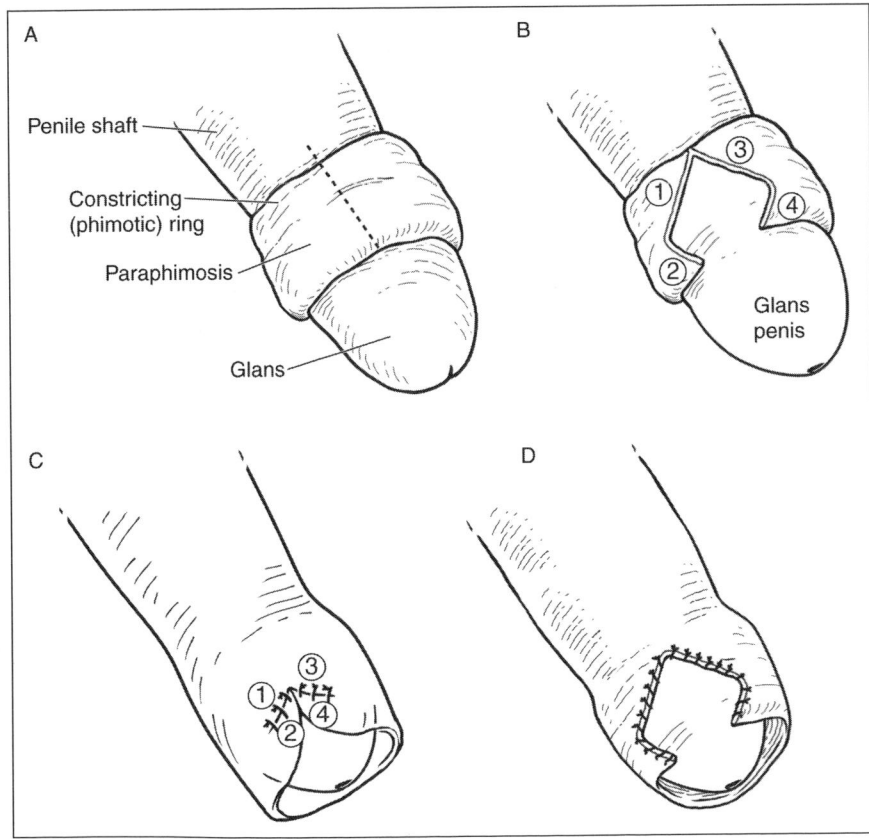

FIGURE 127-8 The dorsal slit of the foreskin. *A.* The dotted line represents the incision line. *B.* The foreskin opens after the incision is made. The numbers represent the edges of the incision. *C.* The foreskin has been reduced and the edges of the incision sewn shut. A small gap should remain in the midline that is free of sutures. *D.* Alternatively, sew the edges closed with a simple running stitch.

This technique can be technically difficult for the non-Surgeon. As an alternative to the two-hemostat technique, a one-hemostat technique may be performed. Place one hemostat over the foreskin and phimotic ring at the 12 o'clock position (Figure 127-8*A*). Remove the clamp after 1 to 2 minutes. Cut the crushed tissue with scissors through the phimotic ring. **Be careful not to cut the skin on the shaft of the penis.** The foreskin will then open up as described above (Figure 127-8*B*).

After the foreskin has been incised and reduced over the glans, approximate the cut edges with 3–0 chromic suture using a simple interrupted stitch (Figure 127-8*C*). Sew edge 1 and edge 2, on the illustration, together. Sew edge 3 and edge 4, on the illustration, together. A gap will remain at the 12 o'clock position that corresponds to the area of the initial incision. Alternatively, sew the cut edges with a simple running stitch (Figure 127-8*D*). Loosely apply petrolatum gauze and gauze squares over the wound. Apply a piece of tape to hold the dressing on the penis. **The tape should not be applied circumferentially as this can cause ischemia to the penis.**

MODIFIED DORSAL SLIT OF THE FORESKIN

A modified dorsal slit technique has been described where only the phimotic ring is cut rather than the entire foreskin.[4,8] Clean, prep, anesthetize, and drape the penis as above. As an alternative to a penile block, infiltrate under the phimotic ring at the 12 o'clock position with local anesthetic solution without epinephrine using a 27 gauge needle. Be sure to raise a wheal both proximally and distally to the phimotic ring (along the dotted line in Figure 127-9*A*). A penile block is the preferred method of anesthesia as injection onto the distal penis is extremely painful.

Incise the phimotic ring with a #15 scalpel blade. **Incise only the phimotic ring. Do not extend the cut more than 3 mm proximally or distally to the phimotic ring.** Once incised, the foreskin will spring open into a diamond-shaped defect (Figure 127-9*B*). Reduce the foreskin. Cover the penis with gauze and allow the cut edges to ooze for 10 to 15 minutes to decompress the foreskin. Approximate the edges of the wound with 3–0 chromic suture in a running pattern. Apply a bandage of petrolatum gauze and gauze squares over the wound. Apply a piece of tape to hold the dressing on the penis. **The tape should not be applied circumferentially as this can cause ischemia to the penis.**

ALTERNATIVE TECHNIQUES

A variety of alternative techniques have been described in the literature.[5,9,13,17,18] These techniques are variations on the basic principles previously discussed. We will briefly review the osmotic (sugar), hyaluronidase, and glans aspiration techniques.

OSMOTIC (SUGAR) TECHNIQUE

An alternative to surgical techniques is the osmotic technique.[9,17,18] It is an innovative, painless, but time-consuming method. The glans and foreskin are immersed in sugar. An osmotic gradient is formed between the edematous foreskin and the sugar. The hypertonicity of the sugar draws the edema fluid out of the foreskin. The deflated foreskin can then be manually reduced over the glans. This technique should not be performed if the foreskin or the gland is infected, gangrenous, or ulcerated.

Place ordinary table sugar into the invaginated thumb of a large surgical glove. Insert the penis into the thumb of the glove, like in the iced glove method described above.[17] The penis may also be wrapped distally to proximally in a gauze square saturated with a 50% dextrose solution.[9,18] In all reports, the sugar was left on the penis for a minimum of 1 hour before manual reduc-

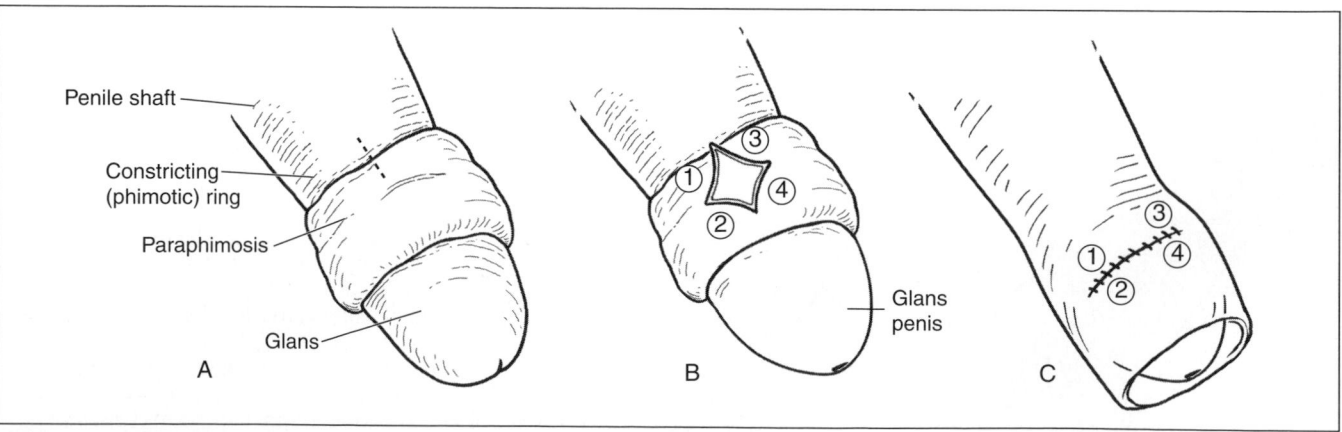

FIGURE 127-9 The modified dorsal slit of the foreskin. *A*. The dotted line represents the incision line. *B*. The foreskin opens after the incision is made. The numbers represent the edges of the incision. *C*. The foreskin has been reduced and the edges of the incision sewn shut.

tion was successful. The maximum time reported before successful reduction was 4 hours.[17]

HYALURONIDASE METHOD

Hyaluronidase (Wydase, Wyeth-Ayerst Laboratories, Philadelphia, PA) is a commercially available mammalian enzyme that degrades the intercellular ground substance of connective tissue. It is widely used in ophthalmologic and plastic surgery as a spreading agent. When injected into an edematous foreskin, hyaluronidase disperses the extracellular edema fluid, facilitating reduction of the paraphimosis.[5,13]

Clean, prep, drape, and anesthetize the penis. Inject hyaluronidase subcutaneously using a tuberculin syringe at various points around the circumference of the foreskin. A total of 150 units, 1 mL, of hyaluronidase should be used. An alternative is to inject the hyaluronidase into the puncture holes previously made from the needle decompression technique.[9,13] The edema should resolve almost immediately. Manual compression may be applied to the foreskin for 1 to 2 minutes to help mobilize the fluid. After the edema has decreased, manually reduce the foreskin.

The advantage of this technique is the rapidity with which the edema resolves. However, hyaluronidase is contraindicated in patients with penile infections or cancer as it may spread bacteria or malignant cells through the tissue planes. It is also contraindicated if the foreskin or glans is gangrenous or ulcerated.

GLANS ASPIRATION TECHNIQUE

Raveenthiran describes this method that is based on techniques used to treat priapism.[19] The author reports using this technique on four patients with paraphimoses with a 100 percent success rate and no complications. He recommended it for use when the foreskin is very friable and not amenable to vigorous manipulation. This technique is described for the sake of completeness but is not recommended.

Clean, prep, drape, and anesthetize the penis. Apply a sterile tourniquet to the penile shaft proximal to the phimotic ring. Use either umbilical tape or a Penrose drain. Insert a 20 gauge needle on a 10 mL syringe into the midline of the glans, halfway between the meatus and the corona. Keep the needle and syringe parallel to the urethra. Advance the needle while aspirating with the syringe. Once blood is encountered, stop advancing the needle. Continue to aspirate blood until the glans collapses completely. It is estimated that approximately 3 to 12 mL of blood will need to be aspirated, depending on the size of the glans. Remove the needle. Grasp and firmly squeeze the glans with the nondominant hand. While maintaining this pressure, release the tourniquet and manually reduce the foreskin over the collapsed glans with the dominant hand.

ASSESSMENT

The successfully reduced paraphimosis should have the general appearance of a normal uncircumcised penis. The patient usually notes immediate pain relief. It is normal for residual edema to be present. Reassure the patient that the edema will spontaneously resolve over hours to days.[3,8] If invasive techniques were utilized, observe the patient in the Emergency Department for 45 to 60 minutes to confirm hemostasis. Observe the patient for full recovery from any sedation or procedural sedation techniques as per hospital policy.

AFTERCARE

Wound care following a surgical reduction is the same as that for any sutured laceration. Many physicians do not dress the site at all. But if desired, the site may be covered with antibiotic ointment or petrolatum gauze and a dry sterile gauze.[6] The patient should be counseled on proper wound care. The patient should inspect the glans and foreskin three to four times a day if Babcock clamps or surgical techniques were used to reduce the paraphimosis. They should return immediately to the Emergency Department if any signs of infection develop. Advise them to avoid intercourse or masturbation for 4 to 6 weeks.[6]

Antibiotics should be prescribed if the foreskin is abraded, infected, ulcerated, or torn by the Babcock clamp technique. They should also be prescribed if the foreskin was reduced by an invasive technique (needle decompression, dorsal slit, modified dorsal slit, hyaluronidase, or glans aspiration). Oral antibiotics whose spectrum covers skin flora should be prescribed. Cephalexin, 500 mg orally four times a day, is usually adequate.

All patients need to follow-up with a Urologist in 1 to 2 days. The definitive treatment is circumcision. This is typically delayed 7 to 10 days until any edema, inflammation, or ulceration has resolved.[7,8]

COMPLICATIONS

Incomplete reduction and pain are possible complications of manual reduction. With that in mind, it is important to allow enough time for adequate dispersion of edema. Manual reduction may also be associated with glans contusion and even glans ischemia if manual pressure is too great.[4] The iced glove method may produce cold injury if not properly monitored during use.[3] Compromised penile skin may be torn during manual or Babcock clamp reduction. The treatment is to suture any tears that occur.[8]

If surgical techniques are performed, bleeding is a common complication in this very vascular tissue. Venous bleeding can be profuse. It is important to have good control of the tissue edges so that adequate hemostatic stitches can be placed. A compressive dressing may aid in hemostasis. If the penile shaft is lacerated during a surgical reduction, it too should be sutured. And as with all invasive procedures, infection may be a complication of the needle decompression, dorsal slit, modified dorsal slit, hyaluronidase, and glans aspiration techniques.

The glans aspiration method runs the risk of transecting the urethra if the needle is not advanced parallel to the urethra. Complications of the hyaluronidase method may range from minor ecchymoses at the injection site to anaphylaxis and shock if the hyaluronidase is inadvertently injected intravascularly.[5,13]

SUMMARY

A paraphimosis is a problem that is best prevented. Replacement of the foreskin after urethral catheterization or glans cleaning is important. Early intervention is necessary and can prevent disastrous tissue loss. Gaining the patient's trust will greatly aid in the reduction. The reduction techniques should be attempted in a stepwise manner beginning with noninvasive techniques and progressing to increasingly invasive techniques.

REFERENCES

1. Hollowood AD, Sibley GN: Non-painful paraphimosis causing partial amputation. *Br J Urol* 1997; 80(6):958.
2. Houghton GR: The "iced-glove" method of treatment of paraphimosis. *Br J Surg* 1973; 60(11):876–877.
3. Green M, Strange GR: Paraphimosis reduction, in Henretig FM, King C, Joffee MD, et al (eds): *Textbook of Pediatric Emergency Procedures.* Baltimore: Williams and Wilkins, 1997:1007–1010.
4. Shaw KN: Reduction of paraphimosis, in Dieckmann RA, Fiser DH, Selbst SM (eds): *Pediatric Emergency and Critical Care Procedures.* St. Louis: Mosby, 1997:435–436.
5. DeVries CR, Miller AK, Packer MG: Reduction of a paraphimosis with hyaluronidase. *Urology* 1996; 48:464–465.
6. Holman JR, Stuessi KA: Adult circumcision. *Am Fam Physician* 1999; 59(6):1514–1518.
7. Dunmire SM, Paris PM: *Atlas of Emergency Procedures.* Philadelphia: Saunders, 1994:187–188.
8. Schneider RE: Urologic procedures, in Roberts JR, Hedges JR (eds): *Clinical Procedures in Emergency Medicine,* 4th ed. Philadelphia: Saunders, 1998:947–952.
9. Olson C: Emergency treatment of paraphimosis. *Can Fam Physician* 1998; 44:1253–1254.
10. Ganti SU, Sayegh N, Addonizio JC: Simple method for reduction of paraphimosis. *Urology* 1985; 25(1):77.
11. Skoglund RW, Chapman WH: Reduction of a paraphimosis. *J Urol* 1970; 104:137.
12. Turner CD, Kim HL, Cromie WJ: Dorsal band traction for reduction of paraphimosis. *Urology* 1999; 54(5):917–918.
13. Fuenfer MM, Najmaldin A: Emergency reduction of paraphimosis. *Eur J Pediatr Surg* 1994; 4(6):370–371.
14. Reynard JM, Barua JM: Reduction of paraphimosis the simple way—the Dundee technique. *Br J Urol* 1999; 83(7):859–860.
15. Barone JG, Fleisher MH: Treatment of paraphimosis using the "puncture" technique. *Pediatr Emerg Care* 1993; 9(5):298–299.
16. Hamdy FC, Hastie KJ: Treatment of paraphimosis using the "puncture" technique. *Br J Surg* 1990; 77:1186.
17. Kerwat R, Shandall A, Stephenson B: Reduction of paraphimosis with granulated sugar. *Br J Urol* 1998; 82:755.
18. Coutts AG: Treatment of paraphimosis. *Br J Surg* 1991; 78(2):252.
19. Raveenthiran V: Reduction of paraphimosis: a technique based on pathophysiology. *Br J Surg* 1996; 83:1247.

Chapter 128
PHIMOSIS REDUCTION

Khursheed A. Mallick
Neil Troost

INTRODUCTION

A phimosis is a condition in which the foreskin cannot be retracted behind the glans of the penis. In males younger than four years of age, it is normal for the foreskin to be unretractable. In older boys and adults, the foreskin can usually be retracted without difficulty.[1] Surgical recourse for a phimosis has been known for hundreds of years.[2] A Byzantine surgeon by the name of Oribasius, in the fourth century AD, gave a seemingly well-acquainted description of a technique involving forced dilation of the constrictive foreskin, scalloping out of its inner surface, then stretching it over a parchment-wrapped lead tube placed between the filleted skin and the glans.[2] Techniques for management of a phimosis in the Emergency Department are simple and remain an important intervention directed to relieving urinary obstruction.

ANATOMY AND PATHOPHYSIOLOGY

At birth there is a physiologic phimosis in the majority of male neonates. This is due to natural adhesions that exist between the foreskin and the glans of the penis. During the first 3 to 4 years of life, as the penis grows, epithelial debris (smegma) accumulates under the foreskin and gradually separates the foreskin from the glans. Intermittent penile erections aid in allowing the foreskin to eventually become retractable. The foreskin of most males will retract easily by the age of four. Forcible retraction should be categorically discouraged as this can result in scarring and constriction.[1] For a nonobstructive phimosis in children, topical steroids and topical conjugated equine estrogen have shown excellent results in releasing the stubborn physiologic adhesions between the foreskin and the glans.[3,4]

A phimosis can be the cause of other problems or be a result of other medical conditions. Once acquired, a phimosis can become a paraphimosis if the foreskin is retracted and not promptly reduced. It can result in urinary tract infections from bacterial colonization of the phimosis or secondary to urinary obstruction. Other complications of a phimosis include recurrent balanitis, local infection, urinary retention, carcinoma of the penis, and easy growth of venereal warts and other sexually transmitted diseases. A phimosis may also be secondary to many of the disease processes just mentioned. It may also be due to local trauma (known as Tristram Shandy syndrome) or the congenital lack of conversion to a mobile foreskin.[5] Penile carcinoma deserves special mention. Coexistent phimosis is seen in up to 52 percent of cases of penile carcinoma. The need for timely follow-up should be impressed upon the patient regardless of the intervention required in the Emergency Department.[6]

INDICATIONS

The sole indication for release of a phimosis is urinary obstruction that cannot be relieved by passing a urethral catheter.

CONTRAINDICATIONS

The ability to pass a urinary catheter (Foley or coudé) into the bladder eliminates the acute need for the reduction of a phimosis. Patients with bleeding disorders, gross infections of the foreskin, who are immunocompromised, or who have lesions of the foreskin should have a urinary catheter placed into the bladder rather than an incision of the phimotic foreskin. If a catheter

ASSESSMENT

Regardless of the technique, observe the patient in the Emergency Department for 45 to 60 minutes to confirm hemostasis. Observe the patient for full recovery from any sedation or procedural sedation techniques as per hospital policy.

AFTERCARE

The patient may be discharged with Urologic follow-up within 48 hours. Instruct the patient to return to the Emergency Department immediately if the wound is red, has a discharge, is swollen, or if fever develops. The patient should be given oral analgesics for pain control. Patients should be discharged on oral antibiotics whose spectrum covers skin flora. Cephalexin, 500 mg orally four times a day, is usually adequate. Between discharge and examination by a Urologist, the patient should practice gentle daily washing of the penis with soap, avoid placing any powders or creams in the area, and check the wound three to four times daily for signs of infection. Sexual intercourse and masturbation should be avoided until the incisions have completely healed.

COMPLICATIONS

Direct mechanical injury to the glans or urethra by inadvertent placement of instruments into the urethra could be devastating but is easily avoidable by following proper technique. Increased bleeding may result if the skin is not crushed by the hemostat before it is cut with the scissors.[5] It is also important to avoid advancing the clamp, and therefore the incision, beyond the comfortable limitation of the coronal sulcus. Otherwise, the skin on the penile shaft will be cut. This can result in a cosmetic defect and possibly skin sloughing requiring a skin graft. Wound infection and dehiscence are a possibility with any incision and greatly reduced in conscientious patients.

SUMMARY

From a variety of disease processes, the endpoint of phimosis causing urinary obstruction lends itself to simple correction by the Emergency Physician. Careful performance of the above techniques will result in excellent functional and aesthetic foreskin repair.

REFERENCES

1. Gillenwater JY, Howards SS, Grayhack JT, et al (eds): *Adult and Pediatric Urology,* 3rd ed. St. Louis: Mosby, 1995:2730–2731.
2. Kostakopoulos A, Lascaratos J, Louras G: Penile surgical techniques described by Oribasius. *Br J Urol* 1999; 84(1):16–19.
3. Caffaratti J, Garat JM, Orsola A: Conservative treatment of phimosis in children using a topical steroid. *Urology* 2000; 56(2):307–310.
4. Baba K, Iwamoto T, Yamagoe M, et al: Conservative treatment of childhood phimosis with topical conjugated equine estrogen ointment. *Int J Urol* 2000; 7(1): 1–3.
5. Schneider RE: Urologic procedures, in Roberts JR, Hedges JR (eds): *Clinical Procedures in Emergency Medicine,* 3rd ed. Philadelphia: Saunders, 1998:947–987.
6. Gillenwater JY, Howard SS, Grayhack JT, et al (eds): *Adult and Pediatric Urology,* 3rd ed. St. Louis: Mosby, 1995:2005.
7. Cheng W, Saing H: A prospective randomized study of wound approximation with tissue glue in circumcision in children. *J Paediatr Child Health* 1997; 33(6):515–516.
8. Baumgartner IM, Forte A, Gallinaro LS, et al: Local anaesthesia with eutectic cream of lidocaine and prilocaine for treatment of cicatrizial phimosis in outpatients. *Eur Rev Med Pharmacol Sci* 1998; 2(5–6):207–208.
9. Dean GE, Ritchie ML, Zaontz MR: La Vega slit procedure for the treatment of phimosis. *Urology* 2000; 55(3):419–421.

Chapter 129

DORSAL SLIT OF THE FORESKIN

Patricia Vidal
Mark Doucette
Andreas Skoubis

INTRODUCTION

A dorsal slit of the prepuce or foreskin is performed primarily in the Emergency Department. This technique is used to relieve strangulation of the glans by a paraphimosis, to release a paraphimosis, or to aid in the visualization of the urethral meatus in patients with a phimosis.[1] This technique is easy to learn, simple to perform, and takes approximately 10 minutes. Performing a dorsal slit of the foreskin requires complete anesthesia of the foreskin and/or penis (Chapter 125).

ANATOMY AND PATHOPHYSIOLOGY

The prepuce, or foreskin, is the skin originating just proximal to the corona that encircles the glans and often extends beyond it.[2] It may be incomplete, primarily at the ventral midline or the frenulum. The frenulum is the fusion site of the preputial and urethral folds. The glans is composed of the corpus spongiosum that enlarges to cover the tips of the corpora cavernosa. It has less erectile tissue than the cavernosa and contains the urethra.[2]

The blood supply to the foreskin and glans is from the left and right superficial penile arteries. The arteries are derived from the inferior external pudendal arteries, which are branches of the femoral arteries. The penile arteries travel in the superficial fascia of the penis and above Buck's fascia.[3] The left and right superficial penile arteries freely communicate over the midline.[4] Superficial veins accompany the arteries and ultimately drain to the saphenous veins in the thighs. The lymphatics travel deep to Buck's fascia and ultimately empty into the inguinal chain of lymph nodes. The somatic nerves to the foreskin are derived from the pudendal nerves.

A more detailed description of the anatomy and pathophysiology of the penis, a paraphimosis, and a phimosis can be found in Chapters 127 and 128.

INDICATIONS

A dorsal slit of the foreskin should be performed to release a paraphimosis or a phimosis. A paraphimosis is the inability to replace the retracted foreskin over the glans. A paraphimosis is considered an emergency since prolonged retraction of the foreskin leads to swelling of the prepuce resulting in strangulation injury to the glans.[1] A phimosis is the inability of the foreskin to retract and expose the glans. A phimosis should be released if it causes urinary retention. A phimosis can be due to true circumferential scar formation. Forceable retraction of a phimotic foreskin will result in tearing of the foreskin. A phimosis may be due to other disease processes such as edema (secondary to congestive heart failure, anasarca), inflammation with or without balanitis, or a malignancy. Refer to Chapters 127 and 128 for further details regarding a paraphimosis or a phimosis.

CONTRAINDICATIONS

There are no absolute contraindications to the reduction of a paraphimosis. Surgical reductions in children should be performed by a Pediatric Urologist, a Urologist, or after consultation with a Urologist. **A surgical reduction of a paraphimosis should be performed only after noninvasive and lesser invasive techniques have been unsuccessfully attempted** (Chapter 127).

The ability to pass a urinary catheter (Foley, coudé, filiforms and followers) into the bladder eliminates the acute need for reduction of a phimosis. Refer to Chapter 121 for the complete details regarding the techniques of urethral catheterization. Patients with bleeding disorders, gross infections of the foreskin, who are immunocompromised, or who have lesions of the foreskin should have a urinary catheter placed into the bladder rather than an incision of the phimotic foreskin. If a catheter cannot be inserted into the urethra in these patients, a Urologist should be consulted prior to any invasive procedures. Patients with a nonobstructing phimosis should be referred for elective circumcision and not have a dorsal slit procedure.

EQUIPMENT

Povidone iodine solution
Local anesthetic solution without epinephrine
5 mL syringe
27 gauge needle
Hemostats, straight or straight Kelly
#15 scalpel blade on a handle
Needle driver
3–0 or 4–0 chromic catgut, Dexon, or Vicryl
Petrolatum gauze
Metzenbaum scissors
Suture scissors
4×4 gauze squares
Sterile gloves
Sterile drapes
Topical antibacterial ointment

The use of tissue glue of the type normally found in Emergency Departments has been studied in children undergoing circumcision.[5] It was shown to increase infection, bleeding, and wound dehiscence when compared to suture. The use of suture must be recommended at this time to close the wound edges after the release of a paraphimosis or a phimosis.

PATIENT PREPARATION

Explain the benefits, risks, potential complications, and aftercare of the procedure to the patient and/or their representative. An informed consent should be obtained and placed in the medical record.

Prepare the penis for any intervention. Clean the penis of any dirt, debris, and discharge. Apply drapes to isolate the penis. Apply povidone iodine solution onto the penis. If possible, apply povidone iodine solution under the foreskin using a cotton-tipped applicator if necessary. If the patient has pain in the area of the foreskin, or if a procedure other than catheter insertion is to be performed, the penis should be anesthetized. Refer to Chapter 125 for the complete details regarding penile anesthesia. Alternatively, infiltration of local anesthetic solution can be used to anesthetize the foreskin. Draw up 5 mL of local anesthetic solution without epinephrine into a syringe armed with a 27 gauge needle. Inject a subcutaneous wheal of local anesthetic solution 2 cm

proximal to the distal end of the foreskin. Continue subcutaneous infiltration circumferentially around the penis with the local anesthetic solution. The patient may require intravenous sedation or procedural sedation prior to the injection of local anesthetic solution into the penis.

The use of topical anesthetics such as lidocaine jelly, prilocaine creams, or combinations (EMLA, LET, LAT) is not recommended.[6] The application of these mixtures requires an occlusive dressing and 60 to 90 minutes for the anesthetic effect, which may then be inadequate.

TECHNIQUES

DORSAL SLIT OF THE PARAPHIMOTIC FORESKIN

One must always be prepared to perform surgical techniques if nonsurgical reduction is unsuccessful. This technique involves the incision of the phimotic ring under strict sterile technique.[7–9] Place the patient supine and anesthetize the penis, if it hasn't been done previously. Apply povidone iodine to the penis and let it dry. Apply sterile drapes to isolate a surgical field. Consider the administration of parenteral sedation prior to performing this procedure to alleviate the patient's anxiety.

Clamp a straight-blade hemostat over the foreskin and phimotic ring at the 11 o'clock and 1 o'clock positions. Place one jaw of each hemostat beneath the phimotic ring and the other jaw on top of it. **Be careful not to clamp the skin on the shaft of the penis.** Pull the foreskin taut between the hemostats. Grasp the hemostats with the nondominant hand or have an assistant hold them. Incise the foreskin and phimotic ring at the 12 o'clock position with a scissors or #15 scalpel blade (Figure 129-1*A*). **Be careful not to cut the skin on the shaft of the penis.** Remove the hemostats. The incision will open into a pentagonal shape (Figure 129-1*B*). Reduce the foreskin over the glans. Cover the penis with sterile gauze and allow the edges of the incision to ooze for 10 to 15 minutes.

This technique can be technically difficult for the non-Surgeon. As an alternative to the two-hemostat technique, a one-hemostat technique may be performed. Place one hemostat over the foreskin and phimotic ring at the 12 o'clock position (Figure 129-1*A*). Remove the clamp after 1 to 2 minutes. Cut the crushed tissue with scissors through the phimotic ring. **Be careful not to cut the skin on the shaft of the penis.** The foreskin will then open up as described (Figure 129-1*B*).

After the foreskin has been incised and reduced over the glans, approximate the cut edges with 3–0 chromic suture using a simple interrupted stitch (Figure 129-1*C*). Sew edge 1 and edge 2, on the illustration, together. Sew edge 3 and edge 4, on the illustration, together. A gap

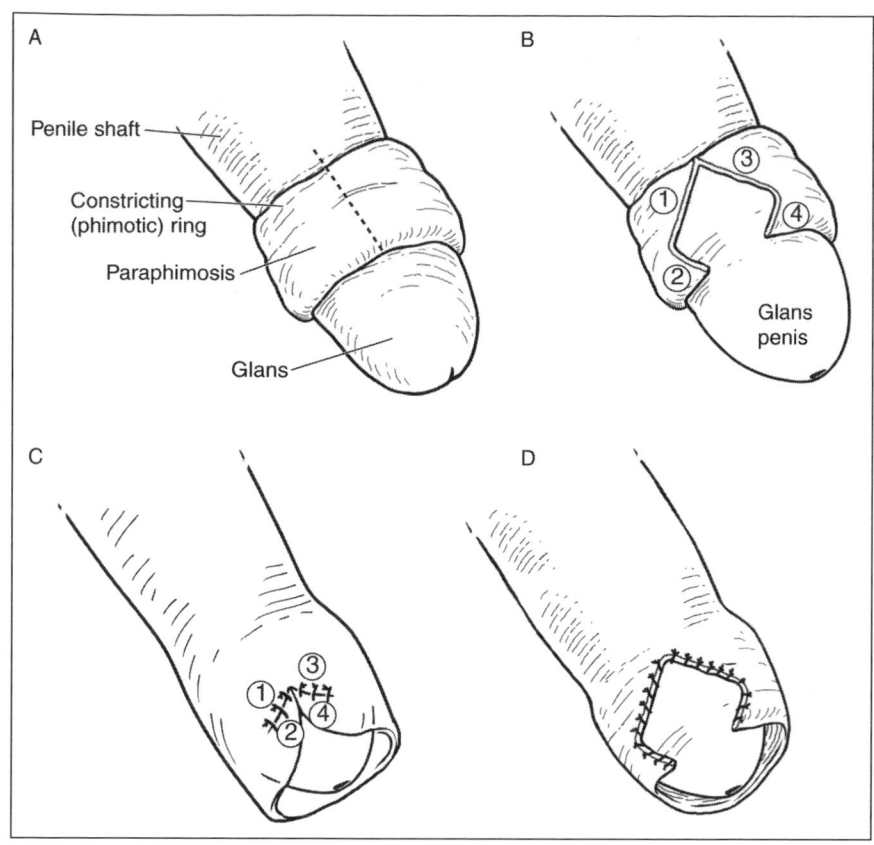

FIGURE 129-1 Dorsal slit of the paraphimotic foreskin. *A.* The dotted line represents the incision line. *B.* The foreskin opens after the incision is made. The numbers represent the edges of the incision. *C.* The foreskin has been reduced and the edges of the incision sewn shut. A small gap should remain in the midline that is free of sutures. *D.* Alternatively, sew the edges closed with a simple running stitch.

will remain at the 12 o'clock position that corresponds to the area of the initial incision. Alternatively, sew the cut edges with a simple running stitch (Figure 129-1*D*). Loosely apply petrolatum gauze and gauze squares over the wound. Apply a piece of tape to hold the dressing on the penis. **The tape should not be applied circumferentially as this can cause ischemia to the penis.**

MODIFIED DORSAL SLIT OF THE PARAPHIMOTIC FORESKIN

A modified dorsal slit technique has been described where only the phimotic ring is cut rather than the entire foreskin.[9,10] Clean, prep, anesthetize, and drape the penis as described previously. As an alternative to a penile block, infiltrate under the phimotic ring at the 12 o'clock position with local anesthetic solution without epinephrine using a 27 gauge needle. Be sure to raise a wheal both proximally and distally to the phimotic ring (along the dotted line in Figure 129-2*A*). A penile block is the preferred method of anesthesia because injection onto the distal penis is extremely painful.

Incise the phimotic ring with a #15 scalpel blade. **Incise only the phimotic ring. Do not extend the cut more than 3 mm proximally or distally to the phimotic ring.** Once incised, the foreskin will spring open into a diamond-shaped defect (Figure 129-2*B*). Reduce the foreskin. Cover the penis with gauze and allow the cut edges

to ooze for 10 to 15 minutes to decompress the foreskin. Approximate the edges of the wound with 3–0 chromic suture in an interrupted or running pattern (Figure 129-2*C*). Apply a bandage of petrolatum gauze and gauze squares over the wound. Apply a piece of tape to hold the dressing on the penis. **The tape should not be applied circumferentially as this can cause ischemia to the penis.**

DORSAL SLIT OF THE PHIMOTIC FORESKIN

The preferred method to correct an obstructing phimosis in the Emergency Department setting is the dorsal slit procedure. The patient's penis should be thoroughly anesthetized prior to performing this procedure. Consideration should also be given to administering intravenous analgesics, intravenous sedation, or procedural sedation.

Insert the bottom jaw of a straight hemostat between the foreskin and glans at the twelve o'clock position (Figure 129-3*A*). For those individual patients or cultural situations where dorsal incision of the foreskin, much less excision, is cosmetically unacceptable, a ventral approach may be substituted which will yield an apparently uncircumcised penis without obstructive symptoms.[9] Advance the hemostat until the tip of the jaw is at the coronal sulcus (Figure 129-3*A*). The coronal sulcus is where the foreskin attaches to the penis. De-

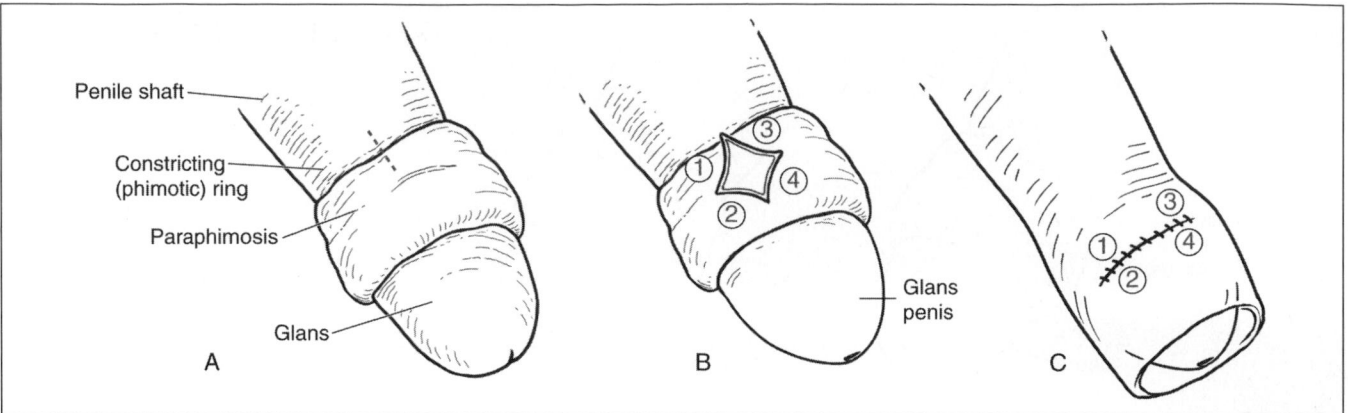

FIGURE 129-2 Modified dorsal slit of the paraphimotic foreskin. *A.* The dotted line represents the incision line. *B.* The foreskin opens after the incision is made. The numbers represent the edges of the incision. *C.* The foreskin has been reduced and the edges of the incision sewn shut.

pending on the cause of the phimosis, adhesions may be encountered. These should be gently broken as the hemostat is advanced. The skin of the prepuce is relatively thin and the jaw of the hemostat should be easily palpated. The tip of the jaw should be seen to tent the skin at the coronal sulcus when properly placed (Figure 129-3*B*). **It cannot be overemphasized that the physician must be confident that the instrument has not been inadvertently placed in the urethra. If the jaw of the hemostat cannot be felt and cannot be seen tenting the skin of the foreskin, remove the hemostat and reinsert it.**

Once properly placed, close the hemostat. Allow the hemostat to remain closed for 2 to 3 minutes to crush the skin. Remove the hemostat. Insert a scissors and advance it with the same attention to position the tip at the coronal sulcus. Incise the crushed tissue to the level of the coronal sulcus (Figure 129-3*C*). If straight scissors are not available, a #15 blade may be used to cut the crushed skin after another instrument is placed underneath the foreskin to protect the glans from injury. **This method of using a scalpel blade is dangerous and not recommended because control is reduced and the potential for error is unnecessarily increased.**

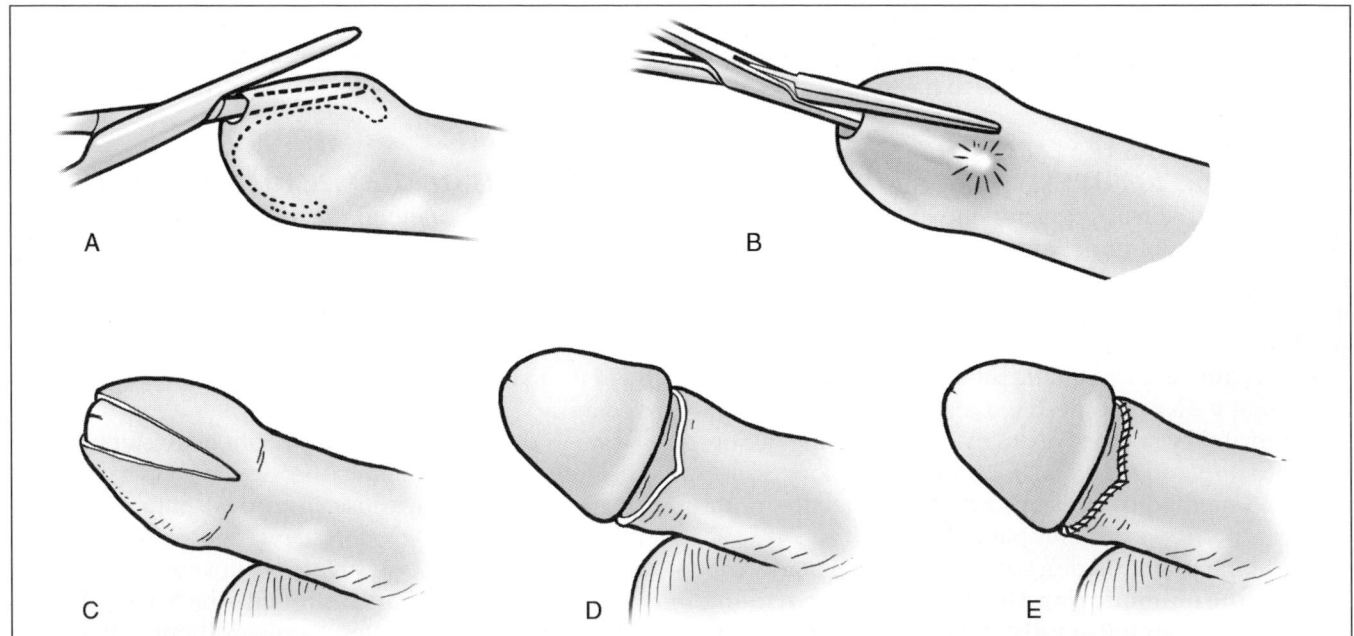

FIGURE 129-3 Dorsal slit of the phimotic foreskin. *A.* A hemostat is inserted under the foreskin and advanced to the coronal sulcus. *B.* The hemostat is elevated to tent the skin and confirm it is properly placed. *C.* The dorsal slit has been made. *D.* The foreskin is retracted. *E.* Interrupted sutures have been placed in the cut edges of the foreskin.

Retract the cut foreskin. This will leave an open wound edge on both sides of the midline (Figure 129-3D). Cover the penis with gauze and allow the cut edges to ooze for 10 to 15 minutes. Approximate the open wound edges using 3–0 or 4–0 chromic gut suture in an interrupted or running pattern. Begin suturing from the midline to the distal end of the incision (Figure 129-3E).[9] Return the foreskin to its "resting" position to guard against a newly acquired iatrogenic paraphimosis. Apply a bandage of petrolatum gauze and gauze squares over the wound. Apply a piece of tape to hold the dressing on the penis. **The tape should not be applied circumferentially as this can cause ischemia to the penis.**

ASSESSMENT

The foreskin should now be retractable to a sufficient degree to allow visualization of the meatus (when performed for a phimosis) or reduced over the glans to relieve pressure (when performed for a paraphimosis). The successfully reduced paraphimosis should have the general appearance of a normal uncircumcised penis. It is normal for residual edema to be present. Reassure the patient that the edema will spontaneously resolve over hours to days. Observe the patient in the Emergency Department for 45 to 60 minutes to confirm hemostasis. Observe the patient for full recovery from any sedation or procedural sedation techniques as per hospital policy.

AFTERCARE

Wound care following a surgical reduction is the same as that for any sutured laceration. Many physicians do not dress the incision site. But if desired, it may be covered with antibiotic ointment or petrolatum gauze and dry sterile gauze.[6] The patient should be counseled on proper wound care. The patient should inspect the glans and foreskin three to four times a day. They should return immediately to the Emergency Department if any signs of infection develop. They should also be advised to avoid intercourse or masturbation for 4 to 6 weeks.[6]

Antibiotics should be prescribed that cover gram-positive organisms. An extended-spectrum penicillin or first-generation cephalosporin is most frequently prescribed. Cephalexin, 500 mg orally four times a day, is usually adequate.

All patients need to follow-up with a Urologist in one or two days. The definitive treatment is circumcision, which is typically delayed 7 to 10 days until any edema, inflammation, or ulceration has resolved.[7,8]

COMPLICATIONS

Direct mechanical injury to the glans or urethra by inadvertent placement of instruments into the urethra could be devastating but is easily avoidable by following proper technique. Increased bleeding may result if the skin is not crushed by the hemostat before it is cut with the scissors. It is also important to avoid advancing the clamp, and therefore the incision, beyond the comfortable limitation of the coronal sulcus. Otherwise, the skin on the penile shaft will be cut. This can result in a cosmetic defect and possibly skin sloughing requiring a skin graft. Wound infection and dehiscence are a possibility with any incision and greatly reduced in conscientious patients. Bleeding is a common complication in this very vascular tissue. Venous bleeding can be profuse and it is important to have good control of the tissue edges so that adequate hemostatic stitches can be placed. A compressive dressing may aid in hemostasis. If the penile shaft is lacerated during a surgical reduction, it too should be sutured. And, as with all invasive procedures, infection may be a complication.

SUMMARY

A dorsal slit is an easy and rapid way to relieve strangulation pressure from a paraphimosis or to allow visualization of the urethral meatus from an obstructing phimosis. This procedure is performed primarily in emergency situations as the cosmetic result is usually suboptimal. Patients with a phimosis who are able to void should be referred to a Urologist before performing a dorsal slit. The dorsal slit procedure should only be performed when a phimosis is obstructing and a urethral catheter cannot be placed. A paraphimosis is always an emergency. Often this will reduce with less invasive techniques that should be attempted first. Severe cases will require a dorsal slit.

REFERENCES

1. Jordan GH, Schlossberg SM, Devine CJ: Surgery of the penis and urethra, in Walsh P, Retik A, Vaughan E, Wein A (eds): *Campbell's Urology*, 7th ed. Philadelphia: Saunders 1998:3317–3394.
2. Maizels M: Normal and anomalous development of the urinary tract, in Walsh P, Retik A, Vaughan E, Wein A (eds): *Campbell's Urology*, 7th ed. Philadelphia: Saunders 1998:1545–1595.
3. Hinman F Jr., Stempen PH: *Atlas of Urosurgical Anatomy*, 1st ed. Philadelphia: Saunders, 1993:422–444.
4. Hinman F Jr., Stempen PH: *Atlas of Urologic Surgery*, 1st ed. Philadelphia: Saunders, 1989:81.

5. Cheng W, Saing H: A prospective randomized study of wound approximation with tissue glue in circumcision in children. *J Paediatr Child Health* 1997; 33(6):515–516.

6. Forte A, Palumbo P, Baumgartner IM, et al: Local anesthesia with eutectic cream of lidocaine and prilocaine for treatment of cicatrizial phimosis in outpatients. *Eur Rev Med Pharmacol Sci* 1998; 2(5–6):207–208.

7. Houghton GR: The "iced-glove" method of treatment of paraphimosis. *Br J Surg* 1973; 60(11):876–877.

8. Holman JR, Stuessi KA: Adult circumcision. *Am Fam Physician* 1999; 59(6):1514–1518.

9. Schneider RE: Urologic procedures, in Roberts JR, Hedges JR (eds): *Clinical Procedures in Emergency Medicine*, 4th ed. Philadelphia: Saunders, 1998:947–952.

10. Shaw KN: Reduction of paraphimosis, in Dieckmann RA, Fiser DH, Selbst SM (eds): *Pediatric Emergency and Critical Care Procedures*. St. Louis: Mosby, 1997:435–436.

Chapter 130
TESTICULAR (MANUAL) DETORSION

Patricia Vidal
Brenna Born

INTRODUCTION

Testicular torsion is a true urologic emergency. It occurs when a testicle rotates on its vascular pedicle resulting in vascular obstruction (Figure 130-1). Torsion is most common between the ages of 12 to 18.[1] Age should not be considered when making the diagnosis, however, as torsion may occur in an antenate, neonate, or geriatric patient.[2] **A history of prior orchiopexy does not negate the possibility of torsion.** Presenting signs and symptoms frequently include acute and diffuse scrotal pain, scrotal swelling, a high-riding testicle, and an absent cremasteric reflex. **If torsion is suspected, a Urologist should be consulted immediately and manual detorsion attempted.**

The differential diagnosis of the acutely swollen or painful scrotum also includes torsion of the testicular appendage, epididymitis, orchitis, hernia, varicocele, tumor, trauma, idiopathic scrotal edema, fat necrosis, viral inflammation, and Henoch-Schönlein purpura.[3,4] **As testicular torsion is the diagnosis requiring the most urgent action, it should be first on the differential diagnosis list.** Testicular torsion may result in irreversible damage to the involved testis. It may also affect the contralateral testicle. Recent studies have examined the possible immunologic mechanism for this global effect on fertility but the exact pathophysiology has not been established.[5,6]

ANATOMY AND PATHOPHYSIOLOGY

Testicular torsion results in the obstruction of the blood supply to the testis. The venous obstruction leads to edema. This is followed by arterial obstruction that leads to testicular ischemia. Because the degree of tor-

sion or vascular compromise cannot be quantified by current methods, the time for torsion to result in irreversible testicular damage cannot be determined.[2] A complete vascular occlusion will cause a testicle to develop permanent and irreversible damage earlier than a testicle with partial vascular occlusion. The literature is variable and cites a range of 6 to 24 hours of vascular occlusion required to cause irreversible ischemic damage to a testicle.[7] Most authors agree that the best outcomes are obtained with detorsion within 6 hours of symptom onset.

Testicular torsion may be classified as extravaginal or intravaginal. Extravaginal torsion occurs primarily in neonates. The testis, epididymis, and tunica vaginalis twist together on their vertical axis because the gubernaculum has not yet become attached to the scrotal wall. It is caused by the free rotation of the testicle around the spermatic cord at a level above the tunica vaginalis. Intravaginal torsion occurs in peri- or postpubertal males and has been associated with the so-called bell-clapper deformity. In the normal scrotum, the tunica vaginalis only partially covers the epididymis and does not cover the spermatic cord. In the bell-clapper deformity, the tunica vaginalis encases the entire testicle, epididymis, and base of the spermatic cord. This allows the contents to twist and move within the tunica vaginalis as a bell-clapper does within a bell.[8] Both intravaginal and extravaginal torsion usually occur in a medial or inward fashion.

The definitive therapy for a torsed testicle is surgery. There is agreement that, at the time of surgery, a necrotic testicle should be removed and a pink, healthy appearing testicle should be left in place. The question remains of what to do with those testicles whose viability is not clear at the time of surgery. Current recommendations are to remove an obviously necrotic testicle or a testicle that

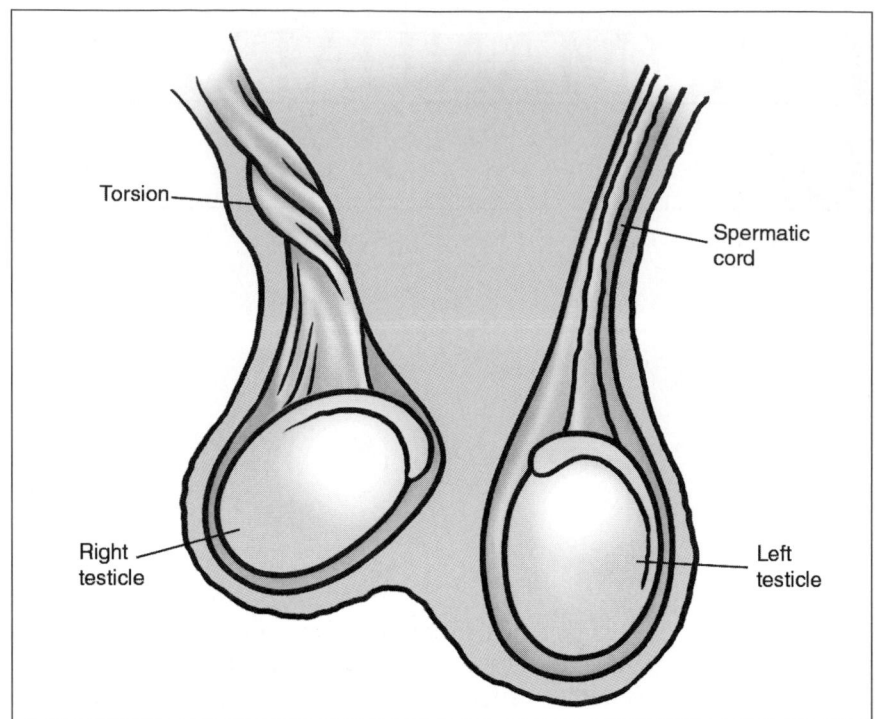

FIGURE 130-1 Torsion of the right testicle. The testicle lies horizontally and in a higher position than the normal testicle.

stays cyanotic after detorsion; but leave in place any testicle which appears viable.[1,3]

Recent research has addressed the issue of immunology and future fertility post-torsion. The blood-testicle barrier has been well established. The theory exists that ischemic damage to the torsed testicle breaks down the blood-testicle barrier allowing the body to produce autoantibodies that attack the contralateral testicle.[6] Another theory has proposed that abnormal or subfertile testicles are more likely to torse and that these differences in fertility may have predated the torsion.[2,9] These subfertile changes may resolve within several months after orchiectomy of the torsed testicle.[5] Studies in sperm-producing rodents have found evidence of immunologic damage to the contralateral testicle after torsion, especially if the torsed testicle is allowed to remain torsed for more than 24 hours.[5,6] These studies and others seem to support the theory of immunologic damage after ischemia.

INDICATIONS

An attempt should be made to manually reduce all suspected testicular torsions.[7] If reduced within 6 to 8 hours of the start of symptoms, the survival rate of the testicle after manual detorsion is near 100 percent.[7] After 8 hours, the risk of testicular atrophy increases but the testis may still be salvageable; especially if the vascu-

lar obstruction is incomplete.[4] Successful manual detorsion after longer periods of time becomes difficult due to edema formation. **However, due to the lack of significant complications, manual detorsion should be attempted regardless of the length of symptoms.**

CONTRAINDICATIONS

There are no absolute contraindications to attempt to manually reduce a testicle that is torsed. There are, however, some situations in which it might not be warranted. If the testis has become fixed to the scrotal wall, it may be necrotic and detorsion outside of the Operating Room is not possible.[7] If the Operating Room and Surgeon are available, an attempt at manual detorsion might delay definitive repair.[10] If the degree of swelling and/or pain preclude the examiner from applying firm pressure on the testicle, detorsion might not be possible. If the clinical picture suggests another cause for the patient's symptoms and the suspicion for a testicular torsion is very low, a radiologic study (testicular scan or Doppler ultrasound) might be warranted prior to an attempt at detorsion. If the testicle has been torsed for more than 24 hours, orchiectomy without detorsion might help to preserve fertility in the contralateral testicle.[6] However, this has not been sufficiently confirmed and is not currently recommended.

EQUIPMENT

No equipment is required to manually detorse a testicle. However, as the testicle is tender and the procedure is bound to be painful, consider the judicious administration of parenteral analgesia, sedation, or procedural sedation. The use of a Doppler stethoscope or color Doppler ultrasound to assist with the diagnosis and determination of a successful detorsion is helpful but not required.

PATIENT PREPARATION

Explain the procedure to the patient and/or their representative. Explain that the procedure will be quick but painful. Explain that giving medicine to relieve the pain may interfere with the determination of success. Inform the patient that there are no risks to attempting to manually reduce the torsed testicle. Potential complications include continued pain, increased pain, and the inability to detorse the testicle. No matter what result is obtained with manual detorsion, an operation will be necessary prior to discharge to prevent future episodes of torsion. If manual detorsion is unsuccessful, emergent operative intervention may be required.

The use of anesthesia is not absolutely contraindicated. It may be required depending on the patient's age, ability to cooperate, and the examiner's preference. In general, the use of irreversible intravenous sedation or a spermatic cord block should be avoided as they interfere with the patient's ability to assess pain and the determination of a successful detorsion.[2] The injection of local anesthetic solution into the spermatic cord may further compromise testicular blood flow.[9] Options for pain relief, when required, include procedural sedation, intravenous analgesics, and/or intravenous sedatives.

TECHNIQUE

The direction of most torsions has been described as inward or medial. To detorse a testicle, it must be rotated outward or lateral (Figure 130-2). This has also been described as "detorse as you would open a book" or "supinate the hand as the testicle is rotated."[2,10] Another way to think of it is if you are looking at the patient from the foot of the bed. Rotate the patient's right testicle counter clockwise and the patient's left testicle clockwise (Figure 130-2).

Place the patient semirecumbent or supine. Stand next to the patient. Place the left hand on the patient's right testicle or the right hand on the patient's left testicle, depending on which is torsed. Grasp the spermatic cord with the other hand to stabilize it from moving. Grasp the testicle gently but firmly. Rotate the testicle within the scrotum 180 degrees outward (Figure 130-2).

The average degree of torsion has been cited as 720 degrees.[4] **Continue to detorse the testicle until the patient experiences pain relief and the normal scrotal anatomy is restored.** If at any point in the procedure the patient experiences an increase in pain or there is resistance to rotating the testicle, stop and attempt to detorse the testicle in the opposite direction. Occasionally, a testicle may be torsed outward or lateral.

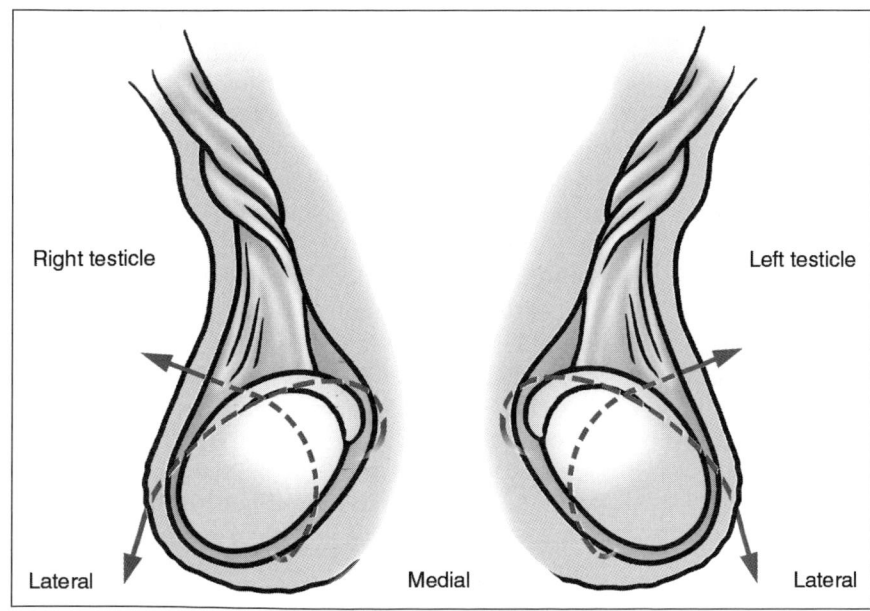

FIGURE 130-2 Manual detorsion of a testicle. The arrows represent the directions to rotate the testicle.

ASSESSMENT

Successful detorsion is marked by the sudden relief of pain and the restoration of the normal scrotal anatomy. The normal anatomy is indicated by a lengthening of the spermatic cord and a vertical lie of the testicle. If available, a Doppler stethoscope or color Doppler ultrasound may be used to monitor the effects of the detorsion. The resolution of edema will depend on the degree and duration of ischemia, but will not be as immediate as the pain relief.[10] If the patient has relief of pain but the testicle is still high riding or horizontal, continue to detorse the testicle in the same direction until there is complete pain relief and a return of the normal scrotal anatomy.

AFTERCARE

All patients with a diagnosis of testicular torsion should be admitted to the hospital with emergent Urological consultation. This is true despite a successful manual detorsion. The timing of the operative intervention will be changed from emergent to urgent if the testicle is detorsed in the Emergency Department or clinic setting.[7] Urgent surgery is still required because, even with pain relief, the torsion may not have been completely reduced. One study found evidence of continued torsion with venous congestion even after successful manual detorsion.[4] Following testicular torsion, the patient must undergo bilateral orchiopexy. **The bell-clapper deformity that is implicated in many testicular torsions is almost always bilateral. Therefore, the contralateral testicle is at increased risk for torsion.** Due to the risk of impaired fertility after torsion, all efforts must be undertaken to preserve the contralateral testicle and future fertility.

COMPLICATIONS

There are few complications to manual detorsion and none that should deter the physician from an attempt at detorsion should it be indicated. The procedure is painful and detorsion in the wrong direction will initially increase the patient's discomfort. There is also the possibility that, despite proper technique, the physician will be unable to detorse the testicle and emergent surgery will be required. If it turns out that testicular torsion is not the correct diagnosis, the patient will have endured an uncomfortable procedure without gain. While some suggest that detorsion in the wrong direction may increase the degree of vascular compromise, others have found no increase in ischemia, even with failure of detorsion.[4] Complications may also arise from a delay in notification of the Urologist.[2]

A more serious potential complication stems from the false sense of security obtained when the patient has pain relief. Manual detorsion may only partially restore blood flow and rapid surgical intervention may still be required. Delaying the trip to the Operating Room due to lack of pain may cause "castration by procrastination."[2]

SUMMARY

Emergency Physicians must be aware of the possibility and urgency of a testicular torsion. They should be prepared to rapidly attempt manual detorsion. Early notification of the Urologist is essential as the ischemia time and testicular salvage are inversely proportional. Manual detorsion may successfully relieve or reduce the ischemia, increasing testicular survival and future fertility. All patients with testicular torsion should receive definitive therapy and repair in the Operating Room.

REFERENCES

1. Rajfer J: Congenital anomalies of the testis and scrotum, in Walsh P, Retik A, Vaughan E, et al (eds): *Campbell's Urology*, 7th ed. Philadelphia: Saunders, 1998:2172–2186.
2. Lindsey D, Stanisic TH: Diagnosis and management of testicular torsion: pitfalls and perils. *Am J Emerg Med* 1988; 6(1):42–46.
3. Rozanski T, Bloom D, Colodny A: Surgery of the scrotum and testis in children, in Walsh P, Retik A, Vaughan E, et al (eds): *Campbell's Urology*, 7th ed. Philadelphia: Saunders, 1998:2193–2206.
4. Cronan KM, Zderic SA: Manual detorsion of the testes, in Henretig FM, King C, Joffe MD, et al (eds): *Textbook of Pediatric Emergency Procedures*. Baltimore: Williams and Wilkins, 1997:1003–1006.
5. Nagler HM, Deitch AD, deVere White R: Testicular torsion: temporal considerations. *Fertil Steril* 1984; 42(2):257–262.
6. Koşar A, Küpeli B, Alçigir G, et al: Immunologic aspect of testicular torsion: detection of antisperm antibodies in contralateral testicle. *Eur Urol* 1999; 36:640–644.
7. Cattolica EV: Preoperative manual detorsion of the torsed spermatic cord. *J Urol* 1985; 6(1):42–46.
8. Garel L, Dubois J, Azzie G, et al: Preoperative manual detorsion of the spermatic cord with Doppler ultrasound monitoring in patients with intravaginal acute testicular torsion. *Pediatr Radiol* 2000; 30(1):41–44.

9. Nagler HM: A clinical approach to testicular torsion, in Seidmon EJ, Hanno PM (eds): *Current Urologic Therapy*, 3rd ed. Philadelphia: Saunders, 1994:480–482.

10. Schneider RE: Urologic procedures, in Roberts JR, Hedges JR (eds): *Clinical Procedures in Emergency Medicine*, 3rd ed. Philadelphia: Saunders, 1998:956–957.

Chapter 131
ZIPPER INJURY MANAGEMENT

Patricia Vidal
Lacy Knight

INTRODUCTION

Zipper injuries frequently occur to the foreskin, the skin of the penis, and the scrotum. Zipper injuries result in entrapment of tissue when the zipper is opened or closed. It primarily occurs in uncircumcised young boys, intoxicated adults, the mentally handicapped, males not wearing underwear, and elderly men suffering from movement or cognitive disorders. The most common type of zipper entrapment compresses the skin between the sliding piece and the teeth of the zipper. Another type of entrapment involves the skin between the teeth of the zipper after the sliding piece has moved beyond the area.[1,2] Multiple methods to extract the entrapped skin have been reported.[1-11] These methods range from manipulation to tooth-by-tooth extraction to circumcision. Treatment should be guided by the type of entrapment.[1] Removal of the zipper can be performed quickly using simple tools to extract the entrapped tissue and thus prevent secondary injury.

ANATOMY AND PATHOPHYSIOLOGY

The zipper is a simple device that is used daily by millions of people (Figure 131-1). It consists of a sliding piece that moves in two directions. The sliding piece is composed of a front and back plate connected by the median bar.[5] The median bar is usually located at the top of the sliding piece. A finger grip is attached to the front plate of the sliding piece and functions as a handle to move the sliding piece. The teeth are two opposing sets of rectangular metal or plastic pieces attached to fabric to keep them aligned. Moving the sliding piece across an open zipper will interlock the teeth and close the zipper. Reversing the sliding piece direction will unlock the teeth and open the zipper.

Although any skin can become entrapped in a zipper, it primarily occurs to the foreskin, penis, and scrotum.

Entrapment often occurs in those who are in a rush to get dressed, not wearing underwear, intoxicated, or in a rush to zip up their pants. Zipper injuries are extremely painful. Patients are often unable to relieve the entrapment themselves and present to the Emergency Department for relief. Because this is an embarrassing injury, patients often present after several attempts at self-extraction and a few hours after the injury. The self-extraction attempts and delay to presentation often result in significant edema that can complicate the removal of the entrapped skin.

INDICATIONS

Skin entrapped between the sliding piece and teeth or between the teeth of the zipper must be extricated. The skin should be extricated as soon as possible to minimize edema and prevent necrosis.

CONTRAINDICATIONS

There are no absolute contraindications to the removal of a zipper, the slider, or the teeth from an entrapped piece of skin. A Urologist should be consulted after releasing the entrapment in cases of significant edema, skin necrosis, urethral involvement, or infection.

EQUIPMENT

Heavy-duty wire cutter or bone cutter
Scissors, bandage or Mayo
Scissors, small or iris
Topical anesthetic, e.g., EMLA cream
Local anesthetic solution without epinephrine
Mineral oil
Miniature hacksaw
27 gauge needle
5 mL syringe

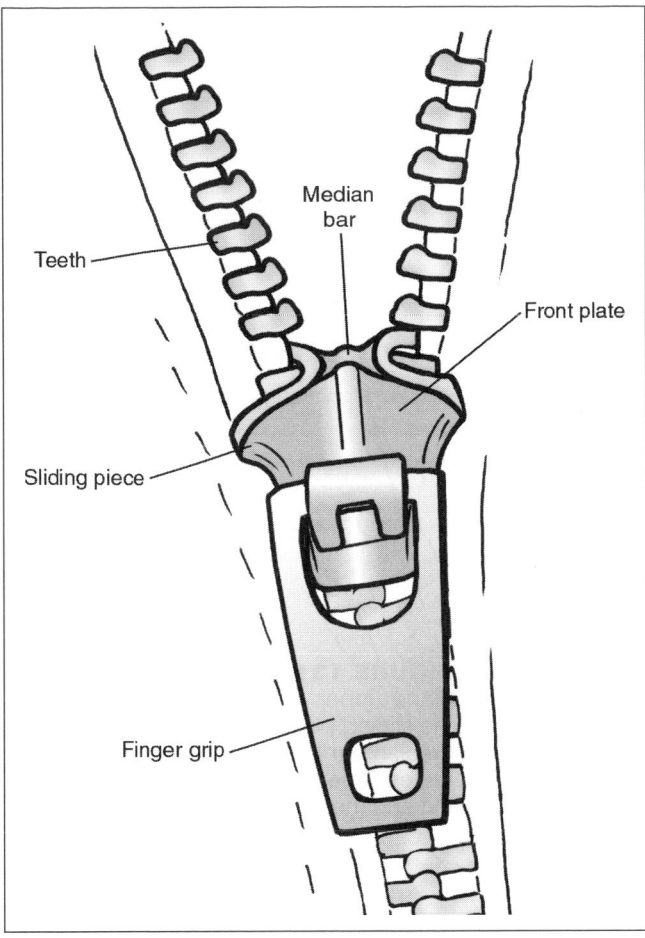

FIGURE 131-1 Anatomy of a zipper.

PATIENT PREPARATION

Explain the procedure and aftercare required to the patient and/or their representative. Obtain a signed consent to perform the procedure. Assess the patient's level of anxiety and pain as they must remain calm during the procedure to avoid secondary injury. The application of a topical anesthetic (EML cream) may be helpful but delays extraction of the entrapped skin. If the patient has significant pain, local anesthetic solution can be subcutaneously infiltrated around the entrapped skin or a penile block (Chapter 125) can be performed. The application of parenteral analgesia, sedation, or procedural sedation may be required in rare instances.

TECHNIQUES

MANUAL REMOVAL

Attempt to dislodge the zipper manually. **Do not forcefully try to unzip it. Excessive force is not neces-**

sary and can result in avulsions and lacerations to the skin. Patients have often unsuccessfully tried this at home multiple times prior to presenting to the Emergency Department. Apply mineral oil liberally to the zipper and entrapped skin. Allow the mineral oil to soak the skin and zipper for approximately 10 minutes. Attempt to gently unzip the zipper with special care taken to avoid further injury.[9]

CUTTING OF THE MEDIAN BAR

The median bar can be cut with a heavy-duty wire cutter or bone cutter.[6,7] If the skin is entrapped between the sliding piece and the teeth (Figure 131-2A), cut the median bar (Figure 131-2B). The front and back plates of the zipper will separate and release the entrapped skin (Figure 131-2C). Occasionally, the skin is entrapped between the teeth of the zipper (Figure 131-3). Cut the median bar of the sliding piece. Manually pull the two rows of teeth apart to release the entrapped skin.

CUTTING OF THE CLOTH SURROUNDING ZIPPER TEETH

Occasionally, the skin is trapped between the teeth of the zipper and a wire cutter or bone cutter is not available.[8] Cut the cloth holding the zipper to the clothes with a bandage or Mayo scissors (Figure 131-4, long dashed lines). Using a small or iris scissors, cut the cloth between the teeth that are entrapping the skin (Figure 131-4, small dashed lines). Separate the teeth and free the entrapped skin.

This technique is less than ideal. Cutting the cloth between the teeth of the zipper will often cause lacerations to the entrapped skin. It is very painful for the patient when the skin is cut. It is worth the additional time to locate and borrow a heavy-duty wire cutter from the Maintenance Department to cut the median bar.

ALTERNATIVE TECHNIQUES

If a wire cutter or bone cutter is not available, or the median bar is not accessible, the previously mentioned techniques for zipper removal cannot be performed. Alternatives do exist but are not ideal. Each has its own risks and contraindications. The first option is to excise the entrapped skin if it is part of a redundant portion of tissue that allows for easy removal. A second alternative is to cut the median bar with a miniature hacksaw blade to divide it.[10] This alternative carries the risk for significant injury to the skin and soft tissues. If the aforementioned alternatives are not effective to remove a zipper entrapped on the foreskin, circumcision may be necessary if cultural beliefs are not a contraindication.[6]

7. Nolan JF, Stillwell TJ, Sands JP: Acute management of the zipper-entrapped penis. *J Emerg Med* 1990; 8:305–307.

8. Oosterlinck W: Unbloody management of penile zipper injury. *Eur Urol* 1981; 7:365–366.

9. Kanegaye JT, Schonfeld N: Penile zipper entrapment: a simple and less threatening approach using mineral oil. *Pediatr Emerg Care* 1993; 9:90–91.

10. Strait RT: A novel method for removal of penile zipper entrapment. *Pediatr Emerg Care* 1999; 15(6):412–413.

11. Schneider R, Williams MA: Pediatric urology in the emergency department. AUA Update Series 1997; Vol XVI, Lesson 20:156.

Section Eleven

OPHTHALMOLOGIC PROCEDURES

Chapter 132
EYE EXAMINATION

Shari Schabowski

INTRODUCTION

Physicians often approach the eye examination with some degree of apprehension. Eye complaints comprise up to 10 percent of Emergency Department visits. A systematic approach to the eye examination can alleviate any discomfort and provide the basis for an accurate diagnosis and treatment. The most common ophthalmologic problems that present to an Emergency Department are injuries, inflammation, infections, and visual disturbances.

A careful history will help to guide the differential diagnosis and the physical examination. It must include a history of the presenting complaint, the mechanism of any injury, exposures to chemicals or infectious agents, baseline visual acuity, known ophthalmologic problems, baseline medical problems, current medications, and any known allergies. The eye examination progresses from the outside and works inward, beginning with the visual acuity to assess the function of the eye. **It is important to routinely inspect all anatomic structures of the eye regardless of the presenting eye complaint.** Secondary problems, such as corneal lesions associated with conjunctivitis, may be missed if a complete examination is not performed on all patients.

EYE ANATOMY

The bony orbit is pyramidal in shape and surrounds the eyeball and its associated neurovascular structures. The blood supply to the structures of the orbit originates from the ophthalmic artery. The anatomy of the eyeball and its surrounding soft tissue structures is demonstrated in Figure 132-1. A detailed discussion of the complex anatomy of the eye is beyond the scope of this chapter. The anatomy relevant to the eye examination will be discussed throughout this chapter.

VISUAL ACUITY

Visual acuity is referred to as the vital sign of the eyes. It provides a means for the functional assessment of this delicate sensory apparatus. **Documentation of the visual acuity is essential when approaching a patient with eye complaints.** Assess the patient's visual acuity as soon as possible, preferably as part of the triage assessment. Test and document the patient's visual acuity before the physical examination begins. There are few exceptions to this rule. Chemical exposures to the eye require irrigation without delay to avoid potential irreversible visual loss. **Eye irrigation after a chemical exposure must precede visual acuity testing. Failure to document visual acuity is a common omission and may have medicolegal ramifications.**

Test and document the visual acuity with the respective annotation to the right eye (OD), the left eye (OS), and both eyes (OU). Test the problematic eye first. Completely cover the eye not being tested. Light shining into the opposite eye may adversely affect the results of visual acuity testing. A list of commonly used abbreviations in the measurement of visual acuity is listed in Table 132-1. Inquire as to the patient's baseline visual acuity and whether they wear corrective lenses for reference. Test the visual acuity using corrective lenses whenever possible. The abbreviations for the documentation of with and without correction are CC and SC, respectively.

Use caution when allowing contact lenses to be used as a visual aid in patients with eye pain, an eye injury, or an eye discharge, as their application may worsen their condition. **Remove all contact lenses before the slit lamp examination and fluorescein staining. Fluorescein will permanently stain soft contact lenses and may stain hard contact lenses.**

An accurate assessment of visual acuity is essential and this cannot be overemphasized. It is common for a clinician to miss a secondary ophthalmologic diagnosis

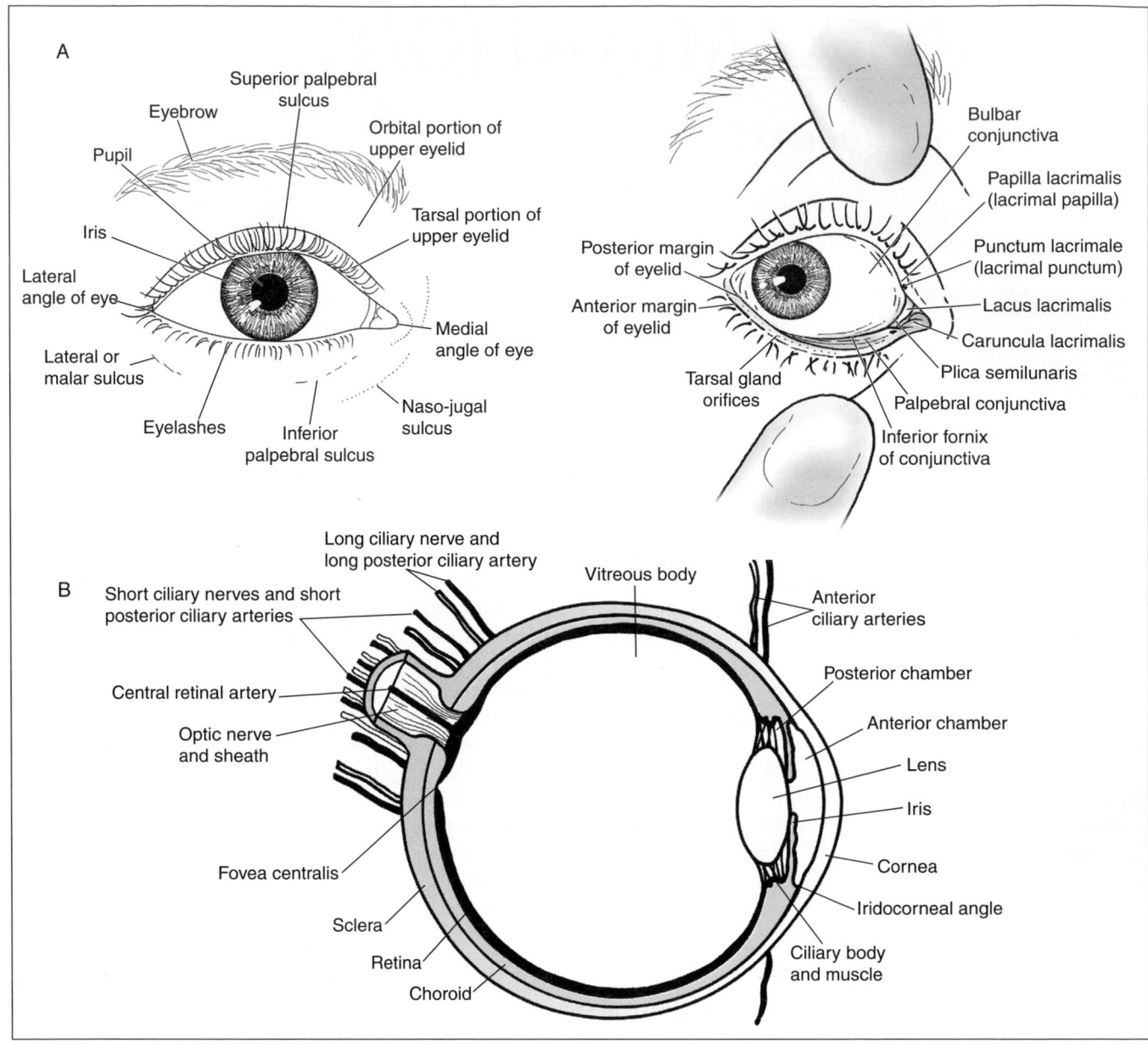

FIGURE 132-1 Anatomy of the eye and its surrounding soft tissues. *A.* Surface anatomy. *B.* Midsagittal section through the eyeball.

TABLE 132-1. COMMONLY USED ABBREVIATIONS FOR THE DOCUMENTATION OF VISUAL ACUITY

OD = right eye
OS = left eye
OU = both eyes
CC = with correction
SC = without correction
CF = counts fingers
HM = hand movement
LP = light perception
NLP = no light perception
+ = positive
− = negative

when they do not recognize a change in visual acuity. As a rule of thumb, a patient with previously normal (20/20) vision with or without correction that has an acute deterioration to 20/50 or less suggests a serious ophthalmologic condition. These cases require emergent consultation and prompt referral to an Ophthalmologist.

VISUAL ACUITY CHARTS

The Snellen eye chart is the most commonly used tool for assessing visual acuity (Figure 132-2). Place the Snellen chart on a flat wall in a well-lit room without obstructions. Place the patient standing 20 feet from the chart. With one eye completely covered, instruct the pa-

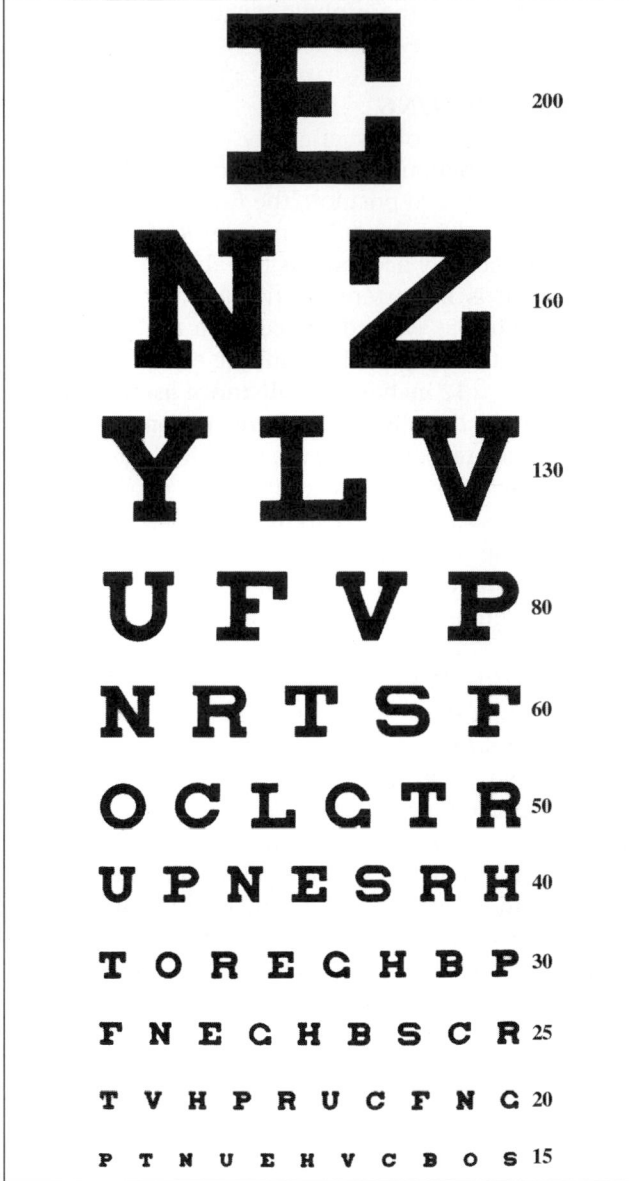

FIGURE 132-2 The Snellen eye chart.

tient to read each line of the chart beginning at the top and proceeding to the bottom or until they are unable to correctly and consistently read the letters. The visual acuity is the fraction corresponding to the last line that the patient identifies at least half of the letters correctly (i.e., 20/40). The numerator corresponds to what the patient is able to see at 20 feet. The denominator corresponds to the distance where a patient with normal vision would be able to read the same line accurately. For example, a patient with a visual acuity of 20/40 sees at 20 feet what a patient with normal vision would see at 40 feet. Document the fraction corresponding to the line minus the number of letters missed if the patient is able to accurately identify more than half of the letters on that line (i.e., 20/40 –3).

Test the patient 10 feet from the chart if they are unable to read any of the letters on the chart at 20 feet. The test is the same at 10 feet as it is at 20 feet. The documentation changes notation. Document 10/200 if the patient is able to read the letter at the line designated 20/200, but from the 10 foot mark. The test can also be performed at 5 feet if necessary. Document a 5 as the numerator if the patient reads the Snellen chart from 5 feet away (i.e., 5/200).

The Snellen chart is the most effective tool for documenting an accurate and reproducible visual acuity. There are circumstances that render this tool less effective and inaccurate. The chart utilizes the English alphabet and effective use requires that the patient can identify all letters. This is difficult, if not impossible, in patients who are illiterate or do not speak and/or read English. The illiterate E chart is an alternative (Figure 132-3). Instruct the patient to identify the direction that each "E" is facing. An alternative is to use a pediatric visual acuity chart (Figure 132-4). Instruct the patient to identify the objects on each line. Both of these visual acuity charts are assessed and documented like that of the Snellen chart.

There are a few circumstances where the standard eye chart may give falsely low and inaccurate readings. Patients with eye pain or photophobia may have difficulty reading the chart in bright light secondary to excessive lacrimation, blepharospasm, or pain. There are several options to provide a more optimal assessment of visual acuity. A Rosenbaum card is the handheld equivalent of the Snellen chart (Figure 132-5). It is viewed at a distance of 14 inches. Its advantages are that it can be used in the patient's room with less-offensive lighting and it can adjust for refractory errors in near-sighted patients who present without correction. A clever idea that some use is to attach a 14 inch string to the Rosenbaum card so that it can be accurately tested at the exact distance each time. A near vision test for children may also be used to assess visual acuity (Figure 132-6).

Photophobia or eye pain, particularly that which results from corneal injuries or lesions, may prevent the patient from complying with the visual examination. They may often have difficulty opening the eye at all. The instillation of a topical ophthalmic anesthetic agent may be remarkably helpful as an adjunct to the visual acuity evaluation as well as for the remainder of the eye examination. A patient with eye pain or photophobia that gets complete relief with a topical ophthalmic anesthetic agent suggests that the etiology of the pain is located on the conjunctiva or the cornea. Persistent pain suggests that the problem originates from a deeper structure, such as an iritis, uveitis, or meningeal irritation. The topical ophthalmic anesthetic agents are toxic to corneal epithelial cells and delay healing. **They are to**

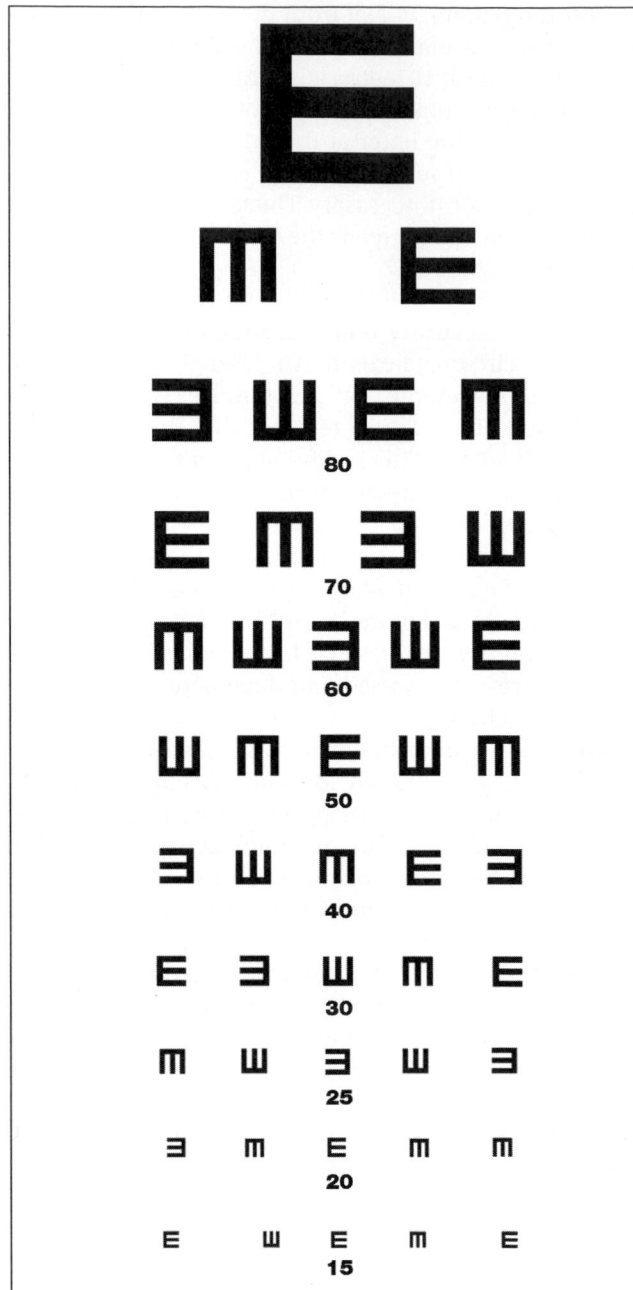

FIGURE 132-3 The illiterate E chart.

be used in the diagnosis and evaluation of the eye. They should never be prescribed for treatment.

PINHOLE DEVICE

The pinhole device can filter out excessive light (Figure 132-7). It may correct refractory errors to 20/30. An index card punctured multiple times with an 18 gauge needle can substitute if the pinhole device is not available. Instruct the patient to place the pinhole device over the eye being tested and close the other eye. Instruct the patient to read the visual acuity chart. Record the patient's visual acuity in each eye. Make a notation in the record that the pinhole device was used in the measurement of the visual acuity.

FINGER COUNTING

Another means of visual acuity assessment must be utilized if the patient is unable to identify the letter or object in the 20/200 position, the first and largest letter in the visual acuity chart. The next level of visual acuity that is traditionally accepted is the ability to count fingers (CF). It is important for documentation that the examiner note at what distance from the eye the patient is able to consistently count the examiner's fingers (e.g., OD CF at 12 inches). **The distance used for counting fingers is the distance where the patient is first able to accurately complete the test.** Documentation of "CF at 2 feet" means that the patient can accurately count fingers at 2 feet. This implies that the patient would not be able to count the fingers with the hand held at a distance greater than 2 feet. Test one eye at a time then both eyes simultaneously.

HAND MOVEMENTS

The next test of visual acuity to perform is hand movements if the patient cannot count fingers. Move or wave a hand back and forth in front of the eye being examined. Document hand movement positive (HM+) or hand movement negative (HM−). Note the distance from the eye that hand movement is first visible (i.e., how close to the eye must the hand be positioned) in the medical record (e.g., HM+ at 12 inches). Test one eye at a time then both eyes simultaneously.

LIGHT PERCEPTION

The next determination of visual acuity is whether the patient has light perception if they are unable to perceive hand movement. Use a penlight or ophthalmoscope to determine the presence or absence of light perception. Shine the light directly into one eye while the opposite eye is covered. Document the patient's ability to correctly identify when the light is on and off. This is noted as light perception positive (LP+) or light perception negative (LP−). Test one eye at a time then both eyes simultaneously. **True blindness is present when the patient has no light perception.**

UNCOOPERATIVE OR UNRESPONSIVE PATIENTS

Unresponsive patients are a challenge for the evaluation of visual acuity. First shine a light into each of the patient's eyes to test for pupillary reactivity. Move the light slowly through all of the cardinal positions to identify if the patient is able to track the light movement. Refer to the evaluation of extraocular movements section below. Perform the doll's eyes maneuver if the patient is unable to track the light. Refer to Chapter 103 for the complete details regarding doll's eyes testing.

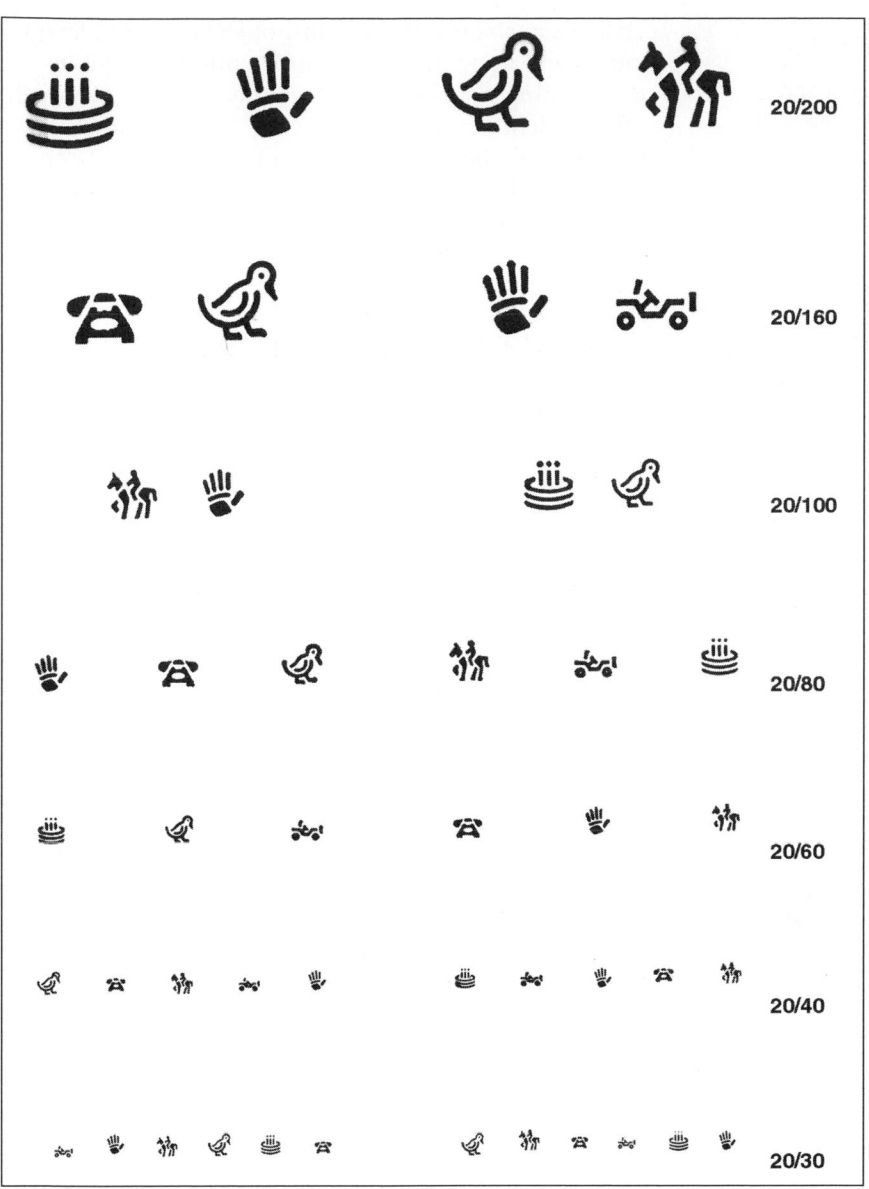

FIGURE 132-4 The pediatric visual acuity chart.

A difficult situation occurs in the patient whose visual acuity is "no light perception or LP–" but has normal pupillary responses and normal responses to the doll's eyes maneuver. This suggests that the visual loss is not anatomic or physiologic, but rather has a psychologic component. Test the optokinetic reflex in order to narrow the differential diagnosis. This uses either a spinning device or a scintoscope. A patient who can see movement will not be able to resist the normal tracking response to the rotating cylinder. A positive response will appear as nystagmus upon examination.

PEDIATRIC VISUAL ACUITY TESTING

It is important to evaluate the vision of infants. There is a critical time during which visual problems must be corrected to avoid permanent visual disturbances. This is optimally before 4 months of age. The eyes continue to develop quickly up to 2 years of age. Refer any questionable visual disturbances to a Pediatric Ophthalmologist.

Infants from term delivery to 3 to 4 months of age are not able to consistently follow and track objects. An infant's eyes may not move in perfect alignment until the age of approximately 3 to 4 months. Infants begin to focus on faces and follow them at approximately 6 weeks of age. They should consistently focus on and follow objects at 4 months of age.

Testing an infant's vision can be quite difficult. Place the infant with their parent holding them in the feeding position. Cover one of the infant's eyes. Ask the parent to move their head from side to side. Note whether the infant's uncovered eye tracks the parent's face. Repeat this

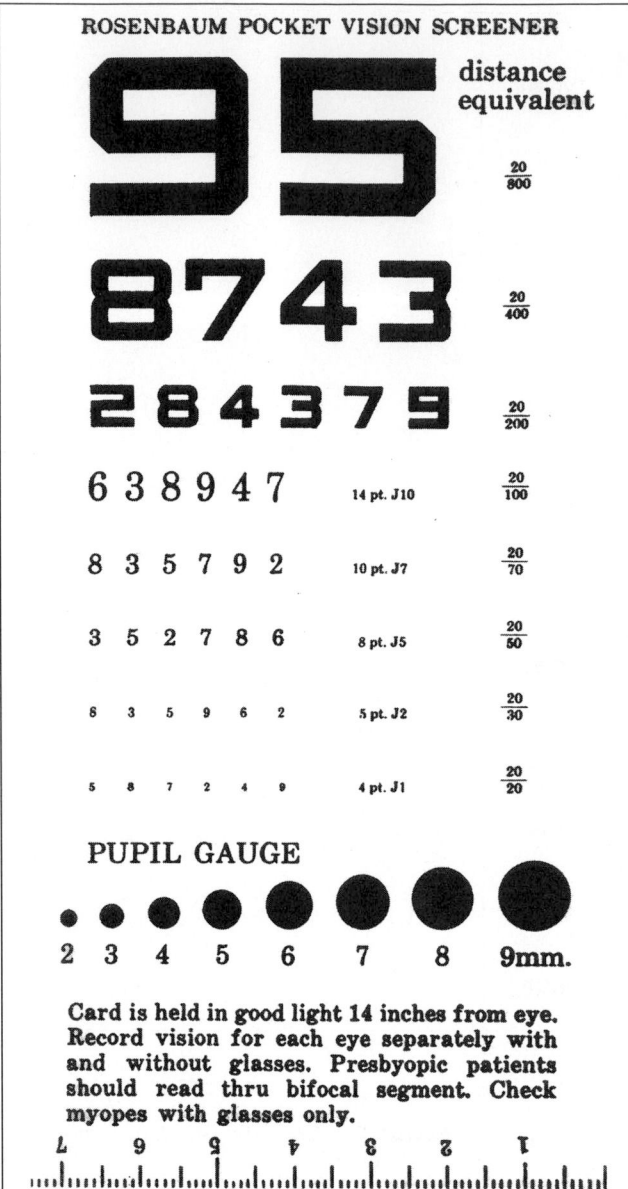

FIGURE 132-5 The Rosenbaum pocket vision screener.

charts use shapes of common objects in the place of letters and apply the same corresponding fractions for determining visual acuity. Have the child identify each of the pictures before beginning the examination to ensure that the child knows what the picture represents. Children may use unexpected words to identify the objects, which may complicate the interpretation of the exam.

GENERAL INSPECTION OF THE EYE

The examination of the eye proceeds from the outside and works inward. Begin with inspecting the external structures. Note the presence of any enophthalmos or exophthalmos. This is best accomplished by viewing the eyes from above and behind the patient. The normal globe position is just within the orbital rim. Enophthalmos is a recession of the globe within the bony orbit. It is an important clue for the presence of a blow-out or orbital floor fracture. Exophthalmos is a protrusion of the globe from the bony orbit. It may be an important clue to the presence of a retrobulbar hemorrhage or an orbital cellulitis. Esotropia refers to an inward or nasal deviation of the globe. Exotropia refers to an outward or temporal deviation of the globe.

Evaluate the eyes and eyelids for symmetry, lid position, obvious injuries, lesions, discoloration, and/or swelling. Ptosis suggests a Horner's syndrome or a third cranial nerve abnormality. **Any evidence of facial trauma or eye trauma raises the possibility of a ruptured globe. Avoid placing pressure directly on the globe if there is the possibility of a ruptured globe. Inadvertent tactile pressure placed on the globe may result in extrusion of intraocular structures through the wound if the globe has been penetrated or lacerated.** This can result in an otherwise avoidable visual loss that is typically not reparable. Manipulate the eyelids by applying pressure over the bony orbit instead of directly on the globe (Figure 132-9).

EVALUATION OF EXTRAOCULAR MOVEMENTS

Extraocular movements are easily assessed in the cooperative patient. Instruct the patient to keep their head still and directed towards the examiner. Instruct the patient to follow the motions of a finger with only their eyes as it follows the pattern of an H (Figure 132-10). This is referred to as the six cardinal positions for testing extraocular muscle movements. It may be helpful to retract the patient's eyelids to better visualize the eye movements. Observe the eyes for symmetric or conjugate gaze as each position is reached. Note whether the

with the opposite eye covered. The inability to track objects suggests that the visual acuity is 20/200 or less.

Children who cannot yet read or identify the letters of the alphabet are at a disadvantage when using the Snellen chart (Figure 132-2). Use the illiterate E chart (Figure 132-3), the pediatric visual acuity chart (Figure 132-4), the pediatric near vision test (Figure 132-6), or the Allen chart (Figure 132-8) to test their visual acuity. The illiterate E chart requires the patient to identify the direction that each variably rotated letter E faces (i.e., up, down, right, and left). Some clinicians find it helpful to describe the E as a table and ask which way the legs are facing. The procedure and documentation is otherwise the same as with the Snellen chart. The pediatric

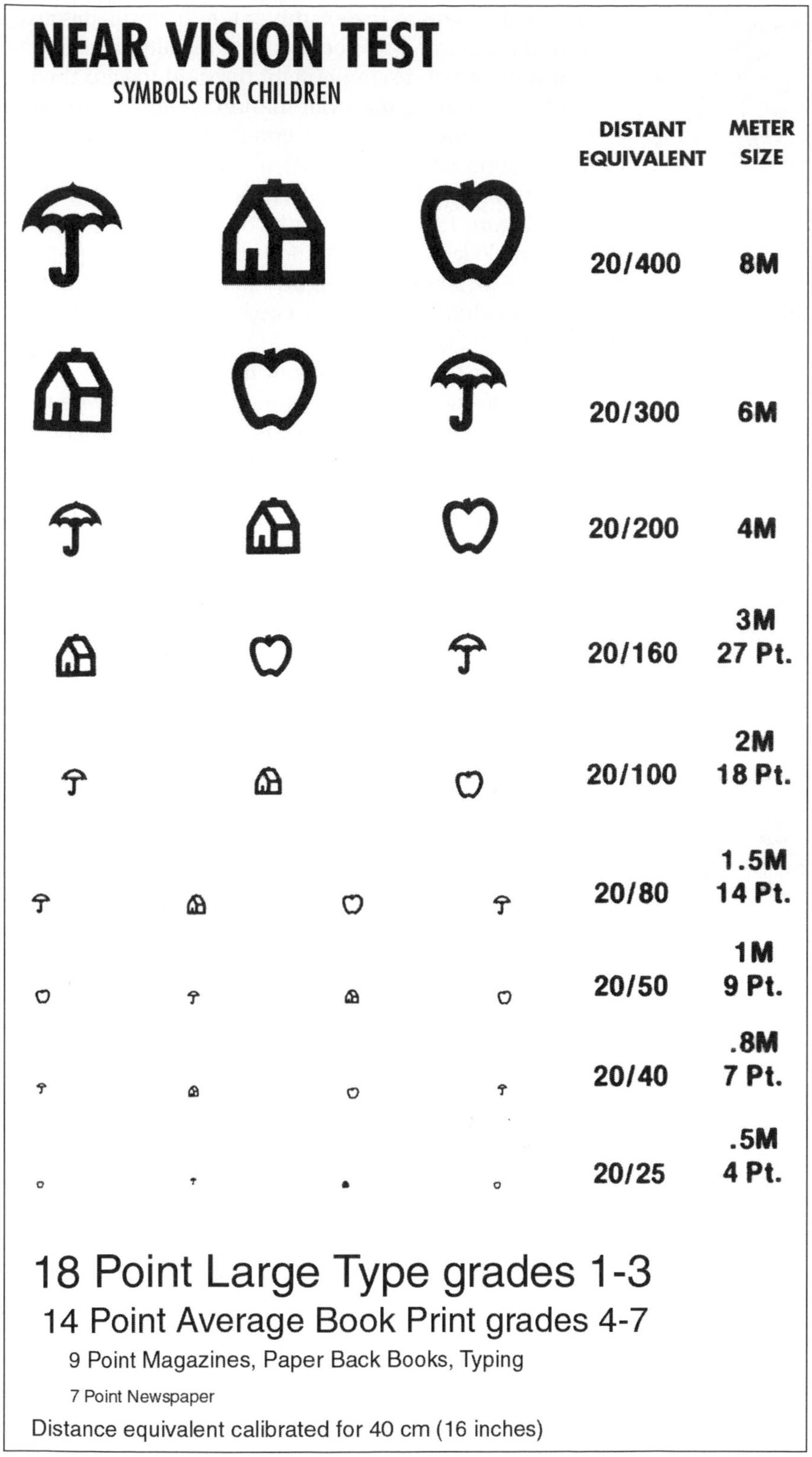

FIGURE 132-6 The near vision visual acuity test uses symbols for children.

patient sees one finger clearly at each position. Ask the patient to describe the orientation of the images (i.e., side to side) if more than one image is noted. Assess the far lateral positions by paying careful attention for evi-

dence of nystagmus. A few beats of nystagmus that quickly extinguishes is within normal limits. Keep in mind that the nose may obstruct the view at extreme points. Move the examining hand into a plane that is a

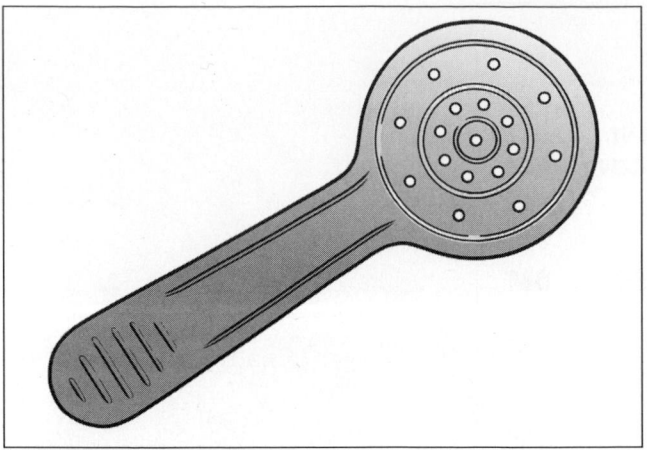

FIGURE 132-7 The pinhole device.

few inches closer to the examiner (i.e., a few inches away from the patient) if this occurs, and repeat the testing.

It is helpful to use a penlight directed toward the patient's eyes during the examination when a question of subtle disconjugate gaze is entertained, particularly in the position where the patient complains of diplopia. Look into the patient's pupils to see the reflection of the light (Figure 132-11). The reflection of the light is symmetrical, located in the same position in each pupil, if the gaze is conjugate (Figure 132-11*A*). Asymmetrical light reflection is noted in cases of disconjugate gaze (Figure 132-11*B*).

Consider the innervation of the extraocular muscles in order to narrow the differential diagnosis when abnormal extraocular movements are identified. The lateral rectus muscle is innervated by the sixth cranial nerve (CN VI). The superior oblique muscle is innervated by the fourth cranial nerve (CN IV). The remaining

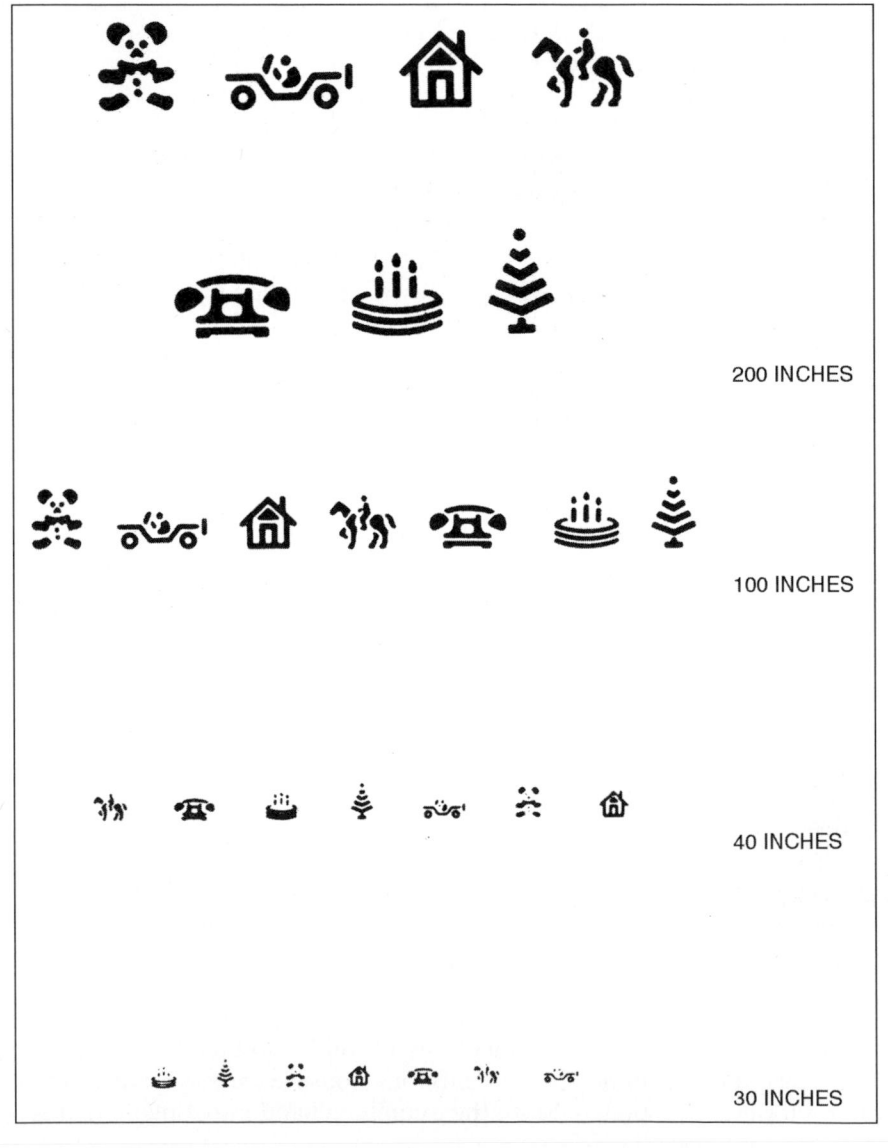

200 INCHES

100 INCHES

40 INCHES

30 INCHES

FIGURE 132-8 The Allen chart to measure pediatric visual acuity.

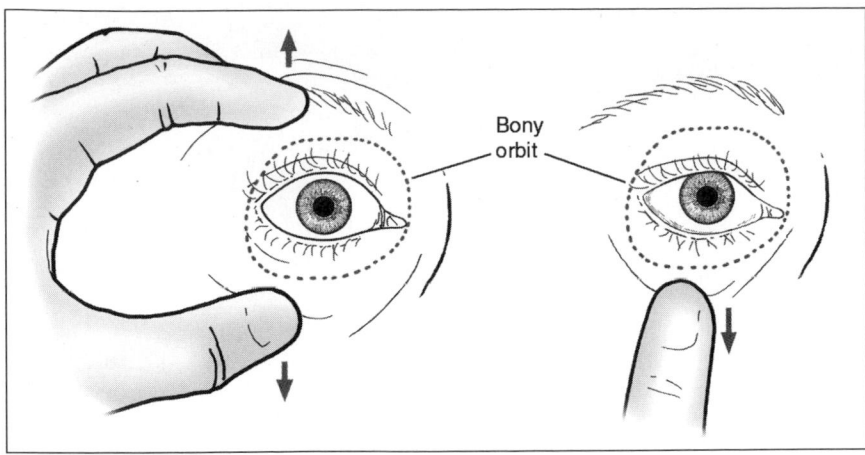

FIGURE 132-9 Open and close the eyelids by applying pressure over the bony orbit in suspected cases of a ruptured globe.

extraocular muscles are innervated by the third cranial nerve (CN III). An isolated sixth cranial nerve palsy, particularly in a child, strongly suggests an intracranial neoplasm. A complete third cranial nerve palsy suggests an intracranial aneurysm pressing on the oculomotor nerve. A physical obstruction originating in the retrobulbar region manifests as restricted extraocular movements in one eye. Consider the presence of an orbital cellulitis or a retrobulbar hemorrhage in the appropriate clinical setting.

Consider the presence of an orbital floor or blow-out fracture if the patient is unable to elevate one of the eyes. The etiology of the restricted movement may be physical entrapment of the inferior rectus and/or inferior oblique muscles within the orbital floor fracture or a contusion of the nerve innervating the inferior oblique muscle. The two must be distinguished as the management, treatment, and follow-up are different. Place two drops of a topical ophthalmic anesthetic agent into the affected eye. Grasp the bulbar conjunctiva with forceps and attempt to gently elevate the eye. A physical cause is ruled out if the eye is able to be elevated and a nerve contusion is likely.

EXAMINATION OF THE PUPILS

Place the patient with their head looking directly forward while retracting the upper eyelid. Complete the pupillary examination and a cursory evaluation of the cornea and anterior chamber simultaneously. Clinicians commonly use the abbreviation "PERRLA" as documentation for the pupillary examination. "PERRLA" means the pupils are equal, round, and reactive to light with normal accommodation. **This abbreviation is inadequate when a patient has eye complaints. It is important to document a detailed pupillary examination.**

Darken the room if possible. Instruct the patient to focus on a distant object. The normal response is symmetric dilation of the pupils. Note the size, in millimeters, of each pupil. Shine a focused beam of light into one eye to test reactivity. The normal pupil will constrict immediately and briskly. Document the direct response to light in millimeters at maximal constriction (e.g., OD = 4 mm → 2 mm). Note if the pupil is not briskly reactive (e.g., OS = 5 mm → 3 mm, sluggish) or if it dilates (e.g., OS = 3 mm → 6 mm). Repeat this test with the contralateral eye.

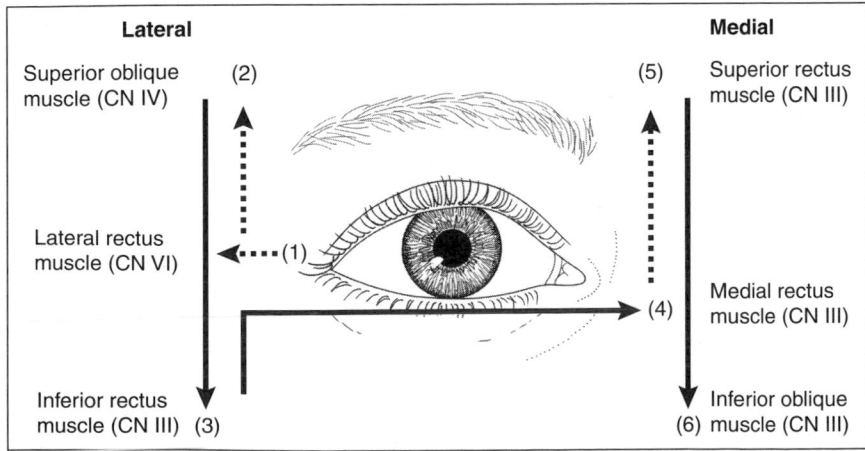

FIGURE 132-10 The six cardinal positions for testing extraocular muscle movements. Note that the testing follows an H-shape.

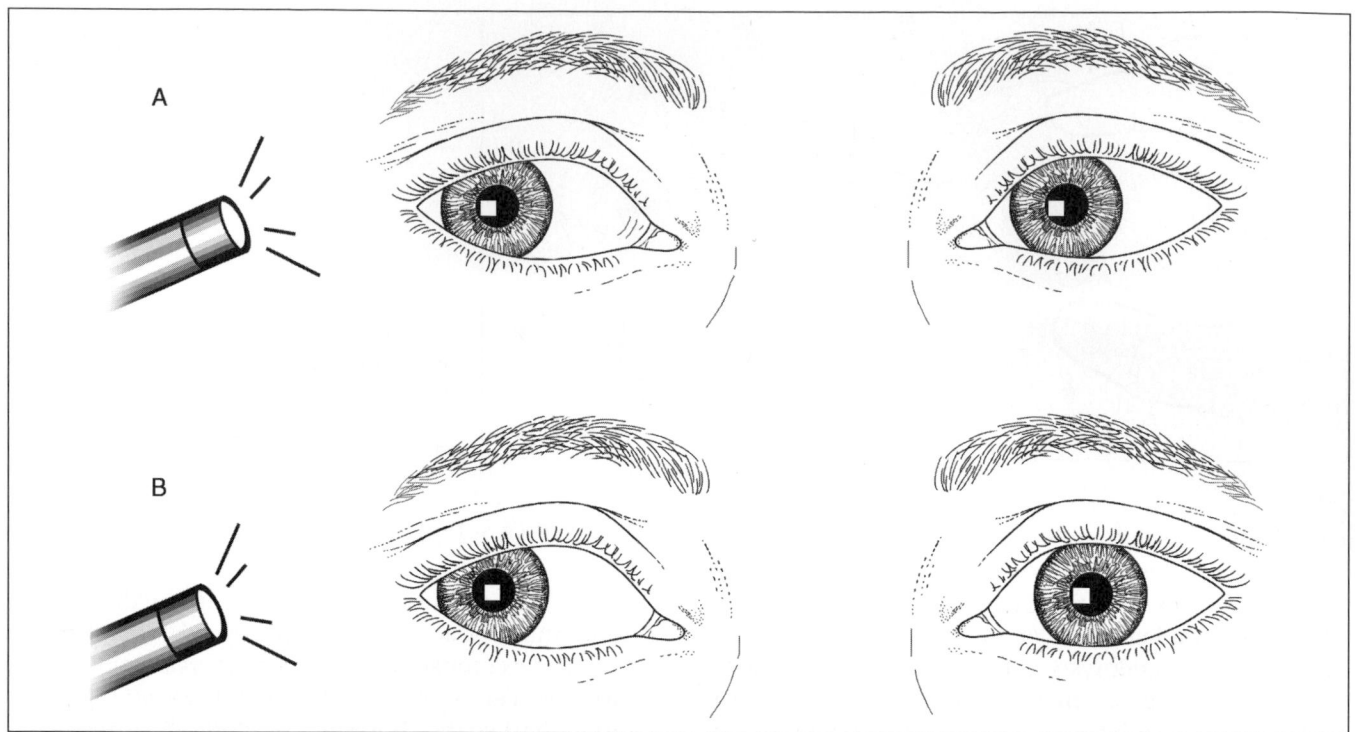

FIGURE 132-11 Shine a penlight into the eyes in the position that the patient complains of diplopia. Observe the light reflection in the pupils. *A.* Conjugate gaze. *B.* Disconjugate gaze.

The consensual pupillary response is the reaction of the contralateral eye to light shined into the opposite eye. The normal consensual pupillary response is constriction of the contralateral pupil when light is shined into the opposite eye. This occurs because some of the efferent optic nerve fibers cross the midbrain to the contralateral optic tract and result in constriction of the contralateral pupil. Be careful to document a normal consensual response if it is present.

A common example of an abnormal pupillary examination illustrates the importance of paying specific attention to the consensual pupillary response. The relative afferent pupillary defect (RAPD) results from the tested eye not perceiving the light. There is no perception of light (LP–) transmitted to the optic tracts. The tested pupil will not constrict to direct light. The pupil may, in fact, inappropriately dilate in response to direct light. There will be no consensual response in the contralateral pupil. The contralateral pupil will constrict appropriately to direct light and the previously unresponsive pupil will demonstrate a normal consensual response. The "swinging flashlight test" is used to test for a RAPD. Shine the light into one eye. Note the direct and consensual responses. Swing the light over to test the opposite eye. Note the direct and consensual responses.

A common problem for the Emergency Physician is the patient with unequal pupils. The primary consideration is typically a "blown pupil" suggesting uncal herni-ation from a mass lesion. This does not occur in a patient who is awake, alert, and cooperating with the eye examination. Physiologic anisocoria is the most common cause. Patients with physiologic anisocoria will have a normal response to light and typically the difference in pupillary size will be no more than 2 to 3 millimeters. **The physician must determine which of the two pupils is abnormal when they are abnormal and unequal.** The normal response to a darkened room is dilation. The pupil that does not dilate is abnormally miotic. The appropriate response to bright light is constriction. The pupil that does not constrict is abnormally mydriatic.

It is important to note and document the shape of each pupil. They should be round and regular. Irregularly shaped pupils may give important clues to otherwise undiagnosed injuries. A D-shaped pupil suggests a disruption of the ciliary muscles in the region adjacent to the flat part of the D. A teardrop-shaped pupil suggests a ruptured globe, with the point of the teardrop directed toward the point of penetration. A quivering and dilated pupil that does not react appropriately to light suggests a lens dislocation partially obstructing the visual axis. An irregularly shaped pupil may be an important diagnostic clue, but don't be misled. The most common cause of an irregularly shaped pupil is a postoperative change. Always inquire about previous eye surgery or old injuries.

EXAMINATION OF THE EXTERNAL STRUCTURES

The examination should proceed from the outside and work inward following an anatomic checklist. Examine the eyelids, lash line, and tarsal plates. Examine them for symmetry, normal position of the eyelashes, injury, infection, or inflammation. Examine the puncta of the lacrimal apparatus for signs of inflammation and obstruction. Examine the bulbar conjunctiva and vasculature for injection, ciliary flush, chemosis, discharge, and foreign bodies. Examine the cornea for clarity, evidence of injury, lesions, or foreign bodies. Examine the palpebral conjunctiva and cul-de-sac for injection, foreign bodies, discharge, and lymphatic (follicular) enlargement. Examine the anterior chamber for clarity, depth, and particulate matter.

Expose the structures of the inner aspect of the upper eyelid. Evert the eyelids (Figures 132-12 and 132-13) or retract the eyelids (Figures 132-14 and 132-15). Place the patient facing forward with their eyes focused downward to evert the upper eyelid (Figure 132-12). **The patient's eyes must remain directed downward as looking up or forward will cause the eyelids to return to their natural position.** This will make it difficult if not impossible to evert the eyelids. This process requires the use of a cotton-tipped applicator. An assistant may be required to aim and focus a light source during the examination as it may require two hands to evert and hold the eyelids in position.

Grasp the midpoint of the upper eyelash line or the tarsal plate between the index finger and thumb (Figure 132-12A). Place a cotton-tipped applicator 0.5 to 1.0 cm superior to the tarsal plate, with the cotton tip in the midplane of the upper eyelid (Figure 132-12A). Apply gentle pressure directed slightly downward against the upper eyelid with the cotton-tipped applicator. Use the other hand to pull the eyelid upward and evert it (Figure 132-12B). The upper eyelid may not completely evert. Sweep the cotton-tipped applicator from left to right while still holding the lash line in one hand and simultaneously applying gentle downward pressure with the applicator within the false pocket to completely evert the upper eyelid (Figure 132-12C).

Eversion of the lower eyelid is much simpler (Figure 132-13). Instruct the patient to look upward. Place the index finger on the patient's lower eyelid. Apply downward traction to evert the lower eyelid.

The use of a Desmarres eyelid retractor is an alternative option, if available, to retract the eyelids. It is very difficult to manually evert the eyelids when they are swollen. Manual eyelid eversion can result in excessive pressure being placed on the potentially injured globe. An eyelid retractor can be used to avoid placing pressure

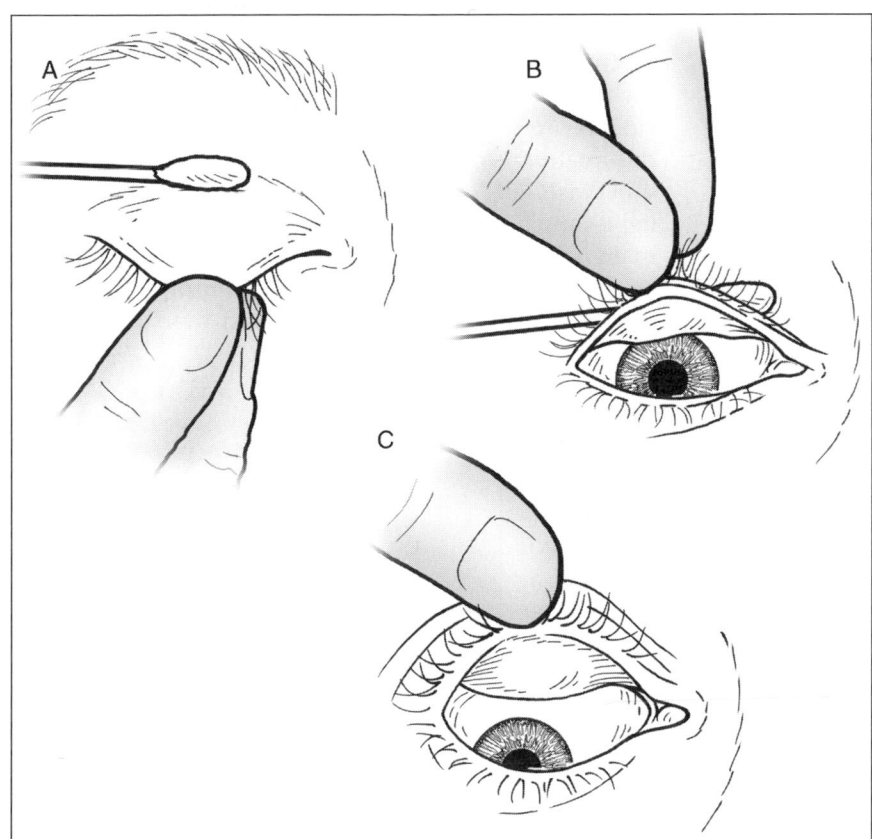

FIGURE 132-12 Eversion of the upper eyelid. *A.* Grasp and pull down the upper eyelashes while simultaneously placing a cotton-tipped applicator at the base of the upper eyelid. *B.* Flip the upper eyelid over the cotton-tipped applicator. *C.* Hold the everted eyelid in place and remove the cotton-tipped applicator.

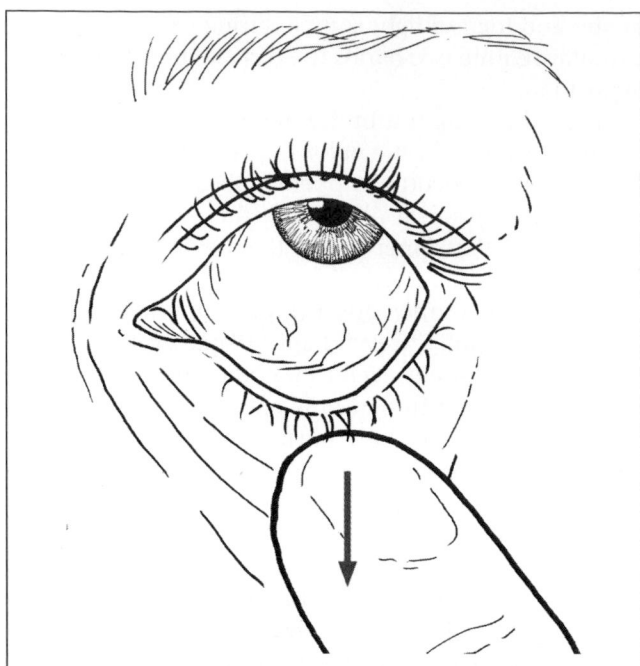

FIGURE 132-13 Eversion of the lower eyelid.

on the globe (Figure 132-14). Place the patient facing forward with their eyes directed downward. Place the eyelid retractor approximately 5 mm above the tarsal plate on the outer surface of the eyelid (Figure 132-14A). Grasp the midpoint of the upper eyelash line or the tarsal plate between the index finger and thumb. Slightly retract the upper eyelid away from the globe. Elevate and retract the tarsal plate upward to evert the eyelid onto the retractor (Figure 132-14B). Lift the retractor upwards to fully expose the undersurface of the eyelid (Figure 132-14C).

This technique allows the eyelid to be retracted with one hand while directing the light with the other hand. It also prevents any pressure from being placed on the globe if a rupture is suspected. It may be necessary to

slide the retractor 0.5 cm to the left and to the right of midline to fully visualize the structures. Use the same technique to retract the lower eyelids. Instruct the patient to direct their gaze and focus upward when retracting the lower eyelid.

A simple method to retract, but not evert, the eyelid with the Desmarres retractor is shown in Figure 132-15. Place the eyelid retractor in front of the upper eyelid (Figure 132-15A). Gently insert the retractor under the upper eyelid (Figure 132-15B). Apply slight outward traction on the retractor to securely grasp the tarsal plate. Rotate the retractor upward to retract the upper eyelid (Figure 132-15B). Elevate the retractor upward to open the eyelid (Figure 132-15C). Use the same technique to retract the lower eyelid. **Never use this technique if a foreign body or ruptured globe is suspected.** It may cause secondary injury by embedding a foreign body, perforating the globe with the foreign body, or expressing the ocular contents if the globe is ruptured.

Eyelid retractors are not uniformly available in all Emergency Departments. They should be part of an "eye kit" (Table 132-2). An alternative used by some is to unfold a paper clip and bend it into shape with a clamp (Figure 132-16). This is not recommended by the editors as the metal coating on the paper clip flakes off and can result in corneal abrasions and foreign bodies.

SLIT LAMP EXAMINATION

The slit lamp is an essential piece of machinery for a thorough eye examination (Figure 132-17). It is an invaluable resource that can be used to identify and aid in the treatment of ophthalmologic problems that might otherwise go unrecognized. It provides an adjustable light source with variable magnification. The eyes remain in a fixed position while the light and microscope are independently adjusted. The result of these attributes is that it can focus precisely on the structures of

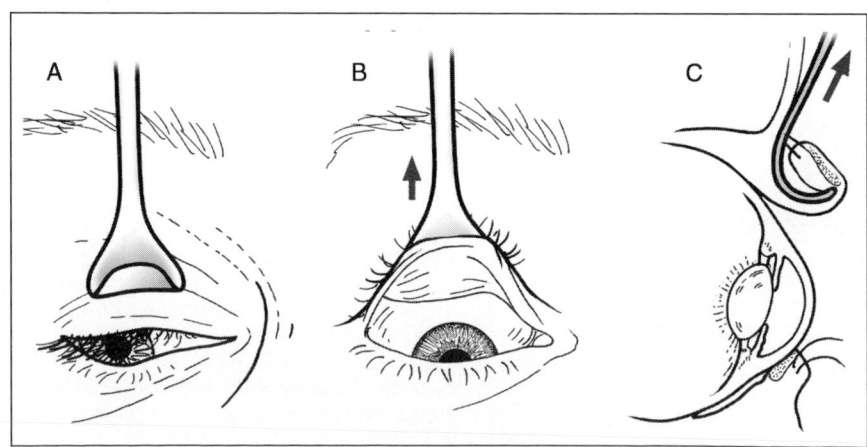

FIGURE 132-14 Eversion of the upper eyelid with a Desmarres retractor. *A.* Place the retractor 5 mm above the tarsal plate. *B.* Grasp the eyelashes and evert the upper eyelid over the retractor. *C.* Elevate the retractor to fully expose the under surface of the eyelid.

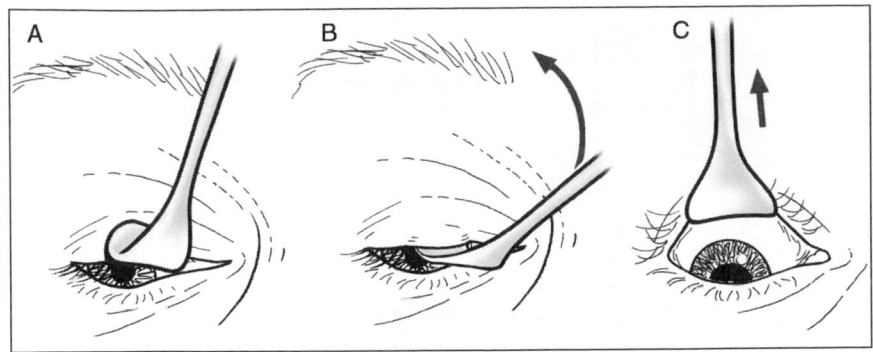

FIGURE 132-15 Retraction of the upper eyelid. *A.* Place the retractor in front of the eyelid. *B.* Insert the retractor and rotate it towards the forehead. *C.* Elevate the retractor to expose the globe.

the eye and provide a three-dimensional image. The slit lamp provides invaluable information, particularly when examining the cornea and the anterior chamber. The three-dimensional microscopic capability is best demonstrated when examining the intricate topography of the iris.

It may be helpful to set up the slit lamp before the patient is in the room until one feels comfortable using the slit lamp. Place one hand against the middle of the forehead bar in the examination plane to help become familiar with the capabilities of the machine and the joystick. Practice focusing the slit lamp on the details of the skin on your hand. Adjust the focus by sliding the joystick to move the entire slit lamp apparatus forward and backward. Slide the joystick side to side to scan across and examine the entire width of the eye. Rotate the joystick clockwise and counterclockwise to move the line of vision up and down.

Place the machine in the standard position. **It takes very few adjustments of the slit lamp to complete the entire examination.** The slit lamp can be focused and locked in position with the knob located on the table base for procedures that require the physician's hands to be free (e.g., foreign bodies embedded within the cornea). This allows one hand to hold the eyelids open while using the appropriate tool in the other hand.

TABLE 132-2. RECOMMENDATIONS FOR A COMPLETE EMERGENCY DEPARTMENT EYE KIT

Snellen chart
Rosenbaum card
"E" chart
Pinhole device
Lid retractor
Fluorescein strips (individually packaged)
Slit lamp
Alcohol swabs
Ophthalmoscope
Topical anesthetic agent, proparacaine or tetracaine
Topical mydriatic agent, phenylephrine
Topical cycloplegic agents
Topical pupillary constrictors, pilocarpine and timolol

SETTING UP THE SLIT LAMP

The slit lamp has many parts, most of which are capable of moving. The slit lamp components are often moved into a complete disarray by others. This is noted when the examiner sits down to use the slit lamp. **It is important to start by readjusting the slit lamp to a "standard operating position."**

The body of the slit lamp has three rotating arms. The examiner's neutral position is designated as 0 degrees and the center of the chin rest is designated 180 degrees. The lower arm rotates the binocular microscope. It is rarely, if ever, necessary to move the rotat-

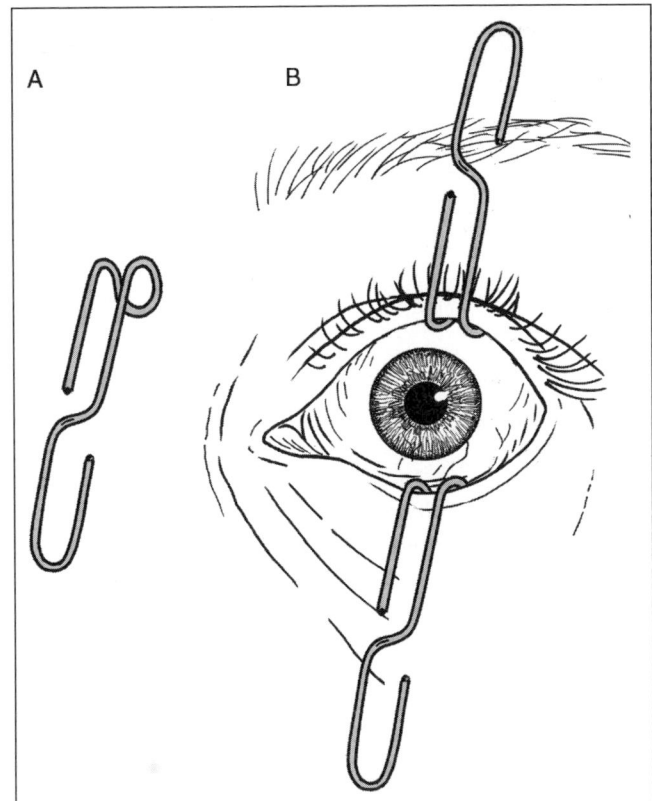

FIGURE 132-16 An alternative to an eyelid retractor. *A.* Unfold a paper clip and bend it into shape with a hemostat. *B.* Paper clips used to retract the eyelids.

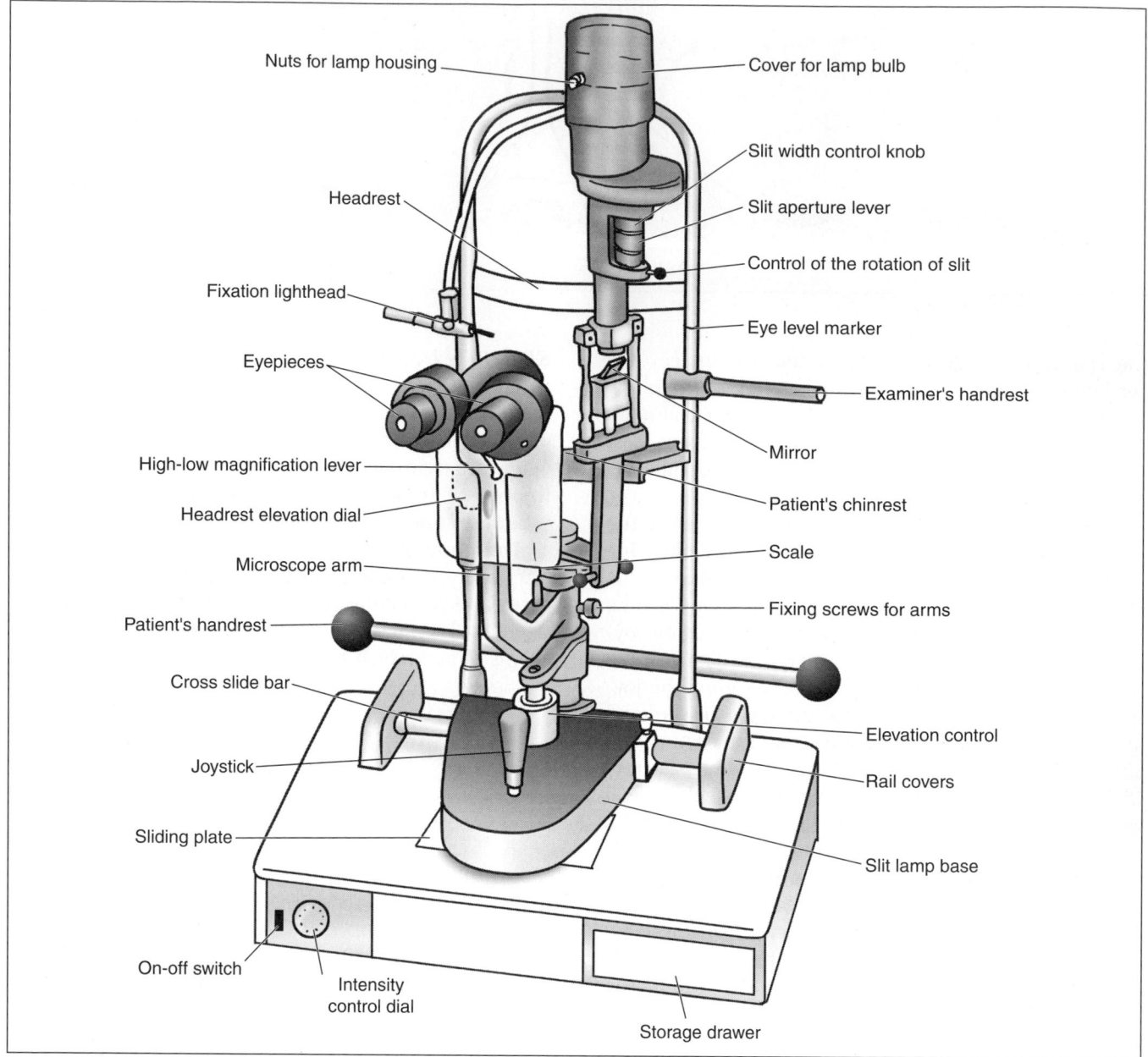

FIGURE 132-17 The slit lamp.

ing binocular microscope from the 0 degrees position for the purposes of an Emergency Department examination. The next two arms are moved as a unit. The lower arm rotates the light 90 degrees in either direction. The light source remains directed toward the structure that is being focused upon. The angle of the light is changed when the arm is rotated up to 90 degrees in either direction. The standard position for the light is to rotate it 45 degrees to the examiner's left to examine the patient's right eye and 45 degrees to the examiner's right to examine the patient's left eye. Rotation of the upper arm independently rotates the slit of light in the coronal plane. Never rotate the two upper

arms independently during the Emergency Department examination.

The eyepieces of the binocular microscope can be adjusted and focused independently in accordance to the examiner's needs. The standard starting position is in the 0 and 0 position. The eyepieces can be adjusted to compensate for refractory errors and to correct for the interpupillary distance of the examiner.

Two levels of magnification are typically available (10× and 16×). The switch to change magnification is located just below the eyepieces. The standard beginning position is low magnification. The higher power may be helpful when examining the details of the cornea or looking for cellular or inflammatory material within the anterior chamber.

The next step is to find the on-off switch. It is typically located just under the table base and on the left. Place one hand in the examination plane against the head-band where it should pick up a focused beam of light to ensure that the light source is functional. Check to ensure that the slit lamp is plugged in if no light is seen. Observe the top of the slit lamp to determine whether light shines through the casing that houses the light source. The bulb will periodically need to be replaced. Remove the casing and replace the bulb as needed. The correct position for the bulb is obvious as it has a notch that fits into a corresponding notch in the housing.

The focused light can be adjusted in intensity, color, vertical width, and horizontal width. The standard position is for the light to be at its maximum size with a circular beam of white light at its greatest intensity. This position is used for scanning the eye and examining the external structures. Some patients will not be able to tolerate the light at maximum intensity. Make adjustments from the starting position as necessary. Three independent adjustment mechanisms interact to create the most appropriate illumination to meet examination needs.

The color of the light and the intensity of the light originate from the same mechanism. Most of the positions represent variations in intensity of a white light. There are two other options for color. The cobalt blue light is used for emphasizing corneal lesions that pick up fluorescein stain. The green light or red filter is helpful for patients who cannot tolerate the white light secondary to photophobia.

The horizontal width of the light can be adjusted with the knob located at the base of the middle arm. The light can be narrowed to 1 to 2 mm or a "slit" for evaluating the depth of corneal lesions (Figure 132-18*A*). The vertical control is used in conjunction with the horizontal control. Narrow the horizontal width to 2 to 3 mm and the vertical width to 2 mm when examining the anterior chamber. This creates a small focused beam. Rotate the light 30 to 60 degrees in order to illuminate the depth of the anterior chamber (Figure 132-18*B*). This orientation is most beneficial when attempting to identify cellular or inflammatory material within the anterior chamber.

PATIENT POSITIONING

Cleanse the chin rest and the forehead bar before the slit lamp is used to examine a patient. The patient must be able to tolerate a seated position, leaning slightly forward with their head placed in the chin rest and their forehead pressed against the bar to use the slit lamp (Figure 132-19). The slit lamp examination cannot be completed in a patient who cannot remain in a seated position.

A motorized chair with the ability to move up and down is optimal for this examination. The slit lamp can be adjusted to match the height of a chair or stretcher if necessary. Press the release bar located below the slit lamp table to move the entire table up and down. Release the bar to lock the slit lamp table in position. The level of the chin bar can be adjusted to account for the subtle differences in the length of individual patient faces. Rotate the knob located at the base of the chin rest apparatus to move it up and down. Raise or lower the chin bar so that the reference mark located below the forehead bar is at the patient's eye level.

The patient must remain in this position to effectively focus upon and examine the eyes (Figure 132-19). A common pitfall of the slit lamp examination is to allow the patient to tilt their head back and away from the forehead bar. The angle created makes focusing very difficult, if not impossible. Check the patient's position if there is any difficulty in focusing the slit lamp.

Use the joystick to move the slit lamp and scan the patient's eye. The patient must keep their eye in a fixed position while the examiner uses the joystick to move the slit lamp and scan the eye. Instruct the patient to focus their right eye on the examiner's left shoulder when scanning the left eye and on the right shoulder when scanning the right eye. It is very difficult for the examiner to focus and complete a thorough examination if the patient's eyes wander.

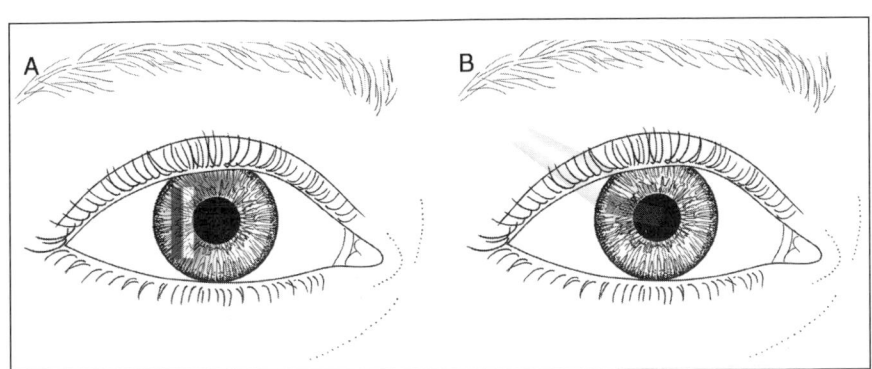

FIGURE 132-18 The light of the slit lamp. *A*. A narrow slit to focus on the cornea. *B*. A focused beam of light directed from a 45 degree angle illuminates the anterior chamber.

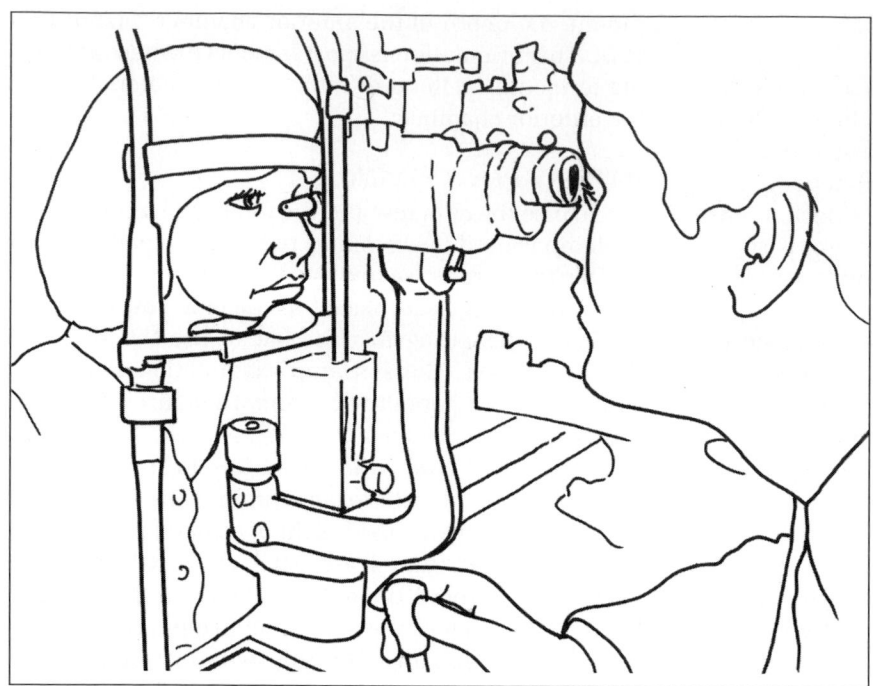

FIGURE 132-19 Patient positioning in the slit lamp.

THE SLIT LAMP EXAMINATION

The slit lamp examination begins with an overall microscope-enhanced evaluation of the external structures of the eye including the lash line, the bulbar conjunctiva, the palpebral conjunctiva, and the puncta. The cornea is best evaluated with a wide beam and with the slit. **Do not focus the light into the pupil for an extended period of time.** It is very uncomfortable for the patient and may result in injury. The normal cornea is perfectly clear and homogeneous. Note any deviation from this if applicable. Specific abnormalities are best documented in writing in addition to a basic schematic diagram.

The anterior chamber should be clear and without particulate matter. It may be difficult initially to identify cells floating in the anterior chamber. They appear like "dust in a sunbeam." The cells, if not clumped, are barely visible with the microscope at the lowest magnification. They do, however, reflect the light slightly, and this may catch the examiner's eye. Take care to pay special attention to the lower one-fourth of the anterior chamber because, in an upright position, cells and inflammatory products tend to settle and may form a meniscus. Flare is the non cellular inflammatory material in the anterior chamber that makes the aqueous humor appear hazy, or gelatinous, and obscure the details of the iris. Use the high-power magnification to identify particulate matter after scanning the anterior chamber with the low-power magnification.

ADMINISTRATION OF FLUORESCEIN

Repeat the corneal examination with the aid of fluorescein stain after the slit lamp examination is com-

pleted without stain. Fluorescein is a hydrophilic substance that stains and illuminates any portion of the cornea where there is a breech in the epithelium. The addition of fluorescein helps to illuminate corneal lesions that might otherwise go unrecognized. This includes corneal abrasions or keratopathy associated with viral infections. Fluorescein is most commonly packaged as two individual single-use strips, one for each eye. There is the potential for infectious agents to be transmitted when one fluorescein strip is used for both eyes or when a multidose vial of fluorescein solution is used. Take care to avoid iatrogenically transmitted infections.

Place a small drop of saline or topical ophthalmic anesthetic solution onto the tip of the fluorescein strip. Retract the lower eyelid by placing pressure on the skin overlying the inferior orbital rim and distracting it downward. Ask the patient to look upward to facilitate the administration of the stain, in addition to avoiding inadvertent corneal injuries caused by the strip itself. Touch the fluorescein strip lightly against the palpebral conjunctiva of the inferior eyelid (Figure 132-20A). Ask the patient to gently open and close their eyelids to distribute the fluorescein across the entire eye. Aqueous fluorescein solution can be used as an alternative to the paper strips. Retract the lower eyelid and instill 2 drops of fluorescein into the cul-de-sac of the lower eyelid (Figure 132-20B). **Take special care when using fluorescein to avoid accidentally staining the patient's skin, clothing, or contact lenses. Contact lenses, particularly soft types, must be removed prior to the application of fluorescein to prevent them from becoming permanently stained.**

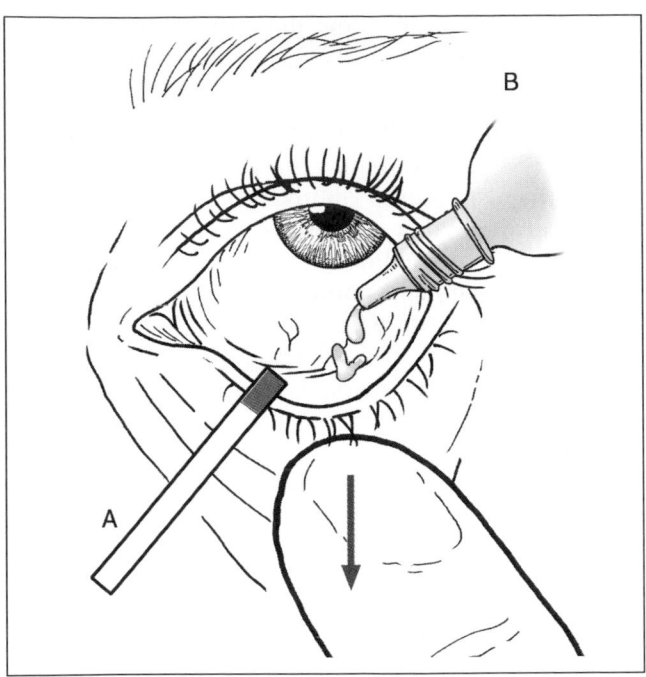

FIGURE 132-20 Instillation of fluorescein stain. *A.* Fluorescein-tipped strips. *B.* Aqueous fluorescein solution.

A small amount of fluorescein is required to adequately stain the cornea. A common mistake is to apply an excessive amount of fluorescein stain. This illuminates the entire tear film and makes it difficult to evaluate subtle lesions on the cornea. Ask the patient to blink

several times to remove the excess fluorescein from the cornea. This maneuver will typically not remove the fluorescein adhering to any corneal defects. Place one or two drops of sterile saline or eyewash onto the eye to remove the excess fluorescein stain if blinking does not remove the excess fluorescein.

The underlying cell layers of the cornea will hold the fluorescein stain if the corneal epithelium is injured. This allows corneal lesions to be visualized. Use the cobalt blue light, preferably in conjunction with the slit lamp, to identify and evaluate any corneal lesions that become apparent. The regions that stain with fluorescein and are visible with the cobalt blue light will appear bright yellow to yellow-green. **The green light on the ophthalmoscope and the slit lamp are not intended to be used to illuminate the fluorescein stain.** The green light will enhance the stain in some circumstances but is not as effective as the cobalt blue light source.

EYEDROP ADMINISTRATION

TRADITIONAL METHODS

Topical ophthalmologic medications are used for examining and treating the eyes. Eyedrops and ophthalmologic ointments are most effectively and accurately instilled within the lower eyelid (Figure 132-21). Instruct the patient to direct their head towards the examiner with their eyes looking upward (Figure 132-21*A*). Patients

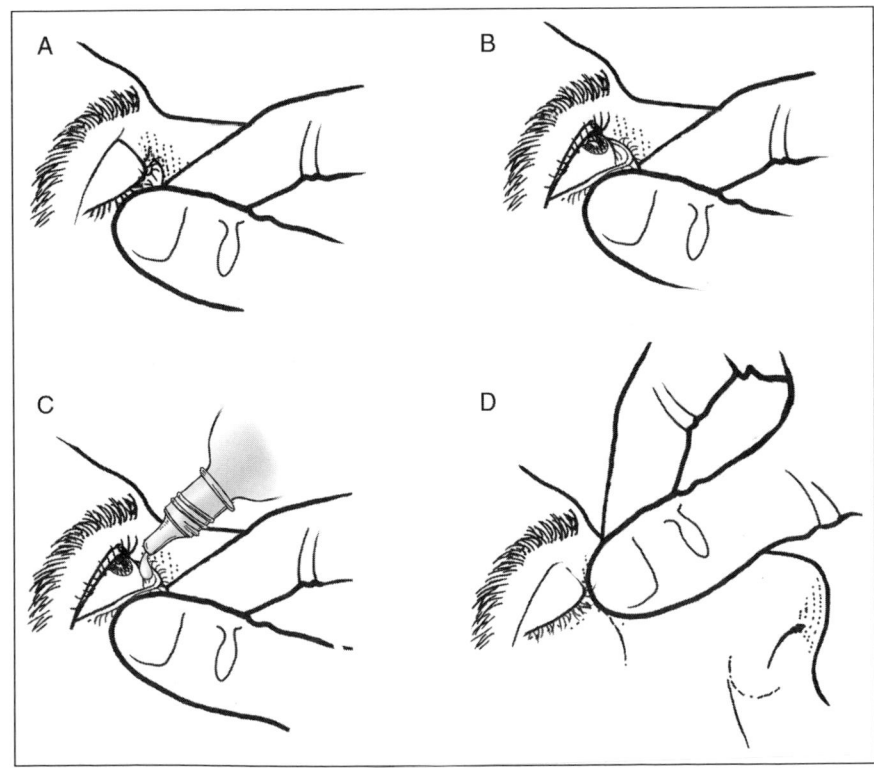

FIGURE 132-21 The installation of eyedrops. *A.* Grasp the lower eyelid. *B.* Pull the lower eyelid downward and outward to expose the cul-de-sac. *C.* Place the drops into the cul-de-sac. *D.* Apply thumb pressure over the lacrimal duct to prevent drainage of the drops into the nose.

often close their eyes at this point. Retract the lower eyelid, without placing pressure on the globe, and expose the inferior cul-de-sac (Figure 132-21B). Apply the drops, or ointment, in the cul-de-sac (Figure 132-21C). Close the eyelid and apply thumb pressure over the lacrimal duct (Figure 132-21D). This prevents the liquid medicine from immediately draining into the nose. Instruct the patient to blink once or twice to quickly distribute the medication across the globe. This last step, applying pressure on the lacrimal duct, is unnecessary if instilling an ophthalmic ointment.

UNCOOPERATIVE PATIENTS

Some patients require but do not want medication in their eyes. The best examples of these challenging patients are infants, small children, and patients with altered mental status. Prying the eyes of these patients open and applying the drops is difficult for both the physician and the patient. **Forcefully opening the eyelids is potentially dangerous because secondary injuries may occur.** The majority of medication is typically applied to the physician's hand or the stretcher, as anyone who has tried this approach knows. An alternative approach in this situation is advisable.

The problem is that the uncooperative patient squeezes their eyes closed tightly. Place the patient supine with an assistant holding the head in a fixed upright position with the eyes facing the ceiling in order to overcome this challenge (Figure 132-22). Note the small anatomic depression created over the medial canthus of each eye when they are closed tightly. Place the eyedrops in this anatomic depression to create a shallow pool (Figure 132-22). Firmly maintain the patient's head in this position until they spontaneously

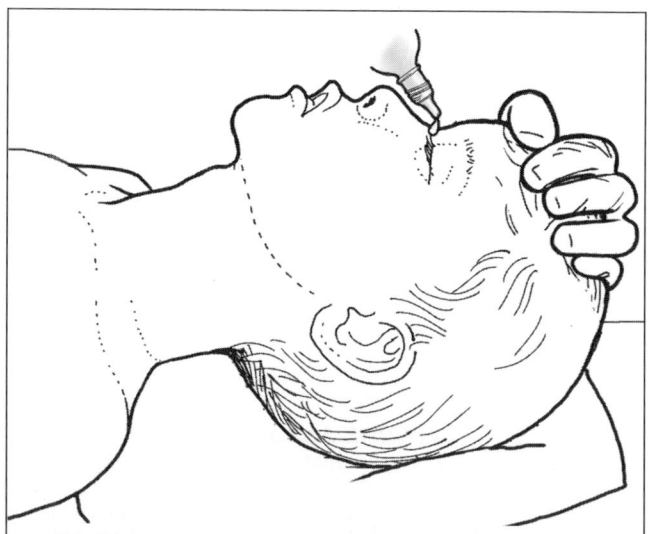

FIGURE 132-22 The instillation of eyedrops in an uncooperative patient.

open their eyes and allow the medication to spread across the globe.

OPHTHALMIC ANESTHETIC AGENTS

Two types of eye medications are required in drop form for most routine ophthalmologic examinations, a topical ophthalmic anesthetic agent and a dilating agent. Topical ophthalmic anesthetic agents provide relief from eye pain and photophobia. This may help the patient to cooperate with the necessary examination. Topical ophthalmic anesthetic agents may be used as adjuncts to fluorescein application and to facilitate the placement of eyelid retractors.

Tetracaine hydrochloride and proparacaine hydrochloride are the most commonly available agents. Their onset of action and duration of action are similar. The onset is within 1 minute and lasts 10 to 15 minutes. Tetracaine hydrochloride (Pontocaine) instillation often results in a transient stinging sensation that lasts 3 to 10 seconds before dissipating. Proparacaine hydrochloride (Ophthetic or Ophthaine) does not result in the stinging sensation.

PUPILLARY DILATING AGENTS

Dilating agents are used as an adjunct to the funduscopic examination. **Perform and document a complete pupillary examination before instilling dilating agents.** It is important to document the use of dilating agents and the time of administration. **Avoid using dilating agents in patients who require serial pupillary examinations to follow their neurologic status. Dilating agents are contraindicated in patients with a known or suspected narrow iridocorneal angle or glaucoma.** Dilating the pupil may result in acute angle-closure glaucoma. Some intraocular lens implants may become dislodged if the pupils are pharmacologically dilated. **Inquire about ocular surgery and glaucoma prior to dilating the pupils.**

Dilating agents are categorized as mydriatics and cycloplegics. **All dilating agents are stocked with red caps.** Mydriatic agents directly dilate the pupil while cycloplegics paralyze the ciliary muscles. **Cycloplegic agents should not be used in patients who require serial neurologic examinations.** Choose a non-cycloplegic mydriatic agent such as phenylephrine to dilate the pupils of a patient requiring serial examinations. The duration of action is significantly shorter than that of a cycloplegic agent. **Phenylephrine is systemically absorbed and should be avoided in patients with hypertension or cardiac conditions.** A combination of a mydriatic agent (e.g., phenylephrine) and a shorter-acting cycloplegic agent (e.g., cyclopentolate) is optimal when maximal dilation is necessary or when a single agent is ineffective.

Most Emergency Departments stock five dilating agents. The choice of agents depends upon the length of time required for dilation, the need for a cycloplegic agent, and the need for a mydriatic agent. Atropine (Isopto Atropine) produces cycloplegia lasting 5 to 10 days and mydriasis lasting 7 to 14 days. Cyclopentolate (Cyclogyl, AK-Pentolate, Pentolair) produces cycloplegia lasting 6 to 24 hours and mydriasis lasting 24 hours. Homatropine (Isopto Homatropine) produces cycloplegia and mydriasis lasting 1 to 3 days. Phenylephrine (Neo-Synephrine, Mydfrin, Relief) produces mydriasis lasting 5 hours. Tropicamide (Mydriacyl) produces mydriasis lasting 4 to 6 hours.

THE FUNDUSCOPIC EXAMINATION

A funduscopic examination is an essential part of every eye evaluation. It is particularly helpful when the patient complains of visual disturbances or visual loss. Examine the patient's right eye first. Hold the ophthalmoscope in the right hand and use the right eye to examine the patient's right eye. The examiner may otherwise find themself in an awkward nose-to-nose position with the patient. Instruct the patient to look over the examiner's right shoulder at a fixed point in the distance. Examine the patient's left eye. Hold the ophthalmoscope in the left hand and use the left eye to examine the patient's left eye.

Set the ophthalmoscope initially at 0. Adjust the dial as the examination begins to adjust for refractory errors. Moving the dial into the red moves the point of focus forward toward the red retina. Approach the eye from a slightly lateral position to quickly identify the medial position of the optic disk. Position the ophthalmoscope as close as possible to the patient's eye without making contact. Imagine looking at the fundus through a peephole. The closer you get, the wider the view on the other side. By the same analogy, the larger the peephole the better the view on the other side.

Dilate the patient's pupils to obtain the best results from the ophthalmoscope examination. Adjust the diameter of the light down to the size of the patient's pupil in order to avoid the bright reflection off of the iris if dilation is not possible. This bright reflection is a common reason for inadequate visualization of the fundus. The patient's eyes are often moving if the structures seem to move in and out of focus. Remind the patient to focus on one point in the distance.

Inspect the eye grounds for uniformity. The normal color of the fundus is creamy peach to pink. A pale fundus with a small cherry-red spot in the region of the macula suggests an infarction generally associated with a retinal artery occlusion. The optic disk is located on the nasal aspect of the fundus. If the optic disk does not come into view, follow the blood vessels that extend from the disk to the periphery of the retina. The disk margin should be sharp with the exception of the nasal aspect that may appear slightly blurred in a normal eye. Papilledema appears as diffusely blurred disk margins. Papilledema may be the result of localized inflammation of the optic nerve or may be the result of elevated intracranial pressure.

The veins will appear darker and wider than the arteries. Evaluate the blood vessels for evidence of hemorrhages and irregularities. Acute hemorrhages may be helpful in the diagnosis of a variety of problems such as a hypertensive emergency or the shaken baby syndrome. Give careful consideration to the clinical setting. A helpful finding in the patient suspected of having increased intracranial pressure is the presence or absence of venous pulsations. Venous pulsations are best seen as the veins cross into the optic cup. The presence of venous pulsations is a normal finding. The first sign as the intracranial pressure rises is a loss of venous pulsations followed later by papilledema. The green light or red filter helps to provide a sharper image when evaluating the retinal vessels in detail.

Examine the fovea and the surrounding macula. This area is located approximately 2 to 3 disk diameters (DD) lateral to the optic disk. Instruct the patient to look directly into the light to bring the fovea and macula into view. The target setting on the ophthalmoscope is helpful for this purpose. Look into the patient's eye with the ophthalmoscope turned to the target. Instruct the patient to look directly into the center of the target. The fovea will be found at the center of the target in your view.

Examine the vitreous chamber for evidence of a vitreous hemorrhage when a retinal detachment is suspected or when the patient complains of floaters. The fluid within the vitreous chamber is gelatinous so blood within it does not dissipate quickly. Blood within this chamber appears as clouds, spots, or veils to the patient and the examiner. Their color is typically described as black or red. Set the ophthalmoscope to +10 to move the point of focus anteriorly toward the examiner's eye to evaluate the vitreous. Dial the ophthalmoscope down as the examination proceeds. Each click results in focusing a little deeper within the vitreous chamber until the point of focus is upon the retina at the posterior aspect of the chamber.

INTRAOCULAR PRESSURE MEASUREMENT

The measurement of intraocular pressure should be included in the eye examination. It is particularly important in patients with eye pain and visual loss. Refer to

Chapter 135 regarding the complete details of ocular tonometry.

SUMMARY

Approach all eye complaints with a detailed history that includes a chief complaint, the duration of symptoms, and the natural history of their evolution. It is important to inquire about exposures and trauma. The past medical history must include the patient's baseline visual acuity and any history of eye problems. Perform a complete examination on all patients with eye complaints. Always document an accurate visual acuity and carefully inspect all of the eye structures. A thorough approach in all patients with eye complaints improves diagnostic accuracy. The end result is decreased morbidity and long-term complications in this vital sensory apparatus.

REFERENCES

1. Palay DA, Krachmer JH: *Ophthalmology for the Primary Care Physician.* St Louis: Mosby, 1997.
2. Vaughn DG, Asbury T, Riordan-Eva P: *General Ophthalmology,* 13th ed. East Norwalk, CT: Appleton & Lange, 1992.
3. Catalano RA: *Ocular Emergencies.* Philadelphia: Saunders, 1992.
4. Handler JA, Ghezzi KT: General ophthalmologic examination. *Emerg Med Clin North Am* 1995; 13(3):521–538.
5. Santen SA, Scott JL: Ophthalmologic procedures. *Emerg Med Clin North Am* 1995; 13(3):681–701.
6. Datner EM, Jolly BT: Pediatric ophthalmology. *Emerg Med Clin North Am* 1995; 13(3):669–679.
7. Barish RA, Naradzay J: Ophthalmologic therapeutics. *Emerg Med Clin North Am* 1995; 13(3):649–667.
8. Newell FW: *Ophthalmology Principles and Concepts,* 8th ed. St. Louis: Mosby, 1996.

Chapter 133
CONTACT LENS REMOVAL

Dino P. Rumoro

INTRODUCTION

The Emergency Physician must be familiar with the proper technique of removing both soft and hard contact lenses from patients who are unable to do so for various reasons. Patients with altered mental status are at particular risk of corneal damage if contact lenses are allowed to remain in place. Healthy individuals who wear contact lenses overnight experience a 4 to 15 fold increase in the risk of corneal injury over those who remove their contact lenses daily.[1] The explanation for this increased risk focuses on corneal hypoxia and an immune response to antigens present on the lens surface, both of which lead to an inflammatory response and susceptibility to infectious organisms.[1] This results in an increased incidence of ulcerative keratitis and *Pseudomonas aeruginosa* infection.[2]

ANATOMY AND PATHOPHYSIOLOGY

Contact lenses rest on a three-layer tear film (outer lipid, middle aqueous, and inner mucus layer) that covers the corneal and conjunctival epithelium. This tear layer provides oxygen and nutrients to the avascular cornea. The cornea also receives nutrition from blood vessels at the limbus and the aqueous humor. It is believed that contact lenses increase tear evaporation and disrupt the three-layer tear film, leading to the lack of corneal oxygenation and the symptoms of dry eye.[3] A dry eye causes discomfort and corneal edema with resultant hazy vision. The normal blinking action causes contact lens movement and a "fresh" flow of oxygenated tears over the cornea in the awake patient. This is obviously not present in the sleeping or comatose patient.

The normal resting position of the contact lens is over the cornea. It may occasionally drift from the center of the eye and relocate over the sclera or in various parts of the eye, including under the upper eyelid. Explore all aspects of the eye, including under the upper and lower eyelid margins, when evaluating an individual for contact lens removal.

INDICATIONS

Contact lenses must be removed from any patient who is unconscious or suffers an ocular injury. Lenses should not be left in place if fluorescein stain is to be used to examine the eye. Fluorescein can permanently stain the lens material. Give patients the opportunity to remove their own contact lenses if there are no contraindications (i.e., immobilization, ocular trauma, etc.).

CONTRAINDICATIONS

The only absolute contraindication to removing a contact lens would be in the case of a ruptured globe. Leave the contact lens in place for the Ophthalmologist to remove at the time of their examination and/or surgical repair. Extreme caution must be exercised to avoid unnecessary pressure on the eye itself so as not to complicate the injury when severe ocular damage has occurred.

EQUIPMENT

Normal saline
Two cups, labeled left and right
Hard lens remover suction cup device, optional
Soft lens remover device, optional
Cotton-tipped applicators

PATIENT PREPARATION

Instruct the patient to remove their contact lenses if there are no contraindications. Patients are usually quite adept at removing their contact lenses. Remove the contact lenses if the patient is unable to remove them or cannot remove them.

Explain to the patient that their contact lenses must be removed (if they are awake). A signed consent is not required to remove a contact lens. Place the patient sitting or supine, whichever is most appropriate for the current clinical situation. Place several drops of a saline solution onto the eye. This maximally moistens the lenses to the point where they can be seen to slide easily over the surface of the eye.

All contact lenses should be centered over the cornea for ease of removal by gentle manipulation of the eyelids. The lenses may often become displaced from the cornea. Care must be taken to search for the lens in other parts of the eye. Shine a penlight at an angle to the eye to aid in the search. A common location for a displaced contact lens to migrate is under the upper eyelid. **Evert the upper eyelid if a contact lens cannot be found elsewhere to complete the search before assuming either that the lens fell out or the patient is not wearing contact lenses.** Instill fluorescein into the eye if the patient still insists that it is present. The fluorescein will pool around the edges of the contact lens and make it easy to locate. **Warn the patient that fluorescein may permanently stain their contact lens.**

Prepare the equipment. Locate the equipment required to remove the contact lenses. Label two cups, left and right, to place the lenses within after they are removed. Fill the cups with enough saline to cover the contact lenses. The person performing the procedure should wear powderless gloves. Wipe powdered gloves clean with a saline or a water-moistened towel to remove the powder. Powdered gloves can also be placed under running water to flush away the powder.

HARD CONTACT LENS REMOVAL TECHNIQUES

The hard contact lens can be identified by its small size (6 to 10 mm). It is smaller than the cornea. Center the hard contact lens on the cornea. Place the index finger (or thumb) of one hand at the base of the eyelashes of the upper eyelid and the index finger (or thumb) of the opposite hand at the base of the eyelashes of the lower eyelid (Figure 133-1*A*). Gently, but firmly, approximate the eyelids by moving them toward the center of the cornea until the margins of the eyelids touch the edges of the hard contact lens (Figure 133-1*B*). Press slightly harder on the lower eyelid until the bottom edge of the hard contact lens lifts off the cornea utilizing the edge of the lower eyelid as a fulcrum (Figures 133-1*C* and *D*). Continue to push the eyelids together until the hard contact lens is lifted completely off the cornea and can be easily grasped.[4,5]

The awake patient may not like the examiner's fingers near their eyes. Pull the skin of the lateral margin of the eyelids laterally with an index finger (Figure 133-2*A*). Alternatively, place one finger on the lateral edge of the upper eyelid and one finger on the lateral edge of the lower eyelid and pull laterally (Figure 133-2*B*). Instruct the patient to look downward and inward toward their nose. The hard contact lens will pop off the cornea. Grasp and remove the contact lens. This technique does not put as much pressure on the globe as the previous technique, an advantage if the patient has ocular trauma.

A commercially produced suction cup-like rubber device, resembling a golf tee, can be used to remove hard contact lenses if available (Figure 133-3). Moisten the surface of the device with a drop of saline or water. Gently touch the suction cup to the center of the hard contact lens. Suction will form and result in the hard contact lens adhering to the device. Lift the device and the attached contact lens from the cornea. **Slide the hard contact lens sideways to remove it from the suction cup. Do not attempt to pull the hard contact lens off the suction cup as this may damage the contact lens.**

A final technique involves the use of a cotton-tipped applicator (Figure 133-4). Moisten the cotton with saline or water. Place the cotton-tipped applicator over the lower edge of the hard contact lens (Figure 133-4*A*). Carefully and gently slide the hard contact lens off the cornea and onto the sclera with the moistened cotton-tipped applicator. Gently press the cotton-tipped applicator into the sclera and under the edge of the hard contact lens (Figure 133-4*B*). Lift the hard contact lens from the sclera. **Do not use the cotton-tipped applicator to elevate the hard contact lens from the cornea. It can result in a corneal abrasion.**[6]

SOFT CONTACT LENS REMOVAL TECHNIQUES

Soft contact lenses can be identified by their larger sizes (12 to 14 mm). They usually extend just to or just beyond the corneal-scleral junction. There are numerous techniques to remove a soft contact lens (Figures 133-5, 133-6, and 133-7). The easiest and simplest method is to remove it manually (Figure 133-5). Retract the lower eyelid with the nondominant index finger (Figure 133-5*A*). The soft contact lens will slide partially onto the conjunctival surface of the lower eyelid. Grasp the soft contact lens between the thumb and index finger. Pinch the fingers together and remove the soft contact lens.

A second technique to remove soft contact lenses is illustrated in Figure 133-5*B*. Gently place the index finger and thumb of the nondominant hand on the upper and lower eyelids, respectively. Retract the eyelids. Grasp the soft contact lens between the thumb and index finger of the dominant hand. Slide the soft contact lens inferiorly. Gently pinch the fingers together to pull the soft contact lens from the eye.[4]

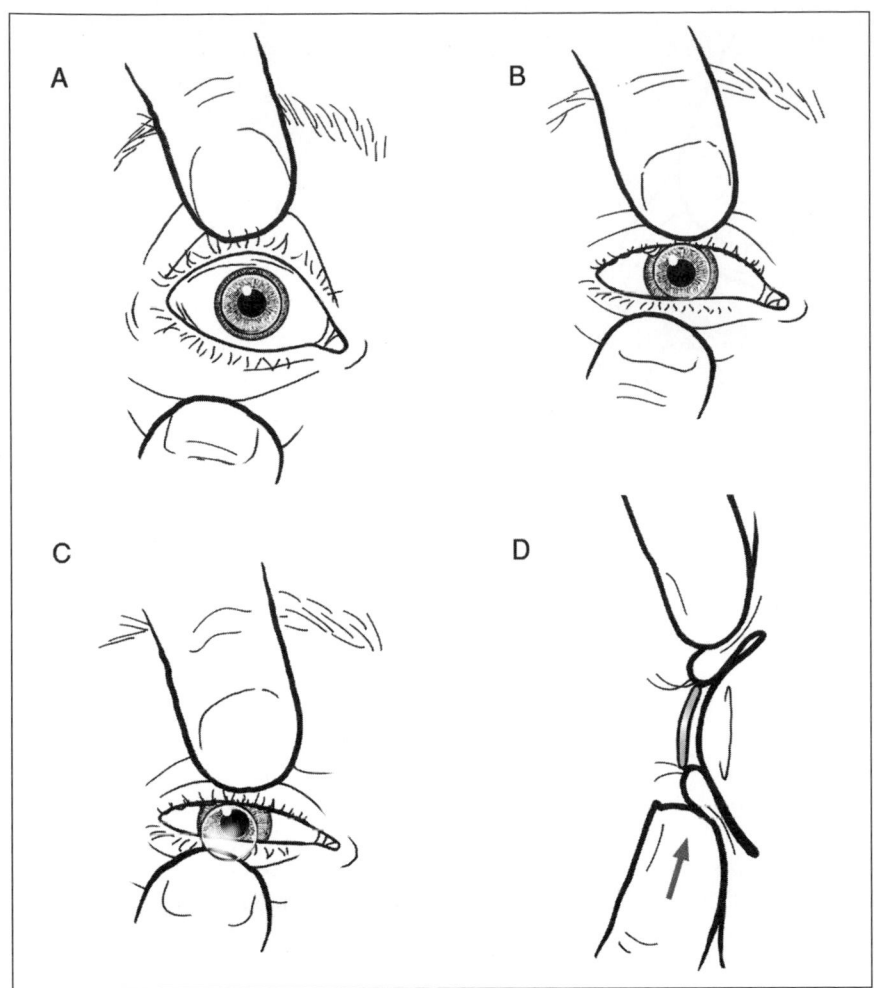

FIGURE 133-1 Hard contact lens removal. *A.* Use both thumbs to open the eyelids. *B.* Close the eyelids until the edges of the eyelids just contact the lens. *C.* Push the edge of the lower eyelid under the edge of the contact lens to pop it off the eye. *D.* Lateral view of the lower eyelid pushing the contact lens off the eye.

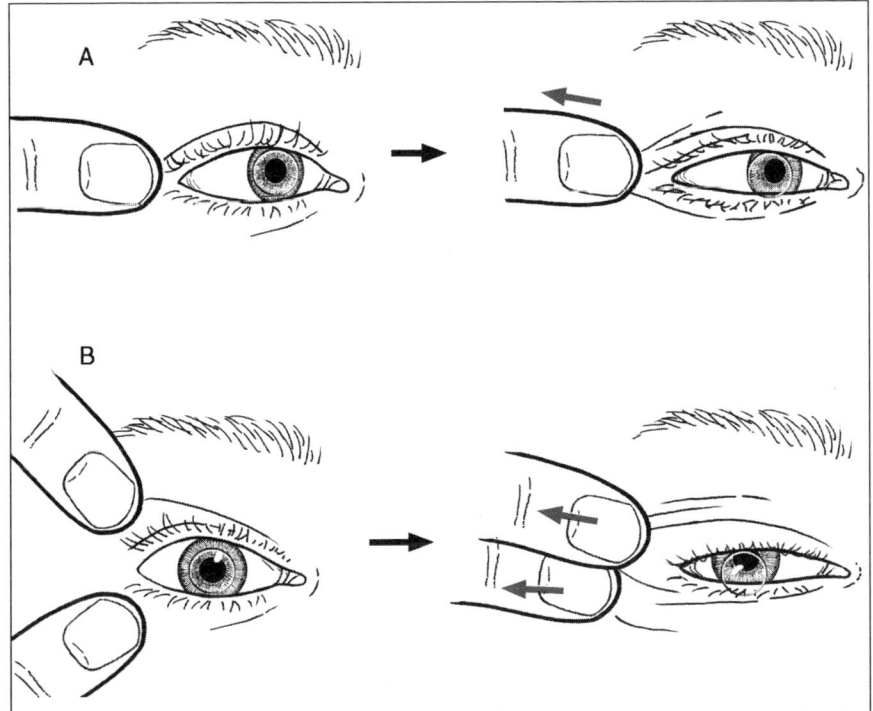

FIGURE 133-2 Alternative hard contact lens removal techniques. These methods do not apply pressure onto the globe. Apply laterally directed pressure to the skin lateral to the eyelids (*A*) or to the eyelids (*B*) to "catch" the contact lens and pop it off the eye.

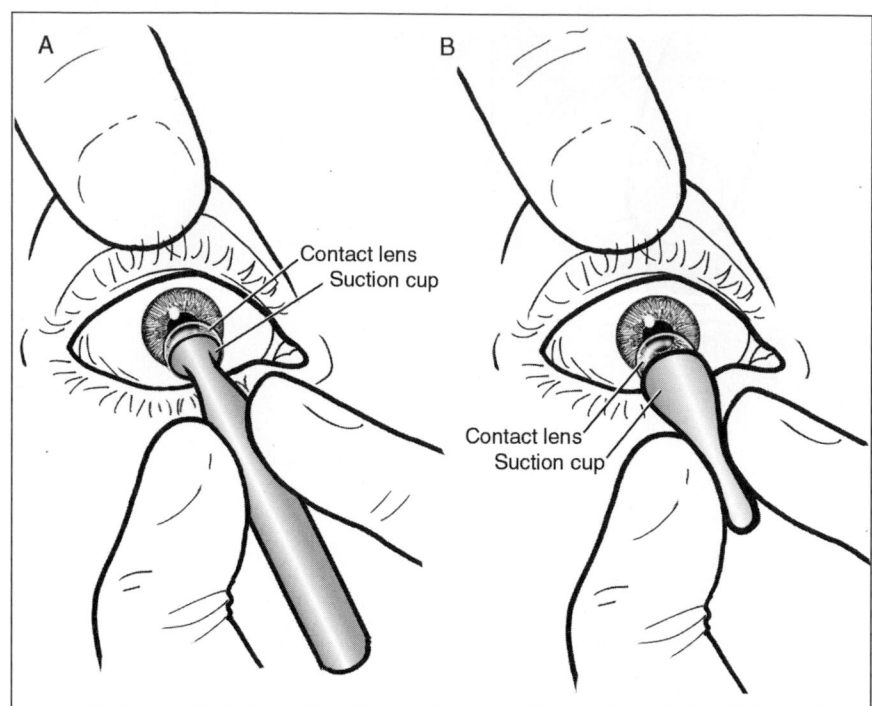

FIGURE 133-3 Suction cup removal of hard contact lenses. *A.* Suction cup on a plastic handle. *B.* Fingertip held suction cup.

A third technique to manually remove a contact lens uses the patient's eyelids (Figure 133-5*C*). Place the thumb of the nondominant hand and dominant hand on the upper and lower eyelid, respectively. Retract the eyelids until the edges of the contact lens are fully visible. Close both eyelids against the superior and inferior edges of the soft contact lens. Continue to close the eyelids until the contact lens pops off the eye. Grasp and remove the soft contact lens with the dominant hand.

A commercially available rubber tweezer-like device can be used to remove soft contact lenses. Place the rubber tips of the device onto the center of the soft contact lenses (Figure 133-6). Gently squeeze the tweezers

closed using minimal pressure. The soft contact lens will fold and lift off the eye. Remove the soft contact lens from the eye.

A commercially available rubber disc on a stick can be used to remove soft contact lenses. Place the rubber disc over the center of the soft contact lens (Figure 133-7). Apply gentle pressure to slide the soft contact lens onto the sclera. Lift the stick to remove the attached soft contact lens. The rubber disc may occasionally not stick to the soft contact lens. Apply a drop of water or saline to the rubber disc and repeat the procedure. The drop of liquid will form a seal between the rubber disc and the soft contact lens.

SCLERAL LENS REMOVAL TECHNIQUES

The scleral lens is essentially a giant soft contact lens. It is approximately the size of a quarter and covers the cornea and sclera. Remove the scleral lens using the same techniques used to remove a soft contact lens.

AFTERCARE

Place removed contact lenses in the appropriately marked container. Ensure that the contact lenses are covered completely with saline solution. Perform an eye examination using fluorescein if the patient complains of eye pain after contact lens removal. The procedure may have resulted in a corneal abrasion.

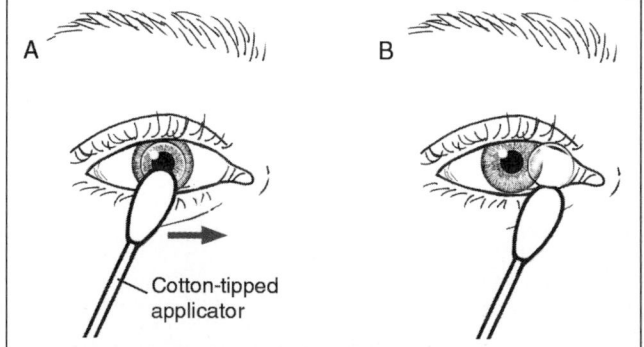

FIGURE 133-4 A cotton-tipped applicator to remove a hard contact lens. *A.* Place a cotton-tipped applicator against the lower edge of the hard contact lens. Push the hard contact lens onto the sclera. *B.* Push the cotton-tipped applicator under the edge of the contact lens to lift it off the eye.

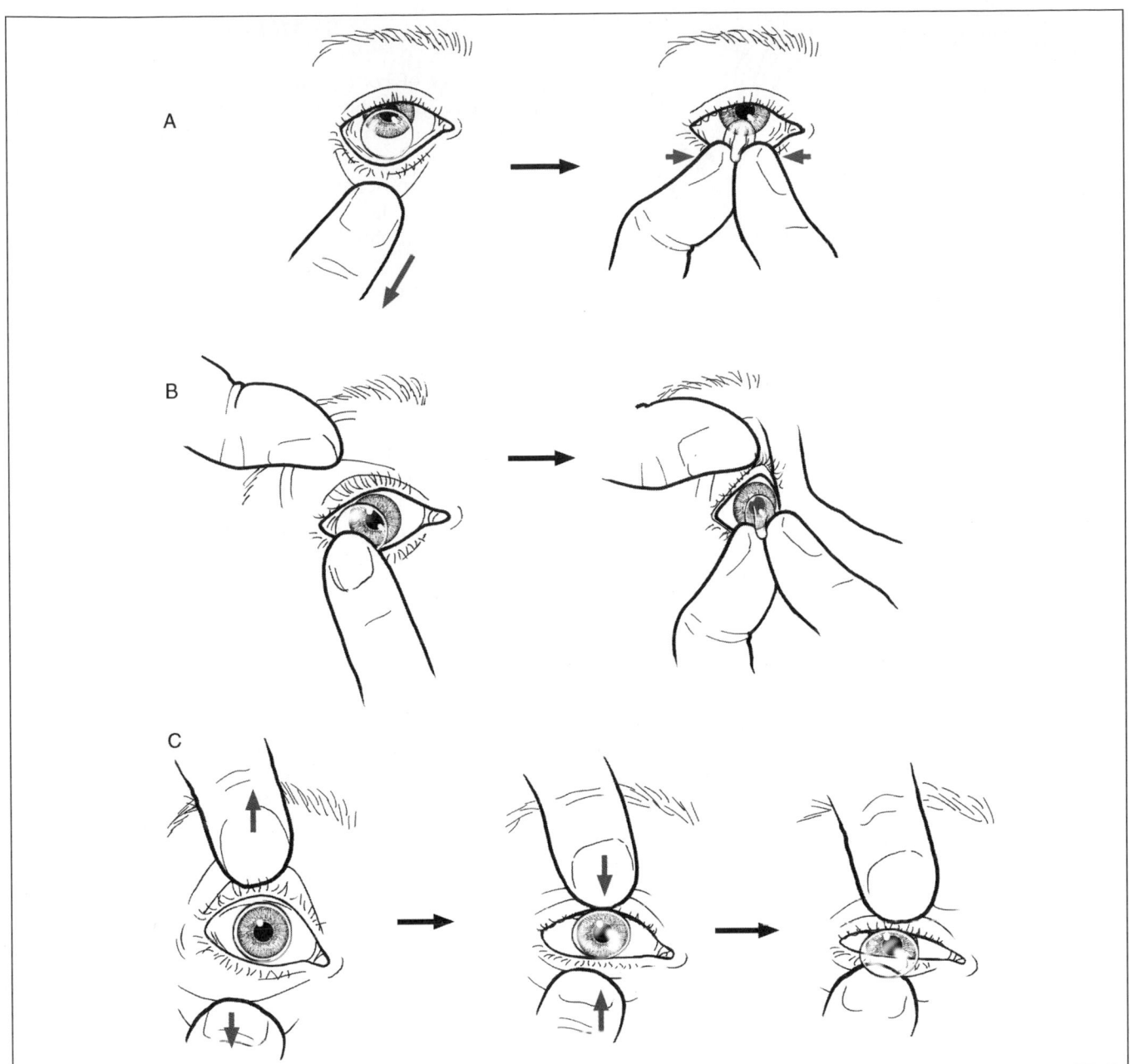

FIGURE 133-5 Manual soft contact lens removal techniques. *A.* Pull the lower eyelid downward and grasp the contact lens. *B.* Retract the eyelids. Slide the soft contact lens off the cornea and onto the sclera. Grasp and remove the contact lens. *C.* Use the patient's eyelids to pop the contact lens off the eye.

COMPLICATIONS

Any attempt to remove contact lenses with fingernails or other solid objects not approved for the removal of contact lenses can cause corneal abrasions. Their use must be avoided. Proper contact lens removal techniques can also result in corneal abrasions. Do not patch corneal abrasions resulting from contact lens removal in order to prevent an infectious process.[6] The

suction cup of the hard contact lens remover may occasionally be inadvertently placed on the cornea. **Do not pull it off the cornea.** Slide it to the lateral corner of the sclera and remove it with a twisting motion.

Never remove a contact lens if there is concern for a potential globe perforation. The techniques described in this chapter are gentle yet put pressure on the globe while removing a contact lens. This pressure on the globe may result in extrusion of the intraocular con-

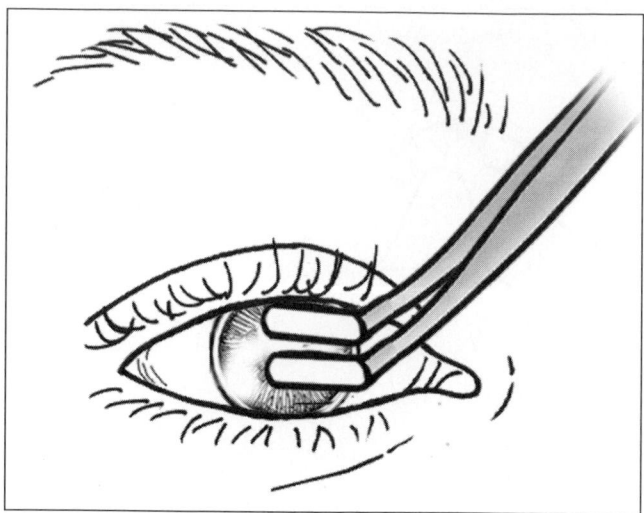

FIGURE 133-6 A tweezer-like device to grasp and remove the soft contact lens.

tents (i.e., lens or vitreous) and permanent blindness. Use a suction cup device (hard contact lens) or a rubber disc (soft contact lens) if the contact lens must be removed before the Ophthalmologist arrives.

Additional complications include the inability to remove the lens and damage to the contact lens itself.[6] Consult an Ophthalmologist or Optometrist if a contact lens cannot be removed from the cornea. Desiccated lenses that are not properly rehydrated prior to removal can result in the removal of the corneal epithelium and a corneal abrasion.[4] A properly hydrated lens will slide easily over the surface of the eye. Apply saline drops onto the eye to hydrate the contact lens prior to removal.

SUMMARY

Removal of contact lenses is a procedure that all physicians must be able to perform on any patient who is unconscious, who has ocular trauma, or who cannot remove their own lenses. Failure to perform this simple procedure appropriately can result in serious ocular damage. The removal of a contact lens is easy, quick, simple, and straightforward. Never remove a contact lens if a globe perforation is suspected unless absolutely necessary.

REFERENCES

1. Levy B, McNamara N, Corzine J, et al: Prospective trial of daily and extended wear disposable contact lenses. *Cornea* 1997; 16(3):274–276.
2. Fonn D, du Toit R, Simpson TL, et al: Sympathetic swelling response of the control eye to soft lenses in the other eye. *Invest Ophth Vis Sci* 1999; 40(13): 3116–3121.
3. Fonn D, Situ P, Simpson T: Hydrogel lens dehydration and subjective comfort and dryness ratings in symptomatic and asymptomatic contact lens wearers. *Optom Vis Sci* 1999; 76(10):700–704.
4. Gould H: How to remove contact lenses from comatose patients. *Am J Nurs* 1976; 76(9):1483–1485.
5. Dunn JL: Removing contact lenses. *Nursing* 1975:58.
6. Santen SA, Scott JL: Ophthalmologic procedures. *Emerg Med Clin North Am* 1995; 13(3):681–701.

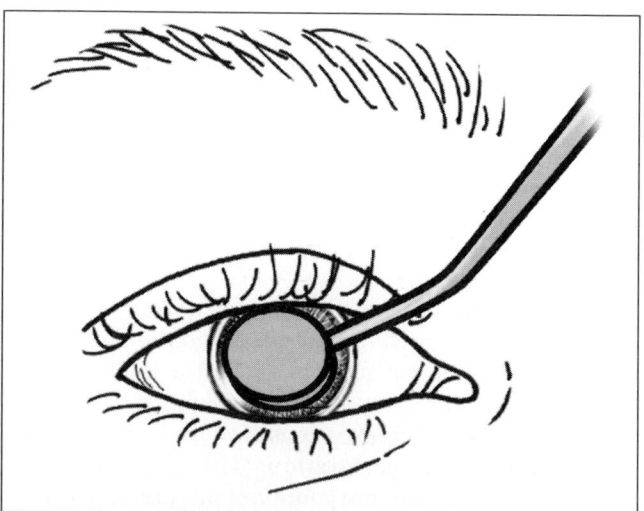

FIGURE 133-7 A rubber pad to remove a soft contact lens.

Chapter 134

OCULAR BURN MANAGEMENT AND EYE IRRIGATION

Steven J. Socransky

INTRODUCTION

Ocular burns are true emergencies and represent a significant minority (7.2 to 9.9 percent) of ocular trauma cases.[1,2] Chemical burns account for the large majority of ocular burns, with thermal burns being the second most common cause.[3] Most victims are young males.[2,4] The industrial workplace is the most common setting, although a significant number of cases occur in the home.[4] Assaults are a significant cause of ocular burns in the lower socioeconomic groups of large cities.[4,5]

Caustic agents are primarily responsible for the most severe chemical ocular burns. Most reports indicate that alkali burns are more frequent than acid burns.[1,3,4] Examples of more common alkalis and acids are listed in Table 134-1.[4,6–13] Ammonia causes the most serious alkali burns, while calcium hydroxide (lime) is the most common cause of alkali burns.[4] Hydrofluoric acid causes the most serious acid burns, while sulfuric acid is the most common cause of acid burns.[4] Fortunately, caustic agents account for only a minority of chemical ocular exposures.[1] Most chemical ocular exposures are due to relatively innocuous noncaustic substances (e.g., shampoos, hair sprays, personal defense sprays) and therefore do not cause significant or lasting damage.[1,14,15]

Ocular irrigation is a simple procedure that is commonly employed in the Emergency Department. It is potentially an eye-saving procedure in the setting of significant chemical ocular burns. Physicians, nurses, and emergency medical personnel who deal with ocular emergencies should be trained in ocular irrigation. When possible, first aid personnel in the workplace should be familiar with the use of ocular irrigation.[16] **Most importantly, ocular irrigation must be employed rapidly.[1,17] Delays in irrigation can limit its effectiveness and increase morbidity.[3]**

ANATOMY AND PATHOPHYSIOLOGY

The anterior surface of the globe is the major target of toxins in ocular burns (Figure 134-1). The eyelids are the most important protective structure for the eye. The orbicularis oculi muscle is innervated by branches of the facial nerve and closes the eyelids in response to noxious stimuli. The cornea provides little in the way of protection from chemical agents. The cornea is composed of five convex and transparent tissue layers. The cornea's major function is the refraction and transmittance of light. Despite its avascularity, the cornea is exquisitely sensitive to pain. Paradoxically, more extensive burns may be less painful due to destruction of corneal nerve endings and resultant anesthesia.[18] The cornea merges with the sclera to form the limbus at its outer margins. Stem cells at the level of the limbus are responsible for regeneration of the corneal epithelium. The corneal epithelium is unable to regenerate when the limbus is damaged. Although tougher than the cornea, the fibrous sclera is also susceptible to chemical injury.

The sclera is covered by the bulbar conjunctiva, which becomes the palpebral conjunctiva as it reflects onto the inner surface of the eyelids. These areas of reflection are referred to as the superior and inferior fornices of the upper and lower eyelids. The spaces between the eyelids and the globe are referred to as the superior and inferior conjunctival sacs (also known as palpebral sulci). Posterior to the cornea lies the anterior chamber, which contains the aqueous humor. The anterior and posterior chambers are separated by the iris, ciliary body, trabecular meshwork, and lens.[19]

The damage produced to the eye by toxins depends on several factors: duration of contact; anion or cation concentration; and amount, pH, and inherent toxicity of the chemical.[17,20] **Alkalis generally produce the most**

TABLE 134-1. COMMON CAUSTIC AGENTS AND THEIR SOURCES

Substance	Class	Source
Ammonium hydroxide	Alkali	Fertilizers, refrigerants, sparklers
Calcium hydroxide	Alkali	Mortar, plaster, cement
Magnesium hydroxide	Alkali	Sparklers, fireworks
Potassium hydroxide	Alkali	Oven and drain cleaners
Sodium hydroxide	Alkali	Lye soaps, airbags, EMLA cream, hair straightener
Sodium hypochlorite	Alkali	Bleaches, drain cleaners
Acetic acid	Acid	High vinegar concentrations
Chromic acid	Acid	Chrome plating
Hydrochloric acid	Acid	Household and pool cleaners
Hydrofluoric acid	Acid	Rust removers, glass, mineral, gasoline, silicone industries
Sulfuric acid	Acid	Industrial cleaners, battery acid
Sulfurous acid	Acid	Bleach, refrigerants

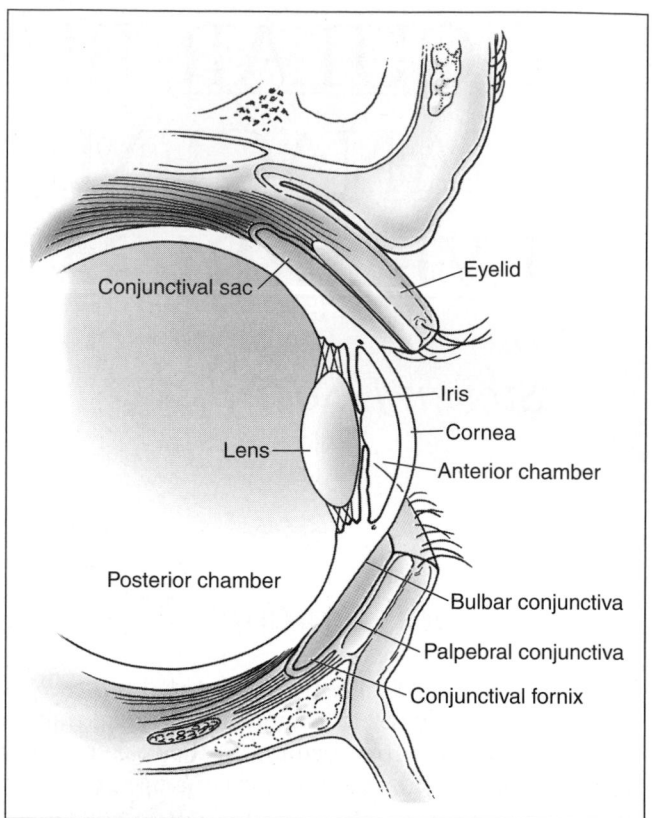

FIGURE 134-1 Cross-sectional anatomy of the eye and surrounding structures.

damage. Alkalis release hydroxyl ions that combine with tissue fatty acids and proteins, causing liquefaction necrosis.[11] The resultant degradation of corneal tissue allows for easy passage of the chemical into the anterior chamber. This causes a rapid rise (within a few seconds to a few minutes of contact) in aqueous humor pH and consequent damage to the iris, lens, ciliary body, and other ocular structures.[4,18,21] Damage to these structures and the cornea results in decreased visual acuity, secondary glaucoma, and cataracts. This damage can continue as the anterior chamber pH may remain elevated for hours. **Measurement of tear film pH immediately after irrigation will often yield a normal pH.[7–8] This may be falsely reassuring.** It may either reflect the pH of the irrigant or a transient neutralization of the tear film pH.[18] Alkalis may diffuse from the anterior chamber to the anterior ocular surface several minutes after irrigation has been discontinued, causing the tear film pH to rise again.

In general, acids cause less damage than alkalis. Acids lead to coagulation necrosis and protein precipitation, which usually prevents penetration beyond the cornea.[11] Exceptions include acids in higher concentration (particularly sulfuric acid) and hydrofluoric acid, which behaves more like an alkali.[4,5,18] These acids, like alkalis, can cause damage to deeper structures. Ocular burns caused by weaker acids can progress if treatment is delayed.[18]

Most noncaustic chemical eye exposures involve nontoxic agents that do not penetrate the cornea and cause only mild and self-limited irritation. Notable exceptions include surfactants and high-concentration lacrimators, both of which can cause damage to deeper structures.[10,18] Lacrimators in low concentration (tear gas) stimulate corneal nerve endings, causing pain and tearing, but they do not cause deeper injury.[18] Surfactants can cause significant damage that is often minimally symptomatic.[10] Although most solvents can cause sizable superficial corneal defects, reepithelialization is the rule and deeper tissues are spared.[10,18]

INDICATIONS

The treatment of chemical exposures to the eye is the primary indication for ocular irrigation. In this setting, irrigation has three principal objectives: immediate dilution of the offending agent, removal of the agent, and normalization of anterior chamber pH.[18] Nonembedded foreign bodies that are too small or too numerous to be removed adequately with a forceps or a cotton-tipped applicator can usually be removed with irrigation. Foreign bodies that are suspected but cannot be visualized may be removed with irrigation. Certain ocular infections are treated with antibiotics delivered by eye irrigation, although this is not a usual indication in the Emergency Department.

CONTRAINDICATIONS

There are no true contraindications to ocular irrigation. **An irrigating lens should not be used if a deep corneal injury or a foreign body is suspected.**[22] **This lens may cause the foreign body to further injure the cornea or penetrate the globe. It is preferable to carefully employ the traditional method of irrigation using intravenous tubing and eyelid retraction rather than commercial devices that contact the globe in the setting of an actual or potential globe penetration or rupture.**

EQUIPMENT

Topical ocular anesthetic, 0.5% proparacaine or 0.5%
    tetracaine
Towels and a basin to collect fluid runoff
Bags of crystalloid solution
Intravenous tubing
Gauze pads
Cotton-tipped applicators
Lid retractors, paper clip or Desmarres
Commercial irrigation device, Morgan Lens or Eye
    Irrigator
Protective eyewear, gloves, and gowns for health care
    personnel

PATIENT PREPARATION

Patients with ocular chemical burns may also have upper respiratory tract injuries, gastrointestinal tract injuries, and facial burns.[1] Nonchemical traumatic injuries are also possible. Airway, breathing, and circulatory problems should take priority. Significant ocular burns will need to be dealt with early and simultaneously with other problems. Initially, irrigation of the periocular skin should be performed with ocular irrigation itself, such that residual toxin does not enter the eye, causing further chemical injury.

Patients with isolated ocular injuries often have severe pain that requires parenteral narcotics. If this is the case, a monitored setting is appropriate. Intravenous sedatives and analgesics may facilitate ocular irrigation in a patient with severe pain and blepharospasm. Place the patient supine. Place towels and a basin under the patient's head to collect the runoff irrigant solution. Due to the speed with which ocular irrigation must be started, an explanation of the risks and benefits of the irrigation procedure should be offered to the patient while preparing for and initiating irrigation. Health care personnel and first-aid workers in the workplace are at risk for injury themselves.

Protective equipment is essential and should be easily and rapidly accessible. Contaminated clothes should be removed and bagged in plastic until they can be cleaned or discarded.[15]

TECHNIQUES

Topical ocular anesthetic solution, if immediately available, should first be instilled into the inferior conjunctival sac. Frequent readministration of the topical anesthetic may be necessary (every 5 to 10 minutes) to ease patient discomfort and facilitate irrigation.

OCULAR IRRIGATION

Hang the bag of crystalloid solution at a height of 70 to 200 cm above the patient's head in order to obtain an adequate flow rate.[23,24] The traditional eye irrigation technique involves directing the flow of crystalloid solution over the globe at a wide open rate (Figure 134-2). Hold the end of the intravenous tubing 3 to 5 cm above the patient's eye to avoid blunt injury to the ocular surface. An assistant is usually needed to hold the eyelids open. Dry gauze pads will facilitate one's ability to maintain a grip on the slippery eyelids and keep them open. Direct the flow of crystalloid solution at the entire surface of the globe, including into the conjunctival sacs and down to the conjunctival fornices.[18,25] Having the patient look in a direction opposite to where the irrigant is directed helps in this regard.[26] Although one can point the stream directly at the conjunctiva, it is better to direct it across the cornea in order to reduce the potential for further corneal injury.[22]

Manual retraction of the eyelids with gauze pads does not always allow for adequate irrigation of the conjunctival fornices. In these instances, eyelid retractors (Desmarres or bent paper clip) must be employed (Figure 134-3). **The eye must be well anesthetized when using eyelid retractors, and care must be taken to avoid further ocular injury.** Desmarres retractors are preferred to paper clips. Many paper clips are coated with nickel or silver that, when the paper clip is bent, can flake off, resulting in iatrogenic foreign bodies.[27] The use of a WaterPik or handheld drench hose has been described but offers no definite advantages over intravenous tubing.[28,29]

Two commercially available devices exist which are less labor-intensive and facilitate ocular irrigation. The Morgan Lens (MorTan Inc., Missoula, MT) is a scleral contact lens-type device that is designed to fit over the anterior ocular surface (Figure 134-4A). Connect the proximal end of the device to intravenous tubing and start a minimal flow of irrigant solution through the Morgan Lens. Retract the upper eyelid and ask the patient to look down. Insert the lens under the upper eyelid

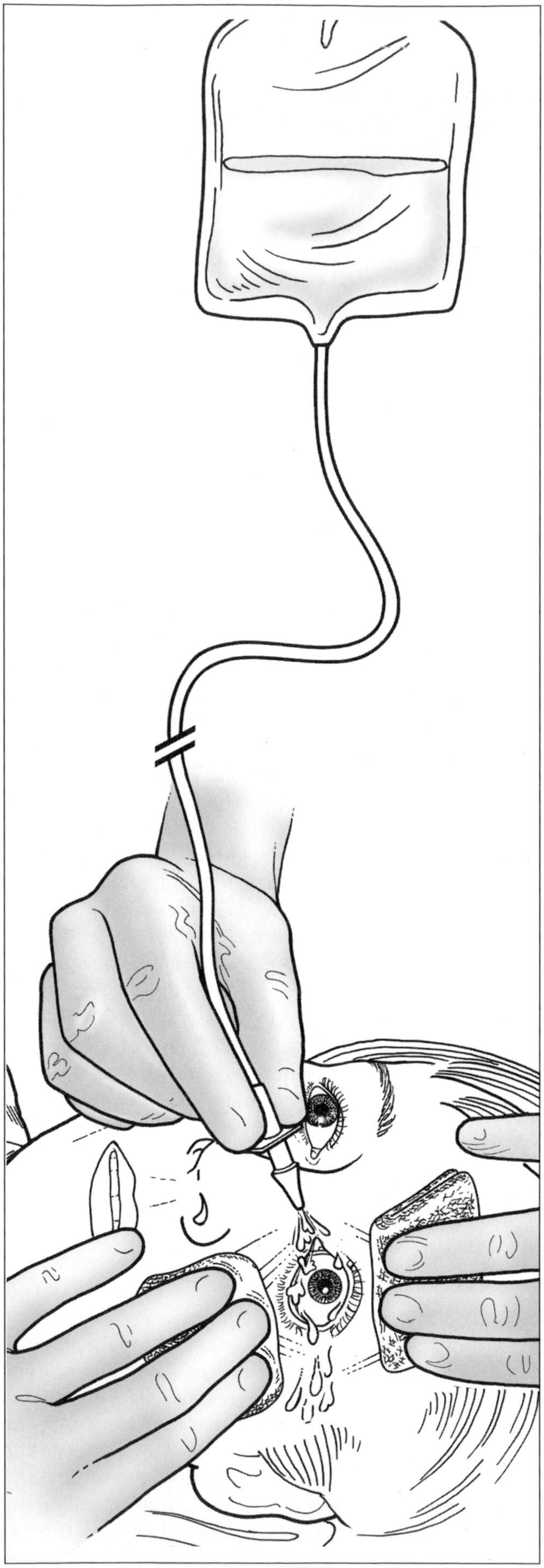

◄── **FIGURE 134-2** Standard ocular irrigation setup using intravenous tubing. An assistant retracts the eyelids using gauze pads or lid retractors. Complete irrigation of the conjunctival sacs is crucial.

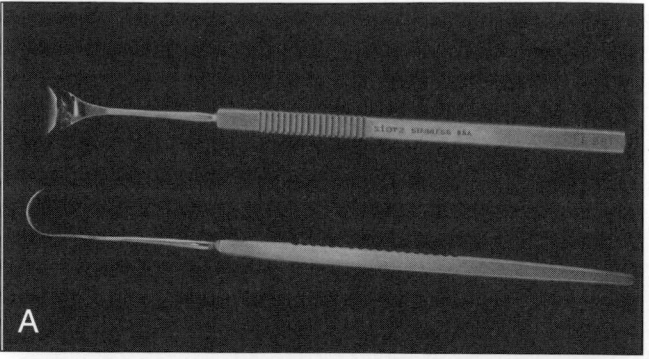

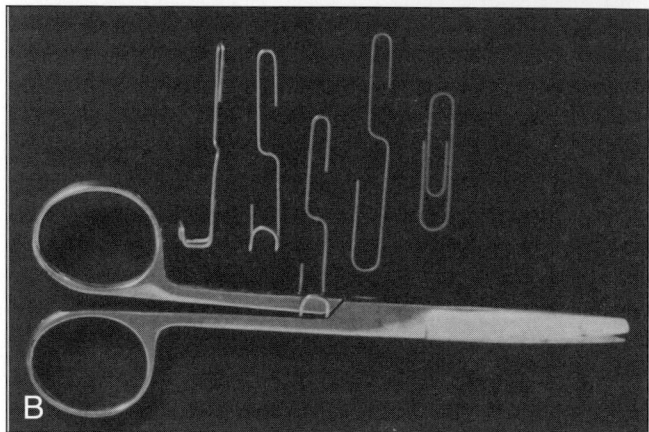

FIGURE 134-3 Eyelid retractors. *A.* The Desmarres eyelid retractor. *B.* An eyelid retractor fashioned from a paper clip.

(Figure 134-4*B*). Retract the lower eyelid and ask the patient to look upward. Insert the lower part of the lens under the lower eyelid (Figure 134-4*C*). The lens is removed by reversing these steps (Figure 134-4*D*). Increase the flow of the irrigant solution through the lens.

The Eye Irrigator (American Health & Safety, Madison, WI) delivers the irrigant via a U-shaped cannula with multiple perforations through which the irrigant flows (Figure 134-5*A*). Insert a speculum into the inferior conjunctival sac and retract the lower eyelid (Figure 134-5*B*). Insert the Eye Irrigator under the upper eyelid (Figure 134-5*B*). These steps are reversed for removal of the device. This device is somewhat similar to irrigating systems reported both by Yamabayashi and Terzidou.[23,24]

SOLID PARTICLES

Ocular burns can be caused by chemicals that are primarily in the solid form (e.g., lime). **Prior to irrigation, attempt to remove as much solid as possible**

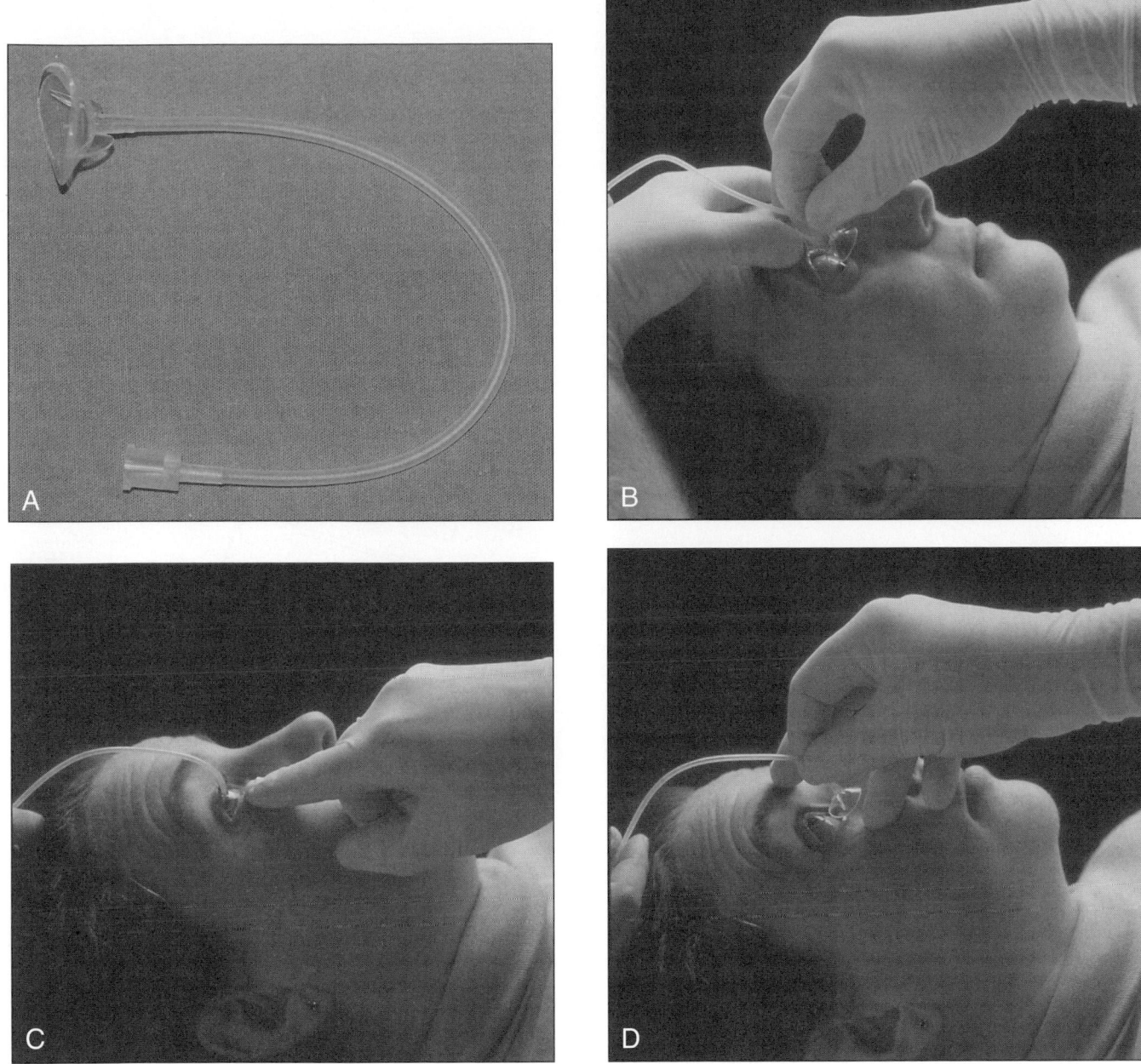

FIGURE 134-4 Eye irrigation with the Morgan Lens. *A.* The Morgan Lens. *B.* Placement of the lens under the upper eyelid. *C.* Placement of the lens under the lower eyelid. *D.* Removal of the lens. (Photos *B, C,* and *D* courtesy of MorTan Inc., Missoula, MT.)

using a moistened cotton-tipped applicator while everting and retracting the eyelids. Quickly proceed to irrigation once most of the solid material has been removed or if removal is limited by blepharospasm. Copious irrigation is often successful in removing any residual solid material.[17] Proceed directly to irrigation when solid material is not suspected in significant quantity and inspect the conjunctival sac for foreign material once the initial irrigation has been completed.

CONTACT LENSES

Concern that contact lenses may trap chemicals between them and the cornea appears to be unfounded. Contact lenses may, in fact, be protective and act as a shield between the toxin and the cornea.[30,31] **Irrigation should not be delayed in order to remove a contact lens unless it appears that a contact lens can be removed easily and quickly.** This is the case even when commercial irrigation devices are used. Contact lenses can be

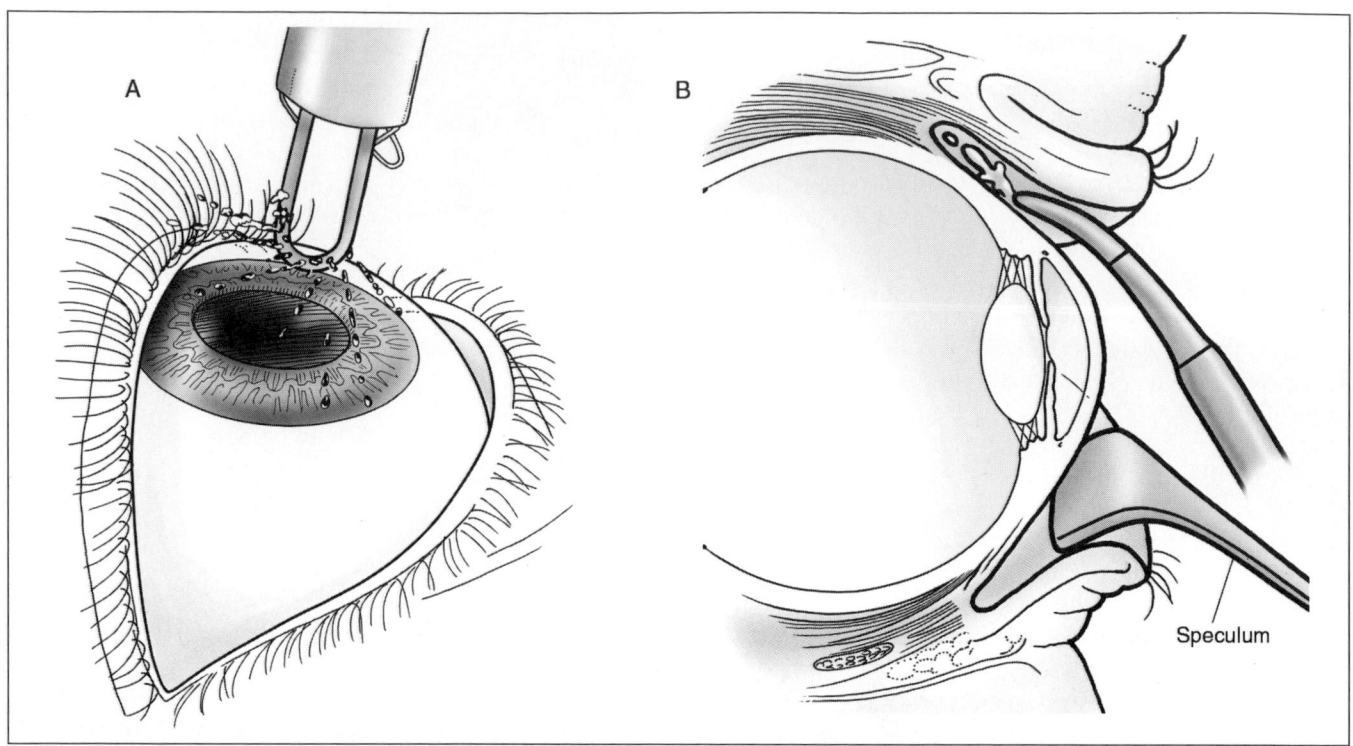

FIGURE 134-5 Eye irrigation with the Eye Irrigator. *A.* The Eye Irrigator. *B.* Cross-section of the orbit with the Eye Irrigator under the upper eyelid and a speculum opening the lower eyelid.

removed once an initial period of irrigation has been completed. Refer to Chapter 133 regarding the details of contact lens removal. The contact lenses should be discarded, as the toxin may be absorbed by the contact lens, only to be released to the surface of the cornea if reused.[15,30]

IRRIGATION FLUID

The choice of irrigation fluid is much less important than the speed with which irrigation is started.[18,21] Tap water is perfectly acceptable at the scene of the chemical exposure, although there may be problems with patient discomfort.[17] Normal saline and Ringer's lactate solution are both acceptable during ambulance transport and in hospital. It has been thought that the more neutral pH of Ringer's lactate solution (pH 6.0 to 7.2) should cause less patient discomfort than normal saline (pH 4.5 to 6.0). Similarly, balanced salt solutions (e.g., BSS Plus, Alcon Laboratories, Fort Worth, TX) should theoretically cause less patient discomfort due to its enhanced buffering capacity, physiologic osmolarity, and physiologic pH. These theories have yet to be clearly substantiated.[14,32,33] **Use the irrigant that is most readily available.** Balanced salt solutions should be used only in patients who require prolonged irrigation and for whom other irrigants are unsuitable due to their expense and time-consuming preparation (requiring reconstitution in glass bottles).[14,32]

The use of warmed irrigation fluid appears to increase patient comfort.[34] Ernst et al have reported an optimal irrigant temperature of 32.2 to 37.8 °C (90 to 100 °F). Werwath et al found that 120 seconds was required to heat 1 L bags of normal saline and Ringer's lactate solution to a temperature of 101 °F in a microwave oven set at the highest cooking intensity.[35] **This cannot be routinely recommended, as microwave ovens vary and overheated irrigant fluid will cause secondary injury. Irrigation should not be delayed while an irrigant fluid is being warmed despite the potential value of warmed fluid.** Commence irrigation with room temperature crystalloid solution and switch to a warmed crystalloid solution once prepared. Although not experimentally validated, Rost has suggested that cooler liquids at the beginning of irrigation may help reduce the heat of the reaction, thus limiting chemical injury.[21]

There is probably no chemical ocular burn for which crystalloid irrigants are contraindicated.[18] Metallic sodium, metallic potassium, and white phosphorus may react violently. Irrigation with copious amounts of crystalloid probably dissipates the heat of the initial reaction more than it initiates a thermochemical reaction.[18]

SPECIFIC ANTIDOTES

The mainstay of treatment for chemical ocular burns is early and copious irrigation. Although specific antidotes usually play little role in the treatment of most toxic ocular exposures, there are some instances where antidotes can be helpful once the initial irrigation has been performed. **Consultation with a poison center should be considered in cases of exposure to unusual toxins.**[22]

EDTA may be helpful in removing adherent calcium hydroxide corneal deposits from lime exposures that cannot be removed with a cotton-tipped applicator or toothless forceps.[1,10,22] A 0.05 M neutral solution of EDTA can be prepared by diluting 20 mL of Endrate disodium (150 mg/mL) with 180 mL of normal saline.[10] A cotton-tipped applicator soaked in the EDTA solution can be used to loosen such deposits. EDTA may also be useful in exposures to potassium permanganate and zinc chloride.[10]

Ascorbic acid may be useful in potassium permanganate exposures. A 5% solution can be prepared by dissolving a 500 mg tablet of ascorbic acid in 25 mL of normal saline. The resultant manganese oxide deposits can be dissolved by dripping the solution into the eyes from a moistened piece of gauze.[36]

Copper sulfate (3% solution) can be used to negate the effects of embedded white phosphorus.[10,22] Polyethylene glycol may be useful in phenol exposures.[37] Mineral oil has been suggested in the removal of cyanoacrylates.[22] Calcium gluconate solutions have no beneficial effect in ocular exposures to hydrofluoric acid.[38]

DURATION OF IRRIGATION

Irrigation should be continued for 20 minutes in the home or workplace prior to patient transport. Emergency medical technicians should continue irrigation during ambulance transport until hospital arrival. The duration of any further irrigation in the Emergency Department depends on the severity of the exposure and the nature of the toxin.

Minor exposures with nontoxic substances need not undergo copious irrigation. Irrigation with crystalloid solution using a squeeze-type bottle may be sufficient. In fact, irrigation that had been performed either in the home or in the workplace may be all that is needed. However, treatment should proceed as for caustic agents if the chemical nature of the substance is unknown. **Assume that any previous irrigation was inadequate and that further irrigation is necessary in the Emergency Department.**[4]

Although no definite standard duration for ocular irrigation is available in the literature, most would agree that patients who are significantly symptomatic or who have received a caustic exposure should have their eyes irrigated with a minimum of 1 to 2 L of crystalloid solution

over 20 to 30 minutes.[17,39] Exposures to noncaustic agents, milder acid burns, and very mild alkali burns will usually not need further irrigation. Moderate to severe acid burns and anything more than a mild alkali burn will likely require more prolonged irrigation.

The duration of irrigation for caustic exposures is in part governed by pH measurement. After the initial irrigation, measure the pH of the inferior conjunctival sac using wide-range pH paper (i.e., accurate in the pH range of at least 2 to 10) or litmus paper.[10] Litmus paper with a narrower range and urine dipsticks may not be adequate. **If the pH is abnormal, continue irrigation and recheck the pH at 10 to 15 minute intervals until it normalizes.**[10,22] If the pH has reached the near-normal range (i.e., 7 to 8), discontinue irrigation and recheck the pH in 10 to 30 minutes to ensure that it continues to remain normal.[18,22] **In clinically severe caustic burns, regardless of the ocular pH, irrigation should be continued until the patient is evaluated by an Ophthalmologist. Alkali burns are more likely to require prolonged irrigation than acid burns.** In fact, several hours of irrigation may be required for severe alkali burns. In this instance, the Ophthalmologist may opt to perform a regional nerve block to incapacitate the orbicularis oculi muscle, thus limiting blepharospasm and improving patient comfort.[11]

ASSESSMENT

Ocular assessment should be limited to observation of gross injury, assessment of ocular pH, and quick verification of visual acuity until irrigation is complete. These assessments should not be prolonged and should not delay initial irrigation. A full ophthalmologic assessment is required once irrigation has been discontinued. This should include a recheck of visual acuity, measurement of intraocular pressures, and a slit lamp examination to evaluate for corneal injury, uveitis, and globe perforation.

AFTERCARE

The extent of aftercare required is dependent upon the severity of the injury. Minor exposures to innocuous agents and very mild caustic exposures without corneal changes should be reevaluated in 24 hours if the patient is symptomatic. Some exposures (e.g., gases, vapors, fumes) can result in delayed evidence of corneal injury on slit lamp and fluorescein exams.[10] Thus, patients with apparently minor exposures should be cautioned to return to the Emergency Department if their symptoms worsen or do not improve.

Patients with mild exposures that result in corneal defects should be treated with topical antibiotics that have antistaphylococcal and antipseudomonal activity.[10] Ascertain the patient's tetanus immune status and administer prophylaxis as indicated. Analgesics or an eye patch may be offered if patient discomfort is significant.[1,10] Cycloplegics should be prescribed in order to decrease the pain resulting from ciliary spasm and to decrease the risk of the formation of posterior synechiae if anterior chamber involvement is suspected.[10,25] Telephone consultation with an Ophthalmologist is recommended. Ophthalmology follow-up should occur within 24 hours.

Moderate to severe ocular burns require admission and acute evaluation by an Ophthalmologist. Medical treatment of secondary glaucoma may be required. Anterior chamber paracentesis and lavage may be needed early in the course of severe alkali burns in order to decrease the anterior chamber pH as well as intraocular pressure.[1,10,22,37] Necrotic tissue will have to be debrided.[4] The goals of longer-term therapy include the prevention of corneal ulceration, prevention of scarring of the anterior ocular structures, prevention of globe perforation, and the promotion of corneal reepithelialization.[22] Steroids, nonsteroidal anti-inflammatory agents, frequent lubrication, and soft contact lenses may help in this regard.[1,4] Ascorbic acid and collagenase inhibitors are experimental. More severe injuries require surgical intervention due to the loss of stem cells at the limbus and thus the loss of potential corneal reepithelialization.[4]

COMPLICATIONS

Pain and discomfort are common after ocular exposure to chemicals. These can be minimized with topical ocular anesthetics, parenteral sedatives, and parenteral narcotics in the Emergency Department. Corneal injury is usually the result of the primary chemical injury. Corneal injury may result from the irrigant or irrigating device, particularly if improper technique is used. Frequent use of topical anesthetics can lead to corneal injury. Extrusion of ocular contents is possible in the setting of globe penetration. The diving reflex is a rare but possibly significant complication. This reflex is mediated by the ophthalmic branch of the trigeminal nerve and the vagus nerve. It is triggered by a cold water stimulus to the face and results in bradycardia without hypotension. The diving reflex is more common in infants and children. Its clinical importance is greatest in patients with significant comorbid disease. Continuous cardiac monitoring is wise in these subsets of patients. Irrigation with warm water may limit this reflex.[40,41]

SUMMARY

Ocular irrigation is an eye-saving procedure in the setting of significant ocular burns. For trained personnel, it is an easy and safe procedure to perform. First-aid workers, emergency medical technicians, and Emergency Department personnel should be trained in its use. Ocular irrigation should be performed rapidly with the most available nontoxic irrigant, as delays of even seconds can limit its effectiveness.

REFERENCES

1. Pfister RR: Chemical corneal burns, in Olson RJ (ed): *Common Corneal Problems.* Boston: Little Brown, 1984:157–168.
2. Edwards RS: Ophthalmic emergencies in a district general hospital casualty department. *Br J Ophthalmol* 1987; 71(12):938–942.
3. Kuckelkorn R, Kottek A, Schrage N, et al: Poor prognosis of severe chemical and thermal eye burns: the need for adequate emergency care and primary prevention. *Int Arch Occup Environ Health* 1995; 67(4):281–284.
4. Wagoner MD: Chemical injuries of the eye: current concepts in pathophysiology and therapy. *Surv Ophthalmol* 1997; 41(4):275–313.
5. Pfister RR: Chemical injuries of the eye. *Ophthalmology* 1983; 90(10):1246–1253.
6. Maudgal PC: Ocular burn caused by soft brown soap. *Bull Soc Belge Ophtalmol* 1996; 263:81–84.
7. Brahma AK, Inkster C: Alkaline chemical ocular injury from EMLA cream. *Eye* 1995; 9(pt 5):658–659.
8. White JE, McClafferty K, Orton RB, et al: Ocular alkali burn associated with automobile air-bag activation. *Can Med Assoc J* 1995; 153(7):933–934.
9. Smith RS, Shear G: Corneal alkali burns arising from accidental instillation of a hair straightener. *Am J Ophthalmol* 1975; 79(4):602–605.
10. Grant WM, Schuman JS: *Toxicology of the Eye,* 4th ed. Springfield, IL: Charles C Thomas, 1993.
11. Linden JA, Renner GS: Trauma to the globe. *Emerg Med Clin North Am* 1995; 13(3):581–604.
12. Swisher L: *Ocular Burns.* 1999. http://www.emedicine.com.
13. Harris LS, Cohn K, Galin MA: Alkali injury from fireworks. *Ann Ophthalmol* 1971; 3(8):849–851.
14. Herr RD, White GL Jr, Bernhisel K, et al: Clinical comparison of ocular irrigation fluids following chemical injury. *Am J Emerg Med* 1991; 9(3):228–231.
15. Lee RJ, Yolton RL, Yolton DP, et al: Personal defense sprays: effects and management of exposure. *J Am Optom Assoc* 1996; 67(9):548–560.

16. Poe CA: Eye-irrigating lens more effective if applied seconds after accident. *Occup Health Safety* 1990; 59(1):43–47.

17. Burns FR, Paterson C: Prompt irrigation of chemical eye injuries may avert severe damage. *Occup Health Safety* 1989; 58(4):33–36.

18. Smilkstein MJ: Ophthalmic principles, in Goldfrank LR, Flomenbaum NE, Lewin NA, et al (eds): *Goldfrank's Toxicologic Emergencies,* 6th ed. New York: McGraw-Hill, 1998:447–456.

19. Snell RS, Smith MS: *Clinical Anatomy for Emergency Medicine.* St. Louis: Mosby, 1998:243–285.

20. Onofrey BE: Management of corneal burns. *Optom Clin* 1995; 4(3):31–40.

21. Rost KM, Jaeger RW, deCastro FJ: Eye contamination: a poison center protocol for management. *Clin Toxicol* 1979; 14(3):295–300.

22. Santen SA, Scott JL: Ophthalmologic procedures. *Emerg Med Clin North Am* 1995; 13(3):681–701.

23. Terzidou C, Georgiadis N: A simple ocular irrigation system for alkaline burns of the eye. *Ophthalm Surg Lasers* 1997; 28(3):255–257.

24. Yamabayashi S, Furuya T, Gohd T, et al: Newly designed continuous corneal irrigation system for chemical burns. *Ophthalmologica* 1990; 201(4):174–179.

25. Hammerton ME: Management of ocular burns. *Aust Fam Physician* 1995; 24(6):1006–1010.

26. Dunmire SM, Paris PM: *Atlas of Emergency Procedures.* Philadelphia: Saunders, 1994: 97–104.

27. Veser FR, O'Connor RE: Corneal abrasion during eyelid retraction. *Ann Emerg Med* 1995; 26(6):758–760.

28. Blumberg EJ: Use of Water-Piks in acute chemical burns of the eye. *Tex Med* 1973; 69(8):92.

29. Watts MT, Mulira A: The use of a new design irrigator for the emergency treatment of chemical eye injuries in an accident and emergency department. *Arch Emerg Med* 1989; 6(2):149–152.

30. Nilsson SE, Andersson L: The use of contact lenses in environments with organic solvents, acids or alkalies. *Acta Ophthalmol (Copenh)* 1982; 60(4):599–608.

31. Guthrie JW, Seitz GF: An investigation of the chemical contact lens problem. *J Occup Med* 1975; 17(3):163–166.

32. Jones JB, Schoenleber DB, Gillen JP: The tolerability of lactated Ringer's solution and BSS plus for ocular irrigation with and without the Morgan therapeutic lens. *Acad Emerg Med* 1998; 5(12):1150–1156.

33. McGary WB, Ernst AA, Nick TG, et al: Normal saline vs lactated Ringer's solution for ocular irrigation. *Acad Emerg Med* 1998; 5(4):371–372.

34. Ernst AA, Thomson T, Haynes M, et al: Warmed versus room temperature saline solution for ocular irrigation: a randomized clinical trial. *Ann Emerg Med* 1998; 32(6):676–679.

35. Werwath DL, Schwab CW, Scholten JR, et al: Microwave ovens. A safe new method of warming crystalloids. *Am Surg* 1984; 50(12):656–659.

36. Sigg T, Leikin JB, Sigg K, et al: Treatment of ocular potassium permanganate exposure with 5% ascorbic acid solution. *Ann Emerg Med* 1998; 32(6):754–755.

37. Brown VKH, Box VL, Simpson BJ: Decontamination procedures for skin exposed to phenolic substances. *Arch Environ Health* 1975; 30:1–6.

38. Beiran I, Miller B, Bentur Y: The efficacy of calcium gluconate in ocular hydrofluoric acid burns. *Hum Exp Toxicol* 1997; 16(4):223–228.

39. Lubeck D, Greene JS: Corneal injuries. *Emerg Med Clin North Am* 1988; 6(1):73–94.

40. Assi A, Casey JH, McGuinness A: Diving reflex induced by ocular irrigation. *Lancet* 1994; 344(8927):952.

41. Arndt GA, Stock C: Bradycardia during cold ocular irrigation under general anaesthesia: an example of the diving reflex. *Can J Anaesth* 1993; 40(6):511–514.

Chapter 135

INTRAOCULAR PRESSURE MEASUREMENT (TONOMETRY)

Michelle M. Verplanck
Mark Rolain

INTRODUCTION

This chapter reviews three reliable techniques used to measure intraocular pressure (IOP). Tonometry is the measurement of IOP. Tonometers commonly used to measure IOP in the Emergency Department include the Goldman tonometer, the Tono-Pen, and the Schiøtz tonometer. The Goldman tonometer is considered the clinical standard used by Ophthalmologists. However, it is difficult to use and requires a slit lamp biomicroscope. For these reasons, many Emergency Departments use the Tono-Pen. The Schiøtz tonometer is mentioned for completeness and historical significance. It is useful to become comfortable with one or more of these techniques as early detection of abnormal IOP can prevent irreversible vision loss. There are multiple traumatic, pathologic, and postsurgical causes for elevated IOP. The clinical signs and symptoms of elevated IOP are similar regardless of the etiology.

ANATOMY AND PATHOPHYSIOLOGY

Aqueous humor is produced by the ciliary body in the posterior chamber of the eye, directly behind the iris (Figure 135-1). Most of the aqueous humor flows forward, through the pupil, into the anterior chamber. It drains out of the eye through the trabecular meshwork located at the angle where the cornea and iris meet. Aqueous humor production equals outflow in a healthy eye at steady state. IOP reflects the pressure of the ocular contents and by convention is expressed in millimeters of mercury or mmHg.[1] The mean IOP in the general population is 16 mmHg with a standard deviation of

3 mmHg.[2] Therefore, normal pressure is considered to range from 10 to 21 mmHg.

Aqueous humor production and outflow can be dramatically affected by disease or injury of the eye. Even small changes in IOP over long time periods can be vision threatening. However, significant increases in pressure can cause rapid and irreversible damage to vision in just a few hours. Nontraumatic conditions that result in an elevation of IOP include primary angle-closure glaucoma and secondary angle-closure glaucoma. Traumatic conditions associated with elevated IOP include retrobulbar hemorrhage, hyphema, and traumatic iritis. Conditions associated with low IOP that threaten vision include penetrating trauma and post-surgical complications.

Patients with primary or secondary acute angle-closure glaucoma often present with ocular pain and decreased vision, usually in one eye. They may describe a headache in the brow region, with or without associated nausea and vomiting. External examination frequently reveals that the conjunctiva is erythematous, the cornea appears milky or hazy, and the pupil is slightly dilated with a sluggish response to light (Figure 135-2).

Traumatic retrobulbar hemorrhage can result in markedly elevated IOP. Patients will present with a painful proptosis and fullness of the periorbital tissues. There is usually restricted movement of the eye in one or more fields of gaze. Acute onset of retrobulbar inflammation will present the same way, but there is no history of trauma. Refer to Chapter 139 regarding the complete details and management of a retrobulbar hemorrhage.

Traumatic iritis may result in an elevated or a reduced IOP. Traumatic iritis presents following blunt, nonpenetrating trauma to the eye. Inflammatory cells

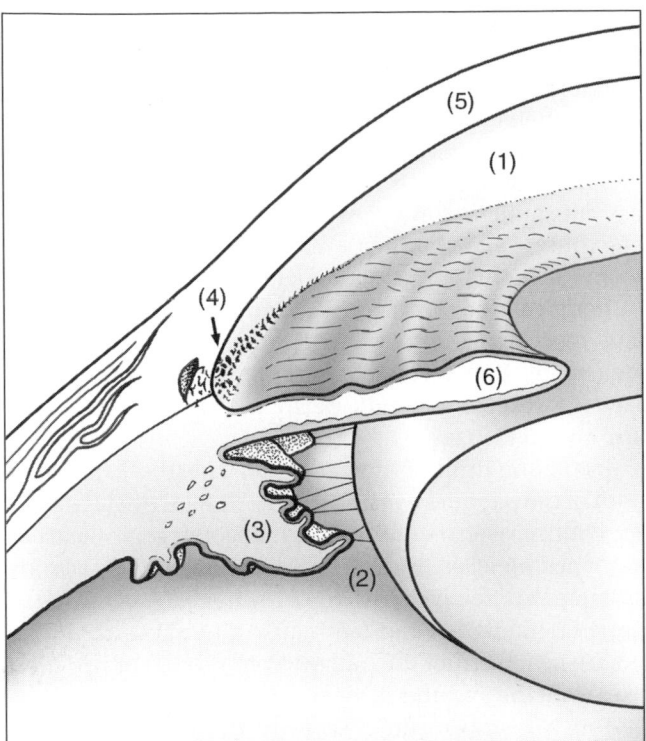

FIGURE 135-1 Anatomy of the anterior segment of the eye: (*1*) anterior segment; (*2*) posterior segment; (*3*) ciliary body; (*4*) trabecular meshwork; (*5*) cornea; (*6*) iris.

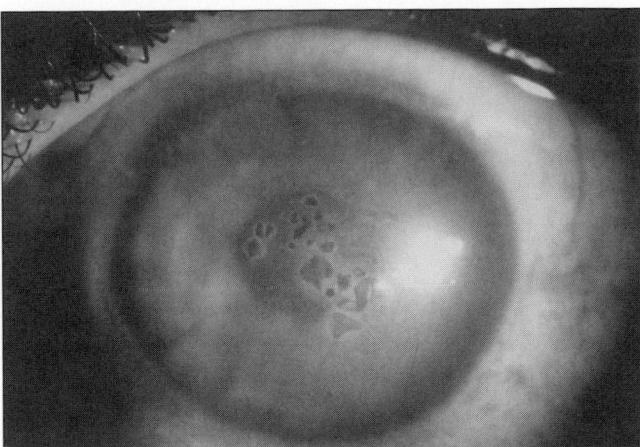

FIGURE 135-2 An eye with angle-closure glaucoma and a markedly elevated IOP. Note the injected conjunctiva, the corneal edema, and the mid-dilated pupil.

circulating in the anterior chamber may impede aqueous outflow resulting in high IOP. Iritis may also affect the ciliary body causing a decrease in the production of aqueous humor and a lower IOP. These patients present with eye pain and photophobia. They usually describe their vision as slightly blurred and give a history of trauma within the last 48 hours. The history of recent trauma and light sensitivity is important given that the external examination of the eye may appear normal. The cornea will be clear and a slit lamp examination is usually necessary to identify the inflammatory cells in the anterior chamber.

INDICATIONS

Patients presenting with a painful eye and/or decreased vision, with no history of ocular trauma, should have their IOP measured and documented. Some of the common presentations that require documentation of the IOP are reviewed in the previous section. This includes confirming the clinical diagnosis of acute angle-closure glaucoma, determining IOP after blunt ocular trauma, and determining IOP in a patient with iritis.

CONTRAINDICATIONS

It is essential to rule out a ruptured globe before tonometry is performed when a patient relays a history of trauma. Tonometry should be strictly avoided if there is evidence of a ruptured globe or the suspicion of a ruptured globe. A ruptured globe from penetrating trauma to the anterior segment of the eye, including corneal or scleral lacerations, is usually obvious upon clinical examination. However, blunt trauma resulting in a ruptured globe may be very difficult to see on examination. Any blunt force (e.g., closed fist) causing an anteroposterior compression of the globe can result in a scleral rupture posterior to the attachment of the extraocular muscles. This is rarely obvious on external examination or a nondilated slit lamp examination. The clue here is that the patient has dramatically reduced vision and prominent swelling of the periorbital tissues.

Avoid tonometry if there is any evidence of blood in the anterior chamber. Compression of the cornea may result in further bleeding and visual complications even though elevated IOP is a major risk associated with a hyphema and a microhyphema. A hyphema is visible blood that layers out in the anterior chamber between the iris and the cornea (Figure 135-3). A microhyphema is diffuse blood circulating in the anterior chamber. These patients present with decreased vision, photophobia, and blood in the anterior chamber. A common cause of blood in the anterior chamber is blunt, nonpenetrating trauma to the eye. A patient with blood in the anterior chamber and a history of sickle cell disease or trait is at a higher risk of elevated IOP.[3] Consult an Ophthalmologist if a sickle cell patient presents with blood in the anterior chamber.

Viral conjunctivitis is one of the most common ocular conditions seen in the Emergency Department. Con-

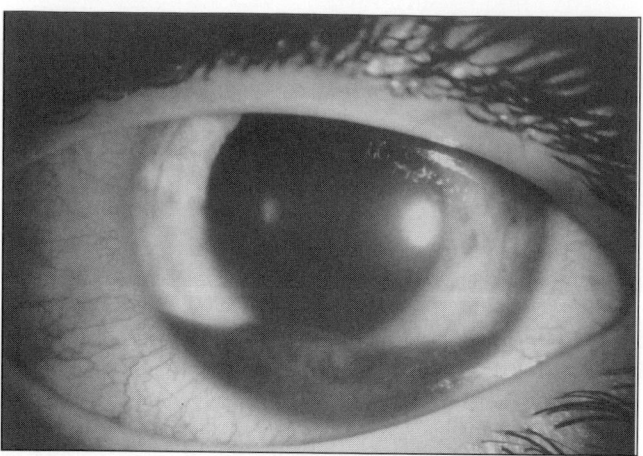

FIGURE 135-3 A traumatic hyphema with 10 to 15 percent layered blood in the anterior chamber.

junctivitis is so highly infectious that it is a relative contraindication to performing tonometry. These patients may present with ocular pain and decreased vision just like patients with angle-closure glaucoma. Conjunctivitis symptoms are usually binocular and the pain is not as severe. Acute angle-closure glaucoma almost always presents in one eye. It is reasonable to proceed with tonometry to rule out increased IOP as an etiology of a painful red eye if the diagnosis of conjunctivitis is uncertain. **Clean the instrumentation carefully to prevent spreading the infection to the contralateral eye.** Proper cleaning of the instrumentation is discussed in the techniques section.

EQUIPMENT

Topical Corneal Anesthesia

Proparacaine hydrochloride 0.5% (Alcaine)
Tetracaine hydrochloride 0.5% (AK-T-Caine)

Stain for Tear Film

Fluorescein sodium 1 mg, individually wrapped sterile
   ophthalmic strips (Fluorets)
Fluorescein sodium 0.25%-benoxinate HCL 0.4%, sterile
   ophthalmic solution (Fluress)

Tonometer

Goldmann applanation tonometer
Mentor Tono-Pen XL electronic digital tonometer
Schiøtz indentation tonometer

Antiseptic

70% isopropyl alcohol solution and swabs

PATIENT PREPARATION

Inform the patient of the need to measure the pressure in their eye. Explain that an instrument will contact their tear film directly over the cornea. Reassure the patient that tonometry is not painful. It is not necessary to have the patient sign a consent form as tonometry is part of a routine eye examination. One may choose to document the discussion with the patient for completeness.

Remove all contact lenses before the instillation of any topical ocular anesthetic agent or fluorescein. Measuring IOP through a contact lens is unreliable. The fluorescein dye will permanently stain clothing and contact lenses.

Instill one drop of topical ocular anesthetic agent in both of the patient's eyes. The contralateral eye is used as the control, even if only one eye is of concern. Topical ocular anesthetic agents begin working within 30 seconds and remain effective for 10 to 15 minutes. The drops may burn when applied and may cause a transient drying of the cornea. Instruct the patient not to touch or rub their eyes until the anesthesia wears off.

Touch a strip of fluorescein to the tear film on the inner layer of each lower eyelid if using the Goldman (applanation) tonometer. Dampen the strip with a drop of the topical ocular anesthetic agent if the eye is extremely dry. Pull the lower eyelid down and instill a drop of fluorescein in the cul-de-sac of each lower eyelid if using liquid fluorescein. Fluorescein is not necessary when using the Tono-Pen or the Schiøtz tonometer.

TECHNIQUES

GOLDMAN (APPLANATION) TONOMETER

The Goldman tonometer is considered the clinical standard for measuring IOP. This method of tonometry is based on the Imbert-Fick principle.[4] It states that the pressure inside an ideal dry, thin-walled sphere equals the force necessary to flatten its surface divided by the area of the flattening ($P = F/A$; where P = pressure, F = force, A = area). The Goldman tonometer determines the force necessary to flatten or applanate an area of the cornea 3.06 mm in diameter. The degree of flattening is determined while viewing the cornea through a split prism device in the tonometer head. Fluorescein is used to stain the tear film in order to distinguish the cornea from the tear film. The eye is viewed through the cobalt blue filter causing the fluorescein stained tear film to appear yellow-green. The technique is described below.[5]

The Goldman tonometer is nonportable. It requires the patient to be cooperative, the patient to sit upright, and a working knowledge of the slit lamp. The Goldman tonometer in combination with a slit lamp examination provides the clinician with the most detailed information about the patient's ocular condition.

Place two drops of a topical ocular anesthetic agent onto each eye. Place fluorescein dye in the eye. Position the tonometer head and cobalt filter on the slit lamp. Set the tension knob at 10 mmHg. It is more accurate to measure IOP by increasing rather than decreasing the force of applanation. Seat the patient in front of the slit lamp. Support the chin in the chin rest and place the forehead firmly against the strap (Figure 135-4). Instruct the patient to look straight ahead and open both eyes as wide as possible. Spread the eyelids with the thumb and forefinger if necessary. **Do not put pressure on the globe while holding the eyelids open.**

Move the tonometer head within one-half inch of the cornea. Use the control stick on the slit lamp to center the applanation head directly over the pupil. Look for two semicircles on the ocular surface as the tonometer head is advanced onto the corneal tear film (Figure 135-5). Ensure that the tension knob is set at 10 mmHg. The semicircles will not be touching if the patient's pressure is above 10 mmHg (Figure 135-5*B*). Turn the tension knob up until the inside borders of the fluorescein rings are touching (Figure 135-5*A*). Read the IOP on the tension knob. The semicircles will overlap if the pressure is below 10 mmHg (Figure 135-5*C*). Turn the tension knob down until the inside borders of the fluorescein rings are touching (Figure 135-5*A*). Read the IOP on the tension knob.

Clean the tonometer head with an alcohol swab immediately after use. Let it air dry 1 to 2 minutes so that the alcohol evaporates and is not transferred to the corneal surface.[6] Repeat the procedure on the contralateral eye.

MENTOR TONO-PEN XL

The Mentor Tono-Pen XL is a handheld tonometer with a strain gauge that creates an electronic signal as the 1.5 mm footplate flattens the cornea.[7] A single microprocessor chip analyzes each application of the footplate and averages 4 to 10 valid readings. The Tono-Pen can record IOP with the patient in any position as the electronic probe is not gravity dependent. **The tip is a very sensitive probe that can be easily damaged. Never touch the tip.** The small tip is useful in patients with

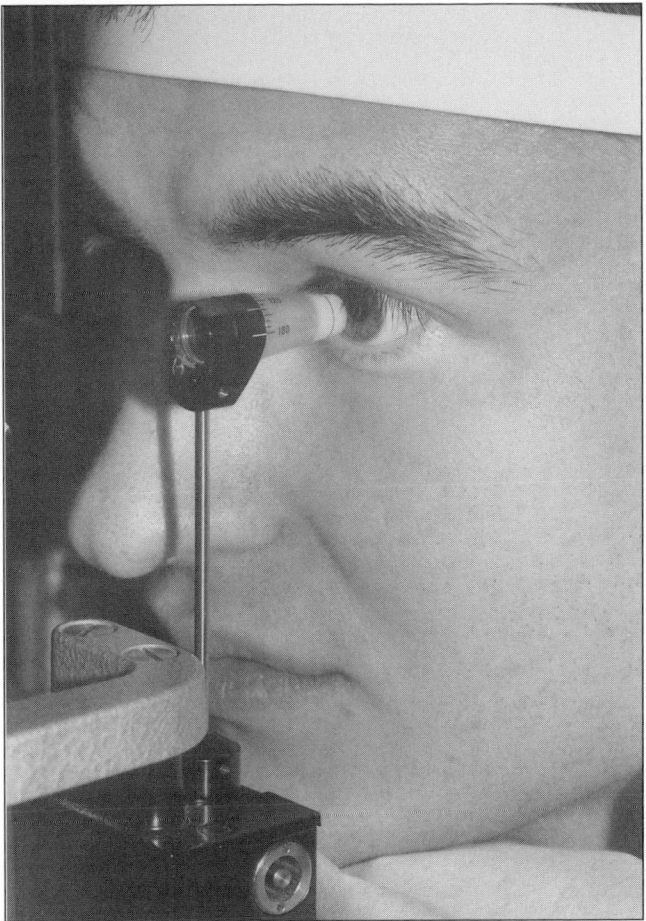

FIGURE 135-4 A patient positioned in the slit lamp with a Goldman tonometer in position on the cornea.

eyelid swelling or when it is difficult to open the eye. The small contact area is also useful when corneal surface irregularities are present. The risk of a corneal abrasion is minimized with a smaller contact area. The Tono-Pen should not indent the cornea if used properly, reducing the risk if there is an unidentified ruptured globe or a hyphema.

Place the patient in a seated or supine position. Instruct the patient to look straight ahead. Place two drops of a topical ocular anesthetic agent onto each eye. Fluorescein is not necessary when using the Tono-Pen. Place a new Ocu-Film tip cover on the instrument for each

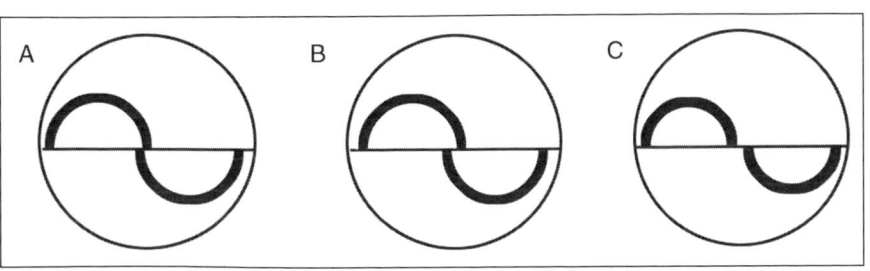

FIGURE 135-5 Semicircles as seen through the Goldman tonometer. *A.* The inner edges of the semicircles are touching signifying the correct IOP reading. *B.* Semicircles are not touching because the pressure reading on the tension knob is too low. *C.* Semicircles are overlapping because the pressure reading is to high.

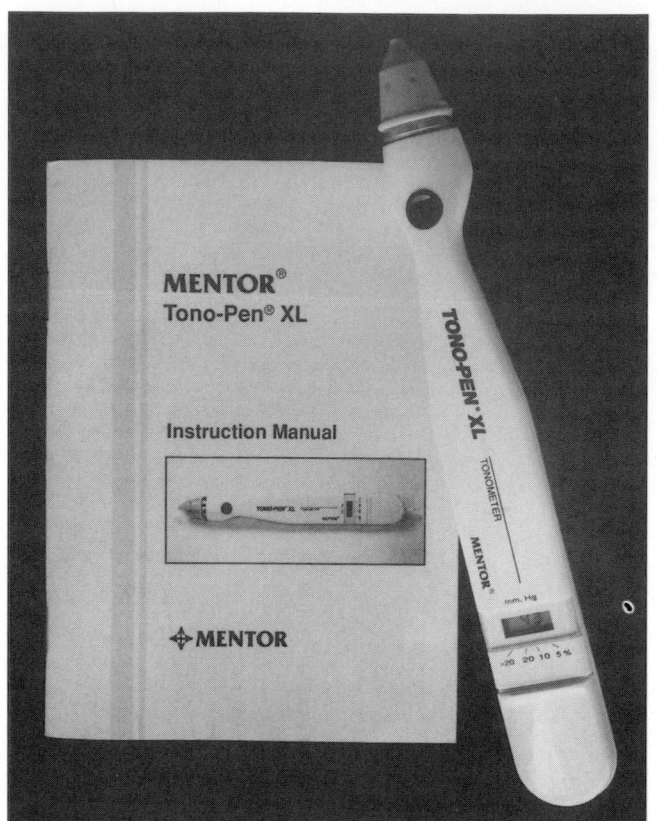

FIGURE 135-6 The Mentor Tono-Pen XL with Ocu-Film cover in place and operation manual.

new patient and when not in use to keep the probe covered (Figure 135-6). **The Ocu-Film tip covers are made of latex. Don't forget to question the patient about allergies.**

Calibrate the instrument each time before it is used. It must also be calibrated whenever the battery is replaced, after an unsuccessful calibration, or if indicated on the liquid crystal display (LCD). Aim the transducer end of the Tono-Pen straight down. Depress the operation button twice within 1.5 seconds. The Tono-Pen will beep and display "CAL" in the LCD window. Wait for the Tono-Pen to beep and display "UP" in the LCD window. This can take as long as 15 seconds. Immediately and quickly invert the Tono-Pen so that the transducer end is pointing straight up. The Tono-Pen will beep and display "Good" in the LCD window if it is functioning properly. Repeat the calibration procedure if "bAd" is displayed in the LCD window.

The display of "Good" in the LCD window indicates that the Tono-Pen is functioning properly. Press the operation button once. The Tono-Pen will display [8.8.8.8] in the LCD window, followed by a single row of dashes [----], and then a double row of dashes [====]. This indicates that the Tono-Pen is ready to measure IOP.

Grasp the Tono-Pen like a pencil and hold it perpendicular to the corneal surface (Figure 135-7). Gently con-

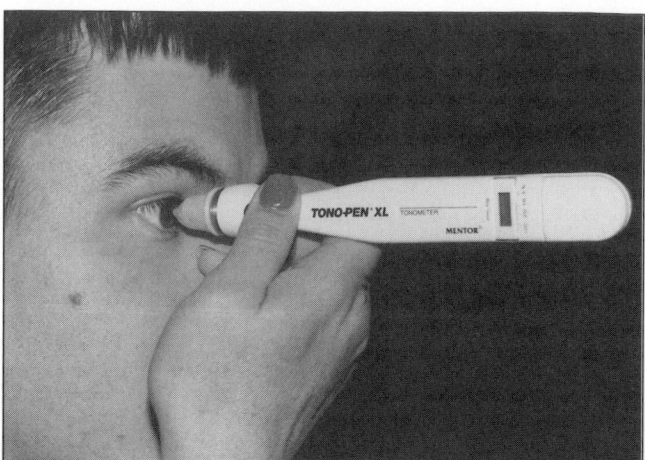

FIGURE 135-7 The Tono-Pen positioned on the cornea.

tact the cornea directly over the pupil or central cornea (Figure 135-7). Make contact with the cornea in a series of light taps. The Tono-Pen chirps each time a valid IOP is obtained. The microprocessor sounds a final beep and displays a mean IOP on the LCD after it receives four valid readings. A single row of dashes [----] in the LCD window indicates that an insufficient number of valid readings was collected. Obtain additional measurements after pressing the operation button.

SCHIØTZ TONOMETER

The Schiøtz tonometer estimates IOP by measuring the indentation of the globe caused by a known weight.[8] The Schiøtz tonometer is a sturdy, low maintenance, and affordable instrument. It is gravity dependent and requires the patient to be supine or have their head fully extended to get an accurate reading. The Schiøtz tonometer case contains the Schiøtz tonometer, a calibration scale, weights, and a calibration platform (Figure 135-8).

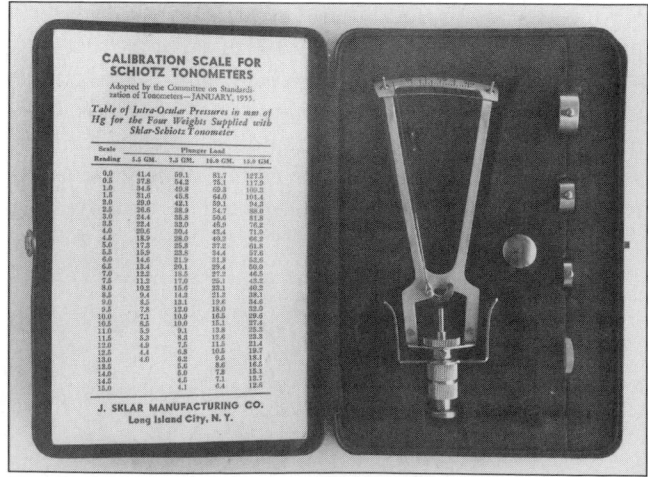

FIGURE 135-8 The contents of the Schiøtz tonometer case.

The tonometer consists of a plunger and a hammer device connected to a needle (Figure 135-9). The needle is calibrated to a scale, with each unit measuring 0.05 mm on the scale. The plunger, the hammer, and the needle weigh 5.5 grams. This can be increased to 7.5 grams, 10 grams, or 15 grams by adding known weights to the tonometer. The weighted plunger is heavy and has a large contact area that causes significant indentation of the cornea with each measurement. **The more weight it takes to move the needle on the scale or indent the cornea, the higher the IOP.** The scale reading is converted to IOP in mmHg by a conversion chart supplied with each Schiøtz tonometer (Figure 135-8).

Place the patient supine or sitting with their head fully extended. Ensure that the patient is comfortable. A tight collar, flexed neck, breath-holding, squeezed eyelids, looking toward the nose, or accommodation results in a falsely elevated reading. Place two drops of a topical ocular anesthetic agent onto each eye. Calibrate the tonometer by placing the footplate of the plunger on the platform provided in the case (Figures 135-8 and 135-9). **The scale reading must be "0" while the footplate is on the platform. The instrument requires repair if it does not read zero while on the platform.**

Instruct the patient to look at a fixation target directly overhead and to open both eyes as wide as possible. Spread the eyelids with the nondominant index finger and thumb if necessary. Grasp the Schiøtz tonometer by its handle. Ensure that the fingers holding the eyelids open are pushing on the orbital rim and not the globe, falsely elevating the IOP. Place the footplate of the Schiøtz tonometer directly over the pupil and gently lower it onto the tear film (Figure 135-10). Note the reading on the scale. Add more weight if the scale reading is less than 3 units. **Do not push down on the cornea with the Schiøtz tonometer. This will cause a false elevation in the IOP reading.** Repeat the measurement several times or until three readings are within 0.5 scale units. Convert the scale reading to IOP with the conversion chart (Table 135-1).

Clean the tonometer immediately after each use. Clean the barrel with two pipe cleaners, the first soaked in 70% isopropyl alcohol and the second one dry. Clean the plunger with an alcohol swab. Allow the instrument to air dry 1 to 2 minutes before being used in the contralateral eye so that the alcohol evaporates and is not transferred to the corneal surface.[7]

ASSESSMENT

The normal range for IOP is 10 to 21 mmHg. IOP in the general population does not follow a gaussian distribution. There is actually a higher distribution of elevated

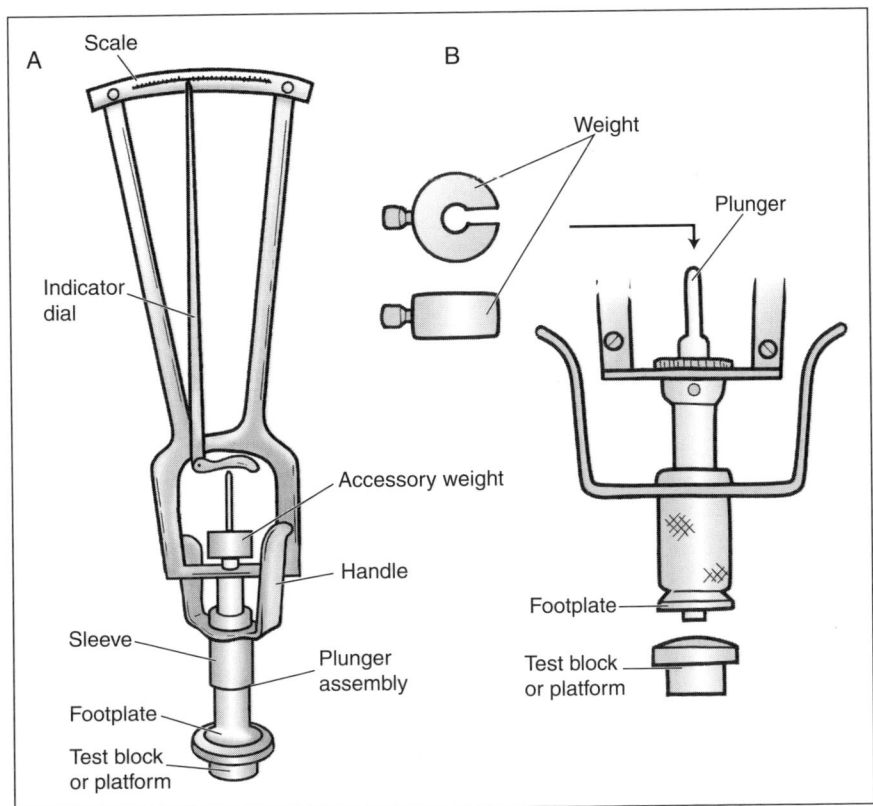

FIGURE 135-9 The Schiøtz tonometer. *A.* Schematic of the tonometer. *B.* Schematic of the plunger assembly.

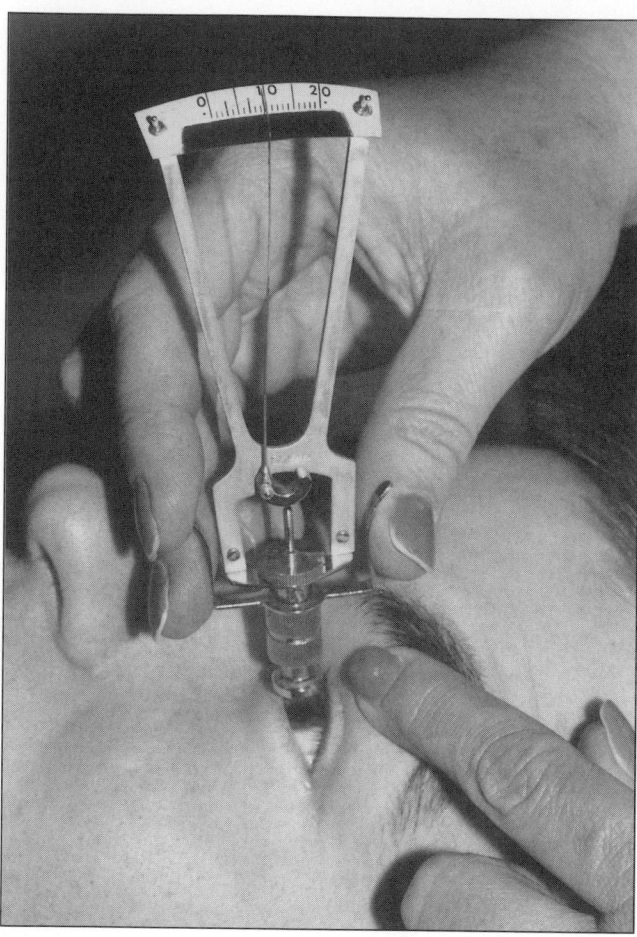

FIGURE 135-10 The Schiøtz tonometer positioned on the cornea.

TABLE 135-1. THE SCHIØTZ TONOMETER SCALE. USE THE TONOMETER SCALE READING AND THE WEIGHT APPLIED TO THE PLUNGER (GRAM LOAD) TO DETERMINE THE IOP READING IN mmHg.

Tonometer reading	5.5 gram load	7.5 gram load	10 gram load	15 gram load
0.0	41.5	59.1	81.7	127.5
0.5	37.8	54.2	75.1	117.9
1.0	34.5	49.8	69.3	109.3
1.5	31.6	45.8	64.0	101.4
2.0	29.0	42.1	59.1	94.3
2.5	26.6	38.8	54.7	88.0
3.0	24.4	35.8	50.6	81.8
3.5	22.4	33.0	46.9	76.2
4.0	20.6	30.4	43.4	71.0
4.5	18.9	28.0	40.2	66.2
5.0	17.3	25.8	37.2	61.8
5.5	15.9	23.8	34.4	57.6
6.0	14.6	21.9	31.8	53.6
6.5	13.4	20.1	29.4	49.9
7.0	12.2	18.5	27.2	46.5
7.5	11.2	17.0	25.1	43.2
8.0	10.2	15.6	23.1	40.2
8.5	9.4	14.3	21.3	38.1
9.0	8.5	13.1	19.6	34.6
9.5	7.8	12.0	18.0	32.0
10.0	7.1	10.9	16.5	29.6
10.5	6.5	10.9	15.1	27.4
11.0	5.9	9.0	13.8	25.3
11.5	5.3	8.3	12.6	23.3
12.0	4.9	7.5	11.5	21.4
12.5	4.4	6.8	10.5	19.7
13.0	4.0	6.2	9.5	18.1
13.5		5.6	8.6	16.5
14.0		5.0	7.8	15.1
14.5		4.5	7.1	13.7
15.0		4.0	6.4	12.6
15.5			5.8	11.4
16.0			5.2	10.4
16.5			4.7	9.4
17.0			4.2	8.5
17.5				7.7
18.0				6.9
18.5				6.2
19.0				5.6
19.5				4.9
20.0				4.5

pressures than would be predicted. This means that an abnormal IOP is defined somewhat empirically. Baseline IOP is specific to each patient.[10] Use the patient's contralateral eye as a control.

We can make general assumptions about certain ranges of IOP in order to make rapid clinical assessments and facilitate patient care. Readings of 0 to 9 mmHg should be discussed with an Ophthalmologist, especially if there is a history of recent eye surgery or recent eye trauma. Readings of 10 to 21 mmHg are normal. Readings of 22 to 25 mmHg should be followed up with an Ophthalmologist within 2 to 3 days. IOP readings greater than 26 mmHg require an emergent consultation with an Ophthalmologist.

COMPLICATIONS

Infectious agents can be transferred via tonometer heads.[9] **It is essential to properly clean each instrument before use, before using it on the contralateral**
eye, and after use. The use of a 70% isopropyl alcohol swab is an effective disinfectant for the Goldman[9] and the Schiøtz tonometers.[6] The Tono-Pen has single-use disposable latex covers.

Corneal abrasions can occur while using contact tonometers. It is very important to have a cohesive tear film to avoid cornea abrasions. Instruct the patient to blink several times just prior to tonometry to spread the tear film. Apply artificial tears in patients with extremely dry eyes. The Schiøtz tonometer puts significant weight on the cornea and must be applied very gently. Warn the patient that their eye may be uncomfortable when the anesthetic wears off if a small abrasion is suspected after measuring the IOP. Instruct the patient to instill artificial tears every 4 to 6 hours. Treat larger abrasions with a topical ocular antibiotic of choice and schedule a follow-up visit.

SUMMARY

The practice of tonometry is essential in guiding appropriate eye care. The Goldman, Tono-Pen, or Schiøtz contact tonometers are readily available in most Emergency Departments. The literature frequently debates the comparative accuracy of each instrument. The Goldman applanation tonometer is generally considered the clinical standard.[11,12] However, all three instruments are useful for screening IOP in the Emergency Department. Factors such as the patient's ability to ambulate and the presence of periorbital swelling will influence the operator's choice of an instrument. The Emergency Physician should select a tonometer that feels comfortable and use it routinely. The physician will be able to measure IOP rapidly and reliably with repcated use of the tonometer.

REFERENCES

1. Moses RA, Hart WM: *Adler's Physiology of the Eye Clinical Application,* 8th ed. St. Louis: Mosby, 1987:223.

2. The American Academy of Ophthalmology: *Basic Science Course Section 10.* San Francisco: The American Academy of Ophthalmology, 1996:18.

3. The American Academy of Ophthalmology: *Basic Science Course Section 6.* San Francisco: The American Academy of Ophthalmology, 1994–1995:207.

4. The American Academy of Ophthalmology: *Basic Clinical Science Course Section 10.* San Francisco: The American Academy of Ophthalmology, 1996:19.

5. Hoskins HD, Kass M: *Becker-Shaffer's Diagnosis and Therapy of the Glaucomas,* 6th ed. St. Louis: Mosby, 1989:67–71.

6. American Academy of Ophthalmology Clinical Alert Program: Updated recommendations for ophthalmic practice in relation to the human immunodeficiency virus. *Ophthalmology* 1989; 96:1–4.

7. Mentor Tono-Pen XL. Mentor Massachusetts Incorporated, Norwell, Massachusetts, 1999, sections 1–8.

8. Hoskins HD, Kass M: *Becker-Shaffer's Diagnosis and Therapy of the Glaucomas,* 6th ed. St. Louis: Mosby, 1989:76–78.

9. Pepose JS, Linette G, Lee SF, et al: Disinfection of Goldman tonometers against human immunodeficiency virus type I. *Arch Ophthalmol* 1989; 107:983–985.

10. Hoskins HD, Kass M: *Becker-Shaffer's Diagnosis and Therapy of the Glaucomas,* 6th ed. St. Louis: Mosby, 1989:79.

11. Frenkell RE, Hong YJ, Shin DH: Comparison of the Tono-Pen to the Goldman applanation tonometer. *Arch Ophthalmol* 1988; 106:750–753.

12. Bengtsson B: Comparison of Schiøtz and Goldman tonometry in a population. *Acta Ophthalmol* 1972; 50:445–453.

Chapter 136
CORNEAL FOREIGN BODY REMOVAL

Dino P. Rumoro

INTRODUCTION

Corneal foreign bodies are a common complaint confronting Emergency Physicians and account for approximately 35 percent of all eye injuries seen.[1] Many objects have been implicated as a source of corneal foreign bodies including, but not limited to: glass, metal, wood, dirt, dust, insects, and plant particles.[1] The majority of ocular foreign bodies require prompt removal. More than 75 percent of retained foreign bodies present on the eye surface are corneal in nature, and if left in place for more than 3 days will result in a keratitis.[2]

The prevailing symptom that forces patients to seek treatment is the sensation of an ocular foreign body or simply the pain associated with the foreign body. A variety of techniques exist for removal of ocular foreign bodies. A discussion of each of these techniques is necessary to determine the proper technique for a given situation.

ANATOMY AND PATHOPHYSIOLOGY

Many foreign bodies are diverted from the surface of the eye by the rapid blinking action of the eyelids and the eyelashes. A foreign body may not necessarily lodge itself into the cornea or the surrounding scleral surface if it is able to get past the eyelids and eyelashes. It may be washed to the inner canthus by a combination of blinking and tear flow. The foreign body may occasionally be carried away via drainage through the lacrimal ducts.[2] Objects that resist these means of diversion may be found in the upper or lower fornices, the channels created by the fold of the inner surfaces of the eyelids in communication with the conjunctival surface of the eye. The foreign body in the upper fornix is typically found lodged in the subtarsal groove on the inner surface of the upper eyelid, inferior to the tarsal plate.[2] Foreign bodies may also travel deeper into the respected fornices where they may be difficult to find. Foreign bodies may lodge themselves into the surface of the conjunctiva overlying the sclera or into the cornea itself, which obviously carries the most risk of serious injury or permanent scarring.

The cornea is only millimeters thick. It is comprised of five layers (from outer to inner layer): epithelium, Bowman's membrane, stroma, Descemet's membrane, and the endothelial layer that lies directly over the anterior chamber.[3] The surface epithelium itself has five layers of squamous cells. Most superficial corneal foreign bodies become embedded in this layer and do not result in scarring. Bowman's membrane has no regenerative capacity, and if injured, may result in scarring and permanent injury.[4] Foreign bodies that violate Bowman's membrane are considered deep corneal injuries. The stroma is composed of collagen and accounts for the largest portion of the cornea. Descemet's membrane is a basement membrane that can be regenerated if injured. The final component of the cornea is the endothelial layer that is composed of a single row of cuboidal cells that can regenerate if damaged.

Healthy cells adjacent to the injury slide over the damaged site and eventually replicate to the previous number of cells present when the corneal epithelium is injured.[3] Conjunctival epithelium migrates over the cornea to aid in its repair, even if the entire surface epithelium of the cornea is removed.

Corneal innervation is provided by sensory nerve fibers located in the surface epithelium. These are concentrated primarily in the center of the cornea and sparsely located in the periphery.[5,6] Injuries to the corneal epithelium produce pain, tearing, photophobia, and the sensation of a foreign body.[6] More pain occurs when the central portion of the cornea is affected due to the distribution of the sensory nerves.[6]

Patients are fairly adept at identifying the location of an embedded foreign body due to the corneal innervation. A study evaluated 50 patients with corneal foreign bodies and their accuracy in identifying the foreign body location.[7] Eighteen patients (36 percent) were unable to identify the foreign body location, 14 (44 percent) were able to identify the exact location, and 18 (56 percent) were partially correct in identifying the location based upon vertical and horizontal components. **Acknowledge the patient's sensation of a foreign body location and evaluate the area thoroughly.**

The presence of a metallic foreign body in the cornea can result in a rust ring. This is identified as a brownish ring surrounding the foreign body. **The rust ring, and the metallic foreign body, must be removed from the cornea.** The rust ring may be removed at the time of the foreign body removal or within 24 hours by an Ophthalmologist. Refer to Chapter 137 for the complete details of rust ring removal.

INDICATIONS

In general, foreign bodies involving the eye must be removed. Foreign bodies that are superficial and located on the cornea, sclera, eyelid, upper fornix, or lower fornix can safely be removed. Metallic foreign bodies require prompt removal to avoid the formation of a rust ring. The upper eyelid must be everted to evaluate for the presence of a foreign body under the eyelid, especially if vertical abrasions appear on the surface of the cornea.

CONTRAINDICATIONS

Corneal foreign bodies located in the direct axis of vision can cause permanent visual disturbances if improperly removed.[4] Consult an Ophthalmologist before removing these foreign bodies, as they often prefer to remove them. Deeply embedded objects or multiple foreign bodies that would require extensive debridement can result in significant scarring.[1] Consult an Ophthalmologist before attempting to remove these foreign bodies. **Avoid any manipulation of the eye if a perforated globe is suspected based upon direct examination of the eye or upon the mechanism of injury.** Foreign bodies embedded deeply within the cornea may be left in place if they are composed of an inert substance such as glass.[1] This will avoid the possibility of additional scarring from extensive debridement as long as the object is well below the corneal surface to allow for healing of the epithelium over the object. This decision must be made in conjunction with an Ophthalmologist. Refer injuries to an Ophthalmologist that are old, those in which the foreign body has been covered by epithelium, and foreign bodies resistant to removal. Do not attempt to extract a corneal foreign body if the patient is confused or uncooperative as this can result in a perforated globe. Consider the use of intravenous sedation, procedural sedation, or general anesthesia to extract the foreign body after consulting an Ophthalmologist.

EQUIPMENT

Slit lamp
Cotton-tipped applicator
Corneal spud
Ringer's lactate solution or normal saline
Intravenous tubing
25 to 27 gauge needle
Tuberculin syringe with needle
Topical ocular anesthetic solution
Topical ophthalmic antibiotic
Cycloplegic agents
Fluorescein strips or liquid
Electric burr drill and burrs
Eye patches
Adhesive tape
Benzoin solution

PATIENT PREPARATION

Perform a complete eye examination prior to removing a foreign body. Measure visual acuities prior to any ocular procedure and following the procedure to document any changes. Refer to Chapter 132 for the complete details regarding the eye examination. Apply a topical ocular anesthetic agent into the affected eye. Note any irregularities in the contour of the eye, any loss of anterior chamber depth, prolapse of the iris through a corneal laceration, focal injection, hyphema, and lens opacification. All of these signs may indicate a ruptured globe that requires an emergent Ophthalmology consultation.[4] Vary the beam of light from the slit lamp in its direction of illumination from direct exposure to indirect exposure, and even tangential exposure, to highlight any surface defects.[8] Examine the anterior chamber for cells and flare that occurs in older injuries as a result from a secondary iritis. The patient typically suffers from the discomfort of an anterior uveitis rather than the foreign body itself.[1]

Stain the eye with fluorescein dye. Fluorescein can permanently stain contact lenses and should not be used in their presence. Illuminate the eye with a cobalt blue light, looking for the green reflection of a corneal abrasion. Observe the site for the flow of fluorescein stain away from the site of a corneal puncture as anterior chamber fluid flows forth, otherwise known as Seidel sign.[4,8] A positive Seidel sign indicates a ruptured globe. Irrigate the fluorescein stain from the eye after the examination is complete to avoid chemical-induced irritation.

Explain the process of ocular foreign body removal to the patient and/or their representative. Discuss the benefits and risks of the procedure. Obtain a signed informed consent to perform this procedure. Instill additional topical ophthalmic anesthetic solution as necessary.

TECHNIQUES

EYELID FOREIGN BODIES

Evert the upper eyelid.[8] Instruct the patient to look downward as a cotton-tipped applicator is used to gently press on the upper eyelid over the tarsal plate. Grasp the eyelashes with the thumb and index finger. Pull the upper eyelid outward, downward, and upward to evert it over the applicator. Examine the undersurface of the eyelid for foreign bodies. Remove any foreign bodies by sweeping the area with a saline moistened cotton-tipped applicator (Figure 136-1). Double evert the eyelid by lifting the inferior edge of the eyelid created by the initial eversion. This is best accomplished by using a cotton-tipped applicator or an appropriate lid retractor. Examine the sclera and conjunctiva for foreign material. Allow the upper eyelid to return to normal. Release the eyelid and instruct the patient to blink their eyes. Refer to Chapter 132 and Figures 132-12 through 132-15 for the complete details regarding the eyelid eversion.

Evert the lower eyelid by pulling the lower eyelashes forward while the patient looks upward.[4] Examine the area in similar fashion to the upper eyelid. Sweep the scleral and palpebral (eyelid) conjunctival area with a saline soaked cotton-tipped applicator if the patient experiences a foreign body sensation but no debris can be visualized.

IRRIGATION

Superficial foreign bodies on the conjunctiva or the cornea can sometimes be removed by using an irrigation technique. A brief description is presented in this section. Refer to Chapter 134 for the complete details regarding eye irrigation.

The most appropriate solution to use is Ringer's lactate solution followed by normal saline. Tap water can

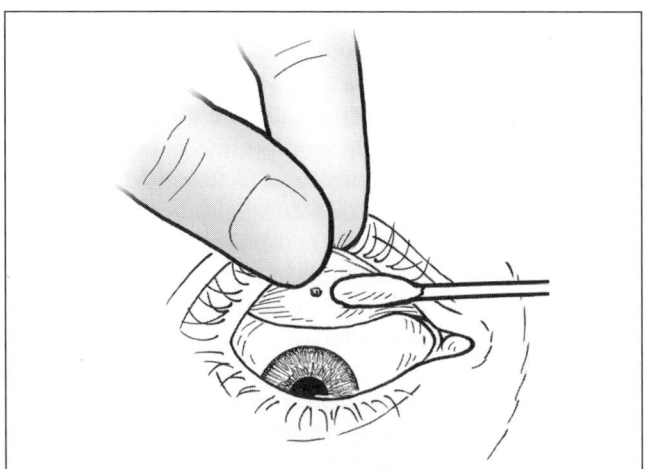

FIGURE 136-1 Evert the eyelids and remove the foreign body with a moistened cotton-tipped applicator.

be used in the prehospital setting. Ringer's lactate solution causes less irritation because the range of its pH (6.0 to 7.2) is closer to the normal pH (7.4) of the eye in comparison to the pH (4.5 to 6.0) of normal saline.[4] **Never use Morgan or Mediflow lenses for eye irrigation in the face of a foreign body as it may lodge the object further into the cornea.**

Place the patient supine with their head tilted toward the side being irrigated to aid in proper runoff of the irrigant. Flush sterile solution through the open end of intravenous tubing while holding the patient's eye open. Flush from the scleral surface with the flow of solution directed over the cornea, thus washing the object out of the eye.[1,4,8] **Never direct the solution onto the object in order to avoid embedding it deeper into the soft underlying tissues. Never direct the flow directly onto the surface of the cornea to avoid secondary injury.** Use a forceps or cotton-tipped applicator to remove objects flushed onto the palpebral conjunctiva.[4] **Never use a forceps on the eye itself.**

COTTON-TIPPED APPLICATOR

Use a cotton-tipped applicator premoistened with saline to remove a foreign body from the conjunctiva overlying the sclera or the eyelids.[8] Gently touch the premoistened tip to the conjunctival surface and lift off the foreign body. **Do not use the cotton-tipped applicator to remove a foreign body from the cornea.[8]** It can result in a large corneal abrasion by removing the surface epithelium.

MANUAL EXTRACTION TECHNIQUE

Extract the foreign body with a corneal spud or hypodermic needle if it is not removed via irrigation or if it is embedded superficially into the corneal surface. A corneal spud is a stainless steel device that comes in a variety of shapes. It generally consists of a sharpened metal tip attached to a handle.[1] It is used to lift off or to carve out a corneal foreign body.[1] Many physicians prefer to use a tuberculin syringe. It allows for better control of the needle by using the syringe portion as the grip. One editor (EFR) always uses a saline-filled tuberculin syringe. This allows the physician to apply saline drops to moisten the eye as well as to flush away the foreign body after it is dislodged from the cornea. An 18 gauge needle has been described for the removal of large foreign bodies because of its wide diameter.[1] This is physician dependent. **Proper explanation of the extraction procedure using a needle will ease a nervous patient and ensure better compliance by limiting unexpected movements.**

Perform the procedure under direct visualization with the slit lamp. Place the patient seated at the slit lamp with their head firmly in place against the forehead rest to avoid any unexpected movement (Figure 136-2*A*).

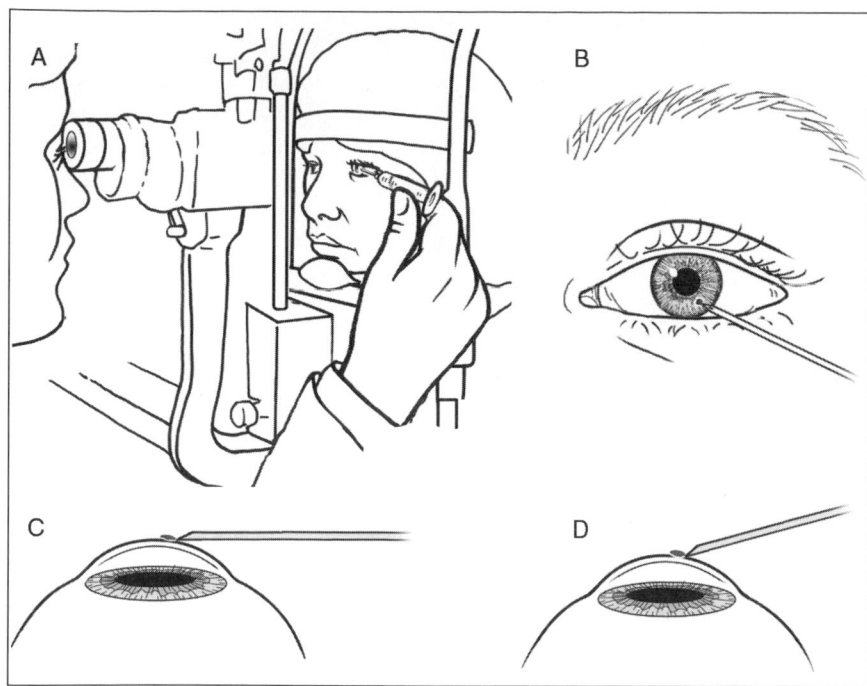

FIGURE 136-2 A hypodermic needle to remove a corneal foreign body. *A.* Position the patient in the slit lamp. Stabilize the hand holding the needle. *B.* Approach the foreign body from the periphery. *C.* Hold the needle tangential to the cornea to remove the foreign body. *D.* Slightly angle the needle to pry a foreign body off the cornea.

Hold the needle, or spud, between the thumb and index finger of the dominant hand as one would a pencil with the bevel facing the examiner. Stabilize the dominant hand on the patient or the slit lamp apparatus with the remaining fingers. Instruct the patient to focus their vision on a given point to avoid eye movement.

Approximate the tip of the needle, or spud, to the foreign body with the naked eye before utilizing the slit lamp microscope in order to avoid inadvertent injury. Approach the foreign body from the periphery and not across the patient's field of vision (Figure 136-2*B*). Gently tease out the foreign body using the beveled edge of the needle, or spud, in a tangential direction in relation to the eye to avoid inadvertent deep puncture if the patient suddenly moves (Figure 136-2*C*). Use the tip to gently pry the foreign body loose if absolutely necessary, but extreme care must be exercised (Figure 136-2*D*). Remove the loose foreign body with a moistened cotton-tipped applicator or with gentle irrigation.

ELECTRIC BURR DRILL TECHNIQUE

An electric battery powered drill equipped with various sized diamond dental burrs, if available, can be used for foreign body removal (Figure 136-3). Its use is typically associated with an increased tissue defect when compared to using a needle or a spud.[9] **Use caution as the burr drill can also embed the foreign body deeper into the cornea.**

Choose a burr size that is slightly larger than the diameter of the foreign body. Grasp the device in a similar fashion to the tuberculin syringe. Press the finger bar to turn on the drill and rotate the burr bit. Approach the foreign body tangentially to the eye (Figure 136-4). Gently place the rotating burr bit on the area to be debrided using short applications of 2 to 3 seconds in duration. Lift the burr from the cornea after each application to examine the area for removal of the foreign body.

ASSESSMENT

Carefully examine the cornea under the slit lamp with and without the use of fluorescein dye. Ensure that the foreign body is completely removed. Consult an Ophthalmologist if the foreign body has broken off or is deeply embedded within the cornea. Measure and record the patient's visual acuity after the extraction procedure. Compare this to the preextraction visual acuity. Consult an Ophthalmologist if there is a difference in the preextraction and postextraction visual acuity.

AFTERCARE

A corneal abrasion will be present upon removal of the foreign body. The defect is usually larger than the original foreign body and should be treated as a typical corneal abrasion. Place a broad-spectrum ophthalmic antibiotic ointment (e.g., an aminoglycoside) in the eye followed by patching the eye closed if the defect is large and painful. Avoid pressure patching in the case of small,

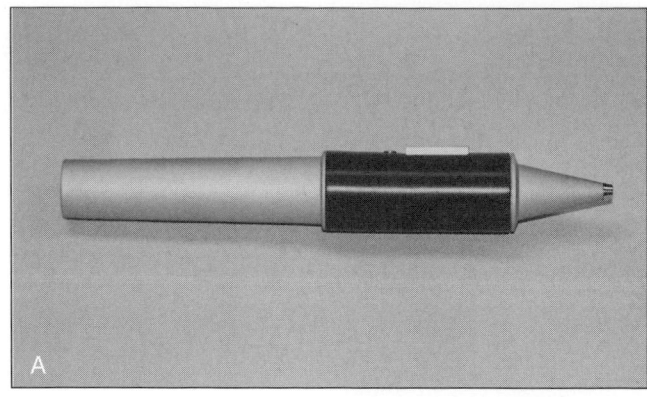

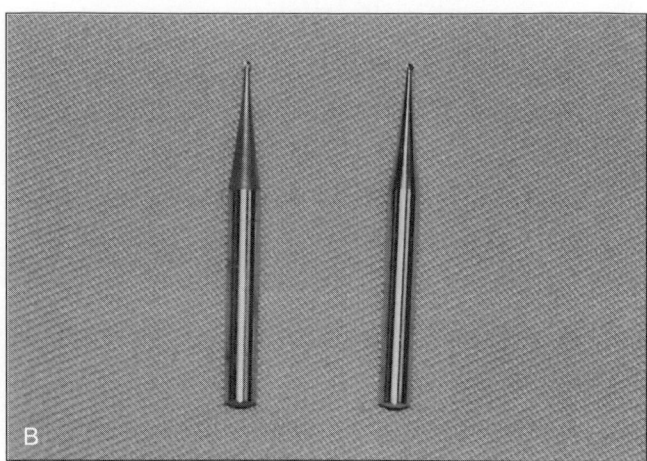

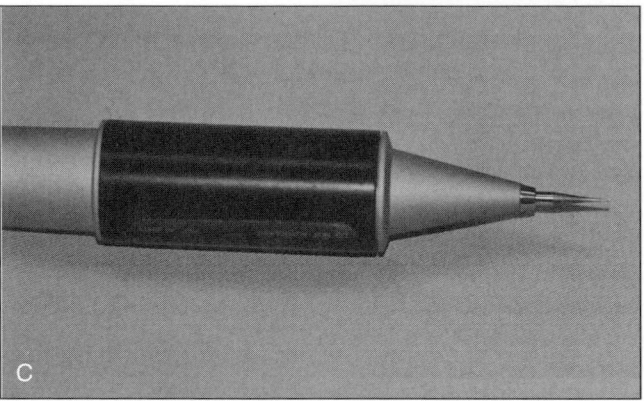

FIGURE 136-3 The burr drill used to remove a corneal foreign body. *A.* The drill. *B.* The burr bits. *C.* The burr drill with a burr bit inserted.

superficial abrasions that are painless. Instruct the patient to instill topical broad-spectrum antibiotics every 4 hours if the eye is not patched.[1,4,5,8]

The use of pressure patches should be considered cautiously as they may be associated with additional discomfort and delayed healing.[10] Avoid the use of patches in cases of organic foreign bodies and in patients who wear contact lenses, as the bacterial milieu is favorable for the development of local infection.[4] The use of an eye patch is controversial and usually not required. Refer to Chapter 138 regarding the complete details of eye patching.

The proper method of applying an eye patch is to first administer all necessary medications. Instruct the patient to close both eyes. Apply a folded patch to the affected eye (rounded edge pointed downward) over which is placed an unfolded patch. Prep the skin with a benzoin solution to aid with tape adherence. Apply strips of tape from the medial aspect of the forehead, over the patch, to the lateral cheek. Apply the tape tightly enough to prevent eye opening but lightly enough to not cause discomfort. Apply strips of tape repeatedly over the patch until it is entirely covered. Apply the final pieces of tape over the center of the patch while holding the cheek

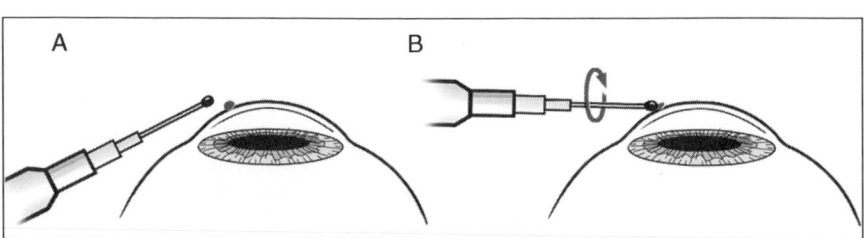

FIGURE 136-4 Removal of a corneal foreign body with a burr drill.

soft tissue superiorly. This will ensure that the cheek, when released, will pull the bandage taut and avoid loosening.[4,8]

Cycloplegics (e.g., 1% cyclopentolate) can also be used to alleviate pain or in cases of significant corneal defects or an anterior uveitis.[1] Topical steroids have no place in the treatment of traumatic corneal defects.[1] Oral analgesics are appropriate in cases of persistent discomfort. **Do not prescribe topical ocular anesthetic agents due to their abusive potential and the direct deleterious effects of the anesthetic on the corneal epithelium.**[4] Refer all patients to an Ophthalmologist for reexamination in 24 hours, especially if a patch has been applied. Instruct the patient not to operate a vehicle if the eye is patched closed. These instructions also hold true if the eye is not patched but an ocular procedure was performed to remove a foreign body.

Many eye injuries occur while at work due to failure to comply with wearing eye protection, resulting in a significant loss of working hours.[6,7,11] Take the time necessary to explain the importance of wearing safety goggles if the injury occurred while at work, gardening, or participating in hobbies (e.g., woodworking, drilling, auto repair, etc.).

COMPLICATIONS

A foreign body will occasionally not be able to be removed in the Emergency Department. Refer the patient to an Ophthalmologist for definitive treatment before further attempts at removal result in severe ocular injury and the potential for violation of the anterior chamber. **Notify an Ophthalmologist immediately if inadvertent puncture of the globe occurs from attempts at foreign body removal because a surgical emergency now exists.**

Improper placement of eye patches can cause delayed corneal healing.[8] Caution the patient against driving while the eye is patched due to impaired depth perception.[8]

Continued discomfort at the 24 hour follow-up may indicate the foreign body was not completely removed, a corneal rust ring from a metallic object has formed, a penetrating eye injury, anterior uveitis, or an infection.[1] Contaminated corneal foreign bodies or those consisting of vegetative material can also lead to corneal ulceration from the introduction of bacteria.[1]

Corneal defects will not always be completely healed at the 24 hour follow up. The eye may require one additional day of patching if the defect is still a significant size. Treat the defect by applying a topical antibiotic for several more days if the defect is markedly smaller than the original injury.[1]

Care must be taken to avoid further damage to the eye when treating children or patients who are uncoop-

erative. Intravenous sedation and analgesia can be used in these situations. Consult an Ophthalmologist for treatment under general anesthesia if sedation is contraindicated or if the physician is not comfortable with removing the foreign body under sedation.[4]

SUMMARY

Corneal foreign bodies are routinely encountered in the Emergency Department. They must be definitively treated in order to avoid long-lasting ocular disability. A complete and exhaustive history and physical examination of the eye are mandatory for proper documentation. The most reliable method of corneal foreign body removal is the use of a hypodermic needle or corneal spud, taking care to avoid additional ocular trauma. Administer appropriate antibiotics and/or cycloplegics after removal of the foreign body. Decide whether or not to patch the eye. Refer the patient to an Ophthalmologist in 24 hours for evaluation of proper healing and the immediate treatment of any evolving complications.

REFERENCES

1. Augeri PA: Corneal foreign body removal and treatment. *Optom Clin* 1991; 1(4):59–70.
2. Roper-Hall MJ: Foreign bodies of the eye and their treatment. *Nurs Mirror Midwives J* 1966; 123(7):7–8.
3. Wolf MA: The management of corneal abrasions and corneal foreign bodies. *Occup Health Nurs* 1981; 29(6):32–33.
4. Santen SA, Scott JL: Ophthalmologic procedures. *Emerg Med Clin North Am* 1995; 13(3):681–701.
5. Kaiser PK: A comparison of pressure patching versus no patching for corneal abrasions due to trauma or foreign body removal. *Ophthalmology* 1995; 102(12):1936–1942.
6. Shah S, Brahma AK, Sabala A: Pain and corneal foreign bodies. *J R Soc Med* 1995; 88:406P–408P.
7. Kaye-Wilson LG: Localisation of corneal foreign bodies. *Br J Ophthalmol* 1992; 76:741–742.
8. Knoop K, Trott A: Ophthalmologic procedures in the emergency department—part III: slit lamp use and foreign bodies. *Acad Emerg Med* 1995; 2(3):224–230.
9. Liston RL, Olson RJ, Mamalis N: A comparison of rust-ring removal methods in a rabbit model: small-gauge hypodermic needle versus electric drill. *Ann Ophthalmol* 1991; 23:24–27.
10. Hulbert MFG: Efficacy of eye pad in corneal healing after corneal foreign body removal. *Lancet* 1991; 337:643.
11. Janda AM: Ocular trauma: triage and treatment. *Postgrad Med* 1991; 90(7):51–60.

Chapter 137
CORNEAL RUST RING REMOVAL

Dino P. Rumoro

INTRODUCTION

Corneal rust rings occur commonly when metallic foreign bodies become embedded in the cornea. Removal of the rust ring is imperative to avoid permanent staining of the cornea, persistent inflammation, or disruption of corneal integrity (necrosis) with loss of stromal substance.[1-3] Two techniques for the removal of rust rings are discussed: hypodermic needle extraction and corneal burr drill removal. The use of topical deferoxamine as a chemical chelator is mentioned only for the sake of completeness.

ANATOMY AND PATHOPHYSIOLOGY

The cornea is approximately 0.5 mm thick. It is comprised of five layers (from outer to inner layer): epithelium, Bowman's membrane, stroma (largest layer), Descemet's membrane, and the endothelial layer which lies directly over the anterior chamber. Corneal rust rings are formed from the oxidation of iron present in metallic foreign bodies. As little as 3 hours of corneal contact are required to form the brown stain of a rust ring.[1]

INDICATIONS

All corneal metallic foreign bodies require prompt removal to avoid the possibility of rust ring formation. A rust ring requires complete removal in a timely fashion in order to avoid the damaging effects of rust on the cornea.

CONTRAINDICATIONS

Corneal foreign bodies and rust rings that are located in the direct axis of vision can cause permanent visual disturbances if improperly removed.[2] Consult an Oph-
thalmologist before removing these, as they often prefer to remove them. Do not attempt to extract a rust ring if the patient is confused or uncooperative as this can result in a perforated globe. Consider the use of intravenous sedation, procedural sedation, or general anesthesia to extract the rust ring.

EQUIPMENT

Slit lamp
25 or 27 gauge needle
Tuberculin syringe with a needle
Burr drill
Burr bits
Topical ocular anesthetic agent
Topical ophthalmic antibiotic
Cycloplegic agents
Ringer's lactate solution or normal saline

PATIENT PREPARATION

Explain the procedure, its risks, and benefits to the patient and/or their representative. Obtained a signed informed consent to perform this procedure. Apply a topical ocular anesthetic agent into the affected eye. Determine the patient's visual acuity in the affected eye. Seat the patient at the slit lamp with their head firmly in place to avoid any unexpected movement (Figure 137-1). Examine the eye via the slit lamp and rule out the possibility of an intraocular foreign body with a corneal perforation. Perform a complete eye examination to rule out any other ocular problems. Remove the foreign body, if still present, with the hypodermic needle or tuberculin syringe. Refer to Chapter 136 for the complete details regarding corneal foreign body removal. The rust ring will often be removed simultaneously with the metallic foreign body. Make an attempt to

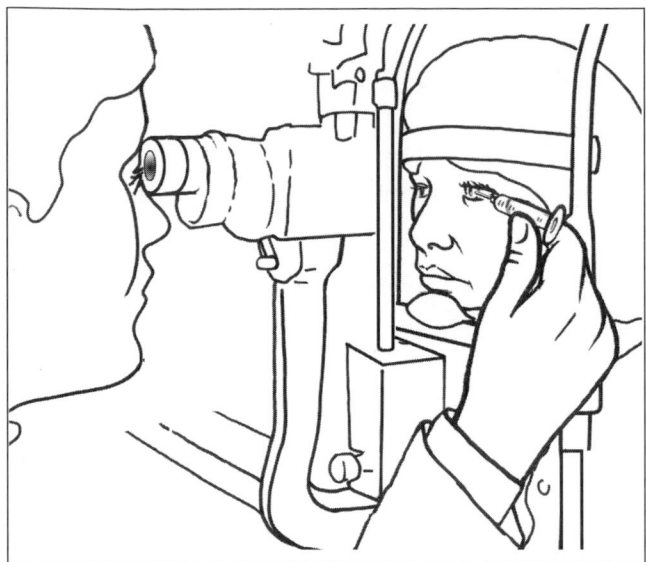

FIGURE 137-1 Positioning of the patient and the examiner's hand.

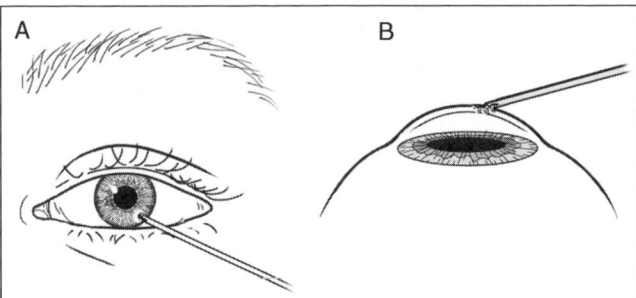

FIGURE 137-2 Manual extraction of the rust ring.

remove the rust ring if it remains after removal of the foreign body.

TECHNIQUES

MANUAL TECHNIQUE

Scrape out the rust ring in a similar fashion to the removal of a metallic foreign body (Figure 137-2). Refer to Chapter 136 for the complete details regarding corneal foreign body removal. Use the beveled edge of the needle to remove the rust ring. **The entire area of rust stained epithelium must be completely removed without any residual rust.**

ELECTRIC DRILL TECHNIQUE

An electric battery-powered drill equipped with diamond burrs, if available, can be used for rust ring removal (Figure 136-3). The burr bit cuts away corneal tissue very slowly. Corneal rust rings were induced in rabbits and comparisons were made between manual extraction versus electric drill extraction.[1] Both were equally effective for rust ring removal. The burr was shown to cause a deeper corneal defect. **Use caution when using an electric burr device.** There was no difference in corneal scarring between the two techniques. The burr drill can also be used to extract rust in the bulbar conjunctiva.[4]

Choose a burr size that is slightly larger than the diameter of the rust ring. Grasp the device in a similar fashion to a pen. Press the finger bar to turn on the drill and rotate the burr bit. Approach the rust ring tangen-

tially to the eye (Figure 137-3). Gently place the rotating burr bit on the area to be debrided using short applications of 2 to 3 seconds in duration. Lift the burr from the cornea after each application to examine the area for removal of the rust ring. **Thoroughly inspect the base of the crater to ensure that it is free of rust.**[4] Continue the process until the rust ring is removed. Use a slightly larger burr bit if rust still remains along the periphery of the crater.

DELAYED REMOVAL

The rust ring may be removed after it ages.[2,8] Allow the rust ring to remain for 24 to 48 hours. During this time the iron deposits will kill the surrounding corneal epithelial cells. The rust ring will "soften" and be easily removed in one piece with a needle, spud, or burr drill. **Do not allow the rust ring to remain for longer than 24 to 48 hours, ideally 24 hours, as it can cause significant damage to the cornea.**

CHEMICAL CHELATION

Topical deferoxamine has been used experimentally for the nonsurgical removal of rust stains on the cornea.[6] It has been shown to remove rust, though perhaps not as reliably as the methods previously described. The potential exists for resultant eye irritation, corneal ulceration, or persistence of the rust stain.[6] The clinical use of deferoxamine should be limited for use only in very select situations such as children with multiple lesions or when the central axis of vision is involved.[7] This technique is reserved for the Ophthalmologist and is therefore not described in this text.

ASSESSMENT

Measure and document visual acuities before and after the procedure. Consult an Ophthalmologist if the post-procedural visual acuity is different from the pre-procedural visual acuity.

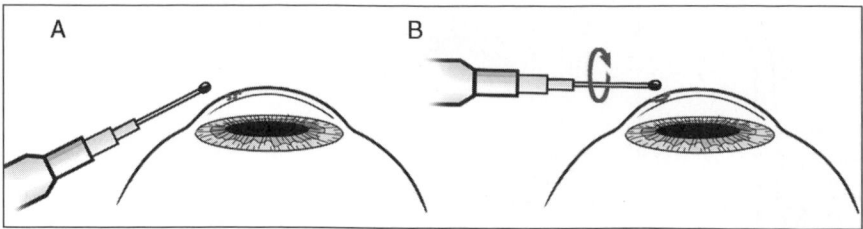

FIGURE 137-3 Burr drill extraction of the rust ring.

AFTERCARE

A corneal defect resembling a corneal abrasion will be present after the rust ring is removed. The defect is usually larger than the original foreign body and should be treated as a typical corneal abrasion. Apply topical ocular antibiotic ointment in the eye. The use of an eye patch is controversial but considered by most as unnecessary. Instruct the patient not to operate a vehicle. Administer cycloplegics to alleviate pain from an actual or potential anterior uveitis.[2] Oral analgesics are appropriate in cases of persistent discomfort. Refer the patient to an Ophthalmologist for reexamination in 24 hours.

Instruct the patient on the importance of safety goggles.[5] Many eye injuries occur while at work due to failure to comply with wearing eye protection, resulting in a significant loss of working hours.[5,9,10] Take the time that is necessary to explain the importance of wearing safety goggles if the injury occurred while at work, gardening, or participating in hobbies (e.g., woodworking, drilling, and auto repair).

COMPLICATIONS

Abandon multiple attempts at removal of the rust ring to avoid severe ocular injury and the potential for violation of the anterior chamber if the depth of the rust cannot be determined or if repeated debridement is unable to completely remove the rust ring. The eye can be patched closed, or left open, for 24 hours and the patient referred to an Ophthalmologist for definitive removal the following day in these situations or in cases of hesitancy in removing a rust ring. Delayed removal is often easier than the initial attempts due to further oxidation and injury of the corneal epithelium resulting in "softening" of the rust. The "softened" rust ring is easily scraped out in 24 to 48 hours.[2] The disadvantage of this approach is that the patient's eye may be patched twice, first on the initial presentation and again 24 hours later after the rust ring is removed.

SUMMARY

Removal of corneal rust rings is imperative in order to avoid permanent ocular injury. It is best accomplished with a small gauge hypodermic needle or with an electric burr device. An alternative approach is to leave the rust for delayed removal by an Ophthalmologist in 24 hours when the rust has "softened."

REFERENCES

1. Liston RL, Olson RJ, Mamalis N: A comparison of rust-ring removal methods in a rabbit model: small-gauge hypodermic needle versus electric drill. *Ann Ophthalmol* 1991; 23(1):24–27.
2. Santen SA, Scott JL: Ophthalmologic procedures. *Emerg Med Clin North Am* 1995; 13(3):681–701.
3. Brown N, Clemett R, Grey R: Corneal rust removal by electric drill: clinical trial by comparison with manual removal. *Br J Ophthal* 1975; 59:586–589.
4. Hardesty HH: Electric rust-ring remover technique. *Am J Ophthalmol* 1965; 60(3):526–527.
5. Janda AM: Ocular trauma: triage and treatment. *Postgrad Med* 1991; 90(7):51–60.
6. North PJ: Treatment of corneal rust rings with desferrioxamine. *Br J Ophthalmol* 1970; 54:498–499.
7. Removal of corneal rust stains. *Med J Aust* 1971; 2(16):786.
8. Newell FW: *Ophthalmology Principles and Concepts.* St. Louis: Mosby, 1978:186.
9. Shah S, Brahma AK, Sabala A: Pain and corneal foreign bodies. *J R Soc Med* 1995; 88:406P–408P.
10. Kaye-Wilson LG: Localization of corneal foreign bodies. *Br J Opthalmol* 1992; 76:741–742.

Chapter 138
EYE PATCHING AND EYE SHIELDS

Rebecca R. Roberts

INTRODUCTION

Eye shields are used to protect the eye from further injury when the integrity of the globe is compromised or potentially compromised. The best results are obtained when early repair of globe disruption occurs, before any contents leak out or change position.[1,2] In contrast, eye patches are intended to prevent movement of the eyelid over an injured but intact cornea. Eye patching is often performed to protect the eye from bright light or to facilitate healing of a corneal abrasion. While there have been no substantial changes in the indications for eye shields and their method of application, eye patching has recently become controversial.

EYE PATCHING

INDICATIONS
Patches are indicated for corneal injuries due to abrasions as well as to thermal, light, or chemical burns.[3] Patches are believed to promote healing and provide pain relief by decreasing movement of the eyelid across the recovering cornea.[3,4] Secondarily, patches block light in photophobic patients with ciliary spasm or reactive iritis due to a corneal injury.[4-6]

Some of these assumptions have now been questioned. Patching is believed to decrease corneal oxygenation, increase temperature, and increase infection risk.[5-7] Several trials have randomized patients with corneal abrasions to receive patching versus no patching.[6-8] They have found no difference in pain scores or healing time for small abrasions less than 10 mm in diameter. There was a significant decrease in healing time for patched patients with abrasions greater than 10 mm in diameter. Therefore, patching is still recommended for those with large defects.[6,7] More recently, soft contact lens bandages have been used for patients who must maintain binocular vision.[8,9]

CONTRAINDICATIONS
Absolute contraindications to patching are corneal abrasions in patients due to the wearing of contact lenses because of the increased incidence of infection and more pathogenic bacteria harbored by contact lens wearers.[6] **Any patient considered at risk for penetration or rupture of the globe should not be patched.** Patching will increase intraocular pressure and may cause extravasation of the contents of the globe. Patients must be carefully assessed for the presence of corneal ulcers masquerading as abrasions.[3] Patching of a corneal ulcer may place pressure on the ulcer and deepen the ulcer or perforate the cornea.

Relative contraindications are related to abrasion size and individual patient needs. Small abrasions are felt to heal well without patching. Patients requiring the use of binocular vision may benefit from not patching.[6,7] Patches that come loose and allow eyelid movement are more painful for patients than no patch.[3,4] Contraindications to ophthalmoplegics used in conjunction with patches are patients with known glaucoma or narrow angles on physical examination.[3] Paradoxically, the contraindication to contact lens bandages is an abrasion in a patient who was wearing contact lenses, again because of the risk of infection.[10]

EQUIPMENT
Cycloplegic drops to reduce photophobia,[4-6]
    1% cyclopentolate or 5% homatropine
Broad-spectrum antibiotic ointment or drops, gentamicin or erythromycin
Eye patches
1 inch tape
Contact bandage, soft (Acuvue) lens with minus 0.5 diopters of power[9]
Elastic-strapped pressure patch

PATIENT PREPARATION
Conduct a complete eye exam to ensure the integrity of the globe and the absence of an infection or foreign body. Document the visual acuity for both eyes.[12] Patients should receive tetanus prophylaxis if their immunizations are not up to date.[4] Apply cycloplegic drops and antibiotic ointment to the affected eye.[3,4] Refer to Chapter 132, on the examination of the eye, for complete details regarding the instillation of drops

and ointment into the eyes. For patients with small corneal abrasions, no further treatment is required.

EYE-PATCHING TECHNIQUE

After patient preparation as above, instruct the patient to close both eyes and to keep them both shut for the rest of the procedure. Tear off 4 to 6 strips of 1 inch tape, each 4 to 5 inches long, and have them at the bedside. Obtain two cotton eye patches. Fold the first patch in half. Apply it to the affected eye (both eyes remaining closed). Place the second patch, unfolded, over the first patch (Figure 138-1A). Apply the pretorn strips of tape diagonally from the center of the forehead to the cheek above the mandible[3,4] (Figure 138-1B). To ensure the correct amount of pressure, lift the lower cheek up slightly before securing the first two strips of tape.[3,4] The patch will hold the eye more securely if the nasal and temporal strips are placed in a slight arc concave toward the center of the eye. Care must be taken to avoid taping the nasolabial folds, lips, mustache (if any), and the skin near the mandible.[3,4] Otherwise, eating and speaking will be uncomfortable for the patient and the patch will rapidly loosen. If the

patient has a significant amount of facial hair, the tape may not stick. An elastic-strapped pressure patch may be applied instead.

SOFT CONTACT BANDAGE TECHNIQUE

For patients who require immediate use of both eyes, soft contact lenses can be applied as a corneal bandage.[8,9] Prepare the patient as described previously. Apply ophthalmic antibiotic drops rather than ointment to the affected eye. Remove the contact lens from the storage bottle. Rinse the storage solution from the contact lens. Place the contact lens on the index finger of the dominant hand. Using the nondominant hand, open the patient's eyelids. Instruct the patient to look straight ahead. Gently apply the contact lens directly to the cornea. The patient should remain in the Emergency Department for a recheck in 15 to 30 minutes to make sure that the contact lens fits properly and they are able to tolerate it.[9]

ASSESSMENT

Make sure that the patient with a patch does not feel the lid of the injured eye moving when they blink the

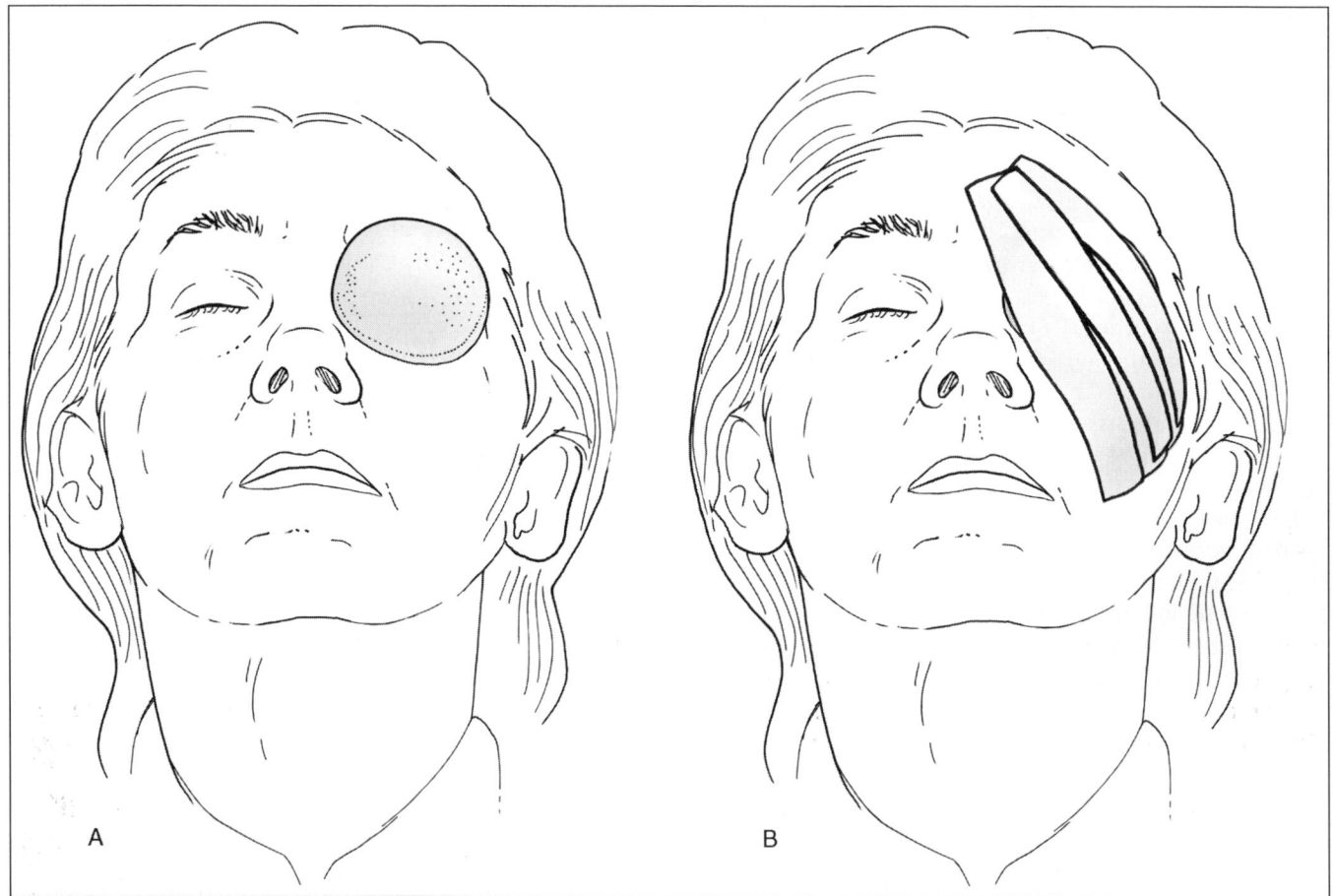

FIGURE 138-1 Eye patching. *A.* A patch is applied over the eyelid. *B.* The patch is secured with tape.

unaffected eye.[4] Ensure that the tape is not interfering with the patient's speech or chewing movements.

AFTERCARE

The patient should remove the patch if it becomes loose. Patches should be changed or removed after 24 hours to reduce the risk of infection.[3,4] Most patients will need oral pain medications for the first 24 hours in addition to the patch.[4] Ketorolac (0.5%) ophthalmic drops have been useful alone or in conjunction with a contact lens bandage for pain relief.[5,9] The patient must be reexamined in 24 hours by an Ophthalmologist for healing progress as well as infection and other complications. They can expect complete resolution in 2 to 3 days. Instruct the patient not to drive or operate dangerous equipment due to the loss of binocular depth perception.[3,7] The elderly may need assistance even for walking, especially up or down stairs.[3] Discourage the patient from reading, as this will cause involuntary movement of the patched eye.

COMPLICATIONS

Infection is rare but is most likely to occur in contact lens wearers or in patients who have used a patch for a prolonged period.[3,4,10] Patches applied too tightly can raise intraocular pressure high enough to cause retinal artery occlusion, leading to retinal ischemia, infarct, and blindness. Allergy to ophthalmic medications, the patch, or the tape materials can occur. Accidents due to lack of binocular depth perception can occur.[3,4] Healing times may be prolonged with loose patches that allow movement of the eyelid over the cornea.[3,4] With pressure patches, the eyelashes may get caught between the eyelids and the cornea and further abrade the cornea.[3] Contact lens bandages can cause infective ulcerative keratitis or corneal revascularization.[9] For these reasons, eye patching has fallen out of favor.

EYE SHIELDS

INDICATIONS

Eye shields serve as temporary protection for patients in whom a penetrated or ruptured globe is suspected.[10] The purpose is to prevent any further injury, with resultant extravasation of the contents of the globe and resultant outcome of poor vision.[2,5] Signs associated with a ruptured globe include bloody chemosis, increase or decrease in the depth of the anterior chamber, irregular or peaked iris, positive Seidel test, vitreous hemorrhage, low intraocular pressure, hyphema, and loss of visual acuity.[10,13–15] **If a ruptured globe is suspected, further examination is contraindicated.** Instead, an eye shield is applied immediately and to remain in place while other injuries are managed, tests are obtained (e.g.,

orbital computed tomography scans), and the consulting Ophthalmologist is contacted.[2]

CONTRAINDICATIONS

The only contraindication to the application of an eye shield arises when the surrounding face and orbits are so extensively damaged that the metal shield or its edges will directly injure the globe. The protective function of the shield relies on its edges being supported by the orbital rim, frontal bone, and maxillary bone.

EQUIPMENT

Metal or plastic eye shield
1 inch tape

If commercially available eye shields are not available, a clean, disposable paper drinking cup may be used.[4,12] Using a scissors, make ¾ to 1 inch deep cuts around the open end of the cup (Figure 138-2). Approximately 6 to 8 cuts should be made. Fold the flaps on the open end of the cup outward.

PATIENT PREPARATION

The first procedure in patients with suspected globe disruption is the application of the eye shield.[14] There should be no preparations except to dry the area of skin that will receive the securing tape. Specifically, the eye should not be irrigated, no gauze or patch should touch the eye, and no antibiotic or anesthetic ointments or drops should be applied. All of these are likely to cause further injury to the exposed globe.[2,11] Contact an Ophthalmologist immediately to expedite globe repair.[10,14]

TECHNIQUE

Apply the commercial eye shield (Figure 138-3*A*) or the one improvised from a paper cup (Figure 138-3*B*)

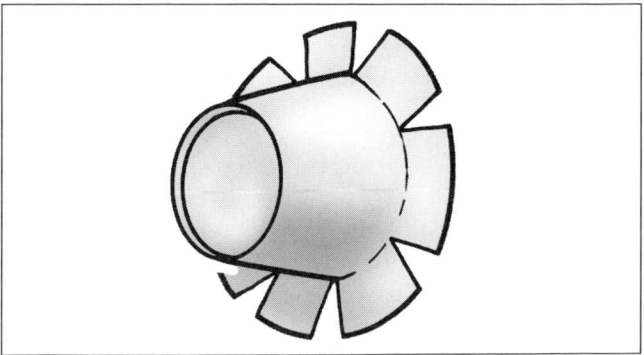

FIGURE 138-2 A Styrofoam or paper cup may be used if a commercial eye shield is not available. The top of the cup is cut in multiple places and the "flaps" are bent down to create a flat surface.

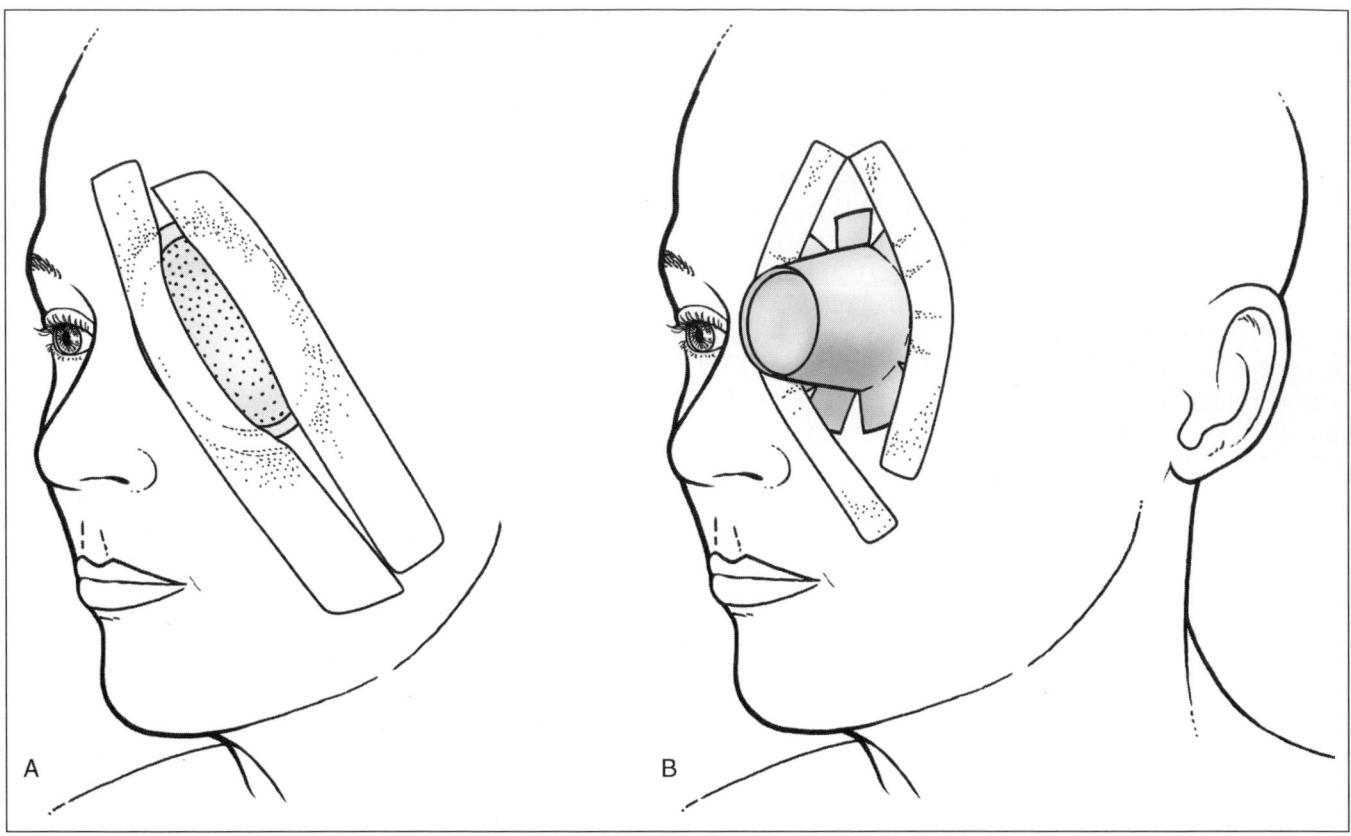

FIGURE 138-3 Eye shields. *A.* A commercial eye shield is applied. *B.* An improvised eye shield is applied.

over the injured eye. Ensure that its edges do not contact structures any closer to the eye than the orbital rim. Tear off 4 to 6 strips of 1 inch tape, each 4 to 5 inches long. Apply the strips of tape diagonally from the center of the forehead to the cheek above the mandible to hold the shield in place[12] (Figures 138-3*A* and *B*). Care must be taken to avoid taping the nasolabial folds, lips, mustache (if any), and skin over the mandible. Otherwise, mandibular movement may cause the shield to move and potentially injure the eye. If the patient requires the use of an oxygen mask, it should be trimmed around the eye shield to prevent it from displacing the eye shield and causing further eye injury.[2]

AFTERCARE

The shield position should frequently be checked for any movement in position or loosening of the tape due to blood, perspiration, or other fluids. The shield must remain in place until tests demonstrate that the globe is intact or the consulting Ophthalmologist arrives. The patient should not be allowed to eat or drink. Additional therapy includes tetanus prophylaxis, prophylactic intravenous antibiotics, and parenteral antieme-

tics for nausea, because vomiting will cause extrusion of the contents of the globe.[1,2,11,14,15]

COMPLICATIONS

Poor positioning or shield movement can further injure the eye or cause extravasation of the contents of the globe. The patient must be handled gently during the entire procedure because even wincing or squinting of the eye can increase intraocular pressure sufficiently to cause the extravasation of the contents of the globe.

SUMMARY

The eye is one of the most delicate and complex structures of the body. It is injured more frequently than would be predicted based on its relative size.[16] Preservation of vision is essential to maintaining quality of life. In addition, the cornea is one of the most sensitive organs of the body, and tiny injuries to it can result in significant pain and loss of function. It is therefore essential that Emergency Physicians be skilled in eye injury management. The application of an eye patch or eye shield is a simple, rapid, and straightforward procedure. Despite this, the improper application of these devices can result in significant morbidity.

REFERENCES

1. Lubeck D: Penetrating ocular injuries. *Emerg Med Clin North Am* 1988; 6(1):127–146.
2. Colvin J, Langford S, Emonson D, et al: Initial management and transport of patients with perforating eye injuries. *Aust Fam Physician* 1995; 24(6):1017–1020.
3. Scott-Brown WG, Kerr AG: *Scott-Brown's Otolaryngology*, 6th ed. Oxford, England: Butterworth-Heinemann, 1997.
4. Santen SA, Scott JL: Ophthalmologic procedures. *Emerg Med Clin North Am* 1995; 13(3):681–701.
5. Kaiser PK, Pineda R: A study of topical nonsteroidal anti-inflammatory drops and no pressure patching in the treatment of corneal abrasions. Corneal Abrasion Patching Study Group. *Ophthalmology* 1997; 104(8):1353–1359.
6. Patterson J, Fetzer D, Krall J, et al: Eye patch treatment for the pain of corneal abrasion. *South Med J* 1996; 89(2):227–229.
7. Kaiser PK: A comparison of pressure patching versus no patching for corneal abrasions due to trauma or foreign body removal. Corneal Abrasion Patching Study Group. *Ophthalmology* 1995; 102(12):1936–1942.
8. Hulbert MF: Efficacy of eyepad in corneal healing after corneal foreign body removal. *Lancet* 1991; 337(8742):643.
9. Donnenfeld ED, Selkin BA, Perry HD, et al: Controlled evaluation of a bandage contact lens and a topical nonsteroidal anti-inflammatory drug in treating traumatic corneal abrasions. *Ophthalmology* 1995; 102(6):979–984.
10. Linden JA, Renner GS: Trauma to the globe. *Emerg Med Clin North Am* 1995; 13(3):581–605.
11. Colvin J: Penetrating eye injury. *Med J Aust* 1980; 2(11):630.
12. Garcia GE: Management of ocular emergencies and urgent eye problems. *Am Fam Physician* 1996; 53(2):565–574.
13. Kylstra JA: Management of suspected ocular laceration or rupture. *Can J Ophthalmol* 1991; 26(4): 224–228.
14. Weisman RA, Savino PJ: Management of patients with facial trauma and associated ocular/orbital injuries. *Otolaryngol Clin North Am* 1991; 24(1):37–57.
15. Edwards MG, Pieramici DJ, Fekrat S, et al: Corneoscleral lacerations and ruptures, in MacCumber MW (ed): *Management of Ocular Injuries and Emergencies.* Philadelphia: Lippincott-Raven, 1998: 207–226.
16. Biehl JW, Valdez J, Hemady RK, et al: Penetrating eye injury in war. *Mil Med* 1999; 164(11):780–784.

Chapter 139

ACUTE ORBITAL COMPARTMENT SYNDROME (RETROBULBAR HEMORRHAGE) MANAGEMENT

Eric Savitsky

INTRODUCTION

Emergency Physicians must be able to promptly recognize and manage an acute orbital compartment syndrome, which is defined as an acute elevation of intraorbital pressure with resultant ocular dysfunction. The diagnosis of an orbital compartment syndrome is based on clinical signs and symptoms. Patients typically present with ocular pain, proptosis, afferent pupillary defects, and diminished visual acuity. Clinical signs of an acute orbital compartment syndrome include chemosis, elevated intraocular pressure, mydriasis, diminished retropulsion of the affected globe to direct manual pressure, ophthalmoplegia, and fundoscopic signs of retinal ischemia (rare).

Orbital compartment syndromes have been described in multiple clinical settings. The presentation that Emergency Physicians will most likely encounter is an acute post-traumatic retrobulbar hemorrhage leading to an orbital compartment syndrome.[1,2] Orbital compartment syndromes have been documented following blepharoplasty, retrobulbar anesthesia, orbital and sinus surgery, orbital fractures with intraorbital emphysema, spontaneous subperiosteal hemorrhages, and spontaneous retrobulbar hemorrhages.[3–9] Orbital compartment syndromes may also occur as the result of chronic and progressive disease processes.[10]

Acute orbital compartment syndromes demand prompt recognition because irreversible loss of vision occurs without rapid treatment.[11] The exact etiology of vision loss in orbital compartment syndromes remains speculative. Possible causes include optic nerve ischemia, direct optic nerve damage, and retinal artery occlusion.[12,13] Once the diagnosis of an acute orbital compartment syndrome is made, emergent surgical intervention is indicated. Immediate lateral canthotomy and cantholysis are indicated within 1 hour of injury and ocular dysfunction. **The primary therapy for an acute orbital compartment syndrome is surgical intervention.** Medical interventions aimed at reducing intraocular pressure (e.g., mannitol, acetazolamide, topical beta-blockers, etc.) should be considered adjunctive therapy and not a substitute for surgical intervention.

ANATOMY AND PATHOPHYSIOLOGY

The orbit of the eye is a closed space posterior to the orbital septum and contained within the bony orbit. The lateral wall of the orbit is formed by the zygomatic bone. The posterior wall is formed by the sphenoid bone. The medial wall is·formed by the ethmoid bone. The roof is formed by the frontal bone. The floor is formed by the maxillary bone. The globe is enclosed in a fascial envelope.

The medial and lateral canthal tendons provide structural fixation of the eyelids to the orbital rim. The lateral canthal tendon (LCT) is located posterior and inferior to the lateral canthal fold (Figure 139-1). The LCT originates from the lateral tarsal plates (Figure 139-1) and attaches to the lateral orbital tubercle of the zygoma (Figure 139-2). The LCT measures 10.6 mm (SD +/− 0.9 mm) in length from its attachment site to the lateral canthal angle. It is 10.2 mm (SD +/− 0.8 mm) in width at its origin at the lateral ends of the tarsal plates. It attaches 1.5 mm (SD +/− 0.3 mm) behind the orbital margin and approximately 9.7 mm (SD +/− 0.8 mm) below the frontozygomatic suture at the lateral orbital tubercle.[14]

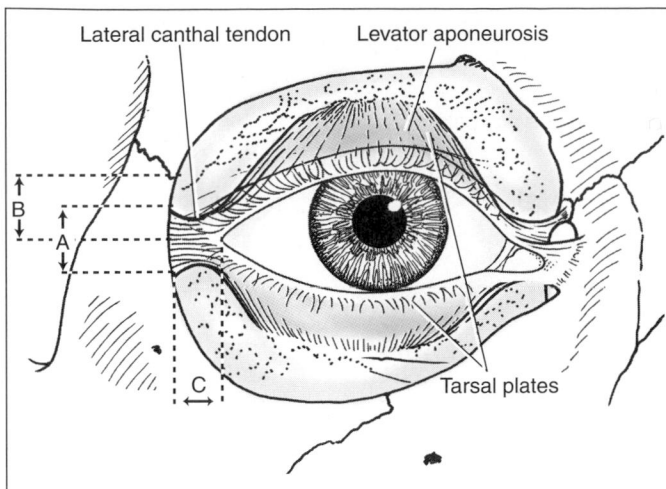

FIGURE 139-1 The lateral canthal tendon, or LCT (A = the vertical height of the LCT, B = the distance from the frontozygomatic suture to the midpoint of the LCT origin, C = the length of the LCT as measured from the canthal margin to its origin).

Immediately anterior to the LCT is Eisler's pocket, a collection of adipose tissue. Posterior to the LCT, at its attachment site to the lateral orbital tubercle is the check ligament of the lateral rectus muscle (Figure 139-2).

Any increase in intraorbital contents (e.g., retrobulbar hematoma, intraorbital emphysema, retrobulbar abscess) will result in an elevation of intraorbital pressure because the orbit is a closed space. The globe itself may partially accommodate some of the elevation in intraorbital pressure by prolapsing forward (Figure 139-3). This will result in ocular pain and proptosis. The intraorbital pressure rises dramatically as the orbit approaches maximal distention. This rise in intraorbital pressure may result in a chemosis, elevated intraocular pressures, and dysfunction of the pupillary sphincter. An ophthalmoplegia may arise when the extraocular muscles or the nerves innervating them are damaged. The damage may be in the form of a mass effect (e.g., retrobulbar hemorrhage) or from direct trauma.

The exact mechanisms by which orbital compartment syndromes result in blindness remain speculative. A common theory is that as the intraorbital pressure increases, orbital venous outflow is impeded and leads to diminished retinal and optic nerve arterial perfusion pressures.[15–17] This results in an afferent pupillary defect, diminished visual acuity, and, rarely, fundoscopic signs of retinal ischemia. Over time, the elevated intraorbital pressure leads to irreversible optic nerve and/or retinal ischemia. Experimental studies have demonstrated that irreversible ischemic injury to the retina may occur within 90 minutes of vascular insufficiency.[18–21] Additional theories suggest that direct mechanical compression or longitudinal traction on the optic nerve may contribute to the loss of vision in orbital compartment syndromes.[22,23]

A history of progressive loss of vision following orbital trauma suggests a reversible disease process (e.g., retrobulbar hemorrhage). If loss of vision is immediate and complete following orbital trauma, the chance of recovery of vision is poor.[24] This is because the loss of vision in the latter case is due to direct optic nerve, reti-

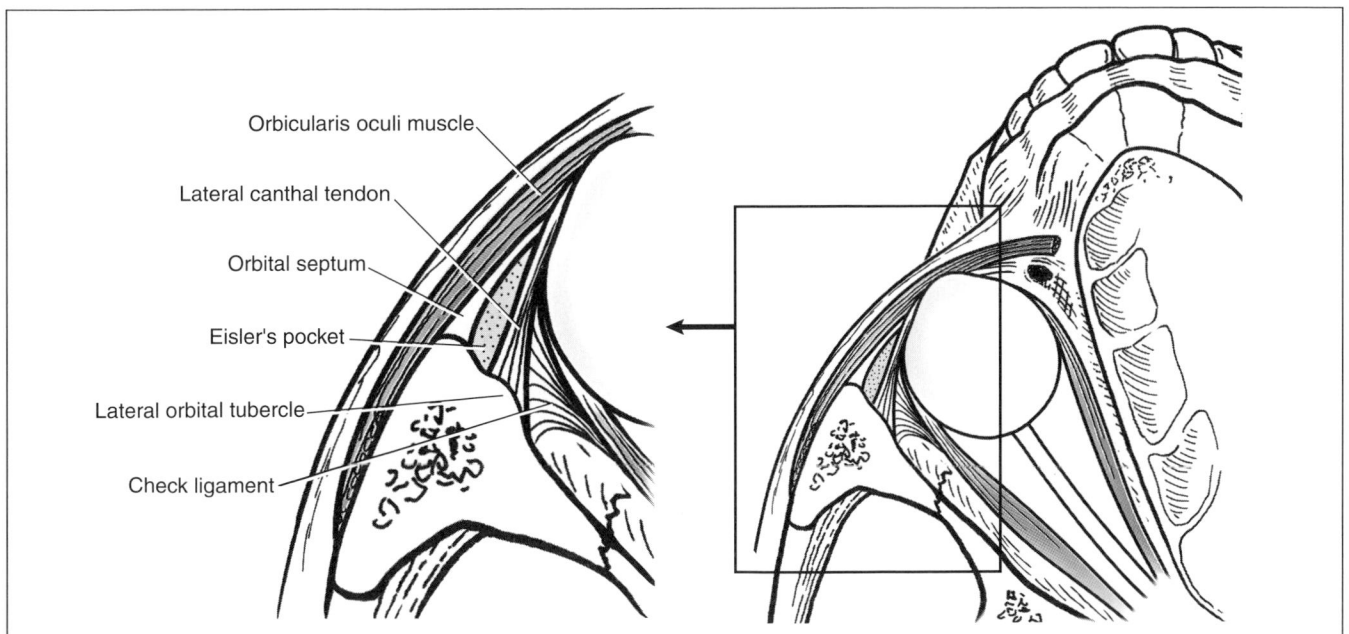

FIGURE 139-2 An axial view of the orbital contents. Identification of the LCT will require dissection of the conjunctiva and fascial tissues with a hemostat and iris scissors. A pocket of adipose tissue (Eisler's pocket) will be encountered beneath the superficial tissue layers. The LCT lies just posterior to this adipose tissue collection.

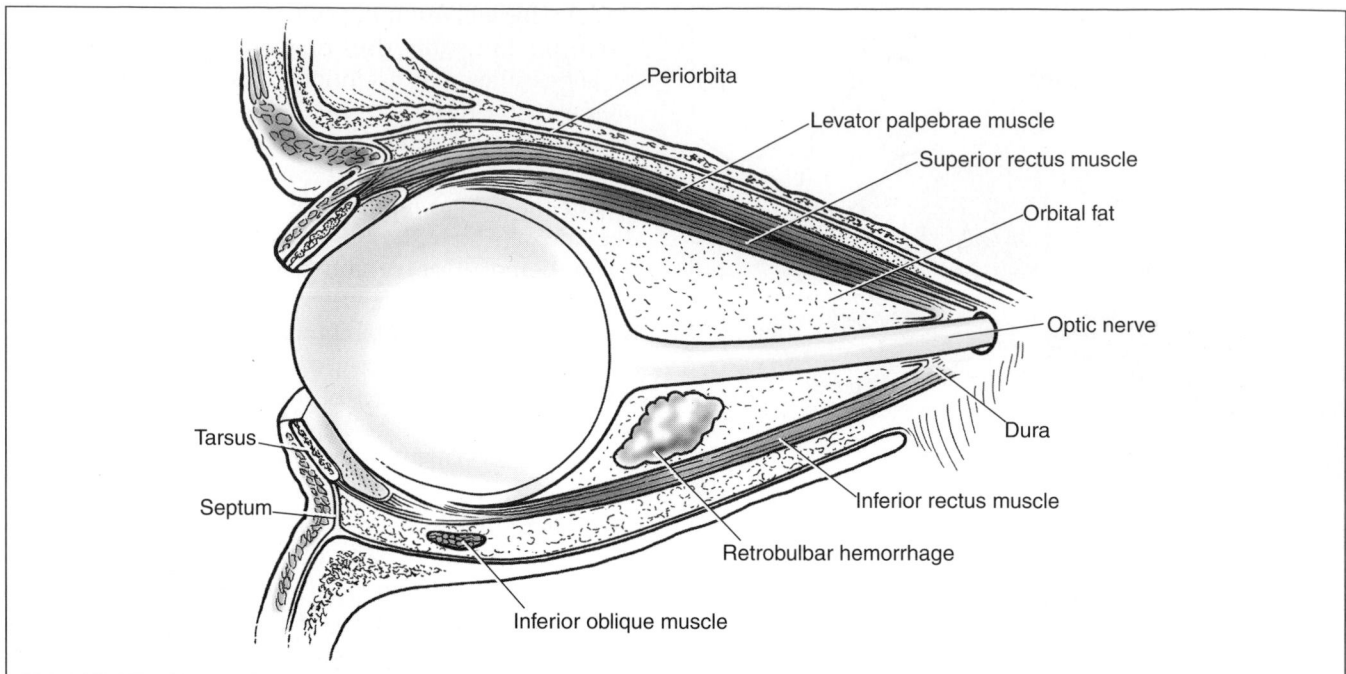

FIGURE 139-3 A sagittal view of the orbital contents. Note the location of the retrobulbar hemorrhage.

nal, or vascular injury rather than an orbital compartment syndrome.

INDICATIONS

An acute orbital compartment syndrome is an indication for immediate orbital decompression.[25] Multiple case series have documented the efficacy of immediate orbital decompression in restoring visual acuity to affected patients.[26–28]

CONTRAINDICATIONS

There are no definite contraindications to performing this procedure, as permanent loss of vision may result from untreated acute orbital compartment syndromes. The patient's airway, breathing, circulation, and any life-threatening injuries must be addressed prior to performing this procedure. If the patient is confused or uncooperative or has an altered sensorium, sedation and restraint will be required to prevent iatrogenic injury to the globe.

EQUIPMENT

Topical ocular anesthetic solution, proparacaine or tetracaine
Ocular tonometer (applanation, Schiøtz, or Tono-Pen)
Sterile saline or sterile water
Local anesthetic solution with epinephrine
Straight mosquito hemostat

Iris scissors
Tissue forceps
2×2 gauze squares
Topical ocular antibiotic ointment (bacitracin, ciprofloxacin, erythromycin, gentamicin, neosporin, polysporin, or sulfacetamide)

PATIENT PREPARATION

Explain the procedure to the patient and/or their representative, including the risks, benefits, and outcome if it is not performed. This is a painful procedure for the awake and alert patient. Consider the administration of procedural sedation. Lucid patients will require parenteral medications for analgesia and sedation in addition to local anesthetics. Measure and record the visual acuity. Perform a brief ophthalmologic examination. Apply topical ocular anesthetic solution to the conjunctiva of the affected eye. Measure and record the intraocular pressure.

TECHNIQUE

Place the patient supine. Irrigate the lateral canthal fold region with sterile saline or sterile water. Avoid the use of povidone iodine solution, as inadvertent ocular exposure could easily occur. Using sterile technique, identify the lateral canthal fold (Figure 139-4). Inject 1 mL of local anesthetic solution with epinephrine subcutaneously along the lateral canthal fold. The goal is to anesthetize the tissue extending laterally from the can-

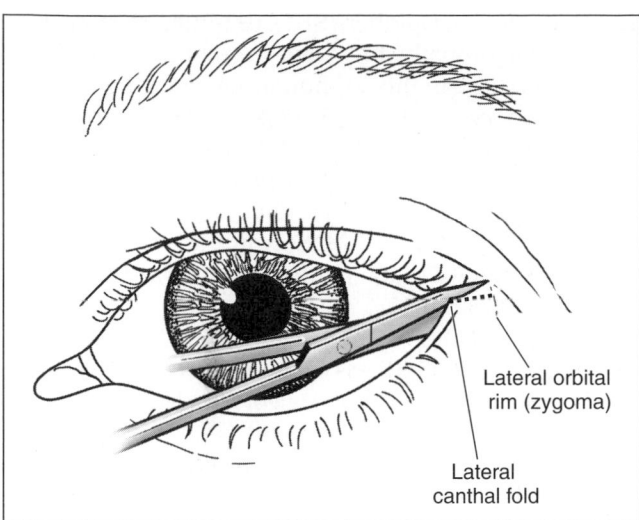

FIGURE 139-4 Illustration of lateral canthotomy. Iris scissors are used to cut all tissue layers along the lateral canthal fold up to the orbital rim.

thal fold to the orbital rim. **Caution must be exercised to avoid inadvertent needle puncture of the globe.**

Insert a straight mosquito hemostat at the lateral canthal fold. Place one jaw of the hemostat anterior and one jaw posterior to the lateral canthal fold. Advance the tips of the hemostat laterally until the orbital rim is encountered. Clamp and compress the intervening tissue for approximately 1 minute. This will minimize any bleeding precipitated by the lateral canthotomy. Remove the hemostat. Cut all the tissue layers along the lateral canthal fold up to the orbital rim (lateral canthotomy) with an iris scissors (Figure 139-4). All tissue layers, from the skin to conjunctiva, must be incised down to the orbital rim.

Grasp the lower eyelid with a hemostat or forceps and retract it outward. Identify the lateral canthal tendon located just posterior and inferior to the lateral canthal fold (Figures 139-1 and 139-2). Dissect the conjunctiva and fascial tissues with a hemostat or iris scissors. A pocket of adipose tissue (Eisler's pocket) will be encountered beneath the superficial fascial planes (Figure 139-2). The lateral canthal tendon lies just posterior to this adipose tissue collection (Figure 139-1). Completely divide the lateral canthal tendon at its midportion with an iris scissors (lateral cantholysis).

ASSESSMENT

A successful lateral canthotomy and cantholysis will cause an immediate decrease in intraocular pressure. Recheck the intraocular pressure. **If the intraocular pressure remains elevated, reexplore the lateral canthal tendon region to make sure that it has been completely transected.** Occasionally, the intraorbital and intraocular pressures will remain elevated despite successful cantholysis. These refractory cases necessitate emergent

decompression of the deep orbital wall.[7] Such decompressions call for operative techniques that are to be performed by Ophthalmologists and Otolaryngologists.

The resolution of proptosis, afferent pupillary defects, and restoration of visual acuity will usually not occur immediately. Patients who respond to surgical intervention will gradually regain their visual acuity over a period of hours to days.

AFTERCARE

Apply a topical antibiotic ointment along the canthotomy site. In orbital compartment syndromes, elevated intraocular pressures merely reflect elevated intraorbital pressures. Therefore, any attempts to decrease intraocular pressures will not reliably reduce retrobulbar optic nerve compression. Medical interventions decreasing intraocular pressure may be used following, or in conjunction with, a lateral canthotomy and cantholysis. These interventions are similar to those employed for the management of elevated intraocular pressures in patients with acute angle-closure glaucoma. They include the use of topical beta-blockers, mannitol, acetazolamide, and centrally acting alpha agonists. **These medications are not a substitute for surgical orbital decompression.**

Most patients with an orbital compartment syndrome are critically ill and will be admitted to the intensive care unit following their Emergency Department evaluation and treatment. Ensure a timely Ophthalmologic consultation for a complete eye exam and possible repair of the canthotomy and cantholysis sites once the orbital compartment syndrome resolves. Repair of the lateral canthal fold and lateral canthal tendon is controversial. Many Ophthalmologists do not advocate suture repair, as a majority of wounds heal without complication by secondary intention. Patients with no other acute medical or traumatic conditions, restored vision, a normal ophthalmologic examination, and normal post-procedural intraocular pressures may be discharged after evaluation by an Ophthalmologist.

COMPLICATIONS

Time constraints, abnormal anatomy (resulting from traumatized tissue), and lack of familiarity with the lateral canthotomy and cantholysis techniques can make this a challenging procedure. Hemorrhage is often minimal and can be controlled with direct pressure. Mechanical injuries include globe perforation, injury of the lacrimal gland and artery, injury of the lateral rectus muscle, scleral lacerations, and secondary ectropions. Most of these complications can be prevented by knowing and identifying the anatomic landmarks, reviewing the procedure before it is performed, and using extreme care in performing the canthotomy and cantholysis. Despite the use of sterile technique, infections at the canthotomy and cantholysis sites can occur. They should be treated with parenteral antibiotics that cover typical skin flora.

SUMMARY

Emergency Physicians must be able to promptly recognize and manage an acute orbital compartment syndrome, defined by an acute elevation of intraorbital pressure with resultant ocular dysfunction. Patients will present with ocular pain, proptosis, an afferent pupillary defect, and diminished visual acuity. An acute orbital compartment syndrome requires emergent treatment to preserve vision. Immediate lateral canthotomy and cantholysis are indicated, preferably within 1 hour of injury and ocular dysfunction. The primary therapy is surgical intervention. Medical management should be considered adjunctive therapy.

REFERENCES

1. Fry HJH: Orbital decompression after facial fractures. *Med J Aust* 1967; 1:264–267.
2. Hislop WS, Dutton GN, Douglas PS: Treatment of retrobulbar haemorrhage in accident and emergency departments. *Br J Oral Maxillofac Surg* 1996; 34:289–292.
3. Kersten RC, Rice CD: Subperiosteal orbital hematoma: visual recovery following delayed drainage. *Ophthalm Surg* 1987; 18:423–427.
4. Cartwright MJ, Ginsburg RN, Nelson CC: Tension pneumoorbitus. *Ophthal Plast Reconstr Surg* 1992; 8:303–304.
5. Fleishman JA, Beck RW, Hoffman RO: Orbital emphysema as an ophthalmologic emergency. *Ophthalmology* 1984; 91:1389–1391.
6. Jordan DR, White GL, Anderson RL, et al: Orbital emphysema: a potential blinding complication following orbital fractures. *Ann Emerg Med* 1988; 17:853–855.
7. Hunts JH, Patrinely JR, Stal S: Orbital hemorrhage during rhinoplasty. *Ann Plast Surg* 1996; 37:618–623.
8. Petrelli RL, Petrelli EA, Allen WE: Orbital hemorrhage with loss of vision. *Am J Ophthalmol* 1980; 89:593–597.
9. Anderson RL, Edwards JJ: Bilateral visual loss after blepharoplasty. *Ann Plast Surg* 1980; 5:288–292.
10. Stewart WB, Toth BA: A multidisciplinary approach to orbital neoplasm. *Clin Plastic Surg* 1988; 15:263–272.
11. Hislop WS, Dutton GN: Retrobulbar hemorrhage: can blindness be prevented? *Injury* 1994; 25:663–665.
12. Hargaden M, Goldberg SH, Cunningham D, et al: Optic neuropathy following simulation of orbital hemorrhage in the nonhuman primate. *Ophthalm Plast Reconstr Surg* 1996; 12:264–272.
13. Linberg JV: Orbital compartment syndromes following trauma. *Adv Ophthalm Plast Reconstr Surg* 1987; 6:51–62.
14. Gioia VM, Linberg JV, McCormick SA: The anatomy of the lateral canthal tendon. *Arch Ophthalmol* 1987; 105:529–533.
15. Sacks SH, Lawson W, Edelstein D, et al: Surgical treatment of blindness secondary to intraorbital hemorrhage. *Arch Otolaryngol Head Neck Surg* 1988; 114:801–804.
16. Schabdach DG, Goldberg SH, Breton ME, et al: An animal model of visual loss from orbital hemorrhage. *Ophthalm Plast Reconstr Surg* 1994; 10:200–205.
17. Young VL, Gumucio CA, Lund H, et al: Long-term effect of retrobulbar hematomas on the vision of cynomolgus monkeys. *Plast Reconstr Surg* 1992; 89:70–75.
18. Hayreh SS, Weingest TA: Experimental occlusion of the central retinal artery of the retina: I. Ophthalmoscopic and fluorescein fundus angiographic studies. *Br J Ophthalmol* 1980; 64:896–912.
19. Hamasaki DI, Kroll AJ: Experimental central retinal artery occlusion. *Arch Ophthalmol* 1968; 80:243–248.
20. Kroll AJ: Experimental central retinal artery occlusion. *Arch Ophthalmol* 1968; 79:453–469.
21. Hayreh SS, Weingest TA: Experimental occlusion of the central artery of the retina: IV. Retinal tolerance time to acute ischaemia. *Br J Ophthalmol* 1980; 64:818–825.
22. Mauriello JA, DeLuca J, Krieger A, et al: Management of traumatic optic neuropathy—a study of 23 patients. *Br J Ophthalmol* 1992; 76:349–352.
23. Muthukumar N: Traumatic haemorrhagic optic neuropathy: case report. *Br J Neurosurg* 1997; 11:166–167.
24. Frenkel REP, Spoor TC: Diagnosis and management of traumatic optic neuropathies. *Adv Ophthalmol Plast Reconstr Surg* 1987; 6:71–90.
25. Krausen AS, Ogura JH, Burde RM, et al: Emergency orbital decompression: a reprieve from blindness. *Otolaryngol Head Neck Surg* 1981; 89:252–256.
26. Heinze JB, Hueston JT: Blindness after blepharoplasty: mechanism and early reversal. *Plast Reconstr Surg* 1978; 61:347–354.
27. Jafek BW, Kreiger AE, Morledge D: Blindness following blepharoplasty. *Arch Otolaryngol* 1973; 98:366–369.
28. Goldberg RA, Marmor MF, Shorr N, et al: Blindness following blepharoplasty: two case reports, and a discussion of management. *Ophthalmol Surg* 1990; 21:85–89.

Chapter 140
GLOBE LUXATION REDUCTION

Jeffrey S. Schlab

INTRODUCTION

Luxation of the globe is a rare event whereby the eyelids slip behind the midcoronal plane of the eye in an extremely proptosed eyeball (Figure 140-1). The orbicularis oculi muscle then goes into spasm, which maintains the luxation of the globe. Extraocular eye movements become severely limited. The optic nerve and retinal vasculature are subjected to an abnormal amount of traction, resulting in possible damage to these structures or the retina.[1]

ANATOMY AND PATHOPHYSIOLOGY

There are three major causes of globe luxation: spontaneous, voluntary, and traumatic. Spontaneous luxation tends to occur in individuals with shallow orbits.[2] Structural abnormalities—such as laxity of the supporting muscles and fascia as well as anomalous extraocular muscles—can predispose to spontaneous luxation.[2–4] Pathologic processes that cause proptosis can predispose to luxation. The literature documents cases of luxation associated with orbital tumors, Graves' disease, cerebral gummas, histiocytosis X, and craniofacial dysostosis.[1,5,6] Voluntary luxation occurs in individuals who learn to cause globe propulsion by using a digit or use of their extraocular muscles. Some patients use a Valsalva maneuver to luxate their globe(s) voluntarily. Traumatic luxation results from trauma to the globe or the surrounding bony orbit. It can occur from motor vehicle accidents or even relatively minor trauma to the face.[7,8] Traumatic luxation can also occur from intentional eye gouging or even during the forceps-assisted delivery of a neonate.[9,10]

The normal anatomic relationship of the globe to the surrounding structures is seen in Figure 140-2. The midcoronal plane of the eye is a transverse section through the eye in the coronal plane. It is through the widest portion of the eye and divides the eye into anterior and posterior halves. When the eyelids get behind the midcoronal plane, the orbicularis oculi muscle is pulled taut and begins to go into spasm. This spasm prevents spontaneous reduction of the globe.

INDICATIONS

Globe reduction is indicated to relieve traction on the optic nerve and retinal vessels. The patient's visual acuity has the potential of being compromised without prompt reduction. Sustained globe luxation is physically and psychologically uncomfortable for the patient, may result in permanent loss of vision, and is difficult to reduce without general anesthesia.

CONTRAINDICATIONS

Obvious rupture of the globe and extensive orbital fractures that require immediate surgical intervention are relative contraindications to globe reduction. Edema and retrobulbar hemorrhage can make reduction outside the Operating Room impossible.[1,6]

EQUIPMENT

Topical ocular anesthetic (0.5% proparacaine or 0.5% tetracaine)
Sterile gauze and gloves
Sutures or eyelid retractors
Local anesthetic solution (1% lidocaine), if eyelid retaining sutures need to be placed
3 mL syringe
27 gauge needle

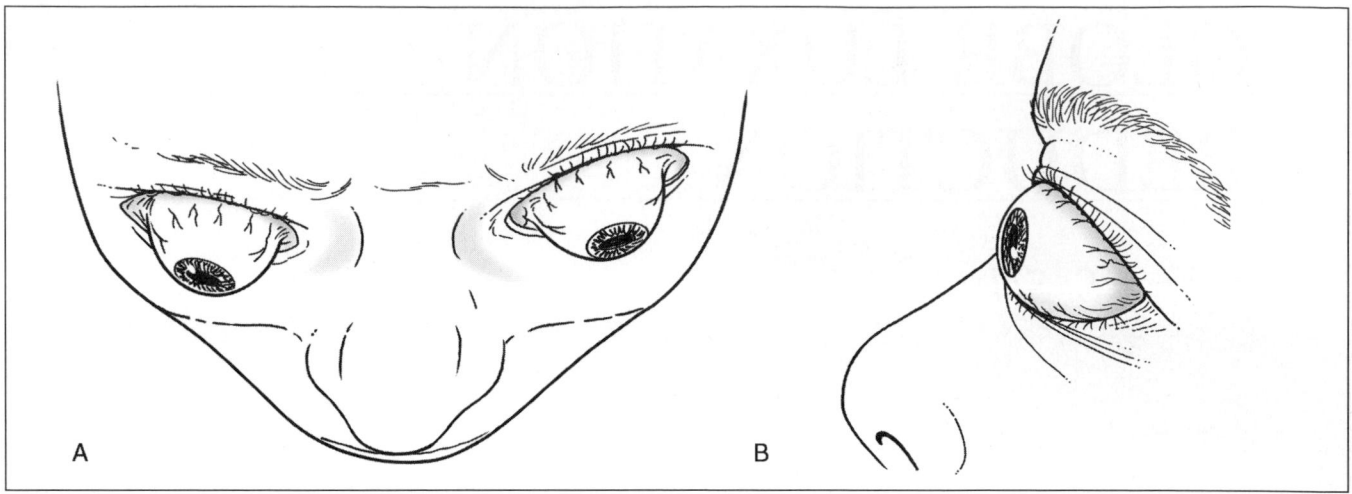

FIGURE 140-1 The luxated globe. *A.* Superior view. *B.* Lateral view.

PATIENT PREPARATION

Prior to any attempt at reduction, a directed eye exam addressing the integrity of the globe, visual acuity, pupillary reactivity, and range of ocular motion should be performed. Describe the procedure to the patient and/or their representative. Answer any questions about the procedure and obtain an informed consent for the procedure. Place the patient supine. Instill a topical ocular anesthetic agent into the affected eye. Allow 1 to 2 minutes for the anesthetic to take full effect.

TECHNIQUE

Reduction of a globe luxation ideally requires two people (Figure 140-3). Instruct an assistant to apply steady upward and outward traction on the upper eyelid and downward and outward traction on the lower eyelid by grasping and pulling on the eyelashes. While traction is being applied to the eyelids, apply steady and gentle pressure with a gloved thumb to the globe until it is manipulated back into the orbit.[1,6]

If the eyelashes are not accessible or an assistant is not available, an eyelid retractor may be placed behind the eyelids to provide countertraction. Other authorities have recommended the placement of a suture through the anesthetized skin of the eyelids to help retract them.[1,4,6] **Extreme care must be taken to prevent penetration of the globe by the anesthetic needle or the suture needle if retaining stitches are placed in the eyelids.**

ASSESSMENT

After the procedure, a repeat and complete eye examination must be performed and documented. Pay special attention to visual acuity and range of extraocular muscle movement.[1,6,10] Full visual acuity may not return to baseline for several days or longer.[4] A search for possible causes of luxation should be initiated in the Emergency Department.[1] This includes but is not limited to thyroid function testing and orbital imaging to rule out a tumor. This evaluation should be performed after consultation with an Ophthalmologist.

AFTERCARE

Patients with spontaneous luxations that reduce without difficulty and who are without visual impairment may be discharged home after consultation with an Ophthalmologist. These patients require follow-up with the Ophthalmologist within 24 hours.[1,6] They should be instructed to avoid Valsalva maneuvers.[1] All patients with traumatic luxation require emergent Ophthalmologic consultation and imaging of the orbits.[1,6]

COMPLICATIONS

It is not uncommon for eyelashes to be retained in the conjunctival fornices after this procedure.[10] A thorough evaluation and removal of any free eyelashes is warranted to prevent corneal abrasions or injury.[1,6,10] If one

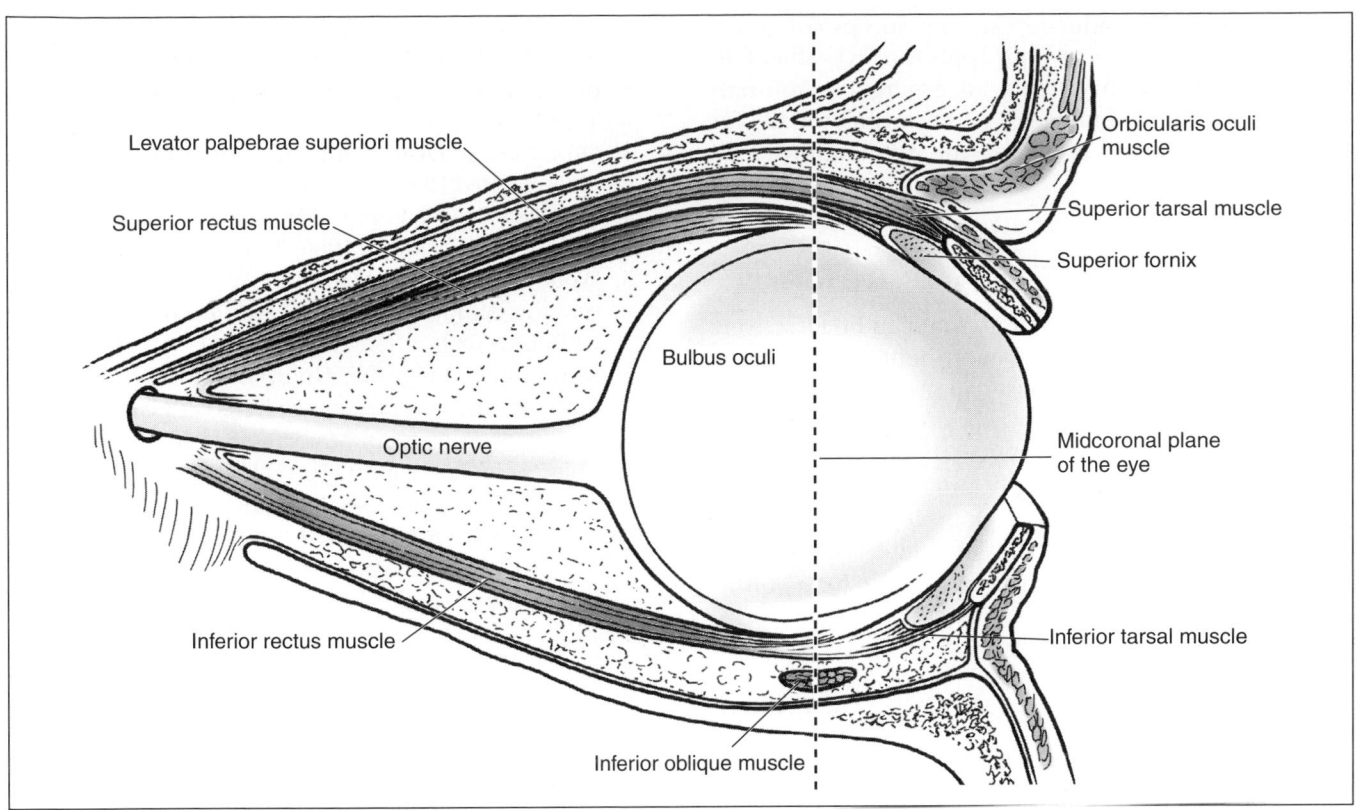

FIGURE 140-2 Anatomy of the eye and orbit.

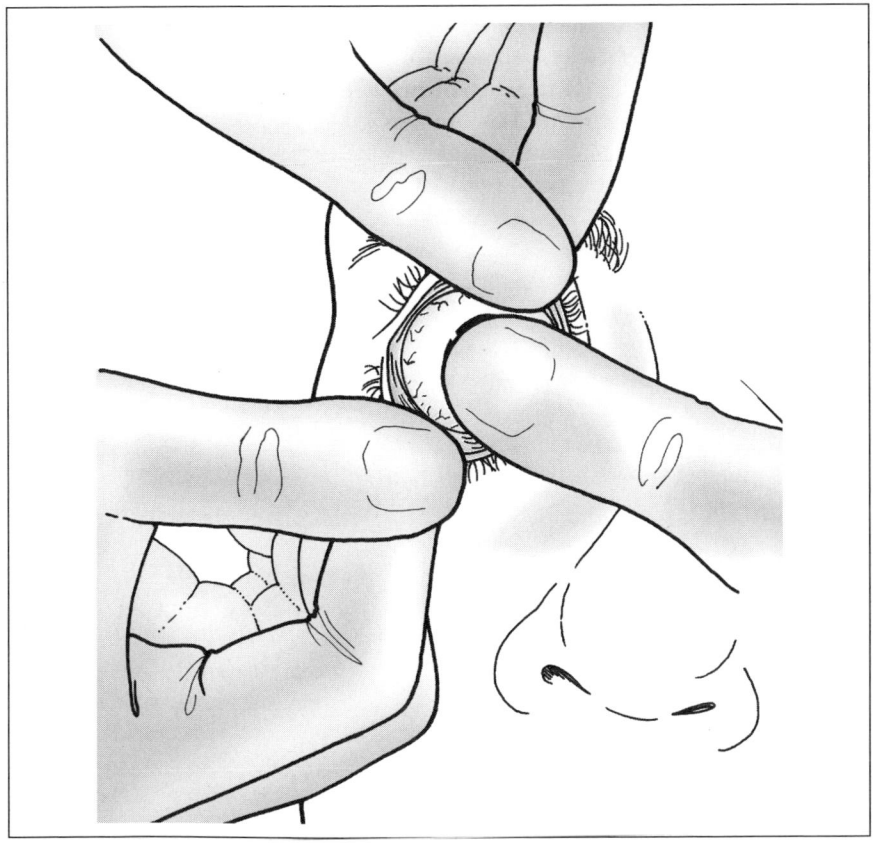

FIGURE 140-3 Reduction of a globe luxation.

or two attempts at reduction are not successful, instill saline drops to the eye and apply an eye shield to prevent further injury while an emergent Ophthalmologic consult is obtained.[1,6] Refer to Chapter 138 for the complete details regarding the application of an eye shield.

SUMMARY

Globe luxation is a rare entity that can be effectively dealt with in the Emergency Department. Prompt intervention by an Emergentologist can result in the preservation of visual acuity. After a brief initial eye examination, uncomplicated cases can be reduced by the Emergency Physician. Complicating factors—such as the presence of trauma, open globe injury, or inability to reduce the globe—warrant emergent Ophthalmologic consultation. Predisposing factors for spontaneous luxation should be investigated.

REFERENCES

1. Love JN, Bertram-Love NE: Luxation of the globe. *Am J Emerg Med* 1993; 11(1):61–63.

2. Alexandrakis G, Tse DT, Chang WJ: Spontaneous globe luxation associated with floppy eyelid syndrome and shallow orbits. *Arch Ophthalmol* 1999; 117(1):138–139.

3. Offenbach B: Dislocation (luxation) of the eyeball. *N Engl J Med* 1954; 251(9):338–339.

4. Chhabra HN, Kawuma AMS: Luxation of the eyeball. *Br J Ophthalmol* 1986; 70:150–151.

5. Wood CM, Pearson ADJ, Craft AW, et al: Globe luxation in histiocytosis X. *Br J Ophthalmol* 1988; 72(8):631–633.

6. Samples JR, Hedges JR: Ophthalmologic procedures, in Roberts JR, Hedges JR (eds): *Clinical Procedures in Emergency Medicine,* 3rd ed. Philadelphia: Saunders, 1998:1116–1119.

7. Reuling FH, Hadlund RL: Traumatic luxation of the globe. *EENT Monthly* 1970; 49(3):129–130.

8. Van Der Wal KGH, Van Der Pol BAE: Traumatic luxation of the eyeball. *J Craniomaxillofac Surg* 1991; 19(5):205–207.

9. Fowler JG: Spontaneous luxation of the eyeball. *JAMA* 1941; 116:1206–1208.

10. Zengin N, Karakurt A, Gültan E, et al: Traumatic globe luxation. *Acta Ophthalmol* 1992; 70(6):844–846.

Section Twelve

OTOLARYNGOLOGIC PROCEDURES

Chapter 141
EXTERNAL AUDITORY CANAL FOREIGN BODY REMOVAL

Rebecca R. Roberts

INTRODUCTION

Foreign bodies are commonly found in the external auditory canal (EAC) of children and mentally impaired adults. Children commonly place small objects such as food (beans, peas, corn, seeds) or small round objects (beads, rocks, toys) in the EAC.[1-4] Adults are more likely to suffer from items used to clean or scratch the ear (cotton, paper, pencil lead) and insects that crawl into the ear, especially cockroaches.[3] The EAC and tympanic membrane are exquisitely sensitive and delicate.[2,5] Foreign bodies in the EAC are extremely irritating to patients and, unless proper care is taken in removal, can cause injuries.

ANATOMY

The EAC is S-shaped and 2.5 cm long in adults.[6] The lateral or distal third is cartilaginous, with thick skin; it has more hair follicles, glands, and subcutaneous tissue than the medial or proximal two-thirds, which is bony, with a thinner, more fragile layer of skin.[6,7] The narrowed isthmus is located between the cartilaginous and bony portions.[1,6] The canal ends medially at the tympanic membrane, which is situated obliquely to increase the surface area for carrying sound energy to the middle ear.[7] The anteroinferior EAC is 0.6 mm longer than the posterosuperior portion.[6] Auriculotemporal branches of cranial nerves V, VII, IX, and X and the greater auricular nerve of the cervical plexus supply sensation to the EAC.[6]

INDICATIONS

All EAC foreign bodies should be removed. The need to remove the foreign body is individualized to the patient, type of foreign body, physician preference and experience, and availability of an Otolaryngologist. The only question is how quickly this must be done, who should do it, and which is the safest of available techniques. Some foreign bodies are very easily and safely removed with the equipment available in any Emergency Department. Others—due to impaction, large size, sharp edges, location in the canal, involvement of the tympanic membrane or middle ear structures, or patient age—will require removal under general anesthesia or even an approach to removal from outside the canal.[1,5,8]

The most urgent indication for immediate removal is an alkaline button battery because of the extensive and severe damage it may cause in a very short time. These are most commonly found in the EAC of a young child. There are two mechanisms for the rapid destruction of surrounding tissues by the batteries. The moisture and cerumen in the EAC have a high conductivity, which causes conduction of electric current from the battery and results in localized electrical burns. Local inflammation from burns will cause a fluid exudation into the EAC. This increases the electrical conduction injury and causes the battery to begin leaking alkaline electrolyte solution, which can penetrate deeply into underlying tissues, with resultant liquefaction necrosis.[2,9]

CONTRAINDICATIONS

Rather than contraindications to removal, these can also be thought of as indications for referral to an Otolaryngologist for removal of the foreign body. The major contraindication to removal in the Emergency Department is probable injury with direct removal. Examples are foreign bodies that have perforated or impaled the tympanic membrane. Removal will cause further damage to the tympanic membrane as well as potential disruption of the middle ear ossicles and loss of hearing. These foreign bodies require removal under general anesthesia with the aid of an operating microscope.[1,2,4,8] Another contraindication is a large object that has impaled itself in the wall of the EAC. Direct removal will require anesthesia and possibly an approach from outside the canal to avoid denuding the skin of the EAC.[2] Finally, objects that are difficult to remove and a patient (usually a young child) who cannot hold still or be held still for the procedure should be referred to an Otolaryngologist.[1,4,8] These cases are likely to result in injury to the patient if the foreign body is removed in the Emergency Department.

Irrigation is almost always safe to attempt. The most important contraindication for irrigating the EAC is an acute or chronically ruptured tympanic membrane.[8,10–12] Water forced into the middle ear can lead to otitis media, labyrinthitis, mastoiditis, disruption of the ossicles, and loss of balance or hearing. Some authors recommend alternate methods for any patient who has never had an ear exam to document the integrity of the tympanic membrane.[8,10] Completely impacted foreign bodies, leaving no space that would allow the irrigant to flow behind it, will only be driven deeper into the canal, making subsequent removal even more difficult.[13] A relative contraindication for irrigation with water is an organic object, such as a bean or rice, which will absorb water and swell, making removal more difficult.[13] If the object is very small and irrigation is expected to rapidly succeed in removal before swelling occurs, it can be attempted. Otherwise, the object can be irrigated with alcohol, removed with instruments, or extracted with suction.

Directly grasping the foreign body with forceps is contraindicated for large or spherical objects that will not allow clear passage of the forceps jaws along its sides. Attempts to grab this type of object will only drive it further back into the EAC.[8,13]

EQUIPMENT

Anesthesia

Local anesthetic solution, 1% lidocaine
1 mL syringe
5 mL syringe
27 or 30 gauge needle
EAC speculum

Irrigation

10 to 20 mL syringe
Butterfly catheter with any size needle
Kidney basins
One Chux or other water barrier
Tap water or saline at or slightly above body
    temperature[5,11,12]

Alternate Irrigation Equipment[7]

Plastic portion of 18 gauge angiocatheter
Oral jet-irrigation device (Water-Pik)
deVillbiss irrigator (requires a compressed air source)
Metal ear syringe

Instruments to Pass behind Object and Pull It Out (Figure 141-1)

Ear curettes or cerumen spoon, metal or disposable
    plastic
Wire loop
Blunt or ball right-angle hook

Instruments Used to Grasp Object Directly (Figure 141-1)

Alligator forceps
Hartman forceps

Suction

Frazier suction tips
Intravenous tubing with flange created at tip using heat
    source
Vacuum/suction source
Connection tubing
Hemostat

Cyanoacrylate Glue[15]

Ear speculum
Cyanoacrylate glue or Superglue
Paper clip or other small stick-shaped object
Superglue removal equipment

Cyanoacrylate Glue Removal[16]

Acetone to debond glue from skin
Cotton balls
Cotton-tipped applicators
Irrigation or instruments for final removal

Commercially Available Devices

Hognose otoscope tip
Oto-Nasal Extractor

PATIENT PREPARATION

Explain the procedure and potential complications to the patient and/or their representative. The most convenient position for adult patients is to remain seated

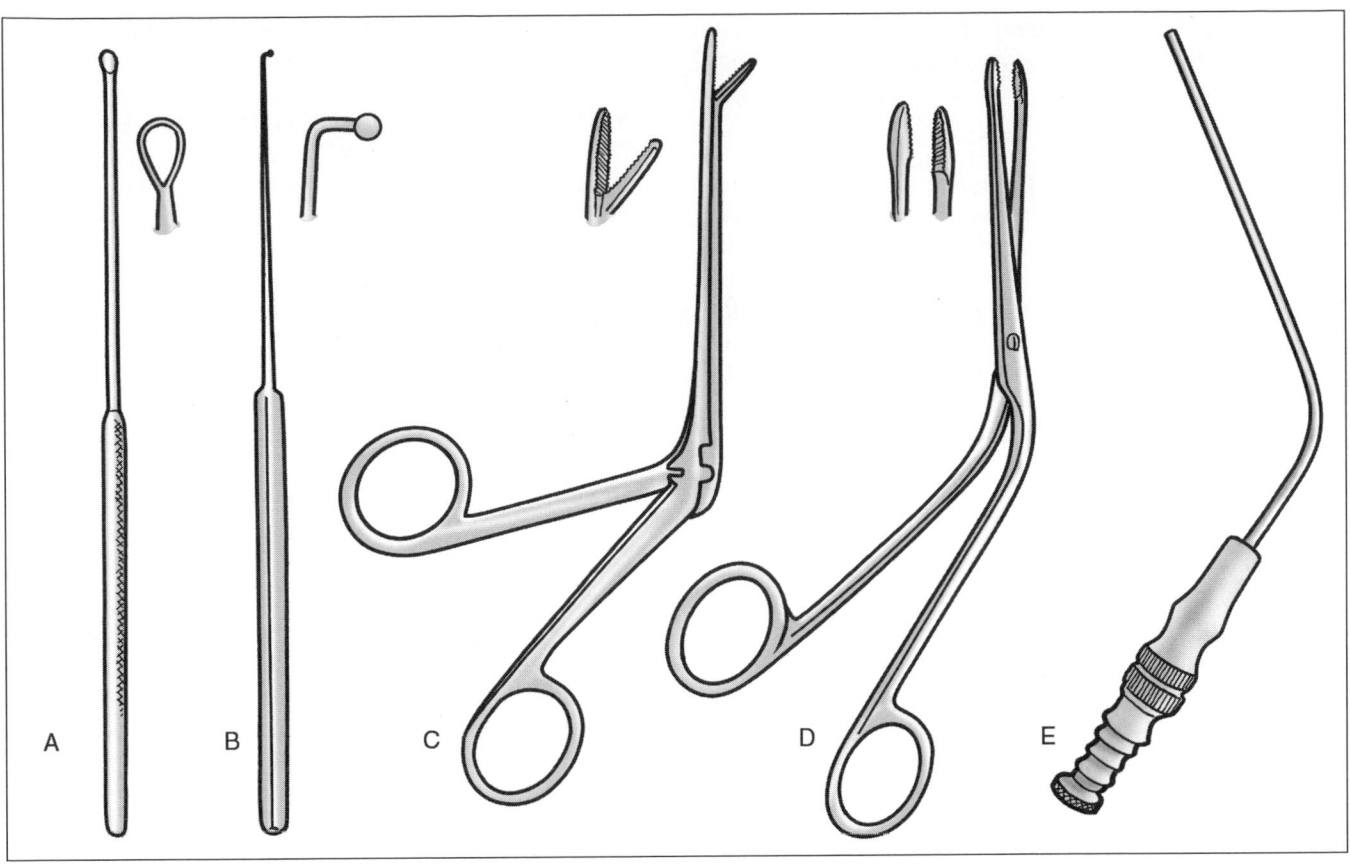

FIGURE 141-1 Instruments used for removal of foreign bodies from the external auditory canal. *A.* Cerumen loop. *B.* Right-angle ball hook. *C.* Alligator forceps. *D.* Hartman forceps. *E.* Frazier suction catheter.

with the affected ear facing the physician. Children can sit on the lap of a parent or attendant with the affected ear facing the physician. The parent or attendant should wrap one arm around the child's body and arms while the other stabilizes the head.[2] Smaller children can be swaddled in a papoose made from a sheet and tape or a commercial immobilization device.[2] The child may be placed supine with their head facing the ceiling. The child should not be placed with the affected ear facing up, as this may cause the foreign body to move farther into the canal. All techniques require the EAC to be straightened. In the adult, this is accomplished by pulling the pinna up and back while simultaneously pulling it slightly out from the head.[7] In the small child, pull the pinna down, back, and slightly out from the head.[5,7]

The patient may require anesthesia of the EAC. Turn the affected ear toward the ceiling and fill the EAC with 5 to 10 mL of lidocaine using the syringe tip, an angiocatheter, or a butterfly catheter with the needle cut off. This will result in substantial but short-lived topical anesthesia for the procedure. If the effect wears off before the procedure is complete, the topical application of lidocaine can be repeated as needed or longer-acting

agents may be used. Although usually not necessary, local anesthetic solution may be injected to provide analgesia. Fill a 1 mL syringe with local anesthetic solution and apply a 27 to 30 gauge needle. Position a plastic or metal EAC speculum in the EAC. Insert the needle through the speculum and inject 0.25 mL subcutaneously in the superior and inferior quadrants distal to the isthmus. If needed, all four quadrants can be injected.[14] Refer to Chapter 144 for a complete discussion of EAC anesthesia.

TECHNIQUES

PRECAUTIONS FOR USING INSTRUMENTS IN THE EAC

There are two major precautions the physician must take to avoid pushing the foreign body further into the ear or causing damage to the EAC and tympanic membrane. First, the procedures must be performed under direct vision.[7] Second, the hand holding the instruments must remain firmly in contact with the patient's head at all times to stabilize the hand and avoid abrading or puncturing the canal wall or damaging the tympanic membrane should the patient move.[1,7] Even a very co-operative patient may move due to an involuntary reflex cough.[5]

IRRIGATION

Irrigation is the safest method of foreign body removal.[1,7,8,17] It is most successful for nonimpacted, smaller foreign bodies. Tuck a water barrier into the patient's gown or collar. Place a kidney basin under the ear and against the cheek to catch the irrigation solution and the foreign body. The patient or an assistant can hold the basin in place. Attach a butterfly needle to a 10 to 20 mL syringe. Cut off the needle and most of the tubing, leaving only 1 to 2 cm of the tubing. This remaining tubing will usually be curved, which is optimal for directing the irrigation stream.

Draw up body temperature tap water or saline from another kidney basin into the syringe. Insert the butterfly tubing 1 cm into the EAC with the tip aimed upward and away from the foreign body[11] (Figure 141-2). Rapidly inject the irrigating solution. This will cause the water to shoot past the foreign body, bounce off the tympanic membrane, and carry the foreign body along with it as it exits the EAC.[1,8]

Care must be taken to make sure that the irrigation stream can easily exit the EAC, so as to prevent increased hydrostatic pressure resulting in damage to the tympanic membrane.[10] Sometimes irrigation will not completely remove the object but force an object located

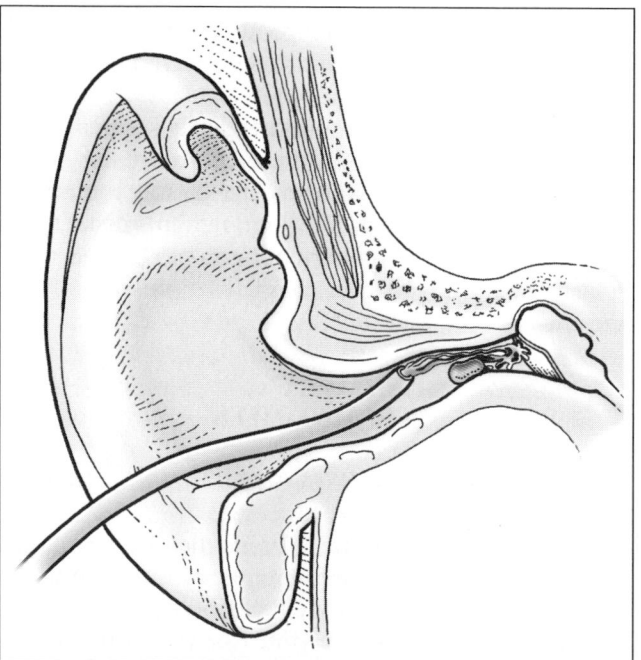

FIGURE 141-2 Irrigation with butterfly catheter tubing attached to a syringe. The stream of fluid is aimed toward the top of the external auditory canal and above the foreign body.

very deeply more laterally, where an instrument can be safely used to grasp and remove it.

SLIDING FOREIGN BODY OUT WITH AN INSTRUMENT FROM BEHIND

This technique requires either a cerumen spoon or wire loop for small objects or a right-angle hook for larger ones (Figures 141-1A and B). Pass the tip of the instrument over and behind the foreign body with the spoon, loop, or hook in the same plane as the EAC wall. Rotate the instrument 90 degrees to bring the loop or hook directly in contact with the back (medial) side of the object. Gently pull the instrument out of the EAC, pulling the foreign body out with it.[1,7]

GRASPING FOREIGN BODIES WITH FORCEPS

If this maneuver is to be successful, there must be sufficient space between the EAC wall and the foreign body, or a projecting edge, that can be grasped, so as to avoid pushing it further into the canal.[1,3,8] This technique is contraindicated if the object is spherical and located against the tympanic membrane, which can be injured during the removal.[3] The most commonly used instruments include the alligator forceps (Figure 141-1C) and the Hartman forceps (Figure 141-1D). Insert the forceps into the EAC and grasp the foreign body (Figure 141-3). Withdraw the instrument and the foreign body gently in order to avoid abrading the EAC wall.

SUCTION REMOVAL

Frazier suction catheters are most useful with small foreign bodies (Figure 141-1E). Otherwise, this technique will be unsuccessful or will push the object farther into the EAC. Attach the Frazier suction catheter to the suction tubing. Turn on the suction source. Insert the catheter into the EAC. Place a thumb over the hole in the catheter handle to direct the suction through the tip of the catheter. Gently advance the suction catheter until the tip is in contact with the foreign body. Withdraw the suction catheter and foreign body from the EAC.

For impacted smooth, spherical objects, suction with plastic intravenous tubing can be used.[18] Cut a short length of plastic intravenous tubing and attach one end to the negative pressure source. Fashion the other end into a small flange shape using a heat source and any metal object with a rounded end, such as the tip of a hemostat or larger clamp. Heat the jaws of the hemostat and insert them into the plastic tubing just enough to create a flange. Turn on the suction source. Place a hemostat onto the tubing to temporarily clamp the suction tubing. Gently advance the flange tip into the EAC until it contacts the foreign body, taking care not to push it inward (Figure 141-4). Remove the hemostat from the tubing to activate the suction. Gently but quickly remove the tubing and attached foreign body from the EAC.

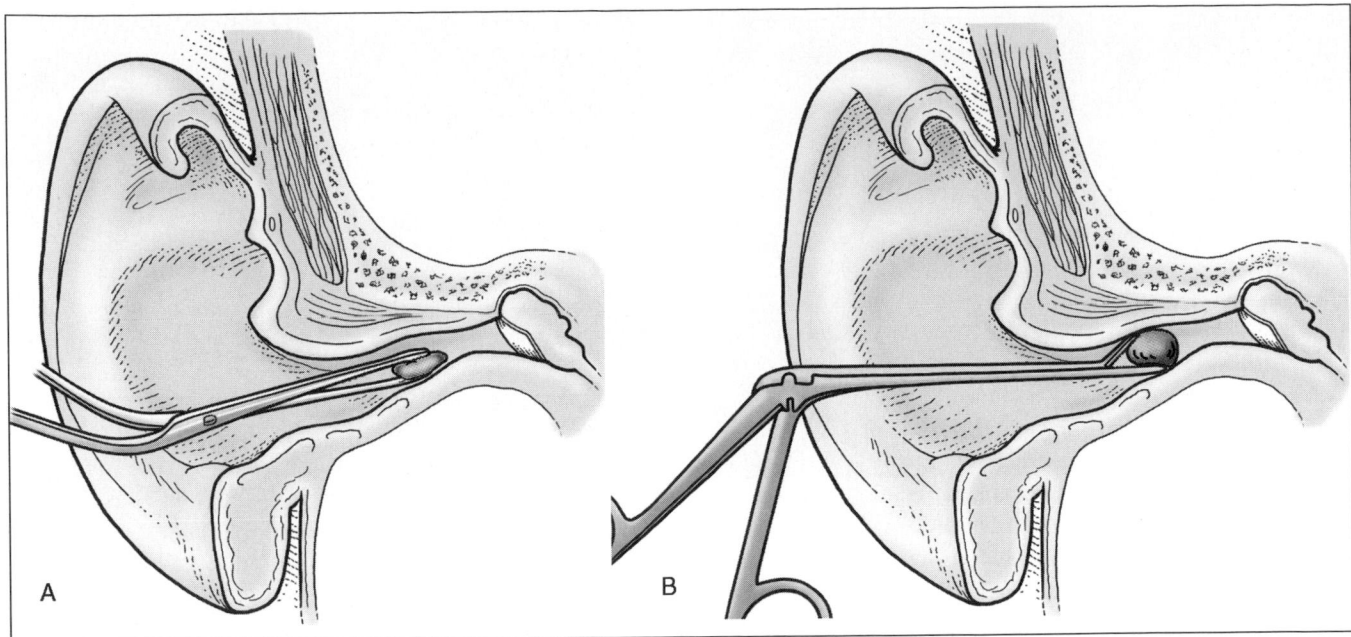

FIGURE 141-3 Forceps removal of a foreign body. *A.* Hartman forceps. *B.* Alligator forceps.

CYANOACRYLATE GLUE–ASSISTED REMOVAL

Cyanoacrylate glue can be used to extract impacted spherical objects that allow no space for irrigation or instrument removal and are located laterally or distally in the EAC.[15] Insert an ear speculum into the EAC with the tip near the foreign body. Do not touch the foreign body with the speculum so as to prevent it from being impacted. The ear speculum will prevent the physician from touching the EAC with glue.

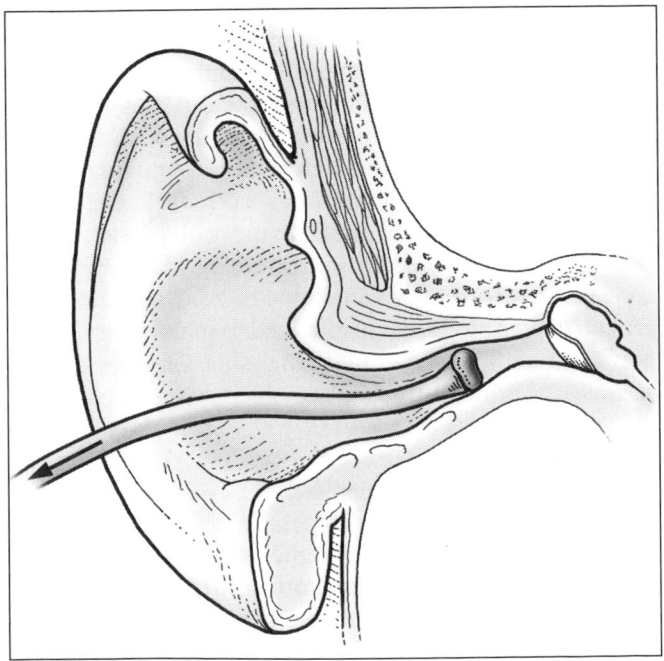

FIGURE 141-4 Suction removal of a foreign body.

Obtain a long, thin object (straightened paper clip or cotton-tipped applicator stick). Moisten the tip of the paper clip or applicator stick with a very tiny amount of cyanoacrylate glue. A larger amount can drop off into the EAC. Quickly insert the paper clip or applicator stick through the ear speculum, before the glue dries, until it just touches the foreign body. Maintain this position for 15 to 20 seconds to allow bonding of the glue to the foreign body. Remove the paper clip or applicator stick with the foreign body attached.

REMOVAL OF CYANOACRYLATE GLUE

For either iatrogenic or patient-introduced cyanoacrylate glue, debonding from the patient's tissues by acetone must precede the removal.[16] Failure to do this will result in tearing of the skin or tympanic membrane. Infuse acetone into the EAC using cotton balls or swabs. Allow it to remain in the EAC for 5 minutes. Since acetone evaporates rapidly, several applications may be necessary. Once the glue mass is free, it can be removed by irrigation, instruments, or suction.

HOGNOSE OTOSCOPE TIP

The Hognose (IQDr. Incorporated, Austin, TX) is a disposable single-use device that attaches to a standard otoscope (Figure 141-5). The tip is soft, self-molding, and looks like the nose of a hog. It has an insufflation port and suction tubing attached to its side.

Attach the Hognose to the otoscope. Turn on the otoscope's light source. Attach the tubing to a suction source. Turn on the suction source to low or medium. Insert the Hognose into the EAC while visualizing the

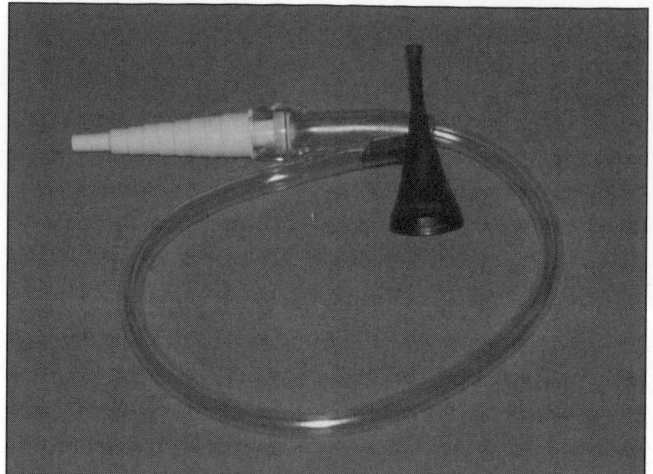

FIGURE 141-5 The Hognose otoscope tip.

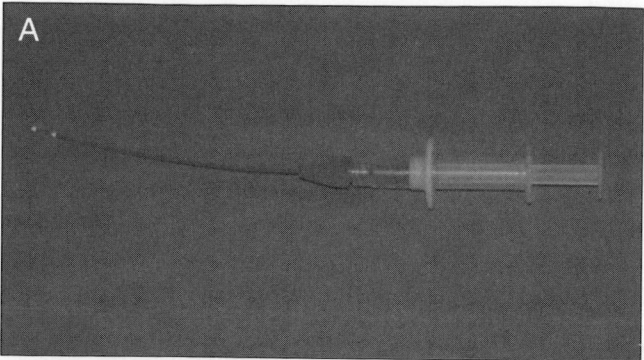

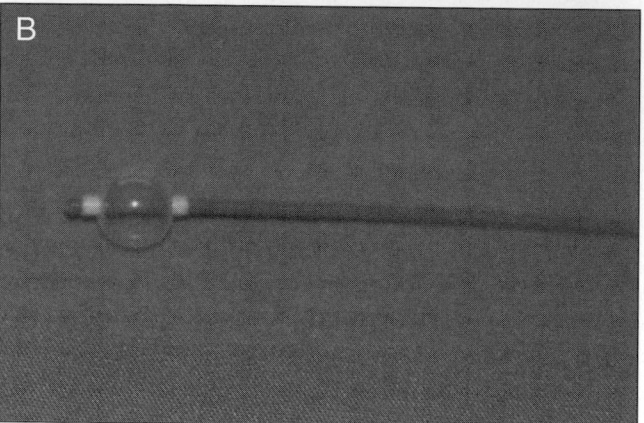

FIGURE 141-6 The Oto-Nasal Extractor. *A.* Overview of the unit with the balloon deflated. *B.* The distal end with the balloon inflated.

foreign body. When the tip of the Hognose is just next to the foreign body, place a finger over the insufflation port to engage the suction. Gently advance the otoscope until the tip of the Hognose is against and attached to the foreign body. While maintaining suction, withdraw the Hognose with the foreign body attached.

OTO-NASAL EXTRACTOR

The Oto-Nasal Extractor (Inhealth Technologies, Carpinteria, CA) is a device designed to extract foreign bodies from the nasal and auditory passages (Figure 141-6). It is a disposable single-use device consisting of a balloon-tipped catheter attached to a syringe.

Inflate the balloon and inspect it for any air leaks. Deflate the balloon. Insert the catheter along the wall of the EAC until the balloon is just past the foreign body. Inflate the balloon by depressing the plunger on the syringe. Withdraw the catheter and foreign body from the EAC while maintaining the balloon in the inflated state. If the foreign body has a central hole (e.g., candy or bead), insert the catheter through the hole rather than around it.

LIVE INSECT REMOVAL

A live insect in the EAC is one of the most painful and upsetting foreign bodies. Patients suffer as the insect moves, vibrates, and claws the sensitive tympanic membrane in an effort to escape.[2] In the past, mineral oil was infused to smother and kill the insect prior to removal.[3,13,19] However, this method has several disadvantages. A significant time passes while the patient is still suffering and the insect dies. Due to being stuck in the viscous oil, the insect is more difficult to remove and frequently breaks into multiple pieces. The EAC is now impossible to anesthetize with a local infusion of lidocaine, which is repelled by the oil.

A preferred technique is to immobilize the insect with an infusion of 1% lidocaine into the EAC.[19] A topical anesthetic composed of benzocaine and antipyrine (Auralgan) may also be used to provide anesthesia. In this way the insect becomes inert more quickly than with oil. The EAC and tympanic membrane are thus anesthetized for patient comfort and the insect is more likely to be removed in a single piece than with mineral oil.

The insect can then be easily removed by irrigation or instrument removal. Sometimes both techniques are used. Irrigation can be used to move the dead insect more distally in the EAC, followed by instrument removal. It is recommended that the EAC be inspected and irrigated after the insect is removed to make sure that no tiny parts of the insect remain in the EAC, as they can be a cause of otitis externa.[2]

ASSESSMENT

After the foreign body has been removed, it is crucial to reexamine the ear to confirm that the EAC, tympanic membrane, and hearing are all normal and have not been damaged.[2,3,17] In children, but also adults with psychiatric problems, it is prudent to examine the other ear, nose, and any other orifice that may be harboring an unsuspected foreign body.[2–4] Remaining irrigation fluid in the EAC should be removed to prevent otitis externa.[7]

AFTERCARE

Most authors recommend prescribing several days of topical otic drops to prevent or treat subclinical otitis externa, which is often precipitated by abrasion of the canal or inflammation due to foreign body impaction.[2] Commonly recommended drops include Cortisporin Otic, Domeboro Otic, Otobiotic, Pediotic, and VoSol Otic. Consult an Otolaryngologist for patients with injuries, hearing deficits, severe otitis externa, or in whom removal of the object was unsuccessful. All other patients can receive follow-up with a primary care physician in 48 to 72 hours. Patients should be instructed in the proper application of ear drops and told to return to the Emergency Department immediately if they develop ear pain, fever, decreased hearing, vertigo, headache, or a stiff neck.

COMPLICATIONS

Numerous complications can result from the removal of a foreign body from the EAC.[2–4,7,10,12,13,17] The complication rate for irrigation is 1 per 1000 cases.[12,17] It is higher for all other techniques.[7] Irrigation can push a foreign body further into the EAC. If the irrigating solution is cold, caloric stimulation can result in vomiting, vertigo, bradycardia, and syncope. Middle ear debris can be forced through a preexisting or iatrogenic tympanic membrane defect, resulting in otitis media, damage to the ossicles, labyrinthitis, mastoiditis, loss of hearing and balance, or central nervous system infection. Otitis externa can result from abrasions to the EAC. Butterfly tubing is less likely than the angiocatheter to damage the EAC or tympanic membrane because of its more pliable nature, larger diameter, and curved tip.

It is known that Water-Pik irrigation, even at low pressures, can rupture the tympanic membrane. For this reason, it cannot be recommended for the removal of foreign bodies from the EAC.

Instrumentation and suction should be used with caution to prevent secondary injury. This includes EAC lacerations or abrasions, tympanic membrane rupture, pushing of foreign bodies further into the EAC, and disruption or removal of the ossicles. Abrasions or lacerations to the EAC can result in otitis externa.

Cyanoacrylate glue can also cause problems. The physician may glue their fingers together or to the instruments. The foreign body may be glued to the skin of the EAC or the tympanic membrane. Removal of the glue can abrade and irritate the skin and/or tympanic membrane.

SUMMARY

Foreign bodies in the EAC are common. With adequate anesthesia, careful planning, and gentle handling, most foreign bodies can be successfully removed from the EAC. The removal techniques require equipment that is already available in the Emergency Department. The removal techniques are easy to perform, quick, and simple to learn. An impacted button battery is a true emergency and requires immediate removal. An emergent consultation with an Otolaryngologist is required if the button battery cannot be removed or if any evidence of injury is present after the button battery has been removed.

REFERENCES

1. Ballenger JJ, Snow JB: *Otorhinolaryngology: Head and Neck Surgery.* Baltimore: Williams & Wilkins, 1996:978–980.
2. Ansley JF: Treatment of aural foreign bodies in children. *Pediatrics* 1998; 101(4 pt 1):638–641.
3. Bressler K, Shelton C: Ear foreign-body removal: a review of 98 consecutive cases. *Laryngoscope* 1993; 103(4):367–370.
4. Balbani APS, Sanchez TG, Ossamu B, et al: Ear and nose foreign body removal in children. *Int J Pediatr Otorhinolaryngol* 1998; 46:37–42.
5. Burke M: Small things from small places. *Aust Fam Physician* 1999; 28(2):132–133.
6. Linstrom CJ, Lucente FE: Infections of the external ear, in Bailey BJ: *Head and Neck Surgery—Otolaryngology.* Philadelphia: Lippincott, 1993:1542–1544.
7. Manthey DE, Harrison BP: Otolaryngologic procedures, in Roberts JR, Hedges JR (eds): *Clinical Procedures in Emergency Medicine.* Philadelphia: Saunders, 1998:1120–1149.
8. Ballenger JJ: *Diseases of the Nose, Throat, Ear, Head, and Neck,* 14th ed. Philadelphia: Lea & Febiger, 1991.
9. McRae D, Premachandra DJ, Gatland DJ: Button batteries in the ear, nose, and cervical esophagus: a destructive foreign body. *J Otolaryngol* 1989; 18(6):317–319.
10. Ballachanda BB, Peers CJ: Cerumen management. Instruments and procedures. *ASHA* 1992; 34(2):43–46.
11. Carne S: Ear syringing. *Br Med J* 1980; 280(6211): 374–376.
12. Hanger HC, Mulley GP: Cerumen: its fascination and clinical importance: a review. *J R Soc Med* 1992; 85(6):346–349.

13. Scott-Brown WG, Kerr AG: *Scott-Brown's Otolaryngology,* vol 3, 6th ed. Oxford, England: Butterworth-Heinemann, 1997:11–12.

14. Scott-Brown WG, Kerr AG: *Scott-Brown's Otolaryngology,* 6th ed. Oxford, England: Butterworth-Heinemann, 1997.

15. Thompson MP: Removing objects from the external auditory canal. *N Engl J Med* 1984; 311(25):1635.

16. Abadir WF, Nakhla V, Chong P: Removal of superglue from the external ear using acetone: case report and literature review. *J Laryngol Otol* 1995; 109:1219–1221.

17. Sharp JF, Wilson JA, Ross L, et al: Ear wax removal: a survey of current practice. *Br Med J* 1990; 301(6763): 1251–1253.

18. Jensen JH: Technique for removing a spherical foreign body from the nose or ear. *Ear Nose Throat J* 1976; 55(8):270–271.

19. Schittek A: Insect in the external auditory canal—a new way out. *JAMA* 1980; 243(4):331.

Chapter 142

CERUMEN IMPACTION REMOVAL

Rebecca R. Roberts

INTRODUCTION

Removal of impacted cerumen is one of the most common otolaryngologic procedures performed by non-otolaryngologists. This procedure is also believed to be the most common cause of iatrogenic otolaryngologic complications referred to specialists.[1] In the United States, an estimated 150,000 ears are irrigated each week to remove cerumen.[2]

ANATOMY AND PATHOPHYSIOLOGY

The S-shaped external auditory canal (EAC) is 2.5 cm long in adults.[3] The lateral or distal third is cartilaginous, with thicker skin, more hair follicles, glands, and subcutaneous tissue than the medial or proximal two-thirds, which is bony and has a thinner, more fragile layer of skin.[3,4] The narrowed isthmus is located between the cartilaginous and bony portions.[3] The canal ends medially at the tympanic membrane, which is situated obliquely to increase the surface area for carrying sound energy to the middle ear.[4] The anteroinferior EAC is 0.6 mm longer than the posterosuperior portion.[3] Auriculotemporal branches of cranial nerves V, VII, IX, and X and the greater auricular nerve of the cervical plexus supply sensation to the EAC.[3]

Cerumen is a mixture comprising secretions of the ceruminous glands of the lateral two-thirds of the EAC, the pilosebaceous glands located at the roots of canal hairs, and sloughed squamous epithelial cells.[3,5] It is generally expelled naturally by migration assisted by chewing movements.[5,6]

There are many reasons for cerumen to become impacted.[4,5] The most common is self-cleaning with cotton-tipped applicator swabs that can push cerumen farther into the external auditory canal. Abundant hairs in the EAC, more commonly seen in males than females, can obstruct the migration of cerumen. Small (especially in children), tortuous, or scarred external auditory canals will obstruct cerumen migration. Some

people produce large quantities of cerumen. Diseases such as Parkinson's can alter the consistency of the cerumen and inhibit its migration. Hearing aids, stethoscope earpieces, or any other objects worn in the EAC may compact the cerumen. Deficits in the substance that causes sloughed squamous epithelial cells to separate will inhibit the movement of cerumen. Non-impacted cerumen exposed to water can swell and obstruct the EAC.

INDICATIONS

The primary indication for removal of impacted cerumen is symptomatology of significant impaction.[1] The most common complaint is hearing loss, which is often abrupt and expressed as a "blocked ear." Hearing remains normal or nearly so as long as there is a small space in the EAC through which sound can pass to reach the tympanic membrane. The hearing loss becomes subjectively significant when the canal is completely obstructed or the tympanic membrane is compressed by cerumen.[4,6] Other typical symptoms of cerumen impaction include pain, tinnitus, vertigo, unsteady gait, or reflex cough due to vagus nerve stimulation.[4,5] Other reasons to remove cerumen include the need to examine the ear canal and tympanic membrane or to test hearing.[6,7]

CONTRAINDICATIONS

The contraindications to cerumen removal are different for each of the techniques discussed. Nearly all cerumen can be safely removed by using one of the techniques listed. Often, two or more techniques can be used together with increased success.[4,7]

The most important contraindication for irrigating the EAC is an acute or chronically ruptured tympanic membrane.[5–8] Water forced into the middle ear can lead to otitis media, labyrinthitis, mastoiditis, disruption of the ossicles, and loss of balance or hearing.[8] Some authors recommend alternate methods for any patient who has never had an ear exam to document the integrity of the tympanic membrane.[7,8] Most patients can give you this information. A relative contraindication is moderate to severe otitis externa.[5,6]

The major contraindication to instrument removal is a patient, usually pediatric, who is so uncooperative that injury to the EAC or tympanic membrane is likely to occur with movement.[4] The second contraindication is cerumen pushed directly against the tympanic membrane. In these circumstances, the tympanic membrane can be abraded or perforated during the removal of cerumen.

The major contraindication to suction removal is a single, hard, irregular, and impacted cerumen plug. Suction will be unsuccessful. Suction works best if there are multiple tiny fragments or very soft cerumen.[7]

Cerumen softening agents should not be used if the patient has a ruptured tympanic membrane. Other contraindications to softening agents are an allergy to the agent or coexisting otitis externa.[5,9,10]

EQUIPMENT

Anesthesia

Local anesthetic solution or suspension (e.g., viscous lidocaine, lidocaine solution, or Auralgan)
3 mL syringe

Irrigation

10 to 20 mL syringe
Butterfly catheter with any size needle
Kidney basins
Chux or other water barrier
Tap water or saline at or slightly above body
temperature[5,6]

Alternate Irrigation Equipment[4]

Plastic portion of 18 gauge angiocatheter
Oral jet irrigation (Water-Pik); no longer recommended
(see "Complications," below)
deVillbiss irrigator, requires a compressed air source
Metal ear syringe

Instruments to Separate and Loosen Cerumen (Figure 142-1)

Ear curettes or cerumen spoon, metal or disposable
plastic
Wire loop
Blunt or ball right-angle hook

Instruments to Grasp Cerumen Directly (Figure 142-1)

Alligator forceps
Hartman forceps

Suction

Frazier suction catheters
Suction source
Connection tubing
Hemostat

Cerumen Softening Agents

Water
Olive or almond oil
5% sodium bicarbonate solution
Commercial agents (e.g., Cerumenex)

PATIENT PREPARATION

Explain the procedure and potential complications to the patient and/or their representative. The most convenient position for adult patients is to remain seated with the ear facing the physician. Children can sit on the lap of a parent or attendant with the affected ear facing the physician. The parent or attendant should wrap one arm around the child's body and arms while the other stabilizes the head.[11] Smaller children can be swaddled in a papoose made from a sheet and tape or a commercial immobilization device.[11]

Turn the affected ear toward the ceiling and fill the EAC with 5 to 10 mL of local anesthetic solution or suspension using the syringe tip, an angiocatheter, or a butterfly catheter with the needle cut off. This will result in substantial but short-lived topical anesthesia for the procedure.[12] If the effect wears off before the procedure is complete, the topical application of local anesthetic solution or suspension can be repeated as needed or longer-acting agents may be used. All cerumen removal techniques require the EAC to be straightened. In the adult, this is accomplished by pulling the pinna up and back while simultaneously pulling it slightly out from the head.[4] In the small child, the pinna is pulled down, back, and slightly out from the head.[4,13]

TECHNIQUES

PRECAUTIONS FOR USING INSTRUMENTS IN THE EAC

There are two major precautions the physician must take to avoid pushing cerumen further into the ear or causing damage to the EAC and tympanic membrane.

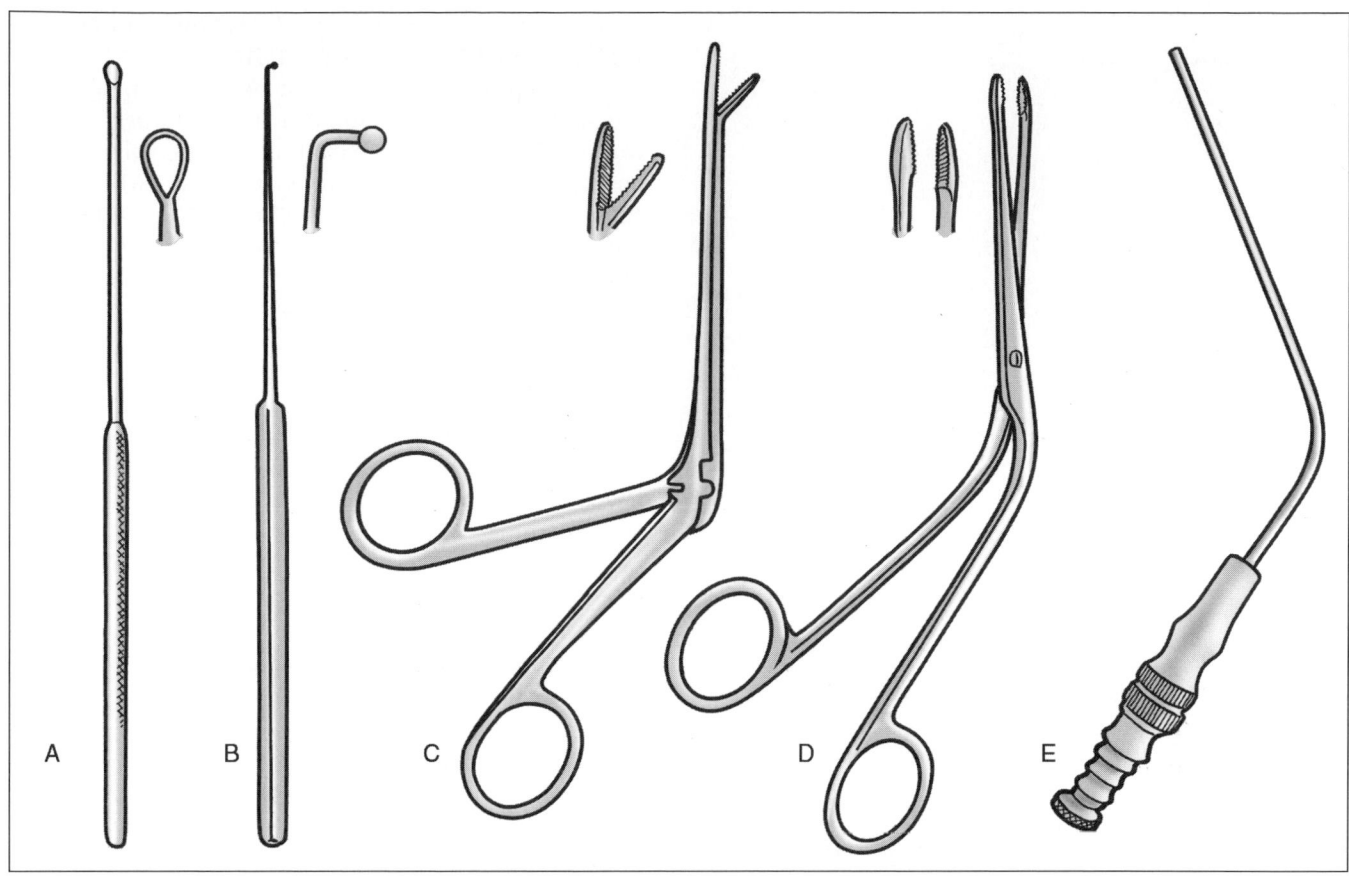

FIGURE 142-1 Instruments used for removal of cerumen from the external auditory canal. *A.* Cerumen loop. *B.* Right-angle ball hook. *C.* Alligator forceps. *D.* Hartman forceps. *E.* Frazier suction catheter.

First, the procedures must be performed under direct vision.[4] Second, the hand holding the instrument must remain firmly in contact with the patient's head at all times to stabilize the hand and avoid scrapping the canal wall or puncturing the tympanic membrane should the patient move.[4,10] Even a very cooperative patient may move due to an involuntary reflex cough.[13]

IRRIGATION

Irrigation is the safest and easiest method of removing cerumen, and it is usually successful.[1,4,8,10] It is less likely to lacerate or damage the EAC or tympanic membrane than other techniques. It is also the technique most commonly used by non-otolaryngologists.

Place a kidney basin under the affected ear and against the patient's cheek to catch the irrigation solution and the cerumen. Instruct the patient or an assistant to hold the basin in place. Attach a butterfly needle to a 10 to 20 mL syringe. Cut off the needle and most of the tubing, leaving only 1 or 2 cm. This remaining tubing will usually be curved, which is optimal for directing the irrigation stream. Draw up body temperature tap water or saline from another kidney basin into the syringe. In-

sert the butterfly tubing 1 cm into the EAC with the tip aimed in a direction opposite to the location of the cerumen[6] (Figure 142-2). This will cause the water to shoot past the cerumen, bounce off the tympanic membrane, and force the cerumen out of the EAC along with the irrigating solution.[8] If there is no obvious break in the cerumen, the stream should be directed superiorly.[8]

Care must be taken to make sure that the irrigation stream can easily exit the EAC, so as to prevent an increase in hydrostatic pressure, which could cause damage to the tympanic membrane.[7] Often, irrigation will have to be repeated numerous times, but persistence is usually rewarded with success.[4] Irrigation will sometimes have to be combined with either cerumen softening agents, manual separation of cerumen from the EAC wall, or direct grasping of the cerumen for removal.[4]

INSTRUMENT REMOVAL: SEPARATION OF CERUMEN FROM THE EAC WALL

This technique is a useful adjunct to irrigation and/or instrument removal.[10] Sometimes the cerumen is firmly pressed against the EAC wall in all directions. Irrigation will not work or may even worsen the situation by push-

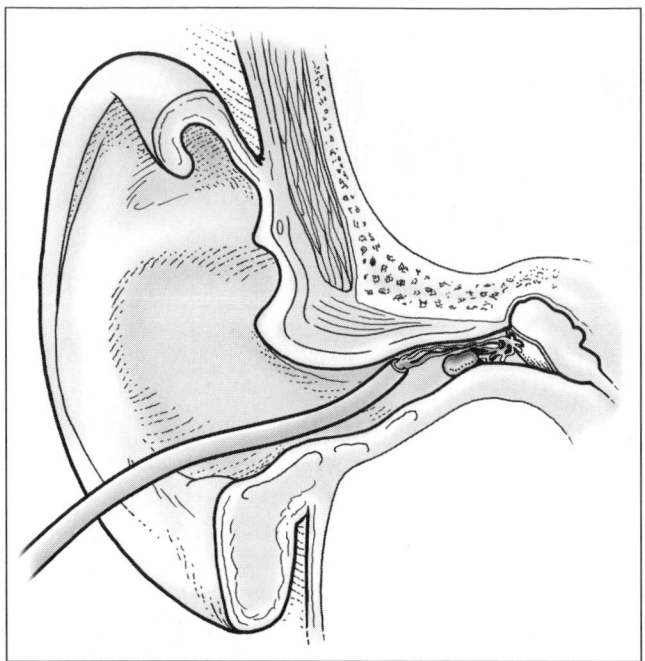

FIGURE 142-2 Irrigation with butterfly catheter tubing attached to a syringe. The stream of fluid is aimed toward the top of the external auditory canal and above the cerumen.

ing the cerumen further into the EAC. In this case, cerumen curettes, loops (Figure 142-1A), right-angle hooks (Figure 142-1B), or wires are used to gently separate the cerumen from the EAC wall and compress it into the center of the EAC lumen.[7]

The best place to start is superiorly. The cerumen should not be pulled out with the same movement, as this can abrade the EAC.[10] Once there is a free passage to the tympanic membrane, irrigation as described above is highly successful and safe. Alternatively, separation of the cerumen from the EAC wall can be performed all the way around the cerumen (circumferentially). This results in a cerumen plug freely suspended in the EAC, which can easily be removed by irrigation, pulled out with a right-angle hook, or grasped with forceps.[10]

INSTRUMENT REMOVAL: SLIDING CERUMEN OUT WITH INSTRUMENTS FROM BEHIND

This technique requires either a cerumen spoon (Figure 142-1A) or wire loop for small cerumen particles or a right-angle hook (Figure 142-1B) for larger amounts. After separating the cerumen from the canal wall, as described above, position the instrument with the loop or hook in the same plane as the EAC wall. Insert the tip of the instrument into the EAC above and just beyond the cerumen to be removed. Rotate the instrument 90 degrees to bring the loop or hook behind and directly in contact with the back (medial) side of the cerumen. Gently pull the instrument out of the EAC, pulling the cerumen out with it.[4]

INSTRUMENT REMOVAL: GRASPING CERUMEN WITH FORCEPS FOR REMOVAL

To be successful, there must be sufficient space for the jaws of the forceps on both sides between the EAC wall and the cerumen or a leading edge laterally that can be grasped. Once the cerumen is separated from the canal wall, as described above, insert the forceps into the EAC. Grasp the cerumen with the jaws of the Hartman (Figure 142-3A) or alligator (Figure 142-3B) forceps. Gently withdraw the forceps, taking care not to abrade the EAC wall. If the cerumen is located too far medially and instrumentation would cause pain or damage to the tympanic membrane, irrigation can move the cerumen plug laterally for subsequent grasping by the forceps.

Note that for optimal outcome, one may need to alternate irrigation and instrument removal to remove all of the cerumen plugs safely and completely.[4] For example, irrigation may gently soften or loosen the plug. Then a cerumen loop can be used to separate it from the canal wall. Irrigation can be used again to move it more laterally. Finally, a forceps or hook can be used to remove the cerumen plug from the EAC.

SUCTION REMOVAL

This technique requires soft cerumen or multiple small flakes. Use the same preparations and precautions described above. Attach the Frazier suction catheter or suction tubing to the suction source. Turn on the suction source. Insert the catheter into the EAC. Place the thumb over the hole to direct the suction through the tip of the catheter. Gently advance the suction catheter until the tip is in contact with the cerumen (Figure 142-4). Withdraw the suction catheter and cerumen from the EAC. Usually the tip must be withdrawn and cleaned continuously, because most cerumen will plug the suction tip.

CERUMEN SOFTENING AGENTS

If the cerumen is so impacted and hard that the above techniques are likely to cause pain and/or injury or if the cerumen cannot be removed, apply a cerumen softening agent. After the cerumen has softened, it can be removed using the techniques described above. Most of the agents are surprisingly comparable in their effectiveness.[5,9] In fact, plain water is quite effective for cerumen softening and disintegration.[5,9] This explains why persistent irrigation with water is so often successful.

Fill the EAC with olive oil, almond oil, 5% sodium bicarbonate, or a commercially available agent. Most authors recommend waiting 15 to 30 minutes before attempting to remove the cerumen.[6] Some recommend using the agents at home for up to a week before further attempts at removal.[6,7] Because prolonged exposure to these agents can precipitate otitis externa or allergic reactions, they must be removed and the canal dried after their use.[4]

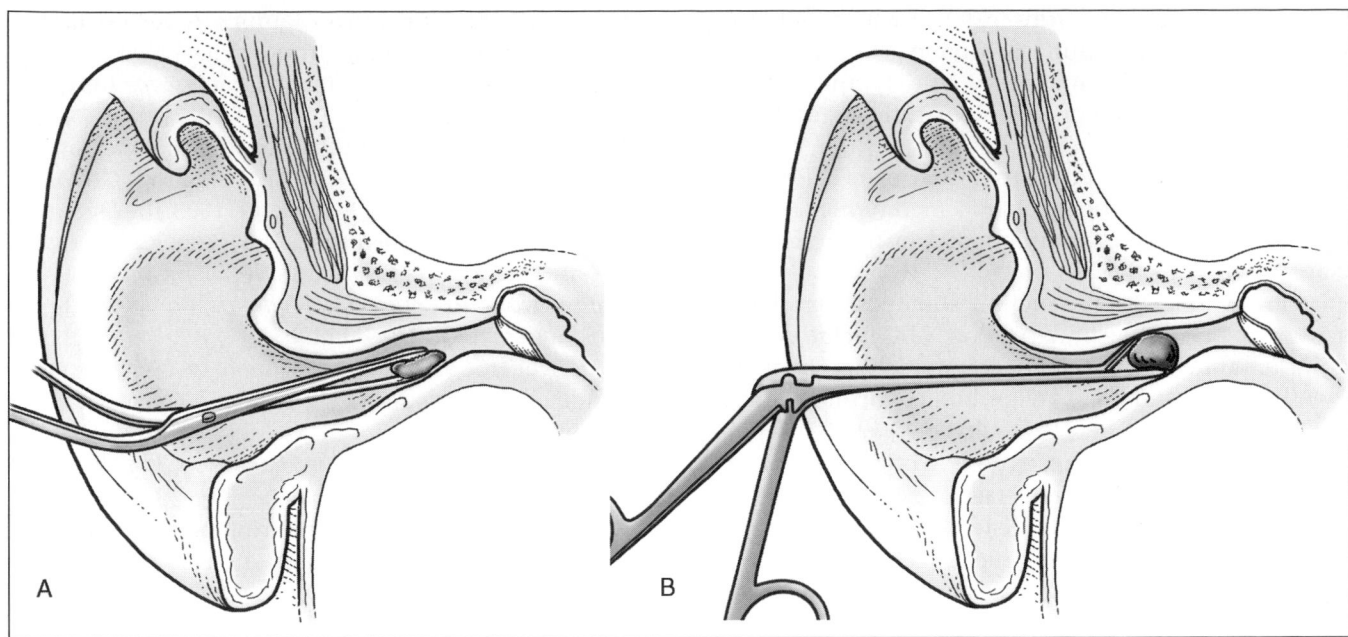

FIGURE 142-3 Forceps removal of cerumen. *A.* Hartman forceps. *B.* Alligator forceps.

ASSESSMENT

After cerumen has been removed, it is critical to re-examine the ear to confirm that the EAC, tympanic membrane, and hearing are all normal.[1] Remaining water and softening agents should be removed to prevent otitis externa.[4]

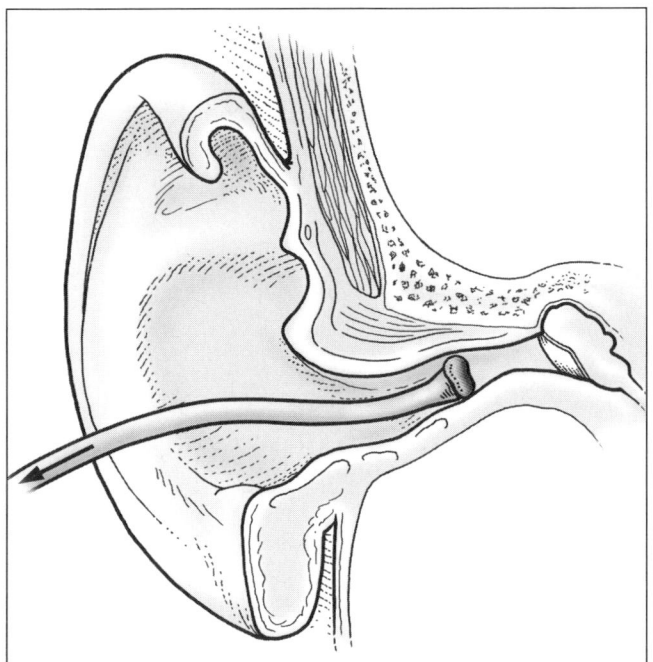

FIGURE 142-4 Suction removal of cerumen.

AFTERCARE

Many authors recommend prescribing several days of topical otic drops to prevent or treat subclinical otitis externa, which is frequently present in these patients. Commonly recommended are Cortisporin Otic, Otic Domeboro, Otobiotic, Pediotic Suspension, and VoSol. Consult an Otolaryngologist for patients with injuries, hearing deficits, or severe otitis externa or in whom cerumen removal was unsuccessful. Otherwise, the patient can receive follow-up with a primary care physician in 48 to 72 hours. Patients should be instructed in the proper application of ear drops. They should return to the Emergency Department if they develop ear pain, fever, decreased hearing, vertigo, headache, or a stiff neck. They should also be cautioned against future use of cotton swabs or other instruments in the EAC.

COMPLICATIONS

Numerous complications can result from the removal of cerumen from the EAC.[1,2,5,7,14,15] The complication rate for irrigation is 1 per 1000 cases.[1,5] It is higher for all other techniques. Irrigation can push cerumen further into the EAC. If the irrigating solution is cold, caloric stimulation can result in vomiting, vertigo, bradycardia, and syncope. Middle ear debris can be forced through a preexisting or iatrogenic tympanic membrane defect, resulting in otitis media, ossicle damage, labyrinthitis, mastoiditis, loss of hearing and balance, or central nervous system infection. Otitis externa can result from abrasions to the EAC. Butterfly tubing is less likely than the angiocatheter to damage the EAC or tympanic membrane because of its more pliable nature, larger diameter, and curved tip.

It is known that Water-Pik irrigation, even at low pressures, can rupture the tympanic membrane. For this reason, it cannot be recommended in the removal of cerumen from the EAC.

Instrumentation and suction should be used with caution to prevent secondary injury. This includes lacerations or abrasions of the EAC, rupture of the tympanic membrane, pushing of foreign bodies further into the EAC, and disruption or removal of the ossicles. Abrasions or lacerations to the EAC can result in otitis externa.

Cerumen softening agents can cause a contact reaction in the EAC, which may lead to an otitis externa. If the tympanic membrane is ruptured, the agents may cause permanent middle ear damage. Do not use these agents if the tympanic membrane is ruptured acutely or by history.

SUMMARY

Successful cerumen removal will often require using multiple techniques in sequence, adapted to the individual patient's situation. With adequate anesthesia, careful planning of the procedural sequence, and gentle handling, those who have been relieved of cerumen impaction will be among your most grateful patients.

REFERENCES

1. Sharp JF, Wilson JA, Ross L, et al: Ear wax removal: a survey of current practice. *Br Med J* 1990; 301(6763):1251–1253.

2. Dinsdale RC, Roland PS, Manning SC, et al: Catastrophic otologic injury from oral jet irrigation of the external auditory canal. *Laryngoscope* 1991; 101(1 Pt 1):75–78.

3. Linstrom CJ, Lucente FE: Infections of the external ear, in Bailey BJ: *Head and Neck Surgery—Otolaryngology.* Philadelphia: Lippincott, 1993:1542–1544.

4. Manthey DE, Harrison BP: Otolaryngologic procedures, in Roberts JR, Hedges JR (eds): *Clinical Procedures in Emergency Medicine.* Philadelphia: Saunders, 1998:1120–1149.

5. Hanger HC, Mulley GP: Cerumen: its fascination and clinical importance: a review. *J R Soc Med* 1992; 85(6):346–349.

6. Carne S: Ear syringing. *Br Med J* 1980; 280(6211): 374–376.

7. Ballachanda BB, Peers CJ: Cerumen management. Instruments and procedures. *ASHA* 1992; 34(2): 43–46.

8. Ballenger JJ: *Diseases of the Nose, Throat, Ear, Head, and Neck,* 14th ed. Philadelphia: Lea & Febiger, 1991.

9. Bellini MJ, Terry RM, Lewis FA: An evaluation of common cerumenolytic agents: an in vitro study. *Clin Otolaryngol* 1989; 14(1):23–25.

10. Ballenger JJ, Snow JB: *Otorhinolaryngology: Head and Neck Surgery.* Baltimore: Williams & Wilkins, 1996: 978–980.

11. Ansley JF: Treatment of aural foreign bodies in children. *Pediatrics* 1998; 101(4 pt 1):638–641.

12. Scott-Brown WG, Kerr AG: *Scott-Brown's Otolaryngology,* 6th ed. Oxford, England: Butterworth-Heinemann, 1997.

13. Burke M: Small things from small places. *Aust Fam Physician* 1999; 28(2):132–133.

14. Scott-Brown WG, Kerr AG: *Scott-Brown's Otolaryngology,* vol 3, 6th ed. Oxford, England: Butterworth-Heinemann, 1997: chap 6:11–12.

15. Bailey BJ: Impacted ear wax and a water-pick instrument. *JAMA* 1983; 250(11):1456.

Chapter 143
TYMPANOCENTESIS

Paul J. Jones

INTRODUCTION

Tympanocentesis is a diagnostic and therapeutic procedure in which a needle is inserted through the tympanic membrane to aspirate fluid from the middle ear space. The procedure is considered diagnostic when the material obtained is sent for laboratory and/or microbiological analysis. It is considered therapeutic in most instances because it relieves pressure, thereby reducing pain, and many times shortens the course of an acute otitis media. The procedure is quick, simple, and not as frequently performed as it should be. Note also that authors are calling for culture-directed antibiotic therapy for otitis media to reduce the need for broad-spectrum antibiotics and prevent, as much as possible, the emergence of multiresistant organisms.[1–4]

ANATOMY AND PATHOPHYSIOLOGY

The ear is divided into the external, middle, and inner parts. The external ear is comprised of the auricle, the external auditory canal, and the external auditory meatus. The middle ear contains an air space and mastoid cells ventilated by the eustachian tube, the tympanic membrane, and the three ossicles. The inner ear is made up of the cochlea, semicircular canals, fluids, and cranial nerve VIII. The facial nerve courses through the middle ear space and mastoid process. It can be affected by a severe infection in these areas. Facial asymmetry during an acute ear infection is an indication of an unusually severe infection.

Inspection of the tympanic membrane will usually show it to be bulging during an acute infection with loss of mobility on pneumatic otoscopy. Conditions that are more chronic may show color changes of the tympanic membrane, with or without associated scarring and distortion.

INDICATIONS

Tympanocentesis is performed to obtain fluid for microbiological culture and antibiotic sensitivity testing to determine the infectious cause of a middle ear effusion. Tympanocentesis is warranted for patients with otitis media that is severe, unresponsive to conventional antimicrobial therapy, or in a child less than 8 weeks of age to rule out gram-negative organisms. Tympanocentesis is warranted for patients with an acute otitis media and either an acquired or congenital immunodeficiency as they will often require directed therapy. Patients who develop acute otitis media while taking appropriate antimicrobial therapy should be evaluated for the organism responsible and its sensitivity to antibiotics. Tympanocentesis is also performed when the patient has an otitis media associated with unusually severe pain, signs of toxicity, bullous myringitis, facial nerve palsy, mastoiditis, meningitis, encephalitis, brain abscess, or dural sinus thrombosis.

CONTRAINDICATIONS

There are no absolute contraindications to tympanocentesis. It should not be performed in a patient who is uncooperative, as secondary injury may result. Uncooperative patients will require sedation, procedural sedation, or general anesthesia to perform this procedure. Tympanocentesis should be performed by an Otolaryngologist if the landmarks on the tympanic membrane are obscured.

EQUIPMENT

21 gauge spinal needle
3 mL aspirating syringe
Ear speculum
Ear wax curette
Culture swabs and media
Laboratory tubes for fluid cell count and differential
Topical anesthetic solution
Intravenous extension tubing
Headlamp or overhead surgical light source
Frazier suction catheters
Suction tubing
Suction source

PATIENT PREPARATION

Explain the risks, benefits, and potential complications of the procedure to the patient and/or their representative. The post-procedural care should also be discussed. Obtain a signed consent for the procedure.

Place the patient supine on a gurney. View the tympanic membrane with an otoscope. Remove any cerumen from the external auditory canal using a curette. The cerumen may also be flushed from the external auditory canal. Refer to Chapter 142 for the complete details regarding cerumen removal. Again, view the tympanic membrane with an otoscope. While the administration of topical or local anesthesia is often not helpful in the presence of an acute infection, it is not harmful. Apply a topical anesthetic solution into the external auditory canal followed by a cotton ball. Allow the solution to remain for 5 to 10 minutes. Topical anesthetic solutions include benzocaine-antipyrine (Auralgan), viscous 4% lidocaine, or cocaine. Refer to Chapters 106 and 144 for the details regarding regional anesthesia of the ear. Children and uncooperative patients must be restrained and/or sedated so that the head is immobile. This may require intravenous sedation, procedural sedation, or general anesthesia.

TECHNIQUE

Bend a 21 gauge spinal needle at the hub to approximately 60 degrees. Attach the spinal needle to a 3 mL aspirating syringe. Insert the ear speculum into the external auditory canal (Figure 143-1A). View the tympanic membrane through the ear speculum using a headlight or overhead surgical light source for illumination.

Insert the spinal needle through the speculum and into the inferior half of the tympanic membrane (Figures 143-1A and B). **Avoid inserting the needle through the posterior superior quadrant of the tympanic membrane. This location is near the ossicles. Any movement of the needle near the ossicles could result in disarticulation of the ossicles requiring surgical repair.** Aspirate the middle ear fluid into the syringe (Figure 143-1A). Withdraw the syringe and ear speculum. Transfer the fluid into appropriate laboratory medium and containers as quickly as possible. Label the containers and have them transported to the laboratory for a Gram's stain, culture and sensitivities, cell count, and differential of the cells present.

ALTERNATIVE TECHNIQUE

An alternative method involves attaching intravenous extension tubing between the spinal needle and the syringe. The physician can observe the tympanic membrane, insert the spinal needle, and have a hand available for manipulation of the ear speculum or a suction catheter. An assistant is required to hold the syringe and aspirate the middle ear fluid. The remainder of the technique is as described previously.

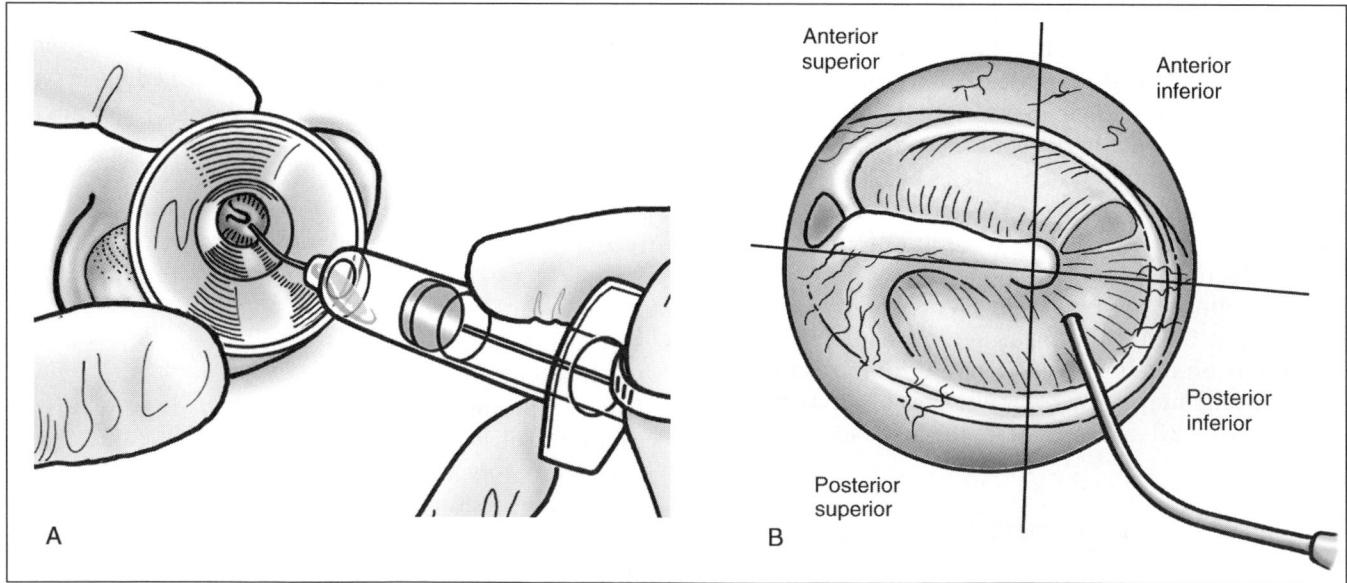

FIGURE 143-1 Tympanocentesis of the right ear. The patient is lying supine with their head directed to the left. *A.* An ear speculum is inserted into the external auditory canal. A needle is inserted through the posterior inferior quadrant of the tympanic membrane to aspirate middle ear fluid. *B.* Magnified view of the tympanic membrane.

AFTERCARE

Most patients will have immediate improvement in their pain and, in many cases, their hearing. Because there is a small opening in the tympanic membrane, further drainage may occur and should be expected for 48 to 72 hours. Instruct the patient and/or caregivers to keep the ear dry for 2 to 3 days. This is especially true during bathing or hair washing. A cotton earplug coated with a thin film of petroleum jelly (e.g., Vaseline) works well. The tympanic membrane usually spontaneously heals within 48 to 72 hours. Follow-up for laboratory results and documentation of antimicrobial change or appropriateness is necessary in 48 to 72 hours.

COMPLICATIONS

Common complications include persistent perforation with or without otorrhea, development of a scar on the tympanic membrane, and an otitis externa. Pain and bleeding are usually minimal and self-limited. One of the most significant complications is the disruption of the ossicles of the middle ear. Disruption of the ossicles can be avoided by inserting the needle into the inferior half of the tympanic membrane and preventing patient movement during the procedure. Rare complications include injury to the chorda tympani, facial nerve, or internal carotid artery.

SUMMARY

Acute otitis media is one of the most common infections seen in children. Most episodes respond quickly, with or without antimicrobial therapy. Tympanocentesis can be used to direct antimicrobial therapy in patients when a clinical response is delayed, host immunosuppression exists, or unusual organisms are suspected. Tympanocentesis can be used to provide immediate pain relief from a severe middle earache. The procedure is quick and simple to perform in the Emergency Department.

REFERENCES

1. Bluestone CD: Role of surgery for otitis media in the era of resistant bacteria. *Pediatr Infect Dis J* 1998; 17(11):1090–1100.
2. Green M, Wald ER: Emerging resistance to antibiotics: impact on respiratory infections in the outpatient setting. *Ann Allergy Asthma Immunol* 1996; 77(3):167–173.
3. Poole MD: It's time to bring back diagnostic tympanocentesis. *ENT J* 1994; 73(1):49–50.
4. Potsic WP, Cotton RT, Handler SD: *Surgical Pediatric Otolaryngology*. New York: Thieme Medical, 1997: 10–11.

Chapter 144
AURICULAR HEMATOMA EVACUATION

Eric F. Reichman

INTRODUCTION

Blunt trauma to the auricle can cause abrasions, ecchymosis, hematoma formation, and lacerations. Abrasions and ecchymosis of the auricle require no therapy other than oral analgesics and observation for infection.[1] Some authors recommend the application of topical antibiotics to all abrasions as prophylaxis for infection.[2] Lacerations to the auricle are addressed in Chapter 80. This chapter addresses the management of an auricular hematoma.

Injuries to the auricle are common due to its exposed position and lack of protection from surrounding structures.[3] The most common cause for an auricular hematoma formation is blunt trauma while participating in the contact sports of wrestling or boxing.[1,2,4–6] Such trauma may occur in other situations, including assaults, falls, fights, and motor vehicle crashes. Auricular trauma and hematomas are common in children due to the high incidence of head injuries during playtime.[2,4] Blood dyscrasias may also cause an auricular hematoma.

An auricular hematoma presents as a firm and painful swelling that obscures the normal convolutions on the lateral aspect of the auricle. It can develop within minutes to hours of the blunt trauma. **An auricular hematoma must be evacuated to prevent the cosmetic disfigurement known as cauliflower ear. The sooner it is evacuated, the less chance of permanent disfigurement.**[4,5] After evacuation, the patient requires a pressure dressing to the auricle, oral antibiotics, and close follow-up to prevent complications.[2,5,7,8]

ANATOMY AND PATHOPHYSIOLOGY

The auricle is that portion of the external ear that projects from the side of the head. It functions to augment sound delivery to the tympanic membrane and assist in sound localization. It is fixed in position by both ligaments and muscles.[9] It has an underlying cartilaginous framework that is 0.5 to 1.0 mm thick and provides the auricle with its unique shape. The cartilage is a single, thin sheet of flexible yellow elastic cartilage with many convolutions on the lateral surface.[10] The only portion of the auricle without cartilage is the lobule in which fibrofatty tissue replaces the cartilage.[9] **The cartilage is avascular and derives its blood supply and nutrients from the adjacent perichondrium.**[11]

The skin covering the auricle is similar to that elsewhere on the body.[12] It contains sebaceous glands and a varying number of hair follicles. The skin on the lateral surface of the auricle is tightly adherent to the perichondrium and lacks a subcutaneous layer (Figure 144-1). The skin on the medial surface of the auricle is loosely attached and has a layer of subcuticular tissue between the skin and perichondrium.

Trauma may cause the perichondrium to be torn off the underlying cartilage due to the tight attachment of the skin to the perichondrium on the lateral surface of the auricle. This traumatic avulsion of the perichondrium causes hemorrhage into the space between it and the cartilage, allowing a hematoma to form (Figure 144-2). Bleeding into this potential subperichondral space causes dissection of the perichondrium from the underlying cartilage. Auricular hematomas can be painful due to the rich sensory innervation to the area and the accumulation of blood in this relatively closed space.[11] **Failure to adequately evacuate a hematoma may lead to cartilage necrosis and a deformed ear.** The necrosis is due to a combination of separating the cartilage from its blood supply and direct pressure effects from the hematoma.

The cauliflower ear is a purely cosmetic deformity that results from an auricular hematoma not being evacuated and allowing the auricle to spontaneously heal. The hematoma is invaded by fibroblasts and slowly replaced by fibrous tissue. This organization of the hematoma causes irregular thickening of the auricle. The perichondrium, elevated from the cartilage by the

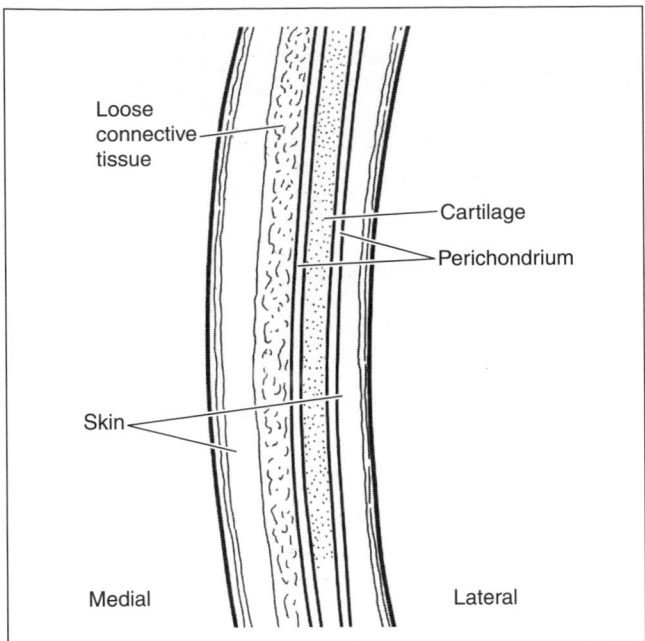

FIGURE 144-1 Cross-section of the auricle. The skin on the medial surface has a layer of loose connective tissue that is lacking on the lateral surface.

hematoma, senses the lack of adjacent cartilage and activates chondroblasts. New cartilage is deposited on the surface of the hematoma causing further thickening and deformity of the auricle.

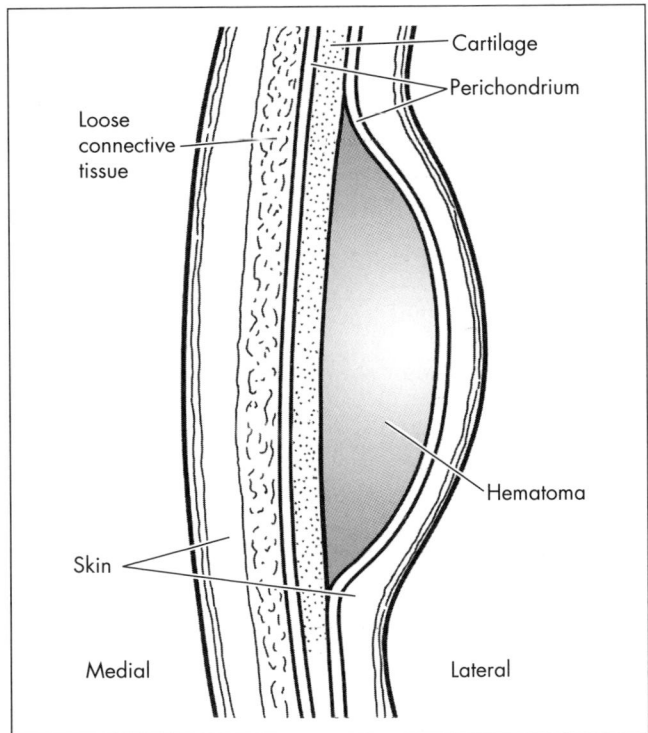

FIGURE 144-2 An auricular hematoma. The blood collects between the perichondrium and the cartilage.

INNERVATION OF THE AURICLE

A brief review of the innervation of the auricle will later aid in understanding the technique of regional anesthesia. Three nerves contribute to the sensory enervation of the auricle (Figure 144-3).[8,11–15] The auriculotemporal branch of the mandibular division of the trigeminal nerve supplies sensation to the upper, lateral surface of the auricle. This nerve emerges subcutaneously just anterior to the auricle at the level of the external auditory canal. Two branches of the cervical plexus become subcutaneous at the posterior border of the midportion of the sternocleidomastoid muscle and ascend to the auricle. The lesser occipital nerve provides sensory innervation to the upper medial surface of the auricle. The great auricular nerve provides sensory innervation to most of the medial surface and the lower half of the lateral auricular surface.

INDICATIONS

Any auricular hematoma requires evacuation. The indication for evacuation is to prevent the cosmetic deformity known as the cauliflower ear.[7] It is preferable to evacuate the hematoma within 12 to 24 hours after its occurrence. Although there is no urgency to immediately evacuate the hematoma, the longer it remains the higher the chance of clot organization and new cartilage deposition.[7,16]

CONTRAINDICATIONS

There are no absolute contraindications to the evacuation of an auricular hematoma. If the skin overlying the hematoma is cellulitic, or if purulent material is drained from the hematoma, the patient will require hospital admission and intravenous antibiotics.[1,8] An Otolaryngologist or Plastic Surgeon should be immediately consulted on these patients. The auricular hematoma should be evacuated by a consultant if it has been present more than 5 to 7 days. These hematomas have already begun organization and new cartilage has developed requiring curettage associated with the evacuation.[7,16]

EQUIPMENT

Auricular Anesthesia

Povidone iodine solution
10 mL syringe
25 or 27 gauge needle, 2 inches long
10 to 20 mL of local anesthetic solution without
  epinephrine

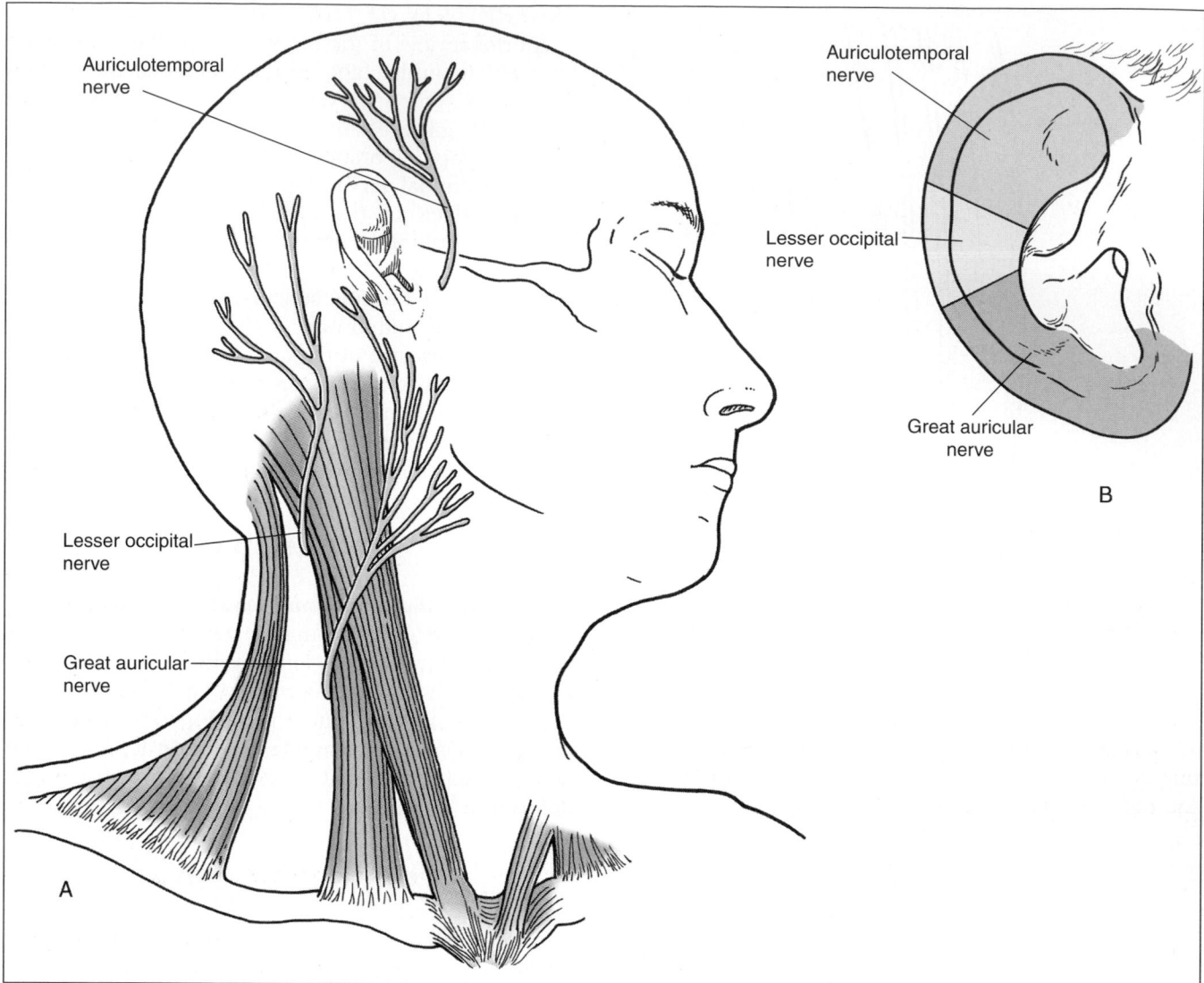

FIGURE 144-3 The sensory innervation of the auricle. *A.* The distribution of cutaneous nerves surrounding the auricle. *B.* An enlarged view of the auricle demonstrating the cutaneous innervation.

Auricular Hematoma Aspiration

Antiseptic solution
Tuberculin or insulin syringe
0.25 mL of local anesthetic solution without
    epinephrine
10 mL syringe
18 gauge needle
Topical antibiotic ointment

Auricular Hematoma Incision and Drainage

Auricular anesthesia as above
15 surgical scalpel blade on a handle
Curved hemostat

Sterile drain (optional)
10 mL syringe
18 gauge angiocatheter without the needle
Sterile saline
Topical antibiotic ointment
Forceps

Mastoid Pressure Dressing

Petrolatum gauze
Cotton balls soaked in sterile saline
Dry cotton balls
4×4 gauze squares
4 inch elastic gauze bandage
Scissors

Surgical Pressure Dressing

Cotton bolsters or dental rolls
Needle driver
4–0 monofilament nylon suture

PATIENT PREPARATION

Explain the risks, benefits, and potential complications of the procedure to the patient and/or their representative. The post-procedural care should also be discussed. Obtain a signed consent for the procedure. Some physicians omit the signed consent and place the following statement in the procedure note: "The risks, benefits, and complications were described and discussed with the patient. They understood this and gave verbal consent for the procedure."

Remove any dirt and debris from the auricle and surrounding skin. Apply povidone iodine solution to the same areas. Follow aseptic technique for the remainder of the procedure.[4] In patients who are anxious and without other associated injuries, the administration of intramuscular lorazepam (Ativan) or oral diazepam (Valium) may be beneficial.[15]

AURICULAR ANESTHESIA

The local anesthetic solution used for auricular anesthesia should contain no epinephrine.[2,13,14,17] Epinephrine is not used for fear of intense vasoconstriction of end arterioles resulting in decreased perfusion with possible ischemia and necrosis of the auricle. Some authors recommend the use of 1/100,000 epinephrine mixed with the local anesthetic solution.[1,15,16] The epinephrine may decrease bleeding by its vasoconstrictive action. It may also prevent reaccumulation of the hematoma after it has been evacuated. Authors who advocate using epinephrine state that the auricle has a rich blood supply and that, based on anecdotal evidence, there is no danger of ischemia or necrosis from the use of epinephrine in healthy patients without evidence of traumatized vascularity. **Although many physicians will use epinephrine, it has not been proven safe to use or proven to prevent reaccumulation of the hematoma.** It may be wiser to be conservative and not use epinephrine than to use it and have to deal with the complications to the patient and potential litigation.

The choice of which local anesthetic to use is physician-dependent. Lidocaine (1%) is the most commonly used local anesthetic. Long-acting local anesthetic solutions, such as bupivacaine (Marcaine) or etidocaine (Duranest), may be used to provide analgesia for several hours after the procedure is completed.[14]

The methods of anesthesia for evacuation of an auricular hematoma range from none to a superficial skin wheal to a regional block. Some authors advocate using no anesthesia if needle aspiration of a small and fresh hematoma is performed.[2] This is not generally recommended as the pain from an 18 gauge needle aspiration is more uncomfortable than local anesthesia infiltration.

If using the aspiration technique to evacuate the hematoma, local anesthetic solution can be infiltrated directly over the hematoma. Place a skin wheal, using 0.25 mL of local anesthetic solution without epinephrine, over the hematoma in the area of maximum fluctuance. **When placing the skin wheal, be careful not to inject the local anesthetic solution into the hematoma.** This will cause expansion of the hematoma and increase the separation of the perichondrium from the underlying cartilage.[17] It may also cause new bleeding, which can increase the possibility of hematoma reaccumulation.

A regional auricular block is the preferred method to obtain anesthesia.[13] It prevents distortion of the auricle from direct injection and further separation of the perichondrium from the underlying auricular cartilage.[17] Subcutaneous infiltration of the surrounding skin is less painful than injection directly into the sensitive auricular skin.[15] The landmarks for regional anesthesia are simple to locate, consistent, and predictable. The greatest reason for failure of an auricular block is incorrect needle placement.[14] A regional auricular block can be done prior to using the aspiration technique or the incision and drainage technique to evacuate the hematoma. If the aspiration technique fails (i.e., hematoma reaccumulates), then there is no need to reprep and perform an auricular block prior to performing the incision and drainage.

There are three methods to perform a regional auricular block (Figures 144-4 and 144-5). Each method blocks the lesser occipital, great auricular, and auriculotemporal nerves. Some physicians prefer to subcutaneously inject local anesthetic solution circumferentially around the attachment of the auricle to the head (Figure 144-4).[2,11,13,17] An alternative method is based on blocking the sensory supply to the ear in a more anatomic distribution (Figure 144-5).[8,14] This latter method uses half the anesthetic and half the number of subcutaneous injections than the former method. For these reasons, this author prefers the second method, which is described in the following paragraph.

To perform a regional auricular block, first cleanse the auricle and surrounding skin of any dirt and debris. Apply povidone iodine solution. Place a skin wheal of local anesthetic solution 0.5 cm below the pinna of the auricle (Figure 144-5A). Insert a 2 inch, 25 or 27 gauge needle through the skin wheal, aimed just posterior to

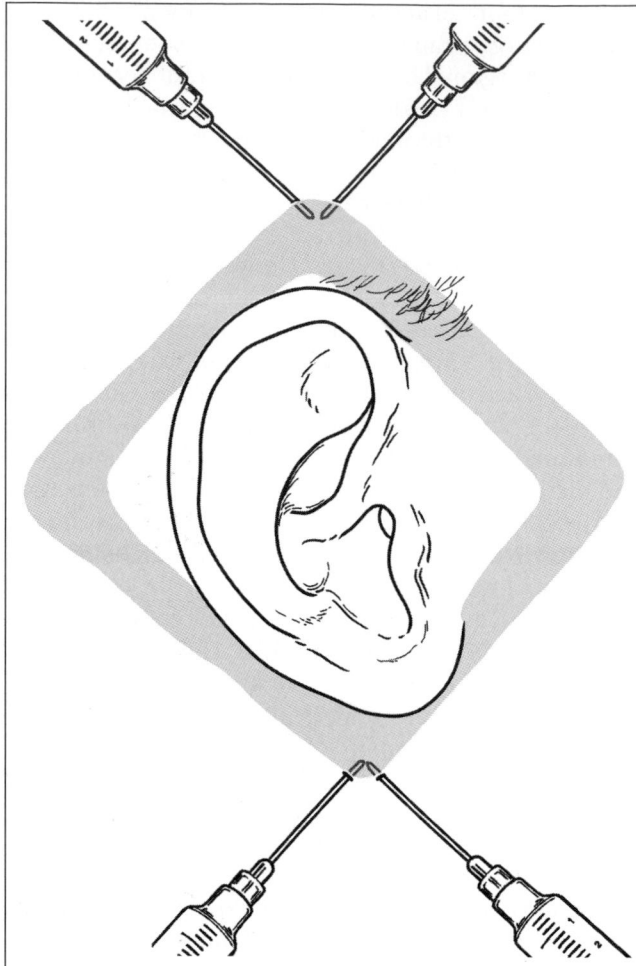

FIGURE 144-4 Regional anesthesia of the auricle. The technique of circumferential application of local anesthetic solution. Shaded areas represent subcutaneous infiltration of local anesthetic solution.

the attachment of the auricle to the head. Infiltrate subcutaneously, in a superior direction, always remaining 0.5 to 1.0 cm posterior to the auricular attachment to the head. Stop infiltrating at the level of the superior attachment of the auricle to the head. This infiltration requires 5 to 8 mL of local anesthetic solution. Withdraw the needle almost completely. Redirect the needle through the skin wheal and aimed just anterior to the attachment of the auricle to the head. Infiltrate subcutaneously, in a superior direction, always remaining 0.5 to 1.0 cm anterior to the auricular attachment to the head. Stop infiltrating at the level of the superior attachment of the auricle to the head. This infiltration requires 5 to 8 mL of local anesthetic solution. Care must be taken not to inject too deeply anterior to the auricle as it can cause temporary paralysis of the facial nerve. An alternative to the anterior infiltration is the injection of 3 to 4 mL of local anesthetic solution just superior and anterior to the tragus (Figure 144-5B).[1,18] This

injection blocks the auriculotemporal nerve at its origin. **Allow 10 to 15 minutes for the full anesthetic effect prior to beginning the procedure.**[17]

TECHNIQUES

The methods for treating and managing an auricular hematoma require the evacuation of the hematoma and replacing the perichondrium onto the underlying cartilage. The techniques include aspiration, incision and drainage, and closed suction drainage. The first two techniques will be described in detail. The closed suction technique requires inpatient admission and is not a procedure to be performed in the Emergency Department. It will therefore not be described here.

ASPIRATION

Some consider the aspiration technique to be the primary method to evacuate an auricular hematoma.[2,3,5,6] They reserve the incision and drainage technique for incomplete aspiration or recurrence of the hematoma. Unfortunately, the hematoma frequently recurs after using the aspiration technique and the patient requires a second procedure to evacuate the hematoma.[1,3,6,19] Because of the high rate of recurrence, this author and others prefer to use the incision and drainage technique as the primary procedure.[16]

Clean and prep the skin. Anesthesia is achieved by performing a regional auricular block or by placing a skin wheal of local anesthetic over the hematoma. Attach an 18 gauge needle onto a 10 mL syringe. Insert the needle into the area of maximum fluctuance (Figure 144-6). Apply negative pressure to the syringe, by withdrawing the plunger, to evacuate the hematoma. Express the hematoma between the thumb and index finger of the opposite hand while applying negative pressure with the syringe to ensure complete evacuation of the hematoma.

Remove the needle and apply manual pressure to the area of the former hematoma for 3 to 5 minutes. If the hematoma recurs or if complete aspiration is not possible, perform the incision and drainage technique. If the hematoma is completely evacuated and does not recur, apply topical antibiotic ointment and a pressure dressing.

There are several disadvantages to this technique. First, the hematoma frequently recurs.[1,3,6,19] This means that the patient often needs a second drainage procedure. Even if the hematoma is adequately evacuated, the elimination of the dead space is problematic.[19] The dead space may fill with blood or serous fluid requiring a second procedure. A surgically applied pressure dressing may alleviate the dead space and make the aspiration technique more successful. Finally, the aspiration

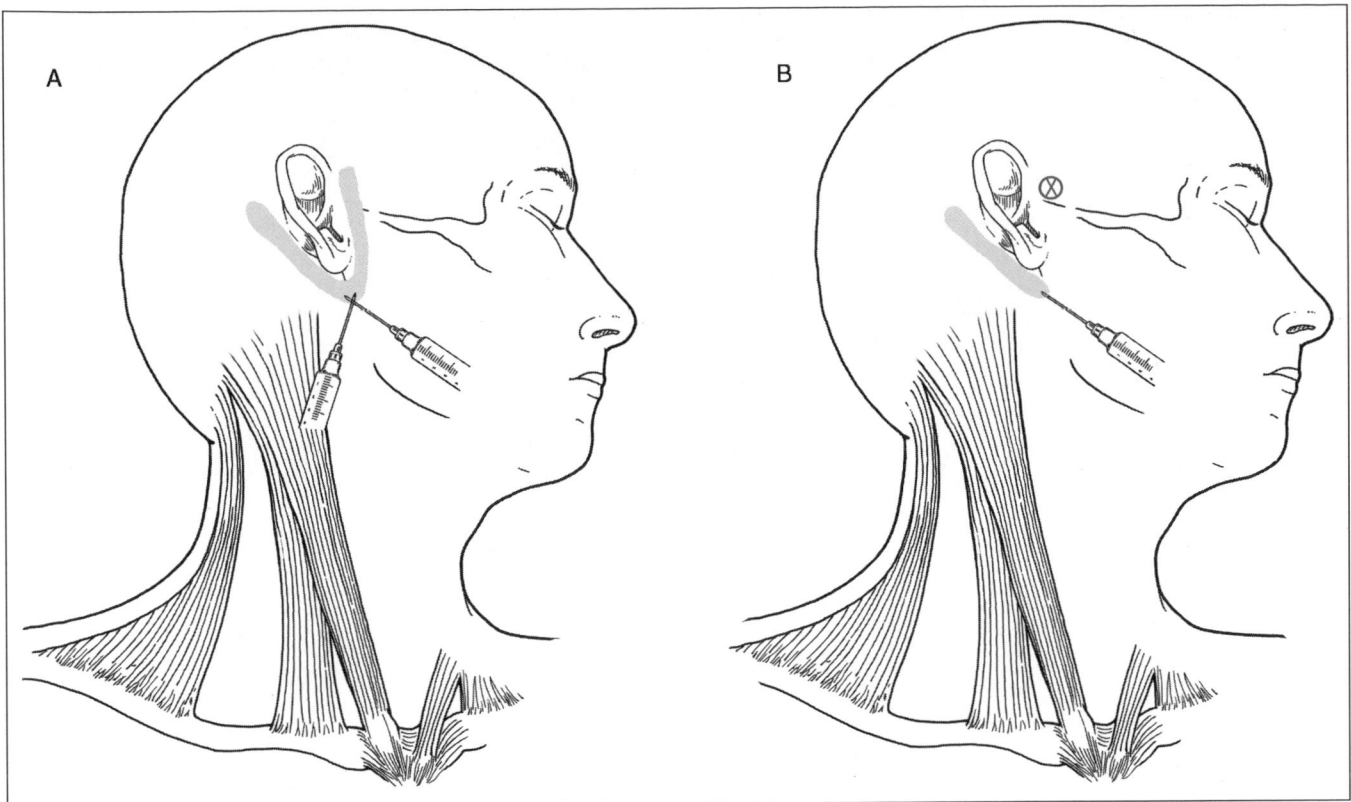

FIGURE 144-5 Regional anesthesia of the auricle. *A*. A more anatomical auricular block. *B*. An alternative regional block that anesthetizes the auriculotemporal nerve at its origin. Local anesthetic solution is injected at the ⊗ symbol. Shaded areas represent subcutaneous infiltration of local anesthetic solution.

technique may not remove all of the hematoma.[1] Again, the patient will need a second procedure. For these above stated reasons, the aspiration technique is not the preferred method to drain an auricular hematoma.

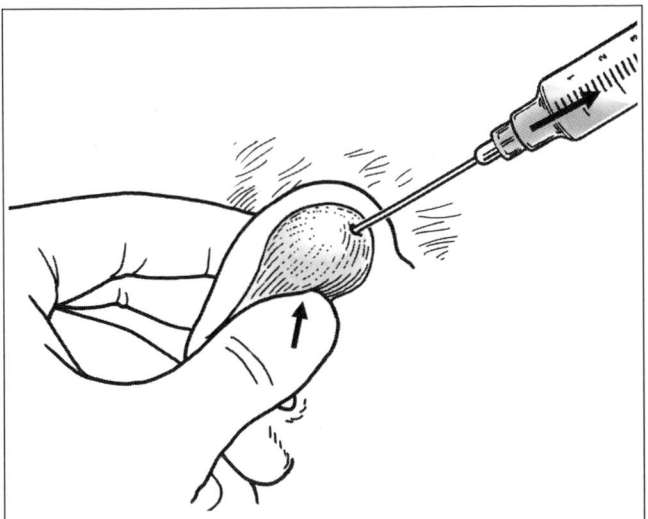

FIGURE 144-6 The aspiration of an auricular hematoma. The hematoma is expressed with the thumb and index finger as negative pressure is applied to the syringe.

INCISION AND DRAINAGE

This is the preferred technique to evacuate an auricular hematoma.[16] It requires a regional auricular block for anesthesia. This technique takes more time to perform than the aspiration technique.

As noted previously, the skin should be cleaned and prepped in the usual manner. Perform a regional auricular block to provide adequate analgesia. Allow the block 10 to 15 minutes to achieve maximal effect.[17] Incise the auricular skin with a #15 surgical scalpel blade at the edge of the hematoma (Figure 144-7*A*). **When making the incision, it should follow the curvature of the pinna and be no longer than 1 centimeter.** Gently peel this skin and attached perichondrium off the hematoma using forceps. Express the hematoma with the thumb and index finger of the opposite hand. Insert a curved hemostat and gently loosen any remaining blood clot (Figure 144-7*B*). Fill a 10 mL syringe with sterile saline and attach a plastic 18 gauge angiocatheter. Gently flush out the area of the hematoma (Figure 144-7*C*). Reapproximate the skin and perichondrium on the cartilage. Compress the tissue to eliminate any fluid and dead space. Some authors apply a small rubber drain through the incision to prevent accumulation of blood or serous fluid.[4,8] The use of a drain is optional. A drain can be

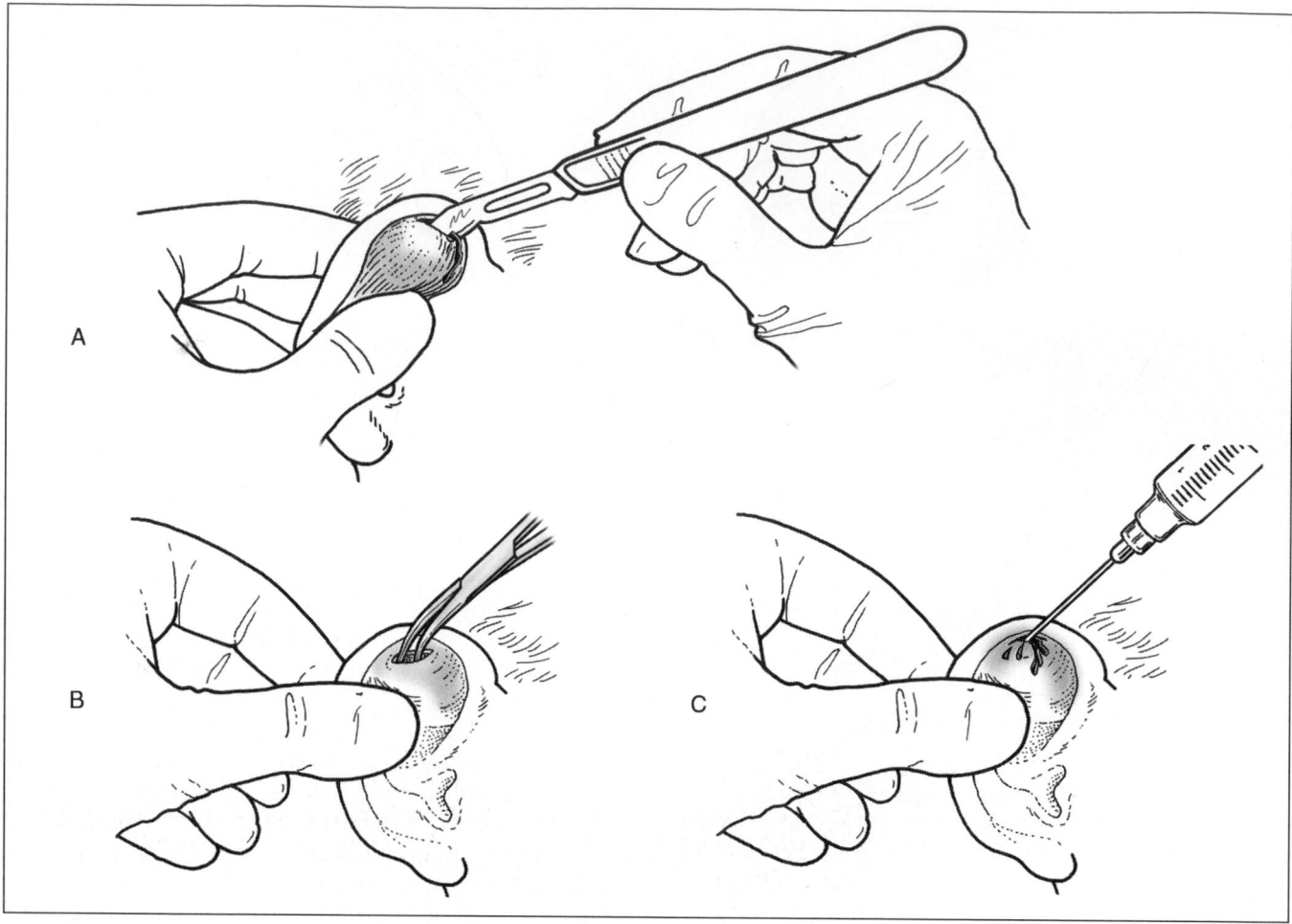

FIGURE 144-7 Incision and drainage of an auricular hematoma. *A.* An incision is made along the helical rim. *B.* The hematoma is evacuated with the aid of a hemostat. The thumb and index finger express the hematoma from the subperichondral space. *C.* The subperichondral pocket is flushed with normal saline to remove any residual blood and clot.

made by cutting a small strip from a sterile Penrose drain.

Apply manual pressure to the area of the former hematoma for 3 to 5 minutes. If the hematoma or serous fluid does not reaccumulate, apply topical antibiotic ointment and a pressure dressing as described below. If the hematoma or serous fluid does reaccumulate, consider inserting a rubber drain or applying a surgical pressure dressing.

PRESSURE DRESSINGS

A pressure dressing must be applied to the auricle after the successful drainage of an auricular hematoma. It prevents reaccumulation of the hematoma or serous fluid; it also supports the auricle while the perichondrium reattaches to the cartilage.[3,6,10] The pressure dressing must be applied for at least 48 hours.[4] The pressure dressing can be the traditional mastoid dressing or a surgically applied dressing.[16,17,19,20] These

pressure dressings apply even pressure over the entire auricle without compromising the blood flow while simultaneously eliminating the dead space within the wound.[17]

MASTOID PRESSURE DRESSING

The most commonly applied dressing is the mastoid pressure dressing (Figure 144-8). Although simple to place, it has many disadvantages when compared to the surgically applied pressure dressing. It is bulky and hard to keep in place. It is very conspicuous. Patients must keep it dry and remain relatively inactive to prevent it from coming off.

Place a piece of sterile dry cotton in the external auditory canal and level with the base of the auricular cartilage. Mold a sterile material that conforms easily onto all the convolutions of the auricle until it is level with the lateral helical rim (Figure 144-8*A*). The choices of material include cotton balls soaked in mineral oil, cotton balls soaked in saline, or petrolatum gauze. The material chosen is left to physician preference and what

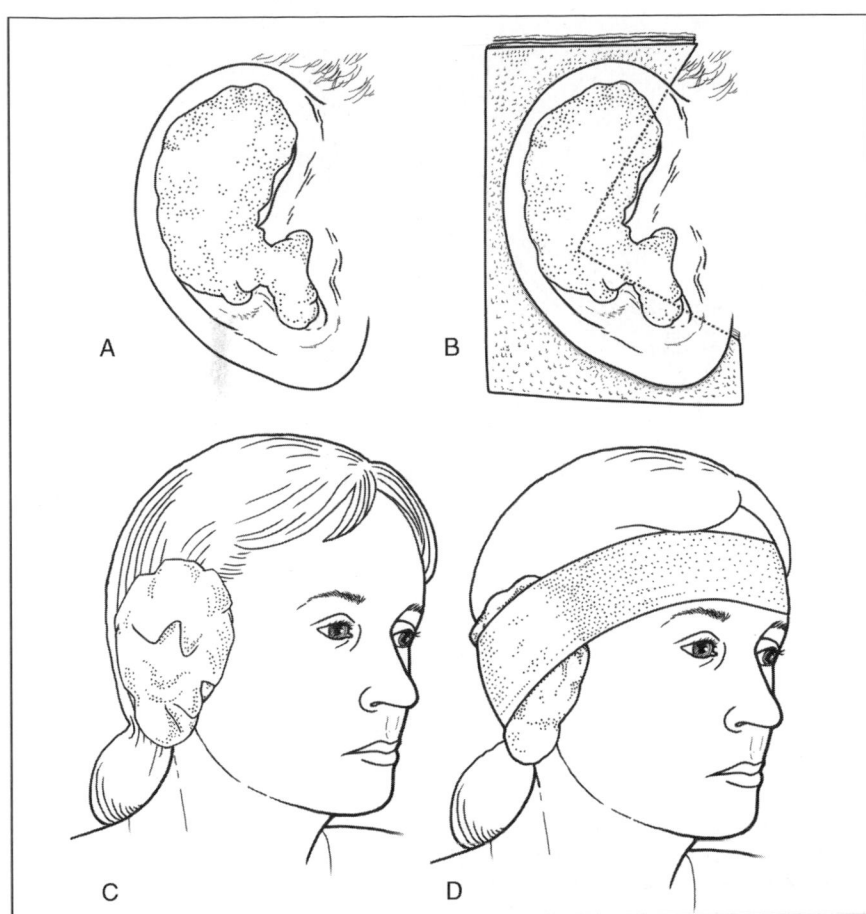

FIGURE 144-8 The traditional mastoid dressing. The convolutions are covered with a layer of petroleum gauze. *A.* Saline-soaked cotton balls are packed over the convolutions, level with the helical rim. *B.* Trimmed gauze squares are placed between the auricle and the head. *C.* Fluffed gauze is placed over the auricle. *D.* The circumferential application of an elastic gauze bandage to the head. The bandage should cover the injured auricle and not the contralateral auricle.

is available in the Emergency Department. This author prefers to use petrolatum gauze. The petrolatum gauze allows the dressing to be removed with minimal trauma to the ear. Pack the auricle with saline-soaked cotton balls. **All the convolutions of the auricle must be thoroughly packed. The packing of the auricular convolutions assures even application of pressure to all portions of the auricle.**

Cut out and discard a semicircle or a V-shaped section from a pile of gauze squares. Place the remaining C-shaped gauze pads behind the auricle (Figure 144-8*B*). The gauze pads should be built up until they completely fill the area between the auricle and the head. This padding is used to support the auricle as well as prevent undue contortion or uneven pressure from the compression dressing.[2]

Unfold and fluff several gauze squares or open a roll of gauze. Place the fluffed gauze over the lateral surface of the auricle (Figure 144-8*C*). Wrap an elastic gauze snugly over the auricle and around the head to hold the dressing in place (Figure 144-8*D*). The circumferential head dressing should not encompass the opposite auricle. The elastic gauze bandage is used to compress the auricle between the two layers of gauze padding.

SURGICAL PRESSURE DRESSING

A surgically applied pressure dressing may be used instead of the traditional mastoid dressing (Figure 144-9).[1,7,16,19] This dressing applies even pressure over the former hematoma site to prevent reaccumulation. It takes more skill to apply than the traditional mastoid dressing. Aseptic technique is mandatory to prevent infection and perichondritis.

The surgically applied pressure dressing has many advantages over the traditional mastoid dressing. It produces pressure exactly where it is needed. The wound is not obscured with a bulky dressing. This allows the patient to easily observe and monitor the site for reaccumulation of fluid and possible infection. This dressing is comfortable and well tolerated by the patient. It is unlike the bulky and conspicuous mastoid dressing that is difficult to keep in place, especially when sleeping. The dressing can remain in place while monitoring the auricle, unlike the mastoid dressing that must be removed and replaced daily. The patient can remain active, including taking a shower, without fear of the dressing coming undone. The surgical pressure dressing is adaptable to any location or a variety of hematomas.

Trim a cotton dental bolster or cotton roll to fit the convolution of the auricle over the site of the drained

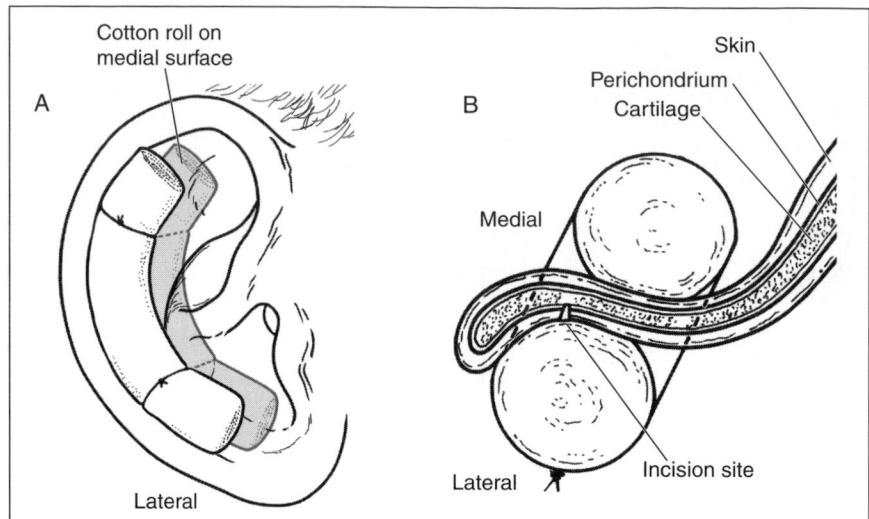

FIGURE 144-9 A surgically applied pressure bandage. *A.* A cotton roll is applied to the lateral surface of the auricle, over the site of the evacuated hematoma. A second cotton roll is applied on the medial surface of the auricle directly beneath the first cotton roll. The cotton rolls are secured with 4–0 monofilament nylon suture. *B.* Cross-sectional illustration of the surgical pressure dressing. The position of the cotton rolls and suture is seen in relation to the incision site. Note that the perichondrium is apposed to the cartilage and the dead space is eliminated.

hematoma. Place the cotton roll over the site of the former hematoma (Figure 144-9*A*). Place a second dental roll on the medial surface of the auricle opposite the first dental roll (Figures 144-9*A* and *B*). Place the needle of a 4–0 monofilament nylon suture immediately adjacent to the first cotton bolster. Pass the suture through the entire thickness of the auricle and out the medial surface. Pass the needle over the second cotton bolster and back through the auricle. Snugly tie the suture over the anterior cotton bolster (Figure 144-9*B*). The suture should be snug enough to allow the cotton bolsters to firmly hold the perichondrium to the cartilage without causing vascular compromise. Apply additional sutures using the same technique until the cotton bolsters are firmly attached and any dead space is eliminated.

Monofilament nylon is the preferred suture material for this procedure.[7] It causes less tissue reaction than silk, cotton, gut, or absorbable sutures. It has less of a tendency to cut the ear tissues when tied over the cotton bolsters. Monofilament nylon is less likely to wick bacteria into the auricle and cause an infection than multifilament nylon. The suture may be safely left in place for up to 3 weeks without any complications.

AFTERCARE

The post-procedural care of the auricle is as important as the initial hematoma evacuation. Proper follow-up and care can minimize or prevent any cosmetic deformities. All patients should be seen within 12 to 24 hours to reevaluate the auricle for infection or reaccumulation of the hematoma or serous fluid. Analgesia can be provided by the use of nonsteroidal anti-inflammatory agents. Determine the patient's tetanus immune status and provide prophylaxis as required.

Provide all patients with oral and written instructions regarding the signs and symptoms of cellulitis and perichondritis. This includes the immediate return to the Emergency Department for increasing pain, progressive swelling, redness, tenderness, and warmth. Prophylaxis with oral antibiotics is indicated with any laceration, incision, or puncture of the auricular skin.[4] Antibiotics should be taken for five days.[4,5,16] Recomendations include a range of first-generation cephalosporins, antistaphylococcal antibiotics, or antipseudomonal antibiotics.[4,5,16]

Apply the pressure dressing for a minimum of 48 hours.[4] A pressure dressing is recommended for a total of 4 to 5 days. A mastoid dressing must be removed daily to evaluate the auricle, then reapplied. A surgically applied dressing will avoid daily visits to the physician.

Drain any residual clot or serous fluid at the follow-up visit. This can easily be accomplished by needle aspiration and replacement of the pressure dressing.[6,20] If necessary, a sterile drain can be inserted.[8] All drains must be removed within 48 hours of placement to decrease the risk of infection.

COMPLICATIONS

The complications are primarily related to incomplete evacuation of the hematoma or reaccumulation of the hematoma. Incomplete evacuation of the hematoma, if by the aspiration technique, requires an incision and drainage of the hematoma. If necessary, gentle curettage of the cartilage with a hemostat should dislodge the clot. Reaccumulation of the hematoma, or serous fluid, must be evacuated. Consider placing a sterile drain into the incision.[8] Another option is to place a surgical pressure dressing.[7]

Infection may complicate any surgical procedure. This may be due to reaccumulation or incomplete evacuation of the hematoma, which then becomes infected. Strict adherence to aseptic technique will usually prevent infection. Since patients are prophylactically placed on antibiotics, any cellulitis of the auricle at the follow-up visits requires hospital admission and intravenous antibiotics.

Perichondritis is the most feared complication. It is an aggressive and rapidly progressive infection. The auricle will become red, hot, and exquisitely tender if perichondritis develops. This is followed by diffuse swelling and abscess formation. This infection can lead to significant cartilage necrosis and a deformed ear if not promptly treated. *Pseudomonas aeruginosa* is isolated in 95 percent of patients with perichondritis.[1] Over 50 percent of cases are polymicrobial with *Staphylococcus aureus* associated with *Pseudomonas aeruginosa*. These patients require Otolaryngology or Plastic Surgery consults for surgical debridement, broad spectrum intravenous antibiotics, and hospital admission.[1,8]

SUMMARY

An auricular hematoma forms in minutes to hours after blunt trauma to the ear. An auricular hematoma presents as a firm and painful swelling that obscures the normal convolutions on the lateral aspect of the auricle. It requires drainage to restore the normal convolutions of the auricle and prevent future deformity. Complete evacuation can be accomplished by needle aspiration or by incision and drainage. After the procedure, oral antibiotics are given prophylactically to prevent infection. Follow-up is required within 12 to 24 hours of the procedure to evaluate the patient for reaccumulation of the hematoma and infection. Patients should be educated about the signs and symptoms of perichondritis. Frequent wound evaluation is required until the auricle is healed.

REFERENCES

1. Templer J, Renner GJ: Injuries of the external ear. *Otolaryngol Clin North Am* 1990; 23(5):1003–1018.
2. Pierce MC: External ear procedures, in Henretig FM, King C (eds): *Textbook of Pediatric Emergency Procedures.* Baltimore: Williams & Wilkins, 1997:651–657.
3. Barwick WJ, Klein HW: Soft tissue injuries of the face, in Serafin D, Georgiade NG (eds): *Pediatric Plastic Surgery,* vol. 2. St. Louis: Mosby, 1984: 633–677.
4. Austin DF: Diseases of the external ear, in Ballenger JJ, Snow JB (eds): *Otorhinolaryngology: Head and Neck Surgery,* 15th ed. Baltimore: Williams & Wilkins, 1996:974–988.
5. Dunmire SM, Paris PM: *Atlas of Emergency Procedures.* Philadelphia: Saunders, 1994:77–81.
6. Spira M, Hardy SB: Management of the injured ear. *Am J Surg* 1963; 106:678–684.
7. Eade GG: Preventing cauliflower ears. *Northwest Med* 1964; 63:99.
8. Liston SL, Cortez EA, McNabney WK, et al: External ear injuries. *JACEP* 1978; 7(6):233–236.
9. Austin DF: Anatomy of the ear, in Ballenger JJ, Snow JB (eds): *Otorhinolaryngology: Head and Neck Surgery,* 15th ed. Baltimore: Williams & Wilkins, 1996:838–857.
10. Kotler HS, Tardy ME: Reconstruction of the outstanding ear (otoplasty), in Ballenger JJ, Snow JB (eds): *Otorhinolaryngology: Head and Neck Surgery,* 15th ed. Baltimore: Williams & Wilkins, 1996: 989–1002.
11. Snell RS, Smith MS: *Clinical Anatomy for Emergency Medicine.* St. Louis: Mosby, 1993.
12. Hollinshead WH, Rosse C: *Textbook of Anatomy,* 4th ed. Philadelphia: Harper & Row, 1985.
13. Adriani J: *Regional Anesthesia: Techniques and Clinical Applications,* 4th ed. St. Louis: Warren H. Green, 1985.
14. Murphy TM: Somatic blockade of head and neck, in Cousins MJ, Bridenbaugh PO (eds): *Neural Blockade in Clinical Anesthesia and Management of Pain,* 3rd ed. Philadelphia: Lippincott-Raven, 1998: 489–514.
15. Bumsted RM, Ceilley RI: Surgical gems: local anesthesia of the auricle. *J Dermatol Surg Oncol* 1979; 5(6):448–449.
16. Manthey DE, Harrison BP: Otolaryngologic procedures, in Roberts JR, Hedges JR (eds): *Clinical Procedures in Emergency Medicine,* 3rd ed. Philadelphia: Saunders, 1998:1120–1149.
17. Trott AT: *Wounds and Lacerations: Emergency Care and Closure,* 2nd ed. St. Louis: Mosby, 1997.
18. Simon RR, Brenner BE: *Emergency Procedures and Techniques,* 3rd ed. Baltimore: Williams & Wilkins, 1994:102–104.
19. Scarcella JV: Tie-over dressing to prevent recurrence of a hematoma of the ear: case report. *Plast Reconstr Surg* 1978; 61(4):610–611.
20. Peacock WF: Otolaryngologic emergencies, in Tintinalli JE, Ruiz E, Krome Rl (eds): *Emergency Medicine: A Comprehensive Study Guide,* 4th ed. New York: McGraw-Hill, 1996:1068–1081.

Chapter 145
NASAL FOREIGN BODY REMOVAL

Margaret J. Provenza

INTRODUCTION

Young children are naturally curious creatures and spend a great deal of time investigating themselves and the world around them. This involves handling, tasting, and smelling whatever they get their hands on. When these investigations go too far, the Emergency Physician is faced with a foreign body in a youngster's nose. Adult patients with mental retardation or psychiatric conditions may also present with nasal foreign bodies. Several methods are available for removing these objects, including manual removal under direct vision, catheter removal, or positive pressure.

ANATOMY AND PATHOPHYSIOLOGY

The nasal cavity consists of two passages on either side of the nasal septum. The superior, middle, and inferior bony turbinates project into each passage and are covered by a mucous membrane overlying a venous plexus. The cartilaginous septum is covered by a thin mucosa and receives its blood supply from the muco-perichondrium. Sensory nerves of the nasal cavity are branches of the greater palatine nerve and sphenopalatine ganglion.[1] These nerves are easily numbed with topical anesthetics. The nasal cavity is separated from the orbit by the thin lamina papyracea and from the anterior cranial fossa by the cribriform plate of the ethmoid bone.

A foreign body in the nasal cavity sets off an inflammatory response and the venous plexus becomes congested. This swelling may eventually obscure the object from view. The longer the object remains in the nasal cavity, the more likely the patient is to develop pressure necrosis, granulation tissue, and a purulent discharge. A unilateral malodorous discharge and/or epistaxis from a child's nose is the hallmark of a foreign body.

The presence of a disk or button battery in the nasal cavity requires urgent removal. The moisture in the nasal cavity may cause leakage of the battery and a low-voltage direct current between the anode and cathode. This may cause tissue electrolysis and destruction of the mucosa, cartilage, and bone within hours.[1] These patients need to be seen and followed by an Otolaryngologist after the battery is removed. An electrical burn may cause damage to the nasal tissues that is more extensive than is visible initially in the Emergency Department. Patients may develop a delayed septal perforation and alar collapse from extensive tissue damage.[2]

INDICATIONS

The presence of a foreign body in the nasal cavity is an indication for its removal. All nasal foreign bodies must be removed to prevent erosion of the nasal tissues and possible aspiration.

CONTRAINDICATIONS

There are only a few contraindications to the removal of a nasal foreign body in the Emergency Department. One contraindication is if the airway is in danger. This might be due to a posteriorly placed foreign body or an uncooperative patient. An impacted foreign body should be removed under general anesthesia. If a larger object has entered the nose traumatically, the object should be removed by the appropriate consultant, as it may have penetrated the cranial cavity, the orbit, or a sinus cavity.[3,4]

EQUIPMENT

Nasal Anesthesia and Vasoconstriction

4% cocaine solution
4% lidocaine solution with 0.25% phenylephrine
5 mL syringe
Atomizer device, optional

Manual Removal of Foreign Body (Figure 145-1)

Headlight or head mirror
Nasal speculum
Alligator forceps
Hartman forceps
Bayonet forceps
Frazier suction catheter
Ear curette
Blunt mastoid hook
Wire loop

Catheter Removal of Foreign Body

Fogarty vascular catheter, #4 or #5
Foley catheter, 5 to 6 French
5 mL syringe
Oto-Nasal Extractor (InHealth Technologies,
    Carpinteria, CA)

Positive Pressure

Cooperative parent
Bag-valve device
Face mask, various sizes

PATIENT PREPARATION

The physician should obtain appropriate consent for the procedure. The procedure will have to be discussed with the parent or guardian, as these patients are usually children or retarded adults. The physician should observe universal precautions, especially eye protection, while working in close proximity to the mucous secretions in the airway. Both nasal cavities should be carefully inspected for foreign bodies before and after the

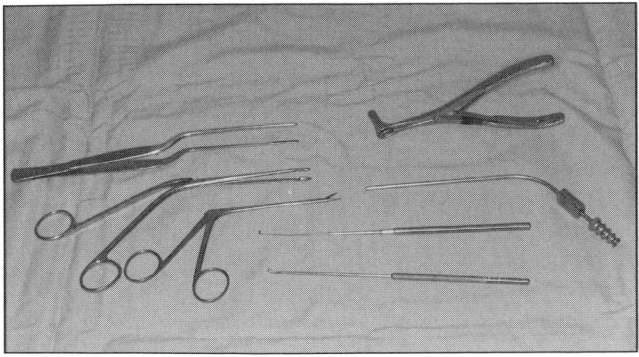

FIGURE 145-1 Equipment for manual removal of nasal foreign bodies. Starting at the upper right and moving clockwise: nasal speculum, Frazier suction catheter, mastoid hook, wire loop, alligator forceps, Hartman forceps, and bayonet forceps.

mucosa is decongested. A child will sometimes insert objects up both nostrils. A good light source is indispensable for examining the nasal cavity and removing the foreign object.

Anesthesia of the nasal mucosa is obtained by the topical application of lidocaine or cocaine. Cocaine has the added benefit of vasoconstriction and decongestion of the nasal mucosa. The maximum dose of cocaine to administer is 3 mg/kg. If lidocaine is used, a vasoconstrictive agent such as epinephrine or phenylephrine should be added. A syringe can be used as a dropper to apply the medication intranasally. This is best done by administering several drops at a time and then reassessing visibility in the airway before adding more. If the entire dose is added at one time, the child is more apt to blow the medication out the nose before it can take effect. An anatomizer device may also be used. Commonly available are either devices that attach to a syringe or a nasal decongestant container. Allow 5 to 10 minutes for the medication to work.

If the patient is cooperative, it would be appropriate to have them attempt to blow the object out of their nostril. Have the patient sit up and lean forward. Have the patient blow forcefully through their nose while covering the uninvolved nostril with a finger. Even if this has failed at home, it may work with the nasal mucosa swelling alleviated by the decongestants.[2]

Most children will need to be restrained while the foreign body is being removed. Even the child who appears cooperative and is adequately anesthetized may move suddenly while instruments are in the nasal cavity. One method is for the child to sit on their parent's lap (Figure 145-2). The adult should cross their legs over the child's legs, using one arm to restrain the child's arms and trunk and the other arm to hold the child's forehead. Alternatively, instruct an assistant to hold the patient's head while the parent controls the body and limbs. Another alternative is to wrap the child in a sheet or use a papoose board.[2] Severely uncooperative patients may require sedation, procedural sedation, or general anesthesia prior to removal of the foreign body.

TECHNIQUES

MANUAL REMOVAL

The most straightforward method is to remove the foreign body under direct vision. Insert the nasal speculum to hold the nostril open. Adjust the headlight or head mirror to illuminate the nasal cavity. **It cannot be overemphasized how crucial adequate light and visibility are to successfully remove the object.** Remove any mucus or blood with the Frazier suction. Grasp an irregularly shaped object with a Hartman or alligator forceps. Forceps may only cause an object that is round

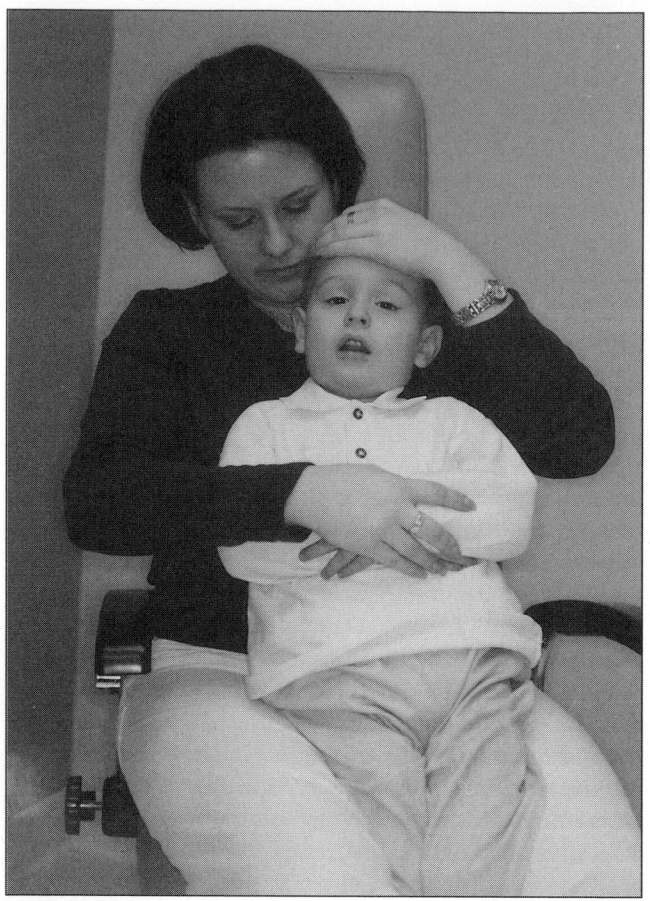

FIGURE 145-2 Restraining the child. The adult crosses their legs over the child's legs. Restrain the arms and torso with one hand. Restrain the head with the other hand.

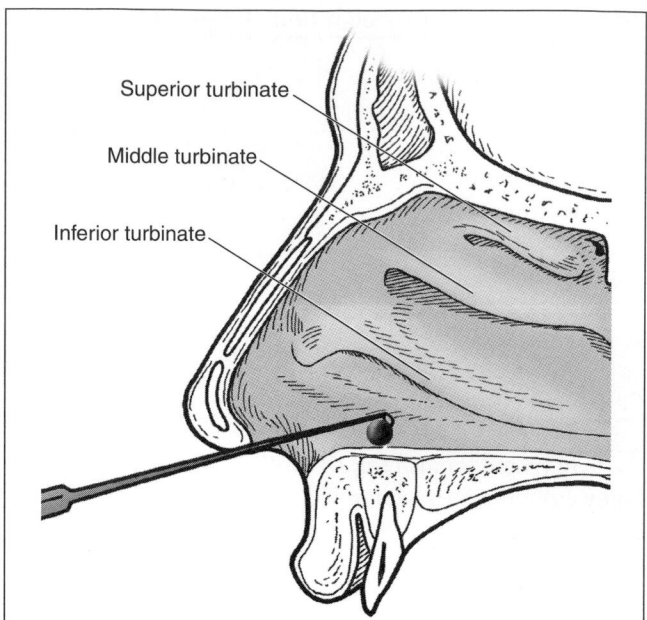

FIGURE 145-3 Removing a round, smooth object from the nasal cavity. The mastoid hook or wire loop is passed through the nares and behind the foreign body. The hook is used to pull the object out.

or smooth to slip farther posteriorly when the jaws close. In these cases, pass the wire loop or mastoid hook behind the object and pull the object out[2] (Figure 145-3). If the object is a bead and the opening is facing the examiner, the jaws of a small alligator forceps can be passed through the opening (Figure 145-4). Open the jaws when they are beyond the lumen of the bead and pull the bead from the nasal cavity.

CATHETER REMOVAL

Some physicians prefer to use a catheter with a balloon to pull foreign bodies from the nasal cavity. Authors describe using a variety of catheters. This includes a #4 to 8 Fogarty vascular catheter, a #6 Fogarty biliary catheter, and a 5 to 6 French Foley balloon catheter.[2,6,7] Lubricate the catheter. Insert the catheter until the balloon is beyond the object. The catheter may be placed either above or below the foreign body.[2] Inflate the balloon with 2 to 3 mL of air. Pull the catheter, and the balloon will push the foreign body out of the front of the nostril. A balloon catheter can also be used to stabilize a

foreign body from behind while it is removed with a forceps. The disadvantage to this method is that it is more traumatic and epistaxis is more common.[7] If the catheter is not passed under direct vision, the physician risks pushing the object posteriorly and dislodging it into the airway.

OTO-NASAL EXTRACTOR

The Oto-Nasal Extractor (Inhealth Technologies, Carpinteria, CA) is a device designed to extract foreign bodies in the nasal and auditory passages (Figures 141-6). It is a disposable single-patient-use device consisting of a balloon-tipped catheter attached to a syringe. Inflate the balloon and inspect it for any air leaks. Deflate the balloon. Insert the catheter into the nasal cavity until the balloon is just past the foreign body. Inflate the balloon by depressing the plunger on the syringe. Withdraw the catheter and foreign body from the nose while maintaining the balloon in the inflated state. If the foreign body has a central hole, such as a candy or bead, insert the catheter through the hole in the foreign body rather than around it. The main disadvantage of this single-patient-use device is its high cost.

POSITIVE PRESSURE

Positive pressure from a blower, an Ambu-bag, or even a parent can be applied to the airway to blow the object out of the nasal cavity when the patient is not able to blow their nose voluntarily. The advantage to this into the mouth, lungs, and out the nose.[9] A variant of this method uses an anesthesia bag connected to high-flow oxygen (10 to 15 L/min). Cover the mouth with the mask, close the thumb hole, and allow the bag to expand and gradually increase the airway pressure. If this does not expel the foreign body, compress the bag.[7]

Another variation of this method uses the parent to blow into the child's mouth, as though performing cardiopulmonary resuscitation, while covering the uninvolved nostril with a finger. Tell the child to open their mouth widely for a "big kiss." The parent should make a tight seal over the child's mouth with their mouth while giving a quick brisk breath of air. The advantage to this technique is that it "can be entirely atraumatic, physically and emotionally."[10]

ALTERNATIVE TECHNIQUES

Some physicians use "superglue" to aid in the removal of a foreign body. Apply a small drop of the glue to the tip of a wooden applicator stick. Press the tip of the wooden stick against the foreign body. Maintain the wooden stick against the foreign body for 20 to 30 seconds to form a bond. **Do not allow the drop of glue to fall from the stick, as it will bond to the nasal mucosa. Do not touch the tip of the wooden applicator stick to the nasal mucosa, as it will bond to the mucosa.** Slowly withdraw the wooden applicator stick with the foreign body bonded to the tip. The main disadvantages of this technique are potential bonding of the nasal mucosa and the time it takes for the glue to bond to the foreign body.

ASSESSMENT

The nasal cavity should be inspected for any ulcerations, bleeding, or a second foreign body. A gray precipitate may be noted if a disk battery has been removed. After a battery is removed, the nasal cavity should be irrigated with saline to remove any electrolyte solution or precipitate to prevent further damage.[3] Bleeding can be controlled with topical phenylephrine or epinephrine.

AFTERCARE

The patient can be discharged home with nasal saline spray to the affected nostril until secretions are clear of blood or pus. Patients with ulcerations on opposing sides of the nasal cavity must be followed up to prevent obstructive synechiae or adhesions from forming. The caretakers should be educated to remove any small objects from the child's reach, supervise children when they have access to small objects, and childproof the house.

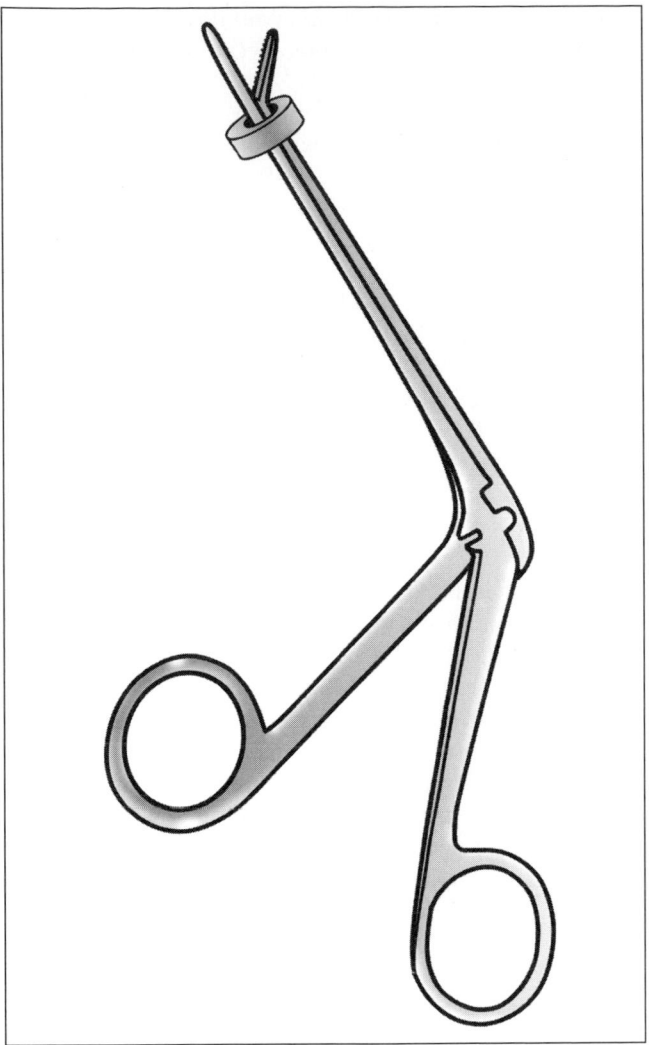

FIGURE 145-4 An alligator forceps is used to remove a bead or other object with a hollow center.

technique, if it is successful, is that no instruments are placed into the nose. The disadvantage is that the foreign body becomes a flying body. Eye protection is advised.

If an SMR cabinet or other blower with a nasal tip is available, place the nasal tip in the unobstructed nasal cavity. This method is contraindicated if there are foreign bodies in both nasal passages. **It is important to be sure that the nasal tip is placed in the open nasal cavity or the object could be blown into the trachea or esophagus.** Blow short puffs of air during the child's cries. The soft palate will close when the child is vocalizing and direct both the air and the foreign body out the other nostril.[8]

A bag-valve-mask device (Ambu-bag) can also be used to blow the foreign body out the nostril. Cover the patient's mouth tightly with the mask. Close the unobstructed nostril with a finger. Squeeze the bag to force air

COMPLICATIONS

The most significant complication would be to dislodge the foreign body into the airway. This is most likely to occur in an uncontrolled situation. Placing the patient supine and in the Trendelenburg position may prevent accidental aspiration of the foreign body.[11] **Consider the use of sedation, procedural sedation, or general anesthesia if the patient is uncooperative.** Complications related to manipulation within the nasal cavity include bleeding or subsequent infection. In rare instances, an anterior nasal pack may be required to tamponade bleeding. The longer the object has been in the nasal cavity, the more likely there is to be ulceration and granulation tissue. This will spontaneously resolve once the foreign body is removed. Toxic doses of cocaine and/or lidocaine may result in cardiac arrhythmias and seizures.

SUMMARY

There are multiple techniques for removing foreign bodies from the nasal cavity. Each has its own advantages and disadvantages. These methods include the use of forceps, balloon catheters, and positive pressure. The physician should chose a method according to the shape and location of the object, the tools available, and the cooperation of the patient.

REFERENCES

1. Anon JB, Rontal M, Zinreich SJ: *Anatomy of the Paranasal Sinuses.* New York: Thieme, 1996:38–39.
2. Shapiro RS: Foreign bodies of the nose, in Bluestone CD, Stool SE (eds): *Pediatric Otolaryngology,* 2nd ed. Philadelphia: Saunders, 1990:752–759.
3. Tong MCF, van Hasselt CA, Woo JKS: The hazards of button batteries in the nose. *J Otolarygol* 1982; 21(6):458–460.
4. Fallon MJ, Plante DM, Brown LW: Wooden transnasal intracranial penetration: an unusual presentation. *J Emerg Med* 1992; 10:439–443.
5. Alsarraf R, Bailet JW: Self-inserted sphenoid sinus foreign bodies. *Arch Otolaryngol Head Neck Surg* 1998; 124:1018–1020.
6. Rotello L: Removal of foreign bodies from the nose, in Jastremski MS, Dumas M (eds): *Emergency Procedures.* Philadelphia: Saunders, 1992:130–133.
7. Kadish HA, Corneli HM: Removal of nasal foreign bodies in the pediatric population. *Am J Emerg Med* 1997; 15:54–58.
8. Tong MCF, Ying SY, van Hasselt CA: Nasal foreign bodies in children. *Int J Pediatr Otorhinolaryngol* 1996; 35:207–211.
9. Finkelstein JA: Oral Ambu-bag insufflation to remove unilateral nasal foreign bodies. *Am J Emerg Med* 1996; 14:57–58.
10. Backlin SA: Positive-pressure technique for nasal foreign body removal in children. *Ann Emerg Med* 1995; 25:554–555.
11. Simon RR, Brenner BE: *Emergency Procedures and Techniques,* 3rd ed. Baltimore: Williams & Wilkins, 1994:266.

Chapter 146
NASAL FRACTURE REDUCTION

Joseph P. Allegretti

INTRODUCTION

Nasal fractures due to blunt trauma are a common occurrence. Fights, auto accidents, and sports accidents account for most fractures in an urban setting. Work, farm, sports, or leisure activity accidents account for most of these injuries in rural areas.[1] Males aged 15 to 25 years old make up the majority of the population, with fights being their major etiology.[2–5] These fractures are often missed on initial evaluation, especially when there are many more urgent trauma concerns. Perform closed or open reduction of these fractures within the first 2 weeks, when it is easiest to avoid the need for more elaborate operations later to correct the disfigurement and nasal airway obstruction. Perform the reduction in children within 3 to 7 days, as fracture fixation occurs faster than in adults.[6]

The clinical indications of a nasal fracture include a history of epistaxis, new onset nasal blockage, or a change in nasal appearance. Determine whether the patient has a prior history of a nasal bone fracture, as repeat nasal bone fractures will be more difficult to reduce. An old photograph of the patient may aid this determination. One study revealed that 30 percent of injured noses had a preexisting nasal deformity.[7] At least 48 percent of the general population has a nasal septal deviation.[8] Physical examination may demonstrate skin lacerations, nasal tenderness and mobility, internal mucoperichondrial tears, ecchymosis, or a septal hematoma. A septal hematoma must be drained to avoid cartilage necrosis and a resulting saddle nose deformity. Refer to Chapter 147 regarding the complete details of nasal septal hematoma management.

ANATOMY AND PATHOPHYSIOLOGY

The mechanism of injury, force of impact, direction of impact, and the history of any prior nasal deformity must be ascertained from the patient in order to understand the potential magnitude of the fracture. Photographic documentation is crucial before one attempts any nasal manipulation. Obtain radiographs, Waters and lateral nasal, to support the physical findings of a nasal fracture (Figure 146-1). Many surgeons recommend radiographs as part of medical legal documentation, although all Otolaryngologists do not agree. Radiographs can have a high false-negative rate due to the lack of fine resolution or a high false-positive rate from the misinterpretation of the normal bony sutures.[9,10]

The direction of the force to fracture the nasal bone is variable. There are several lateral and frontal force injury classifications, but no consensus exists.[5,11,12] One study demonstrated that 66 percent of nasal fractures were due to lateral forces, 13 percent from frontal forces, and 21 percent from mixed forces.[3] This predominance of lateral force fractures is due to several factors.[13] It takes more than twice the force, in cadavers, to cause a frontal impact fracture than to cause a lateral impact fracture.

Always rule out associated maxillofacial injuries, especially when the patient presents with ocular hypertelorism and lid lateral-pull laxity.[14] Thoroughly evaluate the patient for the presence of other head or neck injuries if they have a nasal fracture. Associated head and neck injuries take priority for management and evaluation as they can result in significant morbidity. Subcutaneous emphysema may be found in nasal trauma cases, as well as with simple lamina papyracea fractures and nose blowing. Scleral chemosis, subconjunctival hemorrhage, eyelid edema, periorbital ecchymosis, or subconjunctival hemorrhage may be associated with a complex facial fracture or an isolated nasal fracture. A history of anosmia indicates a possible cribriform plate fracture. Evaluate the patient for cerebrospinal fluid rhinorrhea and the presence of beta$_2$-transferrin.[1] Consider obtaining axial and coronal computed tomography scans of the paranasal sinuses with possible cisternography.

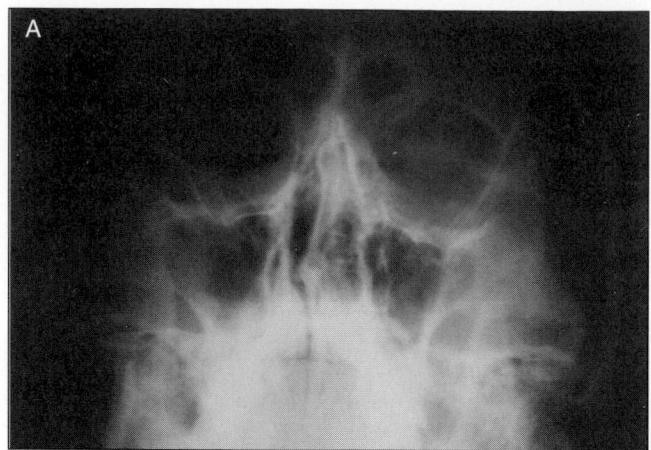

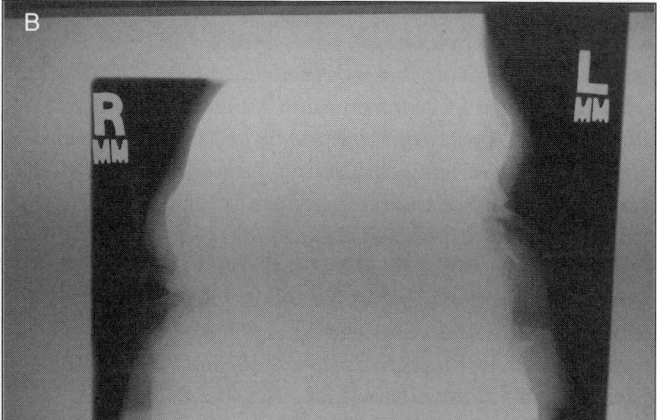

FIGURE 146-1 Radiographs demonstrating a nasal fracture. *A.* Waters view of a deviated nasal septum and right nasal bone fracture. *B.* Lateral view of a fracture from a frontal and inferior force having driven the lower aspect of the nasal bones in.

The nose consists of the external nose and the septum. The external nose consists of the bony upper third, cartilaginous lower third, and surrounding soft tissue and skin (Figure 146-2). The bony part consists of the paired nasal bones, the frontal processes of the maxillary bones, and the nasal processes of the frontal bones. The inferior nasal bones are thinner than the superior nasal bones. Thus, the lower bony portion is the most common area of the external nose to be fractured.

The cartilaginous components consist of the arched paired upper lateral cartilages and the horseshoe-shaped paired lower lateral cartilages. The former articulates with the cartilaginous septum and nasal bones, while the latter has ligamentous attachments to each other in front of the cartilaginous septum. The lower and upper lateral cartilages articulate with each other and form a crucial part of the nasal valve, the critical control point of nasal resistance and obstruction. Any of these relationships can become dislocated from a traumatic impact and will require repair for an optimal functional and aesthetic outcome. The more lateral sesamoid cartilages are relatively unimportant in these regards.[15]

The bony nasal septum consists of the perpendicular plate of the ethmoid bone, the vomer, the anterior nasal spine, the maxillary crest, and the palatine bone (Figure 146-3). The perpendicular plate of the ethmoid bone is thin, except at its articulation with the vomer and cartilaginous septum. **The perpendicular plate of the ethmoid bone is the most common location for a septal fracture.** The quadrangular cartilage of the septum is anteriorly located on the maxillary crest. It can be dislocated into either nostril with a significant force, especially from an inferior direction, and result in nasal airway obstruction.[5]

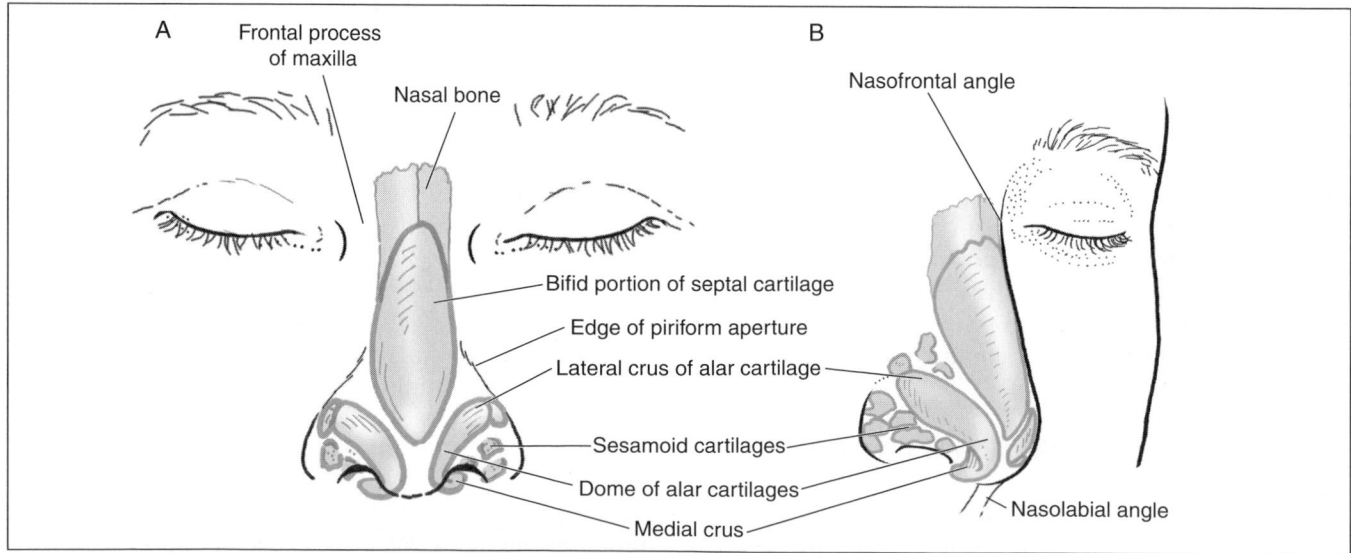

FIGURE 146-2 Anatomy of the external nasal cartilages. *A.* Frontal view. *B.* Lateral view.

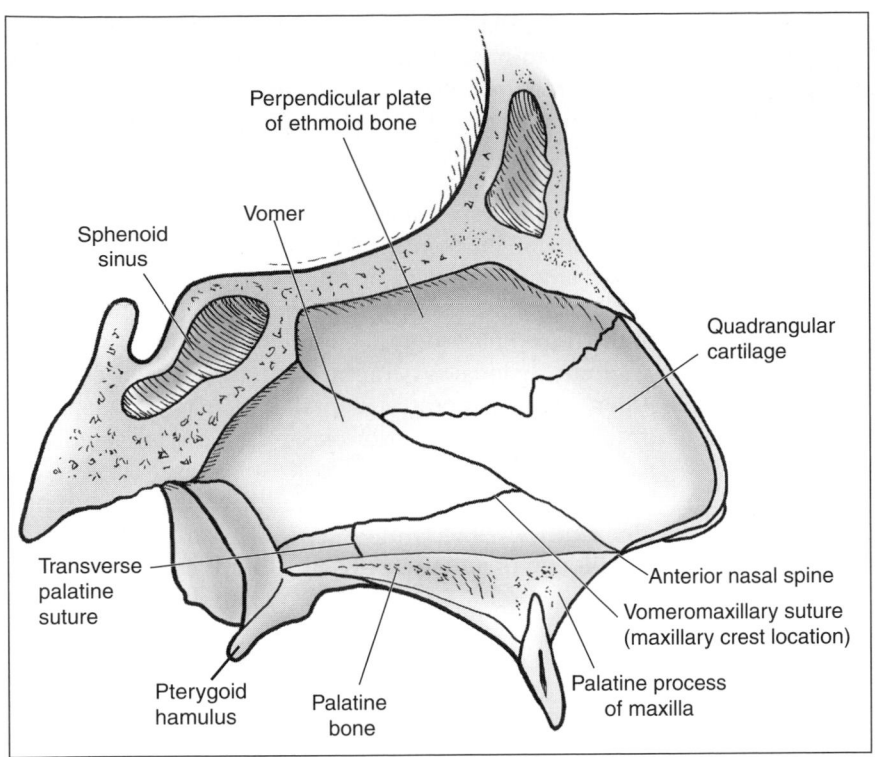

Perpendicular plate
of ethmoid bone

Vomer

Sphenoid
sinus

Quadrangular
cartilage

Transverse
palatine
suture

Anterior nasal spine

Vomeromaxillary suture
(maxillary crest location)

Pterygoid
hamulus

Palatine
bone

Palatine process
of maxilla

FIGURE 146-3 Anatomy of the nasal septum.

The septal fracture is often similar, regardless of whether a frontal or lateral impact is sustained (Figure 146-4). It usually begins just posterior to the nasal spine, at or just above the maxillary crest. The fracture can progress through this area and straight into the vomer where it curves like a C, vertically upward and into the perpendicular plate of the ethmoid bone.[16]

Nasal fractures increase in severity from a unilateral depression without a septal fracture, to a nasal twist or deviation, to a significantly comminuted nasal fracture as the frontal or lateral force of impact increases (Figure 146-5). Between these extremes are the moderately severe bilateral fractures with the contralateral side being driven outward and more significantly impacted traumas, such as the previously described C-shaped septal fracture with overriding and interlocked fragments. This latter condition often appears as the classically shortened and twisted nose with tip ptosis from columellar retraction. There is often significant nasal airway obstruction as the quadrangular cartilage telescopes over the perpendicular plate of the ethmoid, causing thickening at this point and the appearance of a bilaterally deviated nasal septum.[17]

The more common lateral force shifts the bony pyramid laterally (Figure 146-5), while a frontal impact broadens the nose. "Open book fractures" may occur in pediatric patients due to the open, midline suture of the nasal bones. This results in each of the nasal bones being

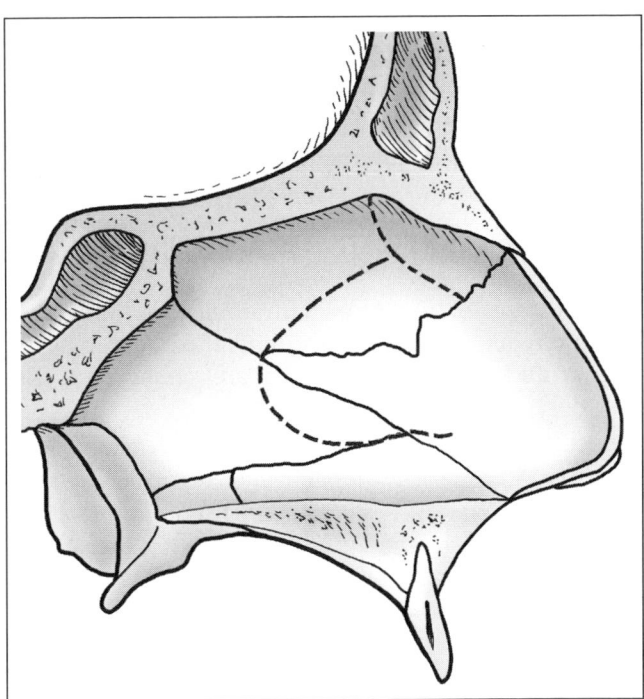

FIGURE 146-4 Schematic illustration of a common nasal septal fracture pattern. The fracture proceeds from the area of the maxillary crest through the vomerine bone and up into the perpendicular plate of the ethmoid like a backwards C shape going up into a T.

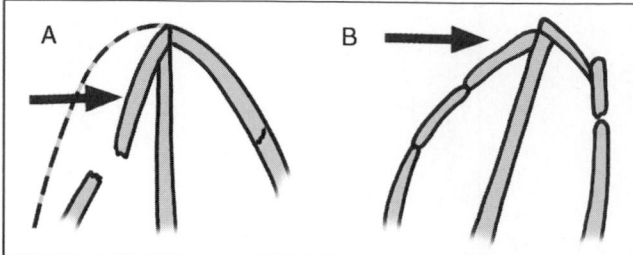

FIGURE 146-5 Nasal fractures resulting from lateral forces. *A.* Unilateral nasal fracture. *B.* Bilateral nasal fracture. The arrows depict the direction of the force of impact.

shifted laterally (Figure 146-6). Children have fewer nasal fractures because of their smaller and more cartilaginous (i.e., more elastic) noses.[18,19] Greenstick fractures are more likely in children, because of their resilient noses, than complete fractures, and can be present when it is not apparent externally.[20,21]

INDICATIONS

Attempt to reduce nasal fractures within the first 3 hours after the trauma, before the edema develops. Otherwise, perform the reduction 3 to 10 days after the injury when the edema subsides. The indications for a closed nasal reduction include unilateral or bilateral nasal bone fractures, with or without a nasal septal fracture. Interestingly, one study found that 30 percent of nasal fractures that underwent closed nasal reduction were still malaligned postoperatively.[17] Strongly consider reduction under general anesthesia for pediatric nasal fractures.

CONTRAINDICATIONS

There are no absolute contraindications for nasal fracture reduction as long as timing, the patient's health status, and associated injuries are considered. The proper approach varies by the extensiveness of the fracture. Open nasal reduction is required for more severe nasal fractures, especially those with C-shaped septal fractures and cartilage telescoping over the perpendicular plate of the ethmoid bone.[3] Some authors have defined the indications for this more aggressive approach as being a nasal pyramid deviation exceeding one-half of the width of the nasal bridge.[17] Consider using an open approach, either during the same setting or within a few days, if deformities persist after closed reduction. Relative indications for the open approach include dislocation-fractures of the caudal septum, open septal fractures, septal hematomas, displaced fractures of the anterior nasal spine, associated alar cartilage deformities, or recent intranasal surgery. An open approach may be required if an extensive septal deformity exists.[2] Otherwise, the nasal deformity will be difficult to reduce against the interlocked forces.[2]

EQUIPMENT

Headlight with light source, or overhead light
5 mL syringe
27 gauge needle, 1.5 inches long
25 gauge spinal needle
Local anesthetic solution containing
    1:100,000 epinephrine
Oxymetazoline nasal spray
4% cocaine, 4 mL
Surgical cotton paddies, 0.5 × 2 inches
Bayonet forceps
Walsham forceps (Figure 146-7)
Asch forceps (Figure 146-7)
Rubber tubing
Boies nasal fracture elevator (Figure 146-7)
Killian nasal speculum
Silastic nasal splints or Goldsmith splints
Antibiotic impregnated strip gauze or nasal tampon
Plaster of Paris splinting/casting material
5–0 plain gut suture
Paper tape, 1 inch wide
Benzoin solution

PATIENT PREPARATION

Explain the procedure, its risks, and benefits to the patient and/or their representative. Significant complications include patient dissatisfaction, the possible need for open reduction within 2 weeks, and formal nasal reconstruction months later. Other potential complications (all of much lower probability) include reactions to anesthesia, excessive bleeding, infection, saddle nose deformity, septal perforation, CSF rhinorrhea, and/or

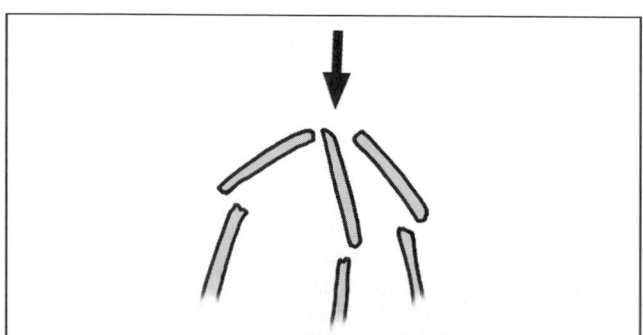

FIGURE 146-6 An open book nasal fracture resulting from a frontal impact.

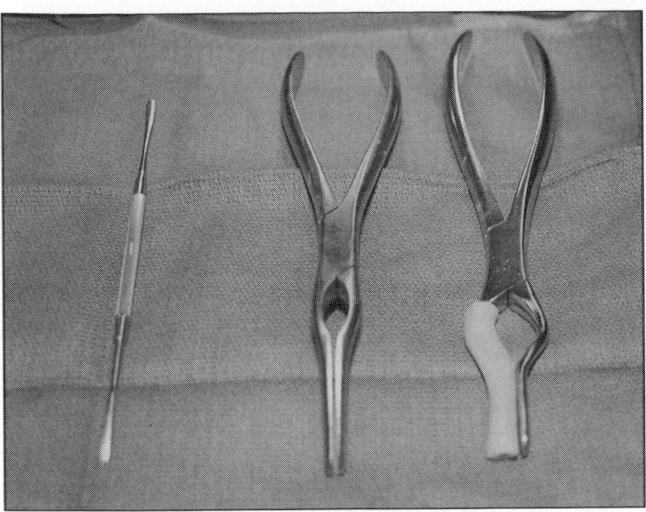

FIGURE 146-7 Nasal fracture reduction instruments. From right to left: Asch forceps (with rubber tubing on one tong), Walsham forceps, and an elevator.

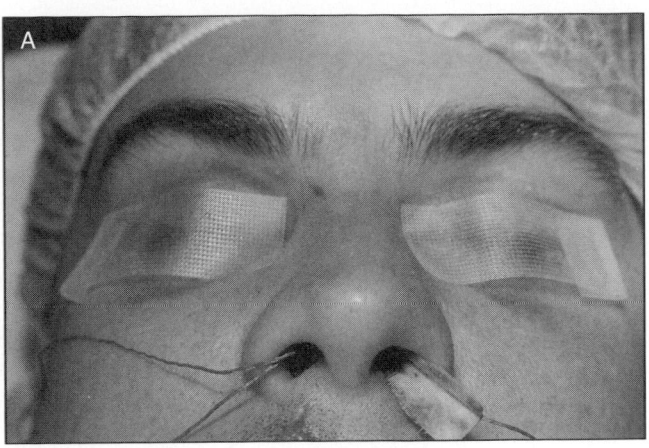

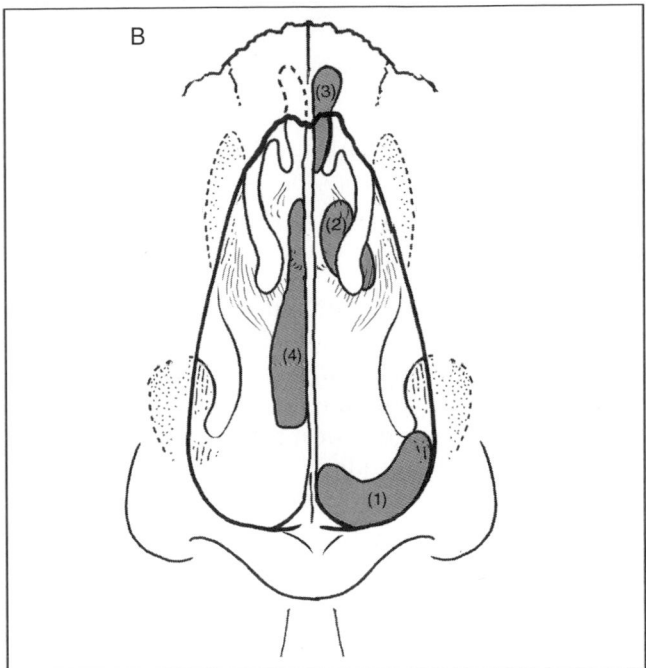

FIGURE 146-8 Topical anesthesia of the nasal mucosa. A. Surgical cotton patties soaked with cocaine placed in the nares. B. Typical sites for placement of the pledgets: (1) nasal floor, (2) posterior aspect of middle and inferior turbinate, (3) intranasal dorsum, and (4) along the nasal septum.

visual disturbances. Obtain an informed consent for the procedure.

Place the patient sitting upright in a multiposition procedure chair, or on a stretcher, with the head elevated to decrease blood flow and bleeding. Obtain an objective measure of the degree of lateral displacement. Draw a perpendicular line from the midpoint of the interpupillary line and extending downward to the base of the nasal columella. A point one-third of the way down from the cephalic end is the reference point for any deviation.[22] Consider the administration of parenteral analgesics, sedatives, or procedural sedation. Refer to Chapter 109 regarding the details of procedural sedation and analgesia. Obtain a pre-reduction photograph of the patient's face and nose, if possible.

NASAL ANESTHESIA

Anesthetize the nasal mucosa. Insert a nasal speculum. Apply oxymetazoline nasal spray bilaterally to decongest the nasal mucosa. Place 4 mL of 4% cocaine onto cotton pledgets. Cocaine is a vasoconstrictor, a decongestant, and an anesthetic. Insert the nasal speculum and pack the cocaine soaked pledgets into the nose using a bayonet forceps (Figure 146-8A). Ideally, place four pledgets in each nostril at the strategic points of the neurovascular supply (Figure 146-8B). These areas include the posterior edge of the middle turbinate (sphenopalatine ganglion and artery), the anterior to middle turbinate and opposing septum (anterior ethmoid nerve and artery), the nasal floor (branches of both nerves and arteries), and the mid-septum (branches of both nerves and arteries)[6,15] (Figures 146-9 and 146-10). Allow the cocaine pledgets to remain in the nasal cavity for 10 minutes.

Inject local anesthetic solution to anesthetize the remainder of the nose. The usual agent is 1 to 2% lidocaine containing 1:100,000 epinephrine.[23] Acidosis from the injured tissues can make local anesthesia less effective. The addition of sodium bicarbonate, at a 1:10 dilution, will counteract the acidosis and lessen the discomfort from the injection.[24]

Perform the local anesthetic injections intranasally to avoid the added pain of transgressing the skin (Figure 146-11). Infiltrate subcutaneously to anesthetize the external, nasal, infratrochlear, and infraorbital branches of the trigeminal nerve[3,4] (Figure 146-12). Insert the nee-

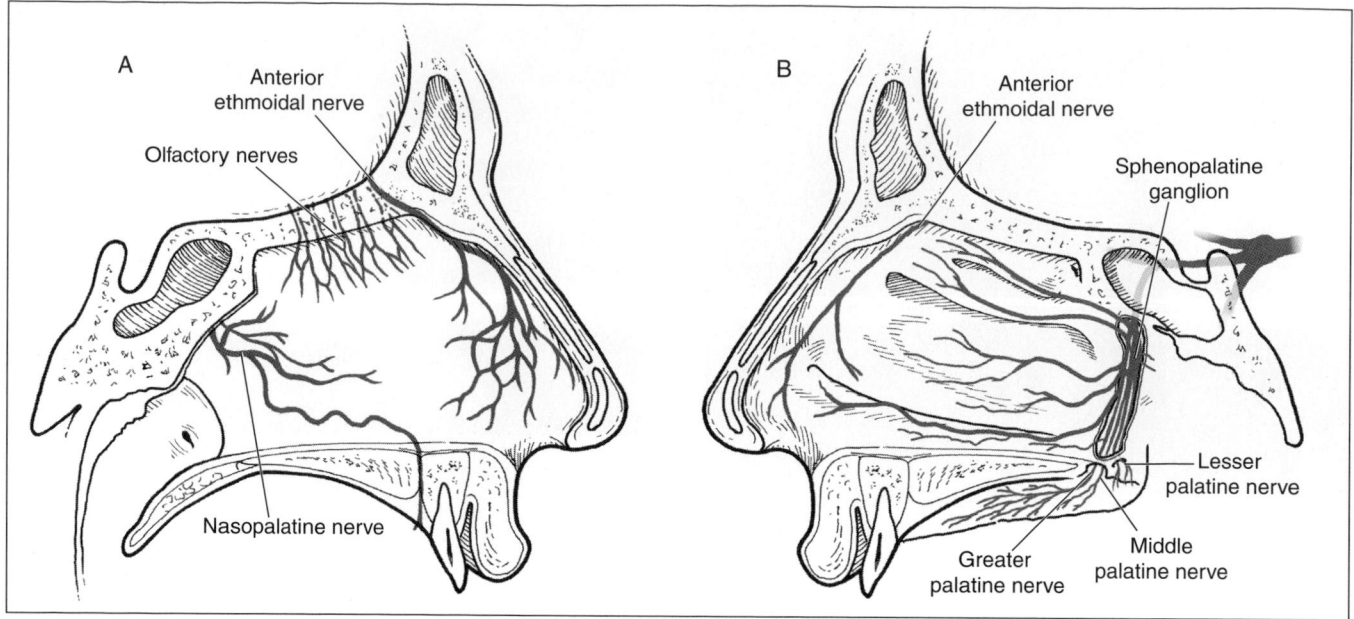

FIGURE 146-9 Nerve supply of the nasal mucosa. *A.* The nasal septum. *B.* The lateral nasal wall.

dle into the nasal cavity. Infiltrate along the nasal floor to anesthetize the superior alveolar nerve and ganglion. Infiltrate posterior to the inferior and middle turbinates to block the sphenopalatine nerve and ganglion. Allow 10 to 15 minutes for the local anesthetic agent to take effect. Assess the adequacy of the anesthesia using pinprick of the nasal mucosa. If intranasal injections are performed properly, in a patient who is under pro-

cedural sedation and analgesia, the rare but potentially serious complications of using topical cocaine may be avoided. One paper proposed using EMLA (eutectic mixture of local anesthetics) cream externally and cocaine intranasally.[25] This has yet to become a broadly accepted technique. The Emergency Physician may not feel comfortable with the technique of intranasal injection. The nerves may be anesthetized percutaneously.

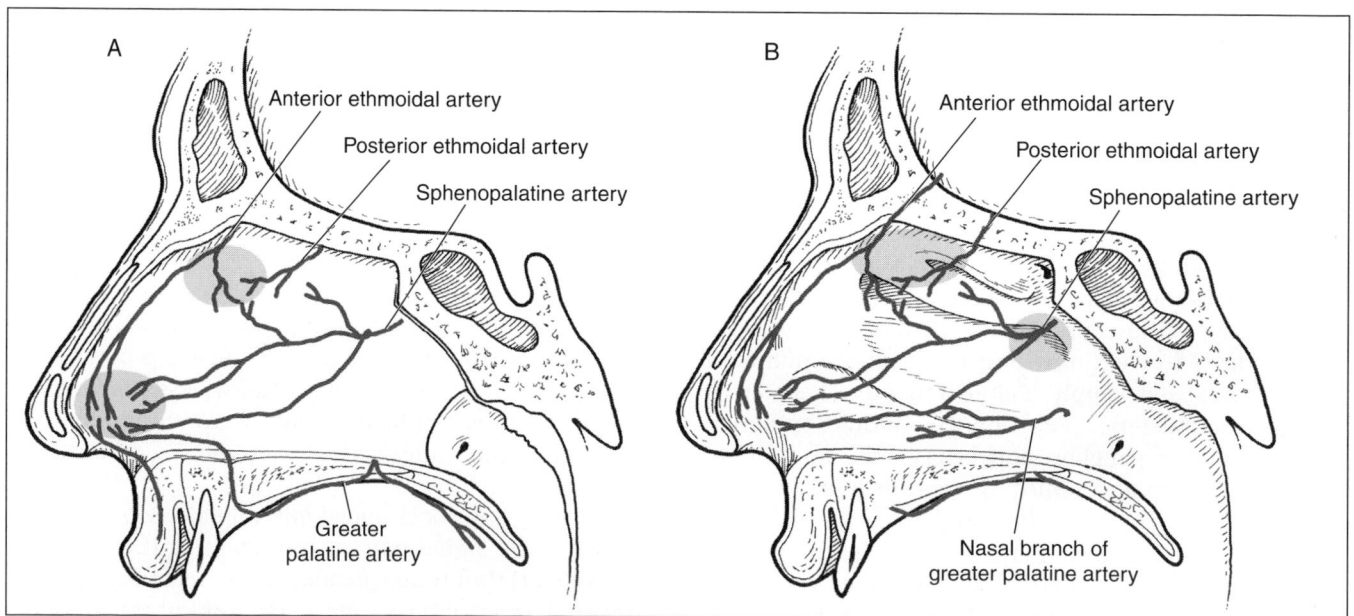

FIGURE 146-10 Blood supply of the nasal mucosa. *A.* The nasal septum. *B.* The lateral nasal wall.

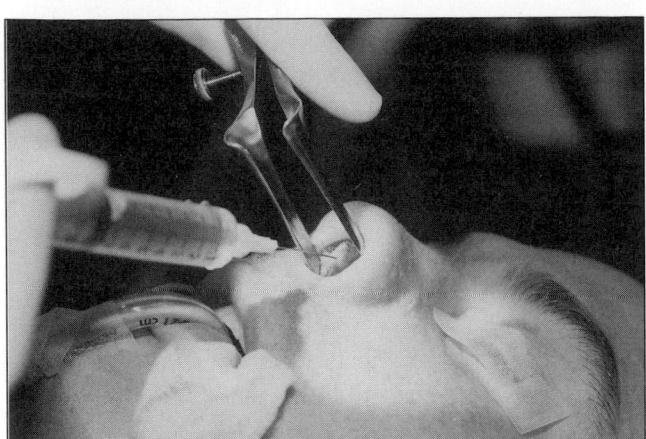

FIGURE 146-11 Intranasal injection with speculum exposure and a fine needle.

TECHNIQUES

NASAL BONE REDUCTION

Several studies have demonstrated that closed nasal reduction is 80 to 95 percent successful.[8,26] Measure the distance from the nostril rim to the nasofrontal angle in order to avoid putting the blade in too far (Figure 146-13*A*). Insert one blade of the Asch forceps, one blade of the Walsham forceps, or a Boies nasal fracture elevator into the nostril to the measured distance. Place the instrument against the depressed nasal bone. Apply a gentle upward and outward force while simultaneously applying digital counterpressure to guide the bone into reduction (Figure 146-13*B*). Alternatively, cover the other blade of the Asch or Walsham forceps with rubber tubing

so that it can provide counterpressure to the intranasal blade during outward reduction[6] (Figure 146-14). Repeat the procedure on the contralateral side if there is a bilateral nasal bone fracture.

NASAL SEPTAL REDUCTION

A nasal septal fracture is often present if bilateral pyramidal fractures exist. **Always reduce the nasal bone fracture(s) before manipulating the septum.** Insert a nasal speculum and determine whether the reduction of the nasal bones results in a straightening of the septum. If not, withdraw the nasal speculum and reduce the septum with the Asch or Walsham forceps (Figure 146-15). Insert the forceps with one blade in each nostril. Gently close the blades of the forceps to grasp the septum. Elevate the septum upward and anteriorly to disimpact any interlocked fragments. Reinsert the nasal speculum and visualize the nasal septum. Insert a Boies or Freer elevator under direct visualization and straighten it more precisely.

ASSESSMENT

Thoroughly evaluate the nasal cavity and nose. Determine the adequacy of the reduction procedure. Determine visually whether the nasal bones and the nasal septum are reduced. Consult an Otolaryngologist if the manipulations fail to provide a satisfactory reduction, if the fracture appears too comminuted, or if the nose or septum is too deviated for a closed approach. The patient may require open reduction 2 weeks from the day of trauma. Perform a thorough examination to rule out

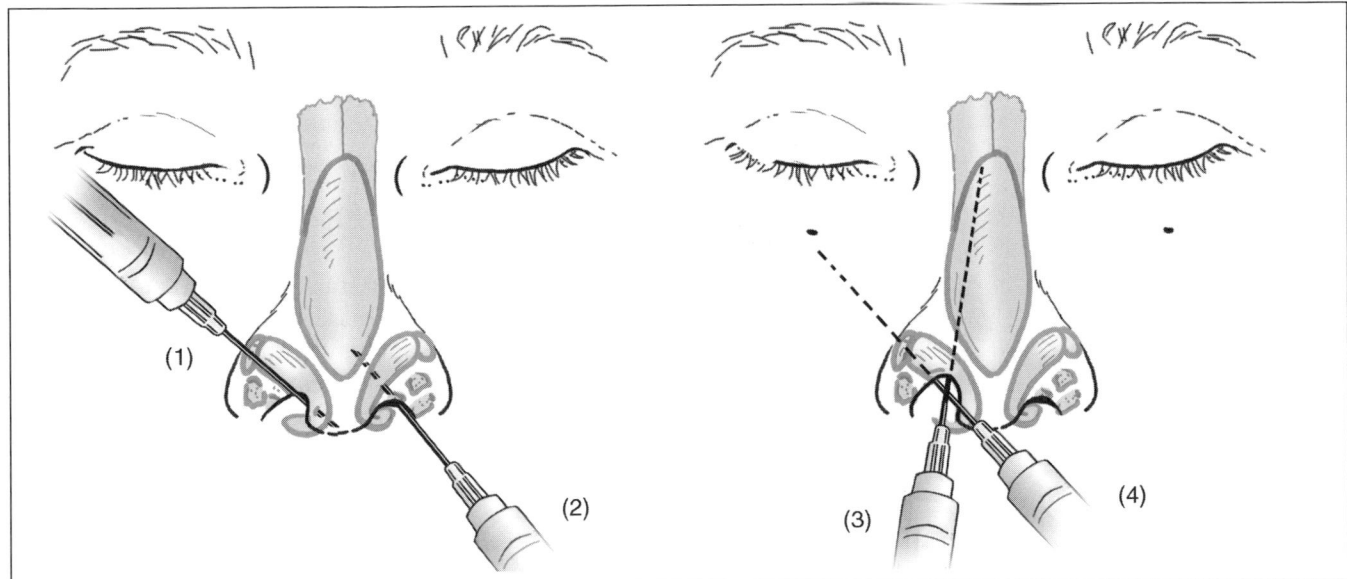

FIGURE 146-12 Intranasal injection of local anesthetic solution: (*1*) nasal spine, (*2*) nasal tip, (*3*) nasal dorsum along outside of nasal bones, and (*4*) infraorbital nerve.

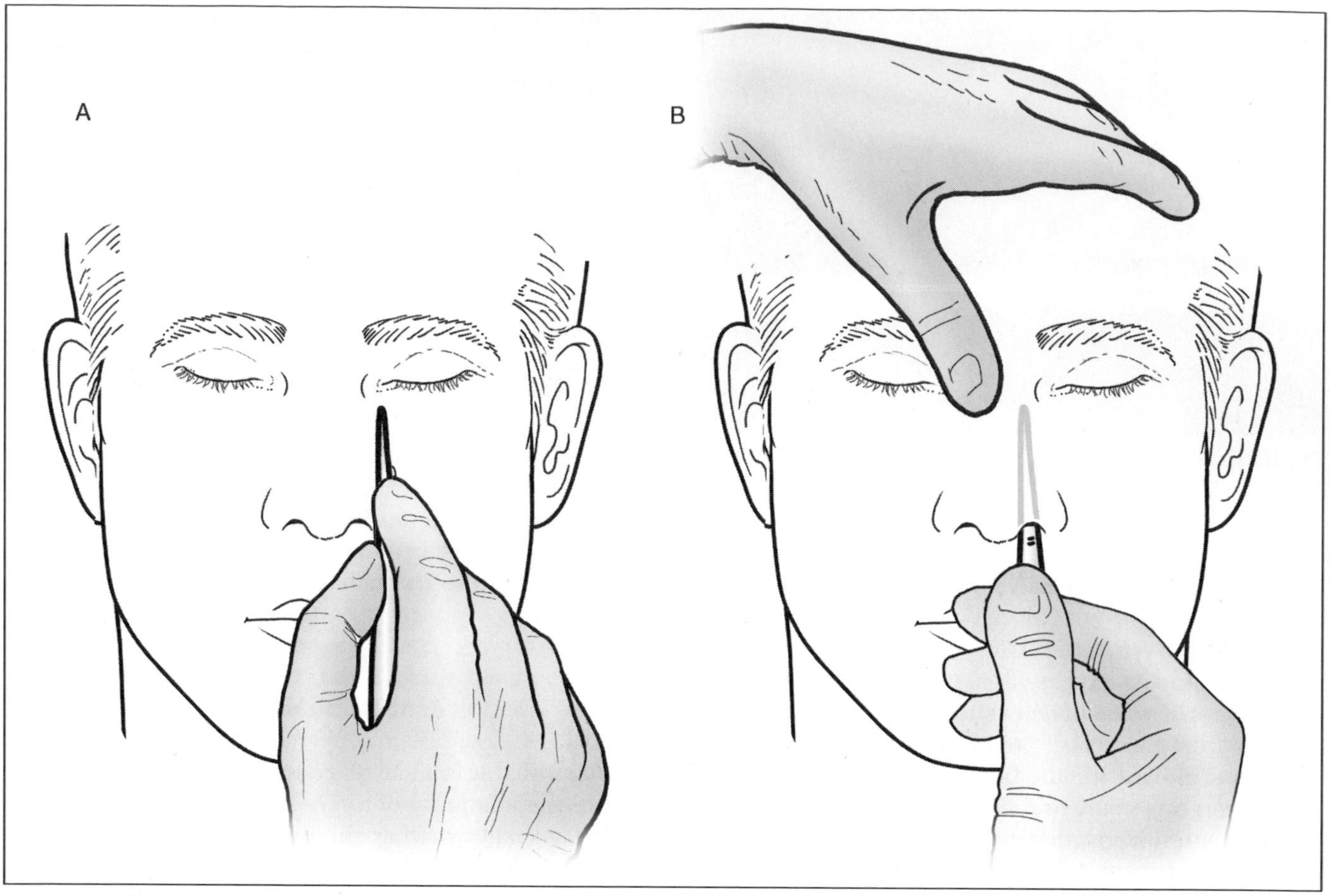

FIGURE 146-13 Closed reduction of a nasal fracture. *A.* Measure the nostril to nasofrontal angle (N-NFA) distance with the Boies elevator or another instrument. *B.* Place the elevator or forceps intranasally, just less than the N-NFA distance, and elevate the depressed bone. Reduce the contralateral nasal bone downward.

an associated septal hematoma. This must be evacuated and managed to prevent complications. Refer to Chapter 147 regarding the details of nasal septal hematoma management. Attempt to suture any nasal septal mucosal

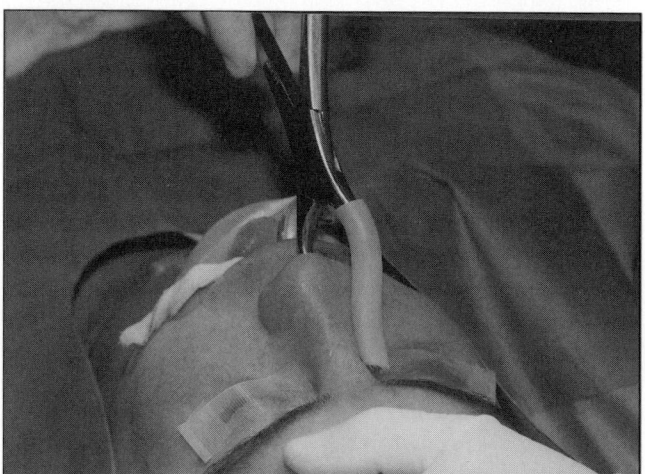

FIGURE 146-14 Placement of nasal reduction forceps. Note the rubber tubing over the outer tong to protect the skin.

tears that exist from the fracture or the reduction procedure using 5–0 plain gut suture. Warn the patient of the potential for a septal perforation that can lead to chronic crusting, bleeding, or an audible whistling. Obtain post-reduction photographs of the nose. Place the pre-reduction and post-reduction photographs in the patient's medical record.

AFTERCARE

Brace the septum for stability with bilateral Silastic splints for 5 to 10 days. This also helps to prevent the formation of a nasal septal hematoma. Doyle or Goldsmith septal splints have lumens that allow the patient to nasally breath in the postoperative period. These splints must be kept open by the patient applying 6 drops of hydrogen peroxide to each nostril three times a day, while avoiding swallowing this solution. An alternative is bilateral anterior nasal packing. The equipment is readily available in every Emergency Department. This is especially useful in cases of epistaxis. Apply antibiotic impregnated gauze ribbon, iodinated gauze ribbon, or

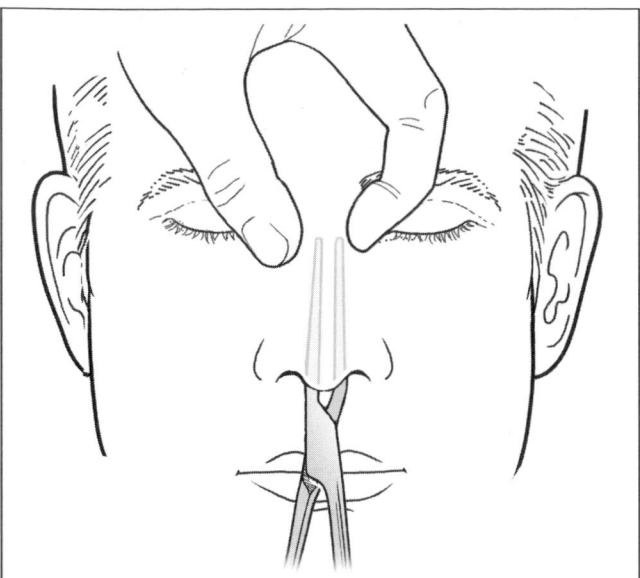

FIGURE 146-15 The Asch forceps to elevate a frontal/inferior force fracture and straighten the associated deviated nasal septum.

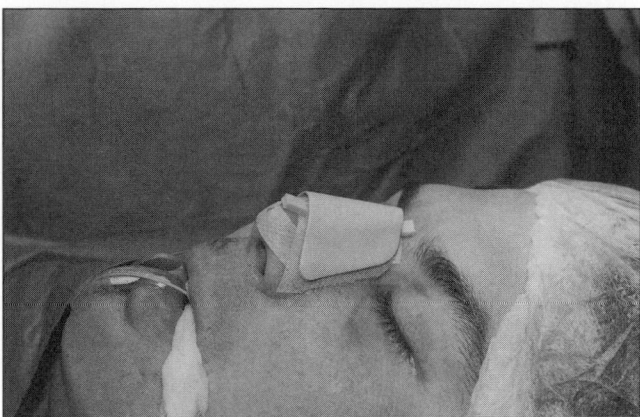

FIGURE 146-16 Post-reduction Denver splint applied after appropriate taping and midline vertical foam rubber placement.

a nasal sponge/tampon. Avoid overpacking as this can splay out the fractured nasal bones.[6]

All patients with nasal packing must be placed on oral antibiotics with gram-positive coverage, such as cefazolin (Keflex), for the duration of the packing. Leave the nasal packing in place for 1 to 7 days depending upon the amount of manipulation, the amount of bleeding, and physician preference. Avoid nasal splinting and packing in patients with nasal fractures requiring a minor degree of manipulation, especially when patients are assessed to have a low probability of follow-up and compliance.

Consider applying an external splint in addition to the internal splint or nasal packing. Some authors do not advocate external splinting and its use is based on physician preference. It serves to support the healing fracture and to remind the patient to keep their nose protected. Cleanse the skin of the nose and the surrounding area with alcohol. Apply benzoin solution to the nose and surrounding area. Apply 1 inch wide paper tape in horizontal strips, layered downwards from the nasofrontal angle to the tip of the nose. Apply benzoin solution over the tape. Apply 3 to 5 layers of 2 inch wide orthopedic plaster of Paris over the tape. Alternatively, apply an appropriately sized Denver aluminum or Thermoplast splint over the tape (Figure 146-16). Ensure that the foam rubber strut is placed vertically over the midline length of the nose to prevent any skin necrosis. Place tape over the splint to secure it.

Instruct the patient to return to the Emergency Department if excessive bleeding occurs post-reduction. Prescribe acetaminophen supplemented with narcotic analgesics as needed. Instruct the patient to avoid aspirin containing products and nonsteroidal anti-inflammatory drugs as they can increase the risk of bleeding.

COMPLICATIONS

Pack (or repack) the nasal cavity, after providing adequate local anesthesia, if bleeding occurs. A septal hematoma is likely if a patient complains of persistent or excessive pain, has noticeable nasal widening, and has an ecchymotic septum. This must be evacuated as described in Chapter 147. Infection, cartilage necrosis, and disfiguring nasal dorsal saddling may occur if the septal hematoma is not evacuated. A nasal dorsal hematoma can occur as well and must be recognized and evacuated. Cerebrospinal fluid rhinorrhea and visual impairment are rare complications of the nasal manipulation, but more likely complications of the original trauma. Cerebrospinal fluid rhinorrhea can be delayed from the initial trauma until the edema has subsided.

SUMMARY

Nasal fractures may be reduced and repaired in the Emergency Department using a closed technique. Perform the reduction, ideally within 3 hours of the injury, before significant edema occurs. It is otherwise best to wait until the swelling subsides in approximately 1 week. Repair nasal septal fractures at the same time as the nasal reduction. Severe fractures sometimes require an open reduction. Photographic and radiographic documentation can be important medicolegally as part of the preoperative evaluation. Drain any septal or nasal dorsal hematomas. Internal and external splinting are useful to help insure good postoperative healing. Antibiotics are essential if nasal packing is applied.

REFERENCES

1. Bailey BJ: Nasal fractures, in Bailey BJ, Johnson JT, Kohut RI, et al (eds): *Head and Neck Surgery-Otolaryngology,* 1st ed. Philadelphia: Lippincott 1993:991–1007.
2. Dickson MG, Sharpe DT: A prospective study of nasal fractures. *J Laryngol Otol* 1986; 100:543–551.
3. Illum P, Kristensen S, Jorgensen K, et al: Role of fixation in the treatment of nasal fractures. *Clin Otolaryngol* 1983; 8:191–195.
4. Murray JAM: Management of acute nasal trauma, in Daniel RK (ed): *Aesthetic Plastic Surgery: Rhinoplasty,* 1st ed. Boston: Little Brown, 1993:643–656.
5. Colton JJ, Beekhuis GJ: Management of nasal fractures. *Otolaryngol Clin North Am* 1986; 19(1):73–85.
6. Arden RL, Mathog RH: Nasal fractures, in Cummings CW, Fredrickson JM, Harker LA, et al (eds): *Otolaryngology—Head and Neck Surgery,* 2nd ed. St. Louis: Mosby, 1993:737–753.
7. Mayell MF: Nasal fractures: their occurrence, management, and some late results. *J R Coll Surg Edinb* 1973; 18(1):31–36.
8. Illum P: Long-term results after treatment of nasal fractures. *J Laryngol Otol* 1986; 100:273–277.
9. Clayton MI, Lesser THJ: The role of radiography in the management of nasal fractures. *J Laryngol Otol* 1986; 100:797–801.
10. De Lacey GJ: The radiology of nasal injuries: problems of interpretation and clinical relevance. *Br J Radiol* 1977; 50(594):412–414.
11. Clark WD: Nasal and nasal septal fractures. *Ear Nose Throat J* 1983; 62:25–32.
12. Stranc MF, Robertson GA: A classification of injuries of the nasal skeleton. *Ann Plast Surg* 1979; 2(6): 468–474.
13. Murray JAM, Maran AGD: A pathological classification of nasal fractures. *Injury* 1986; 17(5):338–344.
14. Mathog RH: Post-traumatic telecanthus, in Mathog RH (ed): *Maxillofacial Trauma.* Baltimore: Williams & Wilkins, 1984:303–318.
15. Gross CW, Parks SS: Nasal fractures, in English GM (ed): *Otolaryngology,* vol 4. Philadelphia: Lippincott-Raven 1997:1–14.
16. Harrison DH: Nasal Injuries: their pathogenesis and treatment. *Br J Plast Surg* 1979; 32(1):57–64.
17. Murray JAM, Muran AGD, Mackenzie IJ, et al: Open vs. closed reduction of the fractured nose. *Arch Otolaryngol* 1984; 110:797–802.
18. Grymer LF, Gutierrez C, Stoksted P: Nasal fractures in children: influence on the development of the nose. *J Laryngol Otol* 1985; 99:735–739.
19. Stucker FJ, Bryarly RC, Shockley WW: Management of nasal trauma in children. *Arch Otolaryngol* 1984; 110:190–192.
20. Moran W: Nasal trauma in children. *Otolaryngol Clin North Am* 1977; 10(1):95–101.
21. East CA, O'Donaghue G: Acute nasal trauma in children. *J Pediatr Surg* 1987; 22(4):308–310.
22. Houghton DJ, Hanafi Z, Papakostas K, et al: Efficacy of external fixation following nasal manipulation under local anesthesia. *Clin Otolaryngol* 1998; 23:169–171.
23. El-Kholy A: Manipulation of the fractured nose using topical local anesthesia. *J Layngol Otol* 1989; 103:580–581.
24. Arndt KA, Burton C, Noe JM: Minimizing the pain of local anesthesia. *Plast Reconstr Surg* 1983; 72(5):676–679.
25. Kurihara K, Kim K: Open reduction and interfragment wire fixation of comminuted nasal fractures. *Ann Plast Surg* 1990; 24(2):179–185.
26. Kaban LB, Mulliken JB, Murray JE: Facial fractures in children. *Plast Reconstr Surg* 1977; 59(1):15–20.

Chapter 147
NASAL SEPTAL HEMATOMA EVACUATION

Michael Friedman
Roy Landsberg
George Chiampas

INTRODUCTION

Soft tissue and bony injuries of the nose are common because the nose is centrally located and the most anteriorly protruding structure of the face.[1] **Suspect a nasal septal hematoma, although an uncommon complication of nasal trauma, in any individual who has sustained a nasal injury.[2,3] All individuals who have sustained nasal trauma must undergo a careful examination of the septum and nasal passages, regardless of the mechanism of injury or the findings on external examination.[2]**

Blunt trauma, either intentional or unintentional, is the most common cause of a nasal septal hematoma. Consider a bleeding diathesis if the hematoma develops after a seemingly trivial injury.[2,4,5] Other etiologies for a septal hematoma include sports injuries and child abuse.[5,6] Iatrogenic septal hematomas following nasal septal surgery are probably more common than reported in the literature. Evaluate patients who have had recent nasal surgery and present with complaints of pain and nasal obstruction for a possible septal hematoma.

Septal hematomas are characterized by severe localized nasal pain, tenderness on palpation of the nasal tip, and a cherry-like swelling or bluish discoloration of the nasal mucosa emanating from the septum that obstructs all or a portion of the nasal passage[1–3,7] (Figure 147-1). Evacuation must be performed to prevent complications.[1,2,4,5] Patients require bilateral nasal packing, oral antibiotics, and close follow-up with an Otolaryngologist to prevent complications following the evacuation of the hematoma.[2,4,8]

Distinguishing an uncomplicated septal hematoma from one that has become infected is difficult, particularly if there has been a delay of several days in seeking medical attention following the injury.[2] Nasal septal abscesses are a rare complication of septal hematomas

that occur following nasal trauma. Nasal septal abscesses generally are larger and more painful than uncomplicated septal hematomas. The overlying nasal mucosa is inflamed and occasionally has an inflammatory exudate.[2] Local extension of the infection, if left untreated, into the cavernous sinus with subsequent intracranial infection is the most important potential complication.[5,8] The most common complication of a septal abscess is cartilage necrosis that results in nasal structural collapse and a saddle nose deformity.

ANATOMY AND PATHOPHYSIOLOGY

The nose is both a sensory organ and a respiratory organ. It performs an important function for the entire body by providing both physical and immunologic protection from the environment.[9] The nose aids in the formation of basic speech sounds.[9] The supporting structure of the nose consists of bone, cartilage, and connective tissue. The nose, on frontal view, is in the shape of a pyramid of which approximately the upper two-fifths comprise the bony vault and the lower three-fifths comprise the cartilaginous vault. The upper narrow end joins the forehead at the glabella and is referred to as the root of the nose. The two nares are separated from each other by a skin-cartilage septum known as the columella.[9,10] The cartilaginous framework of the nose provides both its structure and function. **The septal cartilage is avascular and receives its blood supply from the adherent mucoperichondrium.**

The skin covering the external nose is thin and contains an areolar type of subcutaneous tissue. The skin is loosely attached over the upper half. The skin over the lower half of the nose is intimately bound to the lower lateral cartilage and may sometimes be thick, fatty, and contain sebaceous glands.[9,10]

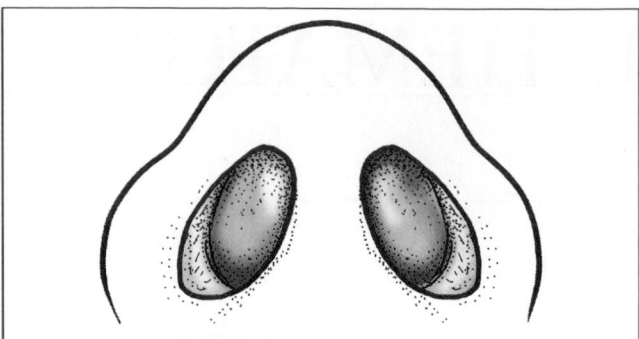

FIGURE 147-1 Bilateral nasal septal hematomas creating a partial obstruction.

The precise mechanism for a nasal septal hematoma formation following nasal trauma is not known. Nasal septal hematomas are thought to occur when a mechanical force to the nasal cartilage results in rupture or leakage from the perichondrial blood vessels of the nasal septum. In instances where the nasal cartilage is fractured, blood may dissect through the fracture line and form bilateral septal hematomas. Accumulation of the extravasated blood strips the perichondrium from the cartilage, forming a closed space in which the blood accumulates (Figure 147-2). **The hematoma, when not recognized initially and evacuated promptly, can expand and mechanically obstruct the blood vessels that supply the nasal cartilage. Pressure induced avascular necrosis of the nasal septal cartilage can develop rapidly because there is no alternative blood supply to the cartilage.**[1–3,7] The accumulated blood and necrotic tissue can form a nidus for infection from bacteria that colonize the nasal mucosa.[1–3,7]

Cartilage necrosis subsequently leads to the saddle nose deformity. The term "saddle nose deformity" is a nonspecific description of a nose with a depression over its dorsal surface[9] (Figure 147-3). The deformity results from a septal hematoma or abscess not being evacuated. Necrosis with subsequent fibrosis may develop causing a permanent thickening or absorption of the nasal septum with partial obstruction of the nasal airway.[7–9]

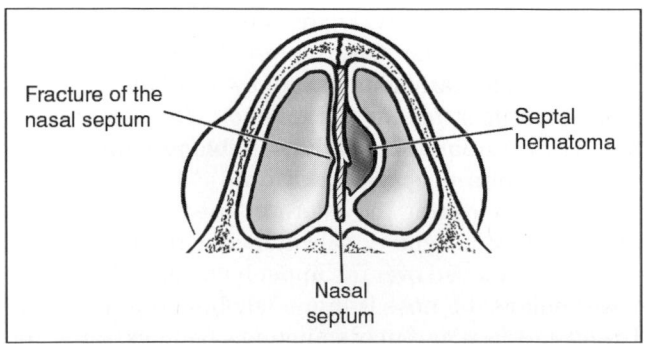

FIGURE 147-2 A small left-sided nasal septal hematoma.

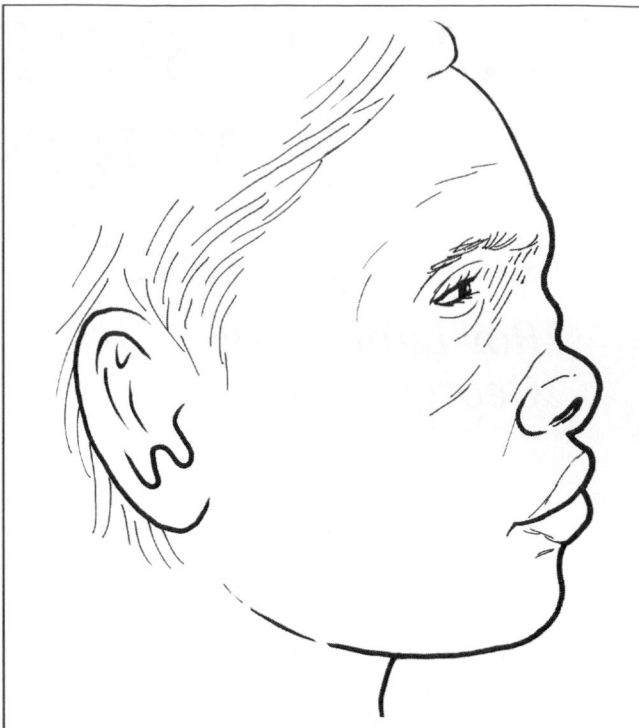

FIGURE 147-3 The saddle nose deformity.

The sphenopalatine branches of the internal maxillary artery and the ethmoidal arteries from the ophthalmic artery supply the internal nose. The veins terminate in the anterior facial and ophthalmic veins.[10] Venous drainage is clinically important in understanding the complications of a septal abscess. Branches of the trigeminal nerve provide sensory innervation to the nose.[9,10]

INDICATIONS

Any significant septal hematoma requires evacuation. A nasal septal hematoma may progress to form an abscess with associated complications of avascular necrosis of the nasal septum, meningitis, or cavernous sinus thrombosis in as little as 3 to 4 days.[7,8] It is not urgent to evacuate a simple hematoma in the Emergency Department as complications occur over a period of days. It is essential, however, to identify a hematoma so that a treatment plan is initiated and to rule out a septal abscess that does require immediate evacuation.[5]

CONTRAINDICATIONS

There are no absolute contraindications to the evacuation of a nasal septal hematoma.

EQUIPMENT

Headlight
Nasal speculum
2% ephedrine
Cotton-tipped applicators
10 ml syringe
25 or 27 gauge needle, 1½ inches long
Local anesthetic solution containing epinephrine
4% cocaine
2% pontocaine
#15 surgical blade on a handle
Frazier suction catheter
Suction source and tubing
Nasal speculum
Bayonet forceps
Nasal tampon or sponge
Iodoform gauze

PATIENT PREPARATION

Explain the risks, benefits, complications, and after-care of the procedure to the patient and/or their representative. Obtain a signed consent for the procedure. Aseptic technique should be followed and maintained throughout the procedure. The procedure is considered clean, but not sterile, as the nasal mucosa can never be sterilized. It is crucial, however, that the instruments are sterile.

Administer anesthesia for the evacuation of a nasal septal hematoma by one of two routes: topical application with supplemental infiltration and regional block. Some authors recommend using both techniques. However, most nasal septal hematomas can be adequately evacuated with topical anesthesia supplemented by local infiltration.[7] Dampen the swabs of four cotton-tipped applicators with either a solution of 2% pontocaine with ephedrine or cocaine. Insert a nasal speculum to expose one nostril. Gently insert the applicator beneath the roof of the nose so that it reaches the branches of the anterior ethmoidal nerve. Pause until some vasoconstriction and anesthesia takes place, if it meets resistance on insertion, and advance the applicator further (Figure 147-4). Pass an applicator into the nasal fossa and move it from the floor of the nasal vestibule, across the midportion of the inferior turbinate, and reaching the posterior aspect of the middle turbinate in the region of the sphenopalatine foramen.[11] Infiltrate local anesthetic solution containing epinephrine, if additional anesthesia is desired, through the mucoperichondrium and circumferentially around the hematoma.

An atomizer or nasal spray bottle can provide an alternative and commonly used method for septal anesthesia. Mix equal amounts of 2% pontocaine with ephedrine

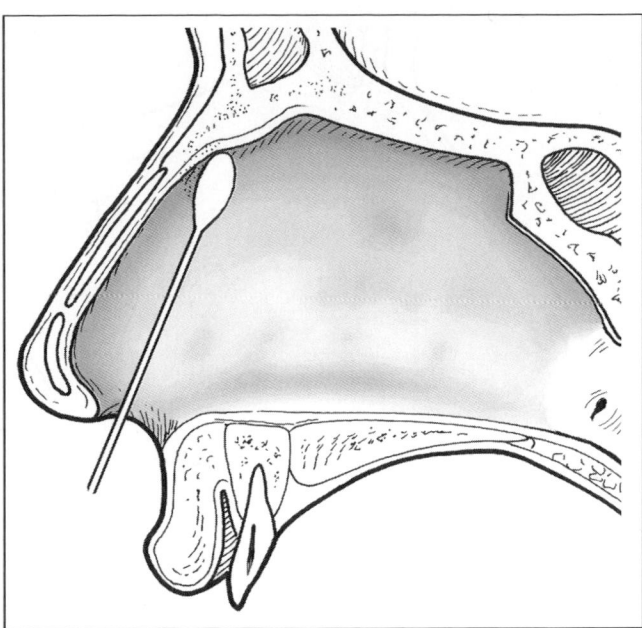

FIGURE 147-4 Cotton swab technique for septal anesthesia

and place this in the atomizer or nasal spray bottle. Insert the nasal speculum to gain access to the entire nasal cavity. Insert the atomizer or nasal spray bottle into the nostril. Instill two puffs of solution into the nostril. Allow 5 to 10 minutes for the anesthetic to take affect. Infiltrate local anesthetic solution containing epinephrine, if additional anesthesia is desired, through the mucoperichondrium and circumferentially around the hematoma.

Confirm the presence of a septal hematoma. Compress the area with a cotton-tipped applicator. The bulge from the hematoma is compressible with the applicator. It should not shrink with the application of a topical vasoconstrictor.[2,6]

TECHNIQUES

ASPIRATION

Some authors feel that simple aspiration with an 18 gauge needle may be adequate for a small, early hematoma. Most patients require a more extensive evacuation as clotted blood cannot be removed with aspiration. Simple aspiration may, however, be used to diagnosis a septal hematoma.[6–8] Insert an 18 gauge needle, attached to a 10 mL syringe, into the septal hematoma. Aspirate the contents of the hematoma. No additional procedure is necessary if the hematoma can be completely evacuated by aspiration. Simple clinical assessment of the septum is the guide to determine if the hematoma has been evacuated. Apply a nasal pack as described below.

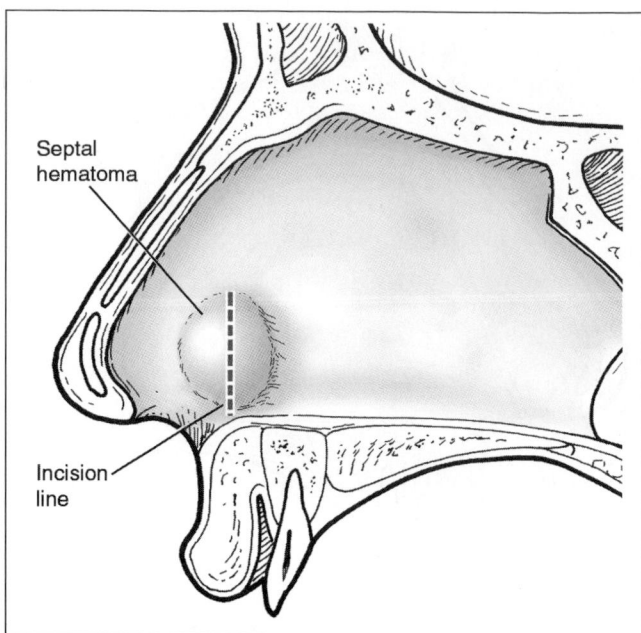

FIGURE 147-5 Septal hematoma with markings for a vertical incision through the mucoperichondrium.

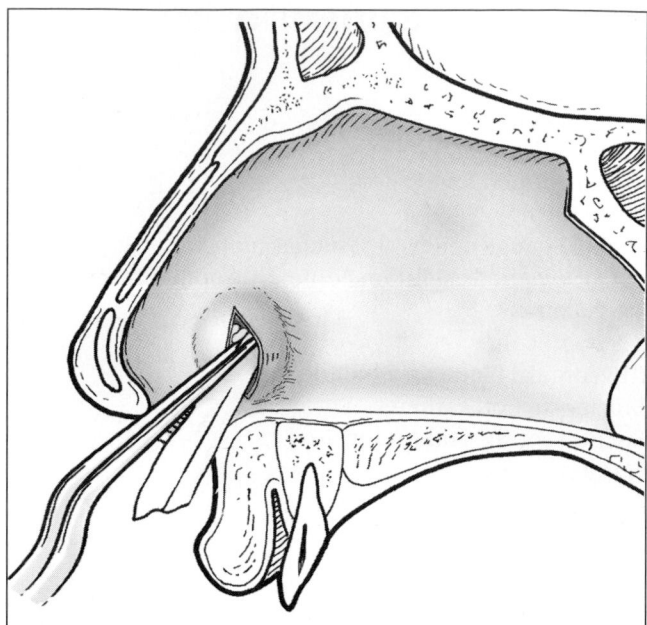

FIGURE 147-6 Iodoform gauze is placed between the separated mucoperichondrium and the cartilaginous septum.

INCISION AND DRAINAGE

The incision and drainage technique is the primary procedure to drain a septal hematoma. Cleanse the skin surrounding the nares of any dirt and debris. Apply alcohol or povidone iodine to the area and allow it to dry. Make a 0.75 to 1.0 cm long vertical incision, with a #15 scalpel blade, in the septal mucoperichondrium overlying the hematoma (Figure 147-5). **Do not cut into the cartilaginous septum.** The length of the incision depends upon the size of the septal hematoma. Some authors prefer to use an L-shaped incision in the mucoperichondrium.[12–16] These authors feel that this incision allows the mucoperichondrium to reposition flat against the cartilaginous septum. The choice of incision type is left to physician preference.

Use the Frazier suction catheter to gently evacuate any clot or necrotic debris. Always send a sample of the fluid or hematoma to the laboratory for Gram's stain, anaerobic cultures, and aerobic cultures.[2,7,8] Apply topical antibiotic ointment over the incision and nasal packing as described below.

A bilateral septal hematoma can, almost always, be evacuated from one side. Apply gentle pressure to the contralateral hematoma to express it out the incision. Make a second vertical incision contralaterally, either anterior or posterior to the first incision to prevent septal perforation, if complete evacuation is not achieved unilaterally.

WICK INSERTION

Insert a wick of 1/8 inch iodoform gauze through the incision (Figure 147-6). Allow 1 inch of the wick to extend into the nasal cavity for easy removal. **Be careful to ensure that the wick is flat between the mucoperichondrium and the cartilaginous septum. Do not pack the cavity with the wick.** This will allow continuous drainage, prevent premature reapproximation of the mucoperichondrium onto the septum, and prevent reaccumulation of the hematoma. Some authors recommend inserting a Penrose drain, or a piece of one, instead of the iodoform gauze.[6] This has not been found to be beneficial when compared to iodoform gauze.[6] The Penrose drain can be a substitute if iodoform gauze is not available or the patient is allergic to iodine.

NASAL PACKING

Apply bilateral nasal packs following the successful drainage of a septal hematoma. Packing inhibits reaccumulation of the hematoma, or serous fluid, thereby preventing the severe complications associated with a septal hematoma. The use of commercially available nasal packing devices, such as nasal tampons or sponges, provides adequate protection against reaccumulation. Patients report such devices to be significantly more comfortable than traditional gauze packing. This, coupled with the ease of insertion when compared to gauze packing, has made such devices very popular.

Place the patient's head in the sniffing position. Coat a nasal tampon with a water-soluble antibiotic ointment. Insert the nasal speculum to obtain adequate visualization of the nasal septum. Grasp the nasal tampon with a bayonet forceps. Introduce the forceps with the nasal tampon in a horizontal position through the speculum. **Be careful to not tear the incision in the**

mucoperichondrium open or to dislodge the wick. Place the nasal tampon on the floor of the nasal cavity and against the nasal septum.[8] Withdraw the bayonet forceps and the nasal speculum. Repeat the nasal packing procedure on the contralateral side. Both nasal cavities must be packed to maintain the septum in the midline, prevent bowing of the septum into the contralateral nasal cavity, and reaccumulation of the hematoma. Refer to Chapter 148 regarding the complete details of nasal packing.

AFTERCARE

Proper follow-up is vital to prevent any infectious process or cosmetic deformity. All patients must be reevaluated within 24 hours and again in 48 hours for removal of the nasal packs. Prescribe acetaminophen and narcotic analgesics for pain control. Prescribe broad-spectrum antibiotics, specifically those with staphylococcal coverage, as prophylaxis against infection and the development of a septal abscess.[6] Instruct the patient to avoid nonsteroidal anti-inflammatory drugs as they increase the risk of bleeding. Provide all patients with proper discharge instructions. They should return to the Emergency Department immediately if they experience increased pain, bleeding, or a fever. Refer all patients to an Otolaryngologist within 24 hours.

COMPLICATIONS

The most common acute complication of a nasal septal hematoma is an abscess or cosmetic deformity. Complications are primarily related to incomplete evacuation or reaccumulation of the hematoma. This may be avoided by adequate removal of the hematoma with suction, placement of an iodoform gauze drain, and bilateral nasal packing. An abscess may result in ascending infections including meningitis and cavernous sinus thrombosis. *Staphylococcus aureus* is the primary pathogen isolated from the majority of reported cases, regardless of age. Prescribe appropriate prophylactic antibiotics.[2,5,6]

Complications of septal hematoma drainage are rare and include nasal bleeding, inadequate evacuation, and septal perforation. Nasal bleeding can usually be controlled with the prescribed packing. Incomplete removal of the hematoma is not a serious problem if identified. A septal hematoma may reoccur if the incision is made on opposite sides of the septum. Limit the incision to one side if possible. The second incision, if required, on the contralateral side must not oppose the first incision.

SUMMARY

A nasal septal hematoma is a rare but potentially serious complication of nasal trauma. Proper manage-ment consists primarily of early recognition and prompt evacuation. Administration of antimicrobial therapy is necessary to prevent or treat a secondary nasal abscess. Follow-up with an Otolaryngologist is required within 24 hours of the procedure to evaluate for the reaccumulation of the hematoma and/or an abscess. These patients require continual follow-up until the nasal septum is healed.

REFERENCES

1. Ballenger JJ, Snow JB: *Otorhinolaryngology: Head and Neck Surgery.* Baltimore: Williams & Wilkins, 1996:30–32.
2. Ginsburg CM: Nasal septal hematoma. *Pediatr Rev* 1998; 19(4):142–143.
3. Ginsburg CM, Leach JL: Infected nasal septal hematoma. *Pediatr Infect Dis J* 1995; 14(11):1012–1013.
4. Krespi YP, Ossoff RH: *Complications in Head and Neck Surgery.* Philadelphia: Saunders, 1993:341–342.
5. Feinberg AN, Gushurst CA, Purdy WK, et al: Bilateral nasal septal hematomas. *Arch Pediatr Adolesc Med* 1998; 6:601–602.
6. Canty PA, Berkwitz RG: Hematoma and abscess of the nasal septum in children. *Arch Otolaryngol Head Neck Surg* 1996; 122(12):1373–1376.
7. Becker W, Naumann HH, Pfaltz CR: *Ear, Nose and Throat Diseases: A Pocket Reference,* 2nd ed. New York: Thieme, 1994:260–262.
8. Waters TA, Peacock WF IV: Nasal emergencies and sinusitis, in Tintinalli JE, Kelen GD, Stapczynski JS (eds): *Emergency Medicine, A Comprehensive Study Guide,* 5th ed. New York: McGraw-Hill, 2000:1532–1539.
9. Gates GA: *Current Therapy in Otolaryngology: Head and Neck Surgery,* 6th ed. St. Louis: Mosby, 1998:133–134, 168.
10. Williams PL: *Grays' Anatomy,* 38th ed. New York: Churchill Livingstone, 1995:1631–1633.
11. Hinderer KH: *Fundamentals of Anatomy and Surgery of the Nose.* Birmingham: Aesculapius, 1978:104–107.
12. Chan TC: Septal hematoma drainage, in Rosen P, Chan TC, Vilke GM, et al (eds): *Atlas of Emergency Procedures.* St. Louis: Mosby, 2001:198–199.
13. Dunmire SM, Paris PM: *Atlas of Emergency Procedures.* Philadelphia: Saunders, 1994:94–95.
14. Isaacman DJ, Post JC: Drainage and packing of a nasal septal hematoma, in Henretig FM, King C, Joffe MD, et al (eds): *Textbook of Pediatric Emergency Procedures.* Baltimore: Williams & Wilkins, 1997:675–680.

15. Votey S, Dudley JP: Emergency ear, nose, and throat procedures. *Emerg Med Clin North Am* 1989; 7(1):117–154.

16. Simon RR, Brenner BE: *Emergency Procedures and Techniques,* 4th ed. Philadelphia: Lippincott Williams & Wilkins, 2002:401–402.

Chapter 148
EPISTAXIS MANAGEMENT

Stephen M. Kelanic
David D. Caldarelli

INTRODUCTION

Epistaxis is an extremely common condition in the United States with an incidence estimated at 10 per 10,000 people per year.[1] It is a common reason for patient visits to the Emergency Department. Epistaxis usually is the result of well-localized intranasal trauma. However, it may be the initial sign of a more serious underlying systemic illness. Epistaxis is often self-limited and can be managed conservatively. Epistaxis can also manifest itself as a profuse spontaneous hemorrhage that is extremely difficult to control and result in aspiration, hypotension, cardiovascular collapse, syncope, and airway compromise.

The proper management of epistaxis and the prevention of adverse consequences depend on a timely and thorough evaluation of the patient as well as the appropriate intervention. The Emergency Physician must be familiar with a variety of techniques that can be used to control intranasal hemorrhage.

ANATOMY AND PATHOPHYSIOLOGY

An understanding of the vascular anatomy of the nasal cavity is essential to efficient and immediate control of nasal bleeding. The blood supply to the sinonasal cavity arises from both the internal and external carotid artery system (Figure 148-1). The sphenopalatine artery arises as one of the terminal branches of the internal maxillary artery, a branch of the external carotid system, and is the primary blood supply to the sinonasal cavities. The anterior and posterior ethmoid arteries, terminal branches of the internal carotid system, supply blood to the superior straits of the nose. The superior labial branch of the facial artery supplies the anterior nasal cavity and anastomoses with branches from the anterior ethmoid artery and the sphenopalatine artery in an area of the anterior nasal septum known as Kiesselbach's plexus or Little's area (Figure 148-2). It has been esti-

mated that 90 percent of all nasal bleeding occurs in this area.[2] This is particularly true for children and young adults. Older adults tend to bleed from the posterior nasal cavity, from branches of the sphenopalatine and posterior ethmoidal arteries. This has been attributed to arteriosclerosis.[2]

Epistaxis may result from numerous local and/or systemic factors that damage the delicate mucosal lining of the nasal cavity and expose the underlying vasculature. The most common cause of epistaxis is accidental or self-inflicted trauma, often from digital manipulation of the nasal mucosa (i.e., nose picking). This eventually heals and crusts over but is subject to repeated irritation and bleeding when the patient sneezes or blows their nose. The anterior source of this bleeding makes it very easy to treat. High-velocity trauma to the region of the midface and skull base may be manifest as a severe, life-threatening hemorrhage that may be extremely difficult to control.

Local inflammatory reactions due to acute upper respiratory infections, allergic rhinitis, and chronic sinusitis may cause epistaxis.[3] The mucosa becomes inflamed, hypervascular, and is easily disrupted with forceful nose blowing. The presence of an intranasal foreign body may inflame the nasal mucosa, with consequent granulation tissue and bleeding. This should be expected if the bleeding is unilateral and associated with nasal obstruction and foul rhinorrhea.

Epistaxis may be attributed to a nasal septal deformity.[4] The deflected nasal septum creates turbulent airflow that desiccates the mucosa and leads to crusting and bleeding. Epistaxis attributed to nasal septal deviation presents just posterior to the deflection and may be difficult to control. Nasal septal perforations bleed frequently and easily from mucosal irritation and granulation tissue.

Postoperative bleeding as the result of sinonasal surgery—such as septoplasty, rhinoplasty, turbinectomy, and endoscopic sinus surgery—may also be encountered. Blood-tinged nasal secretions are to be expected

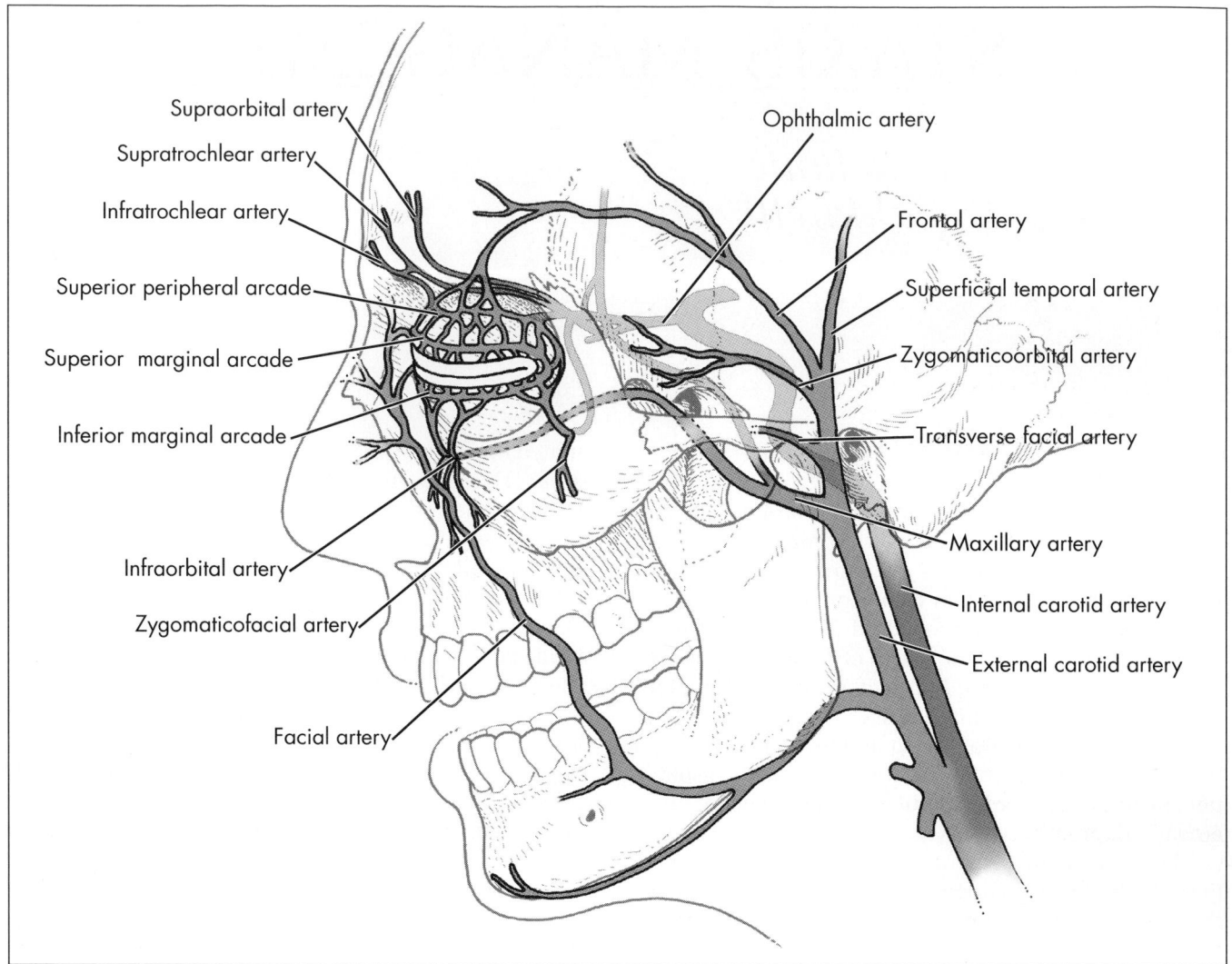

FIGURE 148-1 The blood supply of the nasal cavity arises from the internal and external carotid artery systems.

for the first 2 weeks after surgery. Severe epistaxis may occur during the first postoperative week, with an estimated incidence ranging from 0.9 to 8.9 percent.[5] The bleeding is usually posterior, brisk, and may be difficult to control. Consult the Otolaryngologist who performed the procedure in all cases of postoperative bleeding.

Nasal bleeding may be the first sign of a sinonasal neoplasm. The bleeding is usually intermittent and often accompanied by nasal obstruction and pain. Severe bleeding is unusual except in the case of juvenile nasal angiofibromas, which should be suspected in adolescent males.

Patients without identifiable local causes for epistaxis most likely suffer from an underlying systemic process. Consider the possibility of a defect in the coagulation cascade. Hypertension is often cited as a significant factor for epistaxis. Studies have been unable to demonstrate a significant difference in the prevalence of epistaxis in patients with hypertension versus patients without hypertension.[6,7] Nonsteroidal anti-inflammatory drugs and aspirin containing products have been associated with epistaxis.[8,9] Osler-Weber-Rendu disease is an autosomal dominant inherited condition in which the blood vessel walls lack contractile elements. Consequently, prolonged heavy bleeding occurs from relatively minor insults, as the vessels are unable to contract and allow clotting to take place. The patient's coagulation profile is normal and the diagnosis is made by the family history. Other systemic etiologies include alcoholism, blood dyscrasias, liver disease, malnutrition, and pregnancy.

INDICATIONS

A patient with epistaxis must be evaluated expediently. All patients with epistaxis require a thorough

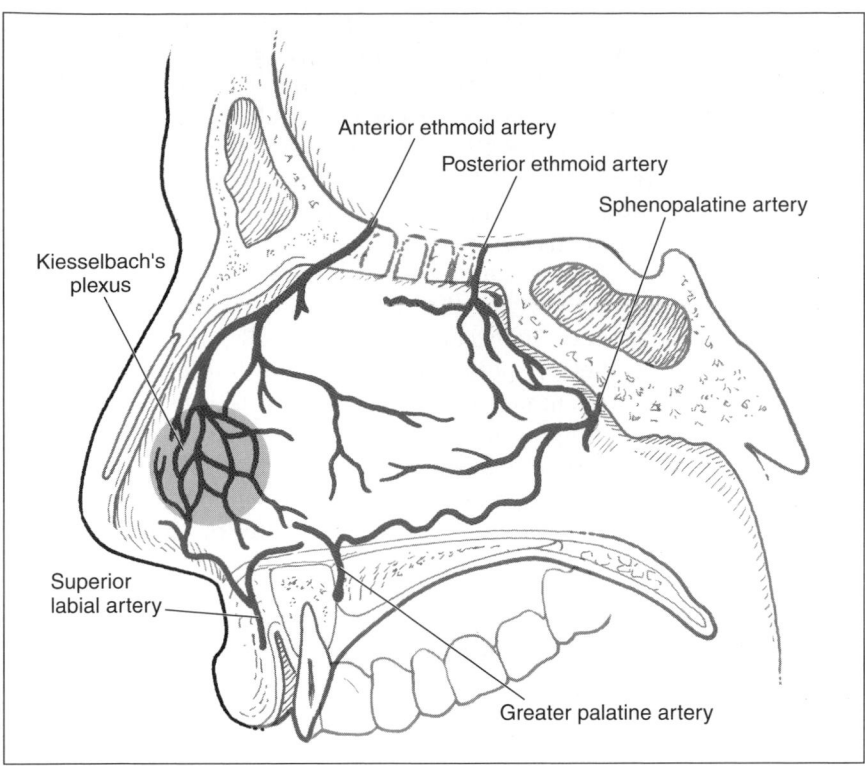

FIGURE 148-2 The anterior ethmoid artery and the sphenopalatine arteries supply the anterior nasal septum and Kiesselbach's plexus.

examination and control of the bleeding. Epistaxis that has resolved still requires management to prevent rebleeding.

CONTRAINDICATIONS

There are no contraindications to the management of epistaxis. Manage any unstable vitals signs, unstable airway, life- or limb-threatening injuries, or any complications related to blood loss (e.g., hypotension, chest pain, syncope, etc.) before managing the epistaxis. In the interim, apply a nose clip or a nasal sponge/tampon to control the bleeding. A thorough examination and more definitive means of control can be performed at a later time.

EQUIPMENT

Nose clip
Headlight or overhead light source
Yankauer suction catheter
Frazier suction catheters, #5 and #7
Nasal speculum, short and medium lengths
Bayonet forceps
Kidney basin
Weeder metal tongue blade or wooden tongue
    depressors

Gown, gloves, and face shield
Cotton balls
Topical anesthetics and vasoconstrictors (Table 148-1)
Silver nitrate applicator sticks
Petroleum (Vaseline)-impregnated gauze ribbon,
    0.5 inches wide
Synthetic nasal sponges/tampons, various lengths
Nasal balloons (anterior, posterior, anterior and
    posterior)
14 French Foley catheter with a 30 mL balloon
Gelfoam
4×4 gauze squares
Surgicel
ENTaxis nasal packing
3 inch long dental rolls or tonsil packs, or 3×36 inch
    Vaseline gauze
Umbilical tape or 0 silk suture
Red rubber catheters
Lubricant

PATIENT PREPARATION

Explain the procedure, its risks, and its benefits to the patient and/or their representative. Obtain a signed informed consent for the procedure. Ensure that the patient has a thorough understanding of the post-procedural care instructions and follow-up requirements.

TABLE 148-1. ANESTHETICS AND
VASOCONSTRICTORS OF THE NASAL MUCOSA

Anesthetics	Vasoconstrictors
Lidocaine (4%)	Phenylephrine (0.5–1.0%)
Cocaine (4%)	Cocaine (4%)
Pontocaine (2%)	Oxymetazoline (0.05%)
	Epinephrine (1:1000)
	Xylometazoline
	Ephedrine (3%)

Anesthetic and vasoconstrictor combinations
Cocaine
Lidocaine and phenylephrine (50:50)
Lidocaine and oxymetazoline (50:50)
Epinephrine (0.25 mL of 1:1000) and lidocaine (20 mL)

Position the patient sitting in an upright multipositional procedure chair. Alternatively, place the patient sitting upright on a gurney with the back elevated. Prepare the wall suction unit to make sure that it is working. Apply suction tubing and a suction catheter to the suction source.

The importance of good lighting cannot be overemphasized. Apply a headlamp if one is available. An alternative is an overhead adjustable light source. Position the light so that it is aimed in the patient's mouth. The overhead light often hits the examiner in the head, casts shadows, and is too bright for the patient's eyes. It is also difficult to position properly as both of the examiner's hands must be used for the procedure.

Inspect the posterior oropharynx for active bleeding using the Weeder tongue blade or a wooden tongue blade. Insert a short nasal speculum to evaluate each side of the anterior nasal cavity. Open the speculum vertically. Suction out any blood and blood clots with the Frazier suction catheter. Instruct the patient to blow their nose firmly, one nostril at a time, in order to evacuate the nasal cavities. This allows the anterior nasal septum, Kiesselbach's plexus, the nasal vestibule, the inferior turbinate, and the floor of the nasal cavity to be examined. Consider a posterior site of bleeding if the source is difficult to localize. A patient will occasionally present with bilateral epistaxis. It is sometimes difficult to determine from which side the bleeding is originating. Ask the patient which side started bleeding first. This is usually the side where the bleeding point can be found.

Vasoconstrict and anesthetize the nasal mucosa (Table 148-1). Decongest the nasal mucosa with an aerosolized agent. Instruct the patient to sniff in deeply after the spray is applied. Allow 3 to 5 minutes to pass for the vasoconstriction to occur. Apply a topical anesthetic spray to the nasal passageway. Spraying achieves excellent vasoconstriction and anesthesia as the agents diffuse through the entire nasal cavity and pharynx. It is possible to anesthetize and vasoconstrict the nasal mucosa in one step by using cocaine or a combination of an anesthetic and vasoconstrictor agent (Table 148-1). Alternatively, place cocaine soaked pledgets into the nasal cavity. Direct the pledgets along the floor of the nose, against the nasal septum, and toward the superior straits of the nose. Monitor the patient's vital signs when vasoconstrictors are applied.

There are numerous techniques to manage epistaxis. These include the use of absorbable packs, electrocautery, Foley catheters, gauze rolls, intranasal balloon catheters, petrolatum (Vaseline)-impregnated ribbon gauze, nasal tampons or sponges, and silver nitrate. The technique and material of choice depend upon the location of the bleeding (anterior versus posterior) and physician preference. Different techniques and equipment are required to control anterior versus posterior bleeding.

ANTERIOR EPISTAXIS MANAGEMENT TECHNIQUES

Anterior nasal packing is required when local measures fail to control epistaxis. This may be due in part to anterior or structural problems in which the bleeding source cannot be identified. It may also be due to heavy or profuse bleeding. The premise behind placing nasal packing is that it provides mechanical pressure and tamponades the bleeding site.[10] Note that this is an uncomfortable procedure; therefore the previously described steps for applying topical anesthesia should be undertaken.

ABSORBABLE PACKING

Diffuse bleeding is frequently encountered in patients with coagulopathies and blood dyscrasias. The trauma of inserting the nasal packing (tampon or Vaseline gauze) can lead to more serious bleeding. A piece of Gelfoam sponge or oxidized cellulose (Surgicel) is often effective. These substances, coated with an antibiotic ointment (e.g., Bacitracin) provide adequate pressure and hemostasis without extreme trauma to the nasal mucosa. This packing does not need to be removed and will slowly dissolve with the use of a topical saline spray, which may be started within 24 hours of the packing being placed.

The two most commonly used absorbable dressings are Gelfoam and Surgicel. Gelfoam is an absorbable gelatin sponge that is readily available and inexpensive. It forms a scaffold for the formation of a blood clot. Surgicel is composed of oxidized and regenerated cellulose. It promotes coagulation better than Gelfoam. Unfortunately, Surgicel results in delayed healing; its use should be reserved for persistent bleeding or when Gelfoam is not available.

Absorbable packs may be used for primary and secondary hemostasis. Apply a piece of Gelfoam or Surgicel directly over the site of discrete bleeding or diffuse oozing. The material may be used for secondary hemostasis and be placed over an area that has clotted and stopped bleeding. This can serve as a "Band-Aid" to help prevent the clot from dislodging prematurely and the bleeding to restart. It can be placed over areas that have been chemically or electrically cauterized. An absorbable pack can be placed prior to packing the nasal cavity with a sponge/tampon or gauze. The absorbable pack will prevent the clot from becoming dislodged when the sponge/tampon or gauze is removed.

Insert the nasal speculum and identify the scabbed or bleeding site. Apply a piece of Gelfoam or Surgicel over the site. Allow a clot to form onto the absorbable packing. The nasal cavity may be packed with a sponge/tampon or Vaseline gauze if the physician chooses.

Two additional absorbable dressings are topical thrombin and collagen. They are expensive, not usually available in the Emergency Department, and should be limited to circumstances where other hemostasis methods have failed. Topical thrombin is made from bovine thrombin. Place a piece of Gelfoam saturated with thrombin over the bleeding site. Thrombin converts fibrinogen to fibrin, bypassing the coagulation cascade, to form a clot. Collagen is available in multiple forms from a variety of sources. It promotes platelet aggregation and forms a scaffold for the formation of a clot. Cover the bleeding site with collagen followed by a piece of Gelfoam.

CHEMICAL CAUTERIZATION

The location of the bleeding is usually within the anterior nasal cavity, specifically on the anterior nasal septum. Sometimes no active bleeding is found at the time of the evaluation. Suctioning of the nasal cavity will remove clots and may allow the site to bleed and be visualized. A scabbed excoriation or an exposed blood vessel may be found along the nasal septum. Chemically cauterize these areas using silver nitrate applicators.

Insert the nasal speculum and identify the scabbed site or the exposed vessel. Apply the silver nitrate under direct vision by rubbing the applicator on the area immediately surrounding the scab or blood vessel. Apply the silver nitrate for 3 to 10 seconds. **Do not apply the applicator in any one spot for more than 10 seconds. This may cause mucosal necrosis and damage to the underlying cartilaginous septum. Do not apply the silver nitrate too excessively or in the same spot on both sides of the septum, as this may result in a septal perforation.** Apply a topical antibiotic ointment to the area. Place a piece of Gelfoam or Surgicel over the site to help stabilize the clot.

A relatively dry field is required to use the silver nitrate applicator. Moderate to severe bleeding results in the silver nitrate coagulating the blood. It will not contact the mucosal tissue and bleeding will continue. Attempt to simultaneously suction the blood while using the silver nitrate applicator. Unfortunately, the suction often pulls off the coagulum and the bleeding continues. A final technique is to apply the silver nitrate centripetally around the bleeding site. This will cauterize the feeder vessels and may stop the bleeding. **Do not cauterize an area over 0.75 cm in diameter, as this can result in damage to the underlying cartilaginous septum.** Pack the nasal cavity with a sponge/tampon or Vaseline gauze if these techniques fail.

ELECTRICAL CAUTERIZATION

Electrocautery can effectively control bleeding if the site is identified. **This technique is reserved for the experienced Otolaryngologist.** It can cause significant damage to the mucosa and cartilage in inexperienced hands. The technique of electrocautery is not discussed for these reasons.

RIBBON GAUZE PACKING

The traditional technique of anterior nasal packing consists of using 0.5 inch wide petrolatum (Vaseline)-impregnated gauze ribbon (Figure 148-3). This technique is extremely effective but not often used as it is cumbersome, time-consuming, and simpler methods exist (e.g., silver nitrate cautery, sponges/tampons).

Insert the nasal speculum. Grasp one end of the Vaseline gauze with a bayonet forceps. Insert the Vaseline gauze into the nasal cavity and along the floor (Figure 148-3A). Tightly pack the nasal cavity in a layered fashion from bottom to top, extending as far back as possible toward the choanal arch (Figure 148-3B). **Be careful to avoid injuring the mucosa overlying the septum and the turbinates.** Cut the Vaseline gauze so that it protrudes approximately 2 cm from the nostril. Tape this loose end to the patient's cheek so that it does not accidentally pull the packing out. The packing is later removed by gently pulling on this free end of gauze ribbon protruding from the nostril.

The pressure of one-sided anterior nasal packing can bow the septum contralaterally, allowing the packing to "loosen" and the bleeding to restart. Pack the contralateral anterior nasal cavity to maintain the septum in the midline and exert pressure on the bleeding site.

EXPANDABLE NASAL SPONGES/TAMPONS

One of the easiest, quickest, and most effective techniques to control anterior epistaxis is to insert an expandable sponge or tampon (e.g., Merocel packing). These packs are particularly useful when the bleeding is diffuse, a specific site cannot be clearly identified, or

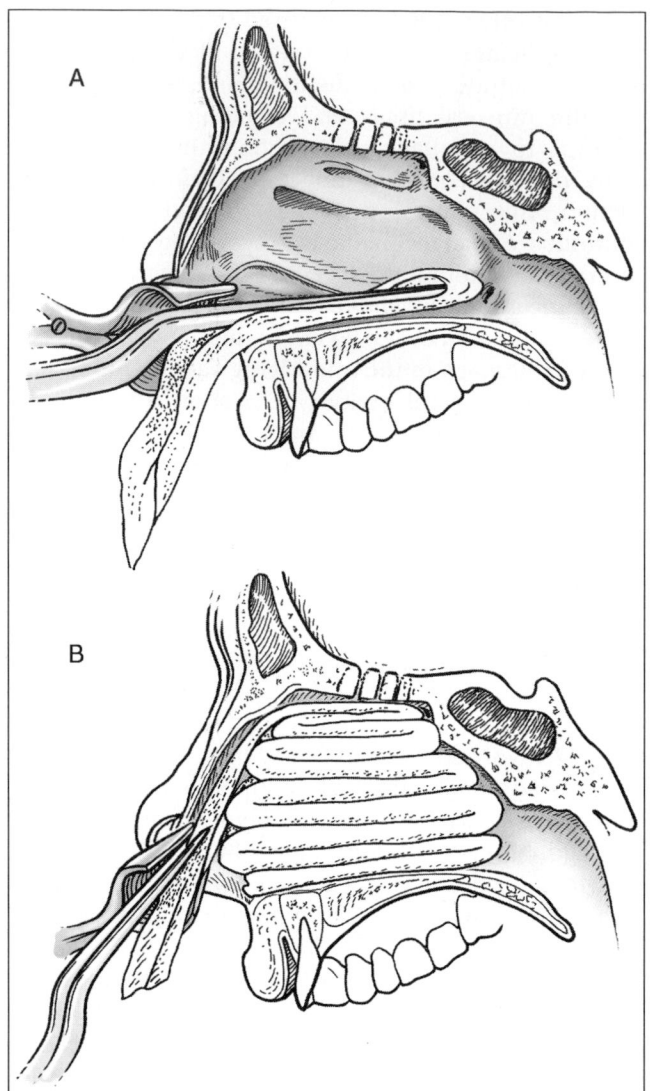

FIGURE 148-3 Anterior nasal packing using petrolatum (Vaseline)-impregnated gauze ribbon. *A.* Insert a nasal speculum and begin packing inferiorly to superiorly. *B.* The gauze-packed anterior nasal cavity.

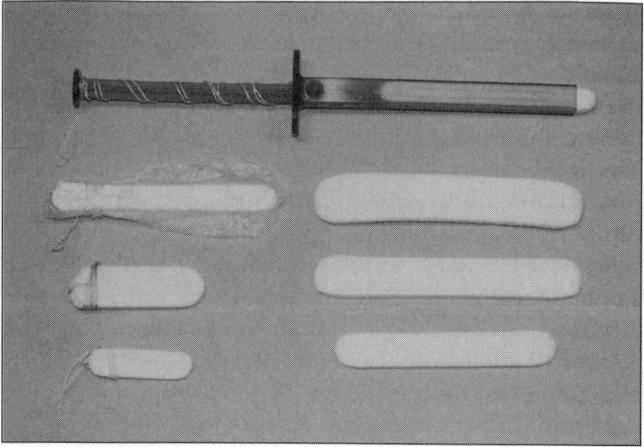

FIGURE 148-4 Various sizes, shapes, and styles of nasal sponges/tampons.

the bleeding is heavy. The packs come in various sizes (4.5, 6, 8, and 10 cm), shapes, and styles (Figure 148-4). Initially quite rigid, they soften and expand with the absorption of saline or surrounding blood. A 4.5 or 6 cm sponge is generally adequate for anterior epistaxis.

Prepare the sponge/tampon. Cut the string from the sponge/tampon. It is not necessary to remove the packing. The sponge/tampon is barely visible when properly inserted. The string hanging from the nostril is irritating to the patient and not cosmetically appealing. Lightly coat the sponge/tampon with a non-water-soluble lubricant (e.g., Vaseline) or antibiotic ointment (e.g., Neosporin). This will prevent premature expansion of the tampon from a water-soluble lubricant or antibiotic ointment, nasal secretions, or blood.

Insert and open the nasal speculum within the affected nasal cavity. Grasp the sponge/tampon with a bayonet forceps or the dominant thumb and index finger. Insert and advance the sponge/tampon just lateral to the nasal septum, in a vertical position, with the length of the pack directed along the floor of the nose (Figure 148-5A). Advance the sponge/tampon until it is completely within the nasal cavity. The sponge/tampon will expand from the blood and secretions within the nasal cavity (Figure 148-5B). Slowly drip 1 to 3 mL of tap water or saline onto the tip of the sponge/tampon to help it expand more rapidly.

Inspect the oropharynx for bleeding. Persistent bleeding may be due to the septum bowing contralaterally. Pack the contralateral anterior nasal cavity with a sponge/tampon of equal length and size. Observe the patient for oozing or bleeding anteriorly or posteriorly. Continued bleeding requires removal of the sponge/tampon from the bleeding nasal cavity and insertion of a larger one, two small ones, or Vaseline gauze packing.

Keep several helpful hints in mind when using the nasal sponges/tampons. Trim large sponges/tampons to 5 to 6 cm in length. The extra length is not required for anterior epistaxis, is uncomfortable for the patient, and is more difficult to remove. The Rhino Rocket is a sponge/tampon within a plastic syringe-like device. Remove the sponge/tampon from the syringe-like device before inserting it. The device can generate significant force and result in mucosal tears, septal injuries, and turbinate injuries. Insert and advance the sponge/tampon rapidly to prevent premature expansion. There is no advantage to using a non-water-soluble antibiotic ointment versus a lubricant. The antibiotic ointment is more expensive and its antibacterial activity lasts only 2 to 4 hours. Insert two sponges/tampons side by side if the patient has a large nasal cavity.

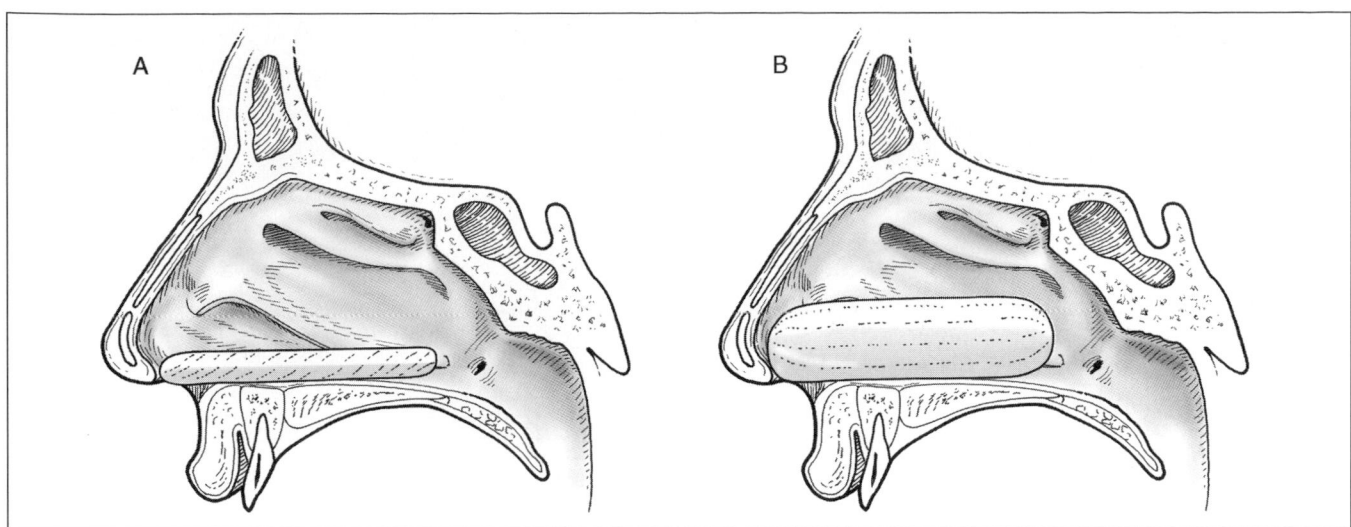

FIGURE 148-5 The expandable nasal sponge/tampon. *A.* Insertion along the floor of the nasal cavity. *B.* The expanded state.

Removal of the sponge/tampon is simple and quick. Apply 1 to 2 mL of tap water, saline, or a vasoconstrictor in a dropwise fashion to the tip of the sponge/tampon in the nostril. This will thoroughly hydrate the packing and ensure that it can be withdrawn atraumatically. Allow 5 to 10 minutes to ensure that the packing is completely hydrated. Grasp the string or the end of the sponge/tampon with a hemostat. Place a kidney basin under the patient's nose. Pull quickly and parallel to the floor of the nasal cavity to remove the packing. Epistaxis after removal is often due to dislodgement of the clot. Use an absorbable pack or silver nitrate to stop the bleeding. Look at the sponge/tampon to identify the blood spot and the location of the bleeding.

INFLATABLE NASAL BALLOON CATHETERS

The development of plastic inflatable balloon catheters has simplified the management of epistaxis. The nasal balloons are easy to use and quick to place. They are available in a variety of sizes and shapes (Figure 148-6). They are available with anterior balloons, posterior balloons, or dual balloons. The anterior balloon fills the nasal cavity and acts as an anterior pack. The posterior balloon occludes the nasopharynx and acts as a posterior pack. The inflatable balloons are much more expensive than other methods used to manage epistaxis. The increased cost is offset by decreased physician contact time as compared with that required for petrolatum (Vaseline) gauze packing. The balloons have a maximal inflatable volume that is manufacturer-specific, noted on the packaging, and noted on the balloon's inflation hub.

Prepare the equipment. Select an anterior balloon catheter. A dual-balloon catheter may be used if an anterior balloon catheter is not available. Inflate the balloon with air to just below its maximum capacity. Observe and palpate the balloon for leaks. It may also be inflated in a cup of water to look for leaks. Completely deflate the balloon. Apply a lubricant over the catheter and balloon.

Insert the nasal speculum. **Insert the catheter with the distal bevel toward the nasal septum.** This prevents the distal end of the catheter from getting caught on the turbinates, damaging the mucosa overlying the turbinates, and causing a second source of epistaxis. Advance the catheter along the floor of the nasal cavity until just the inflation hub is protruding from the nostril (Figure 148-7). Inflate the balloon with 10 mL under the maximum volume of air (Figure 148-7). **Do not use saline or water to inflate the balloon.** Rupture of the balloon can result in aspiration if it is filled with liquid. **Do not inflate the balloon with more than the manufacturer's recommended volume.** If the patient complains of pain, the balloon may have been inflated larger than the nasal cavity. Deflate the balloon until the pain subsides.

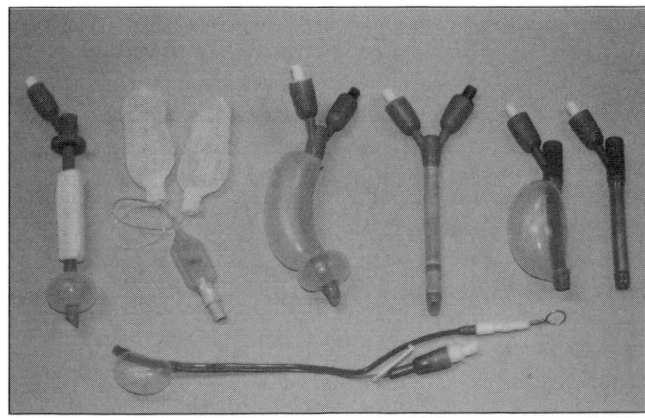

FIGURE 148-6 Examples of some inflatable nasal balloon catheters.

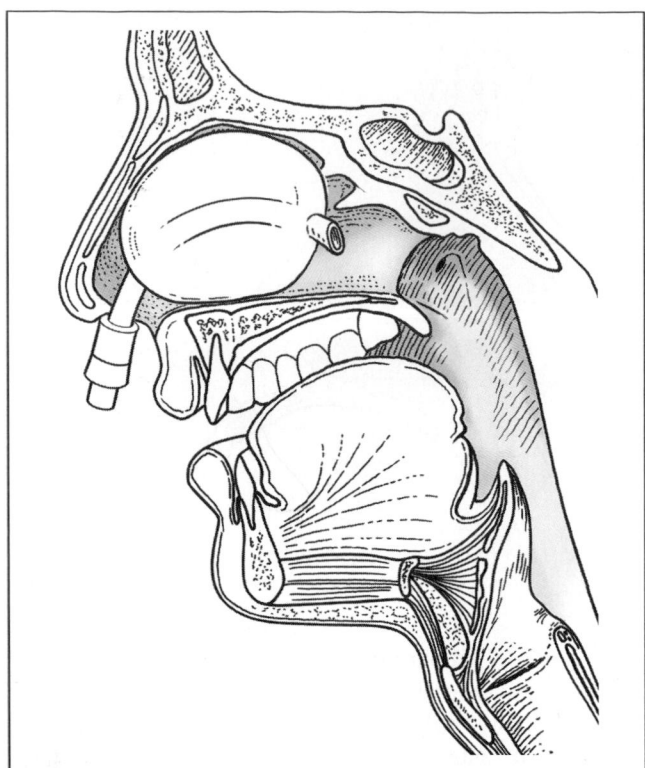

FIGURE 148-7 Inflation of an anterior balloon catheter to control anterior epistaxis.

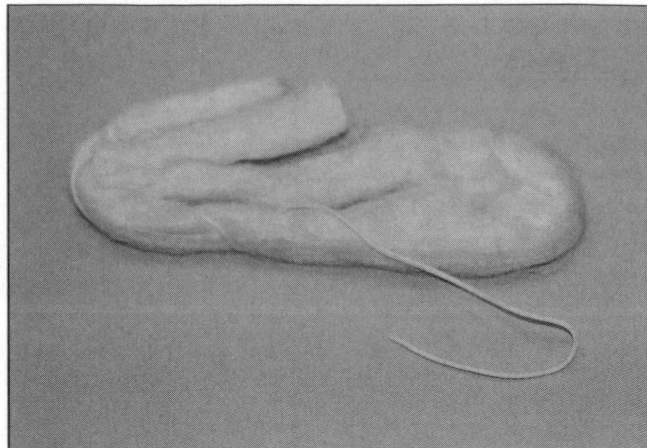

FIGURE 148-8 The ENTaxis nasal packing (Boston Medical Products, Westborough, MA).

Observe the patient for continued bleeding. Increase the volume of the balloon to the maximum volume if the patient does not complain of pain. The balloon may cause a bowing of the septum to the contralateral side. If the bleeding continues, pack the contralateral anterior nasal cavity to keep the septum in the midline. Observe the patient for further bleeding from the nostril or into the nasopharynx. Continued bleeding suggests that the source is high in the nasal cavity or posterior. **The inflatable balloons do not always fill the upper portion of the nasal cavity.** Deflate the balloon, pack the high anterior nasal cavity with Vaseline gauze and reinflate the balloon. Observe the patient for continued bleeding that would require a posterior pack, as described in the following sections.

ENTAXIS NASAL PACKING

A relatively new anterior nasal packing is the ENTaxis (Figure 148-8). It is a natural polymer derived from seaweed and contains calcium alginate.[11] The packing provides hemostasis, has healing properties, and is atraumatically inserted and removed. Hydration with normal saline activates the calcium alginate and makes it pliable. The packing expands 300 percent and conforms to the anterior nasal cavity. It activates platelet aggregation to provide hemostasis, keeps the nasal mucosa moist, and gels into a smooth surface that allows easy removal.

Prepare the packing. The ENTaxis is packaged in a plastic tray with a tear-off paper lid. Peel the lid completely off the tray. Fill the tray with normal saline to saturate the packing. Remove the hydrated packing from the tray. Squeeze out the excess saline from the packing.

Insert a nasal speculum. Grasp the packing on the end opposite the string with a bayonet forceps. Insert the packing along the floor of the nasal cavity. Continue to insert the packing in an accordion-like fashion until the entire packing is within the nasal cavity. The packing will expand and gel to fill the nasal cavity. Secure the string to the patient's cheek or nose with a piece of tape.

Removal of the packing is simple and quick. The packing remains hydrated and in a gelled state while within the nasal cavity. Place a kidney basin under the patient's nose. Untape the string from the patient's face. Grasp the packing with a bayonet forceps. Gently withdraw the packing from the nasal cavity.

POSTERIOR EPISTAXIS MANAGEMENT TECHNIQUES

A posterior source of the bleeding must be sought when epistaxis is bilateral, brisk, and not controlled with anterior nasal packing. It is estimated that 5 percent of all cases of epistaxis originate from a posterior source.[12] **The placement of a posterior nasal pack is extremely uncomfortable.** The patient may require, on some occasions, intravenous sedation and analgesia in addition to the topical anesthesia previously described. The rationale behind placing a posterior pack is that the occlusion of the choanal arch provides a semirigid buttress against which anterior nasal packing may be placed, allowing adequate hemostasis to be achieved. This buttress may be formed from either a gauze pack, a 30 mL Foley catheter, an expandable nasal sponge/tampon, or an inflatable nasal balloon catheter. From a practical standpoint, the Foley catheter and inflatable nasal balloon catheter are most easily tolerated by the patient. The inflatable nasal balloon catheter is definitely the easiest to place, as it has two balloons that serve as both anterior and posterior packs. **An anterior nasal pack is always required on the side of a posterior pack.** Strongly consider inserting a contralateral anterior nasal pack to maintain the septum in the midline.

TRADITIONAL (GAUZE ROLL) PACKING

The traditional technique of posterior nasal packing involves using rolled gauze, dental rolls, or tonsil packs placed through the oropharynx (Figure 148-9). This technique is difficult, time-consuming, messy, requires many supplies, and is not well tolerated by the patient. Easier and quicker techniques exist. For these reasons, this technique is not often performed.

Prepare the equipment. Gather the required equipment on a bedside procedure table. Use 3 inch long dental rolls or tonsil packs. An alternative is to use 3 inch wide and 36 inch long petrolatum gauze. Form a tight cylindrical roll with the gauze (Figure 148-9A). Tie two pieces of umbilical tape or 0 silk suture around the pack to divide it into thirds (Figure 148-9A).

Anesthetize and vasoconstrict both nasal cavities. Apply a topical anesthetic spray to the soft palate, uvula, and oropharynx. Lubricate a red rubber catheter. Pass the red rubber catheter through one nostril and along the floor of the nasal cavity. Advance the catheter so that the tip is visible in the patient's oropharynx. Grasp the tip of the catheter with a hemostat and pull it out the patient's mouth (Figure 148-9B). Clamp the free ends of the catheter together. Pass a second red rubber catheter through the other nostril and out the patient's mouth.

Insert the posterior pack. Tie the free end of one piece of the umbilical tape or silk surrounding the packing to the distal end of one red rubber catheter exiting the patient's mouth (Figure 148-9C). **Tie the knots tightly.** Tie the second piece of umbilical tape or silk to the second red rubber catheter. Pull the proximal ends of both red rubber catheters until the packing is against the choanae (Figure 148-9D). It may be necessary to place a finger into the patient's mouth and push the pack behind the soft palate and uvula if it gets caught (Figure 148-9D). Place a hemostat on both pieces of umbilical tape exiting the nostrils. Apply slight traction with the hemostat to maintain the posterior pack against the choanae. Instruct an assistant or the patient to hold the hemostat.

Place an anterior pack and secure the posterior pack. **An anterior nasal pack is always required when placing a posterior nasal pack.** The anterior pack may be

an expandable sponge/tampon or Vaseline gauze (Figure 148-9E). Tie the umbilical tape or silk exiting each nostril together (Figure 148-9F). **Always place a piece of cotton or gauze between the knot and the columella to prevent pressure necrosis (Figure 148-9F). Tie the umbilical tape or silk snugly but not too tight to hold the posterior pack in place and not apply pressure to the choanae or the columella.** Tape the umbilical tape or silk exiting the patient's nostril and mouth to their face (Figure 148-9F).

Removal of this packing is simple and requires several stages. Remove the anterior packing. Thoroughly examine the mucosa to make sure that the epistaxis has not restarted. Suction any clots and blood from the nasal cavity. Rebleeding requires the placement of a new anterior pack if it cannot be controlled with an absorbable dressing or silver nitrate. Cut the knot, securing the umbilical tape or silk around the columella. Pull the pieces of umbilical tape or silk exiting the patient's mouth to remove the posterior pack completely.

FOLEY CATHETER TECHNIQUE

A Foley catheter may be used to provide a posterior buttress. Using a Foley catheter is easy, quick, and simple. Select a 14 French Foley catheter with a 30 mL balloon. Inflate the balloon with air. Ensure the integrity of the balloon. Some physicians cut off the portion of the Foley catheter distal to the balloon. They believe that the distal tip is irritating to the patient and may stimulate their gag reflex. The practice of cutting off the distal tip is based purely on physician preference.

Lubricate the distal third of the Foley catheter. Insert the Foley catheter into the nostril and along the floor of the nasal cavity. Advance the catheter until the tip is visible in the patient's oropharynx. Inflate the balloon with 7 to 10 mL of air. **Do not use saline, as the fluid can result in aspiration if the balloon ruptures.** Withdraw the catheter to lodge the balloon against the choanal arch (Figure 148-10A). If the balloon withdraws into the nasal cavity, advance it back into the nasopharynx. Add an additional 3 to 5 mL of air and withdraw the catheter. Continue the process by adding 3 to 5 mL aliquots of air until the balloon lodges against the choanal arch. Inflate the balloon with an additional 5 mL of air and the soft palate just begins to bulge. The balloon is overinflated if the soft palate bulges or the patient experiences pain.

Place an anterior pack and secure the Foley catheter. Apply slight traction to maintain the balloon against the choanal arch. Instruct an assistant or the patient to hold the Foley catheter. Place the anterior pack using an expandable sponge/tampon or Vaseline gauze. **Place a piece of cotton or gauze against the columella and nasal ala to prevent pressure necrosis.**[13] Place an umbilical clamp on the Foley catheter and over the

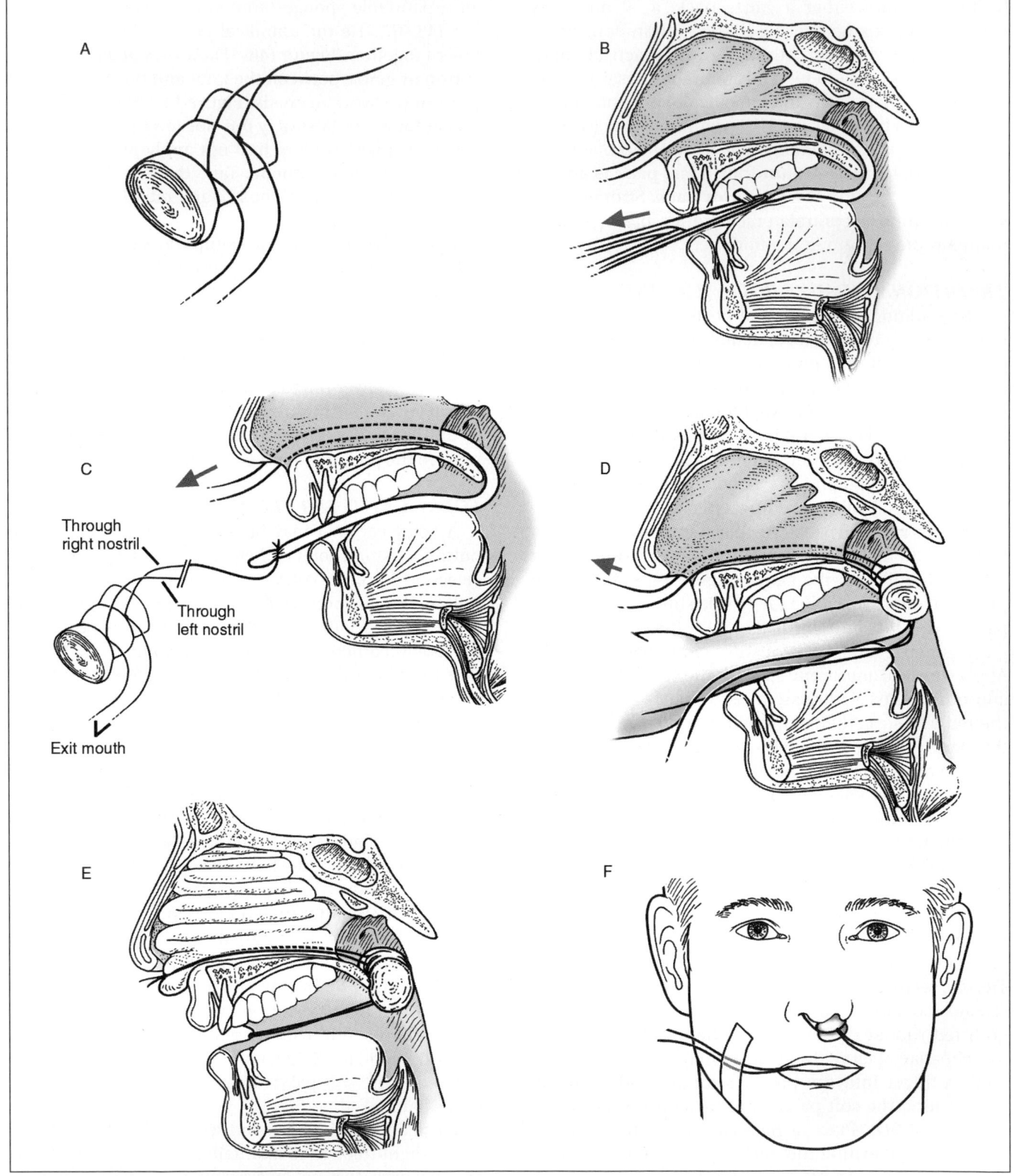

A

B

C

Through
right nostril

Through
left nostril

Exit mouth

D

E

F

FIGURE 148-9 The traditional technique of placing a posterior nasal pack. *A.* Preparation of the pack. *B.* A red rubber catheter inserted through the nostril and pulled out the mouth. *C.* The pack is attached to the red rubber catheters. *D.* The pack is pulled into place. Use a finger to pass the pack around the soft palate and uvula. *E.* An anterior nasal pack has been placed. *F.* The ties of the posterior pack are secured.

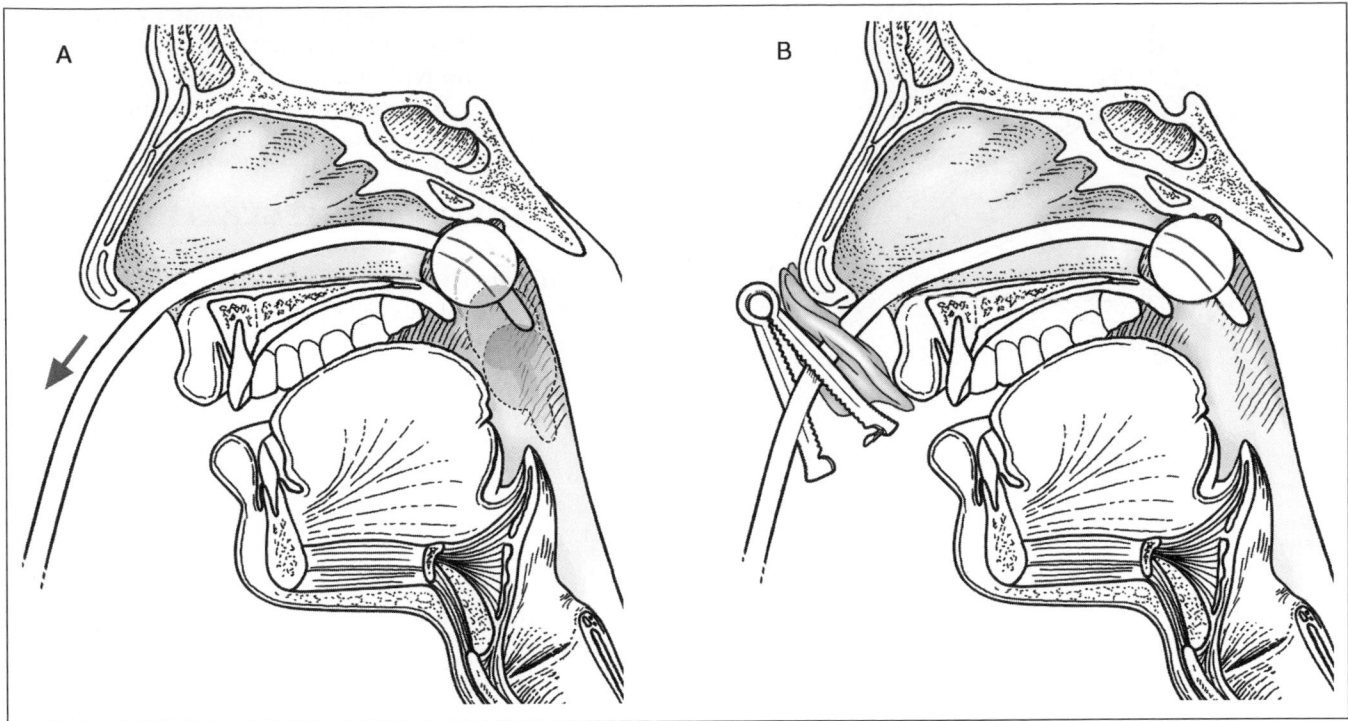

FIGURE 148-10 The Foley catheter technique. Insert a Foley catheter along the floor of the nasal cavity until the tip is visible in the patient's oropharynx. *A.* Inflate the balloon and withdraw the catheter to lodge the balloon against the choanal arch. *B.* Secure the Foley catheter.

protective padding (Figure 148-10*B*). **The clamp must hold the balloon against the choanal arch without applying pressure to the choana or columella.**

Removal of this packing is simple and requires several stages. Cut the open loop of the umbilical clamp with a scissors. Open the jaws of the clamp and remove them from the Foley catheter. Remove the anterior packing. Thoroughly examine the mucosa to make sure that the epistaxis has not restarted. Suction any clots and blood from the nasal cavity. Rebleeding requires the placement of a new anterior pack if it cannot be controlled with an absorbable dressing or silver nitrate. Deflate the balloon and pull the catheter out the patient's nostril.

EXPANDABLE NASAL SPONGES/TAMPONS

Many physicians prefer to use an 8 or 10 cm sponge/tampon rather than the other techniques of posterior packing. This technique is easy, quick, simple, and inexpensive. The technique for insertion and removal is exactly the same as for the anterior technique described previously.

INFLATABLE NASAL BALLOON CATHETERS

A dual-balloon catheter can be used when a posterior pack is required. These catheters come in many types and styles (Figure 148-6). They are expensive but easy to use and quickly placed. The smaller distal balloon ob-structs the choanal arch and acts as a posterior pack (Figure 148-11). The larger proximal balloon fills the nasal cavity and acts as an anterior pack (Figure 148-11). The distal balloon holds 10 mL and the anterior balloon holds 30 mL in most dual-balloon systems. Note the manufacturer's maximum volume recommendations on the package and on the inflation ports of the balloons.

Prepare the equipment. Fully inflate both balloons with air. Observe and palpate the balloons for leaks. They may also be inflated in a cup of water to look for leaks. Completely deflate both balloons. Apply a lubricant over the catheter and balloons.

Insert the catheter with the distal bevel toward the nasal septum. This prevents the distal end of the catheter from getting caught on the turbinates, damaging the mucosa overlying the turbinates, and causing a second source of epistaxis. Advance the catheter along the floor of the nasal cavity until the distal tip is visible in the patient's oropharynx.

Inflate the distal balloon with 4 to 5 mL of air. **Do not use saline or water to inflate the balloon.** Rupture of the balloon can result in aspiration if it is filled with liquid. Withdraw the catheter to lodge the balloon against the choanal arch (Figure 148-11). If the balloon withdraws into the nasal cavity, advance it back into the nasopharynx. Add an additional 2 to 3 mL of air and withdraw the catheter. Continue this process until the balloon lodges or the maximum balloon volume is

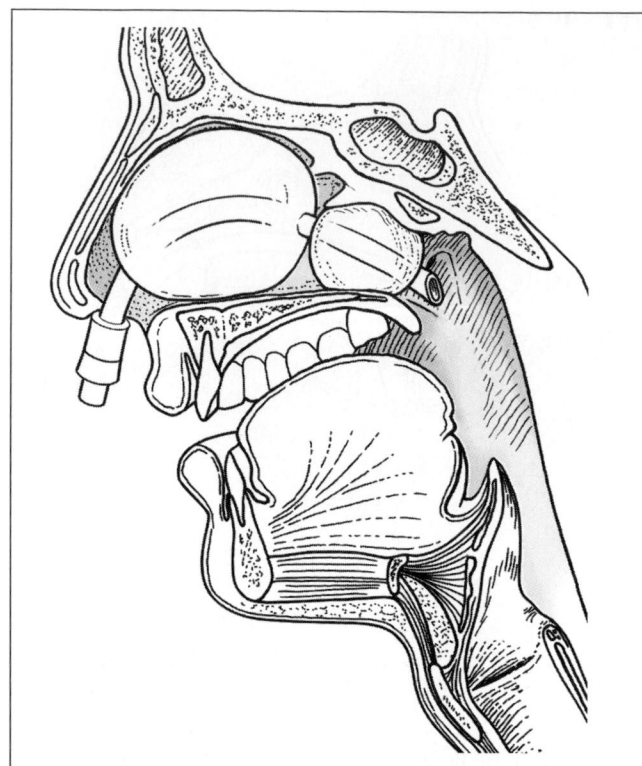

FIGURE 148-11 Placement of a dual-balloon catheter.

reached. Inflate the anterior balloon with 20 to 25 mL of air.

Observe the patient for bleeding. Inflate both balloons with additional aliquots of air until the bleeding stops or the maximum balloon volume is reached. The balloon does not always fill the high anterior nasal cavity. Deflate the anterior balloon, pack the high anterior nasal cavity with Vaseline gauze, and reinflate the anterior balloon. Place an anterior pack contralaterally if the bleeding continues to maintain the septum in the midline and apply pressure to the ipsilateral nasal cavity.

SPHENOPALATINE ARTERY BLOCK

This technique is a last resort when an Otolaryngologist is not available, the hemorrhage is unremitting, and other methods to control the hemorrhage have failed. Local anesthetic solution is injected into the pterygopalatine canal to occlude the sphenopalatine artery. The local anesthetic solution can cause pressure necrosis of the adjacent nerves.

Place the patient supine with their mouth open. Apply a topical anesthetic spray to the hard palate. Identify the greater palatine foramen. Insert a 27 gauge needle into the mucosa of the hard palate, 1 cm medial to the gum line between the junction of the second and third maxillary molars. Probe this area with the needle until it falls into the greater palatine foramen. Inject 0.25 mL of local anesthetic solution containing epinephrine into the mucosa overlying the greater palatine foramen. Arm a 3 or 5 mL syringe containing local anesthetic solution with epinephrine with a 22 or 24 gauge needle. Insert the needle 28 mm into the greater palatine foramen. Inject 3 mL of the local anesthetic solution.

SURGICAL INTERVENTION

Consult an Otolaryngologist when the epistaxis is difficult to control by the described methods, as surgical intervention is then indicated. Surgical therapy may include septoplasty, endoscopic cauterization, arterial ligation (internal maxillary artery, sphenopalatine artery, anterior and posterior ethmoid arteries, external carotid artery), or embolization.

AFTERCARE

The post-procedural care of patients with anterior epistaxis is just as important as the initial control of bleeding. All patients with nasal packing require prophylactic oral antibiotic therapy with adequate coverage for *Staphylococcus aureus*, *Streptococcus pneumoniae*, *Haemophilus influenzae*, and *Moraxella catarrhalis*. This is due to the significant risk of developing sinusitis and toxic shock syndrome. Arrange follow-up with an Otolaryngologist within 24 to 48 hours. Remove the packing in 48 to 72 hours if the patient experienced only minimal blood loss and was hemodynamically stable.

Inform the patient that the anterior pack is "uncomfortable." Acetaminophen will provide any required analgesia. Avoid aspirin containing compounds and nonsteroidal anti-inflammatory drugs, as they can contribute to further bleeding. Instruct the patient to apply saline nasal spray to the packing or each nostril three or four times per hour while awake. The use of a humidifier at home will aid in preventing drying of the packing or the nasal mucosa. The patient must avoid nose picking and nose blowing. Instruct the patient on the proper technique to apply pressure on the nose if bleeding restarts. Such pressure should be maintained for 20 minutes. Continued bleeding calls for a return to the Emergency Department. The patient should also return for increased nasal pain, fever, or any symptoms related to blood loss (chest pain, dyspnea on exertion, dizziness, light-headedness, presyncope, shortness of breath, and syncope).

Patients with unstable vital signs, uncontrollable bleeding, posterior packing, or serious concomitant medical problems will require hospitalization. Patients with posterior nasal packs require consultation with an Otolaryngologist and admission to an intensive care unit. They must be monitored for respiratory distress, hypoxia, hypotension, anemia, and cardiac sequelae. It has been estimated that 40 percent of patients with posterior nasal packing eventually require intubation.[12] The nasal ala and columella must be evaluated continually in order to prevent pressure necrosis.

Patients with a posterior nasal pack may experience hypoxemia and hypercarbia. The etiology of these phenomena, called the nasopulmonary reflex, is unknown. The PaO_2 may decrease 7.5 to 15 mmHg. The $PaCO_2$ may increase 7 to 15 mmHg. The nasopulmonary reflex is more worrisome in patients with underlying lung disease or comorbid conditions.

COMPLICATIONS

The complications associated with epistaxis are variable, wide-ranging, and estimated to be from 2 to 69 percent.[14] Epistaxis may be complicated by hemorrhage, hypoxemia, hypovolemia, circulatory collapse, and airway compromise. Complications resulting from the treatment of epistaxis include nasal septal perforation, sinusitis, otitis media, toxic shock syndrome, aspiration, alar necrosis, and hypoxia from intrapulmonary shunting due to the stimulation of the nasopulmonary reflex.[15]

The majority of complications can be prevented by using proper technique, providing supplemental oxygen when not contraindicated, ordering appropriate prophylactic antibiotics, arranging appropriate hospitalization if indicated, obtaining an Otolaryngology consultation, and arranging for adequate follow-up.

SUMMARY

Epistaxis is a common condition that affects 10 to 13 percent of the general population. The key to successful management includes a prompt and thorough evaluation of the patient, an accurate diagnosis of the problem, and rapid control of the bleeding. Ninety percent of cases of epistaxis stem from an anterior source and can be controlled with either chemical cautery or nasal packing. Posterior bleeding requires the use of both a posterior pack and anterior packing. All patients with nasal packing require prophylactic antibiotics to prevent sinusitis and toxic shock syndrome. Follow-up is required in 24 to 72 hours with an Otolaryngologist or the Emergency Department to remove the nasal packing.

REFERENCES

1. Small M, Maran AGD: Epistaxis and arterial ligation. *J Laryngol Otol* 1984; 98:281–284.
2. Grandis JR, Parnes SM, Dibiase PA, et al: *The Management of Epistaxis*. Self-instructional package (SIPac) number 77399. Alexandria, VA: American Academy of Otolaryngology-Head and Neck Surgery Foundation Inc., 1977:11–28.
3. Murray AB, Milner RA: Allergic rhinitis and recurrent epistaxis in children. *Ann Allergy Asthma Immunol* 1995; 74:30–33.
4. O'Reilly BJ, Simpson DC, Dharmeratnam R: Recurrent epistaxis and septal deviation in young adults. *Clin Otolaryngol* 1996; 21:12–14.
5. Garth RJN, Cox HJ, Thomas MR: Haemorrhage as a complication of inferior turbinectomy: a comparison of anterior and radical trimming. *Clin Otolaryngol* 1995; 20:236–238.
6. Weiss NS: Relation of high blood pressure to headache, epistaxis and selected other symptoms. The United States health examination survey of adults. *N Engl J Med* 1972; 287(13):631–633.
7. Mitchell JRA: Nose bleeding and high blood pressure. *Br Med J* 1959; 1:25–27.
8. Watson MG, Shenoi PM: Drug-induced epistaxis? *J R Soc Med* 1990; 83:162–164.
9. Shaheen OH: Arterial epistaxis. *J Laryngol Otol* 1975; 89(1):17–34.
10. Pringle MB, Beasley P, Brightwell AP: The use of merocel nasal packs in the treatment of epistaxis. *J Laryngol Otol* 1996; 110:543–546.
11. Boston Medical Products: *ENTaxis nasal packing*. Boston: Boston Medical Products.
12. Viducich RA, Blanda MP, Gerson LW: Posterior epistaxis: clinical features and acute complications. *Ann Emerg Med* 1995; 25(5):592–596.
13. Wurtele P: How I do it: emergency nasal packing using an umbilical cord clamp to secure a Foley catheter for posterior epistaxis. *J Otolaryngol* 1996; 25(1):46–47.
14. Elahi MM, Parnes LS, Fox AJ, et al: Therapeutic embolization in the treatment of intractable epistaxis. *Arch Otolaryngol Head Neck Surg* 1995; 121:65–69.
15. Cassisi NJ, Biller HF, Ogura JH: Changes in arterial oxygen tension and pulmonary mechanics with the use of posterior packing in epistaxis: a preliminary report. *Laryngoscope* 1971; 81:1261–1266.

Chapter 149
LARYNGOSCOPY

Steven Charous

INTRODUCTION

Evaluation of the larynx can be crucial in the diagnosis and management of common and life-threatening disorders. The approach to the patient with laryngeal dysfunction begins with taking a complete history. Symptoms may be related to any of the three primary functions of the larynx, which are protection of the lower airway from aspiration, a conduit of the airway, and phonation. Symptoms may include aspiration, cough, dysphagia, odynophagia, dyspnea, or hoarseness. Otalgia may be a referred symptom from the larynx and transmitted by a branch of the vagus nerve. Information regarding patient age, onset, duration, severity, and progressive nature of the process is necessary. Determine the patient's past medical history including prior intubations, neck trauma, reflux esophagitis, similar previous episodes, and other systemic diseases. The social history, including smoking and alcohol usage, needs to be investigated. Medications, allergies, and over-the-counter drugs should be reviewed.

Perform a physical examination, including a complete head and neck examination, once a history has been obtained.[1] Listen for stridor and watch for accessory muscle breathing. Consciously and critically evaluate the patient's voice to hear breathiness, clarity, and volume. Inspect the ears, nose, oral cavity, oropharynx, and nasopharynx. Careful palpation of the neck is extremely important. Note any lymphadenopathy and neck masses. This must include their size, location, tenderness, and mobility. Palpate the larynx and note any crepitus (the lack of crepitus on lateral movement of the larynx over the vertebral bodies can be indicative of a laryngeal or hypopharyngeal mass), movement with swallowing, and asymmetry. This can help in determining the extent of a disease process.

Visualize the larynx after performing a complete history and physical examination, with the exception of true airway emergencies. This allows the physician to examine the larynx in context to the patient's symptoms and other physical findings. It also allows a rapport to develop between the patient and physician prior to undergoing a mildly invasive procedure.

There are four methods of performing indirect laryngoscopy: mirror laryngoscopy, nasal flexible fiberoptic laryngoscopy, oral flexible fiberoptic laryngoscopy, and rigid telescopic laryngoscopy. The following is a complete description of the procedure involved in performing each of these techniques. An excellent pictorial source for viewing normal and pathological conditions of the larynx may be found in Bruce Benjamin's *Diagnostic Laryngoscopy: Adults and Children*.[2] Table 149-1 reviews the advantages and disadvantages of each procedure. Each method allows visualization of the larynx with different degrees of distortion (Figure 149-1).

ANATOMY AND PATHOPHYSIOLOGY

The larynx occupies the central neck and is located within the hypopharynx[3,4] (Figure 149-2). Lateral to the larynx are the pyriform sinuses, the pharyngeal recesses that are the primary route for food to pass into the esophagus. The basic framework of the larynx consists of the thyroid cartilage, cricoid cartilage, epiglottic cartilage, arytenoid cartilage, and the hyoid bone. The shield-like thyroid cartilage supports the soft tissues of the larynx. It is connected to the hyoid bone via the thyrohyoid membrane and is attached to the cricoid cartilage via the cricothyroid membrane and at the cricothyroid joint. The signet ring shaped cricoid cartilage is the only complete cartilaginous ring in the larynx. On top of its posterior portion sits the paired arytenoid cartilages. The arytenoid cartilages are somewhat shaped like an inverted T. Each has a body, a muscular process, and a vocal process. The aryepiglottic folds connect the epiglottis to the top portion of the arytenoid body, the vocal ligament attaches the vocal process to the thyroid cartilage, and the cricoarytenoid muscles attach to the muscular process. The epiglottic cartilage is leaf-shaped and forms the anterior wall of the laryngeal entranceway. Its main portion projects posterior to the tongue base. It folds downward over the

TABLE 149-1 SUMMARY OF THE ADVANTAGES AND DISADVANTAGES OF THE DIFFERENT TECHNIQUES USED TO PERFORM INDIRECT LARYNGOSCOPY

	Hand-held mirror	Per-oral flexible endoscopy	Per-oral rigid endoscopy	Nasal flexible endoscopy
Gag reflex	Moderate	Moderate	Moderate	Minimal
Visual clarity	Good	Good–distorted	Superior	Good–distorted
Anesthetic	Occasionally	Yes	Occasionally	Yes
Observe larynx during speech	No	No	No	Yes
Patient cooperation	Necessary	Necessary	Necessary	Not necessary
Approximate equipment cost	Minimal	$4500	$4500	$4500
Documentation possible?	No	Yes	Yes	Yes

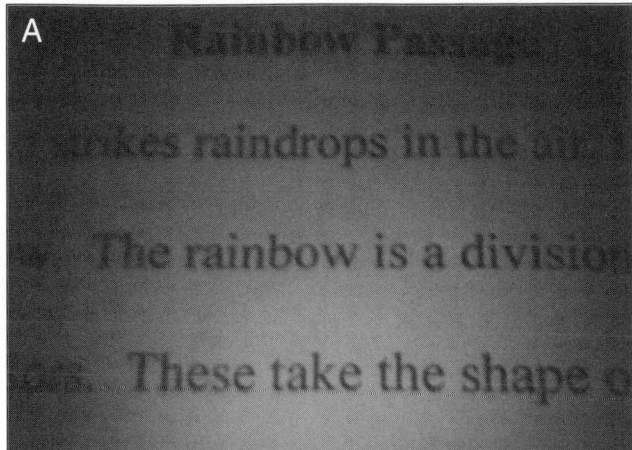

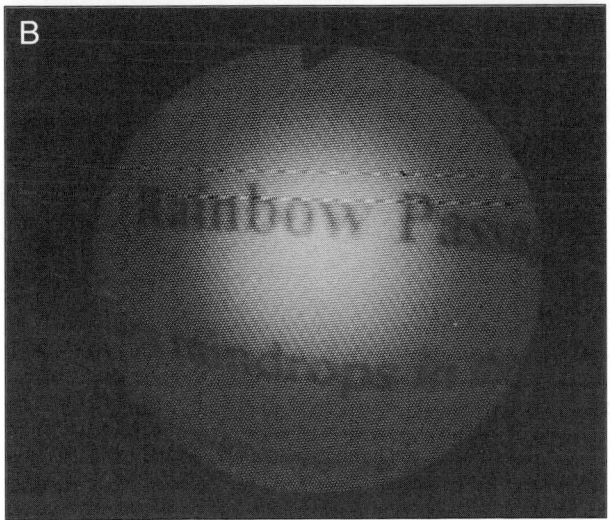

FIGURE 149-1 Visualization through the endoscopes. *A.* Endoscopic view through the 90-degree rigid telescope. Note the magnification, clarity, and breadth of view. *B.* Endoscopic view through flexible fiberoptic scope. Note the distortion and limited view as compared to the view through the rigid scope.

larynx during swallowing to aid in protecting the laryngeal opening from aspiration.

The muscles associated with the larynx may be divided into extrinsic muscles and intrinsic muscles. The extrinsic muscles move the larynx as a unit and can be further subdivided into those muscles that elevate the larynx (stylohyoid, digastric, geniohyoid, stylopharyngeus) and those that depress the larynx (omohyoid, sternohyoid, sternothyroid). The intrinsic muscles are involved with vocal cord mobility and all cause adduction with the exception of the cricoarytenoid muscle that causes abduction. Innervation to the intrinsic laryngeal muscles is via the recurrent laryngeal nerve, a branch of the vagus nerve (cranial nerve X). The cricothyroid muscle is the only muscle innervated by the external branch of the superior laryngeal nerve, a branch of the vagus nerve. All of the laryngeal muscles and cartilages are covered with respiratory epithelium.

Just superior to the vocal cords is a recess called the laryngeal ventricle. Just superior to the ventricle are the false vocal folds. These are rounded protrusions rich in mucous secreting glands. The supraglottic larynx is defined as that portion of the larynx extending from the tip of the epiglottis to the laryngeal ventricle. The glottic larynx contains the true vocal cords and extends approximately 5 to 7 mm inferiorly. The subglottis extends from the inferior glottis to the inferior edge of the cricoid cartilage.

The primary function of the larynx is to protect the airway from the aspiration of food particles. A complex reflex arc, with the glossopharyngeal nerve (cranial nerve IX) mediating the sensory arm and the vagus nerve (cranial nerve X) mediating the motor arm, occurs with swallowing. With each swallow the larynx elevates, the aryepiglottic folds squeeze medially, the epiglottis folds posteriorly over the larynx, and the true and false vocal folds close tightly. This allows the food bolus to pass around the larynx, into the pyriform sinuses, and subsequently into the esophagus. Any alteration or disturbance in the reflex arc may predispose a patient to aspiration.

Phonation occurs with adduction of the vocal cords as air passes from the trachea through the vocal cords. The mucosa overlying the muscles of the vocal cords

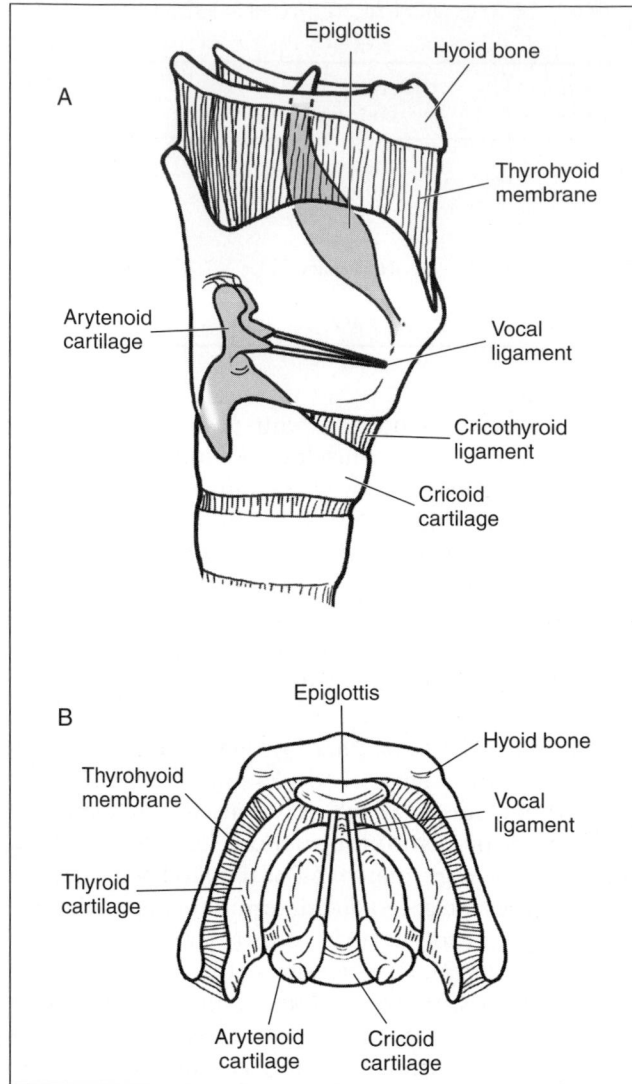

FIGURE 149-2 The laryngeal framework. *A.* Lateral view. *B.* Superior view.

undulates and the two vibrating vocal cords produce sound. Anything that alters the mucosal wave of the vocal cords, impairs adduction, or changes the configuration of vocal cord alignment will result in decreased phonatory performance. Note that mucosal wave abnormalities can only be observed with videostroboscopy of the larynx. Many things, such as inflammation to thick mucous or from vocal cord paralysis to tumors, can change a person's voice. Be careful and define hoarseness as a change in the patient's vocal quality. What may be normal for one patient may not be for another.

The larynx also is crucial in respiratory activity. Inspiration signals the recurrent laryngeal nerve to stimulate vocal cord abduction. Impairment in abduction, unilaterally or bilaterally, can lead to respiratory compromise.

INDICATIONS

Have a very low threshold for examining the larynx. The diagnostic value of laryngoscopy greatly outweighs the minimal discomfort associated with the quick procedure. Any patient presenting with hoarseness, symptoms of aspiration, shortness of breath, a foreign body sensation, hemoptysis, or any other symptom that may be related to the larynx should have laryngoscopy performed as part of a complete physical examination.

CONTRAINDICATIONS

There are no absolute contraindications for laryngoscopy. Patients with severe respiratory compromise, such as a child with suspected epiglottitis, should have laryngoscopy performed in the Operating Room (or in a controlled area) with an Anesthesiologist, intubation equipment, and tracheotomy instrumentation ready for use. Performing laryngoscopy in the respiratory distressed patient can lead to increased distress and ventilatory collapse if laryngospasm ensues. Use caution when performing laryngoscopy in a patient with a high-grade airway obstruction, a supraglottic expanding hematoma, or significant laryngeal trauma.

EQUIPMENT

Anesthesia and Vasoconstriction

10% lidocaine spray
20% benzocaine spray
2% tetracaine spray
4% cocaine
3% ephedrine or Neo-Synephrine spray
Cotton pledgets

Scopes

#4 or #5 dental mirror, with or without magnification
3 to 5 mm diameter flexible fiberoptic laryngoscope;
   3 mm is better for children
90 degree rigid laryngoscope

Light Sources

Headlight for mirror examinations
125 to 250 watt halogen or xenon light sources for
   fiberoptic laryngoscopes

Miscellaneous

Alcohol lamp, heated beads, or glass of warm water for
   mirror examination

4×4 gauze squares
Water-soluble lubricant
Antifog solution
Video camera and equipment for teaching and
    photodocumentation, optional

Set up all of the required equipment on a bedside procedure table (Figure 149-3). Prepare several different endoscopes, if available. If one fails, or is inadequate, another will be immediately available. The availability of multiple endoscopes allows the physician to choose the scope and technique of their choice.

PATIENT PREPARATION

Explain the risks, benefits, and potential complications of the procedure to the patient and/or their representative. **Patient reassurance and relaxation is of the utmost importance in obtaining excellent visualization of the larynx.** This can be achieved by reviewing what can be expected from the patient's perspective, by reassuring them of the minimal discomfort, and by reassuring them of the short duration of the procedure.

Patient positioning is crucial in obtaining laryngeal visualization in any per-oral technique. Place the patient sitting upright in a multipositional procedure chair or on a gurney with their legs together. Instruct the patient to lean slightly forward and to draw their chin forward. This aligns the larynx and the oropharynx in a vertical plane to allow visualization of the anterior portion of the larynx. Raise or lower the multipositional chair, or the gurney, so that the patient's mouth is at the examiner's eye level.

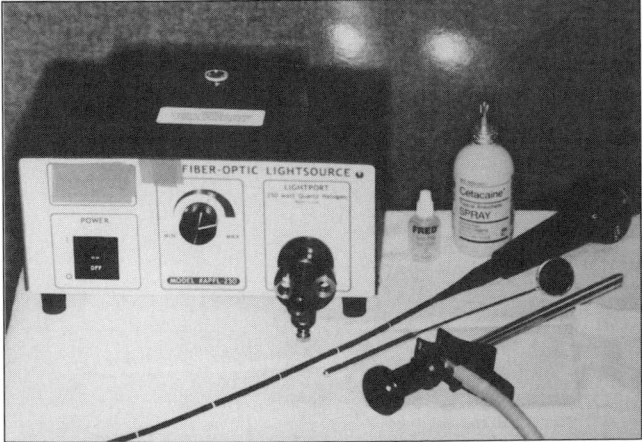

FIGURE 149-3 Basic equipment required for examination of the larynx in the ambulatory setting. Included are the rigid 90 degree telescope, dental mirror, flexible fiberoptic scope, gauze, oral anesthetic, antifog solution, and a light source. Not included is topical spray for nasal decongestion and anesthesia.

Patient cooperation and positioning is not crucial for flexible fiberoptic examination of the larynx performed through the nose. Place the patient, optimally, sitting upright with their head against a headrest. The headrest will prevent the common occurrence of the patient's head backing away from the examiner. Examination with the patient in the supine position is technically more challenging as gravity pushes the tongue posteriorly and the scope falls against the posterior pharyngeal wall; both of which make visualization of the anteriorly placed larynx more difficult. However, in most instances, it can still be performed without significant problems.

The use of good lighting cannot be overemphasized when performing a mirror examination. Apply a headlamp if one is available. An alternative is an overhead adjustable light source. Position the light so that it is aimed in the patient's mouth. The overhead light often hits the examiner in the head, casts shadows, and is too bright for the patient's eyes. It is also difficult to properly position as both of the examiner's hands must be used for the procedure.

TECHNIQUES

THE MIRROR EXAMINATION

Determine whether the patient has a significant gag reflex. If so, apply topical anesthesia. Spray a topical local anesthetic agent (benzocaine, lidocaine, or tetracaine) onto the patient's palate, tonsillar pillars, posterior pharyngeal wall, and base of the tongue. The application of a topical anesthetic agent is optional if the patient does not have a significant gag reflex. Instruct the patient to keep their eyes open and focus on a distant object to diminish the gag reflex. Practicing the entire procedure once with the patient, without inserting the mirror, is often a more reassuring and efficient manner of performing indirect laryngoscopy.

Instruct the patient to protrude their tongue. Grasp the tongue firmly, between the nondominant thumb and index finger, with a neatly folded gauze square (Figure 149-4). **Do not apply excessive traction on the tongue.** This is counterproductive as it elevates the tongue and makes the patient uncomfortable. Place the nondominant middle finger against the upper teeth as a brace. It may also be used to elevate the upper lip if needed. Instruct the patient to breathe through their mouth in a slow "panting-like" manner and to try to relax their tongue. This maneuver diminishes the gag reflex, elevates the palate, and lowers the tongue giving better access and visualization of the oropharynx.

Warm the mirror over an alcohol lamp, in heated beads, or in a cup of warm water to prevent fogging during the examination. Test the mirror back, if any type of heat is used, on the examiner's wrist for exces-

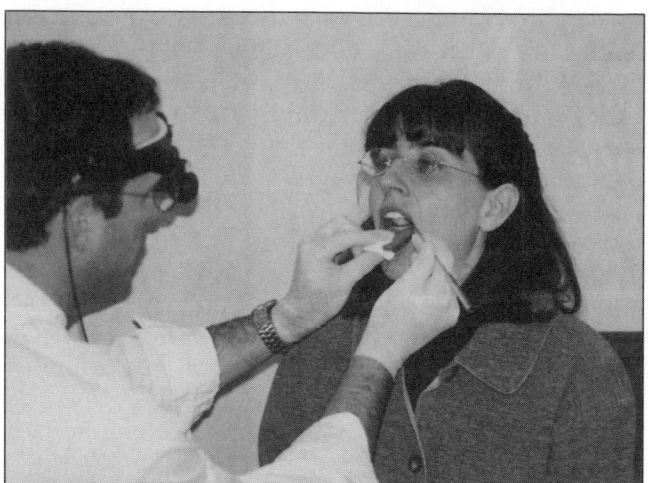

FIGURE 149-4 Proper positioning for an indirect mirror examination of the larynx. Both of the examiner's hands are braced against the patient for stability. Some patients require elevation of the upper lip with the examiner's left, or nondominant, middle finger.

sive heat that can injure the patient. An alternative is to use a mirror that has antifog solution placed on it to prevent fogging during the examination. Grasp the mirror with the dominant hand midway down the shaft like a pen (Figure 149-4). Brace the dominant fifth finger against the patient's cheek.

Introduce the mirror into the oral cavity with the glass surface parallel to the tongue (Figure 149-4). Instruct the patient to say a high-pitched "e-e-e" and hold it for 5 seconds just before the mirror touches and elevates the uvula and soft palate. The high-pitched "e-e-e" tilts the epiglottis forward and brings the vocal cords into view and apposition. Inform the patient that the "e-e-e" may sound like "ahhhhhh" while their tongue is held. This is helpful to them as they try to cooperate fully with the instructions. The examiner should simultaneously demonstrate the high-pitched sound as patients invariably will phonate in too low of a pitch for too short of a time period. Prevent gagging by asking the patient to phonate before the mirror actually touches the soft palate, avoiding touching the base of the tongue, and avoid touching the anterior tonsillar pillars.

Focus the headlight (or overhead light), as the patient phonates, on the mirror. Gently and slightly maneuver the mirror until the larynx is visualized. **Remember the orientation through the mirror. Left and right are the same but anterior and posterior have reversed orientation.**

Perform a quick and systematic evaluation of the larynx and hypopharynx. Assess the airway structures including the base of the tongue, vallecula, epiglottis, aryepiglottic folds, true and false vocal cords, arytenoids, posterior pharyngeal wall, and pyriform sinuses. Visualize adduction and abduction of the vocal cords

during phonations and inspirations. Several reinsertions of the mirror are often required to obtain a complete examination.

PER-ORAL FLEXIBLE FIBEROPTIC LARYNGOSCOPY

The examiner will often have a more leisurely view of the larynx with this technique, as compared to the mirror exam. Patients usually gag less and can tolerate this examination for longer periods of time.

Position the patient the same as for the mirror examination. All patients undergoing this procedure, in contrast to the mirror examination, must be topically anesthetized with an aerosolized local anesthetic agent as described above. Connect the light source to the fiberoptic scope and turn it on. Turn off the overhead room lights, if possible, to provide better contrast.

Instruct the patient to protrude their tongue and to grasp it with a gauze square (Figure 149-5). Hold the eyepiece of the scope in the dominant hand. Use the dominant thumb to manipulate the tip controller. Grasp and hold the middle portion of the fiberoptic scope with the thumb and index finger of the nondominant hand. Brace the remaining fingers of the nondominant hand against the patient's cheek (Figure 149-5). Instruct the patient to breathe slowly through their mouth in a "panting-like" manner.

Advance the scope with both hands until the tip is situated within the middle of the mouth and over the base of the tongue. Use the hand control to direct the tip of the scope downwards. Look through the scope and visualize the base of the tongue, the vallecula, and the tip of the epiglottis. Direct the scope posteriorly

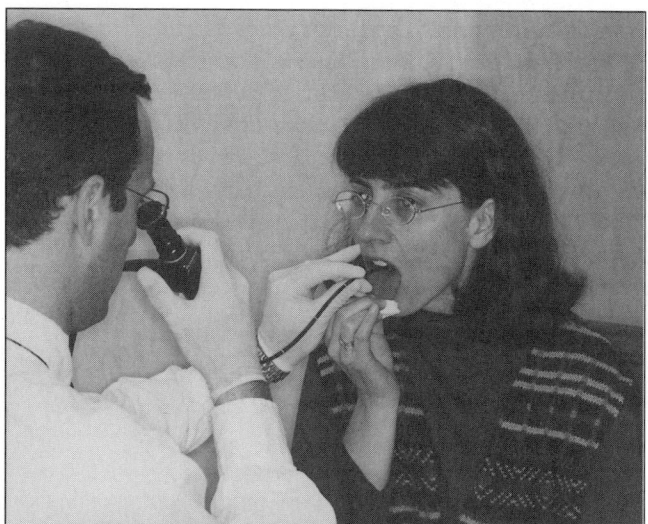

FIGURE 149-5 Positioning for an oral flexible fiberoptic examination of the larynx. The patient grasps their tongue. The examiner's left hand is braced against the patient's cheek.

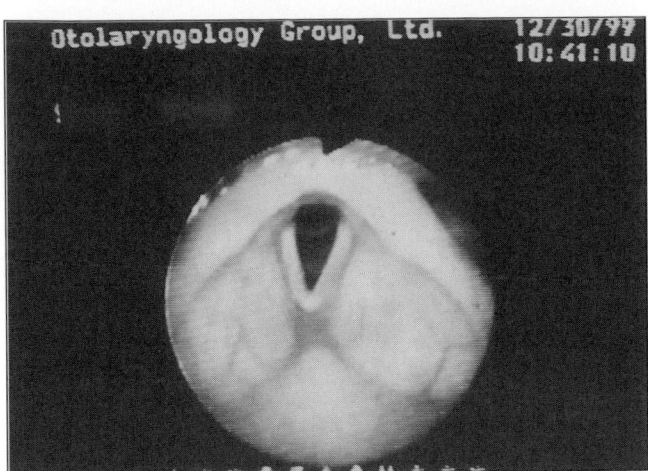

FIGURE 149-6 Endoscopic view of larynx through a flexible fiberoptic scope.

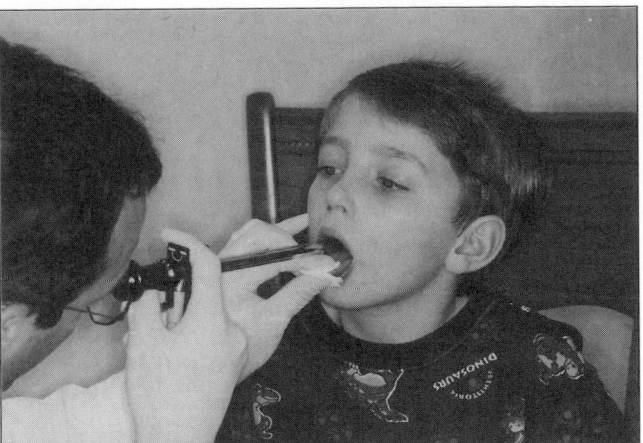

FIGURE 149-7 Positioning for a rigid telescopic examination of the larynx. Note that the telescope is stabilized on the left index finger and the left fifth finger braces against the patient's cheek.

over the epiglottis. The larynx and hypopharynx will come into view (Figure 149-6). Adjust the eyepiece, if necessary, to focus the scope. **Avoid touching the epiglottis as this may induce gagging.** Entry into the laryngeal vestibule will allow a more detailed examination, but may also induce laryngospasm if the vocal cords are touched. Perform a systematic examination of the laryngeal and hypopharyngeal anatomy. Instruct the patient to say "e-e-e" while viewing abduction and adduction of the vocal cords.

PER-ORAL RIGID FIBEROPTIC LARYNGOSCOPY

Position the patient the same as for the mirror examination. All patients undergoing this procedure, in contrast to the mirror examination, must be topically anesthetized with an aerosolized local anesthetic agent as described above. Connect the light source to the fiberoptic scope and turn it on. Turn off the overhead room lights, if possible, or dim them to provide better contrast. Apply antifog solution onto the laryngoscope lens.

Instruct the patient to protrude their tongue. Either the patient or the examiner may grasp the patient's tongue with gauze as it protrudes (Figure 149-7). Hold the scope with both hands while stabilizing the non-dominant hand against the patient's cheek if the patient holds their own tongue. Hold the scope with the dominant index finger and thumb if the examiner is grasping the patient's tongue (Figure 149-7). Stabilize the scope with the dominant fifth finger against the patient's cheek. Instruct the patient to breathe slowly through their mouth in a "panting-like" manner.

Insert the laryngoscope into the center of the mouth. Advance it straight backwards and over the tongue. Stop advancing the scope when the circumvallate papillae are reached. Instruct the patient to phonate as described above. Advance the scope until the larynx is

visualized (Figure 149-8). Tilt and gently rotate the scope to visualize the entire larynx and hypopharynx during phonation and quiet breathing.

FLEXIBLE NASOPHARYNGOSCOPY OR NASOLARYNGOSCOPY

Patient positioning is not crucial with this technique. Anesthetize the nasal passage so that the procedure is best tolerated. Visualize both nasal cavities with a nasal speculum to determine which nasal passageway will be easier to pass the scope through. Decongest the nasal mucosa with aerosolized oxymetazoline, 3% ephedrine, or cocaine. Instruct the patient to sniff in deeply after the spray is applied. Allow 3 to 5 minutes to pass for the vasoconstriction to occur. Apply a topical anesthetic spray to the nasal passageway. Spraying achieves excellent vasoconstriction and anesthesia as the agents

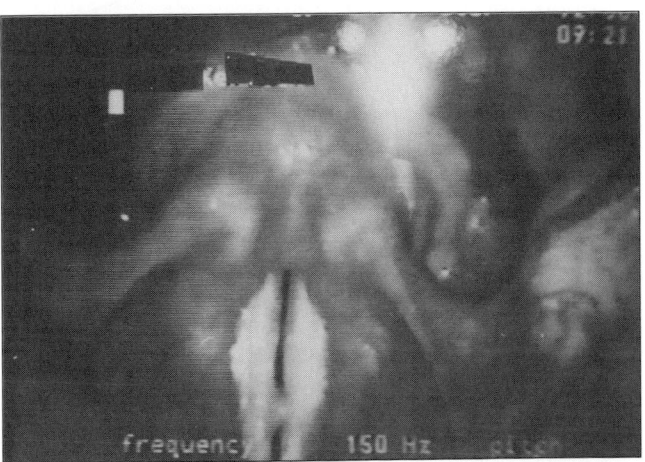

FIGURE 149-8 Endoscopic view of the larynx through a rigid 90 degree telescope.

diffuse through the entire nasal cavity and pharynx. Alternatively, place cocaine-soaked pledgets into the nasal cavity inferior and superior to the inferior turbinate for 10 minutes to achieve excellent anesthesia and vasoconstriction.

Connect the light source to the fiberoptic scope and turn it on. Turn off the overhead room lights, if possible, to provide better contrast. Hold the eyepiece of the scope in the dominant hand (Figure 149-9). Use the dominant thumb to manipulate the tip controller. Grasp and hold the middle portion of the fiberoptic scope with the thumb and index finger of the nondominant hand. Brace the remaining fingers of the nondominant hand against the patient's cheek (Figure 149-9).

Insert the tip of the scope into the nose. Advance the scope with both hands and directed either along the floor of the nose or along the superomedial aspect of the inferior turbinate, depending upon the nasal anatomy (Figure 149-10). Instruct the patient to breathe through their nose as the nasopharynx is encountered. This lowers the soft palate and opens the nasopharynx. Direct the tip of the endoscope downward and advance it past the oropharynx. Slide the tip of the scope

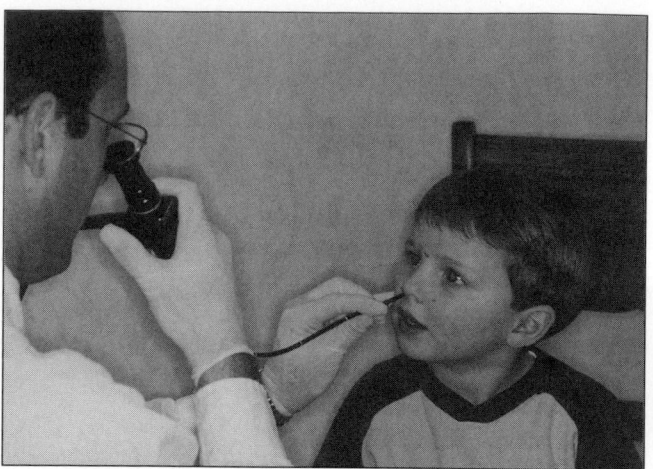

FIGURE 149-9 Positioning for a nasal flexible fiberoptic examination of the larynx. Note that the left, nondominant, hand is stabilized against the patient's cheek.

behind the epiglottis, along the posterior pharyngeal wall, and into the hypopharynx and larynx. **Avoid touching the epiglottis to prevent gagging and the vocal cords to prevent laryngospasm.** Almost all pa-

Superior turbinate

Middle turbinate

Inferior turbinate

Sphenoid sinus

Routes for flexible scope

Auditory tube opening

Choana

Hard palate

Soft palate

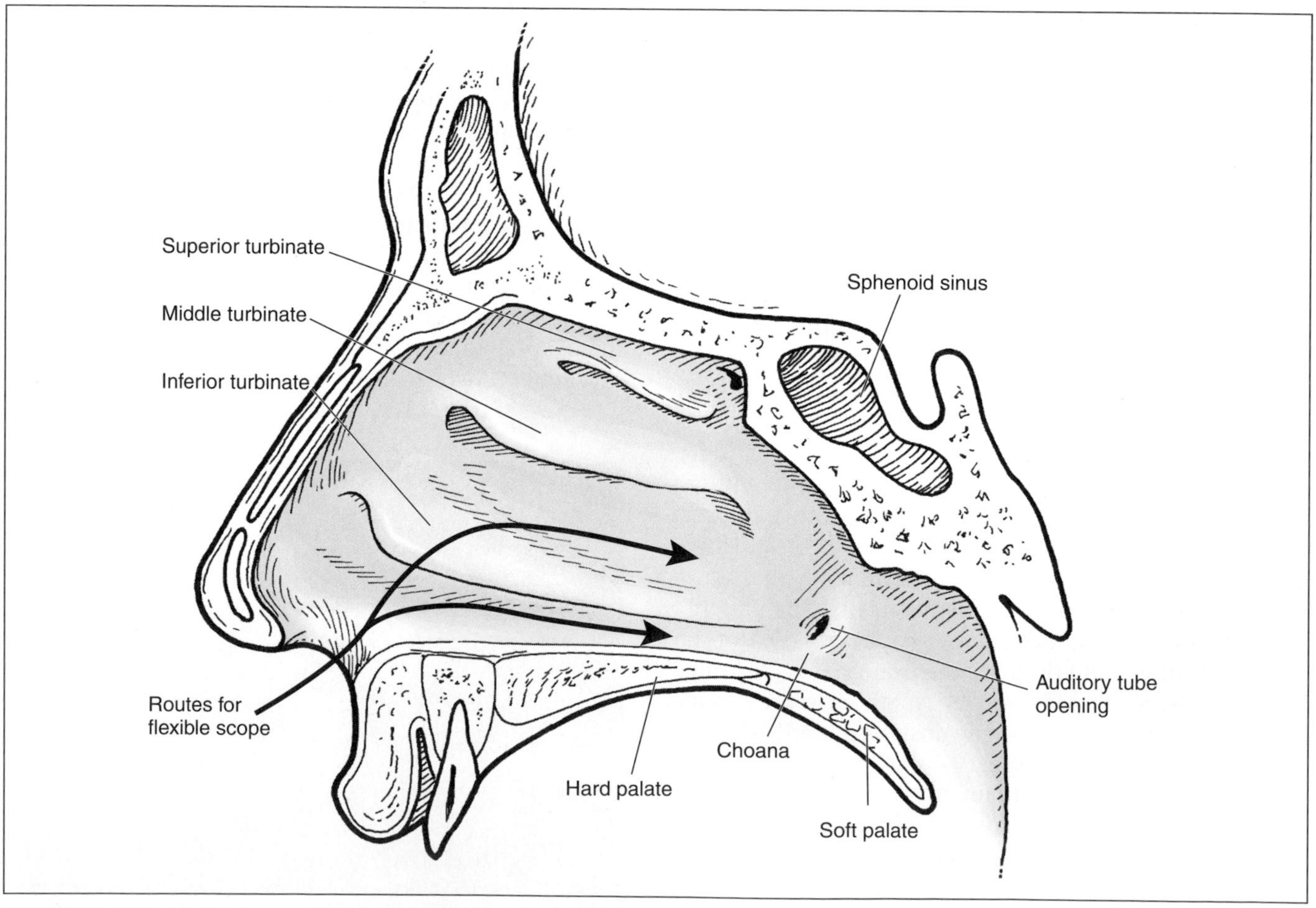

FIGURE 149-10 Anatomy of the lateral nasal wall and the two routes that the flexible scope can follow to gain access to the nasopharynx and subsequently the larynx.

tients can tolerate this procedure. Gagging is unusual. Apply a topical anesthetic agent to the oral cavity and oropharynx if the patient gags. Perform a leisurely and thorough examination of the airway. This is the only technique in which normal speech can be observed.

AFTERCARE

Inform the patient that the effects of the topical anesthetic persist an average of 30 to 45 minutes. Alert the patient that they may experience symptoms of aspiration, such as coughing or choking, when swallowing. Liquids are more likely to cause problems than solids. Instruct the patient not to ingest any solid or liquid substances until the topical anesthetic agent wears off.

COMPLICATIONS

Few complications arise from laryngoscopy. Epistaxis is possible with nasal endoscopy. It is uncommon when using vasoconstrictive agents and careful manipulation of the scope. Emesis is rare, even in the patient with an extremely sensitive gag reflex. Laryngospasm can be avoided as long as care is taken to avoid direct contact with the vocal cords.

SUMMARY

Visualization of the larynx is a basic and often crucial component in the physical examination of the patient. A variety of techniques have been described, all of which are adequate in evaluating the larynx and hypopharynx. Risks and complications are rare. Maintain a very low threshold when deciding whether or not to perform laryngoscopy. Patient education and preparation are as, if not more, important than equipment and instrumentation in obtaining a thorough examination.

REFERENCES

1. Saunders WH: Physical examination, in Schuller DE, Schleuning AJ (eds): *DeWeese and Saunders' Otolaryngology: Head and Neck Surgery,* 8th ed. St. Louis: Mosby, 1994:3–27.
2. Benjamin B: *Diagnostic Laryngoscopy: Adults and Children.* Philadelphia: Saunders, 1990.
3. Fried MP, Meller SM: Adult laryngeal anatomy, in Fried MP (ed): *The Larynx: A Multidisciplinary Approach,* 2nd ed. St. Louis: Mosby, 1996:33–45.
4. Asher VA, Sasaki CT, Gracco CL: Laryngeal physiology: normal and abnormal, in Fried MP (ed): *The Larynx: A Multidisciplinary Approach,* 2nd ed. St. Louis: Mosby, 1996:33–45.

Chapter 150
AIRWAY FOREIGN BODY REMOVAL

David L. Walner

INTRODUCTION

The death toll in the United States from foreign body aspiration among all age groups has remained at approximately 3000 per year for the past 20 years.[1] The mortality rate following foreign body aspiration is estimated at 1 to 2 percent. The most likely cause of death is complete airway obstruction, generally at the level of the larynx or trachea. Globular objects such as hot dogs, candies, nuts, and grapes are the most commonly aspirated food objects.[2] Rubber balloons and toys are the most commonly aspirated nonfood objects.[2] The majority of foreign body aspirations (> 70 percent) occur in children, most of whom are younger than 3 years of age.[1]

The management of airway foreign bodies requires specific expertise and training. Airway foreign bodies must be managed by an Otolaryngologist or other qualified physician, depending on the institution, with experience in airway endoscopy and the knowledge to deal with potential complications related to airway obstruction. The morbidity and mortality associated with airway foreign body retrieval has greatly declined due to the development of safe endoscopic techniques, rod-lens telescopes, and optical forceps.

The burden of proof lies in the physician's hands in order to diagnose airway foreign bodies. Keep in mind that information gained from the history, physical examination, and radiologic studies may not clearly define the presence of a foreign body.[3] Thirty-three percent of airway foreign body cases are neither observed nor suspected. The physical examination may be normal in up to 39 percent of patients. Radiographic studies may be normal in up to 20 percent of the patients. The only definitive test when considering the diagnosis of an airway foreign body is endoscopy to evaluate the entire laryngotracheobronchial tree.

ANATOMY AND PATHOPHYSIOLOGY

The airway is divided into three anatomic regions: the larynx, the trachea, and the bronchi. The laryngeal aditus is formed by the epiglottis anteriorly, the aryepiglot-tic folds laterally, and posteriorly by the corniculate cartilages and upper border of the arytenoid muscle. The larynx extends from the level of the aditus to the lower border of the cricoid cartilage, where it is continuous with the trachea.[4] The infant larynx is located higher in the neck than the adult larynx. The cricoid cartilage descends in the neck through childhood. Due to the superior position of the infant larynx, the epiglottis is located with the tip often resting on the soft palate.[5] The infant larynx is approximately one-third the size of the adult larynx. Laryngeal foreign bodies are most common in infants due to the small size of the inlet.

The trachea begins at the lower border of the cricoid cartilage, extending downward from about the level of the sixth cervical vertebra in adults or the fourth cervical vertebra in infants. The trachea extends inferiorly to the level of the carina. The inferior end of the trachea is located at the level of the fifth thoracic vertebra or the sternal angle. The trachea is 4 cm long in a full-term newborn infant and 11 to 13 cm long in an adult. The diameter of the trachea is 3.6 mm in a newborn and 12 to 23 mm in an adult.[6]

The trachea divides into two mainstem bronchi.[6] The right mainstem bronchus is shorter, straighter, and larger in diameter than the left mainstem bronchus. This explains why right mainstem foreign bodies are more common than left mainstem foreign bodies. The mainstem bronchi divide into three lobar bronchi on the right and two on the left. The lobar bronchi divide into segmental bronchi. There are, usually, 10 segmental bronchi on the right, and 8 on the left.[6]

Airway foreign bodies commonly become lodged in one of three locations: the larynx, the trachea, or the bronchi. Laryngeal foreign bodies account for 4 to 5 percent of airway foreign bodies.[7] Laryngeal foreign bodies have a mortality rate of 45 percent due to complete airway obstruction.[8] Approximately one-third of survivors of transient airway obstruction suffer from hypoxic encephalopathy.

Most choking victims are able to generate a forceful cough to expel the foreign body. Some patients are unable to relieve the obstruction themselves. The use of the Heimlich maneuver has further decreased mortality.[9] **It** should be emphasized that the relief of an airway obstruction should only be attempted if signs of a complete airway obstruction are observed.[10] Only perform oral cavity finger sweeps if a foreign body is seen within the oral cavity.[10] Immediate intervention is not only unnecessary, but may be potentially dangerous if a patient is able to breathe, speak, or cough.[11]

Laryngeal foreign bodies can present with only mild or moderate respiratory distress. They may be located, or wedged, between the laryngeal ventricles, the true vocal folds, or the immediate subglottis (Figure 150-1A). Plain radiographs of the neck will detect radiopaque foreign bodies (Figures 150-1B and C). Flexible awake fiberoptic laryngoscopy allows visualization of the larynx and supraglottic structures.

Tracheal foreign bodies account for 9 percent and bronchial foreign bodies account for 81 percent of airway foreign bodies.[7] The classic diagnostic triad of a tracheobronchial foreign body consists of the sudden onset of paroxysmal coughing, wheezing, and diminished breath sounds on the affected side. However, these symptoms may only be present in 50 percent of cases. Approximately 33 percent of cases of airway foreign bodies are neither observed nor suspected.[12] Tracheal foreign bodies may present with audible biphasic or expiratory stridor. Audible expiratory wheezing is more likely associated with a main bronchus obstruction. Tachypnea and cyanotic episodes may occur, generally when larger obstructing objects are present. Small foreign bodies may travel distally to a secondary bronchus and produce the more subtle symptoms of mild wheezing, cough, pneumonia, or fever. No abnormalities are found in up to 39 percent of patients.[3] It is estimated that only 70 percent of patients with a foreign body aspiration seek treatment within the first week of the aspiration.[13]

The most common airway foreign bodies are food items. Peanuts account for nearly 40 percent of tracheobronchial foreign bodies[14] (Figure 150-2). Other common foreign bodies include plastic toys, pins, tacks, watermelon seeds, sunflower seeds, nails, screws, carrots, and popcorn. More than 80 percent of airway foreign bodies are radiolucent and can be difficult to diagnose. The most common radiologic findings are identified using both inspiratory and expiratory chest radiographs. This can be in the form of a check valve with postobstructive hyperinflation and mediastinal shift to the contralateral side (Figure 150-3). It may also be seen in the form of a ball valve with atelectasis, collapse of the distal airways, and mediastinal shift to the ipsilateral side. Pneumonia can be present in 9 percent of cases, generally when the foreign body has been present for weeks or months. Chest radiographs can be normal in up to 11 to 20 percent of patients with tracheobronchial foreign bodies.[3]

Suspect an airway foreign body based upon the history, physical examination, and radiologic findings. However, the diagnosis is not always clear-cut. It is the responsibility of the physician suspecting an airway foreign body to confer with the appropriate specialist and to strongly suggest endoscopy consisting of laryngoscopy and bronchoscopy. Endoscopy remains the gold standard to rule in or rule out an airway foreign body.

INDICATIONS

The indications for airway endoscopy must take into account the patient's history, physical examination, radiologic findings, and the suspected location of the foreign body. An accurate history is of the utmost importance in the diagnosis of foreign body aspiration as the remainder of the assessment, physical examination, and radiographic studies can be deceptively unremarkable. The characteristic history consists of an incipient choking or gagging episode. Caretakers often describe subsequent coughing spells when the event was witnessed. Aspiration must be assumed if the patient was eating peanuts, seeds, or beans during the episode. All witnessed aspirations with nuts or nondissolvable food matter require endoscopy and removal if the foreign material is identified.

CONTRAINDICATIONS

The majority of patients presenting to the Emergency Department with airway foreign bodies are in stable condition. This allows time to adequately access the patient and formulate the best possible treatment plan. Infants and children with airway foreign bodies require an institution with the capability for comprehensive pediatric care. This includes a physician who is experienced with airway endoscopy and foreign body retrieval in children, a facility with pediatric endoscopic equipment, pediatric anesthesia capabilities, and pediatric intensive care capabilities. This often will require transfer to a specialized pediatric center. Attempting removal of airway foreign bodies in a less-than-adequate environment can be catastrophic for the patient and is not advised. This same philosophy applies to adult airway endoscopy and to having qualified personal who are experienced in this area.

Stabilize the patient first if their airway is stable, if an airway foreign body is suspected or known, and has other medical issues prior to proceeding with airway foreign body retrieval. Follow basic life support protocols, including the section on a choking victim, in the rare situation of an acutely obstructed airway. Any patient with a suspected laryngeal foreign body or impending airway

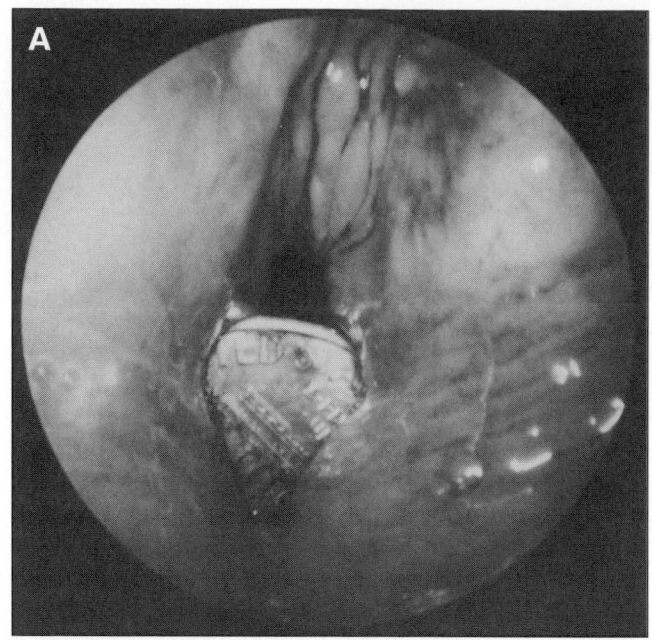

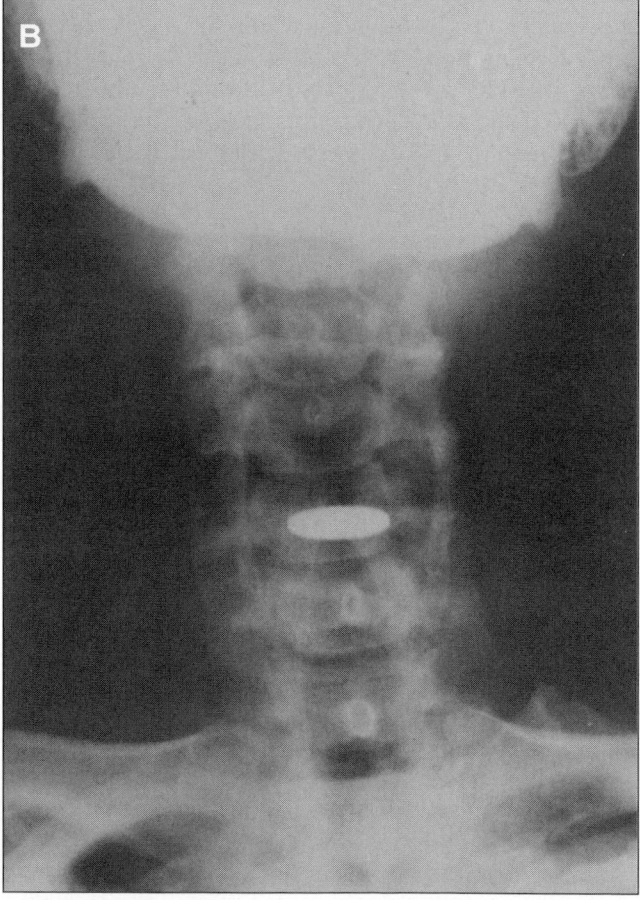

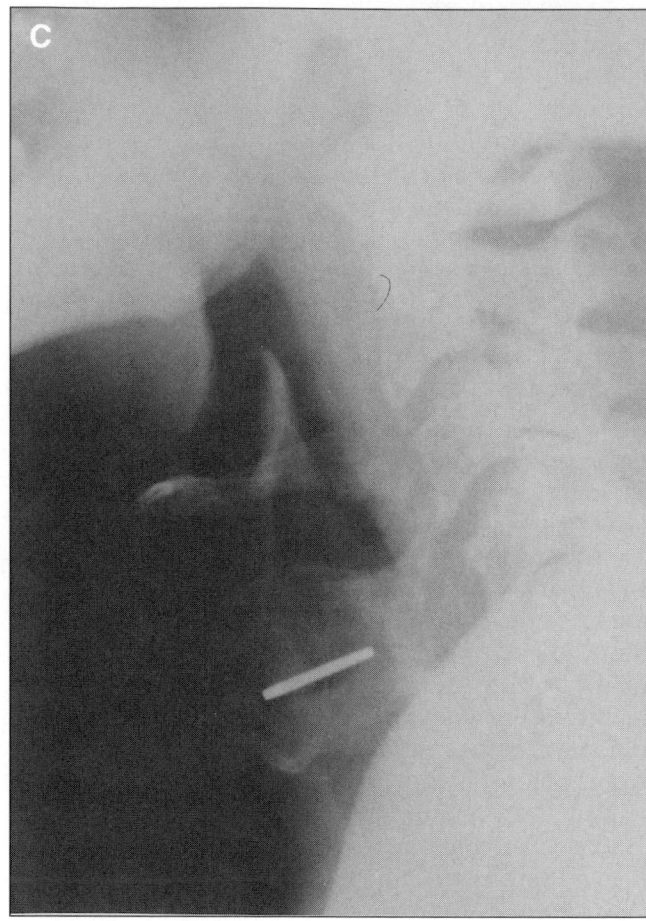

FIGURE 150-1 Laryngeal foreign body. *A.* Coin lodged within the laryngeal ventricles resulting in a partial airway obstruction. *B.* Anteroposterior neck radiograph. *C.* Lateral neck radiograph.

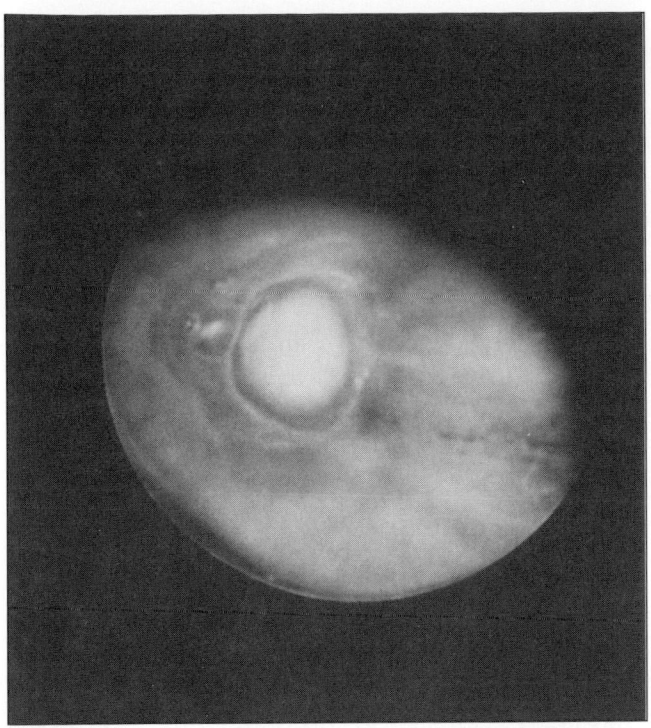

FIGURE 150-2 Endoscopic view of a nut in the left mainstem bronchus.

obstruction requires emergent endoscopy and control of the airway in the Operating Room, if possible. A cricothyrotomy will be required as a lifesaving measure if attempts at resuscitation are unsuccessful.

EQUIPMENT

Emergency Department Equipment

Intubation equipment
Percutaneous transtracheal jet ventilator
Cricothyroidotomy kit
Suction source, tubing, and catheter
Magill forceps
Laryngoscope with Miller blades
Topical anesthetic spray
Fiberoptic nasopharyngoscope

Operating Room Equipment

The proper equipment must be selected based upon the patient's age and size, as well as the suspected composition of the foreign body. Laryngoscopes are selected to allow visualization of the larynx and the passage of a bronchoscope. Rigid, ventilating bronchoscopes with fiberoptic telescopes provide optimal visualization (Figure 150-4A). This allows direct access to

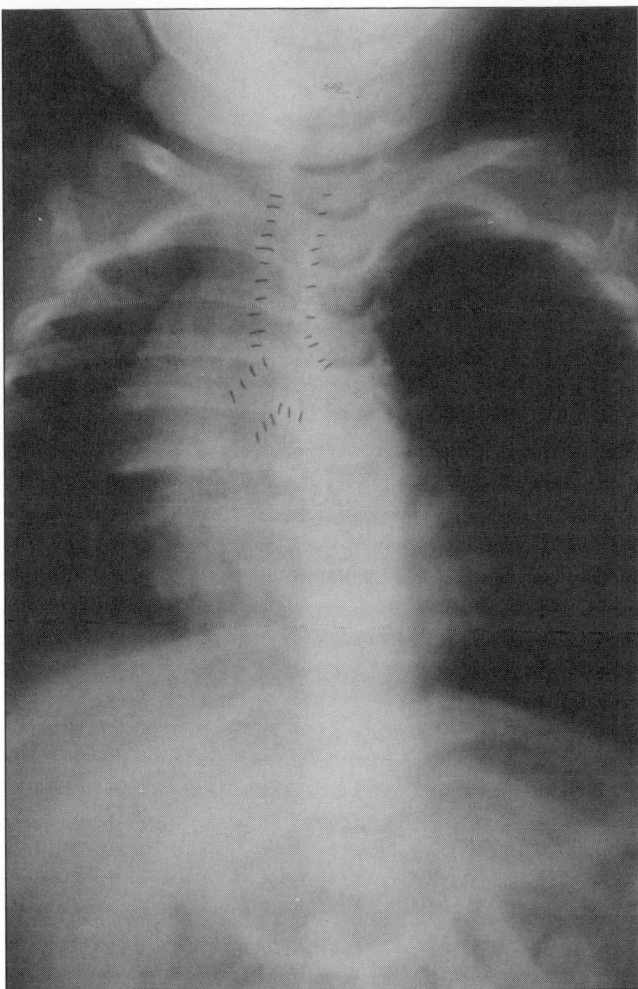

FIGURE 150-3 Chest radiograph of a patient with a left mainstem bronchus foreign body and a check valve-type of obstruction. Marks delineate the trachea and the mainstem bronchi.

the airway, excellent visualization, continuous administration of anesthetic agent and oxygen, and a conduit for the introduction of instruments (forceps) to retrieve the foreign object. Numerous extraction instruments are available and include smooth, toothed, cupped, angled, open mouth, and optical forceps (Figures 150-4B and C). The forceps allow a magnified and direct view through the forceps.

PATIENT PREPARATION

Timing of endoscopy and airway foreign body retrieval must be based upon each individual patient. Do not waste time if impending airway obstruction exists. Immediately notify and mobilize an Anesthesiologist, Otolaryngologist, and the Operating Room as this is an emergent situation. It is appropriate to wait for NPO

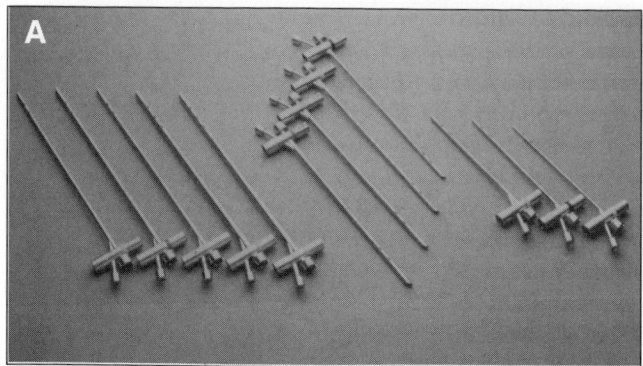

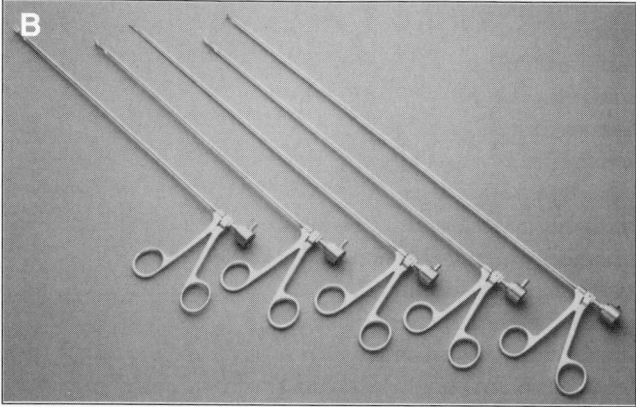

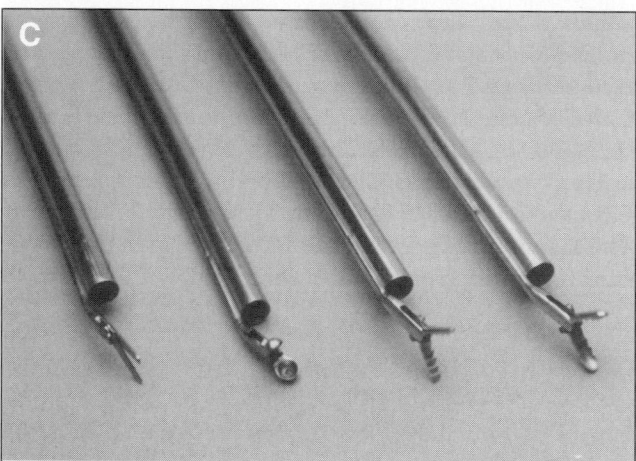

FIGURE 150-4 Equipment for operative removal of an airway foreign body. *A.* Karl Storz rigid ventilating broncho-scopes. *B.* Karl Storz foreign body retrieval forceps. *C.* Close-up view of various foreign body retrieval forceps.

status to be present and the stomach empty prior to proceeding to the Operating Room if the diagnosis of an airway foreign body is highly suspected and the patient is stable. This is considered a timely approach and may take up to 6 hours for children or 8 hours for adults. Waiting this time in the stable patient decreases the risk of aspiration and further compromising the situation. It is also appropriate to wait, in a stable patient, in order to assemble the appropriate and best nursing and anesthe-

sia team to care for the patient. Using personnel who are unfamiliar with endoscopy can create a compromised and stressful situation.

TECHNIQUES

EMERGENCY DEPARTMENT TECHNIQUES

The foreign body airway obstruction protocol based upon the pediatric basic life support textbook treats conscious infants (younger than 1 year of age) with four back blows while the infant is in a prone position on the rescuer's forearm, face down, and the head lower than the trunk. This is combined with four rapid chest thrusts (as in infant CPR), if the obstruction persists, while the infant is supine with the head lower than the body.[10] Treat unconscious infants by opening the airway and attempting rescue breathing based on basic life support protocols.[10] Treat children and adults with the standard Heimlich maneuver, using gentle thrusts in smaller children to decrease the likelihood of injury to the abdominal organs.

Attempt orotracheal intubation in the Emergency Department if the airway obstruction progresses rapidly. Intubation can be used to force the foreign body into one mainstem bronchus and allow ventilation of one lung. Intubate the patient. Grasp an upper airway foreign body that is visualized with a McGill forceps and remove it. Insert and advance the endotracheal tube as far as it will advance if the foreign body is not visualized or unable to be grasped. Withdraw the endotracheal tube to the proper position and begin ventilation. **Always be prepared to perform a cricothyrotomy or transtracheal jet ventilation.** Transtracheal jet ventilation allows for short-term oxygenation, is temporary, and may allow time for safe transport to the Operating Room so that endoscopy and foreign body retrieval can be performed in a more controlled environment with appropriate equipment at hand. Refer to Chapters 5, 14, and 13 regarding the details of orotracheal intubation, cricothyroidotomy, and transtracheal jet ventilation, respectively.

Direct laryngoscopy and bronchoscopy in a child or adult with an airway foreign body is a dangerous situation. The procedure may result in a partial airway obstruction becoming a complete airway obstruction. **Always have a cricothyroidotomy tray immediately available.** All equipment must be selected, assembled, and ready for use.

It is possible to remove foreign bodies located within the hypopharynx in the Emergency Department. Typical foreign bodies that may be removed include pieces of food and fishbones. **The patient must be stable and in no risk of airway compromise.** Obtain anteroposterior and lateral soft tissue radiographs of the neck to localize, if possible, the foreign body. Perform indirect laryngoscopy to identify the foreign body and its location. Refer to Chapter 149 regarding the complete details of laryngoscopy. Obtain intravenous access.

Place the patient in full monitoring (pulse oximeter, cardiac monitor, noninvasive blood pressure cuff). Apply a topical anesthetic spray to the oropharynx and the base of the tongue. Place the patient supine. Administer a small dose of an intravenous sedative if required. Gently insert a #3 Miller laryngoscope blade. Elevate the patient's tongue and jaw. Grasp the foreign body with a McGill forceps. Withdraw the McGill forceps followed by the laryngoscope.

OPERATING ROOM TECHNIQUES

The procedure begins with the induction of general anesthesia. It cannot be overemphasized that anesthesia should only be administered by an Anesthesiologist who is competent and comfortable with the situation. Pediatric patients require an Anesthesiologist with pediatric airway experience if the patient is stable. Full monitoring and mask induction allows the patient to maintain spontaneous respiration. Muscle relaxants are avoided as they can induce complete airway obstruction.

The Otolaryngologist begins the procedure. Place the patient supine with a shoulder roll to position the airway. Insert the laryngoscope into the larynx. Expose the larynx by elevating the laryngoscope. Topical anesthetic is applied to the larynx to avoid laryngospasm. The bronchoscope with telescope is then passed under direct vision through the mouth and into the laryngeal introitus. Ventilation can continue via a port on the scope. The foreign body is visualized. Forceps are inserted through the scope and used to grasp the foreign body. Small objects can be removed directly through the scope, whereas larger objects require removing the bronchoscope along with the forceps and foreign body. The bronchoscope is passed again, after removal of the foreign body, to identify any mucosal injury or second foreign body that may occur in as many as 5 percent of patients.[3]

A specific type of foreign body, such as a tack or sharp object, may become lodged in the larynx or upper trachea. Extraction with the forceps using standard endoscopic techniques may not be possible. Patients may require a tracheotomy and an open approach (laryngotomy) to remove the foreign body.

ALTERNATIVE TECHNIQUE

The use of a flexible fiberoptic bronchoscope to retrieve bronchial foreign bodies may be acceptable for physicians who are well trained with this technique. The mainstay of tracheobronchial foreign body retrieval remains to be rigid bronchoscopy.

AFTERCARE

After the retrieval of an airway foreign body, most patients should be breathing spontaneously. An endotracheal tube may rarely, in the presence of significant laryngeal or tracheobronchial edema, need to remain in place temporarily. This would require admission to an intensive care unit. Humidified oxygen is helpful to keep the airway moist and prevent mucous crusts from forming. A postoperative radiograph will help to determine any changes to the lung fields following extraction.

All patients who have undergone foreign body removal require at least a few hours of airway observation in a monitored setting. Racemic epinephrine treatments and intravenous Decadron can be administered as needed. Discharge from the hospital is acceptable when the patient is breathing comfortably and no longer in danger of airway compromise. Some patients may be discharged home the same day as surgery, while others may require multiple days of airway support and observation.

COMPLICATIONS

Complications from the foreign bodies themselves include hypoxia leading to cerebral anoxia if not identified. Intraoperative complications can occur in the hands of an inexperienced endoscopist who loses control of a foreign body in the airway and is faced with obstruction or respiratory arrest. Cardiac arrhythmias can occur from hypoxia or direct pressure on the left mainstem bronchus. Postoperative problems can include laryngeal or tracheobronchial edema from the foreign body or the instrumentation of the airway. Mucosal irritation can instigate a tracheitis or bronchitis. Pneumonia can develop. Pneumomediastinum has been reported in as many as 13 percent of aspirations and a pneumothorax slightly less frequently.[15]

A foreign body pulled up from a main stem bronchus can become dislodged in the larynx or trachea and cause a complete airway obstruction. A foreign body in the hypopharynx can be pushed distally and result in an airway obstruction. The foreign body needs to be quickly removed, pushed back down into one of the mainstem bronchi to allow ventilation of at least one lung, or a surgical airway performed. Failure to react appropriately in this situation can result in asphyxiation and death.

SUMMARY

Airway foreign bodies pose a diagnostic and therapeutic challenge. The initial encounter in the physician's office or Emergency Department must uncover any historical fact, physical abnormality, or radiographic abnormality that may lead to a definitive or presumed diagnosis of an airway foreign body. Endoscopy must be performed by a skilled team to allow safe and efficient removal of the foreign body. Hypopharyngeal foreign bodies may be safely removed in the Emergency Department by a trained physician.

REFERENCES

1. Darrow DH, Holinger LD: Foreign bodies of the larynx, trachea, and bronchi, in Bluestone CD, Stool SE, Kenna MA (eds): *Pediatric Otolaryngology,* 3rd ed. Philadelphia: Saunders, 1996:1390–1401.

2. Ryan CA, Yacoub W, Paton T, et al: Childhood deaths from toy balloons. *Am J Dis Child* 1990; 144:1221–1224.

3. McGuirt WF, Holmes KD, Feehs R, et al: Tracheobronchial foreign bodies. *Laryngoscope* 1988; 98:615–618.

4. Hollinshead WH: *Anatomy for Surgeons: The Head and Neck,* 3rd ed. Philadelphia: Harper & Row, 1982:389–441.

5. Holinger PH, Johnson KC, Schiller F: Congenital anomalies of the larynx. *Ann Otol Rhinol Laryngol* 1954; 63:581–606.

6. Holinger LD, Green CG: Anatomy, in Holinger LD, Lusk RP, Green CG (eds): *Pediatric Laryngology and Bronchoesophagology.* Philadelphia: Lippincott-Raven, 1997:19–33.

7. Dayan SH, Portugal LG, Walner DL, et al: Laryngeal obstruction after inhalation of a penny from a metered-dose inhaler. *Otolaryngol Head Neck Surg* 1999; 120(4):548–551.

8. Lima JA: Laryngeal foreign bodies in children: a persistent, life-threatening problem. *Laryngoscope* 1989; 99:415–420.

9. Heimlich H: A lifesaving maneuver to prevent food choking. *JAMA* 1975; 234(4):398–401.

10. Chameides L, Hazinski MF: *Textbook of Pediatric Advanced Life Support.* Dallas, TX: American Heart Association, 1994.

11. Committee on Accident and Poison Prevention: First aid for the choking child. *Pediatrics* 1988; 81(5):740–742.

12. Gibson SE, Shott SR: Foreign bodies of the upper aerodigestive tract, in Myer CM, Cotton RT, Shott SR (eds): *The Pediatric Airway.* Philadelphia: Lippincott, 1995:195–222.

13. Mu L, He P, Sun D: Inhalation of foreign bodies in Chinese children: a review of 400 cases. *Laryngoscope* 1991; 101:657–660.

14. Hughes CA, Baroody FM, Marsh BR: Pediatric tracheobronchial foreign bodies: historical review from the Johns Hopkins hospital. *Ann Otol Rhinol Laryngol* 1996; 105:555–561.

15. Burton EM, Riggs W, Kaufman R, et al: Pneumomediastinum caused by foreign body aspiration in children. *Pediatr Radiol* 1989; 20:45–47.

Chapter 151
PERITONSILLAR ABSCESS INCISION AND DRAINAGE

Julio C. Silva

INTRODUCTION

Emergency Department visits for peritonsillar abscesses are quite frequent. One recent study cited an incidence of approximately 45,000 cases of this disease process per year.[1] The mean age of affected patients is 25 years. It is a relatively rare finding before the age of 5 years. There remains a fair amount of controversy in the literature regarding the optimal antibiotic choice and the mechanism of drainage. The objective for the Emergency Physician remains to make an accurate diagnosis, to institute appropriate care, and to arrange adequate follow-up.

ANATOMY AND PATHOPHYSIOLOGY

The anatomy of the oral cavity is relatively simple (Figure 151-1). The peritonsillar abscess can be found posterolateral to the palatine tonsil and posterior to the palatoglossal fold (or arch). **Note the close proximity of the internal carotid artery and the facial artery to the peritonsillar abscess (Figure 151-2).** Use extreme care to not penetrate too deeply and lacerate these arteries.

Most patients will have had symptoms for approximately 4 days by the time abscess formation has occurred. The most common symptoms include fever, sore throat, dysphagia, and trismus. Physical examination will reveal a nonexudative pharyngitis in the majority of cases, soft palate edema, a bulging prominent tonsil, and uveal deviation away from the abscessed tonsil (Figure 151-3). The differential diagnosis includes infectious mononucleosis, leukemias, odontogenic infections, and aneurysms of the internal carotid artery.

The peritonsillar abscess has been attributed to progression and direct extension of an acute exudative pharyngitis. More recent work has described a group of salivary glands, Weber's glands, located in the supratonsillar space as the actual site of bacterial invasion and subsequent abscess formation.[2] The bacterial inoculum results in tissue necrosis and pus formation typically located between the tonsillar capsule and the lateral pharyngeal wall and/or the supratonsillar space. Progression of pus formation and cellulitis within the supratonsillar space results in a gradual involvement of the surrounding musculature, particularly the internal pterygoids, leading to spasm and the classic trismus seen with this disease.

The most common isolate found on culture remains group A beta-hemolytic streptococci.[3] The abscess is often polymicrobial and includes group A beta-hemolytic streptococci, *Staphylococcus aureus, Bacteroides fragilis,* and *Bacteroides melaninogenicus.* There is an increasing prevalence of beta-lactamase producing organisms.[3]

Treatment options for peritonsillar abscess drainage have undergone a significant amount of debate in the literature. These range from simple or single aspiration of the abscess, repeated aspirations, and incision and drainage. Patients treated with aspiration alone have success rates ranging from 85 to 100 percent.[1,4,5] The overall recurrence rate is less in patients undergoing incision and drainage.[1,4,5]

INDICATIONS

All peritonsillar abscesses require either aspiration or incision and drainage. The decision regarding the choice of technique is left to physician preference and, when possible, in consultation with an Otolaryngologist.

CONTRAINDICATIONS

There are no absolute contraindications to draining a peritonsillar abscess. Patients with severe trismus limiting visibility and access may require intravenous analgesics and muscle relaxants, procedural sedation, or

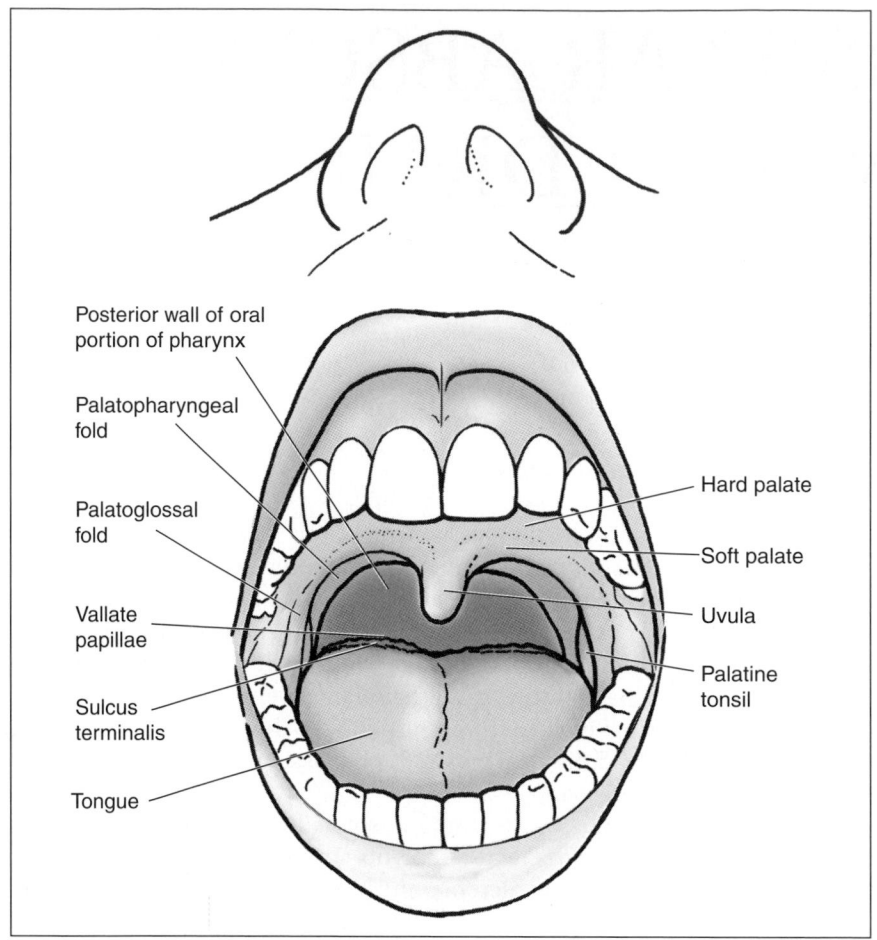

FIGURE 151-1 Anatomy of the oropharynx as seen through the open mouth.

Posterior wall of oral portion of pharynx

Palatopharyngeal fold

Palatoglossal fold

Vallate papillae

Sulcus terminalis

Tongue

Hard palate

Soft palate

Uvula

Palatine tonsil

intraoperative drainage. Consult an Otolaryngologist for all patients who are coagulopathic, taking oral anticoagulants, or with a known bleeding disorder. These patients are at risk for significant bleeding and associated complications. Admit children to the hospital for intravenous antibiotics, incision and drainage under general anesthesia, and possible tonsillectomy.

EQUIPMENT

#11 scalpel blade on a handle
Curved hemostat
Frazier suction catheter
Suction source and tubing
Tongue depressor
Topical anesthetic spray (lidocaine, tetracaine, or benzocaine)
Syringe, 3 or 5 mL
25 or 27 gauge needle, 2 inches long
Local anesthetic solution with epinephrine
10 mL syringe
18 gauge needle

Culturettes or culture bottles
Headlamp
Gloves and mask for the physician
Oral rinse solution, hydrogen peroxide or Peridex

PATIENT PREPARATION

Explain the procedure, its risks, and benefits to the patient and/or their representative. Obtain a signed informed consent for the procedure. Ensure that the patient has a thorough understanding of the postprocedural care instructions and follow-up requirements.

Position the patient sitting in an upright multipositional procedure chair. Alternatively, place the patient sitting upright on a gurney with the back elevated. Prepare the wall suction unit to ensure it is working. Apply suction tubing and a suction catheter to the suction source.

The use of good lighting cannot be overemphasized. Apply a headlamp if one is available. An alternative is an overhead adjustable light source. Position the light so that it is aimed in the patient's mouth. The overhead

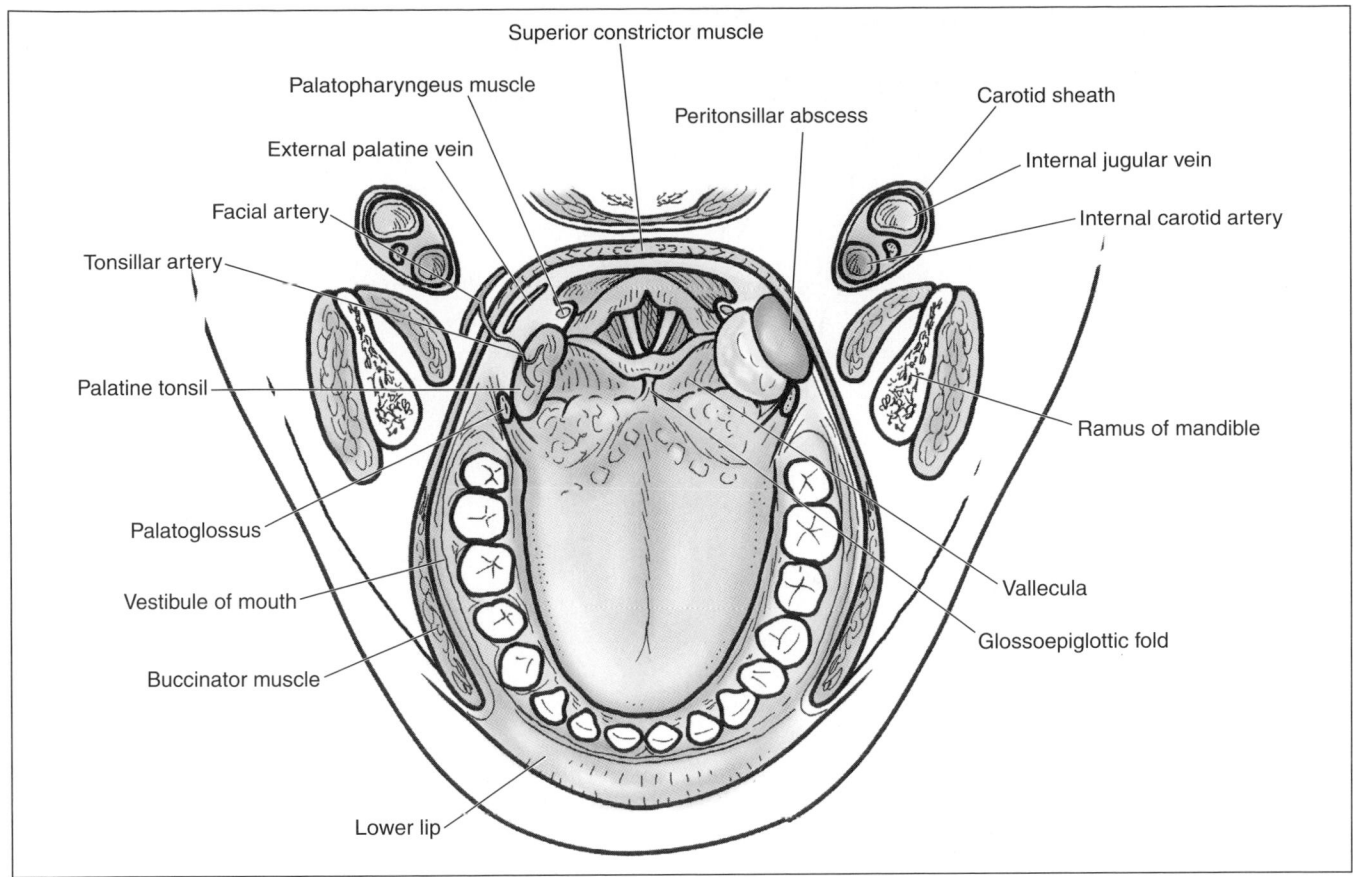

FIGURE 151-2 Horizontal section through the mouth and oropharynx. Note the close proximity of the peritonsillar abscess to the internal carotid artery and the facial artery.

light often hits the examiner in the head, casts shadows, and is too bright for the patient's eyes. It is also difficult to properly position because both of the examiner's hands must be used for the procedure.

Incision and drainage must be preceded by adequate anesthesia to the abscess site. Determine the most fluctuant region of the abscess. Anesthetize this area. Spray topical anesthetic over the abscess (Figure 151-4*A*). Dry the mucosa overlying the peritonsillar abscess with a gauze square. Arm a 3 mL syringe with a 25 or 27 gauge needle. Inject 1 mL of local anesthetic solution containing epinephrine through the area of topical anesthesia and just under the mucosal surface (Figure 151-4*B*). Allow 3 to 5 minutes for the anesthetic to work.

TECHNIQUES

ASPIRATION

Identify the area of maximal fluctuance at the upper pole of the abscess. Anesthetize the area as mentioned previously. Prepare the equipment. Apply an 18 gauge

needle onto a 10 mL syringe. **A smaller needle may not allow thick pus to be aspirated.** Break the seal of the syringe. Trim the needle cap and place it over the needle to act as a depth gauge (Figure 151-5*A*). The needle should project only 1 cm from the distal end of the needle cap. Alternatively, apply a piece of tape onto the needle to mark a point 1 cm from the tip of the needle (Figure 151-5*B*). The guard (cap or tape) serves as a marker for the maximum allowable depth to insert the needle during the procedure. **Limiting of the depth of insertion of the needle will prevent injury to the carotid artery that is located approximately 1.5 to 2 cm posterior and lateral to the tonsil.**

Depress the tongue with a tongue depressor held in the nondominant hand (Figure 151-6*A*). Insert the prepared needle attached to the syringe into the upper pole of the abscess, into the point of maximal fluctuance[6–9] (Figures 151-6*A* and *B*). Hold and advance the needle parallel to the floor and directly posterior. **Do not direct the needle laterally where it can injure the carotid artery.** Aspirate while advancing the needle. Approximately 85 to 90 percent of abscesses occur in the upper pole of the tonsil.[6,9] If purulent fluid is obtained,

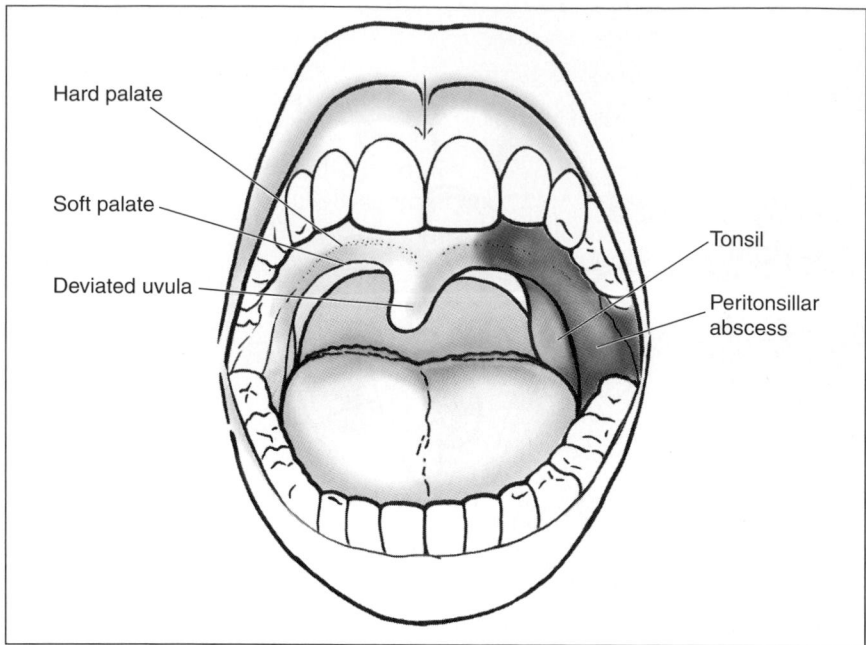

FIGURE 151-3 A peritonsillar abscess. The abscess displaces the tonsil forward and medially. The uvula is deviated towards the contralateral side.

continue to aspirate and remove as much material as possible. Obtain a culture and sensitivity of the aspirated material. Allow the patient to rinse and spit several times with Peridex solution or half-strength hydrogen peroxide solution.

If the initial aspirate is negative, reattempt the procedure by inserting the needle into the middle pole and then the inferior pole of the abscessed tonsil until purulent material is obtained (Figure 151-6A). **A completely negative aspiration, while more consistent with a tonsillar cellulitis, does not rule out the exis-tence of an abscess.** Gentle palpation will reveal fluctuance when an abscess if present.

INCISION AND DRAINAGE

One of the editors (E.F.R.) recommends to always perform a needle aspiration prior to the incision and drainage technique. Aspiration will localize the collection of pus and allow a more accurate incision and drainage. **A negative aspiration at all three sites (Figure 151-6A) is a contraindication for an incision and drainage procedure.** It may be too early and an

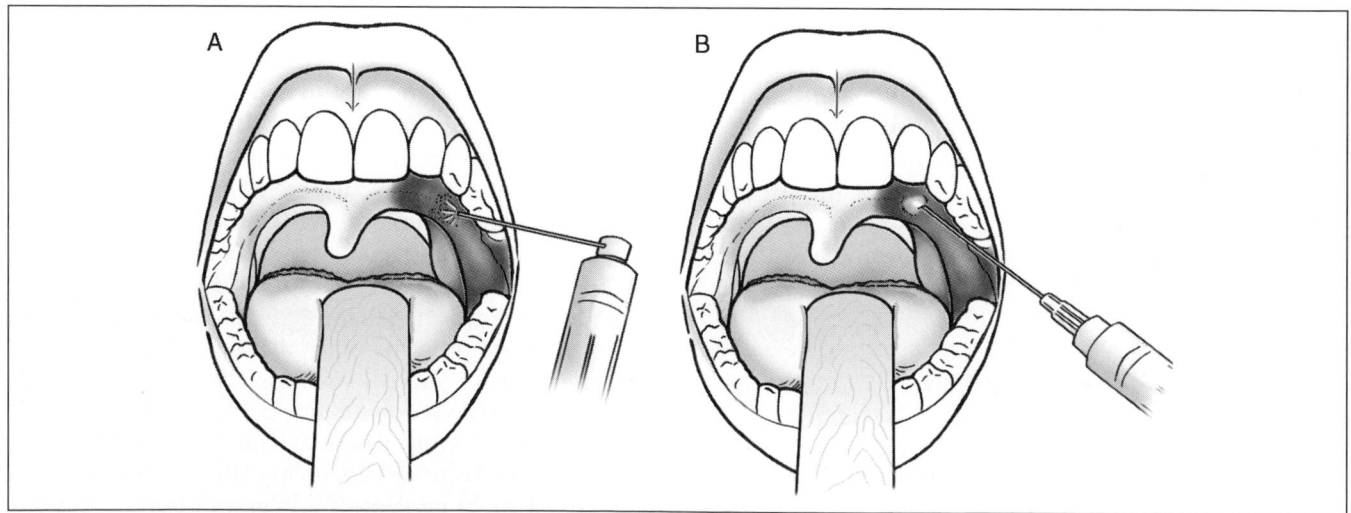

FIGURE 151-4 Anesthesia techniques. *A.* Topical spray anesthesia. *B.* Infiltrative anesthesia.

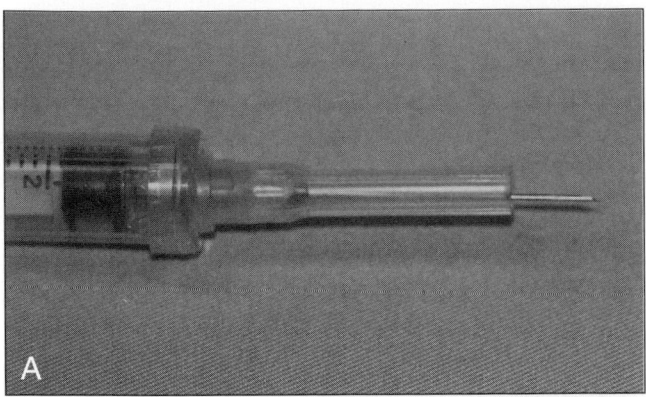

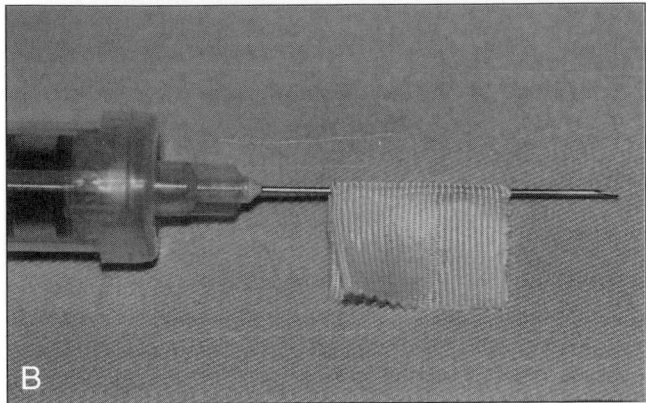

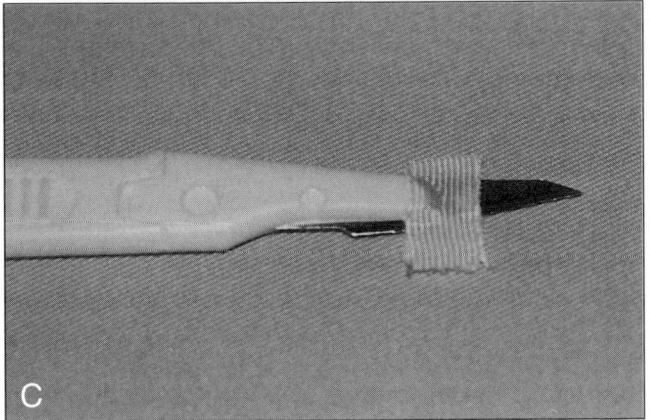

FIGURE 151-5 Safety techniques to prevent injury to the internal carotid artery. *A*. The needle cover is cut and placed over the needle as a guard. *B*. Tape applied to an 18 gauge needle. *C*. Tape applied to a #11 scalpel blade.

abscess has not yet formed. A negative aspiration at all three sites suggests the patient has a tonsillar cellulitis requiring oral antibiotics, gargles with hydrogen peroxide, and follow-up in 24 hours for reevaluation.

Identify the area of maximal fluctuance at the upper pole of the abscess. Anesthetize the area as mentioned previously. Prepare the equipment. Place a piece of tape on the #11 scalpel blade so that only 0.75 to 1 cm is ex-

posed (Figure 151-5*C*). Place the Frazier suction catheter near the incision site. Insert the scalpel blade to make a horizontal stab wound to a maximum depth of 1 cm in the same area noted for the aspiration technique (Figures 151-7*A* and *B*). The Frazier suction catheter will remove any blood and purulent material to prevent the patient from aspirating. **The depth of the stab should be no more than 1 centimeter. Extend the length of the incision to a maximum of 1.0 to 1.5 centimeters.**

Insert a curved hemostat into the wound (Figure 151-7*C*). Gently spread apart the jaws of the hemostat to break up any loculations in the abscess. Continue to simultaneously suction the area during the procedure. Packing of the abscess cavity is not required. Obtain a culture and sensitivity of the purulent material. Allow the patient to rinse and spit several times with Peridex solution or half-strength hydrogen peroxide solution. Leave the suction in the patient's hand so they can use it as needed.

ASSESSMENT

Allow the patient to rinse and spit with either water or saline solution. Observe the patient for any evidence of continued bleeding or upper airway symptomatology. Assess the patient's ability to tolerate oral fluids prior to discharge.

AFTERCARE

Discharge the patient with oral antibiotics and analgesics. Penicillin is still the drug of choice. Many Otolaryngologists will either add clindamycin or metronidazole due to the increasing incidence of penicillin-resistant organisms.[1,10] An alternative is to substitute clindamycin or amoxicillin-clavulanate for penicillin.[1,10] Nonsteroidal anti-inflammatory drugs will adequately control any pain and fever. Recommend to the patient to follow a soft diet and drink plenty of fluids during the first 48 hours after the intervention. Instruct the patient to gargle with half-strength hydrogen peroxide or Peridex after each meal, at a minimum, and several other times per day. Arrange follow-up within 48 hours, or sooner if they do not improve. Instruct the patient to return to the Emergency Department immediately if they develop bleeding, shortness of breath, difficulty swallowing, drooling, or have any concerns.

Admission is generally required for patients who appear toxic, pediatric patients, dehydrated patients, immunocompromised patients, recurrent abscesses, and for patients who are unable to tolerate oral fluids. These patients require observation for 23 hours and intravenous antibiotics.

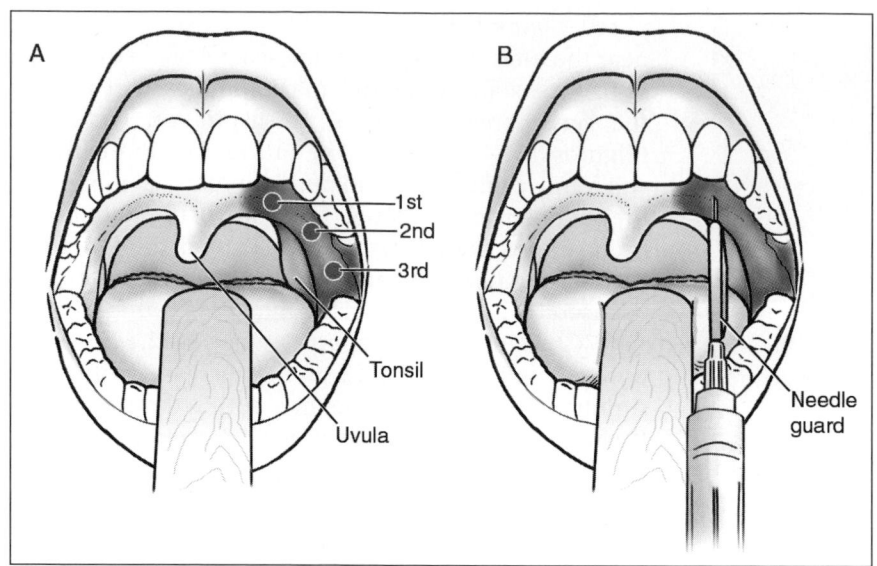

FIGURE 151-6 Needle aspiration of a peritonsillar abscess. *A.* Recommended sites for needle aspiration. *B.* Aspiration in the first area.

COMPLICATIONS

There are few complications associated with the management of a peritonsillar abscess. Potential complications include aspiration. This is usually not a concern as the patient has not often eaten for hours. Protect against aspiration of purulent material and subsequent pulmonic infection by having the patient sit upright during the procedure and using suction as the abscess is opened. Too large or deep of an incision can injure the carotid artery (or a carotid artery aneurysm) or result in prolonged bleeding. Always limit the depth of the needle or scalpel.

SUMMARY

A peritonsillar abscess is commonly encountered in the Emergency Department. Diagnosis and treatment results in rapid symptom resolution in the majority of patients. Admission may be required in a few instances for observation and intravenous antibiotics.

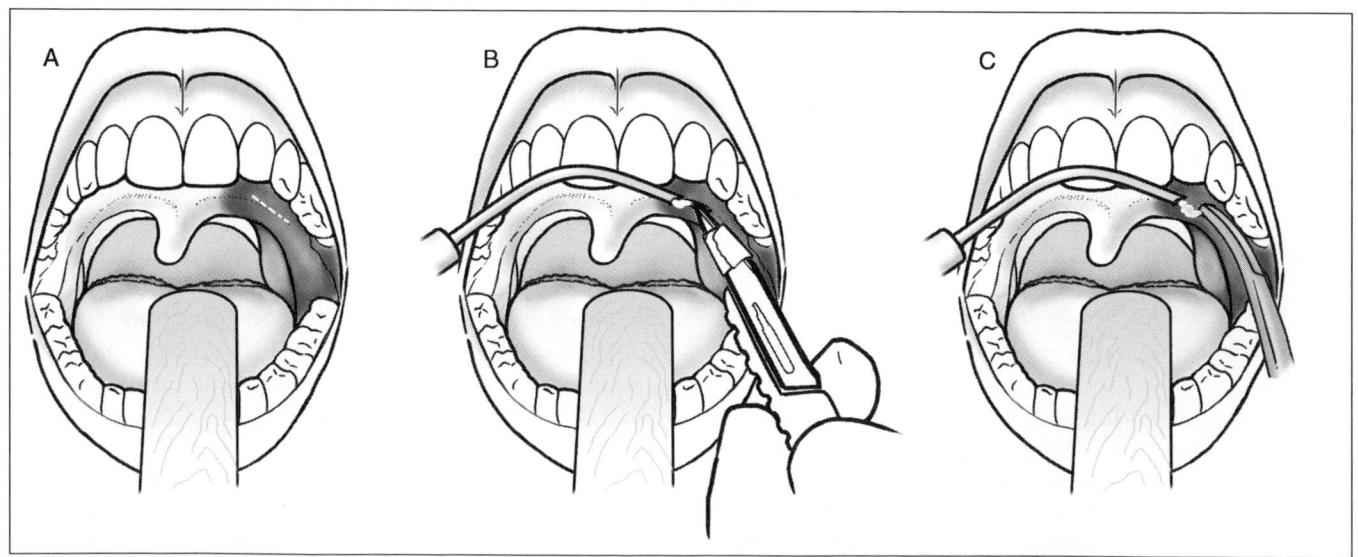

FIGURE 151-7 Incision and drainage of a peritonsillar abscess. *A.* The incision site is also the same site for the first aspiration. *B.* Incision with a #11 scalpel blade. Note the tape marking the maximum insertion depth of the scalpel blade. Suction any bloody or purulent fluid that escapes from the incision. *C.* Hemostat gently inserted to break any loculations.

REFERENCES

1. Herzon FS: Peritonsillar abscess: incidence, current management practices, and a proposal for treatment guidelines. Mosher award thesis. *Laryngoscope* 1995; 105(8 Pt 3):1–17.
2. Passy V: Pathogenesis of peritonsillar abscess. *Laryngoscope* 1994; 104(2):185–190.
3. Kieff DA, Bhattacharyya N, Siegel NS, et al: Selection of antibiotics after incision and drainage of peritonsillar abscesses. *Otolaryngol Head Neck Surg* 1999; 120(1):57–61.
4. Wolf M, Even-Chen I, Kronenberg J: Peritonsillar abscess: repeated needle aspiration versus incision and drainage. *Ann Otol Rhinol Laryngol* 1994; 103(7):554–557.
5. Maharaj D, Rajah V, Hemsley S: Management of peritonsillar abscess. *J Laryngol Otol* 1991; 105(9):743–745.
6. Weinberg E, Brodsky L, Stanievich J, et al: Needle aspiration of peritonsillar abscesses in children. *Arch Otolaryngol Head Neck Surg* 1993; 119:169–172.
7. Maisel RH: Peritonsillar abscess; tonsil antibiotic levels in patients treated by acute abscess surgery. *Laryngoscope* 1982; 92:80–87.
8. Zalzal GH, Cotton RT: Pharyngitis and adenotonsillar disease, in Cummings CS, Fredrickson JM, Hanker CA, et al (eds): *Otorhinolaryngology—Head and Neck,* 2nd ed. St. Louis: Mosby, 1993:1180–1198.
9. Spires JR, Owens JJ, Woodsen GE, et al: Treatment of peritonsillar abscess. A prospective study of aspiration versus incision and drainage. *Arch Otolaryngol Head Neck Surg* 1987; 11:984–986.
10. MacDougall G, Denholm SW: Audit of the treatment of tonsillar and peritonsillar sepsis in an ear, nose and throat unit. *J Laryngol Otol* 1995; 109(6):531–533.

Chapter 152
SUBLINGUAL ABSCESS INCISION AND DRAINAGE

Julio C. Silva

INTRODUCTION

Odontogenic infections are frequently evaluated in the Emergency Department. The vast majority of odontogenic infections require minimal intervention. The spread of such infections from the mandibular premolars and first molar can lead to the development of a sublingual abscess.

ANATOMY AND PATHOPHYSIOLOGY

The topographical anatomy of the anterior oral cavity is rather simple (Figure 152-1). The sublingual space is located between the oral mucosa and the mylohyoid muscle (Figure 152-2). The posterior boundary of this space is open, allowing communication with the submandibular space. **It is important to remember that the posterolateral regions on each side of the floor of the mouth contain the lingual artery, vein, and nerve. These areas must be avoided when draining a sublingual abscess.**

Patients will usually complain of swelling of floor of the mouth. There may be significant tongue elevation in cases of bilateral involvement. The accumulation of purulence in this area of the mouth is typically a result of the spread of an infection from the mandibular premolars and the first molar (Figure 152-3). The most common organisms involved are *Streptococcus, Peptostreptococcus, Eubacterium, Porphyromonas, Prevotella,* and *Fusobacterium.* Antibiotics typically used post-procedurally include penicillin, clindamycin, or metronidazole.[1]

INDICATIONS

All patients presenting with a sublingual abscess require intraoral incision and drainage.

CONTRAINDICATIONS

There are no absolute contraindications to draining a sublingual abscess. Patients with severe trismus limiting visibility and access may require intravenous analgesics and muscle relaxants, procedural sedation, or intraoperative drainage.[2] Consult an Otolaryngologist for all patients who are coagulopathic, taking oral anticoagulants, or with a known bleeding disorder. These patients are at risk for bleeding and associated complications. Admit children to the hospital for intravenous antibiotics, incision and drainage under general anesthesia, and observation.

EQUIPMENT

Gauze 4×4 squares
Suction source
Yankauer or Frazier suction catheter
#11 scalpel blade on a handle
Mosquito hemostat
Sterile Penrose drain
Ribbon gauze
Headlight or overhead spotlight
Culturette or culture bottles
4–0 silk suture
Suture scissors
Oral rinse solution, hydrogen peroxide or Peridex
Topical anesthetic spray (lidocaine, tetracaine, or benzocaine)
Local anesthetic solution containing epinephrine
5 mL syringe
25 to 27 gauge needle, 2 inches long

PATIENT PREPARATION

Explain the procedure, its risks, and benefits to the patient and/or their representative. Obtain a signed in-

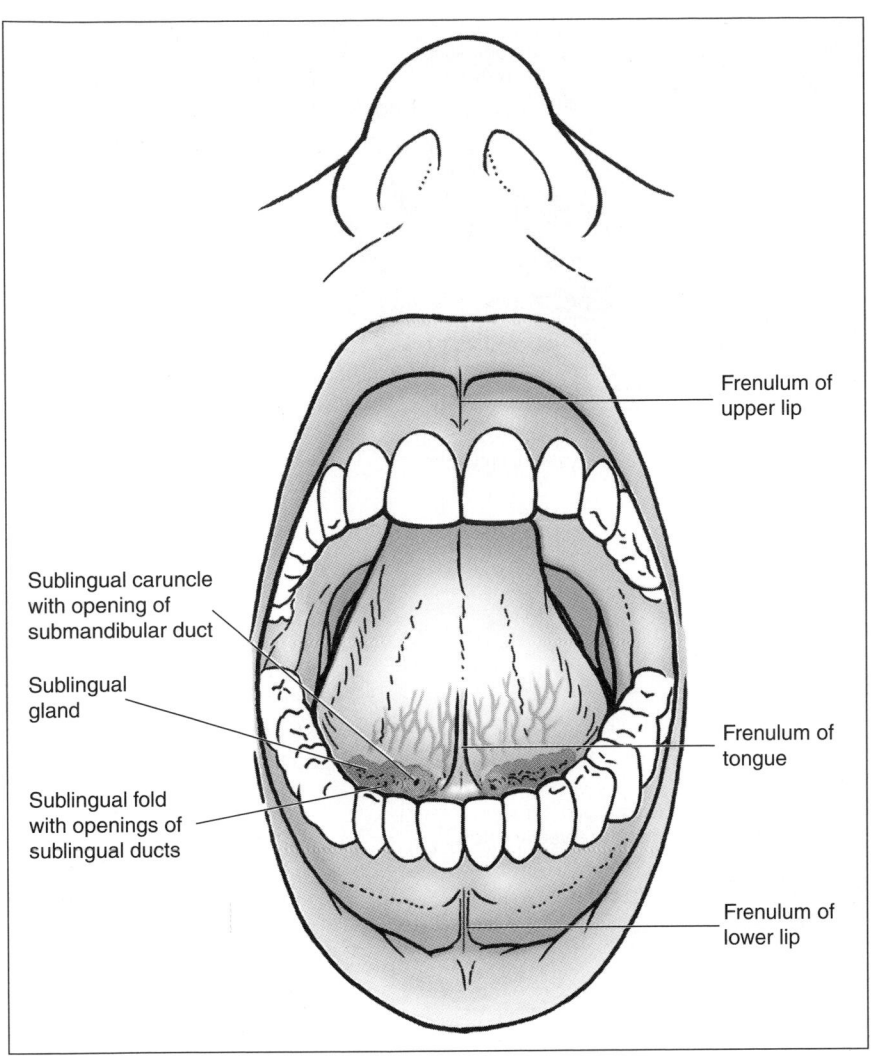

FIGURE 152-1 Topographical anatomy of the anterior oral cavity.

Frenulum of upper lip

Sublingual caruncle with opening of submandibular duct

Sublingual gland

Sublingual fold with openings of sublingual ducts

Frenulum of tongue

Frenulum of lower lip

formed consent for the procedure. Ensure that the patient has a thorough understanding of the post-procedural care instructions and follow-up requirements.

Position the patient sitting in an upright multipositional procedure chair. Alternatively, place the patient sitting upright on a gurney with the back elevated. Prepare the wall suction unit to ensure it is working. Apply suction tubing and a suction catheter to the suction source.

The use of good lighting cannot be overemphasized. Apply a headlamp if one is available. An alternative is an overhead adjustable light source. Position the light so that it is aimed in the patient's mouth. The overhead light often hits the examiner in the head, casts shadows, and is too bright for the patient's eyes. It is also difficult to properly position as both of the examiner's hands must be used for the procedure.

Incision and drainage must be preceded by adequate anesthesia to the abscess site. Determine the most fluctuant region of the abscess on the floor of the mouth. Anesthetize this area. Spray a topical anesthetic agent over the abscess. Dry the mucosa overlying the abscess with a gauze square. Arm a 3 mL syringe with a 25 or 27 gauge needle. Inject 1 mL of local anesthetic solution containing epinephrine through the area of topical anesthesia and just under the mucosal surface. Allow 3 to 5 minutes for the anesthetic to work.

TECHNIQUE

Make a stab incision at the point of maximal fluctuance with a #11 scalpel blade. Allow the abscess cavity to drain into the suction catheter. Gently insert a mosquito hemostat to assist in the drainage of the purulent material. **Do not spread the tip of the hemostat as if opening a subcutaneous abscess. Injury to surrounding neurovascular structures can result.** Obtain a

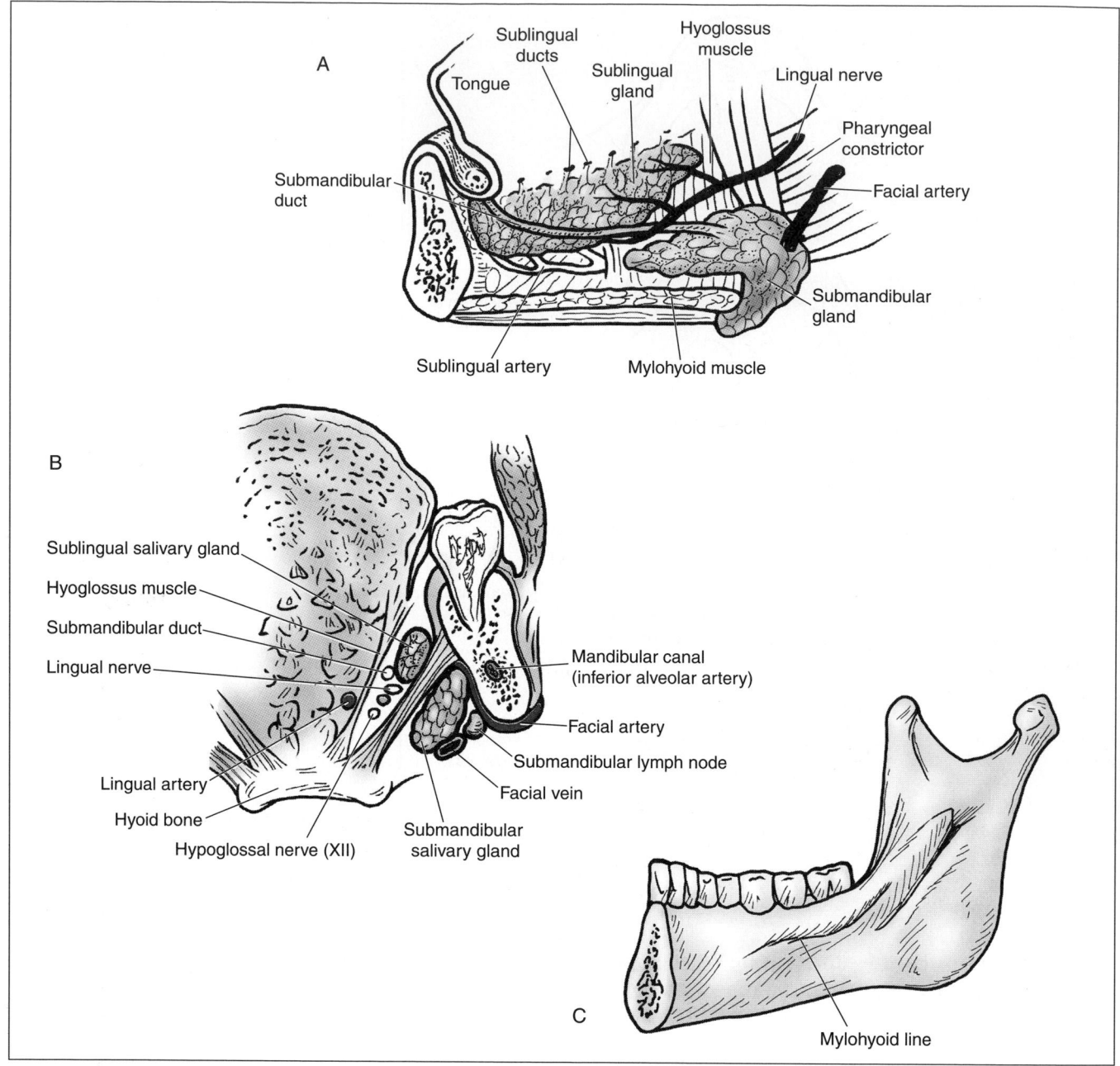

FIGURE 152-2 Anatomy of the sublingual space and the surrounding structures. *A.* Midsagittal view. *B.* Anterior view of a coronal section between the first and second molar. *C.* The medial surface of the mandible.

specimen of the abscess fluid for culture and sensitivity. Allow the patient to rinse and spit several times with Peridex solution or half-strength hydrogen peroxide solution.

Gently pack the abscess cavity with a strip of ribbon gauze.[3] Use caution not to injure any surrounding structures. Alternatively, cut a piece from a sterile Penrose drain and insert it into the abscess cavity. Throw one silk suture through the mucosa and through the drain or ribbon gauze. This will allow the drain or

ribbon gauze to remain in place until removed by the Otolaryngologist.

ASSESSMENT

Allow the patient to rinse and spit with either water or saline solution. Observe the patient for any evidence of continued bleeding or upper airway symptomatology. Assess the patient's ability to tolerate oral fluids prior to discharge.

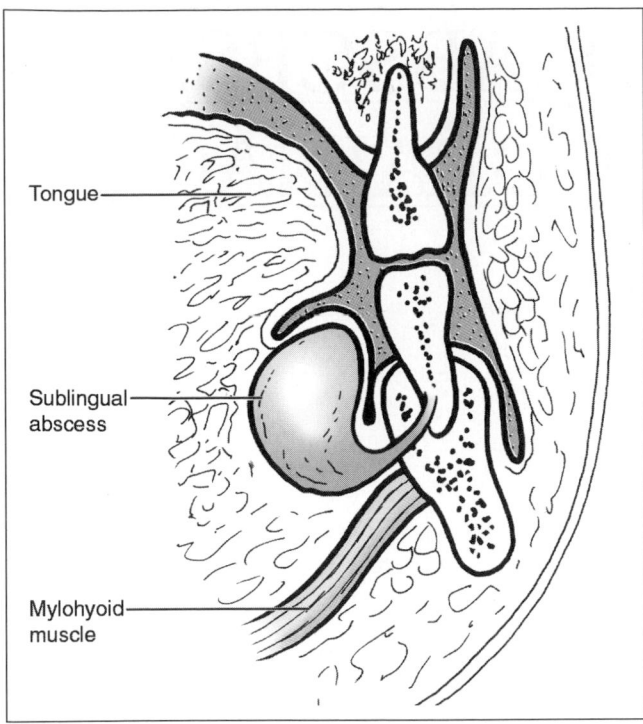

FIGURE 152-3 A sublingual space, between the oral mucosa and the mylohyoid muscle, abscess originating from a mandibular tooth.

AFTERCARE

Instruct the patient to gargle with half-strength hydrogen peroxide or Peridex solution five times per day (after each meal, at a minimum, and several other times) until the abscess cavity is healed.[3] Recommend to the patient to follow a soft diet and drink plenty of during the first 48 hours after the intervention. Arrange follow-up with an Otolaryngologist within 24 to 48 hours for reevaluation and removal of the drain or ribbon gauze. Arrange follow-up with a Dentist within 24 hours for evaluation of the teeth. Instruct the patient to return to the Emergency Department immediately if they develop bleeding, shortness of breath, difficulty swallowing, drooling, or have any concerns.

Discharge the patient with oral antibiotics and analgesics. Penicillin is still the drug of choice. Many Otolaryngologists will add either clindamycin or metronidazole due to the increasing incidence of penicillin-resistant organisms.[4,5] An alternative is to substitute clindamycin or amoxicillin-clavulanate for penicillin.[4,5] Nonsteroidal anti-inflammatory drugs will adequately control any pain and fever.

Admission is generally required for patients who appear toxic, pediatric patients, dehydrated patients, immunocompromised patients, and for patients who are unable to tolerate oral fluids. These patients require observation for 23 hours and intravenous antibiotics.

COMPLICATIONS

Potential complications are minimal. Prolonged bleeding from the incision site can occur if a vein or small arteriole is cut. The application of pressure usually resolves any bleeding. **Do not tie off the bleeding vessel with a suture or use cautery unless absolutely necessary! A branch of the lingual or hypoglossal nerve may be nearby and injured, resulting in paralysis of some muscles or loss of taste sensation.** Aspiration is usually not a concern because often the patient has not eaten for hours. Protect against aspiration of purulent material and subsequent pulmonic infection by having the patient sit upright during the procedure and using suction as the abscess is opened. Do not penetrate too deeply with the scalpel blade and do not spread the jaws of the hemostat within the abscess cavity to prevent injury to any neurovascular structures.

SUMMARY

Sublingual abscesses can result from the spread of odontogenic infections. Diagnosis and treatment results in rapid resolution in the majority of patients. Admission may be required in a few instances for observation and intravenous antibiotics.

REFERENCES

1. Peterson LJ: Odontogenic infections, in Cummings CW, Fredrickson JM, Harker LA, et al (eds): *Otolaryngology Head and Neck Surgery,* 3rd ed. St. Louis: Mosby, 1998:1354–1361.
2. Levitt GW: The surgical treatment of deep neck infections. *Laryngoscope* 1971; 81(3):403–411.
3. Simon RR, Brenner BE: *Emergency Procedures and Techniques,* 3rd ed. Baltimore: Williams & Wilkins, 1994:272–273.
4. Herzon FS: Peritonsillar abscess: incidence, current management practices, and a proposal for treatment guidelines. Mosher award thesis. *Laryngoscope* 1995; 105(8 pt 3):1–17.
5. MacDougall G, Denholm SW: Audit of the treatment of tonsillar and peritonsillar sepsis in an ear, nose, and throat unit. *J Laryngol Otol* 1995; 109(6):531–533.

Chapter 153

PAROTID DUCT ABSCESS INCISION AND DRAINAGE

Julio C. Silva

INTRODUCTION

Patients with pathologic conditions of the parotid gland and/or duct often present to the Emergency Department prior to formal evaluation by an Otolaryngologist. These conditions include obstruction of the duct, abscesses, infections, and tumors. The Emergency Physician can provide temporary relief of a parotid duct abscess until the patient receives definitive care.

ANATOMY AND PATHOPHYSIOLOGY

The parotid gland is the largest salivary gland. It is located on the face between the ramus of the mandible and mastoid process[1,2] (Figure 153-1). The parotid duct travels across the surface of the masseter muscle and crosses the anterior aspect of the mandible, approximately 1 cm below the zygomatic arch. The duct turns medially to penetrate the buccinator muscle and the buccal fat pad to enter the oral cavity (Figure 153-2). The ostium of the parotid duct is located at the level of the second maxillary molar (Figure 153-3). Abscesses of the parotid duct are often seen in patients with strictures of the parotid duct or a sialolith causing proximal dilatation.[3]

INDICATIONS

Parotid duct abscesses require intraoral incision and drainage.

CONTRAINDICATIONS

There are no absolute contraindications to the incision and drainage of a parotid duct abscess. **Consult an Otolaryngologist prior to proceeding with the procedure.** There are a large number of important structures

in the area adjacent to the parotid duct. The procedure has the potential to result in complications. Patients with severe trismus limiting visibility and access may require intravenous analgesics and muscle relaxants, procedural sedation, and intraoperative drainage. Consult an Otolaryngologist for all patients who are coagulopathic, taking oral anticoagulants, or with a known bleeding disorder. These patients are at risk for bleeding and associated complications. Admit children to the hospital for intravenous antibiotics, incision and drainage under general anesthesia, and observation.

EQUIPMENT

Gauze 4×4 squares
Suction source and tubing
Yankauer or Frazier suction catheter
#11 scalpel blade on a handle
Mosquito hemostat
Sterile Penrose drain
Ribbon gauze
Headlight or overhead spotlight
Culturette or culture bottles
4–0 silk suture
Suture scissors
Oral rinse solution, hydrogen peroxide or Peridex
Topical anesthetic spray (lidocaine, tetracaine, or benzocaine)
1 to 2 mL of local anesthetic solution with epinephrine
5 mL syringe
25 or 27 gauge needle, 2 inches long

PATIENT PREPARATION

Explain the procedure, its risks, and benefits to the patient and/or their representative. Obtain a signed informed consent for the procedure. Ensure that the

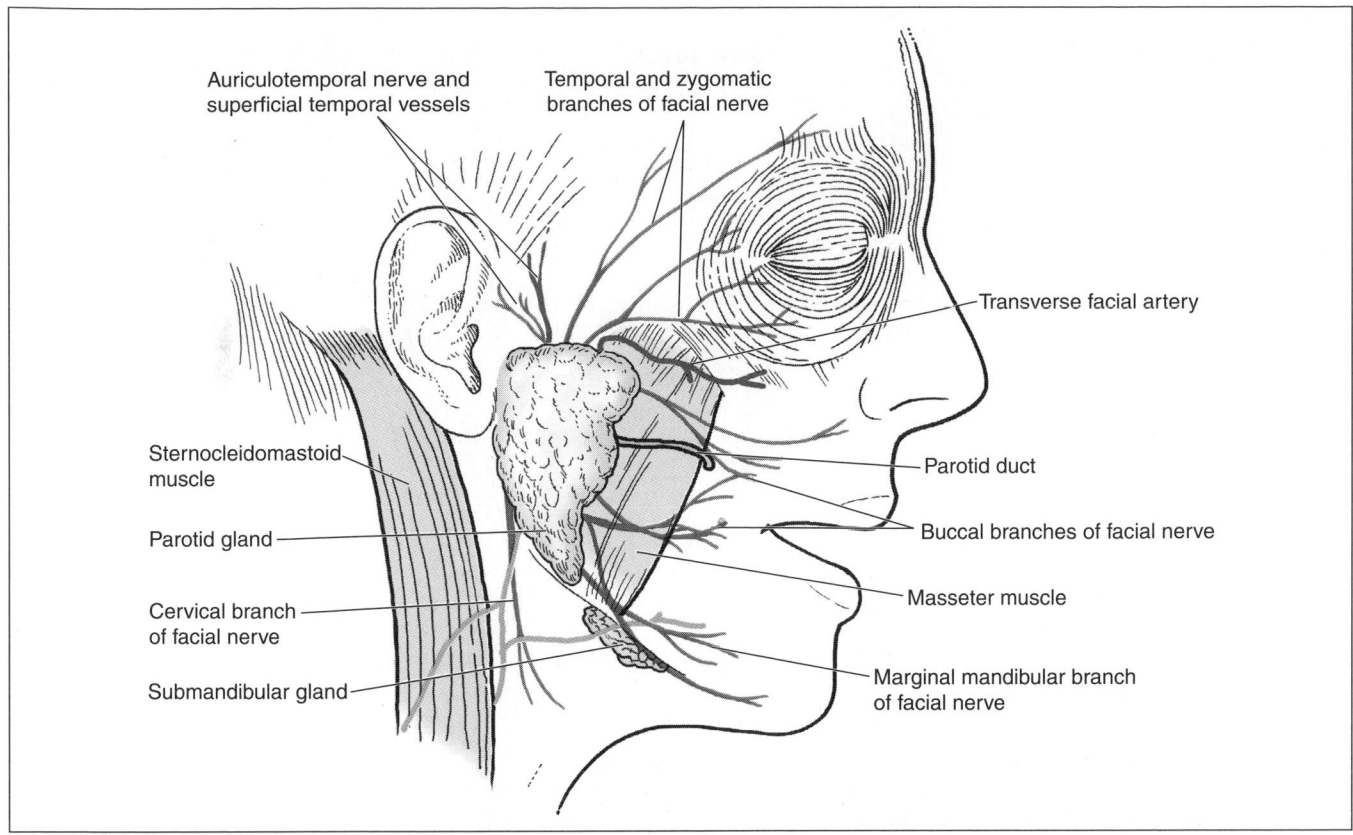

FIGURE 153-1 Anatomy of the parotid gland and surrounding structures.

patient has a thorough understanding of the postprocedural care instructions and follow-up requirements.

Position the patient sitting in an upright multipositional procedure chair. Alternatively, place the patient sitting upright on a gurney with the back elevated. Prepare the wall suction unit to ensure it is working. Apply suction tubing and a suction catheter to the suction source.

The use of good lighting cannot be overemphasized. Apply a headlamp if one is available. An alternative is an overhead adjustable light source. Position the light so that it is aimed in the patient's mouth. The overhead light often hits the examiner in the head, casts shadows, and is too bright for the patient's eyes. It is also difficult to properly position as both of the examiner's hands must be used for the procedure.

Incision and drainage must be preceded by adequate anesthesia to the abscess site. Determine the most fluctuant region of the abscess. Spray a topical anesthetic agent over the abscess. Dry the mucosa overlying the abscess with a gauze square. Arm a 3 mL syringe with a 25 or 27 gauge needle. Inject 1 mL of local anesthetic solution containing epinephrine through the area of topical anesthesia and just under the mucosal

surface. Allow 3 to 5 minutes for the anesthetic to take effect.

TECHNIQUE

Make a stab incision at the point of maximal fluctuance with a #11 scalpel blade (Figure 153-4). Allow the abscess cavity to drain into the suction catheter. Gently insert a mosquito hemostat to assist in the drainage of the purulent material. **Do not spread the tip of the hemostat as if opening a subcutaneous abscess. Injury to surrounding neurovascular structures can result.** Obtain a specimen of the abscess fluid for culture and sensitivity. Allow the patient to rinse and spit several times with Peridex solution or half-strength hydrogen peroxide solution.

Gently pack the abscess cavity with a strip of ribbon gauze.[3] Use caution not to injure any surrounding structures. Alternatively, cut a piece from a sterile Penrose drain and insert it into the abscess cavity. Throw one silk suture through the mucosa and through the drain or ribbon gauze. This will allow the drain or ribbon gauze to remain in place until removed by the Otolaryngologist.

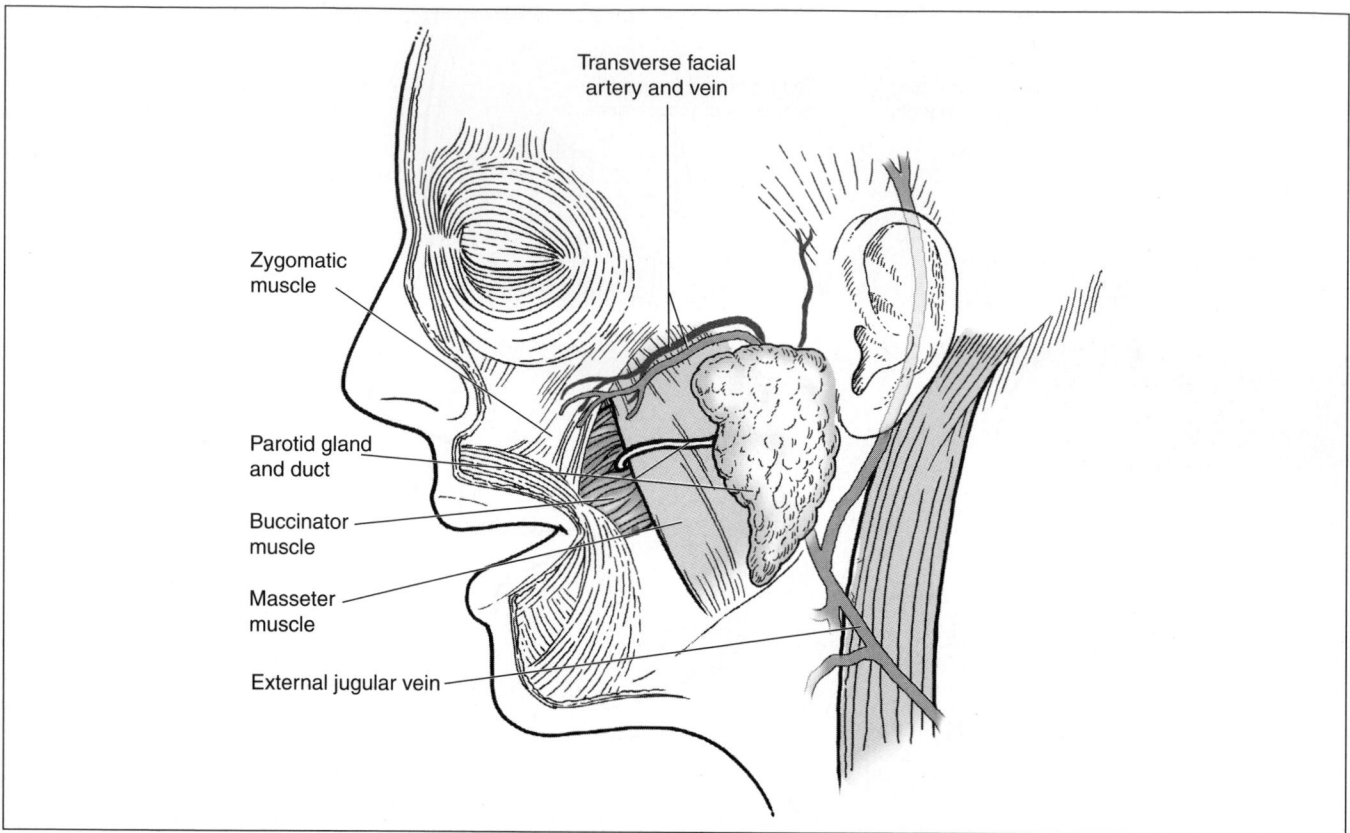

FIGURE 153-2 Anatomy of the parotid gland and duct. Note that the duct travels over the masseter muscle and through the buccinator muscle to gain access into the oral cavity.

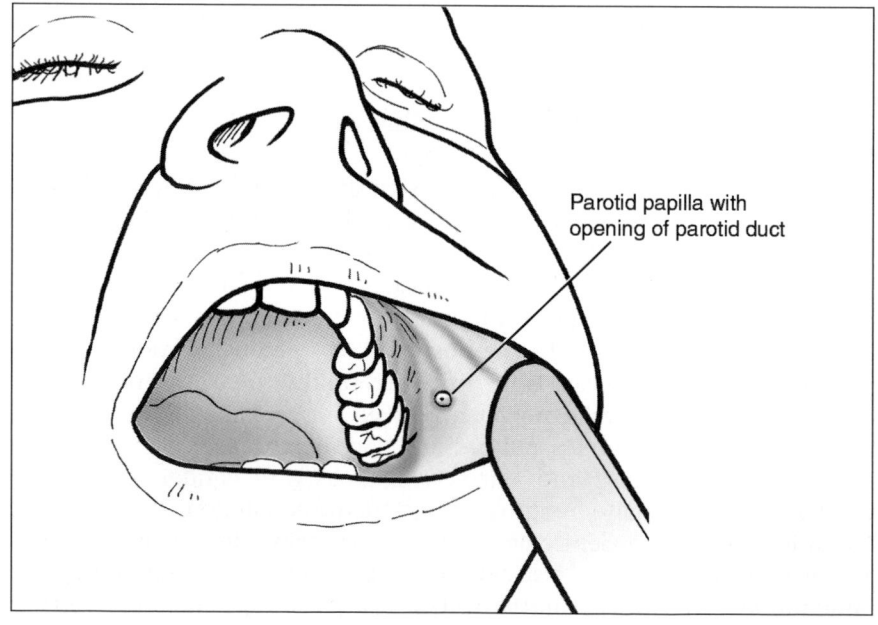

FIGURE 153-3 The ostium of the parotid duct is located on the buccal mucosa at the level of the second maxillary molar.

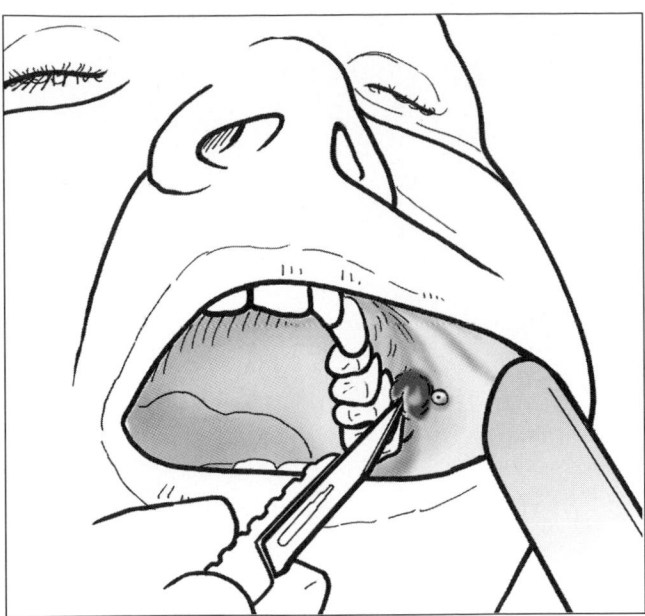

FIGURE 153-4 Incision of a parotid duct abscess.

ASSESSMENT

Allow the patient to rinse and spit with either water or saline solution. Observe the patient for any evidence of continued bleeding or upper airway symptomatology. Assess the patient's ability to tolerate oral fluids prior to discharge.

AFTERCARE

Instruct the patient to gargle with half-strength hydrogen peroxide or Peridex solution five times per day (after each meal, at a minimum, and several other times) until the abscess cavity is healed.[3] Recommend to the patient to follow a soft diet and drink plenty of fluids during the first 48 hours after the intervention. Arrange follow-up with an Otolaryngologist within 24 hours for reevaluation and removal of the drain or ribbon gauze. Instruct the patient to return to the Emergency Department immediately if they develop bleeding, shortness of breath, difficulty swallowing, drooling, or have any concerns.

Discharge the patient with oral antibiotics and analgesics. Penicillin is still the drug of choice. Many Otolaryngologists will add either clindamycin or metronidazole due to the increasing incidence of penicillin-resistant organisms.[4,5] An alternative is to substitute amoxicillin-clavulanate or clindamycin for penicillin.[4,5] Nonsteroidal anti-inflammatory drugs will adequately control any pain and fever.

Admission is generally required for patients who appear toxic, pediatric patients, immunocompromised patients, and for patients who are unable to tolerate oral fluids. These patients require observation for 23 hours and intravenous antibiotics.

COMPLICATIONS

Potential complications are minimal. Prolonged bleeding from the incision site can occur if a vein or small arteriole is cut. The application of pressure usually resolves any bleeding. **Do not tie off the bleeding vessel with a suture or use cautery unless absolutely necessary! A nerve or blood vessel may be nearby and injured resulting in paralysis of some muscles or loss of sensation.** Aspiration is usually not a concern because often the patient has not eaten for hours. Protect against aspiration of purulent material and subsequent pulmonic infection by having the patient sit upright during the procedure and using suction as the abscess is opened. Do not penetrate too deeply with the scalpel blade and do not spread the jaws of the hemostat within the abscess to prevent injury to any neurovascular structure.

SUMMARY

Parotid duct abscesses can develop in patients with pathologic conditions of the parotid gland or duct. Drainage of this particular abscess should be performed in consultation with an Otolaryngologist who will provide follow-up care. Admission may be required in a few instances for observation and intravenous antibiotics.

REFERENCES

1. Graney DO, Jacobd JR, Kern RC: Anatomy, in Cummings CW, Fredrickson JM, Harker LA, et al (eds): *Otolarnygology Head and Neck Surgery,* 3rd ed. St. Louis: Mosby, 1998:1354–1361.
2. Hollinshead WH, Rosse C: *Textbook of Anatomy,* 4th ed. Philadelphia: Harper & Row, 1985:881–888.
3. Simon RR, Brenner BE: *Emergency Procedures and Techniques,* 3rd ed. Baltimore: Williams & Wilkins, 1994:272–273.
4. Herzon FS: Peritonsillar abscess: incidence, current management practices, and a proposal for treatment guidelines. Mosher award thesis. *Laryngoscope* 1995; 105(8 pt 3):1–17.
5. MacDougall G, Denholm SW: Audit of the treatment of tonsillar and peritonsillar sepsis in an ear, nose and throat unit. *J Laryngol Otol* 1995; 109(6):531–533.

Section Thirteen
DENTAL PROCEDURES

Chapter 154
DENTAL ANESTHESIA AND ANALGESIA

Eric F. Reichman
Kevin P. Kern

INTRODUCTION

Dental anesthesia techniques are used by Emergency Physicians for a variety of intraoral and extraoral pathologies, including dental caries, jaw fractures, dry sockets, laceration repair, and tooth fractures. These techniques are simple to learn, easy to perform, and provide temporary pain relief for the patient. The Emergency Physician can provide pain-free intraoral manipulations, extraoral manipulations, facial manipulations, and simple pain control until the patient receives definitive evaluation and treatment by a Dentist or Oral Surgeon. The fundamental principles of dental anesthesia and anatomy will be discussed so that the Emergency Physician will feel knowledgeable and comfortable performing dental anesthetic techniques.

ANATOMY AND PATHOPHYSIOLOGY

An understanding of the anatomy of the fifth cranial nerve is essential to performing dental nerve blocks[1] (Figure 154-1). The fifth cranial nerve is also referred to as CN V or the trigeminal nerve. It is the largest cranial nerve. It is a mixed cranial nerve containing primarily sensory fibers to the skin of the face and scalp, the nasal cavity, and the oral cavity. The motor fibers innervate the muscles of mastication.

The trigeminal nerve originates in the brainstem as a small motor root and a large sensory root. These roots fuse as they leave the brainstem. The trigeminal nerve travels forward into the middle cranial fossa where it expands into a large and crescent-shaped trigeminal ganglion. The trigeminal ganglion divides to give rise to the three divisions of the trigeminal nerve: the ophthalmic nerve (V_1), the maxillary nerve (V_2), and the mandibular nerve (V_3). Each of these nerves leaves the middle cranial fossa through its own foramen.

OPHTHALMIC NERVE

The ophthalmic nerve is the smallest branch of the trigeminal nerve. It travels forward in the lateral wall of the cavernous sinus and enters the orbit via the superior orbital fissure. It provides sensory innervation to the forehead, scalp, upper eyelid, cornea, nasal cavity, sinuses, and the orbit. This nerve is not discussed further because it does not innervate any oral or dental structures.

MAXILLARY NERVE

The maxillary nerve is purely sensory. It travels forward in the lateral wall of the cavernous sinus and exits the cranial vault via the foramen rotundum into the pterygopalatine fossa. It then enters the orbit through the inferior orbital fissure to continue on as the infraorbital nerve and emerge on the face. The infraorbital nerve terminates as a sensory nerve to the lower eyelid, upper cheek, nose, and upper lip. The infraorbital nerve gives off the anterior superior alveolar nerves prior to its termination. These nerves supply the maxillary sinus, the maxillary incisors, the maxillary canine teeth, and the maxillary premolar teeth. The anterior superior alveolar nerve occasionally crosses the midline to supply the contralateral maxillary incisors.

The maxillary nerve forms numerous branches in the pterygopalatine fossa. The zygomaticofacial and zygomaticotemporal nerves are cutaneous to the face and temple. The nasal and nasopalatine nerves supply the nasal cavity and floor of the nasal cavity. The nasopalatine nerve exits the nasal canal through the midline incisive foramen, just posterior to the central incisors. It provides sensory innervation to the anterior hard palate and associated soft tissues. The greater palatine nerve exits the greater palatine foramen to provide sensory innervation to the posterior two-thirds of the hard palate. The lesser palatine nerve exits the lesser palatine foramen to provide sensory innervation to the soft palate. The greater and lesser palatine nerves exit 1 cm medial to the junction of the second

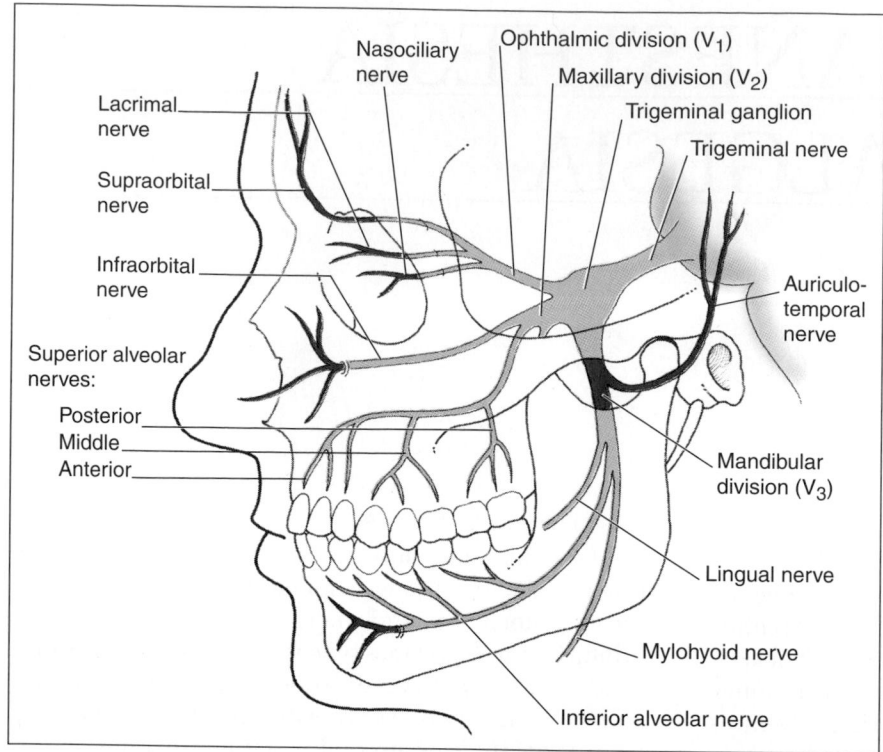

FIGURE 154-1 The anatomy of the trigeminal nerve.

and third molar on the hard palate. The middle superior alveolar nerve provides sensory innervation to the premolars, and occasionally the canine and the first molar teeth. The posterior superior alveolar nerve provides sensory innervation to the molars and, occasionally, the premolars.

MANDIBULAR NERVE

The mandibular nerve is the largest division of the trigeminal nerve. It is the only division of the trigeminal nerve to contain motor fibers. The mandibular nerve exits the middle cranial fossa via the foramen ovale. It provides branches to the meninges and the small muscles of the palate and the medial pterygoid muscle. It divides into a small anterior division and a large posterior division.

The anterior division of the mandibular nerve is primarily motor. It innervates the muscles of mastication (masseter, temporalis, and lateral pterygoid). The sensory portion of the anterior division is the buccal nerve. This nerve travels between the two heads of the lateral pterygoid muscle, under the masseter muscle, and emerges from the anterior border of the masseter muscle. It travels forward to innervate a small and variable portion of the skin of the cheek. It primarily innervates the mucous membranes of the cheek.

The posterior division of the mandibular nerve is purely sensory. It divides into the auriculotemporal, inferior alveolar, and lingual nerves. The auriculotemporal nerve supplies sensory innervation to the skin of the auricle, external auditory canal, scalp, and temporomandibular joint. It conveys postganglionic parasympathetic fibers to the parotid gland.

The lingual nerve descends into the mouth and travels along the lateral surface of the tongue. It supplies sensory innervation to the anterior two-thirds of the tongue and the floor of the mouth. The lingual nerve receives, near its origin, and conveys the chorda tympani from the facial nerve. The chorda tympani provides taste sensation to the anterior two-thirds of the tongue and preganglionic fibers to the submandibular ganglion for the submandibular and sublingual glands.

The inferior alveolar nerve descends immediately posterior and adjacent to the lingual nerve. It enters the upper one-third of the ramus of the mandible, posterior to the lingula, to enter the mandibular canal. It provides sensory innervation to the mandible, the mandibular teeth, and the adjacent mucous membranes. The inferior alveolar nerve gives origin to the mental nerve. The mental nerve exits the mental foramen located on the outer surface of the mandible between the first and second premolars. It supplies sensory innervation to the lower lip, the skin of the chin, and the mucous membrane of the chin.

INDICATIONS

Dental nerve blocks can be performed to provide temporary relief of pain. They are often used to provide relief from alveolar ridge fractures, dental caries, dry sockets, mandible fractures, and tooth fractures. Nerve blocks can be performed prior to painful intraoral procedures such as incision and drainage of dental abscesses and laceration repair to the cheek, lips, oral mucosa, and tongue. Nerve blocks do not distort the local anatomy, when compared to infiltration of the surrounding soft tissue with local anesthetic solution, and allow better approximation of the wound edges during suturing. Nerve blocks are an excellent alternative if narcotic analgesics are contraindicated or to be avoided. Local anesthetic solutions containing epinephrine can be utilized to provide longer pain relief (Table 154-1).

CONTRAINDICATIONS

The two absolute contraindications to dental anesthesia include a known hypersensitivity to the anesthetic agent and gross distortion of the anatomic landmarks required to perform the nerve block. Other relative contraindications include an uncooperative patient, such as an anxious adult, scared child, or any patient with altered mental status. These patients place themselves and the physician at significant risk for injury. It may be most prudent to abort the procedure and perform procedural sedation and analgesia or general anesthesia prior to the procedure to ensure the safety of the patient and the physician.

The needle used to inject local anesthetic solution should not traverse infected tissue. Injection of the local anesthetic solution into or through infected tissue is also a relative contraindication. These processes may result in spread of the infection into other adjacent tissues or tissue planes. It is possible to cause bacteremia when injecting into infected tissues. Local anesthetic solutions are less effective when injected into areas of infection or inflammation. An infection that tracks along a nerve and into a bone of the face and/or skull is extremely difficult to treat. Evaluate the risks and benefits of injecting through infected tissue and attempt an alternative method of anesthesia if possible.

EQUIPMENT

Nonsterile gloves
Antiseptic mouth rinse, any of the following:
　Hydrogen peroxide
　Ethanol (7%) with chlorhexidine (0.5%)
　Povidone iodine
　0.12% chlorhexidine or Peridex
4×4 gauze squares
Cotton-tipped applicators
Aspirating dental syringe
Local anesthetic solution (Table 154-1)
Syringes, 1 mL and 3 mL
Suction source and tubing
Yankauer suction catheter
Topical anesthetic (viscous lidocaine, viscous benzocaine, or aerosolized benzocaine)
Overhead light source
22 to 27 gauge needles, 2 inches long

The above-listed supplies are required to provide dental anesthesia. They are contained in every Emergency Department. An aspirating dental syringe and anesthetic cartridges, if available, are ideal to perform the nerve blocks (Figure 154-2). Standard 1 to 3 mL syringes armed with a 25 or 27 gauge, 2 inch long needle will also work. The aspirating dental syringe allows better control of the syringe and the ability to simultaneously aspirate and insert the needle with one hand. This allows the nondominant hand to be used to identify landmarks, retract the cheek or tongue, adjust the light source, and/or use the suction catheter. A dental or multipositional procedure chair would be preferred to the use of a standard cart or gurney.[2,3] Unfortunately, this may not be available in many Emergency Departments.

PATIENT PREPARATION

Perform a thorough history and a directed physical examination, dependent on the clinical situation, in any patient undergoing dental anesthesia. Give special at-

TABLE 154-1. LOCAL ANESTHETIC SOLUTIONS COMMONLY USED IN DENTAL ANESTHESIA PROCEDURES [2-4]

Anesthetic solution	Proprietary name	Time of onset (minutes)	Duration of action (minutes)	Maximum adult dose (mg)	Maximum pediatric dose (mg/kg)
1% procaine	Novocaine™	2–5	15–90	500	7.0
1% procaine with epinephrine		2–5	15–120	600	9.0
2% lidocaine	Xylocaine™	2–5	90–120	300	4.5
2% lidocaine with epinephrine		2–5	90–180	500	7.0
0.5% bupivacaine	Marcaine™	5	240–280	175	2.0
0.5% bupivacaine with epinephrine		5	240–280	225	3.0

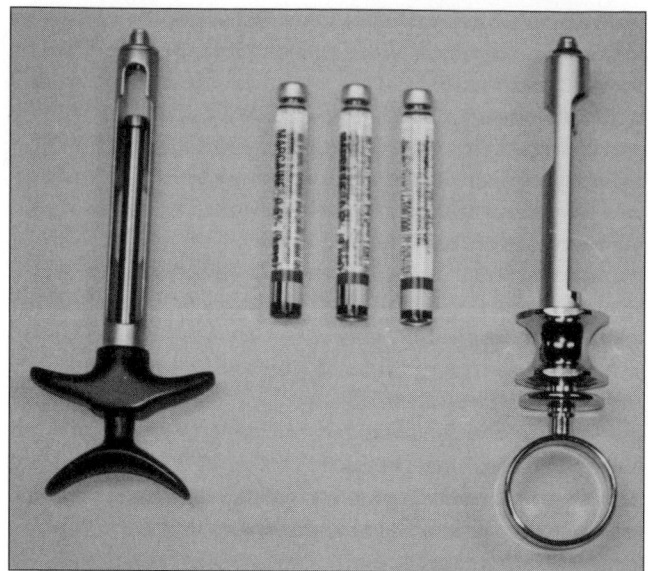

FIGURE 154-2 The aspirating dental syringe and local anesthetic cartridges.

tention to the past medical history, past surgical history, current medications, and any history of allergic or adverse reactions to an anesthetic agent. A patient with severe systemic disease may be better served by rescheduling the procedure after appropriate consultation or referral. This will clarify functional reserve and treatment limitations.[2,3] Any patient with cardiac valvular disease, congenital heart anomalies, artificial heart valves, or any previous cardiac surgery must receive antibiotic prophylaxis to help prevent bacterial endocarditis caused from transient bacteremia.

Explain the procedure, its risks, and benefits to the patient and/or their representative. Obtain an informed consent for the specific technique to be performed. A formal consent may exist depending upon the institution in which one practices. Some physicians desire a formal signed and dated consent form. Other physicians choose to chart: "All the risks, benefits, and complications were described and discussed with the patient. They understood the procedure described and gave verbal consent for the procedure." This is physician and institution dependent. Place the patient in a well-lighted environment. Reassurance often alleviates a patient's anxiety regarding injections or manipulations and puts them at ease.[2]

Prepare the mucosa at the injection site. Completely dry the mucosa with gauze squares. Apply an antiseptic solution [7% ethyl alcohol (ETOH) with 0.5% chlorhexidine solution, povidone iodine, 0.12% chlorhexidine solution, hydrogen peroxide, or weak iodine] to the working area with a cotton ball or gauze square for 15 seconds. Alternatively, the patient can swish 0.12% chlorhexidine mouth rinse or hydrogen peroxide for 30 seconds and then spit it out.

Apply a topical anesthetic agent (viscous lidocaine or benzocaine with a cotton-tipped applicator, or 20% benzocaine spray) for added patient comfort. **Never use TAC (tetracaine, adrenalin, and cocaine) or other topical anesthetic combinations that are used for cutaneous laceration repair on mucosal surfaces.** They may lead to significant systemic toxicity. Fatalities have been described with the administration of TAC to mucous membranes.[5]

TECHNIQUES

The general procedure of a dental nerve block will be described. The specific details are contained within each nerve block described below. Identify the anatomic landmarks required to perform the nerve block. Clean the mucous membrane at the injection site with a gauze square. Apply an antiseptic solution. Apply a topical anesthetic and allow it to work for 2 to 3 minutes. Reidentify the anatomic landmarks. Insert a 25 or 27 gauge needle into the appropriate area to deliver the local anesthetic agent. **If the patient experiences paresthesias, do not inject the local anesthetic solution. Paresthesias signify that the tip of the needle is within the nerve bundle.** Withdraw the needle 1 to 2 mm and allow the paresthesias to resolve. This usually takes 5 to 20 seconds. Inject the local anesthetic solution. Allow up to 10 minutes for the local anesthetic solution to take effect. Some Dentists prefer to apply pressure to the area immediately next to the site of the anesthetic injection with a cotton-tipped applicator. This aids in distracting the patient from the pain of injection. Other Dentists "jiggle" the mucous membrane to and fro rapidly as they simultaneously introduce the needle.[2–4]

SUPRAPERIOSTEAL INFILTRATION (FIELD BLOCK)

This technique is commonly used in dentistry. Excellent anesthesia can be achieved with this technique when it is used to anesthetize a branch of the anterior or middle superior alveolar nerve.[3,4] This technique deposits local anesthetic agent against the periosteum of the alveolar ridge adjacent to a tooth (Figure 154-3A). The local anesthetic agent then infiltrates through the periosteum, the cortical plate of the maxilla, and the medullary bone to anesthetize the nerve root as it leaves the apex of the tooth. This technique works best for teeth with associated thin cortical bone. This includes the maxillary incisor, canine, and premolar teeth. The molars of the maxilla in an adult are less likely to be anesthetized with this technique as the cortical bone in which they lie is relatively thick and a poor conduit for the anesthetic. Supraperiosteal infiltration is also a poor technique for anesthesia of mandibular teeth in the adult patient for the same reasons. In children, the corti-

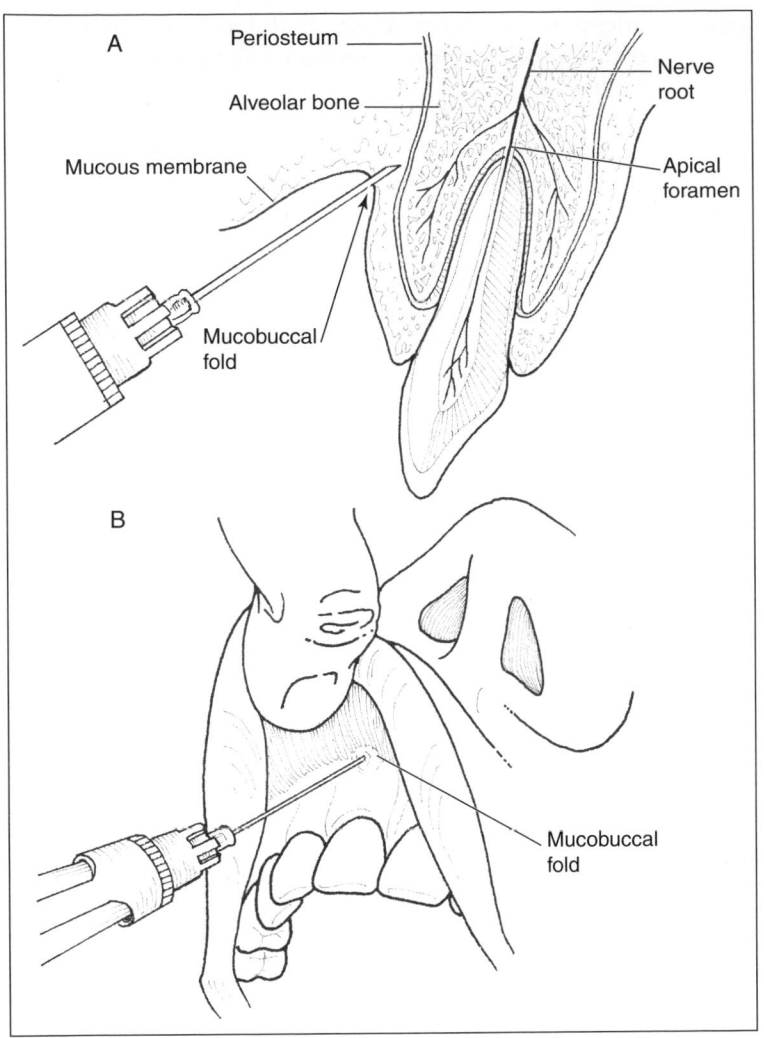

FIGURE 154-3 Supraperiosteal infiltration of local anesthetic solution. *A.* Illustration of the correct needle position. *B.* Elevate the upper lip and insert the needle through the mucobuccal fold.

cal bone of the maxillary molars and the mandible is thin and may allow this technique to be effectively utilized to anesthetize a tooth.[6]

Anatomy: The middle superior alveolar nerve provides sensory innervation to the ipsilateral premolars, canine, and first molar teeth. The anterior superior alveolar nerve provides sensory innervation to the ipsilateral medial and lateral incisors, canine, and sometimes the first premolar teeth.

Patient positioning: Place the patient recumbent in a dental chair with their neck extended 45 degrees. Alternatively, position the patient sitting upright with their back and head firmly set against an examination chair or table.

Landmarks: Use the nondominant hand to grasp and pull the upper lip outward and upward (Figure 154-3*B*). Identify the mucobuccal fold above the tooth to be anesthetized.[3,4]

Needle insertion and direction: Clean, prep, and apply a topical anesthetic agent to the mucobuccal fold above the tooth to be anesthetized. Firmly grasp the upper lip. Pull it outward and upward to tighten the tissues and allow a clear identification of the maxillary mucobuccal fold (Figure 154-3*B*). Insert a 27 gauge needle through the mucobuccal fold over the center of the tooth to be anesthetized (Figure 154-3*B*). Aim the tip of the needle toward the maxilla. Advance the needle 1.0 to 1.5 cm until it contacts the maxilla (Figure 154-3*A*). Withdraw the needle 1 mm. Aspirate to confirm that the tip of the needle is not within a blood vessel. Inject 1 to 2 mL of local anesthetic solution.

Remarks: The anesthetic will be deposited in a non-optimal location if the needle is too deep or too shallow. It may take as long as 10 minutes to achieve anesthesia as the local anesthetic solution diffuses through the cortical bone and to the nerve root. **Be careful when using this technique for anesthesia of the incisor or canine**

teeth because advancing the needle too far may breach the nasal cavity or maxillary sinuses.

INFRAORBITAL NERVE BLOCK

Anatomy: The infraorbital nerve is the terminal branch of the maxillary nerve. It exits the maxilla via the infraorbital foramina and supplies sensation to the ipsilateral upper lip, cheek, lateral nose, and lower eyelid. It may be blocked by either an extraoral or intraoral approach.

Patient positioning: Place the patient recumbent in a dental chair with their neck extended 30 degrees. Alternatively, position the patient sitting upright with their head and back against an examination chair or table with the neck extended 30 degrees. Instruct the patient to slightly open their mouth.

Landmarks: Identify the infraorbital foramen by palpation. It is located below the infraorbital ridge in the mid-pupillary line (Figure 154-4). The mid-pupillary line is a line drawn in the sagittal plane (vertical) through the pupil while the patient is staring straight ahead.

Needle insertion and direction (extraoral approach): Identify the infraorbital foramen as above. Clean and prep the skin over the infraorbital foramen with povidone iodine solution. Instruct the patient to close their eyes. Insert a 25 or 27 gauge needle through the skin overlying the infraorbital foramen (Figure 154-5). Advance the needle to just beneath the subcutaneous tissue. **Do not enter the infraorbital canal as this may damage the nerve.** Aspirate to confirm that the tip of the needle is not within a blood vessel. Inject 1 to 2 mL of local

anesthetic solution. Massage the area over the infraorbital foramen for a few seconds to ensure optimal infiltration.[4]

Needle insertion and direction (intraoral approach): Clean, prep, and apply a topical anesthetic agent to the mucosa opposite the first maxillary premolar. Place the nondominant index finger over the infraorbital foramen (Figure 154-6). Retract the upper lip using the nondominant thumb. Identify the mucobuccal fold above the first premolar. Insert a 25 or 27 gauge needle through the mucobuccal fold. Advance the needle towards the nondominant index finger situated over the infraorbital foramen. Stop advancing the needle when the tip is felt beneath the index finger. The estimated depth of penetration of the needle tip is 1.0 to 1.5 cm in an older child or an adult and 0.5 to 1.0 cm in a younger child. Aspirate to confirm that the tip of the needle is not within a blood vessel. Inject 1 to 2 mL of local anesthetic solution.

Remarks: **Be careful not to penetrate too deeply when performing the intraoral approach.** The infraorbital venous plexus may be disrupted and result in a hematoma. The globe may also be accidentally penetrated. Avoid these complications by positioning the nondominant index finger over the infraorbital foramen and using it to palpate and track the advancing needle tip. The intraoral approach is the preferred technique.

NASOPALATINE NERVE BLOCK

Anatomy: The nasopalatine nerve provides sensory innervation to the anterior one-third of the hard palate (Figure 154-7*A*). It exits the maxilla via the incisive fora-

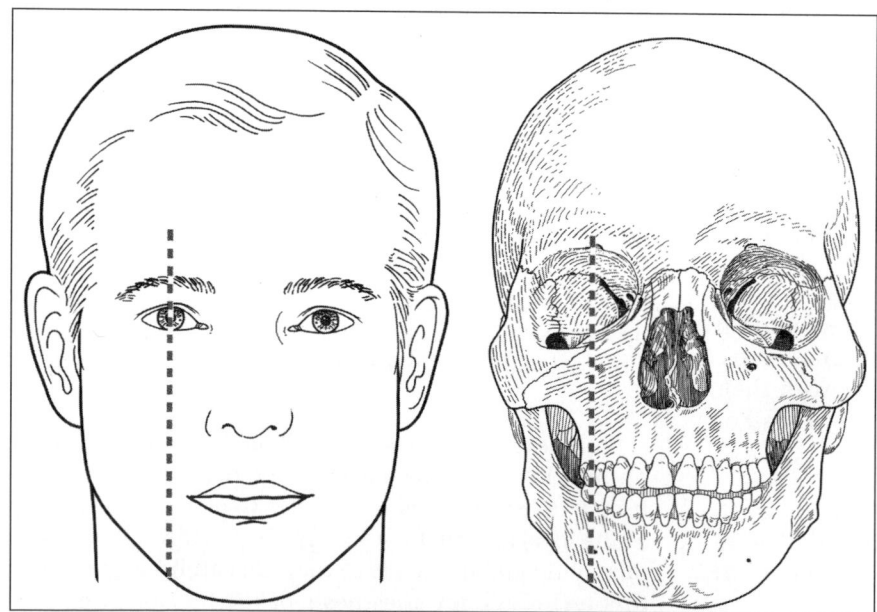

FIGURE 154-4 The supraorbital foramen, infraorbital foramen, and the mental foramen all lie along a straight line drawn through the pupil in the midposition.

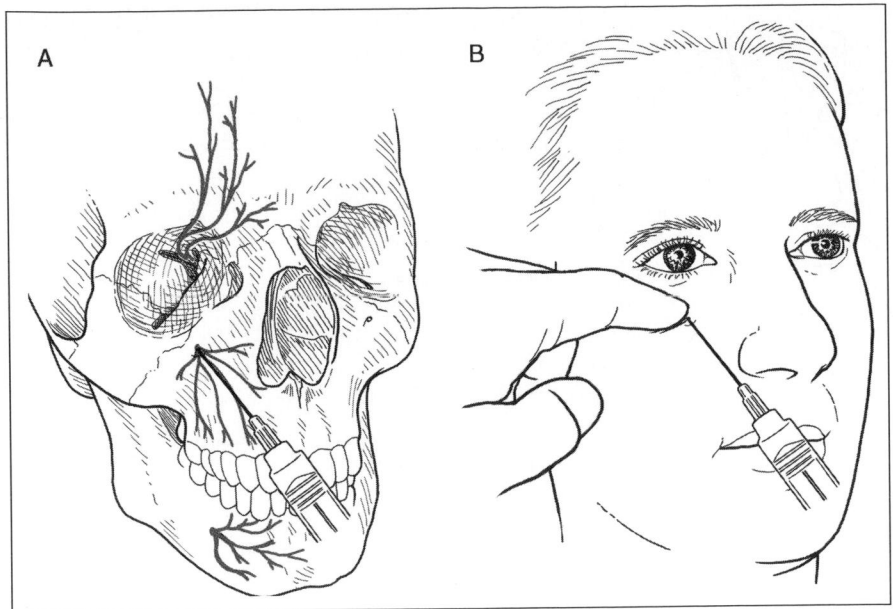

FIGURE 154-5 The extraoral approach to the infraorbital nerve block. *A.* Location of the nerve. *B.* Insertion of the needle.

men in the midline and 0.5 cm posterior to the central incisors.

Patient positioning: Place the patient recumbent in a dental chair with their head extended 45 degrees. Alternatively, place the patient supine with a rolled sheet beneath their shoulder blades to assist in neck extension. Instruct the patient to fully open their mouth.

Landmarks: The incisive foramen lies in the midline and approximately 5 mm posterior to the central incisors of the maxilla. Overlying the incisive foramen is the incisive papilla, a soft tissue elevation.

Needle insertion and direction: Clean, prep, and apply a topical anesthetic agent to the mucosa on the anterior one-third of the hard palate. Identify the incisive foramen by first identifying the incisive papilla. Insert a 27 gauge needle, with the bevel facing the hard palate, from a position immediately lateral to the edge of the incisive papilla (Figure 154-7B). Advance the needle 3 to 4 mm towards the midline or until bone is identified. Aspirate to confirm that the tip of the needle is not within a blood vessel. Inject 0.25 to 0.40 mL of local anesthetic solution. The area surrounding the injection site will blanch upon deposition of the local anesthetic solution.[2,3]

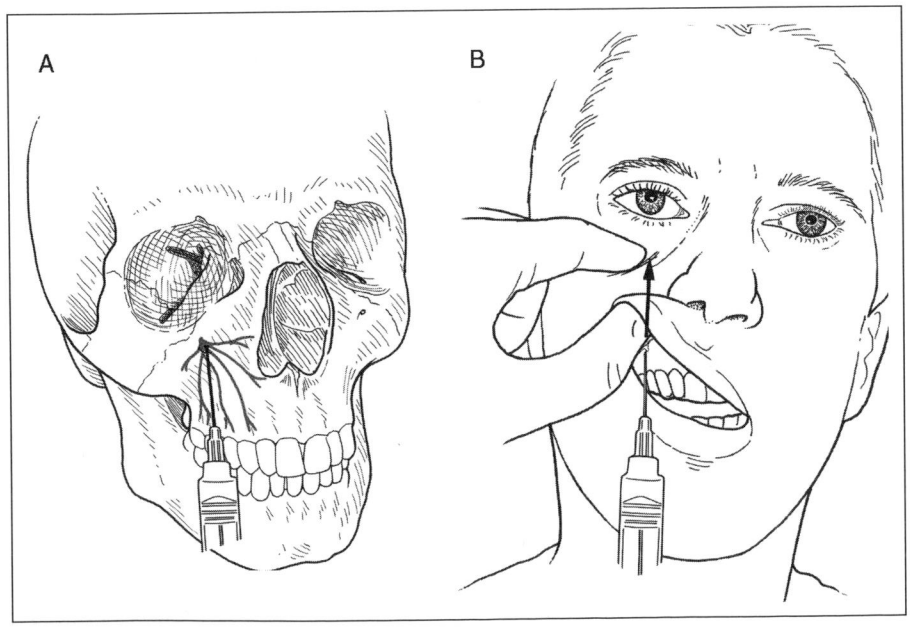

FIGURE 154-6 The intraoral approach to the infraorbital nerve block. *A.* Location of the nerve. *B.* Insertion of the needle.

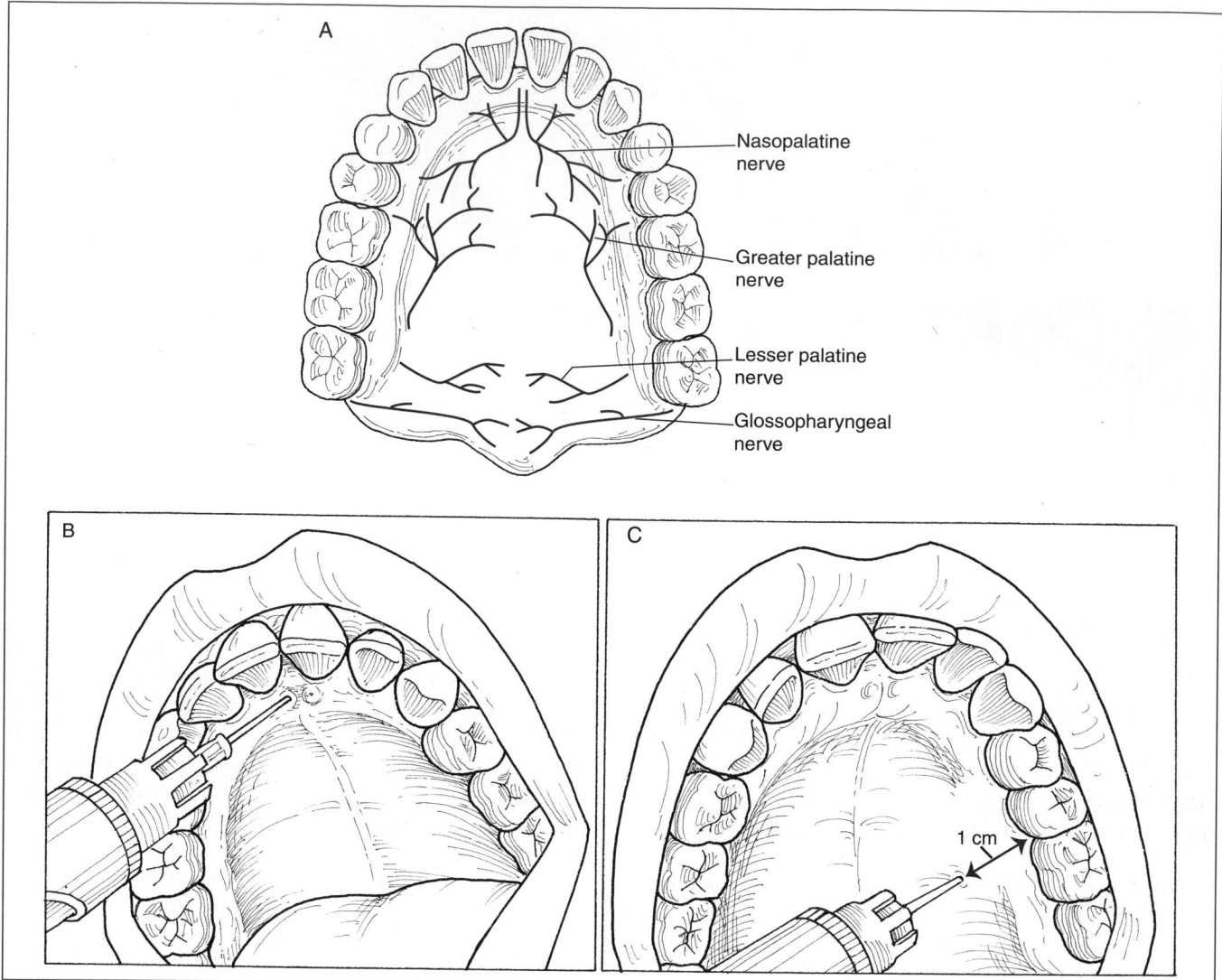

FIGURE 154-7 Anesthesia of the palate. *A.* Sensory innervation of the palate. *B.* Nasopalatine nerve block. *C.* Greater palatine nerve block.

Remarks: This is a particularly painful injection due to the adherent nature of the mucosa to the underlying hard palate. Topical anesthetics will provide adequate preinjection anesthesia. Some clinicians use a cotton-tipped applicator or a blunt instrument to put pressure on the incisive papilla for 30 seconds prior to and during the injection.[3] This seems to defer the attention of the patient and make the injection more bearable. **Be careful not to penetrate too deeply with the needle and enter the incisive foramen.** Insertion into the incisive foramen will cause severe pain. **Injection into the incisive foramen can result in permanent nerve damage**.[2,3] The mucosa of the hard palate receives its blood supply from the hard palate. Injection of more than 0.4 mL will elevate the mucosa from the hard palate and result in mucosal necrosis. This block may be performed to repair lacerations of the mucosa of the anterior hard palate.

GREATER PALATINE NERVE BLOCK

Anatomy: The greater palatine nerve provides sensory innervation to the ipsilateral posterior two-thirds of the hard palate (Figure 154-7*A*). It enters the oral cavity via the greater palatine foramen. The greater palatine foramen lies between the second and third maxillary molar and approximately 1 cm onto the hard palate.

Patient positioning: Place the patient recumbent in a dental chair with their head extended 45 degrees. Alternatively, place the patient supine with a rolled sheet beneath their shoulder blades to assist in neck extension. Instruct the patient to fully open their mouth.

Landmarks: The greater palatine foramen lies 1 cm medial to the gingival junction of the second and third maxillary molar.

Needle insertion and direction: Clean, prep, and apply a topical anesthetic agent to the hard palate adjacent to the second and third maxillary molars. Insert a 27 gauge needle 1 cm medial to the junction of the second and third maxillary molars (Figure 154-7*C*). Ensure that the tip of the needle is held at 90 degrees to the curve of the palate. Aspirate to confirm that the tip of the needle is not within a blood vessel. Inject 0.3 to 0.5 mL of local anesthetic solution. The area surrounding the injection site will blanch upon deposition of the local anesthetic solution.[2,3]

Remarks: This block may be performed to repair lacerations of the mucosa of the hard palate. The mucosa of the hard palate receives its blood supply from the hard palate. Injection of more than 0.4 mL will elevate the mucosa from the hard palate and result in mucosal necrosis. The position of the lesser palatine foramen is 2 to 4 mm posterior to the greater palatine foramen. The lesser palatine nerve provides sensory innervation to the soft palate and uvula. If anesthetized, as it often is when blocking the greater palatine nerve, the patient may experience a feeling of dysphagia or throat closure. Reassurance is usually adequate to alleviate the patient's anxiety.

POSTERIOR SUPERIOR ALVEOLAR NERVE BLOCK

Anatomy: The maxillary nerve exits the skull via the foramen rotundum. It then courses anteriorly into the pterygopalatine fossa and divides into its constituent branches. The posterior superior alveolar nerve provides sensory innervation to the maxillary molar teeth and their associated mucosal tissues.

Patient positioning: Place the patient semi-recumbent in a dental chair with their head extended 30 degrees. Alternatively, place the patient sitting upright with their head and back firmly against the examination chair or table and their head extended 30 to 45 degrees. Instruct the patient to fully open their mouth.

Landmarks: Pull the buccal mucosa laterally and identify the inferior-most posterior portion of the zygoma. It lies posterior, lateral, and superior to the third maxillary molar. The pterygomaxillary fissure lies posterior, medial, and superior to the vestibule between the third maxillary molar and the posterior zygoma. The pterygopalatine fossa can be reached by following the pterygomaxillary fissure superiorly and medially.[2,3]

Needle insertion and direction: Clean, prep, and apply a topical anesthetic agent to the recess posterior and lateral to the maxilla. Insert the nondominant index finger between the maxillary molars and the cheek (Figure 154-8*A*). Palpate the zygomatic process of the maxilla with the index finger. Rotate the index finger 180 degrees so that the pad is against the patient's cheek (Figure 154-8*B*). Apply outward pressure to move the cheek away from the teeth. Place the needle along the middle of the nail plate of the index finger. Aim the needle and syringe along the index finger (Figure 154-8*B*). The needle and syringe should be aimed posteriorly, superiorly, and medially (Figure 154-8*C*). Insert and advance the needle 2.5 cm along the index finger. If the needle contacts bone, withdraw the needle completely and direct it more laterally.[2,3] Aspirate to confirm that the tip of the needle is not within a blood vessel. Inject 3 mL of local anesthetic solution.

Remarks: Bend the needle 30 degrees at the hub to assist in achieving a medial direction of the needle. **Do not bend the needle more than 30 degrees as the needle may fracture. It is extremely important to never change the direction of a needle once it is inserted.** This is associated with an increased risk of needle breakage requiring an operative procedure to recover the needle segment. **Never force the needle.** The needle is inappropriately positioned if it is meeting resistance. Abort the procedure, reidentify the landmarks, and reattempt the procedure.[2,3] Occasionally, the first molar is only partially anesthetized by this block. Consider supplementation of this block with a supraperiosteal infiltration of the first molar.

MENTAL NERVE BLOCK, INTRAORAL APPROACH

Anatomy: The mental nerve is one of the two terminal divisions of the inferior alveolar nerve. It provides sensory innervation to the ipsilateral skin and mucosa of the lower lip and chin. It exits the bony mandible at the mental foramen.

Patient positioning: Place the patient recumbent in a dental chair. Alternatively, place the patient sitting upright or supine with their head against the examination table and in the neutral position. Instruct the patient to slightly open their mouth.

Landmarks: The mental foramen lies in the same plane as the infraorbital foramen and the mid-pupillary line (Figure 154-4). The mental foramen is located approximately 1 cm beneath the gum line, between the first and second premolar.

Needle insertion and direction: Clean, prep, and apply a topical anesthetic agent to the oral mucosa overlying the mental foramen. Grasp the lower lip with the nondominant hand. Pull it outward and downward (Figure 154-9). Insert a 27 gauge needle into the mucobuc-

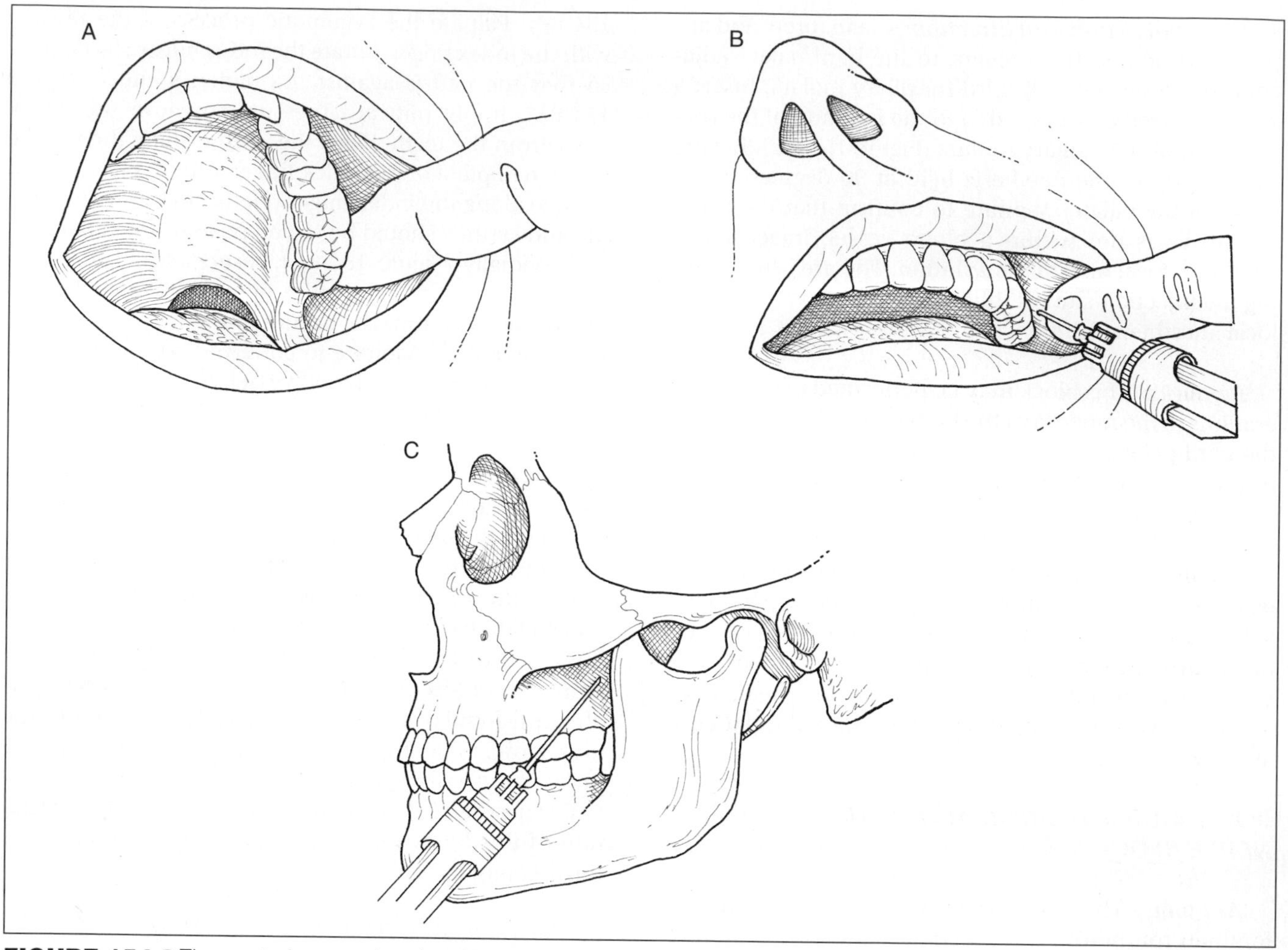

FIGURE 154-8 The posterior superior alveolar nerve block. *A.* Insert the nondominant index finger. *B.* Retract the cheek. *C.* The proper direction for insertion and advancement of the needle.

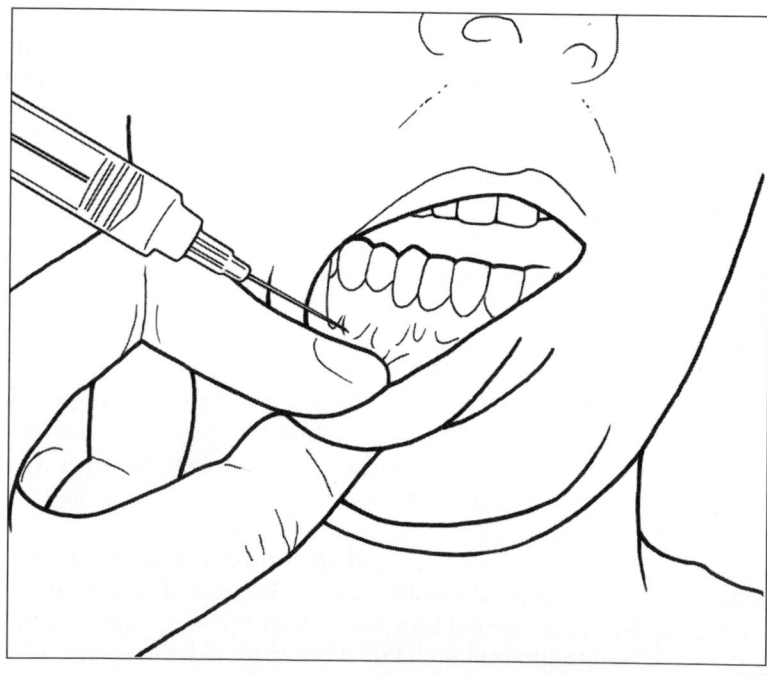

FIGURE 154-9 The intraoral approach to the mental nerve block.

cal fold between the first and second premolar (Figure 154-9). Advance the needle medially until it contacts the mandible. Aspirate to confirm that the tip of the needle is not within a blood vessel. Inject 1.5 to 2.0 mL of local anesthetic solution.

Remarks: The mental nerve block, as the infraorbital nerve block, has an intraoral and an extraoral approach. The extraoral approach will not be discussed as it is more painful and there is no benefit to its use over the intraoral approach. A description of the extraoral approach to the mental nerve block is found in Chapter 106. A near midline lower lip or chin injury may necessitate bilateral mental nerve blockade due to the midline crossover from each of the mental nerves.[2]

BUCCAL NERVE BLOCK

Anatomy: The buccal nerve is one of the main branches of the mandibular nerve. It travels down the medial aspect of the ramus of the mandible, anterior to the inferior alveolar neurovascular bundle. It crosses from the medial mandible into the soft tissue of the cheek at the level of the occlusive plane. It supplies the sensory innervation to the mucous membrane of the cheek and vestibule.[1] It innervates, to a variable degree, a small patch of skin over the cheek.

Patient positioning: Place the patient recumbent in a dental chair with their head extended 30 degrees. Alternatively, place the patient sitting with their head and back firmly against an examination chair or upright table with their head extended 30 to 45 degrees. Instruct the patient to fully open their mouth.

Landmarks: Visually identify the third mandibular molar. Palpate the anterior border of the ramus of the mandible. The buccal nerve traverses the anterior border of the ramus of the mandible, posterior and slightly lateral to the third molar at the level of the occlusive plane.

Needle insertion and direction: Clean, prep, and apply a topical anesthetic agent to the oral mucosa over the anterolateral border of the ramus of the mandible. Place the thumb of the nondominant hand on the inner surface of the cheek. Pull the cheek outward. Insert a 27 gauge needle 1 mm lateral to the anterior border of the ramus of the mandible and at the level of the occlusal plane (Figure 154-10). Advance the needle 3 to 4 mm into the soft tissues. Aspirate to confirm that the tip of the needle is not within a blood vessel. Inject 2 mL of local anesthetic solution.

Remarks: Buccal nerve blocks are used when extensive intraoral manipulation is anticipated, when buccal

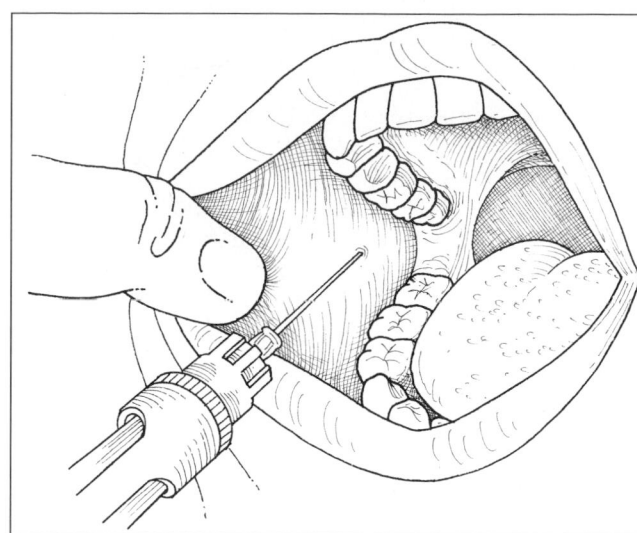

FIGURE 154-10 The buccal nerve block.

manipulation or repair is required, or for the incision and drainage of an abscess. It provides additional patient comfort. The block is nearly always performed as an adjunct to an inferior alveolar, maxillary, or posterior superior alveolar nerve block.[3]

INFERIOR ALVEOLAR NERVE BLOCK

Anatomy: The lingual and inferior alveolar nerves are two of four branches of the mandibular nerve. The nerves initially travel together and inferiorly on the medial side of the mandibular ramus (Figure 154-11*A*). The lingula is a palpable bony landmark immediately anterior to the mandibular foramen. The inferior alveolar nerve courses posterior to the lingula and enters the mandibular canal via the mandibular foramen. It continues to travel anteriorly within the mandible to provide sensory innervation to the body of the mandible, the mandibular teeth, and the overlying oral mucosa. One of the terminal branches of the inferior alveolar nerve is the mental nerve. The inferior alveolar nerve may be blocked by the classic, open-mouth approach or the closed-mouth approach.

Patient positioning: Place the patient in a dental chair with their head neutral, such that the occlusive surface is parallel to the floor. Alternatively, place the patient sitting upright in an examination chair or on a gurney with their head positioned firmly against the back of the gurney or chair. Instruct the patient to fully open their mouth. Perform the open-mouth approach if the patient can fully open their mouth. Perform the closed-mouth approach if the patient has trismus or cannot fully open their mouth.

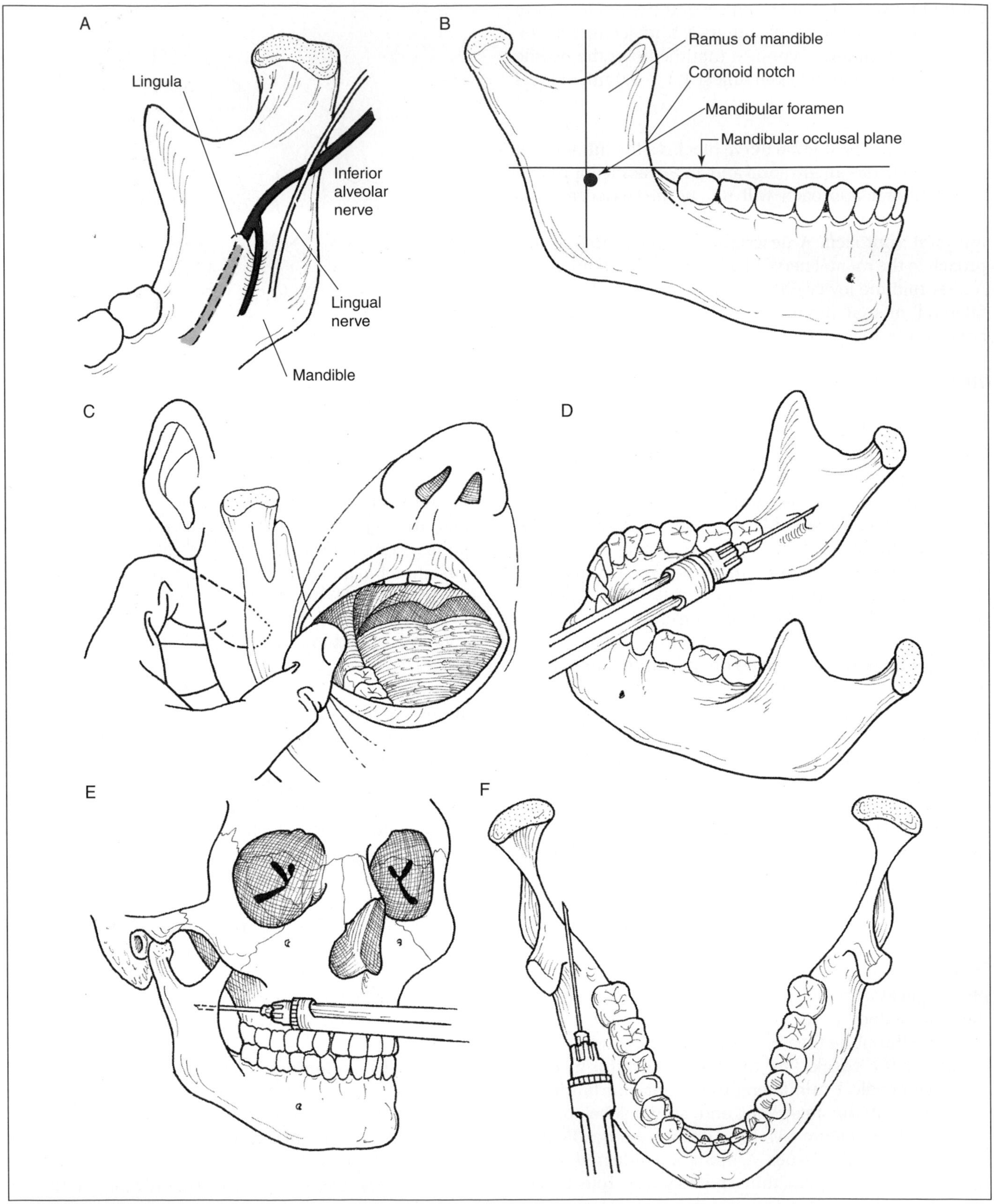

FIGURE 154-11 The inferior alveolar nerve block. *A.* The course of the inferior alveolar nerve and the lingual nerve along the ramus of the mandible. *B.* The anatomy of the external surface of the mandible. *C.* Positioning for the open-mouth approach. *D.* Proper needle insertion and direction for the open-mouth approach. *E.* The closed-mouth approach. *F.* Superior view of the closed-mouth approach demonstrating the proper needle direction.

Landmarks: Identify by palpation the anterior border of the ramus of the mandible within the mouth, the coronoid notch within the mouth, and the posterior border of the ramus of the mandible externally (Figure 154-11*B*). Approximately equidistant from these two points lie the lingual and the inferior alveolar nerves. Palpate the lingula of the ramus of the mandible. It is a bony projection on the medial surface of the ramus of the mandible and 1 cm above the occlusive plane.

Needle insertion and direction (open-mouth approach): Clean, prep, and apply a topical anesthetic agent to the inner surface of the ramus of the mandible. Stand opposite the side to be blocked. Place the thumb of the nondominant hand on the anterior border of the ramus of the mandible. Move the thumb posteromedially to identify the lingula. Place the index finger of the nondominant hand against the extraoral border of the mandibular ramus, just above the angle of the mandible. Grasp the ramus between the thumb and the forefinger (Figure 154-11*C*). Pull the cheek outward using the nondominant thumb as a lever. Place a 27 gauge, 2 inch needle on a 3 mL syringe that contains local anesthetic solution. A 5 mL syringe is too large for this approach. A syringe smaller than 3 mL will not carry enough anesthetic.

Introduce the needle from the opposite side (Figure 154-11*D*). Align the tip of the needle towards the lingula with the barrel of the syringe between the contralateral first and second premolars. Hold the syringe parallel to the occlusal plane and 3 to 4 mm above the premolars. Insert the needle into the oral mucosa just superior and posterior to the lingula. Advance the needle until the tip contacts the ramus of the mandible. Aspirate to confirm that the tip of the needle is not within a blood vessel. Inject 2 mL of local anesthetic solution.

The above technique is optimal if the operator is right-handed and a right-sided inferior alveolar block is attempted. If the operator is right-handed and attempting a left-sided inferior alveolar nerve block, it is still necessary to stand opposite the side to be anesthetized with the syringe in the dominant hand. Place the nondominant arm over and around the patient's head so that the thumb of the nondominant hand can contact the anterior border of the mandibular ramus and the index finger can grasp the posterior border above the angle of the mandible. The remainder of the technique is the same.

Needle insertion and direction (closed-mouth approach): This method can be used when the patient cannot fully open their mouth due to an abscess, edema, mandible fractures, trismus, or if the mandible is wired-closed to the maxilla. This approach deposits the local anesthetic solution superior to the site of the classic, open-mouth approach. The local anesthetic solution will descend, due to gravity, to bathe the inferior alveolar nerve and provide adequate anesthesia.

Place the nondominant thumb on the inner surface of the cheek. Pull the cheek outward. Place a 27 gauge needle on a 3 mL syringe that contains local anesthetic solution. Place the needle and syringe parallel to the occlusal plane and aligned along the junction of the maxillary molars and their gingiva (Figure 154-11*E*). Direct the needle just medial to the ramus of the mandible (Figures 154-11*E* and *F*). Advance the needle 3 cm through the mucosa. Aspirate to confirm that the tip of the needle is not within a blood vessel. Inject 2 mL of local anesthetic solution.

Remarks: **It is crucial that the tip of the needle contacts the mandible in the open-mouth approach.** The needle is usually advanced 0.5 to 1 cm before the mandible is encountered. The needle is most likely inappropriately placed and deposition of anesthesia will not produce the desired results if the mandible is not encountered. Remove the needle, reidentify the appropriate anatomic landmarks, and reattempt the procedure if the mandible is not encountered.[4] The buccal, inferior alveolar, and lingual nerves must be blocked on one side to achieve complete anesthesia of the hemimandible.

LINGUAL NERVE BLOCK

Anatomy: The lingual nerve is a branch of the mandibular division of the trigeminal nerve. It travels with the inferior alveolar nerve until the inferior alveolar nerve enters the mandible. The lingual nerve leaves the medial aspect of the mandibular ramus and penetrates the posterior tongue at the level of the occlusive plane, just medial to the third mandibular premolar. It courses anteriorly to provide sensory innervation to the anterior two-thirds of the tongue, the floor of the mouth, and the lingual mucous membrane.[1]

Patient positioning: Place the patient in a dental chair with their head neutral, such that the occlusive surface is parallel to the floor. Alternatively, place the patient sitting upright in an examination chair or on a gurney with their head firmly against the back of the gurney or chair. Instruct the patient to fully open their mouth.

Landmarks: Identify the lingual side of the second mandibular molar. The injection site is 1 cm medial to the second mandibular molar.

Needle insertion and direction: Approach the patient from the contralateral side. Move the tongue upward or toward the contralateral side with a tongue blade. Insert a 27 gauge, 2 inch needle into the mucosa 1 cm medial to the second mandibular premolar (Figure 154-12). Advance the needle posteriorly 1 cm. Aspirate

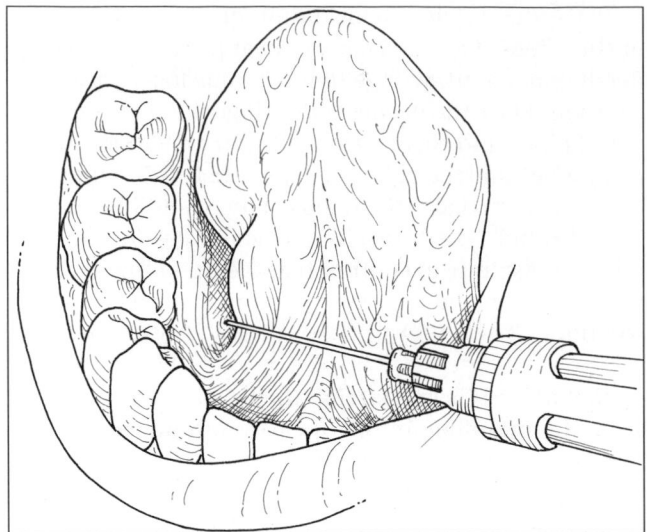

FIGURE 154-12 The lingual nerve block.

to confirm that the tip of the needle is not within a blood vessel. Inject 1.0 to 1.5 mL of local anesthetic solution.

Remarks: The inferior alveolar nerve and the lingual nerve can be, and usually are, blocked simultaneously during an inferior alveolar nerve block. The lingual nerve, however, can be blocked in an isolated fashion. Perform an isolated lingual nerve block only when the initial combined block has failed or for isolated tongue lacerations.[1,3] This is an optimal block for tongue laceration repair. However, bilateral lingual nerve blocks may be necessary.

ASSESSMENT

Anesthesia is usually achieved within 5 minutes of the injection. However, depending upon the particular injection and the local anesthetic used, anesthesia can be achieved anywhere from 20 seconds to 10 minutes. The block was properly performed if the patient experiences anesthesia. Repeat the block if anesthesia is not achieved by 10 minutes.

AFTERCARE

The aftercare of dental anesthesia is minimal. Re-examine the area of the local anesthetic injection before the patient is discharged to ensure that a hematoma has not developed. **Instruct the patient to use caution as there is no sensation in the area anesthetized.** Encourage them to refrain from meals, chewing gum, hot beverages, aggravated scratching, placing foreign bodies in the mouth, or anything that may cause injury to the anesthetized area. Parents must be informed to discourage children from testing the anesthetized area by biting or chewing. Many Dentists and Physicians place a cotton roll, or rolled 2×2 gauze, between the area anesthetized and the teeth to provide added protection from a self-inflicted bite injury.[2,3]

COMPLICATIONS

Any patient receiving dental anesthesia has the potential to develop complications. The key is to have knowledge of these complications and be prepared to deal with them should they occur. Most severe complications will declare themselves in a rapid fashion. These severe complications include intravascular injection of local anesthetic, allergic reactions to the local anesthetic, and unintentional overdosage. These can be avoided by aspiration before injection, obtaining an appropriate history of prior anesthesia, and cautious calculation of anesthetic dosages, respectively.[2,3]

Late complications of dental anesthesia include hematomas, neuropathy, infection, and trismus.[2,3] Hematomas after dental anesthesia occur after the inadvertent puncture of an artery or vein. Arterial hematomas enlarge more rapidly and are usually more painful than venous hematomas. They can cause a significant facial deformity. Hematomas following dental anesthesia are usually of little significance, require no intervention, and resolve spontaneously with time. Treatment initially involves applying cold packs. Heat in the form of an externally placed heating pad should be used to help disintegrate the clot after 24 hours.[2,3]

A peripheral neuropathy can occur in the form of prolonged anesthesia, paresthesias (burning or itching sensation), hyperesthesias (increased sensitivity to noxious stimuli), and dysesthesias (painful sensation to non-noxious stimuli). This is a result of direct damage to the nerve from traumatic needle insertion, deposition of local anesthetic into a foramen or canal causing pressure injury to the nerve, or chemical injury to the nerve. Reduce the risk of causing a neuropathy by avoiding injections into a foramen, using a small gauge needle, and withdrawing the needle slightly before injection if the patient should feel a shock or paresthesias with needle insertion.[2,3]

Infection due to dental anesthesia is rare, but does exist. Follow several simple measures to minimize potential infections. Never inject through an infected area. Doing so may carry bacteria through facial planes into deeper compartments. Refrain from multiple injections (needle misadventures) as this increases the risk of iatrogenic infection. This is easily resolved by appropriately identifying the anatomic landmarks prior to needle insertion.

Needle breakage can occur as a result of manufacturing defects or operator imprudence. **To prevent needle breakage, never exert force against resistance.** Resistance signifies that the tip of the needle is against bone or a tooth. Withdraw the needle and reattempt insertion if this occurs. **Never advance the needle to the hub.** The greatest percentage of needle breaks occur when the needle is inserted to the hub.[2,3] **Never redirect the needle after it is inserted through the skin or mucosa.** This puts abnormal force on the needle and potentiates breakage. The needle may inadvertently be in an undesired anatomic location. Withdraw the needle completely, identify the appropriate anatomic landmarks, and reinsert the needle.

SUMMARY

Dental anesthetic techniques are easy to learn, simple to perform, and effective in providing temporary pain relief. The required equipment is readily available in every Emergency Department. Consider using local anesthetic agents that contain epinephrine because they provide significantly longer analgesia than those without epinephrine. A rapidly performed local anesthetic injection goes a long way towards patient satisfaction.

REFERENCES

1. Wilson-Pauwels L, Akesson EJ, Stewart PA: *Cranial Nerves Anatomy and Clinical Comments.* Philadelphia: Decker, 1988:49–69.
2. Howe GL, Whitehead FIH: *Local Anesthesia in Dentistry,* 3rd ed. London: Butterworth, 1990:81–93.
3. Jastak JT, Yagiela JA, Donaldson D: *Local Anesthesia of the Oral Cavity.* Philadelphia: Saunders, 1995.
4. Amsterdam JT: Regional anesthesia of the head and neck, in Roberts JR, Hedges JR (eds): *Clinical Procedures in Emergency Medicine,* 3rd ed. Philadelphia: Saunders, 1998:497–510.
5. Orlinski M, Dean E: Anesthetic and analgesic techniques, in Roberts JR, Hedges JR (eds): *Clinical Procedures in Emergency Medicine,* 3rd ed. Philadelphia: Saunders, 1998:454–473.
6. Kassuto Z, Helpin ML: Orofacial anesthesia techniques, in Henretig FM, King C, Joffe MD, et al (eds): *Textbook of Pediatric Emergency Procedures.* Baltimore: Williams & Wilkins, 1997:713–723.

Chapter 155
DENTAL ABSCESS INCISION AND DRAINAGE

Daniel J. Ross

INTRODUCTION

Patients frequently present to the Emergency Department complaining of a "toothache." The common causes of toothache pain are multiple.[1] Several of these conditions present with clinical evidence of inflammation or intraoral swelling. Similarly, there are multiple etiologies for a dental abscess (Table 155-1). Distinguishing a pulpal abscess from a periodontal abscess and simple pericoronitis can impact treatment, prognosis, and morbidity.[2–5] The Emergency Physician must have a basic understanding of dental anatomy, pathophysiology, and treatment protocols in order to accurately diagnose and treat these conditions. Many of these conditions can initially be managed through the Emergency Department. The Emergency Physician must also know when dental infections require consultation or referral to a higher level of care.[3,5,6]

ANATOMY AND PATHOPHYSIOLOGY

Teeth are essentially composed of three layers (Figure 155-1). These layers, from the outside and working inward, are the enamel, the dentin, and the pulp. The dentin and pulp are living tissues that are sensitive to noxious stimuli. The crown is covered with enamel, while the root is covered with a substance known as cementum. Cementum helps attach the tooth to the surrounding alveolar bone via the periodontal ligament (PDL). The neurovascular supply enters the pulp through the apical foramen at the root apex. The pulp contains only pain-transmitting neuronal fibers, while the PDL contains both pain- and pressure-sensitive fibers.[7] Dental abscesses arise when bacteria penetrate the normal anatomic and physiologic barriers of the tooth and surrounding structures. This can lead to a pulpal abscess, periodontal abscess, or a pericoronitis (Figure 155-2).

PULPAL ABSCESSES

Dental abscesses often arise from pulpal necrosis secondary to dental caries or a defective dental restoration.[1,3,4,6,7] Dental caries is commonly known as dental decay or "cavities." This is the direct destruction of the tooth substance by the acidic bacterial products of normal oral flora. A carious tooth may not initially be painful. The products of inflammation eventually reach the dental pulp as the disease process progresses and the tooth will become sensitive.[1–3,7–9] This is known as pulpitis. Patients will report non-localizable and intermittent symptoms. This process may initially be reversible by routine dental treatment (e.g., a filling). The pulp will rapidly necrose and die once the pulp tissues actually become infected. Products from the necrotic pulp may escape the confines of the tooth via the apical foramen and involve the PDL. This makes the affected tooth easily localizable by percussion and spontaneously, or constantly, sensitive.[1–3,5–7,9]

Bacterial products and the host's immune response can lead to destruction of alveolar bone and tooth mobility once the infection involves the PDL.[1,3,5,7] The infection will follow the path of least resistance as it penetrates the alveolar plate. It may perforate laterally to form a vestibular abscess (Figure 155-3A). It may perforate medially to form a palatal abscess (Figure 155-3B). Further spread will be dictated by the proximity of muscle attachments and fascial planes as the infection penetrates the soft tissues.[3,5–7,9–11] The appropriate treatment for an abscessed tooth may include endodontic treatment, incision and drainage, or extraction. An incision and drainage procedure is warranted if the infectious process extends outside the alveolus and involves the soft tissues.[5,9,10]

Penetration of infectious products outside the root apex can lead to a multitude of clinical signs throughout the head and neck. Swelling, fluctuance, and spontaneous drainage of purulence may be seen intraorally or extraorally. A localized or generalized cellulitis may be

TABLE 155-1. COMMON ETIOLOGIES FOR A
DENTAL ABSCESS

Cysts that become infected
Gingival infections
Mixed periodontal/periapical infections
Periapical infections
Periodontal infections
Postoperative infections
Root fracture that becomes infected

present. The patient may develop trismus. There is often a foul odor.[1,5,6,10] A reactive maxillary sinusitis can occur due to the proximity of the maxillary root apices. Sinusitis can develop by direct extension of an infection as draining purulence follows the path of least resistance.[5,11] One or more of the various dental spaces may become infected via extension.[5,6,10] A sinus tract may eventually form and allow purulence to drain either through the tooth, the intraoral soft tissues, or extraorally. Patients with chronic dental abscesses often complain of swelling, a foul odor, and a foul taste, but not pain.[12] Systemic symptoms may be present including fever, malaise, anorexia, and leukocytosis.[5,6,10,12]

Dental infections extending into the fascial compartments of the head and neck are immediately considered complicated infections.[3,5,6,10] Patients often have a rapidly progressing cellulitic process that can quickly lead to airway compromise. They typically have a toxic appearance and present with dysphagia, dysphonia, or dyspnea. The classic example is Ludwig's angina or a concurrent bilateral involvement of the sublingual, submental, and submandibular spaces. Infectious extensions into the lateral pharyngeal, retropharyngeal, and prevertebral spaces are rare and can lead to disastrous complications such as aspiration, mediastinitis, and airway compromise.[10,11] A retropharyngeal space of greater than 3 to 5 mm on lateral soft tissue neck radiographs or CT scans is indicative of airway compromise.[10] **Consider rapid and aggressive management with early airway intervention, intravenous antibiotics, and immediate surgical consultation in patients who are suspected of manifesting any of these processes.[3,10,11]**

PERIODONTAL ABSCESSES

Poor dental hygiene and poor nutrition lead to local inflammation of the tissues surrounding and attaching the tooth to its socket, allowing bacterial penetration. Early periodontal disease is isolated to the gingiva and known as gingivitis.[5,13] Alveolar bone may be destroyed as the disease progresses, leading to gingival pockets and tooth mobility.[1,5,12] Food debris or plaque may become trapped within these pockets and create a localized infection known as a periodontal abscess.[4,5,13] Periodontal disease is very common in pregnant women.[5]

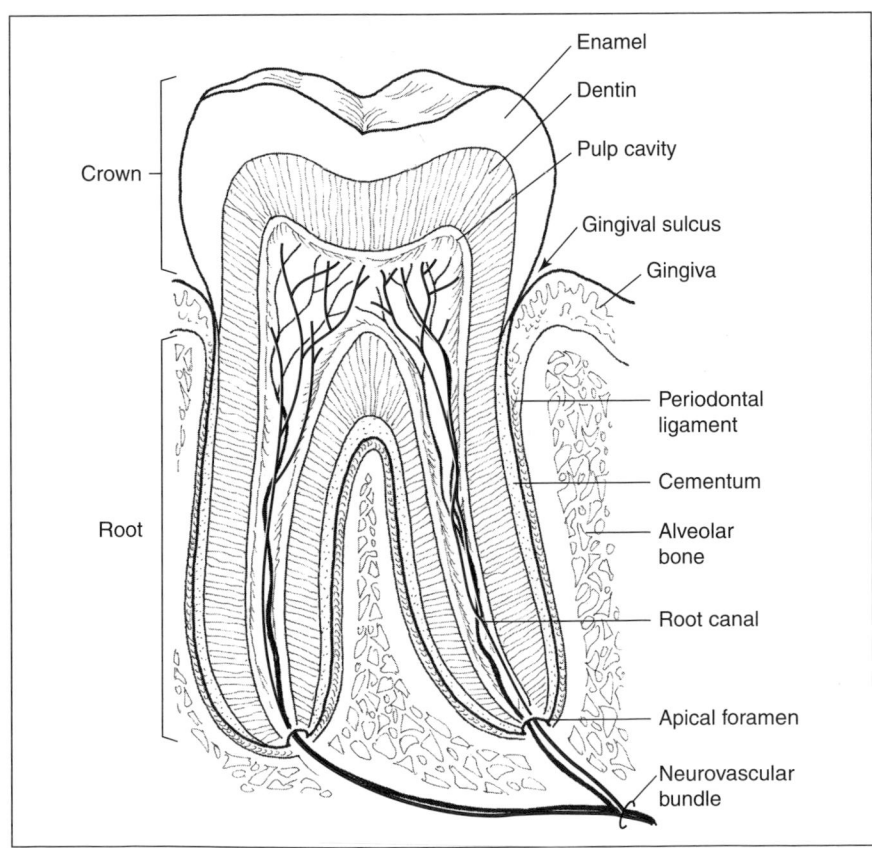

FIGURE 155-1 The anatomy of a tooth.

Labels (top to bottom, right side): Enamel, Dentin, Pulp cavity, Gingival sulcus, Gingiva, Periodontal ligament, Cementum, Alveolar bone, Root canal, Apical foramen, Neurovascular bundle

Labels (left side): Crown, Root

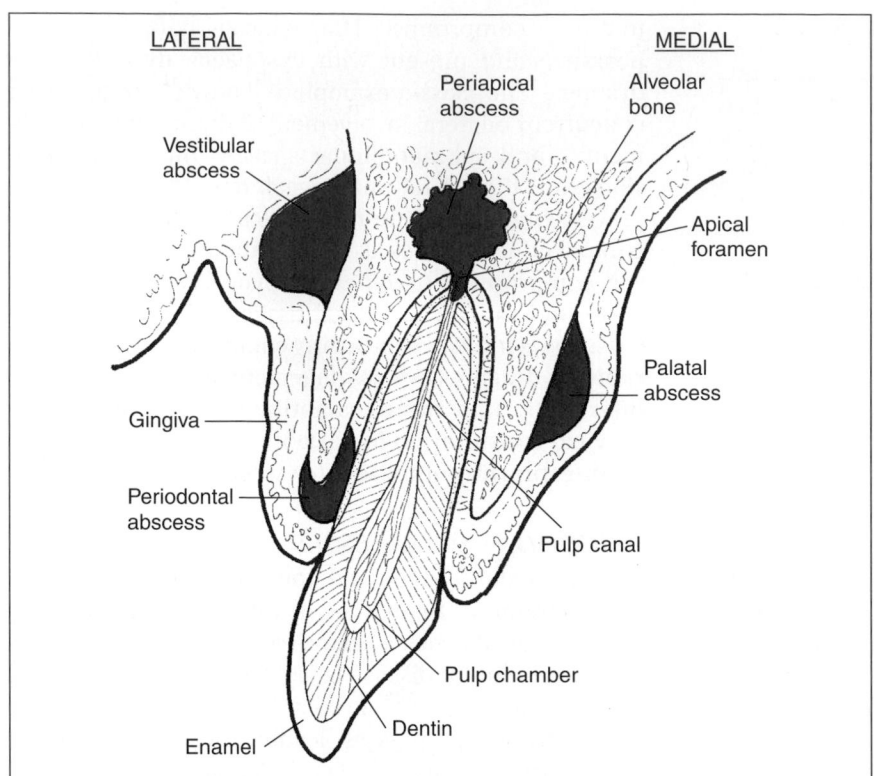

FIGURE 155-2 Locations of common dental abscesses.

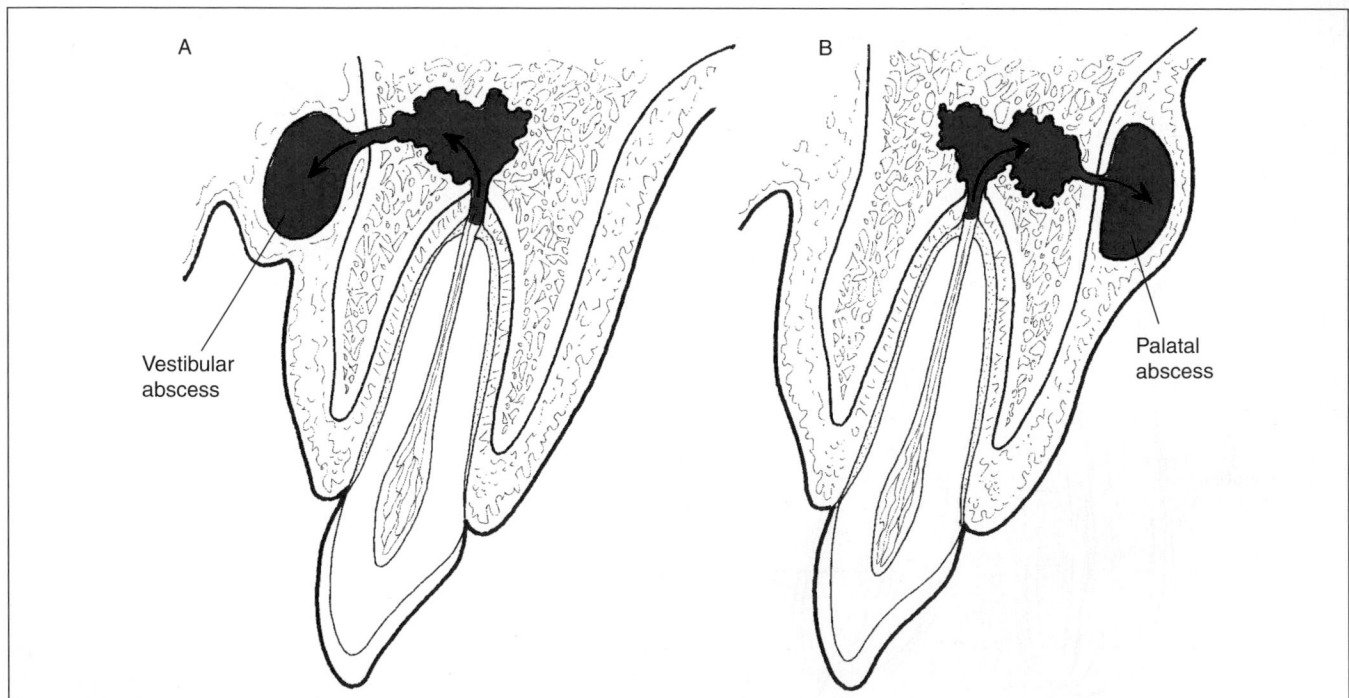

FIGURE 155-3 The spread of a dental abscess. A pulpal abscess progresses to a periapical abscess that perforates the alveolar plate. *A.* Labial or buccal perforation leads to a vestibular abscess. *B.* Palatal or lingual perforation leads to a palatal or lingual abscess, respectively.

Patients may complain of bleeding, foul odor, bad taste, loose teeth, pain, or swelling. The physical examination reveals gingival tissue that may be erythematous or necrotic and bleed easily. Heavy accretions of dental plaque and calculous may be present. An abscess may present as a focal swelling, tooth mobility, pain on percussion, and purulence that is expressible from the gingival sulcus.[1,5,12,13] It may be impossible, with concurrent dental caries, to differentiate a dental abscess from a periodontal abscess without radiographs.[3,5] In fact, both lesions may occur together.[12] A periodontally diseased tooth may be so mobile that it cannot be salvaged and requires extraction.[5]

Periodontal abscesses rarely spread beyond the local dentoalveolar structure and rarely require an urgent referral.[3,4] Treat an isolated periodontal abscess with dental anesthesia, incision and drainage, and dilute peroxide (1:5 dilution or 5%) or chlorhexidine rinses. Prescribe oral antibiotics for evidence of spread, if there is a delay to definitive care, or for systemic manifestations.[1,3–5,12] Appropriate antibiotics include penicillin, clindamycin, or erythromycin. Refer patients with these lesions to a Dentist within 24 to 48 hours for definitive follow-up care to avoid recurrence.[1,3,5]

PERICORONITIS

Inflammation can occur around the crown of any erupting tooth and is common around impacted teeth, especially the third molars.[1,3,4,14] This condition is known as pericoronitis. It is often exacerbated by the impaction of food under the soft tissue. Progression or overzealous treatment can easily lead to extension of the infection posteriorly to multiple contiguous spaces, including the retropharyngeal space.[1,3,14,15] Simple cases are easily managed in the Emergency Department. Always maintain a very low threshold for consultation and referral of patients with complicated presentations.

Treatment of pericoronitis may include dental anesthesia, direct saline irrigation, warm salt water rinses, dilute peroxide or chlorhexidine rinses, and oral analgesics. The presence of swelling, trismus, and inflammation may be severe enough to warrant a course of oral antibiotics.[1] Some authors advocate antibiotic coverage in essentially all cases.[1,10,14] Definitive treatment is completed eruption or extraction of the tooth. Refer the patient to a Dentist for follow-up and definitive care within 24 to 48 hours.

INDICATIONS

The indications for dental abscess incision and drainage include a pulpal or periodontal abscess with clinical evidence of alveolar penetration and soft tissue spread.[9,10] Some authors recommend incision and drainage for purely cellulitic processes.[4,5,11] Extraoral incision and drainage is indicated for dental infections progressing toward inevitable spontaneous extraoral drainage.[3,10]

CONTRAINDICATIONS

A review of the current literature reveals no direct contraindications. Maintain a low threshold for consultation and referral to a Dentist for any patient with rapidly progressing infections, difficulty breathing, difficulty swallowing, fascial space involvement, temperature greater than 101 °F (38.3 °C), white blood cell count greater than 10,000, severe trismus (manifested by mandibular opening less than 10 mm or inability to adequately visualize the hypopharynx), a toxic appearance, compromised host defenses, or who are children.[3,6,10,16]

EQUIPMENT

#15 scalpel blade on a handle
#11 scalpel blade on a handle
Minnesota retractor
Weider tongue retractor
Fraser suction catheter
Suction source and tubing
Needle driver
Hemostat
Suture, 4–0 and 5–0 silk
Gelfoam
Light source, overhead or headlamp

PATIENT PREPARATION

Explain the procedure, its risks, and benefits to the patient and/or their representative. Obtain dental radiographs if the infection is from a dental source.[5,6,10] Obtain an informed consent for the procedure. Provide adequate anesthesia; ideally, in the form of a dental block. Obtain a separate informed consent for the dental block. Direct infiltration into an area of purulence does not achieve adequate anesthesia and risks spreading the infection by inoculation.[3,5] Dental blocks may require augmentation with direct infiltration anterior and posterior to the abscess. Anesthetize areas adjacent to the abscess last to avoid seeding. Refer to Chapter 154 for a complete discussion of dental analgesia and anesthesia. The application of procedural sedation may be required if adequate local anesthesia is not possible.[10] Refer to Chapter 109 for the complete details regarding procedural sedation and analgesia. Address endocarditis prophylaxis where appropriate (Table 155-2).

TABLE 155-2. PROPHYLACTIC REGIMENS FOR ENDOCARDITIS IN PATIENTS UNDERGOING DENTAL OR ORAL SURGICAL PROCEDURES[a]

Standard general prophylaxis:
Amoxicillin orally 1 hour prior to procedure
    Adults 2000 mg, children 50 mg/kg

Unable to take oral medications:
Ampicillin intramuscularly or intravenously 30 minutes prior to procedure
    Adults 2000 mg, children 50 mg/kg

Penicillin allergic patients:
Clindamycin orally 1 hour prior to procedure
    Adults 600 mg, children 20 mg/kg
Cephalexin or Cefadroxil orally 1 hour prior to procedure
    Adults 2000 mg, children 50 mg/kg
Azithromycin or Clarithromycin orally 1 hour prior to procedure
    Adults 500 mg, children 15 mg/kg

Penicillin allergic patient unable to take oral medications:
Clindamycin intravenously 30 minutes prior to procedure
    Adults 600 mg, children 20 mg/kg
Cefazolin intramuscularly or intravenously 30 minutes prior to procedure
    Adults 1000 mg, children 25 mg/kg

[a]American Heart Association Recommendations, 1997.

TECHNIQUES

SIMPLE INTRAORAL INCISION AND DRAINAGE

There are two techniques for intraoral incision and drainage. The first technique is to make a simple stab incision with a #11 scalpel blade in the area of greatest fluctuance and in the area that best facilitates dependent drainage (Figure 155-4*A*). **Do not make the incision more than 1 cm in length.** Insert a closed, curved hemostat into the incision (Figure 155-4*B*). Gently spread the jaws of the hemostat in several different directions to break up any loculations (Figure 155-4*C*). Express and suction any remaining purulence. Insert a sterile rubber drain cut from a 0.25 inch wide Penrose drain or from a sterile surgical glove (Figure 155-4*D*). Place 1 to 2 silk sutures through the drain and the oral soft tissues. This will ensure that the drain does not fall out and result in premature closure of the incision or aspiration of the drain.

The second technique for simple intraoral incision and drainage differs only in the location of the incision. Make an incision with a #15 scalpel blade at the alveolar crest within the gingival sulcus, scalloping around the teeth. Extend the incision one tooth medial and distal to the tooth in question or the area of the abscess. Gently elevate the attached gingiva from the bone with a blunt instrument. Continue the blunt dissection until the abscess cavity is penetrated. This typically occurs just with the level of unattached gingiva. The remainder of the

procedure is as described above. This technique affords some mechanical advantages to the operator and is well tolerated by the patient postoperatively. It can be performed in both arches, buccally, palatally, and lingually. It is often useful for draining a periodontal abscess.[3,5,10]

EXTRAORAL INCISION AND DRAINAGE

Extraoral incision and drainage is indicated when a dental infection appears to be progressing toward inevitable extraoral drainage.[10] This procedure requires more attention and skill because of the numerous underlying vital structures and the possible cosmetic consequences.[3,10] Make every effort to avoid extraoral incision and drainage.[3] Consider consulting a Dentist before performing an extraoral incision and drainage.

Extraoral incision and drainage differs from the intraoral approach.[3,10,11] **Advise the patient that they will almost certainly have a visible scar after the incision heals.[3,10]** Extraoral incision and drainage requires the use of sterile technique. Prepare the area with povidone iodine and allow it to dry. Apply sterile drapes to isolate a field. Perform local subcutaneous infiltrative anesthesia of the skin. Use a separate needle and syringe for any intraoral anesthetic techniques.

Make a 1.0 to 1.5 cm long incision with a #15 scalpel blade in an area of healthy skin, proximal to the site of expected breakdown and in a location that facilitates dependent drainage (Figure 155-5). Extend the incision into the subcutaneous tissues. This is another critical difference from the intraoral technique. Insert a hemostat to penetrate and drain the abscess cavity. Spread the hemostat in several directions to break up any loculations. The remainder of the procedure is performed as described above. Scarring with extraoral incisions is virtually universal.[3,10]

ASSESSMENT

Basic postoperative assessment includes inspecting the operative site for the minor complications described below. **Assure adequate drain retention. A loose intraoral drain may represent an aspiration risk.** Observe the patient for post-procedural bleeding. It can be controlled with the application of pressure, a local anesthetic agent containing epinephrine, or Gelfoam.

AFTERCARE

The application of warm moist compresses, oral fluids, rest, and good nutrition are mainstays in the treatment of any inflammatory process. Patients may benefit from a soft, bland diet and frequent oral rinses with a warm saltwater solution. All patients require postoperative oral analgesics.[3,5,10,11] Patients with an ex-

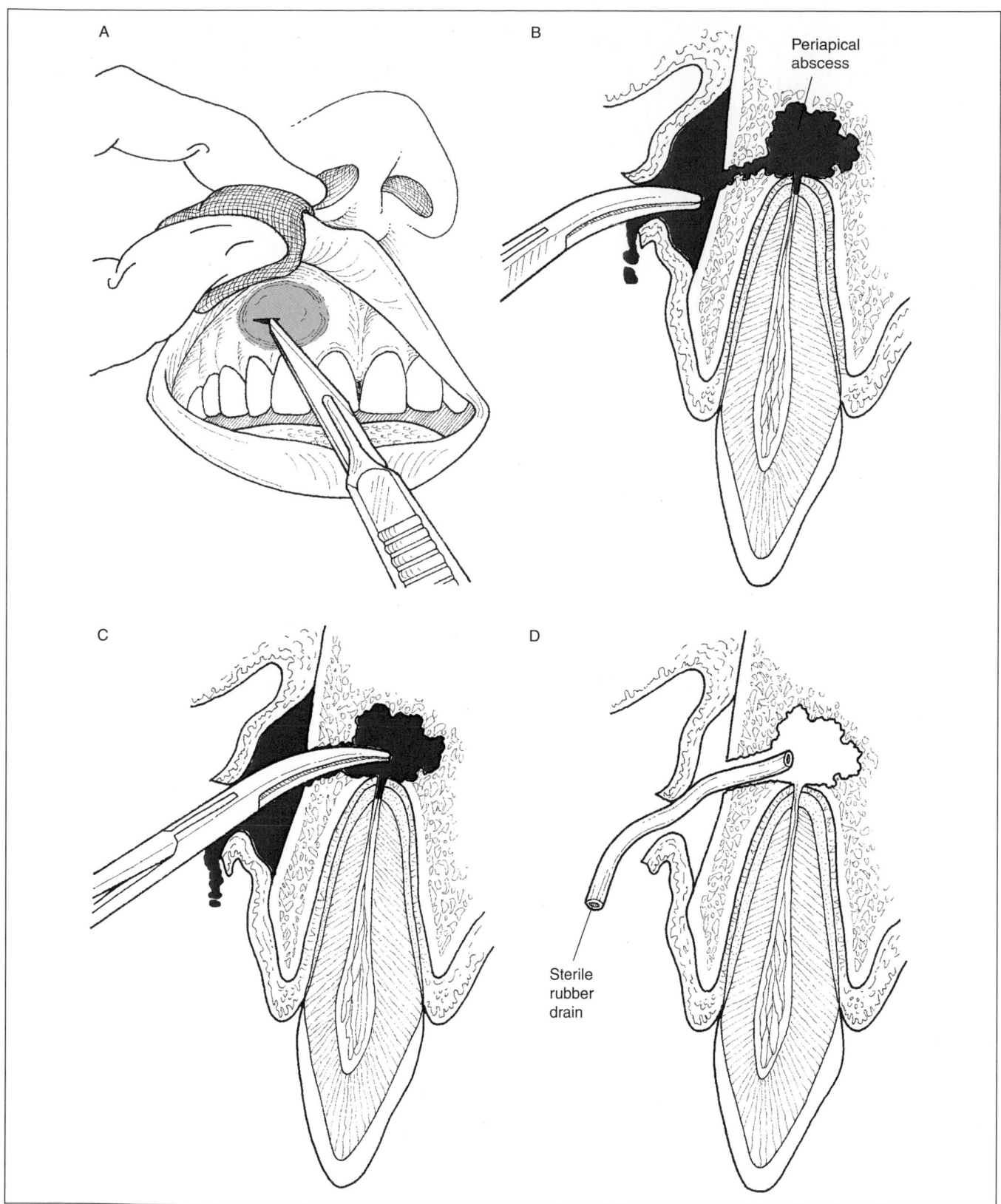

FIGURE 155-4 Incision and drainage of a periapical abscess that has extended into a vestibular abscess. *A*. Make a stab incision with a #11 scalpel blade. *B*. Insert a hemostat into the incision. *C*. Advance the hemostat into the abscess cavity to lyse any adhesions. *D*. Place a sterile drain into the abscess cavity.

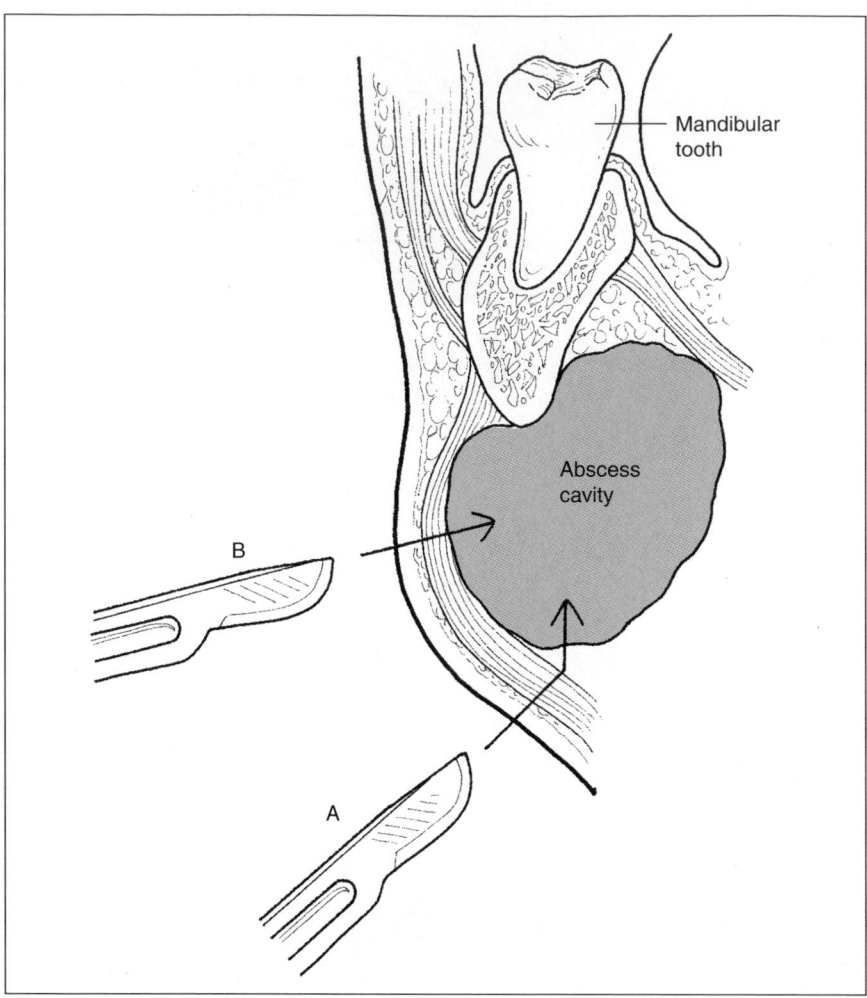

Mandibular
tooth

Abscess
cavity

B

A

FIGURE 155-5 Extraoral drainage of a dental abscess. Choose a location that has healthy skin and that will allow dependent drainage.

traoral incision require dressing changes.[3,5,10,11] Provide the patient with adequate supplies and teaching. Instruct the patient on the application of pressure if postprocedural bleeding occurs.

The use of antibiotics in light of adequate drainage is somewhat controversial. Clear-cut indications for oral antibiotics in orofacial infections include cellulitis, extraoral incision, systemic symptoms, persistent infection, pericoronitis, fascial space involvement, and immunocompromised patients.[10] The prudent clinician is advised to err on the side of caution while the academics quarrel over antibiotic indications. Penicillin is the drug of choice for the empiric treatment of dental-related infections. Alternatives to penicillin include erythromycin, clindamycin, or a cephalosporin. Clindamycin is very useful when anaerobes are suspected or in recalcitrant infections where sensitivities are lacking.[3,5,6,10]

Allow the intraoral drain to remain in place until the swelling has resolved and purulent drainage has ceased. Evaluate the patient for drain removal or advancement in 24 to 48 hours. Prescribe oral antibiotics and anal-

gesics during this time. Refer the patient to a Dentist within 24 hours.

COMPLICATIONS

Minor postoperative pain, swelling, bleeding, drainage, and possibly bruising can be expected following incision and drainage of a dental abscess. Significant post-procedural bleeding can be controlled with pressure, a vasoconstricting local anesthetic agent, or Gelfoam.[5,6,12,13] An incision or drainage tract that communicates freely between the oral cavity and the external face represents a significant complication. Refer these patients to a Plastic or Oral Surgeon.

SUMMARY

The recognition of common dental-related infections (pericoronitis, periodontal abscesses, and dental abscesses) can impact patient prognosis and morbidity. The diagnosis and treatment of these maladies, and their complications, requires knowledge of dental anatomy and pathophysiology. The Emergency Department management of these infections is quick and simple. Refer all patients to a Dentist or Oral Surgeon for definitive care of their teeth.

REFERENCES

1. Hicks JL, Vaughan GG: Odontogenic and periodontal sources of oral pain, in Montgomery MT, Redding SW (eds): *Orofacial Emergencies: Diagnosis and Management.* Portland, OR: JBK Publishing, 1994:1–39.
2. Montgomery S, Ferguson CD: Endodontics: diagnostic, treatment planning, and prognostic considerations. *Dent Clin North Am* 1986; 30(3):533–547.
3. Amsterdam JT: Emergency dental procedures, in Roberts JR, Hedges JR (eds): *Clinical Procedures in Emergency Medicine,* 3rd ed. Philadelphia: Saunders, 1998:1045–1064.
4. Morris JA Jr, Swiontkowski MF, Herrmann HJ: Wilderness trauma emergencies, in Auerbach PS (ed): *Wilderness Medicine,* 3rd ed. St. Louis: Mosby, 1995:343–352.
5. Ross DJ, Kirsch T: Dental emergencies, in Vanrooyen M, Kirsch T, Clem K, et al (eds): *Emergent Field Medicine.* New York: McGraw-Hill, 2001.
6. Peterson LJ: Principles of management and prevention of odontogenic infections, in Peterson LJ, Ellis E, Hupp JR, et al (eds): *Contemporary Oral and Maxillofacial Surgery.* St. Louis: Mosby, 1988:383–408.
7. Cohen S, Burns RC: *Pathways of the Pulp,* 6th ed. Philadelphia: Mosby, 1994.
8. Amsterdam JT: Dental disorders, in Rosen, P, Barkin R, Danzl DD, et al (eds): *Emergency Medicine: Concepts and Clinical Practice,* 4th ed. St. Louis: Mosby, 1998:2680–2697.
9. Antrim DD, Bakland LK: Treatment of endodontic urgent care cases. *Dent Clin North Am* 1986; 30(3):549–572.
10. King RC: Orofacial infections, in Montgomery MT, Redding SW (eds): *Orofacial Emergencies: Diagnosis and Management.* Portland, OR: JBK Publishing, 1994:40–87.
11. Peterson LJ: Complex odontogenic infections, in Peterson LJ, Ellis E, Hupp JR, et al (eds): *Contemporary Oral and Maxillofacial Surgery.* St. Louis: Mosby, 1988:409–424.
12. Klokkevold P: Common dental emergencies: evaluation and management for emergency physicians. *Emerg Med Clin North Am* 1989; 7(1):29–63.
13. Ahl DR, Hilgeman JL, Snyder JD: Periodontal emergencies. *Dent Clin North Am* 1986; 30(3):459–472.
14. Gibson DE, Verono AA: Dentistry in the emergency department. *J Emerg Med* 1987; 5(1):35–44.
15. Peterson LJ: Principles of management of impacted teeth, in Peterson LJ, Ellis E, Hupp JR, et al (eds): *Contemporary Oral and Maxillofacial Surgery.* St. Louis: Mosby, 1988:223–256.
16. Josell SD, Abrams RG: Managing common dental problems and emergencies. *Pediatr Clin North Am* 1995; 38(5):1325–1342.

Chapter 156

POST-EXTRACTION PAIN AND DRY SOCKET (ALVEOLAR OSTEITIS) MANAGEMENT

Austen Chai

INTRODUCTION

Post-extraction pain, or periosteitis, begins as the local anesthetic agent wears off. The pain begins to diminish, most of the time, within 12 hours. The prescription of nonsteroidal anti-inflammatory drugs will provide analgesia and comfort while the pain subsides over 1 to 2 days. Narcotic analgesics may occasionally be required for the first 24 to 48 hours.

Pain that develops 2 to 4 days after the tooth extraction most likely indicates a localized alveolar osteitis or a dry socket. A dry socket occurs most commonly with the extraction of the third mandibular molar, but can be associated with any tooth that has been extracted. The pain is quite severe in nature. The signs of an infection are absent.

ANATOMY AND PATHOPHYSIOLOGY

The etiology or the pathogenesis of a dry socket is not clear.[1-6] It is believed to be caused by an increased level of fibrinolysis of the blood clot in the socket before the clot has had the time to be replaced by granulation tissue. The clot falls out of the socket and exposes the bony surface of the socket to the oral cavity. The exposed bone is extremely sensitive, resulting in severe pain.[1-4] The extraction site may emit a foul odor and the patient often complains of a bad taste in their mouth.[1,2]

INDICATIONS

The single and utmost therapeutic goal of alveolar osteitis is to relieve the patient's pain during the healing process. This procedure should be performed on all patients with a dry socket.

CONTRAINDICATIONS

There are no contraindications to the management of a dry socket.

EQUIPMENT

Dental mirror
2×2 gauze squares
Scissors
Dry socket paste
Gelfoam
Irrigating syringe
Normal saline solution
Frazier suction catheter
Suction source and tubing
Forceps
Iodoform ribbon gauze
Eugenol-impregnated ribbon gauze
Oil of cloves

PATIENT PREPARATION

Explain the risks, benefits, potential complications, and aftercare to the patient and/or their representative. A signed consent is not required for this procedure. Place the patient sitting upright or supine. A multipositional dental chair is ideal and allows for a variety of positions to visualize the affected tooth. This procedure may be accomplished with no anesthesia. Consider performing a dental block to temporarily alleviate the patient's pain and allow the procedure to be accomplished with minimal discomfort, and increase the level of patient satisfaction. Refer to Chapter 154 for the complete details regarding dental anesthesia and analgesia. Consider obtaining radiographs to rule out a retained root tip or other foreign material.

TECHNIQUES

Identify the defective tooth. Gently and thoroughly irrigate the socket with normal saline to remove any debris. Pack dry socket paste into the socket. Dry socket paste is composed of balsa wood fragments saturated with eucalyptol and looks like chewing tobacco. Com-

pletely fill the socket with the dry socket paste. The patient will experience almost instant pain relief if a dental block was not performed. Place a piece of Gelfoam on top of the dry socket paste. Compress the Gelfoam and dry socket paste into the socket. Instruct the patient to bite down against a 2×2 gauze square placed over the socket for 5 to 10 minutes.

Unfortunately, few Emergency Departments stock dry socket paste. An alternative is ribbon gauze impregnated with eugenol, iodine, or oil of cloves. Pack the socket completely with ribbon gauze (Figures 156-1A, B, and C). Place a piece of Gelfoam on top of the ribbon gauze (Figure 156-1D). Compress the Gelfoam and ribbon gauze into the socket. Instruct the patient to bite down against a 2×2 gauze square placed over the socket for 5 to 10 minutes.

AFTERCARE

The patient may be discharged immediately after the procedure. Nonsteroidal anti-inflammatory drugs are usually adequate to provide analgesia. Narcotic analgesics are not needed nor required. Arrange follow-up as soon as possible with the Dentist or Oral Surgeon

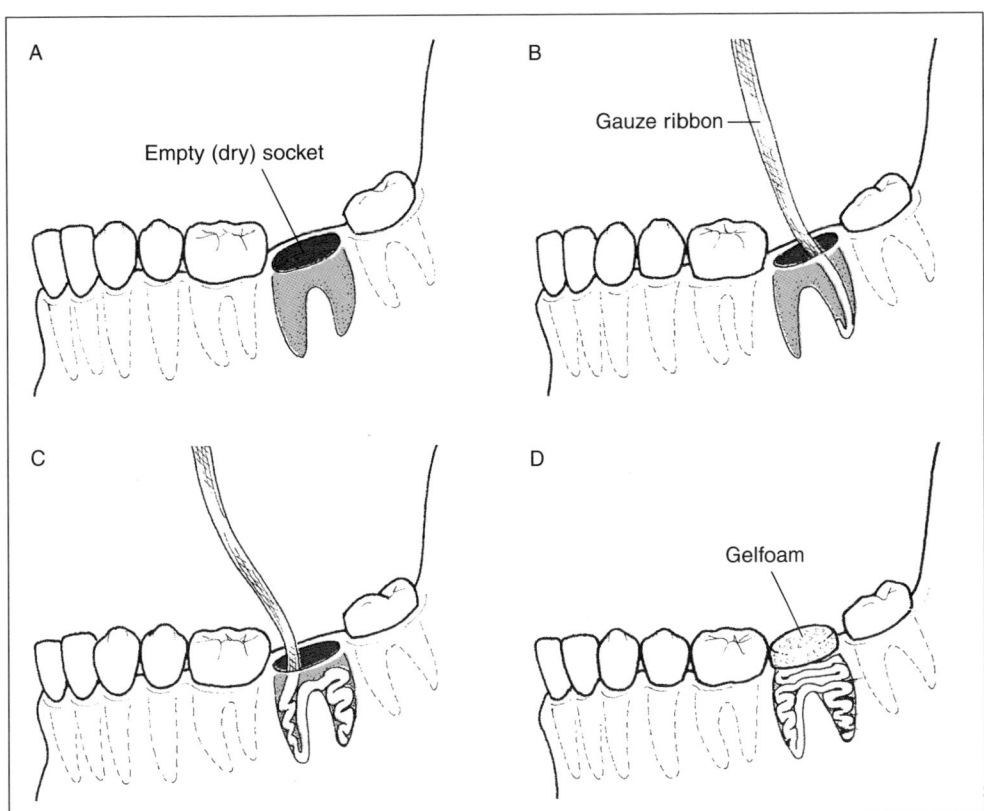

FIGURE 156-1 Packing a dry socket with ribbon gauze. *A.* The empty socket. *B.* Pack the socket starting inferiorly and working upwards. *C.* Completely fill the socket. *D.* Apply Gelfoam over the socket and the ribbon gauze.

who performed the extraction procedure. Replace the dressing daily, or as needed, until the patient is pain free. Prescribe antibiotics to cover the oral flora. Oral penicillin VK (500 mg QID) is the preferred antibiotic. Clindamycin (300 mg QID) is an alternative for patients allergic or intolerant to penicillin. Instruct the patient to begin a soft diet, to not ingest extremely hot or cold substances, and to not play with the packing with their tongue.

COMPLICATIONS

There are no complications associated with this procedure. A potential complication is the aspiration of the material used to pack the socket. This has never been reported in the literature. The packing may fall out and result in the patient's pain recurring. Instruct the patient to return to the Emergency Department if the packing falls out prior to their follow-up appointment.

SUMMARY

A dry socket can be extremely painful. Packing an empty socket is easy, quick, simple, and provides the patient with significant relief. The packing needs to be changed daily for several days and then less frequently after that, until the patient is free of pain. Prescribe antibiotics to cover oral flora and analgesics to manage pain.

REFERENCES

1. Peterson LJ: Prevention and management of surgical complications, in Peterson LJ, Ellis E III, Hupp JR (eds): *Contemporary Oral and Maxillofacial Surgery,* 3rd ed. St. Louis: Mosby-Year Book, 1998:257–275.
2. Neville BW, Damm DD, Allen CM: *Oral and Maxillofacial Pathology.* Philadelphia: Saunders, 1995:119–121.
3. Hermesch CB, Hilton TJ, Biesbrock AR, et al: Perioperative use of 0.12% chlorhexidine gluconate for the prevention of alveolar osteitis: efficacy and risk factor analysis. *Oral Surg Oral Med Oral Path Oral Radiol Endod* 1998; 85(4):381–387.
4. Birm H: Etiology and pathogenesis of fibro alveolitis (dry socket). *Int J Oral Surg* 1973; 2:241–246.
5. Colby RC: The general practitioner's perspective of the etiology, prevention, and treatment of dry socket. *Gen Dent* 1997; 45(5):461–467.
6. Garibaldi JA, Greenlaw J, Choi J, et al: Treatment of post-operative pain. *J Calif Dental Assoc* 1995; 23(4):71–74.

Chapter 157
POST-EXTRACTION BLEEDING MANAGEMENT

Austen Chai
Eric F. Reichman

INTRODUCTION

Post-extraction bleeding occurs after removal of a tooth. It is a common problem. It is often seen in the Emergency Department in the late evening or night when the patient is unable to contact their Dentist. The application of direct pressure over the bleeding site by having the patient bite down on a folded piece of moist gauze almost always controls post-extraction bleeding. Many patients, however, will report that they have been doing this prior to coming to the Emergency Department and request additional assistance.

ANATOMY AND PATHOPHYSIOLOGY

A careful history may reveal that the patient inadvertently caused the extraction site to bleed by drinking through a straw, spitting, gargling, or smoking. All these activities will produce negative pressure within the oral cavity and remove the clot from the extraction site. Ask the patient if they are touching the extraction site with their tongue, causing a mechanical disruption of the clot. Obtain information about any significant medical history, any history of bleeding, and current medications. This includes use of aspirin products, anticoagulants, broad-spectrum antibiotics, alcohol, and antineoplastic medications, all of which may contribute to prolonged bleeding. Ask about the symptoms and examine for the signs of liver disease, hypertension, or hematologic disorders.[1,2] Post-extraction bleeding may be a sign of an underlying and undiagnosed coagulopathy.

INDICATIONS

All post-extraction bleeding must be managed carefully and methodically. The techniques are easy to perform, simple, and straightforward.

CONTRAINDICATIONS

There are no contraindications to the management of post-extraction bleeding.

EQUIPMENT

2×2 gauze squares
Irrigating syringe
Dental mirror, optional
Local anesthetic solution containing
    1:100,000 epinephrine
23 to 25 gauge, 1.5 inch needle
5 mL syringe
Silk or plain gut sutures, 4–0 or 5–0
Absorbable gelatin sponge (Gelfoam)
Oxidized regenerated cellulose (Surgicel)
Suture set
Dental forceps
Tea bag, optional
Bone rongeur
Bone wax
Headlamp
Yankauer suction catheter
Suction source and tubing
Silver nitrate matchsticks
Electrocautery unit

PATIENT PREPARATION

Explain the risks, benefits, potential complications, and aftercare to the patient and/or their representative. Document this discussion in the medical record. A signed consent form is usually not required for these procedures. Consider obtaining a radiograph of the affected area to rule out a retained root or a bony spur.

Position the patient to visualize the extraction site. Place the patient in a multipositional dental chair, if available, or on a gurney. Do not place the patient in a chair as they may become pre-syncopal and require being placed supine to prevent injury. An overhead light source or a headlamp is ideal to illuminate the field. Suction any blood and oral secretions from the mouth. Visualize the extraction site for any signs of bleeding. Thoroughly irrigate the site with saline and remove all clots with the aid of suction. It may be necessary to perform a dental block if the patient complains of pain upon irrigation. Refer to Chapter 154 for the complete details regarding dental anesthesia and analgesia.

TECHNIQUES

Management of post-extraction bleeding is simple. Numerous methods to control the bleeding have been described and tested (Table 157-1). These techniques are often performed in a sequential manner as described below. The techniques may, of course, be performed in any order, depending on the physical examination and physician preference.

MECHANICAL PRESSURE

Place saline-moistened 2×2 gauze squares within the socket. Apply firm pressure by having the patient bite down on the gauze for 20 minutes. Instruct the patient to maintain pressure for 20 minutes despite initial bleeding. Place the suction catheter, intermittently, into the vestibule of the mouth to remove any blood and secretions. The application of pressure will control most post-extraction bleeding. It may be necessary to perform a dental block, if not performed during the irrigation phase, if the patient cannot bite down due to pain.

TEA BAG APPLICATION

Place a saline-moistened tea bag in the socket if mechanical pressure does not control the bleeding. The tannins in the tea leaves will assist with the coagulation process. Instruct the patient to bite down on the tea bag for 15 minutes.

TABLE 157-1. METHODS TO CONTROL POST-EXTRACTION BLEEDING

Absorbable dressing into socket and mechanical pressure with gauze squares
Absorbable dressing into socket and stitch gingival tissue closed
Cauterize bleeding granulation tissue
Cauterize or stitch bleeding blood vessels
Gingival infiltration with local anesthetic containing epinephrine
Mechanical pressure with gauze squares
Moist tea bag and pressure
Rongeur or apply bone wax to bone spurs
Stitch gingival tears

ABSORBABLE DRESSINGS

The two most commonly used absorbable dressings are Gelfoam and Surgicel. Gelfoam is an absorbable gelatin sponge that is readily available and inexpensive. It forms a scaffold for the formation of a blood clot. Surgicel is composed of oxidized and regenerated cellulose. It promotes coagulation better than Gelfoam and can be packed into the socket under pressure. Unfortunately, Surgicel results in delayed healing of the socket and its use should be reserved for persistent bleeding or when Gelfoam is not available.

Place an absorbable dressing (Gelfoam or Surgicel) in the socket if the extraction site continues to bleed.[1-3] The authors prefer to use Gelfoam because it is easier to manipulate and because it absorbs more rapidly than Surgicel. Work the Gelfoam in your fingers until it resembles the shape of the socket. Insert the Gelfoam into the socket and compact it with a dental forceps. Insert additional pieces of Gelfoam into the socket, as necessary, to obtain a solid mass of Gelfoam filling the socket. An alternative is to pack the socket with Surgicel. Apply a 2×2 gauze square over the socket. Instruct the patient to bite down for approximately 30 minutes. The editors prefer to place a figure-of-eight stitch using 4–0 or 5–0 silk suture or plain gut suture over the socket (Figure 157-1). The suture applies pressure over the socket and ensures that the Gelfoam or Surgicel will not prematurely fall out of the socket. This technique will usually stop most post-extraction bleeding.

Two additional absorbable dressings are topical thrombin and collagen. They are expensive, not usually available in the Emergency Department, and their use should be limited to circumstances where other hemostasis methods have failed. Topical thrombin is made from bovine thrombin. Place a piece of Gelfoam saturated with thrombin into the socket. Thrombin converts fibrinogen to fibrin, bypassing the coagulation cascade, to form a clot within the socket. Collagen is available in multiple forms from a variety of sources. It promotes platelet aggregation and forms a scaffold for the formation of a clot. Pack the socket with collagen and cover it with a piece of Gelfoam. Place a figure-of-eight suture over the thrombin or collagen filled socket to secure it in place.

LOCAL ANESTHETIC INFILTRATION

Infiltrate the soft tissue surrounding the socket with local anesthetic solution containing epinephrine if the bleeding is not controlled by the above methods. The most commonly used local anesthetic solutions are lidocaine and bupivacaine. Infiltrate the soft tissues surrounding the socket with the local anesthetic solution until the tissue blanches. This usually requires 2 to 3 mL of the local anesthetic solution. Irrigate the socket. Apply a piece of moist gauze over the socket. Instruct the patient to bite down and to exert pressure on the socket. The patient is often able to bite down much harder on

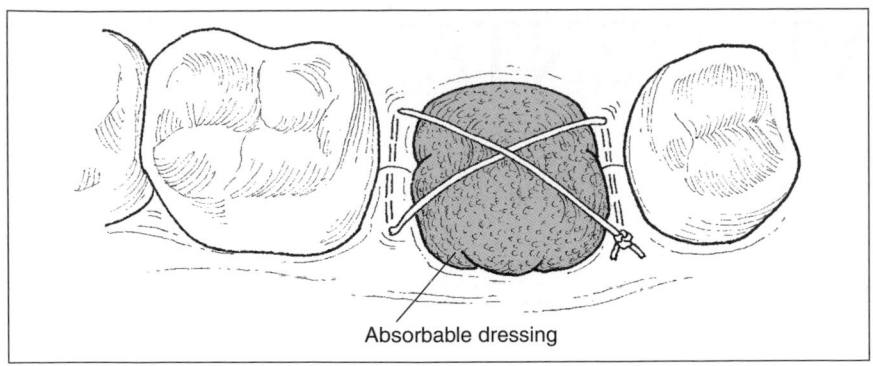

FIGURE 157-1 Pack the socket with Gelfoam followed by a figure-of-eight stitch to control the bleeding.

Absorbable dressing

the tissues after the infiltration of the local anesthetic solution.

The effect of mechanical pressure combined with the vasoconstrictive effects of epinephrine control the bleeding. Occasionally, after the vasoconstrictive effect of epinephrine wears off, there is a rebound effect and the persistence of bleeding. This may be prevented by routinely placing Gelfoam or Surgicel into the socket.

MISCELLANEOUS TECHNIQUES

Reexamine the extraction site if the bleeding is not controlled by the above methods. The source of bleeding may be new granulation tissue, gingival tears, a bone spur, or a partially transected vessel. Cauterization of granulation tissue with silver nitrate or electrocautery will control the bleeding. Use a blunt instrument to feel for the presence of a bone spur. This may be a source of significant bleeding. Remove the bone spur with a rongeur or cover it with bone wax to control the bleeding. An exposed and bleeding arteriole or venule can be controlled with cauterization (silver nitrate or electrocautery) or the application of a plain gut suture through the vessel. Suture any tears in the gingiva.

ASSESSMENT

Observe the patient for 30 to 60 minutes after the bleeding has terminated. Do not give the patient anything by mouth (NPO). Reevaluate the socket for signs of bleeding. Continued bleeding requires further attempts at termination.

AFTERCARE

Discharge the patient home after the bleeding has been terminated and a brief observation period. Instruct the patient to avoid any liquids or solids for 2 hours. Stress the importance of not spitting, gargling, drinking through a straw, smoking, using aspirin-containing products, or playing with the site with their tongue. Instruct the patient to apply gauze squares and bite down for 20 minutes if the bleeding returns. Additional in-

structions should include a soft diet, avoidance of extremely hot or cold substances, avoidance of chewing gum, and avoidance of other such "sticky" foods. They should return promptly to the Emergency Department if the bleeding continues after 20 minutes. Arrange follow-up as soon as possible with the Dentist or Oral Surgeon who performed the extraction.

COMPLICATIONS

There are no documented complications associated with the termination of post-extraction bleeding. The complications are associated with the bleeding itself. Obtain screening labs (PT, PTT, platelet count, and bleeding times) if hemostasis is not achieved by any of the aforementioned methods. Early consultation with a Dentist or Oral Surgeon and a Hematologist should be considered if the patient is coagulopathic or has a bleeding disorder.

SUMMARY

A careful history and physical examination will often provide the reasons for most post-extraction bleeding that presents to the Emergency Department. Most patients without complicating medical conditions will be easily managed in a simple and systematic manner with a minimal amount of equipment. All patients should follow-up with their Dentist or Oral Surgeon after the bleeding is terminated.

REFERENCES

1. Peterson LJ: Prevention and management of surgical complications, in Peterson LJ, Ellis E III, Hupp JR (eds): *Contemporary Oral and Maxillofacial Surgery,* 3rd ed. St. Louis: Mosby-Year Book, 1998:257–275.
2. Souis S: *Principles and Practice of Oral Medicine,* 2nd ed. Philadelphia: Saunders, 1995:249–261.
3. Simon RR, Brenner BE: *Emergency Procedures and Techniques,* 3rd ed. Baltimore: William & Wilkins, 1994:283.

Chapter 158
DEFECTIVE DENTAL RESTORATION MANAGEMENT

Daniel J. Ross

INTRODUCTION

Management of defective dental restorations may seem initially like a daunting task to the Emergency Physician. The treatment of common dental emergencies is published in the *Emergency Medicine Clinics of North America* under the heading "Difficult and Advanced Procedures."[1] The urgent management of these conditions can be relatively simple for the clinician armed with a modicum of knowledge of dental anatomy, pathophysiology, and various treatment modalities.[1,2] The astute clinician must also recognize the inherent limitations of treating these problems in the Emergency Department.

Patients frequently present to the Emergency Department with some sort of dental complaint.[1-4] They typically complain of discomfort.[1,2] They may or may not be aware of the etiology of the discomfort. The patient's chief complaint may be directed at a particular tooth. Be diligent in searching the entire mouth for alternative primary, comorbid, or secondary problems. The recognition of frequently encountered comorbid problems such as root fractures, periapical abscesses, and dentofacial trauma are beyond the scope of this chapter.

The perioral tissues are exceptionally sensitive to noxious stimuli. This is particularly true for the oral mucosa, the periodontal ligament, and the dentin. This concept is paramount to the effective management of any dental-related complaint. The management of defective dental restorations is essentially as simple as relieving the patient's discomfort and employing temporizing measures until they can be followed-up by the appropriate specialist.

ANATOMY AND PATHOPHYSIOLOGY

A meaningful discussion of the management of defective dental restorations requires a brief outline of the available types of dental appliances. In general, dental appliances are either fixed or removable. Fixed dental appliances are considered permanently attached to the teeth. They include crowns, bridges, implants, some forms of dentures, orthodontic bands and brackets, interdental wiring, and any type of filling (silver amalgam, gold, porcelain, or tooth-colored composite material). Removable dental appliances are those that are not permanently attached to the teeth and include partial dentures, complete dentures, space-maintenance devices, and other orthodontic devices.

A few basic principles will help guide the nondental practitioner in treating patients with a defective dental restoration. Know your limitations. A defective dental restoration is rarely, if ever, a true emergency.[2] Refer the patient to a Dentist if you are unfamiliar with an appliance or a presentation, or if there is any hesitancy to treat. Always consider a secondary or comorbid process. Obtain dental radiographs when in doubt. Treat the tooth for dental trauma if a restoration is determined to be defective secondary to trauma. Never remove a fixed appliance without first discussing it with a specialist, preferably the one who placed it. Always treat pain, inflammation, and evidence of infection. Always consider ingestion or aspiration when dealing with a multiply fragmented appliance. Obtain neck, chest, and abdominal radiographs if all appliance fragments cannot be accounted for. It is probably best to do as little as possible if a patient is actively involved in an ongoing treatment process. Always use caution and tact when discussing the possibility of a defective dental restoration with a patient. Remember that you are not an expert. The treating specialist may have insight into the patient's current condition that you are unaware exist. Always arrange follow-up within 24 to 48 hours with a dental specialist.

Removable appliances can predispose patients to easily treatable mucosal conditions.[5-7] Exposure to broad-spectrum antibiotics or chemotherapeutic agents, compromised cellular immunity, xerostomia, lack of good oral hygiene measures, and trauma from poorly fitting dentures can lead to oral candidal overgrowth.[5,8] Patients often complain of burning pain. Treat the oral cavity with nystatin or clotrimazole troches. The appliance itself may harbor the organism and must be treated. Instruct the patient to take the appliance out of their mouth for 24 to 48 hours and soak it overnight in a nystatin suspension [5 mL nystatin in 250 mL (8 ounces) of tap water]. Instruct the patient to scrub the denture daily with an approved product to clean it.[5–7]

Oral candidiasis must be differentiated from other mucosal ulcerating conditions such as simple traumatic ulcers, aphthous ulcers, and oral herpes. Herpetic lesions occur on attached mucosa only, whereas aphthous ulcers occur on unattached mucosa.[5–8] Traumatic ulcers, minor aphthae, and major aphthae can be treated with topical corticosteroid ointment, such as triamcinolone, applied with a cotton-tipped applicator. The symptoms associated with herpetic outbreaks can be diminished if treated with acyclovir.[5–7] Orthodontic or interdental wiring that is impinging upon the oral mucosa may lead to traumatic ulcerations. Apply soft dental wax directly to the irritating appliance to relieve the impingement. This can be easily removed or replaced and is available over the counter at many local pharmacies.

In general, all patients with painful mucosal conditions may benefit from soft and bland diets, frequent use of ice chips for comfort, and frequent warm saltwater rinses to avoid superinfection.[5,6] A stomatitis cocktail or BMX solution may be helpful for patients with severe mucosal pain. Mix equal amounts of Benadryl (12.5mg/ 5 mL), Maalox, and Xylocaine (2% viscous lidocaine). Instruct the patient to swish 30 mL in their mouth for 1 minute and then spit it out.

The repair of defective or broken removable appliances in the Emergency Department is not recommended even though over-the-counter products are available for the home repair of broken dentures (Figure 158-1). These procedures can be tedious, time-consuming, and fraught with complications—even for the trained dental professional. The appliances are expensive, highly technical, and required multiple hours by both the Dentist and the dental lab technician to fabricate. An inappropriate repair attempt can result in patient discomfort, morbidity, and irreversible damage to an otherwise salvageable appliance. **In this light, it seems best to recommend referral or a home repair product to the patient seeking care for a defective removable appliance.**

The temporary and urgent repair of defective fixed dental restorations by nondental personnel is advocated throughout the literature.[2–4,6,9–11] Use caution because sensitivity from recent dental procedures can occur from pulpal or periodontal ligament (PDL) irritation. This may be expected sequelae of the dental procedure and not necessarily an indication that the restoration is defective.[1,12] **Do not alter a fixed restoration if it is firmly in place.** Trauma from occlusion can result if a new dental restoration is left "too high" and does not fit properly with the opposing dentition.[6,9–12] These patients complain of pain with mastication and are sensitive to percussion secondary to PDL irritation. Simple temporizing measures include dental blocks (Chapter 154), oral analgesics, a soft diet, and possibly removing the tooth from occlusion by placing a small amount of soft dental wax (or something similar) between the teeth on the opposite side.[9]

Long-standing fixed dental restorations may be defective secondary to microleakage or recurrent decay around the margins of the restoration.[1,12] Estimates suggest that approximately 1 of 3 restorations in existence may be defective in some fashion.[12,13] A faulty restoration that sits within or upon a tooth can lead to dentinal exposure regardless of the etiology. **Exposed dentin is highly sensitive and prone to further decay.** Dentinal sensitivity (also known as reversible pulpitis) is typically nonspontaneous and fleeting.[1,8,10,14] Patients who complain of spontaneous and lasting sensitivity have an

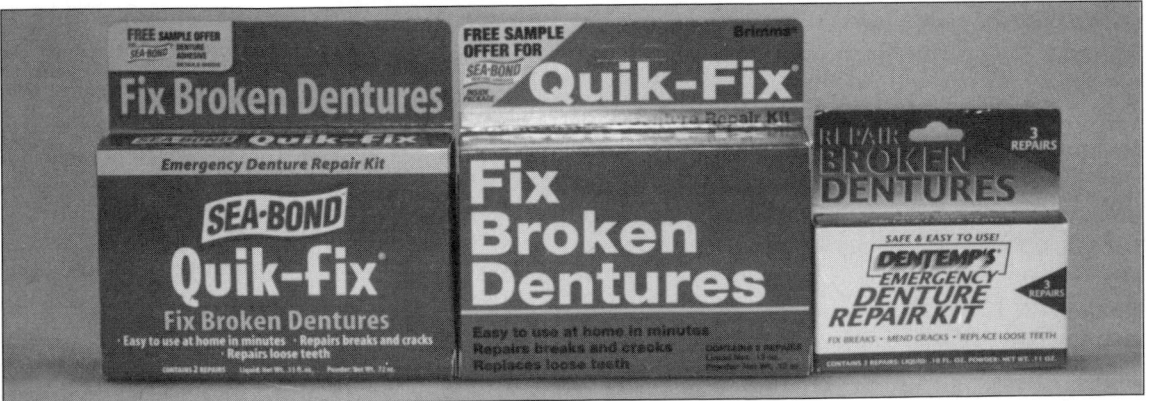

FIGURE 158-1 Commercially available home repair kits for the fractured denture.

irreversible pulpitis that is most likely due to recurrent decay. Sensitivity to percussion is indicative of periapical involvement and suggests the possibility of a periapical periodontitis or an abscess.[1,6,8,10,14]

Evaluate the tooth and its restoration for recurrent decay or a possible dentinal exposure if a patient presents complaining of sensitivity associated with a tooth that has a long-standing restoration. **A temporary restoration can easily be fabricated in the Emergency Department if the restoration in question is missing, broken, or easily removed.**

Consideration should be given to a possible pulpal pathology, as outlined above, if a restoration is firmly in place. Provide dental anesthesia, oral analgesics, antibiotics as necessary, and a referral to a Dentist. Refer to Chapter 155 for the details regarding the management of dental abscesses.

INDICATIONS

Replace any previously fixed, permanent or temporary, dental restoration that has completely or partially fallen out or that is easily removed with a dental explorer. Replace any previously fixed, permanent or temporary, crown that has fallen out or is easily removed with a dental explorer and is in the patient's possession.

CONTRAINDICATIONS

Relative contraindications for the placement of a temporary dental filling include patients who are involved with an extensive ongoing dental treatment plan, have a consulting specialist readily available, are at a significant aspiration risk, or have obvious extensive comorbid or secondary processes including antecedent trauma.

EQUIPMENT

10 mL syringe
18 gauge angiocatheter
Normal saline solution
Local anesthetic solution that contains epinephrine
Dental mirror
Dental explorer
2×2 gauze squares
Sterile cotton rolls
Dental floss
Cavit-G
IRM (zinc oxide and eugenol)
Dycal (calcium hydroxide paste)
Copalite (cavity varnish) or clear acrylic nail polish
Tin foil
Cotton-tipped applicators

Discoid-cleoid dental carver
Articulating paper
Fraser suction catheters
Suction source and tubing
Petrolatum-based lubricant (Vaseline)
Good overhead lighting

PATIENT PREPARATION

Explain the procedure, its risks, complications, and aftercare to the patient and/or their representative. Obtain an informed consent for the procedure. The simple placement of a temporary filling does not usually require local anesthesia. However, consider the use of a dental block if the patient is uncomfortable. Refer to Chapter 154 for the complete details regarding dental anesthesia and analgesia.

Prepare the patient. Seat the patient in a multipositional procedure chair. Gently irrigate the area with a syringe that contains normal saline and is armed with an 18 gauge angiocatheter to remove any food debris. Warm saline is usually less sensitive to the exposed dentin.[1] Gently remove any debris that does not irrigate away with a dental explorer. **Do not attempt to remove any decay because doing so may lead to a complicating pulpal exposure.**[1] Remove the loose portion of the restoration. **Do not remove any firmly fixed portion of the restoration.**

It is mandatory to have a dry field when performing this procedure. Dry the area to be filled with sterile cotton pellets or compressed air. Remember that the tooth may be sensitive.

TECHNIQUES

REPLACING A TEMPORARY OR PERMANENT FILLING

Treatment of defective fillings depends upon the relative size of the defect. There are no specific guidelines of what size (i.e., how many millimeters) the defect must be to perform each of these techniques. Paint small dentinal exposures with calcium hydroxide paste followed by cavity varnish or clear acrylic nail polish to relieve sensitivity.[1,3,6,11] Alternatively, place a simple tin foil dressing over the tooth to act as a bandage following placement of the calcium hydroxide paste.[3,6,11]

Larger defects require a filling to avoid food impaction and other sequelae. Cavit-G is an excellent choice for temporary filling material, especially in inexperienced hands.[1,3,4,15] This material is premixed, nonirritating, and sets quickly (approximately 30 minutes) upon contact with saliva. IRM, or a mixture of zinc oxide and eugenol, is a similar material with the benefit of pulpal sedative properties. The use of IRM is operator dependent and requires a longer setting time.[15] Oddly enough, multiple mixtures of zinc oxide and eugenol are available over-the-counter for home use (Dentemp, Tempanol, Thin Set; Figure 158-2).

Cavit-G is recommended for Emergency Department use. Determine whether the missing filling exposes an open endodontically treated root (i.e., root canal). Place a small sterile cotton pellet into the canal prior to placing the filling material if the pulp cavity is exposed.[15] Express a small amount of Cavit-G from the container. Apply it onto the cavity and condense it into the cavity with the moistened end of a cotton-tipped applicator or a dental explorer (Figure 158-3*A*). A temporary restoration placed by nondental personnel is always better "short" and out of occlusion with the opposing tooth for patient comfort. **Work quickly because Cavit-G can set rapidly and it may be difficult to remove once it sets.** Remove any excess Cavit-G with the stick end of the cotton-tipped applicator. Instruct the patient to fully occlude on the new restoration and grind their teeth back and forth in all directions for 5 to 10 minutes. This will form the occlusal aspect of the filling to fit the opposing teeth.

Remove any excess material with the stick end of the cotton-tipped applicator. Use the discoid-cleoid dental carver to remove excess material once it begins to harden (Figure 158-3*B*). Use dental floss to contour a proper embrasure and clear excess material from the gingival tissues. **Use the dental floss in a downward direction only. Never bring the dental floss back up toward the occlusal surface because doing so risks dislodging the new restoration.** Simply pull the dental floss through after one downward pass around the tooth.

REPLACING A TEMPORARY OR PERMANENT CROWN

The patient preparation required for this procedure is essentially the same as that for replacing a temporary filling. However, avoid dental anesthesia if possible to allow better patient proprioception. This will provide the clinician with a crucial aid in assessing the orientation and occlusion of the final restoration.[1] The same over-the-counter mixtures for repairing a filling may be used to temporarily replace a crown (Figure 158-2).

Reapply the crown to ensure that it fits properly. It is often necessary to remove a small amount of the existing cement from within the patient's existing restoration in order to provide an adequate seal and a proper occlusion.[1] This may or may not be possible to do with the discoid-cleoid dental carver. The nondental clinician is advised against the use of rotary instruments for this purpose, as these may irreversibly damage the inside of the coping. Reinsert the patient's crown after removing some of the cement to assure a proper fit and proper occlusion. Make an attempt using the alternative technique described below if sufficient preexisting cement cannot be removed and the crown seats properly. Treat dentinal sensitivity as outlined above (i.e., as replacing a filling) if the appliance does not seat at all.

Proceed with this technique if the restoration appears to fit and a small amount of preexisting cement can be removed from the inside. Prepare the area. Apply a thin layer of petrolatum-based lubricant (Vaseline) to the mucosal tissues surrounding the tooth to aid in the cleanup. **Do not contaminate the prepared tooth with the lubricant.**

Prepare or mix a thin consistency of zinc oxide and eugenol cement. Place a very small amount of the mixture into the preexisting crown with a cotton-tipped applicator.[6,9,10] Place the crown on the tooth and in the proper orientation. Firmly and fully seat the crown with firm finger pressure. Remove any excess cement material from around the margin of the newly cemented restoration. This may be easier once the material has hardened. Instruct the patient to gently and fully occlude on the restoration. **Ensure proper occlusion.** Ask the patient to provide a subjective report if their occlusion feels like baseline (i.e., does their bite feel funny). Con-

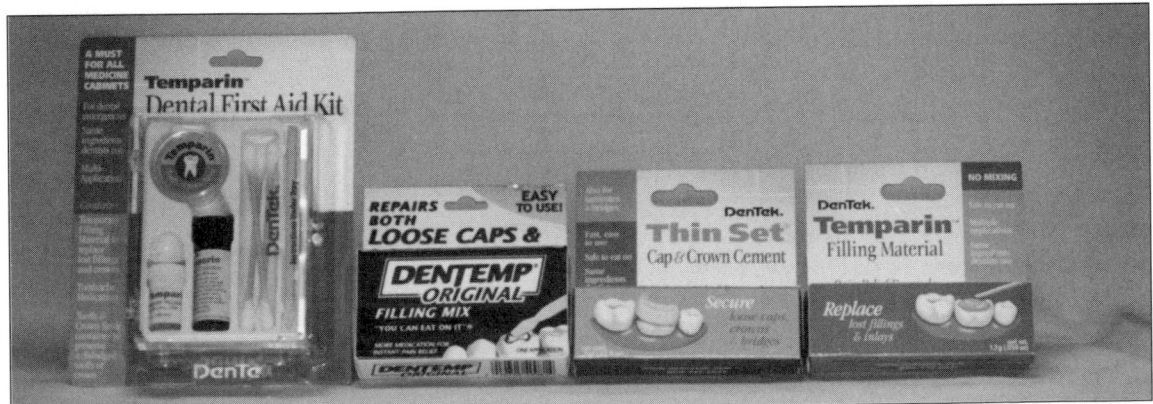

FIGURE 158-2 Commercially available home use products for temporary dental filling and crown restoration.

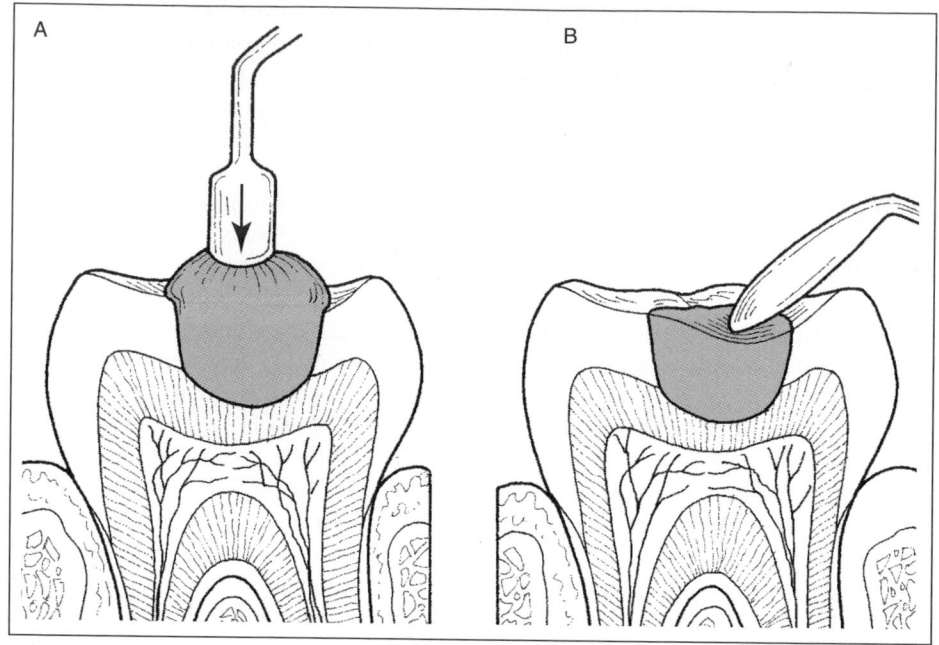

FIGURE 158-3 Application of temporary restorative material. *A.* Pack the material into the defect and condense it. *B.* Remove any excess material.

firm this using articulating paper to ensure that the contact marks are light or minimal. Wipe the petrolatum-based lubricant from the mucosal tissues.

A simpler, alternative, and far more temporary method of replacing a crown involves using Vaseline as the cementing agent.[1] Apply a thin layer of Vaseline to the inside of the coping. It may be necessary to remove a small amount of the preexisting cement. Seat the crown on the tooth in the proper orientation. Ensure proper occlusion. Warn the patient that the crown may come off again and about the risk of aspiration. Instructions may be given to the patient for repeating the procedure at home.

ASSESSMENT

Check the patient's occlusion. It may be necessary to use articulating paper to ensure minimal or no contact with the opposing teeth with the temporary filling. The newly cemented crown restoration must primarily be assessed for proper occlusion. The patient's subjective opinion is invaluable in this regard. Seal the restoration's margins to prevent continued dentinal sensitivity.

AFTERCARE

Instruct the patient not to eat or chew on their new restoration for at least 1 hour. Additional instructions should include a soft diet, avoidance of extremely hot or cold substances, avoidance of chewing gum, and avoidance of other such "sticky" foodstuffs. They may brush their teeth normally but should not floss adjacent to the new restoration. Warn them that they may experience some continued sensitivity. Nonsteroidal anti-inflammatory drugs will provide any needed analgesia. Arrange follow-up within 24 to 48 hours.

COMPLICATIONS

Typical complications of replacing a filling include improper occlusion and poor retention of the restoration. The solution for both problems is replacing the restoration. Adjust the occlusion with the discoid-cleoid dental carver. Treat the restoration as a dental restoration that is "too high" if using the discoid-cleoid dental carver is not effective. Treat the tooth as a simple dentinal exposure if a temporary restoration is continually falling out. An unlikely complication would be a pulpal exposure, manifested as minimal bleeding from within the tooth defect.[1,3,4] Manage this as a dental trauma or fractured tooth.

Typical complications for replacing a crown are similar to those listed in replacing a temporary filling. These restorations are often easily removed with a slight twisting motion. A restoration that is seated "too high" should be replaced. Treat the tooth as a simple dentinal exposure if a restoration is consistently "too high."

SUMMARY

Management of the patient with a dental complaint may initially seem intimidating to the nondental clinician. The recognition and treatment of dental pain, minor defective dental restorations, and painful mucosal conditions can be relatively simple provided a minimal understanding of basic dentistry. Emergency Physicians must be cognizant of the inherent limitations involved in treating these patients in the Emergency Department. Have a low threshold for referral. Pain, inflammation, and infection should always be treated. Refer patients to the appropriate specialist within 24 to 48 hours.

REFERENCES

1. Klokkevold P: Common dental emergencies: evaluation and management for emergency physicians. *Emerg Med Clin North Am* 1989; 1:29–63.
2. Gibson DE, Verono AA: Dentistry in the emergency department. *J Emerg Med* 1987; 5(1):35–44.
3. Antrim DD: Treatment of traumatic dental injuries by nondental personnel. *US Navy Med* 1983; 74(3):18–23.
4. Amsterdam JT: Emergency dental procedures, in Roberts JR, Hedges JR (eds): *Clinical Procedures in Emergency Medicine*, 3rd ed. Philadelphia: Saunders, 1998:1045–1064.
5. Glass BJ, Kuel RF, Langlais RP: Treatment of common orofacial conditions. *Dent Clin North Am* 1986; 30(3):421–446.
6. Ross DJ, Kirsch T: Dental emergencies, in Vanrooyen M, Kirsch T, Clem K, et al (eds): *Emergent Field Medicine*. New York: McGraw-Hill, 2001: 276–302.
7. Neville BW, Damm DD, White, DK, et al: *Color Atlas of Clinical Oral Pathology*, 1st ed. Philadelphia: Lea & Febiger, 1991.
8. Regezi JA, Sciubba JJ: *Oral Pathology: Clinical Pathologic Correlations*, 1st ed. Philadelphia: Saunders, 1989.
9. Morris JA Jr, Swiontkowski MF, Herrmann HJ: Wilderness trauma emergencies, in Auerbach PS (ed): *Wilderness Medicine*, 3rd ed. St. Louis: Mosby, 1995:343–352.
10. Blank LW, Charbeneau GT: Urgent treatment in operative dentistry. *Dent Clin North Am* 1986; 30(3):489–501.
11. Dickson M: *Where There Is No Dentist*, 1st ed. Berkley: The Hesperian Foundation, 1983.
12. Robertello FJ, Taybos GM, Cotton WR: Complications and prognostic considerations in operative dentistry. *Dent Clin North Am* 1986; 30(3):473–488.
13. Elderton RJ: The prevalence of failure of restorations: a literature review. *J Dent* 1976; 4(5):207–210.
14. Hicks JL, Vaughan GG: Odontogenic and periodontal sources of oral pain, in Montgomery MT, Redding SW (eds): *Orofacial Emergencies: Diagnosis and Management*. Portland, OR: JBK Publishing, 1994:1–39.
15. Segerdal MJN: *Temporary Dentistry*, 1st ed. LaCanada, CA: P.I.B.L., 1993.

Chapter 159
SUBLUXED AND AVULSED TOOTH MANAGEMENT

Suneel Upadhye
Daniel J. Ross

INTRODUCTION

Traumatic dental injuries are a common presentation to the Emergency Department. They can have significant cosmetic, functional, and psychological consequences for the patient. Studies estimate the incidence of Emergency Department visits for dentoalveolar trauma to be as high as 10 percent.[1] Approximately 50 percent of children will sustain traumatic dental injuries, the majority of these to the permanent teeth.[1-4]

The appropriate Emergency Department management of dental trauma depends heavily upon the type of tooth (permanent versus primary), the age of the tooth, the time elapsed since the incident, and the extent of the damage. Successful treatment of dental injuries requires a basic understanding of dental anatomy, terminology, and pathophysiology. Violence of a suspicious nature must always be considered when evaluating dental injuries. The goals of the emergent treatment of dental trauma are to maintain patient comfort and tooth vitality, while ensuring prompt dental follow-up for definitive care.

ANATOMY AND PATHOPHYSIOLOGY

TOOTH ANATOMY

There are significant differences in the adult and pediatric dentitions that impact their treatment in the Emergency Department (Figure 159-1). The pediatric dentition is known as the primary or deciduous dentition and consists of 20 teeth. These include 8 incisors, 4 canines, and 8 molars. The adult dentition consists of 32 teeth and is composed of 8 incisors, 4 canines, 8 premolars, and 12 molars. The variable absence of a tooth or the addition of an extra tooth is common in either dentition. The teeth in both the pediatric and adult dentitions erupt in a predictable sequence, albeit with considerable individual variation (Figure 159-1). Treat-

ment strategies differ for permanent versus deciduous (primary) teeth as well as by the age of the adult tooth. **Exercise great care when evaluating patients with a "mixed" dentition, roughly between the ages of 6 and 12 years.**

The anatomy of a tooth is rather simple (Figure 159-2). The tooth itself consists of a neurovascular pulp surrounded by supportive dentin, which is surrounded by a hard thick crown of enamel. The crown portion lies above the gum line or gingiva. The root portion lies embedded within the alveolar bone of the jaw, anchored by a thin layer of cementum and the periodontal ligament. The alveolar bone, periodontal ligament fibers, and fragile cementum cell layer taken together are considered a functional unit known as the attachment apparatus. A complete attachment apparatus requires an intact cementum cellular layer and a fully formed root apex. Immature adult teeth do not have a fully formed apex and necessitate special attention to maintain pulpal viability.[2,4,5]

TOOTH INJURY

Mechanisms of tooth injury include direct trauma (i.e., a blow) or occlusive trauma (i.e., biting on a hard object or a seizure). These mechanisms can result in a spectrum of injury patterns that vary from simple sensitivity to complete tooth avulsion. Crown and root fractures are discussed in Chapter 160. This chapter focuses on the diagnosis and management of dental subluxations and avulsions.

Appropriate treatment of dental injuries requires a thorough history and meticulous examination of the oral cavity, including subsequent radiographs after ruling out more serious injuries. Historically, important points include the age of the patient, the time of the trauma, the mechanism of injury, teeth or tooth pieces at the scene, subjective disturbance of bite, and treatments provided since the time of the incident. The physical examination must include an assessment of the

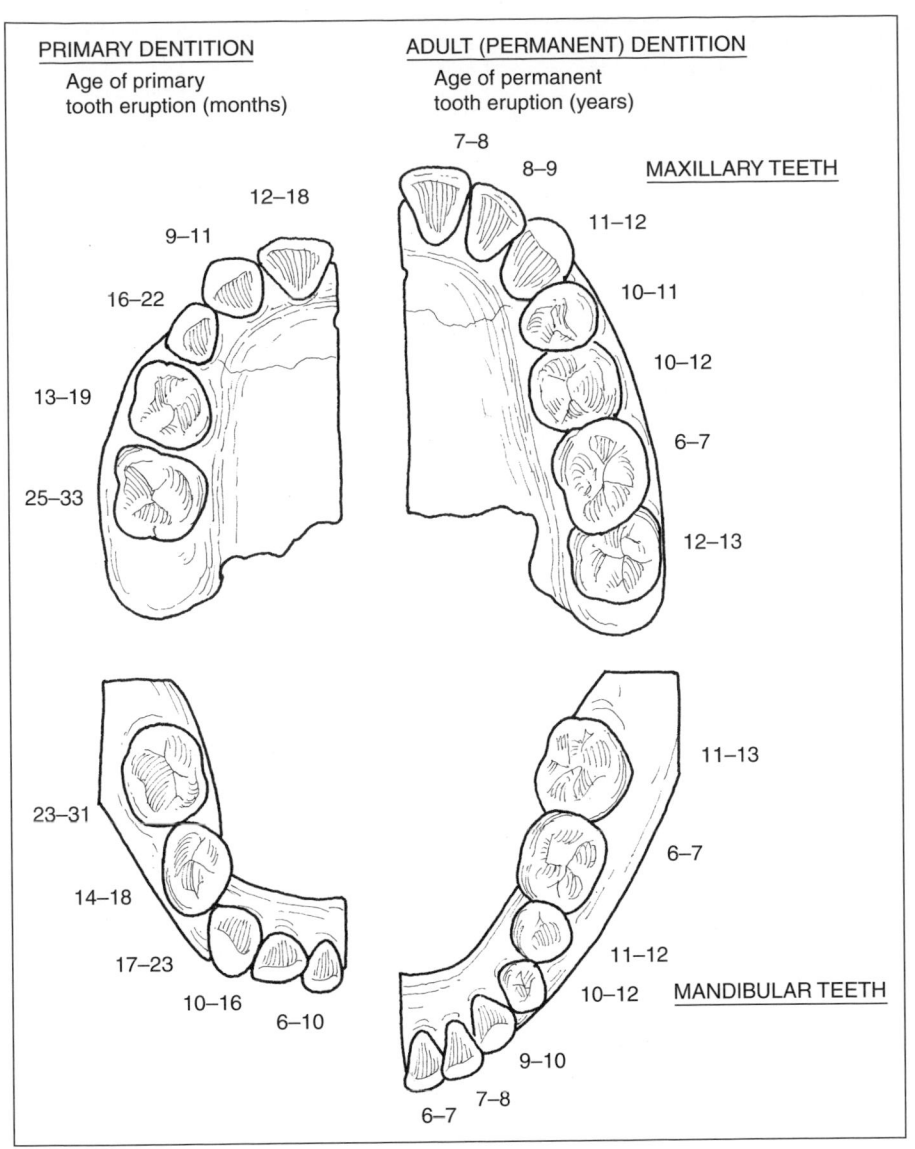

PRIMARY DENTITION
Age of primary
tooth eruption (months)

ADULT (PERMANENT) DENTITION
Age of permanent
tooth eruption (years)

MAXILLARY TEETH

MANDIBULAR TEETH

FIGURE 159-1 The normal eruptive patterns of the pediatric and adult dentition.

extraoral and intraoral soft tissues, bony displacement, missing teeth, crown fractures, pulp exposures, tooth sensitivity, and tooth mobility.

The need for radiographs with dental trauma is worth emphasizing. A tooth that is missing, both by history and physical examination, may be found completely intruded below the gum line, floating within the maxillary sinus or stomach, or even aspirated. **Obtain facial films if a tooth, or portion of a tooth, cannot be unequivocally located by history or physical examination. Strongly consider obtaining chest and abdominal radiographs if the tooth, or the portion in question, is not visualized on the facial films.**[1,2,6]

CONCUSSED AND SUBLUXED TEETH

Concussed teeth are essentially injured, nonmobile, and nonfractured teeth. These teeth have suffered a direct blow and are sensitive with no concrete clinical or radiographic evidence of injury. Subluxed teeth may or may not be sensitive, are not displaced, but are perceptively mobile when manipulated between two cotton applicators or other instruments. Mild gingival bleeding may be present. Both concussion and subluxation imply an injury to the attachment apparatus. Pain control, soft diet instructions, and follow-up with a Dentist are all that is required in the management of most of these injuries. Excessive mobility from a severe subluxation may be irritating, painful, and damaging. These injuries require a temporary splint for relief.[1,2,4–7] Subluxed and concussed primary and permanent teeth are treated in the same manner.[1,8]

LUXATED TEETH

Luxated teeth are displaced or dislocated from their usual position within the alveolus. They are commonly associated with other injuries such as alveolar fractures,

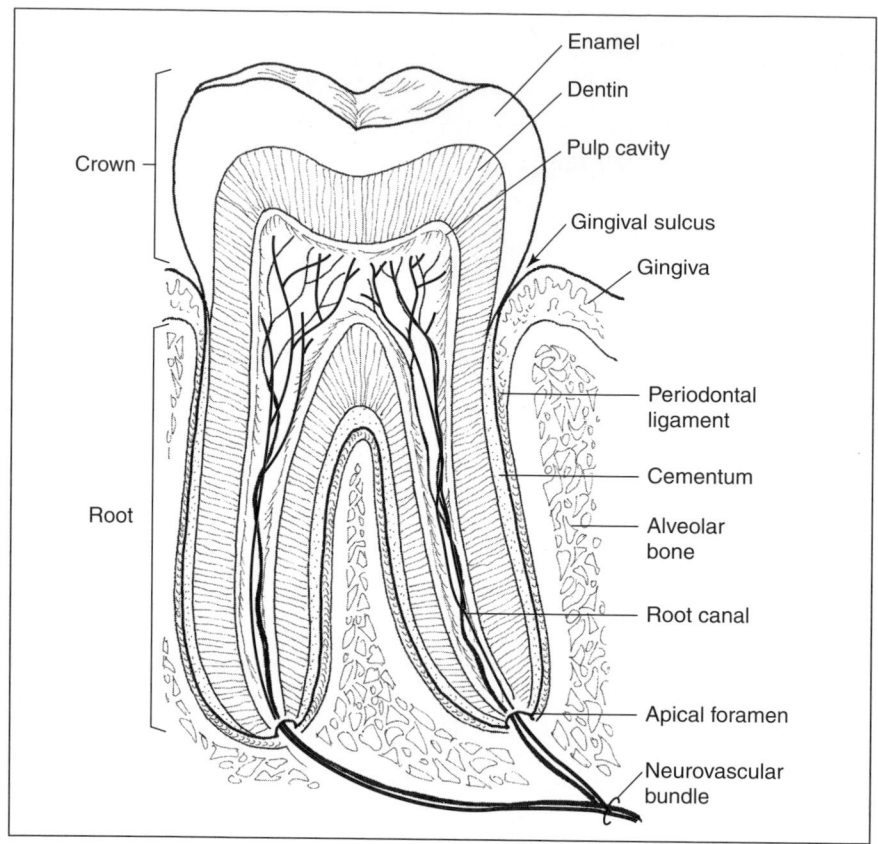

FIGURE 159-2 The dental anatomic unit (i.e., the tooth) and its supporting structures.

Labels: Enamel, Dentin, Pulp cavity, Gingival sulcus, Gingiva, Periodontal ligament, Cementum, Alveolar bone, Root canal, Apical foramen, Neurovascular bundle, Crown, Root

root fractures, and gingival lacerations.[1,7] Subcategories of injury within this class are described by the direction of the dislocation. Luxated teeth may be displaced laterally, intruded, or extruded (Figure 159-3). Lateral luxations may be mesial, distal, buccal, or lingual in direction. An alveolar fracture is self-evident when several teeth are luxated in a solid segment.

Extruded teeth represent a partial avulsion from the alveolar socket and a damaged attachment apparatus. They typically appear clinically longer than the surrounding teeth (Figure 159-3B). Patients may complain of an occlusal prematurity. There may be associated gingival bleeding. A hematoma surrounding the apex may preclude complete repositioning. These injuries are treated in the same manner as lateral luxations.[1,2,4] Extract any extruded primary teeth.[1]

Intrusion is a severe form of luxation injury with the tooth driven inward in an axial direction. These injuries are manifested by displacement of the tooth into the alveolar socket with a corresponding fracture of the alveolar bone surrounding the apex (Figure 159-3A). Adjacent structures, such as the floor of the nose or maxillary sinus, may be involved or damaged. These injuries may be so profound that the tooth is not visible within the oral cavity and believed to be avulsed. **It is worth reiterating that a tooth that cannot be unequivocally located on physical examination requires radiographic localization.** Immature adult teeth suffering intrusion injuries generally have the best prognosis. They are often left alone and allowed to re-erupt. Mature adult teeth often require surgical or orthodontically assisted re-eruption and root canal therapy. The intrusion of primary teeth frequently leads to damage of the developing permanent tooth buds and requires close dental follow-up. Rule out more serious injuries, arrange an expedited appointment for definitive care, prescribe appropriate analgesics, and give strong consideration to the prescription of antibiotics.[1,2,4,9]

AVULSED TEETH

Avulsed teeth are teeth that have been completely torn from their alveolar sockets. **The teeth have suffered profound attachment and neurovascular damage that progresses in a time-dependent fashion.** There is a high likelihood of associated injuries with this type of trauma. Perform a thorough evaluation of the entire oral cavity after any dried blood, clots, and debris have been removed. Bleeding can generally be controlled with firm digital pressure or local infiltration of an epinephrine-containing local anesthetic solution. Patients may present with the tooth in hand or may not be aware of the location of the tooth. **The onus is on the physician to**

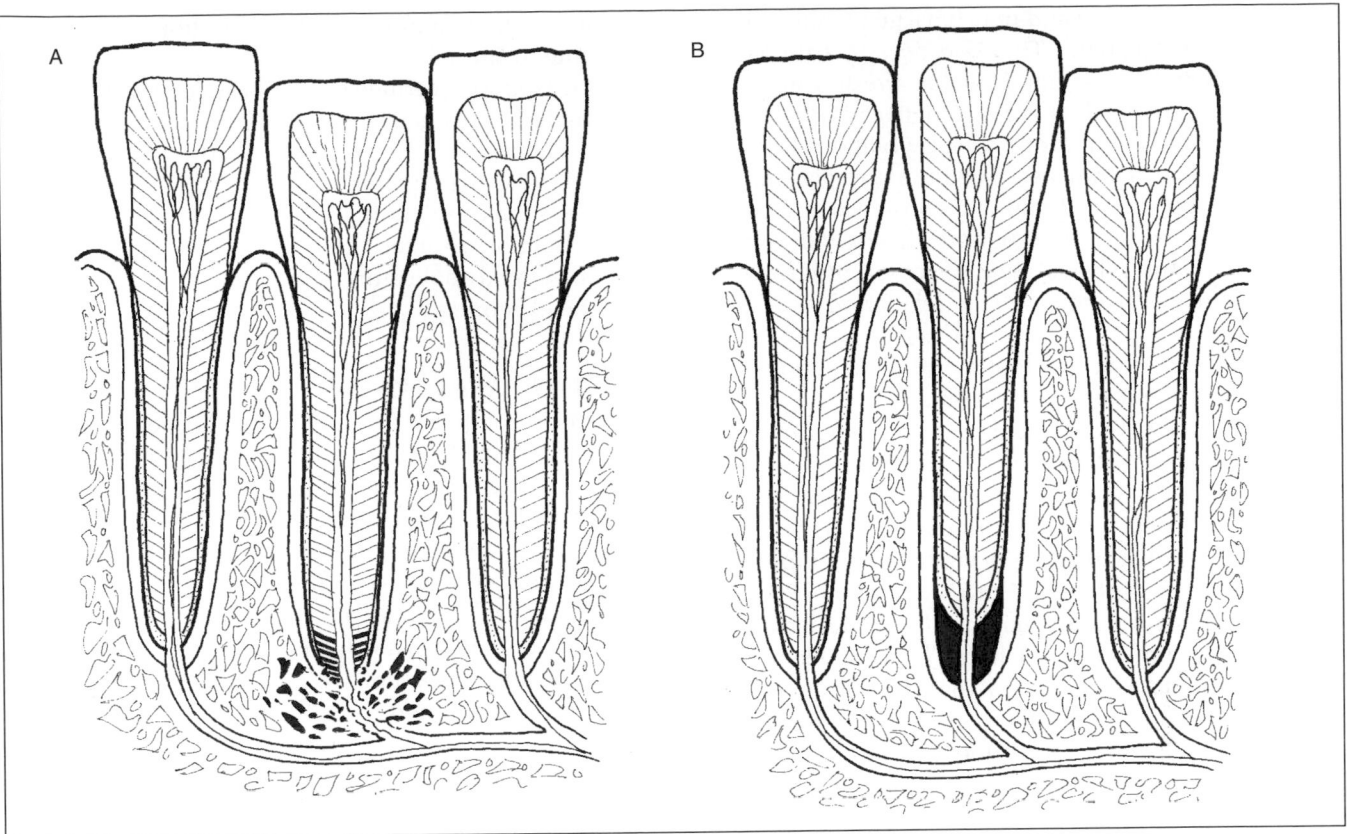

FIGURE 159-3 Luxation injuries with neurovascular damage at the apex. *A.* Intrusive luxation injury. *B.* Extrusive luxation injury.

determine the exact whereabouts of the tooth. Treat the patient for pain, control the bleeding, and provide tetanus prophylaxis if the tooth is lost. Prescribe antibiotics for these patients if there are significant concomitant injuries or as the situation warrants. Arrange follow-up with a Dentist at their convenience. As a rule, primary teeth are not replanted to avoid damage to the developing permanent teeth and possible growth disturbances. Exercise great care in evaluating patients in the mixed dentition stage, roughly between the ages of 6 and 12 years.[1,2,4]

Make an attempt at replantation in order to preserve patient comfort, cosmesis, and function when a permanent avulsed tooth is available. The objective for the emergency treatment of these injuries is to maintain viability of the torn periodontal ligament fibers on the external root surface as pulpal necrosis is inevitable for the majority of these teeth.[1] A successfully replanted tooth may be fully functional with little or no cosmetic impact following root canal therapy. **Periodontal ligament fibers are extremely sensitive to desiccation. The most critical factor in the successful replantation of avulsed teeth is the speed with which the tooth is replanted.**[1,2,7,10] Patients, parents, or Emergency Med-

ical Service (EMS) personnel may be instructed to replant an avulsed tooth in the field in order to improve the prognosis.[1,2]

Take great care in the handling of an avulsed tooth. They should be handled minimally and only by the crown. The root surface should not be manipulated in any way other than gentle cleansing with sterile saline, or tap water as a substitute. This will prevent further damage to the cementum and periodontal ligament. Treat the socket in a similar fashion (i.e., cleansed of any obstructing clots or debris with gentle irrigation and suction only) following anesthesia.[2,10]

A tooth can be transported or stored in such a way as to prevent desiccation of the fragile periodontal ligament fibers and to improve salvage rates when it is not possible to immediately replant an avulsed tooth.[1] The best possible transport and storage solutions are Hank's balanced salt solution and Viaspan (a solution used in preserving transplant tissues). Successful results have been reported for up to 96 hours post-trauma when these media are employed.[2] Commercially available products, Save-a-Tooth and EMT Tooth Saver (Smart Practice, Phoenix, Arizona) or Emergent Tooth Preservation System (Omega Dental Systems, North Little Rock,

Arkansas), contain Hank's solution in a small container for transport or storage and may have great utility in the Emergency Department. This is especially true where definitive dental care is not available. Fresh whole milk and sterile normal saline are alternatives but carry diminishing returns for tooth salvageability. Saliva can be employed as a transport medium (by placing the tooth in the buccal vestibule of a conscious and cooperative adult) for very brief periods, again with diminishing hopes for salvage. Tap water or plastic wrap may prevent desiccation for a brief period if all else fails.[2,4,9]

The literature indicates that irreversible periodontal ligament cell damage occurs within 30 minutes of dry storage and 100 percent of cells are dead after 60 minutes of dry storage.[2,4,10] An esthetic and functional, albeit less than ideal, result may be possible through a process known as ankylosis if appropriately and aggressively treated by a Dentist. **It is not acceptable to simply discard these teeth.** Soaking in Hank's solution for 30 minutes prior to replantation has yielded good results in teeth with dry times up to 1 hour.[10] Acceptable results for teeth with dry times longer than 1 hour have been reported after treatment with a regimen consisting of soaks in citric acid, stannous fluoride, and doxycycline prior to replantation.[10] Consult a Dentist before using these soaking solutions.

REDUCTION OF SEVERELY SUBLUXED, LATERALLY LUXATED, AND EXTRUDED TEETH

The emergent treatment of a severely subluxed tooth, a laterally luxated tooth, or an extruded tooth involves obtaining adequate anesthesia, reduction of the tooth, and a temporary splint for stabilization.

INDICATIONS

Any severely subluxed, laterally luxated, or extruded tooth is a candidate for reduction.

CONTRAINDICATIONS

There are no absolute contraindications to the reduction of a severely subluxed, laterally luxated, or extruded tooth. Laterally luxated and extruded primary teeth can be repositioned and splinted. However, their manipulation may damage the permanent tooth bud growing beneath the primary tooth root. Therefore, extract all luxated and extruded primary teeth.[4,7,8] Consult a Dentist or Oral Surgeon if there is a significant alveolar bone fracture. Do not attempt to reduce teeth that are fractured or grossly carious.

EQUIPMENT

Local anesthetic solution, with and without epinephrine
Dental aspirating syringe or a 3 mL syringe with a 2 inch, 25 to 27 gauge needle
Sterile saline
Sterile 2×2 gauze squares
Suction source and tubing
Fraser suction catheter
Cotton-tipped applicators
Overhead lighting

PATIENT PREPARATION

Explain the procedure, its risks, and benefits to the patient and/or their representative. Obtain a signed informed consent for the procedure. Place the patient on a multipositional procedure chair with good overhead lighting. Administer dental anesthesia. Refer to Chapter 154 regarding the details of dental anesthesia and analgesia. Cleanse the oral cavity with saline or tap water and gentle suction. Thoroughly examine the entire oral cavity. Obtain radiographs as indicated. Provide tetanus prophylaxis if required.

TECHNIQUES

Severely Subluxed Tooth Reduction

A severely subluxed tooth is not displaced from its socket but is excessively mobile. Ensure that the tooth is in its proper anatomic location. Apply a temporary dental splint, as described below.

Laterally Luxated Tooth Reduction

A laterally luxated tooth has its roots displaced laterally and out of the socket (Figure 159-4). It is often associated with a fracture of the surrounding alveolar bone. Place the dominant thumb over the medial surface of the tooth and the index finger overlying the root end of the tooth (Figure 159-4). Apply downward and inward pressure with the index finger (Figure 159-4*A*) followed by the application of outward pressure with the thumb (Figure 159-4*B*) to reduce the tooth. Apply a temporary dental splint, as described below.

Extruded Teeth Reduction

An extruded tooth is a partially avulsed tooth that protrudes above the adjacent teeth. Apply gentle pressure to the crown of the tooth to reduce the tooth. **Do not force the tooth into the socket.** Consult a Dentist if the tooth will not reduce. A hematoma in the base of the socket often prevents reduction.

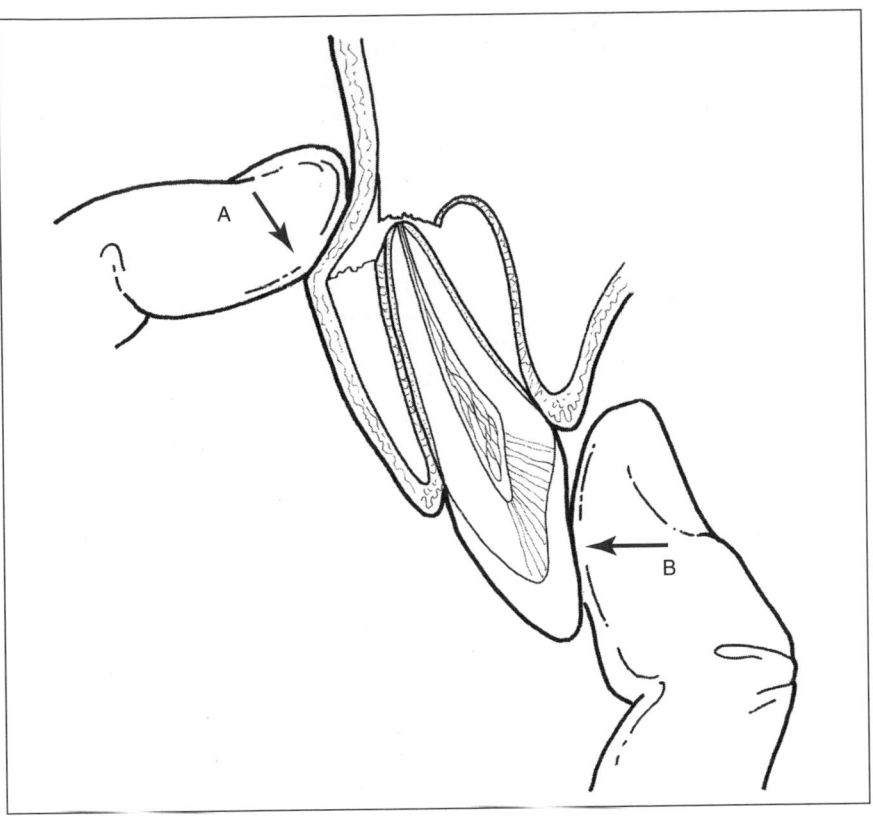

FIGURE 159-4 Manually repositioning a laterally luxated tooth. Apply downward and inward pressure with the index finger (*A*) followed by outward pressure with the thumb (*B*).

ASSESSMENT

Obtain post-reduction radiographs to verify the correct tooth position. Radiographs may be delayed until after splinting. Reassess the patient for pain, occlusal discrepancies, and stability of the reduction. Manage any soft tissue injuries.

AFTERCARE

Prescribe appropriate analgesics. Nonsteroidal anti-inflammatory drugs supplemented with an occasional narcotic analgesic will provide adequate analgesia. Prescribe empiric antibiotics (penicillin or clindamycin). Instruct the patient to avoid extremely hot or cold substances, to eat a liquid/soft diet, and to avoid chewing in the area of the injury. Provide specific instructions regarding interim dental splint care as discussed below. Arrange follow-up with a Dentist or Oral Surgeon within 24 hours. Remind the patient that any dental injury can result in the loss of tooth vitality and, ultimately, the loss of the tooth despite the best of efforts to maintain it.[1,2,9]

COMPLICATIONS

Immediate complications of any dental trauma include pain and cosmetic deformity. Additionally, instability may be an issue following the application of a temporary splint. Delayed complications can be variable and include root resorption, pulpal necrosis, infection, and abscess formation. Extension of untreated infections into alveolar bones may cause osteomyelitis and/or systemic infectious complications. A permanent tooth may develop abnormally in a younger child if injured. Bleeding is minimal and often self-limited. Refer to Chapter 157 for the details of post-extraction bleeding management. Ensuring prompt dental follow-up, adequate outpatient analgesics, and empiric antibiotics can abate most of these complications.

REPLANTATION OF AN AVULSED TOOTH

Permanent teeth that have been avulsed should be handled gently and only by the crown. Time is a critical factor in the successful treatment of these injuries and every effort should be made to expedite the care of these patients. Replantation consists of gently reinserting the tooth in the proper orientation and fully seating it with gentle pressure.

INDICATIONS

Any intact and avulsed permanent tooth is a candidate for replantation.

CONTRAINDICATIONS

There are no absolute contraindications to the replanting of permanent teeth by nondental personnel.

Concerns for the ABCs (airway, breathing, and circulation), concomitant major morbidity, and aspiration risk in acutely or chronically debilitated patients should be considered prior to tooth replantation. Primary teeth are never replanted. Do not attempt to replant teeth that are fractured or grossly carious.

EQUIPMENT

Local anesthetic solution, with and without epinephrine
Dental aspirating syringe or a 3 mL syringe with a 2 inch, 25 to 27 gauge needle
Sterile saline
Hank's balanced salt solution
Sterile 2×2 gauze squares
Sterile cotton rolls
Suction source and tubing
Fraser suction catheter
Cotton-tipped applicators
Overhead lighting

PATIENT PREPARATION

Explain the procedure, its risks, and benefits to the patient and/or their representative. Obtain a signed informed consent for the procedure. Place the patient in a multipositional procedure chair with good overhead lighting. Administer dental anesthesia. Refer to Chapter 154 regarding the details of dental anesthesia and analgesia. Cleanse the oral cavity gently with saline or tap water. Use gentle suction but never near the injured tooth. Thoroughly examine the entire oral cavity. Obtain radiographs as indicated. Provide tetanus prophylaxis if required. Gently irrigate the avulsed tooth and socket with sterile saline or Hank's solution. Remove any clots and debris using a Frazier suction catheter. **Take great care to avoid touching or contaminating the tooth root.** Soak the tooth in Hank's solution for 30 minutes prior to replantation if the extraoral dry time exceeds 30 minutes.

TECHNIQUE

Grasp the avulsed tooth gently and only by the crown. Replace the avulsed tooth into the socket in an anatomically correct position. Seat the tooth fully with gentle but firm digital pressure. **Never force the tooth into the socket.** Evaluate the patient's occlusion. Instruct the patient to gently bite together several times while observing for any prematurity. Occasionally, a tooth cannot be completely seated or its position is uncertain. Instruct the patient to temporarily bite on a gauze roll until the dental specialist arrives or store the tooth in a storage/transport media until definitive dental care can be rendered.[2,9] Address any soft tissue injuries once the tooth's position has been verified. Apply a temporary dental splint, as described below.

ASSESSMENT

Obtain post-replantation radiographs to verify the correct tooth position. Radiographs may be delayed until after splinting. Reassess the patient for pain, occlusal discrepancies, and stability of the replanted tooth prior to discharge. Manage any soft tissue injuries.

AFTERCARE

Prescribe appropriate analgesics. Nonsteroidal anti-inflammatory drugs supplemented with an occasional narcotic analgesic will provide adequate analgesia. Prescribe empiric antibiotics (penicillin or clindamycin). Instruct the patient to avoid extremely hot or cold substances, to eat a liquid/soft diet, and to avoid chewing in the area of the injury. Provide specific instructions regarding interim dental splint care as discussed below. Arrange follow-up with a Dentist or Oral Surgeon within 24 hours. Remind the patient that any dental injury can result in the loss of tooth vitality and, ultimately, the loss of the tooth despite the best of efforts to maintain it.[1,2,9]

COMPLICATIONS

Immediate complications of any dental trauma include pain and cosmetic deformity. Additionally, instability may be an issue following the application of a temporary splint. Delayed complications can be variable and include root resorption, pulpal necrosis, infection, and abscess formation. Extension of untreated infections into alveolar bones may cause osteomyelitis and/or systemic infectious complications. A permanent tooth may develop abnormally in a younger child if injured. Bleeding is minimal and often self-limited. Refer to Chapter 157 for the details of post-extraction bleeding management. Ensuring prompt dental follow-up, adequate outpatient analgesics, and empiric antibiotics can abate most of these complications.

PREPARING A TEMPORARY DENTAL SPLINT

Concussed teeth, subluxed primary teeth, and subluxed permanent teeth usually do not require splinting. A temporary splint may prevent further damage and improve patient comfort if severe mobility, or subluxation, is present. Manually reposition laterally luxated and extruded permanent teeth using gentle and firm digital manipulation following adequate anesthesia. A Dentist or Oral Surgeon will typically extract laterally luxated or extruded primary teeth. Intruded teeth, both primary and adult, are associated with considerable comorbidity and complications. These injuries require consultation with a Dentist or an Oral Surgeon after defining the extent of the injuries with appropriate radiographs.

INDICATIONS

Any severely traumatized and grossly mobile, luxated, repositioned, or replanted tooth requires temporary splinting. This will prevent further damage, promote patient comfort, preserve form, and preserve function.

CONTRAINDICATIONS

There are no absolute contraindications to the temporary splinting of mobile teeth. The aspiration risk in acutely or chronically debilitated patients should be considered prior to tooth splinting.

EQUIPMENT

Local anesthetic solution, with and without epinephrine
Dental aspirating syringe or 3 mL syringe with a 2 inch, 25 to 27 gauge needle
Sterile saline
Coe-Pak or Perio-Pack
Dental utility wax or beeswax
Sterile 2×2 gauze squares
Sterile cotton rolls
Applicator sticks; tongue depressors or the wooden end of cotton swabs will substitute
Fraser suction catheter
Suction source and tubing
Overhead lighting

PATIENT PREPARATION

Explain the procedure, its risks, and benefits to the patient and/or their representative. Obtain a signed informed consent for the procedure. Place the patient in a multipositional procedure chair with good overhead lighting. Administer dental anesthesia. Refer to Chapter 154 regarding the details of dental anesthesia and analgesia. Cleanse and thoroughly examine the entire oral cavity. Obtain radiographs as indicated. Provide tetanus prophylaxis if required. Manually reposition any luxated and avulsed teeth. **Manage any soft tissue injuries prior to splint placement to avoid wound contamination by the splint material.**

TECHNIQUES

Cold-curing periodontal packing material (i.e., Coe-Pak or Perio-Pack) is an ideal splinting material for practitioners without dental experience. Measure out equal amounts of the catalyst and the epoxy (Figure 159-5A). Thoroughly mix the catalyst and epoxy compounds together to form a putty-like consistency (Figure 159-5B).

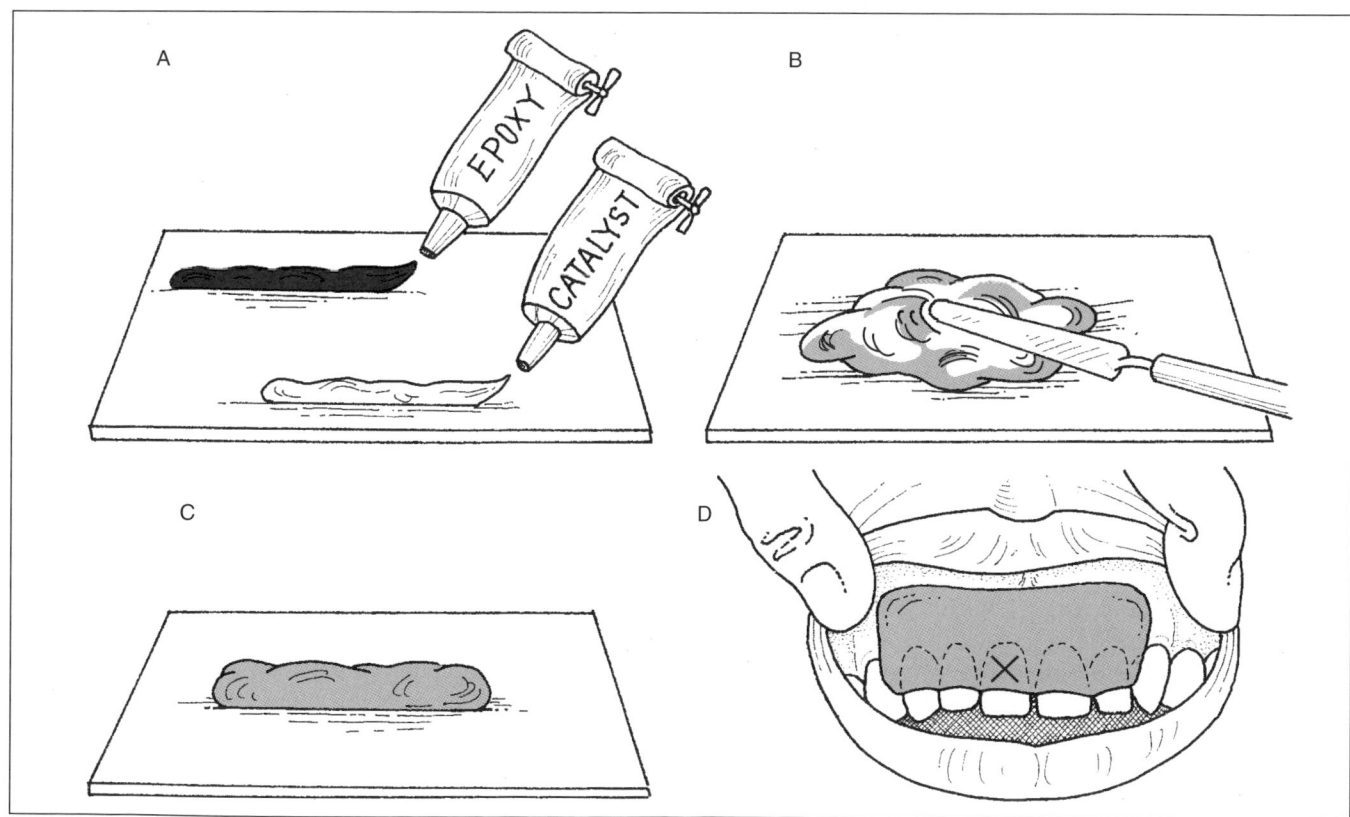

FIGURE 159-5 Preparation of the dental bonding resin and repair of the injured tooth. *A.* Equal amounts of the epoxy and catalyst are measured. *B.* The epoxy and catalyst are mixed together. *C.* The hardening dental paste is molded into a supportive bridge. *D.* The dental bridge is applied over the injured tooth and adjacent two uninjured teeth (both sides) for support while hardening.

Roll the material into a log (Figure 159-5*C*). Apply the material to frame both aspects, medial and lateral, of the injured tooth and two to three adjacent stable teeth on either side of the injured tooth (Figure 159-5*D*). **To allow proper occlusion, do not place the packing material on the masticatory surfaces of the teeth. The material must be kept dry and uncontaminated to cure, which is achieved within minutes.**

Numerous alternative techniques have also been used to temporarily splint a tooth. A simpler technique employs softened dental utility wax or beeswax in a similar fashion. The wax splint is not nearly as stable as the cold-curing periodontal packing. Both the medial and lateral surfaces of the teeth can be splinted in this fashion. Ligature splinting with suture material has been described but rarely provides any significant stability. Advanced techniques include acid-etched composite resin, direct interdental wiring, resin-wire combinations, arch bars, and stabilization with a figure-of-eight stitch to the adjacent tooth. These are excellent materials in experienced hands. Unfortunately, they are difficult to use, fraught with complications, and cost prohibitive for routine Emergency Department use.[1,2,4-9]

ASSESSMENT

Allow the patient to wait in the Emergency Department until the splinting material has hardened. The splint material should impinge minimally on the soft tissues. The patient must be able to open and close their mouth and lips freely, without any obstruction. Reassess the patient for pain, occlusal discrepancies, and stability of the replanted or subluxed tooth prior to discharge. Obtain post-splint radiographs to verify the proper tooth position.

AFTERCARE

Prescribe appropriate analgesics. Nonsteroidal anti-inflammatory drugs supplemented with an occasional narcotic analgesic will provide adequate analgesia. Prescribe empiric antibiotics (penicillin or clindamycin). Instruct the patient to avoid extremely hot or cold substances, to eat a liquid/soft diet, and to avoid chewing in the area of the injury. Provide specific instructions regarding interim dental splint care. Arrange follow-up with a Dentist or Oral Surgeon within 24 hours. Remind the patient that any dental injury can result in the loss of tooth vitality and, ultimately, the loss of the tooth despite the best of efforts to maintain it.[1,2,9]

COMPLICATIONS

The complications of temporary splinting are minimal. The splint material may not stabilize the tooth. A tooth allowed to move within the socket may result in damage to the cementum or the periodontal ligament. An improperly splinted tooth may fall out and result in

an aspiration risk. To prevent irritation and bleeding, do not apply splinting material over the soft tissues.

SUMMARY

Traumatic dental injuries are a common presentation to the Emergency Department, especially in pediatric patients during the mixed dentition stage. These injuries may have significant cosmetic, functional, and psychological consequences for the rest of the patient's life. The appropriate Emergency Department management of dental trauma depends heavily upon the type of tooth involved (primary versus permanent), the time elapsed since the incident, and the extent of the damage. A basic understanding of dental anatomy, terminology, pathophysiology, and treatment protocols will facilitate an accurate description of the extent of injuries to the dental consultant and be of great aid in providing temporizing emergent dental care when no specialist is readily available.

REFERENCES

1. Dale RA: Dentoalveolar trauma. *Emerg Med Clin North Am* 2000; 18(3):521–538.
2. Camp JH, Stewart C, Winograd SM: Dental trauma: diagnostic considerations, emergency procedures and definitive management. *Emerg Med Rep* 1995; 16(9):79–86.
3. Gibson DE, Verono AA: Dentistry in the emergency department. *J Emerg Med* 1987; 5(1):35–44.
4. Beaudreau RW: Oral and dental emergencies, in Tintinalli JE, Kelen GD, Stapczynski JS (eds): *Emergency Medicine: A Comprehensive Study Guide*, 5th ed. New York: McGraw-Hill, 2000:1539–1556.
5. Amsterdam JT: Dental disorders, in Rosen P, Barkin R, Danzl DF, et al (eds): *Emergency Medicine: Concepts and Clinical Practice*, 4th ed. St. Louis: Mosby, 1998:2680–2697.
6. Ross DJ, Kirsch T: Dental emergencies, in Vanrooyen M, Kirsch T, Clem K, et al (eds): *Emergent Field Medicine*. New York: McGraw-Hill, 2001:276–302.
7. Klokkevold P: Common dental emergencies: evaluation and management for emergency physicians. *Emerg Med Clin North Am* 1989; 7(1):29–63.
8. Antrim DD, Bakland LK, Parker MW: Treatment of endodontic urgent care cases. *Dent Clin North Am* 1986; 30(3):549–573.
9. Amsterdam JT: Emergency dental procedures, in Roberts JR, Hedges JR (eds): *Clinical Procedures in Emergency Medicine*, 3rd ed. Philadelphia: Saunders, 1998:1045–1064.
10. Trope M: Clinical management of the avulsed tooth. *Dent Clin North Am* 1995; 39(1):93–112.

Chapter 160
FRACTURED TOOTH MANAGEMENT

Suneel Upadhye
Daniel J. Ross

INTRODUCTION

Traumatic dental injuries are a common presentation to the Emergency Department. It has been estimated that approximately 50 percent of children will sustain traumatic dental injuries.[1-3] The appropriate Emergency Department management of dental trauma depends upon the extent of the damage and the age of the patient. This requires a basic understanding of dental anatomy, terminology, and pathophysiology. Violence of a suspicious nature such as potential domestic or child abuse must always be considered when evaluating dental injuries, especially if there is conflicting physical evidence given the clinical history. The goals of the emergent treatment of dental trauma are to maintain patient comfort and tooth vitality while ensuring prompt dental follow-up for definitive care.

ANATOMY AND PATHOPHYSIOLOGY

TOOTH ANATOMY

There are significant differences in the adult and pediatric dentitions that impact their treatment in the Emergency Department (Figure 160-1). The pediatric dentition is known as the primary or deciduous dentition and consists of 20 teeth, which includes 8 incisors, 4 canines, and 8 molars. The adult dentition consists of 32 teeth and is composed of 8 incisors, 4 canines, 8 premolars, and 12 molars. The variable absence of a tooth or the addition of an extra tooth is common in either dentition. The teeth in both the pediatric and adult dentitions erupt in a predictable sequence, albeit with considerable individual variation. Treatment strategies differ for permanent versus deciduous teeth as well as by the age of the adult tooth. **Exercise great care when evaluating patients with a "mixed" dentition, roughly between the ages of 6 and 12 years.**

The anatomy of a tooth is rather simple (Figure 160-2). The tooth itself consists of a neurovascular pulp surrounded by supportive dentin, which is surrounded by a hard thick crown of enamel. The crown portion lies above the gum line or gingiva. The root portion lies embedded within the alveolar bone of the jaw, anchored by a thin layer of cementum and the periodontal ligament. The alveolar bone, periodontal ligament fibers, and fragile cementum cell layer taken together are considered a functional unit known as the attachment apparatus. A complete attachment apparatus requires a fully formed root apex. Immature adult teeth do not have a fully formed apex and necessitate special attention to maintain pulpal viability.[1,3,4]

TOOTH INJURY

Mechanisms of tooth injury include direct trauma (i.e., a blow) or occlusive trauma (i.e., biting on a hard object or a seizure). These mechanisms can result in a spectrum of injury patterns that vary from simple sensitivity to complete tooth avulsion. The fracture of any portion of the tooth, whether the crown or the root, falls in the middle of this spectrum and is frequently seen in the Emergency Department.[3]

Appropriate treatment of dental injuries requires a thorough history and meticulous examination of the oral cavity, including subsequent radiographs after ruling out more serious injuries. Historically, important points include the age of the patient, the time of the trauma, the mechanism of injury, teeth or tooth pieces at the scene, subjective disturbance of bite, and treatments provided since the time of the incident. The physical examination must include an assessment of the extraoral and intraoral soft tissues, bony displacement, missing teeth, crown fractures, pulp exposures, tooth sensitivity, and tooth mobility. This chapter focuses primarily on tooth fractures, while luxation and avulsion injuries are dealt with in Chapter 159.

The need for radiographs with dental trauma is worth emphasizing. A tooth that is missing, by both history and physical examination, may be found completely intruded below the gum line, floating within the maxillary sinus or stomach, or even aspirated. **Obtain**

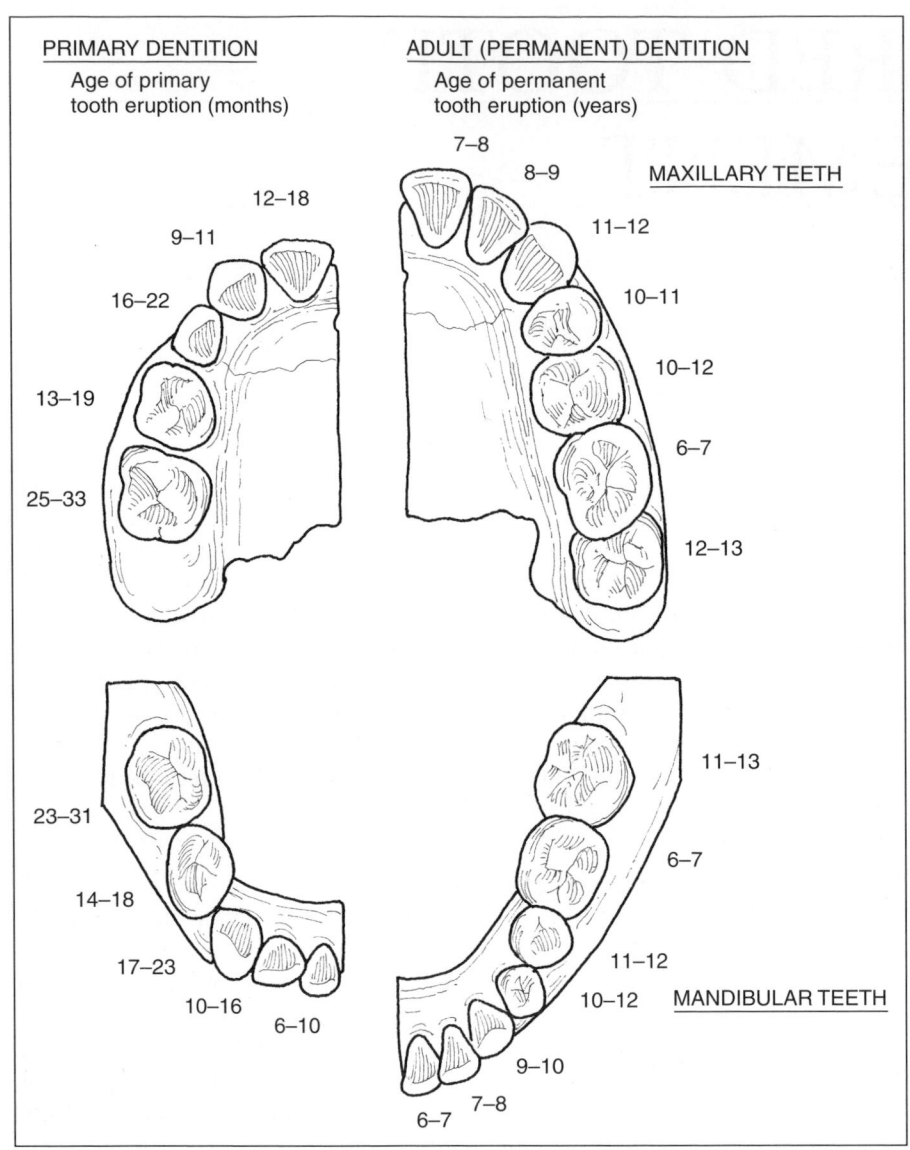

PRIMARY DENTITION
Age of primary
tooth eruption (months)

ADULT (PERMANENT) DENTITION
Age of permanent
tooth eruption (years)

MAXILLARY TEETH

MANDIBULAR TEETH

FIGURE 160-1 The normal eruptive patterns of the pediatric and adult dentition.

facial films if a tooth, or portion of a tooth, cannot be unequivocally located by history or physical examination. Strongly consider obtaining chest and abdominal radiographs if the tooth, or portion in question, is not visualized on facial films.[1,5]

TOOTH FRACTURES

Fractures involving the crown of the tooth are commonly described in the emergency literature by the Ellis classification system[1,3–7] (Figure 160-3). **An Ellis I fracture involves only the enamel portion of the tooth.** These injuries typically are not sensitive or painful. They can result in a sharp edge of enamel that may irritate the tongue and other soft tissues. Emergency treatment may be as simple as smoothing the rough edge with an emery board or similar instrument.[1,4,10] These injuries frequently involve the prominent anterior teeth and may be cosmetically unappealing. Reassure patients with these concerns that aesthetic restorations are possible by their Dentist.[3–6,8] **Forewarn patients with even minor trauma and sensitivity that unseen or undiagnosed trauma at the apex of any traumatized tooth, even with an appropriately treated crown fracture, can compromise the blood flow to the pulp and obviate the need for root canal therapy.[3,8]**

The Ellis II fracture involves the dentin. It can be recognized by the yellow to pink hue of the dentin in contrast to the white of enamel. This fracture allows for potential contamination of the dentin microtubular networks by oral bacteria that may eventually compromise the pulp if not treated. Dentin is alive and formed by the pulp. It is sensitive to temperature, osmotic gradients, and mechanical forces. Dentin is laid down concentrically from within the pulp chamber as the tooth ages. Therefore, children have less dentin than pulp (as compared to adults) and their pulp is less insulated against

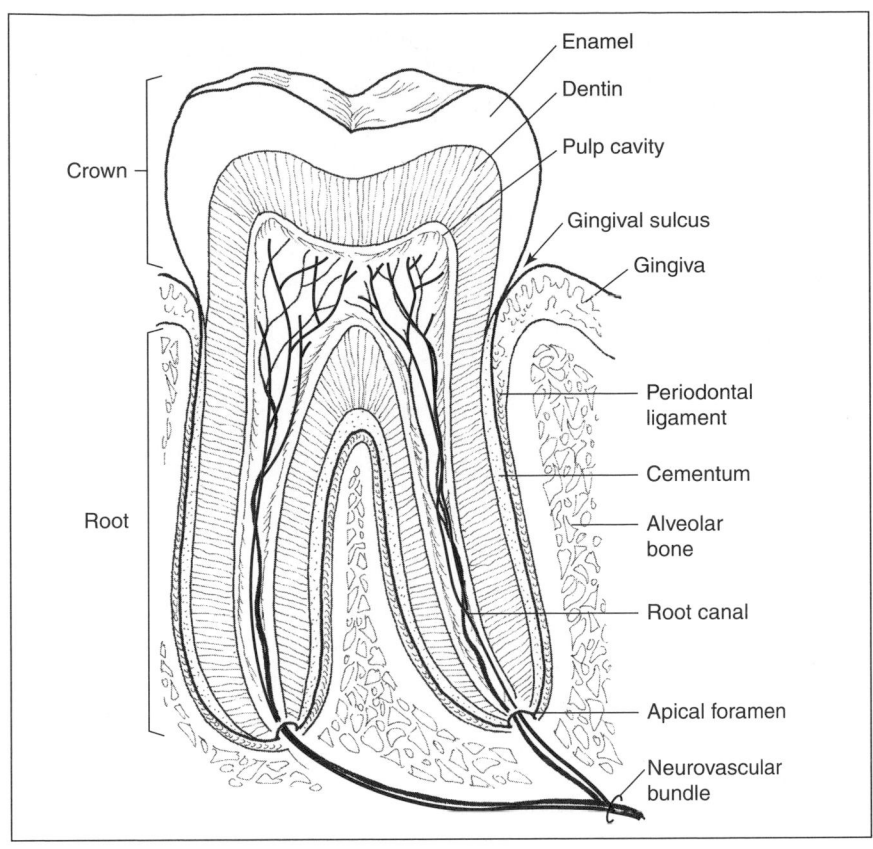

FIGURE 160-2 The dental anatomic unit (i.e., the tooth) and its supporting structures.

trauma and subsequent infection. Children under the age of 12 years with Ellis II fractures have a higher risk of complications and require more expeditious follow-up.[1,4,8] **Refer these patients to a General or Pediatric Dentist as soon as possible.**

Ellis II fractures in mature teeth essentially require the same care as immature teeth with a less urgent follow-up. Emergency treatment in both cases consists of applying a protective dressing which is also sedative to the pulp, such as Dycal or zinc oxide and eugenol, followed by a sealant such as Copalite, clear acrylic nail polish, or a dental bonding resin.[1,2,4–6,8,9] Emergency Physicians should probably avoid attempting to bond small tooth fragments to a fractured crown due to the risk of bond failure, subsequent aspiration, and occlusal discrepancies. Recently, it was suggested that a single-step, glass ionomer cement replace the long-held standard of Dycal followed by Copalite.[3] This material has definite advantages but can be quite tricky to use in unskilled (nondental) hands.

The Ellis III fracture involves exposure of both the dentin and the pulp. This is identified as a reddish tinge or subtle bleeding from the exposed dentin. Frank pulpal exposures are obvious. The pulp is highly vascular and exquisitely sensitive due to exposed nerve endings. The pulp is exceedingly vulnerable to bacterial infection if exposed. **These fractures constitute a true dental emer-**

gency and should be evaluated immediately by a Dentist for possible emergent root canal therapy. Although less than ideal, minimal pulp exposures (less than 1 to 2 mm) may be treated as Ellis II fractures with a Dentist follow-up within 24 hours.[1–6,8] Complete coverage of the fractured crown may be difficult in these cases. Dental dry foil or tin foil may provide adequate coverage. Any root canal manipulation is fraught with complications, even in the hands of Endodontists. Emergency Physicians are well advised to avoid these procedures.[1,6,8]

Fractures of the root are much less common than crown fractures and occur in less than 7 percent of dental injuries.[1,3] Root fractures are uncommon in primary teeth as they have short roots.[1] Root fractures may be described as either horizontal or vertical. Horizontal root fractures are described according to their location along the tooth root (Figure 160-4). Vertical root fractures occasionally extend into the crown. All root fractures are prone to infection and impaired healing, and may ultimately lead to pulpal necrosis and tooth loss.

The clinical diagnosis of root fractures is challenging at best, even with the aid of radiographs readily available in the typical Emergency Department setting (i.e., Panorex). Root fractures classically present with pain, mobility, and sometimes displacement of a tooth fragment. However, these fractures are often insidious and found only on dental radiographs after follow-up re-

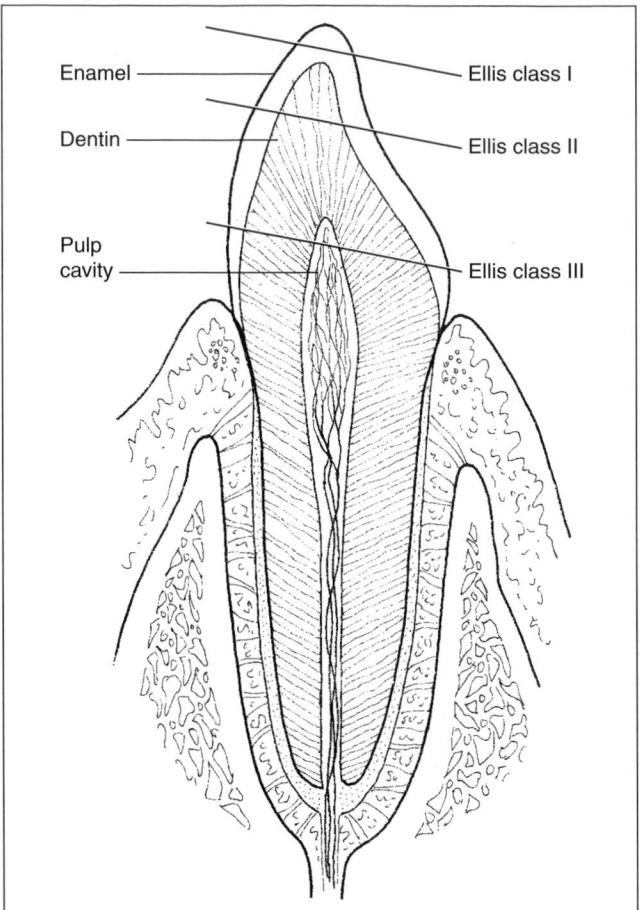

FIGURE 160-3 The Ellis classification scheme of dental fractures through the crown.

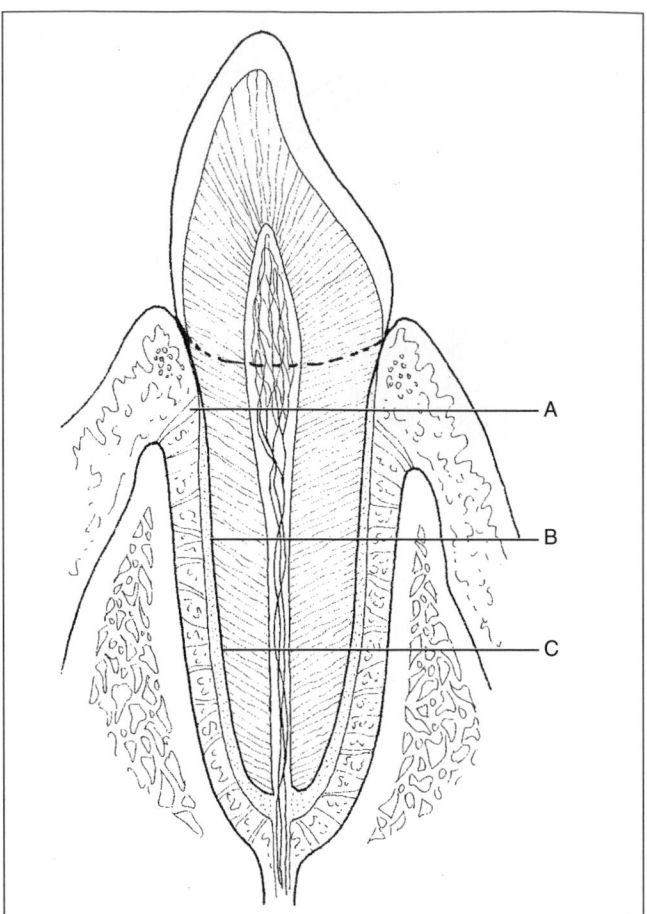

FIGURE 160-4 Classification of root fractures according to their location. *A.* Incisal or coronal third fracture. *B.* Mid-root fracture. *C.* Apical third fracture.

veals continued sensitivity. **Emergency Physicians must maintain a high level of clinical suspicion for these injuries and probably err on the side of cautious overtreatment.[1,3]**

Vertical root fractures and root fractures in the coronal portion of the root have a poor prognosis. Horizontal root fractures elsewhere along the tooth root have a good prognosis if treated before a coagulum can develop between the fragments, generally within 24 to 72 hours.[1,6] Immediate reduction and immobilization with one of the various splinting techniques is the treatment of choice.[1,6,7] Refer to Chapter 159 for the details regarding dental splinting techniques.

INDICATIONS

Fractured teeth may require no treatment or a significant amount of treatment based upon the type of injury as described by the Ellis classification system. Fractured roots must be treated based upon the level of clinical suspicion.

CONTRAINDICATIONS

There are no absolute contraindications to the temporary repair of a fractured tooth or tooth root. Concerns for the ABCs (airway, breathing, and circulation), concomitant major morbidity, and aspiration risk in acutely or chronically debilitated patients should be considered prior to tooth repair.

EQUIPMENT

Local anesthetic solution, with and without epinephrine
Dental aspirating syringe, or a 3 mL syringe with a
   2 inch, 25 to 27 gauge needle
Dental explorer
Discoid-cleoid carver
Dental drill or emery board
Sterile saline
Sterile 2×2 gauze squares
Sterile cotton rolls

Applicator or molding sticks; tongue depressor or the wooden end of cotton swabs will substitute

Zinc-eugenol paste or other commercial dental filling material

Copalite (cavity varnish) or clear acrylic nail polish

Zinc oxide-eugenol (ZOE or IRM)

Dycal (calcium hydroxide paste)

Dental dry foil or tin foil

Fraser tip suction catheter

Suction source and tubing

Good overhead lighting

Dental floss

PATIENT PREPARATION

Explain the risks, benefits, and aftercare to the patient and/or their representative. Obtain an informed consent for the procedure. Position the patient upright in a multipositional examination chair in a well-lighted environment. Provide tetanus prophylaxis as required. Provide anesthesia to the patent. Refer to Chapter 154 for the complete details regarding dental anesthesia and analgesia.

Irrigate the oral cavity and dental repair region with saline to remove any gross contaminants or clotted blood. Warm gentle irrigation is usually less sensitive to exposed dentin.[6] **A dry and uncontaminated field is mandatory.** This can be achieved via dabbing with sterile cotton pellets or gently blowing with compressed air. Maintain a dry working environment by isolating the traumatized tooth with sterile cotton rolls on either side. Inject a small amount of local anesthetic solution containing epinephrine directly into the pulp if continued bleeding from a large pulpal exposure is problematic.[5]

TECHNIQUES

ELLIS I FRACTURES

Ellis I fractures are clinically minor injuries. The management includes smoothing of any sharp edges with a dental drill or a nail file to prevent injury or irritation to the soft tissues of the oral cavity. **Use care to avoid overaggressive smoothing and exposure of the dentin (i.e., iatrogenic Ellis II injury).**

ELLIS II FRACTURES

Ellis II fractures are clinically more important than Ellis I fractures. They require coverage of the exposed dentin to prevent infection and reduce sensitivity. Paint small or large dentinal exposures with calcium hydroxide paste followed by several coats of cavity varnish or clear acrylic nail polish to relieve sensitivity.[5,6,10] Apply the calcium hydroxide paste in a thin layer with any small, blunt instrument. Apply cavity varnish or clear nail polish with a small, disposable brush or with a sterile cotton pellet. Apply three to four coats. Allow adequate drying time between coats. Alternatively, place a simple tin foil dressing over the tooth to act as a bandage following placement of the calcium hydroxide.[5,6,10]

ELLIS III FRACTURES

Ellis III fractures are true dental emergencies and should be treated by a Dentist or Oral Surgeon. Treat pulpal exposures, if no specialist is immediately available, by applying a saline-moistened cotton pledget over the exposed pulp and holding it there until the bleeding stops. This may take 2 to 5 minutes. Apply a thick mixture of calcium hydroxide paste (Dycal) over the exposed pulp and dentin. Apply the calcium hydroxide paste over an adjacent tooth to form a temporary hold. Contour the calcium hydroxide paste so that it does not irritate the surrounding tissue. The majority of these injuries will require root canal therapy. Refer the patient to a Dentist within 24 hours if they are not seen in the Emergency Department.

ASSESSMENT

Reassess the patient for pain and any occlusal discrepancies prior to discharge.

AFTERCARE

Most of these patients will have some degree of sensitivity until definitive treatment by a Dentist. Prescribe appropriate outpatient analgesics. Nonsteroidal anti-inflammatory drugs supplemented with a narcotic analgesic will provide adequate pain control for Ellis II and III fractures. Antibiotics are generally not necessary unless the initial presentation has been significantly delayed, suppuration is present, or a significant delay is expected in obtaining dental follow-up. Instruct the patients to avoid extremely hot or cold substances, to begin a liquid/soft diet until seen by a Dentist, to avoid chewing in the area of the injured tooth, and to avoid topical analgesics (such as oil of cloves) due to the propensity for sterile abscess formation.[1,3,6] Always warn patients about continued sensitivity.

COMPLICATIONS

Complications of dental trauma include pain, cosmetic deformity, loss of tooth viability, and unsuspected or unrecognized injury to adjacent teeth with later complications. Extension of untreated infections into alveolar bones may cause osteomyelitis, abscess formation, and/or systemic infectious complications. A permanent tooth may develop abnormally in a younger child if injured. Ensuring prompt follow-up with a Dentist can abate the majority of these complications. It goes without saying that Emergency Physicians must be ever vigilant for cases suspicious for child abuse or neglect.

SUMMARY

Dental fractures are relatively common traumatic injuries. Appropriate clinical assessment and treatment requires an understanding of basic dental anatomy, terminology, and pathophysiology. Management includes addressing patient discomfort, stabilization, and coverage of exposed vulnerable tooth components. Arrange prompt follow-up with a Dentist for definitive care for any dental injury.

REFERENCES

1. Camp JH, Stewart C, Winograd SM: Dental trauma: diagnostic considerations, emergency procedures and definitive management. *Emerg Med Rep* 1995; 16(9):79–86.
2. Gibson DE, Verono AA: Dentistry in the emergency department. *J Emerg Med* 1987; 5(1):35–44.
3. Beaudreau RW: Oral and dental emergencies, in Tintinalli JE, Kelen GD, Stapczynski JS (eds): *Emergency Medicine: A Comprehensive Study Guide*, 5th ed. New York: McGraw-Hill, 2000:1539–1556.
4. Amsterdam JT: Dental disorders, in Rosen P, Barkin R, Danzl DF, et al (eds): *Emergency Medicine: Concepts and Clinical Practice*, 4th ed. St. Louis: Mosby, 1998:2680–2697.
5. Ross DJ, Kirsch T: Dental emergencies, in Vanrooyen M, Kirsch T, Clem K, et al (eds): *Emergent Field Medicine.* New York: McGraw-Hill, 2001:276–302.
6. Klokkevold P: Common dental emergencies: evaluation and management for emergency physicians. *Emerg Med Clin North Am* 1989; 7(1):29–63.
7. Antrim DD, Bakland LK, Parker MW: Treatment of endodontic urgent care cases. *Dent Clin North Am* 1986; 30(3):549–573.
8. Amsterdam JT: Emergency dental procedures, in Roberts JR, Hedges JR (eds): *Clinical Procedures in Emergency Medicine*, 3rd ed. Philadelphia: Saunders, 1998:1045–1064.
9. Morris JA Jr, Swiontkowski MF, Herrmann HJ: Wilderness trauma emergencies, in Auerbach PS (ed): *Wilderness Medicine*, 3rd ed. St. Louis: Mosby, 1995:343–352.
10. Antrim DD: Treatment of traumatic dental injuries by nondental personnel. *US Navy Med* 1983; 74(3):18–23.

Chapter 161
TEMPOROMANDIBULAR JOINT DISLOCATION REDUCTION

Suneel Upadhye

INTRODUCTION

Mandible or temporomandibular joint (TMJ) dislocations usually occur in the setting of prior musculoskeletal problems of the jaw.[1-3] This includes joint laxity, prior injury or dislocation, inherent hypermobile syndromes (e.g., Marfan, Ehlers-Danlos), or neuromuscular problems (e.g., dystonic reactions) that pull the mandible out of its joint. The mandibular dislocation typically results from TMJ hyperextension or trauma. The Emergency Physician must be able to reduce a TMJ dislocation. The procedure is easy, simple, and straightforward.

ANATOMY AND PATHOPHYSIOLOGY

The TMJ is an unusual joint (Figure 161-1). It is composed of two joints separated by an articular disk. The TMJ functions as a hinge and gliding joint. A discussion of the mechanics of the TMJ is beyond the scope of this chapter. Anterior dislocations are most commonly seen in the Emergency Department. The etiology of the dislocation includes laughing, chewing, opening the mouth wide (eating, for procedures, yawning, vomiting), seizures, and trauma. All of these actions can result in the mandibular condyle sliding forward and anterior to the articular eminence of the temporal bone. The muscular attachments of the mandible result in a pulling of the condyle superiorly and in front of the articular eminence (Figure 161-2). This causes the mandible to become fixed in dislocation and rarely spontaneously reduce.

TMJ dislocations are commonly anterior, but may be in any direction. Anterior TMJ dislocations may occur spontaneously in normal individuals and can occasionally reduce spontaneously. Dislocations of the TMJ are usually bilateral, but can occur unilaterally. Posterior, superior, and lateral dislocations are much more rare. They are seen in the context of direct trauma to the mandible, with or without an associated mandible fracture.

The diagnosis can often be made clinically in a cooperative patient with a nontraumatic history. The patient will present in pain with an open mouth, protruding mandible, and malocclusion. A unilateral dislocation will cause the mandible to protrude towards the nondislocated side. A depression, palpable and visible, will be noted in the preauricular area. Mandibular radiographs are indicated when trauma is involved to rule out an associated fracture. The dislocation is often best seen on the Panorex view of the mandible. TMJ views, if available, are also useful. Computed tomography (CT) scanning is warranted if an associated basilar skull fracture, intracranial injuries, or facial fractures are suspected.

INDICATIONS

Attempt to reduce a closed anterior TMJ dislocation without a concomitant mandible fracture in an alert, cooperative, and consenting patient.

CONTRAINDICATIONS

Mandibular dislocations that are open, superior in direction, lateral in direction, or posterior in direction require an Oral Surgeon or Otolaryngology consultation prior to reduction attempts. Dislocations, regardless of the direction, associated with mandible fractures require consultation prior to reduction attempts. The inability to reduce an anterior mandible dislocation by the

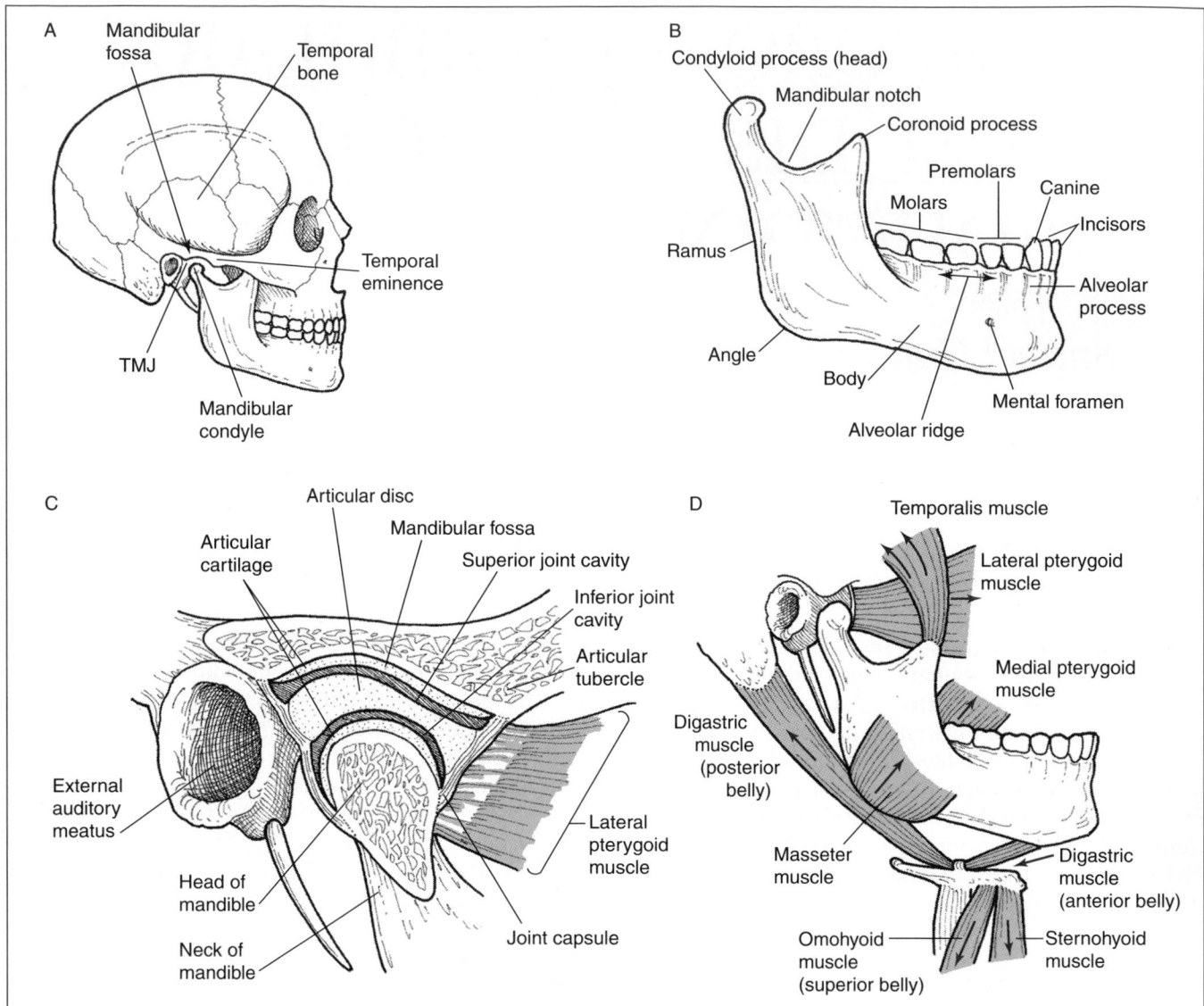

FIGURE 161-1 Anatomy. *A.* Lateral view of the head and temporomandibular joint. *B.* Anatomy of the mandible. *C.* Sagittal section through the temporomandibular joint. *D.* The attachment of the muscles of mastication to the mandible. The arrows represent the direction of pull of the muscles.

closed method requires consultation and reduction under general anesthesia. Patients presenting with cranial nerve injuries associated with the dislocation require emergent consultation prior to the reduction.

EQUIPMENT

25 gauge needle
3 mL syringe
Gauze squares or rolls
Gloves
Povidone iodine solution
Local anesthetic solution without epinephrine
Equipment and supplies for procedural sedation

PATIENT PREPARATION

Explain the procedure, its risks, and benefits to the patient and/or their representative. Obtain a signed informed consent for the procedure. Place the patient sitting in a multipositional procedure chair with a solid headrest to support their head. Alternatives include placing the patient supine on a gurney or in a chair with an assistant standing behind the patient to stabilize their head (Figure 161-3).

The mandible can often be reduced without anesthesia. This is not recommended. **Adequate analgesia and muscle relaxation will allow easier manipulation of the mandible back into its anatomic position.** Strongly consider the use of parenteral analgesics,

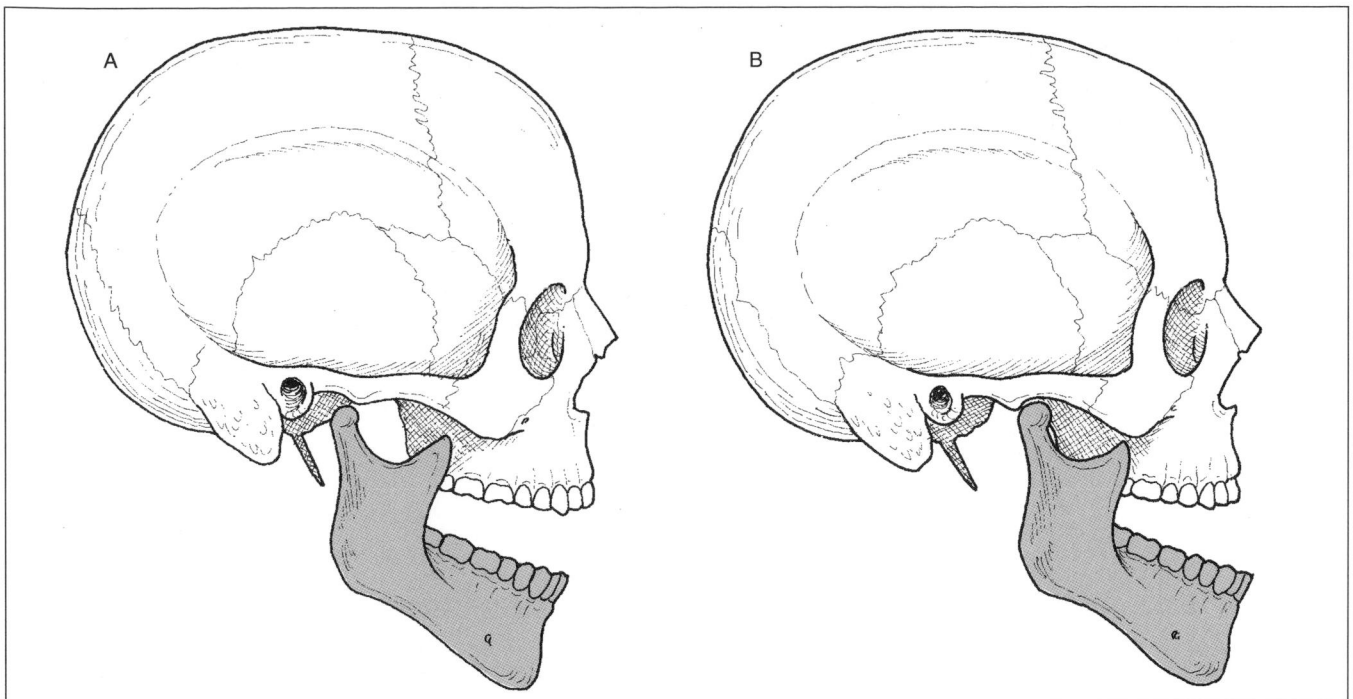

FIGURE 161-2 Anatomic relationships of the mandible. *A.* The fully opened mandible. *B.* The anteriorly dislocated mandible.

sedatives, and/or muscle relaxants. Procedural analgesia and sedation may be required to overcome the patient's pain and masticatory muscle spasm. This is especially true to relax the muscles of mastication and allow reduction if the mandible has been dislocated for more than 6 to 8 hours. Refer to Chapter 109 for the complete details regarding procedural analgesia and sedation.

An alternative, or adjunct, to the administration of parenteral medications is to inject local anesthetic solution into the TMJ space (Figure 161-4). This injection is simple, quick, and relieves significant discomfort. Locate the depression 2.5 cm anterior to the tragus of the pinna and just above the head (condyle) of the mandible. This is the location of the TMJ space. Clean the skin of any dirt and debris. Apply povidone iodine solution to the skin over the TMJ space and allow it to dry. Insert a 25 gauge needle perpendicular to the skin and directed medially. Advance the needle 0.5 cm and into the TMJ space. Inject 1 mL of local anesthetic solution without epinephrine. Inject the contralateral TMJ space if the dislocation is bilateral. Consider injecting the contralateral TMJ space in a unilateral TMJ dislocation. The patient may experience pain in their contralateral TMJ from muscle spasm due to the increased pressure on it from the dislocation.

TECHNIQUE

The actual reduction requires no specialized equipment beyond nonsterile gloves and gauze 4×4 squares. Position the patient as mentioned previously. Apply gloves and then wrap several layers of gauze around each thumb. **The gauze squares on the thumbs are to prevent possible lacerations to the examiner's thumbs when the mandible reduces.**

Stand or sit in front of the patient (Figure 161-3). Place both thumbs into the patient's mouth and onto the most posterior molars of the mandible bilaterally (Figure 161-5A). Wrap the index, middle, ring, and little fingers below the mandible, with the index fingers behind the angles of the mandible (Figures 161-5A and B). Slowly apply downward and backward pressure to allow the muscles of mastication to stretch and overcome the muscle spasm (Figure 161-5A). The downward pressure releases the mandibular condyle from the articular eminence of the temporal bone. Instruct the patient to further open their jaw to accentuate the deformity. This may disengage the impacted mandibular condyle from the anterior articular eminence of the TMJ. The masseter muscle will cause a rapid and sudden closing of the patient's jaw when the condyle of the mandible is eased back and over the articular eminence.

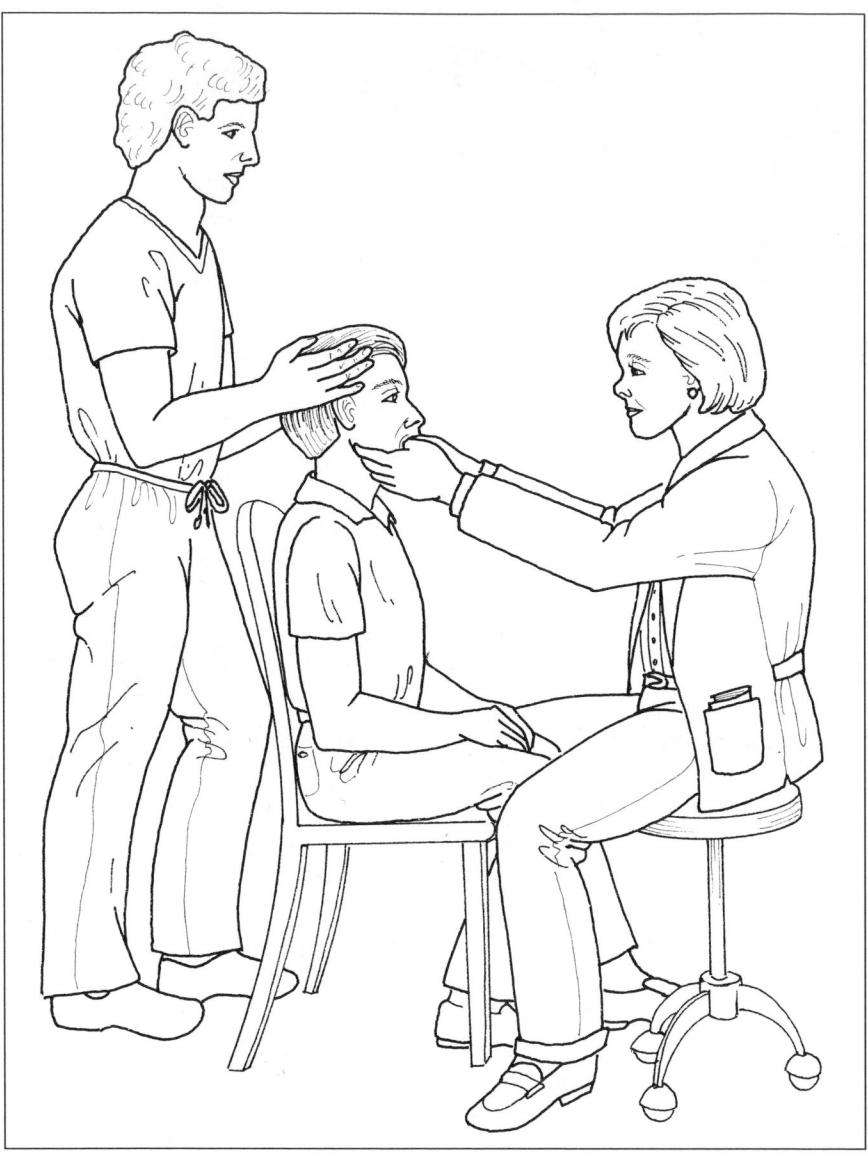

FIGURE 161-3 Alternative positioning of the patient.

Numerous alternative techniques have been developed to reduce a TMJ dislocation. One technique is to place the thumbs on the buccal aspect of the molars. This avoids the potential injury to the thumbs when the mandible relocates. This method limits the force placed upon the mandible and may not result in a reduction. Another technique requires the physician to stand behind the patient and place downward and backward pressure on the lower molars.

ASSESSMENT

The patient should be able to open and close their mandible without any difficulty after a successful reduction. Postreduction radiographs are not necessary unless a fracture was present or suspected on prereduction radiographs.

AFTERCARE

Refer the patient to an Oral Surgeon or Otolaryngologist within 24 to 48 hours. Chronic or recurrent dislocations may require surgical fixation. Instruct the patient to avoid excessive jaw opening (over 2 cm), to avoid "gummy" foods and hard foods, and to begin a soft diet to avoid excessive strain on the TMJ. Instruct the patient to support their mandible with their hand when yawning so that it does not open widely and dislocate. Nonsteroidal anti-inflammatory drugs will provide adequate analgesia, if needed at all.

COMPLICATIONS

Complications of the initial injury include fractures, intrusion of the mandibular condyle into the external au-

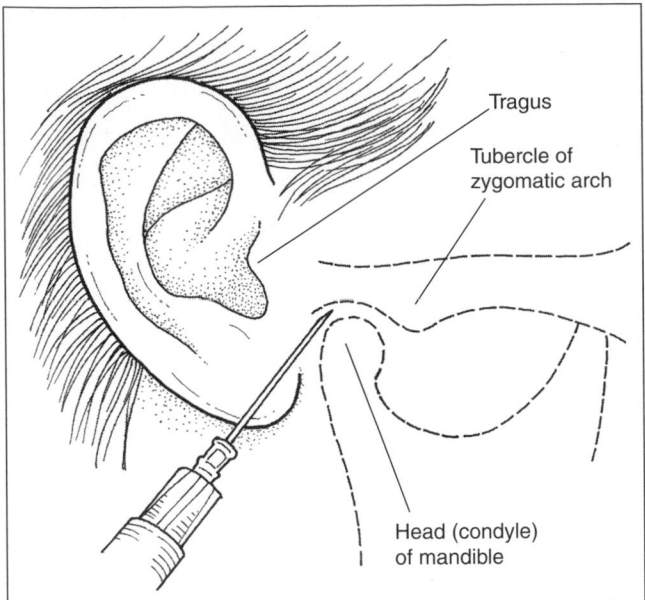

FIGURE 161-4 Anesthesia of the temporomandibular joint. Insert the needle 2.5 cm anterior to the tragus of the auricle and just above the mandibular condyle.

Tragus

Tubercle of zygomatic arch

Head (condyle) of mandible

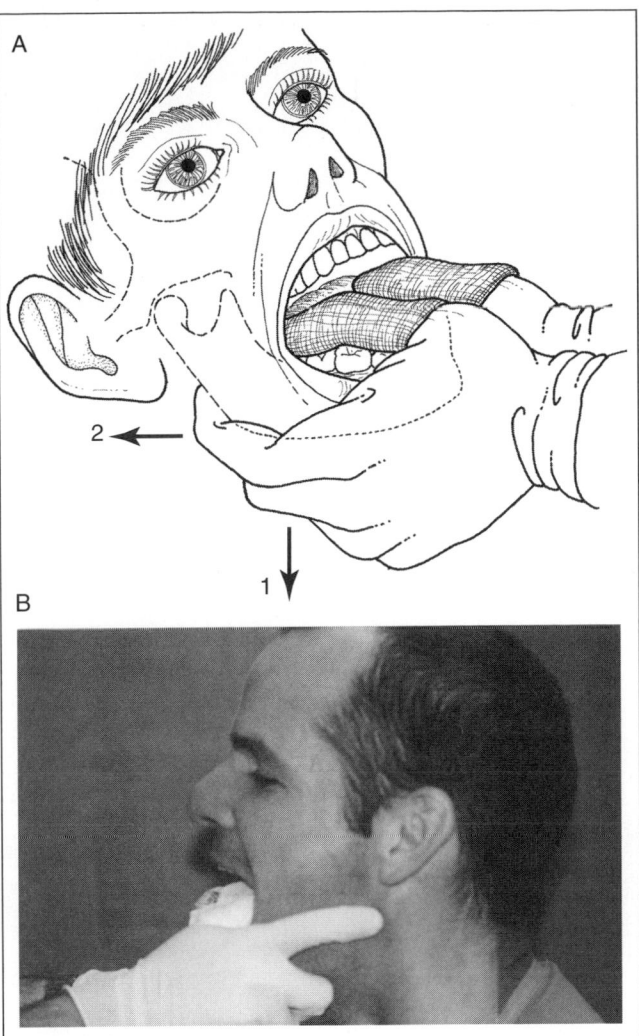

A

B

2

1

FIGURE 161-5 Proper thumb and hand placement for the reduction of an anteriorly dislocated mandible. *A.* Illustration of the reduction technique. Apply downward pressure with the thumbs (1) followed by posteriorly directed pressure (2) to reduce the dislocation. *B.* Reduction of a dislocated mandible.

ditory canal (posterior dislocation) or basal skull (superior dislocation), cerebral contusions, facial nerve injuries, and middle or inner ear injuries with hearing and balance impairments. Recurrent dislocation is possible in the future after the mandible has been dislocated once.

The reduction technique is rarely associated with complications. Significant pain after a successful reduction may signify a fracture or articular cartilage avulsion. Fractures are rarely iatrogenic. They are often present on initial radiographs but not identified until retrospectively examined. A fracture may be displaced during the reduction. The physician's thumbs can be crushed and/or lacerated by the patient's teeth.

Closed reduction may be unsuccessful. The patient will require reduction under general anesthesia. This is particularly true of chronic dislocations, dislocations for longer than 12 hours, and recurrent dislocations. An avulsed articular cartilage or articular disc may be interposed and prevent closed reduction.

SUMMARY

Uncomplicated anterior mandible dislocations can be managed with basic anesthesia and sedation techniques. A gentle and progressive reduction will allow the mandibular condyle to relocate into the TMJ space without significant complications. Dislocations that are complicated by fractures, overlying skin damage, nonanterior in location, or have associated neurological injuries require an emergent consultation and reduction by an Oral Surgeon or an Otolaryngologist.

REFERENCES

1. Peacock WF IV: Face and jaw emergencies, in Tintinalli JE, Kelen GD, Stapczynski JS (eds): *Emergency Medicine: A Comprehensive Study Guide,* 5th ed. New York: McGraw-Hill, 2000:1526–1532.
2. Kruger G-O: *Textbook of Oral and Maxillofacial Surgery.* St. Louis: Mosby, 1984.
3. Amsterdam JT: Dental disorders, in Rosen P, Barkin R, Danzl DD, et al (eds): *Emergency Medicine: Concepts and Clinical Practice,* 4th ed. St. Louis: Mosby, 1998:2680–2697.

Section Fourteen

PODIATRIC PROCEDURES

Chapter 162
INGROWN TOENAIL REMOVAL

Jeff Schaider

INTRODUCTION

An ingrown toenail (onychocryptosis) is a common affliction that can occur in any toe. It most commonly afflicts the great toe, occurring when the lateral edge of the nail plate penetrates the soft tissue of the lateral nail fold. There are three stages of ingrown toenails. Stage I includes erythema, slight edema, and pain when pressure is applied to the lateral nail fold. Stage II includes the stage I findings, drainage, and infection. Stage III is a magnification of the two previous stages with the addition of granulation tissue and lateral nail fold hypertrophy. Most ingrown toenails can be definitively managed in the Emergency Department.

ANATOMY AND PATHOPHYSIOLOGY

The toenail usually does not grow into the soft tissue; instead, the soft tissue overgrows and obliterates the nail sulcus in response to external pressure and irritation.[1-5] The nail itself is usually normal, although some older patients have incurved nails. The causes of an ingrown toenail are multiple and include trimming the nails too short, using sharp tools to clean the nail gutters, wearing improperly fitted (too tight) shoes, rotated digits, and bony deformities. Improper toenail trimming results in a small nail spike that continues to grow and irritate the soft tissue (Figure 162-1). The end result is a chronic infection.

INDICATIONS

Warm soaks, oral antistaphylococcal antibiotics, and shoes with an adequate toe box may be curative in mild cases (stages I and II). Elevate and maintain the nail edge above the soft tissues or trim the edge of the nail. More severe cases (stage III) require partial toenail removal. Have a lower threshold for toenail removal in diabetic patients to prevent a more severe infection from forming. Other indications for removal of an ingrown toenail include chronic or recurring ingrown toenails, failure of optimal conservative therapy, fungal infections of the toenail, and severe pain.

CONTRAINDICATIONS

The only relative contraindication to toenail removal is a decreased vascular supply to the toe. Trim the toenail edge if possible and minimize any injury to the adjacent soft tissues. These patients require an evaluation by a Podiatrist and a Vascular Surgeon to minimize future complications.

EQUIPMENT

General Supplies

Povidone iodine solution
Sterile drapes
Sterile gloves
Curved hemostat
Cotton
Scissors or nail splitter
Tourniquet or sterile Penrose drain
Curette
Topical antibacterial ointment
4×4 gauze squares
Tape, 1 inch wide

Chemical Matrix Ablation

Cotton-tipped applicators
Phenol solution (89%)
Isopropyl alcohol (70%)
Silver nitrate matchsticks

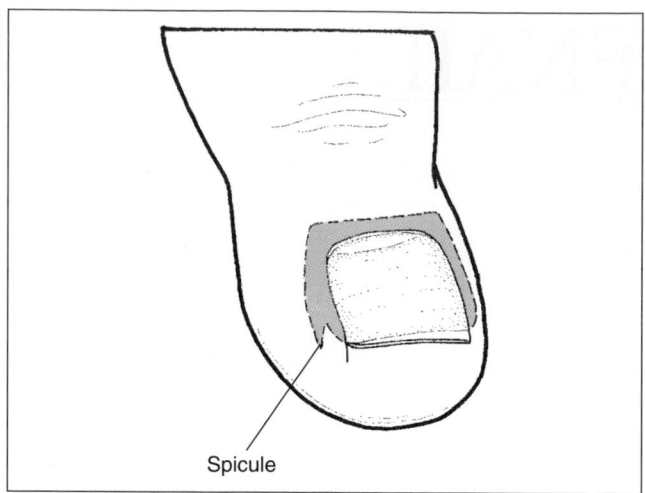

FIGURE 162-1 An ingrown toenail. Note the nail spicule and the overgrowth of the adjacent soft tissues.

Surgical Matrix Excision

#15 scalpel blade on a handle
Needle driver
5–0 nylon suture

Nail Matrix Cauterization

Electrocautery unit, disposable

PATIENT PREPARATION

Explain the risks, benefits, complications, and aftercare of the procedure to the patient and/or their representative. Obtain an informed consent for the procedure. Place the patient supine on a gurney or procedure table. Flex the patient's hip and knee so that the plantar surface of the foot is flat against the gurney. An overhead light source is essential to provide appropriate illumination. Perform a digit block using aseptic technique. Refer to Chapter 106 regarding the details of digital anesthesia. Apply povidone iodine solution over the involved toe and allow it to dry. Apply a sterile drape to delineate a sterile field.

TECHNIQUES

Manage early ingrown toenails (stages I and II) with conservative therapy. Remove the medial or lateral one-quarter of the toenail along with the germinal matrix at the base of the toenail for stage III ingrown toenails. The entire nail may be removed if both sides are ingrown. It may be necessary to prevent any new nail growth in the area once the nail has been removed. Three options include chemical ablation of the matrix, surgical excision of the matrix, and electrocautery of the nail matrix.

TOENAIL ELEVATION AND TRIMMING

Ingrown toenails in the first two stages can be trimmed or elevated to relieve the patient's symptoms (Figure 162-2). Trim the distal edge of the nail plate to remove the ingrown portion (Figure 162-2A). Remove the distal one-third to one-half of the nail plate. Smooth the nail plate edge so that it will grow out freely. Remove any debris along the lateral nail fold (paronychia) or nailbed.

An alternative is to elevate the edge of the nail plate (Figure 162-2B). Insert the jaws of the hemostat so that

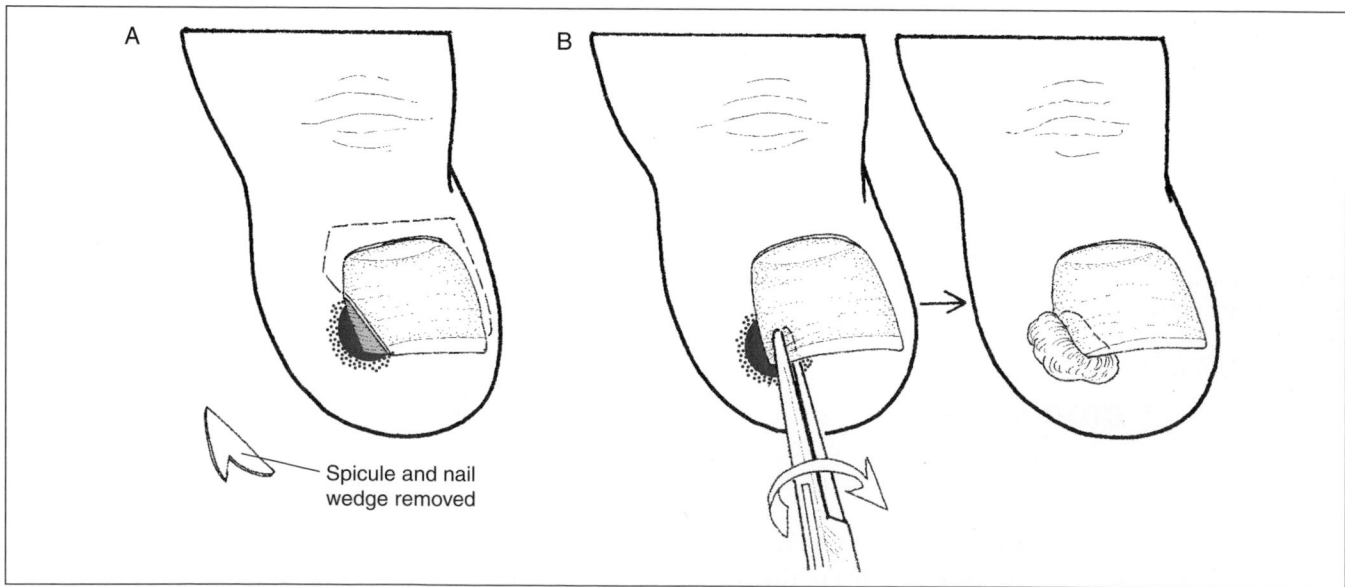

FIGURE 162-2 Management of stage I and II ingrown toenails. *A.* Trimming the lateral nail edge. *B.* Elevation of the lateral nail edge.

one is above and the other is below the ingrown nail edge. Clamp the jaws of the hemostat onto the nail plate. Elevate the edge of the nail plate above the adjacent soft tissues. Insert a wad of cotton under the nail edge to maintain it above the adjacent soft tissues. Release the hemostat. Teach the patient this technique so that they can replace the cotton wad daily until the nail plate grows out and past the soft tissues. The main disadvantage of this technique is that the patient must maintain the nail plate elevation for 3 to 6 weeks.

TOENAIL REMOVAL

Apply a tourniquet along the base of the afflicted toe (Figure 162-3A). The tourniquet may be a commercially available product for the digits or a Penrose drain. Separate the nail from the underlying nail bed. Grasp and stabilize the toe with the nondominant hand. Insert one jaw of a curved hemostat under the distal toenail margin and along the medial or lateral side of the nail plate, depending upon which side is ingrown (Figure 162-3B). Advance the hemostat until the jaw is at the proximal corner of the involved side of the ingrown nail (Figure 162-2C). Grasp the nail by clamping the jaws of the curved hemostat on the toenail.

Dislodge the ingrown nail from the skin, the nail bed, and the nail matrix by rotating the hemostat away from the ingrown portion (Figure 162-3D). Continue to rotate the hemostat until the entire ingrown portion of the nail is separated from the skin, the nail bed, and the nail matrix. A large and complete portion of the underlying toenail will emerge from under the skin fold (Figure 162-3E). The nail plate might have broken and a significant piece may still be under the inflamed skin border if only a small amount of the nail is visible after rotating the hemostat. Expose this area and use the curved hemostat to remove any remaining nail plate.

Cut away the ingrown portion of the toenail, from distal to proximal, with a heavy scissors or nail splitter (Figure 162-3F). The granulation tissue overlying the nail bed must be removed to prevent another ingrown toenail (Figure 162-3G). Trim the granulation tissue using a #15 scalpel blade or a curette (Figure 162-3H).

CHEMICAL NAIL MATRIX ABLATION

Chemical ablation of the nail matrix with phenol has several advantages. The procedure is easy, quick, and simple to perform. No special equipment is required. The use of an incision or electrocautery, and their associated complications, is avoided.

Chemical ablation of the matrix with phenol is the author's preferred method. Remove any obvious remaining nail matrix and nail bed with a blunt instrument such

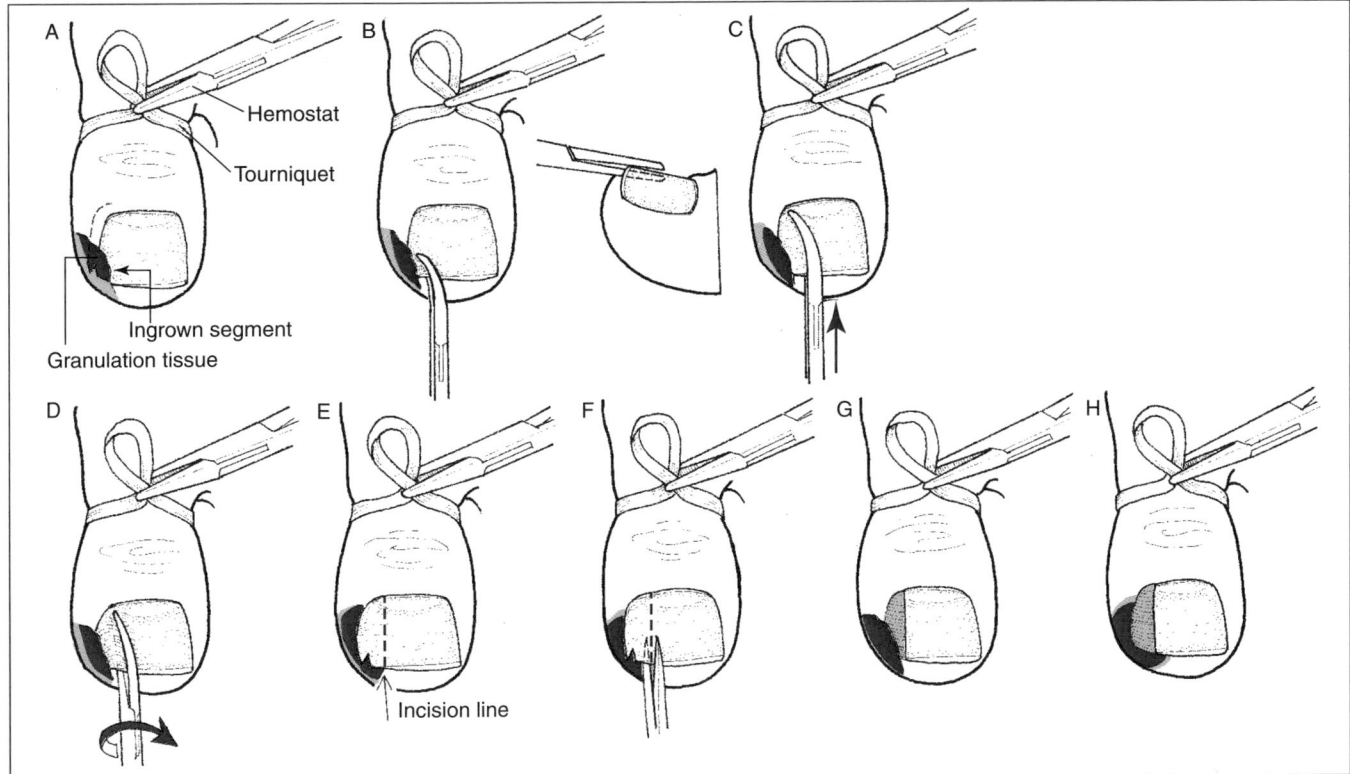

FIGURE 162-3 Ingrown toenail removal. *A.* Placement of a tourniquet. *B.* Place one jaw of the hemostat above the nail plate and one jaw beneath the nail plate. *C.* Advance the hemostat toward the base of the nail plate. *D.* Rotate the hemostat to elevate the edge of the toenail. *E.* Determine where to cut the nail plate. *F.* Cut the nail plate with a heavy scissors or a nail splitter. *G.* The lateral one-fourth of the nail plate has been removed. *H.* The granulation tissue has been trimmed away.

as a curette. **Completely dry the field of any blood and fluid.** Dip a cotton-tipped applicator in a phenol solution. **Avoid excessive saturation of the swab.** Introduce the swab between the roof and the root matrix (i.e., under the eponychium) of the removed nail section (Figure 162-4). Rotate the cotton-tipped applicator slowly for 30 seconds (20 seconds for children) and then remove it. Repeat the phenol application two additional times using a fresh phenol-soaked cotton-tipped applicator. **Do not allow the phenol to contact normal skin. Immediately wipe off any phenol that contacts the skin.** Dip a cotton-tipped applicator in isopropyl alcohol. Swab the area in similar fashion as the phenol swab. The isopropyl alcohol neutralizes the necrotizing effect of the phenol.

An alternative to phenol is silver nitrate. The preferred technique is a phenol matrixectomy. Silver nitrate may be used if phenol is not available. The main disadvantage of silver nitrate is that it turns the tissues black. Insert the silver nitrate matchstick under the eponychium (Figure 162-4). Roll the matchstick around for 5 to 10 seconds to ablate the matrix.

SURGICAL NAIL MATRIX ABLATION

Surgical excision of the toenail matrix requires more time and experience than chemical ablation.[4] This technique is usually reserved for the Podiatrist or the Orthopedic Surgeon. Expose the nail matrix by retracting the adjacent overlying skin. Make an oblique proximal incision from the proximal corner of the nail if necessary to fully expose the nail matrix in the ingrown area (Figure 162-5A). Make an incision with a #15 scalpel blade to sep-

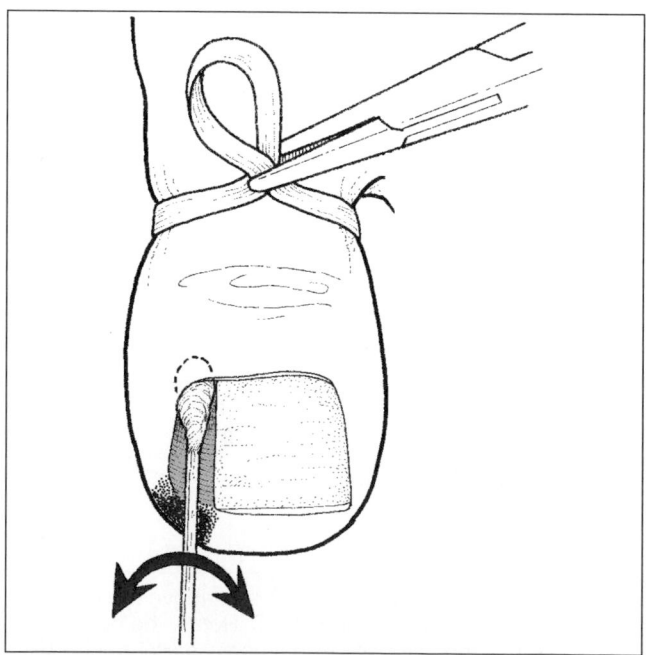

FIGURE 162-4 Chemical nail matrix ablation.

arate the nail matrix to be removed from the remaining nail and matrix (Figure 162-5B). Grasp the corner of the matrix with a hemostat. Use the scalpel blade to separate the matrix from the underlying tissues. Remove the nail matrix. Do not forget to remove the dorsal and deep matrix that envelops the base of the toenail under the skin fold. Remove any remaining nail matrix and nail bed with a curette. Close the skin incision with 5–0 nylon suture.

ELECTROCAUTERY NAIL MATRIX ABLATION

Electrocauterization of the nail matrix is rapidly performed but requires access to an electrocautery instrument. Apply electrocautery between the roof and the root matrix of the removed nail section to destroy the matrix in this area. Avoid excessive burning of the surrounding tissues. This technique can cause significant damage to normal tissue and should be reserved for the Podiatrist or the Orthopedic Surgeon.

AFTERCARE

Apply a topical antibiotic ointment and a small compressive gauze dressing over the toe. The patient requires follow-up in 24 to 48 hours for a dressing change and evaluation of the wound. Saturate the dressing with saline or sterile water to make the removal process less painful. Instruct the patient to elevate the foot for the first 2 to 3 days to prevent bleeding and edema. Large shoes, sandals, or cast shoes are best used in the immediate post-procedure days. The use of oral antibiotics is restricted for patients who are immunocompromised, have an associated cellulitis, or whose vascular supply to the toe is decreased. Prescribe nonsteroidal anti-inflammatory drugs supplemented with narcotic analgesics as needed for pain control. Instruct the patient to return to the Emergency Department immediately if they experience increased pain, develop a fever, or notice increased redness of the toe or foot. Demonstrate the proper method to trim toenails (Figure 162-6).

Chemical ablation of the matrix with phenol induces a chemical burn. The patient may experience a serous drainage for a few days up to two weeks.[1] The use of nonsteroidal anti-inflammatory drugs can limit the duration and the amount of drainage.[1] Instruct the patient to soak the foot in warm water three times a day for 10 to 15 minutes each time. Apply a topical antibiotic ointment after each soak. Prolonged drainage may be due to a superficial infection and requires evaluation.

COMPLICATIONS

The most common complication is the persistence of toenail horns or spikes due to incomplete ablation of the

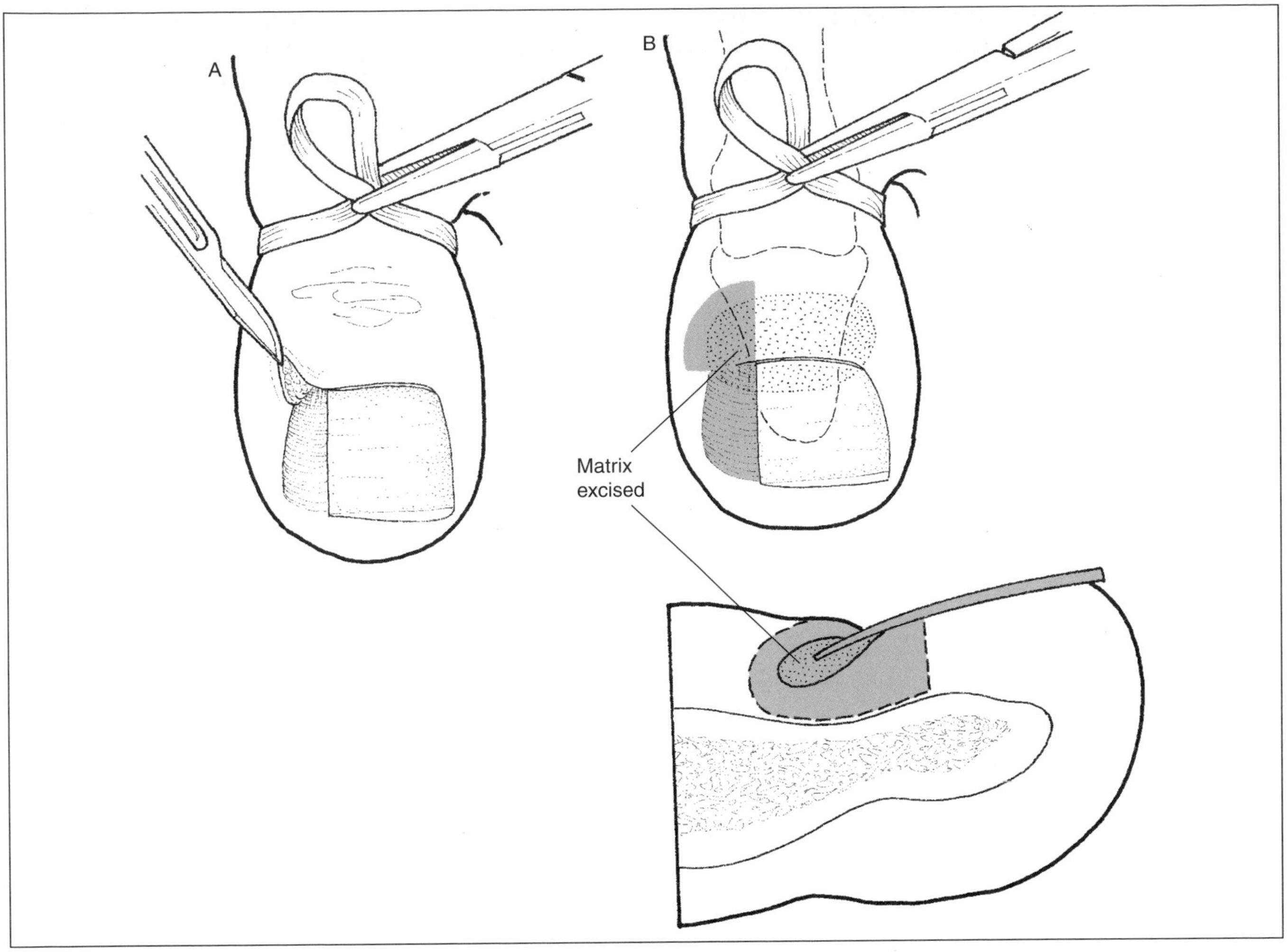

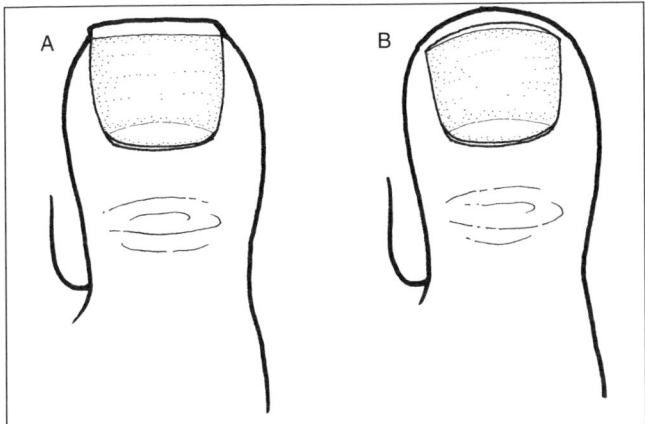

FIGURE 162-5 Surgical nail matrix ablation. *A.* An incision in the eponychium to expose the matrix. *B.* Removal of the matrix. The pink shading represents the areas of tissue to be removed.

nail and matrix. These can be managed with nail trimming if mild or en bloc excision of the area if severe. Ensure that the portion of the nail is completely removed and that no fragments remain under the nail folds.

FIGURE 162-6 The technique of toenail trimming. *A.* Correct. *B.* Incorrect.

Phenol will deteriorate if it is exposed to air or light. Store the phenol solution in a cool, dark place. Replace the solution frequently. The field must be dry before applying phenol. Phenol mixed with blood results in an alteration of the pH of the phenol, decreasing its effectiveness and turning the tissues black. The ingrown toenail will recur if the phenol is old or exposed to light before it is used, if the phenol is not properly applied, or if fragments of the toenail or matrix remain. The patient may experience a chemical burn if too much phenol is applied or it is not neutralized with isopropyl alcohol.

SUMMARY

An ingrown toenail can be managed easily, quickly, and definitively in the Emergency Department. Perform a partial toenail removal on patients with clinical stage III toenails characterized by pain, overgrowth of inflamed and infected tissue, and drainage. Remove the lateral or medial one-quarter of the nail. Apply phenol solution to the nail matrix to prevent further growth of the nail and a recurrence.

REFERENCES

1. Bliss IL: Phenol matrixectomy, in Johnson KA (ed): *Master Techniques in Orthopedic Surgery: The Foot and Ankle.* New York: Raven Press, 1994:15–20.

2. Eisele SA: Conditions of the toenails. *Orthop Clin North Am* 1994; 25(1):183–188.

3. Mercier LR, Pettid FJ, Tamisiea DF, et al: *Practical Orthopedics,* 4th ed. St. Louis: Mosby, 1995:252–254.

4. Sanders M: Marginal toenail ablation, in Johnson KA (ed): *Master Techniques in Orthopedic Surgery: The Foot and Ankle.* New York: Raven Press, 1994:3–13.

5. Zuber TJ, Pfenninger JL: Management of ingrown toenails. *Am Fam Physician* 1995; 52(1):181–190.

Chapter 163
PLANTAR PUNCTURE WOUND MANAGEMENT

Justin Onzuka

INTRODUCTION

Plantar puncture wounds are encountered quite frequently in the Emergency Department. They are often incurred while walking barefoot or in the course of work. Nails produce the majority of such wounds. Various other objects such as wood, metal, and glass are also common causes. There is very little data regarding the proper management of plantar puncture wounds, but it is clear that complications can and do arise.[1–4] Infection and retained foreign bodies remain the most serious of these complications.

One of the difficulties with plantar puncture wounds is that patients do not always present to the Emergency Department. Most patients remove the offending foreign body and never seek medical treatment. The true risk of infection and osteomyelitis remains unknown. The infection rate is estimated to be approximately 2 to 8 percent, with only a fraction of these complications proceeding to osteomyelitis.[1] There are seasonal variations, with the warm months, from May through October, being the peak times for plantar puncture wounds.[1]

The pathophysiology and management of plantar puncture wounds is dependent on a host of factors, including the location of the wound, the penetrating material, the depth of penetration, the footwear at the time of injury, the time to presentation, and any concomitant illnesses. This chapter summarizes the approach to and management of the plantar puncture wound.

ANATOMY AND PATHOPHYSIOLOGY

The foot is a complex structure (Figures 163-1 and 163-2). The plantar surface is composed of the skin and a thin subcutaneous layer. The skin has a thickened stratum corneum layer, making it one of the thickest areas of epidermis in the body. This thickened epidermal layer gives the plantar surface protection against mechanical forces. The plantar aponeurosis extends over the base of the foot and forms the plantar fascia. Deep to the fascia are various muscles and tendons and their sheaths. The longitudinal arch of the foot extends from the metatarsal heads to the calcaneus. The dorsal surface of the foot has a thin skin layer without much subcutaneous tissue. Under the thin subcutaneous layer is the superior dorsal fascia and the dorsal aponeurotic layer, which encompasses the extensor tendon sheaths.

The thickened plantar epidermal layer prevents minor mechanical insults from penetrating the skin. An object can puncture the plantar surface of the foot and compromise the deeper layers of the foot. The impaling object may just breach the plantar fascia or even go through the foot, depending on the depth of penetration.

INDICATIONS

Determine if the penetrating object is small, such as a needle or pin, and if a portion may still be within the foot. If the patient was able to remove the object intact, no further treatment is required and the patient may be discharged with a wound care sheet and asked to return if there are any signs of infection. **Obtain soft tissue radiographs if the impaling object is broken off or the possibility of a retained foreign body exists.** Most metallic and glass foreign bodies are visible on plain radiographs. Wood and plastic foreign bodies are not visible on plain radiographs. They require evaluation by computed tomography (CT) scanning, magnetic resonance imaging (MRI), ultrasound, or wound exploration[3] (Figure 163-3). Large penetrating objects are an indication for wound irrigation and exploration (Figure 163-4).

CONTRAINDICATIONS

There are a few relative contraindications to the exploration of a plantar puncture wound. Evidence of deep

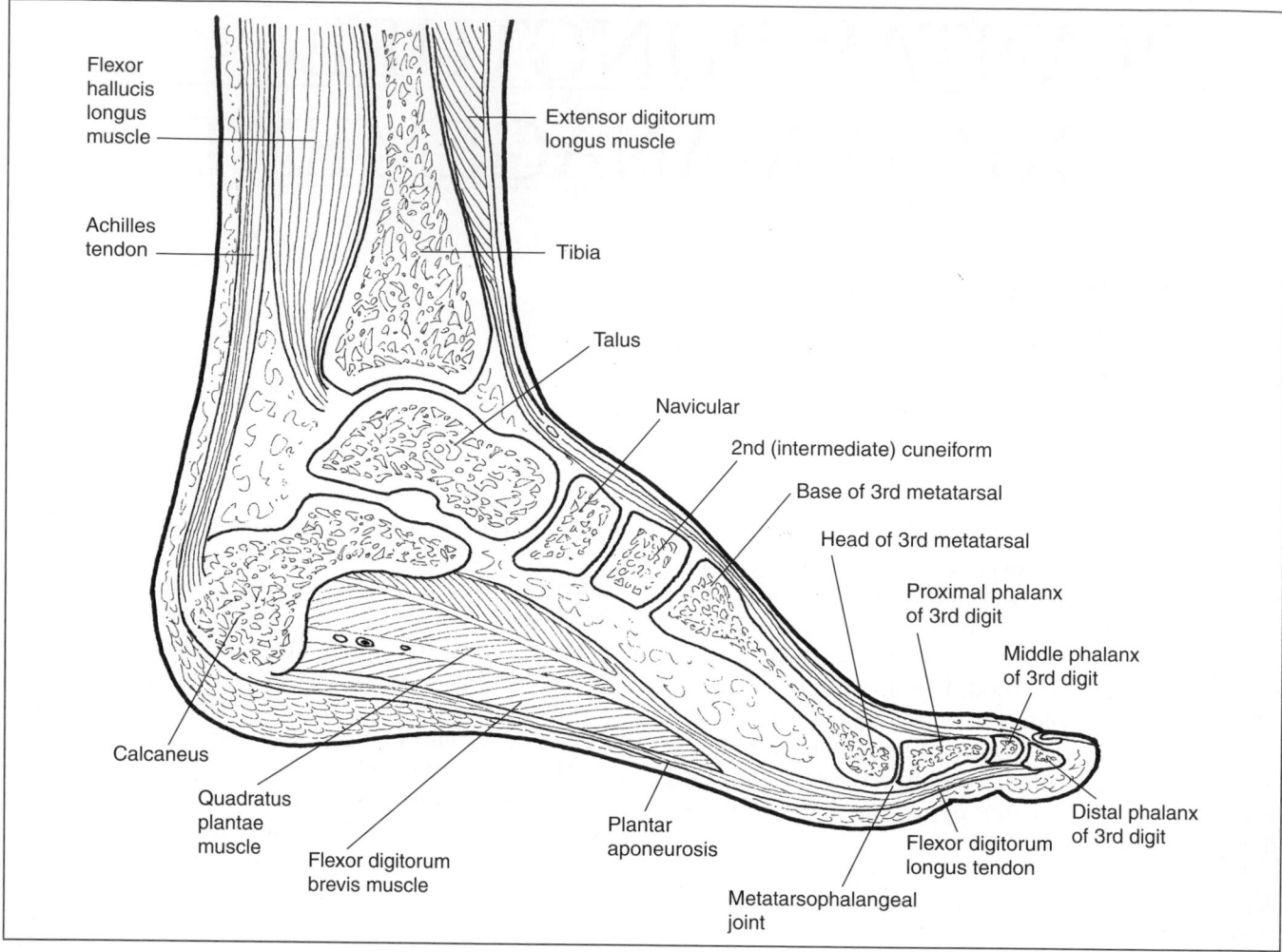

FIGURE 163-1 The anatomy of the foot in midsagittal section.

penetration, extensive penetration, or multiple retained foreign bodies should be evaluated in consultation with a Podiatrist or Orthopedic Surgeon. Manage patients who present more than 72 hours after the injury with evidence of infection while taking antibiotics, a draining tract, or dorsal foot symptoms (pain, erythema, or swelling) in consultation with a foot specialist. Surgical exploration and irrigation is required for penetration of any joint space or wounds overlying the metatarsal heads. Do not explore plantar puncture wounds if you are not experienced in or comfortable with the procedure.

EQUIPMENT

Povidone iodine solution
10 mL syringe
Local anesthetic solution without epinephrine
23 to 27 gauge needle
4×4 gauze squares
Eye protection or splash guard

Gloves
15 mL syringe
Sterile normal saline for irrigation
18 gauge plastic angiocatheter without the needle
#15 surgical scalpel blade on a handle
Cuticle clippers or fine iris scissors
Curved mosquito hemostat
Blunt probe
Toothed forceps
Circular corn pad
Tubular cling
Tape, 1 inch wide

PATIENT PREPARATION

Prior to deciding how to manage a plantar puncture wound, one must first assess the situation. Identify the penetrating object and determine whether it may still be embedded in the foot. Determine if it is possible for the patient to have a retained foreign body. Deter-

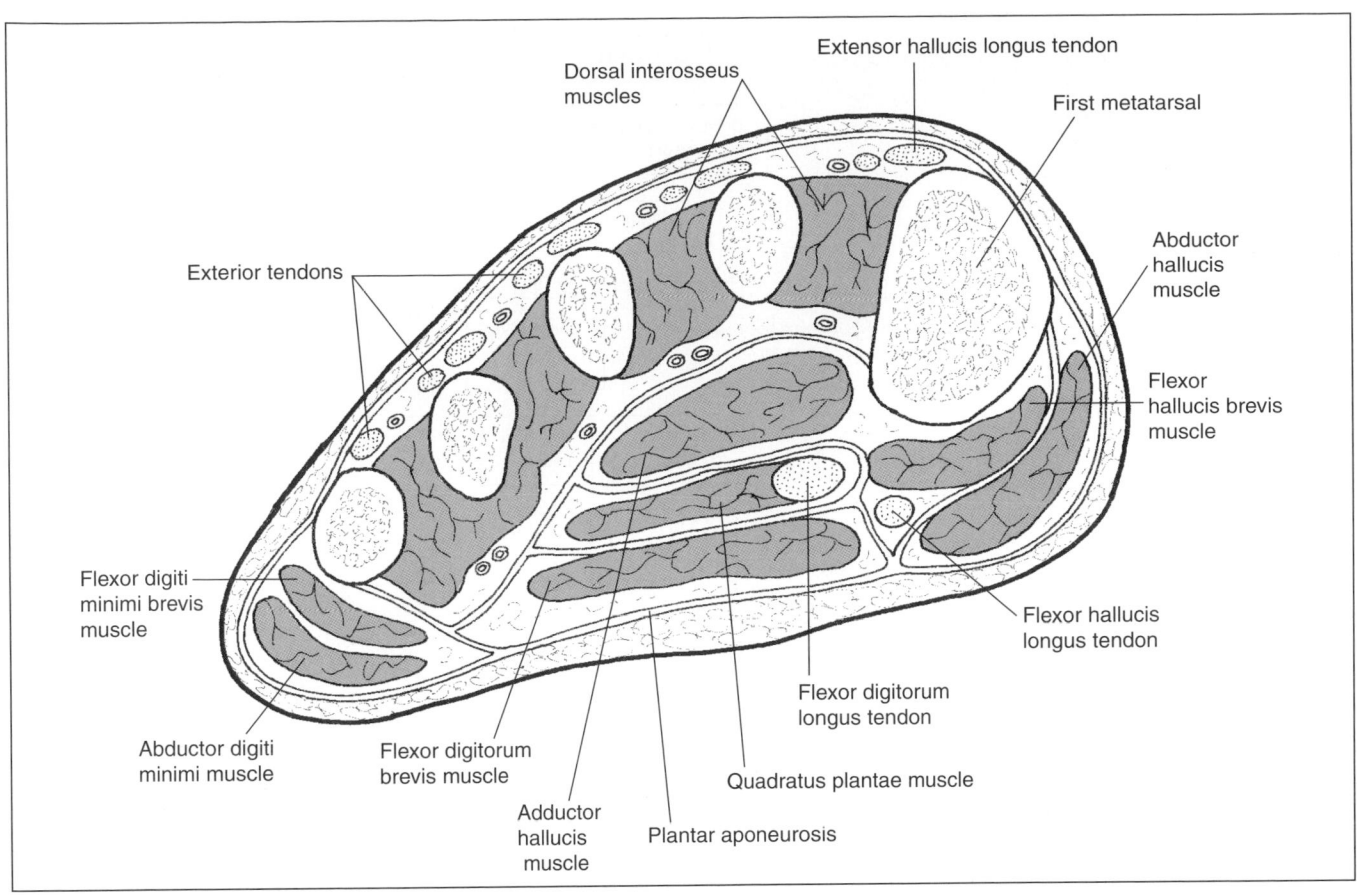

FIGURE 163-2 The anatomy of the foot. Cross-section just proximal to the metatarsal heads.

mine the cleanliness of the penetrating object. Was it contaminated or rusty? Identify the site of the incident. Was it outdoors or indoors? What type of footwear was worn at the time of the incident? Estimate the depth of penetration. Ascertain if the patient has any comorbid health conditions that may affect wound healing.[2] Does the patient need tetanus immune globulin or a booster?

Obtain plain radiographs if a foreign body may be retained, if an infection is present, if the patient presents more than 72 hours after incurring the injury, if the patient stepped on glass, or if the patient feels that a foreign body is present. Glass is radiopaque and visible upon plain radiographs.[5–10] The patient is often correct if they have a foreign body sensation and feel that a foreign body is "still there."[10] Patients were correct 15 of 41 times when they felt that a foreign body was present.

Explain the risks, benefits, and potential complications of the procedure to the patient and/or their representative. Obtain a signed informed consent for the procedure. Place the patient supine or prone on a gurney. Remove any superficial foreign bodies. Clean the skin overlying the wound of any dirt and debris. Clean the skin posterior to the medial malleolus if a posterior tibial nerve block is to be performed. Apply povidone iodine

solution to the skin and allow it to dry. Apply sterile drapes to delineate a sterile field.

Anesthetize the area. **Do not inject directly into the plantar surface of the foot!** This would be extremely painful for the patient. Perform a posterior tibial nerve block.[4] The posterior tibial nerve is superficial at the ankle, midway between the medial malleolus and the heel (Figure 163-5A). It lies between the tendons of the flexor digitorum longus and flexor hallicus longus muscles. It travels with and slightly posterior to the posterior tibial artery. The posterior tibial nerve divides at the inferior border of the calcaneous to form the medial and lateral plantar nerves. The posterior tibial nerve provides motor innervation to the intrinsic foot muscles. The lateral plantar nerve provides sensory innervation to the lateral one-third of the sole and plantar surface of the lateral 1½ toes (Figure 106-27). The medial plantar nerve provides sensory innervation to the medial two-thirds of the sole and the plantar surface of the medial 3½ toes (Figure 106-27).

Place the patient supine with the ankle supported on a pillow or blanket and the leg externally rotated. Identify, by palpation, the medial malleolus and the posterior tibial artery by its pulsation. Place a skin wheal of local

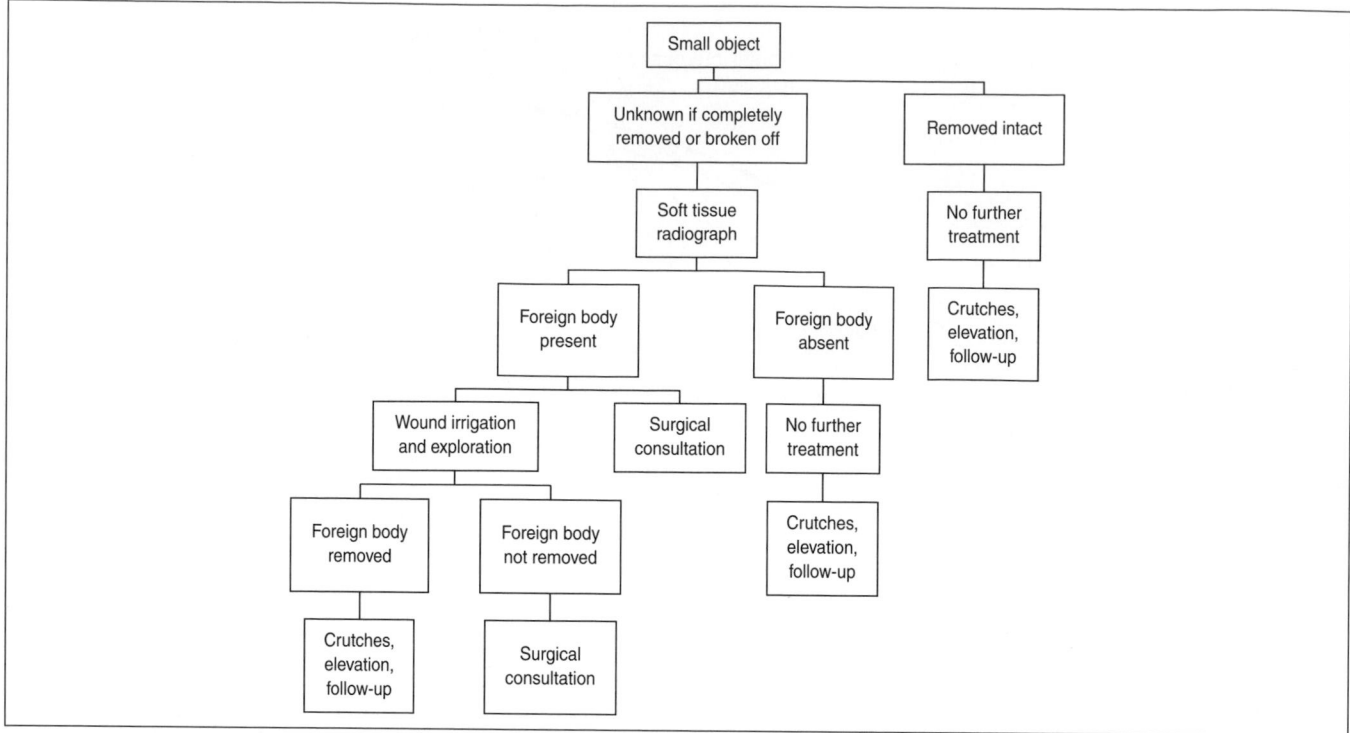

FIGURE 163-3 Management algorithm for small object plantar puncture wounds. (Adapted from Chisholm and Schlesser.[3])

anesthetic solution at the level of the upper border of the medial malleolus and just posterior to the posterior tibial artery or medial to the Achilles tendon. Insert a 25 gauge needle through the skin wheal and perpendicular to the skin (Figure 163-3*B*). Advance the needle to the tibia or until paresthesias are elicited. If paresthesias are elicited, withdraw the needle 2 mm and allow them to resolve. Inject 3 to 5 mL of local anesthetic solution. If paresthesias are not elicited, infiltrate 5 to 7 mL of local anesthetic solution, starting against the posterior tibia as the needle is withdrawn.

TECHNIQUES

Carefully debride any devitalized skin and callused edges (stratum corneum) overlying the wound with a pair of fine scissors or cuticle clippers. Obtain a culture swab of the wound. Gently probe the puncture site. Assess its depth using a blunt probe and fine atraumatic forceps. Up to 3 percent of probed plantar puncture wounds have a retained foreign body.[1]

It is often difficult to determine whether a joint space has been breached by the foreign body. **Assume any puncture wound in the metatarsophalangeal joint area involves a joint space and consider a surgical consulta-**tion. **Make every effort to remove a foreign body within the wound. Avoid extensive exploration to prevent secondary injury to a joint space or tendon sheath. Refer deeply embedded foreign bodies to a Surgeon for exploration and removal in the operating room.**

Irrigate the wound if no foreign body is palpable. Arm a 15 mL syringe containing sterile saline with an 18 gauge plastic angiocatheter. Insert the tip of the catheter into the wound. Take care not to place the tip of the irrigating catheter deep into the wound so as not to drive contaminants deeper. Copiously irrigate the wound with the normal saline. Thoroughly dry the skin. Apply a donut-shaped corn pad around the puncture site. Apply topical antibiotic gel followed by a gauze dressing. The gauze may be held in place with tubular gauze or a gauze roll wrapped about the foot.

AFTERCARE

The use of prophylactic antibiotics is controversial. **There is currently no good evidence supporting the prophylactic treatment of plantar puncture wounds with antibiotics.** Institute empiric antibiotic coverage for *Staphylococcus* and *Streptococcus* if this is a late presentation and there is evidence of cellulitis. Pre-

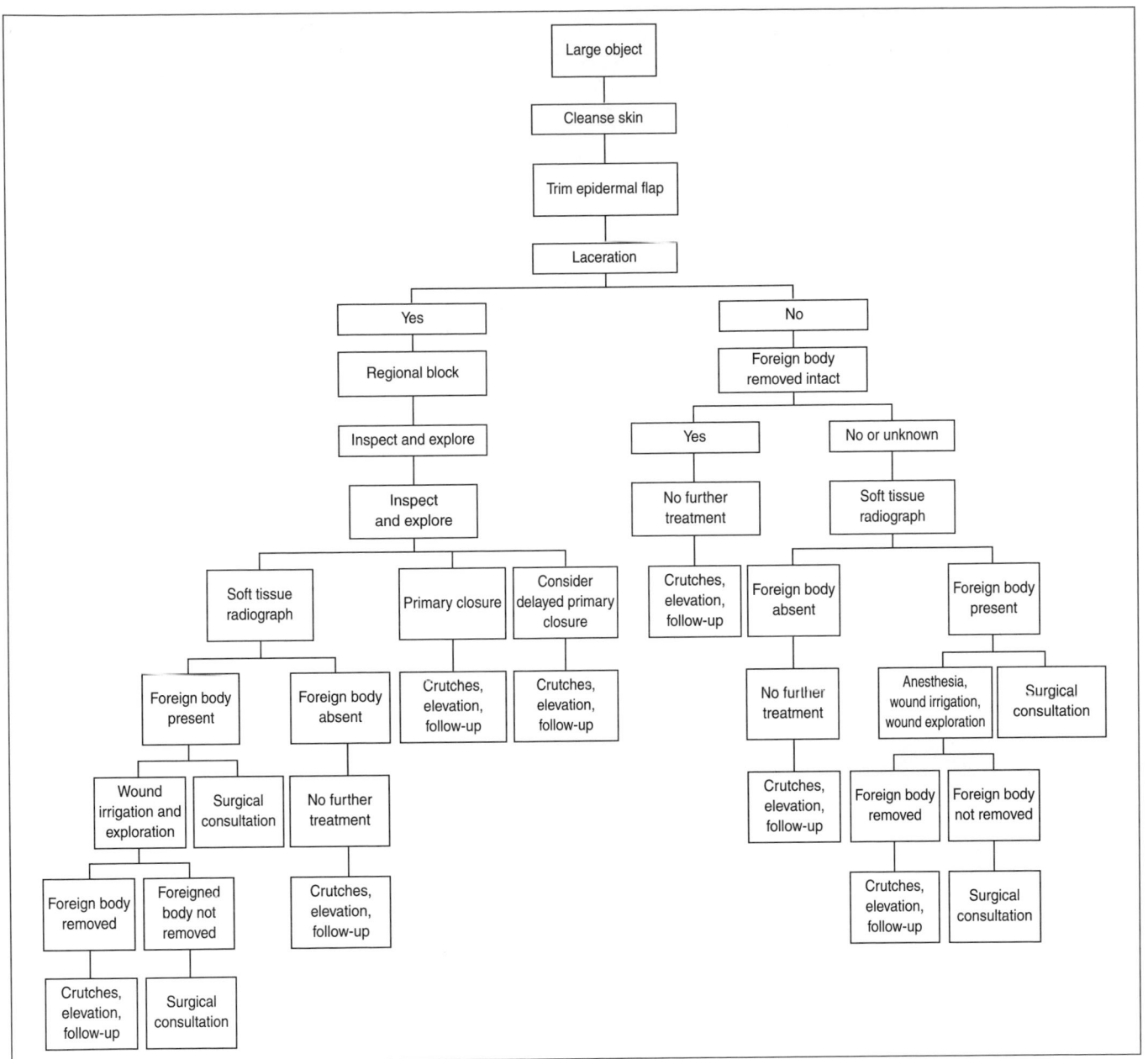

FIGURE 163-4 Management algorithm for large object plantar puncture wounds. (Adapted from Chisholm and Schlesser.[3])

scribe penicillinase-resistant antibiotics for 7 to 10 days, guided by sensitivities. Patients who have diabetes or who are immunocompromised require broad-spectrum antibiotics, such as a third-generation cephalosporin or levofloxacin, and close follow-up.

Prescribe nonsteroidal anti-inflammatory drugs for analgesia. Instruct the patient to elevate the foot as much as possible in the next 48 hours. Adjunctive treatments such as epsom salts or tepid water soaks may have some benefit, but this has not been proven in clini-

cal trials. Give the patient the option of crutches. Instruct them to refrain from placing pressure over the site of the puncture wound. The affected foot should be rested and elevated above heart level whenever possible.

Give the patient a wound care sheet. Instruct them to return to the Emergency Department if they experience worsening pain, swelling, erythema along the dorsal surface of the foot, or a draining sinus. Arrange follow-up within 48 hours with a Primary Care Physician, Podiatrist, or Orthopedist.

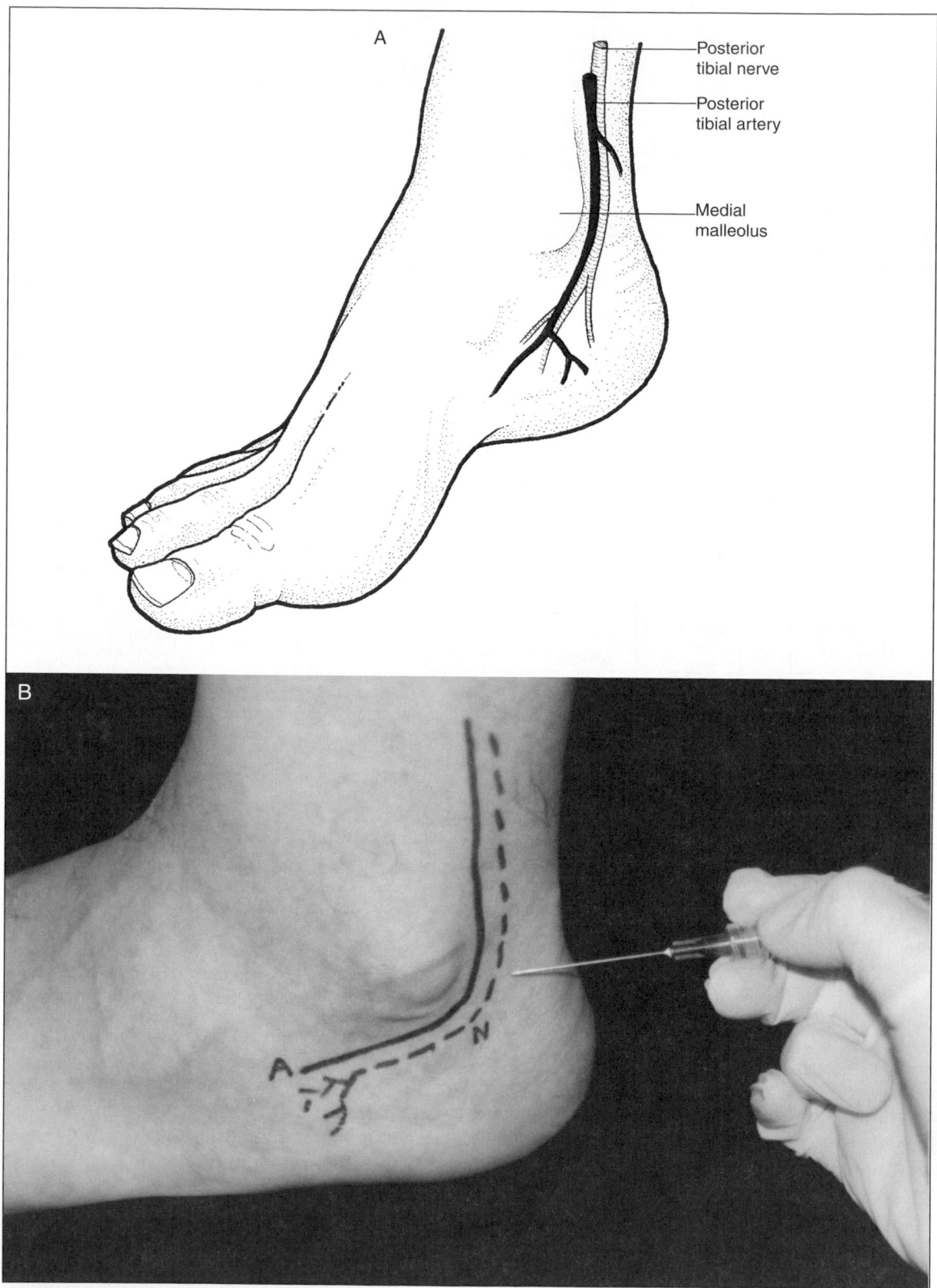

FIGURE 163-5 The posterior tibial nerve block. *A.* The course of the posterior tibial nerve. *B.* Needle insertion and direction.

COMPLICATIONS

The most frequently encountered complications of a puncture wound to the foot are cellulitis, soft tissue abscesses, osteomyelitis, and foreign body granulomas. Symptoms persisting beyond 24 hours of the injury increase the possibility that complications will develop.[4] Late presenters who showed signs of cellulitis despite appropriate antibiotics had retained foreign bodies in more than 50 percent of cases.[1] It is estimated that 8 to 15 percent of all puncture wounds of the foot progress to cellulitis or localized abscesses.[1] Cellulitis is often due to normal skin flora. Approximately 0.6 to 1.8 percent of patients develop osteomyelitis within 6 to 16 months of the injury.[1]

Osteomyelitis is a rare complication and difficult to treat. *Pseudomonas aeruginosa* is the most common organism isolated. It is thought that the use of prior prophylactic antibiotics, increased regional humidity from wearing shoes, or the presence of a serous exudate from the wound may facilitate the growth of *Pseudomonas*.[2] The diagnosis of osteomyelitis can be made from clinical features such as a draining sinus visualized to bone or radiographic evidence of disruption of the bony cortex. Consider obtaining a CT scan, a bone scan, or radio-labeled white blood cell (WBC) scan to make the diagnosis. Treatment involves surgical debridement and/or intravenous antibiotics, fluoroquinolones or ceftazidime, for 4 to 8 weeks.[2]

SUMMARY

The paucity of clinical trials in this area of Emergency Medicine makes the management of plantar puncture wounds controversial. Simple and small plantar puncture wounds have a low incidence of complications. The presence of retained foreign bodies and unknown depths of penetration make puncture wounds vulnerable to complications. A thorough history and physical examination are crucial to stratify patients for risk and to start initial therapy. Basic cleansing and debridement of devitalized tissue along with copious sterile irrigation are the cornerstones of treatment. Careful blunt probe exploration and radiography help to decrease the incidence of retained foreign bodies. Tetanus prophylaxis should be reviewed with all patients. Prophylactic antibiotics are discouraged unless the wound is grossly contaminated. Most important of all is appropriate follow-up within 24 to 48 hours.

Late presenters often have established wound infections requiring antibiotic treatment and appropriate referrals. Retained foreign bodies are a common cause of infections and require a thorough search. Osteomyelitis is a rare complication. Frequent and timely follow-up remains the current standard of care to avoid infectious complications until further studies of antibiotic prophylaxis and initial puncture wound management can resolve the controversies.

REFERENCES

1. Fitzgerald RH Jr, Cowan JDE: Puncture wounds of the foot. *Orthop Clin North Am* 1975; 6(4):965–972.
2. Verdile VP, Freed HA, Gerard J: Puncture wounds to the foot. *J Emerg Med* 1989; 7:193–199.
3. Chisholm CD, Schlesser JF: Plantar puncture wounds: controversies and treatment recommendations. *Ann Emerg Med* 1989; 18:1352–1357.
4. Schwab RA, Powers RD: Conservative therapy of plantar puncture wounds. *J Emerg Med* 1995; 13(3):291–295.
5. Tandberg D: Glass in the hand and foot. Will an x-ray film show it?. *JAMA* 1982; 248(15):1872–1874.
6. de Lacey G, Evans R, Sandin B: Penetrating injuries: how easy is it to see glass (and plastic) on radiographs? *Br J Radiol* 1985; 58(685):27–30.
7. Gron P, Anderson K, Vraa A: Detection of glass foreign bodies by radiography. *Injury* 1987; 17(6):404–406.
8. Ginsburg MJ, Ellis GL, Flom LL: Detection of soft tissue foreign bodies by plain radiography, xerography, computed tomography, and ultrasonography. *Ann Emerg Med* 1990; 19(6):701–703.
9. Avner JR, Baker MD: Lacerations involving glass: the role of routine roentgenograms. *Am J Dis Child* 1992; 146(5):600–602.
10. Montano JB, Steele MT, Watson WA: Foreign body retention in glass-caused wounds. *Ann Emerg Med* 1992; 21(11):1360–1363.

INTRODUCTION

Toe fractures result from a direct blow (from an object falling on an unprotected toe) or a "stubbing" injury. The significance of toe fractures depends upon which digit is affected. Most important is the great toe, as it is the main propulsive segment of the forefoot. Many patients do not present to the Emergency Department, as they consider the injury trivial. Those who do present to the Emergency Department often do so because of severe pain and/or a large subungual hematoma.

Toe fractures are common injuries that rarely require surgical treatment. They may be completely and definitively managed in the Emergency Department. Most toe fractures require only a properly placed splint. An intra-articular fracture with severe displacement of the great toe may require open reduction and internal fixation to prevent deformity and arthritis in the joint. Complications of a toe fracture include damage to cartilage, hypermobility of fracture segments, malposition, and malunion.

ANATOMY AND PATHOPHYSIOLOGY

The foot can be anatomically divided into the forefoot, the midfoot, and the hindfoot (Figure 164-1). The forefoot is composed of the metatarsals and their respective phalanges. Sesamoid bones often lie along the plantar surface of the metatarsal heads. The sesamoid bones of the great toe lie in a groove on the plantar surface of the metatarsal head and within the tendon of its respective flexor hallucis brevis muscle belly.

Each toe has two pairs of digital nerves that course along the superior and inferior aspects of the digit. The digital artery and vein accompany the nerve. The great toe often receives superficial cutaneous nerves along its dorsal surface.

Obtain radiographs of the affected toe(s). Antero-posterior and oblique views will demonstrate most fractures. Lateral views may be necessary to identify phalangeal fractures of the great toe. Obtain the lateral projection with toes 2 to 5 passively dorsiflexed to avoid overlap. An alternative method to achieve adequate radiographic views of the great toe in the lateral projection is to insert dental x-ray film between the first and second toes and direct the x-ray beam laterally.[1]

INDICATIONS

The indications for simple splinting of toe fractures are to relieve pain and allow for healing. The management of closed fractures depends on the digit involved. Manage nondisplaced phalangeal fractures of the great toe with buddy taping to the adjacent normal toe as a splint. Mildly displaced phalangeal fractures of the great toe can be reduced using local anesthesia, gentle traction, and buddy taping. Manage nondisplaced phalangeal fractures of toes 2 to 5 with buddy taping. Mildly displaced phalangeal fractures of toes 2 to 5 can be reduced using local anesthesia, gentle traction, and buddy taping. Exact anatomic reduction of toes 2 to 5 is not a concern as long as the general alignment of the toe is satisfactory.[2]

CONTRAINDICATIONS

Consult an Orthopedic Surgeon or Podiatrist for open fractures, extensive crush injuries to the forefoot, injuries with the potential to develop a compartment syndrome, intraarticular fractures, or severely displaced toe fractures (especially of the great toe). The incidence of

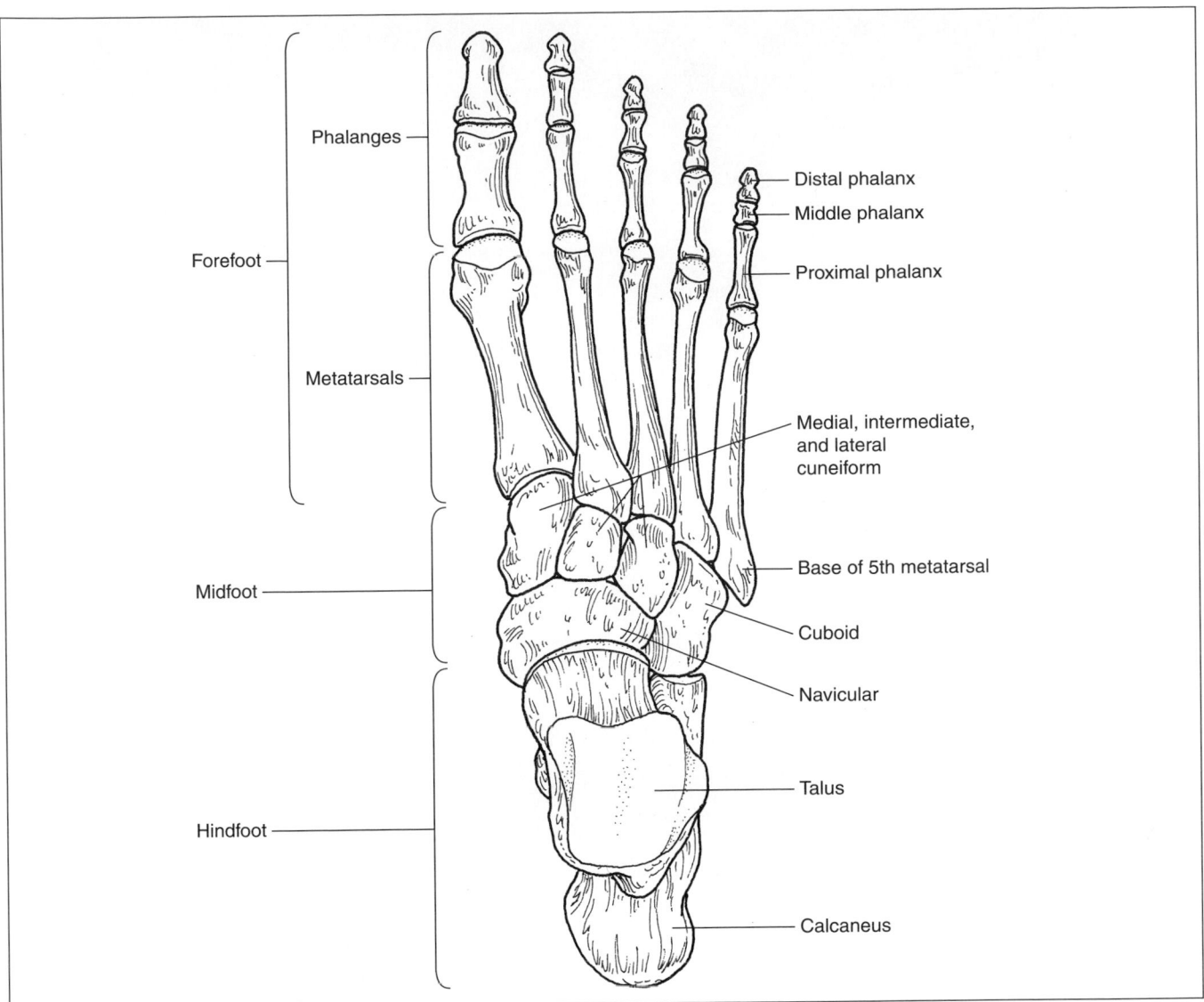

FIGURE 164-1 The bony anatomy of the foot.

arthritis and malunion is quite high with these injuries. Fractures of multiple toes on one foot cannot be treated with buddy taping.

EQUIPMENT

Povidone iodine solution or isopropyl alcohol swabs
Local anesthetic solution without epinephrine
25 or 27 gauge needle
5 mL syringe
2×2 gauze squares or a soft corn pad
Chinese finger trap, optional
Bunion pad
Metatarsal bar or wooden tongue depressors
Permeable tape, ½ inch wide
Fluoroscopy unit, optional

PATIENT PREPARATION

Explain the risks, benefits, and potential complications of the procedure to the patient and/or their representative. Obtain a signed informed consent for the procedure. Obtain radiographs or a fluoroscopic image to assess the severity of the injury. Place the patient sitting upright so that the affected foot is suspended above the floor in order to allow adequate space for manipulation and splinting of the toe. An alternative is to place the patient supine with the hip and knee flexed, so that the sole of the foot is flat against the gurney. If a subungual hematoma presents with a great toe fracture or a significant crush injury, it should be drained to relieve pressure and improve patient comfort. Refer to Chapter 85 for complete details regarding the management of a subungual hematoma.

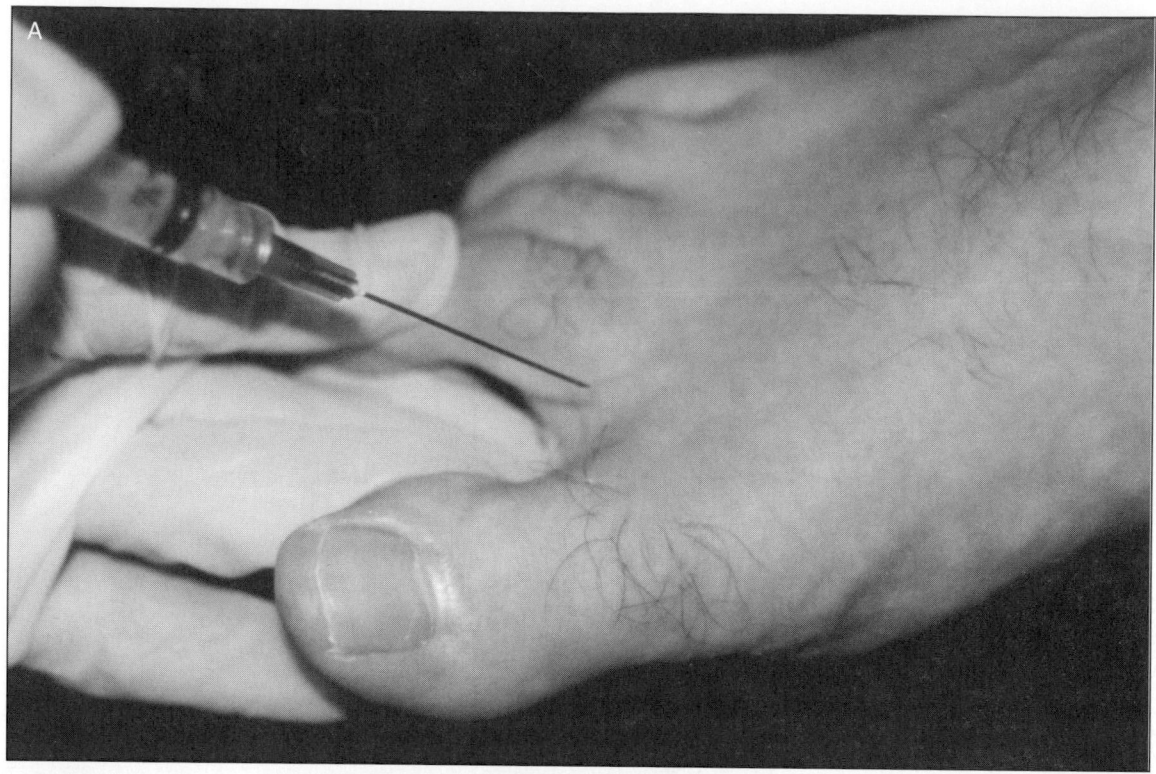

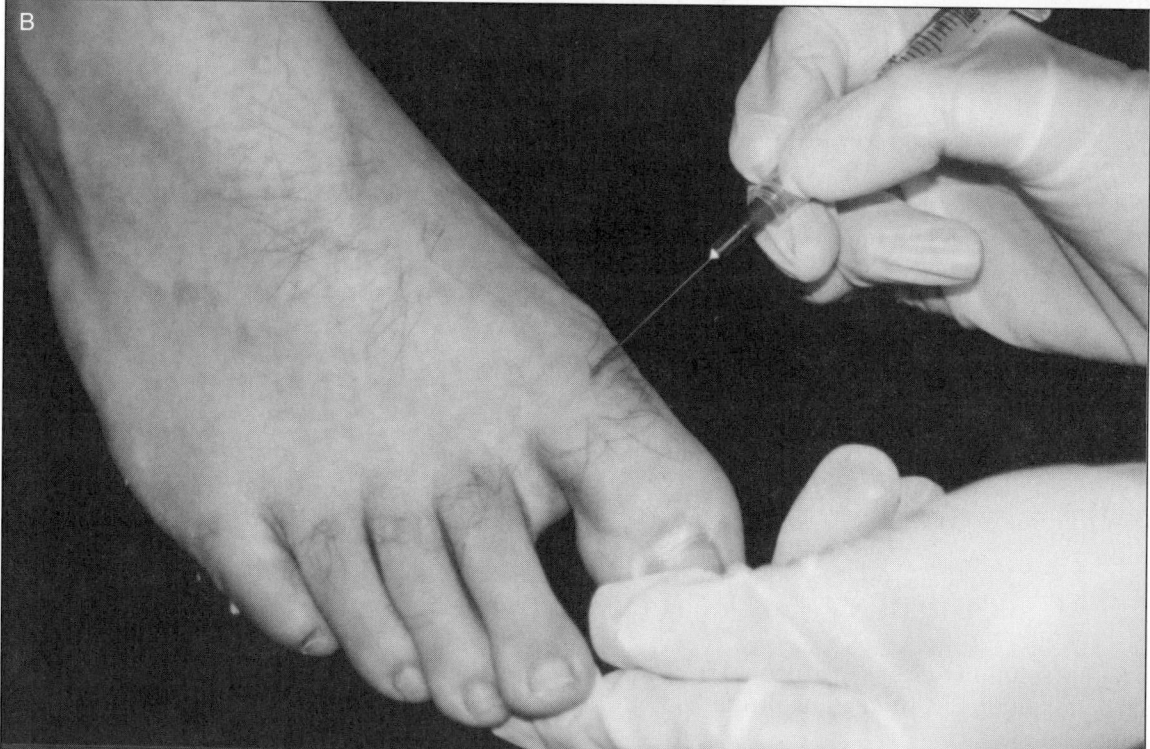

FIGURE 164-2 Digital block of the toe. *A.* Needle position and direction for infiltration of the lateral surface. *B.* Needle position and direction for infiltration of the dorsal surface.

The use of anesthesia is physician-dependent and patient-dependent. Buddy taping of nondisplaced fractures of toes 2 to 5 or minimally displaced fractures of toes 2 to 5 requires no anesthesia. Consider performing a digital block if the patient is significantly tender and a displaced fracture must be reduced. Clean the web spaces of the affected toe of any dirt or debris. Apply povidone iodine solution or isopropyl alcohol to the web space and allow it to dry. Arm a 5 mL syringe containing local anesthetic solution without epinephrine with a 25 or 27 gauge needle.

Insert the needle into the dorsal surface of the web space. Aim the needle 45 degrees downward and toward the posterior aspect of the phalanx (Figure 164-2A). Advance the needle while injecting 1 to 2 mL of local anesthetic solution. **Do not puncture the plantar surface of the toe.** The local anesthetic solution will easily inject into the areolar tissue of the web space. Withdraw the needle. Shift the needle so that it is aimed along the dorsal surface of the toe (Figure 164-2B). Advance the needle while injecting 1 to 2 mL of local anesthetic solution over the dorsal surface. Completely withdraw the needle. Inject local anesthetic solution into the contralateral side of the affected toe in the same way as in the first web space. Allow 5 to 10 minutes for the block to take effect. Reassess the patient to determine whether the block was successful. An additional injection along the plantar surface of the toe may be required to provide total anesthesia, especially of the great toe. Refer to Chapter 106 for additional details regarding digital injection anesthesia.

An alternative is to perform a hematoma block by injecting local anesthetic solution directly into the fracture site. Clean and prepare the skin. Insert the needle over the fracture site. Advance the needle until it enters the fracture. Aspirate a small amount of blood to confirm that the tip of the needle is properly positioned. Inject 2 to 3 mL of local anesthetic solution into the hematoma. Allow 5 to 10 minutes for the local anesthetic to take effect before proceeding.

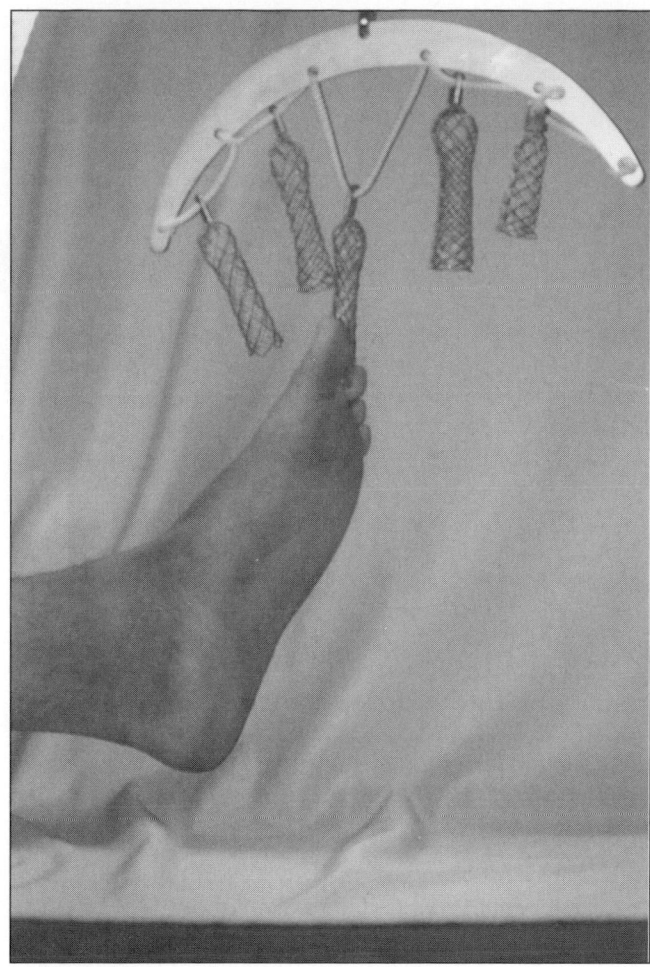

FIGURE 164-3 Use of the Chinese finger trap to aid fracture reduction. Place the affected toe in the Chinese finger trap. Suspend the foot by the affected toe.

TECHNIQUES

FRACTURE REDUCTION

Closed reduction can be achieved with the use of the Chinese finger trap or straightforward axial traction. Place the affected toe in the Chinese finger trap (Figure 164-3). Elevate and suspend the foot by the affected toe in the Chinese finger trap. Allow the weight of the leg to distract the fracture site. Reduce the fracture as described below. Remove the toe from the Chinese finger trap. Obtain a radiograph or fluoroscopic image to confirm the reduction. Buddy tape the toe.

The alternative is to reduce the fracture manually without the use of a Chinese finger trap (Figure 164-4). Grasp the base of the affected toe or fractured phalanx with the nondominant index finger and thumb. Grasp the distal aspect of the fractured phalanx with the dominant index finger and thumb. Apply distally directed inline traction with the dominant hand and simultaneous countertraction with the nondominant hand to distract the fracture site. Reduce the fracture. Obtain a

radiograph or fluoroscopic image to confirm the reduction. Buddy tape the toe.

BUDDY TAPING

Buddy tape the toe after the reduction (Figure 164-5). Place a piece of folded 2×2 gauze or a corn pad between the fractured toe and its neighboring toe (Figure 164-5A). The gauze or corn pad will prevent maceration and pressure necrosis of the skin. Tape the toes together (Figure 164-5B).

ASSESSMENT

Reassess the toe's perfusion by checking the capillary refill time after any attempt at reduction. Obtain a postreduction radiograph or fluoroscopic image to verify proper alignment. Mild to moderate displacement in phalangeal fractures of toes 2 to 5 is quite acceptable. Repeat the reduction process as necessary to reduce the

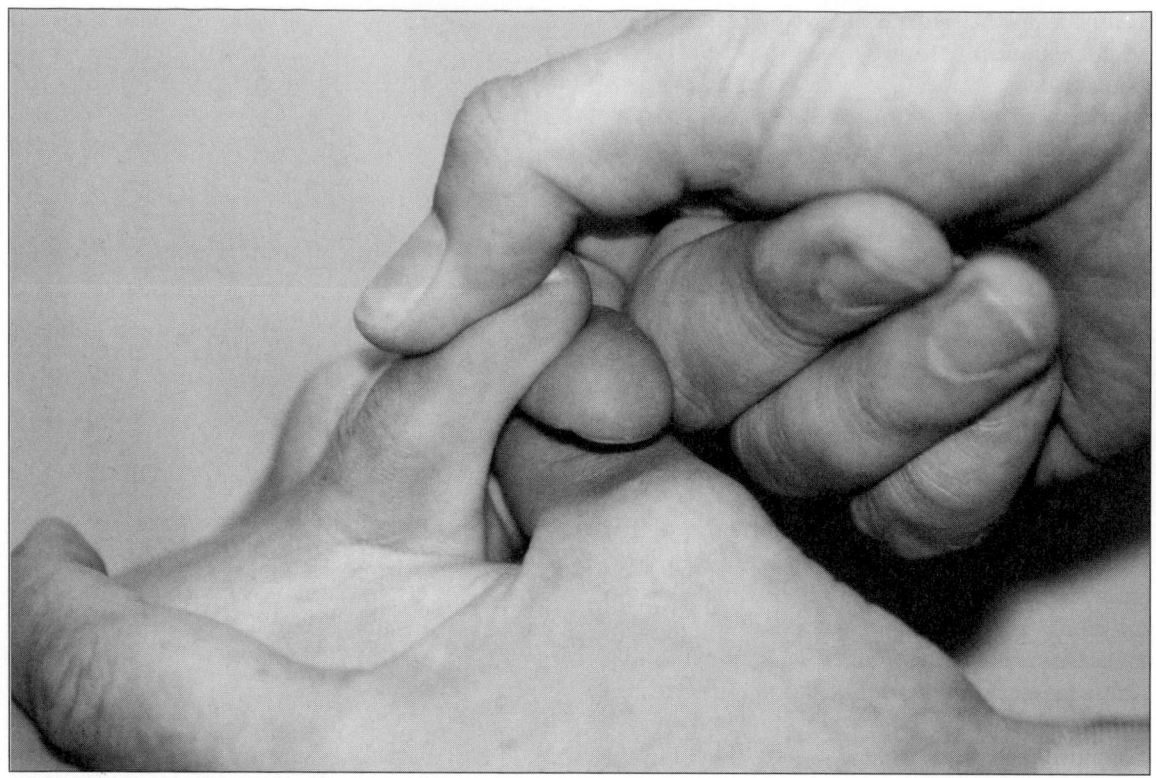

FIGURE 164-4 Manual fracture reduction.

fracture. Consult an Orthopedic Surgeon or Podiatrist if the fracture cannot be adequately reduced.

AFTERCARE

All toe fractures are persistently painful. They require analgesia and splinting for 2 to 3 weeks. Prescribe non-steroidal anti-inflammatory drugs supplemented with narcotic analgesics. Provide the patient with a hard-soled shoe, wooden-soled shoe, or Reese orthopedic shoe. It is felt that dorsiflexion of the forefoot in walking causes the most pain in toe fractures.[1]

An alternative to the orthopedic shoe is to place a metatarsal bar for patient comfort. Use a commercially available unit or make a metatarsal bar by taping wooden tongue depressors together[1] (Figure 164-6). Obtain four tongue depressors and cut one in half (Figure 164-6A). Place two tongue depressors side by side (Figure 164-6B). Place the third tongue depressor to cover the seam of the adjacent tongue depressors (Figure 164-6B). Tape the tongue depressors together to form the longitudinal sup-

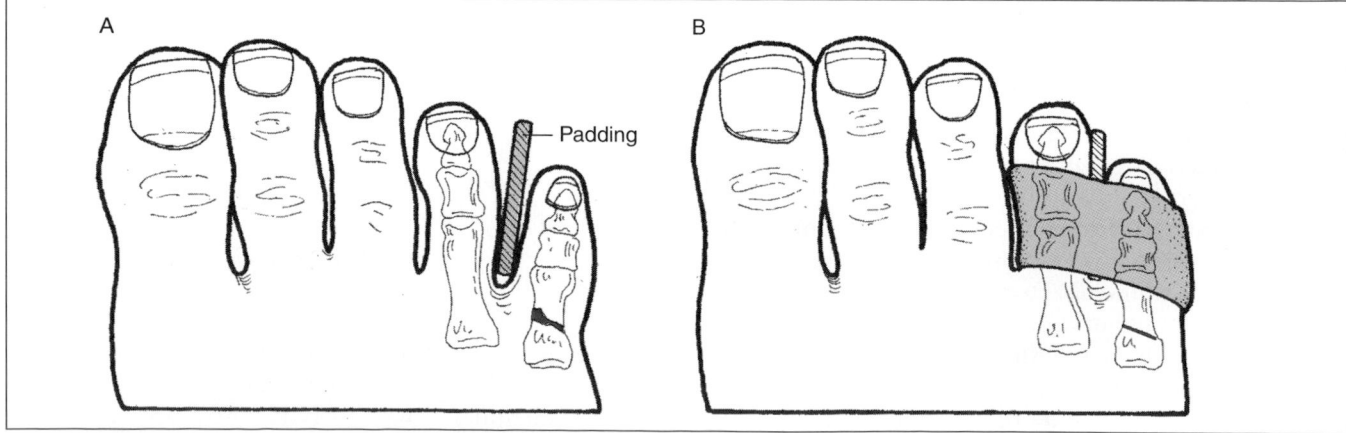

FIGURE 164-5 Buddy taping the fractured toe. *A.* Place gauze or a corn pad between the fractured toe and an adjacent toe. *B.* Tape the toes together.

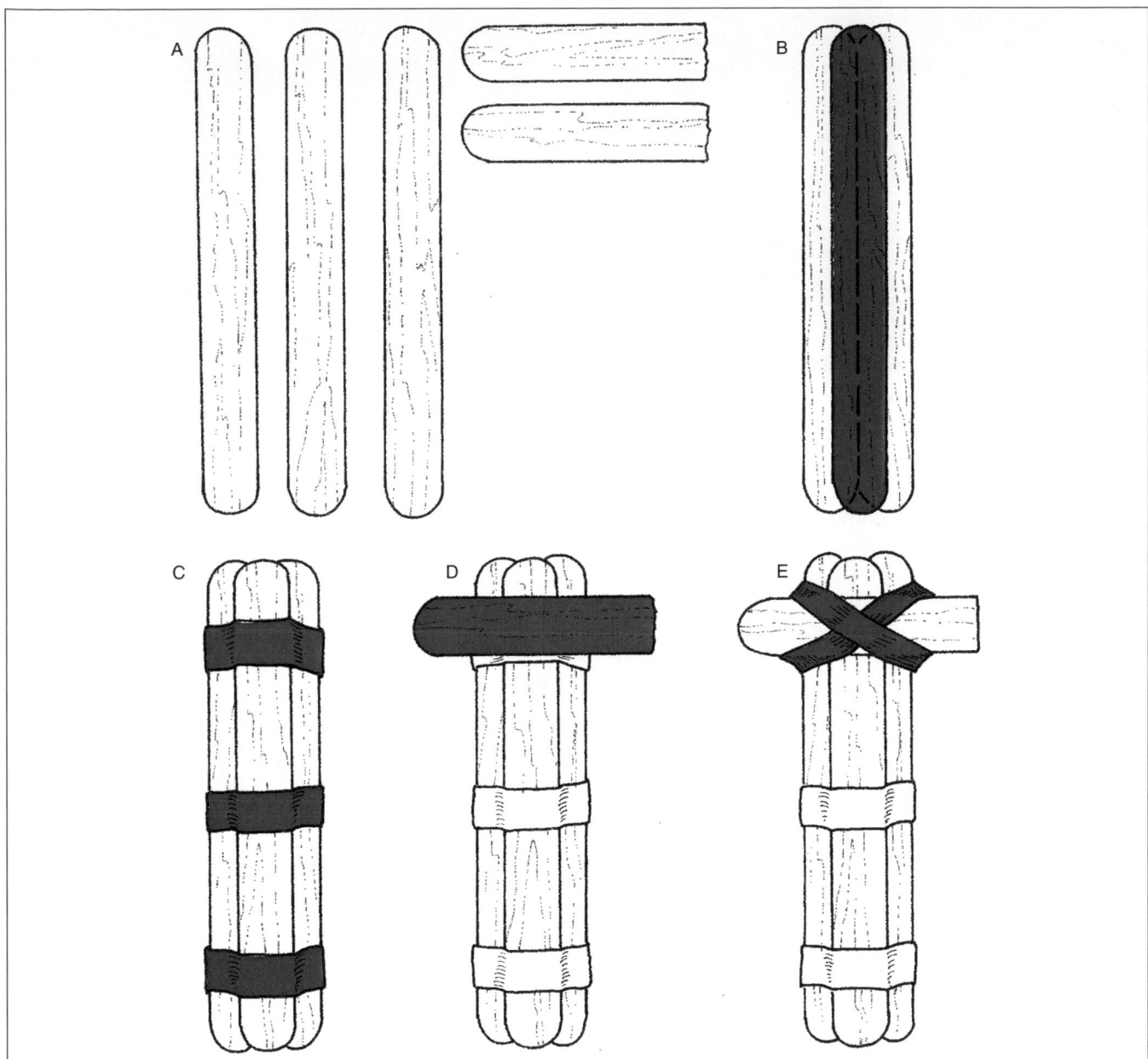

FIGURE 164-6 Fabricating a metatarsal bar from tongue depressors. *A.* Lay out four tongue depressors, one of which is cut in half. *B.* Place two tongue depressors side by side. Place the third depressor to cover the seam between the first two. *C.* Tape the tongue depressors together to form the longitudinal support. *D.* Apply the cut tongue depressor to form the transverse support. *E.* Tape the transverse support to the longitudinal support.

port (Figure 164-6*C*). Apply the cut tongue depressor to form the transverse support (Figure 164-6*D*). Tape the transverse support to the longitudinal support (Figure 164-6*E*). Apply the metatarsal bar to the to the sole of the patient's shoe (Figure 164-7). Additional support and pain control can be achieved by immobilizing the foot in a short leg walking cast with a toe plate for no more than 1 to 2 weeks if the patient complains of persistent pain.[2]

Instruct the patient to continue weight bearing as tolerated and, when not walking, to elevate the foot above heart level so as to minimize swelling. Teach the patient how to reapply the buddy splint, as it must be changed every 2 to 3 days for up to 6 weeks, as necessary.

COMPLICATIONS

Long-term sequelae from toe fractures are rare. Persistent angulation at the fracture site with malunion may result in a "sore area" on the plantar surface of the

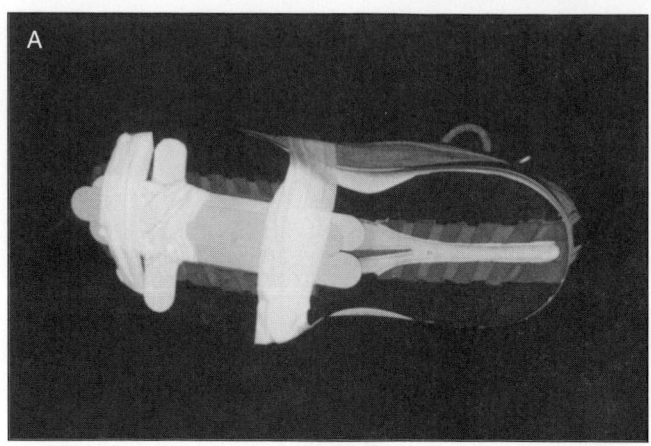 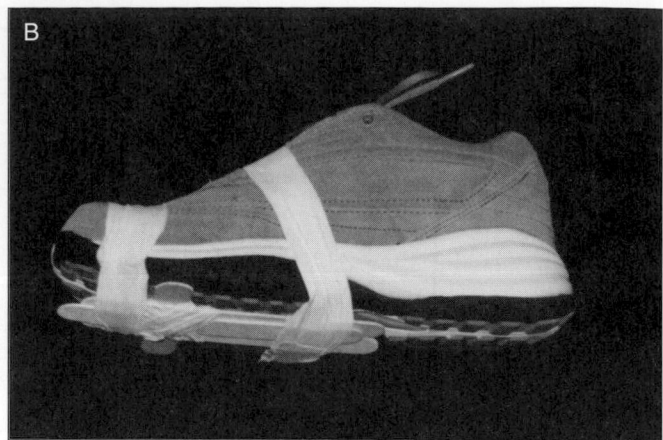

FIGURE 164-7 Application of the metatarsal bar to the patient's shoe. *A.* Inferior view. *B.* Lateral view.

toe. Refer the patient to an Orthopedic Surgeon or Podiatrist if such areas remain symptomatic and functionally disabling. A simple surgery can correct the problem. Any fractures involving the joint space will result in some degree of arthritis. Warn the patient of this possible complication before they are discharged.

Few complications are associated with the management of toe fractures. Persistent angulation can result in the toe pushing against adjacent toes, skin irritation, and possible skin ulceration. Always place a pad between the toes before buddy taping to prevent irritation, pressure necrosis, ulceration, and maceration of the skin.

SUMMARY

Toe fractures are common. They may cause the patient significant pain and discomfort. Simple conservative management with the use of buddy taping and appropriate footwear helps the fracture heal in 3 to 6 weeks. Closed reduction of phalangeal fractures may be required to achieve proper reduction. Most toe fractures can be satisfactorily and rewardingly managed in the Emergency Department with a minimum of complications.

REFERENCES

1. Early JS: Fractures and dislocations of the midfoot and forefoot, in Bucholz RW, Heckman JD (eds): *Rockwood and Green's Fractures in Adults.* Philadelphia: Lippincott Williams & Wilkins, 2001:2235–2239.
2. Mann RA, Coughlin MJ: *Surgery of the Foot and Ankle.* Toronto: Mosby, 1993:1642.

Chapter 165
PLANTAR WART MANAGEMENT

Justin Onzuka

INTRODUCTION

Plantar warts are caused by the human papillomavirus (HPV). Plantar warts were discussed as far back as the ancient Greeks and Romans. They were subsequently identified as being caused by infectious agents in the late 1800s. HPV, a member of the Papovaviridae family, was identified in 1949 and is composed of double-stranded DNA. The peak incidence of plantar warts occurs in the teenage years.[1] They are estimated to occur in 10 percent of children and young adults.[1] Little is known about how the HPV enters the host cell. It is found in the upper epidermis and results in squamous epithelial cell hyperplasia. Numerous types of HPV exist. Simple plantar warts are mainly due to HPV types 1, 2, or 4.

Two-thirds of untreated common warts in children regress spontaneously within 2 years.[1] Patients seek treatment despite these high remission rates, partly because of their location. Large warts on weight-bearing areas can be painful and disabling. If left untreated, they can be transmitted to adjacent or distant body areas. Patients often present with the plantar wart and request its removal. This chapter summarizes the pathogenesis of plantar warts and two techniques for their removal.

ANATOMY AND PATHOPHYSIOLOGY

One must recall the layers of the skin in order to understand the pathogenesis of the HPV (Figure 165-1). The skin is composed of the epidermis, the dermis, and the subcutaneous tissue or hypodermis. The epidermis on the sole of the foot consists mainly of stratified squamous epithelium. The thickness of the epidermis ranges from 0.05 mm on the dorsal surface of the foot to 1.5 mm on the plantar surface.[2] HPV replication occurs in the most superficial epidermal layer. The dermis is composed of connective tissue and serves as a scaffold for the skin. The blood vessels, nerves, glands, and hair follicles are located in the dermis.

HPV is a DNA virus. It gains access to host cells and uses the host's replicating cell proteins to manufacture viral proteins and DNA. This replication process induces epithelial cell hyperplasia, resulting in the mound of thickened skin observed in a plantar wart. The HPV remains in the epidermis but spreads laterally from the mound of verrucous tissue into what appears to be normal-looking epidermis. Intracellular HPV can remain in the dormant state so long as the host's cell mediated immunity holds it in check. Untreated, solitary, and small to mid-sized warts have a remission rate of approximately 70 percent in 2 years, with only 20 percent of the initial lesions persisting in immunocompetent individuals.[3]

INDICATIONS

The task force of the American Academy of Dermatology's Committee on Guidelines of Care has evaluated the indications for treatment of any wart.[3] They include patient request for therapy, symptomatic warts (pain, bleeding, itching, or burning), lesions that are disabling or disfiguring, many or large-sized lesions, to prevent spread to other body areas, and warts in patients who are immunocompromised.

CONTRAINDICATIONS

There are few contraindications to the removal of a plantar wart. **Any lesion whose diagnosis is uncertain requires a biopsy and/or an evaluation by a Dermatologist prior to any ablative removal.** An asymptomatic plantar wart should not be treated in the Emergency Department simply based on its presence. Relative contraindications for cryotherapy include patients who suffer from cold urticaria, cold intolerance, cryofibrinogenemia, cryoglobulinemia, diabetes, or peripheral vascular disease. Patients with diabetes or peripheral vascular

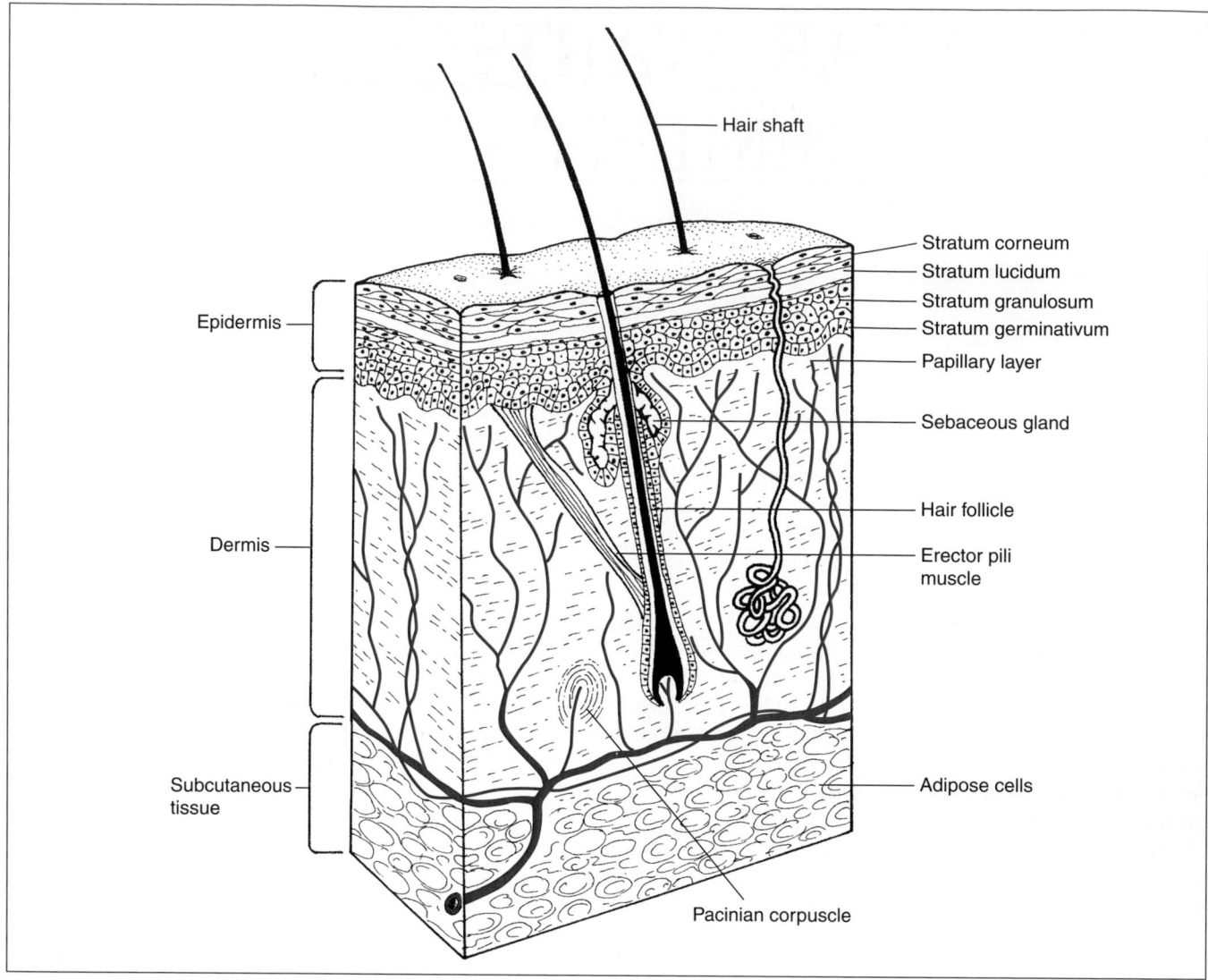

FIGURE 165-1 The anatomy of the skin.

disease have poor plantar blood circulation, may take longer to heal, and are at increased risk of developing a subsequent infection. Patients with hepatitis B, inflammatory bowel disease, or active collagen vascular disease may have an exaggerated freeze response and poor wound healing.[2] Patients who are taking corticosteroids or are immunocompromised may also have an exaggerated freeze response and poor wound healing.[2]

EQUIPMENT

General Supplies

Povidone iodine solution
25 or 27 gauge needle
3 mL syringe

Local anesthetic solution without epinephrine
EMLA cream
#15 surgical scalpel blade on a handle or straight razor blade
Nonsterile gloves
4×4 gauze squares
Pumice stone
Petroleum-based lubricant (i.e., Vaseline)

Cryotherapy

Liquid nitrogen stored in a Dewer tank
Handheld, self-contained spray devices (i.e., CRY-AC in 300 or 500 mL canisters)
Cotton-tipped applicators
Foam cup
Otoscope earpiece/cone

Salicylic Acid Therapy

Cotton-tipped applicators
15% to 40% salicylic acid ointment in collodion, with optional 20% lactic acid
Clear nail polish or petroleum-based lubricant
Occlusive dressing, Band-aid or Tegaderm

PATIENT PREPARATION

Explain the risks, benefits, and potential complications of the procedure to the patient and/or their representative. Obtain a signed informed consent for the procedure. Mention that the patient might experience a "burning" discomfort with the liquid nitrogen application and a possibility of throbbing for up to 24 hours. Consider administering acetaminophen or a nonsteroidal anti-inflammatory drug before or after the procedure.

The area of the wart must be clean, dry, and well exposed. Place the patient in a position of comfort. This may be prone, supine, or standing with the ipsilateral knee and leg resting on a chair. Clean the plantar surface of the foot of any dirt and debris. There is no need for sterile preparation or draping of the foot. Position an overhead light so that the beam is focused onto the wart. **Adequate lighting is essential.**

Anesthesia is rarely required for cryotherapy or the application of salicylate acid to plantar warts. Children, nervous adults, or persons with large warts may require anesthesia. One option is to apply EMLA cream to the wart followed by an occlusive dressing for 1 hour if time permits.

Local injection anesthesia is an alternative. Clean the skin overlying and surrounding the wart site of any dirt and debris. Apply povidone iodine solution and allow it to dry. Inject a small volume (1 to 2 mL) of local anesthetic solution to create a wheal under the plantar wart. One of the editors (E.F.R.) believes this to be cruel and unusual punishment for the patient. Local infiltration is extremely painful as there are numerous sensory nerve fibers in the sole. The tough and tight skin of the plantar surface quickly comes under tension with the injection of the local anesthetic solution and results in undue discomfort.

Perform a posterior tibial nerve block if injection anesthesia is required. The posterior tibial nerve is superficial at the ankle, midway between the medial malleolus and the heel (Figure 106-40). It lies between the tendons of the flexor digitorum longus and flexor hallucis longus muscles. It travels with and slightly posterior to the posterior tibial artery. The posterior tibial nerve divides at the inferior border of the calcaneous to form the medial and lateral plantar nerves. The nerves provide motor innervation to the intrinsic foot muscles. The lateral plantar nerve provides sensory innervation to the lateral one-third of the sole and plantar surface of the lateral 1½ toes (Figure 106-27). The medial plantar nerve provides sensory innervation to the medial two-thirds of the sole and the plantar surface of the medial 3½ toes (Figure 106-27).

Place the patient supine with the ankle supported on a pillow or blanket and the leg externally rotated. Identify, by palpation, the medial malleolus and the posterior tibial artery by its pulsation. Place a skin wheal of local anesthetic solution at the level of the upper border of the medial malleolus and just posterior to the posterior tibial artery or medial to the Achilles tendon. Insert a 25 gauge needle through the skin wheal and perpendicular to the skin (Figure 165-2). Advance the needle to the tibia or until paresthesias are elicited. If paresthesias are elicited, withdraw the needle 2 mm and allow them to resolve. Inject 3 to 5 mL of local anesthetic solution. If paresthesias are not elicited, infiltrate 5 to 7 mL of local anesthetic solution starting against the posterior tibia as the needle is withdrawn.

TECHNIQUES

WART PREPARATION

The plantar wart often has a thicker epidermal layer than the adjacent normal epidermis. Trim the wart to allow easier and more efficient penetration of the liquid nitrogen or salicylic acid. Use a #15 blade or a straight razor blade to shave the wart's surface. Place a 4×4 gauze square under the patient's foot to catch the shavings (Figure 165-3). Approach the plantar wart at its base and at a 30 to 45 degree angle to the skin (Figure 165-3). Gently move the blade in a smooth sawing motion. Trim the wart to reduce it to a flat structure contiguous with the adjacent normal epidermis. It may take several passes of the blade to trim the wart. Soak the affected foot in lukewarm water for 5 to 10 minutes if the wart is very hard and difficult to trim. **Thoroughly dry the wart and the surrounding skin after the soak. The skin must be dry before the application of liquid nitrogen or salicylic acid.** Proceed with the cryotherapy or salicylic acid treatment as these agents can now easily penetrate through the trimmed plantar wart.

CRYOTHERAPY

Cryotherapy can be achieved using one of two methods. A self-contained liquid nitrogen spray can (i.e., CRY-AC) makes the job very easy (Figure 165-4A). Use a spot-freeze technique. Hold the spray tip 1 to 2 cm from the skin surface and tangential to the wart (Figure 165-4B). Gently pull the spray trigger to form a circular "ice field" overlying the wart (Figure 165-4C). **Avoid spraying**

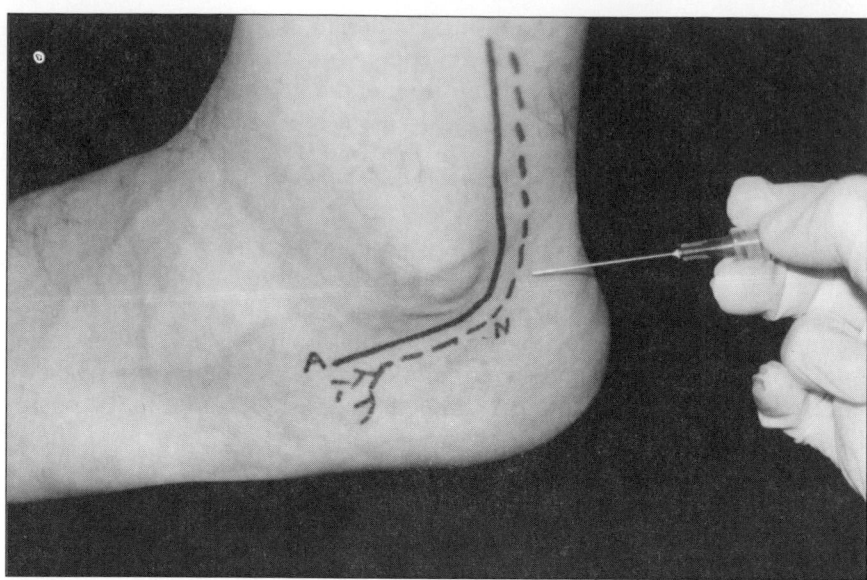

FIGURE 165-2 The posterior tibial nerve block. Note the course of the posterior tibial artery (A), the course of the nerve (N), and the needle position.

liquid nitrogen onto the normal epidermis. A spot-freeze of approximately 30 seconds will form a circular ice field of roughly 2 to 3 mm in diameter (Figure 165-4D). This corresponds to a depth of freeze of approximately 2 to 3 mm and epidermal temperatures of –25 to –150 °C.[4] Place an otoscope earpiece/cone over the wart to zone in a more concentrated cryospray for thicker or irregularly shaped plantar warts. This also prevents a "blast" effect and freeze damage to the surrounding normal tissue. The cure rates approach 97 percent depending upon the type and number of treatments used.[2]

The lack of liquid nitrogen spray should not impede the use of liquid nitrogen if it is available at your institu-tion. Obtain 5 to 10 mL of liquid nitrogen from the stock tank and place it into a foam cup. Dip a cotton-tipped applicator into the liquid nitrogen. Firmly apply the liquid-nitrogen-soaked cotton-tipped applicator to the plantar wart. Hold the applicator to the wart until a narrow halo of white ice forms around the swab, much as in the spray technique. Larger warts require multiple dips of the cotton-tipped applicator into liquid nitrogen followed by application onto the wart. **Do not place the cotton-tipped applicator onto the same spot more than once.** Apply the cotton-tipped applicator to cover the entire wart. This technique reaches a tissue temperature of only −20 °C. It is not as effective as the liquid nitrogen spray at eliminating the plantar wart.

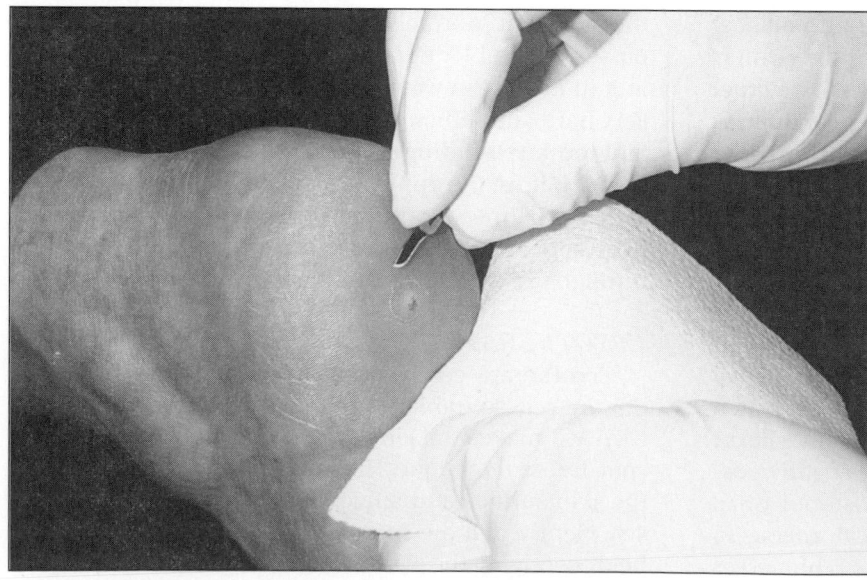

FIGURE 165-3 Trimming the wart with a #15 scalpel blade.

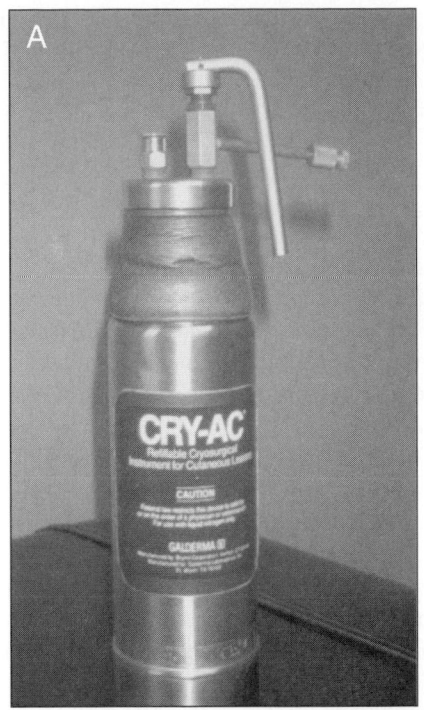

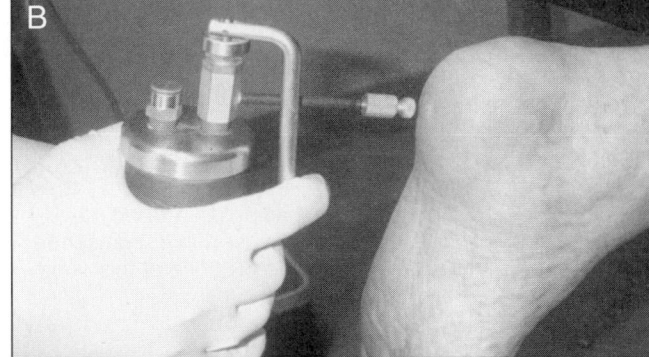

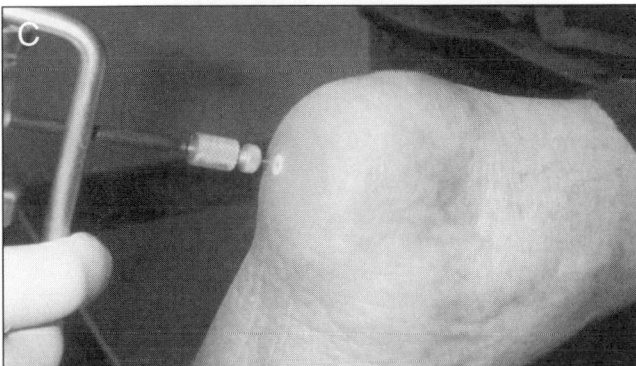

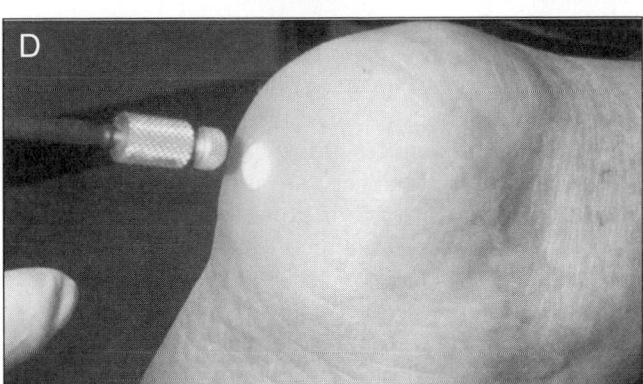

FIGURE 165-4 Cryotherapy for plantar warts. *A.* A self-contained liquid nitrogen spray can. *B.* Positioning of the spray tip 1 to 2 cm from the skin surface. *C.* Spray liquid nitrogen to form a circular ice field over the wart. *D.* A 2 to 3 mm ice field after a 30 second spray.

SALICYLIC ACID THERAPY

Place a rim of petroleum-based lubricant (Vaseline) or clear nail polish around the wart (Figure 165-5). This will protect the surrounding normal skin from the effects of the salicylic acid. Allow the nail polish to dry.

Salicylic acid ointment is available in a variety of concentrations ranging from 15% to 40%. Salicylic acid ointments can be made in any concentration. The ideal concentration is 40%, with or without 20% lactic acid. The lactic acid serves to lower the pH of the ointment and increase the penetration of the salicylic acid into the plantar wart.[3] Topical salicylic acid ointment is recommended over the liquid as it is easy to store and more accurate to apply.

Apply a coat of salicylic acid ointment up to 2 mm beyond the margins of the plantar wart with a cotton-tipped applicator (Figure 165-6). Completely cover the wart so that the underlying skin does not show through. Apply an occlusive dressing on top of the wart. A clear dressing (i.e., Tegaderm) is useful, as it is thin, so that it does not affect the foot on walking. Daily treatments have an 84 percent cure rate at 3 months follow-up.[5]

AFTERCARE

A clear or hemorrhagic blister may form at the site of cryotherapy. The blister is sterile. Leave it intact if it does not interfere with function. It may be punctured with a sterile needle, covered with topical antibiotic ointment, and bandaged if the patient finds the blister a nuisance. Instruct the patient to not pick at the blister. Arrange

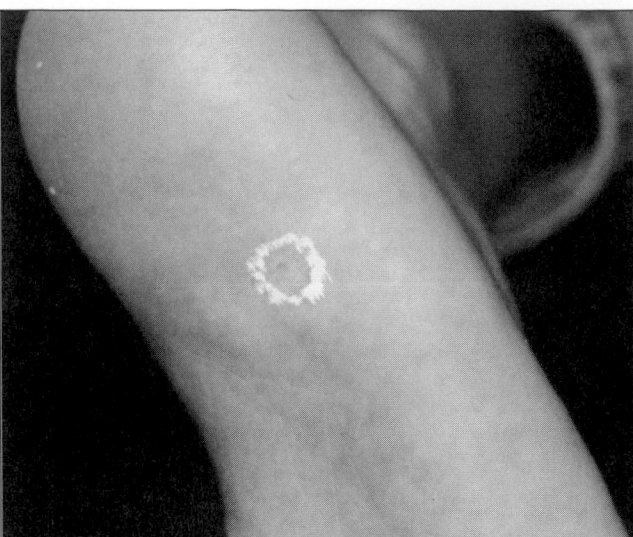

FIGURE 165-5 Application of nail polish around the plantar wart. A white nail polish was used to circumscribe the region of the plantar wart for the purpose of this photograph.

follow-up in 2 to 3 weeks, after healing has occurred by secondary intention.

Salicylic acid therapy does not produce any pain. The patient's complaints of pain indicate excessive irritation or infection that requires prompt assessment. Teach the patient or their caretaker the application procedure. The application procedure must be performed daily until the wart is gone and for at least a week after that.

General instructions include advising the patient to return to the Emergency Department if any signs of an infection develop or there is persistent pain. Mild pain can be managed with acetaminophen or nonsteroidal anti-inflammatory drugs. Educate the patient on the prevention of future warts and the possibility of recurrence.

COMPLICATIONS

One must understand the normal process of healing after cryotherapy before the complications can be understood. The wound is initially raw and erythematous. It may develop a clear or hemorrhagic bulla. Edema and exudate is expected in the first 24 hours. The use of nonadherent gauze or a bandage is often helpful. Cryotherapy pain lasts no more than 24 hours after the procedure.

The main complications of cryotherapy are pain, delayed bleeding, and infection. Hypertrophic scar formation is rare. Discuss this prior to the procedure if the patient is prone to developing hypertrophic scars. The healing process results in mild skin contractures and depigmentation.[2] This is less of an issue with the plantar warts compared to lesions in other, more visible body parts.

Both techniques have the potential to damage normal skin. Do not allow the liquid nitrogen or salicylic acid to extend more than 1 to 2 mm onto the adjacent tissue. Consider using an otoscope cone to prevent blast damage from liquid nitrogen spray. The use of a protective barrier with petrolatum-based lubricant or nail polish will prevent salicylic acid runoff.

SUMMARY

Plantar warts are extremely common. They can be readily managed in the Emergency Department. Treatment consists of a one-time liquid nitrogen application or daily salicylic acid ointment applications. The key to success is patient education so that they know the entire aftercare plan and their expectations are answered in light of the possible complications and recurrence.

REFERENCES

1. Siegfried EC: Warts on children: an approach to therapy. *Pediatr Ann* 1996; 25(2):79–90.
2. Jester DM: Cryotherapy of dermal abnormalities. *Primary Care* 1997; 24(2):269–279.
3. Landow K: Nongenital warts: when is treatment warranted? *Postgrad Med* 1996; 99(3):245–249.
4. Jackson AD: Cryosurgery: a guide for GPs. *Practitioner* 1999; 243:131–136.
5. Goldfarb MT, Gupta AK, Gupta MA, et al: Office therapy for human papillomavirus infection in nongenital sites. *Dermatol Clin* 1991; 9(2):287–296.

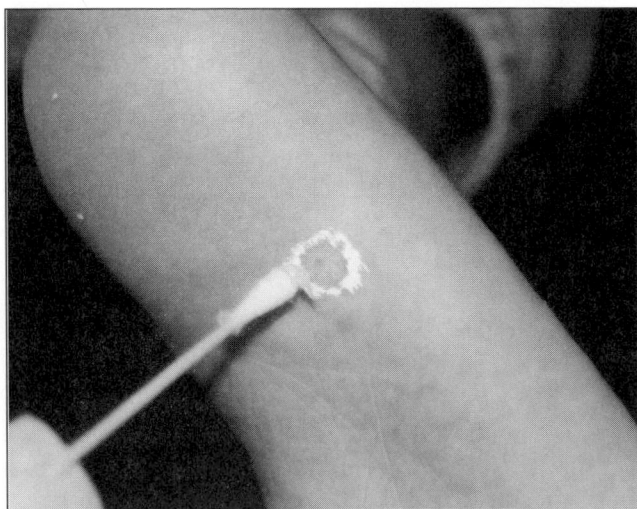

FIGURE 165-6 Application of a salicyclic acid ointment to the plantar wart.

Chapter 166
NEUROMA MANAGEMENT

Stephen E. Miller
Eric R. Snoey

INTRODUCTION

Morton's neuroma, also referred to as an interdigital neuroma, is one of the most common painful disorders of the forefoot. It was first described in 1845 by Dulacher and is named after Thomas Morton, who presented, in 1876, a case series of patients afflicted with this disorder. Patients with an established Morton's neuroma are usually cared for by a Podiatrist or an Orthopedist. They may present to the Emergency Department with a previously undiagnosed neuroma or with a painful exacerbation of known neuroma.

The term neuroma is actually a misnomer. Histologic investigation does not reveal the proliferation of axons found in true neuromas. Instead, in Morton's neuroma, there is a progressive fibrosis and thickening of the perineural tissue with degeneration of the underlying nerve. This most commonly affects the third plantar common digital nerve located between the third and fourth metatarsal heads. It may occur between the second and third metatarsals. A neuroma is rarely seen between the first and second or the fourth and fifth metatarsals.

Morton's neuroma is most commonly found in women in their fourth to sixth decades.[1] It is especially common in those who wear high-heeled shoes or shoes that are narrow at the forefoot. It is more commonly seen in persons with pronated or pes cavus feet.[2] Neuromas do not become symptomatic until their transverse diameter reaches more than 5 mm.[3]

ANATOMY AND PATHOPHYSIOLOGY

Neuromas form just proximal to the bifurcation of the plantar common digital nerves (Figure 166-1) and below the deep transverse intermetatarsal ligament (Figure 166-2). The deep transverse intermetatarsal ligament connects the plantar aspects of the metatarsal heads (Figure 166-2). The neuroma is made up of branches from both the medial and lateral plantar nerves (Figure 166-1). Most commonly affected is the third interdigital nerve. It is the largest of the interdigital nerves and may explain the increased frequency of neuroma formation in this location.

Morton and others postulated that the increased mobility of the fourth and fifth metatarsal heads relative to the others results in disproportionate trauma to the third interdigital nerve. These mechanical factors, combined with the impingement and stretching from a tight transverse intermetatarsal ligament, result in repetitive microtrauma. Histologic evaluation reveals perineural fibroma formation consistent with compression-induced trauma.[1] There is a progression from edema of the endoneurium, fibrosis beneath the perineurium, axonal degeneration, and neuronal necrosis.

Some authors believe that a more significant contributor to neuroma formation is enlargement of the interphalangeal component of the intermetatarsophalangeal bursa, leading to microvascular trauma.[4] Movements of the bursa result in minor obliterative effects on the adjacent digital arteries, leading to ischemia of local neural tissue.

The diagnosis of a Morton's neuroma is usually made clinically, based upon classic historical features and physical examination findings. The pain of a neuroma usually begins intermittently, becoming more frequent with time and eventually constant. The involved intermetatarsal space of the forefoot may have pain, burning, or tingling. Attacks typically occur suddenly after a period of walking, running, or standing.[4] Some patients may complain of pain disturbing their sleep.[4] Hyperesthesia or hypoesthesia in the involved toes and web space is common. Patients often complain of the unilateral feeling of "walking on a lump." Symptoms are aggravated by walking and wearing narrow shoes. Symptoms are relieved by rest and shoe removal.

Physical examination localizes the pain to the involved interspace with minimal involvement of the adja-

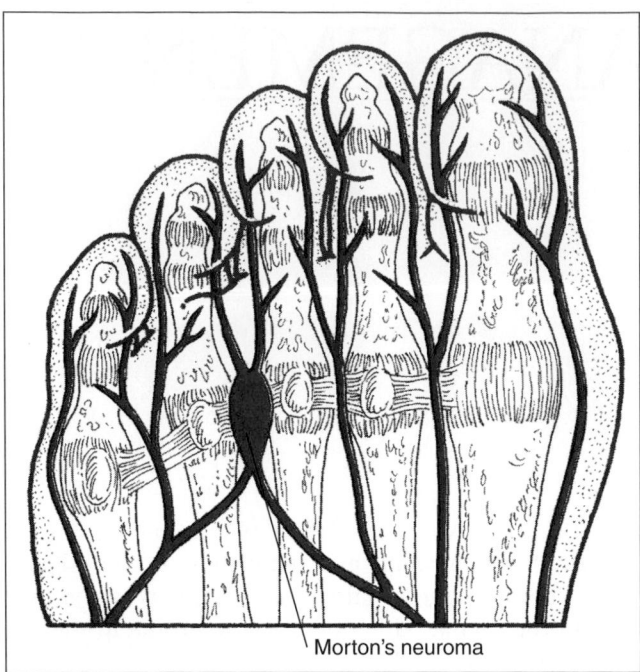

FIGURE 166-1 Morton's neuroma most commonly occurs in the third intermetatarsal space beneath the transverse metacarpal ligament.

cent metatarsal heads. Moderate pressure applied proximally in the affected web space reproduces the pain. A small mass, representing the neuroma, can be palpated in approximately one-third of the cases. A positive Mulder's sign is diagnostic. This is a click felt in the interspace with medial and lateral compression of the metatarsal heads (Figure 166-3).

Radiographic imaging may be helpful in confirming the diagnosis and exploring alternative etiologies. Plain radiographs will not demonstrate a neuroma. They may reveal splaying of the involved toes when the neuroma is especially large or other osseous pathology, such as stress fractures or arthritis. Ultrasound represents the most efficient and effective imaging modality.[1,5] An experienced operator may identify hypoechoic neuromas as small as 2.9 mm.[6] Magnetic resonance imaging (MRI) is quite effective at identifying the presence of a neuroma, but cost and access issues make it a less practical choice. Computed tomography (CT) may be useful if an MRI is contraindicated. The sensitivity of CT scanning is not as good as that of MRI or ultrasound.[1]

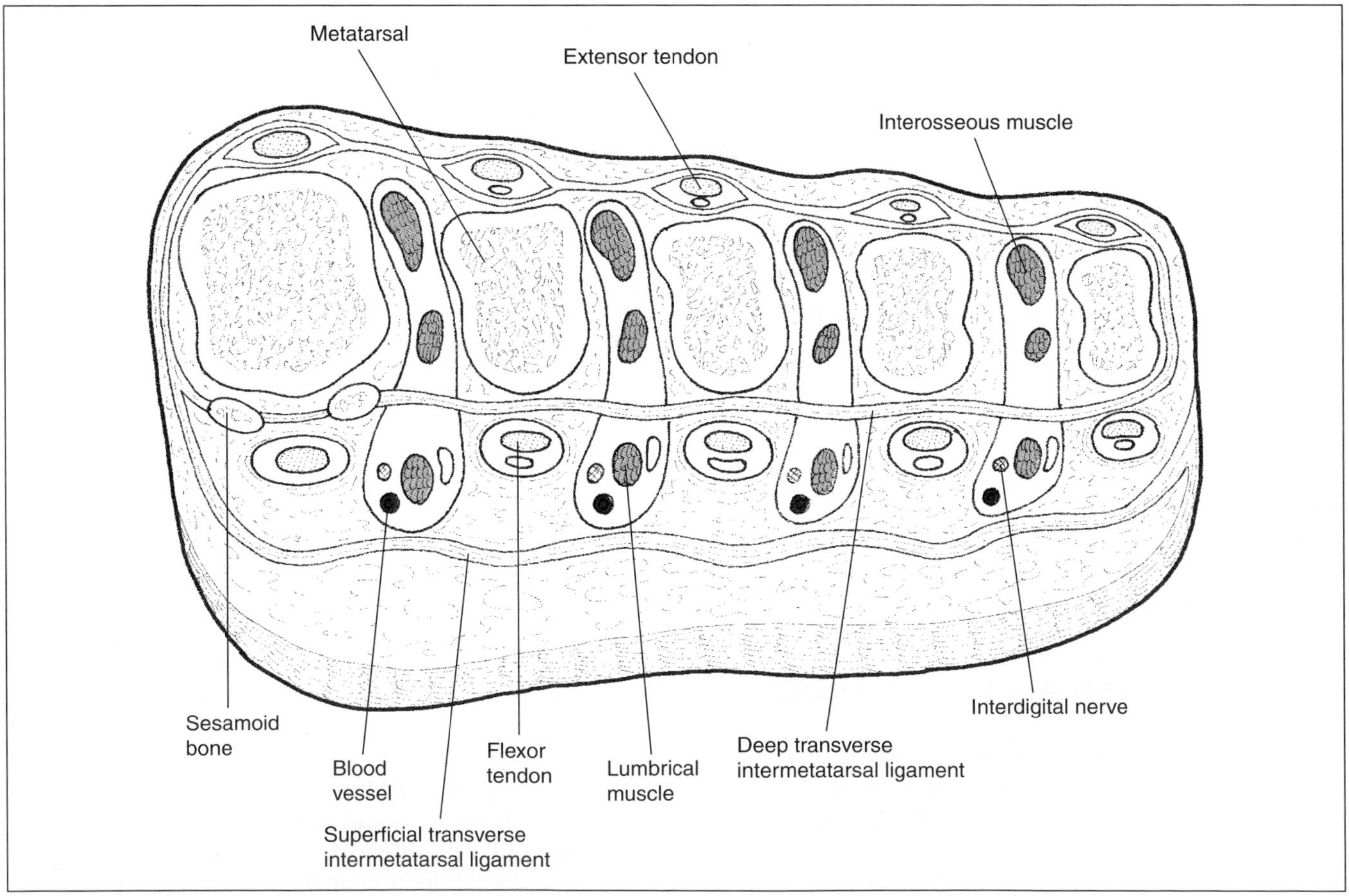

Metatarsal

Extensor tendon

Interosseous muscle

Interdigital nerve

Deep transverse intermetatarsal ligament

Lumbrical muscle

Flexor tendon

Blood vessel

Superficial transverse intermetatarsal ligament

Sesamoid bone

FIGURE 166-2 Anatomy of the forefoot. Cross-section through the distal metatarsals.

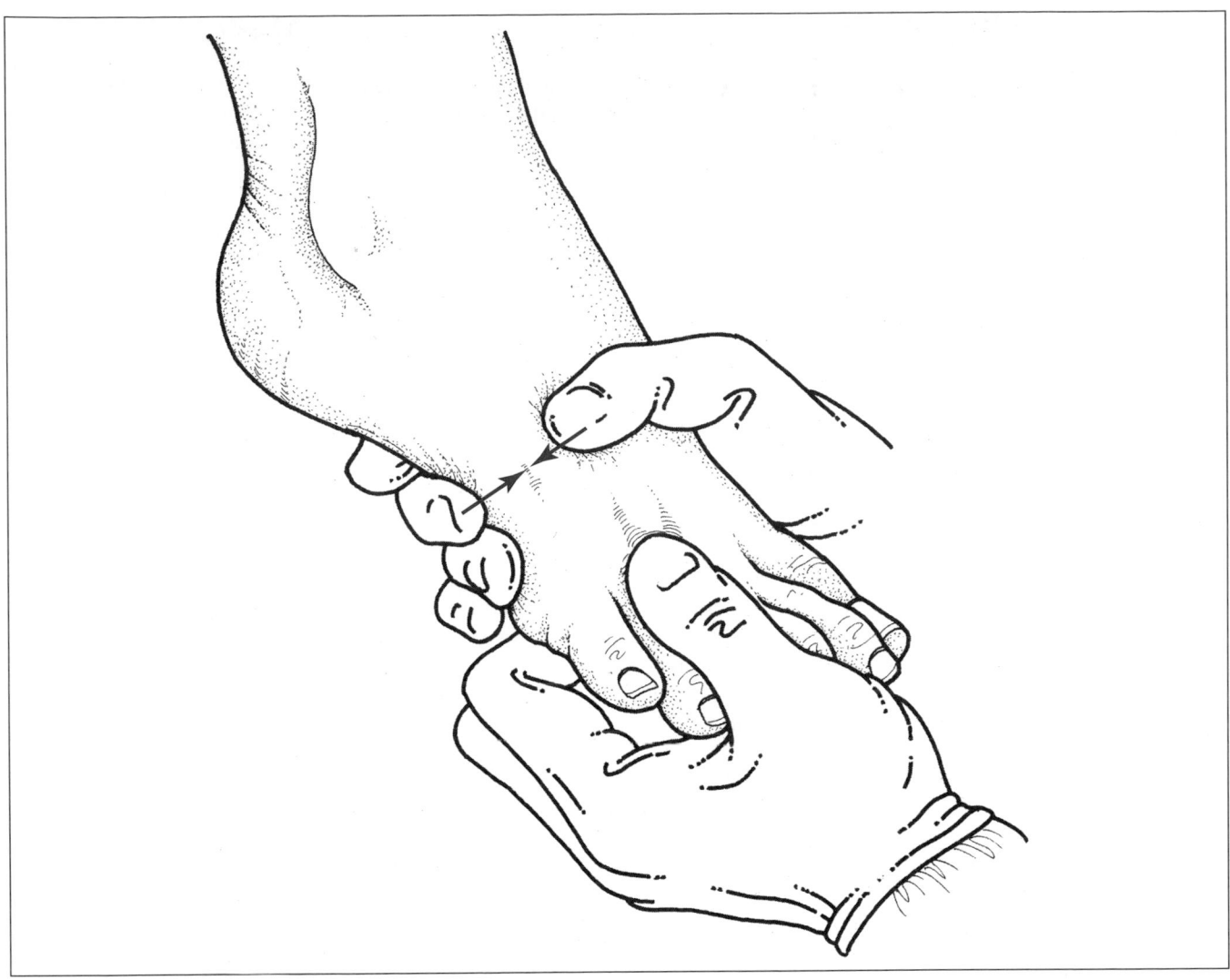

FIGURE 166-3 Examination for Mulder's click. The thumb and forefinger of the examiner's dominant hand are used to compress the interdigital space. The nondominant hand then performs medial and lateral compression of the metatarsal heads (*arrows*). A palpable click is diagnostic, while pain alone is suggestive of a neuroma.

INDICATIONS

Injection of the presumed neuroma will provide significant relief to the patient and confirm a Morton's neuroma as the etiology of the patient's complaints.

CONTRAINDICATIONS

The primary contraindication to injection of a Morton's neuroma is failure to make a correct initial diagnosis. The differential diagnosis for forefoot pain includes a wide variety of pathologies, many of which may closely mimic the presentation of a neuroma. Alternative diagnoses include tarsal tunnel syndrome, peripheral neuropathy, capsulitis, bursitis, rheumatoid arthritis, foreign bodies, avascular necrosis, stress fractures, and ischemia. A careful history and physical examination with discretionary use of imaging modalities will lead to a correct diagnosis.

Some specialists believe injection therapy to be contraindicated in serious athletes.[2] They propose that steroid injection may result in fat pad atrophy, degeneration of the volar plate, and degeneration of the collateral ligaments. A discussion of alternative therapies to injection therapy is provided later in this chapter.

EQUIPMENT

Povidone iodine solution
3 mL syringe
22 or 25 gauge needle
0.5% bupivacaine without epinephrine
Methylprednisolone
Sterile bandage

PATIENT PREPARATION

Explain the risks, benefits, complications, and after-care of the procedure to the patient and/or their representative. Place the patient supine on a gurney with the hip and knee flexed so that the sole of the affected foot is flat on the gurney. Clean the skin overlying the neuroma of any dirt and debris. Apply povidone iodine solution and allow it to dry.

Prepare the injection solution. Mix 1 mL of 0.5% bupivacaine in a 3 mL syringe with 10 mg of methylprednisolone. Another local anesthetic agent, with or without epinephrine, may be used instead of bupivacaine. Long-acting local anesthetic agents provide the patient with longer pain relief after the injection.

TECHNIQUE

Instruct the patient to moderately dorsiflex the toes to separate the metatarsal heads. **Use a dorsal approach to the neuroma, as this is less painful than penetrating the sole with a needle.** Insert the needle into the skin overlying the neuroma if it is palpable. Advance the needle perpendicular to the skin and into the neuroma or into its fascial plane (Figure 166-4). Inject the affected interspace with 1 to 2 mL of a combination long-acting local anesthetic agent and steroid. Insert and direct the needle into the interspace between the deep and superficial transverse metatarsal ligaments in the absence of a palpable neuroma (Figure 166-2). The patient will experience a rapid resolution of symptoms if the injection is successful.

ALTERNATIVE TECHNIQUES

Various types of conservative treatment can be initiated once a Morton's neuroma is diagnosed. A wide range of success rates have been reported (20 to 80 percent) using a combination of injections with other conservative therapy, including orthoses, metatarsal pads,

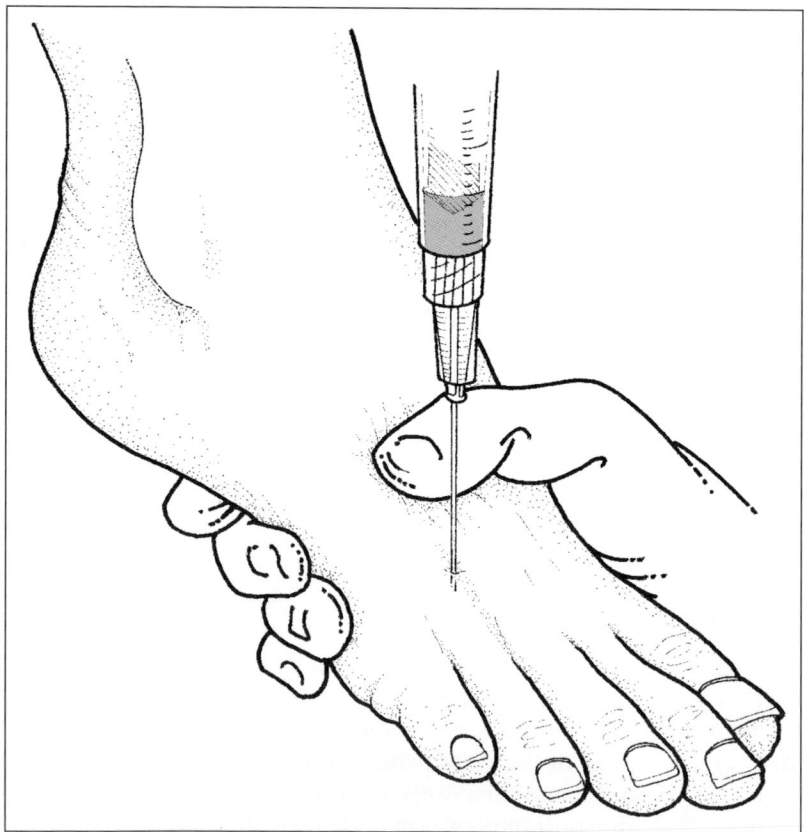

FIGURE 166-4 Injection of the neuroma.

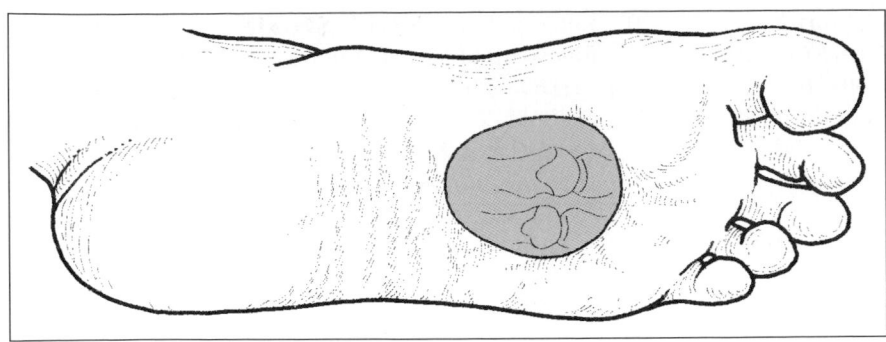

FIGURE 166-5 Placement of a metatarsal pad.

shoes with wider toe boxes, and physical therapy.[7,8] Orthoses are used to help control abnormal pronation, although some studies have shown this to be ineffective.[8] Metatarsal pads serve to spread the metatarsal heads at the involved interspace and decrease compressive trauma (Figure 166-5). The types of physical therapy employed include massage, ultrasound, electrical stimulation, and whirlpool immersion. A trial of acetaminophen or nonsteroidal anti-inflammatory drugs may be helpful in the short term.

Podiatrists and Orthopedists may offer more aggressive and definitive therapy when conservative measures fail. Surgical excision using a dorsal approach has success rates as high as 84 to 93 percent.[9–11] There has recently been increasing support for endoscopic decompression of the deep transverse intermetatarsal ligament, leaving the nerve intact. The advantage is a shorter recovery time, which may make this especially desirable for athletes. No long-term results have been reported, but short-term results appear quite promising.[2] Excision using a carbon dioxide laser has recently been introduced to the field. This may allow for even shorter recovery periods, but only a few case reports have been cited.[5]

AFTERCARE

Pain may be controlled with the use of acetaminophen or nonsteroidal anti-inflammatory drugs. Instruct the patient to wear flat shoes, to wear shoes with flat toe boxes, and to avoid shoes whose heel is elevated above the metatarsals. Apply a metatarsal pad to decrease compressive forces on the neuroma. Place the dome of the pad between the third and fourth metatarsals and just posterior to the metatarsal heads (Figure 166-5). Refer the patient to a Podiatrist or Orthopedic Surgeon for follow-up, orthoses, physical therapy, and possible surgical management.

COMPLICATIONS

Complications associated with neuroma injection are exceedingly rare. They include the introduction of infection, damage to neurovascular structures, or local atrophy secondary to the effects of the steroid. It is common for the pain to recur in days to weeks, even when the injection is successful.

SUMMARY

Morton's neuroma is one of the most common causes of forefoot pain. Injection therapy is useful in alleviating the symptoms of a neuroma and in confirming the diagnosis. Arrange Podiatric or Orthopedic follow-up for all patients given this diagnosis, as more invasive procedures may be needed for long-term resolution of symptoms.

REFERENCES

1. Mendicino SS, Rockett MS: Morton's neuroma—update on diagnosis and imaging. *Clin Podiatr Med Surg* 1997; 14(2):303–311.
2. Nunan PJ, Giesy BD: Management of Morton's neuroma in athletes. *Clin Podiatr Med Surg* 1997; 14(3):489–501.
3. Zanetti M, Strehle JK, Zollinger H, et al: Morton neuroma and fluid in the intermetatarsal bursae on MRI images of 70 asymptomatic volunteers. *Radiology* 1997; 203(2):516–520.
4. Helal B, Wilson D: *The Foot*. Philadelphia: Churchill Livingstone, 1988:493–499.
5. Wasserman G: Treatment of Morton's neuroma with the carbon dioxide laser. *Clin Podiatr Med Surg* 1992; 9(3):671–686.
6. Kaminsky S, Griffin L, Milsap J, et al: Is ultrasonography a reliable way to confirm the diagnosis of Morton's neuroma? *Orthopedics* 1997; 20(1):37–39.

7. Bennett GL, Graham CE, Mauldin DM: Morton's interdigital neuroma: a comprehensive treatment protocol. *Foot Ankle Int* 1995; 16(12):760–763.

8. Kilmartin TE, Wallace WA: Effect of pronation and supination orthosis on Morton's neuroma and lower extremity function. *Foot Ankle Int* 1994; 15(5):256–262.

9. Okafor B, Shergill G, Angel J: Treatment of Morton's neuroma by neurolysis. *Foot Ankle Int* 1997; 18(5):284–287.

10. Keh RA, Ballew KK, Higgins KR, et al: Long-term follow-up of Morton's neuroma. *J Foot Surg* 1992; 31(1):93–95.

11. Diebold PF, Daum B, Dang-Vu V, et al: True epineural neurolysis in Morton's neuroma: a 5-year follow up. *Orthopedics* 1996; 19(5):397–400.

Chapter 167
MANAGEMENT OF SELECT PODIATRIC CONDITIONS

Martin Ehrlich
Jacqueline A. Nemer

INTRODUCTION

Socrates once said "To him whose feet hurt, everything hurts." Patients with foot pain and deformities are commonly seen in the Emergency Department complaining of compromised mobility. The frequency of these disorders increases with age. This chapter addresses common presentations and procedures for the management of the painful foot. A number of other podiatric procedures (e.g., local anesthesia, ingrown toenails, plantar warts, puncture wounds, toe fractures) are addressed in other chapters of this book.

MANAGEMENT OF PLANTAR LESIONS

INTRODUCTION

The skin on the sole of the foot is the thickest skin on the entire body. It is especially adapted to protect the internal structures from environmental demands. A 150-lb person has dissipated 60 tons of force with each foot after walking a mile.[1] Hyperkeratosis (callosity) occurs when the process of keratinization, which maintains the outer layer of epithelium as a horny protective cover, becomes overactive due to shearing forces and pressure points over bony prominences. This is a normal protective response as the body attempts to protect the irritated skin. It may be seen on the hands of a laborer or on the plantar surfaces of feet in those who walk barefoot. Over time, a vicious cycle begins. The hyperkeratotic area becomes a prominence, increases the pressure in a tight shoe, produces further discomfort, and results in further keratinization.

The ubiquitous verruca virus can invade the plantar skin of the foot and produce a wart or a hyperkeratotic response. It is sometimes difficult to differentiate this condition from other hyperkeratoses (calluses or corns).

Warts may occur at any site on the plantar skin, unlike a pressure or friction-induced callus or corn. Warts are less likely to occur on the digits and seldom occur on the dorsal skin. **The surface appearance of all of these conditions may be identical, yet their treatment strategies are radically different.** The wart is treated with epidermal eradication (Chapter 165), whereas other hyperkeratoses are treated with simple paring and rebalancing of the weight-bearing surfaces.

A corn, also known as a helomata or a clavus, represents a well-circumscribed traumatic hyperkeratosis caused by friction or pressure on the skin. It has a visibly translucent core that presses deeply into the dermis. Corns may be so painful as to be disabling.[2] A hard corn (heloma durum) forms primarily on the exposed surfaces of the toes from extrinsic pressure of footwear.[3-6] It is commonly found on the dorsolateral aspect of the fifth toe or the dorsum of the interphalangeal joints of toes 2 to 5.

Hammertoes occur when the intrinsic muscles of the foot lose their stabilizing effect on the interphalangeal joints, allowing the extrinsic muscles of the leg to overpower and flex the interphalangeal joints. This deformity may be associated with the formation of painful hyperkeratotic lesions. These lesions may be overlying or adjacent to any or all of the interphalangeal joints or on the distal tip of the digit.[7]

Soft corns (heloma molle), which are extremely painful, are often misdiagnosed as warts or fungal infections. They are essentially macerated and whitish-appearing hard lesions resulting from the corn's absorption of large amounts of sweat. They occur interdigitally, usually in the fourth web space, as a result of wearing tight shoes that press the condyle of a metatarsal against its neighbor. A soft corn will reveal its central "core" if pared.

Another skin lesion that mimics a wart is porokeratosis plantaris discreta. This small cyst-like lesion is a sweat duct filled with a keratin plug. It is located on the plantar surface of the foot. This lesion often goes by the misnomer "seed wart."

Calluses (tylomata) are broad-based, poorly circumscribed, diffuse areas of hyperkeratosis that develop at pressure sites under the metatarsal heads.[2] Calluses are usually larger than corns, do not have a central core, and may or may not be painful. A large area of hyperkeratosis that occurs in combination with a centrally located plug of keratin is called an intractable plantar keratosis (IPK). These lesions usually require podiatric evaluation for debridement, protective padding, and rebalancing of the weight-bearing surfaces with orthotics.

The first step in treating a patient with a plantar skin lesion is to differentiate a wart (verruca) from a plantar hyperkeratosis. Warts and plantar corns are best distinguished by paring the outer layer of epidermis with a sharp scalpel blade. Warts may or may not be localized under a bony prominence. Apply alcohol to the plantar lesion to enhance the skin lines. **The skin lines of a hyperkeratosis pass through the lesion, whereas those from a wart pass around the lesion. End arteries are visible when a wart is pared.** These appear as multiple black dots that hurt and bleed if cut. Paring the hyperkeratotic lesion reveals only yellowish, translucent, firm keratin; even after many shaves. A firm keratin core is a corn and not a wart. The patient's pain response to pressure on the lesion may help in differentiating a wart from a corn. Pain is elicited with direct pressure on the hyperkeratotic lesion. Squeezing the wart side to side with a similar force elicits maximal pain.

INDICATIONS

Perform paring to provide temporary relief of pain associated with corns and calluses. **Make the patient aware that paring is not a permanent treatment. The first step in treatment is to suggest a better-fitting shoe.** Identify the lesion type by shaving the outer layers of keratinized epidermis. Examine the shaved surface looking for the identifying characteristics of a wart versus a corn or callus. Trimming the callused hyperkeratotic surface will provide temporary relief from the discomfort of a corn, a callus, and even a wart. Definitive treatment of a wart or porokeratosis requires curettage, acid, freezing, or podiatric referral. Perform a more definitive shaving if a corn or callus is identified.

CONTRAINDICATIONS

Severe peripheral vascular disease and overlying cellulitis are the only contraindications to shaving a plantar lesion. Keep in mind that a variety of neoplasms may appear as a callused plantar lesion. **Biopsy is mandatory if there is any question about the nature of the lesion.**[2]

EQUIPMENT

#10 or #15 surgical scalpel blade on a handle
Isopropyl alcohol swabs
18 gauge needle
25 or 27 gauge needle
Local anesthetic solution without epinephrine
Cotton ball or 2×2 gauze square
Tape, 1 inch wide
Lamb's wool
Aperture pads

Podiatrists and Orthopedic Surgeons have specialized equipment to debride warts and hyperkeratotic lesions. This includes curettes, Beaver miniblades, Gill chisel blades, and tissue nippers. This equipment is not commonly available in Emergency Departments, clinics, or offices. The techniques described below use commonly available equipment to manage foot lesions.

PATIENT PREPARATION

Explain the procedure, its risks, and benefits to the patient and/or their representative. Obtain an informed consent to perform the procedure. Soak the foot in warm water for 10 to 15 minutes. Place the patient supine or prone on a gurney. Heel lesions are often best addressed with the patient in the prone position. Sit on a stool so that the lesion is at eye level. Visualize the hyperkeratotic lesion under a bright light. Anesthesia is usually not required. Consider the use of a posterior tibial nerve block (Chapter 106) if the patient is significantly sensitive.

TECHNIQUES

Support the foot to be debrided with the nondominant hand. Wipe the hyperkeratotic area with an alcohol swab. Grasp the skin surrounding the lesion. Place the index finger of the nondominant hand above the hyperkeratotic area and the thumb below it (Figure 167-1). Grasp a #10 or #15 scalpel blade on a handle with the dominant hand. Rest the base of the dominant hand against the patient's foot. This allows a measure of safety for both the practitioner and the patient. If the patient jerks, all materials move in mass with the patient. Place the scalpel blade almost parallel to the lesion (Figure 167-1). Remove superficial amounts of the hyperkeratotic lesion using a semicircular slicing motion.[8] Continue this process of debriding repeatedly until healthy pink tissue is noted.[8]

A central core, if uncovered during the debridement, must be removed to relieve the patient's symptoms. Insert the tip of the scalpel blade into the core. Carefully twist the scalpel blade in a circular motion to remove the core. **Avoid injury to the underlying and adjacent healthy tissue.** Treat the common corn with periodic debridement. Adjunctive therapy includes felt

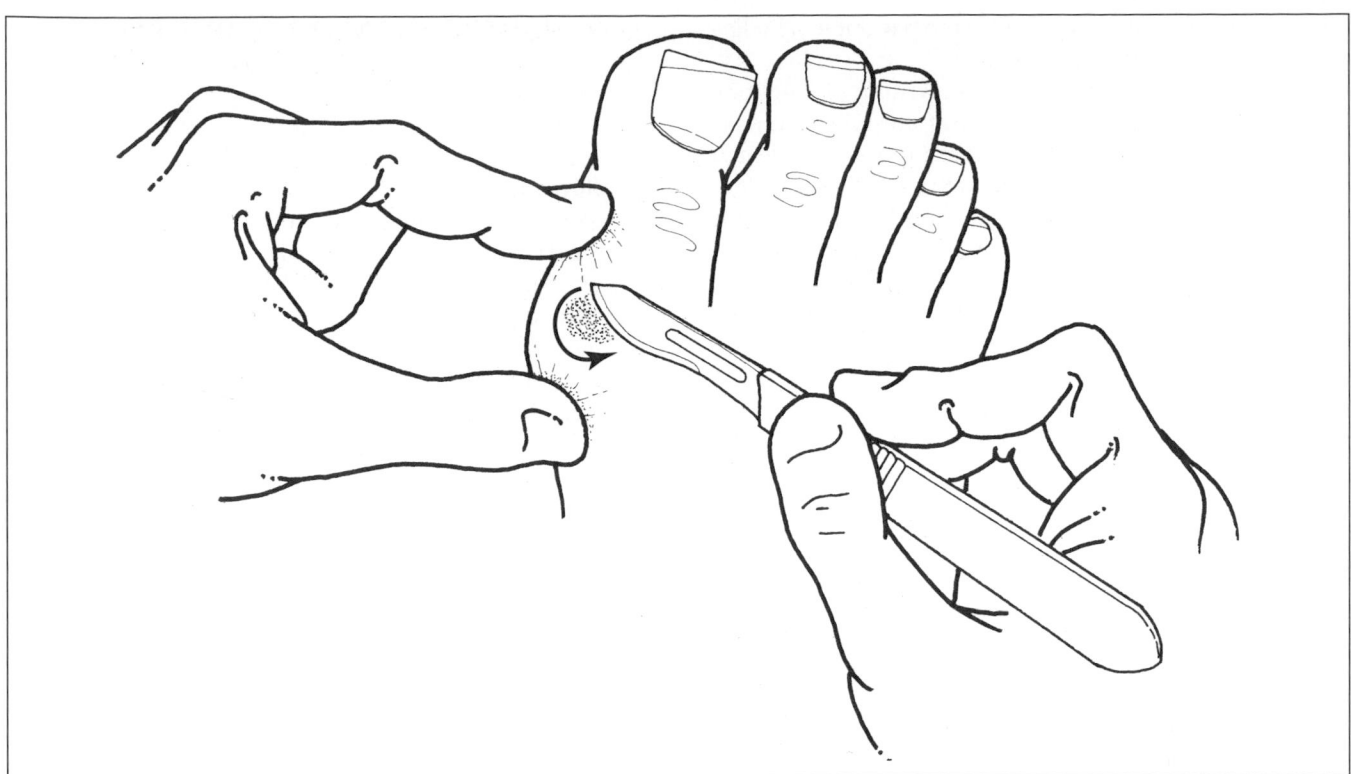

FIGURE 167-1 Technique for using a scalpel blade in the paring of a hyperkeratotic lesion. The scalpel is held almost parallel to the lesion. The epidermis is pared with semicircular shaving motions (*curved arrow*).

corn pads with a central aperture or a horseshoe to relieve pain and disperse pressure at bony prominences to the surrounding skin (Figure 167-2). Place pads under the metatarsals for protection and pressure dispersal from any or all of the metatarsal heads.

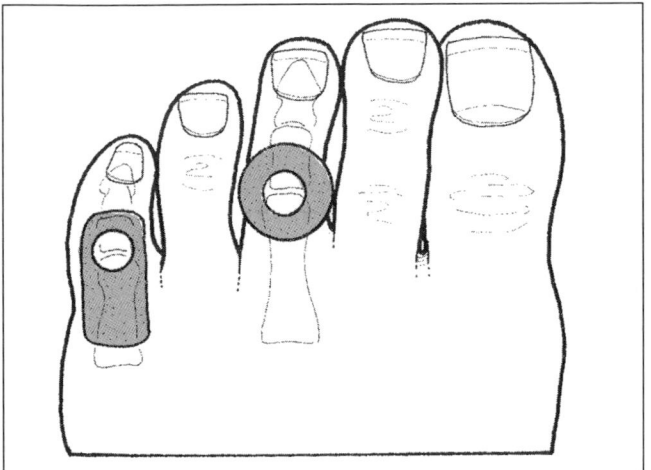

FIGURE 167-2 The use of self-adherent aperture pads to relieve pressure from a pared hyperkeratotic lesion overlying a bony prominence. Pads protecting digital hyperkeratotic lesions are placed on the dorsal surface. Pads protecting the metatarsal heads are placed on the plantar surface. Pads are further secured to the skin with tape.

The macerated soft corn is frequently misdiagnosed on visual inspection as an interdigital fungal infection or wart. Superficial debridement will aid in the diagnosis. Perform a digital or metatarsal block using local anesthetic solution without epinephrine.[9] The digital arteries are end arteries, and local anesthetics containing epinephrine can theoretically induce digital ischemia. Pare the hyperkeratotic lesion with a #10 scalpel blade to provide pain relief and a diagnosis.

The toes must be separated while the lesion is healing. Place a cotton ball or a small gauze square between the toes, either distal or proximal to the lesion. Tape the dressing in place. **Never circumscribe the digit with tape, due to the risk of circulatory impairment from constriction.** Apply lamb's wool around the affected digit. The advantage of lamb's wool is that adhesives are avoided and the patient can change the dressing daily. A foam interdigital cushion is a good choice for pressure dispersion at a later time.

AFTERCARE

The patient can expect 6 to 8 weeks of pain relief after a corn or callus is pared. The procedure may be repeated after this period. Patients must realize that hyperkeratotic lesions are a result of lifestyle choices, such as cramming their feet into constricting, improperly fitted, and/or high-heeled shoes.[10] Refer the patient to a Podiatrist if conservative therapy fails.

Provide all patients with oral and written instructions regarding the signs of infection and lifestyle modification. This includes immediate return to the Emergency Department for increasing pain, progressive swelling, redness, tenderness, and warmth. Follow-up treatment consists of frequent trimming of the keratotic lesion. Consider using shock-absorbing inserts. Metatarsal pads are an excellent choice for submetatarsal pressure dispersion and the protection of pared calluses (Figure 167-3D). Recommend lifestyle modification and the use of appropriate footwear. Home care of the macerated corn includes daily astringent soaks with boric acid solution and a topical antibiotic applied with dressing changes.

PADDING

Padding offers temporary and immediate relief for many patients with foot pain associated with bursitis, fasciitis, and tendonitis. Padding relieves pressure around bony prominences by dispersing it to the surrounding skin. The type of pad and its placement depends on the underlying problem (Figure 167-3). Many commercial pads are available and useful for the management of hyperkeratosis secondary to hammer toes, corns, and calluses (Figure 167-2). The following section discusses the use of padding for common forefoot and hindfoot disorders.

BUNIONS AND BUNIONETTE DEFORMITIES

The bunion affects the first metatarsal head and is known as hallux abducto valgus. The bunionette affects the fifth metatarsal head and is known as the tailor's bunion. Deformities are identified as painful prominent metatarsal heads and surrounding soft tissues (Figure 167-4). Common causes of the bunion and bunionette deformities are complex and multifactorial. These include anatomic and physiologic abnormalities, hereditary conditions, and extrinsic footwear elements.[11] Biomechanical abnormalities lead to dysfunction of the metatarsal phalangeal (MTP) joint.

The bunion deformity consists of lateral deviation of the great toe and medial deviation of the first metatarsal (Figure 167-4). The bunionette deformity is a bunion on the lateral aspect of the foot overlying the fifth metatarsal head. The fifth digit is medially deviated with lateral deviation of the fifth metatarsal (Figure 167-4). Pain results from shoes causing pressure against the bony deformity and the surrounding soft tissues. This can result in subsequent pressure hyperkeratosis. Clinical examination reveals pain upon palpation along the border of the metatarsal head.

The differential diagnosis of a bunion includes bursitis of the first MTP joint, which commonly occurs over the medial bunion bump.[12] Other conditions such as infectious and inflammatory diseases should also be considered. Associated foot complaints may include les-

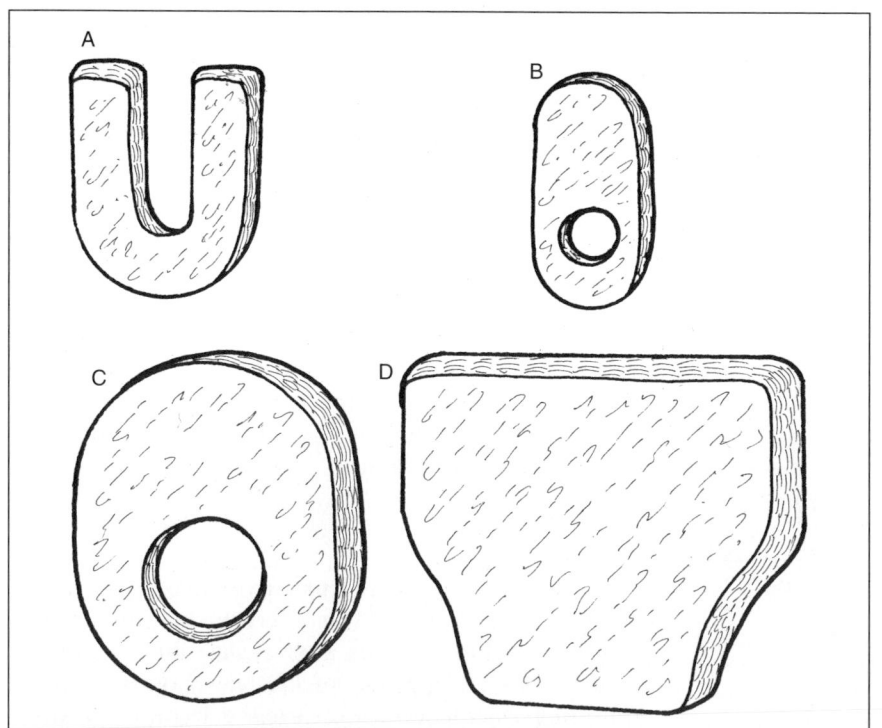

FIGURE 167-3 Examples of padding. *A.* Commercial self-adherent ⅛ inch horseshoe felt digital corn pad. *B.* Commercial self-adherent ¼ inch felt interdigital soft corn pad. *C.* Commercial self-adherent ¼ inch felt bunion shield. *D.* Commercial self-adherent ¼ inch felt submetatarsal pad.

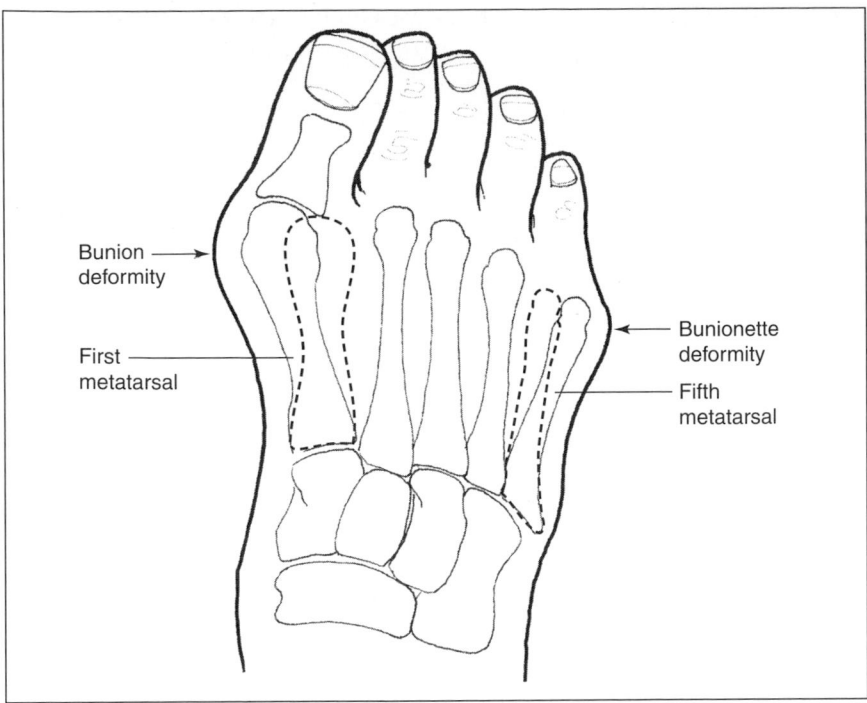

FIGURE 167-4 The bunion and bunionette deformity. The dotted lines represent the normal metatarsal positions.

ser metatarsalgia, intermetatarsal neuroma, hammertoes, corns, and calluses.

EQUIPMENT
Povidone iodine solution
#10 or #15 scalpel blade on a handle
22 gauge needle
3 or 5 mL syringe
Local anesthetic solution without epinephrine
Dexamethasone

TREATMENT
The initial treatment consists of removing the offending footwear. Shoes with a roomy toe box minimize pressure against the inflamed soft tissues and bony prominences. Carefully pare any hyperkeratotic lesions while avoiding injury to surrounding healthy tissue. Padding and accommodative shields help to disperse pressure and may be beneficial. Precut bunion shields are available or may be fashioned from 1 cm thick felt (Figure 167-5). Prescribe nonsteroidal anti-inflammatory drugs (NSAIDs) for analgesia.

A painful bursa overlying the medial aspect of the first metatarsophalangeal (MTP) joint is common. Local aspiration of bursal fluid followed by the injection of a local anesthetic agent and a short-acting steroid may relieve pain and decrease the size of the bursa. Clean the skin overlying the bursa of any dirt and debris. Apply povidone iodine solution to the skin and allow it to dry. Aspirate the bursal fluid with a 22 gauge needle on a 3 or 5 mL syringe. Inject the bursa with a mixture containing 0.5 mL of local anesthetic solution and 4 mg of dexamethasone. Apply a bunion shield (Figure 167-5). Refer the patient to a Podiatrist or Orthopedic Surgeon when conservative measures fail. Surgical techniques can correct the underlying bony deformity.

METATARSALGIA

Metatarsalgia is a general term used to describe a diffusely painful area directly beneath the metatarsal heads. The patient usually complains of forefoot pain that is insidious in onset with walking, worsens throughout the day, and is relieved with rest. The pathophysiology of metatarsalgia is complex. A common denominator is weight transfer from the first ray during ambulation to the lesser metatarsals. This may promote a bursitis, tendonitis, tenosynovitis, and capsulitis of the lesser MTP joints. The patient can usually point to the painful spot. The second metatarsal head is most commonly involved, followed by the third and fourth metatarsal heads.

The clinical diagnosis can be made with direct palpation of each individual metatarsal head. Repetitive force induces a capsulitis (metatarsalgia) beneath the metatarsal head that may progress to a stress fracture of the metatarsal. Radiographs may be negative initially with stress fractures. Repeat the radiographs in 2 to 4 weeks. A hyperkeratotic lesion may be associated with this syndrome. It can be located either directly beneath a

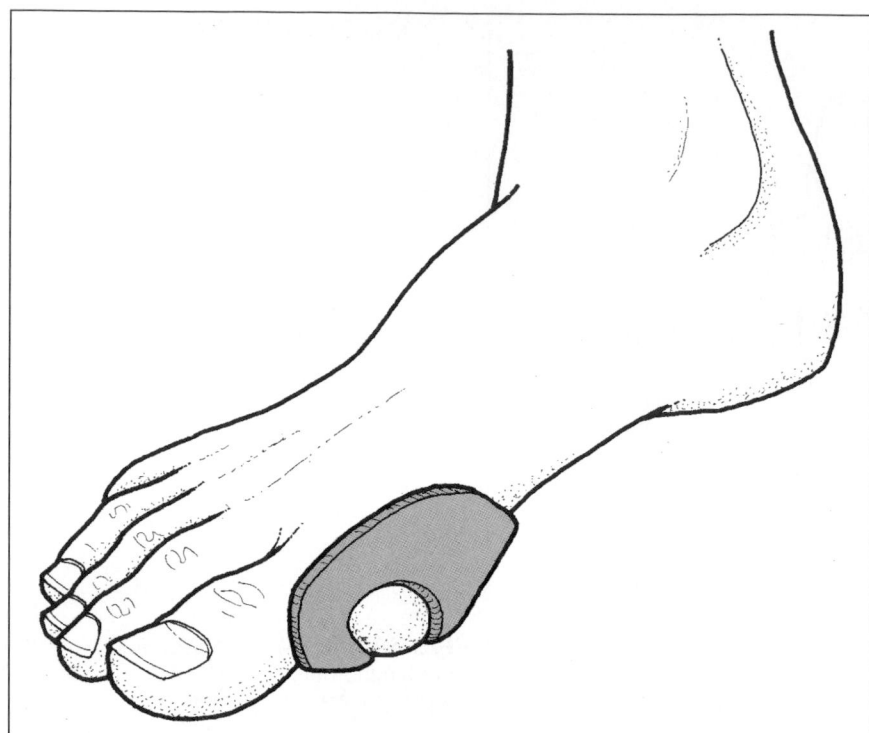

FIGURE 167-5 The application of a commercially available bunion shield.

metatarsal head or diffusely under the lesser metatarsal heads. Paring of the lesion (discussed earlier) is important for diagnosis and treatment. Sufficient debridement may provide immediate pain relief in the Emergency Department.

TREATMENT

All hyperkeratotic lesions require debridement for both diagnosis and treatment. Pad the lesion to disperse pressure to the surrounding tissues. Place a 1 cm thick pad beneath an inner sole under the first metatarsal for discrete pain just beneath the second metatarsal head or second proximal phalangeal shaft (Figure 167-6). This helps to redistribute the weight-bearing surface and protect the second metatarsal. NSAIDs may provide analgesia. Instruct the patient to wear a well-cushioned good-quality athletic or walking shoe. Arrange follow-up with a Podiatrist or Orthopedic Surgeon to address the underlying reason for the hyperkeratotic reaction.

SESAMOIDITIS

Two sesamoid bones lie beneath the first metatarsal. Their structure and function are similar to those of the patella. The clinical examination reveals pain with palpation beneath the sesamoid bones. This may develop into the more painful conditions of chondromalacia, osteoarthritis, and stress fractures. Initial radiographs

may be negative. Serial radiographs taken 2 to 4 weeks later may reveal a fracture. Pressure from the sole of the shoe can irritate the skin, causing painful callus formation.

TREATMENT

Pare any hyperkeratotic lesions. Instruct the patient to wear a well-cushioned good-quality athletic or walking shoe. Apply padding with a central aperture cut out beneath the sesamoid bones to help disperse pressure to the surrounding skin and away from the sesamoid bones. NSAIDs will provide analgesia. Arrange follow-up with a Podiatrist or Orthopedic Surgeon if the patient experiences persistent symptoms.

HEEL PAIN SYNDROMES

The painful heel is a common complaint of the middle-aged and elderly. An in-depth discussion on the myriad of etiologies for heel pain is beyond the scope of this chapter. Patients most often have no associated disease other than obesity. Consider screening young men for ankylosing spondylitis or reactive arthritis. The majority of cases respond to modification of physical activities, the use of NSAIDs, injection of local anesthetic agents and steroids, and the use of specially designed insoles. The use of heel padding as adjunctive therapy is addressed later.

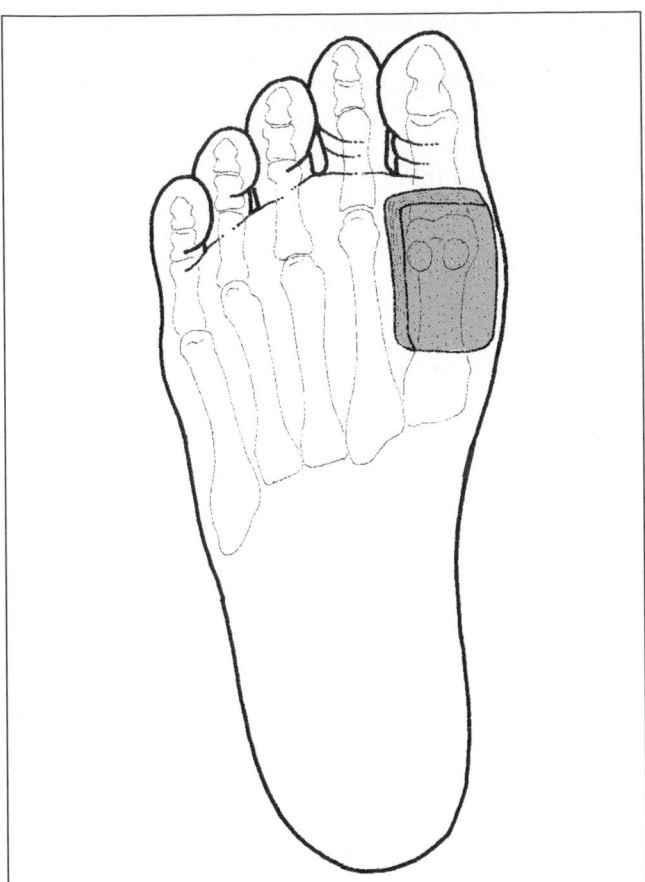

FIGURE 167-6 A ¼ inch-thick felt pad placed beneath the inner sole of a shoe under the first metatarsal to redistribute weight, protecting the second metatarsal in metatarsalgia.

HEEL SPUR SYNDROME

The process of spur formation is termed heel spur syndrome. The etiology is presumed to be chronic traction on the plantar fascia and intrinsic muscles. This results in repeated microtrauma along the medial calcaneal tuberosity, periostitis, and calcification. The patient complains of heel pain progressing over months. Palpation reproduces the pain along the medial border of the calcaneus. Radiographs reveal the spur emanating from the calcaneal tuberosity (Figure 167-7). Absence of a spur suggests plantar fasciitis as the etiology of the pain.

EQUIPMENT
Povidone iodine solution
3 mL syringe
25 gauge needle, 1¼ inches long
Ethyl chloride spray
Local anesthetic solution (without epinephrine), lidocaine, and bupivacaine
Dexamethasone
Felt pad, 1 cm thick
Tape, 2 inches wide

TREATMENT
Treatment is aimed at conservative measures. NSAIDs will provide analgesia. Padding can temporarily relieve heel pain by reducing central pressure on the more painful part of the heel. Apply a 1 cm thick felt pad or

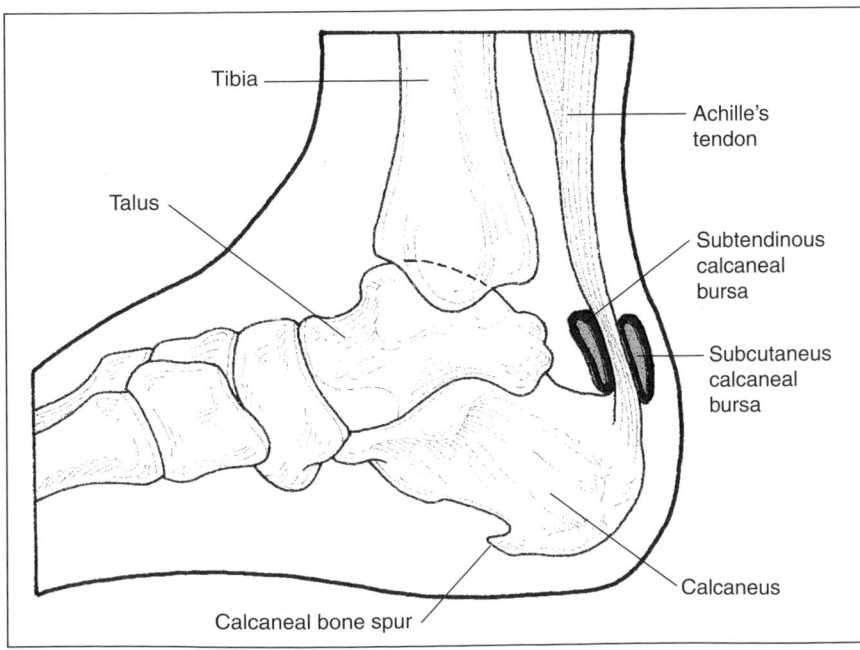

FIGURE 167-7 Sites of potential heel pain.

high-grade foam rubber of similar character cut in the form of a horseshoe directly to the affected heel (Figure 167-8). Secure the pad in place with two or three strips of 2 inch wide tape. Instruct the patient to wear the pad for 1 to 3 days. Remove the pad if it becomes wet to avoid skin maceration.

The patient's shoes may be modified to help provide pain relief. Place a self-adherent sponge pad into the heel of the shoe to decrease pressure on the calcaneus. Have a cobbler place a cut-out into the heel of the patient's shoe if the patient still experiences pain (Figure 167-9). Place a self-adherent sponge pad over the cut-out before the patient wears the shoe.

Injection of local anesthetic solution and corticosteroids is useful in reducing acute inflammation. Mix 1 mL of 1% lidocaine hydrochloride, 1 mL of 0.5% bupivacaine hydrochloride, and 0.8 to 1.0 mg of dexamethasone in a 3 mL syringe. Thoroughly mix the contents of the syringe together. Clean the skin overlying the medial border of the calcaneus of any dirt and debris.

Apply povidone iodine solution and allow it to dry. Spray ethyl chloride to anesthetize the skin. Insert a 25 gauge needle perpendicular to the skin and at the level of the heel spur. Advance the needle in a dart-like motion. Infiltrate the local anesthetic-steroid mixture along the medial calcaneal tubercle and the central plantar calcaneus beneath the spur-fascia junction. **Avoid infiltration into the plantar fat pad, as this area is extremely sensitive and the steroid can cause fat pad atrophy.** The injection procedure can be repeated in 2 to 4 weeks. Refer the patient to a Podiatrist or Orthopedic Surgeon for persistent symptoms despite repeated steroid injections or for an anatomically supinated or pronated foot.

PLANTAR FASCIITIS

Plantar fasciitis is one of the most common causes of heel pain. It is an overuse syndrome, like the heel spur syndrome. Excessive traction on the plantar fascia results in localized inflammation and acute pain at its origin on the calcaneus (Figure 167-10). The inflammation may eventually result in the formation of a heel spur. In the chronic form, the pain can progress distally along the fascial course.

The patient generally describes an insidious onset of heel pain that is characteristically worst first thing in the morning and eases after the first few steps. Plantar fasciitis is common in obese patients. Women—generally in the 40 to 60 year age group—are afflicted more than men. **Clinical examination reveals pain upon palpation along the plantar fascia in the midfoot but not over the area of a heel spur, if present.** Radiographs are generally not helpful at the initial presentation but rather 4 to 6 weeks after the onset if symptoms persist. Radiographs will often confirm the presence of a heel spur that may or may not be involved in plantar fasciitis. One study demonstrated that 46 percent of patients with plantar fasciitis had no spur and 50 percent of patients who had bilateral spurs had pain in only one heel.[13]

TREATMENT

Treatment is aimed at conservative measures. NSAIDs will provide analgesia. Instruct the patient to obtain well-fitted and cushioned footgear that supports the medial longitudinal arch, supports the plantar fascial band, and has good heel shock absorbing qualities. Demonstrate a regimen of active stretching of the medial fascial band (Figure 167-11A). It is important to perform this daily. Stand facing a wall and approximately 2 to 3 ft from the wall. Lean forward and place both palms on the wall. Keep both heels firmly pressed on the ground. The

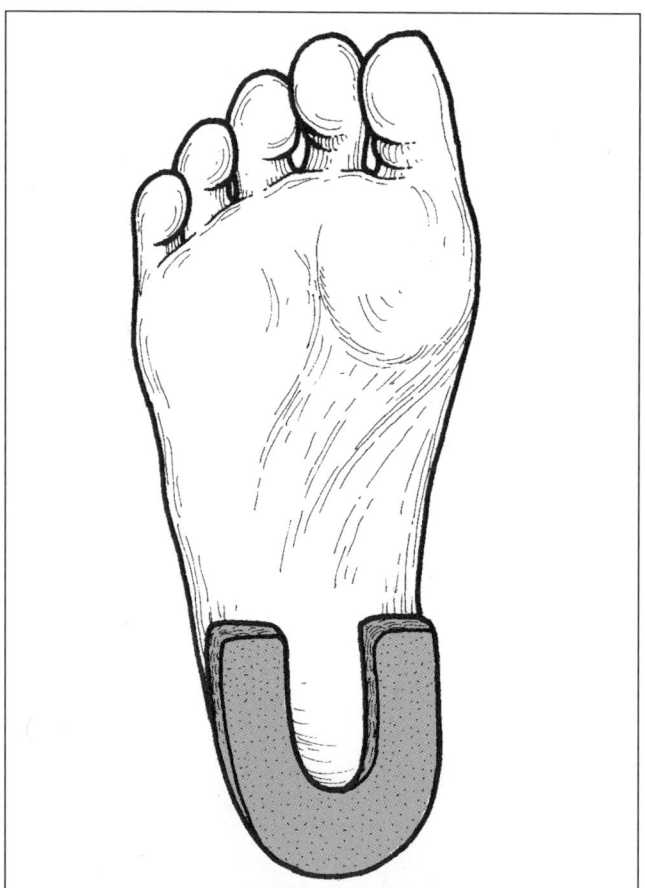

FIGURE 167-8 Relief of heel pain from a heel spur. A ¼ inch thick felt pad or high-grade foam rubber is cut in the form of a horseshoe and applied directly to the affected heel. Secure the pad with two or three strips of 2 inch wide tape.

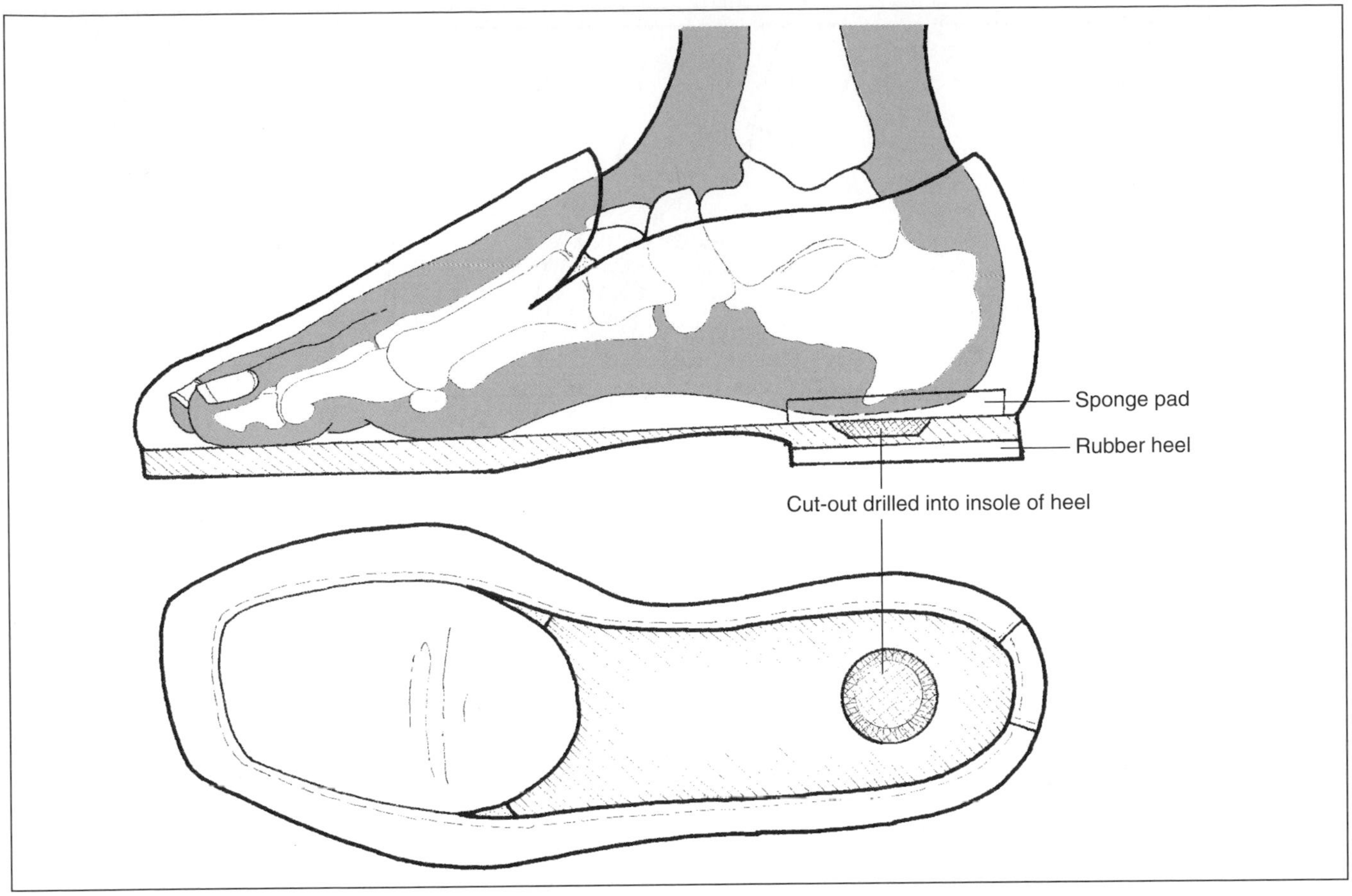

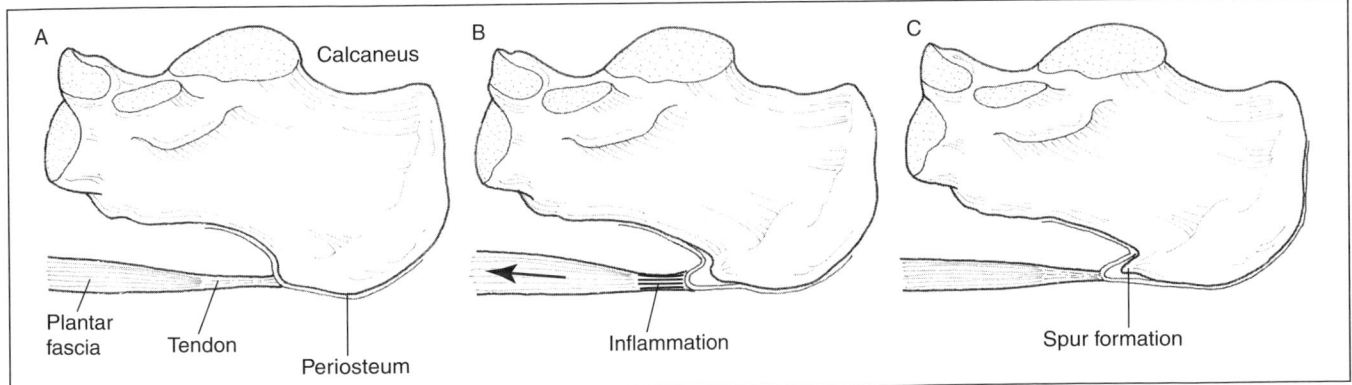

FIGURE 167-9 Shoe modification to relieve heel spur pain.

stretch should be felt in the Achilles tendon and longitudinal arch. Instruct the patient to stretch three times a day for 3 to 5 minutes.

The use of padding can provide relief for some patients. Place medial longitudinal pads to unload the anteromedial aspect of the heel and support the medial longitudinal arch (Figure 167-11*B*). Make the pad from 0.2 inch thick felt and fashion it to fit the patient's longitudinal arch. Secure the pad in place with two or three strips of 2 inch wide tape. Instruct the patient to wear the pad for 1 to 3 days. Remove the pad if it becomes wet so as to avoid skin maceration.

Injection of corticosteroids and local anesthetic agents will control any pain that is not relieved with con-

FIGURE 167-10 The mechanism of plantar fasciitis. *A.* Normal anatomic relationships. *B.* Traction on the tendon elevates the periosteum from the calcaneus and promotes the invasion of inflammatory tissue. *C.* The inflammatory tissue and periosteal elevation can result in the formation of a heel spur.

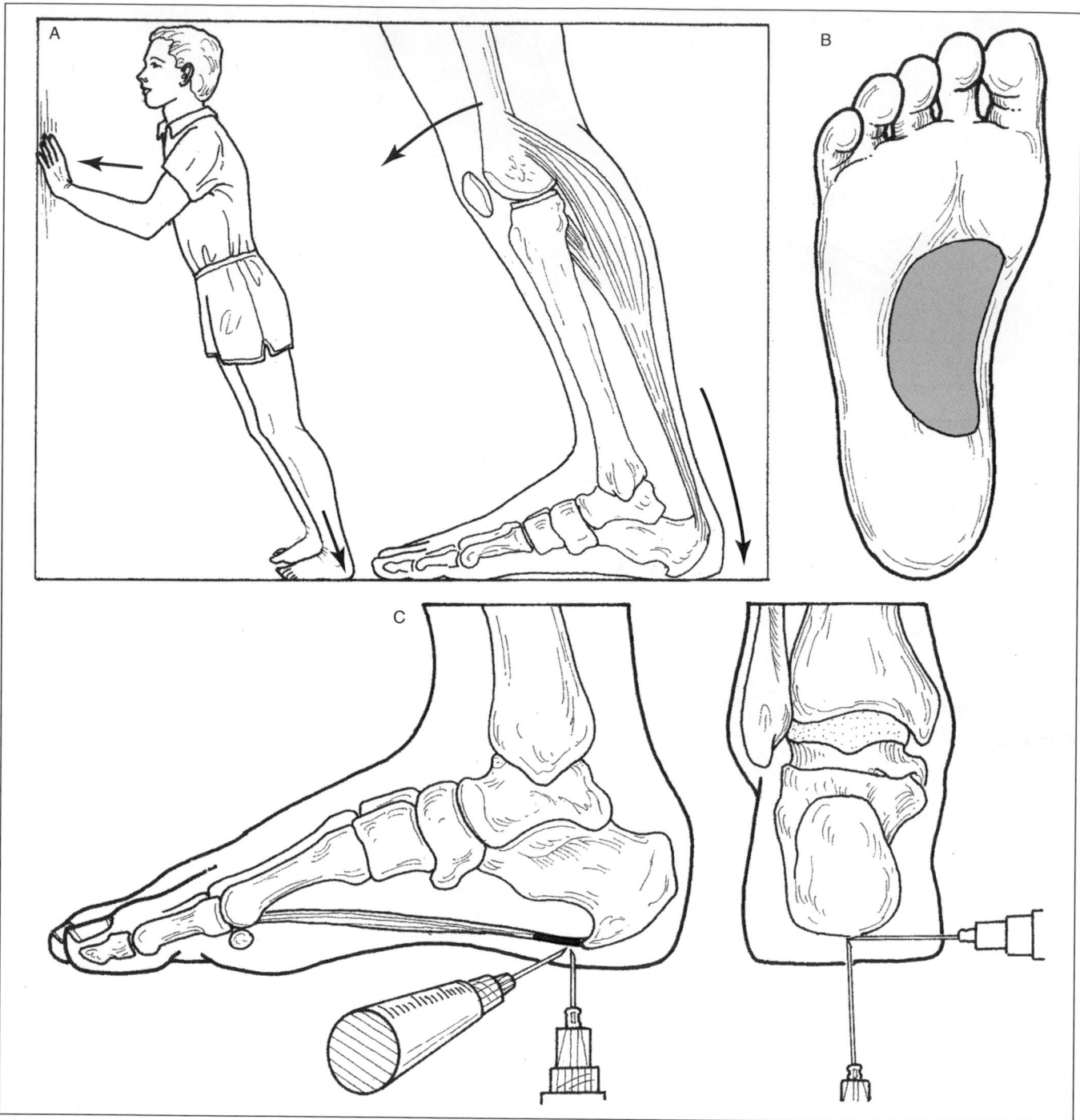

FIGURE 167-11 The treatment of plantar fasciitis. *A.* Active stretching of the medial fascial band. *B.* Placement of a medial longitudinal arch pad. *C.* Injection therapy.

servative measures and help to relieve severe pain (Figure 167-11*C*). Prepare the skin and the injection solution as described with the heel spur syndrome. Inject the solution deep into the plantar fascia.

The injection procedure can be repeated in 2 to 4 weeks if required. **Do not inject more than two or three times into the plantar fascia. Multiple injections can lead to rupture of the plantar fascia. Avoid injection into the plantar fat pad.** This area is extremely sensitive. Steroids injected into the fat pad can cause atrophy and loss of its intrinsic shock-absorbing qualities. Apply a medial longitudinal pad as described above. Relief from a combination treatment may last 6 to 8 weeks. Refer the patient to a Podiatrist or Orthopedic Surgeon for persistent symptoms lasting more than several months and if conservative therapy fails.

RETROCALCANEAL BURSITIS

Retrocalcaneal bursitis is a painful condition. It results from inflammation of one or both of the bursae at the Achilles tendon insertion on the calcaneus (Figure 167-7). The pain in the posterior heel is insidious in onset; it is aggravated by increased activity and shoes with tight heel counterpoints. Palpate the bursae. Place the patient's foot in plantarflexion to relax the Achilles tendon. Squeeze the anterior part of the tendon just proximal to its bony insertion site in the depression above the calcaneus. Tenderness elicited with a squeezing force applied anterior to the Achilles tendon reveals inflammation of the anterior, retrocalcaneal, or subtendinous bursae. Tenderness elicited with pressure on the posterior surface of the Achilles tendon insertion site reveals inflammation of the posterior or subcutaneous calcaneal bursa. Erythema and swelling may be evident at the lateral borders of the Achilles tendon.

TREATMENT

Treatment is conservative and mirrors the treatment for heel spurs. NSAIDs and local steroid injections are recommended. Inject the solution containing steroids and local anesthetic agents directly into the inflamed bursae, avoiding the Achilles tendon. **Never perform more than one or two injections; this will reduce the risk of tendon atrophy at the Achilles tendon insertion site.** Apply a horseshoe-shaped heel pad made from 0.25 inch thick felt or foam rubber to the affected heel.

CALCANEAL APOPHYSITIS (SEVER'S DISEASE)

This condition is a common cause of heel pain, particularly in 8 to 14 year old active males. It results from excessive traction on the calcaneal apophysis by the Achilles tendon, especially during running and jumping. Clinical examination reveals tenderness at the Achilles tendon insertion site on the posterior calcaneus.

TREATMENT

Treatment is aimed at conservative measures. Rest, NSAIDs, and heel lifts fashioned like the pads for heel spurs are recommended. Instruct the patient to perform Achilles tendon stretching exercises, as discussed earlier for plantar fasciitis, three times a day for 3 to 5 minutes (Figure 167-11A). **Steroid injections are not recommended.** Instruct the parent to obtain well-fitted and cushioned athletic footwear; this should be worn by an active adolescent at all times.

ACHILLES TENDINITIS

Repeated trauma to the Achilles tendon from faulty footwear, faulty landing techniques, hard landings, or the use of fluoroquinolone antibiotics can lead to inflammation of the tendon and its sheath due to prolonged friction. Patients complain of pain with prolonged standing and with climbing stairs that is relieved with rest. Clinical examination reveals erythema and localized pain upon palpation just proximal to the Achilles tendon insertion site on the calcaneous.

TREATMENT

Treatment is aimed at conservative measures. It consists of NSAIDs, adequate periods of rest, activity modification, and well-fitting athletic or walking shoes. **Steroid injections of the Achilles tendon are absolutely contraindicated.** Inform the patient regarding shoe modifications, including cutting out the heel counter point (Figure 167-9) or recommending an open-backed shoe. Apply a 0.25 inch thick felt pad fashioned to fit the heel or a commercial cushioned heel lift as appropriate adjunctive therapy. Refer the patient to a Podiatrist or Orthopedic Surgeon for recalcitrant or severe cases.

ACHILLES TENDON RUPTURE

Achilles tendon rupture is one of the most common tendon failures affecting the lower extremity. The Achilles tendon is a source of difficulty for both the serious athlete and the weekend athlete. Typically, the majority of Achilles tendon ruptures occur in the serious athlete during competition or in the relatively sedentary former athlete during demonstrations of former skills on the basketball or volleyball court. Rupture of the Achilles tendon involves a significant force, such as a push-off, a forceful drive, a direct blow, or landing in sudden dorsiflexion with the foot plantarflexed and extended. Rupture of the Achilles tendon can occur at its attachment to the calcaneus, along the tendon, or more commonly at the musculotendinous junction.

Patients typically report a history of sudden pain associated with an audible snap and difficulty tiptoeing or climbing stairs. Clinical findings include a positive Thompson squeeze test, a positive heel resistance test (easy dorsiflexion of the heel and foot against plantarflexion), and a positive gap sign (a palpable, tender gap in the tendon). The Thompson squeeze test is performed with the patient in the prone position and the examiner squeezing the calf. It normally produces plantarflexion. The Thompson test produces markedly decreased motion or none at all if the Achilles tendon is ruptured. Active range of motion and plantarflexion are preserved due to intact extrinsic muscles of the foot.

Obtain radiographs to rule out a fracture. Mammography of the Achilles tendon will detect a partial or complete rupture. This is especially useful when the differential diagnosis includes tendonitis versus a partial tendon rupture.

TREATMENT

Treatment in the Emergency Department is aimed at conservative measures. It consists of NSAIDs, RICE (rest, ice, compression, and elevation), crutch use, and non-weight bearing. Apply a posterior long leg splint with the foot in 20 to 25 degrees of plantarflexion to oppose the tendon ends. Most Achilles tendon ruptures require surgical repair. Arrange follow-up with a Podiatrist or Orthopedic Surgeon within 24 to 28 hours.

INTERDIGITAL NEUROMAS

An interdigital plantar neuroma, also known as a Morton's neuroma, is a common cause of metatarsal pain. This painful condition classically affects adults 20 to 50 years of age, typically women who wear tight shoes or high heels. This painful syndrome usually occurs in the third intermetatarsal space but may occur in the second interspace and rarely in the first or fourth interspace. It is most often unilateral but may be bilateral.

The pathophysiology of this syndrome is complex. The main cause of a Morton's neuroma is an entrapment-type neuropathy that occurs beneath the transverse metatarsal ligament, with anatomic, traumatic, and extrinsic factors all playing a role[14] (Figure 167-12). It has been postulated that the reason for the preponderance of neuroma formation in the third space stems from its dual innervation from the medial and lateral plantar nerves.[15] This leads to an increased nerve thickness, and the area is therefore more subject to trauma and neuroma formation.[15] The fourth metatarsal is the most mobile ray, producing increased mobility of the third web space. This too may result in trauma to the nerve or possibly the development of an enlarged bursa, which can secondarily place extrinsic pressure on the nerve.

Although the reasons for the development of this syndrome are varied, chronic irritation leads the perineural covering to become thickened and fibrotic, with degeneration of the nerve fibers. The damaged sensory nerve no longer conducts normal impulses, producing a burning, neuralgic type pain or numbness limited to the sole beyond the necks of the third and fourth metatarsals and corresponding digits. Pain is aggravated by activities on the foot and most frequently occurs when the patient applies tight-fitting, high-heeled shoes. A common diagnostic clue is the patient's statement that they had to sit down and massage the foot for relief of pain. The pain crises are initially intermittent, but they become more chronic over time.

The clinical examination is often unremarkable. **The patient with an interdigital neuroma does not have pain over the metatarsal heads.** Palpation of the forefoot looking for pain from arthritis, metatarsalgia, capsulitis, or a stress fracture of a metatarsal head is unrewarding. Palpation of the interspace usually reproduces the patient's pain and suggests a neuroma. Mediolateral compression of the metatarsal heads may produce a clicking or crunching feeling (Mulder's sign) and repro-

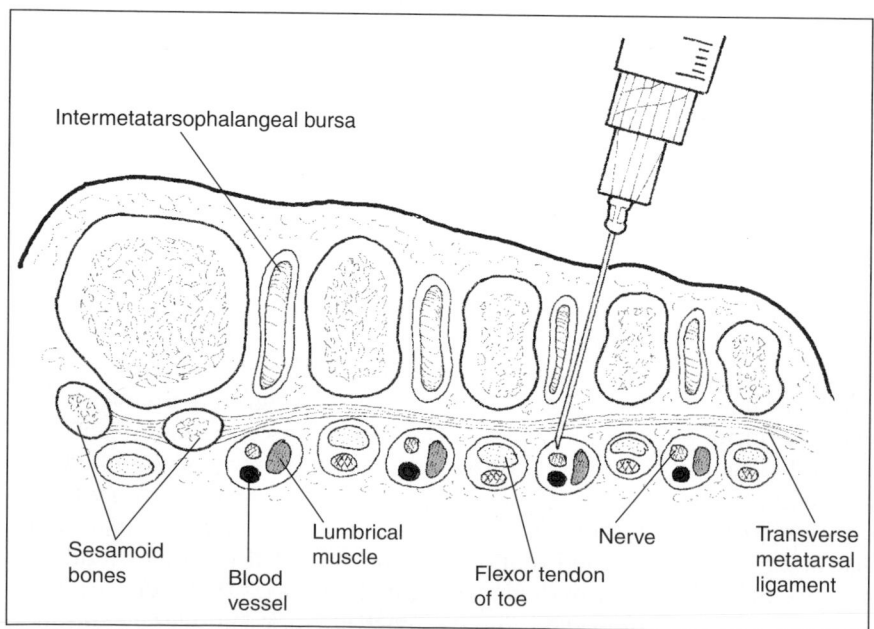

FIGURE 167-12 Cross-section of the foot at the level of the metatarsals demonstrating the anatomy of a Morton's neuroma. The digital nerve lies deep or plantar to the transverse ligament. The third intermetatarsal space is most often involved. The diagram also demonstrates the area of the local steroid/anesthetic needle injection from a dorsal to plantar direction and just deep to the transverse ligament. Prompt relief of pain is both diagnostic and therapeutic of a Morton's neuroma.

Intermetatarsophalangeal bursa

Sesamoid bones

Blood vessel

Lumbrical muscle

Flexor tendon of toe

Nerve

Transverse metatarsal ligament

duce the patient's pain as the swollen nerve is forced between the metatarsal heads (Figure 166-3). A small tumor may rarely be palpable in the affected area. Radiographic studies are unremarkable. A common diagnostic maneuver is to inject 1 to 2 mL of 1% or 2% lidocaine into the intermetatarsal space in a dorsal-to-plantar direction, just deep to the transverse metatarsal ligament (Figure 167-12). Resolution of pain with repeat palpation suggests a Morton's neuroma.

TREATMENT

The majority of interdigital neuromas respond to conservative therapy. Recommend the purchase of shoes with a roomy toe box and a reduction in heel height. Apply a commercially available cushioned inner sole or a 0.25 inch thick felt pad beneath the fourth metatarsal shaft to reduce pressure on the neuroma (Figure 167-13). A trial of NSAIDs may provide adequate analgesia. Instruct the patient to modify their physical activities (i.e., briefer periods of walking or running). Inject a mixture containing 1 mL of 0.25% bupivacaine and 1 mL (5 to 10 mg) of methylprednisolone directly into

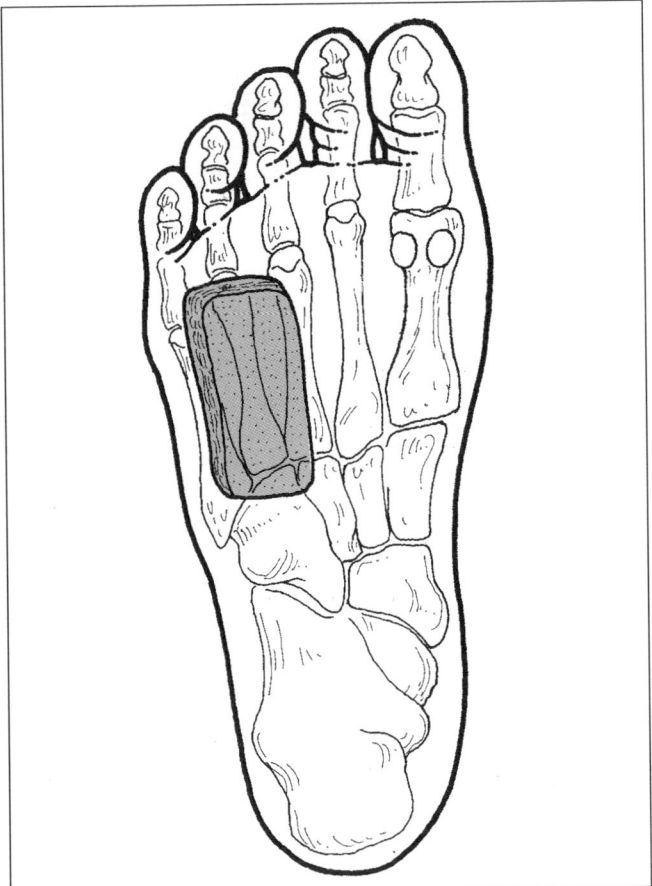

FIGURE 167-13 A commercial cushioned inner sole or a ¼ inch sub-fourth metatarsal felt shaft raise may reduce pressure on a neuroma.

the lesion or indirectly into its fascial plane. Refer to Chapter 166 for complete details regarding injection therapy for a neuroma. The steroid begins to work within 24 to 36 hours to decrease inflammation and edema. Inform the patient that postinjection ecchymosis is common. Repeat injections spaced 1 week apart may be necessary. Refer the patient to a Podiatrist or an Orthopedic Surgeon for surgical therapy if conservative measures fail.

GANGLION CYSTS

A ganglion is a thin-walled, fluid-filled, cystic soft tissue mass histologically similar to a synovial sheath. It frequently contains fluid resembling synovial fluid that ranges in color from clear to amber. Ganglions arise from joint capsules and tendon sheaths, although they do not have a direct open communication with the joint or tendon sheath. The wrist is the most common location of ganglions in the body. Most lower extremity ganglions are located on the dorsal foot and ankle.[16] It is easy to distinguish a ganglion when it occurs over a tendon on the dorsum of the foot, but it can be a challenging diagnosis when it is located in the forefoot. The cystic lesion is painful due to pressure from a shoe or compression of the ganglion against adjacent superficial nerves. The lesion can mimic an interdigital neuroma or MTP joint capsulitis. A higher incidence of ganglions occurs in women. A large percentage of patients will relate a history of trauma prior to the appearance of the ganglion.

The key to an accurate diagnosis is a thorough examination of the foot. The location of the swelling is the key to a correct diagnosis if the clinical examination reveals edema of the forefoot. An interdigital neuroma generally does not cause edema in an intermetatarsal space unless it is unusually large. The typical examination of an interdigital neuroma reveals point tenderness upon palpation over the intermetatarsal space. Capsulitis generally causes swelling and pain with palpation at the MTP joint. The subcutaneous cystic lesion of a ganglion occurs directly beneath the flexor sheath of the involved digit or possibly beneath a metatarsal head. As the ganglion grows, it may move into the intermetatarsal space, where it can compress adjacent structures and cause pain. Generalized swelling is not a common feature of a ganglion. A radiating neuritic type of pain can be present due to pressure on the nerve by the cyst. A number of patients will present asymptomatically with only a cosmetic concern or curiosity as to the nature of the lesion. A ganglion will roll under the examiner's fingers. Consider a soft tissue neoplasm if the lesion is immobile and painless. Arrange follow-up with a Podiatrist or an Orthopedic Surgeon for these suspicious lesions. Consider magnetic resonance imaging (MRI) to better elucidate the nature of the lesion.

EQUIPMENT

Povidone iodine solution
3 mL syringe
1 mL syringe
25 gauge needle, 1¼ inches long
18 gauge needle
Local anesthetic solution without epinephrine
Triamcinolone, injectable
Felt pad, 1 cm thick
Tape, 2 inches wide

TREATMENT

Simple aspiration of the synovial fluid from the cystic lesion can be both diagnostic and therapeutic. Cleanse the skin of any dirt and debris. Apply povidone iodine solution and allow it to dry. Place a subcutaneous wheal of local anesthetic solution overlying the ganglion. Insert an 18 gauge needle attached to a 3 mL syringe into the ganglion. Apply negative pressure to the syringe to aspirate the fluid. The contents of the ganglion are often thick and gelatinous. It is imperative—in terms of the patient's future expectations—to inform them that the ganglion may recur. Arrange follow-up with a Podiatrist or an Orthopedic Surgeon for recurrences.

Some physicians will inject the ganglion cavity with a mixture of a steroid and anesthetic solution. Refer to Chapter 88 for complete details regarding the injection of ganglion cysts. The cystic lesion may reexpand somewhat, but the solution is generally absorbed within 24 hours.

DIABETIC FOOT CARE

Diabetic patients are vulnerable to many systemic complications of their disease. The pathogenic effects of diabetes in the foot are complex and interrelated. The three main risk factors leading to the development of serious cutaneous injury and infection include microcirculatory insufficiency, neuropathic changes, and an altered immune system.

The diabetic patient faces a much higher likelihood of complications from the development of usually benign conditions such as corns, calluses, paronychia, ingrown toenails, and ulcers. The diabetic patient may not appreciate the development of these conditions because of the loss of protective sensory functions. The impact of these complications to the diabetic foot is staggering, to the point where 14 to 24 percent of diabetics with a foot ulcer will require an amputation.[17] **Early and aggressive diagnosis and treatment of common diabetic foot dis-** **orders is essential to maximize the chances for wound healing and reduce the likelihood of complications.**

Radiographic evaluation is mandatory if osteomyelitis is suspected. Characteristic changes include soft tissue swelling, osteolysis, and periosteal elevation. The formation of a sequestrum may be seen as a highly opaque and smooth island of bone surrounded by areas of decreased bone density. Radiographic evaluation often lags behind clinical evidence. A bone scan or MRI is more sensitive than plain radiographs in making an early diagnosis.

The medical history and clinical examination are the most important aspect of evaluating the diabetic foot. **A careful dermatologic, neurologic, orthopedic, and vascular examination must be performed as well as an assessment of the patient's footwear.** A thorough review of the physical examination and assessment of the diabetic foot is beyond the scope of this chapter.

TREATMENT

It is highly important to educate the diabetic patient regarding foot care. Instruct the patient on proper footwear, including good fit, high toe box, a round toe, good support of the heel and arch, inserts to accommodate any plantar lesions, and soft leather. Instruct the patient to check their shoes for any foreign bodies or rough spots at the time of purchase and daily before donning the shoe. Caution the patient to avoid extreme temperatures from the environment or when cleansing the feet. Limit standing to 20 to 30 minutes at a time if a foot lesion is present.

Hyperkeratotic lesions should be treated the same as for nondiabetics, with periodic debridement. Apply a felt corn pad with a central aperture or a horseshoe-shaped pad to relieve pain and disperse pressure at bony prominences to the surrounding skin. Cut a hole in the patient's shoe over any non-weight-bearing bony prominence to prevent irritation of the surrounding soft tissue. Apply a felt pad to cover the tops of any hammer toes. Apply a commercially available adhesive bunion pad or cut a bunion shield from 1 cm thick felt over a bunion or bunionette deformity.

Diabetic patients must be extra vigilant in caring for their toenails. Some authors recommend that diabetics should not cut their own nails, corns, or calluses. Ingrown toenails are treated the same as for nondiabetics. Refer to Chapter 162 for complete details regarding the management of ingrown toenails. Treat mycotic infections (discussed below) aggressively. These conditions are often unnoticed by diabetic patients because of their peripheral neuropathy and the loss of protective sensation. These lesions, therefore, often present at an advanced stage. A simple but thorough vascular examination is mandatory if an infected or advanced lesion is present. Absent or diminished pedal pulses (posterior tibial and dorsalis pedis) may indicate lower extremity ischemia. This requires further vascular evaluation, either through noninvasive testing or by a Vascular Surgeon.

The most common location for foot ulcers is the plantar surface of the forefoot. These are essentially pressure ulcers. Instruct the patient to avoid mechanical stress on the injured extremity, as ongoing trauma prevents healing. Treatment from the Emergency Department is simple and consists of the application of a wound dressing, antibiotics if there is infection, bed rest or the use of crutches, and referral to a Podiatrist or Orthopedic Surgeon. The consultant may use sharp debridement of devitalized tissue from the wound area to promote wound healing.

A moist wound environment is important for wound healing. There are many commercially available foot care products with little proven efficacy, and they may confuse the patient. A simple and clear-cut discharge strategy is wet-to-dry dressing changes twice a day. This can be continued in the home. There is controversy regarding the use of topical agents and foot soaks. Neither one, to date, has been shown to be beneficial in the healing of a diabetic foot ulcer. Cover the lesions with an aperture pad to disperse pressure to the surrounding skin and protect the ulcer. Instruct the patient to place a pillow under the calf and allow the heel to overhang if there is a heel ulcer.

Treat infected ulcers aggressively with systemic antibiotics. Hospital admission is often required. With an appropriate candidate (reliable patient and good home support), mild and most moderate infections can be treated with oral antibiotics on an outpatient basis. The selected antibiotic must achieve good tissue levels and sufficiently cover most skin pathogens, especially aerobic gram-positive cocci. Commonly used antibiotics include cephalexin, clindamycin, amoxicillin-clavulanate, and some of the newer fluoroquinolones. These patients require follow-up within 24 to 72 hours for a wound check and a review of antibiotic therapy when the culture and sensitivity results are available.

Severe infections, with or without systemic symptoms, require hospital admission for parenteral antibiotics and surgical consultation. An experienced consultant will decide if the wound can be debrided at the bedside or necessitates a trip to the operating room. Administer broad-spectrum intravenous antibiotics immediately after wound and blood cultures are obtained. The antibiotic regimen must cover aerobic and anaerobic gram-positive cocci as well as gram-negative organisms. Examples include imipenem-cilastin or vancomycin plus aztreonam plus metronidazole. A beta-lactamase inhibitor (ampicillin-sulbactam) or clindamycin plus a fluoroquinolone is recommended for less severe infections.

Osteomyelitis is a difficult infection to cure, requiring a long course of antibiotics. A 6 week course of antibiotics is recommended, including 1 to 2 weeks of parenteral therapy. Surgical treatment may include debridement of the infected bone if this will not compromise long-term foot function. Debridement will increase the likelihood of a cure and shorten the course of required antibiotics. If the infected bone is located at a bony prominence, removal of the infected bone may correct any underlying bony deformity that may have originally caused the ulcer. Vascular reconstruction and/or amputation are considered for appropriate candidates.

Adjunctive medical therapy includes improving blood glucose, control of comorbid conditions, and medical nutrition to improve the healing potential of foot wounds. A discussion of these topics is beyond the scope of this chapter.

ONYCHOMYCOSIS (FUNGAL TOENAIL INFECTIONS)

Approximately 20% of the U.S. population between the ages of 40 and 60 have fungal nail disease.[18] Onychomycosis is most often caused by dermatophytes, most frequently members of the *Trichophyton* genus. Nondermatophytes (molds or yeasts), however, are also causative organisms. Onychomycosis may occur post-traumatically. It is commonly seen in the first and fifth toenails, where the greatest shoe friction occurs. The infection occurs under or within the nail plate, causing proliferation of keratinized debris under the nail. The nail will become opaque, discolored, thickened, and brittle if the infection is allowed to progress. Formal diagnosis is made by identifying hyphal fragments upon microscopic examination of nail scrapings placed in a potassium hydroxide solution. Onychomycosis is usually diagnosed based upon the clinical examination; therapy is often empiric. "Skipped" normal nails are often seen in fungal toenail infections. In contrast, psoriasis or other inherited nail dystrophies involve all 10 nails.

Four major types of mycotic nail infection have been identified. These include distal subungual onychomycosis, white superficial onychomycosis, proximal white subungual onychomycosis, and candidal onychomycosis. These various entities differ in the pattern of fungal invasion of the nail plate and the causative organism.

Clinical symptoms of mycotic toenail infections include onycholysis (separation of the nail from its bed), hyperkeratosis, brittleness, paronychial inflammation, and color changes. Distal subungual onychomycosis is the most common type. It affects the most distal part of the nail bed and nail plate. White superficial onychomycosis is seen mainly in toenails. It produces a white, brittle appearance due to direct invasion of the nail plate's surface. Proximal white subungual onychomycosis is very rare. It is due to fungus invading the cuticle and turning the proximal nail plate white.

TREATMENT

Treatment of onychomycosis may be divided into topical, systemic, and surgical therapies. Topical agents have been found to be effective if the fungal infection is limited to the distal portion of the nail plate. Simple mechanical filing of the nail plate, curettage of the necrotic subungual tissue, trimming of the nail plate, and topical antimycotic therapy are often effective.

Treatment of more advanced infections begins with an empiric trial of an oral antifungal agent. Itraconazole (Sporanox), a newer member of the azole family, has a very broad antimycotic spectrum of action. It is effective in the treatment of dermatophytes, yeasts, and some nondermatophyte molds. Terbinafine (Lamisil) is an orally active allylamine active against dermatophytes but not yeast. Both itraconazole and terbinafine are associated with a significantly shorter treatment time and higher clinical cure rate over the older systemic agents such as griseofulvin. Studies have shown that pulse therapy is an effective treatment regimen for both itraconazole and terbinafine.[19–23] This consists of 1 week of daily treatment each month for 3 to 4 consecutive months. Inform patients of any potential symptoms, side effects, and drug reactions. Obtain a baseline liver profile, chemistry panel, and complete blood count. There is a small risk of hepatotoxicity from oral antifungal agents. Any patient receiving long-term antifungal therapy for onychomycosis must undergo laboratory monitoring approximately every 4 to 6 weeks.

More extensive involvement or failure of outpatient therapy may require removal of the nail plate in addition to an oral antifungal agent and local wound care. Apply a topical antifungal agent twice daily while the new nail plate develops. Refer the patient to a Podiatrist for refractory chronic onychomycosis, especially the patient who has diabetes or vascular disease. Surgical treatment may include nail plate removal with nail bed debridement (with or without chemical destruction of the nail bed matrix). Close follow-up is mandatory.

SUMMARY

Foot complaints are commonly encountered in the Emergency Department. Many of these conditions can be managed using easy, simple, and straightforward techniques. Refer the patient to a Podiatrist or Orthopedic Surgeon for conditions requiring continued care, chronic conditions, or acute injuries.

REFERENCES

1. Silfverskiold JP: Common foot problems. *Postgrad Med* 1991; 89(5):183–188.

2. Omura EF, Rye B: Dermatologic disorders of the foot. *Clin Sports Med* 1994; 13(4):825–841.

3. Duvries HI: New approach to the treatment of intractable verruca plantaris (plantar wart). *JAMA* 1953; 152(13):1202–1203.

4. Duvries H: *Surgery of the Foot,* 2nd ed. St. Louis: Mosby–Year Book, 1965:456–462

5. Pedowitz WJ: Distal oblique osteotomy for intractable plantar keratosis of the middle three metatarsals. *Foot Ankle* 1988; 9(1):7–9.

6. Winson IG, Rawlinson J, Broughton NS: Treatment of metatarsalgia by sliding distal metatarsals osteotomy. *Foot Ankle* 1988; 9(1):2–6.

7. American College of Foot and Ankle Surgeons: Hammer toe syndrome. *J Foot Ankle Surg* 1999; 38(2):166–178.

8. Della Corte MP, Grisafi PJ, Birrer RB: General treatment guidelines, in Birrer RB, Dellacorte MP, Grisafi PJ (eds): *Common Foot Problems in Primary Care,* 2nd ed. Philadelphia: Hanley & Belfus, 1998:185–187.

9. McGlamry ED, Banks AS, Downey MS: *Fundamentals of Foot Surgery.* Baltimore: Williams & Wilkins, 1987:330–332.

10. Montgomery R, Foot complaints of the elderly. *Cutis* 1976; 18:462–463.

11. Mann RA, Coughlin MJ: *Surgery of the Foot and Ankle,* 6th ed. St. Louis: Mosby–Year Book, 1993: 181–185.

12. Malusky LP: Podiatric procedures, in Roberts JR, Hedges JR (eds): *Clinical Procedures in Emergency Medicine,* 3rd ed. Philadelphia: Saunders, 1998:873–889.

13. Lapidus PW, Guidotti FP: Painful heel: report of 323 patients with 364 painful heels. *Clin Orthop* 1965; 39:178–186.

14. Mann RA, Baxter DE: Diseases of the nerves, in Mann RA, Coughlin MJ (eds): *Surgery of the Foot and Ankle,* 6th ed. St. Louis: Mosby–Year Book, 1993:544–547.

15. Jones JR, Klenerman L: A study of the communicating branch between the medial and lateral plantar nerves. *Foot Ankle* 1984; 4(6):313–315.

16. Wu KK: Intraosseous ganglion cyst of the middle cuneiform bone of the foot. *J Foot Ankle Surg* 1994; 33(6):633–635.

17. American Diabetes Association: Consensus Development Conference on Diabetic Foot Wound Care, Boston, Massachusetts. *Diabetes Care* 1999; 22(8): 1354–1360.

18. Zaias N: Onychomycosis. *Dermatol Clin* 1985; 3(3): 445–460.

19. Havu V, Brandt H, Heikkila H, et al: A double-blind, randomized study comparing itraconazole pulse therapy with continuous dosing for the treatment

of toenail onychomycosis. *Br J Dermatol* 1997; 136: 230–234.

20. De Doncker P, Decroix J, Pierard GE, et al: Antifungal pulse therapy for onychomycosis: a pharmacokinetic and pharmacodynamic investigation of monthly cycles of 1-week pulse therapy with itraconazole. *Arch Dermatol* 1996; 132:34–41.

21. Alpsoy E, Yilmaz E, Basaran E: Intermittent therapy with terbinafine for dermatophyte toe onychomycosis: a new approach. *J Dermatol* 1996; 23(4):259–262.

22. De Backer M, De Keyser P, De Vroey C, et al: A 12-week treatment for dermatophyte toe onychomycosis: terbinafine 250 mg/day vs itraconazole 200 mg/day—a double blind comparative trial. *Br J Dermatol* 1996; 134(suppl 46):16–17.

23. Arenas R, Dominguez-Cherit J, Fernandez LMA: Open randomized comparison of itraconazole versus terbenafine in onychomycosis. *Int J Dermatol* 1995; 34(2):138–143.

Section Fifteen

MISCELLANEOUS PROCEDURES

Chapter 168
ASEPTIC TECHNIQUE

John S. Rose

INTRODUCTION

The proper use and an understanding of aseptic technique is critical for the care of patients in the Emergency Department. Aseptic technique dovetails with prescribed universal precautions and is central to our practice. Knowledge of proper aseptic technique ensures that procedures performed in the Emergency Department provide maximal protection for both the patient and the physician while keeping the risk of contamination as low as possible.[1-8]

Wound infection and sepsis are the two major complications resulting from poor and improper aseptic technique. Other complications that may contribute to the patient's morbidity and mortality include increased length and cost of hospital stay, patient discomfort, scarring, and even death. With this is mind, it is clear that aseptic technique is warranted except in the most dire circumstances.

Numerous terms are used to describe the establishment and maintenance of a "sterile" environment. These include aseptic, sterile technique, and disinfection, to name a few. Many people often, and incorrectly, interchange these terms. The proper definitions of the terms used to describe aseptic technique or associated with it can be found in Table 168-1.

ANATOMY AND PATHOPHYSIOLOGY

The skin and hair are colonized with various organisms. The stratum corneum layer of the epidermis is colonized with a polymicrobial flora. This includes *Staphylococcus aureus, Staphylococcus epidermidis,* various *Streptococcus* species, viruses, yeasts, and molds. Many of these organisms are nonpathogenic, even when placed in environments considered appropriate for infection. *S. aureus* is the most common cause of wound infections. It can result in an infection when introduced into deeper skin layers. Some species, such as *S. epidermidis,* are pathologic only when inoculated into deeper layers of the skin and soft tissue. For most infections, a significant inoculation is required to create a critical level for microbial growth to occur. **Aseptic technique decreases bacterial exposure and reduces the level of potentially pathologic organisms.**

INDICATIONS

The role of aseptic technique in the Emergency Department is primarily for invasive procedures. Invasive procedures require varying degrees of aseptic technique. Placement of a small peripheral intravenous catheter may require no more than a brief wiping of the skin. In contrast, a diagnostic peritoneal lavage requires operating room–level disinfection and strict sterile technique.

Routine and adequate provider disinfection involves careful hand washing, the use of clean and disinfected personal diagnostic equipment (e.g., stethoscopes), and wearing appropriately cleaned coats and clothing. This is critical in preventing iatrogenic infections in the Emergency Department. Aseptic technique in the Emergency Department can be referred to as clinical aseptic technique, since it is virtually impossible to achieve an operating room level of asepsis in the Emergency Department. Clinical aseptic technique involves the combining of adequate disinfection with sterile techniques and protocols at the bedside.

CONTRAINDICATIONS

There are very few contraindications to the maintenance of adequate procedural aseptic technique. One exception would be that extreme clinical circumstance in which time simply does not allow proper aseptic

TABLE 168-1. DEFINITIONS OF TERMS USED FOR DESCRIBING ASEPTIC TECHNIQUE

Term	Definition
Aseptic	Freedom from infection. Prevention of contact with microorganisms. Involves the use of sterile technique and skin disinfection.
Sterile technique	The practice of utilizing sterile equipment and procedures to maintain an aseptic environment.
Sterile field	The zone in which strict sterile technique is maintained. Generally consists of an area 3 to 10 times larger than the area of the primary procedure.
Super aseptic	Ultra-high state of an aseptic environment. Usually, this is achievable only in the operating room.
Disinfection	The cleaning of an area to make it free of pathogenic organisms and microbes.
Clean technique	The practice of using nonsterile equipment to perform procedures. This is considered as part of the universal body fluid precautions.

technique, as in an emergent thoracotomy. Even in such situations, however, the physician can still use sterile gloves and a quick application of an aseptic solution.

Always inquire about allergies and sensitivities to latex and antiseptic solutions. This information will affect the equipment that is chosen to properly prepare the patient.[8] Most if not all hospitals have a latex-free cart that contains equipment for use with latex-allergic patients. Do not use povidone iodine solution in patients allergic to iodine. Alternative agents include chlorhexidine and hexachlorophene preparations.

EQUIPMENT

Povidone iodine solution
Chlorhexidine or hexachlorophene preparations for iodine-allergic patients
70% isopropyl alcohol
Sterile 4×4 gauze squares or applicator sticks
Sterile gloves
Face mask and eye protection
Sterile drapes
Adequate lighting
Sterile gowns
Bedside procedure table

PATIENT PREPARATION

Inform the patient of what the procedure entails before performing any procedure in the Emergency De-

partment. This should include an explanation of sterile technique and a request that the patient not touch the drapes or sterile equipment. Obtain an informed consent before the patient is draped. The only exception to this is if an emergent and lifesaving procedure must be immediately performed.

Place the patient in the most comfortable position possible. Patient discomfort frequently results in movement and the potential loss of the sterile field. Utilize sedation and/or analgesia as necessary to facilitate proper patient positioning. The provider must be comfortably positioned and have adequate lighting.

TECHNIQUES

Aseptic technique can be divided into skin disinfection and sterile technique. Skin disinfection removes any microorganisms found on the skin and decreases potential contamination during the procedure. Sterile technique is performed for the same reason. There are different levels of aseptic technique, ranging from full aseptic technique (mask, gown, gloves, and drapes) to simple sterile gloves. The physician must use their judgment to determine which level is most appropriate to the task at hand.[8]

SKIN DISINFECTION

Disinfection involves the application and scrubbing of a disinfectant preparation onto the skin (Figure 168-1). Simple procedures, such as injections or venipunctures, may require little disinfection. Wipe the skin with gauze that has been impregnated with 70% isopropyl alcohol for simple procedures. The alcohol has an antibacterial effect. The mere force of wiping the skin reduces bacterial counts. No disinfection is used for simple venipunctures in some countries. More comprehensive skin preparation involves the use of a disinfectant agent such as povidone iodine solution.

Povidone iodine and 2% iodine tincture solution are the most commonly used skin antiseptic solutions. Povidone iodine solution is highly germicidal for gram-positive and gram-negative bacteria, viruses, fungi, protozoa, and yeasts.[7] It rapidly reduces bacterial counts on the skin surface.[7] Allow the iodine solution to dry and then wipe it from the skin with 70% alcohol prior to beginning the procedure. The iodine solutions work by killing bacteria as they dry. Isopropyl alcohol can be applied to the skin and scrubbed vigorously for 2 minutes to achieve disinfection, though this may cause skin irritation. Chlorhexidine or hexachlorophene preparations may be used as substitutes in iodine-allergic or sensitive patients. These agents provide good bactericidal activity against gram-positive bacteria but some-

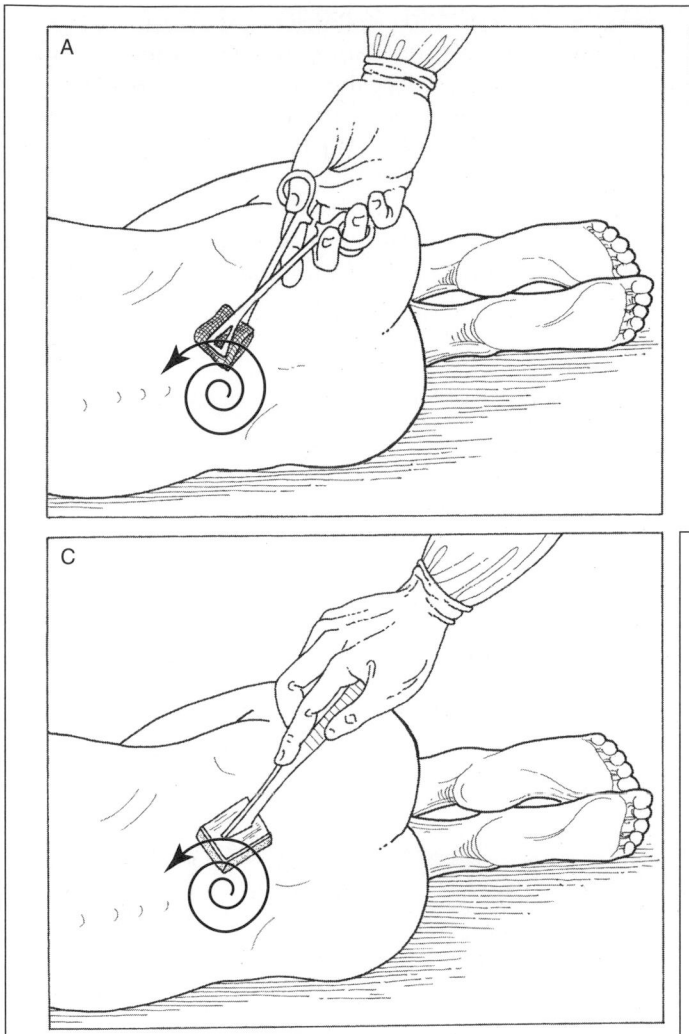
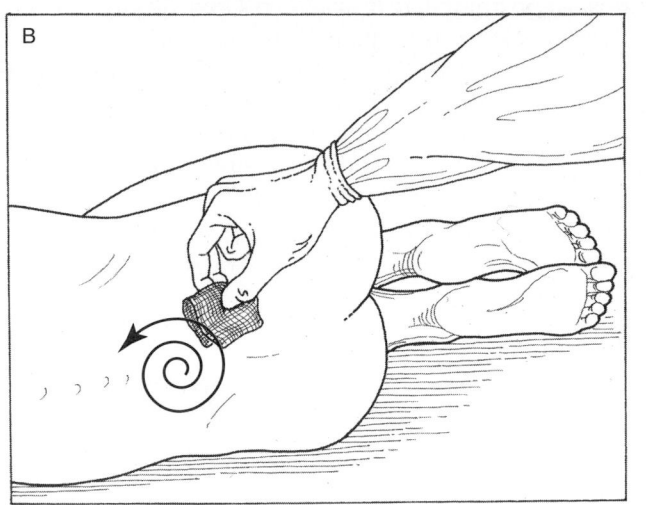

FIGURE 168-1 Preparation of the skin. Disinfectant solution is applied in a concentric circular pattern starting from the procedure site and working outward. Apply the disinfectant solution with sterile gauze held in a clamp (*A*), with sterile gauze held in a sterile gloved hand (*B*), or with a sponge on a stick (*C*).

what less activity against gram-negative organisms.[8] Apply all of these solutions with the technique described below.

Use a skin disinfectant for procedures other than simple venipuncture. Place the disinfectant solution onto either a sterile sponge or sterile gauze. Apply the disinfectant to the skin in a circular motion, beginning with the central area of the procedure and working out toward the periphery of the sterile field (Figure 168-1). Repeat the process three or four times using a new sponge or gauze each time.[8] This technique ensures that the central area where the procedure is to be performed is the most sterile area of the field. The number of organisms increases toward the periphery of the prepped area. The area of disinfection must be much larger than the primary area of the procedure.

STERILE TECHNIQUE

General sterile technique is described, followed by specific details for each step of the procedure. Strict ster-

ile technique is virtually impossible in the Emergency Department. **However, make every effort to maintain a sterile field in order to minimize infection.** Assemble all equipment necessary and place it on a small procedure stand. Avoid having different components scattered around the procedure area. Open all sterile items, using proper sterile protocol, so as to have them available once the provider has donned sterile gloves. Use anesthetic solution containers with removable caps. This allows the provider to draw up anesthetic without having an assistant and minimizes the risk of occupational needle exposure. Perform a thorough hand washing before the procedure.

Apply sterile gloves. Place sterile drapes to form a field wide enough to allow for a comfortable work space. Drape the area near the patient closest to the bedside procedure table. This will minimize inadvertent contamination in moving from the table to the patient. Make a small flat sterile area near the procedure site to allow for placement of important items that must be immediately available. Open all caps, position stopcocks, and prepare all devices prior to starting the procedure. The likelihood of contamination increases if devices are not adequately prepared, thus requiring manipulation during the critical portion of a procedure. **Adhere to universal precautions guidelines.** Use eye and face protection during the procedure. This should be applied before donning gowns and gloves.

OPENING A STERILE PACK

Always make sure that the outer wrapping is intact, the sterility expiration date has not passed, and the sterility indicator tape is the appropriate color before opening a sterile pack.[2] Wash your hands and remove the outer wrap if applicable. Remove the sterility indicator tape (Figure 168-2A). Place the sterile pack on a dry and level surface with the outermost flap facing away from you (Figure 168-2B). Grasp the corners of the outer-

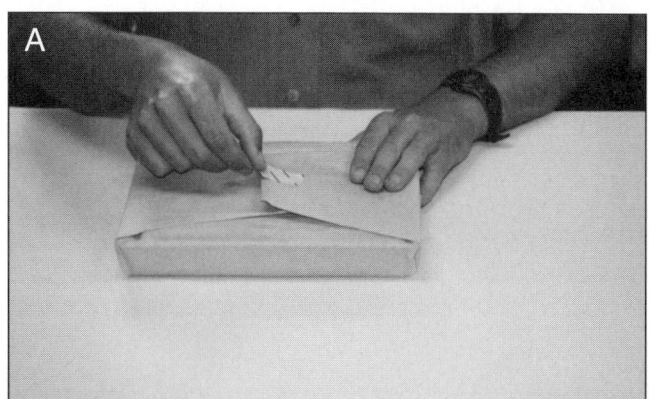

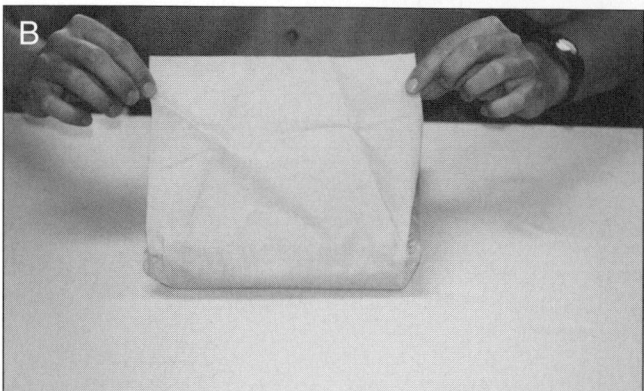

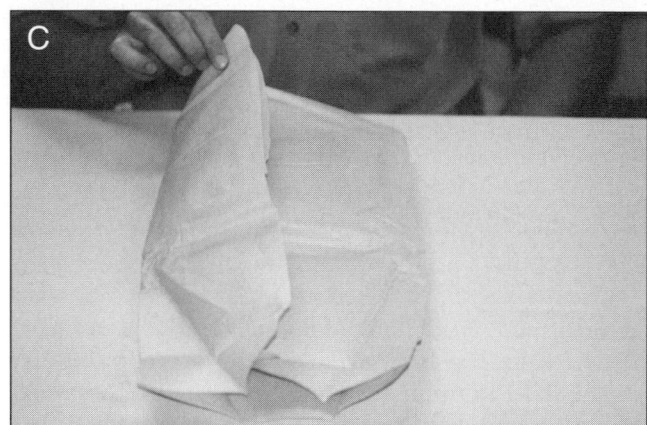

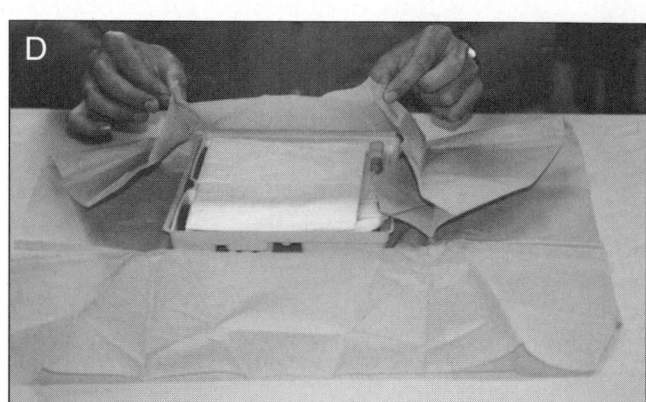

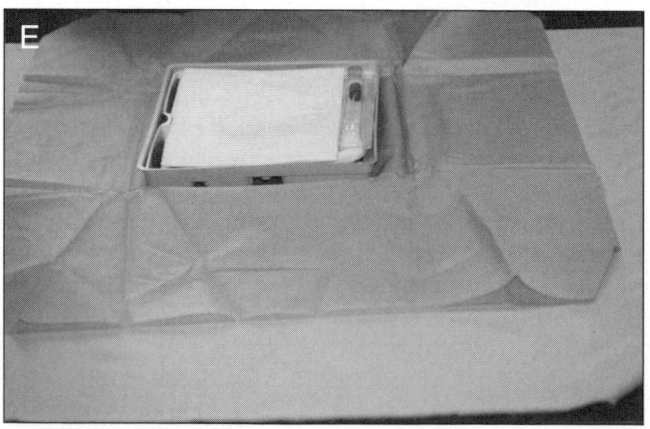

FIGURE 168-2 Opening a sterile pack. *A.* Remove the sterility indicator tape. *B.* Grasp the edges of the outermost flap and open it away from you. *C.* Open the side flaps. *D.* Open the remaining flap toward you. *E.* The open pack.

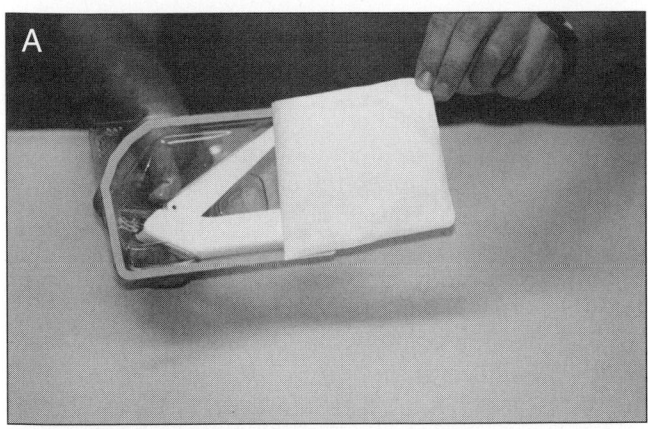

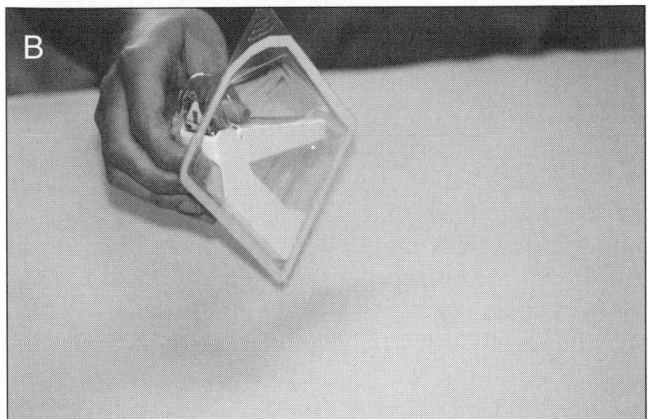

FIGURE 168-3 Opening a hard peel-back container. *A.* Grasp the container with the flap facing the sterile field. Remove the flap. *B.* Drop the contents of the hard container onto the sterile field.

most flap (Figure 168-2*B*). Hold your arms to the sides of the pack to avoid reaching over the sterile area. Lift the flap up and away from you (Figure 168-2*B*). Open the side flaps by grasping the folded corner with a thumb and index finger and pulling the flap to the side (Figure 168-2*C*). Open the bottom flap (Figure 168-2*D*). Grasp and open the bottom flap while stepping back to prevent contaminating the wrap on your clothing. **Make sure that your arms and clothes do not contaminate the contents of the pack when opening the flaps.** Repeat the procedure if the pack has an inner wrap.

PLACING STERILE SUPPLIES ON A STERILE FIELD

Sterile supplies are generally packaged in either a hard or a soft peel-back container. The general principle of opening these is the same, though there are subtle differences. Hold the hard peel-back container in the non-dominant hand with the flap facing the sterile field (Figure 168-3*A*). Pull the flap toward you with the dominant hand so that the open end of the pack will be facing the

field (Figure 168-3*A*). Hold the container 15 to 20 cm above the sterile field. Drop the contents of the sterile pack onto the sterile field, taking care not to contaminate the field with the container itself (Figure 168-3*B*).

Gloves and syringes are wrapped in soft peel-back containers. Grasp both sides of the unsealed edge of the soft pack and pull them apart slightly (Figure 168-4*A*). Hold the open end facing the sterile field (away from you). Continue to open the container. Fold the sides of the sterile packing back and over your hands to keep the contents sterile (Figure 168-4*B*). Gently drop the contents of the soft pack onto the sterile field.

APPLICATION OF A MASK

Surgical masks serve a dual role in the performance of aseptic technique. Masks have been shown to decrease contamination of the sterile field that may result from aerosolized droplets from the mouth and nose. Masks protect the caregiver's mucous membranes from exposure and possible splashing during the procedure. Wear a mask with an eye shield during high-risk procedures.

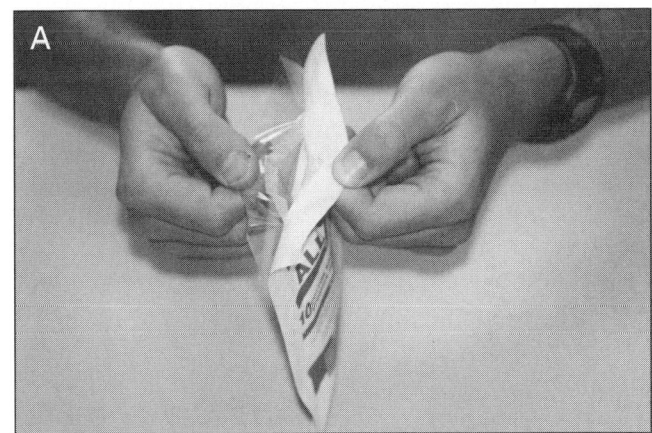

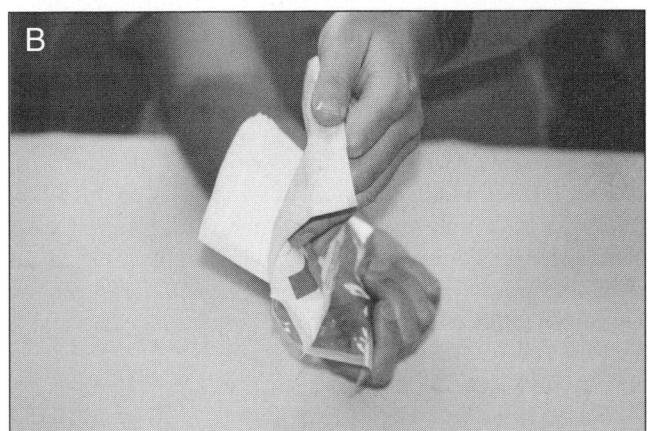

FIGURE 168-4 Opening a soft peel-back container. *A.* Grasp both sides of the unsealed edge and pull them apart. *B.* Face the pack toward the sterile field. Continue to open the edges until the contents fall onto the sterile field.

Apply the mask before donning gloves and other sterile equipment. Secure the mask either by placing the elastic straps around the ears, placing the elastic straps around the head, or tying the mask securely to the face with ties around the head and neck. Pinch the metal nose clip securely to the bridge of the nose for a tighter fit and to minimize the gap between the mask and the nose.

HAND WASHING

Despite the fact that sterile gloves are worn for all sterile procedures, hands must still be thoroughly washed. A full surgical scrub is neither necessary nor feasible in the Emergency Department. Good hand washing technique should not be overlooked.

Remove any watches and rings before hand washing. Rinse your hands in warm water prior to applying antiseptic soap. Apply soap, lather your hands, and rub them together vigorously for approximately 10 seconds. Wash each wrist with the opposite hand. Interlace the fingers and slide them back and forth to clean the web spaces. Clean around the nails with the fingertips and nails of the opposite hand. Completely rinse each hand from the fingers down. Repeat the procedure a second time if the hands were grossly contaminated. Dry your hands with a disposable towel. Turn off the faucet, using the towel with which you dried your hands.

APPLICATION OF A CLEAN GOWN

A clean (nonsterile) gown is often used as an additional barrier to contamination of both the field and the provider's clothing. Simply place your arms into the sleeves and pull on the gown with the opening toward the back. Secure the gown at the back of the neck and the lower back by tying the strings.

APPLICATION OF A STERILE GOWN

A sterile gown is worn for those procedures requiring a stricter sterile technique (i.e., central venous access, diagnostic peritoneal lavage). To open a sterile gown, use the procedure described to open a sterile pack. Grasp and pick up the gown just below the neckline, touching only the inner surface of the gown. Hold the gown up and let it unfold with the inside facing you. Do not allow the gown to touch any nonsterile surfaces. Insert your arms into the sleeves until the gown is in place. Have an assistant grasp the back of the gown, pull it completely on, and tie the strings securely.

APPLICATION OF STERILE GLOVES

Wash your hands thoroughly before putting on sterile gloves. Open the outer wrap of the sterile gloves and remove the inner wrap (Figure 168-5A). Place the inner wrap on a clean surface with the gloves' wrists facing toward you. Unfold the inner wrap, touching only the outside edges (Figure 168-5B). Open the inner wrap according to the procedure for opening a sterile pack (Figure 168-5C). Use the dominant hand to grab the opposite glove at the inner edge of its folded cuff (Figure 168-5D). Slip the nondominant hand into the glove, being careful not to touch the outer surface of the glove (Figure 168-5E). Pull the glove further onto the nondominant hand using the inner edge of the cuff (Figure 168-5F). Place the fingers of the gloved nondominant hand into the folded cuff of the other glove (Figure 168-5G). Slip the dominant hand into the glove (Figure 168-5H). Pull this glove over the dominant hand using the cuff (Figure 168-5I). Carefully unfold the cuff of each glove, taking care not to touch the fingers and palms of the gloves to nonsterile skin. Adjust each glove to ensure a snug fit over the fingers and hand.

REMOVAL OF PROTECTIVE CLOTHING

Remove protective clothing in a systematic manner in order to protect yourself and others from the contaminants on your gown and gloves (Figure 168-6). Place all removed garments into appropriate waste containers. The first step is to untie the gown (Figure 168-6A). Untie the neck strings of the gown. Take off the gown by turning it inside out as it is removed (Figure 168-6B). Roll up the gown with the contaminated surface facing inward (Figure 168-6C). Dispose of the gown. Remove the gloves by turning them inside out, making sure that you do not touch the outside part with your ungloved hands. Use the dominant hand to grasp the cuff of the glove on the nondominant hand (Figure 168-6D). Pull the glove inside out as your remove it and throw it away. Place the ungloved fingers into the inside edge of the gloved dominant hand and remove it by pulling the glove inside out (Figure 168-6E). Dispose of the glove. Remove the mask by untying its ties or removing the elastic straps from behind your ears. Dispose of the mask. Finally, wash your hands.

COMPLICATIONS

Properly performed aseptic technique has very few complications. The primary risk is in patients with sensitivities or allergies to latex or the disinfectant preparations. Although povidone iodine preparations are much less irritating than tincture of iodine, it is a good policy to clean all disinfectant off the patient at the end of the procedure so as to minimize any skin irritation. This is especially true of small children. Use alternate products for those patients with histories of iodine allergies. The main complication of improper aseptic technique is infection at the site of the procedure.[8] This only serves to underscore the need to perform aseptic technique properly.

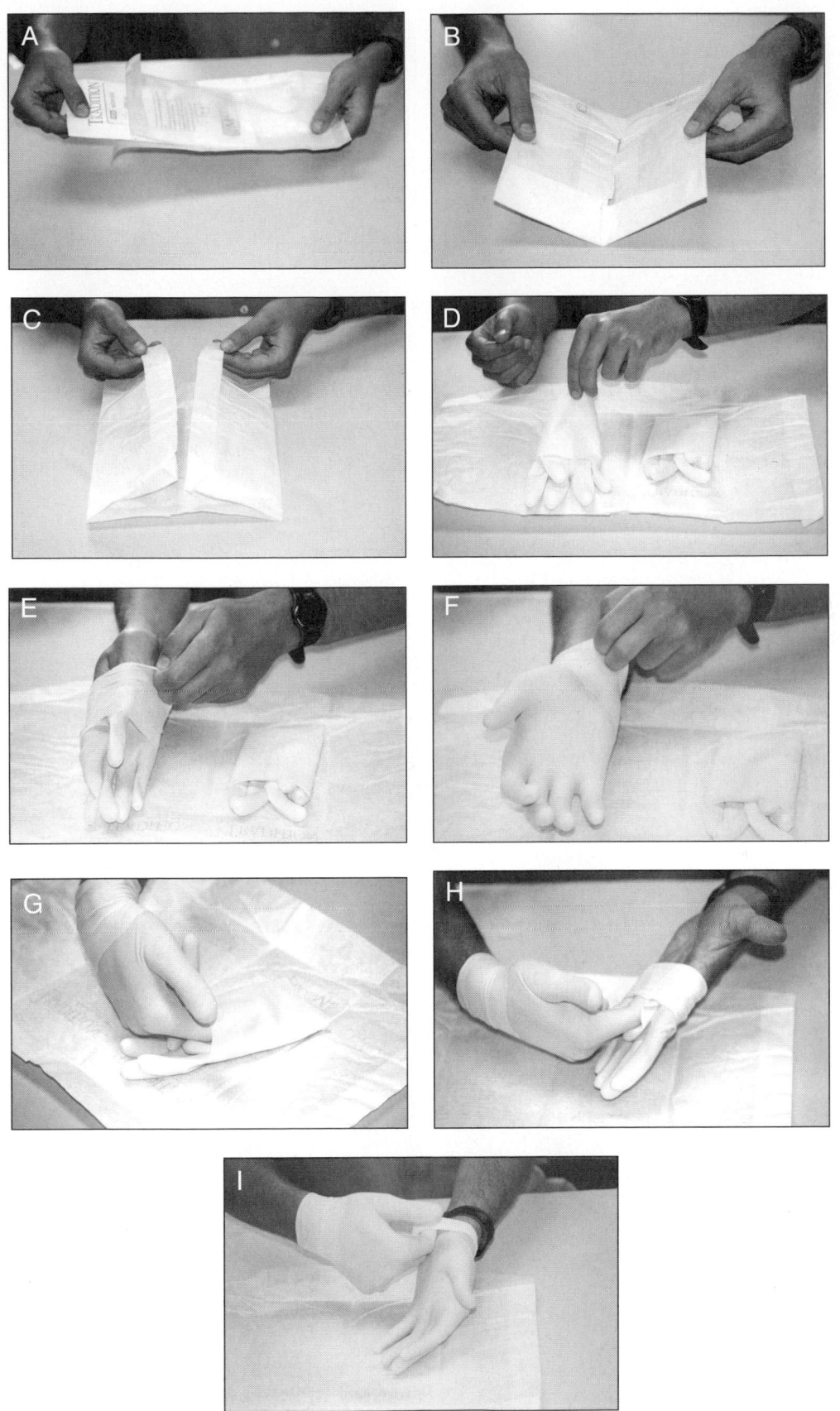

FIGURE 168-5 Application of sterile gloves. *A.* Open the outer wrap and remove the inner wrap. *B.* Unfold the inner wrap. *C.* Completely open the inner wrap. *D.* Grasp the cuff of a glove. *E.* Slip the glove onto the hand. *F.* Pull the glove onto the hand. *G.* Slip the gloved hand into the folded cuff of the second glove. *H.* Slip the glove onto the hand. *I.* Pull the glove onto the hand.

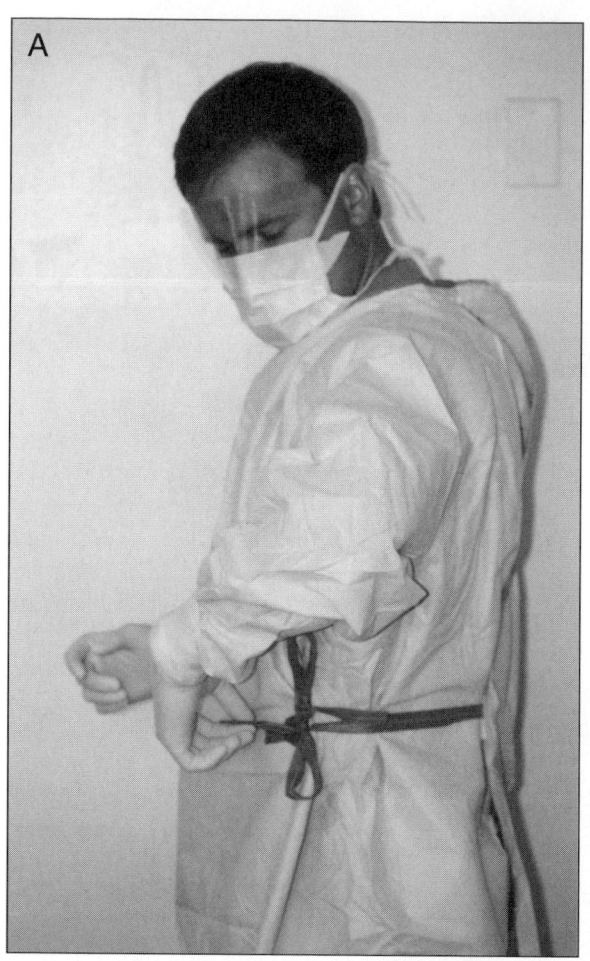

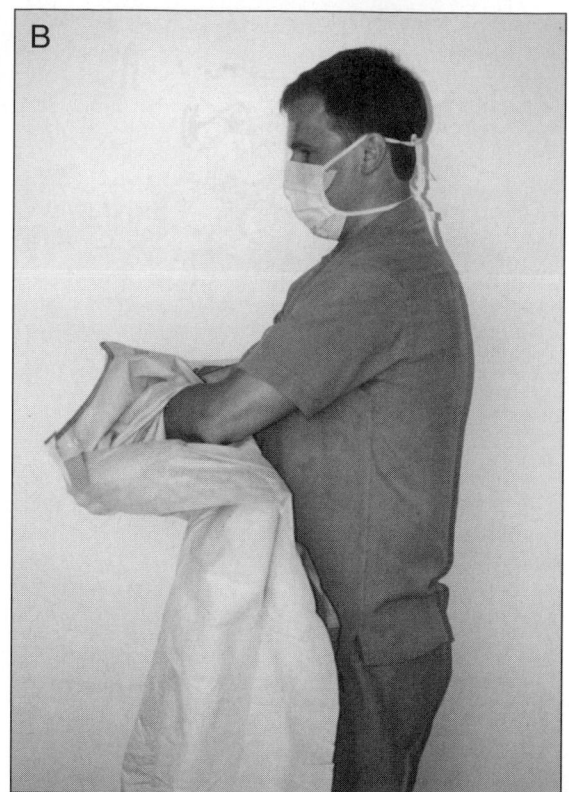

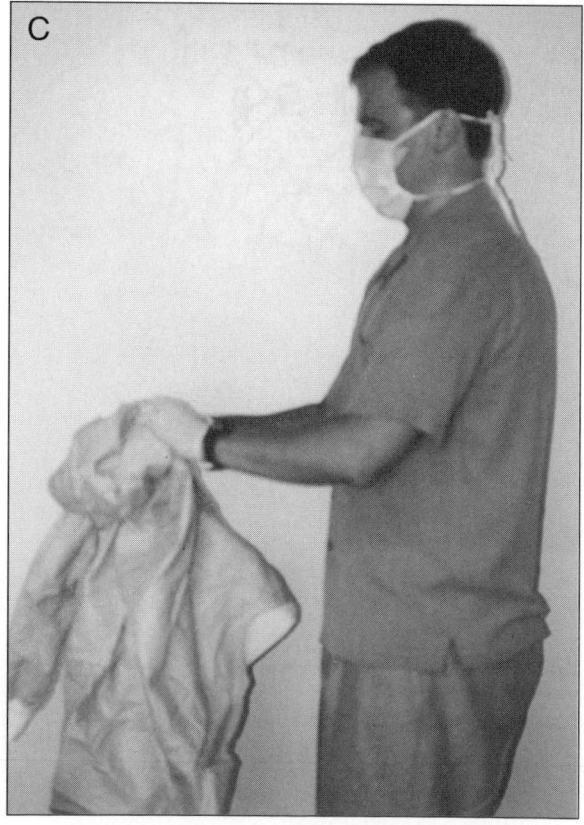

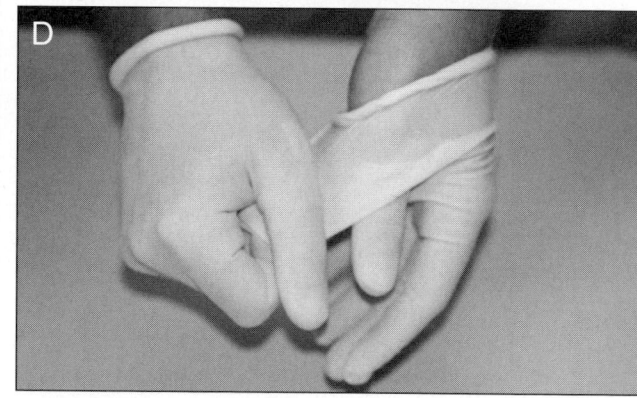

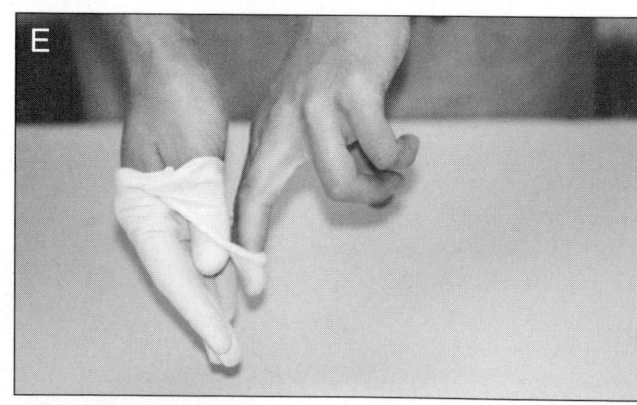

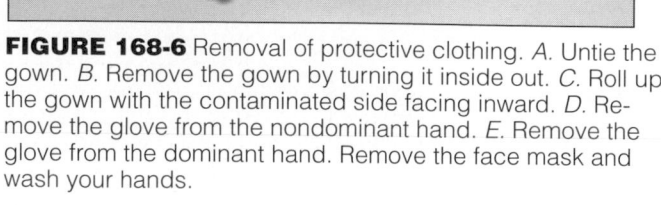

FIGURE 168-6 Removal of protective clothing. *A.* Untie the gown. *B.* Remove the gown by turning it inside out. *C.* Roll up the gown with the contaminated side facing inward. *D.* Remove the glove from the nondominant hand. *E.* Remove the glove from the dominant hand. Remove the face mask and wash your hands.

SUMMARY

Aseptic technique is an important component of all invasive procedures performed in the Emergency Department. Adequate skin disinfection and the proper use of sterile technique will greatly decrease the risk of iatrogenic infections and complications from these procedures. Aseptic technique allows a degree of protection for the caregiver as well as the patient.

REFERENCES

1. Volk WA, Benjamin DC, Kadner RJ: *Essentials of Medical Microbiology,* 3rd ed. Philadelphia: Lippincott, 1987:359–379.
2. Pierce L: Basic principles of aseptic technique. *Plast Surg Nurs* 1997; 17(1):48–49.
3. Adal KA, Farr BM: Central venous catheter related infections—a review. *Nutrition* 1996; 12(3):208–213.
4. Tait AR, Tuttle DB: Preventing perioperative transmission of infection: a survey of anesthesiology practice. *Anesth Analg* 1995; 80(4):764–769.
5. Maki DG: Yes Virginia, aseptic technique is very important: maximal barrier precautions during insertion reduce the risk of central venous catheter related bacteremia. *Infect Control Hosp Epidemiol* 1994: 15:227–230.
6. Belkin NL: Surgical gowns and drapes as aseptic barriers. *Am J Infect Control* 1988; 16(1):14–18.
7. Harden WD, Nichols RL: Aseptic technique in the operating room, in Fry DE (ed): *Surgical Infections.* Boston: Little Brown, 1995:109–118.
8. Alessandrini EA, Maller JS: Aseptic technique, in Henretig FM, King C, Joffe MD, et al (eds): *Textbook of Pediatric Emergency Procedures.* Baltimore: Williams & Wilkins, 1997:43–49.

Chapter 169
HYPOTHERMIC PATIENT MANAGEMENT

Gary An

INTRODUCTION

Hypothermia is defined as a core body temperature below 35 °C. The normal physiologic thermoregulatory responses start to fail once the core body temperature reaches this level, leading to the body's inability to generate enough heat to maintain bodily functions. Hypothermia can be subdivided into primary and secondary hypothermia.[1] Primary accidental hypothermia occurs when a previously normal individual is subjected to an environmental stress. Secondary accidental hypothermia occurs when a predisposing factor leads to disruption of temperature homeostasis and increases the individual's susceptibility to lesser environmental stresses (e.g., drug intoxication, trauma, and endocrine disorders). Drug intoxication and trauma are acquired conditions that are highly associated with the development of hypothermia.[1-6]

Hypothermia can progress after arrival in the Emergency Department. Studies in the trauma population have reported a significant percentage of patients to have a decrease in their core body temperature during their stay in the Emergency Department.[2] This recognition has led to the development of multidisciplinary approaches to maintaining normothermia as the patient moves through the hospital.[3] **The importance of continuity and communication in dealing with this problem cannot be overstated.**

ANATOMY AND PATHOPHYSIOLOGY

Hypothermia can be characterized as mild, moderate, and severe. Mild hypothermia is defined as a core temperature of 32.2 to 35 °C or 90 to 95 °F. Moderate hypothermia is defined as a core temperature of 28 to 32 °C or 82.4 to 90 °F. Severe hypothermia is defined as a core temperature of less than 28 °C or 82.4 °F. The scale can be amended in the trauma patient to 34 to 36 °C

or 93.2 to 96.8 °F for mild hypothermia, 32 to 34 °C or 89.6 to 93.2 °F for moderate hypothermia, and < 32 °C or < 89.6 °F for severe hypothermia.[1]

Mild hypothermia causes the body to increase heat production by shivering and increasing its metabolic rate. The heart rate increases and the patient may become tachypneic. Peripheral vasoconstriction may result in acrocyanosis. Neurologic symptoms may include confusion, dysarthria, and impaired judgment.

Moderate hypothermia is associated with a further decrease in the mental status. This includes lethargy, hallucinations, and loss of the pupillary reflex. The heart rate changes from tachycardia to bradycardia.[4] The cardiac rhythm commonly converts from normal sinus to atrial fibrillation.[4] The respiratory pattern becomes depressed, with a decreasing respiratory rate and tidal volume. The patient stops complaining of "feeling cold" and shivers less.

The patient is usually comatose by the time severe hypothermia is present, often with evidence of cardiorespiratory collapse. Ventricular irritability becomes evident. Ventricular fibrillation becomes refractory to conversion below 28 °C. Asystole occurs at 20 °C. The characteristic electrocardiographic (ECG) finding of an Osborne J wave occurs at approximately 32 °C (Figure 169-1). This is a positive deflection between the QRS and the ST segment.[4-6] It is often best seen in ECG leads aV_L, aV_F, and the left chest leads.[4-6]

Metabolic problems associated with hypothermia include hyperglycemia (mild hypothermia), hypoglycemia (moderate and severe hypothermia), and impaired oxygen consumption (severe hypothermia). It is recommended that uncorrected values be used to guide therapy due to the complexities of the acid-base balance associated with hypothermia.[5] These derangements are reversible with rewarming.

Coagulopathy is one of the most clinically significant metabolic derangements seen with hypothermia. Evidence suggests that significantly increased clotting

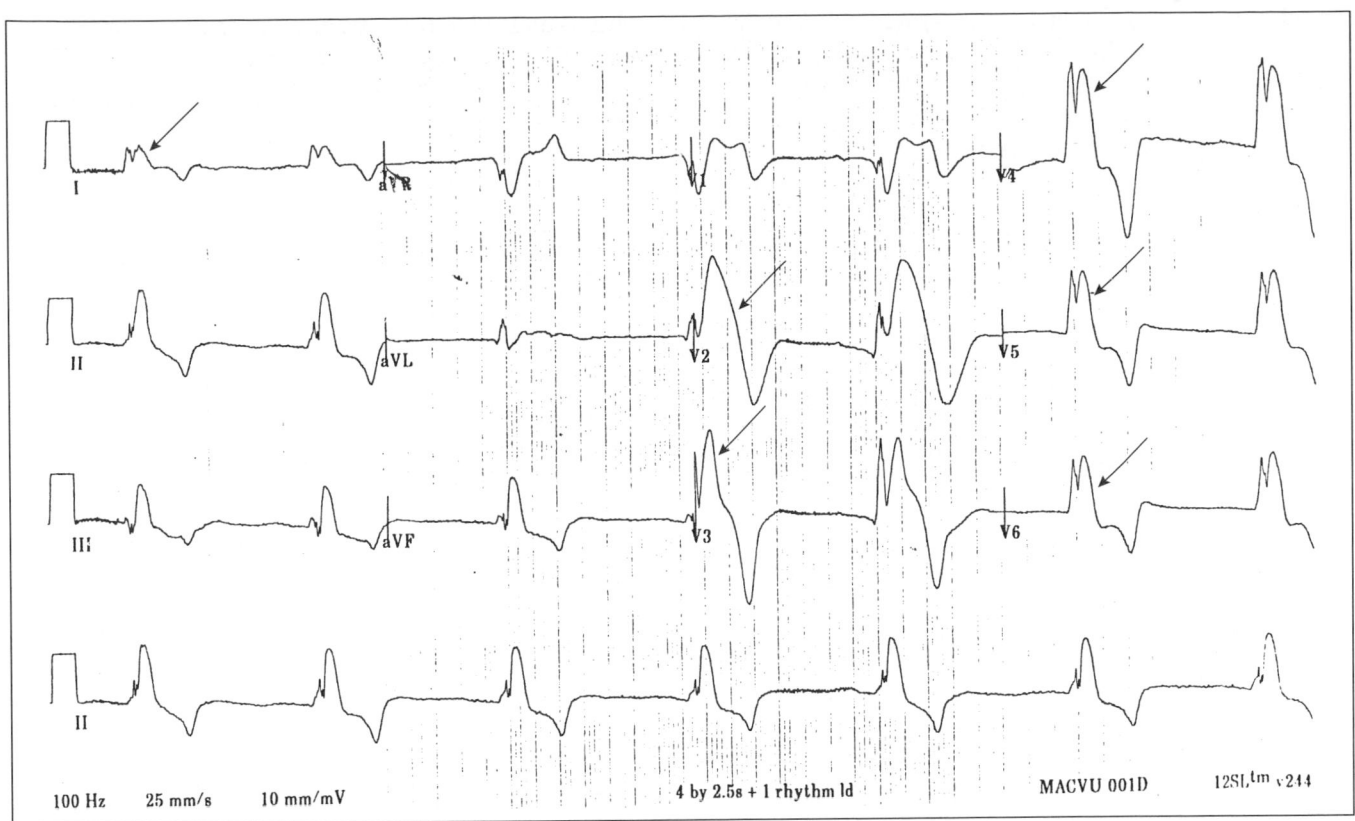

FIGURE 169-1 The Osborne or J wave associated with hypothermia is indicated by the arrows. This patient had a core temperature of 34 ºC.

times occur at core temperatures less than 35 °C.[1,2] Temperatures less than 32 °C lead to severe platelet dysfunction despite normal platelet counts.[1,2] These derangements are reversible with rewarming.

The heat deficit of a hypothermic patient can be calculated using the formula $Q = mc\,(t_2 - t_1)$, where Q is the heat loss (in kcal), m is the patient's body mass (in kg), c is the specific heat of the body (0.83 kcal/kg/°C), and $(t_2 - t_1)$ is the change in body temperature (°C). Application of this formula will allow the calculation of the amount of heat (in kcal) that must be transferred to a hypothermic patient to regain normothermia, assuming no additional losses. Knowing that the specific heat of water is 1.0 kcal/kg/°C allows one to calculate the expected rate of rewarming given the particular method used.[1]

INDICATIONS

Patients presenting with core body temperatures in the ranges of hypothermia must be identified and treated. **Hypothermia should be easily identified, since a temperature evaluation is a vital sign checked in every pa-tient that comes to the Emergency Department.** Treat all patients who present to an Emergency Department with an awareness of the potential that they can develop hypothermia, especially if they are trauma patients or have an altered mental status. **Cover all patients with sheets or blankets as soon as their initial evaluation and any necessary procedures are completed.**

CONTRAINDICATIONS

There are no contraindications to the treatment of accidental hypothermia. There are, however, circumstances in which induced hypothermia may be of medical benefit.[8] These situations are beyond the scope of this chapter.

SPECIAL RESUSCITATION CONSIDERATIONS

Certain components of the initial resuscitation of the hypothermic patient deserve mention. **All patients with hypothermia are identified by measurement of core body temperature on admission.** The following recommendations were made in a review article.[6] Poor peripheral perfusion may result in difficulty assessing the pulse and blood pressure. Use a Doppler ultrasound if necessary. Cutaneous probes for temperature and pulse oximetry will have difficulty picking up signals in hypothermic patients. Oral and auricular temperature probes are often inaccurate in the hypothermic patient. Consider using a rectal or esophageal temperature probe.

Airway management is often required in patients with moderate and severe hypothermia due to a decreased mental status. Standard orotracheal intubation may be difficult due to jaw muscle rigidity. Neuromuscular blocking agents are not recommended for patients with core body temperatures less than 30 °C. The use of topical vasoconstricting agents, smaller endotracheal tubes, and blind orotracheal intubation has been suggested. Fiberoptic guided orotracheal intubation can be utilized if available. Management of ventilated patients must include close monitoring of the endotracheal cuff pressure, as the volume and pressure may increase with patient rewarming. Ventilate patients at rates no greater than 8 to 12 breaths per minute to avoid respiratory alkalosis.[6]

Management of the circulatory system in those with moderate to severe hypothermia often requires fluid resuscitation, as these patients are volume depleted. Dextrose in the initial resuscitation fluid is not contraindicated. **Ringer's lactate solution is not recommended due to concerns about decreased hepatic metabolism of lactate in the hypothermic patient.** Dehydration results in hemoconcentration. Therefore, a low hematocrit suggests an underlying anemia and/or blood loss. The heart is susceptible to arrhythmias. Avoid transthoracic central venous catheters and pulmonary artery catheters until rewarming has been achieved.

Treat nonperfusing cardiac rhythms (ventricular fibrillation, asystole, and junctional ventricular rhythms) using Advanced Cardiac Life Support (ACLS) guidelines. The presence of bradycardia, atrial fibrillation, and other dysrhythmias that do not reduce perfusion do not require pharmacologic support, as these will reverse with rewarming. **Defibrillation at core body temperatures less than 30 to 32 °C may not be effective; resuscitative efforts should be maintained in conjunction with rewarming.[5,6]**

Resuscitation drugs are often ineffective at core body temperatures below 30 °C. Lidocaine has decreased efficacy at these temperatures.[5,6] Procainamide has been suggested to increase ventricular fibrillation.[5,6] Bretylium has been demonstrated to be effective in animal studies, though information regarding optimal clinical dosage is not known in this patient group.[5,6] **Use caution when administering and dosing all resuscitation drugs, due to their decreased metabolism in hypothermic patients,**

which can lead to toxicity. It is recommended that medications be administered at one-half the normal dose during the resuscitation of a moderately or severely hypothermic patient.[6] Avoid vasopressors due to their potential to cause arrhythmias.[6] Repeat the resuscitation cycle with every increase in core body temperature of 1 to 2 °C until a core temperature of 32 °C is achieved.[5] **Patients should not be pronounced dead until they are warm (> 32 °C) and dead.[6]**

FLUID MANAGEMENT

The administration of fluids or blood products can result in hypothermia or worsen it. Infusion of 1 L of crystalloid solution kept at room temperature (21 °C) results in a decrease in core body temperature of 0.3 °C.[1] **When patients are receiving large volumes of resuscitation fluid, active measures to prevent hypothermia must be taken.** This is even more important in patients receiving blood products, which are kept at 4.0 °C. Transfusion of 1 L of blood products leads to a decrease in core body temperature of 0.54 °C.[1] **A normothermic patient can be rendered hypothermic quickly when subjected to an aggressive fluid resuscitation.**

One of the mainstays in the prevention of hypothermia during resuscitation is to use fluid warmers to infuse intravenous fluids. Unfortunately, conventional fluid warmers use a coil/sleeve system in a water bath and pose problems at both slow and rapid infusion rates.[7] With a slow infusion rate, there is time for the fluid to reach room temperature in the tubing between the warmer and the patient. With a fast infusion rate, the length of time the fluid is exposed to the water bath is too short to effectively warm the fluid.

These problems have been addressed with two devices, both of which are useful in the Emergency Department. They both warm infused fluid to a temperature of 40 °C. The first uses a jacket in which circulating warmed fluid covers the entire length of the intravenous tubing, from the warming device to the patient (Hotline, Sims Level 1, Rockland, MA). This device is more effective than conventional fluid warmers at flow rates between 50 and 6000 mL/hr.[7] The second device uses an inline heating unit that warms the fluid rapidly and allows for substantially higher infusion rates (Systems 250/500/1000, Sims Level 1, Rockland, MA). This device can infuse crystalloid solutions or blood products at rates up to 2200 mL/min and is extremely useful in the resuscitation of patients in severe hemorrhagic shock.[7] **Use these devices to administer intravenous fluid to hypothermic patients or to those at risk for developing hypothermia.** These devices may be used as components in some of the methods described below.

PASSIVE EXTERNAL REWARMING

Perform passive external warming on all patients who are mildly hypothermic or who have normal body temperatures and are undressed. Cover the patient with sheets and blankets as soon as they have been examined and any necessary procedures have been performed.

TECHNIQUES

Remove any wet clothing and dry the patient before applying blankets (Figure 169-2). Blankets and sheets may be kept in a blanket warmer as insulating material cooler than the patient will extract heat. **Prevent secondary injury to the patient from blankets and sheets that are too hot.** There is no reason for the blankets to be any warmer than normal body temperature for passive external rewarming.

ASSESSMENT

An otherwise healthy and normal patient will increase their core body temperature by 0.5 to 2.0 °C/hr with passive external rewarming. The body attempts to regain normothermia by increasing its metabolic rate. The patient may manifest evidence of increased cardiopulmonary stress and lactic acidosis during this time.[1]

COMPLICATIONS

Complications occur if attempts are made to place inappropriately heated objects directly on the patient. **Under no circumstances should heated intravenous fluid bags be placed in the axilla or groin, or in any other prolonged contact with the skin.** This may result in thermal injuries ranging from superficial blistering to full-thickness burns. Blankets and sheets that are too warm will also cause damage to the skin.

SUMMARY

Use passive external rewarming as a sole agent in otherwise healthy patients with normothermia who are undressed, patients with mild hypothermia, and as an adjunct to more aggressive rewarming techniques. Always be aware of the possibility of a patient developing hypothermia during their Emergency Department stay.

ACTIVE EXTERNAL REWARMING

INDICATIONS

Perform these maneuvers as sole therapy for patients with mild hypothermia, on awake and otherwise stable patients with moderate hypothermia, and in conjunction with more aggressive rewarming techniques.

CONTRAINDICATIONS

Do not use active external rewarming as the sole therapy for patients with moderate hypothermia who have altered mental status or hemodynamic instability. Active external rewarming is contraindicated as the sole therapy for patients with severe hypothermia (core temperature < 28 °C). **The use of radiant heaters and heating**

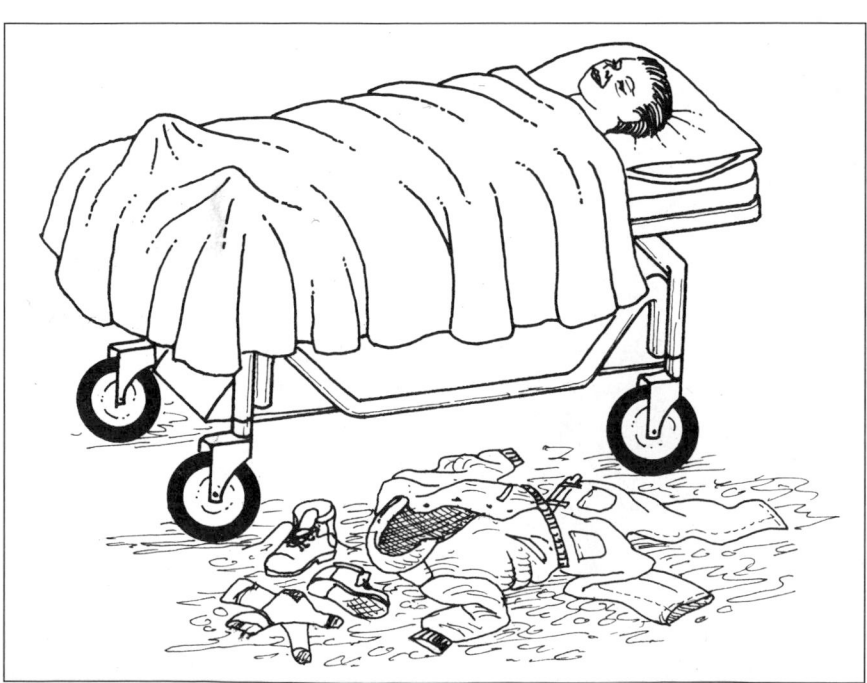

FIGURE 169-2 Passive external rewarming. Remove any wet and/or cold clothes. Cover the patient with blankets.

packs is not currently recommended due to the risk of potential complications and limited efficacy.

EQUIPMENT

Blankets
Forced air rewarming blankets
Fluid circulating rewarming blankets
Water bath and associated supplies

TECHNIQUE

Examine the patient. Determine if the patient is a candidate for active external rewarming. Place a forced air rewarming blanket or a fluid circulating rewarming blanket on the patient (Figure 169-3). **Do not place these blankets, particularly the fluid circulating ones, underneath the patient.** Placing the blanket under the patient may lead to excessive thermal transfer to areas with decreased blood flow due to pressure and prolonged time of contact. A thin sheet may be placed between a fluid circulating blanket and the skin. This is not necessary with forced air blankets. Standard blankets or sheets may be placed over the warming blankets.

Active external rewarming can be accomplished by immersion of the patient in a warm water bath (Figure 169-4). This technique is easy, effective, and simple. Immersion therapy of the hypothermic patient is not performed in the Emergency Department for several reasons. The equipment is bulky, not portable, and oc-

cupies a fixed space. It is difficult to monitor the patient when immersed. Monitoring leads (electrocardiography and pulse oximetry) will not adhere to wet skin. The use of electrical monitoring equipment in a water bath should be avoided.

ASSESSMENT

Care must be taken to reassess any wounds for recurrent bleeding, any catheters or monitors for placement, and any pressure areas that might be in prolonged contact with the heating elements, since the patient is covered with the warming device. With respect to the forced air blankets, check the air source connection to the blanket to make sure that the hot air is not blowing directly on the patient. A directed flow of hot air onto the patient under the blanket may lead to thermal injury.

COMPLICATIONS

Thermal injuries are associated with active external rewarming. They result from improper use of the devices. Maintain vigilance regarding prevention of a focused delivery of heat to a region of skin, particularly one poorly perfused, to essentially eliminate these burns.

Afterdrop refers to a decrease in core temperature that occurs 15 to 20 minutes after active external rewarming begins.[5] This is thought to be due to vasodilatation of the peripheral tissues as they rewarm and a subsequent washout of cooler peripheral blood back to

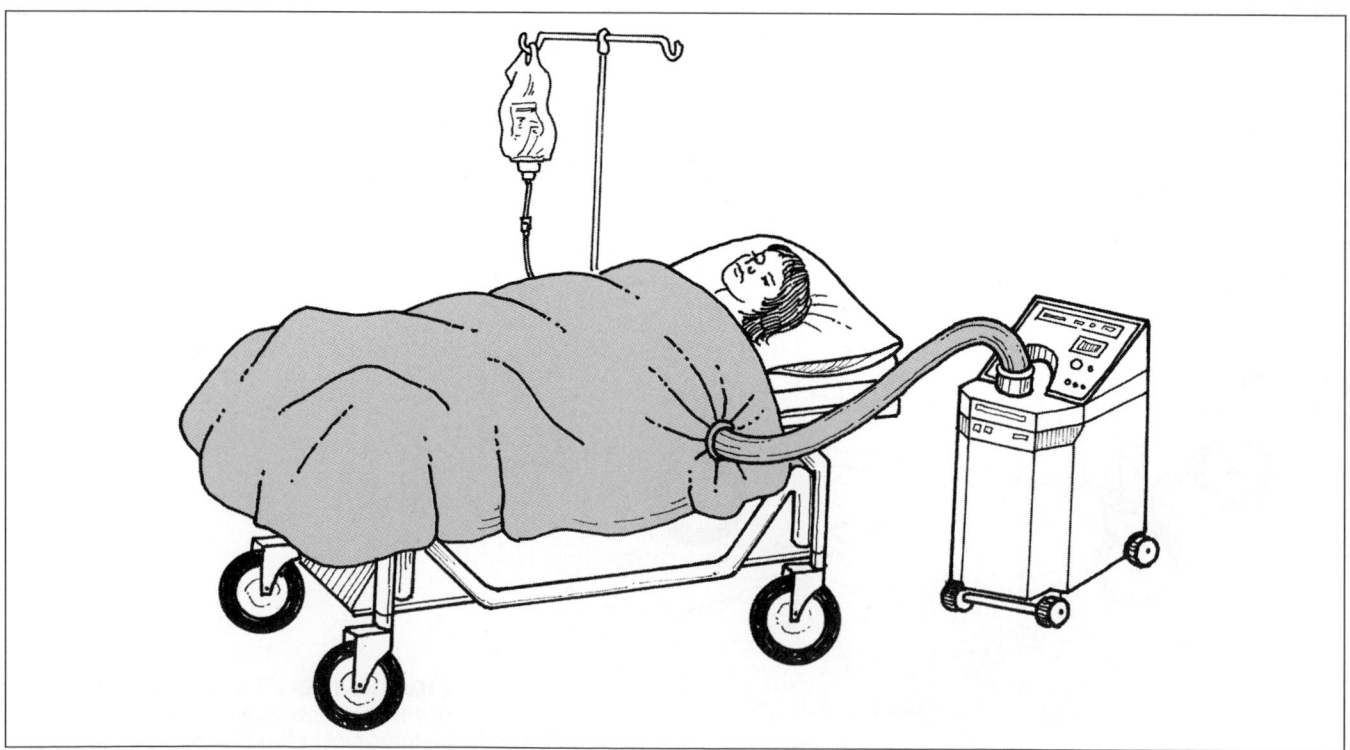

FIGURE 169-3 Active external rewarming with a heating blanket.

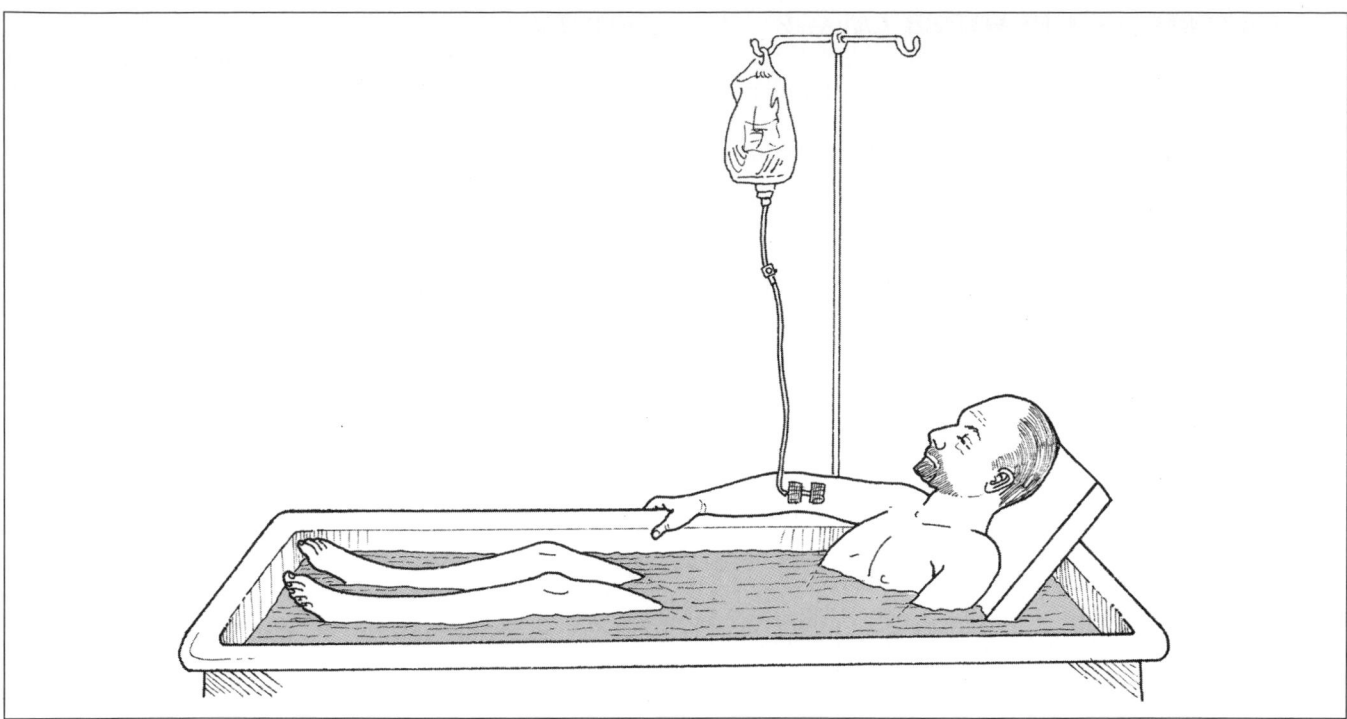

FIGURE 169-4 Active external rewarming with a water bath.

the central areas. Peripheral vasodilatation can lead to hypotension if fluid resuscitation is inadequate or the patient has cardiovascular compromise. Afterdrop can be attenuated by the concomitant use of core rewarming techniques.

SUMMARY

Active external rewarming is useful in treating moderately hypothermic patients who are awake and alert. Warming rates of 1.0 to 2.5 °C/hr have been reported.[6] When these devices are being used, frequent monitoring for potential thermal injuries is required in order to prevent secondary injury. This monitoring is easier when the patient is a cooperative partner who can participate in the process. Active external rewarming, like passive external rewarming, is often used in conjunction with more aggressive techniques or core rewarming. The problem of afterdrop is lessened when active external rewarming is used in conjunction with core warming techniques.

AIRWAY REWARMING

Airway rewarming with warmed and humidified oxygen is safe and easily achieved. However, it is never used as a sole means of rewarming.

INDICATIONS

The technique of airway rewarming may be used in any patient with hypothermia and in conjunction with other techniques. Any patient receiving supplementary oxygen can receive warmed and humidified oxygen. Its efficacy via endotracheal tube is greater than via mask or nasal prongs.

CONTRAINDICATIONS

There are no contraindications to airway rewarming.

EQUIPMENT

Nasal cannula
Face mask
Endotracheal tubes
Humidifier tank
Heating circuit
Oxygen source

TECHNIQUES

The more severely hypothermic patient will often need their airway controlled by orotracheal intubation due to a depressed level of consciousness. **Intubation for the sole purpose of airway rewarming is contraindicated.** Connect the humidifier tank and heating circuit in line with the oxygen source. Humidify and warm the inhaled oxygen to 40 to 45 °C. A rewarming rate of 1.0 to 2.5 °C/hr has been reported.[6]

GASTRIC AND BLADDER LAVAGE

These techniques, based on techniques familiar to most practitioners, are minimally invasive and can be readily performed with minimal interruption of continued resuscitative efforts.

INDICATIONS

These techniques are usually reserved for patients with severe hypothermia. They are rarely used in stable patients and generally reserved for situations where extracorporeal warming is not available.

CONTRAINDICATIONS

The only contraindications to these techniques are the contraindications to the placement of a urethral catheter (Chapter 121) and a nasogastric tube (Chapter 47). Do not perform gastric lavage concurrently with cardiac compressions. Gastric and bladder lavage are of limited value in the management of the hypothermic patient. They are generally bypassed in favor of peritoneal lavage, pleural lavage, and extracorporeal warming.

EQUIPMENT

Warmed (40 °C) saline or sterile water
See Chapter 121 for urethral catheterization supplies
See Chapter 47 for nasogastric intubation supplies

TECHNIQUES

Place the Foley catheter (Chapter 121) and/or the nasogastric tube (Chapter 47). Confirm proper placement of the appropriate tube. Instill sterile saline or sterile water warmed to 40 °C. Inject 60 mL into the tube using the catheter-tip syringe. Instill a total of 300 to 400 mL into the stomach and 200 to 250 mL into the bladder. **Do not overdistend the respective organ.** Gastric overdistention can result in rupture or aspiration. Bladder overdistention can result in rupture and extravasation of fluid. Clamp the Foley catheter or nasogastric tube. Allow the fluid to dwell within the organ for 5 to 10 minutes. Remove the fluid by gravity drainage from the bladder or suction from the stomach. Repeat the process as necessary until the core body temperature increases.

COMPLICATIONS

Gastric lavage may be complicated by perforation of the stomach by either the nasogastric tube or overdistention. Aspiration is a potential complication with gastric lavage. Refer to Chapters 47 and 49 for a more complete discussion of the complications associated with nasogastric intubation and gastric lavage, respectively. Bladder irrigation is safe as long as the bladder is not overdistended. The small surface area of the bladder makes it an inefficient means of rewarming.

SUMMARY

Perform gastric or bladder irrigation only if other types of body cavity rewarming are contraindicated. These techniques are easily initiated using standard equipment in an Emergency Department. These organs have relatively small surface areas, making these techniques inefficient. Overdistention can result in serious complications.

PERITONEAL LAVAGE

This technique is invasive, based on techniques familiar to most practitioners, and can be readily performed with minimal interruption of continued resuscitative efforts.

INDICATIONS

This technique is usually reserved for patients with severe hypothermia. It is rarely used in stable patients and generally reserved for situations where extracorporeal warming is not available.

CONTRAINDICATIONS

Suspicion of injury to a hollow viscus is a contraindication to this technique. The presence of a previous laparotomy scar is a strong relative contraindication. The use of an open peritoneal lavage technique does not mesh well with the continuous infusion of fluid required for this procedure. Other contraindications are those associated with performing a diagnostic peritoneal lavage (Chapter 55).

EQUIPMENT

Warm (40°C) intravenous fluid, normal saline, or
  Ringer's lactate solution
Warm (40°C) peritoneal dialysis fluid
Fluid infuser device, optional
Peritoneal lavage kits
See Chapter 47 for nasogastric tube supplies
See Chapter 121 for Foley catheter supplies

A commercially available, disposable, single-patient use peritoneal lavage kit is available from numerous manufacturers. The kit includes all the material required to perform a closed or semi-open diagnostic peritoneal lavage except lavage fluid. An example is the Arrow kit (Arrow International, Reading, PA). It contains 10% povidone iodine swabs, gauze squares, fenestrated drape, tubing for the administration of intravenous fluid, 1% lidocaine, 5 mL syringes, 22 and 25 gauge needles, an 18 gauge × 2.5 inch introducer needle, an 0.89 mm × 45 cm J-tipped guidewire, an 8 French lavage catheter, and a #11 scalpel blade on a handle. Refer to Chapter 55 for a more complete list of equipment.

TECHNIQUE

Prepare the patient by placing a nasogastric tube (Chapter 47) and a Foley catheter (Chapter 121). Place two peritoneal lavage catheters, one supraumbilical and one infraumbilical (Figure 169-5). Refer to Chapter 55 for complete details regarding placement of the peritoneal lavage catheters. Confirm the position of the catheters. Clamp the infraumbilical catheter. Infuse warm (40 °C) intravenous fluid or peritoneal dialysis fluid through the supraumbilical catheter using the Level 1 infuser or a Hotline fluid warmer. The use of dialysate has the added benefit of potentially correcting some electrolyte abnormalities.[5,6] The fluid may be infused manually, but this technique is much less efficient.

Infuse 1 to 2 L of fluid. Allow the fluid to bathe the peritoneal cavity for 10 minutes. Remove the clamp on the infraumbilical catheter and allow the fluid to drain from the peritoneal cavity. Repeat the procedure. Up to 10 L/hr of fluid may be infused in this fashion.[6] An alternative technique is to allow the fluid to flow continuously through the supraumbilical catheter, into the peritoneal cavity, and out the infraumbilical catheter.

COMPLICATIONS

The potential complications are primarily associated with the placement of the peritoneal dialysis catheter. Refer to Chapter 55 for details regarding these complications. The infusion and removal of the fluid are safe. Avoid

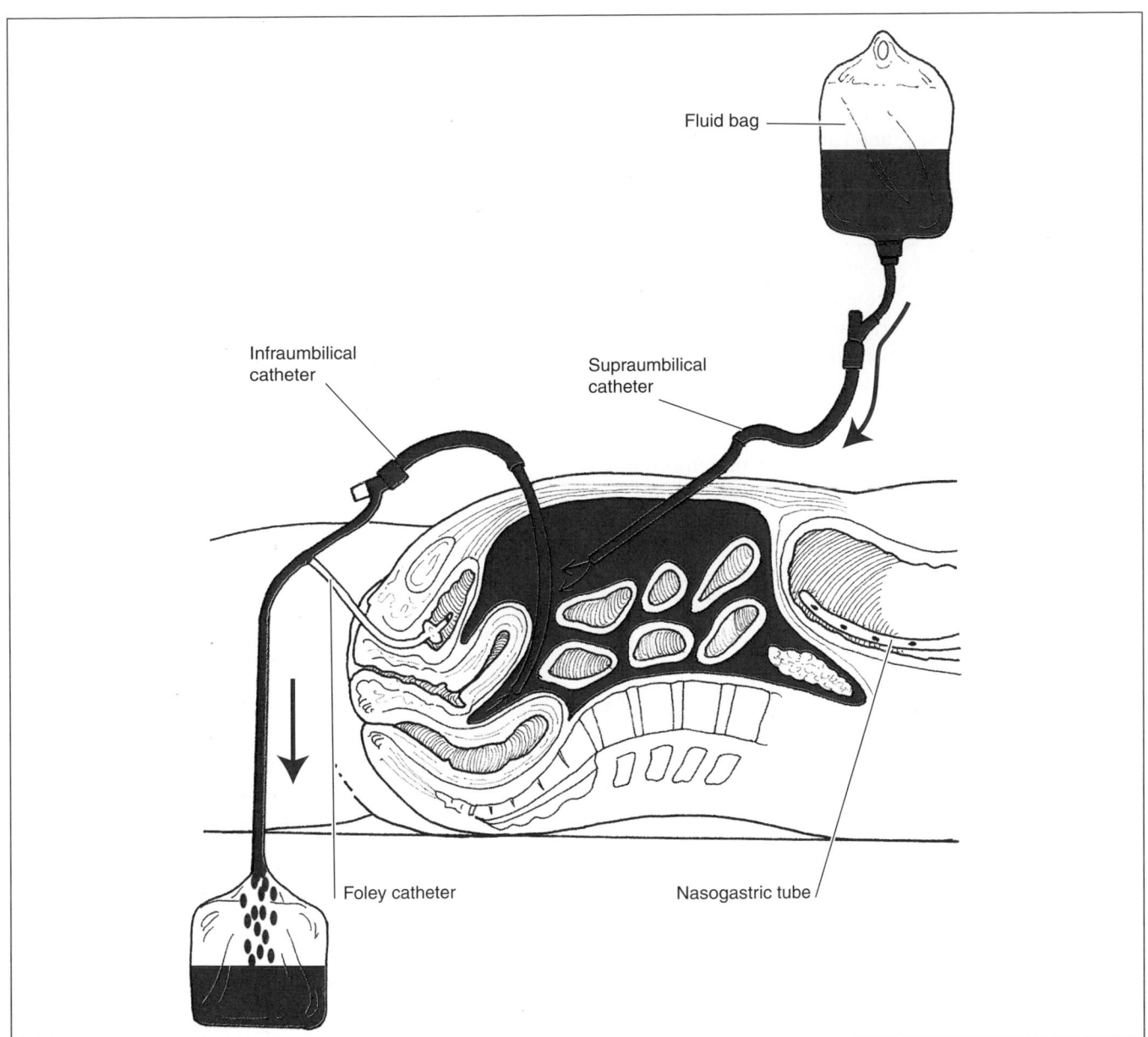

FIGURE 169-5 Active core rewarming with peritoneal lavage.

using highly hyperosmolar peritoneal dialysates in patients with persistent hypovolemia or with a questionable perfusion status as this may worsen existing hypovolemia. Do not use water, as it can result in significant electrolyte shifts.

SUMMARY

Peritoneal lavage is the most widely recognized means of body cavity lavage. This is due in part to the familiarity of many Emergency Physicians with the diagnostic peritoneal lavage procedure. It has the advantage of being able to be performed concurrently with chest compressions and other resuscitative efforts. This technique can raise the core body temperature by 1 to 3 °C/hr.

PLEURAL LAVAGE

This technique is invasive, based on techniques familiar to most practitioners, and can be readily performed with minimal interruption of continued resuscitative efforts. Pleural lavage can be performed closed (tube thoracostomy) or open (via a thoracotomy incision).

INDICATIONS

This technique is usually reserved for patients with severe hypothermia. It is rarely used in stable patients and generally reserved for situations where extracorporeal warming is not available.

CONTRAINDICATIONS

The presence of a pneumothorax and/or hemothorax is the only contraindication to pleural lavage.

EQUIPMENT

See Chapter 28 for tube thoracostomy supplies
Warm (40 °C) intravenous fluid, normal saline, or
   Ringer's lactate solution
Warm (40 °C) peritoneal dialysate
Fluid infuser device, optional

TECHNIQUE

Place two chest tubes into the same pleural space, either the left or the right side, to perform closed pleural lavage (Figure 169-6). The left side is preferred by some physicians who believe that the heart, aorta, and blood within the aorta will be warmed quicker than with right sided chest tubes. Refer to Chapter 28 for full details regarding chest tube placement. Place one tube anteriorly in the second or third intercostal space at the midclavicular line. Place the other tube posteriorly in the fifth or sixth intercostal space at the posterior axillary line. Secure the tubes to the chest wall with suture and tape. Attach the fluid infuser to the anterior chest

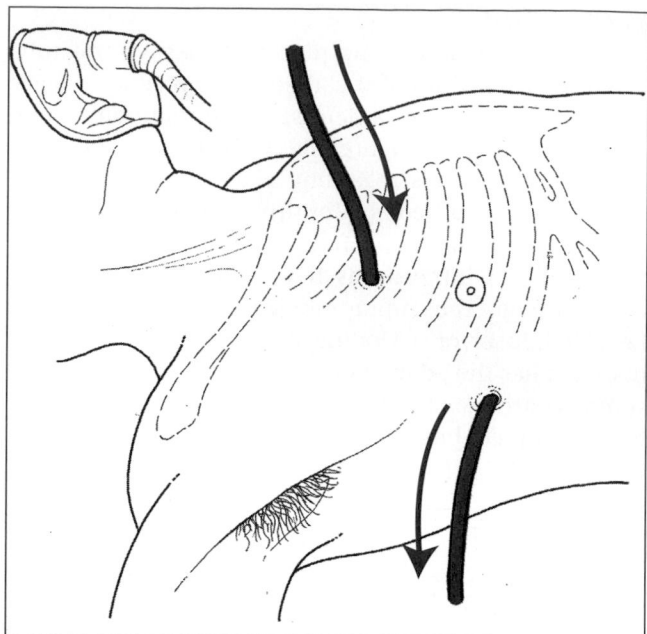

FIGURE 169-6 Active core rewarming with closed pleural lavage.

tube using a Christmas tree adapter. Apply a pleural drainage device to the posterior chest tube in the usual fashion. Infuse warm (40 °C) fluid via the fluid infuser device at a rate of 180 to 550 mL/min.[5] Allow the fluid to exit into the pleural drainage device. The fluid will flow into the anterior chest tube, bathe the structures in the hemithorax (great vessels, heart, lung, and mediastinum), and exit via the posterior chest tube.

Pleural lavage may be performed using an open technique (Figure 169-7). This technique is used when a thoracotomy is indicated for other purposes, such as penetrating trauma or to perform open cardiac massage. Refer to Chapter 31 for full details regarding a thoracotomy. Do not use this technique for the sole purpose of rewarming if other, less invasive or extracorporeal techniques are available. The advantage of open pleural lavage is that it allows direct cardiac rewarming and open cardiac massage.

COMPLICATIONS

The complications are primarily associated with the placement of the chest tube. Refer to Chapter 28 for full details regarding these complications. Maintain free drainage of the irrigation fluid to avoid increasing the intrathoracic pressure.

SUMMARY

Closed pleural lavage is an effective means of rewarming. It can increase the core body temperature by 1 to 5 °C/hr. It is very similar in efficacy to peritoneal lavage. Chest tube placement is slightly more challenging than

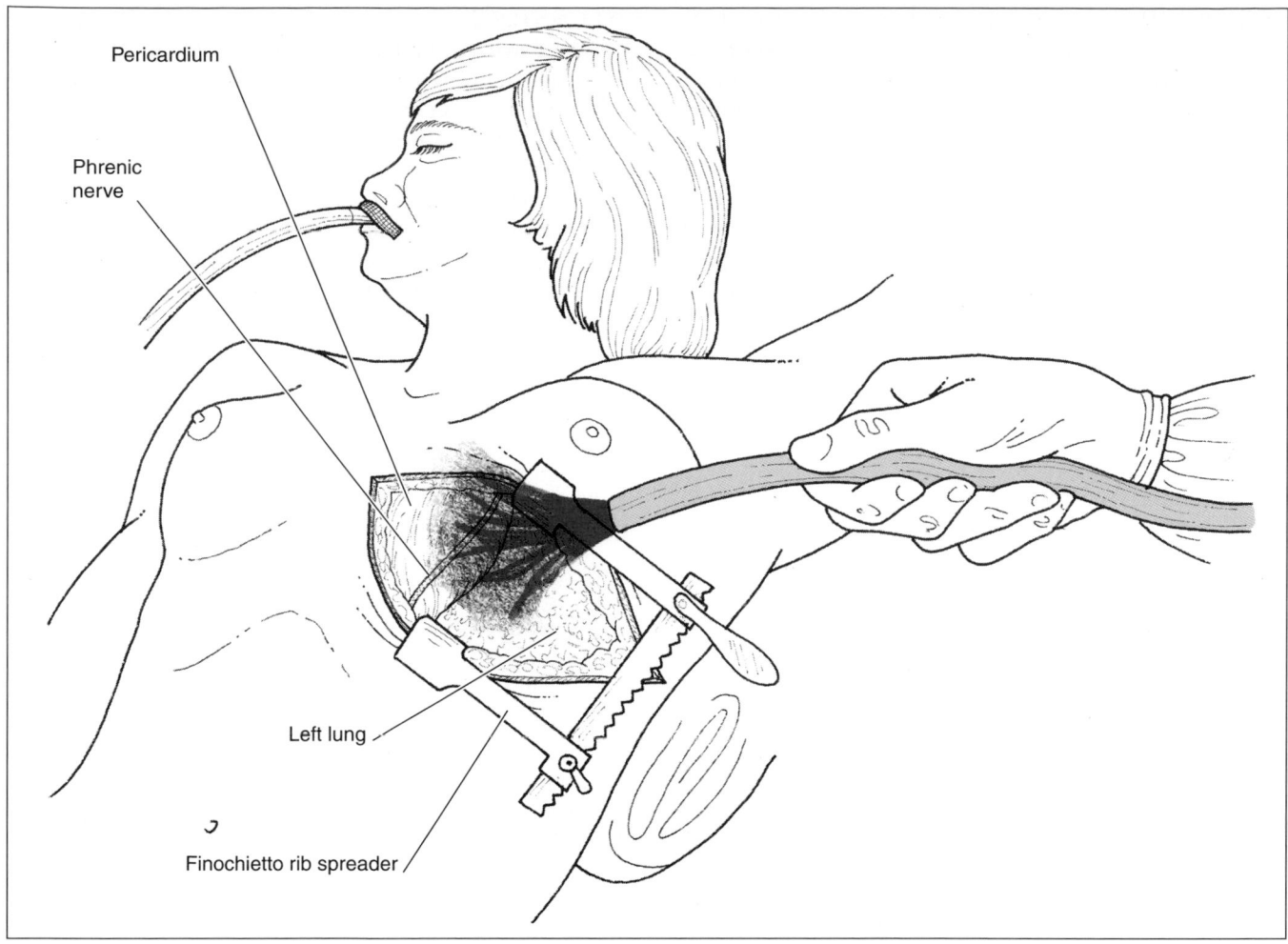

Pericardium

Phrenic nerve

Left lung

Finochietto rib spreader

FIGURE 169-7 Active core rewarming with open pleural lavage.

placement of a peritoneal lavage catheter. Free drainage is usually easier to achieve and maintain with a chest tube than with a peritoneal lavage catheter. The two techniques may be employed simultaneously and carried out in conjunction with other resuscitative measures.

EXTRACORPOREAL REWARMING

Extracorporeal rewarming is the most aggressive, effective, and efficient technique to correct severe hypothermia. It includes the use of hemodialysis, arteriovenous rewarming, venovenous rewarming, and cardiopulmonary bypass. The choice between the first three techniques is made on the basis of available resources and the physician's familiarity with each technique. The fourth technique, cardiopulmonary bypass, is discussed but should not be performed by anyone who is not a surgeon familiar with the procedure.

HEMODIALYSIS

Hemodialysis is readily available in most institutions. It requires the placement of a central venous line. The only contraindications to hemodialysis are those associated with central venous line placement (Chapter 38) and hemodialysis. An advantage of hemodialysis is that associated drug toxicity or significant electrolyte abnormalities can be simultaneously managed as the patient is being rewarmed.

EQUIPMENT
See Chapter 38 for central line equipment
Dual-lumen percutaneous hemodialysis (Quinton or Mahukar) catheter
Dialysis machine
Dialysis nurse or technician
Warmed (40 °C) dialysis fluid

TECHNIQUE

Place a hemodialysis catheter into a femoral vein. Refer to Chapter 38 for full details regarding the placement of a double-lumen central venous line. The catheter may be placed into a subclavian vein if femoral vein access is contraindicated. Femoral vein placement decreases the risk of inducing an arrhythmia with the guidewire.[6] There is a tendency to have fewer problems related to the positioning of the catheter and achieving appropriate flow rates with femoral catheters. Instruct the hemodialysis technician to set the temperature control on the dialysis machine to deliver a blood temperature of 40°C. Attach the dialysis machine tubing to the lumens of the catheter. Begin hemodialysis.

COMPLICATIONS

The potential complications are primarily associated with the placement of the central venous line. Refer to Chapter 38 for details regarding these complications. The hemodynamic status of hypotensive patients may become worse upon initiation of hemodialysis, but this technique has been successfully used on such patients.[6]

SUMMARY

Hemodialysis is available at most institutions and is effective in rewarming a patient. The limitations of this technique include the need to have a dialysis technician or nurse available, the time required to obtain on-call personnel, and the time required to set up the equipment. Hemodialysis is a viable option for the rewarming of a hypothermic patient when other forms of extracorporeal warming are not available.

ARTERIOVENOUS REWARMING

This technique was initially described in 1992.[9] The authors described placing one large-bore catheter in the femoral artery and another in a central vein (femoral, internal jugular, or subclavian). This method allows for rewarming in the Emergency Department without the need for specialized equipment (dialysis or bypass machine) and personnel.

CONTRAINDICATIONS

The lack of a blood pressure makes this method moot. Known occlusive arterial disease, particularly in the iliofemoral region, is a relative contraindication.

EQUIPMENT

See Chapter 38 for central line equipment
Two 8.5 French introducer catheters
Two 10 French single-lumen arteriovenous hemofiltration catheters
Sims Level 1 System 250/500/1000 Fluid Rewarmer
Luer-lock adapter, male-to-male
Warmed (40 °C) saline

TECHNIQUE

Place two catheters, one in the femoral artery and one in a central vein. Refer to Chapter 38 regarding the placement of a central venous catheter. The placement of the arterial catheter is similar to that of the venous catheter.

The tubing for the Level 1 rapid infuser consists of two intravenous spike-tipped lengths that come together in a Y. The Y then runs to a countercurrent warming chamber and then to the patient. Cut off the spike tip from one of the limbs of the Y and attach the male-to-male Luer-lock adapter. Note that if the rapid fluid infuser is a Sims Level 1 System 500, an additional length of wide-bore intravenous tubing may be needed to bridge the distance between the arterial catheter and the fluid-warmer tubing. This version of the Level 1 may be too tall to allow direct connection of one of the limbs to the arterial catheter. Connect this limb to the arterial catheter. Connect the other arm of the Y to a bag of intravenous fluid with the roller clamp closed.

Allow the system to prime with blood under arterial pressure. Connect the primed distal end of the tubing to the central venous catheter. The blood will travel via the arterial catheter to the extracorporeal circuit and through the proximal limb of the tubing to the warming chamber of the Level 1 infuser, through the heating elements to the distal tubing, and back to the patient via the venous catheter (Figure 169-8).

The driving force in this circuit is the patient's systemic blood pressure. Low-flow states will limit the efficacy of the system. However, you may use a pressure infusion of intravenous fluid via the other limb of the Y to augment flow. This fluid will be warmed as it reaches the patient, since this other limb of the Y is proximal to the warming element. Systemic anticoagulation is not required, as the tubing for the Level 1 infuser is heparin-bonded.

COMPLICATIONS

The complications outlined in the initial description of the procedure include the inability to achieve vascular access, a small hematoma at the arterial puncture site, and ischemia of the limb distal to the arterial catheter.[9] Refer to Chapter 38 for a full description of the complications that may arise in placing a catheter.

SUMMARY

Arteriovenous rewarming is an innovative means by which severely hypothermic patients may be rapidly rewarmed without the resources of a dialysis or bypass pump technician. Flow rates of 225 to 375 mL/min are achieved when the patient's systolic blood pressure is greater than 90 mmHg.[9] This technique transfers 94 to 157 kcal/hr back to a patient with core temperature of 32 °C.[9]

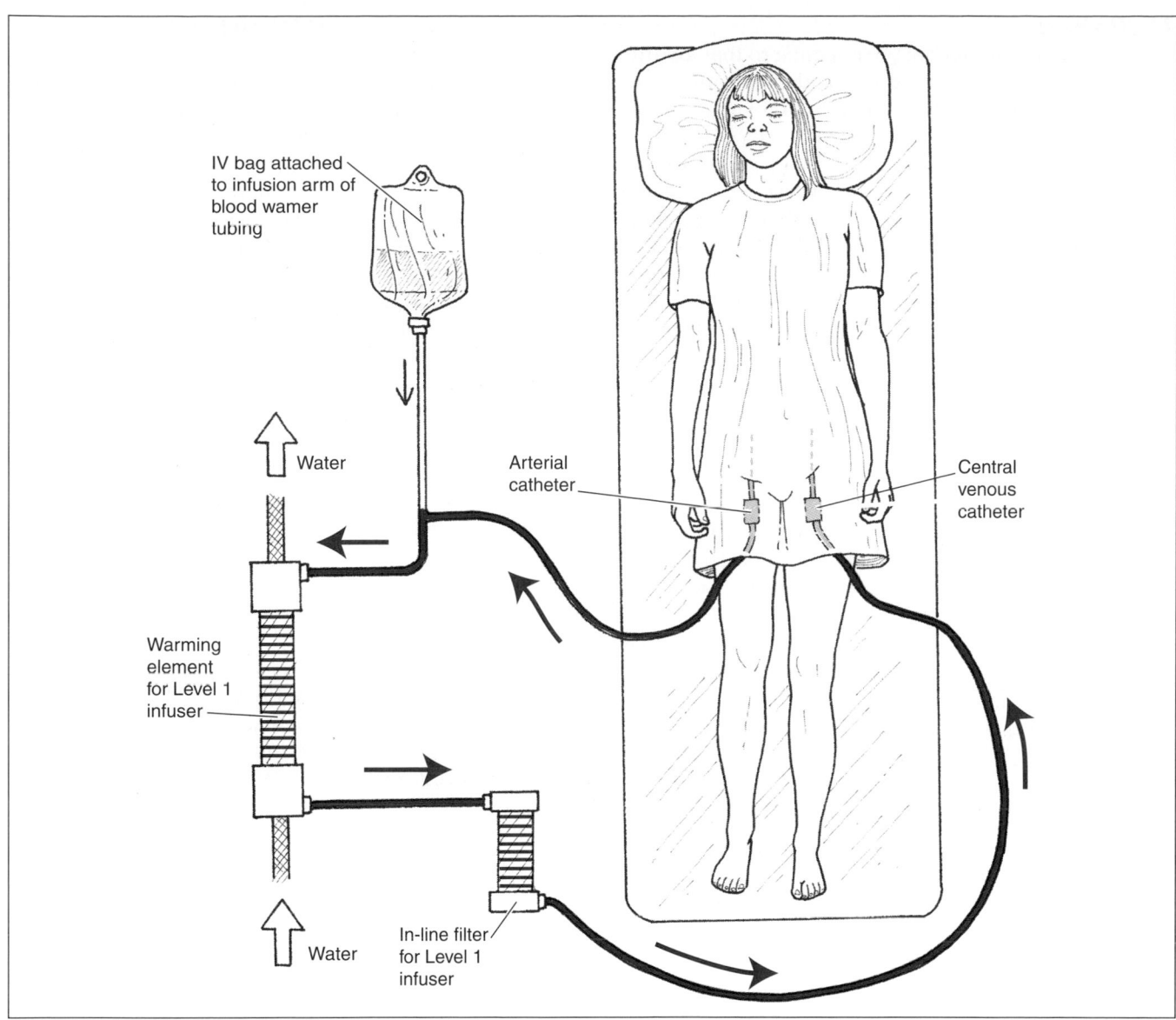

FIGURE 169-8 Arteriovenous rewarming.

VENOVENOUS REWARMING

This technique is rarely utilized by Emergency Physicians due to the lack of a venous roller pump and inexperience with this piece of equipment. The technique is briefly described for the sake of completeness. The venovenous technique has two main advantages over arteriovenous rewarming. First is the lack of arterial cannulation, with its potential for limb ischemia. The second is nonreliance on systemic blood pressure/perfusion to drive the system. Flow may be independently determined and delivered by the roller pump. This may be particularly important in the severely hypothermic patient who presents in full cardiorespiratory arrest. The primary disadvantage of this technique is the re-

quirement of expertise in using the roller pump, though advances in design may obviate this in the future.

CONTRAINDICATIONS
Persons not familiar with the function and operation of a venous roller pump should not attempt this technique.

EQUIPMENT
See Chapter 38 for central line equipment
Two 8.5 French introducer catheters
Two 10 French single-lumen arteriovenous hemofiltration catheters
Sims Level 1 System 250/500/1000 Fluid Rewarmer
Luer-lock adapter, male-to-male
Venous roller pump
Warmed (40 °C) saline

TECHNIQUE

The setup for this technique is similar to that for arteriovenous rewarming. Place two catheters, one in the femoral vein and one in another central vein. Refer to Chapter 38 for details regarding the placement of a central venous catheter. Alternatively, place a dual-lumen hemodialysis catheter.[10] However, if the latter course is to be followed, make sure that the "outflow" port of the catheter is upstream and that the "inflow" port is downstream. This helps to reduce the amount of warmed fluid returning from the circuit that is immediately withdrawn by the roller pump. Place the venous roller pump in line with this circuit, usually between the patient and the warming elements. Adjust the flow rate within the tolerances of the particular device being used.

COMPLICATIONS

The primary complication associated with use of venous roller pumps is an air embolus. This usually happens when the roller pump is operated by a person unfamiliar with it. Recent advancements in roller-pump technology have made their operation simpler and safer. Refer to Chapter 38 for a complete description of the complications that may arise due to the placement of a central venous catheter.

SUMMARY

Venovenous rewarming is one step away from cardiopulmonary bypass. Its use in the Emergency Department is limited due to lack of equipment availability and familiarity. It is a viable option if a roller pump is available as well as a physician familiar with this procedure.

CARDIOPULMONARY BYPASS

Discussion of this technique is limited to some basic properties of rewarming with cardiopulmonary bypass (CPB). This technique should not be attempted by anyone who does not regularly use bypass modalities and without the support of an experienced pump technician. This technique represents the last resort of rewarming techniques. Bypass is usually achieved using femoral-femoral bypass. The CPB pump can provide complete hemodynamic and respiratory support during the resuscitation. Core body temperatures can be raised 1 to 2 °C every 3 to 5 minutes with flow rates of 2 to 3 L/min.[6] If available, use heparin-bonded tubing to avoid systemic anticoagulation, which can worsen existing coagulopathies. The limitations of this technique are that it is extremely resource-intensive, not readily available in many institutions, and requires specific expertise with respect to surgical and mechanical techniques.

SUMMARY

The management and prevention of hypothermia in the Emergency Department is a challenging and perpetual task. The resuscitation of a severely hypothermic patient in full cardiorespiratory arrest can push the practitioner and the department to the limit of their abilities and resources. The real challenge in dealing with hypothermia lies in recognizing and managing the risk of hypothermia in the "routine" patient who presents every day. It is not possible to overstate the importance of continuity of care and the necessity of good communication as the patient is moved from the Emergency Department to either the operating theater or the intensive care unit, so that rewarming efforts may continue.

REFERENCES

1. Gentilello LM: Advances in the management of hypothermia. *Surg Clin North Am* 1995; 75(2): 243–256.
2. Peng RY, Bongard FS: Hypothermia in trauma patients. *J Am Coll Surg* 1999; 188(6):685–696.
3. Aragon D: Temperature management in trauma patients across the continuum of care: the TEMP group. *AACN Clin Issues* 1999; 10(1):113–123.
4. Lee-Chiong TL, Stitt JT: Accidental hypothermia. *Postgrad Med* 1996; 99(1):77–88.
5. Jolly BT, Ghezzi KT: Accidental hypothermia. *Emerg Med Clin North Am* 1992; 10(2):311–327.
6. Hanania NA, Zimmerman JL: Accidental hypothermia. *Crit Care Clin* 1999; 15(2):235–249.
7. Young CC, Sladen RN: Temperature monitoring. *Int Anesth Clin* 1996; 34(3):149–174.
8. Marion DW, Leonov Y, Ginsberg M, et al: Resuscitative hypothermia. *Crit Care Med* 1996; 24(2): S81–S89.
9. Gentilello LM, Cobean RA, Offner PJ, et al: Arteriovenous rewarming: rapid reversal of hypothermia in critically ill patients. *J Trauma* 1992; 32(3):316–327.
10. Josephs JD, Farmer JC: Hypothermia and extra-corporeal rewarming: the journey toward a less invasive, more accessible methodology. *Crit Care Med* 1998; 26(12):1944–1945.

Chapter 170

HYPERTHERMIC PATIENT MANAGEMENT

Eileen F. Couture

INTRODUCTION

The heatstroke victim can be difficult and challenging, even after a successful resuscitation and stabilization in the Emergency Department. Heatstroke is a multisystem insult. More than 300 people die of heat-related illness in the United States each year.[1] This number was surpassed in a single week in 1995 during a heat wave in Chicago.[2–6] This heat wave resulted in more than 400 deaths and 3300 Emergency Department visits. Heatstroke is a very uncommon medical emergency and considered by some as the most important of all the environmental heat illnesses because of its potential for high morbidity and mortality. Major complications of heatstroke include seizures, adult respiratory distress syndrome (ARDS), acute renal failure, liver disease, rhabdomyolysis, and disseminated intravascular coagulation.[7] Survival is possible for the great majority of patients with appropriate recognition and rapid treatment.

The most effective means of cooling remains controversial. The techniques rely upon prompt recognition of symptoms, immediate intervention in the field, and immediate intervention in the Emergency Department. Begin cooling the patient in the prehospital setting by removing the patient from the heat stress, keeping the skin wet, and fanning the patient in transport. **The patient must be exposed adequately and cooling must be initiated in the quickest and most efficient manner possible as stabilization is occurring.**

Cooling measures must be modified to avoid hypothermia once the core temperature reaches 39 °C or 102 °F. Decreasing the core body temperature to less than 39 °C or 102 °F within 30 minutes of presentation improves survival.[4] **Cooling must precede investigation for the cause. Evaporation and convection are the simplest and most efficient means of cooling victims of heatstroke or heat exhaustion.** Evaporation of 1 g of water dissipates approximately seven times more heat than melting the same quantity of ice.[4] Skin blood flow is preserved as compared with the use of ice, because evaporation and convection are much more efficient modes of heat exchange.[8]

ANATOMY AND PATHOPHYSIOLOGY

Heat-related illness comprises a spectrum of symptoms ranging from mild heat edema to heatstroke. Heat edema is self-limited. The patient presents with edema of the hands, feet, and ankles. This usually occurs in the first few days of heat acclimatization. Heat cramps occur most often in individuals who sweat profusely and are exercising or walking. The patient consumes water without salt, resulting in hyponatremia and muscle cramps. Heat syncope is dizziness or syncope after exposure to high temperatures. It is caused by vasodilatation and consequent postural hypotension. Heat exhaustion results from the excessive loss of body water, electrolytes, or both. The patient may complain of headache, nausea, vomiting, malaise, and myalgias. Heat exhaustion is distinguished from heatstroke by a normal mental status and, generally, a temperature below 39 °C or 102 °F.[2,7]

Heatstroke must be suspected in any patient who has acute mental status changes or other signs of central nervous system dysfunction in the setting of a high temperature and a history of heat exposure. The initial temperature is usually above 40 to 42 °C or 104 to 108 °F. Central nervous system dysfunction may manifest as varying degrees of confusion, obtundation, seizures, delirium, or focal deficits.

Core body temperature is maintained within close limits by a balance between heat production and heat dissipation. Muscular and metabolic activity generates heat. Most fevers encountered are a response to microbial invasion. Some fevers are due to exposure to high temperatures or abnormalities in the thermoregulatory apparatus.[9] Heatstroke may occur in previously healthy individuals who are subjected to severe environmental thermal stress, usually during extreme physical exertion. It may occur in patients with compromised homeostatic mechanisms who are subjected to lesser degrees of exposure (classic heatstroke). Factors that may compromise protective thermoregulatory mechanisms include chronic illness, medications, drug abuse, poor judgment, or extreme youth or age[7] (Table 170-1).

It has been speculated that oxidative phosphorylation becomes uncoupled and enzyme systems cease to function when temperature regulation is lost and the core body temperature exceeds 42 °C or 108 °F. Energy stores become depleted as maximum metabolic demands escalate. This causes the cell membranes to become increasingly permeable, thus increasing sodium influxes. These phenomena have been postulated to be part of a positive feedback loop involving progressive depletion of ATP, increased ion flux, increased rates of membrane depolarization and neurotransmitter activity, and a subsequent increase in heat production. Cell membranes eventually lose their integrity. Heat production accelerates, proteins denature, and widespread necrosis occurs as temperature-control mechanisms fail, leading to organ failure. Cellular damage occurs as a result of the elevated temperatures and the length of exposure to heat.[7,10,11] Tissues at greatest risk for heat damage include the vascular endothelium, neural tissue, hepatocytes, and kidneys.

Heat is dissipated by a combination of radiation, convection, conduction, and evaporation.[9] Radiation is the transfer of heat to objects not in direct contact with the subject. Radiation accounts for approximately 65 percent of heat loss in cool environments. It is a major source of heat gain in hot climates. Convection is the transfer of heat to circulating fluid or gas. The amount of heat dissipated by convection becomes minimal as ambient temperature rises. Convective heat loss varies directly with wind velocity. Conduction is the direct transfer of heat to another object by direct contact. Evaporation is the conversion of a liquid to the gaseous phase. Evaporation becomes the dominant mechanism of heat loss as ambient temperatures rise.[4,10]

INDICATIONS

Cooling will not harm patients who are hyperthermic, regardless of the etiology. Cooling can be lifesaving in those with true heatstroke. Heatstroke may be difficult to identify if cooling was initiated in the field and the patient's mental functioning is intact. **Initiate cooling immediately if there is any doubt.**[7] Iced gastric lavage is contraindicated in patients with altered mental status or depressed airway reflexes unless the patient is endotracheally intubated. It is also contraindicated if nasogastric intubation is contraindicated. Iced peritoneal lavage is contraindicated if the placement of a peritoneal lavage catheter is contraindicated.

CONTRAINDICATIONS

Patient stabilization always remains the top priority. Assess the patient's airway, breathing, and circulation first, despite the need for immediate cooling. Any life-threatening or limb-threatening conditions must be addressed simultaneously or before proceeding to cooling measures.

EQUIPMENT

Core thermometer, rectal or esophageal
Large fans
Mist spray bottles
Water
Ice
Immersion tub
Ice packs
Wet sheets and towels
Cooling blanket
Peritoneal lavage kits
Nasogastric tubes
Iced saline

PATIENT PREPARATION

Immediately remove the patient from the heat-stress environment. Remove the patient's clothes. Stabilize the patient's airway, breathing, and circulation as necessary. **Patient outcome is directly related to the length of time the tissues are exposed to the thermal challenge.** Cooling rates should not exceed 0.1 to 0.2 °C per minute. Monitor core body temperature with a rectal or esophageal probe (if the patient is intubated).

TECHNIQUES

EVAPORATION

Wet the exposed patient with tepid water. Place large and powerful fans to strategically direct high-flow air currents toward the patient's head, feet, and torso (Figure 170-1). Spray the patient with water from the mist spray bottles. Keeping the patient "wet and windy" provides a state-of-the-art cooling method for even the smallest Emergency Department without the need to purchase new equipment. Place ice packs wrapped in wet towels on the patient's groin, axilla, and neck. This technique is simple and causes very little to no discomfort to the con-

TABLE 170-1. FACTORS RELATED TO HEAT ILLNESS

Illness	Medications	Behaviors	Groups	Toxins
Autonomic neuropathies	Anticholinergics	Confining garments	Athletes	Alcohol
Cardiovascular disease	Antihistamines	Hot environments	Elderly	Amphetamines
CNS tumors	Diuretics	Inability to care for self	Infants	Cocaine
Dehydration	Lithium	Injudicious exertion	Military recruits	Hallucinogens
Delirium tremors	MAO inhibitors	Poor fluid intake	Neonates	
Diabetes	Phenothiazines	Social isolation	Prior heatstroke	
Hyperthyroidism	Sympathomimetics			
Major burn scarring	Tricyclic antidepressants			
Parkinson's disease				
Pheochromocytoma				
Psychosis				
Thyroid storm				

CNS = central nervous system; MAO = monoamine oxidase.

scious patient. An additional benefit is access to the patient should other interventions be necessary.[4]

Discontinue evaporative cooling when the core body temperature reaches 39 °C or 102 °F. Continued cooling can result in hypothermia as the core temperature continues to decrease after evaporative cooling is discontinued. Monitor the patient to ensure that their core body temperature does not increase.

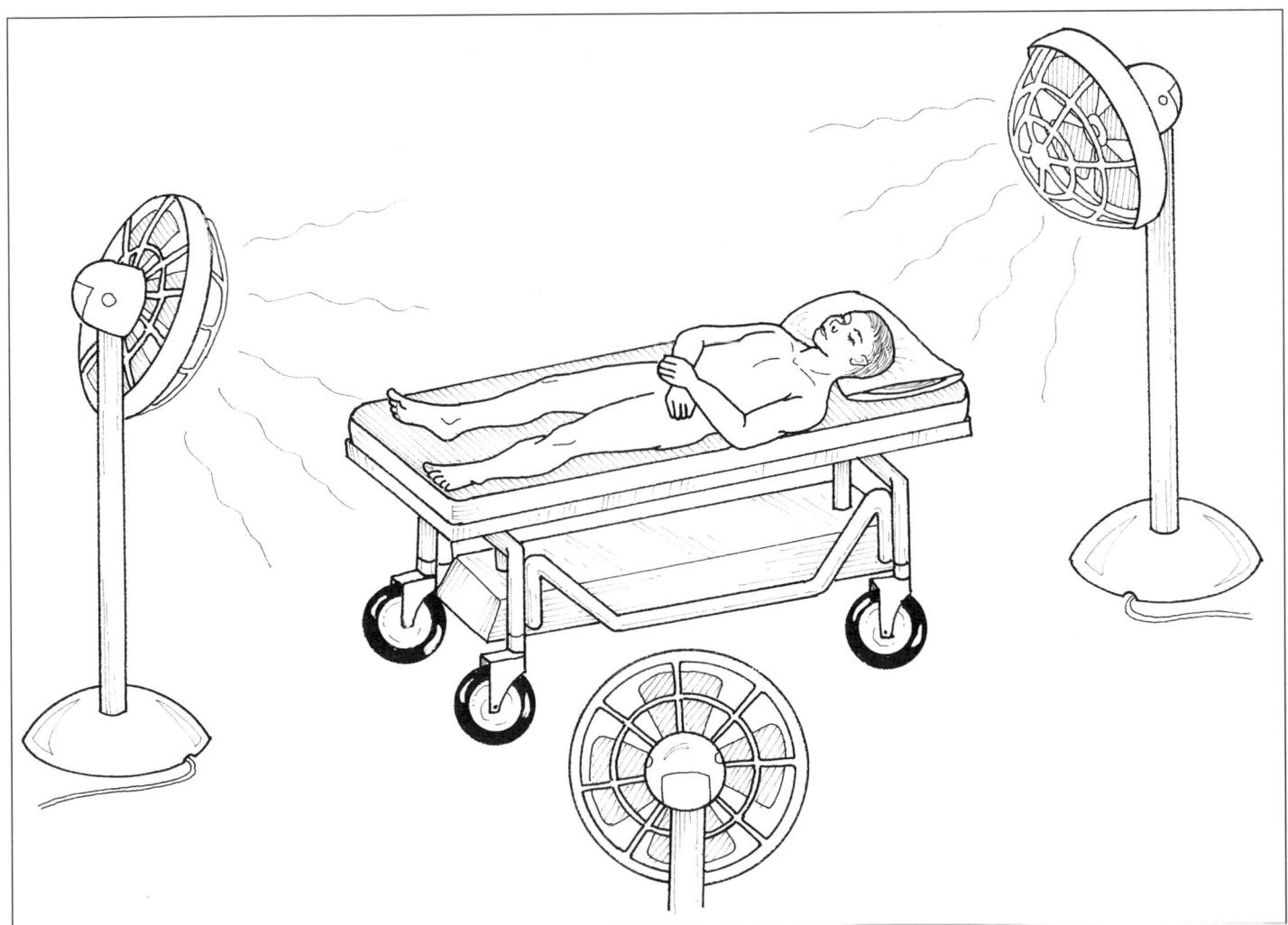

FIGURE 170-1 Large fans at the head, foot, and side of the bed to direct high-flow air currents.

This concept of cooling gained popularity with the Makkah Body Cooling Unit (BCU). The BCU is used today to provide field treatment for people participating in the annual pilgrimage to Mecca who may develop heatstroke. The BCU has been found to provide the fastest core temperature cooling rates of 0.31 °C/min.[10]

ICE WATER IMMERSION

Immersion in an ice water bath is a common method of cooling heatstroke patients. Place the patient in a tub of ice water for 10 to 40 minutes (Figure 170-2). Briskly massage the patient's extremities to maintain peripheral circulation and promote heat loss. Monitor the patient's core temperature carefully. Rectal temperatures will decrease approximately 0.16 to 0.21 °C/min.[7,10]

Ice water immersion is recommended by some authors as the initial technique for hyperthermia management.[6] Unfortunately, it has limited use in the Emergency Department.[4,10] Preparing an ice bath can result in a delay in cooling the patient. Contact with the ice water results in intense vasoconstriction, which blocks heat exchange, paradoxically increases core body temperature, induces shivering, and is uncomfortable for the patient. Heat transfer from the core to the surface is reduced. The practical issues of impairing access to the patient, monitoring the airway, and initiating resuscitative measures are challenging when the patient is in an ice water bath.[4,10,12] The tub and patient lift device are large, bulky, and not often available in the Emer-

gency Department. Multiple caregivers are required to prevent the patient from drowning and to maintain their head above water.

ICE PACKING

Packing the heatstroke patient in ice is an alternative to ice water immersion. It can result in conductive heat loss that is as effective as evaporative cooling. Patients who are awake and alert do not often tolerate ice packing. Its use may require parenteral sedation. The complications and practical limitations are similar to those of ice water immersion.

Place the undressed patient in the center of the gurney. Completely cover the patient with ice. This technique requires a large quantity of ice, which may be unavailable in the Emergency Department. Consider placing plastic sheets or trash bags, with the edges curved upward, under the patient to prevent the ice and water from spilling onto the floor, as health care personnel may otherwise slip on the wet floor, fall, and sustain injuries. Discontinue cooling when the core temperature reaches 39 °C or 102 °F.

ICE PACKS

The placement of ice packs over select body areas is a more reasonable option than ice water immersion or ice packing. It may be used as the sole cooling method or in conjunction with evaporative cooling. Place plastic bags filled with ice or ice water in the patient's axilla and

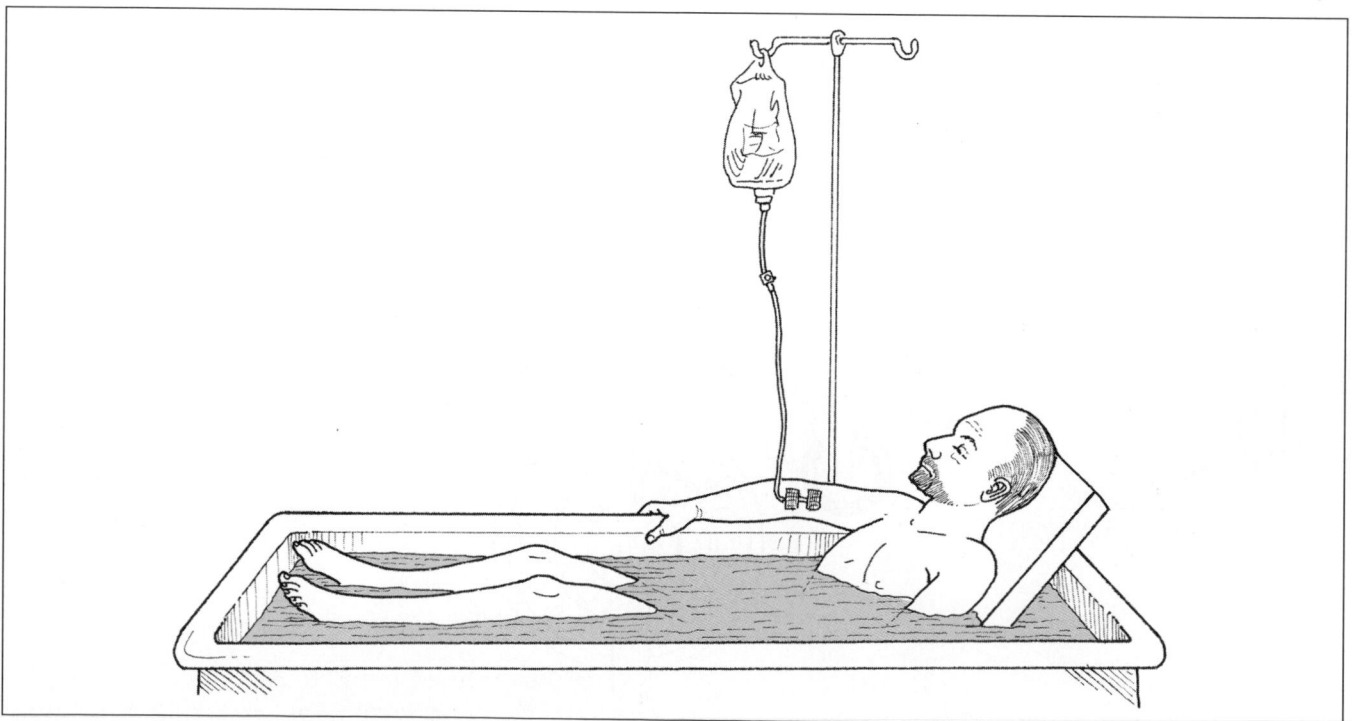

FIGURE 170-2 Ice water immersion to cool a hyperthermic patient.

groin. Remove the ice packs when the core temperature reaches 39 °C or 102 °F.

ICED PERITONEAL LAVAGE

Peritoneal lavage in hyperthermia has been investigated in canine models but used infrequently in humans. The advantages of this technique include the large surface area exposed to iced saline and direct cooling of the core. This technique is invasive, time-consuming, requires significant equipment and expertise, and is associated with significant complications. A case report indicated that iced peritoneal lavage with 2 L of normal saline was successful in decreasing the rectal temperature to 39.5 °C or 103 °F.[8] The patient had responded only partially to external evaporative cooling and iced gastric lavage. Place 1 L bags of Saline or Ringer's lactate solution into an ice water bath to cool down. The technique is similar to that used for hypothermia (Chapter 169). This technique cannot be recommended except for patients who are not responding to other methods of cooling.

ICED GASTRIC LAVAGE

Central cooling techniques have not been studied extensively. An alternative core cooling technique may be iced gastric lavage. This method has been compared to room-air cooling in an anesthetized canine heatstroke model.[9] Gastric lavage with iced tap water cooled the canine models rapidly and safely. The technique yielded cooling rates five to six times faster than in controls. Significant differences in hemodynamic parameters were noted to return to baseline more quickly in the iced gastric lavage group than in the control group. The technique is similar to that used for hypothermia (Chapter 169). Instill 10 mL/kg of iced sterile saline, allow it to dwell for 30 to 60 seconds, and suction out the fluid. Repeat the procedure as necessary. Potential hazards using this technique include aspiration, gastric mucosal injury, electrolyte imbalances with water lavage, and dysrhythmias.[9]

ASSESSMENT

Monitor core body temperature closely with a rectal temperature probe. Monitor the patient's vital signs, neurologic function, urine output, and laboratory measurements (arterial blood gases and serum electrolytes). Consider monitoring central venous pressure and pulmonary artery pressure, especially in patients with heatstroke and limited cardiac reserve. Volume deficits may not be more than 2 to 3 L, especially in patients with classic heatstroke. Hypotension usually responds to intravenous fluids. If required, use an inotrope that produces little vasoconstriction, such as dobutamine. The

use of H_2 blockers may decrease the incidence of gastrointestinal bleeding.[11] Treat rhabdomyolysis aggressively with saline diuresis, alkalinization of the urine, and an infusion of 0.5 gm/kg of mannitol with or without furosemide.[11] Treat seizures with benzodiazepines.[11]

AFTERCARE

Patients with minor heat-related illnesses may be safely discharged home after cooling. Instruct the patient to rest, drink plenty of fluids, and avoid the heat. Discuss with the patient the methods to remain cool if they are exposed to heat. Arrange follow-up within 24 hours for a reevaluation.

Admission is required in several circumstances. Admit patients with heat exhaustion for 23 hour observation if they have abnormal vital signs, abnormal laboratory investigations, or if they remain symptomatic after fluid therapy. Admit all patients with heatstroke to an intensive care unit. Permanently altered and unstable thermoregulatory mechanisms in the survivors of heatstroke increase their susceptibility to future heat illness. Prevention through education should be a part of every discharge plan.

COMPLICATIONS

Further management of the heatstroke victim can be difficult, even after successful initial resuscitation and stabilization. Heatstroke is a multisystem insult that affects virtually every organ. Neurologic complications of hyperthermia include seizures, cerebral edema, and localized brain hemorrhages. Irreversible brain damage often occurs above 42 °C or 108 °F. Cerebellar impairment may persist after recovery. Cardiac complications include tachyarrhythmias, high cardiac output heart failure, and myocardial infarction. Pulmonary edema may be cardiogenic in patients with a limited cardiac reserve or secondary to ARDS. Pulmonary aspiration can be encountered in obtunded patients. Acute renal failure may be due to direct heat damage, renal hypoperfusion, or rhabdomyolysis. Mucosal ulceration of the gastrointestinal tract is common and can lead to gastrointestinal hemorrhage. Liver damage and dysfunction are common. The extent of hepatic necrosis and cholestasis may not be apparent until 48 to 72 hours after heat injury. Hematologic complications include hemolysis, thrombocytopenia, and disseminated intravascular coagulation. Megakaryocytes are especially sensitive to heat injury. Disseminated intravascular coagulation is triggered by diffuse endothelial and organ damage. Its onset is usually delayed 2 to 3 days and is associated with a high mortality.[13,14]

Complications can occur during the cooling of the hyperthermic patient. Discontinue evaporative cooling when the core body temperature reaches 39 °C or 102 °F. Continued cooling can result in hypothermia as the core temperature continues to decrease after evaporative cooling is discontinued. Monitor the patient to ensure that their core body temperature does not increase. Ice water immersion and ice packing make patient monitoring and management difficult if not impossible. Iced peritoneal lavage and iced gastric lavage are invasive procedures associated with significant potential complications. Refer to Chapters 55 and 47 regarding the complications associated with the placement of the peritoneal lavage catheter and the nasogastric tube, respectively.

SUMMARY

The best intervention for heat-related illness is prevention. If caught early, heat illness responds to rest, exposure to shade and a breeze, and the ingestion of cool liquids. External evaporative cooling is acknowledged to be the safest means of cooling a hyperthermic patient. The tragedy of heatstroke is that it so frequently strikes highly motivated young individuals under the discipline of work, military training, or sporting endeavors. The prevention of heatstroke requires adequate rest, hydration before physical exertion, periods of rest during exertion when the individual can cool off, and adequate oral fluid intake. Such precautions should be implemented even in temperate zones during the hot summer months.

REFERENCES

1. Center for Disease Control and Prevention: Heat related deaths—Dallas, Wichita, and Cooke Counties, Texas, and U.S. 1996. *MMWR* 1997; 46(23):528–531.

2. Hett HA, Brechtelsbayer DA: Heat related illness. *Postgrad Med* 1998; 103(6):107–120.

3. Costrini A: Emergency treatment of exertional heatstroke and comparison of whole body cooling techniques. *Med Sci Sports Exerc* 1990; 22(1):15–18.

4. Weiner JS, Khogali M: A physiological body-cooling unit for treatment of heat stroke. *Lancet* 1980; 1:505–509.

5. Semenza JC, Rubin CH, Falter KH, et al: Heat related deaths during the July 1995 heat wave in Chicago. *N Engl J Med* 1996; 335(2):84–90.

6. Dematte JE, O'Mara K, Buescher J, et al: Near fatal stroke during the 1995 heat wave in Chicago. *Ann Intern Med* 1998; 129(3):173–181.

7. Wyndham CH, Strydom NB, Cooke HM, et al: Methods of cooling subjects with hyperpyrexia. *J Appl Phys* 1959; 14:771–776.

8. Horowitz BZ: The golden hour in heat stroke: use of iced peritoneal lavage. *Am J Emerg Med* 1989; 7(6):616–619.

9. Syverud S, Barker WJ, Amsterdam JT, et al: Iced gastric lavage for treatment of heatstroke: efficacy in a canine model. *Ann Emerg Med* 1985; 14(5):424–432.

10. Yarbrough B, Vicario S: Heat illness, in Marx JA, Hockberger RS, Walls RM, et al (eds): *Rosen's Emergency Medicine: Concepts and Clinical Practice*, 5th ed. St Louis: Mosby, 2002:1997–2009.

11. Marini J, Wheeler A: *Critical Care Medicine: The Essentials*, 2nd ed. Baltimore: Williams & Wilkins, 1997:459–464.

12. Magazanik A, Epstein Y, Udassin R, et al: Tap water, an efficient method for cooling heat stroke victims—a model in dogs. *Aviat Space Environ Med* 1980; 51(9):864–867.

13. Mikhail MS, Thangathurai D: Hyperthermia, in Grenvik A, Ayres SM, Holbrook PR, et al (eds): *Textbook of Critical Care*, 4th ed. Philadelphia: Saunders, 2000:217–222.

14. Tek D, Olshaker JS: Heat illness. *Emerg Med Clin North Am* 1992; 10(2):299–310.

Chapter 171
HELMET REMOVAL

Lukas Kolm
Eric F. Reichman

INTRODUCTION

The helmeted person who becomes injured presents unique challenges to prehospital health care providers, athletic trainers, and Emergency Department personnel in providing initial stabilization and management. Greater numbers of people are wearing helmets due to the increasing public awareness for the prevention of head injuries associated with recreational and athletic activities. This practice will limit the most severe outcomes from head trauma. However, the helmeted patient is not immune from life-threatening head and neck injuries. **Secondary injury due to improper helmet removal can adversely affect patient outcome.**[1]

Helmets vary in size, type, and accessories on the basis of the user's activity. They consist of a hard plastic and/or fiberglass shell over a layer of foam that is covered by material. Motorcyclists and racers wear full-face helmets with or without retractable or removable visors. Football, lacrosse, and hockey players use open-faced helmets. These may have clear visors and/or face cages whose bases are screwed into the helmets. Bicyclists, kayakers, roller bladers, skateboarders, and skaters wear simple skull helmets. These helmets cover the top of the skull like a hat and have a strap that is snapped or clipped under the chin to maintain the helmet in position.

Athletes playing football and hockey wear protective shoulder padding in addition to protective helmets. Their facial injuries tend to be less severe.[2] With the helmets and shoulder padding, their cervical spines, in comparison to those of helmeted motorcyclists without shoulder padding, are more adequately stabilized.[2,3] Helmet removal with and without shoulder pad removal has been shown to result in cervical spine movement. This can increase the risk of spinal cord damage in the helmeted patient with a cervical spine injury.[2,3]

Current recommendations for motorcycle helmet removal are to leave the helmet in place until the patient arrives in the Emergency Department or Trauma Unit.[2–5] **The only exception permitting the removal of a helmet in the field is when it significantly delays lifesaving** measures or if airway access is obstructed.[2–4] This may occur in the unconscious and/or apneic patient. Prehospital health care providers should be able to maintain an adequate airway, stabilize a patient's cervical spine, and control associated hemorrhage with removal of only the face plate, guard, and chin strap of the helmet.[4,5]

ANATOMY AND PATHOPHYSIOLOGY

The type and fit of protective equipment, the mechanism of injury, the patient's age, and the patient's physical development all influence cervical spine injury. There is a greater risk of injury when the helmet is too loose. It has been noted that most people wear helmets that are too large for their heads. Inertia is defined as a body's ability to resist change of position and motion. A 4 pound helmet can exert a 200 pound force on the wearer's head and neck when impact occurs at 50 mph. Injury is often more serious when inertial forces cause excessive extension and flexion of the cervical spine without adequate protection for the lower head and neck.[5,6]

The anatomic location of cervical spine injuries tends to differ between children and adults. The immature pediatric spine is more susceptible to flexion and extension injuries in the upper cervical (C2 to C3) segments due to the child's proportionally larger head size, shorter neck with immature development, weak neck muscles, and the neck's higher degree of flexion and extension.[5–7] The relative amount of cartilaginous tissue in comparison to bone makes the pediatric patient more prone to spinal cord injury when subjected to high inertial forces. These injuries may be more difficult to detect on plain radiographs, since cartilaginous injuries are radiolucent.[6,7]

Similar conditions of disproportionate head-to-neck size are artificially created in the helmeted patient. The motorcycle helmet will often cause hyperflexion of the neck. Flexion and extension injuries without adequate lower neck protection result in an increased incidence of upper cervical spine (atlantoaxial, C1, and C2) injuries in comparison to lower cervical spine segments.[7,8] There is a greater incidence of lower cervical spine (C5 and C6) injury among football and hockey players.[8] The shoulder padding offers support to the lower head and upper neck. It decreases the amount of flexion and extension at the time of impact.

Flexion and distraction while removing a helmet may cause spinal cord compression, as demonstrated in unstable C1 to C2 injuries with helmet removal in cadaveric models.[8] Similar unfavorable results were demonstrated with neck flexion and extension during helmet and shoulder pad removal.[8] The properly fitting helmet is tight enough that a significant force must be applied to remove it in the field, thus increasing the chance of cervical spine movement. **Apply proper in-line cervical immobilization before helmet removal or medical intervention while avoiding in-line traction. In-line traction increases the risk of subluxation or distraction at the site of injury.**

It is recommended that the helmet and padding not be removed in the field. Overzealous manipulation of the patient or improper helmet and/or padding removal can complicate an underlying injury. The helmet can be secured to a long backboard with supplemental neck stabilization provided by use of neck immobilizers, foam-Velcro fitted supports, or sandbags. If shoulder pads or helmets are removed in the field, the posterior aspect of the neck and shoulders must be adequately supported while in-line immobilization is maintained to avoid further spinal cord injury. Cervical immobilization with and without helmet removal is best accomplished with at least two people to assure that the patient's head and neck remain stable.

INDICATIONS

Under most circumstances, the helmeted patient can be assessed and stabilized in the field without removing their helmet or shoulder pads. The patient can often be managed, radiographed, and the cervical spine "cleared" prior to removal of the helmet in the Emergency Department.[9] Helmet removal is warranted emergently in patients who are apneic, without an adequately sustainable airway, those at risk for airway compromise from a helmet being left in place, and those who have uncontrollable hemorrhage.[9]

CONTRAINDICATIONS

Adhere to spinal cord injury precautions throughout the prehospital period. Do not remove the helmet unless absolutely necessary. It is not possible to completely exclude a spinal cord injury or vertebral fractures in the field.

Do not remove the helmet until the cervical spine has been "cleared" of any injury in the Emergency Department. Delay removal if the patient is unconscious, has an abnormal mental status, is under the influence of ethanol or drugs, is intoxicated or potentially intoxicated, has distracting injuries, if there is evidence of a spinal cord injury, if a complete physical examination cannot be performed, if the cervical spine has not been radiographically cleared, or if the patient has neck pain. The only exception is if the patient's airway and breathing cannot be supported with the helmet in place.

EQUIPMENT

Long backboard
Head and neck immobilizer
Adjustable cervical collar
Scissors or shears suitable to cut the face mask
Cast saw with spare blades
Screwdrivers, flat head and Phillips head
Towels

PATIENT PREPARATION

The hemodynamically stable and helmeted patient should have radiographs of the neck, be physically assessed, be determined not to be intoxicated, and have a normal mental status prior to removal of the helmet.[9,10] This includes a complete neurologic examination. If the patient is alert and responsive, explain the procedure and its possible complications. Explain the procedure to the patient's family and/or guardian if time permits. Explain all potential risks involved in helmet removal, including the possibility of worsening an underlying spinal cord injury. The risk of permanent central nervous system damage should be stated as well as the fact that the precautions to avoid such injury are not foolproof but will be observed as carefully as possible. Answer any questions or concerns of the patient or family.

Remove any removable parts if they were not detached from the helmet prior to arrival in the Emergency Department. The face mask, face shield, and/or visor can often be removed with a flat or Phillips head screwdriver. **Carefully look for any damage to the patient's helmet.** External damage to the helmet may be the only initial indication of the severity of the impact. Inspect the integrity of the helmet shell for fit and structural breaks. The patient may be wearing eyeglasses or sunglasses under the helmet. Remove the glasses before helmet removal begins. Contact lenses may remain in place until the helmet is removed.

The helmet will cause flexion of the cervical spine when a patient is placed supine. This flexion is even more pronounced in a child due to their large occiput. Place rolled towels or sheets under the patient's shoulders to eliminate the excessive flexion of the cervical spine. Such flexion is minimal and requires no towels under the shoulders if the patient is wearing shoulder pads in addition to a helmet.

TECHNIQUES

MANUAL ONE-PERSON TECHNIQUE

Helmet removal can be performed by one or two people. Reserve the one-person technique for extreme interventions (Figure 171-1). With only one person present, it is necessary to pad voids behind the patient's neck and shoulders (Figure 171-1A). **The goal is to keep the head and neck in the neutral position as much as possible while removing the helmet.**

Stand above the patient's head looking down toward their feet. Place the heels of both hands on the sides of the helmet (Figure 171-1B). Insert the index, middle, ring, and little fingers into the space between the patient's head and the helmet. Gently spread open the helmet with both hands to create clearance between the helmet padding and the patient's face and ears (Figure 171-1B). Slowly and gently remove the helmet (Figure 171-1C). If the helmet is of the full-face type, gently tilt it posteriorly and continue to pull the helmet off until the nose is cleared. Return the helmet to a neutral position after the nose is cleared. **Avoid cervical spine hyperextension during this stage of helmet removal.**

Stop removing the helmet when the bottom of the helmet is just above the patient's occiput. Move the fingers of both hands onto the patient's occiput while keeping the heels of both hands on the helmet (Figure 171-1D). The fingers will now maintain stabilization and immobilization of the head and neck. Push the helmet off the patient's head using the heels of both hands while maintaining immobilization of the patient's head and neck with the fingers (Figures 171-1E and F). Maintain the head manually in-line until immobilization can be accomplished with a cervical collar, backboard, sandbags, and tape.[9–11]

MANUAL TWO-PERSON TECHNIQUE

The two-person technique has the same goals as the one-person technique (Figure 171-2). The assistant provides in-line immobilization while the helmet is removed.[9–11] Instruct an assistant to stand at the patient's side, at the level of the patient's neck and shoulders. Place one of the assistant's hands under the patient's occiput and upper neck. Place the assistant's other hand under the patient's mandible so that the mental process (chin) rests in the assistant's first web space (Figure 171-2B). Place the tip of the assistant's thumb on the angle of the patient's mandible. Place the index and long finger of the assistant's hand on the contralateral angle of the patient's mandible. Instruct the assistant to hold this position and maintain in-line immobilization of the patient's head and neck.[11,12]

The procedure to remove the helmet is similar to that described for the one-person technique. Stand above the patient's head looking down toward their feet. Place the heels of both hands on the sides of the helmet (Figure 171-2B). Insert the index, middle, ring, and little fingers into the space between the patient's head and the helmet. Gently spread open the helmet with both hands to create clearance between the helmet padding and the patient's face and ears (Figure 171-2B). Slowly and gently remove the helmet (Figure 171-2C). If the helmet is of the full-face type, gently tilt it posteriorly and continue to pull it off until the nose is cleared. Return the helmet to a neutral position after the nose is cleared. **Avoid cervical spine hyperextension during this stage of helmet removal.** Completely remove the helmet (Figure 171-2D).

Maintain the head manually in-line until immobilization can be accomplished with a cervical collar, backboard, sandbags, and tape.[9–11] The physician's hands should be applied to the patient's head and neck to maintain in-line immobilization (Figure 171-2E). Instruct the assistant to remove their hands (Figure 171-2F). Instruct the assistant to apply a cervical collar and secure the patient's head with sandbags and tape. The physician can now release hold of the patient.

CAST SAW (BIVALVE) TECHNIQUE

Cast saws can effectively be used to cut through the shells of most helmets (Figure 171-3). This technique allows for removal of the helmet without cervical spine movement.[9,10,13] **Cut the helmet off any patient with neurologic injury or abnormal cervical spine radiographs—also if there is a concern for head and neck trauma or if the helmet is extremely snug-fitting to prevent cervical spine movement.** This technique requires the presence of two providers.[9,10,13]

Protect the patient from secondary injury from the cast saw and the sharp edges of the helmet. Instruct the responsive patient to keep their eyes closed throughout the cutting and removal process to prevent corneal foreign bodies, corneal abrasions, and globe penetration. Place a towel over the patient's face for protection. Explain that there may be sounds of material or Velcro being torn or pulled with the helmet and not to be alarmed. Warn the patient about the noise associated with cutting the helmet with the cast saw. Protect the patient's eyes from exposure to foreign body penetration or abrasions if they are unresponsive. This includes taping the eyelids closed and placing a towel over the face.

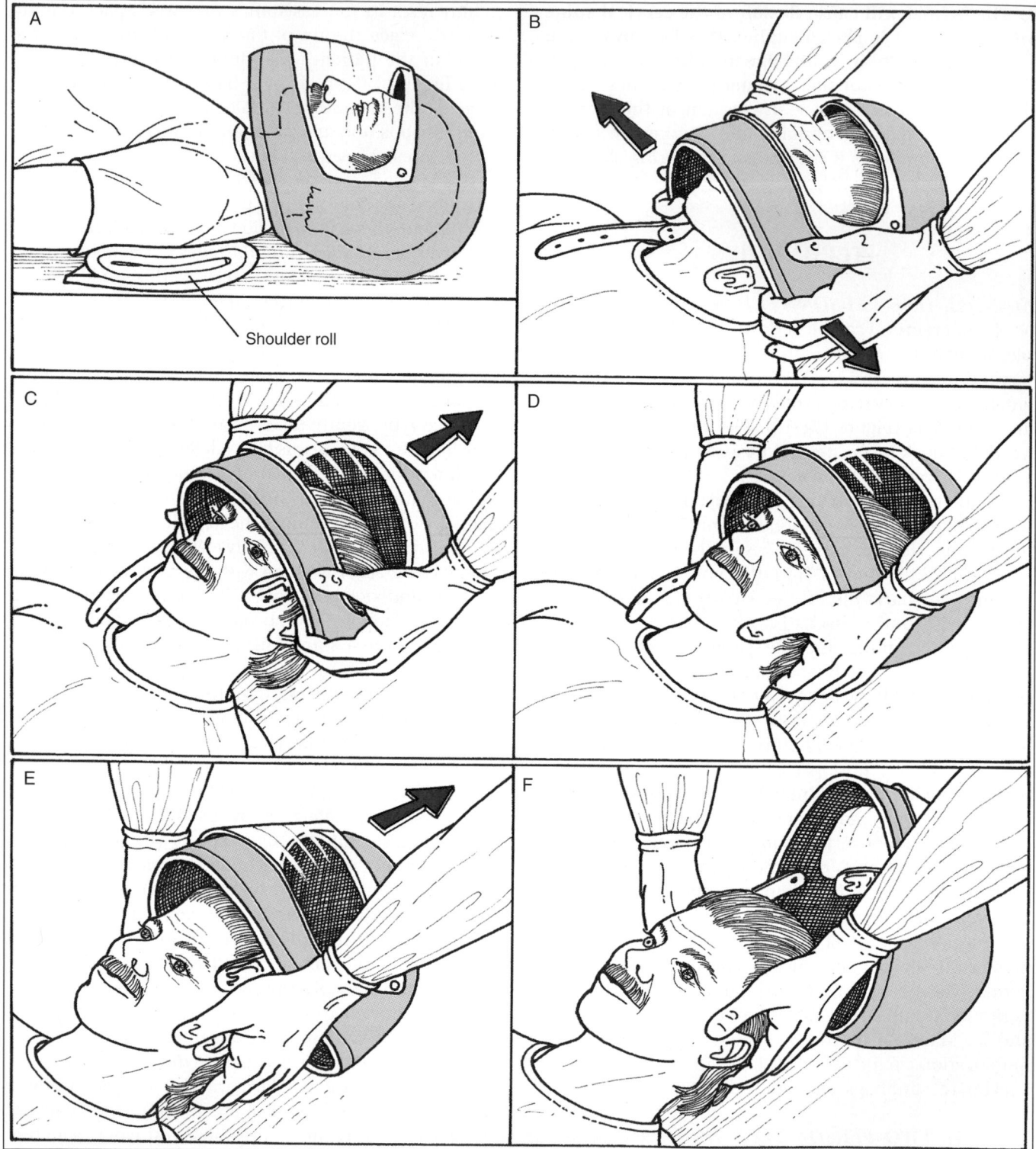

FIGURE 171-1 The one-person helmet removal technique. *A.* Patient positioning. *B.* The base of the helmet is spread open. *C.* The helmet is removed to expose the occiput. *D.* In-line immobilization is applied with the fingers. *E.* The helmet is pushed off with the heels of the hands. *F.* The helmet is removed while in-line immobilization is maintained.

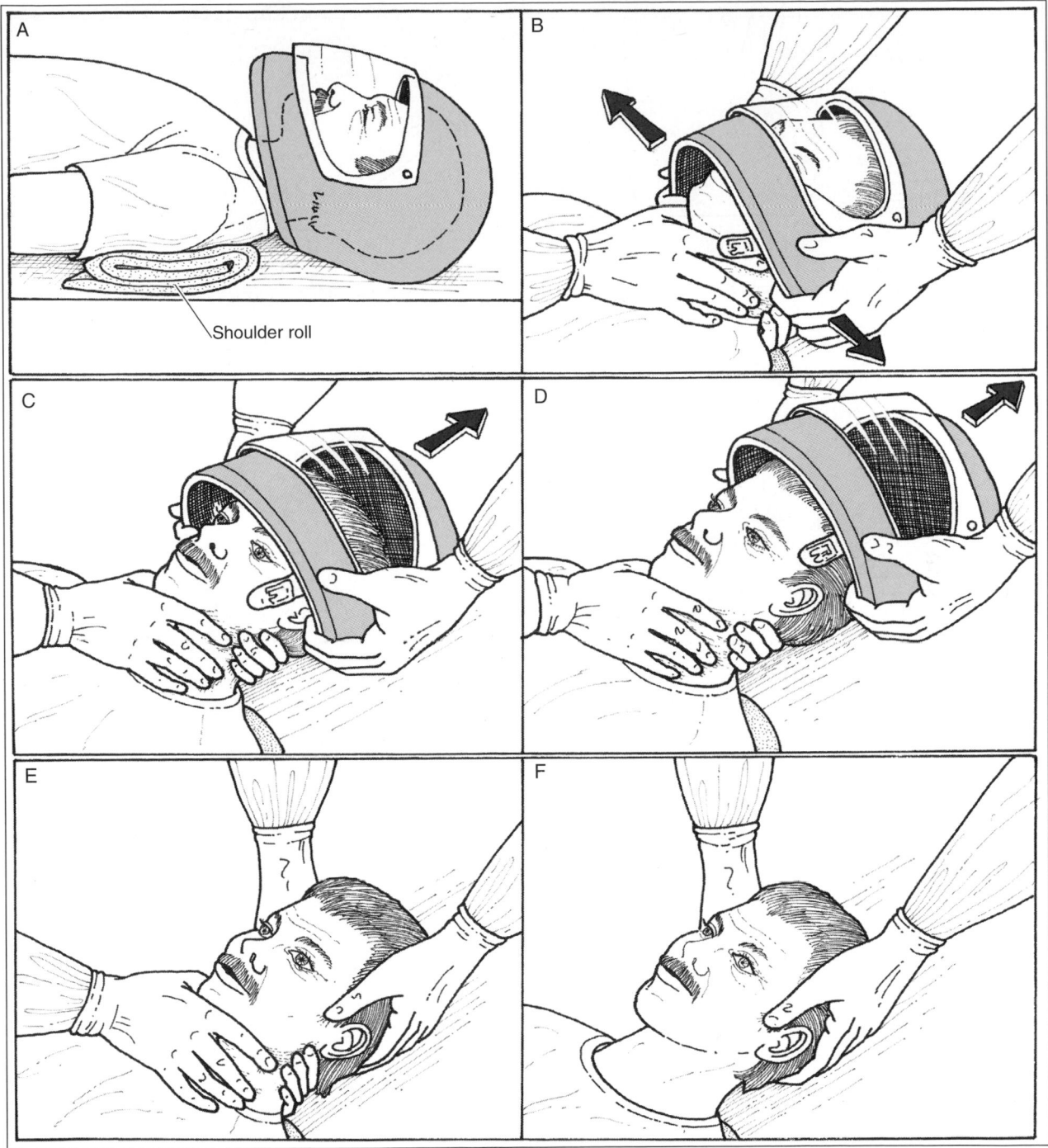

FIGURE 171-2 The two-person helmet removal technique. *A.* Patient positioning. *B.* An assistant provides in-line immobilization. The base of the helmet is spread open. *C.* Remove the helmet to clear the nose. *D.* The helmet is removed while the assistant continues in-line immobilization. *E.* The physician provides in-line immobilization, in addition to the assistant. *F.* The assistant removes their hands and the physician maintains the in-line immobilization.

Instruct the assistant, as described above for the two-person technique, to stabilize and immobilize the patient's head and neck (Figure 171-3*B*). Cut the helmet from ear to ear in a coronal plane with the cast saw (Figure 171-3*C*). Cut the padding and straps with a heavy scissors. Remove the anterior portion of the helmet (Figure 171-3*D*). Gently slide out the posterior portion of the helmet while the assistant maintains in-line immobilization of the head and neck (Figure 171-3*E*). The physician should then support the patient's head and maintain in-line immobilization (Figure 171-3*F*). Instruct the assistant to slowly and carefully remove their hands (Figure 171-3*G*). Instruct the assistant to apply a cervical collar and secure the patient's head with sandbags and tape. The physician can now release hold of the patient.

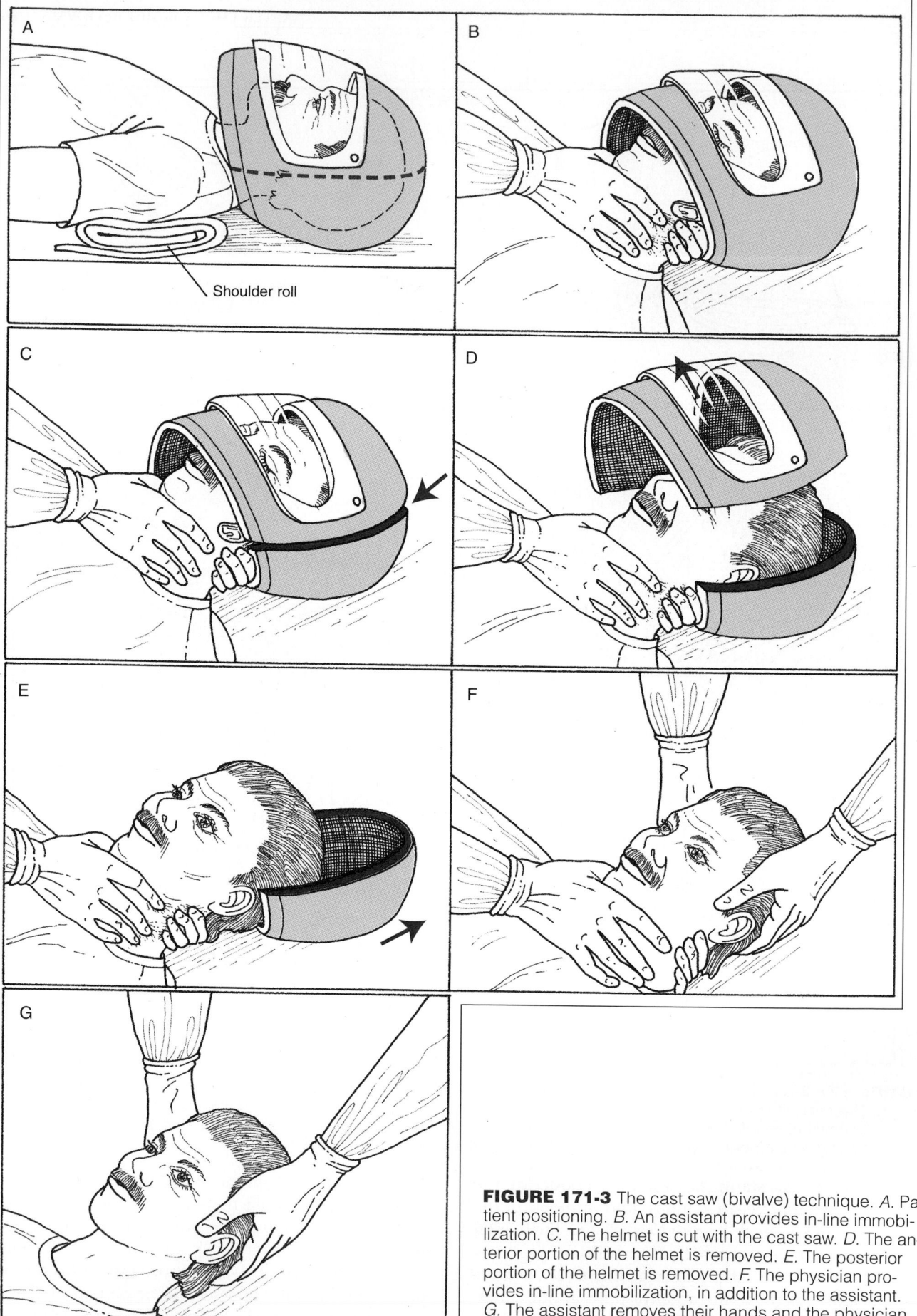

FIGURE 171-3 The cast saw (bivalve) technique. *A*. Patient positioning. *B*. An assistant provides in-line immobilization. *C*. The helmet is cut with the cast saw. *D*. The anterior portion of the helmet is removed. *E*. The posterior portion of the helmet is removed. *F*. The physician provides in-line immobilization, in addition to the assistant. *G*. The assistant removes their hands and the physician maintains the in-line immobilization.

Shoulder roll

ASSESSMENT

Reassess the patient after removing the helmet and securing their head and neck.[14] Examine the patient for secondary injury due to the helmet removal procedure. These include lacerations and avulsions to the ear and nose, corneal abrasions, and corneal foreign bodies. Perform a complete head, eyes, ears, nose, and throat examination looking for injury. Perform and document a complete neurologic examination.

COMPLICATIONS

The most concerning aspect of helmet removal is adequate immobilization of the patient's head and neck during the procedure. Gross movement of the head and neck can result in displacement of fractures, spinal cord injury, or exacerbation of a partial spinal cord injury. **Avoid any movement of the head and neck when there is strong suspicion of spinal cord injury or severe head trauma.** Some movement of the patient's head or neck is likely to occur during helmet removal. **Minimizing the amount of motion is paramount.**

Secondary injury to the ears, eyes, and nose can be avoided by using careful technique. Spreading open the sides of the helmet before removal in the one-person or two-person techniques will eliminate traction injuries to the scalp and ears. Tilting the helmet posteriorly will allow the chin portion of the helmet to clear the nose and avoid traction injuries to the nose.

A separate set of complications is applicable to the cast saw (bivalve) technique. Proper education of the patient is required to prevent them from moving because of the noise and vibration associated with this technique. Covering the patient's eyes with a towel (or gauze squares) will prevent corneal abrasions, corneal foreign bodies, and globe penetration from foreign bodies. Use caution to prevent cutting the patient's ears when cutting the helmet padding. The cut edges of the helmet are extremely sharp. Careful removal will prevent cutting the patient's ears or scalp.

SUMMARY

Health care personnel who care for trauma victims must be aware of the different types of helmets available and the means to safely remove them. Proper assessment of the helmeted patient will determine the need for emergent helmet removal. A thorough physical assessment and radiographic studies may take place prior to removing the helmet if the patient is stable upon initial assessment. By using proper techniques, helmets may safely be removed without causing secondary injury.

REFERENCES

1. Daya MR, Mariani RJ: Out-of-hospital splinting, in Roberts JR, Hedges JR (eds): *Clinical Procedures in Emergency Medicine,* 3rd ed. Philadelphia: Saunders, 1998:792–797.
2. Donaldson WF III, Lauerman WC, Heil B, et al: Helmet and shoulder pad removal from a player with suspected cervical spine injury. *Spine* 1998; 23(16):1729–1733.
3. Max W, Stark B, Root S: Putting the lid on injury costs: the impact of the California motorcycle helmet law. *J Trauma* 1998; 45(3):550–556.
4. Meyer R, Daniel WW: The biomechanics of helmets and helmet removal. *J Trauma* 1985; 25(4):329–332.
5. Roberts WO: Helmet removal in head and neck trauma. *Phys Sports Med* 1998; 26(7):77–78.
6. Swenson TM, Lauerman WC, Blanc RO, et al: Cervical spine alignment in the immobilized football player: radiographic analysis before and after helmet removal. *Am J Sports Med* 1997; 25(2):226–230.
7. American Heart Association: *Pediatric Advanced Life Support Manual.* Austin, TX: American Heart Association, 2002.
8. Palumbo MA, Hulstyn MJ, Fadale PD, et al: The effect of protective football equipment on alignment of the injured cervical spine: radiographic analysis in a cadaveric model. *Am J Sports Med* 1996; 24(4):446–453.
9. Koenig WJ: Helmet removal, in Dieckman RA, Fiser DH, Selbst SM (eds): *Illustrated Textbook of Pediatric Emergency and Critical Care Procedures.* St Louis: Mosby, 1997:602–603.
10. Kelly KP: Helmet removal, in Henretig FM, King C (eds): *Textbook of Pediatric Emergency Procedures.* Baltimore: Williams & Wilkins, 1997:343–349.
11. Gastel J, Palumbo MA, Hulstyn MJ: Emergency removal of football equipment. A cadaveric cervical spine injury model. *Ann Emerg Med* 1998; 32(4):411–417.
12. Budassi SA: Helmet removal from injured patients. *J Emerg Nurs* 1981; 7:290.
13. Aprahamian C, Thompson BM, Darin JC: Recommended helmet removal techniques in a cervical spine injured patient. *J Trauma* 1984; 24(9): 841–842.
14. American College of Surgeons Committee on Trauma: Skills station IX: head and neck trauma assessment and management, in *Advanced Trauma Life Support for Doctors,* 6th ed. Chicago: American College of Surgeons, 1997:205–213.

Chapter 172
PNEUMATIC ANTISHOCK GARMENT

Moses S. Lee

INTRODUCTION

The pneumatic antishock garment (PASG) is commonly used in the prehospital setting to transport patients with hypovolemic shock. It has also been used for nontraumatic causes of hemorrhage (pelvic fractures, ruptured ectopic pregnancy, and ruptured aortic aneurysms) and to stabilize extremity fractures. The most common PASG is the Military/Medical Antishock Trousers (MAST trousers). The PASG was initially designed in 1903 but did not see routine use until the Vietnam War.[1]

The PASG was primarily used for trauma victims with hypovolemic shock. Several studies have demonstrated an elevation of blood pressure and control of bleeding with the application of the PASG.[2,3] The largest series reviewed the use of the PASG in 1120 patients. Approximately 84 percent of these responded with an increase in systolic blood pressure greater than 20 mmHg, a decrease in heart rate, or evidence of enhanced tissue perfusion.[4] Recent controlled studies have questioned the efficacy of the PASG, especially in penetrating abdominal injuries and thoracic injuries.[5,6] The Advanced Trauma Life Support course sponsored by the American College of Surgeons states that "the efficacy of PASG in-hospital or in the rural setting remains unproven and, in the urban prehospital setting, controversial."[7] The criteria for the application of the PASG have been revised and are noted in the "Indications" section below.

ANATOMY AND PATHOPHYSIOLOGY

The mechanism of action of the PASG has been the focus of numerous experimental studies. The increase in blood pressure from the application of the PASG is due to enhanced venous return (autotransfusion), increased total peripheral vascular resistance, and reduced volume loss from hemorrhage control. Recent studies have demonstrated that the patient receives only a 4 mL/kg autotransfusion effect from the inflated PASG.[8] Previous studies had suggested an autotransfusion up to 2000 mL.[9]

The predominant effect of the PASG is an increase in peripheral vascular resistance.[10,11] The decreased diameter of blood vessels under the suit leads to increased preload, improved stroke volume, and increased cardiac output. This temporarily improves cerebral and coronary blood flow.

Control of hemorrhage is the third effect of the PASG. The compressive effect decreases blood flow, minimizes tears in the vessels, and allows clot formation to occur. Use of the PASG has been recommended as part of the initial management of major pelvic fractures prior to definitive intervention.[12] The PASG offers several advantages in the treatment of pelvic fractures.[12,13] It compresses the pelvic area and tamponades bleeding, immobilizes pelvic fractures, reduces bony displacement, and improves pelvic bone alignment. The PASG has been used in nontraumatic pelvic hemorrhage in the obstetric and gynecologic patient.[13] Hemostasis is likely a result of the compressive effect on the blood vessels under the garment.

INDICATIONS

There are no absolute indications for the use of the PASG. Its original use as an adjunct to support a failing circulatory system still holds, even though it may be only minimally effective. The PASG can serve as a splint for lower extremity fractures and tamponade intraabdominal bleeding. Its use in penetrating trauma of the abdomen and in thoracic injuries is controversial.[5] It may be helpful in hypotensive patients with blunt abdominal trauma, penetrating abdominal trauma, long prehospital transport times, and in patients with signs of hypovolemic shock regardless of the etiology. The PASG is most useful in the management of pelvic fractures with persistent retroperitoneal hemorrhage.

The National Association of EMS Physicians published their recommendations regarding medically directed prehospital use of the PASG in 1997.[14] The report suggests that the PASG is "usually indicated, useful, and effective" for only one indication: hypotension due to a ruptured aortic aneurysm. The association considered the use of the PASG as "acceptable" but with uncertain efficacy in suspected pelvic fractures, anaphylactic shock unresponsive to standard therapy, otherwise uncontrollable lower extremity hemorrhage, and severe traumatic hypotension (pulse without blood pressure). Other uses with uncertain efficacy include application in the elderly, in paroxysmal supraventricular tachycardia, uncontrolled hemorrhage (gynecologic, urologic, and lower extremity), hypothermia-induced hypotension, ruptured ectopic pregnancy, septic shock, spinal shock, and to assist in intravenous cannulation.

CONTRAINDICATIONS

The use of counterpressure devices is temporizing at best; definitive care is the final goal. Absolute contraindications to the use of the PASG are congestive heart failure and pulmonary edema. Relative contraindications include cardiogenic shock, cardiac tamponade, myocardial infarction, penetrating thoracic injuries, diaphragmatic injuries, pregnancy, abdominal evisceration, impaled foreign bodies, lower extremity compartmental injury, lumbar spine instability, and uncontrolled hemorrhage in any area not covered by the garment.

EQUIPMENT

The PASG is currently available through emergency medical services (EMS) product distributors. The most commonly known PASG is the Military/Medical Antishock Trousers[15] (Figure 172-1). This suit is composed of three compartments, each of which is individually inflatable. There are two leg compartments and an abdominal compartment. Each compartment has its own pop-off valve and stopcock. The pop-off valve is preset at the factory to 104 mmHg to prevent overinflation of the compartment. The stopcock is a lever positioned to regulate the flow of air into and out of the compartment. The PASG is inflated with a foot pump. It is currently available in three sizes (David Clark Co., Inc., Worcester, MA).

PATIENT PREPARATION

Thoroughly examine the patient prior to the application of the PASG. Examination after its application can be difficult. If the patient is clothed in shorts or long

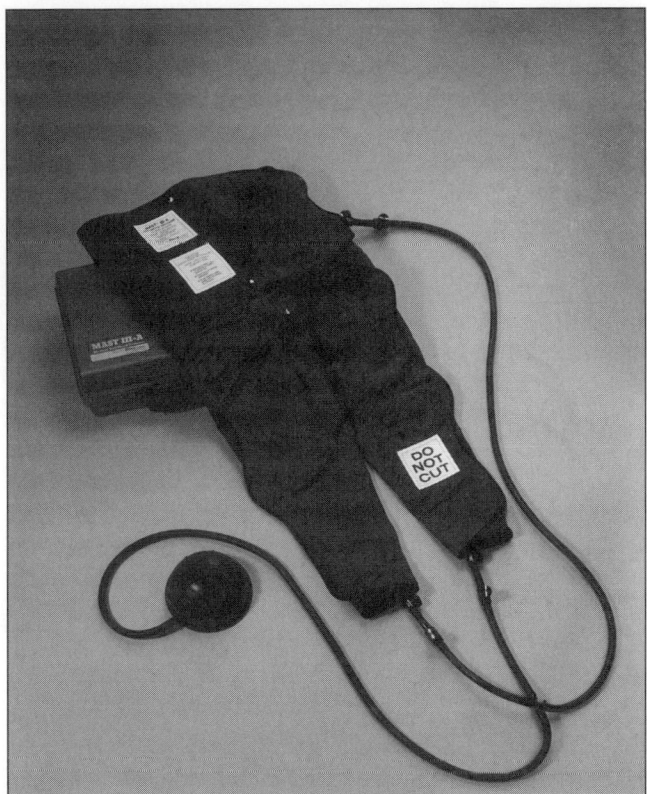

FIGURE 172-1 The Military/Medical Antishock Trousers. (Photo courtesy of David Clark Co., Inc., Worcester, MA.)

pants, remove any sharp objects in their pockets to avoid a penetrating injury to the suit and/or the patient. Reduce any gross bony deformities of the lower extremity whenever possible.

TECHNIQUE

PASG APPLICATION AND INFLATION

Lay out and open the PASG (Figure 172-2). Place the patient supine and on top of the open PASG. Fasten the PASG with the Velcro closures around the patient's legs and abdomen (Figure 172-3). The PASG may be slid under the patient if they cannot be transferred to another gurney. Connect the inflation hoses for the compartments to the foot pump. Determine which of the compartments are to be inflated. Open the stopcock(s) to the compartment(s) to be inflated. Close the stopcock(s) to the compartment(s) not to be inflated. Apply a blood pressure cuff to one of the upper extremities to monitor the response to the inflated PASG.

Inflation of all three compartments requires two steps. **Always inflate the leg compartments before the abdominal compartment if all three are to be inflated.** Close the stopcock to the abdominal compartment and

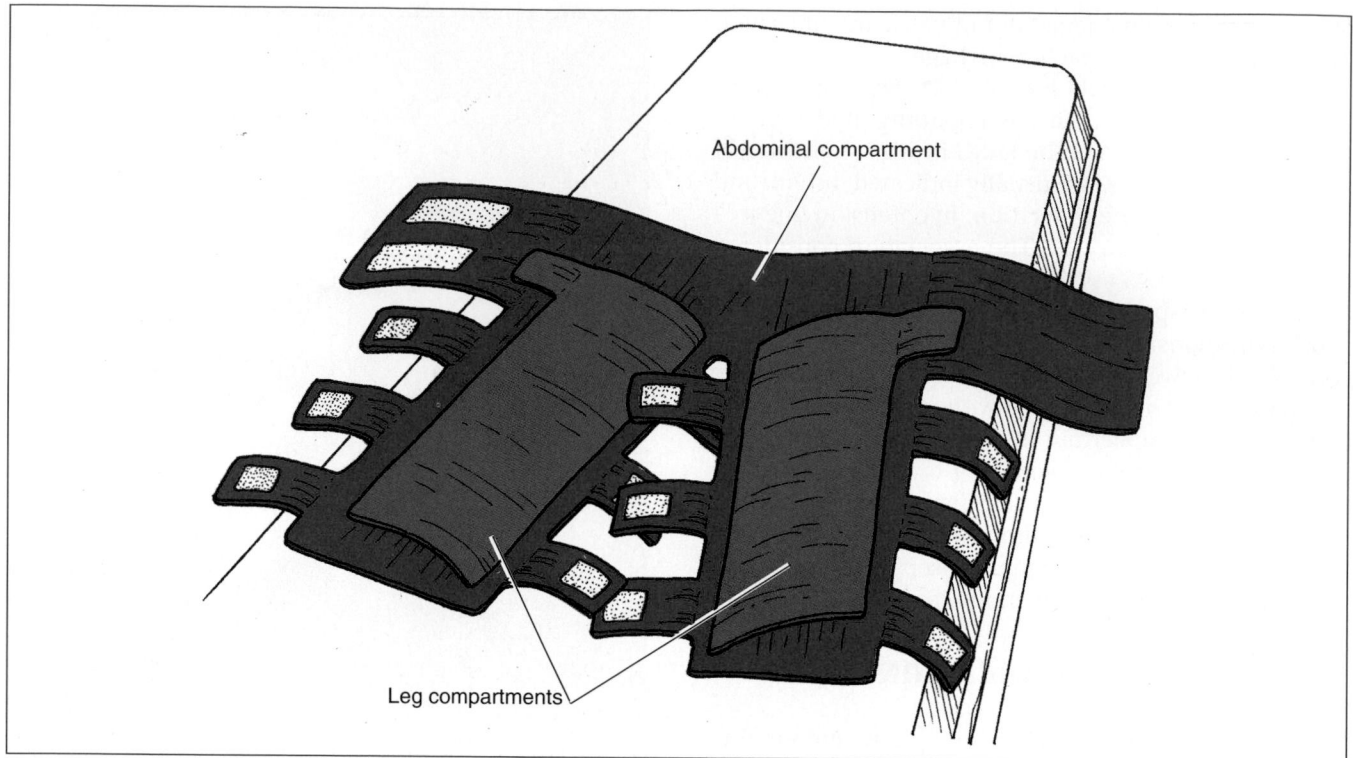

FIGURE 172-2 The three compartments of the PASG positioned on a gurney.

open the stopcocks to the leg compartments. Inflate the leg sections. Close the stopcocks to the leg compartments and open the stopcock to the abdominal compartment. Inflate the abdominal compartment. Close the stopcock to the abdominal compartment.

Inflate the compartments with the foot pump (Figure 172-3). The operator may want to initially inflate the compartments by blowing into them. This may provide volume more quickly than the pump during the low-resistance initial phase.[16] Partially inflate the leg compartments.[17] Assess the patient's blood pressure. **The goal is to achieve a systolic blood pressure of approximately 100 mmHg in the hypotensive patient with the lowest inflation pressure possible.** This is not important if the goal is to inflate the PASG to stabilize an extremity or pelvic fracture. Continue to incrementally inflate the compartments and monitor the blood pressure until the systolic blood pressure reaches 100 mmHg. Do not inflate the abdominal compartment if a systolic blood pressure of 100 mmHg is achieved with inflation of the leg compartments. Always close the stopcock to the inflated compartment so that it does not deflate.

PASG DEFLATION

Deflation can take place in two settings. This can occur in the Emergency Department once resuscitative efforts have restored a satisfactory blood pressure or

a complication (e.g., pulmonary edema) develops. If emergency surgery is indicated, the PASG can be left on until the patient is on the operating table and the Surgeon and Anesthesiologist have established appropriate patient monitoring.

Deflate the compartments gradually. It is critical to constantly monitor the patient's blood pressure if the PASG was placed for the management of hypotension or exsanguination. Deflate the abdominal compartment first if all three compartments were inflated. Open the abdominal compartment stopcock and release a small amount of air. Assess the patient's blood pressure. A systolic blood pressure drop of more than 5 mmHg requires a bolus of intravenous fluid to restore the systolic blood pressure. Continue incremental deflation of the abdominal compartment with alternating blood pressure assessments. Deflate the leg compartments in a similar fashion.

COMPLICATIONS

Several complications can occur from the use of the PASG. The most common are hypotension, respiratory compromise, and the development of a compartment syndrome. Hypotension is often the result of precipitous removal of the PASG without adequate fluid resuscita-

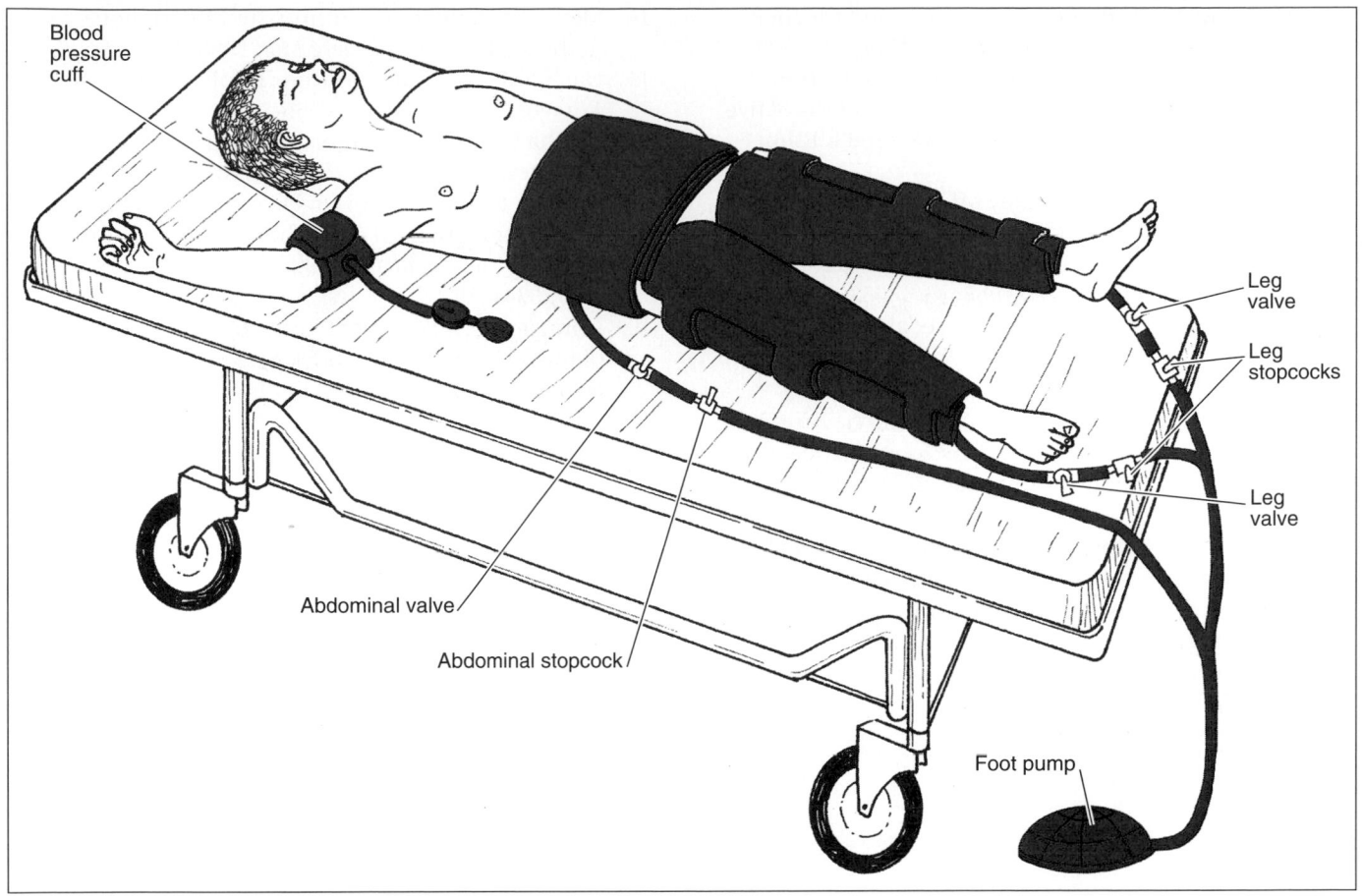

Blood
pressure
cuff

Leg
valve

Leg
stopcocks

Leg
valve

Abdominal valve

Abdominal stopcock

Foot pump

FIGURE 172-3 The PASG secured around the patient with Velcro straps.

tion. Respiratory distress is often subjective, especially in an alert patient. Suspect a diaphragmatic rupture if respiratory distress occurs after the inflation of the abdominal compartment. Deflate the abdominal compartment and see whether the respiratory distress resolves. A compartment syndrome can occur with prolonged application of the PASG in a patient with extremity trauma. This is a rare complication.[4,6] Other complications include metabolic acidosis, renal hypoperfusion, pulmonary edema, congestive heart failure, stimulation of urination, stimulation of defecation, vomiting, lumbar spine instability, and skin breakdown.

There are several limitations to the use of the PASG. These include the limited ability to perform a physical examination, limited vascular access, the inability to perform a peritoneal lavage, and the inability to perform a urethral catheterization. Another consideration is the effect of environmental factors. This is relevant only in aeromedical transport, where Boyle's law (the volume of gas is inversely proportional to its pressure) takes effect. Modify the inflation pressures if the patient is transported aeromedically.[18]

SUMMARY

The pneumatic antishock garment has been used as an adjunct to hypovolemic shock for a number of years. It can increase venous return, tamponade hemorrhage, splint pelvic fractures, and splint long bone fractures. Use caution when removing the garment to avoid abrupt hypotension. Use of the PASG has significantly decreased over the years due to short transport times in the urban prehospital setting and limited use in penetrating trauma.

REFERENCES

1. Cutler BS, Daggett W: Application of the "g-suit" to the control of hemorrhage in massive trauma. *Ann Surg* 1971; 173(4):511–517.
2. Pelligra R, Sandberg EC: Control of intractible abdominal bleeding by external counterpressure. *JAMA* 1979; 241(7):708–713.

3. McSwain NE Jr: Pneumatic trousers and the management of shock. *J Trauma* 1977; 17(9):719–724.

4. Wayne MA, MacDonald SC: Clinical evaluation of the antishock trouser. Retrospective analysis of five years of experience. *Ann Emerg Med* 1983; 12(6): 342–347.

5. Bickell WH, Pepe PE, Bailey ML, et al: Randomized trial of pneumatic antishock garments in the prehospital management of penetrating abdominal injuries. *Ann Emerg Med* 1987; 16(6):653–658.

6. Mattox KI, Bickell WH, Pepe PE, et al: Prospective MAST study in 911 patients. *J Trauma* 1989; 29(8): 1104–1112.

7. American College of Surgeons: *Advanced Trauma Life Support (ATLS) Course.* Chicago: American College of Surgeons Committee on Trauma, 1983: 68–69, 87–88.

8. Niemann JT, Stapczynski JS, Rosborough P, et al: Hemodynamic effects of pneumatic external counterpressure in canine hemorrhagic shock. *Ann Emerg Med* 1983; 12(11):661–667.

9. Abernathy C, Dickinson TC, Lokey TH: A military anti-shock trousers program in the small hospital setting. *Surg Clin North Am* 1979; 59(3):461–470.

10. McSwain NE: Pneumatic anti-shock garment: state of the art 1988. *Ann Emerg Med* 1988; 17(5):506–525.

11. Davis SM: Antishock trousers: a collective review. *J Emerg Med* 1986; 4:145–155.

12. Mucha P, Welch TJ: Hemorrhage in major pelvic fractures. *Surg Clin North Am* 1988; 68(4):757–773.

13. Mud HJ, Schattenkerk ME, Devries JE, et al: Non-surgical treatment of pelvic hemorrhage in obstetric and gynecologic patients. *Crit Care Med* 1987; 15(5):534–535.

14. Domeier RM, O'Connor RE, Delbridge TR, et al: Use of the pneumatic anti-shock garment (PASG). National Association of EMS Physicians. *Prehosp Emerg Care* 1997; 1(1):32–35.

15. MAST. 1999. http://www.davidclark.com/medical.shtml

16. Dick T: Putting the pressure on shock: a look at the antishock fashions. *J Emerg Med Serv* 1982; 7(6): 26–32.

17. Kaback KR, Sanders AB, Meislin HW: MAST suit update. *JAMA* 1989; 252(18):2598–2603.

18. Sanders AB, Meislin HW: Effect of altitude change on MAST suit pressure. *Ann Emerg Med* 1983; 12(3): 140–144.

Chapter 173

HAZMAT PATIENT MANAGEMENT

Atilla B. Üner

INTRODUCTION

Hazardous materials (hazmat) incidents occur most often during the transport of chemicals or at industrial site accidents. Hazmat incidents may strike any community at any time.[1] Every Emergency Department must be prepared to respond to victims of a hazmat exposure.

Decontamination is the procedure of eliminating or reducing to a safe level any harmful substances on persons and equipment.[2] **Decontamination of victims in the field should always be performed by Emergency Medical Service (EMS) providers or before the patient enters the Emergency Department.** However, this does not always occur. Patients may be too ill for lengthy decontamination procedures prior to transport. Exposed patients may leave the scene and present to the Emergency Department on their own.[3,4] Basic decontamination by Emergency Department personnel can be safely performed outdoors in a designated decontamination area.[5]

Exposure to a hazmat exposed patient who has been inadequately decontaminated or not decontaminated at all is a real possibility. This can result in exposure and secondary injury to health care personnel, other patients, and visitors. The Emergency Department may be closed in part or in whole until the facility can be decontaminated. The panic and fear induced by rumors or odors can lead to unnecessary facility closure, delayed or inadequate patient treatment, and psychogenic illness in both health care personnel and bystanders.[3,4]

The three primary goals for the Emergency Department are to isolate and contain the contamination; decontaminate and treat exposed patients while protecting staff, other patients, and visitors; and maintain normal services, or reestablish them, as soon as possible.[3]

Early recognition of potentially hazmat contaminated patients will aid in preventing secondary contamination and Emergency Department closures. Numerous clues may identify a patient for hazmat contamination at triage.[3,4] These include accidents at agricultural or industrial sites, accidents involving chemical transports, suspected mass casualty incidents, a cholinergic toxidrome, mucous membrane irritation, chemical burns, soiling with unidentified liquids or powders, intentional overdose with chemicals, unexplained unconsciousness or cardiac arrest, and symptoms occurring in Paramedics or Emergency Medical Technicians (EMTs) after patient transport.

Information management is critical to the response.[4] Designate a person to obtain as much information as possible on the involved substance. Even preliminary and general information is useful and should be immediately conveyed to the treating physician.[1] The maintenance of material safety data sheets (MSDS) is mandatory for each chemical used or stored at an industrial site or during transport. Request information on the MSDS from fire or EMS services at the scene. Further information resources are listed after the "References" section of this chapter. Verify all information for accuracy by cross-referencing several sources.[4]

This chapter describes a general approach to the management of the hazmat contaminated patient. The Emergency Department response and patient management will have to be tailored to specific agents and circumstances, such as number of patients and facility resources. All Emergency Departments are strongly encouraged to conduct regular inservice training sessions and drills on hazmat decontamination procedures. Information and training materials are available free of charge from the U.S. Department of Health and Human Services Agency for Toxic Substances and Disease Registry. These materials are highly recommended.

ANATOMY AND PATHOPHYSIOLOGY

Hazardous materials can enter the body through inhalation, absorption, and ingestion.[6] The total dose is a function of the concentration and properties of the substance, the exposure time, and the exposure route. There is a dose-response relationship between the absorbed dose and toxic effects for most toxic chemicals.[6] The effects can be local, systemic, and quite variable for different agents.

Inhalation is the most common route of exposure. It may lead to local irritation, airway obstruction, and/or pulmonary systemic absorption. Absorption through intact skin is facilitated by fat solubility, open wounds, burns, exposure of the eyes and mucous membranes, and by dermal contamination underneath soiled clothing leading to an occlusive dressing effect.[2,4] The axillae, groin, and skin folds have a thin epidermal layer that facilitates the absorption of a contaminant. Ingestions can be accidental or intentional.

Patients exposed to hazardous materials may show any or all of the following: local effects such as chemical burns, respiratory tract effects of inhaled toxins, systemic effects of absorbed toxins, associated trauma, psychiatric reactions (agitation and anxiety), or contamination without apparent injury.[4]

The hazard to personnel, or risk of secondary contamination, is determined by the dose of the hazardous material that is carried by the victim and absorbed by the caregiver.[7] Toxic liquids and solids can pose a dermal contact hazard.[3] Solids or volatile liquids can pose an inhalational hazard.[3] Most gases or vapors dissipate quickly and are unlikely to pose a secondary contamination hazard.[7] However, the risk to emergency personnel is real.[4,8] Contamination with corrosives or pesticides may indeed cause illness in personnel.[4,7,8] Toxins can rarely be emitted from vomitus (such as hydrogen cyanide after cyanide salt ingestion) or exhaled breath after ethylene oxide exposure.[2]

INDICATIONS

Decontaminate any potentially contaminated patient prior to their entry into the Emergency Department.[8] The more toxic the substance, the more rapidly the decontamination should be performed. Pesticides and corrosives are common and worrisome contaminants.[7] Asymptomatic contaminated patients can be triaged for decontamination before those with symptoms to prevent toxicity if the risk of toxicity is high. Decontaminate symptomatic patients before asymptomatic patients if the risk of toxicity is low.[4] Initiate any life support measures simultaneously with decontamination.[4] Patients who have been decontaminated or exposed to gases or vapors without signs of skin or eye irritation do not require further decontamination.[2,4,5]

The absence of a system to isolate waste water is not a contraindication to water decontamination. **When in doubt, decontaminate the patient.** Dilution will suffice to reduce the hazardous substance to a safe level.

CONTRAINDICATIONS

Contraindications to water decontamination include contamination with metallic sodium, lithium, calcium, potassium, cesium, and rubidium.[1,9] Other contraindications to water decontamination include exposure to dusts of pure magnesium, sulfur, strontium, titanium, uranium, yttrium, zinc, and zirconium.[1,9] These substances react violently with water and can cause secondary injury.[1,9] Cover the patient and/or substance with mineral oil, remove the substance with forceps, and store it in a container with mineral oil.[4,9] However, many of these substances may already have reacted with moisture on the patient's skin.[1,9] Rapid removal of the chemical agent is better than allowing continuing injury to occur.[5] Adding large amounts of water to the small amount of residual chemical on the patient's body poses little risk of creating a serious reaction hazard.[10]

Patients soaked in flammable liquids pose special problems. Water decontamination may be inadequate to completely remove the substance from the patient's skin. Do not cardiovert or defibrillate the patient until the material is completely removed from the skin, so as to prevent an explosion or a fire.[5]

The use of chemical agents for neutralization is contraindicated. These substances may cause secondary injury or toxicity or they may react with another substance in an adverse manner. Use large quantities of water for decontamination rather than a neutralization agent.[5]

EQUIPMENT

Personal Protective Equipment (per Person)

Scrub suit and closed shoes
Plastic shoe covers
Protective goggles
Water resistant face mask
Latex gloves
Chemical resistant (i.e., nitrile) gloves
Chemical resistant coverall suit with booties and hood
Duct tape
Rubber apron
Butyl rubber gloves
Chemical resistant rubber boots or shoe covers
Respiratory protection

The regulations of the Occupational Safety and Health Administration (OSHA) require level B protection for responders to an unknown chemical hazard, with a positive-pressure self-contained breathing apparatus and chemical resistant clothing.[3,6,8] The high cost of such equipment and constant skills retraining required to use it may prohibit hospitals from purchasing it.[6]

Hospital gowns, standard Tyvek suits, surgical masks, and latex gloves are not considered adequate protection.[4,7,9] Personal protective equipment is available through specialized dealers and requires training to provide reliable protection.[4,6,8,9] The minimum protection recommended for hospital decontamination personnel includes a scrub suit, a chemical resistant suit with booties and hood, plastic shoe covers, at least two layers of gloves (surgical and nitrile) taped at the sleeve, protective eyewear, and respiratory protection.[4,6]

There is no consensus on how to provide respiratory protection. The required level, if any, will depend upon the agent, the dose, prior training, and decontamination circumstances.[4,6,8] Respiratory protection is rarely necessary if decontamination is performed oudoors.[7] Information obtained about the contaminant will aid in determining the level of protection needed.

Patient Decontamination

Decontamination unit located outside of the hospital
Designated decontamination facility inside the hospital
Decontamination stretchers, if applicable
Portable wading pools for ambulatory patients
Warm running water source with a hose and soft-
    stream nozzle
Portable barriers to assure privacy and protect from
    wind
Liquid hand or dishwashing soap
Liquid shampoo
Soft-bristled brushes
Devices to decontaminate hands and nails (e.g., surgi-
    cal scrub sets)
Eye irrigation equipment

Miscellaneous Supplies

Polyethylene plastic bags
Name tags
Yellow tape and signs to mark decontamination zones
Scissors to cut clothing
Scrub suits, towels, and blankets for patients after
    decontamination

PATIENT PREPARATION

Patients should be initially received in a secured area outside of the Emergency Department. Clearly mark the area with yellow tape or other similar device. This is considered a contaminated "hot zone." Triage, a primary survey, and required immediate lifesaving basic life support may be performed here by appropriately protected personnel.[4,6]

The decontamination area is also considered a contaminated "hot zone."[4] **Perform basic life support and immediate life saving measures only in the decontamination area.**[9] However, the extent of medical treatment in the decontamination area will need to be decided from case to case. Treatment of cardiac dysrhythmias and wounds or administration of toxin-specific antidotes may have to be initiated prior to complete decontamination.[9] **Keep in mind that invasive procedures prior to decontamination may provide a percutaneous route of contamination with the hazardous substance.** Devices, such as monitors, used in the decontamination area will have to be decontaminated after use.[9] Use long leads, if available, that extend into the clean support area to prevent having to decontaminate monitoring devices.[9]

Patients are considered safe to move into the contamination reduction area ("warm zone") and then the Emergency Department (support area, "cold zone") only when decontamination is completed. Perform a secondary survey, including a search for any toxidromes, and begin definitive medical treatment after decontamination.[4]

DECONTAMINATION TECHNIQUE FOR CHEMICAL AGENTS

Don personal protective equipment before approaching the contaminated patient.[4] Suggested minimum personal protective equipment and its application is described here. Wear standard work attire, such as a scrub suit, and closed shoes (no clogs or slippers). Place plastic shoe covers over shoes. Don goggles and a water resistant face mask. This is for splash protection only. Don latex gloves followed by nitrile or other chemical resistant gloves. Don a chemical resistant coverall suit with booties and a hood. Tape the sleeves to the gloves with duct tape. Don a butyl rubber apron and butyl rubber gloves for protection against water and chemicals. This protocol provides no respiratory protection.

Perform a primary survey and treat any life-threatening conditions with basic life support interventions.[4] Remove all of the patient's clothing. This includes shoes and jewelry. Cut off the clothing if necessary. Place the clothing in a plastic bag and seal it with duct tape. Place this bag into another bag and seal it to "double bag" the clothing. Double bag any jewelry and watches separately if time and circumstances permit. This allows for possible later decontamination and salvage. Label the bags with the patient's name or medical record number.

Patients may assist with their own decontamination. **Do not irrigate the patient prior to complete clothing removal.** Chemicals on clothing will soak through wet clothing and onto the skin, resulting in additional injury or absorption.[2,5]

Remove any visible chemicals on the patient's body by gently washing off liquids or brushing off solids. Avoid skin irritation or injury, as both will lead to increased absorption of any remaining chemicals. Avoid aerosolization of the contaminant. Blot any heavy liquids with absorbent towels.[2,5]

Patients with open wounds require the area surrounding the wound to be gently washed with water. Irrigate the wound with clean water. Cover large wounds with plastic wrap to prevent runoff into the wound during the remaining decontamination procedure.[2] **Do not delay copious water irrigation if this wound care cannot be accomplished rapidly.**

Begin copious water irrigation with warm water using low water pressure (normal shower pressure) for 3 to 5 minutes. Use liquid soap, shampoo, and soft brushes to gently cleanse the skin and any body hair.[5] Thoroughly rinse the patient after soaping and shampooing. Repeat the procedure until all visible contamination is removed. **Do not forget to thoroughly clean any mucous membranes, the nails, the external auditory canals, the axillae, the groin, and any other skin folds.** Use cleaning devices such as surgical scrub sets for nail folds or syringes to flush the external auditory canals.

Irrigate the eyes, if contaminated, for 5 minutes. Remove any contact lenses and place them in a double bag. A Morgan lens may be used if the globe is intact. Irrigation with running water is also an option but may be less thorough than with a Morgan lens. A nasal oxygen cannula may be placed on the bridge of the nose if both eyes are affected.[2] Allow water to flow through the cannula and direct it from the medial canthus outward. Refer to Chapter 134 for the details regarding eye irrigation.

The nonambulatory contaminated trauma patient or a patient with altered mental status may need to be decontaminated on a specialized stretcher that is equipped to catch waste water. Autopsy tables from the morgue may be used after covering the surface with plastic. Enough decontamination personnel must be available to maintain cervical spine immobilization while log-rolling the patient as the decontamination process is performed.

DECONTAMINATION TECHNIQUE FOR BIOLOGICAL WEAPONS AGENTS

Biological weapons agents include bacteria, spores, viruses, and toxins. Chemical decontamination renders biological weapons agents harmless by the use of disinfectants.[10] **Most biological warfare agents are transmitted by inhalation; therefore respiratory protection is highly recommended.** Treat dermal exposures immediately with soap-and-water decontamination using a soft brush followed by rinsing with copious amounts of water. This alone is often sufficient to avert contact infection. Wash with a dilute bleach (hypochlorite) solution to eradicate any remaining biological agent.

Mix 1 part Clorox bleach and 9 parts water, as standard stock Clorox is a 5% solution, to make a 0.5% sodium hypochlorite solution. The diluted bleach solution must be made fresh daily with a pH in the alkaline range. Diluted and undiluted bleach solutions evaporate quickly. Store the bleach solution in closed and distinctly marked containers to avoid confusing the 5% and the 0.5% solutions. Wash the contaminated areas with a soaked cloth or swab for 10 to 15 minutes with the 0.5% sodium hypochlorite solution. **A contact time of 10 to 15 minutes is required.**[10] Rinse thoroughly with water.

The dilute bleach solution is contraindicated for application into the eyes, into open brain and spinal cord injuries, or for surgical irrigation of the abdomen. However, it may be used for lavage of other noncavity wounds and removed by suction to an appropriate disposal container. Within 5 minutes, the now contaminated bleach solution will be neutralized and considered non-hazardous.

Use a 5% hypochlorite solution (undiluted Clorox) to decontaminate fabric, clothing, and equipment. **A contact time of 30 minutes prior to normal cleaning is required for the decontamination of equipment.** The 5% bleach solution is corrosive to most metals and injurious to most fabrics. Thoroughly rinse and oil metal surfaces after completion.

Physical methods to render biological weapons agents harmless include heat and radiation. Dry heat requires 2 hours of treatment at 160 °C to render biological agents completely harmless. Autoclaving is effective. Steam at 121 °C and 1 atmosphere of overpressure (15 psi) will reduce the required time to approximately 20 minutes, depending upon volume.

Rooms in fixed spaces that become contaminated are best decontaminated with gases or liquids in aerosol form (e.g., formaldehyde). This is combined with surface disinfectants, in most cases, to ensure complete decontamination. Solar ultraviolet radiation that reaches the earth's surface has a certain disinfectant effect, often in combination with drying, and will aid in the decontamination of outdoor decontamination facilities. Chlorine-calcium or lye may be used if it is necessary to decontaminate terrain.

ASSESSMENT

Move the patient after decontamination to the contamination reduction zone ("warm zone"). Assess the patient and initiate any required advanced life support measures. **There are no objective criteria to assess whether decontamination was sufficient.** There is, however, evidence that copious water irrigation and soap cleansing are highly effective in removing many chemical contaminants.[4] Measure the tear film pH if the eyes were exposed to corrosive agents. Continue eye irrigation until the pH is neutral. This may take up to 15 minutes. Assess all wounds. Thoroughly irrigate any wounds. **Transfer the patient into the support zone (Emergency Department or "cold zone") when deemed decontaminated.**

HEALTH CARE PERSONNEL DECONTAMINATION TECHNIQUE

Health care personnel must remove their personal protective equipment in an organized fashion to prevent self-contamination after decontamination of the patient.[6] This is a suggested protocol for the minimum personal protective equipment, which may need to be altered if more sophisticated equipment is to be decontaminated and recycled.

Remove the tape securing the gloves to the suit. Place the tape in a plastic bag. Remove the outer gloves, turning them inside out as they are removed. Place the gloves in the plastic bag. Remove the suit, turning it inside out as it is removed. Place the suit in the plastic bag. Seal the bag with duct tape. Remove the plastic shoe cover from one foot and step over the "clean line." Remove the other shoe cover and put that foot over the line. Place both shoe covers in a plastic bag at the line. Remove the goggles and mask. Place them in the plastic bag. Seal the plastic bag. Remove the inner gloves. Place them in a plastic bag and seal it. Close off the dirty area until the level of contamination is established and the area is properly decontaminated. Move to a shower area. Remove the scrub suit and seal it in a plastic bag. Shower thoroughly with soap and water. Dress in normal work attire.

AFTERCARE

Further patient management will depend on the type of exposure and other circumstances. Perform a thorough secondary survey to detect occult trauma or medical illness. Monitoring for cardiac dysrhythmias or for noncardiogenic pulmonary edema may be necessary after exposure to certain chemicals.[2,5] Some toxins necessitate treatment with specific antidotes, which should be initiated as soon as possible.

Dilute ingested chemicals with 4 to 8 ounces of water. Activated charcoal (1 gm/kg) may be given to prevent further absorption.[5] Ingestion of corrosive agents may necessitate early endoscopy, in which case charcoal should be withheld.[5] Induction of emesis is rarely indicated and may pose a hazard to the patient (corrosives, hydrocarbons) and to personnel (cyanide).[2,5]

COMPLICATIONS

Hypothermia may be caused or worsened by the decontamination procedures.[2,5] This must be anticipated and treated accordingly.[2,5] Residues of highly toxic chemicals remaining in skin folds or under nails may pose a risk to the patient and caregivers.[5] This should be searched for and removed. Toxic vomitus may pose a risk to health care personnel, even after adequate decontamination.[2,5] Emesis must be contained and discarded appropriately.

SUMMARY

Emergency Departments must be prepared to decontaminate and treat victims of hazardous materials exposures at any time. Procedures must be developed, practiced, and incorporated into the hospital's mass casualty incident plan. Lack of preparation and practice will expose medical personnel to greater risks and lead to less than optimal patient care. This chapter presents a general approach to decontamination procedures, which must be adapted to the individual circumstances and type of exposure.

REFERENCES

1. Leonard RB: Hazardous materials accidents: initial scene assessment and patient care. *Aviat Space Environ Med* 1993; 64(6):546–551.
2. Hau ML: Emergency care in acute chemical exposure. *AAOHN J* 1995; 43(4):276–284.
3. Burgess JL, Kirk M, Borron SW, et al: Emergency department hazardous materials protocol for contaminated patients. *Ann Emerg Med* 1999; 34(2): 177–182.
4. Kirk MA, Cisek J, Rose SR: Emergency department response to hazardous materials. *Emerg Med Clin North Am* 1994; 12(2):461–481.
5. Agency for Toxic Substances and Disease Registry: *Managing Hazardous Materials Incidents:* Vol III: *Medical Management Guidelines for Acute Chemical Exposures.* Atlanta, GA, 2001, ATSDR: 33–42.
6. Agency for Toxic Substances and Disease Registry: *Managing Hazardous Materials Incidents:* Vol II: *Hospital Emergency Departments: A Planning Guide for the Management of Contaminated Patients.* Atlanta, GA, 2001, ATSDR: 23–39.

7. Olson KR: Hazmat-o-phobia. Why aren't hospitals ready for chemical accidents? *West J Med* 1998; 168: 32–33.

8. Levitin HW, Siegelson HJ: Hazardous materials. Disaster medical planning and response. *Emerg Med Clin North Am* 1994; 12(2):327–348.

9. Cox RD: Decontamination and management of hazardous materials exposure victims in the emergency department. *Ann Emerg Med* 1994; 23(4): 761–770.

10. Handbook on the medical aspects of NBC defensive operations FM 8–9. United States Army Military Research Institute for Infectious Diseases (USAMRIID), 1999, http://www.usamriid.army.mil/Content/FMs/amedp6/index.htm

INFORMATION RESOURCES

1. Local Poison Control Centers will provide detailed medical information for any hazardous material.

2. U.S. Department of Health and Human Services, Agency for Toxic Substances and Disease Registry (ATSDR). 1600 Clifton Road, N.E., Atlanta, GA, 30333. Phone (404) 639-6360 for information and educational material. Phone (404) 639-0616 for advice during business hours. 24-hour telephone number: (404) 639-0615. The ATSDR will provide extensive medical and patient decontamination protocols for any hazardous material.

3. CHEMTREC. Information Service of the Chemical Manufacturers Association. 24-hour telephone number: (800) 424-9300. CHEMTREC will provide chemical information and assist in obtaining medical information and site decontamination.

4. National Pesticide Telecommunications Network (NPTN). Oregon State University/Environmental Protection Agency. Phone (800) 858-7378, 7 days per week, 6:30–16:30 Pacific Time, excluding holidays. Will provide chemical information on pesticide products.

5. Nuclear Regulatory Commission (NRC) Emergency Center. 24-hour telephone number: (301) 816-5100. Will coordinate assistance for nuclear accidents or releases by one of four national NRC centers, including information, advice, and personnel if needed.

6. National Response Center. 24-hour telephone number: (800) 424-8802. Takes reports on any chemical or nuclear release or spill, or suspected terrorist attack, and coordinates response of federal agencies, including but not limited to the FBI and the Chemical/Biological Defense Command of the U.S. Army.

7. United States Army Military Research Institute on Infectious Diseases (USAMRIID). Phone (301) 619-2833. Homepage: http://www.usamriid.army.mil/html/Home/home.asp. Publications: http://www.usamriid.army.mil/html/Publications/publications.html. Information on diagnostics, medical management, and vaccines relating to biological weapons can be obtained by contacting the commander of the USAMRIID.

8. Selected Computerized Databases. Chemical Hazard Response Information System (CHRIS), CIS, Inc., (800) 247-8737. Poisindex, Tomes, Meditext, and Hazardtext Micromedex, Inc., (800) 525-9083. Toxicology Data Network (ToxNet), The National Library of Medicine, (301) 496-6531.

INDEX

Page references followed by *f* and *t* indicate figures and tables, respectively.